WORLD *of* HEALTH

WORLD *of* HEALTH

Brigham Narins, *Editor*

GALE GROUP

Detroit
San Francisco
London
Boston
Woodbridge, CT

STAFF

The Gale Group
27500 Drake Rd.
Farmington Hills, MI 48331-3535

ISBN: 0-7876-3649-5 (hc.)
Printed in the United States of America
10 9 8 7 6 5 4 3 2 1

I(T)P™

Library of Congress Cataloging-in-Publication Data
World of health / Brigham Narins, editor.
p. cm.
Includes bibliographical references and index.
Summary: An alphabetical collection of articles on health and medical topics, theories, discoveries, concepts, and the people behind them.
ISBN 0-7876-3649-5 (hc.)
1. Medicine Juvenile literature. 2. Health Juvenile literature.
[1. Health Encyclopedias. 2. Medicine Encyclopedias.] I. Narins, Brigham, 1962-
R130.5.W67 1999
610–dc21 99-31918
CIP

CONTENTS

Introduction

Welcome to the ***World of Health***. We hope you will find this collection interesting and useful. The 1,400 individual entries in this volume provide an up-to-date overview of the various medical sciences and allied health-related disciplines. The entries explain in concise, detailed, and jargon-free language some of the most important topics, principles, and recent discoveries in medicine and health. Brief biographies of the people who made those discoveries and shaped our understanding of the body, diseases, and treatments are also included; for example, users will find here biographical sketches of many winners of the Nobel Prize in Physiology or Medicine.

From abortion, barber-surgeons, and Marie and Pierre Curie to x-ray machine, yellow fever, and Rolf M. Zinkernagel, this book covers a broad spectrum of the most significant procedures, historical events, disorders, therapies, devices, and people in medical history. *World of Health* has been designed and written with the student and non-expert in mind. In so doing, we have compiled a vast array of entries that will be useful to students who need accessible and concise information for school-related work, as well as to others who want reliable and informative introductions to the numerous aspects of the world of health.

It becomes increasingly important for all citizens to have a practical, theoretical, and historical understand of the major health-related issues—how their bodies work, what happens when they get sick, and what kinds of treatments and institutions are available to help, as well as the issues and problems that arise from the rapid growth of medical knowledge and technologies. We hope that the essays and articles contained in this book will help you understand some of these important issues and how they affect you and the world in which you live.

How to Use the Book

This first edition of ***World of Health*** has been designed with ready reference in mind.

- **Entries are arranged alphabetically**, rather than by chronology or scientific field.
- **Bold-faced terms** direct reader to related entries.
- **Cross-references** at the end of entries alert the reader to related entries that may not have been specifically mentioned in the body of the text.
- A **Sources Consulted** section lists many worthwhile print and electronic materials encountered in the compilation of this volume. It is there for the inspired reader who wants more information on the people and discoveries covered in this volume.
- The **Historical Chronology** includes well over 500 important events in the medical sciences and health-related fields spanning the period from 5,000 B.C. through 1999.
- A **comprehensive general index** guides the reader to all topics and persons mentioned in the book. Bolded page references refer the reader to the term's full entry.

Special Thanks

In compiling this edition, we have been fortunate in being able to call upon the following people—our panel of advisors—who contributed to the accuracy of the information in this premier edition of *World of Health*, and to them we would like to express sincere appreciation:

Rosalyn Carson-DeWitt, MD
Physician and medical writer
Durham, North Carolina

James Lauritsen
Librarian
Gettysburg High School
Gettysburg, Pennsylvania

Larry I. Lutwick, MD, FACP
Director of Infectious Diseases
VA New York Harbor Health Care System

Professor of Medicine
SUNY—Health Science Center
Brooklyn, New York

Ralph M. Myerson, MD, FACP
Clinical Professor of Medicine
MCP-Hahnemann School of Medicine
Philadephia, Pennsylvania

A

ABORTION

Therapeutic abortion is the intentional ending of a **pregnancy** before the fetus can live independently. Abortion has been legal in the United States since 1973. Women have abortions because continuing a pregnancy would cause hardship, endanger their life or health, or because the fetus has severe abnormalities. Pre-abortion counseling is important to resolve any questions about having the procedure.

A doctor must know the stage of a woman's pregnancy before performing an abortion. The doctor asks questions about the woman's menstrual cycle and does a **physical examination**. This may be done at an office visit before the abortion or on the day of the abortion. Some states require a waiting period before an abortion can be performed. Others require parental or court consent for a child under age 18 to receive an abortion.

The first trimester of pregnancy includes the first 13 weeks after the last menstrual period. In the United States, about 90% of abortions are performed during this period. It is the safest time in which to have an abortion. Although an abortion during the first trimester is safer, some second trimester abortions are unavoidable. The results of genetic testing are often unavailable before 16 weeks. Also, some women, especially teens, may not recognize a pregnancy or come to terms with it soon enough to have an earlier abortion. Abortions performed between 13-24 weeks have a higher rate of complications. Abortions after 24 weeks are extremely rare and are usually limited to the mother's life being in danger.

Serious complications resulting from abortions performed before 13 weeks are rare. Of the 90% of women who have abortions in this time period, 2.5% have minor complications that can be handled without hospitalization. Less than 0.5% have complications that require a hospital stay. The rate of complications increases as the pregnancy progresses.

Very early abortions cost $200-$400. Later abortions cost more because they involve more risk, more services, anesthesia, and sometimes a hospital stay. Insurance carriers and HMOs may or may not cover the procedure. Federal law prohibits federal funds, including Medicaid funds, from being used for an elective abortion.

Early in pregnancy, most women can have abortions at clinics or outpatient facilities. Between five and seven weeks, a pregnancy can be ended by menstrual extraction, sometimes called menstrual regulation, mini-suction, or preemptive abortion. The contents of the uterus are suctioned out through a thin (3-4 mm) plastic tube inserted through the undilated cervix. Suction is applied by a bulb syringe or a small pump. Menstrual extraction is safe, but because the amount of fetal material is so small, it is easy to miss. An incomplete abortion means the pregnancy continues.

Another type of abortion, medical abortion, involves taking medications. There are two methods. In the first, a woman receives an injection of methotrexate at her doctor's office. Methotrexate stops the fetal cells from dividing. About a week later, she is given misoprostol (Cytotec), which stimulates contractions of the uterus. Within two weeks, the woman expels the contents of her uterus. This method is 90-96% effective. A follow-up visit to the doctor is necessary.

In the other method, a woman is given Mifepristone (RU-486). This drug blocks the action of progesterone, a hormone needed to continue a pregnancy. On the first doctor's visit, a woman takes a mifepristone pill. Two days later, she returns to take two misoprostol pills. Ninety percent of women complete the abortion within four days; 95-97% of women, within 14 days. A follow-up visit to the doctor is necessary. If the procedure is incomplete, a surgical abortion is performed.

First trimester surgical abortions are performed using vacuum aspiration, also called dilation and evacuation (D & E), suction dilation, vacuum curettage, or suction curettage. During a vacuum aspiration, the woman's cervix is gradually dilated by expanding rods inserted into the cervix. Once dilated, a tube is inserted and the contents of the uterus are suctioned out. The procedure is 97-99% effective. The amount of discomfort involved varies considerably. Local anesthesia is often given to numb the cervix, but it does not mask uterine cramping. The woman may return home after a few hours.

Some second trimester abortions are performed as a D & E. The procedures are similar to those in a first trimester, but the risk is higher. For some women, it is not safe. An alternative is an abortion by induced labor. Induced labor may require an overnight hospital stay. The day before, the woman visits her doctor for tests and has rods inserted in her cervix to dilate it or receives medication to speed up labor. On the day of the abortion, drugs to induce contractions and a salt water solution are injected into the uterus. Within 8-72 hours, the fetus is delivered.

Regardless of the abortion method, a woman is observed for a period of time to make sure her blood pressure is stable and that bleeding is controlled. The doctor may prescribe **antibiotics** to reduce chance of infection. Women who are Rh negative (lacking genetically determined proteins in their red blood cells that produce immune responses) are given a human RH immune globulin (RhoGAM) after the procedure if the father of the fetus is Rh positive.

Bleeding continues for about five days after a surgical abortion and longer after a medical abortion. To decrease the risk of infection, a woman should avoid intercourse and not use tampons and douches for two weeks after the abortion. A follow-up visit is a necessary part of the woman's aftercare. **Contraception** will be offered to women who wish to avoid future pregnancies, because menstrual periods normally resume within a few weeks.

Abscess

An abscess is a pus-filled sore, usually caused by a bacterial infection. It results from the body's defensive reaction to foreign material. Abscesses are often found in the soft tissue under the skin, such as the armpit or the groin. However, they may develop in any organ, and are commonly found in the breast and gums. Abscesses are far more serious and call for more specific treatment if they are located in deep organs such as the lung, liver, or brain.

Most abscesses are caused by an infection. In response to an invading germ, white blood cells gather at the infected site and begin producing chemicals called enzymes that attack the germ. These enzymes act like acid, killing the germs and breaking them down into small pieces to be picked up by the circulation and eliminated from the body. These chemicals also digest body tissues. In most cases, the germ produces similar chemicals. The result is a thick, yellow liquid—pus—containing digested germs, digested tissue, white blood cells, and enzymes.

Sterile abscesses are a milder form of the same process. They are not caused by germs but rather by non-living irritants such as drugs. If an injected drug like penicillin is not absorbed, it stays where it was injected and may cause enough irritation to generate a sterile abscess—sterile because there is no infection involved. Sterile abscesses are quite likely to turn into hard, solid lumps as they scar, rather than remaining pockets of pus.

Many different agents cause septic abscesses. The most common are the pus-forming (pyogenic) bacteria like *Staphylococcus aureus*, which are nearly always the cause of skin abscesses. Abscesses near the large bowel, particularly around the anus, may be caused by any of the numerous bacteria found within the large bowel. Brain and liver abscesses can be caused by any organism that can travel there through the circulation. Bacteria, amoeba, and certain fungi can travel in this fashion. Abscesses in other parts of the body are caused by organisms that normally inhabit nearby structures or that infect them.

An abscess can damage surrounding tissue. If an abscess ruptures into neighboring areas or permits the infectious agent to spill into the bloodstream, serious consequences may follow. Blood **poisoning** describes a local infection that has spilled into the blood stream and spread throughout the body. Blood poisoning, known to physicians as septicemia, is life threatening. Abscesses in and around the nasal sinuses, face, ears, and scalp may work their way into the brain. Abscesses within an abdominal organ such as the liver may rupture into the abdominal cavity with life-threatening results.

Superficial abscesses are easily identified by local inflammation. Deeper abscesses may produce symptoms such as fever and discomfort. If the patient's symptoms and **physical examination** do not help, a physician may have to do tests to locate an abscess. An imaging technique such as a computed tomography scan may be used to locate an abscess and confirm its size.

Some abscesses can be treated with antibiotics, but often the lining of the abscess cavity blocks the drug from getting to the source of infection. In this case, the cavity must be drained. A doctor will cut into the lining of the abscess, which allows pus to escape. Once the abscess is opened, the doctor cleans and irrigates the wound thoroughly with saline. If it is not too large or deep, the doctor may simply pack the abscess wound with gauze for 24-48 hours to absorb the pus and discharge. Most abscesses heal after drainage alone; others require drainage and antibiotic drug treatment.

If it is a deep abscess, the doctor may insert a drainage tube after cleaning out the abscess. Once the tube is in place, the surgeon closes the incision with simple stitches, and applies a sterile dressing. Drainage is maintained for several days to help prevent the abscess from reforming. Much of the **pain** around the abscess will be gone after the surgery. Healing is usually very fast. After the tube is taken out, antibiotics may be continued for several days.

Abstinence

Webster's Dictionary defines abstinence as ''voluntary refraining'' from particular behaviors. Many sexuality educators argue that a key goal of adolescent sex education is helping to postpone sexual intercourse until the individuals involved are physically and emotionally ready for mature relationships including the associated consequences. Abstinence is among the topics most often covered in educating individuals and families, along with **sexually transmitted diseases**, including

AIDS. Found to be effective in encouraging the postponement of sexual intercourse are the development of strong interpersonal skills and self-esteem. Individuals are encouraged to accept responsibility for their bodies and actions, and they are urged to avoid situations that could lead to a lack of self-control, such as those involving drug or alcohol use. A peer group that shares and respects such values is also helpful. Commitment to abstinence, proponents argue, allows for peace of mind and freedom from worries about unwanted **pregnancy**, birth control, sexually transmitted diseases, and the emotional stress of failed relationships.

Studies have found that 10% of American teenager girls become pregnant each year and more than 80% of those who give birth and keep their babies end up on welfare. Three million new cases of sexually transmitted diseases are documented annually in the teen population, and up to 29% of sexually active girls are diagnosed with **chlamydial infections**. However, studies have also shown that more than half of American teens refrain from sexual activity until they are at least 17. Moreover, by the time they reach the age of 20, 20% of boys and 24% of girls have not had sexual intercourse. The Sexuality Information and Education Council of the United States (SIECUS) cites a key goal of comprehensive sexuality education is to help teens postpone sexual activity until they are ready for mature relationships.

See also Chlamydial infections; Sexually transmitted diseases

Accidents

Nearly 37 million Americans visit hospital emergency rooms each year for treatment of injuries attributed to accidents. Of these, 147,000 persons die from their injuries, making accidents the fifth leading cause of death in the United States. For persons under the age of 65, automobile accidents (accounting for nearly 29% of all injury deaths) are the number one cause of accidental deaths in the United States. In second place are falls, which occur mainly in the home; this type of accident is the leading cause of accidental death for persons over 75.

By taking adequate precautions, many deaths due to accidents could be avoided. Many deaths occurring as the result of automobile accidents, for example, could be avoided if adults and children would use safety restraints, e.g., seat belts and restraint seats; it is estimated that one half of all adult fatalities and 90% of the deaths of children under five could have been prevented by the use of suitable restraints.

Drinking alcohol raises the risk of accidental injury and death. A relatively small amount of alcohol can impair a person's judgment, concentration, and reaction time. In 1996, 17,000 people died and more than 321,000 (for an average of one injury every two minutes) were injured in automobile accidents where police determined that alcohol was a factor. The injured included, besides the drivers, pedestrians, motorcyclists, and bicyclists who had been drinking.

Each year about one third of all adults over the age of 65 sustain falls. Falls are the leading cause of nonfatal injury to elderly persons. Deaths from falls, or from complications arising as the result of a fall, are responsible for more than half of all accidental deaths of older persons. In addition, up to 25% of those who fall end up restricting their activities to prevent another fall. Although many falls can be attributed to an older person's unsteady gait, mobility problems, diminished vision, or use of multiple medications, there may also be contributing factors in the environment such as poor lighting, loose rugs, slippery surfaces, and objects on the floor that can be addressed before an accident occurs.

First degree **burns** (which involve damage to the epidermis, or outer layer of skin) frequently result from minor household accidents such as touching a hot object, a corrosive chemical (acids or alkalis), or uninsulated electrical wiring. Burns of this type can easily be prevented by exercising care when cooking or ironing, handling chemicals, or dealing with electricity.

In the case of accidents that leave the outer skin barrier scraped, cut, or punctured, it is essential that the injury be dealt with immediately to prevent infection.

Some authorities on childhood injuries prefer not to use the term accidents because most of these injuries are preventable and occur in predictable patterns. Children are particularly susceptible to preventable accidents, such as **poisoning**s. A disproportionate number of childhood accidents are associated with stressful life events, such as the arrival of a new baby, **divorce**, death of a family member, or marriage of a parent. Parents can take appropriate measures to prevent their children from suffering accidental injury by noting that these accidents all too often involve chemicals stored in kitchen and dining areas; overheated bath water; electrical appliances; stairways; walkers; swimming pools; portable heaters; burning cigarettes; disposable lighters; toothpicks; firearms; microwave ovens; automatic garage doors; hazards associated with playpens, high chairs, or cribs; swings, slides, and other outdoor play equipment; windows; plastic bags; toy balloons and other toys; and discarded freezers and refrigerators.

The increasing emphasis on **exercise** and sports accounts for many injuries. An estimated 50 million Americans suffer at some point in their lives from knee pain or injuries, and at least one in four sports injuries involves the knee. Types of knee injuries include sprains (i.e., torn ligaments such as frequently occur in skiing, hockey, or soccer accidents), runner's knee (i.e., a degeneration of cartilage that affects nearly 30% of all runners but also shows up among skiers, cyclists, soccer players, and people who participate in high impact aerobics), and **tendinitis** (i.e., an inflammation of the tendons prevalent among dancers, hikers, and cyclists).

Muscle strains and sprains are typical of the types of accidents that result from a single, abrupt incident; they are particularly common among weekend athletes don't know or have ignored the physical limitations of their muscles and joints.

See also Emergency medical services; Sports medicine

Acetaminophen

Acetaminophen is used to relieve minor aches and pains such as **headache**s, muscle aches, backaches, toothaches, menstrual cramps, arthritis, and the aches and pains that often accompany colds. It is also used to reduce **fever**.

Acetaminophen is available without a prescription and is sold under various brand names, including Tylenol, Panadol, Aspirin Free Anacin, and Bayer Select Maximum Strength Headache Pain Relief Formula. Many multi-symptom cold, flu, and sinus medicines also contain acetaminophen.

Studies have shown that acetaminophen relieves pain and reduces fever about as well as aspirin. But differences between these two drugs exist. Acetaminophen is less likely than aspirin to irritate the stomach. However, unlike aspirin, acetaminophen does not reduce the redness, stiffness, or swelling that accompany arthritis.

Acetaminophen has few side effects. The most common one is lightheadedness. Some people experience trembling and pain in the side or the lower back. Allergic reactions are rare. Anyone who develops symptoms such as a rash, swelling, or difficulty breathing after taking acetaminophen should stop taking the drug and get immediate medical attention. Other rare side effects include yellow skin or eyes, unusual bleeding or bruising, weakness, fatigue, bloody or black stools, bloody or cloudy urine, and a sudden decrease in the amount of urine.

The usual dosage for anyone over age 12 is 325-650 mg every 4-6 hours as needed. No more than 4000 mg should be taken in 24 hours. Anyone who drinks three or more alcoholic beverages a day should check with a physician before using this drug because there is a risk of liver damage from combining large amounts of alcohol and acetaminophen. People who already have kidney or liver disease or liver infections should also consult a physician before using the drug, as should women who are pregnant or breastfeeding. For children ages 6-11 years, the usual dose is 150-300 mg, three to four times a day. For younger children, a physician's advice should be asked.

Patients should not use acetaminophen for more than 10 days to relieve pain (5 days for children) or for more than 3 days to reduce fever, unless directed to do so by a physician. If symptoms do not go away—or if they get worse—medical attention is necessary.

Patients must avoid using two different acetaminophen-containing products at the same time. Overdoses of acetaminophen may cause nausea, vomiting, sweating, and exhaustion. Very large overdoses can cause liver damage. In case of an overdose, get immediate medical attention.

Acetaminophen may interact with several other medicines. If this happens, the effects of one or both of the drugs may change or the risk of side effects may be greater. Among the drugs that may interact with acetaminophen are alcohol, **nonsteroidal anti-inflammatory drugs** (NSAIDs) such as Motrin, **oral contraceptives**, the antiseizure drug phenytoin (Dilantin), the blood-thinning drug warfarin (Coumadin), the cholesterol-lowering drug cholestyramine (Questran), the antibiotic Isoniazid, and zidovudine (Retrovir, AZT). Check with a physician or pharmacist before using acetaminophen with any other medicine. Smoking cigarettes may also interfere with the effectiveness of acetaminophen. Smokers may need to take higher doses of the medicine, but should not take more than the recommended daily dosage unless told by a physician to do so.

Acetaminophen interferes with the results of some medical tests. Before having medical tests done, check to see whether taking acetaminophen will affect the results. Avoiding the drug for a few days before the tests may be necessary.

ACNE

Acne is a common skin disease characterized by pimples on the face, chest, and back. It occurs when the pores of the skin become clogged with oil, dead skin cells, and bacteria. Acne affects nearly 17 million people in the United States. While it can arise at any age, acne usually begins at **puberty** and worsens during adolescence. Nearly 85% of people develop acne at some time between the ages of 12-25 years.

The face, chest, and back are most affected because those areas have the most sebaceous glands. These glands produce sebum, an oily natural moisturizer. The glands are found in hair follicles and open onto the skin through pores. At puberty, sebum production increases. Excess sebum can combine with dead skin cells and form a hard plug, or comedo, which blocks the pore. Mild noninflammatory acne consists of the two types of comedones, whiteheads and blackheads.

Moderate and severe inflammatory types of acne result if the plugged follicle is invaded by *Propionibacterium acnes*, bacteria that normally live on the skin. A pimple forms when the damaged follicle releases sebum, bacteria, and skin and white blood cells into the surrounding tissues. The most severe acne consists of cysts (closed sacs) and nodules (hard swellings). Scarring occurs when new skin cells replace damaged cells.

Due to hormonal changes, teenagers often develop acne. Usually, boys are more severely affected than girls. However, acne can flare up before menstruation, during **pregnancy**, and **menopause**. Individuals with a family history of acne are more likely to have acne. No foods cause acne, but certain ones may trigger flare-ups. Acne can be a side effect of drugs including tranquilizers, antidepressants, **antibiotics**, **oral contraceptives**, and anabolic steroids. Abrasive soaps, hard scrubbing, or picking at pimples will make them worse, as will oil-based makeup and hair sprays. Sweating in hot weather and exposure to oils, greases, and polluted air aggravate acne. Emotional **stress** may contribute to acne.

Acne patients are often treated by family doctors, but some cases are handled by a dermatologist, a skin disease specialist, or an endocrinologist, a specialist who treats diseases of the endocrine (hormones and glands) system. Acne is not difficult to diagnose. The doctor takes a complete medical history and asks about skin care, diet, flare-ups, medication use, and prior treatment. **Physical examination** includes the face, upper neck, chest, shoulders, back, and other affected areas. Treatment choices depend on whether the acne is mild, moderate, or severe.

Treatment for mild to moderate acne consists of topical medications (medications that go on the skin) and oral antibiotics. These drugs may be used for months to years to control flare-ups. Topical medications are cream, gel, lotion, or pad preparations that include antibiotics (agents that kill bacteria) or comedolytics (agents that loosen hard plugs and open pores). Possible side effects include mild redness, peeling, irritation, dryness, and an increased sensitivity to sunlight. Oral antibiotics may also be prescribed for mild to moderate acne. The drugs are taken daily for two to four months. Possible side effects include allergic reactions, stomach upset, vaginal yeast infections, **dizziness**, and tooth discoloration.

For severe acne with cysts and nodules, oral isotretinoin (Accutane) is used. It may be prescribed with topical or oral antibiotics. It reduces sebum production and cell stickiness and is taken for four to five months. Side effects include temporarily worse acne, dry skin, **nosebleeds**, vision disorders, and elevated liver enzymes, blood fats, and cholesterol. This drug cannot be taken during pregnancy because it causes **birth defects**. Women who are unresponsive to other therapies may be prescribed anti-androgen drugs, certain types of oral contraceptives, or female sex hormones.

Oral corticosteroids, or anti-inflammatory drugs, are used for an extremely severe, but rare type of destructive inflammatory acne called acne fulminans, found mostly in adolescent males. Acne conglobata, a more common form of severe acne, is characterized by numerous, deep, inflammatory nodules that heal with scarring. It is treated with oral isotretinoin and corticosteroids.

Surgical or medical treatments are available to treat acne or acne scars. In comedone extraction, the comedo is removed from the pore with a special tool. Chemical peels involve applying glycolic acid to peel off the top layer of skin to reduce scarring. Another technique in which the top layer of skin is removed is dermabrasion. In this procedure, the affected skin is frozen with a chemical spray, and removed by brushing or planing. If scars are deep, a procedure called punch grafting may be an option. Deep scars are excised and the area repaired with small skin grafts. Drug injection is another option for some people. With intralesional injection, corticosteroids are injected directly into inflamed pimples. Collagen injection elevates shallow scars.

Acne is not curable, but it can be controlled by proper treatment. Acne tends to reappear when treatment stops, but spontaneously improves over time.

ACROMEGALY AND GIGANTISM

Acromegaly is characterized by excess growth hormone (GH) production, leading to increased growth in bone and soft tissue and other disturbances throughout the body. In children, excess GH causes exceptional growth of long bones. This variant is called gigantism, because the additional bone growth causes unusual height. When too much GH is produced after a person has already reached adult height, the disorder is called acromegaly. Acromegaly is rare, affecting approximately 50 out of every 1 million people. Both men and women are affected. Because symptoms occur gradually, most patients are not identified until they are middle aged.

GH is one of several hormones produced by the pituitary gland, which is located in the brain. Pituitary hormones are in-

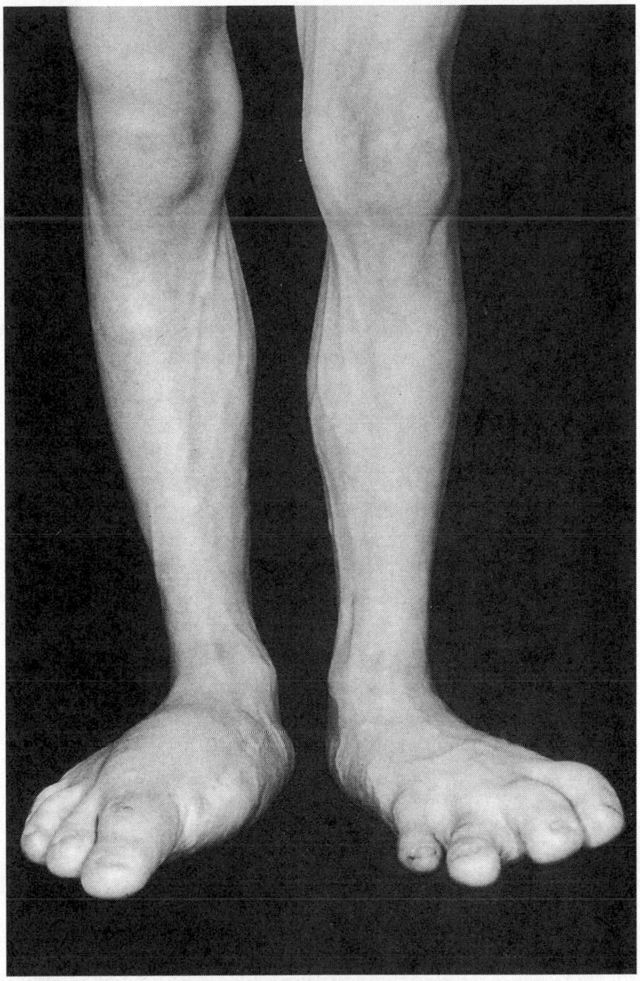

Enlarged feet is one deformity caused by acromegaly. ***(Custom Medical Stock Photo. Reproduced by permission.)***

volved in many activities throughout the body, including growth regulation and reproductive functions. Under normal conditions, the pituitary's activity is directed by the hypothalamus, a small structure located at the base of the brain. In acromegaly, the pituitary ignores signals from the hypothalamus to stop releasing GH. As a result, bones, soft tissue, and organs throughout the body begin to enlarge, and the body changes its ability to process and use nutrients like sugars and fats.

The hands and feet of an individual with acromegaly grow larger. The jaw line, nose, and forehead also grow, and facial features are described as ''coarsening.'' The throat and sinuses can swell, causing the voice to become deeper, and patients may also develop loud snoring. Hormonal changes cause heavy sweating, oily skin, and increased coarse body hair. The metabolism is also affected, as demonstrated by problems processing sugars from the diet (sometimes leading to diabetes), high blood pressure, increased calcium in the urine (possibly causing **kidney stones**), and increased risk of gallstones. Swelling of the thyroid gland in the neck may also be apparent.

People with acromegaly have more skin tags, or outgrowths on the skin, than normal. They may also develop growths, called polyps, in the large intestine which may become **cancer**ous. Patients with acromegaly often suffer from **headache**s and arthritis. Swellings and enlargements throughout the body may press on nerves, causing local tingling or burning, and sometimes result in muscle weakness.

In 90% of patients, acromegaly is caused by a noncancerous tumor within the pituitary, called an adenoma. The adenoma may press on nearby structures within the brain, causing headaches and changes in vision. It may also interfere with the release of other pituitary hormones. These disruptions can change the menstrual cycle of women, decrease sexual drive in men and women, and cause abnormal production of breast milk in women. In rare cases, excess GH production in the pituitary is linked to tumors elsewhere in the body or abnormalities in the hypothalamus.

Because acromegaly produces changes slowly, diagnosis is often delayed. The characteristic coarsening of facial features is usually not recognized by family members, friends, or long-time family physicians. Often, the diagnosis is suspected by a new physician who sees the patient for the first time.

Demonstrating high levels of GH in the blood is not sufficient to diagnose acromegaly; however, other blood tests are useful. Normal patients show decreased GH production when given a large dose of sugar (glucose). Patients with acromegaly don't show this decrease and often show an increase. **Magnetic resonance imaging** (MRI) can be used to view the pituitary and to identify an adenoma. If no adenoma is found, the search for a tumor elsewhere begins.

Typically, the first step in treating acromegaly is surgical removal of a pituitary adenoma. While surgery can rapidly improve several symptoms, most patients also require medication. Bromocriptine (Parlodel) is a medication that can be taken by mouth, while octreotide (Sandostatin) must be injected every eight hours. Both of these medications help reduce GH production, but often are taken for life and have side effects. Patients who cannot undergo surgery may be treated with **radiation therapy** to shrink the adenoma. Radiating the pituitary may take up to 10 years, however, and may also injure/destroy normal parts of the pituitary.

Without treatment, patients with acromegaly will most likely die early because of the disease's effects on the heart, lungs, brain, or due to the development of cancer in the large intestine. With treatment, however, a patient with acromegaly may be able to live a normal lifespan.

ACUPUNCTURE AND ACUPRESSURE

Acupuncture and acupressure are based on ancient Japanese and Chinese medicine. In acupuncture, special needles are inserted into points just under the skin to promote **pain** relief and healing. In acupressure, pressure is placed on similar points for the same purposes. Both systems are based on a belief that health relies on maintaining a balanced flow of *qi*, (also referred to as *chi*), a vital life energy present in all living organisms. *Qi* supposedly circulates along 12 major energy pathways in the body, called meridians. Each is linked to specific organs and systems in the body. Within the meridian system there are over one thousand acupoints, which are specific anatomical locations that can be stimulated to control the flow of *qi*.

Millions of people have used acupuncture and acupressure for many health conditions. The treatment is often used in conjunction with more conventional methods and has gained wide acceptance. The most studied mechanism is the stimulation of acupoints using needles, which are manipulated manually or with electrical stimulation. Other stimulation techniques include pressure (acupressure), heat, lasers, and moxibustion (the burning of an herb at or near certain sites on the body).

The purpose of acupuncture and acupressure is to promote the body's own healing power. Conditions that are said to benefit from these treatments include the effects of daily **stress**, **headache**s, neck and shoulder pain, aches and pains, **allergies**, menstrual difficulties, fatigue, **anxiety**, **insomnia**, digestive problems, nausea, and back pain. Acupuncture and acupressure may work by stimulating the release of the body's natural pain-killing chemicals, called endorphins.

Acupuncture involves the insertion of fine needles, made of stainless steel, gold, or other metals, into acupoints. The needles can be heated, attached to a mild electric current, or twirled continuously with the hand. Some needles are left in place for only a few minutes, while others remain for days. Pain during treatment should be minimal. There may be a slight pricking sensation when a needle is inserted but this does not last long. If there is some discomfort, it can be relieved by a slight change in the position of the needle.

During acupressure, light to medium pressure is applied to an acupoint and it is rotated in a tight circle. Primarily, this is done with the fingers, thumbs, and hands. Sometimes the elbows or knees are used for key pressure points. Since the most reactive points are tender or sensitive when pressed, this response helps to determine the right location. If the response cannot be felt, the pressure point location may not be correct or the pressure may not be strong enough. The sensations felt during an acupressure treatment should fall somewhere between pleasure and pain. Acupressure on a single point can last thirty seconds, five minutes, or be continued for twenty minutes in one-minute sequences with rests in between. The length of the massage depends on the tolerance of the patient and on the type of acupressure.

There are instances where more traditional Western medicine is the treatment of choice, including life threatening infection, severe trauma, or the need for surgical procedures, such as open heart surgery. This understanding has led to the practice of both systems side by side in some places, with the strengths of each system complementing the weaknesses of the other.

Before the first treatment, an acupuncturist obtains a thorough medical history and studies the patient carefully. All aspects of the individual are considered. The practitioner will observe the person's tone of voice and body language, as well as discussing many aspects of health, including eating habits, sensitivity to temperature, emotional distress, and urine color.

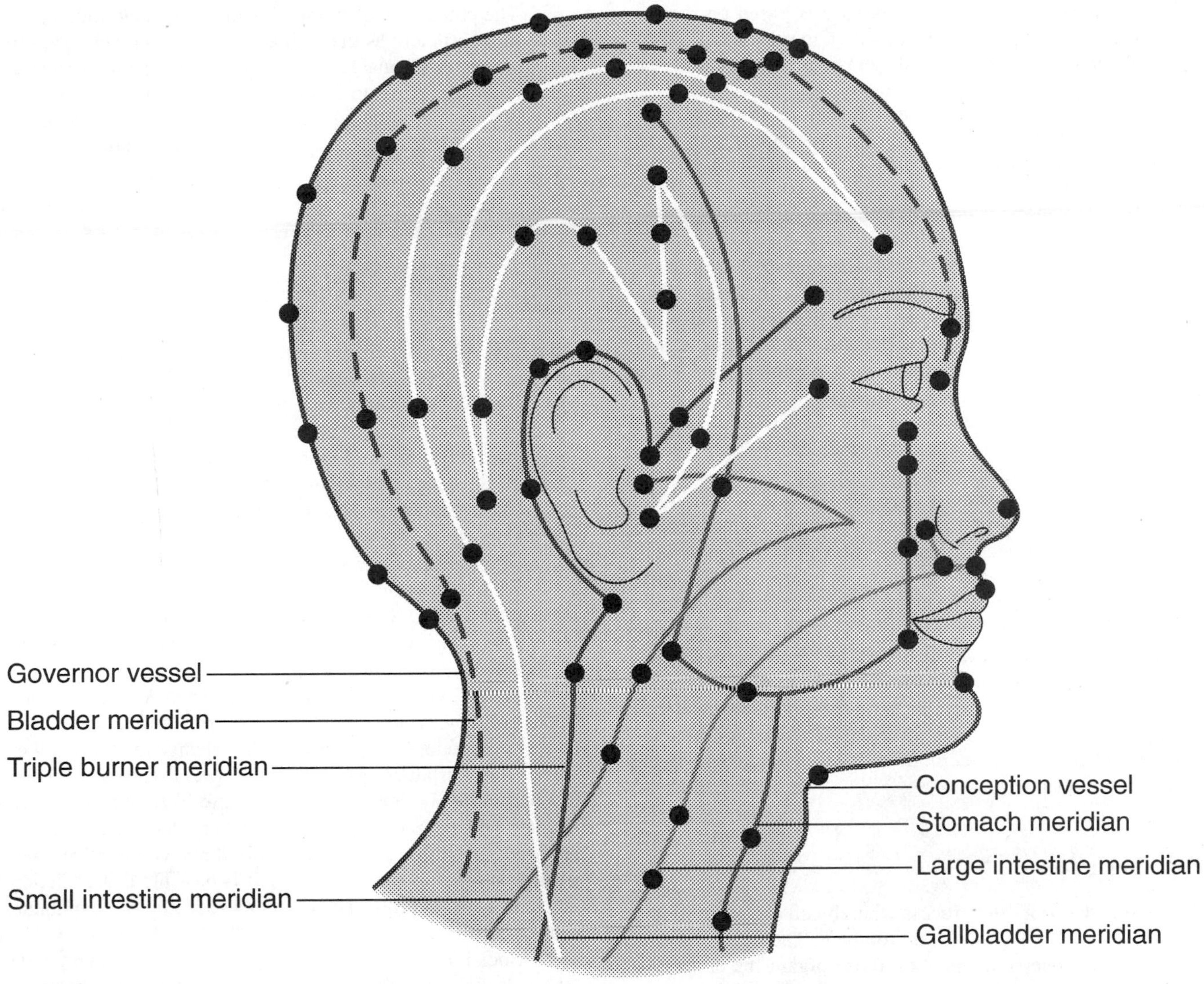

Acupuncture sites and meridians on the face and neck. ***(Illustration by Hans & Cassady, Inc.)***

Before receiving acupressure, patients are usually asked why they want acupressure, and are also asked about their current physical condition, medical history, and any areas of specific pain.

Since acupuncture and acupressure treatments are individualized to each patient, care afterwards will depend on the condition being treated and the patient's response. The practitioner may recommend changes in diet, **exercise**, and lifestyle to improve the patient's condition. The number of treatments depend on the patient and the skills of the practitioner.

While acupuncture and acupressure may be used in combination with other forms of therapy, they should not be used as a replacements for necessary medical treatment. Serious side effects are unusual, but with acupuncture localized congestion is frequently reported after needle insertion. Less commonly reported adverse effects may include **fainting**, black and blue marks (hematoma formation), and a collapsed lung.

ACUTE STRESS DISORDER

Acute stress disorder is an **anxiety disorder** that occurs within one month of a traumatic event. Trauma is defined as a stressful situation that causes intense fear. The stress often arise from a life-threatening or dangerous situation such as rape, mugging, combat, or natural disasters. **Post-traumatic stress disorder** is a similar disorder, but the symptoms occur months or years after the trauma takes place.

Acute stress disorder is characterized by dissociative and anxiety symptoms. Dissociation is a psychological reaction to trauma in which the mind tries to deal with the trauma by ''sealing off'' some details from conscious awareness. Dissociative symptoms include emotional detachment, temporary loss of memory, depersonalization, and derealization. Anxiety symptoms connected with acute stress disorder include irritability, physical restlessness, sleep problems, inability to concentrate, and being easily startled.

Diagnosis of acute stress disorder is based on the patient's history and a physical examination to rule out any physical problems. The key clue to diagnosis is a traumatic event within one month of the onset of symptoms. The diagnosis is supported by symptoms that significantly interfere with a person's normal ability to socialize or to work. Some symptoms of acute stress disorder result from biochemical changes in the central nervous system, muscles, and digestive tract that are not subject to conscious control. Symptoms last between two days and four weeks.

Treatment for acute stress disorder usually includes antidepressant medications and short-term psychotherapy. **Acupuncture** has been recommended as a treatment, and other alternative approaches include **meditation**, breathing exercises, and **yoga**. These alternative approaches may be helpful when combined with short-term psychotherapy.

Recovery depends on the severity of the trauma and how long it lasted. Other important factors include a person's closeness to the trauma and his or her previous level of functioning. Recovery is usually quicker when only a short time period has passed between the trauma and onset of symptoms. Immediate treatment and good social support improve the chances of a good recovery. If the patient's symptoms interfere with normal life and have lasted longer than one month, the diagnosis may be changed to post-traumatic stress disorder. Without treatment, a person with acute stress disorder is at increased risk for substance abuse or major **depressive disorders**.

Traumatic events usually cannot be predicted, so it is difficult to prevent acute stress disorder. However, professional help soon after a trauma might reduce the likelihood or severity of the disorder.

ADAPTATION

Adaptation describes the process whereby an organism adapts to, or learns to survive in, its environment. The process is crucial to natural selection, enabling those organisms or species best suited to a particular environment to survive. Ethologists, scientists who study the behavior of animals in their natural habitats from an evolutionary perspective, document adaptive behavior.

Adaptation occurs in individual organisms as well as in species. Sensory adaptation consists of physical changes in sense organs in response to the presence or cessation of stimuli. Examples include the adjustment by pupils of the eyes when moving from bright light into a darkened room, or the way in which the sense of touch becomes accustomed to the sensation of cold after an initial plunge into water. Once a steady level of stimulation (such as light, sound, or odor) is established, the organism's sensors adjust, and no longer respond actively to it. However, any abrupt changes in stimulus require further adaptation.

The adrenalin-produced reactions to environmental dangers, including rapid breathing, increased heart rate, and sweating, are collectively referred to as the "fight or flight" response. These reactions are considered a form of adaptation. The ability to learn new responses, as in classical and operant **conditioning**, is another form of adaptation.

The process of adaptation begins in infancy. Infants become more efficient as they nurse and with each year acquire behavior that will enable them to succeed. In the preschool years, the child learns to function or adapt to his environment by emulating and imitating the behavior of others. These adaptive behavior skills are vital to a child's successful development.

See also Conditioning

ADDICTION

Addiction is a dependence, on a behavior or substance, that a person is powerless to stop. The term has been partially replaced by the word *dependence* for substance abuse. Addiction has been extended, however, to include mood-altering behaviors or activities. Some researchers speak of two types of addictions: substance addictions such as **alcoholism**, drug abuse, and smoking; and process addictions such as gambling, spending, shopping, eating, and sexual activity. Many addicts are addicted to more than one substance or process.

Addiction is one of the most costly public health problems in the United States. It is a progressive syndrome, which means that it becomes a more severe problem over time unless it is treated.

Addiction to substances results from several factors. Some substances are more addictive than others, either because they produce a rapid and intense change in mood; or because they produce painful withdrawal symptoms when stopped suddenly. Some people are more likely than others to become addicts because their body chemistry increases their sensitivity to drugs. Some forms of **substance abuse and dependence** seem to run in families. It is possible that addiction is due to genes, family and social environment, or a combination of both.

Social learning is considered the most important single factor. It includes patterns of use in the addict's family or social environment, peer pressure, and advertising or media influence. Inexpensive or readily available tobacco, alcohol, or drugs produce marked increases in rates of addiction.

Before the 1980s, the so-called addictive personality was used to explain addiction. A person with an addictive personality was described as escapist, impulsive, dependent, devious, manipulative, and self-centered. Many doctors now believe that these traits develop in addicts as a result of the addiction, rather than the traits being a cause of the addiction.

In addition to a preoccupation with using and acquiring the abused substance, the diagnosis of addiction is based on five criteria. Those criteria are a loss of willpower; harmful consequences; unmanageable lifestyle; tolerance or escalation of use; and withdrawal symptoms upon quitting.

Treatment requires both medical and social approaches. Substance addicts may need hospital treatment to manage withdrawal symptoms. Individual or group psychotherapy is often helpful, but only after substance use has stopped. Antiaddiction medications, such as methadone and naltrexone, are also commonly used. The most frequently recommended social form of outpatient treatment is twelve-step programs such as Alcoholics Anonymous. Such programs are also frequently combined with psychotherapy. There are twelve-step groups for all major substance and process addictions.

The prognosis for recovery from any addiction depends on the substance or process, the individual's circumstances, and his or her personality. People who are addicted to several substances or activities have the most difficulty in breaking their addictions.

The most effective form of prevention appears to be a stable family that models responsible attitudes toward mood-altering substances and behaviors. Prevention education programs are also widely used to inform the public of the harmfulness of substance abuse.

ADENOVIRUS INFECTIONS

Adenoviruses are a class of DNA viruses (small infectious agents) that can cause upper respiratory tract infections, **conjunctivitis**, and other infections in humans. Infants and children are most commonly affected by adenoviruses. Adenovirus infections can occur throughout the year, but seem to be most common from fall to spring.

Adenoviruses are responsible for 3-5% of acute respiratory infections in children and 2% of respiratory illnesses in civilian adults. They are more apt to cause infection among people who live in close contact. Outbreaks among children are frequently reported at boarding schools and summer camps. Most children have been infected by at least one adenovirus by the time they reach school age. Most adults have acquired immunity to many adenoviruses due to infections they had as children.

An adenovirus infection can either be acute or chronic. In acute infections, adenoviruses use healthy cells in the body to replicate up to one million new viruses per cell. Once the new viruses are produced, the infected cell bursts open and releases them. People with this kind of infection feel sick. In chronic or latent infection, a much smaller number of viruses are released and healthy cells can multiply more rapidly than they are destroyed. People who have this kind of infection don't feel sick.

In children, adenoviruses most often cause acute upper respiratory infections with **fever** and runny nose. Occasionally more serious lower respiratory diseases, such as **pneumonia**, may occur.

Adenoviruses also cause acute pharyngoconjunctival fever in children. Symptoms, which appear suddenly, usually disappear in less than a week. The symptoms include inflammation of the lining of the eyelid (conjunctivitis), fever, **sore throat**, runny nose, and swollen lymph glands in the neck.

Other adenoviruses also cause fever and acute **diarrhea** in young children. This condition can last as long as two weeks. Another type of adenovirus can cause hemorrhagic cystitis (inflammation of the bladder and of the tubes that carry urine to the bladder from the kidneys). A child who has hemorrhagic cystitis has bloody urine for about three days, and invisible traces of blood can be found in the urine a few days longer. The child will feel the urge to urinate frequently, but will have difficulty doing so, for about the same length of time.

In adults, the most frequently reported adenovirus infection is acute respiratory disease. This disease often strikes military recruits. Symptoms include fever, sore throat, runny nose, and **cough**. Other symptoms that may appear are weakness, chills, **headache**, and swollen lymph glands in the neck. The symptoms typically last three to five days.

Another illness caused by an adenovirus is epidemic keratoconjunctivitis. This inflammation of tissues lining the eyelid and covering the front of the eyeball can be caused by using contaminated contact lens solutions or by drying the hands or face with a towel used by someone who has this infection. The inflamed, sticky eyelids characteristic of conjunctivitis develop 4-24 days after exposure and last between one and four weeks. Only 5-8% of patients with epidemic keratoconjunctivitis experience respiratory symptoms. One or both eyes may be affected. As symptoms of conjunctivitis subside, eye pain and watering and blurred vision develop. These symptoms of **keratitis** may last for several months, and about 10% of these infections spread to at least one other member of the patient's household.

Specific adenovirus infections can be traced to particular sources and produce distinctive symptoms. In general, however, adenovirus infection is caused by:

- Inhaling airborne viruses
- Getting the virus in the eyes by swimming in contaminated water, using contaminated eye solutions or instruments, wiping the eyes with contaminated towels, or rubbing the eyes with contaminated fingers.
- Not washing the hands after using the bathroom, and then touching the mouth or eyes.

Although symptoms may suggest the presence of adenovirus, distinguishing these infections from other viruses can be difficult. A definitive diagnosis is based on culture or detection of the virus in eye secretions, sputum, urine, or stool.

Treatment of adenovirus infections is usually aimed at relieving symptoms. Bed rest may be recommended along with medications to reduce fever and/or pain. (**Aspirin** should not be given to children because of concerns about **Reye's syndrome**.) Eye infections may benefit from topical **corticosteroids** to relieve symptoms and shorten the course of the disease. Hospitalization may be required for certain severe infections. No effective **antiviral drugs** have been developed.

Adenovirus infections are rarely fatal and most patients recover fully. Practicing good personal hygiene and avoiding people with infectious illnesses can reduce the risk of developing adenovirus infection. Proper handwashing can prevent the spread of the virus by oral-fecal transmission. Sterilization of instruments and solutions used in the eye can prevent eye infections, as can adequate chlorination of swimming pools.

ADOLESCENT HEALTH

Adolescents are young people between the ages of 12 and 20. Traditionally, this group has been cared for either by pediatricians or family physicians. In recent years a new specialty of adolescent medicine has been created, but specialists administering these medications for adolescents are not available in many locations. Although adolescent care facilities and school-based clinics are becoming more common, most adolescents are still cared for in traditional health care settings.

Adolescence, which is the progression from childhood to adulthood, is a time of great physical and emotional change. Adolescent health care addresses both these areas. Frequently, families whose children reach adolescence in good health tend to take this for granted. Medical checkups may become brief and infrequent. Many teens only see a doctor for quick checkups required by their schools for participation in sports. The American Academy of Pediatrics recommends yearly checkups for adolescents with complete evaluations every two years. Immunizations required during adolescence include vaccination against hepatitis B, a diphtheria/tetanus booster, and revaccination against measles for those who have not received a second booster during elementary school.

Adolescents often have the worst eating habits of any age group. Teenage diets tend to be heavy in salt, saturated fats, and cholesterol, a typical fast food diet. They are likely to be deficient in calcium, iron, and vitamins A and C. A nutritional assessment and nutritional counseling should be a part of every checkup for this age group, as eating habits change at puberty. To accommodate the rapid growth that occurs at this age, teens need more calories than adults of the same size. Girls ages 16-18 need about 2,100 calories daily to maintain their weight. Boys of the same age need about 3,200 calories daily. It is not unusual for a 70 lb., 56 in. tall 11-year-old boy to grow into a 150 lb., 70 in. eighteen-year-old.

About one in 20 adolescents is obese (more than 20% above his or her ideal weight), and another 10-20% are moderately overweight. Since **obesity** increases the risk of cardiovascular disease, and can cause isolation from peers, adolescents should be encouraged to lose weight or maintain a healthy weight using a moderate, common sense approach to eating and exercise. However, excessive concern about appearance can lead to fad dieting, anorexia, bulimia, or **anabolic steroid** use.

Sexual maturation is another hallmark of adolescence. For boys, as puberty begins, the hormone testosterone causes growth of the testes and penis, accompanied by the development of pubic hair. Later, boys also develop facial hair and their voices begin to deepen. An increase in testosterone stimulates muscle growth, so that boys not only grow taller during puberty but also develop bulkier muscles in the arms, shoulders, and thighs that give them their distinctly masculine shape. Ejaculations usually start between the ages of 11-15 in response to sexual fantasies or masturbation.

Girls enter puberty about a year earlier than boys. In response to the secretion of estrogen, the female hormone, they develop enlarged breasts, pubic hair, and reach menarche. The average age of first **menstruation** in the United States is 12.5, although initially menstruating between the ages of 8-16 is considered normal. During adolescence, girls also grow taller and start to accumulate the fat deposits at the breasts, hips, and buttocks that give them a typical female shape. It is recommended that girls have a pelvic examination by age 18, or earlier if they are sexually active.

Sexual activity in adolescents is a major health care concern. It is estimated that by age 19, 80% of boys and 75% of girls have had sexual intercourse, with about 1 million teenage girls becoming pregnant each year. Keeping adolescents healthy involves not only birth control counseling, but educating both sexes on the dangers of **sexually transmitted diseases** such as **AIDS**, **gonorrhea**, chlamydia, and **genital herpes**. In addition, up to 10% of teens explore issues of sexual identity and gender orientation.

Adolescence can be a time of emotional turmoil. Although some mood swings and rebellious behavior are a normal part of establishing an individual adult identity, continued **depression**, a high level of risk-taking behavior, talk of **suicide** or excessive violence, and extreme alienation and isolation are not normal and should be brought to the attention of a mental health professional. Adolescents are often concerned about issues of confidentiality, particularly on the subjects of mental health and sexual behavior. For this reason they often fail to seek medical advice when they need it.

See also Adolescent pregnancy; Eating disorders; Gender identity

ADOLESCENT PREGNANCY

The United States has the highest teenage **pregnancy** rate of any Western nation, with approximately 560,000 girls giving birth every year. The rate is twice that of Canada and England and seven times that of the Netherlands. Although that rate has been declining in recent years, teenage pregnancy still extracts a tremendous toll on family and government financial resources, on the hopes and dreams of the young people involved and on the future of their baby.

Physically, a woman is able to bear a child once she has gone through **puberty**. However, pregnancy and parenthood can be more emotionally, physically, and financially taxing than expected.

Pregnancies can be unexpected, resulting, for instance, from the failure of a contraceptive method. However, many teens do not have the facts regarding teenage pregnancy, and instead of asking their doctor, they ask their friends—who can be a tremendous source of misinformation. Among the common beliefs that teens hold is that urinating or douching after sex will prevent pregnancy (they won't) and that "you can't get pregnant the first time" (you can). Teens are often embarrassed to visit the doctor and ask questions, and will have conflicting feelings about having sex: on the one hand, they may feel that "everybody else is having sex"; on the other, they may feel too shy to even talk about it. Add to that the sexual messages presented by the media and it is no wonder that teens feel pressured to have sex even though they may not be emotionally ready to handle it.

The first sign of a pregnancy is often a missed menstrual period. Pregnancy should be confirmed with a pregnancy test, first a home kit and then a test in the doctor's office. Unfortunately, pregnant teens often delay seeking **prenatal care**; seven out of 10 teenage mothers don't see a doctor during the first three months of pregnancy. However, the first three months of a pregnancy is a vital time in the development of the baby. Unless the mother receives proper care and nutrition, there can be health risks for the baby. Most common (and often a result of poor prenatal care) among teenage mothers is the risk of having a **low birthweight** baby, a baby born too small and too soon. Low-birthweight babies are at special risk for having immature hearts, lungs, and brains, and mental retardation. Besides the lack of prenatal care, other maternal factors that can affect the baby's health include poor **nutrition**, cigarette **smoking**, **iron deficiency anemia**, drug and alcohol abuse, and **sexually transmitted diseases** (STDs).

Teenage mother face higher risks than older mothers, too. During their pregnancy, they are more vulnerable to having toxemia, anemia and preeclampsia without proper care. Also, they may go into labor too early or face especially long labor.

It is estimated that about half of the teenage girls who get pregnant opt for **abortion**s. Of the girls who give birth, most decide to keep their babies. Between 1982 and 1988, only three percent of Caucasian girls gave their babies up for adoption, compared to 19% between 1965 and 1972. That figure is even smaller for African-American girls.

Raising a baby, even with the support of a family and the baby's father, is often difficult. The teenage mother must adjust to having her freedom curtailed in a way she never before imagined, and to having the baby dependent upon her 24 hours a day. Teenage mothers are less likely than their peers to finish high school or attend college.

However, many states and localities have teenage-parent support programs that will help teenage mothers and fathers adjust to their new responsibilities. Some programs, like Women, Infants and Children (WIC), make sure that the teenage parent will have the necessities available to take care of the baby, such as access to a pediatrician and baby food and formula. Other programs, such as those offered by some local hospitals, will teach young parents what they need to know to take care of an infant, and provide guidance and reassurance.

Teenage mothers are also more likely to become pregnant again within two years of their baby's birth.

Sexually active teens should be certain to get the facts about pregnancy and **contraception**. Family doctors and obstetrician-gynecologists are excellent sources of information, as are organizations such as Planned Parenthood. Birth control methods such as the Pill and **Depo-Provera/Norplant** are almost 100% effective in preventing pregnancy; they are available through prescription. Sexual **abstinence** is also 100% effective. Barrier methods of contraception are also effective, but only the **condom** can protect against the passage of STDs and **AIDS**.

See also Adoption; Contraception; Low birthweight; Pregnancy; Premature labor; Prenatal care

ADOPTION

An adult assumes the role of parent for a child other than his or her own biological offspring in the process of adoption. Legally recognized adoptions require a court or other government agency to award permanent custody of a child (or, occasionally, an older individual) to adoptive parents. Specific requirements for adoption vary among states and countries. Adoptions can be privately arranged through individuals or agencies, or arranged through a public agency such as a state's child protective services. Adoptees may be adopted singly or as sibling groups; and they may come from the local area or from other countries. Adoptive parents may be traditional married couples, they may also be single men or women, or they may be non-traditional couples. Parents may be childless or already have children.

Adoption is a practice that dates to ancient times. The Romans, for example, saw adoption as a way of ensuring male heirs to childless couples so that family lines and religious traditions could be maintained. In contrast, modern American adoption laws are written in support of the best interests of the child, not of the adopter.

Adoption arrangements are typically thought of as either closed or open. Actually, they may involve many varying degrees of openness about identity and contact between the adoptive family and the birth family. The move to open records led to an increase in open adoptions in which information is shared from the beginning. Open adoptions may be completely open, as is the case when the birth parents (usually the mother) and adoptive parents meet beforehand and agree to maintain contact while the child is growing up. The child then has full knowledge of both sets of parents. Other open adoptions may include less contact, or periodic letters sent to an intermediary agency, or continued contact with some family members but not others. It can be a complex issue.

The desire to provide children with permanent homes and the resulting sense of security and attachment as soon as possible gives rise to another type of adoption, the legal risk adoption. This involves placement in the prospective adoptive home prior to the legal termination of parental rights and subsequent freeing of the child for adoption. In these cases, child protective services are generally involved and relatively certain that the courts will ultimately decide in favor of the adoptive placement.

Whether the child is free for adoption or a legal risk placement, there is generally a waiting period before the adoption is finalized or recognized by the courts. Although estimates vary, about 10% of adoptions "disrupt," that is, the child is removed from the family before finalization. Interestingly, many children who have experienced disruption go on to be successfully adopted, suggesting that disruption is often a bad fit between parental expectations, skills, or resources and the child's needs.

Estimating the total number of children adopted in the United States is difficult because private and independent adoptions are reported only voluntarily to census centers. According to the National Committee for Adoption, there were just over 100,000 domestic adoptions in the US in 1986, roughly an even split between related and unrelated adoptions. Of unrelated domestic adoptees, about 40% were placed by public agencies, 30% by private agencies, and 30% by private individuals. Almost half of these adoptees were under the age of two, and about one-quarter had special needs. There were also just over 10,000 international adoptions, the majority of these children under the age of two and placed by private agencies.

The American Public Welfare Association has collected data through the Voluntary Cooperative Information System on children in welfare systems across the US who are somewhere in the process of being adopted. Of children in the public welfare systems, about one-third had their adoptions finalized in 1988, one-third were living in their adoptive home waiting for finalization, and one-third were awaiting adoptive placements. Key statistics on these adoptions appear below.

Characteristic Percent of Total Adoptees

- White, 60%
- Black, 23%
- Hispanic, 9%
- Adopted by foster family, 40%
- Adopted by unrelated families, 37%
- Adoptees with special needs, 60%
- Adoptees median age, 4.8 years

Although adopting parents may have certain expenses if the adoption is privately arranged, adoptions are assumed to be a gratuitous exchange by law. No parties may profit improperly from adoption arrangements and children are not to be brokered. The objectives of public and private agencies can differ somewhat. Private agencies generally have prospective adoptive parents as their clients and the agency works to find a child for them. Public agencies, on the other hand, have children as their clients and the procurement of parents as their primary mission.

There is general agreement that children who are adopted and raised in families do better than children raised in institutions or raised with birth parents who are neglectful or abusive. Compared to the general population, however, the conclusions are less robust and the interpretation of the statistics is not clear. Adopted adolescents, for example, receive mental health services more often than their non-adopted peers, but this may be because adoptive families are more likely to seek helping services or because once referring physicians or counselors know that a child is adopted they assume there are likely to be problems warranting professional attention.

When adjustment problems are manifested by adoptees, they tend to occur around school age or during adolescence. D. M. Brodzinsky and his colleagues have conducted a series of studies from which they conclude that adopted infants and toddlers generally do not differ from non-adopted youngsters, but greater risks for problems such as aggression or depression emerge as the 5- to 7-year-old child begins to understand the salience and implications of being adopted. Still, it should be noted that the absolute incidence of adjustment problems in adoptees is low even though it may be statistically higher than the corresponding figures for non-adoptees.

Problems associated with adoption may not always be the result of psychological adjustment to adoption status or a reflection of less than optimal family dynamics. Attention Deficit/Hyperactivity Disorder (ADHD) was found to be more prevalent in adoptees than non-adoptees, both among children adopted as infants and children removed from the home at older ages. C. K. Deutsch suggests that ADHD in children adopted as infants may be genetically inherited from the birth parents. In the case of children who have been removed from the home because of the trauma of abuse, the hypervigilance used to cope with a threatening environment may compromise the child's ability to achieve normal attention regulation.

These are complex issues and adoptees are a heterogeneous group. One certainty is that it is as important to understand their individual differences as it is their commonalities.

See also Child care; Child development

ADRENAL DISORDERS

The adrenal glands are a pair of small organs located just above the kidney. These glands contain two types of tissue. The adrenal cortex produces hormones that affect water balance and metabolism in the body. The adrenal medulla produces adrenaline and noradrenaline (also called epinepherine and norepinepherine).

Release of some of these hormones is stimulated by adrenocorticotropic hormone (ACTH). ACTH is produced in the pituitary gland. ACTH levels rise in response to **stress**, emotions, injury, infection, **burns**, surgery, and decreased blood pressure. ACTH causes the release of the hormones hydrocortisone (cortisol), aldosterone, and androgen.

If the body produces too much or too little of the adrenal hormones, it could be an indication of a disease. Cushing's syndrome is caused by an abnormally high level of hydrocortisone. The high level may be the result of an adrenal gland tumor; enlargement of both adrenal glands due to a pituitary tumor; or the result of taking corticosteroid drugs for a long time.

Addison's disease is a rare disorder in which symptoms are caused by a deficiency of hydrocortisone and aldosterone. The most common cause of this disease is an autoimmune disorder, in which the immune system attacks the adrenal gland. Addison's disease generally progresses slowly. However, acute episodes, called Addisonian crises, are brought on by infection, injury, or other stresses.

Adrenal virilism is the development or premature development of male secondary sexual characteristics caused by male sex hormones (androgens) excessively produced by the adrenal gland. This disorder can occur before birth and can lead to sexual abnormalities in newborns. It can also occur in girls and women later in life. The cause is usually genetic, but in rare cases adrenal virilism is caused by an adrenal gland tumor.

Adrenal gland cancers are rare **cancer**s occuring in the endocrine tissue of the adrenals. A cancer that arises in the adrenal cortex is called an adrenocortical carcinoma and can produce high blood pressure, weight gain, excess body hair, weakening of the bones and diabetes. A cancer in the adrenal medulla is called a pheochromocytoma and can cause high blood pressure, **headache**, **palpitations**, and excessive perspiration. Although these cancers can happen at any age, most occur in young adults.

Adrenoleukodystrophy (ALD) is a rare genetic disease characterized by a loss of myelin, a substance that surrounds and insulates nerve cells in the brain. Progressive adrenal gland dysfunction is another symptom of the disease. The childhood form of the disease is the classical form and is the most severe. It is progressive and usually leads to total disability or **death**. It affects only boys because the genetic defect is sex-linked (carried on the X chromosome).

Diagnosis of adrenal gland disorders involves performing laboratory tests to measure the amounts of hormones in a patient's blood. ALD diagnosis is made based on observed symptoms, a biochemical test, and a family history. An adrenal gland scan is done when too much adrenaline and noradrenaline are produced in the body and a tumor in the adrenal gland is suspected. One such situation in which a tumor might be suspected is when high blood pressure (**hypertension**) does not respond to medication.

The adrenal gland scan takes several days. On the first day, a radiopharmaceutical is injected intravenously into the patient. On the second, third, and fourth day the patient is positioned under the camera for imaging for approximately 30 minutes each day. The area scanned extends from the hips to the lower chest. Sometimes the upper legs and head are also included. Follow-up tests might include a nuclear scan of the bones or kidney, a computed tomography scan (CT) of the adrenals, or an ultrasound of the pelvic area.

If a tumor is causing the disorder, the treatment will depend on the type and location of the tumor. If the tumor is benign, then surgically removing the tumor may be the best option. Surgery may be done by laparoscopy in some cases. It may be followed by **chemotherapy** and/or **radiation therapy**.

Sometimes the doctor must remove the adrenal gland and the surrounding tissues. Adrenalectomy is the surgical removal of one or both glands. It is usually performed by conventional (open) surgery, but in selected patients surgeons may use **laparoscopy**.

Adrenal virilism may be treated with daily doses of a glucocorticoid, but there are no drug treatments for ALD. Treatment for ALD consists of treating the symptoms and supporting the patient with physical therapy, psychological counseling, and special education in some cases. There is no cure for this disease. Death usually occurs between one and ten years after onset of symptoms.

ADRIAN, EDGAR DOUGLAS (1889-1977)

English physiologist

What physical changes occur within an organism's body when it sees, hears, smells, tastes, or feels some outside stimulus? That question has intrigued scientists for at least a century. By

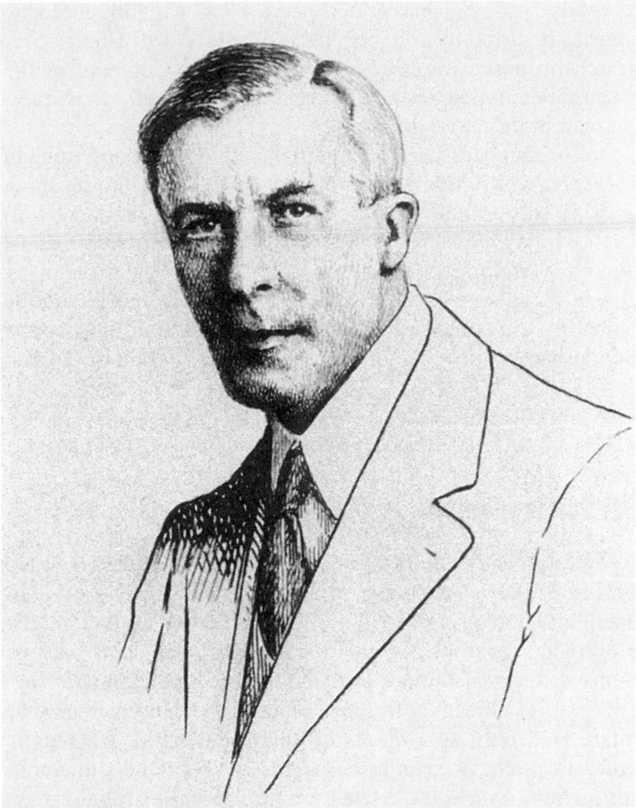

Edgar Douglas Adrian

the early 1870s, some initial answers to the puzzle had begun to appear. Research showed that an electrical impulse causes heart muscle to contract in an ''all-or-nothing'' manner. That is, after stimulation, the muscle either responds in a specific manner independent of the stimulus's intensity and frequency or not at all. By the turn of the century, the all-or-nothing response was shown to be characteristic of all smooth muscle. This research also suggested that neurons (nerve cells) might behave similarly to muscle cells.

Confirmation of this view was provided over the next two decades by the work of a number of scientists, particularly by that of Edgar Douglas Adrian. Adrian was born in London, England, on November 30, 1889. He entered Trinity College, Cambridge, in 1908 and became a student of the physiologist Keith Lucas (1879-1916). Lucas had already completed some of the most critical research on the effect of electrical stimulation on muscle action.

Using sophisticated techniques of detection and analysis, Adrian was able to discover a number of facts about nerve transmission. He confirmed, first of all, that neurons, like muscle cells, respond in an all-or-nothing mode. He also showed that the electrical impulse traveling through a neuron does not change if the kind or the strength of the stimulus changes. In addition, he found that some sense organs eventually adapt to a stimulus that is applied steadily, while others do not.

Much of Adrian's research was inspired by or had significant impact on practical medical problems. For example, his early work on muscle and nerve cells was influenced by injuries incurred by soldiers during World War I. His later research on nerve transmission led to the development of the **electroencephalogram** and the treatment of deafness, paralysis, and other nerve disorders.

Adrian became a lecturer in physiology at Cambridge in 1919 and was promoted to professor in 1937. He left teaching in 1951 to become Master of Trinity College. From 1950 to 1955 he was president of the Royal Society. His two highest honors were creation as a hereditary baron of the realm by Queen Elizabeth II (1926-) in 1955 and his receipt of the Nobel Prize for physiology or medicine (shared with **Charles Scott Sherrington**) in 1932. Adrian died in London on August 4, 1977.

AGGRESSION

Aggression is a form of behavior in which an attack, directed against either an opponent or an inanimate object, is threatened, attempted, or carried out to completion. It may be displayed as a verbal assault or a physical one, and may be motivated out of offense or defense. One's perception of aggression is subjective. In some cultures a raised voice may be interpreted only as a means of getting attention, whereas in others it might be seen as an aggressive act. One's tolerance for aggression may be related to one's moral or religious beliefs. In times of war, for example, opposing sides may feel morally or religiously justified in inflicting acts of aggression upon the enemy. Views about the origin of aggression are also influenced by religious and moral values. For instance, one's personal views about the existence of original sin may affect one's opinion about whether aggression is an innate or learned form of behavior. During the past century, social scientists have attempted, through research with human and animal subjects, to learn more about the relative roles played by nature and nurture in the development of aggression. Certain chromosomal abnormalities in humans appear to be associated with an increased tendency toward aggressiveness, though the interpretation of these correlates is controversial. Correlates also exist between early abuse in childhood and later tendencies toward criminal violence.

Social scientists have examined animal and human aggression from an evolutionary perspective, by looking at the relative costs and benefits incurred by the opponents in an aggressive encounter. When resources such as food, mates and territory are limited, the competition over them usually takes on a more aggressive quality. In cases of human conflict, the exact nature of costs and benefits is often difficult to define objectively.

Among animals, aggressive encounters rarely lead to death. Humans, however, are capable of killing one another, and over the course of history have done so on a grand scale. The invention of sophisticated weapons now makes it possible for humans to annihilate their perceived enemies without seeing them. Why humans take part in aggressive acts that have such extreme consequences has been the subject of considerable research and debate, as have questions concerning the nature of factors that elicit aggression. Because aggression is a form of behavior and because the biological and cultural origins of behaviors are difficult to separate from one another, it is likely that definitive answers to these and other questions will remain somewhat elusive.

AGING

Aging is the series of biological changes, involving a variety of processes, that over time lead to the functional impairment and eventual death of an organism. Although the simple passage of time determines chronological age, it does not determine biological age. Each species has a unique life span, and the speed of aging is paced by the length of the life span.

As complex organisms such as mammals age, reproductive capacity declines and is eventually lost, muscular strength decreases, reflexes are diminished and slowed, senses such as vision and hearing lose acuity, pulmonary and cardiovascular capacity decreases, and organs such as the liver, stomach, and intestine lose some of their capacity to perform their usual functions. In humans, some of the most marked changes of aging are external. Aging humans often have graying or loss of hair, wrinkled skin, and stooped posture. Although there are many processes involved in aging, not all affect every organism.

Most explanations for how and why aging occurs begin on the cellular level. Although not all is understood, when cells group together into complex organisms, control of cell growth and differentiation is important, and aging processes may be a byproduct of this control.

The strands of deoxyribonucleic acid (DNA) that guide a cell's physiologic process can be damaged during the normal function of generating ribonucleic acid (RNA), the cell's messengers. The presence of repair mechanisms confirms this idea because if the DNA were not properly repaired, cellular functions would be impaired. Thus, it is thought that by either wear and tear or through improper repair, over time the DNA may be destroyed and cellular reproduction function impaired.

One of the most important sources of possible cellular damage arises from metabolism, the process involved in acquiring the energy necessary for cellular function. Energy for cellular function is secured by building and storing adenosine triphosphate (ATP). In this process, oxygen leaves its usual paired molecule to form single charged molecules that are highly reactive. If they break free of the usual metabolic process, these so-called "free radicals" can cause anything from disruption of cell membranes, broken or malformed enzyme molecules, or damage in the cell nucleus. Free radicals can be neutralized by anitoxidants such as vitamins C or E, or can be captured and destroyed by one of the enzymes specifically evolved for this purpose. Cellular repair mechanisms repair the damage unless it is severe enough to cause cell death. The cell lives as long as the organism in which it resides.

Since the term "organ" covers a wide variety of structures as different as the skin and liver, it is difficult to make specific descriptions of changes brought about by aging. In general, the organs diminish in size and often have a decreased number of cells. However, those cells remaining may still show exhibit good functional ability. One change that is universal but has varying effects depending on the tissue is the stiffening observed in collagen. Collagen is part of skin, arteries, cartilage, tendons, and many other parts of the body. In the aging process, this stiffening of collagen makes the skin more fragile, the **cardiovascular system** less resilient (resulting in high blood pressure) and the muscles and joints stiffer and more prone to injury.

In whole organisms, the various tissues are interdependent for continued function, so as various systems age, the entire organism becomes impaired. For example, all the cells of the body are affected to some extent by the amount of hormones circulating in the blood. If levels of those hormones are altered, as in the aging process, all the tissues of the body are affected to some degree.

Older animals are poorer in agility, balance, and in their ability to regulate body temperature. In addition, the **immune system** is less able to respond quickly, vigorously, and with as accurate an attack in older organisms, leaving the older animal more vulnerable to disease. Of equal concern is the loss of ability of the immune system to make specific identification of a foreign antigen (a substance that produces an antibody when introduced directly into the body), leading to the possibility of mounting an immune attack that may include tissues of the host or not recognizing cancer cells.

In human beings, the maximum potential life span is about 115 years and appears to have remained constant for about the past 100,000 years. Life expectancy, on the other hand, has increased dramatically in the twentieth century. This increase is due to many factors, including improved economic status, better living conditions, and improvements in the diagnosis and treatment of many diseases.

The average life expectancy at birth has grown from 40 years in the mid-ninteenth century to 75 years at the end of the twentieth century. Some experts, however, believe it is unlikely that the average life expectancy will exceed 85 years, most likely because of a biological limit inherent in human cells. Certain factors can, however, exert positive effects on human life expectancy, such as moderate exercise, a relaxed lifestyle, and a balanced diet.

See also Immune system; Metabolism; Nutrition

AIDS

Acquired immune deficiency syndrome (AIDS) is an infectious disease caused by the human immunodeficiency virus or HIV. It was first recognized in the United States in 1981. AIDS is the advanced form of infection with the HIV virus.

AIDS is considered one of the most devastating public health problems in recent history. In 1996, the Centers for Disease Control and Prevention (CDC) estimated that one million persons in the United States are HIV-positive, and nearly a quarter of a million are living with AIDS. Approximately 16,700 people died from AIDS in the United States in 1997. The World Health Organization (WHO) estimates that 18 million adults and 1.5 million children worldwide were infected with HIV as of 1995.

HIV can be transmitted through heterosexual or homosexual intercourse, from mother to child during pregnancy or through breastfeeding, and through exposure to contaminated blood or blood products. Shared needle use among intravenous drug users or needle stick injuries among healthcare workers can also transmit the virus. HIV is not transmitted by handshakes or other casual contact, coughing or sneezing, or by bloodsucking insects such as mosquitoes. HIV attacks the body through three disease processes: immunodeficiency, autoimmunity, and nervous system dysfunction.

Immunodeficiency means that the immune system is weakened or does not work properly. Infections and cancers can take advantage of the situation and cause disease. Autoimmunity is a condition in which the immune system works against the body's own cells. Researchers do not know precisely how HIV attacks the nervous system. One theory is that, once infected with HIV, one type of immune system cell, called a macrophage, releases a toxin that harms the nervous system.

The course of AIDS generally progresses through three stages. The first stage of AIDS is usually acute retroviral syndrome. During this stage, symptoms may include **fever**, fatigue, muscle aches, loss of appetite, digestive disturbances, weight loss, skin **rashes**, **headache**, and chronically swollen lymph nodes. Acute retroviral syndrome develops between one and six weeks after infection and lasts for two to three weeks.

During the acute retroviral syndrome stage, the HIV virus enters a patient's lymph nodes. The disease then enters the second stage and becomes latent for many years. However, the virus continues to replicate in the lymph nodes. Chronic painless swellings in the lymph nodes occur during the latency period. Many patients develop low-grade fevers, chronic fatigue, and general weakness. HIV may also cause food malabsorption, loss of appetite, and increased metabolism that contribute to the so-called AIDS wasting or wasting syndrome.

At any time during HIV infection, patients may suffer from a yeast infection in the mouth called thrush or other mouth infections; **diarrhea** and other gastrointestinal symptoms; diseases of the lungs and kidneys; and degeneration of nerve fibers in the arms and legs. HIV infection of the nervous system leads to loss of strength and reflexes and feelings of numbness or burning in the feet or lower legs.

Late-stage AIDS is usually marked by a sharp decline in the number of CD4+ lymphocytes (a type of immune system cell), followed by a rise in infections and cancers. Once the patient's CD4+ lymphocyte count falls below 200 cells/mm^3, the risk for opportunistic infections increases sharply. AIDS patients easily develop bacterial infections and are highly vulnerable to viral infections. A common fungal disease associated with AIDS is *Pneumocystis carinii* **pneumonia** (PCP). Other fungal infections include **candidiasis** or thrush. Toxoplasmosis is caused by a protozoan, as are amebiasis and **cryptosporidiosis**.

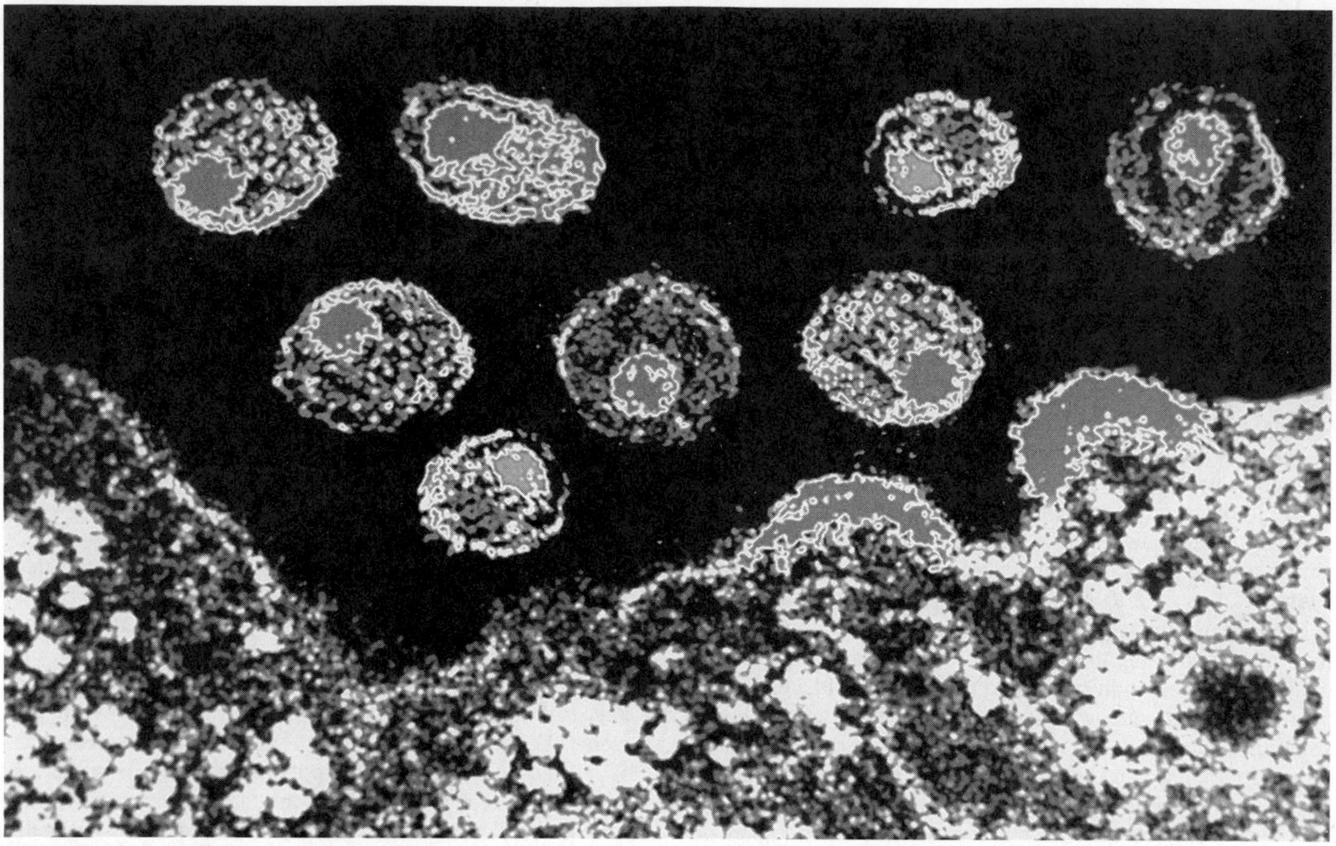

HIV-1 virus.

AIDS **dementia** complex is a late complication. It is marked by loss of reasoning and memory, inability to concentrate, apathy, and unsteadiness or weakness in walking. Some patients also develop seizures. There are no specific treatments for AIDS dementia complex. Patients in late-stage AIDS may develop inflammations of the muscles and may have arthritis-like pains in the joints.

Patients with late-stage AIDS may develop **Kaposi's sarcoma**, a type of skin tumor. It is the most common AIDS-related cancer. The second most common form of cancer in AIDS patients is a tumor of the lymphatic system (lymphoma).

Because HIV infection produces such a wide range of symptoms, a doctor looks for the overall pattern of symptoms rather than any one finding. Blood tests can be more than 99.9% accurate in detecting HIV infection within four to eight weeks following exposure. In addition to diagnostic blood tests, other blood tests are used to track the course of AIDS in patients that have already been diagnosed. Doctors use many tests to diagnose opportunistic infections, cancers, or other disease conditions in AIDS patients.

Most AIDS patients require complex long-term treatment with medications to treat or prevent infectious diseases. AIDS-related malignancies in the central nervous system are usually treated with **radiation therapy**. Cancers elsewhere in the body are treated with **chemotherapy**.

Researchers have developed drugs that suppress replication of the HIV virus in the body. Treatment guidelines for these agents are in constant change as new medications are developed and introduced. However, at the present time, there is no cure for AIDS.

AIDS TESTS

AIDS tests, short for acquired immunodeficiency syndrome tests, cover a number of different procedures used to diagnose and treat HIV patients. Some AIDS tests are used to diagnose patients or confirm a diagnosis; others are used to measure the progression of the disease or the effectiveness of specific treatment regimens. Some AIDS tests can also be used to screen blood donations for safe use in **transfusions**.

Diagnostic blood tests for AIDS are usually given to persons in high-risk populations who have been exposed to HIV or who have the early symptoms of AIDS. Most persons infected with HIV will develop a detectable level of antibody within three months of infection. Public health experts recommend testing all children born to mothers with HIV.

It is possible to diagnose HIV infection by isolating the virus itself from a blood sample or by demonstrating the presence of HIV antigen in the blood. (An antigen is a protein that causes the immune system to produce antibodies against it.)

Isolating the virus itself is expensive, not widely available, and slow. More common are blood tests that work by detecting the presence of antibodies to the HIV virus.

The enzyme-linked immunosorbent assay (ELISA) test involves HIV antigens that are attached to a plastic surface. A sample of the patient's blood serum is added. If there are any HIV antibodies in the blood, they will attach to the HIV antigens. After rinsing off excess blood factors, a second antibody is added. This antibody binds with any HIV antibodies that are attached to the HIV antigens. The second antibody also contains a chemical that changes color, indicating the presence of HIV antibodies in the patient's blood.

Occasionally, the ELISA test will be positive for a patient without symptoms of AIDS from a low-risk group. This result may be a false positive. The Western blot or immunoblot test is used to confirm the diagnosis of AIDS. In Western blot testing, HIV antigens are suspended in a flat slab of gel. An electric current run through the gel causes the proteins to separate from one another and move varying distances depending on their molecular size. Afterwards, the gel is pressed against a nylon or nitrocellulose filter, transferring the proteins to the filter. The patient's blood is reacted against the filter, followed by treatment with developing chemicals. If HIV antibodies are present, they show up as a colored patch or blot on the filter.

Immunofluorescent assay (IFA) is sometimes used to confirm ELISA results instead of Western blotting. An IFA test detects the presence of HIV antibody in a sample of the patient's serum by mixing HIV antigen with a fluorescent chemical, adding the blood sample, and observing the reaction under a microscope with ultraviolet light.

Polymerase chain reaction (PCR) is used to evaluate the very small number of AIDS patients with false-negative ELISA and Western blot tests. The PCR test can measure the presence of viral nucleic acids in the patient's blood even when there is no detectable antibody to HIV. However, the overwhelming majority of infected persons will be detected by ELISA screening within one to three months of infection.

Blood tests to evaluate patients already diagnosed with HIV infection are also important. Doctors can measure the number or proportion of certain types of cells in an AIDS patient's blood to see whether and how rapidly the disease is progressing, or whether certain treatments are helping the patient. These cell count tests include:

- Complete **blood count** (CBC).
- Absolute CD4+ lymphocytes. A lymphocyte is a type of white blood cell that is important in an immune response.
- CD4+ lymphocyte percentage. A white blood cell count that is broken down into categories in this way is called a WBC differential.

The most recent type of blood test for monitoring AIDS patients is the viral load test. It can tell the doctor the speed at which HIV is replicating in the body. The viral load test is based on PCR techniques.

Another test measures beta$_2$-microglobulin (β_2M), a protein found on the surface of all human cells with a nucleus. It is released into the blood when a cell dies. Although rising blood levels of β_2M are found in patients with **cancer** and other serious diseases, a rising β_2M blood level can be used to measure the progression of AIDS. Finally, found in the viral core of HIV, p24 is a protein that can be measured by the ELISA technique. Doctors can use p24 assays to measure the antiviral activity of the patient's medications. However, p24 is consistently present in only 25% of persons infected with HIV.

If the test results indicate that the patient is HIV- positive, he or she will need counseling, information, referral for treatment, and support. Doctors can either counsel the patient themselves or invite an experienced HIV counselor to discuss the results with the patient. They will also assess the patient's emotional and psychological status.

ALBINISM

Albinism is an inherited condition present at birth, characterized by a lack of pigment that normally gives color to the skin, hair, and eyes. It is a rare disorder and it occurs in fewer than five people per 100,000 in the United States and Europe. Other parts of the world have a much higher rate. Many types of albinism exist, all of which involve lack of pigment in varying degrees. The condition, which is found in all races, may be accompanied by eye problems and may lead to skin **cancer** later in life.

In most types of albinism, a child inherits flawed genes for making pigment from both parents. Because making pigment is complex, there are many genes that direct it. Every cell in the body contains a matched set of genes, one inherited from each parent. These genes act as a blueprint that guides the development of a fetus. Albinism is an inherited problem caused by a flaw in one or more of the genes that are responsible for the eyes and skin to make pigment. As a result, little or no pigment is made, and the child's skin, eyes and hair may be colorless.

It's also possible to inherit one normal gene and one albinism gene. In this case, the one normal gene provides enough information in its cellular blueprint to make some pigment, and the child will have normal skin and eye color. About one in 70 people are albinism carriers; that is, they have one flawed gene, but no symptoms. Carriers have a 50% percent chance of passing the albinism gene to their child. However, if both parents are carriers, there is a 1 in 4 chance for each of their children to have albinism.

Although people with albinism may experience eye problems, one of the myths about albinism is that it causes people to have pink or red eyes. In fact, people with albinism can have irises varying from light gray or blue to brown. (The iris is the colored portion of the eye.) If people with albinism seem to have reddish eyes, it's because light is being reflected from the back of the eye (retina) in much the same way as happens when people are photographed with an electronic flash.

People with albinism may be very far-sighted or near-sighted, and may have other defects in the curvature of the lens of the eye (**astigmatism**) that cause images to appear un-

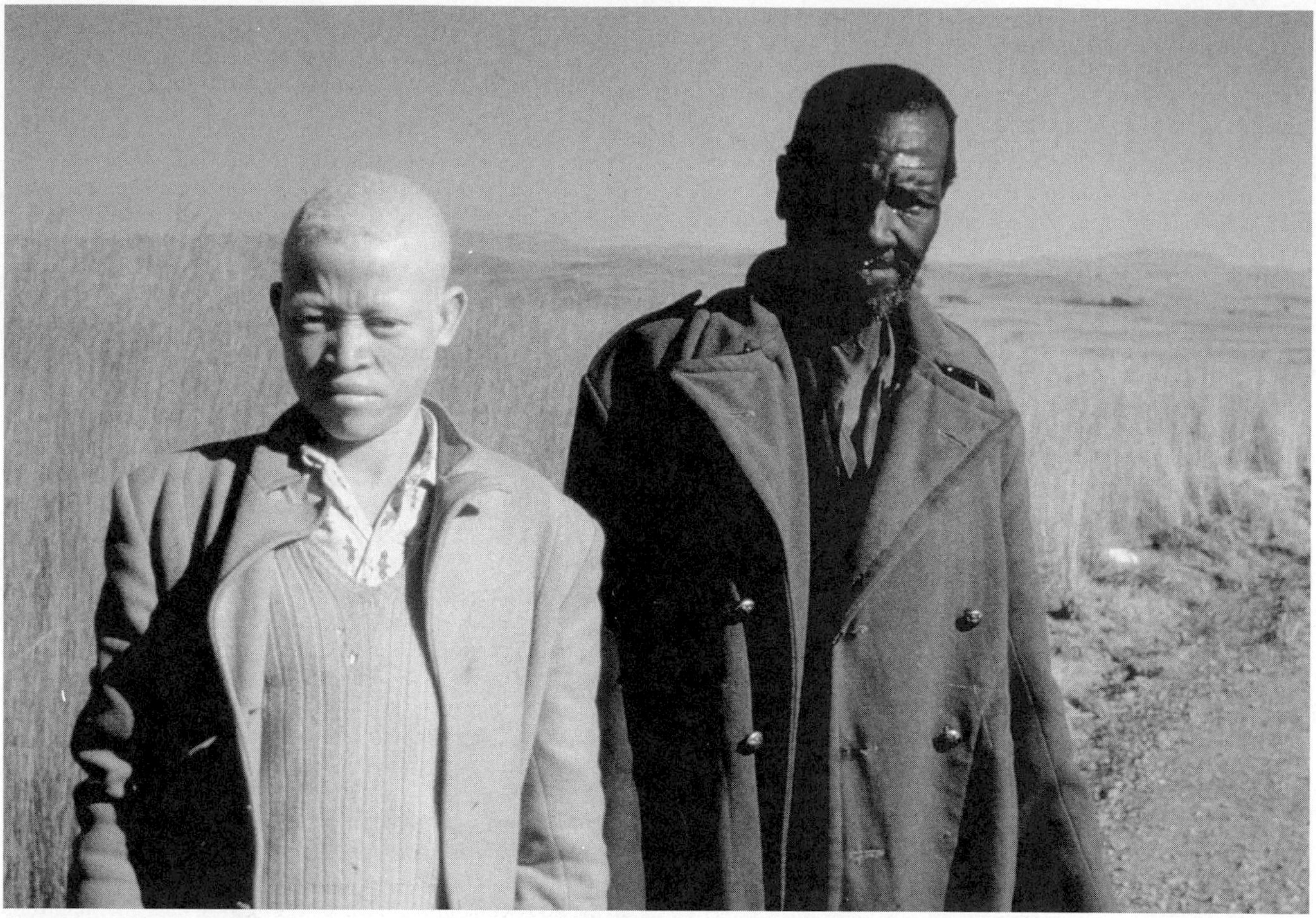

A man with albinism (left) and his normally pigmented father. ***(Photograph by Norman Lightfoot, Photo Researchers, Inc. Reproduced by permission.)***

focused. Another potential problem is nystagmus, a constant, involuntary movement of the eyeball. It may be difficult for some people with albinism to coordinate the eyes in fixing and tracking objects, which may lead to an appearance of having crossed eyes (strabismus). Their eyes may be very sensitive to light because their irises allow too much light to enter their eyes.

In addition to the characteristically light skin and eye problems, people with a rare form of albinism called Hermansky-Pudlak Syndrome (HPS) also have a greater tendency to have bleeding disorders, inflammation of the large bowel (colitis), lung (pulmonary) disease, and kidney (renal) problems.

It's not always easy to diagnose the exact type of albinism a person has. Recently, a blood test has been developed that can identify carriers of the gene for some types of albinism. Similar tests during pregnancy can diagnose some types of albinism in an unborn child. The specific type of albinism a person has can be determined by taking a good family history and examining the patient and several close relatives.

There is no treatment to replace the lack of pigment caused by albinism. Also, doctors can only treat, not cure, eye problems. Glasses are usually needed and can be tinted to ease **pain** from too much sunlight. There is no cure for nystagmus, and treatments for focusing problems (surgery or contact lenses) are not effective in all cases. Crossed eyes can be treated during infancy, using eye patches, surgery or medicine injections.

Patients with albinism should avoid excessive exposure to the sun. If exposure can't be avoided, they should use UVA-UVB sunblocks with an SPF of at least 20. Taking betacarotene may help provide some skin color, although it doesn't protect against sun exposure.

In the United States, people with this condition can expect to have a normal lifespan. People with albinism may experience some social problems because of a lack of understanding on the part of others.

ALCHEMY

In a general sense, alchemy is perceived as the transformation of a common substance to something rare and valuable. Medieval alchemists are often portrayed as little more than quacks attempting to make gold from lead. This depiction is not entirely correct. To be sure, there were such characters, but for real alchemists, called adepts, the field was an almost divine mixture of science, mystery, and philosophy.

Alchemy has existed for more than two thousand years. The first mentions of it can be found in ancient Chinese, Indian, and Middle Eastern texts as early as the fourth and fifth centuries B.C. Some historians believe that alchemy arose independently in each culture. Because of common ideas, however, other historians argue that it arose from a single source. They suggest that alchemy began in China or India and gradually spread westward. Whatever its origins, alchemy came to Europe via Egypt during the Alexandrian era, starting in the fourth century B.C.

The overall goal of alchemy was to make sense of the nature of matter. **Aristotle** promoted the idea that there are four principle elements of matter: air, fire, earth, and water. He claimed that all physical matter is composed of these elements in varying amounts. An Arab alchemist, Jabir (also called Geber), refined this theory in the eighth century A.D. with a focus on metals. He suggested that metals were composed of sulphur and mercury. Much later, the Swiss physician, Paracelsus (1493-1541), added a third element to the theoretical composition of metal: salt. It should be stressed that these three elements—mercury, sulphur, and salt—were different from the ordinary substances of the same names.

Because metals were all composed of the same elements, it was thought possible to transform one type of metal into another by altering the relative amounts of constituent elements. To accomplish such a transformation, it was necessary to have what was called the philosopher's stone. Not only could this stone transform lead into gold, but it could also act as a powerful medicine. If used for this purpose, it was called the elixir vitae or elixir of life. In addition to curing any disease, the elixir vitae could supposedly increase a person's lifespan, potentially conferring immortality. The trick was to find the philosopher's stone, which, despite its name, was supposed to have been a red powder.

The futile search for the philosopher's stone endured for centuries and involved countless people. Alchemists believed that it was composed of a superfine form of gold. Base metals such as tin or lead were supposed to be composed of impure sulphur and mercury; gold of more purified sulphur and mercury; and the philosopher's stone of super-purified, or quintessentialized sulphur and mercury. Just a few grains of philosopher's stone would be sufficient to transform a base metal into pure gold.

It was thought that the philosopher's stone could be derived from mixing a metal ore such as iron, lead, or mercury, and some type of organic acid. The resultant mixture would be heated, dissolved in acid, distilled or evaporated, oxidized, and sealed in a special container. The container would be gently warmed and allowed to cool. If everything were done properly, the philosopher's stone would be found. However, each stage required the perfect combination of factors. Not only did measurable factors such as quantity of materials, temperature, and elapsed time have to be on target, but astrological influences and other intangibles had to be in place. Experiments could last for years, during which time alchemists exposed themselves to poisonous fumes and a near-constant danger of fire.

To aid in their search for the philosopher's stone, alchemists looked to ancient texts for clues. One of the most influential was called the Emerald Tablet. According to legend, it had been discovered in the tomb of Hermes—for which reason, alchemists often referred to themselves as Sons of Hermes—and it laid out 13 principles of alchemy. These principles, like most alchemical writings, were profoundly cryptic. For example, the second principle of the Emerald Tablet read: "What is below is like that which is above, and what is above is like that which is below, to accomplish the miracles of one thing."

The use of symbolism and allegory was widespread in alchemical texts. They were intended to be mystifying, because adepts were very keen to keep their secrets hidden. They did not want them to be understood by anyone with lesser motives. The adepts' pursuit of the philosopher's stone was based on the lofty ideal of uncovering the nature of matter. They did not want their work misused by people who were only motivated by greed for gold. Such people were dismissed as puffers or bellows-blowers.

Regardless of motive, neither the puffers nor the adepts had any luck discovering the philosopher's stone. Along the way, however, they developed novel experimental procedures, discovered new substances, and built laboratory equipment. These accomplishments aided in the development of a science that is still successfully practiced today: namely, chemistry.

For a time, the terms chemistry and alchemy were used interchangeably. As a result, some of the biggest names in chemistry from the medieval and Renaissance periods were also associated with alchemy. Paracelsus, who was mentioned previously, brought alchemy into the medical arena with his theory that chemical cures were effective against disease. Robert Boyle, considered the father of chemistry, was involved in alchemy from 1646 until the end of his life. His influential book, *The Skeptical Chymist* (1661), defined the differences between chemistry and alchemy and introduced the concept of element known today. Alchemy's last gasp was fueled by Isaac Newton, physicist and founder of calculus, in the late 17th century.

ALCOHOL USE AND ABUSE

Alcoholism refers to alcohol abuse and alcohol dependence. Both of these disorders involve repeated life problems that are directly tied to a person's use of alcohol. Alcoholism has serious consequences, affecting an individual's health and personal life, as well as having an impact on society at large. For example, alcohol is a contributing factor in 50% of all **death**s from motor vehicle accidents.

Alcohol exerts a depressive effect on the brain, creating difficulty walking, poor balance, slurring of speech, and generally poor coordination. At higher alcohol levels, breathing and heart rates become slower, and vomiting may occur. Still higher alcohol levels may result in **coma** and death.

Long-term alcohol use affects virtually every organ system. Effects on the nervous system include blackouts and sleep disturbances. Further, numbness and tingling may occur in the arms and legs. Two nervous system syndromes are associated with alcoholism. Wernicke's syndrome results in disordered eye movements, very poor balance, and difficulty walking; Korsakoff's syndrome severely affects memory, preventing new learning from taking place.

Alcohol causes stomach acid to enter the esophagus, causing **pain** and bleeding. Stomach inflammation can also result in bleeding and pain, and decreased appetite. **Diarrhea** is common, due to alcohol's effect on the pancreas. Additionally, inflammation of the pancreas (**pancreatitis**) is serious and painful. Throughout the intestinal tract, alcohol interferes with nutrients being absorbed.

The liver is severely affected by constant alcohol use. Alcohol interferes with the liver's chemical processes, and the liver begins to enlarge and fill with fat. Fibrous scar tissue develops and interferes with the liver's normal structure and function (cirrhosis). Eventually, the liver may become inflamed (hepatitis).

Alcohol alters blood cells. White blood cells (important for fighting infections) decrease in number, weakening the immune system. As a result, alcoholics are at increased risk for infections, and may experience an increased risk of **cancer**. Effects on platelets and blood clotting factors cause an increased risk of bleeding.

With excessive alcohol, blood pressure becomes dangerously high. High levels of fats in the bloodstream increase the risk of heart disease. Heavy drinking results in increased heart size, weakened heart muscle, abnormal heart rhythms, and a greatly increased risk of **stroke**.

Heavy drinking has a negative effect on fertility in both men and women. Alcoholism in **pregnancy** may lead to **fetal alcohol syndrome**, which causes distinctive facial defects, lowered IQ, and behavioral problems in the child.

There are two types of alcoholism. In *alcohol dependence*, a person becomes accustomed to a certain amount of alcohol (tolerance) and must constantly increase the amount to obtain the desired effect. Another aspect of alcohol dependence is withdrawal. Withdrawal refers to the unpleasant symptoms experienced by an alcoholic when alcohol is not used. People dependent on alcohol tend to drink more than intended and are unable to stop once started. Large blocks of their time are taken up by alcohol. Their drinking continues regardless of negative effects on their health, relationships, education, or job. With *alcohol abuse*, a person repeatedly fails to live up to his or her most important responsibilities; physically endangers him or herself, or others; gets into trouble with the law; and experiences difficulties in relationships or jobs.

Diagnosis often occurs when family members alert an alcoholic's physician to the problem. A physician may suspect alcoholism if a patient suffers repeated injuries or experiences medical problems related alcohol use. Diagnosis is aided by administering questionnaires. Determining the exact quantity of alcohol that a person drinks is less important than determining how drinking affects relationships, jobs, educational goals, and family life.

Treatment of alcoholism has two parts. The first step is detoxification, which involves helping the person stop drinking and ridding his or her body of the harmful (toxic) effects of alcohol. An alcoholic needs support to get through withdrawal. Withdrawal can range from mild to life-threatening. Mild withdrawal symptoms include nausea, achiness, diarrhea, difficulty sleeping, sweatiness, **anxiety**, and trembling. More severe withdrawal can include **hallucinations**, seizures, unbearable craving for alcohol, confusion, **fever**, fast heart rate, high blood pressure, and **delirium**. Patients at highest risk for the most severe symptoms of withdrawal (referred to as delirium tremens) often have other medical problems.

After detoxification, the next treatment phase is **rehabilitation**. Rehabiliatation helps the patient avoid alcohol and change the behaviors that led to alcoholism. Sessions led by peers are considered among the best methods of preventing a return to drinking (relapse). Perhaps the most well-known such group is Alcoholics Anonymous, which uses a 12-step model to help people avoid drinking. These steps involve recognizing the destructive power that alcohol has held over the alcoholic's life, looking to a higher power for help, and reflecting on the ways in which the use of alcohol has hurt others and, if possible, making amends.

There are also medications that may help an alcoholic avoid drinking. Disulfiram (Antabuse) is a drug which, when mixed with alcohol, causes **nausea and vomiting**, diarrhea, and trembling. Naltrexone and acamprosate seem to be helpful in limiting the effects of a relapse. However, medications alone are not helpful; an alcoholic must work very hard to achieve recovery.

ALEXANDER, HATTIE (1901-1968)

American microbiologist and pediatrician

Hattie Alexander, a dedicated pediatrician, medical educator, and researcher in microbiology, won international recognition for deriving a serum to combat influenzal **meningitis**, a common disease that previously had been nearly always fatal to infants and young children. Alexander subsequently investigated microbiological genetics and the processes whereby bacteria, through genetic mutation, acquire resistance to antibiotics. In 1964, as president of the American Pediatric Society, she became one of the first women to head a national medical association.

Hattie Elizabeth Alexander was born on April 5, 1901, in Baltimore, Maryland. She was the second of eight children born to Elsie May (Townsend) Alexander and William Bain Alexander, a merchant. Alexander attended Baltimore schools and then enrolled in Goucher College in Baltimore on a partial scholarship. She excelled at sports but was only an average student in her course work, which included bacteriology and physiology. Alexander graduated from Goucher with an A.B. degree in 1923. For the next three years she worked as a bacteriologist for the U.S. Public Health Service laboratory in Washington, D.C., and at a branch laboratory of the Maryland Public Health Service. Impressed with her research experience, Johns Hopkins University in Baltimore admitted her to their medical program. Alexander performed exceptionally at Johns Hopkins, earning her M.D. in 1930.

As an intern at the Harriet Lane Home of Johns Hopkins Hospital from 1930 to 1931, Alexander became interested in influenzal meningitis. The source of the disease was *Hemophilus influenzae,* a bacteria that causes inflammation of the meninges, the membranes surrounding the brain and spinal cord. In 1931 Alexander began a second internship at the Babies Hospital of the Columbia-Presbyterian Medical Center in New York City. There, she witnessed first-hand the futility of medical efforts to save babies who had contracted influenzal meningitis.

Beginning in 1933, with her medical training complete, Alexander held a series of pediatric, teaching, and research positions at the Babies Hospital, the Vanderbilt Clinic of the Columbia-Presbyterian Medical Center, and Columbia University's College of Physicians and Surgeons. She was appointed an adjunct assistant pediatrician in 1933 and an assistant attending pediatrician in 1938 by the Babies Hospital, and she held parallel posts at the Vanderbilt Clinic; she would be promoted to attending pediatrician at the Babies Hospital and the Vanderbilt Clinic in 1951. At Columbia, she held a fellowship in children's diseases from 1932 to 1934 and became an assistant in children's diseases in 1933 and an instructor in children's diseases in 1935.

Alexander's early research focused on deriving a serum (the liquid component of blood, in which antibodies are contained) that would be effective against influenzal meningitis. Serums derived from animals that have been exposed to a specific disease-producing bacterium often contain antibodies against the disease and can be developed for use in immunizing humans against it. Alexander knew that attempts to develop an anti-influenzal serum from horses had been unsuccessful. The Rockefeller Institute in New York City, however, had been able to prepare a rabbit serum for the treatment of pneumonia, another bacterial disease. Alexander therefore experimented with rabbit serums, and by 1939 she was able to announce the development of a rabbit serum effective in curing infants of influenzal meningitis.

In the early 1940s, Alexander experimented with the use of drugs in combination with rabbit serum in the treatment of influenzal meningitis. Within the next two years, she saw infant deaths due to the disease drop by 80%. With improvements in diagnosis and the standardization of treatment, the mortality rate fell still further in later years. In recognition of her research on influenzal meningitis, Alexander received the E. Mead Johnson Award for research in pediatrics from the American Academy of Pediatrics in 1942 and the Elizabeth Blackwell Award from the New York Infirmary in 1956; and, in 1961, she became the first woman recipient of the Oscar B. Hunter Memorial Award of the American Therapeutic Society.

Alexander's research in supplementary drug treatment for influenzal meningitis led her to the study of **antibiotics** (antibacterial substances generally produced by a bacterium or a fungus). As was evident from the cultures of influenza bacilli utilized in Alexander's research, antibiotics do not provide a permanent defense against bacteria. Alexander was among the first to recognize that it was through genetic mutation that bacteria are able to develop resistance to antibiotics, and she became a pioneer in research on DNA, the nucleic substance that bears an organism's genetic blueprint. By 1950, due to lab work conducted in association with Grace Leidy, Alexander was able to alter the genetic code of *Hemophilus influenzae* by manipulating its DNA. Alexander subsequently extended this line of research to other bacteria and to viruses.

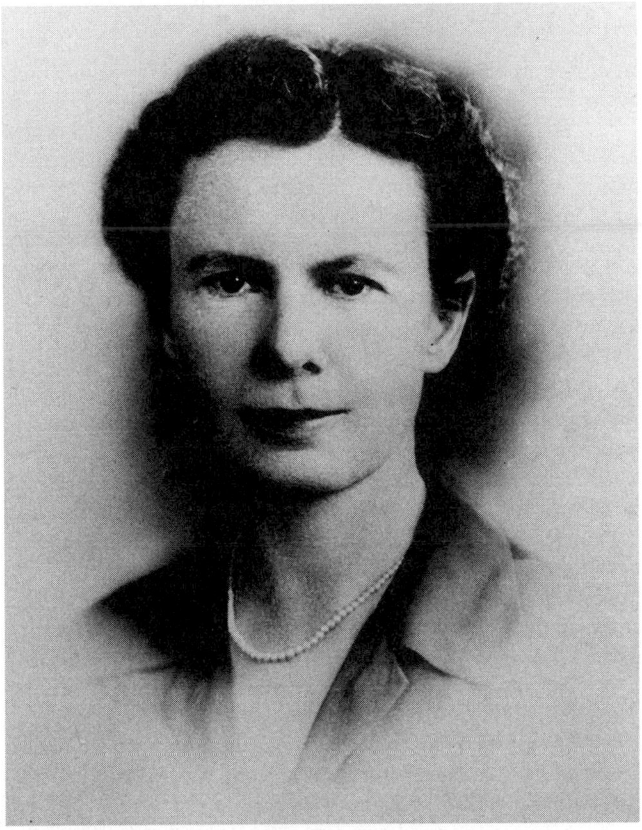

Hattie Alexander

In addition to her hospital service, research, and teaching duties, Alexander also served on the influenza commission under the United States Secretary of War from 1941 to 1945, served as consultant to the New York City Department of Health from 1958 to 1960, and joined the medical board of the Presbyterian Hospital of the Columbia-Presbyterian Medical Center in 1959. After chairing the governing council of the American Pediatric Society from 1956 to 1957 and serving as vice president from 1959 to 1960, she became president of the society in 1964.

During her career she published some 150 papers as well as chapters in textbooks on microbiology and pediatrics and delivered many honorary lectures at medical and academic institutions. Alexander lived with her companion, Dr. Elizabeth Ufford, in Port Washington, N.Y. In her spare time, Alexander enjoyed music, boating, travel, and growing exotic flowers. She died from cancer on June 24, 1968, at the age of 67.

Allergies

Allergies are abnormal reactions of the immune system which occur in response to otherwise harmless substances.

Allergies are among the most common of medical disorders. It is estimated that 60 million Americans, or more than one in every five people, suffer from some form of allergy, with similar proportions throughout much of the rest of the world. Allergy is the single largest reason for school absence and is a major source of lost productivity in the workplace.

An allergy is a type of immune reaction. Normally, the immune system responds to foreign microorganisms or particles, like pollen or dust, by producing specific proteins called antibodies that are capable of binding to identifying molecules, or antigens, on the foreign particle. This reaction between antibody and antigen sets off a series of reactions designed to protect the body from infection. Sometimes, this same series of reactions is triggered by harmless, everyday substances. This is the condition known as allergy, and the offending substance is called an allergen.

Allergens enter the body through four main routes: the airways, the skin, the gastrointestinal tract, and the circulatory system.

- Airborne allergens cause the sneezing, runny nose, and itchy, bloodshot eyes of **hay fever** (allergic rhinitis). Airborne allergens can also affect the lining of the lungs, causing **asthma**, or the conjunctiva of the eyes, causing **conjunctivitis** (pink eye).
- Allergens in food can cause **itching** and swelling of the lips and throat, cramps, and **diarrhea**. When absorbed into the bloodstream, they may cause **hives** (urticaria) or more severe reactions involving recurrent, non-inflammatory swelling of the skin, mucous membranes, organs, and brain (angioedema). Some food allergens may cause **anaphylaxis**, a potentially life-threatening condition marked by tissue swelling, airway constriction, and drop in blood pressure.
- In contact with the skin, allergens can cause reddening, itching, and blistering, called contact dermatitis. Skin reactions can also occur from allergens introduced through the airways or gastrointestinal tract. This type of reaction is known as atopic dermatitis.
- Injection of allergens, from insect **bites and stings** or drug administration, can introduce allergens directly into the circulation, where they may cause system-wide responses (including anaphylaxis), as well as the local ones of swelling and irritation at the injection site.

People with allergies are not equally sensitive to all allergens. Some may have severe allergic rhinitis but no food allergies, for instance, or be extremely sensitive to nuts but not to any other food. Allergies may get worse over time. For example, childhood ragweed allergy may progress to year-round dust and pollen allergy. On the other hand, a person may lose allergic sensitivity. Infant or childhood atopic dermatitis disappears in almost all people, for example. More commonly, what seems to be loss of sensitivity is instead a reduced exposure to allergens or an increased tolerance for the same level of symptoms.

Mast cells, one of the major players in allergic reactions, capture and display a particular type of antibody, called immunoglobulin type E (IgE) that binds to allergens. Inside mast cells are small chemical-filled packets called granules. Granules contain a variety of potent chemicals, including histamine.

Immunologists separate allergic reactions into two main types: immediate hypersensitivity reactions, which are mainly mast cell-mediated and occur within minutes of contact with allergen, and delayed hypersensitivity reactions, mediated by T cells (a type of white blood cells) and occurring hours to days after exposure.

Inhaled or ingested allergens usually cause immediate hypersensitivity reactions. Allergens bind to IgE antibodies on the surface of mast cells, which spill the contents of their granules out onto neighboring cells, including blood vessels and nerve cells. Histamine binds to the surfaces of these other cells through special proteins called histamine receptors. Interaction of histamine with receptors on blood vessels causes increased leakiness, leading to the fluid collection, swelling and increased redness. Histamine also stimulates **pain** receptors, making tissue more sensitive and irritable. Symptoms last from one to several hours following contact.

In the upper airways and eyes, immediate hypersensitivity reactions cause the runny nose and itchy, bloodshot eyes typical of allergic rhinitis. In the gastrointestinal tract, these reactions lead to swelling and irritation of the intestinal lining, which causes the cramping and diarrhea typical of food allergy. Allergens that enter the circulation may cause hives, angioedema, anaphylaxis, or atopic dermatitis.

Allergens on the skin usually cause delayed hypersensitivity reaction. Roving T cells contact the allergen, setting in motion a more prolonged immune response. This type of allergic response may develop over several days following contact with the allergen, and symptoms may persist for a week or more.

While allergy to specific allergens is not inherited, the likelihood of developing some type of allergy seems to be, at least for many people. If neither parent has allergies, the chances of a child developing allergy is approximately 10-20%; if one parent has allergies, it is 30-50%; and if both have allergies, it is 40-75%.One source of this genetic predisposition is in the ability to produce higher levels of IgE in response to allergens. Those who produce more IgE will develop a stronger allergic sensitivity.

The most common airborne allergens are the following:

- Plant pollens
- Animal fur and dander
- Body parts from house mites (microscopic creatures found in all houses)
- House dust
- Mold spores
- Cigarette smoke
- Solvents
- Cleaners.

Common food allergens include the following:

- Nuts, especially peanuts, walnuts, and Brazil nuts
- Fish, mollusks, and shellfish

- Eggs
- Wheat
- Milk
- Food additives and preservatives.

The following types of drugs commonly cause allergic reactions:

- Penicillin or other **antibiotics**
- Flu vaccines
- **Tetanus** toxoid vaccine
- Gamma globulin.

Common causes of contact dermatitis include the following:

- Poison ivy, oak, and sumac
- Nickel or nickel alloys
- Latex.

Insects and other arthropods whose bites or stings typically cause allergy include the following:

- Bees, wasps, and hornets
- Mosquitoes
- Fleas
- **Scabies**.

Symptoms depend on the specific type of allergic reaction. Allergic rhinitis is characterized by an itchy, runny nose, often with a scratchy or irritated throat due to post-nasal drip. Inflammation of the thin membrane covering the eye (allergic conjunctivitis) causes redness, irritation and increased tearing in the eyes. Asthma causes **wheezing**, **cough**ing, and **shortness of breath**. Symptoms of food allergies depend on the tissues most sensitive to the allergen and whether it is spread systemically by the circulatory system. Gastrointestinal symptoms may include swelling and tingling in the lips, tongue, palate or throat; nausea; cramping; diarrhea; and gas. Contact dermatitis is marked by reddened, itchy, weepy skin blisters.

Whole body or systemic reactions may occur from any type of allergen, but are more common following ingestion or injection of an allergen. Skin reactions include the raised, reddened, and itchy patches called hives. A deeper and more extensive skin reaction, involving more extensive fluid collection, is called angioedema. Anaphylaxis is marked by airway constriction, blood pressure drop, widespread tissue swelling, heart rhythm abnormalities, and in some cases, loss of consciousness.

Allergies can often be diagnosed by a careful medical history, matching the onset of symptoms to the exposure to possible allergens. Allergy tests can be used to identify potential allergens. These tests usually begin with prick tests or patch tests, which expose the skin to small amounts of allergen to observe the response. Reaction will occur on the skin even if the allergen is normally encountered in food or in the airways. RAST testing is a blood test that measures the level of reactive IgE antibodies in the blood. Provocation tests, most commonly done with airborne allergens, present the allergen directly through the route normally involved. Food allergen provocation tests require abstinence from the suspect allergen for two weeks or more, followed by ingestion of a measured amount. Provocation tests are not used if anaphylaxis is is a concern due to the patient's medical history. For a complete description, see the article on allergy testing.

A large number of prescription and over-the-counter drugs are available for treatment of immediate hypersensitivity reactions. Most of these work by decreasing the ability of histamine to provoke symptoms. Other drugs counteract the effects of histamine by stimulating other systems or reducing immune responses in general.

Antihistamines block the histamine receptors on nasal tissue, decreasing the effect of histamine released by mast cells. They may be used after symptoms appear, though they may be even more effective when used preventively, before symptoms appear. A wide variety of antihistamines are available.

Older antihistamines often produce drowsiness as a major side effect. Such antihistamines include the following:

- Diphenhydramine (Benadryl and generics)
- Chlorpheniramine (Chlor-trimeton and generics)
- Brompheniramine (Dimetane and generics)
- Clemastine (Tavist and generics).

Newer antihistamines that do not cause drowsiness are available by prescription and include the following:

- Astemizole (Hismanal)
- Loratidine (Claritin)
- Fexofenadine (Allegra)
- Azelastin HCl (Astelin).

Hismanal has the potential to cause serious heart **arrhythmias** when taken with the antibiotic erythromycin, the antifungal drugs ketoconazole and itraconazole, or the antimalarial drug quinine. Taking more than the recommended dose of Hismanal can also cause arrhythimas. Seldane (terfenadine), the original non-drowsy antihistamine, was voluntarily withdrawn from the market by its manufacturers in early 1998 because of this potential and because of the availability of an equally effective, safer alternative drug, fexofenadine.

Decongestants constrict blood vessels to counteract the effects of histamine. Nasal sprays are available that can be applied directly to the nasal lining and oral systemic preparations are available. Decongestants are stimulants and may cause increased heart rate and blood pressure, **headache**s, and agitation. Use of topical decongestants for longer than several days can cause loss of effectiveness and rebound congestion, in which nasal passages become more severely swollen than before treatment.

Topical **corticosteroids** reduce mucous membrane inflammation and are available by prescription. Allergies tend to become worse as the season progresses because the immune system becomes sensitized to particular antigens and can produce a faster, stronger response. Topical corticosteroids are especially effective at reducing this seasonal sensitization because they work more slowly and last longer than most other medication types. As a result, they are best started before allergy season begins. Side effects are usually mild, but may include headaches, **nosebleed**s, and unpleasant taste sensations.

Cromolyn sodium prevents the release of mast cell granules, thereby preventing the release of histamine and other chemicals contained in them. It acts as a preventive treatment if it is begun several weeks before the onset of the allergy season. It can also be used for year round allergy prevention. Cromolyn sodium is available as a nasal spray for allergic rhinitis and in aerosol (a suspension of particles in gas) form for asthma.

Immunotherapy, also known as desensitization or allergy shots, alters the balance of antibody types in the body, thereby reducing the ability of IgE to cause allergic reactions. Immunotherapy is preceded by allergy testing to determine the precise allergens responsible. These tests are described in full in the article on allergy testing. Injections involve very small but gradually increasing amounts of allergen, over several weeks or months, with periodic boosters. Full benefits may take up to several years to achieve and are not seen at all in about one in five patients. Individuals receiving all shots will be monitored closely following each shot because of the small risk of anaphylaxis, a condition that can result in difficulty breathing and a sharp drop in blood pressure.

Because allergic reactions involving the lungs cause the airways or bronchial tubes to narrow, as in asthma, **bronchodilators**, which cause the smooth muscle lining the airways to open or dilate, can be very effective. Some bronchodilators used to treat acute asthma attacks include adrenaline, albuterol, or other ''adrenoceptor stimulants,'' most often administered as aerosols. Theophylline, naturally present in coffee and tea, is another drug that produces brochodilation. It is usually taken orally, but in a severe asthma attack is may be given intravenously. Other drugs, including steroids, are used to prevent asthma attacks and in the long-term management of asthma.

Calamine lotion applied to affected skin can reduce irritation somewhat. Topical corticosteroid creams are more effective, though overuse may lead to dry and scaly skin.

The emergency condition of anaphylaxis is treated with injection of adrenaline, also known as epinephrine. People who are prone to anaphylaxis because of food or insect allergies often carry an ''Epi-pen'' containing adrenaline in a hypodermic needle. Prompt injection can prevent a more serious reaction from developing.

Allergies can improve over time, although they often worsen. While anaphylaxis and severe asthma are life-threatening, other allergic reactions are not. Learning to recognize and avoid allergy-provoking situations allows most people with allergies to lead normal lives.

Avoiding allergens is the best means of limiting allergic reactions. For food allergies, there is no effective treatment except avoidance. By determining the allergens that are causing reactions, most people can learn to avoid allergic reactions from food, drugs, and contact allergens such as poison ivy or latex. Airborne allergens are more difficult to avoid, although keeping dust and animal dander from collecting in the house may limit exposure. Cromolyn sodium can prevent mast cell degranulation, thereby limiting the allergic response.

ALTERNATIVE MEDICINE

Alternative medicine is a broad category of approaches to healing that encompasses a wide variety of techniques, modalities, and medical systems that, for the most part, are considered outside the mainstream of traditional Western medicine. The use of the terms ''alternative'' versus ''complementary'' medicine reflect a shift in public and professional consciousness. While ''alternative'' has been used to suggest substitution, an either/or relationship, implying modalities used instead of conventional medicine, ''complementary'' or ''integrative'' medicine are terms increasingly used to suggest modalities used in conjunction with conventional medicine.

With its growing popularity among health care consumers and professionals worldwide, however, alternative medicine is becoming less ''alternative'' with each passing year. In the 1990s an increasing number of medical schools began offering courses in alternative medicine, and some hospitals began creating departments of alternative medicine. According to a report published in the *New England Journal of Medicine* in 1993, the estimated number of annual visits to providers of alternative medicine (425 million) in the United States in 1990 exceeded the number of visits to all primary care physicians (388 million).

Most alternative medical techniques are founded on a holistic perspective of health. That is, when diagnosing and treating a patient, consideration is given to the whole person, including the physical, emotional, mental, and spiritual aspects of the individual. However, much of what is called alternative medicine is derived from the healing practices of other cultures or ancient traditions. For example, for centuries many cultures around the world have used herbs for medicinal purposes, including the Native Americans, and the use of **acupuncture**, which has been used in China 2697 B.C.

Alternative therapies may be divided into seven major categories, according to the Office of Alternative Medicine, a branch of the **National Institutes of Heath** established in 1992 by Congress for the purpose of investigating the efficacy of alternative therapies:

- Mind-body interventions refer to the mind's role in the cause and course of illness. This role has been substantially reinforced by the discovery of the complex interactions between the mind and the neurological, hormonal, and **immune system**. Meditation, **guided imagery**, **hypnosis**, **biofeedback**, and **yoga** are a few examples of these therapies.
- Bioelectromagnetic applications in medicine (BEM), an emerging science, studies how living organisms interact with electromagnetic fields. The most important BEM modalities in alternative medicine are nonthermal applications of nonionizing radiation, such as those emitted by power lines. Additional applications of BEM fields are bone repair, nerve stimulation, wound healing, treatment of **osteoarthritis**, electroacupuncture, tissue regeneration, and immune system stimulation.
- Traditional and folk remedies is a category that includes the following five modalities: Traditional **Chinese medicine** refers to acupuncture, vaccines not yet accepted by mainstream medicine, including antineoplastons, cartilage products, ethylene diamine tetracetic acid (EDTA), immunoaugmentive therapy, coleys toxins, neural therapy, apitherapy, iscador, and biologically guided chemotherapy.

- Herbal medicine includes the use of plants and plant products found in the folk medicine traditions of all cultures. The World Health Organization estimates that four billion people—80% of the world's population—use herbal medicine for some aspect of primary health care.
- Diet and nutrition in the prevention and treatment of chronic disease represents a continuum of philosophies ranging from the idea that supplementing the typical American diet lies somewhat beyond the recommended daily allowance (RDA) necessary to promote optimum health, to the idea that supplementation well beyond the RDA is often required to reverse the effects of long-term deficiencies.

In the 1990s leading drug companies around the world worked on projects to find plants in the jungles of South and Central America that may yield more effective medicines than those produced in their laboratories. The United States National Cancer Institute also developed a $20.5 million program for the study of medicinal plants. The increased popularity of alternative and complementary medicine has become a challenge and opportunity that health professionals, scientists, policy makers, and health related industries could not afford to ignore.

See also Ayurvedic medicine; Biofeedback; Chinese traditional herbal medicine; Chinese traditional medicine; Chiropractic; Herbal medicine; Homeopathic medicine; Massage; National Institutes of Health; Nutrition; Naturopathic medicine

Altitude sickness

Altitude sickness is a general term encompassing several disorders that occur high altitudes. High altitude is greater than 8,000 feet; medium altitude is between 5,000 and 8,000 feet; and extreme altitude is greater than 19,000 feet. There are groups of people who have lived at high altitudes for generations, and they are simply accustomed to living at such altitudes. However, people who are accustomed to lower altitudes are at risk of developing altitude sickness.

Most healthy individuals suffer altitude sickness at very high altitudes. About 20% of people ascending above 9,000 feet in one day will develop altitude sickness. Individuals with preexisting medical conditions—even a minor respiratory infection—may become sick at more moderate altitudes.

Altitude sickness occurs because the air contains less oxygen at higher altitudes. Therefore, there is a lower amount of oxygen for an individual to breathe. This is known as hypoxia. Furthermore, since there is less oxygen to inhale, less oxygen reaches the blood. This is known as hypoxemia. These two conditions are the major factors that form the basis for all the medical problems associated with altitude sickness.

Acute mountain sickness (AMS) is a mild form of altitude sickness that results from ascent to altitudes higher than 8,000 feet. Some individuals are affected at even lower altitudes. AMS tends to be most severe on the second or third day after reaching the high altitude, and it usually lessens after three to five days if the person remains at the same altitude. Symptoms include **dizziness**, **headache**, **shortness of breath**, nausea, vomiting, loss of appetite, and **insomnia**.

High-altitude pulmonary edema (HAPE) is a life-threatening condition that afflicts a small percentage of those who suffer from AMS. In this condition, fluid leaks from blood vessels into the lung tissue. As this fluid accumulates within the lung tissue (pulmonary edema), the individual begins to become more and more short of breath.

Typically, the individual with HAPE ascends quickly to a high altitude and almost immediately develops shortness of breath, rapid heart rate, **cough** productive of a large amount of sometimes bloody sputum, and rapid breathing. Without medical assistance, the patient goes into a **coma** and dies within hours.

High-altitude cerebral edema (HACE), the rarest and most severe form of altitude sickness, involves cerebral edema. The symptoms often begin with those of AMS, but neurologic symptoms such as an altered level of consciousness, speech abnormalities, severe headache, loss of coordination, **hallucinations**, and even seizures. Without medical intervention, **death** results.

Diagnosing altitude sickness relies on the individual's symptoms during travel to higher altitudes. Mild AMS requires no treatment other than an **aspirin** or ibuprofen for headache, and avoidance of further ascent. Narcotics should be avoided because they may blunt the respiratory response. Oxygen may also be used to alleviate symptoms of mild AMS.

As for HAPE and HACE, the most important course of action is to descend to a lower altitude as soon as possible. Even a 1,000-2,000-foot descent can improve symptoms. If descent is not possible, **oxygen therapy** should be started. Additionally, dexamethasone (a steroid) has been suggested in order to reduce cerebral edema.

The prognosis for mild AMS is good, if appropriate measures are taken. As for HAPE and HACE, the prognosis depends upon the rapidity and distance of descent and medical intervention.

To prevent altitude sickness, a person should spend at least one night at an intermediate altitude before going to higher elevations. In general, climbers should take at least two days to go from sea level to 8,000 feet. After reaching that point, healthy climbers should allow one day for each additional 2,000 feet, and one day of rest should be taken every two or three days. Should mild symptoms begin to surface, further ascent should be delayed.

Attention to diet can also help prevent altitude sickness. Water loss is a problem at higher altitudes, so climbers should drink ample water and avoid alcohol and large amounts of salt. Eating frequent small, high-carbohydrate snacks, such as fruits and starchy foods, can help.

Alzheimer's disease

Alzheimer's disease (AD) is the most common form of **dementia**, a neurologic disease characterized by loss of mental

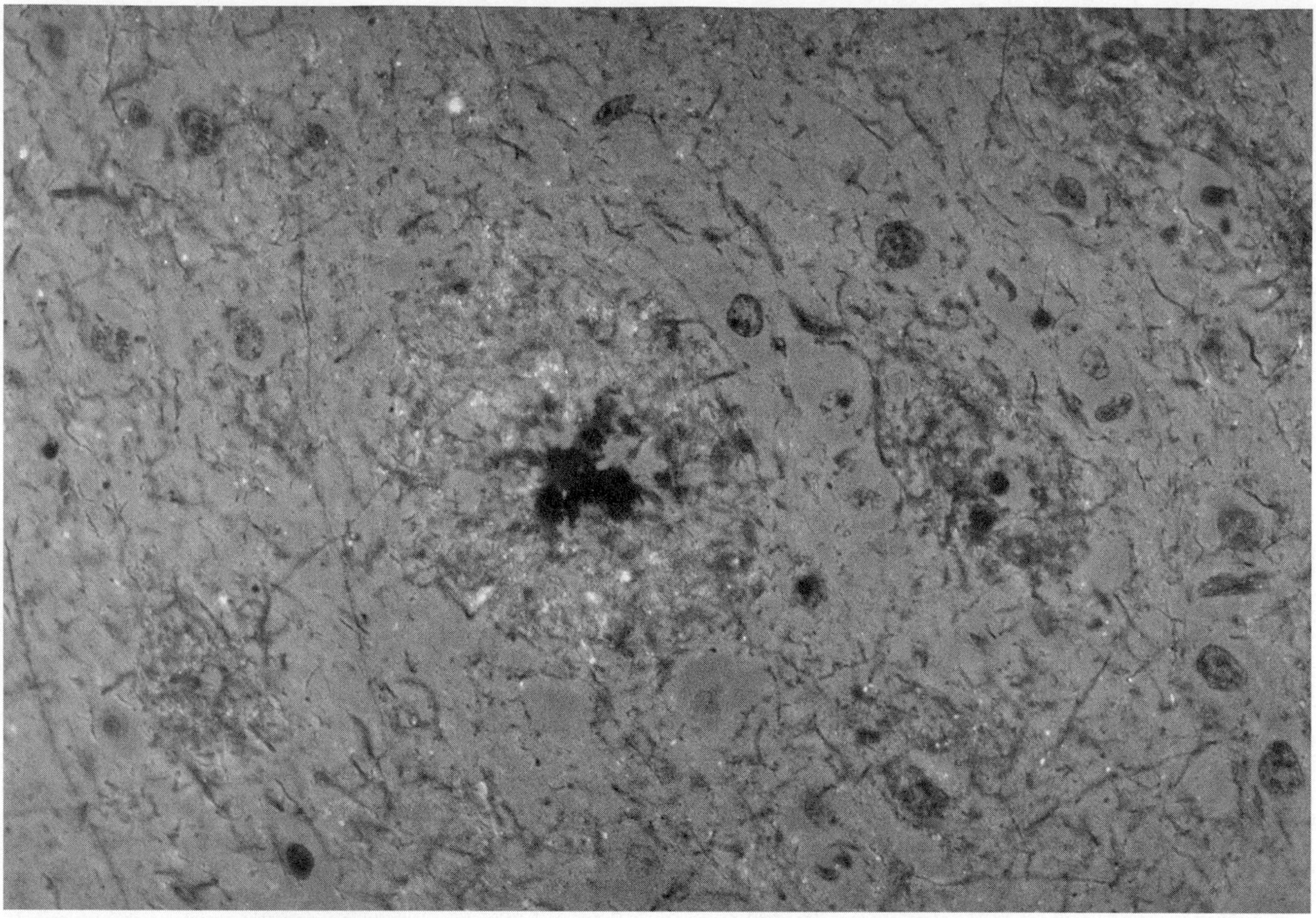

Diseased tissue from the brain of an Alzheimer's patient showing senile plaques within the brain's gray matter. ***(Photograph by Cecil Fox, Photo Researchers, Inc. Reproduced by permission.)***

ability severe enough to interfere with normal activities of daily living, lasting at least six months, and not present from birth. AD usually occurs in old age, and is marked by a decline in cognitive functions such as remembering, reasoning, and planning.

A person with AD usually has a gradual decline in mental functions, often beginning with slight memory loss, followed by losses in the ability to maintain employment, to plan and execute familiar tasks, and to reason and exercise judgment. Communication ability, mood, and personality may also be affected. Most people who have AD die within eight years of their diagnosis, although that interval may be as short as one year or as long as 20 years. AD is the fourth leading cause of **death** in adults after heart disease, **cancer**, and **stroke**.

Between two and four million Americans have AD; that number is expected to grow to as many as 14 million by the middle of the 21st century as the population as a whole ages. While a small number of people in their 40s and 50s develop the disease (called early-onset AD), AD predominantly affects the elderly. AD affects about 3% of all people between ages 65 and 74, about 19% of those between 75 and 84, and about 47% of those over 85. Slightly more women than men are affected with AD, but this may be because women tend to live longer, and so there is a higher proportion of women in the most affected age groups.

The costs for caring for a person with AD is considerable, and has been estimated at approximately $174,000 per person over the course of the disease. Most people with AD are cared for at home; the cost of extended nursing home care adds substantially to this estimate.

The cause or causes of Alzheimer's disease are unknown. Some strong leads have been found through recent research, however, and these have also given some theoretical support to several new experimental treatments.

AD affects brain cells, preferentially those in brain regions responsible for learning, reasoning, and memory. **Autopsy** of a person with AD shows that these regions of the brain become clogged with two abnormal structures, called neurofibrillary tangles and senile plaques. Neurofibrillary tangles are twisted masses of protein fibers inside nerve cells, or neurons. Senile plaques are composed of parts of neurons surrounding a group of brain proteins called beta-amyloid deposits. While it is not clear exactly how these structures cause problems, some researchers now believe that their formation is in fact responsible for the mental changes of AD, presumably by interfering with the normal communication between neurons in the brain. Two drugs approved by the Food and Drug Administration (FDA) as of January 1998 both act to increase the level of chemical signaling molecules in the brain, known as neurotransmitters, to make up for this decreased communication ability.

What triggers the formation of plaques and tangles is unknown, although there are several possible candidates. Inflammation of the brain may play a role in their development, and use of **nonsteroidal anti-inflammatory drugs** (NSAIDs) seems to reduce the risk of developing AD. Restriction of blood flow may be part of the problem, perhaps accounting for the beneficial effects of estrogen, which increases blood flow in the brain, among its other effects. Highly reactive molecular fragments called free radicals damage cells of all kinds, especially brain cells, which have smaller supplies of protective antioxidants thought to protect against free radical damage. Vitamin E is one such antioxidant, and its use in AD may be of possible theoretical benefit.

Several genes have been implicated in AD, including the gene for amyloid precursor protein, or APP, responsible for producing amyloid. Mutations in this gene are linked to some cases of the relatively uncommon early-onset forms of AD. Other cases of early-onset AD are caused by mutations in the gene for another protein, called pre-senilin. AD eventually affects nearly everyone with Down syndrome, caused by an extra copy of chromosome 21. Other mutations on other chromosomes have been linked to other early-onset cases.

Potentially the most important genetic link was discovered in the early 1990s on chromosome 19. A gene on this chromosome, called apoE, codes for a protein involved in transporting lipids into neurons. ApoE occurs in at least three forms, called apoE2, apoE3, and apoE4. Each person inherits one apoE from each parent, and therefore can either have one copy of two different forms, or two copies of one. Compared to those without apoE4, people with one copy are about three times as likely to develop late-onset AD, and those with two copies are almost four times as likely to do so. Despite this important link, not everyone with apoE4 develops AD, and people without it can still have the disease. Why apoE4 increases the chances of developing AD is not known.

While the ultimate cause or causes of Alzheimer's disease are still unknown, there are several risk factors that increase a person's likelihood of developing the disease. The most significant one is, of course, age; older people develop AD at much higher rates than younger ones. Another risk factor is having a family history of AD, Down syndrome, or **Parkinson's disease**. People who have had head trauma or hypothyroidism may manifest the symptoms of AD more quickly. No other medical conditions have been linked to an increased risk for AD.

Many environmental factors have been suspected of contributing to AD, but population studies have not borne out these links. Among these have been pollutants in drinking water, aluminum from commercial products, and metal dental fillings. To date, none of these factors has been shown to cause AD or increase its likelihood. Further research may yet turn up links to other environmental culprits, although no firm candidates have been identified.

The symptoms of Alzheimer's disease begin gradually, usually with memory lapses. Occasional memory lapses are of course common to everyone, and do not by themselves signify any change in cognitive function. The person with AD may begin with only the routine sort of memory lapse—forgetting where the car keys are—but progress to more profound or disturbing losses, such as forgetting that he or she can even drive a car. Becoming lost or disoriented on a walk around the neighborhood becomes more likely as the disease progresses. A person with AD may forget the names of family members, or forget what was said at the beginning of a sentence by the time he hears the end.

As AD progresses, other symptoms appear, including inability to perform routine tasks, loss of judgment, and personality or behavior changes. Some patients have trouble sleeping and may suffer from confusion or agitation in the evening (''sunsetting''). In some cases, people with AD repeat the same ideas, movements, words, or thoughts, a behavior known as perseveration. In the final stages people may have severe problems with eating, communicating, and controlling their bladder and bowel functions.

The Alzheimer's Association has developed a list of ten warning signs of AD. A person with several of these symptoms should see a physician for a thorough evaluation:

- Memory loss that affects job skills
- Difficulty performing familiar tasks
- Problems with language
- Disorientation of time and place
- Poor or decreased judgment
- Problems with abstract thinking
- Misplacing things
- Changes in mood or behavior
- Changes in personality
- Loss of initiative.

Other types of dementing illnesses, including some that are reversible, can cause similar symptoms. It is important for the person with these symptoms to be evaluated by a professional who can weigh the possibility that his or her symptoms may have another cause. Approximately 20% of those originally suspected of having AD turn out to have some other disorder; about half of these cases are treatable.

Diagnosis of Alzheimer's disease is complex, and may require office visits to several different specialists over several months before a diagnosis can be made. While a confident provisional diagnosis may be made in most cases after thorough testing, AD cannot be definitively diagnosed until autopsy examination of the brain for senile plaques and neurofibrillary tangles.

The diagnosis of AD begins with a thorough physical exam and complete medical history. Except in the disease's earliest stages, accurate history from family members or caregivers is essential. Since there are both prescription and over-the-counter drugs that can cause the same mental changes as

AD, a careful review of the patient's drug, medicine, and alcohol use is important. AD-like symptoms can also be provoked by other medical conditions, including tumors, infection, and dementia caused by mild strokes (multi-infarct dementia). These possibilities must be ruled out as well through appropriate blood and urine tests, brain **magnetic resonance imaging** (MRI) or **computed tomography scans** (CT), tests of the brain's electrical activity (electroencephalographs or EEGs), or other tests. Several types of oral and written tests are used to aid in the AD diagnosis and to follow its progression, including tests of mental status, functional abilities, memory, and concentration. Still, the neurologic exam is normal in most patients in early stages.

One of the most important parts of the diagnostic process is to evaluate the patient for depression and **delirium**, since each of these can be present with AD, or may be mistaken for it. (Delirium involves a decreased consciousness or awareness of one's environment.) Depression and memory loss are both common in the elderly, and the combination of the two can often be mistaken for AD. Depression can be treated with drugs, although some antidepressants can worsen dementia if it is present, further complicating both diagnosis and treatment.

A genetic test for the ApoE4 gene is available, but is not used for diagnosis, since possessing even two copies does not ensure that a person will develop AD.

Alzheimer's disease is currently incurable, and as of 1997 only two drugs—tacrine (Cognex) and donepezil hydrochloride (Aricept)— have been approved by the FDA for its treatment. Several other drugs are being prescribed more often as their benefits are demonstrated in wider testing. Nonetheless, the mainstay of treatment for a person with AD continues to be good nursing care, providing both physical and emotional support for a person who is gradually able to do less and less for himself, and whose behavior is becoming more and more erratic. Modifications of the home to increase safety and security are often necessary. The caregiver also needs support to prevent anger, despair, and burnout from becoming overwhelming. Becoming familiar with the issues likely to lie ahead, and considering the appropriate financial and legal issues early on, can help both the patient and family cope with the difficult process of the disease. Regular medical care by a practitioner with a non-defeatist attitude toward AD is important so that illnesses such as urinary or respiratory infections can be diagnosed and treated properly, rather than being incorrectly attributed to the inevitable decline seen in AD.

There is currently no sure way to prevent Alzheimer's disease, though some of the drug treatments discussed above may eventually be proven to reduce the risk of developing the disease. The most likely current candidates are estrogen, NSAIDs, vitamin E, and selegiline, although this list may grow or shrink with further research.

Amblyopia

Amblyopia is a decrease in vision in one or both eyes in which there are no structural defects. It is a diagnosis of exclusion, meaning that when a decrease in vision is detected, other causes must be ruled out. Once no other cause is found, amblyopia is the diagnosis.

Lazy eye is a common non-medical term used to describe amblyopia because the eye with poorer vision doesn't seem to be doing its job of seeing. Amblyopia is the most common cause of impaired vision in children, affecting nearly 3 out of every 100 people or 2-4% of the population.

Vision is a combination of the clarity of the images of the eyes (visual acuity) and the processing of those images by the brain. If the images produced by the two eyes are substantially different, the brain suppresses the blurrier image. This suppression can lead to amblyopia. During the first few years of life, preferring one eye over the other may lead to poor visual development in the blurrier eye.

There are several causes of amblyopia. **Strabismus**, or crossed eyes, is the most common cause of functional amblyopia. The brain receives two different images and this causes confusion. Images from the misaligned or crossed eye are turned off to avoid double vision. Anisometropia is another type of functional amblyopia. In this case, the two eyes do not have the same ability to focus on an image. For example, one eye may be more nearsighted than the other eye. Clouding of the lens of the eye, or cataract, will cause the image to be blurrier than the other eye. Ptosis is the drooping of the upper eyelid. If light cannot enter the eye because of the drooping lid, the eye is essentially not being used. Nutritional deficiencies or chemical toxicity may result in amblyopia. Alcohol, tobacco, or a deficiency in the B **vitamins** may result in toxic amblyopia. Amblyopia can also run in families.

Because children with outwardly normal eyes may have amblyopia, it is important to have regular vision screenings. While there is some controversy regarding the age children should have their first vision examination, their eyes can, in actuality, be examined at any age, even at one day of life.

There is a critical period in vision development, and amblyopia may not be treatable after age eight or nine. The earlier amblyopia is found, the better the outcome. Most physicians test vision as part of a child's medical examination. If there is any sign of an eye problem, they may refer a child to an eye specialist.

The primary treatment for amblyopia is occlusion therapy, or eye patching. It is important to alternate patching the good eye and the amblyopic eye. The treatment plan should be discussed with the doctor to fully understand how long the patch will be on. Eye exercises may be prescribed to force the amblyopic eye to focus and work. This is called vision therapy or **vision training**. Even after vision has been restored in the weak eye, part-time patching may be required over a period of years to maintain the improvement.

While patching is necessary to get the amblyopic eye to work, it is just as important to correct the reason for the amblyopia. Glasses may also be worn. Surgery or vision training may be necessary in the case of strabismus. Better nutrition is indicated in some toxic amblyopias. Occasionally, amblyopia is treated by blurring the vision in the good eye with eye drops or lenses.

The younger the person, the better the chance for improvement with occlusion and vision therapy. However, treatment may be successful in older children—even adults. Success also depends upon how severe the amblyopia is, the specific type of amblyopia, and patient compliance. It is important to diagnose and treat amblyopia early because significant vision loss can occur if left untreated.

Ambulatory Health Care

Ambulatory care covers a wide range of health care services that are provided for patients who are not admitted overnight to a hospital. These services are performed at outpatient clinics, urgent care centers, emergency rooms, ambulatory or same-day surgery centers, diagnostic and imaging centers, primary care centers, community health centers, occupational health centers, mental health clinics, and group practices.

Ambulatory health care has grown tremendously since the early 1980s. Its growth has been driven by a desire for insurers and the United States government to control health care costs. In addition, advances in technology make many tests and surgeries that were formerly done as inpatient procedures in hospital settings safe to do in freestanding clinics or centers. The development of expensive specialty equipment such as **magnetic resonance imaging** (MRI) has lead to the establishment of specialty centers for diagnostic testing. Some **health maintenance organizations** (HMOs) have developed their own freestanding ambulatory health care centers. Other insurers encourage patients to use ambulatory care centers by limiting their reimbursement to specific centers and refusing to cover the full cost of certain procedures when done in hospital inpatient settings.

The growth of ambulatory surgical centers, also called outpatient or same-day surgery centers illustrates the shift in procedures away from hospitals. In 1970 the first ambulatory surgery center in the United States opened in Phoenix, Arizona. The next year, the **American Medical Association** (AMA) passed a resolution supporting outpatient surgery under general or local anesthesia for low risk patients needing selected procedures. By 1976 there were 67 outpatient surgery centers in the United States.

Outpatient surgery has grown with extraordinary rapidity since 1982 when the United States government approved Medicare reimbursement for surgeries performed in ambulatory surgery centers. By 1998, there were over 2,400 outpatient surgery centers performing over 5 million surgeries annually in the United States.

Cost is the primary factor driving the expansion of ambulatory health care services. It is estimated that a procedure performed in an outpatient surgery center costs 30-60% less than the identical surgery performed in an inpatient hospital setting. Convenience is another factor in the rise of ambulatory care. Many patients find it more convenient and less stressful to recover at home rather than in a hospital. Advances in microsurgery have made it safe for many procedures that once required a hospital stay to be done as day surgery.

All ambulatory care facilities that receive Medicare reimbursement are regulated and inspected by the federal government. Forty-one states also regulate some types of ambulatory care centers. Centers can also seek voluntary accreditation from organizations such as the Accreditation Association for Ambulatory Health Care (AAAHC) or the Joint Commission on Accreditation of Healthcare Organizations (JCAHO). Individuals associated with ambulatory care centers may join the Society for Ambulatory Care Professionals, an organization that promotes standards and education for ambulatory care workers.

In choosing an ambulatory care facility, clients should inquire about licensing or certification from the appropriate state agency and certification by Medicare. The center's physicians should be board certified in the area in which they practice. Other questions that might be asked when selecting high quality ambulatory care could include: Is the center associated with a hospital? Does the center have a hospital transfer plan in case of emergencies? How is anesthesia administered and monitored? What is done to insure confidentiality of patient information, and under what circumstances is patient information released? Will the insurance company reimburse for services provided at this center? How much experience does the center have with the particular procedure or test the client needs done?

Ambulatory health care is an increasingly important source of health care services in the United States. Since 1973, the National Center for Health Statistics has conducted the National Ambulatory Medical Care Survey to collect information on who uses ambulatory care and for what reasons. This survey shows a steady increase in the use of ambulatory care facilities.

American Medical Association

The American Medical Association (AMA) is the professional organization of physicians in the United States. Besides providing a group voice to physicians, it promotes the art and science of medicine and improve public health.

To reach this goal, the AMA devotes much of its resources to gathering, synthesizing and distributing current information on health and the practice of medicine, to setting standards for medical ethics, to fostering medical education, and to serving as an advocate for physicians and patients.

The AMA was founded in 1847, and today encompasses approximately 297,000 members in 54 state groups. Its headquarters are in Chicago, with additional offices in New York City and Washington, D.C.

In today's complex medical world, ethical issues confront practitioners almost daily. As technology speeds ahead, the need for ethical guidance becomes even more important. The AMA provides ethical guidance to physicians through its "Principals of Medical Ethics" and "Fundamental Elements of the Patient-Physician Relationship." In addition, the AMA's Code of Medical Ethics is regarded as the standard for professional conduct for physicians in the United States, both by the physicians themselves and by the courts.

Through these standards, the AMA places the patients' interests first and protects the patients' right to full disclosure while guiding physicians on such technological advances as genetic engineering.

The AMA monitors and supports technological advances in medicine. In addition to working with government agencies to make effective treatments quickly available, the AMA is active in disseminating information about new drug development. It co-sponsors the council that names all new US-developed drugs, and also has a programs that monitors any discrepancies between scientific findings and drug use in practice.

Through its many publications, the AMA can quickly and easily disseminate information about current advances. The *Journal of the American Medical Association* (JAMA) is the world's most widely read medical journal, published in 11 languages. In addition to JAMA, the AMA publishes *American Medical News,* a weekly update on social and economic health news, and 10 monthly medical journals in such specialties as family medicine, internal medicine, opthamology, surgery, otolaryngology, and pediatrics.

With such a wealth of information available, it makes sense then that the AMA also has an extensive library available to members. It also provides a great deal of current medical information on its web sits (www.ama-assn.org). The web site can be accessed by physicians, medical students and patients who are seeking information about particular conditions.

The AMA is also a powerful lobbying force in Washington, D.C. Among the issues that the AMA takes special interest in are the reform of Medicare, monitoring the development of managed care, and funding medical education. The AMA is also active in the courts, both providing legal assistance to physicians at the local level and working at the national level to influence medicine-related laws. For example, in 1993 the AMA blocked a movement to increase physicians' DEA registration fees four-fold (the DEA registration is what allows a physician to prescribe drugs), and in 1983 worked to force the recognition of a person's right to refuse medical treatment.

Members of the AMA meet twice a year to discuss concerns and set policy as delegates to the national convention. Delegates are elected to represent specialty medical societies, state medical societies, the armed forces, the US public health service, medical students, organized medical staff, medical schools, residents, women physicians, young physicians, international medical graduates, minority physicians, and older physicians.

The decisions made at these national conventions have tremendous impact on American health care practices. For example, at the 1999 national conference, members voted to "unionize." Although not strictly intended as a movement to form a labor organization such as the AFL-CIO, the members decided it was necessary that they band together to present an solid front in dealing with managed care providers. Since the advent of managed care, physicians' salaries have flattened out, and many physicians believe it is managed care that is cutting into their earnings.

On another front, AMA action through the national convention forced insurers from imposing so-called "drive-through deliveries," which sent a woman home too soon after having a baby, the physicians believed. Now new mothers and their infants receive at least a two-day stay in the hospital after birth.

In addition to professional education and a powerful group voice, the AMA offers physicians resources for managing their practices and their personal lives, ranging from medical and pharmaceutical supplies to hospital indemnity insurance to personal financial services.

The AMA's home office is located at 515 North State St., Chicago, IL, 60610.

AMERICANS WITH DISABILITIES ACT

The Americans with Disabilities Act was passed in 1990 to protect the civil rights of people with disabilities. Just as previous laws had made it illegal to discriminate against people on the basis of their gender, race or religion, the ADA made it illegal to discriminate against people with disabilities, whether physical or mental. It was signed into law by President George Bush on July 26, 1990.

The ADA protects people who have disabilities from discrimination in employment and in access to such public places as shopping malls, theaters, restaurants, doctors' offices, and pharmacies or to such public services as public transportation and telecommunications.

The act defines a disability as a physical or mental impairment that "substantially limits" one or more major life activities, such as walking, seeing, learning, speaking, hearing, breathing, taking care of oneself, performing manual tasks, or working. Examples of impairments that would constitute disabilities are blindness, paralysis, AIDS, or a learning disability. A temporary condition, such as a broken arm, would not be considered a disability under the law, nor would the use of illegal drugs. However, a person who has recovered from cancer would be protected as a person with a record of a disability, and in some cases, alcoholics would also be protected under the ADA. However, the definition of "disability" under the ADA is being refined almost daily as new cases crop up.

Under this law, an employer cannot ask a job applicant if he or she has any physical or mental impairments. However, this does not mean that the employer must hire an applicant simply because the applicant is disabled; rather, it means that if the disabled applicant is equally as qualified as a nondisabled applicant and can fulfill the requirements of the job, the employer may not refuse to hire the applicant because of his or her disability. For example, two people apply for a job in a pharmacy as a pharmacy technician. One applicant uses a wheelchair. If both applicants have sufficient training and experience to do the job, they both must be considered. However, if the applicant in the wheelchair has no experience as a pharmacy technician while the other applicant has three years' experience, the pharmacy can hire the other applicant without fear of being accused of discrimination.

A long-standing excuse for not hiring people in wheelchairs or with other disabilities was that they would not, for instance, be able to get up and down stairs and so on. However, the ADA requires that employers with 15 or more employees make "reasonable accommodations" for employees with disabilities. A "reasonable accommodation" might mean building a ramp so an employee in a wheelchair can get up the two steps into the building, or purchasing a blind employee a Braille keyboard for his computer. There are several caveats here, however: the disability must be known to the employer (generally, by having been brought up by the employee), and the employee must ask for a reasonable accommodation. In many cases where an employee does request an accommodation, he or she often has a suggestion for fulfilling that need. Employers are not required to lower performance standards (of quality of work expected or quantity of output expected) as an accommodation. Nor must they provide a personal item such as a hearing aid, or make an accommodation that would create an undue hardship for the business—for example, installing an elevator at an employee's request when doing so would financially strap the company. In such a case, however, the employer is expected to make an effort to find another option, or give the disabled employee the option of paying the part of the cost of the accommodation that the company says is an undue hardship.

Besides ensuring the rights of the disabled in the workplace, the ADA also protects their rights in the enjoyment of public facilities. For example, shopping malls are required to provide a sufficient number of handicapped-only parking spaces. Restaurants must have tables that are positioned in such a way that a person in a wheelchair can sit at them. Public telephones must be lowered so that a person in a wheelchair can use them as well.

In addition, state and local governments are also subject to the standards of the ADA, and may not discriminate against disabled persons. This includes public transportation systems whether or not they receive federal funding. Buses, streetcars and subway cars must be accessible to persons in wheelchairs, for example, either from raised platforms or by being equipped with wheelchair lifts.

New construction of public buildings, whether for government offices or for such public areas as a shopping mall, must also be handicapped accessible, with elevators, ramps, and doorways sufficiently large for the passage of a wheelchair.

For more information on the Americans with Disabilities Act, you can contact the Equal Employment Opportunity Commission (800/669-3362), the President's Committee on employment of People with Disabilities (202-376-6200), or the U.S. Justice Department (202/366-1656).

AMNESIA

Amnesia refers to the loss of memory. Memory loss may result from damage to parts of the brain vital for memory storage, processing, or recall (the limbic system, including the hippocampus in the medial temporal lobe). Amnesia can also be a symptom of neurodegenerative diseases. People whose primary symptom is memory loss (amnesiacs), typically retain their sense of self. They may even be aware that they suffer from a memory disorder.

Amnesia has several root causes. Most are traceable to brain injury related to physical trauma, disease, infection, drug and alcohol abuse, or reduced blood flow to the brain. In Wernicke-Korsakoff syndrome, for example, damage to the memory centers of the brain results from the use of alcohol or **malnutrition**. Infections that damage brain tissue, including **encephalitis** and herpes, can also cause amnesia. If the amnesia is thought to be of psychological origin, it is termed psychogenic. There are at least three general types of amnesia.

Anterograde amnesia follows brain trauma and is characterized by the inability to remember new information. Recent experiences and short-term memory disappear, but victims can easily recall events prior to the trauma. *Retrograde amnesia* is the opposite of anterograde amnesia: the victim can recall events that occurred after a trauma, but cannot remember previously familiar information from before the trauma. *Transient global amnesia* has no consistently identifiable cause, but researchers have suggested that migraines or transient ischemic attacks may be the trigger. (A transient ischemic attack is sometimes called a small **stroke**.) A victim experiences sudden confusion and forgetfulness. Attacks can be as brief as 30-60 minutes or can last up to 24 hours. In severe attacks, a person is completely disoriented and may experience retrograde amnesia that extends back several years.

In diagnosing amnesia, doctors look at several factors. During a **physical examination**, the doctor inquires about recent traumas or illnesses, drug and medication history, and checks the patient's general health. Psychological exams may be ordered to determine the extent of amnesia and the memory system affected. The doctor may also order imaging tests such as **magnetic resonance imaging** (MRI) to reveal whether the brain has been damaged, and blood work to exclude treatable metabolic causes or chemical imbalances.

Treatment depends on the root cause of amnesia and is handled on an individual basis. Regardless of cause, cognitive **rehabilitation** may be helpful in learning strategies to cope with memory impairment.

Some types of amnesia, such as transient global amnesia, are completely resolved and there is no permanent loss of memory. Others, such as Korsakoff syndrome, associated with prolonged alcohol abuse or amnesias caused by severe brain injury, may be permanent. Depending on the degree of amnesia and its cause, victims may be able to lead relatively normal lives. Amnesiacs can learn through therapy to rely on other memory systems to compensate for what is lost.

Amnesia is only preventable in so far as brain injury can be prevented or minimized. Common sense approaches include wearing a helmet when bicycling or participating in potentially dangerous sports, using automobile seat belts, and avoiding excessive alcohol or drug use. Brain infections should be treated swiftly and aggressively to minimize the damage due to swelling. Victims of strokes, brain aneurysms, and transient ischemic attacks should seek immediate medical treatment.

Amputation

Amputation is the intentional surgical removal of a limb or body part. It is performed to remove diseased tissue or to relieve **pain**. Amputation is performed to remove tissue that no longer has an adequate blood supply; to remove malignant tumors; and because of severe trauma to the body part. About 65,000 amputations are performed in the United States each year. More than 90% of the amputations are due to circulatory complications of diabetes, and most of these operations involve the legs.

Amputations can be either planned or emergency procedures. Injury and arterial embolisms are the main reasons for emergency amputations. Amputations cannot be performed on patients with uncontrolled diabetes mellitus, **heart failure**, or infection. Patients with blood clotting disorders are also not good candidates for amputation.

The operation is performed under regional or general anesthesia by a general or orthopedic surgeon in a hospital operating room. Details of the operation vary slightly depending on what part is to be removed. The goal of all amputations is twofold: to remove diseased or damaged tissue so that the wound will heal cleanly, and to construct a stump that will allow the attachment of a prosthesis or artificial replacement part.

The surgeon makes an incision around the part to be amputated. The part is removed, and the bone is smoothed. A flap is constructed of muscle, connective tissue, and skin to cover the raw end of the bone. The flap is closed over the bone with sutures (surgical stitches) that remain in place for about one month. Often, a rigid dressing or cast is applied that stays in place for about two weeks.

Before an amputation is performed, extensive testing is done to determine the proper level of amputation. Other tests measure the blood flow through the area. The greater the blood flow, the more likely healing is to occur. The goal of the surgeon is to find the place where healing is most likely to be complete, while allowing the maximum amount of limb to remain for effective **rehabilitation**.

After amputation, medication is prescribed for pain, and patients are treated with **antibiotics** to prevent infection. The stump is moved often to encourage good circulation. Physical therapy and rehabilitation are started as soon as possible, usually within 48 hours. There is a positive relationship between early rehabilitation and effective functioning of the stump and prosthesis. Length of stay in the hospital depends on the severity of the amputation and the general health of the amputee, but ranges from several days to two weeks.

Rehabilitation can be a long, difficult process. Twice daily physical therapy is not uncommon. Additionally, psychological counseling is an important part of rehabilitation. Many people feel a sense of loss and grief when they lose a body part. Others are bothered by phantom limb syndrome, where they feel as if the amputated part is still in place. They may even feel pain in this missing limb. Many amputees benefit from joining self-help groups and meeting other amputees.

Amputation is major surgery. All the risks associated with anesthesia exist, along with the possibility of heavy blood loss and the development of blood clots. Infection is a special concern. Infection rates in amputations average 15%. If the stump becomes infected, it is necessary to remove the prosthesis and sometimes to amputate a second time at a higher level. Failure of the stump to heal is another major complication. Nonhealing is usually due to an inadequate blood supply. Centers that specialize in amputation usually have the lowest rates of complication.

Anabolic Steroids

Anabolic steroids are a group of synthetic drugs that are related in chemical structure to the male hormone testosterone. ''Anabolic'' means to build up protein and muscle tissue, and that is what these drugs do. Anabolic steroids have legitimate medical uses, but they are more commonly known for their abuse by athletes seeking to enhance their performance by increasing their muscle mass and strength.

In 1935 scientists discovered that under certain conditions giving anabolic steroids to dogs increased the dogs' muscle mass. However, it was not until the 1950s that athletes began using steroids to give them what they believed to be a competitive edge. The first athletes to abuse steroids competed in areas such as weightlifting, bodybuilding, football, discus, and other events where success was highly dependent on strength. Presently, anabolic steroids abuse has spread to virtually every sport at every level of competition. A 1997 study by the National Institute on Drug Abuse estimated that 0.8-1.5% of all eighth, tenth, and twelfth graders in the United States had tried anabolic steroids. Men, however, are many times more likely to use steroids than women.

More than 20 anabolic steroids have been banned by the International Olympic Committee and most other organizations sponsoring national and international athletic competitions. The ban is enforced through drug testing, which at times is considered controversial. In 1983, 19 athletes were disqualified for their use of banned steroids. In 1988, the United States Congress passed legislation making non-medical distribution or possession of anabolic steroids a Federal offense. Following in 1990, anabolic steroids were reclassified as a controlled substance. This legislation lead to an increase in the black market sale of steroids, which in 1997 was estimated at $400 million annually.

Anabolic steroids are administered either orally by pill or intramuscularly through injection. Steroids taken in pill form remain in the body several weeks, while injected steroids can be detected for months. Abusers normally take large doses of steroids, hundreds of times stronger than would be prescribed for legitimate medical use, hoping to increase the muscle building effects of these drugs. This also increases the severity of side effects. Degree of side effects range from mild and annoying to serious and life-threatening.

Anabolic steroids have different effects on men and women and on adolescents and adults. In all people, they may lead to increased **acne**, **baldness**, **jaundice**, trembling, the swelling of the feet, bad breath, high blood pressure, liver damage, increased risk of some cancers, aching joints, and increased chance of injury to tendons, ligaments, and muscles. They may also be psychologically or physically addicting and produce depression and withdrawal symptoms when stopped.

In men, anabolic steroid use also causes a decrease in the production of natural testosterone. Long term use leads to shrinking of the testicles, reduced sperm production, **impotence**, development of breasts, and the enlargement of the prostate gland. Steroids also may produce psychological effects, such as increased aggression, extreme irritability, and delusions of invincibility.

Anabolic steroid use causes women to become more masculine in appearance. Women may grow facial hair and see a reduction in their breast size. Their voices permanently deepen, they may stop menstruating, and their clitorises may enlarge. In adolescents, anabolic steroids, even in small doses, can irreversibly stop growth, forcing the body to unknowingly complete growth. As a result, the growth plates of the long bones of the arms and legs permanently close, preventing further increases in height.

Anabolic steroids, however, are also powerful drugs with legitimate medical uses. They have been approved by the U.S. Food and Drug Administration in treating specific types of **anemia**, some types of cancer such as **testicular cancer**, some cases of **osteoporosis**, **endometriosis**, and a few rare hereditary diseases involving pituitary malfunctions. Anabolic steroids are also given to female transsexuals to masculinize them as part of the gender change process.

Anabolic steroids have been successfully used by patients diagnosed with **AIDS** who are experiencing muscle deterioration and severe weight loss as a side effect of the disease. Two steroids in particular, naldrolone and oxandrolone, have been shown to be successful in reversing weight and muscle loss for those AIDS. With this reversal has come an improvement in quality of life for many patients.

Anabolic steroids are powerful drugs with the potential for serious side effects if abused. They must be prescribed by a medical doctor for limited use to treat specific conditions. People using anabolic steroids should be monitored regularly for adverse effects.

ANAEROBIC INFECTIONS

An anaerobic infection is caused by bacteria which cannot grow in the presence of oxygen. These bacteria are called anaerobic bacteria or anaerobes. Anaerobic bacteria can infect deep **wounds**, deep tissues, and internal organs where there is little oxygen. These infections are characterized by **abscess** formation, foul-smelling pus, and tissue destruction.

Anaerobic bacteria grow in places which completely, or almost completely, lack oxygen. They are normally found in the mouth, gastrointestinal tract, and vagina, and on the skin. Anaerobic bacteria can cause an infection when a normal barrier, such as skin, gums, or intestinal wall, is damaged due to surgery, injury, or disease. Usually, the immune system kills any invading bacteria, but sometimes the bacteria are able to grow and cause an infection.

Commonly known diseases caused by anaerobic bacteria include gas **gangrene**, **tetanus**, and **botulism**. Nearly all dental infections are caused by anaerobic bacteria.

There are many different kinds of anaerobic bacteria which can cause an infection. Indeed, most anaerobic infections are mixed infections which means that there are several different bacteria growing. The anaerobic bacteria that most frequently cause infections are *Bacteroides fragilis*, *Peptostreptococcus*, and *Clostridium* species.

The signs and symptoms of anaerobic infection vary depending on the location of the infection. In general, anaerobic infections result in tissue destruction, an abscess which drains foul-smelling pus, and possibly **fever**.

The diagnosis of anaerobic infection is based primarily on symptoms, the patient's medical history, and location of the infection. A foul-smelling infection or drainage from an abscess is diagnostic of anaerobic infection. This foul smell is produced by anaerobic bacteria and occurs in one third to one half of patients late in the infection. Other clues to anaerobic infection include tissue necrosis and gas production at the infection site. A sample from the infected site may be obtained, using a swab or a needle and syringe, to determine which bacteria are causing the infection. Because these bacteria can be easily killed by oxygen, they rarely grow in the laboratory cultures of tissue or pus samples.

The recent medical history of the patient is helpful in diagnosing anaerobic infection. A patient who has or recently had surgery, dental work, tumors, blood vessel disease, or injury are susceptible to this infection. The failure to improve following treatment with **antibiotics** that aren't able to kill anaerobes is another clue that the infection is caused by anaerobes. The location and type of infection also help in the diagnosis.

Diagnostic tests may include blood tests to see if bacteria are in the bloodstream and x rays to look at internal infections. Serious infections may require hospitalization for treatment. Immediate antibiotic treatment of anaerobic infections is necessary. Laboratory tests may identify the bacteria causing the infection. Every antibiotic does not work against all anaerobic bacteria but nearly all anaerobes are killed by chloramphenicol (Chloromycetin), metronidazole (Flagyl or Protostat), and imipenem (Primaxin). Other antibiotics which may be used are clindamycin (Cleocin) or cefoxitin (Mefoxin).

Surgical removal or drainage of the abscess is almost always required. This may involve drainage by needle and syringe to remove the pus from a skin abscess (called "aspiration"). The area would be numbed prior to the aspiration procedure. Also, some internal abscesses can be drained using this procedure with the help of ultrasound (a device which uses sound waves to visualize internal organs). This type of abscess drainage may be performed in the doctor's office.

Complete recovery should be achieved with the appropriate surgery and antibiotic treatment. Untreated or uncontrolled infections can cause severe tissue and bone destruction, which would require plastic surgery to repair. Serious infections can be life threatening.

Analgesics

Analgesics are medicines used to relieve pain such as **headaches**, backaches, joint pain, sore muscles, menstrual cramps, and pain that results from surgery, injury, or illness. While these drugs do not treat whatever is causing the pain, they can provide enough relief to make people more comfortable and to allow them to carry out their daily routines.

Pain is the body's signal that something is wrong. Pain can result from an injury, such as a broken bone, a burn or a sprain; from overuse of muscles (including muscle tension due to **stress**); from infections, such as sinus infections or **meningitis**; or from natural events, such as **childbirth**.

Pain begins at the level of the cells. In response to injury or inflammation, cells release chemical messengers. These chemical messengers alert other specialized cells called pain receptors. The pain receptors send signals to the brain. The brain interprets the signals, and we perceive pain. Analgesics work by either blocking the signals that go to the brain or by interfering with the brain's interpretation of the signals.

Among the most common analgesics are **aspirin**, choline salicylate, magnesium salicylate, and sodium salicylate. Ibuprofen, naproxen sodium, and ketoprofen are all in the general category known as **nonsteroidal anti-inflammatory drugs** (NSAIDs). NSAIDs relieve pain and also reduce inflammation. Another common analgesic, **acetaminophen**, provides pain relief but does not reduce inflammation.

Determining the best pain reliever depends, in part, on the type of pain. The two main categories are acute pain and chronic pain. Acute pain is usually temporary and results from something specific, such as a surgery, injuries, or infections. Chronic pain is any pain that lasts more than three months and may disrupt daily life. Sometimes chronic pain is just a nagging discomfort, but it can flare up into severe pain. Narcotic analgesics are used to treat some kinds of serious, chronic pain. But for most types of chronic pain, a combination of non-narcotic medication and lifestyle changes is recommended.

Severe, sudden, or lingering pain can be a sign of a serious medical condition. Medical attention is necessary for any pain that comes on suddenly; is more frequent or more severe than ever before; does not go away, or gets worse; or interferes with daily activities. If pain is accompanied by **fever**, stiff neck, weakness, swelling, redness, nausea, vomiting, numbness, confusion, vision problems, speech problems, poor coordination, medical attention should also be sought.

Overuse of pain relievers can actually make some types of pain worse. To manage long-term pain, such as recurring headaches, chronic backache, or arthritis pain, many pain treatment specialists recommend an approach that helps people cope without depending on large or frequent doses of drugs. Relaxation techniques, **biofeedback**, **massage**, **exercise**, proper diet, and good sleep habits can all be helpful. Psychological counseling may also help patients and their families deal with the **anxiety** and depression that often accompany long-term pain.

Side effects are one reason to be careful about frequent or long-term use of pain relievers. Narcotic analgesics are very effective, but can cause **addiction**. Aspirin and ibuprofen can irritate the stomach. Acetaminophen (Tylenol, Panadol) does not produce the side effects that aspirin ibuprofen do, but high doses can cause liver damage, especially in people who drink alcohol regularly. Some pain relievers contain **caffeine**, which enhances their effectiveness. Taking these drugs near bedtime can interfere with sleep. Anyone who gets edgy or jittery from caffeine should also be careful about using them during the day.

Analgesics, opioid

Opioid analgesics are used to relieve pain from a variety of conditions. Some are used before or during surgery (including dental surgery) both to relieve pain and to make anesthetics work more effectively. They may also be used for the same purposes during labor and delivery.

Opioid analgesics relieve pain by acting directly on the central nervous system. However, this can also lead to unwanted side effects, such as drowsiness, **dizziness**, breathing problems, and physical or mental dependence.

Among the drugs in this category are codeine, propoxyphene (Darvon), propoxyphene and **acetaminophen** (Darvocet N), meperidine (Demerol), hydromorphone (Dilaudid), morphine, oxycodone, oxycodone and acetaminophen (Percocet, Roxicet), and hydrocodone and acetaminophen (Lortab, Anexsia). These drugs come in many forms—tablets, syrups, suppositories, and injections, and are sold only by prescription. For some, a new prescription is required for each new supply—refills are prohibited according to federal regulations.

Anyone who uses opioid analgesics—or any narcotic—over a long time may become physically or mentally dependent on the drug. Physical dependence may lead to withdrawal symptoms when the person stops taking the medicine. Building tolerance to these drugs is also possible when they are used for a long period. Over time, the body needs larger and larger doses to relieve pain.

These drugs should be taken exactly as directed. The recommended dose should never be exceeded, not should they be taken more often than directed. If the drugs do not seem to be working, the doctor should be consulted. It's important not to share these or any other prescription drugs with other people because the drug may have different effects on different people.

Children and older people are especially sensitive to opioid analgesics and may have serious breathing problems after taking them. Children may also become unusually restless or agitated when given these drugs.

Opioid analgesics increase the effects of alcohol. Anyone taking these drugs should not drink alcoholic beverages.

People with certain medical conditions or who are taking other medicines can have problems if they take opioid analgesics. Side effects can be dangerous in people with certain medical conditions such as **allergies**; heart, kidney, or liver disease; history of convulsions; or **asthma**, emphysema, or any chronic lung disease. Women who are pregnant, plan to become pregnant, or are breastfeeding should let their physicians know. It is important that the physician knows about any current or past alcohol or drug abuse.

Opioid analgesics should not be taken with other medications without the physician's approval. Drug interactions can be severe and possibly fatal.

Some people experience drowsiness, dizziness, lightheadedness, or a false sense of well-being after taking opioid analgesics. Anyone who takes these drugs should not drive, use machines, or do anything else that might be dangerous until they know how the drug affects them. **Nausea and vomiting** are common side effects, especially when first beginning to take the medicine. If these symptoms do not go away after the first few doses, check with the physician or dentist who prescribed the medicine.

Dry mouth is another common side effect. Patients who must use opioid analgesics over long periods and who have dry mouth should see their dentists, as the problem can lead to **tooth decay** and other dental problems.

Anaphylaxis

Anaphylaxis is a rapidly progressing, life-threatening allergic reaction.

Anaphylaxis is a type of allergic reaction, in which the immune system responds to otherwise harmless substances from the environment. Unlike other allergic reactions, however, anaphylaxis can kill. Reaction may begin within minutes or even seconds of exposure, and rapidly progress to cause airway constriction, skin and intestinal irritation, and altered heart rhythms. In severe cases, it can result in complete airway obstruction, **shock**, and **death**.

Like the majority of other allergic reactions, anaphylaxis is caused by the release of histamine and other chemicals from mast cells. Mast cells are a type of white blood cell and they are found in large numbers in the tissues that regulate exchange with the environment: the airways, digestive system, and skin.

On their surfaces, mast cells display antibodies called IgE (immunoglobulin type E). These antibodies are designed to detect environmental substances to which the immune system is sensitive. Substances from a genuinely threatening source, such as bacteria or viruses, are called antigens. A substance that most people tolerate well, but to which others have an allergic response, is called an allergen. When IgE antibodies bind with allergens, they cause the mast cell to release histamine and other chemicals, which spill out onto neighboring cells.

The interaction of these chemicals with receptors on the surface of blood vessels causes the vessels to leak fluid into surrounding tissues, causing fluid accumulation, redness, and swelling. On the smooth muscle cells of the airways and digestive system, they cause constriction. On nerve endings, they increase sensitivity and cause **itching**.

In anaphylaxis, the dramatic response is due both to extreme hypersensivity to the allergen and its usually systemic distribution. Allergens are more likely to cause anaphylaxis if they are introduced directly into the circulatory system by injection. However, exposure by ingestion, inhalation, or skin contact can also cause anaphylaxis. In some cases, anaphylaxis may develop over time from less severe **allergies**.

Anaphylaxis is most often due to allergens in foods, drugs, and insect venom. Specific causes include:

- Fish, shellfish, and mollusks
- Nuts and seeds
- Stings of bees, wasps, or hornets
- Papain from meat tenderizers
- Vaccines, including flu and **measles** vaccines
- Penicillin
- **Cephalosporins**
- Streptomycin
- Gamma globulin
- Insulin
- Hormones (ACTH, thyroid-stimulating hormone)
- **Aspirin** and other NSAIDs
- Latex, from exam gloves or **condom**s, for example.

Exposure to cold or **exercise** can trigger anaphylaxis in some individuals.

Symptoms may include:

- Urticaria (**hives**)
- Swelling and irritation of the tongue or mouth
- Swelling of the sinuses
- Difficulty breathing
- **Wheezing**
- Cramping, vomiting, or **diarrhea**
- **Anxiety** or confusion
- Strong, very rapid heartbeat (**palpitations**)
- Loss of consciousness.

Not all symptoms may be present.

Anaphylaxis is diagnosed based on the rapid development of symptoms in response to a suspect allergen. Identification of the culprit may be done with RAST testing, a blood test that identifies IgE reactions to specific allergens. Skin testing may be done for less severe anaphylactic reactions.

Emergency treatment of anaphylaxis involves injection of adrenaline (epinephrine) which constricts blood vessels and counteracts the effects of histamine. Oxygen may be given, as well as intravenous replacement fluids. **Antihistamines** may be used for skin rash, and aminophylline for bronchial constriction. If the upper airway is obstructed, placement of a breathing tube or tracheostomy tube may be needed.

The rapidity of symptom development is an indication of the likely severity of reaction: the faster symptoms develop, the more severe the ultimate reaction. Prompt emergency medical attention and close monitoring reduces the likelihood of death. Nonetheless, death is possible from severe anaphylaxis. For most people who receive rapid treatment, recovery is complete.

Avoidance of the allergic trigger is the only reliable method of preventing anaphylaxis. For insect allergies, this requires recognizing likely nest sites. Preventing food allergies requires knowledge of the prepared foods or dishes in which the allergen is likely to occur, and careful questioning about ingredients when dining out. Use of a Medic-Alert tag detailing drug allergies is vital to prevent inadvertent administration during a medical emergency.

People prone to anaphylaxis should carry an ''Epi-pen'' or ''Ana-kit,'' which contain an adrenaline dose ready for injection.

Andersen, Dorothy (1901-1963)

American physician and pathologist

Dorothy Andersen was the first medical researcher to recognize the disorder known as **cystic fibrosis**. She devoted much of her life to the further study of this disease, as well as to the study of congenital defects of the heart. During World War II, Anderson was asked to develop a training program in cardiac embryology and anatomy for surgeons learning techniques of **open-heart surgery**.

Dorothy Hansine Andersen was born on May 15, 1901, in Asheville, North Carolina. She was the only child of Hans Peter Andersen and the former Mary Louise Mason. Hans Peter Andersen was a native of Denmark and was employed by the Young Men's Christian Association (YMCA) in Asheville. Andersen was forced to take responsibility for her own upbringing early in life. Her father died when she was thirteen years old, leaving behind an invalid wife dependent on her daughter's care. They moved to Saint Johnsbury, Vermont, where Mary Andersen died in 1920.

Andersen put herself through Saint Johnsbury Academy and Mount Holyoke College before enrolling in the Johns Hopkins School of Medicine, from which she received her M.D. in 1926; while still a medical student, Andersen published two scientific papers dealing with the reproductive system of the female pig in the prestigious journal *Contributions to Embryology*. After graduating from Johns Hopkins, Andersen accepted a one-year position teaching anatomy at the Rochester School of Medicine. She then did her internship in surgery at the Strong Memorial Hospital in Rochester, New York. For medical students an internship is normally followed by a residency, which ultimately leads to certification as a physician. However, Andersen was unable to find a hospital that would allow her to do a residency in surgery or to work as a pathologist because she was a woman.

Denied the opportunity to have a medical practice, Andersen turned instead to medical research. She took a job as research assistant in pathology at Columbia University's College of Physicians and Surgeons that allowed her to begin a doctoral program in endocrinology, the study of glands. She completed the course in 1935 and was granted the degree of doctor of medical science by Columbia University. From 1930 to 1935 Andersen also served as an instructor in pathology at the Columbia Medical School. Andersen later accepted an appointment as a pathologist at Babies Hospital of the Columbia-Presbyterian Medical Center in New York City, where she stayed for more than twenty years, eventually becoming chief of pathology in 1952. By 1958 she had become a full professor at the College of Physicians and Surgeons.

Andersen's research interests fell into two major categories. The first of these involved a long and careful study of congenital (existing from birth) heart problems based on the examination of infants who had died of cardiac conditions. She began that study during her first year at Babies Hospital and was still publishing her findings on the subject in the late 1950s. Andersen's experience with cardiac problems was put to use during World War II when she was asked to teach courses for physicians who wanted to learn how to conduct open-heart surgery.

Her second area of research, and the one for which Andersen is probably best known, evolved out of her discovery in 1935 of cystic fibrosis. That discovery came about during the postmortem examination (**autopsy**) of a child who had supposedly died of **celiac disease**, a nutritional disorder. Eventually she realized that she had found a disease that had never been described in the medical literature, to which she gave the name cystic fibrosis. Cystic fibrosis is a congenital disease of the mucous glands and pancreatic enzymes that results in abnormal digestion and difficulty in breathing; it is believed to affect approximately one in fifteen hundred people. Over the next twenty-six years, Andersen was successful in developing diagnostic tests for cystic fibrosis, but she was less successful in her efforts to treat and cure the disease.

Andersen, a heavy smoker, died of lung cancer in New York City on March 3, 1963. Among the honors she received were the Mead Johnson Award for Pediatric Research in 1938, the Borden Award for Research in Nutrition from the American Academy of Pediatrics in 1948, the Elizabeth Blackwell Citation for Women in Medicine from the New York Infirmary in 1954, a citation for outstanding performance from Mount Holyoke College in 1952, and, posthumously, the distinguished service medal of the Columbia-Presbyterian Medical Center.

See also Cystic fibrosis

Androgens

Androgens are a group of chemically-related male sex hormones. They can be produced naturally by the body or be manufactured synthetically and then administered to the individual. Androgens belong to a group of hormones called steriod hormones. Testosterone is the most abundant androgen in the male body.

Testosterone is responsible for the development of male sexual characteristics. In normal males, it is produced at the onset of **puberty** by the testes in response to stimulation by hormones called gonadotrophins that originate in the anterior pituitary gland and the hypothalamus, a part of the brain.

Testosterone causes boys to acquire the sexual characteristics of men. In response to testosterone, the penis, testes, and scrotum grow and the voice deepens. Hair grows on the body and face and the skin becomes coarser. Androgens also stimulate growth. Not only do boys grow taller during puberty, they also develop larger, bulkier muscles in the arms, shoulders and thighs that give them their distinctly masculine shape.

Androgens allow ejaculations to begin, usually between the ages of 11-15, in response to sexual fantasies or masturbation. After puberty, the testes produce testosterone for the rest of a man's life, but in decreasing amounts as men reach their late 40s or early 50s.

Testosterone is not the only androgen in the body, but it is by far the most important one. The adrenal cortex, or outer part of the adrenal gland, a small gland located above the kidney, also produces androgens as well as hormones that help regulate water balance in the body. These adrenal androgens cause the same effects as testosterone, but are produced in much smaller quantities.

Women produce androgens in the ovaries and adrenal cortex. Almost all of a woman's androgens are immediately converted by the body into estrogens, the hormones that give women their female sexual characteristics. The small amount of androgens that remain unconverted play a role in determining the sex drive of women and in slowing bone loss or **osteoporosis**. In Cushing's disease, the adrenal cortex overproduces hormones. This excess of androgens may cause some women with Cushing's disease to develop male characteristics such as facial hair or a deep voice.

Androgens have legitimate therapeutic medical uses. They are prescribed for men when testosterone is not naturally produced by the body. Synthetic androgens come in the forms of a pill, a patch, and injectable forms. They are prescribed more commonly for male children to make **undescended testes** descend, or to bring about male puberty when it is seriously delayed. In adult men, androgens are used to correct natural hormone deficiencies and to reduce "male menopause" symptoms such as lack of sex drive, anxiety, and depression. Some androgens are used to treat **dwarfism** because of their ability to stimulate growth.

Legitimate medical uses of androgens in women include their use in treating some kinds of **breast cancer** and **anemia**. Sometimes androgens are given after childbirth to reduce breast pain and fullness in women who choose not to breast feed. Women who undergo gender change are also given androgens to increase their male characteristics.

Androgens are part of a group of drugs known as anabolic steriods that are used illegally by some athletes in an attempt to increase their muscle bulk and strength. These black market androgens are usually taken in doses many times higher than would be prescribed for medical reasons. Their use has been outlawed by the International Olympic Committee and most other national and international organizations regulating sports competitions.

Serious, sometimes life-threatening side effects may occur when androgens are taken. They may cause **liver disease**, stimulate **prostate cancer**, interfere with sperm production if taken in high doses, cause **acne**, irregular menstrual cycles in women, **dizziness**, **headache**, **nausea**, weight gain, **jaundice**, and swelling of the feet in both men and women. Androgens interact with many common medications and should never be taken without medical supervision.

See also Anabolic steroids

Anemias

Oxygen is distributed throughout the body by red blood cells, which contain an oxygen-carrying molecule called hemoglobin. Hemoglobin's ability to carry oxygen depends on iron. Red blood cells live for about 120 days. When they die, their iron is re-used to create new red blood cells. Anemia develops when heavy bleeding causes significant iron loss, if red blood cell production slows down, or if red blood cells are destroyed more rapidly than normal.

Poor diet can contribute to vitamin and iron deficiency anemias in which fewer red blood cells are produced. Hereditary disorders and certain diseases can cause increased blood cell destruction. However, excessive bleeding is the most common cause of anemia. Anemia can be mild, moderate, or severe enough to lead to life-threatening complications. More than 400 different types exist.

Iron deficiency anemia is the most common form of anemia. The deficiency occurs when the body loses more iron than it gets from food and other sources. The body tries to compensate for the iron deficiency by producing more red blood cells, which are characteristically small in size.

Folic acid deficiency anemia is the most common type of megaloblastic anemia (red blood cells are bigger than normal). It is caused by a deficiency of folic acid, a vitamin needed to produce normal cells. Although this condition usually results from a dietary deficiency, it is sometimes due to an inability to absorb enough folic acid from foods.

Less common is vitamin B_{12} deficiency anemia. This anemia develops when the body doesn't absorb enough vitamin B_{12} from foods. The most common form of B_{12} deficiency is **pernicious anemia**, which is caused by the body not absorbing vitamin B_{12} properly.

Some people are born with hemolytic anemia. An inherited form of hemolytic anemia is **thalassemia**. Thalassemia stems from the body's inability to manufacture enough normal hemoglobin. There are two categories of thalassemia. Alpha-thalassemias most commonly affect people of African ancestry; beta-thalassemias affect people of Mediterranean ancestry and Southeast Asians.

Sickle-cell anemia is hereditary. It affects people of African or Mediterranean ancestry. A child who inherits the sickle cell gene from each parent will have the disease. Sickle-cell anemia causes the body to produce defective hemoglobin, which forces red blood cells to assume an abnormal crescent shape. The blood cells do not work well and do not live as long as normal cells. The deformed cells can block narrow blood vessels, possibly causing a life-threatening condition called sickle cell crisis.

Aplastic anemia is characterized by decreased production of red and white blood cells and platelets (disc-shaped cells that allow the blood to clot). This disorder may be inherited or acquired due to recent severe illness; long-term exposure to industrial chemicals; or use of **anticancer drugs** and certain other medications.

Weakness, fatigue, and a run-down feeling are signs of mild anemia. Skin that is pasty or sallow or pale gums, nail beds, or eyelid lining are other signs of anemia. Someone who is weak, tires easily, is often out of breath, and feels faint or dizzy may be severely anemic.

Other symptoms of anemia are:

- **Angina** pectoris
- Cravings for ice, paint, or dirt
- **Headache**
- Inability to concentrate, memory loss
- Inflammation of the mouth (**stomatitis**) or tongue
- **Insomnia**
- Irregular heartbeat
- Loss of appetite
- Dry, brittle, or ridged nails
- Rapid breathing
- Sores in the mouth, throat, or rectum
- Sweating
- Hand and feet swelling
- Thirst
- **Tinnitus**
- Unexplained bleeding or bruising.

Personal and family health history may suggest certain anemias. Laboratory blood tests that measure the percentage of red blood cells or the amount of hemoglobin are used to confirm diagnosis and determine the type of anemia. X rays and examinations of bone marrow may also be used.

Anemia due to nutritional deficiencies can be treated with iron, folic acid, or other supplements or with injections of vitamin B_{12}. Surgery may be necessary to treat anemia caused by excessive loss of blood. **Transfusion**s may be used to increase red blood cells.

Although pernicious anemia is considered incurable, regular B_{12} shots will alleviate symptoms and reverse complications. Some symptoms will disappear almost as soon as treatment begins.

Treatment for aplastic anemia may involve blood transfusions or bone marrow transplant. If the condition is due to immunosuppressive drugs, symptoms may disappear once drugs are discontinued. This type of anemia rarely becomes severe. If it does, transfusions or hormone treatments to stimulate red blood cell production may be prescribed.

Although sickle cell anemia cannot be cured, effective treatments enable patients to enjoy more normal lives. Treatment involves regular **eye examination**s, immunizations for pneumonia and infectious diseases, and prompt treatment for sickle cell crises and infections of any kind.

People with mild thalassemia lead normal lives and do not require treatment. Those with severe thalassemia may require bone marrow transplantation.

Anyone with anemia caused by poor nutrition should modify the diet to include more vitamins, minerals, and iron. Vitamin C can stimulate iron absorption. The following foods are good sources of iron:

- Almonds
- Broccoli
- Dried beans
- Dried fruits
- Enriched breads and cereals
- Lean red meat
- Liver
- Potatoes
- Poultry
- Rice
- Shellfish
- Tomatoes.

ANESTHESIA

The term ''anesthesia'' refers to insensibility to pain. Efforts to ease or eliminate pain are as old as pain itself. The early Chinese used both acupuncture and Indian hemp to dull the perception of pain. Ancient Hindu civilizations used henbane and wine as well as hemp. The Romans experimented with mechanical methods of producing unconsciousness: pressing on the carotid artery in the neck or controlled bleeding from arteries in the wrist. In the first century A.D. the Greek physician Dioscorides (40-90 A.D.) described the use of wine of mandragora (mandrake) to produce a deep sleep in surgical patients and used the Greek ''anesthesia'' to describe the phenomenon. Pliny (23-79 A.D.) also mentioned the use of mandragora. The Greek poet Homer referred to the pain-killing effects of nepenthe, and the Greek hisotrian Herodotus wrote of hemp fumes. Alcohol—wine and brandy—was widely used by early peoples for its numbing effects. So was the opium poppy. Its seeds have been found in prehistoric Swiss lake dwellings, and it had found its way to Egypt by the second century A.D. Opium remained in use and was praised by Avicenna (980-1037) in the eleventh century as the most powerful of stupor-producing substances. It was promoted for many medical uses by **Thomas Sydenham** in the 1600s.

Early Arab writings mention anesthesia by inhalation. This idea was the basis of the ''soporific sponge'' (''sleep sponge''), introduced by the Salerno school of medicine in the late twelfth century and by Ugo Borgognoni (Hugh of Lucca) in the thirteenth century. The sponge was promoted and described by Hugh's son and fellow surgeon, Theodoric Borgognoni (1205-1298; Theodoric of Bologna). In this anesthetic method, a sponge was soaked in a dissolved solution of opium, mandragora, hemlock juice, and other substances. The sponge was then dried and stored; just before surgery the sponge was moistened and then held under the patient's nose. When all went well, the fumes rendered the patient unconscious.

Mechanical methods of inducing anesthetic effects were also used. Guy de Chauliac (1300-1368) employed compression of the nerve trunk in the 1300s, and **Ambroise Paré** did the same in the 1500s. Bleeding patients into unconsciousness, the ancient Roman practice, was recommended in 1777 by Alexander Munro II of Edinburgh, Scotland, and put into practice around 1800 by Philip Syng Physick (1768-1837) of Philadelphia.

The modern era of anesthesia began in the late eighteenth century when chemists began to investigate the nature of many substances. Joseph Priestley discovered nitrous oxide in 1772, and in 1800 Humphry Davy discovered the gas's anesthetic properties when inhaled. Davy's student, Michael Faraday, showed in 1818 that inhalation of ether had the same effect. Henry Hill Hickman (1800-1830) experimented with both carbon dioxide and nitrous oxide on animals to carry out painless surgery in the early 1820s.

The anesthetic effects of these substances were first put to practical use by several American dentists and doctors. Georgia physician Crawford Long (1815-1878) performed the first operation under ether anesthesia in 1842. Two years later, a Hartford, Connecticut, dentist named Horace Wells (1815-1848) used inhaled nitrous oxide to extract a tooth painlessly. Boston dentist William T. G. Morton (1819-1868) arranged the first public demonstration of ether-anesthetized surgery in 1846. News of the technique leaped across the Atlantic; in London, two months after Morton's surgery, Dr. Robert Liston (1794-1847) performed an amputation using ether anesthetic. The technique soon spread worldwide.

After Morton's demonstration, the question arose of what to call the new phenomenon. Oliver Wendell Holmes suggested the term *anesthesia.* Although Holmes is often credited with inventing the term, in fact it had appeared in Bailey 's 1721 *Dictionary Britannicum* and had been mentioned as long ago as the first century A.D.

Scottish obstetrician James Young Simpson (1811-1870) introduced chloroform to childbirth (after first experimenting with ether) in 1847. Queen Victoria's use of chloroform for her own labors in 1853 and 1857 firmly established the procedure as standard in childbirth. Dr. John Snow (1813-1858), who administered the chloroform to the queen, became the foremost authority on anesthesia and is recognized today as the world's first professional anesthetist, a pioneer of a new medical specialty. *Local anesthesia* also became important, especially after the invention of the hypodermic syringe by Charles Gabriel Pravaz (1791-1853) in 1853. Alexander Wood (1817-1884) of Edinburgh used the syringe to inject pain-relieving **morphine** soon after. Dr. B. W. Richardson (1828-1896) of Glasgow, Scotland, introduced ether spray for freezing tissue in 1866. Carl Koller (1857-1944) demonstrated the use of cocaine as a local anesthetic in 1884. Baltimore surgeon **William Halsted** developed the technique of conduction anesthesia by blocking nerve impulses with injections of cocaine. The addictive cocaine was replaced by synthetics beginning with **Novocain** in 1904. *Intratracheal anesthesia*—introducing an anesthetic through a tube in the trachea—was pioneered by New York surgeon George Fell (1850-1918) and perfected in 1909 by Samuel Meltzer and John Auer of the Rockefeller Institute. *Spinal anesthesia* to numb the lower half of the body was experimented with in 1885 by New York neurologist Leonard Corning (1855-1923) when he injected a cocaine solution into the spinal region. The German doctor August Bier (1861-1949) refined the technique in 1898, and Rudolph Matas (1860-1957) of New Orleans introduced it to the United States in 1899. By the 1920s the use of spinal anesthesia was widespread in the United States. *Intravenous anesthesia* was first attempted by Robert Boyle and the renowned architect Christopher Wren (1632-1723) around 1659. An injected warm solution of opium in sherry stupified their subject, a dog. Johann Major of Germany tried the same technique in a human subject in 1667. The idea, however, was abandoned until about 1874, when Pierre Oré used chloral hydrate intravenously on a dog and then, in 1875, on a human patient. Once **barbiturates** were discovered in the early 1900s, and especially after improved substances were developed in the 1920s, the use of intravenous anesthetics became firmly established.

Early in the 1900s the surgeons Harvey Cushing (1869-1939) and George Crile (1864-1943) contributed to the safety of anesthesia by promoting monitoring of the patient's blood pressure during operations. Crile and Cushing also combined local or regional with general anesthetics, dosing surgical patients with morphine and scopolamine or local infiltration anesthesia to block nerve impulses that can reach the brain even during deep ether anesthesia. Relaxants such as atropine and curare also came into use to lessen the involuntary resistance of a patient to the application of anesthetics such as ether or the spinal needle.

Today's anesthetist is a highly trained specialist who administers several anesthetics at the same time and uses sophisticated equipment to monitor a patient's blood pressure; rate of respiration; heartbeat; and blood levels of oxygen, carbon dioxide, and anesthetic vapors. Although current anesthetics are highly effective, they do pose a certain amount of risk. As a result, continued research focuses on developing safer and more effective anesthetics. For example, researchers at the University of Pennsylvania Medical Center have demonstrated that giving an anesthetic to patients prior to surgery (called pre- emptive analgesia) appears successful in stopping post-surgical pain before it begins. Researchers are also using gene therapy in an animal model which may lead to new discoveries about the brain's reaction to anesthesia. By using a virus-mediated gene that appears to affect the chemical receptors in lab animals' brains, investigators have developed the ability to study the pharmacological responses of genetically altered receptors. With this approach, it may be possible to learn more about how brain receptors react to general anesthesia, which, in turn, could lead to improved and new approaches to anesthesia.

ANEURYSMS

An aneurysm occurs at a weak point in the wall of a blood vessel (artery). Because of the flaw, the artery wall bulges outward. This bulge is called an aneurysm. An aneurysm can rupture, spilling blood into the surrounding body tissue. A particularly dangerous type of aneurysm is a cerebral aneurysm. A common form of cerebral aneurysm is a berry aneurysm, so-called because of its shape. If a cerebral aneurysm ruptures, it can cause permanent brain damage, disability, or **death**.

A ruptured aneurysm spills blood into the brain or into the fluid-filled area that surrounds the brain tissue. Bleeding into this area, called the subarachnoid space, is referred to as subarachnoid hemorrhage (SAH). Cerebral aneurysms can be caused by brain trauma, infection, hardening of the arteries (**atherosclerosis**), or cancer, but most seem to arise from a congenital, or developmental, defect.

Some aneurysms may have a genetic link and run in families. Better evidence links aneurysms to certain rare diseases of the connective tissue. Polycystic kidney disease is also associated with cerebral aneurysms.

Cigarette smoking, excessive alcohol consumption, and recreational drug use (for example, use of cocaine) have been linked with an increased risk of aneurysm rupture. High blood pressure may be a risk factor but not the most important one. **Pregnancy**, labor, and delivery may increase the possibility of an aneurysm rupturing, but not all doctors agree.

Most aneurysms go unnoticed until they rupture. However, 10-15% are found because of their size or their location. Common warning signs include symptoms that affect only one eye, such as an enlarged pupil, a drooping eyelid, or **pain** above or behind the eye. Other symptoms are a localized **headache**, unsteady gait, a temporary problem with sight, double vision, or numbness in the face.

Some aneurysms bleed without rupturing, but symptoms may develop gradually. The symptoms include headache, nausea, vomiting, neck pain, black-outs, ringing in the ears, **dizziness**, or seeing spots.

Nearly 50% of patients who have aneurysmal SAHs experience "the warning leak phenomenon." Persons with warning leak symptoms have sudden, atypical headaches that occur days or weeks before the actual rupture. These headaches are referred to as sentinel headaches. Nausea, vomiting, and dizziness may accompany sentinel headaches.

When an aneurysm ruptures, most victims experience a sudden, extremely severe headache. **Nausea and vomiting** commonly accompany the headache. The person may experience a short loss of consciousness or prolonged **coma**. Other common signs of a SAH include a stiff neck, **fever**, and a sensitivity to light. About 25% of victims experience problems linked to specific areas of the brain, swelling of the brain (**hydrocephalus**), or seizure.

Based on symptoms, a doctor will run several tests to confirm an aneurysm or an SAH. A computed tomography scan (CT or CAT) of the head is the initial procedure. The scan is most useful when it is done within 72 hours of a rupture.

If the CT scan is negative for a hemorrhage or if the diagnosis is unclear, the doctor will order a **cerebrospinal fluid (CSF) analysis**. Cerebral **angiography** can be used to map the brain's blood vessels and the damaged area.

The primary treatment for a ruptured aneurysm involves stabilizing the victim's condition. The patient may require mechanical ventilation, oxygen, and fluids. Medications may be given to prevent major secondary complications such as seizures, rebleeding, and vasospasm (narrowing of the affected blood vessel). Vasospasm decreases blood flow to the brain and causes the death of nerve cells.

In general, surgical procedures are performed as soon as possible to prevent rebleeding. The chances that aneurysm will rebleed are greatest in the first 24 hours, and vasospasm usually does not occur until 72 hours or more after rupture. The preferred surgical method is a clip ligation in which a clip is placed around the base of the aneurysm to block it off from circulation.

Fifteen to twenty-five percent of people who experience a ruptured aneurysm do not survive. An additional 25-50% die as a result of complications associated with the hemorrhage. Of the survivors, 15-50% suffer permanent brain damage and disability. These conditions are caused by the death of nerve cells. Immediate medical treatment is vital to prevent further complications and brain damage in those who survive the initial rupture.

ANGINA

The term angina describes chest pain caused by too little oxygen to the heart muscle. An angina episode is not the same as a **heart attack**, because the pain is temporary and it seldom causes permanent damage to heart muscle.

Angina is divided into two categories: angina of effort and variant angina. Angina of effort is caused by the narrowing of the arteries (**atherosclerosis**). The narrowed arteries don't allow enough blood through to the heart muscle during periods of exercise, **stress**, or excitement. Due to atherosclerosis, people with angina of effort have an increased risk of heart attack.

Variant angina is uncommon and occurs independently of atherosclerosis. Variant angina is not related to excessive work by the heart muscle. Research indicates that it is caused by heart artery muscle spasm that is too brief or too weak to cause an actual heart attack.

Angina causes a pressing pain or sensation of heaviness, usually in the chest under the breast bone. Sometimes the pain is felt in the shoulder, arm, neck, or jaw. Angina episodes occur when the heart's need for oxygen increases beyond what is available. Emotional stress, extreme temperatures, heavy meals, cigarette smoking, and alcohol can cause or contribute to an episode of angina.

Physicians can usually diagnose angina based on symptoms and what causes them. However, other diagnostic testing is used to confirm the diagnosis. This testing can also reveal any underlying heart disease.

An electrocardiogram is a test that records electrical impulses from the heart. The resulting graph shows if the heart muscle isn't functioning properly. Electrocardiograms are also useful in investigating other possible heart abnormalities.

Because angina often occurs during stress, the heart may need to be tested during exercise. The **stress test** is an electrocardiogram done before, during, and after exercise. Blood pressure is also measured and any angina symptoms are noted.

A more complex stress test, called an angiogram, may be used to picture the blood flow in the heart muscle during the most intense time of exercise and after rest. In this procedure, a long, thin, flexible tube (catheter) is placed in an artery located in the forearm or groin. This catheter is threaded through the artery into a heart artery. A dye is injected through the catheter so x rays can clearly detect the heart and arteries. Many brief x rays are made to create a movie of blood flowing through the coronary arteries.

Angina is first treated by controlling factors that put a person at risk. Risk factors include cigarette smoking, high blood pressure, high cholesterol levels, and **obesity**. Angina is often controlled by medication, usually nitroglycerin. This drug relieves angina pain by increasing the diameter of the blood vessels carrying blood to the heart muscle. Nitroglycerin is taken whenever discomfort occurs or is expected. It may be taken by mouth by placing the tablet under the tongue or through the skin with a medicated patch. In addition, **beta blockers** or calcium channel blockers may be prescribed.

If these treatments don't work, physicians may recommend surgery or **angioplasty**. Coronary artery bypass surgery is an operation in which a blood vessel (often a long vein taken from the leg) is grafted onto the blocked artery to bypass the blocked portion. This newly formed pathway allows blood to flow to the heart muscle.

Another procedure to improve blood flow is balloon angioplasty. In this procedure, the physician inserts a catheter with a tiny balloon at the end into a forearm or groin artery. The catheter is then threaded into the coronary arteries and the balloon is inflated to open narrowed sections of the blood vessel.

Long-term treatment for angina usually involves treating atherosclerosis. This treatment requires diet and lifestyle changes such as regular exercise, reducing dietary sugar and saturated fats, and increasing dietary fiber. Medications to decrease blood pressure or cholesterol may be prescribed.

The prognosis for a patient with angina depends on its origin, type, severity, and the person's general health. Someone with angina has the best outsome if he or she gets prompt medical attention and learns what causes the attacks, what they feel like, how long episodes usually last, and whether medication relieves the attacks. If symptom patterns change significantly, or if symptoms resemble those of a heart attack, immediate medical help is vital.

Angiography

Angiography is the x-ray study of blood vessels. An angiogram uses a dye to make the blood vessels visible under x ray. Angiography is used to detect abnormalities or blockages in the blood vessels (occlusions) throughout the circulatory system and in some organs.

The procedure is commonly used to identify atherosclerosis; to diagnose heart disease; to evaluate kidney function and detect kidney cysts or tumors; to detect an aneurysm (an abnormal bulge of an artery that can rupture), tumor, blood clot, or arteriovenous malformations (abnormals tangles of arteries and veins) in the brain; and to diagnose problems with the retina. It is also used to map the heart or the brain prior to surgery.

Angiography is performed at a hospital. It requires injecting a contrast dye into the blood vessels, making them visible to x ray. The dye is injected by *arterial puncture*. The puncture is usually made in the groin area, armpit, inside elbow, or neck. After being cleaned with an antiseptic agent and injected with a local anesthetic, a small incision is made in the skin. A needle containing an inner wire called a stylet is inserted through the incision. When the radiologist has punctured the artery with the needle, the stylet is removed and replaced with another long wire called a guide wire.

The guide wire is fed through the outer needle and threaded through the artery to the area requiring angiographic study. Once it is in position, the needle is removed and a catheter is slid over the length of the guide wire until it to reaches the area of study. The guide wire is removed and the catheter is left in place in preparation for the injection of the dye.

The dye is either injected with a syringe or with an automatic injector connected to the catheter. The injection causes some mild to moderate discomfort, but it is usually brief. To view the area of study from different angles or perspectives, the patient may be asked to change positions, and subsequent dye injections may be administered.

Throughout the dye injection procedure, x-ray pictures and/or fluoroscopic pictures (moving x rays) are taken. Because of the high pressure of arterial blood flow, the dye dissipates quickly, so pictures must be taken rapidly.

Once x rays are complete, the catheter is carefully removed. Pressure is applied to the puncture site for 10-20 minutes so the arterial puncture can reseal itself. A pressure bandage is then applied.

Most angiograms follow the general procedures outlined above, but vary slightly depending on the area of the vascular system being studied.

After an angiography, a person may stay in the hospital overnight. Otherwise, the patient is kept under close observation for at least 6-12 hours before being released. The patient's blood pressure and vital signs are monitored and the puncture site observed closely. Pain medication may be prescribed, and a cold pack is applied to the puncture site to reduce swelling. The puncture site is normally sore and bruised for several weeks. A hematoma, a hard mass created by broken blood vessels, may develop. It should be watched carefully, as it may indicate continued bleeding of the puncture site.

Because angiography involves puncturing an artery, internal bleeding or hemorrhage are possible complications of the test. As with any invasive procedure, infection of the puncture site or bloodstream is a risk, but this is rare.

A **stroke** or **heart attack** may be triggered by an angiogram if blood clots or plaque on the inside of the arterial wall are dislodged. The heart may also become irritated by the movement of the catheter through its chambers during lung and heart angiography procedures.

Patients who are allergic to the dye used in angiography may experience symptoms such as swelling, difficulty breathing, **heart failure**, or a sudden drop in blood pressure.

Angiography involves minor exposure to radiation. Unless the patient is pregnant, or multiple tests are required, the small dose of radiation from a single procedure poses little risk.

Angiography patients should rest for 2-3 days after the procedure. Patients who experience continued bleeding or abnormal swelling of the puncture site, sudden dizziness, or chest pains should seek medical attention immediately.

ANGIOPLASTY

Angioplasty is a medical procedure used to widen an artery that is narrowed or blocked. A narrowed or blocked artery prevents blood from getting to where it is needed. It is usually caused by an accumulation of fatty deposits within the artery (**atherosclerosis**). The accumulation of fatty deposits is called a plaque. The goal of angioplasty is to return adequate blood supply to regions that are deprived.

There are two conditions that can be treated with angioplasty. The first is **coronary artery disease**, which is characterized by decreased blood flow to the heart. The second is peripheral vascular disease, which results from blocked arteries in the limbs, especially the legs.

Coronary angioplasty is performed by a cardiologist, a physician who specializes in heart disorders. The procedure consists of inserting a catheter, or very thin tube, through the artery to the plaque's location. (The blockage is located by **angiography**.) Once the catheter is in place, a balloon at its tip is inflated. The balloon stretches the artery narrowed by the plaque. Sometimes prop, called a stent, is placed in the spot to help keep the artery open. The physician then removes the catheter and balloon.

Angioplasty of blocked arteries in the extremities or supplying organs, such as the kidneys is performed by a physician specializing in interventional radiologic procedures. The procedure is similar to coronary angioplasty.

The individual undergoing an angioplasty enters the hospital the morning of the procedure. They shouldn't eat or drink anything after midnight of the night before, but a clear liquid breakfast is sometimes allowed. Blood tests, an electrocardiogram, and a **chest x ray** may be done prior to procedure.

The area where the catheter is inserted (arm or groin) is shaved and cleaned with antibacterial soap to prevent infection. Electrode patches are placed on the individual's chest to monitor heart pattern, rate, and rhythm during the procedure. A local anesthetic is injected into the site where the catheter is inserted. As the x-ray dye is injected into the blood stream, the patient may feel a warm flush feeling. Medications may be given intravenously to decrease the patient's anxiety.

After angioplasty, an observation period is required in a cardiac care unit or a hospital room for several hours up to two days. If the angioplasty catheter is inserted into the femoral artery in the groin, the individual is instructed to lie flat and keep the affected leg straight for at least six hours. The arm or groin puncture site is closely observed for any problems, and peripheral pulses of the affected extremity are frequently checked. A pressure dressing may be applied to the puncture site to prevent excess bleeding. A cardiac monitor is used to monitor the patient's heart pattern, rate, and rhythm after coronary angioplasty.

Individuals undergoing angioplasty have a remote risk of an allergic reaction to the local anesthetic or the x-ray dye, which can also be harmful to the kidneys. There is also a risk of excessive bleeding at the site of the catheter entry. If there is damage to the artery, an emergency situation could arise resulting in bypass surgery or surgery. Because of the nature of the procedure, there is a risk of a disturbance of the heart's rhythm or, rarely, a heart attack or **stroke**.

Once completed, the angioplasty will result in a return of adequate blood supply to the region that was previously deprived of blood and oxygen. The individual is allowed to return home with scheduled follow-up by the physician.

ANTACIDS

Antacids are medicines that neutralize stomach acid. They are used to relieve acid **indigestion**, upset stomach, sour stomach, and heartburn.

Antacids are taken by mouth and work by neutralizing excess stomach acid. They contain ingredients such as aluminum hydroxide, calcium carbonate, magnesium hydroxide, and sodium bicarbonate, alone or in various combinations. Antacid products may also contain other ingredients such as simethicone, which relieves gas.

Antacids differ in how quickly they work and how long they provide relief. Those that dissolve rapidly in the stomach, such as magnesium hydroxide and sodium bicarbonate, bring the fastest relief. Antacids that contain calcium carbonate or aluminum dissolve more slowly and can take up to 30 minutes to begin working. The longer an antacid stays in the stomach, the longer it works. Those that contain calcium carbonate or aluminum work longer than those that contain sodium bicarbonate or magnesium. Also, taking any kind of antacid after a meal, instead of on an empty stomach, provides longer-lasting relief because the medicine stays in the stomach.

Among the brands of antacid products on the market are Alka-Seltzer, Maalox, Mylanta, Tums, and Rolaids. Generic forms are also available. These products can be bought without a prescription and come in tablet (regular and chewable), lozenge, and liquid forms.

Antacids are meant to be used only occasionally. They should not be taken continuously for more than two weeks unless under a physician's directions. Taking antacids over long periods could mask the symptoms of a serious stomach or intestinal problem, such as peptic ulcer disease. Older people should be especially careful, as they may have **ulcers** without showing the typical symptoms.

If any signs of **appendicitis** or inflamed bowel are present, antacids should not be taken. Symptoms of appendicitis include cramping, **pain**, and soreness in the lower abdomen, bloating, and nausea and vomiting.

Anyone whose symptoms do not improve after taking antacids or who has black, tarry stools should call a physician. These symptoms could be signs of a serious condition that needs medical attention.

Antacids may interact with many other medicines. When this happens, the effects of one or both drugs may change, or the risk of side effects may be greater. Anyone taking a prescription drug should check with his or her physician before taking antacids. Antacids may affect the results of some medical tests. When scheduling a medical test, ask whether it is all right to take antacids before the test.

Side effects are very rare when antacids are taken as directed. They are more likely when the medicine is taken in large doses or over a long time. Minor side effects include a chalky taste, mild constipation or diarrhea, thirst, stomach cramps, and whitish or speckled stools. These symptoms do not need medical attention unless they do not go away or they interfere with normal activities.

Other uncommon side effects may occur. Anyone who has unusual symptoms after taking antacids should get in touch with his or her physician.

ANTHRAX

Anthrax is a bacterial infection caused by *Bacillus anthracis*. It primarily affects livestock but can occasionally spread to humans, affecting the skin, intestines, or lungs. In humans, the infection can be treated, but it is almost always fatal in animals.

Anthrax is often fatal to cattle, sheep, and goats, and their hides, wool, and bones are often heavily contaminated. In humans, the disease is almost always an occupational hazard, contracted by those who handle animal hides (farmers, butchers, and veterinarians) or sort wool. It is also possible to become infected with anthrax by eating meat from contaminated animals. There are no reports of the disease spreading between people.

Symptoms vary depending on how the disease was contracted. They usually appear within one week of exposure. In humans, anthrax most frequently occurs when the bacteria enter a cut or abrasion. Cutaneous anthrax, as this infection is called, is the mildest form of the disease. The first symptom is an itchy, raised area like an insect bite. Within one to two days, the area becomes inflamed. Next, a blister forms around the dying tissue which becomes black in the center. Other symptoms may include shivering and chills. The bacteria usually remain within the sore. In rare cases, they may spread to nearby lymph nodes or escape into the bloodstream), causing fatal blood **poisoning**.

Inhaling the bacteria can lead to a rare, fatal form of anthrax known as pulmonary or inhalation anthrax that attacks the lungs, sometimes spreading to the brain. Inhalation anthrax begins with flu-like symptoms: **fever**, fatigue, **headache**, and **shortness of breath**. Symptoms progress to **bronchitis**, and it becomes difficult to breathe. Finally, the patient enters **shock**. This form of anthrax is usually fatal.

Intestinal anthrax is rare and often fatal. It is caused by eating meat from an animal that died of anthrax. Intestinal anthrax causes stomach and intestinal inflammation and sores or lesions. The first signs of disease are **nausea and vomiting**, loss of appetite, and fever, followed by abdominal **pain**, vomiting of blood, and severe bloody **diarrhea**.

Anthrax is diagnosed by detecting *B. anthracis* in blood, **skin lesions**, or respiratory secretions. The bacteria may be positively identified using biochemical methods. Blood samples will indicate elevated antibody levels (increased amounts of a specific protein produced in response to anthrax infection).

In the early stages, anthrax is curable with high doses of penicillin. Other commonly used **antibiotics** are also effective.

Death is unlikely with appropriate care. Ten to twenty percent of patients will die from cutaneous anthrax if it is not properly treated. All patients with inhalation anthrax will die if untreated. Intestinal anthrax is fatal 25-75% of the time.

Anthrax is relatively rare in the United States because of widespread animal vaccination and practices used to disinfect hides or other animal products. For those in high-risk professions, an anthrax vaccine is available that is 93% effective in protecting against infection.

Other means of preventing the spread of infection include carefully handling dead animals suspected of having the disease and providing good ventilation when processing hides, fur, wool, or hair. Anyone visiting a country where anthrax is common or where herd animals are not vaccinated should avoid contact with livestock or animal products and avoid eating meat that has not been properly prepared and cooked.

ANTIACNE DRUGS

Anti-acne drugs are medicines that help clear up pimples, blackheads, whiteheads, and more severe forms of **acne**. Acne is a skin condition in which pores or hair follicles become blocked. This allows a waxy material, sebum, to collect inside the pores or follicles. As a result, small swellings develop on the skin surface. Bacteria and dead skin cells can collect, causing inflammation. Swellings that are small and not inflamed are whiteheads or blackheads. When they become inflamed, they turn into pimples. Pimples that fill with pus are called pustules.

People who have certain medical conditions or who are taking other medicines may have problems if they use antiacne drugs. Before using these products, be sure to let the physician know about any allergies, pregnancy, breastfeeding, eczema, or any other conditions such as alcoholism, diabetes, or high cholesterol or high triglyceride levels.

Benzoyl peroxide and tretinoin work by mildly irritating the skin. This encourages skin cells to slough off, which helps open blocked pores. Benzoyl peroxide also kills bacteria, which helps prevent whiteheads and blackheads from turning into pimples.

Benzoyl peroxide is found in many over-the-counter acne products that are applied to the skin. Some benzoyl peroxide products are available without a physician's prescription; others require a prescription. Tretinoin (Retin-A) requires a physician's prescription and comes in liquid, cream, and gel forms, which are applied to the skin.

Anti-acne drugs such as benzoyl peroxide and tretinoin may irritate the skin slightly. The face should only be washed with mild soap and water two or three times a day, unless the physician says otherwise. Abrasive soaps should be avoided, as should cleansers and products that dry the skin or make it peel, such as medicated cosmetics, cleansers that contain alcohol, or other acne products. Tretinoin may increase sensitivity to sunlight, so it is best to avoid exposure to the sun and not use tanning beds, tanning booths, or sunlamps.

The most common side effects of anti-acne drugs applied to the skin are slight redness, dryness, peeling, and stinging, and a warm feeling to the skin. These problems usually go away as the body adjusts to the drug and do not require medical treatment.

Other side effects should be brought to a physician's attention:

- Blistering, crusting or swelling of the skin
- Severe burning or redness of the skin
- Darkening or lightening of the skin
- Skin rash.

Patients using anti-acne drugs on their skin should tell their physicians if they are using any other prescription or nonprescription (over-the-counter) medicine that they apply to the skin in the same area.

Isotretinoin (Accutane), which is taken by mouth in capsule form, is available only with a physician's prescription. Isotretinoin shrinks the glands that produce sebum. This medicine cannot be used during pregnancy, because it causes birth defects. Patients who use isotretinoin usually take the medicine for a few months, then stop for at least two months. If the condition is still severe, the physician may prescribe a second course of treatment.

Isotretinoin may cause a sudden decrease in night vision. This medicine may also make the eyes, nose, and mouth very dry. Isotretinoin may also increase sensitivity to sunlight, and patients should avoid exposure to the sun and should not use tanning beds, tanning booths, or sunlamps.

In the early stages of treatment with isotretinoin, some people's acne seems to get worse before it starts getting better. If the condition becomes much worse or if the skin is very irritated, check with the physician who prescribed the medicine.

Bowel inflammation is not a common side effect, but it may occur with isotretinoin use. If any of the following signs occur, stop taking isotretinoin immediately and check with a physician:

- Pain in the abdomen
- Bleeding from the rectum
- Severe **diarrhea**.

Other side effects of isotretinoin that require medical attention include:

- Burning, redness, or itching of the eyes
- **Nosebleed**s
- Signs of inflammation of the lips, such as peeling, burning, redness or pain.

ANTIANGINA DRUGS

Antiangina drugs are medicines that relieve the symptoms of **angina** pectoris (severe chest **pain**). The dull, tight chest pain of angina occurs when the heart muscle is not getting enough oxygen. By relaxing blood vessels, antiangina drugs reduce the heart's work load and increase the amount of oxygen-rich blood that reaches the heart. These drugs come in different forms, and are used in three main ways.

Taken regularly over a long period, some antiangina medicines reduce the number of angina attacks. Others are taken just before some activity that usually brings on an attack, such as climbing stairs, to prevent attacks. The third type is taken when an attack begins to relieve the pain and pressure. Not every type of antiangina drug can be used in every way. Some work too slowly to prevent attacks that are about to begin or to relieve attacks that have already started.

Antiangina drugs, also known as nitrates, come in many different forms: tablets and capsules that are swallowed; tablets that are held under the tongue, inside the lip, or in the cheek until they dissolve; stick-on patches; ointment; and in-the-mouth sprays. Commonly used antiangina drugs include isosorbide dinitrate (Isordil, Sorbitrate, and other brands) and nitroglycerin (Nitro-Bid, Nitro-Dur, Nitrolingual Spray, Nitrostat Tablets, Transderm-Nitro, and other brands).

These medicines are available only with a physician's prescription. The recommended dosage depends on the type and form of antiangina drug and may be different for different patients. Changes in medication and doses should only be done with physician approval.

These medicines make some people feel lightheaded, dizzy, or faint when they get up after sitting or lying down. Antiangina drugs may also cause **dizziness**, lightheadedness, or **fainting** in hot weather or when people stand for a long time or **exercise**. Drinking alcohol while taking antiangina drugs may cause the same problems.

Other side effects may occur. Anyone who has unusual symptoms after taking an antiangina drug should get in touch with his or her physician. Antiangina drugs may interact with other medicines. This may increase the risk of side effects or change the effects of one or both drugs. Anyone who takes antiangina drugs should let the physician know all other medicines he or she is taking.

If the person is taking the form of nitroglycerin that is placed under the tongue and symptoms are not relieved within three doses taken about 5 minutes apart, the person should go to the hospital emergency room as soon as possible. A **heart attack** may be in progress.

Some people develop tolerance to antiangina drugs over time. That is, the drug no longer produces the desired effects. Anyone who seems to be developing a tolerance to this medicine should check with his or her physician.

ANTIANXIETY DRUGS

Antianxiety drugs are medicines that calm and relax people with excessive anxiety, nervousness, or tension. Everyone feels nervous or anxious once in awhile. Usually, the feeling is related to something happening in the person's life, such as a job interview, and it goes away when life is back to normal again. This type of anxiety does not need medical treatment. But some people feel anxious almost all the time, or they respond to slightly stressful events with feelings that are out of proportion. Constant anxiety, irrational worries, and sense of impending doom can seriously interfere with their daily lives. For people with such intense or prolonged anxiety, antianxiety drugs can help bring their feelings under control and reduce bothersome symptoms such as pounding heartbeat, breathing problems, irritability, nausea, and faintness.

Antianxiety drugs are prescribed for severe general anxiety and for specific **anxiety disorders**, such as **phobias**, **panic disorder**, **obsessive-compulsive disorder** (OCD), and **post-traumatic stress disorder**. Physicians may sometimes prescribe these drugs for other conditions, such as **sleep disorders**, epilepsy, and other seizure disorders.

There are two main types of antianxiety drugs, also known as anxiolytics or minor tranquilizers. The family of antianxiety drugs known as **benzodiazepines** includes alprazolam (Xanax), chlordiazepoxide (Librium), diazepam (Valium), and lorazepam (Ativan). The other widely used antianxiety drug is buspirone (BuSpar), which is not a benzodiazepine.

Benzodiazepines take effect fairly quickly, starting to work within an hour after they are taken. The effects of buspirone are not felt until the drug has built up to certain levels in the body. People must take it every day for 2-3 weeks before they will notice any effects. These medicines are available only with a physician's prescription and are sold in tablet, capsule, liquid, rectal, and injectable forms.

Seeing the physician regularly while taking antianxiety drugs is important. The physician will check to make sure the medicine is working as it should and will note unwanted side effects. Some people feel drowsy, dizzy, lightheaded, or less alert. Anyone who takes these drugs should not drive, use machines or do anything else that might be dangerous until they have found out how the drugs affect them.

Antianxiety drugs may add to the effects of alcohol and other drugs that slow down the central nervous system (CNS), such as **antihistamines**, cold medicine, allergy medicine, sleep aids, medicine for seizures, tranquilizers, some pain relievers, and **muscle relaxants**.

People with certain medical conditions can have problems if they take antianxiety drugs. A physician should also be warned of any medical conditions such as current or past drug abuse and kidney or liver disease. Anyone who has had unusual reactions to these medications in the past should let his or her physician know. The physician should also be told about any **allergies** to foods, dyes, preservatives, or other substances.

Common side effects of antianxiety drugs are nausea, **dizziness**, lightheadedness, **headache**, restlessness, nervousness, or unusual excitement. These problems usually go away as the body adjusts to the drug and do not require medical treatment unless they persist or they interfere with normal activities.

More serious side effects are rare, but may occur. Anyone who has unusual symptoms during or after treatment with antianxiety drugs should get in touch with his or her physician.

ANTIARRHYTHMIC DRUGS

Antiarrhythmic drugs are medicines that correct irregular or too fast heartbeats. Normally, the heart beats at a steady, even pace. The pace is controlled by electrical signals that begin in one part of the heart and quickly spread through the whole heart. If something goes wrong with this control system, the result may be an irregular heartbeat, or an arrhythmia. Antiarrhythmic drugs correct irregular heartbeats, restoring the normal rhythm. If the heart is beating too fast, these drugs will slow it down. By correcting these problems, antiarrhythmic drugs help the heart work more efficiently.

Antiarrhythmic drugs are available only with a physician's prescription and are sold in capsule, tablet, and injectable forms. Commonly used antiarrhythmic drugs are disopyramide (Norpace, Norpace CR), procainamide (Procan SR, Pronestyl, Pronestyl-SR), and quinidine (Cardioquin, Duraquin, Quinidex, and other brands).

Persons who take these drugs should see their physician regularly. The physician will check to make sure the medicine is working as it should and will note any unwanted side effects.

Some people feel dizzy, lightheaded, or faint when using these drugs. This medicine may cause blurred vision or other vision problems. Because of these possible problems, anyone who takes these drugs should not drive, use machines or do anything else that might be dangerous until they have found out how the drugs affect them. Anyone taking this medicine should not drink alcohol without his or her physician's approval.

Some antiarrhythmic drugs may change the results of certain medical tests. Before having medical tests, anyone taking this medicine should alert the health care professional in charge. Anyone who is taking antiarrhythmic drugs should be sure to tell the health care professional in charge before having any surgical or dental procedures or receiving emergency treatment.

Antiarrhythmic drugs may cause dry mouth. Mouth dryness that continues over a long time may contribute to **tooth decay** and other dental problems.

People taking antiarrhythmic drugs may sweat less, which can cause the body temperature to rise. Anyone who takes this medicine should be careful not to become overheated during **exercise** or hot weather and should avoid hot baths, hot tubs, and saunas.

People with certain medical conditions may have problems if they take antiarrhythmic drugs. For example, antiarrhythmic drugs may cause low blood sugar, which can be a particular problem for people with congestive heart disease or diabetes. Before prescribing these drugs, the physician should be warned of any existing medical conditions.

Antiarrhythmic drugs may interact with other medicines. When this happens, the effects of one or both of the drugs may change or the risk of side effects may be greater. Anyone who takes antiarrhythmic drugs should let the physician know all other medicines he or she is taking.

Anyone who has had unusual reactions to an antiarrhythmic drug in the past should let his or her physician know before taking this type of medicine again. Patients taking procainamide should let their physicians know if they have ever had an unusual or allergic reaction to procaine or any other ''caine-type'' medicine, such as xylocaine or lidocaine. Patients taking quinidine should mention any previous reactions to quinine. The physician should also be told about any **allergies** to foods, dyes, preservatives, or other substances.

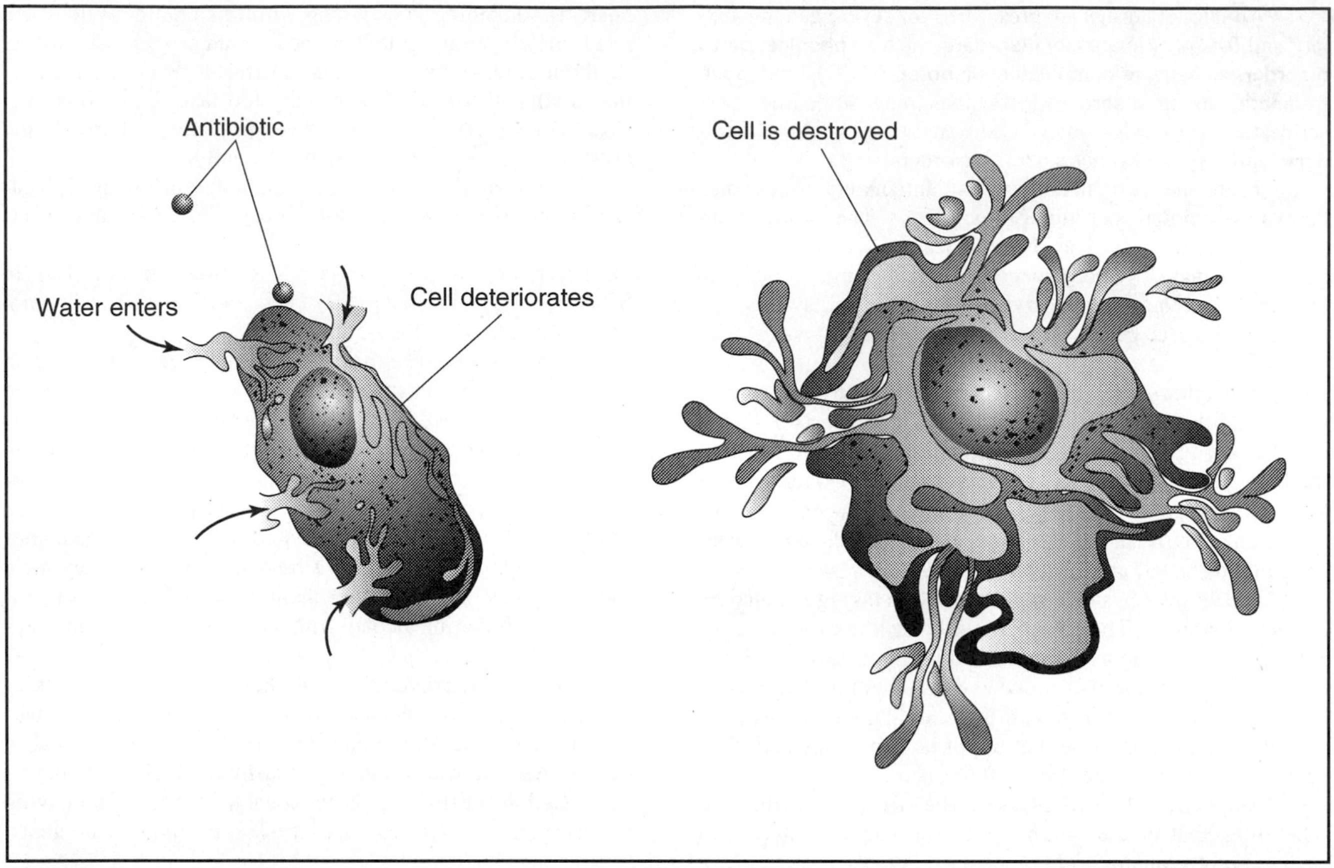

Different antibiotics destroy bacteria in different ways. Some short-circuit the processes by which bacteria receive energy. Others disturb the structure of the bacterial cell wall, as shown in the illustration above. Still others interfere with the production of essential proteins. *(Illustration by Electronic Illustrators Group.)*

The effects of taking antiarrhythmic drugs in **pregnancy** have not been studied in humans. In studies of laboratory animals, this medicine increased the risk of miscarriage. Antiarrhythmic drugs pass into breast milk. Women who are pregnant or breastfeeding should check with their physicians before taking this medicine.

Serious side effects are not common, but may occur. Anyone who has unusual symptoms after taking antiarrhythmic drugs should get in touch with his or her physician.

ANTIBIOTICS

Antibiotics are medicines that kill the bacteria that cause infections. Antibiotics have been used since the 1930s to treat or prevent a wide variety of infections. Before then, there were few effective ways of combating bacterial infections. Illnesses such as **pneumonia**, **tuberculosis**, and **typhoid fever** were essentially untreatable. Even minor infections could be deadly.

Since the introduction of antibiotics in the mid 1930s, physicians and patients have come to depend on these drugs to treat everything from **sore throat**s and urinary tract infections to meningitis and tuberculosis. These drugs are also used to prevent infections before, during, and after surgery.

Different antibiotics kill bacteria in different ways. Some short-circuit the processes by which bacteria get energy, others disturb the structure of the bacterial cell wall, and still others interfere with the production of essential proteins. Antibiotics do not work against viral diseases such as colds or influenza.

Some 150 antibiotics are available. These include **tetracyclines**, aminoglycosides, **penicillins**, **cephalosporins**, fluoroquinolones, streptogramins, **sulfonamides**, and erythromycins.

In recent years, health experts have noticed that certain antibiotics are becoming less effective. The reason is due to antibiotic resistance, a problem that develops when antibiotics are overused or misused. Sometimes a few bacteria in a population can resist the effects of an antibiotic. Because bacteria reproduce so quickly, the trait can be rapidly passed on through generations until almost all the bacteria of that species are immune to a particular antibiotic. The more antibiotics are used, the more rapidly the process happens. As a result, almost every disease-causing bacterium is resistant to at least one antibiotic.

Health experts are particularly concerned about antibiotic resistance in bacteria that cause certain serious infections.

For example, some strains of *Staphylococcus aureus*, that may cause **boils**, pneumonia, or bloodstream infections, are resistant to almost all antibiotics, making those conditions very difficult to treat. Many strains of tuberculosis, also an infectious disease, also are now resistant to one or more of the agents used to control tuberculosis.

Everyone can help keep antibiotic resistance from becoming an even bigger problem. For example, do not use an antibiotic for a cold or flu. Such illnesses are due to viral infections, which cannot be treated with antibiotics. Taking an antibiotic when it is not needed will only encourage the spread of resistant bacteria. When an antibiotic is prescribed, be sure to take all the medicine, for as long as directed. When a patient stops taking the medicine too soon, only the most vulnerable bacteria are killed, leaving the tougher ones alive and well.

Antibiotics are classified as narrow-spectrum drugs when they work against only a few types of bacteria. Broad-spectrum antibiotics attack many types of bacteria. However, broad-spectrum antibiotics are more likely to promote antibiotic resistance. For that reason, narrow-spectrum antibiotics, which often cost less, are used whenever possible. Broad-spectrum antibiotics should be reserved for infections that do not respond to narrow-spectrum drugs.

To completely clear up infections and to help prevent antibiotic resistance, antibiotics should be taken exactly as directed. Do not stop taking the medicine just because symptoms begin to improve.

People who have certain medical conditions or who are taking certain other medicines may have problems if they take antibiotics. Antibiotics may cause a number of side effects. Anyone who has unusual or disturbing symptoms after taking antibiotics should call the physician as soon as possible.

Antibiotics may interact with other medicines as well as with foods. When this happens, the effects of the antibiotic or the risk of side effects may be greater. Anyone who takes antibiotics should let the physician know all other medicines he or she is taking.

ANTICANCER DRUGS

Anticancer drugs are medicines used to treat various kinds of **cancer**. Cancer is the uncontrolled growth of cells that interfere with the growth of healthy cells. The approach to treating cancer depends on where in the body it occurs, the type of cells making up the cancer, and how advanced the cancer is. The usual treatments are surgery, **chemotherapy** (treatment with anticancer drugs), radiation, or some combination of these methods.

Anticancer drugs interfere with the growth of tumor cells, eventually causing their **death**. However because these drugs are so powerful, they may also affect the growth of normal body cells, causing many side effects, some of which may be serious. Anticancer drugs come in different forms, depending on the type of drug. Some are given only as injections; others are taken by mouth in tablet or liquid form.

The recommended dosage depends on many factors, such as body weight or kidney function, and is different for different patients. Patients who take anticancer drugs at home should follow their physician's orders or the directions on the label. Always take anticancer drugs exactly as directed. Never take smaller or larger, more frequent or less frequent doses. Take the drug for as long as it has been prescribed—no more and no less. Some drugs need to be taken at a specific time of day to be most effective and to reduce the chance of side effects. Be sure to follow these directions carefully.

Anticancer drugs are sometimes given together with other medicines.When using a combination of medicines, be sure to take each at the correct time. Do not mix the drugs together. Anyone who has trouble remembering when to take each drug should ask his or her health care team for tips on ways to keep track.

Anticancer drugs may cause a variety of side effects, some very serious; others not as serious, but still troubling. In addition, some unwanted effects may not appear until months or years after the drugs were used. It is important to understand what side effects are possible and to weigh the advantages of using this medicine with the risks of side effects. Health care professionals can help patients sort out the relative risks and benefits. It is also very important to see the physician as often as directed so that he or she can make sure the medicine is working and check for unwanted effects that may not be obvious to the patient.

Nausea and vomiting are common side effects of anticancer drugs. However, other drugs may be given along with them to reduce these often incapacitating side effects. Unless a physician has said to stop taking the medicine, patients should always keep taking their anticancer drugs, even if they feel ill. A patient who vomits just after taking a dose of an anticancer drug should check with the health care professional in charge to find out whether to take another dose immediately or to wait until the next scheduled dose. Some anticancer drugs cause loss of hair, which may include eyebrows, eyelashes, and pubic hair. This is a temporary effect. The hair should grow back normally after the treatment ends, but the color or texture of the new hair may be slightly different.

Anticancer drugs may interact with a number of other medicines. When this happens, the effects of one or both of the drugs may change or the risk of side effects may be greater. Anyone who takes anticancer drugs should let the physician know all other prescription or non-prescription (over-the-counter) medicines he or she is taking. The physician should also be told if the patient has been treated with radiation or has taken other anticancer drugs.

Many anticancer drugs cause sterility, which may be permanent. Anyone taking anticancer drugs (or who has recently taken the drugs) should not have any vaccinations (immunizations)without the approval of the physician who is overseeing the cancer treatment. These patients must also avoid contact with anyone who has recently taken oral polio vaccine, as there is a chance the polio virus could be passed on. No one in the patient's household should take oral polio vaccine. All these precautions are necessary because anticancer drugs may lower the body's resistance to infection.

ANTICOAGULANT AND ANTIPLATELET DRUGS

Anticoagulant drugs help prevent harmful clots from forming in blood vessels by decreasing the blood's ability to clot. Although these drugs are sometimes called blood thinners, they do not actually thin the blood. Furthermore, this type of medicine will not dissolve clots that already have formed, although the drug stops an existing clot from worsening.

Anticoagulant drugs are used in several situations. For example, they may be given to prevent blood clots from forming after the replacement of a heart valve or to reduce the risk of a **stroke** or another **heart attack** after a first heart attack. They are also used to reduce the chance of blood clots forming during open heart surgery or bypass surgery. Low doses of these drugs may be given to prevent blood clots in patients who must stay in bed for a long time after certain kinds of surgery.

Anticoagulant drugs, also called antiplatelet drugs, anticlotting drugs, and blood thinners, are available only with a physician's prescription. They come in tablet and injectable forms. Some commonly used anticoagulant drugs are dicumarol, warfarin (Coumadin), dipyridamole (Persantine), enoxaparin (Lovenox) and heparin.

A physician must know about any existing medical conditions before prescribing anticoagulant drugs, because they can be dangerous in combination with certain conditions. Persons who take anticoagulants should see a physician regularly while taking these drugs. The physician will order periodic blood tests to check the blood's clotting ability.

These drugs can increase the risk of severe bleeding and heavy blood loss. Because of this risk, anyone taking an anticoagulant drug must take care to avoid injuries. Sports and other potentially hazardous activities should be avoided. Any falls, blows to the body or head, or other injuries should be reported to a physician, as internal bleeding may occur without any obvious symptoms.

The most common minor side effects of anticoagulant medicines are bloating or gas. These problems usually go away as the body adjusts to the drug and do not require medical treatment. More serious side effects may occur, especially if too much of this medicine is taken. Anyone who has unusual symptoms while taking anticoagulant drugs should get in touch with his or her physician.

People who are taking anticoagulant drugs should tell all medical professionals who provide medical treatments or services to them that they are taking this medicine. They should also carry identification stating that they are using an anticoagulant drug.

Other prescriptions or over-the-counter medicine—especially **aspirin**—should not be taken without checking with the physician who prescribed the anticoagulant drug.

Diet also affects the way anticoagulant drugs work in the body. The reason that diet is so important is that vitamin K affects how the anticoagulant drugs work. Vitamin K is found in meats, dairy products, leafy, green vegetables, and some multiple **vitamins** and nutritional supplements. For the drugs to work properly, it is best to have the same amount of vitamin K in the body all the time.

Alcohol can change the way anticoagulant drugs affect the body. Anyone who takes these drugs should not have more than 1-2 drinks at any time and should not drink alcohol every day.

Anyone who has had unusual reactions to anticoagulants in the past should let his or her physician know before taking the drugs again. The physician should also be told about any **allergies** to foods; dyes; preservatives; or other substances.

Anticoagulants may cause many serious problems if taken during **pregnancy**. **Birth defects**, severe bleeding in the fetus, and other problems are possible. The mother may also experience severe bleeding if she takes anticoagulants during pregnancy, during delivery, or even shortly after delivery. Some anticoagulant drugs may pass into breast milk.

ANTICONVULSANT DRUGS

Anticonvulsant drugs are medicines used to prevent or treat convulsions (seizures)in people with epilepsy. Epilepsy is not a single disease — it is a set of symptoms that may have different causes in different people. There is an imbalance in the brain's electrical activity which causes seizures. These may affect part or all of the body and may or may not cause a loss of consciousness. Anticonvulsant drugs act on the brain to reduce the frequency and severity of seizures.

Anticonvulsant drugs are an important part of the treatment program for epilepsy. Different kinds of drugs may be prescribed for different types of seizures. In addition to taking medicine, patients with epilepsy should get enough rest, avoid **stress**, and practice good health habits. Some physicians believe that giving the drugs to children with epilepsy may prevent the condition from getting worse in later life. However, others say the effects are the same, whether treatment is started early or later in life. Determining when treatment begins depends on the physician and his assessment of the patient's symptoms.

Anticonvulsant drugs include such medicines as carbamazepine (Tegretol), phenytoin (Dilantin), and valproic acid (Depakote, Depakene). The drugs are available only with a physician's prescription and come in tablet, capsule, liquid, and ''sprinkle'' forms. The recommended dosage depends on the type of anticonvulsant, its strength, and the type of seizures for which it is being taken. Check with the physician who prescribed the drug or the pharmacist who filled the prescription for the correct dosage. Do not stop taking this medicine suddenly after taking it for several weeks or more. Gradually tapering the dose may reduce the chance of withdrawal effects. Do not change brands or dosage forms of this medicine without checking with a pharmacist or physician. If a prescription refill does not look like the original medicine, check with the pharmacist who filled the prescription.

Patients on anticonvulsant drugs should see a physician regularly while on therapy, especially during the first few months. The physician will check to make sure the medicine is working as it should and will note unwanted side effects. The physician may also need to adjust the dosage during this period.While taking anticonvulsant drugs, do not start or stop taking any other medicines without checking with a physician. The other medicines may affect the way the anticonvulsant medicine works.

Anticonvulsant drugs may interact with medicines used during surgery, dental procedures, or emergency treatment. These interactions could increase the chance of side effects. Anyone who is taking anticonvulsant drugs should be sure to tell the health care professional in charge before having any surgical or dental procedures or receiving emergency treatment. Some people feel drowsy, dizzy, lightheaded, or less alert when using these drugs, especially when they first begin taking them or when their dosage is increased. Anyone who takes anticonvulsant drugs should not drive, use machines or do anything else that might be dangerous until they have found out how the drugs affect them. This medicine may increase sensitivity to sunlight. Even brief exposure to sun can cause a severe **sunburn** or a rash. While being treated with this medicine, avoid being in direct sunlight, especially between 10 a.m. and 3 p.m.; wear a hat and tightly woven clothing that covers the arms and legs; use a sunscreen with a skin protection factor (SPF) of at least 15; protect the lips with a sun block lipstick; and do not use tanning beds, tanning booths, or sunlamps.

People with certain medical conditions or who are taking certain other medicines can have problems if they take anticonvulsant drugs. Before taking these drugs, be sure to let the physician know about any of these conditions. The physician should also be told about any **allergies** to foods, dyes, preservatives, or other substances.

Birth defects have been reported in babies born to mothers who took anticonvulsant drugs during **pregnancy**. Women who are pregnant or who may become pregnant should check with their physicians about the safety of using anticonvulsant drugs during pregnancy. Some anticonvulsant drugs pass into breast milk and may cause unwanted effects in babies whose mothers take the medicine. Women who are breastfeeding should check with their physicians about the benefits and risks of using anticonvulsant drugs.

Anticonvulsant drugs may affect blood sugar levels. Patients with diabetes who notice changes in the results of their urine or blood tests should check with their physicians. Taking anticonvulsant drugs with certain other drugs may affect the way the drugs work or may increase the chance of side effects. The most common side effects are **constipation**, mild nausea or vomiting, and mild **dizziness**, drowsiness, or lightheadedness. These problems usually go away as the body adjusts to the drug and do not require medical treatment. Less common side effects may occur and do not need medical attention unless they persist or are troublesome. Anyone who has unusual symptoms after taking anticonvulsant drugs should get in touch with his or her physician.

ANTIDEPRESSANT DRUGS

Antidepressant drugs are medicines that relieve symptoms of mental depression. They are used to treat serious, continuing mental depression that interferes with a person's ability to function. Everyone feels sad, ''blue,'' or discouraged occasionally, but usually those feelings do not interfere with everyday life and do not need treatment. However, when the feelings become overwhelming and last for weeks or months, professional treatment can help. Although depression is one of the most common and serious mental disorders, it is also one of the most treatable. According to the American Psychiatric Association, 80-90% of people with depression can be helped. If untreated, depression can lead to social withdrawal, physical complaints, such as fatigue, sleep problems, and aches and **pain**s, and even suicide.

The first step in treating depression is an accurate diagnosis by a physician or mental health professional. The physician or mental health professional will ask questions about the person's medical and psychiatric history and will try to rule out other causes, such as thyroid problems or side effects of medicines the person is taking. Lab tests may be ordered to help rule out medical problems. Once a person has been diagnosed with depression, treatment will be tailored to the person's specific problem. The treatment may consist of drugs alone, counseling alone, or drugs in combination with counseling methods such as psychotherapy or cognitive behavioral therapy.

Antidepressant drugs help reduce the extreme sadness, hopelessness, and lack of interest in life that are typical in people with depression. These drugs also may be used to treat other conditions, such as obsessive compulsive disorder, **premenstrual syndrome**, chronic pain, and eating disorders.

Antidepressant drugs, also called antidepressants, are thought to work by influencing communication between cells in the brain. The drugs affect chemicals called neurotransmitters, which carry signals from one nerve cell to another. These neurotransmitters are involved in the control of mood and in other responses and functions, such as eating, sleep, pain, and thinking.

The main types of antidepressant drugs in use today are: Tricyclic **antidepressants**, such as amitriptyline (Elavil), imipramine (Tofranil), nortriptyline (Pamelor); Selective serotonin reuptake inhibitors (SSRIs or serotonin boosters), such as fluoxetine (Prozac), paroxetine (Paxil), and sertraline (Zoloft); Monoamine oxidase inhibitors (MAO inhibitors), such as phenelzine (Nardil), and tranylcypromine (Parnate); Lithium (used mainly to treat manic depression, but also sometimes prescribed for recurring bouts of depression).

Selective serotonin reuptake inhibitors act only on the neurotransmitter serotonin, while tricyclic antidepressants and MAO inhibitors act on both serotonin and another neurotransmitter, norepinephrine, and may also interact with other chemicals throughout the body. Because the neurotransmitters involved in the control of moods are also involved in other processes, such as sleep, eating, and pain, drugs that affect these neurotransmitters can be used for more than just treating depression. **Headache**, eating disorders, **bed-wetting**, and other problems are now being treated with antidepressants.

All antidepressant drugs are effective, but certain types work best for certain kinds of depression. For example, people who are depressed and agitated do best when they take an antidepressant drug that also calms them down. People who are depressed and withdrawn may benefit more from an antidepressant drug that has a stimulating effect.

Recommended dosage depends on the kind of antidepressant drug, the type and severity of the condition for which it is prescribed, and other factors such as the patient's age. Check with the physician who prescribed the drug or the pharmacist who filled the prescription for the correct dosage. Always take antidepressant drugs exactly as directed. Never take larger or more frequent doses, and do not take the drug for longer than directed.

While antidepressant drugs help people feel better, they cannot solve problems in people's lives. Some mental health professionals worry that people who could benefit from psychotherapy rely instead on antidepressant drugs for a "quick fix." Others point out that the drugs work gradually and do not produce instant happiness. The best approach is often a combination of counseling and medicine, but the correct treatment for a specific patient depends on many factors. The decision of how to treat depression or other conditions that may respond to antidepressant drugs should be made carefully and will be different for different people.

Most antidepressant drugs do not begin working right away. The effects may not be felt for several weeks. Continuing to take the medicine is important, even if it does not seem to be working at first. There may be side effects depend on the type of antidepressant drug.

Antidepressant drugs may interact with a variety of other medicines. When this happens, the effects of one or both of the drugs may change or the risk of side effects may be greater. Some interactions may be life-threatening. Anyone who takes antidepressant drugs should let the physician know all other medicines he or she is taking.

Antidepressants, tricyclic

Tricyclic antidepressants are medicines that relieve mental depression. Since their discovery in the 1950s, tricyclic antidepressants have been used to treat mental depression. Like other antidepressant drugs, they reduce symptoms such as extreme sadness, hopelessness, and lack of energy. Some tricyclic antidepressants are also used to treat bulimia, cocaine withdrawal, **panic disorder**, **obsessive-compulsive disorder**s, certain types of chronic **pain**, and **bed-wetting** in children.

Named for their three-ring chemical structure, tricyclic antidepressants work by correcting chemical imbalances in the brain. But because they also affect other chemicals throughout the body, these drugs may produce many unwanted side effects. Tricyclic antidepressants are available only with a physician's prescription and are sold in tablet, capsule, liquid, and injectable forms. Some commonly used tricyclic antidepressants are amitriptyline (Elavil), desipramine (Norpramin), imipramine (Tofranil), nortriptyline (Pamelor), and protriptyline (Vivactil). Different drugs in this family have different effects, and physicians can choose the drug that best fits the patient's symptoms.

The recommended dosage depends on many factors, including the patient's age, weight, general health and symptoms. The type of tricyclic antidepressant and its strength also must be considered. Check with the physician who prescribed the drug or the pharmacist who filled the prescription for the correct dosage. Always take tricyclic antidepressants exactly as directed. Never take larger or more frequent doses, and do not take the drug for longer than directed. Do not stop taking the medicine just because it does not seem to be working. Visit the physician as often as recommended so that the physician can check to see if the drug is working and to note for side effects.

Some people feel drowsy, dizzy, or lightheaded, when taking these drugs. The drugs may also cause blurred vision. Anyone who takes these drugs should not drive, use machines or do anything else that might be dangerous until they have found out how the drugs affect them. Anyone taking tricyclic antidepressants should check with his or her physician before drinking alcohol or taking any drugs that cause drowsiness.

Tricyclic antidepressants may interact with medicines used during surgery, dental procedures, or emergency treatment. These interactions could increase the chance of side effects. Anyone who is taking tricyclic antidepressants should be sure to tell the health care professional in charge before having any surgical or dental procedures or receiving emergency treatment. These drugs may also change the results of medical tests. Before having medical tests, anyone taking this medicine should alert the health care professional in charge. They may increase sensitivity to sunlight. Even brief exposure to sun can cause a severe **sunburn** or a rash. Hence adequate precautions need to be taken. The physician should also be told about any **allergies** to foods, dyes, preservatives, or other substances.

Problems have been reported in babies whose mothers took tricyclic antidepressants just before delivery. Women who are pregnant or who may become pregnant should check with their physicians about the safety of using tricyclic antidepressants. Tricyclic antidepressants pass into breast milk and may cause drowsiness in nursing babies whose mothers take the drugs. Women who are breastfeeding should check with their physicians before using tricyclic antidepressants.

Taking tricyclic antidepressants with certain other drugs may affect the way the drugs work or may increase the chance of side effects. The most common side effects are **dizziness**, drowsiness, dry mouth, unpleasant taste, **headache**, nausea, mild tiredness or weakness, increased appetite or craving for sweets, and weight gain. These problems usually go away as the body adjusts to the drug and do not require medical treatment. If any unusual side effects occur, check with the physician who prescribed the medicine as soon as possible.

Antidiabetic drugs

Antidiabetic drugs are medicines that help control blood sugar levels in people with **diabetes mellitus** (sugar diabetes). Diabetes mellitus is a disorder of metabolism, the processes through which the body uses food that has been broken down by digestion. Most food is broken down into a type of sugar called glucose, which the body can use for energy and growth. Glucose travels through the bloodstream to cells throughout the body. But glucose cannot enter the cells without the help of a hormone called insulin. Insulin is produced by the pancreas, a large gland beneath the stomach. In people with diabetes mellitus, the body does not have enough insulin to move the glucose into the cells. This may be because the pancreas does not produce enough insulin or because the cells do not respond to the insulin, even though plenty is produced. Either way, glucose builds up in the blood and passes out of the body in urine without ever having been used as fuel.

Untreated, diabetes can lead to very serious problems, including heart disease, kidney failure, blindness, nerve damage, and **amputations**. But with proper management, the risk of such problems can be greatly reduced. The management plan depends on the type of diabetes: insulin-dependent diabetes mellitus (IDDM) or noninsulin-dependent diabetes mellitus (NIDDM).

In insulin-dependent diabetes mellitus, also known as Type 1 diabetes, the pancreas produces little or no insulin. People with this type of diabetes must take injections of insulin every day to stay alive. They must also eat properly, following a schedule that helps keep glucose levels in the blood from getting too high or too low, and they must closely monitor their blood sugar levels with blood or urine tests.

People with Noninsulin-dependent diabetes mellitus, also known as Type 2 diabetes, produce enough insulin, but their bodies are unable to use it. Often, this type of diabetes can be controlled through diet and **exercise**. When it cannot, insulin or drugs called oral hypoglycemics may be prescribed.

In addition to insulin, which is taken by injection, four types of medications (oral hypoglycemics) are used to help control noninsulin-dependent diabetes mellitus. Each type of medicine helps lower blood sugar in a different way, and all are available only with a physician's prescription. Some patients may take the pills alone or combined with other pills; others may take pills plus insulin injections. The four types of oral hypoglycemics are Sulfonylureas, such as glipizide (Glucotrol), glyburide (DiaBeta, Glynase, Micronase), chlorpropamide (Diabinese), and tolbutamide (Orinase); Biguanides, such as metformin (Glucophage); Alpha-glucosidase inhibitors, such as acarbose (Precose) and miglitol (Glyset); and Thiazolidinediones, such as troglitazone (Rezulin).

The recommended dosage depends on the type of antidiabetic drug. Check with the physician who prescribed the drug or the pharmacist who filled the prescription for the correct dosage. Always take antidiabetic drugs exactly as directed. Never take larger or more frequent doses, and do not stop taking the medicine even if symptoms of diabetes improve. Patients who use insulin should be trained by a health care professional in the proper way to prepare and inject their insulin.

Seeing a physician regularly while taking antidiabetic drugs is important, especially during the first few weeks. The physician will check to make sure the medicine is working as it should and will watch for unwanted side effects. The physician may also need to adjust the dosage or change medicines. For this medicine to be effective, doses must be carefully balanced with meals and daily activity. Health care professionals can teach patients how to achieve this balance and what to do if blood sugar levels get too high or too low. Following all guidelines for diet, exercise, regular blood sugar testing, use of alcohol and tobacco, sick days, and preparation for emergencies is extremely important.

Antidiabetic drugs do not cure diabetes, but they do help keep the condition under control and reduce the risk of serious complications. People with diabetes may need to take this medicine for the rest of their lives. Sulfonylureas may increase sensitivity to sunlight. While being treated with this medicine, avoid being in direct sunlight, especially between 10 a.m. and 3 p.m.; wear a hat and tightly woven clothing that covers the arms and legs; use a sunscreen with a skin protection factor (SPF) of at least 15; protect the lips with a sun block lipstick; and do not use tanning beds, tanning booths, or sunlamps.

People with diabetes should wear a medical identification necklace or bracelet at all times and should carry a medical ID card listing all their medicines. People with certain medical conditions or who are taking certain other medicines can have problems if they take antidiabetic drugs. Blood sugar may need to be tested more often, and different combinations of drugs and insulin may be necessary. Before taking antidiabetic drugs, be sure to let the physician know about all of the medical conditions. The physician should also be told about any **allergies** to foods, dyes, preservatives, or other substances.

Uncontrolled diabetes during **pregnancy** can lead to **birth defects** and other problems in the baby. In general, it is easier to control blood sugar levels during pregnancy with insulin than with sulfonylureas. Women who become pregnant or plan to become pregnant while taking antidiabetic drugs should check with their physicians about the best way to control their blood sugar levels. Women who want to breastfeed their babies should check with their physicians if they are using oral hypoglycemics.

Some of the side effects of these drugs, such as **dizziness**, mild drowsiness, **heartburn**, changes in taste, changes in appetite, mild nausea, vomiting, stomach **pain**, fullness or discomfort in the stomach, **constipation**, frequent urination or increased urine output, usually go away as the body adjusts to the drug and do not require medical treatment unless they continue. Other side effects are possible when taking insulin or sulfonylureas. Anyone who has unusual symptoms after taking antidiabetic drugs should get in touch with his or her physician.

Antidiabetic drugs may interact with a number of other medicines. When this happens, the effects of one or both of the drugs may change or the risk of side effects may be greater. It is therefore important to check with a physician or pharmacist before combining antidiabetic drugs with any other prescription or nonprescription (over-the-counter) medicine.

ANTIDIARRHEAL DRUGS

Antidiarrheal drugs are medicines that relieve **diarrhea**. Antidiarrheal drugs help control diarrhea and some of the symptoms that go along with it. An average, healthy person has anywhere from three bowel movements a day to three a week, depending on that person's diet. Normally the stool (the material that is passed in a bowel movement) has a texture something like clay. With diarrhea, bowel movements may be more frequent, and the texture of the stool is thin and sometimes watery. Diarrhea is not a disease, but a symptom of some other problem. The symptom may be caused by eating or drinking food or water that is contaminated with bacteria, viruses, or parasites, or by eating something that is difficult to digest. People who have trouble digesting lactose (milk sugar), for example, may get diarrhea if they eat dairy products. Some cases of diarrhea are caused by **stress**, while others are brought on by taking certain medicines.

Antidiarrheal drugs work in several different ways. The drug loperamide, found in Imodium A-D, for example, slows the passage of stools through the intestines. This allows more time for water and salts in the stools to be absorbed back into the body. Adsorbents, such as attapulgite (found in Kaopectate) pull diarrhea-causing substances from the digestive tract. However, they may also pull out substances that the body needs, such as enzymes and nutrients. Bismuth subsalicylate, the ingredient in Pepto-Bismol, decreases the secretion of fluid into the intestine and inhibits the activity of bacteria. It not only controls diarrhea, but relieves the cramps that often accompany diarrhea. It not only controls diarrhea, but relieves the cramps that often accompany diarrhea. These medicines come in liquid, tablet, caplet, and chewable tablet forms and can be bought without a physician's prescription. The dose depends on the type of antidiarrheal drug. Read and follow the directions on the product label. For questions about dosage, check with a physician or pharmacist. Never take larger or more frequent doses, and do not take the drug for longer than directed.

Diarrhea usually improves within 24-48 hours. If the problem lasts longer or if it keeps coming back, diarrhea could be a sign of a more serious problem. and medical attention as soon as possible. Severe, long-lasting diarrhea can lead to dehydration. In such cases, lost fluids and salts, such as calcium, sodium, and potassium, must be replaced.

Anyone who has a history of liver disease or who has been taking **antibiotics** should check with his or her physician before taking the antidiarrheal drug loperamide. A physician should also be consulted before anyone with acute ulcerative colitis or anyone who has been advised to avoid constipation uses the drug. Loperamide should not be used by people whose diarrhea is caused by certain infections, such as salmonella or shigella. To be safe, check with a physician before using this drug. Before taking antidiarrheal drugs, be sure to let the physician know about all medical conditions. The physician should also be told about any **allergies** to foods, dyes, preservatives, or other substances.

Women who are pregnant or breastfeeding should check with their physicians before using antidiarrheal drugs. They should also ask advice on how to replace lost fluids and salts.

Taking antidiarrheal drugs with certain other drugs may affect the way the drugs work or may increase the chance of side effects. The most common side effects of attapulgite are constipation, bloating, and fullness. Bismuth subsalicylate may cause ringing in the ears, but that side effect is rare. Possible side effects from loperamide include skin rash, constipation, drowsiness, dizziness, tiredness, dry mouth, nausea, vomiting, and swelling, **pain**, and discomfort in the abdomen. Some of these symptoms are the same as those that occur with diarrhea, so it may be difficult to tell if the medicine is causing the problems. Children may be more sensitive than adults to certain side effects of loperamide, such as drowsiness and dizziness. Other rare side effects may occur with any antidiarrheal medicine. Anyone who has unusual symptoms after taking an antidiarrhea drug should get in touch with his or her physician.

ANTIFUNGAL DRUGS

Antifungal drugs are of two kinds, systemic and topical. Systemic antifungal drugs are medicines taken by mouth or by injection to treat infections caused by a fungus. Topical antifungal drugs are medicines applied to the skin to treat skin infections caused by a fungus.

A fungus is a one-celled form of life. Unlike a plant, which makes its own food, or an animal, which eats plants or other animals, a fungus survives by invading and living off other living things. Because fungi thrive in moist, dark places, fungal infections are especially likely to be found in the mouth, armpits, groin, and genital areas. But they can also occur on the scalp, neck, trunk, and other parts of the body. Common fungal infections include **athlete's foot**, jock itch, **candidiasis** (also called thrush or yeast infection), and **ringworm**, which is not caused by a worm, but by a fungus. Topical antifungal drugs not only relieve the symptoms of fungal infection, such as **itching**, burning, and cracked skin, but they also eliminate the fungus. However, those that occur inside the body or that do not clear up after treatment with creams or ointments may need to be treated with systemic antifungal drugs. These drugs are used, for example, to treat a type of fungal infection called candidiasis also known as thrush or yeast infection), which can occur in the throat, in the vagina, or in other parts of the body. They may also be used to treat fungal infections such as **histoplasmosis**, **blastomycosis**, and aspergillosis, which can affect the lungs and other organs.

Systemic antifungal drugs, such as fluconazole (Diflucan), itraconazole (Sporanox), ketoconazole (Nizoral), and miconazole (Monistat I.V.) are available only by prescription. They are available in tablet, capsule, liquid, and injectable forms. Topical antifungal drugs are available without a physician's prescription and come in many forms, including creams, ointments, liquids, powders, aerosol sprays, and vaginal suppositories. Creams and liquids are usually the most effective for treating fungal infections on the skin, because they can get into the cracks and crevices where fungi grow. But because powders absorb moisture, they are good to use in moist areas of the body, such as between the toes. Commonly used topical antifungal drugs include ciclopirox, clotrimazole, econazole, miconazole, nystatin, oxiconazole, terconazole, and tolnaftate.

Among the brands of products that contain topical antifungal drugs are Absorbine Jr., Desenex, Gyne-Lotrimin, Loprox, Lotrimin, Micatin, Monistat, Mycelex, Mycolog-II, Oxistat, Spectazole Cream, Terazol, and Tinactin.

The recommended dosage depends on the type of antifungal drug and the medical problem for which the drug is being taken. Doses may also be different for different patients. Check with the physician who prescribed the drug or the pharmacist who filled the prescription for the correct dosage. Always take systemic antifungal drugs exactly as directed. Itraconazole and ketoconazole should be taken with food. Fungal infections can take a long time to clear up, so it may be necessary to take the medicine for several months, or even for a year or longer. It is very important to keep taking the medicine for as long as the physician says to take it, even if symptoms begin to improve. If the drug is stopped too soon, the symptoms may return. Systemic antifungal drugs work best when the amount of medicine in the body is kept constant. This means that the medicine has to be taken regularly. Try to take the medicine at the same time every day, and do not miss any doses. While taking this medicine, visit the physician as often as the physician recommends. The physician needs to keep checking for side effects throughout the antifungal therapy.

Topical antifungal drugs are meant to be used only on the skin or in the vagina. Be careful not to get the medicine in the eyes. Wash the hands with soap and water after applying antifungal drugs to the skin. Stop using the topical antifungal drug and call a physician if the infection has not cleared up in the amount of time given for each type of infection.

Women who are pregnant or who plan to become pregnant should check with their physicians before taking systemic antifungal drugs. Any woman who becomes pregnant while taking systemic antifungal drugs should let her physician know immediately. Similarly, some antifungal drugs pass into breast milk. Women who are breastfeeding should check with their physicians before using systemic antifungal drugs.

Liver problems, stomach problems and other problems may occur in people who drink alcohol while taking systemic antifungal drugs. Do not drink alcohol or use any prescription or nonprescription (over-the-counter) medicines that contain alcohol while using this medicine. (Medicines that may contain alcohol include some **cough** syrups, tonics, and elixirs.) Continue to avoid alcohol for at least a day after you stop taking an antifungal drug. Taking systemic antifungal drugs with certain other drugs may affect the way the drugs work or may increase the chance of side effects. The most common minor side effects of systemic antifungal drugs are **constipation**, diarrhea, nausea, vomiting, **headache**, drowsiness, **dizziness**, and flushing of the face or skin. These problems usually go away as the body adjusts to the drug and do not require medical treatment. Less common side effects, such as menstrual problems in women, breast enlargement in men, and decreased sexual ability in men also may occur and do not need medical attention unless they do not improve in a reasonable amount of time.

Systemic antifungal drugs may cause serious and possibly life-threatening liver damage. Patients who take these drugs should have liver function tests before they start taking the medicine and as often as their physician recommends while they are taking it. More serious side effects are not common, but may occur. If any unusual symptoms are noted, check with the physician who prescribed the medicine immediately.

Serious and possibly life-threatening side effects can result if the oral forms of itraconazole or ketoconazole or the injectable form of miconazole are taken with certain drugs. *Anyone who takes systemic antifungal drugs should let the physician know all other prescription and nonprescription (over-the-counter) medicines he or she is taking.* Be sure to check with a physician or pharmacist before combining systemic antifungal drugs with any other medicine.

Antigas agents

Antigas agents are medicines that relieve the uncomfortable symptoms of too much gas in the stomach and intestines. Excess gas can build up in the stomach and intestines for a number of reasons. Eating high-fiber foods, such as beans, grains, and vegetables is one cause. Some people unconsciously swallow air when they eat, drink, chew gum, or smoke cigarettes, which can lead to uncomfortable amounts of gas in the digestive system. Surgery and certain medical conditions, such as irritable colon, peptic ulcer, and diverticulosis, can also lead to gas build-up. Certain intestinal parasites can contribute to the production of severe gas—these parasites need to be treated separately with special drugs. Abdominal **pain**, pressure, bloating, and flatulence are signs of too much gas. Antigas agents help relieve the symptoms by preventing the formation of gas pockets and breaking up gas that already is trapped in the stomach and intestines.

Antigas agents are sold as capsules, liquids, and tablets (regular and chewable) and can be bought without a physician's prescription. Some commonly used brands are Gas-X, Flatulex, Mylanta Gas Relief, Di-Gel, and Phazyme. The ingredient that helps relieve excess gas is simethicone. Simethicone does not relieve acid **indigestion**, but some products also contain **antacids** for that purpose. Check the product container for dosing information. Typically, the doses should be taken after meals and at bedtime. Chewable forms should be chewed thoroughly. Check with a physician before giving this medicine to children under age 12 years.

Some anti-gas medicines may contain sugar, sodium, or other ingredients. Anyone who is on a special diet or is allergic to any foods, dyes, preservatives, or other substances should check with his or her physician or pharmacist before using any of these products. In addition, anyone who has had unusual reactions to simethicone—the active ingredient in antigas medicines—should check with his or her physician before taking these drugs.

No common or serious side effects have been reported in people who use this medicine. Antigas agents are not known to interact with any other drugs. However, anyone who has unusual symptoms after taking an antigas agent should get in touch with his or her physician.

ANTIHELMINTHIC DRUGS

Antihelminthic drugs are medicines that rid the body of parasitic worms. People can become infected with parasitic worms in a number of ways. The eggs of pinworms, for example, can be transferred from person to person through contaminated food, drinking glasses, clothing, or linens. Tapeworms and roundworms may enter the body when people eat undercooked meat or fish. The worms then live inside the body and may go unnoticed if they cause no troublesome symptoms. However, if they multiply rapidly or invade a vital organ, they can cause serious and sometimes life-threatening problems. The body has no natural means of getting rid of parasitic worms, but antihelminthic drugs do the job very well. Some kill the worms on contact. Others starve or paralyze the worms, which then pass out of the body in the feces.

Each type of antihelminthic drug is effective against particular kinds of worms. For example, niclosamide is effective against tapeworms, but will not work for treating pinworm or **roundworm infections**. Antihelminthic drugs are available only with a physician's prescription. They are sold as liquids and tablets (regular and chewable). Some commonly used antihelminthics are mebendazole (Vermox), niclosamide (Niclocide), praziquantel (Biltricide), pyrantel (Antiminth), and thiabendazole (Mintezol).

The proper dose depends on the patient, the type of antihelminthic drug, and the condition for which it is being taken. The number of doses per day, the time between doses, and the length of treatment may also depend on these factors. To completely rid the body of parasitic worms, take the medicine exactly as directed, for as long as directed. A second round of treatment a few weeks later may be necessary to make sure the infection is completely cleared.

Some antihelminthic medicines work best when taken with fatty foods, such as whole milk or ice cream. Others should be taken after a light meal. Be sure to follow directions about when to take the medicine and what to take with it. People who cannot follow the directions because they are on low-fat or other special **diets** should check with their physicians about how to take the medicine. Some people feel drowsy, dizzy, or less alert when using certain antihelminthic drugs. Anyone who takes these drugs should not drive, use machines or do anything else that might be dangerous until they have found out how the drugs affect them.

Because some kinds of worms, such as pinworms, can be passed from one person to another, everyone in the household may need to take medicine when one person is infected. While under treatment with an antihelminthic drug, see the physician as often is recommended. The physician will check to see if the infection is clearing and will make sure no unwanted side effects exist. The physician may also suggest ways to help keep the infection from coming back. Be sure to follow these suggestions. Check with the physician if symptoms do not improve or if they get worse.

Patients being treated for hookworm or whipworm infections may need to take iron supplements. Ask the physician about this. People with certain medical conditions or who are taking certain other medicines can have problems if they take antihelminthic drugs. Before taking these drugs, be sure to let the physician know about any of these conditions.Anyone who has had unusual reactions to antihelminthic drugs in the past should let his or her physician know before taking the drugs again. The physician should also be told about any **allergies** to foods, dyes, preservatives, or other substances.

Women who are pregnant or who plan to become pregnant should check with their physicians before taking antihelminthic drugs. Some antihelminthic drugs pass into breast milk and may cause unwanted effects in nursing babies whose mothers take the medicine. Breastfeeding mothers who need to take antihelminthic drugs should ask their physicians whether they need to stop breastfeeding.

Taking antihelminthic drugs with certain other drugs may affect the way the drugs work or may increase the chance of side effects. The most common side effects of antihelminthic drugs are **dizziness**, drowsiness, **headache**, sweating, dry mouth, dry eyes, and ringing or buzzing in the ears. These problems usually go away as the body adjusts to the drug and do not require medical treatment. Less common side effects of antihelminthic drugs, such as loss of appetite, **diarrhea**, nausea, vomiting, or stomach or abdominal **pain** or cramps, also may occur and do not need medical attention unless they do not go away or they interfere with normal activities. If more serious side effects are not common, but may occur. Call a physician immediately should any of unusual side effects occur. Antihelminthic drugs may interact with other medicines. When this happens, the effects of one or both drugs may change, or the risk of side effects may be greater. Anyone who takes antihelminthic drugs should therefore tell the physician about all other medicines he or she is taking.

ANTIHISTAMINES

Antihistamines are medicines that relieve or prevent the symptoms of hay fever and other kinds of allergy. An allergy is a condition in which the body becomes unusually sensitive to some substance, such as pollen, mold spores, dust particles, certain foods, or medicines. These substances, known as allergens, cause no unusual reactions in most people. But in people who are sensitive to them, exposure to allergens causes the immune system to overreact. The main reaction is the release of a chemical called histamine from specialized cells in the body tissues. Histamine causes such familiar and annoying allergy symptoms as sneezing, **itching**, runny nose, and watery eyes.

As their name suggests, antihistamines block the effects of histamine, reducing allergy symptoms. When used for this purpose, they work best when taken before symptoms are too severe. Antihistamine creams and ointments may be used to temporarily relieve itching. Some antihistamine products are available only with a physician's prescription. Others can be bought without a prescription. These drugs come in many forms, including tablets, capsules, liquids, injections and suppositories. Some common antihistamines are astemizole (Hismanal), brompheniramine (Dimetane, Dimetapp), chlorpheniramine (Deconamine), clemastine (Tavist), diphenhydramine (Benadryl), doxylamine (an ingredient in sleep aids such as Unisom and Vicks NyQuil), loratadine (Claritin), and promethazine (Phenergan).

Recommended dosage depends on the type of antihistamine. Check with the physician who prescribed the drug or the pharmacist who filled the prescription for the correct dosage, and always take antihistamines exactly as directed. If using non-prescription (over-the-counter) types, follow the directions on the package label. Never take larger or more frequent doses, and do not take the drug longer than directed. For best effects, take antihistamines on a schedule, not just as needed. Histamine is released more or less continuously, so countering its effects requires regular use of antihistamines.

People who have seasonal **allergies** should take antihistamines before allergy season starts or immediately after being exposed to an allergen. Even then, however, antihistamines do not cure allergies or prevent histamine from being released. They can only be expected to reduce allergy symptoms by only about 50%. In some people antihistamines become less effective when used over a long time. Switching to another type of antihistamine may help.

People with asthma, emphysema, chronic **bronchitis**, or other breathing problems should not use antihistamines unless directed to do so by a physician. Some antihistamines make people drowsy, dizzy, uncoordinated, or less alert. For this reason, anyone who takes these drugs should not drive, use machines or do anything else that might be dangerous until they have found out how the drugs affect them. Antihistamines can interfere with the results of skin and blood tests. Anyone who is taking antihistamines should notify the health care provider in charge before scheduling medical tests.

Because children are often more sensitive to antihistamines, they may be more likely to have side effects and to suffer from accidental overdoses. Check with a physician before giving antihistamines to children under 12 years. Older people may also be more likely to have side effects, such as nervousness, irritability, dizziness, sleepiness, and low blood pressure from antihistamines. People with certain medical conditions or who are taking certain other medicines can have problems if they take antihistamines. Before taking these drugs, be sure to let the physician or pharmacist know about all medical conditions. Anyone who has had unusual reactions to antihistamines in the past should let his or her physician know before taking the drugs again. The physician should also be told about any allergies to foods, dyes, preservatives, or other substances.

Pregnant women should not use antihistamines unless directed to do so by a physician. Antihistamines pass into breast milk and may cause side effects in nursing babies. Women who are breastfeeding should check with their physicians before using antihistamines.

Taking antihistamines with certain other drugs may affect the way the drugs work or may increase the chance of side effects. Antihistamines may increase the effects of other drugs that slow down the central nervous system (CNS), such as alcohol, tranquilizers, **barbiturates**, and sleep aids. Avoid drinking alcohol while taking antihistamines, and check with a physician before combining antihistamines with any other drugs. Common side effects of antihistamines include drowsiness, dizziness, poor coordination, restlessness, excitability, nervousness, and upset stomach. These problems usually go away as the body adjusts to the drug and do not require medical treatment. Less common side effects, such as dry mouth, nose, and eyes, irritability, difficulty urinating, and blurred vision, also may occur and do not need medical attention unless they do not go away or they interfere with normal activities. Other rare side effects may occur. Anyone who has unusual symptoms after taking antihistamines should get in touch with his or her physician.

ANTIHYPERTENSIVE DRUGS

Antihypertensive drugs are medicines that help lower blood pressure in people whose blood pressure is too high. Blood pressure is a measurement of the force with which blood moves through the body's system of blood vessels. Although everyone's blood pressure goes up and down in the course of a typical day, some people have blood pressure that stays high all the time. This condition is known as **hypertension**. Hypertension is not the same as nervous tension. People who have high blood pressure are not necessarily tense, high-strung, or nervous. They may not even be aware of their condition. Being aware of high blood pressure and doing something to control it are extremely important, however. Untreated, high blood pressure can lead to diseases of the heart and arteries, kidney damage, or **stroke**, and can shorten life expectancy.

Treatments for high blood pressure depend on the type of hypertension. Most cases of high blood pressure are called essential or primary hypertension, meaning that the high blood pressure is not caused by some other medical condition. For most people with primary hypertension, it is difficult to figure out the exact cause of the problem. However, such hypertension usually can be controlled by some combination of antihypertensive drugs and changes in daily habits(such as diet, **exercise**, and weight control). Controlling primary hypertension is however a lifelong commitment. Although people may be able to reduce the amount of medicine they take as their blood pressure improves, they usually must continue taking it for the rest of their lives.

In people with secondary hypertension, the high blood pressure may be due to medical problems such as kidney disease, narrowing of certain arteries, or tumors of the adrenal glands. Correcting these problems often cures the high blood pressure, and no further treatment is needed.

Many different types of drugs are used, alone or in combination with other drugs, to treat high blood pressure. The major categories are:

- Angiotensin-converting enzyme (ACE) inhibitors, such as benazepril (Lotensin), captopril (Capoten), enalapril (Vasotec), lisinopril (Prinivil, Zestril), quinapril (Accupril), and ramipril (Altace). ACE inhibitors work by preventing a chemical in the blood, angiotensin I, from being converted into a substance that increases salt and water retention in the body. These drugs also make blood vessels relax, which further reduces blood pressure.

- Angiotensin II receptor antagonists, such as losartan (Cozaar) and losartan with hydrochlorothiazide (Hyzaar). These drugs act at a later step in the same process that ACE inhibitors affect. Like ACE inhibitors, they lower blood pressure by relaxing blood vessels.
- **Beta blockers**, such as atenolol (Tenormin), metoprolol (Lopressor), nadolol (Corgard), propranolol (Inderal), and timolol (Blocadren). Beta blockers affect the body's response to certain nerve impulses. This, in turn, decreases the force and rate of the heart's contractions, which lowers blood pressure.
- Blood vessel dilators (**vasodilators**), such as hydralazine (Apresoline) and minoxidil (Loniten). These drugs lower blood pressure by relaxing muscles in the blood vessel walls.
- Calcium channel blockers, such as amlopidine (Norvasc), diltiazem (Cardizem), isradipine (DynaCirc), nifedipine (Adalat, Procardia), and verapamil (Calan, Isoptin, Verelan). Drugs in this group slow the movement of calcium into the cells of blood vessels. This relaxes the blood vessels and lowers blood pressure.
- **Diuretics**, such as chlorthalidone (Hygroton), furosemide (Lasix), hydrochlorothiazide (Esidrix, HydroDIURIL), and metolazone (Zaroxolyn). These drugs control blood pressure by eliminating excess salt and water from the body.
- Nerve blockers, such as alpha methyldopa (Aldomet), clonidine (Catapres), guanabenz (Wytensin), guanadrel (Hylorel), guanethidine (Ismelin), prazosin(Minipress), rauwolfia derivatives (Reserpine), and terazosin (Hytrin). These drugs control nerve impulses along certain nerve pathways. This allows blood vessels to relax and lowers blood pressure.

The recommended dosage depends on the type, strength, and form of antihypertensive drug. Check with the physician who prescribed the drug or the pharmacist who filled the prescription for the correct dosage. Always take antihypertensive drugs exactly as directed. Never take larger or more frequent doses, and do not miss any doses. Some antihypertensive drugs may take several weeks to noticeably lower blood pressure. Once it begins to work and symptoms improve, continuing to take the medicine is just as important. Stopping some hypertensive drugs suddenly may cause serious problems. Check with the physician who prescribed the medicine to find out if it is necessary to gradually taper down before stopping the medicine completely.

Antihypertensive drugs will not cure high blood pressure, but will help control the condition. To avoid the serious health problems that high blood pressure can cause, patients may have to take medicine for the rest of their lives. Furthermore, medicine alone may not be enough. People with high blood pressure also may need to avoid certain foods and keep their weight under control. The health care professional who is treating the condition can offer advice on what measures may be necessary.

Anyone taking antihypertensive drugs should not take any other prescription or over-the-counter medicine without first checking with his or her physician. Some medicines may increase blood pressure. Most patients who take antihypertensive drugs are not bothered by side effects. However, antihypertensive drugs may interact with many other medicines. When this happens, the effects of one or both of the drugs may change or the risk of side effects may be greater. *Anyone taking antihypertensive drugs should not take any other prescription or nonprescription (over-the-counter)medicine without first checking with his or her physician.*

ANTI-INSOMNIA DRUGS

Anti-insomnia drugs are medicines that help people fall asleep or stay asleep. Physicians prescribe anti-insomnia drugs for short-term treatment of **insomnia**. Insomnia is a problem in which people have trouble falling asleep, staying asleep, or waking too early and not being able to go back to sleep. These drugs are used for occasional treatment of temporary sleep problems and should not be taken for more than a week or two at a time. People whose sleep problems last longer than this should see a physician.

The anti-insomnia drug described here, zolpidem (Ambien), is a classified as a central nervous system (CNS) depressant. CNS depressants are medicines that slow the nervous system. Physicians also prescribe medicines in the benzodiazepine family, such as flurazepam (Dalmane), quazepam (Doral), triazolam (Halcion), estazolam (ProSom), and temazepam (Restoril), for insomnia. Zolpidem is available only with a physician's prescription and comes in tablet form.

The medicine works quickly, often within 20 minutes, so it should be taken right before going to bed. Some people feel drowsy, dizzy, confused, lightheaded, or less alert the morning after they have taken some anti-insomnia drugs. The medicine may also cause clumsiness, unsteadiness, double vision, or other vision problems the next day.

Zolpidem and other sleep medicines may cause a special type of temporary memory loss, in which the person does not remember what happens between the time they take the medicine and the time its effects wear off. This is usually not a problem, because people go to sleep right after taking the medicine and stay asleep until its effects wear off. But it could be a problem for anyone who has to wake up before getting a full night's sleep (7-8 hours).

Because these medicines work on the central nervous system, they may add to the effects of alcohol and other drugs that slow down the central nervous system, such as **antihistamines**, cold medicine, allergy medicine, medicine for seizures, tranquilizers, some pain relievers, and **muscle relaxants**. *The combined effects of zolpidem and alcohol or other CNS depressants (drugs that slow the central nervous system) can be very dangerous, leading to unconsciousness or even death. Anyone who shows signs of an overdose or of the effects of combining zolpidem drugs with alcohol or other drugs should have immediate emergency help.* Warning signs include severe drowsiness, severe nausea or vomiting, breathing problems, and staggering.

Before taking this medicine, be sure to let the physician know about any allergies; pregnancy or breastfeeding; chronic lung diseases such as emphysema, **asthma**, or chronic **bronchitis**; liver or kidney disease; current or past alcohol or drug abuse; depression; or **sleep apnea**.

The most common minor side effects are daytime drowsiness or a ''drugged'' feeling, vision problems, memory problems, nightmares or unusual dreams, vomiting, nausea, abdominal or stomach pain, **diarrhea**, dry mouth, **headache**, and general feeling of discomfort or illness. These problems usually go away as the body adjusts to the drug and do not require medical treatment.

More serious side effects are not common, but may occur. Anyone who has unusual symptoms after taking anti-insomnia drugs should get in touch with his or her physician.

Anti-itch drugs

Anti-itch drugs are medicines taken by mouth or by injection to relieve **itching**. The medicine described here, hydroxyzine, is a type of antihistamine used to relieve itching caused by allergic reactions. An allergic reaction occurs when the body is unusually sensitive to some substance, such as pollen, dust, mold, or certain foods or medicine. The body reacts by releasing a chemical called histamine that causes itching and other symptoms, such as sneezing and watery eyes. **Antihistamines** reduce the symptoms by blocking the effects of histamine.

Anti-itch drugs, also called antipruritic drugs, are available only with a physician's prescription and come in tablet and injectable forms. Some commonly used brands of the anti-itch drug hydroxyzine are Atarax and Vistaril. This medicine should not be used for more than four months at a time because its effects can wear off. See a physician regularly while taking the medicine to determine whether it is still needed.

Hydroxyzine may add to the effects of alcohol and other drugs that slow down the central nervous system, such as other antihistamines, cold medicine, allergy medicine, sleep aids, medicine for seizures, tranquilizers, some pain relievers, and **muscle relaxants**. Anyone taking hydroxyzine should not drink alcohol and should check with his or her physician before taking any other medicines.

Some people feel drowsy or less alert when using this medicine. Anyone who has had unusual reactions to hydroxyzine in the past should let his or her physician know before taking the medicine again. The physician should also be told about any **allergies** to foods, dyes, preservatives, or other substances.

A woman who is pregnant or who may become pregnant should check with her physician before taking this medicine. In studies of laboratory animals, hydroxyzine has caused **birth defects** when taken during **pregnancy**. Although the drug's effects on pregnant women have not been fully studied, physicians advise against taking it in early pregnancy. The medicine may pass into breast milk and may cause problems in nursing babies whose mothers take it.

The most common side effect, drowsiness, usually goes away as the body adjusts to the drug. If it does not, reducing the dosage may be necessary. Other side effects, such as dry mouth, also may occur and do not need medical attention unless they continue.

More serious side effects are not common, but may occur. Twitches, **tremors**, or convulsions (seizures) signal a need for medical attention.

Antinausea drugs

Antinausea drugs are medicines that control nausea—a feeling of sickness or queasiness in the stomach with an urge to vomit. These drugs also prevent or stop vomiting. Drugs that control vomiting are called antiemetic drugs.

The drug described here, prochlorperazine (Compazine), controls both **nausea and vomiting**. Prochlorperazine is also sometimes prescribed for symptoms of mental disorders, such as **schizophrenia**. Prochlorperazine is available only with a physician's prescription. It is sold in syrup, capsule, tablet, injection, and suppository forms.

Prochlorperazine may cause a movement disorder called tardive dyskinesia. Signs of this disorder are involuntary twitches and muscle spasms in the face and body and jutting or rolling movements of the tongue. The condition may be permanent. Older people, especially women, are particularly at risk of developing this problem when they take prochlorperazine. Some people feel drowsy, dizzy, lightheaded, or less alert when using this medicine. The drug may also cause blurred vision, and movement problems. For these reasons, anyone who takes this drug should not drive, use machines or do anything else that might be dangerous until they have found out how the drug affects them.

Prochlorperazine makes some people sweat less, which can allow the body to overheat. The drug may also make the skin and eyes more sensitive to the sun. People who are taking prochlorperazine should try to avoid extreme heat and exposure to the sun. When going outdoors, they should wear protective clothing, a hat, a sunscreen with a skin protection factor (SPF) of at least 15, and sunglasses that block ultraviolet (UV) light. Saunas, sunlamps, tanning booths, tanning beds, hot baths, and hot tubs should be avoided while taking this medicine. Anyone who must be exposed to extreme heat while taking the drug should check with his or her physician.

Do not stop taking this medicine without checking with the physician who prescribed it. Stopping the drug suddenly can cause **dizziness**, nausea, vomiting, **tremors**, and other side effects. When stopping the medicine, it may be necessary to taper down the dose gradually.

Prochlorperazine may cause false **pregnancy** tests. Women who are pregnant (or planning to become pregnant) or breast feeding should check with their physicians before using this medicine.

Before using prochlorperazine, people should make sure that their physicians are aware of all their meidcal conditions. Many side effects are possible with this drug, including, but not limited to, **constipation**, dizziness, drowsiness, decreased sweating, dry mouth, stuffy nose, movement problems, changes in menstrual period, increased sensitivity to sun, and swelling or pain in breasts. Anyone who has unusual or troublesome symptoms after taking prochlorperazine should get in touch with his or her physician.

This medicine adds to the effects of alcohol and other drugs that slow down the central nervous system, such as **antihistamines**, cold and flu medicines, tranquilizers, sleep aids, anesthetics, some pain medicines, and **muscle relaxants**. Do not drink alcohol while taking prochlorperazine. Prochlorperazine may interact with other medicines. When this happens, the effects of one or both of the drugs may change or the risk of side effects may be greater. Be sure to check with a physician or pharmacist before taking any other prescription or nonprescription (over-the-counter) drug with Prochlorperazine.

ANTIPARKINSON DRUGS

Antiparkinson drugs are medicines that relieve the symptoms of **Parkinson's disease** and other forms of parkinsonism.

Parkinsonism is a group of disorders that share four main symptoms: tremor or trembling in the hands, arms, legs, jaw, and face; stiffness or rigidity of the arms, legs, and trunk; slowness of movement (bradykinesia); and poor balance and coordination. Parkinson's disease is the most common form of parkinsonism.

All types of parkinsonism occur when nerve cells in a particular part of the brain die or lose the ability to function. These cells normally produce a chemical called dopamine, that helps relay signals to different parts of the brain. This process is important in producing smooth, coordinated movement throughout the body. When dopamine-producing cells are lost, normal movement becomes impossible. In people with late-stage Parkinson's disease, 80% or more of these important cells are dead or impaired.

There is no cure for Parkinson's disease or other forms of parkinsonism but several drugs help relieve the symptoms. Some drugs, such as levodopa, replenish dopamine in the brain. Others mimic the role of dopamine or block the effects of other chemicals that cause problems in the brain when dopamine levels drop. Levodopa is one of the drugs used. It can either be used alone or in combination with carbidopa, to restore dopamine levels in the brain. Carbidopa helps make levodopa more effective and reduces some of the side effects that occur. In addition, antidyskinetics and anticholinergics, such as benztropine and trihexyphenidyl, are also used. These block the effects of other brain chemicals, thereby reducing some of the involuntary **tremors**.

All antiparkinson drugs are available only with a physician's prescription. They are sold in tablet (regular and extended-release), liquid, extended-release capsule, and injectable forms. The recommended dosage depends on the type of antiparkinson drug. Finding the correct dose for a particular patient is a process that may take time and patience. The physician tries to tailor the treatment to the patient, taking into account what symptoms the patient has and how much the symptoms interfere with normal life. No two patients react the same to a particular drug, so a person may need to try different drugs and different dosages before finding the best treatment.

Always take antiparkinson drugs exactly as directed. Never take larger or more frequent doses. Do not stop taking this medicine without first checking with the physician who prescribed it. Gradually tapering the dose may reduce the chance of side effects and prevent symptoms from getting worse.

Antiparkinson drugs may interact with medicines used during surgery, dental procedures, or emergency treatment. These interactions could increase the chance of side effects. Anyone who is taking antiparkinson drugs should be sure to tell the health care professional in charge before having any surgical or dental procedures or receiving emergency treatment. In addition, a physician should be consulted regarding any special dietary requirements for the patient.

Taking levodopa over a long time can lead to a problem called the ''on-off'' effect, in which a patient suddenly becomes unable to move. The effect may last only a few minutes or as long as several hours. When it ends, the patient is able to move normally again, but the effect may occur again and again without warning. A patient who experiences this problem should check with a physician. Another possible problem with long-term use of levodopa is called the ''wearing-off'' effect. With this effect, patients notice more pronounced symptoms as each dose wears off. Changing the dose of the medicine and the frequency with which it is taken may help prevent this effect. Patients who have this problem should check with their physicians and should not change the dose of their medicine themselves.

Antiparkinson drugs may cause false results on some urine tests for sugar or ketones. Persons with diabetes who take this medicine should check with their physicians. Women who are pregnant or who may become pregnant should check with their physicians before using any antiparkinson drug. Women who are breastfeeding should check with their physicians before using any antiparkinson drug.

Antiparkinson drugs may add to the effects of alcohol and other drugs that slow down the central nervous system. Taking antiparkinson drugs with certain other drugs may affect the way the drugs work or may increase the chance of side effects. Be sure to check with a physician or pharmacist before combining antiparkinson drugs with any other prescription or nonprescription (over-the-counter) medicine. The most common side effects of antidyskinetics are drowsiness; **nausea and vomiting**; **constipation**; difficult or painful urination; dry mouth, nose, or throat; blurred vision; increased sensitivity of the eyes to light; and decreased sweating. These problems usually go away as the body adjusts to the drug and do not require medical treatment unless they continue or they interfere with normal activities.

More serious side effects are rare, but may occur. Check with the physician who prescribed the medicine as soon as possible if confusion, eye pain, or skin rash occur.

ANTIPROTOZOAL DRUGS

Antiprotozoal drugs are medicines that are used to treat a variety of diseases caused by protozoa. Protozoa are one-celled organisms, such as amoebas. Some are parasitic and cause infections in the body. African **sleeping sickness**, giardiasis, amebiasis, *Pneumocystis carinii* **pneumonia** (PCP), and **malaria** are examples of diseases caused by protozoa.

Antiprotozoal drugs come in liquid, tablet, and injectable forms and are available only with a doctor's prescription. Some commonly used antiprotozoal drugs are metronidazole (Flagyl), eflornithine (Ornidyl), furazolidone (Furoxone), hydroxychloroquine (Plaquenil), iodoquinol (Diquinol, Yodoquinol, Yodoxin), and pentamidine (Pentam 300). The recommended dosage depends on the type of antiprotozoal drug, its strength, and the medical problem for which it is being used. Check with the physician who prescribed the drug or the pharmacist who filled the prescription for the correct dosage. Always take antiprotozoal drugs exactly as directed.

Some people feel dizzy, confused, lightheaded, or less alert when using these drugs. The drugs may also cause blurred vision and other vision problems. For these reasons, anyone who takes these drugs should not drive, use machines or do anything else that might be dangerous until they have found out how the drugs affect them. The antiprotozoal drug furazolidone may cause very dangerous side effects when taken with certain foods or beverages. Likewise, metronidazole (Flagyl) can cause serious liver damage if taken with alcohol. Check with the physician who prescribed the drug or the pharmacist who filled the prescription for a list of products to avoid while taking these medicines.

Anyone who has ever had unusual reactions to antiprotozoal drugs or related medicines should let his or her physician know before taking the drugs again. The physician should also be told about any **allergies** to foods, dyes, preservatives, or other substances.

Some antiprotozoal drugs may cause problems with the blood. This can increase the risk of infection or excessive bleeding. Patients taking these drugs should be careful not to injure their gums when brushing or flossing their teeth or using a toothpick. They should check with the physician before having any dental work done. Care should also be taken to avoid cuts from razors, nail clippers, or kitchen knives, or household tools. Anyone who has any of these symptoms while taking antiprotozoal drugs should call the physician immediately:

- **Fever** or chills
- Signs of cold or flu
- Signs of infection, such as redness, swelling, or inflammation
- Unusual bruising or bleeding
- Black, tarry stools
- Blood in urine or stools
- Pinpoint red spots on the skin
- Unusual tiredness or weakness.

Children are especially sensitive to the effects of some antiprotozoal drugs. *Never give this medicine to a child unless directed to do so by a physician, and always keep this medicine out of the reach of children. Use safety vials.* Women who are pregnant or who plan to become pregnant should check with their physicians before taking antiprotozoal drugs. Mothers who are breastfeeding should also check with their physicians about the safety of taking these drugs.

Before using antiprotozoal drugs, people with any medical problems should make sure their physicians are aware of their conditions. The most common side effects are **diarrhea**, nausea, vomiting, and stomach pain. These problems usually go away as the body adjusts to the drug and do not require medical treatment. Other rare side effects may occur. Anyone who has any unusual symptoms after taking an antiprotozoal drug should get in touch with his or her physician immediately.

Antiprotozoal drugs may interact with other medicines. When this happens, the effects of one or both of the drugs may change or the risk of side effects may be greater. Anyone who takes antiprotozoal drugs should let the physician know of all other medicines he or she is taking. Be sure to check with a physician or pharmacist before combining antifungal drugs with any other prescription or nonprescription (over-the-counter) medicine.

ANTIPSYCHOTIC DRUGS

Antipsychotic drugs are medicines used to treat **psychosis** and other mental and emotional conditions. Psychosis is a severe mental illness in which people lose touch with reality. They may hear voices, see things that aren't really there, and have strange or untrue thoughts, such as believing that other people can hear their thoughts or are trying to harm them. They may also neglect their appearances and may stop talking or talk only "nonsense."

Antipsychotic drugs do not cure mental illness, but can reduce some of the symptoms or make them milder. The medicine may improve symptoms enough for the person to undergo counseling and live a more normal life. The type of antipsychotic medicine prescribed depends on the type of mental problem the patient has. Antipsychotic drugs are also known as neuroleptics or major tranquilizers. Several types of these drugs are available, such as haloperidol (Haldol), lithium (Lithonate), chlorpromazine (Thorazine), and thioridazine (Mellaril). The newer antipsychotics include risperidone (Risperdal), quetiapine (Seroquel) and olanzapine (Zyprexa). These medicines are available only with a physician's prescription. The recommended dosage depends on the type of antipsychotic drug, the condition for which it is prescribed, and other factors. Check with the physician who prescribed the medicine for the correct dosage. Always take antipsychotic drugs exactly as directed. Never take larger or more frequent doses, and do not take the drug for longer than directed. This is important for all patients, but especially for older people and children, who may be more sensitive to this type of medicine.

Do not stop taking this medicine suddenly after taking it for several weeks or more. Gradually tapering the dose may be necessary to reduce the chance of withdrawal symptoms. If it is necessary to stop taking the drug, check with the physician who prescribed it for instructions on how to stop. See a physician regularly while taking antipsychotic drugs, especially during the first few months. The physician will check to make sure the medicine is working as it should and will watch for unwanted side effects. The physician may also need to adjust the dosage during this period. The physician will advise the patients if any major changes in diets are needed.

Antipsychotic drugs may interact with medicines used during surgery, dental procedures, or emergency treatment. These interactions could increase the chance of side effects. Anyone who is taking antipsychotic drugs should be sure to tell the health care professional in charge before having any surgical or dental procedures or receiving emergency treatment. Some antipsychotic drugs may change the results of certain medical tests. Before having medical tests, anyone taking this medicine should alert the health care professional in charge.

Some people feel drowsy, dizzy, or less alert when using these drugs, especially as doses increase. Antipsychotic drugs may also cause blurred vision and other vision changes and may affect judgment. Because of these possible problems, anyone who takes these drugs should not drive, use machines or do anything else that might be dangerous until they have found out how the drugs affect them. The drugs may increase sensitivity to sunlight. Even brief exposure to sun can cause a severe **sunburn** or a rash. Hence appropriate precautions need to be taken.

People taking antipsychotic medicines may sweat less, which can cause the body temperature to rise. Anyone who takes this medicine should be careful not to become overheated during exercise or hot weather and should avoid hot baths, hot tubs, and saunas. Overheating could lead to heat **stroke**. Some antipsychotic drugs make people more sensitive to cold. Anyone who takes this medicine should dress warmly in cold weather and take care to avoid long exposure to the cold.

Children may be especially sensitive to the effects of antipsychotic drugs. This sensitivity may increase the chance of side effects, especially muscle spasms and involuntary movements. Lithium may weaken the bones of children who take it. Consult with a physician if this is a concern.

People with certain medical conditions or who are taking certain other medicines can have problems if they take antipsychotic drugs. Before taking these drugs, be sure to let the physician know about all the medical conditions. Anyone who has had unusual reactions to antipsychotic drugs in the past should let his or her physician know before taking the drugs again. The physician should also be told about any **allergies** to foods, dyes, preservatives, or other substances.

Women who are pregnant or who may become pregnant should check with their physicians before using antipsychotic drugs. Some antipsychotic drugs pass into breast milk and may cause drowsiness and other problems in nursing babies whose mothers use the drugs. Breastfeeding is not recommended during treatment with antipsychotic drugs.

Some of the side effects of antipsychotic drugs will go away as the patient's body adjusts to the medicine and do not need medical attention unless they continue or they interfere with normal activities. If more serious side effects occur, stop taking the medicine and check with a physician immediately. Some side effects, such as trembling of the fingers and hands or involuntary movements of the mouth, tongue, and jaw, may occur even after treatment with this medicine has ended. Check with a physician if any unusual symptoms occur after stopping the drug. Patients who are taking lithium should make sure that they and their families know the signs of taking too much of the medicine and should check with a physician immediately if any unusual symptoms occur.

Antipsychotic drugs may interact with a number of other medicines. When this happens, the effects of one or both of the drugs may change or the risk of side effects may be greater. Because antipsychotic drugs work on the central nervous system, they may add to the effects of alcohol and other drugs that slow down the central nervous system. Anyone who takes antipsychotic drugs should let the physician know of all other medicines that he or she is taking. Be sure to check with a physician or pharmacist before combining antipsychotic drugs with any other prescription or nonprescription (over-the-counter) medicine.

Antiretroviral drugs

Antiretroviral drugs prevent the reproduction of a type of virus called a retrovirus. The human immunodefiency virus (HIV), that causes acquired immune deficiency syndrome (**AIDS**), is a retrovirus. These drugs are therefore used to treat HIV infections. These medicines cannot prevent or cure HIV infection, but they help to keep the virus in check.

Viruses are tiny, disease-causing particles that are unable to reproduce on their own. They must invade the cells of other living things and take over the cells' machinery in order to multiply. In the process, they cause illness. HIV is a specific type of virus called a retrovirus. It slowly weakens the immune system by invading and destroying special immune cells that help defend the body against infections.

Antiretroviral drugs do not kill viruses, because that could also damage or kill the cells the viruses have infected. Instead, these drugs block the reproduction of the viruses. However, they do not eliminate HIV and restore the immune system completely. Hence, people who take these drugs may still get serious infections and have other health problems. Furthermore, antiretroviral drugs do not prevent the spread of HIV from an infected person to someone else. People taking these drugs must still observe all precautions to avoid infecting others.

There are three main types of antiretroviral drugs:

- Nucleoside analogs, or nucleoside reverse transcriptase inhibitors (NRTIs), such as didanosine (ddI, Videx), lamivudine (3TC, Epivir), stavudine (d4T, Zerit), zalcitabine (ddC, Hivid), and zidovudine (AZT, Retrovir).
- Non-nucleoside reverse transcriptase inhibitors (NNRTIs), such as delavirdine (Rescriptor), loviride, and nevirapine (Viramune)
- **Protease inhibitors**, such as indinavir (Crixivan), nelfinavir (Viracept), ritonavir (Norvir) and saquinavir (Invirase).

Many of these drugs became available only in the mid- to late-1990s, and their introduction changed the way physicians treat HIV. Instead of being limited to just a few drugs, physicians now carefully choose combinations of these drugs for patients to take together. In the past, antiretroviral drugs were prescribed only when patients became very ill. But increasingly, they are being given earlier to keep people infected with HIV from getting so sick.

These medicines are available only with a physician's prescription and come in liquid, tablet, capsule, and injectable forms. Physicians consider many factors when deciding the correct dosage for each patient, such as body weight and overall general health. Patients using this medicine must carefully follow all instructions, making sure to take the medicine at the proper time and to schedule meals as directed. Always take antiretroviral drugs exactly as directed. Never take larger or more frequent doses, and do not take the drug for longer than directed. Take only the medicine that has been prescribed, and do not share this medicine with anyone else. Because these drugs can cause serious side effects, patients must pay close attention to their health and must make regular visits to their physicians. Anyone considering taking antiviral drugs should be sure to understand all the risks, benefits and requirements of this treatment.

Do not stop taking this medicine without checking with the physician who prescribed it. The only exception is for patients who have severe nausea, vomiting, and stomach **pain**. These symptoms could be signs of inflammation of the pancreas. Patients who have these symptoms should stop taking the medicine and call their physicians immediately. In all other cases, it is very important to keep taking the drugs, even if symptoms improve.

People with certain medical conditions or who are taking certain other medicines may have problems if they take antiretroviral drugs. Before using antiretroviral drugs, people should make sure their physicians are aware of all their medical conditions. Anyone who has had unusual reactions to antiretroviral drugs in the past should let his or her physician know before taking the drugs again. The physician should also be told about any **allergies** to foods, dyes, preservatives, or other substances. Women infected with HIV, who are either pregnant or are breast feeding their infants, should discuss the use of these drugs with their physicians.

Taking antiretroviral drugs with certain other drugs may affect the way the drugs work or may increase the chance of side effects. Some side effects occur early in treatment, but usually go away as the body adjusts to the drug. Among these are **anxiety**, irritability, restlessness, **diarrhea**, **headache**, sore muscles, dry mouth, and sleep problems. These side effects do not require medical treatment unless they continue or are troublesome. More serious side effects may also occur. If any unusual symptoms occur, check with a physician immediately. Anyone who develops new or unusual symptoms while taking antiretroviral drugs should get in touch with his or her physician. *Be sure to check with a physician before taking any other prescription or nonprescription (over-the-counter) medicine.*

ANTISEPTICS

Antiseptics are medicines that slow or stop the growth of germs and help prevent infections in minor cuts, scrapes, and **burns**.

Antiseptics are applied to the skin to keep bacteria from getting into **wounds** and causing infection. Although antiseptics do not usually kill bacteria, they do weaken them and slow their growth.

Simply applying an antiseptic to a wound is not adequate treatment. The wound should be cleaned first, and in most cases it should be covered with a bandage or other type of dressing to keep it clean and moist while it heals. However, some antiseptics, such as phenol, can damage the skin if the wound is covered after they are applied. Others, such as hydrogen peroxide and iodine, should be allowed to dry completely before the wound is covered.

Because antiseptics can irritate the skin and even interfere with the healing process, they should be used sparingly. Some medical experts advise people to use antibiotic ointments instead of antiseptics because they can actually kill the bacteria that may cause a wound to become infected. Rule of thumb: if hydrogen peroxide or another antiseptic is the only thing available to use at the time of injury, use it. If an antibiotic ointment or cream is available, use one of them instead.

Some commonly used antiseptics are isopropyl alcohol, hydrogen peroxide, iodine, phenol, methyl salicylate, and thymol. Most of the antiseptic products on the market contain one or more of these ingredients. These products can be bought without a doctor's prescription.

The correct amount to use depends on the product. Check the directions on the package or container or ask a pharmacist how to use the antiseptic.

Antiseptics are meant to be used for no more than one week. If the wound has not healed in that time, stop using the antiseptic and call a doctor.

Only minor cuts, scrapes, and burns should be treated with antiseptics. Certain kinds of injuries may need medical care and should not be self-treated with antiseptics. These include:

- Large wounds
- Deep cuts
- Cuts that continue bleeding
- Cuts that may need stitches
- Burns any larger than a small red spot
- Scrapes imbedded with particles that won't wash away
- Animal bites
- Punctures
- Eye injuries.

Antiseptics also should not be used to treat **sunburn** or existing infections

Anyone who has **allergies** of any kind should check with a doctor or pharmacist before using an over-the-counter antiseptic product.

Because some antiseptics can irritate the skin, check with a doctor before using these products on children under 2 years of age. Older people and people with sensitive skin should also check with a doctor or pharmacist before using an antiseptic.

When hydrogen peroxide is applied to a wound, it fizzes as oxygen is released. This fizzing action helps loosen and remove dead tissue and is not harmful. After the fizzing stops, the edges of the wound may be white—another harmless effect. When treating children or others who might be frightened by these effects, explain what is going to happen and assure them that the fizzing will not be painful.

Iodine may stain the skin. The stain can be removed with a compound called sodium thiosulfate. Ask the pharmacist for help in obtaining this compound.

Hydrogen peroxide solutions that contain more than 20% hydrogen peroxide can damage the skin and mucus membranes and can even lead to infection, rather than preventing it. Solutions this strong should be used only occasionally and in small amounts, if at all. Care should also be taken if hydrogen peroxide is used in the mouth, as a mouthwash or a gargle. Spit out the hydrogen peroxide after gargling. Do not swallow it.

Iodine can cause a lasting stinging sensation called iodine burn. Burning is especially likely if the wound is covered with a bandage before the iodine has had time to dry. It is also more likely with iodine solutions that contain 7% iodine or more. Iodine solutions this strong should not be used as antiseptics.

Some people develop an allergy to iodine when they use it repeatedly. Anyone who has a rash, a lasting burning sensation, or an unusually warm feeling in the area where the iodine was applied should contact a physician or pharmacist.

Antiseptics are not known to interact with any other medicines. However, they should not be used together with any other topical cream, solution, or ointment.

ANTISPASMODIC DRUGS

Antispasmodic drugs relieve cramps or spasms of the stomach, intestines, and bladder. The drug described here, dicyclomine (Bentyl), is prescribed to treat a condition called **irritable bowel syndrome**. In some people, the main symptom is abdominal **pain**. In others, it is **diarrhea** or alternating bouts of diarrhea and **constipation**.

Dicyclomine is available only with a prescription and is sold as capsules, tablets (regular and extended-release forms), and syrup. The usual dosage for adults is 20 mg, four times a day. However, the physician may recommend starting at a lower dosage and gradually increasing the dose to reduce the chance of unwanted side effects. The dosage for children depends on the child's age. Check with the child's physician for the correct dosage.

Dicyclomine makes some people sweat less, which allows the body to overheat and may lead to heat prostration (**fever** and heat **stroke**). Anyone taking this drug should try to avoid extreme heat. If that is not possible, check with the physician who prescribed the drug. This medicine can cause drowsiness and blurred or double vision. People who take this drug should not drive, use machines, or do anything else that might be dangerous until they have found out how the medicine affects them.

Dicyclomine should not be given to infants or children unless the physician decides the use of this drug is necessary. Diclyclomine should not be used by women who are breast feeding. Women who are pregnant or plan to become pregnant should check with their physicians before using this drug.

Anyone with the following medical conditions should not take dicyclomine unless directed to do so by a physician:

- Previous sensitivity or allergic reaction to dicyclomine
- **Glaucoma**
- **Myasthenia gravis**
- Blockage of the urinary tract, stomach, or intestines
- Severe ulcerative colitis
- Reflux esophagitis.

In addition, patients with these conditions should check with their physicians before using dicyclomine:

- Liver disease
- Kidney disease
- High blood pressure
- Heart problems
- **Enlarged prostate** gland
- Hiatal **hernia**
- Autonomic neuropathy (a nerve disorder)
- Hyperthyroidism.

Dicyclomine may interact with other medicines. When this happens, the effects of one or both of the drugs may change or the risk of side effects may be greater. The most common side effects are **dizziness**, drowsiness, lightheadedness, nausea, nervousness, blurred vision, dry mouth, and weakness. Other side effects may occur. Anyone who has unusual symptoms after taking dicyclomine should get in touch with his or her physician. Be sure to check with a physician or pharmacist before combining dicyclomine with any other prescription or nonprescription (over-the-counter) medicine.

ANTIVIRAL DRUGS

Antiviral drugs are medicines that cure or control virus infections. There are several different drugs in the antiviral family, and each is used for specific kinds of viral infections. For example, acyclovir (Zovirax) is used to treat **chickenpox**, **shingles**, and the symptoms of herpes virus infections of the genitals, lips, mouth, skin, and brain. The medicine does not cure the infections, but it relieves the discomfort and speeds healing of sores, when they are present. Similarly, valacyclovir (Valtrex) and famciclovir (Famvir) can also be used to relieve the symptoms of shingles. Another antiviral, ganciclovir (Cytovene) is prescribed for cytomegalovirus (CMV) eye infections in people whose immune systems are weakened. Ganciclovir does not cure the CMV infection, but it may keep the symptoms from getting worse. Ganciclovir may also help prevent CMV infections in people who are going to be given drugs or treatments that will weaken their immune systems, such as organ or bone marrow transplant patients.

Other types of antiviral drugs, such as amantadine (Symmetrel) and rimantadine (Flumadine) are used to prevent or treat certain kinds of **influenza** (flu). They are given either alone or in combination with flu shots. Still another class of drugs, **antiretroviral drugs**, targets a specific type of virus called a retrovirus. Human immunodeficiency virus (HIV), the virus that causes **AIDS**, is a retrovirus.

Viruses are tiny structures that are too small to be seen with a regular microscope. The powerful electron microscope invented in the 1940s revealed that a virus is nothing more than a core of genetic material (RNA or DNA), wrapped in a protective protein coat. These tiny agents of disease are not considered living things, because they cannot reproduce on their own. They must invade the cells of other living things and take over the cells' machinery to make more copies of themselves. Once inside their hosts' cells, viruses reproduce wildly, spread through the body and cause illness. Some illnesses caused by viruses come and go — common colds, flu, **measles**, **mumps**, and chicken pox, for example. Others, such as cytomegalovirus and Epstein-Barr virus, linger in the body for life.

Developing antiviral medicines has been difficult, because most drugs that kill viruses also damage the host's cells, where the viruses hide. However, since the 1980s, when the virus that causes AIDS began to receive attention, medical researchers have focused on the problem of treating viral infections, and encouraging progress has been made. Rather than killing the viruses, antiviral drugs block steps in the process through which viruses reproduce. Some may also stimulate the immune system so that the body can fight the viruses itself.

Antiviral drugs are available only with a physician's prescription and are sold in capsule, tablet, liquid, ointment, and injectable forms. The recommended dosage depends on the type of antiviral drug and the kind of infection for which it is being used. Dosage may be different for different people. Check with the physician who prescribed the drug or the pharmacist who filled the prescription for the correct dosage.

Some antiviral drugs work best when they are at constant levels in the blood. To help keep levels constant, take the medicine in doses spaced evenly through the day and night. Do not miss any doses. To make sure the infection clears up completely, take this medicine for as long as it has been prescribed. Do not stop taking the drug just because symptoms begin to improve, and do not miss any doses. Do not to take the medicine for longer than the physician orders. When taken by mouth, these medicines should be taken with a full glass of water. Some must be taken with food. Check package directions or ask the physician or pharmacist for instructions on how to take the medicine.

When taking an antiviral drug to prevent flu, start taking the medicine before, or as soon as possible after, being exposed to people who have the flu. When taking an antiviral medicine for chickenpox, shingles, or herpes infection, start taking the medicine as soon as possible after the symptoms appear. The medicine may not be as effective if too much time passes. Patients who are taking an antiviral drug for herpes should keep in mind that the medicine will not prevent them from spreading the infection to other people. They must still take precautions to avoid passing the virus through sexual contact.

People with certain other medical conditions or who are taking certain other medicines can have problems if they take antiviral drugs. Before taking these drugs, be sure to let the physician know about any of these conditions. Drinking alcoholic beverages while taking certain antiviral drugs may increase the chance of side effects. Anyone who takes these drugs should check with a physician before drinking alcohol or taking medicines that contain alcohol. Anyone who has had unusual reactions to antiviral drugs in the past should let his or her physician know before taking the drugs again. The physician should also be told about any **allergies** to foods, dyes, preservatives, or other substances.

Women who are pregnant or who may become pregnant should check with their physicians before using antiviral drugs. Women who are breastfeeding should also check with their physicians before using any antiviral drug. If the medicine is needed, avoiding breastfeeding while under treatment may be necessary.

Taking antiviral drugs with certain other medicines may affect the way the drugs work or may increase the chance of side effects. Antiviral drugs may also interact with a number of other medicines. When this happens, the effects of one or both of the drugs may change or the risk of side effects may be greater. The most common minor side effects are **diarrhea**, nausea or vomiting, **dizziness**, lightheadedness, **headache**, sleep problems, concentration problems, and irritability or nervousness. These problems usually go away as the body adjusts to the drug and do not require medical treatment unless they do persist or they interfere with normal activities. More serious side effects are possible and if any do occur, check with a physician. Anyone who takes antiviral drugs should let the physician know all other medicines he or she is taking.

ANXIETY DISORDERS

The anxiety disorders are a group of mental disturbances characterized by anxiety as the main symptom. Although anxiety is common, not everyone who experiences it has an anxiety disorder. Anxiety is associated with a wide range of physical illnesses, medication side effects, and other psychiatric disorders.

Anxiety disorders are the most common form of mental disturbance in the United States population. It is estimated that 28 million persons suffer from an anxiety disorder every year. These disorders are a serious problem for the entire society because of their interference with patients' work, schooling, and family life. They also contribute to the high rates of alcohol and substance abuse in the United States. Anxiety disorders are an additional problem for health professionals because the physical symptoms of anxiety frequently bring people to primary care doctors or emergency rooms.

The revisions of the *Diagnostic and Statistical Manual of Mental Disorders (DSM)* that took place after 1980 brought major changes in the classification of the anxiety disorders. Prior to 1980, psychiatrists classified patients on the basis of a theory of causality that defined anxiety as the outcome of unconscious conflicts in the patient's mind. *DSM-III* (1980), *DSM-III-R* (1987), and *DSM-IV* (1994) introduced and refined a new classification that took into consideration recent discoveries about the biochemical and post-traumatic origins of some types of anxiety. The present definitions are based on the external and reported symptom patterns of the disorders rather than on theories about their origins.

DSM-IV defines twelve types of anxiety disorders in the adult population. They can be grouped under seven headings:

- **Panic disorders** with or without agoraphobia. The chief characteristic of panic disorder is the occurrence of panic attacks coupled with fear of their recurrence. Patients with agoraphobia are afraid of places or situations in which they might have a panic attack and be unable to leave or to find help.
- **Phobias**. These include specific phobias and social phobia. A phobia is an intense irrational fear of a specific object or situation that compels the patient to avoid it. Some phobias concern activities or objects that involve some risk (for example, flying or driving) but many are focused on harmless animals or other objects. Social phobia involves a fear of being humiliated, judged, or scrutinized. It manifests itself as a fear of performing certain functions in the presence of others, such as public speaking or using public lavatories.
- Obsessive-compulsive disorder (OCD). This disorder is marked by unwanted, intrusive, persistent thoughts or repetitive behaviors that reflect the patient's anxiety or attempts to control it. It affects between 2-3% of the population and is much more common than was previously thought.
- **Stress** disorders. These include **post-traumatic stress disorder** (PTSD) and **acute stress disorder**. Stress disorders are symptomatic reactions to traumatic events in the patient's life.
- Generalized anxiety disorder (GAD). GAD is the most commonly diagnosed anxiety disorder and occurs most frequently in young adults.
- Anxiety disorders due to known physical causes. These include general medical conditions or substance abuse.
- Anxiety disorder not otherwise specified. This last category is not a separate type of disorder, but is included to cover symptoms that do not meet the specific *DSM-IV* criteria for other anxiety disorders.

DSM-IV defines one anxiety disorder as specific to children, namely, separation anxiety disorder. This disorder is defined as anxiety regarding separation from home or family that is excessive or inappropriate for the child's age. In some children, separation anxiety takes the form of school avoidance. Children and adolescents can also be diagnosed with panic disorder, phobias, generalized anxiety disorder, and the post-traumatic stress syndromes.

The causes of anxiety include a variety of individual and general social factors, and may produce physical, cognitive, emotional, or behavioral symptoms. The patient's ethnic or cultural background may also influence his or her vulnerability to certain forms of anxiety. Genetic factors that lead to biochemical abnormalities may also play a role. Anxiety in children may be caused by suffering from abuse, as well as by the factors that cause anxiety in adults.

The diagnosis of anxiety disorders is complicated by the variety of causes of anxiety and the range of disorders that may include anxiety as a symptom. Many patients who suffer from anxiety disorders have features or symptoms of more than one disorder. Patients whose anxiety is accounted for by another psychic disorder, such as **schizophrenia** or major depression, are not diagnosed with an anxiety disorder. A doctor examining an anxious patient will usually begin by ruling out diseases that are known to cause anxiety and then proceed to take the patient's medication history, in order to exclude side effects of prescription drugs. Most doctors will ask about **caffeine** consumption to see if the patient's dietary habits are a factor. The patient's work and family situation will also be discussed. Laboratory tests for blood sugar and thyroid function are also common.

There are no laboratory tests that can diagnose anxiety, although the doctor may order some specific tests to rule out disease conditions. Although there is no psychiatric test that can provide definite diagnoses of anxiety disorders, there are several short-answer interviews or symptom inventories that doctors can use to evaluate the intensity of a patient's anxiety and some of its associated features. These measures include the Hamilton Anxiety Scale and the Anxiety Disorders Interview Schedule (ADIS).

For relatively mild anxiety disorders, psychotherapy alone may suffice. In general, doctors prefer to use a combination of medications and psychotherapy with more severely anxious patients. Most patients respond better to a combination of treatment methods than to either medications or psychotherapy in isolation. In many cases the doctor will need to try a new medication or treatment over a six- to eight-week period in order to assess its effectiveness.

Although anxiety disorders are not always easy to diagnose, there are several reasons why it is important for patients with severe anxiety symptoms to get help. Anxiety doesn't always go away by itself; it often progresses to panic attacks, phobias, and episodes of depression. Untreated anxiety disorders may eventually lead to a diagnosis of major depression, or interfere with the patient's education or ability to keep a job. In addition, many anxious patients develop **addictions** to drugs or alcohol when they try to "medicate" their symptoms. Moreover, since children learn ways of coping with anxiety from their parents, adults who get help for anxiety disorders are in a better position to help their families cope with factors that lead to anxiety than those who remain untreated.

Alternative treatments for anxiety cover a variety of approaches. **Meditation** and mindfulness training are thought beneficial to patients with phobias and panic disorder. **Hydrotherapy** is useful to some anxious patients because it promotes general relaxation of the nervous system. **Yoga**, aikido, **tai chi**, and dance therapy help patients work with the physical, as well as the emotional, tensions that either promote anxiety or are created by the anxiety.

The prognosis for recovery depends on the specific disorder, the severity of the patient's symptoms, the specific causes of the anxiety, and the patient's degree of control over these causes. Anxiety is an unavoidable feature of human existence. However, humans do have some power over their reactions to anxiety-provoking events and situations. Cognitive therapy and meditation or mindfulness training appear to be beneficial in helping people lower their long-term anxiety levels.

APGAR, VIRGINIA (1909-1974)

American Pediatrician

Apgar was an American pediatrician who created a scale for assessing newborn infant health. She graduated from Mount Holyoke College in 1929 and earned her M.D. degree from the College of Physicians and Surgeons at Columbia University in 1933. Although she spent her first two years in a surgical internship, Dr. Apgar elected to enter the growing field of anesthesiology. In 1949 she was appointed the first full professor of anesthesiology at Columbia. That same year, after building the department and training program, Dr. Apgar gave up her administrative duties as head of the anesthesiology department and turned to the study of anesthesia and its role in **childbirth**, assisting in the births of more than 17,000 infants during her career at Columbia.

Apgar published a system for the assessment of newborn health status in 1953. The scoring system that bears her name employs a ten point score based on two points each for healthy heart rate, respiration, muscle tone, reflexes, and color. Typically assessed at one and five minutes after birth, a low Apgar score serves as a quantified signal for further attention or evaluation. For over 40 years the Apgar score has remained the standard method of newborn assessment, prompting one physician to remark, "Every baby born in a modern hospital anywhere in the world is looked at first through the eyes of Virginia Apgar."

During a sabbatical year in 1959, Apgar received a master's degree in public health from Johns Hopkins University. Rather than returning to academic medicine, however, she began working with the National Foundation March of Dimes and devoted the remainder of her life to the prevention of **birth defects** through public education and fund raising for research. She continued to lecture in the area of birth defects at Cornell University Medical College and Johns Hopkins School of Public Health. She received many honors and awards for her work, including the Gold Medal for Distinguished Achievement in Medicine from the Columbia College of Physicians and Surgeons' Alumni Association, the first woman to be so honored. She published a popular book for parents with Joan Beck in 1972 entitled *Is My Baby Alright?*

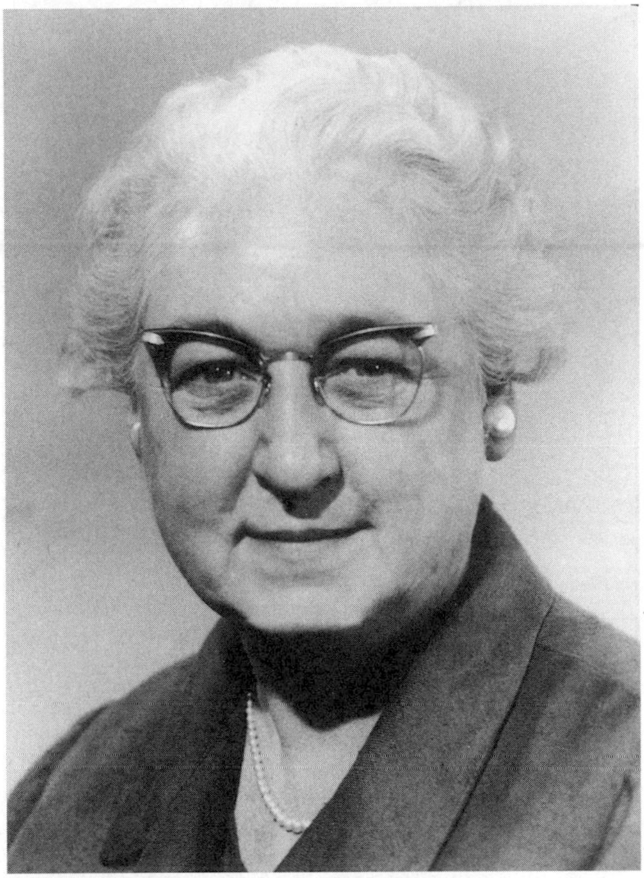

Virginia Apgar

APHASIA

Aphasia is condition characterized by either partial or total loss of the ability to communicate verbally or using written words. A person with aphasia may have difficulty speaking, reading, writing, recognizing the names of objects, or understanding what other people have said. Aphasia is caused by a brain injury, as may occur during a traumatic accident or when the brain is deprived of oxygen during a **stroke**. It may also be caused by a **brain tumor**, a disease such as Alzheimer's, or an infection, like **encephalitis**. Aphasia may be temporary or permanent.

Stroke is the most common cause of aphasia in the United States. Approximately 500,000 individuals suffer strokes each year, and 20% of these individuals develop some type of aphasia. Other causes of brain damage include head injuries, brain tumors, and infection. About half of the people who show signs of aphasia have what is called temporary or transient aphasia and recover completely within a few days. An estimated one million Americans suffer from some form of permanent aphasia.

According to the traditional classification scheme, each form of aphasia is caused by damage to a different part of the left hemisphere of the brain.

The traditional classification scheme includes eight types of aphasia:

- Broca's aphasia, also called motor aphasia, results from damage to the front portion or frontal lobe of the language-dominant area of the brain. Individuals with Broca's aphasia may either be completely unable to use speech (**mutism**) or they may be able to use single-word statements or even full sentences. However, these sentences are construct with great difficulty. Hearing com-

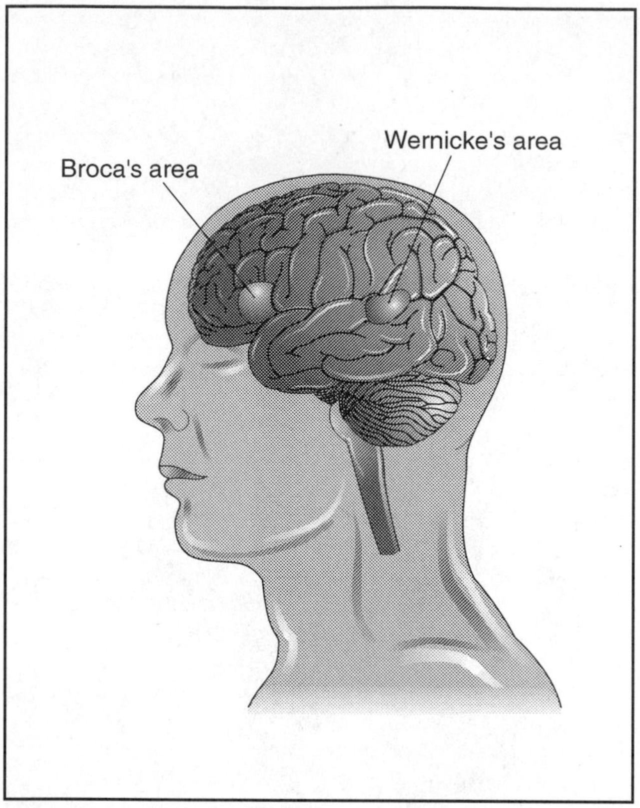

Areas in the brain associated with Broca's aphasia and Wernicke's aphasia.

prehension is usually not affected, so they are able to understand other people's speech and conversation and can follow commands. Often, weakness on the right side of their bodies makes it difficult to write. Reading ability is impaired. Individuals with Broca's aphasia may become frustrated and depressed because they are aware of their language difficulties.

- Wernicke's aphasia is caused by damage to the side portion or temporal lobe of the language-dominant area of the brain. Individuals with Wernicke's aphasia speak in long, uninterrupted sentences; however, the words used are frequently unnecessary or even made-up. They may be unable to understand other people's speech. Reading ability is diminished, and although writing ability is retained, what is written may be abnormal. No physical symptoms, such as the right-sided weakness seen with Broca's aphasia, are typically observed. Also, in contrast to Broca's aphasia, individuals with Wernicke's aphasia are not aware of their language errors.
- Global aphasia is caused by widespread damage to the language areas of the left hemisphere. As a result, all basic language functions are affected, but some areas may be more affected than others. For example, an individual may have difficulty speaking but may be able to write well. The individual may experience weakness and loss of feeling on the right side of their body.
- Conduction aphasia, also called associative aphasia, is rather uncommon. Individuals with conduction aphasia are unable to repeat words, sentences, and phrases. Speech is fairly unbroken, although individuals may frequently correct themselves and words may be skipped or repeated. Although able to understand spoken language, it may also be difficult for the individual with conduction aphasia to find the right word to describe a person or object. The impact of this condition on reading and writing ability varies. As with other types of aphasia, right-sided weakness or sensory loss may be present.
- Anomic or nominal aphasia primarily influences an individual's ability to find the right name for a person or object. As a result, an object may be described rather than named. Hearing comprehension, repetition, reading, and writing are not affected, other than by this inability to find the right name. Speech is fluent, except for pauses as the individual tries to recall the right name. Physical symptoms are variable, and some individuals have no symptoms of one-sided weakness or sensory loss.
- Transcortical aphasia is caused by damage to the language areas of the left hemisphere outside the primary language areas. There are three types of aphasia: transcortical motor aphasia, transcortical sensory aphasia, and mixed transcortical aphasia. Transcortical aphasias are distinguished from other types by the individual's ability to repeat words, phrases, or sentences. Other language functions may also be impaired to varying degrees, depending on the extent and particular location of brain damage.

Following brain injury, an initial bedside assessment is made to determine whether language function has been affected. If the individual experiences difficulty communicating, attempts are made to determine whether this difficulty arises from impaired language comprehension or an impaired ability to speak. A typical examination involves listening to spontaneous speech and evaluating the individual's ability to recognize and name objects, comprehend what is heard, and repeat sample words and phrases. A speech pathologist or neuropsychologist may be asked to conduct more extensive examinations using in-depth, standardized tests. The results of these tests indicate the severity of the aphasia and may also provide information regarding the exact location of the brain damage. This more extensive testing is also designed to provide the information necessary to design an individualized speech therapy program.

Initially, the underlying cause of aphasia must be treated or stabilized. To regain language function, therapy must begin as soon as possible following the injury. Although there are no medical or surgical procedures currently available to treat this condition, aphasia resulting from stroke or **head injury** may improve through the use of speech therapy. For most individuals, however, the primary emphasis is placed on making the most of retained language abilities and learning to use other means of communication to compensate for lost language abilities.

The degree to which an individual can recover language abilities is highly dependent on how much brain damage occurred and the location and cause of the original brain injury. Other factors include the individual's age, general health, motivation and willingness to participate in speech therapy, and whether the individual is left or right handed. Language areas may be located in both the left and right hemispheres in left-handed individuals. Left-handed individuals are, therefore, more likely to develop aphasia following brain injury, but because they have two language centers, may recover more fully because language abilities can be recovered from either side of the brain. The intensity of therapy and the time between diagnosis and the start of therapy may also affect the eventual outcome.

Apothecary

Apothecary was the early name applied to individuals who prepared and sold substances for medical use. The forerunner of today's pharmacist, the apothecary procured, mixed, and evaluated medications. The role of the apothecary-pharmacist has undergone many changes over the centuries. Once associated with the supernatural and **alchemy**, the apothecary became a leading health care practitioner whose field of expertise was based on science and who often treated patients directly. Eventually, the traditional apothecary was replaced by pharmacists, as we know them from the local drug store. Today, the pharmacist is primarily a dispenser of drugs already formulated and manufactured by pharmaceutical companies.

The art of the apothecary, that is mixing compounds according to the specific health needs of a patient, goes back to at least to 2200 to 3000 B.C. in ancient China, where the medicinal values of herbs were sought out and investigated. During the latter part of the eighth century, the first apothecaries and apothecary shops appeared in Baghdad. These street market shops sold medicines along with syrups, perfumes, and wines. This approach to **pharmacy** spread throughout Europe. As greater scientific rigor was applied to medicine, alchemists, who relied on herbs and magic, were replaced by apothecaries, who based their medicines on demonstrable physical effects. During Medieval times, the equivalent of today's apothecary-pharmacist were primarily priests, monks, and medicine men.

In 1606, the Society of Apothecaries of London was created through a charter issued by James I (James VI of Scotland) and was associated with the Guild of Grocers. In 1617, a new charter came into being establishing an independent Apothecary Guild recognized as a distinct group of craftsmen. This charter resulted from England's move toward establishing an official pharmaceutical standard, published as the *Pharmacopeiae Londonensis*. The granting of charter to the apoethcaries represents the first independently organized group of pharmacists in the western world. The charter made it illegal for anyone other than an apothecary to prepare or sell medicines.

The first American apothecary store appeared in Philadelphia around 1780 and focused on supplying German immigrants with remedies familiar in their former home country. At that time, the apothecary practiced almost like a doctor. In addition to making and prescribing medicines, they made house calls to treat patients and trained apprentices. Many also performed surgery and served as male midwives during birth. Since there were no regulations regarding drug compounding, the effectiveness of medicines were haphazard and depended on accurate measurements and compounding of the right substances by the individual apothecary. However, the apothecary had many effective substances in his arsenal to treat patients, including chalk for heartburn and calamine for the skin, which are ingredients in some modern medications.

By the turn of the twentieth century, the apothecary as a compounder of medicine who also counseled patients on health, was still the accepted approach to pharmacy. The apothecary-pharmacist still compounded approximately 60 percent of all medications dispensed in the 1930s and 1940s. However, after World War II, the growth of commercial drug manufacturers marked a sharp decline in the need for compounding and the apothecary. In 1951, the Durham-Humphrey amendment to the United States Food, Drug, and Cosmetic Act introduced doctor-prescription only legal status for most medicines, resulting in the development of the modern day pharmacist as a dispenser of pre-manufactured drugs. Still, in the 1960s, about 100 apothecaries practiced the United States. These apothecaries differed from the modern drug store in that they focused solely on medications, including compounding substances for an individual patient's needs.

Throughout the 1970s and the 1980s, the pharmacist as an apothecary became nearly non-existent especially as large chain drug stores took control of the pharmaceutical sales market. However, some community pharmacists continued to compound their own drugs, primarily salves and ointments, from formulas handed down through generations. Today, the apothecary is making a comeback as the need for specific doses and customized medications begins to grow again. Each day, thousands of compounded drug dosages are dispensed by pharmacists who are also compounders or apothecaries. Although most drugs are still dispensed according to manufactured dosages, the modern apothecary may adjust dosages according to a doctor's prescription, prepare medications without dyes or preservatives that may cause allergic reactions in some patients, make a medication more palatable for children, and use many other approaches to meet an individual patient's needs.

See also Alchemy; Pharmacy

Appendicitis

Appendicitis is an inflammation of the appendix, which is the worm-shaped pouch attached to the cecum, the beginning of the large intestine. The appendix has no known function in the body, but it can become diseased. Appendicitis is a medical emergency, and if it is left untreated the appendix may rupture and cause a potentially fatal infection.

Appendicitis is the most common abdominal emergency found in children and young adults. One person in 15 develops appendicitis in his or her lifetime. The main symptom of ap-

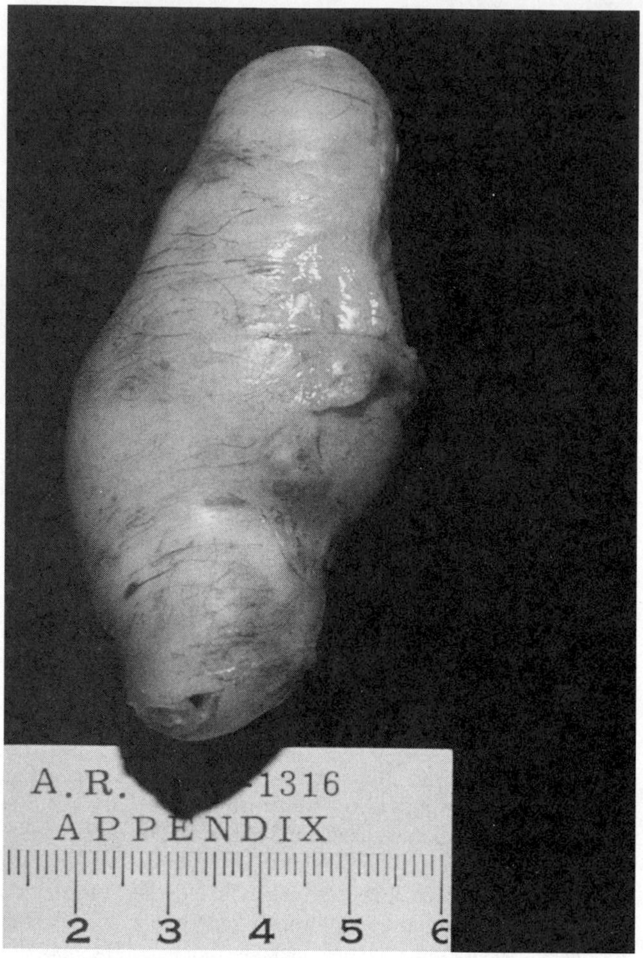

An extracted appendix. ***(Photograph by Lester V. Bergman, Corbis Images. Reproduced by permission.)***

pendicitis is increasingly severe abdominal **pain**. Since many different conditions can cause abdominal pain, an accurate diagnosis of appendicitis can be difficult. A timely diagnosis is important, however, because a delay can result in rupture of the appendix. When this happens, the infected contents of the appendix spill into the abdomen, and could cause a serious infection of the abdomen called **peritonitis**. The treatment for acute (sudden, severe) appendicitis is appendectomy, surgery to remove the appendix. Because the consequences of a ruptured appendix are life-threatening, persons suspected of having appendicitis are often taken to surgery before the diagnosis is certain.

The causes of appendicitis are not well understood, but it is believed to occur as a result of one or more of these factors: an obstruction within the appendix, the development of an ulceration (an abnormal change in tissue accompanied by the death of cells) within the appendix, and the invasion of bacteria. Under these conditions, bacteria may multiply within the appendix. The appendix may become swollen and filled with pus (a fluid formed in infected tissue, consisting of while blood cells and cellular debris), and may eventually rupture. Signs of rupture include the presence of symptoms for more than 24 hours, a **fever**, a high white blood cell count, and a fast heart rate. Very rarely, the inflammation and symptoms of appendicitis may disappear but recur again later.

The distinguishing symptom of appendicitis is pain beginning around or above the navel. The pain, which may be severe or only achy and uncomfortable, eventually moves into the right lower corner of the abdomen. There, it becomes more steady and more severe, and often increases with movement, **cough**ing, and so forth. The abdomen often becomes rigid and tender to the touch. Increasing rigidity and tenderness indicates an increased likelihood of perforation and peritonitis. Loss of appetite is very common. **Nausea and vomiting** may occur in about half of the cases and occasionally there may be **constipation** or **diarrhea**. The temperature may be normal or slightly elevated. The presence of a fever may indicate that the appendix has ruptured.

A careful examination is the best way to diagnose appendicitis. It is often difficult even for experienced physicians to distinguish the symptoms of appendicitis from those of other abdominal disorders. Therefore, very specific questioning and a thorough **physical examination** are crucial. The physician should ask questions, such as where the pain is centered, whether the pain has shifted, and where the pain began. The physician should press on the abdomen to judge the location of the pain and the degree of tenderness.

While laboratory tests cannot establish the diagnosis, an increased white cell count may point to appendicitis. **Urinalysis** may help to rule out a urinary tract infection that can mimic appendicitis. Patients whose symptoms and physical examination are compatible with a diagnosis of appendicitis are usually taken immediately to surgery, where a laparotomy (surgical exploration of the abdomen) is done to confirm the diagnosis. Other tests, such as a computed tomography scan (CT), and an ultrasound examination of the abdomen may be performed to avoid unnecessary surgery. Abdominal x-rays are not of much value except when the appendix has ruptured.

Often, the diagnosis is not certain until an operation is done. To avoid a ruptured appendix, surgery may be recommended without delay if the symptoms point clearly to appendicitis. If the symptoms are not clear, surgery may be postponed until they progress enough to confirm a diagnosis.

Appendicitis is usually treated successfully by appendectomy. Unless there are complications, the patient should recover without further problems. The mortality rate in cases without complications is less than 0.1%. When an appendix has ruptured, or a severe infection has developed, the likelihood is higher for complications, with slower recovery, or death from disease. There are higher rates of perforation and mortality among children and the elderly. Appendicitis is probably not preventable, although there is some indication that a diet high in green vegetables and tomatoes may help prevent it.

ARBER, WERNER (1929-)
Swiss molecular biologist

Werner Arber's discovery of an enzyme that could cleave long strands of deoxyribonucleic acid (DNA) led to a revolution in genetics research, providing the foundation that led to techniques to separate and reassemble basic genetic material. Gene splicing, as it was called, proved invaluable for DNA sequencing and gene mapping, which focuses on genetic organization. The most controversial outcome of this research, however, was the eventual manipulation of DNA structures by geneticists, first in test tubes and then *in vivo,* or within a living organism. Arber received the 1978 Nobel Prize in physiology or medicine for his research on gene splicing, sharing the prize with United States scientists **Hamilton O. Smith** and **Daniel Nathans**, who had also played an essential role in the development of gene splicing. A devoted family man, Werner eschewed politics but was well aware of the implications of genetic manipulation and warned his fellow scientists that such genetic research should be used carefully. As a result, Arber conducted studies and participated in symposia on how to prevent the unintentional release of a genetically altered virus into the environment.

Werner Arber was born in Gränichen, Switzerland, on June 3, 1929. Educated in the Swiss public school system, he entered the Federal Institute of Technology in Zurich in 1949, where he focused on the natural sciences. Arber soon became exposed to experimental research and embarked on studies to isolate and characterize the radioactive isotope of chlorine. After graduation in 1953, he entered the University of Geneva as a graduate student, received an appointment as a research assistant in a laboratory, and studied biophysics. Werner became interested in bacterial viruses (bacteriophages) through the biophysicist Jean J. Weigle's studies of variations in these viruses, which aimed to show that a specific bacteriophage will only infect a specific host. Another biophysicist, **Salvador Edward Luria**, showed that when phages infect a different strain of bacteria, a few survive to plate efficiently with the new host strain. Most of the phages die out, and the surviving phages are no longer capable of infecting an earlier host. The phenomenon was first called host-induced variation and is now commonly known as host-controlled restriction-modification.

During his graduate studies, Arber assisted biophysicists at Geneva in developing high-level magnification techniques in electron microscopy to study bacteriophages. He completed his dissertation on deficiencies of a mutant strain of bacteriophage lambda and received his Ph.D. in 1958. Arber then went to the University of Southern California for further study and to refine his laboratory techniques in genetics and bacteriophage research. While in the United States, Arber also took the opportunity to visit several colleagues who were studying bacteriophages.

Arber returned to Switzerland to join the faculty at the University of Geneva in 1960. With support from the Swiss National Science Foundation, he embarked on studies of the molecular basis of bacteriophage restriction. Working with one of his graduate students, Daisy Dussoix, Arber found in 1962 that restriction was host-controlled and involved changes in the phage's DNA. In effect, the DNA of the invading phages is cut into component parts, although some phages survived the operation. This discovery set in motion a series of studies that jump-started genetics to become the new frontier in biomedical research.

Arber himself formulated a hypothesis presupposing that an endonuclease enzyme in the host severs the DNA of invading phages into component parts, while a methylase enzyme modifies the DNA of the host to make it invulnerable to its own endonuclease enzyme. Although he had yet to discover such an enzyme, Arber hypothesized that an endonuclease recognizes specific sequences of nucleotides, a fundamental building block of DNA and RNA, and cuts the DNA of the invading phages at the specific locations of these nucleotides. Arber called this two-enzyme theory a restriction-modification system. The theory received initial confirmation when Arber, with the biophysicist Urs Kühnlein, isolated phage mutants that were inert to restriction and modification by mutation at specific nucleotide recognition sites. This discovery directly correlated Kühnlein's observation of DNA methylation with host-controlled modification in phages.

In 1965 Arber was appointed extraordinary professor of molecular genetics at the University of Geneva. He continued his research on restriction-modification and discovered, in 1968, the restriction endonuclease of *Escherichia coli* B, a common gut bacterium widely used in genetic studies. (At the same time Matthew Meselson and Robert Yuan identified the endonuclease from *Escherichia coli* K.) Although Arber's enzyme recognized specific nucleotide sequences, it cut the DNA at random spots and would later be known as a Type I restriction endonuclease. Since these Type I endonucleases severed the DNA at areas away from the recognition sites, they were unsuitable for studies of gene splicing. The second part of Arber's theory—that the endonuclease cut the invader's DNA at *specific* sites—was confirmed by the microbial geneticist Hamilton Smith and his colleagues, K. W. Wilcox and Thomas J. Kelley. Working at Johns Hopkins University, they identified what eventually came to be known as Type II, or specific, endonuclease. Daniel Nathans, also at Johns Hopkins, was a cancer researcher who first identified eleven cleaved fragments of a simian (monkey or ape) virus and eventually deduced the order in which individual fragments were replicated, showing that they began at a specific site and went in both directions around a circle, stopping approximately 180 degrees from where they started. Nathans and colleagues went on to isolate messenger RNA (mRNA), a type of RNA that is complementary to the protein-encoding segments of the host strand of DNA and communicates genetic information to proteins. They then began to map transcription sites (the origin and direction of each mRNA transcript during infection) by looking at different stages of infection and testing the RNA's ability to hybridize to the various ''restriction fragments'' due to their nucleotide sequences. This pioneering research led to a barrage of genetic studies aimed at mapping genetic codes, culminating in the international human genome project, which geneticists began in the late 1980s to develop a comprehensive road map of the human genetic system. Over the years, geneticists built upon the work of Arber, Smith, and Nathans to develop techniques to produce enough of a particular gene to study and then to artificially alter DNA through the transfer or insertion of genetic material.

Arber eventually became dissatisfied with what he perceived to be academic politics and the dearth of students devoting themselves to research careers at the University of Geneva. He left the university in 1970 and spent a year at the University of California at Berkeley as a visiting professor in the Department of Molecular Biology. Upon returning to Switzerland, he took an appointment as ordinary professor of molecular biology at the University of Basel and was reserved extensive modern facilities in the Biozentrum research institute, which was then under construction.

In 1978, Arber, Smith, and Nathans won the Nobel Prize for physiology or medicine, Arber being noted for his research showing that the host can alter DNA to prevent invasion by phages and other foreign genes through methylation (combining DNA with two carbons and three hydrogens), which cleaves the DNA. The cumulative efforts of these three scientists were an example of the growing emphasis on interdisciplinary communication and cooperation in scientific research as new discoveries in genetics were made simultaneously at many institutions throughout the world.

Arber's subsequent research has focused on genetic systems and their diversification. With the confirmation in the 1970s of **Barbara Mc Clintock**'s theories of transposable genes that could "jump" to different strands of DNA during the early stages of meiosis (the process of cell division), Arber and other geneticists began to experiment with gene transplantation. Arber has theorized that genetic exchange through transposition may account for the diverse bacterial genetic codes that occur during evolution.

Investigations into recombinant DNA technology, however, also had controversial aspects. Studies of combining eukaryotic DNA (that is, DNA from an organism consisting of more than one cell) with bacterial or viral DNA in a molecule raised concerns about producing pathogens (a micro-organism that can carry disease), especially since these pathogens could be cloned by copying the DNA molecules. Arber participated in discussions that led to a set of guidelines developed by the National Institutes of Health to conduct recombinant DNA research safely. As Arber points out in his introductory paper for the proceedings of the symposium, *Genetic Manipulation: Impact on Man and Society,* the initial risk was faced by the experimenters themselves, who were in direct contact with potential pathogens. What concerned the public, however, was the possibility of potential pathogens being accidentally introduced into the environment. Arber called for a realistic evaluation of the risks, saying that the guidelines had been designed to reduce the risks to a minimum.

Because of these precautions, geneticists have avoided serious mishaps and developed remarkable recombinant DNA studies, including a promising biomedical application known as gene therapy. Gene therapy begins with the splicing of DNA segments from various origins into a vector DNA molecule. Vectors act as "molecular delivery trucks," carrying genes to targeted cell types or organ systems, and are carefully chosen for their ability to colonize certain cell types and tissues in the body and become an inheritable trait. In gene therapy, disease-causing genes (specific nucleotide sequences) are replaced with normal sequences or additional genetic material is inserted to change the genes. This genetic material, for example, could carry a gene that expresses an inhibitor of a certain protein or hormone that causes a disease, such as arthritis. Investigators have also focused on gene therapies for cancer.

Arber married his wife, Antonia, in 1965. They have two daughters. Outside of his scientific pursuits, Arber has devoted his time to his family, who strongly support his scientific efforts.

Aristotle (384 B.C.-322 B.C.)

Greek philosopher and biologist

While he is highly regarded as a philosopher and father of logic and reasoning, Aristotle is also known for accomplishments in and contributions to other sciences. Throughout his life, he wrote several biological works which laid the foundations for *comparative anatomy*, taxonomy (classification), and *embryology*.

Aristotle was born in the northern Greek village of Stagira. His father was the court physician to the king of Macedonia, and it was at the Macedonian court where Aristotle spent much of his early boyhood. His father died before Aristotle was ten years old and the boy was raised by friends of the family.

At age seventeen, Aristotle was sent to the Academy of Plato in Athens where he plunged wholeheartedly into Plato's pursuit of truth and goodness, and soon became Plato's best pupil, earning the nickname "intelligence of the school." In the year 347 BC, twenty years after Aristotle's arrival, Plato died; Aristotle then left the Academy to travel. His journeys led him through the Greek empire and he eventually moved to Assos, a city in Asia Minor where his friend Hermias was the ruler. There, he married Pythias, Hermias' niece and adopted daughter, and began his research into natural history and biology.

In 342 B.C., Philip II invited Aristotle to return to the Macedonian court at Pella and teach his son, Alexander. Aristotle's student later became known in history as Alexander the Great.

After the death of Philip and Alexander's rise to the throne, Aristotle left the court for a brief visit to his hometown; he soon returned to Athens to resume his scientific studies. In 335 B.C., he founded a university called the *Lyceum.* He had renounced some of Plato's theories and began his own style of brilliant teaching at the newly-established school. In the mornings, he would stroll through the Lyceum gardens, discussing problems and theories with his advanced students. Because he walked about while teaching, Athenians nicknamed his school the *Peripatetic*—the Greek term meaning "to walk about." Like their headmaster, Lyceum pupils performed research in nearly every existing field of knowledge. They dissected animals and studied the habits of insects, helping Aristotle to compile data for his classification system.

The school became the basic building block for the great library and museum in the area. Unfortunately, in the year 323 B.C., the ruling emperor Alexander died, forcing Aristotle to leave Athens due to anti-Macedonian sentiment and accusations of impiety. He went to his mother's homeland of Chalcis where he died a year later.

Aristotle contributed much to the field of biology, especially through his early work on classification. He realized that you had to observe an array of characteristics, not just one as a basis for grouping, and scientists consider him to be the first person to group organisms in ways that made sense. He did not believe in evolution, but as a careful student of nature, he separated living things according to their complexity, the scala naturae (''scale of nature''). He assigned each increasingly complex form of life to a step on a ladder, and every step was taken. In the eighteenth century, Carolus Linnaeus (1707-1778) developed binomial nomenclature, whereby all organisms were named according to genus and species. Linnaeus said, ''God Creates, Linnaeus arranges.'' His system of classification remains in use today. Aristotle was a painstaking observer, believing nature never created anything without a reason. He was particularly fascinated by sea creatures, often dissecting them and studying their natural habitats. This approach to anatomy led him to look for correlations between structure and function and to a belief that each biological part has its own special uses. The Judeo-Christian culture was in agreement with Aristotle's view that species are fixed and unchanging, and that the Creator designed each species with a particular purpose. These beliefs remained undisputed until 1859 when Darwin published his theory of natural selection to explain evolution.

In his studies, Aristotle balanced empiricism or observation and formalism, rational deduction. When studying embryology, he observed the change from pupa to adult in insects. Aristotle deducted that the immature stage is trying to express the perfect form of the adult insect. From his observations, he also concluded that certain lower forms of life, such as worms and flies, come from rotting fruit or manure by a process of spontaneous generation. This concept was disproved by the experiments of Francisco Redi in the seventeenth century and Louis Pasteur in the nineteenth century.

Besides his work in the field of biology, Aristotle also was the first to define and classify the various branches of knowledge. He sorted them into physics, metaphysics, rhetoric, poetics, and logic. In doing so, he laid the foundation of most of the sciences.

AROMATHERAPY

Aromatherapy is a branch of herbal medicine that uses the essential oils found in plants for their healing or medicinal properties. Fragrant, concentrated oils from parts of plants, such as their flowers, fruit, stalks, roots, and bark, are used for the purpose of improving a person's health and well-being.

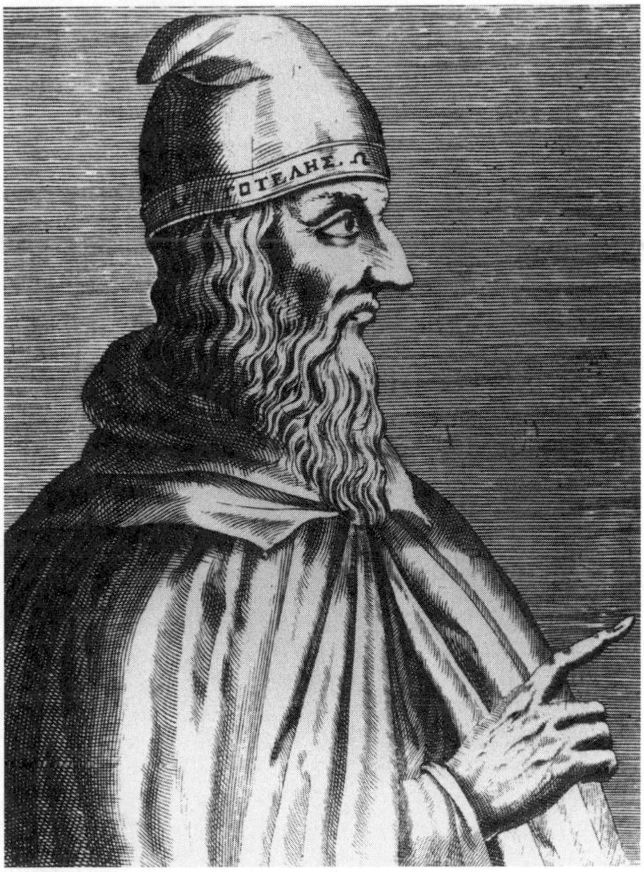

Aristotle

Although its name suggests that it is primarily a form of aroma or smell therapy, the essential oils are, in fact, intended mainly to be absorbed into the body via the skin, through **massage**, and the lungs, through inhalation. Aromatherapy is widely used to reduce **stress**, as well as to rejuvenate and detoxify the body. It is also used to treat a wide variety of other conditions.

There are several things to be concerned about when using essential oils, in addition to the purity of the oils themselves. Some individuals experience a skin reaction (**dermatitis**) to certain oils when they are applied, whereas others suffer skin irritation from overuse. More serious are instances in which oils are incorrectly taken internally. Individuals with conditions like high blood pressure or epilepsy should never treat themselves, and young children and pregnant women should be especially careful.

As a holistic therapy, aromatherapy is believed to benefit both the mind and the body. As far back as the time of the Egyptians, fragrant oils were recommended for bathing and massage, and plant fragrances were used against the **plague** in both ancient and medieval times. However, not until the 1930s was aromatherapy formalized by its advocates as a specialized branch of herbal medicine.

Aromatherapists select particular oils for certain conditions. A plant's essential oils or aromatic essences, (the con-

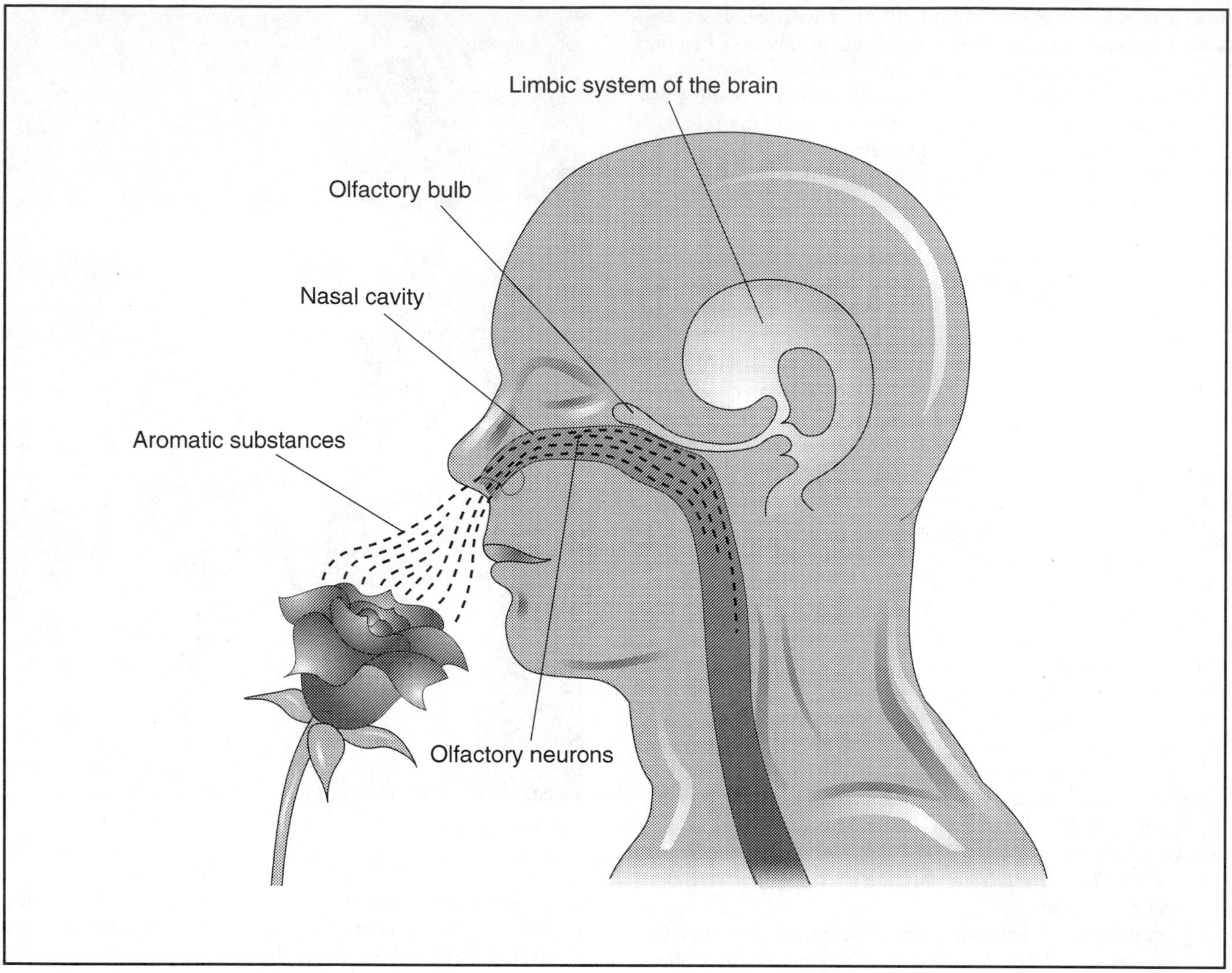

As a holistic therapy, aromatherapy is believed to benefit both the mind and body. Here, the aromatic substances from a flower stimulates the olfactory bulb and neurons. The desired emotional response (such as relaxation) is activated from the limbic system of the brain. ***(Illustration by Electronic Illustrators Group.)***

centrated substances produced by plants) are used for specific purposes such as repelling insects or enemies, storing energy, or attracting pollinating insects. Each oil has its own scent, as well as its own claimed healing characteristics. Some are considered antiseptic, some anti-inflammatory, and others stimulating or relaxing. These oils enter the body through inhalation and absorption. Inhalation can be as simple as putting a drop of oil on a handkerchief (to promote relaxation) or a few drops into steaming water (to relieve congestion). Massage is the most common form of absorbing the oils directly into the body through the skin, and is considered the most effective method.

Proponents of aromatherapy argue that it works on the mind as well as the body. The body is affected directly, since the tiny molecular structure of the oils allows them to penetrate the skin and be absorbed into the bloodstream. Then, depending on the particular ''healing properties'' of the specific oil, the oil produces an internal effect that can be diuretic, anti-inflammatory, or antiviral. Other oils support the immune system or energize, pacify, or detoxify the body.

The mind is affected by aromatherapy via the sense of smell. Whether inhaled directly or as a result of the fragrance emitted by an oil massage, the concentrated aroma is said to initiate a complex chain of events within the body. First, the aroma enters the nose and is received by the cilia or fine hairs that are linked to the olfactory nerve. The converted, electrical message is then transmitted to the limbic area of the brain. Stimulation of the brain's limbic system is believed to influence an individual's mood, emotions, and overall alertness. Aromatherapists emphasize that essential oils can affect the chemical activity of the brain and therefore produce both psychological and physical changes.

Certain scents are known to soothe and relax the body and mind. Aromatherapists claim regular relief for patients with physical conditions like **headache**s and emotional situations like **anxiety** and irritability. However, essential oils can be dangerously toxic if taken internally. Oils applied externally also can have a powerful, unintended effect, such as producing uterine contractions in a pregnant woman. In general, it is important not to overestimate the healing properties of oils. A physician should be consulted if a critical situation occurs.

ARRHYTHMIAS

Arrhythmias are deviations from the normal rhythm or pattern of heartbeats which cause the heart to pump improperly. The heartbeat can be too slow, too fast, have extra beats, skip a beat, or otherwise beat irregularly.

The heart has four chambers or sections. Blood from the body enters the right auricle. It flows to the right ventricle. From there it is pumped out to the lungs where it picks up oxygen. The blood returns to the heart where it enters the left auricle, flows into the left ventricle, and is pumped out to the body where it gives up its oxygen to the cells. The blood then returns to the right auricle where it starts its travels over again. The sequence of contractions of the four chambers (the heartbeat) must be exact, otherwise the effectiveness of the pumping mechanism is decreased.

A normal heartbeat starts in the right auricle. Here the heart's natural pacemaker, the sinus node, sends an electrical signal to the center of the heart. This signal causes the main pumping chambers, the ventricles, to contract. Arrhythmias occur when the heartbeat starts in a part of the heart other than the sinus node, an abnormal rate or rhythm develops in the sinus node, or a heart conduction "block" prevents the electrical signal from traveling down the normal pathway.

More than four million Americans have arrhythmias, most of which are harmless. Middle-aged adults who do not have heart disease commonly experience harmless arrhythmias. As people age, the probability of experiencing an arrhythmia increases. In people with heart disease, it is usually the heart disease that is dangerous, not the arrhythmia.

Arrhythmias often occur during and after **heart attack**s. Some types of arrhythmias, such as ventricular tachycardia, are serious and even life threatening. In the United States, arrhythmias are the primary cause of **sudden cardiac death**, accounting for more than 350,000 **death**s each year. Ventricular fibrillation is the most serious arrhythmia and is fatal unless medical help is immediate.

Slow heart rates (less than 60 beats per minute) are called bradycardias, while fast heart rates (more than 100 beats per minute) are called tachycardias. Bradycardia can result in poor circulation of blood, leading to a lack of oxygen throughout the body, especially the brain. Tachycardias also can compromise the heart's ability to pump effectively because the ventricles do not have enough time to completely fill.

In many cases, the cause of an arrhythmia is unknown. Known causes of arrhythmias include heart disease, **stress**, caffeine, tobacco, alcohol, diet pills, and **decongestants** in **cough** and cold medicines.

Symptoms of an arrhythmia include a fast heartbeat, pounding or fluttering chest sensations, skipping a heartbeat, "flip-flops," **dizziness**, faintness, **shortness of breath**, and chest **pain**s.

Examination with a stethoscope, electrocardiograms, and electrophysiologic studies are all used to diagnose arrhythmias. Sometimes arrhythmias can be identified simply by listening to the patient's heart through a stethoscope. More often, an electrocardiogram (ECG) that shows the heart's activity will reveal an arrythmia. In other cases, cardiac catheterization for electrophysiologic studies is performed in a hospital to identify the origin of serious arrhythmias and determine the heart's response to various treatments.

Many arrhythmias do not require any treatment. For serious arrhythmias, treating the underlying heart disease sometimes controls the arrhythmia. In some cases the arrhythmia itself is treated with drugs, electrical shock, automatic implantable defibrillators, artificial **pacemakers**, or surgery.

Drug therapy can manage many arrhythmias, but finding the right drug and dose requires care and can take time. Common drugs for suppressing arrhythmias include beta-blockers, calcium channel blockers, quinidine, digitalis preparations, and procainamide. All of the drugs used to treat arrhythmias have possible side effects ranging from mild to serious.

In emergency situations, cardioversion or defibrillation (the application of an electrical shock to the chest wall) is used. Cardioversion restores the heart to its normal rhythm. It is followed by drug therapy to prevent recurrence of the arrhythmia.

Artificial pacemakers that send electrical signals to make the heart beat properly can be implanted under the skin during a simple operation. Leads from the pacemaker are anchored to the right side of the heart. Pacemakers are used to correct bradycardia and are sometimes used after surgical or catheter ablation.

Automatic implantable defibrillators correct life-threatening ventricular arrhythmias by recognizing them and then restoring a normal heart rhythm by pacing the heart or giving it an electric shock. They are implanted within the chest wall without major surgery and store information for future evaluation by physicians. Automatic implantable defibrillators have proven to be more effective in saving lives than drugs alone, although they often are used in conjunction with drug therapy.

Ablation, a procedure to alter or remove the heart tissue causing the arrhythmia in order to prevent a recurrence, can be performed through a catheter or surgery. Supraventricular tachycardia can be treated successfully with ablation. Ablation treatments are used when medications fail.

Maze surgery treats atrial fibrillation by making multiple incisions through the atrium to allow electrical impulses to move effectively. This often is recommended for patients who have not responded to drugs or cardioversion.

Advances in diagnostic techniques, new drugs, and medical technology have extended the lives of many patients with serious arrhythmias. Diagnostic techniques enable physicians to accurately identify arrhythmias, while new drugs, advances in pacemaker technology, the development of implantable defibrillators, and progress in ablative techniques offer effective treatments.

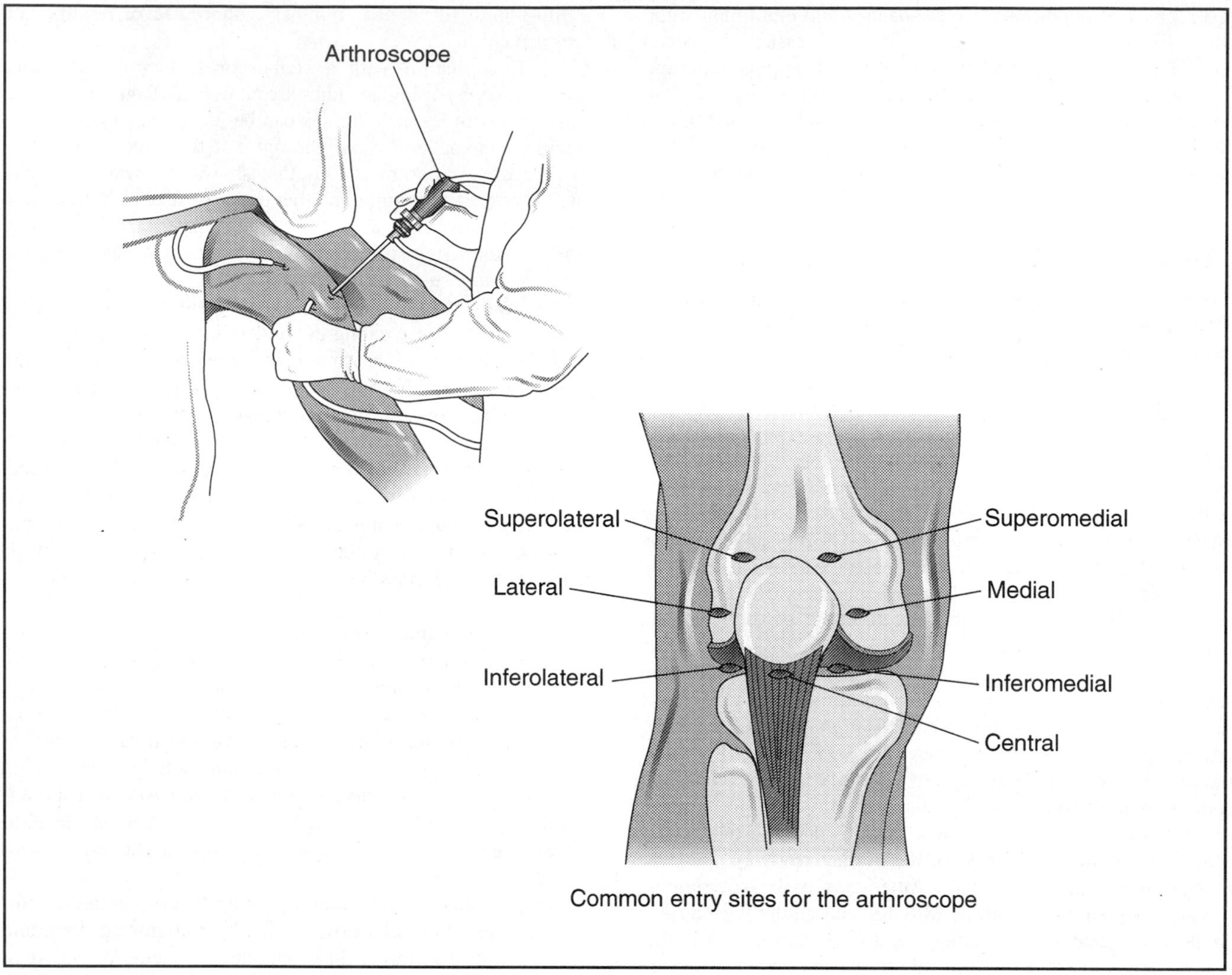

Surgeon performing arthroscopic surgery on patient's knee.

ARTHROSCOPIC SURGERY

Arthroscopic surgery is a procedure used to identify, monitor, and diagnose joint injuries and disease, to remove bone or cartilage, or repair tendons or ligaments. Diagnostic arthroscopic surgery is performed when medical history, physical exam, x rays, and other tests such as MRIs or CTs do not provide a definitive diagnosis.

In arthroscopic surgery, an orthopedic surgeon uses an arthroscope (a fiber-optic instrument) to see the inside a joint. After making an incision about the size of a buttonhole in the patient's skin, a sterile sodium chloride solution is injected to distend the joint. The arthroscope, an instrument the size of a pencil, is then inserted into the joint.

The arthroscope has a lens and a lighting system through which the structures inside the joint are transmitted to a miniature television camera attached to the end of the arthroscope. The surgeon uses irrigation and suction to remove blood and debris from the joint before examining it. Other incisions may be made in order to see other parts of the joint or to insert additional instruments. Looking at the interior of the joint on the television screen, the surgeon can determine the amount or type of injury and, if necessary, take a biopsy specimen or repair or correct the problem.

Arthroscopic surgery can be used to remove floating bits of cartilage and treat minor tears and other disorders. The site of the incision is bandaged.

Arthroscopic surgery is also used to diagnose and treat joint problems, most commonly in the knee, but also in the shoulder, elbow, ankle, wrist, and hip. Some of the most common joint problems seen with an arthroscope are inflammation of the joints injuries to the shoulder (rotator cuff tendon tears, impingement syndrome, and recurrent dislocations), knee (cartilage tears, wearing down of or injury to the cartilage cushion, and anterior cruciate ligament tears with instability), and wrist (**carpal tunnel syndrome**). Loose pieces of bone or cartilage in the knee, shoulder, elbow, ankle, or wrist also show up frequently.

Corrective arthroscopic surgery is performed with instruments that are inserted through additional incisions. Arthritis can sometimes be treated with arthroscopic surgery. Some problems are treated with a combination of arthroscopic and standard surgery.

Also called arthroscopy, the procedure is performed in a hospital or outpatient surgical facility. The type of anesthesia (local, spinal, or general) and the length of the procedure depends on the joint operated on and the complexity of the problem. Arthroscopic surgery rarely takes more than an hour. Most patients are released that same day, although some stay in the hospital overnight.

Considered the most important orthopedic development in the 20th century, arthroscopic surgery is widely used. The use of arthroscopic surgery on famous athletes has been well publicized. It is estimated that 80% of orthopedic surgeons practice arthroscopic surgery. This technique was initially a diagnostic tool used prior to open surgery, but as better instruments were developed, it began to be used to actually treat a variety of joint problems. Recently, lasers were introduced in arthroscopic surgery, and other new energy sources are being explored. Lasers and electromagnetic radiation can repair rather than resect injuries and may be more cost effective than instruments.

Immediately after the procedure, the patient spends several hours in the recovery room. An ice pack will be put on the joint that was operated on for up to 48 hours after the procedure. Pain medicine, prescription or non-prescription, is given. The morning after the surgery, the dressing can be removed and replaced by adhesive strips. The patient should call his/her doctor upon experiencing an increase in pain, swelling, redness, drainage or bleeding at the site of the surgery, signs of infection (**headache**, muscle aches, **dizziness**, **fever**), or nausea and vomiting.

It takes several days for the surface **wounds** to heal, and several weeks for the joint to fully recover. Many patients resume their daily activities, including going back to work, within a few days of the procedure. A **rehabilitation** program, including physical therapy, may be suggested to speed recovery and improve the future functioning of the joint.

Complications are rare in arthroscopic surgery, occurring in less than 1% of patients. These include infection and inflammation, blood vessel clots, damage to blood vessels or nerves, and instrument breakage.

ARTIFICIAL BONE

Bone grafts are second only to blood transfusions on America's list of transplants. Artificial bone is becoming an increasing alternative to the two most common types of bone grafts or repairs: the *autografts*, in which a piece of bone is taken from elsewhere in the patient's body (usually the pelvis), or the *allograft* bone transplanted from cadavers; the Red Cross maintains a bone bank for this purpose. A third type of bone-replacement surgery involves titanium and cobalt chromium alloys. Bone is very alive and constantly rebuilds itself. Its porus framework is a composition of collagen protein fibers running through *hydroxyapatite*, a mineral that makes up about 70% of living bone. Due to the fact that there is little ''spare'' bone in the body for use in autografts, possible rejection by the recipient's immune system and the risk of transmitted diseases from cadaver bones, and to find a substance that more closely resembled real bone than the metal alloys, researchers turned to the artificial production of hydroxyapatite.

In the 1960s, Marshall R. Urist, a professor of orthopedic surgery at the University of California, Los Angeles, uncovered the process of bone formation. Improved diagnostic techniques and research into the structure and composition of bone,has led to the development and FDA approval, or pending approval, of a number of synthetic calcium-based bone repair products. The first FDA approval of a synthetic bone implant (or bone void filler) was granted in 1992 to a product called *Pro Osteon*, a calcium phosphate material that mimics hydroxyapatite manufactured from coral through a thermochemical process developed in the 1970s. Because this material remains porus, it acts as a framework through which cells and blood vessels from the natural bone intertwine. This new bone growth connects both ends of the fracture and the body ultimately reabsorbs the synthetic framework. In over 20,000 procedures using this product, there have been zero rejections. Because of its porosity, however, this material lacks the strength needed for weight-bearing bones.

Richard J. Lagow, a chemist at the University of Texas at Austin, developed a way to synthesize hydroxyapatite into a porous and much stronger form suitable for bone replacement, and a denser form similar to tooth enamel. The finished product, a bioceramic called *Megagraft 1000*, is processed by calcium metal, calcium hydroxide, and phosphoric acid reaction at 700 to 850 degrees Celsius. Not only does its porosity invite invasion by blood vessels and cells that gradually break down the implant as new, natural bone grows, the number of ''pores'' can be adjusted to match that of the graft recipient, encouraging faster regrowth of natural bone. In collaboration with professor Joel W. Barlow, a chemical engineer at the same university, Lagow devised a computer-guided laser to generate different bone shapes and sizes with the intention of providing bone ''blanks'' customized for individual patient needs. Hydroxyapatite is also used as a coating for **artificial joints** and prostheses to encourage bone to grow and bind tightly to the implant.

1993 saw FDA approval of *Collagraft*, a hydroxyapatite/tricalcium phosphate and bovine collagen which is mixed with the patients bone marrow. In 1998, Dr. Jay Lieberman, of the University of California, Los Angeles began clinical trials to treat *osteonecrosis* (bone death) of the hip, by inserting a capsule containing *bone-morphogenetic protein* (BMP), into an allograft. BMP, discovered by Urist in 1965, occurs naturally in small quantities in the bone matrix and imitates the bone development process which occurs during fetal development. John M. Wozney with Genetics Institute in Massachusetts, first cloned BMP in 1988—in 1998, more than 30 BMPs have been cloned. Over the next decade, researchers look to tissue-engineered implants for reconstructive skeletal deformities and cell-based therapies for osteoarthritis and osteoporosis. Carbon fiber composites—materials used in skis and tennis rackets—are also being tested for use because the composites resemble bone in both stiffness and flexibility.

ARTIFICIAL HEART

Because the heart functions primarily as a pump to keep blood circulating through the body, medical researchers have long attempted to develop a mechanical pump to take over its job in the event of damage or disease. In 1935 the French-born surgeon **Alexis Carrel**, and famed American aviator Charles Lindbergh (1902-1974), designed a perfusion pump that kept excised organs, including the heart, alive by circulating blood through them. News reports called this device an ''artificial'' or ''robot'' heart. The first total artificial heart (TAH) was implanted in 1957 in a dog at the Cleveland Clinic by Willem Kolff, a Dutch-born surgeon, and Tetsuzo Akutsu. Kolff later led a medical team at the University of Utah at Salt Lake City in developing the artificial heart. At the urging of another TAH pioneer, **Michael DeBakey**, the United States government, through the National Institutes of Health, established an Artificial Heart Program in 1964 to develop both partial and total artificial heart devices. By 1966, DeBakey had designed and implanted a pneumatically driven component called a Left Ventricular Assist Device (LVAD) to serve the chamber of the heart that pumps blood out into the arteries. This was an important development, for the great majority of severe heart disease is caused by left ventricle failure.

The first human artificial heart implant was carried out by Denton Cooley and his surgical team at the Texas Heart Institute in 1969. The pneumatically driven Dacron-lined plastic heart, designed by Argentine-born Domingo Liotta, was a temporary measure to keep a patient alive until a heart transplant could be performed. Artificial heart implantation captured worldwide headlines in 1982 when the first TAH intended for permanent use was implanted in the chest of a patient on the verge of death—dentist Barney Clark. The procedure was done at the University of Utah by a surgical team headed by William DeVries. The device, called a *Jarvik-7*, was designed by American physician **Robert Jarvik**. The plastic and titanium pump was powered by compressed air delivered by a large external air compressor through two tubes that passed into the body via incisions in the abdomen. Clark survived for 112 days. DeVries then joined the staff at Humana Hospital in Louisville, Kentucky, where he carried out four other Jarvik-7 implants during 1984 and 1985. Each of these patients also died, including William Schroeder, who suffered a repeated series of debilitating setbacks during his 620-day struggle to survive. The results of permanent implantation of the Jarvik-7 revealed its insurmountable limitations: it caused blood clots to form, which traveled to the brain and precipitated stroke; the abdominal incisions provided a pathway for infection-causing bacteria; and the patient's mobility was severely restricted by the cumbersome compressor. These problems and the concurrent development of successful heart transplantation, permanent installation of the Jarvik-7 and any other TAHs rapidly fell out of use, especially after Schroeder's death in 1986.

At the same time as heart transplantation became an established procedure for terminal heart disease, demand for donor hearts outstripped supply. In 1998, more than 50,000 Americans could benefit from a heart transplant while the available number of donor hearts remains steady at approximately 2,000. The mechanical heart thus became a ''bridge for transplantation''—a last resort to keep a patient alive until a donor heart became available. Meanwhile, research focuses on a new generation of electrically powered artificial hearts, both TAHs and LVADs which use portable battery packs to transmit power via radio signals through unbroken skin to an implanted mechanical heart pump. The first of these devices was experimentally implanted in a human subject in 1991. While no significant progress has been made, two groups of researchers are working under the National Heart Lung and Blood Institute contract program. One group—The Texas Heart Institute and ABIOMED, Inc., anticipates clinical trials of a new TAH by the year 2000. The second—Pennsylvania State University College of Medicine and 3M Health Care—foresees formal testing of a long-term (two-year) LVAD beginning in 1998. A third study at the University of Pittsburgh Artificial Heart Program aims at improving fluid dynamics in artificial hearts by minimizing reverse blood flow within the pump which causes blood clots.

See also Barnard, Christiaan

ARTIFICIAL HEART VALVE

Heart valves are flaps of tissue within the heart that open to allow blood to flow from one of the heart's four chambers to the next and then close to prevent any blood from leaking back. When any one of the heart's four valves becomes too diseased or damaged to function adequately, the only effective treatment is valve replacement. This was not possible until the advent of **open-heart surgery** in the 1950s. Researchers then set out to design a valve that could be easily implanted and tolerated by surrounding tissue, would not promote clot formation, and would be durable. A precursor of the artificial heart valve was developed by American surgeon Charles A. Hufnagel (1916-), who inserted a tube-and-float device in a patient's descending *aorta* in 1952, to prevent aortic backflow. An artificial cardiac aortic valve (a caged-ball device) was implanted into a human being in March 1960 by Dwight Harken at Peter Bent Brigham Hospital in Boston. This was followed shortly by a total artificial mitral valve replacement (a flexible-leaflet) performed by Nina Braunwald at the National Institutes of Health.

The first completely successful artificial heart valve, an invention that became, and remains, a standard in the field, was designed and implanted in a fifty-two-year-old man by surgeons Albert Starr (1926-) and M. L. Edwards in Portland, Oregon, in 1961. This Starr-Edwards valve consisted of a silicone-rubber ball enclosed in a stainless steel cage; today, the valve has a hollow metal ball, an alloy cage, and a Teflon base. Later in the 1960s, the tilting-disc valve was developed. Valve design was improved after the space program produced pyrolite carbon, a strong and durable new material. The St. Jude Medical pivoting bileaflet valve, consisting of two leaflets rotating within a ring, was introduced in 1976. Mechanical heart valves made the headlines in 1990 when Shiley Laboratories recalled all its convexo-concave tilting-disk valves from the market because of the risk of strut fractures that could cause sudden cardiac failure; many patients with other types of Shiley valves wrongly believed their implants were also likely to fail suddenly.

Because of the danger of blood clot formation, implantation of a mechanical heart valve requires that the patient take *anticoagulation* medication for life. Alternatives to artificial valves carry a much lower risk of blood clots and reduce the need for anticoagulation therapy. These include both human and animal valve transplants: Human tissue valves are either *allografts* (or homografts)—valves transplanted from a deceased person whose organs have been donated for transplantation, or *autografts*—in which the pulmonic valve is removed from the patient to replace the abnormal aortic valve and the pulmonic valve is then replaced with an allograft. Animal valve transplants are either *porcine* (pig) or *bovine* (cow) tissue, traditinoally held in place by a stent. In 1997, the United States Food and Drug Administration approved the ''Stentless Toronto SPV Valve,'' a porcine tissue valve manufactured by St. Jude Medical, Inc, which is entirely supported by the patient's aorta. With no stent to take up space, a larger valve can be implanted, improving blood flow.

Artificial limb and joint

Almost four million Americans use artificial limbs, the majority necessitated by amputation resulting from poor circulation caused by diabetes or atheroscleroses. Crude artificial limbs have been used since the earliest loss of an extremity; Greek historian Herodotus mentioned a wooden foot in 500 B.C.; a Roman mosaic depicts a peg-leg; and medieval knights had artificial limbs to improve their appearance. Today, prostheses rival natural limbs both in function and appearance.

The modern era of artificial limbs began with the famous French surgeon Ambroise Paré (1517-1590), a barber-surgeon who, in 1536, became a battlefield surgeon. After devising safer, more effective methods of **amputation**, Paré turned his attention to the design of artificial limbs, exercising great ingenuity and striving to simulate some degree of natural movement. An artificial leg pictured in Paré's *Works of 1575* featured a movable knee joint controlled by a string, a flexible foot operated with a strong spring, and an artificial hand with fingers that moved individually by means of tiny internal cogs and levers. As the many nineteenth-century wars created a larger demand, more sophisticated devices were invented. The most significant impetus for improvement in prosthetic design was the birth in the early 1960s of babies with vestiges of arms, a birth defect caused by a drug called *thalidomide* often prescribed to pregnant women. Artificial arms powered by carbon dioxide were developed for these children. Modern limbs include electric arms which use a small battery, others controlled by a tiny switch, and the *myoelectric prostheses* which uses electrical impulses detected by small electrodes placed on the skin over the remaining arm muscles. Artificial legs can be fitted with spring-loaded feet, artificial feet constructed with toes, synthetic coverings made to match skin tone and hair patterns, and electrodes in the artificial limb leading to the natural skin which allows the brain to register ''feeling'' in the prosthesis. Artificial limbs take advantage of plastics and fiberglass for enhanced strength and comfort.

Joints are the movable points where two bones come together—as at the knee or shoulder. Surgical joint replacement-*-joint arthroplasty*—began in the 1950s. Today, more than 500,000 joint repairs and replacements are performed in the U.S. each year, including 20,000 new cases of hip *osteonecrosis* (bone death). The first total knee arthroplasty was performed in 1951; 10 years later the first total hip replacement occurred, and shoulder replacements began in the 1960s. Artificial joints are secured either by cement or ''bone ingrowth,'' a process in which the natural bone grows into the porous surface of the a prosthesis. In 1998, Dr. Jay Lieberman, of the University of California, Los Angeles began clinical trials to treat osteonecrosis of the hip by inserting a capsule containing *bone-morphogenetic protein* (BMP) into an allograft (implant of purified human bone). Total hip replacements are metal and have a limited life span—BMP, which occurs naturally in small quantities in the bone matrix, imitates the bone development process which occurs during fetal development. Researchers believe BMP may reducing the need for total hip replacement. John M. Wozney with Genetics Institute in Massachusetts, first cloned BMP in 1988—in early 1998, more than 30 BMPs were cloned. 1998 also saw results of a seven-year study in which cells from a patient's healthy cartilage are transplanted into the damaged portion of the knee joint, regenerating cartilage and reducing the need for knee replacement. Researchers look ahead to tissue-engineered implants and cell-based therapies for degenerative diseases such as osteoarthritis and osteoporosis. Research is ongoing to improve prosthetic materials, surgical techniques, ways of securing joints, and postoperative mobility.

Artificial skin

Artificial skin, a synthetic equivalent to human skin, can dramatically increase the chance of survival of severely burned patients. The first synthetic skin was invented by John F. Burke, chief of Trauma Services at Massachusetts General Hospital, and Ioannis V. Yannas, chemistry professor at Massachusetts Institute of Technology. Seeing so many burn victims during his career, Burke had long been seeking a replacement for human skin that would prevent infection and dehydration. Meanwhile, Ioannis Yannas had been studying collagen, a protein found in human skin. Teaming up during the 1970s, the two found that collagen fibers and a long sugar molecule (called a polymer) could be combined to form a porous material that resembled skin and, when placed on wounds of lab animals, seemed to encourage the growth of new skin cells around it. The pair then created a kind of artificial skin using polymers from shark cartilage and collagen from cowhide. Using their synthetic material, called *Silastic*, Burke and Yannas continued experimenting and found that artificial skin acts like a framework onto which new skin tissue and blood vessels grow, although these new cells are unable to produce hair follicles or sweat glands normally formed in the dermis. As the new skin grows, the cowhide and shark substances from the artificial skin are broken down and absorbed by the body. In 1979 Burke and Yannas used their artificial skin on their first patient, a woman who had suffered burns over half her body. After peeling away her burned skin, Burke applied a layer of artificial skin and, where possible, grafted to it some of her own unburned skin. Three weeks later, the woman's new skin, the same color as her unburned skin, was growing at an amazingly healthy rate.

Meanwhile, at nearby Harvard University, Howard Green had begun culturing human skin cells under sterile conditions and growing a sheet of human epidermis cells from a tiny piece of a person's skin. However, when the cultured skin was placed on a wound it was rejected by the body's immune system. Green later began work with Eugene Bell of MIT who founded a research group called Organogenesis. The goal of this Boston-based firm was to make artificial skin that would include an epidermis layer and solve the problem of rejection. This research has produced a product called *Graftskin*—a living skin equivalent made of purified bovine collagen into which dermal cells from infant boys' foreskin have been ''seeded.'' On top of that layer is an epidermal layer of the cultured human skin cells. It is formed into 4 × 8 in (10 × 20 cm) sheets that can be sutured or stapled onto a patient during surgery. No rejection was seen in clinical trials. Hospital trials included burn victims, patients needing skin grafts after cancer surgery, and those with chronic nonhealing wounds. In January, 1998, this multilayered, tissue-engineered skin trade marked *Apligraf* received unconditional recommendation from the FDA advisory panel for treating venous leg ulcers, making it the first living manufactured organ ever recommended for approval by the FDA. (A welcome side benefit of this research is that it can be used to test dermatological products without testing on animals.)

Another company in California, Advanced Tissue Sciences, engineers a product called *Dermagraft* using a similar method, producing 250,000 square feet of final product from one foreskin. In a study of 85 burn patients, Dermagraft, used as a temporary skin until permanent skin grafts could be done, cut the need for surgery in half and reduced hospital stays my months. Hy-Gene, Inc. in New Jersey, clones a patient's own skin cells producing an epidermis about 10 layers thick. In three weeks, a small patch of cloned skin can grow enough to cover an entire human from head to toe. This product was patented and went into clinical trials in November, 1997. A fourth company, Integra Life Sciences, does not clone skin but manufactures a matrix from collagen and shark cartilage with appropriate pore size and absorption rate for a wide range of human body parts. The environment of this lattice-like structure ''tricks'' the body into growing replacement tissue.

Aspirin

Aspirin is a medicine that relieves minor aches and pains and reduces **fever**. It is used for **headache**s, toothaches, muscle pain, menstrual cramps, joint pain from arthritis, and in adults for aches associated with colds and flu. Some people take aspirin daily to reduce the risk of **stroke**, **heart attack**, or other heart problems.

Aspirin, also known as acetylsalicylic acid, is sold over the counter and comes in many forms, from the familiar white tablets to chewing gum to rectal suppositories. Coated, chewable, buffered, and extended release forms are available. Many other over-the-counter combination medicines contain aspirin as one of their active ingredients.

Aspirin belongs to a group of drugs called salicylates. Other members of this group include sodium salicylate, choline salicylate, and magnesium salicylate. These drugs are more expensive and no more effective than aspirin. However, they are a little easier on the stomach. Aspirin is quickly absorbed into the bloodstream and provides quick and relatively long-lasting pain relief. Aspirin also reduces inflammation. Researchers believe these effects come about because aspirin blocks the production of pain-producing chemicals called prostaglandins.

Besides relieving pain and reducing inflammation, aspirin also lowers fever by acting on the part of the brain that regulates temperature. The brain then signals the blood vessels to widen, which allows heat to leave the body more quickly.

Although it is a common over-the-counter medication, aspirin, even children's aspirin, should never be given to children or teenagers with flu-like symptoms or **chickenpox**. In children, aspirin can cause **Reye's syndrome**, a life-threatening condition that affects the nervous system and liver. As many as 30% of children and teenagers who develop Reye's syndrome die. Those who survive may have permanent brain damage.

No one should take aspirin for more than 10 days in a row unless told to by a physician. Anyone with fever should not take aspirin for more than 3 days without a physician's consent. Do not to take more than the recommended daily dosage. Check with a physician before giving aspirin to a child under 12 years for arthritis, rheumatism, or any condition that requires long-term use of the drug.

Some people should never use aspirin without first checking with their physician. These include pregnant women, women who are breastfeeding (aspirin can pass into breast milk), people with a history of bleeding problems, people who are taking blood-thinning drugs such as warfarin (Coumadin), people with a history of **ulcers**, and people with a history of **asthma** or nasal polyps. People who are allergic to fenoprofen, ibuprofen, indomethacin, ketoprofen, meclofenamate sodium, naproxen, sulindac, tolmetin, or the orange food-coloring tartrazine may also be allergic to aspirin.

People with **AIDS** or AIDS-related complex who are taking AZT (zidovudine) should avoid aspirin because it can increase the risk of bleeding. People with liver damage or severe kidney failure also should not take aspirin.

Aspirin should not be taken before surgery, as it can increase the risk of excessive bleeding. Because of this risk, do not take aspirin daily over long periods to reduce the risk of stroke or heart attack, for example unless advised to do so by a physician.

The most common side effects or aspirin are stomachache, heartburn, loss of appetite, and small amounts of blood in stools. Less common side effects are **rashes**, **hives**, fever, vision problems, liver damage, thirst, stomach ulcers, and bleeding. People who are allergic to aspirin or those who have asthma, **rhinitis**, or polyps in the nose may have trouble breathing after taking aspirin.

It may increase, decrease, or change the effects of many drugs. Aspirin can make drugs such as methotrexate (Rheumatrex) and valproic acid (Depakote, Depakene) more toxic. If taken with blood-thinning drugs, such as warfarin (Coumadin) and dicumarol, aspirin can increase the risk of excessive bleeding. Aspirin counteracts the effects of other drugs, such as angiotensin-converting enzyme (ACE) inhibitors and **beta blockers** that lower blood pressure, and medicines used to treat **gout** (probenecid and sulfinpyrazone). Blood pressure may drop unexpectedly and cause **fainting** or dizziness if aspirin is taken along with nitroglycerin tablets. Aspirin may also interact with **diuretics**, diabetes medicines, other **nonsteroidal anti-inflammatory drugs** (ibuprofen), seizure medications, and steroids. Anyone who is taking these drugs should ask his or her physician whether they can safely take aspirin.

Assistive Devices

There is a variety of equipment developed specifically for individuals with disabilities to make the activities of their daily living easier. These tools, known as assistive devices, help maintain or improve the ability of a disabled individual to perform regular functions such as bathing, dressing, opening doors, reading, writing, and eating. For example, an individual with impaired use of the upper extremities would benefit from the use of writing grips, jar openers, weighted utensils, or nonslip placemats.

Technological advances make it easier for an individual with a disability to work inside or outside the home or pursue an education. For example, computer equipment such as Braille printers enable the visually impaired to read computer printouts; and touch screens or switches allow computer access through eye blinks or head or neck movements. Vehicle modifications include wheelchair lifts and hand controls for driving. An assistive technology device may be funded by outside agencies if the device is necessary for the individual to achieve his or her vocational goal.

A variety of assistive devices also make life easier for those with **hearing loss**. These devices can be used in conjunction with a hearing aid (or in place of one), and can be grouped into one of three categories: 1) Amplifying devices: These are connected to a sound source, such as a TV or radio, and transmit the sound to a set of headphones; controls allow for adjustment of volume or pitch without interfering with the sound coming from the speaker. Inexpensive models use a long cord to connect to the amplifier and headphones, though wireless systems allow more freedom of movement. An amplifier for the telephone receiver allows for volume adjustment in hearing the caller. 2) Alerting devices: These use a very loud noise, flashing lights, or a vibrator attached to the wrist or bed to communicate; more advanced systems use a built-in microphone to listen for specific sounds that then trigger an alert. These devices can be programmed to flash or sound differently in conjunction with the telephone, doorbell, alarm clock, smoke detector, clothes dryer, or oven. 3) Decoding devices: These convert audio into written text that scrolls across a television screen. All news and prime time programs, as well as many syndicated television shows and videos, are closed captioned in this way. There are also specialized teletypewriters (TTYs) that convert telephone audio into written text to facilitate conversation. Most audiologists and medical supply stores carry or can order assistive devices for individuals with a hearing impairment. Prices range from approximately $25 for a basic telephone amplifier to more than $300 for a TTY.

An evaluation by a competent specialist, conducted whenever possible in the environment where the technology will be used, will help determine the appropriate options from which the person can choose. Evaluators may come from different disciplines. A speech pathologist, or one who specializes in **speech therapy**, may evaluate the need for an augmentative/alternative communication device, while a specialist in **physical therapy** or **occupational therapy** would evaluate the need for a customized, motorized wheelchair. The range of assistive technology devices is constantly expanding to meet the functional needs of individuals with disabilities.

See also Hearing loss; Physical therapy; Speech therapy; Occupational therapy

Asthma

Asthma is a chronic (long-lasting) inflammatory disease of the airways. It causes the airways to narrow periodically. This produces **wheezing** and breathlessness. Obstruction to air flow either stops spontaneously or responds to treatment, but continuing inflammation makes the airways hyper-responsive to stimuli such as cold air, **exercise**, dust mites, air pollution, **stress**, and **anxiety**.

About 10 million Americans have asthma, and the number seems to be increasing. Between 1982-92, the rate rose by 42% and the **death** rate from asthma increased by 35%.

Changes that take place in the respiratory system of an asthmatic person make the airways (the *bronchi* and the smaller *bronchioles*) reactive to stimuli that don't affect healthy people. In an asthma attack, the muscle tissue in the walls of bronchi spasm, and the cells lining the airways swell and secrete mucus into the air spaces. Both these actions cause the airways to narrow which makes breathing more difficult. Many asthmatics react to such as pollen, house dust mites, or animal dander. These are called allergens. On the other hand, asthma affects many people who do not respond to these allergens in this way.

Asthma often begins in childhood or adolescence, but it also may first appear during adult years. When asthma begins in childhood, it often is due to a hereditary sensitivity to allergens. Allergens also play a role when adults become asthmatic. Exposure to toxic fumes or industrial pollution can cause adult onset asthma. Other adults may have asthma caused by **sinusitis**, nasal polyps, or sensitivity to **aspirin** and related drugs.

Because avoiding or minimizing exposure to allergens is the most effective way of treating asthma, it is important to identify which allergen is causing symptoms. In some people, symptoms are worsened by **rhinitis**, sinusitis, acid reflux, or respiratory viral infections (colds). Exposure to tobacco smoke or dust can also trigger an asthma attack. In other people, breathing cold air, exercise, and stress trigger attacks.

Besides wheezing and shortness of breath, the person with asthma may **cough** and feel a tightness in the chest. Wheezing is often loudest when the patient breathes out, in an attempt to expel used air through the narrowed airways. Some asthmatics are free of symptoms most of the time but may occasionally be short of breath (acute asthma). Others spend much time coughing and wheezing or have continual cold-like symptoms (chronic asthma).

Shortness of breath may cause anxiety. The asthmatic may sit upright, lean forward, use the muscles of the neck and chest wall to help breathe and be unable to speak. Confusion and a bluish tint to the skin are signs that emergency treatment is needed immediately.

Asthma is diagnosed by family history of asthma or **allergies** and a physical examination. A test called spirometry measures how rapidly air is exhaled and how much is retained in the lungs. Repeating the test after the patient inhales a drug that widens the air passages (a bronchodilator) shows whether the airway narrowing is reversible, which is a typical finding in asthma.

Often, it is difficult to determine what triggers asthma attacks. Allergy skin testing may be done, although an allergic skin response does not always mean that the allergen is causing the asthma. A **chest x ray** helps rule out other respiratory disorders. People with asthma should periodically have their lung function measured by spirometry to monitor their lung function and response to treatment.

Drugs used to treat asthma include the anti-inflammatory drugs such as theophylline and **bronchodilators** such as albuterol. Steroids are also used to block inflammation and are extremely effective in relieving symptoms of asthma. However, their long-term use can cause numerous unacceptable side-effects

Leukotriene modifiers are a new type of drug that can be used in place of steroids in older children or adults who have a mild degree of asthma that persists. They work by counteracting substances released by white blood cells in the airways that cause the passages to constrict and secrete mucus. Other anti-inflammatory drugs such as cromolyn and nedocromil are used to prevent asthmatic attacks over the long term in children.

Severe asthma attacks should be treated quickly. The patient suffering an acute attack may need extra oxygen. Medication to expand the breathing tubes is inhaled repeatedly or continuously. If the patient does not respond promptly and completely, a steroid is given. Rarely, it may be necessary to use a mechanical ventilator to help the patient breathe.

Long-term asthma treatment is based using an inhaler that meters a dose of medication to expand the airways. Patients should be taught how to monitor their symptoms so that they will know when an attack is starting. Infants, young children, and the elderly may need special help in managing their asthma.

Most patients with asthma respond well when to drug therapy, and lead relatively normal lives. More than half of affected children stop having attacks by the time they reach age 21. Many others have less frequent and less severe attacks as they grow older. A minority of patients have progressively more trouble breathing and run the risk of **respiratory failure** without intensive treatment.

Astigmatism

Astigmatism is the result of the inability of the cornea to properly focus an image on the retina of the eye. The result is a blurred image.

The cornea is the outermost part of the eye. It is a transparent layer that covers the colored part of the eye (iris), pupil, and lens. The cornea bends light and helps to focus it onto the retina where specialized cells (photo receptors) detect light and transmit nerve impulses via the optic nerve to the brain where the image is formed. The cornea is dome shaped. Any incorrect shaping of the cornea results in an incorrect focusing of the light that passes through that part of the cornea.

Astigmatism is an image distortion that results from an improperly shaped cornea. Usually the cornea is spherical, like a baseball. In astigmatism, the cornea is elliptically shaped, more like a football. This causes a point of light will have two points of focus, instead of one nice sharp image on the retina.

This double focus results in blurry vision. What the blur looks like depends upon the amount and the direction of the astigmatism. A person with nearsightedness (myopia) or farsightedness (hyperopia) may see a dot as a blurred circle. A person with astigmatism may see the same dot as a blurred oval or frankfurter-shaped blur. In addition to blurring, people with astigmatism may also experience **headaches** and eyestrain.

Some cases of astigmatism are caused by problems in the lens of the eye. Minor variations in the curvature of the lens can produce minor degrees of astigmatism called lenticular astigmatism. In these patients, the cornea is usually normal in shape. Infants, as a group, have the least amount of astigmatism. Astigmatism may increase during childhood, as the eye is developing.

Regular astigmatism may be caused by the weight of the upper eyelid resting on the eyeball creating distortion, surgical incisions in the cornea, trauma or scarring to the cornea, or the presence of tumors in the eyelid. Irregular astigmatism can be caused by scarring or keratoconus.

Keratoconus is a condition in which the cornea thins and becomes cone shaped. It usually occurs around **puberty**, and is more common in women. Although the causes of keratoconus are unknown, it may be hereditary or a result of chronic eye rubbing, as in people with **allergies**.

Diabetes plays a role in the development of astigmatism. High blood sugar levels can cause shape changes in the lens of the eye. This process usually occurs slowly, and often is noticed only when the diabetic has started treatment to control his blood sugar. The return to more normal blood sugar levels allows the lens to return to normal and this change is sometimes noticed by the patient as farsightedness. Because of this, diabetics should wait until their blood sugar is under control for at least one month to allow vision to stabilize before being measured for eyeglasses.

A variety of tests can be used to detect astigmatism during an eye exam. The patient may be asked to describe the astigmatic dial, a series of lines that radiate outward from a center. People with astigmatism will see some of the lines more clearly than others. One diagnostic instrument used is the keratometer. This measures the curvature of the central cornea. A keratoscope projects a series of concentric light rings onto the cornea. Misshapen areas of the cornea are revealed by noting areas of the light pattern that do not appear concentric on the cornea. Because these instruments are measuring the cornea, it is important to have a refraction in case the lens is also contributing to the astigmatism. A refraction is when the patient looks at an eye chart and the doctor puts different lenses in front of the patient's eyes and asks which one looks better.

Astigmatism can be treated by the use of cylindrical eyeglasse lenses or contact lenses. Lenses are shaped to counteract the shape of the sections of cornea that are causing the difficulty. There is some debate as to whether people with very small amounts of astigmatism should be treated. Generally, if vision is good and the patient experiences no overt symptoms, treatment is not necessary. When treating larger amounts of astigmatism or astigmatism for the first time, the doctor may not totally correct the astigmatism. The cylindrical correction in the eyeglasses may make the floor appear to tilt, thus making it difficult for the patient at first.

Contact lenses that are used to correct astigmatism are called toric lenses. When a person blinks, the contact lens rotates. In toric lenses, it is important for the lens to return to the same position each time. Hard and soft toric lenses are available in a variety of prescriptions, materials, and even in tints.

In 1997, the Food and Drug Administration (FDA) approved laser treatment of astigmatism. Patients considering this should make sure the surgeon has a lot of experience in the procedure and discuss the possible side effects or risks with the doctor. In the case of keratoconus, a corneal transplant is performed if the astigmatism can not be corrected with hard contact lenses.

Astigmatism is a condition that may be present at birth. It may also be acquired if something distorts the cornea. Vision can generally be corrected with eyeglasses or contact lenses. The major risks of surgery (aside from the surgical risks) are over and under correction of the astigmatism. There is no cure for over correction. Under correction can be solved by repeating the operation.

ASTROLOGY AND MEDICINE

Until the last few centuries, astrology was strongly linked with the practice of medicine. Astrology is a type of **divination** in which the stars and planets are thought to reveal the cause of human illness as well as to suggest appropriate cures. The idea that the human body mimics the universe on a smaller scale, and therefore can be influenced by it, is found in many cultures.

In the western world, early references to the influence of the stars and planets on human health date to the fifth century B.C. Ancient Egyptians believed that different body parts were under the influence of different signs of the Zodiac. This belief spread into Europe through Greece, and in the fourth century B.C. were seen in **Hippocrates**' writings. Astrology was an important part of medicine until the end of the 17th century when it began to be replaced by scientific theories of disease.

Astrology is based on observations of 12 constellations, the sun, the moon, and the planets. The constellations correspond with the 12 signs of the zodiac: Aries, Taurus, Gemini, Cancer, Leo, Virgo, Libra, Scorpio, Sagittarius, Capricorn, Aquarius, and Pisces. With regard to medicine, each zodiac sign was said to govern or rule a different part (or parts) of the body. For example, Aries was linked to the head, face, ears, eyes, and mouth. Great significance was attached to the position of the planets and the moon in relation to the zodiac constellations. Interpreting this information involved complex sets of rules that were laid out in the medical texts of the day. In general, to diagnose an illness, a physician would find out in which constellation the moon appeared when his patient first became ill. By figuring out which planets were affecting the moon during that time period, he would consult the astrological rules and make a diagnosis. Some physicians would also predict the outcome of a patient's illness using astrology.

Treatment of an illness could also be determined by the movement of the stars, moon, and planets. Just as zodiac constellations were linked to specific body parts, planets were associated with healing plants and herbs. To be effective, these plants and herbs had to be collected during the times in which their associated planets were visible. These times were calculated from an almanac in which the rising and setting times of planets were given. To gather the plants and herbs at any other times would prevent them from being effective.

Other treatments besides herbal remedies might also be governed by astrological signs. For example, **bleeding**, a common medical procedure until the early 19th century, should only have been done when the moon was in a particular constellation.

The link between astrology and medicine began to loosen when physicians and scientists learned more about the body and the factors that caused disease. However, the relationship of astrology with medicine endures to today, for example, in the field of medical astrology.

ASYLUMS

For centuries, the mentally ill have been treated with a combination of fear, disgust and shame. In many cultures throughout history, a person who was mentally ill was believed to be evil or possessed; punishment, not humane treatment, typically followed.

The earliest known mental hospitals were found in the Middle East in Baghdad and Cairo. By 1247, the notorious British madhouse known as Bedlam was built, in which the mentally ill were routinely shackled and treated as a sort of sideshow for the general public.

As witchcraft hysteria grew and spread throughout Europe and colonial North America between the 15th and 17th centuries, the widespread general suspicion of the times did not bode well for the mentally ill. During this period, their cruel treatment was based on the conviction that the mentally ill were surely possessed. In Bedlam and in the French asylum Bicetre during this time, inmates were considered to be less than human and their treatment was aimed at protecting society from their odd behavior.

In Colonial America before the establishment of any asylums, the insane were often auctioned off to be cared for by farmers, while others were sent to the poorhouse or driven out of town. Eventually, the first mental asylum in Colonial America was established in Williamsburg, Va. in 1773; 20 years later the French social reformer Philippe Pinel horrified sane Frenchmen by removing the shackles from some inmates at Bicetre.

It was not until the 19th century that the personal crusade of American reformer Dorothea Dix led to the establishment of more humane mental asylums in the United States, Canada and England.

While the primary emphasis on these reforms was better care for the mentally ill, the result was the establishment of centralized state-run asylums that still isolated patients from family and friends and too often mistreated and abused patients.

In the beginning of the 20th century, a more modern, humane approach to mental health care began to gather momentum. Following the two world wars and the creation of many post-traumatic mental problems, the mental health movement continued to gather interest throughout the country. The development of a whole new range of drugs to treat mental illness further changed the outlook for mental problems.

Within the past 20 years, laws recognizing the rights of the mentally ill to treatment in the least restrictive environment heralded the close of many of the old, Victorian asylums in favor of outpatient mental health clinics and local treatment centers.

ATELECTASIS

Atelectasis is a collapse of lung tissue affecting part or all of one lung. This condition prevents normal oxygen absorption by the blood as it passes through the lungs.

Atelectasis can result from an obstruction (blockage) of the airways. This causes the tiny air sacs in the lung, called alveoli, to collapse. These sacs are very thin-walled and contain a rich blood supply. Their function is to increase the surface area where the exchange of oxygen for carbon dioxide can take place as blood passes through the lungs. When the airways are blocked by a mucus plug, a foreign object, or tumor, the alveoli are unable to fill with air, and the surface area for oxygen-carbon dioxide exchange is decreased. Collapse of the alveoli can occur in any area of the lung.

Atelectasis is a potential complication following surgery, especially in people who have undergone chest or abdominal operations. Congenital atelectasis can result from a failure of the lungs to expand at birth. This is a special concern in premature babies. The congenital condition may be localized or may affect all of both lungs.

Causes of atelectasis include insufficient attempts at respiration by the newborn, bronchial obstruction, and absence of surfactant (a substance secreted by alveoli that maintains the stability of lung tissue by reducing the surface tension of fluids that coat the lung). The lack of surfactant reduces the surface area available for effective gas exchange.

Pressure on the lung from fluid or air can cause atelectasis. So can obstruction of airways by thick mucus that develops with some infections and lung diseases. Tumors and inhaled objects can also cause obstruction of the airway, leading to atelectasis.

Anyone undergoing chest or abdominal surgery using general **anesthesia** is at risk to develop atelectasis, since breathing is often shallow after surgery to avoid **pain** from the surgical incision. Any significant decrease in airflow to the alveoli allows secretions to collect, which increases the chance of infection. Chest injuries causing shallow breathing, including fractured ribs, can also cause atelectasis.

Common symptoms of atelectasis include **shortness of breath** and decreased chest wall expansion. If atelectasis only affects a small area of the lung, symptoms are usually minimal. If the condition affects a large area of the lung and develops quickly, the individual may turn blue or pale, have trouble breathing, and feel a stabbing pain on the affected side. **Fever** and increased heart rate may occur if infection accompanies atelectasis.

Atelectasis can be diagnosed by a thorough **physical examination**. When the doctor listens to the lungs through a stethoscope, diminished or bronchial breath sounds may be heard. By tapping on the chest while listening through the stethoscope, the doctor can often tell if the lung is collapsed. A **chest x ray** that shows an airless area in the lung confirms the diagnosis. If an obstruction of the airways is suspected, a computed tomography scan (CT) or bronchoscopy may be performed. In a bronchoscopy, a device with a camera is inserted through the airways to detect a blockage.

If atelectasis is due to obstruction of the airway, the first step in treatment is to remove the cause of the blockage. This may be done by coughing, suctioning, or bronchoscopy. If a tumor causes the blockage, surgery may be necessary to remove it. **Antibiotics** are commonly used to fight the infection that often accompanies atelectasis. In cases where recurrent or long-lasting infection is disabling or where significant bleeding occurs, the affected section of the lung may be surgically removed.

If atelectasis is caused by a mucus plug or inhaled foreign object, the patient usually recovers completely when the blockage is removed. If it is caused by a tumor, the outcome depends on the nature of the tumor involved

When recovering from surgery, frequent repositioning in bed along with coughing and deep breathing exercises help keep the lungs clear. Breathing exercises and breathing devices, such as a spirometer that measures air flow, encourage the lungs to expand. Although smokers have a higher risk of developing atelectasis following surgery, stopping smoking six to eight weeks before surgery can help reduce the risk. Increasing fluid intake during respiratory illness or after surgery helps lung secretions to remain loose. Increasing humidity may also be beneficial. Postural drainage techniques can be learned from a respiratory therapist or physical therapist and are a useful tool for anyone affected with a illness that could cause atelectasis.

ATHEROSCLEROSIS

Atherosclerosis is the build up of a waxy plaque on the inside of blood vessels that affects only the inner lining of an artery and is characterized by plaque deposits that block the flow of blood. It is often called arteriosclerosis. Atherosclerosis, a progressive process responsible for most heart disease, is a type of arteriosclerosis or hardening of the arteries.

Plaque is made of fatty substances, cholesterol, waste products from the cells, calcium, and fibrin, a stringy material that helps blood to clot. As the inner layer of the artery wall thickens, the artery's diameter is reduced, and blood flow and oxygen delivery are decreased. Plaques can rupture or crack open, causing the sudden formation of a blood clot (thrombosis). Atherosclerosis can cause a **heart attack** if it completely blocks the blood flow in the heart (coronary) arteries. It can cause a **stroke** if it completely blocks the brain (carotid) arteries. Atherosclerosis can also occur in the arteries of the neck, kidneys, thighs, and arms, causing kidney failure or **gangrene** that leads to **amputation**.

Atherosclerosis can begin in the late teens, but it usually takes decades to cause symptoms. Some people experience rapidly progressing atherosclerosis during their thirties, others during their fifties or sixties. Atherosclerosis is complex. Its exact cause is still unknown, however a person who has high cholesterol, high blood pressure, and smokes cigarettes is eight times more likely to develop atherosclerosis than someone who does not have these risk factors. Physical inactivity, diabetes, and **obesity** also increase the risk of atherosclerosis. Many of these risk factors can be eliminated by lifestyle changes.

Some risk factors cannot be changed. These include heredity, age, gender, and ethnicity. People whose parents have

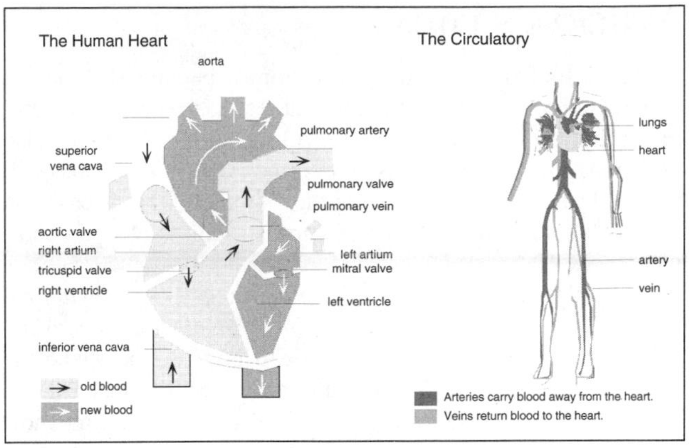

The progression of atherosclerosis. ***(Illustration by Hans & Cassady, Inc.)***

coronary artery disease, atherosclerosis, or stroke at an early age are at increased risk. The high rate of severe **hypertension** among African-Americans puts them at increased risk. Risk is higher in men who are 45 years of age and older and women who are 55 years of age and older.

Symptoms differ depending upon the location of the atherosclerosis, but include chest **pain**, heart attack, or sudden **death, dizziness**, weakness, loss of speech, blindness, disease of the blood vessels in the outer parts of the body (peripheral vascular disease), and high blood pressure that is difficult to treat.

Physicians may be able to diagnose atherosclerosis during a physical exam by means of a stethoscope and gentle probing of the arteries with the hand (palpation). More definite tests are **electrocardiography**, **echocardiography** or ultrasonography of the arteries, radionuclide scans, and **angiography**. Coronary angiography is the most accurate diagnostic method and the only one that requires entering the body (invasive procedure).

Treatment for atherosclerosis includes lifestyle changes, lipid-lowering drugs, coronary **angioplasty** (a non-surgical procedure in which a catheter tipped with a balloon is threaded from a blood vessel in the thigh into the blocked artery), and coronary artery bypass surgery. Atherosclerosis requires lifelong care.

Patients who have less severe atherosclerosis may achieve adequate control through lifestyle changes and drug therapy. Many of the lifestyle changes help prevent the disease and promote good health. Most of the drugs prescribed for atherosclerosis seek to lower cholesterol. Alternative therapies that focus on diet and lifestyle can help prevent, retard, or reverse atherosclerosis. These include some herbal therapies, relaxation techniques, and dietary modifications.

Atherosclerosis can be successfully treated but not cured. Recent clinical studies have shown that atherosclerosis can be delayed, stopped, and even reversed by aggressively lowering cholesterol. New diagnostic techniques enable physicians to identify and treat atherosclerosis in its earliest stages. New technologies and surgical procedures have extended the lives of many patients who would otherwise have died.

Athlete's foot

Athlete's foot is a common condition of peeling skin on the feet caused by a fungal infection that results in the skin becoming itchy, sore, cracked, and peeling. Athlete's foot (also known as foot **ringworm**) is so common that most people will have at least one episode during their lifetime. The disease can be treated, but it can be tenacious and difficult to clear up completely.

Athlete's foot is caused by a the fungi *Trichophyton rubrum*, *T. mentagrophytes*, and *Epidermophyton floccosum*. These fungi live exclusively on dead body tissue (hair, the outer layer of skin, and nails), and grow best in moist, damp, dark places with poor ventilation. The infection occurs most often between the fourth and fifth toes.

Symptoms of athlete's foot include itchy, sore skin on the toes, with scaling, cracking, inflammation, and blisters. Blisters that break, exposing raw patches of tissue, can cause **pain** and swelling. As the infection spreads, **itching** and burning may get worse.

If it's not treated, athlete's foot can spread to the soles of the feet and toenails. Stubborn toenail infections may appear with crumbling, scaling and thickened nails, and nail loss. The infection can spread further if patients scratch and then touch themselves elsewhere (especially in the groin or under the arms). It's also possible to spread the infection to other parts of the body via contaminated bed sheets or clothing.

Many people carry the athlete's foot fungi on their skin. However, these fungi will only grow to the point of causing athlete's foot if conditions are right. Many people believe athlete's foot is highly contagious, especially in public swimming pools and shower rooms. Research has shown, however, that it is difficult to pick up the infection simply by walking barefoot over a contaminated damp floor. Exactly why some people develop the condition and others don't is not well understood.

Sweaty feet, tight shoes, synthetic socks that don't absorb moisture, a warm climate, and not drying the feet well after swimming or bathing, all contribute to the growth of the fungi.

Not all foot **rashes** are athlete's foot, which is why a physician should diagnose the condition before any remedies are used. Using nonprescription products on a rash that is not athlete's foot could make the rash worse.

A dermatologist diagnoses the condition by **physical examination** and by examining a preparation of skin scrapings under a microscope. This test, called a KOH preparation, treats a sample of tissue scraped from the infected area with heat and potassium hydroxide (KOH). This treatment dissolves certain substances in the tissue sample, making it possible to see the fungi under the microscope.

Athlete's foot may be resistant to medication and should not be ignored. Simple cases usually respond well to antifungal creams or sprays (clotrimazole, ketoconazole, miconazole nitrate, sulconazole nitrate, or tolnaftate). If the infection is resistant to treatments placed directly on the skin, the doctor may prescribe oral antifungal drugs. Untreated athlete's foot may lead to a secondary bacterial infection in the skin cracks.

Alternative medical treatments may be appropriate for treating athlete's foot. A footbath containing cinnamon has been shown to slow down the growth of certain molds and fungi, and is said to be very effective in clearing up athlete's foot. Other herbal remedies used externally to treat athlete's foot include a foot soak or powder containing goldenseal (*Hydrastis canadensis*), tea tree oil (*Melaleuca* spp.), or calendula (*Calendula officinalis*) cream to help heal cracked skin.

Athlete's foot usually responds well to treatment, but it is important to use all medication as directed, even if the skin appears to be free of disease. Otherwise, the infection could return. The toenail infections that may accompany athlete's foot, are typically very hard to treat effectively

Good personal hygiene and a few simple precautions such as drying feet thoroughly, avoid tight shoes, shoes worn without socks, wearing bathing shoes in public bathing or showering areas, and using a good quality foot powder can help prevent athlete's foot.

Attention-deficit disorder and Attention deficient hyperactivity disorder

Attention-deficit/hyperactivity disorder (ADHD) is a developmental disorder characterized by distractibility, hyperactivity, impulsive behaviors, and the inability to remain focused on tasks.

ADHD is also known as hyperkinetic disorder (HKD) outside of the United States. It is estimated to affect 3-9% of children, and afflicts boys more often than girls.

Although difficult to assess in infancy and toddlerhood, signs of ADHD may begin to appear as early as age two or three. Children with ADHD have short attention spans, becoming easily bored or frustrated with tasks. Although they may be quite intelligent, their lack of focus frequently results in poor grades and difficulties in school. ADHD children act impulsively, taking action first and thinking later. They constantly move, run, climb, squirm, and fidget, but often have trouble with gross and fine motor skills. Their clumsiness may extend to the social arena, where they are sometimes shunned due to their impulsive and intrusive behavior. Many symptoms, particularly hyperactivity, diminish in early adulthood, but impulsivity and inattention problems remain with up to 50% of ADHD individuals throughout their adult life.

The causes of ADHD are not known. It appears that heredity plays a major role, since children with an ADHD parent or sibling are more likely to develop the disorder themselves. Before birth, ADHD children may have been exposed to poor maternal nutrition, viral infections, or maternal substance abuse. In early childhood, exposure to lead or other toxins can cause ADHD-like symptoms. Traumatic brain injury or neurological disorders may also trigger ADHD symptoms. Although the exact cause of ADHD is not known, an imbalance of certain neurotransmitters, the chemicals in the brain that transmit messages between nerve cells, is believed to be the mechanism behind ADHD symptoms.

The first step in determining if a child has ADHD is to consult with a pediatrician. The pediatrician can make an initial evaluation of the child's developmental maturity compared to other children in his or her age group. The physician should also perform a **physical examination** to rule out any organic causes of ADHD symptoms, such as an overactive thyroid or vision or hearing problems.

If no organic problem can be found, a psychologist, psychiatrist, neurologist, neuropsychologist, or learning specialist is typically consulted to perform a comprehensive ADHD assessment. Public schools are required by federal law to offer free ADHD testing upon request.

Psychosocial therapy, usually combined with medications, is the treatment of choice to alleviate ADHD symptoms. Psychostimulants, such as dextroamphetamine (Dexedrine), pemoline (Cylert), and methylphenidate (Ritalin) are commonly prescribed to control hyperactive and impulsive behavior and increase attention span. They work by stimulating the production of certain neurotransmitters in the brain. Possible side effects of stimulants include nervous tics, irregular heartbeat, loss of appetite, and **insomnia**. However, the medications are usually well-tolerated and safe in most cases.

In children who do not respond well to stimulant therapy, tricyclic antidepressants such as desipramine (Norpramin, Pertofane) and amitriptyline (Elavil) are frequently recommended. Reported side effects of these drugs include persistent dry mouth, sedation, disorientation, and cardiac arrhythmia. Other medications prescribed for ADHD therapy include buproprion (Wellbutrin), fluoxetine (Prozac), and carbamazepine (Tegretol, Atretol). Clonidine (Catapres), an antihypertensive medication, has also been used to control aggression and hyperactivity in some ADHD children, although it should not be used with Ritalin. A child's response to medication will change with age, so symptoms should be monitored and prescriptions adjusted accordingly.

In addition to drugs, behavior modification therapy, which uses a reward system to reinforce good behavior and task completion, can be implemented in the classroom and at home. Behavior modification rewards good behavior until it becomes ingrained. A variation of this technique, cognitive-behavioral therapy, works to decrease impulsive behavior by getting the child to recognize the connection between thoughts and behavior, and to change behavior by changing negative thinking patterns.

A number of alternative treatments exist for ADHD. Although there is a lack of controlled studies to prove their efficacy, proponents report that they are successful in controlling symptoms in some ADHD patients. Some of the more popular alternative treatments include:

- EEG (electroencephalograph) **biofeedback**, dietary therapy, and herbal therapy. The safety of herbal remedies has not been demonstrated in controlled studies. **Homeopathic medicine** is probably the most effective alternative therapy for ADD and ADHD because it treats the whole person at a core level.

Untreated, ADHD negatively affects a child's social and educational performance and can seriously damage his or her sense of self-esteem. ADHD children have impaired relationships with their peers, and may be looked upon as social outcasts. They may be perceived as slow learners or troublemakers in the classroom. Siblings and even parents may develop resentful feelings towards the ADHD child.

Some ADHD children also develop a **conduct disorder** problem. For those adolescents who have both ADHD and a conduct disorder, up to 25% develop antisocial personality disorder and the criminal behavior, substance abuse, and high rate of suicide attempts that are symptomatic of it. Children diagnosed with ADHD are also more likely to have a learning disorder, a mood disorder such as depression, or an anxiety disorder.

Approximately 70-80% of ADHD patients treated with stimulant medication experience significant relief from symptoms, at least in the short-term. About half of ADHD children seem to "outgrow" the disorder in adolescence or early adulthood. The other half will retain some or all symptoms of ADHD as adults.

AUTISM

Autism is a severe disorder of brain function marked by problems with social contact, intelligence, and language, together with ritualistic or compulsive behavior and bizarre responses to the environment. Autism is a lifelong disorder that interferes with the ability to understand what is seen, heard, and touched. This can cause profound problems in personal behavior and in the ability to relate to others.

Autism is a brain disorder that affects the way the brain uses or transmits information. Studies have found abnormalities in several parts of the brain that almost certainly occurred during fetal development. The problem may be centered in the parts of the brain responsible for processing language and information from the senses.

There appears to be a strong genetic basis for autism. Identical twins are more likely to both be affected than non-identical twins. In a family with one autistic child, the chance of having another child with autism is about 1 in 20, much higher than in the normal population.

At least one group of researchers has found a link between an abnormal gene and autism. The gene may be just one of three to five genes that interact in some way to cause the condition. Scientists suspect that a faulty gene or genes might make a person vulnerable to develop autism in the presence of other factors, such as a chemical imbalance, viruses, chemicals, or a lack of oxygen at birth. In a few cases, autistic behavior is caused by a disease.

Autism occurs in as many as 1 or 2 per 1,000 children. It is found four times more often in boys (usually the first-born) and occurs around the world in people of all races and social backgrounds. Autism usually is evident in the first three years of life, although sometimes the condition is not diagnosed until a child enters school.

The severity of the condition varies among individuals, ranging from the most severe (extremely repetitive, self-injurious, and aggressive behavior) to very mild, resembling a personality disorder with some learning disability. About 10% of children with autism have an extraordinary ability in one area, such as in mathematics, memory, music, or art. Such children are known as ''autistic savants'' (formerly ''idiot savants'').

Profound problems with social interaction are the most common symptoms of autism. Infants with the disorder won't cuddle; they avoid eye contact and don't seem to want or need physical affection.

The child with autism may not speak at all. If he does, it is often in single words. He may endlessly repeat words or phrases and may reverse pronouns. Bizarre behavior patterns are very common among autistic children and may include complex rituals, screaming fits, rhythmic rocking, arm flapping, finger twiddling, and crying without tears. Autistic children may play with their own saliva, feces, or urine. They may be self-destructive, biting their own hands, gouging at their eyes, pulling their hair, or banging their head.

Many autistic children seem overwhelmed by their own senses. A child with autism may ignore objects or become obsessed with them. Most autistic children appear to be moderately mentally retarded. They may giggle or cry for no reason, have no fear of real danger, but be terrified of harmless objects.

There is no medical test for autism. Because symptoms are so varied, the condition may go undiagnosed for some time or be confused with other diseases. Autism is diagnosed by observing the child's behavior, communication skills, and social interactions after medical tests have ruled out other possible causes of autistic symptoms.

There is no cure for autism. Treatments are aimed at reducing specific symptoms. Because the symptoms vary widely, there is no single approach that works for every person. A spectrum of interventions include training in music, listening, vision, speech and language, and senses. Special **diets** and medications may also be prescribed.

Studies show that people with autism can improve significantly with proper treatment. A child with autism can learn best with special teachers in a structured program that emphasizes individual instruction, educational, and behavioral treatment.

No single medication has proved highly effective for the major features of autism. A variety of drugs can control self-injurious, aggressive, and other difficult behaviors. Drugs also can control epilepsy, which afflicts up to 20% of people with autism. Most experts recommend a complex treatment regimen that begins early and continues through the teenage years. Behavioral therapies are used in conjunction with medications.

While there is no cure, with appropriate treatment the negative behaviors of autism may improve. Earlier generations placed autistic children in institutions. Today, even severely disabled children can be helped in a less restrictive environment to develop to their highest potential. Many become more responsive to others as they learn to understand the world around them, and some can lead nearly normal lives.

AUTOIMMUNE DISORDERS

Autoimmune disorders are conditions in which a person's **immune system** attacks the body's own cells, causing tissue destruction. Autoimmunity is accepted as the cause of a wide range of disorders and is suspected to be responsible for many more. Autoimmune diseases are classified as either general, in which the autoimmune reaction takes place simultaneously in a number of tissues, or organ specific, in which the autoimmune reaction targets a single organ.

To understand autoimmune disorders, it is helpful to understand the workings of the immune system. The purpose of the immune system is to defend the body against attack by infectious microbes (germs) and **foreign objects**. When the immune system attacks an invader, it is very specific—a particular immune system cell will only recognize and target one type of invader. To function properly, the immune system must not only develop this specialized knowledge of individual invaders, it must also learn how to recognize and not attack cells that belong to the body itself.

Every cell carries protein markers on its surface that identify it in one of two ways: what kind of cell it is (e.g. nerve cell, muscle cell, blood cell, etc.) and to whom that cell belongs. These markers are called major histocompatability complexes (MHCs). When functioning properly, cells of the immune system will not attack any other cell with markers identifying it as belonging to its own body.

If the immune system cells do not recognize the cell as ''self,'' they attach themselves to it and put out a signal that the body has been invaded. This in turn stimulates the production of substances such as antibodies that engulf and destroy the foreign invaders. In the case of autoimmune disorders, the immune system cannot distinguish between ''self'' cells and invader cells. As a result, the same destructive operation is carried out on the body's own cells that would normally be carried out on bacteria, viruses, and other such harmful entities.

The reasons why immune systems become dysfunctional in this way is not well understood. However, most researchers agree that a combination of genetic, environmental, and hormonal factors play a role.

Autoimmune disorders include the **systemic lupus erythematosus**, **rheumatoid arthritis**, Goodpasture's syndrome, Grave's disease, Hashimoto's thyroiditis, pemphigus vulgaris, **myasthenia gravis**, **scleroderma** (also called CREST syndrome), autoimmune hemolytic **anemia**, autoimmune thrombocytopenic purpura, polymyositis, dermatomyositis, **pernicious anemia**, **Sjögren's syndrome**, ankylosing spondylitis, and **vasculitis**. Type I **diabetes mellitus** may be caused by an antibody that attacks and destroys the islet cells of the pancreas that produce insulin. Symptoms these above disorders vary widely.

The principle tool used to diagnose autoimmune diseases is antibody testing. These tests measure the level of antibodies found in the blood and determine if they react with specific antigens that would give rise to an autoimmune reaction.

Treatment of autoimmune diseases is specific to the disease, and usually concentrates on alleviating symptoms rather than correcting the underlying cause. Another aspect of treatment is controlling the inflammatory and proliferative nature of the immune response. This is generally accomplished with two types of drugs. Steroid compounds are used to control inflammation. The proliferative nature of the immune response is controlled with immunosuppressive drugs. These drugs work by inhibiting the replication of cells and, therefore, also suppress non-immune cells. Both drug therapies have potentially serious side effects.

AUTOPSY

An autopsy is an examination of the body after **death** to determine the cause of death. An autopsy is performed by a physician trained in pathology.

Most autopsies advance medical knowledge and provide evidence for legal action. Medically, autopsies determine the exact cause and circumstances of death, discover the pathway of a disease, and provide valuable information to be used in the care of the living. When murder is suspected, a government coroner or medical examiner performs autopsies for legal use. This branch of medical study is called forensic medicine. Forensic specialists investigate deaths resulting from violence or occurring under suspicious circumstances.

Benefits of research from autopsies include the production of new medical information to help understand and better treat diseases such as **toxic shock syndrome** and acquired immunodeficiency syndrome (**AIDS**). Organ donation, which saves the lives of other patients, is also another benefit of autopsies.

When performed for medical reasons, autopsies require formal permission from family members or the legal guardian or the deceased. Autopsies required for legal reasons when a crime is suspected do not need the consent of next of kin. During the autopsy, very concise notes and documentation are made for both medical and legal reasons. Some religious groups prohibit medical autopsies.

An autopsy involves the examination of a deceased's body with a detailed examination of the person's remains. This procedure dates back to the Roman era when few human dissections were performed. Autopsies were utilized, however, to determine the cause of death in criminal cases. At the beginning of the procedure the exterior body is examined, and any scratches, bruises, or penetrations of the skin are noted. Next the internal organs are removed and studied. Tests may be done on the blood to determine if a person was using alcohol, illicit drugs, or prescription medications at the time of death. If poisoning is suspected, additional tests are done. The stomach contents may be analyzed to determine what and when the patient last ate. Conditions such as pregnancy or the presence of diseased tissue are noted. In cases where the person has died by criminal action, the nature of the wounds and their exact location are recorded.

Some pathologists argue that more autopsies are performed than necessary. However, recent studies show that autopsies can detect major findings about a person's health condition that were not suspected when the person was alive. The growing awareness of the influence of genetic factors in disease has also emphasized the importance of autopsies.

Despite the usefulness of autopsies, fewer autopsies have been performed in the United States during the past 10-20 years. A possible reason for this decline is concern about malpractice suits on the part of the treating physician. Other possible reasons are that hospitals are performing fewer autopsies because of the expense or because modern technology, such as **computed tomography** (CT) scans and **magnetic resonance imaging**, can often provide sufficient diagnostic information. Nonetheless, federal regulators and pathology groups have begun to establish new guidelines designed to increase the number and quality of autopsies being performed.

Many experts are concerned that if the number of autopsies increases, hospitals may be forced to charge families a fee for the procedure, as autopsies are not normally covered by insurance companies or Medicare. Yet, according to several pathologists, the benefit of the procedure for families and doctors justified the cost. In medical autopsies, physicians limit the examination to only as much of the body as permitted according to the wishes of the family. In some cases, the findings from autopsies can provide peace of mind for the bereaved family.

Once the autopsy has been completed, the body is prepared for final arrangements according to the family's wishes.

There are some risks to the pathologist of disease transmission from the deceased. Some physicians may refuse to do autopsies on specific patients because of a fear of contracting diseases such as AIDS, **hepatitis**, or **Creutzfeld-Jakob disease**. In most situations the cause of death can be determined from autopsy, although occasionally the results are inconclusive.

AVICENNA (980-1037)

Persian physician

Abu Ali al-Husayn ibn Abd Allah ibn Sina, known in the West as Avicenna, was a highly respected Persian **physician** whose medical treatise, the *Canon of Medicine,* influenced medical practice for centuries. He was born near Bukhara, then the capital of the Persian Samanid dynasty and the intellectual center of Islam. Avicenna's father hired tutors to teach him the Koran and literature, and sent him to the greengrocer to learn arithmetic. So bright that his teachers soon had nothing left to impart to him, Avicenna continued his education on his own, instructing himself in astronomy, mathematics, philosophy, and medicine. At 16 he already had a reputation as an authority in legal and medical matters.

When the Samanid ruler Nuh ibn Mansur fell ill, Avicenna was asked to consult with the court doctors. The ruler recovered, and Avicenna was offered a position at court as a physician, which gave him access to the royal library. Avicenna wrote his first book, a work on philosophy, when he was 21.

Following the death of his father, Avicenna acquired a government post. But in the wake of impending Samanid defeat at the hands of the Turks, Avicenna left Bukhara. He took

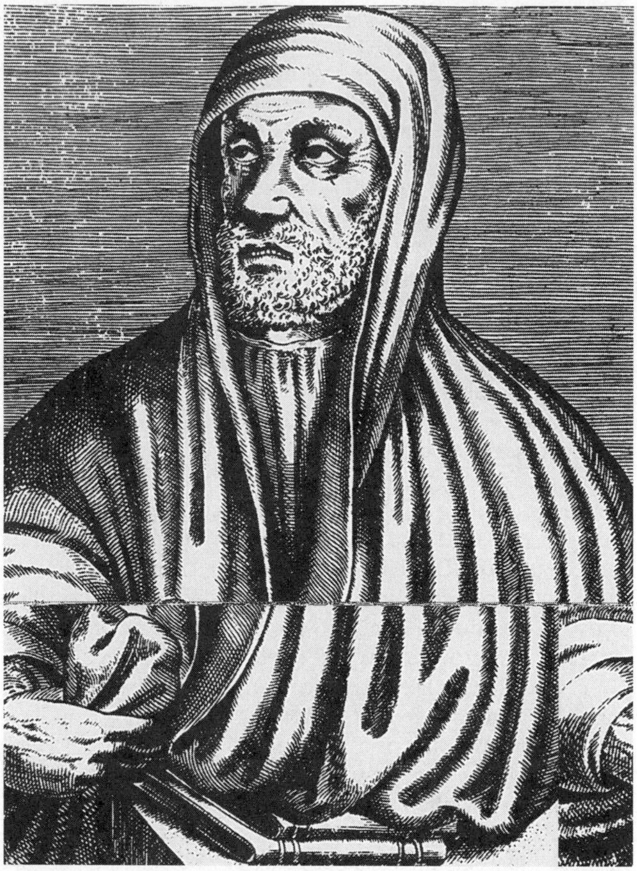

Avicenna

up a series of court appointments in a variety of cities, working as a lawyer, physician, and administrator. He treated the Majd al-Dawla for **depression**, and the Buyid prince Shams al-Dawla for a bowel disorder. Employed by Shams al-Dawla as a physician and vizier, or high executive officer, Avicenna devoted his days to his prince and his nights to discussion sessions with his students that were often also occasions for musical performances and general merriment. Political intrigue shadowed Avicenna. For a time he was forced into hiding, and once he was jailed.

Avicenna began his *Canon of Medicine* in 1012, and completed it a little more than a decade later, in 1023, in Hamadhan, in west-central Iran. His purpose in writing it was put together a clear, concise compendium of Greco-Roman scientific medicine. The *Canon* was translated into Latin by Gerard of Cremona (c.1114-1187) between 1150 and 1187. It became the standard European medical textbook for the duration of the Middle Ages.

The first part of the *Canon* defines the nature of the human body, health, illness, and medical treatment, and the causes and symptoms of disease. Disease is caused by humoral imbalance, bodily malformation, or dysfunction such as obstruction. Urine and pulse are a guide to the inner state of the body, and therapies include drugs, bleeding, and cauterization. Part two of the *Canon* deals with medicinal plants and the conditions they treat. Diseases of individual organs or systems are covered in the third part of the *Canon*. Part four deals with fevers. It also teachers minor **surgery**, and treatment of tumors, dislocations, poisons, and skin conditions, among other afflictions. The fifth and final part of the *Canon* is a guide to preparing medicinal compounds.

Critics of the *Canon* point out that also it was a reliable reference tool for answering certain questions, it did not represent genuine progress. The material on physiology and anatomy was not as well organized as the parts on specific treatments and preparation of pharmaceuticals. In writing his compendium, Avicenna hoped to bring together the best of the ancient texts while correcting their shortcomings, and to provide a working manual that would spare practitioners the need to do original research in physical science. But in discouraging investigation, the *Canon* held back medical progress. And some consider it outdated even at the time of its composition. All the same, Avicenna distinguished between diseases and their causes — a major conceptual leap — and he knew that diseases are spread by water and soil, not only by ''bad air.'' The *Canon*'s materia medica (medical remedies) listed over 760 drugs.

In 1023, the city of Hamadhan was attacked, and Avicenna fled to Isfahan. Lodged and welcomed by the ruler, Ala al-Dawla, Avicenna would spend the last 14 years of his life there in relative peace. He continued his research in practice in medicine, noting that ice compresses effectively relieved **headaches**, and that sugar-rose preserves cured a woman of her **tuberculosis**. In January 1030, Isfahan fell to the Ghaznavids, and Ala al-Dawla and Avicenna evacuated the city. While on a campaign with al-Dawla, Avicenna suffered an acute abdominal attack and died. He was 57 years old.

See also Humors; Pharmacy

AXELROD, JULIUS (1912-)

American biochemist and pharmacologist

Julius Axelrod is a biochemist and pharmacologist whose discoveries relating to the role of neurotransmitters in the sympathetic nervous system earned him the Nobel Prize in physiology or medicine in 1970, together with **Ulf Euler** of Sweden and Sir **Bernard Katz** of Great Britain. As Axelrod himself has said, he was a late starter as a distinguished scientist, due to both the humble circumstances of his birth and his coming of age in the Great Depression of the 1930s. He only began real scientific research in 1946, and earned his Ph.D. in 1955. From then on he compensated for lost time and became the first chief of the pharmacology section of the National Institute of Mental Health, a branch of the prestigious National Institutes of Health.

Axelrod was born on May 30, 1912, in a tenement house in New York City, the son of Isadore Axelrod, a maker of flower baskets for merchants and grocers, and Molly Leichtling Axelrod. His parents had immigrated to the United States from Polish Galicia in the early years of the century, met and married in New York, and settled in the heavily Jewish area of the Lower East Side of Manhattan. Julius Axelrod attended public elementary and high schools near his home but later recalled that he got his real education in the neighborhood public library, reading voraciously through several books a week, everything from pulp novels to Upton Sinclair and Leo Tolstoy. He studied for a year at New York University, but when his money ran out he transferred to the tuition-free City College of New York, from which he graduated in 1933 with majors in biology and chemistry. He later claimed that he did most of his studying on the long subway rides between his home and the uptown Manhattan campus of City College.

Axelrod applied to several medical schools but was not admitted to any. It has been widely reported, in the *New York Times,* for example, that he failed to get into medical school because of quotas for Jewish applicants. It was difficult to find any work in New York in the depths of the Depression, and Axelrod was fortunate to find employment in 1933 as a laboratory assistant at the New York University Medical School at $25 per month. In 1935 he took a position as chemist at the Laboratory of Industrial Hygiene, a nonprofit organization set up by the New York City Department of Public Health to test vitamin supplements added to foods. He married Sally Taub on August 30, 1938, and they eventually had two sons, Paul Mark and Alfred Nathan. Axelrod took night courses and received an M.A. in chemistry from New York University in 1941. In the early 1940s he lost the sight of one eye in a laboratory accident.

Axelrod later speculated that he might have remained at the Laboratory of Industrial Hygiene for the rest of his working life. The work, he said, was moderately interesting, and the pay adequate. However, in 1946, quite by chance, he received the opportunity to do some real scientific research and found it exciting. The laboratory received a small grant to study the problem of why some persons taking large quantities of acetanilide, a non-aspirin pain-relieving drug, developed methemoglobinemia, the failure of hemoglobin to bind oxygen for delivery throughout the body. Axelrod, who had little experience in such work, consulted Dr. Bernard B. Brodie of Goldwater Memorial Hospital of New York. Brodie was intrigued with the problem and worked closely with Axelrod in finding its solution. He also found Axelrod a place among the research staff at New York University. The two men soon discovered that the body metabolizes acetanilide into a substance with an analgesic effect, and another substance that causes methemoglobinemia. They recommended that the beneficial metabolic product be administered directly, without the use of acetanilide. Related analgesics were investigated in the same manner.

In 1949, Axelrod, Brodie, and several other researchers at Goldwater Hospital were invited to join the National Heart Institute of the National Institutes of Health in Bethesda, Maryland. There Axelrod studied the physiology of caffeine absorption and then turned to the sympathomimetic amines, drugs which mimic the actions of the body's sympathetic nervous system in stimulating the body to prepare for strenuous activity. He studied such compounds as amphetamine, mescaline, and ephedrine and discovered a new group of enzymes which allowed these drugs to metabolize in the body. By the mid 1950s, Axelrod decided that he needed a doctorate to advance in his career at the National Institutes of Health. He took a year off to prepare for comprehensive examinations at George Washington University in the District of Columbia, submitted research work he had already done to satisfy the thesis requirements, and received a Ph.D. in pharmacology in 1955, at the age of forty-three. He was then offered the opportunity to create a section in pharmacology within the Laboratory of Clinical Sciences at the National Institute of Mental Health, another branch of the National Institutes of Health. He became chief of the section in pharmacology and held that position until his retirement in 1984.

In 1957 Axelrod began the research which eventually led to the Nobel Prize. He and his colleagues and students studied the manner in which neurotransmitters, the chemicals which transmit signals from one nerve ending to another across the very small spaces between them, operate in the human body. In the 1940s the Swedish scientist Ulf von Euler had discovered that noradrenaline, or norepinephrine, was the neurotransmitter of the sympathetic nervous system. Axelrod was concerned with the way in which noradrenaline was rapidly deactivated in order to make way for the transmission of later nerve signals. He discovered that this was accomplished in two basic ways. First, he found a new enzyme, which he named catechol-O-methyltransferase (COMT), which was essential to the metabolism, and hence the deactivation, of noradrenaline. Second, through a series of experiments on cats, he determined that noradrenaline was reabsorbed by the nerves and stored to be reused later. These seemingly esoteric discoveries in fact had enormous implications for medical science. Axelrod demonstrated that psychoactive drugs such as antidepressants, amphetamines, and cocaine achieved their effects by inhibiting the normal deactivation or reabsorption of noradrenaline and other neurotransmitters, thus prolonging their impact upon the nervous system or the brain. His experiments also pointed the way to many new discoveries in the rapidly growing field of neurobiological research and the chemical treatment of mental and neurological diseases. The 1978 Nobel Prize in physiology or medicine, shared with Ulf von Euler and Bernard Katz, crowned his achievements in this area.

In his later years, Axelrod has worked in many areas of biochemical and pharmacological research, notably in the study of hormones. Especially important to the advancement of medical science was his development of many new experimental techniques which could be widely applied in the work of other researchers. He also had a great impact through his training of and assistance to a long line of visiting researchers and postdoctoral students at the National Institutes of Health. He continued his own research at the National Institute of Mental Health following his formal retirement in 1984. Early in 1993 Axelrod had the unusual experience of having his own life saved through a scientific discovery he had made many years before. At the age of eighty, he suffered a massive heart attack. The cardiologists at Georgetown University Medical

Center soon determined that several of his coronary arteries were almost completely blocked by blood clots and that he must have immediate triple coronary-artery bypass surgery. The complication was that his blood pressure had fallen so dangerously low that he might not survive the operation. The solution to this crisis was to inject a synthetic form of noradrenaline to stimulate the contractions of his heart and thus raise his blood pressure to a more acceptable level. Axelrod survived the operation and within two months was back at work and attending conferences in foreign countries.

AYURVEDIC MEDICINE

Ayurvedic medicine has been the traditional medicine of India and Sri Lanka for at least the past two thousand years. It is a combination of philosophy and science. As such, it takes into account every aspect of a person's life and requires a large degree of patient involvement, and even belief. Because it is a holistic system, it concentrates as much on the individual's mental and spiritual well-being as it does on physical health and seeks to guide individuals to their natural, inner harmony.

Ayurvedic medicine seeks first to prevent disease by keeping an individual's constitution sound and strong, since good health is a means to attain a meaningful life. When a person does get ill, the Ayurvedic practitioner tries to discover what has put his or her constitution out of balance. As a total system of healthcare, Ayurvedic medicine goes far beyond any single type of therapy or treatment and offers instead a complete life regimen.

One of the basic tenets of Ayurvedic medicine is the important principle of "biologic individuality." This means that each person is a unique individual with his or her own special physical and mental constitution, and must, consequently, be treated individually. Therefore, what works for one person does not automatically work for another with the same condition. It is the skill of the practitioner that identifies the exact composition of each person's constitution or his or her psychophysiological type. There are ten major types that are derived from the different combinations of "doshas," or the three vital energies. Since bad health is the result of an imbalance in an individual's dosha, Ayurvedic practitioners first diagnose the exact imbalance and then prescribe some combination of diet, **exercise**, herbal products, and purification procedures to rebalance the patient's dosha.

The primary diagnostic tool for the Ayurvedic physician is simple observation. Doing without most equipment or laboratory testing, the experienced practitioner first asks many questions of the patient, learning details of his health history, as well as that of his family. After those medical questions, he inquires as to the type of child and adolescent the patient was, and learn about the patient's lifestyle, job, likes and dislikes, and habits. During the **physical examination**, the physician observes the patient very closely, first simply noting his overall appearance, especially his coloring. He then studies the eyes, lips, tongue, and nails, looking for signs of doshic imbalance. In addition to palpation, or feeling the body and its internal organs, he listens to intestines, heart, and lungs. The tongue is an especially important diagnostic site, as discoloration and localized sensitivity indicate particular problems with internal organs. Some physicians examine a patient's stools, while most routinely perform an examination of a patient's urine, focusing on color and odor.

Once the Ayurvedic physician completes his diagnosis, he selects therapeutics geared to both the body and the mind. According to the nature of the imbalance, the patient may first undergo some detoxifying or cleansing therapies. These may include sweating in a steam bath or the taking of a laxative or enema.

After the patient is detoxified, the physician may prescribe an herbal remedy to correct the "dosha" imbalance. These are not intended to eliminate any disease, since the disease is the result or symptom of the original imbalance. Essential to this therapy is the physician's advice concerning the patient's lifestyle, food, eating habits, and exercise. Good habits in each of these areas work toward maintaining one's balance following detoxification and therapy.

Meditation is the major tool for **stress** reduction. It consists of several methods, to concentrate the mind using a variety of breathing exercises and/or chanting. Another goal is the elimination of repressed emotions, because Ayurvedic medicine believes that toxins can be produced by repressed and/or negative emotions.

Ayurvedic medicine is not licensed in the United States. The fact that it is a person-specific type of medicine, with no one particular cure appropriate for every disease or patient, makes it especially difficult to assess from a traditional Western medical viewpoint.

As an overall healthcare system, Ayurvedic medicine is safe for most people if they are in the hands of a qualified practitioner. However, certain detoxifying treatments, such as **enemas**, may not be suitable for pregnant women or patients with frail health. Herbal remedies should be taken with care, following the quantity and dosage carefully. Using Ayurvedic medicine in cases of severe trauma, acute **pain**, diseases in an advanced stage, or in place of needed surgery presents a major risk to the patient.

B

Bacteremia

Bacteremia occurs when bacteria enter the bloodstream. This may occur through a wound or infection, or through a surgical procedure or injection. Bacteremia may cause no symptoms and resolve without treatment, or it may produce **fever** and other symptoms of infection. In some cases, bacteremia leads to **septic shock**, a potentially life-threatening condition.

Several types of bacteria live on the surface of the skin or colonize the moist linings of the urinary tract, lower digestive tract, and other internal surfaces. These bacteria are normally harmless as long as they are kept in check by the body's natural barriers and the immune system. People in good health with strong immune systems rarely develop bacteremia. However, when bacteria are introduced directly into the circulatory system, especially in a person who is ill or undergoing aggressive medical treatment, the immune system may not be able to cope with the invasion, and symptoms of bacteremia may develop. For this reason, bacteremia is most common in people who are already affected by or being treated for some other medical problem. In addition, medical treatment may bring a person in contact with new types of bacteria that are more invasive than those already residing in that person's body, further increasing the likelihood of bacterial infection.

Conditions which increase the chances of developing bacteremia include:

- Immune suppression, either due to HIV infection or drug therapy
- Antibiotic therapy which changes the balance of bacterial types in the body
- Prolonged or severe illness
- **Alcoholism** or other drug abuse
- Malnutrition
- Diseases or drug therapy that cause **ulcers** in the intestines, e.g. **chemotherapy** for **cancer**.

Common immediate causes of bacteremia include:

- Drainage of an **abscess**, including an abscessed tooth
- Urinary tract infection, especially in the presence of a bladder catheter
- Decubitus ulcers (pressure sores)
- Intravenous procedures using unsterilized needles, including IV drug use
- Prolonged IV needle placement
- Use of ostomy tubes, including gastrostomy (surgically making a new opening into the stomach), jejunostomy (surgically making an opening from the abdominal wall into the jejunum), and **colostomy** (surgically creating an artifical opening into the colon).

The bacteria most likely to cause bacteremia include members of the *Staphylococcus, Streptococcus, Pseudomonas, Haemophilus,* and *Esherichia coli* (*E. coli*) genera.

Symptoms of bacteremia may include:

- Fever over 101°F (38.3°C)
- Chills
- Malaise
- Abdominal **pain**
- Nausea
- Vomiting
- **Diarrhea**
- Anxiety
- **Shortness of breath**
- Confusion.

Not all of these symptoms are usually present. In the elderly, confusion may be the only prominent symptom. Bacteremia may lead to septic shock, whose symptoms include decreased consciousness, rapid heart and breathing rates and multiple organ failures.

Bacteremia is diagnosed by culturing the blood for bacteria. Samples may need to be tested several times over several hours. Blood analysis may also reveal an elevated number of white blood cells. Blood pressure is monitored closely; a decline in blood pressure may indicate the onset of septic shock.

Antibiotics are the mainstay of treatment, and are often begun before positive identification of the bacteria is made.

Close observation is required to guard against septic shock. Since bacteremia is usually associated with an existing infection elsewhere in the body, finding and treating this infection is an important part of treatment.

Bacteremia may cause no symptoms, but may be discovered through a blood test for another condition. In this situation, it may not need to be treated, except in patients especially at risk for infection, such as those with heart valve defects or whose immune systems are suppressed.

Prompt antibiotic therapy usually succeeds in clearing bacteria from the bloodstream. Recurrence may indicate an undiscovered site of infection. Untreated bacteria in the blood may spread, causing infection of the heart (**endocarditis** or **pericarditis**) or infection of the covering of the central nervous system (**meningitis**).

Bacteremia can be prevented by preventing the infections which often precede it. Good personal hygiene, especially during viral illness, may reduce the risk of developing bacterial infection. Treating bacterial infections quickly and thoroughly can minimize the risk of spreading infection. During medical procedures, the burden falls on medical professionals to minimize the number and duration of invasive procedures, to reduce patients' exposure to sources of bacteria when being treated, and to use scrupulous technique.

BAD BREATH

Bad breath, sometimes called halitosis, is an unpleasant odor of the breath. It is likely to be experienced by most adults at least occasionally. Bad breath, either real or imagined, can have a significant impact on a person's social and professional life.

Bad breath can be caused by a number of problems. Oral diseases, fermentation of food particles in the mouth, sinus infections, and unclean dentures can all contribute to mouth odor. Many non-oral diseases, such as lung infections, kidney failure, or severe liver disease, can also cause bad breath, although this is rare.

Many people think that bad breath originates in the stomach or intestines. This rarely happens. The esophagus is usually closed, and, although a belch may carry odor up from the stomach, the chance of bad breath being caused from air continually escaping from the stomach is remote. Cigarette smoke can cause bad breath, not only in the cigarette smoker, but also in one who is constantly exposed to second-hand smoke.

The easiest way to determine if one has bad breath is to ask someone who is trustworthy and discrete. Another, more private, method of determining if one has bad breath is to lick one's wrist, wait until it dries, then smell the area. Scraping the rear area of the tongue with a plastic spoon, then smelling the spoon, is another method one can use to assess bad breath.

The most effective treatment for bad breath is to treat the cause. Poor **oral hygiene** can be improved by regular brushing and flossing, as well as regular dental checkups. Gentle brushing of the tongue should be part of daily oral hygiene. In addition to good oral hygiene, the use of mouthwash is helpful.

Mouth dryness, experienced at night or during fasting, or due to certain medications and medical conditions, can contribute to bad breath. Dryness can be avoided by drinking adequate amounts of water. Chewing gum may be beneficial.

Some medications, such as some high blood pressure medications, can cause dry mouth, increasing the opportunity to develop bad breath. If this problem is significant, a medication change, under the supervision of one's health care provider, may improve the dry-mouth condition. Oral or sinus infections, once diagnosed, can be treated medically, usually with **antibiotics**. Lung infections and kidney or liver problems will, of course, need medical treatment. Treating the underlying cause will eliminated the problem of bad breath.

Depending on the cause, a multitude of alternative therapeutic remedies can be used. For example, **sinusitis** can be treated with steam inhalation of essential oils and/or herbs.

Most bad breath can be treated successfully with good oral hygiene and/or medical care. Occasionally, for patients who feel that these therapies are unsuccessful, some delusional or obsessive behavior pattern might pertain, and mental health counseling may be appropriate.

BAER, KARL ERNST VON (1792-1876)

Estonian biologist

One of ten children, Von Baer was born in Piep, Estonia, to parents descended from Prussian nobility. Due to the large size of his family, he was sent to live with his childless uncle and aunt until the age of seven. Initially tutored at home, he later spent three years at a school for the children of nobility. Although his father and uncle encouraged him to pursue a military career, from 1810-1814, Von Baer attended the University of Dorpat in Vienna, Austria and obtained an MD degree. From 1814-1817, he studied comparative anatomy at Würzburg. In 1817, he was appointed prosector at the University of Königsberg, where in 1819, he accepted an appointment to teach zoology and anatomy and serve as chief at the new zoological museum that he organized. In 1828, he became a member of the St. Petersburg Academy of Sciences, where he taught zoology from 1829-30. He then returned to Königsberg until 1834. At that time, he became librarian at St. Petersburg Academy of Sciences, and conducted research in anatomy and zoology. In 1846, he was also appointed to the position of Professor of Comparative Anatomy and Physiology at the Medico-Chirugical Academy in St. Petersburg.

Von Baer also took part in other types of scientific projects. In 1837, he led a scientific expedition to Novaya Zemlya in Arctic Russia, and from 1851-6, studied the fisheries of lake Peipus and the Baltic and Caspian Seas. He served as inspector of fisheries for the empire from 1851-1852. He founded the St. Petersburg Society for Geography and Ethnography and the German Anthropological Society. Von Baer died in Dorpat, Estonia, on November 28, 1876.

Von Baer made significant contributions to the world of science. The first of Baer's most famous discoveries grew out of his work at Königsberg. For more than a century, scientists had attempted to determine the exact nature and location of the mammalian egg. In 1673, Regnier de Graaf had discovered follicles in the ovaries that he thought might be eggs. However, he later found structures even smaller than follicles in the uterus, raising doubts about the role of the follicles themselves. During his research at Königsberg, Baer discovered the mammalian egg by identifying a yellowish spot within the follicle visible only with a microscope. He developed this idea in his 1827 treatise, *De ovi mammalium et hominis genesi* (*On the Origin of the Mammalian and Human Ovum*).

Baer's second great accomplishment was his explanation of early embryonic development, a theory that he summarized in his two-volume textbook *Über die Entwicklunggeschichte der Thiere* (*On the Development of Animals*), 1828-1837. Here he set forth the theory that embryos of all animals begin as similar structures that are both simple and homogeneous and develop into complex heterogeneous forms. In fact, he said, it is impossible to distinguish among the early embryos of birds, reptiles, and mammals until their later stages of development. He set forth the germ-layer theory of development which stated that during the early stages of development, embryos ultimately form four (later shown to be three) distinct layers that eventually differentiate into specific organs or body structures. These are the ectoderm, mesoderm and endoderm. While observing embryos, Von Baer discovered the extraembryonic membranes, the chorion, amnion, and allantois and determined their functions. He also discovered the presence of a notochord in early vertebrate embryos. Although the notochord quickly changes into a spinal column, its early presence indicates the evolutionary connection between vertebrates and other organisms now classified together in the phylum *chordata*. For his work, Von Baer was awarded the Copley Medal of the Royal Society in 1876.

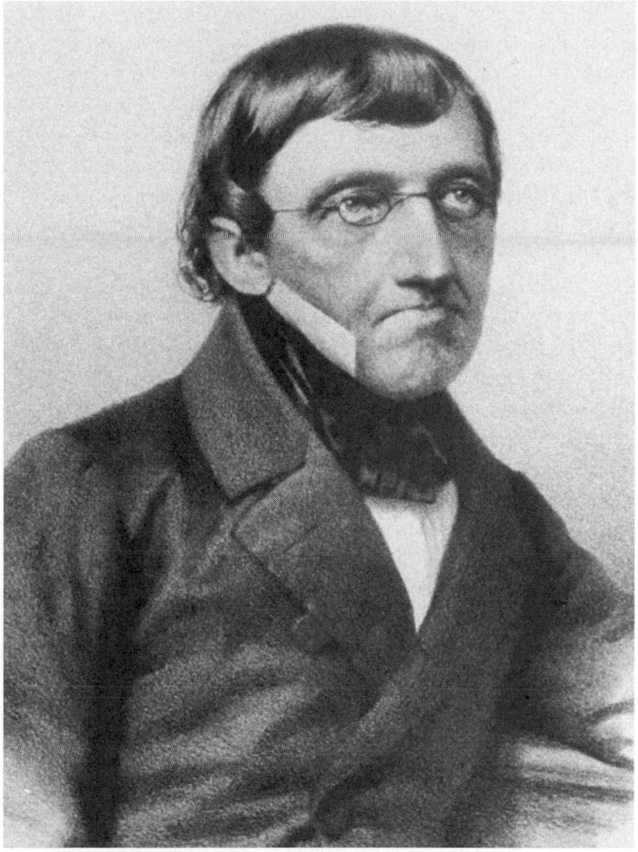

Karl Ernst von Baer

DE BAILLOU, GUILLAUME (1538-1616)
French physician

Guillaume de Baillou was born in 1538, the son of a famous mathematician, architect, and engineer. His affluent family owned an estate at Nogent-le-rotrou. He studied at the University of Paris, concentrating in Latin, Greek, and Philosophy, and later earned a Bachelor of Arts degree in 1568. He continued his studies there, earning a Doctorate in Medicine in 1570.

The first epidemiologist since Hippocrates, Baillou studied the epidemics of Paris between 1570 and 1579. He is known for his descriptions of the **plague**, **measles**, and diphtheria. He also taught the humanities, and later became professor of medicine. Baillou served as a teacher for 46 years, eventually becoming Dean of the Faculty of Medicine. Refusing to leave his medical practice, he declined King Henry IV's invitation to be a **physician** to the Dauphin, the eldest son of the French king, as Baillou was esteemed for his treatment of children. Baillou, however, did later became a physician to Henry IV. He died at the age of 78 in Paris in 1616.

See also Physician; Plague; Diphtheria; Measles; Hippocrates of Cos; Epidemic and pandemic

BAKER, SARA JOSEPHINE (1873-1945)
American physician

Sara Josephine Baker was a pioneer in public health care and preventive medicine in the early part of the twentieth century. Josephine Baker (as she preferred to be called) was born into a wealthy New York family. When her father died, she decided to become a physician, an unheard of ambition for girls of that time. Finding herself ill-prepared for medical school, Baker studied biology and chemistry at home for a year before applying to the Women's Medical College of the New York Infirmary for Women and Children, one of the few colleges that offered women work in medical clinics. She entered school at 18 and received her M.D. in 1898. Baker first served as an intern at the New England Hospital for Women and Children in Boston where she learned the harsh realities of sickness and death in turn-of-the-century slums. Once, while taking care of a sick woman, Baker had to defend herself by kicking a drunk husband down the stairs.

Baker returned to New York and opened a medical practice with a classmate, Dr. Florence M. Laighton. Unfortunately, women doctors were such a rarity at that time that they had few patients and had to close the practice. Baker then became a medical inspector for the City of New York Department of Health. Unlike other medical examiners who never left their offices, Baker went to the people, climbing stairs into slum apartments and entering schools to check on sick children. In the poverty-stricken parts of New York City, she saw first-hand how filthy conditions led to the spread of disease. She went to the Bowery in the middle of the night to vaccinate against smallpox, during the meningitis epidemic in 1905 she worked tirelessly diagnosing and treating the disease, and also helped the Department of Health track down "Typhoid Mary" Mallon, the infamous carrier of that deadly disease. Baker was a crusader in encouraging school children to report and treat common problems of the time such as head lice and eye and skin infections. With Lina Rogers (who may have been the first public health nurse in the country) she started the school nurse program in New York City.

Baker was familiar with the statistics: one-third of the deaths reported in New York City were of children under five years old, and one-fifth were babies less than a year old. Knowing from experience that poor people had little education and knew little about disease prevention, she started a pioneer project in the summer of 1908, sending 30 school nurses into homes of newborns educating mothers on caring for their infants. The results were dramatic—1200 fewer deaths that year—which led the city to form the Division of Child Hygiene, later called the Bureau of Child Health. This was the first taxpayer-supported agency in the world devoted to the health of children. As director of this bureau, Baker spent the next 15 years instituting sound practices that improved the lives of thousands of children. Among her observations, Baker noticed that there were hundreds of children suffering from preventable blindness. She helped design and distribute a dispenser for administering the compound, *silver nitrate* to the eyes of all newborns. This compound helps prevent infection and blindness that results from the mother's infection with the sexually-transmitted disease *gonorrhea.* Baker also created a design for newborn clothing so that babies could be dressed in easily managed layers: underwear and outerwear could be laid out flat so that a baby's arm could be pulled through all layers at once. Sewing companies produced patterns for these clothes which became very popular and affordable.

Despite all of Baker's achievements, some bureaucrats sought to have her dismissed; however, mothers whose children had benefitted marched in protest and her position was saved. Baker was no stranger to gender bias in her professional life. Members of one medical organization narrow-mindedly made comments like "it (her program) was ruining medical practice by keeping babies well." When a group of Brooklyn physicians sought to eliminate the Bureau of Child Hygiene, Baker took it as a compliment and continued about her work. She often wrote using just her initials—Dr. S.J. Baker. When she was invited to present a paper in Philadelphia, the audience of male physicians were shocked and astounded to discover her gender. Despite this lack of support from the medical profession, she wrote numerous respected books on the health of children. She was also an activist for women's right to vote, and a successful fund-raiser for all causes in which she believed.

BALDNESS

Alopecia means hair loss or baldness. Hair loss occurs for many reasons, from pulling hair out to having it killed off by **cancer chemotherapy**. Some causes are considered natural, while others signal health problems. Some conditions are confined to the scalp. Others reflect disease throughout the body.

Often conditions affecting the skin of the scalp result in hair loss. The first clue to the specific cause is the pattern of hair loss, whether it be complete baldness, thinning, or patchy bald spots. Another factor is the condition of the hair and the scalp beneath it. Sometimes only the hair is affected, while sometimes the skin is diseased as well.

Male pattern baldness is considered normal in adult men. Hair loss occurs across the top and front of the head, while the scalp remains healthy. Fungal infections of the scalp usually cause patchy hair loss. The fungus, similar to the ones that cause **athlete's foot** or **ringworm**, often glows under ultra-violet light.

Hair loss may also be caused by mental disorders or from unidentified causes. Complete hair loss is a common result of cancer chemotherapy, due to the toxicity of the drugs used.

Diseases often affect hair growth either selectively or by altering the skin of the scalp. For example, hyperthyroidism (too much thyroid hormone) causes hair to become thin and fine. Hypothyroidism (too little thyroid hormone) thickens both hair and skin.

Dermatologists are skilled in diagnosing the cause of hair loss by sight alone, but also perform a skin biopsy, removing a tiny bit of skin using a local anesthetic so that it can examined under a microscope. Successful treatment of underlying causes is most likely to restore hair growth. Two drugs, minoxidil (Rogaine) and finasteride (Proscar), promote hair growth in a significant minority of patients. When used continuously for long periods of time, minoxidil produces satisfactory results in about one quarter of patients with male pattern baldness and as many as half the patients whose hair loss is caused by unknown causes. Both drugs have so far proved to be quite safe when used for this purpose.

Over the past few decades there have appeared a multitude of hair replacement methods performed by both physicians and non-physicians. They range from simply weaving someone else's hair in with the remains of the client's own to surgically transplanting thousands of hair follicles one at a time.

How successful the outcome of treating baldness is varies with the cause. It is easier to lose hair than to re-grow it. Even when it returns, it is often thin and less attractive than the original crop. However many people who lose hair as the result of chemotherapy or fungal infection are able to grow back normal hair once they stop chemotherapy or are treated for the fungal infection.

Baltimore, David (1938-)

American microbiologist

David Baltimore won the Nobel Prize in physiology or medicine in 1975. He shared the award with the virologist **Renato Dulbecco** and the oncologist **Howard Temin** for the groundbreaking discovery that genetic information doesn't just travel from DNA (deoxyribonucleic acid, which contains genetic information) to RNA (ribonucleic acid, which communicates DNA information to proteins), although that concept had been at the heart of modern genetic theory. Rather, Temin and Baltimore independently discovered that some viruses could replicate their RNA into the DNA of healthy cells, causing tumors. This process is known as reverse transcription and is catalyzed by the enzyme reverse transcriptase. Its implications had a great effect on the study of cancer and the role of viruses in causing the disease. Born March 7, 1938, in New York City to Richard Baltimore and Gertrude Lipschitz, David was a gifted student of science. While still in high school he attended a prestigious summer program for talented students of science at the Jackson Laboratory in Bar Harbor, Maine, where the focus was mammalian genetics. It was there that Baltimore decided to pursue a career in the research sciences and first met his future colleague, Howard Temin, also a student at the time.

Baltimore attended Swarthmore College in Pennsylvania and graduated in 1960 with high honors in chemistry. He started graduate work at the Massachusetts Institute of Technology (M.I.T.) but transferred after one year to the Rockefeller Institute, now called Rockefeller University, in New York. There he studied with Richard M. Franklin, who was a molecular biophysicist specializing in RNA viruses. Baltimore earned his Ph.D. in 1964 and returned to M.I.T. for a postdoctoral fellowship the following year.

Baltimore was interested in a specific group of RNA viruses, the picornaviruses, which include mengovirus and poliovirus, that do not have DNA but nevertheless seemed to reproduce in cells of complex organisms that carry their genetic information in DNA. Since 1964, Temin had been suggesting that RNA viruses could replicate themselves in DNA, but the scientific community disbelieved and even ridiculed him. Baltimore, however, persisted in looking for RNA or DNA enzymes in the genetic material of poliovirus to solve this riddle.

He continued his research in this area as a fellow at the Albert Einstein College of Medicine in the Bronx (1964–65) and as a research associate at the Salk Institute in California (1965–68). At the Salk Institute he met Renato Dulbecco, who had developed innovative techniques for examining animal viruses in the laboratory. He also met Alice Shih Huang, a postdoctoral fellow studying vesicular stomatitis virus.

In 1968, Baltimore returned with Huang to Boston, where they were married. They have one daughter. Baltimore became an associate professor of microbiology at M.I.T. and continued to focus his research on poliovirus. By 1970, however, a number of scientists had suggested that all RNA viruses might not be alike. Baltimore's focus on poliovirus therefore might not reveal clues to the behavior of other viruses. Baltimore began to classify RNA viruses according to their varying replication strategies. It was during his work on this project that he discovered an enzyme that enabled an RNA virus to replicate its single strand of RNA and thus become compatible with the double-stranded DNA in a sample of Rauscher murine leukemia virus. The enzyme was later called reverse transcriptase.

Meanwhile, Temin had independently demonstrated the same thing, using a sample of Rous sarcoma virus. In 1970, both scientists made the initial announcements of reverse transcription within days of each other, at separate conferences. One month later they published an article detailing their findings in the journal *Nature.* The excitement of their news was instantaneous. Many scientists jumped to the conclusion that reverse transcription held the key to a cure for cancer. But Baltimore and Temin were more reserved in their response. They knew that their work did not establish a direct link between viruses and cancer. Their discovery did, however, quickly become a key to the study of cancer. Baltimore immediately began to be recognized for his achievement. In 1972 he was promoted to full professor at M.I.T. and in 1973 he was awarded a lifetime research professorship by the American Cancer Society.

While continuing to study reverse transcriptase, Baltimore and his colleagues at M.I.T. partially synthesized a mammalian hemoglobin gene. Other teams around the country were performing similar experiments at the same time, which raised the specter of genetic engineering. As a prominent figure in the scientific community, Baltimore became outspoken about the risks of genetic engineering. He was concerned that modern science—and biology in particular—might be misused. In 1975, he initiated a conference in which scientists attempted to design a self-regulatory system regarding experiments with recombinant DNA. In 1976, the National Institutes of Health established a committee to oversee federally funded experiments in the field of genetic engineering. After winning the Nobel Prize in 1975, Baltimore continued to be honored for his work. He was elected to the National Academy of Sciences and the American Academy of Arts and Sciences in 1974. In 1983 he became the director of the Whitehead Institute for Biomedical Research, where he remained until 1990. In that position, he made significant advances in the field of immunology and synthetic vaccine research. In 1990 he became President of Rockefeller University.

Baltimore's career took a sudden turn in 1989 when it was revealed that the conclusions of a 1986 paper he had coauthored while still at M.I.T. were based on falsified data. A young scientist, Margaret O'Toole, confronted Thereza Imanishi-Kari, also a coauthor of the article and a supervising scientist in the M.I.T. lab, with suspicions of misconduct. Imanishi-Kari denied any wrongdoing. Baltimore stood by Imanishi-Kari, and O'Toole was subsequently demoted, later claiming that her career had been ruined because she had spoken out against her superiors.

The matter was taken up by a House subcommittee and the Office of Scientific Integrity, which eventually lent credence to O'Toole's suspicions. Baltimore retracted the article but it was too late. Though he was cleared of any wrongdoing and though Imanishi-Kari was not prosecuted, Baltimore's name had been attached to a major breach of scientific ethics. That Baltimore had earlier taken such a strong stand on the ethics of bioengineering was a particular irony not lost on the scientific community. In 1991, under pressure from the faculty, Baltimore resigned as President of Rockefeller University, though he remains a professor there and continues to do research.

Bandages and dressings

In one form or another, bandages and dressings have likely been in use since prehistoric times, with plant materials and strips of animal hide serving the purpose initially and, later, fabrics. Early writings from Mesopotamia, Egypt, China, Greece, and Rome describe wound ointments and dressings, and Homer (c. 900-800 B.C.) mentions bandages for battle wounds, as do Hippocrates (c. 460 B.C.) and the Bible. Ancient Egyptian embalmers were highly skilled in the art of bandaging. The great French surgeon Ambroise Paré (1510-1590) revived and modernized the treatment of wounds by abandoning cauterization in favor of ointments covered with carefully applied bandages. Three hundred years later, English surgeon Joseph Lister (1827-1912) pioneered the use of bandages and dressings soaked in carbolic acid as an antiseptic. Adhesive plasters, the precursors of today's adhesive bandages, were mentioned in an 1830 Philadelphia medical journal, patented in 1845 by Drs. William Shecut and Horace Day of New Jersey, and marketed as *Allcock's Porous Plaster* by Dr. Thomas Allcock. A German pharmacist, Paul Beiersdorf, patented a plaster-covered bandage called *Hansaplast* in 1882.

The adhesive bandage as we know it was the invention of Earl Dickson, an employee of the Johnson & Johnson medical supply company. Dickson's young bride continually cut and burned herself in the kitchen, and the concerned husband repeatedly bandaged her with pieces of gauze and surgical tape. Dickson saw that his wife needed a prepared supply of these dressings she could apply herself, and he began experimenting. He laid out a strip of Johnson & Johnson's surgical tape sticky side up on a table and placed a folded-up gauze pad in the middle of the tape. To keep the gauze clean and the tape sticky, Dickson covered the strip with crinoline. Mrs. Dickson appreciated her husband's invention, and so did Dickson's coworkers and bosses. Johnson & Johnson quickly put the bandages on the market, and, in l920, they became Band-Aids, a name suggested by a Johnson & Johnson mill superintendent, W. Johnson.

A modern wound care dressing widely used in health care facilities has no absorbent pad beneath it's adhesive surface yet does not adhere to the wound. ''SureSkin'' is very thin, transparent *hydrocolloid* dressing in which absorbent materials are built into the adhesive materials. The dressing absorbs excretion from the wound, forming a gel which creates a healing environment for tissue regeneration, and its transparency allows monitoring of the wound without removal. The dressing can remain in place for long periods and, although absorbent and allows penetration of oxygen and water vapor, its protective polyurethane film protects against external bacteria and water, so patients can wear it in the shower or bath without the wound getting wet.

Banting, Frederick Grant (1891-1941)

Canadian physician and medical researcher

Frederick Banting's principal achievement was the first isolation of the hormone insulin in 1921 and its successful use in treating **diabetes**. For this, Banting received the 1923 Nobel Prize for physiology or medicine along with John J. R. Macleod (1876-1935).

Frederick Banting was born in Alliston, Ontario. An average student, he graduated in 1916 from the University of Toronto medical school. After Medical Corps service in World War I, he completed his internship at Toronto's Hospital for Sick Children before beginning a medical practice in London, Ontario. Through an article on diabetes in a medical journal, Banting became interested in the disease, which he began to study at the University of Western Ontario.

By the early 1900s, scientists knew that the pancreas, an organ connected to the small intestine, was involved in diabetes. A pancreas hormone that reduced the blood glucose level was proposed in 1916 by the English physiologist Edward Sharpey-Schäfer. He thought the hormone was produced by cells called *islets of Langerhans* and called it *insuline*, from the Latin word for island. Various scientists tried unsuccessfully to isolate it.

In 1919, Moses Barron, a researcher at the University of Minnesota, showed that blockage of the duct connecting the two major parts of the pancreas caused shriveling of a second cell type, the acinar. It was Barron's article that inspired Banting, who thought that enzymes from the acinar cells digested the islet hormone. By tying off the pancreatic duct to destroy the acinar cells, he believed he could preserve the hormone and extract it from the islet cells.

At the suggestion of a colleague, Banting proposed his experiment to the head of the University of Toronto's Physiology Department, John Macleod, a noted expert on carbohydrate **metabolism**. At first Macleod rejected Banting's proposal, in part because he did not believe the islet hormone existed. Finally, however, Macleod supplied Banting with laboratory space, ten dogs for experimentation, and a medical student who was skilled in glucose measurement named Charles Best (1899-1978). Banting and Best began work in May 1921 while Macleod went on vacation to his native Scotland.

Banting and Best tied off the pancreatic ducts in some dogs so that the acinar cells would atrophy, then removed the pancreases to extract fluid from the islet cells. In the meantime, they removed the pancreases from other dogs to cause diabetes. These dogs were then injected with the islet cell fluid. After many attempts, the procedure was perfected. This required careful measurement of the glucose levels in the diabetic dogs before treatment to be sure they were diabetic and afterward to show that they maintained normal blood glucose levels.

When he returned from vacation in August 1921, Macleod learned of Banting and Best's success. He organized his entire laboratory to isolate and purify insulin from livestock for use in treating human diabetes. Banting and Best initially wanted to name their fluid "isletin," but Macleod insisted on Sharpey-Schäfey's term insuline, shortened to insulin. A major collaborator in the purification work was biochemist James Collip.

At the Hospital for Sick Children in January 1922, fourteen year-old Leonard Thompson became the first human to be successfully treated for diabetes using insulin.

Banting's original theory was incorrect, as Banting and Best later discovered. The digestive enzymes in the acinar cells are inactive and insulin can be extracted from an intact pancreas. What led to their success was their precise method of glucose measurement.

Charles Best received his medical degree in 1925. Banting always insisted that both he and Best be credited for the discovery, and almost turned down his Nobel Prize because Best was not included. Best became head of the University of Toronto's physiology department in 1929 and director of the university's Banting and Best Department of Medical Research after Banting's death.

Frederick Banting also conducted research in cancer and heart disease. He again joined the Medical Corps during World War II, and died in a military air crash in Newfoundland in 1941.

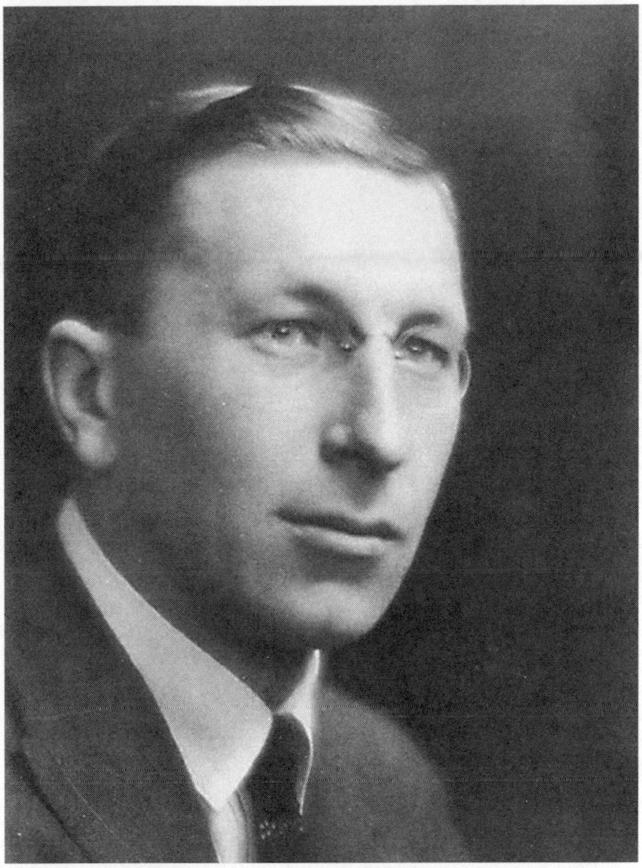

Frederick Grant Banting

Bárány, Robert (1876-1936)

Swedish physician

Robert Bárány made significant contributions to our understanding of the vestibular apparatus, part of the inner ear that plays an important role in maintaining balance. He devised ingenious tests to diagnose inner-ear disease, and he investigated the relationship between the vestibular and nervous systems. Because of his ground-breaking research in this area, he is credited with creating a new field of study, otoneurology. Bárány's achievements were recognized in 1914 with the Nobel Prize in physiology or medicine.

Bárány was born on April 22, 1876, in Rohonc (near Vienna), Austria-Hungary (now Austria), the eldest of six children. His father, Ignaz Bárány, was a bank official. His mother, Marie Hock Bárány, was the daughter of a well-known Prague scientist, and it was her intellectual influence that predominated in the family. When Bárány was young, he contracted tuberculosis of the bones, which left him with a permanent stiffness in his knee but which also first awakened his interest in medicine.

Always a top student, Bárány began attending medical school at the University of Vienna in 1894. In 1900 he received a doctor of medicine degree. He then spent two years studying internal medicine, neurology, and psychiatry at clinics in Frankfurt, Heidelberg, and Freiburg. Next, he returned to Vienna, where he received hospital surgical training. Finally, in 1903, he accepted a post at the Ear Clinic, also in Vienna, which was then directed by Adam Politzer. Bárány's association with Politzer, a leading figure in the history of otology (the study of the ear and its diseases), proved to be highly fruitful.

It was the chance observation that clinic patients often became dizzy after having their ears irrigated that led Bárány to develop one test that still bears his name. The Bárány caloric test involves stimulating each of a patient's inner ears separately by syringing one with hot liquid and the other with cold. Normally, this results in rapid, involuntary movements of the eyeballs, termed nystagmus. Bárány demonstrated that the direction of the nystagmus is determined by the temperature of the water and the position of the head. He also showed that the absence or delay of nystagmus indicates a problem with the balance structures of the ear. The test was an eminently practical technique for diagnosis, since it could easily be performed at a patient's bedside.

Another diagnostic procedure introduced by Bárány was the chair test. The patient is turned in a rotating chair with a specially designed headrest that inclines the head slightly forward. Once again, any deviation from the normal pattern of nystagmus afterward indicates a problem. Yet another of Bárány's inventions during this period was the noise box, a

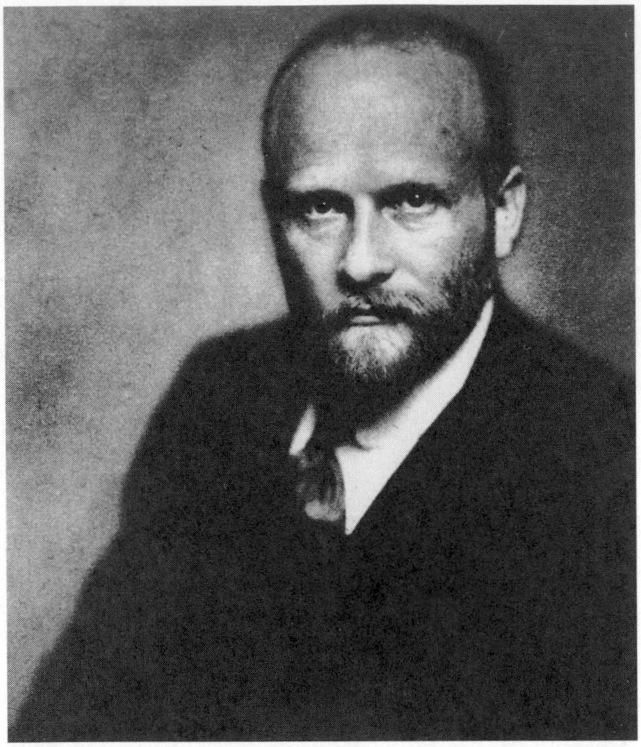

Robert Bárány

much-used device that effectively isolates the hearing performance of one ear by creating a masking noise in the other.

Unfortunately, this phase of great productivity was to be interrupted by the start of World War I. Bárány, who was of Jewish descent, was dispatched by the army to the fortress of Przemysl on the border between Poland and Russia, where he served as a medical officer. While there, Bárány continued to study the connection between the vestibular apparatus and the nervous system. He also developed an improved surgical technique for dealing with fresh bullet wounds to the brain.

However, in April 1915, the Russians occupied Przemysl, and Bárány was transported along with other prisoners by cattle car to Merv in central Asia. Conditions there were unsanitary and difficult, and Bárány came down with malaria. Still, he was relatively fortunate: the medical commander in Merv knew him by reputation and placed him in charge of otolaryngology (the medical specialty concerned with the ear, nose and throat) for both Russian natives and Austrian prisoners. The Russians were grateful patients. Alter Bárány had successfully treated the local mayor and his family, he became a daily dinner guest in their home.

It was while he was still a prisoner of war that Bárány received the news that he had won the Nobel Prize. Thanks to the personal intervention of Prince Carl of Sweden, Bárány was released in 1916. He returned to Vienna that same year, but was bitterly disappointed by the reception he received from colleagues there. They claimed he had inadequately cited their own contributions to his work. These accusations were investigated by the Nobel Prize Committee, which found them groundless. Nevertheless, the attacks prompted Bárány to accept a post as professor at the University of Uppsala in Sweden in 1917, where he remained for the rest of his life. Eventually, he rose to the position of chairman of the department of ear, nose, and throat medicine there.

While at Uppsala, Bárány studied the role of the part of the brain called the cerebellum in controlling body movement. He had previously devised another test for disturbances in cerebellar function, known as the pointing test, in which the patient points at a fixed object with the eyes alternately open and closed. Consistent errors while the eyes are closed indicates a brain lesion.

Bárány also developed a surgical technique for treating chronic sinusitis. For this, he was awarded the Jubilee Medal of the Swedish Society of Medicine in 1925. Among his numerous other awards were the Belgian Academy of Sciences Prize, the ERB Medal from the German Neurological Society, and the Guyot Prize from the University of Groningen in the Netherlands. He also received honorary degrees from several universities, including the University of Stockholm. Austria issued a stamp in his honor in 1976, to commemorate the 100th anniversary of his birth.

Bárány was described as a quiet and solitary man, fanatically devoted to his work. Yet at home, he also enjoyed music and played the piano well; he particularly liked the music of composer Robert Schumann. And despite having had a stiff knee since childhood, he was an avid mountain hiker and tennis player.

Bárány married Ida Felicitas Berger in 1909. They had three children, all of whom went on to become physicians or medical scientists. Their elder son, Ernst, became a professor of pharmacology in Uppsala; their second son, Franz, became a professor of internal medicine in Stockholm; and their daughter, Ingrid, became a psychiatrist in Cambridge, Massachusetts.

Bárány's last years were marred by a series of strokes, which resulted in partial paralysis. He was aware of an international meeting that was organized to celebrate his sixtieth birthday, but, sadly, he died in Uppsala only a few days before the occasion on April 8, 1936. Yet his memory has been kept alive with the Bárány medal, first awarded by the University of Uppsala in 1948, honoring deserving scientists for investigations of the vestibular system. In addition, the Bárány Society was established in 1960 to conduct international symposia on vestibular research.

BARBER, JR., JESSE B. (1924-)

African American neurosurgeon

Jesse B. Barber, Jr. was the first African American to be certified by the American Board of Neurosurgery and became the third black American to practice neurosurgery in the United States. Throughout his career, Barber has made significant contributions to his profession, his school, and his city, holding various positions of importance, including director of the Howard University Medical Stroke Project. He also served as the chief of Neurosurgery at Howard and became the university's first professor of social medicine.

Jesse Belmary Barber, Jr. was born on June 22, 1924 in Chattanooga, Tennessee to the former Mae Fortune and Jesse, Sr., who was a Presbyterian minister and an educator. Although he admired his father deeply and aspired to be a preacher like him, Barber's excellent academic performance led him to begin taking pre-engineering courses. However, after being ranked first in a pre-medical examination, Barber moved toward medicine. After first attending Swift Memorial Junior College and then Hampton Institute and Yale University, Barber received his B.A. from Lincoln University. He was then accepted at the Howard University Medical College where he received his M.D. in 1948.

Barber's practicing career began at Freedman's Hospital where he was an intern and a resident general surgeon from 1948 to 1954. In 1956 he became an instructor of surgery and pathology at Howard, moving two years later to serve as a resident at the McGill University Montreal Neurological Institute. In 1961, however, Barber returned to Howard University to become chief of the division of neurosurgery as well as professor of surgery. He founded the university's Medical Stroke Project in 1968, and in 1983 he became Howard's first professor of social medicine, a field of study which he pioneered.

In addition to his professional contributions, Barber has been a leader as well as a member of many organizations. He was president of both the National Medical Association (1977–1978) and the Washington Academy of Neurosurgery (1973–1974). He also is a member of the National Advisory Committee of the Epilepsy Foundation of America, the Executive Committee for Strokes of the American Heart Association, Kappa Pi and Alpha Omega Alpha. Among the many honors and awards he has received are the Howard University Alumni Federation Award for Meritorious Professional and Community Service (1970), the William Alonzo Warfield Award (1974), the YMCA Century Award (1974), the Distinguished Service Award of the National Medical Association (1974), and the Distinguished Service Award of the Howard University Department of Surgery (1979).

Barber achieved notoriety in 1973 as the neurosurgeon chosen by Hamaas Abdul Khaalis, leader of the Hanafi sect of the Black Muslims, to operate on his wife who had been shot in the head several times during an attack by an opposing sect. Barber also made headlines with his surgical skills when he successfully attempted an extremely rare and difficult transposition of the spinal cord operating procedure in the early 1970s. He performed this operation on a teenager whose scoliosis or curvature of the spine was becoming so severe that it was paralyzing him. Barber literally took the cord out of the spine, straightened it, and reinserted it, resulting in a marked improvement in the boy's paralysis.

Barber attributes his "social medicine perspective," an ideal that has guided his actions throughout his medical career, to the values instilled in him by his missionary parents. He is most proud of his education-oriented efforts, having guided scores of Howard University students toward the field of neurological study. In 1993, he was the facilitator of new exhibit at Howard University that focused on African American neurosurgeons.

Barber married the former Constance Bolling and has four children, Clifton, Jesse III, Charles, and Joye. Retired from active practice, Barber now lives in Washington, DC.

Barber-surgeons

In our time, surgery and medicine are closely allied disciplines. This was also true in ancient Greece and Rome. However, through the Renaissance and until the 18th century in Western Europe, surgery was considered more a trade than a profession, and surgeons had more to do with barbers than with physicians.

This separation between surgery and medicine may have originated in religious attitudes. During the early Middle Ages, most healing (both medical and surgical) was carried out by members of the clergy. However, concern arose about the shedding of blood by priests, and a papal decree (reinforced in 1215 by the Tenth Lateran Council) prohibited priests from doing surgery. As a result, responsibility for surgery passed to monasteries, where it was conducted by barbers who had experience with razors. At first, this was likely done under the supervision of priests. Eventually, surgery spread outside of monasteries, especially during times of war, when military surgeons were in great demand.

The academic and social status of these barber-surgeons was usually considerably less than that of physicians. If medicine was considered a profession practiced by university-trained physicians, then surgery was a trade, sometimes carried out by illiterates.

Barber-surgeon guilds began appearing in Europe around the 13th century. In London, for example, separate trade guilds for barbers and surgeons can be traced at least to 1308, in the case of the Company of Barbers (later known as the Barber-Surgeons' Company, and 1369 for the much-smaller but generally better-educated Fellowship of Surgeons.

Surgery was carried out by both of these guilds. A municipal ordinance issued in 1307 forbade barbers from being "so bold or so hardy as to put blood in their windows, openly or in view of folks, but let them have it privily carried unto the Thames, under pain of paying two shillings to the use of the sheriffs."

Among the guilds, considerable importance was attached to the order in which they were represented in processions. In 1535, the Company of Barbers marched in 17th position, between the pewterers and the cutlers. This was achieved only after considerable lobbying of civic officials, who had demoted the barbers from 17th to 28th place in 1516, followed by 17th place in 1532, 18th place a few years later, 17th place in 1533, and 28th place in 1534.

In 1493, the two competing guilds had started to cooperate on licensing of surgeons, and in 1540 they were amalgamated by an Act of Parliament. This law forbade surgeons from practicing barbery and barbers from practicing surgery, except for the pulling of teeth. There were many more barber-surgeons than physicians, and there is evidence that barber-surgeons sometime ventured beyond their trade into the practice of medicine.

This amalgamation lasted for two centuries, until it was ended by an 18th-century trend that led surgeons across Northern Europe to disassociate from their hair-clipping colleagues.

In England, William Cheselden, a skilled barber-surgeon who could remove bladder stones in less than one minute, led a drive for professional recognition of surgery. London surgeons left the Company of Barber-Surgeons in 1745 to form their own Company of Surgeons, which would evolve into the Royal College of Surgeons of England.

One of the best-known barber-surgeons was Ambroise Paré (1510-1590), who developed new amputation techniques in his work with French army troops, and abandoned the practice of using boiling oil to detoxify gunshot wounds. Paré recorded his knowledge about surgery in a 40-volume work that also summarized the teachings of **Galen**, Hippocrates, and Arabic surgeons.

Barbiturates

Barbiturates are medicines that act on the central nervous system (CNS). As a group, they are known as central nervous depressants or sedative-hypnotic drugs. They cause drowsiness and may control seizures (convulsions).

Barbiturates make people very relaxed, calm, and sleepy. These drugs are sometimes used to help patients relax before surgery. In the past, barbiturates have been used to treat nervousness and sleep problems. Today they have generally been replaced by other medicines for these purposes. Barbiturates may become habit-forming and should not be used to relieve everyday anxiety and tension or to treat sleeplessness over long periods.

Barbiturates are available only with a physician's prescription. The recommended dosage depends on the type of barbiturate and other factors such as the patient's age and the condition for which the medicine is being taken. Some commonly used barbiturates are phenobarbital (Barbita) and secobarbital (Seconal).

Barbiturates should always be taken exactly as directed because of their tendency to become addicting and because of the way then interact with other drugs. Because barbiturates work on the central nervous system, they may add to the effects of alcohol and other drugs that slow the central nervous system, such as **antihistamines**, cold medicine, allergy medicine, sleep aids, medicine for seizures, tranquilizers, some pain relievers, and **muscle relaxants**.

Barbiturates may also add to the effects of anesthetics, including those used for dental procedures. The combined effects of barbiturates and alcohol or other drugs that slow the central nervous system can be very dangerous, leading to unconsciousness or even **death**. Anyone who shows signs of an overdose or a reaction to combining barbiturates with alcohol or other drugs should get emergency medical help immediately.

Barbiturates can change the results of certain medical tests. Before having medical tests, anyone taking this medicine should alert the health care professional in charge so that accurate test results can be obtained.

People may feel drowsy, dizzy, lightheaded, or less alert when using these drugs. These effects may even occur the morning after taking a barbiturate at bedtime. Because of these possible effects, anyone who takes these drugs should not drive, use machines, or do anything else that might be dangerous until they have found out how the drugs affect them.

The most common side effects of barbiturates are **dizziness**, lightheadedness, drowsiness, and clumsiness or unsteadiness. These problems usually go away as the body adjusts to the drug and do not require medical treatment unless they persist or interfere with normal activities. Birth control pills may not work properly when taken while barbiturates are being taken. To prevent pregnancy, use an additional method of birth control.

Barbiturates may also interact with other common prescription and over-the-counter medicines. When this happens, the effects of one or both of the drugs may change or the risk of side effects may be greater. Anyone who takes barbiturates should let the physician know all other medicines he or she is taking.

Bard, Samuel (1742-1821)

American physician

Samuel Bard was a man of great prestige who helped further medical education in the United States. A well known physician in his own right, he helped to found the second medical school in America. Interested in many areas of science, he wrote and taught a variety of subjects, contributing to the educations of most of the great physicians that would come after him.

Samuel Bard was born on April 1st, 1742 in Philadelphia, Pennsylvania. His father was a prominent physician and a good friend of Benjamin Franklin. When Samuel was four, his family moved to New York City where his father set up another successful medical practice.

Little of Bard's life is known until he was fourteen. At that time he enrolled in King's College (later to be renamed Columbia University) to further his education. He was a student of the classics under the guidance of a professor named Leonard Cutting. During Bard's first year at the college he suffered from fever and was sent to the country to spend the summer and restore his health. He was sent to the estate of the man who was at that time lieutenant governor of New York. Bard became friends with the lieutenant governor's daughter and she introduced him to the field of botany. Throughout the rest of his life Bard would be interested in the study of plants.

In 1761, after an apprenticeship with his father, Bard was admitted as a pupil to St. Thomas's Hospital in London. Once his tenure there was complete, he enrolled at Edinburgh University's medical school. During his time in medical school Bard studied much more than medicine. He also studied French, Latin, and drawing. The dissertation that Bard wrote in order to receive his medical degree was a study of the effects of opium on the human body. He received his medical degree in 1765.

After receiving his degree, Bard returned to New York City where he went into practice with his father, and eventually took the practice over. In 1770 Bard married his cousin, Mary, and together they had three children.

Bard had always been interested in medical education, and together with a number of other physicians, he helped to found the second medical school in the United States, the first one in New York State. Bard became a professor of theory and practice of medicine at the college, and also lectured and taught a course on chemistry. The medical school was started as a part of King's College, and when the revolutionary war broke out in 1776 it had to be shut down.

During the war Bard had Loyalist sympathies and moved from New York to New Jersey, leaving his successful medical practice behind. Eventually financial problems forced him to return to New York where he reestablished his medical practice. After the war, Bard served as George Washington's private physician during the time that the new government was centered in New York. At one time he removed a carbuncle (infected boil) from Washington's thigh.

After the war, King's College was renamed Columbia University. When the medical school was reestablished there, Bard again became a professor, and was also named a trustee and dean. In 1813 the medical school became part of the College of Physicians and Surgeons, and Bard was named the new school's first president.

Bard retired and left his practice to his partner, David Hosack, in 1798. He moved to Hyde Park, New York, where he spent twenty-three years of retirement before his death.

During his retirement Bard continued to be very active in the medical field. He had always been interested in obstetrics and midwifery, and during his retirement he found time to write a book on the subject. It was the first textbook of its type written by an American and was used as the standard text on the subject for many years. Bard also wrote a book about the diseases that affect sheep. The effort was spawned by his attempts to raise merino sheep and his concern about the diseases that they suffered from.

Samuel Bard spent much of his retirement serving on boards for various groups in New York that were associated with the science, medicine, and culture of the time. He continued to support the creation of medical schools and tried to spread his theory that experience was the best way a physician could learn. He died at his estate in Hyde Park on May 24th, 1821, just twenty-four hours after his wife passed away.

Barnard, Christiaan (1922-)

South African surgeon

Dr. Christiaan Barnard became internationally famous on December 3, 1967, when he performed the first human-to-human heart transplant. Many other surgeons had been struggling to prepare for this same historic operation, but Barnard's personal drive and fascination with his field propelled him onto the world stage as the first to undertake such ground-breaking surgery. Barnard was born and raised in the arid South African

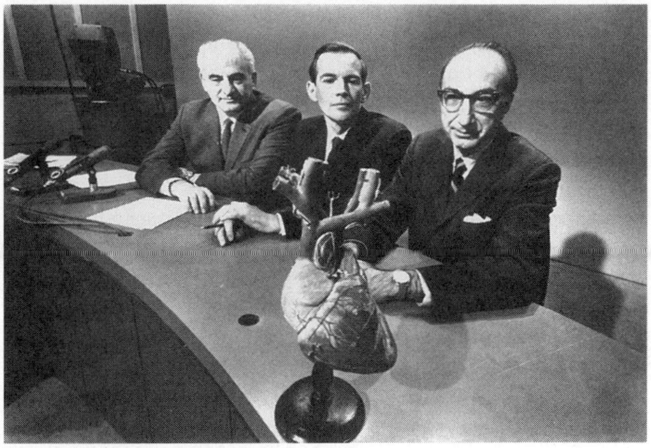

Christiaan Barnard (in the middle)

countryside known for its sheep farms. His father was a Dutch Reformed missionary and the family of six lived very humbly. Barnard, known for his excellent academic performance and photographic memory, graduated from the University of Cape Town medical school in 1946. During his residency, he devoted most of his studies to tubercular meningitis, writing his doctoral thesis on the subject in 1953. When he was transferred to Groote Schuur Hospital—the site of his historic operation—Barnard became interested in surgery. A grant in 1955 to study cardiothoracic surgery at the University of Minnesota enabled him to work under the guidance of the prominent surgeon C. Walton Lillehei, one of the many researchers around the world attempting to develop techniques that would lead to the first human heart transplant. Together, Barnard and Lillehei performed experimental open-heart surgery in animals.

When Barnard returned to South Africa, he and his surgeon brother, Marius, began a rigorous series of heart transplant experiments in dogs using a method called the Shumway technique. By the end of 1967, Barnard felt ready to perform the transplant operation on humans, and it was only a matter of time before the right donor and the right patient appeared. Barnard performed the innovative and, to many, shocking surgery on Louis Washkansky, a fifty-three-year-old grocer with debilitating heart disease. Washkansky received the heart of twenty-five-year-old Denise Darvall, who had been killed by an automobile. Almost immediately, controversy spread, and people worldwide voiced moral, legal, and ethical objections to this operation. Of particular concern was the question of how to define the death of a potential donor, since comatose patients can be maintained by artificial means for an indefinite period. Barnard's reaction to the uproar was one of steely determination to hold his ground; he had no second thoughts and intended to continue with more transplants. When Washkansky first awoke from his surgery, he is reported to have said, "I am the new Frankenstein." He survived with his new heart for eighteen days, at which point the infections that ravaged his body became lethal. It became evident that the surgical methods for accomplishing transplantation had been achieved, but in order to suppress the body's fundamental mechanism of rejecting foreign tissue, powerful antirejection medications had to be administered. These drugs, called immunosuppressants, lower the body's resistance to foreign tissue but simultaneously suppress its overall immune response, or natural ability to fight viral and bacterial infection. Patients are prone to severe infections as a result.

After Barnard's initial heart transplant operation, many other surgeons undertook the same operation in the following weeks, but with very poor results. Survival rates were unacceptably low—doctors still could not control infections which flourished in their patients. Barnard's second heart transplant recipient, Philip Blaiberg, survived a remarkable 593 days, but Barnard recognized that this case was an aberration rather than the rule. After a total of four transplant attempts, he decided to stop until more research could be done. On November 25, 1974, Barnard tried a new technique, the first double-heart transplant, in which he implanted the heart of a ten-year-old girl into a fifty-eight-year-old man without removing the patient's diseased heart. He performed this operation again in 1975, but both patients lived only a few months. Only a handful of centers continued cardiac transplantation after 1969. Many experts felt that research should be directed toward developing the **artificial heart**, since the heart is a simple pumping mechanism and relatively easy to replicate as opposed to other organs, such as the kidney. It remained imperative, however, to develop a successful method for controlling post-transplantation infections. The development in the 1970s of cyclosporin, a specific immunosuppressive agent, once again turned the tide toward organ transplantation. Cyclosporin, which suppresses only certain aspects of the immune system allowing the body to receive a new organ but also fight off the more virulent infections, is by no means a wonder drug but it has clearly reduced the rate of mortality associated with transplants. In the 1990s, investigations into *tolerance induction* and *chimerism* (the coexistence of donor and recipient cells), particularly through simultaneous donor bone marrow infusion with the organ transplant and the role of dendritic cells, hold promise for transplants without the need for immunosuppressive drugs. Barnard's landmark surgery forced many issues surrounding transplantation, legal, ethical, and medical, and he remains a symbol of tenacity and daring in pursuing his goal.

See also Organ transplantation

Barton, Clarissa (Clara)Harlowe (1821-1912)

American teacher, organizer, nurse

Clara Barton was nicknamed ''Angel of the Battlefield'' for her extraordinary work with wounded soldiers during the Civil War. Her most lasting legacy, however, was the establishment of the American Red Cross, a relief organization which still exists today.

Clara Barton was born on December 25, 1821, the youngest of Stephen Barton and Sally Stone's five children. By all accounts, Barton was a painfully shy child, although always stunningly brilliant. Her older brothers and sisters (the next eldest was 10 years older than Barton) coddled her and taught her, so that she was able to read and write at a very early age. Barton's first encounter with nursing occurred at age 11, when her brother slipped from a barn roof and suffered catastrophic injuries. Barton cared for him for two years.

At age 15, Barton began her first career as a schoolteacher. Her family had guided her towards this profession, hoping that it would help her overcome her intense shyness. Indeed, it would appear that teaching had its desired affect, given the strength of Barton's later personality, and her ability to speak publicly, organize, and convince political and governmental officials to address her causes. In 1850, Barton went to Bordentown, New Jersey to teach. At this time, all the schools in New Jersey charged their pupils, a situation Barton found abhorrent. She offered to go without pay at the Bordentown schools, if all children were allowed to attend without cost to them. The school system accepted her offer, and Barton is credited with establishing the first free school in the state. The school grew by leaps and bounds. Unfortunately, the school administrator's chose to hire a male principal to take Barton's place, angering Barton. Perhaps due to the stress of this situation, Barton suffered the first of many ''breakdowns which haunted her life.'' Barton left teaching to recuperate.

After a period of rest, Barton went to Washington D.C., where she became a clerk in the U.S. Patent Office. This was another ''first'' for Barton, as no other American woman had ever held such a governmental post. Barton kept this until 1861, when she resigned in order to pursue her interest in delivering supplies to the troops during the Civil War.

Barton started her Civil War efforts by collecting items ranging from bandages and medical supplies to socks which were needed by the soldiers in the front lines. After a while, she received permission to actually visit the battlefields to deliver these items personally. She began assisting in the care of the wounded, and worked tirelessly through horrific conditions to provide these wounded and ill soldiers with compassionate nursing care.

In 1865, Barton took an interest in identifying the vast numbers of missing and dead soldiers. She ran a missing person's office (the first woman to head a bureau for the U.S. government), lectured on a circuit about her experiences in the war, and worked for the suffragist movement to gain the right to vote for women.

Unfortunately, Barton's feeble health again interrupted her activities, and she had to withdraw from her work and take a rest. In 1869, she ended up seeking a cure in Switzerland, where she began to familiarize herself with the work of the International Red Cross. Although in Europe to bolster her own help, Barton ended up traveling to France to provide aid during the Franco-Prussian War. She also worked in both Strasbourg and Lyon to try to improve the conditions of impoverished women by providing them with work.

In 1873, Barton returned to the U.S., determined to start a branch of the International Red Cross in the United States, and passionate about convincing the U.S. government to ratify the Geneva Convention, which would set policy for the treatment of sick and wounded soldiers by the Red Cross. Although her health sent her to a spa in Danville, NY for a time, Barton was able to convince the U.S. government to ratify the Geneva Agreement. The document was signed in 1882.

See also International Red Cross

Bayley, Richard (1745-1801)

American physician

Richard Bayley was a well known physician of the 18th century. He taught and did research on the most prominent medical problems of the time, and developed a new treatment for diphtheria that helped save many lives. He was also deeply involved in the health of the immigrants that came to the United States through Ellis Island in New York.

Richard Bayley was born in 1745 in Fairfield, Connecticut. As a child he was well educated in a variety of subjects including French and the classics. Little is known about his life until 1766, when he took an apprenticeship with John Charlton. Charlton was a very well known physician who lived and worked in New York. During the time that he was an apprentice, Bayley courted Charlton's sister. Eventually they married and three children. In 1977 his wife died, and a year later he married Charlotte Barclay, with whom he had four children.

Bayley's daughter by first wife, Elizabeth Bayley Seton, converted to Catholicism, became a nun, established the Sisters of Charity of St. Joseph, and established the first Catholic parochial school in the United States. In 1976, she was the first American to be canonized as a Saint.

After three years of apprenticeship, Bayley went to London to continue his study of medicine. There he studied with an anatomist named William Hunter. Bayley studied in London for three years, and in 1772 he returned to America.

When Bailey returned to the United States, he work in research and opened up a medical practice with his old teacher John Charlton. Bayley's research included discovering that diphtheria was different from strep throat. He did pathological observations and autopsies, and eventually found that diphtheria causes death by strangulation, while forms of strep throat do not kill victims in this way. Bayley soon developed a new treatment for diphtheria based on this research. His techniques for helping diphtheria patients rapidly came into wide use across the country.

Bayley kept in touch with his mentor Hunter while he was in the United States, often sharing with him research and new treatment methods. In 1775 Bayley once again sailed to England, returning to America in the spring of 1776 as the Revolutionary War was beginning.

Bayley became a military surgeon for the British in the Revolutionary War, and served under the General William Howe. Bayley was stationed in Newport, Rhode Island for about a year, and then his wife fell ill, and Bayley resigned his post and returned to New York to be with her. She never recovered and passed away only shortly after his return to New York.

Bayley stayed in New York after his wife's death and did not return to military service. He spent much of his time

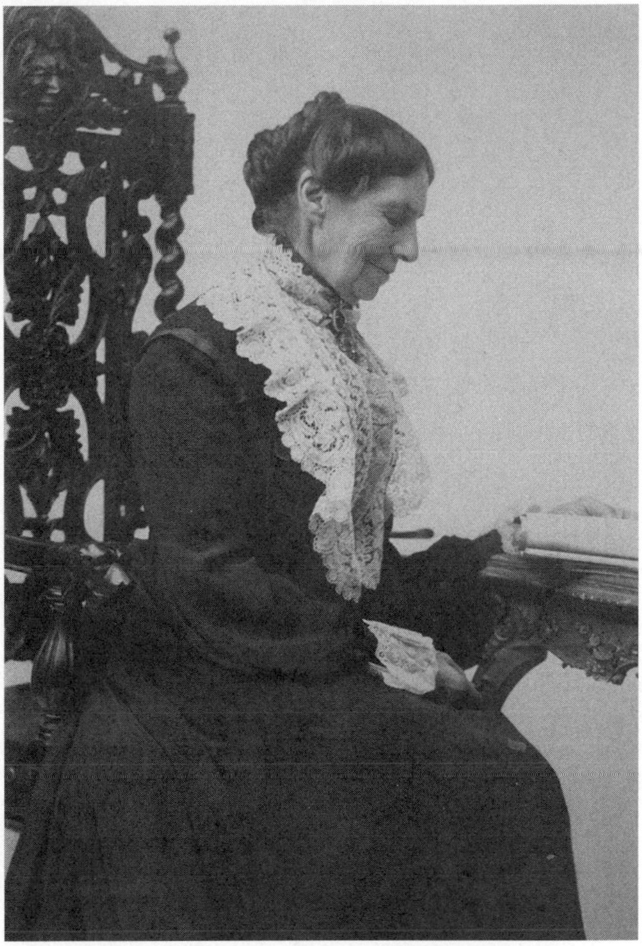

Clara Barton

giving medical lectures and he reestablished the practice that he had once held. In 1788 there were rumors that medical students at the hospital where Bayley lectured were guilty of grave robbing. The mob also believed that Bayley had conducted horrendous and inhumane experiments on the soldiers he had treated during the war. There was a massive riot and a mob destroyed nearly all of Bayley's anatomical collection. Bayley, himself, luckily managed to escape without injury.

Bayley began to become more interested in teaching in his later years. In 1792 he became a professor at Columbia College. He taught a number of subjects including anatomy and surgery. He also continued his research and was innovative in his surgical techniques, developing a new technique of arm amputation at the shoulder joint. Bayley was the first person in the United States to successfully remove an arm at the shoulder joint.

Bayley always had an interest in public health. He helped the cities poor by assisting in the founding of the New York Dispensary. The city was overtaken by a series of yellow fever epidemics that began in 1795. He became interested in the disease and helped to discover how the disease was spread. His discoveries in this area helped to create quarantine laws

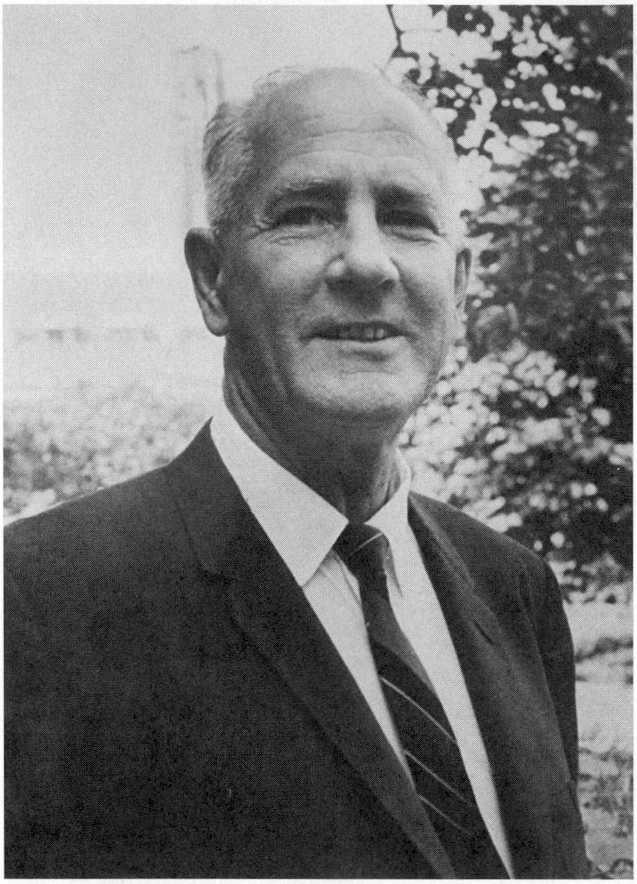

George Wells Beadle

for New York City. Because of his work on yellow fever he was appointed to the position of health physician. His job was to check the ships that were trying to enter the New York harbor and checking the health of their passengers and crew.

Throughout the rest of his life Bayley continued his research and worked as the health physician. Sadly, it was this post that would soon cause his death. He became fatally ill after having checked a ship abroad which a large group of Irish immigrants were dying of yellow fever. He came down with the disease and died of it August 17, 1801.

BEADLE, GEORGE WELLS (1903-1989)

American geneticist

Early in his professional life, George Wells Beadle worked in the laboratory of **Thomas Hunt Morgan**, the geneticist who helped to revolutionize what we know about genetics—the inheritance of characteristics by the deoxyribonucleic acid (DNA) found in the chromosomes of cells. Beadle's innovative research on such diverse living things as corn, fruit flies, and bread mold helped to demystify the activities of genes, making it possible to reduce the inheritance of a particular characteristic to a series of steps needed for the manufacture of biochemicals, notably enzymes. For his work on the ''one gene-one enzyme'' concept, he shared the Nobel Prize for Physiology or Medicine with **Edward Lawrie Tatum** and **Joshua Lederberg** in 1958.

Beadle was born in Wahoo, Nebraska, on October 22, 1903, to Chauncey Elmer and Hattie Albro Beadle. He probably would have worked on the family farm if not for a high school science teacher who advised him to go on to college. At the College of Agriculture at the University of Nebraska, Beadle gained an interest in genetics, especially that of corn. He received his undergraduate degree in biology in 1926, then left for Cornell University in New York where he earned his doctorate in genetics. During this time Beadle married Marion Cecile Hill. They would have one son, David.

In 1931 Beadle went to work in the genetics laboratory of Thomas Hunt Morgan at the California Institute of Technology (Caltech) in Pasadena, California. Morgan had pioneered genetics work on the fruit fly, *Drosophila melanogaster.* Drosophila melanogaster As Beadle studied inherited characteristics such as eye color, he began to think that genes might influence heredity by chemical means. When he left California for Paris in 1935, he continued this line of work with Boris Ephrussi at the Institut de Biologie Physico-Chimique. Carefully transplanting eye buds from the larvae of one type of mutant fruit fly to larvae of another, Beadle showed that eye color in the insects is not a quirk of nature but the result of a long chain of chemical reactions. For all the relative ease of working with fruit flies, however, Beadle sought a simpler organism and a simpler set of chemical reactions to study.

Several years later, Beadle found what he was looking for. When he returned from Paris in 1936 he briefly taught genetics at Harvard and then went on to Stanford University in California, where he remained from 1937 to 1946. As a professor of biology there, he began working with a red bread mold, *Neurospora crassa.* He would work with neurospora for seventeen years. In 1941 he began collaborating with Edward Tatum, and their work eventually won them—with Joshua Lederberg, who later worked with Tatum at Yale—the Nobel Prize.

Neurospora crassa, once the bane of bakers, became a boon for geneticists Beadle and Tatum. Not only does the mold have a short life cycle and grow on a basic sugar medium, but it reproduces both sexually and asexually. Also, the final cell division that produces its reproductive cells, known as ascospores, leaves them in a linear arrangement along the pod-like ascus (spore case), making the trail of inherited characteristics very clear to follow.

Taking a hint from fellow geneticist **Hermann Joseph Muller**, who in the mid–1920s had shown that the rate of mutation increases with exposure to X rays, Beadle and Tatum grew thousand of cultures of molds in which they had induced mutations. The wild strain of the mold can grow on a medium containing very few nutrients. With just some sugar sprinkled with a little biotin (a growth vitamin) and inorganic salts, a wild-type mold can synthesize all the proteins it needs to live. A mold with a mutation, however, loses the ability to make a particular compound it needs to grow, such as a specific amino acid (amino acids are the building blocks of proteins such as those used to construct DNA). Beadle expected that a missing amino acid would have to be supplied to the mold, but found to his surprise the mold was sometimes able to convert a similar compound to the necessary amino acid. Through a process of trial and error, Beadle was able to deduce the sequence of chemical steps involved in the work of conversion.

Once Beadle had pieced together the pathways of chemical production, his ideas could be applied to other molds. One immediate application was to use his techniques to mass-produce the antibiotic penicillin. Penicillin and other antibiotics are derived from compounds produced naturally by certain molds, which use them as a defense against invading bacterial cells.

Beadle also crossed two different mutant strains of mold and found that the resulting hybrid could produce a particular amino acid that neither parent strain could produce alone. This was because one mutant lacked genetic coding for a certain enzyme (a protein that can encourage or inhibit chemical reactions), causing a breakdown in the chemical synthesis along one spot in the sequence, while the other mutant lacked different coding for an enzyme from another spot along the sequence. When crossed, the resulting mold could produce the missing amino acid because it had inherited both genetic patterns, one from each parent. Beadle concluded that specific genes (sequences of protein groups in DNA serving as functional units of inheritance) controlled each step in the sequence. Each gene held the information for the manufacture of a single enzyme, a concept that became known as "one gene, one enzyme."

Extended to other plants and animals, Beadle's theory could be used to explain all of genetic inheritance in terms of chemical reactions. Different genes control the different stages of chemical reactions. For example, cells must be able to produce the pigment that gives an animal's eyes their color. The production of pigment might occur in several steps, with enzymes used to hasten each chemical reaction. If the gene for any one of the enzymes is missing, the cells cannot produce the pigment.

The one gene-one enzyme concept caused a breakthrough in genetic research during the 1940s by shifting the study of genetics away from physical characteristics of organisms to the production of biochemicals. On the heels of this line of research, the compound deoxyribonucleic acid (DNA) was analyzed, and the mechanism of the genetic code was pieced together in the early 1950s. Beadle and Tatum parted ways when Tatum left for Yale University in 1945. Using the same mutation induction techniques on bacteria, Tatum worked along with Joshua Lederberg to show how genetic information can be transferred from one bacterium to another.

Beadle became professor and chairman of the division of biology at Caltech in 1946 and stayed on until 1961. For his work in genetics he won the Lasker Award of the American Public Health Association in 1950. He and his first wife divorced, and he then married Muriel Barnett in 1953. With his second wife he wrote several books on genetics for a general audience. Recognition for years of work came in 1958 when Beadle, Tatum and Lederberg won the Nobel Prize. In that same year Beadle won the Albert Einstein Commemorative Award in Science, and in the following year he received the National Award from the American Cancer Society.

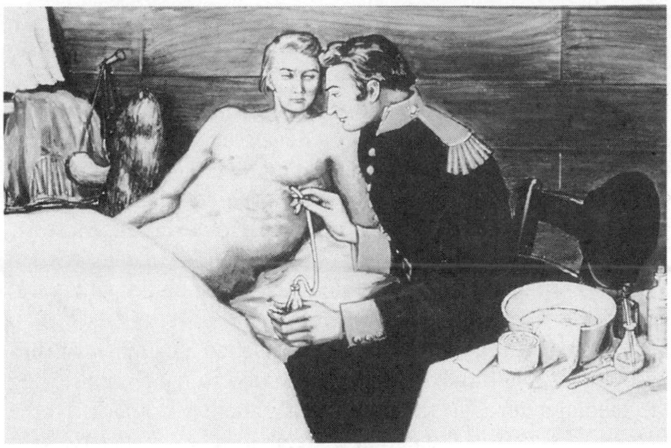

William Beaumont (right) with Alexis St. Martin.

In the 1960s Beadle renewed his interest in the genetics of corn. He became a player in the "corn wars," a debate among geneticists and archaeologists over the domestication of corn or maize in the Americas. Beadle contended that modern corn comes from a Mexican wild grass rather than a now-extinct species of maize. Beadle drew his conclusion from the corn remains that show that domestication occurred at the time of the Mayans and Aztecs.

In 1961 Beadle left California for Chicago, Illinois, where he became the sixth chancellor of the University of Chicago. He remained there until he retired in 1968. By then he had accumulated over thirty honorary degrees from many universities around the country and been awarded memberships into several prestigious academic societies. For their work in popularizing genetics, he and his wife Muriel won the Edison Award in 1967. In the late 1960s Beadle became director of the American Medical Association's Institute for Biomedical Research. He died on June 9, 1989, in Pomona, California, at age eighty-five from complications of Alzheimer's disease.

Beaumont, William (1785-1853)

American surgeon

Beaumont, Connecticut-born and the son of a farmer, worked briefly as a school teacher, then studied medicine at St. Albans, Vermont. He received a license to practice medicine in time to serve as an assistant army surgeon during the War of 1812. Although he left the army in 1815 to start a medical practice in Plattsburgh, New York, he returned in 1820 and remained an Army surgeon, serving at various posts, until 1839.

It was at one of those army posts, Fort Mackinac in northern Michigan, that Beaumont met the patient that was to make both of them famous. The patient was a 19-year-old French Canadian trapper, Alexis St. Martin, who was accidentally shot on June 6, 1822, while visiting the Mackinac branch of the American Fur Company. The bullet wound tore a deep chunk out of the left side of St. Martin's lower chest; and, although Beaumont was sent for immediately, everyone assumed that the young man would never survive. Miraculously, he did—although his wound needed to be rebandaged daily for a year—and in time St. Martin recovered virtually all his strength. (He lived to be 82, in fact.) However, St. Martin's bullet hole never fully closed. An inch-wide opening (called a fistula) remained through which Beaumont could put his finger all the way into the stomach.

About a year later, St. Martin needed a cathartic of rhubarb and sulphur and Beaumont decided to try administering the medicine through the hole in his patient's stomach. To the surgeon's surprise, the cathartic seemed to work exactly as it would have if it had been administered orally—and Beaumont promptly began planning other experiments as well.

Beaumont started by taking small chunks of food, tying them to a string, and inserting them directly into St. Martin's stomach. At varying intervals, he then pulled the food out—and was therefore able to observe, first hand, the results of digestion, hour by hour. Later, by using a hand lens, Beaumont began peering into his patient's stomach, and could actually see how the human stomach behaved at various stages of digestion and under varying circumstances. He was also able to extract and analyze samples of digestive juice.

Over the next few years, Beaumont conducted well over two hundred carefully detailed experiments and, in 1833, published his findings as *Experiments and Observations on the Gastric Juice and the Physiology of Digestion.* The book provided invaluable information on the digestive process and also suggested to other scientists (including **Claude Bernard**) that artificial fistulas might be a practical way to learn more about the body. A year after Beaumont's work was published, St. Martin, probably tiring of the scrutiny Beaumont had subjected him to, refused to cooperate with further studies and returned to Canada.

Although Beaumont resigned from the army in 1840, went into private practice in St. Louis, Missouri, and stayed out of the laboratory, his one classic work earned him lasting fame as one of America's more remarkable pioneer researchers.

BECQUEREL, ANTOINE HENRI (1852-1908)

French physicist

The discovery of radioactivity has been called the most dramatic scientific breakthrough of our time. From the initial experiments came an understanding of the inner workings of the atom and the establishment of a new science, nuclear physics. Though many were to follow him, Henri Becquerel was the first to experiment with radioactivity. Quite by accident, he observed the mysterious energy emitted by uranium, and his research sparked a new wave of scientific theory.

That Becquerel became a scientist was of no surprise to his family—both his father and grandfather before him had

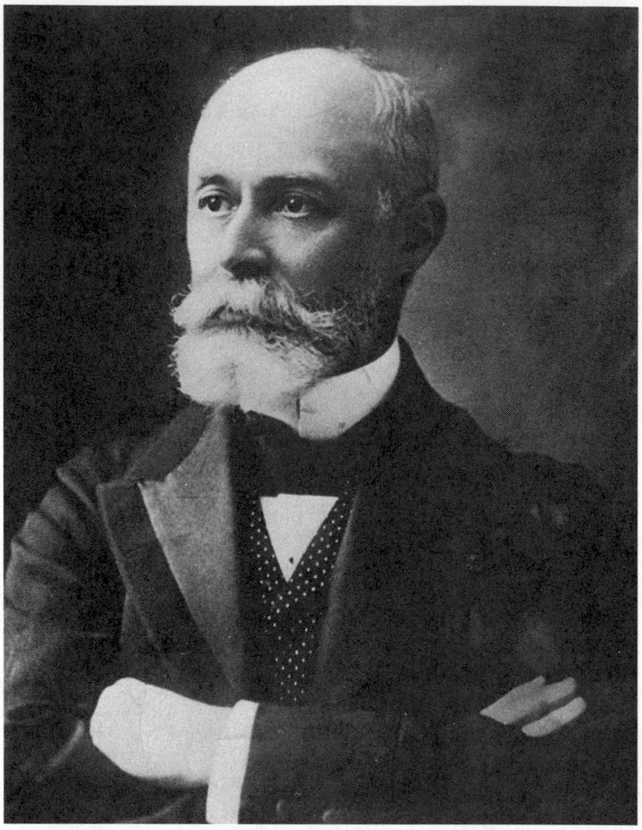

Antoine Henri Becquerel

been physicists. Becquerel's father had specialized in the study of fluorescence, and Henri began his own research in this field while attending college. He received his engineering degree in 1877 from the École des Ponts et Chaussees, after which he entered the Administration of Bridges and Highways. During this time, his wife of four years died shortly after bearing him a son, Jean. Still concentrating on optics, Becquerel pursued his doctorate at the Faculty of Sciences of Paris. He delivered his dissertation in 1888 and was soon elected to the Academy of Sciences. Content to teach at the École Polytechnique, he ceased his experimentation, at least temporarily.

His father Edmond died in 1891, and the following year he was appointed to his father's chairs in the physics departments of the Conservatoire National des Arts et Métiers and the Museum of Natural History, all while continuing to lecture and serve at the Administration of Highways and Bridges. In 1895 he accepted an unprecedented third chair, this time at the École Polytechnique, and at age forty-three he had become one of the most powerful scientists in France, all without offering a major contribution to science. That, however, would soon change.

In the early days of 1896, Becquerel became one of the many scientists fascinated by Wilhelm Röntgen's discovery of **x rays**. Wondering if these "penetrating rays" were related to the luminescence he had studied for years, he experimented with a sample of potassium uranyl sulfate crystal and a photographic plate. Exposing the sample to sunlight (to trigger the luminescent emission), he placed the crystal in a darkroom next to the photographic plate. Though the plate showed developed streaks, indicating the presence of penetrating rays, he noticed the effect whether the crystal had been exposed to light or not. This eliminated the possibility of a luminescent connection, and Becquerel realized he had discovered a new type of penetrating ray. Further research showed that only crystals that contained uranium would develop the plate, and that a disk of pure uranium metal produced penetrating rays nearly four times as intense as his original sample.

Becquerel presented his findings to the world in May of 1896, labeling these new emissions Becquerel rays. Soon, Pierre Curie and Marie Curie, colleagues of Becquerel, found that thorium also emitted Becquerel rays, and they later discovered why: the presence of one of two new *radioactive* (a word coined by Marie Curie) elements, polonium and radium. Becquerel continued his own research, isolating electrons in radiation in 1900 and noting the first evidence of radioactive transformation in 1902.

From this point, the Curies took the leading role in radiation research. Becquerel became their liaison to the scientific world, presenting papers documenting their progress to the Academy of Sciences. For his discovery of radioactivity, Becquerel shared the 1903 Nobel Prize for Physics with the Curies. He was awarded numerous accolades and served as officer of many scientific organizations before his death in 1908.

BEDSORES

Bedsores are also called decubitus ulcers, pressure ulcers, or pressure sores. These tender or inflamed patches develop when skin covering a weight-bearing part of the body is squeezed between bone and another body part, or a bed, chair, splint, or other hard object.

Each year, about one million people in the United States develop bedsores ranging from a mild inflammation to deep **wounds** that involve muscle and bone. This often painful condition usually starts with shiny red skin that quickly blisters and deteriorates into open sores that can harbor life-threatening infection.

Bedsores are not cancerous or contagious. They are most likely to occur in people who must use wheelchairs or who are confined to bed. People over the age of 60 are more likely than younger people to develop bedsores. Risk is also increased by **atherosclerosis** (hardening of arteries), **diabetes**, diminished sensation or lack of feeling, heart problems, inability to control bladder or bowel movements, **malnutrition**, **obesity**, **paralysis**, poor circulation, prolonged bed rest (especially in unsanitary conditions) and **spinal cord injury**.

Bedsores most often develop when constant pressure pinches tiny blood vessels that deliver oxygen and nutrients to the skin. When skin is deprived of oxygen and nutrients for as little as an hour, areas of tissue can die and bedsores can form.

Slight rubbing or friction against the skin can cause minor pressure ulcers. They can also develop when a patient stretches or bends blood vessels by slipping into a different position in a bed or chair. Urine, feces, or other moisture increase the risk of skin infection, and people who are unable to move or recognize internal cues to shift position have a greater than average risk of developing bedsores.

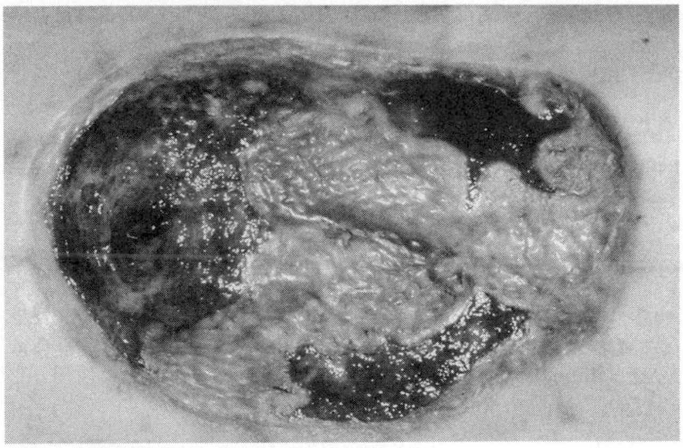

Bedsore. ***(Photograph by Michael English, M.D., Custom Medical Stock Photo. Reproduced by permission.)***

Bedsores are usually recognized by **physical examination**, medical history, and patient and caregiver observations. They usually follow six stages:

- Redness of skin
- Redness, swelling, and possible peeling of outer layer of skin
- Dead skin, draining wound, and exposed layer of fat
- Tissue death through skin and fat, to muscle
- Inner fat and muscle death
- Destruction of bone, bone, infection, fracture, and blood infection.

Prompt medical attention can prevent surface pressure sores from deepening into more serious infections. For mild bedsores, treatment involves relieving pressure, keeping the wound clean, and keeping the area around the ulcer clean and dry. The patient's doctor may prescribe infection-fighting **antibiotics**, special dressings or drying agents, or lotions or ointments to be applied to the wound. Warm whirlpool treatments are sometimes recommended for sores on the arm, hand, foot, or leg.

For more serious bedsores, a procedure called debriding uses a scalpel may be used to remove dead tissue or other debris from the wound. Deep, ulcerated sores that do not respond to other therapy may require skin grafts or plastic surgery.

Immediate medical attention is required whenever the skin turns black or becomes inflamed, tender, swollen, or warm to the touch, the patient develops a **fever** during treatment, or the sore contains pus or has a foul-smelling discharge. With proper treatment, bedsores begin to heal two to four weeks after treatment starts.

To prevent bedsores, the patient should be inspected regularly. A bedridden patient should be repositioned at least once every two hours while awake. A person who uses a wheelchair should shift his weight every 10 or 15 minutes, or be helped to reposition himself at least once an hour. It is important to lift, rather than drag, a person being repositioned, since dragging may aggravate the sores.

If the patient is bedridden, sensitive body parts can be protected by sheepskin pads, special cushions placed on top of a mattress, a water-filled mattress, or a variable-pressure mattress whose sections can be individually inflated or deflated to redistribute pressure.

Bedsores can usually be cured, but can be slow to heal. Without proper treatment, they can lead to infections that slow the healing process, increase the cost of treatment, lengthen hospital or nursing home stays, or cause death. About 60,000 deaths a year are attributed to complications caused by bedsores.

BED-WETTING

Bed-wetting (sometimes called enuresis), is unintentional urination during the night. Most children wet the bed occasionally, and definitions of the age and frequency at which bed-wetting becomes a medical problem vary. Many researchers consider bed-wetting normal until age 6. For a diagnosis of enuresis, wetting must occur twice a week for at least three months with no underlying physiological cause.

Enuresis is divided into two classes. A child with primary enuresis has never established bladder control. A child with secondary enuresis begins to wet after a prolonged dry period. Some children have bladder control problems during both day and night.

The causes of bed-wetting are not entirely known, but it tends to run in families. Most children with primary enuresis have a close relative who also had the disorder. Sometimes bed-wetting can be caused by a serious medical problem such as diabetes, **sickle-cell anemia**, or epilepsy. Snoring and episodes of interrupted breathing during sleep (**sleep apnea**) may contribute to bed-wetting, as do urinary tract infections, severe **constipation**, or **spinal cord injury**.

Recent medical research has found that many children who wet the bed may have a deficiency of an important hormone known as antidiuretic hormone (ADH). ADH helps regulate the level of fluids in the body and helps to concentrate urine. Children who wet the bed, therefore, often produce more urine during the hours of sleep than their bladders can hold. If they do not wake up, the bladder releases the urine and the child wets the bed.

Most children who wet the bed do not have physical or psychological problems. Sometimes emotional **stress**, such as the birth of a sibling, a **death** in the family, or separation from the family, may be a trigger for bedwetting. Daytime wetting, however, may indicate that the problem has a physical cause. While most children have no long-term problems as a result of bed-wetting, some children may develop psychological problems that are aggravated when playmates tease them.

If a child continues to wet the bed after the age of six, parents may wish to seek evaluation and diagnosis by a pediatrician. The child receives a **physical examination**, appropriate laboratory tests, including a urine test (**urinalysis**), and, if necessary other studies.

If the child is healthy and no physical problems are found, which is the case 90% of the time, the doctor may not recommend treatment. Instead he may provide the parents and the child with reassurance, information, and advice.

Occasionally a doctor will determine that the problem is serious enough to require treatment. Standard treatments for bed-wetting include bladder training, **exercise**s, motivational therapy, drug therapy, psychotherapy, and diet therapy. A number of drugs are also used to treat bed-wetting. These medications are usually fast acting, and children often respond to them within the first week of treatment. Among the drugs commonly used are a nasal spray of desmopressin acetate (DDAVP), a substance similar to the hormone ADH, and imipramine hydrochloride, a drug that helps to increase bladder capacity. Studies show that imipramine is effective for as many as 50% of patients. However, children often wet the bed again after the drug is discontinued, and it has some undesirable side effects.

Some bed-wetting with an underlying physical cause can be treated by surgical procedures. These causes include enlarged adenoids that cause sleep apnea, physical defects in the urinary system, or a spinal tumor.

Occasional bed-wetting is not a disease and it does not have a ''cure.'' If the child has no underlying physical or psychological problem that is causing the bed-wetting, in most cases he or she will outgrow the condition without treatment.

BEHAVIORAL SCIENCES

Behavioral science is concerned with human actions, and since behavior is influenced so importantly by people and social settings, the behavioral and social sciences are very closely related. The scientific study of behavior developed in a formal way in the 19th century, and research in the behavioral sciences now makes use of a variety of different research methods that rely on both observation and description as well as statistical modeling and experimentation. The development and testing of general theories that explain behavior is a priority for research that studies social function, development, individual variation, and the various social and biological contexts of behavior.

The core disciplines that contribute to behavioral science include anthropology, psychology, and sociology, but many other disciplines also play an important role, such as the behavioral aspects of biology, economics, geography, law, psychology, and political science. Although behavioral and social sciences have a distinctive focus, considerable overlap may blur the distinctions. Anthropology studies people and their society, but presently and historically; sociology addresses questions that focus on social relations and the essential nature of society. Psychology focuses on mental and cognitive processes of individuals, but ultimately the interdisciplinary links between anthropology, sociology, and psychology are crucial.

Over the course of the 20th century causes of premature death and disability have been changing, and the behavioral and social factors that influence these changes take on added importance. Technological innovation, migration, and civil strife have each contributed to the development of new areas and priorities in medicine, such as occupational health, international health, and specialized health care for migrants and refugees. Environmental factors, chronic disease, and violence each present specialized challenges for health care professionals. With the development and legitimacy of **public health**, primary preventionof disease and health promotion also become more important.

Behavior may be a key factor in determining risk for becoming ill and the various ways that people seek help for their health problems. **Smoking**, sexual promiscuity, diet, risk taking, and other factors under the broad heading of lifestyle may increase the chance of a person acquiring **lung cancer**, **sexually transmitted diseases**, diabetes, and other illness. Behavior may also affect risk for acquiring infectious diseases. For example, poor **sanitation** and hygiene make some people susceptible to **diarrhea**; in contrast, people try in different ways to protect themselves from insects or animals that may transmit disease. Behavioral and social sciences consider how people and societies place themselves at risk for or protect themselves from disease.

Basic research in behavioral and social sciences is not so concerned as epidemiology (the study of patterns of disease in a population) with the relationship of risk factors and disease outcomes, but rather more concerned with the processes that influence risk and protection, and how they operate. It examines the behavioral, psychological, and social processes, such as emotion, motivation, and language development, that contribute to health and disease. Studies under the heading ''biopsychosocial'' research focus on the interdisciplinary interactions between biology and either social or behavioral principles. Psychoneuroimmunology and behavioral cardiology are examples. Another basic research interest examines and develops ways of measuring and analyzing behavior and mental function. Neuropsychological assessment of people's compliance with medical treatment indicates the practical value of applied interests in the field.

The behavioral and social sciences are especially concerned with the question of how specific behavioral and social factors are linked to mental and physical health outcomes (that is, whether a person becomes better or worse), and the ways in which they are related. It also examines the effects of illness or physical condition on human behavior and social relationships. This focus helps to design and evaluate behavioral and social ways of treating a variety of mental and physical diseases and disorders. It also helps to formulate not only strategies for health promotion and disease prevention but also to consider the impact of changes in the structure of health services. Specialty areas of biological and pharmacological research on treatment interventions are becoming more concerned with the behavioral aspects of outcome in their evaluation of these interventions.

Study of behavioral science may provide good training for jobs that require an understanding of the way people act, including administrative, service, or professional positions. For scientists, it also provides a means of taking into account the interactions of behavior and biology, both the practical questions and the scientific issues that researchers try to explain.

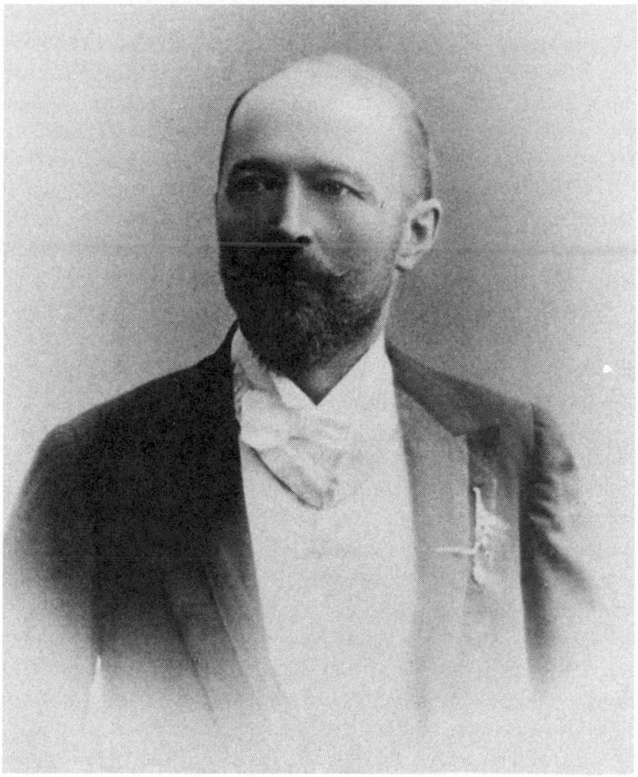

Emil von Behring

See also Environmental health; Health care system; Infection control; Occupation safety and health; Violence and violence prevention

Behring, Emil von (1854-1917)

German bacteriologist

Emil von Behring was one of the founders of the science of immunology. His discovery of the diphtheria and tetanus antitoxins paved the way for the prevention of these diseases through the use of immunization. It also opened the door for the specific treatment of such diseases with the injection of immune serum. Behring's stature as a seminal figure in modern medicine was recognized in 1901 when he received the first Nobel Prize in physiology or medicine.

Emil Adolf von Behring was born on March 15, 1854, in Hansdorf, West Prussia (now Germany). He was the eldest son of August Georg Behring, a schoolmaster with thirteen children, and his second wife, Augustine Zech Behring. Although his father planned for him to become a minister, young Behring had an inclination toward medicine. The family's meager circumstances seemed to put this goal out of his reach, however. Then one of Behring's teachers, recognizing great promise, arranged for his admission to the Army Medical College in Berlin, where he was able to obtain a free medical education in exchange for future military service. He received his doctor of medicine degree in 1878, and two years later he passed the state examination that allowed him to practice.

The army promptly sent Behring to Posen (now Poznan, Poland), then to Bonn in 1887, and finally back to Berlin in 1888. His first published papers, which date from this period, dealt with the use of iodoform as an antiseptic. After completing his military service in 1889, Behring became an assistant at the Institute of Hygiene in Berlin, joining a brilliant team of researchers headed by **Robert Koch**, a leading light in the new science of bacteriology.

It was while working in Koch's laboratory that Behring began his pioneering investigations of diphtheria and tetanus. Both of these diseases are caused by bacilli (bacteria) that do not spread widely through the body, but produce generalized symptoms by excreting toxins. Diphtheria, nicknamed the "strangling angel" because of the way it obstructs breathing, was a terrible killer of children in the late nineteenth century. Its toxin had first been detected by others in 1888. Tetanus, likewise, was fatal more often than not. In 1889, the tetanus bacillus was cultivated in its pure state for the first time by Shibasaburo Kitasato, another gifted member of Koch's team.

The next year, Behring and Kitasato jointly published their classic paper, "Ueber das Zustandekommen der Diphtherie-Immunität und der Tetanus-Immunität bei Thieren" ("The Mechanism of Immunity in Animals to Diphtheria and Tetanus"). One week later, Behring alone published another paper dealing with immunity against diphtheria and outlining five ways in which it could be achieved. These reports announced that injections of toxin from diphtheria or tetanus bacilli led animals to produce in their blood substances capable of neutralizing the disease poison.

Behring and Kitasato dubbed these substances antitoxins. Furthermore, injections of blood serum from an animal that had been given a chance to develop antitoxins to tetanus or diphtheria could confer immunity to the disease on other animals, and even cure animals that were already sick.

The news created a sensation. Several papers confirming and amplifying these results, including some by Behring himself, appeared in rapid succession. In 1893, Behring described a group of human diphtheria patients who were treated with antitoxin. That same year, he was given the title of professor. However, Behring's diphtheria antitoxin did not yield consistent results. It was the bacteriologist **Paul Ehrlich**, another of the talented associates in Koch's lab, who was chiefly responsible for standardizing the antitoxin, thus making it practical for widespread therapeutic use. Working together, Ehrlich and Behring also showed that high-quality antitoxin could be obtained from horses, as well as from the sheep used previously, opening the way for large-scale production of the antitoxin.

In 1894, Behring accepted a position as professor at the University of Halle. A year later, he was named a professor and director of the Institute of Hygiene at the University of Marburg. Thereafter he focused much of his attention on the problem of immunization against tuberculosis. His assumption, unfounded as it turned out, was that different forms of the disease in humans and in cattle were closely related. He tried immunizing calves with a weakened strain of the human tuberculosis bacillus, but the results were disappointing. Although his bovine vaccine was widely used for a time in Germany, Russia, Sweden, and the United States, it was found that the cattle excreted dangerous microorganisms afterward. Nevertheless, Behring's basic idea of using a bacillus from one species to benefit another influenced the development of later vaccines.

Behring did not entirely abandon his work on diphtheria during this period. In 1913, he announced the development of a toxin-antitoxin mixture that resulted in longer-lasting immunity than did antitoxin serum alone. This approach was a forerunner of modern methods of preventing, rather than just treating, the disease. Today children are routinely and effectively vaccinated against diphtheria and tetanus.

However, the first great drop in diphtheria mortality was due to the antitoxin therapy introduced earlier by Behring, and it is for this contribution that he is primarily remembered. The fall in the diphtheria death rate around the turn of the century was one of the sharpest ever recorded for any treatment. In Germany alone, an estimated 45,000 lives per year were saved. It is no wonder, then, that Behring received the 1901 Nobel Prize "for his work on serum therapy, especially its application against diphtheria, by which he... opened a new road in the domain of medical science and thereby placed in the hands of the physician a victorious weapon against illness and deaths." Behring was also elevated to the status of nobility and shared a sizable cash prize from the Paris Academy of Medicine with Émile Roux, the French bacteriologist who was one of the men who had the diphtheria toxin in 1888. In addition, Behring was granted honorary memberships in societies in Italy, Turkey, France, Hungary, and Russia.

There were other, financial rewards as well. From 1901 onward, ill health prevented Behring from giving regular lectures, so he devoted himself to research. A commercial firm in which he had a financial interest built a well-equipped laboratory for his use in Marburg, Germany. Then, in 1914, Behring established his own company to manufacture serums and vaccines. The profits from this venture allowed him to keep a large estate at Marburg, on which he grazed cattle used in experiments. This house was a gathering place of society. Behring also owned a vacation home on the island of Capri in the Mediterranean.

In 1896 Behring married 18-year-old Else Spinola, daughter of the director of a Berlin hospital. They had seven children. Yet despite all outward appearances of personal and professional success, Behring was subject to frequent bouts of serious depression, some of which required sanatorium treatment. In addition, a fractured thigh led to a condition that increasingly impaired his mobility. He was already in a weakened state when he contracted pneumonia in 1917. His body was unable to withstand the added strain, and he died on March 31 in Marburg, Germany.

BÉKÉSY, GEORG VON (1899-1972)

Hungarian American physicist and physiologist

Georg von Békésy was a Hungarian-born scientist who discovered how sound is analyzed and communicated in the cochlea, part of the inner ear. For this work, in 1961 he became the first physicist to receive the Nobel Prize in medicine and physiology in 1961.

The son of a diplomat, Békésy was born in Budapest, Hungary. He studied at the University of Bern in Switzerland, graduating in 1920, and at the University of Budapest, from which he received a doctorate in physics. He then worked at the Hungarian Telephone System Research Laboratory for nearly a quarter of a century. During this same period, he also worked at the central laboratories of Siemens and Halske AC in Berlin as well as serving on the University of Budapest faculty. In 1946, after Soviet forces occupied Hungary, Békésy emigrated to Sweden, and then in 1947, to the United States. There he spent the next 23 years as a professor and researcher, first at Harvard University (1949-1966) and then at the University of Hawaii (1966-1972).

It was Békésy's work as a telecommunications engineer for the Hungarian Telephone System that would prompt his research into the workings of the human ear. In order to determine what frequency range a cable would be able to carry, he decided to investigate how the human ear received sound. His research on the eardrum involved actually attaching two mirrors onto an eardrum and observing the reflections of the membrane's movements as sound waves activated it.

Békésy conducted another series of experiments in which he observed how parts of the middle ear, namely, the hammer, anvil, and stirrup, receive the vibrations transmitted by the eardrum and relay these messages to the cochlea in the inner ear. The fact that nerves in the cochlea pick up sound signals and transmit them along the auditory nerve to the brain for interpretation had long been known. The importance of the basilar membrane, the vibratory tissue most critical for hearing, had also been well established. This membrane stretches the length of the snail-shaped cochlea, partitioning it into two canals, and contains groups of fine fibers, that widen as one moves along the cochlea to its tip.

A widely accepted theory at this time, put forth by Hermann von Helmholtz, held that each fiber on the basilar membrane had a natural period of vibration and responded only to sounds that vibrated at that period. Each group of fibers was claimed to stimulate different nerve endings in this was enabling the brain to differentiate specific frequencies.

Careful work by Békésy disproved the Helmholtz theory. He constructed models of cochlea and worked with cochlea from cadavers to test his ideas. By electrically stimulating the auditory mechanisms of his specimens, he was able to study the function of the cochlea. Békésy had to develop new instruments and techniques for this delicate work. He designed extremely fine drills and probes, which were used to grind a small opening in the skull and then reach the basilar membrane. He used a saline solution containing fine aluminum particles to mimic the cochlea's natural fluid and was able to witness and measure for the first time a phenomenon he called the ''traveling wave.''

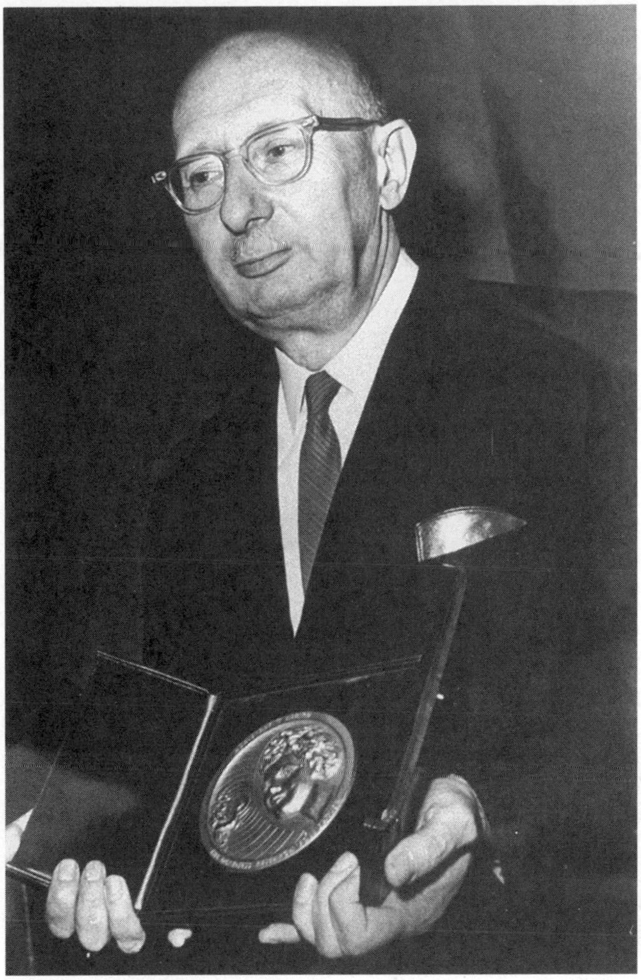

Georg von Békésy

Békésy saw that the stirrup of the middle ear operated much like a lid on an opening in the cochlea, called the oval window. Sound vibrations cause the stirrup to move, exerting pressure on the fluid in the cochlea. The vibrations are transmitted to the basilar membrane in the form of traveling waves. Békésy found that the entire membrane vibrated. Each wave causes maximum vibration at different sections of the membrane according to its frequency. High-pitched sounds produce high-frequency waves that reach their peak on the part of the basilar membrane closest the stirrup, that is, near the cochlea's entrance. Low sounds produce low-frequency waves that reach their maximum amplitude farther along the membrane, near the end of the cochlea. Békésy discovered that pitch and loudness had to do with the location and number of nerve receptors. The shape of the sound wave, along with the varying pitch, loudness, and quality, is what gives the brain the information to interpret.

Later, Békésy would also devise an audiometer to test hearing function and determine whether deafness had been caused by damage to the ear or to the brain, which facilitated proper treatment at an earlier stage.

In addition, Békésy became interested in visual and tactile sensations, which he measured and recorded. He developed a way for the skin to "hear," using equipment consisting of a much larger version of a cochlea. When its membrane was pressed against a person's skin, the skin could feel high and low sounds sent through the tube portion at distinctly different positions along the arm. Such experiments suggested new ways of helping the deaf and improved knowledge about deafness. Békésy passed away in 1972.

BELL'S PALSY

Bell's palsy is an unexplained weakness or **paralysis** of the muscles on one side of the face that affects approximately 40,000-65,000 Americans each year. People with Bell's palsy may be unable to close the eye on the affected side, and may also experience tearing, drooling, and hypersensitive hearing. Bell's palsy can begin quite suddenly, sometimes appearing overnight. Although this disorder is unsettling and inconvenient, it is typically not indicative of a serious health problem. The weakness and paralysis eventually disappear in the majority of cases.

Facial palsies have been linked to conditions such as **Lyme disease**, ear infection, **meningitis**, **syphilis**, German **measles** (**rubella**), **mumps**, **chickenpox**, and infection with Epstein-Barr virus (e.g., **infectious mononucleosis**). Bell's palsy is diagnosed when these other conditions have been eliminated.

The root cause of Bell's palsy has not been identified. Although Bell's palsy is not life-threatening, it can present symptoms similar to truly serious conditions, such as a **stroke**, ruptured aneurysm, or tumors.

Although not considered a serious condition from a health standpoint, Bell's palsy can cause **stress**, embarrassment, and inconvenience for those affected. In the 80-85% of cases, the facial weakness or paralysis is temporary. However, individuals who experience complete paralysis seem to have a poorer recovery rate, with only 60% returning to normal.

The symptoms of Bell's palsy are the result of an inflammation or swelling of the facial nerve that controls the muscles on either side of the face. Swelling increases compression of the nerve. The nerve signal conduction is disrupted, leading the loss of muscle control.

Why the facial nerve becomes inflamed in Bell's palsy is not clear, but it may be related to an infection of the herpes simplex virus (HSV), the virus responsible for **cold sore**s and fever blisters.

Although Bell's palsy is not life-threatening, it shares symptoms with serious conditions, such as stroke. Emergency medical attention is a wise precaution, and extensive testing may be needed to rule out the possibility that the patient is experiencing a more serious condition. Once all other possibilities are exhausted, a diagnosis of Bell's palsy is made. If facial movement, even a small amount, has not returned within 3-4 months, the diagnosis of Bell's palsy may need to be reevaluated.

Many doctors prescribe an antiviral or a steroid drug for Bell's palsy, but there is some controversy about whether these drugs actually help. If drugs are used, they need to be taken as soon as possible following the onset of symptoms. **Antiviral drugs**, such as acyclovir, famciclovir, or valacyclovir destroy actively replicating viruses and prevent further damage to the facial nerve. Steroids such as prednisone reducing swelling and compression of the nerve.

In the past, surgery was performed to relieve the compression on the nerve. However, this treatment option is now used very infrequently because it does not guarantee recovery, and it carries the risk of permanent nerve damage.

The need to protect the affected eye is important. Since the patient may not be able to lower the affected eyelid, the eye may become dry, particularly at night. Excessive dryness can damage the cornea. Daytime treatment includes artificial tears, an eye patch, or other protective measures. Nighttime treatment involves a more intense effort at keeping the eye protected. Eye lubricants or viscous ointments, along with taping the eye shut, are frequently recommended.

In cases of permanent nerve damage, cosmetic treatment options, such as surgery, may be suggested. Practitioners of traditional Chinese medicine have historically used **acupuncture** to treat Bell's palsy.

Most individuals with Bell's palsy begin to notice improvement in their condition within 2-3 weeks of the onset of symptoms. At least 80% of them will be fully recovered within three months. Individuals suffering permanent nerve damage may not regain control of the muscles on the affected side of the face. These muscles may remain weak or paralyzed. If the nerve recovers imperfectly, they may experience involuntary facial twitches or spasms that accompany normal facial expressions.

BENACERRAF, BARUJ (1920-)

Venezuelan American pathologist and immunochemist

Baruj Benacerraf is a Venezuelan-born immunologist whose major contribution to modern immunology was the discovery of the immune-response gene (Ir), which triggers the body's war on disease. For his work linking Ir genes to the major histocompatibility complex or supergene, which controls the nature and vigor of the body's immune response, Benacerraf was awarded the 1980 Nobel Prize in physiology or medicine, which he shared with two other immunologists.

Benacerraf was born on October 29, 1920, in Caracas, Venezuela, to Henriette Lasry and Abraham Benacerraf. His father was a Sephardic Jew who had emigrated from North Africa to Venezuela, working his way to wealth and prominence as a financier and textile importer. When Benacerraf was five, the family moved to France where Benacerraf attended the Lycée Janson and received a classic French education in pre-World War II Paris. In 1938, fearing the outbreak of war in Europe, the family returned to Venezuela; Benacerraf was sent to the United States to follow in his father's footsteps, enrolling as a student in the Textile Engineering School of the Philadelphia Museum of Art. To his family's regret, he left after only two weeks and entered Columbia University to pursue a career in science and medicine.

He graduated in 1942 but was rejected by twenty-five medical schools, including Columbia, Harvard, and Yale, due to his Jewish background and Venezuelan nationality. Eventually, he was accepted by the Medical College of Virginia in Richmond and became a naturalized citizen. In 1943 he married Annette Dreyfus, niece of Nobel laureate **Jacques Lucien Monod** and descendent of Captain Alfred Dreyfus of Devil's Island fame. They had one child, a daughter, Beryl, who would later become a medical radiologist.

Benacerraf interned at Queens General Hospital in New York and then spent two years in the U.S. Army Medical Corps. He was nearly thirty before he began his training in experimental immunology as an unpaid research fellow at the Neurological Institute of Columbia University. The director of the institute, Elvin Kabat, was a pioneer in immunology.

Immunochemistry in the 1950s was an esoteric backwater of biology awaiting the development of powerful electron microscopes, DNA modeling, and a commitment of massive government funding. Only the most general principles of immunity were understood: that proteins called antibodies were manufactured by the body to fight off substances called antigens produced by invading bacteria, viruses, and environmental pollutants. How antibodies were made, by which cells, and how the body distinguished self from nonself were still mysteries.

At Columbia, under Kabat's stern tutelage, Benacerraf learned the importance of precise measurement in immunological research and the value of critical thinking based on firm, empirical evidence. His first experiments dealt with the nature of hypersensitivity, the body's allergic reaction to the overproduction of antibodies. As a child Benacerraf had suffered from bronchial asthma, and his later research would focus on the relationship between allergic diseases and immunological response. In 1949 he moved to Paris to work at the Broussais Hospital with Bernard Halpern, the discoverer of antihistamines. In Paris, Benacerraf studied the action of phagocytes, the cellular scavengers responsible for cleaning the body of diseased cells and foreign contaminants. With Guido Biozzi, an Italian immunologist, Benacerraf developed the equations that describe the amount of particulate matter phagocytes can remove from the liver and spleen.

Due to a heart attack that had crippled his father, Benacerraf was forced to devote considerable time each year to overseeing his family's financial interests in Venezuela. Trips to South America sometimes lasted as long as six months and dealt with such unscientific matters as accounting, high finance, and personnel management. Not until 1956, when he received his first paid appointment as assistant professor of pathology at the New York University School of Medicine, was Benacerraf able to devote his full attention to research and shake the suspicion that he was only a dilettante in science. Later he would come to see that his years of business experience gave him a distinct advantage as an administrator of university departments and government agencies.

In retrospect, Benacerraf came to view the late 1950s and early 1960s as the golden age of his career. His family's finances had been successfully transferred to the United States; he spent only one day a week managing the Colonial Trust Company from its headquarters at Rockefeller Center. At New York University he received a well-equipped laboratory, ample funding, and the support of enthusiastic and innovative colleagues.

With **Gerald M. Edelman** of Rockefeller University, Benacerraf undertook a series of experiments on antibody structure that eventually led Edelman to the 1972 Nobel Prize and Benacerraf to the discovery of a completely unknown gene. Seeking to produce identical immunization in a group of guinea pigs, Benacerraf discovered by accident that when guinea pigs were injected with the same foreign substance, some made antibodies and others did not. By breeding the ''responders'' with the ''nonresponders,'' Benacerraf isolated a gene that appeared to control immune response. He called the gene Ir (for immune response) and traced it to a hitherto unmapped region of the MHC, or major histocompatibility complex, an intricate and ancient supergene located within a specific chromosome.

Scientists were busily mapping the MHC in a variety of mammals and soon 30 Ir genes were identified for the mouse, guinea pig, rat, and rhesus monkey. It was only a matter of time before researchers began mapping the supergene in humans. By then a great deal more was known about the immune response at the cellular level. T-cells (from the thymus) apparently triggered the response and performed a variety of functions. ''Killer'' T-cells moved to neutralize and destroy the invader; ''helper'' T-cells joined with B-cells (from bone marrow) to help manufacture antibodies; and finally ''suppressor'' T-cells slowed and stopped the attack after the enemy had been destroyed. Benacerraf's work had broad medical implications and shed light on why some individuals were more susceptible than others to diseases such as multiple sclerosis and rheumatoid arthritis. His research in the chemistry of suppressor T-cells opened the possibility of controlling the immune response and treating so-called autoimmune diseases, where the body mistakenly mounts an attack against its own tissues.

In 1968 Benacerraf left New York University to become chief of the laboratory of immunology at the National Institute of Allergy and Infectious Diseases in Bethesda, Maryland. Two years later he was appointed chairman of the Department of Pathology at Harvard Medical School and Fabyan Professor of Comparative Pathology. In July 1980 he became president and chief executive officer of the Dana Farber Cancer Institute in Boston.

In October of 1980 it was announced that he would share the 1980 Nobel Prize in physiology or medicine with immunologists **Jean Dausset** and **George Snell** for their joint elucidation of how the immune response was controlled by the MHC supergene. What had begun as an arcane branch of biology had led in barely twenty-five years to a series of genetic discoveries of vital importance to medicine, cancer research, virology, and developmental biology.

Benacerraf is the author of more than five hundred scientific papers, a fellow of the American Academy of Arts and Sciences, and a member of the National Academy of Sciences. He has also been an associate editor of several periodicals, including *American Journal of Pathology, Laboratory Investigation,* and *Journal of Immunology and Immunogenetics.*

A gregarious, cultured man, he has enjoyed a life of rich professional contacts. At home on three continents, he is intimately acquainted with the disparate worlds of immunochemistry, international banking, and classical music. Professionally, he cultivates a skeptical, even pessimistic frame of mind. Well versed in the anecdotal history of science, he believes that accident and error play a far greater role in scientific discovery than historians like to admit.

Benzodiazepines

Benzodiazepines are **antianxiety drugs** that help relieve nervousness, tension, and other symptoms by slowing the central nervous system. The group of drugs known as benzodiazepines includes alprazolam (Xanax), chlordiazepoxide (Librium), diazepam (Valium), and lorazepam (Ativan). These medicines take effect fairly quickly, usually within one hour after they are taken. They are available only with a physician's prescription, and should not be used to relieve the nervousness and tension of normal everyday life. The recommended dosage depends on the type of benzodiazepine, its strength, and the condition for which it is being taken.

While anxiety is a normal response to **stress**, some people have unusually high levels of anxiety that can interfere with everyday life. For these people, benzodiazepines can help bring their feelings under control. The medicine can also relieve troubling symptoms of anxiety, such as pounding heartbeat, breathing problems, irritability, nausea, and faintness.

Physicians may sometimes prescribe these drugs for other conditions, such as muscle spasms, epilepsy and other **seizure disorder**s, **phobias**, **panic disorder**, withdrawal from alcohol, and short-term sleep problems.

People who take benzodiazepines to relieve nervousness, tension, or symptoms of panic disorder should check with their physicians every two to three months to make sure they need to continue taking the medicine. Patients who are taking benzodiazepines for sleep problems should check with their physicians if they are not sleeping better within 7-10 days. Sleep problems that last longer than this may be a sign of another medical problem.

The most common side effects of benzodiazepines are **dizziness**, lightheadedness, drowsiness, clumsiness, unsteadiness, and slurred speech. These problems usually go away as the body adjusts to the drug and do not require medical treatment unless they persist or they interfere with normal activities. More serious side effects are not common, but may occur. Anyone who takes these drugs should not drive, use machines, or do anything else that might be dangerous until they have found out how the drugs affect them.

Benzodiazepines may also cause behavior changes in some people, similar to those seen in people who act differently when they drink alcohol. More extreme changes, such as confusion, agitation, and **hallucinations**, also are possible. Anyone who starts having strange or unusual thoughts or behavior while taking this medicine should get in touch with his or her physician.

Because benzodiazepines work on the central nervous system, they may add to the effects of alcohol and other drugs that slow down the central nervous system, such as **antihistamines**, cold medicine, allergy medicine, sleep aids, medicine for seizures, tranquilizers, some pain relievers, and **muscle relaxants**. They may also add to the effects of anesthetics, including those used for dental procedures. These effects may last several days after treatment with benzodiazepines ends.

The combined effects of benzodiazepines and alcohol or other CNS depressants (drugs that slow the central nervous system) can be very dangerous, leading to unconsciousness or, rarely, even death. Anyone taking benzodiazepines should not drink alcohol and should check with his or her physician before using any CNS depressants.*Taking an overdose of benzodiazepines can also cause unconsciousness and possibly death. Anyone who shows signs of an overdose or of the effects of combining benzodiazepines with alcohol or other drugs should get immediate emergency help.* Warning signs include slurred speech or confusion, severe drowsiness, staggering, and profound weakness.

Some benzodiazepines may change the results of certain medical tests. Before having medical tests, anyone taking this medicine should alert the health care professional in charge.

People with certain medical conditions or who are taking other medicines can have problems if they take benzodiazepines. Benzodiazepines may interact with other medicines. When this happens, the effects of one or both of the drugs may change, or the risk of side effects may become greater. Before taking benzodiazepines, tell the physician if you are taking any other medications, or if you have allergies, are pregnant, breastfeeding, a current or former drug or alcohol abuser, suffering from mental illness, seizures, epilepsy, swallowing problems, chronic lung disease such as emphysema, **asthma**, or chronic **bronchitis**, kidney or liver disease, **glaucoma**, hyperactivity, **myasthenia gravis**, porphyria, or **sleep apnea**.

Berger, Hans (1873-1941)

German psychiatrist and neurologist

Hans Berger was a professor of psychiatry and director of the Jena Psychiatric University Clinic from 1919 until his forced retirement in 1938. But it is his research into the correlation of brain activity and consciousness for which he is remembered. This research led him by a long and frustrating path to the discovery of the electroencephalogram (EEG) of man. The EEG is a graphic representation of electrical waves measured repeatedly between two points of the skull, and though Berger himself did not develop its full potential as a diagnostic tool, the EEG has since come to be invaluable in diagnosing and treating such neurological disorders as epilepsy and brain tumors.

Born on May 21, 1873 in the small northern Bavarian town of Neuses near Coburg, Germany, Berger was the son of Paul Friedrich Berger, a physician, and of Anna Rückert, daughter of a German poet who was well known for his studies in oriental philosophy. In his life and work, Berger combined both sides of this intellectual inheritance, determining early on to become a scientist-philosopher. Berger graduated with honors from the Gymnasium in Coburg and then enrolled at the University of Berlin as an astronomy student in 1892. The next year he volunteered for military service in the German army, and it was as a result of a near fatal accident he had in the army that he set his course to uncover the link between the brain and consciousness. The very day of his accident, Berger's sister informed their parents that she knew Berger had had an accident, so Berger's father sent an urgent telegram to see if his son was all right. This seemed to Berger to be a pure case of telepathic communication with his sister, and he became convinced that he could find the objective proof of such a psychic power.

Released from the army in 1893, Berger began studying medicine, finally earning his doctorate of medicine at Jena in 1897 and becoming a junior staff member at the Psychiatric Clinic of the University of Jena where he would remain until 1938. In 1901 he became Privatdozent, or lecturer at the university and also published his first investigations on the functioning of the brain, recording the change of size as modified by the circulation of blood. He accomplished this by studying brain pulsation in the skull defect of a patient who had undergone a trepanation or surgery through the skull. On the staff of a medical clinic, Berger had access to a wide variety of patients who were willing to participate in his experiments. He continued a variety of experiments searching for some objective, measurable results of psychic or conscious conditions. These included investigations of the influence of heartbeat, vascular measurements, and position of the head on pulsations of the brain, as well as the effects of medications such as caffeine, morphine, camphor, and cocaine on brain activity. As early as 1902 he hit upon recording the electrical activity of the cerebral cortex of a dog in an attempt to measure psychic activity, but by 1910 he had given up on these experiments because they provided such scant results. During these same years, Berger also pursued another line of inquiry: the changes of temperature of the cerebral cortex as measured by introducing minute and precise thermometers into the brains of patients who had undergone cerebral puncture, then a new and popular diagnostic procedure. Searching for the elusive psychic energy (P-energie), these experiments also seemed to lead to a dead end.

Berger served on the western front during the First World War, in a military hospital at Rethel. He came back to a Germany on the brink of revolution. The director of the psychiatric clinic at Jena resigned and returned to his native Switzerland, and Berger was appointed the new director. For the next several years administrative duties deterred Berger's further researches into the correlation between brain and psyche, but in his few private moments he started once again to focus on measuring the electrical activity of the brain. He became known to his colleagues as a punctual and rather strict director, and few of them knew of his researches. His day was strictly defined by the clock of duty, and it was only from 5:00 to 8:00 P.M. that he found time to continue his experiments. As a result of the war, there was a surplus of patients at the clinic with skull defects whose pulsating brain was protected by only a few millimeters of tissue. These patients made excellent subjects for his experiments with electrode stimulation of the brain, specifically of the motor cortex. Berger measured the time between stimulus and corresponding touch sensations in the extremities of his subjects. But soon he hit on a new idea: searching for currents or brain waves in these same patients. Employing rather crude instruments, such as the Edelmann string galvanometer used to record electrocardiograms, he made his first successful EEG on July 6, 1924, when he observed small movements on the galvanometer on a young patient named Zedel. Berger continued these experiments for five more years before publishing his results, using not only patients with skull imperfections or trepanations, but also patients with intact skulls. With this latter group he placed one electrode at the front and another at the back of the skull. In 1929 he published his results in the prestigious *Archiv für Psychiatrie und Nervenkrankheiten.* Entitled ''Über das Elektrenkephalogramm des Menschen,'' it was the first of fourteen such articles published between 1929 and 1938 on the results of his experiments with the EEG. His 1929 article not only shows that regular electrical current oscillations can be recorded from the scalp of humans, but also that these oscillations are not due to blood flow, electrical properties of the skin or any of several other possibilities. His third paper definitely proves the cerebral origin of the waves, yet Berger's findings were largely ignored by the scientific community, and it was not until 1934 when other researches, chief among them neurophysiologist **Edgar Douglas Adrian** and B. C. H. Matthews, finally drew attention to what Berger himself long knew as a certainty: the electrical activity of the brain could be measured.

Berger led a relatively happy domestic life, married in 1911 to a young technical assistant at the clinic, Baroness Ursula von Bulow. They had four children: Klaus, Ruth, Ilse and Rosemarie. Berger continued his studies on the EEG, always balancing research with his administrative duties, installing his increasingly elaborate set of instruments in a tiny annex just off his office. But despite growing international recognition for his achievements, he was largely ignored in Germany. Part of the reason for this was his antipathy for the Nazis and their distrust of him. In 1938, following an International Congress of Psychology in Paris in which he found himself to be something of an international celebrity, he was greeted in Germany by humiliation: his forced retirement. His laboratory was dismantled and he moved to the small town of Bad Blankenburg in Thuringia to live out his days. He could no longer pursue his researches, and on June 1, 1941, following a long depression which he had misdiagnosed as a cardiac condition, Berger took his own life.

In the final analysis, Berger's work on the human electroencephalogram must be viewed as a means to an end. At the back of his mind always was the search for the secret of man's psychophysical nature; of the connection between brain and psyche. Thus his interest in the EEG was towards that end, not in the use of it as a diagnostic tool for which it has become known.

Bergström, Sune Karl (1916-)

Swedish biochemist

Sune Karl Bergström is best known for his research on prostaglandins. These substances, which were first discovered in the prostate gland and seminal vesicles, were found by Bergström and his colleagues to affect circulation, smooth muscle tissue, and general metabolism in ways that can be medically beneficial. Certain prostaglandins, for example, lower blood pressure, while others prevent the formation of ulcers on the stomach lining. For his research, Bergström shared the 1982 Nobel Prize in medicine or physiology with **John R. Vane** and **Bengt Samuelson**.

Sune Bergström was born in Stockholm on January 10, 1916, to Sverker and Wera (Wistrand) Bergström. Upon completion of high school he went to work at the Karolinska Institute as an assistant to the biochemist Erik Jorpes. The young Bergström was assigned to do research on the biochemistry of fats and steroids. Jorpes was impressed enough with his assistant to sponsor a year-long research fellowship for Bergström in 1938 at the University of London. While there, Bergström focused his research on bile acid, a steroid produced by the liver which aids in the digestion of cholesterol and similar substances.

Bergström had planned to continue his research in Edinburgh the following year thanks to a British Council fellowship, but the fellowship was canceled after World War II broke out. He did, however, receive a Swedish-American Fellowship in 1940, which allowed him to study for two years at Columbia University and to conduct research at the Squibb Institute for Medical Research in New Jersey. At Squibb, Bergström researched the steroid cholesterol, particularly its reaction to chemical combination with oxygen at room temperature, a process called auto-oxidation.

Bergström returned to Sweden in 1942, receiving doctorates in medicine and biochemistry from the Karolinska Institute two years later. He was appointed assistant in the biochemistry department of Karolinska's Medical Nobel Institute. While there, he continued experiments with autooxidation, working with linoleic acid, which is found in some vegetable oils. He discovered a particular enzyme was responsible for the oxidation of linoleic acid, and helped attempt to purify the enzyme while working with biochemist **Hugo Theorell**.

While attending a meeting of Karolinska's Physiological Society in 1945, Bergström met the physiologist Ulf von Euler. Von Euler, who was better known as the discoverer of the hormone norepinephrine, had been doing research on prostaglandins. Scientists had observed in the 1930s that seminal fluid used in artificial insemination stimulated contraction and subsequent relaxation in the smooth muscles of the uterus. Von Euler isolated a substance from the seminal fluid of sheep and found it had the same effect in relaxing the smooth muscle of blood vessels. Impressed with Bergström's work on enzyme purification, von Euler gave him some of the extract for further purification.

Bergström began initial experiments but put his work on hold when in 1946 he was named a research fellow at the University of Basel. Returning from Switzerland in 1947, he was appointed professor of physiological chemistry at the University of Lund. His first task was to help revitalize the university's research facilities, which had fallen into disuse during the war. Afterwards, he resumed his research on prostaglandins, assisted by graduate students such as Bengt Samuelson. Working with new large supplies of sheep seminal fluid, Bergström and his colleagues were able to isolate and purify two prostaglandins by 1957. Bergström was appointed professor of chemistry at Karolinska a year later, and brought his research on prostaglandins and his collaboration with Samuelson with him. By 1962, six prostaglandins, identified as A through F, had been identified.

Bergström and Samuelson then worked on determining how prostaglandins are formed. They discovered that prostaglandins are formed from common fatty acids, and further identified specific functions performed by each prostaglandin. Over the next few years, Bergström and Samuelson surmised that certain prostaglandins could be used to treat high blood pressure, blocked arteries, and other circulatory problems by relaxing muscle tissue. These prostaglandins were also shown to prevent ulceration of the stomach lining and to protect against side effects of such drugs as aspirin, long known to irritate the stomach lining. Other prostaglandins could be used to raise blood pressure or stimulate uterine muscle by their contracting effect.

Bergström remained at Karolinska, serving as dean of its medical school from 1963 to 1966 and as rector of the institute from 1969 to 1977. He was chairman of the Nobel Foundation's Board of Directors from 1975 to 1987, and from 1977 to 1982 he served as chairman of the World Health Organization's Advisory Committee on Medical Research. He retired from teaching in 1981, choosing to devote his full time to research at Karolinska.

A modest, reserved man, Bergström's reaction upon learning of his Nobel award was gratitude—first, that his colleagues appreciated his efforts, and second, that his former student Samuelson had also been named. The book *Nobel Prize Winners* reports him as saying that there is ''no greater satisfaction than seeing your students successful.'' His connection with the Nobel Foundation had led some to wonder whether he might be passed over for a prize of his own. But the *New York Times,* reporting on the 1982 awards, noted that ''it was only a matter of time, most scientists agree, before Dr. Bergström's research would be honored by the foundation he directs—for the work was too important to be ignored through any concern over apparent conflicts of interest.''

The scientist married the former Maj Gernandt in Sweden in 1943; the couple has one son. Bergström's memberships include the Royal Swedish Academy of Science (he served as its president from 1983 to 1985), the American Philosophical Society, and the American Academy of Arts and Sciences. Other awards given to Bergström besides the Nobel include the Albert Lasker Award in 1977, Oslo University's Anders Jahre Prize in Medicine in 1970, and Columbia's Louisa Gross Horwitz Prize in 1975.

Beriberi

Beriberi, a disease caused by a thiamine deficiency, is most common in Far Eastern countries where boiled white rice makes up a large part of the daily diet. In other parts of the world, including the United States, the disease is seen today mostly in alcoholics, who often fail to nourish themselves properly. The name *beriberi* is Sinhalese for "I cannot"—an apt description of the patient in later stages of the disease who finds it difficult to perform even simple tasks.

Beriberi occurs in two forms. In the more commonly seen chronic form, the disease is characterized by *polyneuritis*, a generalized inflammation of nerves in the arms and legs. The polyneuritis may soon escalate to severe nerve damage, progressive paralysis of the legs, and a deterioration of muscles. In the more acute form of the disease, the beriberi causes fluid retention, which in turn causes swelling of tissues, including those around the heart. In time, potentially fatal heart problems tend to develop.

Before its cause was discovered, beriberi was almost impossible to treat and caused widespread suffering. In 1896 **Christiaan Eijkman**, a Dutch physician, found that he could give laboratory animals beriberi by feeding them a diet restricted to polished rice and that he could then cure them simply by switching their diet to unpolished rice. Although Eijkman thought a toxin in the rice might be the culprit, his colleague, Gerrit Grijns, correctly deduced that polished rice was lacking an essential substance somehow needed by the nervous system, and that this substance was present in the outer layers of rice and in other foods as well. Reports of Eijkman's and Grijns's work prompted a number of investigators to join the search for the elusive anti-beriberi factor, which in 1934 was finally isolated and identified as thiamine, the first member of the B family of **vitamin**s.

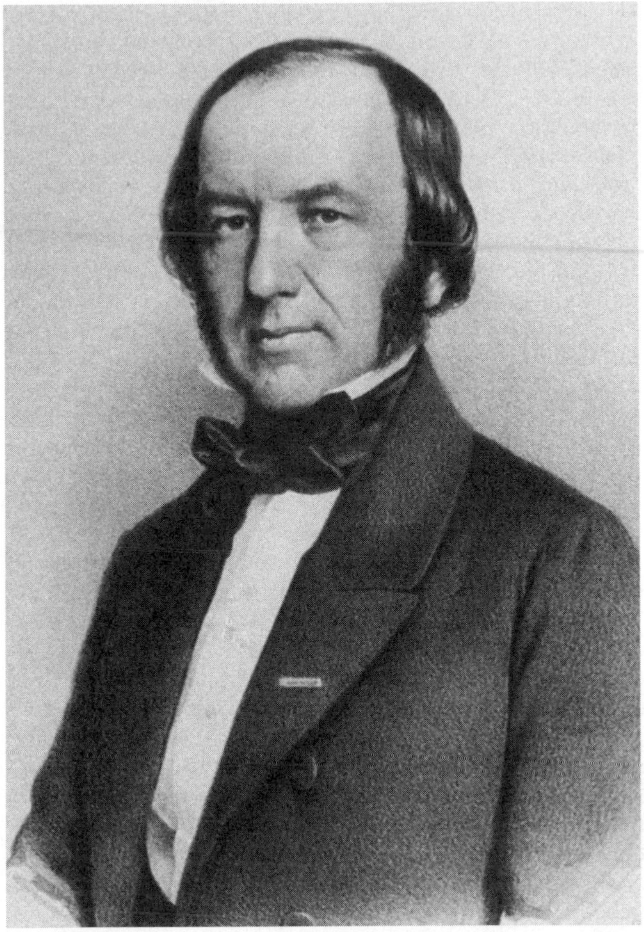

Claude Bernard

Bernard, Claude (1813-1878)

French physiologist

Claude Bernard did not get off to a promising start. Born in 1813 in Saint-Julien, France, this son of poor vineyard workers attended a simple village school and originally dreamed of becoming a writer. At 21, he'd already written several plays and set off to Paris, France, to show them around. A well-known literary critic, however, strongly suggested he try a different career and, after some thought, Bernard took the man's advice. He entered the Faculty of Medicine, finished almost at the bottom of his class, but managed to obtain a medical degree in 1843. Four years later, the young man's fortune changed. He became an assistant to François Magendie, one of France's most prominent—and controversial—physiologists.

Unlike most of his contemporaries, Magendie firmly believed that researchers could study the body's reactions in the same way that they studied the reactions of inorganic material. Bernard agreed, learned a great deal about experimental physiology from his mentor, and then went on to design a number of experimental projects of his own. In 1855, when Magendie died, Bernard took his place as Professor of Experimental Medicine at the College de France. And, because Bernard tended to be more disciplined and organized than Magendie had been, he began attracting more and more scientific attention to the comparatively new discipline.

Many of Bernard's experiments centered around the digestive process. Inspired by **William Beaumont**—who had spent several years peering into the stomach of a patient with an accidentally caused opening (or fistula) in his side—Bernard decided to create artificial fistulas in live animals. Although his experiments infuriated antivivisectionists (including his own wife and daughters), Bernard made a number of discoveries. Among other things, he found that the stomach was not the sole digestive organ, as was then widely believed. While the stomach began the digestive process, much more digestion took place throughout the small intestine, Bernard reported. He also demonstrated the importance of the pancreas, whose secretions were clearly necessary to break down fat molecules, and later went on to identify the various nerves that control gastric secretion.

In 1857, Bernard isolated a starch-like substance in the liver of animals, a substance he named glycogen. Glycogen,

Bernard showed, was a large molecule built up out of numerous tiny molecules of sugar taken from the blood stream. Its primary role was to serve as the body's reserve supply of carbohydrates. When the level of sugar in the blood became low, the stored glycogen broke down again into its components and released more simple sugars back into the blood stream. This continuing process, Bernard pointed out, indicated that the animal's body did not (as was then believed) merely break large molecules down into smaller ones, the way plants did. The animal's body could also take simple molecules and build them up into larger, more complex ones.

In 1851, Bernard devoted some of his attention to the portion of the **nervous system** which governs blood circulation (called the vasomotor system) and discovered that certain specific nerves governed the dilation and constriction of blood vessels. But why did the blood vessels need to keep widening and narrowing? Bernard theorized that, by doing so, the body was better able to control its distribution of heat. On hot days, he suggested, people looked flushed because the skin's blood vessels widened in order to release more excess heat from the body. On cold days, people looked pale because the skin's blood vessels narrowed in order to prevent body heat from escaping. While studying the vasomotor system, Bernard also discovered that the blood's red corpuscles carry oxygen from the lungs to body tissues.

Each of Bernard's findings convinced him that the body is constantly striving to maintain a stable, well-balanced internal environment, one that is not overly affected by outside influences. He therefore concluded that the body must be under the control of one strong and central regulating force. Bernard's theory, although widely accepted today, appeared quite radical in his own time, when most scientists believed that the body's various organs acted quite independently of each other.

Bernard's work brought him worldwide recognition. In 1865, he published the highly influential textbook, *An Introduction to the Study of Experimental Medicine*, which won him election to the prestigious French Academy in 1869. He even served in the French senate under Napoleon III (1808-1873) and, when he died in 1878, Bernard became the first scientist to be given a national funeral, an honor usually reserved for political and military leaders.

BERT, PAUL (1833-1886)

French physiologist

Paul Bert was a French physiologist whose research laid the foundation for understanding how the body reacts to significant changes in air pressure. This work has proved useful both to undersea explorers and divers and those involved in space exploration.

Born in Auxerre, France, Bert originally entered the École Polytechnique in Paris intending to become an engineer. Changing his mind, he first studied law, then became a student of the Claude Bernard, one of the greatest physiologists of the nineteenth century, and the founder of experimental medicine.

Appointed as a professor of physiology, first at Bordeaux in 1866, then at the Sorbonne (1869-86), he studied the effects of altitude on animals. He discovered that altitude sickness in these animals was caused mainly by a lack of oxygen in the air at high altitudes. In addition, he studied hot air balloonists and discovered that the effects of various respiratory gasses dissolved in their blood were proportional to their partial pressures and not to their concentrations in the bloodstream.

Bert was also interested in what happened to blood gasses when people were exposed to greater than normal pressures. This led him to study divers and the phenomenon of decompression sickness. From his studies, he determined that the high external pressures the divers experienced forced large quantities of nitrogen gas from the atmosphere to dissolve in their blood. When the external pressure was relieved as the diver surfaced, this nitrogen came out of the blood stream in the form of bubbles. These bubbles blocked the capillaries (the smallest blood vessels) causing the painful phenomenon that divers called the bends.

In 1875, Bert was awarded a prize of 20,000 francs from the Academy of Sciences for this research. Three years later, he compiled his findings into a book, *La Pression baroméetrique: recherches de physiologie expéerimentale*, called in English *Barometric Pressure: Researches in Experimental Physiology*. Bert's work provided a foundation for the development of aviation medicine, a field of importance during World War II. Still later it served as a starting point in early aerospace research on the effects of changes in pressure on astronauts. In addition to his book on barometric pressure, Bert also wrote several elementary science textbooks.

Bert had other interests besides the effects of air pressure on the body. He experimented with animal tissue grafting and studied the effects of various poisons on the respiration and physiological function of different animals. He also was interested in plant physiology and studied the influence of different colored light on plant growth.

At a time when the Catholic church was deeply involved in education in France, Paul Bert was looked at as a left wing radical, dedicated to providing public education free of church influence. He was elected to the Assembly in 1874, and in 1881 was briefly a cabinet minister of education and worship. His political career was not nearly as successful as his scientific career.

In 1886 Bert was appointed governor-general in Anham and Tonkin (now Vietnam) where the French were a colonial presence. He strove to liberalize French colonial rule and to increase the role the Vietnamese played in the colonial judicial system. Unfortunately, after only a short time as governor-general, he died of dysentery in Hanoi.

BEST, CHARLES HERBERT (1899-1978)

Canadian physiologist

Charles Herbert Best was most renowned as co-discoverer of insulin with **Frederick G. Banting**. Insulin, which is a hormone secreted by the pancreas, regulates the level of sugar in the blood. Its discovery in 1921 led to its use as a treatment for diabetes, which until that time had led swiftly to emaciation, coma, and death. Later in his career, Best assisted in the establishment of associations of diabetics to promote support groups and educational programs for their members. He also did important research on the nutrient choline and the blood anticoagulant heparin.

Best was born on February 27, 1899, in West Pembroke, Maine, a town near the border of the Canadian province of New Brunswick. His parents were Canadian citizens, both originally from Nova Scotia. Best was a direct descendant of Major William Best, who in 1749 was one of the founders of Halifax, Nova Scotia. Best's father, Herbert Huestes Best, was a country doctor whose practice straddled the U.S.-Canadian border. As a teenager, Best often accompanied his father on his rounds in a horse-drawn buggy. Best's mother was Luella Fisher Best.

After finishing high school, Best entered the University of Toronto in a liberal arts program. When World War I interrupted his education, he served as a sergeant in a regiment of the Canadian Tank Corps. He returned to Toronto in 1919 after the war to complete his education, but switched his course of study to physiology and biochemistry in preparation for a medical degree. Best played professional baseball in order to finance his education. He received his B.A. in 1921. In May of 1921, Best's physiology professor, **John James Rickard Macleod**, introduced him to Frederick Grant Banting, a 29-year-old orthopedic surgeon from London, Ontario. Best had worked as a research assistant for Macleod and planned to begin studying for master's degree under him in the fall. Banting would be using Macleod's lab during the intervening summer to do experiments to find out the function of the pancreas in preventing diabetes, and he needed an assistant to help with analyses of blood chemistry. Another of Macleod's students was also interested in the job, so he and Best flipped a coin. Best won. On May 17, 1921, the day after he completed his examinations for his undergraduate degree, Best began working with Banting. It was a collaboration that would set the course of his career.

Experiments done 30 years earlier had shown that when a dog's pancreas was removed by surgery the animal developed the symptoms of diabetes: it would grow insatiably thirsty, begin excreting large amounts of sugar in its urine, and then become listless, go into a coma, and die. Banting's idea was that the pancreas must secrete something in addition to its digestive enzymes in order to prevent this process. He was convinced that the crucial substance would be found in groups of cells on the pancreas called the islets of Langerhans. These cells could be isolated by tying off a dog's pancreatic ducts; the rest of the pancreas would atrophy after several weeks, but the islets of Langerhans would remain intact. An extract could then be made from the cells and injected into a diabetic dog. If Banting's idea was right, such an extract would relieve the symptoms of diabetes.

The way he originally planned the work, Banting would do the surgery, removing the pancreas from some dogs to make them diabetic and tying off the pancreatic ducts in others to isolate the islet cells. Best would do blood and urine tests on the dogs. As the research progressed, however, Best learned

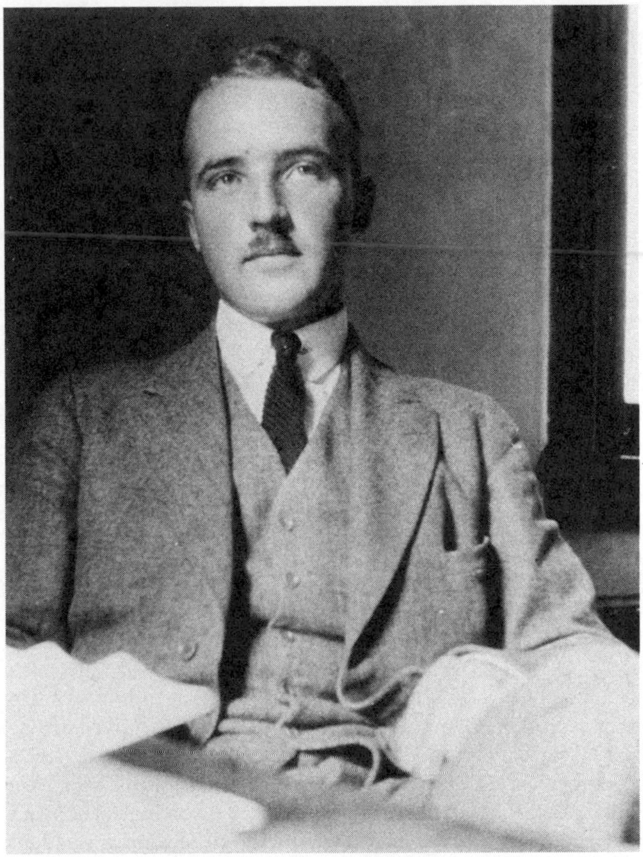

Charles Herbert Best

to do some surgery too. Best, for his part, had a personal interest in diabetes. His father's sister, who had lived with the Best family in West Pembroke, had died in a diabetic coma in 1918.

Banting and Best had expected to spend only eight weeks on their study. But it was July 30 before they were ready to prepare the extract. On that day, Banting removed the shriveled pancreas from a dog whose ducts had been tied. He and Best prepared an extract from it by chopping the pancreas into small pieces, grinding it in a chilled mortar with salt water, and filtering the mixture through cheesecloth. A blood sample from the diabetic dog showed its blood sugar level to be 0.2. Banting and Best injected some of their extract into the dog. An hour later its blood sugar level had dropped to 0.12. After another injection it registered 0.11. This dog died the next day, presumably from an infection. But Banting and Best were encouraged by the result and tested their extract on more diabetic dogs. They called the extract "isletin."

During the following months Banting and Best performed additional experiments to confirm and explain their results. With an injection of their extract they could revive a diabetic dog from its coma and prevent its imminent death. They found ways of obtaining the extract more easily and in larger quantities from the pancreases of fetal calves obtained from a local slaughterhouse. Macleod, who had been vacationing at his home in Scotland during the summer, returned in

September and made suggestions for further studies. He also hired James Bertram Collip, a Ph.D. biochemist, to help purify the active component of the extract. Best continued with the work, but also began his M.A. program at the University of Toronto. That fall Banting and Best wrote their first paper describing the experiments with dogs, titled "The Internal Secretion of the Pancreas." It was accepted for publication in the February 1922 issue of the *Journal of Laboratory and Clinical Medicine.*

By the time the paper was published, however, Banting and Best had already treated a human diabetes patient with the extract. They had also begun to call their extract by the now familiar name of insulin, at the suggestion of Macleod. The word "insulin" is based on the Latin word for island. The first patient to receive insulin was 14-year-old Leonard Thompson, who was so weak after two years of suffering from diabetes that he had been admitted to Toronto General Hospital. Thompson's weight was down to 65 pounds, and his doctors expected him to live for only a few more weeks. Before administering insulin to the boy, Banting and Best performed a perfunctory clinical trial: they injected each other with their extract. Since there seemed to be no side effects other than soreness around the injection, in January 1922 they went ahead and treated the boy. After an initial problem with impurities in the insulin was solved, his condition began to improve. He regained his energy and put on weight. Thompson lived another 11 years, dying in 1935 from pneumonia contracted after a motorcycle accident. This success, a literal pulling back of a diabetic child from the brink of the grave, was repeated again and again in the next months, as insulin became a standard treatment for diabetes.

The 1923 Nobel Prize in physiology and medicine for that year was awarded to Banting and Macleod for the discovery of insulin. Banting was furious. In his opinion, Macleod had done little more than provide laboratory space, whereas Best had shared the work of research. Best was in Boston the day the news arrived, giving an address to medical students at Harvard. Banting immediately sent Best a telegram stating that he would share both the credit for the discovery and the Nobel Prize cash award with Best. Macleod, who considered the work a collaboration, divided his portion of the prize with Collip.

Best continued his studies, receiving his M.A. in 1922 and his M.D. in 1925, while also working on a commercial process for producing insulin. At the same time he received the M.D., Best was also awarded the Ellen Mickle Fellowip for highest standing in the medical course. During the years Best was doing insulin research he had been courting Margaret Mahon, writing her love letters that also included details about the experiments on dogs. She was so well versed in the work that she helped Banting and Best write their first paper about it. Best married Margaret Mahon in 1924, and later they had two sons. In 1926 the couple sailed to England, where Best spent two years doing postgraduate research in the laboratory of Sir Henry Dale in London. This research led Best to the discovery of histaminase, an anti-allergic enzyme. He received his doctorate from the University of London in 1928.

Before the degree was awarded, however, Best had returned to the University of Toronto in 1927 to head the department of physiological hygiene, a post he held until 1941. In 1929, when Macleod retired, Best was also made chair of the department of physiology. He was just 30 years old at the time. He remained in that position until 1965.

Best's study of insulin led him to a related avenue of research. He had noticed that the laboratory dogs whose pancreases had been removed to render them diabetic developed fatty livers, similar to cirrhosis of the liver in alcoholics. Best and his colleagues found that feeding such dogs lecithin prevented this change in the liver. In the 1930s they isolated choline as the active nutritional component of lecithin, a component found in the cells of many plants and animals, and did studies on the role of choline in metabolism. In the 1930s Best also became interested in heparin, which had just been discovered. He recognized that heparin could be an important anticoagulant drug for preventing blood clotting and went to work purifying it for human use. With the outbreak of World War II, Best continued his research interest in blood. He established the Canadian project for supplying dried blood serum to the wounded overseas and personally worked collecting blood from volunteers. This project was a predecessor to the blood transfusion service of the Red Cross. In 1941 Best was appointed director of the medical research unit of the Canadian Navy. In this capacity he coordinated studies to find ways to enhance night vision and to remedy motion sickness.

In 1941, Frederick Banting was killed in a airplane crash en route to a wartime mission. After Banting's death, Best took over his directorship of the Banting and Best department of medical research at the University of Toronto. Best also worked to organize associations of diabetics that provided support groups and educational programs for their members, including summer camps for diabetic children. He was president of the American Diabetes Association from 1948 to 1949 and remained honorary president thereafter. He was also honorary president of the International Diabetes Foundation. In 1953 the University of Toronto named a new building for medical research the Best Institute. The same year, Best became the first president of the International Union of Physiological Sciences.

Best retired from the University of Toronto in 1965. In 1966 friends of Best purchased Best's parents' clapboard house in West Pembroke, Maine and gave it to the American Diabetes Association. Later the home was proposed to the U.S. National Trust for Historic Preservation as a cultural landmark and turned into a museum. Best spent his retirement years traveling around the world with his wife, who was a historian and a botanist, visiting friends and colleagues.

Best received scores of medals, awards, and honorary degrees and was praised by the Pope, the Queen of England, and other heads of state. He wrote numerous scientific articles, and was co-author of a widely used physiology textbook. In March of 1978 one of Best's sons died of a heart attack. Hours after hearing the news, Best himself collapsed from a ruptured blood vessel in his abdomen. He died several days later, on March 31, 1978, at Toronto General Hospital.

BETA BLOCKERS

Beta blockers are medicines that affect the body's response to certain nerve impulses. This, in turn, decreases the force and rate of the heart's contractions, which lowers blood pressure and reduces the heart's demand for oxygen.

The main use of beta blockers is to treat high blood pressure. Some also are used to relieve the type of chest **pain** called **angina** or to prevent **heart attack**s in people who already have had one heart attack. These drugs may also be prescribed for other conditions, such as migraine headache, **tremors**, and irregular heartbeat. As eye drops they are used to treat certain kinds of **glaucoma**.

Beta blockers, also known as beta-adrenergic blockers, are available only with a physician's prescription. Some common beta blockers are atenolol (Tenormin), metoprolol (Lopressor), nadolol (Corgard), propranolol (Inderal), and timolol (Blocadren). Eye drops that contain beta blockers include betaxolol (Betoptic), cartelol (Ocupress), and timolol (Timoptic).

The recommended dosage depends on the type, strength, and form of beta blocker, and the condition for which it is prescribed. Beta blockers may take several weeks to noticeably lower blood pressure. Taking these drugs exactly as directed is important.

Beta blockers will not cure high blood pressure, but they will help control the condition. To avoid the serious health problems that high blood pressure can cause, patients may have to take medicine for the rest of their lives. Anyone taking beta blockers for high blood pressure should not take any other prescription or over-the-counter medicine without first checking with his or her physician. Some medicines may increase blood pressure.

Some beta blockers may change the results of certain medical tests. Before having medical tests, dental work, surgery, or emergency care, anyone taking these drugs should alert the health care professional in charge.

Some people feel drowsy, dizzy, or lightheaded when taking beta blockers. Anyone who takes these drugs should not drive, use machines, or do anything else that might be dangerous until they have found out how the drugs affect them. Beta blockers may increase sensitivity to cold, especially in older people or people who have poor circulation.

People who usually have chest pain when they **exercise** may not have the pain when they are taking beta blockers. This could lead them to be more active than they should be. Anyone taking this medicine should ask his or her physician how much exercise and activity is safe.

People who have certain medical conditions including **allergies**, **diabetes**, emphysema, thyroid problems, who are getting allergy shots, are pregnant or breastfeeding, should discuss their condition with a doctor before starting beta blockers. Effects of these drugs may be greater in people with kidney or liver disease because the medicine is cleared from the body more slowly.

Beta blockers may also worsen heart or blood vessel disease, slow heartbeat (bradycardia), **myasthenia gravis** (chronic disease causing muscle weakness and possibly **paralysis**), **psoriasis** (itchy, scaly, red patches of skin), and depression.

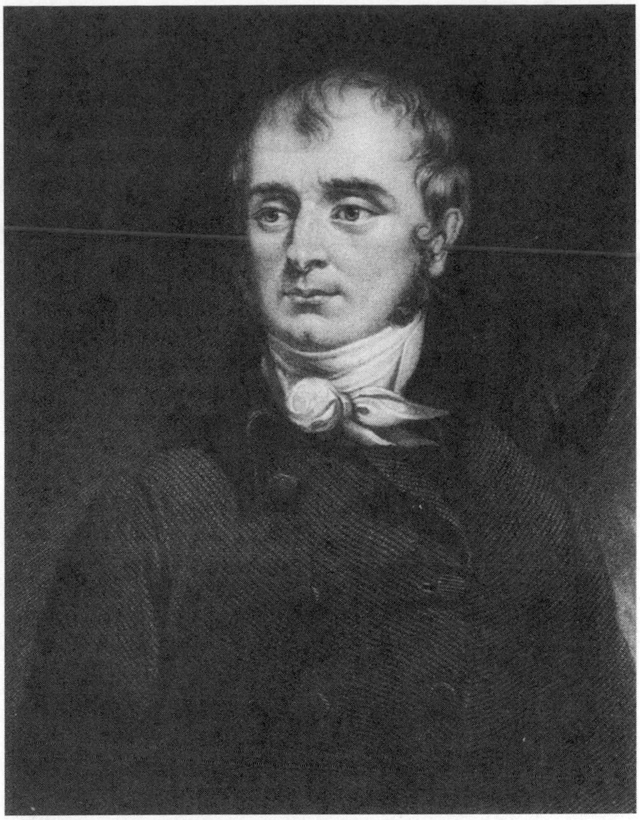

Marie François Xavier Bichat

The most common side effects of beta blockers are **dizziness**, drowsiness, lightheadedness, sleep problems, unusual tiredness or weakness, and decreased sexual ability. In men, this can occur as **impotence** or delayed ejaculation. These problems usually go away as the body adjusts to the drug.

More serious side effects are possible, including breathing problems, slow heartbeat, cold hands and feet, swollen ankles, feet, or lower legs, and depression. If these symptoms appear, a doctor should be consulted promptly.

Beta blockers may interact with a number of other medicines. When this happens, the effects of one or both of the drugs may change, or the risk of side effects may be greater. Anyone who takes beta blockers should let the physician know all other medicines he or she is taking.

BICHAT, MARIE-FRANÇOIS XAVIER (1771-1802)

French physician

Marie François Xavier Bichat was the first person to look beyond the recognizable organ systems and suggest that each part of the body was composed of various kinds of tissues. In addition, he suggested that disease acted upon these tissue is ways that could be seen and studied. For these insights, Bichat is considered the ''father of histology.''

Bichet was born in Thoirette, France, in 1771, the son of a physician. When it came time for Bichat to go to college, the French revolution was underway, and his father, a nervous member of the privileged class, sent his son away to the relative safety of Lyons to study.

In Lyons, Bichat studied mathematics and physical science before settling on the study of anatomy. Political turmoil and the threat of military service forced him to leave Lyons and seek refuge in Paris. There he was befriended by the Pierre-Joseph Desault, a prominent surgeon who served as his mentor and surrogate father until Desault's unexpected death in 1795.

In appreciation of the support Desault had given him, Bichat assembled Desault's journals, added a biographical memoir of Desault, and published the material as *Journal de Chirurgie* (*Journal of Surgery*). This was followed by another work that was a collection of Desault's thoughts on surgery supplemented by Bichat's own ideas.

By this time the political climate had cooled. Bichat took his place in the medical community and continued writing, lecturing, and doing research. Using only a hand-lens, he identified 21 different kinds of tissue, such as fibrous, glandular, or mucus tissue, in the body. He demonstrated that even when these tissue types were found in anatomically different organs or in different parts of the body, they showed physical and chemical similarities.

Bichat also studied the effects of different diseases and therapeutic agents on different tissues. He discovered that like tissues responded in a similar way regardless of where they were located. The idea of looking at tissues and how they were affected by disease, rather than studying whole organs, was a new concept at the time. This eventually led to the branch of medicine known as histology.

Bichat encouraged doctors to autopsy the bodies of their patients to study the physiological effects the their illnesses had on the tissues of the body. It is said that in one six month period, he performed more than 600 autopsies in his drive to understand the connection between disease and observable changes in the tissues.

Besides studying different tissues, Bichat was interested in the distinction between processes such as growth and reproduction, and the processes of self-awareness and interaction with the environment. He recognized that certain nervous diseases that we might consider mental health problems today were different from the other diseases he studied, because they did not cause any physiological changes in the tissues of the body. He supported his opinions with experimental research in which he drowned, smothered, burned, and poisoned a large number of animals.

Bichat was well known as a brilliant teacher during his life. He established the *Société Médicale d'Émulation* to promote professional standards in medicine, and in 1800 was appointed to serve as secretary of a medical advisory board established by the French government. By the age of 31 he had published three well-received books on tissues, general anatomy, and the physiological aspects of life and death.

Unfortunately, Bichat's brilliant career was cut short at the age of 31 by an accident. Standing at the top of a flight of stairs, Bichat staggered, lost his balance and fell. He never recovered from the fall, developed a fever, and died two weeks later. The cause of his fall remained unexplained, even after an autopsy.

Today Bichat is remembered as a physician and teacher who advanced the understanding of the connection between disease and physical changes in the body. He introduced the idea that the body could be studied in ways other than looking at organ systems when studying the disease and healing process. A man of tremendous energy and commitment, he promoted the use of direct experimentation, accurate observation and dissection as ways to learn about the connection between observable physical changes and specific diseases.

BICKERDYKE, MARY ANN BALL (1817-1901)

American nurse

Mary Ann Ball Bickerdyke was a woman of great prestige during the Civil War. She set up army hospitals for the Union forces and traveled with the army improving conditions wherever she went. Both General Ulysses S. Grant and William Tecumseh Sherman were impressed by her devotion and talent, and the entire Union army benefited from her efforts.

Mary Ann Ball Bickerdyke was born on July 19, 1817, in Knox County, Ohio. Her mother passed away in 1818 when Bickerdyke was only one year old. After that she and her siblings were sent to live on their grandparents' farm in Richland County, Ohio.

Little is known about the rest of Bickerdyke's young life. She may have gone to nursing school at Oberlin College, and she may have helped care for the victims of the cholera epidemics that ravaged Cincinnati in both 1837 and 1849.

In 1847 Mary Ann Ball married Robert Bickerdyke who was mechanic, sign painter, and a bass viol player. Together they had two children and lived in Cincinnati. Upon her husbands death in 1859 Bickerdyke was left a poor widow.

Working a laundress, housekeeper, and nurse Bickerdyke managed to support her two children. When the Civil War broke out she soon found a cause that was worthy of her attention. She heard about the dismal living conditions of the Union soldiers, and she quickly acted to help them.

Leaving her children in the care of another family she set off alone to help the soldiers that were stationed in Cairo, Illinois. She brought with her more than a hundred dollars worth of donated food and medical supplies.

When Bickerdyke arrived in Cairo, she had to fight the authorities. Women at that time were not allowed into army encampments without permission. No one wanted to give her the required permission, but when she saw how terrible the living conditions were she persisted and eventually overcame the opposition.

At the time of the Civil War, doctors for the army were more worried about amputations and ways of reducing pain than they were about basic needs such as clean water, fresh air, good meals, and good sanitation. Bickerdyke began making changes that would help the soldiers recover more quickly and help prevent illness. The value of Bickerdyke's work quickly became evident, and when a military hospital was finally opened in Cairo she was named its matron.

Bickerdyke continued to make improvements in the field hospitals. As the Union Army moved from one battle to another, she followed and assisted wherever help was needed most. She began to get more help from officials in the army and in 1862 was officially given a job paying 50 dollars a month as a sanitary field agent. This meant that she was allowed to draw from the Sanitary Commission's stores so she did not have to rely as much on donations and her own ingenuity to obtain supplies. General Grant trusted and valued her work so much that he gave Bickerdyke a pass that allowed her to travel freely through the troops.

Following Grant's army, Bickerdyke traveled to the battle of Shiloh, then to Corinth where she opened another army hospital, to Memphis, and then to the battle of Vicksburg. At Vicksburg Bickerdyke decided to join William Tecumseh Sherman's army for their march to Chattanooga. Along the way she helped to cook and clean and care for the ill soldiers. Once the army reached Chattanooga, Bickerdyke and Sherman argued about whether she would be allowed to travel with the army on their march to Atlanta and then to Savannah. She prevailed and accompanied the army on the first leg of the march, but Sherman would not let her stay with the army past Atlanta.

Throughout the remainder of the war Bickerdyke traveled with different sections of the Union Army helping to set up hospitals and caring for injured soldiers. Even after the war, she stayed on as an army nurse until she was no longer needed. She resigned from her army duty on March 21, 1866.

Eventually Bickerdyke's health began to fail, so she was sent west to San Francisco by her sons in the hope that the climate might improve her health. While there she helped veterans of the war. She received a patronage job with the San Francisco mint. Through her job she could help veterans all over the country receive their pensions. She was always considered an important part of the Union army and was often invited to reunions. She died November 8, 1901 at Bunker Hill, Kansas.

BILLROTH, ALBERT CHRISTIAN THEODOR (1829-1894)

Austrian surgeon

Christian Albert Theodor Billroth was a brilliant surgeon who pioneered new techniques in abdominal surgery and added substantially to what was know at the time about cancers of gastrointestinal tract.

Born in Bergen in 1829 to a family of Swedish origin, Billroth studied at universities in both Sweden and Germany. After receiving a doctor's degree from Berlin in 1852, he visited many of Europe's leading medical schools including those in Vienna, Prague, Paris, Edinburgh, and London, to complete his medical education.

Upon returning to Berlin, Billroth began work as an assistant to B. R. K. Langenbeck at Langenbeck's surgical clinic. In 1860, Billroth was appointed professor of surgery and director of the surgical clinic at the University of Zäurich where he stayed for seven years. He then accepted a similar position at the University of Vienna, where he remained for the remainder of his life.

Billroth was one of the first European surgeons to embrace the need for asepsis (sterility) during operations. He also made full use of the anesthetic chloroform during his during his operations, and was noted for his concern about his patient's well-being. In 1872, he made his first resection of the esophagus, in which he removed a section of esophagus, then sewed the remaining parts back together. Later he performed many similar operations on the stomach and intestines, pancreas, and larynx to remove cancerous growths. These operations were both difficult and dangerous to the patient, but Billroth's success rate was high considering the conditions under which he operated.

By 1890, Billroth had performed 41 gastric resections, of which 19 were a success. His work significantly increased the information available about gastrointestinal cancer tissues, their origin, and their physiology. In addition to his work as a surgeon, he established a training school for nurses in Vienna and a surgical school and clinic that remained open after his death until 1938.

Billroth was also interested in military surgery and volunteered in German hospitals during the Franco-German War. He was celebrated not only for his immense surgical skill, but also for his ability to stay calm under pressure and to improvise new procedures as they were needed. Based on his experience in battlefield hospitals, he advocated successfully for better transportation and treatment for the wounded, noting that the increased accuracy of weapons of war had lead to an increased number of casualties and a greater need for effective medical care at the front.

During his life, Billroth was honored by the Austrian government with a seat in the *Herrnhaus*, an honor rarely given to physicians. He published several books and many papers on surgery and pathology. In addition to being a skilled surgeon, Billroth was an devoted musician and played the piano and violin well. He was a close, life-long friend of the composer Johannes Brahms, who dedicated two string quartets to Billroth. In addition to his writings on surgery, Billroth also wrote a book on the physiology of music. He died at his villa in Abbazia, Yugoslavia, in 1894, having substantially increased the body of knowledge available about diseases of the gastrointestinal system and how to treat them surgically.

BINET, ALFRED (1857-1911)

French psychologist

Alfred Binet was born in Nice, France, on July 8, 1857. He went to Paris to study law, and began a career in law. Around 1878, Binet found himself gripped by the studies of hypnosis performed by Jean Charcot, a French neurologist working at Salpetriere Hospital in Paris. Charcot's work inspired Binet to abandon his law career and enter into further study of medicine and science. Ultimately, he earned a doctorate in natural science, and began work as a research associate in a laboratory at the Sorbonne in 1891. Binet rose through the ranks to become assistant director in 1892, and then director in 1895. He remained director of this Laboratory of Physiological Psychology of the Ecole Pratique Des Hautes Etudes for the rest of his life (from 1895-1911).

Binet's first work was on hypnosis and hysteria, the topics of his mentor, Charcot. Later, he began branching out into studies of subconscious thought, personality, and experimental psychology. Binet's publications from this time period included *La Psychologie du Raisonnement* (*The Psychology of Reason,* 1886); *Le Magnetisme Animal* (*Animal Magnetism,* 1887); and *On Double Consciousness* (1889).

Bored by the prevailing German research of this time period, which primarily studied sensation and perception, Binet found himself captivated by the study of higher reasoning. He explored ways to measure such higher mental functions, attempting to do so utilizing paper, pencil, pictures, inkblots, and other portable objects.

In 1895, Binet founded a laboratory at the Ecole de la Rue de la Grange aux Belles. Here he established his study of the development of intelligence by examining his own young daughters, Armande and Margeurite. In 1903, he published *L'Etude Experimentale de l'Intelligence* (''The Experimental Study of Intelligence''), a well-respected work utilizing data from his work with his daughters. Also in 1895, Binet founded an annual publication called *L'Annee Psychologique.* Much of Binet's work was published in this journal, and he received much acclaim for his innovative methodology. His work included studies of emotion, memory, attention, and problem solving.

Binet became interested in Sir Francis Galton, an English psychologist who was attempting to quantify individual cognitive capacity by administering standardized tests. Binet used Galton's work to examine a variety of famous and brilliant personalities, including writers, artists, mathematicians, and chess players. In 1892, Binet published *Les alterations de la Personnalite* (*Alterations of Personality*), co-authored with C. Fere.

In his study of children's intelligence, Binet compared and contrasted the development of gifted children and retarded (developmentally delayed) children. He attempted to find ways to predict intelligence, examining such parameters as body measurements and handwriting. Binet's study of this area was greatly advanced when the French government approached him in 1904, asking him to make recommendations for the education of children of lesser intellectual capacity. This prompted Binet to renew his efforts to create a diagnostic tool which could quantify an individual child's intellectual ability, in order to place children in classes appropriate to their cognitive abilities. Binet worked on this tool with Theodore Simon, completing the first version in 1905. This Binet-Simon scale was intended to test a child's cognitive capacity, not his or her learned knowledge.

The Binet scale involved testing children on a variety of tasks, especially abstract problem solving, which Binet and Simon determined to be conquered by the majority of children by a particular average age. Binet and Simon tested many, many Parisian school children to determine what problem solving tasks could be expected to be mastered by a given age. Test scores were then reported as a mental age, ranging from 3-13 years. A child's mental age might match his or her chronological age if he or she were perfectly on target for age, or it might differ in either direction from his or her chronological age. A mental age lower than chronological age may indicate mental retardation; a mental age greater than chronological age might indicated giftedness. The scale was also intended to give the tester an indication of other school readiness issues, including social responsibility, self-care, and complexity of play behavior.

In addition to further revisions of the Binet-Simon scale, Binet also published *Les Enfants Anormaux* with Simon (*Abnormal Children,* 1907); as well as *Les Idees Moderne Sur les Enfants* (*Modern Ideas about Children,* 1909). In 1911, Binet died while he was in the process of creating a revised and updated version of the Binet-Simon scale.

The Binet-Simon Scale became known worldwide as a valid and valuable diagnostic tool. In 1908 and 1911, it was revised by Henry H. Goddard in Vineland, New Jersey for American usage. In 1916, Lewis M. Terman of Stanford University further revised the tool for use in the United States. For decades, this Stanford-Binet test was the most commonly utilized intelligence test throughout the United States.

See also Intelligence tests

BIOFEEDBACK

Biofeedback, or biological feedback, is a treatment technique in which individuals are trained to improve their health and well-being by using signals from their own bodies. Its underlying principle is that changes in thinking and emotions can result in corresponding physical changes in the body.

As a type of behavior therapy, biofeedback is used to treat **stress**-related problems by teaching people to consciously regulate mental and physical functions that are not ordinarily under their conscious control. Although results are not always clear-cut or permanent, many people find the technique beneficial.

People of all ages can learn biofeedback. It is a non-invasive, cost-effective, and relatively safe treatment that, if nothing else, makes people more aware of their bodies' functions and gives them an increased sense of responsibility about their health.

As an adjunct to conventional medicine, biofeedback should only be used after patients have undergone a thorough **physical examination**. If a medical consultation reveals serious symptoms or an underlying chronic disease, biofeedback will not prove helpful and can even cause harm in some conditions. In some cases, the failure of biofeedback to achieve the expected results can cause anxiety or lower a person's self-esteem, leading to additional problems. Also, some individuals may fail to transfer biofeedback skills to everyday life and can become dependent upon their trainer.

The term "feedback" was first used in electronics to describe a loop in which information about part of a system is recorded and fed back into that system to adjust its operation. A house thermostat is a common example of a feedback mechanism. It monitors the temperature and sends a signal to the furnace to turn on or shut off to maintain the desired temperature. People react to feedback from their bodies all the time, as they respond to feelings of hunger by eating or to being winded by catching their breath.

As a treatment technique taught by a certified therapist, biofeedback uses various machines that monitor the performance of several body functions, such as heart rate, temperature, muscle tension, skin conductivity, and brain waves. Most people are only slightly aware of these functions since they are part of the autonomic nervous system that normally operates below conscious control. However, once patients are connected to sensors, the machine's readings of their body functions are translated into a signal they can see or hear. Patients are taught, through trial and error and continuous feedback, what they can do to modify a body function. With practice, they can learn, for example, to relax specific muscles.

Ideally, once patients are able to influence a body function by using feedback by using monitoring machines, they will be able to exercise the same control on their own. As a type of relaxation therapy, biofeedback is most effective for stress-related conditions and is used to lower blood pressure, prevent **headaches**, and reduce chronic pain. Biofeedback is often effective when insomnia is caused by an emotional rather than a physical problem. Patients with bruxism and temporomandibular joint syndrome (TMJ) are helped when they learn to relax their facial muscles and jaws.

Once patients with **asthma** learn through biofeedback to control their breathing, their asthma-aggravating fear is reduced. Biofeedback has also been successful in treating chronic **constipation**, fecal and urinary incontinence, and **irritable bowel syndrome**, In controlling high blood pressure, relaxation techniques are best when combined with changes to lifestyle and diet.

Although there is some difference of opinion as to exactly how effective it is and in what circumstances, biofeedback has been thoroughly studied and reported in the scientific literature and has proven to be helpful. It is gaining acceptance in the medical community, and many insurance companies will cover part of its cost. Biofeedback is an additional tool, not a substitute for medical treatment. The duration of treatment depends on the condition of the patient, and can be considered completed when the patient can effectively alter body functions when needed without the assistance of monitoring instruments.

Biofeedback cannot magically erase stress, but in those patients willing to invest the time and effort to achieve results, it often proves beneficial. A positive biofeedback experience often leaves patients with a feeling that of gaining mastery over their bodies. Many find that they gain a real sense of being more responsible for their own health.

Biopsy

A biopsy is a diagnostic procedure used by physicians to obtain a sample of body tissue for laboratory examination. Unhealthy or suspicious looking tissue is biopsied to diagnose disease. Usually, it is done to distinguish between a benign and malignant tumor. Healthy tissue is biopsied in order to test for matches between tissue types, for transplants.

Any part of the body can be biopsied. Depending on whether the part of the body is easily accessible or deep within, there are several different ways to do the biopsy. After the biopsy specimen is obtained by the doctor, it is sent to a laboratory where it is examined microscopically by a pathologist. A pathologist is a physician who is specialized in rendering medical diagnoses by examining fluids and tissues removed from the body. The pathologist prepares a written report, which enables the primary physician to diagnose the patient's condition.

There are several different ways to do biopsies. In an excisional biopsy, the entire organ or lump is removed. This is because, some tumors such as lymphomas (cancer of the lymphatic system) need to be examined in whole in order to get an accurate diagnosis. Another case for an excisional biopsy would be when the organ is small and lies deep within the body (such as the spleen). Cutting into it would be a risky procedure, hence doctors would opt for removal of the whole organ.

In an incisional biopsy, only a small portion of the lump is removed. This is done routinely to distinguish between benign and malignant tumors of the soft tissues (such as muscle, fat, connective tissue).

The parts of the body with natural openings to the surface, such as the intestines, bladder, and the bronchi are biopsied using a procedure known as endoscopy. Endoscopy enables the doctor to view the inside of the body using a long flexible tube known as a scope. There is a lighted source inside the scope and a passage to see the inside of the body. Fiberoptics is used to transmit light and images. A fiberoptic endoscope is inserted through an opening of the body, or a small surgical incision is made on the skin and the scope is inserted. The doctor can visually examine the surface lining the organ and if an abnormality is seen, small pieces of tissue can be pinched off using forceps, attached to the scope. Depending on the organ in the body being examined, the biopsies have different names. An upper GI endoscopy refers to examination of the esophagus, stomach and upper part of the small intestine. A colonoscopy refers to the examination of the entire large bowel, while a sigmoidoscopy examines the lower part of the large bowel and the rectum. A bronchoscopy is used to examine the airways and a cytoscopy to examine the bladder. A colposcopy enables a gynecologist to view the cervix and the uterus.

Fine needle aspiration biopsy was considered a major advance in cancer diagnosis because it was an extremely simple procedure. A fine needle is inserted into a lump or a cyst and cells are aspirated into the syringe. This is especially useful in examining deep set tumors, because the only other alternative to get to them is major surgery. Aspiration biopsy is generally done to see whether a cyst is solid or filled with fluid. Modern imaging techniques such as CT scans and **ultrasounds** are now preferred to determine this difference and aspiration biopsies are used less often.

A punch biopsy is a technique generally used by dermatologists to sample small lumps on the skin. It is a minor procedure where a small biopsy punch is used to cut out a piece of cylindrical skin (approximately 3-4 mm in diameter). A procedure called a "bone marrow biopsy" is used to examine cells of the bone marrow. In adults, the sample is usually taken from the pelvic bone. The biopsy site is numbed with a local anesthetic and a needle is inserted to deaden the membrane covering the bone. A larger rigid needle is then introduced into the marrow of the bone and cells are aspirated into the syringe. Sometimes the aspiration is followed by a "core biopsy," in which a slightly larger needle is used to extract the core of the bone.

For most biopsies, no special preparation is necessary. Local anesthetics may be given and a mild sedative. In case of excisional biopsy, general anesthesia may be used. Biopsies can either be done as an outpatient procedure in a doctor's office or in a local hospital setting. The time for the procedure varies depending on the site and the method of tissue removal. The risks associated with biopsy are small and vary with the procedure used to obtain the tissue sample.

See also Cancer

BIPOLAR DISORDER

Bipolar disorder, also known as manic-depression, is a **mental illness** which causes extreme mood swings between mania (excessive euphoria) and **depression**, negatively impacting an individual's ability to function normally. Typically appearing in early adolescence or young adulthood, it continues throughout life. It affects more than two million people in the United States and as many as two-thirds of these individuals are undiagnosed, misdiagnosed, or receiving inappropriate treatment. Sufferers are at a 30-times greater risk of committing suicide than the general population, which makes accurate diagnosis and effective treatment a priority. A combination of medication, psychotherapy, close observation by an informed individual, and support groups allow most people suffering from this disorder to lead healthy, productive lives.

One early warning sign of bipolar disorder, *hypomania*, usually does not dramatically affect daily functioning and thus often goes unrecognized. During this cycle, the individual has increased energy and activity, racing thoughts and rapid talk, excessive feelings of euphoria, unrealistic belief in their ability, increased sex drive, unrestrained buying sprees, aggressive behavior, decreased need for sleep, extreme irritability and distraction, abuse of drugs, alcohol, or sleeping medication, and denial that anything is amiss. This state must persist for at least four days to be diagnosed as a problem. For a diagnosis of full-blown *mania*, these tendencies must escalate to the degree of severe interference with the ability to function, persist for at least one week, and be unrelated to drug, alcohol, or medication use.

A *major depressive episode* is defined by depression for at least two weeks. Symptoms include persistent anxiety; sadness; feelings of helplessness, hopelessness, worthlessness, pessimism, or guilt; restlessness; irritability; drastic loss of interest in pleasure or daily activities; reduced sex drive; fatigue or feeling 'slowed down;' difficulty concentrating, remembering, or making decisions; body aches not caused by physical illness; weight gain or loss; and suicidal tendencies.

There are several types of bipolar disorder with varying degrees of severity. Some individuals with *Bipolar I* disorder experience depression with few manic episodes while others experience mood swings which progress from severe, to moderate, to "the blues," to normal, moving into hypomania and mania. In *Bipolar II* disorder, some individuals experience extensive depression with infrequent episodes of mania while others experience the reverse. For a *mixed episode* diagnosis, criteria for both mania and major depressive episodes must apply.

Cycles of mania and depression vary greatly. Some individuals cycle only once every few years, *rapid cyclers* experience four or more episodes annually, *ultra-rapid cyclers* have episodes lasting less than a week, and *ultradian cyclers* experience dramatic mood shifts within 24 hours or less.

While there is no known single cause of bipolar disorder, there appears to be some genetic predisposition. Potential causes—such as increased stress or a traumatic emotional event—are many and varied, and experts believe a combination of factors may act as a trigger. The most effective treatment is a combination of appropriate drugs, skilled psychotherapy, and emotional support. Lithium is the most commonly used medication for mania; however, haloperidol or chlorpromazine are also used. **Antidepressants** may be necessary during severe depressive episodes but cautious observation is recommended as this treatment may push a patient into the manic state. In severe cases, hospitalization may be necessary and, as a last resort, Electroconvulsive Therapy (ECT). Because this disorder can be debilitating and deadly, recognition and accurate diagnosis is essential. Sufferers often 'need help to get help,' and observant family and friends can play an important role in this area.

See also Antidepressants; Depressive disorders; Mental illness

BIRTH DEFECTS

Birth defects are physical abnormalities that are present at birth. They are also called congenital abnormalities. More than 3,000 have been identified.

Birth defects are found in 2-3% of all newborn infants. This rate reaches 10% by age five, as more defects become evident. Almost 20% of **death**s in newborns are caused by birth defects.

Abnormalities can occur in any organ or part of the body. Major defects are structural abnormalities that require medical and/or surgical treatment. Minor defects are abnormalities that do not cause serious health or social problems.

The specific cause of many congenital abnormalities is unknown. Any substance that can causes abnormal develop-

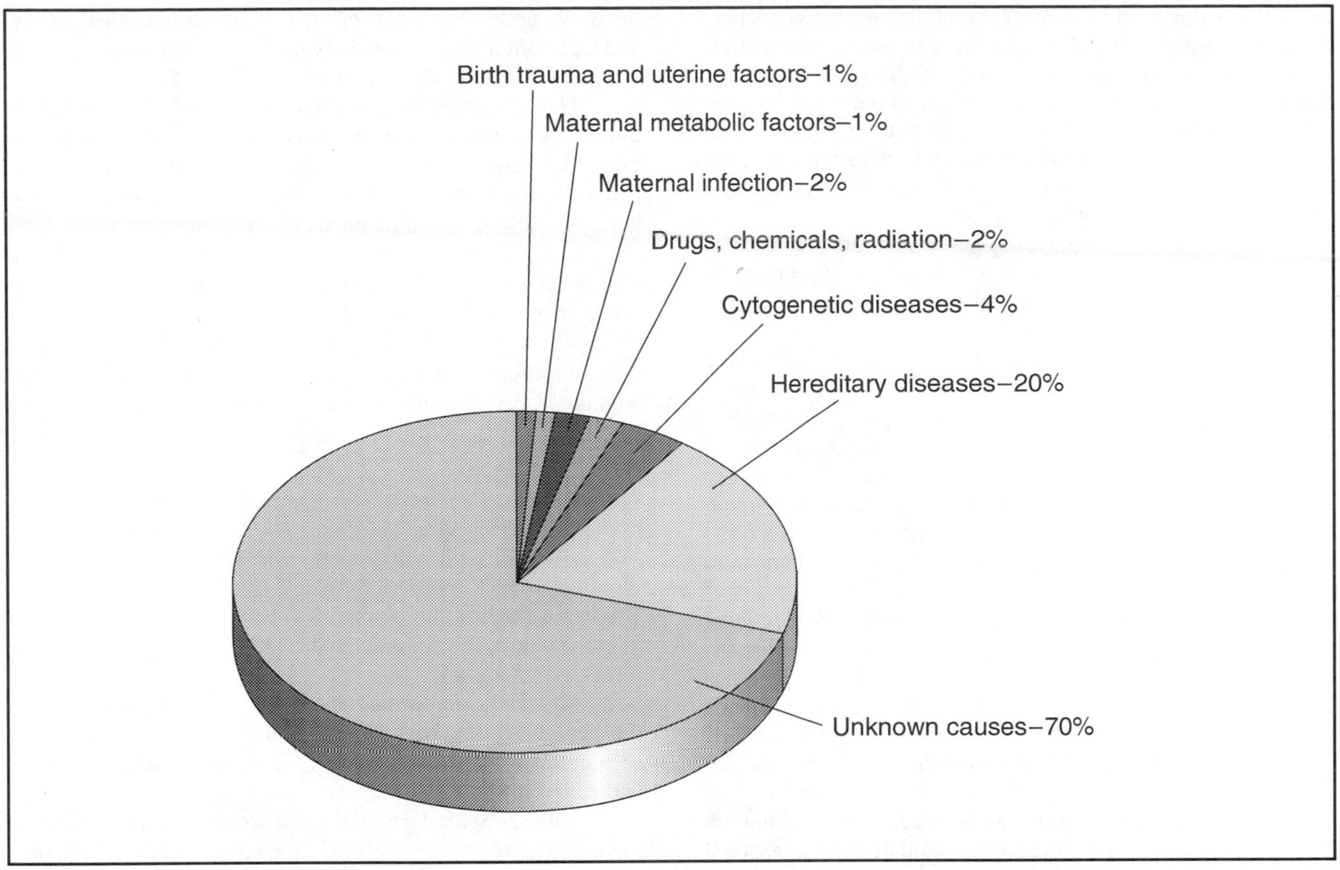

The specific cause of many birth defects is unknown, but several factors associated with pregnancy and delivery can increase the risk of birth defects. These factors include exposure to teratogens, drugs and other chemicals, exposure to radiation, and infections present in the womb. *(Illustration by Electronic Illustrators Group.)*

ment of the egg in the mother's womb is called a teratogen. Growth in the uterus is rapid, and each body organ has a critical period in which it is especially sensitive to outside influences. About 7% of all congenital defects are caused by exposure to teratogens.

Only a few drugs are known to cause birth defects, but all drugs have the potential to cause harm. Thalidomide causes defects of the arms and legs. Drinking large amounts of alcohol while pregnant causes a cluster of defects called **fetal alcohol syndrome** that include **mental retardation**, heart problems, and growth deficiency. Tetracycline, an antibiotic, affects bone growth and discolors the teeth.

Drugs used to treat, sulfa drugs, and some drugs given to treat anxiety and mental illness are known to cause specific defects. Drugs given to treat **cancer** can cause major central nervous system defects. Male hormones may cause masculinization of a female fetus.

Recreational drugs such as LSD have been associated with arm and leg abnormalities and central nervous system problems in infants, as has crack cocaine. Since drug abusers tend to use many drugs and have poor nutrition and prenatal care, it is hard to determine the effects of individual drugs.

Environmental chemicals such as fungicides, food additives, and pollutants are suspected of causing birth defects, although this is difficult to prove. Exposure of the mother to high levels of radiation can cause small skull size (microcephaly), blindness, spina bifida (a malformation of the spinal cord), and cleft palate. How severe the defect is depends on the duration and timing of the exposure.

Three viruses are known to harm a developing baby are **rubella** (German measles), cytomegalovirus (CMV), and herpes simplex. *Toxoplasma gondii*, a parasite that can be contracted from undercooked meat, dirt, or handling the feces of infected cats, causes serious problems. Untreated **syphilis** in the mother is also harmful.

In addition to outside influences, some people carry genes for specific birth defects. A gene is a small unit containing information (DNA) that guides how the body forms and functions. Each person inherits many genes from each parent, arranged on 46 chromosomes. Genes control all aspects of the body, how it works, and all its unique characteristics. Genes can be damaged by chemicals and radiation, but sometimes changes in the genes are unexplained accidents.

Birth defects caused by defective genes include a form of dwarfism called achondroplasia; Huntington's disease, a progressive nervous system disorder; **Marfan syndrome**, which affects connective tissue; some forms of **glaucoma**; and the development of extra fingers or toes.

Other inherited birth defects include **sickle-cell anemia**, a blood disorder found mainly in African-Americans that affects the amount of oxygen the blood can carry and **Tay-Sachs disease**, which causes mental retardation and early death, and is found mainly in people of eastern European Jewish heritage. Two genetic disorders that affect mostly Caucasians are **cystic fibrosis**, a lung and digestive disorder, and **phenylketonuria** (PKU), a metabolic disorder.

Other common genetic birth defects include **hemophilia**, a condition that prevents blood from clotting, Duchenne **muscular dystrophy**, which causes muscle weakness, and **Down syndrome**.

Birth defects whose causes are less understood include cleft lip and palate, **clubfoot**, spina bifida, water on the brain (**hydrocephalus**), **diabetes mellitus**, and some heart defects.

There is no way to prevent all birth defects. If there is a family history of birth defects or if the mother is over age 35, screening tests can be done during early pregnancy to gain information about the likelihood of a birth defect being present. Based on this information, some parents may choose to terminate the pregnancy.

If a birth defect is suspected after a baby is born, confirmation of the diagnosis is necessary. Treatment depends on the type of birth defect and how serious it is. Some abnormalities can be corrected with surgery. Experimental procedures have been used successfully in correcting other defects. Researchers hope that **gene therapy** will eventually correct many birth defects.

The risk of birth defects can be reduced by limiting exposure to chemicals, radiation, alcohol, and drugs (recreational and medicinal) before and during pregnancy. When there is a family history of congenital defects in either parent, **genetic counseling** and testing can help parents plan for future children.

BIRTHMARKS

Birthmarks are benign (noncancerous) skin growths composed of rapidly growing or poorly formed blood vessels or lymph vessels. Found at birth (congenital) or developing later in life (acquired) anywhere on the body, they range from faint spots to dark swellings covering wide areas.

Skin angiomas are composed of either blood vessels (hemangiomas) or lymph vessels (lymphangiomas)that lie beneath the skin's surface. Hemangiomas (strawberry marks) are found on the face and neck (60%), trunk (25%), or the arms and legs (15%). Congenital strawberry marks, 90% of which appear at birth or within the first month of life, grow quickly, and disappear over time. Lymphangiomas are skin bumps caused by enlarged lymph vessels anywhere on the body.

Vascular malformations are poorly formed blood or lymph vessels that appear at birth or later in life. One type, the salmon patch a pink mark composed of dilated capillaries (tiny blood vessels), is found on the back of the neck (also called a stork bite) in 40% of newborns, and on the forehead and eyelids (also called an angel's kiss) in 20%.

Found in fewer than 1% of newborns, port-wine stains are vascular malformations composed of dilated capillaries in the upper and lower layers of the skin of the face, neck, arms, and legs. Often permanent, these flat pink to red marks develop into dark purple bumpy areas in later life.

Hemangiomas acquired later in life include spider angiomas (spider veins), and cherry angiomas. Found around the eyes, cheekbones, arms, and legs, spider veins are red marks formed from dilated blood vessels. They occur during **pregnancy** in 70% of white women and 10% of black women, in alcoholics and liver disease patients, and in 50% of children. Cherry angiomas, dilated capillaries found mainly on the trunk, appear in the 30s, and multiply with aging.

There are no known causes for congenital skin angiomas. Exposure to estrogen causes spider veins in pregnant women or those taking **oral contraceptives**. Spider veins also tend to run in families, and may be associated with liver disease, sun exposure, and trauma.

Hemangiomas first appear as single or multiple white or pale pink marks, ranging from 2-20 cm (average 2-5 cm) in size. Some are symptomless while others cause **pain**, bleed, or interfere with normal functioning because they are numerous, enlarged, infected, or ulcerated. Vision is affected by large marks on the eyelids. Spider and cherry angiomas are unsightly but symptomless.

Vascular malformations (port wine stains, salmon patches, storkbites) may be symptomless or bleed if enlarged or injured. Disfiguring port-wine stains can cause emotional and social problems.

Patients with birthmarks are treated by pediatricians, dermatologists, plastic surgeons, and sometimes ophthalmologists. Angiomas and vascular malformations are not difficult to diagnose. The doctor takes a complete medical history and performs a **physical examination**. Biopsies or specialized x rays or scans of the abnormal vessels and their surrounding areas may be performed. Patients with port-wine stains near the eye may require skull x rays, **computed tomography scans**, vision, and central nervous system tests.

Treatment choices for skin angiomas and vascular malformations depend on their type, location, severity, and whether they cause pain, or disfigurement. Often, no treatment is needed, but the mark is regularly examined until the mark disappears, or requires treatment. This approach is particularly appropriate for the treatment of strawberry marks which often shrink by themselves.

The anti-inflammatory steroid drugs prednisone or prednisolone may be used to treat some birthmarks. The marks begin to subside within 7-10 days, but may take up to 2 months to fully disappear. If no response is seen in 2 weeks, the drug is discontinued. **Corticosteroids** may also be injected directly into the marks with a response usually achieved within a week. These drugs may have substantial undesirable side effects and may not be appropriate for everyone.

Interferon Alpha-2a is used to reduce cell growth for vascular marks that affect vision, and that are unresponsive to corticosteroids. Oral or topical (applied to the skin) **antibiotics** are used on infected marks.

Laser surgery destroys abnormal blood vessels beneath the skin without damaging normal skin. The laser used to treat strawberry marks and port-wine stains penetrates to a depth of 1.8 mm and causes little scarring. Another type of laser that penetrates to a depth of 6 mm is used to treat deep hemangiomas. **Laser surgery** is usually not painful, but can be uncomfortable. Healing occurs within 2 weeks. Side effects include bruising, skin discoloration, swelling, crusting, and minor bleeding.

Surgical excision of the birthmark may be performed under local or general anesthesia. The skin is cut and vascular marks or their scars are removed. The cut is repaired with stitches or skin clips. In cryosurgery, vascular marks are frozen with an extremely cold substance sprayed onto the skin. **Wounds** heal with minimal scarring.

Other treatments include electrodesiccation, where affected vessels are destroyed with current from an electric needle; sclerotherapy, where injection of a special solution causes blood clotting and shrinkage with little scarring; and embolization, where material injected into the vessel blocks blood flow to reduce the size of inoperable growths. Special make-up (Covermark or Dermablend) is also available to cover birthmarks.

BISHOP, J. MICHAEL (1936-)

American molecular biologist

For work in cancer research, J. Michael Bishop shared the 1989 Nobel Prize in physiology or medicine with **Harold Varmus**. He and Varmus found that cancer genes (oncogenes) could be derived from normal cell genes which had not been inherently cancer-causing, as was previously thought; they stopped normal functioning and became cancerous under certain conditions. In presenting the Nobel Prize, Erling Norrby of the Karolinska Institute praised them for their discovery of ''the cellular origin of retroviral oncogenes,'' and claimed they had ''set in motion an avalanche of research on factors that govern the normal growth of cells.''

John Michael Bishop was born February 22, 1936, to John and Carrie Grey Bishop. The family, which included another son and daughter, lived in York, Pennsylvania, where John Bishop was a Lutheran minister. Bishop's early schooling was almost entirely devoid of science, and even when he entered Gettysburg College in 1953 as a premedical student, he had no firm plans for a career. He graduated with a chemistry degree in 1957 and went to Harvard Medical School but took several detours while he was there, first to work in the pathology department of the Massachusetts General Hospital and later to work with the virologist Elmer Pfefferkorn. He obtained his medical degree in 1962 and spent the required amount of time as an intern and resident at Massachusetts General, but his interest had finally focused on investigating the molecular biology of viruses. He worked for three years at the National Institutes of Health as a postdoctoral fellow, learning to do fundamental research. After a year of study in Germany with Gebhard Koch, Bishop took a teaching position in 1968 at the University of California at San Francisco. He was eventually appointed professor in the department of microbiology and immunology, as well as the director of the G. W. Hooper Research Foundation of the University of California Medical Center.

A cancer cell's principal characteristic is unregulated growth and multiplication. Carcinogenesis is a particularly difficult field to study because there appear to be many factors contributing to it (genetics and environment being only two), and also because a cell is an intricate structure with hundreds of different chemical reactions and enzymes controlling and affecting each other. Bishop studied the genetic component of cancer, and of this subject he has written in an article in *Science:* ''Genetic damage remains undetected in the great majority of human tumors. We may have to invent new ways to search for this damage, and we must remain open to the possibility that we will not always find it because it is not always there.''

Many theories of cancer causation already existed when Bishop began his investigations, and new discoveries relevant to the field were made frequently. Robert Huebner and George Todaro had postulated that cancer genes (oncogenes) might lay hidden in cells, the result of viral infection many generations ago, waiting for particular environmental stresses to set them off. **Peyton Rous** had identified a sarcoma virus that caused tumors in chickens. G. Steven Martin found an oncogene, named *src,* src on the Rous sarcoma virus. **Howard Temin** identified the sarcoma virus discovered by Rous as a retrovirus—one that could somehow copy its own RNA information into the DNA of the host cell (which is reverse of the usual process of DNA to RNA reproduction). Temin also participated in David Baltimore's discovery of the enzyme called reverse transcriptase which accomplished that copying.

Bishop, Varmus, and their colleagues Deborah Spector and Dominique Stehelin conducted a search for *src* oncogenes src in different species and found *src-* like genes just about everywhere, apparently as Huebner and Todaro had predicted. They were astonished to find, however, that these genes were not inherently oncogenes but functioned as a regular part of the cellular machinery, performing work for the cell until their normal functioning was somehow changed. Bishop and his colleagues called these genes proto-oncogenes. Retroviruses apparently picked up these normal cellular genes and instigated changes that caused them to become cancerous, although retroviruses were only one possible cause of the transformation; some chemical carcinogens may also convert proto-oncogenes to oncogenes. In a review in *Science,* Bishop uses an analogy to describe proto-oncogenes, though he warns that the analogy is oversimplified: ''The proliferation of cells is governed by an elaborate circuitry that reaches from the surface of the cell to the nucleus. The products of proto-oncogenes may represent some of the junction boxes in that circuitry.... What we now know of oncogenes allows us to view their actions as 'short circuits' at the corresponding junction boxes.''

For this discovery Bishop and Varmus received the 1989 Nobel Prize. Controversy erupted when Stehelin demanded a share of the prize for the work he had done with the two laureates, but the awarding committee remained firm. Stehelin, as well as Spector, had contributed important experiments, but the committee believed that the fundamental intellectual creativity belonged to Bishop and Varmus.

A strong proponent of basic research, in 1993 Bishop coauthored a paper in *Science* which sharply criticized the government's role in the field. The article mentioned ''inadequate funding..., flawed governmental oversight of science, confusion about the goals of federally supported research, and deficiencies in science education,'' and offered a set of guidelines for solving these problems.

Bishop married Kathryn Ione Putnam in 1959; they have two sons. Among his other honors, Bishop won the Gairdner Foundation International Award and the Armand Hammer Cancer Prize in 1984, the American Cancer Society National Medal of Honor in 1985, and the American College of Physicians Award in 1987. He is known as an outstanding teacher and outspoken individual, with a great fondness for music.

BITES AND STINGS

Humans can be injured by the bites or stings of many kinds of animals, including dogs, cats, and fellow humans; arthropods such as spiders, bees, and wasps; snakes; and marine animals such as jellyfish and stingrays.

In the United States, where the dog population exceeds 50 million, dogs surpass all other mammals in the number of bites inflicted on humans. However, most dog-bite injuries are minor. Each year, about 10-20 Americans, mostly children under 10 years old, are killed by dogs.

Cat bites are far less common than dog bites. The tissue damage caused by cat bites is usually limited, but they carry a higher risk of infection. The infection rate for dog bites is 15-20%. For cats it is 30-40%.

Bites from mammals other than dogs and cats are uncommon, with one exception—human bites, of which there are approximately more than 70,000 a year in the United States. Because the human mouth contains a multitude of potentially harmful microorganisms, human bites are more infectious than those of any other animal.

There are more than 700,000 species of arthropods, a group that includes insects, spiders, and crustaceans (crabs). The list of these animals that bite or sting humans is long and encompasses lice, bedbugs, fleas, mosquitoes, black flies, ants, chiggers, ticks, centipedes, scorpions, spiders, bees, and wasps.

In the United States, only two kinds of venomous spider are truly life threatening: black widow spiders and brown (violin or fiddle) spiders. The black widow, which is found in every state but Alaska, prefers dark, dry places such as barns, garages, and outhouses. Brown spiders also prefer sheltered places. Both may bite if disturbed.

Bees and wasps sting to defend their nests or if they are disturbed. Fifty or more Americans a year die after being stung by a bee, wasp, or ant, but almost all of those **death**s are the result of allergic reactions, not exposure to the venom itself.

Venomous snakes, of which there are 20 species in the United States, are found in every state except Maine, Alaska, and Hawaii. Each year about 8,000 Americans are bitten by a venomous snakes, but no more than about 15 die, mostly from rattlesnake bites.

Several varieties of marine animal bite or sting. Jellyfish and stingrays pose the most threat to Americans who live or vacation in coastal communities.

Bites and stings vary in appearance depending on what animal caused the bite. The typical dog bite is a laceration, tear, puncture, or crush injury. Infected bites usually cause **pain**, **cellulitis** (inflammation of the connective tissues), and a pus-filled discharge at the wound site within 8-24 hours. Most infections are confined to the wound site, but some of the microorganisms in dogs' mouths can cause life-threatening infections such as **bacteremia** and **meningitis**.

Cat scratches and bites are also capable of transmitting the *Bartonella henselae* bacterium, which can lead to **cat-scratch disease**, an unpleasant but usually not life-threatening illness.

Humans bites result from fights, sexual activity, medical and dental treatment, and seizures. Children often bite other children, but those bites are hardly ever severe. Human bites are capable of transmitting dangerous diseases, including **hepatitis** B, **syphilis**, and **tuberculosis**.

People do not always feel the black widow spider's bite. The sign may be a mild swelling of the injured area and two red puncture marks. Within a short time, however, some victims experience severe muscle cramps and rigidity of the abdominal muscles. Other possible symptoms include excessive sweating, nausea, vomiting, **headache**s, and vertigo as well as breathing, vision, and speech problems.

A brown spider's bite can cause tissue in an area of up to several inches around the bite to die, producing an open sore that can take months or years to disappear. In most cases, however, the bite simply produces a hard, painful, itchy, and discolored area that heals without treatment in 2-3 days. The bite may also be accompanied by a **fever**, chills, nausea and vomiting, **dizziness**, muscle and joint pain, and a rash.

The familiar symptoms of bee and wasp stings include pain, redness, swelling, and itchiness in the area of the sting. Multiple stings can have much more severe consequences.

Many venomous snake bites fail to poison the victim, or introduce only a small amount of venom into the victim's body. The **wounds** can still become infected by microorganisms that snakes carry in their mouths.

Rattlesnake snake bites usually begin to swell within 10 minutes and sometimes are painful. Other symptoms include skin blisters and discoloration, weakness, sweating, nausea, faintness, dizziness, bruising, and tender lymph nodes. Severe **poisoning** can lead to, muscle contractions, increased heart rate, rapid breathing, large drops in body temperature and blood pressure, vomiting of blood, and **coma**.

Coral snake bites are painful but may be hard to see. After some time has passed, the victim begins to experience the effects of the venom, which include tingling at the wound site, weakness, nausea, vomiting, excessive salivation, and irrational behavior. Nerves in the head can become paralyzed for 6-14 days, causing double vision, difficulty swallowing and speaking, **respiratory failure**, and other problems. Six to eight weeks may be needed before the victim regains muscular strength.

Jellyfish venom is delivered by barbs located on the creature's tentacles. They penetrate the skin of people who brush up against them. Red lesions that are instantly painful and itchy usually result. The pain can continue up to 48 hours. Severe cases may lead to skin death, muscle spasms and cramps, vomiting, nausea, **diarrhea**, headaches, and excessive sweating.

Stingrays deliver their venom through tail spines. They may cause puncture wounds, and pieces of spine can become embedded in the wound. Stingray venom produces immediate, excruciating pain that lasts several hours. Sometimes the victim suffers a severe reaction, including vomiting, diarrhea, hemorrhage (bleeding), a drop in blood pressure, and cardiac arrhythmia (disordered heart action).

Gathering information on the circumstances of the bite is part of bite treatment. This information includes when the bite occurred (the chances of infection increase dramatically, if the wound has been left untreated more than eight hours), the patient's general health, tetanus immunization history, and **allergies**. Laboratory tests for identifying the microorganisms in bite wounds are ordered only if infection has set in. Testing the victim's blood for hepatitis B and other diseases is always necessary after a human bite. Ideally, the biter should be tested as well.

Minor dog bites can be treated at home by washing the wound with soap and water and applying apply antibiotic ointment and a sterile bandage to the wound. Serious dog bites must be looked at by a medical professional promptly. Diabetics, AIDS patients, **cancer** patients, and people who have not had a tetanus shot in five years, should seek medical treatment no matter how minor the bite appears.

Because of the high risk of infection, people who are bitten by a cat should always see a doctor. Experts advise, that cat-bite wounds should always be left open to prevent infection. Cat-bite patients are also more likely to receive antibiotics as a preventive measure.

Human bites should always be examined by a doctor. Such bites are usually treated with antibiotics and left open because of the high risk of infection. The patient may also require immunization against hepatitis B and other diseases.

No spider bite should be ignored. The antidote for severe widow spider bites is a substance called antivenin that contains antibodies to the poison. Doctors exercise caution in using antivenin because it can trigger anaphylactic **shock**, a potentially deadly allergic reaction, and serum sickness, an inflammatory response that can give rise to joint pain, a fever, **rashes**, and other unpleasant consequences.

An antivenin for brown spider bites exists as well, but it is not yet available in the United States. The drug dapsone, used to treat **leprosy**, can sometimes stop the tissue death associated with a brown spider bite

Most bee and wasp stings can be treated at home. Victims who experience an allergic reaction require immediate medical attention. The danger signs, which usually begin 10 minutes after the person is stung, include nausea, chest pain, abdominal cramps, diarrhea, and difficulty swallowing or breathing.

Although most snakes are not venomous, any snakebite should be examined at a hospital. For jellyfish stings, vinegar is used to neutralize jellyfish nematocysts still clinging to the skin. Anesthetic ointments, antihistamine creams, and steroid lotions applied to the skin are sometimes beneficial. Stingray wounds should be washed with saltwater and then soaked in very hot water for 30-90 minutes to neutralize the venom. Afterwards, the wound should be examined by a doctor to ensure that no pieces of spine remain.

BLACK DEATH PANDEMICS

Pandemics of the **plague** have broken out three times in recorded history. A pandemic is a large-scale epidemic. In an epidemic, a disease is confined to certain locations, such as cities or regions. In a pandemic, people are afflicted with a disease over entire countries or continents. Given time, a pandemic can circle the globe. After an initial outbreak that lasts several years, the disease virtually disappears, only to break out in periodic epidemics in the following years. This cycle can be repeated for decades or even centuries before the disease disappears completely.

The first pandemic of plague began in A.D. 542 during the reign of Justinian, Emperor of the Byzantine Empire; for this reason it is called Justinian's plague. It seems to have begun in Egypt and spread northward through the eastern Mediterranean region. In the following years it swept through Europe, central and southern Asia, North Africa, and Arabia, leaving millions dead. The plague struck at a critical time. In Constantinople, the capital of the Byzantine empire, Justinian and his generals were in the midst of battles to rejoin Byzantium to the remains of Western Roman Empire. Justinian's dream was to re-establish the former Roman Empire; and he might have succeeded if not for the plague. Procopius, a historian living in Constantinople at the time, vividly described the plague and its effects. His writings also include an accurate description of what would later be called the bubonic plague. He wrote about agitated, feverish disease victims with painfully enlarged lymph nodes (buboes) under their arms and in their groins. According to Procopius, 300,000 people died within the city alone. It is impossible to verify whether that figure is accurate, but it is certain that Justinian's plague had a dramatic effect on history. Justinian's plans to re-establish the Roman Empire were very likely derailed because of the loss of manpower. In the west, the remnants of the Western Roman empire collapsed into the Dark Ages. Following the initial outbreak in 542, the plague disappeared and reappeared at intervals over the next 200 years. The years 542 to 600 were the most intense plagues years, but local epidemics flared up throughout the Mediterranean region through the mid-eighth century. The population of Europe wasn't able to recover between outbreaks and some historians estimate that the population dropped by half between 542 and 700. After the late-eighth century, plague disappeared from Europe for nearly 600 years.

In 1346, plague was poised to make another sweep through Europe. This pandemic would later be called the Black Death pandemic. Its entry into Europe was through Kaffa, a small Italian trading colony on the shore of the Black Sea in Crimea. Kaffa was besieged by an army and during the siege, plague broke out among the soldiers. According to some sources, the soldiers threw the corpses of those who died over the town walls to spread plague among the men defending the town. Whether that caused plague to break out in the town is unknown, but the defenders were afflicted. They managed to get to their boats and flee to Italy, unknowingly carrying the disease with them. By late 1347, plague was widespread in the Mediterranean region, and in 1348 it spread throughout Italy, France, and England. The Middle East and the Far East were also severely affected. As with Justinian's plague, death rates were appallingly high. From 1346 to 1354, an estimated 20 million people died of plague in Europe. Medieval physicians were at a loss to explain the disease. Some claimed it was due to person-to-person infection, while others said it arose from a poisonous atmosphere. Other explanations put forth by a panicked public blamed astrological influences, divine punishment, and the Jewish community. Tens of thousands of Jewish citizens were burned in Spain, Germany, Switzerland, and France despite protests by Pope Clement VI, Emperor Charles IV, and medical experts who said that they were innocent. However, the authorities were powerless to stop the spread of plague, and they were not believed. Quarantines of plague victims were ordered, but they were largely ineffective because the disease was spread mostly by fleas carried on black rats. Historians estimate that 25-50% of the total population died, and they note that the Black Death undoubtably changed the course of world history. The last major outbreaks of the Black Death pandemic occurred in London in 1665-1666 and in Marseilles in 1720-1722. Each of these outbreaks resulted in approximately 100,000 deaths.

The third pandemic, or Modern pandemic, started in the mid-19th century in central Asia. According to most sources, it continues to the present time. The Modern pandemic began in Yunnan, China, and spread through China and India in the next four years. It reached Bombay in 1896 and is believed to have killed six million people in India alone. From Canton, Hong Kong, and other seaports, plague spread to other continents. Epidemics linked to the Modern pandemic were reported in San Francisco, New Orleans, and other coastal cities throughout the world and millions died. The Modern pandemic also established in areas that previously had been plague free, including North America, South America, and southern Africa. It was during the outbreak in Hong Kong, that the cause of plague, the bacterium was finally identified. Alexandre Yersin, a Swiss bacteriologist, made the discovery that a bacterium caused plague. He named it *Pasteurella pestis* in honor of Louis Pasteur, but it was later renamed *Yersinia pestis* to honor Yersin. With the advent of vaccines and antibiotics and the understanding of how plague spreads, the Modern pandemic has been contained and the plague no longer claims millions of victims. However, health authorities remain vigilant because the plague has not been eradicated. According to **World Health Organization** figures, there were nearly 19,000 cases of plague from 1980 to 1994.

See also Epidemic and pandemic; Plague

BLACK, JAMES (1924-)

English pharmacologist

Sir James Black was one of the founders of a revolution in the way pharmaceutical companies search for medicines. He developed a method of discovering and evaluating new medicines by studying the basic biological mechanisms that underlie disease. His approach led to new, more effective treatments for heart ailments, including heart attack, and to the first successful drug to treat ulcers. For his pioneering efforts, Black shared the 1988 Nobel Prize for physiology or medicine with **George H. Hitchings** and **Gertrude Belle Elion** of Burroughs Wellcome Co. in the United States.

James Whyte Black was born on June 14, 1924, in Uddingston, Scotland, to a working-class family. His father was a Scottish coal miner who worked his way up to mining engineer. Black was the youngest of four sons. One of his older brothers studied medicine and Black soon followed in his footsteps. At age fifteen, he won a residential scholarship to St. Andrew's University, where he received his medical degree in 1946. He remained as an assistant lecturer from 1946 to 1947 before traveling to Malaysia to serve as a senior lecturer in physiology at the University of Malaya from 1947 to 1950. He returned to Scotland in 1950 and lectured in physiology at Glasgow Veterinary School until 1958. During this time he began research on the mechanism of increase in gastric secretions caused by the body's production of histamine. This research formed the basis for his later work on blocking histamine receptors (chemical groups in plasma membrane or cell interior that have an affinity for a specific chemical or compound, in this case histamine) to reduce gastric secretions. During his time in Glasgow, Black also became familiar with the alpha and beta adrenergic receptors, which are responsible for regulating heart beat.

Black joined Imperial Chemical Industries in 1958. There he sought better ways of treating angina pectoris, a painful disease caused by insufficient oxygenation of the heart. The painful episodes suffered by angina patients are caused by increased heart rate, which increases the heart's requirement for oxygen. Black's research led him to theorize that a drug that would neutralize the effects of the hormones adrenaline and noradrenaline, which mediate heart rate, would relieve the symptoms of angina.

The existence of receptors for these hormones had been understood since 1948, when the biochemist Raymond P. Ahlquist first described their action. Black developed a chemically similar but nonfunctional version of the active hormones that would block one of these receptors, the beta receptor. His first studies were with analogs of isoprenaline, a compound similar to noradrenaline. One of these analogs, known as propanolol or the trade name Inderol, had the desired effect. It constricted heart muscle, stopping angina attacks.

In 1964 Black joined the British subsidiary of Smith Kline & French Laboratories. There he worked on new approaches to treating intestinal ulcers. Black knew from his earlier studies that histamine stimulated the secretion of excess acid that causes ulcers. The antihistamines in use at that time inhibited muscle contractions but not acid secretion. Black attacked the problem using the same strategy that worked in the development of the angina treatment—he sought a chemical that would inhibit histamine receptors, blocking the action of the hormone. Many thousands of compounds were tested. Finally in 1972 a partial histamine receptor antagonist was found, guanylhistamine. Unfortunately, it had serious side effects and clinical tests were halted in 1974. After further modification to the chemical structure, Black's group introduced cimetidine, now known as Tagamet (registered trademark), a successful ulcer drug.

Black himself left Smith Kline in 1973. He spent four years as head of the department of pharmacology at University College in London. Then in 1978 he returned to industry, accepting a post as director of therapeutic research at the Wellcome Research Laboratories in Kent. He remained there until 1984, when the lure of academia led him to King's College of Medicine and Dentistry, where he remains today.

In 1988 Black was honored with the Nobel Prize in physiology or medicine, an award he shared with George Hitchings and Gertrude Elion, pharmaceutical researchers from Burroughs Wellcome in the United States. It is unusual for the prize to go to pharmacologists, and the award was a recognition of a truly outstanding contribution to medicine.

Black's success in designing new medicines may be attributed in part to the rational method he employed. Instead of randomly searching for chemicals with a physiological effect, he sought to understand the underlying biological processes and designed drugs that mimic life processes. To test his drugs, he designed "bioassays" that tested how well his drugs would work in the body.

Black is a shy man who does not like to publicize his personal life. He is said to enjoy reading beyond his scientific subjects, music, and the arts. He was married for many years; his wife, Hilary, died in 1987. The couple had one daughter, Stephanie. Black has received several awards and honorary degrees for his work. He was elected to the Royal Society of London in 1976 and received its Mullard Award in 1978. He received the Albert Lasker Clinical Medicine Award in 1976 and was elected a foreign associate of the U.S. National Academy of Sciences in 1991. He was knighted in 1981.

BLACKWELL, ELIZABETH (1821-1910)

Anglo-American physician

Elizabeth Blackwell was born into a family of social activists. The third of nine children, Blackwell was born in Bristol, England on February 3, 1821. Her parents moved the family to New York City when Elizabeth was 12, and her father immediately became active in the abolitionist movement. Unfortunately, after an 1838 move to Cincinnati, Ohio, the family's luck turned sour. Their previously secure finances failed, and Mr. Blackwell died, leaving his family nearly destitute. His daughters opened a young ladies' boarding school in order to provide for the family.

In 1842, Elizabeth Blackwell moved to Henderson, KY to teach, but she found the climate of racism unacceptable and quickly left after only one year. She went back to Cincinnati, and then on to Asheville, NC, where she again began teaching. Here in Asheville, Blackwell began studying medicine on her own. She continued her private medical studies in Charleston, SC, where she also taught at a girls' school.

Blackwell began seeking a medical school which would allow her entrance. Seventeen rejections later, she sent an application to Geneva Medical College (now Hobart and William Smith Colleges). The myth around her eventual acceptance into Geneva Medical College involves the faculty thinking that the idea of a woman applying to medical school was completely preposterous. In fact, they were so convinced that no woman would ever do such a ridiculous thing, that they believed Blackwell's application to be a joke or a hoax. In the spirit of good humor, the faculty went along with the joke by voting "yes" unanimously when her application was presented for vote. Thus was Elizabeth Blackwell's application, neither a joke nor a hoax, accepted for admittance to the Geneva Medical College; the first woman in America ever to attend medical school.

Blackwell endured a lot during her medical studies. The attitudes of her male colleagues and her male teachers ranged from cold to blatantly derisive. She was socially isolated from her all-male peers, and subject to any number of cruel practical jokes. She showed incredible strength, persistence, and determination, graduating at the top of her class on January 12, 1849. She accepted her diploma from the college president, Benjamin Hale, stating: "Sir, by the help of the Most High, it shall be the effort of my life to shed honor on this diploma."

Blackwell attempted to pursue advanced training in surgery in Paris, but was spurned by the male medical establishment. Instead, she was assigned to serve as a midwife at a large maternity hospital. During her time there, Blackwell developed purulent conjunctivitis, and became blind in one eye. Due to this handicap, Blackwell forfeited her plan to study surgery, and left for London. Here she practiced at St. Bartholomew's Hospital until 1851, when she returned to New York.

In New York City, the era's prevailing sexism again thwarted Blackwell's plans, as she was repeatedly denied employment as a physician because she was a woman. Circumventing the male medical establishment, she and her sister Emily (also a physician) worked together to create their own private practice in a tenement building. This practice grew to become the New York Infirmary for Women and Children. The staff was entirely composed of women.

Blackwell established a nurses' training program at the infirmary to help supply medical help for the Union Army during the Civil War. Later, in 1868, the two Blackwell sisters founded Women's Medical College of the New York Infirmary, to provide medical training for women seeking to become physicians.

In 1869, Blackwell returned to London. She established and ran a large practice, and in 1875 helped to found the London School of Medicine for Women, where she served as chair of gynecology. Blackwell also spent a good deal of time writing and lecturing on disease prevention and hygiene. Blackwell was the first woman ever listed in the British Medical Register, and was involved in founding the National Health Society. Scorned and ridiculed in the United States, Blackwell was appreciated in England. Blackwell died in Hastings, England, on May 31, 1910.

BLEEDING

As a medical therapy, bleeding or blood-letting endured for approximately 2,500 years. It was only abandoned at the beginning of the 19th century. The roots of bleeding as a medical therapy can be found in the **Aristotle**an idea that all matter is composed of four elements: air, fire, earth, and water. The ancient Greek physician **Hippocrates** adopted this idea to explain health and disease in humans. In the body, the four elements were represented by four **humors**: blood, phlegm, black bile, and yellow bile. When the humors were ideally balanced, a person enjoyed good health; if the humors were unbalanced, a person suffered an illness. Unbalanced humors were supposed to be caused by an over-accumulation of one of the four humors. Quite reasonably, physicians decided that to regain balance, and therefore health, it was necessary to rid the body of the excess humors. **Galen** (A.D. 130-200) endorsed Hippocrates's theories and medical treatment did not change too much in the following 1,800 years.

The identity of the excess humor was revealed by the symptoms of the ill person. Since blood was thought to be the major humor, nearly any disease could be interpreted as arising from its excess. Through the history, bleeding was used to treat conditions as diverse as inflammation, pain, epilepsy, insanity, pneumonia, syphilis, fractures, and, incredibly, hemorrhage. Bleeding was often used alongside other treatments intended to balance the humors. These other treatments included purging, which meant inducing vomiting or diarrhea, and sweating. Along with bleeding, these treatments made up what was known as heroic medicine. Bleeding was sometimes employed even in the absence of any disease under the assumption that it could maintain health.

Bleeding was done by physicians as well as **barber-surgeons**. There were several ways in which a patient could be bled. The most extreme method was venesection, in which a vein would be opened and a bowl used to catch the blood. In addition to the danger of losing too much blood, the patient also ran the risk of infection or scarring. Local blood-letting was less extreme and was done through cupping or scarification or with leeches. Cupping involved placing a heated glass cup on the skin and allowing it to cool. A partial vacuum would form and when the glass was pulled from the skin, the area would bleed. Scarification required making slight to moderately deep cuts into the skin, but not so deep that veins were opened. **Leeches**, which are blood-sucking parasites, were applied directly to the skin and were thought to be especially useful in treating children and for drawing blood in areas where cupping could not be used.

If they were lucky, patients would recover from their diseases in spite of heroic medicine. In many cases, it's likely that people died from blood loss as there were no rules on how much blood should be removed to restore health. That amount was left to the physician's best judgment. The case of George Washington, first president of the United States, illustrates how that judgment might not lead to the best outcome for the patient. According to his physician's notes, Washington was afflicted with an inflammation of the upper windpipe on a Friday night. As it progressed, he developed a fever and difficulty breathing. Following medical standards of the time, he had someone come to bleed him that night. Twelve to 14 ounces of blood were removed, but he did not improve. The next afternoon, he was bled ''copiously'' twice more. When that proved ineffective, another 32 ounces of blood were removed. In addition to bleeding, his physicians also tried purging. By Saturday night, he was dead.

Through medical history, bleeding had opponents. For example, Erisistratos (300-260 B.C.), an early Greek physician, argued that it was a dangerous practice. He pointed out that the patient could lose too much blood or that the physician might accidentally cut into tendons, arteries, or nerves. However, the practice of bleeding a patient was not given up until the 19th century. Even as late as the 1850s, some physicians still argued passionately for its efficacy against disease. It wasn't until **Louis Pasteur** and **Robert Koch** proved that many diseases arose from infection with microorganisms that bleeding was finally abandoned as a standard medical therapy. Today, bleeding (or therapeutic phlebotomy) is used to treat a very specific set of blood diseases in which certain blood factors are overproduced or produce incorrectly.

See also Humors; Phlebotomy

BLOCH, KONRAD (1912-)

German American biochemist

Konrad Bloch's investigations of the complex processes by which animal cells produce cholesterol have helped to increase our understanding of the biochemistry of living organisms. His research established the vital importance of cholesterol in animal cells and helped lay the groundwork for further research into treatment of various common diseases. For his contributions to the study of the metabolism of cholesterol, he was awarded the 1964 Nobel prize for Physiology or Medicine.

Konrad Emil Bloch was born on January 21, 1912 in the German town of Neisse (now Nysa, Poland) to Frederich (Fritz) D. Bloch and Hedwig Bloch. Sources list his mother's maiden name variously as Steiner, Steimer, or Striemer. After receiving his early education in local schools, Bloch attended the Technische Hochschule (technical university) in Munich from 1930 to 1934, studying chemistry and chemical engineering. He earned the equivalent of a B.S. in chemical engineering in 1934, the year after Adolf Hitler became chancellor of Germany. As Bloch was Jewish, he moved to Switzerland after graduating and lived there until 1936.

While in Switzerland, he conducted his first published biochemical research. He worked at the Swiss Research Institute in Davos, where he performed experiments involving the biochemistry of phospholipids in tubercle bacilli, the bacteria that causes tuberculosis.

In 1936, Bloch emigrated from Switzerland to the United States; he would become a naturalized citizen in 1944. With financial help provided by the Wallerstein Foundation, he earned his Ph.D. in biochemistry in 1938 at the College of Physicians and Surgeons at Columbia University, and then joined the Columbia faculty. Bloch also accepted a position at Columbia on a research team led by Rudolf Schoenheimer. With his associate David Rittenberg, Schoenheimer had developed a method of using radioisotopes (radioactive forms of atoms) as tracers to chart the path of particular molecules in cells and living organisms. This method was especially useful in studying the biochemistry of cholesterol.

Cholesterol, which is found in all animal cells, contains 27 carbon atoms in each molecule. It plays an essential role in the cell's functioning; it stabilizes cell membrane structures and is the biochemical ''parent'' of cortisone and some sex hormones. It is both ingested in the diet and manufactured by liver and intestinal cells. Before Bloch's research, scientists knew little about cholesterol, although there was speculation about a connection between the amount of cholesterol and other fats in the diet and arteriosclerosis (a buildup of cholesterol and lipid deposits inside the arteries).

While on Schoenheimer's research team, Bloch learned about the use of radioisotopes. He also developed, as he put it, a ''lasting interest in intermediary metabolism and the problems of biosynthesis.'' Intermediary metabolism is the study of the biochemical breakdown of glucose and fat molecules and the creation of energy within the cell, which in turn fuels other biochemical processes within the cell.

After Schoenheimer died in 1941, Rittenberg and Bloch continued to conduct research on the biosynthesis of cholesterol. In experiments with rats, they ''tagged'' acetic acid, a 2-carbon compound, with radioactive carbon and hydrogen isotopes. From their research, they learned that acetate is a major component of cholesterol. This was the beginning of Bloch's work in an area that was to occupy him for many years—the investigation of the complex pattern of steps in the biosynthesis of cholesterol.

Bloch stayed at Columbia until 1946, when he moved to the University of Chicago to take a position as assistant professor of biochemistry. He stayed at Chicago until 1953, becoming an associate professor in 1948 and a full professor in 1950. After a year as a Guggenheim Fellow at the Institute of Organic Chemistry in Zurich, Switzerland, he returned to the United States in 1954 to take a position as Higgins Professor of Biochemistry in the Department of Chemistry at Harvard University. Throughout this period he continued his research into the origin of all 27 carbon atoms in the cholesterol molecule. Using a mutated form of bread mold fungus, Bloch and his associates grew the fungus on a culture that contained acetate marked with radioisotopes. They eventually discovered that the two-carbon molecule of acetate is the origin of all carbon atoms in cholesterol. Bloch's research explained the significance of acetic acid as a building block of cholesterol, and

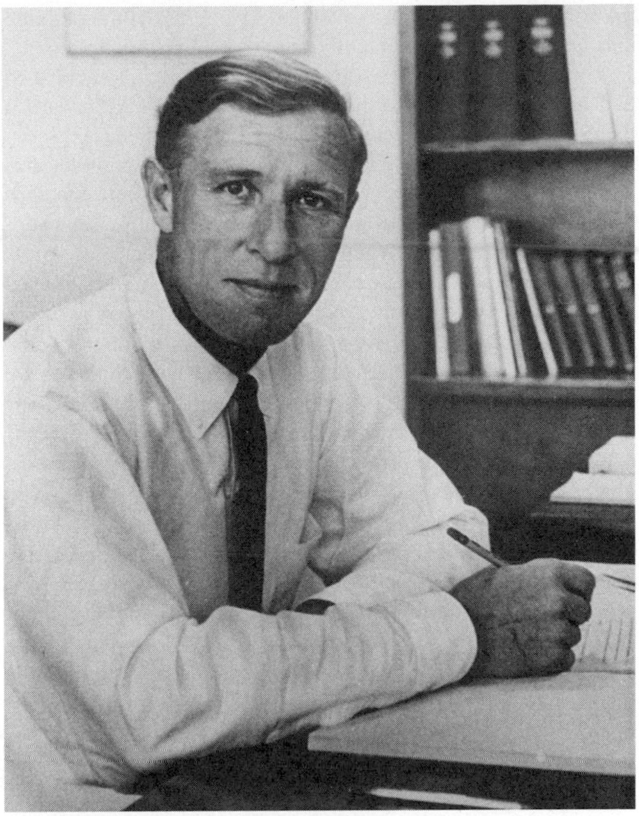

Konrad Bloch

showed that cholesterol is an essential component of all body cells. In fact, Bloch discovered that all steroid-related substances in the human body are derived from cholesterol.

The transformation of acetate into cholesterol takes 36 separate steps. One of those steps involves the conversion of acetate molecules into squalene, a hydrocarbon found plentifully in the livers of sharks. Bloch's research plans involved injecting radioactive acetic acid into dogfish, a type of shark, removing squalene from their livers, and determining if squalene played an intermediate role in the biosynthesis of cholesterol. Accordingly, Bloch traveled to Bermuda to obtain live dogfish from marine biologists. Unfortunately, the dogfish died in captivity, so Bloch returned to Chicago empty-handed. Undaunted, he injected radioactive acetate into rats' livers, and was able to obtain squalene from this source instead. Working with Robert G. Langdon, Bloch succeeded in showing that squalene is one of the steps in the biosynthetic conversion of acetate into cholesterol.

Bloch and his colleagues discovered many of the other steps in the process of converting acetate into cholesterol. **Feodor Lynen**, a scientist at the University of Munich with whom he shared the Nobel Prize, had discovered that the chemically active form of acetate is acetyl coenzyme A. Other researchers, including Bloch, found that acetyl coenzyme A is converted to mevalonic acid. Both Lynen and Bloch, while conducting research separately, discovered that mevalonic acid is converted into chemically active isoprene, a type of hydrocarbon. This in turn is transformed into squalene, squalene is converted into anosterol, and then, eventually, cholesterol is produced.

In 1964, Bloch and his colleague Feodor Lynen, who had independently performed related research, were awarded the Nobel Prize for Physiology or Medicine ''for their discoveries concerning the mechanisms and regulation of cholesterol and fatty acid metabolism.'' In presenting the award, Swedish biochemist **Sune Bergström** commented, ''The importance of the work of Bloch and Lynen lies in the fact that we now know the reactions that have to be studied in relation to inherited and other factors. We can now predict that through further research in this field... we can expect to be able to do individual specific therapy against the diseases that in the developed countries are the most common cause of death." The same year, Block was honored with the Fritzsche Award from the American Chemical Society and the Distinguished Service Award from the University of Chicago School of Medicine. He also received the Centennial Science Award from the University of Notre Dame in Indiana and the Cardano Medal from the Lombardy Academy of Sciences the following year.

Bloch continued to conduct research into the biosynthesis of cholesterol and other substances, including glutathione, a substance used in protein metabolism. He also studied the metabolism of olefinic fatty acids. His research determined that these compounds are synthesized in two different ways: one comes into play only in aerobic organisms and requires molecular oxygen, while the other method is used only by anaerobic organisms. Bloch's findings from this research directed him toward the area of comparative and evolutionary biochemistry.

Bloch's work is significant because it contributed to creating ''an outline for the chemistry of life,'' as E.P. Kennedy and F.M. Westheimer of Harvard wrote in *Science.* Moreover, his contributions to an understanding of the biosynthesis of cholesterol have contributed to efforts to comprehend the human body's regulation of cholesterol levels in blood and tissue. His work was recognized by several awards other than those mentioned above, including a medal from the Societe de Chimie Biologique in 1958 and the William Lloyd Evans Award from Ohio State University in 1968.

Bloch served as an editor of the *Journal of Biological Chemistry,* chaired the section on metabolism and research of the National Research Council's Committee on Growth, and was a member of the biochemistry study section of the United States Public Health Service. Bloch has also been a member of several scientific societies, including the National Academy of Sciences, to which he was elected in 1956, the American Academy of Arts and Sciences, and the American Society of Biological Chemists, in addition to the American Philosophical Society.

Bloch and his wife, the former Lore Teutsch, met in Munich and married in the United States in 1941. They have two children, Peter and Susan. Bloch is known for his extreme modesty; when he was awarded the Nobel Prize, the *New York Times* reported that he refused to have his picture taken in front of a sign that read, ''Hooray for Dr. Bloch!'' He enjoys skiing and tennis, as well as music.

BLOOD COUNT

One of the most commonly ordered clinical laboratory tests, a blood count, also called a complete blood count (CBC), is a basic evaluation of the cells (red blood cells, white blood cells, and platelets) suspended in the liquid part of the blood (plasma). It involves determining the numbers, concentrations, and conditions of the different types of blood cells.

The CBC is a useful screening and diagnostic test that is often done as part of a routine **physical examination**. It can provide valuable information about the blood and blood-forming tissues (especially the bone marrow), as well as other body systems. Abnormal results can indicate the presence of a variety of conditions including anemias, leukemias, and infections, sometimes before the patient experiences symptoms of the disease.

A complete blood count is actually a series of tests in which the numbers of red blood cells, white blood cells, and platelets in a given volume of blood are counted. The CBC also measures the hemoglobin content (important to the transport of oxygen) and the packed cell volume (hematocrit)of the red blood cells. It assesses the size and shape of the red blood cells, and determines the types and percentages of white blood cells.

The blood count is relatively inexpensive and quick. Most laboratories routinely use automated equipment to dilute the blood, sample a measured volume of the diluted suspension, and count the cells in that volume. In addition to counting actual numbers of red cells, white cells, and platelets, the automated cell counters also measure the hemoglobin and calculate the hematocrit and the red blood cell indices (measures of the size and hemoglobin content of the red blood cells). Technologists then examine a stained blood smear under the microscope to identify any abnormalities in the appearance of the red blood cells and to report the types and percentages of white blood cells observed.

The red blood cell (RBC) count determines the total number of red cells (erythrocytes) in a sample of blood. Hemoglobin (Hgb) is the protein-iron compound in the red blood cells that enables them to transport oxygen. Its concentration corresponds closely to the RBC count. Also closely tied to the RBC and hemoglobin values is the hematocrit (Hct), which measures the percentage of red blood cells in the total blood volume. The hematocrit is normally about three times the hemoglobin concentration.

Red blood cell indices are useful in differentiating types of anemias. The indices include four measurements that are calculated using the RBC count, hemoglobin, and hematocrit results. Mean corpuscular volume (MCV) is a measurement of the average size of the red blood cells. The red blood cell distribution width (RDW) is an indication of the variation in RBC size. Mean corpuscular hemoglobin (MCH) measures the average weight of hemoglobin within a red blood cell. A similar measurement, mean corpuscular hemoglobin concentration (MCHC), expresses the average concentration of hemoglobin in the red blood cells.

The white blood cell (WBC) count determines the total number of white cells (leukocytes) in the blood sample. Fewer in number than the red cells, WBCs are the body's primary means of fighting infection. There are five main types of white cells (neutrophils, lymphocytes, monocytes, eosinophils, and basophils). A differential white cell count is done by staining a smear of the patient's blood with a Wright's stain, allowing the different types of white cells to be clearly seen under the microscope. A technologist then counts a minimum of 100 WBCs and reports each type of white cell as a percentage of the total white blood cells counted.

The **platelet count** is an actual count of the number of platelets (thrombocytes) in a given volume of blood. Platelets are involved in blood clotting. Because platelets can clump together, the automated counting method may not be accurate enough for low platelet counts. For this reason, very low platelet levels are often counted manually.

Blood count values vary by age and sex. The normal red blood cell count ranges from 4.2–5.4 million RBCs per microliter of blood for men and 3.6–5.0 million for women. Hemoglobin values range from 14–18 grams per deciliter of blood for men and 12–16 grams for women. The normal hematocrit is 42–54% for men and 36–48% for women. The normal number of white blood cells for both men and women is approximately 4,000–10,000 WBCs per microliter of blood.

Abnormal blood count results are seen in a variety of conditions. One of the most common is anemias, which are characterized by low RBC counts, hemoglobins, and hematocrits. Infections and leukemias are associated with increased numbers of WBCs.

Blood donation

Donating blood is a simple and relatively painless procedure that can help save lives.

According to the American Association of Blood Banks, eight million volunteer donors donate the 14 million pints of blood used in the United States each year. The blood is used to help a variety of people. Donated blood can help restore a person's blood volume after surgery, accident, or childbirth, improve the immunity of a patient suffering from cancer or leukemia and other diseases, and improve the blood's ability to carry oxygen.

Sometimes the donated blood is used as whole blood; that is, the blood from a donor is administered in its entirety to the recipient. In other cases, the blood is separated into its components (platelets, plasma, red and white cells, and clotting factors), and administered to a patient in need of that specific component.

There is no risk of contracting disease if you donate blood, because new, sterile equipment is used for each donor. The U.S. Food and Drug Administration has stringent regulations concerning how blood can be collected, stored and transported, and other organizations, such as the AABB and the American Red Cross, have additional procedures to safeguard both donors and the collected blood.

To protect the nation's blood supply (and blood recipients), each donor is carefully screened to make sure he or she is in good health. At the donation center, a donor will be asked his or her name and address, and this information will be verified. His or her pulse, temperature and blood pressure are taken. The donor is asked if he or she has ever had a condition that might disqualify him or her as a donor; for example, hepatitis, malaria, heart disease, AIDS and most forms of cancer would make someone unsuitable as a donor. If a person's blood pressure is too high or too low, if she is pregnant, or if he or she has had major surgery recently, he or she will be asked to wait some time before donating.

After the screening, the donor is seated in a special reclining chair or lies down on a table. The person drawing the blood wraps a tourniquet around the donor's upper arm; by restricting the flow of blood returning from the hand to the heart, the veins become more prominent and easier to find. The person drawing the blood inserts a needle into the vein. The needle is attached to a collection bag. The donor then lies still and quietly while the blood is collected, which takes only about 10 minutes.

When the unit, or pint, of blood is collected, the needle is removed and an adhesive bandage placed over the spot where the needle had been inserted. The donor is asked to lie still for a few more moments, and then offered fruit juice and perhaps cookies to replenish him or herself. Sometimes donating blood can cause lightheadedness, and it's important to not move too quickly or else dizziness can occur.

The whole procedure takes about an hour.

The donated blood is sealed in a special plastic bag that contains substances that will keep it from clotting (anticoagulants) and will preserve it. Refrigerated, whole blood is useable for 42 days. Blood components, however, can be preserved for much longer—in the case of red blood cells, up to 10 years, if frozen.

A sample of the donated blood is taken for testing. It is checked for infections diseases like AIDS and syphillis, for anemia, and, if the blood type is not already known, for blood typing. Human blood falls into three major groups, A, B, and O; the types get their names from certain molecules found on the surface of the red blood cells. If a person receives a donation of an incompatible blood type, the blood cells can clump together, a dangerous and possibly fatal situation. Type O blood can be received by persons with A, B, or AB blood (which is why type O is sometimes called the ''universal donor''), but a person with Type O blood can only Type O blood. It is also important to match the Rh factor of the blood, which can be positive or negative.

Anyone in good health can donate blood. It is generally recommended that the donor be over age 17 (although some states allow younger persons to donate, with their parent's permission) and weigh at least 110 pounds. The donor's body will replenish the donated blood quickly. However, it's best to not give blood than once every two months.

There are several special donation procedures. Persons who are expecting to undergo surgery may opt to donate several pints of their own blood, which is stored and given back to them during the surgery. This is called an autologus tranfusion.

A donor may give only a specified component of the blood, which is extracted by machine from the donated blood

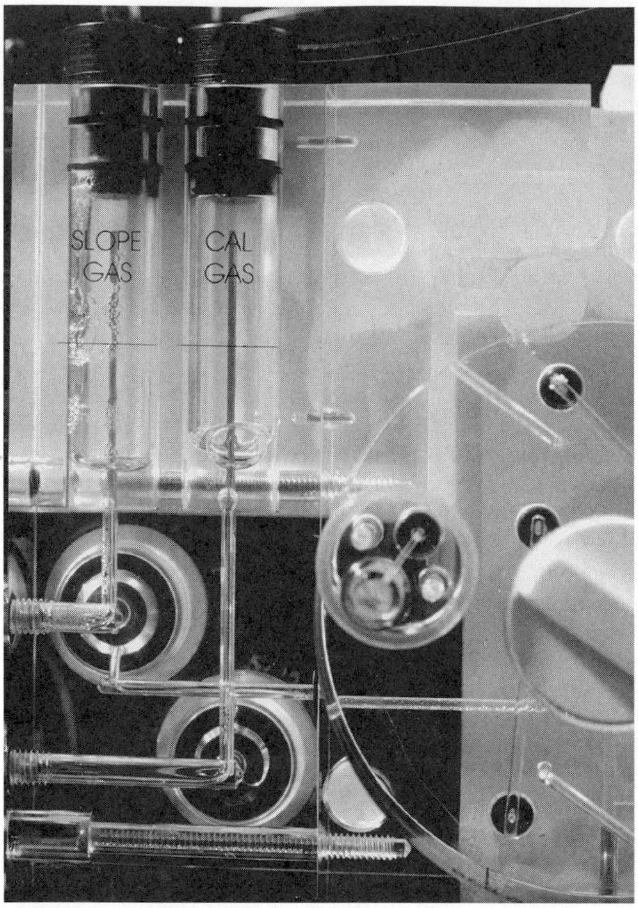

A blood gas analyzer. ***(Photograph by Hank Morgan, Photo Researchers, Inc. Reproduced by permission.)***

before the donated blood is returned to the donor's body. This is a procedure called apheresis. In addition, a patient's family members can donate blood specifically for the patient (as long as their blood type and Rh factors are compatible). This is called a designated or direct donation.

BLOOD GAS ANALYSIS

Blood gas analysis, also called arterial blood gas (ABG) analysis, is a test that measures the amounts of oxygen and carbon dioxide in the blood, and the acidity (pH) of the blood.

An ABG analysis evaluates how effectively the lungs are delivering oxygen to the blood and how efficiently they are eliminating carbon dioxide from it. The test also indicates how well the lungs and kidneys are interacting to maintain normal blood pH (acid-base balance). Blood gas studies are usually done to assess respiratory disease and other conditions that may affect the lungs, and to manage patients receiving **oxygen therapy**. In addition, the acid-base component of the test provides information on kidney function.

Blood gas analysis is performed on blood from an artery. It measures the partial pressures of oxygen and carbon dioxide in the blood, as well as oxygen content, oxygen saturation, bicarbonate content, and blood pH.

Oxygen in the lungs is carried to the tissues through the body attached to red blood cells. Only a small amount of this oxygen can actually dissolve in arterial blood. How much oxygen dissolves depends on the pressure that the gas exerts on the walls of the arteries. This is called the partial pressure. The partial pressure of oxygen tells physicians how much oxygen the lungs are delivering to the blood. Carbon dioxide is released into the blood as a by-product of cell metabolism. The partial carbon dioxide pressure indicates how well the lungs are eliminating this carbon dioxide.

The remainder of oxygen that is not dissolved in the blood combines with hemoglobin, a protein—iron compound found in the red blood cells. The oxygen content measurement in an ABG analysis indicates how much oxygen is combined with the hemoglobin. A related value is the oxygen saturation, which compares the amount of oxygen actually combined with hemoglobin to the total amount of oxygen that the hemoglobin is capable of combining with.

Carbon dioxide dissolves in the blood, primarily forming bicarbonate and smaller amounts of carbonic acid. When present in normal amounts, the ratio of carbonic acid to bicarbonate creates an acid-base balance in the blood, helping to keep the pH at a level where the body's cellular functions are most efficient. The lungs and kidneys both participate in maintaining the carbonic acid-bicarbonate balance. The lungs control the carbonic acid level and the kidneys regulate the bicarbonate. If either organ is not functioning properly, an acid-base imbalance can result. Determination of bicarbonate and pH levels, aids in diagnosing the cause of abnormal blood gas values.

To perform an ABG analysis, blood is obtained by arterial puncture (usually in the wrist, although it could be in the groin or arm) or from an arterial line already in place. A technician then collects the blood with a small sterile needle attached to a disposable syringe. After the blood is drawn, the sample must be transported to the laboratory as soon as possible for analysis.

When the blood has been drawn, the technician or the patient applies pressure to the puncture site for 10–15 minutes to stop the bleeding, and then places a dressing over the puncture. Risks are very low when the test is done correctly, but include bleeding or bruising at the site.

Normal blood gas values are as follows:

- Partial pressure of oxygen (PaO_2): 75–100 mm Hg
- Partial pressure of carbon dioxide ($PaCO_2$): 35–45 mm Hg
- Oxygen content (O_2CT): 15–23%
- Oxygen saturation (SaO_2): 94–100%
- Bicarbonate (HCO_3): 22–26 mEq/liter
- PH: 7.35–7.45.

Values that differ from those listed above may indicate respiratory, metabolic, or kidney disease. These results also may be abnormal if the patient has experienced trauma that affects breathing (especially head and neck injuries). Disorders such as anemia that affect the oxygen-carrying capacity of blood, can produce an abnormally low oxygen content value.

Blood pressure measuring devices

Hypertension, or high blood pressure—also known as the ''silent killer''—affects more than 60 million Americans. Blood pressure measuring devises are the only means through which high blood pressure can be detected. In the course of his pioneering work on blood circulation in the 1600s, William Harvey (1578-1657) noted that blood pulsated out of a severed artery as if it were under rhythmic pressure. Nearly a century later, Stephen Hales (1677-1761), an English clergyman and physiologist, devised a technique to measure the pressure exerted on the vessels as blood was pumped through them. Hales inserted a brass pipe into an animal's blood vessel and used the windpipe of a goose (for its flexibility) to connect the pipe to a long glass tube. The height to which the animal's blood spurted up into the tube gave a measure of the force propelling the blood. One of Hales' most dramatic experiments using this simple manometer involved a white mare, tied flat on the ground to a stable door; the glass tube in this instance was 12 ft. 9 in. (3.8 m) long, and the horse's blood rose in it to a height of 9 ft. 6 in. (2.9 m). Hales began his blood pressure measurement experimentation around 1706, continued around 1712-13, and finally reported his technique in his 1733 book *Haemastaticks*. Another century passed before the Hales manometer was improved upon. In 1828 French physician Jean Leonard Marie Poiseuille (1797-1869) replaced the long glass tube with a U-shaped tube filled with mercury and calibrated to record pressure levels in millimeters of mercury. The German physiologist **Karl Friedrich Wilhelm Ludwig** modified Poiseuille's manometer in 1847, adding a revolving cylinder and float with a revolving drum on which the blood pressure was recorded. This device was called a *kymograph.* It was further refined by Etienne-Jules Marey with his 1863 *sphygmograph*, another blood pressure recorder. The first blood pressure measuring device that required no skin penetration was the *sphygmomanometer* pioneered by Samuel Siegfried von Basch (1837-1905), a German physician, in 1876. This rather inaccurate device was replaced in 1896 by the sphygmomanometer of the Italian physician Scipione Riva-Rocci (1863-1937), the prototype of today's standard instrument which uses an arm band which is inflated until the blood flow through the arteries can no longer be detected. Air is then released from the band, and blood pressure measured on a mercury manometer at the moment when the pulse reappears. While Riva-Rocci's instrument was accurate, it measured only *systolic* pressure—pressure within the artery when the heart is contracting. A Russian physician, Nikolai Korotkoff, added the missing element when he suggested in 1905 that a **stethoscope** be used to listen to the blood flow in the brachial artery of the elbow. Heard through the stethoscope, the tapping that begins when air is released from the band is the systolic pressure; the moment the tapping sound disappears is the *diastolic* (between contractions) pressure.

Wide clinical use of blood pressure measurement using the sphygmomanometer was promoted by American surgeon Harvey Williams Cushing. Standard readings were soon established and became basic indicators of heart and lung health or problems. Today, virtually every visit by an adult to a doctor includes a blood pressure test. Many types of blood pressure measuring devises are now available, even for home use, for which *automated meters* are preferable because of their simplicity. Automated meters are battery-operated electronic or digital devices which measure either sound or force and eliminate the need for a stethoscope, using instead a microphone device. There is even a cuffless *oscillometric* meter, which reads blood pressure from a device in which the patient's finger is placed. Home blood pressure measuring devices offer obvious advantages, even though they provide less accurate readings than those obtained at a physician's office.

Blood typing and crossmatching

Blood typing is a laboratory test done to determine a person's blood type based on the proteins on the surface of blood cells. If the person needs a blood **transfusion**, another test called crossmatching is done to find blood from a donor that the person's body will accept. People must receive blood of the same blood type, otherwise, a serious, even fatal, transfusion reaction can occur.

A child inherits genes from each parent that determine his blood type. This makes blood typing useful in paternity testing. Legal investigations may require typing of blood to identify persons involved in crimes or other legal matters.

Blood typing and crossmatching tests are performed in a blood bank laboratory by technologists trained in blood bank and transfusion services. The tests are done on blood after it has been separated into cells and serum. Serum is the yellow liquid left after the blood clots.

Blood typing and crossmatching tests are based on the reaction between antigens and antibodies. An antigen is a foreign substance that causes the body to launch an attack, known as an immune response, against it. The body builds proteins called antibodies to neutralize each specific antigen.

The antigens found on the surface of red blood cells determine a person's blood type. When red blood cells having a certain blood type antigen are mixed with serum containing antibodies against that antigen, the antibodies attack and stick to the antigen. In a test tube, this reaction is observed as the formation of clumps of cells (clumping).

When blood is typed, a person's blood is mixed in a test tube with commercially-prepared serum and cells. Clumping tells which antigens are present and reveals the person's blood type. When blood is crossmatched, patient serum is mixed with cells from donated blood that might be used for transfusion. Clumping or lack of clumping in the test tube tells whether or not the blood is compatible.

Although there are over 600 known red blood cell antigens organized into 22 blood group systems, routine blood typing and crossmatching is usually concerned with only two systems: the ABO and Rh blood group systems.

A person's ABO blood type—A, B, AB, or O—is based on the presence or absence of the A and B antigens on his red blood cells. The A blood type has only the A antigen, and the

B blood type has only the B antigen. The AB blood type has both A and B antigens, and the O blood type has neither A nor B antigen. Although the distribution of each of the four ABO blood types varies among racial groups, O is the most common and AB is the least common. A person must receive ABO-matched blood for a transfusion. ABO incompatibilities are the major cause of fatal transfusion reactions.

The Rh, or Rhesus system, is also examined during crossmatching. Although there are more than 50 Rh antigens, in routine blood typing and crossmatching tests, only the D antigen, also known as the Rh factor or $Rh_0[D]$, is tested for. If the D antigen is present, the person is Rh-positive; if the D antigen is absent, that person is Rh-negative. In transfusions, the Rh system is next in importance after the ABO system.

Rh incompatibility is the most common and severe cause of hemolytic disease of the newborn (HDN), a type of anemia also known as **erythroblastosis fetalis**. This incompatibility can occur when an Rh-negative woman and an Rh-positive man produce an Rh-positive baby. Cells from the baby can cross the placenta and enter the mother's bloodstream, causing the mother to make anti-D antibodies. These antibodies re-cross the placenta to destroy the baby's red blood cells, causing severe or fatal anemia. This condition can be prevented through injections of a specific immunoglobulin protein if it is recognized early in pregnancy.

When a transfusion is needed, blood from a donor and the recipient are typed and crossmatched. In a test tube, serum from the patient is mixed with red blood cells from the potential donor. If clumping occurs, the blood is not compatible; if clumping does not occur, the blood is compatible. If an unexpected antibody is found in either the patient or the donor, the blood bank does compatibility testing procedures are designed to provide the safest blood product possible for the recipient.

In an emergency, when there is not enough time for blood typing and crossmatching, O red blood cells may be given, preferably Rh-negative. O blood type is called the universal donor because it has no ABO antigens for a patient's antibodies to attack.

To collect the 10 mL blood needed for these tests, a healthcare worker ties a tourniquet above the patient's elbow, locates a vein in the inner elbow region, and inserts a needle into that vein. Vacuum action draws the blood through the needle into an attached tube. Collecting the sample takes only a few minutes. Blood typing and crossmatching must be done three days or less before a transfusion.

BLUE BABY OPERATION

Before 1944, babies born with *cyanosis*—bluish skin caused by lack of oxygen in the blood—either died or lived with painful physical defects. The plight of these ''blue babies'' aroused the interest of Dr. **Helen Taussig** of Johns Hopkins after she became head of that hospital's Children's Heart Clinic in the 1930s. After much pioneering fluoroscopy study, Taussig developed a theory that the cyanosis was due to constriction of the pulmonary artery, the vessel that carries oxygen-depleted bluish blood from the heart to the lungs, where the blood absorbs oxygen and becomes red once again. Next, Taussig visited heart surgeon Robert Gross of Boston, Massachusetts, who had developed an operation to close a baby's blood vessel. This convinced Taussig that a reverse operation—to open a blocked blood vessel—should be possible. In 1941 Dr. Alfred Blalock (1899-1964) became chief surgeon at Johns Hopkins. Taussig, who knew of his reputation as a vascular surgeon and research in blood vessel bypasses, interested Blalock in her theory about cyanosis. Together they experimented on hundreds of dogs to perfect an operation in which a branch of the aorta is joined to the pulmonary artery to create a bypass of the defective portion, assuring adequate flow of blood to the lungs. On November 29, 1944, Blalock performed the first ''blue baby'' operation on a 15-month-old girl, assisted by Taussig. Two more successful operations followed. A paper by Taussig and Blalock reported the procedure in the May 19, 1945, issue of the *Journal of the American Medical Association*. The ''Blalock-Taussig Shunt,'' as the operation came to be called, was soon widely adopted and saved thousands of babies' lives. Surgeons came to Johns Hopkins from around the world to learn the new procedure, and Blalock traveled abroad to further spread knowledge of the operation. This operative technique is still used today for very young children, keeping them alive until they are old enough for **open-heart surgery**. A modified procedure using man-made material for the shunt was first performed in 1963. The Blalock-Taussig procedure was the beginning of the modern era of heart surgery, paving the way for open-heart surgery and surgical correction of many congenital heart defects.

BLUMBERG, BARUCH SAMUEL (1925-)

American research physician

When Baruch Samuel Blumberg was notified on October 14, 1976 that he was a co-winner of the Nobel Prize for physiology or medicine, he made a humorous and low-key comment to the *New York Times:* ''I'm especially pleased that someone from Philadelphia won. It's appropriate in the Bicentennial year and makes up in part for the Phillies not making it to the World Series.'' But there was nothing low-key about the research Blumberg had done to win the prize. In 1963 he had discovered a protein in the blood of Australian Aborigines, the so-called Australia antigen, which he determined to be part of the hepatitis B virus. This discovery has led to the introduction of blood screening programs as well as a successful vaccine against this disease, which has a mortality rate of up to 15 per cent.

Blumberg was born on July 28, 1925, in New York City, one of three children of Meyer Blumberg, a lawyer, and Ida Simonoff. After graduating in 1943 from Far Rockaway High School in Far Rockaway, New York, Blumberg enlisted in the Navy. He was assigned to study physics at Union College in Schenectady, where he earned a B.S. in 1946, and then enrolled at Columbia University graduate school in physics and mathematics. But Blumberg had become more and more interested in medical and biochemical matters, and partly at his father's urging he entered Columbia's College of Physicians and Surgeons in 1947. Four years later he earned his M.D. and completed his internship and residency at Bellevue and Presbyterian hospitals in New York. It was during this period that he met Jean Liebesman, another medical student, whom he married in 1954; they would have four children. Blumberg won a fellowship to Balliol College, Oxford University, in 1955, working toward a Ph.D. in biochemistry. His specific field of interest was hyaluronic acid, one of the major constituents of connective tissue, synovial fluid and the vitreous humor of the eyes. By 1957 he had earned his doctorate and was also hard at work on research which would later win him the Nobel Prize.

As a medical student working in Surinam (then Dutch Guiana), South America, Blumberg had become interested in the manner in which various ethnic groups respond to disease and infection. He began to ask himself a very simple question: why do some people get sick while others do not? It was this question that increasingly guided his work, even while at Oxford. Epidemiologists had already speculated that an answer to this question might lie in the blood, and more specifically in the variations of genetically reproduced proteins in the blood. To study such polymorphisms would necessitate a large variety of blood samples from around the world. Blumberg, on his return from England, took the perfect job for such research as chief of the geographic medicine and genetics section of the National Institutes of Health (NIH). From 1957 to 1964, his travels took him from Alaska, to Africa, the Pacific, South America, Europe and Australia. Often he journeyed to remote areas accompanied only by his blood drawing and testing equipment. It was during this time as well that Blumberg became interested in anthropology.

Soon Blumberg and former Balliol colleague Anthony C. Allison were studying blood samples from patients who had received multiple transfusions, such as hemophiliacs, focusing on the antigen/antibody connection. An antigen is the substance that causes the body to produce a chemical defense, or antibody, against a foreign substance. Their reasoning was that people who had received numerous transfusions might prove to be excellent test cases, producing antibodies other than those they had inherited. The serum of such patients would therefore provide a wide variety of antibody responses once they were tested against other serum samples. Blumberg hypothesized that antibodies created in the serum of hemophiliacs and other transfusion donors would react with unknown antigens in the homogeneous serum of donors from disparate geographic areas.

In 1963, the serum of a New York hemophiliac reacted with that of an Australian Aborigine, and Blumberg labeled the detected antigen the Australia antigen, Au. Initially he and other researchers thought Au, an antigen rare in North America but prevalent in Asia and Africa, might be an indicator of leukemia, because it appeared in many patients suffering from that disease. Later research dealt with groups of patients with Down's syndrome, who also show a high incidence of the antigen.

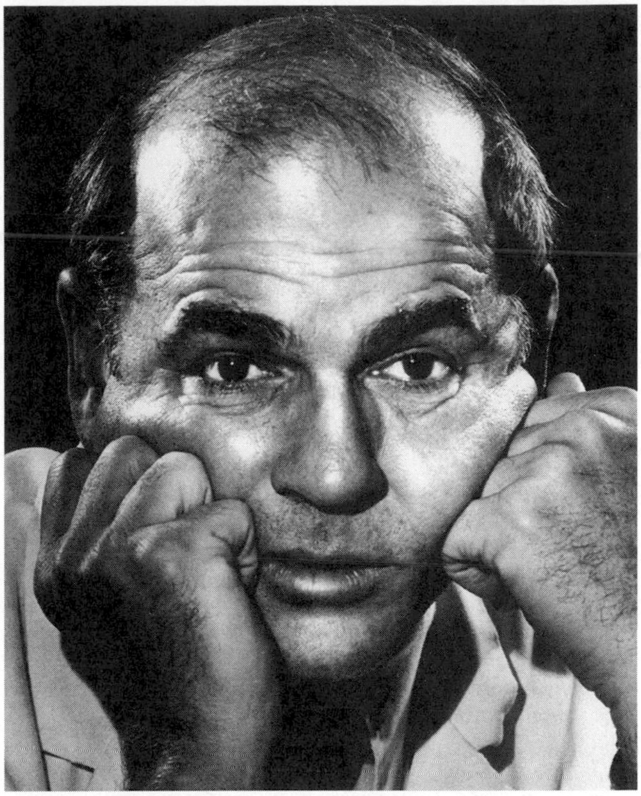

Samuel Baruch Blumberg

In 1964 Blumberg left NIH for the Institute of Cancer Research of the Fox Chase Cancer Center in Philadelphia, where he accepted the position of associate director of clinical research. He continued his researches on the Australia antigen, and in 1966 he discovered the link between Au and hepatitis B. A Down's patient who had previously tested negative for Au suddenly tested positive, and soon developed hepatitis, as did another with a sudden positive test for the antigen. Researchers in Japan and New York began a long series of controlled experiments which finally established the connection between hepatitis B and Au. That same year, the Australia antigen was identified as part of the B virus itself and was renamed HBsAg (hepatitis B virus antigen).

The first practical result of Blumberg's discovery of HBsAg was a blood test which he and others developed to detect and screen out hepatitis B carriers — of which there are approximately one hundred million worldwide, and perhaps one million in the United States — from blood donors, thereby securing a safe blood supply. As early as 1969, such screening was underway at blood banks worldwide. After the American Association of Blood Banks ordered all of its members to use the hepatitis test in 1971, the incidence of hepatitis after transfusions dropped by 25 per cent. In the 1970s, Blumberg, along with Irving Millman, developed a vaccine from the sera of patients with HBsAg which prevents hepatitis B infection. Since becoming commercially available in 1982, it has been widely and successfully used, especially among high-risk professionals such as healthcare workers. Another spin-off from Blumberg's work is research indicating that chronic infection with hepatitis B virus may be a precursor of cancer of the liver, the most common form of cancer in males in parts of Asia, India and Africa. The discovery of a vaccine against the disease may therefore reduce the risk of primary liver cancer. Mass vaccinations of newborns have been undertaken in some Asian and African nations to that effect.

Blumberg shared the Nobel Prize for physiology or medicine in 1976 with Dr. D. Carleton Gajdusek of the National Institute for Neurological Diseases, "for their discoveries concerning new mechanisms for the origin and dissemination of infectious diseases." They shared the $160,000 stipend equally. This is only one of a plethora of awards and honors Blumberg has won. Others include the Eppger Prize from the University of Freiburg (1973), the Distinguished Achievement Award in Modern Medicine (1975), the Gairdner Foundation International Award (1975), the Governor's Award in the Sciences from the Commonwealth of Pennsylvania (1988), and the Gold Medal Award from the Canadian Liver Foundation (1990).

In 1977 Blumberg became a professor of medicine and anthropology at the University of Pennsylvania; soon thereafter he was named vice president of population oncology at the Fox Chase Institute in Philadelphia. He has continued his researches in antigen systems as well as his studies in a wide range of other fields, including virology, physics, history, anthropology and philosophy. With the advent of the AIDS epidemic, Blumberg's antigen/antibody research has taken on new importance. After a long and distinguished career at Fox Chase, Blumberg returned to Oxford as master of Balliol College, becoming, at 64, the first scientist and first American ever to hold that prestigious chair.

Blumberg, known to friends, family and colleagues as Barry, is an avid movie-goer and reader. He also plays squash and enjoys running, hiking, swimming, and canoeing, in addition to his hobbies of carpentry and photography.

Body image

This refers to the perception of one's own body, based chiefly in comparison to socially constructed standards or ideals.

Humans have the unique ability to form abstract conceptions about themselves and to gaze at themselves as both the seer and the object being seen. This can cause conflict when the seer places unrealistic demands on him- or herself, especially on his or her own body. As the advertising and film industries bombard the industrialized world with images of idealized beauty, more and more adolescents are forming negative body images and engaging in self-destructive behaviors to fit an unrealistic ideal.

Children begin to recognize themselves in mirrors in meaningful ways at about 18 months and begin perceiving themselves as physical beings in toddlerhood. School-age children are aware of how their bodies look, though relatively few focus an inappropriate amount of attention on them. Ideally, children learn that their physical appearance is in many ways beyond their control and learn to accept their bodies without judgment. However, children living in the industrialized world are immersed in a culture that creates standards of idealized beauty and then connects those standards to personal worth. Consequently, school-age children can become convinced that they are only worthwhile if they live up to an idealized standard of physical appearance.

Even without the pernicious effects of the media, children face prejudices based on their appearances. Children spend much of their early lives in schools, which are highly social and competitive, with notoriously rigid hierarchies that are often based on physical appearance. Studies have found that teachers are also drawn to the most attractive children, which can further compound a child's poor body image. In a school-age child, a poor body image usually results in social withdrawal and poor self-esteem.

As **puberty** nears, children become increasingly focused on the appearance of their bodies. An adolescent may mature too quickly, too slowly, in a way that is unattractive, or in a way that makes the adolescent stand out in the crowd. Any deviation from the ideal can result in a negative body image, and adolescents may diet or use steroids to counter their own negative self-concept. Distorted body images in adolescence can lead to a number of disorders, **eating disorders** such as anorexia nervosa or bulimia, or dysmorphic disorder (a severe, clinically recognized illusory body image). These disorders are accompanied by psychological problems, such as depression or anxiety, as the victim magnifies a slight flaw to such a degree that all other aspects of personality and appearance are ignored. Body-image disorders such as those mentioned have become prevalent in contemporary society, especially among adolescent girls. In 1982 a study concluded that the incidence of anorexia among adolescent girls, for instance, had doubled every 10 years since the 1950s.

See also Self-esteem

Body odor

The human body produces a variety of odors, in the form of volatile chemical substances that stimulate the sense of smell. While most of these body odors are considered socially unpleasant, there are a few that are considered benign and some that are believed to serve as attractants. Those odors considered to be most noxious are produced in the intestinal tract, the mouth, on the feet and under the arms. Intestinal tract gas, known medically as "flatus," is a normal product of digestion. Flatus is generated when bacteria that reside in the gut process the carbohydrates in food that cannot be broken down by digestive enzymes. The nature of its odor depends on the types of bacteria that colonize the human intestinal tract, as well as the types of food that are consumed. Bad breath, or "halitosis," may be caused by excess bacteria growing on or between teeth, and by gum or gingival disease. When certain food substances such as onions and garlic are eaten, their digestive byproducts produce a characteristic odor on the breath that can linger for many hours. Pharmaceutical drugs can also cause mouth odor. Various disease conditions are associated with bad breath, including certain liver disorders, respiratory tract cancers and infections, and high blood sugar among diabetics. A rare genetic disorder called trimethylaminuria causes individuals to produce a fish-like odor, not only on their breath, but also in their sweat and urine.

Excess sweating, a condition known as ''hyperhydrosis,'' often results in underarm, foot, and general body odor, especially when bathing is not regular. Sweat is a viscous substance, produced by the skin's eccrine glands, distributed across most of the body, and its apocrine glands, found mainly under the arms and in the genital region. Apocrine glands enlarge and become active during puberty. While sweat itself is odorless, its presence, especially in the warm environments under the arm, around the genitals, and between the toes of the feet, encourages the growth of certain bacteria and fungi. These microorganisms digest components of sweat and release volatile chemicals that are responsible for the acrid odor associated with sweat. Some of the common bacteria responsible for body odor include micrococci, staphylococci, aerobic and anaerobic corneforms, and pityrosporum species. ''Bromidrosis'' is the medical term used to describe the condition of unpleasant body odors produced by excess sweating.

Body odors that are considered benign include the scent produced by a mother's breast milk and the individually unique odor of every infant. Scientific studies have demonstrated that human babies and mothers can recognize one another solely on the basis of odor. Genital and anal odors are also emitted by humans. Some people consider strong genital odors to be an attractant. In a famous nineteenth century love letter, Napolean Bonaparte instructed his mistress Josephine that she must not wash, since he would soon be returning from one of his European campaigns and wanted to enjoy her sexual scent.

The act of perceiving an odor, whether it be pleasing or noxious, is called olfaction. At the top of the nasal cavity in humans is a small patch of skin called the olfactory epithelium. Only a few centimeters square, it contains some five million olfactory neurons. When these neurons sense and recognize specific odor molecules, they send signals to the olfactory bulb, which is part of the brain. Individual reaction to the perception of odors is highly variable, and appears to be determined at least somewhat by culture and learning. In previous centuries, when current sanitation and personal hygiene practices differed, humans were presumably more tolerant of bodily odors.

The human nasal cavity also contains a pair of tiny cigar-shaped sacs called the vomeronasal organ. The nerve cells in this organ, like those in the olfactory epithelium, appear able to sense and recognize specific odor molecules. In many animal species, the vomeronasal organ functions as an excessory olfactory system, detecting the presence of volatile chemical substances called pheromones. Pheromones are a type of bodily odor that may advertise the sexual readiness of a potential animal mate. Scientists speculate that human pheromones are involved in sexual attraction, and that the sensory perception of pheromones may occur unconsciously.

Body piercing

The piercing of body parts, also known as 'body modification,' has been practiced since ancient times, often to exhibit virility and courage, and often associated with royalty. For example, Egyptian pharaohs had their navels pierced as a rite of passage into manhood. In Victorian times, members of royal families, both male and female, were known to have their genitals or nipples pierced.

In body piercing, a hollow needle is passed through the body part. This most commonly involves the earlobe or ear cartilage. Other sites that may be pierced include the lip, eyebrows, tongue, nose, nipple, navel, and genitals. After the part is pierced by the needle, a piece of body jewelry other object may be inserted in the resulting hole. Some bleeding may be expected.

In 1999, the American Academy of Dermatology officially discouraged body piercing, pointing out that the practice can lead to chronic infection, nickel allergy problems, formation of granulomas (masses of chronically infected tissues), and other skin problems. Parental consent should be required for anyone under the age of 18 wishing to pierce any part of the body except the earlobes, the dermatologists said, adding that a parent or guardian should be present during the procedure.

By perforating the skin—one of the body's principal protections against disease—piercing can cause life-threatening or disfiguring infections if not conducted safely. According to the U.S. **Centers for Disease Control**, human immunodeficiency virus (HIV), **hepatitis** B virus, and other blood-borne infections may be transmitted if blood-contaminated instruments are not properly sterilized or disinfected. The risk of infection is sufficiently high that the American Red Cross refuses donations of blood from anyone who has undergone body piercing during the previous year. Pierced nipples may also cause infection problems later in life if breast feeding is attempted.

Anyone considering body modification should talk to friends who have undergone a similar procedure, and should visit either their physician, or a number of piercing salons, observing the cleanliness of their establishments and asking about infection control. Reputable piercers take pride in their sterilization practices and equipment. They should be happy to answer your questions. If a piercer refuses to discuss safety issues, go somewhere else.

Never pierce a body part yourself, or allow it to be done by a friend or amateur piercer.

Boerhaave, Hermann (1668-1738)

Dutch physician and botanist

Hermann Boerhaave's primary importance to medicine was as a teacher. He was the first person to develop a modern system of clinical teaching based on bedside observation of the patient. His skills as a teacher drew students from all over Europe who then carried his ideas about medical training back to their native countries.

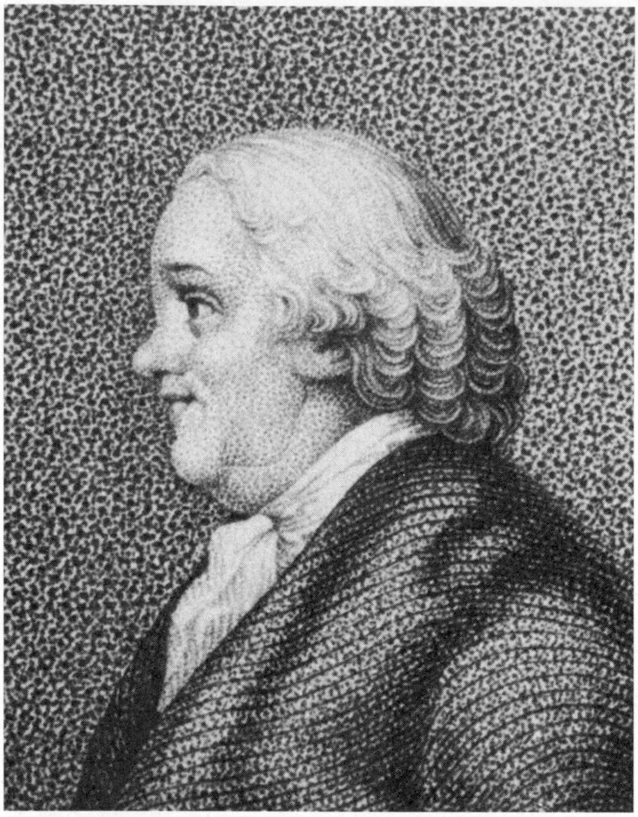

Hermann Boerhaave

Born in Voorhout, Netherlands in 1668, Hermann Boerhaave was a perfect example of the well-educated humanist Renaissance man. He spoke all the major European languages and lectured in Latin. He studied classical literature, mathematics, chemistry, botany, medicine, and anatomy, receiving a doctorate in philosophy from the University of Leiden in 1689 and a doctorate in medicine from Harderwyck in 1693.

Spending his entire professional career at the University of Leiden, Boerhaave served, starting in 1701, as professor of medicine and of botany, rector of the university, professor of practical medicine and professor of chemistry. He almost single-handedly was responsible for the University of Leiden replacing Padua in Italy as the center of medical education in the early eighteenth century.

Boerhaave's teaching methods emphasized bedside instruction, a system still seen today in teaching hospitals where student attend rounds with an instructing physician, visiting each patient and learning through observation and on-the-spot question and answer. He also encouraged students to follow their patients after death through the autopsy procedure so that they could draw a correlation between the symptoms they had observed at bedside and the physical symptoms of disease in the body. Although these methods of understanding disease seem commonplace today, in Boerhaave's time they were a departure from the way medicine was traditionally taught.

Boerhaave's textbooks were translated into many languages and used throughout Europe both during and after his lifetime. His main works included *Institutiones medicae* (*Medical Principals*) written in 1708, *Aphorismi de Cognoscendis et Curandis* (*Aphorisms on the Recognition and Treatment of Disease*) in 1709, and *Elementia Cheminae*(Elements of Chemistry)in 1724. These books brought together and organized masses of information that were available only piecemeal prior to this time. In addition to his contributions to medicine, Boerhaave also published many works describing new species of plants. His work as a professor of botany significantly improved the botanic gardens at the University of Leiden.

In his lifetime, Boerhaave was elected to the French Academy of Sciences and the Royal Society in London. He attracted students from all over Europe including Russia's Peter the Great who studied with him in 1715. Patients also flocked to Leiden hoping for cures. He was so well know that it is reported that a letter from China, addressed only "To the illustrious Boerhaave, physician in Europe" reached him without difficulty.

Hermann Boerhaave died in Leiden in 1738 after a long, painful illness. Through his students, he changed the way medicine was taught, particularly in the medical schools in Edinburgh, Vienna, and in Germany.

Boils

Boils and carbuncles are firm, reddish swellings about 5-10 mm across that are slightly raised above the skin surface. They are formed by bacterial infections of hair follicles and surrounding skin. Boils form pustules (small blister-like swellings containing pus) around the follicle and are sore to the touch. A boil usually has a visible central core of pus; a carbuncle is larger and has several visible drainage points. It is deeper and more extensive than a boil.

Boils occur most commonly on the face, back of the neck, buttocks, upper legs and groin, armpits, and upper torso. Carbuncles are less common than single boils and are most likely to form at the back of the neck.

Boils and carbuncles are common problems especially among adolescents and adults. People who are more likely to develop these skin infections include those with diabetes, **alcoholism** or drug abuse, poor personal hygiene, jobs or hobbies that expose them to greasy or oily substances, especially petroleum products, and **allergies** or immune system disorders such as HIV infection.

Boils and carbuncles are caused by *Staphylococcus aureus*, a bacterium that causes an infection in an oil gland or hair follicle. Although the surface of human skin is usually resistant to bacterial infection, bacteria can enter through breaks in the skin. Hair follicles that are blocked by greasy creams or petroleum jelly are more vulnerable to infection. Bacterial skin infections can be spread by shared cosmetics or washcloths, close human contact, or by contact with pus from a boil or carbuncle.

As the infection develops, an area of inflamed tissue gradually forms a pus-filled swelling or pimple that is painful to touch. As the boil matures, it forms a yellowish head or point. It may either continue to swell until the point bursts open and allows the pus to drain, or it may be gradually reabsorbed into the skin. Boils take between one and two weeks to heal completely after they come to a head and discharges pus. The bacteria that cause the boil can spread to other areas of the skin or even into the bloodstream if the skin around the boil is injured by squeezing. If the infection spreads, the patient will usually develop chills and **fever**, swollen lymph nodes, and red lines in the skin running outward from the boil.

Many patients have repeated episodes of boils that are difficult to treat because their nasal passages carry colonies of *S. aureus*. These bacterial colonies make it easy for the patient's skin to be reinfected. They are most likely to develop in patients with diabetes, HIV infection, or other immune system disorders.

Carbuncles are formed when the bacteria infect several hair follicles that are close together. The abscesses spread until they merge with each other to form a single large area of infected skin with several pus-filled heads. Patients with carbuncles may have a low-grade fever or feel generally unwell.

The diagnosis of boils and carbuncles is usually made by the patient's primary care doctor on the basis of visual examination of the skin. For the most part boils and carbuncles are not difficult to distinguish from other skin disorders. *S. aureus* can easily be cultured in the laboratory if the doctor needs to rule out inclusion cysts or deep fungal infections.

People should not pick at or squeeze boils because of the danger of spreading the infection. It is especially important to avoid squeezing boils around the mouth or nose because infections in these areas can be carried to the brain. Keeping the skin clean, washing hands before and after touching the boil or carbuncle, avoiding greasy cosmetics or creams, and keeping towels and washcloths separate from those of other family members help reduce the spread of bacteria that cause boils.

Boils are usually treated with application of antibiotic creams, such as clindamycin or polymyxin, following the application of hot compresses. The compresses help the infection to come to a head and drain. Carbuncles are usually treated with oral **antibiotics**, usually dicloxacillin (Dynapen) or cephalexin (Keflex), as well as antibiotic ointments. Patients with bacterial colonies in their nasal passages are often given mupirocin (Bactroban) to apply directly to the lining of the nose.

Boils and carbuncles that are very large or that are not draining may be opened with a sterile needle or surgical knife to allow the pus to drain. The doctor will usually give the patient a local anesthetic if a knife is used. Surgical treatment of boils is painful and usually leaves noticeable scars.

In addition to traditional treatment of boils, naturopathic practitioners usually recommend changes in the patient's diet as well as applying herbal poultices to the infected area. The addition of zinc supplements and vitamin A to the diet is reported to be effective in treating boils. The application of a paste or poultice containing goldenseal (*Hydrastis canadensis*) root is recommended by naturopaths on the grounds that goldenseal helps to kill bacteria and reduce inflammation.

Homeopaths maintain that taking the proper homeopathic medication in the first stages of a boil or carbuncle will bring about early resolution of the infection and prevent pus formation. The most likely choices are *Belladonna* or *Hepar sulphuris*. If the boil has already formed, *Mercurius vivus* or *Silica* may be recommended to bring the pus to a head.

Most boils heal without any problems. Some patients, however, suffer from recurrent carbuncles. Although the spread of infection from boils is relatively unusual, there have been **death**s reported from brain infections caused by squeezing boils on the upper lip or in the tissue folds at the base of the nose.

BOIVIN, MARIE GILLAIN (1773-1841)

French midwife

Marie Gillain Boivin was considered to be the most outstanding obstetrician of the nineteenth century. Born in Montreuil, a suburb of Paris, she was educated by nuns whose order ran a hospital at Etampes, and married Louis Boivin at the age of twenty-four. After being widowed, she became a midwife in 1800, practicing in Versailles. When her young daughter was killed in an accident, Boivin returned to Paris where she worked at the Hospice de la Maternité under Maria Louise Dugès La Chapelle (1769-1821), another renowned midwife. Boivin soon became known for her obstetrical skill and knowledge, especially in difficult cases; the leading surgeon of the time said she had an eye at the tip of each finger. She was appointed codirector of the General Hospital for Seine and Oise in 1814, directed a temporary military hospital in 1815, and later directed the Hospice de la Maternité and the Maison Royale de Santé. The king of Prussia invested Boivin with the Order of Merit in 1814, and in 1827 she received an honorary M.D. from the University of Marburg in Germany, one of the few women so honored at the time.

Following her break with Mme. La Chapelle, Boivin turned down lucrative offers and worked instead for minimal pay at a hospital for prostitutes. Her pension was so small she died in severe poverty after one year of retirement. Boivin's contributions to the science of obstetrics included the invention of a new pelvimeter and a vaginal speculum, the use of a **stethoscope** to listen to the fetal heartbeat, and discoveries about causes of miscarriage and diseases of the placenta and uterus. She published a number of widely read treatises on obstetrics, including *Mémorial de l'art des Accouchements* in 1812, which became a textbook for medical students and midwives. Boivin's work on diseases of the uterus, published in 1833, was said to be as modern as was possible at the time.

BOMBAST VON HOHENHEIM (AKA PARACELSUS), PHILIPPUS AUREOLUS THEOPHRASTUS (1493-1541)

Swiss physician, chemist, and philosopher

Philippus Aureolus Theophrastus Bombast von Hohenheim, known as Paracelsus, was a Renaissance physician/scientist who helped revolutionize the theory and practice of medicine. One of his most important contributions was the application of chemistry to medicine, stressing the use of chemical medications rather than the then more popular "magic potions" based on herbs and other substances. Paracelsus maintained an ongoing feud throughout his life with the medical establishment, who considered him a heretic and usurper of their traditions. The word "bombastic" comes from his original name and is an ironic tribute to his aggressive and combative personality.

Paracelsus was born in 1493 in Einsiedeln, Switzerland. His father, Wilhelm of Hohenheim, was a physician and most likely gave Paracelsus his first instruction in medicine. At the age of 16, he enrolled at the University at Basel in Germany to study alchemy, surgery, and medicine. But Paracelsus was already revealing his restlessness and disdain for academic traditions. He soon left the university and became a traveling student, studying and working in Germany, France, Hungary, the Netherlands, and Russia, to name a few. As a result, he never received a complete formal education. He eventually arrived in Italy, where he became an army surgeon and his notoriety for bringing about wonderful cures began.

Paracelsus returned to Basel in 1527 at the age of 32. His cure of the famous printer Johann Froben from a leg infection without the need for amputation led to his appointment as professor of physics, medicine and surgery at the university. However, it did not take the antagonistic Paracelsus long to raise his colleagues' ire. In his lectures, he began to denounce the revered Roman physician **Galen** and his school of thought, going as far as to make a grandiose display of burning this ancient master's written works. Intimidated and angered by Paracelsus, his colleagues were more upset that Paracelsus could often cure people when they could not.

While his colleagues believed that many illnesses were incurable, Paracelsus, a true physician by nature and nurture, wrote, "God has not permitted any disease without providing a remedy." Relying on experimentation and empirical evidence from observing his patients, Paracelsus began a program of research to establish the application of chemistry to medicine. While most medicines of his day were based on plant and animal substances, Paracelsus believed in the curative powers of inorganic materials. As a result, a number of chemical substances, including sulfur, iron, arsenic, and potassium sulfate, became integral to his medical practice. The first to prescribe laudanum for a variety of ailments, Paracelsus developed the concept of therapeutic dosages, emphasizing the need for moderate doses instead of the often toxic amounts given to patients at that time. He is also credited with working toward a systematic classification of chemical substances and for a method of detoxifying dangerous chemical compounds. Known for his management of wounds and chronic ulcers, Paracelsus's description of miners' disease as silicosis and tuberculosis was one of the first occupational disease studies ever performed.

One of Paracelsus's most important contributions was his new concept of what constituted disease. Going against the ancient belief that disease resulted from an upset of humoral balance (based largely on a person's temperament), Paracelsus saw diseases as resulting from specific foreign agents or elements entering the body and causing dysfunction in specific areas of the body, which is similar to the modern concept of disease. As a result, his approach was to treat patients for a specific disease agent instead of using non-specific, antihumoral measures such as sweating, purging, and bloodletting.

When he was forced to leave the University of Basel in 1528, Paracelsus once again took up the life of a nomad, traveling throughout Germany, Switzerland, Bohemia and Austria. He usually stayed in any one place for only a few months, often being run out of town by the medical establishment. However, Paracelsus continued to write extensively on his beliefs and findings in both medicine, surgery, and philosophy. His most famous works included *Paragranum* (1530) and *Opus paramirum* (1531), which outlines his fundamental medical doctrine.

While Paracelsus remained an outcast in the medical profession, his fame and popularity with the public grew. He befriended laborers, trades people, gypsies and other who were considered to be inferior. Known as a glutton and heavy drinker, his enemies berated his association with them and especially his inclination for revelry in lower-class taverns.

Paracelsus eventually grew disenchanted with his inability to establish a position of permanence in medicine. By 1538, he wrote, "If I were permitted to settle down, I would make peace and sit tight even if I were provoked." The Prince Bishop of Salzburg finally offered him asylum in 1540 and Paracelsus spent the rest of his life in a town that had once expelled him for siding with peasants during the Peasants War of 1524-1526. True to his word, Paracelsus wrote little about medicine after his arrival and turned his attention to theology and philosophy. Still, rumors of miraculous cures performed by him spread throughout Europe. He died in September 1541. Even in death, controversy surrounded him. Some said he died of an overdose of a secret elixir of life that he supposedly carried in the pommel of his sword. His enemies attributed it to injuries he received in a tavern brawl.

Like most of his contemporaries, Paracelsus was not strictly scientific in all his beliefs. He placed great faith in many of the occult sciences such as astronomy and alchemy. However, his primary purpose always focused on helping people. While alchemists at that time were looking for ways to turn substances into gold, Paracelsus directed them to "stop making gold; instead, find medicines." In the end, his most important admonition to the medical community of his day may have been his famous battle cry: "The patients are your textbook, the sickbed is your study."

See also Galen

BONE CANCERS

A bone cancer (sarcoma) is a bone tumor that contains **cancer** (malignant) cells. A benign bone tumor is an abnormal growth of noncancerous cells.

A primary bone tumor originates in or near a bone. Most primary bone tumors are benign, and the cells that compose them do not spread (metastasize) to nearby tissue or to other parts of the body.

Malignant primary bone tumors account for fewer than one percent of all cancers diagnosed in the United States. They can infiltrate nearby tissues, enter the bloodstream, and metastasize to bones, tissues, and organs far from the original malignancy. Malignant primary bone tumors are characterized as either bone cancers that originate in the hard material of the bone or soft-tissue sarcomas that begin in blood vessels, nerves, or tissues containing muscles, fat, or fiber.

Osteogenic sarcoma, or osteosarcoma, is the most common form of bone cancer. It accounts for six percent of all instances of the disease, and for about five percent of all cancers that occur in children. Osteosarcomas can grow very rapidly. They often occur along the edge or on the end of one of the fast-growing long bones of the arms and legs.

Ewing's sarcoma is the second most common form of childhood bone cancer. It usually begins in the soft tissue (the marrow) inside bones of the leg, hips, ribs, and arms. It rapidly infiltrates the lungs, and may metastasize to bones in other parts of the body.

Chondrosarcomas are cancerous bone tumors that most often appear in middle age. Usually originating in strong connective tissue (cartilage) in ribs, legs, or hip bones, chondrosarcomas grow slowly taking years to spread to other parts of the body.

Parosteal osteogenic sarcomas, fibrosarcomas, and chordomas are rare. Parosteal osteosarcomas generally involve both the bone and the membrane that covers it. Fibrosarcomas originate in the ends of the bones in the arm or leg, and then spread to soft tissue. Chordomas develop on the skull or spinal cord.

Osteochondromas, which usually develop between age 10-20, are the most common noncancerous primary bone tumors. Giant cell tumors generally develop in a section of the thigh bone near the knee. Giant cell tumors are originally benign, but sometimes become malignant.

The cause of bone cancer is unknown, but the tendency to develop it may be inherited, and the disease seems to be associated with growth spurts that occur during childhood and adolescence. Injuries can make the presence of tumors more apparent but do not cause them.

A bone that has been broken or exposed to high doses of radiation used to treat other cancers (and well above the amount involved in x rays) is more likely than other bones to develop osteosarcoma. A history of noncancerous bone disease also increases bone-cancer risk.

Both benign and malignant bone tumors can distort and weaken bone and cause pain, but benign tumors are more likely to be painless. Pain is the most common early symptom of bone cancer. It is not constant in the early stages of the disease, but it is aggravated by activity and may be worst at night. If the tumor is located on a leg bone, the patient may limp. Swelling and weakness of the limb may not be noticed until weeks after the pain began.

Physical examination and routine x rays may yield enough evidence to diagnose benign bone tumors, but removal of tumor tissue for microscopic analysis (biopsy) is the only sure way to determine malignancy.

Bone cancer is usually diagnosed about three months after symptoms first appear. Twenty percent of malignant tumors have metastasized to the lungs or other parts of the body by that time. Once bone cancer has been diagnosed, the tumor is staged to indicate how far the tumor has spread from its original location. The stage of a tumor suggests which form of treatment is most appropriate, and predicts how the condition will probably respond to therapy.

Bone x rays, computerized axial tomography (CAT scan), **magnetic resonance imaging** (MRI) and radionuclide bone scans are all used to distinguish between the different kinds of benign and malignant bone tumors.

Laboratory tests such as a complete **blood count** (CBC), immunohistochemistry, and reverse transcription polymerase chain reaction (RTPCR) are used to evaluate the type of tumor and the effectiveness of cancer therapies.

Since the 1960s, when **amputation** was the only treatment for bone cancer, new **chemotherapy** drugs and innovative surgical techniques have improved survival with intact limbs. Because osteosarcoma is rare, patients should consider undergoing treatment at a major cancer center staffed by specialists familiar with the disease.

A treatment plan for bone cancer may include chemotherapy, surgery, **radiation therapy**, amputation, or rotationoplasty. Rotationoplasty, sometimes performed after a leg amputation, involves attaching the lower leg and foot to the thigh bone, so that the ankle replaces the knee. A prosthetic is later added to make the leg as long as it should be.

After a patient completes the final course of chemotherapy, CAT scans, bone scans, x rays, and other diagnostic tests may be repeated to determine if any traces of tumor remain. Patients who have received treatment for Ewing's sarcoma are examined often after completing therapy. Regular examinations are recommended to determine whether these tumors have changed in any way.

Benign **brain tumor**s rarely recur, but sarcomas can reappear after treatment was believed to have eliminated every cell.

Likelihood of long-term survival depends on the type and location of the tumor, how much the tumor has metastasized, and on what organs, bones, or tissues have been affected.

Alternative treatments should never be substituted for conventional bone-cancer treatments or used without the approval of a physician. However, some alternative treatments can be used as adjunctive and supportive therapies during and following conventional treatments.

Dietary adjustments, **acupuncture**, **massage**, **reflexology**, and relaxation techniques are said to relieve pain, tension, anxiety, and depression. **Exercise** can be an effective means of reducing mental and emotional **stress**, while increasing physical strength. **Guided imagery**, **biofeedback**, **hypnosis**, body work, and progressive relaxation can also enhance quality of life.

BONE DENSITY TEST

A bone density test or scan measures the strength of an individual's bones and determines the risk of fracture. It is designed to check for **osteoporosis**, a disease that occurs when the bones become thin and weak. Osteoporosis happens when the bones lose calcium and other **minerals** that keep them strong. Osteoporosis begins after **menopause** in many women, and worsens after age 65 in both men and women. It often results in serious **fractures**. These fractures not only bring disability, but may affect longevity. As many as one-fourth of women who fracture their hip after age 50 die within one year.

Most people today will get a bone density scan from a machine using a technology called Dual Energy X-ray Absorptiometry or DEXA for short. This machine takes a picture of the bones in the spine, hip, total body, and wrist, and calculates their density. If a DEXA machine is not available, bone density scans can also be done with dual photon absorptiometry (measuring the spine, hip, and total body) and quantitative **computed tomography scans** (measuring the spine). Bone density scanners that use DEXA technology to just measure bone density in the wrist (called pDEXA scans) are provided at some drugstores. These tests are not as accurate as those that measure density in the total body, spine, or hip where most fractures occur.

To take a DEXA bone density scan, the patient lies on a bed underneath the scanner, a curving plastic arm that emits x rays. These low-dose x rays form a fan beam that rotates around the patient. During the test, the scanner moves to capture images of the patient's spine, hip or entire body. A computer then compares the patient's bone strength and risk of fracture to that of other people in the United States at the same age and to young people at peak bone density. Bones reach peak density at age 30-35 and then start to lose mass. The test takes about 20 minutes to do and is painless. The DEXA bone scan costs about $250. Some insurance companies and Medicare cover the cost. pDEXA wrist bone scans in drugstores are available for about $30.

Not all doctors routinely schedule this test. However a patient may need a bone density scan if she is at risk for osteoporosis, is near menopause, has broken a bone after a modest trauma, has a family history of osteoporosis, uses steroid or antiseizure medications, or has had a period of restricted mobility for more than six months.

The DEXA bone scan exposes the patient to only a small amount of radiation or about one-fiftieth that of a **chest x ray**, or about the amount you get from taking a cross-country airplane flight.

The patient's bone density when compared with people at "young normal bone density" is called the T-score. T scores above 1 mean that a patient has a healthy bone mass. Scores from 0 to –1 mean that the patient has borderline bone mass and should repeat the test in two to five years. If a patient's T score ranges from –1 to –2.5 she has low bone mass and are at risk for osteoporosis. If the T score is below – 2.5 she has osteoporosis and have lost a significant amount of bone. These people have a significantly greater chance of breaking a bone than others with T scores above 0 and should consult with their doctor on ways to slow osteoporosis.

BONE DISORDER DRUGS

Bone disorder drugs are medicines used to treat or prevent **osteoporosis** (brittle bone disease) in women past **menopause** or in elderly men. They also are prescribed for Paget's disease, a painful condition that weakens and deforms bones, and they are used to control calcium levels in the blood.

Bone is living tissue that is constantly being broken down and replaced with new material. Normally, there is a balance between the breakdown of old bone and its replacement with new bone.

In osteoporosis the bones become porous and thin, weaken, and become more likely to break. Osteoporosis is four times more common in women than in men. Women have less initial bone mass than men, tend to live longer, take in less calcium, and need the female hormone estrogen to keep their bones strong. If men live long enough, they too are at risk of getting osteoporosis. Once total bone mass has peaked (around age 35), adults start to lose bone. In women, the rate of bone loss increases substantially during menopause as estrogen levels fall.

The ovaries make estrogen, and bone loss may occur at any age if both ovaries are removed by surgery. **Hormone replacement therapy** is one approach to preventing osteoporosis. However, not all women can use hormone replacement therapy. Bone disorder drugs are a good alternative for people who already have osteoporosis or who are at risk of developing it. Factors increasing the risk of osteoporosis include lack of regular **exercise**, early menopause, being underweight, and a family history of osteoporosis.

Bone disorder drugs are available only with a physician's prescription. Common bone disorder drugs are alendronate (Fosamax), calcitonin (Miacalcin, Calcimar), and raloxifene (Evista). Raloxifene belongs to a group of drugs known as selective estrogen receptor modulators (SERMs). These act like estrogen in some parts of the body but not in others. These drugs are less likely to cause some of the harmful effects that estrogen may cause. Unlike estrogen, raloxifene does not increase the risk of **breast cancer**.

The recommended dose of bone disorder drugs varies with the drug, the reason it is prescribed, and the form it comes in. Bone disorder drug come in tablet, nasal spray, and injectable forms. Treatment usually continues over many years.

Not everyone should take bone disorder drugs. People with low levels of calcium in their blood should not take aldendronaten, nor should women using hormone replacement therapy, or anyone with kidney problems. Before using alendronate, anyone who has digestive or swallowing problems should make sure that his or her physician knows about the condition.

Calcitonin nasal spray may cause irritation or sores in the nose. The injectable form of calcitonin has caused serious allergic reactions in a few people. Before starting treatment with calcitonin, a physician may order an allergy test to make sure there will not be a problem.

A rare but serious side effect of raloxifene is increased risk of blood clots that form in the veins and may break away and travel to the lungs. Because of this possible problem, women with a history of blood clots in their veins should not take raloxifene. Women who have had breast cancer or **cancer** of the uterus should check with their physicians about whether they can safely use raloxifene.

Pregnant or breastfeeding women should check with their physicians before using any bone disorder drugs. Raloxifene should not be used by women who are pregnant or who may become pregnant because of the risk of **birth defects**.

In addition to taking these drugs, people can help maintain strong bones through a well-balanced diet high in calcium. Dairy products and fish such as salmon, sardines and tuna are good sources of both calcium. Dietary supplements may help people when food do not provide enough calcium. Other important bone-saving steps are avoiding smoking and alcohol and getting enough weight-bearing exercise such as walking or lifting weights.

Sometimes bone disorder drugs are prescribed for people who have too much calcium in their blood. These people may need to *limit* the amount of calcium in their diets for the medicine to work properly. Discuss the proper diet with a physician before making dietary changes. The physician should also be told about any **allergies** to foods, dyes, preservatives, medications, or other substances.

Side effects are possible when taking bone disorder drugs. Common side effects of aldendronate include **constipation**, **diarrhea**, **indigestion**, nausea, pain in the abdomen, and pain in the muscles and bones. These problems usually go away as the body adjusts to the medicine and do not need medical attention unless they continue or they interfere with normal activities.

The most common side effects of calcitonin nasal spray are nose problems, such as dryness, redness, **itching**, sores, bleeding and general discomfort. Other side effects include **headache**, back pain and joint pain.

Injectable calcitonin may cause minor side effects such as nausea or vomiting, diarrhea, stomach pain, loss of appetite, flushing of the face, ears, hands or feet, and discomfort or redness at the place on the body where it is injected. Medical attention is not necessary unless these problems persist or cause unusual discomfort. Anyone who gets a skin rash or **hives** after taking injectable calcitonin should check with a physician as soon as possible.

Common side effects of raloxifene include hot flashes, leg cramps, nausea, and vomiting. Women who have these problems while taking raloxifene should check with their physicians.

Bone disorder drugs can interact with many common drugs including **aspirin**, some calcium supplements, and, antacids. Calcitonin may keep certain drugs prescribed for Paget's disease, such as etidronate (Didronel), from working correctly. Raloxifene may affect blood clotting. Patients who are taking other drugs that affect blood clotting, such as warfarin (Coumadin), should check with their physicians before using raloxifene.

BONE GRAFTING

Bone grafting is a surgical procedure by which new bone or a replacement material is placed into spaces between or around broken bone (**fractures**) or holes in bone. Bone grafting is used to repair bone fractures that are extremely complex, pose significant risk to the patient, or fail to heal properly. Bone grafts are also used to help fusion between vertebrae, correct deformities, or provide structural support for fractures of the spine. In addition to fracture repair, bone grafts are used to repair defects in bone caused by **birth defects**, traumatic injury, or surgery for bone **cancer**.

Bone is composed of a matrix, mainly made up of a protein called collagen. It is strengthened by deposits of calcium and phosphate salts, called hydroxyapatite. Within and around this matrix are four types of bone cells. Osteoblasts produce the bone matrix. Osteocytes are mature osteoblasts and maintain the bone. Osteoclasts break down and remove bone tissue. Bone lining cells cover bone surfaces. Together, these four types of cells are responsible for building the bone matrix, maintaining it, and remodeling the bone as needed.

There are three ways in which a bone graft can help repair a defect. The first is called osteogenesis, the formation of new bone by the cells contained within the graft. The second is osteoinduction, a chemical process in which molecules contained within the graft convert the patient's cells into cells that are capable of forming bone. The third is osteoconduction, a physical effect by which the matrix of the graft forms a scaffold on which cells in the recipient are able to form new bone.

New bone for grafting can be obtained from other bones in the patient's own body (an autograft) or from bone taken from other people that is frozen and stored in tissue banks (an allograft). Natural and synthetic replacement materials are also used instead of bone, including natural collagen protein, polymers such as silicone, some acrylics, hydroxyapatite, calcium sulfate, and ceramics. A new material, called resorbable polymeric grafts is also being studied. These resorbable grafts provide a structure for new bone to grow on, then slowly dissolve, leaving only the new bone behind.

To place the graft, the surgeon makes an incision in the skin over the bone defect and shapes the bone graft or replacement material to fit into the defect. After the graft is in place, it is held in place with pins, plates, or screws. The incision is closed with stitches and a splint or cast is used to prevent movement of the bones while healing. The time required for convalescence for fractures or spinal fusion may vary from 1-10 days, and vigorous **exercise** may be limited for up to three months.

Most bone grafts are successful in helping the bone defect to heal. The extent of recovery depends on the size of the defect and the condition of the bone surrounding the graft at the time of surgery. Severe defects take longer to heal and may require additional attention after the initial graft. Less severe bone defects usually heal completely without serious complications.

The drawbacks of autografts include the additional surgical and anesthesia time to obtain the bone for grafting, the

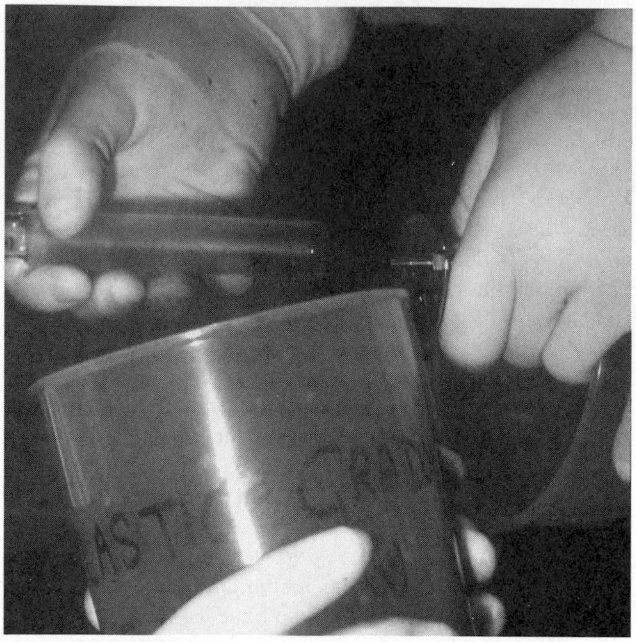

Filtering the bone marrow.

added costs of the additional surgery, **pain** and infection that might occur at the site from which the graft is taken, and the relatively small amount of bone that is available for grafting.

The drawbacks of allografts include variability between lots, since the bone is harvested from a variety of donors. The bone may take longer to incorporate with the host bone than an autograft would, and the graft may be less effective than an autograft. There is the possibility of transferring diseases from the donor to the patient. Other complications may result from the immune response mounted by the patient's immune system against the grafted bone tissue. With the use anti-rejection agents (drugs to combat rejection of grafted bone tissue) immune rejection is less of a problem.

BONE MARROW TRANSPLANTATION

Bone marrow, sponge-like tissue found in the center of certain bones, contains stem cells that are the precursors of white blood cells, red blood cells, and platelets. These blood cells are vital for normal body functions. Blood cells have a limited life span and are constantly being replaced; therefore, healthy stem cells are vital.

In association with certain diseases, stem cells may produce too many, too few, or otherwise abnormal blood cells. Also, medical treatments, particularly **chemotherapy** or radiation treatment, may destroy stem cells or alter blood cell production. The resultant blood cell abnormalities can be life threatening.

Bone marrow transplantation involves extracting bone marrow from a healthy donor and transferring it to a recipient whose body cannot manufacture proper quantities of normal blood cells. The goal of the transplant is to rebuild the recipient's blood cells and immune system and cure the underlying disease. Ailments that may be treated with a bone marrow transplant include both cancerous and noncancerous diseases.

Cancer may or may not specifically involve blood cells, but cancer treatment can destroy the body's ability to manufacture new blood cells. Bone marrow transplantation may be used in conjunction with additional treatments, such as chemotherapy, for various types of leukemia, **Hodgkin's disease**, lymphoma, breast and **ovarian cancer**. Noncancerous diseases for which bone marrow transplantation can be a treatment option include aplastic **anemia**, **sickle-cell anemia**, **thalassemia**, and severe **immunodeficiency**.

Bone marrow transplants are accompanied by a risk of infection, transplant rejection by the recipient's immune system, and other complications. The procedure has a lower success rate the greater the recipient's age. Complications are more likely in people whose health is already impaired. Even in the absence of complications, the transplant and associated treatments are hard on the recipient. A person's ability to withstand the rigors of the transplant is a key consideration in deciding to use this treatment.

Two important requirements for a bone marrow transplant are the donor and the recipient. Sometimes, the donor and the recipient are the same person (an autologous transplant). Typically this happens when a person's bone marrow is healthy but will be destroyed due to medical treatment. If a person's bone marrow is unsuitable for an autologous transplant, the bone marrow must be acquired from another person (an allogeneic transplant).

Allogeneic transplants are more complicated because of proteins called human lymphocyte antigens (HLA) that are on the surface of bone marrow cells. If the donor and the recipient have very dissimilar antigens, the recipient's immune system regards the donor's bone marrow cells as invaders and tries to destroy them. Such an attack negates any benefits offered by the transplant.

HLA matching, a complex procedure, must be done between donor and recipient. A suitable match is more likely if the donor and recipient are related, particularly if they are siblings.

The bone marrow extraction is the same for an autologous or allogeneic transplant. Harvesting is done under general **anesthesia**, and discomfort is usually minimal. Bone marrow is drawn from the hip bone with a special needle and a syringe. Approximately 1–2 quarts of bone marrow is removed from the donor. This amount is only a small percentage of the total bone marrow and is typically replaced within 4 weeks. The donor remains at the hospital for 24–48 hours and can resume normal activities within a few days.

If the bone marrow is meant for an autologous transplant, it is stored frozen until it is needed. Bone marrow for an allogeneic transplant is sometimes treated to remove the donor's T cells (a type of white blood cell) or to remove ABO (blood type) antigens; otherwise, it is transplanted without modification.

The bone marrow is administered to the recipient via a catheter (a narrow, flexible tube) inserted into a large vein in the chest. From the bloodstream, it migrates to the cavities within the bones where bone marrow is normally stored. If the transplant is successful, the bone marrow begins to produce normal blood cells once it is in place.

A bone marrow transplant recipient to spends 4–8 weeks in the hospital. In preparation for receiving the transplant, the recipient undergoes a regimen in which the bone marrow and abnormal cells are destroyed making room for the new marrow to be transplanted. Unfortunately, this treatment also destroys healthy cells and has many side effects such as extreme weakness, nausea, vomiting, and **diarrhea**.

A two- to four-week waiting period follows the marrow transplant before its success can begin to be judged. The marrow recipient is kept in **isolation** during this time to minimize potential infections. The recipient also receives antibiotic medications and blood and platelet **transfusion**s to help fight infection and prevent excessive bleeding.

Following discharge from the hospital, the recipient is monitored through for up to a year. For several months the recipient needs to be careful in avoiding potential infections. Barring complications, the recipient can return to normal activities about 6–8 months after the transplant.

Bone marrow transplants are costly and are accompanied by life-threatening risks. Approximately 30% of people receiving allogeneic transplants do not survive. Autologous transplants have a survival rate near 90%, but are not appropriate in all situations.

There is the danger of **pneumonia** or other infectious disease, excessive bleeding, or liver disorder caused by blocked blood vessels. The transplant may be rejected by the recipient's immune system, or the donor bone marrow may launch an immune-mediated attack against the recipient's tissues. Approximately 25–50% of bone marrow transplant recipients develop long-term, serious complications.

In a successful bone marrow transplant, the donor's marrow migrates to the cavities in the recipient's bones and produces normal numbers of healthy blood cells. Bone marrow transplants can extend a person's life, improve quality of life, and may aid in curing the underlying ailment.

BOOKER, WALTER M. (1907-1988)

African American biologist and pharmacologist

Walter M. Booker was a biologist, physiologist, and pharmacologist who served for twenty years as the chairman of the Department of Pharmacology of the College of Medicine at Howard University, Washington, D. C. As the author of over one hundred scientific papers, Booker studied liver damage in trauma, the effects of anesthesia, and gastrointestinal physiology. He was very active even after his retirement, focusing on such important issues as drug abuse and addiction.

Walter Monroe Booker was born in Little Rock, Arkansas on November 4, 1907. A 1928 graduate of Morehouse College in Atlanta, Georgia, where he obtained a B. A. degree, he received a master's degree from the University of Iowa in 1932, and a doctorate in physiology and chemistry from the University of Chicago in 1943. During those years, he also taught biology and chemistry at Leland College in Louisiana and at Prairie View College. After receiving his Ph.D., he accepted a teaching position at Howard University in 1943, and became an associate professor in 1948, He was appointed Chairman, Department of Pharmacology of the College of Medicine, Howard University in 1954. Booker remained in that position until 1973 when he retired as a full professor.

Booker had done a great deal of research on the heart's response to drugs, and participated in conferences on the subject in nearly a dozen nations. Besides running the pharmacology department at Howard University, Booker was a consultant to the Walter Reed Army Research Institute where he taught during the 1960s and 1970s. He was a consultant to the National Institute on Drug Abuse and the Department of Health, Education and Welfare. His specialization proved useful to the Washington Heart Association, and he was a representative of the American Society for Pharmacology and Experimental Therapeutics to the National Research Council.

Among the many groups to which he belonged were the American College of Clinical Pharmacology and the American Physiological Society. He was a fellow of the American College of Cardiology and a charter member of Sigma Xi, an honorary scientific society. As a senior Fulbright scholar, he studied at the Heymans Institute in Ghent, Belgium during 1957 and 1958.

When he died of cardiac arrest on August 29, 1988, at Howard University Hospital, he was survived by a son, Walter Jr., a daughter, Marjorie Courm, and four grandchildren. His wife, the former Thomye Collins, died in 1986.

BORDET, JULES (1870-1961)

Belgian physician, bacteriologist, and immunologist

Jules Bordet was an important pioneer in the field of immunology. It was his research that made clear the exact manner by which serums and antiserums act to destroy bacteria and foreign blood cells in the body, thus explaining how human and animal bodies defend themselves against the invasion of foreign elements. Bordet was also responsible for developing complement fixation tests, which made possible the early detection of many disease-causing bacteria in human and animal blood. For his various discoveries in the field of biology Bordet was awarded the Nobel Prize in medicine for 1919.

Jules Jean Baptiste Vincent Bordet was born on June 13, 1870, in Soignies, Belgium, a small town situated twenty-three miles southwest of Brussels. He was the second son of Charles Bordet, a schoolteacher, and Célestine Vandenabeele Bordet. The family moved to Brussels in 1874, when his father received an appointment to the École Moyenne, a primary school. Jules and his older brother Charles attended this school and then received their secondary education at the Athénée Royal of Brussels. It was at this time that Bordet became interested in chemistry and began working in a small laboratory which he constructed at home. He entered the medical pro-

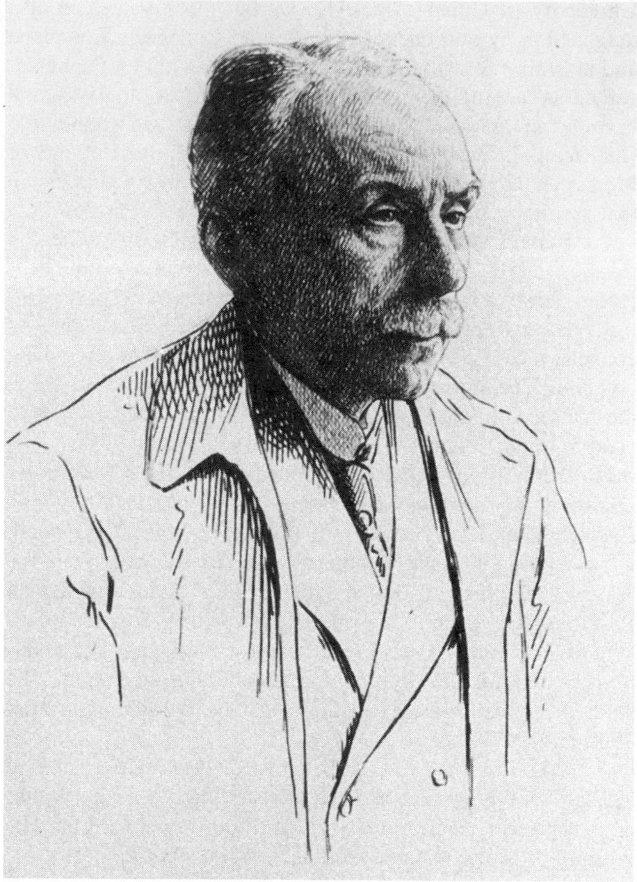

Jules Bordet

gram at the Free University of Brussels at the age of sixteen, receiving his doctorate of medicine in 1892. Bordet began his research career while still in medical school, and in 1892 he published a paper on the adaptation of viruses to vaccinated organisms in the *Annales de l'Institut Pasteur* of Paris. For this work, the Belgian government awarded him a scholarship to the Pasteur Institute, and from 1894 to 1901 he stayed in Paris at the laboratory of the Ukrainian-born scientist Élie Metchnikoff. In 1899 Bordet married Marthe Levoz; they eventually had two daughters and a son, Paul, who also became a medical scientist.

During his seven years at the Pasteur Institute, Bordet made most of the basic discoveries that led to his Nobel Prize of 1919. Soon after his arrival at the Institute, he began work on a problem in immunology. In 1894 Richard Pfeiffer, a German scientist, had discovered that when cholera bacteria was injected into the peritoneum of a guinea pig immunized against the infection, the pig would rapidly die. This bacteriolysis, Bordet discovered, did not occur when the bacteria was injected into a non-immunized guinea pig, but did so when the same animal received the antiserum from an immunized animal. Moreover, the bacteriolysis did not take place when the bacteria and the antiserum were mixed in a test tube unless fresh antiserum was used. However, when Bordet heated the antiserum to 55 degrees centigrade, it lost its power to kill bacteria. Finding that he could restore the bacteriolytic power of the antiserum if he added a little fresh serum from a non-immunized animal, Bordet concluded that the bacteria-killing phenomenon was due to the combined action of two distinct substances: an antibody in the antiserum, which specifically acted against a particular kind of bacterium; and a non-specific substance, sensitive to heat, found in all animal serums, which Bordet called "alexine" (later named "complement").

In a series of experiments conducted later, Bordet also learned that injecting red blood cells from one animal species (rabbit cells in the initial experiments) into another species (guinea pigs) caused the serum of the second species to quickly destroy the red cells of the first. And although the serum lost its power to kill the red cells when heated to 55 degrees centigrade, its potency was restored when alexine (or complement) was added. It became apparent to Bordet that hemolytic (red cell destroying) serums acted exactly as bacteriolytic serums; thus, he had uncovered the basic mechanism by which animal bodies defend or immunize themselves against the invasion of foreign elements. Eventually, Bordet and his colleagues found a way to implement their discoveries. They determined that alexine was bound or fixed to red blood cells or to bacteria during the immunizing process. When red cells were added to a normal serum mixed with a specific form of bacteria in a test tube, the bacteria remained active while the red cells were destroyed through the fixation of alexine. However, when serum containing the antibody specific to the bacteria was destroyed, the alexine and the solution separated into a layer of clear serum overlaying the intact red cells. Hence, it was possible to visually determine the presence of bacteria in a patient's blood serum. This process became known as a complement fixation test. Bordet and his associates applied these findings to various other infections, like typhoid fever, carbuncle, and hog cholera. August von Wasserman eventually used a form of the test (later known as the Wasserman test) to determine the presence of syphilis bacteria in the human blood.

Already famous by the age of thirty-one, Bordet accepted the directorship of the newly created Anti-rabies and Bacteriological Institute in Brussels in 1901; two years later, the organization was renamed the Pasteur Institute of Brussels. From 1901, Bordet was obliged to divide his time between his research and the administration of the Institute. In 1907 he also began teaching following his appointment as professor of bacteriology in the faculty of medicine at the Free University of Brussels, a position which he held until 1935. Despite his other activities, he continued his research in immunology and bacteriology. In 1906 Bordet and Octave Gengou succeeded in isolating the bacillus that causes whooping cough in children and later developed a vaccine against the disease. Between 1901 and 1920, Bordet conducted important studies on the coagulation of blood. When research became impossible because of the German occupation of Belgium during World War I, Bordet devoted himself to the writing of *Traité de l'immunité dans les maladies infectieuses* (1920), a classic book in the field of immunology. He was in the United States to raise money for new medical facilities for the war-damaged Free University of

Brussels when he received word that he had been awarded the Nobel Prize. After 1920, he became interested in bacteriophage, the family of viruses which kill many types of bacteria, publishing several articles on the subject. In 1940 Bordet retired from the directorship of the Pasteur Institute of Brussels and was succeeded by his son, Paul. Bordet himself continued to take an active interest in the work of the Institute despite his failing eyesight and a second German occupation of Belgium during World War II. Many scientists, friends, and former students gathered in a celebration of his eightieth birthday at the great hall of the Free University of Brussels in 1950. He died in Brussels on April 6, 1961.

Botulism

Botulism is a paralyzing and potentially fatal illness caused by one of the most poisonous toxins known. The toxin is produced by a bacteria called *Clostridium botulinum* and manifests in three main forms: infant botulism, foodborne botulism, and wound botulism. Foodborne and wound botulism cause weakness, dizziness, blurred or double vision, slurred speech, nausea, and difficulty swallowing and breathing. Symptoms usually appear 12 to 36 hours after the toxin enters the system but may appear as early as 2 hours or as late as 8 days. While rare—only 34 cases were reported nationwide in 1994—foodborne and wound botulism require emergency medical attention and usually necessitates hospitalization to prevent respiratory failure. In the early stages, injection of an antitoxin produced from horse serum can reduce the severity of the symptoms; however, allergic reaction to the antitoxin can pose a serious risk in itself.

C. botulinum bacteria are harmless, and their spores are found on fruit and vegetables, in seafood, and in soil and marine sediment worldwide. The toxin is produced when these bacteria grow. Growth occurs in the absence of oxygen and at temperatures ranging between 40 and 140° F (4.5-49°C). Home-canned or bottled fruit and vegetables and improperly cooked or reheated food are the most common causes of food botulism. Canned food should be heated to well above 212°F (100°C) for 10 minutes, and boiling food for 10 minutes will kill toxins. Wound botulism, the least common type, occurs when the *C. botulinum* bacteria enters an infected wound.

When the botulism toxin enters the body, it binds to nerve endings where they join the muscles and blocks signals which make the muscles contract. Onset of paralysis can be swift and severe and, before respirators, botulism killed many more people than it does today. From 1910 to 1919, 70% of those infected died. In 1993, the death rate was less than 2%. However, even today, recovery is slow. In 1994, a 47-year-old man was hospitalized for 49 days and required a mechanical ventilator for 42 of those.

Infant botulism, although rare, is the most common form. From 1976, when it was first recognized, until 1993, only 1,206 cases were reported in the United States. About 75 to 100 cases are reported annually. Serious but seldom fatal, it develops when botulism spores are ingested and germinate in the intestinal tract before the baby's system can develop a complete range of beneficial bacteria. All infant cases affect children less than one year old and researchers believe one cause is ingestion of contaminated honey. While honey is perfectly safe for children older than one year, authorities recommend honey not be given to children less than 12 months old. Researchers also suspect a link between infant botulism and **Sudden Infant Death Syndrome** (SIDS).

Of growing concern is avian botulism, which kills millions of birds worldwide each year. The botulism toxin develops in bodies of water with little or no flow and is ingested by the birds.

Purified botulism toxin is now being put to medical use. Its mechanism of action is the same as the poisonous toxin. Licensed by the FDA in 1989 for treatment of blepharospasm and strabismus—both caused by excessive muscle contractions of the eye—it is injected into specific muscles to control those contractions. Researchers are currently studying its use in other muscular disorders.

Bourgeois, Louyse (1563-1636)

French midwife

Louyse Bourgeois was the most famous midwife of her time. As one of the first educated, literate, and medically trained female midwives, she raised her profession to a new level of professional competence and promoted the spread of that competence through her widely read books recounting her observations and experiences.

Bourgeois, a woman of the middle class, acquired her medical knowledge from her husband, an army surgeon. As one of the first graduates of the new school for midwives at the Hotel Dieu hospital in Paris, where she may have studied under the pioneering surgeon Ambroise Paré. Bourgeois developed a very large and successful practice, especially among the French aristocracy. She attended the birth of the future King Louis XIII—reportedly saving the newborn from asphyxia—as well as the five other deliveries of Marie de Medici, wife of Henry IV.

The popularity and reputation of Bourgeois were tarnished when she was accused of responsibility in the death of the queen's daughter-in-law, the Duchesse d'Orleans, from peritonitis following delivery in 1627. Nevertheless, Bourgeois remained influential and successful, although she never received the pension King Henry had promised her.

Bourgeois especially advanced obstetrical knowledge with her observations about detachment of the placenta. She may have been the first midwife to write books about her specialty, the most important of which was *Observations diverses sur la stérilité*, published in 1626. She certainly accustomed child-bearing women to expect a new and higher degree of competence and knowledge from their birth attendant.

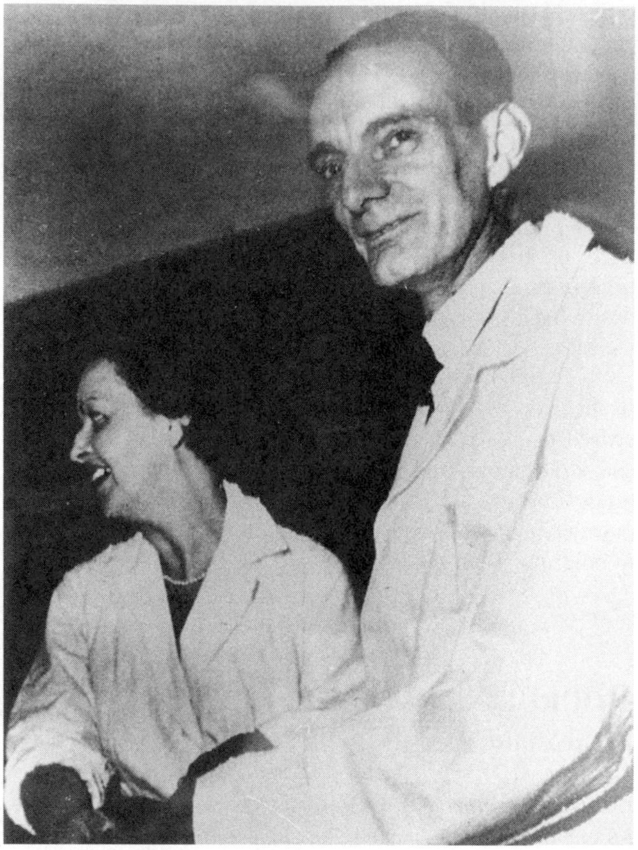
Daniel Bovet

Bovet, Daniel (1907-1992)

Swiss Italian pharmacologist

Daniel Bovet had the distinction of making basic contributions in at least three distinct areas of pharmacology, the science of drugs. His research made possible the commercial development of sulfa drugs, antihistamines, and muscle relaxants. For his accomplishments in pharmacology he was awarded the Nobel Prize in physiology or medicine in 1957.

Bovet was born on March 23, 1907, in Neuchatel, Switzerland, the only son among the four children of Pierre Bovet and Amy Babut Bovet. Pierre Bovet was a professor of experimental education at the University of Geneva and the founder of the Institut J. J. Rousseau. His son later recalled in *Time* that he and his sisters were "guinea pigs" for testing his father's educational theories. Daniel Bovet received his primary and secondary school education in Neuchatel, then studied biology at the University of Geneva, from which he received his *license* in 1927. He did his graduate study in physiology and zoology at the same institution and earned his doctor of science degree in 1929.

Bovet went to Paris in 1929 to become an assistant in the Laboratory of Therapeutic Chemistry at the Pasteur Institute, working under the direction of Ernest Fourneau. In his 1965 article "Role of the Scientist in Modern Society," Bovet declared that being Fourneau's "pupil and collaborator... for nearly twenty years... was the greatest good fortune of my life." Bovet succeeded Fourneau as director of the Laboratory of Therapeutic Chemistry in 1939. It was there that he met Filomena Nitti, a fellow researcher and the daughter of Francesco Saverio Nitti, a former prime minister of Italy who had been driven into exile to Paris following Benito Mussolini's rise to power. Bovet and Filomena Bovet-Nitti, wife and collaborator (as she thereafter identified herself), were married in 1938 and she became his collaborator in nearly all of his research, as well as the coauthor of many of his scientific books and articles. They had two daughters and one son, Danièle Bovet, who became a professor of information science at the University of Rome.

In the early 1930s, the German scientist Gerhard Domagk discovered that Prontosil, a dye product, effectively combated streptococcal infections. Prontosil was a complex chemical, however, and expensive to produce. Bovet and his colleagues at the Pasteur Institute reasoned that the therapeutic action of the substance was probably due to some part of the drug's molecule that was only released when the molecule broke down in the body. After months of work and many experiments, they discovered that the active therapeutic agent was sulfanilamide. This product was much cheaper to produce than Prontosil and was soon being manufactured in quantity, becoming the first of the so-called "wonder drugs." Over the next several years Bovet and his associates went on to synthesize many other sulfanamide derivatives that together formed the group of sulfa drugs that were to save millions of lives during World War II and afterward. Domagk was awarded the Nobel Prize in physiology or medicine in 1939 for his discovery of the therapeutic action of Prontosil, but it was the work of Bovet and his team that had made sulfa drugs a practical reality.

In 1937 Bovet turned his attention to histamine, a hormone that occurs naturally in all body tissues. When an irritant is introduced, an overproduction of free histamine can occur in some localized area of the body. The free histamine in turn causes swelling or an allergic reaction that often leads to severe discomfort, damage to body tissues, or—in extreme cases—to fatal shock. Bovet was struck by the fact that there was no natural product in the human body that would counteract the negative effects of free histamine; he believed that what was needed was an artificial substance which would block them. Bovet and his assistants soon synthesized the first antihistamine, although it had too many problems to be a viable commercial product. Between 1937 and 1941, Bovet and others performed some three thousand experiments to find a practical substitute. Eventually several were developed, including Bovet's own discovery, pyrilamine. These were the first of the many antihistamines now used in modern medicine.

In 1947 Bovet and his family left Paris for Rome, where he was to organize and direct the Laboratory of Therapeutic Chemistry at the Istituto Superiore di Sanità. He also became an Italian citizen. It was about this time that he began to study the muscle relaxant properties of curare, the poison certain South American Indians had long used on their arrows. A chemically pure form of curare had been produced earlier and was used to relax body muscles before surgery, thus allowing the surgeon to use much smaller doses of potentially dangerous anesthetics. However, the effects of the curare itself were very unpredictable, and it was also expensive. Bovet set himself the task of finding a synthetic form of the drug that would have the advantages of predictability and low cost. During eight years of work he produced over four hundred synthetic forms of curare, including gallamine and succinylcholine, the latter becoming widely used. During his research on curare, Bovet spent some time with the Indians of South America to learn how they produced and used the drug. He later remarked humorously that he had done so out of a spirit of adventure; curare was only the pretext.

Bovet left Rome in 1964 to become professor of pharmacology at the University of Sassari on the Italian island of Sardinia. He returned to Rome as director of the Laboratory of Psychobiology and Psychopharmacology of the Italian national research council in 1969. He became professor of psychobiology at the University of Rome in 1971 and remained there as an honorary professor following his retirement in 1982. The positions in Rome reflected still another shift in the focus of his research, indicating an interest in the complex area of mental illness and its treatment through the use of chemicals.

As early as 1957, *Time* had reported Bovet's belief that the key to mental illness lay in chemistry. His studies centered on the effect of various chemical compounds on the central nervous system of the human body. While his work did not produce the kind of dramatic practical breakthroughs that he had achieved in sulfa drugs, antihistamines, and muscle relaxants, he did contribute much important basic research to this field.

Frequently collaborating with his wife, Bovet produced several books and over four hundred articles in the course of his professional life. Before 1947 most of his writings were in French; afterward many appeared in Italian and some in English. However, even this large output does not fully reveal the breadth of his intellectual interests. He was concerned with the impact of scientific discovery on political, social, and economic affairs and with the equally strong impact of those affairs on science. He illustrated this in ''Role of the Scientist in Modern Society.'' ''Unfortunately, in our century,'' he wrote, ''two-thirds of the global population are illiterate and walk barefooted, ten to fifteen per cent suffer from hunger, thirty-three per cent to forty per cent do not have an adequate diet, seventy per cent are not provided with sufficient water supply, and eighty per cent lack adequate hygienic conveniences. Even the best drugs are ineffective for people living in very poor hygienic conditions.'' Science, he concluded, could not solve all of the world's problems. Personally, Bovet was a humble, enthusiastic man who single-mindedly pursued his quest for scientific progress without personal gain in mind. As *Time* noted when he received the Nobel Prize in 1957, Bovet had never taken out a patent in his own name and never made any money from his scientific discoveries. He was the recipient of numerous international awards in addition to the Nobel Prize. He died of cancer in Rome on April 8, 1992.

Bowman, Sir William (1816-1892)

British physician

Sir William Bowman is known as England's ''father of histological anatomy and ophthalmic surgery.'' His work in histology (the study of tissue visible only with the aid of a microscope) produced the most detailed observation and documentation of the structure and function of human and animal tissue. He carried this investigation into ophthalmology—the study of the eye—increasingly devoting his time to eye surgery and eventually founding and becoming the first president of the Ophthalmological Society in 1880. It is said that few people have contributed so greatly to medicine in general as did Bowman. For his contribution, Bowman was knighted (named *Sir* William Bowman) by Queen Victoria in 1884.

Bowman was born in Nantwich, England, the third son and fourth child of John Eddowes Bowman and Elizabeth Eddowes, who were first cousins. His father was a banker who loved nature and was a founding member of the Manchester Geological Society and author of several works in geology and botany. Bowman and his family were extremely close, and his father corresponded with him throughout his career. In 1826 Bowman was sent to Hazelwood School in Birmingham and became an understudy to a house surgeon at the Birmingham Infirmary (small hospital) in 1832 and, at the same time, worked under a distinguished surgeon who later became president of the Royal College of Surgeons. Bowman wanted to become a member of this college, acceptance at which required attendance at a London teaching hospital. He therefore attended the newly founded medical department of King's College in London in 1837. In 1838, he did a study tour of eight European hospitals, and in 1839 qualified for membership! in the Royal College of Surgeons.

In 1840, after being appointed Demonstrator of Anatomy and Curator of the Museum at King's College, he became assistant surgeon at the newly established King's College Hospital. In 1844, he became a fellow at the Royal College of Surgeons, became assistant surgeon to Moorfields Ophthalmic Hospital in 1846, full surgeon in 1851, and full surgeon to King's College Hospital in 1856. He soon resigned that post, however, because of an ever-increasing private practice.

During the course of his career, Bowman sketched and wrote highly detailed and previously undocumented descriptions of the skin, muscle, nerves, sense organs (particularly the eye), kidney, bone, and cartilage. He is probably most famous, however, for his work on the kidney, in which he identified the role of a tiny capsule (now known as Bowman's capsule) in carrying fluid from the kidney to the urinary system. He published his findings in a famous paper called *On the Structure and use of the Malpighian Bodies of the Kidney* (1842). He also composed a measurement table of the diameter of bundles of muscle fibers in 44 animals—including humans—both female and male.

Apart from this and several other famed works, Bowman—together with his instructor, Robert Todd—wrote and illustrated the highly praised *The Physiological Anatomy and Physiology of Man* (1836-1852). This work credited him with ''having no parallel in making so enormous a series of new discoveries while producing material for a book.'' The book has been honored as one of the first documents on histology to contribute significantly to medicine. His histological studies were made possible by the improved design and manufacture process of microscope lenses; however, by modern standards, available methods were extremely primitive, making his detailed observations even more outstanding.

Bowman's work in ophthalmology was as equally precise. He described the cornea, elastic membranes which help the eye to focus (Bowman's membrane), minute fibers in the ciliary muscle of the eye (Bowman's muscle), and other previously unidentified parts of the eye. Bowman also became a top-class ophthalmic surgeon. He developing several surgical techniques including an operation to create an artificial pupil when certain abnormalities caused blindness (Bowman's operation); and probes to clear blocked lacrymal (tear) ducts (Bowman's probes), which are still used today. He performed the first iridectomy, a surgical procedure developed by **Frederick Wilhelm Ernst Albrecht von Graefe** (1828-1870) to ease **glaucoma**, a disease in which pressure builds up in the eyeball ultimately causing blindness; and was one of the first physicians in Britain to become an expert with the ophthalmoscope, invented by **Hermann von Helmholtz** in 1851.

Bowman married Harriet Paget, the daughter of an English surgeon, in 1842. He was popular with his students and known as a ''methodical and kindly practitioner.'' He helped found St. John's Sisterhood of Nursing, and corresponded over many years with distinguished people including Florence Nightingale, Charles Darwin, and Albrecht von Graefe. He was also mentor to **Francis Galton**, who later became the founder of **eugenics**. More than 150 years after his death, most of Bowman's observations have been confirmed as accurate, and his surgical techniques—although improved upon—laid the foundation for modern methods. His contribution to ophthalmology has been called the driving force in understanding eye disease.

See also Glaucoma

BRAILLE, LOUIS (1809-1852)

French teacher

Braille designed a coding system, based on patterns of raised dots, which the blind could read by touch. Born on January 4, 1809, Coupvray, France, Braille was accidentally blinded in one eye at the age of three. Within two years, a disease in his other eye left him completely blind.

In 1819, Braille received a scholarship to the Institut National des Jeunes Aveugles (National Institute of Blind Youth), founded by Valentin Haüy (1745-1822). The same year Braille entered the school, Captain Charles Barbier invented sonography, or nightwriting, a system of embossed symbols used by soldiers to communicate silently at night on the battlefield. Inspired by a lecture Barbier gave at the Institute a few years later, the fifteen-year-old Braille adapted Barbier's system to replace Haüy's awkward embossed type, which he and his classmates had been obliged to learn.

In his initial study, Braille had experimented with geometric shapes cut from leather as well as with nails and tacks hammered into boards. He finally settled on a fingertip-sized six-dot code, based on the twenty-five letters of the alphabet, which could be recognized with a single contact of one digit. By varying the number and placement of dots, he coded letters, punctuation, numbers, diphthongs, familiar words, scientific symbols, mathematical and musical notation, and capitalization. With the right hand, the reader touched individual dots and, with the left, moved on toward the next line, comprehending as smoothly and rapidly as sighted readers. Using the Braille system, students were also able to take notes and write themes by punching dots into paper with a pointed stylus which was aligned with a metal guide.

At the age of twenty, Braille published a monograph describing the use of his coded system. In 1837, he issued a second publication featuring an expanded system of coding text. Despite the students' favorable response to the Braille code, sighted instructors and school board members, fearing for their jobs should the number of well-educated blind individuals increase, opposed his system.

Braille grew seriously ill with incurable tuberculosis in 1835 and was forced to resign his teaching post. He died in Paris on January 6, 1852. The Braille writing system—though demonstrated at the Paris Exposition of Industry in 1834 and praised by King Louis-Philippe—was not fully accepted until 1854, two years after the inventor's death. The system underwent periodic alteration; the standardized system employed today was first used in the United States in 1860 at the Missouri School for the Blind.

BRAIN TUMOR

A brain tumor is an abnormal growth of tissue in the brain. Unlike other tumors, brain tumors spread by local extension and rarely metastasize (spread) outside the brain. A benign brain tumor is composed of non-cancerous cells and does not spread beyond the part of the brain where it originates. A brain tumor is considered malignant if it contains cancer cells, or if it is composed of harmless cells located in an area where it suppresses one or more vital functions.

Each year, more than 17,000 brain tumors are diagnosed in the United States. About half are benign, but may be in life-threatening locations. The rest are malignant and invasive.

Benign brain tumors, composed of harmless cells, have clearly defined borders, can usually be completely removed, and are unlikely to recur. Benign brain tumors do not infiltrate nearby tissues but can cause severe **pain**, permanent brain damage, and **death**. Benign brain tumors sometimes become malignant.

Malignant brain tumors do not have distinct borders. They tend to grow rapidly, increasing pressure within the brain and can spread in the brain or spinal cord beyond the point where they originate. It is highly unusual for malignant brain tumors to spread beyond the central nervous system (CNS).

Primary brain tumors originate in the brain. They represent about 1% of all cancers and 2.5% of all cancer deaths. Approximately 25% of all cancer patients develop secondary or metastatic brain tumors when cancer cells spread from another part of the body to the brain. Metastatic brain tumors can develop on any part of the brain or spinal cord. Brain tumors can develop at any age, but are most common in children between the ages of 3-12, and in adults aged 40-70.

The name of a brain tumor describes where it originates, how it grows, and what kind of cells it contains. A tumor in an adult is also graded or staged according to how malignant it is, how rapidly it is growing, how likely it is to invade other tissues, and how closely its cells resemble normal cells.

Low-grade brain tumors usually have well-defined borders. Some low-grade brain tumors are enclosed in cysts. Low-grade brain tumors grow slowly, if at all. They may spread throughout the brain, but rarely metastasize to other parts of the body.

Mid-grade and high-grade tumors grow more rapidly than low-grade tumors. Described as "truly malignant," these tumors usually infiltrate healthy tissue. Their growth pattern makes it difficult to remove the entire tumor, and these tumors recur more often than low-grade tumors.

A single brain tumor can contain several different types of cells. The tumor's grade is determined by the highest-grade (most malignant) cell detected under a microscope, even if most of the cells in the tumor are less malignant. An infiltrating tumor is a tumor of any grade that grows into surrounding tissue.

The cause of primary brain tumors is unknown, but people who work with rubber and certain chemicals have a greater risk of developing them. There is no evidence that **head injury** causes brain tumors, but researchers are trying to determine the relationship, if any, between brain tumors and viruses, family history, and long-term exposure to electromagnetic fields.

Symptoms do not usually appear until the tumor grows large enough to displace, damage, or destroy delicate brain tissue. When that happens, the patient may experience headaches that become increasingly painful and are most painful when lying down, nausea and vomiting, seizures **dizziness**, loss of coordination or balance, personality changes, sudden loss of vision, memory loss speech problems, sensory changes, mental impairment, and/or weakness or **paralysis** on one side of the body.

When a patient has one or more of these symptoms, a primary care physician will perform a complete **physical examination**, take a detailed medical history, and conduct a basic neurologic examination.

If the results of these examinations suggest a patient may have a brain tumor, a neurologist recommends some or all of these additional diagnostic tests: computed tomography scan (CT scan) to reveal brain abnormalities, magnetic resonance imaging (MRI) to detect tumors beneath the bones of the skull; **electroencephalography** (EEG) to measure electrical activity in the brain; x rays to reveal any distortion in the bones of the skull; **angiography** to outline a tumor and the blood vessels that lead to it; a brain scan to identify and record the location of abnormal cells in the brain; x rays of the spine to detect a spinal cord tumor, or a lumbar puncture (spinal tap) to obtain spinal fluid, which may contain tumor cells.

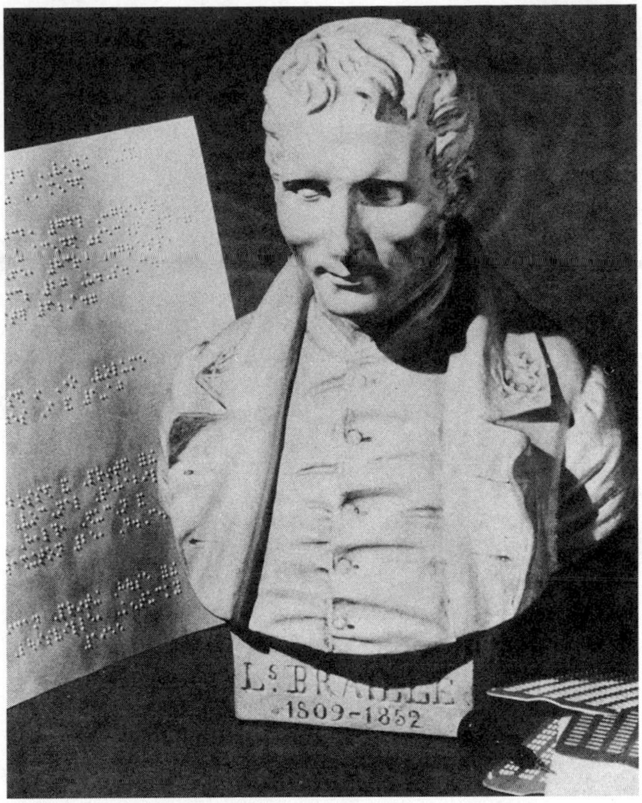

Louis Braille

Interpreting these images and the results of laboratory analysis allows a neurologist to determine whether a tumor is present, but microscopic examination of tumor tissue (a biopsy) is the only way to identify the kind of cells it contains.

Surgery is the treatment of choice for accessible brain tumors that can be removed without causing serious neurologic damage. Patients whose benign brain tumors can be completely removed may not require any additional treatment, although periodic examinations are recommended. Because surgeons cannot be sure that every bit of an infiltrating or metastasizing tumor has been removed, radiation and chemotherapy are used to destroy cells that may have escaped the scalpel.

If a tumor cannot be completely removed, removing a portion of it (debulking) can alleviate the patient's symptoms, enhance the sense of well-being, and increase the effectiveness of other treatments.

Radiation therapy is often a very effective treatment used to help destroy tumor cells. A number of drugs have been developed and found to be effective ways to fight brain tumors. One or more cancer-killing drugs may be taken by mouth or injected into a blood vessel, muscle, or the cerebrospinal fluid. Chemotherapy may be used with radiation and surgery as part of a patient's initial treatment, or used alone to treat tumors that recur.

The chances of a patient's recovery depend on where the tumor is located and what type of cells it contains. A patient

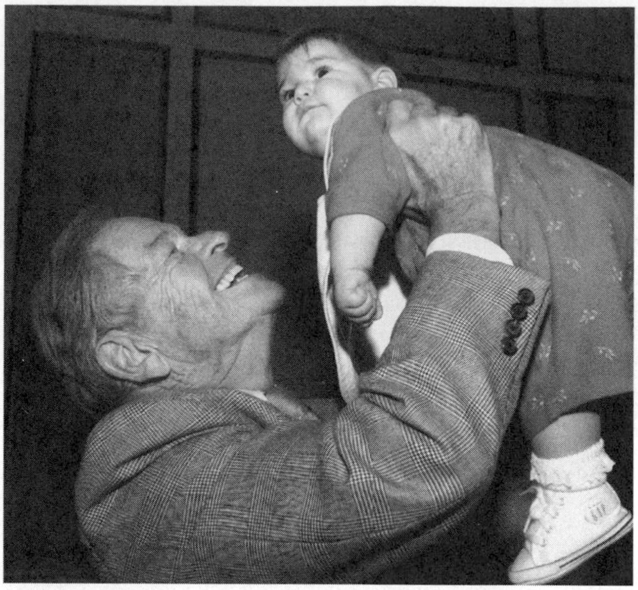

T. Berry Brazelton

whose tumor is discovered early and removed completely may make a full recovery, but the surgery itself can harm or destroy normal brain tissue and cause problems with thought, speech, and coordination, seizures, weakness, or personality changes.

If a brain tumor cannot be cured, treatment is designed to make the patient as comfortable as possible and preserve as much of his neurologic functioning as possible. Brain tumors that cannot be removed can cause irreversible brain damage and death.

Research efforts center on ways to empower chemotherapy drugs to penetrate the blood-brain barrier (which protects the central nervous system by separating the brain from blood circulating throughout the body), and attack cancer cells that have infiltrated tissue inside it.

Brain tumor researchers are also investigating less invasive surgical procedures, methods of incorporating chemotherapy drugs into tumor cells to reduce the need for radiation, and laboratory techniques that enable physicians to select the chemotherapy drugs most likely to kill particular types of tumors. Also being researched is **gene therapy**, in which genetically engineered material is transported to tumor cells by viruses that infect tumor cells and either convert them to normal cells, stop their growth, or kill them.

BRAZELTON, THOMAS BERRY (1918-)

American pediatrician

Well-loved and popular pediatrician, T. Berry Brazelton was born on May 10, 1918 in Waco, Texas, to Thomas Berry Brazelton and Pauline (Battle) Brazelton. His first experiences with babies and children were during his own childhood, when he was frequently put in charge of babysitting his many young cousins at family parties and reunions. It was immediately clear that Brazelton had both a talent for and a love of being with children, including babies. Thanks to these early **child care** experiences, Brazelton was able to decide on a career in pediatrics as early as the sixth grade, abandoning his previously chosen career of veterinarian.

Brazelton left Waco to attend a prep school in Alexandria, Virginia (Episcopal High School). He then attended New Jersey's Princeton University, following the pre-medical curriculum. Brazelton also enjoyed acting in a number of college theatre productions, and even considered accepting a role on Broadway. His parents, however, were tremendously unenthusiastic about this proposal, and recommended that, should he wish them to pay for medical school in the future, he concentrate on his pre-medical studies. Brazelton decided to heed their advice.

After receiving his A.B. from Princeton in 1940, Brazelton went on to earn his M.D. from the College of Physicians and surgeons at New York City's Columbia University. He did his internship year through Columbia University, at Roosevelt Hospital, and then served for a year in the United States Naval Reserve.

In 1945, Brazelton began a medical residency at Massachusetts General Hospital. In 1947, he began his pediatrics training at Boston Children's Hospital. During this time, Brazelton began to recognize that the medical field's emphasis on the study of pathology and disease was of less interest to him than the study of normal development. Brazelton realized that he most wanted the opportunity study and understand human beings, rather than to study and understand disease. In response to these passions, Brazelton decided to enter a residency in child psychiatry, at Putnam Children's Center in Roxbury, MA. He pursued this at a time when child psychiatry had not yet gained respect in the medical field.

In 1950, after having completed his child psychiatry residency, Brazelton began a private practice in Cambridge, MA. In 1951, he was appointed as an instructor at Harvard Medical School.

Also in 1951, Brazelton began doing research with parents and babies. He published a variety of findings, all of which spoke to babies being much more involved with and discerning of their environment than had usually been believed. Brazelton established that, as early as four months into development, a fetus's nervous system was sophisticated enough that a loud noise would evoke a startle response. Other studies revealed that a newborn, only days old, can distinguish between a blank oval and a drawing of a human face. A baby only three weeks of age can distinguish between the voices of its mother and its father. Brazelton honed his powers of observation such that he could observe the behaviors of premature babies and use them to predict recovery time from various illnesses of prematurity.

The Neonatal Behavioral Assessment Scale was published in 1973, with revisions made in 1984. Brazelton designed this scale to utilize information obtained from providing newborns with visual, auditory, and tactile stimuli, in order to study a newborn's response to the environment. This information allows practitioners to obtain very early information about potential developmental problems, as well as helping practitioners and parents characterize the baby's behavioral style as average, quiet, or unusually active. Another advantage of this scale over other evaluative tools is that it allows evaluation to begin during the newborn stage, as opposed to other scales which can't be administered until a baby is several months old. Brazelton created the Neonatal Behavioral Assessment Scale in the hopes that it would also prove helpful for people trying to adopt babies; if newborns could be reliably assessed, and potential adoptive parents could be reassured that the newborns were normal, then perhaps adoptions could be expedited.

Brazelton has also been a tremendously prolific writer, supplying parents with a variety of anecdotally-based books on child development. Brazelton describes his main goals as being to strengthen the parent-child bond by helping parents understand their children as individuals, and by providing reassurance as to the vast range of baby's personalities and responses. Some of his very popular books include *Infants and Mothers: Individual Differences* (1969, revised 1983); *Toddlers and Parents* (1974); *Doctor and Child* (1976); *On Becoming a Family* (1981); *Working and Caring* (1984); *What Every Baby Knows* (1987); *The Earliest Relationship: Parents, Infants and the Dream of Early Attachment* (1990, with Bertrand Cramer); *Touchpoints: Your Child's Emotional and Behavioral Development* (1993).

Through the 1990s, in his 70s and early 80s, Brazelton has maintained an extremely active schedule. He has continued a small pediatric practice, while continuing to teach medical students and residents, researching behavior, lecturing widely, appearing on numerous television programs, writing prolifically for periodicals and websites, and helping lobby the public to push for their parental rights in the form of what ultimately passed as the Family Leave Act of 1993. Brazelton still sees his most important mission as fostering a sense of competent, loving, joyful parenting.

See also Child care; Spock, Benjamin

BREAST CANCER AND CARE

Breast cancer is the second leading cause of cancer death in women. It is characterized by the abnormal growth and uncontrolled division of cells in the breast. **Cancer** cells form a tumor, that is often felt as a lump in the breast. This tumor can invade and destroy surrounding normal tissue, and can spread (metastasize) cancer cells throughout the body via the bloodstream or lymph system.

Every woman is at risk for breast cancer. If she lives to be 85, there is a one out of nine chance that she will develop the condition sometime during the rest of her life. As a woman ages, her risk of developing breast cancer rises dramatically regardless of her family history. The breast cancer risk of a 25-year-old woman is only one out of 19,608; by age 45, it is one in 93. In fact, 80% of all breast cancers are found in women over age 50.

There are a number of risk factors for the development of breast cancer, including: family history of breast cancer in

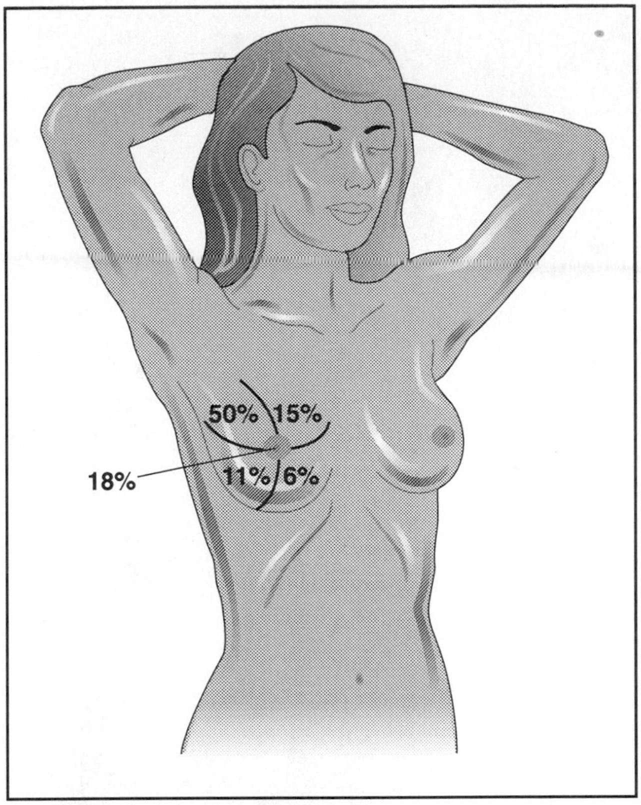

This illustration shows the frequency of breast cancer developing in the four quadrants of the breast and the nipple. *(Illustration by Electronic Illustrators Group.)*

mother or sister, early onset of menstruation, late **menopause**, and history of abnormal breast biopsies. Reproductive history may also be a factor; women who had no children or have children late in life and women who have never breastfed are at increased risk for breast cancer. However, more than 70% of women who get breast cancer have no known risk factors.

The best way to manage breast cancer risk is by doing a *breast self-examination* (BSE) at the same time each month. The entire breast tissue area (which extends up to the collarbone) and both armpits should be checked visually and by hand for changes. The changes in the breast that may be a sign of breast cancer include: a lump or thickening in breast or armpit, nipple turning inward, unusual discharge from the nipple, dimpled or reddened skin on the breast, and a change in breast size or shape. A woman should see her doctor as soon as possible if she observes any of these signs.

Periodic clinical breast examinations by a health care professional are also important in early breast cancer detection. Women between 20 and 39 should have an exam performed at least once every three years; women over 40 should be examined annually.

More than 90% of all breast cancers are detected on a *mammogram* (x ray of the breast). Screening mammograms should be ordered according to the doctor's guidelines. Despite the controversy about the cost-effectiveness of mammo-

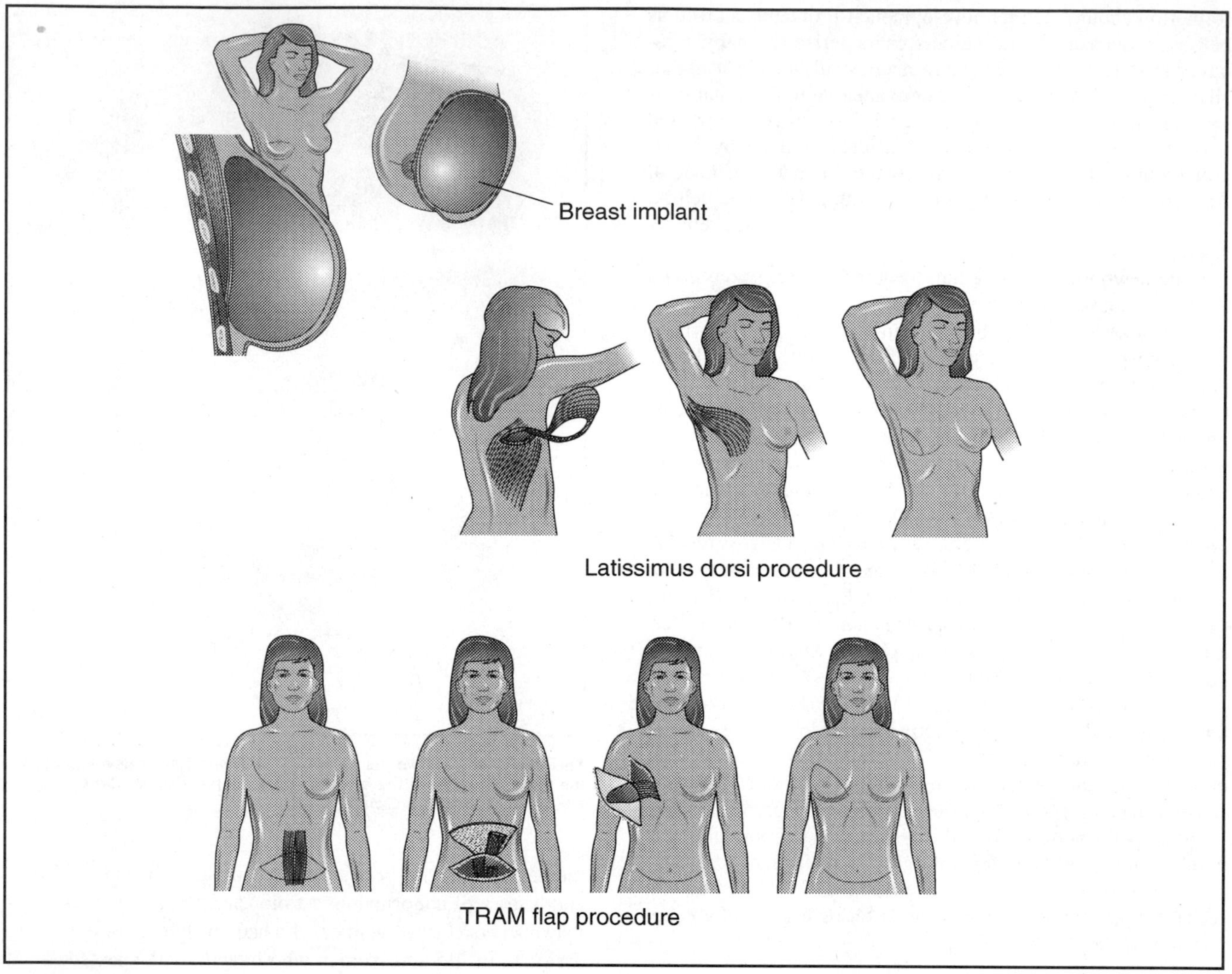

Types of breast reconstruction.

grams for women in their 40s, most doctors agree with the current American Cancer Society guidelines that recommend screening mammograms every year or two for women between 40 and 49, and every year after age 50. Women with a family history of breast cancer may want to have a mammogram every year after age 40. A baseline mammogram should be done by age 35, so that a normal x ray can be used to compare future mammograms, even when there is no reason to believe there is a lump or cyst.

If anything irregular is detected on a mammogram, such as a mass, changes from earlier mammograms, abnormalities of the skin, or enlargement of the lymph nodes, further testing may be recommended. This could include an ultrasound of the breast, a biopsy or needle sampling, or consultation with a breast surgeon.

Biopsy of the breast is a removal of suspicious breast tissue for examination by a pathologist. An excisional biopsy is a surgical procedure in which the entire lump area and some surrounding tissue is removed for examination. If the mass is very large, an incisional biopsy is done where only a portion of the area is removed and analysed. Needle biopsy can be done in two methods. An aspiration needle biopsy uses a very fine needle to withdraw cells and fluid from the mass for analysis. A large core needle biopsy uses a larger diameter needle to remove small pieces of tissue from the mass that can be analyzed. After the tissue sample is removed, a pathologist will examine the cells within it to determine whether the mass is benign (non-cancerous) or malignant (cancerous).

It is important to realize that not all lumps detected in the breast are cancerous. Many are benign and require only the removal of the lump. However, when a malignancy is found, it is important to determine the extent of the disease is so proper treatment can begin as soon as possible.

To find out if the cancer has spread to other parts of the body (metastasized), doctors will also biopsy underarm lymph nodes to test for cancer cells that have spread. Checking to see if there are cancer cells in the lymph nodes is also a way to tell how advanced the cancer is. This is called ''staging'' cancer. Breast cancer is rated from Stage 0 to Stage IV based on the size of the tumor and if the cancer has spread to surrounding lymph nodes and/or organs.

Breast cancer treatment is prescribed and administered by an oncologist (cancer specialist). Treatment options include surgery, **chemotherapy**, and radiation. Breast cancer is treated in two ways, locally to eliminate tumor cells from the breast by surgery and radiation, and systemically to destroy cancer cells that have traveled to other parts of the body. Systemic therapy includes chemotherapy and hormonal treatments.

The extent of surgery depends on the type of breast cancer, whether the disease has spread, and the patient's age and health. If the tumor is less than about 1.6 inches or there isn't much chance it will return, the patient and doctor may opt for removal of the tumor alone (**lumpectomy**) followed by **radiation therapy**. In a lumpectomy, the doctor removes the lump and an area of tissue surrounding it. Some of the lymph nodes under the arm may be removed (axillary dissection) and tested to see if the cancer has spread there.

If the tumor is larger, **mastectomy** may be needed. In a modified radical mastectomy, the doctor removes the entire breast, the underarm (axillary) lymph nodes, and the lining over the chest muscle (but not the muscles themselves. A radical mastectomy is used only when the cancer has invaded the chest muscles; the surgeon removes the breast, the chest muscles, and all of the lymph nodes under the arm.

Surgery can also be combined with breast reconstruction. Breast reconstruction is a series of surgical procedures performed to recreate a breast which looks and feels as natural as possible. It can be performed at the time of masectomy surgery, or at a later date. A breast mound is formed by using artificial materials called breast implants, or by using tissues from other parts of the woman's body, and the nipple and areolar complex (darker area around the nipple) are recreated. Other procedures may be necessary, such as lifting the opposite breast (mastopexy), or making it larger or smaller to match the reconstructed breast.

The presence of cancer cells in the lymph nodes may require more extensive surgery. If the cancer has spread to the nodes, the patient will need either radiation, chemotherapy, hormone therapy, or a combination of all three after surgery. This is called ''adjuvant therapy.''

Radiation stops the cancer cells from dividing. It works especially well on fast-growing tumors. Unfortunately, it also stops some types of healthy cells from dividing. Healthy cells that divide quickly, like those of the skin and hair, are affected the most. This is why radiation can cause fatigue, skin problems, and hair loss.

Breast cancer surgery may be followed by *chemotherapy* in even the earliest stages. Chemotherapy drugs are administered either orally or by injection into a blood vessel. Chemotherapy is usually given in cycles, with a course of drugs followed by a period of time for recovery before another course of drugs. Chemotherapy treatment time may range between four to nine months.

There may be significant side effects with some types of chemotherapy, including **nausea and vomiting**, temporary hair loss, mouth or vaginal sores, fatigue, weakened immune system, and **infertility**. However, chemotherapy for early breast cancer uses medications that cause few side effects.

The growth of some breast cancer cells may be slowed or stopped with the drug *tamoxifen*, an anti-estrogen medication. Research suggests that tamoxifen may lower the chance that a breast cancer can return by between 25% and 35%. It can also prevent the recurrence of new cancer in the opposite breast. Other *hormone treatments* include the use of progestins, estrogens, and androgens. In rare cases, the surgeon may suggest removal of the ovaries (oophorectomy) in premenopausal women as a way of eliminating the main source of estrogen, which can boost the growth of some breast tumors.

Stem cell treatment is used to treat advanced breast cancer. By first removing a woman's stem cells from her bone marrow or blood, the doctor can use very high doses of chemotherapy or radiation to kill cancer cells. Because this also kills healthy white blood cells, leaving the woman vulnerable to infection, the stem cells are then replaced, where they restore the body's ability to fight infection.

It is normal to be depressed or moody, to cry, or to be less interested in sex after breast cancer treatment. Many women have found that joining a support group of breast cancer survivors can help them work through their emotions.

The prognosis for breast cancer depends on the type and stage of cancer. Most patients can return to a normal lifestyle within a month or so after surgery. **Exercise**s can help the patient regain strength and flexibility. Regular follow-up with a physician is important to look for any recurrence of the cancer.

BREAST-FEEDING

Medical anthropologists have argued that that insofar as breast milk has nourished human children since the earliest known humans, breast-feeding must have distinct advantages for mothers, infants, and the whole human species. But whether a mother breast feeds her newborn child has been to a large extent influenced by specific cultural practices in relatively recent times. In much of 18th-century Europe, for example, it was considered unseemly to feed babies at the breast or even to feed them milk. The great Viennese composer Amadeus Mozart insisted that his babies be raised, as he was, on sugar water; not surprisingly, four of his six children died in the first three years of their lives. And medical historians have speculated that Mozart's early and tragic death may have been related to his sugar-water diet as an infant.

Newborn babies need about 50 calories per pound of body weight each day; this requirement drops to 45 calories by the infant's first birthday. But babies are pretty good about signaling when they are hungry or full, so these numbers are of more referential than practical value. The best food for infants is breast milk, and it is the only nutritional substance needed for the first six months of life.

Studies performed in a number of developed countries have shown that breast-fed infants have lower rates of **diar-**

rhea, respiratory infections, allergic problems, **ear infections**, **meningitis**, **urinary tract infections** and other diseases. This is because breast milk carries mother's antibodies in the colostrum and milk that are specific for the human species. Breast milk is also thought to provide protection against allergies later in life.

At birth, a baby carries his mother's immunity but is without a functional immune system of his own. At about 6 weeks, he begins to acquire his own immune system. At the age of 6 months, an immature **immune system** will help keep him healthy and allergy free. Breast milk supplies the baby with all the immunities he needs until his own immune system is developed.

The composition of human milk changes to meet the changing needs of the maturing baby. Even when a baby is able to take solids, human milk remains the primary source of nutrition during the first year. Because it takes between two and six years for a child's immune system to fully mature, human milk continues to boost the immune system as long as it is offered.

The American Academy of Pediatrics has advocated breast-feeding since 1948. This organization has continued to revise its guidelines over the years and urge mothers to use human milk for infant **nutrition**. The Academy bases this recommendation on extensive research covering nutrition, the immune system, economic and psycho-social reasons, development and the environment. The Academy has also reported that the longer children are breast-fed, the better they perform on reading, math, and cognitive tests; and they exhibit superior scholastic performance compared to their non-breast-fed peers. These results were based on a study of more than 1,000 children who were breast-fed for various lengths of time and some who were not breast-fed.

In order to produce breast milk, a *lactating* mother need only consume a healthy diet of vegetables, fruits, grains and proteins. She can obtain calcium from a variety of nondairy foods such as dark green vegetables, seeds, nuts and bony fish. Contrary to a popular misconception, it is not necessary to drink milk to make milk.

Women should not breast-feed their infants if they (the women) are taking medications that pass into breast-milk, or if they have certain infections such as HIV, **chickenpox**, or active **tuberculosis**. If a mother cannot or is unwilling to breast feed her baby, infant formula may provide a satisfactory alternative to breast milk.

Even though breast-feeding is a natural process, many mothers who decide to breast-feed benefit from taking a breast-feeding class. Potential problems associated with breast-feeding include sore, swollen (engorged) breasts and/or cracked nipples. Both the La Leche League and the Nursing Mother's Breast-feeding Council provide information on breast-feeding. Most hospitals now have nurses who specialize in breast-feeding.

Breastfeeding is also advantageous to the mother; for example, it helps her lose weight more easily. A mother burns calories during milk production; and some of the weight gained during **pregnancy** is intended for lactation. Breastfeeding also releases a hormone in a woman's body that causes her uterus to return to its normal size and shape more quickly. Yet another hormone released during breastfeeding acts as a natural tranquilizer, promoting a sense of calm and well-being in the mother while she is breastfeeding.

A doctor's advice should be sought when switching from breast milk (or infant formula) to cow's milk. Some authorities advise waiting until the infant is at least one year old before making this transition.

BREAST SIZE PROCEDURES

Breast size procedures are performed to increase or decrease the size of the breast. The two types of breast size procedures are *breast implantation and breast reduction.* Breast implantation is a surgical procedure for enlarging the breast. Breast-shaped sacks made of a silicone outer shell and filled with silicone gel or saline (salt water), called *implants*, are used. Breast implantation is usually performed to make normal breasts larger for cosmetic purposes. Sometimes a woman having a breast reconstruction after a **mastectomy** will need the opposite breast enlarged to make the breasts more symmetric. Breasts that are very unequal in size due to trauma or congenital deformity may also be corrected with an enlargement procedure.

A cosmetic breast enlargement is usually an outpatient procedure. It may be done under local or general **anesthesia**, depending on patient and physician preference. The incision is made through the armpit, under the breast, or around the areola (the darkened area around the nipple). These techniques create the most inconspicuous scars. The implant is placed between the breast tissue and underlying chest muscle, or under the chest muscle. The operation takes approximately one to two hours. The cost of a cosmetic procedure is rarely covered by insurance. However, if enlargement is part of breast reconstruction after a mastectomy, health plans may pay for some or all of it. The surgeon's fee ranges from $2,700-$4,200 and up. The procedure may also be called breast augmentation or augmentation mammaplasty.

Breast enlargement may result in decreased sensation in the breast, or interference with breast-feeding. Implants can also make it more difficult to read and interpret mammograms, possibly delaying **breast cancer** detection. Also, the implant itself can rupture and leak, or become displaced. A thick scar that normally forms around the implant, called a capsule, can become very hard. This is called capsular contracture, and may result in **pain** and/or an altered appearance of the breast. The older the implant, the greater the chances that these problems will occur.

There has been publicity about possible health risks from breast implants. Most concerns have focused on silicone gel-filled implants. As of 1992, the Food and Drug Administration (FDA) restricted the use of this type of implant, and ordered further studies. Today only saline-filled implants are used for cosmetic breast surgery. Recent studies have shown no evidence long-term health risks from silicone implants. However, research on the possible links between these implants and autoimmune or connective tissue diseases is continuing.

Breast reduction is a surgical procedure performed in order to decrease the size of the breasts. Women with very large breasts (macromastia or mammary hyperplasia) seek breast reduction for relief of **pain** in the back, shoulder, and neck. They may also feel uncomfortable about their breast size and have difficulty finding clothing that will fit properly. Additionally, breast reduction may be needed after reconstructive surgery following the surgical removal of cancerous breast tissue (**mastectomy**), to make the breasts more symmetric.

Men who have enlarged breasts (**gynecomastia**) may also be candidates for breast reduction. However, excessive alcohol intake, smoking marijuana, or using anabolic steroids may cause gynecomastia, and surgery is not recommended for men who continue to use these products.

Breast reduction may also be called reduction mammaplasty. It is most often done in the hospital, under general anesthetic. However, studies have suggested that an outpatient procedure, using local anesthetic and mild sedation may be appropriate for some patients. The operation takes approximately two to four hours. The most commonly made incision encircles the areola (darkened area around the nipple) and extends downward and around the underside of the breast. This produces the least conspicuous scar. The excess tissue, fat, and skin are removed, and the nipple and areola are repositioned. In certain cases, **liposuction** (fat suctioning) is used to remove extra fat from the armpit area. A hospital stay of up to three days may be needed for recovery.

If considered medically necessary, breast reduction is covered by some insurance plans. However, a specified amount of breast tissue may need to be removed in order to qualify for coverage. Surgeon's fees range from $4,800-$6,500 and up.

Before surgery to reduce or increase breast size is performed, the woman should have a clear understanding of what her new breasts will look like. She and her physician should agree about the desired final result. Many surgeons find it helpful to have the patient review before and after pictures, to clarify expectations.

BRECKINRIDGE, MARY (1881-1965)

American nurse

Mary Breckinridge was an American nurse who started the Frontier Nursing Service in the Appalachian region of Kentucky, in order to provide health care to poor people who lived in remote mountain settlements. Breckinridge also founded the first school in America that trained and certified midwifes. Her efforts were instrumental in reducing the high infant and maternal mortality rates in pre World War II Appalachia.

Mary Breckinridge was born in Kentucky on Feb. 16, 1881. Her father, Clifton Breckinridge, was a US Congressman, and a diplomat to Russia under President Cleveland. Her grandfather, John Cabell Breckinridge, had been Vice President of the United States under Buchanan, and Secy. of War under Jefferson Davis. Breckinridge had three siblings, a brother Carson, born in 1878, a sister Lees born in 1884, and brother Clif born in 1895.

Raised amidst wealth and high society, Breckinridge traveled extensively in her youth. She grew up in her mother's ancestral home on a southern plantation in Oasis, Mississippi, in her father's ancestral home, near Lexington, Kentucky, and on her maternal grandmother's estate in Hazelwood, New York. During her teenage years, when her father served as a Russian diplomat, she lived in both Russia and western Europe. Tutored by French and German governesses at first, she later attended the Rosemont Dezaley Boarding School in Lausanne, Switzerland. Upon her return to the United States at the age of seventeen, she enrolled for two years of study at Miss Low's finishing school in Stamford, Connecticut. Several years later she began a brief marriage that ended in her husband's death in 1906. Driven by this loss, she chose to pursue a career in nursing. In 1907 she went to New York to begin her studies at the St. Lukes Hospital Training School. She graduated in 1910, and soon began a second marriage. Her first child, a boy whom she called Breckie, short for Breckinridge, was born on Jan. 21, 1914. A daughter, Polly, was born in 1916, but lived for only a few hours. Then Breckie died, after a brief illness, on Jan. 23, 1918. Shortly after the death of her son, Breckinridge divorced her second husband.

The death of her two children motivated Breckinridge to devote her life to improving the health of others. In 1918 she traveled to the slums of Washington DC, to nurse those fallen ill in the influenza epidemic. A year later she joined the Comité Américain pour les Régions Dévastées de la France. Within a few months of reporting to a small town just north of Paris, she asked permission to organize a visiting nurse program. Two years later, her program a success, she was supervising dozens of women, trained as both nurses and midwifes, who would travel about France caring for young children and pregnant women. In the United States there were as yet no schools of midwifery, and when Breckinridge returned home in 1921, she vowed she would start one. In 1922 she entered the Teachers College of Columbia University in NYC, to study public-health nursing. In the summer of 1923 she conducted a public health survey in the Appalachian Mountains of Kentucky. Riding over 650 miles on mule and horseback she traveled along trails in Appalachia and interviewed the ''granny women'' who attended the delivery of babies. They were largely illiterate and none were trained in nursing. No licensed physicians served the region, which had one of the highest birth rates in the country, as well as the highest infant mortality.

After completing her studies at Columbia University, Breckinridge traveled to England to enroll at the British Hospital for Mothers and Babies in southeast London. In 1924 she obtained her certificate in midwifery, then went on to the Highlands and Islands Medical and Nursing Service in Scotland for additional training. In both England and Scotland, Breckinridge witnessed the correlation between the low incidence of death during childbirth, the low infant mortality, and the high quality of care-giving provided by the nurse midwives. Meanwhile, in America, the death rate for women in childbirth was amongst the highest in the developed world.

Arriving in Leslie County, Kentucky, in May of 1925, Breckinridge announced her intent to bring a nursing and midwifery service to Appalachia. The Kentucky Committee for Mothers and Babies, which in 1928 changed its name to the Frontier Nursing Service, established itself that summer in the town of Hyden. A two-story building with a small medicine dispensary served as headquarters. Breckinridge hired six nurse midwifes trained in England and Scotland, to provide general health care and to attend births on their daily rounds in the county. No reliable transportation existed other than horseback and mule, and the women soon became known as the ''nurses on horseback.'' Within a year, as word of the service spread, American nurses began to arrive in Hyden. Originally funded by the personal wealth of the Breckinridge family, the success of the service eventually attracted large donations. By 1928, enough funds had been raised to establish a small hospital in Hyden, and to hire a medical director with training in obstetrics. The small nursing staff formed the American Association of Nurse-Midwifes that same year. By the early 1930s, the service was reaching one thousand rural families in a seven hundred square mile area, and had established several outpost nursing centers. In addition to delivering babies, the service treated such then-common illnesses as tuberculosis and trachoma. In 1931 while traveling on horseback, Breckinridge suffered a serious fall, crushing a vertebra in the small of her back. For over a year she was unable to mount a horse. The accident left her dependent on a steel brace for the remainder of her life.

As the Frontier Nursing Service grew, Breckinridge began sending American nurses to England for midwife training. Eventually the expense became too high, and plans were made to establish the Frontier School of Midwifery and Family Nursing, the first such school in America. In the early 1940s, the school began graduating Certified Midwives (CM), licensed to practice in Kentucky. Their training included a six-month program of classroom instruction and fieldwork.

Breckinridge died at age of 84, on May 16. 1965. She was buried along side her two children in a Lexington, Kentucky cemetery. In her forty years of work with the Frontier Nursing Service, well over 50,000 registered patients were treated and over a quarter of a million inoculations were administered. Only eleven maternal deaths were recorded.

Bretonneau, Pierre Fidèle (1778-1862)

French physician

Bretonneau was the first person to study and describe fully the symptoms of **diphtheria**, and gave the disease its name. He also believed there was a difference between typhoid fever and **typhus**, which were often mistaken as the same disease. In a time before anyone understood that pathogens (germs) cause disease and infection, Bretonneau suspected that these diseases were contagious, believing that diphtheria was transmitted between individuals from drinking glasses. His suspicion was an entire generation earlier than **Louis Pasteur**'s **germ theory**.

Bretonneau was born in Saint-Georges-sur-Cher in France. His father, Pierre, was a master surgeon and his mother, Elisabeth Lecomte, was from a wealthy, upper-class family. Oddly enough, Bretonneau received virtually no education as a young child and was still unable to read at the age of nine. He was sent to the École de Santé in Paris in 1795 where he attended medical lectures, but left in 1801 after being unfairly failed in an examination. He entered the field of public health, becoming an officer, and his medical skill quickly gained him recognition. He was asked to be chief physician at the hospital of Tours, for which he needed a degree. So he sat for his final exam, wrote his doctoral thesis, and took the position in 1815. He also became director of École de Santé where he lectured to medical students. However, he left both positions in 1838 to devote his time and medical skills to the poor.

Bretonneau gained a reputation as a dedicated and capable physician and therapist whose lectures based on the medical philosophy of **Hippocrates** (460-377 B.C.) earned him a great deal of respect from his students. His close scrutiny of the symptoms of diphtheria when the epidemic swept through Tours from 1818-1820 led him to discover that a leathery parchment-like membrane (the name diphtheria comes from the Greek word for leather) formed in the throat of the patient, ultimately causing asphyxiation (suffocation). His desire to help prevent **death** through asphyxiation led him to invent a device called the double cannula (a small tube for insertion into a body cavity) with which he performed the first successful **tracheotomy** in 1825 on a four year old girl. By cutting an opening into the windpipe through her neck, he saving her life. Four previous attempts to save other children had failed, but as a result of his determination and ultimate success, another physician by the name of Trousseau soon reported performing successful tracheotomies on more than 200 children with diphtheria.

In 1819, Bretonneau also identified typhoid fever as being a different from typhus—the two originally thought to have been the same disease. Also, because these diseases produce lesions, or sores, of the mucous membranes that go through cyclical changes in appearance as the disease progresses, each stage was originally believed to be a different disease when first observed at one of the progressive stages. Because of his keen observation skills, Bretonneau understood the cyclic development of the individual disease.

He was also able to prove that the mucous membranes respond differently to different microorganisms (germs), just as the skin shows many different reactions to different diseases, and firmly believed that a single, contagious agent caused disease to spread from one person to another. In 1829, he described fully the course of the typhoid epidemic at Chenonceaux, giving sound evidence for the way in which it spread. Regardless of all his observation skills, Bretonneau wrote very few monographs; rather, he felt it most important to pass his findings on to his students, upon whom he made a deep and lasting impression.

Bretonneau gained a reputation as ''independent, proud yet modest, and disdainful of honors.'' He also had many interests beside medicine: he constructed hydraulic hammers, thermometers and barometers, was a first-class botanist (he wrote an essay on grafting plants), studied the habits of bees and ants, and his private garden in Palluau was famous throughout all of Europe. He was 25 years younger than his first wife and, at the age of 78, married a young woman of 18. He was 84 when he died.

See also Diphtheria; Germ theory; Tracheotomy; Typhoid fever; Typhus

Broca, Pierre Paul (1824-1880)

French anthropologist and anatomist

Pierre Paul Broca, the son of a Huguenot doctor, was born near Bordeaux, France, in 1824. After studying mathematics and physical science at the local university, he entered medical school at the University of Paris in 1841. He received his M.D. in 1849. Though trained as a pathologist, anatomist, and surgeon, Broca's interests were not limited to the medical profession. His versatility and tireless dedication to science permitted him to make significant contributions to other fields, most notably to anthropology.

The application of his expertise in anatomy outside the field of medicine began in 1847 as a member of a commission charged with reporting on archaeological excavations of a cemetery. The project permitted Broca to combine his anatomical and mathematical skills with his interests in anthropology.

The discovery in 1856 of Neanderthal Man once again drew Broca into anthropology. Controversy surrounded the interpretation of Neanderthal. It was clearly a human skull, but more primitive and apelike than a modern skull and the soil stratum in which it was found indicated a very early date. Neanderthal's implications for evolutionary theory demanded thorough examination of the evidence to determine decisively whether it was simply a congenitally deformed *Homo sapiens* or a primitive human form. Both as an early supporter of Charles Darwin and as an expert in human anatomy, Broca supported the latter view. Broca's view eventually prevailed, though not until the discovery of the much more primitive Java Man (then known as *Pithecanthropus*, but later *Homo erectus*).

Broca is best known for his role in the discovery of specialized functions in different areas of the brain. In 1861, he was able to show, using post-mortem analysis of patients who had lost the ability to speak, that such loss was associated with damage to a specific area of the brain. The area, located toward the front of the brain's left hemisphere, became known as Broca's convolution. Aside from its importance to the understanding of human physiology, Broca's findings addressed questions concerning the evolution of language.

All animals living in groups communicate with one another. Non-human primates have the most complex communication system other than human language. They use a wide range of gestures, facial expressions, postures, and vocalizations, but are limited in the variety of expressions and are unable to generate new signals under changing circumstances. Humans alone possess the capacity for language rather than relying on a body language vocabulary. Language permits humans to generate an infinite number of messages and ultimately allows the transmission of information—the learned and shared patterns of behavior characteristic of human social groups, which anthropologists call culture—from generation to generation. The development of language spurred human evolution by permitting new ways of social interaction, organization, and thought.

Given the importance assigned to human speech in human evolution, scientists began to look for the physical preconditions of speech. The fact that apes have the minimal parts necessary for speech indicated that the shape and arrangement of the vocal apparatus was insufficient for the development of speech. The vocalizations produced by other animals are involuntary and incapable of conscious alteration. However, human speech requires codifying thought and transmitting it in patterned strings of sound. The area of the brain isolated by Broca sends the code to another part of the brain that controls the muscles of the face, jaw, tongue, palate, and larynx, setting the speech apparatus in motion. This area and a companion area that controls the understanding of language, known as Wernicke's area, are detectable in early fossil skulls of the genus *Homo*. The brain of *Homo* was evolving toward the use of language, although the vocal chamber was still inadequate to articulate speech. Broca discovered one piece in the puzzle of human communication and speech, which permits the transmission of culture.

Equally important, Broca contributed to the development of physical anthropology, one of the four subfields of anthropology. Craniology, the scientific measurement of the skull, was a major focus of physical anthropology during this period. Mistakenly considering contemporary human groups as if they were living fossils, anthropologists became interested in the nature of human variability and attempted to explain the varying levels of technological development observed worldwide by looking for a correspondence between cultural level and physical characteristics. Broca furthered these studies by inventing at least twenty-seven instruments for making measurements of the human body, and by developing standardized techniques of measurement.

Broca's many contributions to anthropology helped to establish its firm scientific foundation at a time when the study of nature was considered a somewhat sinister science.

Bronchitis

Bronchitis is an inflammation of the air passages between the nose and the lungs, including the trachea (windpipe) and the larger air tubes of the lung that bring air in from the trachea (bronchi). Bronchitis can either be of brief duration (acute) or a long-term disease (chronic).

Acute bronchitis is most prevalent in winter. It usually follows a viral infection, such as a cold or the flu, and can be accompanied by a secondary bacterial infection. Acute bronchitis usually begins with the symptoms of a cold, such as a runny nose, sneezing, and dry cough. However, the **cough** soon becomes deep and painful. Coughing brings up a greenish yellow phlegm or sputum. These symptoms may be accompanied by a **fever** of up to 102°F (38.8°C). **Wheezing** after coughing is common.

In uncomplicated acute bronchitis, the fever and most other symptoms disappear after three to five days. While acute bronchitis typically resolves completely within two weeks, the cough associated with it may persist for several weeks longer. Like any upper airway inflammatory process, acute bronchitis may increase a person's likelihood of developing **pneumonia**. Acute bronchitis is often complicated by a bacterial infection, in which case the fever and a general feeling of illness may persist. The bacterial infection should be treated with **antibiotics**.

Anyone can get acute bronchitis, but infants, young children, and the elderly are more likely to get the disease because they generally have weaker immune systems. Smokers, people with heart or other lung diseases, and individuals exposed to chemical fumes or high levels of air pollution are also at higher risk of developing acute bronchitis.

Chronic bronchitis is one of a group of diseases that are called chronic obstructive pulmonary disease (COPD). Other diseases in this category include emphysema and chronic asthmatic bronchitis. Chronic bronchitis may progress to emphysema, or both diseases may be present together.

Chronic bronchitis develops slowly over time. A mild cough, sometimes called smokers' cough, is usually the first visible sign of the disease. Coughing brings up phlegm, and wheezing and **shortness of breath** may accompany the cough. Diagnostic tests will show a decrease in lung function. As the disease advances, breathing becomes difficult and activity decreases. To diagnose chronic bronchitis, these symptoms must be present for at least three months in each of two consecutive years.

Chronic bronchitis is caused by inhaling bronchial irritants, especially cigarette smoke. The American Lung Association estimates that 80-90% of COPD cases are caused by smoking. Other irritants include chemical fumes, air pollution, and environmental irritants, such as mold or dust. Until recently, more men than women developed chronic bronchitis, but as the number of women who smoke has increased, so has their rate of chronic bronchitis. Because this disease progresses slowly, middle-aged and older people are more likely to be diagnosed with chronic bronchitis.

Initial diagnosis of bronchitis is based on observing the patient's symptoms and health history. The physician will listen to the patient's chest with a stethoscope for sounds that indicate lung inflammation and narrowing of the airways, such as moist rales, crackling, and wheezing. Moist rales are a bubbling sound caused by fluid in the bronchial tubes.

A **sputum culture** may be performed, particularly if the sputum is green or has blood in it, to determine whether a bacterial infection is present and to identify the disease-causing organism so that an appropriate antibiotic can be selected. Normally, the patient will be asked to cough deeply, then spit the material that comes up from the lungs (sputum) into a cup. This sample is then grown in the laboratory to determine which organisms are present. The results are available in two to three days, except for tests for **tuberculosis**, which can take as long as two months.

A pulmonary function test is important in diagnosing chronic bronchitis and other variations of COPD. This test involves breathing into an instrument called a spirometer. The spirometer measures the amount of air entering and leaving the lungs. The test is painless and is done in the doctor's office.

To better determine what type of obstructive lung disease a patient has, the doctor may also do a **chest x-ray**, electrocardiogram (ECG), and/or blood tests. An electrocardiogram is an instrument that is used to measure the electrical activity of the heart and is useful in the diagnosis of heart conditions.

When no secondary infection is present, acute bronchitis is treated in the same way as the **common cold**. Home care includes drinking plenty of fluids, resting, not smoking, increasing moisture in the air with a cool mist humidifier, and taking **acetaminophen** (Datril, Tylenol, Panadol) for fever and pain. **Aspirin** should not be given to children because of its association with the serious illness **Reye's syndrome**.

Cough suppressant lozenges (drops) or syrups are used only when the cough is dry and produces no phlegm. If the patient is coughing up phlegm, the cough should be allowed to continue. The purpose of the cough it to bring up extra mucus and irritants from the lungs. When coughing is suppressed, the phlegm accumulates in the plugged airways and can become a breeding ground for pneumonia bacteria.

Expectorant cough medicines, unlike cough suppressants, do not stop the cough. Instead they are used to thin the mucus in the lungs, making it easier to cough up. This type of cough medicine may be helpful to individuals suffering from bronchitis. People who are unsure about what type of medications are in over-the-counter cough syrups should ask their pharmacist for an explanation.

If a secondary bacterial infection is present with the bronchitis, the infection is treated with an antibiotic. Patients need to take the entire amount of antibiotic prescribed. Stopping the antibiotic early can lead to a return of the infection.

The treatment of chronic bronchitis is complex and depends on the stage of chronic bronchitis and whether other health problems are present. Lifestyle changes, such as quitting smoking and avoiding secondhand smoke or polluted air, are an important first step. Controlled exercise performed on a regular basis is also important.

Drug therapy begins with **bronchodilators**. These drugs relax the muscles of the bronchial tubes and allow increased air flow. They can be taken by mouth or inhaled using a nebulizer. A nebulizer is a device that delivers a regulated flow of medication into the airways. Common bronchodilators include albuterol (Ventolin, Proventil, Apo-Salvent) and metaproterenol (Alupent, Orciprenaline, Metaprel, Dey-Dose).

Anti-inflammatory medications are added to reduce swelling of the airway tissue. **Corticosteroids**, such as prednisone, can be taken orally or intravenously. Other steroids are inhaled. Long-term steroid use can have serious side effects. Other drugs, such as ipratropium (Atrovent), are given to reduce the quantity of mucus produced.

As the disease progresses, the patient may need supplemental oxygen. There are many complications of COPD that often require hospitalization in the latter stages of the disease.

Alternative practitioners focus on prevention by eating a healthy diet that strengthens the immune system and practicing **stress** management. Bronchitis can become serious if it progresses to pneumonia, therefore, antibiotics may be required. In addition, there are a multitude of botanical and herbal medicines that can be formulated to treat bronchitis. Some examples include inhaling eucalyptus or other essential oils in warm steam. **Homeopathic medicine** and traditional Chinese medicine may also be very useful for bronchitis, and **hydrotherapy** can contribute to cleaning the chest and stimulating immune response.

When treated, acute bronchitis normally resolves in one to two weeks without complications, although a cough may continue for several more weeks. The progression of chronic bronchitis, on the other hand, may be slowed, and an initial improvement in symptoms may be achieved. Unfortunately, however, there is no cure for chronic bronchitis, and the disease can often lead to or coexist with emphysema. Chronic bronchitis is a major cause of disability and **death** in the United States. The American Lung Association estimates that about 14 million Americans suffer from the disease.

The best way to prevent bronchitis is not to begin smoking or to stop smoking. Other preventative steps include avoiding chemical and environmental irritants, such as air pollution, and maintaining good overall health. Immunizations against certain types of pneumonia (as well as **influenza**) are an important preventative measure for anyone with lung or immune system diseases.

BRONCHODILATORS

Bronchodilators are medicines that help open the bronchial tubes (airways) of the lungs, allowing more air to flow through them. They are used by people with the condition **asthma**. People with asthma have trouble breathing, because their airways are inflamed and narrowed.

Normally, air moves smoothly through the airways and into the tiny air sacs of the lungs while a person is breathing in (inhaling). Breathing out (exhaling) happens automatically when the person stops inhaling. In a person with asthma, inhaling is not a problem. Incoming air can slide around the blockage, because the act of inhaling makes the airways expand. The problem comes when the person with asthma tries to exhale. The air can no longer get past the blockage, and it remains trapped in the lungs. The person can then only take shallow breaths. Bronchodilators work by relaxing the smooth muscles that line the airways. This makes the airways open wider and allows air to leave the lungs. These drugs also are used to relieve breathing problems associated with emphysema, chronic **bronchitis**, and other lung diseases.

Some bronchodilators are inhaled, using a nebulizer or an inhalation aerosol. Others are taken as injections or by mouth. Examples of prescription bronchodilators are albuterol (Proventil, Ventolin), epinephrine (Primatene), ipratropium (Atrovent), metaproterenol (Alupent, Metaprel), and terbutaline (Brethine). A few bronchodilators, such as ephedrine, can be bought without a physician's prescription. However, even over-the-counter bronchodilators should only be used as recommended by a physician.

Check with the doctor who prescribed the bronchodilator or the pharmacist who filled the prescription for the correct dosage of the drug. Always use these medicines exactly as directed. Taking larger than recommended doses or using the medicine too often can lead to serious side effects and even **death**.

People with certain medical conditions or who are taking certain other medicines can have problems if they use bronchodilators. In addition, anyone who has had unusual reactions to any bronchodilator or an inhaled form of any other drug in the past should let his or her physician know before taking the drugs again. If symptoms do not improve or if they get worse after using a bronchodilator, call a physician right away.

Some bronchodilators pass into breast milk. Breastfeeding mothers should check with their physicians before using bronchodilators.

Before using bronchodilators, people with any of these medical conditions should make sure their physicians are aware of their conditions:

- **Allergies**—to sulfites, foods, medications, or other substances.
- **Pregnancy**
- **Glaucoma**
- Brain damage
- Convulsions (**seizures**)—recently or anytime in the past
- **Mental illness**
- **Parkinson's disease**
- **Diabetes**
- Heart or blood vessel diseases
- Rapid or irregular heartbeat
- High blood pressure
- Overactive thyroid
- **Enlarged prostate**
- Obstruction of the neck of the bladder.

The most common bronchodilator side effects are nervousness or restlessness and trembling. These problems usually go away as the body adjusts to the drug and do not require medical treatment. Less common side effects, such as dry mouth or throat, bad taste in the mouth, **cough**ing, dizziness or lightheadedness, drowsiness, headache, sweating, fast or pounding heartbeat, muscle cramps or twitches, nausea, vomiting, **diarrhea**, sleep problems and weakness also may occur and do not need medical attention unless they do not go away or they interfere with normal activities.

More serious side effects are not common, but may occur. If any of the following side effects occur, check with the physician who prescribed the medicine as soon as possible:

- Chest **pain** or discomfort
- Irregular heartbeat
- Unusual bruising
- Hives or rash
- Swelling
- Wheezing or other breathing problems
- Numbness in the hands or feet
- Blurred vision

Bronchodilators may interact with a number of other medicines. When this happens, the effects of one or both of the drugs may change or the risk of side effects may be greater. Be sure to check with a physician or pharmacist before combining bronchodilators with any other prescription or nonprescription (over-the-counter) medicine.

Brown, Michael S. (1941-)

American geneticist

Michael S. Brown, a genetics professor and director of the Center for Genetic Diseases at the University of Texas Southwestern Medical School, is one of America's foremost experts on cholesterol metabolism in the human body. In the 1970s, Brown and Joseph Goldstein investigated familial hypercholesterolemia, a dangerous inherited disorder which causes elevated levels of cholesterol in the blood. Their research led them to the discovery of a protein in the membranes of a cell, called the LDL receptor, which plays a central role in the body's ability to lower cholesterol levels. For this discovery and their subsequent research on the LDL receptor, Brown and Goldstein shared the 1985 Nobel Prize in physiology or medicine.

Brown was born in New York City on April 13, 1941, to Harvey and Evelyn Katz Brown. He attended the University of Pennsylvania as an undergraduate, receiving his bachelor's degree in 1962. Following his graduation, Brown enrolled in the medical school at the University of Pennsylvania, where he was awarded the Frederick Packard Prize in Internal Medicine for his research. He earned his M.D. in 1966 and served as an intern and a resident at Massachusetts General Hospital in Boston. It was during his residency that he met Joseph Goldstein, his future research partner, who was also on the staff at Massachusetts General.

In 1968, Brown was made a clinical associate at the National Institutes of Health (NIH) in Bethesda, Maryland. He was assigned to the biochemistry lab, where he worked with Earl Stadtman, head of the laboratory for the National Heart, Lung, and Blood Institute. While at NIH, Brown focused his research on gastroenterology, particularly on the role of enzymes in digestive chemistry. In 1971, while studying a particular enzyme involved in the production of cholesterol, Brown was offered a position as an assistant professor at the University of Texas Southwestern Medical School in Dallas. He accepted, and Goldstein, who had also served at NIH in Bethesda, joined the Texas Southwestern faculty a year later. At this time the two began a collaboration which was to distinguish them as pioneers in genetics.

In Dallas during the 1970s, Brown and Goldstein examined skin samples from people who suffered from hypercholesterolemia, specifically those rare patients whose condition was homozygous, meaning that they had not just one defective gene but two. In these cases, patients often exhibited extremely high levels of low-density lipoprotein, LDL, even during childhood. LDL carries cholesterol to the cells, and in excessive quantities can clog arteries and encourage heart disease. Brown and Goldstein discovered that the cells of these patients were missing a crucial protein, called a receptor, which binds to LDL and regulates its level in the body. Without the protein, the body can not break down LDL, and it accumulates in the blood. Brown and Goldstein's breakthrough was the discovery and isolation of this LDL receptor protein.

Brown and Goldstein not only identified the LDL receptor, they also located the gene responsible for its production. By sequencing and cloning the gene, they were able to localize the gene mutations responsible for familial hypercholesterolemia, as well as other inherited conditions involving cholesterol metabolism. Their findings also led to possible drug therapies for people with cholesterol disorders. By administering a combination of drugs which would inhibit the liver's ability to synthesize cholesterol, Brown and Goldstein increased their patients' need for cholesterol from outside sources. The patients' bodies subsequently produced more LDL receptors, and their cholesterol levels fell sharply. They also found that a liver transplant can correct genetic deficiencies in the production or expression of LDL receptors. In later research, Brown and Goldstein engineered a mouse which, because of its abnormally high numbers of LDL receptors, could eat a high-fat diet and yet show no significant rise in LDL.

In a remarkable series of experiments, Brown and Goldstein were ultimately able to define and analyze each step in the path of cholesterol through the body, from production to dissolution. They also demonstrated a mechanism by which a low-fat diet and regular exercise can decrease cholesterol levels. Brown and Goldstein's work had significant implications not only for genetic defects, but also for nutrition and fitness. In addition, the team's research methods contributed to a greater understanding of cell receptors in general, serving as a model for research on over twenty other receptors. In the words of the Nobel Prize committee, as quoted in the *New York Times,* Brown and Goldstein "revolutionized our knowledge about the regulation of cholesterol metabolism and the treatment of diseases caused by abnormally elevated cholesterol levels in the blood."

In addition to the Nobel Prize, Brown has received several honorary degrees and a number of awards for his research, including the Pfizer Award from the American Chemical Society in 1976, the Albert Lasker Medical Research Award in 1985, and the National Medal of Science in 1988. He has been a member of the National Academy of Sciences since 1980. He was appointed Paul J. Thomas Professor of Genetics and director of the Center for Genetic Diseases at the University of Texas Southwestern Medical School, positions he has held since 1977.

Brown balances his scientific and medial careers, and despite his success as a researcher, he still makes rounds at the hospital. He is also well known for his entertaining style of scientific presentations. While still in medical school at Penn, Brown married Alice Lapin on June 21, 1964, and they have two daughters.

BRUCE, DAVID (1855-1931)

Scottish microbiologist

Bruce is noted for his work in parasitology, especially for his discovery of the cause of brucellosis and **sleeping sickness**. Born in Melbourne, Australia, to Scottish immigrants, Bruce and his parents returned to Scotland when he was five years old. Although Bruce longed to become a professional athlete, he was stricken with **pneumonia** at age 17. Bruce studied natural history and medicine at the University of Edinburgh, and after graduation, he found a job working with a doctor. He later met Mary Elizabeth Steele, whom he married in 1883. The couple subsequently began a lifelong partnership in medical science.

After joining the Army Medical Service, David and Mary Bruce were assigned to Malta in 1884, where Bruce began a study of an often-fatal disease suffered by English soldiers assigned to the Maltese garrison. The disease, known as *Malta, Mediterranean,* or *undulating fever,* caused chills, sweats, and weakness. Using a microscope, Bruce described the cause as a ''micrococcus'' growing in the spleens of patients. Eventually, the organism was isolated by Danish scientist Bernhard L. F. Bang (1848-1932).

In 1905, a scientific team headed by Bruce found that the soldiers were contracting the disease by drinking the milk of infected goats. Goats' milk was thus eliminated from the soldiers' diets, and the disease vanished. Soon, physicians were calling the disease *brucellosis* in honor of Bruce. However, the fight against the disease was not yet over. Almost twenty years passed before physician **Alice Catherine Evans** discovered that brucellosis was often transmitted by the milk of cows as well as goats, leading to a drive to pasteurize all milk products and ultimately a decline in the disease's occurrence in humans.

After leaving Malta in 1889, Bruce was stationed in Africa. He conducted research in Zululand and Uganda on *nagana*, a common disease affecting domestic animals. He found that the infected tsetse flies could transmit the disease to humans. In 1903, after directing a hospital during the Boer War, Bruce was named director of the Royal Society's Sleeping Sickness Commission. With Aldo Castellani (1877-1971), Bruce and his colleagues isolated and described the microorganism that caused the disease, a worm-like parasite called a trypanosome. Bruce was then able to prove that the tsetse fly was the transmitter.

Bruce was knighted in 1908. By 1914, the Bruces had returned to England, where David served as commandant of the Royal Army Medical College. He directed scientific research during World War I and worked on **tetanus** antitoxins. He died in 1931, just four days after his wife's death. Before dying, David Bruce asked that any account of his work should acknowledge his wife's assistance and support.

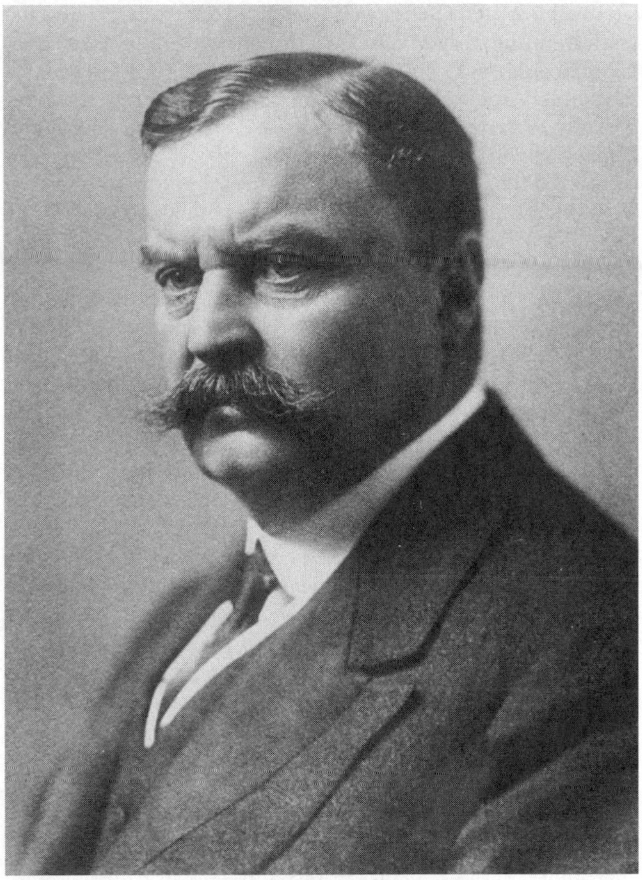

David Bruce

BRUCELLOSIS

Brucellosis is a bacterial disease caused by members of the *Brucella* genus that can infect humans but primarily infects livestock. Symptoms of the disease include intermittent **fever**, sweating, chills, aches, and mental depression. The disease can become chronic and recur, particularly if untreated.

Also known as undulant fever, Malta fever, Gibralter fever, Bang's disease, or Mediterranean fever, brucellosis is most likely to occur among those individuals who regularly work with livestock. The disease originated in domestic livestock but was passed on to wild animal species, including the elk and buffalo of the western United States. In humans, brucellosis continues to be spread via unpasteurized milk obtained from infected cows or through contact with the discharges of cattle and goats during miscarriage. In areas of the world where milk is not pasteurized, for example in Latin America and the Mediterranean, the disease is still contracted by ingesting unpasteurized dairy products. However, in the United States, the widespread pasteurization of milk and nearly complete eradication of the infection from cattle has reduced the number of human cases from 6,500 in 1940 to about 70 in 1994.

Brucellosis is caused by several different species of parasitic bacteria of the genus Brucella. A human contracts the disease by coming into contact with an infected animal and either allowing the bacteria to enter a cut, breathing in the bacteria, or by consuming unpasteurized milk or fresh goat cheese obtained from a contaminated animal. In the United States, the disease is primarily confined to slaughterhouse workers.

Scientists do not agree about whether brucellosis can be transmitted from one person to another. Some people have reportedly been infected with the disease through blood **transfusion** or bone marrow transplant. Newborn babies have also contracted the illness from their mothers during birth. It is believed that brucellosis can also be transmitted sexually.

The disease is not usually fatal, but the fevers can be exhausting. Symptoms usually appear between five days and a month after exposure and begin with a single bout of high fever accompanied by shivering, aching, and drenching sweats that last for a few days. Other symptoms may include **headache**, poor appetite, backache, weakness, and depression. Mental depression can be so severe that the patient may become suicidal.

In rare, untreated cases, the disease can become so severe that it leads to fatal complications, such as **pneumonia** or bacterial **meningitis**. Infection by the Brucella bacteria *B. melitensis* can cause miscarriage, especially during the first three months of **pregnancy**. Brucellosis can also occur in a chronic form, in which symptoms recur over a period of months or years.

Brucellosis is usually diagnosed by detecting one or more *Brucella* species in blood or urine samples. Blood samples will also indicate elevated antibody levels or increased amounts of a protein produced directly in response to infection with brucellosis bacteria.

Early diagnosis and prompt treatment is essential to prevent chronic infection. Untreated, the disease may linger for years, but it is rarely fatal. Prolonged treatment with antibiotic drugs, including **tetracyclines** (with streptomycin), co-trimoxazole, and **sulfonamides**, is effective. Bed rest is also important. In the chronic form of brucellosis, the symptoms may recur, requiring a second course of medication.

There is no human vaccine for brucellosis, but humans can be protected by controlling the disease in livestock. After checking to make sure an animal is not already infected, and destroying those that are, all livestock should be immunized. Butchers and those who work in slaughterhouses should wear protective glasses and clothing, and protect broken skin from infection.

Some experts suggest that a person with the disease refrain from engaging in unprotected sex until free of the disease. The sexual partners of an infected person should also be closely monitored for signs of infection.

Bruises

Bruises, or ecchymoses, commonly refer to bleeding that is confined within a tissue of the body. Healthy people will develop bruising from blunt injury or with **sprains and strains**. In some cases, individuals may just have naturally fragile blood vessels which cause them to bruise easily. However, there are also a number of diseases that cause excessive bruising.

Bruised tissue changes colors as it resolves and is reabsorbed. Initially dark red or purple, it fades through green to orange and then yellow. Sometimes bleeding that happens in one place will appear in another. For instance, retroperitoneal bleeding (into the back of the abdomen) will eventually appear in the groin, and bleeding into the thigh or knee will work its way down to the ankle.

An abnormal tendency to bruise can be due to hereditary bleeding disorders like **hemophilia**, to drugs like coumadin, to diseases of the blood-forming organs like leukemia, or to diseases that increase the fragility of blood vessels. When large bruises develop from minor injuries or reoccur frequently in the same place, they may indicate one of these problems. Easy or unusual brusing should be evaluated by a physician to determine the cause.

A bruise by itself needs no treatment. Ice (ideally a bag with ice and water in it) during the first several hours will reduce the amount of bleeding. Rest, elevation of the injured body part, and applying pressure to the bruised area with an elastic bandage will also slow the accumulation of blood. Twenty-four hours after acquiring the bruise, heat, especially moist heat, will promote healing of the injured tissues.

Eating green, leafy vegetables, a principle dietary source of Vitamin K, may help reduce bruising. Infants receive an injection of Vitamin K at birth to prevent their tendency to develop this deficiency at about two weeks of age. Orange-colored and dark-colored bioflavanoids, from fruits and vegetables (especially blueberries and cherries) can assist in strengthening the connective tissue, slowing the spread of bleeding within the tissue. *Arnica*, a homeopathic remedy, can be used in case of trauma to lessen bruising. Any astringent herb applied to the skin (such as witch hazel) will tighten the tissue, decreasing bruising.

On rare occasions, a bruise is so large the body cannot completely absorb it. It then turns into a lake of old blood that must be surgically removed. Even more rarely, the lake may become subsequently infected and turn into an **abscess**.

Bruxism

Bruxism is the habit of clenching and grinding the teeth. It usually occurs at night during sleep, but it may also occur during the day. Approximately one in four adults experiences it, but because it is an unconscious habit, most people are not aware of it until their teeth have been damaged.

While bruxism is typically associated with **stress**, anger, or anxiety, it may also be caused by abnormal occlusion (the way the upper and lower teeth fit together), or crooked or missing teeth.

Symptoms of bruxism include: dull **headache**s; sore and tired facial muscles; earaches; sensitive teeth; and locking, popping, and clicking of the jaw.

During a dental examination, a dentist may recognize damage resulting from bruxism, including: enamel loss from the chewing surfaces of teeth; flattened tooth surfaces; loosened teeth; and fractured teeth and fillings. Left untreated, bruxism may lead to tooth loss and jaw dysfunction.

Medical and dental histories and examinations are necessary to differentiate bruxism from other conditions that may cause similar **pain**, such as ear infections, dental infections, and temporomandibular joint (TMJ) dysfunction. However, uncommonly worn-down teeth strongly suggest a diagnosis of bruxism.

To prevent further damage to the teeth, bruxism is treated by placing a removable, custom-fitted plastic appliance called a night guard between the upper and lower teeth. Although the clenching and grinding behavior may continue, the teeth wear away the plastic instead of each other.

In some cases, abnormal occlusion may be adjusted and high spots removed so that the teeth fit together in a more comfortable position. Missing teeth may be replaced and crooked teeth may be straightened with orthodontic treatment to eliminate possible underlying causes of bruxism. In cases where jaw muscles are very tight, a dentist may prescribe **muscle relaxants**.

Stress management and behavior modification techniques may be useful to break the habit of clenching and teeth grinding. Tight jaw muscles may be relaxed by applying warm compresses to the sides of the face. Herbal muscle relaxants also can be helpful. **Massage** therapy and deep tissue realignment can assist in releasing the clenching pattern. This is a more permanent alternative treatment for bruxism.

Bruxism may cause permanent damage to teeth and chronic jaw pain unless properly diagnosed and promptly treated. However, the behavior may be eliminated if its underlying causes are found and addressed. Increased awareness in patients prone to anxiety, stress, or anger may prevent the habit of bruxism from developing.

BUDD, WILLIAM (1811-1880)

British physician and epidemiologist

In an era when other physicians were ''noncontagionists'' and believed that infectious diseases were either ''atmospheric'' (airborne), arose from filth and neglect, or developed spontaneously in the soil, William Budd was a firm believer that infectious diseases, particularly **cholera** and typhoid, were contagious—that they were transmitted from one person to another through excrement. This theory was a forerunner to **Louis Pasteur**'s **germ theory**.

Budd was born in the small town of North Tawton, Devon, to Samuel Budd, a surgeon, and Catherine Wreford, who came from an old Devon family. Budd was one of 10 children and the fifth of nine boys. All children received their early education at home; however, after Samuel inherited land from his grandfather, an Anglican minister, they were sent to prestigious universities. Six became doctors—three graduating from Edinburgh and three from Cambridge.

Budd's education was prolonged because of a severe attack of **typhoid fever**, which interrupted his studies at École de Médecine in Paris, where he finally finished in 1837 to attend Edinburgh University to complete his M.D. He graduated in 1838 to practice general medicine in North Tawton, and was appointed assistant physician to the Seaman's Hospital in Greenwich 18 months later. Between 1839 and 1840, he studied more than 80 cases of typhoid at North Tawton, arriving at the conclusion that the ''poisons'' of the disease grew and multiplied in the intestines of the victim and were ''cast off'' in that person's excretions. Whatever these ''poisons'' were, he concluded (correctly) they contaminated water supplies and infected individuals who drank that water. He believed the same to be true of cholera and, against popular opinion, he implemented **public health** measures promoting the importance of disinfection and keeping water supplies clean and uncontaminated with sewage. In this way, he successfully curbed the 1866 outbreak of cholera in Bristol.

Budd applied his contagion theory to many other diseases, including **diphtheria**, **scarlet fever**, **tuberculosis**, and sheeppox. He contended that ''each specific agent of contagion multiplies at certain sites within the sick host, is eliminated and transported by definite routes, and can be destroyed or interrupted in its passage to other susceptible hosts.'' Even after publishing a compilation of his years of study in a classic monograph called *Typhoid Fever* (1873), many of his contemporaries continued to insist his theory was incorrect.

A severe second illness, which he believed to be a return of typhoid, forced Budd's early retirement from Seaman's Hospital. He moved to Bristol and spent the rest of his career at St. Peter's Hospital, Bristol Medical Center, and Bristol Royal Infirmary. He founded the Bristol Microscopical and Pathological societies, and served 10 years as a councilor and ultimately became president of the Bath and Bristol Provincial Medical and Surgical Association. He gave important evidence before the Royal Sanitary Commission in 1869, and was elected a fellow of the Royal Society in 1871 because of his views on epidemics and the spread of infectious diseases.

Budd married Caroline Mary Hilton, the daughter of a landowner, in 1847 and they had nine children. Although otherwise healthy, he suffered from attacks of severe **headaches** and, later in life, from nervous exhaustion believed due to overwork. He became an invalid after a **stroke** in 1873, and he died in a small town called Clevedon by the sea. He was reputed for his warm humanity, sense of obligation to pass on his medical knowledge, and to improve public health. His logic and conviction about disease communication placed him ahead of his time and earned him the praise of John Tyndall as ''a man of highest genius whose doctrines are now everywhere victorious.''

See also Cholera; Germ theory; Louis Pasteur; Typhoid fever

BURNET, FRANK MACFARLANE (1899-1985)

Australian immunologist and virologist

While working at the University of Melbourne's Walter and Eliza Hall Institute for Medical Research in the 1920s, Frank Macfarlane Burnet became interested in the study of viruses and bacteriophages (viruses that attack bacteria). That interest eventually led to two major and related accomplishments. The first of these was the development of a method for cultivating

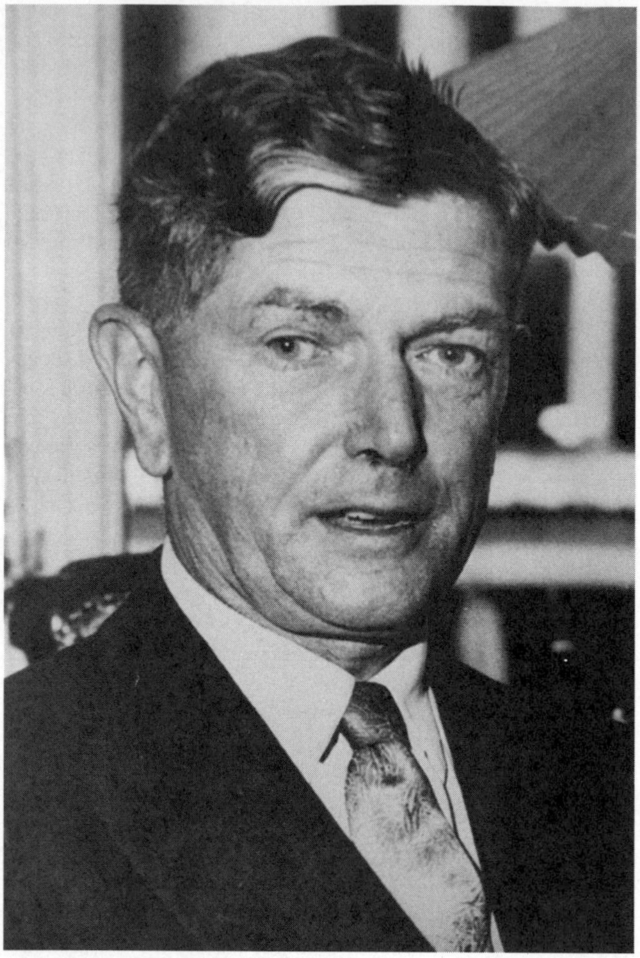

Frank Macfarlane Burnet

viruses in chicken embryos, an important technological step forward in the science of virology. The second accomplishment was the development of a theory that explains how an organism's body is able to distinguish between its own cells and those of another organism. For this research, Burnet was awarded a share of the 1960 Nobel Prize for physiology or medicine (with Peter Brian Medawar).

Burnet was born in Traralgon, Victoria, Australia, on September 3, 1899. His father was Frank Burnet, manager of the local bank in Traralgon, and his mother was the former Hadassah Pollock MacKay. As a child, Burnet developed an interest in nature, particularly in birds, butterflies, and beetles. He carried over that interest when he entered Geelong College in Geelong, Victoria, where he majored in biology and medicine.

In 1917 Burnet continued his education at Ormond College of the University of Melbourne, from which he received his bachelor of science degree in 1922 and then, a year later, his M.D. degree. Burnet then took concurrent positions as resident pathologist at the Royal Melbourne Hospital and as researcher at the University of Melbourne's Hall Institute for Medical Research. In 1926 Burnet received a Beit fellowship that permitted him to spend a year in residence at the Lister Institute of Preventive Medicine in London. The work on viruses and bacteriophages that he carried out at Lister also earned him a Ph.D. from the University of London in 1927. At the conclusion of his studies in England in 1928, Burnet returned to Australia, where he became assistant director of the Hall Institute. He maintained his association with the institute for the next thirty-seven years, becoming director there in 1944. In the same year he was appointed professor of experimental medicine at the University of Melbourne. During his first year back from England, in 1928, Burnet was also married to Edith Linda Druce, a schoolteacher. The Burnets had two daughters, Elizabeth and Deborah, and a son, Ian. When his first wife died in 1973, Burnet was married a second time, to Hazel Jenkin.

Burnet's early research covered a somewhat diverse variety of topics in virology. For example, he worked on the classification of viruses and bacteriophages, on the occurrence of psittacosis in Australian parrots, and on the epidemiology of herpes and poliomyelitis. His first major contribution to virology came, however, during his year as a Rockefeller fellow at London's National Institute for Medical Research from 1932 to 1933. There he developed a method for cultivating viruses in chicken embryos. The Burnet technique was an important breakthrough for virologists since viruses had been notoriously difficult to culture and maintain in the laboratory.

Over time, Burnet's work on viruses and bacteriophages led him to a different, but related, field of research, the vertebrate immune system. The fundamental question he attacked is one that had troubled biologists for years: how an organism's body can tell the difference between ''self'' and ''not-self.'' An organism's immune system is a crucial part of its internal hardware. It provides a mechanism for fighting off invasions by potentially harmful—and sometimes fatal—foreign organisms (antigens) such as bacteria, viruses, and fungi. The immune system is so efficient that it even recognizes and fights back against harmless invaders such as pollen and dust, resulting in allergic reactions.

Burnet was attracted to two aspects of the phenomenon of immunity. First, he wondered how an organism's body distinguishes between foreign invaders and components of its own body, the ''self'' versus ''not-self'' problem. That distinction is obviously critical, since if the body fails to recognize that difference, it may begin to attack its own cells and actually destroy itself. This phenomenon does in fact occur in relatively rare cases of autoimmune disorders.

The second question on which Burnet worked was how the immune system develops. The question is complicated by the fact that a healthy immune system is normally able to recognize and respond to an apparently endless variety of antigens, producing a specific chemical (antibody) to combat each antigen it encounters. According to one theory, these antibodies are present in an organism's body from birth, prior to birth, or an early age. A second theory suggested that antibodies are produced ''on the spot'' as they are needed and in response to an attack by an antigen.

For more than two decades, Burnet worked on resolving these questions about the immune system. He eventually de-

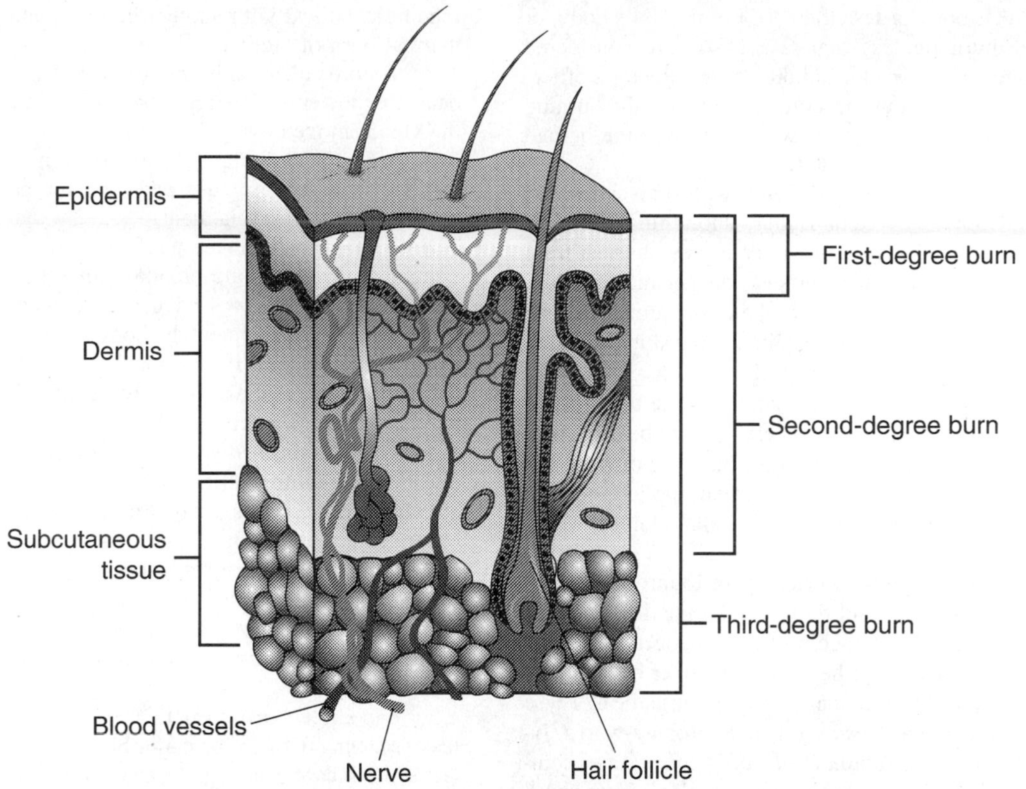

There are three classifications of burns: first-degree, second-degree, and third-degree burns. ***(Illustration by Electronic Illustrators Group.)***

veloped a complete and coherent explanation of the way the system develops in the embryo and beyond, how it develops the ability to recognize its own cells as distinct from foreign cells, and how it carries with it from the very earliest stages the templates from which antibodies are produced. For this work, Burnet was awarded a share of the 1960 Nobel Prize in physiology or medicine. Among the other honors he received were the Royal Medal and the Copley Medal of the Royal Society (1947 and 1959, respectively) and the Order of Merit in 1958. He was elected a fellow of the Royal Society in 1947 and knighted by King George V in 1951.

Burnet retired from the Hall Institute in 1965, but continued his research activities. His late work was in the area of autoimmune disorders, cancer, and aging. He died of cancer in Melbourne on August 31, 1985. Burnet was a prolific writer, primarily of books on science and medicine, during his lifetime.

Burns

Burns are injuries to tissues caused by heat, friction, electricity, radiation, or chemicals. They may be caused by even a brief encounter with heat greater than 120°F (49°C). The source of this heat may be the sun (causing a **sunburn**), hot liquids, steam, fire, electricity, friction (causing rug burns and rope burns), and chemicals (causing a caustic burn upon contact).

Burns are characterized by degree, based on the severity of tissue damage. A first-degree burn causes redness and swelling in the outermost layers of skin (epidermis). A second-degree burn involves redness, swelling and blistering, and the damage may extend beneath the epidermis to deeper layers of skin (dermis). A third-degree burn, also called a full-thickness burn, destroys the entire depth of skin, causing significant scarring. Damage also may extend to the underlying fat, muscle, or bone. The severity of a burn is also judged by the amount of body surface area (BSA) it involves.

Critical, or major, burns are the most serious and should be treated in a specialized burn unit of a hospital. These are defined as first- or second-degree burns covering more than 25% of an adult's body or more than 20% of a child's body, or a third-degree burn on more than 10% BSA.

Signs of a burn are localized redness, swelling, and **pain**. A severe burn will also blister. The skin may also peel, appear white or charred, and feel numb. A burn may trigger a **headache** and **fever**. Extensive burns may induce **shock**, the symptoms of which are faintness, weakness, rapid pulse and breathing, pale and clammy skin, and bluish lips and fingernails.

First- or second-degree burns (those covering less than 15% of an adult's body or less than 10% of a child's body, or a third-degree burn on less than 2% BSA) are considered minor burns and may be treated at home or in a doctor's office. The first act of thermal burn treatment is to stop the burning process by letting cool (not cold) water run over the burned area or by soaking it in cool water.

The burn should be cleaned gently with soap and water. Blisters should not be broken. Butter, shortening, or salve should never be applied to the burn since it prevents heat from escaping and drives the burning process deeper into the skin. If the skin of the burned area is unbroken, the burn should be left exposed to the air to promote healing. If the skin is broken, the burned area should be coated lightly with an antibacterial ointment and covered with a sterile bandage. The burn should also be bandaged if it is on an area where it might be disturbed, such as the sole of the foot or palm of the hand. Cool wet compresses may provide some pain relief when applied to small areas of first- and second-degree burns. Ice should never be applied to the burn.

Aspirin, **acetaminophen** (Tylenol), or ibuprofen (Advil) may be taken to ease pain and relieve inflammation. In addition, several homeopathic remedies, including *Cantharis* and *Causticum*, can assist in burn healing. A number of botanical remedies, applied to the skin, can also help burns heal. These include aloe (*Aloe barbadensis*), oil of St.-John's-wort (*Hypericum perforatum*), calendula (*Calendula officinalis*), comfrey (*Symphytum officinale*), and tea tree oil (*Melaleuca* spp.).

A doctor should be consulted if any signs of infection appear while the burn is healing, including: increased warmth, redness, pain, or swelling; pus or similar drainage from the wound; swollen lymph nodes; or red streaks spreading away from the burn. Minor burns typically heal in 5-10 days with no scarring.

In situations where a person has received moderate or critical burns, lifesaving measures take precedence over burn treatment and emergency medical assistance must be called. Severe burns may cause the victim to stop breathing, and artificial respiration (also called mouth-to-mouth resuscitation or rescue breathing) should be administered immediately. Also, a person with burns covering more than 12% BSA is likely to go into shock; this condition may be prevented by laying the person flat and elevating the feet about 12 in (30 cm). Burned arms and hands should also be raised higher than the person's heart.

In the case of burns from fire, clothes that are smoldering or smoking should be removed. However, any clothing that is embedded in the burn should not be disturbed. Covering the burn victim with a light, cool, wet cloth, such as a sheet but not a blanket or towel, will stop the burning process.

Burns from liquid chemicals must be rinsed with cool water for at least 15 minutes to stop the burning process. In cases of burns from dry chemicals such as lime, the powder should be completely brushed away before the area is washed. Any clothing which may have absorbed the chemical should be removed. The burn should then be loosely covered with a sterile gauze pad and the person taken to the hospital for further treatment. A physician may be able to neutralize the offending chemical with another before treating the burn like a thermal burn of similar severity.

Before electrical burns are treated at the site of the accident, the power source must be disconnected if possible and the victim moved away from it to keep the person giving aid from being electrocuted. Electrical burns should be loosely covered with sterile gauze pads and the person taken to the hospital for further treatment.

At the hospital, the staff will provide further medical treatment. A tube to aid breathing may be inserted if the patient's airways or lungs have been damaged. Also, because burns dramatically deplete the body of fluids, replacement fluids are administered intravenously. The patient is also given **antibiotics** intravenously to prevent infection, and he or she may also receive a **tetanus** shot.

Once the burned area is cleaned and treated with antibiotic cream or ointment, it is covered in sterile bandages, which are changed 2-3 times a day. Surgical removal of dead tissue (**debridement**) also takes place. The burn victim may also be placed in a hyperbaric chamber. In a hyperbaric chamber (which can be a specialized room or enclosed space), the patient is exposed to pure oxygen under high pressure, which can aid in healing if administered in the first 24 hours after the burn injury occurs.

Moderate burns usually heal in 10-14 days and may leave scarring. Critical or major burns take longer to heal, and leave significant scarring. As the burns heal, thick, taut scabs (eschar) form, which the doctor may have to cut to improve blood flow to the more elastic healthy tissue beneath. The patient will also undergo physical and occupational therapy to keep the burned areas from becoming inflexible. In cases where the skin has been so damaged that it cannot properly heal, a skin graft is usually performed. A skin graft involves taking a piece of skin from an unburned portion of the patient's body (autograft) and transplanting it to the burned area. When doctors cannot immediately use the patient's own skin, a temporary graft is performed using the skin of a human donor (allograft), either alive or dead, or the skin of an animal (xenograft), usually that of a pig.

BURSITIS

Bursitis is the painful inflammation of the bursa, a padlike sac that cushions the movement between the bones, tendons and muscles near the joints. Bursitis is most often caused by repetitive movement, and is also known by several common names including weaver's bottom, clergyman's knee, and miner's elbow.

There are over 150 bursae in the human body. Each sac contains a small amount of *synovial fluid*, a clear liquid that acts as a lubricant. Inflammation of the bursae causes pain on movement. The most common site for bursitis to occur is the shoulder (subdeltoid), but it also is seen in the elbows, hips, knees, heels, and toes.

The most common cause of bursitis is repeated physical activity, but it can flare up for no known reason. It can also be caused by trauma, **rheumatoid arthritis**, **gout**, and acute or chronic infection.

Pain and tenderness are common symptoms. If the affected joint is close to the skin, as with the shoulder, knee, elbow, or Achilles tendon, swelling and redness are seen and the area may feel warm to the touch. The bursae around the hip joint are deeper, and swelling is not obvious. Movement may be limited and is painful. In the shoulder, it may be difficult to raise the arm out from the side of the body.

In acute bursitis symptoms appear suddenly; with chronic bursitis, pain, tenderness, and limited movement reappear after **exercise** or strain.

When a patient has joint pain, a careful **physical examination** is needed to determine what type of movement is affected and if there is any swelling present. Bursitis will not show up on x rays, although sometimes calcium deposits in the joint may be visible. Inserting a thin needle into the affected bursa and removing (aspirating) some of the synovial fluid for examination can confirm the diagnosis. In most cases, the fluid will not be clear. It can be tested for the presence of microorganisms, which would indicate an infection, and crystals, which could indicate gout. In instances where the diagnosis is difficult, a local anesthetic (a drug that numbs the area) is injected into the painful spot. If the discomfort stops temporarily, then bursitis is probably the correct diagnosis.

Conservative treatment of bursitis is usually effective. The application of heat, rest, and **immobilization** of the affected joint area is the first step. A sling can be used for a shoulder injury; a cane is helpful for hip problems. The patient can take **nonsteroidal anti-inflammatory drugs** (NSAIDs) like **aspirin**, ibuprofin, and naproxen. They can be obtained without a prescription and relieve the pain and inflammation.

When bursitis does not respond to conservative treatment, an injection into the joint of a long-acting corticosteroid preparation, like prednisone, can bring immediate and lasting relief. A corticosteroid is a hormonal substance that is the most effective drug for reducing inflammation. The drug is mixed with a local anesthetic and works on the joint within five minutes. Usually one injection is all that is needed. In cases where both anti-inflammatory and corticosteroid medications are not effective in relieving bursitis pain, surgery to remove the damaged bursa may be performed

If the bursitis is related to an inflammatory disease like arthritis or gout, or to an infection, then management of that condition is needed to control the bursitis. *Septic* bursitis is caused by the presence of a pus-forming organism, usually *staphylococcus aureus.* This condition requires treatment with **antibiotics**. The bursa will also need to be drained by needle two or three times over the first week of treatment. When a patient has such a serious infection, there may be underlying causes such as diabetes or an inefficient immune system.

Once the pain caused by the bursitis decreases, exercise of the affected area can begin. If the nearby muscles have become weak, a doctor or physical therapist can recommend exercises to build strength and improve movement.

The use of vitamin supplements, herbs, homeopathy, **aromatherapy**, and **hydrotherapy** can help relieve the symptoms of bursitis. Calcium and magnesium supplements may help prevent the condition, and ginger is useful in reducing inflammation. **Acupuncture** has been proven effective in treating hip and shoulder pain caused by bursitis. Other therapies that deal effectively with musculoskeletal problems (relating to the muscles and skeleton), may also be helpful, such as **naturopathic medicine**, **chiropractic**, and applied **kinesiology**.

To prevent a reoccurence of bursitis, overexercising and repetitive movements that trigger the condition should be avoided. When doing repetitive tasks, frequent breaks should be taken. To protect the joints, use cushioned chairs when sitting and foam kneeling pads for the knees. Leaning on the elbows, kneeling or sitting on a hard surface for a long period of time should be avoided. Wearing low heeled shoes can help prevent bursitis in the heel, as can changing to new running shoes as soon as the old ones are worn out.

C

CABRINI, FRANCES XAVIER (1850-1917)

Italian-American missionary and saint

A source of inspiration and comfort to countless people in urban areas worldwide, Frances Xavier Cabrini or Mother Cabrini, as she was later called established over 60 orphanages, schools, and **hospitals** in the United States, England, Italy, France, Spain, Panama, Chile, Argentina, and Brazil. She also founded a religious order, the Missionary Sisters of the Sacred Heart. In 1946, Cabrini was canonized, making her the first American citizen to become a saint in the Roman Catholic Church.

Agostino Cabrini and his 52-year-old wife Stella (Ordini) had already lost nine children when their 13th child was born on July 15, 1850 in Sant'Angelo Lodigiano, the Lombardy region of Italy. The baby was born two months prematurely and was so weak that her parents thought she would not survive. The baby was immediately baptized and named Francesca Maria Cabrini. Throughout her childhood, Frances remained frail and was often too weak to attend school. In her early years, she was tutored by her older sister Rosa who was a local teacher.

Frances continued her education at a school run by the religious order, Daughters of the Sacred Heart, in Arluno. In 1870 she received her teaching certificate, with top honors, at the age of 18. Frances hoped to join the Daughters of the Sacred Heart, but her health was too fragile, and instead taught in Vidardo. In 1874, one year after she had taken religious vows, a local priest urged her to help reorganize a grossly mismanaged orphanage in Codogno. Despite verbal and sometimes physical abuse by the women administrators, Cabrini worked at improving conditions. However, the orphanage was closed in 1880. In that same year, seven of the orphans joined Cabrini in establishing a religious order called the Missionary Sisters of the Sacred Heart. The order was officially sanctioned by Pope Leo XIII in 1888.

Mother Cabrini next traveled to the United States at the urging of Bishop Giovanni Battista Scalabrini. The bishop had observed the plight of Italian immigrants in America and established the Congregation of St. Charles Borromeo and a church in New York. Knowing that more needed to be done for the immigrants, especially for Italian children in America, the bishop asked Cabrini to take charge of an orphanage in New York. Urged also by the Pope, she sailed for New York in 1889 accompanied by six other nuns.

When she arrived in New York, Archbishop Michael Corrigan of New York informed her that the project was discontinued and suggested that she return to Italy. In a bold move, Cabrini challenged the authority of the archbishop and informed him that she would remain in New York. He later recommended that she and the other sisters establish a school at the church of the Scalabrinian Fathers in lower Manhattan. After establishing the school, Cabrini convinced the archbishop to open an orphanage for Italian immigrant girls.

With limited resources, Cabrini created a nurturing environment for the children residing at 59th Street as well as another orphanage she established in lower Manhattan. She supplied both homes with day-old bread provided by local shop keepers and soliciting donations from the rich as well as the poor. The orphanage soon branched out, first to Hoboken, New Jersey, Staten Island, and Brooklyn, all of which had Italian settlements. She then secured a 450-acre estate formerly owned by the Jesuits in West Park, New York, and moved the children there.

During a trip to Italy with several American girls who joined her order, Cabrini founded a teachers college in Rome and had several audiences with Pope Leo XIII, who was very impressed by her accomplishments. In 1891, she expanded her work to Latin America, establishing a private school for young women in Nicaragua. She then turned her attention to the southern United States. Mother Cabrini was drawn to the area because of the desperate plight of Italian immigrants living and working in that region. In less than a month after their arrival in 1892, Mother Cabrini and her Missionary sisters founded

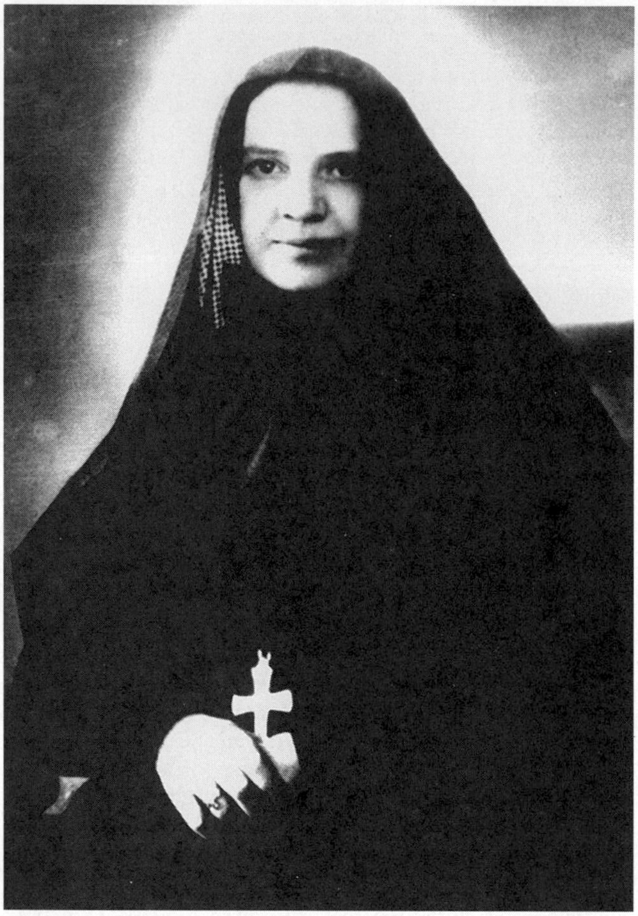

Frances Xaviar Cabrini

an orphanage and school in New Orleans and offered comfort to the city's poor, sick, and dying.

Caring for the sick soon became a priority for Cabrini. In 1891, while visiting New York, Bishop Scalabrini convinced the nuns to take charge of a small, recently opened hospital in an upper Manhattan Italian neighborhood. When the hospital was forced to close in 1892 due to financial difficulties, Mother Cabrini moved the patients to a building on 12th Street, where she and the other sisters cared for the sick in an environment that initially lacked heat and water. Enlisting the aid of doctors of all faiths, Cabrini persuaded them to donate their services to Columbus Hospital while working-class Italians were encouraged to donate money, food, and supplies.

Ironically, the outbreak of typhoid fever on an Italian battleship docked in New York harbor proved a positive development for the hospital. While other hospitals refused to treat victims of the epidemic, Columbus Hospital took them in. With increasing popular support for the hospital after the epidemic, Cabrini secured a bank loan to renovate the facility. In 1885, the completely renovated hospital received approval from the state of New York. Two other branches of the Columbus Hospital were later established: one in Chicago, the other in Seattle, a city where Cabrini also founded a school and became a United States citizen in 1909.

In 1910, Cabrini became Superior for life of the order she founded. For the next few years she traveled to various locations to care for the sick. She tended nuns stricken with a smallpox epidemic in Rio de Janeiro and a yellow fever outbreak in New Orleans required the sisters' nursing skills. By 1917, recurring bouts of malaria contracted in Latin America weakened Cabrini, and she died in Chicago in December of that year.

See also Death; Hospitals

CAFFEINE

Caffeine is a drug that stimulates the central nervous system. It makes people more alert, less drowsy, and improves coordination. When combined with certain pain relievers and medicines for treating migraine headache, caffeine makes those drugs work more quickly and effectively. Caffeine alone can also help relieve **headache**s. **Antihistamines** are sometimes combined with caffeine to counteract the drowsiness that those drugs cause. Caffeine is also used to treat some breathing problems, because it widens the bronchial airways.

Caffeine was first discovered in coffee in 1820. It is also found naturally in tea and chocolate. Colas and some other soft drinks also contain it. Caffeine is sold in tablets and capsules that can be bought without a prescription. Over-the-counter caffeine brands include No Doz, Overtime, Pep-Back, Quick-Pep, Caffedrine, and Vivarin.

People who use large amounts of caffeine over long periods of time build up a tolerance to it. When that happens, they have to use more and more caffeine to get the same effects. Heavy caffeine use can also lead to dependence. If the person then stops using caffeine abruptly, withdrawal symptoms may occur. These can include throbbing headaches, fatigue, drowsiness, yawning, irritability, restlessness, vomiting, or runny nose. These symptoms can go on for as long as a week if caffeine is avoided. Then the symptoms usually disappear.

Caffeine cannot replace sleep and should not be used regularly to stay awake as the drug can lead to more serious **sleep disorders**, like **insomnia**. When determining caffeine dosage, be sure to consider how much caffeine is being taken in from coffee, tea, chocolate, soft drinks, and other foods. Check with a pharmacist or physician to find out how much caffeine is safe to use.

Caffeine may cause problems for people with these medical conditions: food or drug **allergies**, peptic ulcer, heart **arrhythmias** or **palpitations**, heart disease or recent **heart attack**, high blood pressure, liver disease, insomnia (trouble sleeping), anxiety or panic attacks, **Agoraphobia** (fear of being in open places), **Premenstrual syndrome** (PMS).

At recommended doses, caffeine can cause restlessness, irritability, nervousness, shakiness, headache, lightheadedness, sleeplessness, nausea, vomiting, and upset stomach. At higher than recommended doses, caffeine can cause excitement, agitation, anxiety, confusion, a sensation of light flashing before the eyes, unusual sensitivity to touch, unusual sensitivity of other senses, ringing in the ears, frequent urination, muscle twitches or **tremors**, heart arrhythmias, rapid heartbeat, flushing, and convulsions.

Caffeine can pass from a pregnant woman's body into the developing fetus. Although there is no evidence that caffeine causes **birth defects** in people, it does cause such effects in laboratory animals given very large doses (equal to human doses of 12-24 cups of coffee a day). In humans, evidence exists that doses of more than 300 mg of caffeine a day (about the amount of caffeine in 2-3 cups of coffee) may cause **miscarriage** or problems with the heart rhythm of the fetus. Women who take more than 300 mg of caffeine a day during **pregnancy** are also more likely to have babies with low birth weights.

Caffeine passes into breast milk and can affect the nursing baby. Nursing babies whose mothers use 600 mg or more of caffeine a day may be irritable and have trouble sleeping. Women who are breastfeeding should check with their physicians before using caffeine.

Serious side effects are possible when caffeine is combined with certain drugs. For example, taking caffeine with the decongestant phenylpropanolamine can raise blood pressure. And very serious heart problems may occur if caffeine and monoamine oxidase inhibitors (MAO) are taken together. Caffeine also interferes with drugs that regulate heart rhythm, such as quinidine and propranolol (Inderal). Because caffeine stimulates the nervous system, anyone taking other central nervous system (CNS) stimulants should be careful about using caffeine. Always check with a pharmacist or physician about which drugs can interact with caffeine.

Certain drugs interfere with the breakdown of caffeine in the body. These include **oral contraceptives** that contain estrogen, the antiarrhythmia drug mexiletine (Mexitil), the ulcer drug cimetidine (Tagamet), and the drug disulfiram (Antabuse), used to treat alcoholism. Caffeine may also interfere with the body's absorption of iron. Anyone who takes iron supplements should take them at least an hour before or two hours after using caffeine.

CAIUS, JOHN (1510-1573)

English physician and scholar

Caius (the Latin form of his name that he adopted, which has at least 10 alternative spellings) is best known for his 1552 book *A Boke or Counseill against the Disease commonly called the Sweate, or Sweatyng Sicknesse,* considered one of the first original descriptions of an epidemic. He was also noteworthy as a physician to three English monarchs, King Edward VI, Queen Mary, and Queen Elizabeth, and a founder of Gonville and Caius College at Cambridge, England's first school for formal medical education. Caius was a notable man of letters, translating and lecturing and publishing on subjects ranging from British dogs to philosophy, to the origins of universities.

Born in Norwich in 1510, he started studying the humanities at Cambridge University's Gonville Hall at the age of 18. It is believed his initial intention was to become a cleric. He switched to medical studies in 1539 but remained interested in theology and church matters for the rest of his life.

Caius went to Italy and studied at the University of Padua, living for eight months under the same roof as the famed anatomist Andreas Vesalius. He was awarded his M.D. degree at Padua in 1541. Caius traveled throughout Italy, Switzerland, Germany, Holland and France before returning to England. In London, he commenced teaching and practicing medicine in London.

In 1547 Caius became a Fellow of the College of Physicians of London. He was elected president of the group nine times between 1555 and 1571. In that post, he successfully lobbied for the right to dissect the bodies of executed criminals and fought a bid by surgeons to administer internal remedies.

Caius's account of the English "sweating sickness" was the first description of a disease written in the English language. After observing an epidemic at Shrewsbury in 1551 and 1552, he recorded symptoms including difficulty in breathing, severe prostration, delirium, and rapid heartbeat. Death could occur just three hours after symptoms first appeared. Neither physicians nor historians agreed on the illness. Speculation has ranged from influenza to plague, to relapsing fever, and to acute rheumatic fever. Caius originally wrote this account in English to warn "everye personne" about the disease. Later, he revised it and had it published in Latin for his medical colleagues.

Caius is considered a founder of Cambridge's Gonville and Caius College, even though the institution that was then named Gonville Hall was already more than 180 years old at the time of his study. After he became successful and wealthy, Caius learned that his old college had fallen into disrepair. He arranged a new charter from Queen Mary, provided a generous endowment, and enlarged the buildings.

To signify elements of academic excellence, Caius arranged for the symbolic construction of the three famous gates at the college. To this day, newcomers enter the institution through the low-ceilinged Gate of Humility. While studying there, they daily pass through a handsome portico named the Gate of Virtue, and after receiving their degrees, they leave through the Gate of Honor.

In 1559, Caius was named the college's master, a post he continued to occupy until just before his death in 1573. However, his religious beliefs caused him considerable difficulty at Cambridge. Henry VIII had started the English Reformation in 1534 by creating the Church of England, headed by himself. Caius, however, retained sympathy for the Pope. It is believed that Elizabeth I dismissed him as her physician for that reason in 1568. In 1572 the vice-chancellor of Cambridge University (who later become the Archbishop of Canterbury) ordered that Caius's rooms be raided. A variety of "popish" garments and books were seized and burned. After his death in 1573, however, Caius was buried in the chapel at Gonville and Caius College.

CALCIUM IMBALANCE

Calcium is the most abundant mineral in the human body, and iscritical to good health. It is not only a component of bones and teeth, but is also essential for blood clotting and necessary for muscle and nerve functions. If the level of calcium in the body becomes too low (hypocalcemia) or too high (hypercalcemia), serious medical problems can occur.

*Hypercalcemia*is an abnormally high level of calcium in the blood, usually more than 10.5 milligrams per deciliter of blood. Symptoms include loss of appetite, nausea, vomiting, **constipation**, and abdominal **pain**. If the kidneys are involved, the individual will have to urinate frequently during both the day and night and will be very thirsty. As the calcium levels rise, the symptoms become more serious. Stones may form in the kidneys and waste products can build up. Blood pressure rises and the heart rhythm may change. Muscles become increasingly weak. The individual may experience mood swings, confusion, **psychosis**, and eventually, **coma** and **death**.

Ten to twenty percent of all persons with **cancer** have hypercalcemia. In fact, it is the most common life-threatening metabolic disorder associated with cancer. Cancers of the breast, lung, head and neck, kidney, and blood are frequently associated with hypercalcemia. It is seen most often in patients with tumors of the lung (25–35%) and breast (20–40%), according to the National Cancer Institute. Cancer causes hypercalcemia in two ways. First, if a tumor grows into the bone, it destroys calcium-containing bony tissue (osteolysis), which is then reabsorbed by the body. Secondly, substances secreted by cancer cells can increase calcium levels (humoral hypercalcemia of malignancy).

Cancer patients are often dehydrated because they take in inadequate amounts of food and fluids and often suffer from **nausea and vomiting**. **Dehydration** reduces the ability of the kidneys to remove excess calcium from the body. Hormones and **diuretics** that increase the amount of fluid released by the body can also trigger hypercalcemia.

Other conditions can cause hypercalcemia. Hyperparathyroidism, the excessive secretion of parathyroid (the hormone that controls calcium levels) by one or more of the parathyroid glands, is the most common cause of hypercalcemia in the general population. Excessive intake of vitamin D can increase the intestinal absorption of calcium. During therapy for peptic **ulcers**, abnormally high amounts of calcium **antacids** are sometimes taken. Over use of antacids can cause milk-alkali syndrome and hypercalcemia. Diseases or conditions which cause bone loss or deterioration, such as Paget's and **paralysis** of the arms and legs can also lead to hypercalcemia.

Severe hypercalcemia can be life-threatening. If the patient has normal kidney function, fluids can be given by vein (intravenously) to clear the excess calcium from the bloodstream. If the patient's kidneys are not working well, hemodialysis (a blood filtration therapy) is probably the safest and most effective method to reduce dangerous calcium levels.

Drugs such as furosemide, called loop diuretics, can be given after adequate fluid intake is established. These drugs inhibit calcium reabsorption in the kidneys and promote urine production. Drugs that inhibit bone loss, such as calcitonin, biphosphates, and plicamycin, are helpful in achieving long-term control. Phosphate pills help lower high calcium levels caused by a deficiency in phosphate. Anti-inflammatory agents such as steroids are helpful with some cancers and toxic levels of vitamin D. Hyperparathyroidism is usually treated by surgical removal of one or more of the parathyroid glands.

Hypocalcemia, an insufficiency of serum calcium levels, can be caused by hypoparathyroidism, by kidney failure, by low levels of plasma magnesium (hypomagnesia), or by failure to get adequate amounts of calcium or vitamin D in the diet. Hypocalcemia may also result from the consumption of toxic levels of phosphate, found in certain enema formulas.

Symptoms of severe hypocalcemia include numbness or tingling around the mouth or in the feet and hands, as well as in muscle spasms in the face, feet, and hands. Hypocalcemia can also result in depression, memory loss, or **hallucinations**. Severe hypocalcemia occurs when free calcium in the bloodstream is under 3 milligrams per deciliter of blood. Chronic and moderate hypocalcemia can result in **cataracts**. In this case, the term ''chronic'' means lasting one year or longer.

Severe hypocalcemia requires injection of calcium ions (such as calcium gluconate). Long-term treatment of hypocalcemia includes oral calcium supplements (such as calcium carbonate, calcium chloride, calcium lactate, or calcium gluconate) and vitamin D supplements. Where hypocalcemia results from kidney failure, treatment includes injections of 1,25-dihydroxyvitamin D. If hypocalcemia is caused by low serum magnesium levels, the magnesium deficiency must be corrected to effectively treat the hypocalcemia.

CALDICOTT, HELEN (1938-)

Australian pediatrician and antinuclear activist

Helen Caldicott is a pediatrician and an antinuclear activist, who opposes both nuclear weapons and nuclear power. In the early 1970s she spearheaded an antinuclear movement in her native Australia, which forced an end to French nuclear testing in the South Pacific and managed to stop Australian uranium exports from 1975 to 1982. In the late 1970s and early 1980s, she became a leader in the antinuclear movement in the United States through her role in reviving the organization Physicians for Social Responsibility, which expanded rapidly during her presidency (which ran from 1978 to 1983). She helped found several other organizations which have worked to abolish controlled nuclear fission. Relying on her passionate oratory and intensely personal style, which are grounded in a thorough knowledge of the medical effects of exposure to radiation, she was particularly effective in raising grass-roots support and bringing nuclear issues to the forefront in the 1980s.

Caldicott was born on August 7, 1938, in Melbourne, Australia, the daughter of a factory manager, Philip Broinowski, and an interior designer, Mary Mona Enyd (Coffey) Broinowski. She received a public-school education except for four years spent at Fintona Girls School in Adelaide, a private secondary school. She recalls today that she was strongly affected as an adolescent by reading Nevil Shute's *On the Beach,* a novel about nuclear devastation set in Australia. At the age of 17, she enrolled at the University of Adelaide Medical School, graduating in 1961 with a B.S. in surgery and an M.B. in medicine (the equivalent of an American M.D.).

She moved to Boston with her husband in 1966 for a three-year fellowship in nutrition at Harvard Medical School. Returning to Adelaide in 1969, she accepted a position in the renal unit of Queen Elizabeth Hospital. In the early 1970s at the same hospital, she completed a year's residency and a two-year internship in pediatrics. She also set up a clinic for cystic fibrosis.

Both her work with children afflicted with cystic fibrosis, a genetic disorder, and her experience as an expectant mother assuming responsibility for her own children persuaded Caldicott that she had to take a more active role in ensuring a future for human beings. In 1971, she discovered that France had been conducting nuclear tests over its South Pacific colony of Mururoa for the previous five years and had done so in violation of the International Atmospheric Test Ban Treaty of 1962. Fallout from the tests drifted towards Australia and entered the food chain in various ways. A confidential South Australian government report, for instance, confirmed that higher than normal levels of radiation were present in drinking water in 1971 and in rain in 1972. Caldicott organized opposition at a time when few Australians were aware of either the testing or the radioactive fallout that had resulted. She began by sending a letter of protest to a local newspaper. Subsequently, she made radio and television appearances, commenting on the medical risks of radiation. From her work in pediatrics she was acutely aware that children are more sensitive to the effects of radiation than adults. She always emphasized this fact, appealing to her audience as parents responsible for the well-being of their children. She made public the confidential report (passed on to her by a sympathizer within the state government) describing elevated radiation levels in drinking and rain water. Her speeches began a mass movement against the French tests that had thousands taking part in protest marches and resulted in a boycott of French products. When, in December 1972, the Australian Labor Party swept the Liberal Party out of office, the government undertook legal action against France through the International Court of Justice. Although the court ruled ambiguously, the French government ceased atmospheric testing in the face of widespread organized opposition.

Caldicott was less successful in her attempt to organize against the commercial exploitation of uranium, a relatively rare raw material necessary for most nuclear technology. Australia has rich uranium deposits and exported the material to many different countries. Caldicott got union backing for her proposed export ban by organizing among workers. She recalls today that her emphasis on the fact that radiation exposure causes a deformation of sperm cells (and thus a rise in the rate of birth defects) was her most potent argument. The Australian Council of Trade Unions passed a resolution against the mining, transport, and sale of uranium in 1975. In the same year the government imposed the desired export ban. Under international pressure, however, the ban was lifted in 1982.

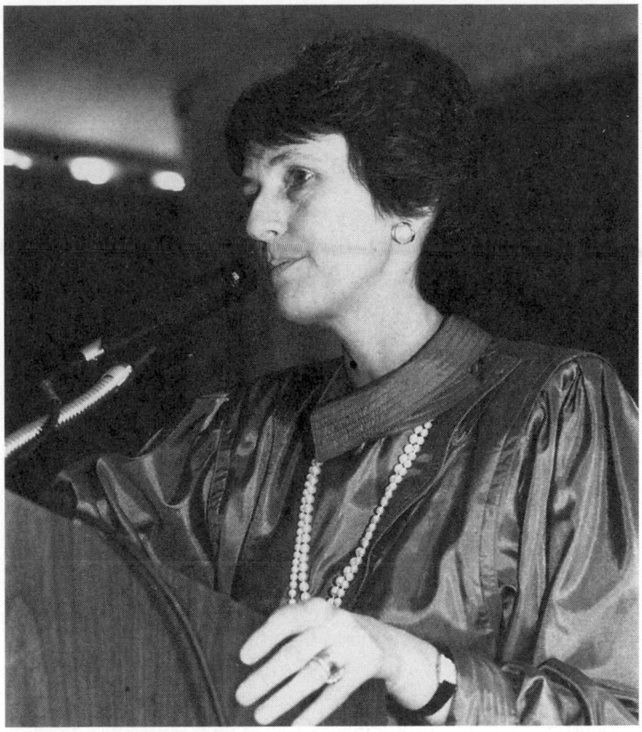

Helen Caldicott

Caldicott returned to Boston in 1975, having received an appointment as a fellow in cystic fibrosis at the Children's Hospital Medical Center. Although she and her family went back to Australia for six months in 1976, they returned to the United States in 1977. At that time, she became an associate in medicine at the Children's Hospital Medical Center and an instructor in pediatrics at Harvard Medical School.

Physicians for Social Responsibility was a group initially formed in 1962. By 1978, when Caldicott became involved with it, its membership had dwindled and its field of action narrowed significantly. It remained a small group until March 28, 1979, when Pennsylvania's Three Mile Island nuclear reactor came within sixty minutes of a possible meltdown. At once, more than five hundred physicians joined Physicians for Social Responsibility. Thereafter, its membership, budget, and size of paid staff continued to grow impressively. With Caldicott at its head, the group fought the nuclear industry, conducted research on the results of nuclear war, worked politically for nuclear disarmament, and conducted numerous symposia and sponsored countless lectures. Caldicott gave up the practice of medicine in 1980 to devote herself to full-time leadership of the organization. Her gifts as a public speaker had a tremendous impact on a great many audiences. Caldicott consciously espouses a feminine ethic of nurturance, exhorting women to become more aggressive in their role as caretakers of humanity and appealing to men to cultivate the elements of nurturing in their lives. Physicians for Social Responsibility also made a powerful documentary film, *Eight Minutes to Midnight,* which was featured on a tour with Caldicott and was nominated for an Academy Award in 1982. In addition to delivering numerous speeches in church, labor, university, and other settings, she wrote *Nuclear Madness: What You Can Do!* with Nancy Herrington and Nahum Stiskin. The book provides detailed descriptions of the medical and environmental results of nuclear war as well as political prescriptions for preventing it.

The growth of the organization brought more diverse membership, which, after becoming unwilling to follow Caldicott in her opposition to nuclear power in addition to nuclear weapons, pushed for a more mainstream position. As a result, she resigned as president in 1983, but continued to serve on the board of directors. She also helped found the Medical Campaign Against Nuclear War, the Women's Action for Nuclear Disarmament, the Women's Party for Survival and a number of other organizations concerned with nuclear and other environmental issues. Her second book, *Missile Envy: the Arms Race and Nuclear War,* came out in 1984.

Caldicott's speeches and writings combine detailed medical descriptions with a highly personal and sometimes emotional approach. She describes the devastating physical results of a nuclear detonation in elaborate detail as it would affect particular individuals according to their geographical location. Medical metaphors and analogies illustrate political and environmental problems, while her personal experiences lend force to the narrative. Her own joy in having and raising her children gave her a heightened concern for the future of the earth. Caldicott's witness to this personal experience often makes her successful in convincing audiences that nuclear dangers are not abstract but threaten every individual human life. Although she makes a particularly strong appeal to women, occasionally arguing that women are particularly suited to save the earth from the warmongers and transnational corporations, she also has a strong following among men.

Her books have gained praise but criticism as well, even at times from those who would seem to be her natural allies. Some critics have pointed to superficial documentation and inaccurate statements in overly polemical presentations. She has also been criticized for failing to recognize that her arguments are essentially middle class and do not address the concerns of working-class people. Yet Caldicott has also been praised for bringing awareness of nuclear dangers to center stage and for offering concrete, grass-roots political programs for combatting those dangers.

Returning to Australia, Caldicott ran for a seat in parliament in 1990, losing by a very narrow margin. Since then, she has published a third book, *If You Love This Planet: A Plan to Heal the Earth* (1992), which focuses more broadly on environmental issues than her previous publications. At home in Canberra, she lives by her environmental convictions. As she told reporter Will Nixon, interviewing her for *E Magazine* in 1992, "I've just planted 400 eucalyptus and rain-forest trees on my land. It was like having a baby, the joy it gave me because I'm replenishing the land." She is also experimenting with systems of self-sustaining agriculture.

Caldicott's numerous awards include the Humanist of the Year Award from the American Association of Humanistic Psychology in 1982, and the International Year of Peace Award from the Australian government in 1986. She was one of the nominees for the Nobel Peace Prize in 1985 and holds many honorary degrees. In 1962, she married William Caldicott, a pediatric radiologist, who has worked with her in her campaigns. They have three children, Philip, Penny, and William Jr.

CAMPER, PIETER (1722-1789)

Dutch anatomist, medical illustrator, obstetrician

From the time he was admitted to Leyden University in the Netherlands as a precocious 11-year-old, this multitalented scientist and artist found no lack of intellectual pursuits to arouse his boundless curiosity. Pieter Camper made several important contributions in the fields of obstetrics, ophthalmology, orthopedics, comparative anatomy, veterinary medicine, anthropology, and medical illustration.

Pieter Camper was born in the city of Leyden in the Netherlands in 1722. Some of his intellectual influence may have come from his father, a cleric, and his grandfather, a physician. He spent a dozen years there at Leyden University, receiving two doctorates at age 24, one in philosophy and the other in medicine. Camper spent most of his working life as a professor at three Dutch universities: Franeker (in the Dutch province of Friesland), Amsterdam, and Groningen.

Concerned that obstetrical training of the day was inadequate, Camper traveled to England to study midwifery. He later wrote a five-volume book about the subject. He pioneered the use of the symphyseotomy, which is the cutting into the bone at the front of the pelvis to widen the birth passage, in place of cesarean sections. Although he did not personally perform this procedure on human patients, he demonstrated its effectiveness in experiments on slaughtered pigs and then on a live animal. He was also an early advocate of allowing the third stage of labor (delivery of the placenta, or afterbirth) to take place naturally whenever possible. Despite his expertise, Camper ironically claimed that obstetrics was merely a hobby. He said that he only accepted payment on one occasion for obstetrical services, regardless of the wealth of the patient.

While in England, he had also undertaken instruction in art at the Painters' Academy in London. He became well known as a medical illustrator, writing a two-volume work on medical illustration, and using a variety of forms including engraving, painting, and sculpture. Unlike many of his contemporaries, he ignored the laws of perspective and made his anatomical depictions architecturally correct using a moving point of view.

Studying the works of earlier painters and manuscript illustrators, he became interested in facial angles and the shapes of skulls. Using these characteristics to compare different ethnic groups, he became a founder of the social science of anthropology.

Camper was a pioneer of comparative anatomy, carefully dissecting animals including the elephant, rhinoceros, and orangutan. He explored the croaking of frogs, air chambers in the bones of birds, and hearing in fish. This work in animal anatomy led to a corresponding interest in veterinary medicine. During an outbreak of cattle pest in 1769, Camper performed 100 autopsies and promoted inoculation of animals against the disease. In human anatomy, he discovered the processus vaginalis peritonaei, a factor in abdominal hernia.

Ophthalmology was an early interest of Camper's. At Leyden University, his doctoral dissertations in both philosophy and medicine dealt with the eyes. He was particularly interested in cataracts, experimenting with cataract surgery and carrying out basic research aimed at pinpointing the cause. He also accurately described how the eye focuses, allowing it to perceive objects at different distances.

In the area of orthopedics, Camper wrote about congenital dislocation of the hip, as well as the structures of the knee and elbow. He also wrote and published an important paper about human locomotion, describing the anatomy of the foot and the best forms of footwear.

In non-medical disciplines, Camper's interests extended to paleontology (acquiring a large collection of fossils), civil engineering (proposing improvements to the design of flood dikes), agronomy (investigating the best methods of clearing land and preparing it for agriculture), botany (combing the countryside, in the company of plant experts, looking for herbs), astronomy (visiting William Herschel and his huge telescope), politics (serving as representative to the Assembly of the General States in The Hague), and technology (studying industrial processes in copper furnaces and glass ovens, personally building many of his tools and instruments).

After a career remarkable for its numerous accomplishments, Camper died in 1789.

CANCER

Cancer is not just one disease, but a large group of almost one hundred diseases. Its two main characteristics are uncontrolled growth of the cells in the human body and the ability of these cells to migrate from the original site and spread to distant sites. If the spread is not controlled, cancer can result in **death**.

Cancer, by definition, is a disease of the genes. A gene is a small part of DNA, which is the master molecule of the cell. Genes make "proteins," which allow our bodies to carry out all the many processes that permit us to breathe, think, move, etc. The genes also produce proteins that are involved in controlling the processes of cell growth and division. An alteration (mutation) to the DNA molecule can disrupt the genes and produce faulty proteins. This causes the cell to become abnormal and lose its restraints on growth. The abnormal cell begins to divide uncontrollably and eventually forms a new growth known as a "tumor" or neoplasm (medical term for cancer meaning "new growth").

In a healthy individual, the immune system can recognize the neoplastic cells and destroy them before they get a chance to divide. However, some mutant cells may escape immune detection and survive to become tumors or cancers. Tumors are of two types, benign or malignant. A benign tumor is slow growing, does not spread or invade surrounding tissue, and once it is removed, it doesn't usually recur. A malignant tumor, on the other hand, invades surrounding tissue and spreads to other parts of the body. If the cancer cells have spread to the surrounding tissues, then, even after the malignant tumor is removed, it generally recurs.

A majority of cancers are caused by changes in the cell's DNA because of damage due to the environment. Environmental factors that are responsible for causing the initial mutation in the DNA are called carcinogens, and there are many types. There are some cancers that have a genetic basis. In other words, an individual could inherit faulty DNA from his parents, which could predispose him to getting cancer.

The major risk factors for cancer are: tobacco, alcohol, diet, sexual and reproductive behavior, infectious agents, family history, occupation, environment and pollution.

Despite the fact that there are several hundred different types of cancers, producing very different symptoms, the American Cancer Society (ACS) has established the following seven symptoms as possible warning signals of cancer:

- Changes in the size, color, or shape of a wart or a mole
- A sore that does not heal
- Persistent **cough**, hoarseness, or **sore throat**
- A lump or thickening in the breast or elsewhere
- Unusual bleeding or discharge
- Chronic **indigestion** or difficulty in swallowing
- Any change in bowel or bladder habits.

Diagnosis of cancer begins with a thorough **physical examination** and a complete medical history. The doctor will observe, feel and palpate (apply pressure by touch) different parts of the body in order to identify any variations from the normal size, feel and texture of the organ or tissue. As part of the physical exam, the doctor will inspect the oral cavity or the mouth. By focusing a light into the mouth, he will look for abnormalities in color, moisture, surface texture, or presence of any thickening or sore in the lips, tongue, gums, the hard palate on the roof of the mouth, and the throat. To detect **thyroid cancer**, the doctor will observe the front of the neck for swelling. He may gently manipulate the neck and palpate the front and side surfaces of the thyroid gland (located at the base of the neck) to detect any nodules or tenderness. As part of the physical examination, the doctor will also palpate the lymph nodes in the neck, under the arms and in the groin. Many illnesses and cancers cause a swelling of the lymph nodes.

The doctor may conduct a thorough examination of the skin to look for sores that have been present for more than three weeks and that bleed, ooze, or crust; irritated patches that may itch or hurt, and any change in the size of a wart or a mole.

Examination of the female pelvis is used to detect cancers of the ovaries, uterus, cervix, and vagina. In the visual examination, the doctor looks for abnormal discharges or the presence of sores. Then, using gloved hands the physician palpates the internal pelvic organs such as the uterus and ovaries to detect any abnormal masses. Breast examination includes visual observation where the doctor looks for any discharge, unevenness, discoloration, or scaling. The doctor palpates both breasts to feel for masses or lumps.

For males, inspection of the rectum and the prostate is also included in the physical examination. The doctor inserts a gloved finger into the rectum and rotates it slowly to feel for any growths, tumors, or other abnormalities. The doctor also conducts an examination of the testis, where the doctor observes the genital area and looks for swelling or other abnormalities. The testicles are palpated to identify any lumps, thickening or differences in the size, weight and firmness.

If the doctor detects an abnormality on physical examination, or the patient has some symptom that could be indicative of cancer, the doctor may order diagnostic tests. Laboratory studies of sputum (sputum cytology), blood, urine, and stool can detect abnormalities that may indicate cancer. Imaging tests such as **computed tomography scans** (CT scans), **magnetic resonance imaging** (MRI), ultrasound and fiberoptic scope examinations help the doctors determine the location of the tumor even if it is deep within the body. Conventional x rays are often used for initial evaluation, because they are relatively cheap, painless and easily accessible.

The most definitive diagnostic test is the biopsy, wherein a piece of tissue is surgically removed for microscope examination. Besides, confirming a cancer, the biopsy also provides information about the type of cancer, the stage it has reached, the aggressiveness of the cancer and the extent of its spread. Since a biopsy provides the most accurate analysis, it is considered the gold standard of diagnostic tests.

The aim of cancer treatment is to remove all or as much of the tumor as possible and to prevent the recurrence or spread of the primary tumor. While devising a treatment plan for cancer, the likelihood of curing the cancer has to be weighed against the side effects of the treatment. If the cancer is very aggressive and a cure is not possible, then the treatment should be aimed at relieving the symptoms and controlling the cancer for as long as possible.

Cancer treatment can take many different forms, and it is always tailored to the individual patient. The decision on which type of treatment is the most appropriate depends on the type and location of cancer, the extent to which it has already spread, the patient's age, sex, general health status and personal treatment preferences. The major types of treatment are: surgery, radiation, **chemotherapy**, immunotherapy, hormone therapy, and bone-marrow transplantation.

Surgery is the removal of a visible tumor and is the most frequently used cancer treatment. It is most effective when a cancer is small and confined to one area of the body.

Radiation kills tumor cells. Radiation is used alone in cases where a tumor is unsuitable for surgery. More often, it is used in conjunction with surgery and chemotherapy. Radiation can be either external or internal. In the external form, the radiation is aimed at the tumor from outside the body. In internal radiation (also known as brachytherapy), a radioactive substance, in the form of pellets or liquid is placed at the cancerous site by means of a pill, injection or insertion in a sealed container.

Chemotherapy is the use of drugs to kill cancer cells. It destroys the hard-to-detect cancer cells that have spread and are circulating in the body. Chemotherapeutic drugs can be taken either orally (by mouth) or intravenously, and may be given alone or in conjunction with surgery, radiation or both.

Immunotherapy uses the body's own immune system to destroy cancer cells.This form of treatment is being intensively studied in clinical trials and is not yet widely available to most cancer patients. The various immunological agents being tested include substances produced by the body (such as the interferons, interleukins, and growth factors), monoclonal antibodies and vaccines. Unlike traditional vaccines, cancer vaccines do not prevent cancer. Instead, they are designed to treat people who already have the disease. Cancer vaccines work by boosting the body's immune system and training the immune cells to specifically destroy cancer cells.

Hormone therapy is standard treatment for some types of cancers that are hormone-dependent and grow faster in the presence of particular hormones. These include cancer of the prostate, breast, and uterus. Hormone therapy involves blocking the production or action of these hormones. As a result the growth of the tumor slows down and survival may be extended for several months or years.

The bone marrow is the tissue within the bone cavities that contains blood-forming cells. Healthy bone marrow tissue constantly replenishes the blood supply and is essential to life. Sometimes, the amount of drugs or radiation needed to destroy cancer cells also destroys bone marrow. Replacing the bone marrow with healthy cells counteracts this adverse effect. A bone marrow transplant is the removal of marrow from one person and the transplant of the blood-forming cells either to the same person or to some one else. Bone-marrow transplantation, while not a therapy in itself, is often used to ''rescue'' a patient, by allowing those with cancer to undergo very aggressive therapy.

Many different specialists generally work together as a team to treat cancer patients. An oncologist is a physician who specializes in cancer care. The oncologist provides chemotherapy, hormone therapy, and any other non-surgical treatment that does not involve radiation. The oncologist often serves as the primary physician and co-ordinates the patient's treatment plan. The radiation oncologist specializes in using radiation to treat cancer, while the surgical oncologist performs the operations needed to diagnose or treat cancer.

There are a multitude of alternative treatments available to help the person with cancer. They can be used in conjunction with, or separate from, surgery, chemotherapy, and radiation therapy. Alternative treatment of cancer is a complicated arena and a trained health practitioner should be consulted.

Most cancers are curable if detected and treated at their early stages. A cancer patient's prognosis is affected by many factors, particularly the type of cancer the patient has, the stage of the cancer, the extent to which it has metastasized and the aggressiveness of the cancer. In addition, the patient's age, general health status and the effectiveness of the treatment being pursued are also important factors.

According to nutritionists and epidemiologists from leading universities in the United States, a person can reduce the chances of getting cancer by following some simple guidelines:

- Eating plenty of vegetables and fruits
- Exercising vigorously for at least 20 minutes every day
- Avoiding excessive weight gain

- Avoiding tobacco (even second hand smoke)
- Decreasing or avoiding consumption of animal fats and red meats
- Avoiding excessive amounts of alcohol
- Avoiding the midday sun (between 11 a.m. and 3 p.m.) when the suns rays are the strongest
- Avoiding risky sexual practices
- Avoiding known carcinogens in the environment or work place.

CANDIDIASIS

Candidiasis is an infection caused by a species of the yeast *Candida*, usually *Candida albicans*. It is a common cause of vaginal infections in women. It may also cause mouth infections in people with reduced immune function, or in patients taking certain **antibiotics**. A more serious form of the condition, known as deep organ candidiasis, can infect nearly all the major organs of the body.

Over one million women in the United States develop vaginal candidiasis, more commonly known as *yeast infections*, each year. Most women with vaginal candidiasis experience severe vaginal **itching**. They also have a discharge that often looks like cottage cheese and has a sweet or bread-like odor. The vulva and vagina can be red, swollen, and painful, particularly during sexual intercourse.

In most cases, vaginal candidiasis can be treated successfully with a variety of over-the-counter antifungal creams or suppositories. These include Monistat, Gyne-Lotrimin, and Mycelex. However, infections often recur, and women may need to take a prescription anti-fungal drug such as terconazole (sold as Terazol) or take other anti-fungal drugs on a preventive basis.

Oral candidiasis, also known as *thrush*, causes white, curd-like patches on the tongue, inside of the cheeks, or the palate. Thrush typically occurs in people with abnormal immune systems. These can include people undergoing **chemotherapy** for **cancer**, people taking immunosuppressive drugs to protect transplanted organs, or people with HIV infection.

Thrush is usually treated with prescription lozenges or mouth washes. Some of the most-used prescriptions are nystatin mouthwashes (Nilstat or Nitrostat) and clotrimazole lozenges. Good **oral hygiene** might reduce problems, but is not a guarantee against candidiasis.

Also known as invasive candidiasis, deep organ candidiasis is a serious infection that can affect the esophagus, heart, blood, liver, spleen, kidneys, eyes, and skin. Like vaginal and oral candidiasis, it is an opportunistic disease that strikes when a person's resistance is lowered, often due to another illness. Anything that weakens the body's natural barrier against colonizing organisms—including stomach surgery, burns, nasogastric tubes, artificial joints and valves, and catheters—can increase a patient's suceptibility to infection. Rising numbers of AIDS patients, organ transplant recipients, and other individuals whose immune systems are compromised help account for the dramatic increase in deep organ candidiasis in recent years. Patients with granulocytopenia (deficiency of white blood cells) are particularly at risk for deep organ candidiasis.

Fungal blood cultures and/or tissue biopsy are usually required to diagnose deep organ candidiasis. Drug treatment is based on a patient's medical history and immune status. If possible, catheters and nasogastric tubes should be removed from patients in whom these devices are still present and anti-fungal chemotherapy started to prevent the spread of the disease.

CANKER SORES

Canker sores are small sores or ulcers that appear inside the mouth, usually on the inside of the lips, cheeks, and/or soft palate. They can also occur on the tongue and in the throat. Often, several canker sores will appear at the same time and may be grouped in clusters. Canker sores appear as a whitish, round area with a red border. The sores are painful and sensitive to touch. The average canker sore is about one-quarter inch in size, although they can occasionally be larger. Canker sores are not infectious.

Canker sores are sometimes confused with **cold sore**s. Cold sores are caused by herpes simplex virus. This disease, also known as oral herpes or fever blisters, can occur anywhere on the body. Most commonly, herpes infection occurs on the outside of the lips and the gums, and much less frequently on the inside the mouth. Cold sores are infectious.

The exact cause of canker sores is uncertain, however, they seem to be related to a localized immune reaction. Other proposed causes for this disease are trauma to the affected areas from toothbrush scrapes, **stress**, hormones, and food **allergies**. Canker sores tend to appear in response to stress. The initial symptom is a tingling or mildly painful **itching** sensation in the area where the sore will appear. After one to several days, a small red swelling appears. The sore is round, it is a whitish color with a grayish colored center. Usually, there is a red ring of inflammation surrounding the sore. The main symptom is pain. Canker sores can be very painful, especially if they are touched repeatedly, e.g., by the tongue. They last for one to two weeks.

Approximately 20% of the U.S. population is affected with recurring canker sores, and more women than men get them. Women are more likely to have canker sores during their premenstrual period. Since canker sores heal by themselves, treatment is not usually necessary. Pain relief remedies, such as topical anesthetics, may be used to reduce the pain of the sores. The use of corticosteroid ointments sometimes speeds healing. Avoidance of spicy or acidic foods can help reduce the pain associated with canker sores.

Alternative therapies for canker sores are aimed at healing existing sores and preventing their recurrence. Several herbal remedies, including calendula (*Calendula officinalis*), myrrh (*Commiphora molmol*), and goldenseal (*Hydrastis canadensis*), may be helpful in the treatment of existing sores. Compresses soaked in teas made from these herbs are applied directly to the sores. The tannic acid in a tea bag can also help dry up the sores when the wet tea bag is used as a compress. Taking dandelion (*Taraxacum officinale*) tea or capsules may help heal sores and also prevent future outbreaks. Since canker sores are often brought on by stress, such stress-relieving techniques as **meditation**, **guided imagery**, and certain **acupressure** exercises may help prevent canker sores or lessen their severity.

CARBOHYDRATE INTOLERANCE

Carbohydrates, which include sugars and starches, are the body's primary source of energy and, along with fats and proteins, one of the three major nutrients in the human diet. Carbohydrate intolerance is the inability of the body to completely process the nutrient carbohydrate into a source of energy for the body, usually because of the deficiency of an enzyme needed for digestion.

Digestion of food begins in the mouth, moves on to the stomach, and then into the small intestine. Along the way, specific enzymes are needed to process different types of sugars. When these enzymes are inadequate, the result is carbohydrate intolerance.

Carbohydrate intolerance can be primary or secondary. Primary deficiency is caused by an enzyme defect present at birth or developed over time. The most common is lactose intolerance. Secondary deficiencies are caused by a disease or disorder of the intestinal tract, and disappear when the disease is treated. These include protein deficiency, **celiac disease**, tropical sprue, and some intestinal infections. In **cancer** patients, treatment with radiation therapy or **chemotherapy** may affect the cells in the intestine that normally secrete lactase, leading to intolerance.

Lactose intolerance, the inability to digest the sugar found in milk, is widespread and affects up to 70% of the world's adult population and is the most common of all enzyme deficiencies. Deficiencies in enzymes other than lactase are extremely rare.

The severity of carbohydrate intolerance symptoms depends on the extent of the enzyme deficiency, and range from a feeling of mild bloating to severe **diarrhea**. In the case of a lactase deficiency, undigested milk sugar remains in the intestine, which is then fermented by the bacteria normally present in the intestine. These bacteria produce gas, cramping, bloating, a "gurgly" feeling in the abdomen, and flatulence. In a growing child, the main symptoms are diarrhea and a failure to gain weight. In an individual with lactase deficiency, gastrointestinal distress begins about 30 minutes to two hours after eating or drinking foods containing lactose. Food intolerances can be confused with food **allergies**, since the symptoms of nausea, cramps, bloating, and diarrhea are similar.

Sugars that aren't broken down by enzymes cause the body to push fluid into the intestines, which results in watery diarrhea. Diarrhea may flush other nutrients out of the intestine before they can be absorbed, causing **malnutrition**.

Carbohydrate intolerance can be diagnosed using oral tolerance and blood tests. To identify lactose intolerance in children and adults, the hydrogen breath test is used to measure the amount of hydrogen in the breath. The patient drinks a beverage containing lactose and the breath is analyzed at regular intervals. If undigested lactose in the large intestine (colon) is fermented by bacteria, it produces hydrogen, which is carried by the bloodstream into the lungs where it is exhaled. Normally there is very little hydrogen detectable in the breath, so its presence indicates faulty digestion of lactose.

No treatment currently exists to improve on the body's ability to produce digestive enzymes, but symptoms can be controlled by diet. Carbohydrate intolerance caused by temporary intestinal diseases disappears when the underlying condition is successfully treated.

Because the degree of lactose intolerance varies so much, treatment should be tailored for the individual. Young children showing signs of intolerance should avoid milk products; infants should switch to soy-based formula. Older children and adults can adjust their intake of lactose depending on how much and what they can tolerate. Generally, small amounts of lactose-containing foods taken throughout the day are better tolerated than a large amount consumed all at once.

For those individuals who are sensitive to even very small amounts of lactose, the lactase enzyme is available without a prescription. It comes in liquid form for use with milk. The addition of a few drops to a quart of milk can reduce the lactose content by up to 90%. Chewable lactase enzyme tablets are also available. Three to six tablets taken before a meal or snack will aid in the digestion of solid foods. Lactose-reduced milk and other products are also available in stores. The milk contains the same nutrients as regular milk.

Because dairy products are an important source of calcium, people who reduce or severely limit their intake of dairy products may need to consider other ways to consume an adequate amount of calcium in their **diets**.

CARBON MONOXIDE POISONING

Carbon monoxide (CO) **poisoning** occurs when carbon monoxide gas is inhaled. CO is a colorless, odorless, highly poisonous gas. It is found in automobile exhaust fumes, faulty stoves and heating systems, fires, and cigarette smoke. Other sources include woodburning stoves, kerosene heaters, improperly ventilated water heaters and gas stoves, and blocked or poorly maintained chimney flues. CO interferes with the ability of the blood to carry oxygen. The result is **headache**, nausea, convulsions, and finally **death** by asphyxiation.

Carbon monoxide, sometimes called coal gas, has been known as a toxic substance since the third century B.C. It was used for executions and suicides in early Rome. Today it is the leading cause of accidental poisoning in the United States. According to the *Journal of the American Medical Association*, 1,500 Americans die each year from accidental exposure to CO, and another 2,300 from intentional exposure (suicide). An additional 10,000 people seek medical attention after exposure to CO and recover.

Anyone who is exposed to CO will become sick, and the entire body is involved in CO poisoning.. A developing fetus can also be poisoned if a pregnant woman breathes CO gas. Infants, people with heart or lung disease, or those with anemia may be more seriously affected. People who are exposed to car exhausts in a confined area, such as underground parking garage attendants, are more likely to be poisoned by CO. Firemen also run a higher risk of inhaling CO.

The symptoms of CO poisoning in order of increasing severity include: headache, **shortness of breath**, dizziness, fatigue, mental confusion and difficulty thinking, loss of fine hand-eye coordination, **nausea and vomiting**, rapid heart rate, **hallucinations**, inability to execute voluntary movements accurately, collapse, lowered body temperature (**hypothermia**), **coma**, convulsions, seriously low blood pressure, cardiac and **respiratory failure**, and death

In some cases, the skin, mucous membranes, and nails of a person with CO poisoning are cherry red or bright pink. Because the color change doesn't always occur, it is an unreliable symptom to rely on for diagnosis.

Although most CO poisoning is acute, or sudden, it is possible to suffer from chronic, or long-term, CO poisoning. This condition exists when a person is exposed to low levels of the gas over a period of days to months. Symptoms are often vague and include (in order of frequency) fatigue, headache, dizziness, sleep disturbances, cardiac symptoms, apathy, nausea, and memory disturbances. Little is known about chronic CO poisoning, and it is often misdiagnosed.

The main reason to suspect CO poisoning is evidence that fuel is being burned in a confined area, for example a car running inside a closed garage, a charcoal grill burning indoors, or an unvented kerosene heater in a workshop. Under these circumstances, one or more persons suffering from the symptoms listed above strongly suggests CO poisoning. In the absence of some concrete reason to suspect CO poisoning, the disorder is often misdiagnosed as migraine headache, **stroke**, psychiatric illness, **food poisoning**, alcohol poisoning, or heart disease.

The presence and extent of CO poisoning is confirmed through various blood tests, including a carboxyhemoglobin test. arterial blood gases and pH, a complete **blood count**, and measurement of other blood components such as sodium, potassium, bicarbonate, urea nitrogen, and lactic acid. An electrocardiogram (ECG) and a **chest x ray** may also be performed.

Victims of CO poisoning should be immediately removed from the source of carbon monoxide gas into fresh air. If the victim is not breathing and has no pulse, **cardiopulmonary resuscitation (CPR)** should be started. Depending on the severity of the poisoning, 100% oxygen may be given with a tight fitting mask as soon as it is available.

Once a patient with CO poisoning is hospitalized, fluids and electrolytes may be administered to correct blood imbalances. In severe cases of CO poisoning, patients are given hyperbaric **oxygen therapy**. This treatment involves placing the patient in a pressurized chamber breathing 100% oxygen. The increased pressure forces more oxygen into the blood.

The speed and degree of recovery from CO poisoning depends on the length of exposure to the gas. Although the symptoms of CO poisoning may subside in a few hours, some patients show memory problems, fatigue, confusion, and mood changes for two to four weeks after their exposure to the gas.

Carbon monoxide poisoning is preventable. Particular care should be paid to situations where fuel is burned in a confined area. Portable and permanently installed carbon monoxide detectors that sound a warning similar to smoke detectors are available for under $50.

CARCINOGENS

Cancer is a mysterious group of diseases which often arouses fearful images of death. There are over one hundred different types of cancer, which can be distinguished by the type of cell or organ which is affected, the treatment plan employed, and the cause of the cancer. Any substance or agent that can cause cancer is called a carcinogen. One of the first people to suspect that certain substances in the environment can cause cancer was Sir **Percivall Pott** (1714-1788), who in 1775 published a paper on cancer occurrence in chimney sweeps. It has since been discovered that benzo(a)pyrene, a chemical found in soot, is a potent carcinogen. Ionizing radiation was first suspected of being carcinogenic around the turn of the twentieth century, when physicians who developed the use of X-rays and radium in medicine showed a high incidence of skin cancer. Later, in 1915, scientists in Japan documented carcinogens when they noticed that rabbits developed tumors when tar was applied to the inside of their ears. By 1930, Ernest Kennaway isolated polycyclic hydrocarbons and proved that they were the carcinogenic agent.

Today, the media rarely misses an opportunity to report on newly discovered carcinogenic substances. Sometimes it seems as if *everything* causes cancer, but very few things are proven carcinogens. The two main categories of carcinogens are genetic and environmental. Specific environmental factors include tobacco, alcohol, diet, infection, sexual practices, occupation, geophysical phenomena, pollution, medications, food additives, and industrial products. Tobacco and diet together account for almost two-thirds of all cancer-related deaths. **Stress** and emotional factors should also be listed as elements that may contribute toward the development of some cancers.

Cigarette smoking is clearly the single most preventable cause of illness and premature death in the United States. The United States Surgeon General estimates that 30% of all cancer deaths are directly attributable to tobacco use. The carcinogens in tobacco include nicotine, tar, carbon monoxide, ammonia, formaldehyde, phenols, creosote, anthracene, pyrene, hydrocyanic acid, arsenic, and lead. Tar is the particulate matter derived from burning organic compounds and is the leading cancer-causing chemical in tobacco smoke. Researchers have also identified 4-(N- nitrosomethylamino)-1-(3-pyridyl)-1butanone (NNK), as a carcinogen that is formed in the production, curing, and aging of tobacco. Studies in animals have shown that it can cause benign and malignant tumors, as well as other forms of cancer. Pipe and cigar smoke contain essentially the same array of poisons although the relative amounts may vary. In 1997, scientists produced the first chemical evidence that an increased risk for lung cancer is associated with passive, second-hand, **smoke inhalation**. The investigators found the metabolite of a tobacco carcinogen in the urine of non-smokers who have been exposed to second-hand smoke. Smokeless tobacco, including chewing tobacco and snuff, are not alternatives to avoid cancer. These products contain large quantities of cancer-causing chemicals called n-nitrosamines. Lip, mouth, tongue, and throat cancers have been positively linked to the use of smokeless tobacco products. Furthermore, the risk of these types of cancers are increased when tobacco is used with alcohol. This phenomenon is known as synergism. While marijuana does not contain nicotine or tobacco, it does contain tar and other carcinogens.

Diet and nutrition have been recognized as major factors that influence the development of many cancers. The National Cancer Institute recommends a low fat, high fiber diet with adequate allowances of vitamin A and vitamin C as a specific way to reduce the risk of developing colon cancer. Cruciferous vegetables like cabbage and brussels sprouts may also help reduce the chances of developing some stomach and colon cancers. Charred foods and alcohol contain carcinogens and should be avoided or consumed in moderation.

Infection may also lead to cancer. This usually occurs when a virus, bacteria, or parasite is contracted. Only about 10 percent of all cancers are believed to be caused by these organisms. Retroviruses such as the herpes virus and the virus that causes **AIDS** have been implicated in certain types of cancer. According to the oncogene theory of virus-mediated cancer, when a virus infects a cell, it may enter the genes of the host cell that control growth and division. The infected cell may begin to divide uncontrollably, resulting in the formation of a tumor. Changes in a single oncogene rarely lead to malignant cancer. Rather, it usually requires many of the more than 100 oncogenes working in concert to initiate this chain of events. Parasitic and bacterial-induced cancer may be due to the chronic irritation, either internal or external, caused by these organisms over long periods of time. It also appears that other co-factors need to be present before many of these cancers can fully develop.

Changes in the body resulting from sexual intercourse, **pregnancy**, and **childbirth** are obviously in a different class of carcinogens than those produced by exposure to chemicals. They are, however, considered environmental since they are not controlled solely by one's own genes. This is not to suggest that childbirth causes cancer. In fact, pregnancy and childbirth may actually help prevent cancer of the uterus, ovary, and breast. However, frequent sexual intercourse with large numbers of partners has been positively linked to an increased risk of **cervical cancer**. Researchers think that the primary carcinogenic agent in this example may actually be an unknown virus.

The percentage of all cancers that can be attributed to work-related influences varies from about 4 percent to as high as 15 percent. Since 1971, the International Agency for Research on Cancer (IARC) has been categorizing carcinogens and occupations associated with high cancer rates. Some chemicals used in shoe, tire, and furniture manufacturing, as well as nickel refining, diesel fuel, and dry cleaning have been identified as ''anticipated'' carcinogens. Arsenic, asbestos, benzene, benzidine, chromium, 2-Naphthylene, oils, and vinyl chloride show occupational exposures causally associated with cancer in humans. Cadmium, DDT, and formaldehyde are other common chemicals that are suspected to cause cancer in humans.

Asbestos is perhaps the most familiar carcinogen in this category. This material, made of small silicate fibers, has been used in construction since the 1800s. Asbestos only becomes a cancer risk when the fibers are set free and inhaled during decomposition or renovation. The fibers irritate the body's alveoli and can lead to lung cancer. Asbestos exposure is now carefully regulated by the Occupational Safety and Health Administration (OSHA).

One of the most infamous carcinogens is PCB or polycholrinated biphenyls. These man-made chemicals encompass 209 individual compounds with various toxicities. PCBs were once widely used as coolants and lubricants before their manufacture was halted in October 1977 due to their accumulations in the environment and resultant health hazards, including their role as carcinogens that can cause cancer. However, PCBs are still widespread throughout the environment, including contaminated water, sediment, and fish. Another group of contaminants that exist worldwide are polychlorinated dibenzo-para-dioxins, or simply dioxins. Dioxins are typically by-products of chemical reactions used for other purposes, like the production of some herbicides. A working group for IARC has determined that one dioxin, 2,3,7,8-tetrachlorodibenzo-para-dioxin (TCDD) is carcinogenic to humans, increasing risk of lung cancer and all cancers combined in those exposed to it. IARC continues to investigate the other dioxins. Benzene, a clear colorless liquid used widely as a solvent and reactant, has also been linked to **leukemia**, which is a type of blood cancer. Radiation refers to energy that is sent through space. It may be in the form of waves such as ultraviolet light, X-rays, and microwaves, or in the form of charged atomic particles including electrons, protons, and neutrons. Radiation can alter genes within chromosomes. **Skin cancer** in early X-ray workers and radium workers, bone sarcoma in luminous dial painters, and **lung cancers** in miners of radioactive ores have all been studied. Ironically, some forms of radiation are used to diagnose and treat cancer.

Radiation from the sun is an increasing concern and may be linked to a depletion of the protective ozone layer in the Earth's upper atmosphere. The sun is the chief cause of non-melanoma skin cancer. The amount of ultraviolet-beta radiation from the sun varies with location, altitude, sky cover, and the time of year. Exposure levels can be reduced by using sun screen products and monitoring prolonged outdoor activities—especially between 11:00 a.m. and 1:00 p.m. during the late summer months.

In recent years, the approval of irradiation of food has raised growing concerns about its possible association with cancer. Food irradiation uses ionizing energy to kill bacteria, mold and insects and can also prolong the food's shelf life. The major concern is that the process forms free radicals, or unidentified radiolytic products, which have been associated with the development of cancer. Those against irradiated foods argue that they contain high levels of carcinogens, including nitrosamines and formaldehyde. However, more than 39 countries, including the United States. approve the controlled use of irradiation for one or more food items, including meats, poultry, seafood, grains, vegetables, nuts, and spices.

Historically, substances have been tested for carcinogenicity by using them on human or animal test subjects. In the late 1970s, however, Bruce Ames of the University of California at Berkeley developed a carcinogenicity test that uses bacteria instead of human or animal subjects. The Ames test yields results in hours or days instead of the years required for human or animal tests, and it has a high rate of consistency with human tests. While this test is not accurate enough to give permanent proof of a substance's carcinogenicity, it does allow for speedy screening of new or previously unsuspected substances. The most difficult aspect of testing substances as potential carcinogens is determining what doses are actually harmful. For example, the Ames test on animals is performed with maximum tolerated doses (MTD), and some scientists question whether testing with MTD accurately reflet a substance's potential carcinogenic effect on humans.

Many environmental carcinogens are avoidable, and early diagnosis and treatment increases the recovery rate for all cancers. Genetically predisposed cancers are more difficult to regulate. They are also less common than many environmentally induced cancers. A growing area of interest are investigations of carcinogens like NNK and their ability to alter genes and cause cancer.

Research conducted by the **World Health Organization** (WHO) has shown that industrialized countries have high cancer rates compared with countries that have little industry. Despite the fact that industrialized countries make up only one-fifth of the world's population, one-half of all the world's cancers are found in people living in these countries. While many people fear the overall increase of chemical and physical carcinogens in the environment, it is especially important to prioritize risk factors of the highest magnitude. For example, smokers should be less concerned about food additives and more concerned about when they will stop smoking.

Cardiac rehabilitation

Cardiac rehabilitation is a comprehensive exercise, education, and behavioral modification program for patients with heart disease. It is designed to control symptoms, improve exercise tolerance, and improve their overall quality of life. **Heart attack** survivors, bypass and **angioplasty** patients, and individuals with **angina**, congestive **heart failure**, and heart transplants are all candidates for a cardiac rehabilitation program.

A cardiac rehabilitation program is designed and supervised by a specialized team of doctors, nurses, and other healthcare professionals. Members of the cardiac rehabilitation team may include a dietician or nutritionist, physical therapist, exercise physiologist, psychologist, vocational counselor, occupational therapist, and social worker. The program usually begins in a hospital setting and continues after the patient is discharged over a period of 6-12 months.

The elements of a cardiac rehabilitation program vary by individual clinical need, and each program is carefully constructed for the patient by his or her **rehabilitation** team.

Exercise programs generally start out slowly, with simple range-of-motion arm and leg exercises. Walking and stair climbing soon follow. Blood pressure is carefully monitored before and after exercise sessions, and patients are taught how to measure their heart rate and recognize symptoms of cardiac distress. Patients with advanced heart disease may require continuous electrocardiogramy (ECG) monitoring during their exercise sessions. After release from the hospital, the patient works with his cardiac team to create an individual exercise plan.

Cardiac patients will also work with a nutritionist or dietician to develop a low-fat, low-cholesterol diet plan. Patients with high blood pressure may be put on a salt-restricted diet and instructed to limit their alcohol intake. Weight loss may also be a goal with overweight cardiac patients.

A psychologist or social worker can help cardiac patients with issues that may be contributing to their heart condition, such as **stress**, **anxiety**, and depression. Counseling and relaxation training can help patients deal with these feelings. In addition, vocational counselors can assist cardiac patients in setting practical goals to return to work.

Encouraging patients to kick the smoking habit is an important part of cardiac rehabilitation. Cardiac patients who smoke are twice as likely to have a heart attack in the following 5 years than non-smoking patients. A smoking cessation program usually includes patient education and behavioral counseling. Nicotine replacement therapy, which uses nicotine patches, nose spray, or gum to wean patients off of cigarettes, is often part of the program. Antidepressants and anti-anxiety medication may also be helpful in some cases.

Patients require ongoing support from their healthcare team, family, and friends to continue the progress they make during the rehabilitation period. The patient and family should be fully educated on the physical limitations of the patient, his recommended diet and exercise plan, his emotional status, and the lifestyle changes required to improve the patient's overall health.

Cardiac tamponade

The heart is surrounded by a sac called the pericardium. When this sac becomes filled with fluid, the liquid presses on the heart, preventing the lower chambers of the heart from properly filling with blood, resulting in a condition called cardiac tamponade. Because the lower chambers (the ventricles) cannot fill with the correct amount of blood, less than normal amounts of blood reach the lungs and the rest of the body. This condition is very serious and can be fatal if not treated.

Blunt or penetrating injury from trauma to the chest or heart can cause large amounts of blood to fill the pericardium, resulting in cardiac tamponade. Fluid can collect inside the pericardium and compress the heart when the kidneys do not properly remove waste from the blood or when the pericardium is damaged by infection or **cancer**. Tamponade can also occur during open-heart surgery.

When tamponade occurs because of trauma, the sound of the heart beats can become faint, and the blood pressure in the arteries decreases, while the blood pressure in the veins increases. In cases of tamponade caused by more slowly developing diseases, **shortness of breath**, a feeling of tightness in the chest, increased blood pressure in the large veins in the neck (the jugular veins), weight gain, and swelling caused by fluid retention can occur.

When cardiac tamponade is suspected, accurate diagnosis can be life-saving. The most accurate way to identify this condition is by using a test called an echocardiogram, or ultrasound of the heart. This test uses sound waves to create an image of the heart and its surrounding sac, making it easy to visualize any fluid that has collected inside the sac.

If the abnormal fluid buildup in the pericardial sac is caused by cancer or kidney disease, drugs used to treat these conditions can help lessen the amount of fluid collecting inside the sac. Drugs that help maintain normal blood pressure throughout the body can also help this condition; however, these drugs are only a temporary treatment. The fluid within the pericardium must be drained out to reduce the pressure on the heart and restore proper heart pumping.

The fluid inside the pericardium is drained by inserting a needle through the chest and into the sac itself, and drawing the fluid out. This procedure is called pericardiocentesis. In severe cases, a tube (catheter) can be inserted into the sac or a section of the sac can be surgically cut away to allow for more drainage.

Cardiac tamponade is life-threatening. However, drug treatments can be helpful, and surgical treatments can successfully drain the trapped fluid, though it may reaccumulate. Some risk of **death** exists with surgical drainage of the accumulated fluid.

CARDIOMYOPATHY

Cardiomyopathy is an ongoing disease process that damages the muscle wall of the lower chambers of the heart. About 50,000 Americans develop cardiomyopathy each year. Congestive cardiomyopathy is the most common form of cardiomyopathy. In congestive cardiomyopathy, also called dilated cardiomyopathy, the walls of the heart chambers stretch (dilate) to hold a greater volume of blood than normal. Another form of cardiomyopathy, hypertrophic cardiomyopathy, causes the walls of the heart's chambers to thicken abnormally.

Congestive cardiomyopathy is the final stage of many heart diseases and the most common condition resulting in congestive **heart failure**. It may be caused by a number of conditions, including **coronary artery disease**, infections, noninfectious inflammatory conditions, alcohol and other drugs or toxins, **hypertension**, nutritional and metabolic disorders, and **pregnancy**.

Infections caused by bacteria, viruses, and other microorganisms can involve the heart, causing inflammation of the heart muscle (**myocarditis**). The inflammation may damage the heart muscle and cause congestive cardiomyopathy. In the United States, the coxsackievirus B is the most common cause of viral congestive cardiomyopathy.

Myocarditis can also be caused by noninfectious disorders. For example, the conditions sarcoidosis, granulomatous myocarditis, and Wegener's granulomatosis cause inflammation and tissue death in the heart muscle.

When the heart muscle is damaged, it cannot pump enough blood to meet the body's needs. Uninjured areas of the walls of the two lower heart chambers (called ventricles) stretch to make up for the lost pumping action. At first, the enlarged chambers allow more blood to be pumped with less force. The stretched muscle can also contract more forcefully. Over time, the heart muscle continues to stretch, ultimately becoming weaker. The heart is forced to work harder to pump blood by beating faster. Eventually it cannot keep up and blood backs up into the veins, legs, and lungs. When this happens, the condition is called congestive heart failure.

Congestive cardiomyopathy usually affects both ventricles. Blood backed up into the lungs from the left ventricle causes fluid to congest the lung tissue. This is called **pulmonary edema**. When the right ventricle fails to pump enough blood, blood backs up into the veins causing **edema** in the legs, feet, ankles, and abdomen.

Congestive cardiomyopathy is usually a chronic condition, developing gradually over time. Patients with early congestive cardiomyopathy may not have symptoms. The most common symptoms are fatigue and **shortness of breath** on exertion. Patients with more advanced congestive cardiomyopathy may also have chest or abdominal **pain**s, extreme tiredness, **dizziness**, and swelling of the legs and ankles. **sudden cardiac death** is not uncommon with this condition. It stems from irregular heart rhythms in the ventricles (ventricular **arrhythmias**).

When a patient is diagnosed with congestive cardiomyopathy, physicians try to find out the cause. If coronary artery disease is not the culprit, in most other cases a cause is not identified. When a condition responsible for the congestive cardiomyopathy is diagnosed, treatment is aimed at correcting the underlying condition. Congestive cardiomyopathy caused by drinking excess alcohol or by drugs or toxins can be treated by eliminating the alcohol or toxin completely. In some cases, the heart may recover after the toxic substance is removed from the body. Bacterial myocarditis is treated with an antibiotic to eliminate the bacteria.

There is no cure for idiopathic congestive cardiomyopathy. Medicines are given to reduce the workload of the heart and to relieve the symptoms. These include digitalis, **diuretics**, **vasodilators**, **beta blockers**, angiotensin converting enzyme inhibitors (ACE inhibitors), and angiotensin receptor blockers. When the heart muscle is damaged so severely that medicines cannot help, a heart transplant may be required.

Hypertrophic cardiomyopathy, also called idiopathic hypertrophic subaortic stenosis and asymmetrical septal hypertrophy, usually appears in young people, often in athletes. For this reason it is sometimes called athletic heart muscle disease. However, people of any age can develop hypertrophic cardiomyopathy.

The cause of hypertrophic cardiomyopathy is not known. In about one-half of cases, the disease is inherited. Hypertrophic cardiomyopathy is the result of abnormal growth of the heart muscle cells. The wall between the heart's chambers (the septum) may become so thickened that it blocks the flow of blood through the lower left chamber (left ventricle). The thickened wall may push on the heart valve between the two left heart chambers (mitral valve), making it leaky. The thickened muscle walls also prevent the heart from stretching as much as it should to fill with blood.

Often people with hypertrophic cardiomyopathy have no symptoms. Unfortunately, the first sign of the condition may be sudden **death** caused by an abnormal heart rhythm. The American Heart Association reports that 36% of young athletes who die suddenly have probable or definite hypertrophic cardiomyopathy. When symptoms do appear, they include shortness of breath on exertion, dizziness, **fainting**, fatigue, and chest pain.

Treatment of hypertrophic cardiomyopathy usually consists of taking medicines and restricting strenuous **exercise**. Drugs called beta blockers and calcium channel blockers are usually prescribed. **Antiarrhythmic drugs** may also be given to prevent abnormal heart rhythms. If the medications do not help relieve symptoms, surgery to help improve blood flow in the heart chambers may help. Some patients have **pacemakers** and/or defibrillators implanted to help control the heart rate and rhythm. Pacemakers and defibrillators provide electrical impulses to the heart, which can return the heart beat to a normal rhythm. If these treatment methods fail and a patient develops heart failure, a heart transplant may be necessary.

Cardiopulmonary resuscitation (CPR)

Cardiopulmonary resuscitation (CPR) is a procedure to support breathing and circulation on a person who has stopped breathing (respiratory arrest) and/or whose heart has stopped (cardiac arrest). It should be performed if a person is unconscious and not breathing in order to maintain oxygen and blood flow to the heart, brain, and other vital organs.

Respiratory and cardiac arrest can be caused by allergic reactions, an ineffective heartbeat, asphyxiation, breathing passages that are blocked, **choking**, drowning, drug reactions or overdoses, electric shock, exposure to cold, severe shock, or trauma.

CPR has been practiced for over 40 years, and is an important part of the emergency cardiac care system designed to save lives. Each year, thousands of **death**s are prevented by prompt notification of the emergency medical system (EMS), followed by early CPR, **defibrillation** (which delivers a brief electric shock to the heart in an attempt to get the heart to beat normally), and advanced cardiac life support measures.

More than five million Americans receive training in CPR through American Heart Association and American Red Cross courses annually. CPR can be performed by trained bystanders or healthcare professionals on infants, children, and adults. It should always be performed by the person on the scene who is most experienced in CPR. When performed by a bystander, CPR is designed to support and maintain breathing and circulation until emergency medical personnel arrive and take over. When performed by healthcare personnel, it is used in conjunction with other basic and advanced life support measures.

To prevent brain damage or death, CPR must be performed within 4-6 minutes of when breathing stopped. It is a two-part procedure that involves rescue breathing and external chest compressions. To provide oxygen to the person's lungs, the rescuer administers mouth-to-mouth breaths, then helps circulate the blood through the heart to vital organs by external chest compressions.

If a person suddenly becomes unconscious, the rescuer should call out for help, and then determine if the person is responsive by shaking him or her gently on the shoulder and asking, loudly, if they are okay. If the person doesn't answer, the rescuer or another bystander should call the emergency medical system (911). The rescuer should kneel near the person's shoulders and check to see whether the person is breathing by looking at the chest and abdomen, and listening and feeling for breath from the person's lips. If no signs of breathing are present after three to five seconds, CPR should be started.

The rescuer opens the person's airway by placing the head face up, with the forehead tilted back and the chin lifted. The rescuer checks again for breathing (three to five seconds), then begins *rescue breathing (mouth-to-mouth artificial respiration)*. He pinches the person's nostrils shut while holding the chin in the other hand. The rescuer places his mouth against the person's mouth with the lips making a tight seal, then gently exhales for about one to one and a half seconds. The rescuer breaks away for an instant to take a breath and then repeats. The person's head is repositioned after each mouth-to-mouth breath.

After two breaths, the rescuer checks the person's pulse by moving the hand that was under the person's chin to the artery in the neck (carotid artery). If the person has a heartbeat, the rescuer continues rescue breathing until help arrives or the person begins breathing on his or her own. If the person is breathing, the rescuer turns the person onto his or her side.

If there is no heartbeat, the rescuer performs chest compressions. The rescuer kneels next to the person, placing the heel of one hand in the spot on the lower chest where the two halves of the rib cage come together (the breastbone). The rescuer puts his other hand on top of the one on the chest and interlocks the fingers. He straightens his arms, leans forward to position the shoulders directly above the hands and presses down, using only the palms, so that the person's breastbone sinks in about 1½-2 in. The rescuer releases without removing the hands, then repeats for 15 times in 10-15 seconds.

The rescuer tilts the person's head and returns to rescue breathing for one or two quick breaths. He then alternates breathing and heart presses for one minute, and checks for a pulse or breathing. If the rescuer finds signs of a heartbeat and breathing, CPR is stopped. If the person is breathing but has no pulse the heart press is continued; if the person has a pulse but is not breathing, rescue breathing is continued.

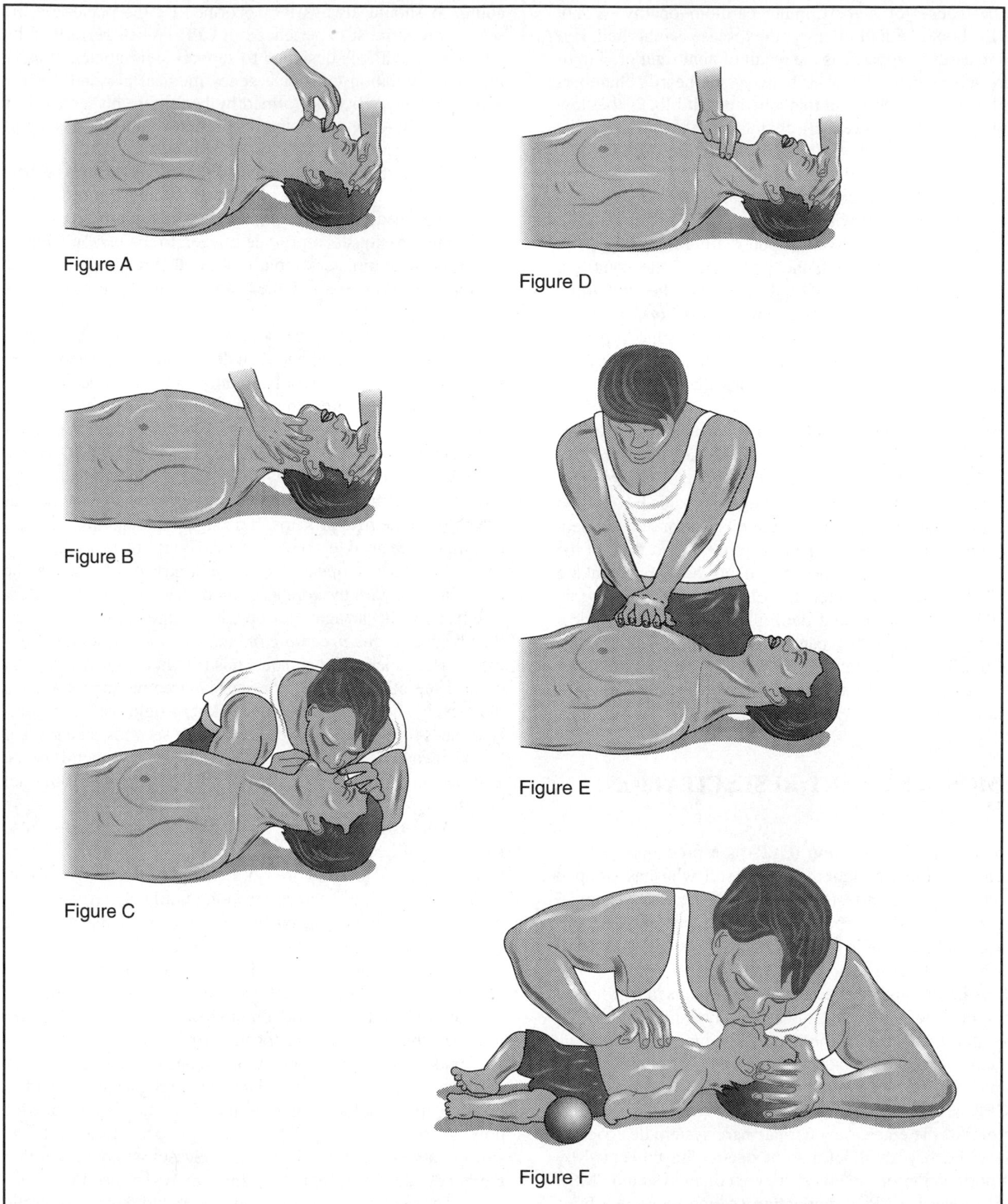

CPR in basic life support. Figure A: The victim should be flat on his back and his mouth should be checked for debris. Figure B: If the victim is unconscious, open airway, lift neck, and tilt head back. Figure C: If victim is not breathing, begin artificial breathing with 4 quick full breaths. Figure D: Check for carotid pulse. Figure E: If pulse is absent, begin artificial circulation by depressing sternum. Figure F: Mouth-to-mouth resuscitation of an infant. *(Illustration by Electronic Illustrators Group.)*

When performing CPR on an infant or child under the age of eight, some slight modifications should be made to the CPR procedure. The rescuer must make a seal around the infant/child's mouth (and nose with infants) and give gentle breaths. The rescuer delivers 20 rescue breaths per minute, taking 1½-2 seconds for each breath. Chest compressions are given with only one hand for a child and with two or three fingers for an infant. The breastbone is depressed only 1-1½ in for a child and ½-1 in for an infant and the rescuer gives at least 100 chest compressions per minute. After administering CPR for one minute, the rescuer should call out for help again if none has arrived, and continue the CPR procedure.

Emergency medical care is always necessary after successful CPR. Once the person's breathing and heartbeat have been restored, the rescuer should make him or her comfortable and stay there until emergency medical personnel arrive. The resucer can continue to reassure the person that help is coming and talk positively until the professionals arrive and take over.

CARDIOVASCULAR SYSTEM

The human circulatory system is termed the cardiovascular system, from the Greek word *kardia*, meaning heart, and the Latin *vasculum*, meaning small vessel. The basic components of the cardiovascular system are the heart, the blood vessels, and the blood. The work done by the cardiovascular system is astounding. Each year, the heart pumps more than 1,848 gal (7,000 l) of blood through a closed system of about 62,100 mi (100,000 km) of blood vessels. This is more than twice the distance around the equator of the Earth. As blood circulates around the body, it picks up oxygen from the lungs, nutrients from the small intestine, and hormones from the endocrine glands, and delivers these to the cells. Blood then picks up carbon dioxide and cellular wastes from cells and delivers these to the lungs and kidneys, where they are excreted. Substances pass out of blood vessels to the cells through the interstitial or tissue fluid that surrounds cells.

The adult heart is a hollow cone-shaped muscular organ located in the center of the chest cavity. The lower tip of the heart tilts toward the left. The heart is about the size of a clenched fist and weighs approximately 10.5 oz (300 g). Remarkably, the heart beats more than 100,000 times a day and close to 2.5 billion times in the average lifetime. A triple-layered sac, the pericardium surrounds, protects, and anchors the heart. A liquid pericardial fluid located in the space between two of the layers, reduces friction when the heart moves.

The heart is divided into four chambers. A partition or septum divides it into a left and right side. Each side is further divided into an upper and lower chamber. The upper chambers, atria (singular atrium), are thin-walled. They receive blood entering the heart, and pump it to the ventricles, the lower heart chambers. The walls of the ventricles are thicker and contain more cardiac muscle than the walls of the atria, enabling the ventricles to pump blood out to the lungs and the rest of the body. The left and right sides of the heart function as two separate pumps. The right atrium receives oxygen-poor blood from the body from a major vein, the vena cava, and delivers it to the right ventricle. The right ventricle, in turn, pumps the blood to the lungs via the pulmonary artery. The left atrium receives the oxygen-rich blood from the lungs from the pulmonary veins, and delivers it to the left ventricle. The left ventricle then pumps it into the aorta, a major artery that leads to all parts of the body. The wall of the left ventricle is thicker than the wall of the right ventricle, making it a more powerful pump able to push blood through its longer trip around the body.

One-way valves in the heart keep blood flowing in the right direction and prevent backflow. The valves open and close in response to pressure changes in the heart. Atrioventricular (AV) valves are located between the atria and ventricles. Semilunar (SL) valves lie between the ventricles and the major arteries into which they pump blood. The ''lub-dup'' sounds that the physician hears through the **stethoscope** occur when the heart valves close. The AV valves produce the ''lub'' sound upon closing, while the SL valves cause the ''dup'' sound. People with a heart murmur have a defective heart valve that allows the backflow of blood.

The heart cycle refers to the events associated with a single heartbeat. The cycle involves systole, the contraction phase, and diastole, the relaxation phase. In the heart, the two atria contract while the two ventricles relax. Then, the two ventricles contract while the two atria relax. The heart cycle consists of a systole and diastole of both the atria and ventricles. At the end of a heartbeat all four chambers rest. The rate of heartbeat averages about 75 beats per minute, and each cardiac cycle takes about 0.8 seconds.

The blood vessels of the body make up a closed system of tubes that carry blood from the heart to tissues all over the body and then back to the heart. Arteries carry blood away from the heart, while veins carry blood toward the heart. Capillaries connect small arteries (arterioles) and small veins (venules). Large arteries leave the heart and branch into smaller ones that reach out to various parts of the body. These divide still further into smaller vessels called arterioles that penetrate the body tissues. Within the tissues, the arterioles branch into a network of microscopic capillaries. Substances move in and out of the capillary walls as the blood exchanges materials with the cells. Before leaving the tissues, capillaries unite into venules, which are small veins. The venules merge to form larger and larger veins that eventually return blood to the heart. The two main circulation routes in the body are the pulmonary circulation, to and from the lungs, and the systemic circulation, to and from all parts of the body. Subdivisions of the systemic system include the coronary circulation, for the heart, the cerebral circulation, for the brain, and the renal circulation, for the kidneys. In addition, the hepatic portal circulation passes blood directly from the digestive tract to the liver.

The walls of arteries, veins, and capillaries differ in structure. In all three, the vessel wall surrounds a hollow center through which the blood flows. The walls of both arteries and veins are composed of three coats. The inner coat is lined with a simple squamous endothelium, a single flat layer of cells. The thick middle coat is composed of smooth muscle that can change the size of the vessel when it contracts or relaxes, and of stretchable fibers that provide elasticity. The outer coat is composed of elastic fibers and collagen. The difference between veins and arteries lies in the thickness of the wall of the vessel. The inner and middle coats of veins are very thin compared to those of arteries. The thick walls of arteries make them elastic and capable of contracting. The repeated expansion and recoil of arteries when the heart beats creates the pulse. We can feel the pulse in arteries near the body surface, such as the radial artery in the wrist. The walls of veins are more flexible than artery walls and they change shape when muscles press against them. Blood returning to the heart in veins is under low pressure often flowing against gravity. One-way valves in the walls of veins keep blood flowing in one direction. Skeletal muscles also help blood return to the heart by squeezing the veins as they contract. The walls of capillaries are only one cell thick. Of all the blood vessels, only capillaries have walls thin enough to allow the exchange of materials between cells and the blood. Their extensive branching provides a sufficient surface area to pick up and deliver substances to all cells in the body.

Blood pressure is the pressure of blood against the wall of a blood vessel. Blood pressure originates when the ventricles contract during the heartbeat. In a healthy young adult male, blood pressure in the aorta during systole is about 120 mm Hg, and approximately 80 mm Hg during diastole. The sphygmomanometer is an instrument that measures blood pressure.

Blood is liquid connective tissue. It transports oxygen-from the lungs and delivers it to cells. It picks up carbon dioxide from the cells and brings it to the lungs. It carries nutrients from the digestive system and hormones from the endocrine glands to the cells. It takes heat and waste products away from cells. The blood helps regulate the body's base-acid balance (pH), temperature, and water content. It protects the body by clotting and by fighting disease through the immune system.

When we study the structure of blood, we find that it is heavier and stickier than water, has a temperature in the body of about 100.4°F (38°C), and a pH of about 7.4. Blood makes up approximately 8% of the total body weight. A male of average weight has about 1.5 gal (5-6 l) of blood in his body, while a female has about 1.2 gal (4-5 l). Blood is composed of a liquid portion (plasma), and blood cells.

Plasma is composed of about 91.5% water, which acts as a solvent, heat conductor, and suspending medium for the blood cells. The rest of the plasma includes plasma proteins produced by the liver, such as albumins, which help maintain water balance; globulins, which help fight disease; and fibrinogen, which aids in blood clotting. The plasma carries nutrients, hormones, enzymes, cellular waste products, some oxygen, and carbon dioxide. Inorganic salts, also carried in the plasma, help maintain osmotic pressure. Plasma leaks out of the capillaries to form the interstitial fluid (tissue fluid) that surrounds the body cells and keeps them moist and supplied with nutrients.

The cells in the blood are erythrocytes (red blood cells), leukocytes (white blood cells), and thrombocytes (platelets). More than 99% of all the blood cells are erythrocytes, or red blood cells. Red blood cells look like flexible biconcave discs about 8 μm in diameter that are capable of squeezing through narrow capillaries. Erythrocytes lack a nucleus and therefore are unable to reproduce. Antigens, specialized proteins on the surface of erythrocytes, determine the ABO and Rh blood types. Erythrocytes contain hemoglobin, a red pigment that carries oxygen, and each red cell has about 280 million hemoglobin molecules. An iron ion in hemoglobin combines reversibly with one oxygen molecule, enabling it to pick up, carry, and drop off oxygen. Erythrocytes are formed in red bone marrow, and live about 120 days. When they are worn out, the liver and spleen destroy them and recycle their breakdown products. Anemia is a blood disorder characterized by too few red blood cells.

Leukocytes are white blood cells. They are larger than red blood cells, contain a nucleus, and do not have hemoglobin. Leukocytes fight disease organisms by destroying them or by producing antibodies. Lymphocytes are a type of leukocyte that bring about immune reactions involving antibodies. Monocytes are large leukocytes that ingest bacteria and get rid of dead matter. Most leukocytes are able to squeeze through the capillary walls and migrate to an infected part of the body. Formed in the white/yellow bone marrow, a leukocyte's life ranges from hours to years depending on how it functions during an infection.

Thrombocytes or platelets bring about clotting of the blood. Clotting stops the bleeding when the circulatory system is damaged. When tissues are injured, platelets disintegrate and release the substance thromboplastin. Working with calcium ions and two plasma proteins, fibrinogen and prothrombin, thromboplastin converts prothrombin to thrombin. Thrombin then changes soluble fibrinogen into insoluble fibrin. Finally, fibrin forms a clot.

See also Angioplasty; Atherosclerosis; Coronary artery bypass graft surgery; Electrocardiography; Endocrine system; Heart attack; Heart-lung machine; Hemophilia; Hypertension; Leukemias; Lymphatic system; Nervous system; Open-heart surgery; Pacemakers; Transfusion; Varicose veins

CARDOZO, W. WARRICK (1905-1962)

African American physician

In 1935, W. Warrick Cardozo was a young pediatrician working at Children's Memorial and Provident hospitals in Chicago under a General Education Board fellowship when, with the aid of a grant from Alpha Pi Alpha fraternity, he began one of the first studies of sickle-cell anemia—a condition in which the majority of red blood cells are crescent-shaped. He found that sickle-cell anemia is inherited. He also established that the disease strikes African Americans almost exclusively, does not cause death among all of the victims of the disease, and that not all persons whose blood contains the sickle cells actually suffer from anemia. These findings arose thirteen years before the nature and characterization of the hemoglobin abnormality that causes sickle-cell anemia was discovered and before the disease became a subject of considerable intensive research.

Born April 6, 1905, in Washington, DC, William Warrick Cardozo was the third generation in his family to attain prominence. His father, Francis L. Cardozo, Jr., was a school principal; his grandfather an educator and politician. William attended Washington public schools, then Hampton Institute in Virginia. At Ohio State University, he received an A.B. degree in 1929 and a M.D. degree four years later. He served his internship at City Hospital in Cleveland, and a residency in pediatrics at Provident Hospital in Chicago.

Cardozo entered private practice in Washington, DC, in 1937, the same year the results of his sickle-cell anemia studies appeared in the Archives of Internal Medicine. He began teaching pediatrics part time at Howard University College of Medicine, where eventually he became a clinical associate professor. He did not stop refining his own learning; in 1942 he sought and gained certification by the American Board of Pediatrics, and in 1948 the American Academy of Pediatrics granted him fellowship. His special interest later turned to children's gastrointestinal disorders.

Despite the demands of a medical practice, Cardozo contributed more than his share of public service. For twenty-four years he served the District of Columbia Board of Health as the school medical inspector. He also served on the Advisory Committee of the District of Columbia Crippled Children's Society. At Howard University College of Medicine, where he taught for many years, he founded Alpha Omega Alpha Honorary Society. On August 11, 1962, Cardozo suffered a fatal heart attack. He was survived by his wife, Julia M. Cardozo, his daughter, Judy, and five sisters.

CARPAL TUNNEL SYNDROME

Carpal tunnel syndrome is a disorder caused by compression at the wrist of the median nerve supplying the hand, causing numbness and tingling. The carpal tunnel is an area in the wrist where the bones and ligaments create a small passageway for the median nerve. The median nerve is responsible for both sensation and movement in the hand, in particular the thumb and first three fingers. When the median nerve is compressed, it cannot function normally, and an individual's hand will feel as if it has "gone to sleep."

Because the carpal tunnel is very narrow, any swelling or fluid accumulation in the area will lead to pressure on the median nerve. **Pregnancy**, **obesity**, arthritis, certain thyroid conditions, diabetes, and certain pituitary abnormalities may cause carpal tunnel syndrome. Various injuries to the arm and wrist (including **fractures**, sprains, and dislocations), can also increase the risk of carpal tunnel syndrome.

Jobs which require an individual to repeatedly bend the wrist inward toward the forearm are a leading cause of carpal tunnel syndrome. Injuries of this type are referred to as "repetitive motion" injuries, and are more frequent among secretaries doing a lot of typing, people working at computer keyboards or cash registers, factory workers, and some musicians. In 1995, about $270 million was spent on sick days taken for **pain** attributed to repetitive motion injuries.

Symptoms of carpal tunnel syndrome include numbness, burning, tingling, and a prickly pin-like sensation over the palm surface of the hand, and into the thumb, forefinger, middle finger, and half of the ring finger. Some individuals notice a shooting pain which goes from the wrist up the arm, or down into the hand and fingers. With continued median nerve compression, an individual may begin to experience muscle weakness, making it difficult to open jars and hold objects with the affected hand. Eventually, the muscles of the hand served by the median nerve may begin to grow noticeably smaller (atrophy), especially the fleshy part of the thumb. Untreated, carpal tunnel syndrome may eventually result in permanent weakness, loss of sensation, or even **paralysis** of the thumb and fingers of the affected hand.

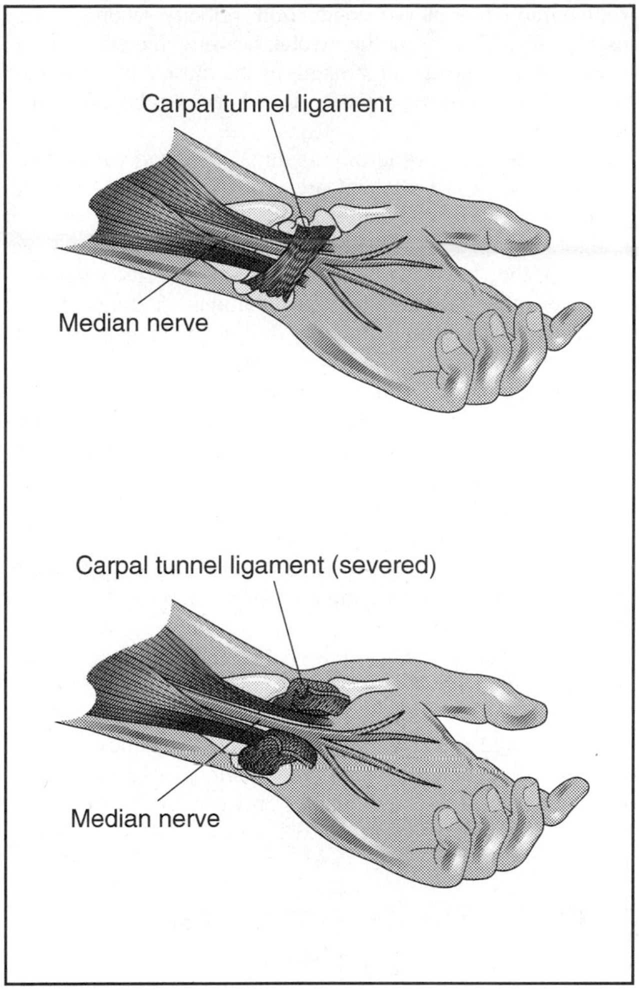

The most severe cases of carpal tunnel syndrome may require surgery to decrease the compression of the median nerve and restore its normal function. This procedure involves severing the ligament which crosses the wrist, thus allowing the median nerve more room and decreasing compression. *(Illustration by Electronic Illustrators Group.)*

To diagnose carpal tunnel syndrome, a doctor will perform a variety of simple tests to measure muscle strength and sensation in the affected hand and arm of the patient. Wrist x rays are often taken to rule out the possibility of a tumor pressing against the median nerve. Further testing may include electromyographic or nerve conduction velocity testing. These tests involve stimulating the median nerve with electricity and measuring the speed and strength of the muscle response and how fast the nerve transmission travels across the carpal tunnel.

Carpal tunnel syndrome is initially treated with splints, which support the wrist and prevent it from flexing inward. Some people get significant relief by wearing splints to sleep at night, while others will need to wear the splints all day, especially if they are performing jobs which stress the wrist. Ibuprofen or other nonsteroidal anti-inflammatory drugs may be prescribed to decrease pain and swelling. When carpal tunnel syndrome is advanced, injection of steroids into the wrist to decrease inflammation may be necessary.

The most severe cases of carpal tunnel syndrome may require surgery. Local anesthesia (numbing medication) or nerve blocks (the injection of anesthetics directly into the nerve) are used to deaden the wrist area, and the ligament which crosses the wrist is cut to decrease compression of the median nerve. Recovery from this type of surgery is typically quick and carpal tunnel symptoms stop completely for about 95% of surgical patients.

Early use of a splint may be helpful for people whose jobs place them at risk of carpal tunnel syndrome. In addition, people who must work long hours at a computer keyboard, can take advantage of recent advances in ''ergonomics,'' which position the keyboard and computer components in a way that increases efficiency and decreases stress.

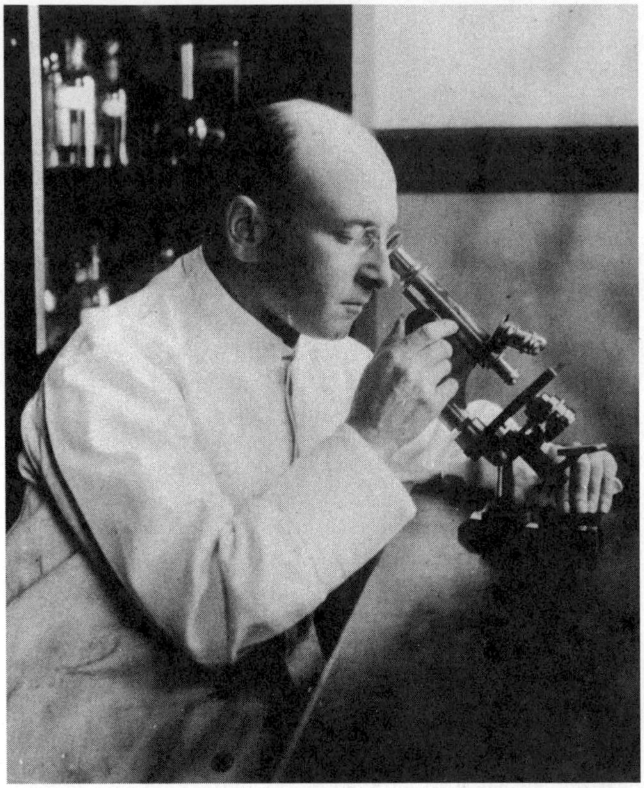

Alexis Carrel

Carrel, Alexis (1873-1944)

French surgeon and physiologist

Alexis Carrel was born in Lyons, France, and brought up by his devout Roman Catholic mother after his father, a **textile** manufacturer, died when Alexis was five. Carrel expressed an early interest in science by dissecting birds and conducting chemistry experiments. He received university degrees in both letters (1890) and science (1891) and then studied medicine at the University of Lyons, earning his medical degree in 1900. As a medical student working at hospitals in Lyons, Carrel displayed a deft talent for dissection and surgery. His interest in blood vessel surgery was aroused in 1894 when the French president, Marie Francois Carnot (1837-1894), was shot. The assassin's bullet severed a major artery, and Carnot bled to death because no techniques existed at the time to repair severed blood vessels. Carrel set out to develop such methods. He learned through embroidery lessons how to use very fine needles and silk thread. He used strict asepsis to avoid infections. To prevent clotting—the major cause of failure in blood vessel suturing—Carrel coated needles, other instruments, and thread with paraffin. To expose blood only to the smooth inner walls of the vessels—thereby further reducing the risk of clotting—Carrel invented the technique of rolling back the vessel ends like cuffs and then stitching the turned-back ends together. Carrel's suturing technique was successfully implemented in 1902. The ability to stitch blood vessels together opened the door to far more sophisticated surgery than had previously been possible, including organ transplantation. Unable to advance professionally at Lyons, Carrel furthered his study of advanced medicine in Paris, France, in 1903 and then moved to Canada, intending to become a cattle rancher. Instead, he became an assistant in physiology at the University of Chicago from 1904 to 1906 and, from 1906 to 1938, was a research member of the Rockefeller Institute for Medical Research in New York City. At both Chicago and the Rockefeller Institute, Carrel expanded his work with blood vessel surgery into the field of organ transplantation, transferring kidneys and other organs in animals. His successful grafting of veins to arteries laid the basis for today's common coronary artery bypass surgery. For his work in suturing and transplantation, Carrel received the 1912 Nobel Prize for medicine or physiology. Carrel also experimented with tissue cultivation. Expanding on the earlier work of Ross Harrison, Carrel kept a piece of tissue from a chick embryo's heart alive and reproducing in his lab for thirty-four years; the tissue culture outlived Carrel! During service for the French army in World War I, Carrel developed a very effective means of irrigating deep wounds with a disinfectant solution. After the war, Carrel collaborated with the famous aviator Charles Lindbergh (1902-1974) to develop a device that would keep entire organs alive outside the body. The Carrel-Lindbergh perfusion pump of the 1930s circulated blood or a nutrient fluid through the organ via the organ's blood vessels. This perfusion pump was also called an artificial heart and was an important early step in the development of methods to maintain circulation when major organs of the body are undergoing surgical intervention. In 1935 Carrel published a best-selling book, *Man, the Unknown*, that promoted an ideal world ruled by an intellectual elite. He returned to Paris in 1939, where he remained during the German occupation, establishing an Institute for the Study of Human Problems. Because Carrel accepted support from the Vichy government and dealt with the Germans in connection with his institute, his reputation was maligned by charges of collaboration at the time of this death in 1944 from heart failure in Paris.

See also Open-heart surgery

CARSON, BENJAMIN S. (1951-)

African American pediatric neurosurgeon

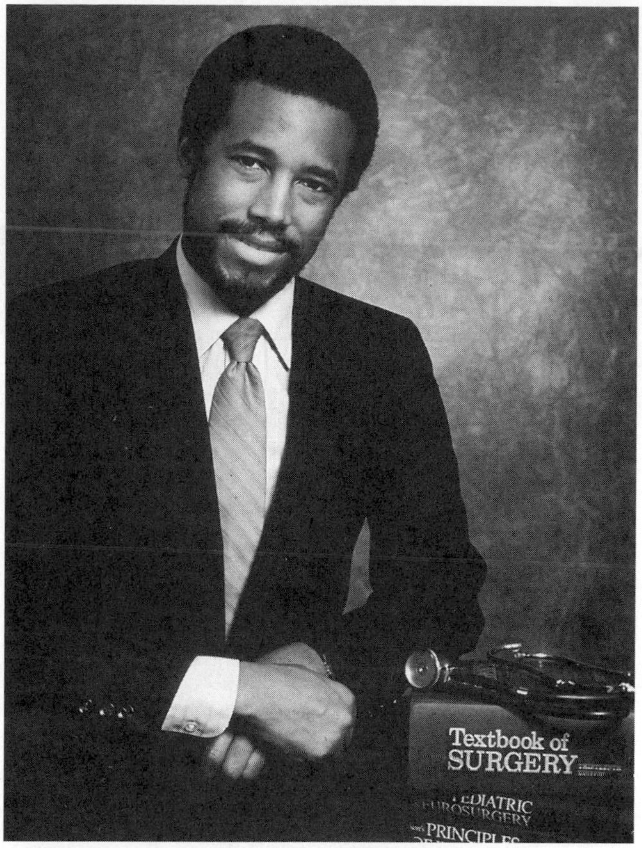

Benjamin S. Carson

Benjamin S. Carson is an internationally acclaimed neurosurgeon best known for leading a surgical team in a successful operation to separate Siamese twins. He is also recognized for his expertise in performing hemispherectomies, where half the brain is removed to stop seizures. He is the director of pediatric neurosurgery at Johns Hopkins University Hospital as well as assistant professor of neurosurgery, oncology, and pediatrics at the School of Medicine.

Born on September 18, 1951, Benjamin Solomon Carson came from a poor family in Detroit. He was the second son of Robert Solomon Carson, a Baptist minister, and Sonya Copeland Carson. His father was twenty-eight when he married, but his mother was only thirteen; she married in order to escape a difficult home situation. When Carson was only eight years old and his brother, Curtis, was ten, their parents divorced and his mother took them to live with relatives in a Boston tenement, while she rented out their house in Detroit. Working as many as three domestic jobs at a time, she earned enough money to move her family back to Detroit two years later.

Both Carson and his brother had a difficult time in school, and their low grades fanned the racial prejudice against them. But their mother took charge of their education, even though she herself had not gone past the third grade. By limiting the television they could watch and insisting they both read two books a week and report on them, she helped them raise their grades considerably. Carson discovered he enjoyed learning, and by the time he reached junior high school he had risen from the bottom to the top of his class.

But even then he continued to face racial prejudice; in the eighth grade, he listened to a teacher scold his class for allowing him, a black student, to win an achievement award. These early difficulties left Carson with a violent temper as a young man. He was often in fights: "I would fly off the handle," he told *People* contributors Linda Kramer and Joe Treen. Once he almost killed a friend in an argument. Carson tried to stab him in the stomach with a knife, but luckily the boy was wearing a heavy belt buckle, which stopped the blade. Only fourteen at the time, Carson was shocked at what he had almost done, and he saw the direction his life could have taken. This experience drove him more deeply into his religion—he is still a Seventh-Day Adventist—and his faith in God helped him control his temper.

He studied hard and did so well during high school that he won a scholarship to Yale University. He received his bachelor's degree from Yale in 1973. He had always dreamed of becoming a doctor and was very interested in psychiatry, but once in medical school at the University of Michigan, he realized he was good with his hands and set his sights on neurosurgery. After completing medical school in 1977, he was one of the few graduates and the first black accepted into the residency program at Johns Hopkins Hospital in Baltimore. In 1983 because of a shortage of neurosurgeons in Australia, Carson was offered a chief neurosurgical residency at Queen Elizabeth II Medical Center in Perth, where he gained a great deal of operating experience. He returned to Johns Hopkins in 1984, and after a year he was promoted to director of pediatric neurosurgery, becoming one of the youngest doctors in the country to head such a division.

One of Carson's accomplishments was reviving the use of a procedure called hemispherectomy—an operation that removes half the patient's brain to cure diseases such as Rassmussen's **encephalitis**, which cause **seizures**. These operations had been stopped because of their high mortality rate, but with Carson's skills the procedure has been highly successful.

But Carson's best known accomplishment was the operation he performed in September 1987 to separate seven-month-old German Siamese twins, who were joined at the head. Carson was the lead surgeon on the team which performed "perhaps the most complex surgical feat in the history of mankind," as he described the operation to *Ebony.* There was a team of seventy medical staff members, including five neurosurgeons, seven pediatric anesthesiologists, five plastic surgeons, two cardiac surgeons, and dozens of nurses and technicians, and it took five months of preparation, including five three-hour dress rehearsals. A crowd of media people waited outside the operating room for Carson and his medical team to emerge, triumphant, at the end of the twenty-two-hour operation.

In 1988 Carson was awarded both the Certificate of Honor for Outstanding Achievement in the Field of Medicine by the National Medical Fellowship and the American Black Achievement Award. He has received honorary doctor of science degrees from several universities, and the Candle Award for Science and Technology from Morehouse College in 1989.

Carson married Lacena Rustin—whom he met at Yale—in 1975; she holds a M.B.A. degree and is an accomplished musician. They have three sons. Carson feels strongly about motivating young people to fulfill their potential, as he did, and he often lectures to students around the nation. He advises young people to "think big," and he has written a book by that title. Carson was also on the editorial advisory board of the Time-Life series *Voices of Triumph,* about the history and achievements of African Americans.

CATARACTS

A cataract is a cloudiness or opacity in the normally transparent crystalline lens of the **eye**. Changes in the proteins, water content, enzymes, and other chemicals of the eye and lens are some of the reasons for the formation of a cataract. This cloudiness can cause a decrease in vision and may lead to eventual blindness.

Cataracts in the elderly are so common that they are thought to be a normal part of the aging process. Between the ages of 52-64, there is a 50% chance of having a cataract, while at least 70% of those 70 and older are affected. Cataracts associated with aging (senile or age-related cataracts) most often occur in both eyes, with each cataract progressing at a different rate. Initially, cataracts may not affect vision. If the cataract remains small or at the periphery of the lens, the visual changes may be minor.

Cataracts that occur in people other than the elderly are much less common. Congenital cataracts occur very rarely in newborns. Genetic defects or an infection or disease in the mother during **pregnancy** are among the causes of congenital cataracts. Traumatic cataracts may develop after a foreign body or trauma injures the lens or eye. Systemic illnesses, such as diabetes, may result in cataracts. Cataracts can also occur with other eye diseases—for example, an inflammation of the inner layer of the eye (uveitis) or **glaucoma**. Such cataracts are called complicated cataracts. Toxic cataracts result from chemical toxicity, such as steroid use. Cataracts can also result from exposure to the sun's ultraviolet (UV) rays.

Both ophthalmologists and optometrists may detect and monitor cataract growth and prescribe prescription lenses for visual deficits. However, only an ophthalmologist can perform cataract extraction. Cataracts are easily diagnosed from the reporting of symptoms, a visual acuity exam using an eye chart, and by examination of the eye itself. Shining a penlight into the pupil may reveal opacities or a color change of the lens even before visual symptoms have developed. An instrument called a slit lamp is basically a large microscope. This lets the doctor examine the front of the eye and the lens. The slit lamp helps the doctor determine the location of the cataract. Other diagnostic tests include a glare test, potential vision test, and contrast sensitivity test.

For cataracts that cause no symptoms or only minor visual changes, no treatment may be necessary. Continued monitoring and assessment of the cataract is needed by an ophthalmologist or optometrist at scheduled office visits. Increased strength in prescription eyeglasses or contact lenses may be helpful. This may be all that is required if the cataract does not reduce the patient's quality of life.

Cataract surgery—the only option for patients whose cataracts interfere with vision to the extent of affecting their daily lives—is the most frequently performed surgery in the United States. There are two types of cataract surgery: intracapsular and extracapsular. Intracapsular surgery is the removal of both the lens and the thin capsule that surround them. This type of surgery was common before 1980, but has since been displaced by extracapsular surgery. Removal of the capsule requires a large incision and doesn't allow comfortable intraocular lens implantation. Thus, people who undergo intracapsular cataract surgery have long recovery periods and have to wear very thick glasses.

Extracapsular cataract surgery is the removal of the lens where the capsule is left in place. Each year in the United States, over a million cataracts are removed this way. Phacoemulsification, a type of extracapsular extraction that uses ultrasonic vibration to break the cataract up into very small pieces which are suctioned out of the eye, needs a very small incision, resulting in faster healing.

A replacement lens is usually inserted at the time of the surgery. A plastic artificial lens called an intraocular lens (IOL) is placed in the remaining posterior lens capsule of the eye. When the intracapsular extraction method is used, an IOL may be clipped onto the iris. Contact lenses and cataract glasses (aphakic lenses) are prescribed if an IOL was not inserted.

Cataract surgery itself is quite safe; over 90% of the time, there are no complications. The success rate of cataract extraction is very high, with a good prognosis. Ordinarily, patients experience improved visual acuity and improved perception of the vividness of colors, leading to increased abilities in many activities, including reading, needlework, driving, golf, and tennis, for example. In addition, sometimes implanted corrective lenses eliminate the need for eyeglasses or contact lenses. A visual acuity of 20/40 or better may be achieved.

Glasses with a special coating to protect against ultraviolet (UV) rays may help to prevent cataracts. Antioxidants may also provide some protection by reducing the free radicals that can damage lens proteins. A healthy diet rich in sources of antioxidants, including citrus fruits, sweet potatoes, carrots, green leafy vegetables, and/or vitamin supplements may be helpful.

CATATONIA

Catatonia is a condition associated with a number of serious mental and physical illnesses. It is characterized by extreme and bizarre changes in muscle tone or activity. There are two specific types of catatonia—*catatonic stupor* and *catatonic excitement*. In catatonic stupor, the motor activity (movement) of an individual drastically slows or stops and the individual "freezes," becoming rigid and/or silent. In catatonic excitement, the individual experiences the opposite, becoming extremely hyperactive and potentially violent.

Symptoms of catatonia include odd ways of walking such as walking on tiptoes or pacing, and rarely, hopping and skipping. Repetitive odd movements of the fingers or hands may also indicate that catatonia is present Echopraxia (imitating the movement of others) and echolalia (parrot-like repetition of words spoken by others), are also common. Other signs and symptoms include selective **mutism**, negativism, facial grimaces, and animal-like noises.

Catatonic stupor is marked by immobility and a behavior known as *cerea flexibilitas* (waxy flexibility) in which the individual assumes bizarre (and sometimes painful) positions that they will maintain for extended periods of time. The individual may refuse food and liquids and become dehydrated and malnourished as a result. In extreme situations, such individuals must be fed through a tube. Catatonic excitement is characterized by excessive movement and violence; the individual may harm him/herself or others. On rare occasions, isolation or restraint may be needed to ensure the individual's safety and the safety of others.

The causes of catatonia are unknown. Medical research indicates that brain structure and function are altered in this condition. A variety of medical conditions also may lead to catatonia including head trauma, cerebrovascular disease, **encephalitis**, and certain metabolic disorders.

Features of catatonia may also be seen in Neuroleptic Malignant Syndrome (NMS), which is an uncommon but serious reaction to some medications used to treat major mental illnesses. NMS is considered a medical emergency since 25% of untreated cases result in **death**. Catatonia can also be present in individuals suffering from a number of other physical and emotional conditions such as drug intoxication, depression, and **schizophrenia**. It is most commonly associated with **mood disorders**.

NMS may occur as a side effect of certain neuroleptic medications (**antipsychotic drugs**) such as haloperidol (Haldol). It comes on suddenly and is characterized by stiffening of the muscles, **fever**, confusion and heavy sweating.

There are no laboratory or other tests that can be used to positively diagnose this condition, but medical and neurological tests are necessary to determine any physical causes of the symptoms observed. Catatonia usually responds quickly to medication, including benzodiazipines (the preferred treatment) and, in some cases, **barbiturates**. Antipsychotic drugs may be appropriate in some cases, but can make catatonia worse. **Electroconvulsive therapy** (ECT) may help those patients who do not respond to medication.

CAT-SCRATCH DISEASE

Cat-scratch disease (also called cat-scratch fever) is an infection caused by the *Bartonella henselae* bacterium, which is found in cats around the world and is transmitted from cat to cat by fleas. It can infect people who are scratched or (more rarely) bitten or licked by a cat that carries the bacterium.

Researchers have discovered that large numbers of North American cats carry antibodies for the disease (meaning that the cats have been infected at some point in their lives). *Bartonella henselae* is uncommon or absent in cold climates, which fleas have difficulty tolerating, but prevalent in warm, humid places such as Memphis, Tennessee, where antibodies were found in 71% of the cats tested. The bacterium, which remains in a cat's bloodstream for several months after infection, seems to be harmless to most cats, and normally an infected cat will not display any symptoms. Kittens (cats less than one year old) are more likely than adult cats to be carrying the infection.

Although cats are popular pets found in about 30% of American households, human infection appears to be rare. One study estimated that for every 100,000 Americans there are only 2.5 cases of cat-scratch disease each year (2.5/100,000).

The first sign of cat-scratch disease may be a small blister at the site of a scratch or bite 3-10 days after injury. The blister (which sometimes contains pus) often looks like an insect bite and is usually found on the hands, arms, or head. Within two weeks of the blister's appearance, lymph nodes near the site of injury become swollen. Often the infected person develops a fever or experiences fatigue or **headache**s. The symptoms usually disappear within a month, although the lymph nodes may remain swollen for several months. Hepatitis, **pneumonia**, and other dangerous complications can arise, but the likelihood of cat-scratch disease posing a serious threat to health is very small. **AIDS** patients and other immunocompromised people face the greatest risk of dangerous complications.

Occasionally, the symptoms of cat-scratch disease take the form of what is called Parinaud's oculoglandular syndrome. In such cases, a small sore develops on the membrane lining the inner eyelid (the palpebral conjunctiva), and is often accompanied by inflammation (conjunctivitis) and swollen lymph nodes in front of the ear. This syndrome may be caused by rubbing one's eyes after handling the cat.

Individuals should see a doctor if a cat scratch or bite fails to heal normally or is followed by a persistent fever or other unusual symptoms such as swollen lymph nodes and long-lasting bone or joint **pain**. When cat-scratch disease is suspected, the doctor will ask about a history of exposure to cats and look for evidence of a cat scratch or bite and swollen lymph nodes. A blood test for *Bartonella henselae* may be ordered to confirm the doctor's diagnosis.

For otherwise healthy people, rest and over-the-counter medications for reducing fever and discomfort (such as **acetaminophen**) while waiting for the disease to run its course are usually all that is necessary. **Antibiotics** are prescribed in some cases, particularly when complications occur or the lymph nodes remain swollen and painful for more than two or three months, but there is no agreement among doctors about when and how they should be used.

Most people recover completely from a bout of cat-scratch disease, and further attacks are rare. Certain common sense precautions can be taken to guard against the disease. Scratches and bites should be washed immediately with soap and water, and it is never a good idea to rub one's eyes after handling a cat without first washing one's hands. Children should be told not to play with stray cats or make cats angry. Immunocompromised people should avoid owning kittens, which are more likely than adult cats to be infectious. Because cat-scratch disease is usually not a life-threatening illness and people tend to form strong emotional bonds with their cats, doctors do not recommend getting rid of a cat suspected of carrying the disease.

Cavell, Edith (1865-1915)

British nurse

Head of a specialized school in Brussels, Belgium, for training nurses, Edith Cavell became part of a group that helped soldiers and other refugees escape from the German army during World War I. She was eventually arrested, tried by a German military court, and sentenced to death. Despite widespread protests, Cavell was executed by a firing squad and became a martyr to the public.

Born in Swardeston, England, Edith Cavell was taught at a young age by her minister father that it was her duty to help others. After working for several years as a governess in England and then Brussels, Cavell returned home in 1895 to care for her father during a brief illness. This experience led her to become a nurse. She trained at London Hospital, during which time she helped care for victims of an epidemic of typhoid fever and subsequently received the Maidstone Medal for her efforts.

After working several years as a nurse, Cavell returned to Brussels and became head of a pioneer training school for lay nurses at the Berkendael Institute beginning in 1907. Shy and retiring, Cavell was strict but fair with her staff and students. By 1914, when World War I began, the school was training top quality **nursing** personnel for **hospitals**, schools, and private **nursing homes**.

Cavell often traveled back to England to visit her mother and was there when she heard of the German invasion of Belgium. Although she knew the dangers involved, she decided to return to her post in Belgium, stating, "At a time like this, I am needed more than ever." The clinic where she trained her nurses became a Red Cross Hospital, where Cavell cared for both German soldiers and troops from the Allied forces. Although the Germans sent most English nurses home, Cavell decided to remain in Brussels and continue with her duties.

Although it was contrary to the Red Cross code of non-involvement in military matters, Cavell helped hide two sick English soldiers in the hospital until they recuperated, eventually finding guides who helped them escape to England. Cavell then joined a small group who helped find and hide fugitive Allied soldiers and refugees from the Germans, who were putting many of those they captured to death. Cavell hid the soldiers until arrangements could be made for their escape. She also supplyed them with money and identification papers and found guides for their escape. She would even take them to secret meetings, choosing crowded streets and other routes so as not to attract attention. Cavell was also careful not to let her staff or students become involved, thus protecting them from danger if she were ever caught.

The German secret police began to suspect Cavell and others at the institute of harboring the fugitives of war. Still, they could find no evidence to support their conviction. Then on July 31, 1915, members of an escape route team that Cavell had worked with were captured. Cavell was arrested five days later. Believing that others had already confessed, Edith admitted to her participation in the escape group and said during her trial that she had "successfully conducted Allied soldiers to the enemy of the German people." Under German law, the penalty was death.

Despite appeals from the American and Spanish ambassadors for clemency, Edith and four others were sent before a firing squad on the morning of October 12, 1915. According to some accounts, the firing squad protested against shooting Cavell, with one soldier being executed for refusing to carry out this duty. Nevertheless, Cavell, still in her nurses uniform, was executed and buried nearby.

Cavell's execution turned out to be a serious blunder by the Germans, who were soon facing a widespread outcry as "murdering monsters." Cavell's death is credited with helping to strengthen Allied morale and doubling recruitment in the Allied army for nearly two months after her death. Cavell's death also may have contributed to the United States entering the war.

Following the war, Cavell's body was exhumed and returned to England in May 1919. With great ceremony, she was taken to Westminster Abbey for a memorial service attended by King George V and then was reburied in Norwich, England. Today a statue stands in her honor at St. Martin's Place near London's Trafalgar Square. The statue is engraved with a statement made by Cavell to her last English visitor before her execution. It reads: "Patriotism is not enough. I must have no hatred or bitterness for anyone." A special service is held there annually near the anniversary of her death. Cavell's heroism was also honored by the naming of Mount Edith Cavell in Jasper National Park in Alberta, Canada, and in a movie and a play about her life and death.

Celiac disease

Celiac disease (also called sprue, nontropical sprue, celiac sprue, and gluten sensitive enteropathy) occurs when the body reacts abnormally to gluten, a protein found in wheat, rye, barley, and oats. Gluten causes an inflammatory response in the small intestine, which damages the tissues and results in impaired ability to absorb nutrients from foods. The inflammation and **malabsorption** create wide-ranging problems in many systems of the body.

The exact cause of celiac disease is not clearly understood, but it is known that both heredity and the immune system play a part. When food containing gluten reaches the small intestine, the immune system begins to attack a substance called gliadin, which is found in the gluten. The resulting inflammation causes damage to the delicate finger-like structures in the small intestine, called villi, where food absorption actually takes place.

The most commonly recognized symptoms of celiac disease relate to the improper absorption of food in the gastrointestinal system. The patient will have **diarrhea** and fatty, greasy, unusually foul-smelling stools. The patient may complain of excessive gas (flatulence), distended abdomen, weight loss, and generalized weakness. A distinctive skin rash, called **dermatitis** herpetiformis, is present in approximately 10% of patients with celiac disease.

Unrecognized and therefore untreated celiac disease may cause or contribute to a variety of other medical conditions. The decreased ability to digest, absorb, and utilize food properly (malabsorption) may cause anemia from iron deficiency or easy bruising from a lack of vitamin K. Poor mineral absorption may result in **osteoporosis**, or ''brittle bones,'' which may lead to bone **fractures**. Vitamin D levels may be insufficient and bring about a ''softening'' of bones (osteomalacia), which produces **pain** and bony deformities, such as flattening or bending. Defects in the tooth enamel, characteristic of celiac disease, may be recognized by dentists. Celiac disease may cause a **failure to thrive** in infants, or lack of proper growth in children and adolescents. People with celiac disease may also experience lactose intolerance.

Many disorders are associated with celiac disease, though the nature of the connection is unclear. One type of epilepsy is linked to celiac disease. Once their celiac disease is successfully treated, a significant number of these patients have fewer or no seizures. Patients with alopecia areata, a condition where hair loss occurs in sharply defined areas, have been shown to have a higher risk of celiac disease than the general population. There appears to be a higher percentage of celiac disease among people with **Down syndrome**, but the link between the conditions is unknown.

People with insulin dependent diabetes (type I) have a much higher incidence of celiac disease. Patients with other conditions where celiac disease may be more commonly found include those with juvenile chronic arthritis, some thyroid diseases, and IgA deficiency.

Because of the variety of ways celiac disease can manifest itself, it is often not discovered promptly. The condition may persist without diagnosis for so long that the patient accepts a general feeling of illness as normal. This leads to further delay in identifying and treating the disorder.

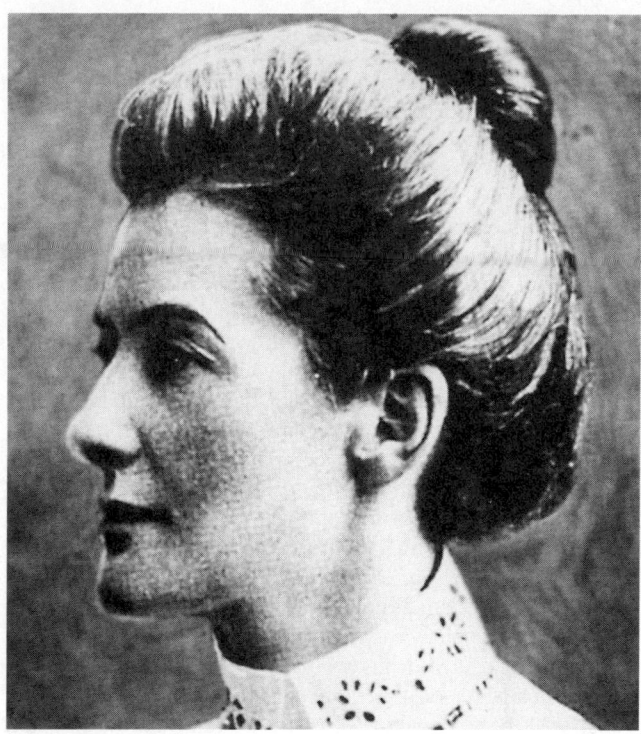

Edith Cavell

If celiac disease is suspected, a blood test can be ordered that looks for the antibodies that the immune system produces in celiac disease. An abnormal result points towards celiac disease, but further tests are needed to confirm the diagnosis. Doctors may order a test of iron levels in the blood because low levels of iron (anemia) may accompany celiac disease. Doctors may also order a test for fat in the stool, since celiac disease prevents the body from absorbing fat from food.

The next step is a biopsy of the small intestine. This is usually done by a gastroenterologist, a physician who specializes in diagnosing and treating bowel disorders. It is generally performed in the office, or in an outpatient department in a hospital. The patient remains awake, but is sedated. A narrow tube is passed through the mouth, down through the stomach, and into the small intestine. A small sample of tissue is taken and sent to the laboratory for analysis. If it shows a pattern of tissue damage characteristic of celiac disease, the diagnosis is established.

The patient is then placed on a gluten-free diet (GFD). Gluten is present in any product that contains wheat, rye, barley, or oats. In addition to the many obvious places gluten can be found in a normal diet, such as breads, cereals, and pasta, there are many hidden sources of gluten. These include ingredients added to foods to improve texture or enhance flavor and products used in food packaging. Gluten may even be present on surfaces used for food preparation or cooking.

Fresh foods that have not been artificially processed, such as fruits, vegetables, and meats, are permitted as part of a GFD. Gluten-free foods can be found in health food stores and in some supermarkets.

Treating celiac disease with a GFD is almost always completely effective. Once the diet has been followed for several years, individuals with celiac disease have similar mortality rates as the general population. Gastrointestinal complaints and other symptoms are alleviated. People who have experienced lactose intolerance related to their celiac disease usually see those symptoms subside. Secondary complications, such as anemia and osteoporosis, resolve in almost all patients, as well. However, about 10% of people with celiac disease develop a cancer involving the lymphatic system (lymphoma).

Experts emphasize the need for lifelong adherence to the GFD to avoid the long-term complications of this disorder. They point out that although the disease may have symptom-free periods if the diet is not followed, silent damage continues to occur. Celiac disease cannot be ''outgrown'' or cured, according to medical authorities.

There are a small number of patients who develop a refractory type of celiac disease, where the GFD no longer seems effective. Once the diet has been thoroughly assessed to ensure no hidden sources of gluten are causing the problem, medications may be prescribed. Steroids or **immunosuppressant drugs** are often used to try to control the disease. It is unclear whether these efforts meet with much success.

Cell therapy

Cell therapy is a treatment intended to regenerate or rejuvenate the body by injecting it with healthy live or freeze-dried cells derived from animal organs or embryos. It is sometimes called fresh or live cell therapy. It is performed to treat specific diseases and disorders, including arthritis, lupus, **cancer**, HIV infection, cardiovascular and neurological disorders, and **Parkinson's disease**. It is also used to stimulate the immune system, revitalize bodily organs, and slow the effects of aging, including memory loss and **sexual dysfunction**.

Cell therapy was developed in Switzerland in the 1930s by Dr. Paul Niehans, following emergency treatment of a dying patient with cells taken from an animal's parathyroid gland. Dr. Niehans then worked with scientists from the Nestle Company, who had successfully developed a method of freeze-drying coffee, to develop a method of freeze-drying cells to guarantee the sterility of preparations as well as preserving the cells.

Studies conducted in German universities found that injected cells migrate to the organ in the human body that corresponds to the organ in the animal from which they were taken. The reasons for the effectiveness of cell therapy, however, are not yet understood. It is thought that live cells may revitalize an ''old'' organ by ''reprogramming'' its genetic material. Another theory proposes that the fresh cells stimulate secretions that restore the proper functioning of the targeted organ.

Cell therapy cannot be practiced within the United States because of Food and Drug Administration (FDA) restrictions. Patients must travel to Mexico, the Bahamas, England, or Germany for treatment. The cost of the therapy is $2,500 for initial injections and $1,500 for follow-up booster treatments.

Before undergoing cell therapy treatment, patients are administered a test injection at the clinic to check for potential allergic reactions. The treatment itself consists of several injections of organ cells into the muscles of the buttocks. Patients are asked to limit alcoholic beverages and smoking during the course of treatment.

After therapy, patients are given instructions regarding lifestyle choices to prolong the effects of cell therapy. Recommendations include diet, **exercise**, adequate rest, and **meditation**.

The cell therapy recovery process is divided into three stages, or phases. The first phase, immediately after treatment, is characterized by marked improvement in skin and general level of well-being. The reaction phase which lasts for approximately two weeks, is marked by tiredness and return of some earlier symptoms. The healing phase, which takes six to nine months after treatment to begin and may last several years, is defined by long-term improvements in stamina, skin tone, and general health. Cell therapy treatments are repeated with ''booster shots'' at one- to three-year intervals.

Patients with kidney or liver disease, short-term infections, or inflammatory disorders should not be treated with cell therapy. In addition, patients who have an allergic reaction to the test injection should not proceed with therapy.

Cellulitis

Cellulitis is a spreading bacterial infection just below the skin surface.

The word ''cellulitis'' actually means ''inflammation of the cells.'' Specifically, cellulitis refers to a bacterial infection of the tissue just below the skin surface. It is most commonly caused by *Streptococcus pyogenes* or *Staphylococcus aureus*. Skin is the first defense against invading bacteria and other microbes. An infection can occur when skin is damaged due to surgery, injury, or a burn and bacteria infects the wound.

Disease-causing bacteria release proteins called enzymes that cause tissue damage. The body's reaction to this damage is inflammation, which is characterized by **pain**, redness, heat, and swelling. An untreated infection may spread to the lymphatic system (acute lymphangitis), the lymph nodes (lymphadenitis), the bloodstream (**bacteremia**), or into deeper tissues. Cellulitis most often occurs on the face, neck, and legs.

A very serious infection, called orbital cellulitis, occurs when bacteria enter and infect the tissues surrounding the eye. In 50-70% of all cases of orbital cellulitis, the infection spreads to the eye(s) from the sinuses or the upper respiratory tract (nose and throat). Twenty-five percent of orbital infections occur after surgery on the face. Other sources of orbital infection include a direct infection from an eye injury, from a dental or throat infection, and through the bloodstream.

Infection of the tissues surrounding the eye causes redness, swollen eyelids, severe pain, and causes the eye to bulge out. This serious infection can lead to a temporary loss of vision, blindness, brain **abscess**es, inflammation of the brain and spinal tissues (**meningitis**), and other complications. Before the discovery of **antibiotics**, orbital cellulitis caused blindness in 20% of patients and **death** in 17% of patients. Antibiotic treatment has significantly reduced the incidence of blindness and death.

Although other kinds of bacteria can cause cellulitis, it is most often caused by *Streptococcus pyogenes* (the bacteria which causes **strep throat**) and *Staphylococcus aureus. Streptococcus pyogenes* is the so-called ''flesh-eating bacteria'' and, in rare caes, can cause a dangerous, deep skin infection called necrotizing fasciitis. These bacteria can be spread through contact with a person who has strep throat or an infected sore. Orbital cellulitis may be caused by bacteria which cannot grow in the presence of oxygen (anaerobic bacteria). In children, *Haemophilus influenzae* type B frequently causes orbital cellulitis following a sinus infection.

Persons who are at a higher risk for cellulitis are those who have a severe underlying disease (such as **cancer**, diabetes, and kidney disease), are taking steroid medications, have a reduced immune system (because of **AIDS**, organ transplant, etc.), have been burned, have insect bites, have reduced blood circulation to limbs, or have had a leg vein removed for coronary bypass surgery. In addition, chicken pox, human or animal bite **wounds**, skin wounds, and recent surgery can put a person at a higher risk for cellulitis.

The characteristic symptoms of cellulitis are redness, warmth, pain, and swelling. The infected area appears as a red patch that gets larger rapidly within the first 24 hours. A thick red line which progresses towards the heart may appear indicating an infection of the lymph vessels (lymphangitis). Other symptoms which may occur include **fever**, chills, tiredness, muscle aches, and a general ill feeling. Some people also experience nausea, vomiting, stiff joints, and hair loss at the infection site.

The characteristic symptoms of orbital cellulitis are eye pain, redness, swelling, warmth, and tenderness. The eye may bulge out and it may be difficult or impossible to move. Temporary loss of vision, pus drainage from the eye, chills, fever, **headache**s, vomiting, and a general ill feeling may occur.

Laboratory tests called *cultures* may be done to determine which kind of bacteria is causing a cellulitis infection, but these tests are not always successful. Cultures check the affected tissue and/or bloodstream for bacteria. In addition, a blood test may be done to count the number of white blood cells in the blood. High numbers of white blood cells suggest that the body is trying to fight a bacterial infection. Patients suspected of having orbital cellulitis may have a computed tomography scan (CT) taken of their head.

A normally healthy person is usually not hospitalized for mild or moderate cellulitis. The condition can be treated with antibiotics such as **penicillins** (Bicillin, Wycillin, Pen Vee, V-Cillin), erythromycin (E-Mycin, Ery-Tab), cephalexin (Biocef, Keflex), cloxacillin (Tegopen), which cure over 90% of all cellulitis cases in 7-10 days. Other general treatment measures include elevation of the infected area, rest, and application of warm, moist compresses to the infected area. Medications such as **acetaminophen** (Tylenol) or ibuprofen (Motrin, Advil) may be taken to relieve pain, and **aspirin** can be taken to decrease fever.

Persons with serious disease and/or those who are taking immunosuppressive drugs may experience a more severe form of cellulitis which can be life threatening. Serious complications include blood **poisoning** (bacteria growing in the blood stream), meningitis (brain and spinal cord infection), tissue death (necrosis), and/or lymphangitis (infection of the lymph vessels). Severe cellulitis caused by *Streptococcus pyogenes* can lead to destructive and life-threatening necrotizing fasciitis.

Persons at high risk for severe cellulitis will probably be hospitalized for treatment and monitoring. Antibiotics may be given intravenously to these patients. Complications such as deep infection, or bone or joint infections, might require surgical drainage. Extensive tissue destruction may require plastic surgery to repair. In cases of orbital cellulitis caused by a sinus infection, surgery may be required to drain the sinuses.

CELSUS, AULUS CORNELIUS (ca. 25 B.C.-ca. 50)

Roman encyclopedist and historian of medicine

Aulus Cornelius Celsus is considered one of the most important contributors to medicine and scientific thought during the Roman Empire, and the most important source of present-day knowledge of Alexandrian medicine. Although apparently not a physician himself, Celsus gathered extensive writings from the Greek Empire, translated them into Roman, and compiled their vast knowledge into an encyclopedia entitled *De artibus* (A.D. 25-35). Originally, this great work contained five books on agriculture, and other books of unknown length on military science, government, history, law, philosophy, rhetoric, and medicine. The only books to survive, however, were *The Eight Books of Medicine*, or *De medicina octo libri*, the most comprehensive medical history and detailed description of medical and surgical procedures ever produced by a Roman writer. They were also the first translation of Greek medical terms into Latin—terms that have remained standard in medicine for 2000 years. However, these books are far more than just simple translations of Greek writings. Celsus clearly formulated his own opinion from the collected knowledge and wrote down his independent theories, involving one that ultimately became-and remains—the basic principle in medicine: ''accurate diagnosis must precede treatment.''

Virtually nothing is known of Celsus' life and work apart from these books. He is thought to have been born on the Mediterranean coast of France around 25 B.C. in the Augustan Age during the rein of Tiberius. It is also believed he came from a wealthy and influential noble family of the ruling class. Although some historians think Celsus may have been a doctor, nowhere in ancient literature is he referred to as such. Also, while the professional practice of medicine was considered beneath the dignity of noble families of the era, knowledge of medicine was usual among educated men, many of whom as head of the household practiced medicine on ill family members, slaves, and livestock. Celsus may have been such a person. Regardless, he read extensively and knew both Greek and Roman. Columella, Quintilian, and Pliny the Elder-great scholars of the first century-wrote with praise of Celsus' work which modern scholars call brilliant and outstanding.

Celsus was a strict adherent to the teachings of the great Greek physician, **Hippocrates** (460-377 B.C.), and some historians believe much *De medicina's* contents came from a vast collection of writings of the school of Hippocrates. In fact, in *De medicina*, Celsus references some 80 Greek medical writers and he has been called both the Roman Hippocrates and the Cicero of Medicine. His medical philosophy was also influenced by Asclepiades, who established Greek medicine in Rome, and by the famous medical school of Alexandria.

Book I of *De medicina* contained a historical overview of medicine; book II dealt with the course and general treatment of diseases; books III and IV with special therapy; books V and VI with pharmacology (drugs and medication); book VII with surgery; and book VIII with bone diseases. In his volumes, Celsus was the first to accurately report symptoms of a number of diseases including epilepsy, **mental illness**es such as **paranoia**, **heart attack**s, and **malaria** (which he described with extreme accuracy); to name the four major signs of inflammation: heat, **pain** swelling, and redness; to describe how flesh reacted (became inflamed) by microbes, recommending cleanliness and washing wounds with solutions such as vinegar; to describe in detail **rabies**, **ulcers**, tumors, **amputation**, removal of part of the skull (which he said should be performed as a last resort), and surgical techniques for un**circumcision**; to use the term ''hydrophobia'' (fear of water); and to recommend for snake bites sucking the poison from the wound, stating (correctly) that the poison is only harmful when absorbed by the wound but not if swallowed.

Also, rather than simply analyzing symptoms, Celsus considered many factors important in diagnosis, such as the patients age, the influence of the seasons, and weather changes. He believed in ''critical days,'' days at which certain diseases peak and the patient begins to recover. He was highly aware of the deadly effect of **gangrene** and therefore concerned with methods for treating wounds. He reported on **plastic surgery** for repair to the nose, lips, and ears; and on dental surgery (suggesting that a badly decayed tooth be filled with lint to prevent it from breaking off as it was extracted) and wiring of the teeth. He recommended a type of surgery (lithotomy) for crushing bladder stones, ligature for tying off arteries to prevent bleeding to death, and various methods to stop hemorrhages (bleeding).

He detailed excellent methods of treating **fractures** and **dislocations**, recommending wooden splints held in place by wax or heavily starched bandages; and advocated **exercise** after the fracture healed, thus becoming the forerunner to modern **physical therapy**. He described the use of painkillers (opium) and **anesthesia** (soaking the root of the mandragora plant in wine as a drink to produce sleep); paid much attention to **headaches**, believing they came from many different sources; and recommended hot oil **massage** to help **insomnia**-for which he gave credit to Asclepiades.

For an understanding of the anatomy, Celsus advocated the value of **dissection** of the human cadaver (dead body)-a practice prohibited by both Greek and Roman religions. (Celsus is credited with reporting rumors of malicious acts of **vivisection** (dissection and dismemberment) having been performed on living criminals for medical research at Alexandria during the reigns of Ptolemy II and III (285-221 BC).) He firmly believed that diagnosis (finding the cause) and prognosis (evaluating the outcome) was essential before effective treatment could be given. Although his treatment recommendations often included drugs, he was a firm advocate of baths, massage, **personal hygiene**, **diet**, and sports.

Perhaps an intellectual whose opinions and recommendations were long before his time, Celsus gained little recognized in his own era and it appears that his works were generally snubbed. They were totally lost until the Middle Ages when the medical portion-the only portion ever found—was discovered in the Vatican Library by Pope Nicholas V in 1426. The Pope arranged for its publication in 1478, a time of medical revival during the Renaissance, and Celsus suddenly gained a reputation as ''a physician of extraordinary merit.''

Celsus is believed to have died in Rome somewhere around AD 50 but not until fourteen hundred years after his death did he gain recognition and praise for both his medical techniques and masterful literary ability.

Centers for Disease Control

The Centers for Disease Control and Prevention (CDC) address current and emerging health risks to help improve public health in the United States and worldwide. Based in Atlanta, Georgia, CDC is an agency of the Department of Health and Human Services. CDC runs programs to prevent and control communicable diseases, develops and implements programs to deal with environmental health problems, directs quarantine activities, and does research on the factors that influence diseases. The agency's mission is to promote health and quality of life by preventing and controlling disease, injury, and disability. Its core values are accountability, respect, and integrity.

CDC was established in 1948 as the Communicable Disease Center to fight malaria, typhus, and other communicable diseases which were then prevalent in several Southern states. In 1970, it was re-named the Center for Disease Control to reflect its broader preventive mission. In 1992, Congress renamed the agency the Centers for Disease Control and Prevention, but kept the initials CDC.

CDC provides a variety of health information for consumers and public health practitioners via its web site, publications, and software. Consumer information covers adolescents and teens, environmental health, foodborne illnesses, infants and children, injuries, men's health, occupational health, senior health, traveler's health, and women's health. For medical practitioners, the agency offers CDC Prevention Guidelines to help prevent and control public health threats such as AIDS, cholera, disaster response, dengue fever, suicide, vaccine-preventable diseases, lung cancer, sexually transmitted diseases, birth defects, and malaria. Immunization recommendations, health information for international travelers, scientific data, surveillance health statistics, and laboratory information are also available.

CDC has approximately 7,800 employees, in nine states and the District of Columbia in the United States, and in other countries. It is comprised of 11 centers, 1 institute, and offices: Office of the Director, Epidemiology Program Office; National Center for Chronic Disease Prevention and Health Promotion; National Center for Environmental Health; National Center for Health Statistics; National Center for HIV, STD, and TB Prevention; National Center for Infectious Diseases; National Center for Injury Prevention and Control; National Immunization Program; National Institute for Occupational Safety and Health; Office of Genetics and Disease Prevention; Office of Global Health; and Public Health Practice Program Office.

Central nervous system stimulants

Central nervous system (CNS) stimulants are medicines that speed up physical and mental processes. They are used to treat **attention-deficit hyperactivity disorder** (ADHD), narcolepsy, and other disorders of the central **nervous system.** Commonly used central nervous system stimulants are amphetamine, dextroamphetamine (Dexedrine, DextroStat), methamphetamine (Desoxyn), pemoline (Cylert), and methylphenidate (Ritalin).

CNS stimulants increase attention, decrease restlessness, and improve physical coordination in people who have ADHD, a condition in which people have unusually high activity levels and short attention spans. The drugs may also curb impulsive behavior related to ADHD. Although central nervous system stimulants are effective in treating ADHD, their use is controversial, especially in children. When used over long periods, CNS stimulants may interfere with growth and cause unwanted behavioral effects. Parents whose children need to take these drugs should thoroughly discuss the risks and benefits with the child's doctor. The doctor may recommend periodic ''drug holidays,'' during which time the child stops taking the medicine.

Narcolepsy, in which people have an uncontrollable desire to sleep or may suddenly fall into a deep sleep, may also be helped by CNS stimulants. The medication is prescribed in an effort to reduce the frequency and severity of attacks of narcolepsy.

Central nervous system stimulants should never be used to increase alertness or as a substitute for sleep. Although they can cause loss of appetite and weight loss, they should not be used as ''diet pills.''

Always take CNS stimulants exactly as directed. Never take larger or more frequent doses, and do not take the drug for longer than directed. This medicine may be habit forming if taken in large doses or over long periods. If it is necessary to stop taking the drug, check with the doctor who prescribed it for instructions on how to stop.

Some people feel drowsy, dizzy, lightheaded, or less alert when using these drugs. The drugs may also give some people a false sense of well-being. Because of these possible effects, anyone who takes these drugs should not drive, use machines, or do anything else that might be dangerous until they have found out how the drugs affect them.

The most common side effects of CNS stimulants are irritability, nervousness, restlessness, loss of appetite, sleep problems, and a false sense of well-being. After these effects wear off, other effects may occur, such as trembling, drowsiness, unusual tiredness or weakness, or depression. These side effects and after effects usually go away as the body adjusts to the drug and do not require medical treatment unless they continue or they interfere with normal activities.

More serious side effects may occur. If chest pain, irregular heartbeat, breathing problems, **dizziness**, faintness, extreme fatigue, weakness, high **fever**, **hives**, involuntary movement, or a rise in blood pressure occur, check with the doctor who prescribed the medicine as soon as possible.

CNS stimulants may cause physical or mental dependence when taken over long periods. Anyone who shows signs of dependence should check with his or her doctor right away. Dependence can be indicated by an unusually strong desire to keep taking the medicine. Other signs include the need to take larger and larger doses of the medicine to get the same effect, and withdrawal symptoms, such as depression, nausea or vomiting, stomach cramps or **pain**, trembling, or unusual tiredness or weakness when the medicine is stopped.

Because of their high potential for abuse, sale of the the CNS stimulants amphetamines and methylphenidates is strictly controlled. Prescriptions cannot be refilled, and patients must get a new prescription from the doctor each time they need a new supply of medicine.

Before using central nervous system stimulants, people with any of these medical conditions should inform their doctors: **pregnancy**, **allergies** to medications, foods, dyes, preservatives, or other substances; current or past alcohol or drug abuse; **psychosis** or other severe mental illness; severe **anxiety**, tension, agitation, or depression; **seizure disorder**s, such as epilepsy; heart or blood vessel disease; high blood pressure; overactive thyroid; **glaucoma**; and Tourette's syndrome or other tics.

Some central nervous system stimulants pass into breast milk. Breastfeeding is not recommended while taking these drugs. Women who want to breastfeed their babies should check with their doctors before using any central nervous system stimulant.

Taking central nervous system stimulants with certain other drugs may affect the way the drugs work or may increase the chance of side effects. Be sure to check with a doctor or pharmacist before combining central nervous stimulants with any other prescription or nonprescription (over-the-counter) medicine.

Cephalosporins

Cephalosporins are medicines that kill bacteria or prevent their growth. They are used to treat infections in different parts of the body, including the ears, nose, throat, lungs, sinuses, and skin. Physicians may prescribe these drugs to treat **pneumonia**, **strep throat**, staph infections, **tonsillitis**, **bronchitis**, and **gonorrhea**. These drugs will *not* work for colds, flu, and other infections caused by viruses.

The structure of cephalosporin C, the first of the cephalosporin family of antibiotics, was discovered in the 1950s by English scientists Edward Abraham and Guy Newton. Examples of currently used cephalosporin drugs are cefaclor (Ceclor), cefadroxil (Duricef), cefazolin (Ancef, Kefzol, Zolicef), cefixime, (Suprax), cefoxitin (Mefoxin), cefprozil (Cefzil), ceftazidime (Ceptaz, Fortaz, Tazicef, Tazideme), cefuroxime (Ceftin) and cephalexin (Keflex). These medicines are available only with a physician's prescription. They are sold in tablet, capsule, liquid, and injectable forms.

Always take cephalosporins exactly as directed by your physician. Never take larger, smaller, more frequent, or less frequent doses. Take all of the medicine to treat the infection for which it was prescribed. The infection may not clear up completely if too little medicine is taken. Taking this medicine for too long, on the other hand, may open the door to new infections that do not respond to the drug. Do not save some doses of the drug to take for future infections. The medicine may not be right for other kinds of infections, even if the symptoms are the same.

Some cephalosporins work best when taken on an empty stomach. Others should be taken after meals. Check with the physician who prescribed the medicine or the pharmacist who filled the prescription for instructions on how to take the medicine.

Certain cephalosporins should not be combined with alcohol or with medicines that contain alcohol. Abdominal or stomach cramps, nausea, vomiting, facial flushing, and other symptoms may result within 15-30 minutes and may last for several hours. *Do not drink alcoholic beverages or use other medicines that contain alcohol while being treated with cephalosporins and for several days after treatment ends.*

People with certain medical conditions can have problems if they take cephalosporins. These include: **allergies**, diabetes, **phenylketonuria** (PKU), pregnancy, stomach or intestinal problems, kidney problems, bleeding problems, and liver disease. Patients with any of these conditions should check with their doctor if they are prescribed cephalosporins.

Cephalosporins may pass into breast milk and may affect nursing babies. Women who are breastfeeding and who need to take this medicine should check with their physicians. They may need to stop breastfeeding until treatment is finished.

Get medical attention immediately if any of these symptoms develop while taking cephalosporins: **shortness of breath**, pounding heartbeat, skin rash or **hives**, severe cramps or **pain** in the stomach or abdomen, **fever**, severe watery or bloody **diarrhea**, and unusual bleeding or bruising.

Taking cephalosporins with certain other drugs may affect the way the drugs work or may increase the chance of side effects. Anyone who takes cephalosporins should let the physician know all other medicines he or she is taking.

Some patients experience diarrhea while taking cephalosporins, and certain diarrhea medicines, such as diphenoxylate-atropine (Lomotil), may make the problem worse. Check with a physician before taking any medicine for diarrhea caused by cephalosporins.

Birth control pills may not work properly when taken at the same time as cephalosporins. To prevent **pregnancy**, use other methods of birth control in addition to the pills while taking cephalosporins.

Taking cephalosporins with certain other drugs may increase the risk of heavy bleeding. Among the drugs that may have this effect when taken with cephalosporins are: anticoagulants such as warfarin (Coumadin), blood viscosity reducing medicines such as pentoxifylline (Trental), and the antiseizure medicines divalproex (Depakote) and valproic acid (Depakene).

CEREBRAL PALSY

Cerebral palsy (CP), or static encephalopathy, is the name for a collection of **movement disorders** caused by brain damage that occurs before, during, or shortly after birth. A person with CP is often also affected by other conditions caused by brain damage.

The affected muscles of a person with CP may become rigid or excessively loose, or the person may lose control of muscles, or have problems with balance and coordination. A combination of these is also possible. The person may be primarily affected in the legs (paraplegia or diplegia), or in the arm and leg of one side of the body (hemiplegia), or all four limbs may be involved (quadriplegia).

A person with CP may also be affected by a number of other problems, including seizure disorder, visual deficits, hearing problems, **mental retardation**, learning disabilities, and attention-deficit/hyperactivity disorder. None of these is necessarily part of CP, however, and a person with CP may have no other impairments except for the movement disorder.

CP affects approximately 500,000 children and adults in the United States, and is diagnosed in more than 6,000 newborns and young children each year. CP is not an inherited disorder, and as of yet there is no way to predict with certainty which children will develop it. It is not a disease, and is not communicable. CP is a nonprogressive disorder, which means that symptoms neither worsen nor improve over time. However manifestation of the symptoms may become more severe over time; for example, rigidity of muscles can lead to contractures and deformities that require a variety of interventions.

Cerebral palsy is caused by damage to the motor control centers of the brain. When the nerve cells (neurons) in these regions die, the appropriate signals can no longer be sent to the muscles under their control. The resulting poor control of these muscles causes the symptoms of CP.

The symptoms of CP are usually not noticeable at birth; as children develop through the first 18 months of life, though, they progress through a predictable set of developmental milestones. Children with CP will develop these skills more slowly because of their motor impairments, and delay in reaching milestones is usually the first symptom of CP. The more severe the CP, the earlier the diagnosis is usually made.

Children do not consistently favor one hand over the other before 18 months, and doing so may be a sign that the child has difficulty using the other hand. This same preference for one side of the body may show up as an asymmetric crawling effort, or continuing to use only one leg for the work of stair climbing after age three.

It must be remembered that children normally progress at somewhat different rates, and slow beginning accomplishment is often followed by normal development. There are also other causes for delay in reaching some milestones, including problems with vision or hearing. Because CP is a nonprogressive disease, loss of previously acquired milestones indicates that CP is not the cause of the problem.

The impairments of CP become recognizable in early childhood. The type of motor impairment and its location are used as the basis for classification. There are five generally recognized types of impairment:

- Spastic—Muscles are rigid, posture may be abnormal, and fine motor control is impaired
- Athetoid—Marked by slow, writhing, involuntary movements
- Hypotonic—Muscles are floppy, without tone
- Ataxic—Balance and coordination are impaired
- Dystonic—Mixed.

The location of the impairment usually falls into one of three broad categories:

- Hemiplegia—One arm and one leg on the same side of the body involved
- Diplegia—Both legs; arms may be partially involved
- Quadriplegia—All four extremities involved.

Therefore, a person with CP may be said to have spastic diplegia, or ataxic hemiplegia, for instance. CP is also termed mild, moderate, or severe, although these are subjective categories with no firm boundaries.

Loss of muscle control, especially of the spastic type, can cause serious orthopedic problems, including **scoliosis** (spine curvature), hip dislocation, or contractures. A contracture is a shortening of a muscle, caused by an imbalance of opposing force from a neighboring muscle. Contractures begin as prolonged contractions, but can become fixed or irreversible without regular range of motion **exercise**s. A fixed contracture occurs when the contracted muscle adapts by reducing its overall length. Fixed contractures may cause postural abnormalities in the affected limbs, including clenched fists, tightly pressed or crossed thighs, or equinus. In equinus, the most common postural deformity, the foot is extended by the strong pull of the rear calf muscles, causing the toes to point. The foot is commonly pulled inward as well, a condition called equinovarus. Contractures of all kinds may be painful, and may interfere with normal activities of daily living, including hygiene and mobility.

As noted, the brain damage that causes CP may also cause a large number of other disorders. These may include:

- Mental retardation
- Learning disabilities
- Attention-deficit/hyperactivity disorder
- Seizure disorder
- Visual impairment, especially **strabismus** (''cross-eye'')
- **Hearing loss**
- Speech impairment.

These problems may have an even greater impact on the child's life than the physical impairment of CP, although not all children with CP are affected by other problems. About one-third of children with CP have moderate-to-severe mental retardation, one-third have mild mental retardation, and one-third have normal to above average intelligence.

The tracking of developmental progress is the most important test the physician has in determining whether a child has cerebral palsy. Most children with CP can be confidently diagnosed by 18 months. However, diagnosing CP is not always easy, since variations in child development may account for delays in achieving milestones, and since even children who are obviously delayed may continue to progress through the various developmental stages, and attain a normal range of skills later on. Serious or prolonged childhood illness may cause delays that are made up later on.

Evidence of other risk factors may aid the diagnosis. The Apgar score, evaluated immediately after birth, measures the newborn's heart rate, cry, color, muscle tone, and motor reactions. Apgar scores of less than 3 out a possible 10 are associated with a highly increased risk for CP. Presence of abnormal muscle tone or movements may signal CP, as may the persistence of infantile reflexes. A child with seizures or congenital organ malformation has an increased likelihood of CP. Ultrasound examination, a diagnostic technique that creates a two-dimensional image of internal body structures, may help to identify brain abnormalities, such as enlarged ventricles (chambers containing fluid) or periventricular leukomalacia (an abnormality of the area surrounding the ventricles), which may be associated with CP.

X rays, MRIs, and CT scans are often used to look for scarring, cysts, expansion of the cerebral ventricles (**hydrocephalus**), or other brain abnormalities that may indicate the cause of the symptoms. Blood tests and genetic tests may be used to rule out other possible causes, including **muscular dystrophy** (a disease characterized by the progressive wasting of muscles), mitochondrial (cellular) disease, other inherited disorders, or infection.

Cerebral palsy cannot be cured, but many of the disabilities it causes can be managed through planning and timely care. Treatment for a child with CP depends on the severity, nature, and location of the impairment, as well as the associated problems the child has. Optimal care of a child with mild CP may involve regular interaction with only a physical therapist and occupational therapist, whereas care for a more severely affected child may include a speech-language therapist, special education teacher, adaptive sports therapist, nutritionist, orthopedic surgeon, and neurosurgeon. Since CP is not a progressive disorder, its symptoms will not worsen with time. Nonetheless, the way in which those symptoms affect the growing child will change over time, and may require new strategies for treatment, adaptation, and compensation.

Cerebral palsy can affect every stage of maturation, from childhood through adolescence to adulthood. At each stage, the person with CP and his or her caregivers must strive to achieve and maintain the fullest range of experiences and education consistent with the person's abilities. The advice and intervention of professionals remains crucial for many people with CP.

Although CP is not a terminal disorder, it can affect a person's lifespan by increasing the risk of infection, especially lung infections. Poor nutrition can contribute to the likelihood of infection. People with mild cerebral palsy may have near-normal lifespans. The lifespan of those with more severe forms, especially spastic quadriplegia, is often considerably shortened. However, over 90% of infants with CP survive into adulthood.

The cause of most cases of CP is unknown, but it has become clear in recent years that birth difficulties are not to blame in most cases. Rather, developmental problems before birth, usually unknown and generally undiagnosable, are responsible for most cases. Although the incidence of CP caused by Rh factor incompatibility has declined markedly, the incidence of CP as a consequence of prematurity has increased, because of the increasing success of medical intervention in keeping premature babies alive.

CEREBROSPINAL FLUID (CSF) ANALYSIS

Cerebrospinal fluid (CSF) analysis is a laboratory test to examine a sample of the fluid surrounding the brain and spinal cord. This fluid is a clear, watery liquid that protects the central nervous system from injury and cushions it from the surrounding bone structure. It contains a variety of substances, particularly glucose (sugar), protein, and white blood cells from the immune system. The fluid is withdrawn through a needle in a procedure called a *lumbar puncture*.

The purpose of a CSF analysis is to diagnose medical disorders that affect the central nervous system. Some of these conditions include: **meningitis**, **encephalitis**, tumors or **cancer**s of the nervous system, **syphilis**, bleeding (hemorrhaging) around the brain and spinal cord, **multiple sclerosis**, and **Guillain-Barré syndrome**.

In some circumstances, a lumbar puncture to withdraw a small amount of CSF for analysis may lead to serious complications. Lumbar puncture should be performed only with extreme caution, and only if the benefits are thought to outweigh the risks. For example, in people who have blood clotting (coagulation) or bleeding disorders, lumbar puncture can cause bleeding that can compress the spinal cord. If there is a large **brain tumor** or other mass, removal of CSF can cause the brain to drop down within the skull cavity (herniate), compressing the brain stem and other vital structures, and leading to irreversible brain damage or **death**. These problems are easily avoided by checking blood coagulation through a blood test and by doing a **computed tomography scan** (CT) or **magnetic resonance imaging** (MRI) scan before attempting the lumbar puncture.

The procedure to remove cerebrospinal fluid is called a lumbar puncture, or spinal tap, because the area of the spinal column used to obtain the sample is in the lumbar spine, or lower section of the back. In rare instances, such as a spinal fluid blockage in the middle of the back, a doctor may perform a spinal tap in the neck.

In order to get an accurate sample of cerebrospinal fluid, it is critical that a patient is in the proper position. The spine must be curved to allow as much space as possible between the lower vertebrae, or bones of the back, for the doctor to insert a lumbar puncture needle between the vertebrae and withdraw a small amount of fluid. The most common position is for the patient to lie on his or her side with the back at the edge of the exam table, head and chin bent down, knees drawn up to the chest, and arms clasped around the knees. It is important to be relaxed and to remain still during the entire procedure. If the patient is anxious or uncooperative, a short-acting sedative may be given.

During a lumbar puncture, the doctor drapes the back with a sterile covering that has an opening over the puncture site and cleans the skin surface with an antiseptic solution. Patients receive a local anesthetic (numbing medication) to minimize any **pain** in the lower back.

The doctor inserts a hollow, thin needle in the space between two vertebrae of the lower back and slowly advances it toward the spine. A steady flow of cerebrospinal fluid will begin to fill the needle as soon as it enters the spinal canal. The doctor measures the cerebrospinal fluid pressure with a special instrument called a manometer and withdraws several vials of fluid for laboratory analysis. The amount of fluid collected depends on the type and number of tests needed to diagnose a particular medical disorder.

Normal CSF is clear and colorless. It may be cloudy in infections; straw- or yellow-colored if there is excess protein, as may occur with cancer or inflammation; blood-tinged if there was recent bleeding; or yellow to brown (xanthochromic) if caused by an older instance of bleeding.

After the procedure, the doctor covers the site of the puncture with a sterile bandage. Patients must avoid sitting or standing and remain lying down for as long as six hours after the lumbar puncture. They should also drink plenty of fluid to help prevent headache.

In most cases, this test to analyze CSF is a safe and effective procedure. Some patients experience pain, difficulty urinating, infection, or leakage of cerebrospinal fluid from the puncture site after the procedure. For most people, the most common side effect after the removal of CSF is a headache. This occurs in 10-30% of adult patients and in up to 40% of children. It is caused by a decreased CSF pressure related to a small leak of CSF through the puncture site. These headaches usually are a dull pain, although some people report a throbbing sensation. A stiff neck and nausea may accompany the headache. Lumbar puncture headaches typically begin within two days after the procedure and persist from a few days to several weeks or months.

Since an upright position worsens the pain, patients with a lumbar puncture headache can control the pain by lying in a flat position and taking a prescription or non-prescription pain relief medication, preferably one containing **caffeine**. In rare cases, the puncture site leak is ''patched'' using the patient's own blood.

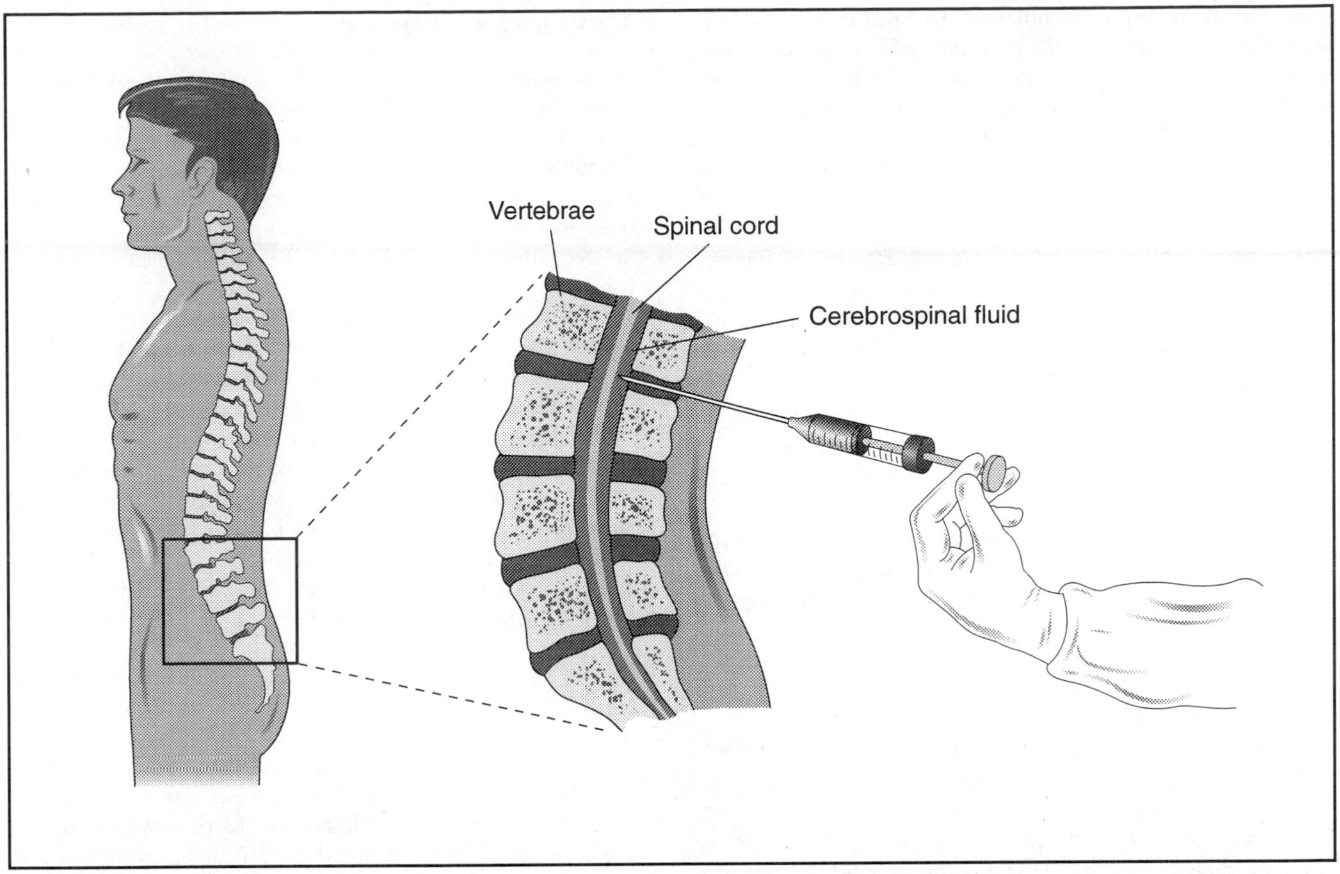

During a lumbar puncture, or spinal tap, a procedure in which cerebrospinal fluid is aspirated, the physician inserts a hollow, thin needle in the space between two vertebrae of the lower back and slowly advances it toward the spine. The cerebrospinal fluid pressure is then measured and the fluid is withdrawn for laboratory analysis. *(Illustration by Electronic Illustrators Group.)*

CERVICAL CANCER

Cervical cancer is a disease in which the cells of the cervix become abnormal and start to grow uncontrollably, forming tumors. The cervix is the lower part or the neck of the uterus (womb). It connects the uterus to the vagina (birth canal). Cervical cancer generally begins as an abnormality in the cells on the outside of the cervix. It is a very slow growing cancer. The change in the cells from normal to pre-cancerous to cancerous is very gradual and may take several years to develop. For this reason, routine screening tests for cervical cancer are very important. When detected early, it is nearly 100% curable.

The cause of cervical cancer is not known. However, certain factors are believed to increase one's risk of developing cervical cancer. Engaging in sexual activity at a young age is one such factor. The cells lining the cervix do not fully mature until the age of 18 and, therefore, are more susceptible to cancer causing-agents and viruses.

More than 90% of women with cancer of the cervix are infected with the human papilloma virus (HPV). Hence, HPV infection is the single most important risk factor for cervical cancer. The HPV belongs to a group of 70 viruses that can cause **warts** (papillomas). HPV usually causes warts in the genital area. The viruses are passed from one person to another during unprotected sex. Having multiple sexual partners increases one's risk of getting this cancer, because the greater the number of sexual partners, the greater is the risk of acquiring HPV infection. Even if a woman has only one sexual partner, but the man has several partners, he is considered a ''high-risk male'' and can transmit HPV to the woman.

Smoking is considered a risk factor, possibly because smoking causes some abnormal changes in the cells and these cells have a higher likelihood of becoming cancerous.

In its early stages, cervical cancer may have no symptoms. Often, the diagnosis is made during a routine pelvic examination. Some women experience symptoms such as bleeding between periods (irregular vaginal bleeding); postmenopausal vaginal bleeding; vaginal bleeding after intercourse; and vaginal discharge with an unpleasant odor. When the cancer is in an advanced stage and has invaded the tissue surrounding the cervix, a woman may have **pain** in the pelvic area, and heavy bleeding from the vagina.

A Pap smear is the best screening test used to detect cancer of the cervix. It is done as a part of a regular pelvic exam. A medical swab or brush is rubbed against the cervix. The tissue sample collected is smeared on a slide and sent to the laboratory for microscopic examination. This test detects cervical abnormalities more than 95% of the time. A negative test means that no abnormalities are present. If a Pap test is positive, an abnormality has been detected in the cell lining the cervix.

Because the Pap test is a screening test, rather than a diagnostic test, the doctor will order a biopsy. The purpose of the biopsy is to check if the abnormality is due to a precancerous change or if cancer is present. During the biopsy, a piece of cervical tissue is removed and examined under a microscope. A cervical biopsy can be performed in several different ways. In a procedure known as **colposcopy**, the doctor uses a magnifying scope to view the surface of the cervix clearly. If any abnormal areas are seen, the doctor can use a pair of biopsy forceps to remove a small piece of the suspicious area for further testing. The tissue is then sent to the laboratory for examination.

Treatment for cervical cancer depends on the stage of the disease and the extent of its spread. The three standard modes of treatment are surgery, **radiation therapy**, and **chemotherapy**.

A radical **hysterectomy** removes the entire uterus, the ovaries, the upper part of the vagina that is next to the cervix, and the lymph nodes from the pelvic region.

Radiation therapy, which involves the use of high energy x rays to kill cancer cells, can also be used for treating cervical cancer. However, radiation therapy to the pelvic region has many effects. It could cause a narrowing of the vagina (vaginal stenosis) that makes intercourse painful. It may also stop the ovaries from releasing eggs and producing the female hormone estrogen. When this happens, it causes **premature menopause** in young women and they will need estrogen replacement therapy. Many women are treated with both surgery and radiation therapy.

Chemotherapy, or the use of **anticancer drugs** to kill the cancer cells, is not a common form of treatment for cervical cancer because it is not as effective as other methods. Nevertheless, the effectiveness of combination chemotherapy, (where more than one drug is used to treat the cancer), is being tested in clinical trials.

The prognosis for cervical cancer is very good. When detected in the early stages, approximately 91% of the women survive 5 years or more.

Most cases of cervical cancers can be prevented, since they start with easily detectable pre-cancerous changes. One of the best ways to prevent cervical cancers is by having regular Pap tests. If pre-cancerous changes are detected, appropriate treatment can prevent them from developing into invasive cancers. Another way to prevent cervical cancers is to avoid the risk factors. Abstaining from sexual relations when one is very young, and using appropriate precautions (**condom**s) when engaging in sexual activity will help to avoid HPV infections. Quitting smoking will also help to reduce the risk for cervical and many other cancers.

CESAREAN SECTION

A cesarean section, or c-section, is a surgical procedure in which incisions are made through a woman's abdomen and uterus to deliver her baby. The procedure is performed in the United States on nearly one of every four babies delivered — more than 900,000 babies each year. C-sections are performed whenever abnormal conditions complicate labor and vaginal delivery, threatening the life or health of the mother or the baby.

The most common reason that a cesarean section is performed (in 35% of all cases, according to the U.S. Public Health Service) is that the woman has had a previous c-section. The ''once a cesarean, always a cesarean'' rule originated back when the incision in the uterus was made vertically; the resulting scar was weak and had a risk of rupturing during later deliveries. Today, the incision is almost always made horizontally across the lower end of the uterus (this is called a ''low transverse incision''), resulting in reduced blood loss and a decreased chance of rupture. This kind of incision allows many women to have a vaginal birth after a cesarean (VBAC).

The second most common reason that a c-section is performed (in 30% of all cases) is difficult **childbirth** due to non-progressive labor (dystocia). Uterine contractions may be weak or irregular, the cervix may not be dilating, or the mother's pelvic structure may not allow adequate passage for birth.

Another 12% of c-sections are performed to deliver a baby in a breech presentation: buttocks or feet first. Breech presentation is found in about 3% of all births. When a c-section is being considered because the baby is in a breech position, the doctor may first attempt to reposition the baby. The doctor may also try a vaginal breech delivery, depending on the size of the mother's pelvis, the size of the baby, and the type of breech position the baby is in.

In 9% of all cases, c-sections are performed in response to fetal distress. Fetal distress refers to any situation that threatens the baby's oxygen supply, such as the umbilical cord getting wrapped around the baby's neck. This may appear on the fetal heart monitor as an abnormal heart rate or rhythm.

The remaining 14% of c-sections are indicated by other serious factors. One is prolapse of the umbilical cord: the cord is pushed into the vagina ahead of the baby and becomes compressed, cutting off blood flow to the baby. Another is **placental abruption**: the placenta separates from the uterine wall before the baby is born, cutting off blood flow to the baby. The risk of this is especially high in multiple births (twins, triplets, or more). A third factor is **placenta previa**: the placenta covers the cervix partially or completely, making vaginal delivery impossible. In some cases requiring c-section, the baby is in a transverse position, lying horizontally across the pelvis, perhaps with a shoulder in the birth canal.

The mother's health may also make delivery by c-section the safer choice, especially in cases of maternal diabetes, **hypertension**, **genital herpes**, Rh blood incompatibility, and preeclampsia (high blood pressure related to **pregnancy**).

There are several ways that obstetricians and other doctors diagnose conditions that may make a c-section necessary.

Ultrasound testing reveals the positions of the baby and the placenta. Fetal heart monitors, in use since the 1970s, transmit any signals of fetal distress. Oxygen deprivation may be determined by testing the pH of a blood sample taken from the baby's scalp, or by checking the amniotic fluid for meconium (feces). A lack of oxygen causes an unborn baby to defecate.

When a c-section becomes necessary, the mother is prepped for surgery. A catheter is inserted into her bladder and an intravenous (IV) line is inserted into her arm. Leads for monitoring the mother's heart rate, heart rhythm, and blood pressure are attached. In the operating room, the mother is given anesthesia — usually a regional anesthetic (epidural or spinal), making her numb from below her breasts to her toes. In some cases, a general anesthetic will be administered. Surgical drapes are placed over the body, except the head; these drapes block the direct view of the procedure.

The first incision opens the abdomen, and is usually made horizontally across and above the pubic bone (informally called a "bikini cut"). The second incision opens the uterus. Once the uterus is opened, the amniotic sac is ruptured and the baby is delivered. The time from the initial incision to birth is typically five minutes.

After the umbilical cord is clamped and cut, the newborn is evaluated. The placenta is removed from the mother, and her uterus and abdomen are stitched, or sutured, closed (surgical staples may be used instead in closing the outermost layer of the abdominal incision). Suturing may take an additional 30-40 minutes.

Following this procedure, a woman commonly experiences gas pains, incision pain, and uterine contractions. A woman who undergoes a c-section requires both the care given to any new mother and the care given to any patient recovering from major surgery. She should be offered pain medication that does not interfere with breastfeeding. She should be encouraged to get out of bed and walk around 8-24 hours after surgery to stimulate circulation (thus avoiding the formation of blood clots) and bowel movement. She should nap when the baby does, limit climbing stairs to once a day, and avoid lifting anything heavier than the baby.

Full recovery may be seen in four to six weeks. As the woman heals, she may gradually increase appropriate **exercises** to regain abdominal tone. She may resume driving after two weeks, although some doctors recommend waiting for six weeks, the typical recovery period from major surgery.

Because a c-section is a surgical procedure, it carries more risk to both the mother and the baby. The mother is at risk for increased bleeding and infection of either incision, the urinary tract, or the tissue lining the uterus (endometritis). Less commonly, she may receive injury to the surrounding organs. When a general **anesthesia** is used, she may experience complications from the anesthesia. Very rarely, she may blood clots leading to pelvic **thrombophlebitis** (inflammation of the major vein running from the pelvis into the leg) or a pulmonary embolus (a blood clot lodging in the lung).

Undergoing a c-section may also cause psychological distress beyond hormonal mood swings and **postpartum depression** ("baby blues"). A woman may feel disappointment and a sense of failure for not experiencing a vaginal delivery. She may feel isolated if the father or birthing coach is not with her in the operating room, and may feel helpless from a loss of control over labor and delivery with no opportunity to actively participate. Women who undergo a c-section should be encouraged to share their feelings with others and seek professional help if negative emotions persist. Hospitals can often recommend support groups for such mothers.

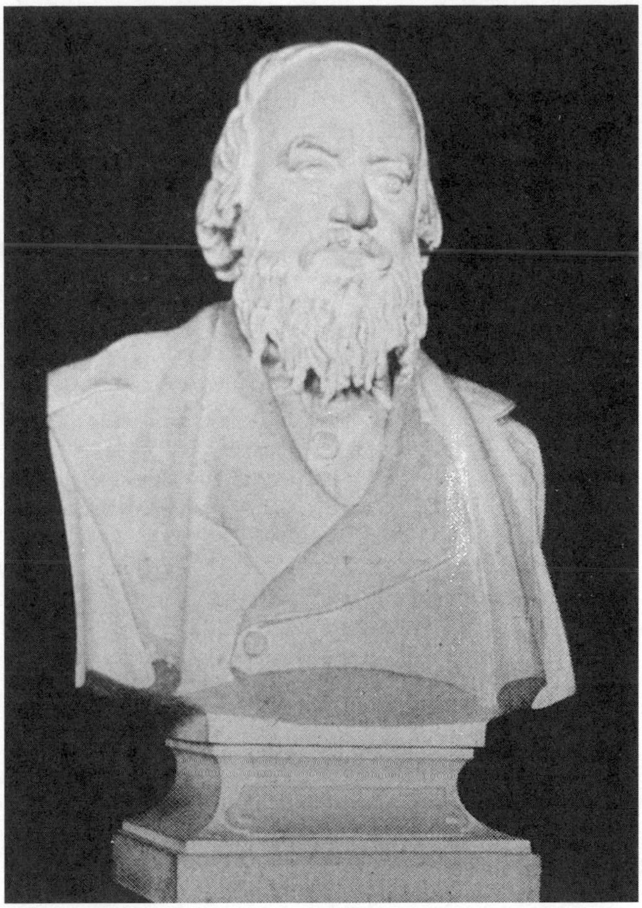

Edwin Chadwick

CHADWICK, EDWIN (1800-1890)

English lawyer and public health reformer

Although trained as a lawyer, Edwin Chadwick earned a place in the history of medicine by encouraging government involvement in health promotion. Reforms introduced during his short-lived public health career included improved sewers and water supply systems needed to accommodate population growth associated with England's Industrial Revolution.

Born in 1800 near Manchester, England, Chadwick moved with his parents to London at the age of 10. There, after studying classical and modern languages, he helped finance his legal training by writing essays for newspapers, including one about life assurance for the *Westminster Review* that attracted considerable attention.

From that beginning, Chadwick developed what became known as the ''sanitary idea,'' assuring health by creating central and local government agencies to regulate nuisances and provide for clean water and removal of sewage. Rejecting the widely held belief that poor health was largely a matter of fate, he argued that disease arose from correctable environmental causes.

Chadwick's philosophy of health reform was heavily influenced by the utilitarian lawyer Jeremy Bentham, for whom he worked as an aide before becoming a lawyer himself. Bentham believed that all reforms should be based on ''the greatest happiness of the greatest number.''

Chadwick's **sanitation** initiatives were rooted in the now discredited belief that disease was caused by unpleasant odors (miasmas) from trash and sewers. Nonetheless, after his reforms were introduced, mortality rates in England decreased and life expectancy increased.

Chadwick's self-flushing sewers, lined with glazed brick, remained in use into the final years of the twentieth century. Prior to his environmental initiatives, English sewers collected surface water and waste in underground receptacles but did not carry it away. For this reason, sewage often decomposed into foul-smelling gases that Chadwick believed caused illness.

In addition, sewers of the day had to be cleaned manually, a job that Chadwick considered inhumane. He proposed building smaller diameter, egg-shaped sewer pipes that could be flushed with pressurized water. Liquid wastes could thus be removed to the countryside to be used as fertilizer. Instead of the existing jumble of individually designed cesspools, Chadwick's sewers were built as an engineered, citywide system.

Chadwick also sponsored legislation requiring government registration of births, deaths, and marriages. Those records, previously maintained by the church, were useful for tracking epidemics and other causes of death. Chadwick correlated such vital statistics with data about living conditions to identify possible factors in disease causation. **Florence Nightingale** provided him with statistics for this work and enthusiastically promoted Chadwick's sanitation proposals. In turn, Chadwick lobbied for sanitary commissioners to ensure the health of soldiers fighting in the Crimea, as Nightingale was setting up her nursing service there.

In addition, Chadwick pushed for government health inspectors, better-ventilated and less-crowded housing, wider streets, workplace health and safety legislation, increased use of indoor plumbing, and limits on the employment of children in factories.

His best-known writing is his *Inquiry into the Sanitary Conditions of the Labouring Population of Great Britain,* a massive survey published in 1842 that vividly described ''open sewers, stagnant pools of liquid refuse, insanitary privies, and the stench of underventilated, overcrowded tenements,'' comparing the urban environments in London, Glasgow, Manchester, Birmingham, Leeds, and other large centers.

To implement recommendations from this report, Chadwick led the campaign for England's first Public Health Act. It nonetheless took the cholera epidemic of 1847 in which 10,000 Londoners die to persuade Parliament to finally pass the legislation the following year.

Chadwick's reforms were met with fear and distrust. He encountered opposition from political foes who balked at centralized government and the cost of his public works projects, as well as engineers who disagreed with his sewer designs and doctors who objected to a nonphysician being responsible for public health. Chadwick's formal career in public health lasted only from 1848 to 1854, when the unpopularity of his reforms forced him and other members of London's Board of Health to resign. They were replaced by a new health-promotion bureaucracy made up of doctors.

Despite this less-than-noble end to his formal career in public health, Chadwick continued to write extensively about health-related issues. A two-volume, summarized compilation of his writings was published in 1887 under the title *The Health of Nations.*

In 1889, Chadwick's contributions to public health were recognized by Queen Victoria, who knighted him as one of the first civilian Knight Commanders of the Most Honourable Order of the Bath (KCB).

See also Public health, Sanitation

Chain, Ernst Boris (1906-1979)

German biochemist

Chain is renowned for his role in the discovery of **penicillin**, a drug that has saved millions of lives and was the first of the **antibiotic** ''wonder drugs.'' The son of a wealthy chemist, Chain was born in Berlin in 1906. He earned his Ph.D. in chemistry in 1930 from the Friedrich-Wilhelm University in Berlin. When Adolf Hitler (1889-1945) came to power in early 1933, Chain immigrated to England, where he worked and studied under **Frederick Gowland Hopkins** at Cambridge University.

At the recommendation of Hopkins, **Howard Florey** invited Chain to join his pathology laboratory at Oxford to pursue studies of antimicrobial agents. While Chain conducted a literature search on lysozyme, an antibacterial enzyme, he came across a paper by Alexander Fleming published in 1929 describing his work with penicillin found in molds. Chain and Florey decided to continue the work, which Fleming had abandoned shortly after his discovery.

Chain conducted the first chemical assay of penicillin. Florey and Chain concluded that penicillin was nontoxic yet effective in destroying a wide range of bacteria, and began conducting clinical trials in humans. The results were so successful that penicillin was quickly put into mass production to treat the infections of wounded soldiers during World War II. In 1945 Chain, Florey, and Fleming were awarded the Nobel Prize in Medicine for discovering penicillin.

Chain went on to discover penicillinase, an enzyme that causes the destruction of penicillin in the body. After World War II, Chain became scientific director of a health institute in Rome, but returned to England in 1961, where he headed a new laboratory at the University of London.

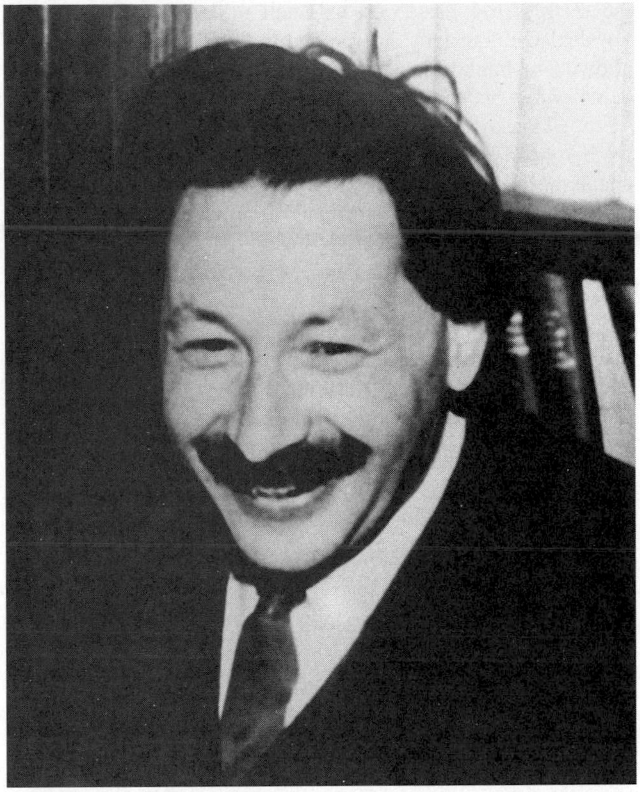

Ernst Boris Chain

Chapman, Nathaniel (1780-1853)

American physician

Nathaniel Chapman was a prominent Philadelphia physician and medical leader in the United States during the early 1800s. As professor of Materia Medica and then professor of the theory and practice of medicine at the University of Pennsylvania, Chapman held what were then the most prestigious medical posts in the country. He authored several important early medical works and was the first president of the American Medical Association.

Chapman was born at Summer Hill in Virginia to George and Amelia Chapman, who had six sons and one daughter. Growing up in a comfortable upper class life, Chapman was a clever child who dabbled in poetry. After graduating from the Alexandria Academy, he began his medical apprenticeship in Maryland at the age of 15. He eventually studied under Benjamin Rush at the University of Pennsylvania in Philadelphia and graduated with honors in 1801. Chapman then went on an academic tour of Europe and returned to the United States in 1804 to begin his career. During the intervening years, Chapman showed an intense interest in politics and patriotism and wrote several articles on European politics that were published in popular magazines of the time.

Known for his wit and winning personality, Chapman established a successful medical practice in Philadelphia (then one of the most populous and scientific cities in the young country) and began the independent teaching of midwifery. Chapman, however, had higher ambitions, namely to join the faculty of the University of Pennsylvania's prestigious medical school. Although not considered to have a brilliant medical mind, Chapman was popular and well respected by his colleagues, who appreciated Chapman's firm grasp of medical science at that time. In 1813, Chapman's former teacher Rush died, leaving vacant Rush's prestigious position as chair of the theory and practice of medicine. That same year, Chapman joined the University of Pennsylvania as chair of Materia Medica. Although much infighting went on to determine who would be appointed to Rush's chair, Chapman finally won out and became chair of the theory and practice of medicine in 1816. Not yet 40 years old, he now held one of the most influential medical positions in America.

In 1817, Chapman founded the Medical Institute of Philadelphia, the first post-graduate medical school in the United States. He also authored several medical works, including his major work, *Discoveries on the Elements of Therapeutics* and *Materia Medica*, in six volumes. Although extremely popular with his students and colleagues, Chapman refused to accept new ideas in medicine during a period of significant advances in the understanding of how the human body functions. By 1820, many of his beliefs, such as the usefulness of ''bleeding'' patients, were considered anachronisms. Chapman, however, held little faith in the new medical discoveries based largely on the growing field of pathology. In the end, his refusal to accept the proven results of medical experimentation cost him many followers.

Despite no longer at the forefront of medical science, Chapman continued to influence the field, primarily through his training of students, his membership in many medical organizations, and his founding of the medical magazine Philadelphia Journal of the Medical and Physical Sciences in 1820. Chapman also maintained his national medical reputation among the populace until the end of his career. He was the attending physician when President James Buchanan's estranged fiance, Ann Caroline Coleman, died and was called to Washington as a consulting physician in 1841 when President William Henry Harrison became ill. In 1848, towards the end of his career, Chapman's colleagues recognized his life-long efforts in medicine by electing him the first president of the American Medical Association. Chapman retired in 1850 due to illness, thus ending the ''Medical Age of Chapman'' in Philadelphia.

Chapman's personal life was marked by a wide acceptance among the young country's most elite and influential personages and by deep personal tragedies. A devoted family man, he and his wife, Rebecca Biddle Chapman, had six children, with only three surviving to adulthood. Then, in 1845, Chapman's son, John, died at the age of 33. His son, George, followed in 1850, and his beloved daughter Emily died in 1852. Crushed by these losses, Chapman lingered on until July 1, 1852, when he died in his Philadelphia home. A long-time patriot and proponent of America's growing importance in the arts and sciences, Chapman was buried on July 4, 1852.

CHARAKA

The *Charaka Samhita* is among the earliest surviving Sanskrit medical manuals, and the most authoritative. *Samhita* is Sanskrit for compendium, and Charaka is a proper name. So translated, the work means ''Charaka's Compendium.'' Although the exact date of composition of the *Charaka Samhita* is unknown, scholars estimate that it was written around 100 A.D. It was eventually supplemented, edited, and partially rewritten by other authors over an extended period up to 800 A.D. *Charaka* reiterates the teachings of the school of Atreya, a famous physician of antiquity, and lengthy passages take the form of a dialogue between Atreya and Agnivesha, Charaka's teacher. *Charaka* was translated into Persion and Arabic in the eighth century, and is still used today. Most of what is known about Indian medical science derives from this text and two others, the *Susruta Samhita* and the *Ashtangahridaya Samhita.*

The *Charaka Samhita* is long, running to 1,000 pages in English translation. It represented a major advance over the supersitious ways of treating medical problems of the *Atharva Veda* (one of the four sacred books of Hinduism, which included songs and spells concerning the healing of diseases). Instead of appeasing deities and making sacrifices, practitioners were now looking at clinical problems and deciding how to treat them based on the specific disease. Perhaps most significant, they developed concepts of health and disease which they applied in practice.

The science of medicine became known as Ayurveda, or science of life. Just as we now seek to explain a disease as a problem of nutrition or genetics, Ayurvedic physicians formed a medical theory that guided the way they evaluated patients and diseases.

Unlike the **germ theory** which developed much later, Ayurveda proposed that human disorders arose from an imbalance of three vital substances, or **humors**, present in every living creature: wind, bile, and phlegm (that is, mucus). Life and health were considered not only a product of karma (the sum of a person's actions in previous states of existence) but also of behavior in this life. The things that upset the balance of the humors included improper food and practices, and accidents. Ayurveda emphasized prevention through cleansing, exercise, diet, and good habits.

By the time *Charaka* was written, doctoring was recognized as a profession, and sons often followed in the footsteps of their fathers. Then, as now, medicine promised a materially and spiritually satisfying life. According to *Charaka,* a **physician** could expect religious merit for relieving suffering, material gain from successful cures, and personal satisfaction from the fame and reputation that a successful practice would bring. The text offers practical advice on medical training and managing patients, and it laid down a code of ethics for physicians. *Charaka* warned against unscrupulous physicians who make phony diagnoses in search of quick money, and emphasized a moral basis of medicine as a public service.

According to *Charaka* the medical profession was reserved for the highest castes (categories of a hereditary social order in South Asia). Because **surgery** was considered to be the work of low-caste persons such as barbers, the text does not deal with surgery. Moreover, Indian physicians were not allowed to handle or to dissect corpses, which limited students' ways of learning about how the human body worked.

Charaka regarded disease as originating either inside the body or from outside. Divided into eight sections and 150 chapters, the text is above all an exhaustive work on therapeutic medicine, that is, the treatment of ailments curable by drugs and modification of diet and lifestyle. It also covers bodily structure and function, the cause, symptoms, and prognosis of disease, and the effect of disease on the body. Physicians are urged to examine patients carefully, and to tailor treatment not just to the disease but also to the person, climate, time of year, and environment. Thus, different people with identical symptoms might receive different treatments. *Charaka* describes more than 600 drugs of animal, plant, and mineral origin, along with formulas for medicines and instructions for making them.

See also Alternative medicine; Ayurvedic medicine; Medical ethics; *Sushruta*

CHARCOT, JEAN-MARTIN (1825-1893)

French physician, neurologist, and teacher

Jean-Martin Charcot was born on November 29, 1825 in Paris, France; he died at Auberge des Settons, near Vézelay, France on August 16, 1893. He is remembered as a physician, neurologist, and teacher who succeeded in relating many neurological disorders to physical causes. He held the position of professor at the University of Paris for 33 years. In 1862, he began an association with the Salpetrière Hospital, an ancient and famous hospital in Paris, that lasted throughout his life (eventually Charcot would become director of this hospital).

Charcot studied medicine in Paris. After failing a competitive examination in 1847, he was elected Interne at the Salpetrière in 1848. Charcot's M.D. thesis (1853) contributed to the understanding of the difference between **rheumatoid arthritis**, and **gout** and other joint diseases. Charcot was the first to describe intermittent claudication (1858). When he began practicing at the Salpetrière in 1862, he found many long-term patients suffering from undiagnosed or unknown chronic afflictions of the nervous system. Over the next eight years, made systematic clinical observations of their physical symptoms, which he succeeded in correlating with actual lesions by conducting autopsies.

Charcot made classical descriptions of multiple or disseminated sclerosis and in 1869 of amyotrophic lateral sclerosis, subsequently known as Maladie de Charcot (Charcot's disease), **Lou Gehrig's disease**, and ALS. (Amyotrophic refers to a loss of muscle mass; lateral refers to the nerve tracks that run down both sides of the spinal cord, where many neurons affected by ALS are found; sclerosis refers to the scar tissue that remains following disintegration of the nerves). Charcot was the first physician to link symptoms of ALS to a group of nerves specifically affected by the disease, i.e., the motor neurons that originate in the spinal cord).

Charcot's important contributions to medicine included his recognition of the importance of small arteries in cerebral hemorrhage (a familial neuropathy now known as Charcot-Marie-Tooth disease involving a progressive degeneration of the muscles in the foot, lower leg, hand and forearm, and a mild loss of sensation in the limbs, fingers and toes. He also made contributions to the understanding of tabes dorsalis (a type of neurosyphilis), as well as of a destructive and painless arththritis know as Charcot's joint. Still other studies focused on **polio**myelitis, cerebral localization and **aphasia**. Charcot never lost his interest in general medicine, however, and wrote about thyroid and **liver disease**.

Although he conducted laboratory experiments, Charcot was opposed to animal experimentation. He did, however, defend Pasteur's **rabies** vaccination. He was a popular lecturer at the Salpetrière, and his Leçons sur les maladies du système nerveux faits à la Salpetrière (1872 to 1873) was translated into many languages. In 1872, he was appointed Professor of Pathologic Anatomy at the Sorbonne; ten years later he became Professor of Disease of the Nervous System at the University of Paris.

Charcot also had a special interest in the malady then known as **hysteria**, which seemed to be a **mental illness** with physical symptoms. He was convinced that hysteria came about because of a weak neurological system, and that the disease had a familial origin. He was intrigued because the malady could be triggered by a traumatic event like an accident, but it then became progressive and irreversible. To study patients, he applied the technique of **hypnosis** to induce and study their symptoms. By using a large accordion-sized camera to capture the "fits" of his patients, Charcot was able to demonstrate that hysteria, like organic diseases, was associated with a set of distinguishing symptoms. Charcot's research on hysteria enhanced his reputation outside his own discipline, but his critics argued that he was using the power of suggestion to bring about his patients' crises. In retrospect, however, it appears that many of Charcot's ideas on hysteria were well founded. Not surprisingly, Charcot attracted students from all over Europe, including Pierre Marie, J. F. F. Babinski, V. M. Bechterew, Alfred Binet, and Pierre Janet, and Sigmund Freud.

Freud, who had applied for and received the University Jubilee Travel Grant to Paris for 1884/5 to study with Charcot, remarked in a letter to his fiancee that Charcot had the air of "a worldly priest from whom one expects a ready wit and an appreciation of good living." Freud was especially struck by Charcot's brilliance, and by his lively interest in all that took place around him. Although Freud was favorably impressed with Charcot's person, he disagreed with Charcot's idea that hypnosis is a neurological phenomenon, and went on to argue that the hypnotic state is a psychological phenomenon.

An accomplished artist, Charcot's drawings and caricatures have been preserved at the Salpetrière. He is also remembered for his books about demons, the deformed, and the sick, and their relationship to art. Charcot's only son, Jean, abandoned medicine after his father's death, and went on to become France's foremost polar explorer.

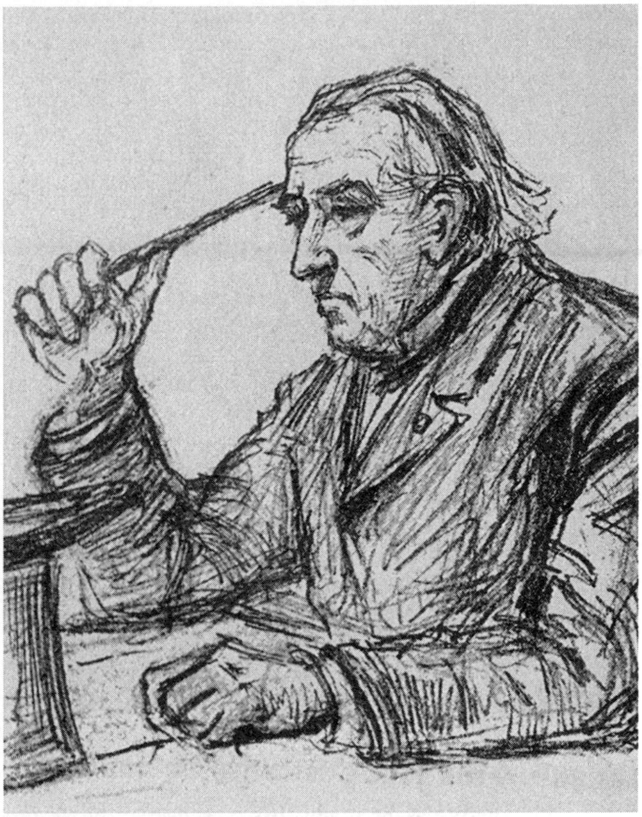

Jean-Martin Charcot

CHARCOT-MARIE-TOOTH DISEASE

Charcot-Marie-Tooth disease (CMT) is the name for a group of inherited disorders of nerve conduction causing weakness and mild loss of sensation in the limbs.

CMT affects the peripheral nerves, those groups of nerve cells carrying information to and from the spinal cord. CMT decreases the ability of these nerves to carry motor commands to muscles, especially those furthest from the spinal cord in the feet and hands. As a result, these muscles are weakened. CMT also causes mild sensory loss.

CMT is named for the three neurologists who first described it, and does not involve the teeth in any way. It is also known as hereditary motor and sensory neuropathy, and is also sometimes called peroneal muscular atrophy, referring to the muscles in the leg affected early on in the disease.

The symptoms grouped together under the name CMT can be caused by any of at least six different genetic defects. Most of the defects, identified as of early 1998, affect myelin, the coating that insulates nerve cells to promote efficient conduction. Myelin defects cause either a reduction in nerve conduction velocities, or a diminished nerve signal.

CMT is currently subdivided into type 1A, type 1B, type 2, and type X, based on the particular genetic defect involved. All but type X exhibit the inheritance pattern known as autosomal dominant. In this pattern, only one defective gene copy is needed to develop the disease, which may be inherited from either parent (who will also have the disease). A person with CMT of this type has a 50% chance of passing the gene along to each offspring. CMT type X is inherited as an X-linked trait, meaning the gene is carried on the X chromosome. Women carry two X chromosomes, while men carry only one. Without a ''backup'' copy of the normal gene, a man with the CMT type X gene is more likely to be seriously affected than is a woman. Expression of the gene does occur in women to a lesser extent, leading to disease of variable severity. Affected men may pass the gene on to their daughters, but not to their sons.

A rare, related disorder, called CMT type 3 or Dejerine-Sottas disease, also involves myelin. It is an autosomal recessive trait, meaning genetic contributions from both parents are needed for a child to express the disease.

CMT causes progressive, symmetrical weakness and muscle atrophy, or wasting. The earliest symptoms include foot deformity and difficulty walking or running. The characteristic deformities of CMT are very high arches and flexed toes, or ''claw-toe.'' Foot deformities may lead to **pain** in poorly-fitted shoes. Foot drop may lead to tripping or require deliberate high steps over curbs and other obstructions. Sports involvement may lead to frequent sprains or **fractures** of the ankles. Symptom onset in type 1 is usually in childhood or adolescence, while for type 2 it may be in the early twenties or later.

Symptoms progress from the feet upward to the calves then thighs, and from leg weakness only to involve the fingers and hands. There may be minor loss of sensation in the feet and hands as well, although this rarely causes difficulty. Complaints of cold legs are common, as are cramps in the legs, especially after **exercise**. Some patients develop tremor in the upper limbs as the disease progresses. Most people with CMT remain able to walk throughout their lives.

Diagnosis of CMT begins with a careful medical history and a detailed neurological exam to determine the extent and distribution of weakness. A nerve conduction velocity test, an electrical test of nerve function, shows characteristic changes. This is often combined with electromyography, an electrical test of the muscles. A nerve biopsy—removal of a small piece of the nerve—may be performed to look for the swelling characteristic of CMT type 1. DNA testing is available for CMT type 1, but not for other types currently. DNA testing may be performed on both the person suspected of having CMT and on family members who may be at risk.

Physical and occupational therapy form an important part of CMT treatment. Physical therapy is used to preserve range of motion and minimize deformity caused by muscle shortening, or contracture. Braces are sometimes used to improve control of the lower extremities. Occupational therapy is used to design compensatory tools and techniques to aid in dressing, feeding, writing, and other activities of daily living.

Tremors may be worsened by **caffeine**, so reducing caffeine use may help minimize them. Beta-blockers may help relieve tremor. Alcohol should be avoided, as should certain drug combinations that can cause muscle damage. Such damage may result from combining gemfibrozil (Lopid) with lovastatin (Mevacor), for instance, both used to treat high cholesterol levels.

CMT causes progressive weakness, but does not usually shorten life expectancy. Most people with CMT are able to lead full and productive lives despite their impairments.

There is no way to prevent CMT in a person who has the gene or genes responsible. **Genetic testing** is available for family planning purposes.

Chelation therapy

Chelation therapy is the administration of a drug that removes toxic metals from the bloodstream. Physicians have used chelation therapy since the 1950s to treat **heavy metal poisoning**—primarily **lead poisoning**—and to remove metals that have built up in tissues as a result of such genetic disorders as Wilson's disease, cystinuria, and hemochromatosis.

In addition to these accepted uses, chelation therapy has also been promoted by some as a non-surgical alternative for the treatment of **atherosclerosis**. However, no controlled scientific study has yet supported these claims and most physicians do not recommend chelation therapy for this purpose.

Chelation therapy is generally only recommmended when high levels of metal are present in the blood, since it does not seem to benefit those with lower levels. Currently, four drugs are used for chelation therapy: edetate calcium disodium (calcium EDTA), dimercaprol (BAL), succimer, and d-Penicillamine. Calcium EDTA is usually injected into a muscle, but it can be administered through a vein. BAL is injected into a muscle and is usually used along with calcium EDTA for the treament of lead poisoning. Because the muscular injection of these two drugs can be painful, they are normally administered with a local anesthetic (numbing medication). Succimer and d-Penicillamine are given in pill form.

The dosage of chelation therapy depends upon which drug is being used, the type and level of metal present in the patient's blood, and the patient's age and general health. If calcium EDTA is given on its own or with BAL, one treatment will last approximately five days with doses being given 4-12 hours apart. A second treatment may be administered after a two-day interval. If BAL is being given on its own, treatment will last approximately two weeks with doses being given 4-12 hours apart. Treatment with succimer takes about 19 days, while treament with d-Penicillamine may last as long as six months, particularly if the drug is being used to remove heavy metals that have accumulated in the blood because of a genetic disorder.

Patients who are pregnant or who have severe kidney problems, very low urine output, or very low blood circulation should not be given edetate calcium disodium (calcium EDTA). Patients with abnormally low levels of the enzyme glucose-6-phosphate dehydrogenase should not be given BAL, since the drug can trigger a breakdown of the red blood cells (hemolysis) in these persons. BAL should also not be given to patients who are allergic to peanuts, since the drug is mixed with peanut oil before it is administered. Finally, patients who are allergic to penicillin should not be given d-Penicillamine.

High doses of calcium EDTA can cause kidney damage. However, this can be reversed when the patient stops taking the drug. High doses may also cause **headache**, **fever**, chills, nausea, and vomiting. An irregular heartbeat may also be experienced when this drug is rapidly injected into a vein. Treament with BAL may produce a mild fever, nausea with occasional vomiting, and an increase in liver enzymes. It also may cause allergy-like symptoms, such as a runny nose and watery eyes, which can be alleviated by **antihistamines**. Succimer can produce mild nausea, fever, chills, and a skin rash. D-Penicillamine can cause an allergic reaction, particularly in persons sensitive to penicillin.

Iron supplements should not be taken while BAL is being administered, since the interaction between the two can cause severe vomiting.

CHEMOTHERAPY

Chemotherapy is treatment of a disease or medical condition with chemicals that attack the cause of the medical condition. The term is most commonly used to describe treatment of **cancer** with **anticancer drugs**. Chemotherapy destroys cancer cells in a tumor. It can also kill cancer cells that have broken off from the main tumor and traveled through the blood or lymph systems to spread (metastasize) to other parts of the body.

Scientists have explored the use of chemicals to treat cancer since the mid-nineteenth century. The sex hormones estrogen and androgen were first used to treat breast and prostate cancer in 1945, and a year later, the first chemotherapy drug developed specifically to treat cancer was introduced by American scientist Cornelius Rhoads.

Today, more than 50 chemotherapy drugs are available to treat cancer and many more are under development. Most chemotherapy drugs interfere with the ability of cells to grow or multiply. They are classified based on how they work. The main types of chemotherapy drugs are alkylating drugs, antimetabolites, antitumor antibiotics, plant alkaloids, and steroid hormones.

Many chemotherapy drugs fight cancer by interfering with DNA, the molecule that encodes, or maps, genetic information in the body. Alkylating drugs (such as cyclophosphamide) kill cancer cells by directly attacking DNA. Antimetabolites (such as 5-fluorouracil) interfere with the production of DNA and keep cells from growing and multiplying. Antitumor interfere with production of DNA and cell proteins. They are made from natural substances such as fungi. Doxorubicin and bleomycin belong to this group of chemotherapy drugs.

Plant alkaloids slow cancer growth by preventing cells from dividing. Vinblastine and vincristine are plant alkaloids obtained from the periwinkle plant. Steroid hormones slow the growth of some cancers that depend on hormones. For example, tamoxifen is used to treat **breast cancer**s that depend on the hormone estrogen for growth.

Chemotherapy can cure some types of cancer. In some cases, it is used to slow the growth of cancer cells or to keep the cancer from spreading to other parts of the body. Chemotherapy can also ease the symptoms of cancer, helping some patients to have a better quality of life. Chemotherapy is usually given in addition to other cancer treatments, such as surgery and **radiation therapy**. When given with other treatments, it is called adjuvant chemotherapy.

Oncologists, doctors who specialize in treating cancer, determine which chemotherapy drugs are best suited for each patient. This decision is based on the type of cancer, the patient's age and health, and other drugs the patient is taking. Some patients should not be treated with certain chemotherapy drugs. Age and medical conditions such as heart disease, kidney disease, and diabetes may affect the drugs with which a person may be treated.

How often and how long chemotherapy is given depends on the type of cancer, how patients respond to the drugs, patients' health and ability to tolerate the drugs, and on the types of drugs given. An oncologist decides which chemotherapy drug or combination of drugs will work best for each patient. The use of two or more drugs together often works better than a single drug for treating cancer. This is called combination chemotherapy.

Chemotherapy drugs are administered in different ways, depending on the drugs to be given and the type of cancer. Oral chemotherapy is given by mouth in the form a pill, capsule, or liquid. Topical chemotherapy is given as a cream or ointment applied directly to the cancer, and is common in treatment of certain types of skin cancer. Intravenous (IV) chemotherapy is injected into a vein, and intramuscular (IM) chemotherapy is injected into a muscle. Chemotherapy may also be injected directly into the cancer. This is called intralesional (IL) injection.

Chemotherapy is frequently given through a catheter or port permanently inserted into a central vein or body cavity. A port is a small reservoir or container that is placed in a vein or under the skin in the area where the drug will be given. This eliminates the need for repeated injections and may allow patients to spend less time in the hospital while receiving chemotherapy.

Chemotherapy drugs are toxic to normal cells as well as cancer cells. Many are also designed to attack fast growing cells in the body. Cancer cells grow more quickly than most other body cells. So do cells of the bone marrow (where blood cells are made), cells in the stomach and intestines, and cells of the hair follicles. Therefore, the most common side effects of chemotherapy are linked to their effects on these other fast growing cells. Some of these side effects include: **nausea and vomiting**, loss of appetite, hair loss, anemia and fatigue, infection, easy bleeding or bruising, sores in the mouth and throat, damage to the nervous system, and kidney damage.

CHESELDEN, WILLIAM (1688-1752)

English surgeon

William Cheselden, a quick and precise surgeon who could remove bladder stones in less than one minute, was instrumental in raising surgery to a profession. Cheselden also was a significant educator on the early teachings of anatomy, and served as court physician to Queen Caroline.

Born in 1688 in Somerby, Leicestershire, England, Cheselden's premedical education consisted of classical Greek and Latin literature. At age 15 he was apprenticed to a Leicester surgeon. Moving to London, he studied under the anatomist William Cowper and James Ferne, a surgeon at St. Thomas's Hospital.

After Cheselden was admitted to the Company of **Barber-Surgeons**, he began lecturing on anatomy at St. Thomas's at age 22. Three years after that, he published *Anatomy of the Human Body,* which was written in English instead of the Latin, which was commonly used for such books. Cheselden's *Anatomy* remained in print for almost a century. Venturing beyond mere structural anatomy, it described the role of saliva in digestion. At the time, digestion was generally believed to result from the mechanical actions of the abdominal muscles and diaphragm on the stomach, but Cheselden argued that other parts of the abdomen especially the fetus in a pregnant woman received more muscular force than the stomach, yet were never digested.

His *Anatomy* was not only appreciated for its scientific merit, but for its artistic quality as well. This was also true of a book later written by Cheselden, *Osteographia, or the Anatomy of the Bones,* also published in numerous editions. The initial pages of *Osteographia* contained much admired illustrations of the skeletons of the crocodile, bear, ostrich, and other animals in action, produced with the help of a camera obscura, a predecessor of the photographic camera.

Led by Cheselden, London surgeons left the Company of Barber-Surgeons in 1745 to form their own Company of Surgeons, which would later evolve into the Royal College of Surgeons of England. The uneasy relationship with barbers had existed since 1540, but by the 1700s surgeons were becoming better educated than their hair-clipping colleagues and Cheselden and others pushed for professional recognition.

In 1727, Cheselden introduced to England the lateral lithotomy procedure for swift removal of bladder stones. Prior to that, stones were removed using instruments inserted through the urethra, which was enlarged by surgical incision. Cheselden's quick method, adopted from the French surgeon Jacques de Beaulieu, involved cutting through the perineum (the area between the anus and the urethral opening). Since surgical anesthesia was not developed until the nineteenth century, Cheselden's patients, with little more than rum to ease their pain, appreciated the speed of his procedures. His average time for performing a lateral lithotomy is estimated between 30 and 90 seconds.Cheselden's innovation remained in use for more than 200 years until it was replaced by a procedure that mechanically crushes the stones.

Another major accomplishment was his restoration of sight to a young man who had been blind since birth. Cheselden performed an iridotomy, using a cataract-extraction knife to create an artificial pupil.

Despite his skill, Cheselden, however, experienced considerable anxiety before his operations. He wrote: ''If I have any reputation in this way I have earned it dearly, for no one ever endured more anxiety and sickness before an operation, yet from the time I began to operate all uneasiness ceased and if I have had better success than some others I do not impute it to more knowledge but to the happiness of mind that was never ruffled or disconcerted and a hand that never trembled during any operation.''

Cheselden was appointed physician to the Court of Queen Caroline in 1727, but appears to have somehow fallen from royal favor during the following decade when the Queen died in 1737 of a strangulated umbilical hernia and was not consulted.

Just before his death in 1752, Cheselden provided surgical training to John Hunter, now considered a founder of pathological anatomy.

See also Barber-surgeons

CHEST PHYSICAL THERAPY

Chest physical therapy is the term for a group of treatments designed to promote expansion of the lungs, strengthen respiratory muscles, and eliminate secretions from the respiratory system. The purpose of chest physical therapy, also called chest physiotherapy, is to help patients breathe more freely and to get more oxygen into the body.

A chest physical therapy program includes postural drainage, chest percussion, chest vibration, turning, deep breathing exercises, and coughing. It is usually done in conjunction with other treatments to rid the airways of secretions. These other treatments include suctioning, nebulizer treatments, and the administration of expectorant drugs.

Turning from side to side permits lung expansion. Patients may turn themselves or be turned by a caregiver. The head of the bed is also elevated to promote drainage if the patient can tolerate this position. Critically ill patients and those dependent on mechanical respiration are turned once every one to two hours around the clock.

Coughing helps break up secretions in the lungs so that the mucus can be suctioned or spit out. Patients sit upright and breath in (inhale) deeply through the nose. Then they breath out (exhale) in short puffs or coughs. Coughing is repeated several times a day.

Deep breathing helps expand the lungs by forcing better distribution of the air into all sections of the lung. The patient either sits in a chair or sits upright in bed and inhales while pushing the abdomen out to force maximum amounts of air into the lung. The patient then exhales while contracting, or pulling in, his abdomen. Deep breathing exercises are done several times each day for short periods.

Postural drainage involves draining secretions from the lungs into the airway where they can either be coughed up or suctioned out. The patient is placed in a head or chest down position and is kept in this position for up to 15 minutes. Critical care patients and those depending on mechanical ventilation receive postural drainage therapy four to six times daily. Percussion and vibration may be performed in conjunction with postural drainage.

Percussion is rhythmically striking the chest wall with cupped hands. It is also called cupping, clapping, or tapotement. The purpose of percussion is to break up thick secretions in the lungs so that they can be more easily removed. Percussion is performed on each lung segment for one to two minutes at a time.

As with percussion, the purpose of *vibration* is to help break up lung secretions. Vibration can be either mechanical or manual. A vibrating device (mechanical) or quickly moving hand (manual) is pressed up against the chest while the patient exhales. The procedure is repeated several times each day for about five breaths.

People who have medical conditions that make it difficult to clear secretions from their lungs can often benefit from chest physical therapy, including those with **cystic fibrosis** or neuromuscular diseases like **Guillain-Barré** syndrome, progressive muscle weakness (**myasthenia gravis**), or **tetanus**. People with lung diseases such as **bronchitis**, **pneumonia**, or chronic obstructive pulmonary disease (COPD) may also benefit from chest physical therapy. People who are likely to aspirate their mucous secretions because of diseases such as **cerebral palsy** or **muscular dystrophy** also receive chest physical therapy, as do some people who are bedridden, confined to a wheelchair, or who cannot breath deeply because of postoperative **pain**.

CHEST X RAY

A chest x ray is a procedure used to evaluate organs and structures within the chest for symptoms of disease. Chest x rays include views of the lungs, heart, small portions of the gastrointestinal tract, thyroid gland and the bones of the chest area. X rays are a form of radiation that can penetrate the body and produce an image on an x ray film. Another name for x ray is radiograph.

Chest x-rays, or films, are frequently ordered to diagnose or rule out **pneumonia**. Other lung disorders such as tuberculosis, emphysema, and **pulmonary edema** (fluid in the lungs) may also be detected or evaluated through the use of chest x ray.

When cancer is suspected, a chest x ray may also be ordered by a physician to check for possible tumors of the lungs, thyroid, lymphoid tissue, or bones of the thorax. These may be primary tumors. X rays also check for secondary spread of **cancer** from one organ to another.

While less sensitive than **echocardiography**, chest x ray can be used to check for cardiac disorders that affect the size and shape of the heart, such as congestive **heart failure**.

Chest x rays may also be used to detect **pneumothorax** (presence of air or gas in the chest cavity), and to see foreign bodies that may have been swallowed or inhaled.

The chest x ray can be an important tool for evaluating the effectiveness of treatment for a diagnosed condition. It is often used to verify the correct placement of chest tubes or catheters. In addition, chest x rays taken at regular intervals (serial x rays) are an important tool to measure how a patient is responding to treatment for lung disease and other medical conditions.

The chest x ray may be performed in a physician's office or referred to an outpatient radiology facility or hospital radiology department. In some cases, a portable x ray machine may be used to take chest films at a patient's bedside. There is no advance preparation necessary for chest x rays, however all jewelry and other metal objects must be removed from the neck and torso before the films are taken. Typically, the patient is asked to wear a hospital gown for the procedure.

Routine chest x rays consist of two views. The frontal view (referred to as posterioranterior or PA), and the lateral (side) view. It is preferred that the patient stand for this exam, particularly when studying collection of fluid in the lungs.

During the actual time of exposure, the technologist will ask the patient to hold his or her breath to ensure there is no motion that could detract from the quality and sharpness of the film image. The procedure will only take a few minutes and the time patients must hold their breaths is a matter of a few seconds.

A radiologist, or physician specially trained in the technique and interpretation of x rays, will view the x ray films and issue a written report of the findings. A normal chest x ray will show normal structures for the age and medical history ofthe patient. Abnormal findings on chest x rays are used in conjunction with physical exam findings, patient medical history and other diagnostic tests to reach a final diagnosis.

Pregnant women, particularly those in the first or second trimester, should not have chest x rays unless absolutely necessary. If the exam is ordered, women who are, or could possibly be, pregnant must wear a protective lead apron. Because the procedure involves radiation, care should always be taken to avoid overexposure, particularly for children. However, the amount of radiation from one chest x ray procedure is minimal.

CHICKENPOX

Chickenpox (also called varicella) is a common and extremely infectious childhood disease that can also affect adults. It produces an itchy, blistery rash that typically lasts about a week and is sometimes accompanied by a **fever**.

Chickenpox has been a typical part of growing up for most children in the industrialized world. About four million Americans contract the disease each year. Chickenpox can strike at any age, but by ages 9 or 10 about 80-90% of American children have already been infected. Because almost every case of chickenpox leads to lifelong protection against further attacks, adults account for less than 5% of all cases in the United States. Adults, however, are much more likely than children to suffer dangerous complications. More than half of all chickenpox deaths occur among adults.

Chickenpox is caused by the varicella-zoster virus (a member of the herpes virus family), which is spread through the air or by direct contact with an infected person. Once someone has been infected with the virus, an incubation period of about 10-21 days passes before symptoms begin. A case of chickenpox usually starts without warning or with only a mild fever and a slight feeling of unwellness. Soon small red spots begin to appear on the scalp, neck, or upper half of the trunk, and 12 to 24 hours later, the spots become itchy, fluid-filled bumps called vesicles. These blisters continue to appear in crops for the next 2-5 days. Although some people develop only a few blisters, in most cases the number reaches 250-500. Blisters can develop anywhere on the skin and inside the mouth, nose, ears, vagina, or rectum. Occasionally a minor and temporary darkening of the skin (called **hyperpigmentation**) is noticed around some of the blisters. The blisters soon begin to form scabs and fall off. Scarring usually does not occur unless they have been scratched and become infected. The degree of itchiness can range from barely noticeable to extreme. Some chickenpox sufferers also have **headache**s, abdominal **pain**, or a fever.

Treatment usually takes place in the home and focuses on reducing discomfort and fever. Because chickenpox is a viral disease, **antibiotics** are ineffective against it.

Applying wet compresses or bathing in cool or lukewarm water once a day can help the itch. Adding four to eight ounces of baking soda or one or two cups of oatmeal to the bath is a good idea. Other recommended remedies to relieve **itching** include applying calamine lotion, aloe vera, witch hazel, or an herbal preparations of rosemary (*Rosmarinus officinalis*) and calendula (*Calendual officinalis*) to the blisters. Because scratching can cause blisters to become infected and lead to scarring, children with chicken pox should have their nails cut short. For babies, light mittens or socks on the hands can prevent scratching.

If mouth blisters make eating or drinking an unpleasant experience, cold drinks and soft, bland foods can ease discomfort. Painful genital blisters can be treated with an anesthetic cream recommended by a doctor or pharmacist. Antibiotics are often prescribed if blisters become infected.

Fever and discomfort can be reduced by **acetaminophen** or another medication that does not contain **aspirin**. *Aspirin and any medications that contain aspirin or other salicylates must not be given to children with chickenpox, for they appear to increase the chances of developing Reye's syndrome.* The best idea is to consult a doctor or pharmacist if one is unsure about which medications are safe.

Children with chickenpox should be kept home from school during the infectious period of the disease, which is usually about a week. The disease can be spread from one or two days before the rash breaks out until all the blisters have formed scabs, which usually happens 4-7 days later.

Some people are at greater risk for developing complications from chickenpox, the most common of which are bacterial infections of the blisters, pneumonia, dehydration, encephalitis, and hepatitis. Children born to mothers who contract chickenpox just prior to delivery may face an increased possibility of dangerous consequences, including brain damage and death. If the infection occurs during early **pregnancy**, there is a small (less than 5%) chance of congenital abnormalities. Children less than one year old, and children whose immune systems have been weakened by a genetic disorder, disease, or medical treatment, may also have complications. Medications which reduce the severity of chicken pox symptoms, including varicella-zoster immune globulin (VZIG) and the antiviral drug acyclovir (Zovirax), or often prescribed to treat immunocompromised children and others at high risk of developing complications.

Medical help should always be sought when anyone in these high-risk groups contracts the disease. In addition, a doctor should be called immediately if an individual with chicken pox experiences a fever which exceeds102°F (38.9°C) or takes more than four days to disappear. Chicken pox blisters that are leaking pus or are excessively red, warm, tender, or swollen may be infected and should be examined by a doctor.

If a child with chicken pox seems nervous, confused, or unusually sleepy; complains of a stiff neck or severe headache; shows signs of poor balance or has trouble walking; finds bright lights hard to look at; is having breathing problems or is coughing a lot; is complaining of chest pain; is vomiting repeatedly; or is having convulsions, get that child to a hospital or medical facility immediately. These may be signs of **Reye's syndrome** or **encephalitis**, two rare but potentially very dangerous conditions.

There is one long-term consequence of chickenpox that strikes about 20% of the population, particularly people 50 and older. Like all herpes viruses, the varicella-zoster virus never leaves the body after an episode of chickenpox, but lies dormant in the nerve cells, where it may be reactivated years later by disease or age-related weakening of the immune system. The result is **shingles** (also called herpes zoster), a very painful nerve inflammation, accompanied by a rash, that usually affects the trunk or the face.

A vaccine for chickenpox became available in the United States in 1995 under the name Varivax. Varivax is a live, attenuated (weakened) virus vaccine. It has been found to prevent the disease in 70-90% of the vaccinated population, and in the remaining cases to reduce the severity of an attack. The U.S. Center for Disease Control (CDC) recommends that the vaccine should be given to all children (with the exception of certain high-risk groups) at 12-18 months of age, preferably when they receive their **measles-mumps-rubella** vaccine. **Vaccination** is also recommended for children over 12 who have not had chickenpox.

Child abuse

Child abuse is the blanket term for four types of child mistreatment: physical abuse, sexual abuse, emotional abuse, and neglect. In many cases children are the victims of more than one type of abuse. The abusers can be parents or other family members, caretakers such as teachers and babysitters, acquaintances (including other children), and (in rare instances) strangers.

Child abuse was once viewed as a minor social problem affecting only a handful of U.S. children. However, in recent years it has received close attention from the media, law enforcement, and the helping professions, and with increased public and professional awareness has come a sharp rise in the number of reported cases. But because abuse is often hidden from view and its victims too young or fearful to speak out, experts suggest that its true prevalence is possibly much greater than the official data indicate. In 1996, more than three million victims of alleged abuse were reported to child protective services (CPS) agencies in the United States, and the reports were substantiated in more than one million cases. Put another way, 1.5% of the country's children were confirmed victims of abuse in 1996. Parents were the abusers in 77% of the confirmed cases, other relatives in 11%. Sexual abuse was more likely to be committed by males, whereas females were responsible for the majority of neglect cases. More than 1,000 U.S. children died from abuse in 1996.

Although experts are quick to point out that abuse occurs among all social, ethnic, and income groups, reported cases usually involve poor families with little education. Young mothers, single-parent families, and parental alcohol or drug abuse are also common in reported cases. Charles F. Johnson remarks that ''More than 90% of abusing parents have neither psychotic nor criminal personalities. Rather they tend to be lonely, unhappy, angry, young, and single parents who do not plan their pregnancies, have little or no knowledge of child development, and have unrealistic expectations for child behavior.'' About 10%, or perhaps as many as 40%, of abusive parents were themselves physically abused as children, but most abused children do not grow up to be abusive parents.

Physical abuse is the nonaccidental infliction of physical injury to a child. The abuser is usually a family member or other caretaker, and is more likely to be male. In 1996, 24% of the confirmed cases of U.S. child abuse involved physical abuse.

A rare form of physical abuse is Munchausen syndrome by proxy, in which a caretaker (most often the mother) seeks attention by making the child sick or appear to be sick.

Charles F. Johnson defines child sexual abuse as ''any activity with a child, before the age of legal consent, that is for the sexual gratification of an adult or a significantly older child.'' It includes, among other things, sexual touching and penetration, persuading a child to expose his or her sexual organs, and allowing a child to view pornography. In most cases the child is related to or knows the abuser, and about one in five abusers are themselves underage. Sexual abuse was present in 12% of the confirmed 1996 abuse cases. An estimated 20-25% of females and 10-15% of males report that they were sexually abused by age 18.

Emotional abuse, according to Richard D. Krugman, ''has been defined as the rejection, ignoring, criticizing, isolation, or terrorizing of children, all of which have the effect of eroding their self-esteem.'' Emotional abuse usually expresses itself in verbal attacks involving rejection, scapegoating, belittlement, and so forth. Because it often accompanies other types of abuse and is difficult to prove, it is rarely reported, and accounted for only 6% of the confirmed 1996 cases.

Neglect—failure to satisfy a child's basic needs—can assume many forms. Physical neglect is the failure (beyond the constraints imposed by poverty) to provide adequate food, clothing, shelter, or supervision. Emotional neglect is the failure to satisfy a child's normal emotional needs, or behavior that damages a child's normal emotional and psychological development (such as permitting drug abuse in the home). Failing to see that a child receives proper schooling or medical care is also considered neglect. In 1996 neglect was the finding in 52% of the confirmed abuse cases.

The usual physical abuse scenario involves a parent who loses control and lashes out at a child. The trigger may be normal child behavior such as crying or dirtying a diaper. Unlike nonabusive parents, who may become angry at or upset with their children from time to time but are genuinely loving, abusive parents tend to harbor deep-rooted negative feelings toward their children.

Unexplained or suspicious **bruises** or other marks on the skin are typical signs of physical abuse, as are **burns**. Skull and other bone **fractures** are often seen in young abused children, and in fact, head injuries are the leading cause of **death** from abuse. Children less than one year old are particularly vulnerable to injury from shaking. This is called **shaken baby syndrome** or shaken impact syndrome. Not surprisingly, physical abuse also causes a wide variety of behavioral changes in children.

John M. Leventhal observes that ''The two prerequisites for this form of maltreatment include sexual arousal to children and the willingness to act on this arousal. Factors that may contribute to this willingness include alcohol or drug abuse, poor impulse control, and a belief that the sexual behaviors are acceptable and not harmful to the child.'' The chances of abuse are higher if the child is developmentally handicapped or vulnerable in some other way.

Genital or anal injuries or abnormalities (including the presence of **sexually transmitted diseases**) can be signs of sexual abuse, but often there is no physical evidence for a doctor to find. In fact, **physical examination**s of children in cases of suspected sexual abuse supply grounds for further suspicion only 15-20% of the time. **Anxiety**, poor academic performance, and suicidal conduct are some of the behavioral signs of sexual abuse, but are also found in children suffering other kinds of **stress**. Excessive masturbation and other unusually sexualized kinds of behavior are more closely associated with sexual abuse itself.

Emotional abuse can happen in many settings: at home, at school, on sports teams, and so on. Some of the possible symptoms include loss of self-esteem, sleep disturbances, **headache**s or stomach aches, school avoidance, and running away from home.

Many cases of neglect occur because the parent experiences strong negative feelings toward the child. At other times, the parent may truly care about the child, but lack the ability or strength to adequately provide for the child's needs because handicapped by depression, drug abuse, **mental retardation**, or some other problem.

Neglected children often do not receive adequate nourishment or emotional and mental stimulation. As a result, their physical, social, emotional, and mental development is hindered. They may, for instance, be underweight, develop language skills less quickly than other children, and seem emotionally needy.

Doctors and many other professionals who work with children are required by law to report suspected abuse to their state's Child Protective Services (CPS) agency. Abuse investigations are often a group effort involving medical personnel, social workers, police officers, and others. Some hospitals and communities maintain child protection teams that respond to cases of possible abuse. Careful questioning of the parents is crucial, as is interviewing the child (if he or she is capable of being interviewed). The investigators must ensure, however, that their questioning does not further traumatize the child. A physical examination for signs of abuse or neglect is, of course, always necessary, and may include x rays, blood tests, and other procedures.

Notification of the appropriate authorities, treatment of the child's injuries, and protecting the child from further harm are the immediate priorities in abuse cases. If the child does not require hospital treatment, protection often involves placing him or her with relatives or in foster care. Once the immediate concerns are dealt with, it becomes essential to determine how the child's long-term medical, psychological, educational, and other needs can best be met, a process that involves evaluating not only the child's needs but also the family's (such as for drug abuse counseling or parental skills training). If the child has brothers or sisters, the authorities must determine whether they have been abused as well. On investigation, signs of physical abuse are discovered in about 20% of the brothers and sisters of abused children.

Child abuse can have lifelong consequences. Research shows that abused children and adolescents are more likely, for instance, to do poorly in school, suffer emotional problems, develop an antisocial personality, become promiscuous, abuse drugs and alcohol, and attempt suicide. As adults they often have trouble establishing intimate relationships. Whether professional treatment is able to moderate the long-term psychological effects of abuse is a question that remains unanswered.

Government efforts to prevent abuse include home-visitor programs aimed at high-risk families and school-based efforts to teach children how to respond to attempted sexual abuse. Emotional abuse prevention has been promoted through the media.

When children reach age three, parents should begin teaching them about ''bad touches'' and about confiding in a suitable adult if they are touched or treated in a way that makes them uneasy. Parents also need to exercise caution in hiring babysitters and other caretakers. Anyone who suspects abuse should immediately report those suspicions to the police or his or her local CPS agency, which will usually be listed in the blue pages of the telephone book under Rehabilitative Services or Child and Family Services, or in the yellow pages. Round-the-clock crisis counseling for children and adults is offered by the Childhelp USA/IOF Foresters National Child Abuse Hotline. The National Committee to Prevent Child Abuse is an excellent source of information on the many support groups and other organizations that help abused and at-risk children and their families. One of these organizations, National Parents Anonymous, sponsors 2,100 local self-help groups throughout the United States, Canada, and Europe. Telephone numbers for its local groups are listed in the white pages of the telephone book under Parents Anonymous or can be obtained by calling the national headquarters.

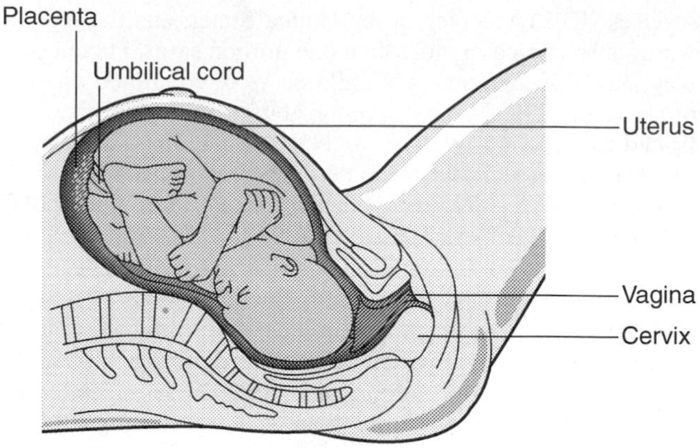

(Illustration by Hans & Cassady, Inc.)

CHILDBIRTH

Childbirth includes both labor (the process of birth) and delivery (the birth itself); it refers to the entire process as an infant makes its way from the womb down the birth canal to the outside world. The average length of labor is about 14 hours for a first pregnancy and about eight hours in subsequent pregnancies. However, many women experience a much longer or shorter labor.

Childbirth usually begins spontaneously, following about 280 days after conception, but it may be started by artificial means if the **pregnancy** continues past 42 weeks gestation. One of the first signs of approaching childbirth may be a ''bloody show,'' the appearance of a small amount of blood-tinged mucus released from the cervix (the opening of the uterus) as it begins to dilate. This is called the ''mucus plug.'' In about 10% of women, labor is signaled by the rupture of the amniotic sac. When a woman's ''water breaks,'' the amniotic fluid is released in a trickle or gush.

The most common sign of the onset of labor is contractions, or labor pains. Sometimes women have trouble telling the difference between ''true'' and ''false'' labor pains. True labor pains are felt high up on the abdomen, radiating to the lower back, and get progressively stronger, longer, and closer together.

Labor can be described in terms of a series of stages. During the first stage of labor, the cervix dilates (opens) from 0-10 cm. This stage has an early, or latent, phase and an active phase. As labor begins, the muscular wall of the uterus begins to contract as the cervix relaxes and expands. During a contraction, the infant experiences intense pressure that pushes it against the cervix, eventually forcing the cervix to stretch open. At the same time, the contractions cause the cervix to thin. Most women are relatively comfortable during the initial latent phase and walking around is encouraged, since it naturally stimulates the labor process.

The active phase of labor is faster and more efficient than the latent phase. Contractions are longer and more regular, usually occurring about every two minutes. They are also

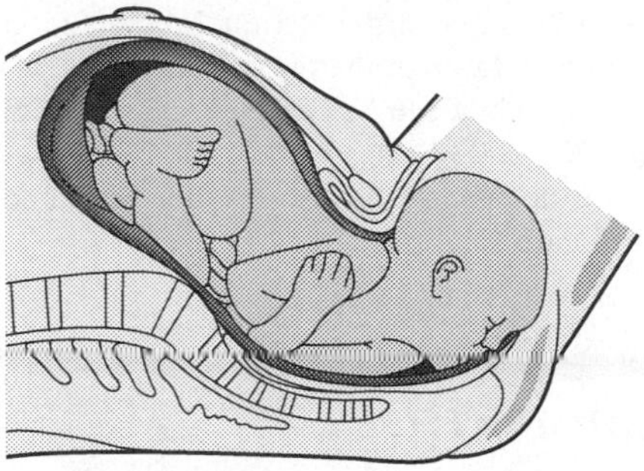

Stage 2: Expulsion of the fetus

(Illustration by Hans & Cassady, Inc.)

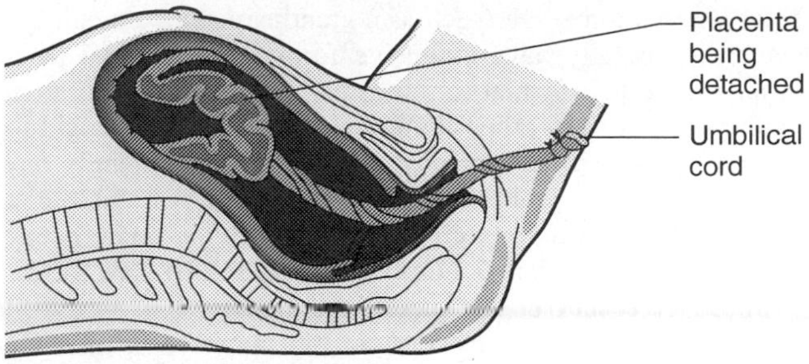

Stage 3: Expulsion of the placenta

(Illustration by Hans & Cassady, Inc.)

more painful. Women may use the breathing exercises learned in childbirth classes to cope with the pain experienced during this phase. Many women also receive pain medication at this point — either a short-term medication, such as Nubain or Numorphan, or an epidural anesthesia that numbs the lower part of the body.

As the cervix dilates to 8-9 cm, the transition phase begins. This is the transition between the first stage (during which the cervix dilates from 0-10 cm) and the second stage (during which the baby is pushed out through the birth canal) of labor. The baby's head begins to descend, and the mother begins to feel the urge to ''push'' or bear down. Active pushing by the mother should not begin until the second phase, since pushing too early can cause the cervix to swell or to tear and bleed.

As the mother enters the second stage of labor, her baby's head appears at the top of the cervix. The infant passes down the vagina, helped along by strong contractions and the mother's pushing. Active pushing by the mother is very important during this phase of labor.

In some cases, when labor does not progress as it should or the baby appears to be in distress, a doctor may use forceps or a vacuum extractor to help the baby out of the birth canal. A forceps is a spoon-shaped device that resembles a set of salad tongs. It is placed around the baby's head so the doctor can pull the baby gently out of the vagina. In vacuum assisted birth, a large rubber or plastic cup is placed against the baby's head, while a pump creates suction that pulls on the cup to ease the baby down the birth canal.

When the top of the baby's head appears at the opening of the vagina, the birth is nearing completion. This position is called *crowning*, since only the crown of the head is visible. As the baby crowns, the perineum (the tissues between the vagina and the rectum) may stretch so tight that the baby's progress is slowed. If there is risk of tearing the perineum, the doctor may choose to make a small incision to enlarge the vaginal opening. This is called an episiotomy.

Once the baby's entire head is out, the shoulders follow. The attending practitioner suctions the baby's mouth and nose to ease the baby's first breath. The rest of the baby usually slips out easily, and the umbilical cord is cut

In the third and last stage of labor, contractions continue to push the placenta out of the vagina by the continuing uterine contractions. The placenta, which has provided nourishment to the fetus throughout the pregnancy, is pancake shaped and about 10 inches in diameter. It is important that all of the placenta be removed from the uterus to prevent excessive bleeding after childbirth.

Approximately 4% of babies are in what is called the *breech position* when labor begins. In breech presentation, the baby's bottom or legs are positioned to enter the birth canal instead of the head. Depending on the type of breech presentation, the mother and attending practitioner will need to weigh the risks and make a decision on whether to attempt a vaginal birth or deliver the baby with a **cesarean section**.

A cesarean section, also called a c-section, is a surgical procedure in which incisions are made through a woman's abdomen and uterus to deliver her baby. Cesarean sections are performed whenever abnormal conditions complicate labor and vaginal delivery, threatening the life or health of the mother or the baby.

There are several popular methods taught to prepare women and their partners for childbirth. Lamaze (or Lamaze-Pavlov), introduced in the 1960s, is the most common in the United States today. It promotes breathing exercises and concentration techniques to allow mothers to control pain while maintaining consciousness. Other instructional techniques include the Read method, the LeBoyer method, and the Bradley method.

CHILD CARE

Each day in the United States, millions of children, ranging from infants to preteens, are in the care of someone who isn't their parent. Child care is no longer a luxury; it is a necessity when two incomes are needed for families to make ends meet. Parents have a variety of options to choose from for child care. Their decision is influenced by cost, convenience, and what they and the child feel comfortable with. They can select from child care in a home setting or out-of-home day care.

Home-setting day care can take place at either the child's home or the caregiver's. In the former case, the in-home caregiver either comes to the child's home to stay with the child all day, or may actually be a live-in employee. Such caregivers are called babysitters, nannies, or au pairs. A babysitter is often a relative (such as a grandparent) or a neighbor. Nannies generally have extensive formal training. Au pairs usually have less formal training than nannies, and are often young women from other countries. If the child is brought to another person's home for day care, this is called family day care. The caregiver takes care of a small group of children at his or her home. Group family day care is similar to family day care, except that a larger number of children to care for requires the presence of additional caregivers.

Many families choose out-of-home day care. In this type of care, children attend child care centers for all or part of each day. These centers may be operated independently, or may be part of a chain of day care centers, or run by a school, community center, or religious group. These centers may also offer part time or occasional care, such as play groups.

Whatever the child care setting, most caregivers (except for babysitting family members) are usually required to be licensed by the state. Cities and towns may have additional certification requirements.

When considering a child care situation, certain standards should be looked for and met. Among them:

Staff members should have training in early childhood education as well as training in first aid and CPR.

Both center staff members and children who are cared for at the center should have proof of up-to-date immunizations.

Snacks and meals, if provided, should be nutritious.

Steps must be taken to minimize the spread of infectious diseases (for example, toys and tables should be disinfected with bleach solutions, rubber gloves are worn when changing diapers, and children who become ill are isolated, cared for, and/or sent home as soon as possible.).

Children must never be left unattended or allowed to leave the facility with someone other than a parent without the parent's written permission.

A variety of age-appropriate toys, games, activities and books should be available for children.

Electrical outlets must be covered.

Smoking is not allowed in the facility.

Caregivers interact with the children.

Children look happy and active, and the setting has a warm, comfortable atmosphere for both children and adults.

Parents are welcome to drop in without prior notice.

The cost of child care varies, depending on the location and type of program and the age of the child. In general, infant care is more expensive than care for an older child (up to $100 a day is not unheard of), because infants are more labor intensive and the teacher-child ratio is lower (three infants per teacher is ideal for an infant up to one year of age, as opposed to four children per teacher at age two). Some facilities will not accept children under the age of two years nine months, or children who have not yet been toilet trained.

It is important to choose a child care giver with whom both the parent and the child feel comfortable and secure. For some families, that caregiver is a family member; for others, it is a teacher at a for-profit center. Choosing a child care option takes time, and sometimes the least expensive option isn't always the best.

For more information, contact the National Association for the Education of Young Children, the organization that accredits child care facilities. They can be reached at 1509 16th St. NW, Washington, DC, 20036 (800-424-2460). The state department of child-care licensing can also provide valuable information about child care facilities.

CHILD DEVELOPMENT

Child development is a general term that takes into account all areas of a child's growth, including physical, intellectual, emotional, moral, social, psychological, and sensory and motor development.

All children develop at different rates in different areas, and the growth of a child is a complex process of becoming older, bigger, and more accomplished. A child may lag behind his peers in physical development, for instance, but function at above average in intellectual or emotional growth. How quickly a child develops physically, mentally and emotionally depends on many things, including economic, social, genetic, and environmental factors.

Physical growth is a continuous process, and occurs at varying rates within discrete stages: infancy (from birth to 3 years), followed by the preschool period (from 3 to 6); early childhood from age 6 to 9, and later childhood from 9 to 12. These periods are followed by early and late adolescence.

Psychologically, an infant grows from total emotional dependence on mother (or a primary caregiver) to an awareness of the self as a separate individual. From this point, the child develops an increasingly more complex range of emotions and a mastery of basic intellectual concepts.

While children develop at various rates, there are some guidelines established as the study of child development progressed during the late 1800s and early 1900s, based on observations of children under controlled conditions.

Medical and child development experts have established some basic milestones of normal development, beginning with infancy when a baby normally will smile at 6 weeks, roll over onto his back at 9 or 10 weeks, raise his head and shoulders from a face-down position at 4 to 6 months, and sit unsupported at 6 months. At 8 months, a normal baby will say simple, two-syllable words such as ''Dada,'' and try to feed himself with a spoon. He'll rise to a sitting position at 9 months, and, at 12 months he'll understand simple commands and be able to stand unsupported for a few seconds. A normal baby will walk unaided and make a three-brick-high tower at 18 months, achieve bowel control at 20 months, and stay dry during the day by 2 years. He'll talk in simple sentences at 3 years, stay dry during the night at 3 and a half, and be able to dress and undress himself at 4 years. At 5 years, he'll be able to hop, skip, and draw a stick figure.

In this way, a child's psychological development is linked to his physical growth and his ability to interact with others in his environment. Guidelines are only suggestions, not hard-and-fast rules; there is no cause for concern if a child's development does not strictly conform to established guide-

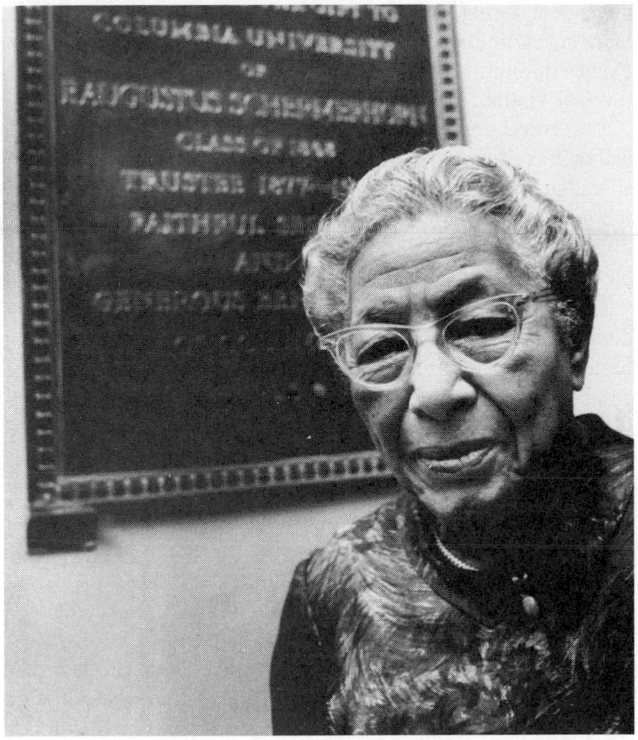

May Edward Chinn

lines. However, a professional probably should be consulted if a child appears to fall short in all areas, or if development in one or more areas is far behind what is considered normal.

CHINN, MAY EDWARD (1896-1980)

African American Native American physician

May Edward Chinn is best remembered for the racial barriers she confronted as one of the first black women physicians in New York City. Denied hospital privileges and research opportunities at New York City hospitals early in her career, she became a family doctor in Harlem, where she was the only practicing black woman physician for several years. For her determination to provide medical care to the disadvantaged and for her work in cancer detection, she received honorary doctor of science degrees from New York University and Columbia University, and a distinguished alumnus award from Columbia Teachers College.

May Edward Chinn was born on April 15, 1896, in Great Barrington, Massachusetts. Her mother, Lulu Ann, was the daughter of a Chickahominy Native American and a slave. Her father, William Lafayette, was the son of a slave and a plantation owner. Chinn went to the Bordentown Manual and Training Industrial School, a boarding school in New Jersey, and spent one year of her childhood on the estate of Charles Tiffany, the jewelry magnate, where her mother was a live-in cook. The Tiffanys treated Chinn like family and took her to classical music concerts in New York City. She later learned to play the piano and became an accompanist to popular singer Paul Robeson in the early 1920s. Chinn played classical music and church music throughout her life and performed for black soldiers during World War I. Although she never completed high school, she was admitted to Columbia Teachers College on the basis of her entrance examination. Originally intending to pursue a degree in music, Chinn quickly abandoned music for science because a music professor who believed that blacks were unsuited for classical music ridiculed her, but another professor praised her for a paper she had written on sewage disposal. In 1921 she received a bachelor's degree in science from Columbia Teachers College, and in 1926 she became the first black woman to graduate from Bellevue Hospital Medical College.

Upon graduation Chinn found that no hospital would allow her practicing privileges. The Rockefeller Institute had seriously considered her for a research fellowship until they discovered that she was black. With her fair skin and last name, many assumed that she was white or Chinese. She later told Muriel Petioni, former president of the Society of Black Women Physicians, that black workers often snubbed her because they assumed she was passing as white, and they did not want to jeopardize her position.

Though she was the first African American woman intern at Harlem Hospital, racial and gender discrimination kept her from obtaining hospital privileges there. Chinn described her early practice in Harlem as akin to an old-fashioned family practice in the rural South a century earlier. She performed major medical procedures in patient's homes, while minor procedures were done in her office. She told George Davis of the *New York Times Magazine* ''that conditions were so bad that it seemed that you were not making any headway.'' To get at the roots of poverty, she earned a master's degree in public health from Columbia University in 1933.

In the 1940s Chinn became very interested in cancer but was still prohibited from establishing formal affiliations with New York hospitals. Instead, she had her patients' biopsies read secretly for her at Memorial Hospital. In 1944 she was invited to join the staff of the Strang Clinic, a premier cancer detection facility affiliated with Memorial and New York Infirmary hospitals. She worked there for twenty-nine years and became a member of the Society of Surgical Oncology.

In her autobiographical paper written in 1977, Chinn noted that the committees established by Mayor LaGuardia after the Harlem riots of 1935 were pivotal in integrating blacks into medicine in New York City. As committee findings were reported in the newspapers, conditions began to change. Chinn saw this firsthand when she became the first black woman granted admitting privileges at Harlem Hospital in 1940.

African American male doctors were another source of discrimination. In a *New York Times* interview with Charlayne Hunter-Gault in 1977, she described three types: ''those who acted as if I wasn't there; another who took the attitude 'what does she think that she can do that I can't do?' and the group that called themselves support[ive] by sending me their night calls after midnight.'' Like other black women physicians of her era, Chinn worked long hours but never got rich from her practice. By 1978 Chinn had given up her practice and begun examining African American students as a consultant to the Phelps-Stokes Fund. In late 1980 she collapsed and died at age eighty-four at a Columbia University reception honoring a friend.

CHINESE TRADITIONAL HERBAL MEDICINE

Chinese traditional herbal medicine is an alternative system of treatment arising from a holistic philosophy of life. It emphasizes the interconnection of the mental, emotional, and physical components within each person, and the importance of harmony between individuals and their social groups, as well as between humanity as a whole and nature. Although Chinese medicine is neither the oldest system recorded by historians nor the only form of herbal therapy practiced today, it is the oldest continuous surviving tradition of herbal medicine. The only other alternative system of treatment that can be traced as far back as Chinese medicine is the Ayurvedic system of India. It should be noted that traditional Chinese herbal medicine did not develop in complete isolation. As early as the second century B.C., Chinese merchants in India came into contact with **Ayurvedic medicine**. In the sixteenth and seventeenth centuries A.D., Chinese trade with the West—especially with the Dutch—led to exchanges of information and observations about the use of herbs in medical treatment.

In 1970 the Chinese Academy of Medical Science published a collection of traditional herbal remedies in common use. It lists 796 prescriptions made from combinations of 248 plant or animal ingredients. A group of American pharmacologists evaluated these prescriptions in 1974 and estimated that 44.7% are useful, measured by present western methods of chemical analysis.

The purpose of Chinese traditional herbal medicine is to restore health through correction of imbalances within the patient's body or between the patient and the larger social and natural order. Chinese medicine regards the human body as a small-scale reflection of the cosmos. The principles of treatment are derived from Taoism, a philosophy or religion that emphasizes following the right path, or Tao, in order to find one's place within the larger universe of being. Taoism's holistic emphasis was reflected in the close correlation between Chinese herbal medicine and daily dietary habits. Foods were eaten with regard to their therapeutic qualities and adjusted to changes in the body. Traditional herbal medicine in China included preventive treatment. It was a customary part of people's lives, not necessarily reserved for acute illness or emergencies.

The specific teachings of Taoism that have had the most profound effect on Chinese medicine are the concept of duality, and the belief in a primordial form of universal energy called *qi*. The terms yin and yang are applied to the two primal opposites that continually interact and produce constant change in the universe. These opposites are regarded as interdependent rather than mutually destructive or antagonistic. Humans participate in *qi*, or the universal life force, which circulates throughout the body and determines the person's basic level of vitality.

Over a period of centuries, Chinese doctors worked out elaborate systems of correlation between yin and yang and the so-called five elements (wood, fire, earth, metal, and water); the ten major internal organs of the body; and meridians, or invisible three-dimensional pathways that circulate *qi* and blood throughout the body. The meridians regulate the yin/yang balance in the body, provide connections between the individual human being and cosmic forces or influences, and protect the body against external sources of disease. There are certain points along the meridians where *qi* is thought to collect or concentrate. These points are used in Chinese medicine for acupuncture treatment as well as diagnosis. Prescriptions for herbal medicines are formulated to correct excesses of yin or yang, blockages or incorrect direction in the flow of *qi*, disorders located in a specific organ, and the emotional problems that accompany physical illness. Chinese herbal medicine does not distinguish between psychiatric and general medical conditions in the manner of western medicine.

Diagnosis in Chinese medicine has four phases. The doctor first makes a visual examination, noting the patient's expression, complexion, and general physique. The distinctive feature of Chinese medicine is the detailed examination of the tongue for color, shape, and coating (if any). Next, the doctor listens to the patient's breathing and looks for any unusual body sounds or odors. A verbal questioning phase follows that is similar to history taking in a western medical examination. And finally, the doctor feels the patient's ten organs through the abdomen, the *qi* points along the meridians, and the pulse. Chinese medicine distinguishes three different pulse points on each wrist and as many as 30 different pulse qualities at each point. Pulse diagnosis takes years to master in the Chinese system and is regarded by patients as an important measure of a doctor's skill.

Traditional Chinese herbal medicine applies herbs to the body externally as well as internally. Dried herbs may be mixed with water and used as poultices to treat arthritis, rheumatism, sprains, **bruises**, **abscess**es, and strained backs. A distinctive technique is the use of moxibustion, which is the application of heat to an area of skin directly over a meridian by burning a wick made of herbs (usually mugwort) a slight distance above the skin. Moxibustion is used to treat many conditions, including **mumps**, vaginal bleeding, pulled nerves, arthritis, and chronic **nosebleed**s.

Acupuncture, **massage**, and the use of suction cups, called cupping, are external treatments that are often used in Chinese medicine in conjunction with internal herbal therapy.

Traditional Chinese medicine uses herbs for preventive treatment as well as for curing illness. Prescriptions are fine-tuned by the herbalist, as well as by the doctor, and formulated according to the individual patient's constitution, as well as the nature of the herbs. When the patient takes the doctor's prescription to the herbalist, it will be made up in one of several traditional forms: broth, pills, wine with herbs steeped in it, gum, fermented dough, or paste. Pills may be made with wax, honey, or flour paste. Pastes can often be used externally as well as internally.

Normal results are recovery from the illness or internal imbalance for which the patient was treated.

CHINESE TRADITIONAL MEDICINE

Traditional Chinese medicine (TCM) is an ancient and still very vital holistic system of health and healing, based on the notion of harmony and balance, and employing the ideas of moderation and prevention.

TCM is a complete system of health care with its own unique theories of anatomy, health, and treatment. It emphasizes diet and prevention and using acupuncture, herbal medicine, **massage**, and **exercise**, and focuses on stimulating the body's natural curative powers.

TCM should not be substituted for contemporary modern trauma practice; it is most useful as an adjunct to the healing regimen. Nor is TCM the first line of treatment for bacterial infection or **cancer**, but may usefully complement contemporary medical treatment for those conditions.

In theory and practice, TCM is completely different from western medicine both in terms of considering how the human body works and how illness occurs and should be treated. As a part of a continuing system that has been in use for thousands of years, it is still employed to treat over one quarter of the world's population. Since the earliest Chinese physicians were also philosophers, their ways of viewing the world and man's role in it affected their medicine. In TCM, both philosophically and medically, moderation in all things is advocated, as is living in harmony with nature and striving for balance in all things. Prevention is also a key goal of Chinese medicine, and much emphasis is placed on educating the patient to live responsibly. The Chinese physician also is more of an advisor than an authority; he or she believes in treating every patient differently based on the notion that one does not treat the disease or condition but rather the individual patient. Thus two people with the same complaint may be treated entirely differently, if their constitutions and life situations are dissimilar. Disease is considered to be evidence of the failure of preventive health care and a falling out of balance or harmony.

There is some confusion in the West about the fundamental philosophical principles upon which traditional Chinese medicine is based—such as the concept of yin and yang, the notion of five elements (wood, fire, earth, metal, and water), and the concept of *chi*—yet each can be explained in a way that is understandable to Westerners.

Yin and yang describe the interdependent relationship of opposing but complementary forces believed to be necessary for a healthy life. Basically, the goal is to maintain a balance of yin and yang in all things.

The five elements, or five-phase theory, is also grounded in the notion of harmony and balance. The concept of *chi* which means something like "life force" or "energy," is perhaps most different from western ideas, and asserts that *chi* is an invisible energy force that flows freely in a healthy person, but is weakened or blocked when a person is ill. Specifically, the illness is a result of the blockage, rather than the blockage being the result of the illness.

Besides these philosophical concepts that differ considerably from infection-based principles of medicine and health, the methods employed by traditional Chinese medicine are also quite different. If mainstream western practitioners could be described as interventionist (doing something to actively treat a disease) and dependent on synthetic pharmaceuticals, TCM methods are mostly natural and noninvasive. For example, where western physicians might employ surgery and **chemotherapy** or radiation for a cancer patient, a TCM physician might use acupuncture and dietary changes. TCM believes in "curing the root" of a disease and not merely in treating its symptoms.

Another major difference is how the patient is regarded. In western medicine, patients with similar complaints or diseases usually will receive virtually the same treatment. In TCM, however, the physician treats the patient and not the condition, believing that identical diseases can have entirely different causes.

During a consultation with a TCM practitioner, the patient will receive a considerable amount of time and attention. During the important first visit, the practitioner will conduct four types of examinations, all extremely observational and all quite different from what patients usually experience.

First the practitioner will ask many questions, going beyond the typical patient history to inquire about such particulars as eating and bowel habits or sleep patterns. Next, the physician looks at the patient, observing his or her complexion and eyes, while also closely examining the tongue. (The tongue is believed to be a barometer of the body's health, and different areas of the tongue can reflect the functioning of different body organs.) After observing, the physician listens to the patient's voice or **cough** and then smells his or her breath, body odor, urine, and even bowel movements. Finally, the practitioner touches the patient, palpating his or her abdomen and feeling the wrist to take up to six different pulses. It is through these different pulses that the well-trained practitioner can diagnose any problem with the flow of the all-important *chi*. Altogether, this essentially observational examination will lead the physician to diagnose or decide the patient's problem. This diagnosis is very different from one in contemporary western medicine. No blood or urine samples are tested in a laboratory. The key to this technique lies in the experience and skill of the practitioner.

After making a diagnosis, the physician will suggest a course of treatment from one or all of the available TCM methods. These fall into four main categories: herbal medicine, acupuncture, dietary therapy, and massage and exercise. A typical TCM prescription consists of a complex variety of many different herbal and mineral ingredients. Chinese herbal remedies are intended to assist the body's own systems so that eventually the patient can stop taking them and never becomes dependent on them. Herbal formulas are usually given as teas, which differ according to the patient.

Traditional Chinese medicine seeks to harmonize and rebalance the entire human system rather than to treat just symptoms. Since proper internal balance is considered to be the key to human health, TCM strives to cure disease by restoring that balance and therefore allowing the body to repair itself. Its continuing medical goal is to detect and correct abnormalities before they cause permanent physical damage.

CHIROPRACTIC

Chiropractic is a therapy that focuses on the relationship of the spinal column to the nervous system and on its effects in maintaining good health. Chiropractic seeks to properly align the vertebrae of the spine in order to restore the normal functioning of the nervous system and thus allow the body to heal itself.

In little more than a century, chiropractic has gone from a curious cult-medicine status to an internationally recognized alternative treatment. Founded in 1895 by a Canadian-American, Donald David Palmer (1845-1913), chiropractic had its origins in Palmer's cure of a deaf janitor by putting one of his vertebrae back into its normal position. Palmer continued to refine his work and eventually based an entire medical philosophy on the notion that the vertebrae of the spine must be properly aligned in order for people to achieve and maintain health.

Misalignments, or what he called ''subluxations,'' interfere with the normal transmission of nerve impulses from the brain to the body's organs and tissues and can affect health. Chiropractic techniques offered many what they considered a safe and economical alternative to conventional medicine. Since Palmer's days, chiropractors have grown into the third largest health-care profession, after physicians and dentists. By the mid-1990s, they were licensed to practice without supervision or referral from medical doctors in every state, and Americans spent nearly $2.5 billion annually on chiropractic care. Also, 1 in 20 Americans visit a chiropractor each year, and some 30 U.S. hospitals have chiropractors on their staff.

The word chiropractic is derived from the Greek word *cheir* meaning hand, and *prakticos* meaning done by or skillful use of. Chiropractic focuses virtually all its efforts on the physical manipulation of spine and joints. It does not use drugs or surgery, and it does not diagnose diseases or ailments or even claim to treat them specifically. Rather, it believes that the body possesses its own innate healing capability and that healing occurs from the inside out. Further, when the body is in balance — and specifically when the vertebrae of the spine are kept in proper alignment — good health ensues because the body's immune system is working properly. Chiropractic attributes a damaged or inefficient immune system to the impairment of normal nerve transmission caused by spinal misalignment.

Within the framework of chiropractic there are several schools or philosophies that differ according to their methods and goals. Two contrasting schools — the ''mixers'' and the ''straights'' — differ in the actual methods employed. As the simpler, more traditional school, straight chiropractic relies exclusively on spinal adjustments to correct vertebral misalignments and therefore restore nerve function. Straights account for only about 15% of all chiropractors. The other chiropractic philosophy, whose proponents are called ''mixers,'' believes in blending or mixing other available therapeutic methods with traditional chiropractic. Thus, these individuals also use other adjunctive therapies such as **massage**, applied **kinesiology**, **acupressure**, nutritional counseling, and ultrasound among many others, seeking to employ whatever works best. A third branch of chiropractic follows the teaching of John McTimoney (1914-1980). This philosophy says that the entire musculoskeletal system of the body is as important as the spine, and it therefore treats the joints of the entire body. A McTimoney chiropractor will examine, and work on if necessary, all areas of the body where joints can become misaligned.

A visit to a chiropractor begins very much like one to an orthodox physician. A detailed medical history precedes a **physical examination**, during which the chiropractor takes the patient's pulse and blood pressure, and checks their reflexes. Blood and urine tests may be ordered. The physical exam concentrates primarily on the spine, and the patient will be instructed to perform a number of movements while the chiropractor both carefully watches and palpates (probes with pressure) certain areas. This allows the chiropractor to focus on detecting muscle strength or weakness, the range of spinal motion available, incorrect posture, or any structural deformities. Most chiropractors now also x-ray the patient's spine if they complain of pain, and these x rays allow them to locate vertebral misalignments.

Treatment for a specific problem is always tailored to the individual's age, weight and build, overall condition, and even level of pain tolerance, and it consists of what are called adjustments. These are hands-on treatments in which the chiropractor manipulates the patient's spine. Depending on what part of the body is being treated, the patient will be asked to stand, sit, or lie down. Manipulation is done quickly, with each adjustment taking only seconds. It is here that the chiropractic technique differs from regular physical therapy and massage, for the practitioner typically performs a special, high-velocity thrust maneuver that places many pounds of force to a part of the spine for only the briefest time. Although this usually does not cause pain, it often results in popping sounds similar to knuckles being cracked. For patients who are not comfortable with high-velocity techniques, indirect thrust may be used. Indirect thrust uses a gentle stretching motion to manipulate the joint over a towel or padded block. Finally, depending upon the nature of the problem being treated, heat or cold may be applied.

Despite the generally wide acceptance of chiropractic health care, there is little solid evidence for its benefits beyond back care. Still, many people simply do not care as long as they get some relief from their problems. Supporters say that it is only a matter of time until such evidence appears, and in the meantime, patients take fewer drugs, have less surgery, and have fewer hospital stays with chiropractic care. This certainly accounts for much of its broad appeal.

Patients with known bone diseases, **fractures**, or bone **cancer** should not see a chiropractor. Pregnant women with back **pain** can be treated, but should never allow themselves to be x-rayed.

CHLAMYDIAL INFECTIONS

Chlamydial pneumonia refers to one of several types of **pneumonia** that can be caused by a variety of the bacteria known as *Chlamydia.*

Pneumonia is an infection of the lungs. The air sacs (alveoli) and tissues of the lungs become swollen, and the alveoli may fill with pus or fluid. This prevents the lungs from taking in sufficient oxygen, which deprives the blood and the rest of the body's tissues of oxygen.

There are three major types of *Chlamydia*: *Chlamydia psittaci*, *Chlamydia pneumoniae*, and *Chlamydia trachomatis*. Each of these has the potential to cause a type of pneumonia.

Chlamydia trachomatis is a major cause of **sexually transmitted diseases** (called nongonococcal urethritis and **pelvic inflammatory disease**). When a woman with an active chlamydial infection gives birth to a baby, the baby may aspirate (suck into his or her lungs) some of the mother's bacteria-laden secretions while passing through the birth canal. This can cause a form of relatively mild pneumonia in the newborn, occurring about two to six weeks after delivery.

Chlamydia psittaci is a bacteria carried by many types of birds, including pigeons, canaries, parakeets, parrots, and some gulls. Humans acquire the bacteria through contact with dust from bird feathers, bird droppings, or from the bite of a bird carrying the bacteria. People who keep birds as pets or who work where birds are kept have the highest risk for this type of infection. This pneumonia, called psittacosis, causes **fever**, **cough**, and the production of sputum containing pus. Psittacosis may be quite severe, and is usually more serious in older patients. The illness can last several weeks.

Chlamydia pneumoniae usually causes a type of relatively mild ''walking pneumonia.'' Patients experience fever and cough. This type of pneumonia is called community-acquired pneumonia because it is easily passed from one member of the community to another.

Laboratory tests indicating the presence of one of the strains of *Chlamydia* are sophisticated, expensive, and performed in only a few laboratories across the country. For this reason, doctors diagnose most cases of chlamydial pneumonia by performing a **physical examination** of the patient, and noting the presence of certain factors. For instance, if the mother of a baby sick with pneumonia is positive for a sexually transmitted disease caused by *Chlamydia trachomatis*, the diagnosis is obvious. History of exposure to birds in a patient sick with pneumonia suggests that *Chlamydia psittaci* may be the culprit. A mild pneumonia in an otherwise healthy person is likely to be a community-acquired walking pneumonia, such as that caused by *Chlamydia pneumoniae*.

Treatment varies depending on the specific type of *Chlamydia* causing the infection. A newborn with *Chlamydia trachomatis* improves rapidly with erythromycin. *Chlamydia psittaci* infection is treated with tetracycline, bed rest, oxygen supplementation, and codeine-containing cough preparations. *Chlamydia pneumoniae* infection is treated with erythromycin.

The prognosis (outlook for recovery) is generally excellent for the newborn with *Chlamydia trachomatis* pneumonia. *Chlamydia psittaci* may linger, and severe cases have a death rate of as high as 30%. The elderly are hardest hit by this type of pneumonia. A young, healthy person with *Chlamydia pneumoniae* has an excellent prognosis. In the elderly, however, there is a 5-10% death rate from this infection.

Prevention of *Chlamydia trachomatis* pneumonia involves recognizing the symptoms of genital infection in the mother and treating her prior to delivery of her baby.

Chlamydia psittaci can be prevented by warning people who have birds as pets, or who work around birds, to be careful to avoid contact with the dust and droppings of these birds. Sick birds can be treated with an antibiotic in their feed. Because people can contract psittacosis from each other, a person sick with this infection should be kept in **isolation**, so as not to infect other people.

Chlamydia pneumoniae is difficult to prevent because it is spread by respiratory droplets from other sick people. Because people with this type of pneumonia do not always feel very sick, they often continue to attend school, go to work, and go to other public places. They then spread the bacteria in the tiny droplets that are released into the air during coughing. Therefore, this pneumonia is very difficult to prevent and often occurs in outbreaks within communities.

CHOKING

Choking is the inability to breathe because the trachea is blocked, constricted, or swollen shut. Choking is a medical emergency. When a person is choking, air cannot reach the lungs. If the airways cannot be cleared, **death** follows rapidly.

Anyone can choke, but choking is more common in children than in adults. Choking is a common cause of accidental death in young children who are apt to put toys or coins in their mouths, then unintentionally inhale them. About 3,000 adults die each year from choking on food.

People also choke because infection causes the throat tissue to swell shut. It is believed that this is what caused George Washington's death. Allergic reactions can also cause the throat to swell shut. Acute allergic reactions are called anaphylactic reactions and may be fatal. Strangulation puts external pressure on the trachea, causing another form of choking.

Finally, people can choke from obstructive **sleep apnea**. This is a condition where tissues of the body obstruct the airways during sleep. Sleep apnea is most common in obese men who sleep on their backs. Smoking, heavy alcohol use, lung diseases such as emphysema, and an inherited tendency toward a narrowed airway and throat all increase the risk of choking during sleep.

Regardless of the cause, choking cuts off the air supply to the lungs. Cardinal signs of a blocked airway include not being able to speak or cry out, turning blue in the face from lack of oxygen, desperately grabbing at one's throat, and coughing or labored breathing that produces a high-pitched sound. Following these symptoms, a person may fall unconscious. When the airway is blocked during sleep, a person may gasp, stop breathing, or awaken suddenly.

Diagnosing choking due to mechanical obstruction is straightforward, since the symptoms are obvious even to an untrained person. In choking due to infection, the person, usually a child, will have a **fever** and signs of illness before labored breathing begins. If choking is due to an allergic reaction to medication or insect bites, the person's earlobes and face will swell, giving an external sign that internal swelling is also occurring.

Choking due to sleep apnea is usually diagnosed on reports of symptoms by the person's sleep partner. There are also alarm devices to detect the occurrence of sleep apnea. Eventually sleep may be interrupted so frequently that daytime drowsiness becomes a problem.

Choking, except during sleep apnea, is a medical emergency. If choking is due to allergic reaction or infection, people should summon emergency help or go immediately to an emergency room. If choking is due to obstructed airways, the **Heimlich maneuver** (an emergency procedure in which a person is grasped from behind in order to forcefully expel the obstruction) should be performed immediately. In severe cases a **tracheotomy** (an incision into the trachea through the neck below the larynx) must be performed.

Patients who suffer airway obstruction during sleep can be treated with a device similar to an oxygen mask that creates positive airway pressure and delivers a mixture of oxygen and air.

Many people are treated successfully for choking with no permanent effects. However, if treatment is unsuccessful, the person dies from lack of oxygen. In cases where the ariway is restored after the critical period passes, there may be permanent brain damage.

Watching children carefully to keep them from putting **foreign objects** in their mouth and avoiding giving young children food like raisins, round slices of hot dogs, and grapes can reduce the chance of choking in children. Adults should avoid heavy alcohol consumption when eating and avoid talking and laughing with food in their mouth. The risk of obstructive sleep apnea choking can be reduced by avoiding alcohol, tobacco smoking, tranquilizers, and sedatives before bed.

CHOLERA

Cholera is an acute illness characterized by watery **diarrhea** that is caused by the bacterium *Vibro cholerae.* Cholera is spread by eating food or drinking water contaminated with the bacteria. Although cholera was a public health problem in the United States and Europe a hundred years ago, modern sanitation and the treatment of drinking water have virtually eliminated the disease in developed countries. In third world countries, however, cholera is still common.

Cholera is spread by eating food or drinking water that has been contaminated with cholera bacteria. Contamination usually occurs when human feces from a person who has the disease seeps into a community water supply. Fruits and vegetables can be contaminated in areas where crops are fertilized with human feces. Cholera bacteria also live in warm, brackish water and can infect persons who eat raw or undercooked seafood obtained from such waters. Cholera is rarely transmitted directly from one person to another.

Cholera often occurs in outbreaks or epidemics. The World Health Organization (WHO) estimates that during any cholera epidemic, approximately 0.2-1% of the local population will contract the disease. Anyone can get cholera, but infants, children, and the elderly are more likely to die from the disease because they become dehydrated faster than adults. There is no particular season in which cholera is more likely to occur.

Because of an extensive system of sewage and water treatment in the United States, Canada, Europe, Japan, and Australia, cholera is generally not a concern for visitors and residents of these countries. People visiting or living in other parts of the world, particularly on the Indian subcontinent and in parts of Africa and South America, should be aware of the potential for contracting cholera and practice prevention. Fortunately, the disease is both preventable and treatable.

Because *V. cholerae* bacteria are sensitive to acid, most cholera-causing bacteria die in the acidic environment of the stomach. However, when a person has ingested food or water containing large amounts of cholera bacteria, some will survive to infect the intestines.

In the small intestine, the rapidly multiplying bacteria produce a toxin that causes a large volume of water and electrolytes (electrically charged molecules in solution) to be secreted into the bowels and then to be abruptly eliminated as watery diarrhea. Vomiting may also occur. Symptoms begin to appear between one and three days after the contaminated food or water has been ingested.

Most cases of cholera are mild, but about 1 in 20 patients experience severe, potentially life-threatening symptoms. In severe cases, fluids can be lost through diarrhea and vomiting at the rate of one quart per hour. This can produce a dangerous state of **dehydration** unless the lost fluids and electrolytes are rapidly replaced. Dehydration occurs most rapidly in the very young and the very old because they have fewer fluid reserves. Immediate replacement of the lost fluids and electrolytes is necessary to prevent kidney failure, **coma**, and **death**.

Rapid diagnosis of cholera can be made in the laboratory by examining a fresh stool sample under the microscope for the presence of *V. cholerae* bacteria. In areas where cholera occurs often, however, patients are usually treated for diarrhea and vomiting symptoms as if they had cholera without laboratory confirmation.

The key to treating cholera lies in preventing dehydration by replacing the fluids and electrolytes lost through diarrhea and vomiting. The discovery that rehydration can be accomplished orally revolutionized the treatment of cholera and other, similar diseases by making this simple, cost-effective treatment widely available throughout the world.

WHO has developed an inexpensive oral replacement fluid containing appropriate amounts of water, sugar, and salts that is used worldwide. In cases of severe dehydration, replacement fluids must be given intravenously.

Adults may be given the antibiotic tetracycline to shorten the duration of the illness and reduce fluid loss. WHO recommends this antibiotic treatment only in cases of severe dehydration. If **antibiotics** are overused, the cholera bacteria organism may become resistant to the drug, making the antibiotic ineffective in treating even severe cases of cholera. Tetracycline is not given to children whose permanent teeth have not come in because it can cause the teeth to become permanently discolored.

Today, cholera is a very treatable disease. Patients with milder cases of cholera usually recover on their own in three to six days without additional complications. They may eliminate the bacteria in their feces for up to two weeks. Chronic carriers of the disease are rare. With prompt fluid and electrolyte replacement, the death rate in patients with severe cholera is less than 1%. Untreated, the death rate can be greater than 50%. The difficulty in treating severe cholera is not in knowing how to treat it, but in getting medical care to ill people in underdeveloped areas of the world where medical resources are limited.

The best form of cholera prevention is to establish good sanitation and waste treatment systems. In the absence of adequate sewage treatment, precautions such as boiling water, eating only well-cooked foods, and peeling fruit and nuts before eating them help to reduce the possibility of infection.

A cholera vaccine exists that can be given to travelers and residents of areas where cholera is known to be active, but the vaccine is not highly effective. It provides only 25-50% immunity, and then only for a period of about six months. The vaccine is never given to infants under six months of age. The United States Centers for Disease Control and Prevention do not currently recommend cholera **vaccination** for travelers. Residents of cholera-plagued areas should discuss the value of the vaccine with their doctor.

CHOLESTEROL-REDUCING DRUGS

Cholesterol-reducing drugs are medicines that lower the amount of cholesterol (a fatlike substance) in the blood.

Cholesterol is a chemical that can do both good and harm in the body. On the good side, cholesterol plays important roles in the structure of cells and in the production of hormones. But too much cholesterol in the blood can lead to heart and blood vessel disease. To complicate matters, not all cholesterol contributes to heart and blood vessel problems. One type, called high-density lipoprotein (HDL) cholesterol, or "good cholesterol," actually lowers the risk of these problems. The other type, low density lipoprotein (LDL) cholesterol, or "bad cholesterol," is the type that threatens people's health. The names reflect the way cholesterol moves through the body. To travel through the bloodstream, cholesterol must attach itself to a protein. The combination of a protein and a fatty substance like cholesterol is called a lipoprotein.

Many factors may contribute to the fact that some people have higher cholesterol levels than others. A diet high in certain types of fats is one factor. Medical problems such as poorly controlled diabetes, an underactive thyroid gland, an overactive pituitary gland, liver disease or kidney failure also may cause high cholesterol levels. And some people have inherited disorders that prevent their bodies from properly using and eliminating fats. This allows cholesterol to build up in the blood.

Treatment for high cholesterol levels usually begins with changes in habits. By losing weight, stopping smoking, exercising more and reducing the amount of fat and cholesterol in the diet, many people can bring their cholesterol levels down to acceptable levels. However, some may need to use cholesterol-reducing drugs to reduce their risk of health problems.

Different types of cholesterol-reducing drugs work in different ways. Not all cholesterol comes from the diet —some is made in the body. So the strategy of some drugs is to prevent the body from making cholesterol. Other cholesterol-reducing drugs interfere with the body's ability to absorb cholesterol from food. A third approach involves drugs that combine with cholesterol and remove it from the bloodstream. Cholesterol-reducing drugs will not cure problems that cause high cholesterol; they will only help control cholesterol levels.

Examples of cholesterol-reducing drugs are cholestyramine (Questran), colestipol (Colestid), gemfibrozil (Lopid), lovastatin (Mevacor), pravastatin (Pravachol) and simvastatin (Zocor). Lovastatin, pravastatin and simvastatin belong to a group of medicines called HMG-CoA (3-hydroxy-3-methylglutaryl-coenzyme A) reductase inhibitors. These drugs prevent the body from making cholesterol by blocking a key enzyme in the process.

People who have certain medical conditions or who are taking certain other medicines may have problems if they take cholesterol-reducing drugs. Before using these drugs, people with any medical conditions, for example, a person with allergies, or a woman who is pregnant or breastfeeding, should make sure their physicians are aware of their conditions as well as any other medicine they may be taking.

Some of the minor side effects of cholesterol-reducing drugs are heartburn, **indigestion**, belching, bloating, gas, nausea or vomiting, stomach pain, **dizziness** and and headache. They usually go away as the body adjusts to the drug and do not require medical treatment unless they continue or they interfere with normal activities. Additional side effects are possible, and should be reported to the patient's physician.

CHOLESTEROL TEST

The cholesterol test is a way of measuring the cholesterol levels in a sample of the patient's blood. Total serum cholesterol (TC) is the measurement routinely taken. Doctors sometimes order a complete lipoprotein profile to better evaluate the risk for **atherosclerosis** (**coronary artery disease**, or CAD). The full lipoprotein profile also includes measurements of triglyceride levels (a chemical compound that forms 95% of the fats and oils stored in animal or vegetable cells) and lipoproteins (high density and low density). Blood fats are also called lipids.

The type of cholesterol in the blood is as important as the total quantity. Cholesterol is a fatty substance and cannot be dissolved in water. It must combine with a protein molecule called a lipoprotein in order to be transported in the blood. There are five major types of lipoproteins in the human body; they differ in the amount of cholesterol that they carry in comparison to other fats and fatty acids, and in their functions in the body. Lipoproteins are classified according to their density. Chylomicrons are normally found in the blood only after a person has eaten foods containing fats. They contain about 7% cholesterol. Very low-density lipoproteins (VLDLs) carry mostly triglycerides, but they also contain 16-22% cholesterol. Intermediate-density lipoproteins (IDLs) are short-lived lipoproteins containing about 30% cholesterol that are converted in the liver to low-density lipoproteins (LDLs).

LDL molecules carry cholesterol from the liver to other body tissues. They contain about 50% cholesterol. LDL particles are involved in the formation of plaques (abnormal deposits of cholesterol) in the walls of the coronary arteries. LDL is known as ''bad cholesterol.'' High-density lipoproteins (HDLs) are made in the intestines and the liver. HDLs are about 50% protein and 19% cholesterol. They help to remove cholesterol from artery walls. Lifestyle changes, including exercising, keeping weight within recommended limits, and giving up smoking can increase the body's levels of HDL cholesterol. HDL is known as ''good cholesterol.''

Because of the difference in density and cholesterol content of lipoproteins, two patients with the same total cholesterol level can have very different lipid profiles and different risk for CAD. The critical factor is the level of HDL cholesterol in the blood serum. Some doctors use the ratio of the total cholesterol level to HDL cholesterol when assessing the patient's degree of risk. A low TC/HDL ratio is associated with a lower degree of risk.

The purpose of the TC test is to measure the levels of cholesterol in the patient's blood. The patient's cholesterol can also be fractionated (separated into different portions) in order to determine the TC/HDL ratio. The results help the doctor to assess the patient's risk for CAD. High LDL levels are associated with increased risk of CAD, whereas high HDL levels are associated with relatively lower risk.

In addition, the results of the cholesterol test can assist the doctor in evaluating the patient's metabolism of fat, or in diagnosing inflammation of the pancreas, liver disease, or disorders of the thyroid gland.

The frequency of cholesterol testing depends on the patient's degree of risk for CAD. People with low cholesterol levels may need to be tested once every five years. People with high levels of blood cholesterol should be tested more frequently, according to their doctor's advice. The National Cholesterol Education Program offers guidelines for testing based on a person's risk factors.

The cholesterol test requires a sample of the patient's blood. Fasting before the test is required to get an accurate triglyceride and LDL level. The blood is withdrawn from one of the patient's veins. The blood test takes between three and five minutes.

The ''normal'' values for serum lipids depend on the patient's age, sex, and race. Normal values for people in Western countries are usually given as 140-220 mg/dL (milligrams per deciliter) in adults, although as many as 5% of the population has TC higher than 300 mg/dL. Among Asians, the figures are about 20% lower. As a rule, both TC and LDL levels rise as people get older.

Some doctors prefer to speak of ''desired'' rather than ''normal'' cholesterol values, on the grounds that ''normal'' refers to statistically average levels that may still be too high for good health.

It is possible for blood cholesterol levels to be too low as well as too high. TC levels less than 160 mg/dL are associated with higher mortality rates from **cancer**, liver disease, respiratory disorders, and injuries. The connection between unusually low cholesterol and increased mortality is not clear, although some researchers think that the low level is a secondary sign of the underlying disease and not the cause of disease or death.

Low levels of serum cholesterol are also associated with **malnutrition** or hyperthyroidism. Further diagnostic testing may be necessary in order to locate the cause.

Prior to 1980, hypercholesterolemia (an abnormally high TC level) was defined as any value above the 95th percentile for the population. These figures ranged from 210 mg/dL in persons younger than 20 to more than 280 mg/dL in persons older than 60. It is now known, however, that TC levels over 200 mg/dL are associated with significantly higher risk of CAD. Levels of 280 mg/dL or more are considered elevated. Treatment with diet and medication has proven to successfully lower risk of **heart attack** and **stroke**.

Elevated cholesterol levels may also result from hepatitis, blockage of the bile ducts, disorders of lipid metabolism, **nephrotic syndrome**, inflammation of the pancreas, or hypothyroidism.

CHRONIC FATIGUE SYNDROME

Chronic fatigue syndrome (CFS) is a condition that causes extreme tiredness. People with CFS have debilitating fatigue that lasts for six months or longer. They also have many other symptoms. Some of these are **pain** in the joints and muscles, **headache**, and **sore throat**. CFS does not have a known cause, but appears to result from a combination of factors.

CFS is the most common name for this disorder, but it also has been called chronic fatigue and immune disorder (CFIDS), myalgic encephalomyelitis, low natural killer cell disease, postviral syndrome, Epstein-Barr disease, and Yuppie flu. CFS has so many names because researchers have been unable to find out exactly what causes it and because there are many similar, overlapping conditions. Reports of a CFS-like syndrome called neurasthenia date back to 1869. Later, people with similar symptoms were said to have **fibromyalgia** because one of the main symptoms is myalgia, or muscle pain. Because of the similarity of symptoms, fibromyalgia and CFS are considered to be overlapping syndromes.

In the early to mid-1980s, there were outbreaks of CFS in some areas of the United States. Doctors found that many people with CFS had high levels of antibodies to the Epstein-Barr virus (EBV), which causes mononucleosis, in their blood. For a while they thought they had found the culprit, but it turned out that many healthy people also had high EBV antibodies. Scientists have also found high levels of other viral antibodies in the blood of people with CFS. These findings have led many scientists to believe that a virus or combination of viruses may trigger CFS.

CFS was sometimes referred to as Yuppie flu because it seemed to often affect young, middle-class professionals. In fact, CFS can affect people of any gender, age, race, or socioeconomic group. Although anyone can get CFS, most patients diagnosed with CFS are 25-45 years old, and about 80% of cases are in women. Estimates of how many people are afflicted with CFS vary due to the similarity of CFS symptoms to other diseases and the difficulty in identifying it. The Centers for Disease Control and Prevention (CDC) has estimated that 4-10 people per 100,000 in the United States have CFS. According to the CFIDS Foundation, about 500,000 adults in the United States (0.3% of the population) have CFS. This probably is a low estimate since these figures do not include children and are based on the CDC definition of CFS, which is very strict for research purposes.

Although what causes CFS is still controversial, many doctors and researchers now think that CFS may not be a single illness. Instead, they think CFS may be a group of symptoms caused by several conditions. One theory is that a microorganism, such as a virus, or a chemical injures the body and damages the immune system, allowing dormant viruses to become active, causing flu-like symptoms. Immune abnormalities have been found in studies of people with CFS, although the same abnormalities are also found in people with allergies, autoimmune diseases, **cancer**, and other disorders.

The role of psychological problems in CFS is very controversial. Because many people with CFS are diagnosed with depression and other psychiatric disorders, some experts conclude that the symptoms of CFS are psychological. However, many people with CFS did not have psychological disorders before getting the illness. Many doctors think that patients become depressed or anxious because of the effects of the symptoms of their CFS.

Having CFS is not just a matter of being tired. People with CFS have severe fatigue that keeps them from performing their normal daily activities, for example, working, attending school, or even taking part in social activities.

CFS is diagnosed by evaluating symptoms and eliminating other causes of fatigue. In the United States, many doctors use the CDC case definition to determine if a patient has CFS.

Diagnosis of CFS is made based on unexplained continuing or recurring chronic fatigue that has lasted for at least six months, that is of new or definite onset (that is, the person has not been tired their whole life), and that seriously interferes with a person's life. In addition, a patient must have four or more of that following symptoms: trouble remembering or concentrating; sore throat; tender lymph nodes; muscle pain; pain in many joints without swelling or redness; headaches; unrefreshing sleep; and postexertional malaise (a vague feeling of discomfort or tiredness following exercise or other physical or mental activity) lasting more than 24 hours. These symptoms must have continued or recurred during six or more consecutive months of illness and must not have started before the fatigue began.

There is no cure for CFS, but treatment is available to help relieve the symptoms. Treatment is usually individualized to each person's particular symptoms and needs. Most doctors recommend a combination of rest, exercise, and a balanced diet. Counseling and **stress** reduction techniques also may help some people with CFS.

Many nutritional supplements and herbal preparations advertised for treatment of CFS are unproven, though others seem to provide some people with relief. People with CFS should discuss their treatment plan with their doctors, and carefully weigh the benefits and risks of each therapy before making a decision. Drugs that sometimes alleviate the symptoms of CFS include **nonsteroidal anti-inflammatory drugs**, low dosages of antidepressants, and antianxiety drugs. Research into the cause and treatment of CFS is continuing.

The course of CFS varies widely for different people. Some people get progressively worse over time, while others gradually improve. Some have periods of illness that alternate with periods of good health. While many people with CFS never fully regain their health, they find relief from symptoms and adapt to the demands of the disorder by carefully following a treatment plan combining adequate rest, nutrition, exercise, and other therapies.

CHRONIC OBSTRUCTIVE LUNG DISEASE

Chronic obstructive lung disease, also known as chronic obstructive pulmonary disease (COPD), is a general term for a group of conditions in which there is persistent difficulty in expelling (or exhaling) air from the lungs. COPD commonly refers to two related, progressive diseases of the respiratory system, chronic **bronchitis** and emphysema. Because smoking is the major cause of both diseases, chronic bronchitis and emphysema often occur together in the same patient.

COPD is one of the fastest-growing health problems. Nearly 16 million people in the United States, 14 million with chronic bronchitis and 2 million with emphysema, suffer from COPD. COPD is responsible for more than 96,000 deaths annually, making it the fourth leading cause of death. Although COPD is more common in men than women, the increase in incidence of smoking among women since World War II has produced an increase in deaths from COPD in women. COPD has a large economic impact on the health-care system and a destructive impact on the lives of patients and their families. Quality of life for a person with COPD decreases as the disease progresses.

In chronic bronchitis, chronic inflammation caused by cigarette smoking results in a narrowing of the openings in the bronchi, the large air tubes of the respiratory system, and interferes with the flow of air. Inflammation also causes the glands that line the bronchi to produce excessive amounts of mucus, further narrowing the airways and blocking airflow. The result is often a chronic **cough** that produces sputum (mainly mucus) and **shortness of breath**. Cigarette smoke also damages the cilia, small hairlike projections that move bacteria and foreign particles out of the lungs, increasing the risk of infections.

Emphysema is a disease in which cigarette smoke causes an overproduction of the enzyme elastase, one of the immune system's infection-fighting biochemicals. This results in irreversible destruction of a protein in the lung called elastin, which is important for maintaining the structure of the walls of the alveoli, the terminal small air sacs of the respiratory system. As the walls of the alveoli rupture, the number of alveoli are reduced and many of those remaining are enlarged, making the lungs of thc paticnt with emphysema less elastic and overinflated. Due to the higher pressure inside the chest that must be developed to force air out of the less elastic lungs, the bronchioles, small air tubes of the respiratory system, tend to collapse during exhalation. Stale air gets trapped in the air sacs, and fresh air cannot be brought in.

In the general population, emphysema usually develops in older individuals with a long smoking history. However, there is also a form of emphysema that runs in families. People with this type of emphysema have a hereditary deficiency of a blood component, an enzyme inhibitor called alpha-1-antitrypsin (AAT). This type of emphysema is sometimes called early onset emphysema because it can appear when a person is as young as 30 or 40 years old. It is estimated that there are between 75,000 and 150,000 Americans who were born with AAT deficiency. Of this group, emphysema afflicts an estimated 20,000-40,000 people (1-3% of all cases of emphysema). The risk of developing emphysema for an AAT-deficient individual who also smokes is much greater than for others.

The first symptoms of chronic bronchitis are cough and mucus production. These symptoms resemble a chest cold that lingers on for weeks. Later, shortness of breath develops. Cough, sputum production, and shortness of breath may become worse if a person develops a lung infection. A person with chronic bronchitis may later develop emphysema as well. In emphysema, shortness of breath on exertion is the predominant early symptom. Coughing is usually minor and there is little sputum. As the disease progresses, the shortness of breath occurs with less exertion, and eventually may be present even when at rest. At this point, a sputum-producing cough may also occur. Either chronic bronchitis or emphysema may lead to **respiratory failure**—a condition in which there occurs a dangerously low level of oxygen or a serious excess of carbon dioxide in the blood.

The first step in diagnosing COPD is a good medical evaluation, including a medical history and a **physical examination** of the chest using a stethoscope. In addition, the doctor may order further tests such as a test of pulmonary function to measure the air taken into and exhaled from the lungs, a chest x ray, and blood gas levels to determine the amount of oxygen and carbon dioxide present in the blood.

The precise nature of the patient's condition determines the type of treatment prescribed for COPD. With a program of complete respiratory care, disability can be minimized, acute episodes prevented, hospitalizations reduced, and some early deaths avoided. On the other hand, no treatment has been shown to slow the progress of the disease, and only **oxygen therapy** increases survival rate.

Medications frequently prescribed for COPD patients include bronchodilaters to open narrowed airways, **corticosteroids** to block inflammation, oxygen replacement (from portable or stationary tanks), and antibiotics to combat respiratory infection, among others.

Surgical procedures for emphysema are very rare. The great majority of patients cannot be helped by surgery, and no single procedure is ideal for those who can be helped.

A structured, outpatient pulmonary **rehabilitation** program helps the lungs to operate more effectively in certain patients with COPD. Services may include general **exercise** training, administration of oxygen and nutritional supplements, intermittent mechanical ventilatory support, continuous positive airway pressure, relaxation techniques, breathing exercises and techniques (such as pursed lip breathing), and methods for mobilizing and removing secretions.

COPD is a disease that can be treated and controlled, but not cured. Survival of patients with COPD is clearly related to the degree of their lung function when they are diagnosed and the rate at which they lose this function. Overall, the median survival is about 10 years for patients with COPD who have lost approximately two-thirds of their lung function at diagnosis. In other words, these patients have a fifty-fifty chance of surviving more than 10 years.

Lifestyle modifications that can help prevent COPD, or improve function in COPD patients, include quitting smoking, avoiding respiratory irritants and infections, avoiding allergens, maintaining good nutrition, drinking lots of fluids, avoiding excessively low or high temperatures and very high altitudes, maintaining proper weight, and exercising to increase muscle tone.

CIGARETTE SMOKING

The **World Health Organization** (WHO) has named tobacco one of the greatest public health threats of the twenty-first century. As of 1999, more than one billion people worldwide smoke, and 3.5 million people are expected to die from causes directly related to tobacco use. This death rate is expected to rise to 10 million by the year 2030. Seventy percent of these deaths will occur in developing countries where the proportion of smokers is growing, particularly among women. Calling tobacco "a global threat," WHO says these figures do not include the enormous physical, emotional, and economic costs associated with disease and disability caused by tobacco use.

In the United States alone, 25.2 million men, 23.2 million women, and 4.1 million teens between 12 and 17 years of age, smoke. Every day, more than three million youths under the age of 18 begin smoking. The gruesome statistics show that more than five million children alive today will die prematurely because, as adolescents, they decided to use tobacco. Nationally, one in five of all deaths is related to tobacco use. It kills more than 430,000 people every year—more than **AIDS**, alcohol, drugs abuse, automobile **accidents**, murders, **suicides**, and fires *combined.* Five million years of potential life is lost *every year* due to premature death caused by tobacco use, medical costs total more than $50 billion annually, and indirect cost another $50 billion.

Of the 4,000 or more different chemicals present in cigarette smoke, 60 are known to cause cancer and others to cause cellular genetic mutations that can lead to **cancer**. Cigarette smoke contains nicotine—a highly addictive chemical—tars, nitrosamines, and polycyclic hydrocarbons, all of which are carcinogenic. It also contains carbon monoxide which, when inhaled, interferes with transportation and utilization of oxygen throughout the body.

Cigarette smoke is called mainstream smoke when inhaled directly from a cigarette. Sidestream smoke is smoke emitted from the burning cigarette and exhaled by the smoker. Sidestream smoke is also called environmental tobacco smoke (ETS) or secondhand smoke. Inhalation of ETS is known as passive smoking. In 1993, the Environmental Protection Agency (EPA) classified ETS as a Group A (known human) carcinogen—the grouping reserved for the most dangerous **carcinogens**. By 1996, the Department of Health and Human Services' **Centers for Disease Control** and Prevention (CDC) found that nine out of 10 non-smoking Americans are regularly exposed to ETS. A study by the American Heart Association reported in 1997 that women regularly exposed to ETS have a 91% greater risk of heart attack and those exposed occasionally a 58% greater risk—rates which are believed to apply equally to men. The EPA estimates that, annually, ETS is responsible for more than 3,000 lung cancer deaths, 35,000-62,000 deaths from heart attacks, and lower respiratory tract infections (such as bronchitis [300,000 cases annually] and asthma [400,000 existing cases]), and middle ear infections in children.

ETS may be more carcinogenic than mainstream smoke as it contains higher amounts of carcinogenic materials with smaller particles. These smaller particles are more likely to lodge in the lungs than the larger particles in mainstream smoke. Researchers found that no safe threshold exists for exposure to ETS. With this information, many municipal governments and workplaces have banned cigarette smoking altogether.

Scientific evidence has proven that smoking can cause cancer of the lung, larynx, esophagus, mouth, and bladder; cardiovascular disease; chronic lung ailments; coronary heart disease; and **stroke**. Smokeless tobacco has equally deadly consequences. When cigarette smoke is inhaled, the large surface area of the lung tissues and alveoli quickly absorb the chemical components and nicotine. Within one minute of inhaling, the chemicals in the smoke are distributed by the bloodstream to the brain, heart, kidneys, liver, lungs, gastrointestinal tract, muscle, and fat tissue. In pregnant women, cigarette smoke crosses the placenta and may effect fetal growth.

Cardiovascular disease, or diseases of the blood vessels and heart, include stroke, **heart attack**, peripheral vascular disease, and aortic **aneurysm**. In 1990 in the United States, one fifth of all deaths due to cardiovascular disease were linked to smoking. Specifically, 179,820 deaths from general cardiovascular disease, 134,235 deaths from heart disease, and 23,281 deaths from cerebrovascular disease (stroke) were directly linked to smoking. In addition, researchers have noted a strong dose-response relationship between the duration and extent of smoking and the death rate from heart disease in men under 65. The more one smokes, the more one is likely to develop heart disease. Researchers have also seen a similar trend in women.

Cigarette smoking leads to cardiovascular disease in a number of ways. Smoking damages the inside of the blood vessels, initiating changes that lead to **atherosclerosis**, a disease characterized by blood vessel blockage. It also causes the coronary arteries (that supply the heart muscle with oxygen) to constrict, increasing vulnerability of the heart to heart attack (when heart muscle dies as a result of lack of oxygen) and cardiac arrest (when the heart stops beating). Smoking also raises the levels of low-density lipoproteins (the so-called ''bad'' cholesterol) in the blood, and lowers the levels of high-density lipoproteins (the so-called ''good'' cholesterol), a situation that has been linked to atherosclerosis. Finally, smoking increases the risk of stroke by 1.5 to 3 times the risk for non-smokers.

Smoking causes 85% of all **lung cancers**, and 14% of all cancers—among them cancers of the mouth, pharynx (throat), larynx (voice-box), esophagus, stomach, pancreas, cervix, kidney, ureter, and bladder. More than 171,500 new diagnoses were expected in 1998. Other environmental factors add to the carcinogenic qualities of tobacco. For example, alcohol consumption combined with smoking accounts for three-quarters of all oral and pharyngeal cancers. Also, persons predisposed genetically to certain cancers may develop cancer more quickly if they smoke. Only 14% of lung cancer patients survive five years after diagnosis.

Smoking is the leading cause of lung disease in the United States. Among the direct causes of death are **pneumonia**, **influenza**, **bronchitis**, emphysema, and chronic airway obstruction. Smoking increases mucus production in the airways and deadens the respiratory cilia, the tiny hairs that sweep debris out from the lungs. Without the action of the cilia, bacteria and inhaled particles from cigarette smoke are free to damage the lungs.

In the smaller airways of the lungs—the tiny bronchioles that branch off from the larger bronchi—chronic inflammation is present in smokers which causes airway to constrict causing cough, mucus production, and shortness of breath. Eventually, this inflammation can lead to **chronic obstructive pulmonary disease** (COPD), a condition in which oxygen absorption by the lungs is greatly reduced, severely limiting the amount of oxygen transported to body tissues.

For the 40 years prior to 1987, breast cancer was the leading cause of cancer death among women in the United States. In 1987, lung cancer took the lead. As well as increased risk of cancer and cardiovascular disease, women smokers are at increased risk of **osteoporosis** (a disease in which bones become brittle and vulnerable to breakage), **cervical cancer**, and decreased fertility. Pregnant women have increased risk for spontaneous abortion, premature separation of the placenta from the uterine wall (a life-threatening complication for mother and fetus), placenta previa (in which the placenta implants much lower in the uterus than normal, which may lead to hemorrhage), bleeding during pregnancy, and premature rupture of the placental membranes (which can lead to infection). Infants born to women who smoke during **pregnancy** are at increased risk for low birth weight (18,600 cases annually), and other developmental problems. In men, smoking lowers testosterone levels, and appears to increase male **infertility**.

Numerous other health problems are caused by smoking such as poor circulation in the extremities due to constricted blood vessels. This not only leads to constantly cold hands and feet, it often requires **amputation** of the lower extremities. Smoking also deadens the taste buds and the receptors in the nasal epithelium, interfering with the senses of taste and smell, and may also contribute to periodontal disease.

In 1992, the Surgeon General of the United States declared nicotine to be as addictive as cocaine. An article published in the December 17, 1997 issue of the *Journal of the National Cancer Institute* stated nicotine addiction rates are higher than for alcohol or cocaine—that of all people trying only one cigarette, 33-50% will ultimately become addicted. The article concluded that simply knowing the harmful effects of tobacco is insufficient to help people kick the **addiction** and that behavioral intervention and support methods similar to those applied in alcohol and drug addictions appear to be most helpful.

The physical effects of cigarette smoke include several neurological responses which, in turn, stimulate emotional responses. When serotonin, a neurotransmitter (substances in the brain used by cells to transmit nerve impulses) is released, a person feels more alert. Nicotine stimulates serotonin release. Soon, however, serotonin release becomes sluggish without the boost from nicotine and the smoker becomes dependent on nicotine to prompt the release of serotonin. Other neurotransmitters released in response to nicotine include dopamine, opioids (naturally occurring, pain-killing substances), and various hormones, all of which have powerful effects on the brain where addiction occurs.

In 1998, scientists found a defective gene which makes the metabolism of nicotine difficult. The normal gene produces a liver enzyme needed to break down nicotine. The defective gene, found in about 20% of nonsmokers, may lessen the likelihood of nicotine addiction.

In 1999, researchers discovered a version of a gene which increases the levels of dopamine in the brain. Because nicotine stimulates the release of dopamine, researchers believe the new-found gene may reduce the individual's desire to ''pump up'' dopamine production with nicotine.

Quitting smoking significantly lowers the risk of cancer and cardiovascular disease. In fact, the risk of lung cancer decreases from 18.83 at 1-4 years after quitting, to 7.73 at 5-9 years, to below 5 at 10-19 years, to 2.1 at 20-plus years. The risk of lung cancer for nonsmokers is 1.

Weight gain is a common side effect of quitting, since smoking interferes with pancreatic function and carbohydrate metabolism, leading to a lower body weight in some people. However, not all people experience this lowered body weight from smoking, thus, not all people who quit gain weight. Taste buds and smell are reactivated in nonsmokers, which may lead to increased food intake.

About 80% of people who quit relapse within the first two weeks. Less than 3% of smokers become non-smokers annually. Nicotine gum and patches, which maintain a steady level of nicotine in the blood, have met with some success but are more successful when combined with other support programs. Researchers now believe that smoking may be linked to depression, the withdrawal symptom causing most people who quit to begin again. In 1997, the FDA approved the **antidepressant** medication bupropion to help treat nicotine dependence.

In 1998, a $206 billion settlement from tobacco companies to 46 states included a ban on all outdoor advertising of tobacco products. In 1999, the CDC appropriated more than $80 million to curtail tobacco use among young people. Coordinated education and prevention programs through schools have lowered the onset of smoking by 37% in seventh-grade students alone. By educating today's youth to the dangers of tobacco use, adults of tomorrow will have a longer, healthier, more productive life.

Circumcision

Circumcision refers to the surgical removal of the foreskin (prepuce) of the penis. In the United States, circumcision in infant boys is usually performed for cultural or religious reasons. In addition, infant circumcision provides some medical advantages. Studies indicate that uncircumcised boys under the age of five are 20 times more likely than circumcised boys to suffer infections of the urinary tract. Older boys undergo circumcision because of inflammation of the penis, for social reasons, to improve hygiene, and for a condition called phimosis (a tightening of the foreskin that may close the opening of the penis.) Often circumcision is done at the same time as other surgery. Beyond childhood, circumcised men are less likely to suffer phimosis. There are also indications that circumcised men are less likely to suffer from **cancer** of the penis or inflammation of the penis. There are also studies indicating that circumcised men have fewer **sexually transmitted diseases**. The medical advantages are considered to be slight, because conditions such as phimosis and cancer of the penis are rare even in men who have not been circumcised. Overall, the minor benefits of circumcision seem balanced by the minor risks, and the preferences of the parents usually determine whether a boy is circumcised or not.

Circumcision should not be performed on infants with certain deformities of the penis that may require a portion of the foreskin for repair. Also, infants with a large hydrocoele or **hernia** may suffer important complications. Premature infants or infants with serious infections are also poor candidates for circumcision. Circumcision should not be performed on infants with hemophilia or other bleeding disorders or on infants whose mothers were taking anticoagulant drugs (drugs that keep blood from clotting). In older boys or men, circumcision is a minor procedure. Therefore, it can be performed in virtually anyone without a serious illness or unusual deformity.

In infants, the foreskin is pulled tightly into a specially designed clamp, and the foreskin pulls away from the broadened tip of the penis (glans). Pressure from the clamp stops bleeding from blood vessels that supplied the foreskin. In older boys or adults, an incision is made around the base of the foreskin, the foreskin is pulled back, and then it is cut away from the tip of the penis. Stitches are usually used to close the skin edges.

Despite a long-standing belief that infants do not experience serious **pain** from circumcision, most authorities now believe that some form of local anesthesia is necessary. In older boys, the doctor will inject local anesthesia at the base of the penis, blocking key nerves.

Complications following newborn circumcision appear to occur 0.2-2% of the time. Most complications are minor. Bleeding accounts for about half of the complications, and it is usually easy to control. Infections are rare. There may be injuries to the penis itself, and in very unusual cases these can be difficult to repair.

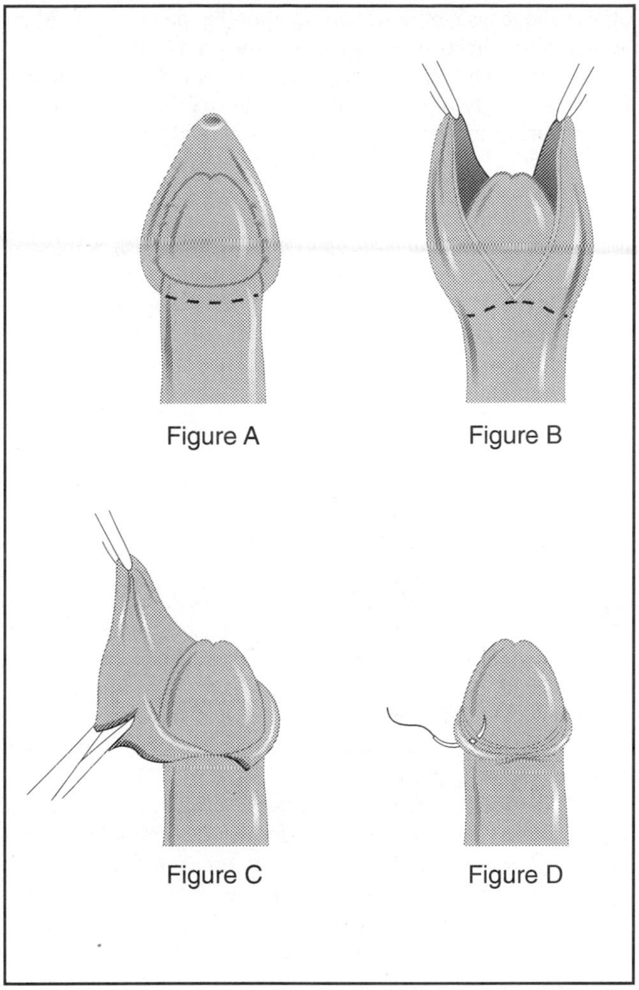

A typical circumcision procedure involves the following steps: Figure A: The surgeon makes an incision around the foreskin. Figure B: The foreskin is then freed from the skin covering the penile shaft. Figure C: The surgeon cuts the foreskin to the initial incision, lifting the foreskin from the mucous membrane. Figure D: The surgeon sutures the top edge of the skin that covers the penile shaft and the mucous membrane. *(Illustration by Electronic Illustrators Group.)*

Cirrhosis

Cirrhosis is a chronic, degenerative disease in which normal liver cells are damaged and are then replaced by scar tissue. Cirrhosis changes the structure of the liver and the blood vessels that nourish it. The disease reduces the liver's ability to manufacture proteins and process hormones, nutrients, medications, and poisons.

Cirrhosis gets worse over time and can become potentially life threatening. It can cause excessive bleeding (hemorrhage),, impotence, **liver cancer**, **coma** due to accumulated ammonia and body wastes (liver failure), and death.

Cirrhosis is the seventh leading cause of disease-related death in the United States. It is twice as common in men as in women. The disease occurs in more than half of all malnourished chronic alcoholics and kills about 25,000 people a year. It is the third most common cause of death in adults between the ages of 45 and 65.

Portal or nutritional cirrhosis is the form of the disease most common in the United States. About 30-50% of all cases of cirrhosis are this type. Nine out of every 10 people who have nutritional cirrhosis have a history of **alcoholism**. Portal or nutritional cirrhosis is also called Laënnec's cirrhosis.

Biliary cirrhosis is caused by diseases within the liver that impede bile flow. Bile is formed in the liver and is carried by ducts to the intestines. Bile then helps digest fats in the intestines. Biliary cirrhosis can scar or block these ducts. It represents 15-20% of all cirrhosis.

Various types of chronic hepatitis, especially **hepatitis** B and hepatitis C, can cause postnecrotic cirrhosis. This form of the disease affects up to 40% of all patients who have cirrhosis.

Disorders like the inability to metabolize iron may cause pigment cirrhosis (hemochromatosis), which accounts for 5-10% of all instances of the disease.

Long-term alcoholism is the primary cause of cirrhosis in the United States. Men and women respond differently to alcohol. Although most men can safely consume two to five drinks a day, one or two drinks a day can cause liver damage in women. Individual tolerance to alcohol varies, but people who drink more and drink more often have a higher risk of developing cirrhosis. In some people, one drink a day can cause liver scarring.

Liver injury, reactions to prescription medications, exposure to toxic substances, and repeated episodes of **heart failure** with liver congestion can cause cirrhosis. The disorder can also be a result of diseases that run in families (inherited diseases) or from poor nutrition. In about 10 out of every 100 patients, the cause of cirrhosis cannot be determined. Many people with cirrhosis do not have any symptoms.

Symptoms of cirrhosis result from the loss of functioning liver cells or organ swelling due to scarring. The liver enlarges during the early stages of illness, and the palms of the hands turn red. Other symptoms include loss of appetite, nausea, weakness, and weight loss.

As the disease progresses, the spleen enlarges and fluid collects in the abdomen (ascites) and legs (**edema**). Spiderlike blood vessels appear on the chest and shoulders bruise easily.

Cirrhosis can cause dry skin and intense **itching**. The whites of the eyes and the skin may turn yellow (**jaundice**), and urine may be dark yellow or brown. Stools may be black or bloody, and the patient may develop persistent high blood pressure (portal **hypertension**).

If the liver loses its ability to remove toxins from the brain, the patient may become forgetful and unresponsive, neglect personal care, have trouble concentrating, and acquire new sleeping habits. High protein intake in these patients can also lead to these symptoms.

A patient's medical history can reveal illnesses or lifestyles likely to lead to cirrhosis. Liver changes can be seen during a **physical examination**. A doctor who suspects cirrhosis may order blood and urine tests to measure liver function. Because only a small number of healthy cells are needed to carry out essential liver functions, test results may be normal even when cirrhosis is present.

Computed tomography scans (CT), ultrasound, and other imaging techniques can be used to determine the size of the liver, indicate healthy and scarred areas of the organ, and detect gallstones. Cirrhosis may also be diagnosed during surgery or by examining the liver with a laparoscope. This viewing device is inserted into the patient's body through a tiny incision in the abdomen.

Liver biopsy is usually needed to confirm a diagnosis of cirrhosis. In this procedure, a tissue sample is removed from the liver and is examined under a microscope in order to learn more about the organ.

The goal of treatment is to cure or reduce the condition causing cirrhosis, prevent or delay disease progression, and prevent or treat complications.

Salt and fluid intake is often limited, and activity is encouraged. A diet high in calories and moderately high in protein can benefit some patients. **Tube feedings** or vitamin supplements may be prescribed if the liver continues to deteriorate. Patients are asked not to consume alcohol. A variety of other drugs are availabe to treat the many symptoms of cirrhosis.

Liver transplants can benefit patients with advanced cirrhosis. However, the new liver will eventually become diseased unless the underlying cause of cirrhosis is removed. Patients with alcoholic cirrhosis must demonstrate a willingness to stop drinking before being considered suitable transplant candidates.

Cirrhosis-related liver damage cannot be reversed, but further damage can be prevented by patients who eat properly, get enough rest, do not consume alcohol, and remain free of infection.

If the underlying cause of cirrhosis cannot be corrected or removed, scarring will continue. The liver will fail, and the patient will probably die within five years. Eliminating alcohol abuse could prevent 75-80% of all cases of cirrhosis. Patients who stop drinking after being diagnosed with cirrhosis can increase their likelihood of living more than a few years from 40% to 60-70%.

CITRIC ACID CYCLE • See Krebs, Hans Adolf

CLAUDE, ALBERT (1898-1983)

American cell biologist

Biologist Albert Claude received the Nobel Prize in 1974 for his discoveries concerning the fine structure of the cell. His early work described the nature of mitochondria as the powerhouse of the cell, paving the way for much groundbreaking research by others. In addition, he demonstrated that the interior of cells were not merely an arbitrary mass of substances, but rather a highly organized space delineated by the net-like endoplasmic reticulum, a formation that he was the first to recognize.

Born in Longlier, Belgium (now Luxembourg), on August 24, 1898, Albert Claude chose to become a U.S. citizen at age 43. Though he maintained dual citizenship, his decision was the logical outcome of a growing research career in the United States, a place of opportunity for an individual who began life with what seemed like limited prospects. Claude's father, Florentin Joseph Claude, was a baker and unable to provide the kind of upbringing one might expect a Nobel Prize winner to have had. His mother, Marie-Glaudicine Wautriquant, and his father evidently provided the right attitude for young Claude, for he overcame the constraints of a limited education and poverty to gain acceptance into the University of Liege. This was possible because of his service in World War I, in which he won the Interallied Medal along with veteran status. The university admitted him under a special program designed for war veterans.

Claude earned an M.D. degree in 1928 under his continuing government scholarship and attended the Kaiser Wilhelm Institute in Berlin for further study. He relocated to the United States in 1929 to join the staff of the Rockefeller Institute in New York City, home to much of the great biomedical research and discoveries of the early twentieth century. There Claude studied the tumor agent of Rous sarcoma, a virus of chickens. Though Claude had not been invited to join the Institute, the director, Simon Flexner, one of the country's leading medical educators, approved his hiring.

In the laboratory of James B. Murphy, Claude began earnest work on isolating the originating factor of the sarcoma, a malignant plasma, first discovered in 1911 at Rockefeller Institute by **Peyton Rous**, that was a type of soft-tissue cancer in chickens. Only recently had microbiologists first suggested that cancers might be caused by newly discovered agents known as viruses. But it was not until 1932 that Rous' work was vindicated by the discovery of transmissible wild rabbit cancers that were proven to be viral in nature.

Diligently pursuing the new field of virology, Claude developed a technique using a high-speed centrifuge to spin fractionated (broken-up) cells infected with viruses in an attempt to isolate their agents. Though his primitive machine was constructed from meat grinders and sieves, Claude was able to fractionate various components of cells that had never been separated before, paving the way for new understanding of their varying functions. Though he never succeeded in fully isolating the virus within the cell mixture (a development that came years later by other investigators), his discoveries nevertheless became crucial to the study of cell biology.

The Rous virus is among those now known as a ribonucleic acid (RNA) virus, that is, its genetic material is derived from RNA rather than the more common deoxyribonucleic acid (DNA). Claude was surprised to find that it was not only virus-infected cells that showed a high RNA content, but also healthy cells. By the early 1940s Claude joined forces with biochemists George Hogeboom and Rollin Hotchkiss in an attempt to determine the origins of this cellular RNA.

Claude, Hogeboom, and Hotchkiss found a variety of different ''granules'' in the cells that they determined were mitochondria, which were first discovered in 1897. However, the purpose of these often abundant cell components, especially in the liver cells, still remained unknown. Claude found that the mitochondria were not the source of the cells' RNA, but they did harbor certain enzymes that seemed to be involved in the cells' energy metabolism, a process dimly understood at the time. Claude and his colleagues, in fact, proved in 1945 that mitochondria are the ''powerhouses'' of all cells, from bacteria to liver, from plants to fungi to animals. The RNA, it turned out, was concentrated in other cell particles that fellow researcher George Palade discovered and called microsomes. Later renamed ribosomes, these particles were shown to be the centers of protein production in all cells of every type of living thing. In 1974 Claude, Palade, and a third researcher, Christian R. Duvé, shared the Nobel Prize for physiology or medicine.

By the early 1940s, Claude had significantly perfected ultracentrifugation (the process of separating cell particles) and was seeking other new technologies with which to probe the cell. In 1942 he became convinced that the newly developed electron microscope would be useful in furthering his studies and secured the use of the device at the Interchemical Corporation, home to the only electron microscope in New York City which was used primarily for metallurgical purposes.

The cells that Claude and his associate, Keith Porter, observed under the microscope showed the presence of a ''lacework'' structure that was eventually proven to be the major structural feature of the interior of all but bacterial cells. This lace-work structure was also responsible in part for providing the shape of cells as well as the location for many granular cell components, including ribosomes. The discovery of this endoplasmic reticulum (derived from the Latin word for ''fishnet'') altered biologists' view of cells as simply bags of ''stuff'' to highly organized biological units.

In 1948 Claude returned to his native Belgium and for a time gave up active research to become an administrator at the Université Libre de Bruxelles, where he spent the next twenty years developing a significant cancer research center. During the same period he headed the Institut Jules Bordet, where he resumed research on the fine structure of cells.

In 1972 the Rockefeller University (formerly Institute) awarded Claude emeritus standing. Other honors accrued over the span of his career include the Medal of the Belgian Academy of Medicine, the Louisa G. Horowitz Prize of Columbia University, and the Paul Ehrlich and Ludwig Darmstaedter Prize of Frankfurt. In addition, Claude was a full member of the Belgian and French academies of science and an honorary member of the American Academy of Arts and Sciences. Other honors included the Order of the Palmes Académiques of France, the Grand Cordon of the Order of Léopold II, and the Prix Fonds National de la Recherche Scientifique from Belgium.

CLEFT LIP AND PALATE

A cleft is a birth defect that occurs when the tissues of the lip and/or palate of a fetus do not properly fuse very early in the **pregnancy**. A cleft lip, sometimes referred to as a harelip, is an elongated opening between the upper lip and the nose. It may involve one or both sides of the lip and may occur with or without a cleft palate. A cleft palate, in which the roof of the mouth abnormally opens into the floor of the nose, may also occur without a cleft lip.

One of every 30 babies is born with some type of birth defect. Approximately one in 700 has a cleft, the fourth most common birth defect in the United States (congenital heart defect is the most prevalent). Twice as many boys as girls are afflicted with a cleft lip, both with and without a cleft palate. However, twice as many girls as boys are afflicted with a cleft palate without a cleft lip. Clefting occurs most often in Asians, Latinos, and Native Americans (one of 500 births) and least often in people of African descent (one of 1000 births).

Babies born with cleft lips or cleft palates may have trouble breathing, as well as swallowing. They cannot adequately suck, so they cannot nurse and must be fed with a special bottle or a bulbar syringe. Later, when their teeth erupt, the upper and lower teeth and jaws are often misaligned, resulting in difficulty chewing. Thus, clefting leaves children vulnerable to **dehydration** and **malnutrition**. A cleft palate also affects a child's speech, since the palate is necessary for speech formation. Even when a cleft palate is surgically repaired, it can permanently affect an individual's speech patterns.

A cleft results when developing facial structures fail to fuse between the fourth and eighth weeks of gestation. This failure may be initiated by either genetic or environmental factors. The genes that cause clefting may be passed from either parent. A parent with a cleft has at least a 5% chance of passing along the trait. However, if the clefting is associated with a recognized genetic syndrome in which the genes are dominant rather than recessive, the chance of inheritance becomes 50%. Clefting may also result from environmental disruptions in development. These disruptions may be triggered by drugs, tobacco, or the **rubella** virus. The mother's diet during pregnancy may also affect the likelihood of clefting. This critical fusion stage takes place very early in the pregnancy, before many women even find out they are pregnant, so they may not yet have stopped using substances that may be harmful to the fetus or begun taking prenatal **vitamins**.

Clefting is apparent upon examination immediately after birth. The extent of the deformity varies with the severity of the cleft lip or palate.

Clefts may be repaired with reconstructive surgery that closes the palate and returns the lip to its normal position. Cleft lip defects may be repaired shortly after birth, but many doctors prefer to operate on infants according to the "rule of 10": when the child is at least 10 weeks old and weighs at least 10 pounds. While repair of the cleft lip is usually successful in one operation, a second operation may be performed later to refine the scar. Repair of a cleft palate is performed in a series of operations not usually completed by the time the child is two years old. If the defect lies primarily in the forward, bony portion of the palate (called the hard palate), doctors may wait to operate until the child is between five and seven years old and has more bone growth.

Nonsurgical treatment of a cleft palate is available for patients who do not want surgery or who are at high risk in surgery. One option is a prosthetic appliance worn as an artificial palate.

Later, the child will need orthodontic treatment to realign the structures of the mouth for proper function. The child may also need speech therapy to produce intelligible sounds with cleft-affected anatomy.

Children with clefts are also vulnerable to frequent ear infections. Their Eustachian tubes do not effectively drain fluid from the middle ear to the mouth, so fluid accumulates, pressure builds, and infection sets in. These children must have drainage tubes inserted into their ears to prevent **hearing loss**.

Children born with cleft lips and palates who become unduly self-conscious of their appearance and speech differences may benefit from psychological therapy. Parents who suffer guilt over their child's birth defect may also find help in professional counseling.

With reconstructive surgery, orthodontic treatment, and speech therapy, the effects of clefting may be minimized. Breathing, eating, and speech are also greatly improved with treatment. With the anatomical structures corrected and their functions restored, a child born with a cleft lip and/or palate may lead a normal life.

No known means of preventing clefting in a developing baby is known, although early pregnancy detection and good prenatal care, including prenatal vitamins and the avoidance of harmful substances appear to reduce the risk. Couples with an incidence of clefting in their families may wish to consult a genetic counselor.

CLINICAL TRIALS

According to the **National Institutes of Health**, a clinical trial is "a research study to answer specific questions about vaccines or new therapies or new ways of using known treatments." These studies allow researchers to determine whether new drugs or treatments are safe and effective. When conducted carefully, clinical trials can provide fast and safe answers to these questions.

Ideas for clinical trials usually originate with medical researchers. After researchers have tested new therapies or procedures in their own laboratories, they begin planning first-phase clinical trials if the new therapies or procedures seem to hold promise. Tests on humans are carried out only if laboratory and animal studies show promising results.

Clinical trials must adhere to a set of rules called protocols. The protocols define the requirements for participating in the trial; the schedules of tests, procedures, medications, and dosages; and the duration of the study. In the course of the clinical trial, the research staff monitors the health of the participants and ascertains the safety and effectiveness of the treatment.

Clinical trials involving experimental drugs proceed through four phases: In Phase I, researchers conduct their first tests on from 20 to 80 volunteers in order to evaluate the drug's safety, determine a safe dosage range, and identify side effects. In Phase II, the drug under study is given to a larger population (100-300 volunteer patients) to test its effectiveness and to acquire further data about its safety. In Phase III, the study drug is administered to an even larger group of patients (1,000-3,000) to further study the drug's effectiveness, monitor its side effects, compare it to other commonly used treatments, and collect data that will allow the drug to be used safely. Phase IV clinical studies are conducted after the drug has been marketed to collect information about its effect in various populations and about any side effects associated with long-term use.

The federal government has established strict guidelines and instituted safeguards to protect participants in clinical trials. All clinical trials carried out in the United States must be approved and monitored by an independent committee of physicians, statisticians, community advocates, and others to ensure that the clinical trial is ethical and that the rights of study participants are protected. Federal regulations require that any institution that conducts or supports biomedical research on human beings have such a committee in place to initially approve and periodically review the research.

Participants in clinical trials must be informed about the key facts of the clinical trial before they decide whether or not to participate. These facts include the purpose of the research; the goal of the research; the plan and duration of the trial; any potential risks; potential benefits; as well as the existence of any alternative treatments. In addition, the participant in the clinical trial must be informed that he or she has the right to withdraw from the trial at any time.

All clinical trials place restrictions on who can participate in the program based on such factors as age, type of disease, medical history, and current medical condition. Some clinical trials need volunteers with illnesses or conditions to be studied in the clinical trial, whereas Phase I trials, vaccine studies, and research on preventive care may seek healthy volunteers.

Clinical trials are sponsored by government agencies such as the National Institutes of Health; pharmaceutical companies; individual physicians; health care institutions; and organizations that develop medical devices or equipment. Trials typically take place in hospitals, universities, doctors' offices, and community clinics.

Controls, i.e., standards by which experimental observations are evaluated, play an important role in clinical research. In many clinical studies, participants in a control group receive an inactive pill, liquid, or powder (a placebo) that has no treatment value instead of an active drug or treatment. This is because experimental treatments are often compared with placebos to assess the treatment's effectiveness. If the clinical trial is blind or masked, participants are not informed whether they are in the experimental or control group. In double-blind or double-masked studies, neither the participants nor the study staff know which participants are receiving the experimental treatment and which ones are receiving either a standard treatment or placebo.

See also Drug safety; Hospitals; Vaccination

Clubfoot

Clubfoot is a deformity in which one or both feet are twisted into an abnormal position at birth. The condition is also known as talipes. True clubfoot is characterized by abnormal bone formation in the foot. There are four variations of clubfoot, known as talipes varus, talipes valgus, talipes equinus, and talipes calcaneus. In talipes varus the foot generally turns inward so that the leg and foot look somewhat like the letter J. In talipes valgus the foot rotates outward like the letter L. In talipes equinus, the foot points downward, similar to a toe dancer. Finally, in talipes calcaneus, the foot points upward, with the heel pointing down. Talipes varus is the most common form of clubfoot.

Clubfoot is relatively common and occurs more often in boys than in girls. It can affect one foot or both. Sometimes a child's feet appear abnormal at birth because of the way the fetus was positioned before birth. If there is no anatomic abnormality of the bone, it is not true clubfoot and can usually be corrected by applying special braces or casts to straighten the foot.

The cause of clubfoot is unclear, but is probably the result of several related factors, not one single cause. A combination of genetic and environmental factors, such as infections or drugs that may affect prenatal growth, seem to be responsible for the condition.

True clubfoot is usually obvious at birth. Uncorrected clubfoot in an adult causes only part of the foot, usually the outer edge, the heel, or the toes, to touch the ground. For a person with clubfoot, walking is difficult or impossible.

True clubfoot is usually obvious on **physical examination**. Diagnosis of clubfoot is confirmed by a routine x ray of the foot that shows the bones are malformed or misaligned. Ultrasonography does not always reveal the presence of club foot prior to the birth of the child.

The sooner the treatment of clubfoot is started after birth the better, since an infant's foot contains large amounts of cartilage and the muscles, ligaments, and tendons are supple. In one common treatment, a series of casts is applied over a period of months to reposition the foot into a normal alignment. In mild cases, splinting and wearing braces at night may correct the deformity. In the most severe cases, surgery may be required, especially when the Achilles tendon needs to be lengthened. When clubfoot is severe enough to require surgery, the condition is usually not completely correctable, although significant improvement is possible. Long-term care by an orthopedist (a doctor who specializes in treatment of the skeletal system and its associated muscles and joints) is required after initial treatment to ensure that the correction of the deformity is maintained. Exercises,corrective shoes, or nighttime splints may be needed until the child stops growing.

With prompt, expert treatment, clubfoot is usually correctable. Most individuals are able to wear regular shoes and lead active lives. If clubfoot is left untreated, the deformity becomes fixed, the growth of the leg and foot is affected, and some level of permanent disability results.

Since the cause is unclear, there is no known prevention for clubfoot.

Coagulation disorders

Coagulation disorders deal with disruption of the body's ability to control blood clotting. The most commonly known coagulation disorder is **hemophilia**, a condition in which patients bleed for long periods of time before clotting. There are other coagulation disorders with a variety of causes.

Coagulation, or clotting, occurs as a complex process involving several components of the blood. Plasma, the fluid component of the blood, carries a number of proteins and coagulation factors that regulate bleeding. Platelets, small colorless fragments in the blood, initiate contraction of damaged blood vessels so that less blood is lost. They also help plug damaged blood vessels and work with plasma to accelerate blood clotting. A disorder affecting platelet production or one of the many steps in the entire process can disrupt clotting.

Coagulation disorders arise from different causes and produce different complications. There are several common coagulation disorders. Hemophilia, or hemophilia A (factor VIII deficiency), an inherited coagulation disorder, affects about 20,000 Americans. This genetic disorder is carried by females but most often affects males. Christmas disease, also known as hemophilia B or factor IX deficiency, is less common than hemophilia A with similar in symptoms. Disseminated intravascular coagulation disorder, also known as consumption coagulopathy, occurs as a result of other diseases and conditions. This disease accelerates clotting, which can actually cause hemorrhage. **Thrombocytopenia** is the most common cause of coagulation disorder. It is characterized by a lack of circulating platelets in the blood. This disease also includes idiopathic thrombocytopenia. Von Willebrand's disease is a hereditary disorder with prolonged bleeding time due to a clotting factor deficiency and impaired platelet function. It is the most common hereditary coagulation disorder. Hypoprothrombinemia is a congenital deficiency of clotting factors that can lead to hemorrhage. Other coagulation disorders include factor XI deficiency, also known as hemophilia C, and factor VII deficiency. Hemophilia C afflicts one in 100,000 people and is the second most common bleeding disorder among women. Factor VII is also called serum prothrombin conversion accelerator deficiency. One in 500,000 people may be afflicted with this disorder that is often diagnosed in newborns because of bleeding into the brain as a result of traumatic delivery.

Some coagulation disorders present symptoms such as severe bruising. Others will show no apparent symptoms, but carry the threat of severe internal bleeding.

Factor XI deficiency, or hemophilia C, occurs more frequently among certain ethnic groups, with an incidence of about 1 in 10,000 among Ashkenazi Jews. Nearly 50% of patients with this disorder experience no symptoms, but others may notice blood in their urine, nosebleeds, or bruising. Patients with factor VII deficiency vary greatly in their bleeding severity.

Several blood tests and other kinds of tests can be used to detect various coagulation disorders. In the case of acquired coagulation disorders, information such as prior or current diseases and medications is important in determining the cause of the blood disorder.

In mild cases, treatment may involve the use of drugs that stimulate the release of deficient clotting factors. In severe cases, bleeding may only stop if the clotting factor that is missing is replaced through infusion of donated human blood in the form of fresh frozen plasma or cryoprecipitate.

The prognosis for patients with mild forms of coagulation disorders is normally good. Many people can lead a normal life and maintain a normal life expectancy. Without treatment of bleeding episodes, severe muscle and joint pain, and eventually damage can occur. Any incident that causes blood to collect in the head, neck, or digestive system can be very serious and requires immediate attention. DIC can be severe enough to cause clots to form, and a stroke could occur. DIC is also serious enough to cause **gangrene** in the fingers, nose, or genitals. The prognosis depends on early intervention and treatment of the underlying condition. Hemorrhage from a coagulation disorder, particularly into the brain or digestive track, can prove fatal. In the past, patients who received regular transfusions of human blood products were subject to increased risk of acquired immunodeficiency syndrome (AIDS) and other diseases. However, efforts have been made since the early 1990s to ensure the safety of the blood supply.

Prevention of coagulation disorders varies. Acquired disorders may only be prevented by preventing onset of the underlying disorder (such as cirrhosis). Hereditary disorders can be predicted with prenatal testing and genetic counseling. Prevention of severe bleeding episodes may be accomplished by refraining from activities that could cause injury, such as contact sports. Open communication with healthcare providers prior to procedures or tests that could cause bleeding may prevent a severe bleeding incident.

CODEPENDENCY

Codependency **personality disorder** is a dysfunctional relationship with the self characterized by living through or for another, attempting to control and blame others, feeling victimized, attempting to ''fix'' others, and feeling intense anxiety around intimacy. It is very common in people raised in dysfunctional families, and in the partners and children of alcoholics and addicts. This pattern of compulsive, self-defeating, learned behaviors may often develop within more than one member of a dysfunctional family (or other social unit) in order to survive in a family that is experiencing great emotional pain and **stress**. Often these behaviors are passed on from generation to generation, continuing the destructive cycle of pain.

The idea of codependency emerged in the early 1970s in the field of chemical addiction first **alcoholism** and later drug **addiction**. Counselors began observing the alcoholic's negative impact on the family unit. In an effort to help the spouses and children of alcoholics, these counselors borrowed heavily from the theories and methods of marriage and family therapy.

Counselors found that in an alcoholic household, the spouse and children may in various ways unknowingly support the alcoholic's dependent behavior. For example, by becoming ''strong'' and responsible, a child may enable an alcoholic father to ''get away'' with irresponsible behavior. These family members were called ''co-alcoholics'' because, like the family member dependent on alcohol, they enabled the alcoholic to continue drinking. They, in fact, became as dependent as the abuser on the abuser's continuing addiction.

The alcoholic's manipulativeness often entangled family members in a web of unspoken and oppressive rules and regulations whose end result stifled open expression of feelings and direct confrontation with personal and interpersonal problems. Frustration and repressed anger was often associated with the seemingly mature and responsible caretaking behavior of the co-alcoholic. Co-alcoholics were viewed as less obviously disturbed than the alcoholic but often also in need of **counseling** or psychotherapy.

In the early 1970s, social scientists also became interested in the area of addiction and began conducting research on the effects of **substance abuse** on the family. These scientists later initiated investigations on compulsions other than chemical addictions, such as physical abuse, **sexual abuse**, extreme religiosity, and work addition, among others, as abusive patterns that could lead to what they labeled ''codependence'' in family members. This research led to the conclusion that individuals raised in such families experience identifiable emotional and behavioral problems in coping with adult life. The adult retains the wounds, the pain, the emotions, and the destructive behaviors that he or she learned as a child. Thus, codependent behaviors were found to arise as a result of any dysfunctional relationship or upbringing and to be caused by deprivation, abuse, or a lack of nurturing in childhood.

Although the term ''codependency'' gained increasing popularity in the 1990s and has even been called ''the most popular nonissue of the 1990s'' some therapists maintained that there was little evidence to support its existence as a bona fide psychiatric disorder.

On the other hand, opponents argued that America is a society largely characterized by emotionally disabling families and people who are inadequately prepared for adulthood. They felt that the term ''codependency'' is merely the effort of contemporary thinkers to describe a phenomenon that has been prevalent in American society for decades.

Although codependency has many identifiable symptoms, because the main symptom involves fixing or controlling others instead of facing internal pain, the codependent many never recognize his or her disease. To amplify the basic definition of the term, the emotional symptoms of codependency may include any of the following: stress, **depression**, anxiety; nervousness; irritability; alternation between lethargy and hyperactivity; loss of **self-esteem**; fear of independence; dysfunctional and entrapping relationships with family members, friends, and coworkers; isolation; emotional pain or emotional numbness; or even **suicidal** thoughts.

In addition to emotional problems, the codependent may also suffer from chronic physical ailments. These may include gastrointestinal disturbances, colitis, ulcers, migraine headaches, nonspecific rashes and skin problems, high blood pressure, and other stress-related physical illnesses.

One irony can be that as much as a codependent feels responsibility for others and needs to take care of them, he or she believes deep down that other people are responsible for him, blaming others for his unhappiness and problems. Another irony is that while he feels controlled by people and events, he himself is overly controlling. He is afraid to allow other people to be unique and independent individuals and to let events unfold naturally and spontaneously. His world is rigid, inflexible, and he takes comfort in routine.

An ''expert'' in knowing best how things should turn out and how people should behave, the codependent person tries to control others through overt or covert threats, coercion, compulsive advice giving, helplessness, guilt, manipulation, or domination.

Aside from compulsive behaviors such as perfectionism or workaholism, individuals suffering from alcohol or drug-related codependency often feel caught up in a kind of treadmill existence. Whether or not they achieve their goals, they feel driven to achieve more and have an anxious feeling of incompleteness or emptiness regardless of what they accomplish.

Most therapeutic approaches to codependency stress awareness as the first step in recovery; the second step is acceptance. Many treatment modalities approach codependency as an addiction, since codependents have as much difficulty accepting their powerlessness over people and events as substance abusers over their drug of choice. Ongoing therapy and a twelve-step program such as that offered by Co-Dependents Anonymous are often recommended.

See also Alcohol use and abuse; Substance abuse and dependence

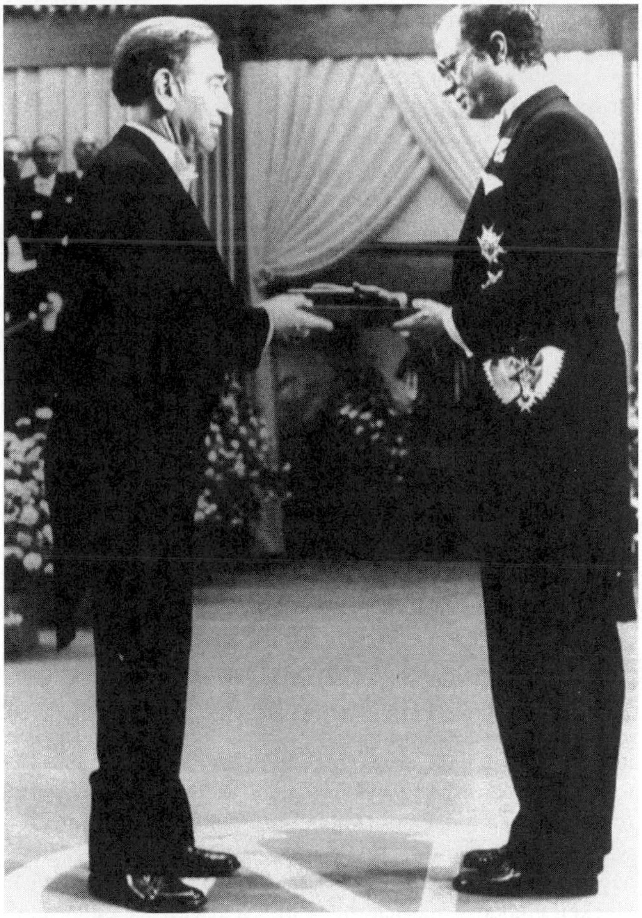

Stanley Cohen (left) accepting the Nobel Prize.

Cohen, Stanley (1922-)

American biochemist

A pioneer in the study of growth factors—the nutrients that differentiate the development of cells—Stanley Cohen is best known for isolating nerve growth factor (NGF), the first known growth factor, and for subsequently discovering and fully identifying the epidermal growth factor (EGF). Cohen shared the 1986 Nobel Prize for physiology or medicine with his colleague, Italian American neurobiologist **Rita Levi-Montalcini**, who first discovered NGF. Research on NGF has led to better understanding of such degenerative disorders as **cancer** and **Alzheimer's disease**, while studies concerning

EGF have proved useful in exploring alternative burn treatments and skin transplants.

Cohen was born in Brooklyn, New York, in 1922 to Russian immigrant parents. Though his father earned only a modest living as a tailor, both parents, Louis and Fannie (Feitel) Cohen, ensured that their four children received quality educations. As a child, Cohen was stricken with **polio**, imparting him with a permanent limp. His illness, however, influenced him to pursue intellectual interests. While a student at James Madison High School he earnestly studied science as well as classical music, learning to play the clarinet. Cohen entered Brooklyn College to study chemistry and zoology, graduating in 1943 with a B.A. Following his undergraduate studies, Cohen received a scholarship to Oberlin college in Ohio, where he earned an M.A. in zoology in 1945. He then attended the University of Michigan on a teaching fellowship in biochemistry, earning his Ph.D. in 1948.

From 1948 until 1952, Cohen worked at the University of Colorado School of Medicine in Denver, holding a research and teaching position in the Department of Biochemistry and Pediatrics. There Cohen earned the respect of his peers for his collaborative studies with pediatrician Harry H. Gordon on the metabolic functions of creatinine (a chemical found in blood, muscle tissue, and urine) in newborn infants. Cohen moved to St. Louis, Missouri, in 1952 to work as a postdoctoral fellow in the radiology department at Washington University. The following year, he was asked to become a research associate in the laboratory of renowned zoologist Viktor Hamburger, who was conducting studies on growth processes. Levi-Montalcini, who had been researching nerve cell growth in chicken embryos that had been injected with the tumor cells of male mice, had just returned from Rio de Janeiro, where she had conducted successful tissue culture experiments that definitively proved the existence of NGF. Working at the lab in St. Louis, Levi-Montalcini relied on Cohen's expertise in biochemistry to isolate and analyze NGF.

The collaboration between Levi-Montalcini and Cohen combined two similar personalities. Both scientists have been characterized by their unassuming manners despite their obvious intellectual abilities and perceptive intuitions. Describing her early recollections of Cohen, Levi-Montalcini wrote in her autobiography *In Praise of Imperfection,* "I had been immediately struck by Stan's absorbed expression, total disregard for appearances—as evidenced by his motley attire—and modesty.... He never mentioned his competence and extraordinary intuition which always guided him with infallible precision in the right direction." Between the years 1953 and 1959, Cohen and Levi-Montalcini conducted intense research, both enthusiastically pursuing thier findings concerning NGF.

By 1956 Cohen had succeeded in extracting NGF from a mouse tumor; however, this proved to be a difficult substance to work with. Upon the suggestion of biochemist Arthur Kornberg, Cohen added snake venom to the extract, hoping to break down the nucleic acids that made the extract too gelatinous. Fortuitously, the snake venom produced more nerve growth activity than the tumor extract itself, and Cohen was able to proceed more rapidly with his studies. In 1958 he discovered that an abundant source of NGF could be found in the salivary glands of male mice—glands not unlike the venom sacs of snakes. Cohen's biochemical advances enabled Levi-Montalcini to study the neurological effects of NGF in rodents.

At a time when Levi-Montalcini and Cohen were advancing rapidly in their collaborative research, funding for Hamburger's laboratory could no longer support Cohen. Before leaving Washington University, Cohen was able to purify NGF as well as produce an antibody for it; however, its complete chemical structure was not fully determined until 1970 when researchers at Washington University completed analysis of NGF's two identical chains of amino acids. Before departing St. Louis, Cohen also observed an unusual occurrence in newborn rodents that had been injected with unpurified salivary NGF. Unlike control mice, whose eyes opened on the thirteenth or fourteenth day, those injected with the unpurified NGF opened their eyes on the seventh day; they also sprouted teeth earlier than did the control group.

Cohen left Washington University in 1959 to join a research group at Vanderbilt University in Nashville, Tennessee; there he continued his work with growth factors, focusing on identifying the unknown factor in unpurified NGF that had caused the mice to open their eyes earlier than normal. By 1962, Cohen had extracted the contaminant in these samples of NGF and was able to purify a second substance, a protein that promoted skin cell and cornea growth which he called epidermal growth factor, or EGF. This protein has found widespread use in treating severe burns; a solution rich in EGF can promote the speedy healing of burned skin, while a skin graft soaked in EGF will quickly bond with damaged tissue. Cohen also isolated the protein which acted as a receptor for EGF—an important step toward understanding the transmission of signals that stimulate normal and abnormal cell growth—that has been particularly crucial in studying cancer development. Cohen was successful in fully identifying the amino acid sequence of EGF by 1972.

Despite his significant contributions, Cohen has never managed a large laboratory, and for many years his work went unacknowledged. He remarked in *Science* that while the scientific community took little notice of his early studies on growth factors, this anonymity proved beneficial. "People left you alone and you weren't competing with the world," he recalled. "The disadvantage was that you had to convince people that what you were working with was real." Cohen's work has subsequently gained wide recognition, and he has received numerous awards in addition to the Nobel, including the Alfred P. Sloan Award in 1982, as well as both the National Medal of Science and the Albert Lasker Award in 1986.

COHN, FERDINAND JULIUS (1828-1898)

German bacteriologist, plant pathologist

Cohn, the first scientist to define and systematically classify bacteria, is considered a founder of modern bacteriology. He is also noteworthy for providing critical support to others in the fledgling science, including the Nobel Prize-winning **Robert Koch**.

Born to Jewish parents in 1828 in the Prussian city of Breslau (now Wroclaw, Poland), Cohn was a child prodigy reportedly able to read and write before his second birthday. He was admitted to the University of Breslau at the age of 14, but because of anti-Semitic feelings in Prussia, he was never granted a degree there even though he successfully undertook four years of studies.

Instead, Cohn completed his studies at the University of Berlin, where he studied under the prominent physiologist Johannes Peter Müller. When revolution swept Europe in 1848, Cohn kept his liberal tendencies to himself and kept involved in his studies. In September, 1849, he wrote a rather anguished entry in his journal: "Germany dead; France dead; Italy dead; Hungary dead; only cholera and court-martials immortal. I have retired from this unfriendly outside world, buried myself in my books and studies; seeing few people, learning much, only inspired by nature." That year, Cohn's immersion in serious study was awarded with a doctorate in botanical studies.

However, continued anti-Semitism and Cohn's liberal politics forced him back to the University of Breslau, where he was allowed to work in the Physiological Institute, and in 1859 became professor of botany.

Cohn's initial research interests were simple forms of plant life: algae and fungi. However, over time his fascination with plant diseases evolved into an interest in bacteria. He noticed that both plant and animal cells consist of protoplasmic material that is essentially identical, and was the first to state that bacteria are plants, not animals, as previously considered.

In 1872, Cohn published *Researches on Bacteria,* a landmark, three-volume treatise that contained the first systematic classification of bacteria. Cohn identified the six classes of bacteria: *Bacillus, Bacterium, Micrococcus, Spirillium, Spirochaete* and *Vibrio.* He discovered spores, tiny reproductive bodies produced by plants and bacteria, which Cohn identified as living bridges between the plant and animal worlds. Another important observation was that bacteria were capable of surviving high temperatures.

Cohn's work, combined with other discoveries by **Louis Pasteur** and the English physicist John Tyndall eventually discredited the theory of spontaneous generation, which held that living organisms could develop from nonliving matter.

In an 1873 publication, *Bacteria, the Smallest of Living Organisms,* Cohn dramatically stated that bacteria "rule with demoniacal power over the weal and woe, and even over the life and death of man." It was highly likely, he said, that "already identified bacteria are in many diseases the conveyors and originators of infection, that they are the ferment of contagion...We have the firm conviction that to a more thorough and clearer knowledge of these facts will be joined the discovery of new methods by which to encounter the fearful enemy with better success than hitherto," Cohn accurately predicted.

In addition to his other accomplishments, Cohn established the world's first plant physiology institute at Breslau in 1866. He also founded a journal, *Contributions on Plant Biology,* that chronicled the earliest years of modern bacteriology.

One of his greatest contributions to science, however, was an indirect one. In 1876, an unknown rural doctor named Robert Koch came to Cohn, convinced he had discovered the cause of anthrax, a livestock disease that can be transmitted to humans, causing pneumonia and skin ulcers. Cohn recognized Koch's work as authoritative. He published the discovery in his new journal and introduced the country physician to the scientific research community. With support from Cohn, Koch went on to discover the bacterial causes for cholera and tuberculosis, receiving the Nobel Prize in 1905.

COHNHEIM, JULIUS FRIEDRICH (1839-1884)

German pathologist

Julius Friedrich Cohnheim, a Prussin-born German pathologist, had solved a medical puzzle that vexed scientists for 13 centuries the origin of pus. Cohnheim discovered that pus is the green/yellow liquid that seeps into injured body tissues that is made up of white blood cells that migrate through the walls of capillaries. Cohnheim wrote upon his discovery that "...The so-called pus cells...are colorless blood corpuscles, which forced their way out of the blood vessels..." adding: "There is no inflammation without the participation of blood vessels."

Born in 1839 in Demmin in northern Prussia (present-day Poland), Cohnheim began his medical studies at the University of Berlin when he was 17. Because pursuing his education.

In Berlin, Cohnheim studied under **Rudolf Virchow**, who was considered the father of cellular pathology. Cohnheim's doctoral dissertation, written under Virchow's supervision, investigated inflammation in serous membranes. He was one of a number of Virchow's students who equaled or surpassed their master. Disproving Virchow's belief that pus originated in nearby connective tissues, Cohnheim found that the thick liquid, made up largely of debris from disintegrated white blood corpuscles, was much more than a local phenomenon. Rather, it was produced by a dynamic process that involved the whole body. "It seems to me that the enormous production of pus-corpuscles will be decidedly easier of comprehension if we be permitted to regard the whole organism as concerned in it, and not merely that portion in which the inflammation has been established," he observed.

From 1868 to 1872, Cohnheim worked in Kiel as a pathology professor, after which he occupied a similar post in Breslau. There, Cohnheim was present when Robert Koch presented his ground-breaking discovery of the **anthrax** germ. This development encouraged Cohnheim to continue his own search for the bacteria behind **tuberculosis** and **cholera**. When Koch eventually discovered the tuberculosis bacillus, he drew on some of Cohnheim's research on rabbit eyes.

Cohnheim's accomplishments included creating and managing a pathology institute at Breslau and writing a popular two-volume textbook, *Lectures on General Pathology.* During the German-Danish War in 1864, he served with the Prussian Army as a surgeon.

Cohnheim also made a variety of important initial contributions to the other related areas of science. He was one of the first pathologists to observe inflammation through the microscope, studying injured blood vessels in transparent membranes from the tongues of frogs and the mesentery, a double-layered membrane connecting the small intestine, stomach, spleen, pancreas and other abdominal organs. Cohnheim made an important contribution to laboratory science, developing the still-in-use technique of freezing fresh body tissues and then slicing them into thin sections for examination under a microscope. His other investigations included studies of nerve endings, coronary arteries, the structure of muscle fibre, cancer of the fibula (a bone in the lower leg), and fatal trichinosis (a disease caused by eating insufficiently cooked meat containing nematode worms). He also provided an early description of a paradoxical phenomenon in which the movement of a blood clot can be influenced by a large hole between the atrial chambers of the heart (atrial septal defect).

In 1878 he moved from Kiel to the University of Leipzig. During the final decade of his life there, Cohnheim suffered from gouty arthritis that resisted treatment and confined him to a chair or bed. He died from complications of the disease in 1884, at the age of 45. A pathologist to the end, he allowed a postmortem dissection of his body to reveal the nature of his gout.

Cold sore

A cold sore is a fluid-filled blister that usually appears at the edge of the lips. Other names for a cold sore are fever blister, oral herpes, labial herpes, herpes labialis, and herpes febrilis. Cold sores do not usually form inside the mouth except for the very first time they occur, which distinguishes them from the common canker sores.

Cold sores are caused by a herpes virus. There are eight different kinds of human herpes viruses. Only two of these, herpes simplex, types 1 and 2, can cause cold sores. It is commonly believed that herpes simplex virus type 1 infects above the waist and herpes simplex virus type 2 infects below the waist. This is not completely true. Both herpes virus type 1 and type 2 can cause herpes lesions on the lips or genitals, but recurrent cold sores are almost always type 1.

Oral herpes is very common. More than 60% of Americans have had a cold sore, and almost 25% of those infected experience recurrent outbreaks. Most people who have had cold sores became infected before age 10. Anyone can become infected by herpes virus and once infected, the virus remains latent for life. Herpes viruses are spread from person to person by direct skin-to-skin contact. The highest risk for spreading the virus is the time period beginning with the appearance of blisters and ending with scab formation. However, infected persons need not have visible blisters to spread the infection to others, since the virus may be present in the saliva without obvious oral lesions.

Viruses are different from bacteria. While bacteria are independent and can reproduce on their own, viruses enter human cells and force them to make more virus. The infected human cell is usually killed and releases thousands of new viruses. The cell death and resulting tissue damage cause the actual cold sores. In addition, herpes virus can infect a cell, and instead of making the cell produce new viruses, it hides inside the cell and waits. Herpes virus hides in the nervous system. This is called latency and may last days, months, or even years. At some future time, the virus ''awakens'' and causes the cell to produce thousands of new viruses, which sparks an active infection.

Active infections that follow periods of latency are called ''recurrent'' infections. Although it is unknown what triggers latent virus to activate, several conditions seem to bring on infections. These include **stress**, illness, tiredness, exposure to sunlight, menstruation, fever, and diet.

While anyone can be infected by herpes virus, not everyone will show symptoms. The first symptoms of herpes occur within 2-20 days after contact with an infected person. Symptoms of the primary infection are usually more severe than those of recurrent infections. The primary infection can cause symptoms like other viral infections including tiredness, **headache**, fever, and swollen lymph nodes in the neck.

Typically, 50-80% of persons with oral herpes experience a prodrome (symptoms of oncoming disease) of pain, burning, **itching**, or tingling at the site where blisters will form. This prodromal stage may last anywhere from a few hours, to one to two days. The herpes infection prodrome occurs in both the primary infection and recurrent infections.

In 95% of the patients with cold sores, the blisters occur at the outer edge of the lips which is called the ''vermilion border.'' Less often, blisters form on the nose, chin, or cheek. Following the prodrome, the disease process is rapid. First, small red bumps appear which quickly form fluid-filled blisters. The painful blisters may either burst and form a scab or dry up and form a scab. Within two days of the first red bumps, all the blisters have formed scabs. The skin heals completely and without scarring within six to ten days.

Some children have a very serious primary (first episode) herpes infection called ''gingivostomatitis.'' This causes fever, swollen lymph glands, and numerous blisters inside the mouth, and on the lips and tongue which may form large, open sores. These painful sores may last up to three weeks and can make eating and drinking difficult. Because of this, young children with gingivostomatitis are at risk for **dehydration**.

Most people experience fewer than two recurrent outbreaks of cold sores each year. Some people never experience outbreaks, whereas some have very frequent outbreaks. In most people, the blisters form in the same area each time and are triggered by the same factors (such as stress, sun exposure, etc.).

Because oral herpes is so common, it is diagnosed primarily by symptoms. Laboratory tests may be performed to confirm the diagnosis.

There is no cure for herpes virus infections. There are **antiviral drugs** available which have some effect in lessening the symptoms and decreasing the length of herpes outbreaks. There is evidence that some may also prevent future outbreaks. Acyclovir (Zovirax) is the drug of choice for herpes infection and can be given intravenously or taken by mouth. It can be applied directly to sores as an ointment but is less effective in this form.

Oral herpes can be painful and embarrassing but it is not a serious infection. There is no cure for oral herpes, but outbreaks usually occur less frequently after age 35. The spread of herpes virus to the eyes is very serious. Herpes virus can infect the cells in the cornea and cause scarring which may impair vision.

The only way to prevent oral herpes is to avoid contact with infected persons. But because many people are not aware that they are infected, they can easily infect others. As of early 1998 there were no herpes vaccines available, although herpes vaccines are being tested. Good health and hygiene, in addition to minimizing contact with infected people, may help to reduce outbreaks of cold sores and herpes.

Colic

Colic is persistent, unexplained crying in a healthy baby between two weeks and five months of age.

Colic, which is not a disease, affects 10-20% of all infants. It is more common in boys than in girls and most common in a family's first child. Symptoms of colic usually appear when a baby is 14-21 days old, reach a crescendo at the age of three months, and disappear within the next eight weeks. Episodes occur frequently but intermittently and usually begin with prolonged periods of crying in the late afternoon or evening. They can last for just a few minutes or continue for several hours. Some babies who have colic are simply fussy. Others cry so hard that their faces turn red, then pale.

No one knows what causes colic. The condition may be the result of swallowing large amounts of air, which becomes trapped in the digestive tract and causes bloating and severe abdominal **pain**. Other possible causes of colic include an immature digestive-tract, intolerance to certain foods, hunger or overfeeding, lack of sleep, loneliness, overheated milk or formula, overstimulation resulting from noise, light, or activity, and tension.

During a colicky episode, babies' bellies often look swollen, feel hard, and make a rumbling sound. Crying intensifies, tapers off, then gets louder. Many babies grow rigid, clench their fists, curl their toes, and draw their legs toward their body. A burp or a bowel movement can end an attack. Most babies who have colic don't seem to be in pain between attacks.

Pediatricians and family physicians suspect colic in an infant who has cried loudly for at least three hours a day at least three times a week for three weeks or longer; is not hungry but cries for several hours between dinnertime and midnight; demonstrates the clenched fists, rigidity, and other physical traits associated with colic.

The baby's medical history and a parent's description of eating, sleeping, and crying patterns are used to confirm a diagnosis of colic. **Physical examination** and laboratory tests are used to rule out infection, intestinal blockage, and other conditions that can cause abdominal pain and other colic-like symptoms.

Medications do not cure colic. Doctors sometimes recommend simethicone to relieve gas pain but generally advise parents to take a practical approach to the problem.

Gently massaging the baby's back can release a trapped gas bubble, and holding the baby in a sitting position can help prevent air from being swallowed during feedings. Bottle-fed babies can swallow air if nipple holes are either too large or too small. Nipple-hole size can be checked by filling a bottle with cold formula, turning it upside down, and counting the number of drops released when it is shaken or squeezed. A nipple hole that is the right size will release about one drop of formula every second. Babies should not be fed every time they cry, but feeding and burping a baby more often may alleviate symptoms of colic. A bottle-fed baby should be burped after every ounce, and a baby who is breastfeeding should be burped every five minutes.

When cow's milk is the source of the symptoms, bottle-fed babies should be switched to a soy-milk hydrolyzed protein formula. A woman whose baby is breastfeeding should eliminate dairy products from her diet for seven days, then gradually reintroduce them unless the baby's symptoms reappear.

Since intolerance to foods other than cow's milk may also lead to symptoms of colic, breastfeeding women may also relieve their babies' colic by eliminating coffee, cocoa, citrus, peanuts, wheat, and broccoli and other vegetables belonging to the cabbage family from their diet.

Rocking a baby in a quiet, darkened room can prevent overstimulation, and a baby usually calms down when cuddled in a warm, soft blanket. Colicky babies cry less when they are soothed by the motion of a wind-up swing, a car ride, or being carried in a parent's arms. Pacifiers can soothe babies who are upset, but a pacifier should never be attached to a string.

A doctor should be notified if a baby who has been diagnosed with colic develops a rectal **fever** higher than 101°F (38.3°C), cries for more than four hours, vomits, has **diarrhea** or stools that are black or bloody, loses weight, or eats less than normal.

Colic is distressing, but it is not dangerous. Symptoms almost always disappear before a child is six months old.

Many doctors believe that colic cannot be prevented. Some alternative practitioners, however, feel that colic can be prevented by an awareness of food intolerances and their impact.

Colombo, Realdo (1516?-1559)

Italian anatomist

Realdo Colombo was one of the first anatomists in the Western world to describe pulmonary circulation, observing that blood travels between the right and left ventricles of the heart by way of the lungs. Previously, it was believed that blood traveled through a hidden passage (or passages) connecting the ventricles.

Although two other Europeans wrote about this phenomenon around the same time, it was Colombo's book, *The 15 Books Written Concerning Anatomy,* that directly influenced seventeenth-century anatomist **William Harvey**'s concept of the heart as a pump circulating blood throughout the body.

Son of a pharmacist based in Cremona, Italy, Colombo initially followed his father's trade before undertaking studies in Milan, Venice and then in Padua. Colombo earned his M.D. degree in 1544. At the University of Padua, he studied medicine under another famed anatomist, Andreas Vesalius, eventually becoming his assistant. In 1544, he succeeded Vesalius as lecturer on anatomy and surgery. From 1545 to 1559, Colombo taught in Pisa and at the Sapienza in Rome. Additionally, in 1550 he was appointed a surgeon to the Pope. Throughout Colombo's career as a lecturer, many distinguished persons, including ambassadors, cardinals, and archbishops, attended his lectures.

The phenomenon of pulmonary circulation, also known as the lesser circulation, was first reported in the thriteenth century by the Syrian doctor Ibn al-Nafis. Some of Ibn al-Nafis' writings were translated into Latin during the Renaissance, but his observations about blood circulation were apparently never read by Colombo or his European counterparts, who subscribed to the ancient Roman belief that a passage existed through the septum, a thick muscular partition separating the ventricles of the heart. Anyone questioning this concept of the heart risked being accused of heresy by religious leaders who considered the organ to have spiritual properties. However, Vesalius wrote in 1543 that the septum appeared to contain no passages, prompting Colombo to wonder how blood actually traveled between the ventricles, if not through the septum.

Much of Colombo's knowledge of anatomy was obtained by the now controversial practice of **vivisection**: he dissected live animals, paying particular attention to the movements of their lungs and heart. He also dissected as many as 14 human cadavers a year.

Through these experiments, Colombo determined that blood traveled between the two sections of the heart through the lungs. Colombo wrote, "Between the ventricles there is a dividing wall... Almost everyone assumes that the blood passes from the right ventricle into the left across this wall....But they are completely wrong. For the blood is conducted to the lungs by the pulmonary artery, where it is diluted and together with air is led from the left ventricle by the pulmonary veins, which no one has noticed until now, nor described in writing, although everyone should take particular notice of this fact."

Colombo's dissections allowed him to make other important observations. The Greek scientist **Aristotle** had taught that the left ventricle contained cold blood, whereas the right ventricle contained warm blood. Contradicting this, Colombo observed: "In the left ventricle you can feel for yourself that the heat is so intense that the hand cannot possibly endure it." He also noticed that the active phase of the heart was in systole (contraction), not in diastole (dilation) as was previously believed. These discoveries were crucial to Harvey, who credited Colombo's work in his landmark book, *On the Motion of the Heart and Blood in Animals.*

However, whether Colombo was actually the first Western anatomist to observe the pulmonary circulation is subject to controversy. Juan Valverde, a former student of Colombo, accurately described pulmonary circulation in a 300-page book published in 1556, three years before Colombo's book. However, it is known that Valverde had attended lectures in Padua between 1544 and 1546 at which Colombo revealed his discovery. Valverde is also accused of heavily plagiarizing Vesalius.

Less easily dismissed is an incidental but quite accurate reference to the lesser circulation in a theological work published by the Spanish theologian and physician Miguel Serveto in 1553. That book, *The Restoration of Christianity,* had actually been written much earlier, as Servetus had sent a manuscript copy to the religious reformer John Calvin in 1546. It is known, however, that Servetus and Vesalius had studied together in Paris during the previous decade.

In any case, Colombo's concept of the pulmonary circulation is considered the fullest and most authoritative of his day.

COLON THERAPY

Colon therapy refers to flushing water through the entire length of the colon or large intestine. It is also called colon hydrotherapy or colonic irrigation.

Colon therapy is performed in order to eliminate wastes that have accumulated in the colon and to promote a better-functioning large intestine. It is believed that colon therapy can relieve a score of symptoms from gas, bloating, and **constipation** to depression, **insomnia**, and **headaches**. Colon therapy also is used to administer therapeutic substances via the mucous membranes of the colon.

Colon therapy is not recommended for people suffering from heart or kidney disease, **cancer**, or diseases of the colon, including diverticulitis, Crohn's disease, or ulcerative colitis. A colon therapist should always use disposable tubing to reduce the risk of infection.

Colon therapy is usually administered by a trained colon hydrotherapist or colon hygiene technician in a clinic or spa. The procedure takes about one hour. The patient lies on their back and the therapist inserts a plastic tube into the anus. Either plain filtered water or water to which herbs, enzymes, oxygen, or other therapeutic agents are added is pumped into the rectum either by relying on gravity or by a mechanical device. The water is kept at body temperature. During a session, a total of 20-35 gallons of water can be flushed through the entire length of the colon through a process of filling and releasing. Sometimes, the water is held inside the colon for a designated period of time while the therapist massages the abdomen to enhance waste removal. Waste is then eliminated. Sometimes it is necessary to undergo several colon therapy sessions for a complete colon cleansing.

There have been reports of significant and sometimes fatal water and salt imbalances resulting from colon therapy. In these cases, people became weak, developed fluid in their lungs, suffered convulsions, and died. Combining **fasting** with colon therapy may increase the risk of a dangerous fluid imbalance. With improper technique, the tubes could tear the colon. If equipment is not properly sterilized, bacterial contamination can result in infection.

Relief from constipation may result. Many clients treated claim their headaches, arthritis, and other aches and **pains** were banished.

COLOR BLINDNESS

Color blindness is the word used to describe mild to severe difficulties with identifying various colors and shades of colors. It is a misleading term because colorblind people are not blind. Rather, they tend to confuse some colors, and a rare few may not see colors at all.

Normal color vision requires the use of special cells, called cones, located in the retina of the eye. There are three types of cones, termed red, blue, and green, which enable people to see a large spectrum of colors. A defect or deficiency of any of the types of cones will result in abnormal color vision.

Red/green color blindness is the most common deficiency, affecting 8% of Caucasian males and 0.5% of females. People with red/green color blindness can often distinguish red or green if they can visually compare the colors. For example, they can pick out red or green from a package of colored pencils. However, if handed a red pencil, they cannot tell what color the pencil is.

Blue color blindness, which is rare, is an inability to distinguish both blue and yellow. Blue and yellow are seen as white or grey. Although as many females as males have this deficiency, it usually appears in people who have physical disorders, such as **liver disease** or **diabetes mellitus**. However, it is not uncommon for young boys to have blue/green confusion that becomes less pronounced in adulthood.

Total color blindness is called achromatopsia. This very rare hereditary disorder results in vision that is black, white, and shades of gray. It affects one person in 33,000 in the United States, males and females equally. People with achromatopsia usually have poor visual acuity and extreme sensitivity to light. Their vision is significantly impaired, and they protect their light-sensitive eyes by squinting in even ordinary light.

The symptom of color blindness is the long-term inability to distinguish colors or notice some colors entirely. Most cases of color blindness are inherited, affecting males almost exclusively. But a number of other causes can also lead to color blindness.

Alzheimer's disease, diabetes, **glaucoma**, leukemia, liver diseases, chronic **alcoholism**, **macular degeneration**, **multiple sclerosis**, **Parkinson's disease**, **sickle cell anemia**, and **retinitis pigmentosa**.

Accidents or **stroke**s that damage the eye can lead to color blindness. Some frequently used medications such as **antibiotics**, **barbiturates**, antitubercular drugs, high blood pressure medications, and a number of medications used to treat nervous disorders and psychological problems may also lead to color blindness.

Strong chemicals, such as those used in industry, can cause loss of color vision. These include carbon monoxide, carbon disulfide, fertilizers, styrene, and lead-based chemicals.

Aging may also play a role in color blindness. After age 60, changes occur in people's capacity to see colors.

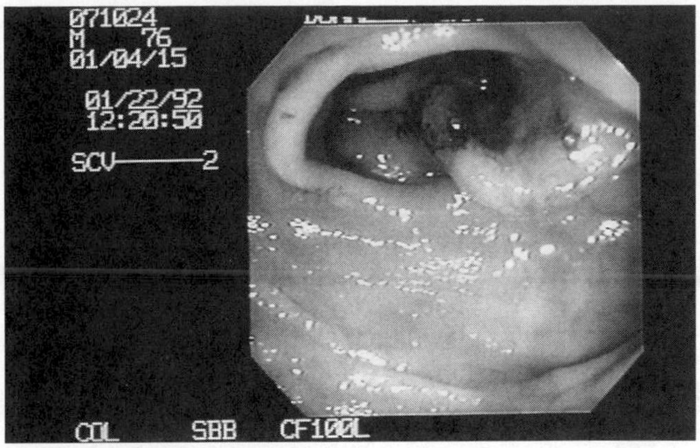

An endoscopic view of a colorectal tumor. ***(Custom Medical Stock Photo. Reproduced by permission.)***

Several tests are available to detect color vision in the general public. The American Optical/Hardy, Rand, and Ritter (AO/H.R.R.) pseudoisochromatic test is the test used most often to detect color blindness. A person with full color vision looking at a sample plate from this test would see a number, composed of blobs of one color, clearly located somewhere in the center of a circle of blobs of another color. A colorblind person is not able to distinguish the number.

The Ishihara test is made up of eight test plates similar to the AO/H.R.R. pseudoisochromatic test plates. The person being tested looks for numbers made up of various colored dots on each test plate.

The Titmus II Vision Tester Color Perception test requires a person to look into a stereoscopic machine. The person's chin rests on a base, and the image comes on only when the forehead touches a pad on the top of the unit. Either a series of plates, or only one plate, can be used to test for color vision. The one most often used in doctor's offices is one that has six samples on it. Six different designs or numbers are on a black background, framed in a yellow border. While Titmus II can test one eye at a time, its value is limited because it only tests for red/green deficiencies and is not highly accurate.

There is no treatment or cure for color blindness. Most color-deficient people compensate well for their defect and may even discover instances in which they can discern details and images that would escape normal-sighted persons.

Color blindness that is hereditary is present in both eyes and remains constant through time. Some cases of acquired color vision loss are not severe and last for only a short time. Other cases tend to be progressive, becoming worse with time.

Hereditary color blindness cannot be prevented. In the case of acquired color blindness, if the cause of the problem is removed, the condition may improve with time. If not, damage may become permanent.

COLORECTAL CANCER

The **digestive system** is made up of the esophagus (food pipe), stomach, and the small and large intestines. The upper 5 - 6 ft (1.5-1.8 m) of the large intestine is called the colon, and the last 6 - 8 in (15-20 cm) of the colon is the rectum. Colorectal cancer is a disease in which the cells of the tissues lining the colon and the rectum start to grow uncontrollably and form tumors.

The main function of the colon is to absorb water and the nutrients from the food already digested by the stomach and the small intestine. The waste material left behind goes into the rectum. From here, it is excreted out of the body through the anus. The colon has four sections: the ascending colon, the transverse colon, the descending colon, and the sigmoid colon which extends to the rectum. Cancer can develop in any of the four sections or in the rectum (the last part of the colon). Cancers beginning in the different sections have different symptoms.

Colorectal cancers have a very high cure rate if found early. Unfortunately, most colorectal cancers are ''silent tumors.'' They grow slowly and often do not produce symptoms until they reach a large size. Therefore, diagnosis is often delayed. The cancer usually begins as a benign growth in the lining of the intestine. These benign growths are called polyps. There are two kinds of polyps, hyperplastic polyps that are small and completely benign. They do not ever develop into cancers. The second kind of polyps, called adenomas, are dangerous and have the potential to become cancerous.

While we do not know the exact cause of most colorectal cancers, the risk factors that makes a person more susceptible to colorectal cancer are:

- Family history: Some rare disease conditions such as Familial Adenomatous Polyps (FAP) and Lynch syndrome (a genetic condition that predisposes certain families to colon cancer. These may make an individual more likely to develop cancer of the colon or the rectum. Inheriting defective genes causes approximately 10% of colorectal cancers.
- History of colorectal cancer: Even when colorectal cancer has been completely removed, new cancers may still develop in other areas of the colon and the rectum.
- Recurrent intestinal polyps: Polyps are benign growths in the colon or rectum. While most polyps are harmless, some particular types do increase the risk of colorectal cancer, especially if they are large and there are many of them.
- Inflammatory bowel disease: Chronic ulcerative colitis, a condition in which the colon is inflamed over a long period of time and causes **ulcers** in the lining, can increase the risk of colon cancer.
- Age: About 90% of colorectal cancers are found in people over the age of 50.
- Diet: Eating foods that are high in fat and low in fiber may increase the risk of colorectal cancer.
- Physical inactivity: A sedentary lifestyle and not enough physical activity has been reported to be associated with a higher risk of colorectal cancer.

The earliest sign of colon cancer may be bleeding. Most of the tumors bleed only small amounts and the bleeding is occasional. Evidence of the blood is found during chemical testing of the feces for hidden (occult) blood. This is called **fecal occult blood test**. When tumors grow to a large size, they may cause a change in the bowel habits. The stools may be very narrow in diameter. There may be other symptoms of general stomach discomfort, such as a feeling of fullness or bloating, stomach cramps, gas **pains**, **diarrhea** or **constipation**. Sometimes the patient complains of a feeling that the bowel does not empty completely. Constant tiredness and weight loss with no known reason may be other warning signs. Many of these symptoms can be caused by conditions other than cancer, however they must be evaluated by a doctor without delay.

If the doctor suspects colon cancer, then he or she may use one of the following tests to find out if the disease is present. A thorough **physical examination** will be conducted to check all symptoms and a complete medical history will be taken to assess any risk factors. A digital rectal examination will be done during the physical. In this procedure, the physician inserts a gloved finger into the rectum to feel for anything abnormal. This simple test can help to detect many rectal cancers. A fecal occult blood test may be ordered, where a sample of stool is examined for blood.

A sigmoidoscopy may be done to enable the doctor to look inside the rectum and part of the colon. A **colonoscopy** will be ordered if the doctor wishes to examine the entire colon lining. If a suspicious mass is detected, then the doctor may cut out a small piece to examine it under a microscope and see if there are any cancer cells. This procedure is called a biopsy.

Another test that is used to diagnose colon cancer is known as a double contrast barium **enema**. The patient is given a barium sulfate enema through the anus. This is a chalky substance that partially fills and opens the colon. When the colon is about half full of barium, the patient is turned on the x-ray table so that the barium spreads throughout the colon. Air is then inserted into the colon to make it expand and x-ray films are taken.

Treatment for colon and rectal cancers depend on the stage of the cancer (the extent to which it has spread). The standard modes of treatment are surgery, **radiation therapy** and **chemotherapy**.

Surgery is the main treatment for colon cancer. If the cancer is found at a very early stage, the doctor may take out the cancer without cutting into the abdomen. Instead the doctor may put a tube through the rectum into the colon and cut the tumor out. If the cancer is larger but confined to a portion of the colon, the abdomen is opened up and the cancerous growth and a small piece of normal tissue from either side of the cancer is removed. If there is any likelihood of the cancer having spread to the nearby lymphnodes, they may be removed as well. The remaining sections of the colon are then attached back together.

If the doctor is not able to sew the colon back together, he will make an opening called the stoma on the outside of the body for the waste material to pass out of the body. This is called a **colostomy**. Sometimes the colostomy is temporary until the colon is healed and then it can be reversed. However, if the surgery involves taking out the entire lower colon, a permanent colostomy is needed.

In the case of rectal cancer, different surgical methods are used. When the cancer is found in the polyps, a procedure known as polypectomy is used. Local excision is used to remove small superficial cancers. If the cancer is in the deeper layers of the rectum, a cut is made through all the layers of the rectum to remove the invasive cancer as well as some surrounding normal rectal tissue. All of these methods can be done without cutting through the abdomen.

Radiation therapy involves the use of high-energy radiation to kill cancer cells. It can be applied to both colon and rectal cancers. Radiation therapy is generally used after the surgery to destroy any cancerous material that may not have been removed during surgery. If the tumor is in a place that makes surgery hard, then radiation may be used before surgery to shrink the tumor. In advanced cancers, where surgery is not an option, radiation may be used to ease the symptoms such as pain, blockage or bleeding.

In colorectal cancers, chemotherapy is generally used after surgery to destroy any cancerous cells that may have migrated from the original site and spread to other parts. The anticancer drugs are either given through a vein in the arm or by mouth, in the form of pills. In the case of advanced cancers, chemotherapy may be given to alleviate symptoms.

The death rate from colorectal cancer has been going down for the past 20 years. This may be because of the advanced methods of early detection and improved treatment modes. If colorectal cancer is detected at an early stage and if treated appropriately, 92% of the people will survive 5 years or more. If the disease has spread to distant sites such as the liver or the lung, the outlook is not good, with only 7% of the patients surviving 5 years after initial diagnosis.

Although the exact cause of colorectal cancer is not known, it is possible to prevent many colon cancers by avoiding the risk factors. By following the screening guidelines, the number of colon cancer cases can be lowered, and by detecting the disease at an earlier stage, the death rate can be lowered.

The American Cancer Society recommends that beginning at age 50, both men and women should follow the schedule for early detection of colorectal cancer. This includes a yearly fecal occult blood test, and an annual digital rectal examination. Flexible sigmoidoscopy should be done every 5 years, and a colonoscopy every 5 - 10 years. A barium enema x ray should also be done every 5 - 10 years.

Proper diet and **exercise** go a long way in preventing colorectal cancer. The American Cancer Society recommends eating at least five servings of fruits and vegetables every day and six servings of food from plant sources such as breads, cereals, grain products, rice, pasta, or beans. Avoiding high-fat, low-fiber foods, such as red meat and processed foods, is also advised. Achieving and maintaining an ideal body weight by at least 30 minutes of physical activity every day is recommended.

COLOSTOMY

Ostomy is a surgical procedure used to create an opening for urine and feces to be released from the body. Colostomy refers to a surgical procedure where a portion of the large intestine is brought through the abdominal wall to carry stool out of the body.

A colostomy is created to treat various disorders of the large intestine, including **cancer**, obstruction, inflammatory bowel disease, ruptured diverticulum, ischemia (compromised blood supply), or traumatic injury. Temporary colostomies are created to divert stool from injured or diseased portions of the large intestine, allowing rest and healing. Permanent colostomies are performed when the distal bowel (bowel at the farthest distance) must be removed or is blocked and inoperable. Although **colorectal cancer** is the most common indication for a permanent colostomy, only about 10-15% of patients with this diagnosis require a colostomy.

Surgery will result in one of three types of colostomies.

In end colostomy, the functioning end of the intestine (the section of bowel that remains connected to the upper gastrointestinal tract) is brought out onto the surface of the abdomen, forming the stoma by cuffing the intestine back on itself and suturing (sewing) the end to the skin. A stoma is an artificial opening created to the surface of the body. The surface of the stoma is actually the lining of the intestine, usually appearing moist and pink. The distal portion of bowel (now connected only to the rectum) may be removed, or sutured closed and left in the abdomen. An end colostomy is usually a permanent ostomy, resulting from trauma, cancer or another pathological condition.

Double–barrel colostomy. This colostomy involves the creation of two separate stomas on the abdominal wall. The proximal (nearest) stoma is the functional end that is connected to the upper gastrointestinal tract and will drain stool. The distal stoma, connected to the rectum and also called a mucous fistula, drains small amounts of mucus material. This is most often a temporary colostomy performed to rest an area of bowel, and to be later closed.

A loop colostomy is created by bringing a loop of bowel through an incision in the abdominal wall. The loop is held in place outside the abdomen by a plastic rod slipped beneath it. An incision is made in the bowel to allow the passage of stool through the loop colostomy. The supporting rod is removed approximately 7-10 days after surgery, when healing has occurred that will prevent the loop of bowel from retracting into the abdomen. A loop colostomy is most often performed for creation of a temporary stoma to divert stool away from an area of intestine that has been blocked or ruptured.

A colostomy pouch will generally have been placed on the patient's abdomen, around the stoma during surgery. During the hospital stay, the patient and his or her caregivers will be educated on how to care for the colostomy. Determination of appropriate pouching supplies and a schedule of how often to change the pouch should be established. Regular checking and meticulous care of the skin surrounding the stoma is important to maintain an adequate surface on which to apply the pouch. Some patients with colostomies are able to routinely irrigate the stoma, resulting in regulation of bowel function; rather than needing to wear a pouch, these patients may need only a dressing or cap over their stoma.

Potential complications of colostomy surgery include excessive bleeding, surgical wound infection, **thrombophlebitis** (inflammation and blood clot to veins in the legs), **pneumonia**, and pulmonary embolism (blood clot or air bubble in the lungs' blood supply).

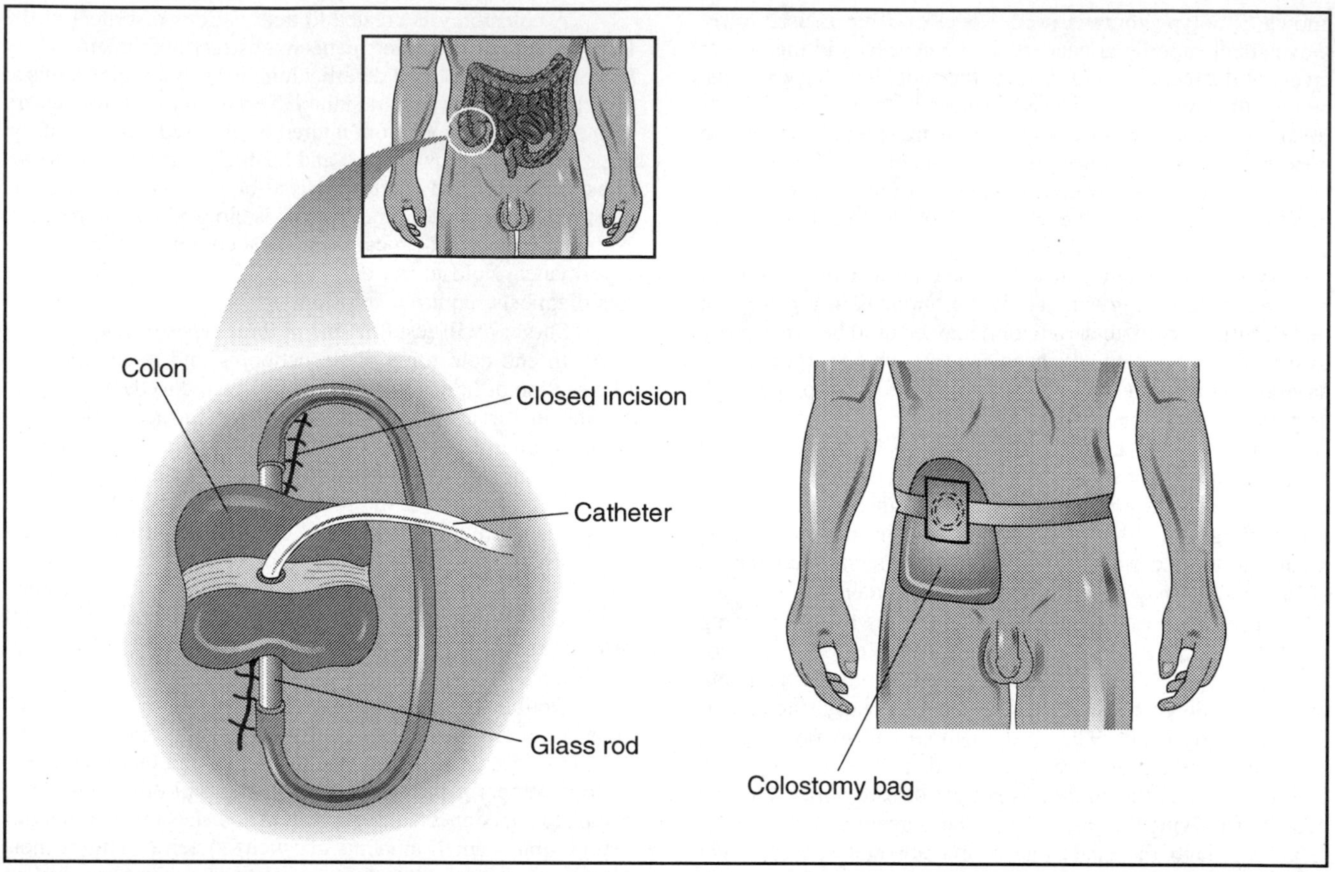

A colostomy is a surgical procedure in which a portion of the large intestine, or colon, is brought through the abdominal wall to carry feces out of the body. There are three types of colostomies: end colostomy, double-barrel colostomy, and loop colostomy. The loop colostomy is featured in the illustration above. *(Illustration by Electronic Illustrators Group.)*

Complete healing is expected without complications. The period of time required for recovery from the surgery may vary depending of the patient's overall health prior to surgery. The colostomy patient without other medical complications should be able to resume all daily activities once recovered from the surgery. The doctor should be made aware of any problems such as increased pain, swelling, or redness in the surgical area, headache, dizziness, or increased abdominal pain.

Stomal complications, such as the stoma moving below the surface of the abdomen or increasing in length above it, or a narrowing of the stomal opening, need to be monitored.

Colposcopy

Colposcopy is a procedure that allows a physician to take a closer look at a woman's cervix and vagina using a special instrument called a colposcope. It is used to check for precancerous or abnormal areas. The colposcope can magnify the area between 10 and 40 times; some devices also can take photographs.

The colposcope helps to identify abnormal areas of the cervix or vagina so that small pieces of tissue (biopsies) can be taken for further analysis.

Colposcopy is used to identify or rule out the existence of any precancerous conditions in the cervical tissue. If a **PAP test** shows abnormal cell growth, further testing, such as colposcopy, often is required. A PAP test is a screening test that involves scraping cells from the outside of the cervix. If abnormal cells are found, the physician will attempt to find the area that produced the abnormal cells and remove it for further study (biopsy). Only then can a diagnosis be made.

Colposcopy is sometimes performed if the cervix looks abnormal during a routine examination. It may also be suggested for women with **genital warts** and for diethylstilbestrol (DES) daughters (women whose mothers took DES when pregnant with them).

Women who are pregnant, or who suspect that they are pregnant, must tell their doctor before the procedure begins. Pregnant women can, and should, have a colposcopy if they have an abnormal PAP test. However, special precautions must be taken during biopsy of the cervix.

A colposcopy is performed in a physician's office and is similar to a regular gynecologic exam. An instrument called a speculum is used to hold the vagina open, and the gynecologist looks at the cervix and vagina through the colposcope instead simply by eye, as in a routine examination.

The colposcope is placed outside the patient's body and never touches the skin. The cervix and vagina are swabbed with dilute acetic acid (vinegar). The solution highlights abnormal areas by turning them white (instead of a normal pink color). Abnormal areas can also be identified by looking for a characteristic pattern made by abnormal blood vessels.

If any abnormal areas are seen, the doctor will take a biopsy of the tissue, a common procedure that takes about 15 minutes. Several samples might be taken, depending on the size of the abnormal area. A biopsy may cause temporary discomfort and cramping, which usually go away within a few minutes. If the abnormal area appears to extend inside the cervical canal, a scraping of the canal may be done. The biopsy results are usually available within a week.

If the tissue sample indicates abnormal growth (dysplasia) or precancer, and if the entire abnormal area can be seen, the doctor can destroy the tissue using one of several procedures, including ones that use high heat (diathermy), extreme cold (cryosurgery), or lasers. Another procedure, called a loop electrosurgical excision (LEEP), uses low-voltage high-frequency radio waves to excise tissue. If any of the abnormal tissue is within the cervical canal, a cone biopsy (removal of a conical section of the cervix for inspection) will be needed.

Occasionally, patients may have bleeding or infection after biopsy. Bleeding is usually controlled with a topical medication. Any unusual symptoms such as heavy vaginal bleeding, fever, or abdominal pain should immediately be brought to the attention of a physician.

If visual inspection shows that the surface of the cervix is smooth and pink, this is considered normal. If abnormal areas are found and biopsied and the results show no indication of **cancer**, a precancerous condition, or other disease, this also is considered normal.

Abnormal conditions that can be detected using colposcopy and biopsy include precancerous tissue changes (cervical dysplasia), cancer, and cervical **warts** (human papilloma virus).

COMA

Coma, from the Greek word *koma,* meaning deep sleep, is a state of extreme unresponsiveness, in which an individual exhibits no voluntary movement or behavior. Furthermore, in a deep coma, even painful stimuli (actions which, when performed on a healthy individual, result in reactions) are unable to effect any response, and normal reflexes may be lost.

Coma lies on a spectrum with other alterations in consciousness. The level of consciousness required by, for example, someone reading this passage lies at one extreme the spectrum, whereas complete brain death lies at the other end. In between are such states as obtundation (dullness), drowsiness, and stupor. All of these are conditions which, unlike coma, still allow the person to respond to stimuli, although such a response may be brief and require stimulus of greater than normal intensity.

Consciousness is defined by two fundamental elements: awareness and arousal. Awareness allows people to take in and process all the information communicated by the five senses, and thus relate to themselves and to the outside world. Awareness has both psychological and physiological components. The psychological component is governed by a person's mind and mental processes. The physiological component refers to the functioning of a person's brain, and therefore that brain's physical and chemical condition. Awareness is regulated by cortical areas within the cerebral hemispheres, the outermost layer of the brain which separates humans from other animals by allowing for greater intellectual functioning.

Arousal is regulated solely by physiological functioning and consists of more primitive responsiveness to the world, for example, reflex (involuntary) responses to stimuli. Arousal is maintained by the reticular activating system (the RAS). This is not an anatomical area of the brain, but rather a network of structures (including the brainstem, the medulla, and the thalamus) and nerve pathways, which function together to produce and maintain arousal.

Coma is the result of something that interferes with the functioning of the cerebral cortex or the functioning of the structures which make up the RAS. In fact, a huge and varied number of conditions can result in coma. A good way of categorizing these conditions is to consider the anatomic and metabolic causes of coma. Anatomic causes of coma are conditions that damage the brain structures responsible for consciousness, either at the level of the cerebal cortex or the brainstem, whereas metabolic causes of coma consist of those conditions that change the chemical environment of the brain, thereby adversely affecting function.

Metabolic causes of coma include a decrease in the delivery to the brain of substances necessary for appropriate brain functioning, such as oxygen, glucose (sugar), and sodium.

Drugs or alcohol in toxic quantities can disrupt the functioning of neurons, as can substances normally found in the body, but that, due to some diseased state, accumulate at toxic levels. Accumulated substances that might cause coma include ammonia due to liver disease, ketones due to uncontrolled diabetes, or carbon dioxide due to a severe **asthma** attack.

Coma may also be caused by changes in chemical levels in the brain due to the electrical derangements caused by seizures (sudden attacks).

As in any neurologic condition (one that originates in the nervous system), history and examination form the cornerstone of diagnosis when the patient is in a coma; however, history must be obtained from family, friends, or mental status examination. The Glasgow Coma Scale provides a means of examining a comatose patient. It assigns a different number of points for exam results in three different categories: opening the eyes, verbal response (using words or voice to respond), and motor response (moving a part of the body). When performed as part of the admission examination, a Glasgow score of 3 to 5 points (out of a total of 15) often suggests that the patient has likely suffered fatal brain damage, whereas 8 or more points indicates that the patient's chances for recovery

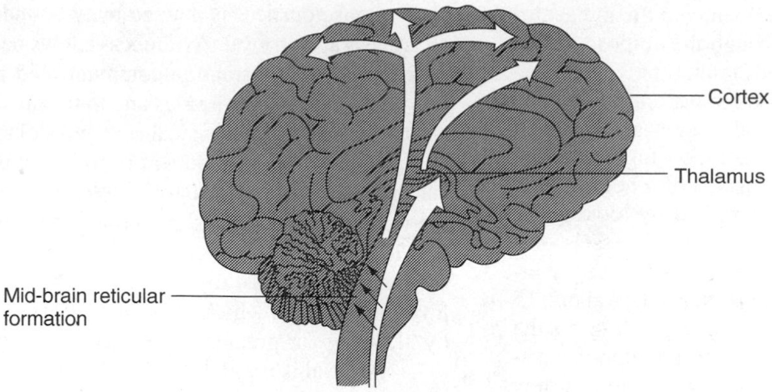

A side-view of the brain, showing movement of the reticular activating substance (RAS) essential to consciousness

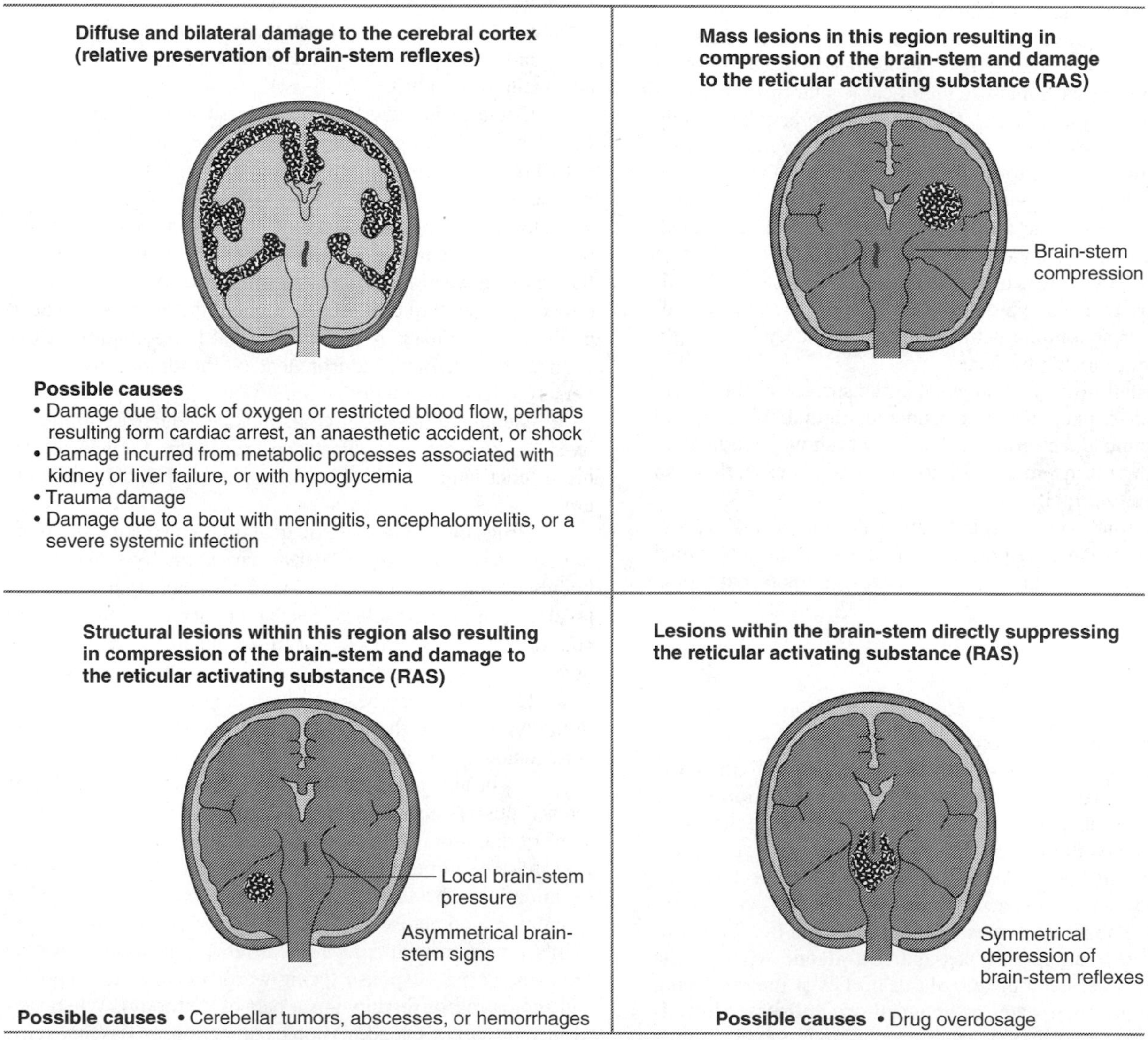
Diffuse and bilateral damage to the cerebral cortex (relative preservation of brain-stem reflexes)
Possible causes
• Damage due to lack of oxygen or restricted blood flow, perhaps resulting form cardiac arrest, an anaesthetic accident, or shock
• Damage incurred from metabolic processes associated with kidney or liver failure, or with hypoglycemia
• Trauma damage
• Damage due to a bout with meningitis, encephalomyelitis, or a severe systemic infection
Mass lesions in this region resulting in compression of the brain-stem and damage to the reticular activating substance (RAS)
Brain-stem compression
Structural lesions within this region also resulting in compression of the brain-stem and damage to the reticular activating substance (RAS)
Local brain-stem pressure
Asymmetrical brain-stem signs
Possible causes • Cerebellar tumors, abscesses, or hemorrhages
Lesions within the brain-stem directly suppressing the reticular activating substance (RAS)
Symmetrical depression of brain-stem reflexes
Possible causes • Drug overdosage

The four brain conditions that result in coma. ***(Illustration by Hans & Cassady, Inc.)***

are good. Metabolic causes of coma are diagnosed from blood work and **urinalysis** to evaluate blood chemistry, drug screen, and blood cell abnormalities that may indicate infection. Anatomic causes of coma are diagnosed from CT (**computed tomography scans**) or MRI (**magnetic resonance imaging**) scans.

Coma is a medical emergency, and attention must first be directed to maintaining the patient's respiration and circulation, using intubation and ventilation, administration of intravenous fluids or blood as needed, and other supportive care. If head trama has not been excluded, the neck should be stablized in the event of fracture. It is obviously extremely important for a physician to determine quickly the cause of a coma, so that potentially reversible conditions are treated immediately. For example, an infection may be treated with **antibiotics**; a **brain tumor** may be removed; and brain swelling from an injury can be reduced with certain medications. Various metabolic disorders can be addressed by supplying the individual with the correct amount of oxygen, glucose, or sodium; by treating the underlying disease in liver disease, asthma, or diabetes; and by halting seizures with medication. Because of their low incidence of side effects and potential for prompt reversal of coma in certain conditions, glucose, the B-vitamin thiamine, and Narcan (to counteract any narcotic-type drugs) are routinely given.

Some conditions that cause coma can be completely reversed, restoring the person to his or her original level of functioning. However, if areas of the brain have been sufficiently damaged due to the severity or duration of the condition which led to the coma, the person may recover from the coma with permanent disabilities, or may even never regain consciousness. Patients who have suffered head injuries tend to do better than do patients whose coma was caused by other types of medical illnesses. Leaving out those people whose coma followed drug poisoning, only about 15% of patients who remain in a coma for more than just a few hours make a good recovery. Adult patients who remain in a coma for more than four weeks have almost no chance of eventually regaining their previous level of functioning. On the other hand, children and young adults have regained functioning even after two months in a coma.

COMMON COLD

Colds, sometimes called rhinovirus or coronavirus infections, are the most common illness to strike any part of the body. It is estimated that the average person has more than 50 colds during a lifetime. Anyone can get a cold, although preschool and grade school children catch them more frequently than adolescents and adults. Repeated exposure to viruses causing colds creates partial immunity.

Although most colds resolve on their own without complications, they are a leading cause of visits to the doctor and of time lost from work and school. Treating symptoms of the common cold has given rise to a multimillion dollar industry in over-the-counter medications.

Cold season in the United States begins in early autumn and extends through early spring. Although it is not true that getting wet or being in a draft causes a cold (a person has to come in contact with the virus to catch a cold), certain conditions such as fatigue and overwork, emotional **stress**, and poor nutrition may lead to increased susceptibility.

Colds make the upper respiratory system less resistant to bacterial infection. Secondary bacterial infection may lead to middle ear infection, **bronchitis**, **pneumonia**, sinus infection, or **strep throat**. People with chronic lung disease, **asthma**, diabetes, or a weakened immune system are more likely to develop these complications.

Colds are caused by more than 200 different viruses. The most common groups are rhinoviruses and coronaviruses. Different groups of viruses are more infectious at different seasons of the year, but knowing the exact virus causing the cold is not important in treatment.

People with colds are contagious during the first two to four days of the infection. Colds pass from person to person in several ways. When an infected person coughs, sneezes, or speaks, tiny fluid droplets containing the virus are expelled. If these are breathed in by other people, the virus may establish itself in their noses and airways.

Colds may also be passed through direct contact. If a person with a cold touches his runny nose or watery eyes, then shakes hands with another person some of the virus is transferred to the uninfected person. If that person then touches his mouth, nose, or eyes, the virus is transferred to an environment where it can reproduce and cause a cold.

Finally, cold viruses can be spread through inanimate objects (doorknobs, telephones, toys) that become contaminated with the virus.

Once acquired, the cold virus attaches itself to the lining of the nasal passages and sinuses. This causes the infected cells to release a chemical called histamine. Histamine increases the blood flow to the infected cells, causing swelling, congestion, and increased mucus production. Within one to three days the infected person begins to show cold symptoms.

The first cold symptoms are a tickle in the throat, runny nose, and sneezing. The initial discharge from the nose is clear and thin. Later it changes to a thick yellow or greenish discharge. Most adults do not develop a **fever** when they catch a cold. Young children may develop a low fever of up to 102°F (38.9°C).

In addition to a runny nose and fever, signs of a cold include coughing, sneezing, nasal congestion, **headache**, muscle ache, chills, **sore throat**, hoarseness, watery eyes, tiredness, and lack of appetite. The cough that accompanies a cold is usually intermittent and dry.

Colds make people more susceptible to bacterial infections such as strep throat, middle ear infections, and sinus infections. A person whose cold does not begin to improve within a week; or who experiences chest **pain**, fever for more than a few days, difficulty breathing, bluish lips or fingernails, a cough that brings up greenish-yellow or grayish sputum, skin rash, swollen glands, or whitish spots on the tonsils or throat should consult a doctor to see if they have acquired a secondary bacterial infection that needs to be treated with an antibiotic.

People who have emphysema, chronic lung disease, diabetes, or a weakened immune system—either from diseases such as **AIDS** or leukemia, or as the result of medications, (**corticosteroids**, **chemotherapy** drugs)—should consult their doctor if they get a cold. People with these health problems are more likely to get a secondary infection.

Colds are diagnosed by observing a person's symptoms. There are no laboratory tests readily available to detect the cold virus. However, a doctor may do a **throat culture** or blood test to rule out a secondary infection.

There are no medicines that will cure the common cold. Given time, the body's immune system will make antibodies to fight the infection, and the cold will be resolved without any intervention. **Antibiotics** are useless against a cold. However, a great deal of money is spent by pharmaceutical companies in the United States promoting products designed to relieve cold symptoms. These products usually contain **antihistamines**, **decongestants**, or pain relievers.

Given time, the body will make antibodies to cure itself of a cold. Most colds last a week to 10 days. Most people start feeling better within 4 or 5 days. Occasionally a cold will lead to a secondary bacterial infection which causes strep throat, bronchitis, pneumonia, sinus infection, or a middle ear infection. These conditions usually clear up rapidly when treated with an antibiotic.

It is not possible to prevent colds because the viruses that cause colds are common and highly infectious. However, using common sense can help to reduce their spread, for example, eating a healthy diet and getting enough sleep, and avoiding close contact with someone who has a cold for the first few days of their infection.

COMMUNICATION DISORDERS

Communication disorders affecting speech and language can afflict children and adults. They can be the result of damage to the brain's language areas, such as when a person suffers a stroke, and affect the way words are spoken and the way they are understood.

Babies begin to understand language when they are just a few months old. By the age of 6 months, some babies understand such simple things as ''no'' and ''bye-bye.'' Between the age of a year and a year-and-a-half, children can say their first words (usually ''Mama'' and ''Dada''), follow simple instructions (such as ''Come here), and even use two-word phrases such as ''all gone.'' Although all children develop language skills at different rates (boys tend to develop them slightly later than girls do), a child who is showing no progress in language may be suffering from a communication disorder. Or, the child may have difficulty hearing. In either case, the child should be examined by a pediatrician. There may be a physical cause to the difficulty, or there may be a psychological or emotional cause.

Some children suffer from articulation problems, that is, pronouncing words clearly. For example, some children hear the difference between the sound of an ''r'' and the sound of a ''w,'' but cannot produce the R sound, so the word ''rock'' may be pronounced ''wock.'' Other children cannot hear the differences in speech sounds, which can make learning to read especially difficult because they cannot associate spoke sounds with the symbols on the page. Unless problems such as these (and as lisping) are corrected, the child may find him or herself sorely disadvantaged in social situations when older.

Stuttering is another common form of communication problem. The stutterer cannot get words to come out in a smooth flow, although he or she knows what he or she wants to say. Some stutterers will grow out of stuttering as they become more expert with spoken language. Others will never shake the problem, and it can get worse when the person is nervous or in an unfamiliar situation. Stuttering affects about 1% of children.

Some speech problems have a physical cause, such as a cleft lip or palate (which can be corrected with surgery), or cerebral palsy, a disease which affects muscle control, including the muscles used for speech.

Speech development can be delayed in some children by hearing loss or deafness (because the child cannot hear, he lacks the model to work with in learning to speak), by mental retardation, or by learning disabilities that can effect the child's ability to understand or order language.

If the language center of the brain suffers an injury (such as a stroke or head injury), communication problems can result, a condition called aphasia. Not always will a person's entire communication ability be knocked out. Some patients may lose the ability to name objects, although they know what the objects are (called anomia). Others may not be able to articulate words properly (dysarthia), which can result if the nerves to the voice box or mouth have been damaged. Some people cannot comprehend written words (ataxia). Persons suffering from Broca's aphasia (or expressive aphasia), are similar to stutterers in that they know what they want to say but have trouble getting the words out. People with Wernicke's aphasia, meanwhile, speak fluently but the words come out garbled and confused (a ''word salad'') because they cannot make sense of what is being said or tell exactly what they themselves are saying. The most damaging language disruption is global aphasia, in which a person can comprehend only a very few words and may be completely unable to speak.

Fortunately, many of these conditions can be helped through speech therapy. Children are often taught language through play, such as with a doll's house. For example, through using a doll's house, the therapist can teach the child the names of objects and then, by asking the child to do certain actions with the objects, about action verbs. Practice is key, and parents must be sure to work with the child in between sessions with the speech therapist.

Speech therapists can also help adults who have suffered brain damage, although the extent of a patient's recovery depends on the extent of the damage. Exercises for the tongue and mouth can help a dysarthria patient, and other patients can be helped through the use of picture boards to communicate. Patients can recover part or all of their speech spontaneously six months to two years after the damage occurs.

See also Aphasia; Dyslexia; Language development; Speech therapy

COMMUNITY HEALTH

While personal health care services deal directly with individuals for the maintenance of health or the control or cure of disease, community health services are directed toward population groups. Those involved in the management of community-based health problems work toward solutions, often geared toward **preventive medicine** and health promotion. Emphasis in community health care often includes measures to increase accessibility.

As early as 1946, the Hill-Burton Act allocated federal funds, in amounts based on population distribution, for new hospital construction. The authors of this legislation and its later revisions believed that because the national government could not know all the needs of people in the country's thousands of cities and towns, planning should take place at the state level. Amendments in 1954 broadened the program to include **nursing homes**, **rehabilitation** facilities, and chronic disease facilities. The Community Health Services and Facilities Act of 1961 made federal grants available to meet identified local health needs. The National Health Planning and Resources Development Act of 1974 assisted in the establishment of Health Systems Agencies, which had the objectives: improve the health of residents of a health service area while restraining increases in the cost of providing residents with health services; increase accessibility, acceptability, continuity, and quality of health services to residents of that area while preventing unnecessary duplication of services; and, preserve and improve competition in the health service areas. These agencies emphasized issues of concern to their local communities, such as programs to address **migrant health** and **minority health** care needs; access to services for the poor and rural residents; management of **environmental health** issues; and, provision for **mental health care** services.

In the '80s and '90s, the high cost of health care has become a major focus of the federal government. Methods of cost containment for the **Medicare and Medicaid** programs continue to be pursued. State government involvement in planning health care services has varied dramatically. Prosperous states, such as New York and Massachusetts, continue to actively pursue solutions to health problems with regulations and state spending, while other states view health services as local and federal issues and provide only the traditional health functions of disease control and maintenance of birth and death records. As public interest in health promotion and prevention continues to increase, local hospitals are often assuming the role in planning, marketing, and providing a wide range of health services in most communities.

See also Medicare and Medicaid; Preventive medicine; Environmental health

COMPUTED TOMOGRAPHY SCANS

Computed tomography (CT) scans are completed with the use of a 360-degree x-ray beam and computer production of images. These scans allow for cross-sectional views of body organs and tissues.

CT scans are used to image a wide variety of body structures and internal organs. Since the 1990s, CT equipment has become more affordable and available. In some diagnoses, CT scans have become the first imaging exam of choice. Because the computerized image is so sharp, focused, and three-dimensional, many tissues can be better differentiated than on standard x rays. The CT scan can show details of **sinusitis**, and bone **fractures**. Physicians may order CT of the sinuses to provide an accurate map for surgery. Brain scans can detect tumors and **stroke**s. The introduction of CT scanning, especially spiral CT, has helped reduce the need for more invasive procedures.

CT scans of the body will often be used to observe abdominal organs, such as the liver, kidneys, adrenal glands, spleen, and lymph nodes, and extremities. CT scans can focus on the thoracic or abdominal aorta to locate aneurysms and other possible aortic diseases. CT scans of the chest are useful in distinguishing tumors and in detailing accumulation of fluid in chest infections.

Computed tomography, also called CT scan, CAT scan, or computerized axial tomography, is a combination of focused x-ray beams and computerized production of an image. Introduced in the early 1970s, this radiologic procedure has advanced rapidly and is now widely used, sometimes in the place of standard x rays.

A CT scan may be performed in a hospital or outpatient imaging center. Although the equipment looks large and intimidating, it is very sophisticated and fairly comfortable. The patient is asked to lie on a gantry, or narrow table, that slides into the center of the scanner. The scanner looks like a doughnut and is round in the middle, which allows the x-ray beam to rotate around the patient. The scanner section may also be tilted slightly to allow for certain cross-sectional angles.

Following the procedure, films of the images are usually printed for the radiologist and referring physician to review. A radiologist can also interpret CT exams on a special computer screen. The procedure time will vary in length depending on the area being imaged. Average study times are from 30 to 60 minutes. Some patients may be concerned about claustrophobia but the width of the "doughnut" portion of the scanner is such that many patients can be reassured of openness.

While traditional x rays image organs in two dimensions, with the possibility that organs in the front of the body are superimposed over those in the back, CT scans allow for a more three-dimensional effect. Some have compared CT images to slices in a loaf of bread. Precise sections of the body can be located and imaged as cross-sectional views. The screen before the technologist shows a computer's analysis of each section detected by the x-ray beam. Thus, various densities of tissue can be easily distinguished.

Contrast agents are often used in CT exams and in other radiology procedures to illuminate certain details of anatomy which may not be easily seen. Some contrasts are natural, such as air or water. Other times, a water-based contrast agent is administered for specific diagnostic purposes. Barium sulfate is commonly used in gastroenterology procedures. The patient may drink this contrast, or receive it in an enema. Oral and rectal contrast are usually given when examining the abdomen or cells, and not given when scanning the brain or chest. Iodine is the most widely used intravenous contrast agent and is given through an intravenous needle.

Spiral CT, also called helical CT, is a newer version of CT scanning which is continuous in motion and allows for three-dimensional recreation of images. For example, traditional CT allows the technologist to take slices at very small and precise intervals one after the other. Spiral CT allows for a continuous flow of images, without stopping the scanner to move to the next image slice. A major advantage of spiral CT is the ability to reconstruct images anywhere along the length of the study area. The procedure also speeds up the imaging process, meaning less time for the patient to lie still. The ability to image contrast more rapidly after it is injected, when it is at its highest level, is another advantage of spiral CT's high speed.

Radiation exposure from a CT scan is similar to, though higher than, that of a conventional x ray. This is a risk to pregnant women, but the exposure to other adults is minimal and should produce no effects. Although severe contrast reactions are rare, they are a risk of many CT procedures.

Normal findings on a CT exam show bone, the most dense tissue, as white areas. Tissues and fat will show as various shades of gray, and fluids will be gray or black. Air will also look black. Intravenous, oral, and rectal contrast appear as white areas. The radiologist can determine if tissues and organs appear normal by the sensitivity of the gray shadows. In CT, the images which can cut through a section of tissue or organ provide three-dimensional viewing for the radiologist and referring physician.

Abnormal results may show different characteristics of tissues within organs. Accumulations of blood or other fluids where they do not belong may be detected. Radiologists can differentiate among types of tumors throughout the body by viewing details of their makeup.

Concussion

Concussion is a trauma-induced change in mental status, with confusion and **amnesia**, and with or without a brief loss of consciousness.

A concussion occurs when the head hits or is hit by an object, or when the brain is jarred against the skull, with sufficient force to cause temporary loss of function in the higher centers of the brain. The injured person may remain conscious or lose consciousness briefly, and is disoriented for some minutes after the blow. According to the Centers for Disease Control and Prevention, approximately 300,000 people sustain mild to moderate sports-related brain injuries each year, most of them young men between 16 and 25.

While concussion usually resolves on its own without lasting effect, it can set the stage for a much more serious condition. ''Second impact syndrome'' occurs when a person with a concussion, even a very mild one, suffers a second blow before fully recovering from the first. The brain swelling and increased intracranial pressure that can result is potentially fatal. More than 20 such cases have been reported since the syndrome was first described in 1984.

Most concussions are caused by motor vehicle accidents and **sports injuries**. In motor vehicle accidents, concussion can occur without an actual blow to the head. Instead, concussion occurs because the skull suddenly decelerates or stops, which causes the brain to be jarred against the skull. Contact sports, especially football, hockey, and boxing, are among those most likely to lead to concussion. Other significant causes include falls, collisions, or blows due to bicycling, horseback riding, skiing, and soccer.

The risk of concussion from football is extremely high, especially at the high school level. Studies show that approximately 1 in 5 players suffer concussion or more serious brain injury during their brief high-school careers. The rate at the collegiate level is approximately 1 in 20. Rates for hockey players are not known as certainly, but are believed to be similar.

Concussion and lasting brain damage is an especially significant risk for boxers, since the goal of the sport is, in fact, to deliver a concussion to the opponent. For this reason, the American Academy of Neurology has called for a ban on boxing. Repeated concussions over months or years can cause cumulative **head injury**. The cumulative brain injuries suffered by most boxers can lead to permanent brain damage. Multiple blows to the head can cause ''punch-drunk'' syndrome or dementia pugilistica, as evidenced by Muhammed Ali, whose parkinsonism is a result of his career in the ring.

Young children are likely to suffer concussions from falls or collisions on the playground or around the home. **Child abuse** is, unfortunately, another common cause of concussion.

Symptoms of concussion include:

- **Headache**
- Disorientation as to time, date, or place
- Confusion
- **Dizziness**
- Vacant stare or confused expression
- Incoherent or incomprehensible speech
- Incoordination or weakness
- Amnesia for the events immediately preceding the blow
- Nausea or vomiting
- Double vision
- Ringing in the ears.

These symptoms may last from several minutes to several hours. More severe or longer-lasting symptoms may indicate more severe brain injury. The person with a concussion may or may not lose consciousness from the blow; if so, it will be for several minutes at the most. More prolonged unconsciousness indicates more severe brain injury.

The severity of concussion is graded on a three-point scale, used as a basis for treatment decisions.

- Grade 1: no loss of consciousness, transient confusion, and other symptoms that resolve within 15 minutes.

- Grade 2: no loss of consciousness, transient confusion, and other symptoms that require more than 15 minutes to resolve.
- Grade 3: loss of consciousness for any period.

Days or weeks after the accident, the person may show signs of:

- Headache
- Poor attention and concentration
- Memory difficulties
- **Anxiety**
- Depression
- Sleep disturbances
- Light and noise intolerance.

The occurrence of such symptoms is called ''post-concussion syndrome.''

It is very important for those attending a person with concussion to pay close attention to the person's symptoms and progression immediately after the accident. The duration of unconsciousness and degree of confusion are very important indicators of the severity of the injury and help guide the diagnostic process and treatment decisions.

A doctor, nurse, or emergency medical technician may make an immediate assessment based on the severity of the symptoms; a neurologic exam of the pupils, coordination and sensation; and brief tests of orientation, memory, and concentration. Those with very mild concussions may not need to be hospitalized or have expensive diagnostic tests. Questionable or more severe cases may require CT or MRI scans to look for brain injury.

The symptoms of concussion usually clear quickly and without lasting effect, if no further injury is sustained during the healing process. Guidelines for returning to sports activities are based on the severity of the concussion.

A grade 1 concussion can usually be treated with rest and continued observation alone. The person may return to sports activities that same day, but only after examination by a trained professional, and after all symptoms have completely resolved. If the person sustains a second concussion of any severity that same day, he or she should not be allowed to continue contact sports until he or she has been symptom-free, during both rest and activity, for one week.

A person with a grade 2 concussion must discontinue sports activity for the day, should be evaluated by a trained professional, and should be observed closely throughout the day to make sure that all symptoms have completely cleared. Worsening of symptoms, or continuation of any symptoms beyond one week, indicates the need for a CT or MRI scan. Return to contact sports should only occur after one week with no symptoms, both at rest and during activity, and following examination by a physician. Following a second grade 2 concussion, the person should remain symptom-free for two weeks before resuming contact sports.

A person with a grade 3 concussion (involving any loss of consciousness, no matter how brief) should be examined by a medical professional either on the scene or in an emergency room. More severe symptoms may warrant a **computed tomography scan** (CT) or **magnetic resonance imaging** (MRI) scan, along with a thorough neurological and physical exam. The person should be hospitalized if any abnormalities are found or if confusion persists. Prolonged unconsciousness and worsening symptoms require urgent neurosurgical evaluation or transfer to a trauma center. Following discharge from professional care, the patient is closely monitored for neurological symptoms which may arise or worsen. If headaches or other symptoms worsen or last longer than one week, a CT or MRI scan should be performed. Contact sports are avoided for one week following unconsciousness of only seconds, and for two weeks for unconsciousness of a minute or more. A person receiving a second grade 3 concussion should avoid contact sports for at least a month after all symptoms have cleared, and then only with the approval of a physician. If signs of brain swelling or bleeding are seen on a CT or MRI scan, the athlete should not return to the sport for the rest of the season, or even indefinitely

For someone who has sustained a concussion of any severity, it is critically important that he or she avoid the possibility of another blow to the head until well after all symptoms have cleared to prevent second-impact syndrome. The guidelines above are designed to minimize the risk of this syndrome.

Concussion usually leaves no lasting neurological problems. Nonetheless, symptoms of post-concussion syndrome may last for weeks or even months.

Studies of concussion in contact sports have shown that the risk of sustaining a second concussion is even greater than it was for the first, if the person continues to engage in the sport.

Many cases of concussion can be prevented by using appropriate protective equipment. This includes seat belts and air bags in automobiles, and helmets in all contact sports. Helmets should also be worn when bicycling, skiing, or horseback riding. Soccer players should avoid heading the ball when it is kicked at high velocity from close range. Playground equipment should be underlaid with soft material, either sand or special matting.

The value of high-contact sports such as boxing, football, or hockey should be weighed against the high risk of brain injury during a young person's participation in the sport. Steering a child's general enthusiasm for sports into activities less apt to produce head impacts may reduce the likelihood of brain injury.

CONDITIONING

Conditioning is a way of establishing new behaviors by providing either a stimulus or a reward for the desired behavior. It has widespread applications in psychology. There is also growing evidence that conditioning might be useful to boost the body's immunity against disease, or to suppress the immune system's tendency to reject transplanted organs.

There are two main types of conditioning: classical and operant.

The best-known examples of classical conditioning are the experiments conducted in the late 1800s and early 1900s by the Russian physiologist Ivan Pavlov. Initially, Pavlov was interested in the functioning of the digestive system (he received the 1904 Nobel Prize in Medicine and Physiology for that work). In experiments with dogs, he developed an experimental apparatus for measuring their saliva formation as they ate, using tubes that redirected secretions from the animals' salivary ducts. While conducting these experiments, Pavlov noticed that some dogs started salivating before they were fed.

New dogs did not salivate in this way, only those that had previously participated in similar laboratory sessions. Pavlov showed that this salivation was initiated by some stimulus associated with the earlier feeding, perhaps the ringing of a bell or just the appearing of the lab worker who fed the animals.

Thus, in classical conditioning, a stimulus not typically associated with a particular response (i.e. the ringing of the bell) is repeatedly presented around the same time as a stimulus that causes the response naturally (in the case of Pavlov's dogs, food), until the initial stimulus evokes the response on its own. This is known as a conditioned reflex.

Continuing to study this phenomenon for more than three decades, Pavlov concluded that a great deal of animal and human behavior resulted from classical conditioning. Although his view of the importance of conditioning was probably exaggerated, subsequent research has uncovered dozens of reflexes that respond to classical conditioning, including blinking of the eyes, the knee-jerk response, and stimulation of the heart, liver, kidneys, and stomach.

More recently, researchers have become interested in the effects of classical conditioning on the immune system, which creates antibodies that fight infection. Studies in mice and humans have demonstrated that when the immune-strengthening drug **interferon** is administered a few times combined with the odor of camphor (an aromatic compound that normally has no effect on the immune system), later exposure to camphor alone increased activity of the body's natural killer cells, which act against tumors and viruses. Similarly, animal research has suggested that classical conditioning might be useful for suppressing the body's immune response that rejects transplanted organs.

Other medical applications of classical conditioning are for combating alcohol and tobacco abuse, and to teach children to stop bedwetting.

Operant conditioning, on the other hand, does not use a stimulus to prompt behavior. Rather, it employs a 'reward' *after* the desired behavior, or sometimes a punishment to discourage inappropriate behavior. Examples of operant conditioning are the 'puzzle box' experiments conducted by the American psychologist Edward Thorndike in the late 1800s. Thorndike placed a hungry cat or other animal in a box that could only be opened if the animal pulled on a string or a latch, or performed a combination of similar actions. The first time the animal was placed in the box, it usually took some time to escape and enjoy some nearby food. But over time, the animal learned to escape within seconds. In these experiments, behavior was modified through the rewards of escape and food.

Operant conditioning can be used, among other things, to shape the behavior of cocaine users or patients with severe behavioral problems.

Many (perhaps doubtful) stories are told of how college and university classes use operant conditioning to shape the behaviors of their professors. In one such story, students in an introductory psychology course agreed to 'reinforce' their professor for each move to the left by nodding approval and paying attention, ignoring him and stopping their note-taking if he moved to the right. According to the story, recounted in a popular textbook about the psychology of learning, the professor got midway through the lecture and then fell off the left side of the stage.

Condom

Male condoms are thin sheaths of latex (rubber), polyurethane (plastic), or animal tissue that are rolled onto an erect penis immediately prior to intercourse. They are commonly called ''safes'' or ''rubbers.'' Female condoms are made of polyurethane, and are inserted into the vaginal canal before sexual relations. The open end covers the outside of the vagina, and the closed ring fits over the cervix (opening into the uterus). Both types of condoms collect the male semen at ejaculation (the release of semen during intercourse), and thus act as a barrier to fertilization. Condoms also perform as barriers to the exchange of bodily fluids between persons involved in a sexual act, whether male-to-male, male-to-female, or female-to-female contact.

Both male and female condoms are used to prevent **pregnancy** and to protect against acquired immunodeficiency syndrome (**AIDS**), **genital warts** and other **sexually transmitted diseases**. To accomplish these goals, the condom must be applied and removed correctly.

Male and female condoms should not be used together as there is a risk that one of them may come off. The male condom should not be snug on the tip of the penis. A space of about 1/2 inch should be left at the end to avoid the possibility of it breaking during sexual intercourse. The penis must be withdrawn quickly after ejaculation to prevent the condom from falling off as the penis softens. So the condom should always be removed while the penis is still erect to prevent the ejaculate (sperm) from spilling into the vagina.

Male condoms made from animal tissue and linen have been in use for centuries. Latex condoms were introduced in the late 1800s and gained immediate popularity because they were inexpensive and effective. At that time, they were primarily used to protect against sexually transmitted diseases. A common complaint made by many consumers is that condoms reduce penis sensitivity and impair orgasm. Both men and women may develop **allergies** to the latex. Consumer interest in female condoms has been slight.

Male condoms may be purchased lubricated, ribbed, or treated with spermicide (a chemical that kills sperm). To be effective, condoms must be removed carefully so as not to ''spill'' the contents into the vaginal canal. Condoms that leak or break do not provide protection against pregnancy or disease.

If used correctly, male condoms have an effectiveness rate of about 90%, but this rate can be increased to about 99% if used with a spermicide. (Several types of spermicides are available; they can be purchased in the form of contraceptive creams and jellies, foams, or films.) Benefits associated with this type of contraceptive device include easy availability (no prescription is required), convenience of use, and lack of serious side effects. The primary disadvantage is that sexual activity must be interrupted in order to put the condom on.

Female condoms have a lower effectiveness rate against pregnancy; but, when used correctly and at every intercourse, during the course of a year they prevented pregnancy in over 75% of the women surveyed.

Checking the expiration date on a condom and examining it for holes before use are additional ways of enhancing its effectiveness. Because petroleum jellies, such as Vaseline, and other oil-based lubricants can weaken latex, any lubricants used during intercourse should be water-soluble.

Conduct disorder

Conduct disorder (CD) is a behavioral and emotional disorder of childhood and adolescence. Children with conduct disorder act inappropriately, infringe on the rights of others, and violate the behavioral expectations of others.

Conduct disorder is present in approximately 9% of boys and 2-9% of girls under the age of 18. Children with conduct disorder act out aggressively and express anger inappropriately. They engage in a variety of antisocial and destructive acts, including violence toward people and animals, destroying property, lying, stealing, skipping school, and running away from home. They often begin using and abusing drugs and alcohol, and having sex at an early age. Irritability, temper tantrums, and low self-esteem are common personality traits of children with conduct disorder.

The Diagnostic and Statistical Manual of Mental Disorders fourth edition, (*DSM-IV*) describes two subtypes of conduct disorder, one beginning in childhood and the other in adolescence. There is no known cause. But researchers and physicians suggest a number of factors that may lead to conduct disorder.

Difficulty in school is an early sign of potential conduct disorder problems. While the patient's IQ tends to be in the normal range, they can have trouble with verbal and abstract reasoning skills and may lag behind their classmates. Consequently, they feel as if they don't "fit in." The frustration and loss of self-esteem resulting from this academic and social inadequacy can trigger the development of conduct disorder.

An emotionally, physically, or sexually abusive home environment, a family history of antisocial personality disorder, or parental substance abuse can damage a child's perceptions of himself and put him on a path toward negative behavior. Other less obvious environmental factors can also play a part in the development of conduct disorder. Long-term studies have shown that maternal smoking during **pregnancy** may be linked to the development of conduct disorder in boys. Animal and human studies suggest that nicotine can have undesirable effects on babies. These include altered structure and function of their nervous systems, learning deficits, and behavioral problems. In a study of 177 boys ages 7-12 years, those with mothers who smoked over one half a package of cigarettes daily while pregnant were more apt to have a conduct disorder than those with mothers who did not smoke.

Other conditions that may cause or co-exist with conduct disorder include **head injury**, substance abuse disorder, major depressive disorder, and **attention deficit hyperactivity disorder** (ADHD). Thirty to 50% of children diagnosed with ADHD, a disorder characterized by a persistent pattern of inattention or hyperactivity, also have conduct disorder.

DSM-IV defines conduct disorder as a repetitive behavioral pattern of violating the rights of others or societal norms. Three of the following criteria, or symptoms, are required over the previous 12 months for a diagnosis of conduct disorder (one of the three must have occurred in the past 6 months): bullying, threatening, or intimidating others; picking fights; using a dangerous weapon; being physically cruel to people; being physically cruel to animals; stealing while confronting a victim (for example, mugging or extortion); forcing someone into sexual activity; deliberately setting a fire with the intention of causing damage; deliberately destroying the property of others; breaking into someone else's house or car; frequently lying to get something or to avoid obligations; stealing without confronting a victim or breaking and entering (e.g., shoplifting or forgery); staying out at night; breaking curfew (beginning before 13 years of age); running away from home overnight at least twice (or once for a lengthy period); often skipping school (beginning before 13 years of age).

Conduct disorder is diagnosed and treated by a number of social workers, school counselors, psychiatrists, and psychologists. Genuine diagnosis may require psychiatric expertise to rule out such conditions as **bipolar disorder** (manic depression) or ADHD. A comprehensive evaluation of the child should ideally include interviews with the child and parents, a full social and medical history, a cognitive evaluation, and a psychiatric exam. One or more clinical inventories or scales may be used to assess the child for conduct disorder—including the Youth Self-Report, the Overt Aggression Scale (OAS), Behavioral Assessment System for Children (BASC), Child Behavior Checklist (CBCL), and Diagnostic Interview Schedule for Children (DISC). The tests are verbal or written and are administered in both hospital and outpatient settings.

Treating conduct disorder requires an approach that addresses both the child and his environment. Behavioral therapy and psychotherapy can help a child with conduct disorder to control his anger and develop new coping skills. Family **group therapy** may also be effective in some cases. Parents should be counseled on how to set appropriate limits with their child and be consistent and realistic when disciplining. If an abusive home life is at the root of the conduct problem, every effort should be made to move the child into a more supportive environment. Parent training programs are increasing in number.

For children with coexisting ADHD, substance abuse, depression, or learning disorders, treating these conditions first is preferred, and may result in a significant improvement to the conduct disorder. In all cases of conduct disorder, treatment should begin when symptoms first appear. Recent studies have shown Ritalin to be a useful drug for both ADHD and CD.

When aggressive behavior is severe, mood-stabilizing medication, including lithium, carbamazepine, and propranolol, may be an appropriate option for treating the aggressive symptoms. However, placing the child into a structured setting or treatment program such as a psychiatric hospital may be just as beneficial for easing aggression as medication.

The prognosis for children with conduct disorder is not bright. Follow-up studies of conduct-disordered children have shown a high incidence of antisocial personality disorder, affective illnesses, and chronic criminal behavior later in life. However, proper treatment of coexisting disorders, early identification and intervention, and long-term support may improve the outlook significantly.

CONFLICT RESOLUTION

Conflict resolution is the process of defusing antagonism and reaching agreement between conflicting parties, especially through some form of negotiation. It can also be thought of as the study and practice of solving interpersonal and intergroup conflict.

A given conflict may be defined in terms of the issues that caused it, the strategies used to address it, or the outcomes or consequences that follow from it. Preschool and early elementary school-aged children tend to have conflict over property issues, and they tend to use physical strategies to resolve them, like taking a toy they want from another child. As children grow older the causes of conflict are more frequently about social order, and they are more likely to use verbal strategies as solutions.

Strategies for resolving or preventing the development of conflict can be classified as avoidance, diffusion, or confrontation. Turning on the TV rather than discussing an argument is a form of avoidance. Two teen athletes talking to their peers or counselors after a dispute on the football field is an example of diffusion. Insulting another student's girlfriend or arranging to meet after school to fight are examples of confrontation. Courtroom litigation, like the trial and indictment of a juvenile who has violated the law, also represents a form of confrontation.

The phrase conflict resolution refers specifically to strategies of diffusion developed during the second half of the 20th century as alternatives to traditional litigation models of settling disputes. Based on the idea that it is better to expose and resolve conflict before it damages people's relationships or escalates into violence, methods of conflict resolution were developed in business management and gradually adopted in the fields of international relations, legal settings, and, during the 1980s, educational settings. According to the principles of conflict resolution, the only true solution to a conflict is one that attempts to satisfy the inherent needs of all the parties involved.

Most conflict resolution programs employ some form of negotiation as the primary method of communication between parties. Negotiation can be distributive, where each party attempts to win as many concessions to his or her own self-interest as possible (win-lose), or integrative, where parties attempt to discover solutions that embody mutual self-interest (win-win). Research on games theory and the decision-making process suggest that the face-to-face conversation involved in direct negotiation may actually influence people to act in the interest of the group (including the opposing party), or some other interest beyond immediate self-interest. Face-to-face negotiation tends to be integrative in its consequences.

The success of a given instance of conflict resolution depends on the attitudes and skills of the disputants and of the mediator or arbitrator. The elementary skills that have been identified as promoting conflict resolution overlap to a high degree with those that reflect social competence in children and adolescents. They include:

- Awareness of others
- Awareness of the (not necessarily obvious) distinctions between self and others
- Listening skills
- Awareness of one's own feelings and thoughts, and the ability to express them
- Ability to respond to the feelings and thoughts of others

A child or adolescent will employ the basic skills of conflict resolution to varying degrees in responding to a conflict. Responses can be graded according to the level of cooperativeness they reflect, i.e., the level of integration the child experiences between his own self-interest and the interest of the opposing party. Thus, threatening the other party reflects a slightly more integrated, constructive response to conflict than an immediately aggressive response such as hitting. Examples of progressively more cooperative responses to conflict are: withdrawing from a conflict; demanding or requesting the opposing party to concede; providing reasons the opposing party should concede (appealing to norms); proposing alternatives to the opposing party; and proposing "if" statements, suggesting willingness to negotiate. Perspective taking, or articulating and validating the feelings and thoughts of the other party ("I see that you want...."), reflects the higher orders of conflict resolution skills. Integration of interests ("We both want...") reflects the highest level, leading to a consensual settlement of negotiations.

Conflict resolution in education includes any strategy that promotes handling disputes peacefully and cooperatively outside of, or in addition to, traditional disciplinary procedures. The rise of violence and disciplinary problems, along with an increasing awareness of the need for behavioral as well as cognitive instruction, spurred the development of conflict resolution programs in schools during the 1980s. These programs received national attention in 1984 with the formation of the National Association for Mediation in Education (NAME). By the late 1990s most major cities had instituted some form of large-scale conflict resolution program. According to a 1994 National School Boards study, 61% of schools had some form of conflict resolution program.

Conflict resolution programs differ widely in terms of who participates, the quantity of time and energy they require, and levels of funding they receive. Funding is usually provided by an outside source such as the state, a university program, or a local non-profit organization. Programs can be classroom-wide, school-wide, or district-wide, and can include any of the following components:

- Curriculum and classroom instruction
- Training workshops for faculty, staff, students, and/or parents in conflict management skills, negotiation, and mediation
- Peer education and counseling programs where students either train each other in conflict resolution skills and/or actually carry out dispute resolution
- Mediation programs in which students, staff, or teachers carry out dispute resolution

Some conflict resolution programs provide a venue for actual dispute resolution, while others only provide only training and instruction. School-wide or district-wide peer counseling and peer mediation programs carry out actual dispute resolution on a larger scale. Peer mediation, where students are trained in a step-by-step mediation process in order to provide ongoing mediation service for other students, is the most popular form of conflict resolution program. While these "applied" programs are more expensive than strictly curriculum-based programs, they appear to be significantly more effective. One study demonstrated that curriculum by itself does not change students' behavior in conflict situations, whereas the structured format of a peer mediation program did change the way students addressed conflict.

See also Violence and violence prevention

Conformity

Conformity can be defined as the tendency of individuals to change their behavior to conform to real or imagined pressure from a group. This tendency is of particular interest in **community health**, where conformity may influence the willingness of people to engage in activities such as drug abuse or high-risk sexual activities, or prompt them to avoid drug rehabilitation programs.

A simple example of conformity is the tendency of pedestrians to cross a street against the light, after other pedestrians have done the same. In such a situation, many people feel pressured to conform to the actions of others, even if it means disregarding a law and risking injury from being hit by an automobile.

Social groups can offer both advantages and disadvantages. They can provide care and support, and are good at collectively solving theoretical problems such as puzzles, etc. However, groups can also have a negative influence. When personalities and emotions enter the mix, groups frequently make poor decisions. Most people are eager to please their friends and acquaintances by conforming, which is far easier than disagreeing with a group that has opinions or behaviors different from our own.

The phenomenon of conformity is of interest to outreach workers because social networks may provide a link to a wide range of people involved in drug abuse and high-risk sexual activity. Drug users are often suspicious of street workers, but networks offer opportunities to discourage needle sharing or promote safer sexual practices, if these messages can be successfully communicated to key members of these groups.

Conjunctivitis

Conjuctivitis is an inflammation or redness of the lining of the white part of the eye and the underside of the eyelid (conjunctiva) that can be caused by infection, allergic reaction, or physical agents like infrared or ultraviolet light.

Conjunctivitis is the inflammation of the conjunctiva, a thin, delicate membrane that covers the eyeball and lines the eyelid. Conjunctivitis is an extremely common eye problem because the conjunctiva is continually exposed to microorganisms and environmental agents that can cause infections or allergic reactions. Conjunctivitis can be acute or chronic depending upon how long the condition lasts, the severity of symptoms, and the type of organism or agent involved. It can also affect one or both eyes and, if caused by infection, can be very easily transmitted to others during close physical contact, particularly among children in a daycare center. Other names for conjunctivitis include pink eye and red eye.

Conjunctivitis may be caused by a viral infection, such as a cold, acute respiratory infection, or disease such as **measles**, herpes simplex, or herpes zoster. Symptoms include mild to severe discomfort in one or both eyes, redness, swelling of the eyelids, and watery, yellow, or green discharge. Symptoms may last anywhere from several days to two weeks. Infection with an adenovirus, however, may also cause a significant amount of pus-like discharge and a scratchy, foreign body type of sensation in the eye. This may also be accompanied by swelling and tenderness of the lymph nodes near the ear.

Bacterial conjunctivitis can occur in adults and children and is caused by organisms such as *Staphylococcus*, *Streptococcus*, and *Hemophilus*. Symptoms of bacterial conjunctivitis include a pus-like discharge and crusty eyelids after awakening. Redness of the conjunctiva can be mild to severe and may be accompanied by swelling. Persons with symptoms of conjunctivitis who are sexually active may possibly be infected with the bacteria that cause either **gonorrhea** or chlamydia. There may be large amounts of pus-like discharge and symptoms may include intolerance to light (photophobia), watery mucous discharge, and tenderness in the lymph nodes near the ear that may persist for up to three months.

Conjunctivitis may also be caused by environmental hazards, such as wind, smoke, dust, and allergic reactions caused by pollen, dust, or grass. Symptoms range from **itching** and redness to a mucous discharge. Persons who wear contact lenses may develop allergic conjunctivitis caused by the various eye solutions and foreign proteins contained in them.

Other less common causes of conjunctivitis include exposure to sun lamps or the electrical arcs used during welding, and problems with inadequate drainage of the tear ducts.

An accurate diagnosis of conjunctivitis centers on taking a patient history to learn when symptoms began, how long the condition has been going on, the symptoms experienced, and other predisposing factors, such as upper respiratory complaints, **allergies**, **sexually transmitted diseases**, herpes simplex infections, and exposure to persons with pink eye. It may be helpful to learn whether an aspect of an individual's occupation may be the cause, for example, welding. Diagnostic tests are usually not indicated unless initial treatment fails or an infection with gonorrhea or chlamydia is suspected. In such cases, the discharge may be cultured and Gram stained to determine the organism responsible for causing the condition. Cultures and smears are relatively painless.

The treatment of conjunctivitis depends on what caused the condition. In all cases, warm compresses applied to the affected eye several times a day may help to reduce discomfort.

Conjunctivitis due to a viral infection, particularly those due to adenoviruses, are usually treated by applying warm compresses to the eye(s) and applying topical antibiotic ointments to prevent secondary bacterial infections.

Viral conjunctivitis caused by herpes simplex should be referred to an ophthalmologist. Topical steroids are commonly prescribed in combination with antiviral therapy.

In cases of bacterial conjunctivitis, a physician may prescribe an antibiotic eye ointment or eye drops containing sodium sulfacetamide (Sulamyd) to be applied daily for 7-14 days. If, after 72 hours, the condition does not improve, a physician or primary care provider should be notified because the bacteria involved may be resistant to the antibiotic used or the cause may not be bacterial.

For cases of conjunctivitis caused by a gonococcal organism, a physician may prescribe an intramuscular injection of ceftriaxone (Rocephin) and a topical antibiotic ointment containing erythromycin or bactracin to be applied four times daily for 2-3 weeks. Sexual partners should also be treated.

With accompanying chlamydia infection, a topical antibiotic ointment containing erythromycin (Ilotycin) may be prescribed to be applied 1-2 times daily. In addition, oral erythromycin or tetracycline therapy may be indicated for 3-4 weeks. Here again, sexual partners should also be treated.

Allergic conjunctivitis can be treated by removing the allergic substance from a person's environment, if possible; by applying cool compresses to the eye; and by administering eye drops 4-6 times daily for four days. Also, the antihistamine diphenhydramine hydrochloride (Benadryl) may help to relieve itchy eyes.

Conjunctivitis caused by gonococcal and chlamydial infection usually requires conventional medical treatment. With bacterial, viral, and allergic conjunctivitis, however, alternative options can be helpful. Internal immune enhancement with supplementation can aid in the resolution of bacterial and viral conjunctivitis. Removal of the allergic agent is an essential step in treating allergic conjunctivitis. As with any of the recommended treatments, however, if no improvement is seen within 48-72 hours, a physician should be consulted.

Homeopathically, there are a number of acute remedies designed to treat conjunctivitis. These include *Pulsatilla* (windflower, *Pulsatilla nigricans*), *Belladonna*, and eyebright (*Euphrasia officinalis*). Eye drops, prepared with homeopathic remedies and/or herbs, can be a good substitute for pharmaceutical eye drops. Eye washes can also be made. Herbal eyewashes made with eyebright (1 tsp. dried herb steeped in 1 pint of boiling water) or chamomile (*Matricaria recutita*; 2-3 tsp. in 1 pint of boiling water) may be helpful. Eyewashes should be strained and cooled before use, and close attention should be paid to make sure that any solution put into the eye is sterile.

Other simple home remedies may help relieve the discomfort associated with conjunctivitis. A boric acid eyewash can be used to clean and soothe the eyes. A warm compress applied to the eyes for 5-10 minutes three times a day can help relieve the discomfort of bacterial and viral conjunctivitis. A cool compress or cool, damp tea bags placed on the eyes can ease the discomfort of allergic conjunctivitis.

If treated properly, the prognosis for conjunctivitis is good. Conjunctivitis caused by an allergic reaction should clear up once the allergen is removed. However, allergic conjunctivitis will likely recur if the individual again comes into contact with the particular allergen. Conjunctivitis caused by bacteria or a virus, if treated properly, is usually resolved in 10-14 days. If there is no relief of symptoms in 48-72 hours, or there is moderate to severe eye pain, changes in vision, or the conjunctivitis is suspected to be caused by herpes simplex, a physician should be notified immediately. If untreated or if treatment fails and is not corrected, conjunctivitis may cause **visual impairment** by spreading to other parts of the eye, such as the cornea.

Conjunctivitis can, in many cases, be prevented, or at least the course of the disease can be shortened by following some simple practices.

- Frequently wash hands using antiseptic soap, and use single-use towels during the disease to prevent spreading the infection.
- Avoid chemical irritants and known allergens.
- If in an area where welding occurs, use the proper protective eye wear and screens to prevent damaging the eyes.
- Use a clean tissue to remove discharge from eyes, and wash hands to prevent the spread of infection.
- If medication is prescribed, finish the course of **antibiotics**, as directed, to make sure that the infection is cleared up and does not recur.
- Avoid contact, such as vigorous physical activities, with other persons until symptoms resolve.

Conscience

The development of conscience, or moral development, involves the formation of a system of values on which to base decisions concerning ''right'' and ''wrong,'' or ''good'' and ''bad.'' Values are underlying assumptions about standards that govern moral decisions.

Although morality has been a topic of discussion since the beginning of human civilization, the scientific study of moral development did not begin in earnest until the late

1950s. Lawrence Kohlberg (1927-1987), an American psychologist building upon Jean Piaget's work in cognitive reasoning, posited six stages of moral development in his 1958 doctoral thesis. Since that time, morality and moral development have become acceptable subjects of scientific research.

There are several approaches to the study of moral development, which are categorized in a variety of ways. Briefly, the social learning theory approach claims that humans develop morality by learning the rules of acceptable behavior from their external environment (an essentially behaviorist approach). Psychoanalytic theory proposes instead that morality develops through humans' conflict between their instinctual drives and the demands of society. Cognitive development theories view morality as an outgrowth of cognition, or reasoning, whereas personality theories are holistic in their approach, taking into account all the factors that contribute to human development.

The differences between these approaches rest on two questions: 1) where do humans begin on their moral journey; and 2) where do we end up? In other words, how moral are infants at birth? And how is ''moral maturity'' defined? What is the ideal morality to which we aspire? The contrasting philosophies at the heart of the answers to these questions determine the essential perspective of each moral development theory. Those who believe infants are born with no moral sense tend toward social learning or behaviorist theories (as all morality must therefore be learned from the external environment). Others who believe humans are innately aggressive and completely self-oriented are more likely to accept psychoanalytic theories (where morality is the learned management of socially destructive internal drives). Those who believe it is our reasoning abilities that separate us from the rest of creation will find cognitive development theories the most attractive. Finally, those who view humans as holistic beings born with a full range of potentialities will most likely be drawn to personality theories.

What constitutes ''mature morality'' is a subject of great controversy. Each society develops its own set of norms and standards for acceptable behavior, leading many to say that morality is entirely culturally conditioned. Does this mean there are no universal truths, no cross-cultural standards for human behavior? The debate over this question fuels the critiques of many moral development theories. Kohlberg's six stages of moral development, for example, have been criticized for elevating Western, urban, intellectual (upper-class) understandings of morality, while discrediting rural, tribal, working-class, or Eastern moral understandings. Feminists have pointed out potential sexist elements in moral development theories devised by male researchers using male subjects only (such as Kohlberg's early work). Because women's experience in the world is different from men's (in every culture), it would stand to reason that women's moral development might differ from men's, perhaps in significant ways.

The rise in crime, drug and alcohol abuse, gang violence, teen parenthood, and suicide in recent years in Western society has also caused a rise in concern over morality and moral development. Parents and teachers want to know how to raise moral children, and they turn to moral development theorists to find the answers.

Overall, democratic family and school systems are much more likely to promote the development of internal self-controls and moral growth than are authoritarian or permissive systems. Permissive systems fail to instill any controls, while authoritarian systems instill only fear of punishment, which is not an effective deterrent unless there is a real chance of being caught (punishment can even become a reward for immoral behavior when it is the only attention a person ever gets). True moral behavior involves a number of internal processes that are best developed through warm, caring parenting with clear and consistent expectations, emphasis on the reinforcement of positive behaviors (rather than the punishment of negative ones), modeling of moral behavior by adults, and creation of opportunities for the child to practice moral reasoning and actions.

As previously stated, there is disagreement as to the exact motivations involved in moral behavior. Whatever the motivations, however, the internal processes remain the same. The Four Component model describes them as follows:

1) moral sensitivity—empathy (identifying with another's experience) and cognition of the effect of various possible actions on others;

2) moral judgment—choosing which action is the most moral;

3) moral motivation—deciding to behave in the moral way, as opposed to other options; and

4) implementation—carrying out the chosen moral action.

Most people in fact have more than one moral ''voice'' and shift among them depending on the situation. In one context, a person may respond out of empathy and place care for one person over concern for social rules. In a different context, that same person might instead insist on following social rules for the good of society, even though someone may suffer because of it. People also show a lack of consistent morality by sometimes choosing to act in a way that they know is not moral, while continuing to consider themselves ''moral'' people. This discrepancy between moral judgment (perceiving an act as morally right or wrong) and moral choice (deciding whether to act in the morally ''right'' way) can be explained in a number of ways, any one of which may be true in a given situation: 1) weakness of will (the person is overwhelmed by desire); 2) weakness of conscience (guilt feelings are not strong enough to overcome tempation); or 3) limited/flexible morality (some latitude allowed in moral behavior while still maintaining a ''moral'' identity).

The Moral Balance model proposes that most humans operate out of a limited or flexible morality. Rather than expecting moral perfection from ourselves or others, we set certain limits beyond which we cannot go. Within those limits, however, there is some flexibility in moral decision-making. Actions such as taking coins left in the change-box of a public telephone may be deemed acceptable (though not perfectly moral), while stealing money from an open, unattended cash register is not. Many factors are involved in the determination of moral acceptability from situation to situation, and the limits on moral behavior are often slippery. If given proper en-

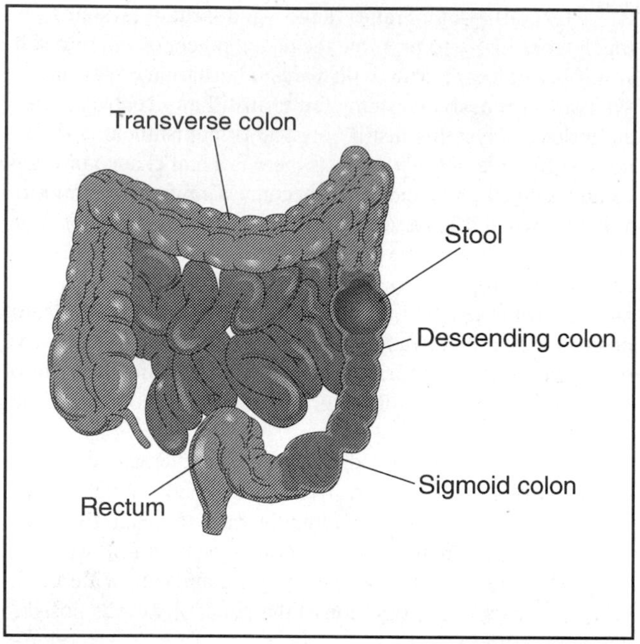

Constipation is an acute or chronic condition in which bowel movements occur less often than usual or consist of hard, dry stools that are painful or difficult to pass. ***(Illustration by Electronic Illustrators Group).***

couragement and the opportunity to practice a coherent inner sense of morality, however, most people will develop a balanced morality to guide their day-to-day interactions with their world.

CONSTIPATION

Constipation is an acute or chronic condition in which bowel movements occur less often than usual or consist of hard, dry stools that are painful or difficult to pass. Bowel habits vary, but an adult who has not had a bowel movement in three days or a child who has not had a bowel movement in four days is considered constipated.

Constipation is one of the most common medical complaints in the United States. Constipation can occur at any age, and is more common among individuals who resist the urge to move their bowels at their body's signal. This often happens when children start school or enter daycare and feel shy about asking permission to use the bathroom.

Constipation is more common in women than in men and is especially apt to occur during **pregnancy**. Age alone does not increase the frequency of constipation, but elderly people (especially women) are more likely to suffer from constipation.

Although this condition is rarely serious, it can lead to bowel obstruction, chronic constipation, **hemorrhoids** (a mass of dilated veins in swollen tissue around the anus), **hernia** (a protrusion of an organ through a tear in the muscle wall), spastic colitis (**irritable bowel syndrome**—(a condition characterized by alternating periods of **diarrhea** and constipation), and laxative dependency.

Chronic constipation may be a symptom of **colorectal cancer**, depression, diabetes, diverticulosis (small pouches in the muscles of the large intestine), **lead poisoning**, or **Parkinson's disease**.

Constipation usually results from not getting enough **exercise**, not drinking enough water, or from a diet that does not include an adequate amount of fiber-rich foods like beans, bran cereals, fruits, raw vegetables, rice, and whole-grain breads.

Other causes of constipation include anal fissure (a tear or crack in the lining of the anus); chronic **kidney failure**; colon or rectal **cancer**; depression; hypercalcemia (abnormally high levels of calcium in the blood); hypothyroidism (underactive thyroid gland); illness requiring complete bed rest; irritable bowel syndrome; and **stress**.

Constipation can also be a side effect of a variety of medications, including **antacids**, blood pressure medications, **diuretics** (drugs that promote the formation and secretion of urine), and iron or calcium supplements.

An adult who is constipated may feel bloated, have a headache, swollen abdomen, or pass rock-like feces; or strain, bleed, or feel pain during bowel movements. A constipated baby may strain, cry, draw its legs toward the abdomen, or arch the back when having a bowel movement.

Everyone becomes constipated once in a while, but a doctor should be notified if significant changes in bowel patterns last for more than a week or if symptoms continue more than three weeks after increasing activity and fiber and fluid intake.

The patient's observations and medical history help a primary care physician diagnose constipation. The doctor uses his fingers to see if there is a hardened mass in the abdomen, and may perform a rectal examination. Other diagnostic procedures include a barium **enema**, which reveals blockage inside the intestine; laboratory analysis of blood and stool samples for internal bleeding or other symptoms of systemic disease; and a sigmoidoscopy (examination of the sigmoid area of the colon with a flexible tube equipped with a magnifying lens).

Physical and psychological assessments and a detailed history of bowel habits are especially important when an elderly person complains of constipation.

If changes in diet and activity fail to relieve occasional constipation, an over-the-counter laxative may be used for a few days. Preparations that soften stools or add bulk (bran, psyllium) work more slowly but are safer than Epsom salts and other harsh **laxatives** or herbal laxatives containing senna (*Cassia senna*) or buckthorn (*Rhamnus purshianna*), which can harm the nerves and lining of the colon.

A woman who is pregnant should never use a laxative. Neither should anyone who is experiencing abdominal pain, nausea, or vomiting.

A warm-water or mineral oil enema can relieve constipation, and a non-digestible sugar (lactulose) or special electrolyte solution is recommended for adults and older children with stubborn symptoms.

If a patient has an impacted bowel, the doctor inserts a gloved finger into the rectum and gently dislodges the hardened feces.

Changes in diet and exercise usually eliminate the problem.

Most Americans consume between 11 and 18 grams (about a half an ounce of fiber a day. Consumption of 30 grams of fiber and between six and eight glasses of water each day can generally prevent constipation.

Sitting on the toilet for 10 minutes at the same time every day, preferably after a meal, can induce regular bowel movements. This may not become effective for a few months, and it is important to defecate whenever necessary.

Fiber supplements containing psyllium (*Plantago psyllium*) usually become effective within about 48 hours and can be used every day without causing dependency. Powdered flaxseed (*Linium usitatissimum*) works the same way. Insoluble fiber, like wheat or oat bran, is as effective as psyllium but may give the patient gas at first.

Consumer protection

In 1998, the White House raised important questions about how and whether the federal government should implement a patient's bill of rights that would strengthen consumer confidence in the health care system by ensuring that the system is fair and responsive to consumers' needs, by reaffirming the importance of the physician-patient relationship, and by setting forth the rights and responsibilities of all Americans in improving their own health.

In the absence of binding federal legislation, laws governing consumer protection in the health arena are implemented on a state-by-state basis; as a medical consumer, your rights and legal protection will be based on laws and guidelines in place in the state in which you live. Federal agencies are available to offer advice to the consumer and to identify health fraud, but for the most part, the advice that they offer is limited to the caveat emptor axiom: let the buyer beware. However, fraud in the health care industry has occurred with sufficient frequency that federal agencies are now able to offer guidelines for avoiding fraudulent health schemes.

The **Food and Drug Administration**, for example, has prepared a list of the top 10 health frauds: these being fraudulent arthritis products, spurious **cancer** clinics, bogus AIDS cures, instant weight-loss schemes, fraudulent sexual aids, quack **baldness** remedies or appearance modifiers, false **nutrition**al schemes, unproven claims for a muscle stimulators, and so-called cures for **Candidiasis** hypersensitivity.

Dishonest promoters seem to be particularly fond of peddling arthritis remedies and cancer cures. They frequently promise quick or painless cures; promote products made from a special or secret formula; present testimonials from satisfied patients, claim their products are effective for a wide variety of ailments; and claim to have the cure for a disease that is not yet understood by medical science.

If you have questions about the claims made for a medical product, you can consult the following agencies for advice: the Food and Drug Administration (for questions about medical devices, medicines, and food supplements that are mislabeled, misrepresented, or in some way harmful); the U.S. Postal Service (in the case of products purchased by mail); the Council of Better Business Bureaus (for publications and advice on products); the Federal Trade Commission (in the case of false advertising); the Cancer Information Service (for answers about questions about cancer-related issues, including foods and products); the National Arthritis, Musculoskeletal and Skin Diseases Information Clearinghouse (for answers about questions related to arthritis); the National Institute on **Aging** (for information on health and aging); and/or the **U. S. Department of Health and Human Services.**

If you want to take legal action, the National Council Against Health Fraud can refer you to an experienced lawyer. This organization also offers a registry of expert witnesses, information on defense witnesses, and maintains a list of unproven, fraudulent, and potentially dangerous treatments. You can also contact your state Attorney General's office.

Contraception

Contraception (birth control) prevents **pregnancy** by interfering with the normal process of ovulation, fertilization, and implantation. There are different kinds of birth control that act at different points in the process.

Every month, a woman's body begins the process that can potentially lead to pregnancy. An egg (ovum) matures, the mucus that is secreted by the cervix (a cylindrical-shaped organ at the lower end of the uterus) changes to be more inviting to sperm, and the lining of the uterus grows in preparation for receiving a fertilized egg.

Birth control (contraception) is designed to interfere with the normal process and prevent the pregnancy that could result. There are different kinds of birth control that act at different points in the process, from ovulation, through fertilization, to implantation. Each method has its own side effects and risks. Some methods are more reliable than others.

Although there are many different types of birth control, they can be divided into a few groups based on how they work.

Hormonal methods use medications (hormones) to prevent ovulation. Hormonal methods include birth control pills (**oral contraceptives**), Depo Provera injections and Norplant.

Barrier methods work by preventing the sperm from getting to and fertilizing the egg. Barrier methods include the **condom**, diaphragm, and cervical cap. The condom is the only form of birth control that also protects against **sexually transmitted diseases**, including HIV (the virus that causes **AIDS**).

Spermicides kill sperm on contact. Most spermicides contain nonoxynyl-9. Spermicides come in many different forms such as jelly, foam, tablets, and even a transparent film. All are placed in the vagina. Spermicides work best when they are used at the same time as a barrier method.

Intrauterine contraceptive devices (**IUD**s) are inserted into the uterus, where they stay from 1-10 years. An IUD prevents the fertilized egg from implanting in the lining of the uterus, and may have other effects as well.

Tubal sterilization is a permanent form of contraception for women. Each fallopian tube is either tied or burned closed. The sperm cannot reach the egg, and the egg cannot travel to the uterus.

Vasectomy is the male form of sterilization, and should also be considered permanent. In vasectomy, the vas defrens, the tiny tubes that carry the sperm into the semen, are cut and tied off. Thus, no sperm can get into the semen.

Unfortunately, there is no perfect form of birth control. Only abstinence (not having sexual intercourse) can protect against unwanted pregnancy with 100% reliability. The failure rates, which means the rates of pregnancy, for most forms of birth control are quite low. However, some forms of birth control are more difficult or inconvenient to use than others. In actual practice, the birth control methods that are more difficult or inconvenient have much higher failure rates, because they are not used faithfully.

All the different forms of birth control have one thing in common. They are only effective if used faithfully. Birth control pills will work only if taken every day; the diaphragm is effective only if used during every episode of sexual intercourse. The same is true for condoms and the cervical cap. Some methods are automatically working every day, no matter what. These methods include **Depo Provera**, **Norplant**, the IUD, and tubal sterilization.

There are many different ways to use birth control. For example, birth control pills must be taken by mouth every day. Depo Provera is a hormonal medication that is given by injection every three months. Norplant is a long-acting hormonal form of birth control that is implanted under the skin of the upper arm. Spermicides and barrier methods work in the vagina. The IUD is inserted into the uterus. Tubal sterilization is a form of surgery. A doctor must perform the procedure in a hospital or surgical clinic.

The methods of birth control also differ from each other in the timing of when they are used. Some methods of birth control must be used specifically at the time of sexual intercourse (condoms, diaphragm, cervical cap, spermicides). All other methods of birth control must be working all the time to provide protection (hormonal methods, IUDs, tubal sterilization).

There are risks associated with some forms of birth control. The hormone (estrogen) in birth control pills can increase the risk of **heart attack** in women over 40 who smoke. The IUD can increase the risk of serious pelvic infection. The IUD can also injure the uterus by poking into or through the uterine wall, which may require surgery to repair. Tubal sterilization (''tying the tubes'') is a surgical procedure and has all the risks of any other surgery, including the risks of anesthesia, infection, and bleeding.

No specific preparation is needed before using contraception. However, a woman must be sure that she is not already pregnant before using a hormonal method or having an IUD placed.

Many methods of birth control have side effects. Knowing the side effects can help a woman to determine which method of birth control is right for her. The hormones in birth control pills, Depo Provera, and Norplant can cause changes in menstrual periods, changes in mood, weight gain, **acne**, and **headaches**. In addition, it may take many months to begin ovulating again once a woman stops using Depo Provera or Norplant. A woman must insert the diaphragm in just the right way to be sure that it works properly. Some women get more urinary tract infections if they use a diaphragm. This is because the diaphragm can press against the urethra, the tube that connects the bladder to the outside. Some women and men are allergic to spermicides or find them irritating to the skin. The IUD is a foreign body that stays inside the uterus, and sometimes the uterus rejects it. A woman may have heavier menstrual periods and more menstrual cramping with an IUD in place. Some women report increased menstrual discomfort after **tubal ligation**. It is not known if this is related to the tubal ligation itself.

There is no perfect form of birth control. Every method has a small failure rate and side effects. Some methods carry additional risks. However, every method of birth control has fewer risks than pregnancy.

Cooling treatments

Cooling treatments lower body temperature in order to relieve **pain**, swelling, constriction of blood vessels, and to decrease the likelihood of cellular damage by slowing the metabolism. Sponge baths, cold compresses, and cold packs are all wet cooling treatments. Dry treatments, such as ice bags and chemical cold packs, are also used to lower body temperature.

The most common reason for cooling a body is **fever** or hyperthermia (extremely high fever). The body can sustain temperatures up to 104°F (40°C) with relative safety; however, when temperatures rise above 104°F (40°C), damage to the brain, muscles, blood, and kidneys is increasingly likely. Cooling treatments are also applied immediately following sprains, **bruises**, **burns**, eye injuries, and muscle spasms to help alleviate the resulting swelling, pain, and discoloration of the skin.

Cooling treatments slow chemical reactions within the body. For this reason, cooling tissues below normal temperature (98.6°F/37°C) can prevent injury from inadequate oxygen or nutrition. Cold water drowning victims suffering from **hypothermia** (cooling of the body below its normal temperature) have been successfully resuscitated after long periods underwater without medical complications because of this effect. For the past 40 years, heart surgeons have been experimenting with hypothermia to protect tissues from lack of blood circulation during an operation. Neurosurgeons are also working with hypothermia to protect the very sensitive brain tissues during periods of absent or reduced blood flow.

Depending on the medical need, various cooling methods are used. Cold packs and ice bags are placed on a localized site and provide topical relief. These compresses should be covered with a waterproof material to protect the skin. Repeated treatments produce the desired pain and swelling relief. Cold treatments are placed on the groin and under the arms to treat hyperthermia. Treatments are refreshed periodically until the appropriate temperature is attained. A tepid sponge bath relieves fever without cooling the body too fast. Eighty degrees Farenheit is still 20°F below body temperature and yet warm enough not to drive blood from the skin, thereby preventing the cooling from getting to the body's core. Limbs are bathed first and then the chest, abdomen, back, and buttocks. Perfusion (bathing) of isolated regions like the brain by using cooled blood is an experimental treatment, offering promising results for the treatment of **stroke**.

Topical treatments are prepared with ice, cold water (59°F/15°C), and chemical cold packs. Tepid baths should be 80-93°F (26.7-34°C).

Small children, adults with circulation problems, and the elderly are all at risk of tissue damage. Rapid cooling causes chills, which in effect raise the body's temperature by raising its metabolism. Blood clots may form from thickened blood caused by the temperature change.

Cori, Carl Ferdinand (1896-1957) Cori, Gerty Theresa Radnitz (1896-1984)

Czech American biochemists

Carl and Gerty Cori were both born in Prague, Austria-Hungary (now the Czech Republic) in 1896. They entered the University of Prague's medical school at roughly the same time, each planning to become a physician. At some point during their student days, they met each other, fell in love, and teamed up to share laboratory research in biochemistry. They decided that they not only enjoyed working together but also preferred biochemical research to medical practice. But in 1920, after they married and obtained their medical degrees, only Carl was able to find a research position. It was in Vienna, Austria, and Gerty joined the staff of a hospital there, but they still longed to work together. In 1922, when Carl was offered a position as a biochemist at the New York Institute for the Study of Malignant Diseases in Buffalo, New York, he immigrated to the United States. Gerty followed him a few months later when a job opened up for her in the same institution.

At the New York Institute, the Coris did some research on the **metabolism** of abnormal growths but spent most of their time investigating the way normal healthy bodies utilize sugars and starches. The research team was particularly intrigued by two hormones—epinephrine and the recently discovered **insulin**—and their roles in carbohydrate metabolism.

In a series of papers published during the 1920s, the Coris provided the scientific world with a great deal of information about what happened to sugars after they were absorbed by experimental white rats. Among other things, they reported, normally about half the absorbed sugar (now called glucose) is converted to glycogen and stored in this form in the liver and muscles, with the rest either stored as fat or burned as fuel. The administration of insulin, however, not only decreases the amount of sugar stored in the liver, but increases its utilization elsewhere.

In 1932, the two scientists joined the faculty of Washington University in St. Louis, Missouri, where they were able

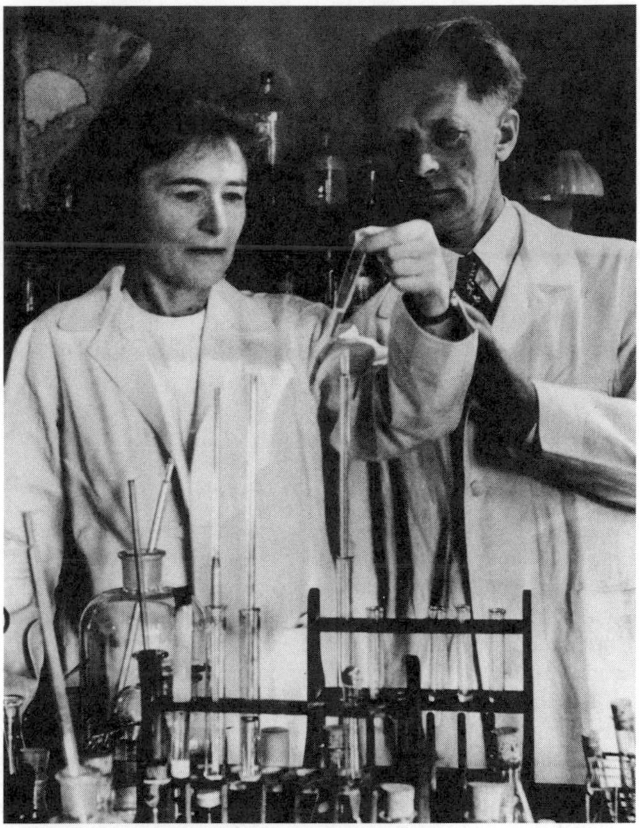

Gerty Theresa Cori and Carl Ferdinand Cori

to probe even more deeply into the mysteries of carbohydrate metabolism. The work of another biochemist, **Otto Meyerhof**, had already established the fact that, when muscles contract, the glycogen stored in them is somehow converted to lactic acid. The Coris wanted to find out exactly how the glycogen is broken down and how, after its conversion to lactic acid, it is then resynthesized into glucose. In their new laboratory, they were able to find the answers.

Using minced frog muscles to help them in their investigations, the Coris were soon able to isolate and identify a sugar and phosphate compound, previously unknown, which they named glucose-1-phosphate (often called Cori ester in their honor.) This discovery, plus their discovery of two new enzymes, helped them disprove a widely held belief—that the highly branched glycogen molecule breaks itself down to glucose molecules by adding water molecules at each of its many links. Although this breakdown process seemed simple and logical, the Coris pointed out it would also lead to a pronounced energy loss that would have impaired the eventual resynthesis. Instead of using water, glycogen—helped by one of the enzymes they discovered—adds inorganic phosphate at each of its links to form the newly-discovered phosphate-containing compound (which involved less energy loss) and then undergoes a long series of chemical changes before it is finally broken down. The Coris patiently detailed each of the changes and then went on to outline the resynthesis process—

in time, actually managing to synthesize the glycogen in a test tube.

For their work on glycogen, the Coris shared—with the Argentinean Bernardo Houssay (1887-1971)—the 1947 Nobel Prize in physiology or medicine. Gerty Cori was the third woman to be awarded a Nobel Prize in a scientific field. The other two were Marie Curie and her daughter, Irène Joliot-Curie. Other honors the couple shared included membership in the American Society of Biological Chemists, the National Academy of Sciences, the American Chemical Society, and the American Philosophical Society. They were joint recipients of the Midwest Award of the American Chemical Society in 1946 and the Squibb Award in Endocrinology in 1947.

CORMACK, ALLAN M. (1924-)

South African American physicist

Allan M. Cormack is a physicist whose theoretical analysis and experiments in the fields of nuclear and particle physics, computer tomography and math led to his invention of a mathematical technique for computer-assisted X-ray tomography. **Computerized axial tomography**, otherwise known as the CAT scan, is a process by which X rays can be concentrated on specific sections of the human body at a variety of angles. Once this information is analyzed by a computer, it is combined to reproduce images of internal structures previously unviewable by medical technology. It is considered the most revolutionary development in the field of radiography since the discovery of the x ray by **Wilhelm Conrad Röntgen** in 1895. Cormack was the first to analyze the possibility of such an examination of a biological system, in 1963 and 1964, and to develop the equations needed for computer-assisted x-ray reconstruction of pictures of the human brain and body. In 1979 Cormack was awarded the Nobel Prize for physiology or medicine, along with **Godfrey Hounsfield**, a British engineer who, independently of Cormack, developed the first commercially successful CAT scanning devices.

Allan MacLeod Cormack was born in Johannesburg, South Africa, on February 23, 1924, the son of George and Amelia (MacLeod) Cormack, a civil service engineer and a teacher respectively, who had emigrated from Scotland to South Africa prior to World War I. Young Cormack attended the Rondebosch Boys High School. At the University of Cape Town, South Africa, Cormack chose the field of engineering, but two years later he changed his major to physics, completing a baccalaureate of science in 1944.

He remained at the University of Cape Town, completing a Master of Science degree in the field of crystallography in 1945. During the years that followed, Cormack became a lecturer in physics at the University of Cape Town and pursued graduate studies in the field of theoretical physics for two years at Cambridge University in England. Working as a research student in the university's Cavendish Laboratory, he studied radioactive helium under the tutelage of Otto Robert Frisch. He also attended lectures on quantum physics given by Nobel Prize winner Paul Dirac.

In 1950 Cormack returned to South Africa from Cambridge to resume his position as a lecturer in physics at the University of Cape Town, where he would remain until 1956. During this period he was asked to serve a six-month service as resident medical physicist in the radiology department at the Groote Schuur Hospital in Cape Town, where he supervised the use of radioisotopes as well as the calibration of film badges used to measure hospital workers' exposure to radiation.

At Groote Schuur, Cormack witnessed first hand how radiation was being used in the diagnosis and treatment of **cancer** patients. Baffled by deficiencies in the technology used for such procedures, Cormack began a series of experiments and analyses, the results of which were two papers published separately between 1963 and 1964 in the *Journal of Applied Physics*. Cormack also conducted theoretical physics research in Boston on subatomic particles, following a 1956 Harvard University sabbatical as a Research Fellow, where he worked in the cyclotron laboratory under director Andreas Koehler.

Following a brief return to Cape Town in 1957, Cormack returned to the United States, accepting a post as assistant professor of physics at Tufts University in Medford, Massachusetts. Between 1956 and 1964, most of his research in connection with the development of computerized axial tomography was conducted on his own time. Neither of his two *Journal of Applied Physics* papers met with significant response, despite the fact that they proved the feasibility of his method for producing images of heretofore unviewable or barely viewable cross sections of the human body.

Cormak was naturalized as a citizen of the United States in 1966, and continued his academic career and his research in particle physics at Tufts. He was eventually promoted to associate and then full professor of physics, serving as chairman of the physics department from 1968 to 1976. Meanwhile, Hounsfield was independently coming to conclusions similar to Cormack's, and developed the first CAT scanner as early as 1972.

In 1979 Cormack and Hounsfield were awarded the Nobel Prize for physiology or medicine for their joint, though independent, development of CAT scan theory and technology. At the time, their selection as recipients of the prize was considered highly unusual. Unlike previous Nobel recipients, neither Cormack nor Hounsfield held a doctorate in medicine or science; further, their discovery was awarded the prize only after the Nobel Assembly vetoed the first choice of the selection committee; and, finally, it was highly unusual that the two men had never met or worked together, yet had worked on the same invention concurrently.

In 1980, Tufts appointed Cormack to university professor, its highest professorial rank, and awarded him with an honorary doctoral degree. In 1990, as one of several scientists receiving the National Medal of Science, Cormack was recognized by President George Bush.Cormack is a member of the National Academy of Science and the American Academy of Arts and Sciences, and is a fellow of the American Physical Society.

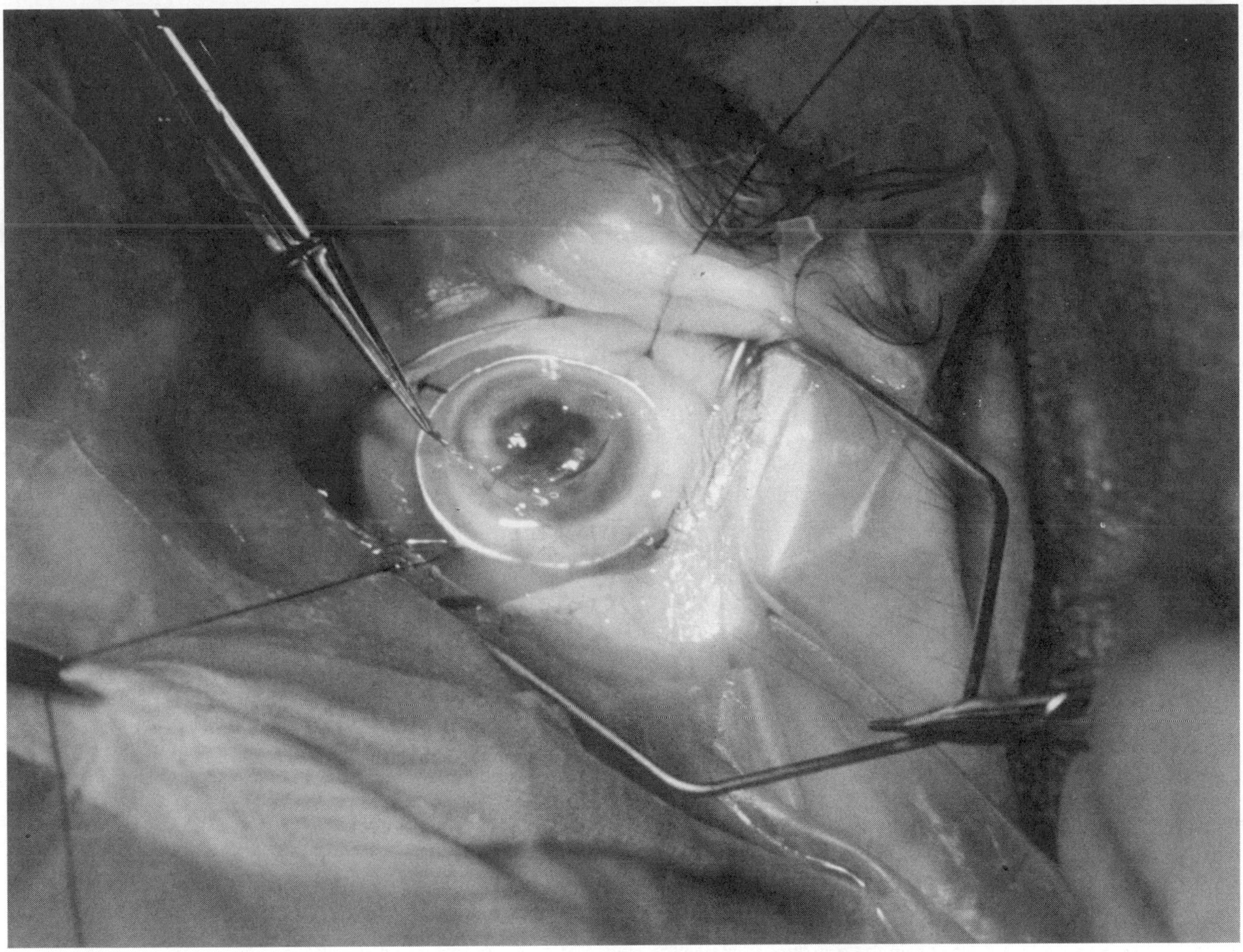

A corneal transplant in progress. *(Photograph by Chet Szymecki, Phototake NYC. Reproduced by permission.)*

CORNEAL TRANSPLANTATION

In corneal transplant, also known as keratoplasty, a patient's damaged cornea is replaced by the cornea from the eye of a human cadaver. This is the single most common type of human transplant surgery and has the highest success rate. Eye banks acquire and store eyes from donor individuals largely to supply the need for transplant corneas.

Corneal transplant is used when vision is lost in an eye because the cornea has been damaged by disease or traumatic injury. Some of the disease conditions that might require corneal transplant include the bulging outward of the cornea (keratoconus), a malfunction of the inner layer of the cornea (Fuchs' dystrophy), and painful swelling of the cornea (pseudophakic bullous keratopathy). Some of these conditions cause cloudiness of the cornea; others alter its natural curvature, which can also reduce the quality of vision.

Injury to the cornea can occur because of chemical **burns**, mechanical trauma, or infection by viruses, bacteria, fungi, or protozoa. Herpes virus is one of the more common infections leading to corneal transplant.

Surgery would only be used when damage to the cornea is too severe to be treated with corrective lenses. Occasionally, corneal transplant is combined with other types of eye surgery (such as cataract surgery) to solve multiple eye problems in one procedure.

Corneal transplant is a very safe procedure that can be performed on almost any patient who would benefit from it. Any active infection or inflammation of the eye usually needs to be brought under control before surgery can be performed.

The cornea is the transparent layer of tissue at the very front of the eye. It is composed almost entirely of a special type of collagen. It normally contains no blood vessels, but because it contains nerve endings, damage to the cornea can be very painful.

In a corneal transplant, a disc of tissue is removed from the center of the eye and replaced by a corresponding disc from a donor eye. The circular incision is made using an instrument called a trephine. In one form of corneal transplant (penetrating keratoplasty), the disc removed is the entire thickness of the cornea and so is the replacement disc. Over 90% of all corneal transplants in the United States are of this type. In lamellar keratoplasty, on the other hand, only the outer layer of the cornea is removed and replaced.

The donor cornea is attached with extremely fine sutures. Surgery can be performed under anesthesia that is confined to one area of the body while the patient is awake (local anesthesia) or under anesthesia that places the entire body of the patient in a state of unconsciousness (general anesthesia.) Surgery requires 30-90 minutes.

Over 40,000 corneal transplants are performed in the United States each year.

A less common but related procedure called epikeratophakia involves suturing the donor cornea directly onto the surface of the existing host cornea. The only tissue removed from the host is the extremely thin epithelial cell layer on the outside of the host cornea. There is no permanent damage to the host cornea, and this procedure can be reversed. It is usually employed in children. In adults, the use of contact lenses can usually achieve the same goals.

Corneal transplants are highly successful, with over 90% of operations in United States achieving restoration of sight. However, there is always some risk associated with any surgery. Complications that can occur include infection, **glaucoma**, **retinal detachment**, cataract formation, and rejection of the donor cornea.

Graft rejection occurs in 5-30% of patients, a complication possible with any procedure involving tissue transplantation from another person (allograft). Allograft rejection results from a reaction of the patient's immune system to the donor tissue. Cell surface proteins called histocompatibility antigens trigger this reaction. These antigens are often associated with vascular tissue (blood vessels) within the graft tissue. Since the cornea normally contains no blood vessels, it experiences a very low rate of rejection. Generally, blood typing and **tissue typing** are not needed in corneal transplants, and no close match between donor and recipient is required. Symptoms of rejection include persistent discomfort, sensitivity to light, redness, or a change in vision.

If a rejection reaction does occur, it can usually be blocked by steroid treatment. Rejection reactions may become noticeable within weeks after surgery, but may not occur until 10 or even 20 years after the transplant. When full rejection does occur, the surgery will usually need to be repeated.

Although the cornea is not normally vascular, some corneal diseases cause vascularization (the growth of blood vessels) into the cornea. In patients with these conditions, careful testing of both donor and recipient is performed just as in transplantation of other organs and tissues such as hearts, kidneys, and bone marrow. In such patients, repeated surgery is sometimes necessary in order to achieve a successful transplant.

Cornea donors are carefully screened. Individuals with infectious diseases are not accepted as donors.

Coronary artery disease

Coronary artery disease, also called coronary heart disease or heart disease, is the leading cause of death for both men and women in the United States.

Coronary artery disease occurs when the coronary arteries become partially blocked or clogged. This blockage limits the flow of blood from the coronary arteries, the major arteries supplying oxygen-rich blood to the heart. The coronary arteries expand when the heart is working harder and needs more oxygen. If the arteries are unable to expand, the heart is deprived of oxygen (myocardial ischemia). When the blockage is limited, chest pain or pressure called **angina** may occur. When the blockage cuts off the flow of blood, the result is heart attack (myocardial infarction or heart muscle death).

Healthy coronary arteries are clean, smooth, and slick. The artery walls are flexible and can expand to let more blood through when the heart needs to work harder. The disease process in arteries is thought to begin with an injury to the linings and walls of the arteries. This injury makes them susceptible to atherosclerosis and blood clots (thrombosis).

Coronary artery disease is usually caused by atherosclerosis. Cholesterol and other fatty substances accumulate on the inner wall of the arteries. They attract fibrous tissue, blood components, and calcium and harden into artery-clogging plaques. Atherosclerotic plaques often form blood clots that can also block the coronary arteries (coronary thrombosis). Congenital defects and muscle spasms, too, can block blood flow. Recent research indicates that infection from organisms such as chlamydia bacteria may be responsible for some cases of coronary artery disease.

A number of major contributing factors increase the risk of developing coronary artery disease. Some of these can be changed and some cannot. People with more risk factors are more likely to develop coronary artery disease.

Risk factors that cannot be changed include heredity, sex, and age. For example, people whose parents have coronary artery disease are more likely to develop it. African-Americans are also at increased risk because they experience a higher rate of severe **hypertension** than whites do. Men are more likely to have heart attacks than women are and to have them at a younger age. Over age 60, however, women have coronary artery disease at a rate equal to that of men. Occasionally, coronary disease may strike a person in the 30s. Older people (those over 65) are more likely to die of a heart attack. Older women are twice as likely as older men to die within a few weeks of a heart attack.

Other risk factors can be changed. For example, smoking increases both the chance of developing coronary artery disease and the chance of dying from it. Smokers are two to four times more likely than are nonsmokers to die of sudden heart attack. Second hand-smoke may also increase risk. Dietary sources of cholesterol are meat, eggs, and other animal products. The body also produces it. Age, sex, heredity, and diet affect one's blood cholesterol. The risk of developing coronary artery disease increases steadily as blood cholesterol levels increase above 160 mg/dL (milligrams per deciliter). When a person has other risk factors, the risk multiplies.

High blood pressure makes the heart work harder and weakens it over time. It increases the risk of heart attack, **stroke**, kidney failure, and congestive **heart failure**. In combination with **obesity**, smoking, high cholesterol, or diabetes, high blood pressure raises the risk of heart attack or stroke several times.

Lack of **exercise** increases the risk of coronary artery disease. Even modest physical activity, like walking, is beneficial if done regularly.

The risk of developing coronary artery disease is seriously increased for diabetics. More than 80% of diabetics die of some type of heart or blood vessel disease.

Other risk factors such as obesity and stress and anger have been linked to coronary artery disease, but their significance is not known yet.

Chest pain (angina) is the main symptom of coronary heart disease but it is not always present. Other symptoms include **shortness of breath**, and chest heaviness, tightness, pain, a burning sensation, squeezing, or pressure either behind the breastbone or in the arms, neck, or jaws. Many people have no symptoms of coronary artery disease before having a heart attack.

Diagnostic tests for coronary artery disease measure weight, blood pressure, blood lipid levels, and fasting blood glucose levels. Other diagnostic tests help to confirm the diagnosis.

An electrocardiogram (ECG) shows the heart's activity and may reveal a lack of oxygen (ischemia). But a definite diagnosis cannot be made from **electrocardiography**. About 50% of patients with significant coronary artery disease have normal resting electrocardiograms. Another type of electrocardiogram, known as the exercise **stress test**, measures how the heart and blood vessels respond to exertion when the patient is exercising on a treadmill or a stationary bike. It sometimes gives a normal reading when the patient has a heart problem or an abnormal reading when the patient does not.

If the electrocardiogram reveals a problem or is inconclusive, the next step is exercise echocardiography or nuclear scanning (angiography), which uses sound waves to create an image of the heart's chambers and valves. It does not reveal the coronary arteries themselves but can detect abnormalities in heart wall motion caused by coronary disease.

Radionuclide angiography enables physicians to see the blood flow of the coronary arteries. Nuclear scans are performed by injecting a small amount of radiopharmaceutical such as thallium into the bloodstream. A scanning camera passes back and forth over the patient who lies on a table. Thallium scanning is usually done in conjunction with an exercise stress test. When the stress test is finished, thallium or sestamibi is injected. The patient resumes exercise for one minute to absorb the thallium.

Coronary angiography is the most accurate method for making a diagnosis of coronary artery disease, but it is also the most invasive. It is a form of cardiac catheterization that shows the heart's chambers, great vessels, and coronary arteries using x-ray technology.

Coronary artery disease can be treated many ways. The choice of treatment depends on the severity of the disease. Treatments include lifestyle changes and drug therapy, percutaneous transluminal coronary **angioplasty**, and coronary artery bypass surgery. Coronary artery disease is a chronic disease requiring lifelong care. Angioplasty or bypass surgery is not a ''cure.''

People with less severe coronary artery disease may gain adequate control through lifestyle changes and drug therapy. Many of the lifestyle changes that prevent disease progression—a low-fat, low-cholesterol diet, weight loss if needed, exercise, and not smoking—also help prevent the disease from developing.

Drugs such as nitrates, beta-blockers, and calcium-channel blockers relieve chest pain and complications of coronary artery disease, but they cannot clear blocked arteries. Nitrates (nitroglycerin) improve blood flow to the heart. Beta-blockers (acebutelol, propranolol) reduce the amount of oxygen required by the heart during stress. One type of calcium-channel blocker (verapamil, diltiazem hydrochloride) helps keep the arteries open and reduces blood pressure. **Aspirin** helps prevent blood clots from forming on plaques, reducing the likelihood of a heart attack. Cholesterol-lowering medications are also indicated in most cases.

Percutaneous transluminal coronary angioplasty and bypass surgery are procedures that enter the body (invasive procedures) to improve blood flow in the coronary arteries. Percutaneous transluminal coronary angioplasty, usually called coronary angioplasty, is a nonsurgical procedure. It is successful about 90% of the time, but for one-third of patients the artery narrows again within six months. The procedure can be repeated. It is less invasive and less expensive than coronary artery bypass surgery.

In coronary artery bypass surgery, a healthy artery or vein from an arm, leg, or chest wall is used to build a detour around the coronary artery blockage. The healthy vessel then supplies oxygen-rich blood to the heart. Bypass surgery is major surgery. It is appropriate for those patients with blockages in two or three major coronary arteries, those with severely narrowed left main coronary arteries, and those who have not responded to other treatments.

Three semiexperimental surgical procedures for unblocking coronary arteries are currently being studied. Atherectomy is a procedure in which the cardiologist shaves off and removes strips of plaque from the blocked artery. In laser angioplasty, a catheter with a laser tip is inserted into the affected artery to burn or break down the plaque. A metal coil called a stent can be implanted permanently to keep a blocked artery open. Stenting is becoming more common.

In many cases, coronary artery disease can be successfully treated. Advances in medicine and healthier lifestyles have caused a substantial decline in death rates from coronary artery disease since the mid-1980s. New diagnostic techniques enable doctors to identify and treat coronary artery disease in its earliest stages. New technologies and surgical procedures have extended the lives of many patients who would otherwise have died. Research on coronary artery disease continues.

A healthy lifestyle can help prevent coronary artery disease and help keep it from progressing. A heart-healthy life-

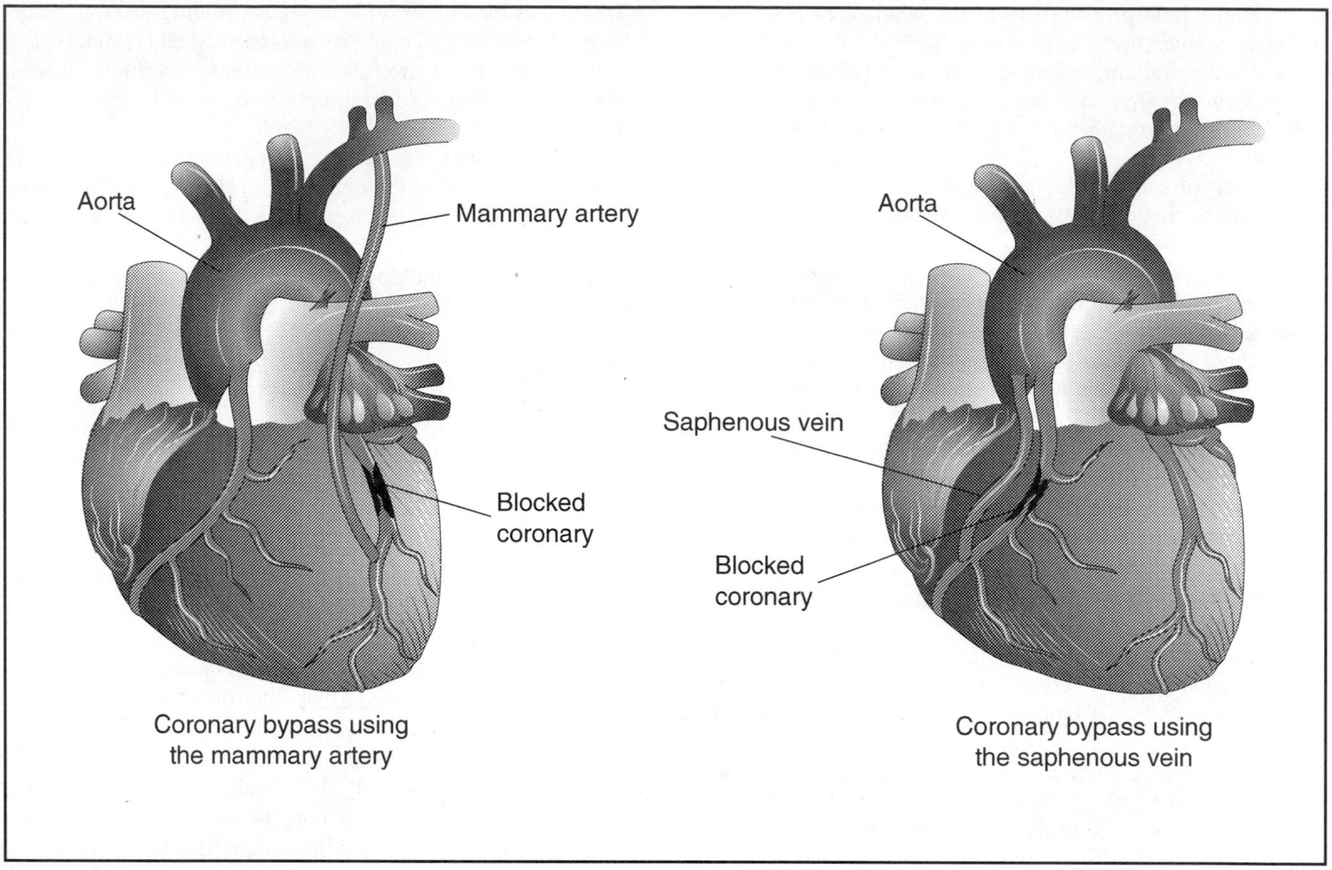

Coronary artery bypass graft surgery builds a detour around one or more blocked coronary arteries with a graft from a healthy vein or artery. The graft goes around the clogged artery (or arteries) to create new pathways for oxygen-rich blood to flow to the heart. ***(Illustration by Electronic Illustrators Group.)***

style includes eating right, regular exercise, maintaining a healthy weight, no smoking, moderate drinking, no recreational drugs, controlling hypertension, and managing stress. Cardiac rehabilitation programs are excellent to help prevent recurring coronary problems for people who are at risk and who have had coronary events and procedures.

CORONARY ARTERY BYPASS GRAFT SURGERY

Coronary artery bypass graft surgery (also called coronary artery bypass surgery, CABG, and bypass operation) is performed to restore blood flow to the heart. This relieves chest **pain** and ischemia (the inability of tissue to function due to insufficient blood supply), improves the patient's quality of life, and in some cases, prolongs the patient's life. The goals of the procedure are to enable the patient to resume a normal lifestyle and to lower the risk of a **heart attack**.

The decision to perform coronary artery bypass graft surgery is a complex one, and there is some disagreement among experts as to when it is indicated. Many experts feel that it has been performed too frequently in the United States. According to the American Heart Association, appropriate candidates or coronary artery bypass graft surgery include patients with blockages in at least three major coronary arteries, especially if the blockages are in arteries that feed the heart's left ventricle; patients with **angina** so severe that even mild exertion causes chest pain; and patients who cannot tolerate other procedures and do not respond well to drug therapy. It is well accepted that coronary artery bypass graft surgery is the treatment of choice for patients with severe **coronary artery disease** (three or more diseased arteries with impaired function in the left ventricle).

Coronary artery bypass graft surgery is major surgery performed in a hospital. The length of the procedure depends upon the number of arteries being bypassed, but it generally takes from 4 to 6 hours—sometimes longer. The average hospital stay is 4 to 7 days. Full recovery from coronary artery bypass graft surgery takes 3 to 4 months.

Coronary artery bypass graft surgery is widely performed in the United States. The American Heart Association estimates that 573,000 coronary artery bypass graft surgeries were performed on 363,000 patients in 1995. Seventy 4% of these procedures were performed on men and 44% on men and women under the age of 65 (1995 data).

The surgery team for coronary artery bypass graft surgery includes the cardiovascular surgeon, assisting surgeons, a cardiovascular anesthesiologist, a perfusion technologist (who operates the heart-lung machine), and specially trained nurses. After general anesthesia is administered, the surgeon removes the veins or prepares the arteries for grafting. If the saphenous vein (long vein in the leg) is to be used, a series of incisions are made in the patient's thigh or calf. More commonly, a segment of the internal mammary artery will be used, and the incisions are made in the chest wall. The surgeon then makes an incision from the patient's neck to navel, saws through the breastbone, and retracts the rib cage open to expose the heart. The patient is connected to a heart-lung machine, also called a cardiopulmonary bypass pump, which cools the body to reduce the need for oxygen and takes over for the heart and lungs during the procedure. The heart is then stopped and a cold solution of potassium-enriched normal saline is injected into the aortic root and the coronary arteries to lower the temperature of the heart, which prevents damage to the tissue.

Next, a small opening is made just below the blockage in the diseased coronary artery. Blood will be redirected through this opening once the graft is sewn in place. If a leg vein is used, one end is connected to the coronary artery and the other to the aorta. If a mammary artery is used, one end is connected to the coronary artery while the other remains attached to the aorta. The procedure is repeated on as many coronary arteries as necessary. Most patients who have coronary artery bypass graft surgery have at least three grafts done during the procedure.

Electric shocks start the heart pumping again after the grafts have been completed. The heart-lung machine is turned off and the blood slowly returns to normal body temperature. After implanting pacing electrodes (if needed) and inserting a chest tube, the surgeon closes the chest cavity.

Long term, symptoms recur in only about 3-4% of patients per year. Five years after coronary artery bypass graft surgery, survival expectancy is 90%, at 10 years it is about 80%, at 15 years it is about 55%, and at 20 years it is about 40%.

Angina recurs in about 40% of patients after about 10 years. In most cases, it is less severe than before the surgery and can be controlled by drug therapy. In patients who have had vein grafts, 40% of the grafts are severely obstructed 10 years after the procedure. Repeat coronary artery bypass graft surgery may be necessary, and is usually less successful than the first surgery.

There are two new types of minimally invasive coronary artery bypass graft surgery: port-access coronary artery bypass (also called PACAB or PortCAB) and minimally invasive coronary artery bypass (also called MIDCAB). These procedures are minimally invasive because they do not require the neck-to-navel incision, sawing through the breastbone, or opening the rib cage to expose the heart. Both procedures enable surgeons to work on the coronary arteries through small chest holes called ports and other small incisions. Port-access coronary artery bypass requires the use of a heart-lung machine but minimally invasive coronary artery bypass does not. Advantages of these procedures over standard coronary artery bypass graft surgery include a shorter hospital stay, a shorter recovery period, and lower costs. Still, the American Heart Association Council on Cardio-Thoracic and Vascular Surgery feels that both procedures appear promising but that further study is needed.

Coronary artery bypass graft surgery is major surgery and patients may experience any of the complications associated with major surgery. The risk of death during coronary artery bypass graft surgery is 2-3%. Possible complications include graft closure and development of blockages in other arteries, long-term development of atherosclerotic disease of saphenous vein grafts, abnormal heart rhythms, high or low blood pressure, blood clots that can lead to a **stroke** or heart attack, infections, and depression. There is a higher risk for complications in patients who are heavy smokers, patients who have serious lung, kidney, or metabolic problems, or patients who have a reduced supply of blood to the brain.

COR PULMONALE

Cor pulmonale is an increase in bulk of the right ventricle of the heart, generally caused by chronic diseases or malfunction of the lungs. This condition can lead to **heart failure**.

Cor pulmonale, or pulmonary heart disease, occurs in 25% of patients with chronic obstructive pulmonary disease (COPD). In fact, about 85% of patients diagnosed with cor pulmonale have COPD. Chronic **bronchitis** and emphysema are types of COPD. High blood pressure in the blood vessels of the lungs (**pulmonary hypertension**) causes the enlargement of the right ventricle. In addition to COPD, cor pulmonale may also be caused by lung diseases, such as **cystic fibrosis**, pulmonary embolism and, pneumoconiosis. Loss of lung tissue after lung surgery or certain chest-wall disturbances can produce cor pulmonale, as can neuromuscular diseases, such as **muscular dystrophy**. A large pulmonary thromboembolism (blood clot) may lead to acute cor pulmonale.

Any respiratory disease or malfunction which affects the circulatory system of the lungs may lead to cor pulmonale. These circulatory changes cause the right ventricle to compensate for the extra work required to pump blood through the lungs. The right ventricle has thin walls and is crescent-shaped. The resulting pressure causes the right ventricle to dilate and bulge, eventually leading to its failure.

Cor pulmonale should be expected in any patient with COPD and other respiratory or neuromuscular diseases. Initial symptoms of cor pulmonale may actually reflect those of the underlying disease. These may include chronic **cough**ing, **wheezing**, weakness, fatigue, and **shortness of breath**. Edema (abnormal buildup of fluid), weakness, and discomfort in the upper chest may be evident in cor pulmonale.

An electrocardiograph (EKG) will show signs such as frequent premature contractions in the atria or ventricles. **Chest x ray**s may show enlargement of the right descending pulmonary artery. This sign, along with an enlarged main pulmonary artery, indicates pulmonary artery **hypertension** in patients with COPD. **Magnetic resonance imaging** (MRI) is often the preferred method of diagnosis for cor pulmonale because it can clearly show and measure the volume of the pulmonary arteries. Other tests used to support a diagnosis of cor pulmonale may include arterial **blood gas analysis** (to measure the level of oxygen in the blood), pulmonary function tests (to measure how effectively the lungs are working), and hematocrit (to measure the percentage of red blood cells in the blood).

Treatment of cor pulmonale is aimed at increasing a patient's **exercise** tolerance and improving oxygen levels of the arterial blood. Treatment is also aimed at the underlying condition that is producing cor pulmonale. Common treatments include **antibiotics** for respiratory infection; anticoagulants to reduce the risk of thromboembolism; and digitalis, oxygen, and **phlebotomy** to reduce red blood cell count. A low-salt diet and restricted fluids are often prescribed.

The prognosis for cor pulmonale is poor, particularly because it occurs late in the process of serious disease.

Cor pulmonale is best prevented by prevention of COPD and other irreversible diseases that lead to heart failure. Smoking cessation is critically important. Carefully following the recommended course of treatment for the underlying disease may help prevent cor pulmonale.

CORTICOSTEROIDS

Corticosteroids are used in several forms, to treat many different conditions. Because they reduce **itching**, swelling, redness, and allergic reactions, they are often used in treating skin problems, severe **allergies**, **asthma**, and arthritis. These drugs also suppress the body's immune response, so they are used in patients who have received organ transplants, to reduce the chance of rejection. In people whose bodies do not produce enough natural corticosteroids, the drugs can raise the levels of those hormones. Corticosteroids also are used to treat certain **cancer**s (along with other drugs), and to reduce inflammation in other medical conditions.

Corticosteroids are medicines that are similar to the natural hormone cortisone. They affect many body processes, including the breakdown of protein, fat, and carbohydrate; the activity of the nervous system; the balance of salt and water; and the regulation of blood pressure. Because of their widespread effects, these drugs are useful in treating many medical conditions, but they can also have undesirable side effects.

These medicines come in a variety of forms, suitable for treating different conditions. For example, inhalant corticosteroids are used to prevent asthma attacks, while corticosteroid ointments, creams and gels are used to treat skin problems. Some examples of corticosteroids are beclomethasone, betamethasone, hydrocortisone, mometasone, prednisone, and triamcinolone.

Corticosteroids are powerful drugs that may cause serious side effects. Anyone taking them should be sure they fully understand the benefits and risks of these drugs.

Inhalant forms of these drugs will reduce the frequency and severity of asthma attacks when taken every day, but will not relieve an asthma attack once it has started.

In children and teenagers, these medicines can stop or slow growth and affect the function of the adrenal glands (small glands located above each kidney, which secrete natural corticosteroids). Another possible problem for children is that corticosteroids may make infections such as **chickenpox** and **measles** more serious. The benefits and risks of giving corticosteroids to children and teenagers should be thoroughly discussed with the child's physician. By adjusting the doses and forms in which corticosteroids are given, the physician may be able to lower the chance of unwanted side effects.

In older people, corticosteroids may increase the risk of high blood pressure and bone disease. Bone problems from corticosteroids are especially likely in older women.

Corticosteroid ointments, creams and gels can be absorbed through the skin and travel into the bloodstream. This is not a problem unless large amounts are absorbed. Then, unwanted side effects in other parts of the body are possible. There are precautions patients can take to avoid that happening.

Patients taking corticosteroids over long periods may need to follow special diets, reducing the amount of sodium or increasing the amount of protein they eat, for example.

People with certain medical conditions or who are taking certain other medicines can have problems if they take corticosteroids. Corticosteroids can also cover up the symptoms of some medical problems. If the condition gets worse, the patient has no way of knowing it. Before taking these drugs, patients need to let their doctors know about any medical conditions they may have, but particularly allergies and diabetes. Pregnant or breastfeeding women also need to alert their doctors to their condition. In addition, taking corticosteroids with certain other drugs may affect the way the drugs work or may increase the chance of side effects. Thus, patients should tell their doctors about any other medications they are taking.

Side effects generally are rare when corticosteroids are used for a short time. However, when they are used over time, they may lower the body's ability to fight off infections or may make infections harder to treat. Other common side effects include changes in appetite (increase or decrease), nervousness, restlessness, sleep problems, and **indigestion**. These problems usually go away as the body adjusts to the drug and do not require medical treatment. Less common side effects may occur with some forms of corticosteroids. Inhalants may cause dry throat, headache, nausea, skin bruising or thinning, and san unpleasant taste. Nasal spray forms may irritate the nose or throat, and ointments, gels, or creams may irritate the skin. Again, these side effects do not need medical attention unless they don't go away or they interfere with normal activities.

More serious side effects are not common, but may occur. Breathing problems, **wheezing**, or tightness in the chest occur, should be immediately reported to a physician. A number of additional side effects, for example, rash, irregular heartbeat, and rapid weight gain, are possible. Anyone who has unusual or bothersome symptoms after taking corticosteroids should get in touch with his or her physician.

Cortisol tests

This test is a measure of serum cortisol (also known as hydrocortisone), or urine cortisol, (also known as urinary free cortisol), an important hormone produced by a pair of endocrine glands called the adrenal glands.

This test is performed on patients who may have malfunctioning adrenal glands. Blood and urine cortisol, together with the determination of adrenocorticotropic hormone (ACTH), are the three most important tests in the investigation of Cushing's syndrome (caused by an overproduction of cortisol) and Addison's disease (caused by the underproduction of cortisol).

Increased levels of cortisol are associated with **pregnancy**. Physical and emotional **stress** can also elevate cortisol levels. Drugs that may cause increased levels of cortisol include estrogen, **oral contraceptives**, amphetamines, cortisone, and spironolactone (Aldactone). Drugs that may cause decreased levels include androgens, aminoglutethimide, betamethasone, and other steroid medications, danazol, lithium, levodopa, metyrapone and phenytoin (Dilantin).

Cortisol is a potent hormone known as a glucocorticoid that affects the metabolism of carbohydrates, proteins, and fats, but especially glucose. Cortisol increases blood sugar levels by stimulating the release of glucose from glucose stores in cells. It also acts to inhibit insulin, thus affecting glucose transport into cells.

The hypothalamus (an area of the brain), the pituitary gland (sometimes called the ''master gland'') and the adrenal glands coordinate the production of cortisol. After corticotropin-releasing hormone (CRH) is made in the hypothalamus, CRH stimulates the pituitary to produce adrenocorticotropic hormone (ACTH). The production of ACTH in turn stimulates a part of the adrenal glands known as the adrenal cortex to produce cortisol. Rising levels of cortisol act as a negative feedback to curtail further production of CRH and ACTH, thus completing an elaborate feedback mechanism.

There are two methods for evaluating cortisol: blood and urine. The most reliable index of cortisol secretion is the 24-hour urine sample collection, but when blood levels are required or requested by the physician, plasma cortisol should be measured in the morning and again in the afternoon. Cortisol levels normally rise and fall during the day in what is called a diurnal variation, so that cortisol is at its highest level between 6-8 A.M. and gradually falls, reaching its lowest point around midnight. One reason for ordering blood cortisol levels versus a 24-hour urine collection is that sometimes the earliest sign of adrenal malfunction is the loss of this diurnal variation, even though the cortisol levels are not yet elevated. For example, individuals with Cushing's syndrome often have upper normal plasma cortisol levels in the morning and exhibit no decline as the day progresses.

When testing for cortisol levels through the blood, a blood specimen is usually collected at 8 A.M. and again at 4 P.M. It should be noted that normal values may be transposed in individuals who have worked during the night and slept during the day for long periods of time.

When testing for cortisol level through the urine, a 24-hour urine sample is collected, refrigerated, and sent to the reference laboratory for examination.

Risks for the blood test are minimal, but may include slight bleeding from the blood-drawing site, **fainting** or feeling lightheaded after venipuncture, or hematoma (blood accumulating under the puncture site).

Reference ranges for cortisol vary from laboratory to laboratory but are usually within the following ranges for blood:

- Adults (8 A.M.): 6-28 mg/dL; adults (4 P.M.): 2-12 mg/dL
- Child 1-6 years (8 A.M.): 3-21 mg/dL; child 1-6 years (4 P.M.): 3-10 mg/dL
- Newborn: 1/24 mg/dL.

Reference ranges for cortisol vary from laboratory to laboratory but are usually within the following ranges for 24-hour urine collection:

- Adult: 10-100 mg/24 hr
- Adolescent: 5-55 mg/24 hr
- Child: 2-27 mg/24 hr.

Increased levels of cortisol are found in Cushing's syndrome, excess thyroid (hyperthyroidism), **obesity**, ACTH-producing tumors, and high levels of stress.

Decreased levels of cortisol are found in Addison's disease, conditions of low thyroid, and **hypopituitarism**, in which pituitary activity is diminished.

Cough

A cough is a forceful release of air from the lungs that can be heard. Coughing protects the respiratory system by clearing it of irritants and secretions.

While people can generally cough on purpose, a cough is usually a reflex triggered when an irritant stimulates one or more of the cough receptors found at different points in the respiratory system. These receptors then send a message to the cough center in the brain, which in turn tells the body to cough. A cough begins with a deep breath in, at which point the opening between the vocal cords at the upper part of the larynx (glottis) shuts, trapping the air in the lungs. As the diaphragm and other muscles involved in breathing press against the lungs, the glottis suddenly opens, producing an explosive outflow of air at speeds greater than 100 mi (160 km) per hour.

In normal situations, most people cough once or twice an hour during the day to clear the airway of irritants. However, when the level of irritants in the air is high or when the respiratory system becomes infected, coughing may become frequent and prolonged. It may interfere with **exercise** or sleep, and it may also cause distress if accompanied by **dizziness**, chest **pain**, or breathlessness. In the majority of cases, frequent coughing lasts one to two weeks and tapers off as the irritant or infection subsides. If a cough lasts more than three weeks it is considered a chronic cough, and physicians will try to determine a cause beyond an acute infection or irritant.

Coughs are generally described as either dry or productive. A dry cough does not bring up a mixture of mucus, irritants, and other substances from the lungs (sputum), whereas a productive cough does. In the case of a bacterial infection, the sputum brought up in a productive cough may be greenish, gray, or brown. In the case of an allergy or viral infection it may be clear or white. In the most serious conditions, the sputum may contain blood.

Coughs are usually caused by respiratory infections, including colds or influenza, the most common causes of coughs; **bronchitis**, an inflammation of the mucous membranes of the bronchial tubes; **croup**, a viral inflammation of the larynx, windpipe, and bronchial passages that produces a bark-like cough in children; **whooping cough**, a bacterial infection accompanied by the high-pitched cough for which it is named; **pneumonia**, a potentially serious bacterial infection that produces discolored or bloody mucus; **tuberculosis**, another serious bacterial infection that produces bloody sputum; fungal infections, such as aspergillosis, **histoplasmosis**, and cryptococcoses.

Environmental pollutants, such as cigarette smoke, dust, or smog, can also cause a cough. In the case of cigarette smokers, the nicotine present in the smoke paralyzes the hairs (cilia) that regularly flush mucus from the respiratory system. The mucus then builds up, forcing the body to removed it by coughing. Postnasal drip, the irritating trickle of mucus from the nasal passages into the throat caused by **allergies** or **sinusitis**, can also result in a cough. Some chronic conditions, such as **asthma**, chronic bronchitis, emphysema, and **cystic fibrosis**, are characterized in part by a cough. A condition in which stomach acid backs up into the esophagus (gastroesophageal reflux) can cause coughing, especially when a person is lying down. A cough can also be a side effect of medications that are administered via an inhaler. It can also be a side effect of beta-blockers and ACE inhibitors, which are drugs used for treating high blood pressure.

To determine the cause of a cough, a physician should take an exact medical history and perform an exam. The appearance of the sputum will also help determine what type of infection, if any, may be involved. The doctor may even observe the sputum microscopically for the presence of bacteria and white blood cells. **Chest x ray**s may help indicate the presence and extent of such infections as pneumonia or tuberculosis. If these actions are not enough to determine the cause of the cough, a bronchoscopy or **laryngoscopy** may be ordered. These tests use slender tubular instruments to inspect the interior of the bronchi and larynx.

Treatment of a cough generally involves addressing the condition causing it. An acute infection such as pneumonia may require **antibiotics**, an asthma-induced cough may be treated with the use of bronchodialators, or an antihistamine may be administered in the case of an allergy. Physicians prefer not to suppress a productive cough, since it aids the body in clearing respiratory system of infective agents and irritants. However, cough medicines may be given if the patient cannot rest because of the cough or if the cough is not productive, as is the case with most coughs associated with colds or flu. The two types of drugs used to treat coughs are antitussives, which suppress a cough, and **expectorants**, which make mucus easier to cough up by thinning it. Some studies have shown that in acute infections, simply increasing fluid intake has the same thinning effect as taking expectorants.

Many health practitioners advise increasing fluids and breathing in warm, humidified air as ways of loosening chest congestion. Others recommend hot tea flavored with honey as a temporary home remedy for coughs caused by colds or flu. Various **vitamins**, such as vitamin C, may be helpful in preventing or treating conditions (including colds and flu) that lead to coughs. Avoiding mucus-producing foods can be effective in healing a cough condition. These mucus-producing foods can vary, based on individual intolerance, but dairy products are a major mucus-producing food for most people.

Because the majority of coughs are related to the **common cold** or influenza, most will end in 7-21 days. The outcome of coughs due to a more serious underlying disease depends on the nature of that disease. It is important to identify and treat the underlying disease and origin of the cough.

Cough suppressants

Cough suppressants are medicines that prevent or stop **coughing**. They act on the center in the brain that controls the cough reflex, and are meant to be used only to relieve dry, hacking coughs associated with colds and flu. They should not be used to treat coughs that bring up mucus or the chronic coughs associated with smoking, asthma, emphysema or other lung problems.

Many cough medicines contain cough suppressants along with other ingredients. Some combinations of ingredients may cancel each other's effects. One example is the combination of cough suppressant with an expectorant — a medicine that loosens and clears mucus from the airways. The cough suppressant interferes with the ability to cough up the mucus that the expectorant loosens.

Dextromethorphan is an ingredient in many cough medicines, such as Vicks Formula 44, Drixoral Cough Liquid Caps, Sucrets Cough Control, Benylin DM and some Robitussin products. These medicines come in capsule, tablet, lozenge, and liquid forms and are available without a physician's prescription.

Dextromethorphan is not meant to be used for coughs associated with smoking, asthma, emphysema, chronic **bronchitis**, or other lung conditions. It also should not be used for coughs that produce mucus.

A lingering cough could be a sign of a serious medical condition. Coughs that last more than 7 days or are associated with fever, rash, sore throat, or lasting headache should have medical attention. Call a physician as soon as possible.

People with **phenylketonuria** (a hereditary inability to metabolize phenylalanine, an amino acid) should be aware that some products with dextromethorphan also contain the artificial sweetener aspartame, which breaks down in the body to phenylalanine.

Anyone who has asthma or liver disease should check with a physician before taking dextromethorphan.

Women who are pregnant or breastfeeding or who plan to become pregnant should check with their physicians before taking dextromethorphan.

The dye tartrazine is an ingredient in some cough suppressant products. This dye causes allergic reactions in some people, especially those who are allergic to aspirin.

Side effects of dextromethorphan are rare, but may include nausea, vomiting, stomach upset, slight drowsiness, and dizziness.

Patients who take monoamine oxidase inhibitors (MAO inhibitors) should be aware that also taking products containing dextromethorphan can cause dizziness, fainting, fever, nausea and possibly coma. Do not take dextromethorphan unless a physician permits the use of the two drugs together.

When dextromethorphan is taken with medicines that cause drowsiness, this effect may be enhanced.

Counseling

Counseling is advice, instruction, or help offered by one person in order to direct the actions, thoughts, or opinions of another. The word ''counseling'' can be used in many ways, but often is used in the context of mental health care. Assistance with mental health issues, either given or received, is commonly known as counseling (or psychotherapy)

Counseling for mental health problems is on the increase in the United States, where it's estimated that one in every five people consult with a **mental health care** professional at some point of their lives. It's also estimated that one of every three people develop some sort of mental disorder at some time during their lives, and that only 28% of those people seek professional help. This reluctance to get counseling is primarily due to the many misconceptions about mental health and the belief that mental health problems are somehow shameful. In the United States today, the stigma against mental health care is still very strong.

Experts recommend that counseling is needed when a problem is interfering with in a person's life. If a particular issue is damaging a person's relationships, or hindering the ability to function in school, at work, or at home, that person should seek counseling.

Mental health care may be included under a person's health insurance policy, although it is almost always covered in a much more limited way that physical illness, with limits on number of visits per year and a fairly small lifetime maximum coverage amount. A person who doesn't have insurance and can't afford to pay out-of-pocket for counseling can contact a local or state agency or a mental health advocacy group to seek assistance. Many community mental health centers offer counseling on a sliding scale based on a person's ability to pay.

Counseling sessions typically last between 45 and 90 minutes. A person suffering from a mental health disorder may require only several counseling sessions, or could be in counseling for many years, depending on the severity of the problem.

Counseling is available from different types of health care professionals, and from others who have received training in counseling. Ministers, priests, and rabbis (called ''pastoral counselors'') serve as counselors but aren't health care professionals.

Because anyone with or without formal training in counseling can advertise themselves as a ''psychotherapist,'' it's important to check a person's credentials before becoming a client. A primary-care doctor often can recommend a health care professional. It's important, however, for a patient to feel comfortable with a counselor before agreeing to work together.

Those seeking counseling should make sure a professional has met state licensing requirements to be certified as either a psychiatrist, psychologist, social worker, nurse-psychotherapist or psychiatric nurse, or marriage and family therapist.

A psychiatrist is a licensed medical doctor with additional training in the specialty of psychiatry, who is qualified to prescribe medications and make medical decisions. A ''board-certified psychiatrist'' is one who has completed extra training and passed national examinations.

Psychologists have completed graduate Ph.D. programs that include clinical training and internships, but they are not medical doctors. Most states require a Ph.D. for licensing as a ''psychologist'' (only a few states allow master's-level graduates to call themselves a psychologist). All have extensive training in psychotherapeutic techniques.

Certified social workers or licensed clinical social workers usually have completed two years of graduate work, specializing in mental health care. Some have doctoral degrees. Most states require social workers to be licensed, and to complete two years of post-graduate clinical work.

Psychiatric nurses and nurse-psychotherapists have nursing degrees and special training in mental health care, and must pass state examinations in order to practice.

Marriage and family therapists usually have completed graduate work, often in psychology. They are licensed in some, but not all states, and usually are required to have completed at least two years of supervised clinical training.

Other types of counselors include pastoral counselors, stress management counselors, sex therapists, and hypnotherapists. There also are counseling groups, self-help groups, and support groups, which some people find useful in dealing with problems.

Counseling (also called ''talk therapy'') is probably most useful if the client's personality and life experiences are the primary cause of the problem.

See also Family therapy; Mental health care; Mental illness; Psychological tests; Psychoanalysis

Cournand, André F. (1895-1988)

French American physician

André F. Cournand shared the 1956 Nobel Prize in physiology or medicine with German surgeon **Werner Forssmann** and American physiologist **Dickinson Woodruff Richards, Jr.** for

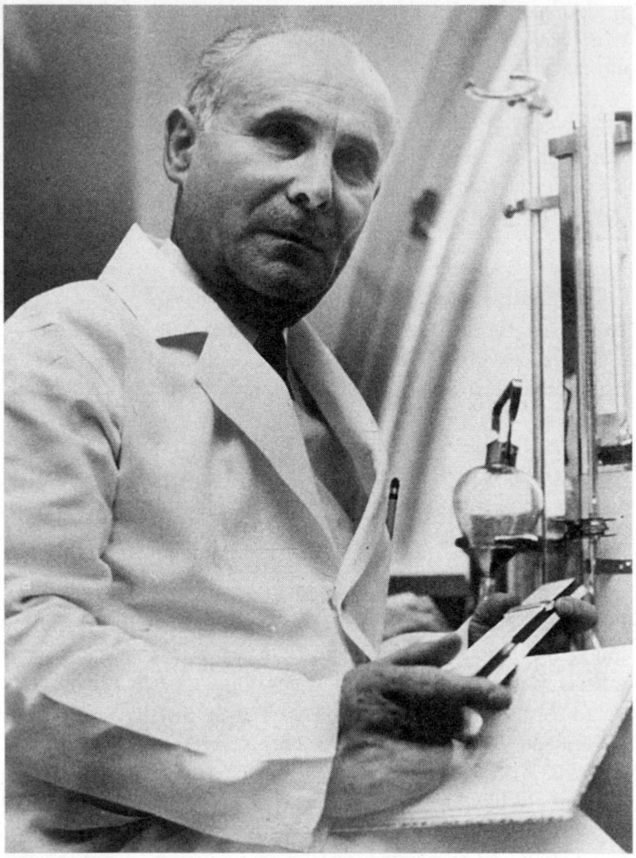

André Frederic Cournand

pioneering work in the field of cardiac and pulmonary physiology. Cournand helped develop the technique of cardiac catheterization, which permits blood samples to be obtained from the heart for determining cardiac abnormalities.

Cournand was born in Paris on September 24, 1895. His father, Jules Cournand, and his grandfather were both dentists. At age 15, young André began to accompany his parents to the salon of a physician friend where many internationally known scientists met and discussed issues of their day.

In 1913, Cournand received his bachelor's degree from the University of Paris-Sorbonne, where he also began his medical studies in 1914. But in that year the first World War broke out, and many medical professors enlisted in the army. In the spring of 1915, Cournand decided to postpone his studies. In July of that year he joined a surgical unit that provided emergency care on the front lines. By 1916 he was trained as an auxiliary battalion surgeon and was serving in the trenches. He didn't return to medical school until 1919. After serving as an intern, he received his M.D. in 1930.

Cournand had decided to specialize in upper respiratory diseases and, delaying his entry into private practice, pursued further training in the United States. He joined a residency program at the Tuberculosis Service of the Columbia University College of Physicians and Surgeons at Bellevue Hospital in New York City. He stayed at Columbia for the remainder of his career, rising from his initial position as investigator to a full professor in 1951. He became a naturalized citizen of the United States in 1941.

At Bellevue Cournand began what would become a long collaboration with Dickinson W. Richards. Together, they investigated the theories of a Harvard physiologist, Lawrence J. Henderson, who had postulated that the heart, lungs, and circulatory system are a functional unit designed to transport respiratory gases from the atmosphere to the tissues in the body and back out again.

In order to study respiratory gases and their concentrations in the blood as it passed through the heart, samples of blood from the heart had to be obtained. At this time, there was no established technique for this task. Catheters—flexible tubes intended to introduce and remove fluids from organs—had been used for the past 100 years, but only in animal experiments. The safety of catheter use in humans was doubtful. But Cournand was aware that in 1929 a German scientist, Werner Forssmann, had dramatically demonstrated the safety of cardiac catheterization by performing it on himself. He had inserted a catheter into one of his arm veins and then threaded it into his right atrium. Cournand became convinced of the safety of catheterization after speaking with one of his professors in Paris who had also performed a type of catheterization on himself, and subsequently scores of others, without any problems.

The Bellevue team experimented on animals for four years, working to standardize the procedure and perfect the equipment they were convinced was necessary for their studies of the cardiac system. When at last cardiac catheterization was used to obtain a sample of mixed venous blood in humans, what could previously be only vaguely determined by clinical observation could be physiologically described. Cardiac catheterization not only allows for samples of mixed venous blood to be collected, but it also measures blood pressure in various parts of the cardiac circulatory system—the right atrium, the ventricles, and the arteries—and measures total blood flow and gas concentrations. In short, the functions of the heart and lungs can be fully specified through cardiac catheterization.

During World War II, Cournand led a team of physicians investigating the use of cardiac catheterization on patients suffering from severe circulatory shock resulting from traumatic injury. Obtaining physiological measurements of cardiac output in these patients helped identify the cause of shock—a fall in cardiac output and return. As a result of these findings, it was determined that the best treatment for shock was a total blood transfusion rather than simply replacing plasma, which had previously been used and was found to cause **anemia**.

After the war, Cournand applied the technique of cardiac catheterization to patients with heart and pulmonary diseases. The team continually worked to improve the technique and was able to obtain simultaneous readings of blood pressure in the right ventricle and the pulmonary artery. This allowed for greater diagnostic accuracy of congenital defects as well as evaluations of treatment. Eventually these investigations led to increased understanding of acquired heart diseases and the relation between diseases of the lungs and cardiac function, thus opening up the field of pulmonary heart diseases.

Cournand began to be recognized for his research in the 1940s, when he was invited to speak at and lead various conferences. In 1949 he won the Lasker Award, and in 1952 he was invited by the National Institutes of Health to screen grant applications for the Lung, Heart and Kidney Study Section. Cournand's increasing recognition culminated in the fall of 1956 when he was awarded the Nobel Prize. In 1958 he was elected to the National Academy of Science.

Cournand retired in 1964 and devoted the years until his death to the study of the social and ethical implications of modern science. He died on February 19, 1988, in Great Barrington, Massachusetts.

Credé, Carl Siegmund Franz (1819-1892)

German obstetrician

Credé saved the eyesight of countless newborns by discovering that a common cause of infant blindness could be prevented by applying silver nitrate eyedrops at birth. He also implemented what was known as "Credé's method" for hastening delivery of the placenta (afterbirth) during the third stage of labor, which is still used in modern obstetrical practice.

Born in Berlin in 1819, where his father was a high-ranking education official, Credé obtained most of his medical training there. He graduated from the University of Berlin in 1842 and spent the next five years studying in and traveling throughout France, Belgium, Italy, and Austria.

Returning to Berlin, Credé then served as obstetrical assistant at a local clinic. He later was recognized as a teacher of obstetrics in 1850. Two years later he became director of the Berlin School of Midwives and physician-in-chief at the lying-in division at Berlin's Charité Hospital.

There, Credé established one of Europe's first outpatient gynecology departments. When he was later appointed professor of obstetrics and director of the Lying-In Hospital in Leipzig, Germany, he established a similar department there in Leipzig.

Credé's method of hastening delivery of the placenta was by no means new. The practice, involving massage applied to the abdomen externally, was previously known to Hippocrates, the people of Old Calabar in southeastern Nigeria, and to numerous aboriginal tribes in North America. Credé credited an Austrian doctor named von Plenck with developing the technique.

But Credé popularized the idea after he became concerned with the standard practice of rushing removal of the placenta by pulling on the umbilical cord and manually invading the vagina and uterus, which increased the risks of bleeding, infection, and inversion of the uterus. He taught his obstetrics students that the less a woman is handled, the lower the risk of infection. For this reason, Credé vigorously opposed the tendency of nineteenth-century doctors and midwives to conduct internal examinations of women in labor.

Massage, applied externally, was nonetheless acceptable to quicken the third stage of labor, to lessen the anxiety of the mother and "to allow the physician to return to his other responsibilities," Credé wrote. His method is still used by doctors and midwives when the mother is unable to push out the placenta herself.

Credé's greatest legacy was his use of silver nitrate to prevent ophthalmia neonatorum, a potentially blinding disease that occurred in as many as 12% of live births. Of those, 3% of infants were blinded and 20% had at least some degree of eye damage. The disease was acquired by the newborns as they passed through an infected birth canal, most commonly when the mother had **gonorrhea**.

Washing an infant's eyes to prevent infection had been tried with various substances including water, chlorine water, and solutions of thymol, carbolic acid, salicylic acid, and potassium permanganate. Silver nitrate had also been previously tried, but Credé refined the technique (a single drop of 2% silver nitrate solution applied with a glass rod) and demonstrated its effectiveness. In a three-year period in the early 1880s, among 1,160 newborns treated by Credé with silver nitrate, only two developed ophthalmia. This compares with 111 infants who developed the disease among 977 untreated births at the same hospital from 1874-1876.

Credé's silver nitrate treatment (the solution was later diluted to 1%) became widely accepted as standard obstetrical practice. It continues to be used in some jurisdictions, although gonorrhea is not as common among mothers and silver nitrate is now frequently replaced by eye drops that are less irritating.

Credé was also a prominent writer, editor, teacher, and administrator. His *Clinical Lectures on Midwifery,* coauthored with son-in-law Gerhard Leopold and published in 1853 and 1854, went through five editions and later was translated into English. He wrote other textbooks and edited a prominent German gynecological journal for almost 40 years.

Due to prostate cancer, Credé was forced to retire in 1887, dying five years later. Sadly, the man who prevented so many cases of blindness was himself rendered sightless in his final months of life by kidney failure.

See also Childbirth

Creutzfeldt-Jakob disease

Creutzfeldt-Jakob disease (CJD) is a transmissible, rapidly progressing, fatal neurodegenerative disorder related to "mad cow disease."

Before 1995, Creutzfeldt-Jakob disease was little-known outside of the medical profession; even within it, most doctors did not know much about it, and hardly any had ever seen a case. But with the discovery of a "new variant" form, the possibility that those with it became infected simply by eating beef, and the radical theory that the infectious agent is a rogue protein, CJD has become one of the most talked-about diseases in the world, and has taken on a significance far beyond the small number of **death**s it currently causes each year.

First described in the 1920s, CJD is a neurodegenerative disease causing a rapidly progressing **dementia** which ends in death, usually within eight months of the onset of symptoms.

It is also a very rare disease, affecting only about one in every million members of the population worldwide. In the United States, CJD is thought to affect about 250 people each year. CJD affects adults of all ages, but is rare in young adults and most common between ages 50 and 75.

The most obvious pathologic feature of CJD is the formation of numerous fluid-filled spaces in the brain (vacuoles), giving it a sponge-like appearance. CJD is one of several human ''spongiform encephalopathies,'' diseases that produce this characteristic change in brain tissue. Others are kuru; Gerstmann-Straussler-Scheinker disease, predominantly characterized by cerebellar ataxia; and fatal familial insomnia, associated with progressive insomnia, autonomic system disfunction, and weakness caused by motor system disfunction.

Six forms of spongiform encephalopathies are known to occur in other mammals: scrapie in sheep, recognized for more than 200 years; chronic wasting disease in elk and mule deer in Wyoming and Colorado; transmissible mink encephalopathy; exotic ungulate encephalopathy in some types of zoo animals; feline spongiform encephalopathy in domestic cats; and bovine spongiform encephalopathy (BSE) in cows.

BSE was first recognized in Britain in 1986. Besides the spongiform changes in the brain, BSE causes dementia-like behavioral changes—hence the name ''mad cow disease.'' BSE is thought to be an altered form of scrapie, transmitted to cows when they were fed sheep offal (slaughterhouse waste) as part of their feed.

The use of slaughterhouse offal in animal feed has been common in many countries and has been practiced for at least 50 years. The trigger for the BSE epidemic in Britain seems to have come in the early 1980s, when the use of organic solvents for preparation of offal was halted there. It seems likely that these solvents had been destroying the scrapie agent, thereby preventing infection, and that the change in preparation procedure opened the way for the agent to ''jump species'' and cause BSE in cows which consumed scrapie-infected meal. The slaughter of infected (but not yet visibly sick) cows at the end of their useful farm lives, and the use of their carcasses for feed, spread the infection rapidly and widely. For at least a year after BSE was first recognized in British herds, infected bovine remains continued to be incorporated into feed, spreading the disease still further. (It is thought that most cows with BSE became infected as a result of eating meal containing offal from other cows, not sheep.) Although milk from infected cows has never been shown to pass the infectious agent, passage from infected mother to calf has occurred through unknown means.

Beginning in 1988, the British government took steps to stop the spread of BSE, banning the use of bovine offal in feed and other products and ordering the slaughter of infected cows. By then, the slow-acting agent had become epidemic in British herds. In 1992, it was diagnosed in over 25,000 animals (1% of the British herd). By mid-1997, the cumulative number of BSE cases in the United Kingdom had risen to more than 170,000. The feeding ban did stem the tide of the epidemic; however, the number of new cases each week fell from a peak of 1,000 in 1993 to less than 300 two years later.

The export of British feed and beef to member countries was banned by the European Union, but cases of BSE had developed in Europe by then as well; however, by mid-1997, only about 1,000 cases had been identified. In 1989, the United States banned import of British beef and began monitoring U.S. herds in 1990. To date, no BSE has been detected in the United States, and only one case has been reported in North America in a cow imported to Canada from Britain.

From the beginning of the BSE epidemic, scientists and others in Britain feared that BSE might jump species again to infect humans who had consumed infected beef. In 1995, this fear seemed to be realized with the first cases of a new variant of Creutzfeldt-Jacob disease, termed nvCJD. Its victims, 23 in all as of early 1998, are much younger than the 60-65 average for CJD, and the time from symptom onset to death has averaged 12 months instead of eight. EEG abnormalities characteristic of CJD are not typically seen in nvCJD.

Evidence is growing stronger that nvCJD is in fact caused by BSE. While definitive proof was still lacking as of early 1998, many researchers now treat the BSE-nvCJD connection as solidly established.

Assuming that BSE is the source, the question that has loomed from the beginning has been is how many people will eventually be affected. Epidemiological models of infectious disease produce estimates ranging from less than one hundred to tens of thousands, depending on the assumptions used by the modelers. The incubation period of nvCJD in humans is not known, nor are the genetic and environmental risk factors which influence susceptibility, nor the quantity of infectious agent needed to cause the disease. It is estimated that between one and two million infected cattle have been eaten by humans, most in the earliest stages of the epidemic. Estimates cannot be based on the very few cases which have developed so far. These cases could represent the very few people with the right combination of exposure and susceptibility to a relatively fast-developing infection, or they could be the first few victims of a slower-acting, more highly infectious agent.

It is clear that Creutzfeldt-Jakob disease is caused by an infectious agent, but it is not yet clear what type of agent that is. Originally assumed to be a virus, evidence is accumulating that, instead, CJD is caused by a protein called a ''prion,'' (PREE-on, for ''proteinaceous infectious particle'') transmitted from victim-to-victim. The other spongiform encephalopathies are also hypothesized to be due to prion infection.

If this hypothesis is proved true, it would represent one of the most radical new ideas in biology since the discovery of DNA. All infectious diseases, in fact all life, uses nucleic acids—DNA or RNA—to code the instructions needed for reproduction. Inactivation of the nucleic acids destroys the capacity to reproduce. However, when these same measures are applied to infected tissue from spongiform encephalopathy victims, infectivity is not destroyed. Furthermore, purification of infected tissue to concentrate the infectious fraction yields protein, not nucleic acid. While it remains possible that some highly stable nucleic acid remains hidden within the purified protein, this is seeming less and less likely as further experiments are done. The ''prion hypothesis,'' as it is called, is now widely accepted, at least provisionally, by most researchers in the field. The most vocal proponent of the hypothesis, Stanley Prusiner, was awarded the Nobel Prize in 1997 for his work in the prion diseases.

The large majority of CJD cases are sporadic, meaning they have no known route of infection or genetic link. Causes of sporadic CJD are likely to be diverse and may include spontaneous genetic mutation, spontaneous protein changes, or unrecognized exposure to infectious agents. It is highly likely that future research will identify more risk factors associated with sporadic CJD.

About one in four people with CJD begin their illness with weakness, changes in sleep patterns, weight loss, or loss of appetite or sexual drive. A person with CJD may first complain of visual disturbances, including double vision, blurry vision, or partial loss of vision. Some visual symptoms are secondary to cortical blindness related to death of nerve cells in the occipital lobe of the brain responsible for vision. This form of visual loss is unusual in that patients may be unaware that they are unable to see. These symptoms may appear weeks to months before the onset of dementia.

Muscle spasms and jerking movements, called myoclonus, are also a prominent symptom of CJD. Balance and coordination disturbance (ataxia), is common in CJD, and is more pronounced in nvCJD. Stiffness, difficulty moving, and other features representing **Parkinson's disease** are seen and can progress to akinetic **mutism**, or a state of being unable to speak or move.

CJD is diagnosed by a clinical neurological exam and **electroencephalography** (EEG), which shows characteristic spikes called triphasic sharp waves. **Magnetic resonance imaging** (MRI) or **computed tomography scans** (CT) should be done to exclude other forms of dementia, and in CJD typically shows atrophy or loss of brain tissue. Lumbar puncture, or spinal tap, may be done to rule out other causes of dementia (as cell count, chemical analysis, and other routine tests are normal in CJD) and to identify elevated levels of marker proteins known as 14-3-3. Another marker, neuron-specific enolase, may also be increased in CJD. CJD is conclusively diagnosed after death by brain **autopsy**.

There is no cure for CJD, and no treatment which slows the progression of the disease. Drug therapy and nursing care are aimed at minimizing psychiatric symptoms and increasing patient comfort. However, the rapid progression of CJD frustrates most attempts at treatment, since ever-worsening cognitive deficits and more prominent behavioral symptoms develop so quickly. Despite the generally grim prognosis, a few CJD patients progress more slowly and live longer than the average; for these patients, treatment will be more satisfactory.

Creutzfeldt-Jakob disease is invariably fatal, with death following symptom onset by an average of eight months. About 5% of patients live longer than two years. Death from nvCJD has averaged approximately 12 months after onset.

There is no known way to prevent sporadic CJD, by far the most common type. Not everyone who inherits the gene mutation for familial CJD will develop the disease, but at present, there is no known way to predict who will and who won't succumb. The incidence of iatrogenic CJD has fallen with recognition of its sources, the development of better screening techniques for infected tissue, and the use of sterilization techniques for surgical instruments, which inactivate prion proteins.

Strategies for prevention of nvCJD are a controversial matter, as they involve a significant sector of the agricultural industry and a central feature of the diet in many countries. The infectious potential of contaminated meat is unknown, because the ability to detect prions within meat is limited. Surveillance of North American herds strongly suggests there is no BSE here, and strict regulations on imports of European livestock make future outbreaks highly unlikely. Therefore, avoidance of all meat originating in North America, simply on grounds of BSE risk is a personal choice unsupported by current data. The ban on the export of British beef continues in countries of the European Union, although some herds in these countries have developed low levels of infection as well.

Crick, Francis Harry Compton (1916-)

British molecular biologist

Francis Crick worked closely with **James Watson** and together they were able to deduce the structure of the deoxyribonucleic acid (DNA) molecule. This was very important because it showed that DNA, not protein as previously believed, was the actual carrier of genetic instructions for the cell. The Watson and Crick model reveals valuable information about the organization and operation of life itself. Their discovery is generally considered to be the most important scientific breakthrough of this century. Their model, originally constructed in 1953, showed the DNA molecule as consisting of two chains, each wrapped around the same axis like a spiral staircase. These helical chains are made of alternating units of phosphate and sugar molecules. Each side of the chain is connected by four base pairs which include adenine, thymine, guanine, and cytosine. Every base is attached at one end to a sugar molecule. The opposite end of the base molecule will only bind to its complementary base. For example, adenine is always chemically bound to thymine, and cytosine is always bound to guanine. This consistent, complementary pairing of the bases revealed how DNA was able to make exact copies of itself and thus pass on hereditary information.

Crick was born in 1916 in Northampton, England. After graduating with a degree in physics from University College, London, he developed radar systems and magnetic mines for the British military during World War II. In 1947, he worked at Strangeways Research Laboratory by day and studied biology in the evenings. He later moved to the Cavendish Laboratory at Cambridge University. It was there that he first met James Watson and began work on the structure of DNA. Although Watson had to initially persuade Crick to work with DNA, it wasn't long before Crick enthusiastically embraced the project. Crick eventually became consumed with this mission and even named his house The Golden Helix after their working hypothesis.

Crick gained his Ph.D. from Caius College, Cambridge, in 1953. That same year several other Cambridge scientists were awarded the Nobel Prize in other areas of research. Nearly 10 years later, Francis Crick shared the Nobel Prize in Phys-

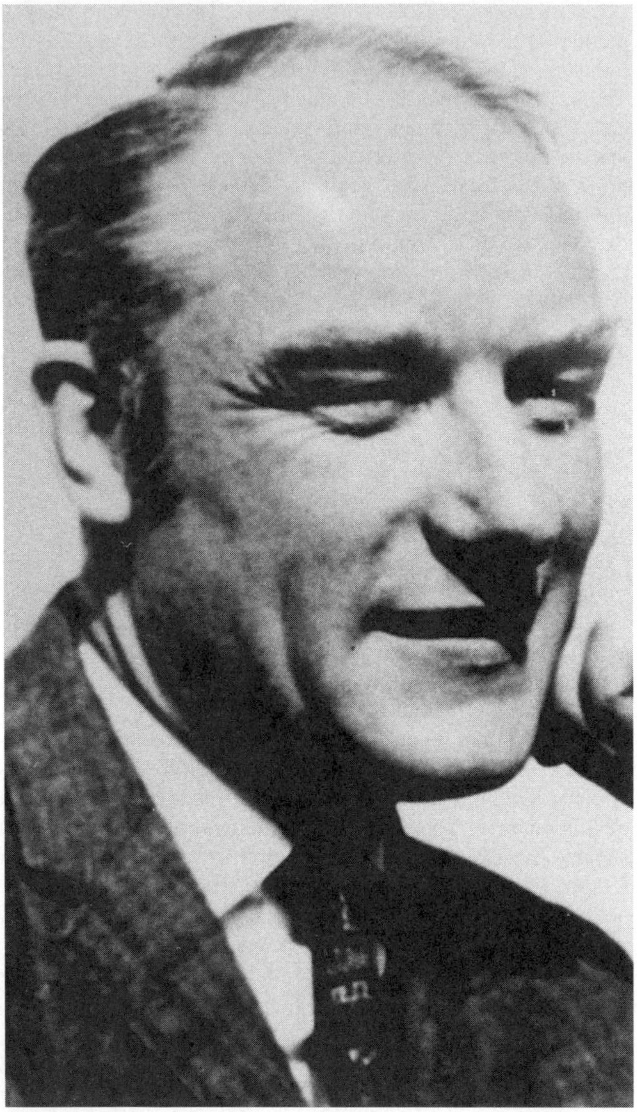

Francis Crick

iology and Medicine with James Watson and **Maurice Hugh Frederick Wilkins** for their work with DNA.

With fellow workers at Cambridge University, Crick later studied the structure and function of the genetic code—the sequence of nitrogen bases in DNA that directs the joining of amino acids to build protein molecules. Crick is credited with developing the term "codon" as it applies to the set of three bases that code for one specific amino acid. These codons are used as "signs" to guide protein synthesis within the cell. As a result of his later work with Drs. Barnett, Brenner, and Watts-Tobin, Crick was able to formulate a set of general properties of the genetic code. He has also used the common *Escherichia coli* bacteriophage to study genetic mutation mechanisms. In 1977, his distinguished status in the scientific community earned him a professorship at the famous Salk Institute for Biological Studies in San Diego, California. He continues to lead an active role in several areas of ongoing research today.

See also Franklin, Rosalind Elsie

Cri du chat syndrome

Newborns with cri du chat (cat's cry) syndrome have a characteristic mewing cry believed caused by abnormal development of the larynx (the organ containing the vocal chords). The syndrome arises from what is known as a deletion—the absence of genetic material from a missing portion of a chromosome. In cri du chat syndrome, the deletion is in chromosome 5. The disorder is also called 5p– (5 p minus) syndrome, in reference to the area where the deletion occurs. Children with this syndrome have physical abnormalities, language and motor skill difficulties, and varying degrees of **mental retardation**.

Although all individuals have two copies of chromosome 5, the normal chromosome does not compensate for the genetic material missing from the flawed chromosome in cri du chat syndrome. The deletion can be inherited through generations of a family or may appear at random. It is estimated that the syndrome occurs in 1 in 50,000 births. According to the 5p– Society, approximately 50-60 children are born with cri du chat syndrome each year in the United States.

The deletion on chromosome 5 has several indicators. The primary sign is the unusual high-pitched mewing cry during the first weeks of life. This is accompanied by low birth weight, slow growth, and a small head (microcephaly). Muscle tone is poor (hypotonia) and possible medical problems include heart disease and **scoliosis** (curvature of the spine). Children with cri du chat syndrome have language difficulties, delayed motor skill development, and mental deficiencies that vary in severity. Behavioral problems, such as hyperactivity, may become apparent as the child matures.

As the child matures, the cat-like cry is lost. A definitive diagnosis is based on karyotyping—a laboratory procedure that separates chromosomes from the infant's cells and demonstrates that genetic material is missing. Cri du chat syndrome can be detected before birth if the mother undergoes amniocentesis testing or chorionic villus sampling. Samples of cells are collected from the fluid surrounding the fetus and are analyzed for genetic defects (amniocentesis) or from the outer membrane (chorion) of the sac that holds both the fetus and the fluid (chorionic villus sampling).

Cri du chat syndrome is a very rare disorder with no cure or known prevention. Treatment consists of supportive care and developmental therapy.

The extent of mental retardation and other symptoms depends on the size of the chromosomal deletion—larger deletions generally translate into more serious symptoms. With intensive early intervention and special schooling, many cri du chat children can develop adequate social, motor, and language skills. Most individuals with cri du chat syndrome have a normal lifespan.

CROUP

Croup is a common childhood ailment. Typically, it arises from a viral infection of the larynx (voice box) and is associated with mild upper respiratory symptoms such as a runny nose and **cough**. The key symptom is a harsh barking cough. Croup is usually not serious and most children recover within a few days. In a small percentage of cases, a child develops breathing difficulties and may need medical attention.

At one time, the term croup was primarily associated with **diphtheria**, a life-threatening respiratory infection. Owing to widespread vaccinations, diphtheria has become rare in the United States, and croup currently refers to a mild viral infection of the larynx.

Parainfluenza viruses are the typical cause, but influenza (flu) and cold viruses may sometimes be responsible. All are highly contagious and easily transmitted via sneezing and coughing. Children between the ages of 3 months and 6 years are usually affected, with the greatest incidence at one to two years of age. Croup can occur at any time of the year, but it is most typical during early autumn and winter. The characteristic harsh barking of a croupy cough can be very distressing but rarely indicates a serious problem. Most children can be treated at home; however, 1-5% may require medical treatment.

Croup may sometimes be confused with more serious conditions, such as **epiglottitis** or bacterial tracheitis, which arise from bacterial infection and must receive medical treatment.

A croupy cough may be preceded by one to three days of symptoms that resemble a slight cold. It is often accompanied by a runny nose, hoarseness, and a low fever. When the child inhales, there may be a raspy or high-pitched noise, called stridor, owing to the narrowed airway and accumulated mucus. In this case, medical attention is required.

However, the airway rarely narrows so much that breathing is impeded. Symptoms usually disappear within a few days. Medical treatment may be sought if the child's symptoms do not respond to home treatment.

Emergency medical treatment is required immediately if the child has difficulty breathing, swallowing, or talking; develops a high fever (103°F/39.4°C or more); seems not alert or confused; or has pale or blue-tinged skin.

Home treatment is the usual method of managing croup symptoms. It is important that the child is kept comfortable and calm as much as possible, because crying can make symptoms seem worse. Humid air can help a child with croup feel more comfortable. Recommended methods include sitting in a steamy bathroom with the hot water running or using a cool-water vaporizer or humidifier. Breathing may also be eased by going outside into cooler air. The child should drink frequently in order to stay well hydrated. To treat any fever, the child may be given an appropriate dose of acetaminophen (Tylenol). Antihistamines and decongestants are ineffective in treating croup. *Children under 18 should not be given aspirin, as it may cause* **Reye's syndrome**, *a life-threatening disease of the brain.*

If the child does not respond to home treatment, medical treatment at a doctor's office or emergency room could be necessary. An x ray of the throat area may be done to assess the possibility of epiglottitis or other blockage of the airway. Based on severity of symptoms and response to treatment, the child may need to be admitted to hospital. Of the 1-5% of children requiring medical treatment, approximately 1% need respiratory support. Such support involves intubation (inserting a tube into the trachea) and oxygen administration.

Botanical/herbal medicines can help heal a croupy cough. Herbs to consider include aniseed (*Pimpinella anisum*), sundew (*Drosera rotundifolia*), thyme (*Thymus vulgaris*), and wild cherry bark (*Prunus serotina*). Homeopathic medicine can also be used to treat croup.

CRYOTHERAPY

Cryotherapy is a technique that uses an extremely cold liquid or instrument to freeze and destroy abnormal skin cells. The technique, also called cryosurgery, has been in use since the turn of the century, but modern techniques have made it widely available to dermatologists and primary care doctors.

Cryotherapy can destroy a variety of skin growths ranging from non-threatening warts to basal cell and squamous cell cancers.

There are three main techniques. In the simplest, usually reserved for warts and other non-threatening skin growths, the doctor will dip a cotton swab or other applicator into a cup containing a "cryogen," such as liquid nitrogen, and apply it directly to the skin growth to freeze it. At a temperature of −320°F (−196°C), liquid nitrogen is the coldest cryogen available. The goal is to freeze the growth as quickly as possible, then let it thaw slowly for maximum effect. A second application may be necessary depending on the size of the growth. In another technique, a small amount of cryogen is sprayed directly onto the growth. Freezing may last from 5-20 seconds. A second freeze-thaw cycle may be required. Sometimes, a small needle connected to a thermometer is inserted into the growth to ensure it is cooled sufficiently to guarantee maximum destruction. In a third option, the cryogen is circulated through a probe to cool it. The probe is then brought into direct contact with the growth to freeze it. This can take two to three times longer than the spray technique.

Cryotherapy is not recommended for certain areas of the body because of the dangers of destroying surrounding tissue or unacceptable scarring. These areas include: skin that overlies nerves, the corners of the eyes, the fold of skin between the nose and lip, skin surrounding the nostrils, and the border between the lips and the rest of the face. Suspected cases of malignant melanoma (a cancer of pigmented skin cells) should not be treated with cryotherapy, but should be removed surgically. Similarly, basal cell or squamous cell tumors that have reappeared at the site of a previously treated tumor should be surgically removed. If it remains unclear whether a growth is benign or malignant, a tissue sample should be removed for analysis (biopsy) before any attempts to destroy it with cryotherapy. Care should be taken in people with diabetes or certain circulation problems when cryotherapy is considered for growths located on their lower legs, ankles, and feet. In these patients, healing can be poor and the risk of infection can be high.

Patients will experience some **pain** at the time of the freezing, but local anesthesia is usually not required. The doctor may want to reduce the size of certain growths, such as warts, prior to the cryotherapy procedure, and may have patients apply salicylic acid preparations to the growth over several weeks. Sometimes, the physician will lightly pare away some of the tissue.

Redness, swelling, and the formation of a blister at the site of cryotherapy are all expected. Wounds on the head and neck may take four to six weeks to heal, but those on the body, arms, and legs can take longer. Some patients experience pain at the site following the treatment. This can usually be eased with **acetaminophen** (Tylenol), though in some cases a stronger pain reliever may be required.

Cryotherapy poses little risk and can be well-tolerated by elderly and other patients who are not good candidates for other surgical procedures. There is some risk of scarring, infection, and damage to underlying skin, tissue, and nerves, but these risks are generally minimal in the hands of experienced users of cryotherapy. Lightening or darkening of the skin may also occur.

Cryotherapy boasts high success rates in permanently removing skin growths; even for squamous cell and basal cell cancers, studies have shown a cure rate of up to 98%. For certain types of growths, such as some forms of warts, repeat treatments over several weeks are necessary to prevent the growth's return.

Cryptococcosis

Cryptococcosis is an infection caused by inhaling the fungus *Cryptococcus neoformans*. It is one of the diseases most often affecting **AIDS** patients. Cryptococcosis may be limited to the lungs, but frequently spreads throughout the body. Although almost any organ can be infected, the fungus is often fatal if it infects the nervous system, where it causes inflammation of the membranes covering the brain and spinal cord (meningitis).

The fungus causing cryptococcus, *C. neoformans*, is found in soil contaminated with pigeon or other bird droppings. It has also been found on unwashed raw fruit. Cryptococcosis is rare in healthy individuals, but is the most common fungal infection affecting people with AIDS.

People with Hodgkin's disease or who are taking large doses of drugs that suppress the immune system (corticosteroids, **chemotherapy** drugs) are more susceptible to cryptococcal infection.

Once the cryptococcal fungus reaches the lungs, three things can happen. The immune system can heal the body without medical intervention, the disease can stay localized in the lungs, or it can spread throughout the body. In healthy people, the body usually heals itself and the infected person notices no symptoms and has no complications.

If the body does not heal itself, the fungus begins to grow in the lungs and forms nodules that can be seen on chest x rays. In the early stages of infection, an individual usually only exhibits symptoms of a respiratory infection, such as a dry **cough**, so the disease is rarely diagnosed.

The fungus can remain dormant in the lungs and produce an active infection later if the immune system is weakened. If the disease becomes active, it can cause cryptococcal pneumonia in the lungs. Unfortunately, cryptococcal pneumonia has symptoms similar to other pneumonias (cough, chest **pain**, difficulty breathing), making it difficult to accurately diagnose.

Most patients are not diagnosed as having cryptococcosis until they show signs of cryptococcal meningitis. Fever and headache, nausea, vomiting, unwanted weight loss, and fatigue are common symptoms. Others may include blurred vision, stiff neck, aversion to light, and seizures.

Cryptococcal infection can spread to the kidneys, bone marrow, heart, adrenal glands, lymph nodes, urinary tract, blood, and skin. Painless **rashes** and lesions that mimic other skin diseases may develop.

Physicians who regularly work with AIDS patients have the most experience in diagnosing cryptococcosis. The preferred methods of diagnosis use simple and very accurate blood and cerebrospinal fluid (CSF) tests. CSF is collected during a procedure called a lumbar puncture, during which an anesthetic is applied near the spine and a needle withdraws fluid from the space between the vertebrae and the spinal cord. Chest x rays are useful in assessing lung damage, but the x ray alone does not lead to a definitive diagnosis of cryptococcosis.

Once cryptococcosis is diagnosed, treatment begins with amphotericin B (Fungizone), sometimes in combination with 5-flucytosine (Ancobon). Amphotericin B is a powerful drug with potentially toxic side effects, such as kidney toxicity and lower concentrations of an important blood component called hemoglobin. This medication can also cause fever, chills, nausea and vomiting, diarrhea, headache, and muscle aches. Patients may receive other medication to minimize the side effects from these drugs.

Amphotericin B, with or without 5-flucytosine, is given for several weeks until the patient is stable, after which the patient receives oral fluconazole (Diflucan). Patients with AIDS must continue taking fluconazole for the rest of their lives to prevent a relapse of cryptococcosis. Sometimes fluconazole is given to patients with advanced AIDS as a preventative measure.

Untreated cryptococcosis is always fatal. For AIDS patients who do not receive continued fluconazole, the relapse rate is 50-60% within six months. Once cryptococcosis infection has been successfully treated, individuals may be left with a variety of neurologic symptoms, such as weakness, headache, and hearing or visual loss. In addition, fluid may accumulate around the brain (**hydrocephalus**).

The best way to prevent cryptococcosis is to stay free of HIV infection. People with suppressed immune systems should stay away from areas contaminated with pigeon or other bird droppings.

Cryptosporidiosis

Dehydration and **malnutrition** are the most common effects of cryptosporidiosis, an infection of the intestine by microscopic parasites known as *Cryptosporidia*.

First identified in 1976 as a cause of disease in humans, *Cryptosporidia* are normally passed in the feces of infected persons and animals in the form of cysts. The cysts can remain in the ground and water for months, and when ingested produce symptoms after maturing in the intestine and the bile ducts. The most common sources of infection are other humans, water supplies, or reservoirs. These are contaminated by animals that defecate in these areas. An outbreak in Milwaukee in 1993 in which over 400,000 persons were affected was traced to the city's water supply. Cysts of *Cryptosporidia* are extremely resistant to disinfectants commonly used in water treatment plants and are incompletely removed by filtration.

Most persons who experience significant symptoms have altered immune systems and diseases such as AIDS or **cancer**. However, as shown in the Milwaukee outbreak, even those with normal immunity can experience symptoms.

Human-to-human transmission (such as occurs in daycare centers or through sexual behavior) is also an important cause.

Many individuals can be infected without any illness, but the major symptom is diarrhea, which is often watery and incapacitating. Dehydration, low-grade fever, nausea, and abdominal cramps are frequent.

In those with a normal immune system, the disease usually lasts about ten days. For patients with altered immunity (immunocompromised), the story is quite different, with diarrhea becoming chronic, debilitating and even fatal.

In about 20% of AIDS patients, bile duct infection also occurs, causing symptoms similar to gallbladder attacks. Eighty percent or more of those with infection of the bile ducts die from the disease. The lungs and pancreas are also sometimes involved. *Cryptosporidia* are just one cause of the diarrhea wasting syndrome in AIDS, which results in severe weight loss and malnutrition.

Diagnosis is based on either finding the characteristic cysts in stool specimens, or on tissue samples from an infected organ, such as the intestine.

The first aim of treatment is to avoid dehydration. Oral rehydration solution or intravenous fluids may be needed. Medications used to treat diarrhea by decreasing intestinal movement, such as loperamide or diphenoxylate, are also useful but should only be used with the advice of a physician.

Treatment aimed directly at *Cryptosporidia* is only partially effective, and rarely eliminates the organism. The medication most commonly used is paromomycin (Humatin), but others are presently under evaluation.

Cryptosporidia rarely cause a serious disease in persons with normal immune systems. Replacement of fluids is all that is usually needed. On the other hand, those with altered immune systems often suffer for months to years. Paramomycin and other drugs have been able to improve symptoms in over half of those treated. Unfortunately, many organisms are resistant, and subsequent infections are common.

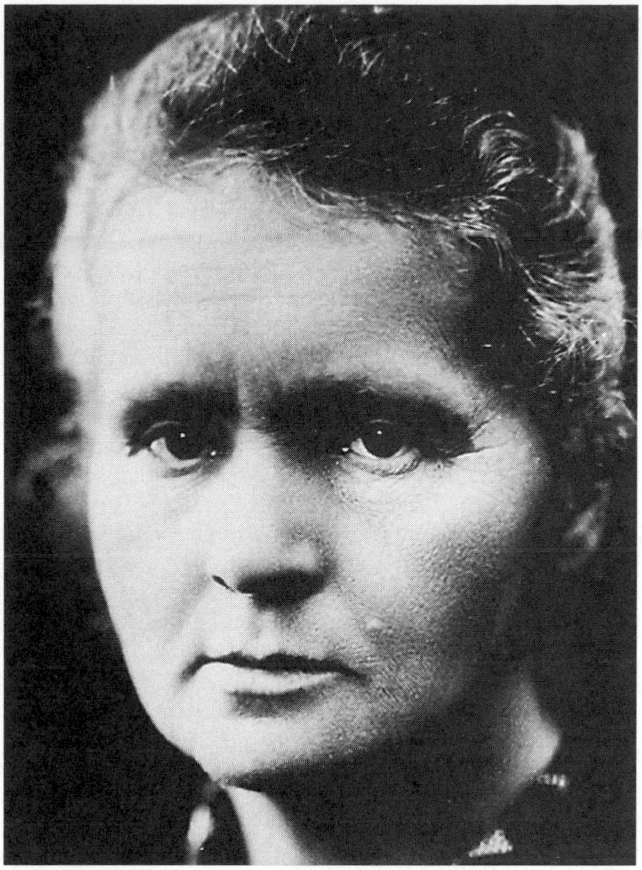

Marie Curie

The best way to prevent cryptosporidiosis is to minimize exposure to cysts from infected humans and animals. Proper hand washing technique, especially in day care centers is recommended.

Curie, Marie (1867-1934)

Polish French physicist

The story of Marie Curie's rise to prominence is one of perseverance and triumph over tremendous obstacles. The legacy of scientific knowledge she left resulted from some of the most important research ever conducted, most before she was thirty-five years old—a tremendous accomplishment for any scientist, let alone a young woman at the turn of the century.

Curie was born Marie Sklodowska in Warsaw, Poland, in 1867. Her mother was principal of a local girls' school, and her father a physics teacher. Curie showed early signs of following in her parents' footsteps, excelling in both primary and high schools. Unfortunately, Poland was under Russian rule, and the Polish intelligentsia was not favored by the Russian authorities. Although her record was outstanding, Curie was barred from her homeland's universities. After working for several years, during which time she subsidized her sister's education in Paris, Curie left Poland for France, where she enrolled at the Sorbonne in 1891. Her meager savings barely covered tuition and rent for her one-room apartment; she often went for long periods without food and once fainted from hunger during class. Her enthusiasm for learning did not waver, however, and in 1893 she received a degree in physics, graduating first in her class.

The next year, while pursuing a second degree, she met **Pierre Curie** at a colleague's house. He—who, with his brother, had made a name for himself by discovering piezoelectricity a few years earlier—was studying for his dissertation at the Sorbonne. They formed a friendship that quickly became love, and the two were married on July 26, 1895, soon after Pierre Curie earned his doctorate.

Marie Curie, too, was working toward her own dissertation, but had not decided on a subject. Their contemporary, **Henri Becquerel**, had just discovered that uranium salts emitted energy (called, at that time, Becquerel rays). At Becquerel's suggestion, Marie Curie set out to find other substances that emitted such rays. It was known that the ore pitchblende possessed properties similar to those of uranium, and the Curies chose this ore as the starting point of what would prove to be a long scientific journey.

Studying the pitchblende, the Curies detected the presence of a substance that was much more *radioactive* (a word Marie Curie had coined) than even pure uranium. They extracted this new element in 1898 and named it polonium, after Marie Curie's homeland. However, it was evident that pitchblende contained another new element, one that was thousands of times more radioactive than uranium, but that existed in amounts so small as to be nearly undetectable. Another French chemist confirmed the presence of this element, which the Curies had named radium, by examining pitchblende's spectral lines. This did not convince many scientists, nor did it satisfy the Curies, who were determined to prove the existence of radium by extracting a measurable amount. This would be no small task, since, in order to produce even a gram of radium, several tons of pitchblende would have to be refined.

At this time, Pierre Curie abandoned his teaching position in order to assist his wife's research. Though Marie Curie was the engine and mastermind of the project, they worked as one; in fact, all of the notes in her dissertation refer to the experimenters as "we"—neither she nor her husband are mentioned individually.

The Curies spent the bulk of their life savings to purchase waste ore from Czechoslovakian mines. They rented a leaky wooden shed in which they could refine the raw ore, and for the next four years they refined and purified the pitchblende, producing smaller and smaller samples that were more and more radioactive. The exhausting process, ordinarily performed by a team of several mine workers, took a dire physical toll upon the couple, and this, along with the arrival of their daughter, Irene, was nearly too much for them. Only Marie's intense determination held them together. By 1902 they had extracted one-tenth of a gram of radium, enough for Marie to base her dissertation upon (eight tons of pitchblende would eventually be required to extract one ounce of the new element).

The Curies and Becquerel shared the 1903 Nobel Prize for Physics for their contributions to the new science of radioactivity, but the couple did not attend the ceremony, for they were too ill to make the trip. Pierre Curie was also offered a professorial position in the Sorbonne's research laboratory, with his wife as his lab superintendent. In 1906, Pierre Curie was killed in a traffic accident, and his wife took over his position, continuing his lectures at the exact point at which they were interrupted. She was the first woman to teach at the Sorbonne.

In the years after her husband's death, Marie Curie conducted extensive work at the new Paris Institute of Radium; because of its mysterious properties, radium was used as a medicinal aid. Though it was often used indiscriminately, Curie's assistance proved that there were certain illnesses for which radium was an effective therapy. In particular, radium played an important role in the treatment of **cancer**, and still does. Marie Curie also introduced the use of radium and x-ray technology in medicine. For the discovery of radium and polonium, she was awarded the 1911 Nobel Prize for Chemistry, the only person to hold two Nobel laureates in the sciences.

Except for World War I, during which she drove an ambulance, Curie spent the remainder of her life studying the role of radium therapy. Though the process was wildly successful for many years, she received no royalties from its use, since she and her husband had chosen not to besmirch the scientific purity of their discovery by patenting it. Instead, she lived—rather comfortably—on the Nobel Prize money, as well as on income from other accolades.

Late in her life, the dangerous nature of radioactivity became tragically evident: her long years of exposure to radium had resulted in leukemia, leading to her death in 1934. She is historically recognized as an outstanding female scientist, as well as one of the greatest researchers.

Curie, Pierre (1859-1906)

French physicist

The name "Curie" is most often associated with **Marie Curie**, and with good reason. However, her husband Pierre had made a name for himself years before Marie began her epic work, and he assisted in the research that won the couple two Nobel Prizes.

Thinking his introverted son to be a slow learner, Curie's father chose to educate him at home. He proved to be an exceptional student once directed—so much so that he earned his bachelor's degree from the Sorbonne at the age of sixteen. He worked as a laboratory assistant there during his post-graduate studies, which gave him an opportunity to work with his older brother, Jacques. During this time, the two brothers did intense research in crystallography. In 1880, they discovered that certain crystals, such as quartz, would produce a small electric current when pressure was applied to them. They called this effect piezoelectricity (from a Greek work meaning "to press"). This discovery gained the Curie brothers international notice and earned Pierre an appointment at the Municipal School of Industrial Physics and Chemistry, where he taught until 1904.

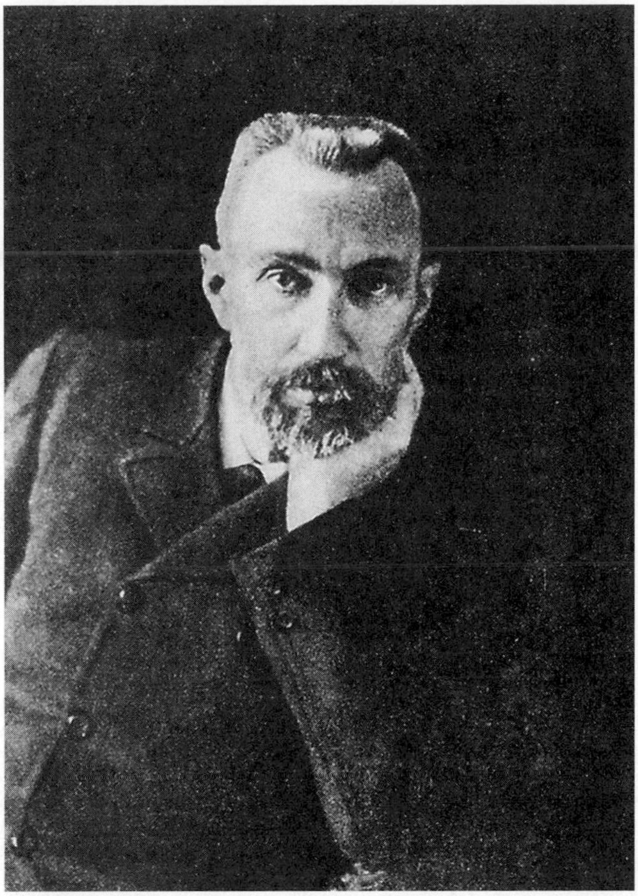

Pierre Curie

During the early 1890s, Curie became interested in the effects of temperature upon magnetism, and he began his doctoral studies in this area; he would eventually formulate a correlation between these properties that is still known as Curie's law. While researching at the Sorbonne, he met Marie Sklodowska, a young Polish woman working on her physics degree. They soon fell in love and in July 1895 were married shortly after the completion of Curie's doctoral dissertation.

In 1896 the Curies' mutual colleague **Henri Becquerel** had discovered the presence of radiation (at that time called Becquerel rays) emanating from samples of uranium. Marie Curie chose this as the subject of her own dissertation, and for the next six years the husband and wife team conducted exhaustive research to determine the source of this radioactivity, a term Marie Curie coined. Acting as one, the Curies discovered polonium and then radium. For their efforts, the Curies shared the 1903 Nobel Prize for Physics with Becquerel. Though proud of his work, Pierre Curie acknowledged the tremendous power contained in radioactive substances and the destructive potential that power held.

In 1904, Curie was given a professorship at the Sorbonne, with his wife as superintendent of his laboratory. Though they finally had scientific freedom and financial stability, their contentment was short-lived. On April 19, 1906, Curie slipped on a rain-slicked street and was crushed under the wheel of a horse-drawn cart. He died instantly. Marie Curie was given her husband's position at the Sorbonne and in 1911 won an unprecedented second Nobel Prize (this time in chemistry) for the work she and her husband had begun a decade earlier.

Cyclosporiasis

Cyclosporiasis refers to infection by *Cyclospora,* a microscopic, single-celled parasite that infects the human intestine. This parasite is a member of the group of protozoa known as coccidia, to which *Cryptosporidia* also belongs. This group of parasites infects the human intestine, and causes chronic recurrent infections in those with altered immunity or **AIDS**. Even in people with normal immune function, *Cyclopsora* can cause prolonged bouts of **diarrhea** and other gastrointestinal symptoms.

Until recently, *Cyclospora* was considered to be a form of algae. The parasite causes a common form of waterborne infectious diarrhea throughout the world. Just how the parasite gets into water sources is not yet clear. It is known that ingestion of small cysts in contaminated water leads to disease.

Symptoms begin after an incubation period of about a day or so following ingestion of cysts. A brief period of flu-like illness characterized by weakness and low-grade fever is followed by watery diarrhea, nausea, loss of appetite and muscle aches. In some patients symptoms may wax and wane for weeks, and there are those in whom nausea and burping may predominate. It is also believed that infection can occur without any symptoms at all.

In patients with altered immune systems, such as those with AIDS and **cancer**, prolonged diarrhea and severe weight loss often become major problems. The bile ducts are also susceptible to infection in AIDS patients.

The disease should be suspected in anyone with a history of prolonged or recurrent diarrhea. The parasite can be identified from stool specimens. Using an endoscope to obtain tissue samples from an infected organ such as the intestine is another way to make the diagnosis.

The first aim of treatment, as with any severe diarrheal illness, is to avoid **dehydration** and **malnutrition**. Oral rehydration solution or intravenous fluids are sometimes needed. Medications used to treat diarrhea by decreasing intestinal movement, such as loperamide or diphenoxylate, are also useful but should only be used with the advice of a physician.

The use of the medication trimethoprim-sulfamethoxazole (Bactrim) for one week can be successful in treating intestinal infections and prevents relapse in those with a normal immune system. The same medicine can be prescribed to treat infections of both the intestine or bile ducts in individuals with impaired or weakened immune systems, but maintenance or continuous treatment is often needed.

Even without treatment, symptoms usually do not last much more than a month or so except in cases with altered immunity. Fortunately, treatment is usually successful even in those patients.

Aside from a waterborne source as the origin of infection, little else is known about how the parasite is transmitted. Therefore, little can be done regarding prevention, except to maintain proper hand washing techniques and hygiene.

CYSTIC FIBROSIS

Almost everyone has experienced the congestion that accompanies a bad cold. The thick mucus that forms in the nose and throat makes breathing difficult. Luckily, this congestion dissipates in a few days as the body fights off the cold.

However, individuals afflicted with cystic fibrosis must constantly cope with the mucus which accumulates in the lungs, pancreas, and intestine. Cystic fibrosis, or mucoviscidosis, is an inherited disease that affects the exocrine glands. It is expressed only in the homozygous state without X chromosomal linkage. This genetic disease is often referred to as autosomal recessive. This means that children born to parents who each carry one recessive gene for the disease have a 25% chance of inheriting both copies of the defective gene—and with them the disease. This common disorder mainly effects about 1 out of every 2,000 caucasians of European descent, and it is the leading fatal genetic disease in the United States. The disease is less common in African Americans and very rare in Asians and Native Americans.

Cystic fibrosis was not classified as a separate disease until 1938. In 1989, scientists at the University of Michigan and the Hospital for Sick Children in Toronto, Ontario, Canada, announced that they had identified the defective gene that causes cystic fibrosis. The gene is found on chromosome 7, and over 600 mutations have been identified. Depending on the mutation, the symptoms and pathologies can range from mild to extremely severe. In 1992, scientists at the Cystic Fibrosis Center at the University of North Carolina were able to breed mice that showed human symptoms of cystic fibrosis. This newest achievement provided researchers with a model with which to study the disease.

Cystic fibrosis can be fatal if the mucus blocks the lungs. Patients may suffer from **pneumonia** caused by bacterial infections. Other serious complications include respiratory failure, **diabetes**, enlarged heart, liver cirrhosis, intestinal blockage, pancreatic disfunction, sodium deficiency, and sterility.

Abdominal cramps, malnutrition, growth retardation, and coughing are all symptoms associated with cystic fibrosis. However, the increased salinity of sweat is the most useful test to diagnose the disease. It is difficult to predict when any of these symptoms will appear or how severe they will be. While the disease used to be fatal to nearly all children who developed it, more than 50% of cystic fibrosis patients now live longer than thirty years.

Treatments are available for cystic fibrosis, but there is no cure. Often, **antihistamines** and decongestants are prescribed to open air passages. Cough suppressants are avoided since coughing helps to loosen the mucus in the trachea and lungs. **Antibiotics** help to treat pneumonia, and studies of the over-the-counter anti-inflammatory drug ibuprofen indicate that it can slow pulmonary decline. Physical therapy and surgery have also been used.

In 1990, researchers used laboratory cell cultures to correct the genetic defect that causes cystic fibrosis. They knew that the accumulation of mucus was caused by a blockage of the cell channel used to regulate the flow of sodium and chloride ions (Na^+ and Cl^-) in and out of the cell. The proper balance of these ions maintains the water balance of the mucus outside the cell. This equilibrium is controlled by a specific protein produced by two copies of a single gene. If both genes are defective, cystic fibrosis occurs.

Scientists are currently investigating gene therapy as an approach to treating cystic fibrosis. The process involves inserting a copy of the normal cystic fibrosis gene into a virus that has been altered not to cause disease. The virus is then inserted into lung cells removed from a cystic fibrosis patient. Researchers have found that the normal gene reaches the DNA of the lung cells and begins producing the correct protein, leading to decreased mucus secretion. A unique approach to apply this technology to human use is the development of an aerosol spray. However, since viruses can cause problems in cystic fibrosis patients like inflamed lungs and swollen nostrils which make breathing more difficult, the spray approach uses liposomes (a sphere spontaneously formed when fat molecules are in solution) to act as the gene carrier, or vector. The liposomes are coated with the healthy cystic fibrosis genes and then sprayed in the nostrils. Scientists have found that some of the genes do make it to cell nuclei in the lungs. Research continues into the effectiveness of this approach.

In 1996, scientists discovered that cystic fibrosis patients have a genetic defect that hinders the proper absorbtion of salt into lung epithelial cells. In turn, the resultant excess salt content inhibits a naturally occurring antimicrobial agent produced by these epithelial cells. With this natural defense system disabled, the immune system compensates by mounting a strong attack on bacteria. Unfortunately, this immune response is so overwhelming that it causes inflammation of the lung's minute branching airways, which further exacerbates the formation of mucus.

Rapid discoveries concerning the genetic factors in cystic fibrosis have led to research into new therapeutic approaches. Researchers at the National Institutes of Health, for example, have developed a ''gene-assist'' drug called CPX that helps promote chloride ion transport. With the development of new genetic testing technologies, physicians are able to test for a wider variety of the most common cystic fibrosis mutations known. As a result, a National Institutes of Health consensus panel has recommended that genetic testing should be offered to couples expecting a baby or to become pregnant, especially if they have a family history of cystic fibrosis. Many scientific and ethical concerns are associated with genetic testing of cystic fibrosis. **Genetic testing** sensitivity for cystic fibrosis can vary greatly, which carries the risk of not identifying a carrier or fetus with the disease. In addition, genetic counseling should be offered to couples at risk, but there is a shortage of genetic counselors. Finally, information about a person's genetic predisposition to cystic fibrosis and other diseases could lead to discrimination by employers and insurance companies.

D

DALE, HENRY HALLETT (1875-1968)

English physiologist

Henry Hallett Dale was a British physiologist who devoted his scientific career to the study of how chemicals in the body regulate physiological functions. In 1936 Dale and German pharmacologist **Otto Loewi** were jointly awarded the Nobel Prize in physiology or medicine for research demonstrating that nerve cells communicate with one another primarily by the exchange of chemical transmitters. In addition to his scientific work, Dale was a prominent figure in science and medicine in England at critical junctures in that nation's history. He was knighted in 1932.

Born June 9, 1875, in London, Henry Hallett Dale was the second son of seven children born to Charles Dale, a London businessman, and his wife, Frances Hallett Dale. After graduating from Tollington Park College, London, and the Leys School, Cambridge, Dale entered Trinity College at Cambridge University in 1894. His academic skills gained him first honors in the natural sciences and the Coutts-Trotter studentship at Trinity College.

Dale left Cambridge in 1900 to finish his clinical work in medicine at St. Bartholomew's Hospital in London. He received his bachelor's degree in 1903, and his medical doctorate in 1909. During this time, he also was awarded the George Henry Lewes studentship, which allowed him to pursue further physiological research. Later, Dale also received the Sharpey studentship in physiology at University College, London. Dale used these opportunities for research from 1902 to 1904, studying with Ernest Henry Starling and William Maddock Bayliss at University College. Starling and Bayliss identified secretin—a substance secreted by the small intestine—as the first hormone, and Dale collaborated with the pair in further studies on the impact of secretin on cells in the pancreas. Dale's work with Starling and Bayliss instilled in him the idea that physiological functions could be affected by such chemicals as hormones. It was also in this laboratory that Dale first met Otto Loewi, who at the time was visiting University College from Germany. Dale and Loewi would go on to become lifelong friends, collaborators, and co-recipients of the 1936 Nobel Prize.

In 1904 Dale spent three months working in the laboratory of the chemist **Paul Ehrlich** in Germany. Members of Ehrlich's laboratory were studying the relationship between the chemical structure of biological molecules and their effect on immunological responses, research that would garner for Ehrlich the 1908 Nobel Prize in physiology or medicine. As did the experience at Starling's laboratory in London, Ehrlich's research introduced Dale to the potential impact that chemicals can have on mediating biological and physiological processes.

After Dale returned to Starling's London laboratory, he was recommended to chemical manufacturer Henry Wellcome for a position with London's Wellcome Physiological Research Laboratories, a commercial laboratory. Established in the 1890s to produce an antitoxin for **diphtheria**, the laboratories, by the first decade of the 1900s, had begun to promote and pursue basic scientific research.

Once Dale had settled at Wellcome, the company suggested that he consider examining the therapeutic properties of ergot, a fungus being used by obstetricians to induce and promote labor. For the next decade, Dale devoted his research efforts to studying the properties of the drug, leading to the accidental discovery of the phenomenon of adrenaline (or epinephrine) reversal, in which the normally excitatory effects of these drugs are neutralized.

Dale's research on the effects of ergot also introduced him to ongoing efforts to study the central nervous system. Dale showed, with the chemist George Barger, that epinephrine is one chemical in a class of such chemicals that has ''sympathomimetic'' properties.

Dale's accomplishments drew the attention of Henry Wellcome, and Dale was promoted in 1906 to the directorship of the Wellcome Laboratories. Dale began studies of the chemicals that operate in the posterior pituitary lobe of the brain.

Dale resigned from the Wellcome Laboratories in 1914, and joined the scientific staff of the Medical Research Committee; after 1920 this group came to be known as the Medical Research Council. During World War I Dale joined the war effort by engaging in physiological studies of shock, dysentery, gangrene, and the effects of inadequate diet.

After the war, the Medical Research Council evolved to become the National Institute for Medical Research, and Dale served as the organization's first director from 1928 until 1942. His research efforts during the 1920s continued the work he began during the war—studying how histamine contributes to the swelling of tissue after traumatic shock. Dale demonstrated that histamine leads to the loss of plasma fluid into the tissues and produces swelling. This could lead to more serious problems, including decreased blood circulation, shock, and death.

Dale's study of histamine also contributed to his subsequent work on the nervous system. Histamine, like the neurotransmitter acetylcholine, dilates vascular tissue in the human body.

In 1927 Dale collaborated with H. W. Dudley to isolate acetylcholine from the spleen of an ox and a horse. Having isolated the crucial compound, Dale sought to understand how and where acetylcholine plays its role in vasodilatation, or the widening of the cavities of blood vessels. Over the next decade, Dale worked with colleagues at the National Institute for Medical Research and concluded that acetylcholine serves as a neurotransmitter and that this is the chemical mediator involved in the transmission of nerve impulses. Dale's findings disproved the proposition of John Carew Eccles and other neurophysiologists who maintained that nerve cells communicate with one another via an electrical mechanism. Dale demonstrated that a chemical process and not an electrical one was the underlying mechanism for nerve transmission. A similar conclusion had been reached by **Otto Loewi**: As early as 1921 Loewi suggested that a chemical mediator was responsible for the conduction of nerve impulses; it would be Dale who would identify the mediator.

For their work, Dale and Loewi were jointly awarded the 1936 Nobel Prize in physiology or medicine. During the 1930s, Dale continued collaborative research with G. L. Brown, W. Feldberg, J. H. Gaddum, and M. Vogt at the National Institute for Medical Research. Their efforts produced more evidence that acetylcholine is a neurotransmitter involved in nerve impulses.

During World War II, Dale served as chair of the Scientific Advisory Committee to the War Cabinet. Having been elected a fellow of the Royal Society in 1914, he served as secretary from 1925 to 1935, and as president from 1940 to 1945. His many other public affiliations included serving as president of various organizations, such as the Royal Institution of Great Britain during the mid–1940s, the British Association for the Advancement of Science in 1947, the Royal Society of Medicine from 1948 to 1950, and the British Council during the 1950s.

Other distinctions bestowed upon Dale include receiving the Copley Medal from the Royal Society in 1937 and being knighted with the Grand Cross Order of the British Empire in 1943. He also garnered the Order of Merit in 1944. Since 1959 the Society for Endocrinology has awarded the Dale Medal for the kind of excellence in research exemplified by Dale; and since 1961 the Wellcome Trust he chaired from 1938 until 1960 has endowed the Henry Dale professorship with the Royal Society.

In later years Dale worked with Thorvald Madsen of Copenhagen directing an international campaign to standardize drugs and vaccines. The 1925 conference of the Health Organization of the League of Nations adopted such standards for insulin and pituitary products largely because of Dale's efforts. He repeated these efforts to see into law the Therapeutic Substances Act in England. His other political activities included promoting both the peaceful use of nuclear energy and the value of scientific research. He died on July 23, 1968, after a brief illness.

DAM, HENRIK (1895-1976)

Danish biochemist

Henrik Dam is best known for his discovery of **vitamin K**, which gives **blood** the ability to clot, or coagulate. The discovery of vitamin K dramatically reduced the number of deaths by bleeding during surgery, and for the discovery Dam received the 1943 Nobel Prize in medicine and physiology. (**Edward A. Doisy**, the American biochemist who isolated and synthetically produced vitamin K, shared this prize with Dam.)

Carl Peter Henrik Dam was born in Copenhagen, Denmark, on February 21, 1895. His father, Emil Dam, was a pharmaceutical chemist who wrote a history of pharmacies in Denmark. His mother, Emilie Peterson Dam, was a schoolteacher. He attended the Polytechnic Institute in Copenhagen, from which he received his master of science degree in 1920. He was associated with the Royal School of Agriculture and Veterinary Medicine in Copenhagen for the next three years, after which he spent five years as an assistant at the University of Copenhagen's physiological laboratory. He became assistant professor of biochemistry in 1928 and associate professor in 1929 (a post he held until 1941).

During these years Dam studied microchemistry under Fritz Pregl in Austria (1925) at the University of Graz, and collaborated with biochemist Rudolf Schoenheimer in Freiburg, Germany (on a Rockefeller Fellowship) from 1932 to 1933. He was awarded a doctorate in biochemistry by the University of Copenhagen in 1934. Afterwards, he worked with the Swiss chemist Paul Xarrer at the University of Zurich in 1935. Dam specialized in nutrition, which became his area of expertise.

While Dam was studying in Copenhagen he became interested in what would become the vitamin K factor. In the late 1920s he began experimenting with hens in an attempt to discover how the animals synthesized cholesterol. Providing them with a synthetic diet, Dam discovered that they developed internal bleeding in the form of hemorrhages under the skin—lesions similar to those found in the disease **scurvy**. He added lemon juice to the diet (citrus fruits, high in **vitamin C**, had been found by the18th-century Scottish physician James Lind to cure scurvy in sailors), but the supplement did little to reverse the hens' condition.

After experimenting with a variety of food additives, Dam came to the conclusion that some vitamin must exist to give blood the ability to clot—and that this vitamin was what was missing from his synthetic hen diet. He made his findings known in 1934, naming the vitamin ''K'' from the German word *Koagulation*. Dam's continued research, along with the work of Doisy and other biochemists, led to the isolation of vitamin K and its synthetic production.

Dam's discovery proved vitally important in two areas: in surgical procedures and in treatment of newborn babies. Prior to surgery, patients are given vitamin K to assist in clotting the blood and reduce the risk of death by hemorrhage. Newborns are born deficient in vitamin K. Normally, beneficial bacteria that exist in the environment enter the intestinal tracts of infants and induce production of vitamin K. Modern hospitals are disinfected to such an extreme, however, that they kill these good bacteria along with the harmful ones. Mothers are injected with vitamin K shortly before giving birth to ensure that adequate amounts of the vitamin will be in the newborn's system.

Dam's discovery led not only to the Nobel Prize but also the Christian Bohr Award in Denmark in 1939. Dam came to the United States in 1940 for a series of lectures in the U.S. and Canada under the auspices of the American-Scandinavian Foundation. During his visit Nazi Germany invaded Denmark. Dam chose not to return to his native country and accepted a position as senior research associate at the University of Rochester's Strong Memorial Hospital. Because of the war, the Nobel Prize Committee decided to present the awards in New York in 1943. The Nobel recipients of that year, including Dam, were the first to be awarded their prize in the United States. In 1945, Dam became an associate member of the Rockefeller Institute for Medical Research.

After Denmark was liberated, Dam returned in 1946 to accept the position of head of the biology department at the Polytechnic Institute (the position had been awarded to him in absentia in 1941). He returned to the U.S. in 1949 for a three-month lecture tour, this time to discuss vitamin E. In 1956, he was named head of the Danish Public Research Institute. He was a member of numerous organizations including the American Institute of Nutrition, the Society for Experimental Biology and Medicine, the Royal Danish Academy of Science, the Société Chimique of Zurich, and the American Botanical Society. During his career he published more than 100 articles in scientific journals on vitamin K, vitamin E, cholesterol, and a variety of other topics. Dam married Inger Olsen in 1925. Dam died in Copenhagen at the age of 81 on April 17, 1976.

DAUSSET, JEAN (1916-)

French immunologist

Jean Dausset was born in Toulouse, France, and moved with his family to Paris at age eleven. After having earned an undergraduate degree in mathematics, he enrolled in the University of Paris medical school. When World War II broke out in 1939, Dausset joined the French medical corps. After France fell to the Germans in 1940, Dausset went to North Africa to fight with the Free French army. Before leaving Paris, Dausset gave all his identification papers to a Jewish colleague, who was therefore able to survive the Nazi occupation.

After the war ended, Dausset completed his studies at the university, receiving his medical degree in 1945. From 1946 to 1958 Dausset was director of laboratories at the French National Blood Transfusion Center, although he left for two years (1948-49) to study hematology under a fellowship at Harvard Medical School.

Dausset's work at the blood center, and earlier experiences during the war with transfusions, drew him into studies of abnormal transfusion reactions. In 1952 he discovered an antigen on certain people's white blood cells. By 1958, when he joined the medical faculty at the University of Paris, he had found more variants of the antigen. In 1965, Dausset suggested that these and other newly discovered antigens were all part of a single set of linked genes, which constituted the human MHC (major histocompatibility complex). He called this the human leucocyte antigen group (HLA) and, in 1967, showed that tissue transplants are more successful when donor and recipient have matching HLA types. In 1967 Dausset was the first researcher to investigate possible links between an individual's HLA types and the person's risk for disease. For all of these findings about HLA, Dausset shared the 1980 Nobel Prize for physiology or medicine with George Snell and **Baruj Benacerraf**. Dausset had become head biologist of Paris's city hospital system in 1963 and also headed the Institute for Research into Diseases of the Blood. In 1968 he assumed directorship of the French National Institute for Scientific Research and became a professor of medicine at the University of Paris and, since 1978, the College of France. He remained at the university through the 1980s, continuing his studies of HLA. He has since founded the Human Polymorphism Study Center in Paris and has helped organize a collaboration to map the human genome. As his personal motto he chose ''*Vouloir pour valoir,*'' or, roughly translated, ''To achieve a lofty goal, you must aspire to it. ''

DAVIS, MARGUERITE (1887-1967)

American chemist

Marguerite Davis is best known as co-discoverer of vitamins A and B. Her research at the University of Wisconsin in Madison with biochemist **Elmer Verner Mc Collum** led to definitive identification of both vitamins and paved the way for later research in **nutrition**.

Davis was born on September 16, 1887, in Racine, Wisconsin. Her father, Jefferson J. Davis, was a physician and botanist who taught at the University of Wisconsin. Her grandmother, Amy Davis Winship, was a social worker and an early champion of women's rights. Her background, coupled with her own interest in science, led her to enroll at the

University of Wisconsin in 1906. She transferred to the University of California at Berkeley in 1908 and received her bachelor of science degree there in 1910. Upon graduation, she returned to the University of Wisconsin and pursued graduate studies, although she never completed the master's program. She worked briefly for the Squibbs Pharmaceutical Company in New Brunswick, New Jersey, but returned to Wisconsin.

It was during her time at the University of Wisconsin that she began her work with McCollum, who had been studying nutrition for several years. The Dutch physician **Christiaan Eijkman** and the British biochemist Sir **Frederick Gowland Hopkins** had determined that traces of as-yet unidentified elements in foods were essential for adequate nutrition. The Polish-American biochemist Casimir Funk, believing the substances were amines, proposed the name "vitamine"—literally, "life-giving amine" (when it later became clear that not all the substances were amines the "e" was dropped). McCollum was trying to create simple mixtures that could replace natural food in animal diets. Although his efforts were unsuccessful, he wanted to find out whether natural food contained some special substance like that proposed by Eijkman and Hopkins.

Davis and McCollum worked with various food components and in 1913 discovered a factor in some fats that apparently was essential to life. Because the substance differed chemically from one described earlier by Eijkman, Davis and McCollum named theirs fat-soluble A and Eijkman's water-soluble B. These were later called vitamins A and B. The identification of A and B led later to the discovery of the other vitamins and their specific roles in nutrition, as well as which foods contain them.

Davis joined the University of Wisconsin's chemical research staff and founded its nutrition laboratory. She later went on to Rutgers University in New Jersey and organized a similar lab for its school of pharmacy. She retired and moved back to Racine in 1940 but continued to serve as a chemistry consultant for many years. She became active in Racine civic affairs and pursued other interests, including history and gardening. In 1958 Racine's Women's Civic Council recognized Davis for her contributions as a civic leader. Davis died in Racine on September 19, 1967, three days after her eightieth birthday.

Davis, Nathan Smith (1817-1904)

American medical educator, editor

Nathan Smith Davis was founder of the **American Medical Association** (AMA), serving twice as that organization's president, and also as founding editor of the *Journal of the American Medical Association (JAMA).*

Unlike most nineteenth-century American physicians, Davis was not born to wealthy parents. Instead, he was born in a log cabin, in Chenango County, New York. He had only six months of higher education before starting a medical apprenticeship in 1834. Davis helped pay for this apprenticeship by taking care of his instructor's cow and horse. In 1837, he graduated from The College of Physicians and Surgeons of the Western District of New York. His thesis challenged the common belief at that time that oxygen combined with carbon in the lungs.

Following graduation, Davis entered general practice in the New York communities of Vienna and Binghamton. It was in Binghamton that Davis started his lifelong involvement in professional societies, beginning with his appointment to the Broome County Medical Society.

Davis worked to improve the quality and duration of medical education. Elected in 1844 to the New York Medical Society, he introduced a resolution calling for a national medical association to "elevate... the standard of medical education in the United States." Others had proposed such an association before him, but Davis's resolution was the first to succeed.

The fledgling organization met in New York City on May 5, 1846, with delegates agreeing that a national group was needed to establish both uniform educational requirements and a medical code of ethics. After another preliminary meeting in Philadelphia in 1847, the AMA held its first meeting in Baltimore the following year. Although he was barely 30 at the time of founding, Davis remained the AMA's central figure for the remainder of his career. Of the association's first 50 annual meetings, he was present at 47.

In 1849, Davis moved to Chicago's Rush Medical College as professor of physiology and general pathology. At the time, Chicago was a frontier community with no sewer system or general hospital. Davis was involved in establishing Chicago's Mercy Hospital and also created the Chicago Medical Society and the Illinois Medical Society. In 1859, Davis and some colleagues left Rush to start the Medical Department of Lind University, which was reorganized in 1864 into the Chicago Medical College, and in 1870 into the medical school at Northwestern University. Davis served as president of the Chicago Medical College and as dean of Northwestern's medical department.

In 1870, he donated $3,000 to found the Dean's Dispensary, which provided free medical treatment to those unable to afford it. In addition, Davis helped establish Chicago's Washingtonian Home for Inebriates. Less lofty, however, were Davis's attitudes towards women and blacks. He argued that both should be excluded from the AMA.

In 1883, when Davis was 66, he became the first editor of *JAMA,* when that weekly periodical was introduced to replace the AMA's yearly *Transactions.*

Davis was also involved in editing the *Chicago Medical Journal, Chicago Medical Examiner, American Medical Temperance Quarterly, Northwestern Medical and Surgical Journal,* and the *Annalist,* as well as the *Ecletic Journal of Education and Literary Review.*

He authored a number of books: *A Textbook on Agriculture* (1848), *History of Medical Education and Institutions in the United States* (1851), *Clinical Lectures on Various Important Diseases* (1873), *Lectures on the Principles and Practice of Medicine* (1884), and *The History of Medicine, With the Code of Ethics* (1903). The latter work covered the history of American medicine more extensively that any other earlier attempt.

Throughout his career, Davis campaigned against consumption of alcohol, which he described as "a positive protoplasmic poison, directly impairing every natural structure and function of the living body in proportion to the quantity used, and the length of time its use is continued.'' At the time, whiskey and cod liver oil were commonly used as a treatment for tuberculosis, but research by Davis and a colleague found that patients treated with alcohol actually fared worse than those who did not receive it. In 1891, he founded the American Medical Temperance Society. He made controversial bids to ban alcohol from the AMA's annual banquets. When a testimonial dinner was held for him in 1901, Davis, then 84, proposed a toast to: ''Pure water...it disorders no man's brain; it fills no asylums or prisons; it begets no anarchy, but it sparkles in the dew drop.''

He continued to practise medicine until he died at the age of 87.

DEATH

Death is defined as the stopping of all vital functions of thebody including heartbeat, brain activity (including the brain stem), and breathing.

Death comes in many forms, sometimes expected during a terminal illness, sometimes unexpected from accident or medical condition. When a terminal illness is diagnosed, the patient, family, friends, and caregivers are all able to prepare for the impending death. The terminally ill patient goes through several levels of emotional acceptance while in the process of dying. First, there is denial and isolation. Second, comes anger and resentment. Thirdly, the patient tries to escape the inevitable, and then with the realization that death is eminent, suffers depression. Finally, the reality of death is realized and accepted.

As of 1997, the top three causes of death in the United States were heart disease, **cancer**, and **stroke**. These were followed by chronic obstructive pulmonary diseases, **accidents**, pneumonia and **influenza**, **diabetes mellitus**, and **suicide**.

In recent years, the development of **organ transplantation**, together with new technologies that can support life even when major organ systems fail, have made it necessary to develop precise legal definitions of death.

In addition to lack of breathing or heartbeat, signs of death may include:

- No pupil reaction to light.
- No jaw reflex (the jaw will react like the knee if hit with a reflex hammer).
- No gag reflex (touching the back of the throat induces vomiting).
- No response to **pain**.

Current ability to resuscitate patients who have ''died'' has produced some remarkable stories. Drowning in cold water (under 50°F/10°C) so effectively slows **metabolism** that victims may be revived after a half hour under water.

Only recently has there been concerted public effort to improve care of the dying. Hospice care represents one of the greatest advances ever made in this direction. There has also been a liberalization of the use of narcotics and other drugs for symptomatic relief and improvement in the quality of life for the dying.

One of the most difficult issues surrounding death is that life-support technology has created an opportunity for choice, not of the event itself but of its timing. When to die, or when to let a loved one die, is coming within our power to determine. This is both a blessing and a dilemma. Insofar as the decision can be made ahead of time, a legal document known as a **living will** may be used to address this dilemma. By outlining the conditions under which one would rather be allowed to die, a person can contribute significantly to that final decision, even if not competent to do so at the time. The problem is that there are uncertainties surrounding every severely ill patient. Each instance presents a greater or lesser chance of survival, and it is often greater than zero. The best living will follows an intimate discussion with decision-makers covering the many possible scenarios surrounding the end of life. This discussion is difficult, for few people like to contemplate their own demise. However, the benefits of a living will are substantial, both to physicians and to the loved ones who are faced with that final decision. Most states have passed living will laws, honoring instructions on artificial life support that were made while the patient was still competent.

Another issue that has become front-page news in the United States is assisted suicide (**euthanasia**), largely because of the activities of Dr. Jack Kevorkian, a pathologist from Michigan who has become one of euthanasia's most fervent advocates. The issue highlights the many new problems generated by increasing ability to intervene effectively in the final moments of life and unnaturally prolong the process of dying. Fortunately, the public appearance of euthanasia has also stimulated discussion about more compassionate care of the dying.

After death, an **autopsy** can precisely determine cause of death. A specialist known as a pathologist extensively examines the body and submits a detailed report to the attending physician. Although an autopsy can do nothing for the individual after death, it can benefit the family and, in some cases, medical science. Hereditary disorders and disease may be found—knowledge that could be used to prevent illness in family members. Information culled from an autopsy can further medical research. For example, the link between **smoking** and **lung cancer** was confirmed from data gathered through autopsy. Early information about **AIDS** was also compiled through autopsy reports.

DEBAKEY, MICHAEL ELLIS (1908-)

American surgeon and inventor

Michael Ellis DeBakey is a world renowned cardiovascular surgeon, medical inventor, medical statesperson, and teacher who is chancellor of the Baylor College of Medicine in Houston, chair and Olga Keith Weiss Professor of its department of surgery, and director of the DeBakey Heart Center. He is the recipient of the America's highest civilian honor, the Medal of Honor with Distinction (awarded in 1969), and of the country's highest scientific award, the National Medal of Science (1987). DeBakey is best known for his landmark cardiovascular surgeries, including the first successful implantation

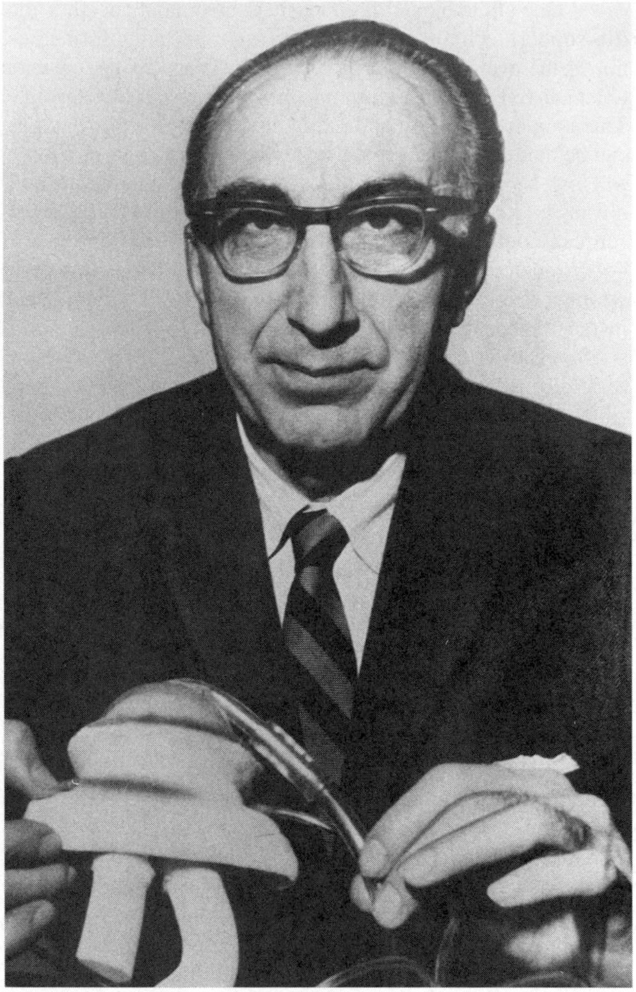

Michael DeBakey

of an **artificial heart** in 1966. He also pioneered the use of artificial arteries and coronary bypass, invented new equipment and instruments, and conducted important research on the causes of arteriosclerosis.

Born on September 7, 1908, in Lake Charles, Louisiana, to Shaker Morris and Raheega (Zorba) DeBakey, Michael DeBakey was the oldest of five children. His father was a successful pharmacist and businessperson, his mother "a compassionate person who was always trying to help someone," according to DeBakey in the *Tulanian.* His keen intellect was obvious at an early age: as a reward for doing well in his schoolwork, DeBakey's parents would let him read the *Encyclopedia Britannica;* he had completed the whole set before entering high school. His ingenuity, however, was not limited to academics; he played several musical instruments, participated in sports, sewed, and maintained a garden with his brother.

The variety in DeBakey's life did not change when he entered Tulane University in 1926. In college, he became an accomplished billiards player and played saxophone in the Tulane University band and orchestra. DeBakey had earned enough credits to enter medical school by the time he was a sophomore, but he also wanted a baccalaureate degree. He therefore persuaded the university to let him complete his degree while concurrently attending medical school. While still a medical student, DeBakey created his first invention: a modified roller pump for blood transfusions which did not damage the blood during the procedure. Twenty years later, this device became a major component of John H. Gibbon's **heart-lung machine**, used in the first **open-heart surgery**. While at Tulane, DeBakey met his mentor, the surgeon Alton Ochsner.

With his medical degree in hand in 1932, DeBakey completed two years of surgical residency training at Charity Hospital in New Orleans. He then went to Europe to study under two prominent surgeons: Rene Leriche of the University of Strasbourg, France, and Martin Kirschner of the University of Heidelberg, Germany. Upon his return to the United States, DeBakey completed his master's of science degree at Tulane.

In 1937, DeBakey returned to Tulane to serve on its faculty until, at the beginning of World War II, he volunteered for military service; after serving four years in the U.S. Surgeon General's office, he was appointed director of the Surgical Consultants' Division there. His work led to the establishment of the mobile army surgical hospitals (MASH units). He also helped organize a specialized medical center system to treat soldiers returning from the war; that system later became the Veterans' Administration (VA) Medical Center System. DeBakey also proposed a systematic follow-up of veterans with certain medical problems, which eventually became the VA's Medical Research Program. He received the Legion of Merit Award in 1945 for his wartime achievements.

In 1946, DeBakey again returned to Tulane as an associate professor of surgery. Two years later, he was named chair of the department of surgery at Baylor University College of Medicine. He remained at Baylor for the rest of his academic career, becoming first the president of the College of Medicine in 1969 and, a decade later, its chancellor.

DeBakey's record is filled with many firsts, all targeting the diagnosis and treatment of arteriosclerosis (hardening of the arteries). When Debakey began his research, the prognosis for patients with arteriosclerosis was poor—individuals with the disease usually died by age fifty. Now, in large part due to DeBakey's work, such patients can live well into their eighties. During the 1950s, DeBakey was the first to classify arterial disease by location, characteristic, and pattern, making diagnosis much easier. The cause, however, was still unknown.

Between 1950 and 1953, DeBakey developed the Dacron and Dacron-velour artificial grafts to replace diseased arteries—a process which is now commonly practiced worldwide. Though DeBakey sewed his first Dacron graft on his wife's sewing machine, subsequent Dacron artificial arteries were created using a special knitting machine developed by the Philadelphia College of Textiles. In 1953, DeBakey performed the first successful removal and graft replacement of an aneurysm (a swelling caused by a weakness in a vessel wall) of the thoracic aorta; this procedure, too, is now widely used around the world. Also in 1953, DeBakey performed the first successful removal of a blockage of the main (carotid) artery of the neck, a procedure known as an endarterectomy. This procedure has become the standard method for treating stroke.

Beginning in 1953, DeBakey pioneered four different kinds of operations for the treatment of aneurysms in different areas of the aorta: the removal (resection) and graft replacement of an aneurysm in the downward section of the aortic arch, which curves like a cane handle over the top of the heart; the resection of an aneurysm in the muscle layer of the aorta; the resection and graft replacement of an aneurysm of the upper part of the aorta; and the resection of an aneurysm of the portion of the aorta between the chest and the abdomen. In 1958, DeBakey also performed the first successful patch-graft **angioplasty** to reverse the narrowing of an artery caused by an endarterectomy.

By the early 1960s DeBakey had established the standard procedure of therapy in arterial disease, for which he received the Albert Lasker Clinical Research Award in 1963. A year later, DeBakey was the first to successfully perform an aortocoronary artery bypass, now commonly referred to as "bypass surgery." Using a large vein removed from the patient's leg, he re-routed blood around any damaged area between the aorta and coronary arteries, leaving healthy areas intact. Since the 1960s, DeBakey has also tested different artificial- and partial-artificial heart devices, and in 1966 conducted the landmark operation in which the first partial-artificial heart was successfully transplanted. In 1968, DeBakey was one of the first surgeons to perform heart transplantations; however, rejection problems led him to suspend this practice until 1984, when better anti-rejection drugs (such as cyclosporine) and other technological advances became available.

From 1983 to 1987, DeBakey teamed with Dr. Joseph Melnick and other colleagues to study more closely the causes of arteriosclerosis. They found that the cytomegalovirus (known as CMV), a common virus which causes arterial lesions when first contracted early in life, could lay dormant for years after initial infection. Those individuals with arteriosclerosis were found to have high levels of antibodies to the virus, and it was suggested that CMV might play a role in the development of arteriosclerosis. In 1987, DeBakey and his research team announced that high cholesterol levels, long thought to be one of the major causes of heart disease, were in fact not related to how quickly arteries became blocked. In another study, they also showed that while smoking, a high fat diet, and high blood pressure may put an individual at high risk, they do not themselves cause arteriosclerosis.

In order to apply the specialized medical center system to the civilian sector, DeBakey (with the help of federal funding) founded the Cardiovascular Research and Training Center at the Texas Medical Center in the early 1970s. Later, in 1985, Baylor established the DeBakey Heart Center for research and public education in the prevention and treatment of heart disease.

While his reputation as a surgeon grew, DeBakey continued teaching, writing research papers, attending medical symposia and consulting governments on different aspects of health care. As a member of the Medical Task Force of the Hoover Commission on Organization of the Executive Branch, DeBakey helped establish the National Library of Medicine in Washington, DC, in the early 1950s. It is now the world's largest and most prestigious repository of medical archives. He has served as an advisor to almost every president over the past 50 years, works to improve international health standards, and consults for European, Eastern block, and Middle and Far East countries to establish better health care systems. DeBakey has performed almost 50,000 cardiovascular procedures, trained almost 1,000 surgeons, and has written 1,200 medical articles, chapters, books, research papers on surgery, medicine, health, medical research and education, ethics and social issues. He corresponds regularly with many of his patients, from princes to paupers, is the editor of many professional publications, and holds the rank of colonel in the United States Army Reserves. He has received numerous awards, honorary degrees and appointments.

By 1976, DeBakey had trained so many surgeons and physicians that they decided to form the Michael E. DeBakey International Surgical Society, which offers medical symposia biennially. His former students describe him as a workaholic, single-minded, focused, and expecting the highest standards of excellence from everyone with whom he deals. "He didn't ask more of anyone else than he asked of himself," recalled pulmonary and vascular surgeon Daniel Mahaffey in the *Tulanian.* Ochsner, DeBakey's mentor, told the *Tulanian,* "I've never known anyone who works harder and with less apparent strain. His capacity for work is almost unlimited."

In 1936, DeBakey married Diane Cooper, a Texas native, with whom he had four sons; two became businessmen, one a restaurateur, and one an attorney. His wife died of a massive heart attack in 1972; DeBakey, who had been performing cardiac surgery at the time, rushed to his wife's bedside, but was unable to keep her alive. Two years later, he married Katrin Fehlhaber, a German artist and actor. In 1977, they had a daughter.

Debridement

Debridement is the process of removing dead tissue from pressure ulcers, **burns**, and other wounds, to speed healing.

Wounds that contain non-living tissue take longer to heal. This tissue may become colonized with bacteria, producing an unpleasant odor. Though the wound is not necessarily infected, the bacteria can cause inflammation and strain the body's ability to fight infection. Necrotic tissue may also hide pockets of pus called **abscess**es, which can develop into a general infection that may in turn lead to **amputation** or **death**.

Not all wounds need debridement. Sometimes it is better to leave a hardened crust of dead tissue, than to remove it and create an open wound, particularly if the crust is stable and the wound is not inflamed. Before performing debridement, the physician will take a medical history with attention to factors that might complicate healing, such as medications being

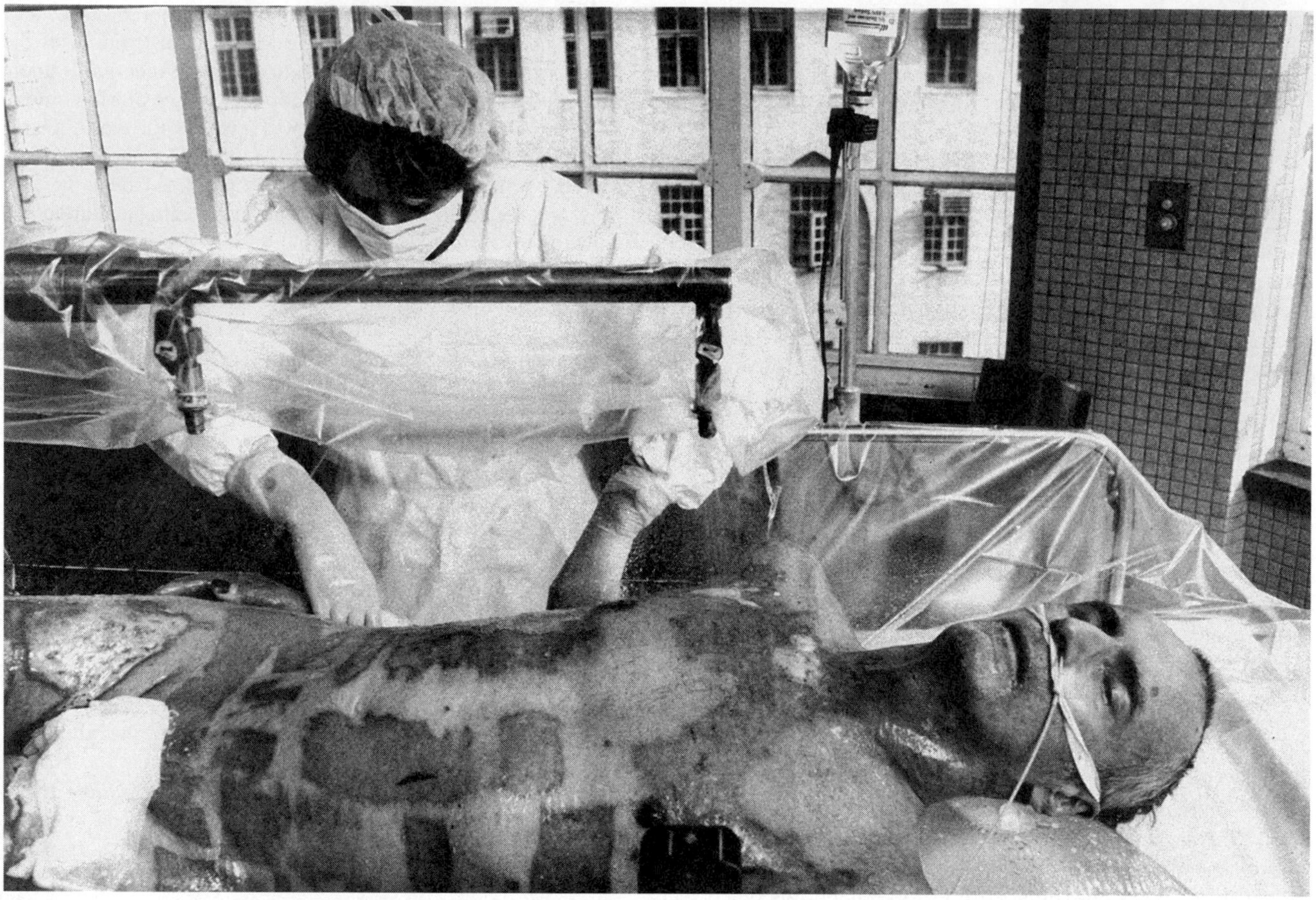

A burn sufferer undergoes debridement (the removal of dead skin). The patterns on his chest are from skin grafts. ***(Photograph by Ann Chawatsky, Phototake NYC. Reproduced by permission.)***

taken and **smoking**. Some ulcers and other wounds occur in places where blood flow is impaired. In such cases, the physician or nurse may decide not to debride the wound because blood flow may be insufficient for proper healing.

The four major debridement techniques are surgical, mechanical, chemical, and autolytic.

Surgical debridement uses a scalpel, scissors, or other instrument to cut dead tissue from a wound. It is the quickest and most efficient method, and is preferred if there is rapidly developing inflammation of the body's connective tissues (**cellulitis**) or a more generalized infection (**sepsis**) that has entered the bloodstream.

The physician will begin by flushing the area with a saline (salt water) solution, and then will apply a topical anesthetic gel to the edges of the wound to minimize pain. Using forceps to grip the dead tissue, the physician will cut it away bit by bit with a scalpel or scissors. Sometimes it is necessary to leave some dead tissue behind rather than disturb living tissue.

In mechanical debridement, a saline-moistened dressing is allowed to dry overnight and adhere to the dead tissue. When the dressing is removed, the dead tissue is pulled away too. This process is one of the oldest methods of debridement. It can be very painful because the dressing can adhere to living as well as nonliving tissue. Because mechanical debridement cannot select between good and bad tissue, it is unacceptable for clean wounds where a new layer of healing cells is already developing.

Chemical debridement makes use of certain enzymes and other compounds to dissolve necrotic tissue. It is more selective than mechanical debridement. The body makes its own enzyme, collagenase, to break down collagen, one of the major building blocks of skin. A pharmaceutical version of collagenase is available and is highly effective as a debridement agent. As with other debridement techniques, the area first is flushed with saline. Any crust of dead tissue is etched in a cross-hatched pattern to allow the enzyme to penetrate. A topical antibiotic is also applied to prevent introducing infection into the bloodstream. A moist dressing is then placed over the wound.

Autolytic debridement takes advantage of the body's own ability to dissolve dead tissue. The key to the technique is keeping the wound moist, which can be accomplished with a variety of dressings. These dressings help to trap wound fluid that contains growth factors, enzymes, and immune cells that promote wound healing. Autolytic debridement is more selective than any other debridement method, but it also takes the longest to work. It is inappropriate for wounds that have become infected.

Risks of debridement include the possibility that underlying tendons, blood vessels, or other structures will be damaged during the examination of the wound or during surgical debridement. Surface bacteria may also be introduced deeper into the body, causing infection.

Although debridement procedures cause some **pain**, they are generally well tolerated by patients. It is not uncommon to debride a wound again in a subsequent session.

Decompression sickness

Decompression sickness (DCS) is a dangerous and occasionally lethal condition caused by nitrogen bubbles that form in the blood and other tissues of scuba divers who surface too quickly.

According to the Divers Alert Network, a worldwide organization devoted to safe-diving research and promotion, less than 1% of divers fall victim to DCS or the rarer bubble problem called gas embolism, air embolism, or arterial gas embolism. A study of the U.S. military community in Okinawa, where tens of thousands of sport and military dives are made each year, identified 84 DCS and 10 arterial gas embolism cases in 1989–95, including 9 deaths. This translated into one case in every 7,400 dives and one **death** in every 76,900 dives. But DCS symptoms can be quite mild, and many cases go unnoticed.

The air we breathe is mostly a mixture of two gases, nitrogen (78%) and oxygen (21%). Unlike oxygen, nitrogen is not converted into other substances by the body. For this reason, most of the nitrogen we inhale is expelled when we exhale, but some is dissolved into the blood and other tissues. During a dive, however, the lungs take in more nitrogen than usual. This happens because the surrounding water pressure is greater than the air pressure at sea level (twice as great at 33 ft [10 m], for instance). As the water pressure increases, so does the pressure of the nitrogen in the compressed air inhaled by the diver. Because increased pressure causes an increase in gas density, the diver takes in more nitrogen with each breath than at sea level. But instead of being exhaled, the extra nitrogen safely dissolves into the tissues, where it remains until the diver begins returning to the surface (under some circumstances the extra nitrogen can cause **nitrogen narcosis**, but that condition is distinct from DCS). On the way up, the water pressure drops, and with this decompression the extra nitrogen gradually diffuses out of the tissues and is delivered by the bloodstream to the lungs, which expel it from the body. But if the diver surfaces too quickly, potentially dangerous nitrogen bubbles can form in the tissues and cause DCS. These bubbles can compress nerves, obstruct arteries, veins, and lymphatic vessels, and trigger harmful chemical reactions in the blood. The precise reasons for bubble formation remain unclear.

How much extra nitrogen enters the tissues varies with the dive's depth and duration. Dive tables prepared by the U.S. Navy and other organizations specify how long most divers can safely remain at a particular depth. If the dive table limits are exceeded, the diver must pause on the way up to allow the nitrogen to diffuse into the bloodstream without forming bubbles. DCS can occur, however, even when a diver obeys safe-diving rules. These cases may involve as contributing factors fatigue, **obesity**, **dehydration**, **hypothermia**, and recent alcohol use. As well, people who fly or travel to high-altitude locations without letting 12–24 hours pass after their last dive are at risk for DCS, because their bodies undergo further decompression. This is true even when flying in commercial aircraft. Many travelers are unaware that to save money the cabin pressure in commercial aircraft is set much lower than the pressure at sea level. Exactly how long a diver should wait before flying or traveling to a high-altitude location depends on how much diving he or she has done and other considerations. If there is uncertainty about the appropriate waiting period, the sensible course of action is to let the full 24 hours pass.

Because the nitrogen bubbles that cause DCS can affect any of the body's tissues, a wide range of symptoms is possible. Symptoms can appear minutes after a diver surfaces, and in about 80% of cases do so within eight hours. **Pain** is often the only symptom. It ranges from mild to severe, and is usually limited to the joints but can be felt anywhere. Severe **itching**, skin **rashes**, and skin mottling are other possible symptoms. All of these are sometimes classified as manifestations of Type 1 or "mild" DCS. Type 2 or "serious" DCS can lead, among other things, to **paralysis**, brain damage, **heart attack**s, and death. Many DCS victims, however, experience both Type 1 and Type 2 symptoms.

DCS is treated by giving the patient oxygen and placing him or her in a hyperbaric chamber, an enclosure in which the air pressure is first gradually increased and then gradually decreased. This shrinks the bubbles, allowing nitrogen to safely diffuse out of the tissues. Hyperbaric chamber facilities exist throughout the United States. No matter how mild one's symptoms may appear, immediate transportation to a facility is essential. Treatment is necessary even if the symptoms clear up before the facility is reached, because bubbles may still be in the bloodstream and pose a threat. The Divers Alert Network maintains a list of facilities and a 24-hour hotline that can provide advice on handling DCS and other diving emergencies.

DCS sufferers who undergo chamber treatment within a few hours of first experiencing symptoms usually enjoy a full recovery. If treatment is delayed the consequences are less predictable, although many people have been helped even after several days have passed. A 1992 report on diving accidents indicated that full recovery following chamber treatment was immediate for about 50% of divers. Some people, however, suffer numbness, tingling, or other symptoms that last weeks, months, or even a lifetime. In the Okinawa study, 6 of the 94 patients experienced "long-lasting" symptoms even after repeated chamber treatments.

The obvious way to minimize the risk of DCS is to follow the rules on safe diving and air travel after a dive. People who are obese, suffer from lung or heart problems, or are otherwise in poor health should not dive. And because the effect of nitrogen diffusion on the fetus remains unknown, diving while pregnant is not recommended.

Decongestants

Decongestants are medicines used to relieve nasal congestion (stuffy nose), a common symptom of colds and **allergies**. Congestion results when membranes lining the nose become swollen. Decongestants relieve this swelling by narrowing blood vessels that supply the nose. This reduces blood supply to the swollen membranes, causing them to shrink.

These medicines do not cure colds or reverse the effects of histamines — chemicals released as part of the allergic reaction. They relieve only the stuffiness. When considering whether to use a decongestant for cold symptoms, keep in mind that most colds go away with or without treatment and that taking medicine is not the only way to relieve a stuffy nose. Drinking hot tea or broth or eating chicken soup may help.

Decongestants are sold in many forms, including tablets, capsules, caplets, gelcaps, liqui-caps, liquids, nasal sprays, and nose drops. These drugs are sometimes combined with other medicines in cold and allergy products designed to relieve several symptoms. Some decongestant products require a physician's prescription, such as Claritin and Allegra, but there are also many nonprescription (over-the-counter) products.

Commonly used decongestants include oxymetazoline (Afrin and other brands), phenylpropanolamine, and pseudoephedrine (Sudafed, Actifed, and other brands).

Decongestant nasal sprays and nose drops may cause a problem called rebound congestion if used repeatedly over several days. When this happens, the nose remains stuffy or gets worse with every dose. The only way to stop the cycle is to stop using the drug. The stuffiness should then go away within about a week. Anyone showing signs of severe rebound congestion should see a doctor.

Do not share droppers or spray bottles with anyone else, as this could spread infection. Do not let droppers and bottle tips touch countertops or other surfaces.

Some decongestants cause drowsiness. People who take these drugs should not drive, use machines, or do anything else that might be dangerous until they know how the drugs affect them.

The decongestant phenylpropanolamine has caused serious side effects, including **death**, when taken in large amounts. Phenylpropanolamine may interact with **caffeine**, causing symptoms that include disorientation, confusion, and talking incoherently. Anyone taking phenylpropanolamine should avoid anything that contains caffeine. This includes coffee, tea, cola, chocolate, and many prescription and nonprescription (over-the-counter) medicines. Older people are especially vulnerable to this problem.

In general, older people may be more sensitive to the effects of decongestants and may need to take lower doses. They should not take long-acting (extended release) forms of decongestants unless they have previously taken a short-acting form with no ill effects.

Children may also be more sensitive to the effects of decongestants. Call a physician or poison center immediately if they are given large amounts of these drugs or if they swallow nose drops, nasal spray or eye drops.

Some phenylpropanolamine products also contain the dye tartrazine, which causes an allergic reaction in some people. People who are allergic to aspirin are particularly likely to be allergic to tartrazine.

In studies of laboratory animals, some decongestants have had unwanted effects on fetuses. However, it is not known whether such effects also occur in people. Women who are pregnant or who plan to become pregnant should check with their physicians before taking decongestants. Women who take the decongestant phenylpropanolamine after delivery may have mood or mental changes.

Some decongestants pass into breast milk and may have unwanted effects on nursing babies. Women who are breastfeeding should check with their physicians before using decongestants. If they need to take the medicine, it may be necessary to bottle feed the baby with formula.

Anyone with heart or blood vessel disease, high blood pressure, diabetes, **enlarged prostate**, or overactive thyroid should not take decongestants unless under a physician's supervision. The medicine can increase blood sugar in people with diabetes. It can be especially dangerous in people with high blood pressure, as it may increase blood pressure. Before using decongestants, people with glaucoma or a history of mental illness should make sure their physicians are aware of their conditions.

The most common side effects from decongestant nasal sprays and nose drops are sneezing and temporary burning, stinging, or dryness. These effects are usually temporary and do not need medical attention. If any of the following side effects occur, stop using the drops or spray immediately and call the physician:

- Increased blood pressure
- Headache
- Fast, slow, or fluttery heartbeat
- Nervousness
- **Dizziness**
- Nausea
- Sleep problems.

The most common side effects of decongestants taken by mouth are nervousness, restlessness, excitability, dizziness, drowsiness, headache, nausea, weakness, and sleep problems. Anyone who has these symptoms while taking decongestants should stop taking them immediately.

Patients who have any of the following symptoms while taking decongestants should call the doctor immediately:

- Increased blood pressure
- Fast, irregular, or fluttery heartbeat
- Severe headache
- Tightness or discomfort in the chest
- Breathing problems
- Fear or anxiety
- **Hallucinations**
- Trembling or shaking
- Convulsions (**seizures**)
- Pale skin
- Painful or difficult urination.

Decongestants may interact with a variety of other medicines. Do not take decongestants at the same time as **Mono-**

amine oxidase inhibitors (MAO inhibitors) such as phenzeline (Nardil) or tranylcypromine (Parnate), or within two weeks of stopping treatment with an MAO inhibitor unless a physician approves.

Other drugs that may interact with decongestants include:

- **Tricyclic antidepressants** such as imipramine (Tofranil) or desipramine (Norpramin)
- Maprotiline (Ludiomil)
- Amantadine (Symmetrel)
- Amphetamines
- Medicine to relieve asthma or other breathing problems
- Methylphenidate (Ritalin)
- Appetite suppressants
- Other medicine for colds, sinus problems, hay fever or other allergies
- **Beta blockers** such as atenolol (Tenormin) and propranolol (Inderal)
- Digitalis glycosides, used to treat heart conditions.

Be sure to check with a physician or pharmacist before combining decongestants with any other prescription or nonprescription (over-the-counter) medicine.

DEFIBRILLATION

Ventricular fibrillation is a state of cardiac arrhythmia in which the individual heart muscles contract in a random, uncoordinated way. The heart appears to shiver, and blood circulation ceases. Ventricular fibrillation is fatal unless an electric shock is applied within minutes to restore normal heart contraction. As early as 1899, French physiologists, Jean Louis Prevost and Frederic Battelli were able to stop ventricular fibrillation in a dog by applying an electric shock to the animal's exposed heart. In 1930, William B. Kouwenhoven, an American electrical engineer at Johns Hopkins University, developed with colleagues a closed-chest defibrillator that sent **alternating current** (AC) electrical shocks to the heart through electrodes placed on a dog's chest. In 1947, Claude Beck, professor of surgery at Case Western Reserve University, first successfully resuscitated a human patient by internal cardiac massage and electrical defibrillation; American cardiologist Paul Zoll applied AC defibrillator to human patients in 1961; and the **direct current** (DC) defibrillator introduced by Lown and Neuman in 1962 provided greater reliability and safety.

Defibrillators greatly improved the ability of patients to survive heart surgery, invasive cardiac diagnostic and treatment techniques, and heart attacks, all of which can send the heart into ventricular fibrillation. Since the 1970s, most hospital emergency rooms have been equipped with electric defibrillators, and portable devices have become standard equipment for **ambulances**. Most recently, automated external defibrillators (AEDs), light-weight, portable, user-friendly devices about the size of a lunch box, can be found at sports stadiums, hotels and casinos, in coast guard marine vehicles and police cars, and many other places where people gather. These devices can be used by operators with much less training than paramedics, and are intended for use by on-site personnel like fire fighters until paramedics arrive. Sometimes called the ''smart'' defibrillator, they provide audio instructions and visual prompts to walk the operator through the defibrillating process, as well as recording the sequences of events such as when the operator connected the analyzer and pushed the shock button.

An implantable device, called the *automatic implantable cardioverter defibrillator* (AICD) was invented by Mieczyslaw Mirowski of the Johns Hopkins University Medical School to stop heart arrhythmias. Approved for use by the Food and Drug Administration in October 1985, Mirowski's AICD senses two kinds of abnormal heart rhythms—ventricular fibrillation and ventricular tachycardia—automatically sending an electric shock to the heart to correct the disturbance. As a defibrillator, the device jolts the heart out of ventricular fibrillation; as a cardioverter, it shocks the heart out of an abnormally fast heartbeat called ventricular tachycardia, restoring normal heart rate. Because the AICD requires a heftier power pack than the standard cardiac **pacemaker**, the battery pack for the AICD is separately implanted in the patient's abdomen. The lithium batteries can deliver 100-150 shocks during their three-year lifetime. The AICD is a potential lifesaver for the 700,000 people in the United States who survive heart attacks each year and are therefore at risk for potentially fatal **arrhythmias**. The AICD is also routinely used for patients whose arrhythmias cannot be treated with medication or surgery.

DEHYDRATION

Dehydration is the loss of water and salts essential for normal body function. It occurs when the body loses more fluid than it takes in.

Young and middle-aged adults who drink when thirsty generally maintain fluid balance. Children need more water because they expend more energy, but most children who drink when thirsty get as much water as they need. Adults over the age of 60 who drink only when thirsty probably get only about 90% of the fluid they need.

Dehydration is a major cause of infant illness and **death**. Dehydration can occur in children who have stomach flu characterized by vomiting and **diarrhea**, or who cannot or will not take enough fluids to compensate for excessive losses associated with **fever** and **sweating** of acute illness. An infant can become dehydrated only hours after becoming ill.

When the body's fluid supply is severely depleted, hypovolemic shock is likely to occur. This condition, which is also called physical collapse, is characterized by pale, cool, clammy skin; rapid heartbeat; and shallow breathing. Blood pressure sometimes drops so low it cannot be measured, and skin at the knees and elbows may become blotchy. Anxiety, restlessness, and thirst increase. After the patient's temperature reaches 107°F (41.7°C), damage to the brain and other vital organs occurs quickly.

Strenuous activity, excessive sweating, high fever, and prolonged vomiting or diarrhea are common causes of dehydration. So are staying in the sun too long, not drinking enough fluids, and visiting or moving to a warm region where it doesn't often rain. Alcohol, **caffeine**, and **diuretics** or other medications that increase the amount of fluid excreted can cause dehydration.

Reduced fluid intake can be a result of appetite loss associated with acute illness, excessive urination, nausea, bacterial or viral infection or inflammation of the pharynx, or inflammation of the mouth caused by illness, infection, irritation, or vitamin deficiency.

Other conditions that can lead to dehydration include disease of the adrenal glands, **diabetes mellitus**, eating disorders, kidney disease, and chronic lung disease.

An infant who does not wet a diaper in an eight-hour period is dehydrated. The soft spot on the baby's head (fontanel) may be depressed. Symptoms of dehydration at any age include cracked lips, dry or sticky mouth, lethargy, and sunken eyes. A person who is dehydrated cries without shedding tears and does not urinate very often. The skin is less elastic than it should be and is slow to return to its normal position after being pinched. Dehydration can cause confusion, **constipation**, discomfort, drowsiness, fever, and thirst. The skin turns pale and cold, the mucous membranes lining the mouth and nose lose their natural moisture. The pulse sometimes races and breathing becomes rapid. Significant fluid loss can cause serious neurological problems.

Increased fluid intake and replacement of lost electrolytes are usually sufficient to restore fluid balances in patients who are mildly or moderately dehydrated. In these cases, just drinking water may be all that is needed. Adults who need to replace lost electrolytes may drink sports beverages (e.g. Gatorade or Recharge) or consume a little additional salt. Parents should follow label instructions when giving children Pedialyte or other commercial products recommended to relieve dehydration. Children who are dehydrated should receive only clear fluids for the first 24 hours.

A child who is vomiting should sip one or two teaspoons of liquid every 10 minutes. A child who is less than a year old and who is not vomiting should be given one tablespoon of liquid every 20 minutes. A child who is more than one year old and who is not vomiting should take two tablespoons of liquid every 30 minutes. A baby who is being breast-fed should be given clear liquids for two consecutive feedings before breast-feeding is resumed. A bottle-fed baby should be given formula diluted to half its strength for the first 24 hours after developing symptoms of dehydration.

Children and adults can gradually return to their normal diet after they have stopped vomiting and no longer have diarrhea. Bland foods should be reintroduced first, with other foods added as the digestive system is able to tolerate them. Milk, ice cream, cheese, and butter should not be eaten until 72 hours after symptoms have disappeared.

Severe dehydration can require hospitalization and intravenous fluid replacement. If an individual's blood pressure drops enough to cause **shock**, medical treatment is usually required. A doctor should be notified whenever an infant or child exhibits signs of dehydration or a parent is concerned that a stomach virus or other acute illness may lead to dehydration.

A doctor should also be notified if:

- A child less than three months old develops a fever higher than 100°F (37.8°C)
- A child more than three months old develops a fever higher than 102°F (38.9°C)
- Symptoms of dehydration worsen
- An individual urinates very sparingly or does not urinate at all during a 6-hour period
- **Dizziness**, listlessness, or excessive thirst occur
- A person who is dieting and using diuretics loses more than 3 lbs (1.3 kg) in a day or more than 5 lbs (2.3 kg) a week.

If dehydration is caused by vomiting or diarrhea, medications may be prescribed to resolve these symptoms. Patients who are dehydrated due to diabetes, kidney disease, or adrenal gland disorders must receive treatment for these conditions as well as for the resulting dehydration.

Mild dehydration rarely results in complications. If the cause is eliminated and lost fluid is replaced, mild dehydration can usually be cured in 24–48 hours.

Vomiting and diarrhea that continue for several days without adequate fluid replacement can be fatal. The risk of life-threatening complications is greater for young children and the elderly. However, dehydration that is rapidly recognized and treated has a good outcome.

DELAYED HYPERSENSITIVITY SKIN TEST

A delayed hypersensitivity test is an immune function test measuring the presence of activated T cells that recognize a certain substance.

The immune system protects against infection by viruses, bacteria, fungi, and parasites. After initial exposure to a foreign substance, or antigen, the immune system creates both antibodies and sensitized T cells. Both these immune agents respond when the body is reexposed to the antigen. Antibodies, which are circulating proteins, respond within minutes, to give what is termed an immediate hypersensitivity reaction. T cells responses occur over several days, and are thus called delayed hypersensitivity reactions. The cascade of events initiated by the T cells leads to hardening (induration) and redness (erythema) at the injection site.

A delayed hypersensitivity test (DHT) is performed for one of three reasons:

- To test for exposure to specific diseases, such as **tuberculosis** (TB). Tuberculosis testing is done by injecting into the skin a small volume of TB antigen, which contains no organisms (live or dead) but can still provoke an immune response.
- To test for allergic sensitivity to potential skin irritants, such as poison ivy. Skin allergy testing is usually done by placing a series of adhesive patches on the skin containing potential allergens, or allergy-causing substances.
- To assess the vitality of the T cell response as part of the evaluation of immune system health in infection,

cancer, immune disorders, pre-transplantation screening, **aging**, and **malnutrition**. DHT can help predict survival in immunocompromised patients, and evaluate the success of restorative therapy. Antigens used for these tests must be ones the patient has been exposed to before, and, therefore, include inactivated antigens from common infectious agents to which the patient might have been exposed, such as **mumps**, *Candida albicans*, **tetanus** toxoid, and trichophyton (a skin fungus).

The most accurate TB test is the Mantoux test, in which a small amount of TB antigen is injected into the skin. The area is examined 48–72 hours after the injection.

In the patch test, 20–30 adhesive patches are usually placed on the upper back. The patches are kept in place and the area is kept dry for 48 hours. The patches are then removed, and the skin is examined 24 hours afterward, and possibly again a day or more following that. Patch testing is usually performed following a patient complaint of skin irritation from an unknown substance. Testing may suggest several candidates; identifying the right one requires careful review of the patient's possible exposure.

The test of overall T cell responsiveness is performed with several injections. Each area injected is circled and marked. Results are read 48 hours after the injection.

Absence of exposure to TB is indicated by absent or very little skin reaction; redness or hardness smaller than 5 mm (about a quarter of an inch) is considered normal for a person not exposed or infected with TB. TB exposure is indicated by a reaction of 10 mm or more. The degree of redness is not important. A 5–10 mm area could indicate exposure if there is an underlying risk to TB.

Patch test sites should be normal or only slightly red. Patch test areas that become reddened and irritated indicate reaction to the substance in the patch.

T cell responsiveness tests should be positive; that is, the injected areas should be reddened and hard. Two affected areas of 2 mm or more is considered a positive result. Absence of any reaction to injected areas indicates lack of T cell responsiveness, a condition called anergy. T cell anergy is seen in immune deficiency diseases including **AIDS**, some cases of infectious diseases, malignancies, immunosuppressive therapy (including corticosteroid treatment), some autoimmune diseases, **malnutrition**, major surgery, and some viral immunizations.

No special precautions or preparations before the test are necessary for most patients. Those with known hypersensitivity to certain skin irritants should alert the clinician performing the test. Some commercial preparations of fungal antigens contain mercury, a source of irritation to some patients.

After the test, patches should be kept dry. Injection sites may be washed, but excessive rubbing should be avoided. Patches and injection sites may become reddened or irritated. If a patch causes severe **itching** or discomfort, the patient should remove it immediately.

DHT is quite safe for virtually all people. There is no risk of infection from the agents injected, since they are purified antigens, not whole organisms. Life threatening, hypersensitive reactions (**anaphylaxis**) are a very small risk; patients should notify the administering physician immediately if signs of **wheezing**, swelling, or diffuse redness of the skin develops.

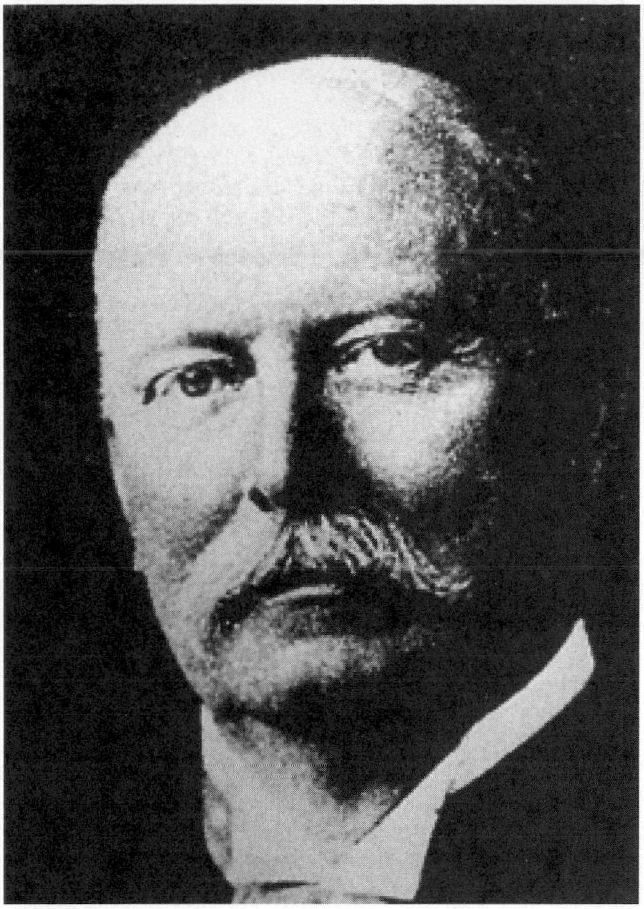

Max Delbrück

DELBRÜCK, MAX (1906-1981)

German American molecular biologist

Max Delbrück, the youngest of seven children, was born in Berlin, Germany on September 6, 1906. In 1924 he began university studies in astronomy and astrophysics and in 1930 received a Ph.D. in physics from the University of Göttingen. As a post-doctoral student, he traveled to Copenhagen, Denmark, where he worked with Niels Bohr, the theorist who proposed the model of the atom. After further work in Zurich, Switzerland, and Berlin, Delbrück left Germany for the United States in 1937, following Hitler's takeover.

In the United States, Delbrück studied biology and genetics at the California Institute of Technology under a Rockefeller Foundation grant and, while studying the genetics of fruit flies, became interested in the genetics of bacteriophages, large viruses that infect bacteria. Along with Emory Ellis, a biologist, Delbrück developed experimental methods to investigate bacteriophages and mathematical systems to analyze the results of the experiments. They published their results in 1939. In 1940, Delbrück met **Salvador Luria**, an Italian-American biologist conducting bacteriophage research at Columbia University. The two found that they shared interests and thus began a collaboration of research focused on mutations in bacteria that produced resistance to bacteriophages. Together, Delbrück and Luria published their work in 1943. They presented the first evidence that bacterial heredity is controlled by genes, and in doing so, overturned prevailing ideas about how genetic traits are acquired. Their work began the sciences of bacterial **genetics** and molecular biology.

Delbrück's work with Luria and **Alfred Hershey**, a microbiologist, standardized bacteriophage research. In 1946 Delbrück and Hershey independently demonstrated that genetic material from different viruses could be combined to form a virus different from either. They called this phenomenon genetic recombination, and their groundbreaking work paved the way for other geneticists to make further discoveries about bacteriophages, culminating with the discovery that deoxyribonucleic acid, or DNA, is the genetic material. By the early 1950s Delbrück received a letter from his friend **James Watson**, detailing the double helix structure of DNA. Delbrück's casual manner and wit provided a relaxed atmosphere, and thus his laboratory became a meeting place for many molecular biologists working on problems in genetics. His contributions were recognized in 1969 when he, Hershey, and Luria shared the Nobel Prize in physiology or medicine for work in replication and genetic structure of viruses.

DELIRIUM

Delirium is a state of mental confusion which develops quickly and usually fluctuates in intensity. Rather than being a specific disease, delirium is a syndrome, or group of symptoms, caused by a disturbance in the normal functioning of the brain. The delirious patient has a reduced awareness of and responsiveness to the environment, which may be manifested as disorientation, incoherence, and memory disturbance. Delirium is often marked by **hallucinations**, **delusions**, and a dream-like state.

Delirium affects at least one in ten hospitalized patients, and is a common part of many terminal illnesses. Delirium is more common in the elderly than in the general population. While it is not a specific disease itself, patients with delirium usually fare worse than those with the same illness who do not have delirium.

There are a large number of possible causes of delirium. Metabolic disorders are the single most common cause, accounting for 20–40% of all cases. This type of delirium, termed "metabolic encephalopathy," may result from organ failure, including liver or **kidney failure**. Other metabolic causes include **diabetes mellitus**, **hyperthyroidism** and **hypothyroidism**, vitamin deficiencies, and imbalances of fluids and electrolytes in the blood. Severe **dehydration** can also cause delirium.

Drug intoxication ("intoxication confusional state") is responsible for up to 20% of delirium cases, either from side effects, overdose, or deliberate ingestion of a mind-altering substance. Medicinal drugs with delirium as a possible side effect or result of overdose include:

- Anticholinergics, including atropine, scopolamine, chlorpromazine (an antipsychotic), and diphenhydramine (an antihistamine)
- Sedatives, including **barbiturates**, **benzodiazepines**, and ethanol (drinking alcohol)
- **Antidepressant drugs**
- **Anticonvulsant drugs**
- **Nonsteroidal anti-inflammatory drugs** (NSAIDs), including ibuprofen and **acetaminophen**
- **Corticosteroids**, including prednisone
- **Anticancer drugs**, including methotrexate and procarbazine
- Lithium
- Cimetidine
- **Antibiotics**
- L-dopa.

Delirium may result from ingestion of legal or illegal psychoactive drugs, including:

- Ethanol (drinking alcohol)
- Marijuana
- LSD (lysergic acid diethylamide) and other hallucinogens
- Amphetamines
- Cocaine
- Opiates, including heroin and morphine
- PCP (phencyclidine)
- Inhalants.

Drug withdrawal may also cause delirium. Delirium tremens, or "DT's," may occur during alcohol withdrawal after prolonged or intense consumption. Withdrawal symptoms are also possible from many of the psychoactive prescription drugs.

Poisons may cause delirium ("toxic encephalopathy"), including:

- Solvents, such as gasoline, kerosene, turpentine, benzene, and alcohols
- Carbon monoxide
- Refrigerants (Freon)
- Heavy metals, such as lead, mercury, and arsenic
- Insecticides, such as Parathion and Sevin
- Mushrooms, such as *Amanita* species
- Plants such as jimsonweed (*Datura stramonium*) and morning glory (*Ipomoea* spp.)
- Animal venoms.

Other causes of delirium include:

- Infection
- **Fever**
- Head trauma
- Epilepsy
- Brain hemorrhage or infarction
- **Brain tumor**
- Low blood oxygen (hypoxemia)
- High blood carbon dioxide (hypercapnia)
- Post-surgical complication.

The symptoms of delirium come on quickly, in hours or days, in contrast to those of **dementia**, which develop much more slowly. Delirium symptoms typically fluctuate through the day, with periods of relative calm and lucidity alternating with periods of florid delirium. The hallmark of delirium is a fluctuating level of consciousness. Symptoms may include:

- Decreased awareness of the environment
- Confusion or disorientation, especially of time
- Memory impairment, especially of recent events
- Hallucinations
- Illusions and misinterpreted stimuli
- Increased or decreased activity level
- Mood disturbance, possibly including anxiety, euphoria or depression.
- Language or speech impairment.

Treatment of delirium begins with recognizing and treating the underlying cause. Delirium itself is managed by reducing disturbing stimuli, or providing soothing ones; use of simple, clear language in communication; and reassurance, especially from family members. Physical restraints may be needed if the patient is a danger to himself or others, or if he insists on removing necessary medical equipment such as intravenous lines or monitors. Sedatives or **antipsychotic drugs** may be used to reduce anxiety, hallucinations, and delusions.

Persons with delirium usually have a worse prognosis for the underlying disease than the person without delirium. Nonetheless, those without terminal illness usually recover from delirium. They may not, however, regain all their original cognitive abilities, and may be left with some permanent impairments, including fatigue, irritability, difficulty concentrating, or mood changes.

DEMENTIA

Dementia is a loss of mental ability severe enough to interfere with normal activities of daily living, lasting more than six months, not present since birth, and not associated with a loss or alteration of consciousness. Dementia is a group of symptoms caused by gradual **death** of brain cells. Dementia is usually caused by degeneration in the cerebral cortex, the part of the brain responsible for thoughts, memories, actions and personality. Death of brain cells in this region leads to the cognitive impairment which characterizes dementia.

The loss of cognitive abilities that occurs with dementia leads to impairments in memory, reasoning, planning, and personality. While the overwhelming number of people with dementia are elderly, it is not an inevitable part of **aging**. Instead, dementia is caused by specific brain diseases. **Alzheimer's disease** (AD) is the most common cause, accounting for three quarters of all cases, followed by vascular or multi-infarct dementia. The brain of a person with AD becomes clogged with two abnormal structures, called neurofibrillary tangles and senile plaques. Neurofibrillary tangles are twisted masses of protein fibers inside nerve cells, or neurons. Senile plaques are composed of parts of neurons surrounding a group of proteins called beta-amyloid deposits. Why these structures develop is unknown. Vascular dementia is estimated to cause from 5–30% of all dementias. It occurs from decrease in blood flow to the brain, most commonly due to a series of small **stroke**s (multi-infarct dementia).

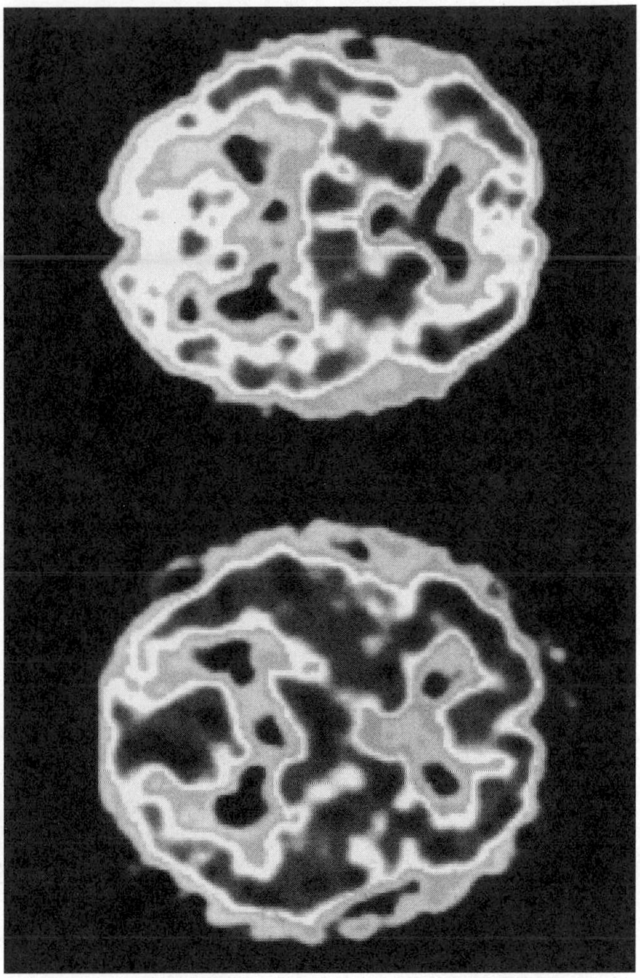

A colored positron emission tomography (PET) scan of the brain of an AIDS patient suffering from dementia (top). Compared to the scan of a normal brain (bottom), the dark areas of the brain in the AIDS patient are much smaller, reflecting a decrease in the brain's ability to function. ***(Photo Researchers, Inc. Reproduced by permission.)***

Dementia is marked by a gradual impoverishment of thought and other mental activities. Losses eventually affect virtually every aspect of mental life. The slow progression of dementia is in contrast with **delirium**, which involves some of the same symptoms, but has a very rapid onset and fluctuating course with alteration in the level of consciousness.

Symptoms include:

- Memory losses
- Impaired abstraction and planning
- Language and comprehension disturbances
- Poor judgment
- Impaired orientation ability
- Decreased attention and increased restlessness
- Personality changes and **psychosis**

Treatment of dementia begins with treatment of the underlying disease, where possible. The underlying causes of nutritional, hormonal, tumor-caused and drug-related dementias may be reversible to some extent. Treatment for stroke-related dementia begins by minimizing the risk of further strokes, through smoking cessation, **aspirin** therapy, and treatment of **hypertension**, for instance. There are no therapies which can reverse the progression of Alzheimer's disease. Aspirin, estrogen, vitamin E, and selegiline are currently being evaluated for their ability to slow the rate of progression.

Care for a person with dementia can be difficult and complex. The patient must learn to cope with functional and cognitive limitations, while family members or other caregivers assume increasing responsibility for the person's physical needs. In progressive dementias such as Alzheimer's disease, the person may ultimately become completely dependent. Education of the patient and family early on in the disease progression can help them anticipate and plan for inevitable changes.

Symptoms of dementia may be treated with a combination of psychotherapy, environmental modifications, and medication. Drug therapy can be complicated by forgetfulness, especially if the prescribed drug must be taken several times daily.

Two drugs, tacrine (Cognex) and donepezil (Aricept), are commonly prescribed for Alzheimer's disease. These drugs inhibit the breakdown of acetylcholine in the brain, prolonging its ability to conduct chemical messages between brain cells. They provide temporary improvement in cognitive functions for about 40% of patients with mild-to-moderate AD. Hydergine is sometimes prescribed as well, though it is of questionable benefit for most patients.

Long-term institutional care may be needed for the person with dementia, as profound cognitive losses often precede death by a number of years. Early planning for the financial burden of nursing home care is critical. Useful information about financial planning for long-term care is available through the Alzheimer's Association.

Family members or others caring for a person with dementia are often subject to extreme **stress**, and may develop feelings of anger, resentment, guilt, and hopelessness, in addition to the sorrow they feel for their loved one and for themselves. Depression is an extremely common consequence of being a full-time caregiver for a person with dementia. Support groups can be an important way to deal with the stress of caregiving. The location and contact numbers for caregiver support groups are available from the Alzheimer's Association; they may also be available through a local social service agency or the patient's physician. Medical treatment for depression may be an important adjunct to group support.

The prognosis for dementia depends on the underlying disease. On average, people with Alzheimer's disease live eight years past their diagnosis, with a range from one to twenty years. Vascular dementia is usually progressive, with death from stroke, infection, or heart disease.

DENTAL INSTRUMENTS

Cavities in teeth have been filled since earliest times with a variety of materials: stone chips, turpentine resin, gum, metals. Arculanus (Giovanni d'Arcoli) recommended gold-leaf fillings in 1484. The renowned physician **Ambroise Paré** used lead or cork; in the 1700s, Pierre Fauchard, the father of modern dentistry, favored tin foil or lead cylinders; and Philip Pfaff, dentist to Frederick the Great of Prussia, used gold foil. Gold leaf as a filling became popular in the United States in the early nineteenth century; Marcus Bull of Hartford, Connecticut, began producing beaten gold for dental use in 1812 which was replaced in 1853 in the United States and England by sponge gold. This was followed by cohesive, or adhesive, gold introduced by American dentist Robert A. Arthur in 1855 and, by 1847, gutta percha was being used.

The invention of the power-driven dental drill led to increased demand for fillings and so for an inexpensive filling material. In 1826, Auguste Taveau of Paris, France, used silver coins to developed what was probably the first dental amalgam—a solution of one or more metals mixed with mercury. The French Crawcour brothers emigrated to the United States in 1833, introducing Taveau's amalgam; however, the poor quality of the amalgam led to its condemnation by many dentists, kicking off the so-called "amalgam war," a 10-year period from 1840 to 1850 of bitter controversy about the merits and deficiencies of mercury amalgam. Numerous experiments were made from the 1860s through the 1890s to develop improved amalgam filling materials, and Chicago, Illinois, dentist G. V. Black finally standardized both cavity preparation and amalgam manufacture in 1895.

After truly effective dental cement was developed, baked porcelain inlays became popular for filling large cavities. These were first described by B. Wood in 1862. In 1897 an Iowa dentist, B. F. Philbrook, described his method of casting metallic fillings from a wax impression that matched the shape of the cavity perfectly. Dr. William H. Taggart of Chicago described a similar method for casting gold inlays in 1907. This technique made possible the modern era of accurate filling and inlay fitting. Amalgams—"silver fillings"—are still used, even though periodic controversies arise regarding the possibility of mercury toxicity. "White fillings," however, are gaining in popularity as they give a more aesthetic and natural look. Several types of cosmetic fillings are available today: *Direct composites* consist of quartz resin usually containing a light-sensitive agent which allows them to be hardened, or bonded, into place by shining an intense light for about 40 seconds; *indirect composite/porcelain inlays*, specifically designed for strength as well as aesthetics, are usually fabricated in a laboratory then bonded in the dentist's office. Available in a variety of shades to match natural teeth, composites are extremely strong and can withstand the 40,000 pounds of pressure per square inch exerted when chewing with the back teeth.

Crowns (used to replace and cover missing portions of teeth) and bridges (mountings for artificial teeth anchored to and bridging the gap between the natural tooth at either side) were made of gold and used by the Etruscans at least 2,500 years before modern dentistry. Crowns and bridges fell from popularity during the Middle Ages and were only gradually rediscovered. The gold shell crown, described by Pierre Mouton of Paris, France, in 1746, was not patented until 1873 by

Beers. The Logan crown, patented in 1885, used porcelain fused to a platinum post, replacing the unsatisfactory wooden posts previously used. In 1907 the detached-post crown was introduced, which was more easily adjustable. Bridge work developed along with crowns; dentists would add extra facing to a crown to hold a replacement for an adjacent missing tooth. The major advance came with the detachable facings patented by Dr. Walter Mason of New Jersey in 1890 and the improved interchangeable facings introduced by Mason's associate Dr. Thomas Steele in 1904. Today, crowns and bridges can be made from full porcelain, porcelain-fused-to-metal, polymer glass, or all metal. Cement and bonding materials for metal-free restorations—called *adhesive dentistry*—utilize zinc phosphate or glass ionometer cements. Cosmetic dentistry—reproducing a tooth for aesthetic reasons—is now popular and widely practiced: a dental implant is a metal screw placed into the jaw bone providing an anchor for a permanent false tooth or a set of false teeth; veneers are porcelain laminates which cover the natural tooth to mask and strengthen discolored or fractured teeth; and full caps (similar to crowns) are permanently placed over the original tooth to give an attractive appearance to a misshaped tooth or to narrow gaps between natural teeth.

DEPO-PROVERA/NORPLANT

Norplant is a long-acting hormone that is inserted under the skin and prevents conception for up to five years. Depo-Provera is also a hormone, but it is injected into a muscle and provides protection against **pregnancy** for three months. The hormone in Norplant and Depro-Provera is progestin, a synthetic hormone similar to one found naturally in a woman's body.

Both hormones are about 99% effective in preventing pregnancy. Neither of these methods provide protection from **AIDS** or other **sexually transmitted diseases**.

Given as a shot, Depo-Provera works in several ways to prevent conception. First, it prevents the egg (ovum) from maturing and being released, and it causes the mucous in the cervix (opening into the uterus or womb) to thicken, making it difficult for the sperm to enter. Depo-Provera also causes the lining of the uterus to become thinner, making implantation of a fertilized egg unlikely. The injection must be given within the first five days of a normal period and provides protection against pregnancy for three months. It is recommended that a second contraceptive device be used for two weeks after the first injection.

Norplant capsules contain a synthetic hormone that is slowly released over a period of up to five years. It functions like Depo-Provera in that it prevents the ovaries from producing ova (eggs) and also results in thicker mucous in the cervix, which prevents the sperm from passing through the cervix. Norplant can be inserted at any time.

The woman being considered for Depo-Provera will have a pelvic and breast examination, a Pap test, blood pressure check, weight check, and a review of her medical history.

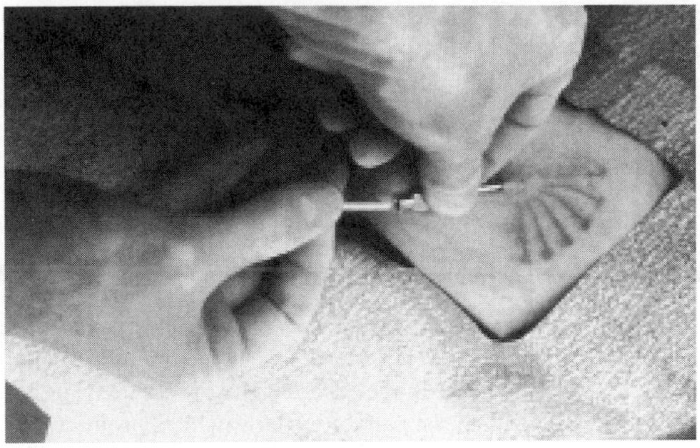

A physician inserts a contraceptive implant under the skin of a woman's arm. ***(Photo Researchers, Inc. Reproduced by permission.)***

Women who have **diabetes mellitus**, major depression, blood-clotting problems, **liver disease**, or weight problems should use this approach only under strict medical supervision. It should not be used if the woman is pregnant, has unexplained vaginal bleeding, suffers from severe liver disease, has breast cancer, or desires to become pregnant within 18–24 months. Advantages of this approach may include a decreased risk of **cancer** of the lining of the uterus (endometrial cancer) and stopping menstrual periods.

Individuals who select Norplant will receive the same basic **physical examination** as for Depo-Provera. If approved for this method, an implantation site will be selected (usually the inside of the upper arm), and the area prepared for minor surgery. The physician will use a local anesthetic to numb the area, a small incision will be made, the six Norplant capsules will be inserted, and the incision sewn up. Protection against pregnancy normally begins within 24 hours. If necessary, the implants can be removed in 15–20 minutes. Norplant should not be used by women who are pregnant, have blood clotting problems, or have unexplained vaginal bleeding. Advantages include light periods with less cramping and decreased anemia. This form of birth control may also protect against endometrial cancer.

Because Depo-Provera and Norplant use only the hormone progestin, they may provide an alternative for women who cannot use estrogen-containing birth control pills.

The most common side effects associated with Depo-Provera are yellowing of the skin, headache, nervousness, **dizziness**, abdominal **pain**, hair loss, rash, increase in number of migraine headaches, increased or decreased interest in sexual intercourse, the development of dark spots on the skin, depression, and weakness. Danger signs that need to reported immediately include weight gain, heavy vaginal bleeding, frequent urination, blurred vision, fainting, severe abdominal pain, and coughing up blood. Because the effects of Depo-Provera may last up to 12 weeks, it may take a longer time for women trying to become pregnant after discontinuing the injections.

The main reactions to Norplant include headache, weight gain, irregular periods or no period at all, breast tenderness, **acne**, gain or loss of facial hair, color changes of the skin over the area of insertion, and ovarian cysts. The doctor should be notified immediately of lumps in the breast, heavy vaginal bleeding, yellowing of the skin or eyes, or infection of the incision. Women who use Norplant are discouraged from **smoking**.

DEPRESSIVE DISORDERS

Depression is an illness caused by biochemical imbalance in the brain. It is characterized by persistent feelings of anxiety; sadness; helplessness; hopelessness; worthlessness; pessimism; guilt; restlessness; irritability; drastic loss of interest in pleasurable or routine activities; reduced sex drive; fatigue; difficulty concentrating, remembering, or making decisions; body aches not caused by physical illness; weight gain or loss; and often suicidal tendencies. In clinical depression, these and other negative emotions are out of proportion to the individual's life situation and can be so profound that the sufferer loses interest in life. In severe or prolonged depression, the individual may be unable to get out of bed for days at a time, and their ability to perform even the most routine activities is drastically impaired. Depressive illness differs drastically from the usual moods and emotions experienced by most people, such as sadness, ''the blues,'' or grief after losing a loved one. It is one of the most common and destructive illness in the United States. Often misunderstood by sufferers and their families alike, it is highly treatable with modern medications by well-trained experts.

Official diagnosis of a major depressive illness is based on the *Diagnostic and Statistical Manual* (DSM) published by the American Psychiatric Association. Now in its fourth version, this handbook officially recognizes the following types of clinical depression: normal depressed mood and grief, adjustment disorder with depressed mood, mild depression (dysthymia), major depression, **bipolar disorder** (manic-depression), atypical depression, **seasonal affective disorder** (SAD), and post-partum depression. Disorders can be short- or long-term and range from relatively mild to severe. Researchers estimate that associated costs, which include loss of productivity at work, hiring new personnel, medical expenses, and stress placed on families, may range from $15-35 billion a year.

Unrecognized and untreated depression can cause extreme suffering, not only to the patient, but to his or her loved ones. It can begin for no apparent reason and plunge the individual into a downward spiral of despair. It is a true illness, like **cancer**, diabetes, or high blood pressure, which can become incapacitating. An estimated 35-40 million people in the United States are expected to suffer a major depressive illness during their life-time; 25% of these will attempt suicide within five years of onset. Anyone talking about suicide should be taken seriously and medical assistance sought immediately. Depression in children often goes unrecognized: suicide is the second greatest cause of death in children and adolescents.

One truly unfortunate aspect of depression is that, frequently, sufferers tend to blame themselves, and neither they nor their families recognize it as an illness. Even if they do, they may not realize the necessity of appropriate treatment. This lack of understanding can cause alienation, which only adds to the **pain** loss of self-esteem, and feelings of guilt already caused by the depression. Depressed individuals cannot ''pull themselves up by the bootstraps,'' and this lack of understanding only increases the patient's suffering.

Causes of depression are many and varied. Researchers believe hereditary factors predispose certain individuals to depressive illness. In some individuals, traumatic life situations such as the break-up of a relationship, loss of a loved one, or loss of employment, is the trigger. Lack of light in winter brings about seasonal affective disorder, the severity of which ranges from mild to debilitating, and biochemical or hormonal changes appear to trigger **postpartum depression** in some women following childbirth. Cyclic **antidepressants**, MAO inhibitors, and ''third generation'' medications help more than 80% of people treated and, in difficult cases, **electroconvulsive therapy** (ECT) can be useful. Appropriate psychotherapy and counselling combined with medication is often extremely helpful.

DERMATITIS

Dermatitis is a general term used to describe inflammation of the skin, usually characterized by a pink or red rash that itches.

Contact dermatitis is an allergic reaction to something that irritates the skin and is manifested by one or more lines of red, swollen, blistered skin that may itch or weep. It usually appears within 48 hours after touching a substance to which the skin is sensitive. The condition is more common in adults than in children.

Contact dermatitis can occur on any part of the body, but it usually affects the hands, feet, and groin. It usually does not spread from one person to another, nor does it spread beyond the area exposed to the irritant unless affected skin comes into contact with another part of the body. However, in the case of some irritants, such as poison ivy, contact dermatitis can be passed to another person or to another part of the body.

Allergic reactions are genetically determined, and different substances cause contact dermatitis to develop in different people. A reaction to resin produced by poison ivy, poison oak, or poison sumac is the most common source. Flowers, herbs, and vegetables can also affect the skin of some people. **Burns** and **sunburn** increase the risk of dermatitis, and chemical irritants that can cause the condition include chlorine, cleansers, detergents and soaps, fabric softeners, glues used on artificial nails, perfumes, and topical medications. Contact dermatitis can develop when the first contact occurs or after years of exposure.

Stasis dermatitis is characterized by scaly, greasy looking skin on the lower legs and around the ankles. A consequence of poor circulation, it occurs when leg veins can no longer return blood to the heart as efficiently as they once did. When that happens, fluid collects in the lower legs and causes them to swell. Stasis dermatitis can also result in a rash that can break down into sores known as stasis ulcers, in which case a doctor should be notified immediately.

Nummular dermatitis generally affects the hands, arms, legs, and buttocks of men and women older than 55 years of age. This stubborn inflamed rash forms circular, sometimes itchy, patches and is characterized by flares and periods of inactivity. The cause of nummular dermatitis is not known, but it usually occurs in cold weather and is most common in people who have dry skin. Hot weather and **stress** can aggravate this condition, as can allergies, fabric softeners, soaps and detergents, wool clothing, and bathing more than once a day.

Atopic dermatitis is characterized by **itching**, scaling, swelling, and sometimes blistering. In early childhood it is called infantile eczema and is characterized by redness, oozing, and crusting. It is usually found on the face, inside the elbows, and behind the knees. It can be caused by **allergies**, **asthma**, or stress, and there seems to be a genetic predisposition for atopic conditions.

There may also be a genetic predisposition to seborrheic dermatitis, which may be dry or moist and is characterized by greasy scales and yellowish crusts on the scalp, eyelids, face, external surfaces of the ears, underarms, breasts, and groin. In infants it is called ''cradle cap.'' Seborrheic dermatitis is usually caused by overproduction of the oil glands. In adults it can be associated with **diabetes mellitus** or gold allergy. In infants and adults it may be caused by a biotin deficiency.

To diagnose dermatitis, the doctor may scrape off a small piece of affected skin for microscopic examination, or perform patch tests—dabbing small amounts of a suspected irritant onto skin on the patient's back. The doctor will ask about potential irritants that have recently come into contact with the affected area.

Treating contact dermatitis begins with eliminating the source of irritation. If the irritant cannot be avoided completely, the patient should wear gloves and other protective clothing whenever exposure is likely to occur. Prescription or over-the-counter corticosteroid creams can lessen inflammation and relieve irritation. Creams, lotions, or ointments not specifically formulated for dermatitis can intensify the irritation. Oral **antihistamines** are sometimes recommended to alleviate itching, and **antibiotics** are prescribed if the rash becomes infected.

Patients who have a history of dermatitis should remove their rings before washing their hands. They should use bath oils or glycerine-based soaps and bathe in lukewarm saltwater. Patting rather than rubbing the skin after bathing and thoroughly massaging lubricating lotion or nonprescription cortisone creams into still-damp skin can soothe red, weepy nummular dermatitis. Highly concentrated cortisone preparations should not be applied to the face, armpits, groin, or rectal area. Periodic medical monitoring is necessary to detect side effects in patients who use such preparations on **rashes** covering large areas of the body.

Coal-tar salves can help relieve symptoms of nummular dermatitis that have not responded to other treatments, but these ointments have an unpleasant odor and stain clothing.

Patients who have stasis dermatitis should elevate their legs as often as possible and sleep with a pillow between the lower legs. Tar or zinc paste may also be used to treat stasis dermatitis. Because these compounds must remain in contact with the rash for as long as two weeks, the paste and bandages must be applied by a nurse or a doctor.

Coal-tar shampoos may be used for seborrheic dermatitis that occurs on the scalp. Sun exposure after the use of these shampoos should be avoided because the risk of sunburn of the scalp is increased.

A number of botanical and homeopathic therapies can be useful for skin conditions These include burdock root (*Arctium lappa*), calendula (*Calendula officinalis*) ointment, and chamomile (*Matricaria recutita*) ointment.

A patient who has dermatitis should notify a doctor if **fever** develops, the skin oozes or other signs of infection appear, if symptoms do not begin to subside after seven days' treatment, or if he/she comes into contact with someone who has a wart, **cold sore**, or other viral skin infection.

DES EXPOSURE

DES (diethylstilbestrol) is a hormone that was prescribed for pregnant women in the 1950s and early 1960s. Many years later, doctors discovered that the daughters of the women who received DES were at high risk for a variety of problems, including **infertility**, **premature labor**, and **cancer** of the vagina and cervix.

In the 1950s and early 1960s, several drug companies claimed that DES could prevent miscarriages. DES is a synthetic hormone, related to estrogen. Since up to 20% of all pregnancies end in miscarriage, this seemed an important breakthrough and DES was prescribed for many women who had bleeding in early **pregnancy**. Ultimately, it was found to have no effect on miscarriages and the practice of prescribing DES was stopped in the 1960s. Almost 10 years later, the daughters of women who had taken DES during pregnancy began to develop unusual symptoms.

Doctors discovered that when these young women reached their teens, they were at higher risk for a variety of problems, including a rare cancer known as clear cell adenocarcinoma of the vagina and cervix, infertility, premature labor, and other problems in pregnancy.

DES has affected a very specific group of women who were exposed to DES in the womb before 18 weeks of pregnancy. In other words, their mothers must have taken DES within the first 4–5 months of pregnancy, when the female reproductive organs are formed. DES appears to interfere with proper growth and development of the uterus, cervix, vagina, and fallopian tubes.

In the early 1970s, there was an increase in clear cell adenocarcinoma of the vagina and cervix. Up until that time, doctors had seen these cancers only in elderly women. Suddenly, the disease began to appear in young women.

This was so unusual that researchers studied these women to see if they had anything in common. After a great deal of questioning and examination, it was found that all had been exposed to DES in the womb during the early weeks of pregnancy.

Today, it is difficult to imagine how shocking this discovery was. Doctors had only recently recognized that medications and exposure to chemicals during pregnancy could cause birth defects. This defect had gone undetected for almost two decades.

Since then, doctors have studied DES daughters very carefully. Fortunately, the risk of clear cell adenocarcinoma is actually quite low. In fact, it appears that if a DES daughter has not developed this cancer by age 30, she will not develop it. Since all DES daughters are now over age 30, there should be no further cases related to DES exposure. However, there are a number of other symptoms and problems associated with DES exposure:

- DES daughters often have distinctive changes of the cervix and vagina that can be seen during a pelvic exam. These changes include a cervical hood (a vaginal fold draped over the cervix), cockscomb cervix (an abnormally shaped cervix), and adenosis (glandular cells normally located within the cervix that appear on the outside of the cervix and in the vagina).
- Some DES daughters have fallopian tube abnormalities that lead to infertility.
- Many DES daughters have a uterus that is abnormal in size and shape. The classic sign is the T-shaped uterus. In the normal uterus, the cavity (hollow space inside) is rounded. The abnormal T shape makes it harder for a woman to get pregnant and leads to a higher risk of premature labor and birth.

Women who have been exposed to DES should have a pelvic exam at least once a year. In addition to the usual pelvic exam and Pap smear, DES daughters should also have Pap smears of the vagina and, if possible, **colposcopy**, in which the cervix and vagina are examined through a special magnifying scope. In this way, tiny areas of abnormal cells can be seen. This procedure is easily performed in the doctor's office.

When DES daughters get pregnant, they may be at high risk for premature labor and birth and should be monitored very carefully.

Not all women who were exposed to DES develop problems in pregnancy. However, if problems like infertility or miscarriage do occur, the doctor may recommend a special x ray to check the woman's fallopian tubes and uterus. This special test is called a hysterosalpingogram.

There is no treatment for the abnormalities of the fallopian tubes and uterus caused by DES exposure. Fortunately, there are treatments that can help with infertility or premature labor. Clear cell adenocarcinoma of the vagina or cervix must be treated with surgery and, possibly, **chemotherapy**.

DETOXIFICATION THERAPY

Detoxification is the process of eliminating or neutralizing toxins from the body. By eliminating harmful toxins, it seeks to enable the body to heal itself and return to health.

One of the oldest known medical treatments, detoxification historically was achieved by **fasting**—deliberately abstaining from food for a time. In modern times, with concern over environmental contaminants, detoxification is advocated by some as a necessary means of staying healthy. Naturopaths, who hold that illness can be healed by the natural processes of the body, are the most vigorous supporters of detoxification, since they believe the primary cause of disease is accumulation of uneliminated wastes.

A toxin is anything that causes an irritation in the body or has a harmful effect on it. In addition to the effect of pesticides, industrial chemicals, food additives, and heavy metals, many people add to their toxic intake by ingesting legal and illegal drugs. Naturopaths and other **alternative medicine** practitioners fear an epidemic they call bioaccumulation—a buildup of toxic substances in the body that weakens the organs of elimination as well as the **immune system**, gradually eroding health. Naturopaths and practitioners of traditional medicine agree that the body has its own natural processes for eliminating and neutralizing toxins (via perspiration, urination, exhalation, and bowel movements). However, they disagree on whether those processes are capable of handling the nature and amount of toxins in today's world. Those who believe that the body's systems are unable to cope with these daily poisonous assaults argue that toxins are the primary cause of disease.

Proponents of detoxification say everyone should detoxify at some point. Benefits, they say, include increased vitality, reduced blood pressure and blood fats, and improved assimilation of **vitamins** and **minerals**.

Among the several therapies available for detoxification, some are more intrusive than others. It is recommended that professional advice be obtained when selecting a particular program. The major detoxification therapy categories are: fasting, specific diets, vitamin therapy, **colon therapy**, **chelation therapy**, and hyperthermia.

Fasting is the least expensive and easiest therapy, but it should always be preceded by a visit to a doctor or qualified health professional. Fasting is generally done for a limited, specific number of days. All fasting regimens permit water to be consumed to prevent **dehydration**. Others allow juice as well, although purists consider this a food. The main rationale for fasting is that since far fewer toxins are taken in, the body is able to rid itself of those already present.

As opposed to fasting, detoxification diets can be undertaken for extended periods. Although there are many different types of 'detox' diets, most are based on eating organic rather than processed foods, minimizing meats and maximizing fruits and vegetables, and drinking filtered water. Advocates of traditional Chinese medicine also hold that certain foods (including radishes, turnips, soybeans, swiss chard, and vinegar) can counteract toxins.

Some feel that vitamin therapy (for example, vitamins C and E) can neutralize certain toxins called free radicals.

Colon therapy (cleansing the large intestine with purified water, herbs, or other cleansing agents) is sometimes combined with fasting to flush toxins from the body. A step beyond a simple enema, this procedure is performed by a trained therapist who introduces from 5–25 gal (19–941 l) of water, or other cleansing agents, directly into the rectum using a tube and nozzle. This technique is supposed to remove toxic stool that remains in the folds of the intestine. If performed improperly or too frequently, it can be dangerous.

The most common type of chelation therapy involves using a chemical agent to treat **heavy-metal poisoning** (such as lead or mercury). The synthetic drug ethylenediaminetetraacetic acid (EDTA) is administered intravenously or orally and binds to heavy metals in the blood. The toxic metals are then flushed out naturally through the kidneys. Doctors also use natural chelating agents like zinc, garlic, vitamin C, and amino acids like cysteine. Oral chelation, while less expensive and more convenient, has been reported to be considerably slower than the intravenous method. Chelation therapy has also been used to treat artherosclerosis, or hardening of the arteries. It has been theorized that chelation removes calcium, which is part of the plaque that coats arteries. While some patients have reported remarkable results with this treatment, no reliable scientific data exists to support these claims. Research is also needed to confirm reports of success with treating heart and cancer patients with chelation therapy.

Hyperthermia, also known as heat-stress detoxification, uses a sauna or a steam bath to sweat toxic chemicals from fat cells.

Detoxification therapies should not be undertaken without medical supervision. There is limited research data available to prove that detoxification therapies work, and more scientific studies need to be done to demonstrate that particular therapies are beneficial.

Some detoxification methods are potentially dangerous, with side effects ranging from dehydration to bowel perforation. Unsupervised detoxification should not be tried by anyone who is underweight, pregnant, recovering from substance abuse, nor by those suffering from diabetes mellitus, thyroid problems, or an eating disorder.

DEVIATED SEPTUM

The nasal septum is a thin structure separating the two sides of the nose. If it is not in the middle of the nose, it is considered deviated.

The nasal septum has two parts. Toward the back of the head the nasal septum is rigid bone, but further forward it is cartilage. By placing one finger in each nostril, this cartilage can easily be bent back and forth. If the nasal septum is sufficiently displaced to one side, it will impede the flow of air and mucus through the nose. This condition, called a deviated septum, can cause symptoms and disease.

A deviated septum can be a simple variation in normal structure or the result of a broken nose. Any narrowing of the nasal passageway caused by a deviated septum will threaten the drainage of secretions from the sinuses, which must pass through the nose. It is a general rule of medicine that when flow is obstructed, whether it is mucus from the sinuses or bile from the gall bladder, infection results. People with **hay fever** are at greater risk of obstruction because their nasal passageways are already narrowed by the swollen membranes lining them. The result is **sinusitis**, which can be acute and severe or chronic and lingering.

It is easy to see that a septum is deviated. It is more difficult to determine whether that deviation needs correction. It is common for a patient to complain that he/she can breathe through only one nostril. Then the diagnosis is easy. A deviated septum may also contribute to snoring, **sleep apnea**, and other breathing disorders.

The definitive treatment is surgical repositioning of the septum, accomplished by breaking it loose and fixing it in a proper place while it heals. **Decongestants** like pseudoephedrine or phenylpropanolamine will shrink the membranes and thereby enlarge the passages. **Antihistamines**, nasal cortisone spray, and other allergy treatments may also be temporarily beneficial.

Alternative treatments may include saline drops and sprays, which are very helpful in loosening mucus in the obstructed side and preventing drying in the other side, where all the air blows. Hot peppers, such as jalapenos, can produce enough tears and discharge to flush out many a stopped-up nose. An even more effective treatment is called a nasal lavage, often done using a small pot with a spout. Saline solution is poured into one nostril and allowed to flow out the other nostril. Then, the process is repeated in reverse. These therapies are all useful to take care of symptoms, but do not correct the problem. A procedure known as a nasospecific, in which a deflated balloon is inserted in the nostril and inflated to adjust the septal deviation, can be an alternative to surgery. A trained practitioner in the nasospecific procedure is necessary.

Surgical repair is curative and carries little risk. Chronic infection can be painful and lead to complications until it is resolved. If there is continued obstruction, the infection will very likely return.

Avoidance of virus colds, airborne dusts, air pollution and known allergens will minimize the irritation and swelling of the membranes lining the nasal passages.

DIABETES MELLITUS

Diabetes is a metabolic disease caused by the body's inability to use the hormone insulin to effectively convert carbohydrates into the simple sugar glucose that cells store and use to perform vital functions. Without glucose to fuel their activity, the cells use fat instead, producing ketones as a waste product. Ketones build up in blood and disrupt brain functions. Common signs of diabetes are excessive thirst, urination, and fatigue. The disease can also cause vision loss, decreased blood supply to hands and feet, pain, and skin infections. If left untreated diabetes can induce **coma** and cause **death**.

There are two main types of diabetes. *Juvenile* diabetes (also called Type I) occurs when the pancreas, a gland attached to the small intestine, fails to produce enough insulin; as a result, it is also referred to as insulin dependent diabetes mellitus (IDDM). *Maturity-onset*diabetes, or Type II non-insulin dependent diabetes mellitus (NIDDM), occurs when the body produces insulin but cannot use it efficiently. Juvenile diabetes is usually controlled by doses of insulin and a strict diet. Maturity-onset diabetes, which is often accompanied by obesity, is usually controlled by diet alone.

Diabetes often runs in families. In the United States about ten percent of the caucasian population suffers from diabetes, and it is even more common among African-American, Mexican-American, and certain Native American groups.

The symptoms of diabetes were identified 3,500 years ago in Egypt and were also known in ancient India, China,

Japan, and Rome. The Persian physician **Avicenna** (980-1037) described the disease and its consequences. Thomas Willis (1621-1675), an English epidemiologist, was the first modern western physician to discover that the urine of diabetics tasted sweet. In 1815, the French chemist Michel Eugène Chevreul discovered that the sweetness came from "grape sugar" or glucose. The disease's formal name *diabetes*, meaning a siphon or running through, and *mellitus*, relating to sweetness or honey, was first used in 1860.

Injury to the pancreas was linked to diabetic symptoms by several scientists from the seventeenth to the nineteenth centuries. The existence of a pancreas hormone to reduce the blood glucose level was first proposed in 1916 by the English physiologist Edward Sharpey-Schäfer. Insulin was isolated in 1921 by the Canadians **Frederick Banting** and **Charles Best** (1899-1978), and in 1922 they used it for the first time to successfully treat fourteen-year-old Leonard Thompson of Toronto.

Diabetes is an autosomal dominant disease, but its expression is also thought to be influenced by other conditions, such as aging. Research on Type I diabetes shows that dominant genes either protect against the disease or increase susceptibility to it. Advances in molecular genetics have led to large-scale studies to identify the genes responsible for diabetes. The American Diabetes Association has established a national database that contains information and genetic material from families with Type II diabetes that will help investigators conduct genetic linkage studies to locate the specific genes involved. Scientists have already established that a gene on chromosome 7 is linked to Type II diabetes. When mutated, the gene produces a faulty enzyme that is unable to stimulate the pancreas to produce insulin.

Scientists are developing tests to accurately predict whether someone will develop diabetes or not by observing whether the immune system attacks the pancreas cells that make insulin. The research may also lead to a vaccine against diabetes and drugs to keep the immune system from identifying the pancreas as an enemy, similar to drugs that keep the body from rejecting transplanted organs. New therapies for diabetes are continually under development. For example, studies of a combination drug therapy using metformin and troglitazone has been shown to significantly lower blood glucose levels in Type II diabetes patients by reducing glucose secretion by the liver (metformin) and enhancing the body's use of insulin (troglitazone). Another area under investigation is the use of islet cell transplantation, a promising approach for replacing whole organ transplantation by extracting and replacing only those cellular components that are needed to restore normal function. Islet cell transplantation could be a key to the successful replacement of the insulin-producing islets of Langerhans.

The seventh leading cause of death in the United States, diabetes remains a major health problem. Approximately 10.3 million people in the United States were diagnosed with diabetes in 1997, representing a six-fold increase over four decades. By the early 1990s, the costs associated with treating and caring for diabetes patients was estimated at over $90 billion a year.

DIALYSIS, KIDNEY

The kidneys perform the vital function of filtering waste materials out of the blood. When the kidneys stop functioning, death due to waste buildup occurs quickly. As early as 1861 a Scottish chemist, Thomas Graham (1748-1843), described a procedure he called *dialysis* to purify the blood in cases of **kidney failure**. The blood would be diffused across a membrane that allowed wastes to pass into a balanced fluid, while replenishing substances would pass from the fluid into the blood. Practical application of dialysis was developed by John Jacob Abel, the first professor of pharmacology at Johns Hopkins University School of Medicine. In 1912 Abel was investigating byproducts in the blood, and needed a device to filter these substances out. With colleagues Benjamin Turner and Leonard Rowntree, he built a machine that circulated blood through celloidin tubing immersed in a saline-dextrose solution and wrapped around a rotating drum. Urea and other toxins passed out into the solution, and oxygen passed into the blood. Abel tested this process, which he called *vividiffusion*, on rabbits and dogs, and published the findings in 1914. A major problem, however, was the tendency of the blood to clot while circulating through the tubes. Abel had used *hirudin*, an anticoagulant obtained from leeches, to prevent clotting. Once the effective anticlotting agent *heparin* became widely available, dialysis was ready for clinical use.

Several pioneers developed early versions of dialysis machines during World War II when many injured soldiers and civilians suffered kidney damage and died. In 1937, a young Dutch physician, **Willem Kolff**, working in Groningen, Holland, had already put together a crude dialyzing machine and worked to refine it. After the Germans occupied the Netherlands in 1941, Kolff moved to Kampen where, in spite of wartime shortages, he constructed a dialysis machine using cellophane tubing and beer cans. He first used his device on a human patient in March 1943 and, although all but one of the 15 patients he treated from 1943 to 1944 died, he persevered. By the end of the war, Kolff had refined his machine and began to promote its use, bringing dialyzers to The Hague, Amsterdam, and London. Meanwhile, with no knowledge of Kolff's work, Nils Alwall of Sweden and G. Murray of Canada were also developing a dialysis machine. In 1947 Kolff brought blueprints for his latest machine to doctors at Peter Bent Brigham Hospital at Harvard Medical School in Boston. These doctors, along with John Merrell, Karl Walter, and George Thorn, developed kidney dialysis into a standard treatment, using it to support patients in their pioneering kidney transplantations in 1954. Kidney transplants, the first organs ever to be transplanted, were made possible because of dialysis, which kept the patient alive until the transplanted kidney began functioning or by maintaining patients awaiting a donor organ. Long-term dialysis was not possible, however, until 1960, because each time a patient was attached to a dialysis machine, both an artery and a vein had to be punctured, leading to eventual vessel deterioration. Dr. Belding Scribner of Seattle overcame this problem when he designed a Teflon and Silastic shunt (two parallel tubes with a U-connection) that could be inserted into a patient's artery and vein and left in place for months or even years.

Today, *hemodialysis*, a refined version of this technique, allows the patient the option of home treatment with the aid of a family member or friend, or by specialists at a dialysis center. Patients also have the option of using *Peritoneal* dialysis, in which the abdomen lining (peritoneal membrane) filters waste from the blood into a cleansing solution called *dialystate*. *Continuous Ambulatory Peritoneal Dialysis*, the most common of three types, requires no machine and can be done by the patient. The dialystate, contained in a plastic bag, is transported through a permanent catheter inserted into the abdomen. The catheter is then plugged and, after four to six hours, the patient removes the plug, draining the solution containing waste matter back into the bag, which is then disposed of. This process is repeated continuously. *Continuous Cyclic Peritoneal Dialysis* is a similar function done by a machine connected to the catheter and performed at night while the patient sleeps. This procedure lasts from 10 to 12 hours every night. *Intermittent Peritoneal Dialysis* can also be done at home with a similar machine, but is usually done in hospital several times a week for a total of 36 to 42 hours. Some sessions may last 24 hours.

Diaphragm (birth control)

Diaphragms are dome-shaped barrier methods of **contraception** that block sperm from entering the uterus. They are made of latex (rubber) and formed like a shallow cup. Since vaginas vary in size, each patient needs to be fitted by a doctor or nurse with a diaphragm that conforms to the shape of the vagina as well as the strength of the muscles in the vaginal walls. Diaphragms must be used with spermicidal cream or jelly. The device should cause no discomfort and neither the woman nor her partner should feel that it is there. The level of effectiveness is about 95%.

Before receiving a diaphragm, patients must undergo a **physical examination** and a **Pap test**. If these are normal, the physician will fit the patient for the device and give instructions on how to insert, remove, and clean it. She will also be taught the signs and symptoms of potential complications.

Prior to insertion, the inside of the dome and the rim are covered with a thick layer (perhaps a tablespoon) of a spermicide that is compatible with the diaphragm being used. The domed area covers the opening into the uterus (cervix) and keeps the spermicide in place. As a result, any sperm that might get under the diaphragm will be destroyed.

Diaphragms may be inserted 2–3 hours prior to intercourse, and must be left in place for 6–8 hours following sexual relations. During this time the woman may not swim, bathe, or douche, but she may shower. If she desires to have intercourse again before the 6–8 hours have passed, the diaphragm should not be removed. Instead, an applicator full of spermicide should be deposited into the vagina.

A diaphragm will last for a year or more. It should be examined weekly for holes. This can be done by holding it up to the light or filling it with water.

Before inserting the diaphragm, the woman should empty her bladder and wash her hands with soap and water. The device should be checked for leaks by filling it with water or holding it to the light. A spermicidal jelly is then applied to the inside and outside, and especially around the rim. While standing with one foot elevated on a chair or step, lying down, or squatting, the woman folds the diaphragm inward toward the middle and inserts it into the vagina as far as it will go.

When removed, the diaphragm should be washed with a mild soap and water. After being dried, it can be dusted with corn starch before being returned to its container. The diaphragm should always be stored away from sunlight and heat in a cool, dry place. It should not be washed with harsh or perfumed soaps or used with perfumed powders because either of these substances can damage it.

Although rare, wearing the diaphragm longer than the recommended time can result in toxic shock syndrome. The signs and symptoms of this serious illness include sudden onset of high fever, vomiting, diarrhea, dizziness, faintness, weakness, aching muscles and joints, and rash. The doctor must be notified immediately if any of these conditions appear. An allergic reaction to the spermicide or the material from which the device is made is also possible. Diaphragm use is also associated with an increased risk of bladder infections.

It should be noted that the diaphragm can become dislodged during intercourse, which could result in an unwanted **pregnancy**. To ensure a secure fit, a woman should be examined for a refitting if she gains or loses more than 10 lbs (4.5 kg), or after she gives birth.

Using a male **condom** in conjunction with the diaphragm decreases the potential for pregnancy. Diaphragms provide no protection against AIDS or other sexually transmitted diseases.

Diarrhea

To most individuals, diarrhea means an increased frequency or decreased consistency of bowel movements; however, the medical definition is more exact than this. In many developed countries, the average number of bowel movements is three per day. However, researchers have found that diarrhea best correlates with an increase in stool weight; stool weights above 300 grams per day generally indicates diarrhea. This is mainly due to excess water, which normally makes up 60–85% of fecal matter. In this way, true diarrhea is distinguished from diseases that cause only an increase in the number of bowel movements (hyperdefecation), or **incontinence** (involuntary loss of bowel contents). Diarrhea is also classified by physicians into acute, which lasts 1–2 weeks, and chronic which continues for longer than 23 weeks. Viral and bacterial infections are the most common causes of acute diarrhea.

In many cases, acute infectious diarrhea is a mild, limited annoyance. However, worldwide, acute infectious diarrhea has a huge impact, causing over five million deaths per year. While most deaths are among children under five years of age in developing nations, the impact, even in developed countries, is considerable. For example, over 250,000 individuals are admitted to hospitals in the United States each year because of one of these episodes. Rapid diagnosis and proper treatment can prevent much of the suffering associated with these devastating illnesses. Chronic diarrhea also has a considerable effect on health, as well as on social and economic well being. Patients with **celiac disease**, **inflammatory bowel disease**, and other prolonged diarrheal illnesses develop nutritional deficiencies, which diminish growth and immunity. They affect social interaction and result in the loss of many working hours.

Diarrhea occurs because more fluid passes through the large intestine (colon) than that organ can absorb. As a rule, the colon can absorb several times more fluid than is required on a daily basis. However, when this reserve capacity is overwhelmed, diarrhea occurs. Diarrhea is caused by infections or illnesses that either lead to excess production of fluids or prevent absorption of fluids. Also, certain substances in the colon, such as fats and bile acids, can interfere with water absorption and cause diarrhea. In addition, rapid passage of material through the colon can also do the same. Symptoms related to any diarrheal illness are often those associated with any injury to the gastrointestinal tract, such as **fever**, **nausea**, vomiting, and abdominal **pain**. All or none of these may be present depending on the disease causing the diarrhea. The number of bowel movements can vary—up to 20 or more per day. In some patients, blood or pus is present in the stool. Bowel movements may be difficult to flush (float) or contain undigested food material. The most common causes of acute diarrhea are infections (the cause of traveler's diarrhea), **food poisoning**, and medications. Medications are a frequent and often over-looked cause, especially **antibiotics** and **antacids**. Less often, various sugar free foods, which sometimes contain poorly absorbable materials, cause diarrhea. Chronic diarrhea is frequently due to many of the same things that cause the shorter episodes (infections, medications, etc.); symptoms just last longer. Some infections can become chronic. This occurs mainly with parasitic infections (such as *Giardia*), or when patients have altered immunity (**AIDS**). The following are the more usual causes of chronic diarrhea:

- AIDS
- Colon **cancer** and other bowel tumors
- Endocrine or hormonal abnormalities (thyroid, diabetes mellitus, etc.)
- Food allergy
- Inflammatory bowel disease (Crohn's disease and ulcerative colitis)
- Lactose intolerance
- **Malabsorption syndromes** (celiac and Whipple's disease)
- Other (alcohol, microscopic colitis, radiation, surgery).

The major effects of diarrhea are **dehydration**, **malnutrition**, and weight loss. Signs of dehydration can be hard to notice, but increasing thirst, dry mouth, weakness or lightheadedness (particularly if worsening on standing), or a darkening/decrease in urination are suggestive. Severe dehydration leads to changes in the body's chemistry and could become life-threatening. Dehydration from diarrhea can result in **kidney failure**, neurological symptoms, arthritis, and skin problems.

Treatment is ideally directed toward correcting the cause; however, the first aim should be to prevent or treat dehydration and nutritional deficiencies. The type of fluid and nutrient replacement will depend on whether oral feedings can be taken and the severity of fluid losses. Oral rehydration solution (ORS) or intravenous fluids are the choices; ORS is preferred if possible. A physician should be notified if the patient is dehydrated, and if oral replacement is suggested then commercial (Pedialyte and others) or homemade preparations can be used. The **World Health Organization** (WHO) has provided this easy recipe for home preparation, which can be taken in small frequent sips:

- Table salt—3/4 teaspoon.
- Baking powder—1 teaspoon.
- Orange juice—1 cup.
- Water—1 quart or liter.

When feasible, food intake should be continued even in those with acute diarrhea. A physician should be consulted as to what type and how much food is permitted. Anti-motility agents (loperamide, diphenoxylate) are useful for those with chronic symptoms; their use is limited or even contraindicated in most individuals with acute diarrhea, especially in those with high fever or bloody bowel movements. They should not be taken without the advice of a physician. Other treatments are available, depending on the cause of symptoms. For example, the bulk agent psyllium helps some patients by absorbing excess fluid and solidifying stools; cholestyramine, which binds bile acids, is effective in treating bile salt induced diarrhea. Low fat **diets** or more easily digestible fat is useful in some patients. New **antidiarrheal drugs** that decrease excessive secretion of fluid by the intestinal tract is another approach for some diseases. Avoidance of medications or other products that are known to cause diarrhea (such as lactose) is curative in some, but should be discussed with a physician.

Prognosis is related to the cause of the diarrhea; for most individuals in developed countries, a bout of acute, infectious diarrhea is at best uncomfortable. However, in both industrialized and developing areas, serious complications and death can occur. For those with chronic symptoms, an extensive number of tests are usually necessary to make a proper diagnosis and begin treatment; a specific diagnosis is found in 90% of patients. In some, however, no specific cause is found and only treatment with bulk agents or anti-motility agents is indicated.

Proper hygiene and food handling techniques will prevent many cases. Traveler's diarrhea can be avoided by use of Pepto-Bismol and/or antibiotics, if necessary. The most important action is to prevent the complications of dehydration, as outlined above.

Dick, George (1881-1967) and Dick, Gladys (1881-1963)

American physicians

This husband-and-wife team made major contributions to our knowledge of **scarlet fever** and later found themselves at the center of an international controversy over alleged commercialization of medical advances.

Born in Fort Wayne, Indiana, where his father was a railroad engineer, George Dick studied at Rush Medical College in Chicago. Graduating in 1905, he spent two years treating iron mine workers in Buhl, Montana, after which he studied pathology in Vienna and Munich. In 1909 he joined the faculty at the University of Chicago, also practicing medicine at several Chicago hospitals.

Dick met Gladys Henry in 1911, when both were working as University of Chicago research pathologists. Henry had been born in Pawnee City, Nebraska. Her father was a seller of grain, and a former Civil War cavalry soldier who raised carriage horses. After studying science at the University of Nebraska, Henry went to Johns Hopkins University School of Medicine in Baltimore, where she graduated in 1907 and undertook postgraduate studies (experimental surgery, hematology, and pathochemistry) in Baltimore and Berlin.

The two married in 1914 and became research collaborators at the John R. McCormick Institute for Infectious Diseases, an arrangement that lasted until 1953, when Gladys was forced to retire by debilitating cerebral arteriosclerosis.

The Dicks published a landmark series of articles about scarlet fever in 1923 and 1924 in the *Journal of the American Medical Association.* They determined that the disease was caused by hemolytic streptococci bacteria, which had previously been thought to play only a minor role in scarlet fever. They also discovered that the red rash associated with scarlet fever is caused by a toxin released by the streptococcus bacterium. The Dicks used this toxin to immunize patients and to develop what is now known as the "Dick test," a skin test that determines susceptibility to scarlet fever.

The Dicks found themselves at the center of an international controversy over commercialization of medical research after they patented some of their scarlet fever methods, and sued a pharmaceutical company for patent infringement. They said the purpose of their patents was not to enrich themselves, but solely to ensure quality of scarlet fever toxins and antitoxins. In 1935, the Dicks were criticized by the League of Nations, which said that their patents were restricting medical research. By the 1940s, antibiotics had largely replaced toxins and antitoxins for scarlet fever, and the Dicks decided to abandon their patent-infringement lawsuit. Over the years, scarlet fever has become less common and less severe due to a decrease in streptococcal infections, to better environmental conditions, and to prompt and adequate antibiotic treatment.

DIETARY SUPPLEMENTS

A visit to your local health food store reveals aisles of vitamins, minerals, and herbs that make a variety of claims to improve overall health. While some dietary supplements may hold medicinal value, Americans are spending over $700 million a year on various products that not only provide limited health benefits, but may pose significant health risks. The American Dietetic Association, the National Academy of Sciences, the National Research Council, and other major medical societies agree that most people can get all the vitamins and minerals they need from eating a healthy, well-balanced diet. Dietary supplements cannot replace the hundreds of additional nutrients, called phytochemicals, provided in whole foods.

There are, however, situations in which taking supplements may be appropriate. The elderly or those on a strict weight loss diet may benefit from a multivitamin. Postmenopausal women, especially those not taking estrogen, may need to increase their intake of calcium and Vitamin D to protect against **osteoporosis**. Care should be taken not to take doses higher than the recommended daily allowances (RDA); doses above that amount do not give extra protection, but can increase the risk of encountering toxic side effects. For example, large amounts of Vitamin D can indirectly cause kidney damage, and large amounts of Vitamin A can cause liver damage. Herbal supplements can also have serious side effects. Those herbal supplements containing ephedrine have been linked with abnormal heart rhythms, **stroke**, **hepatitis** and even death.

Consideration of even the most popular supplements should include weighing the benefits against the possible side effects. Beta Carotene (Vitamin A) is an antioxidant (along with **Vitamins** C and E) that neutralizes harmful substances, called free radicals, resulting from cell **metabolism**. Some believe that antioxidants prevent the damage from free radicals that may contribute to cardiovascular disease or **cancer**. Some studies, however, found an increased risk of **lung cancer** in smokers who took beta carotene supplements. Folic acid, one of the B vitamins that helps prevent certain spinal cord birth defects, is also linked to cardiovascular benefits. Intake of folate can, however, mask a vitamin B_{12} deficiency if intake is over 1,000 micrograms per day.

Niacin is another B vitamin that reduces the fats (lipids) in the blood and potentially slows the progression of **atherosclerosis** when combined with diet and exercise. At doses higher than 2,000 micrograms, serious side effects may include liver damage, high blood pressure, and irregular heart beats.

In addition to the antioxidant effects described above, Vitamin C is thought to strengthen resistance to viral infection and act as a mild antihistamine to help relieve cold symptoms. There is no evidence, however, to support the beliefs that high doses of Vitamin C can cure a cold; amounts above 500 milligrams are excreted in the urine. Vitamin E also functions as a potent antioxidant, which may slow the progression of atherosclerosis. Regular intake of Vitamin E may also slow the effects of **Parkinson's disease** and **Alzheimer's disease**. High doses of Vitamin E can cause gastrointestinal side effects and bleeding, especially for individuals on blood thinners (anticoagulants).

Caution should also be taken with use of the various minerals offered as dietary supplements. Chromium is thought to work with insulin for blood sugar utilization. There are no studies that support claims of increased muscle mass, weight loss, or prevention of osteoporosis. Selenium is another antioxidant claimed to prevent cancer and cardiovascular disease. Taking excessive amounts of selenium may cause hair and nail loss. Zinc has been shown in some studies to increase the immune response, reducing the severity of cold symptoms. Excess zinc, however, has been shown to interfere with the body's utilization of essential minerals, such as iron and copper.

While herbs are the basis for many of our medicines, there is no guarantee that the many herbal supplements on the market are worth the millions of dollars Americans spend on them annually. Ginkgo biloba is thought to dilate blood vessels and improve blood flow to the brain and legs. Side effects of this herb include gastrointestinal problems, headaches, and allergic reactions. St. John's Wort may be effective for mild to moderate depression; however, studies are still in progress for possible side effects. Any individual with a known health problem, or any one taking prescribed medications, should consult a doctor before using any nutritional supplements

Consumers cannot assume that these products are safe, pure, or that the quantities of active ingredients are listed on their labels—the nutritional supplement industry is largely unregulated. The Dietary Supplements Health and Education Act of 1994 altered the **Food and Drug Administration**'s (FDA) ability to assess the safety of nutritional supplements before they go out on the market. As a result, the FDA can act only after an illness or injury has been reported through a ''consumer complaint coordinator'' at FDA district offices in cities across the country.

See also Vitamins

DIETS AND WEIGHT MANAGEMENT

Diets are regulated selections of foods, specially designed and prescribed for medical and/or general nutritional reasons.

Diets promote a balanced selection of foods vital for good health. By combining foods appropriate for each individual and drinking the proper amount of water, one can help maintain the best possible health. Eating the proper diet is critical for the health of individuals, groups with special medical and dietary needs, and entire populations afflicted with **malnutrition**.

The Food and Nutrition Board of the National Research Council of the National Academy of Sciences has determined dietary standards called Recommended Dietary Allowances (RDA). These standards explain the daily amounts of energy, protein, minerals, and fat-soluble and water-soluble vitamins needed by healthy males and females, from infancy to old age. Experts in **nutrition** recommend a variety of foods and the maintenance of an ideal weight. Large amounts of fat, saturated fat, and cholesterol should be avoided. Individuals should consume adequate starch and fiber and avoid excess sugar and sodium.

The U.S. Department of Agriculture and the **U.S. Department of Health and Human Services** have developed official dietary guidelines that include these seven basic recommendations:

- Eat a variety of foods.
- Control your weight.
- Eat a low-fat, low-cholesterol diet.
- Eat plenty of vegetables, fruits, and grains.
- Eat sugar in moderation.
- Use salt in moderation.
- If you drink alcohol, do so in moderation.

The food pyramid, developed by nutritionists, provides a visual guide to healthy eating. At its base are those foods that should be eaten numerous times each day, while at its apex are those foods that should be used sparingly. The pyramid suggests a range of servings in each group so that the number of servings can be adjusted to suit each individual's caloric requirements. The daily recommendations (from bottom to top) of the food pyramid include:

- Bread, cereal, rice, and pasta: 6–11 servings
- Vegetables: 3–5 servings
- Fruits: 2–4 servings
- Milk, yogurt, and cheese: 2–3 servings
- Meat, poultry, fish, dried beans, eggs, and nuts: 2–3 servings
- Fats, oils, and sweets: use sparingly.

Carbohydrates, proteins, and fats provide energy in the form of calories to fuel body functions. An older adult or sedentary woman needs about 1,600 calories daily, while children, teenage girls, active women, and sedentary men need about 2,200 calories daily. Active men, teenage boys, and very active women need about 2,800 calories daily. When an individual consumes as many calories each day as his body uses, he is in a state of energy balance and neither gains nor loses weight. When more calories are eaten than the body uses, the excess calories are stored as fat and weight increases. On the other hand, when fewer calories are consumed than the body needs, stored fat is burned and weight decreases.

Calorie-modified diets are prescribed to correct weight problems with a healthy diet. Low-calorie diets are designed for weight reduction and are prescribed for people who are overweight or obese. High-calorie diets are recommended for people with greatly increased energy needs such as athletes in training or individuals fighting diseases such as cancer, **AIDS**, or **cystic fibrosis**. High-calorie diets are also prescribed to treat anorexia nervosa.

Calorie-modified diets are planned by dieticians and prescribed following a complete physical examination and dietary history. A low-calorie diet provides enough energy (usually 1,000–1,800 calories) to meet the person's metabolic needs and activity level. It includes a balanced variety of foods, but limits carbohydrates and alcohol. A low-calorie diet aims to promote a weight loss of 1–2 lb per week. A high-calorie diet usually provides an extra 500–1,000 calories, leading to a weight gain of about 1 lb per week for most people. It has a high protein content, normal fat content, and emphasizes foods that pack many calories into a small volume. Snacking between meals is encouraged as a way to increase the calories consumed.

Fruits and vegetables are excellent sources of fiber. Fiber has important nutritional benefits such as facilitating the movement of food through the digestive tract, helping to prevent **constipation**. Recent evidence suggests low dietary fiber may be responsible for increasing the incidence of diverticulosis and may also be associated with **cancer** of the colon.

High-fiber diets, including whole grains (especially bran), raw vegetables, unpeeled fresh fruits, nuts, and seeds, are recommended to:

- Increase fecal bulk
- Increase intestinal movement
- Prevent or treat constipation, **diverticulosis**, Crohn's disease, or **irritable bowel syndrome**
- Help lower cholesterol
- Assist with weight loss in people who are overweight and improve sugar tolerance in diabetics.

Low-fiber diets exclude raw fruits and vegetables, whole grains, nuts, and seeds, while emphasizing soft, mild foods. They are recommended to:

- Decrease fecal bulk
- Slow intestinal movement
- Decrease stomach acid secretion
- Treat a variety of disorders including indigestion, **diarrhea**, bowel inflammation, and **heart attack**.

High-protein diets are designed to provide about 1.5 g of protein for each kilogram of a person's body weight, and a total of about 2,500 calories daily. Complex proteins, such as milk and meats, should make up one-half to two-thirds of the daily protein requirement. High-protein diets are recommended for people who:

- Have an increased need for protein due to protein-calorie malnutrition, severe stress, or conditions such as AIDS, cancer, or **burns** with high metabolic rates that lead to the loss of large amounts of protein
- Have **malabsorption syndromes**, **celiac disease**, or other disorders characterized by poor food absorption.

A low-protein diet excludes dairy products and meats, and requires that about three-fourths of the daily allowance of protein come from high-value protein sources. Supplements may be prescribed to prevent amino acid deficiencies. Low-protein diets are used in treatment of cirrhosis and kidney disease.

Dietary modification is the first weapon in the fight against the high cholesterol levels that contribute to heart disease and atherosclerosis. Doctors usually prescribe one of the three low-cholesterol diets recommended by the American Heart Association. In the preventive diet, total cholesterol intake is less than 300 milligrams per day. The phase 2 diet, recommended for people with mild elevations of blood cholesterol, restricts cholesterol intake to 200 milligrams per day. For anyone with severely elevated blood cholesterol levels, the most restrictive diet is recommended, which limits cholesterol intake even further. Low-cholesterol diets are prescribed to reduce the risk of heart disease and to treat **atherolsclerosis**, **diabetes**, high cholesterol (which may be hereditary and also require cholesterol-reducing drugs), and high blood pressure. A low-cholesterol diet is not a cure for the conditions it is prescribed to treat, so most people must stay on the diet for the rest of their lives.

Most American diets contain too much fat. Fat often makes up about 40% (about 160 grams) of total calories consumed each day. Most doctors and other experts recommend limiting fat to 30% (about 120 grams) of daily calories, since consumption of too much fat has been linked to obesity, heart disease, and several types of cancer. A low-fat diet usually limits daily fat intake to 50 grams, while an extremely low-fat diet limits fat consumed each day to 25–30 grams. Low-fat diets are recommended to:

- Help prevent heart disease
- Help prevent colon, prostate, and **breast cancers**
- Help treat a variety of conditions including gout, AIDS, gallbladder disease, liver disease, celiac disease, inflammatory bowel disease, and heartburn.

Gluten and gliadin are proteins found in certain grains and grain-containing products. These proteins are toxic to cells within the intestinal tract of an individual who is ''intolerant'' and cause difficulty in food absorption. Celiac disease is caused by intolerance to these proteins. This intolerance causes patients with celiac disease to suffer weight loss, **diarrhea**, malnutrition, and bloating. By eliminating foods containing gluten from the diet, further damage to the intestines can be prevented, symptoms are relieved, and malabsorption of nutrients is corrected. A gluten-free diet eliminates all foods containing wheat, rye, barley, and malt, and must be followed for life.

This diet restricts food, such as sardines, liver, and eggs, that cause the body to produce uric acid. It is usually prescribed as part of a treatment program for **gout** (a disease usually caused by having too much uric acid in the body) and kidney stones, which also includes exercise and medication. In addition to excluding organ meats (sweetbreads, liver, and kidney) and certain types of fish (anchovies, sardines, mackerel) and limiting the amount of other purine-containing foods such as shrimp, meats, and dairy products, this diet emphasizes drinking about 2 qt of water and fruit juice daily, to promote the excretion of uric acid, and eating fruits and vegetables that increase urine alkalinity and the solubility of uric acid.

On the average, Americans consume about 5,000 milligrams of salt or sodium daily. New guidelines suggest that 2,400 milligrams of sodium should be the upper limit, even if there are no signs of heart disease. Most people with heart disease should limit their sodium intake to less than 2,000 milligrams a day, and some low-salt diets restrict sodium to as little as 250 milligrams per day. The amount of salt in the diet is important for people who have high blood pressure or congestive **heart failure**.

Some experts believe excessive intake of salt is a major reason for high blood pressure, especially in Western countries. Excess sodium encourages the body to retain fluid, thereby increasing fluid pumped by the heart and circulating in the bloodstream. Diets high in salt also can be harmful to people with congestive heart failure because the excess fluid backs up into the lungs, causing congestion.

Potassium chloride is a common ingredient in salt substitutes. But too much potassium can be harmful for people with kidney problems. One way to enhance the flavor of food while eliminating salt is to add lemon juice, herbs, spices, or flavored vinegar.

Digestive system

The digestive system is a group of organs responsible for the conversion of food into absorbable chemicals that are then used to provide energy for growth and repair. The digestive system is also known by a number of other names, including the gut, the digestive tube, the alimentary canal, the gastrointestinal (GI) tract, the intestinal tract, and the intestinal tube. The digestive system consists of the mouth, esophagus, stomach, and small and large intestines, along with several glands, such as the salivary glands, liver, gall bladder, and pancreas. These glands secrete digestive juices containing enzymes that break down the food chemically into smaller, more absorbable molecules. In addition to providing the body with the nutrients and energy it needs to function, the digestive system also separates and disposes of waste products ingested with the food.

Food is moved through the alimentary canal by a wavelike muscular motion known as peristalsis, which consists of the alternate contraction and relaxation of the smooth muscles lining the tract. In this way, food is passed through the gut in much the same manner as toothpaste is squeezed from a tube. *Churning* is another type of movement that takes place in the stomach and small intestine, which mixes the food so that the digestive enzymes can break down the food molecules.

Food in the human diet consists of carbohydrates, proteins, fats, **vitamins**, and **minerals**. The remainder of the food is fiber and water. The majority of minerals and vitamins pass through to the bloodstream without the need for further digestive changes, but other nutrient molecules must be broken down to simpler substances before they can be absorbed and used.

Food taken into the mouth is first prepared for digestion in a two step process known as mastication. In the first stage, the teeth tear the food into smaller pieces. In the second stage, the tongue rolls these pieces into balls (boluses). Sensory receptors on the tongue (taste buds) detect taste sensations of sweet, salt, bitter, and sour, or cause the rejection of bad-tasting food. The olfactory nerves contribute to the sensation of taste by picking up the aroma of the food and passing the sensation of smell on to the brain.

The sight of the food also stimulates the salivary glands. Altogether, the sensations of sight, **taste**, and **smell** cause the salivary glands, located in the mouth, to produce saliva which then pours into the mouth to soften the food. An enzyme in the saliva called amylase begins the breakdown of carbohydrates (starch) into simple sugars, such as maltose. Ptyalin is one of the main amylase enzymes found in the mouth; ptyalin is also secreted by the pancreas.

The bolus of food, which is now a battered, moistened, and partially digested ball of food, is swallowed, moving to the throat at the back of the mouth (pharynx). In the throat, rings of muscles force the food into the esophagus, the first part of the upper digestive tube. The esophagus extends from the bottom part of the throat to the upper part of the stomach.

The esophagus does not take part in digestion. Its job is to get the bolus into the stomach. There is a powerful muscle (the esophageal sphincter), at the junction of the esophagus and stomach which acts as a valve to keep food, stomach acids, and bile from flowing back into the esophagus and mouth.

Chemical digestion begins in the stomach. The stomach, a large, hollow, pouched-shaped muscular organ, is shaped like a lima bean. When empty, the stomach becomes elongated; when filled, it balloons out.

Food in the stomach is broken down by the action of the gastric juice containing hydrochloric acid and a protein-digesting enzyme called *pepsin*. Gastric juice is secreted from the linings of the stomach walls, along with *mucus,* which helps to protect the stomach lining from the action of the acid. The 3 layers of powerful stomach muscles churn the food into a fine semiliquid paste called *chyme*. From time to time, the chyme is passed through an opening (the pyloric sphircler), which controls the passage of chyme between the stomach and the beginning of the small intestine.

There are several mechanisms responsible for the secretion of gastric juice in the stomach. The stomach begins its production of gastric juice while the food is still in the mouth. Nerves from the cheeks and tongue are stimulated and send messages to the brain. The brain in turn sends messages to nerves in the stomach wall, stimulating the secretion of gastric juice before the arrival of the food. The second signal for gastric juice production occurs when the food arrives in the stomach and touches the lining. This mechanism provides for only a moderate addition to the amount of gastric juice that was secreted when the food was in the mouth.

Gastric juice is needed mainly for the digestion of protein by pepsin. If a hamburger and bun reach the stomach, there is no need for extra gastric juice for the bun (carbohydrate), but the hamburger (protein) will require a much greater supply of gastric juice. The gastric juice already present will begin the breakdown of the large protein molecules of the hamburger into smaller molecules—polypeptides and peptides. These smaller molecules in turn stimulate the cells of the stomach lining to release the hormone *gastrin* into the bloodstream.

Gastrin then circulates throughout the body, and eventually reaches the stomach, where it stimulates the cells of the stomach lining to produce more gastric juice. The more protein there is in the stomach, the more gastrin will be produced, and the greater the production of gastric juice. The secretion of more gastric juice by the increased amount of protein in the stomach represents the third mechanism of gastric juice secretion.

While digestion continues in the small intestine, it also becomes a major site for the process of absorption, that is, the passage of digested food into the bloodstream, and its transport to the rest of the body.

The small intestine is a long, narrow tube, about 20 ft (6 m) long, running from the stomach to the large intestine. The small intestine occupies the area of the abdomen between the diaphragm and hips, and is greatly coiled and twisted. The small intestine is lined with muscles that move the chyme toward the large intestine. The mucosa, which lines the entire small intestine, contains millions of glands that aid in the digestive and absorptive processes of the digestive system.

The small intestine, or small bowel, is subdivided by anatomists into three sections, the duodenum, the jejunum, and the ileum. The duodenum is about 1 ft (0.3 m) long and connects with the lower portion of the stomach. When fluid food reaches the duodenum it undergoes further enzymatic digestion and is subjected to pancreatic juice, intestinal juice, and bile.

The pancreas is a large gland located below the stomach that secretes pancreatic juice into the duodenum via the pancreatic duct. There are three enzymes in pancreatic juice that digest carbohydrates, lipids, and proteins. Amylase, (the enzyme that is also found in saliva) breaks down starch into simpler sugars such as maltose. The enzyme maltase in intestinal juice completes breaks maltose down into glucose.

Libases in pancreatic juice break down fats into fatty acids and glycerol, while proteinases continue the break down of proteins into amino acids. The gall bladder, located next to the liver secretes bile into the duodenum. While bile does not contain enzymes, it contains salts and other substances that help to emulsify (dissolve) fats that are otherwise insoluble in water. The fats so broken down into small globules allow the lipase enzymes a greater surface area for their action.

Chyme passing from the duodenum next reaches the jejunum of the small intestine, which is about 3 ft (0.91 m) long. Here the digested breakdown products of carbohydrates, fats, proteins, and most of the vitamins, minerals, and iron are absorbed. The inner lining of the small intestine is composed of up to five million tiny, finger-like projections called *villi.* The villi increase the rate of absorption of the nutrients into the bloodstream by extending the surface of the small intestine to about five times that of the surface area of the skin.

There are two transport systems that pick up the nutrients from the small intestine. Simple sugars, amino acids, glycerol, and some vitamins and salts are conveyed to the liver in the bloodstream. Fatty acids and vitamins are absorbed and then transported through the lymphatic system, the network of vessels that carry lymph and white blood cells throughout the body. Lymph eventually drains back into the bloodstream and so circulates throughout the body.

The last section of the small intestine is the ileum. It is smaller and thinner-walled than the jejunum, and it is the preferred site for vitamin B_{12} absorption and bile acids derived from the bile juice.

The large intestine, or colon, is wider and heavier then the small intestine, but much shorter-only about 4 ft (1.2 m) long. It rises up on one side of the body (the ascending colon), crosses over to the other side (the transverse colon), descends (the descending colon), forms an s-shape (the sigmoid colon), reaches the rectum and anus, from which the waste products of digestion (feces or stool) are passed out, along with gas. The muscular rectum, about 5 in (13 cm) long, expels the feces through the anus, which has a large muscular sphincter that controls the passage of waste matter.

The large intestine extracts water from the waste products of digestion and returns some of it to the bloodstream, along with some salts. Fecal matter contains undigested food, bacteria, and cells from the walls of the digestive tract. Certain types of bacteria of the large intestine help to synthesize the vitamins needed by the body. These vitamins find their way to the bloodstream along with the water absorbed from the colon, while excess fluids are passed out with the feces.

See also William Beaumont; Lymphatic system; Smell; Taste

DIGITALIS

An extremely valuable drug in the treatment of heart disease, digitalis is derived from the leaves of the foxglove plant (*Digitalis purpurea*), a popular garden flower. Herb doctors and ''old wives'' had used foxglove for centuries, but the plant's efficacy was unknown to the physicians of early modern times.

In 1775, the eminent English physician **William Withering** (1741-1799) began studying digitalis. Withering's keen interest in botany led him to collect plant specimens, as did his love for one of his patients (whom he married), a flower painter. Withering noted that old country women used foxglove to treat dropsy (**edema**), an accumulation of fluids caused by a failing heart. Willing to consider these ''old wives' tales,'' Withering embarked on a detailed study of digitalis. He determined the most effective treatment form—a powder made from dried leaves picked just before the plant blossomed—and, of critical importance, the correct dosage for different cardiac conditions. Equally important, Withering established clear standards for when to discontinue administration of the drug, which can be toxic.

Withering published a monograph on his findings, *Account of the Foxglove*, in 1785, but he had spread knowledge about the ''new'' drug before then, because digitalis became part of the Edinburgh *Pharmacopoeia* in 1783. In spite of Withering's clear warnings about overdoses of digitalis, the drug was commonly prescribed in dangerously large doses for a host of medical conditions. Finally, in the early twentieth century, investigators clarified the effect digitalis had on the heart and the correct circumstances for the drug's use.

The active principles of digitalis eluded researchers until the mid-1800s. E. Homolle and Theodore Ouevenne won a cash prize in 1841 from the Societe de Pharmacie in Paris when they isolated digitalin. Oscar Schmiedeberg (1838-1921) isolated the highly potent digitoxin in 1875. The English chemist Sydney Smith obtained digoxin from woolly foxglove (*Digitalis lanata*) in 1930.

When used correctly digitalis increases the circulatory power of the heart without increasing the heart rate. It remains a widely prescribed heart medicine today, especially for heart failure.

DILATATION AND CURETTAGE

Dilatation and curettage (D & C) is a gynecological procedure in which the lining of the womb (endometrium) is scraped away. It is commonly used to obtain tissue for microscopic evaluation to rule out **cancer**. D & C may also be used to diagnose and treat heavy menstrual bleeding, and to diagnose growths such as endometrial polyps and uterine fibroids. A D

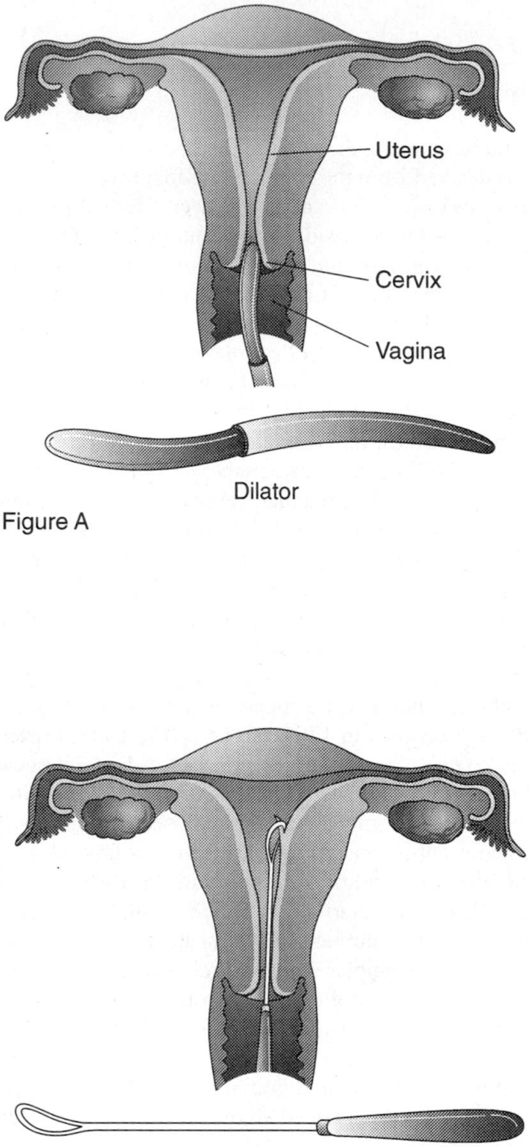

Dilatation and curettage (D & C) is used primarily to diagnose and treat heavy menstrual bleeding and to diagnose endometrial polyps, uterine fibroids, uterine cancer, and cervical cancer. When performing a D & C, the physician inserts a speculum to separate and hold the vaginal walls, then stretches open the cervix with a dilator. Once the cervix is dilated, the physician will insert a curette into the uterus and scrape away small portions of the uterine lining for laboratory analysis. *(Illustration by Electronic Illustrators Group.)*

& C can be used as a treatment as well, to remove **pregnancy** tissue after a miscarriage, incomplete **abortion**, or **childbirth**. Endometrial polyps may be removed, and sometimes non-threatening uterine tumors (fibroids) may be scraped away. D & C can also be used as an early abortion technique, up to 16 weeks.

D & C is usually performed under general anesthesia, although local or epidural anesthesia can also be used. A local anesthetic lessens risk and costs, but the woman will experience cramping during the procedure. The type of anesthesia used often depends on the reason for the D & C.

In the procedure (which takes only minutes to perform), the doctor inserts an instrument to hold open the vaginal walls, and then stretches the opening of the uterus to the vagina (the cervix) by inserting a series of tapering rods, each thicker than the previous one, or by using other specialized instruments. This process of opening the cervix is called dilation.

Once the cervix is dilated, the physician inserts a spoon-shaped surgical device called a curette into the womb. The curette is used to scrape away the uterine lining. One or more small tissue samples from the lining of the uterus or the cervical canal are sent for analysis by microscope to check for abnormal cells.

Although simpler, less expensive techniques such as a vacuum aspiration are quickly replacing the D & C as a diagnostic method, it is still often used to diagnose and treat a number of conditions.

Because opening the cervix can be painful, sedatives may be given before the procedure begins. Deep breathing and other relaxation techniques may help ease cramping during cervical dilation.

A woman who has had a D & C performed in a hospital can usually go home the same day or the next day. Many women experience backache and mild cramps after the procedure, and may pass small blood clots for a day or so. Vaginal staining or bleeding may continue for several weeks.

Most women can resume normal activities almost immediately. Patients should avoid sexual intercourse, douching, and tampon use for at least two weeks to prevent infection while the cervix is closing and to allow the endometrium to heal completely.

The primary risk after the procedure is infection. Signs of infection include heavy bleeding, severe cramps, and foul-smelling vaginal discharge. A woman should report any of these symptoms to her doctor, who can treat the infection with antibiotics before it becomes serious.

D & C is a surgical operation, which carries certain risks associated with general anesthesia. Rare complications include puncture of the uterus (which usually heals on its own) or puncture of the bowel or bladder (which require further surgery to repair).

Removal of the uterine lining causes no side effects, and may be beneficial if the lining has thickened so much that it causes heavy periods. The uterine lining soon grows again normally, as part of the menstrual cycle.

Dioscorides, Pedanius (40-ca. 90)

Greek physician and pharmacologist

In the first century A.D., Dioscorides collected all the available information of his time about every animal, vegetable, mineral, and insect substance that could be used to treat human health problems. He published this information, which included descriptions of nearly 600 plants and almost a thousand drugs, in five volumes known as *De materia medica.* Two later volumes on poisons were also attributed to Dioscorides. His books were often illustrated with precise drawings, and they were translated into many languages, including Latin, Arabic, Italian, French, Spanish, German, and Persian. They were widely distributed throughout the western world in antiquity. Beginning in the sixth century A.D., some editions were alphabetized for quick reference, which made his works into early medical dictionaries.

Although Dioscorides was Greek, he spoke his native tongue with an accent because he was born in Cilicia, an ancient state located in modern-day Turkey. The Roman Empire had conquered much of the Western world in his day, and Dioscorides served in the Roman army of Nero as a physician. As a result of his wide travels, his practical experience, and his extensive reading, he was able to collect the information that went into *De materia medica.*

In *De materia medica,* Dioscorides deliberately attempted to create an exhaustive, structured account of every known substance that could help people with their medical problems. His entries were very practical and plainly written, and some of his descriptions of plants are recognizable today. He described a plant or mineral so that people could recognize it when they looked for it in the field. He explained the properties of each medical material and how they acted on the human body. He also explained how to prepare the material and administer it to a patient. In his entry on opium, for example, he explained that it could be used to reduce **pain**, to make a person sleepy, and to treat a chronic **cough**. He also said that overdoses of opium could put patients into a deep sleep. He explained that the juice from the opium seed capsules was different from the extract from the entire plant, and he detailed how the opium seed capsules should be cut open properly.

In addition to describing and explaining the uses of opium, Dioscorides also mentioned such plants as cannabis (marijuana), peppermint, water hemlock, and wild blackberries. He discussed how minerals like mercury, arsenic, copper oxide, and lead acetate could be used for remedies. He showed how some medicines could be prepared by blending them into milk or honey. He wrote on a number of antidotes for snakebites, and he had a description of how the clay from the island of Lemnos could be used to heal wounds and ulcers. He had remedies for over 950 health problems, including pain, roundworms, and the common cough. He taught his readers how to determine if a drug was watered down, and he was one of the first writers to accurately describe the disease symptoms of the **Black Death pandemics**, which were to ravage Europe for centuries. Such practical information was to make his work important to doctors for 16 centuries.

In spite of the usefulness of some of Dioscorides' writing, many of the healing powers that he claimed for his medical materials are little more than superstition. For example, he recommended applying bedbugs to treat patients with malaria. Much of his work has been superseded and is today considered to be an historical curiosity.

See also Black Death pandemics

Diphtheria

Diphtheria is a potentially fatal, contagious disease that usually involves the nose, throat, and air passages, but may also infect the skin. Its most striking feature is the formation of a grayish membrane covering the tonsils and upper part of the throat.

Like many other upper respiratory diseases, diphtheria is most likely to occur during winter months. At one time it was a major cause of childhood death, but it is now rare in developed countries because of widespread immunization.

People who have not been immunized may get diphtheria at any age. The disease is spread most often by the coughing or sneezing of an infected person or carrier. It is vital to seek medical help at once when diphtheria is suspected.

The symptoms of diphtheria are caused by toxins produced by the diphtheria bacillus, *Corynebacterium diphtheriae.* These toxins destroy healthy tissue in the throat around the tonsils, or in open wounds in the skin, causing the telltale gray or grayish green membrane to form. Inside the membrane, the bacteria produce an exotoxin—a poisonous secretion that causes the life-threatening symptoms of diphtheria. The exotoxin is carried throughout the body in the bloodstream, destroying healthy tissue in other parts of the body.

The most serious complications caused by the exotoxin are inflammations of the heart muscle (myocarditis) and damage to the nervous system. Disturbances in the heart rhythm may culminate in heart failure. Symptoms involving the nervous system can include seeing double, painful or difficult swallowing, and slurred speech or loss of voice. The exotoxin may also cause severe swelling in the neck (''bull neck'').

The signs and symptoms of diphtheria vary according to the location of the infection:

Nasal diphtheria produces few symptoms other than a watery or bloody discharge. Nasal infection rarely causes complications by itself, but is a public health problem because it spreads the disease more rapidly than other forms of diphtheria.

Pharyngeal diphtheria gets its name from the pharynx—the part of the upper throat connecting the mouth and nasal passages with the voice box. This is the most common form of diphtheria, causing the characteristic throat membrane. The membrane often bleeds if it is scraped or cut. It is important not to try to remove the membrane because the trauma may increase the body's absorption of the exotoxin. Other signs and symptoms of pharyngeal diphtheria include mild sore throat, fever of 101–102°F (38.3–38.9°C), a rapid pulse, and general body weakness.

Laryngeal diphtheria, involving the voice box or larynx, is the form most likely to produce serious complications. The fever is usually higher than in other forms of diphtheria (103–104°F or 39.4–40°C) and the patient is very weak. Patients may have severe cough, difficulty breathing, or lose their voices. The development of a ''bull neck'' indicates a high level of exotoxin in the bloodstream. Obstruction of the airway may result in respiratory problems and **death**.

The skin accounts for about 33% of diphtheria cases. It is found chiefly among people with poor hygiene. A diphtheria membrane may form over the wound but is not always present.

Because diphtheria must be treated quickly, doctors usually make the diagnosis based on visible symptoms without waiting for test results. The patient's eyes, ears, nose, and throat are examined to rule out other diseases that may cause fever and sore throat. The most important single symptom suggesting diphtheria is the membrane. When a patient develops skin infections during a diphtheria outbreak, the doctor will consider the possibility of cutaneous diphtheria and take a smear to confirm the diagnosis.

Diphtheria is a serious disease requiring hospital treatment in an intensive-care unit if the patient has developed respiratory symptoms. The most important step is prompt administration of diphtheria antitoxin, without waiting for laboratory results. The antitoxin is made from horse serum and works by neutralizing any circulating exotoxin. The doctor must first test the patient for sensitivity to animal serum. Patients who are sensitive (about 10%) must first be desensitized with diluted antitoxin.

Antibiotics (penicillin, ampicillin, or erythromycin) are given to wipe out the bacteria, prevent spread of the disease, and to protect the patient from developing pneumonia, but they are not a substitute for treatment with antitoxin.

Cutaneous diphtheria is usually treated by cleaning the wound with soap and water, and giving the patient antibiotics for 10 days.

Diphtheria patients need bed rest with intensive nursing care. Patients with laryngeal diphtheria are kept in a **croup** tent or high-humidity environment; they may also need throat suctioning or emergency surgery if their airway is blocked.

Patients recovering from diphtheria should rest at home for a minimum of two to three weeks, especially if they have heart complications. In addition, patients should be immunized against diphtheria after recovery, because having the disease does not always protect against re-infection.

Diphtheria patients who develop myocarditis may be treated with oxygen and with medications to prevent irregular heart rhythms. An artificial pacemaker may be needed. Patients with difficulty swallowing can be fed through a tube inserted into the stomach through the nose. Patients who cannot breathe are usually put on mechanical respirators.

The prospects for recovery depends on the size and location of the membrane and on early treatment with antitoxin; the longer the delay, the higher the death rate. The most vulnerable patients are children under age 15 and those who develop **pneumonia** or **myocarditis**. Nasal and cutaneous diphtheria are rarely fatal.

Universal immunization is the most effective means of preventing diphtheria. The standard course of immunization for healthy children is three doses of DPT (diphtheria-tetanus-pertussis) preparation given between two months and six months of age, with booster doses given at 18 months and at entry into school. Adults should be immunized at 10 year intervals with Td (tetanus-diphtheria) toxoid.

To prevent spread of the disease, diphtheria patients must be isolated for one to seven days or until two successive cultures show that they are no longer contagious. Because diphtheria is highly contagious and has a short incubation period, family members and other contacts of diphtheria patients must be watched for symptoms and tested to see if they are carriers. They are usually given antibiotics for seven days and a booster shot of diphtheria/tetanus toxoid.

DISEASE CONTROL

Clinicians have always intuitively understood the value of disease control and prevention. Early intervention in the course of a disease or even before disease develops has saved the lives of millions of people. Although immunization and screening tests remain important for controlling and preventing diseases, the most promising role for disease control may lie in educating people and changing the personal health behaviors before clinical disease develops.

Screening tests such as the Pap smear (for **cervical cancer**), **mammography** (for **breast cancer**), and the Prostate Specific Antigen (PSA) level (for **prostate cancer**) have all been successful in dramatically reducing the incidence of many cancers. Routine physical examinations and screening for **hypertension** and other risk factors for heart disease have significantly brought down the mortality from **stroke** and **heart attack**s. Similarly, because of very rigid rules for childhood immunizations, once-common childhood infections (e.g. **diphtheria**, pertussis, **measles**) have now become a rare thing in the USA.

Besides controlling and preventing chronic diseases and childhood diseases, infectious diseases can also be controlled by educating people about the risk factors and giving them information on steps they can take to prevent it. The **Centers for Disease Control** (CDC) and many institutions such as the **National Institutes of Health** (NIH) distribute fact sheets on several infectious diseases. These fact sheets give information about the symptoms of the disease, the causative agent, the mode of disease transmission, drugs used to treat the disease and how the disease can be prevented.

In order to control the spread of food and water borne infections, such as **cholera**, **typhoid**, and amebiasis, the following precautions can be taken. When visiting areas where these infections are prevalent, drink only bottled water, carbonated water, and canned or bottled sodas. Boiling water for 1 minute will kill parasites, bacteria, or viruses that may be present. E. histolytica is not killed by low doses of chlorine or iodine; do not rely on chemical water purification tablets, such as halide tablets to prevent amebiasis. Food should be cooked thoroughly to kill parasites, bacteria, or viruses that may be present. If you plan to eat raw vegetables that may be contaminated, they should first be washed with a strong detergent soap and then soaked in vinegar for 10-15 minutes. Do not eat fruit that already has been peeled or cut. Drink only pasteurized milk or da! iry products. Avoid eating dairy products or drinking raw milk. They can be contaminated with unclean water.

In order to prevent African trypanosomiasis and other insect bites, wear protective clothing, including long-sleeved shirts and pants. The tsetse fly can bite through thin fabrics, so clothing should be made of thick material. Wear khaki or olive colored clothing. The tsetse fly is attracted to bright colors and very dark colors. Use insect repellant. Though insect repellants have not proven effective in preventing tsetse fly bites, they are effective in preventing other insects from biting and causing illness. When sleeping, use bednets. Inspect vehicles for tsetse flies before entering. Do not ride in the back of jeeps, pickup trucks, or other open vehicles. The tsetse fly is attracted to the dust that moving vehicles and wild animals create. Avoid bushes. The tsetse fly is less active during the hottest period of the day. It rests in bushes but will bite if disturbed.

Similarly, the spread of all types of invasive group A **streptococcal infections** may be reduced by good handwashing, especially after coughing and sneezing, before preparing foods and before eating. All wounds should be kept clean and watched for possible signs of infection: increasing redness, swelling, drainage, and pain at the wound site. A person with signs of an infected wound, especially if **fever** develops, should seek medical care.

Group B Streptococcal (GBS) infections can be detected during pregnancy by taking a swab of both the vagina and rectum for special culture. A positive culture result means that the mother carries GBS—not that she or her baby will definitely become ill. Carriage of GBS, in either the vagina or rectum, becomes important at the time of labor and delivery—when antibiotics are effective in preventing the spread of GBS from mother to baby.

In order to control hospital-induced (nosocomial) infections such as **Legionnaire's disease**s, diagnostic tests for legionellosis should be used in patients with nosocomial **pneumonia** who are at high risk of developing the disease. In addition, an investigation for a hospital source of Legionella spp. should be initiated immediately. Routinely maintaining cooling towers and using only sterile water for filling and terminal rinsing of nebulization devices is also advised.

HIV and **AIDS** are also preventable. The prevention strategies include practicing abstinence or monogamy (with an uninfected partner), and use of barrier protection (condoms). People who use IV drugs should try to get off drugs. If they cannot they should always use new needles or should clean needles and works with bleach and water. People who use IV drugs should try to get off drugs. If they cannot, they should always use new needles or should clean needles with bleach and water. It is recommended that people who have HIV or AIDS should discuss their serostatus with their doctors and dentists, and inform their sex and needle-sharing partners. Women who are pregnant or planning a pregnancy are encouraged to talk with their doctor about being tested for HIV. If a mother is known to be infected with HIV, treatment is available to decrease the baby s chance of infection. Practices called Universal Precautions and Standard Precautions such as the use of gloves, goggles, gowns, etc., are used by health care practitioners for prevention of transmission of any communicable disease including HIV.

Getting vaccinated against diseases is another way through which one can prevent diseases. If you are traveling to a country where typhoid is common, you should consider being vaccinated against typhoid. Visit a doctor or travel clinic to discuss your **vaccination** options. Remember that you will need to complete your vaccination at least 1 week before you travel so that the vaccine has time to take effect. Some vaccines may lose effectiveness after several years; if you were vaccinated in the past, check with your doctor to see if it is time for a booster vaccination.

See also Preventive medicine

DISEASE PREVENTION

Less than one hundred years ago, one out of every 10 babies born in the United States died before its first birthday. Major advances in hygiene, and development of vaccines led to giant strides being taken in the prevention of disease. Doctors have always intuitively understood the value of disease prevention. When faced with the hard and often unsuccessful task of treating advanced stages of disease, the benefits of incorporating prevention into medical practice have become apparent.

One of the most obvious ways to prevent disease especially among children is through routine childhood immunizations. As a result of widespread vaccination among children over the past several decades, a number of diseases such as **diphtheria**, pertussis, **tetanus**, poliomyelitis, **measles**, **mumps**, **rubella**, and congenital rubella syndrome have become remarkably less common. Several other diseases such as infection by Hemophilus influenzae type B have been shown to cause **meningitis**, **pneumonia**, arthritis, and epiglottitis in one out of every 200 children in the USA before age 5. Similarly, children account for 20 - 30% of the chronic **Hepatitis** B infections in the USA. Hence, new childhood vaccines such as H. influenzae type b (Hib), hepatitis B, hepatitis A, and varicella (for chicken pox) have also been introduced. Although chicken pox is generally mild in healthy children, it accounts for missed school days for the children, missed work days for parents and visits to health care providers. Occasionally it leads to serious complications such as encephalitis, pneumonia, bacterial superinfections, which may require hospitalization and may eventually result in death.

Disease prevention has now become a very challenging medical specialty. The physicians or preventive medicine specialists are trained in epidemiology, biostatistics, environmental and occupational health services, administration, as well as clinical prevention. They are therefore uniquely qualified to work with both individuals and the community to prevent disease. They initiate several programs in infectious disease prevention and control, **sexually transmitted diseases** and in the prevention of chronic diseases. They seek to identify health hazards in the work place and the community. They are active in patient care and like to say that their patient is their community.

There are several steps in the disease prevention program. In order to prevent disease, the prevention technologies have to be first delivered to the patient, in this case the community at large. In the clinical prevention model, which is the traditional model for disease prevention, the health care provider and the patient have to interact. Early detection and treatment rely on that interaction. Screening for diseases, vaccination and early diagnosis all occur within this setup.

The second component of this preventive program is ''behavioral prevention strategies.'' The preventive medicine specialists have to try and use a broad array of strategies to encourage lifestyle changes such as exercise, quitting smoking and adopting healthful diets. To accomplish these behavioral changes, the person's knowledge and attitudes may require changing.

Environmental prevention strategies form the third component of the preventive program. Providing safe drinking water, fluoridation, lead abatement, regulations on public smoking, seat-belt laws, and safer highways all come under this banner. In order to incorporate these changes into the community, societal commitment is required. However once these changes are made, they require very little effort from the individual and can have far-reaching effect.

Primary disease prevention is aimed at reducing risk factors or controlling the causative factors for a health problem. These include risk factors such as smoking in order to prevent lung cancer, environmental exposure to lead to prevent mental retardation in children, and sex education to reduce sexually transmitted diseases. Health services such as **vaccinations**, routine **physical examinations** and providing preventive therapy tools such as fluoridated water also fall under this category. Secondary disease prevention involves early detection and treatment such as **mammography** for detecting **breast cancer** or ''contact tracing'' for detecting and treating persons with **AIDS** and other sexually transmitted diseases.

Tertiary disease prevention involves providing appropriate supportive and rehabilitative services to prevent secondary complications, minimize morbidity and maximize quality of life such as rehabilitation from injuries.

Having a safe environment and a hazard-free workplace, all the appropriate vaccinations, and regular physical examinations are all very important towards preventing disease. In addition, many diseases such as heart disease (which is the number one killer in the United States), **hypertension**, **stroke**, and many **cancer**s can be prevented by adopting a healthful diet, incorporating physical **exercise** as a part of everyday routine, ceasing unhealthy habits such as **smoking**, drug use, overuse of alcohol, reducing **stress**, and maintaining a positive outlook on life.

See also Disease control; Preventive medicine

DISLOCATIONS AND SUBLUXATIONS

The terms dislocation and subluxation refer to the displacement from their normal position of bones that form a joint. These displacements most often result from injury, causing adjoining bones to no longer align with each other. A partial or incomplete dislocation is called a subluxation.

In a healthy joint, the bones are held together with tough, fibrous bands called ligaments, attached to each bone. Surrounding the joint is a fibrous sac called the articular capsule or joint capsule. The ligaments and joint capsule permit movement within a normal range for each joint. In dislocation, one of the bones making up the joint is forced out of its natural alignment by excessive stretching and tearing of the ligaments and capsule. Muscles and tendons surrounding the joint are usually stretched and injured to some degree.

A violent movement at the joint that exceeds normal limits usually causes a joint dislocation. Although dislocations often result from injury, they sometimes occur because of disease affecting the joint structures. Following a dislocation, the bones affected are often immobile and the affected limb may be locked in an abnormal position; **fractures** are also a concern with severe dislocations.

Immediately after the dislocation, the joint almost always swells significantly and feels painful when pressure is applied. If trauma to the joint is violent, small chips of bone can be torn away with the supporting structures. Further dislocations may take place without severe pain because of the slack condition of surrounding muscles and other supporting tissues. A first-time dislocation is treated as a possible fracture. Some infants are born with a hip dislocation, or shallow or abnormally formed joint surfaces that increase possibility of joint dislocation and subluxation.

X rays of the joint and adjacent bones can locate and help determine the extent of dislocated joints. Immediately after the dislocation, application of ice helps to control swelling and decrease pain. If the patient needs to be transported, it is important to prevent the joint from moving (**immobilization**). At times, a cast or splint may be used to immobilize the joint and ensure proper alignment and healing. The realigning of bones following a dislocation is called reduction. This may include simple manipulating of the joint to reposition the bones, or surgical procedures. A general anesthetic or **muscle relaxant** may be used to relax surrounding muscles in spasm. **Acetaminophen** or **aspirin** are sometimes used to control moderate pain, and narcotics may be prescribed for severe **pain**. Recurring dislocation may require surgical reconstruction or replacement of the joint. It is not recommended to reset a dislocated joint without medical personnel, because a fracture may be present.

Chiropractic care may be effective for joint subluxation and dislocation, especially in the spine. Swelling can be addressed using botanical therapies. Bromelain, a pineapple enzyme, and tumeric (*Curcuma longa*) are the most potent botanical remedies for this purpose. **Homeopathic** care with *Arnica* (*Arnica montana*) can reduce the trauma to the body. Ligament and tendon strengthening may be assisted both botanically and homeopathically.

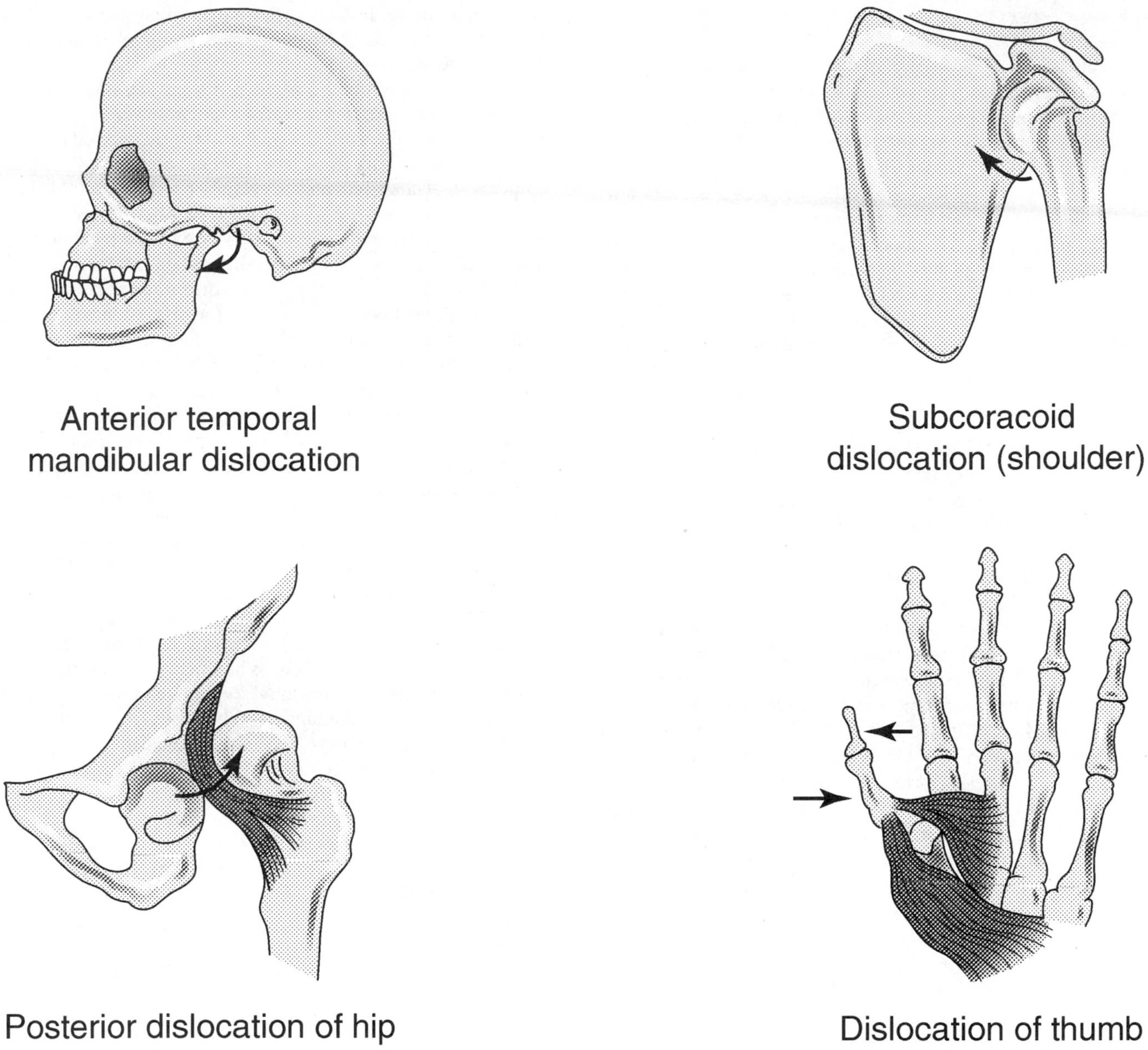

Dislocations and subluxations refer to the displacement of the bones that form a joint. Such conditions most often result from trauma causing adjoining bones to no longer touch each other. A partial or incomplete dislocation is called a subluxation. The illustrations above indicate dislocation of the jaw bone, shoulder blade, hip bone, and the thumb. ***(Illustration by Electronic Illustrators Group.)***

Joint ligaments have poor blood supply and, therefore, heal slowly. This process continues long after the symptoms of the dislocation injury have diminished. Once a joint has been either subluxated or completely dislocated, the connective tissue is stretched to such an extent that the joint becomes extremely vulnerable to repeated dislocations. However, this chance of recurrent dislocation and subluxation will decrease if a proper **rehabilitation** program is implemented to strengthen surrounding muscles. Most joint dislocations are curable with prompt treatment. After the dislocation has been corrected, the joint may require immobilization with a cast or sling for two to eight weeks.

When an individual is involved in strenuous sports or heavy work, joints may be protected by elastic bandage wraps, tape wraps, knee and shoulder pads, or special support stockings. Keeping the muscles surrounding the joint strong will also help prevent dislocations. Long-term problems may also be prevented by allowing an adequate amount of time for an injured joint to rest and heal prior to resuming full activity.

Dissection

Dissection is the act of separating into parts or pieces. Dissection has been called "the way of discovery" in understanding **human anatomy** (form) and **human physiology** (function). Dissection of human and animal cadavers (dead bodies) has produced a vast pool of knowledge, not only of the gross anatomy (muscles, organs, skeletal structure and such), but has ultimately led to understanding the very essence of life at the molecular and genetic level of cells, genes, and DNA. Dissection was, and is, highly controversial. Human dissection was prohibited in ancient Greek and Roman religions and in many countries in the mid-twentieth century. By the turn of the twentieth century, animal dissection was still being strongly opposed by many individuals and organizations worldwide.

The first recorded human dissection was in the sixth century B.C. in the era of the Greek philosopher Alcmaeon (535-? B.C.). By 275 B.C., **Herophilus** of Chalcedon (335 B.C.-280 B.C.) founded the first school of anatomy in Alexandria where he openly encouraged the practice of human cadaver dissection, leading to some of the greatest medical knowledge of ancient times. Herophilus is credited with describing the duodenum, liver, spleen, **circulatory system**, eye, brain tissue, and genitals, and as the first to distinguish between nerves of the sensory (feeling) and motor (movement) **nervous system**.

Roman encyclopedist and physician, **Aulus Cornelius Celsus** (A.D. 3-64), reported rumors of dismemberment and **vivisection** of living criminals in Alexandria during the reigns of Ptolemy II and III (285-221 B.C.). Celsus also published a now famous collection of Greek medical writings around A.D. 30 in which he suggested that opening the bodies of the dead was essential "to learners," even though such practices were still forbidden. Even so, in A.D. 180, the Greek physician **Galen** (A.D. 130-201) published his great works on anatomy, primarily from knowledge gained while performing two secret dissections.

The practice of human dissection was again prohibited by the Roman church in 1163; it was 1315 before the first manual on dissection was published publically by Italian surgeon, Mondino de Luzzi. Regardless of religious prohibition and superstition in the general population, scientific interest in the human anatomy continued. It made a major resurgence in the 1500s due largely to the drawings of muscular structures by Leonardo da Vinci (1452-1519). Even so, in 1564, **Andreas Vesalius** (1514-1564), a founder of modern anatomy, was sentenced to death for performing dissections and publishing his famous seven-volume *De corporis humani fabrica* which depicts the first accurate drawings of the human anatomy.

In 1565, after the Reformation had freed protestants from Catholic rule, the Royal College of Physicians in London, England was given permission to perform dissections on human cadavers. However, as research grew, so did the need for cadavers. By the 1700s, England was using bodies of criminals and the "unclaimed" poor. During an era when people believed being dissected after death was even worse than being hanged, the threat of eventual dissection acted as a deterrent to crime. In cases where prisoners were executed, however, public emotion against dissection ran so high that the bodies were saved from the surgeon's scalpel by angry crowds who attended the public executions.

Thus, grave-robbing became big business as surgeons hired body-snatchers to rob graves of their newly buried occupants. Even in New York City, a three-day riot ensued in 1788 after children peeking through a hospital window saw medical students dissecting human cadavers. The children told their parents, one of whom discovered his wife's body missing from her grave. Subsequently, New York passed a law the following year to allow doctors to more readily obtain cadavers for dissection. Similarly, in England, the Anatomy Act of 1832 allowed unclaimed bodies to be used for dissection. As late as 1829, however, the scarcety of human cadavers resulted in one William Burke of Edinburgh being hanged for asphyxiating victims and selling their bodies to surgeons.

By the twentieth century, **autopsy** and dissection were a widely-accepted practice. By the end of the century, even undergraduate biology students at certain universities in the United States could dissect human cadavers donated as anatomical gifts, wile many individuals were designating their organs upon their death for research or **organ transplantation**.

However, the dissection controversy persists. Millions of healthy animals such as frogs, fetal pigs, mink, cats, and others, are killed each year for dissection in biology classrooms around the world; as are mice, rats, dogs, apes and other primates, for medical research. While many life scientists believe dissection remains essential to the pursuit of knowledge and understanding of the human body, protests from students, parents, and organizations have led to legislation in several U.S. states and other countries allowing students the right to refuse dissecting animals without harming their grades. Also, interactive and three-dimensional computer technology such as CD-ROMs and internet web sites provide "graphics which give the user the ability to peel off layers, just like in a dissection," said Stephen Loomis, professor of zoology at Connecticut College in New London in an article entitled "Instructors Reconsider Dissection's Role in Biology Classes" in *The Scientist*, vol. 11, no. 22 (November 10, 1997): 13-14.

See also Organ transplantation; Vivisection

Dissociative disorders

Dissociative disorders are a group of mental disorders defined as "... a disruption in the usually integrated functions of consciousness, memory, identity, or perception of the environment." All dissociative disorders cause significant interference with the patient's general functioning, including social relationships and employment.

Dissociation is a mechanism that allows the mind to separate or compartmentalize certain memories or thoughts from normal consciousness. These split-off mental contents are not erased. They may resurface spontaneously or be triggered by objects or events in the person's environment.

The dissociation process occurs along a spectrum of severity. It does not necessarily mean that a person has a dissociative disorder or other mental illness. A mild degree of dissociation can occur with physical stress; people who have gone without sleep for a long period of time, have had "laughing gas" for dental surgery, or have been in a minor accident often have brief dissociative experiences. Another commonplace example of dissociation is a person becoming involved in a book or movie so completely that surroundings or the passage of time go unnoticed. Dissociation is related to **hypnosis**, which also involves a temporarily altered state of consciousness.

People in other cultures sometimes have dissociative experiences in the course of religious (in certain trance states) or other group activities. These occurrences should not be judged in terms of what is considered "normal" in the United States.

Moderate or severe forms of dissociation are caused by such traumatic experiences as childhood abuse, combat, criminal attacks, brainwashing in hostage situations, or involvement in a natural or transportation disaster. Patients with acute **stress** disorder, **post-traumatic stress disorder**, or conversion disorder and somatization disorder may develop dissociative symptoms.

In dissociative **amnesia**, the patient is unable to remember important personal information, to a degree that cannot be explained by normal forgetfulness. In many cases, it is a reaction to a traumatic accident or witnessing a violent crime. Patients with dissociative amnesia may develop depersonalization or trance states but do not experience a change in identity.

In dissociative fugue, a person temporarily loses sense of personal identity and travels to another location where he/she may assume a new identity. Again, this condition usually follows a major stress or trauma. Apart from inability to recall past or personal information, patients with dissociative fugue do not behave strangely or appear disturbed to others. Cases of dissociative fugue are more common in wartime or in communities disrupted by a natural disaster.

In depersonalization disorder, the primary symptom is a sense of detachment from self. Depersonalization as a symptom (not as a disorder) is quite common in college-age populations. It is often associated with sleep deprivation or "recreational" drug use. It may be accompanied by "derealization" (where objects in an environment appear altered). Patients sometimes describe depersonalization as feeling like a robot or watching themselves from the outside. Depersonalization disorder may also involve feelings of numbness or loss of emotional "aliveness."

Dissociative identity disorder (DID) is the newer name for multiple personality disorder (MPD). DID is considered the most severe dissociative disorder and involves all of the major dissociative symptoms.

DDNOS (dissociative disorder not otherwise specified) is ascribed to patients with dissociative symptoms that do not meet the full criteria for a specific dissociative disorder.

The moderate to severe dissociation that occurs in patients with dissociative disorders is understood to result from a set of causes:

- An innate ability to dissociate easily
- Repeated episodes of severe physical or sexual abuse in childhood
- The lack of a supportive or comforting person to counteract abusive relative(s)
- The influence of other relatives with dissociative symptoms or disorders.

The relationship of dissociative disorders to childhood abuse has led to intense controversy and lawsuits concerning the accuracy of childhood memories. The brain's storage, retrieval, and interpretation of memories are still not fully understood. Controversy also exists regarding how much individuals presenting dissociative disorders have been influenced by books and movies to describe a certain set of symptoms (scripting).

The major dissociative symptoms are:

Amnesia—marked by gaps in a patient's memory for long periods of time or for traumatic events.

Depersonalization—in which the patient feels that his or her body is unreal, is changing, or is dissolving. Some patients experience this as being outside their bodies or watching a movie of themselves.

Derealization—the external environment is perceived as unreal. The patient may see walls, buildings, or other objects as changing in shape, size, or color. In some cases, the patient may feel that other persons are machines or robots, though the patient is able to acknowledge the unreality of this feeling.

Patients with dissociative fugue, DDNOS, or DID often experience confusion about their identities or even assume new identities. After a stressful experience, the patient may act differently, answer to a different name, or appear confused by his or her surroundings.

Treatment of the dissociative disorders can involve psychotherapy, medications, hypnosis, or a combination of these approaches.

In psychotherapy, patients often require treatment by a therapist with some specialized understanding of dissociation. This background is particularly important if the patient's symptoms include identity problems.

Some doctors will prescribe tranquilizers or antidepressants for the anxiety and/or depression that often accompany dissociative disorders. Patients with dissociative disorders are, however, at risk for abusing or becoming dependent on medications.

Hypnosis is frequently recommended as a method of treatment for dissociative disorders, partly because hypnosis is related to the process of dissociation. Hypnosis may help patients recover repressed ideas and memories. Therapists treating patients with DID sometimes use hypnosis in the process of "fusing" the patient's alternate personalities.

The prospects for recovery from dissociative disorders vary. Recovery from dissociative fugue is usually rapid. Dissociative amnesia may resolve quickly, but can become a chronic disorder in some patients. Depersonalization disorder, DDNOS, and DID are usually chronic conditions. DID usually requires five or more years of treatment for recovery.

DIURETICS

Diuretics, also known as water pills, are medicines that help reduce the amount of water in the body. They treat the buildup of excess fluid in the body that occurs with some medical conditions such as congestive **heart failure**, liver disease, and kidney disease. Some diuretics are also prescribed to treat high blood pressure. They act on the kidneys to increase urine output, reducing fluid in the bloodstream, in turn lowering blood pressure.

There are several types of diuretics. Loop diuretics, such as bumetanide (Bumex) and furosemide (Lasix), get their name from the loop-shaped part of the kidneys where they have their effect. Thiazide diuretics include such commonly used diuretics as hydrochlorothiazide (HydroDIURIL, Esidrix), chlorothiazide (Diuril), and chlorthalidone (Hygroton). Potassium-sparing diuretics prevent the loss of potassium, a problem with other type pes of diuretics. Examples are amiloride (Midamor) and triamterene (Dyrenium). In addition, some medicines contain combinations of two diuretics.

Some nonprescription (**over-the-counter**) medicines contain diuretics. However, the medicines described here cannot be bought without a physician's prescription. Seeing a physician regularly while taking a diuretic is important.

Some people feel unusually tired when they first start taking diuretics. This effect usually becomes less noticeable over time, as the body adjusts to the medicine. Because diuretics increase urine output, users may need to urinate more often.

For patients taking the kinds of diuretics that rob potassium from the body, physicians may recommend adding potassium-rich foods or drinks, such as citrus fruits and juices, to the diet. Or they may suggest a potassium supplement or another medicine that reduces potassium loss. Do not make diet changes without checking with the physician. People who are taking potassium-sparing diuretics should not add potassium to their diets, as too much potassium may be harmful.

People who take diuretics may lose too much water or potassium when they get sick, especially if they have severe vomiting and diarrhea. They should check with their physicians if they become ill.

These medicines make some people feel lightheaded, dizzy or faint when they get up after sitting or lying down. Older people are especially likely to have this problem. Drinking alcohol, exercising, standing for long periods or being in hot weather may make the problem worse.

Anyone who is taking a diuretic should be sure to tell a health care professional before having surgical or dental procedures, medical tests or emergency treatment.

Some diuretics make the skin more sensitive to sunlight. Even brief exposure to sun can cause a severe **sunburn**, itching, a rash, redness, or other changes in skin color.

Anyone who has had unusual reactions to diuretics or sulfonamides (sulfa drugs) in the past should let his or her physician know before using a diuretic. The physician should also be told about any **allergies**.

Diuretics will not help the swelling of hands and feet that some women have during **pregnancy**. In general, pregnant women should not use diuretics unless a physician recommends their use. Women who are breastfeeding and need to use a diuretic should check with their physicians.

Side effects of some diuretics may be more likely in people who have had a recent heart attack or who have liver disease or severe kidney disease. Other diuretics may not work properly in people with liver disease or severe kidney disease. Diuretics may worsen certain medical conditions, such as gout, **kidney stones**, **pancreatitis**, lupus erythematosus and hearing problems. In addition, people with **diabetes** should be aware that diuretics may increase blood sugar levels. People with heart or blood vessel disease should know that some diuretics increase cholesterol or triglyceride levels. The risk of an allergic reaction to certain diuretics is greater in people with bronchial **asthma**. Also, people who have trouble urinating or who have high potassium levels in their blood may not be able to take diuretics.

Some side effects, such as loss of appetite, **nausea and vomiting**, stomach cramps, **diarrhea** and **dizziness**, usually lessen or go away as the body adjusts to the medicine. These problems do not need medical attention unless they continue or interfere with normal activities.

Patients taking potassium-sparing diuretics should know the signs of too much potassium and should check with a physician if any of these symptoms occur:

- Irregular heartbeat
- Breathing problems
- Numbness or tingling in the hands, feet or lips
- Confusion or nervousness
- Unusual tiredness or weakness
- Weak or heavy feeling in the legs.

Patients taking diuretics that cause potassium loss should know the signs of too little potassium and should check with a physician if they exhibit:

- Fast or irregular heartbeat
- Weak pulse
- Nausea or vomiting
- Dry mouth
- Excessive thirst
- Muscle cramps or **pain**
- Unusual tiredness or weakness
- Mental or mood changes.

Anyone who takes a diuretic should let the physician know all other medicines he or she is taking and should ask about possible interactions. Among the drugs that may interact with diuretics are:

- Angiotensin-converting enzyme (ACE) inhibitors such as benazepril (Lotensin), captopril (Capoten) and enalapril (Vasotec).
- Cholesterol-lowering drugs such as cholestyramine (Questran) and colestipol (Colestid).
- Cyclosporine (Sandimmune), a medicine that suppresses the **immune system**.
- Potassium supplements, other medicines containing potassium, or salt substitutes that contain potassium.
- Lithium.
- **Digitalis** heart drugs, such as digoxin (Lanoxin).

The list above does not include every drug that may interact with diuretics. Check with a physician or pharmacist before combining diuretics with any other prescription or nonprescription (over-the-counter) medicine.

DIVERTICULOSIS AND DIVERTICULITIS

Diverticulosis refers to a condition in which the inner lining of the large intestine bulges out through the outer, muscular layer. These outpouchings are called diverticula. Diverticulitis refers to the development of inflammation and infection in one or more diverticula.

The chance of developing diverticula increases with age, so that by the age of 50, about 20–50% of people will have some diverticula. By the age of 90, virtually everyone will have some. Most diverticula measure about 3 mm to just over 3 cm in diameter. Larger diverticula, termed giant diverticula, are quite infrequent, but may measure as large as 15 cm in diameter.

Diverticula are believed caused by overly forceful contractions of the intestine's muscular wall. They are most common in the developed countries of the West (North America, Great Britain, northern and western Europe). This is thought to be due to the diet of these countries, which tends to be low in fiber. A low-fiber diet results in the production of smaller volumes of stool. In order to move this smaller stool, the colon must narrow itself significantly, and does so by contracting down forcefully. This causes an increase in pressure, which, over time, weakens the muscular wall of the intestine and allows diverticular pockets to develop.

The origin of giant diverticula development is not completely understood, although one theory involves gas repeatedly entering and becoming trapped in an already-existing diverticulum, causing stretching and expansion.

The great majority of people with diverticulosis are symptom-free. Many diverticula are accidentally discovered during examinations for other conditions of the intestinal tract.

Some people with diverticulosis have symptoms such as **constipation**, cramping, and bloating. It is unclear whether these symptoms are actually caused by the diverticula themselves, or whether some other gastrointestinal condition might be responsible. One serious risk of diverticulosis is **bleeding**. Although an infrequent complication, the bleeding can be quite severe.

Diverticulitis is believed to occur when a hardened piece of stool, undigested food, and bacteria (called a fecalith) becomes lodged in a diverticulum. This blockage interferes with the blood supply to the area, and infection sets in.

An individual with diverticulitis will experience **pain** and fever. In response to the infection and the irritation of nearby tissues, the abdominal muscles may begin to spasm. Walled-off pockets of infection, called **absccess**es, may appear within the wall of the intestine, or even on the exterior surface of the intestine. When a diverticulum weakens sufficiently, and is filled to bulging with infected pus, a perforation in the intestinal wall may develop. When infected contents of the intestine spill out into the abdomen, the severe infection called **peritonitis** may occur. Other complications of diverticulitis include the formation of abnormal connections between two organs that normally do not connect (fistulas; for example, between the intestine and the bladder), and scarring outside of the intestine, which obstructs it.

When diverticula are suspected because a patient begins to have sudden rectal bleeding, the location of the bleeding can be studied by performing an **angiography**, which involves inserting a tiny tube through an artery in the leg, and moving it up into one of the major arteries of the gastrointestinal system. A chemical that shows up on x-ray films is injected, and the area of bleeding is located by looking for an area where the chemical leaks into the interior of the intestine.

In another procedure called endoscopy, a small, flexible scope (endoscope) is inserted through the rectum and into the intestine. The scope usually bears a fiber-optic camera, which allows the view to be projected onto a television screen.

For cramping pain and constipation believed to be due to diverticulosis, the usual prescription involves increasing fiber in the diet. This can be done by adding supplements of bran or psyllium seed to increase stool volume. Bleeding diverticula can usually be treated by bed rest, with blood **transfusion** needed for more severe bleeding. In cases of very heavy bleeding, medications that encourage clotting can be injected during the course of a diagnostic angiography.

While there are almost no situations when uncomplicated diverticulosis requires surgery, giant diverticula always require removal. The usual treatment involves removing that portion of the intestine.

Treatment for uncomplicated diverticulitis usually requires hospitalization. ''Resting the bowel'' is a mainstay of treatment, and involves keeping the patient from eating or sometimes even drinking. Therefore, the patient will receive fluids and antibiotics through a needle in the vein (intravenous or IV fluids).

The various complications of diverticulitis need to be treated aggressively, because the death rate from such things as perforation and peritonitis is quite high. Abscesses can be drained of their infected contents by inserting a needle through the skin and into the abscess. When this is unsuccessful, open abdominal surgery will be required to remove the piece of the intestine containing the abscess. Fistulas require surgical repair, including removal of the length of intestine containing the origin of the fistula, followed by immediate reconnection of the two free ends of intestine. Peritonitis requires open surgery. Obstructions require immediate surgery to prevent perforation. Massive, uncontrollable bleeding, while rare, may require removal of part or all of the intestine.

When the amount of intestine removed is great, it may be necessary to perform a **colostomy**, which involves pulling the end of the remaining intestine through the abdominal wall, to the outside. This end is fashioned so a bag can fit over it. The patient's waste (feces) collect in the bag. A colostomy may be temporary, in which case another operation will be required to reconnect the intestine. Other times, the patient will have to adjust to living permanently with the colostomy bag. Most people with colostomies can have a very active life.

The prospects for recovery for patients with diverticula are excellent, with only 20% of patients ever seeking any medical help for their condition. While diverticulitis can be a difficult and painful disease, it is usually quite treatable. The prospects are worse for individuals who have other medical problems, particularly those requiring the use of steroid medications. Recovery prospects are also worse in the elderly.

While there is no certain way to prevent the development of diverticula, it is believed that high-fiber diets can help.

Divination

The term divination covers a wide array of methods that supposedly aid a person in discovering hidden knowledge. The hidden knowledge may be a prediction of future events, an explanation of current happenings, or an insight into past events. The techniques range from flashes of insight, to attempting to tap into supernatural powers, to interpreting the significance of omens or other signs. Divination is found in virtually every civilization and culture.

There are three basic types of divination: intuitive divination, possession divination, and wisdom divination.

Intuitive divination occurs when a person, or diviner, has a hunch or a sudden awareness about someone or something. Certain people, such as spiritual leaders, saints, or gurus, are said to be able to gain such insights at will by simply peering at another person or into that person's eyes.

In possession divination, either a nonhuman agent or a diviner is used by supernatural beings as an intermediary to communicate hidden knowledge. Nonhuman agents include nearly everything that is not human such as the weather, fire, water, birds, dice and insects. Another term for nonhuman possession divination is augury. There are many health omens that are interpreted through this type of divination. These omens, such as bats flying over a person's home or crows hovering and cawing over a person, supposedly mean that the person will soon become ill. Other health omens, such as a crow flying away, are interpreted to mean that a person will soon recover from an illness. In human possession divination, knowledge is imparted through dreams or trances. The diviner may or may not be aware of what occurs. There is a long tradition of dream interpretation throughout history. In folk medicine, to dream of howling dogs is an indication that someone close will soon die. However, to dream of the dead is a sign of continuing or renewed good health. In some cultures, healers deliberately seek a trance state through psychoactive substances to gain insight into a patient's illness and the best course of treatment.

Wisdom divination is conducted by people who believe they have the ability to decode or interpret meaning from patterns around them. These patterns may exist in nature, such as the patterns created by earth formations, or may be more personal, such as the patterns formed by the lines on a person's palm. The diviner interprets the patterns according to rules that are sometimes surprisingly complex. For example, the practice of **astrology**, a type of wisdom divination, is directed by the relative positions of stars, planets, the moon, and the sun. Other types of wisdom divination rely on more subjective measures.

Divorce

Statisticians have found that the divorce rate in the United States has remained fairly stable since 1988. Data for 1996 show this rate is 4.3 divorces per 1,000 persons per year. The numbers show that the likelihood of a new marriage ending in divorce is 43% (1988), and that the divorce rate per 1,000 married women (ages 15 and up) is 20.9 (1990). First marriages ending in divorce last an average of 11 years for both men and women, while remarriages ending in divorce last an average of 7.4 years for men and 7.1 years for women.

The number of divorces in this country has been found to be highest among men aged 30-34 years and women aged 25-29 years. One explanation for this is that men in their early 30s frequently place higher priorities on their work than on their families, with the result that their heavy investment in activities outside the home often obscures their investments in family life. It is not surprising, therefore, that conflict between work and family obligations often becomes a point of contention in the marriages of many men in this age group, and that there are large numbers of divorces for these men. At the same time, age 25 seems to be a turning point in the lives of many women. By this age, most women are able to recognize problems in their marriages quite clearly. If a woman perceives that she and her husband do not have enough common ground for continuing their marriage, a woman may opt for divorce.

The *divorce rate* is highest among men aged 20-24 years and women aged 15-19 years. This can be understood by noting that young men in their early 20s are apprentices with respect to their living, husbanding, and fathering, and in other aspects of their lives. Loving frequently means impersonal pleasure seeking and indulging in macho power games. When a young man just out of adolescence chooses to marry, he may seek out a dream woman. If it turns out that his chosen spouse cannot or proves unwilling to fulfill this roll, he may opt for ending the marriage. Men in this age category frequently marry adolescent women, who themselves may not be emotionally prepared for marriage. Many adolescent women marry men they scarcely know in order to escape conflicts with their parents or to achieve greater independence. Unfortunately, these forays into greater independence frequently fail, leading to the observed peak rates in divorce for women in the 15-19 year age group.

National statistics show that the average age for men divorcing from their second marriage is 42; for women it is 39. This has been explained by noting that men in their early 40s who undergo second divorces are frequently those who enter new marriages without having resolved the issues that kept them from forming successful relationships with their first wives. Often, after trying for several years to develop a new kind of relationship with a second partner, familiar hurtful themes reemerge, and the second marriage ends. On the other hand, as women approach 40, they often wish to expand their own horizons and start new enterprises outside of the home. And even if the woman is not motivated to seek a divorce, her increasing independence may contribute to preexisting tensions in the family.

Divorce also represents a pivotal and often traumatic shift in a child's life. Even when a marriage ends on friendly terms, a divorce is not only the end of their parent's marriage, but also the loss of a child's family. The divorce may initially trigger feelings of **grief**, anger, and depression. Investigators have found that children who have very negative views of their parent's divorce have higher rates of depression, anxiety, isolation and acting-out behaviors compared to children with more positive reactions, the trend being especially strong among children aged 11-12. To help children cope with divorce, the **American Medical Association** advises divorcing parents to try to work together to make coparenting, custody arrangements, and transitions from one household to the other as smooth as possible.

Dix, Dorothea Lynde (1802-1887)

American social reformer

Dorothea Dix is known for her pioneering work in the field of mental health. Horrified at the abusive conditions in which the mentally ill were kept, Dix campaigned to have hospitals built to treat the mentally ill.

Born on April 4, 1802, Dix was the only daughter of Joseph Dix and Mary Bigelow Dix. The Dix family, which included Dorothea's two younger brothers, was very poor, and Dorothea was often sent to Boston to live with her grandparents. At age 14, Dix took a job as a teacher in Worcester, Massachusetts. At age 19, Dix founded a school for young ladies in Boston. Unfortunately, Dix suffered from **tuberculosis**, and by 1927, her health become perilous. She was forced to stop teaching, and spent a good deal of time during her recuperation writing. She had a number of works published, including a science textbook called *Conversations on Common Things* (1824); *Ten Short Stories for Children* (1827); *Meditations for Private Hours* (1828); *The Garland of Flora* (1829); and *The Pearl or Affection's Gift: A Christmas and New Year's Present* (1829).

In 1830, believing herself to be fully recovered, Dix resumed teaching, at the same time caring for her ill grandmother. Over the next five years, she worked a grueling schedule as a teacher and a nurse to her grandmother, culminating in a severe relapse of her lung disease. Over the course of the next 18 months, Dix again tried to rest and recuperate, this time at the home of a friend in London.

While in England, Dix read of the French doctor **Philippe Pinel**, who had worked towards prison reform at the end of the 1700s. Dix also studied about the Englishman William Tuke, who had opened a sanitorium for mentally ill called the Retreat at York. The activism of Pinel and Tuke served as a template for Dix, and she returned to the United States in 1837, committed to examining how the mentally ill were being treated. As it turned out, her health was still not sufficiently strong enough for this undertaking, and her recovery took until 1841. During this time, her grandmother died, leaving Dix an inheritance which relieved her of the need to continue teaching in order to support herself.

Finally, in 1841, Dix paid a visit to an East Cambridge, Massachusetts, jail, where she intended to teach Sunday school. She inquired as to where the mentally ill (then referred to as the ''insane'') were kept, and she was escorted into a horrifying underground chamber, where mentally ill women were housed in frigid, filthy conditions.

Dix was ignited by what she saw. She began to lobby various community leaders, imploring them to join her in her

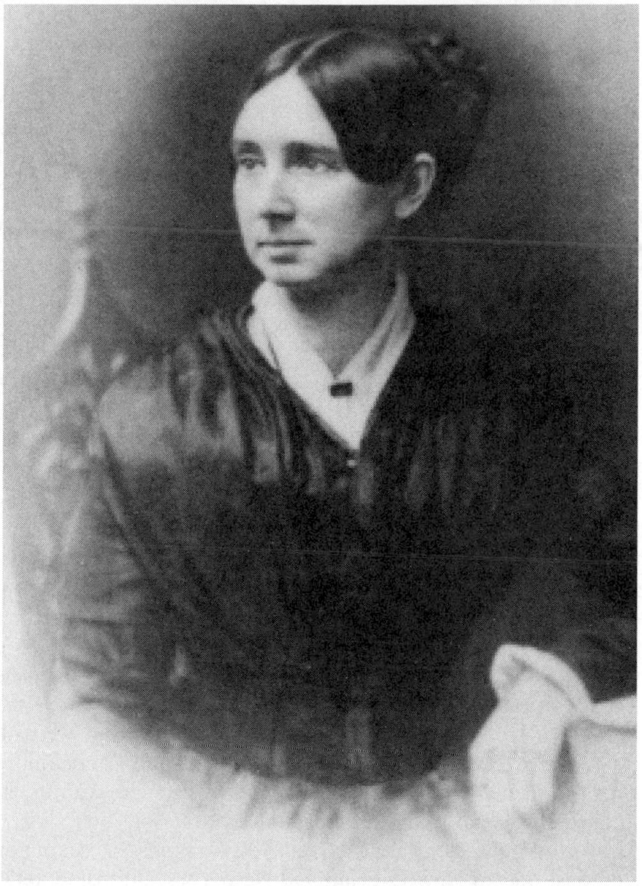

Dorothea Dix

mission to improve conditions for the mentally ill. Three famous activists joined her cause: Horace Mann, the famous educator; Charles Sumner, the abolitionist; and Samuel Gridley Howe, head of the Perkins Institute for the blind. These three were colloquially referred to as the ''three horsemen of reform'' in Massachusetts. Dix spent the next 18 months visiting various Massachusetts poorhouses and prisons, and documenting the circumstances in which she found the mentally ill. Over and over again, Dix was horrified to find these poor unfortunates caged, chained, bound, inadequately fed, abused, and tortured by the very people who should have been their protectors, but who had instead become their captors. With the help of Mann, Howe, and Greely, Dix was able to secure legislation and funding to appropriately house and care for the mentally ill at Worcester State Hospital.

Dix then reached out beyond Massachusetts, again investigating and documenting the conditions in which the mentally ill were housed in New York, New Jersey, Pennsylvania, Maryland, Ohio, Kentucky, and Tennessee. Over time, Dix was successful in most of these states, and new state hospitals for the mentally ill were established in Rhode Island, New Jersey, and Pennsylvania. Her successes in these states sent her further afoot to states in the Midwest and South, and to parts of eastern Canada. Dix had a variety of successes in these locations, but failed at getting federal legislation passed to set aside money to support the mentally ill, blind, deaf, and mute nationwide.

Unable to gain support for this federal fund, in 1854 Dix turned her attention to Scotland and England, where she was able to convince both Queen Victoria and then Parliament of the need to improve the **asylums** in Scotland. Dix traveled the European continent in 1855, visiting France, Switzerland, Italy, Greece, Turkey, Russia, Sweden, Norway, Denmark, Holland, and Germany. Her strong, persuasive convictions, coupled with her talent for dramatically conveying the horror of the plight of the mentally ill, won support for her cause at many stops.

In 1861, Dix undertook a new cause, and accepted an appointment to superintendent of U.S. Army nurses. This put Dix into the position of training the women who would serve as nurses during the Civil War. Dix's tenure in this role was somewhat controversial. She (as always) felt very strongly about how this training should be undertaken, and by whom. This cost her a good deal of criticism, among other reasons because Dix made a mandatory rule that she would only accept middle-aged, homely women into the program. Still, her tireless commitment also won her praise and awards.

After the Civil War, Dix returned to championing the cause of the mentally ill. She continued to travel the United States, investigating and documenting, lobbying and persuading. She even met with an official from Japan about conditions for the mentally ill in his country, and was successful in encouraging Japan to build a hospital in 1875.

In 1881, Dorothea Dix was 79 years old. She set out on her last tour of New England and New York, ultimately retiring to Trenton, New Jersey. Here she lived on the grounds of the New Jersey State Hospital, the very first hospital for which she had lobbied, until her death on July 17, 1887.

See also Mental health care

DIZZINESS

Dizziness is classified in three categories—vertigo, syncope, and nonsyncope nonvertigo—each with symptoms related to the sense of balance. In general, syncope is defined by a brief loss of consciousness (**fainting**) or by dimmed vision and feeling uncoordinated, confused, and lightheaded. Many people experience a sensation like syncope when they stand up too fast. Vertigo is the feeling that either the individual or the surroundings are spinning. Individuals with nonsyncope nonvertigo dizziness feel as though they cannot keep their balance.

The brain coordinates information from the eyes, inner ear, and the body's senses to maintain balance. If any of these information sources is disrupted, the brain may not be able to compensate. For example, people sometimes experience **motion sickness** because the information from their body tells the brain that they are sitting still, but information from the eyes indicates they are moving. The messages don't correspond and dizziness results.

Problems in the inner ear are the most frequent cause of dizziness. The inner ear contains fluid that helps fine-tune the information the brain receives from the eyes and the body. When fluid volume or pressure in one inner ear changes, information about balance is altered. The discrepancy gives conflicting messages to the brain about balance and induces dizziness.

Episodes of dizziness increase with age. Among people aged 75 or older, dizziness is the most frequent reason for seeing a doctor. More than one type of dizziness can be experienced at the same time and symptoms may be mixed. Episodes of dizziness may last for a few seconds or for days.

A person may experience dizziness for many reasons. Syncope is associated with low blood pressure, heart problems, and disorders in the autonomic nervous system. Syncope may also arise from emotional distress, **pain**, and other reactions to outside stress. Nonsyncope nonvertigo dizziness may be caused by rapid breathing, low blood sugar, or migraine **headache**, as well as by more serious medical conditions.

Vertigo is often associated with inner ear problems called vestibular disorders. A particularly intense vestibular disorder, **Méniére's disease**, interferes with the volume of fluid in the inner ear. This disease, which affects approximately one in every 1,000 people, causes intermittent vertigo over weeks, months, or years. Méniére's disease is often accompanied by ringing or buzzing in the ear, hearing loss, and a feeling that the ear is blocked. Damage to the nerve that leads from the ear to the brain can also cause vertigo. Such damage can result from head injury or a tumor. Vertigo can also be caused by disorders of the central **nervous system** and the circulation, such as hardening of the arteries (arteriosclerosis), **stroke**, or **multiple sclerosis**.

Some prescription medications cause changes in blood pressure or blood flow, which in turn cause dizziness in some people. Even common drugs such as **caffeine** or nicotine can cause dizziness. Certain **antibiotics** can damage the inner ear and cause **hearing loss** and dizziness.

Diet may cause dizziness. The role of diet may be direct (as through alcohol intake), or indirect (as through arteriosclerosis caused by a high-fat diet). Some people experience a slight dip in blood sugar and mild dizziness if they miss a meal, but this condition is rarely dangerous unless the person is diabetic. Food sensitivities or allergies can also cause dizziness.

For diagnostic purposes, a patient's sense of balance may be assessed by moving the head to various positions or by tilt-table testing, in which the person lies on a table that is shifted into different positions, reporting any dizziness that occurs. Hearing tests help assess ear damage. X rays, **computed tomography scan** (CT scan), and **magnetic resonance imaging** (MRI) can pinpoint evidence of nerve damage, tumor, or other structural problems. If a vestibular disorder is suspected, a technique called electronystagmography (ENG) may be used. ENG measures electrical impulses generated by eye movements. Blood tests can determine diabetes, high cholesterol, and other diseases. In some cases, a heart evaluation may be useful. Despite thorough testing, an underlying cause cannot always be determined.

Treatment is determined by the underlying cause. If an individual has a cold or **influenza**, a few days of bed rest is usually adequate. Other causes of dizziness, such as mild vestibular system damage, may resolve without medical treatment.

If dizziness continues, drug therapy may prove helpful. Because circulatory problems often cause dizziness, medication may be prescribed to control blood pressure or to treat arteriosclerosis. Sedatives may be useful to relieve tension that can trigger or aggravate dizziness. Low blood sugar associated with diabetes sometimes causes dizziness and is treated by controlling blood sugar levels. An individual may be asked to avoid caffeine, nicotine, alcohol, and any substances that cause allergic reactions. A low-salt diet may also help some people.

When other measures have failed, surgery may be suggested to relieve pressure on the inner ear. If the dizziness is not treatable by drugs, surgery, or other means, **physical therapy** may be used and the patient may be taught coping mechanisms for the problem.

Because dizziness may arise from serious conditions, it is advisable to seek medical treatment. Alternative treatments can often be used alongside conventional medicine without conflict. Relaxation techniques, such as **yoga** and **massage** therapy are widely recommended for reducing stress. Aromatherapists suggest a warm bath scented with essential oils of lavender, geranium, and sandalwood. Homeopathic therapies may be applicable when no organic cause can be identified. An osteopath or chiropractor may suggest adjustments of the head, jaw, neck, and lower back to relieve pressure on the inner ear. Acupuncturists and nutritionists also offer alternative care options.

Outcome depends on the cause of dizziness. Controlling or curing the underlying factors usually relieves dizziness. In some cases, dizziness disappears without treatment. In a few cases, dizziness can become a permanent disabling condition and a person's options are limited.

DOHERTY, PETER C. (1940-)

Australian immunologist and virologist

Peter C. Doherty was born to a piano teacher and a government employee in Brisbane, Australia, on October 15, 1940. A fine student, he earned his bachelor's degree from the University of Queens a year early. He went on to pursue a veterinary (agricultural) career, obtaining his B.V.Sc. from Queensland in 1962, and an M.V.Sc. in 1966.

Later, though, Doherty's career took an unexpected turn. By reading the books of Sir Frank Macfarlane Burnet, a countryman who had won the 1960 Nobel in medicine for his work on immune tolerance, Doherty became interested the immune system. Doherty went to the University of Edinburgh, Scotland, earning a Ph.D. there in 1970 for his studies of viral infection of sheep brains. In 1972 he returned to Australia as a research fellow at the John Curtin School of Medical Research, Australian National University, Canberra—setting the stage for his seminal discovery.

At the Curtin school, space was at a premium. Doherty had his own laboratory for a project studying killer T cells—white blood cells that destroy virus-infected cells in the body

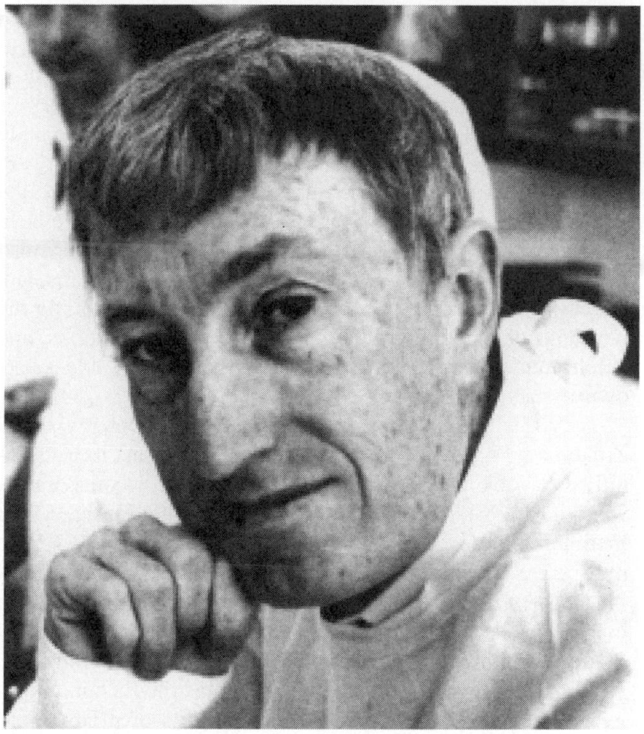

Peter C. Doherty

by recognizing viral proteins on the cells' surfaces. In the nearby laboratory of Robert Blanden, which was working on a similar project, space was so short that they needed to export a worker. That worker, **Rolf Zinkernagel**, moved into Doherty's lab; together the two began studying how killer T cells know which cells to attack.

At the time, immunologists were very interested in a group of genes collectively called the major histocompatibility complex, or MHC. These genes, clustered together in the DNA sequence, encode a series of proteins called the MHC antigens, which determine whether a transplanted organ will be accepted or rejected by a recipient. If the MHC genes of the donor and the recipient match, the organ survives; if they do not, the organ is attacked by the recipient's **immune system** and dies.

A number of researchers had guessed that the rejection of MHC-mismatched organs was essentially the same process as the killing of virus-infected cells by killer T cells. Doherty and Zinkernagel demonstrated that this was true, and that the MHC antigens were necessary for killer T cells to tell friend from foe. When they investigated further, they found something unexpected. Most immunologists had expected that when virus-infected cells and killer cells were poorly MHC matched, the immune cells' killing response would be strongest, much as in badly matched transplants. But the opposite was true. In order to get proper T-cell killing of the virus-infected cells, Doherty and Zinkernagel discovered, the cells' MHC regions had to match.

The two had discovered that T cells—indeed, the immune response in general—can only recognize viral proteins when they are displayed in the context of properly matched MHC antigens. The immune system, which had evolved to recognize "self" from "other" did not react most strongly to "other," but to a third state, "altered self." This discovery finally put transplant rejection into biological context: the body does not purposely reject mismatched organs because they are different, it rejects them because it mistakenly identifies the mismatched MHC antigens as "self" antigens that have been altered by interaction with viral proteins. The finding also opened the way to better methods for heading off transplant rejection, for creating vaccines, and for further unraveling the workings of immunity; vulnerability to certain infections; and autoimmune disease, where the body mistakenly attacks its own tissues.

While immunologists recognized that Doherty's and Zinkernagel's 1973-1974 discovery was important, its true significance took time to sink in. The successful collaborators went their separate ways, with Doherty heading for the Wistar Institute in Philadelphia, as an associate professor in 1975. He returned to the Curtin school in 1982 as professor and head of the Department of Experimental Pathology, leaving once again in 1988 to be chairman of the Department of Immunology at St. Jude Children's Research Hospital, Memphis, Tennessee. At St. Jude's, in addition to heading the hospital's immunology research program, he has maintained his own laboratory work on viruses that cause cancer as well as the Epstein-Barr virus, which causes severe infections in the compromized immune systems of **AIDS** patients.

Along the way, international recognition of Doherty's work grew. In 1983 he was given the Paul Ehrlich Prize in Germany; in 1986, he gained the International Award of the Gairdner Foundation of Canada; and in 1995 he received the Albert Lasker Medical Research Award, often a prelude to a Nobel. Finally, in 1996, for his collaborative work with Zinkernagel, the two were awarded the 1996 Nobel Prize in Physiology or Medicine.

DOISY, EDWARD A. (1893-1986)

American biochemist

Edward Adelbert Doisy was an acclaimed biochemist whose contributions to research involved studying how chemical substances affected the body. In addition to research on **antibiotics**, insulin, and female hormones, he is noted for his successful isolation of vitamin K, a substance that encourages blood clotting. Because he was able to synthesize this substance, many thousands of lives are saved each year. For this research, Doisy shared the 1943 Nobel Prize in medicine or physiology with Danish scientist **Henrik Dam**.

Doisy, one of two children, was born November 13, 1893, in Hume, Illinois, to Edward Perez Doisy, a traveling salesman, and Ada (Alley) Doisy. Doisy received his baccalaureate degree in 1914 from the University of Illinois at Champaign and then obtained his master's in 1916. The advent of World War I interrupted his schooling for two years, during which time he served in the Army. After the war, Doisy received his Ph.D. from Harvard University Medical School in 1920. Beginning in 1919 he rapidly rose through the academic ranks, achieving the position of associate professor of biochemistry in the Washington University School of Medicine, St. Louis. He left this position in 1923 to go to the St. Louis University School of Medicine, and a year later he was appointed to the chair of biochemistry, where he engaged in research and teaching. He also was named the biochemist for St. Mary's Hospital. Doisy held these positions until his retirement in 1965.

For 12 years—from 1922 until 1934—Doisy worked with biologist Edgar Allen to study the ovarian systems of rats and mice. During this time he participated in research that isolated the first crystalline of a female steroidal hormone, now called oestrone. He later isolated two other related products, oestriol and oestradiol–17β. When Doisy administered these in tiny quantities to female mice or rats whose ovaries had been removed, the creatures acted as if they still had ovaries. Many women have benefitted from this research, as these compounds and their derivatives have been used to treat several hormonally-related problems, including menopausal symptoms.

Doisy, in 1936, turned from this line of research to trying to isolate an antihemorrhagic factor that had been identified by Danish researcher Henrik Dam. Dam had discovered a chemical in the blood of chicks that decreased hemorrhaging; he called this substance *Koagulations Vitamine*, or vitamin K. Using Dam's work as a springboard, Doisy and his co-workers spent three years researching this new vitamin. They discovered that the vitamin had two distinct forms, called K1 and K2, and successfully isolated each—K1 from alfalfa, K2 (which differs in a side chain) from rotten fish. Alter Doisy had isolated these two compounds he successfully determined their structures, and was able to synthesize the extremely delicate vitamin K1.

Synthesizing vitamin K enabled large quantities of it to be produced relatively inexpensively. It has since been used to treat hemorrhages that would previously have been fatal, especially in newborns and other individuals who lack natural defenses; it is estimated that the use of vitamin K saves almost 5,000 lives each year in the United States alone. For these research advances, Doisy shared the 1943 Nobel Prize for medicine or physiology with Dam. Some of this research was funded by the University of St. Louis and some of the funds were contributed by the pharmaceutical manufacturer Parke-Davis and Co.—a financial arrangement that Doisy saw as a model for future industry-university research relations.

Over the course of his career, most of Doisy's research focused on how various chemical substances worked in the human body. In addition to vitamin K, his team studying the effects of certain antibiotics, sodium, potassium, chloride, and phosphorus. He also developed a high-potency form of insulin, for use in treating diabetes.

Doisy was made St. Louis University's distinguished service professor in 1951, and later was named emeritus professor of biochemistry. As a sign of his contributions, the university's department of biochemistry was named in his honor in 1965, and he was made its emeritus director. Because of his prominence and his loyalties to the University, there are numerous plaques and buildings bearing his name.

Doisy's contributions to the field of biochemistry are recognized by the numerous honorary awards he held and the scientific societies to which he belonged. He was member of the League of Nations Committee on the Standardization of Sex Hormones from 1932 to 1935, and in 1938 was elected to the National Academy of Sciences. In 1941 he was honored with the Willard Gibbs Medal of the American Chemical Society, which is perhaps the highest distinction in chemical science. He served as both the vice president and then president, from 1943 to 1945, of the American Society of Biological Chemists, and was the 29th president of the Endocrine Society in 1949. Doisy died October 23, 1986.

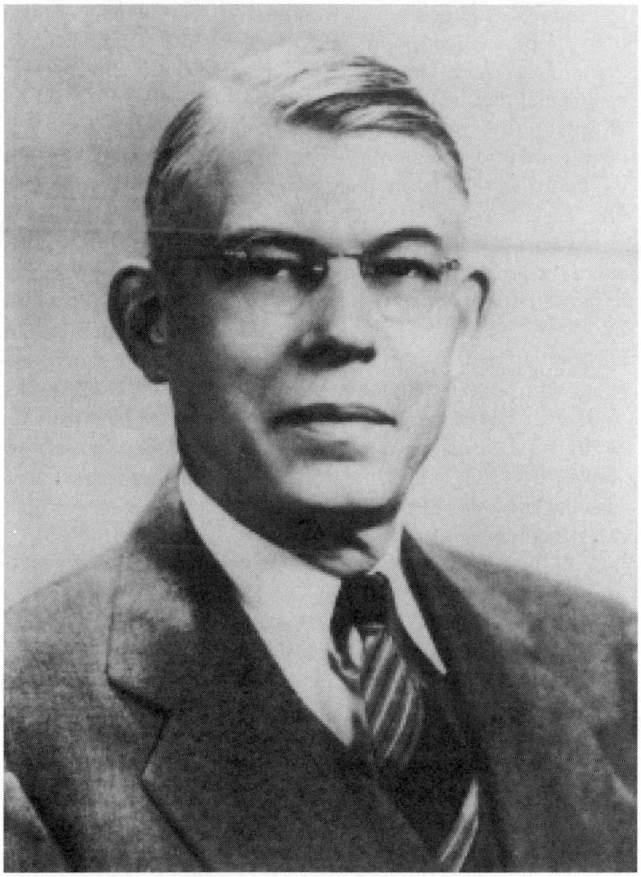

Edward Adelbert Doisy

DOLE, VINCENT P. (1913-)

American biologist

In the 1960s Vincent P. Dole pioneered human studies on the biological basis of heroin **addiction**. He discovered that methadone can quell an addict's craving and that maintenance doses can return narcotics users to productive lives. Dole's innovative approach to studying addiction as a medical problem was conducted at the Rockefeller University Hospital in New York, a unique clinical research center where a scientific approach to this problem was possible. Dole has spent fifty years in biomedical research at Rockefeller and opened several areas of scientific medicine. His early contributions to understanding metabolic disturbances in patients with kidney disease, high blood pressure, and obesity provided the underpinnings of his seminal work in the biology and pharmacology of addiction.

Vincent Paul Dole, Jr., born in Chicago, Illinois on May 8, 1913, was named after his father, an importer of olive oil and olives. His mother, Anne Dowling, once taught school in the rural Wisconsin village where she grew up. Dole's only brother died in childhood. Young Vincent often went on long trips with his parents to visit his father's business interests. He spent the first two years of secondary school at Loyola Academy in Chicago and the final two years at Culver Military Academy in Indiana.

In 1934, he received a bachelor's degree in mathematics from Stanford University. While fascinated by math, Dole really wanted to explore the interplay of living systems. His aunt, a physician, introduced him to the dean of the University of Wisconsin's medical school, and Dole mastered seven semesters of biology that summer in time to enroll. Two years later, he decided to complete a more research-oriented program and transferred to Harvard Medical School. His M.D. from Harvard in 1939 included both clinical research in psychiatry and rheumatoid arthritis as well as laboratory studies in anatomy. His first scientific publication was on the regeneration of nerves.

Following an internship at Massachusetts General Hospital, Dole was invited to join the Rockefeller Institute for Medical Research in 1941. In the laboratory of Donald D. Van Slyke, a founder of clinical chemistry, Dole participated in hundreds of patient investigations. The clinical scientists in this group observed the effects of various **diets** on levels of albumin and lipids in the blood, measured the **metabolism** of proteins, amino acids and fats, and monitored the balance of salts in the body and its effects on **edema**. The team's work established the standard knowledge about nephrosis (kidney disease) for medical students and physicians.

When the institute's hospital became a naval research unit during World War II, Dole helped develop the copper sulfate method, a test that measures blood density in shock victims, and indicates how much fluid they need to have replaced. Blood banks continue to use this test to determine whether potential donors have sufficient hemoglobin to give blood.

After the war, Dole spent one year at the Massachusetts General Hospital arthritis clinic and another year in Europe studying kidney diseases. He returned to Rockefeller in 1947 to establish his own laboratory devoted to the study of hypertension. Using the hospital's resources to study selected patients, he monitored their metabolic state with many elaborate analyses. He tested the low-salt, low-protein diet recommended for kidney disease on these patients, and discovered that sodium was the salt ion contributing to elevated blood pressure. He also found that the diet's low-protein element contributed to diminished appetite and weight loss. Other studies related to hypertension led to Dole's characterization of human sweat gland physiology. Dole became curious about whether the experimental diet he used for **hypertension** could also treat **obesity**. In further studies of patients, he discovered that obese people are not consistent overeaters and that their metabolism is abnormal when they lose weight. Dole's work pointed to obesity as a symptom of an underlying metabolic disease.

As he studied obese patients, Dole began to wonder about the function of their fat, whether it was needed, and how it moves from tissues to muscles where it is burned. In the mid–1950s, he made a significant contribution when he isolated free fatty acids from blood plasma. Despite their low concentration, he found their exceptionally rapid turnover was due to their role as the major carrier of energy in the blood stream. He traced their origin to triglyceride molecules in fat cells and showed how they interact with insulin and carbohydrates, findings that are basic to understanding mechanisms of arteriosclerosis (hardening of the arteries).

In 1963, Dole turned his attention to the epidemic of drug addiction he saw growing around him in New York City. At the time addiction had no place in organized medicine, and was assumed to be a sign of moral weakness that was often relegated to practitioners of psychopathology.

However, Dole persuaded Rockefeller president Detlev Bronk to establish the world's first research program on addiction at the university's hospital. This involved getting permission to treat addicts with long criminal records, administering illegal drugs to them without legal interference, and performing medical studies with an unprecedented degree of thoroughness.

Dole approached this novel problem as a physician and as a scientist. He was profoundly influenced by psychiatrist Marie Nyswander and her book *The Drug Addict as Patient* (1956). Her twenty years of working with addicts suggested that conventional psychotherapy, detoxification, or lock-up programs for chronic narcotic users failed, not through lack of motivation by the addict but for want of effective medical treatment. Physicians Dole and Nyswander (who were married in 1965) admitted tough, hard-core addicts to the Rockefeller Hospital and studied them as sick people. They learned from these patients that they suffered from an organic disease, one needing a medicine that would abolish the pathological craving for narcotics. They needed to restore the addict's neurochemical imbalance before social rehabilitation could even be addressed.

As clinical scientists, Dole, Nyswander, and Mary Jeanne Kreek traced metabolic factors and mechanisms of heroin's action to learn about the body's chemical appetite, tolerance, and physical dependence. They tested many drugs and discovered that a synthetic opiate called methadone—a narcotic in limited use as an analgesic and **cough suppressant**—had a normalizing effect and eliminated the compulsive narcotic hunger without producing euphoria. They later established that methadone acts as a buffer, and that its stabilizing effect is due to its slow elimination from the body.

Dole's initial studies were successful in treating addicts with daily doses of methadone. Like insulin for diabetes, methadone maintenance only corrects, but does not cure, and must be taken for life. More than two-thirds of those who discontinue methadone treatment return to illegal drugs. However, methadone is life saving, as it makes patients alert, healthy, and helps them resume fulfilling and socially productive lives, free of heroin use.

Within a year, Dole expanded his small clinical study, first to Beth Israel Hospital in New York City and then to the city's municipal hospitals. Methadone maintenance programs continue to have a major impact on reducing both crime and the spread of such **epidemic** infectious diseases as **tuberculosis**, **hepatitis**, and Acquired Immunodeficiency Syndrome (**AIDS**). "The simple fact is that it works," Dole told contributor Carol Moberg in an interview, and that this "treatment has survived challenge by professional skeptics, by ideologically hostile agencies, and by competitive modalities." Three decades after its beginning, 115,000 heroin addicts are being treated with methadone in 750 clinics in the United States, as well as thousands more in clinics worldwide.

In 1983, Dole broadened his research to study alcoholism, often a complicating factor in narcotic addiction, that afflicts an even greater segment of the population. Until Dole retired from lab work in 1991, he searched for a model of alcoholism in mice so that potential medicines could be tested that would benefit human alcoholics. However, his detailed report in 1986 discusses why he believes mouse metabolic data cannot be correlated with human alcoholism. He discovered that mice burn alcohol eight times faster than humans, so they cannot reproduce the high blood levels and symptoms of intoxication found in humans; also, mice prefer fats or sugars to alcohol when all are offered in their diets.

Dole's family includes three children from his first marriage in 1942 to Elizabeth Ann Strange: the oldest, Vincent, continues to run the family's olive oil business, Susan heads the Vermont Bar Association, and Bruce manages an electronics business. Marie Nyswander, his second wife and research collaborator, died in 1986. He married Margaret MacMillan Cool in 1992.

Dole was appointed a member of the Rockefeller Institute in 1951 and professor in 1954 when the institute became a graduate university. He has published nearly 200 scientific papers during his career and served as editor of *The Journal of Experimental Medicine* from 1953 to 1965. Dole has received many awards for his work on methadone and for his earlier lipid studies. He was elected a member of the National Academy of Sciences in 1972 and received an Albert Lasker Medical Research Award in 1988. Research into the biology of addictive diseases continues at Rockefeller, where Dole remains active in lecturing and writing.

DOMAGK, GERHARD (1895-1964)

German biochemist

Gerhard Domagk discovered the first synthetic drug that could be used to battle the effects of many bacterial diseases. He was born in Lagow, Brandenburg (which is now Poland, but was then Germany) on October 30, 1895. Domagk began his studies at the University of Kiel but abruptly stopped at the outbreak of World War I during which he served in the military and was wounded in action. He returned to school to study medicine and was awarded a medical degree in 1921.

After his schooling, Domagk began working for I.G. Farbenindustrie, a large company that manufactured industrial dyes. Because of his medical training, he did research on dyes with an eye toward their medical applications. One newly manufactured dye, called Prontosil Red, was of particular interest to Domagk. In 1932, Domagk found that when he injected dye into mice infected with *Streptococcus* bacteria, it cured the animals of the usually fatal effects and seemed to have few side effects. More dramatically, when his daughter Hildegarde contracted a serious *Streptococcus* infection after pricking herself with a knitting needle infected with a virulent bacteria in the laboratory, Domagk, in desperation, administered large doses of Prontosil to her, judging the dosage based only on his experiments with mice. In 1935, the story of her recovery spread like wildfire all over the world. Prontosil was later used by Franklin D. Roosevelt's son who was dying of an infection.

Domagk and many others quickly followed up on his discovery. The same year, a French researcher, Daniele Bovet, discovered that it was just one portion of the Prontosil molecule that was effective against bacteria—a **sulfonamide** called sulfanilamide. This portion of the molecule blocks coenzyme action in bacteria and kills them. In England it was found that the chemical was effective in controlling bacterial **meningitis**, **pneumonia** and **gonorrhea**. In rapid order, other sulfonamide drugs, dubbed ''sulfa'' drugs, were developed which saved many lives and gave the world community hope of curing infectious disease during the 1930s. These drugs included sulfanilamide, sulfapyridine, sulfathiazole, and sulfadiazine.

In 1939 Domagk was recognized for his contribution with a Nobel Prize in medicine and physiology. He initially accepted the award but later was forced to refuse it because Adolf Hitler coerced German scientists into refusing awards by threatening them with arrest and even jailing. After Hitler's death and the end of World War II, Domagk accepted his medal and went on to do further research in the area of **chemotherapy** and its application to **tuberculosis** and **cancer**.

See also Ehrlich, Paul

Domestic Violence

Each year in the United States, male partners abuse an estimated 2 to 4 million women. Domestic violence has been identified as one of the major causes for emergency room visits by women. Studies have shown that one half of all injuries presented by women were the result of a partner's aggression. More than one half of all rapes to women over the age of 30 were partner rapes. Eighty-six percent of the victims had suffered at least one previous incident of abuse, and 40% had previously required medical care for the abuse. Ten percent of the victims were pregnant at the time of the abuse, and ten percent reported that their children had also been abused by the batterer.

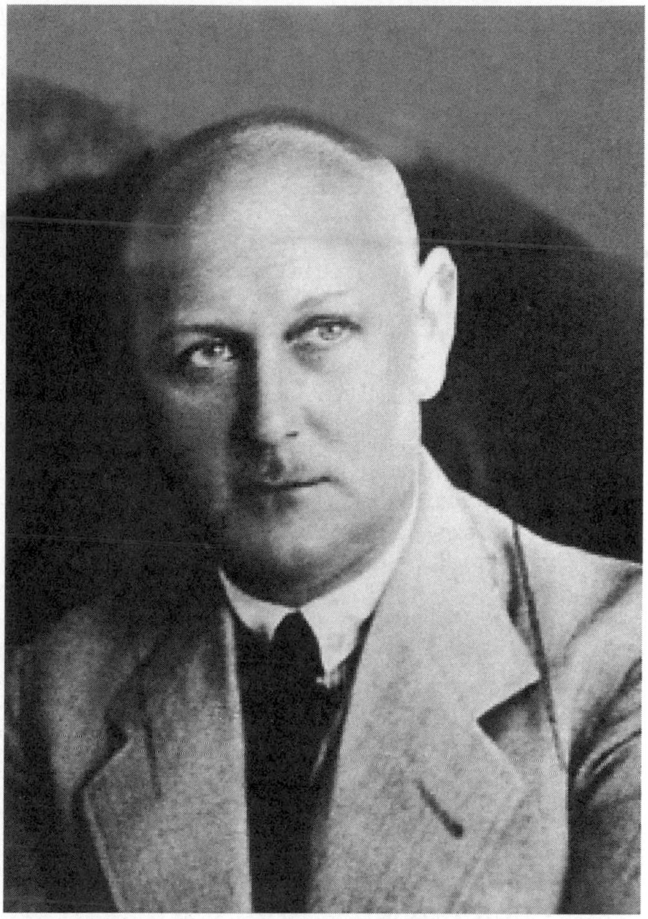

Gerhard Domagk

Domestic violence is a learned pattern of behaviors used by one person in a relationship to control the other. Criminal forms of domestic violence may include stalking, physical assaults, such as hitting, pushing or shoving, or **sexual abuse**, such as unwanted, forced sexual activity. Emotional abuse is another form of domestic violence, which may include intimidation, mind games or insults, or economic abuse, such as withholding money or being prevented from getting or holding a job. The abuse may occur all the time or on a sporadic basis.

In an established cycle of violence, the abusive episode is often followed by apologies and promises that things will get better. Loving behavior and gifts may precede an even more severe episode of violence. The cycle becomes shorter with each occurrence. For abusers and victims who have grown up in abusive situations, recognition that this pattern is abnormal may be difficult.

When attempting to help a victim of abuse, it is important to recognize that the self esteem of the victim is often low, and the abuser may be perceived as the victim¤s main source of love and affection. It is important to help the victim understand that they are not to blame for the abuse and do not deserve this type of treatment. It is also important to recognize that breaking away from the cycle of violence is often a long and difficult process.

Studies have shown that the average battered woman leaves the relationship seven times before making a permanent change.

Stereotypes of the perpetrators of domestic violence may portrait them as having been abused as a child, from a particular socioeconomic group, affected by mental illness or chemical dependency, however these are all myths. Similarly, there is no typical profile of domestic violence victims, except that they are female. What is known is that life in this setting can be dangerous and even deadly. FBI statistics relate 1400 deaths annually in United States women to domestic violence.

Recognizing that the most dangerous time in situations of domestic violence is when the victim tries to leave home, a safety plan should be established. Knowing where they can go and transportation to get therc will allow the victim to leave the home quickly with the appropriate necessities. Quick accessibility to money, important papers and contact phone numbers, and a change of clothing for themselves and their children should be a part of the safety plan. When not in an emergency situation, the best place to call is the National Domestic Violence **Hotline**, staffed 24 hours a day by individuals who can assist the victim in accessing resources within the local community. The phone number is 1-800-799-SAFE(7233) or 1-800-787-3224 (TDD, for the hearing impaired).

See also Child Abuse; Hotline; Rape; Sexual Abuse

Doppler ultrasonography

Doppler ultrasonography is a noninvasive, non-x ray, painless diagnostic procedure that can detect the direction, velocity, and turbulence of blood flow. It is frequently used to detect problems with heart valves or to measure blood flow through the arteries. For instance, disrupted or obstructed blood flow through the neck arteries may indicate that a person is at risk of having a **stroke**. Doppler ultrasonography is also useful for assessing blood flow in the abdomen or legs and viewing the heart to detect and monitor disease. The newest addition to Doppler ultrasound technology is the use of color, which shows the direction and rate of blood flow more clearly.

Doppler ultrasonography makes use of two different, but complementary, principles. The **ultrasound** principle is this: when a high-frequency sound is produced and aimed at a target, the sound will bounce off the target and be detected back at its origin. The Doppler principle is simply that sound pitch increases as the source moves toward the listener and decreases as it moves away.

Medical science utilizes these two principles in the following way. A transducer (sometimes called a probe) sends a series of short sound pulses into the body and pauses between each pulse to listen for the returning sounds. The machine then determines the direction and depth of each returning sound and converts this into a point of light on a television monitor. Thousands of these pulses are computed and displayed every second to produce a detailed image of the object being studied.

During a Doppler ultrasonography procedure, a technician applies special gel to the skin over the area being studied in order to slide the transducer smoothly. He or she will then move the transducer over the skin at various angles to produce different views of the target area for the physician.

Down's syndrome

Records about the existence of Down's syndrome date back to the Saxons, from whom we have anecdotal reports of the disorder. The first medical report of the condition was not published, however, until 1866. In that year, the British physician, J. Langdon Down (1828-1896) wrote a paper dealing with "Ethnic classification of idiots." In this paper, Down described children with the disorder as "representative[s] of the great mongolian race: when placed side by side," he continued, "it is difficult to believe that the specimens compared are not children of [Mongols]." Down based his comparison on the presence of vertical folds of skin above a patient's eyelids, giving him or her an Oriental appearance. Edouard Séguin's (1812-1880) text on *Idiocy and Its Treatment by Physiological Means*, published in the same year, also carried a detailed discussion of the disorder, then known as mongolism. The preferred name for the condition today is *Down's syndrome*.

Credit for the most complete early description of the disorder is usually given to two British physicians, John Fraser and Arthur Mitchell. Fraser and Mitchell discussed 62 cases of the condition, known to them as kalmuc idiocy, and suggested that it occurred as the result of bad health conditions during pregnancy. They found no evidence to suggest that the disorder was hereditary.

Over the next half century, however, the condition did indeed prove to be hereditary. In 1932 the Dutch physician P. J. Waardenberg suspected that it occurred as a result of a chromosomal abnormality. That hypothesis was confirmed in 1959 by the French pediatrician, Jerome Lejeune (1926-). Lejeune and his colleagues found that Down's patients have 47 chromosomes instead of the usual 46. The 47th chromosome is a third copy of chromosome 21. Because of this characteristic, Down's syndrome is also known as trisomy 21. Although 95 percent of all Down's syndrome cases have trisomy 21, there are two other major types of the syndrome. Approximately four percent of Down's syndrome patients have translocation, in which the extra chromosome 21 has broken off and attached to another chromosome. In Mosaicism, which accounts for one percent of the cases, only certain cells have trisomy 21.

Scientists believe that Down's syndrome is a contiguous gene syndrome, meaning that most of the Down's syndrome phenotypic features are unlikely to develop from a single chromosomal region. Chromosome 21, itself, contains nearly 800 genes. Although scientists have yet to isolate all the chromosomes and genes involved in Down's syndrome, they are working on mapping of regions which play a role in determining specific syndrome traits. New methods for karyotyping, including one that uses spectrally classified chromosomes, are being used for identifying chromosomal abnormalities.

Down's syndrome results in retarded physical and mental growth and is, in fact, the most common identifiable form of mental retardation. Patients tend to develop **Alzheimer's disease**-like **dementia** and die by the age of 35. In recent years, research and educational organizations have been very successful in helping the general public understand more about the nature and diversity of Down's syndrome patients and to see that many can lead long and productive lives.

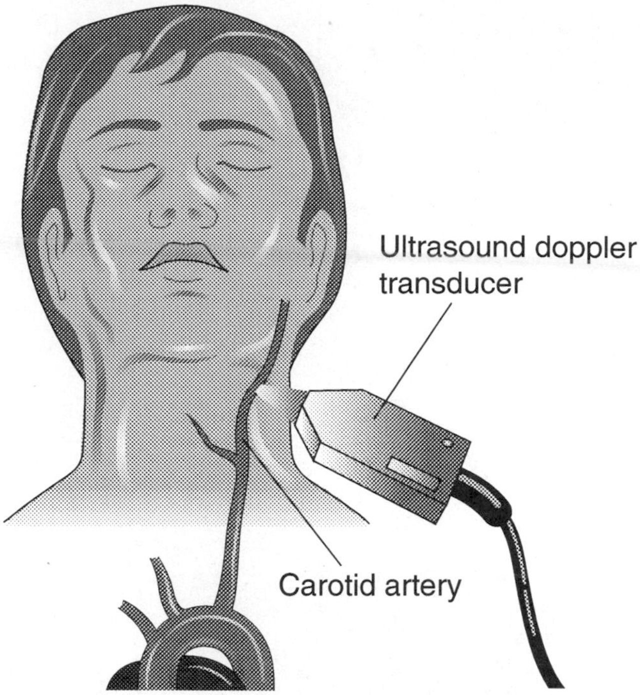

Doppler ultrasonography

DREW, CHARLES RICHARD (1904-1950)

American physician

Charles Drew, noted authority on hematology and human blood **transfusion**, developed a method for storing blood plasma and thus became known as the ''Father of the Blood Bank.'' Drew also exerted his influence on the American Medical Association to rid its affiliates of racism. Born the eldest of five children on June 3, 1904 in Washington, D. C., he was the son of Richard Thomas Drew, a carpet installer, and Nora Rosella Burrell Drew, a teacher. As a child, Drew earned money with a paper route, expanding his territory by hiring other boys to help him deliver papers. He won swimming medals in elementary school and graduated from Paul Laurence Dunbar High School in 1922 as star halfback with honors in football, basketball, track, and baseball. On an athletic scholarship, Drew waited tables so that he could complete undergraduate work at Amherst College where he earned the Mossman and Thomas W. Ashley trophies, Canadian Championship, and Pentathlon Award for athletic prowess in track and football.

An indifferent student in his early years, he was so taken by his studies in biology that he resolved to become a doctor, although he lacked the funds for medical training. Following graduation in 1926, he taught chemistry and biology and directed the sports program at Baltimore's Morgan State College. In 1933, paying his way by working as a referee, he enrolled at McGill University in Montreal, where he earned medical and surgical degrees, a Rosenwald Fellowship, the Williams Prize, a prize in neuroanatomy, and membership in the medical honor society. Drew completed an internship at the Royal Victoria Hospital, followed by a year of surgical residency at Montreal General, where he concentrated on blood typing, surgery, and transfusion. He taught pathology at Freedmen's Hospital and was a professor of surgery at Howard University in Washington, D. C. In 1938 he received a Rockefeller fellowship at New York's Presbyterian Hospital. While serving as a General Education Board Fellow at Columbia-Presbyterian Medical Center, Drew married teacher Minnie Lenore Robbins and began a family. Professionally, Drew concentrated on surgical shock, blood preservation, and the use of plasma in transfusion. He also opened Columbia's first blood bank. Drew completed a Sc.D. in medical science in 1940. His dissertation described the preservation of banked blood, which he learned about from work done at the Cook County Hospital in Chicago. He published his findings in ''Plasma Potassium Content of Cardiac Blood at Death'' (1939) and ''Studies in Blood Preservation: Some Effects of Carbon Dioxide'' (1940).

At the beginning of World War II, Drew took a leave of absence from Howard University to perfect plasma use and blood processing and storage methods for both England and France. During the height of Hitler's assault on England, he directed the ''Blood for Britain'' drive and organized a local civil defense team. His interest in trauma medicine led to the creation of lifesaving blood banks and an appointment with the American Red Cross. In 1941, he directed Red Cross blood collection and the use of dried plasma for the U. S. military. Because of a regulation requiring that blood from non-white donors be stored separately from Caucasian blood and not be administered to military wounded, he spoke out against the absurdity of blood segregation. He was forced to resign his post after he took a firm stand on the fact that blood cannot be identified by race in the laboratory. Returning to Howard University, Drew, humiliated and despairing, gave up research and returned to the classroom, where he distinguished himself through warm, personable relationships with students. He rose to head of surgery at Freedmen's Hospital and, in 1942, became the first African-American to serve as examiner for the American Board of Surgery. This honor was followed by the NAACP's Spingarn Medal, honorary doctorates from Virginia State College and Amherst College, and a consultancy with the army surgeon general, during which he upgraded European medical facilities. He performed community service at local hospitals, spoke against racial bias in medical hiring, and published articles on hematology.

On April 1, 1950, while traveling with three associates to deliver a speech at the Andrew Memorial Clinic of Tuskegee Institute, the car Drew was driving crashed when he fell asleep at the wheel and ran off the road outside Burlington, North Carolina. He was turned away from a nearby hospital that refused to treat African-Americans and died, in dire need

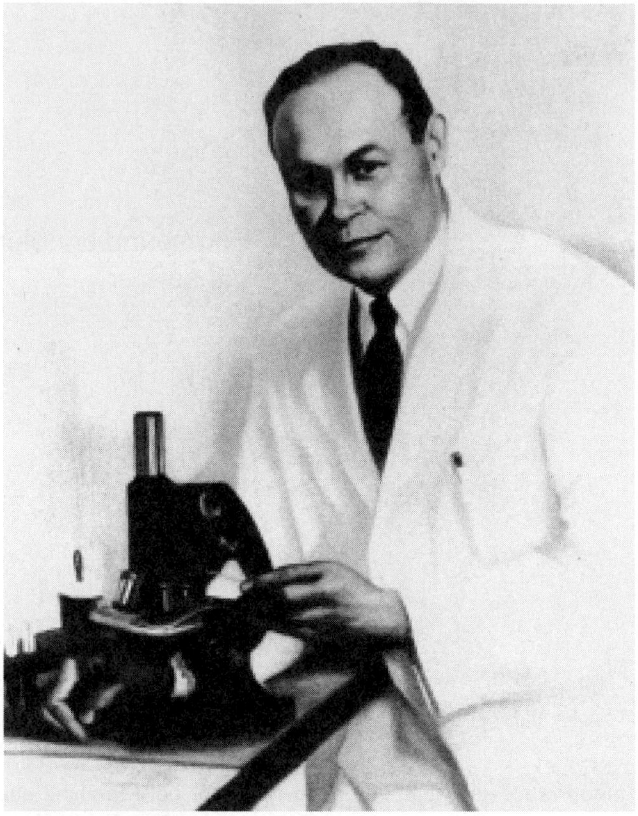

Charles Richard Drew

of a blood transfusion, en route to another hospital. His colleagues honored him with the Charles R. Drew Memorial Fund, which maintains scholarships and lectures. Schools in eight states have been named for him, a Drew clinic operates in Brooklyn, and Howard University boasts a Drew Hall.

DRUG LABELING

Drug labeling includes all labels and any other written, printed, or graphic material that appears on any drug, or on the containers, wrappers, or anything else that accompanies the drug. Drug labeling is regulated by the **Food and Drug Administration**'s (FDA) Division of Drug Marketing, Advertising, and Communications. These regulations apply to both prescription and **over-the-counter drugs**.

The Food and Drug Administration (FDA) requires that drug labeling be balanced and not misleading. The label must be accurate and provide clear instruction to health care practitioners for prescription drugs and to consumers for over-the-counter drugs. Labeling requirements require that the statement of ingredients must include all ingredients, in the order in which they are used in the drug. These ingredients must also be identified by their established name.

FDA has been working to make drug labels better, to promote safer and more effective use of drugs, particularly with regard to prescription drugs used in children and over-the-counter drugs. In 1994, a final rule was established to revise requirements on the pediatric use subsection of professional labeling requirements for prescription drugs. The rule allows more complete information about the use of drugs in children to be included. On March 27, 1999, FDA published a final rule to require a new label format on nearly all over-the-counter drug labels. The new format makes the main messages of the labeling more prominent, includes easier-to-read type, presents information in a standard order, and includes other requirements to make it easier to read labels. The new labels were required starting April 16, 1999.

See also Food and Drug Administration; Over-the-counter drugs

DRUG OVERDOSE

A drug overdose is the accidental or intentional use of a drug or medicine in an amount that is higher than normally used. All drugs have the potential to be misused, whether legally prescribed by a doctor, purchased over the counter at the local drug store, or bought illegally on the street. Taken in combination with other drugs or alcohol, even drugs normally considered safe can cause **death** or serious long-term consequences.

Children are particularly at risk for accidental overdose and account for over 1 million **poisoning**s each year. People who suffer from depression and who have suicidal thoughts are also at high risk for drug overdose. Accidental overdose may even result from misuse of prescription medicines or commonly used medications like **pain** relievers and cold remedies.

Symptoms of overdose differ depending on the drug taken. Some of the most common drugs involved in overdoses are **acetaminophen** (i.e., Tylenol); anticholinergic drugs, which block the action of the neurotransmitter acetylcholine (such as atropine, scopolamine, belladonna, **antihistamines**, and **anti-psychotic** agents); **antidepressant drugs** such as amitriptyline, desipramine, and nortriptyline); cholinergic drugs, which stimulate the parasympathetic **nervous system** (carbamate, pilocarpine, etc.); cocaine and crack cocaine; depressant drugs (tranquilizers, **antianxiety drugs**, sleeping pills); digoxin, a drug used to regulate the heart; narcotics or opiates (heroin, morphine, codeine, etc.); and salicylates (**aspirin**).

Diagnosis of a drug overdose may be based on the symptoms that develop, although the drug may do extensive damage to the body before significant symptoms develop. If the patient is conscious, he or she may be able to tell what drugs and amounts are involved. The patient's recent medical and social history may also help in a diagnosis. For example, a list of medications that the patient takes, whether or not he or she recently consumed alcohol, and even if the patient has eaten in the last few hours before the overdose can be valuable in assessing the situation.

Different drugs have varying effects on the body's crucial acid/base balance and on certain elements in the blood such as potassium and calcium. Blood tests are useful for detecting changes in body chemistry that may give clues as to what drugs were taken. Blood can also be screened for various drugs in the system. Once the overdose drug is identified, blood tests can monitor how fast the drug is clearing out of the body. Urine tests can also screen for some drugs and detect changes in the body's chemistry. Blood and urine tests may show if there is damage to the liver or kidneys as a result of the overdose.

If a drug overdose is discovered or suspected and the person is unconscious, having convulsions, or not breathing, call for emergency help immediately. If the person who took the drug is not having symptoms, call a poison control center immediately anyway. Providing as much information as possible to the poison control center can help determine what the next course of action should be.

Emergency medical treatment may include:

- Assessment of the patient's airway and breathing to make sure that the trachea, the passage to the lungs, is not blocked. A tube may be inserted through the mouth and into the trachea to help the patient breath. This procedure is called intubation.
- Assessment of the patient's heart rate, blood pressure, body temperature, and other physical signs. These might indicate the effects of the drug.
- Blood and urine sample collection. Laboratories will test these for the presence of the suspected overdose drug and any other drugs or alcohol that might be present.
- Elimination of the drug that has not yet been absorbed. Vomiting may be induced using ipecac syrup or other substances that cause vomiting. Ipecac syrup should not be given to patients who overdosed with **tricyclic antidepressants**, theophylline, or any drug that causes a significant change in mental status. If a patient vomits while unconscious, there is a serious risk of **choking**. Activated charcoal is also sometimes given to absorb the remaining drugs.
- Gastric lavage, or ''pumping'' the stomach. For this procedure a flexible tube is inserted through the nose, down the throat, and into the stomach. The contents of the stomach are then suctioned out through the tube. A solution of saline (salt water) is injected into the tube to rinse out the stomach. This solution is then also suctioned out.
- Medication to stimulate urination or defecation. This may flush any remaining drug out of the body faster.
- Intravenous (IV) fluids. An intravenous line (a needle inserted into a vein) may be put into the arm or back of the hand. Fluids, either sterile saline (salt water solution) or dextrose (sugar-water solution) can be administered through this line. Increasing fluids can help to flush the drug out of the system and reestablish balance of fluids, acids/bases, and **minerals** in the body.
- Hemodialysis (a form of blood ''washing'') to filter some drugs out of the blood.

Antidotes are available for some drug overdoses. An antidote is another drug that counteracts or blocks the overdose drug. For example, an acetaminophen overdose can be treated with an oral medication, N-acetylcysteine (Mucomyst), if the level ophen found in the blood is extremely high. Naloxone is an antinarcotic drug that is given to counteract narcotic poisoning. Nalmefen or methadone may also be used. Psychiatric evaluation may be recommended if the drug overdose was deliberate.

While many victims of drug overdose recover without long-term effects, there can be serious consequences. Some drug overdoses cause the failure of major organs like the kidneys or liver, or failure of whole systems like the **respiratory** or circulatory systems. Patients who survive drug overdose may need kidney dialysis, kidney or liver transplant, or ongoing care as a result of **heart failure**, **stroke**, or **coma**. Death can occur in almost any drug overdose situation, particularly if treatment does not begin immediately.

To protect children from accidental drug overdose, all medications should be stored in containers with child-resistant caps. All drugs should be out of children's sight and reach—preferably in a locked cabinet. Prescription medications should be used according to directions and only by the person whose name is on the label. Threats of **suicide** need to be taken seriously and appropriate help sought for people with depression or other **mental illness** that may lead to suicide.

Drug safety

Drug safety refers to the process by which the **Food and Drug Administration** (FDA) learns about the safety profile of a drug before approving it to be marketed to the public and monitors its safety once it is in the marketplace. All medicines have risks. According to FDA, injuries from approved medicines are one of the top 10 causes of death in the United States.

FDA uses state-of-the-art tools and techniques to detect rare and unexpected risks more rapidly and take corrective action more quickly. These include testing and surveillance of drugs, and developing policies, guidance and standards for drug labeling, current good manufacturing practices, clinical and good laboratory practices, and industry practices that demonstrate that drugs are safe. Drug risks include product quality defects, known side effects, medication errors, and uncertainties. Product quality defects are controlled through good manufacturing practices, monitoring and surveillance. Most injuries and deaths are due to known side effects which are identified in the drug's labeling; these can be avoidable (by appropriate use of the drug) or unavoidable (e.g., some drugs have side effects even when used appropriately, such as nausea from antibiotics). Medication errors occur when the drug is given incorrectly or the wrong drug or dose is given. Risks from uncertainties includes unexpected side effects, long-term effects, and uses of the drugs in groups of people (e.g., children or seniors) who were not studied in the **clinical trials** (e.g., a rare event which occurs in fewer than 1 in 10,000 people would not be identified by normal pre-market testing).

In order for a new drug to be approved, the drug's sponsor (usually a pharmaceutical company) submits a new drug application (NDA) with detailed reports on the drug's properties, development, manufacture, and testing results. The sponsor must conduct clinical trials in three phases (I, II, and III) to show that the drug is safe and effective. These trials have many goals. The safety goals are as follows. Phase I seeks to assess safety in healthy volunteers. Phase II and Phase III seek to establish long-term safety in a larger group of people, this time patients with the target disease. During these trials, adverse reactions are closely monitored. When FDA believes that the benefits of a drug outweigh its risks, the agency approves it.

Since it is impossible for FDA to learn everything about a drug's safety profile before approval, the agency uses a postmarketing surveillance system to monitor the safety of marketed drugs. FDA uses MedWatch, a medical product reporting program, to gather information about adverse drug and biologic events and drug quality problems. The agency uses this information, and information it gathers from other sources, to reassess drug risks and recommend ways to manage those risks.

See also Clinical trials; Food and Drug Administration

DRUNK DRIVING

Although the number of deaths attributed to drunk driving has shown a slight decrease over the past few years, alcohol impairment continues to be a major factor in motor vehicle crashes. In 1996, 34% of the drivers of passenger vehicles and 41% of the motorcyclists who died in highway accidents had blood alcohol levels of 0.10% or above, according to the Insurance Institute for Highway Safety. (Although many factors affect blood alcohol levels, on average a 170-pound man would reach a blood alcohol level of 0.10 by having four or five drinks in one hour, and 137-pound woman having three drinks in the same period.) However, alcohol has been observed to affect driving ability and the likelihood of an accident at blood alcohol levels as low as 0.02%. And the probability of a crash begins to increase significantly at a blood alcohol level of 0.05 and rises sharply at 0.08 and above.

Among teenagers, the rates of drinking and driving may actually be rising (after several years of showing a decline). According to surveys of high school students conducted by researchers at the University of Michigan, 31.2% of the seniors surveyed reported driving after drinking in 1984, compared to 15% in 1995. But in 1997, 18.3% of seniors reported driving after drinking.

Because the extent of impairment after drinking alcohol varies from person to person, depending on body weight, gender, mood, whether the drinker is taking any prescription drugs, and on other factors, the most reliable maxim for avoiding an alcohol-related motor-vehicle injury remains: if you drink, don't drive. Even the best driver can become sufficiently impaired by alcohol to injure or kill someone on the highway.

Experts advise that you offer a variety of beverages (some of them nonalcoholic) if you decide to serve alcohol at a party you are hosting. It is also advisable to serve food, even if it's only light snacks because food helps to helps offset (but not eliminate) the effects of alcohol. If a guest ends up drinking too much, common sense says that you should find someone to drive that person home, or offer to let him or her spend the night in your home. And it is understandably better to risk an argument by taking away the keys if an alcohol-impaired guest insists on driving home.

The same rules apply if you are attending someone else's party. And because not all hosts will play by these rules, authorities are insistent that you protect yourself and your passengers from drunk drivers in other cars by always wearing seat belts.

Safe-driving organizations point out that there are steps you can take to reduce the danger of encountering drunk drivers on the highways. For example, if your state does not prohibit drivers from consuming alcoholic beverages while operating a motor vehicle, you can write to your legislators asking that they propose an amendment to your state's law. Some states have lowered the legal blood alcohol content to 0.08% (from 0.10%); you can encourage legislators in your state to do the same if they have not already done so.

See also Adolescent health; Alcohol use and abuse; Metabolism; Motor vehicle safety

DUCHENNE, GUILLAUME-BENJAMIN-AMAND (1806-1875)

French neurologist

Guillaume-Benjamin-Amand Duchenne is best known for his research in disorders related to the nerves and muscles. In 1868, he provided the most comprehensive description to date of what is now known as Duchenne **muscular dystrophy**. He is also credited with identifying tabes dorsalis (a neurological form of syphilis), adult spinal muscular atrophy (Aran-Duchenne type), and facioscapulohumeral muscular dystrophy. In addition, Duchenne is considered the inventor of electrotherapy (the stimulation of nerves and muscles with electric current) and of the **biopsy** (the technique used to remove samples of living body tissues for examination).

Born to a family of seafarers in the French coastal village of Boulogne-sur-Mer, Duchenne was pressured to follow the family tradition and become a seafarer himself. Instead, he studied medicine in Paris. Graduating in 1831 after a rather mediocre academic performance, Duchenne returned home and practiced medicine on the local fishermen, sailors, and their families.

After his return, Duchenne encountered a series of life-changing events: his wife died from puerperal infection shortly after giving birth to a son, a second marriage failed, and Duchenne fell victim to depression. As a result, he neglected his medical practice and turned his infant son over to his mother-in-law.

However, in the midst of his melancholy, Duchenne made an observation that fascinated him: the ability of electricity to make a muscle fiber contract. This seemed to pull him out from his depression and he resumed medical practice in Boulogne.

In 1842 he returned to Paris, where he sought out nerve and muscle disorder cases in local hospitals that caught his interest. Using principles recently developed by the English scientist Michael Faraday, Duchenne continued experimenting with the diagnostic and healing powers of electricity, carrying a homemade induction coil and batteries with him on his rounds.

Another innovative technique Duchenne introduced was the biopsy. In order to obtain biopsy samples of muscle tissue, Duchenne developed a "harpoon" instrument, which distinctly resembled maritime devices he saw as a boy in Boulogne.

These unique types of experimental practices exposed him to derision from some of his medical colleagues, which might explain in part why Duchenne was never appointed to a hospital or university. He was awkward and eccentric, but eventually his private practice in Paris became richly rewarding.

His study of 13 cases of Duchenne muscular dystrophy, published in 1868, was not the first to report the disorder, which had previously been noticed by the Scottish surgeon Charles Bell and, in England, by the medical doctor Edward Meryon. Duchenne called it pseudohypertrophic dystrophy, referring to the apparent overdevelopment of the calf muscle in afflicted boys. A century later, the disorder was named after Duchenne.

Duchenne's mapping of the facial muscles in 1862 led to his discovery of the Duchenne marker—the movement of the pars lateralis muscle near the eyes when a person smiles with genuine delight. This movement is not present during a false or halfhearted smile.

When Duchenne died of a cerebral hemorrhage in Paris in 1875, he had still not attained respect from the local medical community. The esteemed British medical journal, *The Lancet*, nonetheless wrote: "His reputation has come out clear and bright as an honest, hard-working, acute and ingenious observer, an original discoverer, a skillful professional man and a kind-hearted, benevolent gentleman." Several decades after his death, Parisians finally erected a monument to honor the eccentric country doctor.

Dulbecco, Renato (1914-)

Italian American virologist

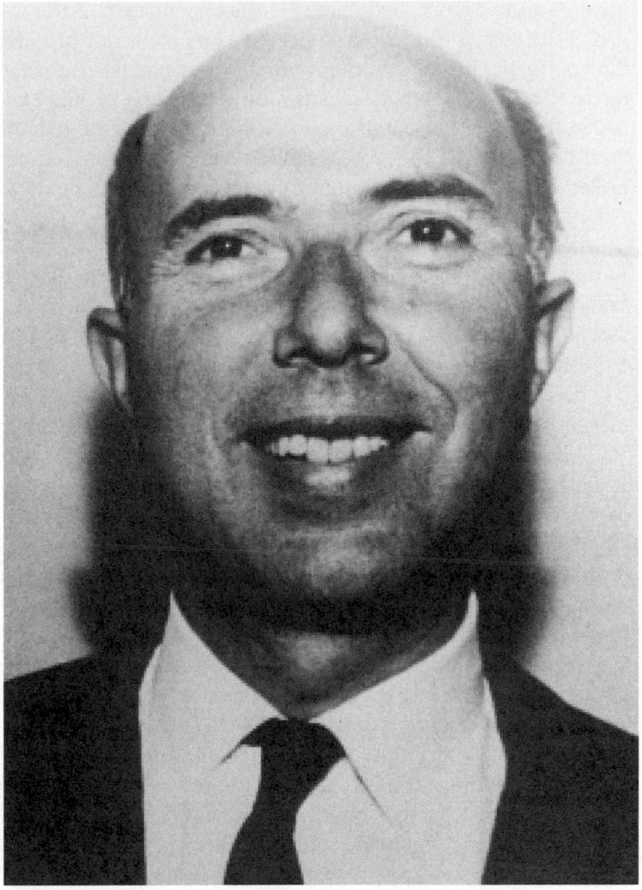

Renato Dulbecco

Renato Dulbecco was a pioneer in the field of virology, the study of viruses. Dulbecco developed the plaque assay technique which allowed scientists to quantify the number of viral units in a laboratory culture, thus making possible most of the later major discoveries in virology. For his work in the study of viruses that could cause **cancer** in animals and humans, Dulbecco shared the 1975 Nobel Prize in medicine or physiology with microbiologist **David Baltimore** and oncologist **Howard Temin**.

Dulbecco was born in Catanzaro, Italy, on February 22, 1914, the son of Leonardo Dulbecco, a civil engineer, and Maria Virdia Dulbecco. During World War I he lived with his mother and siblings in Turin and Cuneo after his father was called into military service. After the war, the family relocated to Imperia, where Dulbecco received his primary and secondary education. His interest in physics led him to build an electronic seismograph, one of the earliest of its kind. He entered the University of Turin in 1930 at the age of 16 to study medicine. By the end of his first year of study, his interests turned to biology and he went to work as a laboratory assistant for Giuseppe Levi, a professor of anatomy and an expert on nerve tissue, where he learned histology and the techniques of cell culture. His fellow students included microbiologist **Salvador Edward Luria** and neurologist **Rita Levi-Montalcini**, both of whom were to be Nobel Prize winners and were to influence Dulbecco's scientific career.

Dulbecco received his doctorate of medicine in 1936 and was drafted into the Italian army as a physician. He was discharged in 1938 but was recalled in 1939 at the outset of World War II. After Italy, led by dictator Benito Mussolini, became a belligerent in 1940, Dulbecco served in France and then in Russia. A serious wound in Russia in 1942 hospitalized him for several months, after which he went home. Following the fall of Mussolini's government, Dulbecco went into hiding in a small village near Turin and became a physician to the local partisan units resisting the German occupation. After the end of the war in 1945, he was elected a city councilor of Turin but soon gave up the position to return to scientific study and research at the University of Turin. In 1946 Luria invited Dulbecco to join his research group at the University of Indiana at Bloomington. Dulbecco and Levi-Montalcini both immigrated to the United States the following year. He became an American citizen in 1953.

At Indiana, Dulbecco experimented with bacteriophage, viruses that invade and kill bacteria cells. His principal discovery at this time was that bacteriophage previously rendered inactive by exposure to ultraviolet light could be reactivated by exposure to white light of short wavelength. This work attracted the attention of **Max Delbrück**, a German-born physicist-turned-microbiologist. In 1949, Delbrück invited Dulbecco to join him at the California Institute of Technology (Caltech) in Pasadena. Dulbecco became a research fellow and later a professor of biology at Caltech, where he remained until 1963.

In the early 1950s, Dulbecco developed a method for determining the number of units of a given virus in a culture of animal cell tissue. This method, called the plaque assay technique, enabled the researcher to count the viral units in a culture by examining the number of plaques, or clear spots, in the culture, where the viruses had killed the host cells. This method was the basis for many of the later important advances made in animal virology. One spectacular practical result of the use of the plaque assay technique was the development of physician **Albert Sabin**'s **polio** vaccine, developed from a living virus, used to prevent poliomyelitis, a paralyzing and sometimes lethal disease. This vaccine eventually superseded the vaccine produced earlier by physician **Jonas Salk**, which was made with a virus killed by formaldehyde.

In the late 1950s Dulbecco's interest shifted to the study of animal viruses that could cause cancerous tumors. His research over the next 20 years was devoted to an investigation of the precise manner in which particular viruses could transform host cells in such ways that the cell was either killed or multiplied indefinitely (that is, became cancerous). While working on the polyoma virus, which causes tumors in mice, Dulbecco and his colleagues discovered that the virus's DNA (deoxyribonucleic acid) combined with the DNA of the host cell and remained there as a provirus (a virus that is integrated with a cell's genetic material and that can be transmitted without causing disintegration when the cell reproduces) which controlled the genetic mechanism of the cell. In a process called cell transformation, the virus could induce a **cancer**-like state, causing the cell to multiply endlessly in a tissue culture environment in the laboratory. In an animal body, the same process of cell transformation and subsequent cell multiplication led to the growth of cancerous tumors.

In 1963 Dulbecco left Caltech to become one of the original fellows of the Salk Institute, a research organization founded by Salk in La Jolla, California. There Dulbecco continued his research on animal tumor viruses.

In 1972 Dulbecco moved to London to become assistant (later deputy) director of research at the Imperial Cancer Research Fund. He was by then involved in the study of breast cancer in human beings. While in London, Dulbecco, Baltimore, and Temin were jointly awarded the Nobel Prize in medicine or physiology for their work on tumor virology. In his Nobel Prize lecture Dulbecco made a strong plea for the governments of the world to ban or otherwise remove cancer-causing substances from the environment.

Dulbecco returned to southern California in 1977 to become a distinguished research professor at the Salk Institute. He became president of the institute in 1982 and held that position until his retirement in 1992. In addition, during the late 1970s Dulbecco taught at the University of California in San Diego.

Dunant, Jean Henri (1828-1910)

Swiss philanthropist

With his life's work dedicated to the needs of others, the Swiss humanitarian Jean Henri Dunant is best known as the founder of the **International Committee of the Red Cross** (ICRC). Born in Geneva into an affluent family who considered religion and charity a priority, Dunant's father and grandfather held important positions in Geneva, including member of Geneva's governing council, director of a Geneva hospital and mayor of nearby Avully.

Dunant began shaping his future with early interests in finance, religion, and public service. A student of economics during the day, he dedicated his evenings to the poor and sick as a representative of the League of Alms. Following in the footsteps of his Calvinist family, Dunant attended church regularly on Sundays, and then brought the message of religion to a local prison. He pursued his religion further when Dunant joined the Réveil (Awakening) evangelical movement at the age of 18. Eager to become a catalyst for new ideas, Dunant began to support the abolition of slavery after meeting American writer Harriet Beecher Stowe in 1853, and he became active in the newly formed Young Men's Christian Academy (YMCA), which opened its first European branch in Paris in 1855.

At the age of 26 years old, Dunant began a position with one of Geneva's largest banking houses in North Africa and Sicily. While knowing this position would produce his income, Dunant continued to work for charitable causes and established a YMCA outpost in Algeria. As a writer, he published his travel observations of North Africa in *Notice sur la régence de Tunis* (An Account of the Regency in Tunis). Dunant's interest in slavery was called to attention when one long chapter was published separately from *Notice* as *L'Esclavage chez les musulmans et aux États-Unis d'Amérique* (Slavery Among the Mohammedans and in the United States of America, 1863.)

In 1859, Dunant's world would change as he left his profession in finance and purchased a large amount of land in the French colony of Algeria with plans of raising cattle and grain. He solicited 100 million Swiss francs by organizing a company supported by investments from family and friends to make his farm a reality but Dunant was missing one key ingredient: water that must be piped from government-owned land.

His appeal to Algerian officials went unanswered, and Dunant decided to personally receive a direct answer from Emperor Napoleon III of France. Upon visiting Napoleon on June 24, 1859 in Solferino, Italy where he was leading the French army and its Italian allies against the Austrians, Dunant witnessed one of nineteenth-century Europe's bloodiest battles. When arriving in nearby Castiglione at the Battle of Solferino, Dunant witnessed the killings and woundings of 40,000. Described by Dunant as ''indescribably hideous,'' he immediately joined the 6,000 people who streamed into Solferino to remove the wounded to Castiglione.

Caring for the wounded in temporary hospitals that were set up in houses, army barracks and the town church and cloister, Dunant became an aid to soldiers from both sides of the war. When he came upon a group of Italian soldiers about to throw several wounded Austrian soldiers down the steps of a church, called the Chiesa Maggiore, in Castiglione he was alarmed. ''Stop,'' Dunant yelled. ''You must not! They are brothers!'' The Austrians were released, and Sono fratelli (They Are Brothers) was the name given to the relief effort.

As the director at the Chiesa Maggiore, Dunant gathered food, organized first aid workers, and recruited tourists, priests, and journalists to help the wounded. With only two badly injured doctors available and three days of relentless care to those in need, Dunant went to the French army headquarters to request the release of all medically trained prisoners into his custody. Charitable organizations in Geneva also sent supplies from Dunant's requests and he organized additional relief efforts at battle sites in Brescia and Milan.

Shortly after Solferino's unforgettable plight, Dunant wrote *Un Souvenir de Solferino* (A Memory of Solferino, 1862) where he told of battle's cruelty to humanity, described the relief effort in Castiglione, and made a proposal to ''take advantage of a special congress to formulate some international principle, with the sanction of an inviolable Convention which, once accepted and ratified, might constitute a basis for Societies for the relief of the wounded in various countries of Europe.'' His book received praise from journalists and Europe's high society.

The first to act on Dunant's idea of cooperative national war relief organizations was the Geneva Public Welfare Society, a private humanitarian organization of leading citizens. By February of the following year, they created a five-member committee that included Dunant. He stressed the importance of approaching the entire world with their mission to gain support. Dunant's public campaign turned to influential public figures, including Victor Hugo, Charles Dickens, and **Florence Nightingale**, to help organize an international conference that would become responsible for arranging the work of national war relief groups.

Dunant's efforts were successful as 39 delegates from 16 countries met at Geneva on October 26, 1863. The delegates' work was swift in drafting a treaty which guaranteed the neutrality of relief workers and adopting the Swiss flag with the colors reversed, a red cross on white, as their emblem, and as a way to honor Dunant and his government. This meeting marked the creation of the ICRC, and the beginning of the Red Cross movement. In 1864, representatives from 12 nations signed the treaty, known as the Geneva Convention, in Paris.

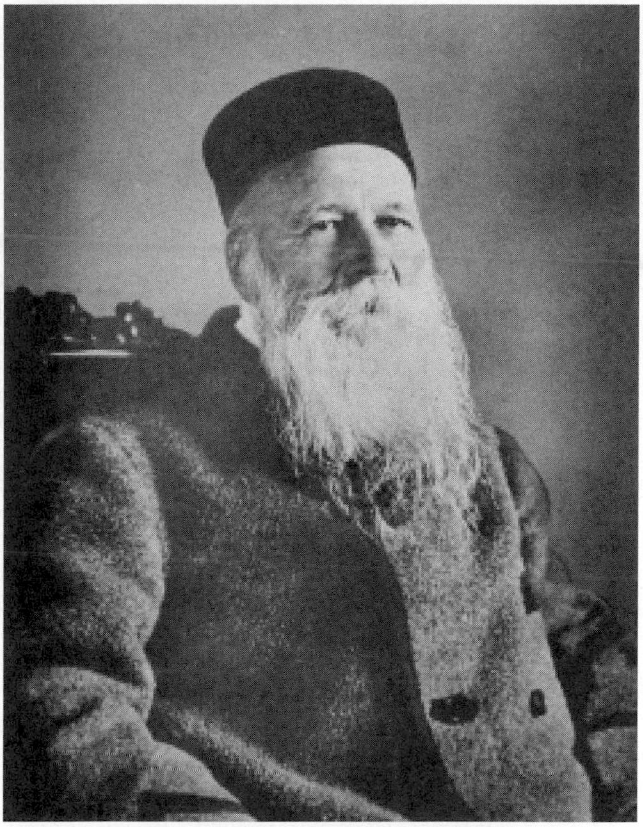

Jean Henri Dunant

While personal triumphs were being celebrated by Dunant, his neglected business in Algeria forced him to declare bankruptcy in 1867. His good deeds were overlooked by several investors, and he was shunned by the Geneva society who had once applauded him. Dunant soon fell into poverty. Although financially ruined, Dunant continued to make great strides at the 1867 general meeting of the Red Cross, where he proposed the same inviolable status as the sick and wounded to the prisoners of war. To help make this a reality, he founded the Provident Society during the Franco-Prussian War in 1871. With a mission to pursue the official neutrality of prisoners, the Provident Society (which came to be known as the World Alliance for Order and Civilization in 1872) established chapters in Britain and France to spread their message. The rights of prisoners were addressed at the first conference in Brussels in 1874 as the rules of war and the treatment of prisoners were outlined. These were eventually acknowledged by other countries as Red Cross chapters were established throughout the world.

With all efforts turned towards the World Alliance from 1871 to 1874, Dunant then became vocally involved with the slave trade as he campaigned against it. While slavery was illegal in Europe, regulations drafted by the British Admiralty stated that naval vessels must surrender runaway slaves who looked for British protection aboard the ships when docking at the fugitive's home ports. Dunant organized such a powerful protest against these orders as a member of the Anti-Slavery Society in Britain and France that they were soon revoked.

Once again showing love for his neighbor, Dunant supported the European Jews who yearned to return to their homeland in Palestine. To help make this a reality, he founded the International Society for the Revival of the Orient in 1864 whose main goal was to establish a European colony in Palestine. While financing was planned by the Syrian and Palestine Colonization Society in 1876, Dunant's plans were stopped when the war between Turkey and Russia in the same year kept the Turkish sultan, Abdul-Hamid from providing land grants for the cause.

No longer acknowledged by family or friends, Dunant chose a solitary life after 1876 that allowed only short public appearances to raise funds for the World Alliance. Living in a garret in southern England, his last brief position was as secretary for Frèdèric Passy's French Society of the Friends of Peace in Paris. He wandered home to Switzerland, surviving as a beggar from village to village, but always keeping a meticulous appearance by using ink to blacken his coat and chalk to whiten his shirt. Time found him entering a hospice in the village of Heiden in 1892, where he spent his remaining years.

Three years later, a journalist named Wilhelm Sondregger found Dunant and published his interview with the humanitarian throughout Europe. Personal interest in his lifelong cause became apparent from the dowager empress of Russia, who provided him a small pension, and editor Bertha von Suttner asked him to contribute regularly to her pacifist periodical.

In 1901, the first Nobel Peace Prize was presented to Dunant and Frèdèric Passy. While unable to attend due to illness, Dunant's life work that instigated peaceful cooperation among nations was respectfully honored. Because he never married, Dunant left the entire proceeds of his prize to philanthropic organizations in Norway and Sweden upon his death in 1910. A free bed for the poor in Heiden at the hospice was also granted from his last requests.

See also Hospices; International Red Cross; Florence Nightingale

Dupuytren, Guillaume (1777-1835)

French surgeon and anatomist

Best remembered for the development of a surgical technique to correct a tissue defect later named after him, Dupuytren conquered early poverty to become a royal surgeon and one of his country's most famous and wealthy people.

Dupuytren was born in Pierre-Buffière, a suburb of the city of Limoges, and endured abject conditions during his early years. However, despite his background and a protracted struggle with **tuberculosis**, his superior intellect earned him a scholarship at the Collège de la Marche. In 1795, when he was just 18 years old, Dupuytren outperformed many others in a competitive examination for the position of anatomy professor at Paris's new School of Medicine. His career received a major boost when he accepted an appointment in 1803 as assistant chief surgeon at the prestigious Hôtel Dieu, where he would remain for three decades, becoming professor of operative surgery there in 1811 and chief surgeon in 1815. In the meantime, in 1810 he invented an early type of stomach tube. In addition, he worked as professor of clinical surgery at the School of Medicine beginning in 1815. He was a popular lecturer, and many of his lectures were featured in the prominent medical publications of the period.

When King Louis XVIII ascended to the throne in 1814, he not only made Dupuytren a baron, but also appointed the **physician** as his royal surgeon. By this time, Dupuytren had made a name for himself as a brilliant anatomist, having performed the first successful removal of a lower jaw and ligation of the subclavian artery in 1812. Subsequently, he discovered an effective way to treat **aneurysms** using compression, invented the cutting forceps (enterotome), and developed a surgical treatment for wry neck, in which muscles of the neck contract spasmodically or continually, producing a crooked neck.

As Dupuytren continued his work under King Louis, he persisted in his intense investigation of new surgical tools and techniques. In 1824, Charles X became king, and he also appointed Dupuytren as his royal surgeon. Much of the physician's most famous work occurred during this period, including his creation of the first good description of the **pathology** of congenital hip dislocation and a new classifying system for **burns** and development of a surgical treatment for **cervical cancer** and invention of an artificial anus.

In 1831, Dupuytren evolved a surgical technique to fix a debilitating problem now known as Dupuytren's contracture. The ailment afflicts perhaps 2-3% of the global population and its etiology is unknown, although it has been associated with liver disease. Dupuytren's contracture involves fibrosis of deep tissues in the palm (and, rarely, the feet). These fibers contract, which causes little or no pain, but results in the permanent retraction of one or more fingers (most often the ring and little fingers) toward the palm. Dupuytren's technique for resolving the deformity centered on the removal of the tissue causing the contracture.

Despite his reputation for having a quick temper and a somewhat sour disposition, by the last years of his life Dupuytren had one of the largest and most lucrative surgical practices in history. He was devoted to his profession and to those who practiced surgery, even donating part of his $1.5 million fortune to start a home for physicians who had fallen on hard times. He also sent aid to King Charles, who by then was in exile, and willed some of his estate to organizations performing medical research. Dupuytren died of tuberculosis in Paris in 1835.

Durable Power of Attorney for Health Care

Modern technology has made it possible for physicians to save lives that even just a few years ago would have been lost. Although such medical advances have given us many reasons for celebration, they have also rasied a variety of questions about whether the essence of life should be maintained if the quality of life is lacking. That is, are patients whose bodies are being kept alive by machine, although they will never recover to lead a normal life, truly enjoying life?

In response to cases such as that of Karen Ann Quinlan, a New Jersey woman who lingered in a **coma** for 10 years after drinking alcohol mixed with a small amount of Valium and Librium, the medical and legal communities devised the advance directive. An advance directive allows a person—before he or she enters surgery or even before falling ill—to make his or her wishes regarding life-sustaining care known. The durable power of attorney for health care (DPAHC) is one form of an advance directive. The other is the **living will**.

The two types of advance directive are similar in that, as stated, they allow a person to tell his or her doctor and family what kind of care they want to have and what measures they would consider too extreme. For example, a termanilly ill **cancer** patient may not want his doctor or hospice nurses to administer **cardiopulmonary resuscitation** (CPR) if he goes into cardiac arrest. He could use either the living will or the durable power of attorney to inform his caregivers and his family.

However, by using the durable power of attorney for health care, this cancer patient could go beyond just stating his wishes: he can name someone he trusts to make medical decisions for him if he becomes unable to do so for himself. This decision-maker—usually a spouse, adult child, or a sibling—is called the ''agent.'' Should the cancer patient unexpectedly fall into a coma, for example, the agent would advise the patient's caregivers about what to do for him—whether he would want to be maintained on a respirator, for example, or receive nourishment through a feeding tube.

The durable power of attorney for health care is more thorough and more flexible than the living will. The living will allows the patient to state the action to be taken in specific cases; however, if the unexpected occurs, the living will does not cover it and the caregivers and family are left to guess at what to do. By naming an agent, the patient will be sure that someone will act on his or her behalf even in the most unexpected of cases—if a stroke leaves the person unable to talk or walk, for example, or on life support with dim prospects for recovery.

The key for making this agent-patient relationship work, of course, is for the patient to discuss his or her thoughts and feelings about extraordinary lifesaving measures with the agent. Among the questions the patient first needs to ask him- or herself, and then talk over with the selected agent, are:

- How important is it for me, in terms of quality of life, to be able to communicate?
- Does quality of life, for me, mean being kept alive on a respirator, or fed through a feeding tube?
- How important is it for me to be able to feed myself, bathe myself, or dress myself? Would I be willing to accept help with these everyday tasks?
- Would I be willing to live with a **colostomy**, or a **pacemaker**?
- Does quality of life, for me, mean being in touch with reality?

Of course, there are many other aspects of care to consider, and for information it's best for a patient to turn to his or her doctor. Like most people, doctors find it uncomfortable to bring up the subject of **death**, and a survey of physicians showed that many physicians won't mention advance directives until the patient brings them up. However, discussing and preparing a durable power of attorney for health care doesn't mean that you'll soon be needing it, despite what supersition might say!

Doctors' offices and hospitals can provide forms on which to base a durable power of attorney for health care, and computer programs that include personal legal forms may also include a form to use for a DPAHC. It may also be worthwhile to speak to an attorney, although the DPAHC is not a complicated document to create.

The agent should understand that this document gives him or her influence only over medical decisions; financial or other legal issues are outside of its scope.

DE DUVÉ, CHRISTIAN (1917-)

English Belgian biochemist and cell biologist

Christian René de Duvé's ground-breaking studies of cellular structure and function earned him the 1974 Nobel Prize in physiology or medicine (shared with **Albert Claude** and **George Palade**). His discovery of the two key cellular organelles—lysosomes and peroxisomes—earned him an honor from the Swedish Academy. This work, along with that of his fellow recipients, established the field of cell biology. De Duvé introduced techniques that have enabled other scientists to better study cellular anatomy and physiology and his research has also been of great value in helping clarify the causes of and treatments for a number of diseases.

Christian René de Duvé was born on October 2, 1917 in England after his parents, Alphonse and Madeleine (Pungs) de Duvé, fled Belgium after the German army invaded it during World War I. De Duvé returned with his parents to Belgium in 1920, where they settled in Antwerp. (De Duvé later became a Belgian citizen.) In 1934, intending to become a physician, de Duvé entered the medical school of the Catholic University of Louvain.

De Duvé joined J. P. Bouckaert's group, where he studied physiology, concentrating on the hormone insulin and its effects on uptake of the sugar glucose. De Duvé's experiences in Bouckaert's laboratory convinced him to pursue a research career when he graduated with an M.D. in 1941. During World War II De Duvé spent time in a prison camp, but managed to escape and returned to Louvain to resume his investigations of insulin. Before obtaining his Ph.D. from the Catholic University of Louvain in 1945, de Duvé published several works, including a 400-page book on glucose, insulin, and **diabetes**. The dissertation topic for his *Agrégé de l'Enseignement Supérieur* was also insulin. De Duvé then obtained an M.Sc. degree in chemistry in 1946.

After graduation, de Duvé studied with **Hugo Theorell** at the Medical Nobel Institute in Stockholm for 18 months, then spent six months with **Carl Ferdinand Cori**, **Gerty Cori**, and **Earl Sutherland** at Washington University School of Medicine in St. Louis. Thus, in his early postdoctoral years he worked closely with no less than four future Nobel Prize winners. De Duvé returned to Louvain in 1947 to take up a faculty post at his alma mater teaching physiological chemistry at the medical school. In 1951, de Duvé was appointed full professor of biochemistry. As he began his faculty career, de Duvé's research was targeted at unraveling the mechanism of action of the anti-diabetic hormone, insulin and his early experiments opened new avenues of research.

As a consequence of investigating how insulin works in the human body, de Duvé and his students also studied the enzymes involved in carbohydrate metabolism in the liver. Duvé separated liver cell components by spinning them in a centrifuge, a machine that rotates at high speed. De Duvé assumed that particular enzymes are associated with particular parts of the cell. These parts, called cellular organelles (little organs) can be seen in the microscope as variously shaped and sized grains and particles within the body of cells. It had long been recognized that there existed several discrete types of these organelles, though little was known about their structures or functions at the time.

Using a technique called differential centrifugation, developed some years earlier by fellow-Belgian Albert Claude at the Rockefeller Institute for Medical Research, in which cells are ground up slightly by hand prior to being spun to separate various components, de Duvé got better separation of liver cell organelles, and was able to isolate certain enzymes to certain cell fractions. One of his first findings was that his target enzyme, glucose–6-phosphatase, associated with the cellular organelles, microsomes, were the site of key cellular metabolic events. This was the first time a particular enzyme had been clearly associated with a particular organelle.

De Duvé and his students also applied the differential centrifugation technique to the enzyme acid phosphatase, which in cells acts to remove phosphate groups from sugar molecules under acidic conditions. He and his students observed that the cell fraction initially showed a lower level of enzyme than expected, but when allowed to sit in the refrigerator for several days, the enzyme activity increased to expected levels. This phenomenon became known as enzyme latency.

De Duvé found an organelle devoted to cellular digestion. With this research, de Duvé identified lysosomes and elucidated their pivotal role in cellular digestive and metabolic processes. Later research in de Duvé's laboratory showed that lysosomes play critical roles in a number of disease processes as well.

De Duvé eventually uncovered more associations between enzymes and organelles. His research on monoamine oxidase showed that the enzyme was associated with a separate cellular organelle, the peroxisome. Further investigation led to more discoveries about this previously unknown organelle. It was discovered that peroxisomes contain enzymes that use oxygen to break up certain types of molecules. They are vital to neutralizing many toxic substances, such as alcohol, and play key roles in sugar **metabolism**.

Using the technique that he had used in these early experiments, de Duvé pioneered its use to answer questions of both basic biological interest and immense medical application. His group discovered that certain diseases result from cells' inability to properly digest their own waste products. Disorders of glycogen storage, including **Tay-Sachs disease**, result from malfunctioning lysosomal enzymes.

In 1962 de Duvé joined the Rockefeller Institute (now Rockefeller University) while keeping his appointment at Louvain. Working with research groups at both institutions, he has studied inflammatory diseases such as arthritis and arteriosclerosis, genetic diseases, immune dysfunctions, tropical maladies, and cancers, leading to the creation of new drugs used in combatting some of these conditions. In 1971 de Duvé formed the International Institute of Cellular and Molecular Pathology, affiliated with the University at Louvain. Research at the institute focuses on incorporating the findings from basic cellular research into practical applications.

De Duvé helped found the American Society for Cell Biology. He has received awards and honors from many countries, including more than a dozen honorary degrees. In 1974, de Duvé, along with Albert Claude and George Palade, both also of the Rockefeller Institute, received the Nobel Prize in physiology or medicine, and were credited with creating the discipline of scientific investigation that became known as cell biology. De Duvé was elected a foreign associate of the United States National Academy of Sciences in 1975, and has been acclaimed by Belgian, French, and British biochemical societies. He has also served as a member of numerous prestigious biomedical and health-related organizations around the globe.

Dwarfism

The condition of being abnormally short or small, dwarfism has numerous causes. Some of these are hereditary, but all concern hormone disturbances, bone or deficiency diseases, and/or organ dysfunction. Two ailments—achondroplasia and pituitary dwarfism—are the most common causes of dwarfism.

Achondroplasia is a condition in which the development of cartilage, and therefore bone, is disturbed. The disorder appears in approximately one in every 10,000 births. The bones (especially those in the limbs) do not grow as long as they should, and simultaneously become abnormally thick. The bones in the trunk of the body and the skull are mostly unaffected, although the skull opening through which the spinal cord passes (foramen magnum) is often narrower than normal, and the opening through which the spinal cord runs (spinal canal) becomes abnormally small as it goes down the length of the spine.

Achondroplasia is caused by a genetic defect. It is a dominant trait, so anybody with the genetic defect will display all the symptoms of the disorder. A parent with it has a 50% chance of passing achondroplasia on to his or her child. Although the disorder can also be passed on to that child's offspring, the majority of cases occur due to a new mutation (change) in a gene. Interestingly, the defect caused by achondroplasia is one of only a few that are known to become more frequent as the father ages. (Many genetic defects are linked to the mother's increasing age.)

People with achondroplasia have abnormally short arms and legs, although because their torsos and heads are usually of normal size, their heads appear to be too big. The bridge of the nose often has a scooped-out appearance due to a characteristic trait called "saddle nose," while the lower back is overly curved, producing "sway back." The face of a dwarf often displays an excessively prominent forehead and a relatively undeveloped upper-jaw area. Because the foramen magnum and spinal canal are too narrow, nerve damage may occur if these openings become compressed. The narrowed foramen magnum may also disrupt the normal flow of fluid between the brain and the spinal cord, resulting in **hydrocephalus** (the accumulation of too much fluid in the brain). Children with achondroplasia have a very high risk of serious and repeated middle-ear infections, which can result in **hearing loss** if left untreated. The disorder does not affect either mental capacity or reproductive ability.

As of the late 1990s, there is no treatment to reverse the defect present in achondroplasia, and the only form of prevention is through **genetic counseling**, which could help parents assess their risk of having a child with achondroplasia. Treatment primarily addresses some of the complications of the disorder, including problems due to nerve compression, hydrocephalus, bowed legs, and abnormal curves in the spine. However, most dwarves enjoy good health and can have a normal lifespan.

The other main cause of dwarfism, pituitary dwarfism, is a rare condition of growth retardation characterized by patients who are very short in stature but have normal body proportions (unlike the achondroplasic dwarves). Thus, they are sometimes referred to as "proportionate dwarves." Some children with this condition go through delayed but normal **puberty** and have normal reproductive capabilities, while others never become sexually mature.

In most cases where children fail to attain a normal height, it is not possible to identify a specific pituitary or genetic disorder. Children born with **cleft palate**s or who suffer serious head trauma, severe environmental deprivation, tumors of the pituitary gland, or brain infections or bleeding are all more likely to have pituitary dwarfism. Endocrinologists (doctors who specialize in the functioning of hormones) have the most experience in diagnosing and treating this disorder.

Pituitary dwarfism is caused by a dysfunction of the pituitary gland, a pea-sized mass of tissue at the base of the brain that has two sections (anterior and posterior). Each of these secretes hormones essential for regulating the body's processes, including growth. Pituitary dwarfism occurs only in children. (Low hormonal output from the pituitary in adults produces different disorders.)

There are two categories of pituitary dwarfism. The first is panhypopituitarism, which is caused by a deficit of all the anterior pituitary hormones. These patients, who account for about two-thirds of pituitary dwarfism cases, have generalized slow growth and do not go through puberty. They also have many other medical disorders, including problems in metabolic regulation and water balance and failure to develop secondary sexual characteristics.

The second category involves an isolated deficiency of growth hormone (GH), which accounts for about one-third of cases. These patients do mature sexually and may reproduce. When there is a deficit of only GH, children grow very slowly and reach sexual maturity long after their peers. These children are below the third percentile in height, and their rate of growth is less than 1.5 in (4 cm) per year. GH deficiency is hereditary in about 10% of pituitary dwarfism cases. Pituitary dwarfism with sexual maturity has been linked to an inherited recessive gene.

Untreated pituitary dwarfs who lack multiple pituitary hormones often die. The success of multiple **hormone replacement therapy** depends on which hormones are absent, the severity of the deficit, and the age at which replacement begins. Treatment becomes a complex balancing act in which combinations of GH and the other missing hormones are replaced. As the child grows, the dosages of replacement hormones are frequently changed to reflect his or her changing metabolic state.

Treatment for GH-only pituitary dwarfism focuses on replacement GH therapy for children with documented GH deficiency. (This therapy must be started early, while the long bones can still grow. For this reason, replacement GH therapy is ineffective in adults.) The long-term effectiveness of GH replacement therapy is still being studied. Research in this area continues, and gene replacement therapy may be a possible solution for some forms of pituitary dwarfism.

DYSLEXIA

Dyslexia is a **learning disability** characterized by problems in reading, spelling, writing, speaking, or listening. In many cases, dyslexia appears to be inherited.

The word "dyslexia" is derived from the Greek word, "dys" (meaning poor or inadequate) and the word "lexis" (meaning words or language).

Dyslexia is not a disease, but describes rather a different kind of mind that learns in a different way from other people. Many people with the condition are gifted and very productive; dyslexia is not at all linked to low intelligence. In fact, intelligence has nothing to do with dyslexia.

The **National Institutes of Health** estimates that about 15% of the U.S. population is affected by learning disabilities, mostly with problems in language and reading. The condition appears in all ages, races and income levels.

The underlying cause of dyslexia is not known, although research suggests the condition is often inherited. New research suggests a possible link with a subtle visual problem that affects the speed with which affected people can read.

Other experts believe that dyslexia is related to differences in the structure and function of the brain that manifests differently in different people.

In any case, research suggests that dyslexic children seem to have trouble learning early reading skills, problems hearing individual sounds in words, analyzing whole words in parts, and blending sounds into words. Letters such as "d" and "b" may be confused.

When a person is dyslexic, there is often an unexpected difference between achievement and aptitude. However, each person with dyslexia has different strengths and weaknesses, although many have unusual talents in art, athletics, architecture, graphics, drama, music or engineering. These special talents are often in areas that require the ability to integrate sight, spatial skills and coordination.

Often, a person with dyslexia has a problem translating language into thought (such as in listening or reading), or translating thought into language (such as in writing or speaking).

Common symptoms include problems with:

- Identifying single words
- Understanding sounds in words, sound order, or rhymes
- Spelling
- Transposing letters in words
- Handwriting
- Reading comprehension
- Delayed spoken language
- Confusion with directions, or right/left handedness
- Confusion with up/down, early/late, and so on
- Mathematics.

Anyone who is suspected to have dyslexia should have a comprehensive evaluation, including hearing, vision and intelligence testing. The test should include all areas of learning and learning processes, not just reading.

Unfortunately, in many schools, a child is not identified as having dyslexia until after repeated failures.

If a child is diagnosed with dyslexia, the parents should find out from the school or the diagnostician exactly what the problem is, what method of teaching is recommended and why. No single method will work with every child, and experts often disagree as to the best method to use.

The primary focus of treatment is aimed at helping the specific learning problem of each affected person. Most often, this may include modifying teaching methods and the educational environment, since traditional educational methods will not always work with a dyslexic child.

People with dyslexia need a structured language program, with direct instruction in the letter-sound system. Teachers must give the rules governing written language. Most experts agree that the teacher should emphasize the association between simple phonetic units with letters or letter groups, rather than an approach that stresses memorizing whole words.

It is important to teach these students using all the senses: hearing, touching, writing and speaking, provided by an instructor who is specifically trained in a program which is effective for dyslexic students.

Many successful and even famous people have dyslexia. How well a person with dyslexia functions in life depends on the way the disability affects that person. There is a great deal of variation among different people with dyslexia, producing different symptoms and different degrees of severity.

Prognosis is usually good if the condition is diagnosed early, and if the person has a strong self image with supportive family, friends and teachers. It is imperative for a good outcome that the person be involved in a good remedial program.

See also Language development

Dyspepsia

Dyspepsia is basically a chronic upset stomach—painful, difficult, or disturbed digestion that might be accompanied by symptoms such as **nausea and vomiting**, **heartburn**, bloating, or stomach discomfort.

This digestive problem may have an identifiable cause, such as bacterial or viral infection, peptic ulcer, gallbladder, or **liver disease**. The bacteria *Helicobacter pylori* is often present in individuals suffering from duodenal or gastric **ulcers**. Investigation of recurrent **indigestion** should rule out these possible causes.

Often, there is no organic cause for dyspepsia, in which case it is classified as functional or nonulcer dyspepsia. There is evidence that functional dyspepsia may be related to a state known as dysmotility, in which the esophagus, stomach, and upper intestine contract spontaneously. These patients may respond to a group of drugs called prokinate agents.

In terms of external causes, a review of the patient's eating habits (e.g. chewing with the mouth open, gulping food, or talking while chewing) could reveal a tendency to swallow air. This may contribute to feeling bloated or excessive belching or gas. **Smoking**, **caffeine**, alcohol, or carbonated beverages sometimes contribute to the discomfort. Sensitivity or allergy to certain food substances may cause gastrointestinal distress, while some medications are associated with indigestion. In addition, stomach problems may also be a response to **stress** or emotional unrest.

Treatment of dyspepsia might begin with a **physical examination** to rule out internal bleeding. If blood is found through a rectal exam, laboratory studies, including a **blood count**, may be ordered. A physician might also order upper-gastrointestinal **x-ray studies** using barium so he or she can see any abnormalities. Endoscopy, a technology for examining the inside of body cavities, permits collection of tissue and culture specimens that could help reach a diagnosis.

The treatment of dyspepsia is based on assessing symptoms and suspected causes. Clinical evaluation is aimed at distinguishing those patients who require immediate testing from those who can safely benefit from more conservative initial treatment. Some of the latter may require only reassurance, dietary modifications, or antacid use. Medications to block production of stomach acids, prokinate agents, or antibiotic treatment might be in order. However, further diagnostic investigation is necessary if there is severe abdominal pain, pain radiating to the back, unexplained weight loss, difficulty swallowing, a palpable mass, or anemia. Additional testing is also required if a patient does not respond to prescribed medications.

Typically, about half of patients with dyspepsia will be found to have either duodenal/gastric ulcer disease or **irritable bowel syndrome**. Very few are shown to have **cancer**. Meanwhile, many people suffering from functional dyspepsia are found to have **gastritis**.

E

E. COLI 0157:H7 INFECTION

Enterohemorrhagic *E. coli* is one of several intestinal types of *E. coli* that infect animals and humans. The O157:H7 strain is the member of the group most often associated with a particularly severe form of **diarrhea** and the most common cause of a unique, sometimes fatal syndrome (hemolytic-uremic syndrome [HUS]) that causes **kidney failure** (although this happens mainly in the very young and old). The bacteria was discovered in 1977, and first reports of infections followed in 1982.

E. coli accounts for about 2% of all cases of diarrhea in the Western world and at least one-third of cases of hemorrhagic colitis, a potentially deadly inflammation of the colon. The bacteria also accounts for the majority of episodes of HUS, especially in children. Ten percent of individuals with *E. coli* O157:H7 infection develop HUS; 5% of those will die of the disease. Some who recover from HUS will be left with kidney damage.

The bacteria produces toxins that are lethal for intestinal cells and also damage the linings of blood vessels. Experts believe that this damage to blood vessels results in the formation of clots, which eventually leads to HUS. After an incubation period of about 3-4 days, watery diarrhea begins. This rapidly progresses to bloody diarrhea in many victims, in which case the bowel movement may be mostly blood. **Nausea and vomiting**, along with low-grade **fever**, are also frequently present. Gastrointestinal symptoms last for about one week, and recovery is often spontaneous.

When a patient complains of bloody diarrhea, **stool culture**s can tentatively identify the bacteria. Further tests at specialized laboratories are usually needed, however, for confirmation of infection. Unfortunately, cultures are often negative or inconclusive if they are collected past 48 hours of the onset of symptoms.

Uncomplicated cases of the infection usually clear up within ten days. It is uncertain whether **antibiotics** are helpful in treating *E. coli* O157:H7, and there is some evidence that they may actually be harmful. **Dehydration** resulting from diarrhea must be treated. Antimotility agents, which decrease the intestines' ability to contract, should not be used in any patient with bloody diarrhea.

E. coli O157:H7 is commonly found in cattle and poultry. Reports of apple cider contamination have occurred. Contaminated hamburger meat has been the most common source of infection, but other sources exist. Human-to-human transmission, mainly through contact with fecal matter, has also been identified in daycare centers.

Thorough cooking of all meat and poultry products and adhering to proper food preparation practices is the most effective way to avoid infection. Food irradiation methods are also being developed to sanitize food.

EAR

The human ear is the anatomical structure responsible for hearing and balance. The ear consists of three parts, the outer, middle, and inner ears.

The outer ear collects sounds from the environment and funnels them through the auditory system. The outer ear is composed of three parts, the pinna (or auricle), the external auditory canal (or external auditory meatus), and the tympanic membrane (or eardrum).

The two flap-like structures on either side of the head commonly called ears are actually the pinnas of the outer ear. Pinnas are skin-covered cartilage, not bone, and are therefore flexible. The lowest portion of the pinna is called the lobe or lobule and is the most likely site for earrings. The pinnas of most humans cannot move, but these structures are very mobile in other mammals, such as cats and dogs.

The external auditory canal is a passageway in the temporal lobe of the skull that begins at the ear and extends inward and slightly upwards. In the adult human it is lined with skin and hairs and is approximately one inch (2.5 cm) long.

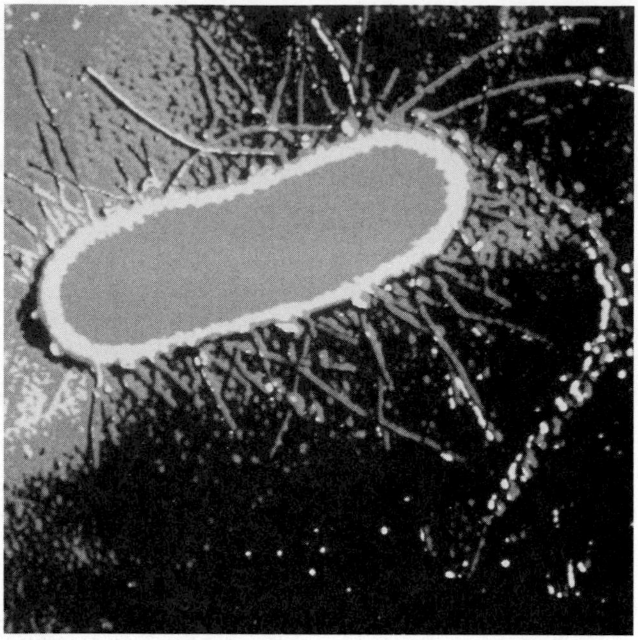

A photo of the *E. coli* bacterium.

The outer 1/3 portion of the canal is lined with a membrane containing ceruminous (ear wax producing) cells and hair cells. The purpose of the cerumen and hairs is to protect the eardrum (which lies at the end of the canal) by trapping dirt and foreign bodies and keeping the canal moist. In most individuals, cleaning of the external auditory canal (with Q-tips for example) is not needed. The inner portion of the external auditory canal contains no glands or hair cells.

The human tympanic membrane or eardrum is a thin, concave membrane stretched across the inner end of the external auditory canal much like the skin covering the top of a drum. The eardrum marks the border between the outer ear and middle ear. The eardrum serves as a transmitter of sound by vibrating in response to sounds traveling down the external auditory canal; it begins sound conduction in the middle ear.

In the adult human, the tympanic membrane has a total area of approximately 63 square mm. It consists of three layers that contribute to the membrane's ability to vibrate while maintaining a protective thickness. The middle point of the tympanic membrane (the umbo) is attached to the stirrup, the first of three bones contained within the middle ear.

The middle ear transmits sound from the outer ear to the inner ear. The middle ear consists of an oval, air-filled space approximately 2 cubic cm in volume. The middle ear can be thought of as a room, the outer wall of which contains the tympanic membrane. The back wall, separating the middle ear from the inner ear, has two windows, the oval window and the round window. There is a long hallway leading away from the side wall of the room, known as the eustachian tube. The brain lies above the room and the jugular vein lies below. The middle ear is lined entirely with mucous membrane (similar to the nose) and is surrounded by the bones of the skull.

The eustachian tube connects the middle ear to the nasopharynx. This tube is normally closed, opening only as a result of muscle movement during yawning, sneezing, or swallowing. The eustachian tube allows for air pressure equalization, permitting the air pressure in the middle ear to match the air pressure in the outer ear. The most noticeable example of eustachian tube function occurs when there is a quick change in altitude, such as when a plane takes off. Prior to takeoff, the pressure in the outer ear is equal to the pressure in the middle ear. When the plane gains altitude, the air pressure in the outer ear decreases, while the pressure in the middle ear remains the same, causing the ear to feel ''plugged.'' In response to this the ear may ''pop.'' The popping sensation is actually the quick opening and closing of the eustachian tube, and the equalization of pressure between the outer and middle ear.

Three tiny bones (the ossicles) in the middle ear form a chain that conducts sound waves from the tympanic membrane (outer ear) to the oval window (inner ear). The three bones are the hammer (malleus), the anvil (incus), and the stirrup (stapes). These bones are connected and move as a link chain might, causing pressure at the oval window and the transmission of energy from the middle ear to the inner ear. Sound waves cause the tympanic membrane to vibrate, which sets up vibrations in the ossicles, which amplify the sounds and transmit them to the inner ear via the oval window. In addition to bones, the middle ear houses the two muscles, the stapedius and the tensor tympani, which respond reflexively (that is, without conscious control) to sounds.

The inner ear is responsible for interpreting and transmitting sound (auditory) sensations and balance (vestibular) sensations to the brain. The inner ear is small (about the size of a pea) and complex in shape; its series of winding interconnected chambers has been compared to (and called) a labyrinth. The main components of the inner ear are the vestibule, semicircular canals, and the cochlea.

The vestibule, a round open space that accesses various passageways, is the central structure within the inner ear. The outer wall of the vestibule contains the oval and round windows (which are the connection sites between the middle and inner ear). Internally, the vestibule contains two membranous sacs, the utricle and the saccule, which are lined with tiny hair cells and attached to nerve fibers, and which serve as the vestibular (balance/equilibrium) sense organs.

Attached to the utricle within the vestibular portion of the inner ear are three loop-shaped, fluid filled tubes called the semicircular canals. The semicircular canals are named according to their location (''lateral,'' ''superior,'' and ''posterior'') and are arranged perpendicularly to each other, like the floor and two corner walls of a box. The semicircular canals are a key part of the vestibular system and allow for maintenance of balance when the head or body rotates.

The cochlea is the site of the sense organs for hearing. The cochlea consists of a bony, snail-like shell that contains three separate fluid-filled ducts or canals. The upper canal, the scala vestibuli, begins at the oval window; the lower canal, the scala tympani, begins at the round window. Between the two canals lies the third canal, the scala media. The scala media is separated from the scala vestibuli by Reissner's membrane and from the scala tympani by the basilar membrane. The scala media contains the organ of Corti, (named after the 19th-century anatomist who first described it). The organ of Corti lies along the entire length of the basilar membrane. The organ contains hair cells and is the site of the conversion of sound waves into nerve impulses, which are sent to the brain for auditory interpretation along Cranial Nerve VIII, also known as the Auditory Nerve.

See also Hearing aids and cochlear implants; Hearing loss; Hearing tests

EAR EXAM WITH AN OTOSCOPE

Used to examine the ear canal and the eardrum, an otoscope is a hand-held instrument with a tiny light and a cone-shaped attachment called an ear speculum. An ear examination is a normal part of most **physical examinations** by a doctor or nurse. It is also done when an ear infection or other type of ear problem is suspected due to **fever**, ear pain, or **hearing loss**.

Some otoscopes blow a small puff of air at the eardrum to see if it will vibrate (a normal response). This type of ear examination with an otoscope can also detect a buildup of wax in the ear canal, or a rupture or puncture of the eardrum.

Prior to an otoscope exam, the patient will often be asked to tip his or her head slightly toward the shoulder so the ear to be examined is pointing up. The doctor or nurse may hold the ear lobe as the speculum is inserted into the ear, and may adjust the position of the otoscope to get a better view of the ear canal and eardrum. Both ears are usually examined, even if there seems to be a problem with just one ear.

The ear canal is normally skin-colored and covered with tiny hairs. A healthy eardrum is usually thin, shiny, and pearly-white to light gray in color. However, an ear infection will cause the eardrum to look red and swollen. In cases where the eardrum has ruptured, there may be fluid draining from the middle ear. A doctor may also see scarring, retraction of the eardrum, or bulging of the eardrum, indicating damage to this delicate structure.

If an ear infection is present, the patient may require treatment with **antibiotics**. If there is a buildup of wax in the ear canal, it might be rinsed or scraped out with special instruments. (It is normal for the ear canal to have some yellowish-brown wax, however.)

EAR INFECTIONS

Otitis externa, a common ear infection, refers to an infection of the ear canal, or the tube leading from the outside opening of the ear in toward the ear drum. The external ear canal is a tube approximately 1 in (2.5 cm) in length. It runs from the outside opening of the ear to the start of the middle ear, designated by the ear drum or tympanic membrane. The canal is partly cartilage and partly bone. In early childhood, the first two-thirds of the canal is made of cartilage, and the last one-third is made of bone. By late childhood, and lasting throughout all of adulthood, this proportion is reversed. The lining of the ear canal is skin, which is attached directly to the covering of the bone. Glands within the skin of the canal produce a waxy substance called cerumen (popularly called earwax). Cerumen is designed to protect the ear canal, repel water, and keep the ear canal too acidic to allow bacteria to grow.

Bacteria, fungi, and viruses have all been implicated in causing ear infections called otitis externa. The most common cause of otitis externa is bacterial infection. Occasionally, fungi may cause otitis externa, and two types of viruses have also been identified as causes.

Otitis externa occurs most often in the summer months, when people are frequenting swimming pools and lakes. Continually exposing the ear canal to moisture may cause significant loss of cerumen. The delicate skin of the ear canal, unprotected by cerumen, retains moisture and becomes irritated. Without cerumen, the ear canal stops being appropriately acidic, which allows bacteria to multiply.

Other conditions predisposing to otitis externa include the use of cotton swabs to clean the ear canals. This pushes cerumen and normal skin debris back into the ear canal, instead of allowing the ear canal's normal cleaning mechanism to work, which would ordinarily move accumulations of cerumen and debris out of the ear. Also, putting other items into the ear can scratch the canal, making it more susceptible to infection.

The first symptom of otitis externa is often **itching** of the ear canal. Eventually, the ear begins to feel extremely painful. Any touch, movement, or pressure on the outside structure of the ear (auricle) may cause quite severe pain. If the canal is sufficiently swollen, hearing may become muffled. The canal may appear swollen and red, and there may be evidence of greenish-yellow pus.

In severe cases, otitis externa may have an accompanying **fever**. Often, this indicates that the outside ear structure (auricle) has become infected as well. It will become red and swollen, and there may be enlarged and tender lymph nodes in front of, or behind, the auricle.

A serious and life-threatening otitis externa is called malignant otitis externa. This is an infection which most commonly affects patients who have diabetes, especially the elderly. It can also occur in other patients who have weakened immune systems. In malignant otitis externa, a patient has usually had minor symptoms of otitis externa for some months, with pain and drainage. The causative bacteria is usually *Pseudomonas aeruginosa*. In malignant otitis externa, this bacteria spreads from the external canal into all of the nearby tissues, including the bones of the skull. Swelling and destruction of these tissues may lead to damage of certain nerves, resulting in spasms of the jaw muscles or **paralysis** of the facial muscles. Other, more severe, complications of this very destructive infection include **meningitis** (swelling and infection of the coverings of the spinal cord and brain), brain infection, or brain abscess (the development of a pocket of infection with pus).

Diagnosis of uncomplicated otitis externa is usually quite simple. The symptoms alone, of ear pain worsened by any touch to the auricle, are characteristic. Attempts to examine the ear canal will usually reveal redness and swelling. It may be impossible (due to pain and swelling) to see much of the ear canal, but this inability itself is diagnostic.

If there is any confusion about the types of organisms causing otitis externa, the canal can be gently swabbed to obtain a specimen. The organisms present in the specimen can then be cultured (allowed to multiply) in a laboratory, and then viewed under a microscope to allow identification.

If the rare disease malignant otitis externa is suspected, **computed tomography scans** (CT scans) or **magnetic resonance imaging** (MRI) scans will be performed to determine how widely the infection has spread within bone and tissue. A swab of the external canal will not necessarily reveal the actual causative organism, so some other tissue sample (**biopsy**) will need to be obtained. The CT or MRI will help the practitioner decide where the most severe focus of infection is located, in order to guide the choice of a biopsy site.

Antibiotics which can be applied directly to the skin of the ear canal (topical antibiotics) are usually excellent for treatment of otitis externa. These are often combined in a preparation which includes a steroid medication. The steroid helps cut down on the inflammation and swelling within the ear canal. Some practitioners prefer to insert a cotton wick into the ear canal, leaving it there for about 48 hours. The medications are applied directly to the wick, enough times per day to allow the wick to remain continuously saturated. After the wick is removed, the medications are then put directly into the ear canal three to four times each day.

In malignant otitis externa, antibiotics will almost always need to be given through a needle in the vein (intravenously or IV). If the CT or MRI scan reveals that the infection has spread extensively, these IV antibiotics will need to be continued for six to eight weeks. If the infection is in an earlier stage, two weeks of IV antibiotics can be followed by six weeks of antibiotics by mouth.

The prognosis is excellent for otitis externa. It is usually easily treated, although it may tend to recur in certain susceptible individuals. Left untreated, malignant otitis externa may spread sufficiently to cause **death**.

Keeping the ear dry is an important aspect of prevention of otitis externa. Several drops of a mixture of alcohol and acetic acid can be put into the ear canal after swimming to insure that it dries adequately.

The most serious complications of malignant otitis externa can be avoided by careful attention to early symptoms of ear pain and drainage from the ear canal. Patients with conditions that put them at higher risk for this infection (diabetes, conditions which weaken the immune system) should always report new symptoms immediately.

EATING DISORDERS

Eating disorders, one of the most difficult **mental illnesses** to diagnose and cure, are divided into three categories: *anorexia nervosa, bulimia nervosa,* and *binge eating*. Frequently, sufferers flatly deny they have a problem, and treatment by doctors and psychiatrists produces little success. There appears to be a connection between anorexia and bulimia, and affective disorders (depression). Thus, **antidepressants** are often used in treating eating disorders. In February 1998, researchers identified a pair of hormones which influence eating habits in rats. These hormones—*orexin A* and *orexin B*, bind to two receptors in the lateral hypothalamus, the region of the brain believed to regulate appetite. Whether these hormones produce a similar activity in humans is yet unknown; however, researchers appear optimistic that the development of drugs imitating these hormones may aid in the treatment of eating disorders by stimulating or depressing appetite.

The psychological driving force behind anorexia and bulimia has been defined as ''the relentless pursuit of thinness.'' Described in a paper for the first time in 1694 by Richard Morton, *anorexia nervosa*, translated as ''nervous loss of appetite,'' was given its name by Sir William Gull 1870s. The fact is, patients do not usually lose their appetite until the disease is well developed. The anoretic has such an overwhelming need to be thin they virtually starve themselves to death. Diagnosis consists of refusal to hold body weight above 85% of normal based on age and height; an intense fear of gaining weight; the inability to see one's shape or body weight as it truly is; and, in females past the age of puberty, the absence of at least three consecutive menstrual cycles. Unusual behavior displayed by some anoretics include collection of recipes, cooking for others while not eating themselves, hiding food, cutting food into small pieces, obsessively counting calories, avoiding eating in public, and secretly exercising—perhaps for an entire night—so family members can't stop them. A common connection between anoretics is overly-protective or strict parents; excessive dieting may give them a sense of control over their own lives. Anorexia commonly begins between 13 and 30 years, is more prevalent in countries where ''thin is beautiful,'' in the middle and upper classes, and in single females. An increasing number of young males are presenting with the disorder, however. Anorexia is particularly difficult to treat, and sufferers develop serious medical complications. Between five and 18 percent die from **starvation**, cardiac arrest, or **suicide**.

Bulimia—Greek for ''ox-like hunger''—appeared in publications during the 18th century but was not classified as an illness until 1979. In 1987, English psychiatrist Gerald Russell gave it the name Bulimia nervosa. Diagnostic criteria include ''binge'' eating at least twice a week for three months or longer accompanied by frequent ''purging,'' such as induction of vomiting; misuse of **laxatives**, **diuretics** or **enemas**; **fasting**; and excessive **exercise**. Evidence links two brain biochemicals—serotonin and norepinephrine—to the binge/purge cycle, chemicals that have also been identified in depression and other psychological illnesses.

While anorexia and bulimia are separate entities, they have considerable overlap: both occur primarily in adolescents and young adults, are long-running and difficult to treat, interfere with social development, are commonly accompanied by depression and obsessive behaviors, and show a family or personal history of major depression, **obsessive-compulsive disorder**, or **anxiety**. Mood elevators and/or **antidepressants** can be helpful in treatment.

Binge eating is similar to bulimia except purging does not occur. Up to two percent of the population has a serious problem with binge eating, and approximately 30 percent of people in medically-supervised weight control programs are diagnosed as binge eaters. Diagnosis includes recurring episodes of overeating and feelings of loss of control when eating until uncomfortably full. Problems with **obesity** and a history of dramatic weight fluctuations are characteristic, and associated medical problems include high cholesterol, **diabetes**, heart disease, gallbladder disease, and depression. Treatment through psychotherapy and antidepressants affecting serotonin levels can be helpful.

See also Antidepressant drugs; Antidepressants, tricyclic; Depressive disorders; Mental illness

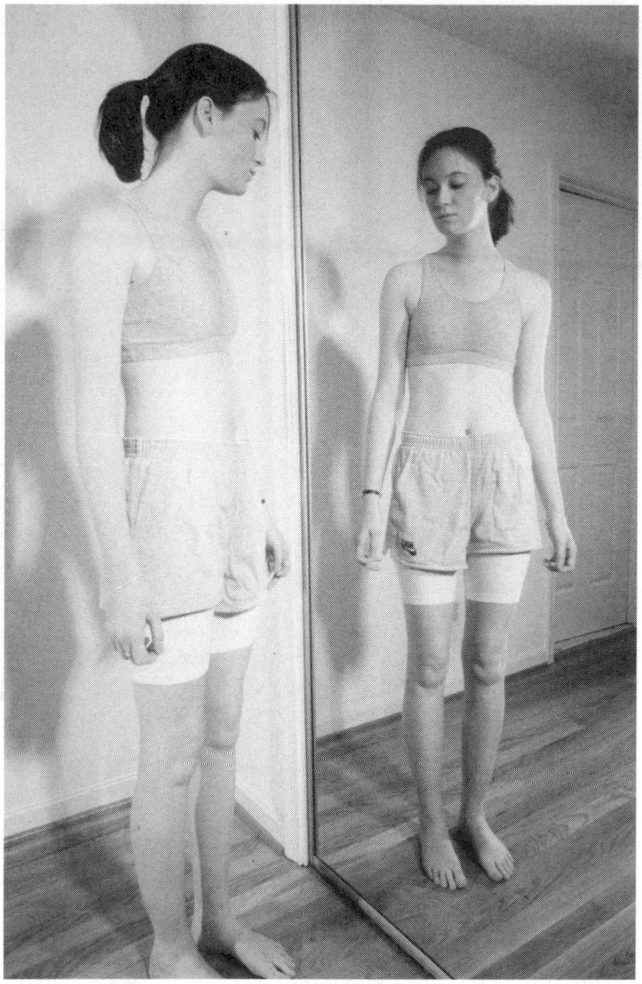

A young woman with an eating disorder.

ECCLES, JOHN CAREW (1903-1997)

Australian neurophysiologist

In 1962, John Carew Eccles was awarded the Nobel Prize for Physiology or Medicine, an award he shared with **Alan Hodgkin** and **Andrew Huxley** for their research in the mechanisms of control and communication between nerve cells.

Born in Melbourne on January 27, 1903, Eccles received his early education from his parents, both of whom were teachers. As a medical student at Melbourne University, he won first-class honors and was also known as an a widely talented athlete in tennis, pole vaulting and cross-country running. Eccles' combined athletic and academic abilities won him a Rhodes Scholarship when he graduated in 1925, allowing him to study under **Charles Scott Sherrington** at Magdalen College, Oxford. There, he became one of Sherrington's research assistants and coauthored eight scientific papers with his superior. His Ph.D. thesis, accepted in 1929, dealt with excitation and inhibition in nerve cells. After receiving his doctorate, Eccles spent 1932–1934 at Exeter College, Oxford.

In 1937 he returned to Australia to head the Kanematsu Memorial Institute of Pathology, a small medical research facility at Sydney Hospital. From 1941–1943, Eccles was a medical adviser for the Australian Army, in charge of collecting and processing blood serum and also working on military issues related to aviation medicine, vision, and hearing. In 1944, he became professor of physiology at the University of Otago in Dunedin, New Zealand. In 1952, Eccles moved again, this time to the Australian National University in Canberra.

Compelled by the University of Canberra policy to retire in 1966, Eccles moved to the United States, where he headed the Institute for Biomedical Research in Evansville, Illinois. In 1968, he switched to State University of New York in Buffalo, where he spent the remainder of his career.

It was at Oxford that Eccles began applying new methods of electrophysiology, which involves the use of electronic amplifiers and cathode-ray oscilloscopes, to study the brief electrical impulses in nerve fibers.

Based on Huxley and Hodgkin's studies on giant squid nerve cells, Eccles demonstrated the ionic mechanisms involved in excitation and inhibition in the peripheral and central portions of the nerve cell membrane. At the time, there was considerable difference of opinion about whether transmission between nerve cells was primarily chemical or electrical in nature. Eccles argued for electrical transmission, although chemical transmission was eventually proven to predominate. His research nonetheless advanced medical knowledge of nervous disorders, heart and kidney disease, and brain function.

Eccles' published books include *The Physiology of Nerve Cells* (1957), *The Physiology of Synapses* (1964), *The Understanding of the Brain* (1973), and *The Human Psyche* (1980).

In addition to his scientific interests in the brain, Eccles developed a broader philosophy of the human person, arguing that the mind and brain are distinct and that consciousness consists of more than just nerve impulses.

Among many awards recognizing his research, Eccles held a few distinguished appointments. He became a knight of the British Empire in 1958. Eccles was president of the Austra-

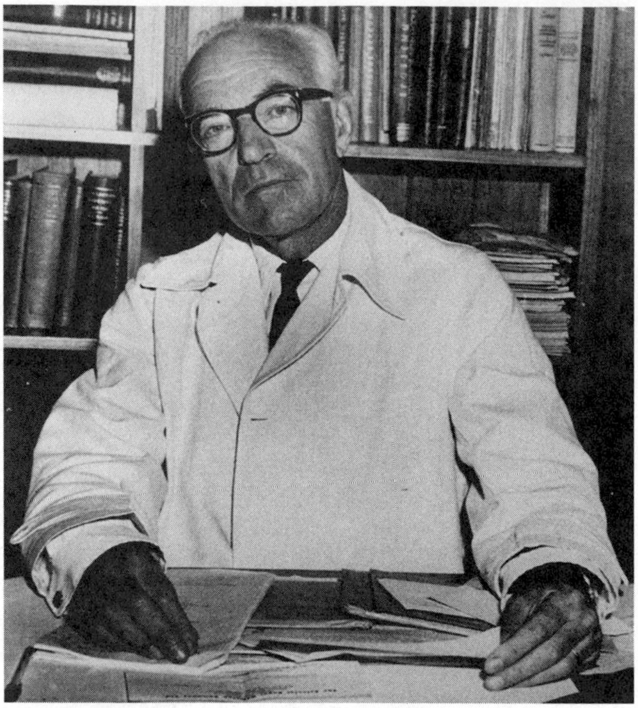
John Carew Eccles

lian Academy of Sciences from 1957 to 1961. He later died in 1997.

ECHOCARDIOGRAPHY

Echocardiography is a diagnostic technique that can provide a wealth of helpful information, including the size and shape of the heart, its pumping strength, and the location and extent of any damage to its tissues. It is especially useful for assessing diseases of the heart valves. Echocardiography can reveal such abnormalities as poorly functioning heart valves or damage to the heart tissue from a past **heart attack**. However, a normal echocardiogram does not rule out the possibility of coronary heart disease.

Echocardiography creates an image of the heart using ultra-high-frequency sound waves that cannot be heard by the human ear. The technique is very similar to the **ultrasound tests** commonly used to see the fetus during **pregnancy**. A big advantage of echocardiography is that it does not involve breaking the skin or probing body cavities and has no known risks or side effects.

Echocardiography is used to diagnose certain cardiovascular diseases. In fact, it is one of the most widely used diagnostic tests for heart disease. By showing the motion of the heart wall, echocardiography can help physicians detect the presence and assess the severity of **coronary artery disease**, as well as help determine whether any chest **pain** is related to heart disease. Echocardiography can also help diagnose hypertrophic cardiomyopathy, in which the walls of the heart thicken to compensate for heart muscle weakness.

An echocardiography examination generally lasts no more than 30 minutes. The transducer, a small, hand-held device at the end of a flexible cable, is placed against the patient's chest. This directs the harmless ultrasound waves into the chest. Some of the waves get echoed (or reflected) back to the transducer. Since different tissues and blood all reflect ultrasound waves differently, the echoed sound waves can be translated into an image of the heart, which the physician can see and evaluate on a monitor.

There a several variations of echocardiogram. One is the Doppler echocardiogram, which can detect abnormalities in the pattern of blood flow, such as the backward flow of blood through partly closed heart valves (''regurgitation''). An **exercise** echocardiogram is performed during physical effort such as walking briskly, when the heart muscle must work harder to supply blood to the body. This allows doctors to detect heart problems that might not be evident when the body is at rest and needs less blood. For patients who are unable to exercise, certain drugs can be used to mimic the effects of exercise by dilating the blood vessels and making the heart beat faster.

ECHOLOCATION • See Spallanzani, Lazzaro

ECTOPIC PREGNANCY

In an ectopic pregnancy, the fertilized egg implants in a location outside the uterus and tries to develop there. The word ''ectopic'' means ''in an abnormal place or position.'' The most common site is the fallopian tube, the tube that normally carries eggs from the ovary to the uterus. However, ectopic pregnancy can also occur in the ovary, the abdomen, and the cervical canal (the opening from the uterus to the vaginal canal). The phrases ''tubal pregnancy,'' ''ovarian pregnancy,'' ''cervical pregnancy,'' and ''abdominal pregnancy'' refer to the specific area of an ectopic pregnancy. More than 95% percent of all ectopic pregnancies occur in the fallopian tube. Only 1.5% develop in the abdomen; less than 1% develop in the ovary or the cervix.

Ectopic pregnancy was first described in the eleventh century and was often a fatal condition until the advent of surgery and blood **transfusion**s in the early twentieth century. The sophisticated diagnostic tools and surgical procedures developed since the 1970s have equipped modern medicine with the tools not to only save a woman's life from this still-deadly condition, but also to preserve her future fertility.

Ectopic pregnancies are the leading cause of pregnancy-related deaths in the first trimester and account for 9% of all pregnancy-related deaths in the United States. More than 1% of pregnancies are ectopic and they are becoming more common. The reason for this increase is not clearly understood, although the dramatic increase in **sexually transmitted diseases** (STD), which can damage the structures required for a normal pregnancy, is at least partly responsible.

Normally, a woman's body produces one egg a month, which is released and travels down the fallopian tube. There it can meet sperm and be fertilized. In a healthy **pregnancy**, the fertilized egg (zygote) continues its passage down the fallopian tube and enters the uterus in three to five days. It continues to grow, implanting itself securely in the wall of the uterus. The zygote's cells develop into the embryo (the organism in its first two months of development) and placenta (a spongy structure that lines the uterus and nourishes the developing organism).

In a tubal ectopic pregnancy, the fertilized egg fails to get all the way down the tube because of scarring or obstruction, so remains in the fallopian tube as it begins growing. Eventually the thin walls of the tube stretch and may burst, resulting in severe bleeding and possibly the **death** of the mother.

As many as 50% of women with ectopic pregnancies have a history of **pelvic inflammatory disease** (PID), an infection of the fallopian tubes that can spread to the uterus or ovaries, but other conditions increase the risk of ectopic pregnancy. These include: **endometriosis**, a benign growth of uterine tissue outside the uterus; exposure to diethylsilbestrol (DES) as a fetus; taking the hormones estrogen and progesterone for birth control or other reasons, which can slow the movement of the fertilized egg down the tube; use of an intrauterine device (**IUD**); and surgery on a fallopian tube. Ectopic pregnancy is also more likely when the ovaries are artificially stimulated with hormones to produce eggs for in vitro fertilization (a procedure in which eggs are taken from a woman's body, fertilized, and then placed in the uterus in an attempt to conceive a child).

In an ectopic pregnancy, all the hormonal changes associated with a normal pregnancy may occur. The early symptoms include: fatigue, nausea, a missed period, breast tenderness, **low back pain**, mild cramping on one side of the pelvis, and abnormal vaginal bleeding (usually spotting). If the fallopian tube has ruptured, blood may irritate the diaphragm and cause shoulder pain. Other warning signs are lightheadedness and **fainting**.

To confirm an early diagnosis of ectopic pregnancy, the doctor must determine first that the patient is pregnant and that the location of the embryo is outside the uterus. If an ectopic pregnancy is suspected, the doctor will perform a pelvic examination, possibly using ultrasound, to locate the source of pain and to detect a mass in the abdomen. After pregnancy is confirmed, several laboratory tests of the patient's blood will provide information for diagnosis. Other tests include a culdocentesis to detect blood from a ruptured tube and a **laparoscopy**, which allows the doctor to see the patient's reproductive organs through a small incision in the abdomen.

Ectopic pregnancy requires immediate treatment. The earlier the condition is treated, the better the chance to preserve the fallopian tube for future normal pregnancies. If the ectopic pregnancy is discovered at less than six weeks, the drug methotrexate may be given to inhibit the growth of rapidly growing cells.

When the pregnancy has already ruptured, a surgical incision into the abdomen, or laparotomy, is performed to stop the immediate loss of blood and to remove the embryo. This usually requires general **anesthesia** and a hospital stay. Every effort is made to preserve and repair the injured fallopian tube. However, if the fallopian tube has already ruptured, repair is extremely difficult and the tube is usually removed.

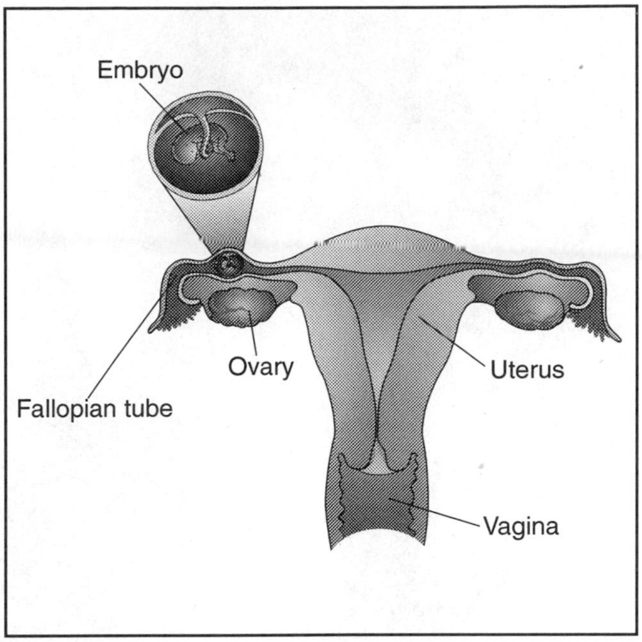

Ectopic pregnancy.

The earlier an ectopic pregnancy is diagnosed and treated, the better the outcome. The chances of having a successful pregnancy are lower after an ectopic pregnancy, but depend on the extent of permanent fallopian tube damage. If the tube has been spared, chances are as high as 60% of having a normal pregnancy. The chances of a successful pregnancy after the removal of one tube are 40%.

In terms of alternative treatments, there are herbal remedies for the temporary relief of the common symptoms of **anxiety** and abdominal discomfort. However, prompt medical treatment is the only sure remedy for ectopic pregnancy.

EDELMAN, GERALD M. (1929-)

American biochemist

Gerald M. Edelman and his associate **Rodney Porter** received the 1972 Nobel Prize in physiology or medicine for their discoveries concerning the chemical structure of antibodies. Edelman used these discoveries to draw conclusions not only about the **immune system** but about the nature of consciousness as well.

Born in New York City on July 1, 1929, to Edward Edelman, a physician, and Anna Freedman Edelman, Gerald Maurice Edelman attended New York City public schools through high school. After graduating, he entered Ursinus College, in Collegeville, Pennsylvania, where he received his B.S. in chemistry in 1950. Four years later, he earned an M.D. de-

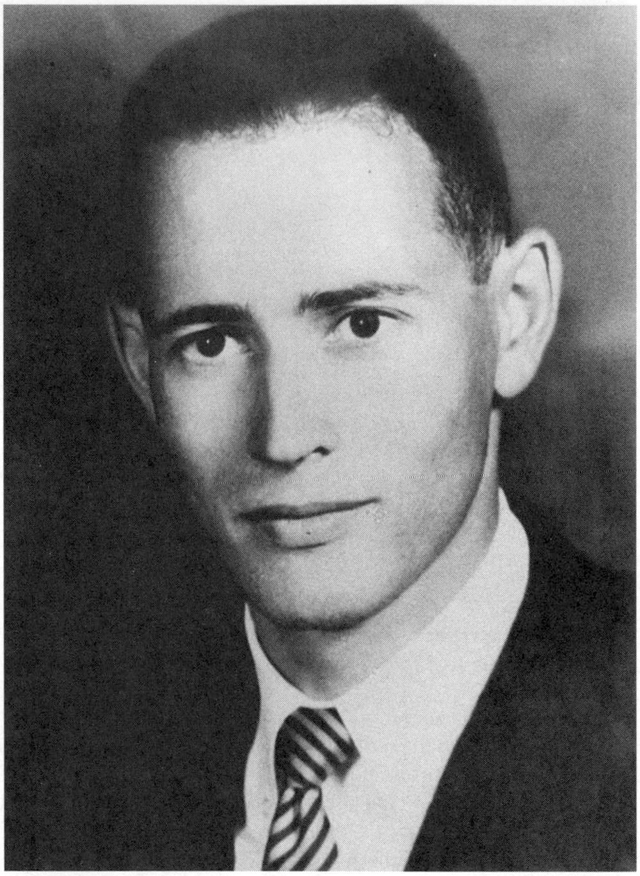

Gerald M. Edelman

gree from the University of Pennsylvania's Medical School, spending a year as medical house officer at Massachusetts General Hospital.

In 1955 Edelman joined the United States Army Medical Corps, practicing general medicine while stationed at a hospital in Paris. Following his 1957 discharge from the Army, Edelman returned to New York City to take a position at Rockefeller University studying under Henry Kunkel. Kunkel, with whom Edelman would conduct his Ph.D. research, was examining the unique flexibility of antibodies at the time.

In 1967, while a debate raged between two schools of scientists to explain antibody synthesis, Edelman and his associate, Joseph Gally proposed a radical theory that would later be confirmed as essentially correct. It depended on the vast diversity that can come from chance in a system as complex as the living organism. Each time a cell divided, they theorized, tiny errors in the transcription—or reading of the code—could occur, yielding slightly different proteins upon each misreading. Edelman and Gally proposed that the human body turns the advantage of this variability in immunoglobulins to its own ends. Many strains of antigens when introduced into the body modify the shape of the various immunoglobulins in order to prevent the recurrence of disease.

Edelman's doctoral thesis investigated several methods of splitting immunoglobulin molecules, and, after receiving his Ph.D. in 1960 he remained at Rockefeller as a faculty member, continuing his research.

In 1961 Edelman and his colleague, M.D. Poulik succeeded in splitting IgG—one of the most studied varieties of immunoglobulin in the blood—into two components by using a method known as ''reductive cleavage.'' The technique allowed them to divide IgG into what are known as light and heavy chains. Data from their experiments and from those of the Czech researcher, Frantisek Franek, established the intricate nature of the antibody's ''active sight.'' The sight occurs at the folding of the two chains which forms a unique pocket to trap the antigen. Porter, who was the first to split an immunoglobulin, combined these findings with his, and, in 1962, announced that the basic structure of IgG had been determined.

In 1965, Porter and Edelman began studying the amino acid sequence in subsections of different myeloma, cancers of the immunoglobulin-producing cells. The project, completed in 1969, determined the order of all 1,300 amino acids present in the protein, the longest sequence determined at that time.

By the end of the 1970s, the principle Edelman and Poulik uncovered led him to conceive a radical theory of how the brain works.

Rather than an incoming sensory signal triggering a predetermined pathway through the **nervous system**, Edelman theorized that it leads to a selection from among several choices. Edelman envisioned the nervous system as a fluid system based on three interrelated stages of functioning.

In the formation of the nervous system, cells receiving signals from others surrounding them fan out like spreading ivy—not to predetermined locations, but rather to regions determined by the concert of these local signals. The signals regulate the ultimate position of each cell by controlling the production of a cellular glue in the form of cell-adhesion molecules and anchoring neighboring groups of cells together. Once established, these cellular connections are fixed, but the exact pattern is different for each individual.

The second feature of Edelman's theory allows for an individual response to any incoming signal. While the vast complexity of these connections allows for some of the variability in the brain, it is in the third feature of the theory that Edelman made the connection to immunology. The neural networks are linked to each other in layers. An incoming signal passes through and between these sheets in a specific pathway. The pathway, in this theory, ultimately determines what the brain experiences, but just as the immune system modifies itself with each new incoming virus, Edelman theorized that the brain modifies itself in response to each new incoming signal. In this way, Edelman sees all the systems of the body being guided in one unified process, a process that depends on organization but that accommodates the world's natural randomness.

Dr. Edelman has received honorary degrees from a number of universities, including the University of Pennsylvania, Ursinus College, Williams College, and others. Besides his Nobel Prize, his other academic awards include the Spenser Morris Award, the Eli Lilly Prize of the American Chemical

Society, Albert Einstein Commemorative Award, California Institute of Technology's Buchman Memorial Award, and the Rabbi Shai Schaknai Memorial Prize.

A member of many academic organizations, including New York and National Academy of Sciences, American Society of Cell Biologists, Genetics Society, American Academy of Arts and Sciences, and the American Philosophical Society, Dr. Edelman is also one of the few international members of the Academy of Sciences, Institute of France. In 1974 he became a Vincent Astor Distinguished Professor, serving on the board of governors of the Weizmann Institute of Science and is also a trustee of the Salk Institute for Biological Studies.

EDEMA

Edema is a condition of abnormally high fluid volume in the circulatory system or in tissues between the body's cells. It is a sign of an underlying problem or problems, rather than a disease unto itself.

Normally, the body maintains a balance of fluid in tissues by ensuring that the same of amount of water entering the body also leaves it. The circulatory system (also called the **cardiovascular system**) transports fluid within the body via its network of blood vessels. The fluid, which contains oxygen and nutrients needed by the cells, moves from the walls of the blood vessels into the body's tissues. After its nutrients are used up, fluid moves back into the blood vessels and returns to the heart. The **lymphatic system** (a network of channels in the body that carries lymph, a colorless fluid containing white blood cells to fight infection) also absorbs and transports this fluid. In edema, either too much fluid moves from the blood vessels into the tissues, or not enough fluid moves from the tissues back into the blood vessels. This fluid imbalance can cause mild to severe swelling in one or more parts of the body.

Many ordinary factors can upset the balance of fluid in the body to cause edema, including immobility (when muscles are inactive for long periods, fluids tend to remain in one place); heat and humidity, which make it easier for fluid to cross into surrounding tissues; medications (steroids, hormone replacements, **nonsteroidal anti-inflammatory drugs** (NSAIDs), and some blood pressure medications can affect how fast fluid leaves blood vessels); salty foods (the body dilutes excess salt by retaining fluid); **menstruation**; and **pregnancy**.

Some medical conditions may also induce edema, including left-sided **heart failure**, which can cause **pulmonary edema** as fluid shifts into the lungs; right-sided heart failure, which can cause swelling in the tissue of the lower legs and feet; kidney disease, because the accompanying decrease in sodium and water excretion can result in fluid retention and overload; thyroid or **liver disease**, which change fluid movement in and out of the tissues; and **malnutrition**.

Edema may occur in a single leg because of blood clots, which cause pooling of fluid; weakened veins that allow blood to gather; inflammatory diseases such as **gout** or arthritis; **lymphedema** (blocked lymph channels that prevent proper draining); and tumors that compress leg vessels and lymph channels.

Symptoms vary depending on the cause of edema. In general, weight gain, puffy eyelids, and swelling of the legs may occur as a result of excess fluid volume. Pulse rate and blood pressure may be elevated, while hand and neck veins may appear swollen.

Treatment of edema depends on its cause, but generally the patient may be told to reduce sodium intake; maintain proper weight (extra weight slows fluid circulation and puts pressure on the veins); **exercise** to stimulate circulation; elevate the legs; use support stockings to promote circulation and decrease pooling of fluid due to gravity; get regular **massages**, unless blood clots are a problem; and stand and/or walk at least every hour or two during travel.

In addition, physicians frequently prescribe the three "Ds"—**diuretics**, **digitalis**, and **diet**—for medical conditions that result in excess fluid volume. Diuretics are medications that promote urination of sodium and water. Digoxin is a digitalis preparation that can decrease heart rate and increase the strength of the heart's contractions. Adequate non-animal-source protein intake is also important, and patients should avoid alcohol, **caffeine**, sugar, dairy products, soy sauce, animal protein, chocolate, olives, and pickles.

In terms of alternative treatments, diuretic herbs can also help relieve edema. One of the best herbs for this purpose is dandelion (*Taraxacum mongolicum*), since, in addition to its diuretic action, it is a rich source of potassium. (Diuretics flush potassium from the body and it must be replaced to avoid a deficiency of this essential element mineral.) **Hydrotherapy** using daily contrast applications of hot and cold (either compresses or immersion) may also be helpful.

EGAS MONIZ, ANTONIO (1874-1955)

Portuguese neurologist

Egas Moniz was born in Avança, Portugal, on November 29, 1874. He received his early education from his uncle, an abbot, and later entered the University of Coimbra in 1891 where he pursued a degree in mathematics. He eventually changed his mind, however, and entered the medical degree program. He received his M.D. from Coimbra in 1899.

For much of his life, Egas Moniz divided his time between political action and medical research. The first decade of the twentieth century was a period of revolutionary upheaval in Portugal and Egas Moniz was active in the Republican movement that led to the overthrow of the monarchy in 1910. He went on to serve as a deputy in the new parliament, ambassador to Spain, foreign minister, and Portuguese delegate to the 1918 Paris Peace Conference. He retired from politics in 1919 after becoming involved in a duel over a political disagreement.

Egas Moniz's scientific research focused on neurology, especially pertaining to the brain. His first major contribution was the development of a technique for studying the brain. Previously, the use of X-rays in studying the brain had met with little success. However, Egas Moniz developed a technique in which he injected solutions into the brain that are opaque to X-rays. With this approach, X-rays could be used to identify the precise location and size of brain tumors and brain injuries. This technique of cerebral **angiography** is still widely used today.

Later in life, Egas Moniz began to explore brain surgery and its possible use in treating **mental illness**. In 1935, he attended a conference in which he learned about the experimental removal of the prefrontal lobe of the brain of two monkeys. After this surgery, symptoms of **anxiety** and frustration could no longer be induced in the monkeys, although the animals had also lost the ability to learn.

Despite the fact that scientists knew nothing about the function of the prefrontal lobes, Egas Moniz saw a possible application of the monkey experiment to human mental disorders. He proposed the use of a surgical procedure for mental patients in which the prefrontal lobes were severed from the rest of the brain, a process now known as prefrontal lobotomy.

Because of a serious case of gout, Egas Moniz was unable to carry out this surgery himself. A colleague, Pedro de Almedia Lima (1903-1983), performed the actual operations under Egas Moniz's direction. Of the first 20 operations performed, seven patients were said to be cured of their disorder, eight experienced some improvement, and five were unchanged. For his development of this technique, Egas Moniz was awarded a share of the 1949 Nobel Prize for physiology or medicine.

Prefrontal lobotomy has occupied a controversial place in medicine. In the late 1940s and early 1950s, lobotomies became popular in the United States for the treatment of a variety of mental disorders. By one estimate, an average of 5,000 operations were performed annually between 1949 and 1952. Opposition to the procedure grew in the 1960s, however, as it became clear that lobotomies often turned humans into ''vegetables.'' Lobotomies eventually fell into disfavor as other methods for treating mental disorders became available. Much more sophisticated versions of Egas Moniz's original procedure have been developed and currently are in use for the treatment of highly specialized conditions, such as intractable **pain**.

EHRLICH, PAUL (1854-1915)

German bacteriologist

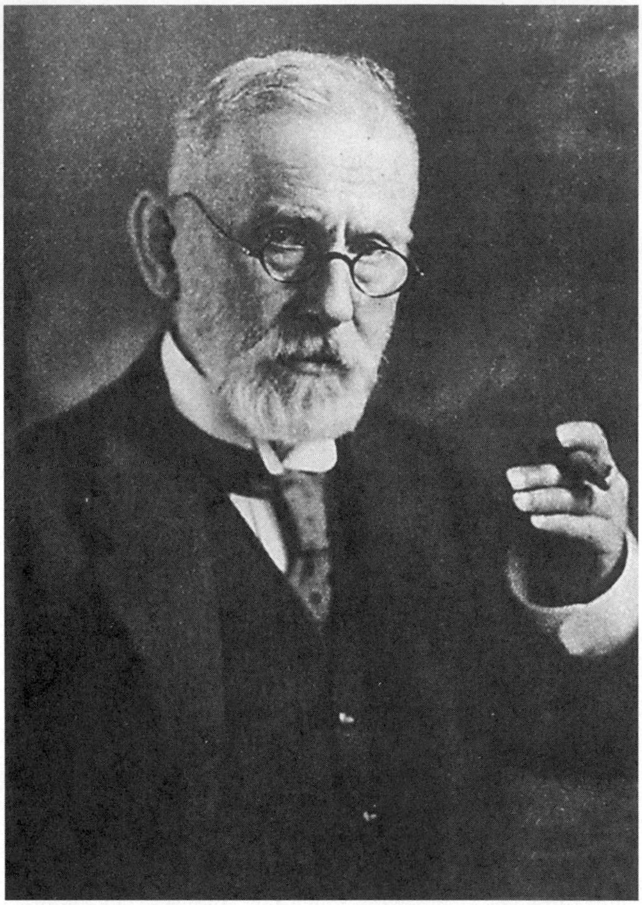

Paul Ehrlich

Through his comprehensive study of the effects of chemicals in the human body, Ehrlich fathered the fields of **chemotherapy** (the treatment of disease with chemical agents) and hematology (the study of blood). He also made important contributions to the understanding of immunity and discovered Salvarsan, the first effective treatment for **syphilis**.

Ehrlich was born on March 14, 1854, in Strehlen, Silesia (then part of Germany), to a prosperous Jewish family. He was the son of Ismar Ehrlich and his wife, Rosa, the aunt of bacteriologist Karl Weigert. Ehrlich's interest in biology and chemistry led him to study medicine. He attended universities in Breslau, Strasbourg, Frieberg-im-Briesgau, and Leipzig, earning his medical degree in 1878. Ehrlich was fascinated by the reactions of cells and tissues to dyes. Using aniline dyes, for example, Ehrlich investigated white blood cells. In the process, he developed new ways of staining cells for research, including the methylene blue stain for bacteria. Heinrich Koch used this stain when he discovered the bacillus that causes **tuberculosis**.

In 1890, Ehrlich became a professor at the University of Berlin, where he worked with **Emil von Behring** and Shibasaburo Kitasato on the study of immunity, or the body's own defense against disease. The group searched for a substance that would give immunity against **diphtheria** using antitoxins. Antitoxins are antibodies produced by the body's immune system to fight poisons invading the body. Ehrlich worked on the chemical aspects of the study and, in 1892, the group announced the development of a diphtheria antitoxin for medical use. Ehrlich also pioneered the production of large quantities of the antitoxin using horses. He shared the 1908 Nobel Prize in Physiology or Medicine with Soviet biologist **Elie Metchnikoff** (1845-1916) for his work on immunity and serum therapy.

In 1894, Ehrlich was made director of a new institute for serum research in Frankfurt, where he studied the concepts of *active* and *passive* immunity and developed his ''side-chain'' theory of immunity to explain how antitoxins work at the cellular level in response to toxins. Ehrlich also continued his study of blood using staining techniques. Realizing that stains colored bacteria but not surrounding cells, he looked for a way to combine the stain with a substance that could kill the bacteria. This, he reasoned, could be a "magic bullet" in the fight against bacterial diseases. He also identified dyes, such as trypan red, that had the ability to destroy microorganisms on their own.

Ehrlich began working with organic compounds containing arsenic because he felt its properties were similar to those of the nitrogen atoms that gave trypan red its effectiveness. He studied literally hundreds of arsenic compounds and, by 1907, he had reached number 606, which he put aside because it was not effective against trypanosomes. However, two years later, Ehrlich's assistant, Sahachiro Hata (1872-1938), discovered that the compound number 606 was effective against the dread disease syphilis. Caused by a microorganism called a *spirochete*, syphilis meant a slow and painful death for thousands of people. In 1910, Ehrlich announced that chemical 606, which he called Salvarsan, could cure syphilis.

For several years, Ehrlich suffered personal and professional attacks because of his work with syphilis. Some felt the disease was a just punishment for sinful sexual behavior and attacked Ehrlich for searching for a cure. The administration of the drug was also complicated, even risky at first, and when a few patients died because doctors administering the drug failed to follow Ehrlich's instructions, Ehrlich was accused of fraud. The attacks finally ceased in 1914, when the German parliament at last endorsed his cure as authentic.

Ehrlich was married in 1883 to Hedwig Pinkus. The couple had two daughters. Unfortunately, the strain surrounding Ehrlich's controversial efforts to cure syphilis took its toll on his health and he suffered a series of strokes during his last year, which led to his death in Bad Homburg, Germany, in 1915.

EIJKMAN, CHRISTIAAN (1858-1930)

Dutch physician

Born in the Netherlands in 1858, Eijkman received his medical degree from the University of Amsterdam in 1883, then went to Germany to study under the famous bacteriologist, Robert Koch. Encouraged by Koch, in 1887 Eijkman joined a commission sent to the Dutch East Indies (now Indonesia) to investigate **beriberi**—and began the work that was to make him famous.

At the time, beriberi was a widely prevalent disease, characterized by polyneuritis, the kind of nerve damage that causes numbness, **paralysis** and, in many cases, **death**. Because **Louis Pasteur**'s **germ theory** of disease had already led to so many successful cures, physicians now assumed that all diseases must be caused by microorganisms. The scientific commission sent to investigate beriberi, therefore, was primarily searching for its causative organism—an organism they failed to find. Disappointed, most of the group returned home in 1887, but Eijkman remained behind to serve as director of

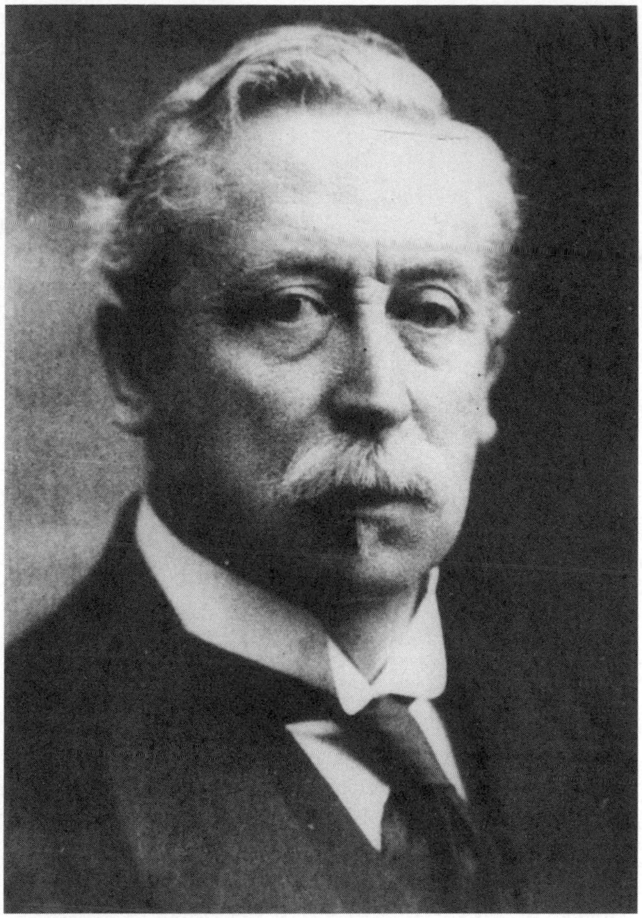

Christiaan Eijkman

a new bacteriology lab set up in a medical school constructed for native doctors. It was there that, around 1890, Eijkman helped solve the problem of beriberi, at least partly by accident.

When a group of laboratory chickens suddenly developed a strange disease—one with symptoms that resembled polyneuritis—Eijkman promptly commandeered the chickens and once again tried to find the causative germ, without success. Moreover, he was unable to transfer the disease from sick chickens to healthy ones. And then, to add to his frustration, the disease vanished as suddenly as it had started.

Fortunately Eijkman refused to give up. He stubbornly continued to delve into every aspect of the peculiar vanishing disease. Before long, he learned that, for a brief period of time, one of the cooks had been feeding the lab chickens boiled rice from the hospital's own stores. A second cook, however, decided it was wrong to feed rice meant for people to mere chickens, and switched back to cheaper unpolished rice. Oddly enough, Eijkman learned that the chickens had developed their illness while eating the "better" polished rice.

To determine whether the polished rice was actually responsible for causing the sickness, Eijkman began feeding it to other chickens which quickly developed the beriberi-like illness. And even more intriguing, Eijkman could then cure this new illness simply by switching the sick chickens back to the unpolished rice. Eijkman, therefore, became the first researcher to pinpoint a dietary-deficiency disease. At first, he didn't fully understand the meaning of his findings, assuming that there must be a toxin in rice grains that could be neutralized by something in the hulls. But others would quickly clarify his results.

A younger colleague, Gerrit Grijns, took over the nutrition studies when an illness compelled Eijkman to go home in 1896, and in 1901 he proposed that beriberi was caused, not by germs, but by the lack of some natural substance present in rice hulls and other foods (this substance turned out to be thiamine). Over the next decade, a number of investigators—most notably, England's **Frederick Gowland Hopkins**—came to similar conclusions about a number of diseases and a new era in medicine was underway. Eijkman, whose work served as the basis for the modern theory of **vitamin**s, shared the Nobel Prize in physiology or medicine with Hopkins in 1929.

Elder Care

Healthier **diets** and lifestyles, combined with advances in medical care are allowing people to live longer. In 1999, 12.5 percent of the U. S. population was made up of adults over the age of 65, and by 2050, an increase to 23% is expected by the Census Bureau. Many of these individuals may develop chronic health conditions, including arthritis, heart/circulatory diseases, such as **hypertension**, and/or brain impairments, such as **Alzheimer's disease**. More than 40% of **hospital** stays and 20% of physician expenses are accounted for by the elderly. These individuals often become unable to live independently or care for themselves without assistance.

Caregiving to the elderly may involve a wide range of responsibilities, including everything from checking in on a parent every day at their home to providing 24 hour a day attention in the caregiver's home. Studies have found that 80 percent of all long term care for the elderly is provided by friends and family. There are a multitude of health services also available to assist in caring for the elderly, depending on the level of medical care they require and the other types of assistance they need. Retirement centers, assisted living centers, day care, **home health care**, **respite care**, **foster care**, and **nursing homes** are available to support and assist families in providing the appropriate level of assistance to the elderly.

Setting up advance directives while the elder is competent can provide peace of mind for family and the elder, as preferences for health care and life support can be spelled out in a **living will**. Selecting a trusted individual to serve as their power of attorney will facilitate decisions about care and finances if the elder becomes unable to make decisions for themselves.

See also Aging; Home health care; Long term care Nursing homes

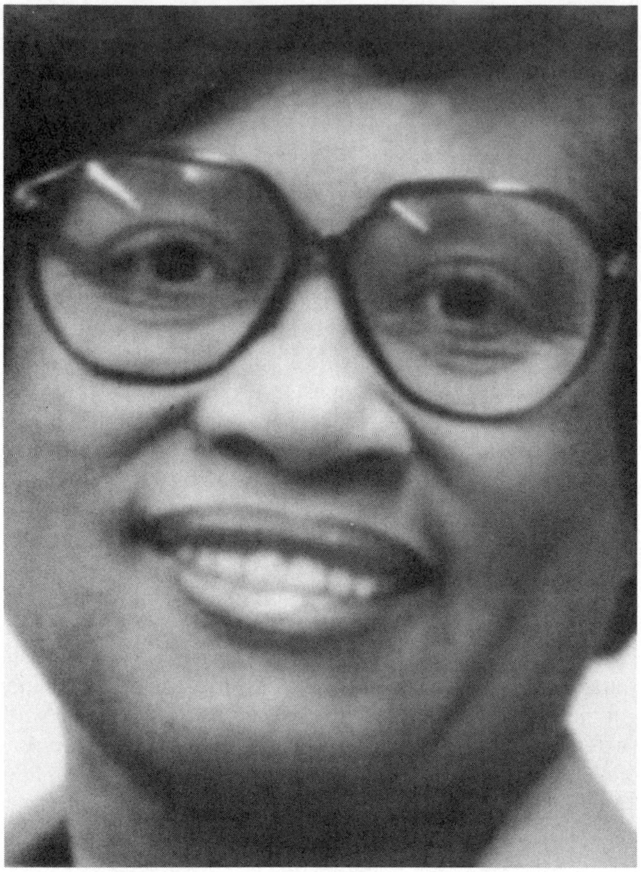

Joycelyn Elders

Elders, Joycelyn (1933-)

American physician (pediatric endocrinologist); former U.S. Surgeon General

Joycelyn Elders held the position of U.S. Surgeon General from 1993 through 1994, when she was forced to resign amidst intense controversy.

Joycelyn Elders was born Minnie Lee Jones on August 13, 1933, the oldest of her parents' eight children. As was the case for many poor black families of the time, Elders was born at home in Schaal, Arkansas. Her parents were sharecroppers, who picked cotton. Her father also supported the family by killing raccoons. This supplied the family with a source of food, as well as bringing in a little money when he could sell the pelts to Sears. Elders's family home was a three-room cabin that lacked indoor plumbing and electricity.

Elders showed her intelligence early on, as her mother taught her to read by age four. By age five, Elders was picking cotton in the fields in the early morning, and then walking five miles to catch a schoolbus. The bus then drove 13 miles away to the black school, a dingy building supplied with the cast-off textbooks of white schools.

Elders had no exposure to medical care as a child. **Childbirth** (her mother had eight children) was accomplished at home. Elders'ss brother once suffered a ruptured appendix, and was transported into town for medical care on a mule.

Elders's parents and brothers and sisters worked extra hard in the cotton fields to support Elders attendance at Philander Smith College in Little Rock, Arkansas. She started college at only fifteen, working as a maid scrubbing floors to help put herself through. Amazingly, Elders was still able to graduate in only three years. It was during her years in college that she first saw a doctor. She also heard Edith Irby Jones speak. Jones was the first black woman to graduate from the University of Arkansas Medical School. Until this point, Elders had thought she'd become a laboratory technician. After hearing Jones speak, Elders became determined to become a physician.

First, however, Elders served in the Army as a physical therapist. The G.I. bill, then, financed her attendance at University of Arkansas Medical School. Elders faced challenges, both as the only woman in the class of 1960, and as an African-American at a school with segregated dining halls and social clubs.

After graduation, Elders did her internship year at the University of Minnesota Hospital in Minneapolis, returning to train in pediatrics at Arkansas Medical Center in Little Rock. Elders was appointed chief of the pediatric residency in 1963, and continued her training with a research fellowship in 1964. In 1967, Elders earned an M.S. in biochemistry, and accepted a position at University of Arkansas Medical School as an assistant professor. By 1976, she was full professor; by 1978 she became a board certified pediatric endocrinologist. Elders name is on about 147 published research papers.

In 1987, Elders was appointed by Arkansas governor Bill Clinton to the position of Arkansas's chief **public health** director. Elders was thrilled at the opportunity to have an impact on such issues as teenage pregnancy, **infant mortality**, and children's health. Under her administration, early childhood screening increased by ten times; the immunization rate by 2 years of age increased from 34 to 64%; and the number of women receiving prenatal care from the state increased by 17% (thereby also concomitantly decreasing the infant mortality rate). Elders also focused efforts on improving statewide HIV testing and **counseling** services, improving **home health care** for the severely chronically and terminally ill, and increasing mammogram rates among low-income women.

Elders was attacked by conservative groups in Arkansas for her policy of creating school-based clinics. Her intention had been that these clinics would provide health care, education, and contraceptives (in particular, **condom**s) to high school students throughout Arkansas. Yet only four of these clinics ever actually handed out condoms. Conservative Christian and right-to-life groups claimed that Elders was pushing **abortion**s. While Elders was forthright about her pro-choice stance, she tried repeatedly to explain that her real goal was simple prevention of **pregnancy**. Still, she was vilified by conservatives, and her efforts sometimes thwarted by their interference.

In 1993, after Bill Clinton was inaugurated as president of the United States, he chose Elders as his Surgeon General. After grueling confirmation hearings, in which Elders's opponents attempted to derail her appointment, Elders was finally confirmed. Surgeon General of the U.S. is both an administrative position (serving as head of the Public Health Service Corps' six thousand doctors, nurses, pharmacists, and scientists) and an educational position. The Surgeon General is expected to choose particular public health problems, and to bring them to the attention of the American public. Elders was excellent at this role, speaking out in her inimitably honest fashion on such topics as teen pregnancy, tobacco use, **AIDS**, drug and alcohol abuse, gun control, and legalization of marijuana for medical purposes. Yet her detractors were many, and she was constantly under barrage for her forthright opinions.

In 1994, Elders spoke at the United Nations' World AIDS Day. A psychologist in the audience proposed a question to her, asking if she thought that **masturbation** could serve as a useful tool to help discourage school children from becoming sexually active too early. Elders responded by saying: ''With regard to masturbation, I think that is something that is part of human sexuality and a part of something that perhaps should be taught.'' Her conservative opponents jumped with both feet on the issue, and her words were twisted and splashed across the media, making it sound as if Elders had advocated teaching masturbation techniques to grade schoolers. In the wake of the controversy, Elders was forced to resign from her post as Surgeon General.

Since her resignation, Elders returned to the University of Arkansas, where she has continued her practice of medicine, as well as teaching and lecturing widely about public health care issues.

See also Koop, C. Everett; Public health

ELECTRIC SHOCK INJURIES

Electric shock injuries are caused by lightning or electric current from a mechanical source passing through the body. Electric shocks cause about 1,000 deaths in the United States each year; about 3–15% of cases are fatal. Injuries range from barely noticeable tingling to instant death, and can affect every part of the body. The severity depends on the current's pressure (voltage), the amount (amperage) and type of current (direct vs. alternating), the body's resistance to the current, the current's path through the body, and how long the body remains in contact with the current. Injuries from household appliances and other low-voltage sources are less likely to produce extreme damage. Many survivors require amputation or are disfigured by burns. How electric shocks affect the skin is determined by how wet, thick, and clean the skin is. Thin or wet skin is much less resistant than thick or dry skin. When skin resistance is low, the current may cause little or no skin damage but severely burn internal organs and tissues. High skin resistance can produce severe skin **burns** but prevent the current from entering the body. The nervous system (the brain, spinal cord, and nerves) is easily injured by electric shocks. Some of this damage is minor and clears up on its own or with medical treatment, but some is severe and permanent. Neurological problems may be apparent immediately after the accident, or gradually develop over up to three years. Damage to the respiratory and cardiovascular systems is worst at the moment of injury. Electric shocks can paralyze the respiratory system or disrupt heart action, causing instant death. Smaller veins and arteries can develop blood clots. Damage to the smaller vessels is probably one reason why **amputation** is often required after high-voltage injuries. Other injuries possible after an electric shock include: **cataracts**, **kidney failure**, substantial destruction of muscle tissue, falling or getting hit by debris from exploding equipment, fire on clothing or nearby flammable substances, and broken or dislocated bones.

Electric shock injuries are diagnosed through information about the accident, a thorough **physical examination**, and watching cardiovascular and kidney activity. The victim's neurological condition can change rapidly and requires close observation. A **computed tomography scan** (CT scan) or **magnetic resonance imaging** (MRI) may be used check for brain injury. When an electric shock accident happens at home or work, immediately shut off the main power. If that cannot be done, and current is still flowing, push the victim away from the source of the current by standing on a dry, nonconducting surface such as a folded newspaper, or plastic or rubber mat and using a nonconducting object such as a wooden broomstick. Do not touch the victim or the source while the current is flowing. Call emergency medical help as quickly as possible. People who are trained to perform **cardiopulmonary resuscitation (CPR)** should, if appropriate, begin first aid while waiting for help to arrive. Burn victims usually need to go to a burn center. Fluid replacement therapy restores lost fluids and electrolytes. Severely injured tissue is repaired surgically, which can involve **skin grafting** or amputation. **Antibiotics** and antibacterial creams are used to prevent infection. Victims may also require treatment for kidney failure. Following surgery, physical therapy to facilitate recovery, and psychological counseling to cope with disfigurement, may be necessary.

Many electric shocks can be prevented. Parents and other adults should know about possible electric dangers in the home. Damaged electric appliances, wiring, cords, and plugs should be repaired only by people with the proper training or replaced. Hair dryers, radios, and other electric appliances should never be used in the bathroom or anywhere else they might accidentally come in contact with water. Young children need to be kept away from electric appliances and taught early about the dangers of electricity. Electric outlets need safety covers in homes with young children. During thunderstorms, people should go indoors immediately, and boaters should return to shore as quickly as possible. People who cannot reach indoor shelter should move away from metallic objects such as golf clubs and fishing rods and lie down in low-ground areas. Standing or lying under or next to tall or metallic structures is unsafe. An automobile is appropriate cover, as long as the radio is off. Telephones, computers, hair dryers, and other appliances that can act as conduits for lightning should not be used during thunderstorms.

ELECTROCARDIOGRAPHY

In the late 1700s medical researchers learned that muscles produce tiny electric impulses now known as "action potentials." Italian biophysicist, Carlo Matteucci (1811-1868), identified action potentials in a pigeon's heart in 1843 and, in 1856, German scientists Rudolf Albert von Kölliker (1817-1905) and Heinrich Müller (1820-1864) recorded these electric currents from a frog's heart. Reasoning that these recordings could reveal irregularities and, hence, heart disease, researchers attempted to develop accurate measuring devices. The French physiologist, Augustus Waller (1856-1922), found that cardiac currents could be recorded by placing surface electrodes on the body. In 1887, Waller developed a capillary electrometer—tubes of mercury that rose and fell with the changes in heart muscle current—which, however, was imprecise and difficult to use. So Dutch physiologist Willem Einthoven set out to design an improved apparatus. In 1903 he described the result, his string galvanometer consisting of a thin, silver-coated quartz wire stretched between the poles of a magnet. As the heart's electric impulse flowed through, the wire was deflected and motion was magnified and projected onto moving photographic film. The extreme sensitivity of the device, which weighed 600 lbs (272.4 kg), allowed it to detect the tiny cardiac currents very accurately. Einthoven called his machine the electrocardiograph and the recorded electrical impulses an electrocardiogram. He devised the standard positioning of the electrodes and described the regular heart waves and the triangle used to interpret electrocardiograms. Through clinical studies, Einthoven identified a number of heart problems with his galvanometer. Einthoven won the Nobel Prize in 1924 for inventing the ECG. In 1942, Emanuel Goldberger added three augmented limb leads to Einthoven's three limb leads and the six chest leads making the 12-lead electrocardiogram that is used today, and English physician Sir Thomas Lewis (1881-1945) established the electrocardiogram as a standard clinical tool.

With refinements in instrumentation and technique, electrocardiography became one of the most useful diagnostic tools in medicine. This highly accurate, easy to interpret, and relatively inexpensive device permits diagnosis of heart conditions without needle or incision and even portable devices are now available: the "HeartMirror," weighing only 3.3 lbs (1.5 kg) operates on four AA NiCad batteries and will record 12 selectable leads. Housed in a carrying case, it is ideal for a physician's office. The "HeartVision" portable emergency device weighing only 13.4 oz (380 gr.) and using four AA batteries, fits into a pocket. Four built-in emergency electrodes eliminate contact leads—the device is simply placed on a patient's chest and displays the reading on a liquid crystal display (LCD). It also stores the reading, which can be printed out later on an analog ECG recorder or personal computer.

ELECTROCONVULSIVE THERAPY

Electroconvulsive therapy (ECT) is a controversial medical treatment to relieve the signs and symptoms of mental illnesses by introducing a small, carefully controlled amount of electricity into the brain. This electrical stimulation, used with **anesthesia** and **muscle relaxant** medications, produces a mild generalized seizure or convulsion. It is used to treat many psychiatric disorders, and is most effective in treating severe depression. ECT is used when patients need to get better fast because they are suicidal, may hurt themselves, refuse to eat or drink, cannot or will not take medication as prescribed, or present some other danger to themselves. The most common risks associated with ECT are disturbances in heart rhythm. ECT is offered on both an inpatient and outpatient basis. Hospitals have specially equipped rooms with oxygen, suction, and **cardiopulmonary resuscitation (CPR)** in order to deal with the rare emergency.

Approximately 30 minutes before the treatment time, the patient may receive a needle containing a medicine (such as atropine) that keeps the pulse rate from decreasing too much during the convulsion. Next, the patient is placed on a cot and hooked up to a machine that automatically takes and displays temperature, pulse, respiration and blood pressure. A mild anesthetic is injected into a vein, followed by a medicine (such as Anectine) that relaxes all of the muscles so that the seizure is mild, and the risk of broken bones is virtually eliminated. When the patient is relaxed and asleep, an airway is placed in the mouth to aid with breathing. Electrodes are placed on the sides of the head. An electric current is passed through the brain with a machine designed for this purpose. In the first stage of the seizure, the muscles in the body that have not been paralyzed by medication contract for 5–15 seconds. In the second stage, which lasts approximately 10–60 seconds, the patient twitches. The entire procedure lasts about 30 minutes. The number of treatments a patient receives depends upon factors such as age, diagnosis, the history of illness, family support, and response to therapy. Patients with depression, for example, usually require 6–12 treatments. Treatments are usually administered every other day, three times a week. Confusion and forgetfulness are common after ECT treatment, particularly elderly patients. These symptoms usually go away with time, but a small minority of patients say they never fully recovered. With the introduction of antipsychotics in the 1950s, the use of ECT became less frequent. For patients who do not respond to medicine or who have severe allergic reactions, ECT may be the only treatment that will help.

Before ECT, the patient is shown videotapes that explain the procedure, has a chance to ask the doctor questions, and signs an ''Informed Consent Form.'' The doctor does a complete **physical examination**, and orders tests such as a **chest x ray**, an electrocardiogram (ECG), **urinalysis**, spinal x ray, brain wave (EEG) and complete **blood count** (CBC) to help identify any potential problem. The patient is told to stop taking some medications, such as lithium and a type of **antidepressant** known as **monoamine oxidase inhibitors**, before treatment, and not to eat or drink for at least eight hours before the procedure. After the treatment, the patient is moved to a recovery area where vital signs are monitored and given mild medications such as **aspirin** for **headache**, muscle pain, or back pain.

ELECTROENCEPHALOGRAPHY

An electroencephalogram (EEG) is a graphic picture of the electrical activity of the brain. This visual image is created when electrodes are placed on a subject's scalp and connected by wires to an *electroencephalograph*, a devise which records the patterns of brain waves—the rhythmic changes in electric potentials in the brain—by tracing them with a fine, inked needle or nib onto a sheet of paper. EEGs are useful in diagnosing epilepsy, **brain tumors**, **strokes**, brain damage caused through head trauma, and other neurological conditions characterized by distinctive, abnormal brain wave patterns. They are also used in investigating psychiatric disorders such as schizophrenia, and in determining brain death—an important process for use in conjunction with organ donation for surgical transplant recipients. The founder of electroencephalography was **Hans Berger** (1873-1941), a German psychiatrist who made the first human EEG in 1924. Interested primarily in psychophysiology—that is, the relationship between the mind and the brain—Berger set about measuring the brain's electrical activity in the hope that a physiological record of this kind would provide insight into mental processes. He found inspiration for his work in the electrocardiograph (ECG) invented by Willem Einthoven in 1900, and in work done earlier on the brain waves of animals. In 1875, Richard Caton (1842-1926), an English physiologist and surgeon, had measured electrical activity in the exposed brains of rabbits and monkeys but had been unable to make a graphic recording; the first recording of this kind was made in 1913 by a scientist named Vladimir Pravdich-Neminskii, who used the Einthoven string galvanometer to record from the intact skulls of dogs. Using a galvonometer much like the one Pravdich-Neminskii had used a decade earlier, Berger began his search for the human EEG by experimenting with the exposed brains of dogs. He then started placing needle electrodes under the scalp of patients who had lost some of their skull bones in surgery. It was while working with one of these patients—a seventeen-year-old who had been operated on because of a suspected brain tumor—that Berger recorded the first human EEG in 1924. He was initially uncertain whether the electrical oscillations he recorded originated in the brain. It was not until after conducting many other experiments—including experiments on the intact skulls of healthy people and of people with brain disorders—that he published his first paper on the human electroencephalogram in 1929. The initial reaction of other scientists to Berger's work was one of disbelief; like Berger himself, the scientific world at first doubted whether the workings of an organ as complex as the brain could be recorded through the skull. Berger did not achieve an international reputation until 1934, when **Edgar Douglas Adrian** (1889-1977), a renowned English neurophysiologist, confirmed his findings. Even then, however, Berger remained unappreciated in his own country. In the late 1930s, the Nazis forced him to retire from the University of Jena, where he had been professor and director of psychiatry since 1919. With his laboratory dismantled and no facilities to carry on his work, Berger fell into a depression and committed suicide in 1941.

Despite his reputation as a reserved and inflexible man, Berger would no doubt be pleased to know that, over the years, research scientists have used the EEG to identify the parts of the brain involved in the mental processes of reasoning, memory, and feeling. He would also, no doubt, be interested in a system that has simplified EEG interpretation. Known as BEAM (brain electrical activity mapping), this system was invented by Frank Duffy of the Harvard Medical School in the early 1980s. It uses computer technology to combine the signals from the individual electrodes into a overall, color-coded map of the brain's electrical activity. BEAM can store large amounts of EEG data, compare healthy profiles with abnormal ones, and provide detailed analyses that have been used to accurately diagnose such conditions as dyslexia and schizophrenia, which are usually difficult to detect. Efforts are currently underway to use BEAM in matching EEG patterns to specific brain functions. For example, research scientists at Johns Hopkins University have used BEAM to map the electrical activity involved in the movement of a monkey's arm; their studies have shown that when the monkey anticipates moving its arm, the pattern of electrical activity in its brain changes. If efforts like these are successful, it may one day be possible to use computers and the electrical activity of the brain not only to control artificial limbs but in many other revolutionary applications as well.

The use of EEGs in neurofeedback (or biofeedback) is becoming increasingly popular; for example, in helping children cope with **Attention Deficit/Hyperactivity Disorders**. In 1997, Neuropathways EEG Imaging system became the first U.S. patented digital EEG neurofeedback device, displaying brain wave voltages and frequencies in *real time*, (there is less than one thousandth of a second delay between when the brain wave begins and its display on a computer screen). This allows interventional feedback when the event is occurring, not after it has passed, and has produced improvement in concentration and other cognitive functions of both ADD clients and head trauma victims. Meanwhile, Mind Media in The Netherlands is marketing *The BrainTracer*, a non-medical device which allows individuals to see their real time brain wave activity on standard home computer screens and print them on standard printers.

ELECTRONIC FETAL MONITORING

The fetal monitor records an unborn baby's heart rate during pregnancy and labor and graphs it on a piece of paper. The fetal monitor is the best way to evaluate an unborn baby, and it is almost the only test to make sure that a baby is doing well during labor. During **pregnancy**, fetal monitoring can be used as a part of antepartum testing. If the practitioner feels that a baby may be at increased risk of problems toward the end of pregnancy, a baby can be checked every week or every other week with a non-stress test. Fetal monitoring is used on and off during early labor. As labor progress, more monitoring is often needed. Usually, as the time for delivery nears, the monitor is left on continuously since the end of labor tends to be

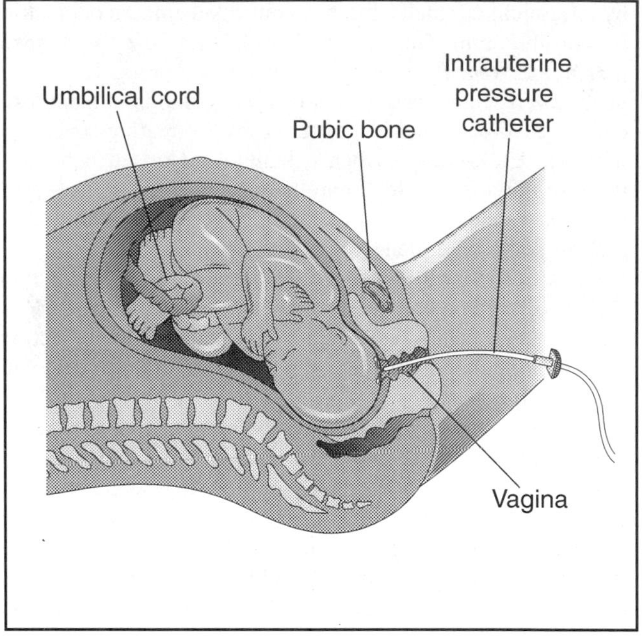

Diagram of EFM.

the most stressful time for the baby. A baby who is having trouble in labor will show changes in heart rate after a contraction. If a baby is not receiving enough oxygen to withstand the stress of labor and delivery is many hours away, a **cesarean section** (C-section) may be necessary.

Using the fetal monitor is simple and painless. Two elastic belts are placed around the mother's abdomen. One belt holds a listening device in place while the other belt holds the contraction monitor. The nurse or midwife adjusts the belts to get the best readings from each device. Sometimes, it is difficult to hear the baby's heartbeat with the monitoring device. Other times, the monitor may show subtle signs of a developing problem. In either case, the doctor or midwife may recommend using an internal belt instead of the external belt. The internal monitor, an electronic wire that is placed on the baby's head during an internal exam, is more accurate but it can only be used when the cervix is already open.

An unborn baby's heart rate normally ranges from 120–160 beats per minute (bpm). A baby who is getting enough oxygen through the placenta moves around. The monitor shows the baby's heart rate rising briefly as he/she moves (just as an adult's heart rate rises when he/she moves). The baby's monitor strip is considered to be reactive when the baby's heart rate rises at least 20 bpm above the baseline heart rate for at least 20 seconds. This must occur at least twice in a 20-minute period. A reactive heart rate tracing means that the baby is doing well. If the baby's heart rate drops very low or rises very high, this signals a serious problem. In either of these cases it is obvious that the baby is in distress and must be delivered soon. However, many babies who are having problems do not give such clear signs. During a contraction, the flow of oxygen (from the mother) through the placenta (to the baby) is temporarily stopped. It is as if the baby has to hold its breath during each contraction. Both the placenta and the baby are designed to withstand this condition. Between contractions, the baby should be receiving more than enough oxygen to do well during the contraction. The first sign that a baby is not getting enough oxygen between contractions is often a drop in the baby's heart rate after the contraction. The baby's heart rate recovers to a normal level between contractions, only to drop again after the next contraction. This is also a more subtle sign of distress. These babies will do fine if they are delivered in a short period of time. Sometimes, these signs develop long before delivery is expected. In that case, a C-section may be necessary. Fetal monitoring is not a perfect test but it is the best test available to diagnose increased risks to an unborn baby at the end of pregnancy and during labor.

Elephantiasis

Elephantiasis is a severely disfiguring and disabling condition in which the arms, legs, or genitals swell so much that they can resemble an elephant's foreleg in size, texture, and color. True elephantiasis is caused by a parasitic infection from three kinds of round worms. These worms block the body's **lymphatic system**—a network of channels, lymph nodes, and organs that helps maintain proper fluid levels in the body by draining lymph from tissues into the bloodstream. This blockage causes fluids to collect in the tissues, which can lead to great swelling, called "**lymphedema**." Elephantiasis is also called Barbados leg, elephant leg, morbus herculeus, mal de Cayenne, and myelolymphangioma. Most cases of elephantiasis are caused by filarial worms found in tropical and subtropical places and transmitted by mosquitoes. They occur in the poor in underdeveloped regions of South America, Central Africa, Asia, the Pacific Islands, and the Caribbean. Elephantiasis is more intense in people who don't live in these areas, because many native people have built up some immunity. Other causes of elephantiasis are: A protozoan disease called **leishmaniasis**, a repeated streptococcal infection, the surgical removal of lymph nodes (usually to prevent the spread of **cancer**), or a hereditary birth defect. Symptoms of elephantiasis include repeated episodes of **fever**, shaking chills, sweating, **headache**s, vomiting, and **pain**. Enlarged lymph nodes, swelling of the affected area, skin ulcers, bone and joint pain, tiredness, and red streaks along the arm or leg also may occur. **Abscess**es can form in lymph nodes or in the lymphatic vessels. They may appear at the surface of the skin as well. Long-term infection with lymphatic filariasis can lead to lymphedema, hydrocele (a buildup of fluid in any saclike cavity or duct) in the scrotum, and elephantiasis of the legs, scrotum, arms, penis, breasts, and vulvae. The most common site of elephantiasis is the leg. It typically begins in the ankle and progresses to the foot and leg. The swollen leg eventually becomes hard and thick. The skin may appear darkened or warty and may even crack, allowing bacteria to infect the leg and complicate the disease.

The only sure way to diagnose lymphatic filariasis is to find the parasite. Examining the person's blood under a microscope may show microfilariae. But many times, people who have been infected for a long time do not have microfilariae in their bloodstream. In these cases, it's necessary to examine the urine or hydrocele fluid or perform other tests. Elephantiasis is treated with diethylcarbamazine (DEC), which is known as Hetrazan in the United States. DEC kills the microfilariae quickly and injures or kills the adult worms slowly, if at all. If all the adult worms are not killed, they may continue to produce more larvae. Therefore, several courses of DEC treatment over a long time period may be necessary to get rid of the parasites. DEC reduces the size of enlarged lymph nodes and, when taken long-term, reduces elephantiasis. In India, DEC has been used in a medicated salt to help prevent spread of the disease. Side effects of DEC may include fever, chills, headache, **dizziness**, **nausea and vomiting**, **itching**, and joint pain. They usually occur within the first few days of treatment and go away as the person continues taking DEC. An alternate treatment, different doses of DEC and steroids, is designed to kill the parasites slowly (to reduce allergic reactions to the dead microfilariae and dying adult worms within the body). Another drug, Ivermectin, has been shown to be excellent in killing microfilariae in early research studies, but its effects on the adult worms are still being investigated. It is probable that patients will need to continue using DEC to kill the adult worms. Mild side effects of Ivermectin include headache, fever, and myalgia. Other ways to manage lymphatic filariasis are pressure bandages to wrap the swollen limb and elastic stockings to help reduce the pressure. Exercising and elevating a bandaged limb also can help reduce its size. Surgery can be performed to reduce elephantiasis by removing excess fatty and fibrous tissue, draining the swelled area, and removing the dead worms. With DEC treatment, the prognosis is good for early and mild cases of lymphatic filariasis. The prognosis is poor, however, for heavy parasitic infestations. Elephantiasis can be controlled by taking DEC preventively and reducing the number of carrier insects in the area. Avoiding mosquito bites by using insecticides and insect repellent, wearing protective clothing, and using bed netting are helpful. Before visiting countries where lymphatic filariasis is found, consult a travel physician to learn about current preventative measures.

Elion, Gertrude Belle (1918-)

American biochemist

Gertrude Belle Elion's innovative approach to drug discovery furthered the understanding of cellular metabolism and led to the development of medications for **leukemia**, **gout**, herpes, **malaria**, and the rejection of transplanted organs. Azidothymidine (AZT), the first drug approved for the treatment of **AIDS**, came out of her laboratory shortly after her 1983 retirement. One of the few women who has held a top post at a major pharmaceutical company, Elion worked at Wellcome Research Laboratories for nearly five decades. Her work, with colleague **George H. Hitchings**, was recognized with the Nobel Prize for physiology or medicine in 1988. Her Nobel award was notable for several reasons: few winners have been women, few have lacked the Ph.D., and few have been industrial researchers.

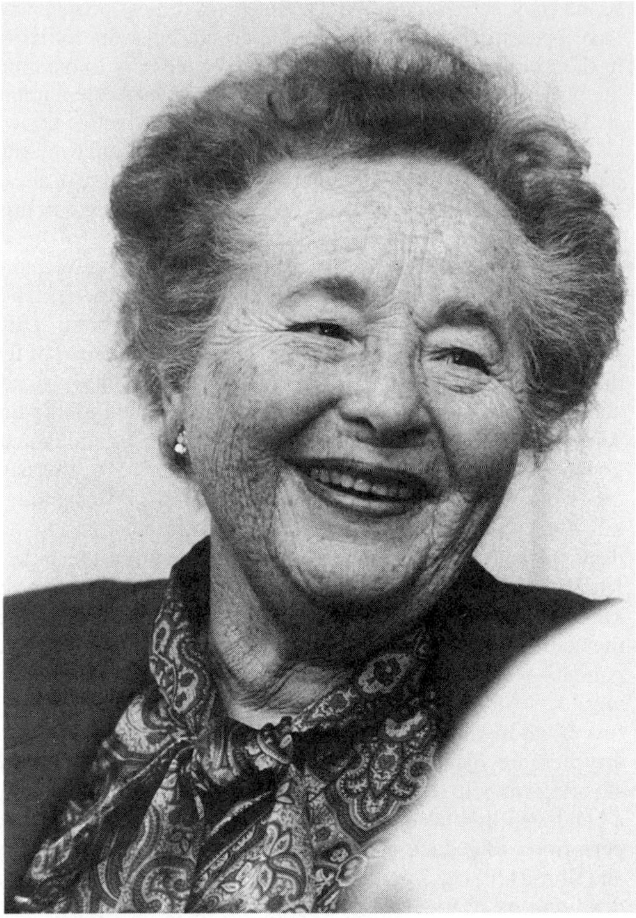

Gertrude Belle Elion

Elion was born on January 23, 1918, in New York City, the first of two children, a daughter and a son, of Robert Elion and Bertha Cohen. Robert, a dentist, immigrated to the United States from Lithuania as a small boy. Bertha came to the United States from Russia at the age of 14. Elion, an excellent student who was accelerated two years by her teachers, graduated from high school at the height of the Great Depression. As a senior in high school, she had witnessed the painful death of her grandfather from **stomach cancer** and vowed to become a **cancer** researcher. She was able to attend college only because several New York City schools, including Hunter College, offered free tuition to students with good grades. In college, she majored in chemistry because that seemed the best route to her goal.

In 1937 Elion graduated Phi Beta Kappa from Hunter College with a B.A. at the age of 19. Despite her outstanding academic record, Elion's early efforts to find a job as a chemist failed. One laboratory after another told her that they had never employed a woman chemist. Her self-confidence shaken, Elion began secretarial school. That lasted only six weeks, until she landed a one-semester stint teaching biochemistry to nurses and then took a position in a friend's laboratory. With the money she earned from these jobs, Elion began graduate school. To afford tuition, she continued to live with her parents and to work as a substitute science teacher in the public schools. In 1941, she graduated summa cum laude from New York University with a M.S. degree in chemistry.

Upon her graduation, Elion again faced difficulties finding work appropriate to her experience and abilities. The only job available to her was as a quality control chemist in a food laboratory, checking the color of mayonnaise and the acidity of pickles for the Quaker Maid Company. After a year and a half, she was finally offered a job as a research chemist at Johnson & Johnson. Unfortunately, her division closed six months after she arrived. The company offered Elion a new job testing the tensile strength of sutures, but she declined.

As it did for many women of her generation, the start of World War II ushered in a new era of opportunity for Elion. As men left their jobs to fight the war, women were encouraged to join the workforce. "It was only when men weren't available that women were invited into the lab," Elion told the *Washington Post.*

For Elion, the war created an opening in the research lab of biochemist George Herbert Hitchings at Wellcome Research Laboratories in Tuckahoe, New York, a subsidiary of Burroughs Wellcome Company, a British firm. When they met, Elion was 26 years old and Hitchings was 39. Their working relationship began on June 14, 1944, and lasted for the rest of their careers. Each time Hitchings was promoted, Elion filled the spot he had just vacated, until she became head of the Department of Experimental Therapy in 1967, where she was to remain until her retirement 16 years later. Hitchings became vice president for research. Over the years, they have written many scientific papers together.

Settled in her job and thrilled by the breakthroughs occurring in the field of biochemistry, Elion took steps to earn a Ph.D., the so-called "union card" that all serious scientists are expected to have as evidence that they are capable of doing independent research. Only one school offered night classes in chemistry, the Brooklyn Polytechnic Institute (now Polytechnic University), so that's where Elion enrolled. Attending classes meant taking the train from Tuckahoe into Grand Central Station and transferring to the subway to Brooklyn. Although the hour-and-a-half commute each way was exhausting, Elion persevered for two years, until the school accused her of not being a serious student and pressed her to attend full-time. Forced to choose between school and her job, Elion had no choice but to continue working. Her relinquishment of the Ph.D. haunted her, until her lab developed its first successful drug, 6-mercaptopurine (6MP).

In the 1940s, Elion and Hitchings employed a novel approach to fighting the agents of disease. By studying the biochemistry of cancer cells, and of harmful bacteria and viruses, they hoped to understand the differences between the metabolism of those cells and normal cells. In particular, they wondered whether there were differences in how the disease-causing cells used nucleic acids, the chemicals involved in the replication of DNA, to stay alive and to grow. Any dissimilarities discovered might serve as a target point for a drug that could destroy the abnormal cells without harming healthy, normal cells. By disrupting one crucial link in a cell's biochemistry, the cell itself would be damaged. In this manner, cancers and harmful bacteria might be eradicated.

Elion's work focused on purines, one of two main categories of nucleic acids. Their strategy, for which Elion and Hitchings would be honored by the Nobel Prize 40 years later, steered a radical middle course between chemists who randomly screened compounds to find effective drugs and scientists who engaged in basic cellular research without a thought of drug therapy. The difficulties of such an approach were immense. Very little was known about nucleic acid biosynthesis. Discovery of the double helical structure of DNA still lay ahead, and many of the instruments and methods that make molecular biology possible had not yet been invented. But Elion and her colleagues persisted with the tools at hand and their own ingenuity. By observing the microbiological results of various experiments, they could make knowledgeable deductions about the biochemistry involved. To the same ends, they worked with various species of lab animals and examined varying responses. Still, the lack of advanced instrumentation and computerization made for slow and tedious work. Elion told *Scientific American,* "if we were starting now, we would probably do what we did in 10 years."

By 1951, as a senior research chemist, Elion discovered the first effective compound against childhood **leukemia**. The compound, 6-mercaptopurine (6MP) (trade name Purinethol), interfered with the synthesis of leukemia cells. In clinical trials run by the Sloan-Kettering Institute (now the Memorial Sloan-Kettering Cancer Center), it increased life expectancy from a few months to a year. The compound was approved by the Food and Drug Administration (F.D.A.) in 1953. Eventually 6MP, used in combination with other drugs and radiation treatment, made leukemia one of the most curable of cancers.

In the next two decades, the potency of 6MP prompted Elion and other scientists to look for more uses for the drug. Robert Schwartz, at Tufts Medical School in Boston, and Roy Calne, at Harvard Medical School, successfully used 6MP to suppress the **immune systems** in dogs with transplanted kidneys. Motivated by Schwartz and Calne's work, Elion and Hitchings began searching for other **immunosuppressants**. They carefully studied the drug's course of action in the body, an endeavor known as pharmacokinetics. This additional work with 6MP led to the discovery of the derivative azathioprine (Imuran), that prevents rejection of transplanted human kidneys and treats **rheumatoid arthritis**. Other experiments in Elion's lab intended to improve 6MP's effectiveness led to the discovery of allopurinol (Zyloprim) for gout, a disease in which excess uric acid builds up in the joints. Allopurinol was approved by the F.D.A. in 1966. In the 1950s, Elion and Hitchings's lab also discovered pyrimethamine (Daraprim and Fansidar) a treatment for **malaria**, and trimethoprim (Bactrim and Septra) for urinary and respiratory tract infections. Trimethoprim is also used to treat Pneumocystis carinii **pneumonia**, the leading killer of people with **AIDS**.

In 1968, Elion heard that a compound called adenine arabinoside appeared to have an effect against DNA viruses. This compound was similar in structure to a chemical in her own lab, 2,6-diaminopurine. Although her own lab was not equipped to screen antiviral compounds, she immediately began synthesizing new compounds to send to a Wellcome Research lab in Britain for testing. In 1969, she received notice by telegram that one of the compounds was effective against herpes simplex viruses. Further derivatives of that compound yielded acyclovir (Zovirax), an effective drug against herpes, **shingles**, and **chicken pox**. An exhibit of the success of acyclovir, presented in 1978 at the Interscience Conference on Microbial Agents and Chemotherapy, demonstrated to other scientists that it was possible to find drugs that exploited the differences between viral and cellular enzymes. Acyclovir (Zovirax), approved by the F.D.A. in 1982, became one of Burroughs Wellcome's most profitable drugs. In 1984 at Wellcome Research Laboratories, researchers trained by Elion and Hitchings developed azidothymidine (AZT), the first drug used to treat AIDS.

Although Elion retired in 1983, she continued at Wellcome Research Laboratories as scientist emeritus and keeps an office there as a consultant. She also accepted a position as a research professor of medicine and pharmacology at Duke University, where she works with a third-year medical student each year on a research project. Since her retirement, Elion has served as president of the American Association for Cancer Research and as a member of the National Cancer Advisory Board, among other positions. Hitchings, who retired in 1975, also remains active at Wellcome Research Laboratories.

In 1988, Elion and Hitchings shared the Nobel Prize for physiology or medicine with Sir **James Black**, a British biochemist. Although Elion had been honored for her work before, beginning with the prestigious Garvan Medal of the American Chemical Society in 1968, a host of tributes followed the Nobel Prize. She received a number of honorary doctorates and was elected to the National Inventors' Hall of Fame, the National Academy of Sciences, and the National Women's Hall of Fame. Elion maintained that it was important to keep such awards in perspective. "The Nobel Prize is fine, but the drugs I've developed are rewards in themselves," she told the *New York Times Magazine.*

Elion never married although she was engaged once. Sadly, her fiance died of an illness. After that, Elion dismissed thoughts of marriage. She is close to her brother's children and grandchildren, however, and on the trip to Stockholm to receive the Nobel Prize, she brought with her 11 family members. Elion has said that she never found it necessary to have women role models. "I never considered that I was a woman and then a scientist," Elion told the *Washington Post.* "My role models didn't have to be women—they could be scientists." Her interests are photography, travel, and music, especially opera. Although her home is in North Carolina, she still keeps her subscription to the Metropolitan Opera in New York.

EMBOLISMS

An embolism is an obstruction in a blood vessel due to a bloodclot or other foreign matter that gets stuck while traveling through the bloodstream. The plural of embolism is emboli.

Emboli have moved from the place where they were formed through the bloodstream to another part of the body, where they obstruct an artery and block the flow of blood. The emboli are usually formed from blood clots but are occasionally comprised of air, fat, or tumor tissue. Embolic events can be multiple and small, or single and massive. They can be life-threatening and require immediate emergency medical care. There are three general categories of emboli: arterial, gas, and pulmonary. Pulmonary emboli are the most common.

In arterial emboli, blood flow is blocked at the junction of major arteries, most often at the groin, knee, or thigh. Arterial emboli are generally a complication of heart disease. An arterial embolism in the brain (cerebral embolism) causes **stroke**, which can be fatal. An estimated 5–14% of all strokes are caused by cerebral emboli. Arterial emboli to the extremities can lead to tissue death, and **amputation** of the affected limb if not treated effectively within hours. Intestines and kidneys can also suffer damage from emboli.

Gas emboli result from the compression of respiratory gases into the blood and other tissues due to rapid changes in environmental pressure, for example, while flying or scuba diving. As external pressure decreases, gases (like nitrogen) which are dissolved in the blood and other tissues become small bubbles that can block blood flow and cause organ damage.

In a **pulmonary embolism**, a common illness, blood flow is blocked at a pulmonary artery. When emboli block the main pulmonary artery, and in cases where there are no initial symptoms, a pulmonary embolism can quickly become fatal. According to the American Heart Association, an estimated 600,000 Americans develop pulmonary emboli annually and 60,000 die from it.

A pulmonary embolism is difficult to diagnose. Less than 10% of patients who die from a pulmonary embolism were diagnosed with the condition. More than 90% of cases of pulmonary emboli are complications of deep vein thrombosis, blood clots in the deep vein of the leg or pelvis.

Arterial emboli are usually a complication of heart disease where blood clots form in the heart's chambers. Gas emboli are caused by rapid changes in environmental pressure that could happen when flying or scuba diving. A pulmonary embolism is caused by blood clots that travel through the blood stream to the lungs and block a pulmonary artery. More than 90% of the cases of pulmonary embolism are a complication of deep vein thrombosis, which typically occurs in patients who have had **orthopedic surgery**, in patients with **cancer** and other chronic illnesses like congestive **heart failure**.

Risk factors for arterial and pulmonary emboli include: prolonged bed rest, surgery, **childbirth**, **heart attack**, stroke, congestive heart failure, cancer, **obesity**, a broken hip or leg, **oral contraceptives**, **sickle-cell anemia**, chest trauma, certain congenital heart defects, and old age. Risk factors for gas emboli include: scuba diving, amateur plane flight, **exercise**, injury, obesity, **dehydration**, excessive alcohol, colds, and medications such as narcotics and **antihistamines**.

Common symptoms of a pulmonary embolism include:

- Labored breathing, sometimes accompanied by chest **pain**
- A rapid pulse
- A **cough** that may produce sputum
- A low-grade **fever**
- Fluid build-up in the lungs.

Less common symptoms include:

- Coughing up blood
- Pain caused by movement or breathing
- Leg swelling
- Bluish skin
- **Fainting**
- Swollen neck veins.

Symptoms of an arterial embolism include:

- Severe pain in the area of the embolism
- Pale, bluish cool skin
- Numbness
- Tingling
- Muscular weakness or **paralysis**.

An embolism can be diagnosed through the patient's history, a physical exam, and diagnostic tests. For arterial emboli, cardiac ultrasound and/or arteriography are ordered. For a pulmonary embolism, a **chest x ray**, lung scan, pulmonary **angiography**, **electrocardiography**, arterial blood gas measurements, and venography or venous ultrasound could be ordered.

Patients with emboli require immediate hospitalization. They are generally treated with clot-dissolving and/or clot-preventing drugs. Thrombolytic therapy to dissolve blood clots is the definitive treatment for a very severe pulmonary embolism. Streptokinase, urokinase, and recombinant tissue plasminogen activator (TPA) are used. Heparin is the **anticoagulant** drug of choice for preventing formation of blood clots. Warfarin, an oral anticoagulant, is sometimes used concurrently and is usually continued after the hospitalization.

In the case of an arterial embolism, the affected limb is placed in a dependent position and kept warm. Embolectomy is the treatment of choice in the majority of early cases of arterial emboli in the extremities. In this procedure, a balloon-tipped catheter is inserted into the artery to remove thromboembolic matter.

With a pulmonary embolism, **oxygen therapy** is often used to maintain normal oxygen concentrations. For people who can't take anticoagulants and in some other cases, surgery may be needed to insert a device that filters blood returning to the heart and lungs.

Of patients hospitalized with an arterial embolism, 25–30% die, and 5–25% require amputation of a limb. About 10% of patients with a pulmonary embolism die suddenly within the first hour of onset of the condition. The outcome for all other patients is generally good; only 3% of patients die who are properly diagnosed early and treated. In cases of an undiagnosed pulmonary embolism, about 30% of patients die.

Embolism can be prevented in high risk patients through antithrombotic drugs such as heparin, venous interruption, gradient elastic stockings, and intermittent pneumatic compression of the legs. The combination of graduated compression stockings and low-dose heparin is significantly more effective than low-dose heparin alone.

Gradient elastic stockings, also called anti-embolism stockings, decrease the risk of blood clots by compressing superficial leg veins and forcing blood into the deep veins. They can be knee- thigh-, or waist-length. Many physicians order the use of stockings before surgery and until there is no longer an elevated risk of developing blood clots. The risk of deep vein thrombosis after surgery is reduced 50% with the use of these stockings. The American Heart Association recommends that the use of graduated compression stockings be considered for all high-risk surgical patients.

Intermittent pneumatic compression involves wrapping knee- or thigh-high cuffs around the legs to prevent blood clots. The cuffs are connected to a pump which inflates and deflates, mimicking the heart's normal pumping action and reducing the pooling of blood. Intermittent pneumatic compression can be used during surgery and recovery and continues until there is no longer an elevated risk of developing blood clots. The American Heart Association recommends the use of intermittent pneumatic compression for patients who cannot take anticoagulants, for example, spinal cord and brain trauma patients.

EMERGENCY MEDICAL IDENTIFICATION

Emergency Medical Identification is a system that alerts physicians and emergency medicine personnel of a health condition, medical history, or other factors that may impact **emergency medical services**. More than 100 million people are admitted to an emergency room each year in the United States. Many of them are unconscious or otherwise unable to communicate to the physician. As a result, the physician may lack important information on other medical problems the patient may have, such as **diabetes**, which must be taken into consideration when providing care. With the proper information, for example, physicians can avoid giving medications that could interact adversely with other medications a patient may be taking.

One of the first emergency medical identification systems was developed by Dr. Marion Collins and his wife, Chrissie Collins. In 1956, the Collins's daughter nearly died after suffering an allergic reaction from a **tetanus** shot. As a result, the couple designed a bracelet for their daughter to wear that contained information about her allergic condition. They then began producing bracelets from their home for other people and eventually built a not-for-profit organization that provides emergency medical identification services for 2.4 million people in the U.S. and 1.7 million people in other countries. According to an organization survey, the system has saved more than 80,000 lives. The Collins's contributions to the development of the system have been recognized with the 1998 **C. Everett Koop** Health Advocate Award presented by the Society for Healthcare Strategy and Market Development of the American Hospital Association and the 1998 Medaille d'Excellence for Health from the World Wins Corporation.

Many private companies now offer emergency medical identification services. These services may include bracelets and other jewelry, identification cards, and computerized back-up information on the patient's medical conditions. According to the **American Medical Association** and the Academy of American Family Physicians, an emergency identification system should include a clearly visible, durable tag with the universal medical symbol (the caduceus, a staff with two oppositely twined serpents and surmounted in wings) and a medical information card that contains pertinent medical information and the identity of family, friends, and personal physicians.

People should carry an emergency medical identification card when they have a medical condition, allergy, implant, or medication that could be life threatening in an emergency situation. It is estimated that that at least 60 million Americans have a medical condition that should be known in times of emergency. Considering that, in the United States, an accident occurs every six seconds and that every six minutes a fatality occurs as a result of an accident, emergency medical identification can certainly help save lives and play an important role in improving health care during an emergency situation.

See also C. Everett Koop

EMERGENCY MEDICAL SERVICES

Emergency medical services have become a method relied upon for timely transportation and treatment of the injured during the twentieth century, but the modern rescue squad did not become a reality until shortly before this time. The idea of a specially trained group of people who could initiate immediate treatment to the wounded and deliver them to safety originated during Napoleon's rule, when his surgeon Dominique Jean Larrey, directed the Grand Armee to develop mobile field **hospitals**, or ambulances volantes (flying ambulances), in addition to a corps of trained and equipped soldiers to aid those on the battlefield. Before Larrey's initiative in the 1790s, wounded soldiers were either left amid the fighting until the combat ended or their comrades would carry them to the rear lines. The Battle of Solferino in 1859, which wounded and killed 40,000 French, Italian, and Austrian soldiers, led Swiss businessman **Jean Henri Dunant** who witnessed the massacre to coordinate a group of civilians to deliver aid to wounded soldiers. Dunant would forever be known for the creation of the **International Red Cross**, and this group would in turn instigate the training of lay people in the techniques of **first aid**. With inspiration from the French military, the American Civil War prompted a system of railroad ambulance cars and base hospitals that were created during the conflict, but these existed only on the Union side of combat.

Following the Civil War, the reform of medical care delivery and the creation of civilian ambulance service throughout the United States began to take precedence. With the northern states leading the way, Cincinnati's (Ohio) Commercial Hospital established what has been documented as the first regular ambulance operation in the country in 1865. Soon after, New York City, with direction from physician Edward B. Dalton, developed an alliance between public agencies and hospitals and private hospitals in Manhattan to create a system that divided the city into ambulance zones, with each hospital held responsible for its zone. Most large cities would begin organizing some type of ambulance service before World War I. In 1899, Chicago used the first motorized ambulance and St. Vincent's Hospital in New York City introduced electric vehicles a year later.

The concept of emergency medical services was organized further by Julian Stanley Wise, who in 1928 formed the Roanoke Life Saving and First Aid Crew consisting of 10 trained volunteers who delivered emergency care to those in need. His foresight became the model that helped organize squads of volunteers that provide ambulance and rescue service throughout much of the United States. Historically, civilian volunteers have been looked to for emergency care, with the oldest continuously active group being the Misericordia di Firenze. Founded in 1240 A.D., this group aided the sick and transported the dead of medieval Florence, and hundreds of branches have remained active in northern Italy throughout the twentieth century. Keeping with Wise's idea that the standard of all emergency work is speed, the Roanoke squad prompted national attention in the volunteer rescue movement as they reached the scene of a drowning 16-year-old boy in 11 minutes, and effectively revived him. Twenty-six thousand members of emergency medical care teams were participating in 850 squads around the world by 1956.

Although interest in the formation of emergency medical care began to surface, the changes came slowly during the first 65 years of the twentieth century. Transportation before the automobile consisted of horse-drawn wagons, then many communities looked to undertakers and their hearses as the main service for carrying patients. By the early 1960s, undertakers still dominated half of the United States ambulance service, and in many places including large cities, ambulances provided only a driver, leaving the patient to ride alone in the back. During this time, fewer than half of the 200,000 ambulance and rescue personnel were trained to the level of Red Cross advanced first aid. Education for this career was limited, with only six states offering standard courses for rescuers, and only four regulated ambulances. Opposition from physicians and the medical establishment that was determined to prevent laypeople from practicing medicine without a license stunted proper development of guidelines for rescue workers this led to their motto of ''Load and go,'' leaving proper medical treatment waiting at the doors of the hospital.

The modern convenience of increased automobiles on the highways during the late '60s and early '70s, and the escalated number of motor-vehicle deaths that resulted from their existence led to John F. Kennedy's label of ''the greatest of the nation's public health problems,'' with his words forever changing the future of emergency medical services in the United States. A seminal report in 1966 from the National Academy of Sciences catalogued the inadequacies of the country's emergency medical care and encouraged solutions in terms of training and standards for the service. This led to the Highway Safety Act of 1966 which set federal standards for training, equipment, and procedures for all states to comply with, leading to the organization of emergency services that was subsidized with government funding throughout the 1970s. As the 911 telephone system came into use and ambulances acquired proper communication equipment, information regarding the patient reached the hospital more efficiently, and adequate care en route became a priority.

Staffing ambulances with highly trained emergency medical technicians took precedence, and a comprehensive 81-hour course was established by the National Highway Traffic Safety Administration by the end of the 1960s to ensure this. The first 200 people to be trained to a national standard occurred in 1969. Another major modification to the EMS system in the United States came from a physician in Belfast, Northern Ireland. J. Frank Pantridge, head of the cardiology department of the Royal Victoria Hospital, converted an ambulance into a mobile cardiac-care unit with modern resuscitation techniques, medications, and an electric defibrillator he powered from two car batteries. Pantridge's idea saved countless lives, and as the United States began training their emergency medical technicians with techniques that included interpreting electrocardiograms and establishing intravenous lines, the title of **paramedic** became formally recognized as an essential part of a rescue squad. Their presence has attributed to a 40% decrease in mortality from **coronary artery disease** in the United States since the 1960s.

Additional advances in emergency medical services throughout the twentieth century include: the Jaws of Life, a machine that generates five tons of force to remove drivers from the tangled metal resulting from a car accident; automated defibrillation; and air transport of patients by helicopter, an idea that originated from the Vietnam War and became useful to civilians in the 1980s.

See also Ambulatory care; Cardiopulmonary resuscitation (CPR); Coronary artery disease; Defibrillation; Dunant, Jean Henri; Electrocardiography; First aid; Hospitals; Paramedics

EMOTIONAL DEVELOPMENT

The study of the emotional development of infants and children is relatively new, having been studied empirically only during the past few decades. Researchers have approached this area from a variety of theoretical perspectives, which differ mainly on the question of whether emotions are learned or biologically predetermined.

Between six and ten weeks, a social smile emerges, usually accompanied by other pleasure-indicative actions and sounds, including cooing and mouthing. This social smile occurs in response to adult smiles and interactions. As infants become more aware of their environment, smiling occurs in response to a wider variety of contexts. Smiles are considered to serve a developmental function.

Laughter, which begins at around three or four months, requires a level of cognitive development because it demonstrates that the child can recognize incongruity. That is, laughter is usually elicited by actions that deviate from the norm, such as being kissed on the abdomen or a caregiver playing peek-a-boo. Because it fosters reciprocal interactions with others, laughter promotes social development.

During the last half of the first year, infants begin expressing fear, disgust, and anger. Anger serves an adaptive function, signalling caregivers of the infant's discomfort or displeasure, letting them know that something needs to be changed or altered. Although some infants respond to distressing events with sadness, anger is more common.

Fear emerges as children become able to compare an unfamiliar event with what they know. The degree to which a child reacts with fear to new situations is dependent on a variety of factors. One of the most significant is the response of its mother or caregiver. Infants repeatedly check with their caregivers for emotional cues regarding safety and security of their explorations, and they look to caregivers for facial cues for the appropriate reaction to unfamiliar adults.

During the second year, infants express emotions of shame, embarrassment, and pride. The reasons for the shame or pride are learned. Different cultures value different actions. One culture may teach its children to express pride upon winning a competitive event, whereas another may teach children to dampen their cheer, or even to feel shame at another person's loss.

During this stage of development, toddlers acquire language and learn to verbally express their feelings. In 1986, Inge Bretherton and colleagues found that 30% of American 20-month-olds correctly labeled a series of emotional and physiological states, including sleep-fatigue, **pain**, distress, disgust, and affection. This ability, rudimentary as it is during early toddlerhood, is the first step children take in the development of emotional self-regulation skills.

Although there is debate concerning an acceptable definition of emotion regulation, it is generally thought to involve the ability to recognize and label emotions, and to control emotional expression in ways that are consistent with cultural expectations. Being able to articulate an emotional state in itself has a regulatory effect. Speech also enables children to self-regulate, using soothing language to talk themselves through difficult situations.

Empathy, a complex emotional response to a situation, also appears in toddlerhood, usually by age two. The development of empathy requires that children read others' emotional cues, understand that other people are entities distinct from themselves, and take the perspective of another person (put themselves in the position of another).

Parents help preschoolers acquire skills to cope with negative emotional states by teaching and modeling the use of verbal reasoning and explanation. Children learn at about age three that expressions of anger and aggression are to be controlled in the presence of adults. Around peers, however, children are much less likely to suppress negative emotional behavior. It appears that these differences are the results of the consequences children have experienced when expressing emotions. Further, this socially contextual distinction demonstrates that preschoolers have begun to internalize society's rules governing the appropriate expression of emotions.

Beginning at about age four, children acquire the ability to alter their emotional expressions, a skill of high value in cultures that require frequent disingenuous social displays. Psychologists call these skills emotion display rules. As such, one's external emotional expression need not match one's internal emotional state. For example, in Western culture, we teach children that they should smile and say thank-you when receiving a gift, even if they don't like it. The ability to use display rules is complex. It requires that children understand the need to alter emotional displays, take the perspective of another, know that external states need not match internal states, have the muscular control to produce emotional expressions, be sensitive to social contextual cues that alert them to alter their expressivity, and have the motivation to enact such discrepant displays in a convincing manner.

Carolyn Saarni has identified two types of emotional display rules, prosocial and self-protective. Prosocial display rules involve altering emotional displays in order to protect another's feelings. On the other hand, self-protective display rules involve masking emotion in order to save face or to protect oneself from negative consequences. In 1986 research findings were mixed concerning the order in which prosocial and self-protective display rules are learned. Some studies demonstrate that knowledge of self-protective display rules emerges first; others show the opposite.

Children ages seven to 11 display a wider variety of self-regulation skills. Sophistication in understanding and enacting cultural display rules has increased dramatically by this stage, such that children begin to know when to control emotional expressivity as well as have a sufficient repertoire of behavioral regulation skills to effectively mask emotions in socially appropriate ways. Several factors influence their emotion management decisions, including the type of emotion experienced, the nature of their relationship with the person involved, age, and gender. Moreover, it appears that children have developed a set of expectations concerning the likely outcome of expressing emotion to others. In general, children report regulating anger and sadness more to friends than mothers and fathers because they expect to receive a negative response such as teasing or belittling from friends. With increasing age, however, older children report expressing negative emotions more often to their mothers than their fathers, expecting dads to respond negatively to an emotional display. These emotion-regulation skills are considered to be adaptive and deemed essential to establishing, developing, and maintaining social relationships.

Children at this age also demonstrate rudimentary cognitive and behavioral coping skills that serve to lessen the impact of an emotional event. For example, when experiencing a negative emotional event, children may respond by employing rationalization or minimization cognitive coping strategies, in which they re-interpret or reconstruct the scenario to make it seem less threatening or upsetting.

During middle childhood, children begin to understand that the emotional states of others are not as simple as they imagined in earlier years, and that they are often the result of complex causes, some of which are not externally obvious. They also come to understand that it is possible to experience more than one emotion at a time, although this ability is somewhat restricted and evolves slowly. It is not until age ten that children are capable of understanding that one can experience two seemingly contradictory emotions, such as feeling happy that they were chosen for a team but also nervous about their responsibility to play well.

Displays of empathy also increase in frequency during this stage. Children from families that regularly discuss the complexity of feelings will develop empathy more readily than those whose families avoid such topics. Furthermore, parents who set consistent behavioral limits and who themselves show high levels of concern for others are more likely to produce empathic children than parents who are punitive or particularly harsh in restricting behavior.

An important factor in the ways adolescents regulate emotional displays is their heightened sensitivity to others' evaluations of them, a sensitivity that can result in acute self-awareness and self-consciousness as they try to blend into the dominant social structure. David Elkind has described adolescents as operating as if they were in front of an imaginary audience in which every action and detail is noted and evaluated by others. As such, adolescents become very aware of the impact of emotional expressivity on their social interactions and, fundamentally, on obtaining peer approval. Because guidelines concerning the appropriateness of emotional displays are highly culture-specific, adolescents have the difficult task of learning when and how to express or regulate certain emotions.

As expected, gender plays a significant role in the types of emotions displayed by adolescents. Boys are less likely than girls to disclose their fearful emotions during times of distress. This reluctance was similarly supported by boys' belief that they would receive less understanding and, in fact, probably be belittled, for expressing both aggressive and vulnerable emotions.

ENCEPHALITIS

Encephalitis is an inflammation of the brain, usually caused by a direct viral infection or a hypersensitivity reaction to a virus or foreign protein. The inflammation is a reaction of the body's **immune system** to infection or invasion. During the inflammation, the brain's tissues become swollen. The combination of the infection and the immune reaction to it can cause **headache** and a **fever**, as well as more severe symptoms in some cases.

There are more than a dozen viruses that can cause encephalitis, spread by either human-to-human contact or by animal **bites**. Encephalitis may occur with several common viral infections of childhood. Viruses and viral diseases that may cause encephalitis include:

- **Chicken pox**
- **Measles**
- **Mumps**
- Epstein-Barr virus (EBV)
- Cytomegalovirus infection
- HIV
- Herpes simplex
- Herpes zoster (**shingles**)
- Herpes B
- **Polio**
- **Rabies**
- Mosquito-borne viruses (arboviruses).

Mosquitoes spread viruses responsible for equine encephalitis (eastern and western types), St. Louis encephalitis, California encephalitis, and Japanese encephalitis. **Lyme disease**, spread by ticks, can cause encephalitis, as can Colorado tick fever. Rabies is most often spread by animal bites from dogs, cats, mice, raccoons, squirrels, and bats and may cause encephalitis.

Equine encephalitis is carried by mosquitoes that do not normally bite humans but do bite horses and birds. It is occasionally picked up from these animals by mosquitoes that do bite humans. Japanese encephalitis and St. Louis encephalitis are also carried by mosquitoes. The risk of contracting a mosquito-borne virus is greatest in mid- to late summer, when mosquitoes are most active, in those rural areas where these viruses are known to exist. Eastern equine encephalitis occurs in eastern and southeastern United States; western equine and California encephalitis occur throughout the West; and St. Louis encephalitis occurs throughout the country. Japanese encephalitis does not occur in the United States, but is found throughout much of Asia. The viruses responsible for these diseases are classified as arbovirus and these diseases are collectively called arbovirus encephalitis.

Herpes simplex encephalitis, the most common form of sporadic encephalitis in western countries, is a disease with significantly high mortality. It occurs in children and adults and both sides of the brain are effected. It is theorized that brain infection is caused by the virus moving from a peripheral location to the brain via two nerves, the olfactory and the trigeminal (largest nerves in the skull).

Herpes simplex encephalitis is responsible for 10% of all encephalitis cases and is the main cause of sporadic, fatal encephalitis. In untreated patients, the rate of death is 70% while the mortality is 15–20% in patients who have been treated with acyclovir. The symptoms of herpes simplex encephalitis are fever, rapidly disintegrating mental state, headache, and behavioral changes.

The symptoms of encephalitis range from very mild to very severe and may include:

- Headache
- Fever
- Lethargy (sleepiness, decreased alertness, and fatigue)
- Malaise
- **Nausea and vomiting**
- Visual disturbances
- Tremor
- Decreased consciousness (drowsiness, confusion, **delirium**, unconsciousness)
- Stiff neck
- **Seizures.**

Symptoms may progress rapidly, changing from mild to severe within several days or even several hours.

Diagnosis of encephalitis includes careful questioning to determine possible exposure to viral sources. Tests which can help confirm the diagnosis and rule out other disorders include:

- Blood tests. These are to detect antibodies to viral antigens, and foreign proteins.
- **Cerebrospinal fluid analysis** (spinal tap). This detects viral antigens, and provides culture specimens for the virus or bacteria that may be present in the cerebrospinal fluid.
- **Electroencephalogram** (EEG)
- **CT** and **MRI scans.**

A brain biopsy (surgical gathering of a small tissue sample) may be recommended in some cases where treatment to date has been ineffective and the cause of the encephalitis is unclear. Definite diagnosis by biopsy may allow specific treatment that would otherwise be too risky.

Choice of treatment for encephalitis will depend on the cause. Bacterial encephalitis is treated with **antibiotics**. Viral encephalitis is usually treated with **antiviral drugs** including acyclovir, ganciclovir, foscarnet, ribovarin, and AZT. Viruses that respond to acyclovir include herpes simplex, the most common cause of sporadic (non-epidemic) encephalitis in the United States.

The symptoms of encephalitis may be treated with a number of different drugs. **Corticosteroids**, including prednisone and dexamethasone, are sometimes prescribed to reduce inflammation and brain swelling. **Anticonvulsant drugs**, including dilantin and phenytoin, are used to control seizures. Fever may be reduced with **acetamlnophen** or other fever-reducing drugs.

A person with encephalitis must be monitored carefully, since symptoms may change rapidly. Blood tests may be required regularly to track levels of fluids and salts in the blood.

Encephalitis symptoms may last several weeks. Most cases of encephalitis are mild, and recovery is usually quick. Mild encephalitis usually leaves no residual neurological problems. Overall, approximately 10% of those with encephalitis die from their infections or complications such as sccondary infection. Some forms of encephalitis have more severe courses, including herpes encephalitis, in which mortality is 15–20% with treatment, and 70–80% without. Antiviral treatment is ineffective for eastern equine encephalitis, and mortality is approximately 30%.

Because encephalitis is due to infection, it may be prevented by avoiding the infection. Minimizing contact with others who have any of the viral illness listed above may reduce the chances of becoming infected. Most infections are spread by hand-to-hand or hand-to-mouth contact; frequent hand washing may reduce the likelihood of infection if contact cannot be avoided.

Mosquito-borne viruses may be avoided by preventing mosquito bites. Mosquitoes are most active at dawn and dusk, and are most common in moist areas with standing water. Minimizing exposed skin and use of mosquito repellents on other areas can reduce the chances of bcing bitten.

Vaccines are available against some viruses, including polio, herpes B, Japanese encephalitis, and equine encephalitis. Rabies vaccine is available for animals; it is also given to people after exposure. Japanese encephalitis vaccine is recommended for those traveling to Asia and staying in affected rural areas during transmission season.

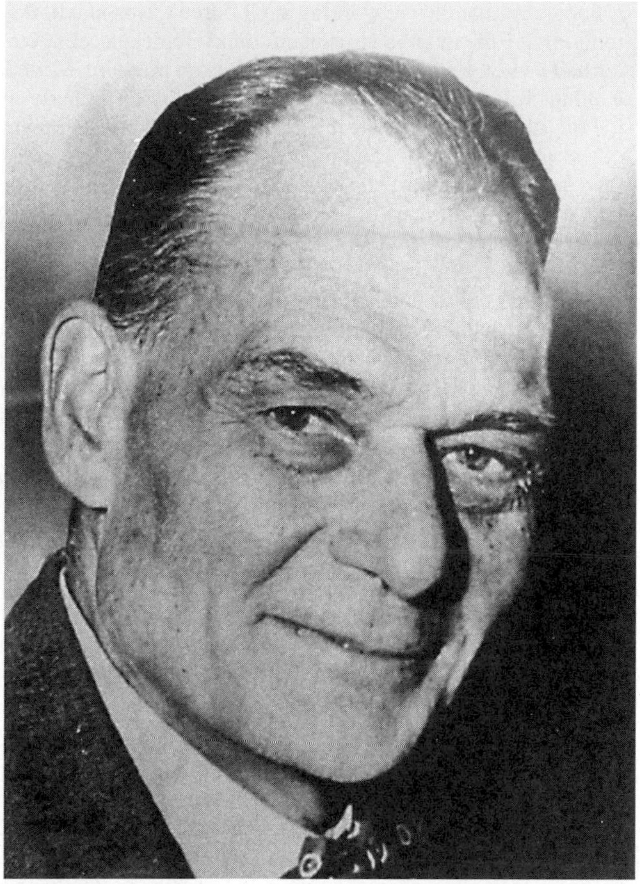

John Franklin Enders

Enders, John F. (1897-1985)

American bacteriologist and virologist

John Franklin Enders was born in Connecticut and graduated from Yale University in 1920. After beginning a career as a real estate agent, Enders decided that business was not for him and enrolled at Harvard University, completing a master's degree in English literature. While pursuing further graduate studies, a roommate introduced him to **Hans Zinsser**, a well-known microbiologist who was head of Harvard's Department of Bacteriology and Immunology. Zinsser's enthusiasm for scientific pursuits was contagious, and this meeting proved fateful to Enders, who then began working in Zinsser's laboratory.

Enders received a Ph.D. from Harvard in 1930 and began research on how the **immune system** fights bacterial disease. However, by 1937 his attention was drawn to the herpes simplex virus. During this time, the study of viruses was hampered by the inadequacy of microscopes and by the fact that viruses can grow only in live tissue. This led Enders to work in the area of tissue culture technique. By 1940 he and his assistant, **Thomas Weller**, worked on developing viral vaccines. World War II interrupted their tissue culture work but by 1947, Enders, Weller and Frederick C. Robbins, (Weller's medical school roommate) were working at Children's Hospital in Boston growing the **mumps** virus in cultures of chicken cells. Weller had been working on cultivating **chicken pox** viruses while Robbins was trying to isolate the virus that causes infantile epidemic **diarrhea**. Together, this team of three innovated methods of tissue culture by adding new medium to the cells rather than transferring the cells to a new medium. They had the added advantage of using newly available **antibiotics** which could be added to the medium to prevent bacterial contamination. Successful in growing mumps viruses, the trio cultivated chicken pox virus and then poliomyelitis virus. Techniques they developed for growing **polio** virus were essential to the later development of the life-saving vaccines of **Jonas Salk** and **Albert Sabin** and for this innovation, Enders, Weller and Robbins received the Nobel Prize for physiology or medicine in 1954. Enders continued working in the area of virus cultures and successfully grew the measles virus which was used in the first measles vaccine. After retirement from Harvard, Enders kept an active interest in virology and, at the time of his death, was studying the **AIDS** virus.

ENDOCARDITIS

Endocarditis is an infection in the endocardium (the inner lining of the heart muscle, which also covers the heart valves) in which the endocardium becomes damaged and bacteria stick to the heart valves or heart lining. The endocardium lines all four chambers of the heart which blood passes through as the heart beats. It also covers the four valves, which normally open and close to allow the blood to flow in only one direction through the heart during each contraction. For the heart to pump blood efficiently, the four chambers must contract and relax, and the four valves must open and close, in a well coordinated fashion. Endocarditis can interfere with the heart's ability to do its job. The endocardium can be damaged and made more susceptible to infection by heart defects that are present at birth, such as mitral valve **prolapse**, in which blood leaks through a poorly functioning mitral valve back into the heart; scarring of the heart muscle, such as **rheumatic fever**; or replacement of a heart valve. Bacteria can get into the blood stream (a condition known as **bacteremia**) in many ways: by spreading from a local infection such as a urinary tract infection, **pneumonia**, or skin infection; as a result of certain medical conditions, such as severe **periodontal disease**, colon **cancer**, or **inflammatory bowel disease**; during minor surgery, such as periodontal surgery, **tooth extraction**s, teeth cleaning, tonsil removal, prostate removal, or endoscopic examination; and through catheters used for intravenous medications and feeding, or dialysis. In people who use intravenous drugs, the bacteria can enter the blood stream through unsterilized, contaminated needles and syringes.

If not discovered and treated, infective endocarditis can permanently damage the heart muscle, especially the valves. It can lead to **heart failure**, a chronic condition in which the heart is unable to pump blood well enough to adequately supply the body. The vegetation formed by bacteria colonizing on heart valves may break off and form **emboli**, which can travel through the circulation, get stuck in blood vessels, and block blood flow. This can damage tissues, and affect the brain or the kidneys. Most cases of infective endocarditis occur in people between the ages of 15–60. Men are affected about twice as often as women. The most common symptom of endocarditis is a mild **fever**. Other symptoms include chills, weakness, **cough**, trouble breathing, **headache**s, aching joints, and loss of appetite. Emboli may also cause Osler's nodes (small, reddish, painful bumps usually found on the inside of fingers and toes); petechiae (tiny purple or red spots on the skin); tiny hemorrhages resembling splinters under the fingernails or toenails; coughing; **shortness of breath**; symptoms of a mini-**stroke** (numbness, weakness, or **paralysis** on one side of the body or sudden vision loss or double vision); kidney damage; or an enlarged spleen. Anyone experiencing any of these symptoms should seek medical help immediately.

Doctors diagnosis endocarditis through a medical history, a **physical examination**, a blood test, and usually **echocardiography**. When doctors suspect infective endocarditis, they admit the patient to a hospital and treat the infection with antibiotics. In recent years, it has become harder to treat endocarditis because of people's resistance to antibiotics. Doctors may need to try a few different types of **antibiotics**—or even a combination of antibiotics—to successfully treat the infection. Antibiotics are usually given for about one month, but may need to be given longer if the infection is resistant to treatment. Once the fever and the worst of the symptoms have gone away, the patient may be able to continue antibiotic therapy at home but should regularly visit his/her doctor to make sure that the antibiotic therapy is working and is not causing adverse side effects, and that there are no complications. The patient should immediately tell the doctor about any symptoms that could indicate serious complications: trouble breathing or swelling in the legs, headache, joint pain, blood in the urine, or stroke symptoms, fever, chills, **diarrhea**, **rash**, **itching**. In cases of heart failure, recurring emboli, infection that doesn't respond to treatment, poorly functioning heart valves, and endocarditis involving prosthetic (artificial) valves, the most common surgical treatment cuts away (debriding) damaged tissue and replacing the damaged valve.

If left untreated, infective endocarditis continues to progress and is always fatal. If it is diagnosed and properly treated within the first six weeks of infection, it can be completely cured in about 90% of cases. The outcome depends on the patient's age and overall physical condition, the severity of the disease involved, the exact site of the infection, how well the antibiotics work, and what kind of complications the endocarditis may be causing. People who are prone to endocarditis should tell health-care professionals before any surgical or dental procedures. They must be treated with antibiotics before these procedures to minimize the risk of infection.

ENDOCRINE SYSTEM

The endocrine system is the body's network of nine glands and over 100 hormones that maintain and regulate numerous events throughout the body. The glands of the endocrine system include the pituitary, thyroid, parathyroids, thymus, pancreas, pineal, adrenals, and ovaries or testes; in addition, the hypothalamus, in the brain, regulates the release of pituitary hormones. Each of these glands secrete hormones (chemical messengers) into the blood stream. Once hormones enter the blood, they travel throughout the body and are detected by receptors that recognize specific hormones. These receptors exist on target cells and organs. Once a target site is bound by a particular hormone, a cascade of cellular events follows that culminates in the physiological response to a particular hormone.

Most endocrine hormones are maintained at specific concentrations in the plasma, the non-cellular, liquid portion of the blood. Receptors at set locations monitor plasma hormonal levels and inform the gland responsible for producing that hormone if levels are too high or too low for a particular time of day, month, or other life period. When excess hormone is present, a negative feedback loop is initiated such that further hormone production is inhibited. Most hormones have this type of regulatory control. However, a few hormones operate on a positive feedback cycle such that high levels of the particular hormone will activate release of another hormone. With this type of feedback loop, the end result is usually that the second hormone released will eventually decrease the initial hormone's secretion. An example of positive feedback regulation occurs in the female menstrual cycle, where high levels of estrogen stimulate release of the pituitary hormone, luteinizing hormone (LH).

All hormones are influenced by numerous factors. The hypothalamus can release inhibitory or stimulatory hormones that determine pituitary function. And every physiological component that enters the circulation can effect some endocrine function. Overall, this system uses multiple bits of chemical information to hormonally maintain a biochemically balanced organism.

The pituitary gland has long been called "the master gland" because it secretes multiple hormones that, in turn, trigger the release of other hormones from other endocrine sites. The pituitary is roughly situated behind the nose and is anatomically separated into two distinct lobes, the anterior pituitary (AP) and the posterior pituitary (PP). The entire pituitary hangs by a thin piece of tissue, called the pituitary stalk, beneath the hypothalamus in the brain. The AP and PP are sometimes called the adenohypophysis and neurohypophysis, respectively.

The PP secretes two hormones, oxytocin and antidiuretic hormone (ADH), under direction from the hypothalamus. AP cells are categorized according to the hormones that they secrete. The hormone-producing cells of the AP include: somatotrophs, corticotrophs, thyrotrophs, lactotrophs, and gonadotrophs. Somatotrophs secrete growth hormone; corticotrophs secrete adrenocorticotropic hormone (ACTH); thyrotrophs secrete thyroid stimulating hormone (TSH); lactotrophs secrete prolactin; and gonadotrophs secrete LH and follicle stimulatory hormone (FSH). Each of these hormones sequentially signals a response at a target site. While ACTH, TSH, LH, and FSH primarily stimulate other major endocrine glands, growth hormone and prolactin primarily coordinate an endocrine response directly on bones and mammary tissue, respectively.

The pineal gland is a small cone-shaped gland believed to function as a body clock. The pineal is located deep in the brain just below the rear-most portion of the corpus callosum (a thick stretch of nerves that connects the two sides of the brain). The pineal gland, also called the pineal body, has mystified scientists for centuries. The 17th-century philosopher Rene Descartes speculated that the pineal was the seat of the soul. However, its real function is somewhat less grandiose than that.

The pineal secretes the hormone melatonin, the level of which fluctuates on a daily basis, with the levels highest at night. Although its role is not well understood, some scientists believe that melatonin helps to regulate other daily events. Exactly what controls melatonin levels is not well understood either; however, visual registration of light may regulate the cycle.

The thyroid is a butterfly-shaped gland that wraps around the back of the esophagus. The two lobes of the thyroid are connected by a band of tissue called the isthmus. An external covering of connective tissue separates each lobe into another 20-40 follicles. Between the follicles are numerous blood and lymph vessels in another connective tissue called stroma. The epithelial cells around the edge of the follicles produce the major thyroid hormones.

The major hormones produced by the thyroid are triiodothyronine (T3), thyroxine (T4), and calcitonin. T3 and T4 are iodine-rich molecules that fuel **metabolism**. The thyroid hormones play several important roles in growth, metabolism, and development. The thyroids of pregnant women often become enlarged in late **pregnancy** to accommodate metabolic requirements of both the woman and the fetus.

Thyroid hormones accelerate metabolism in several ways. They promote normal growth of bones and increase growth hormone output. They increase the rate of lipid synthesis and mobilization. They increase cardiac output by increasing rate and strength of heart contractions. They can increase respiration, the number of red blood cells in the circulation, and the amount of oxygen carried in the blood. In addition, they promote normal nervous system development including nerve branching.

While most people have four small parathyroid glands poised around the thyroid gland, about 14% of the population have one or two additional parathyroid glands. Because these oval glands are so small, the extra space occupied by extra glands does not seem to be a problem. The sole function of these glands is to regulate calcium levels in the body. Although this may seem like a simple task, the maintenance of specific calcium levels is critical. Calcium has numerous important bodily functions. Calcium makes up 2-3% of adult weight with roughly 99% of the calcium in bones. Calcium also plays a pivotal role in muscle contraction and neurotransmitter secretion.

In young children, the thymus extends into the neck and the chest, but after puberty, it begins to shrink. The size of the thymus in most adults is very small. Like some other endocrine glands, the thymus has two lobes connected by a stalk. The thymus secretes several hormones that promote the maturation of different cells of the immune system in young children. In addition, the thymus oversees the development and "education" of a particular type of immune system cell called a T lymphocyte, or T cell.

Although many details of thymal hormonal activity are not clear, at least four thymal products have been identified: thymosin, thymic humoral factor (THF), thymic factor (TF), and thymopoietin. Because **AIDS** is characterized by T cell depletion, some AIDS treatment approaches have tried administering tymosin to boost T cell production.

The pancreas is a large endocrine and exocrine gland situated below and behind the stomach in the lower abdomen. The pancreas is horizontally placed such that its larger end falls to the right and its narrower end to the left. Clusters of exocrine pancreatic cells called acini secrete digestive enzymes into the stomach; endocrine cells secrete hormones responsible for maintaining blood glucose levels.

The endocrine cells of the pancreas are contained in the islets of Langerhans which are themselves embedded in a rich network of blood and lymph vessels. Insulin is secreted in response to high plasma glucose levels. Insulin facilitates glucose uptake into blood cells thus reducing plasma glucose levels. Glucagon has the opposite effect; low plasma glucose triggers the breakdown of stored glucogen in the liver and glucose release into the blood. By balancing these two hormones, the islets continually regulate circulating glucose levels.

One of the two adrenals sit atop each kidney and are divided into two distinct regions, the cortex and the medulla. The outer area makes up about 80% of each adrenal and is called the cortex. And the inner portion is called the medulla. The adrenals provide the body with important buffers against stress while helping it adapt to stressful situations.

Cells of the adrenal medulla, called chromaffin cells, secrete the hormones, epinephrine (adrenaline) and non-epinephrine (nor-adrenaline). Chromaffin cells are neuroendocrine cells which function like some nerve fibers of the sympathetic nervous system. However, these cells are endocrine, because the neurohormones that they release target distant organs. Although the effects of these two medullary hormones are the same whether they originate in the endocrine or the **nervous system**, endocrine hormonal effects are prolonged, because they are removed more slowly from blood than from a nerve terminal. Both cortical and medullary hormones work together in emergencies, or stressful situations, to meet the physical demands of the moment.

The ovaries are located at the end of each fallopian tube in the female reproductive tract, and they produce the female reproductive hormones estrogen, progesterone, and relaxin. Although the fluctuation of these hormones is critical to the female menstrual cycle, they are initially triggered by a hormone from the hypothalamus, called a releasing factor, that enables gonadotrophs in the pituitary to release LH and FSH that, in turn, regulate part of the menstrual cycle. All of these hormones work together as part of the endocrine system to ensure fertility. They are also important for the development of sexual characteristics during puberty.

The two testes are located in the scrotum, which hangs between the legs behind the penis. Most of the testes is devoted to sperm production, but the remaining cells, called Leydig cells, produce testosterone. Testosterone caries out two very important endocrine tasks in males: it facilitates sexual maturation, and it enables sperm to mature to a reproductively competent form. Healthy men remain capable of fertilizing an egg throughout their post-pubertal life. However, testosterone levels do show a gradual decline after about the age of 40 with a total drop of around 20% by age 80.

See also Acromegaly and gigantism; Adrenal disorders; Cardiovascular system; Diabetes mellitus; Dwarfism; Lymphatic system; Menopause; Menstruation; Nervous system; Pregnancy; Reproductive system, female; Reproductive system, male

ENDOMETRIOSIS

Endometriosis is a condition in which bits of the tissue similar to the lining of the uterus (endometrium) grow in other parts of the body. Like the uterine lining, this tissue builds up and sheds in response to monthly hormonal cycles. The blood discarded from these implants falls onto nearby organs, causing swelling and inflammation which lead to scar tissue and adhesions. Endometriosis is estimated to affect 7% percent of women of childbearing age in the United States. It is most common between the ages 25–40. **Pregnancy** may slow the progress of endometriosis. A woman's risk of endometriosis is increased if her female relatives have endometriosis or her periods last longer than a week with an interval of less than 27 days between them.

Endometrial implants are often found on the pelvic organs—the ovaries, uterus, fallopian tubes, and in the cavity behind the uterus. Occasionally, they grow in more distant parts of the body. Implants appear as small bumps on the surfaces of the organs and supporting ligaments. **Ovarian cysts** (endometriomas), ranging from pea to grapefruit size, may form around endometrial tissue. Endometriosis usually advances slowly, over many years. Doctors rank cases from minimal to severe based on the number and size of the endometrial implants, their appearance and location, and the extent of the scar tissue and adhesions in the area of the growths. The cause of endometriosis is unknown. While many women with endometriosis experience severe weakness, others have the disease without knowing it. There is no relation between the severity of the symptoms and the extent of the disease. The most common symptoms are: menstrual **pain**, pain during sex, abnormal bleeding, and **infertility**. There is a strong association between endometriosis and infertility.

If a doctor suspects endometriosis, he/she will do a **pelvic exam** to try to feel implants. Often this does not provide strong evidence of endometriosis. The only way to make a definitive diagnosis is through minor surgery called a **laparoscopy**. A laparoscope, a slender scope with a light on the end, is inserted into the woman's abdomen through a small cut near her belly button. This allows the doctor to examine the internal organs. Often, a sample of tissue is taken for laboratory examination.

Endometriosis is sometimes discovered when a woman has abdominal surgery for another reason. Imaging tests such as **ultrasound**, **computed tomography scan** (CT scan), or **magnetic resonance imaging** (MRI) offer more information but don't help with the initial diagnosis. A blood test to determine the level of the blood protein CA125 can predict a recurrence of the disease. How endometriosis is treated depends on the woman's symptoms, her age, the extent of the disease, and her preferences. It cannot be fully resolved without surgery. Treatment focuses on managing the pain, preserving fertility, and delaying the progress of the condition. **Over-the-counter** pain relievers such as **aspirin** and **acetaminophen** (Tylenol) are used for mild cramping and menstrual pain. Prescription-strength and over-the-counter **nonsteroidal anti-inflammatory drugs** (NSAIDs), such as ibuprofen (Motrin, Advil) and naproxen (Naprosyn), are also effective. Narcotics are occasionally used for severe pain. Hormonal therapies effectively relieve endometriosis but they are also contraceptives. **Oral contraceptives** trick the body into thinking it's pregnant, reducing pain and temporarily withering endometrial implants. Danazol (Danocrine) and gestrinone are synthetic male hormones that lower estrogen levels, prevent menstruation, and shrink endometrial tissues, but they lead to weight gain and **menopause**-like symptoms, and cause some women to develop masculine characteristics. Progestins such as Medroxyprogesterone (**Depo-Provera**) and related drugs minimize pain and stop the condition's progress, but are rarely used because of side effects. Gonadotropin-releasing hormone (GnHR) agonists limit pain and prevent the growth of endometrial implants, but they can cause menopause symptoms and possible bone loss. Removing the uterus, ovaries, and fallopian tubes is the only permanent way to eliminate endometriosis. This is an extreme measure that means that a woman cannot have children and forces her body into menopause. Endometrial implants can be removed with laparoscopic **laser surgery**. For women with minimal endometriosis, this is usually successful in reducing pain and slowing the condition's progress. It may also help infertile women increase their chances of becoming pregnant. Although severe endometriosis should not be self-treated, many women help their condition through alternative therapies such as taking vitamin B complex with **vitamins** C, E, and the **minerals** calcium, magnesium, and selenium; a macrobiotic diet or a less extreme **diet** that cuts out sugar, salt, and processed foods; mind-body therapies such as relaxation and visualization, **acupuncture**, and **biofeedback**; and treatment with chiropractors or homeopathic doctors. Most women with endometriosis have minimal symptoms and do well. Symptoms come back in about 40% of women over the five years following treatment. There is no proven way to prevent endometriosis.

Enemas

An enema is the insertion of a solution into the rectum and lower intestine given to remove feces when an individual is constipated or impacted or in preparation for an examination or surgery, or to give drugs or anesthetic agents. The rectal tube used to give the enema should be smooth and flexible to decrease the possibility of damage to the lining of the rectum. Tap water is commonly used for adults but should not be used for infants because of the danger of electrolyte (substance that conducts electric current within the body and is essential for sustaining life) imbalance. The colon absorbs water, and repeated tap water enemas can cause cardiovascular overload and electrolyte imbalance. Repeated saline enemas can cause increased absorption of fluid and electrolytes into the bloodstream, resulting in overload. Individuals receiving frequent enemas should be observed for overload symptoms that include **dizziness**, sweating, or vomiting. Soap suds and saline used to clean enemas can irritate the lining of the bowel, with repeated use or a solution that is too strong. Only white soap not previously used should be used. The commercially prepared castile soap is preferred, in a concentration no greater than 5 cc soap to 1,000 cc of water.

Cleansing enemas stimulate bowel activity by irritating the lower bowel, and by stretching with the volume of fluid given. When the enema is given, the individual is usually on the left side-lying position, which facilitates absorption of fluid. The length of time it takes to administer an enema depends on the amount of fluid to be absorbed. This varies depending on the age and size of the person receiving the enema, however, general guidelines would be: 250 cc or less for an infant, 500 ml or less for a toddler or preschooler, 500–1,000 cc for a school-aged child, and 750–1,000 cc for an adult. A high enema, given to cleanse as much of the large bowel as possible, is usually administered at higher pressure and with larger volume (1,000 cc), and the individual changes position several times in order for the fluid to flow up into the bowel. A low enema, intended to cleanse only the lower bowel, is administered at lower pressure, using about 500 cc. of fluid. Oil retention enemas lubricate the rectum and lower bowel, and soften the stool. For adults, about 150–200 cc of oil is instilled, while in small children, 75–150 cc of oil is enough. Salad oil or liquid petrolatum are commonly used at a temperature of 91°F (32.8°C). There are also commercially prepared oil retention enemas. The oil is usually retained for one to three hours before it is expelled.

The rectal tube used for infusion of the solution, usually made of rubber or plastic, has two or more openings at the end through which the solution can flow into the bowel. The distance to which the tube must be inserted is dependent upon the age and size of the patient. To prepare an enema, the solution is measured, mixed, and warmed. Afterward, if necessary, a specimen is collected for diagnostic evaluation. Enemas should be used only as a last resort for treatment of constipation and with a doctor's recommendation. Enemas should not be given to individuals who have recently had colon or rectal surgery, a heart attack, or who suffer from an unknown abdominal condition or an irregular heartbeat.

Enlarged prostate

Enlarged prostate is a non-cancerous condition that narrows the urethra (a tube running from the bladder through the prostate gland) and makes eliminating urine more difficult. It affects many men over 50 years old and can be effectively treated by surgery and drugs. The common term for enlarged prostate is BPH, which stands for benign (non-cancerous) prostatic hyperplasia or hypertrophy. BPH is part of the aging process. Symptoms generally appear between ages 55–75. About 10% of all men eventually will require treatment for BPH. BPH is less common in blacks and Asians. The cause of BPH is unknown, but age-related hormonal changes may be a factor. An enlarging prostate gradually obstructs the flow of urine and in time, prevents the bladder from emptying completely at each urination. The urine that collects in the bladder can become infected and lead to stone formation or kidney damage. A man will have to urinate more often, perhaps two or three times at night. The need to urinate can become very urgent and, in time, urine may dribble out to stain clothing. Other symptoms of BPH are a weak and sometimes split stream, and general aching or **pain** in the perineum (the area between the scrotum and anus). Some men have considerable enlargement of the prostate before symptoms develop.

When a man's symptoms point to BPH, the physician will do a digital rectal examination, inserting a finger into the anus to feel whether—and how much—the prostate is enlarged. A smooth prostate surface suggests BPH, whereas a lump in the gland might mean **prostate cancer**. The next step is a blood test for a substance called prostate-specific antigen or PSA. Between 30–50% of men with BPH have an elevated PSA level. This does not mean **cancer**, but other tests are needed to make sure that the prostate enlargement is benign. An **ultrasound** exam of the prostate can show whether it is enlarged and may show that cancer is present. If there's a suspicion of cancer, most urologists will recommend a prostatic tissue biopsy. This is usually done using a lance-like instrument that is inserted into the rectum to obtain prostatic tissue for laboratory examination. To measure how severe the obstruction is, a catheter can be placed through the urethra and into the bladder, the man can urinate into a uroflowmeter, or a special viewing instrument called a cystoscope can be passed into the bladder. It is routine to check a urine sample for an increase in white blood cells, which may mean there is infection of the bladder or kidneys. The same sample could show what type of bacterium is causing the infection, and which **antibiotics** will work best. The kidneys can be checked through imaging by ultrasound or injecting a dye (the intravenous urogram, or pyelogram); or a blood test for creatinine. Drugs to treat BHP include alpha-adrenergic blockers, such as phenoxybenzamine and doxazosin, which improve obstructive symptoms but do not keep the prostate from enlarging; and others such as finasteride which shrink the prostate and may delay the need for surgery. It may take three months or longer for symptoms to improve. Antibiotics are given for infections. Some medications, including **antihistamines** and some **decongestants**, can make the symptoms of BPH worse and cause urinary retention and should be avoided. When drugs don't control symptoms but the physician doesn't believe that surgery is needed, transurethral needle ablation can be tried. In the office and using local **anesthesia**, a needle is inserted into the prostate and radiofrequency energy destroys the tissue that is obstructing urine flow. Microwave hyperthermia, done at an outpatient surgery center, uses a device called the Prostatron to deliver microwave energy to the prostate through a catheter. The standard operation for BPH is transurethral resection (TUR) of the prostate. Under general or spinal anesthesia, a cystoscope is passed through the urethra and prostate tissue surrounding the urethra is removed using either a cutting instrument or a heated wire loop. The small pieces of prostate tissue are washed out through the scope. No incision is needed. Alternatives to TUR include: laser ablation of the prostate done in an operating room; transurethral incision of the prostate which is less invasive than standard TUR and may work well in men whose prostate is not grossly enlarged; transurethral vaporization of the obstructing prostatic tissue; and if the prostate is greatly enlarged an open prostatectomy to remove the entire gland. An extract of the saw palmetto (*Serenoa repens* or *S. serrulata*) stops or decreases the hyperplasia of the prostate. In a man without symptoms whose prostate is enlarged, it is hard to predict when symptoms will develop and how fast they will progress. For this reason, some specialists (urologists) advise "watchful waiting." When BPH is treated by TUR, urinary symptoms will be relieved and quality of life improved for the great majority of men. There is no known way of preventing BPH.

Enterobacterial infections

Enterobacterial infections are disorders of the digestive tract and other organ systems produced by a group of bacteria called Enterobacteriaceae. They can be produced by bacteria that normally live in the human digestive tract without causing serious disease, or by bacteria that enter from the outside. In many cases people get these infections in the hospital. *Klebsiella* and *Proteus* sometimes cause **pneumonia**, ear and sinus infections, and urinary tract infections. *Enterobacter* and *Serratia* often cause bacterial infection of the blood (**bacteremia**), particularly in patients with weakened **immune systems**. **Diarrhea** caused by enterobacteria is common in the United States and can range from a minor nuisance to a life-threatening disorder, especially in infants, elderly persons, **AIDS** patients, and malnourished people. Enterobacterial infections are one of the two leading killers of children in developing countries. Enterobacterial infections of the digestive tract usually start when the organisms invade its lining. These bacteria may be present in the stomach and intestines, transmitted by contaminated food and water, or spread by person-to-person contact. The usual incubation period is 12–72 hours. Escherichia coli infections cause most of the enterobacterial infections in the United States. Noninvasive types of ***E. coli*** include enteropathogenic *E. coli*, or EPEC, and enterotoxigenic *E. coli*, or ETEC. EPEC and ETEC types produce a bacterial poison (toxin) in the stomach that interacts with the digestive juices and causes the patient to lose large amounts of water through the intestines. Invasive types of *E. coli* are called enterohemorrhagic *E. coli*, or EHEC, and enteroinvasive *E. coli, or EIEC.* These subtypes invade the stomach tissues directly, causing tissue destruction and bloody stools. EHEC can produce complications leading to hemolytic-uremic syndrome (HUS), a potentially fatal disorder marked by the destruction of red blood cells and **kidney failure**. EHEC has become a growing problem in the United States because of outbreaks caused by contaminated food. One type of EHEC known as O157:H7 has been identified in undercooked hamburgers, unpasteurized milk, and apple juice. The symptoms of enterobacterial infections are sometimes classified according to the type of diarrhea they produce: Bloody diarrhea (sometimes called dysentery) usually requires antibiotics while watery diarrhea does not. Necrotizing enterocolitis (NEC) is a disorder in newborns, primarily premature newborns.

The diagnosis of enterobacterial infections is complicated because viruses, protozoa, and other types of bacteria can also cause diarrhea. In most cases of mild diarrhea, it is not critical to identify the organism because the disorder is self-limiting. Patients who should have stool tests include those with: bloody diarrhea, watery diarrhea who have become dehydrated, watery diarrhea that has lasted longer than three days, and disorders of the immune system. The patient history helps the doctor determine what type of enterobacterium may be causing the infection. The most important parts of the **physical examination** are checking for signs of severe fluid loss and examining the abdomen to rule out typhoid fever. The doctor will look for signs of **dehydration**. The most common test to identify the cause of diarrhea is examining a stool sample under a microscope. Routine **stool culture**s, however, will not identify any of the types of *E. coli* that cause intestinal infections. ETEC, EPEC, and EIEC can usually be identified only by research laboratories. Because of concern about EHEC outbreaks, however, most laboratories in the United States can now screen for O157:H7 with a test that identifies its toxin. All patients with bloody diarrhea should have a stool sample tested for *E. coli* O157:H7.

Enterobacterial diarrhea is usually treated by fluids to restore the electrolyte balance and paregoric to relieve abdominal cramping. Newborn infants and patients with immune system disorders will be given **antibiotics** intravenously once the organism has been identified. Gentamicin, tobramycin, and amikacin are frequently used to treat enterobacterial infections because many of the organisms are becoming resistant to ampicillin and cephalosporin. Alternative treatments can relieve the discomfort of abdominal cramping, but most alternative practitioners advise consulting a medical doctor if the patient has sunken eyes, dry eyes or mouth, or other signs of dehydration. Herbalists may recommend cloves, ginger, peppermint (*Mentha iperita*), or chamomile (*Matricaria recutita*) tea. Homeopathic practitioners frequently recommend *Arsenicum album*, *Belladonna*, *Veratrum album*, and *Podophyllum*. The prognosis for most enterobacterial infections is good; most patients recover in about a week or 10 days without antibiotics. HUS has a death rate of 3–5%. About a third of the survivors have long-term kidney problems, and another 8% develop high blood pressure, **seizure disorders**, and blindness. The **World Health Organization** (WHO) offers these suggestions for preventing enterobacterial infections: Cook ground beef or hamburgers until the meat is thoroughly done; do not drink unpasteurized milk or use products made from raw milk; wash hands thoroughly and frequently, especially after using the toilet; wash fruits and vegetables carefully, or peel them; keep all kitchen surfaces and serving utensils clean; if drinking water is not known to be safe, boil it or drink bottled water; and keep cooked foods separate from raw foods, and avoid touching cooked foods with utensils that have been used with raw meat.

ENTEROBIASIS

Enterobiasis or pinworm infection, as it is commonly called, is an intestinal infection caused by the parasitic roundworm called *Enterobius vermicularis*. The most common symptom of this irritating, but not particularly dangerous, disease is **itching** around the anal area.

Enterobiasis is also called seatworm infection or oxyuriasis. It can affect people of any age, but is most common among children ages 5 and under and particularly affects those in the daycare setting.

The disease is highly contagious and is caused by a parasitic worm called *Enterobius vermicularis*. The adult female worm is about the size of a staple (approximately 1 cm long and 0.5 mm wide) and has a pointed tip. The disease is transmitted by ingesting the eggs of the pinworm. These eggs travel to the small intestine where, after approximately one month, they hatch and mature into adult worms. During the night, the female adult worms travel to the area around the anus and deposit eggs in the folds of the anal area. A single female pinworm can lay 10,000 eggs and, after laying eggs, dies. The eggs are capable of causing infection after six hours at body temperature.

Significant itching in the anal region is caused by the movement of the adult worm as the eggs are deposited. When an individual scratches the anal region, the tiny eggs get under the finger nails and in the underwear and night clothes. Anything the individual touches with the contaminated fingers, for example, toys, bedding, blankets, bathroom door knobs, or sinks, becomes contaminated. The eggs are very hardy and can live on surfaces for two to three weeks. Anyone touching these contaminated surfaces can ingest the eggs and become infected.

Many individuals with enterobiasis exhibit no symptoms. When present, however, symptoms of the infection begin approximately two weeks after ingesting the pinworm eggs. The main symptom is itching around the anus. Because the itching intensifies at night, when the female worms comes to the anus to lay eggs, it often leads to disrupted sleep and irritability. Poor sleeping at night in small children can be related to pinworms. Occasionally, the itching causes some bleeding and bruising in the region, and secondary bacterial infections can occur. In females, the itching may spread to the vagina and sometimes causes an infection of the vaginal region (vaginitis). Enterobiasis usually lasts one to two months.

First, a physician will rule out other potential causes of the itching, such as **hemorrhoids**, lice, or fungal or bacterial infection. Once these have been ruled out, an accurate diagnosis of enterobiasis will require that either the eggs or the adult worms are detected.

In order to collect a specimen of the eggs for laboratory diagnosis, the physician may provide a paddle with a sticky adhesive on one side, or an individual may be instructed to place a piece of shiny cellophane tape sticky side down against the anal opening. The best time to perform this test is at night or as soon as the individual wakes up in the morning, before having a bowel movement or taking a bath or shower. The pinworm eggs will stick to the tape, which can then be placed on a specimen slide. When under a microscope in the laboratory, the eggs will be clearly visible.

In order to treat the disease, either mebendazole (Vermox) or pyrantel pamoate (Pin-X) will be given in two oral doses spaced two weeks apart. These medications eradicate the infection in approximately 90% of cases. Re-infection is common and several treatments may be required. Because the infection is easily spread through contact with contaminated clothing or surfaces, it is recommended that all family members receive the therapeutic dose. Sometimes a series of six treatments are given, each spaced two weeks apart.

To relieve the rectal itching, a shallow warm bath with either half a cup of table salt, or Epsom salts is recommended. Also, application of an ointment containing zinc oxide or regular petroleum jelly can be used to relieve rectal itching.

Pinworms cause little damage and can be easily eradicated with proper treatment. The disease can be prevented by treating all the infected cases and thus eliminating the source of infection. Some ways to keep from catching or spreading the disease include the following recommendations:

- Wash hands thoroughly before handling food and eating.
- Keep finger nails short and clean.
- Avoiding scratching the anal area.
- Take early morning showers to wash away eggs deposited overnight.
- Once the infection has been identified, and treatment is started, change the bed linen, night clothes, and underwear daily.
- Machine wash linens in hot water and dry with heat to kill any eggs.
- Open the blinds or curtains since eggs are sensitive to sunlight.

ENTEROVIRUS INFECTIONS

Enteroviruses reproduce in the gastrointestinal tract after an infection but don't lead to intestinal symptoms; they causes disease by spreading to organs such as the **nervous system**, heart, and skin. There are four groups of enteroviruses: Coxsackievirus, Echovirus, ungrouped Enterovirus, and **Polio** virus; the first three are covered here. Enteroviruses are found worldwide, but are more common in areas of poor hygiene and overcrowding. Although most cases do not produce symptoms, 5–10 million people in the United States each year suffer from an enteroviral disease. Illness is more common in the very young, including fetuses. The virus is usually transmitted by fingers or objects contaminated by human waste material; it can also be transmitted through contaminated food or water. The incubation period for most enteroviruses ranges from 2–14 days. Enteroviruses are believed to be the cause of at least 10 illnesses. Once they enter the body, they multiply in the lining of the gastrointestinal tract, and eventually reach lymphatic tissue (such as the tonsils). While most don't last long and cause no significant injury, some can make the person severely ill. The most common syndrome caused by enteroviruses is summer grippe (nonspecific febrile illness), which has flu-like symptoms of **fever**, **headache**, and weakness, and typically lasts three to four days. Many patients also develop upper respiratory symptoms and some **nausea and vomiting**. Generalized disease of the newborn is a potentially serious infection with symptoms of fever, irritability, and decreased responsiveness or excessive sleepiness, which is difficult to distinguish from a severe bacterial infection. Inflammation of the heart muscle (**myocarditis**), low blood pressure, hepatitis, and **meningitis** sometimes complicate the illness. Aseptic meningitis **encephalitis**, most often in children and young adults, causes headache, fever, avoidance of light, eye **pain**, drowsiness, and possibly **sore throat**, **cough**, muscle pain, and rash. Occasionally, the brain tissue is affected, producing encephalitis. The illness goes away after a week or so, and permanent damage is unusual. Enteroviruses can also produce the Guillian-Barré syndrome, which involves weakness and **paralysis** of the extremities and the muscles of respiration. Pleurodynia (Bornholm's disease) is due to viral infection and inflammation of the chest and abdominal muscles used for breathing. Pain occurs as acute episodes, lasting 30 minutes or so. Myocarditis and/or **pericarditis** involves infection of the heart muscle (myocardium) and the covering around the heart (pericardium). Infants and young adults are the most susceptible. The disease usually begins as an upper respiratory tract infection with cough, **shortness of breath**, and fever. Chest pain, increasing shortness of breath, irregularities of cardiac rhythm and **heart failure** sometimes develop. Some patients wind up with long-term heart failure. Enterovirus **rashes** are the number one cause of exanthems (rashes) in the summer and fall. They occur anywhere on the body, and often resemble diseases such as **measles**.

In most cases, diagnosis is based on the symptoms that the virus produces. It is not usually necessary to identify a specific strain of virus causing the illness. Cultures are only helpful when obtained from areas that indicate recent infection, such as from swollen joints, cerebrospinal fluid, or blood. New techniques to identify viral genetic material (PCR) are useful in certain cases, but are not routinely used. Enterovirus can attack many different organs and produce a variety of symptoms. Most infections are mild, improve without complications, and require no specific therapy. When the virus attacks critical organs such as the heart, respiratory muscles, or nervous system, specialized care is often needed. There is no effective antiviral medication for enterovirus. In some patients antibodies (hypogammaglobunemia) are given. The outlook for enterovirus infection depends on the organs involved and the immune condition of the patient. Infection causes few problems unless vital organs are involved, immunity is abnormal, or patients have diseases that affect antibody production. In the hospital setting, the best way to avoid transmitting infection is good hand-washing practices and gowns and gloves for hospital staff. Precautions which isolate waste material will help decrease the chance of spreading the illness.

ENVIRONMENTAL HEALTH

Environmental health is concerned with the medical effects of chemicals, pathogenic (disease-causing) organisms, or physical factors in our environment. Because our environment affects nearly every aspect of our lives in some way or other, environmental health is related to virtually every branch of medical science. The special focus of this discipline, however, tends to be health effects of polluted air and water, contaminated food, and toxic or hazardous materials in our environment. Concerns about these issues make environmental health one of the most compelling reasons to be interested in environmental science.

For a majority of humans, the most immediate environmental health threat has always been pathogenic organisms. Improved **sanitation**, **nutrition**, and modern medicine in the industrialized countries have reduced or eliminated many of the communicable diseases that once threatened us. But for people in the less developed countries where nearly 80% of the world's population lives, bacteria, viruses, fungi, parasites, worms, flukes, and other infectious agents remain major causes of illness and death. Hundreds of millions of people suffer from major diseases such as **malaria**, gastrointestinal infections (**diarrhea**, dysentery, **cholera**), **tuberculosis**, **influenza**, and **pneumonia** spread through the air, water, or food. Many of these terrible diseases could be eliminated or greatly reduced by a cleaner environment, inexpensive **dietary supplements**, and better medical care.

For the billion or so richest people in the world—including most of the population of the United States and Canada—diseases related to lifestyle or longevity tend to be much greater threats than more conventional environmental concerns such as dirty water or polluted air. **Heart attack**s, **stroke**s, **cancer**, depression and **hypertension**, traffic **accidents**, trauma, and **AIDS** lead as causes of sickness and death in wealthy countries. These diseases are becoming increasingly common in the developing world as people live longer, exercise less, eat a richer diet, and use more drugs, tobacco, and alcohol. Epidemiologists predict that by the middle of the next century, these diseases of affluence will be leading causes of sickness and death everywhere.

Although a relatively minor cause of illness compared to the factors above, toxic or hazardous synthetic chemicals in the environment are becoming an increasing source of concern as industry uses more and more exotic materials to manufacture the goods we all purchase. There are many of these compounds to worry about. Somewhere around five million different chemical substances are known, about 100,000 are used in commercial quantities, and about 10,000 new ones are discovered or invented each year. Few of these materials have been thoroughly tested for toxicity. Furthermore, the process of predicting what our chances of exposure and potential harm might be from those released into the environment remains highly controversial. Toxins are poisonous, which means that they react specifically with cellular components or interfere with unique physiological processes. A particular chemical may be toxic to one organism but not another, or dangerous in one type of exposure but not others. Because of this specificity, they may be harmful even in very dilute concentrations. Ricin, for instance, is a protein found in castor beans and one of the most toxic materials known. Three hundred picograms (trillionths of a gram) injected intravenously is enough to kill an average mouse. A single molecule can kill an individual cell. If humans were as sensitive as mice, a few teaspoons of this compound, divided evenly and distributed uniformly could kill everyone in the world. By the way, this points out that not all toxins are produced by industry. Many natural products are highly toxic.

Toxins that have chronic (long-lasting) or irreversible effects are of special concern. Among some important examples are neurotoxins (attack nerve cells), mutagens (cause genetic damage), teratogens (result in **birth defects**), and carcinogens (cause cancer). Many pesticides and metals such as mercury, lead, and chromium are neurotoxins. Loss of even a few critical neurons can be highly noticeable or may even be lethal, making this category of great importance. Chemicals or physical factors such as radiation that damage genetic material can harm not only cells produced in the exposed individual, but also the offspring of those individuals as well.

The German physician Paracelsus said in 1540 that "The dose makes the poison." It has become a basic principle of toxicology that nearly everything is toxic at some concentration but most materials have some lower level at which they present an insignificant risk. Sodium chloride (table salt), for instance, is essential for human life in small doses. If you were forced to eat a kilogram all at once, however, it would make you very sick. A similar amount injected all at once into your blood stream would be lethal.

Some of our most convincing evidence about the toxicity of particular chemicals on humans has come from experiments in which volunteers (students, convicts, or others) were deliberately given measured levels under controlled conditions. Because it is now considered unethical to experiment on living humans, we are forced to depend on proxy experiments using computer models, tissue cultures, or laboratory animals. These proxy tests are difficult to interpret. We can't be sure that experimental methods can be extrapolated to how real living humans would react. The most commonly used laboratory animals in toxicity tests are rodents like rats and mice. However, different species can react very differently to the same compound. Of some 200 chemicals shown to be carcinogenic in either rats or mice, for instance, about half caused cancer in one species but not the other. How should we interpret these results? Should we assume that we are as sensitive as the most susceptible animal, as resistant as the least sensitive, or somewhere in between?

It is especially difficult to determine responses to very low levels of particular chemicals, especially when they are not highly toxic. The effects of random events, chance, and unknown complicating factors become troublesome, often resulting in a high level of uncertainty in predicting risk. The case of the sweetener saccharin is a good example of the complexities and uncertainties in risk assessment. Studies in the 1970s suggested a link between saccharin and bladder cancer in male rats. Critics pointed out that humans would have to drink 800 cans of soft drink per day to get a dose equivalent to that given to the rats. Furthermore, they argued, most people are not merely large rats.

The **Food and Drug Administration** uses a range of estimates of the probable toxicity of saccharine in humans. At current rates of consumption, the lower estimate predicts that only one person in the United states will get cancer every 1,000 years from saccharine. That is clearly inconsequential considering the advantages of reduced weight, fewer cases of diabetes, and other benefits from this sugar substitute. The upper estimate, however, suggests that 3,640 people will die each year from this same exposure. That is most certainly a risk worth worrying about.

An emerging environmental health concern with a similarly high level of uncertainty but potentially dire consequences is the disruption of endocrine hormone functions by synthetic chemicals. About ten years ago, wildlife biologists began to report puzzling evidence of reproductive failures and abnormal development in certain wild animal populations. Alligators in a lake in central Florida, for instance, were reported to have a 90% decline in egg hatching and juvenile survival along with feminization of adult males including abnormally small penises and lack of sperm production. Similar reproductive problems and developmental defects were reported for trout in the Great Lakes, seagulls in California, panthers in Florida, and a number of other species. Even humans may be effected if reports of global reduction of sperm counts and increases of hormone-dependent cancers prove to be true.

Both laboratory and field studies point to a possible role of synthetic chemicals in these problems. More than 50 chemicals, if present in high enough concentrations, are now known to mimic or disrupt the signals conveyed by naturally occurring endocrine hormones that control almost every aspect of development, behavior, immune functions, and **metabolism**. Among these chemicals are dioxin, polychlorinated biphenyl, and several persistent pesticides.

In spite of the seriousness of the concerns expressed above, the Environmental Protection Agency warns that we need to take a balanced view of environmental health. The risks associated with allowable levels of certain organic solvents in drinking water or some pesticides in food are thought to carry a risk of less than one cancer in a million people in a lifetime. Many people are outraged about being exposed to this risk, yet they cheerfully accept risks thousands of times as higher from activities they enjoy such as smoking, driving a car, or eating an unhealthy diet. According to the EPA, the most important things we as individuals can do to improve our health are to reduce smoking, drive safely, eat a balanced diet, exercise reasonably, lower stress in our lives, avoid dangerous jobs, lower indoor pollutants, practice safe sex, avoid sun exposure, and prevent household accidents. Many of these factors over which we have control are much more risky than the unknown, uncontrollable, environmental hazards we fear so much.

EPIDEMIC AND PANDEMIC

Epidemic, from the Greek meaning ''prevalent among the people,'' is most commonly used to describes an outbreak of an illness or disease in which the number of individual cases significantly exceeds the usual or ''expected'' number of cases in any given population. In the United States, the **Centers for Disease Control** (CDC) takes the average cases of, let's say, **influenza**, in 122 cities nationwide over the preceding five years. If influenza cases in any area significantly exceed that percentage baseline, it is said to be of epidemic proportions. The term is also used to describe almost any occurrence which increases drastically or becomes rampant—for example, auto thefts from parking lots or a significant increase in gang-related violence. *Pandemic*, which means ''all the people,'' describes and epidemic which occurs in more than one country or population simultaneously. An excellent example of a disease which has reached pandemic proportions is the **AIDS**/HIV virus. Human **obesity**, certainly less fatal than AIDS but which causes numerous health problems, has risen so drastically worldwide that it is now being considered a pandemic.

Diseases which reach epidemic proportions thrive in dense populations. Person-to-person contact is often necessary to spread the bacteria or virus, and groups of people, such as school children and service men and women, are particularly vulnerable. One of the most notorious viruses world-wide is the influenza virus, serious strains of which have killed tens of millions of people over the course of human history. Greek physician, **Hippocrates**, produced the first known record of a flu epidemic in 412 B.C. Just before the end of World War I, a pandemic of ''Spanish Flu'' killed more than 20 million people world-wide—more than the number of people killed by the war—and a half-million people in the United States alone. In 1968, the ''Hong Kong Flu'' pandemic infected more than 50 million people in the United States alone, causing an estimated 20,000 deaths.

In Europe during the 14th century, a pandemic of the bubonic **plague**, or Black Death, killed approximately 40 million people. Outbreaks in the 1990s in India, Zaire, Madagascar, Brazil, Peru, and China have raised concern among some epidemiologists of new pandemics. Frank Fenner, at Canberra's John Curtain School of Medical Research in Australia, believes the ease of modern transportation world-wide, a rising number of refugees from Third World countries, and changing sexual habits in First World countries, create fertile ground for the spread of this and other killer diseases today.

In the study of epidemiology, medical scientists attempt to determine the circumstances in which infectious diseases thrive, then track and attempt to regulate their occurrence and distribution. In 1942, the United Nations formed an agency called the **World Health Organization** (WHO) in an effort to help control epidemics and pandemics of diseases like **tuberculosis**, venereal disease, and **malaria**, as well as establish purified water and **sanitation** systems, **public health** education, health planning, and the training of health workers. Today, WHO's responsibilities include "1) the development of national and international infrastructure and resources to recognize, monitor, prevent, and control communicable diseases and emerging health problems, including antibiotic resistance, and 2) research and training on the diagnosis, epidemiology, prevention, and control of communicable diseases and emerging health problems." Nationally, the Public Health Service plays a major role in research and prevention of epidemics and pandemics.

See also Black death pandemics; Influenza; Influenza pandemic of 1918; Plague

EPIGLOTTITIS

Epiglottitis is an infection of the epiglottis, a leaf-like piece of cartilage extending upwards from the larynx, which can lead to severe airway obstruction. When air is breathed in (inspired), it passes through the nose and the nasopharynx or through the mouth and the oropharynx. These are both connected to the larynx. The air continues down the larynx to the trachea. The trachea then splits into two branches, the left and right bronchi (bronchial tubes). These bronchi branch into smaller air tubes which run within the lungs, leading to the small air sacs of the lungs (alveoli). Food, liquid, or air may be taken in through the mouth. While air goes into the larynx and the **respiratory system**, food and liquid are directed into the tube leading to the stomach, the esophagus. Because food or liquid in the bronchial tubes or lungs could cause a blockage or lead to an infection, the airway is protected by the epiglottis. In epiglottitis, the epiglottis may swell considerably and there is a danger that the airway will be blocked off by the very structure designed to protect it. Air is then unable to reach the lungs. Without medical care, epiglottitis can be fatal. It generally strikes two to seven-year-old children, although older children and adults can also get it. Boys are twice as likely as girls to develop this infection. Because epiglottitis involves swelling and infection of tissues which are all located at or above the level of the epiglottis, it is sometimes referred to as supraglottitis (*supra,* meaning above). About 25% of all children with this infection also have **pneumonia**.

The most common cause of epiglottitis is infection with the bacteria called *Haemophilus influenzae type b.* Other types of bacteria are also occasionally responsible, including some types of *Streptococcus* bacteria and the bacteria responsible for causing **diphtheria**. A patient with epiglottitis typically experiences a sudden **fever**, and begins having severe throat and neck **pain**. Because the swollen epiglottis interferes significantly with air movement, every breath creates a loud, harsh, high-pitched sound referred to as stridor. Because the vocal cords are located in the larynx just below the area of the epiglottis, the swollen epiglottis makes the patient's voice sound muffled and strained. Swallowing becomes difficult, and the patient may drool. The patient often leans forward and juts out his or her jaw, while struggling for breath. Epiglottitis strikes suddenly and progresses quickly. A child may begin complaining of a **sore throat**, and within a few hours be suffering from extremely severe airway obstruction.

Diagnosis begins with a high level of suspicion that a quickly progressing illness with fever, sore throat, and airway obstruction is very likely to be epiglottitis. If epiglottitis is suspected, no efforts should be made to look at the throat, or to swab the throat in order to obtain a culture for identification of the causative organism. These actions may cause the larynx to go into spasm (laryngospasm), completely closing the airway. These procedures should only be performed in a fully equipped operating room, so that if laryngospasm occurs, a breathing tube can be immediately placed in order to keep the airway open. An instrument called a laryngoscope is often used in the operating room to view the epiglottis, which will appear cherry-red and quite swollen. An x-ray picture taken from the side of the neck should also be obtained. The swollen epiglottis has a characteristic appearance, called the "thumb sign." Treatment almost always involves the immediate establishment of an artificial airway: inserting a breathing tube into the throat (intubation); or making a tiny opening toward the base of the neck and putting a breathing tube into the trachea (tracheostomy). Because epiglottitis is caused by a bacteria, **antibiotics** such as cefotaxime, ceftriaxone, or ampicillin with sulbactam should be given through a needle placed in a vein (intravenously). This prevents the bacteria which are circulating throughout the bloodstream from causing infection elsewhere in the body. With treatment, only about 1% of children with epiglottitis die. Without the artificial airway, this figure jumps to 6%. Most patients recover from the infection, and can have the breathing tube removed (extubation) within a few days. Prevention involves the use of a vaccine against H. influenzae type b (called the Hib vaccine). It is given to babies at two, four, six, and 15 months. Use of this vaccine has made epiglottitis rare.

ERASISTRATUS (304 B.C.-250 B.C.)

Greek physician and anatomist

Erasistratus, considered the father of physiology, was born on the island of Chios in ancient Greece. His father and brother were doctors, and his mother was the sister of a doctor. He studied medicine in Athens and then, around 280 B.C., enrolled in the University of Cos, a center of the medical school of Praxagoras. Erasistratus then moved to Alexandria, where he taught and practiced medicine, continuing the work of **Herophilus**. In his later years, he retired from medical practice and joined the Alexandrian museum, where he devoted himself to research.

Although Erasistratus wrote extensively in a number of medical fields, none of his works survive. He is best known for his observations based on his numerous **dissections** of

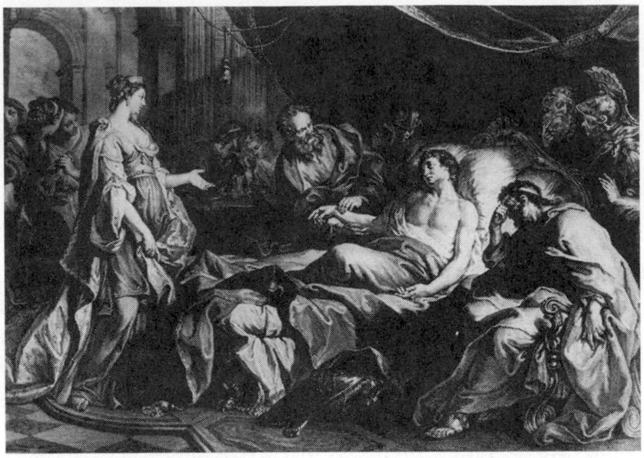

Erasistratus

human cadavers (and, it was rumored, his **vivisection** of criminals, a practice allowed by the Ptolemy rulers). Erasistratus accurately described the structure of the brain, including the cavities and membranes, and made a distinction between its *cerebrum* and *cerebellum* (larger and smaller parts). Contrary to popular belief at the time, he viewed the brain, not the heart, as the seat of intelligence. By comparing the brains of humans and other animals, Erasistratus rightly concluded that a greater number of brain convolutions resulted in greater intelligence. He also accurately described the structure and function of the gastric (stomach) muscles and observed the difference between motor and sensory nerves. Erasistratus promoted hygiene, **diet**, and **exercise** in medical care.

In his understanding of the heart and blood vessels, Erasistratus came very close to working out the circulation of the blood (not actually discovered until **William Harvey** in the seventeenth century A.D.), but he made some crucial errors. Erasistratus understood that the heart served as a pump, thereby dilating the arteries, and he found and explained the functioning of the heart valves. He theorized that the arteries and veins both spread from the heart, dividing finally into extremely fine capillaries that were invisible to the eye. However, he believed that the liver formed blood and carried it to the right side of the heart, which pumped it into the lungs and from there to the rest of the body's organs. He also believed that *pneuma*, a vital spirit, was drawn in through the lungs to the left side of the heart, which then pumped the pneuma through the arteries to the rest of the body. The nerves, according to Erasistratus, carried another form of pneuma, animal spirit.

After Erasistratus, anatomical research through dissection ended, due to the pressure of public opinion. Egyptians believed in the need of an intact body for the afterlife—hence mummification. Scientific anatomical studies were not resumed until the thirteenth century.

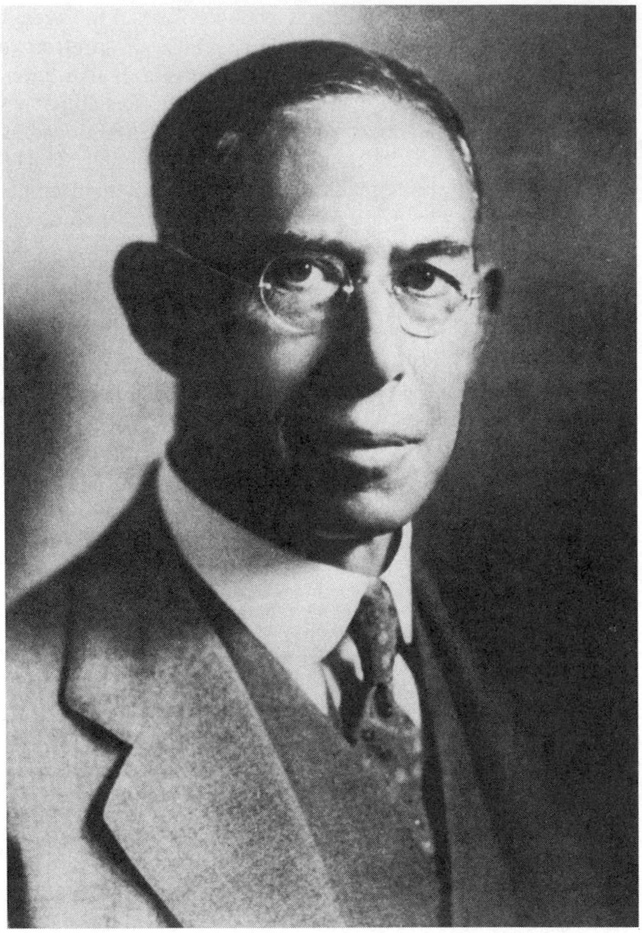

Joseph Erlanger

ERLANGER, JOSEPH (1874-1965)

American physiologist

Joseph Erlanger was an American physiologist whose pioneering work with his collaborator, **Herbert Spencer Gasser**, helped to advance the field of neurophysiology. For their work on "the highly differentiated functions of single nerve fibers" Erlanger and Gasser shared the 1944 Nobel Prize in medicine or physiology. The awarding of the Nobel Prize to Erlanger and Gasser also recognized their roles in developing the most basic tool in modern neurophysiology: the amplifier with cathode-ray oscilloscope. The prize culminated for Erlanger a distinguished career in medical education and physiological research.

Erlanger was born on January 5, 1874 in San Francisco, California, the sixth of seven children, to Herman Erlanger and Sarah Galinger, both immigrants from Southern Germany.

In 1889, Joseph Erlanger entered the classical Latin curriculum at the San Francisco Boys' High School. After graduating in 1891, he began studies in the College of Chemistry at the University of California at Berkeley, receiving a bachelor's degree in 1895. At Berkeley Erlanger performed his first research—studying the development of newt eggs. He then enrolled at the Johns Hopkins University School of Medicine in Baltimore and earned a medical degree in 1899, graduating second in his class. This distinction allowed Erlanger to work as an intern in internal medicine for **William Osler**, the renowned physician and teacher.

In Baltimore, in the summer of 1896, he worked in the histology laboratory of Lewellys Barker, studying the location of horn cells in the spinal cord of rabbits; the following summer, he undertook a project to study the digestive process of dogs. This study led to Erlanger's first published paper in 1901, and to his appointment as assistant professor of physiology at Johns Hopkins by William H. Howell, one of America's most important physiologists and head of the department. He was later promoted to associate professor of physiology.

In 1904, at Johns Hopkins, Erlanger designed and constructed a sphygmomanometer—a device that measures blood pressure. Erlanger improved on previous designs by making it sturdier and easier to use. Later that year, he used the device to find a correlation between blood pressure and orthostatic albuminuria, wherein proteins appear in the urine when a patient stands. His last few years at Johns Hopkins were spent studying electrical conduction in the heart, particularly the activity between the auricles and the ventricles that is responsible for the consistent beating of the heart. Using a clamp of his own design, he was able to determine that a conduction blockage, or heart block, in the bundle of His, a connection between the auricles and ventricles, was responsible for the reduced pulse and fainting spells associated with Stokes-Adams syndrome.

In 1906, Erlanger left Johns Hopkins and moved to the University of Wisconsin, where he became the first professor of physiology at the university's medical school. The following year Erlanger left Wisconsin for the Washington University School of Medicine in St. Louis, where he worked for the remainder of his career, serving as professor of physiology and department chairman.

In 1917, the United States' entry into World War I presented him with the opportunity to return to the laboratory and to his research on cardiovascular physiology. He participated with other physiologists in the study of wound shock and helped to develop therapeutic solutions that were used by the U.S.Army in Europe. He also continued the work that he had begun at Johns Hopkins, studying the sounds of Korotkoff, the sound one hears in an artery when measuring blood pressure with a stethoscope.

In the early 1920s, Erlanger turned to neurophysiology. The arrival at Washington University of Herbert Spencer Gasser, a student of Erlanger's from Wisconsin and a fellow Johns Hopkins graduate, spurred this change. Erlanger and Gasser would collaborate at Washington University until Gasser's departure in 1931 for the Cornell Medical College. Understanding how nerves transmit electrical impulses preoccupied Erlanger and Gasser during the 1920s. The difficulty in studying nerves was that the electrical impulses were too weak and too brief to measure them accurately. In 1920, one of Gasser's former classmates, H. Sidney Newcomer, developed a device that would amplify nerve impulses by some 100,000 times, allowing physiologists to measure and study the subtle changes that occur during nerve transmission. A year later, Erlanger and Gasser, based on advances made at the Western Electric Company, constructed a cathode-ray oscilloscope that could record the nerve impulse. The cathode-ray oscilloscope with amplifier was a technological breakthrough that permitted neurophysiologists to overcome the barrier posed by the subtlety and brevity of nerve activity. Erlanger and Gasser went on to study the details of nerve transmission. Their most significant contribution derived from these researches was their conclusion that larger nerve fibers conducted electrical impulses faster than smaller ones. Also, they demonstrated that different nerve fibers can have different functions.

Erlanger's wholly American education, consisting of a full-time research effort, represented a new generation of American physiologists. For his scientific efforts, Erlanger was elected a member of the National Academy of Sciences, the Association of American Physicians, the American Philosophical Society, and the American Physiological Society. He also received honorary degrees from universities of California, Michigan, Pennsylvania, Wisconsin, and Johns Hopkins University, Washington University, and the Free University of Brussels. His highest honor came when he shared, with Gasser, the 1944 Nobel Prize for physiology or medicine. After his retirement in 1946, Erlanger continued to work part-time performing research and helping graduate students in their work. Erlanger died of **heart failure** on December 5, 1965, one month before his 92nd birthday.

ERYTHROBLASTOSIS FETALIS

Erythroblastosis fetalis is two potentially disabling or fatal-blood disorders in infants: Rh incompatibility disease and ABO incompatibility disease. These disorders are caused by incompatibility between a mother's blood and her unborn baby's blood and may be apparent before birth. Because of the incompatibility, the mother's **immune system** destroys the baby's blood cells, and the baby suffers severe **anemia** (deficiency in red blood cells), brain damage, or **death**. A person's blood type is determined by genes inherited from parents: proteins called antigens in red blood cells and the presence or absence of the Rh-factor. Blood is classified as A, B, AB, or O and positive or negative (e.g., A-positive or B-negative). Blood type doesn't affect health, but the immune system accepts only the individual's blood type or a close match. Introduction of a radically different blood type causes the immune system to produce antibodies that attack and destroy cells carrying the foreign antigen. In a pregnant woman, blood cells from the unborn baby can cross over into the mother's bloodstream, especially at delivery. If the blood types are incompatible, the mother's immune system makes antibodies against the baby's blood. Usually, this doesn't happen in a first **pregnancy**.

Rh incompatibility disease and ABO incompatibility disease have similar symptoms, but Rh disease is much more severe because more of the baby's blood cells are destroyed.

Both incompatibility diseases are uncommon in the United States. Rh disease only occurs if a mother is Rh-negative and her baby is Rh-positive, which happens only when the baby inherits the Rh factor gene from the father. Most people are Rh-positive. ABO incompatibility disease is almost always limited to babies with A or B antigens whose mothers have type O blood. Approximately one third of these babies show evidence of the mother's antibodies in their bloodstream, but only a small percentage develop symptoms of ABO incompatibility disease. The baby's body tries to compensate for the anemia caused by the mother's antibodies by releasing immature red blood cells, called erythroblasts. The overproduction of erythroblasts can cause the liver and spleen to become enlarged, potentially causing liver damage or a ruptured spleen. Excess erythroblast production means that fewer of other types of blood cells are produced, such as platelets and other factors important for blood clotting. Excessive bleeding can be a complication. The destroyed red blood cells release the blood's red pigment (hemoglobin) which degrades into a yellow substance called bilirubin. Bilirubin is normally produced as red blood cells die, but the body can only handle a low level of bilirubin. In erythroblastosis fetalis, high levels of bilirubin accumulate and cause hyperbilirubinemia, a condition in which the baby becomes **jaundice**d, a yellowish tone of the eyes and skin. If hyperbilirubinemia cannot be controlled, the baby develops kernicterus, in which bilirubin is deposited in the brain and may cause permanent damage. Other symptoms include high levels of insulin and low blood sugar, as well as a condition called hydrops fetalis. Hydrops fetalis causes fluids to accumulate within the baby's body, making it look swollen. This inhibits normal breathing and can interfere with lung growth if it continues for an extended period. Hydrops fetalis and anemia can also contribute to heart problems.

Erythroblastosis fetalis can be predicted before birth by determining the mother's blood type. If she is Rh-negative, the father's blood is tested to determine whether he is Rh-positive. If the father is Rh-positive, the mother's blood will be checked for antibodies against the Rh factor. A blood test that demonstrates no antibodies is repeated at week 26 or 27 of the pregnancy. Blood incompatibility is uncovered through blood tests such as the Coombs test, and others. When a mother has antibodies against her unborn infant's blood, the antibodies are monitored and if levels increase, amniocentesis, fetal umbilical cord blood sampling, and ultrasound are used to assess any effects on the baby. If the baby is in danger, and the pregnancy is at least 32–34 weeks along, labor is induced. Under 32 weeks, the baby is given blood **transfusions** while in the mother's uterus. After birth, the severity of the baby's symptoms is assessed. Transfusions may be necessary to treat anemia, hyperbilirubinemia, and bleeding. Hyperbilirubinemia is also treated with **phototherapy**, oxygen and intravenous fluids, or drugs. Treatment of minor symptoms is typically successful and the baby will not suffer long-term problems. Erythroblastosis is a serious condition for approximately 4,000 babies annually, 15% of whom die before birth. Babies who survive pregnancy may develop kernicterus, which can lead to deafness, speech problems, **cerebral palsy**, or **mental retardation**. Extended hydrops fetalis can inhibit lung growth and contribute to **heart failure**. These serious complications are life threatening, but with good medical treatment, the fatality rate is very low. With any pregnancy, **blood typing** is a universal precaution against blood incompatibility disease. If an Rh-negative woman gives birth to an Rh-positive baby, she is injected with immunoglobulin G, a type of antibody protein, within 72 hours of the birth, to destroy fetal blood cells in her bloodstream before her immune system can react to them.

Esophageal cancer

Esophageal cancer is an often fatal malignancy (something that progresses and becomes worse with time) that develops in tissues lining the hollow, muscular canal (esophagus) along which food and liquid travel from the throat to the stomach. It starts in the inner layers of the lining of the esophagus and grows outward. In time, it can block the passage of food and liquid, making swallowing painful and difficult. Squamous cell carcinoma, the most common type of esophageal cancer, can develop at any point along the esophagus. Adenocarcinoma starts in glandular tissue not normally present in the lining of the esophagus. Esophageal cancer is three times more common in men than in women, and among blacks than among whites. Men and women between the ages of 45 and 70 are at the greatest risk. The cause of esophageal cancer is unknown. Risk factors include heavy drinking or **smoking**, especially, when combined; a diet low in fruits, vegetables, zinc, riboflavin, and vitamin A; swallowing household cleansers containing chemicals that can burn and destroy cells; a condition called achalasia; a rare inherited disease called tylosis; and a condition called esophageal webs. Patients with early esophageal cancer may be hoarse and have **hiccups** or elevated calcium levels, but symptoms generally don't appear until the tumor has grown so large that the patient cannot be cured. Dysphagia (trouble swallowing or a sensation of having food stuck in the throat or chest) is the most common symptom. Painful swallowing usually means that a large tumor is blocking the opening of the esophagus.

A barium swallow is usually the first test performed if esophageal cancer is suspected. This special x-ray highlights bumps or flat raised areas on the normally smooth surface of the esophageal wall and detects large, irregular areas that narrow the esophagus in patients with advanced **cancer**, but it can't provide information about disease spread beyond the esophagus. A double contrast study is a barium swallow with air blown into the esophagus to improve the way the barium coats the esophageal lining. In esophagoscopy, a thin lighted tube (esophagoscope) is passed through the mouth, down the throat, and into the esophagus to remove abnormal cells for biopsy. Once a diagnosis of esophageal cancer has been confirmed, tests are performed to determine whether the disease has spread (metastasized) to tissues or organs near the original tumor or in other parts of the body. This is called staging. In Stage 0, cancer cells are confined to the inner lining of the esophagus. Stage I esophageal cancer involves only a small part of the esophagus. In Stage IIA, cancer has invaded the thick, muscular layer of the esophagus that propels food into the stomach and may involve connective tissue covering the outside of the esophagus. In Stage IIB, cancer has spread to lymph nodes near the esophagus and may have invaded deeper layers of esophageal tissue. Stage III esophageal cancer has spread to tissues or lymph nodes near the esophagus or to the trachea (windpipe) or other organs near the esophagus. Stage IV cancer has spread to distant organs like the liver, bones, and brain. Recurrent esophageal cancer develops, after treatment, in the esophagus or another part of the body. Endoscopy and CAT scans provide images of tumors and the extent of disease and indicate the chances that all cancer can be surgically removed. Endoscopic ultrasound determines how deep cancer cells are in the esophagus and may measure disease spread and predict surgical outcomes better than CAT scans. Treatment for esophageal cancer is determined by the stage of the disease and the patient's health. The most common operations are: Esophagectomy, which removes the cancerous part of the esophagus and nearby lymph nodes and is performed only on patients with very early cancer that has not spread to the stomach; and esophagogastrectomy, which removes the cancerous part of the esophagus, nearby lymph nodes, and the upper part of the stomach. These procedures significantly relieve symptoms and improve the nutritional status of more than 80% of patients with dysphagia. Surgery can cure some patients whose disease has not spread beyond the esophagus, but more than 75% of esophageal cancers have spread to other organs before being diagnosed. Patients too ill for surgery may be treated with radiation, delivered by machine or implanted near cancer cells inside the body. Radiation alone won't cure esophageal cancer, but it relieves dysphagia almost as effectively as surgery. Post-operative radiation kills cancer cells that couldn't be surgically removed. Radiation is also used to control bleeding and relieve symptoms in patients who can't be cured. Oral or intravenous **chemotherapy** alone will not cure esophageal cancer, but pre-operative treatments can shrink tumors and increase the probability that cancer can be surgically eradicated. Regular barium swallows and other imaging studies detect recurrence or spread of disease or new tumor development. An experimental treatment, photodynamic therapy (PDT), kills cancer cells by laser beam. PDT cured some early esophageal cancers during preliminary studies. Although esophageal cancer carries a poor prognosis, recent advances in multiple therapies for this disease offer some hope. There is no known way to prevent esophageal cancer.

EUGENICS

The term ''eugenics'', which from its Greek roots means ''good in birth'', originated from the mind of Englishman **Francis Galton** who first introduced his ''science'' of heredity to the public in 1883. A wealthy cousin of Charles Darwin with a fascination for the emerging field of statistics, Galton began research that supported his belief that society's sympathy for the weak prevented proper evolution. He claimed humanity required a form of artificial selection, to eliminate the weak's ability to reproduce. This idea of superiority by one ''race'' over another was the driving force within the early history of eugenics, which in turn led to the justification of atrocities to human beings, including involuntary sterilization in the United States and racial hygiene of Nazi Germany, throughout the early half of the twentieth century.

Historically, nearly every culture dating back to ancient times has implemented the ideas that prompted modern eugenics. Customs and laws dictated prohibition against inbreeding such as the breeding between brother and sister and assured the death of infants born with deformities. Those who were feeble, diseased, or otherwise inferior were sentenced to die, while those who were intellectually superior were brought together to produce offspring. Science brought attention to eugenics with Galton's correlation that intelligence and other admired traits were inherited completely independent of any environmental consideration or influence. With a determination to maximize brilliance and prevent ''feeblemindedness,'' Galton encouraged ''good'' marriages that would produce highly intelligent males and ultimately assure the stock of the next generation.

Galton's presentation of eugenics came on the heels of Charles Darwin's 1859 book, *The Origin of Species.* Revered by many as the end of any scientific justification for the existence of a Creator God, Darwin's theory of evolution dismissed natural equality and promoted the creation of a group called ''Social Darwinists,'' who optimistically preached the survival of the fittest. Evolutionary theory took precedence as the human race was divided into the ''fit'' and ''unfit,'' and eugenics became the scientific community's calling as it promoted ways in which, according to Galton, ''social control may improve or impair the racial qualities of future generations whether physically or mentally.'' Rising fear by some in the Social Darwinist community was also linked to the increased ability medical care was giving to the ''weak'' in terms of survival, instead of the ''natural'' process of eliminating those who would otherwise not survive. This fear traveled through Germany, and in a direct response to the rapid increase of help that was being given to the growing number of impoverished and the weak by medical intervention and welfare policies, the German Social Darwinist Alfred Ploetz wrote his document on ''racial hygiene,'' a term introduced by the author. Ploetz attacked those who helped the weak survive, and declared that racial hygiene was not just for the good of the individual, both also for the good of the race.

Support for eugenics and racial hygiene surfaced across seas with support from **Margaret Sanger** in the United States. As a leader in the movement for global birth control, Sanger declared ''more children from the fit, less from the unfit that is the chief issue of birth control,'' a theory that was readily accepted by the community, during this period. Eugenicists began to unite and ignite public concerns that society was becoming afflicted by the ''unfit,'' and they demanded support from the government which resulted in a number of state legislatures to take direct responsibility to protect its citizens from the financial cost of maintaining those deemed unfit, and the results their breeding would have on society. Policy emerged that brought 34 states to pass laws which denied the insane the right to marry by 1912, nine states restricted marriage from those who were epileptic, and 15 banned the marrying of the mentally retarded to each other. Legislatures continued to be motivated by economic considerations and arguments for eugenics, in addition to the lacking parenting abilities of the "feebleminded," a trait assumedly passed on to their children.

With the "mental defectives" labeled by various American organizations, the public "menace" were institutionalized by increasing numbers that would result in overcrowding of mental **asylums**. As a result, a more radical approach to eliminating the "unfit" came to fruition. Sterilization was supported widely in the United States, and several nations, including Great Britain and Germany, with Pennsylvania becoming the first state to enact a coercive sterilization statute in 1907, which led to laws being passed in 24 states that encouraged sterilization of those who were mentally retarded, insane, or had criminal records. This type of involuntary sterilization led to the infamous 1927 Supreme Court case of Buck v. Bell, which charged that social prejudice was the primary motive behind the decision to perform a coerced surgical procedure on a "feebleminded" young woman from an indigent family in Virginia named Carrie Buck. After further argument that Buck would be denied her due process as guaranteed by the Fourteenth Amendment, the sterilization, however, remained to found legal. Buck's attorney appealed, which ultimately led to the Supreme Court's ruling against Buck. This decision, based on eugenic theory, was not reversed for four decades.

The "betterment" of mankind attempting a utopic world caused the eugenics movement to reach its climax in the early twentieth century, with American biologist Charles Davenport championing the cause that believed certain "racial stock" was superior to others in such areas as intelligence, hard work, and cleanliness. Davenport's theories of human evolution were born from the rediscovered work of Austrian monk Gregor Mendel who discovered the transmission of dominant and recessive traits (**genetics**) by breeding peas a finding that to many was the answer to all of human heredity's mysteries. Eugenic movements continued to grow with the founding of several societies, including the Society for Racial Hygiene by Ploetz in 1905, the Eugenic Society of Great Britain in 1908, and in 1923 The American Eugenics Society, with 29 chapters quickly growing across the country. Promoting better breeding while preventing poor breeding became the eugenics movement creed as they hosted "fitter family" and "better baby" competitions at fairs and exhibitions throughout the United States.

As fear from World War I continued to invade society, the Immigration Act of 1924 set strict quotas limiting immigrants from countries with "inferior" stock into the United States, and Adolf Hitler began to take notice of America's interest in eugenics. With Germany in economic turmoil after the war, Hitler exploited the needy population and gained control with his first command to change the country's sterilization law from voluntary to mandatory. From 1934 to 1937, an astronomical 400,000 sterilizations took place in Germany, compared to 30,000 sterilized on eugenics grounds in the United States by 1939. Hitler began a **euthanasia** program in 1939 by secretly authorizing doctors to grant merciful deaths to the incurably ill this led to the killing of more than 70,000 patients in less than three years. While the mercy killing of euthanasia was not limited to Germany, with support from Britain and the United States appearing at this time, the Nazi regime's "necessary" extermination of inferior races was their mission alone. Leading biologists and physicians in Germany welcomed Hitler's idea of placing race at the center of building a new state, which resulted in the concentration camps and genetic research of humans that define the Holocaust.

As the world began to realize the actual steps Hitler was taking to create his "super-race." opposition to the Nazis and eugenics surfaced. Sterilization laws in the United States decreased in the 1940s with the practice almost nonexistent by the 1950s, and also when IQ tests came under intense scrutiny. The term eugenics became phased out of society, with a shift in the scientific community toward behaviorism and true genetics. Genetic counseling centers became widespread between the 1950s and 1980s in several countries as a way to detect a pattern of disease among families, and the amniocentesis was developed in the late 1960s as a technique to discover irregularities in the fetus. This test became critical after 1973, when the U.S. Supreme Court decision of Roe v. Wade allowed a women to choose **abortion** of a fetus with defects discovered by amniocentesis. Other genetic tests of the late twentieth century include screenings for **sickle-cell anemia** in the African American community, and in 1976 the National Genetic Disease Act provided research, screening, counseling, and education of Cooley's anemia, **Tay-Sachs disease**, **cystic fibrosis**, **Huntington's disease**, and **muscular dystrophy**. While the term eugenics remains to reflect negatively on the modern science of genetics, a more positive enforcement of prevention of disease is taking its place.

See also Abortion; Cystic fibrosis; Euthanasia; Galton, Francis; Genetics; Huntington's disease; Intelligence and intelligence tests; Mental retardation; Muscular dystrophy; Sanger, Margaret Louise; Sickle-cell anemia; Tay-Sachs disease;

EULER, ULF VON (1905-1983)

Swedish physiologist

Ulf von Euler devoted his life to searching for the chemical signals that control physiological processes. In a career spanning six decades and during which he published four hundred and sixty-five scientific papers, von Euler achieved remarkable success. While still in his twenties, he discovered both substance P and prostaglandin, two important compounds that have since been studied extensively. Prostaglandins have become valuable to doctors for the treatment of many disorders, and may be used to treat blood pressure problems, infertility, peptic ulcers, and asthma. Martin A. Wasserman, in *American Pharmacy,* wrote on the significance of prostaglandins to modern medicine, stating that "Prostaglandin' signifies more to scientists today than any medical term since cortisone. For millions of people around the world, prostaglandins hold the promise of relief from an extraordinary range of physical discomforts and life-threatening illnesses.'' In addition, von Euler became the first person to isolate and identify noradrenaline, a key transmitter of nerve impulses which control such involuntary functions as the heartbeat. For the later accomplishment, he was awarded the 1970 Nobel Prize in physiology or medicine.

Ulf Svante von Euler was born on February 7, 1905, in Stockholm, Sweden. From the beginning, he seemed destined for scientific greatness. His father, Hans Euler-Chelpin, was a chemist who received the 1929 Nobel Prize for research into the role of enzymes in sugar fermentation. Von Euler's mother, Astrid Cleve von Euler, was a professor of botany, and his grandfather, Per Teodor Cleve, was a chemist who discovered the elements holmium and thulium. Moreover, von Euler was also a distant relative of the famous eighteenth-century mathematician, Leonhard Euler.

With the help of his father, von Euler coauthored his first scientific paper when he was just seventeen years old. He went on to receive a medical degree from the Karolinska Institute in Stockholm in 1930. That same year, with the aid of a Rockefeller Fellowship, von Euler traveled to London to work in the laboratory of **Henry Hallett Dale**, who would himself win a Nobel Prize in 1936 for discoveries relating to the chemical transmission of nerve impulses. At the time von Euler arrived, one particular compound—acetylcholine—was the focus of most of the study in Dale's laboratory.

It was while von Euler was conducting an experiment involving acetylcholine that he made his first significant observation. He noticed that a section of rabbit intestine would contract whenever it was exposed to an intestinal extract. Surprisingly, though, the addition of atropine to the extract fluid did not suppress the contraction, as was expected. Young von Euler exuberantly declared that he had discovered a new biologically active substance—a bold claim that was soon borne out.

Along with John H. Gaddum, a senior assistant at the lab, von Euler spent the next few months systematically studying the effects of this newly identified compound. The two men demonstrated that extracts of brain would also contract the rabbit gut, and that the extracts that accomplished this result also had the effect of lowering the blood pressure as well. In order to carry out their investigations, the men used a purified preparation, abbreviated ''P.'' Thus, quite unintentionally, the chemical agent causing these effects became known as Substance P. Back in Sweden, von Euler established that this substance had the properties of a polypeptide, a molecular chain of amino acids (the building blocks of proteins).

Von Euler returned to the Karolinska Institute, where he was made an assistant professor of pharmacology and physiology. In 1939, he was named professor and chairman of the physiology department there, a position in which he remained until his retirement in 1971.

In 1934, von Euler made the second most important discovery of his career. While continuing his tests on different kinds of tissue extracts, he found that extracts of sheep vesicular gland dramatically lowered blood pressure when injected into animals. He realized that some unknown factor in the extracts was exerting a powerful physiological effect. Human seminal fluid also seemed to contain this unidentified substance. Soon it became clear that the factor was a fatty acid. Von Euler dubbed it prostaglandin, in the mistaken belief that it originated in the prostate gland.

During the 1930s, von Euler followed up this finding, describing methods for extracting the compound, as well as defining its basic properties. However, it was not until the late 1950s that von Euler's protegé at the Karolinska Institute, **Sune Karl Bergström**, used newly developed technology to achieve the first purification of a prostaglandin. Von Euler later wrote in the scientific journal *Progress in Lipid Research,* that ''a discovery is in principle like an invention, or even a piece of art, in the sense that the result is greater than the sum of its parts.... It is sometimes said that the prostaglandins lay dormant for some 20 years after their discovery. This is not exactly true, since Sune Bergström took over in 1945 where I left it, and with consummate skill and perseverance conducted the chemical work to isolation and identification, thus starting the second stage of the prostaglandin history.'' Subsequent research revealed that prostaglandins are not a single substance, but a group of chemical compounds that perform a variety of jobs throughout the body, including playing a major role in reproduction. For his contributions to the field, Bergström was one of the recipients of the 1982 Nobel Prize in medicine or physiology.

Meanwhile, von Euler continued the search for chemical transmitters that allow nerve cells to communicate. The idea that such neurotransmitters might exist had been proposed as early as 1905, but it was not until forty-one years later that von Euler succeeded in detecting a critical one in the sympathetic nervous system, which controls such automatic actions as the body's response to stress. He had already observed that certain biological extracts seemed to contain a substance that was similar to adrenaline, yet different in some of its actions. Von Euler set about pinpointing this substance, which he soon established to be noradrenaline (also called norepinephrine).

Later, von Euler investigated the way certain nerve endings store and release noradrenaline. Other of his studies dealt with the role of chemical agents in regulating respiration, circulation, and blood pressure. It was for his ground-breaking experiments involving noradrenaline that von Euler shared the 1970 Nobel Prize with **Julius Axelrod** of the United States and **Bernard Katz** of Great Britain, two other prominent figures in the study of chemical transmitters.

Von Euler was not only an eminent researcher, however; he was also known as a fine teacher who nurtured the curiosity of his pupils. An editorial which he wrote for the American journal *Circulation* sums up his approach to teaching and to science: ''There are few things as rewarding for a scientist as having young students starting their research work and finding that they have... made an original observation.... the pleasure of witnessing the progress of the young starting fresh is one, which [the scientist] has every reason to feel happy about and where he can assist by means of his experience.... We must always guard the liberties of the mind and remember that some degree of heresy is often a sign of health in spiritual life.''

Von Euler was a member of the Swedish Academy of Sciences, as well as chief editor of the journal *Acta Physiologica Scandinavica* for many years. His international reputation was solidified by numerous awards, including the Order of the North Star in Sweden, the Cruzeiro do Sul in Brazil, the Pahnes Academiques in France, and the Grand Cross Al Merito Civil in Spain, as well as the Nobel Prize. Few scientists have been as closely identified with the Nobel Prize as von Euler; not only did he win one himself but so did his father, his mentor, and his protegé. Von Euler served as president of the Nobel Foundation from 1966 until 1975.

Von Euler married his first wife, the former Jane Sodenstierna, on April 12, 1930. They were divorced in 1957, and he subsequently married Dagmar Cronstedt on August 20, 1958. He was the father of four children: two sons, Leo and Christopher, and two daughters, Ursula and Marie. Von Euler died of complications following open heart surgery on March 10, 1983, in Stockholm.

Eustachio, Bartolomeo (ca. 1524-1574)

Italian anatomist

Eustachio was one of the Italian anatomists of the sixteenth century who laid the foundation for modern studies of the human body. The Eustachian tube, which extends from the middle ear to the pharynx, was named after him.

Eustachio was born in San Severino in eastern Italy. Scholars have placed his birthdate as early as 1510 and as late as 1524. His father, Mariano, was a physician, and he gave his son an excellent classical education, studying Greek, Hebrew, and Arabic. He studied to be a doctor at the Archiginnasio della Sapienza in Rome, and began his practice around 1540. He became the physician to Cardinal Giulio della Rovere in 1547. In 1549, Eustachio went with Cardinal Rovere to Rome. There he became a professor of anatomy at the Archiginnasio della Sapienza. Because of his position, he was able to obtain human cadavers for dissections.

Religious reverence for the body made human anatomical studies difficult, and doctors could not legally dissect human corpses for many centuries. The problem began to ease during the first of the **Black Death pandemics**, which arrived in Europe in 1348. The popes wanted to know what caused the devastating disease, and they permitted postmortem examinations of plague victims. But it was almost 200 years later, in 1537, before Pope Clement VII allowed human **dissections** in anatomy classes.

Making use of his access to human cadavers, in 1552 he and an artist relative, Pier Matteo Pini, developed a series of 47 copper engraved plates, which illustrated the results of many of Eustachio's dissections. Unfortunately, only eight of these plates were published in his lifetime. In the early 1560s, Eustachio published works on the human kidney, the organs associated with hearing, and human teeth. His book on the kidney, *De renum structura*, was the first dedicated to that organ. The book presented several important discoveries, and introduced the idea of anatomical variation in organs. Many earlier published accounts of dissections had been performed on animals (dogs, for example), and animal organs varied from human organs in significant ways. His book on teeth, *De dentibus*, was the result of dissections of human fetuses, newborn babies, and older humans, and he described the number, arrangement, and types of teeth in babies and adults. He also described the soft inner parts of the teeth and their hard outer structure.

Eustachio's place in the history of anatomy would have been more prominent if the copperplate engravings that he developed with Pier Matteo Pini had not disappeared after his death. Eight of the plates were published in 1564 in *Opuscula anatomica*. Those plates illustrated, among other things, the kidneys, heart, and veins of the arm. But 39 plates of anatomical illustrations could not be found after his death, even though people searched for years. Finally, the plates were discovered early in the eighteenth century. Eustachio had willed them to Pier Matteo Pini upon his death, and one of Pini's descendants had them. Pope Clement XI purchased the lost plates and gave them to his physician, who published them in 1714. The illustrations were very modern looking, and they provided some of the best descriptions of the base of the brain, the sympathetic **nervous system** (the nerves that control the constriction of blood vessels, among other things), the vascular system, and the structure of the larynx. If those plates had been published in the 1550s, the study of human anatomy would have progressed much more rapidly, and Eustachio would have been as famous as **Vesalius**.

The entire time Eustachio taught anatomy in Rome, he was the physician of Cardinal Rovere. Even after he retired from teaching because of **gout**, he continued to serve the Cardinal. When Cardinal Rovere summoned Eustachio from Rome to his home in Fossombrone in 1574, Eustachio set out north on the road known as the Via Flaminia towards the Adriatic Sea. Eustachio died on the road to the Cardinal on August 27, 1574.

See also Black Death pandemics, Vesalius

Euthanasia

Euthanasia is the act of either painlessly causing the **death** or failing to prevent death from occurring from natural causes in an individual with a terminal illness or in an irreversible **coma**. The term is derived from the Greek words *eus* (good) and *thanatos* (death). Although advances in medical technology have made it possible to prolong the life of patients with no hope of recovery, at times the quality of life of the terminally ill individual is called into question.

The term ''negative'' or ''passive euthanasia'' is used to describe the practice of withholding or withdrawing extraordinary means of preserving life. The term ''positive'' or ''active euthanasia'' involves any direct intervention to cause death, such as injecting a lethal drug or participating in a form of assisted suicide in which another person provides the means for the patient to die. Active euthanasia is sometimes called mercy killing.

The right to refuse life support has been a widely accepted concept among the general public and **physicians** alike. There is no law in the United States that requires a competent person to receive life support involuntarily. In 1976, the New Jersey Supreme Court ruled that doctors could disconnect a mechanical respirator keeping a comatose patient alive because being connected to a machine prevented the patient from dying with dignity.

Beginning in 1977, all states recognized advance directives after California became the first to pass a state law the Death with Dignity statute legalizing the **living will**, a document prepared while an individual is alive and competent. It provides guidance to the health care team in the event the person is no longer capable of making decisions. The directive states the individual's preferences concerning life support measures and **organ donation** and may give authority to another person to make decisions for the terminally ill patient who may be comatose.

In 1990, the United States Supreme Court ruled that individuals who make their wishes known have the right to have life-sustaining treatment discontinued, even such routine ones as **antibiotics**, ventilation, **nutrition**, and hydration. In most states, family members or court-appointed surrogates can make all decisions for individuals whose expressed wishes are unknown.

Passive euthanasia raises many legal issues, as in cases in which parents and doctors decide not to pursue extraordinary life-saving measures for children born with severe birth defects. The problem is intensified because machines that can artificially maintain breathing and heart function have altered the definition of death. Since the advent of advanced medical technology, the definition of death was broadened to include brain death lack of electrical activity for a period long enough to preclude a return to functioning.

Even more controversial than passive euthanasia is active euthanasia, which remains illegal worldwide. However, societies advancing the cause of positive euthanasia have existed since 1935 in England and in 1938 in the United States.

Australia's Northern Territory legalized active euthanasia in the mid-1990s, but the law was overturned. Active euthanasia has been widely accepted in the Netherlands, where physicians are not prosecuted if they follow strict procedures and patients persistently and voluntarily request to die.

In the United States, while doctors have sometimes assisted terminally ill patients commit **suicide** without punishment, the Michigan authorities sought to halt the highly publicized suicides assisted by Dr. Jack Kevorkian, retired Michigan pathologist and right-to-die advocate.

The United States Supreme Court upheld laws forbidding physician-assisted suicide in 1997 but left the door open for states, such as Oregon, to pass legislation permitting the practice. The Hemlock Society is one controversial group that has lobbied for right-to-die legislation on a national level.

Defenders of active euthanasia and assisted suicide point out that many people suffer uncontrollable pain that can only be relieved by active intervention. In these cases, they argue, the results are the same as forgoing life support. Opponents argue that active euthanasia brings with it the risk that society may become more tolerant of killing, eventually making involuntary killing and killing for societal convenience acceptable. They also claim that active killing is intrinsically different from withholding treatment, since the disease rather than human action causes death.

The euthanasia issue has sparked much debate in the United States among physicians, religious leaders, lawyers, and the general public over the question of what constitutes actively causing death and what constitutes merely allowing death to occur naturally. The physician is faced with deciding whether the measures used to keep patients alive are extraordinary on a case-by-case basis.

See also Coma; Death; Living will; Physician; Suicide

EVANS, ALICE CATHERINE (1881-1975)

American microbiologist

Evans was born in Neath, Pennsylvania, on January 29, 1881. After completing her primary education and studying for one year at the Susquehanna Institute in Tonawanda, she began teaching in a local elementary school. Four years later, she decided to pursue a college education and entered Cornell University for a two-year nature study course. She became so interested in science that she decided to remain at Cornell for a bachelor of science degree in agriculture.

With the support of her bacteriology professor at Cornell, Evans received a scholarship to the University of Wisconsin and, in 1910, received a master's degree from that institution. She often thought about studying for a doctoral degree, but became so involved in her own research that she never attained that goal.

After graduation from Wisconsin, Evans accepted a research job with the Department of Agriculture, working first in Wisconsin and later in the Dairy Division Laboratories in Washington, D.C. One of her early projects was the study of bacteria in dairy products. She was intrigued to discover a close similarity between two types of bacteria, *Bacillus abortus* and *Micrococcus melitensis*. The former caused spontaneous abortions in cows and was not thought to be transmitted to humans. The latter organism caused a disease in humans originally known as Malta fever, but latter referred to as undulating fever.

Evans' research was of significance for two reasons. First, spontaneous abortion among cows was a serious problem for the dairy industry. The development of a vaccine for *B. abortus* eventually proved to be of enormous benefit to the industry. Second, the similarity of *B. abortus* to *M. melitensis* raised the possibility that, popular opinion to the contrary, harmful bacteria might be transferred from cows to humans.

In 1918, Evans discovered the first confirmed case in which **brucellosis**—a common disease in cows—was transmitted to humans. The agent responsible was yet a third microorganism, *Brucella suis*. Evans was able to demonstrate that this serious disease in cows could be transmitted to humans. Bacteriologists were at first dubious of Evans's work. Some rejected her findings on irrelevant grounds: that she was a woman or that she had no Ph.D., but others wondered how the transmission of brucellosis from cow to human had escaped scientists' notice for so long.

Gradually the answer to that question became clear. First, Evans began to collect more and more reports of brucellosis in humans from countries around the world. Apparently the disease was more common than anyone had imagined. Second, she discovered that the disease can occur in two forms: *acute*, in which the symptoms occur quickly and are easy to recognize, and *chronic*, in which symptoms develop slowly and over many years. It soon became obvious that chronic brucellosis was relatively common among families exposed to raw milk, but that it was typically diagnosed as another condition.

Evans herself developed chronic brucellosis as a result of her research. She experienced a number of devastating attacks of the disease, but survived them all. She lived a long and productive life, serving in 1928 as the first female president of the American Society for Microbiology. She died in Alexandria, Virginia, on September 5, 1975, at the age of 94. As a result of her work, vaccination of cows and pasteurization of milk are now routine and are responsible for dramatic declines in both bovine and human diseases.

EXERCISE

Exercise is physical activity that is planned, structured, and repetitive to condition the body. Exercise is used to improve health, maintain fitness and for physical **rehabilitation**. It is used to prevent or treat heart disease, **osteoporosis**, weakness, diabetes, **obesity**, and depression. Range of motion exercise increases or maintains joint function. Strengthening exercises provide appropriate resistance to the muscles to increase endurance and strength. **Cardiac rehabilitation** exercises improve the cardiovascular system to prevent and rehabilitate heart disorders and diseases. A well-balanced exercise program can improve general health, build endurance, delay many aging effects, and enhance emotional well-being. Before beginning any exercise program, evaluation by a physician is recommended. Some exercise programs should be supervised by a health care professional, especially if used for rehabilitation. If symptoms of **dizziness**, **nausea**, excessive **shortness of breath**, or chest **pain** are present while exercising, stop the activity and inform the physician.

Range of motion exercise improves movement of a specific joint and includes passive, active, and active assists exercises. Passive range of motion is joint movement by another person or a passive motion machine. When passive range of motion is applied, the joint of the person receiving exercise is completely relaxed while the outside force takes the body part, such as a leg or arm, throughout the available range. Injury, surgery, or **immobilization** of a joint may affect the normal joint range of motion. Active range of motion is movement of the joint by the person exercising. In active assist range of motion, the joint receives partial assistance from an outside force and is applied by the exerciser or by the person assisting the individual. Strengthening exercise increases muscle strength and mass, bone strength, and metabolism. A certain level of muscle strength is needed for daily activities, such as walking, running, and climbing stairs. Weight training provides immediate feedback, through observation of progress in muscle growth and improved muscle tone. Strengthening exercise can be isometric, isotonic or isokinetic. Isometric exercise is effective in developing total strength of a particular muscle or group of muscles and is usually performed against an immovable surface or object, such as pressing the hand against the wall. It is often used for rehabilitation since the exact area of muscle weakness can be isolated and strengthened. It can provide a relatively quick and convenient method for overloading and strengthening muscles without any special equipment and with little chance of injury. In isotonic exercise, which includes weight training, calisthenics, chin-ups, push-ups, and sit-ups, the joint is moved during the muscle contraction. Isokinetic exercise combines the best features of isometrics and weight training by using machines that control the speed of contraction within the range of motion. It provides muscular overload at a constant preset speed while the muscle mobilizes its force through the full range of motion.

Exercise can be very helpful in preventing and rehabilitating heart disorders and disease. With an exercise program set at a level considered safe for that person, **heart failure** patients can improve their fitness levels substantially. The increase in endurance should also translate into a more active lifestyle. Endurance or aerobic routines, such as running, brisk walking, cycling, or swimming, increase the strength and efficiency of the heart muscles. Before exercising, proper stretching is important to prevent the possibility of soft tissue injury resulting from tight muscles, tendons, ligaments, and other joint related structures. Proper cool down after exercise reduces painful muscle spasms and may decrease frequency and intensity of muscle stiffness the next day. Overexertion can also lead to muscle strains and stress **fractures** are possibile if activities are too strenuous.

EXPECTORANTS

Expectorants are drugs that loosen and clear mucus and phlegm from the respiratory tract. The expectorant described here, guaifenesin, is a common ingredient in **cough** medicines. Some cough medicines contain other ingredients that may cancel out guaifenesin's effects. Guaifenesin is an ingredient in many cough medicines, such as Anti-Tuss, Dristan Cold & Cough, Guaifed, GuaiCough, and some Robitussin products. Some products that contain guaifenesin are available only with a physician's prescription; others can be bought **over-the-counter**. They come in several forms, including capsules, tablets, and liquids. The recommended dose is 200–400 mg every 4 hours, with no more than 2,400 mg in 24 hours, for adults

THREE TYPES OF EXERCISE

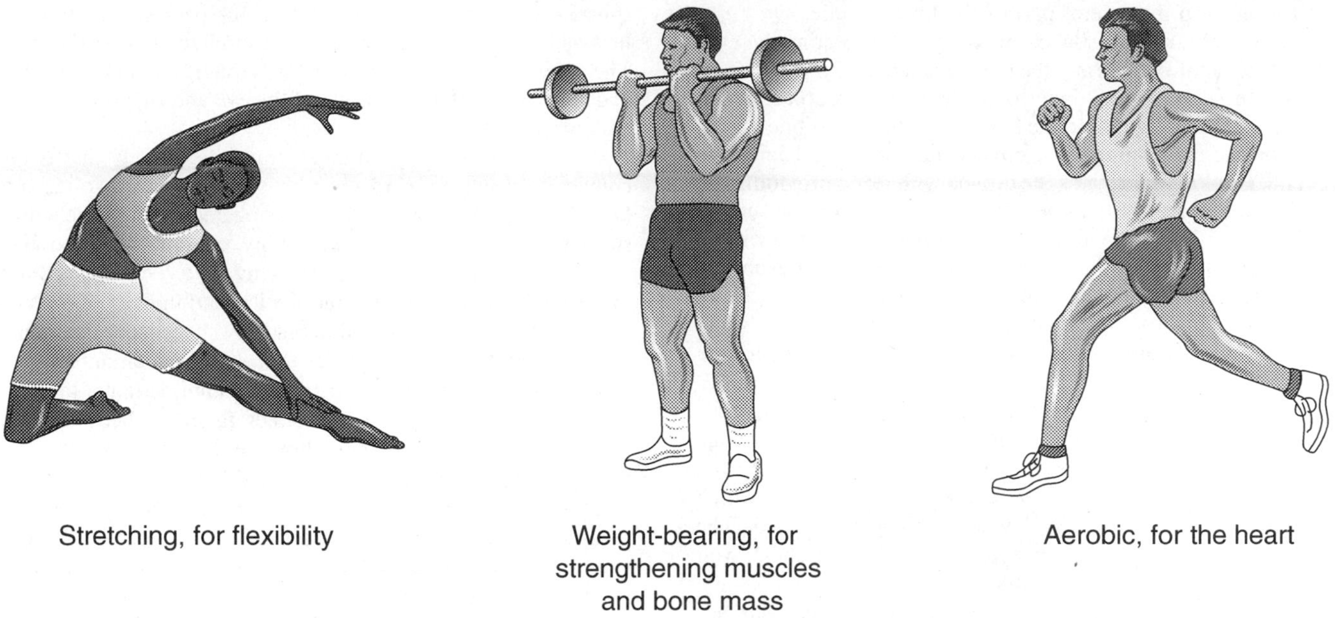
Stretching, for flexibility
Weight-bearing, for strengthening muscles and bone mass
Aerobic, for the heart

Exercise is used to improve health, maintain fitness, and as an important means for physical rehabilitation. ***(Illustration by Electronic Illustrators Group.)***

and children 12 and over; 6–11, 100– 200 mg every 4 hours, with no more than 1,200 mg in 24 hours, for children 6–11; 50– and 100 mg every 4 hours, with no more than 600 mg in 24 hours, for children 2–5. It is not recommended for children under 2. Do not take more than the recommended daily dosage. Guaifenesin is not meant to be used for coughs associated with **asthma**, emphysema, chronic **bronchitis**, or **smoking**; or for coughs that produce a lot of mucus. A lingering cough could be a sign of a serious medical condition. Coughs that last more than 7 days or are associated with **fever**, **rash**, **sore throat**, or lasting **headache** should have medical attention. Call a physician as soon as possible.

Some studies suggest that guaifenesin causes **birth defects**. Women who are pregnant or plan to become pregnant should check with their physicians before using products with guaifenesin. Whether guaifenesin passes into breast milk is not known. Side effects are rare, but may include vomiting, **diarrhea**, stomach upset, headache, skin rash, and **hives**. Guaifenesin is not known to interact with any foods or other drugs. However, cough medicines that contain guaifenesin may contain other ingredients that do interact with foods or drugs. Check with a physician or pharmacist for details about specific products.

EYE

The eye is the organ of sight in humans and animals. It transforms light waves into visual images and provides 80% of all information received by the human brain. These remarkable organs are almost spherical in shape and are housed in the orbital sockets in the skull. Sight begins when light waves enter the eye through the cornea (the transparent layer at the front of the eye), pass through the pupil (the opening in the center of the iris, the colored portion of the eye), then through a clear lens behind the iris. The lens focuses light onto the retina, which functions like the film in a camera. Photoreceptor neurons in retinas, called rods and cones, convert light energy into electrical impulses, which are then carried to the brain via the optic nerves. At the visual cortex in the occipital lobe of the cerebrum of the brain, the electrical impulses are interpreted as images.

Many invertebrate animals have simple light-sensitive eye spots, consisting of a few receptor cells in a cup-shaped organ lined with pigmented cells, which detect only changes in light and dark regimes. Arthropods (insects, spiders, and crabs) have complex compound eyes with thousands of cells that construct composite pictures of objects. They are very sensitive to detecting movement.

The human eyeball is about 0.9 in (24 mm) in diameter and is not perfectly round, being slightly flattened in the front and back. The eye consists of three layers: the outer fibrous or sclera, the middle uveal or choroid layer, and the inner nervous layer or retina. Internally the eye is divided into two cavities: the anterior cavity filled with the watery aqueous fluid, and the posterior cavity filled with gel-like vitreous fluid. The internal pressure inside the eye (the intraocular pressure) exerted by the aqueous fluid supports the shape of the anterior cavity, while the vitreous fluid holds the shape of the posterior chamber. An irregularly shaped eyeball results in ineffective focusing of light onto the retina and is usually correctable with eye glasses or contact lenses. The ophthalmic arteries provide the blood supply to the eyes, and the movement of the eyeballs is facilitated by six extraocular muscles that run from the bony orbit and insert into the sclera, part of the fibrous tunic.

The outer fibrous layer encasing and protecting the eyeball consists of two parts—the cornea and the sclera. The front one-sixth of the fibrous layer is the transparent cornea, which bends incoming light onto the lens inside the eye. A fine mucus membrane, the conjunctiva, covers the cornea and lines the eyelid. Blinking lubricates the cornea with tears, providing the moisture necessary for its health. The cornea's outside surface is protected by a thin film of tears produced in the lacrimal glands located in the lateral part of orbit below the eyebrow. Tears flow through ducts from this gland to the eyelid and eyeball, and drain from the inner corner of the eye into the nasal cavity. A clear watery liquid, the aqueous humor, separates the cornea from the iris and lens. The cornea contains no blood-vessels or pigment and gets its nutrients from the aqueous humor. The remaining five-sixths of the fibrous layer of the eye is the sclera, a dense, tough, opaque coat visible as the white of the eye. Its outer layer contains blood vessels, which produce a "blood-shot eye" when the eye is irritated. The middle or uveal layers of the eye are densely pigmented, well supplied with blood, and include three major structures—the iris, the ciliary body, and the choroid. The iris is a circular, adjustable diaphragm with a central hole (the pupil), sited in the anterior chamber behind the cornea. The iris gives the eye its color, which varies depending on the amount of pigment present. If the pigment is dense, the iris is brown, if there is little pigment the iris is blue, if there is no pigment the iris is pink, as in the eye of a white rabbit. In bright light, muscles in the iris constrict the pupil, reducing the amount of light entering the eye. Conversely, the pupil dilates (enlarges) in dim light, so increasing the amount of incoming light. Extreme fear, head injuries, and certain drugs can also dilate the pupil.

The iris is the anterior extension of the ciliary body, a large, smooth muscle that also connects to the lens via suspensory ligaments. The muscles of the ciliary body continually expand and contract, putting on suspensory ligaments changing the shape of the lens, thereby adjusting the focus of light onto the retina, facilitating clear vision. The choroid is a thin membrane lying beneath the sclera and is connected the posterior section of the ciliary body. It is the largest portion of the uveal tract. Along with the sclera the choroid provides a light-tight environment for the inside of the eye, preventing stray light from confusing visual images on the retina. The choroid has a good blood supply and provides oxygen and nutrients to the retina.

The front of the eye houses the anterior cavity, which is subdivided by the iris into the anterior and posterior chambers. The anterior chamber is the bowl-shaped cavity immediately behind the cornea and in front of the iris, which contains aqueous humor. This is a clear watery fluid that facilitates good vision by helping maintain eye shape, regulating the intraocular pressure, providing support for the internal structures, supplying nutrients to the lens and cornea, and disposing of the eye's metabolic waste. The posterior chamber of the anterior cavity lies behind the iris and in front of the lens. The aqueous humor forms in this chamber and flows forward to the anterior chamber through the pupil.

The posterior cavity is lined entirely by the retina, occupies 60% of the human eye, and is filled with a clear gel-like substance called vitreous humor. Light passing through the lens on its way to the retina passes through the vitreous humor. The vitreous humor consists of 99% water, contains no cells, and helps to maintain the shape of the eye and support its internal components.

The lens is a crystal-clear, transparent body that is biconvex (curving outward on both surfaces), semi-solid, and flexible, shaped like an ellipse or elongated sphere. The entire surface of the lens is smooth and shiny, contains no blood vessels, and is encased in an elastic membrane. The lens is sited in the posterior chamber behind the iris and in front of the vitreous humor. The lens is held in place by suspensory ligaments that run from the ciliary muscles to the external circumference of the lens. The continual relaxation and contraction of the ciliary muscles cause the lens to either fatten or became thin, changing its focal length, and allowing it to focus light on the retina. With age, the lens hardens and becomes less flexible, resulting in far-sighted vision, which necessitates glasses, bifocals, or contact lenses to restore clear, close-up vision. Clouding of the lens also often occurs with age, creating a cataract that interferes with vision. Clear vision is restored by a relatively simple surgical procedure in which the entire lens is removed and an artificial lens implanted.

The retina is the innermost layer of the eye. It is a thin, delicate, extremely complex sensory tissue composed of layers of light sensitive nerve cells. The retina begins at the ciliary body and encircles the entire posterior portion of the eye. Photoreceptor cells in the rods and cones convert light first to chemical energy and then electrical energy. Rods function in dim light, allowing limited nocturnal (night) vision: it is with rods that we see the stars. Rods cannot detect color, but they are the first receptors to detect movement. There are about 126 million rods in each eye and about 6 million cones. Cones provide acute vision, function best in bright light and allow color vision. Cones are most heavily concentrated in the central fovea, a tiny hollow in the posterior part of the retina and the point of most acute vision. Dense fields of both rods and cones are found in a circular belt surrounding the fovea, the macula lutea. Continuing outward from this belt, the cone density decreases and the ratio of rods to cones increases. Both rods and cones disappear completely at the edges of the retina.

The optic nerve connects the eye to the brain. The fibers of the optic nerve run from the surface of the retina and converge and exit at the optic disc (or blind spot), an area about 0.06 in (1.5 mm) in diameter located at the lower posterior portion of the retina. The fibers of this nerve carry electrical impulses from the retina to the visual cortex in the occipital lobe of the cerebrum. If the optic nerve is severed, vision is lost permanently.

The last two decades have seen an explosion in ophthalmic research. Today, 90% of corneal blindness can be rectified with a corneal transplant, the most frequently performed of all human transplants. Eye banks receive eyes for sight-restoring corneal transplantation just as blood banks receive blood for life-giving **transfusions**. Many people remain blind, however, because of the lack of eye donors.

See also Cataracts; Eyelid disorders; Eye injuries; Eye glasses and contact lenses; Eye examination; Glaucoma; Nearsightedness and farsightedness; Visual impairment and blindness

EYE EXAMINATION

An eye examination is a series of tests that measure a person's ocular health and visual status, to detect abnormalities in the visual system, and to determine how well the person can see. It is performed by an ophthalmologist (M.D. or D.O.—doctor of **osteopathy**) or an optometrist (O.D.) to determine if there are any pre-existing or potential vision problems. Eye exams may also reveal the presence of many non-eye diseases. The frequency of eye exams differs with age and the health of the person. Eye exams can be performed in infants, and if a problem is noted the infant can be seen by a pediatric ophthalmologist. A child with no symptoms should have an eye exam at age three. Early exams are important because permanent decreases in vision (e.g., **amblyopia**, also called lazy eye) can occur if not treated early (usually by ages 6–9). With no symptoms, the second exam should take place before first grade. After first grade, the American Optometric Association recommends that healthy people with no risk factors have an eye exam every two years; for ages 19–40, every two-to-three years; for ages 41–60, every two years; and annually after that. Patients with risk factors for eye disease (e.g., people with diabetes or a family history of eye disease; African Americans, who are at higher risk for **glaucoma**) and children who have trouble in school, problems with reading, rub their eyes when reading, etc. may need more frequent checkups. An eye examination costs about $100 and may or may not be covered by insurance. It includes a patient history, primary tests, and additional specialized tests as needed. Primary tests evaluate the physical state of the eyes and surrounding areas and measure the ability to see.

Most exams will include the following procedures. The eye and medical histories include complaints, past eye disorders, medications, blood relatives with eye disorders, any systemic disorders the patient may have, and hobbies and work conditions. If the patient has glasses, he/she should bring them. The visual acuity examination measures each eye to determine how clearly the patient can see. An eye chart, usually a Snellen eye chart, is used. These charts are placed at a distance from the person being tested at which people with normal vision can read the 20/20 line; these people are said to have 20/20 vision. For people who can't read the smallest line, the examiner assigns a ratio based on the smallest line they can read. When a patient can't read any line, the chart is moved closer until he/she can read the line with the largest letters. When a patient can't read the chart at all, the examiner may hold up some fingers, move a hand, or use a penlight. In eye movement examination and cover tests, the examiner asks the patient to look up and down, and to the right and left to see if the patient can move the eyes to their full extent. The examiner asks the patient to stare at an object, then quickly covers one eye and notes any movement in the eye that remains uncovered. The doctor may have the patient look at a pen and follow it as it is moved close to the eyes to check convergence. The examiner checks the pupil's response to light and views the iris for symmetry and physical appearance. For people whose visual acuity is less than 20/20, the examiner will determine the refractive error and obtain a prescription for corrective lenses. An instrument called a phoropter, which the patient sits behind, is generally used. The examiner tests combinations of corrections to learn which allows the patient to see the eye chart best. The exam will check vision at distance and near. A prescription for corrective lenses can also be supplied by automated refracting devices or through a hand-held retinoscope. Sometimes drops will be put in the patient's eyes so that the refraction will be more accurate; this is helpful in children and people who are farsighted.

Next, the examiner checks the health of the eyes and surrounding areas. After dilating the pupils, the examiner uses an ophthalmoscope to view the retina, blood vessels, optic nerve, and other structures. The slit lamp is used to examine the lid and lid margin, cornea, iris, pupil, conjunctiva, sclera, and lens, and in contact lens evaluations. A tonometer may be used to check eye pressure, after using a colored eyedrop. A perimeter measures visual field. A tonometer measures intraocular pressure (IOP). Other tests could include binocular indirect ophthalmoscopy, gonioscopy, color tests, contrast sensitivity testing, ultasonography, and others.

Seeing clearly does not necessarily mean the eyes are healthy or that the eyes are working together as a team. Regular checkups can detect abnormalities, hopefully before a problem arises. The eye doctor can suggest ways to help protect the eyes and vision (e.g., safety goggles, ultraviolet (UV) coatings on lenses). A person should also have an eye exam if he/she notices a change in vision, eyestrain, blur, flashes of light, a sudden onset of floaters (little dots), distortion of objects, double vision, redness, **pain**, or discharge.

EYEGLASSES AND CONTACT LENSES

Eyeglasses are corrective lenses mounted in frames that help those with vision problems see clearly. The lenses are shaped in order to bend light rays so that they will focus at the back of the eye, the retina. Some people who can see distant objects clearly but to whom near objects look blurry suffer from hyperopia or farsightedness. As explained by Franciscus Donders (1818-1889), a Dutch physiologist, the cause of farsightedness is that the eyeball is too shallow and that the image actually focuses beyond the eye. To correct hyperopia, convex corrective lenses are used to make the light rays converge or come together on the retina. Some people suffer from myopia or **nearsightedness**, in which the image is focused in front of the retina so that only near objects can be seen clearly. Concave lenses can be worn to diverge the light rays and permit light from far away objects to focus directly on the retina. A condition called presbyopia occurs when the lens of the eye loses it elasticity and it can no longer change shape. The condition is usually associated with age and becomes evident after 40.

Presbyopia causes people to be somewhat farsighted. Sometimes this is corrected by wearing bifocals, or eyeglasses that have a second lens below the top lens. A person with presbyopia can look through the bottom lens while reading and use the top lens for distant objects.

The invention of eyeglasses has a long and colorful history. It is said that during the days of the Roman Empire, the emperor Nero watched exhibitions in the Coliseum holding a jewel with curved facets up to one eye, but this cannot be verified. However, Roger Bacon, an English scholar, is said to have suggested the use of eyeglasses in the 1200s. An Italian physicist, Salvino degli Armati probably invented eyeglasses in around 1285. He shared the design of his new device with an Italian monk, Allesandro della Spina, who made public the invention and is often given credit for inventing eyeglasses.

In the 14th century Venetian craftsmen, known for their work in glass, were making ''disks for the eyes.'' The finely ground glass disks were given the name lenses by the Italians because of their similarity in shape to lentils. For hundreds of years thereafter, **lenses** were called glass lentils. The earliest lenses were convex—that is they bulged outward in the middle and aided people who were far-sighted. Wearing spectacles became common enough so that a 1352 portrait of St. Hugh showed him wearing them, although he had died some hundred years before. By the fifteenth century, eyeglasses had found their way to China. But long before, Chinese judges had worn smoky quartz spectacles, but it is thought they were worn so the judges could remain impartial and not show expression in their eyes when they heard cases rather than correct vision.

In 1451, Nicholas of Cusa in Germany invented eyeglasses to correct nearsightedness using concave lenses. Rather than bulging in the middle like convex lenses, concave lenses are thinner at the center and thicker at the ends. Pope Leo X was one of the first to wear them.

Early eyeglasses had glass lenses mounted on heavy frames of wood, lead or copper. Natural materials of **leather**, bone and horn were later used and then lighter frames of steel were made by the early seventeenth century. Tortoiseshell frames came into use in the eighteenth century. In 1746, a French optician named Thomin invented actual eyeglass frames that could be placed over the ears and nose.

In the United States, Benjamin Franklin, statesman and scientist, designed the first bifocals in 1760. In this way he could use the top lens to see distant objects and peer down into the bottom lens when he read without needing two pair of glasses. The two lenses were joined in a metal frame. In England in 1827, Sir George Biddle Airy (1801-1892), an English astronomer and mathematician made the first glasses to correct astigmatism, a condition he himself had. **Astigmatism** is blurry vision caused by irregular curves in the cornea, the transparent covering of the eye. The irregular curvature makes it impossible for light rays to focus on a single point. To correct this, the exact area of the irregularity of the cornea is located, and a corresponding area on the eyeglass lens is ground to bring light rays passing through that area into proper focus.

Today eyeglasses come in a wide array of styles and designs. Frames are generally made of metal or plastic, and lenses are made of glass or plastic. Polycarbonate is a type of very hard plastic used for lenses. Robust and lightweight, it is scratch-resistant and provides 100% protection from ultraviolet radiation that can contribute to cataract formation. Along with lightweight frames, such lenses are commonly used in sports glasses and childrens' glasses.

In 1955 the first unbreakable lenses were made and in 1971 a new lens came out which combined the properties of plastic with glass. During the 1950s the Varilux was invented, corrective lenses of variable strength that can be used in place of bifocals. Testing the eyes for visual acuity and examining the eye with a retinoscope are routine before determining the strength, or refractive index, of the lenses prescribed.

Eyewear has been revolutionized with the invention of the contact lens, corrective lenses without the frames, which put a tiny corrective lens directly on the cornea of the eye. However the idea dates back to Leonardo da Vinci who described a way of correcting vision using a water-filled tube, and to a number of scientists who experimented with layers of gelatin to correct vision during the seventeenth and eighteenth centuries. Contact lenses were first made in Europe near the turn of the twentieth century using glass. In 1936 IG Farben, a German company, made the first contact lens from Plexiglas—still used today for ''hard'' contact lenses. An American inventor named Tuohy began use of a lens that covers only the cornea and in 1964 a Czech named Wichterle made the first flexible or ''soft'' lens. Today there is an array of hard and soft lenses, extended wear lenses, tinted lenses, lenses that can correct astigmatism, and lenses to correct **color blindness**.

EYE INJURIES

The cornea, the clear front part of the eye through which light passes, is subject to many infections and to injury from exposure and from **foreign objects**. Infection and injury cause inflammation of the cornea—a condition called **keratitis**. Tissue loss because of inflammation produces an ulcer. The ulcer can either be centrally located, thus greatly affecting vision, or peripherally located. There are about 30,000 cases of bacterial corneal ulcers in the United States each year.

A corneal abrasion is basically a superficial cut or scrape on the cornea. A corneal abrasion is not as serious as a corneal ulcer, which is generally deeper and more severe than an abrasion.

The most common cause of corneal ulcers is germs, but most of them cannot invade a healthy cornea with adequate tears and a functioning eyelid. They gain access because injury has impaired these defense mechanisms. A direct injury from a foreign object inoculates germs directly through the outer layer of the cornea, just as it does to the skin. A caustic chemical can inflame the cornea by itself or so damage it that germs can invade. Improper use of contact lenses has become a common cause of corneal injury. Eyelid or tear function failure is the other way to make the eye vulnerable to infection. Tears and the eyelid together wash the eye and prevent foreign material from settling in. Tears contain enzymes and other substances to help protect against infection. Certain diseases dry up tear production, leaving the cornea dry and defenseless. Other diseases paralyze or weaken the eyelids so that they cannot effectively protect and cleanse the eyes.

A corneal abrasion is usually the result of direct injury to the eye, often from a fingernail scratch, makeup brushes, contact lenses, foreign body, or even twigs. Patients often complain of feeling a foreign body in their eye, and they may have **pain**, sensitivity to light, or tearing.

Viruses, bacteria, fungi, and a protozoan called *Acanthamoeba* can all invade the cornea and damage it under suitable conditions.

- Bacteria from a common **conjunctivitis** (pink eye) rarely spread to the cornea, but can if untreated.
- Fecal bacteria are more likely to be able to infect the cornea.
- A bacterium called *Pseudomonas aeruginosa*, which can contaminate eyedrops, is particularly able to cause corneal infection.
- A group of incomplete bacteria known as *Chlamydia* can be transmitted to the eye directly by flies or dirty hands. One form of chlamydial infection is the leading cause of blindness in developing countries and is known as Egyptian ophthalmia or trachoma. Another type of *Chlamydia* causes a sexually transmitted disease.
- Other **sexually transmitted diseases**—for example, **syphilis**—can affect the cornea.

The most common viruses to damage the cornea are adenoviruses and herpes viruses. Viral and fungal infections are often caused by improper use of topical **corticosteroids**. If topical corticosteroids are used in a patient with Herpes simplex keratitis, the ulcer can get much worse and blindness could result.

Symptoms are obvious. The cornea is intensely sensitive, so corneal ulcers normally produce severe **pain**. If the corneal ulcer is centrally located, vision is impaired or completely absent. Tearing is present and the eye is red. It hurts to look at bright lights.

The doctor will take a case history to try to determine the cause of the ulcer. This can include improper use of contact lenses; injury, such as a scratch from a twig; or severe dry eye. An instrument called a slit lamp will be used to examine the cornea. The slit lamp is a microscope with a light source that magnifies the cornea, allowing the extent of the ulcer to be seen. Fluorescein, a yellow dye, may be used to illuminate further detail. If a germ is responsible for the ulcer, identification may require scraping samples directly from the cornea, conjunctiva, and lids, and sending them to the laboratory.

Ophthalmologists and optometrists, who treat eye disorders, are well qualified to diagnose corneal abrasions. The doctor will check the patient's vision (visual acuity) in both eyes with an eye chart. A patient history will also be taken, which may help to determine the cause of the abrasion. A slit lamp, which is basically a microscope and light source, will allow the doctor to see the abrasion. Fluorescein, a yellow dye, may be placed into the eye to determine the extent of the abrasion. The fluorescein will temporarily stain the affected area.

A corneal ulcer needs to be treated aggressively, as it can result in loss of vision. The first step is to eliminate infection. Broad spectrum **antibiotics** will be used before the lab results come back. Medications may then be changed to more specifically target the cause of the infection. A combination of medications may be necessary. Patients should return for their follow-up visits, so that the doctor can monitor the healing process. The cornea can heal from many insults, but if it remains scarred, corneal transplantation may be necessary to restore vision. If the corneal ulcer is large, hospitalization may be necessary.

The cornea has a remarkable ability to heal itself, so treatment is designed to minimize complications. If an abrasion is very small, the doctor might just suggest an eye lubricant and a follow-up visit the next day. A very small abrasion should heal in 1-2 days; others usually in one week. However, to avoid a possible infection, an antibiotic eye drop may be prescribed. Sometimes additional eye drops may make the eye feel more comfortable. Depending upon the extent of the abrasion, some doctors may patch the affected eye. It is very important to go for the follow-up checkup to make sure an infection does not occur. Use of contact lenses should not be resumed without the doctor's approval.

Treated early enough, corneal infections will usually resolve, perhaps even without the formation of an ulcer. However, left untreated, infections can lead to ulcers and the corneal ulcer can result in scarring or perforation of the cornea. Other problems may occur as well, including **glaucoma**. Patients with certain systemic diseases that impede healing (such as diabetes mellitus or **rheumatoid arthritis**) may need more aggressive treatment. The later the treatment, the more damage will be done and the more scarring will result. Corneal transplant is standard treatment with a high probability of success.

In typical abrasion cases, the prognosis is good. The cornea will heal itself, usually within several days. A very deep abrasion may lead to scarring. If the abrasion does not heal properly, a recurrent corneal erosion (RCE) may result months or even years later. The symptoms are the same as for an abrasion (e.g., tearing, foreign body sensation, and blurred vision), but it will keep occurring. Similar or additional treatment for the RCE may be necessary.

Attentive care of contact lenses will greatly reduce the incidence of corneal damage and ulceration. Germs that cause no problems in the mouth or on the hands can damage the eye, so contact lens wearers must wash their hands before touching their lenses and must not use saliva to moisten them. Tap water should not be used to rinse the lenses. Contacts should be removed whenever there is irritation and left out until the eyes are back to normal. It is not advisable to wear contact lenses while swimming or in hot tubs. Daily wear contact lenses have been found to be less of a risk than contacts for overnight wear (extended wear). Organisms have been cultured from contact lens cases, so the cases should be rinsed in hot water and allowed to air dry. Cases should be replaced every three months. Patients should follow their doctors' schedules for replacement of the contacts.

Eye protection in the workplace, or wherever tiny particles are flying around, is essential. Ultraviolet (UV) coatings on glasses or sunglasses can help protect the eyes from the sun's rays. Goggles with UV protection should be worn when skiing or in suntanning salons, to protect against UV rays. Prompt attention to any red eye should prevent progressive damage.

For people with inadequate tears, use of artificial tears eyedrops will prevent damage from drying. Eyelids that do not close adequately may temporarily have to be sewn shut to protect the eye until more lasting treatment can be instituted.

EYELID DISORDERS

An eyelid disorder is any abnormal condition that affects the eyelids. The eyelids, which consist of thin folds of skin, muscle, and connective tissue, protect the eyes and spread tears over the front of the eyes. Some common lid problems include: stye, blepharitis, chalazion, entropion, ectropion, eyelid **edema**, and eyelid tumors. A stye is an infection of eyelid glands near the lid margins, at the base of the lashes. A chalazion is an enlargement of a meibomian gland, usually not infectious. Initially, a chalazion may resemble a stye, but it usually grows larger and may also be located in the middle of the lid and be internal. Blepharitis is the inflammation of the eyelid margins, often with scales and crust. It can lead to eyelash loss, chalazia, styes, ectropion, corneal damage, excessive tearing, and chronic **conjunctivitis**. Entropion is a condition where the eyelid margin is turned inward; the eyelashes touch the eye and irritate the cornea. Ectropion is a condition where one or both eyelid margins turn outward, exposing the conjunctiva that covers the eye and lines the eyelid. Eyelid edema is a condition where the eyelids contain excessive fluid. Eyelids are susceptible to the same skin tumors as the skin over the rest of the body, including noncancerous tumors and cancerous tumors. Eyelid muscles are susceptible to sarcoma.

Styes are usually caused by bacterial **staphylococcal infections**. The symptoms are **pain** and inflammation near the eyelid margin. A chalazion is caused by a blockage in the outflow duct of a meibomian gland. Symptoms are inflammation and painful swelling. Blepharitis can be caused by bacterial infection, head lice, an overproduction of oil by the meibomian glands, or an unknown cause. It can be a chronic lifelong condition. Symptoms include **itching**, burning, a feeling of something in the eye, inflammation, and scales or crusts surrounding the eyelashes. Entropion usually results from aging, but is sometimes due to a congenital defect, a spastic eyelid muscle, or a scar inside the lid. Symptoms are excessive tearing, redness, and discomfort. The usual cause of ectropion is aging, but it can also be caused by a spastic eyelid muscle, a scar, or **allergies**. Symptoms are excessive tearing and hardening of the eyelid conjunctiva. Eyelid edema is usually caused by allergic reactions, for example, to eye makeup, eyedrops or other drugs, or plants. **Trichinosis**, a disease caused by eating undercooked meat, also causes eyelid edema. Swelling can also be due to infection and lead to orbital **cellulitis** which can threaten vision. Symptoms include swelling, itching, redness, or pain. Eyelid tumors are caused by **AIDS** (**Kaposi's sarcoma**) or increased exposure to ultraviolet (UV) rays. They are usually painless and may or may not be pigmented.

To diagnose eyelid disorders, the doctor uses a slit lamp is used to magnify the eyes. He/she may press on the lid margin to express oil from the meibomian glands or invert the lid to see inside it. **Biopsy** is used to diagnose cancerous tumors. Styes are treated with warm-hot compresses and sometimes topical antibiotics. About 25% of chalazia disappears on its own, but hot compresses may speed the process. Medication may need to be injected or the chalazion may need to be cut out. If a chalazion recurs on the same site, the possibility of sebaceous gland carcinoma should be investigated. Blepharitis is treated with hot compresses and antibiotic ointment, and by cleaning the eyelids. If the blepharitis doesn't clear up with treatment or is a chronic problem, the patient may have **acne** rosacea and need to see a dermatologist. Entropion and ectropion can be surgically corrected and treated with lubricating drops to keep the cornea moist. Patients with swollen eyelids should contact their eye doctor. A severely swollen lid can press on the eye and increase the intraocular pressure. An infection needs to be ruled out. The best treatment for allergic eyelid edema is to find and remove the substance causing the allergy. When that isn't possible, cold compresses and immunosuppresesive drugs such as corticosteroid creams are helpful. For edema caused by trichinosis, the trichinosis must be treated. Cancerous tumors should be removed upon discovery, and noncancerous tumors before they grow enough to interfere with vision or eyelid function. Eyelid reconstruction sometimes accompanies tumor excision.

The prognosis for styes and chalazia is good to excellent. With treatment, blepharitis, ectropion, and entropion usually have good outcomes. The prognosis for nonmalignant tumors is good after proper removal. The survival rate for malignant melanoma depends upon how early it was discovered and if it was completely removed. Sebaceous carcinomas are difficult to detect, so poor outcomes are more frequent. All eyelid disorders, if not treated, can lead to vision problems. Eyelid washing with baby shampoo and not rubbing the eyes and eyelids helps prevent styes, chalazia, blepharitis, and eyelid edema. Blepharitis is associated with dandruff, which can be controlled by washing the hair, scalp, and eyebrows with shampoo containing selenium sulfide. Avoiding allergens helps prevent allergic eyelid edema. Staying inside when pollen counts are high, and eliminating or removing eye makeup, or using hypo-allergenic makeup, helps in some cases. Sunscreen, UV-blocking sunglasses, and wide brimmed hats helps prevent eyelid tumors. Entropian and ectropian are unpreventable.

F

Fabiola, Saint (Unknown-399)

Italian hospital founder

A member of a wealthy Roman family, Fabiola became a Christian ascetic, selling all her belongings and founding the first hospital in the Western world. Despite her aristocratic background, she was known for treating patients herself, even those whose wounds and injuries were so repulsive that they would have been rejected by others.

Before she turned to asceticism (the practice of self-denial and spiritual discipline), Fabiola caused considerable scandal in Rome by divorcing her first husband and marrying another while he was still alive. Later writing the primary information about Fabiola, St. Jerome suggested that Fabiola's first marriage was marked by spousal abuse: "So terrible were the faults imputed to her former husband that not even a prostitute or a common slave could have put up with them." Her remarriage, however, violated the ordinances of the Church and she was forced to remove herself from communion. After her second husband died, Fabiola put on sackcloth during the Easter season, publically confessed her error in the basilica of Lateranus, and was received back into communion by the pope.

Under the influence of St. Jerome, she then sold all her property and devoted herself to practising asceticism and serving the poor and sick.

"She was the first person to found a hospital, into which she might gather sufferers out of the streets, and where she might nurse the unfortunate victims of sickness and want," wrote St. Jerome. "Often did she carry on her own shoulders persons infected with jaundice or with filth," Jerome explained. "Often too did she wash away the matter discharged from wounds which others, even though men, could not bear to look at. . . . I know of many wealthy and devout persons who, unable to overcome their natural repugnance to such sights, perform this work of mercy by the agency of others, giving money instead of personal aid."

In 395, Fabiola travelled to Bethlehem. She returned to Rome after an invasion of the Huns made remaining in Bethlehem dangerous. "Fabiola, used as she was to moving from city to city and having no property other but what her baggage contained, returned to her native land; to live in poverty where she had once been rich, to lodge in the house of another. . . ." Jerome wrote. Back in Rome, Fabiola worked with Pammachius, a former senator, to establish a hospice for pilgrims visiting the city. She also continued her medical work until her death on December 27, 399. All of Rome is said to have attended her funeral. A feast for Fabiola is celebrated on December 27.

Face lift

Face lift surgery is a cosmetic procedure to improve the appearance of the face by redirecting some of the skin and muscle tissue of the face and neck to counter sagging and looseness caused by gravity as the patient ages. Also known as facialplasty, rhytidoplasty, or cervicofacial rhytidectomy, the procedure won't erase all facial wrinkles, for example, wrinkles around the mouth and eyes may benefit little from face lift surgery. Other procedures, such as blepharoplasty, chemical peel, or dermabrasion, also may be necessary. Patients with other medical conditions should consult their primary physician before undergoing face lift surgery. Lung problems, heart disease, and certain other conditions can lead to a higher risk of complications. Patients who take medications that can alter the way their blood clots (including female hormones, **aspirin**, and some non-aspirin pain relievers) should stop these medications prior to surgery to lower the risk that a hematoma, a pocket of blood below the skin and the most frequent complication of face lift surgery, will form.

Face lift surgery can be performed on an outpatient basis with local anesthetics. Patients typically also receive an intravenous sedative that helps to lower their awareness of the procedure. There are many variations of face lift surgery. Which

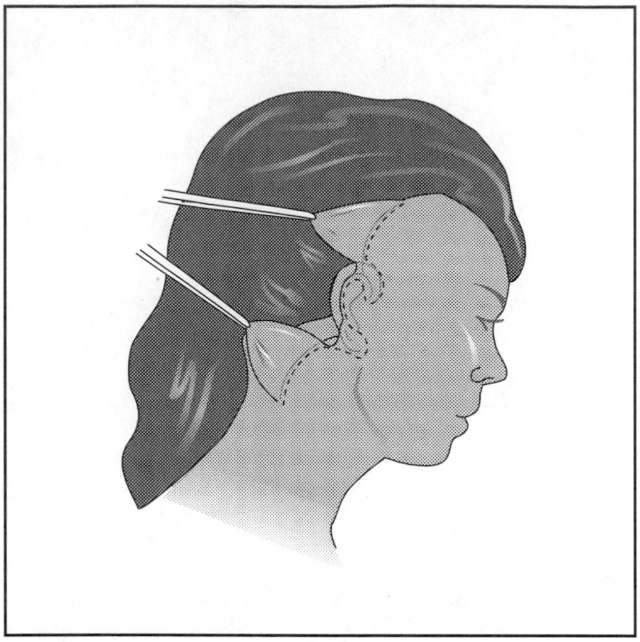

In a typical face lift surgery, the surgeon begins by making an incision within the hairline just above the ear. The incision continues down along the front of the ear, around the earlobe, and then up and behind the ear extending back into the hairline, as shown above. The same procedure is repeated on the other side of the face. The surgeon will then separate the skin from the tissue, remove fat deposits over the cheeks and neck, tighten up muscles and tissues below the chin and upwards behind the neck. The surgeon then trims excess skin from the original incision, pulls the skin back, and sutures it into place. *(Illustration by Electronic Illustrators Group.)*

one is used depends on the patient's facial structure, how much correction is needed, and the preferences of the surgeon. In a typical face lift surgery, the surgeon begins by making an incision within the hairline just above the ear. The incision continues down along the front edge of the ear, around the earlobe, and then up and behind the ear extending back into the hairline. The location of this incision is designed to hide any sign of the procedure later. This is repeated on the other side of the face. The surgeon separates the skin of the face from its underlying tissue, moving down to the cheek and into the neck area and below the chin. Fat deposits over the cheeks and in the neck may be removed surgically or with **liposuction**. The surgeon frees up and tightens certain bands of muscle and tissue that extend up from the shoulder, below the chin, and up and behind the neck. If these muscles and tissue are not tightened, the looseness and sagging appearance of the skin will return. The surgeon trims excess skin from the edges of the original incision, pulls the skin back, and staples or sutures it into place.

Before the procedure, patients meet with their surgeon to discuss the surgery, and clarify the results that can be achieved and the potential problems that can occur. Some physicians prescribe vitamin C and K in the belief that this promotes healing. Patients will also be advised to stop smoking and to avoid exposure to passive smoke before the procedure and afterward. Some surgeons also recommend **antibiotics** be taken beforehand to limit the risk of infection. Some also use a steroid injection before or after the procedure, to reduce swelling. After the surgery, a pressure bandage will be applied to the face to reduce the risk of hematoma. The patient may spend a few hours resting in a recovery room to ensure no bleeding has occurred, then returns home. Some surgeons recommend that the patient lie down for the next 24 hours, consume a liquid diet, and avoid any movements that lead the neck to flex. Ice packs for the first few days can help to reduce swelling and lower the risk of hematoma. Patients continue taking an antibiotic until the first stitches come out about 5 days after the procedure. The balance are removed 7–10 days later. Many patients return to work and limited activities within two weeks of the procedure. The major complication following face lift surgery is a hematoma, which might require the patient to return to have the stitches reopened to find the source of the bleeding. Most hematomas form within 48 hours of surgery. The typical sign is pain or swelling affecting one side of the face but not the other. Another risk of face lift surgery is nerve damage which can affect the patient's ability to raise an eyebrow, distort his smile, or leave him with limited feeling in his earlobe. Most nerve injuries repair themselves within 2–6 months. Some swelling and bruising is normal following face lift surgery. Other complications of face lift surgery include infection, scarring, and hair loss near incision lines.

Factitious disorders

Factitious disorders are a group of mental disturbances in which patients intentionally act physically or mentally ill without obvious benefits. The name factitious comes from a Latin word that means artificial. These disorders are not **malingering**, which is defined as pretending illness when the ''patient'' has a clear motive, such as financial gain. Patients with factitious disorders produce or exaggerate the symptoms of a physical or mental illness by contaminating urine samples with blood, taking **hallucinogens**, injecting themselves with bacteria to produce infections, and other similar behaviors. There are no reliable statistics on the frequency of factitious disorders, but they are more common in men than in women. Several conditions are sometimes classified as factitious disorders: **Munchausen syndrome**, Munchausen by proxy, and Ganser's syndrome. In Munchausen syndrome, which starts in early adulthood, patients dramatize and exaggerate their factitious symptoms. Many go so far as to undergo major surgery repeatedly, at several locations to avoid detection. Many have been employed in hospitals or in health care professions. Munchausen by proxy is factitious disorders in children produced by parents or other caregivers. The parent may falsify the child's medical history or tamper with laboratory tests in order to make the child appear sick. Occasionally, he/she may actually injure the child to assure that the child will be treated. Ganser's syndrome is an unusual reaction to extreme **stress** in which the patient gives absurd or silly answers to simple questions. It has sometimes been labeled as psychiatric malingering, but is more often classified as a factitious disorder.

Factitious disorders are attributed to many causes: **personality disorders**; **child abuse**; the wish to repeat a satisfying childhood relationship with a doctor; the desire to deceive or test authority figures; and the wish to assume the role of patient and be cared for. In many cases, the person has suffered a major personal loss. Indications of a factitious disorder include: Dramatic but inconsistent medical history, extensive knowledge of medicine and/or hospitals, negative test results followed by further symptom development, symptoms that occur only when the patient is not being observed, few visitors, arguments with hospital staff or similar acting-out behaviors, and eagerness to undergo operations and other procedures. When patients with factitious disorders are confronted, they usually deny that their symptoms are intentional. They may become angry and leave the hospital. In many cases they enter another hospital.

Diagnosis of factitious disorders is usually based on the exclusion of bona fide medical or psychiatric conditions, together with a combination of the signs listed earlier. In some cases, the diagnosis is made on the basis of records from other hospitals. Treatment is usually limited to prompt recognition of the condition and the refusal to give unnecessary medications or to perform unneeded procedures. Factitious disorder patients do not usually remain in the hospital long enough for effective psychiatric treatment. Some clinicians have tried psychotherapeutic treatment for factitious disorder patients, and there are anecdotal reports that **antidepressant** or **antipsychotic** medications are helpful in certain cases. Some patients have only one or two episodes of factitious disorders; others develop a chronic form that may be lifelong. Successful treatment of the chronic form appears to be rare.

Failure to thrive

Failure to thrive (FTT) describes a delay in a child's growth or development. It is usually applied to infants and children up to two years of age who do not gain or maintain weight as they should. Shortly after birth most infants lose some weight. After that expected loss, babies should gain weight at a steady and predictable rate. When a baby does not gain weigh as expected, or continues to lose weight, it is not thriving. Failure to thrive is not a specific disease, but rather a group of symptoms which may come from many sources. Organic failure to thrive (OFTT) implies that the organs involved with digestion and absorption of food are malformed or incomplete so the baby cannot digest its food. Non-organic failure to thrive (NOFTT), the most common type, implies the baby is not receiving enough food due to economic factors, parental neglect, or psychosocial problems. Occasionally, there may be a physical condition that limits the baby's ability to take in, digest, or process food. These defects can occur in the esophagus, stomach, small or large intestine, rectum or anus. Usually the defect is an incomplete development of the organ, and it must be surgically corrected. Most physical defects can be detected shortly after birth. Failure to thrive may also result from lack of available food or the quality of the food offered. This can be due to economic factors in the family, parental beliefs and concepts of nutrition, or neglect. If the baby is being breast fed, the quality or quantity of the mother's milk may be the source of the problem. Psychosocial problems, often stemming from a lack of nurturing parent-child relations, can lead to a failure to thrive. The child may exhibit poor appetite due to depression from insufficient attention from parents.

Most babies are weighed at birth and that weight is used as a baseline for future well-baby check-ups. If the baby is not gaining weight at a predictable rate, the doctor will do a more extensive examination. If there are no apparent physical deformities in the digestive tract, the doctor will examine the child's environment. As part of that examination, the doctor will look at the family history of height and weight. In addition, the parents will be asked about feedings, illnesses, and family routines. If the mother is **breastfeeding** the doctor will also evaluate her diet, general health, and well being as it affects the quantity and quality of her milk. Diagnosis of FTT is confirmed by a positive growth and behavioral response to increased nutrition. If there's a physical reason for failure to thrive, correcting that problem should reverse the condition. If the condition is caused by environmental factors, the physician will suggest ways to provide adequate food for the child. Maternal education and parental counseling may also be recommended. In extreme cases, hospitalization or a more nurturing home may be necessary. The first year of life is important as a foundation for future growth and physical and intellectual development. Children with extreme failure to thrive in the first year may never catch up to their peers even if their physical growth improves. In about one third of these extreme cases, mental development remains below normal and roughly half will continue to have psychosocial and eating problems throughout life. When failure to thrive is identified and corrected early, most children catch up to their peers and remain healthy and well developed. Initial failure to thrive caused by physical defects cannot be prevented but can often be corrected before it becomes dangerous to the child. Maternal education and emotional and economic support systems all help to prevent failure to thrive in those cases where there is no physical deformity.

Fainting

Fainting is loss of consciousness caused by a temporary lack of oxygen to the brain. Known by the medical term ''syncope,'' fainting may be preceded by **dizziness**, **nausea**, or a feeling of extreme weakness. When a person faints, the loss of consciousness is brief and he/she will wake up as soon as normal blood flow is restored to the brain. Blood flow is usually restored by lying flat for a short time, which puts the head on the same level as the heart so that blood flows more easily to the brain. A fainting episode may be completely harmless, but it can also be a symptom of a serious underlying disorder. Fainting should be treated as a medical emergency until the cause is determined.

Fainting can be caused by extreme **pain**, fear, or **stress**, standing still or erect for too long, **osteoarthritis** of the neck bones, a disease such as Stokes-Adams syndrome, weakness in the limbs or a temporary problem in speaking caused by obstructed blood flow in vessels passing through the neck to the brain, pregnancy, or low blood sugar. Fainting can also be caused by: Prolonged **cough**ing, straining to defecate or urinate, blowing a wind instrument too hard, remaining in a stuffy environment with too little oxygen, or a temporary drop in the blood supply to the brain caused by a transient ischemic attack (sometimes called a mini-**stroke**). Seek help immediately if a fainting spell is followed by any of these symptoms: Numbness or tingling in any body part, blurred vision, confusion, difficulty speaking, or loss of movement in arms or legs. A few seconds before fainting, a person may sweat or become pale, feel nauseated or dizzy, and have blurred vision or racing heartbeat. Once the person loses consciousness, the pupils may dilate as the heart rate slows down. There may be abnormal movements. Muscles may tighten or the back may arch. These movements do not last long and they are not violent. In most cases, the patient regains consciousness within a few minutes, but the fainting spell may be followed by nervousness, **headache**, nausea, dizziness, pallor or sweating. The person may faint again, especially if he or she stands up within 30 minutes.

Most episodes of fainting are a one-time occurrence. When a person repeatedly faints, a physician should be called. Most of the time, a person who faints ends up lying on the floor. If this happens, the patient should be rolled onto his or her back. Because someone who faints often vomits, bystanders should keep the airway open. A person who is fainting should not be held upright or in a sitting position. These positions prevent blood flow to the brain and may bring on a seizure. Bystanders should check the patient's breathing and pulse rate. The pulse may be weak and slow. If there are no signs of breathing or heart rate, the problem is more serious than fainting, and **cardiopulmonary resuscitation (CPR)** must begin. If breathing and pulse rates seem normal, the person's legs should be raised above the level of the head so that gravity can help the blood flow to the brain. Belts, collars or any other constrictive clothing should be loosened. If the person does not regain consciousness within a minute or two after fainting, medical help should be summoned. After a fainting spell, the person should regain normal color but may continue to feel weak for a short time. Lying down quietly for a few moments may help. In most cases, an attack of fainting is not serious. As soon as the underlying pain or stress passes, the danger of repeated episodes also is eliminated. If a person is feeling faint, unconsciousness may be prevented by sitting with the head between the knees or lying flat with the legs raised. A person who has fainted should lie flat for 10–15 minutes after regaining consciousness to give the system a chance to regain its balance. Standing up too soon may bring on another fainting spell.

FAITH HEALING

Faith Healing is the curing of disease or healing of injuries through prayer and divine intervention. Faith healing dates back to our most ancient societies. Primitive cultures, for example, sometimes relied on medicine men, or witch doctors, to pray to the spirits for healing. The ancient Greeks and Romans also prayed to various gods to cure their illnesses and repair the body. For example, infertile couples who wanted to conceive a child would pray for intervention at the temple of **Imhotep** (ca. 2700 BC), who was a vizier to the Egyptian King Djoser and achieved divine status after his death. Perhaps the most famous examples of faith healing are the Biblical descriptions of Jesus Christ healing lepers and curing the insane.

Although scientists have made phenomenal advances during the twentieth century in understanding and curing sickness and disease, faith healing continues to flourish in modern society. The most obvious examples are the television evangelists who claim to heal through prayer and touch. While many believe that these evangelists ''stage'' their miraculous cures, the debate continues to rage over the effectiveness of faith healing. However, the line of demarcation between ''believers'' and ''non-believers'' is not clear cut. A 1997 survey of physicians at a meeting of the Academy of Family Physicians found that 99% of them believed that religious faith plays a role in patients' recoveries. Not all of these physicians believed in divine intervention but rather that belief can reduce **stress** and have other psychological effects that help to improve patients' **immune system** and the ability to fight disease. Another theory regarding faith healing is that patients recover because of the ''placebo effect,'' that is, when a patient improves in response to a treatment (such as a sugar pill) that has no proven therapeutic value.

More than 200 scientific studies have focused on the role of faith and religion in health. One of the most noted studies took place at the San Francisco General Medical Center in 1982 and 1983. The researchers found that the 192 heart patients who were prayed for were five times less likely to develop further complications than the 201 who were not. In this study and others, patients were picked at random and not according to their religious beliefs, and they did not know whether or not others were praying them for them.

In 1998, researchers at Duke University also studied 4,000 people over the age of 65. They found that those who participated in religious activities were 40% less likely to have high blood pressure and showed faster recoveries from physical illnesses and depression. Scientific explanations for statistically significant better health and faster recoveries in religious people include healthier lifestyles and a stronger social support that bolsters mental well being However, no studies have proven that an individual ''faith healer'' has the ability to cure disease.

While many physicians and scientists agree that faith can play a role in healing, most concur that relying on faith healing to the exclusion of modern medicine can be dangerous. A University of California, San Diego, School of Medicine study looked at 172 pediatric patients who had died over a ten year period. They found that 140 of the of these children would have had survival rates of more than 90% if they had received medical care for their illnesses, which included appendicitis, pneumonia, and diabetes. In some cases, parents who have relied on faith healing alone to cure their sick child have been convicted of involuntary manslaughter due to medical neglect when a child died.

Scientists may never be able to prove conclusively the effectiveness of faith healing. Nevertheless, many physicians and lay people believe that faith healing has a role in modern day treatment of illnesses and disease. A 1996 survey of the general population by *Time* magazine found that 82% of the respondents believed in the healing power of personal prayer. At the same time, only 28% believed in the ability of ''faith healers'' to make people well. If there is any scientific consensus on the matter, it is one of caution.

Falloppio, Gabriele (1523-1562)

Italian physician and scientist

Born in Modena, Falloppio was a famous doctor and surgeon, an academic, and an author. The uterine tubes were named after him (fallopian tubes) for his work in describing them. With **Andreas Vesalius** and **Bartolemeo Eustachio**, Falloppio is considered one of the three heroes of anatomy (the science dealing with the structure of animals and plants). Falloppio first studied medicine at the Medical College of Modena. After dissecting a body in 1545, he earned the right to practice medicine in Modena as a surgeon.

Falloppio treated prominent patients from as far away as Florence and Rome. His patients included members of the Venetian authorities and Pope Julius III's brother, Baldovine del Monte. Known as one of the great surgeons of the age, he established new surgical procedures. He worked extensively in medicine and pharmacology and was an early expert on syphilis. Falloppio was appointed chair of pharmacy in Ferrara in 1548, and professor of anatomy at the University of Pisa in 1549. While in Pisa, he was wrongfully accused of practicing human **vivisection**. During this period, he also disproved Aristotle's statement that the bones of lions are solid and have no marrow by dissecting the bodies of lions in the Medici zoo. In 1551, he was appointed professor of anatomy and surgery at the University of Padua. In 1561, he was offered the position at Professor of Practical Medicine at the University of Bologna, but died before he could start. Falloppio was a member of the Medical College of Venice.

Many works have been attributed to Falloppio, but the only one which was proven to be authentic was *Observationes anatomicae*, published in 1561. This was considered an anatomy work of great originality which contributed to knowledge about bones, the muscles, the vascular system, the kidneys, and the physiological uses of various features.

See also Bartolemeo Eustachio; Andreas Vesalius

False teeth

Replacements for decayed or lost teeth have been produced for millennia. The Etruscans made skillfully designed false teeth out of ivory and bone, secured by gold bridgework, as early as 700 B.C. Unfortunately, this level of sophistication for false teeth was not regained until the 1800s. During medieval times, the practice of dentistry was largely confined to **tooth extraction**; replacement was seldom considered. Gaps between teeth were expected, even among the rich and powerful. Queen Elizabeth I (1533-1603) filled the holes in her mouth with cloth to improve her appearance in public. When false teeth were installed, they were hand-carved and tied in place with silk threads. If not enough natural teeth remained, anchoring false ones was difficult. People who wore full sets of dentures had to remove them when they wanted to eat. Upper and lower plates fit poorly and were held together with steel springs; disconcertingly, the set of teeth could spring suddenly out of the wearer's mouth. Even George Washington (1732-1799) suffered terribly from tooth loss and ill-fitting dentures. The major obstacles to progress were finding suitable materials for false teeth, making accurate measurements of a patient's mouth, and getting the teeth to stay in place. These problems began to be solved during the 1700s. Since antiquity, the most common material for false teeth was animal bone or ivory, especially from elephants or hippopotami. Human teeth were also used, pulled from the dead or sold by poor people from their own mouths. These kinds of false teeth soon rotted, turning brown and rancid. Rich people preferred teeth of silver, gold, mother of pearl, or agate. In 1774 the French pharmacist Duchateau enlisted the help of the prominent dentist Dubois de Chemant to design hard-baked, rot-proof porcelain dentures. De Chemant patented his improved version of these ''Mineral Paste Teeth'' in 1789 and took them with him when he emigrated to England shortly afterward. The single porcelain tooth held in place by an imbedded platinum pin was invented in 1808 by the Italian dentist Giuseppangelo Fonzi. Inspired by his dislike of handling dead people's teeth, Claudius Ash of London, England, invented an improved porcelain tooth around 1837. Porcelain teeth came to the United States in 1817 via the French dentist A. A. Planteau. The famous artist Charles Peale (1741-1847) began baking mineral teeth in Philadelphia, Pennsylvania, in 1822. Commercial manufacture of porcelain teeth in the United States was begun, also in Philadelphia, around 1825 by Samuel Stockton. In 1844 Stockton's nephew founded the S. S. White Company, which greatly improved the design of artificial teeth and marketed them on a large scale. Fit and comfort, too, gradually improved. The German Philip Pfaff (1715-1767) introduced plaster of paris impressions of the patient's mouth in 1756. Daniel Evans of Philadelphia also devised a method of accurate mouth measurement in 1836. The real breakthrough came with Charles Goodyear's discovery of vulcanized rubber in 1839. This cheap, easy-to-work material could be molded to fit the mouth and made a good base to hold false teeth. Well-mounted dentures could now be made cheaply. The timing was fortuitous. Horace Wells (1815-1848) had just introduced painless tooth extraction using **nitrous oxide**. The number of people having teeth removed skyrocketed, creating a great demand for good, affordable dentures, which Goodyear's invention made possible. After 1870, another cheap base, celluloid, was tried in place of rubber, but it too had drawbacks.

Today dentures are primarily made of plastic or ceramic. However, research continues into new and better materials to make dentures longer lasting and more resistant to stain. One such material is cobalt chromium, which is a hard metal that does not rust or change shape. A more recent development in dentistry is the dental implant. Dental implants are constructed from biocompatible materials, such as titanium, which are not recognized by the body's immune system as foreign. Endosteal implant are placed into the bone to replace the root portion of a tooth. A subperiosteal implant—used when there is not enough bone left—fits in a framework fashion over the remaining bone. These implants are then used to support a natural looking artificial tooth, which is usually attached with a dental adhesive.

FAMILY THERAPY

Family therapy is a form of psychotherapy that involves all the members of a nuclear or extended family. It may be conducted by a pair or team of therapists. In many cases the team consists of a man and a woman in order to treat gender-related issues or serve as role models for family members. Although some forms of family therapy are based on behavioral or psychodynamic principles, the most widespread form is based on family systems theory. This approach regards the family, as a whole, as the unit of treatment, and emphasizes such factors as relationships and communication patterns rather than traits or symptoms in individual members.

Family therapy is a relatively recent development in psychotherapy. It began shortly after World War II, when doctors, who were treating schizophrenic patients, noticed that the patients' families communicated in disturbed ways. The doctors also found that the patients' symptoms rose or fell according to the level of tension between their parents. These observations led to considering a family as an organism or system with its own internal rules, patterns of functioning, and tendency to resist change. The therapists started to treat the families of schizophrenic patients as whole units rather than focusing on the hospitalized member. They found that in many cases the family member with **schizophrenia** improved when the ''patient'' was the family system. (This should not be misunderstood to mean that schizophrenia is caused by family problems, although family problems may worsen the condition.) This approach of involving the entire family in the treatment plan and therapy was then applied to families with problems other than the presence of schizophrenia.

Family therapy is becoming an increasingly common form of treatment as changes in American society are reflected in family structures. It has led to two further developments: couples therapy, which treats relationship problems between marriage partners or gay couples; and the extension of family therapy to religious communities or other groups that resemble families.

Family therapy is often recommended in the following situations:

- Treatment of a family member with schizophrenia or **multiple personality disorder** (MPD). Family therapy helps other family members understand their relative's disorder and adjust to the psychological changes that may be occurring in the relative.
- Families with problems across generational boundaries. These would include problems caused by parents sharing housing with grandparents, or children being reared by grandparents.
- Families that deviate from social norms (common-law relationships, gay couples rearing children, etc.). These families may not have internal problems but may be troubled by outsiders' judgmental attitudes.
- Families with members from a mixture of racial, cultural, or religious backgrounds.
- Families who are scapegoating a member or undermining the treatment of a member in individual therapy.
- Families where the identified patient's problems seem inextricably tied to problems with other family members.
- Blended families with adjustment difficulties.

Most family therapists presuppose an average level of intelligence and education on the part of adult members of the family.

Some families are not considered suitable candidates for family therapy. They include:

- Families in which one, or both, of the parents is psychotic or has been diagnosed with antisocial or paranoid personality disorder.
- Families whose cultural or religious values are opposed to, or suspicious of, psychotherapy.
- Families with members who cannot participate in treatment sessions because of physical illness or similar limitations.
- Families with members with very rigid personality structures. Here, members might be at risk for an emotional or psychological crisis.
- Families whose members cannot or will not be able to meet regularly for treatment.
- Families that are unstable or on the verge of breakup.

Family therapy tends to be short-term treatment, usually several months in length, with a focus on resolving specific problems such as **eating disorders**, difficulties with school, or adjustments to bereavement or geographical relocation. It is not normally used for long-term or intensive restructuring of severely dysfunctional families.

In family therapy sessions, all members of the family and both therapists (if there is more than one) are present at most sessions. The therapists seek to analyze the process of family interaction and communication as a whole; they do not take sides with specific members. They may make occasional comments or remarks intended to help family members become more conscious of patterns or structures that had been previously taken for granted. Family therapists, who work as a team, also model new behaviors for the family through their interactions with each other during sessions.

Family therapy is based on family systems theory, which understands the family to be a living organism that is more than the sum of its individual members. Family therapy uses "systems" theory to evaluate family members in terms of their position or role within the system as a whole. Problems are treated by changing the way the system works rather than trying to "fix" a specific member. Family systems theory is based on several major concepts:

The identified patient (IP) is the family member with the symptom that has brought the family into treatment. The concept of the IP is used by family therapists to keep the family from scapegoating the IP or using him or her as a way of avoiding problems in the rest of the system.

The concept of homeostasis means that the family system seeks to maintain its customary organization and functioning over time. It tends to resist change. The family therapist can use the concept of homeostasis to explain why a certain family symptom has surfaced at a given time, why a specific member has become the IP, and what is likely to happen when the family begins to change.

The extended family field refers to the nuclear family, plus the network of grandparents and other members of the extended family. This concept is used to explain the intergenerational transmission of attitudes, problems, behaviors, and other issues.

Differentiation refers to the ability of each family member to maintain his or her own sense of self, while remaining emotionally connected to the family. One mark of a healthy family is its capacity to allow members to differentiate, while family members still feel that they are "members in good standing" of the family.

Family systems theory maintains that emotional relationships in families are usually triangular. Whenever any two persons in the family system have problems with each other, they will "triangle in" a third member as a way of stabilizing their own relationship. The triangles in a family system usually interlock in a way that maintains family homeostasis. Common family triangles include a child and its parents; two children and one parent; a parent, a child, and a grandparent; three siblings; or, husband, wife, and an in-law.

In some instances the family may have been referred to a specialist in family therapy by their pediatrician or other primary care provider. It is estimated that as many as 50% of office visits to pediatricians have to do with developmental problems in children that are affecting their families. Some family doctors use symptom checklists or psychological screeners to assess a family's need for therapy.

Family therapists may be either psychiatrists, clinical psychologists, or other professionals certified by a specialty board in marriage and family therapy. They will usually evaluate a family for treatment by scheduling a series of interviews with the members of the immediate family, including young children, and significant or symptomatic members of the extended family. This process allows the therapist(s) to find out how each member of the family sees the problem, as well as to form first impressions of the family's functioning. Family therapists typically look for the level and types of emotions expressed, patterns of dominance and submission, the roles played by family members, communication styles, and the locations of emotional triangles. They will also note whether these patterns are rigid or relatively flexible.

Preparation also usually includes drawing a genogram, which is a diagram that depicts significant persons and events in the family's history. Genograms also include annotations about the medical history and major personality traits of each member. Genograms help in uncovering intergenerational patterns of behavior, marriage choices, family alliances and conflicts, the existence of family secrets, and other information that sheds light on the family's present situation.

The chief risk in family therapy is the possible unsettling of rigid personality defenses in individuals, or couple relationships that had been fragile before the beginning of therapy. Intensive family therapy may also be difficult for psychotic family members.

Fasting

Fasting is the voluntary abstinence from eating for an extended period of time. It is a controversial procedure. Many people believe that fasting is an easy way to give the **digestive system** a rest to allow the body to rid itself of toxins and wastes. It is also thought to stimulate the **metabolism** and promote healing by strengthening the **immune system**. Under no conditions should pregnant or **breast-feeding** women, or anyone who is diabetic or has kidney or liver problems, has an **eating disorder**, **asthma**, or **tuberculosis**, fast. Fasting's history goes back to Biblical times, where it was a way to purify the body and the mind. It can be found in cultures as diverse as the ancient Greeks and the Native Americans, and was often used as part of a rite or religious exercise. In modern times, many people fast for health, rather than spiritual, reasons. Those who advocate fasting argue that it is a way to get rid of natural waste and environmental chemicals that build up in our bodies. The other major justification for fasting is that it stimulates the metabolism and the immune system, promoting healing and renewal. Both arguments for fasting are based on the belief that by stopping the digestive tract from having to work continuously, a major obstacle to the body's natural healing powers is removed. This is based on the idea that it takes a lot of energy to break down and convert food, energy which can be better spent healing ourselves. Proponents of fasting argue that it provides better overall health and improves vitality. The possible loss of unwanted body fat is a bonus.

There are many types and degrees of fasting. The most popular is the juice fast in which only fresh fruit and vegetable juice is consumed. Some also drink vegetable broth and herbal teas. Since all of these liquids are high in **vitamins**, **minerals**, amino acids, and natural sugars, some consider this to be a restricted diet instead of a real fast. Others say that a true fast consists of consuming only distilled water. A fast can last for 24 hours or for as long as one month. Anything more than a couple of days should be considered a prolonged fast, and be supervised by a physician.

Fasting is controversial. Medical school trained physicians argue that science has yet to prove that fasting actually eliminates toxins from the body, and that, since the body undergoes a series of changes during a fast, it should never be done without prior medical consultation. They also argue that in addition to the minor side effects, like fatigue and **dizziness**, even modified fasting on juices can sometimes cause the formation of **kidney stones** or gallstones. Proponents say that fasting can provide a sense of control of one's life. Self-prescribed fasting of any kind can be dangerous to varying degrees. Some people become light-headed, dizzy, and develop **headache**s. Extended fasting can even lead to sodium and potassium depletion, and a fatal alteration of electrolyte balance.

FATTY LIVER

Fatty liver is the collection of excessive amounts of triglycerides, a form of fat stored by the body and used for energy and new cell formation, and other fats inside liver cells. Also called steatosis, fatty liver can be a temporary or long-term condition, which is not harmful itself, but may indicate some other type of problem. Left untreated, it can contribute to other illnesses. It is usually reversible once the cause of the problem is diagnosed and corrected. The liver changes fats eaten in the diet to types of fat that can be stored and used by the body. The break down of fats in the liver can be disrupted by alcoholism, **malnutrition**, **pregnancy**, or **poisoning**. In fatty liver, large droplets of fat, containing mostly triglycerides, collect within cells of the liver. The condition is generally not painful and may go unnoticed for a long time. In severe cases, the liver can increase to over three times its normal size and may be painful and tender.

The most common cause of fatty liver in the United States is alcoholism. In alcoholic fatty liver, over consumption of alcohol changes the way that the liver breaks down and stores fats. Often, people with chronic alcoholism also suffer from malnutrition by eating irregularly and not having a balanced diet. Other forms of malnutrition (especially when there is not enough protein in the diet), **obesity**, **diabetes mellitus**, and **Reye's syndrome** in children can also cause fatty liver. Pregnancy can cause a rare, but serious, form of fatty liver that starts late in pregnancy and may be associated with **jaundice** and liver failure. Some **drug overdose**s or toxic chemical poisonings, such as carbon tetrachloride, can also cause fatty liver. Often, fatty liver has no symptoms. If there are symptoms, they can include pain under the rib cage on the right side of the body, swelling of the abdomen, jaundice, and **fever**. Symptoms that occur less often in alcoholic fatty liver, but more often in pregnancy related fatty liver, are **nausea**, vomiting, loss of appetite, and abdominal pain. Fatty liver is diagnosed by a **physical examination**, when a doctor notices that the liver is enlarged and tender when the abdomen is examined; through blood tests to determine if the liver is functioning properly; and through a liver **biopsy**, where a small sample of liver tissue removed with a long needle or though a very small incision is examined. In pregnant women, fatty liver is usually associated with another serious complication, preeclampsia or eclampsia. In this condition, the mother has seriously high blood pressure, swelling, and possibly, **seizures**.

Treatment involves correcting the condition that caused fatty liver and providing supportive care. In fatty liver caused by alcoholism, the treatment is to give up drinking alcohol and to eat a healthy, well balanced diet. In fatty liver associated with pregnancy, the recommended treatment is to deliver the baby, if the pregnancy is far enough along. Vitamin and mineral supplements along with nutritional support may be useful. Fatty liver is usually reversible if recognized and treated. There may be some long-term tendency toward other types of liver problems depending on how long and how severe the fatty liver condition was. In pregnant women, the situation can be life threatening for both the mother and the infant. Left untreated, there is a high risk of **death** for both. Severe liver damage that may require a liver transplant can occur in the mother if the condition is not recognized early. Prevention consists of maintaining a well-balanced diet and healthy lifestyle with moderate or no alcohol consumption. Pregnant women require good prenatal care so that symptoms can be recognized and treated as early as possible.

FAUCI, ANTHONY S. (1940-)

American immunologist

Early in his career, Anthony S. Fauci carried out both basic and clinical research in immunology and infectious diseases. Since 1981, Fauci's research has been focused on the mechanisms of the human immunodeficiency virus (HIV), which causes acquired immunodeficiency syndrome (**AIDS**). His work has lead to breakthroughs in understanding the virus's progress, especially during the latency period between infection and full-blown AIDS. As director of both the National Institute of Allergy and Infectious Diseases (NIAID) and the Office of AIDS Research at the **National Institutes of Health** (NIH), Fauci is involved with much of the AIDS research performed in the United States and is responsible for supervising the investigation of the disease mechanism and the development of vaccines and drug therapy.

Anthony Stephen Fauci was born on December 24, 1940, in Brooklyn, New York, to Stephen A. Fauci, a pharmacist, and Eugenia A. Fauci, a homemaker. He attended a Jesuit high school in Manhattan and had a successful academic and athletic career there. After high school, Fauci entered Holy Cross College in Worcester, Massachusetts, as a premedical student, graduating with a B.A. in 1962. He then attended Cornell University Medical School, from which he received his medical degree in 1966 and where he completed both his internship and residency.

In 1968, Fauci became a clinical associate in the Laboratory of Clinical Investigation of NIAID, one of the eleven institutes that comprise the NIH. Except for one year spent at the New York Hospital Cornell Medical Center as chief resident, he has remained at the NIH throughout his career. His earliest studies focused on the functioning of the human **immune system** and how infectious diseases impact the system. As a senior staff fellow at NIAID, Fauci and two other researchers delineated the mechanism of Wegener's granulomatosis, a relatively rare and fatal immune disease involving the inflammation of blood vessels and organs. By 1971, Fauci had developed a drug regimen for Wegener's granulomatosis that is ninety-five percent effective. He also found cures for lymphomatoid granulomatosis and polyarteritis nodosa, two other immune diseases.

In 1972, Fauci became a senior investigator at NIAID and two years later he was named head of the Clinical Physiology Section. In 1977, Fauci was appointed deputy clinical director of NIAID. Fauci shifted the focus of the Laboratory of Clinical Infection at NIAID towards investigating the nature of AIDS in the early 1980s. It was his lab that demonstrated the type of defect that occurs in the T4 helper cells (the immune cells) and enables AIDS to be fatal. Fauci also orchestrated early therapeutic techniques, including bone-marrow transplants, in an attempt to save AIDS patients. In 1984, Fauci became the director of NIAID, and the following year the coordinator of all AIDS research at NIH. He has worked not only against the disease but also against governmental indifference to AIDS, winning larger and larger budgets for AIDS research. When the Office of AIDS Research at NIH was founded in 1988, Fauci was made director; he also decided to remain the director of NIAID. He and his research teams have developed a three-fold battle plan against AIDS: researching the mechanism of HIV, developing and testing drug therapies, and creating an AIDS vaccine.

In 1993, Fauci and his team at NIH disproved the theory that HIV remains dormant for approximately ten years after the initial infection, showing instead that the virus attacks the lymph nodes and reproduces itself in white blood cells known as CD4 cells. This discovery could lead to new and radical approaches in the early treatment of HIV-positive patients. Earlier discoveries that Fauci and his lab are responsible for include the 1987 finding that a protein substance known as cytokine may be responsible for triggering full-blown AIDS and the realization that the macrophage, a type of immune system cell, is the virus's means of transmission. Fauci demonstrated that HIV actually hides from the body's immune system in these macrophages and is thus more easily transmitted. In an interview with Dennis L. Breo published in the *Journal of the American Medical Association,* Fauci summed up his research to date: ''We've learned that AIDS is a multiphasic, multifactorial disease of overlapping phases, progressing from infection to viral replication to chronic smoldering disease to profound depression of the immune system.''

In drug therapy work, Fauci and his laboratory have run hundreds of clinical tests on medications such as azidothymidine (AZT), and Fauci has pushed for the early use of such drugs by terminally ill AIDS patients. Though no truly effective antiviral drug yet exists, drug therapies have been developed that can prolong the life of AIDS victims. Potential AIDS vaccines are still being investigated, a process complicated by the difficulty of finding willing research volunteers and the fact that animals do not develop AIDS as humans do, which further limits available research subjects. No viable vaccine is expected before the year 2000.

Fauci married Christine Grady, a clinical nurse and medical ethicist, in 1985. They have three daughters: Jennifer, Megan, and Alison. Fauci is an avid jogger, a former marathon runner, and enjoys fishing. Widely recognized for his research, he is the recipient of numerous prizes and awards, including a 1979 Arthur S. Flemming Award, the 1984 U.S. Public Health Service Distinguished Service Medal, the 1989 National Medical Research Award from the National Health Council, and the 1992 Dr. Nathan Davis Award for Outstanding Public Service from the American Medical Association. Fauci is also a fellow of the American Academy of Arts and Sciences and holds a number of honorary degrees. He is the author or coauthor of over 800 scientific articles and has edited several medical textbooks.

FECAL OCCULT BLOOD TEST

Fecal occult blood tests (FOBT) use chemical indicators on stool samples to detect the presence of blood not otherwise visible. Blood originating from or passing through the gastrointestinal tract can signal many conditions requiring further tests and, possibly, medical intervention. These include, but are not limited to: Colorectal and gastric **cancer**s; **ulcers**; **hemorrhoids**; **polyps**; **inflammatory bowel disease**; and irritations or lesions of the GI tract caused by medications, such as **nonsteroidal anti-inflammatory drugs** (NSAIDs) or **aspirin**, or by stomach acid disorders, such as reflux esophagitis. FOBT are used routinely (in conjunction with a rectal examination performed by a physician) to screen for **colorectal cancer**, particularly after age 50; the ordering of this test should not be taken as an indication that cancer is suspected. Certain foods and medicines can influence the test results. For 48 hours prior to collecting samples, avoid red meats, NSAIDs (including aspirin), **antacids**, steroids, iron supplements, and vitamin C, including citrus fruits and other foods containing large amounts of vitamin C.

In most cases, stool samples can be collected at home, using a kit supplied by the physician. Another name for this procedure is the hemoccult test. The standard kit contains a specially prepared card on which a small sample of stool will be spread, using a stick provided in the kit. The sample is placed in a special envelope and either mailed or brought in for analysis. When hydrogen peroxide is applied to the back of the sample, the paper will turn blue if an abnormal amount of blood is present. Many factors can result in false-positive and false-negative findings, and it is important to note that a true-positive finding only signifies the presence of blood; it is not an indication of cancer. The National Cancer Institute has found that less than 10% of all positive results were caused by cancer. Alternatively, a negative result (meaning no blood was detected) does not guarantee the absence of colon cancer, which may bleed only occasionally or not at all. The physician will want to follow up on a positive result with further tests.

FEMALE GENITAL MUTILATION

Female genital mutilation is the cutting, or partial or total removal, of the external female genitalia for cultural, religious, or other non-medical reasons. It is usually performed on girls between the ages of four and 10. It is also called female **circumcision**. Female genital mutilation cuts or removes the tissues around the vagina that give women pleasurable sexual feelings. This procedure is used for social and cultural control of women's sexuality. In its most extreme form, infibulation, where the girl's vagina is sewn shut, the procedure ensures virginity. In some cultures, this procedure is considered a rite of passage for young girls. Families fear that if their daughters are left uncircumcised, they may not be marriageable, or that the girl might bring shame to the family by being sexually active and becoming pregnant before marriage. It is illegal to perform female genital mutilation in many countries, including the United States, Canada, France, Great Britain, Sweden, Switzerland, Egypt, Kenya, and Senegal. This procedure is usually done in the home or somewhere other than a medical setting. Often, it is performed by a family member or by a local ''circumciser,'' using knives, razor blades, or other tools that may not be sterilized before use.

Female circumcision includes a wide range of procedures. The simplest form involves a small cut to the clitoris or labial tissue. A Sunna circumcision removes the prepuce (a fold of skin that covers the clitoris) and/or the tip of the clitoris. A clitoridectomy removes the entire clitoris and some or all of the surrounding tissue. The most extreme form of genital mutilation is excision and infibulation, in which the clitoris and all of the surrounding tissue are cut away and the remaining skin is sewn together. Only a small opening is left for the passage of urine and menstrual blood. The **World Health Organization** (WHO) estimates that over 120 million girls and women have undergone some form of genital mutilation. As a very deeply rooted cultural and religious tradition still practiced in over 26 African, Middle Eastern, and Asian countries, up to two million girls per year are at risk. As more people move to Western countries from countries where female circumcision is performed, the practice has come to the attention of health professionals in the United States, Canada, Europe, and Australia. In an effort to integrate old customs with modern medical care, some immigrant families have requested that physicians perform the procedure. While trying to be sensitive to cultural traditions, health care providers are sometimes put in the difficult position of choosing to perform this procedure in a medical facility under sanitary conditions, or refusing the request, knowing that it may be done anyway with no medical supervision. Some families take their daughters back to the country they immigrated from in order to have the girls circumcised. Many national and international medical organizations including the **American Medical Association**, Canadian medical organizations, and the World Health Organization oppose the practice of female genital mutilation. The United Nations considers female genital mutilation a violation of human rights.

A girl or young woman who has recently had the procedure performed may require supportive care to control bleeding and **antibiotics** to prevent infection. Women who were circumcised as children may require medical care to treat complications. Pregnant women who have been infibulated may have to have the labial tissue cut open to allow the baby to be delivered. Aftercare should be provided with a supportive and nonjudgmental approach towards the girls and women who have undergone this procedure. The immediate risks after the procedure are hemorrhage (excessive **bleeding**), severe **pain**, and infection (including **abscess**es, **tetanus**, and **gangrene**). The most severe consequence is **death** due to excessive blood loss. Long-term complications include scarring, interference with the drainage of urine and menstrual blood, chronic urinary tract infections, pelvic and back pain, and **infertility**. Sexual intercourse can be painful. Complications of **childbirth** are also a risk.

FERNEL, JEAN FRANCOIS (1497-1558)

French physician

Known for his intellectual versatility and depth of knowledge, Fernel became a physician only after spending much of his life studying philosophy, astronomy, and mathematics. He is widely regarded as one of the leading figures of 16th century science and medicine, and is remembered especially for his work in the area of physiology and for dispelling some of the period's reliance on astrology and magic in matters of health. Fernel is also reputed to have coined the Latin words that eventually became our modern ''pathology'' and ''physiology.''

Born in Mondidier, France, Fernel was the son of a successful innkeeper and furrier. He attended the College de Ste. Barbe in Paris, from which he earned his master's degree in 1519. He spent until 1524 in virtual seclusion as he sought to learn all he could about his favored academic disciplines. However, he was forced to leave Paris for a period of convalescence in the country when he contracted a serious illness (possibly **malaria**). Soon afterward, Fernel's father stopped financially supporting his son's studies because his younger children needed the money.

Obliged to find a source of income, Fernel returned to Paris and began working as a lecturer on philosophy. It was at this point that he started studying medicine for the first time. In the late 1520s, he published two books on astronomy and mathematics, but his new father-in-law criticized Fernel for subjugating medicine to his other less lucrative academic interests, so Fernel began concentrating his efforts in that area and obtained his license to practice medicine in 1530. Guided loosely by the orthodox teachings of Claudius **Galen**, a Greek physician regarded as the father of experimental physiology (130-200 A.D.), Fernel sought to reestablish the somewhat tarnished field of medicine as an honorable, worthwhile, and helpful profession. He opened an office in Paris, from which he developed a reputation as an excellent medical practitioner. Meanwhile, he was appointed professor of medicine at the University of Paris in 1534. The Flemish anatomist and physician **Andreas Vesalius** was one of Fernel's most distinguished students.

Fernel published his famous *On the Natural Part of Medicine* in 1542. The text discussed **human anatomy**, which he termed ''physiology,'' and—in agreement with the thinking of his day—outlined the **humors**, temperaments, innate heat, spirits, and faculties of man. The book would be regarded as the definitive work on physiology until **William Harvey** discovered the circulation of the blood in 1628.

In about 1547, the dauphin (later King Henry II) appointed Fernel as his royal **physician**. When Fernel managed to save the life of the dauphin's mistress, his already exalted position in French society became even more prominent. During this period, he did much of his important work on exploring and defining the human **nervous system**. Some historians believe that he had achieved an understanding of the reflex system a century before René Descartes announced his own findings on the subject.

Part of the value of Fernel's contribution to our body of medical knowledge came from his skill as a writer. Combining his own knowledge of medicine with astute observations at patients' bedsides, he wrote many works on pathology, medical therapy, and anatomy. In doing so, he helped to synthesize the medical knowledge of the 16th century. Meanwhile, he encouraged his colleagues and contemporaries to begin eschewing their widespread belief in magic and astrology as determining factors in human health in favor of objective, clinical science. A former adherent of astrology, as were many of the period's well-to-do people, Fernel came to believe toward the end of his life that ''the whole book of healing was nothing other than a copy of inviolable laws observable in Nature.''

Some of Fernel's better known publications were *On the Hidden Causes of Things* (1548) and *J. Fernelii Medicina* (1554), which quickly became one of the late 16th century's standard references and went through 30 editions despite its largely traditional restating of Galen's physiology. Fernel's most comprehensive work was his *Universa medicina,* published posthumously in 1567, which he wrote during breaks from accompanying King Henry II to the battlefield as wars with England and Spain raged. In it, he described his observations of peristalsis and the heart's systole and diastole, among other revelations. The physician died in Paris in 1558.

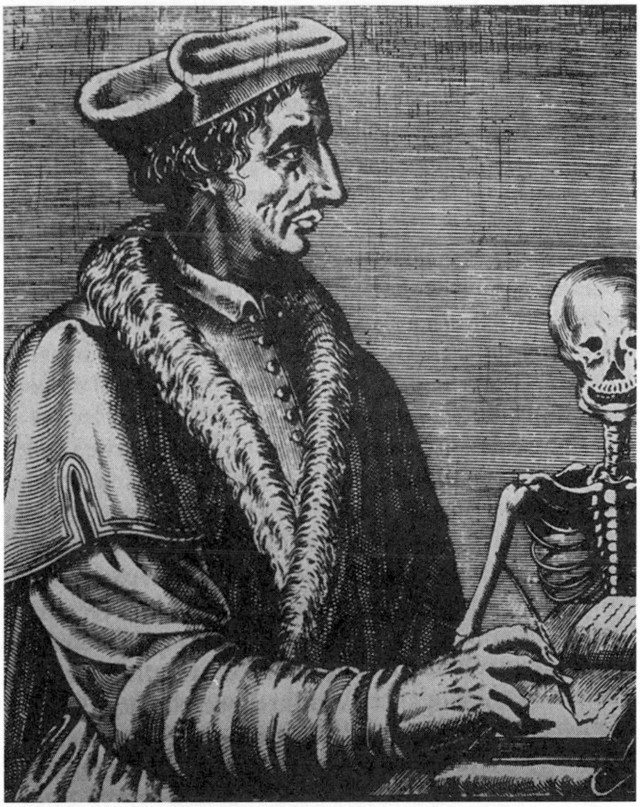

Jean Francois Fernel

FETAL ALCOHOL SYNDROME

Fetal alcohol syndrome (FAS) is a pattern of clinical abnormalities found specifically in some children whose mothers ingested alcohol during **pregnancy**. Alcohol is a teratogenic drug; that is, it can cause birth defects which manifest as physical malformations of the face and head, growth deficiency, **mental retardation**, and—in particular—central **nervous system** dysfunction. FAS results in more babies being born mentally retarded than any other known factor—including **Down's syndrome** and **spina bifida**—yet is completely preventable as simply as abstaining from alcohol during pregnancy. Although FAS sometimes causes embriotic or fetal death, it tragically and devastatingly interferes with the normal development of the fetus. Even though studies have revealed that, although not all children born to alcoholic mothers are affected, every child born with FAS had a mother who drank during pregnancy. Although use of illicit drugs both alone and in combination with alcohol can cause birth defects, more unborn babies are in greater danger from alcohol use alone than from any illegal drug, even cocaine.

Infants, young children, and young adults whose mothers abused alcohol during pregnancy and who suffer from FAS display lower than average birthweight and height, physical abnormalities which may include low muscle tone, smaller than normal skull, irregularities of the face including small eye sockets, mid-face hypoplasia (arrested development of the nose, or ''flat-face'' syndrome), and a very thin upper lip with either an elongated or absent mid-lipline indentation. Neurologic or central nervous system disorders such as hyperactivity, learning and intellectual deficits, distractibility, temper tantrums, short attention and memory span, perceptual problems, impulsive behavior, inability to concentrate, seizures, and abnormal electroencephalogram (EEG, or brain wave patterns) become apparent after the infant stage. Usually, the more severe the physical manifestations of the syndrome, the more severe the intellectual deficits.

Even for FAS-affected children with almost normal intelligence, learning problems become evident by second grade. By grades three and four, affected children experience increasing difficulty with arithmetic, organization, abstract thinking, and attention. Because they have difficulty regulating themselves, children with FAS are often considered problematic behaviorally by the time they reach middle school or junior high where increased independence of judgement and self-control are expected. Behavioral problems then become social adjustment problems around the time the child leaves school and enters the larger environment. Impaired judgement and decision-making abilities and incompetence in independent living become troublesome by this age.

The affects of FAS range from severe to mild and correlate to the amount and frequency of alcohol consumed by the pregnant woman, stage of pregnancy in which drinking takes place, and variability—or changing patterns—of alcohol ingestion. It appears that higher rates of abnormalities are caused by mothers who binge drink than among women who steadily drink consistent quantities, and in whom the most severe physical manifestations of alcoholism are obvious. Also, drinking in the first three months of pregnancy, often before pregnancy is determined, has more serious consequences than drinking the same quantities later in the pregnancy. The possibility of FAS affecting the child of an alcoholic woman is 6%, but the risk increases drastically to 70% for children born after one child is born with FAS. The most severe cases seem to be children of long-term, chronic alcoholic mothers. There is no data so far established which suggests there is a ''risk-free'' level or period of alcohol ingestion during pregnancy, which means there is always the risk that even one or two drinks will damage the development of the extremely vulnerable fetus.

Until the early 1970s, maternal alcohol use was not even considered a risk to the unborn child. As late as the 1960s, federally funded studies into prenatal causes of mental retardation and neurologic abnormalities did not even consider alcohol a possibility. Intravenous alcohol drips were even being used to help prevent premature birth. However, by the 1970s, awareness began to grow about the adverse effects of toxic substances and diet during pregnancy: cigarette **smoking** was known to produce babies of **low birth weight** and diminished size; malnutrition in pregnant women seriously impaired fetal development. When the affects of maternal alcohol use on the fetus were discovered, studies were set in motion worldwide to determine its long-term effects. It is now clear that, even though many infants do not manifest full-fledged signs of FAS, maternal alcohol use causes neurological and behavioral problems which affect the quality of life for the child yet may go relatively unnoticed. Children in this category are diagnosed as having Fetal Alcohol Effect (FAE).

In 1974, the results of one U.S. study were published which compared offspring of 23 alcoholic mothers and 46 non-drinking mothers in matched control groups (participants were from the same general geographic region, socioeconomic group, age, race, marital status, etc.). By the age of seven years, children of alcoholic mothers earned lower scores on math, reading, and spelling tests, and lower IQ scores (an average of 81 versus 95). Although 9% of the children born to non-drinking mothers tested 71 or lower (the level considered as borderline or actual mental inadequacy), 44% of children of alcoholic mothers fell into this range. Similar percentages of reduced weight, height, and head circumference were also observed. A 1982 study from Berlin was the first report indicating FAS caused hyperactivity, distractibility, and speech, eating, and sleeping problems, while a 1990 Swedish study found that as many as 10% of all mildly retarded school-age children in that country suffered from FAS. An early study undertaken in Russia in 1974 of siblings born before and after their mothers became alcoholics reported serious disabilities in many children born after, primarily due to central nervous system damage. Fourteen of the 23 children in this category were mentally retarded. A 1988 study confirmed earlier findings that the younger child of an alcoholic mother is more likely to be adversely affected than the older child. In a study which began in 1974 and followed until the age of 11 years, children of ''low risk'' mothers who simply drank ''socially''—most not even consuming one drink a day after becoming pregnant—found deficits in attention, intelligence, memory, reaction time, learning ability, and behavior were often evident. On average, these problems were more severe in children of women who drank through their entire pregnancy than those who stopped drinking.

Until this decade, most studies regarding FAS have been with children. In 1991, a major report done in the United States on FAS among adolescents and adults aged between 12 to 40 years with an average chronological age of 17 years revealed that physical abnormalities of the face and head as well as size and weight deficiencies were less obvious than in early childhood. However, intellectual variation ranged from severely retarded to normal. The average level of intelligence was borderline or mildly retarded, with academic abilities ranging between the second and fourth grade level. Adaptive living skills averaged that of a seven-year-old, with daily living skills rating higher than social skills.

Accurate diagnosis of FAS is extremely important because affected children require special education to enable them to integrate more fully into society. Because FAS defects can closely mimic those of other birth defects, and because this subject is still relatively new, many physicians are unequipped to recognize FAS-specific birth defects. It is important, therefore, that children with abnormalities, especially whose mothers used alcohol during pregnancy, be fully evaluated by a professional specially trained in birth defects. The most favorable time frame for accurate diagnosis is between the ages of eight months and eight years, although some FAS newborns are so obviously affected that the condition can be recognized much earlier.

Alcohol is a legal psychoactive drug with a high potential for abuse and **addiction**. Because it crosses the placenta (enters the blood stream of the unborn baby), the level of blood alcohol in the baby is directly related to that of the mother, and occurs within just a few short minutes of ingestion. FAS is now considered to be a serious health problem, one which seems extremely difficult to stem. Even though warnings about alcohol consumption by pregnant women were placed on labels of alcoholic beverages in the early 1980s, more than 70,000 children in the ensuing 10 years were born with FAS in the United States alone. The use of alcohol by adolescent women across the nation, and apparently throughout the world, continues to escalate. And, even though there has been an increase in public awareness and education programs regarding

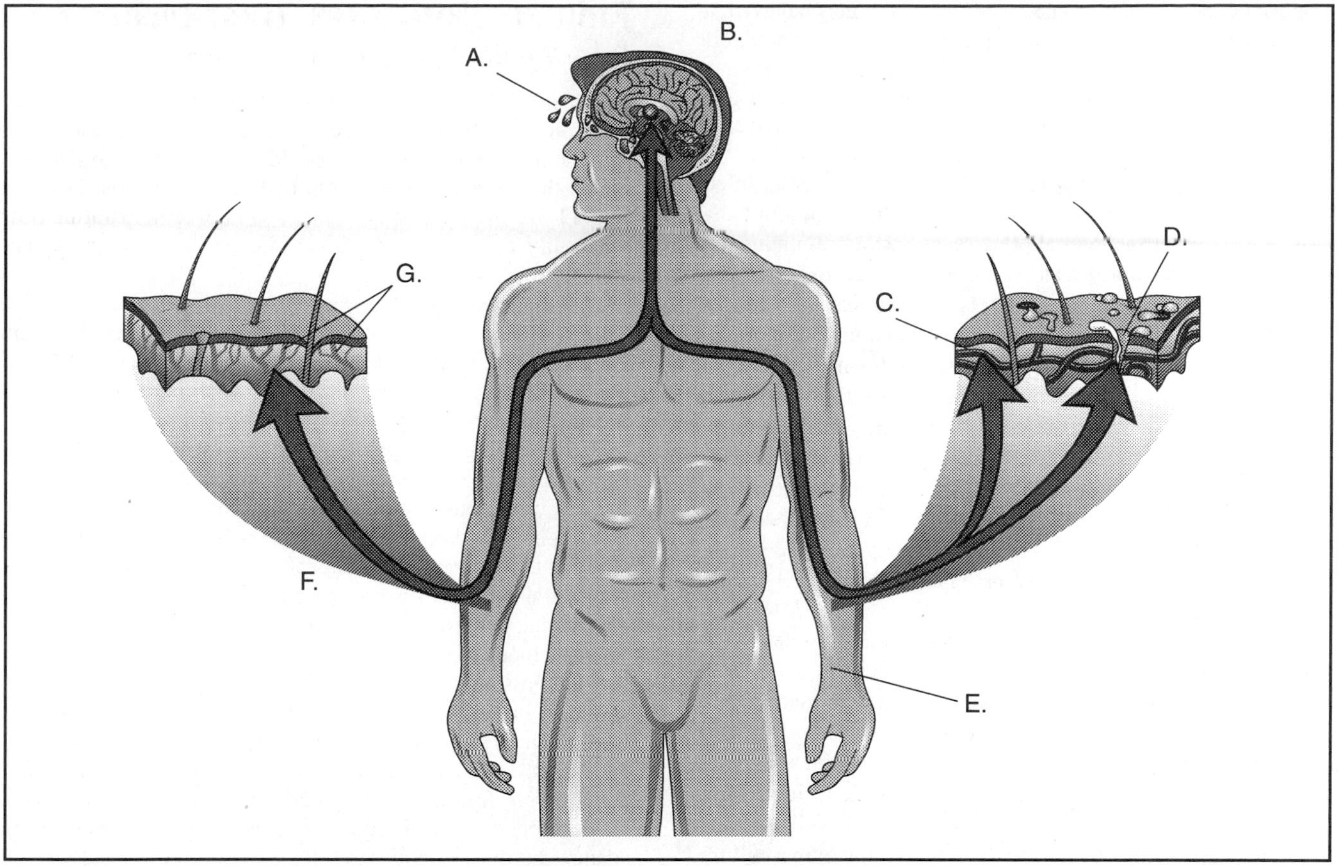

A dramatic rise in body temperature often includes the following symptoms: A. Loss of fluid results in dehydration. B. The hypothalamic set-point is increased, raising metabolism. C. Blood vessels in skin dilate. D. Sweat glands produce excess perspiration. E. Increased pulse rate. F. Increased hypothalmic set-point may introduce chills and shivering to promote heat production from muscles. G. Skin becomes more heat-sensitive. *(Illustration by Electronic Illustrators Group.)*

the tragic yet totally preventable incidence of FAS-related birth defects on the life being formed in utero, large numbers of women still use and abuse alcohol during pregnancy.

Although heavy alcohol use is known to cause FAS, there is absolutely no guarantee that babies will remain unaffected even by moderate ''social'' drinking. Genetic differences in an individual's liver function or ability to metabolize alcohol may cause birth defects in one woman who ingests moderate amounts of alcohol while the offspring of another woman who drinks the same amount or more remain unaffected. The only sure way to prevent FAS is for the mother to take responsibility for the new life developing inside her body and totally abstain from alcohol during the entire pregnancy.

FEVER

A fever is any body temperature elevation over 100°F (37.8°C). A healthy person's body temperature fluctuates between 97°F (36.1°C) and 100°F (37.8°C), with the average being 98.6°F (37°C). The body maintains stability within this range by balancing the heat produced by the metabolism with the heat lost to the environment. The ''thermostat'' that controls this process is located in the hypothalamus, a small structure deep within the brain. The nervous system constantly relays information about the body's temperature to the thermostat, which activates different physical responses to cool or warm the body. These responses include: decreasing or increasing the flow of blood from the body's core, where it is warmed, to the surface, where it is cooled; slowing down or speeding up the rate at which the body turns food into energy (metabolic rate); inducing shivering, which generates heat through muscle contraction; and inducing sweating, which cools the body through evaporation. A fever occurs when the thermostat resets at a higher temperature, primarily in response to an infection. To reach the higher temperature, the body moves blood to the warmer interior, increases the metabolic rate, and induces shivering. The ''chills'' that often accompany a fever are caused by the movement of blood to the body's core, leaving the surface and extremities cold. Once the higher temperature is achieved, the shivering and chills stop. When the infection is overcome or drugs such as **aspirin** or **acetaminophen** (Tylenol) are taken, the thermostat resets to normal and the body's cooling mechanisms switch on: the blood moves to the surface and sweating occurs. Fever is an important part of the immune response. Physicians believe that an elevated body temperature increases the production of cells that fight off bacteria or viruses; inhibits the growth of some bacteria, while speeding up the chemical reactions that help the body's cells repair themselves; and speeds the arrival of white blood cells to the sites of infection.

Fevers are primarily caused by viral or bacterial infections, such as **pneumonia** or **influenza**. Other conditions that can cause a fever include: allergic reactions; autoimmune diseases; trauma, such as breaking a bone; **cancer**; excessive exposure to the sun; intense **exercise**; hormonal imbalances; certain drugs; and damage to the hypothalamus. How long a fever lasts and how high it may go depends on its cause, the age of the patient, and his or her overall health. Most fevers caused by infections appear suddenly and then go away as the **immune system** defeats the infectious agent. An infectious fever may also rise and fall throughout the day, reaching its peak in the late afternoon or early evening. A low-grade fever that lasts for several weeks is associated with autoimmune diseases such as lupus or with some cancers, particularly **leukemia** and **lymphoma**.

A fever is usually diagnosed using a thermometer. Determining the cause of the fever is important. The presence or absence of accompanying symptoms, a patient's medical history, and information about what he or she may have ingested, any recent trips taken, or possible exposures to illness help the physician make a diagnosis. Blood tests can help identify an infectious agent by detecting the presence of antibodies against it or providing samples for growth of the organism in a culture. Blood tests can also provide the doctor with white blood cell counts. **Ultrasound tests**, **magnetic resonance imaging** (MRI) tests, or **computed tomography** (CT) scans may be ordered if the doctor cannot determine the cause of a fever. The most effective treatment for a fever is to address its cause, such as through the administration of antibiotics. Also, because a fever helps the immune system fight infection, it usually should be allowed to run its course. Drugs to lower fever such as aspirin, acetaminophen (Tylenol), and ibuprofin (Advil) can be used if a patient (particularly a child) is uncomfortable. Do not give aspirin to a child or adolescent; it has been linked to an increased risk of **Reye's syndrome**. Bathing a patient in cool water can also help alleviate a high fever. A fever requires emergency treatment: in a newborn (three months or younger) with a fever over 100.5°F (38°C), in an infant or child with a fever over 103°F (39.4°C), or if it's accompanied by severe **headache**, neck stiffness, mental confusion, or severe swelling of the throat. A very high fever in a small child can trigger **seizures** and should be treated immediately. A fever accompanied by the above symptoms can indicate the presence of a serious infection, such as **meningitis**, and should be brought to the immediate attention of a physician. Most fevers caused by infection end as soon as the immune system rids the body of the pathogen and do not produce any lasting effects. The prognosis for fevers associated with more chronic conditions, such as autoimmune disease, depends upon the overall outcome of the disorder.

FIBIGER, JOHANNES (1867-1928)

Danish pathologist and bacteriologist

Johannes Fibiger was a Danish bacteriologist whose early work on childhood **diphtheria** and **tuberculosis** demonstrated the vital role medical research could play in controlling diseases that threatened public health. In 1926, Fibiger received the Nobel Prize in physiology or medicine for demonstrating how cancer-like tissues could be induced experimentally in the laboratory.

Johannes Andreas Grib Fibiger was born on April 23, 1867, in the Danish village of Silkeborg. His father, Christian Fibiger, was a district physician; his mother, Elfride Muller, was a writer and the daughter of a Danish politician. Fibiger attended the University of Copenhagen at age 16 and studied medicine, biology, and zoology. After earning his medical degree in 1890, he undertook several years of medical apprenticeship in various hospitals and with the Danish army.

While working as an assistant in a bacteriological laboratory at the University of Copenhagen Fibiger was persuaded to undertake doctoral work on diphtheria, a virulent childhood disease that caused its victims to suffocate. Fibiger discovered better methods of growing diphtheria bacteria in the laboratory and demonstrated that there were two distinct forms of the bacillus, an important step in identifying carriers of the disease who frequently displayed no symptoms. At the turn of the century, diphtheria was a major public health problem, and epidemics were frequent in Denmark and throughout the rest of the developed world. Fibiger produced an experimental serum against the disease and carefully monitored the results of an inoculation program. In 1897, the International Medical Congress published his report, a model of its kind, which brought Fibiger international attention and confirmed the effectiveness of the serum. The young scientist had received his Ph.D. only two years earlier.

In 1900, at age 33, he joined the faculty of the Institute of Pathological Anatomy, one of a number of young professors hired by the University of Copenhagen. He was also appointed director of the institute and launched a successful program to construct a modern research facility for pathology and anatomy. Within its walls, Fibiger and another faculty member, C.O. Jenson, conducted research on tuberculosis in cattle and humans. Flying in the face of popular opinion, they demonstrated that humans could contract tuberculosis from infected cattle, especially by drinking their milk. Supported by the research of other investigators in Europe, these findings led to the passage of strict regulations governing the sale of raw milk, resulting in fewer adolescent deaths due to tuberculosis.

Fibiger's experiments on tubercular rats led him to the discovery for which he won the Nobel Prize. In 1907 Fibiger became the first researcher to induce what at the time was thought to be **cancer** in a laboratory setting. Fibiger reported his achievement in the *Journal of Cancer Research* and was awarded the 1926 Nobel Prize in medicine or physiology for his discovery of *Spiroptera carcinoma*, the parasitic worm that he thought had produced the cancer. Yet, in his acceptance speech, Fibiger expressed doubt that parasites played any great role in gastric cancer in humans.

Later investigators would find a number of weaknesses in Fibiger's research. Like most scientists of the period, Fibiger had not thought to check his findings against a control group of rats fed on a diet of only white bread. Nor was it easy to reproduce Fibiger's findings in other laboratories due to the lack of a standard strain of laboratory rats in the 1920s; Fibiger's animals had all been caught in the wild. Other investigators expressed doubt that the **abscesses** described by Fibiger were truly cancerous. There was some evidence that the abscesses might have been caused by a diet deficient in vitamin A. Nonetheless, the lasting effect of Fibiger's prize-winning discovery—later refuted by other researchers—was the great impetus it gave to other investigators to pursue laboratory research on the causes of cancer.

Fibiger abandoned parasitology after World War I to follow the work of two Japanese scientists who induced skin cancer in rabbits by painting their ears with coal tar. Conducting his own experiments by painting the backs of rats with the irritant, Fibiger reported two valuable insights: that cancer did not occur with the same frequency in all species or even within the same species, and that individual predisposition played an important role in susceptibility to cancer. At the time of his death, he was working with two colleagues on a vaccine for cancer, hoping to demonstrate that inoculating laboratory animals with matter drawn from malignant tumors would induce immunity to the disease.

During his long career as director of the Institute of Pathological Anatomy at the University of Copenhagen, Fibiger divided his time between research and teaching. He published 79 scientific papers and served as secretary and then president of the Danish Medical Society, and as president of the Danish Cancer Commission. He was co-editor and founder of *Acta Pathologica et Microbiologica Scandinavica*. In 1927, he was awarded the Nordhoff-Jung Cancer Prize

On January 30, 1928, Fibiger died in Copenhagen of a massive heart attack at the age of 60; he had recently learned that he had colon cancer.

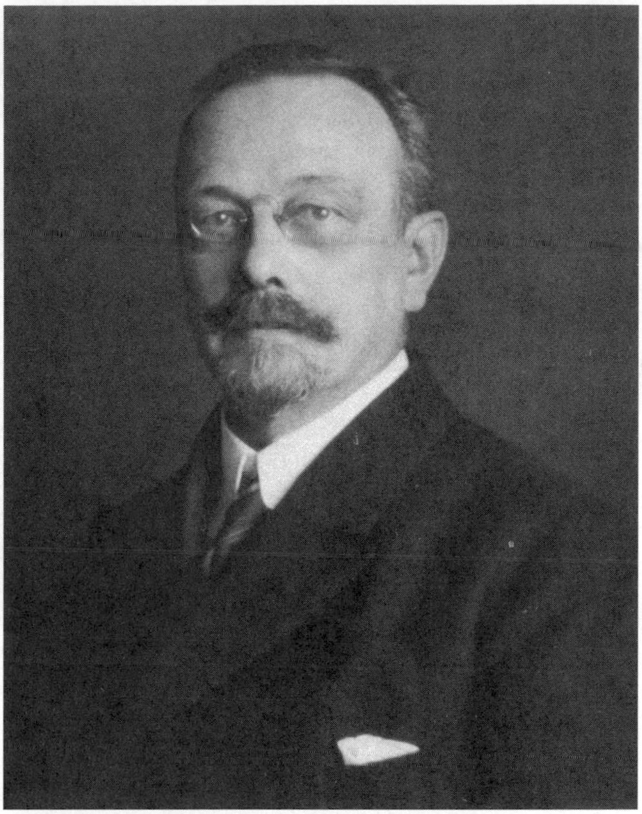

Johannes Grib Fibiger

FIBROCYSTIC CONDITION OF THE BREAST

Fibrocystic condition of the breast refers to many vaguely defined benign breast conditions and symptoms. Breasts come in all shapes and sizes, with varying textures from smooth to lumpy. The tissues of the breast change in response to hormone levels, normal aging, nursing (lactation), weight shifts, or injury; different types of breast tissue respond differently to changes in body chemistry. Fibrocystic breast condition may be called fibrocystic disease, although it is not a single, specific disease process. Variations or changes in the way the breast feels or looks on x-ray may cause the condition to be called "fibrocystic change," mammary dysplasia, mastopathy, chronic cystic mastitis, indurative mastopathy, mastalgia, lumpy breasts, or physiologic nodularity. Between 40–90% of all women have some evidence of "fibrocystic" condition, change, or disease. It is most common among women ages 30–50. This discussion focuses on the tenderness, enlargement, and/or changing "lumpiness" that many women experience before or during their menstrual periods, when female hormones are preparing the breasts for **pregnancy** by stimulating the milk-producing cells and storing fluid. Swelling, with increased sensitivity or **pain**, may result. If pregnancy does not occur, the body reabsorbs the fluid, and the discomfort is relieved. Symptoms range from mild to extremely painful and can vary from month to month. This cycle of breast sensitivity, pain and/or enlargement can also result from medications like **hormone replacement** therapies, and others. Breast pain unrelated to hormone shifts is called "noncyclic" or "trigger-zone breast pain" and may be continuous, or cyclic. Trauma, such as a blow to the area or a previous breast **biopsy**, or sensitivity to certain medications may also underlie this pain. The fibrocystic condition may be cited as the cause of otherwise unexplained breast pain.

Lumps which stand out from enlarged general breast tissue and aren't associated with hormone cycles may also be called fibrocystic condition. The concern with such lumps is **cancer**. Noncancerous lumps are discussed here. Fibroadenomas are tumors of unknown cause which form in the tissues outside the milk ducts and aren't attached to surrounding tissue. They are most common in adolescents and women in their early twenties. Cysts are often painful fluid-filled sacs in the breast that are most common in women between the age of 30 and 50. Sometimes one area of breast tissue feels thicker or

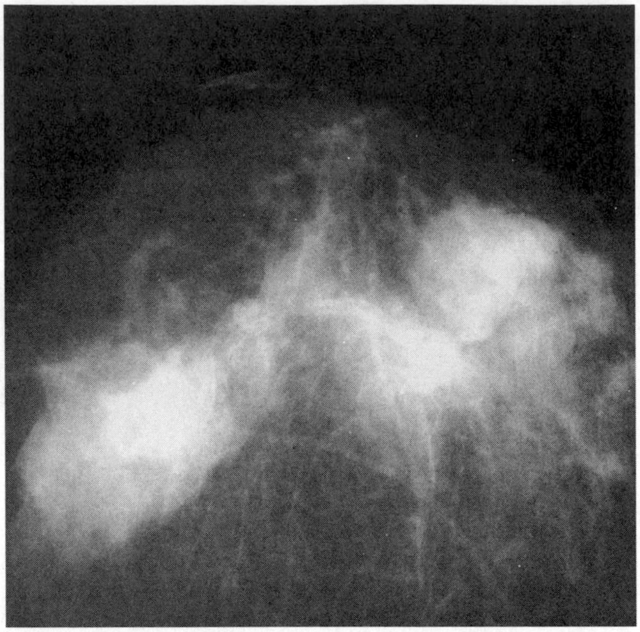

A mammogram of a female breast indicating multiple cysts. ***(Custom Medical Stock Photo. Reproduced by permission.)***

more prominent than the rest of the breast due to old hardened scar tissue and/or dead fat tissue from surgery or trauma; often the cause is unknown. Many other breast problems which are benign or noncancerous may be called ''fibrocystic condition'': disorders which lead to breast inflammation (mastitis), infection, and/or nipple discharge, dilated milk ducts, milk-filled cyst, wart-like growth in the duct, and excess growth of fibrous tissue around the glands.

Breast cancer is the concern in most abnormal breast symptoms. Tell a physician about any new breast lump. A **physical examination** is performed and the patient is usually referred for tests such as **mammography** and breast **ultrasound**. A cyst can be diagnosed by ultrasound. To relieve discomfort, the patient may have the cyst suctioned or drained. The fluid is sometimes sent for analysis. In a breast biopsy, tissue is removed through a needle and examined under a microscope by a pathologist. A ductogram evaluates nipple discharge by threading a very fine tube into the duct, injecting dye into the area, and examining it. A positive response to appropriate therapies supports the diagnosis.

A lump which is benign can be left in the breast. Some women may choose to have a lump surgically removed. Infections are treated with warm compresses and **antibiotics**. Lactating women are encouraged to continue breastfeeding to promote drainage and healing. A serious infection may form an **abscess** which may need surgical drainage. Once a specific disorder is identified, treatment can be prescribed. Symptoms of cyclic breast sensitivity and engorgement can be treated with diet, medication, and/or physical modifications. Over the counter **analgesics** such as **acetaminophen** (Tylenol) or ibuprofen (Advil), hormones or hormone blockers, or birth control pills may be recommended. Warm soaks or ice packs, a well-fitted support bra, and breast massage can relieve symptoms. Many women report relief by reducing or eliminating **caffeine**. Decreasing salt before and during the period when breasts are most sensitive; **Vitamins** A, B complex and E and mineral supplements; a low-fat diet; elimination of dairy products; and evening primrose oil (*Oenothera biennis*), flax oil, and fish oils also help. Most benign breast conditions carry no increased risk for the development of breast cancer. However, a small percentage of biopsies will uncover a tissue pattern in some women that indicates a 15–20% risk of them developing breast cancer over the next 20 years. Strict attention to early detection measures, such as annual mammograms, is especially important for these women. There is no way to prevent fibrocystic condition. Some alternative practitioners believe that eliminating foods high in methyl xanthines (primarily coffee and chocolate) can decrease or reverse fibrocystic breast changes.

FIBROMYALGIA

Fibromyalgia is an inflammation of the fibrous or connective tissue of the body which causes widespread muscle **pain**, fatigue, and multiple tender points. Fibrositis, fibromyalgia, and fibromyositis are a set of symptoms believed to be caused by the same general problem. Fibromyalgia affects 3–6% of the population. It is more common in adults than children, and in women than men, particularly women of childbearing age. The cause of fibromyalgia is not known. Sometimes it occurs in several family members, suggesting that it may be inherited. The primary symptoms of fibromyalgia are muscle and joint pain, stiffness, and fatigue. Pain is the major symptom with aches, tenderness, and stiffness of multiple muscles, joints, and soft tissues. The pain moves from one part of the body to another and is most common in the neck, shoulders, chest, arms, legs, hips, and back. Pain is present most of the time and may last for years, but the severity changes. Symptoms of fatigue may result from chronic pain and **anxiety** about the problem. The inflammatory process also produces chemicals that cause fatigue. Other common symptoms are tension **headaches**, difficulty swallowing, recurrent abdominal pain, **diarrhea**, and numbness or tingling of the extremities. **Stress**, anxiety, depression, or lack of sleep can increase symptoms. Symptoms vary from gradual improvement to episodes of recurrent symptoms.

Diagnosis is difficult because symptoms of fibromyalgia are vague and generalized. Coexisting nerve and muscle disorders such as **rheumatoid arthritis**, spinal arthritis, or **Lyme disease** may further complicate diagnosis. There are no tests to diagnose fibromyalgia. The diagnosis is usually made after ruling out other medical conditions with similar symptoms. In 1990, the American College of Rheumatology developed standards to help diagnose fibromyalgia. According to these standards, a person is thought to have fibromyalgia if he or she has widespread pain in combination with tenderness in at least 11 of the 18 sites known as trigger points, including the base of the neck, along the backbone, in front of the hip and elbow, and at the rear of the knee and shoulder. There is no cure for fibromyalgia. The goal of treatment is to manage the symptoms through **exercise**, proper rest, and diet. A patient's clear understanding of his or her role in the recovery process is imperative for successful management. Helpful treatments include heat and occasionally cold applications, a regular stretching program, and aerobic activities which increase the heart rate. Exercise programs need to include good warm-up and cool-down sessions, with attention to avoiding exercises causing joint pain. The diet should include a variety of fruits and vegetables which provide trace elements and **minerals** necessary for healthy muscles. Adequate rest is essential and avoiding stimulating foods or drinks (such as coffee) and medications like **decongestants** before bedtime is advised. If diet, exercise, and adequate rest do not relieve the symptoms of fibromyalgia, medications such as **antidepressant drugs**, **muscle relaxants**, and anti-inflammatory drugs may be prescribed. People with fibromyalgia often need to see a rheumatologist (a doctor who specializes in disorders of the joints, muscles, and soft tissue) to decide the cause of the symptoms, to learn about fibromyalgia and its treatment, and to exclude other rheumatic diseases. Treatment programs must be individualized to each patient. **Massage** therapy and attention to mental health, including psychological consultation, may be important. Other alternative therapies include hellerwork, rolfing, **homeopathic medicine**, **Chinese traditional medicine** (both acupuncture and herbs), polarity therapy, and Western botanical medicine. Fibromyalgia is a chronic problem with symptoms that improve and worsen. There is no way to prevent fibromyalgia. Staying as healthy as possible with a good diet, safe exercise, and adequate rest is the best prevention.

Filariasis

Filiariasis is a group of tropical diseases caused by thread-like parasitic round worms (nematodes) and their larvae. The larvae transmit the disease to humans through a mosquito bite. Filariasis is characterized by **fever**, chills, **headache**, and **skin lesions** in the early stages and, if untreated, can progress to include gross enlargement of the limbs and genitalia in a condition called **elephantiasis**. Approximately 170 million people in the tropical and subtropical areas of southeast Asia, South America, Africa, and the islands of the Pacific are affected by this debilitating parasitic disease. Filariasis is occasionally found in the United States, especially among immigrants from the Caribbean and Pacific islands. While filariasis is rarely fatal, it is the second leading cause of permanent and long-term disability in the world. The **World Health Organization** (WHO) has named filariasis one of only six ''potentially eradicable'' infectious diseases. In all cases, a mosquito bites an infected individual then bites another uninfected individual, transferring some of the worm larvae to the new host. Once within the body, the larvae migrate to a particular part of the body and mature to adult worms. There are three types of filariasis: lymphatic filariasis affects the circulatory system that moves tissue fluid and immune cells (**lymphatic system**) and is the most common type, subcutaneous filariasis infects the areas beneath the skin and whites of the eye, and serous cavity filariasis infects body cavities but does not cause disease.

Lymphatic filariasis is caused by the adult worms living in the lymphatic vessels near the lymph nodes where they distort the vessels and cause local inflammation. In advanced stages, the worms can obstruct the vessels, causing the surrounding tissue to become enlarged. In Bancroftian filariasis, the legs and genitals are most often involved, while the Malayan variety affects the legs below the knees. Repeated episodes of inflammation lead to blockages of the lymphatic system, especially in the genitals and legs. This causes the affected area to become grossly enlarged, with thickened, coarse skin, leading to a condition called elephantiasis. In conjunctiva filariasis, the worms' larvae migrate to the eye and can sometimes be seen moving beneath the skin or the white part of the eye (conjunctiva). If untreated, this disease can cause blindness. Symptoms vary, but filariasis usually begins with chills, headache, and fever between three months and one year after the insect bite. There may also be swelling, redness, and **pain** in the arms, legs, or scrotum. Areas of pus (**abscess**es) may appear as a result of dying worms or a secondary bacterial infection. The disease is diagnosed by a patient history, a **physical examination**, and by screening blood specimens for proteins produced by the **immune system** in response to this infection. Early diagnosis may be difficult because, in the first stages, the disease mimics other bacterial skin infections.

Filariasis is treated with ivermectin, albendazole, or diethylcarbamazine to eliminate the larvae, impair the adult worms' ability to reproduce, and kill adult worms. Much of the tissue damage may not be reversible. The medication is started at low doses to prevent reactions caused by large numbers of dying parasites. These medications can cause severe side effects in up to 70% of patients. These side effects can be controlled with **antihistamines** and anti-inflammatory drugs (**corticosteroids**). Rarely, treatment with diethylcarbamazine may lead to a fatal inflammation of the brain (**encephalitis**). Other common drug reactions include **dizziness**, weakness, and nausea. Symptoms caused by the death of the parasites include fever, headache, muscle pain, abdominal pain, **nausea and vomiting**, weakness, dizziness, lethargy, and **asthma**. Reactions usually begin within two days of starting treatment and last between two and four days. No treatment can reverse elephantiasis. Surgery can remove surplus tissue, drain the fluid around the damaged lymphatic vessels, and ease massive enlargement of the scrotum. Elephantiasis of the legs can also be helped by elevating the legs and using elastic bandages. The outlook is good in early or mild cases, especially if the patient can avoid being infected again. The disease is rarely fatal, and with continued WHO medical intervention, even gross elephantiasis is now becoming rare. The best way to prevent filariasis is to prevent being repeatedly bitten by the mosquitoes that carry the disease by: limiting outdoor activities at night, particularly in rural or jungle areas; wearing long sleeves and pants and avoiding dark-colored clothing that attracts mosquitoes; avoiding perfumes and colognes; treating clothing ahead of time with permethrin (Duranon, Permanone); wearing

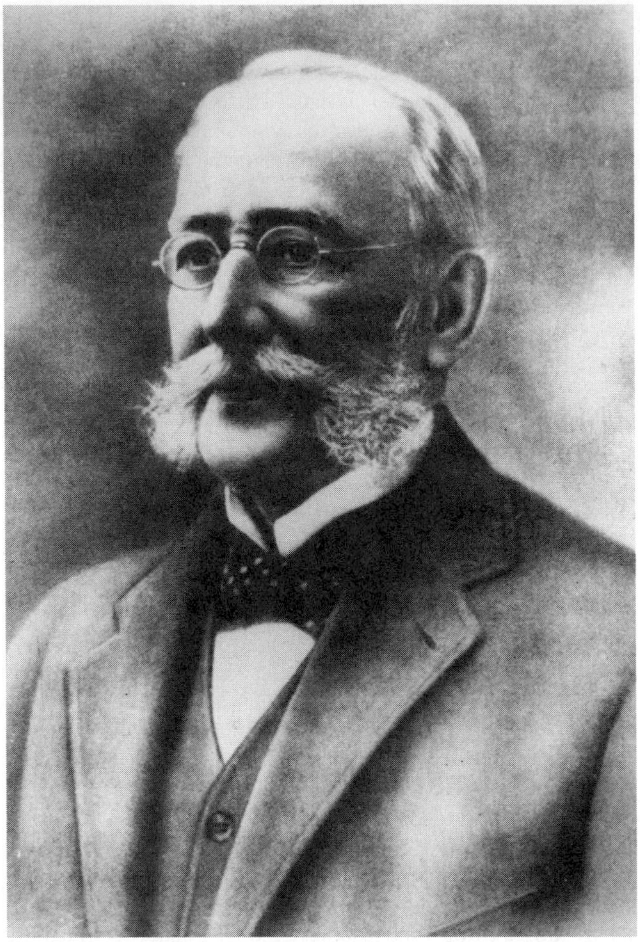

Carlos Juan Finlay

DEET insect repellent, citronella or lemon eucalyptus to repel insects; if sleeping in an open area or in a room with poor screens, use a bed net to avoid being bitten while asleep; using air conditioning; and in highly infested areas, taking ivermectin preventatively. Scientists are working on a vaccine.

FINLAY, CARLOS JUAN (1833-1915)

Cuban physician

Carlos Juan Finlay was a Cuban physician and biologist, who, in 1881, suggested that yellow fever, an acute febrile illness fatal to half its victims, was transmitted by mosquitoes. His theory, confirmed in 1900 by the American surgeon **Walter Reed**, led to widescale control of the disease. Finlay also made important contributions toward the understanding of infant **tetanus** and of **cholera**.

Carlos Juan Finlay was born in Camagüey, Cuba, on December 3, 1833. He was one of seven children born to Edward Finlay, a Scottish physician who had fought alongside Simon Bolivar, and Eliza Isabel, née deBarrés, a French woman. The family owned a large coffee plantation in Guanimar, in the Alquizar region of Cuba. Finlay spent his early childhood on this plantation and in a family home in Havana. He received his schooling from his paternal aunt, Ana, who had started a school in Edinburgh, Scotland, but had returned to Cuba to live with her brother's family. In 1844 Finlay was sent to La Havre, France, to begin his formal education. Two years later, suffering from an attack of chorea, a condition in which facial and limb muscles contract spasmodically, he returned to Cuba. After extensive therapy in his father's medical institute, he returned to Europe in 1848, intending to complete his education in France. Political turmoil across the European continent forced him to remain in England for two years. When he finally entered the lycée in Rouen, his studies were interrupted once again, this time because he had contracted **typhoid fever**. After a period of convalescence in Cuba, he attempted to enroll in a medical training program at the University of Havana. It was not possible to transfer his European credits, and the only program he could enter without prerequisite courses was in Philadelphia, at the Jefferson Medical College. His decision to study in Philadelphia was to have a major impact on his future career, for it was here that he met and befriended the family of John Kearsly Mitchell. Mitchell was an outspoken proponent of the **Germ Theory** of disease, which held that illness was caused by micro-organisms. He and his son S. Weir Mitchell were professors at Jefferson Medical College. The younger Mitchell directed Finlay's studies for three years, and was to become a lifelong friend. Finlay received his medical degree on March 10, 1855.

Although Mitchell attempted to convince Finlay to remain in America and set up a practice for the Spanish community in New York City, Finlay decided to return to Havana and work alongside his father. Together they made several trips to South America, treating a wide diversity of patients. It is likely that while on these trips, the younger Finlay encountered many victims of yellow fever. The disease was also endemic in the Caribbean. In 1857, after obtaining certification in Cuba, he set up a practice in ophthalmology. From 1860 to 1861, he went to Paris for additional clinical study. In 1865 Finlay married Adela Shine, from the island of Trinidad. Together they had three sons, Charles, George and Frank. The family was regarded highly in Cuban society and Finlay distinguished himself as a dedicated and caring physician. In the 1860s and 1870s there were frequent outbreaks of **yellow fever**, and Finlay observed that the disease seemed to be transmitted from one person to another. He postulated that the agent of transmission was the mosquito. In 1881 he was invited to speak before the International Sanitary Conference in Washington DC, as a representative of the Cuban colonial government. European scientists had begun to identify the infectious agents of several other illnesses and Germ Theory had now gained hold. Finlay's notion that yellow fever could be transmitted to humans by mosquitoes was well received.

In June of 1881 Finlay began a series of experiments to test his theories. He bred *Aedes aegypti* mosquitoes in captivity, and allowed them to feed on blood drawn from victims of yellow fever during the early stage of their illness. He then transported the mosquitoes to human volunteers, who were bitten by the insects. His goal was to see if he could induce a mild form of yellow fever that could confer immunity on the volunteers. In 1888, when the Spanish American War broke out, Finlay offered his services to the United States government. He befriended the director of military health, who sent him to work with American troops in Santiago de Cuba. He continued his experimentation, using soldiers as subjects, and by 1898 had collected a wealth of data which he presented to the military officials. It is unlikely, in light of what is now known about the length of incubation of yellow fever in the *Aedes aegypti* mosquito, that many of Finlay's early human experiments were successful. Nonetheless, his research laid the foundation for the success of others. In 1900, when Walter Reed (1851-1902), a major in the United States Army Medical Corps, began the definitive studies of yellow fever transmission, Finlay supplied him with the mosquitoes he had bred.

The pioneering studies that Finlay conducted and Reed was to successfully complete led to the eventual control of yellow fever around the world. In 1902, the government of Cuba honored Finlay by naming him the Chief of Health of the Republic and the President of the Superior Commission of Health. Finlay began, the next year, to tackle a new medical problem. Alarmed at the high rate of infant mortality from tetanus, he examined the pieces of cotton cording traditionally used for tying the umbilicus at birth. Finding them to be a nest for tetanus bacteria, he implemented a new sterile process. The mortality from tetanus was cut in half almost immediately. Finlay went on to make advances in the study of filarial illnesses and cholera. He was a prolific writer on the topics of **pathology** and therapeutics. As a hobby, he spent time deciphering antique Latin manuscripts, and enjoyed playing chess. In his seventies he began a study of immunology. Finlay died in 1915, at the age of eighty two.

FINSEN LIGHT

The finsen light, named for its inventor, Niels Tyberg Finsen, was a powerful light used to cure people of a skin disorder. Niels Finsen was born in 1860 in the Faroe Islands, Danish islands in the North Atlantic Ocean. His parents were of Icelandic origin, so young Niels spent his early schooling in the capital of Iceland. He was a frail and sickly youth. Living so close to the Arctic Circle where the days are short in winter, Niels became aware of the effects of sunlight on his disposition and health. Later Finsen went to Denmark to study for his medical degree at the University of Copenhagen. While at the university he was incorrectly diagnosed as having heart disease, but actually he suffered from Pick's disease, a condition that affects the liver and the lining around the heart. (He later developed ascites, fluid accumulation in the abdominal cavity, and was confined to a wheelchair.) After receiving his medical degree in 1891, Finsen became very interested in how light affects disease as he himself found a benefit from exposure to sunlight. He was familiar with the work of a Swedish researcher who in 1889 had discovered that ultraviolet light (short waves) irritates biological tissue more than infrared light (longer waves such as heat waves). So Finsen began recording the effects of sunlight on insects and amphibians, becoming ever convinced that light could be used to treat human disease. He found that ultraviolet light from the sun or from electric lights could kill bacteria. Finsen was convinced that it was the effect of the light and not the heat it caused and wrote several papers in 1893 and 1894 on the beneficial use of phototherapy. He also thought that red light was helpful in curing **smallpox** but this idea was later abandoned. In 1895 Finsen made an arrangement with Copenhagen Electric Light Works to treat patients two hours each day with ultraviolet light. His patients were diagnosed with lupus vulgaris, a skin disease associated with the **tuberculosis** bacteria. He designed a powerful lamp (the finsen light) for this purpose, a bright artificial light generated by electrical carbon arcs. In 1896 Finsen founded the Finsen Institute for Phototherapy in Copenhagen dedicated to studying effects of light and curing people of disease. At the Institute 800 lupus patients were treated. Half were cured of the disease and nearly the rest showed improvement in their conditions. For this achievement he was awarded the 1903 Nobel Prize in medicine and physiology. Finsen donated half the prize money to the Institute. In failing health, he died the next year at only 43 years old. During Finsen's era both X rays and gamma rays were discovered by **Wilhelm Röntgen** (1845-1923) and **Antoine-Henri Becquerel** (1852-1908) respectively. With Finsen's success with light therapy leading the way, the idea of radiotherapy was born. Since his time, X rays and gamma rays have been used for the diagnoses and treatment of disease. Even today some foods are irradiated with UV light to kill bacteria (although this practice is sometimes controversial). Finsen was also ahead of his time in his concept of the effect of sunlight on disposition and health. In is only fairly recently that **Seasonal Affective Disorder** (SAD) has been recognized as a type of depression caused by a lack of sunlight in winter. People diagnosed with SAD can be treated by sitting under lights to extend exposure to light on short days.

FIRST AID

At the outset of a serious illness or when an injury has been sustained, there are signs and symptoms that can be recognized and a first aid procedure initiated to prevent complications, pain, or discomfort. The ability of individuals who first render care to remain calm and respond appropriately can make a significant difference in the outcome for the victim.

First aid courses or training in **cardiopulmonary resuscitation** are offered by many local fire companies and organizations, such as the American Heart Association and the American Red Cross. Initial priorities can be remembered as A-B-C, that is, opening the Airway, then assessing Breathing and Circulation. Efforts should be made to stop any heavy bleeding by applying pressure to the affected area. If the injured individual is conscious, they should be reassured and made as comfortable as possible. Efforts should be made to prevent further injury, keeping in mind that anyone who has lost consciousness or complains or neck or back pain should not be moved. If you are in doubt about the appropriate action, call for help.

First aid supplies should be kept readily available and replenished promptly after use. In addition to being kept in a designated place in the home and the car, first aid supplies should be carried by campers, hikers, and bikers. A waterproof first aid kit should also be kept on all boats. Although preassembled first aid kits are widely available, items to be kept on hand should include: tweezers, elastic bandages, medical tape, fever thermometer, precut triangular bandages for slings or splints, safety pins, scissors, tongue depressors, antiseptic spray or cream, **antidiarrheal drugs**, **antihistamine drugs**, and assorted **bandages and dressings**. In the car or a boat, additional first aid supplies should include: flares, a clean folded sheet, a flashlight with extra batteries, a folded lightweight blanket, a large waterproof cover (tarp), and a tightly capped plastic bottle of water.

Individuals with special medical conditions or serious allergies should wear a Medic-Alert bracelet or necklace. For information on how to obtain one, call collect in the U. S.: (209)634-4917. Individuals who are hypersensitive to bee or insect stings should have special kit containing adrenaline, an antihistamine, and a hypodermic needle. These insect sting kits must be prescribed by and used under the direction of a physician.

See also Accidents; Bandages and dressings; Choking; Electric shock injuries; Frostbite and frostnip; Head injury; Immobilization; Near drowning; Smoke inhalation; Sports injuries; Traumatic amputations

FISCHER, EMIL HERMANN (1852-1919)

German chemist

The son of a successful businessman, Emil Fischer, at the urging of his father, reluctantly joined the family firm when he left high school. But the young man yearned to be a mathematician or physicist and, after a few years, his father gave in and allowed him to attend the University of Bonn. A year later, in 1872, Fischer transferred to Strasbourg to study with the well-known chemist, Adolf von Baeyer, and decided to make organic chemistry his career.

After earning his doctorate in 1874 Fischer followed Baeyer to Munich, Germany to continue his studies which, at that time, centered around the organic derivatives of hydrazine (a compound of nitrogen and hydrogen). Many of his hydrazine derivatives later proved highly useful to Germany's dye industry, then in its infancy. More importantly, Fischer discovered that his compounds—phenylhydrazine, in particular—reacted chemically with carbohydrates in such a way that they could be used to separate and identify sugars that, until then, were almost impossible to isolate.

In 1882, Fischer joined the faculty of the University of Erlangen, then moved to Würzburg in 1885. There, he attracted worldwide attention through his continued work with carbohydrates. Using phenylhydrazine as a chemical tool, Fischer was able to isolate a number of pure sugars and to study their structures. He synthesized glucose (the most important simple sugar) and 30 other sugars as well. In addition, Fischer began to study the three-dimensional shape (stereochemistry) of these sugars and showed that the shapes of the best-known sugar molecules (and perhaps, by extension, the shapes of other classes of molecules) played a greater role in their biochemical activity than their chemical compositions.

Also during the 1880s, Fischer began a study of uric acid and its derivatives. This resulted in the synthesis of a number of important compounds, including the alkaloids caffeine and theobromine. In 1897, Fischer suggested that uric acid and similar substances—substances that were often found in natural products such as urine and feces—might all be derived from a hypothetical parent compound he named purine. A year later, he went on to synthesize purine itself—and, by so doing, opened up a whole new field of research, that of purine chemistry. (Interestingly, purines proved to be part of a group of substances called the nucleic acids, today considered the key compound of living tissues.)

For his work with carbohydrates and purines, Fischer received the Nobel Prize in chemistry in 1902. By then, however, he had already moved on to an investigation into the highly complex, chain-like molecules of proteins. After synthesizing many of the 13 amino acids known, at the time, to be the "building blocks" of protein, Fischer then identified three more amino acids and went on to describe the various ways amino acids combined with each other inside protein molecules. (In general, the amino group of one amino acid becomes tied to the acidic carboxyl group of a second amino acid by a peptide bond.) Moreover, Fisher developed a method for artificially linking amino acids together and, by 1907, succeeded in forming a remarkably authentic polypeptide made up of 18 amino acid units.

In 1903, Fischer also synthesized 5,5-diethylbarbituric acid—the first **barbiturate**. Barbituric acid, a hypnotic and sedative, found use in the treatment of **insomnia** and **anxiety**. Its modern derivatives include the prescription drugs Barbital, Veronal, and Dorminal.

Although he had become one of the world's best-known and most widely respected scientists, Fisher's last years were marked by tragedy. Suffering from **cancer**, exhausted by the work he did for the German government during World War I, and deeply depressed by the loss of two of his three sons to that war, Fischer took his own life in 1919.

FISH AND SHELLFISH POISONING

Fish and shellfish poisoning is a common but often unrecognized group of illnesses related to food which includes ciguatera, scombroid, and paralytic shellfish poisoning. Ciguatera is a food-related illness that causes abdominal and neurological symptoms. It is caused by eating fish that have a toxin called ciguatoxin, usually red snapper, grouper, and barracuda. Ciguatera is common on many of the islands in the Pacific Ocean. Most cases occur one to six hours after eating the contaminated fish. Initial symptoms are abdominal cramps, **nausea**, vomiting, or watery **diarrhea**. The most common symptoms involve the **nervous system** and include numbness and tingling around the lips, tongue, and mouth; **itching**; dry mouth; metallic taste in the mouth; and blurry vision. In more prominent cases, patients may complain of temporary blindness, a slow pulse, and a feeling of loose teeth. Patients may also have the strange symptom of reversal of hot and cold skin sensations. In very severe cases, there may be breathing difficulties or low blood pressure. Ciguatera is diagnosed by the symptoms after eating fish. There are no tests to detect the poisoning in people, but researchers have developed a test for the toxin left on remaining fish. The treatment for this illness is fluids (by mouth or through a vein) and medications to decrease the itching or to treat vomiting and/or diarrhea. Neurological symptoms may be treated with amitriptyline and other medications. Although **death** can occur, most patients with ciguatera recover. Recovery can be slow and some symptoms can last for weeks or months. Knowing the kinds of fish linked to ciguatera can help a person avoid eating high-risk fish.

Scombroid is a fish-associated illness caused by eating improperly refrigerated fish. Fish linked to this disease include yellowfin tuna, skipjack, bonito, and mackerel. Bacteria that are normally found in fish act directly on a chemical (called histidine) in the flesh of fish that are not properly cooled when stored, producing histamine and other chemicals that cause the illness when the fish is eaten. Symptoms occur as soon as 10 minutes after eating the fish, and can be confused with a fish allergy. Scombroid causes flushing of the face, sweating, a burning feeling in the mouth or throat, vomiting, diarrhea, and **headaches**. A rash that looks like a **sunburn** may occur, and a small number of patients have **hives**. Some patients have a metallic or peppery taste in their mouths. In more severe cases, rapid pulse, blurred vision, and difficulty breathing can occur. Symptoms usually last about four hours. Scombroid poisoning is diagnosed on symptoms occurring after eating fish. There are usually no tests to detect it. Experimentally, however, elevated levels of histamine-related products have been found in the urine. It may be possible to test remaining fish flesh for histamine levels. Scombroid goes away on its own, but **Antihistamines** like diphenhydramine (Benadryl) shorten its duration. Some doctors have found that cimetidine (Tagamet) given through a vein may also be helpful. In rare, more severe cases, epinephrine (adrenaline) may be used. Sombroid is usually not serious. Adequate storage of the target fish prevents scombroid. Since the fish does not appear spoiled or smell bad, the consumer cannot detect the risk before eating it.

Paralytic shellfish poisoning (PSP) is a nervous system disease caused by eating cooked or raw shellfish that contain environmental toxins. These toxins are produced by a group of algae (dinoflagellates). It is unclear whether these toxins are related to the ''blooming'' of the algae, also called red tide. PSP occurs mostly in May through November. PSP develops usually within minutes after eating a contaminated shellfish, most commonly a mussel, clam, or oyster. Symptoms include headache, a floating feeling, **dizziness**, lack of coordination, and tingling of the mouth, arms, or legs. Symptoms include muscle weakness causing difficulty swallowing or speaking, difficulty breathing related to weakness or **paralysis** of the breathing muscle, nausea, vomiting, and diarrhea. The symptoms last 6–12 hours, but a patient may feel weak for a week or more. PSP diagnosis is based on symptoms after eating shellfish. No diagnostic test is available, but tests in mice to detect the toxin from the eaten fish can be done. PSP can have a serious outcome. If early symptoms of PSP are recognized, the doctor will try to flush the toxin from the gastrointestinal tract with medications that create diarrhea. Vomiting may be induced if the patient is not weak. In severe cases, the patient may be placed on a respirator or a machine to clean the blood (dialysis). The prognosis is quite good, especially if the patient passes the first 12 hours, when most deaths occur, without needing breathing support. Controlling PSP requires detecting rising numbers of algae in coastal waters by microscopic examination. By law, shellfish beds are closed when levels of the toxin-producing organisms are above acceptable standards.

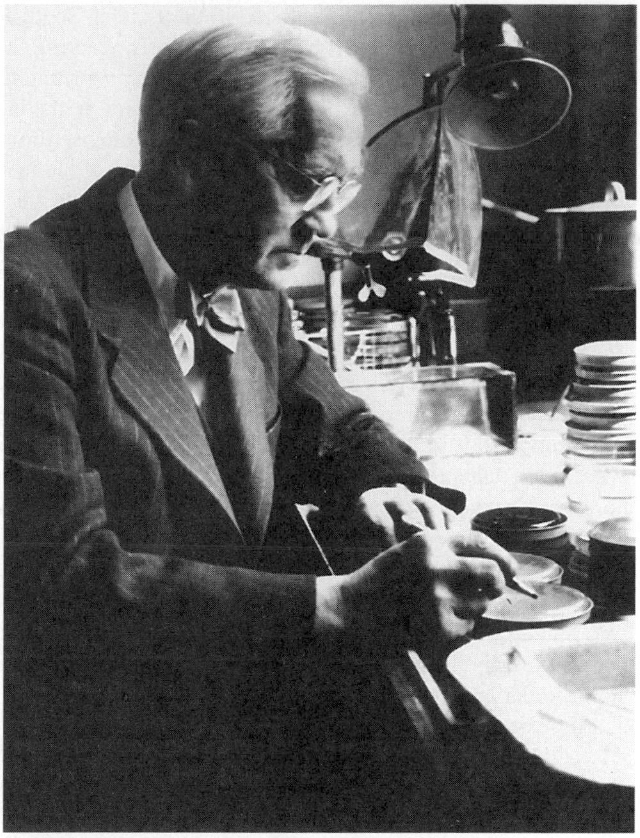

Alexander Fleming

FLEMING, ALEXANDER (1881-1955)

Scottish bacteriologist

With the experienced eye of a scientist, Alexander Fleming turned what appeared to be a spoiled experiment into the discovery of the first of the ''wonder drugs,'' **penicillin**.

Fleming was born on August 6, 1881, to a farming family in Lochfield, Scotland. Following school, he worked as a shipping clerk in London and enlisted in the London Scottish Regiment. In 1901, he began his medical career, entering St. Mary's Hospital Medical School, where he was a prizewinning student. After graduation in 1906, he began working at that institution with Sir Almroth Edward Wright, a pathologist. From the start, Fleming was innovative and became one of the first to use **Paul Ehrlich**'s arsenical compound, Salvarsan, to treat **syphilis** in Great Britain.

Wright and Fleming joined the Royal Army Medical Corps during World War I. They studied wounds and infection-causing bacteria at a hospital in Boulogne, France. At that time, **antiseptics** were used to treat bacterial infections, but Wright and Fleming showed that, especially in deep **wounds**, bacteria survive treatment by antiseptics while the protective white blood cells in the wound are destroyed. This creates an even worse situation in which infection can spread rapidly. Forever affected by the suffering he saw during the war, Fleming decided to focus his efforts on the search for safe antibacterial substances. He studied the antibacterial power of the body's own leukocytes contained in pus. In 1921, he discovered that a sample of his own nasal mucus destroyed bacteria in a petri dish. He isolated the compound responsible for the antibacterial action, which he called lysozyme, in saliva, blood, tears, pus, milk, and egg whites.

Fleming made his greatest discovery in 1928. While he was growing cultures of bacteria in petri dishes for experiments, he accidentally left certain dishes uncovered for several days. Fleming found a mold growing in the dishes and began to discard them, when he noticed, to his astonishment, that bacteria near the molds were being destroyed. He preserved the mold—a strain of Penicillium—and made a culture of it in a test tube for further investigation. He deduced an antibacterial compound was being produced by the mold, and named it penicillin. Through further study, Fleming found that penicillin was nontoxic in laboratory animals. He described his findings in research journals but was unable to purify and concentrate the substance. Little did he realize that the substance produced by his mold would save millions of lives during the twentieth century.

Fleming dropped his investigation of penicillin and his discovery remained unnoticed until 1940. It was then that Oxford University-based bacteriologists **Howard Florey** and **Ernst Chain** stumbled upon a paper by Fleming while researching antibacterial agents. They had better fortune than Fleming, for they were able to purify penicillin and test it on humans with outstanding results. During World War II, the drug was rushed into mass-production in England and the United States and saved thousands of injured soldiers from infections that would otherwise have been fatal.

Accolades began pouring in for Fleming. He was elected to fellowship in the Royal Society in 1943, knighted in 1944, and shared the Nobel Prize in Physiology or Medicine with Florey and Chain in 1945. Fleming continued working at St. Mary's Hospital until 1948, when he moved to the Wright-Fleming Institute. He died in London on March 11, 1955.

FLESH-EATING DISEASE

Flesh-eating disease is more properly called necrotizing fasciitis, a rare, sometimes fatal condition in which bacteria destroy tissues underlying the skin. This tissue death, called necrosis or **gangrene**, spreads rapidly. Flesh-eating disease is an infection that appears to devour body tissue. Media reports increased in the mid-1990s, but the disease was described by **Hippocrates** more than 3,000 years ago and reported during the Civil War. There are two types of flesh-eating disease: Type I, which is caused by anaerobic bacteria, with or without the presence of aerobic bacteria; and Type II, also called hemolytic streptococcal gangrene, which is caused by group A streptococci and may include other bacteria. It may also be called synergistic gangrene. Flesh-eating disease most often affects arms and legs, but can appear anywhere. In nearly every case, a skin injury precedes the disease. As bacteria grow beneath the skin's surface, they produce toxins which destroy superficial fascia, subcutaneous fat, and deep fascia. In some cases, the dermis and the underlying muscle are also affected. Initially, the infected area appears red and swollen, and feels hot and painful. Over the course of hours or days, the skin may become blue-gray, fluid-filled blisters may form, and the area becomes numb. An individual may go into **shock** and develop dangerously low blood pressure. Multiple organ failure may occur, quickly followed by death.

The appearance of the skin, paired with pain and **fever**, raises the possibility of flesh-eating disease. An x ray, **magnetic resonance imaging** (MRI), or **computed tomography scans** (CT scans) of the area reveals a feathery pattern in the tissue, caused by gas in the dying tissue. Necrosis is seen during surgery to collect samples to identify the bacteria. Rapid, aggressive medical treatment, specifically, antibiotic therapy and surgical **debridement**, is critical. **Antibiotics** include a penicillin, an aminoglycoside or third-generation cephalosporin, and clindamycin or metronidazole. **Analgesics** are used to control pain. During surgical debridement, dead tissue is stripped away. After surgery, patients are rigorously monitored for continued infection, shock, or other complications. If available, hyperbaric **oxygen therapy** can also be used. Flesh-eating disease has a fatality rate of about 30%. **Diabetes**, arteriosclerosis, immunosuppression, kidney disease, **malnutrition**, and **obesity** are connected with a poor prognosis. Older individuals and intravenous drug users may also be at higher risk. The infection site also has a role. Survivors may require **plastic surgery** and may have permanent physical disability. Flesh-eating disease cannot be prevented.

FLEXNER, SIMON (1863-1946)

American pathologist and bacteriologist

Simon Flexner pioneered in field investigations where infectious diseases were potentially **epidemic**. He discovered the Flexner bacillus, the cause of a common form of dysentery, and the Flexner serum for treating **meningitis**. His research expertise was already legend when he was selected as the organizing director of the Rockefeller Institute for Medical Research in New York City. For thirty-five years he cultivated the spirit and guided the work of the new institute, while implementing John D. Rockefeller's vision of bringing medicine into the realm of science.

Flexner, the fourth of nine children, was born in Louisville, Kentucky, on March 25, 1863, to Jewish immigrants. His father, Morris, emigrated from Bavaria, first to Strasbourg, France, where he taught school, then eventually to Louisville. He became a peddler and eventually a wholesale merchant of dry goods. Flexner's mother, Esther Abraham, grew up in Alsace and was a dressmaker in Paris before immigrating with her sister to live with relatives in Louisville.

When Morris Flexner's business failed in 1873, the future of his nine children seemed bleak. Young Simon failed to finish sixth grade and his delinquent behavior prompted his father to arrange a tour of the town jail, where, he warned, Simon might end up if he did not change his ways. Young Flexner drifted from one menial job to another until he fell victim to **typhoid fever** at the age of sixteen. But his near-fatal illness transformed him into a self-directed student of science. He began work as a drugstore apprentice while he earned a degree and a medal for excellence at the Louisville College of Pharmacy.

Flexner then taught himself to use a microscope while tending to prescriptions in his brother Jacob's pharmacy. Without books or teachers, he mastered the basics of histology and pathology as he examined tissue specimens given to him by doctors who patronized the store. Flexner found his calling when he realized that his observations on patients' tissues could aid physicians in their diagnoses of diseases. So, at 26, Flexner earned his medical degree at the University of Louisville, a two-year medical school, although this rudimentary education provided no opportunities to perform either physical examinations or laboratory studies. A year later, after publishing two papers based on his microscopic observations, Flexner was sent to Johns Hopkins University by his younger brother Abraham, a recent graduate of the school.

In Baltimore, Flexner joined other young physicians studying **pathology** under William Henry Welch, a chief architect of scientific medicine in the United States. During the next thirteen years Flexner studied many pathological problems, advancing from Welch's personal assistant to full professor. He became familiar with a wide range of infectious diseases and left behind a harvest of original reports.

In 1893, Johns Hopkins, at the behest of the Maryland Board of Health, sent Flexner to diagnose an epidemic of cerebrospinal meningitis raging among Cumberland coal miners. Tracking the dying men to their cabins on precipitous hillsides to conduct autopsies and collect tissues samples, Flexner quickly determined that the disease was caused by a diplococcus bacteria. In another case, he led an 1899 commission from Johns Hopkins to study the diseases in the Philippines just after the Spanish-American War. While learning about epidemics of typhoid fever, **malaria**, dengue, **leprosy**, and **tuberculosis**, Flexner made a thorough investigation of dysentery. He succeeded in isolating the bacillus that causes a prevalent form of the disease, an organism now known as the Flexner bacillus. Upon his return to the States, he became professor of Pathology at the University of Pennsylvania. Two years later, the federal government sent Flexner to investigate an epidemic in San Francisco's Chinatown and, within a month, he had confirmed original suspicions that the disease was bubonic **plague**.

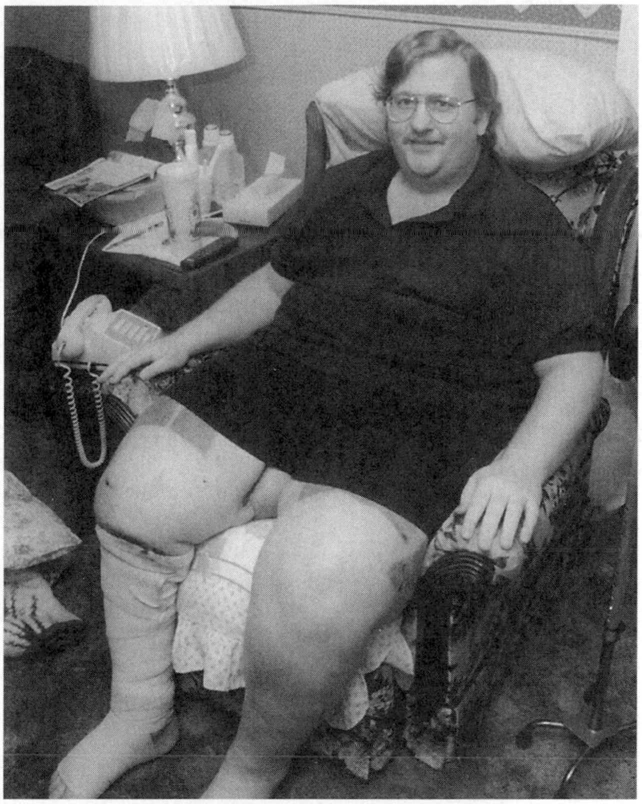

This man survived a bout with a rare, flesh-eating strep bacteria. The patches on his thighs are where physicians removed healthy skin and grafted it to his calves. ***(Photograph by Terry Duennes, AP/Wide World Photo. Reproduced by permission.)***

At the turn of the century, no medical research centers existed in the United States comparable to the **Pasteur**, **Koch**, **Pavlov**, and Kitasato institutes of Europe and Japan. Most American laboratories were only for instructing students and were primitively equipped. A pioneering effort to correct this situation came in 1901 with the founding of the Rockefeller Institute for Medical Research, created through an endowment by John D. Rockefeller. A year later, its board, headed by William Welch, chose Flexner to head the new institute, one devoted to investigations into human disease. He relinquished his professorship in Pennsylvania to pursue that for which there was no assurance of permanence or success.

For over thirty years, Flexner gave the Institute its unique scientific direction. His special genius resided in his respect for individuality and his understanding of the scientific temperament. Although his career had been concerned with pathology of infectious diseases, he established a broad scientific scope and pressed for the application of biochemistry and the physical sciences to studies of human biology.

Flexner brought together a distinguished group of scientists, including Hideyo Noguchi, his protegee from Pennsylvania, S. J. Meltzer, Phoebus Aaron Theodor Levene, **Alexis Carrel**, Jacques Loeb, **Karl Landsteiner**, Eugene Opie, Rufus Cole, and **Peyton Rous**. Attracted by the promise of unlimited experimental freedom and the finest available laboratory equipment, plus an independent endowment from Rockefeller to finance their work, these researchers came from all over the world. John D. Rockefeller's experiment in scientific philanthropy, under Flexner's leadership, created one of the world's greatest biomedical research institutions.

In 1906, soon after the institute's laboratories opened, an epidemic of cerebrospinal meningitis enveloped New York City. Flexner quickly furthered the institute's new mission by developing an antimeningococcus serum from the blood of inoculated horses. Injected directly into the spinal canal of the victims, the serum reduced fatalities by fifty percent. Flexner continued to supervise the manufacture of thousands of bottles a year, and the Flexner serum remained the best therapy for meningitis until the emergence of sulfa drugs in the 1930s. Four years later, poliomyelitis was epidemic in New York. Flexner and his assistants proved its viral origins and postulated one mode of transmission, but they found no cure. However, because Flexner showed how to transfer the virus from one monkey to another, he enabled scientists in the 1950s to maintain a pool of the virus for use in successful **polio** vaccines.

In 1903, Flexner married Helen Whitall Thomas, author of the autobiographical memoir *Quaker Childhood.* Her father, a physician and leading aristocrat in Baltimore, was instrumental in the founding of both Johns Hopkins Medical School and Bryn Mawr College. Helen, whose older sister was president of Bryn Mawr, was teaching English there when she first met Simon Flexner. Their first year of marriage was spent in Europe, where Flexner scouted for scientists to recruit to the Rockefeller Institute, and studied biochemistry in the Berlin laboratory of Emil Fischer. The Flexners had two sons, William Welch, a physicist, and James Thomas, an author of American history, biography, and art. Two of Flexner's own brothers were noted intellectuals. Bernard was a well known lawyer, and Abraham, author of the 1910 report that reformed American medical education, was director of the Institute for Advanced Study at Princeton.

Although Rockefeller Institute's welfare was uppermost in his mind, Flexner undertook other activities on behalf of medical education, research, and public health. A charter trustee of the Rockefeller Foundation, he contributed to the establishment of National Research Council fellowships and to the founding of the Peking Union Medical College. When Welch relinquished all interest in *The Journal of Experimental Medicine* in 1902, Flexner moved it to the Rockefeller, where he served as editor from 1905 until his death in 1946.

Still at the height of his powers, Flexner relinquished his duties as director in 1935 and spent ten good years in retirement. As Eastman Professor at Oxford University in 1937, he wrote *The Evolution and Organization of the University Clinic*. Later, he and his son James wrote a biography of William Welch, chronicling the history of medical science in America. During his long career, Flexner published several hundred scientific papers and essays. His contributions were rewarded with honorary degrees from eighteen universities and membership in numerous scientific societies. He was elected a member of the National Academy of Sciences (1908), the American Philosophical Society (1901), and the Royal Society of London (1919). On his eightieth birthday, an editorial in *The New York Times* called Flexner a guiding genius of American medical science, noting that ''a man of this scientific caliber belongs to the world.'' He died three years later on May 2, 1946, in New York City, of a coronary occlusion following an operation.

FLOREY, HOWARD WALTER (1898-1968)

Australian biochemist

Born in Adelaide, Australia, Florey became a leading researcher of the disease process. With colleague **Ernst Chain**, he isolated **penicillin**, making possible its wide production and use in treating bacterial diseases.

The son of a boot maker, Florey showed no interest in learning the family business. Instead, his natural curiosity and scholastic ability led him to pursue medical research. Florey attended the University of Adelaide, and after earning his medical degree in 1921, he received a Rhodes Scholarship to study at Oxford University. He also studied at Cambridge University and in the United States as a Rockefeller Foundation traveling fellow before returning to Oxford to earn his Ph.D. in **pathology** and biochemistry.

Florey had been interested in antibacterial agents for years, and in 1930 he began studying a natural antibacterial substance called lysozyme which had been discovered by **Alexander Fleming** almost a decade earlier. Florey was the first to purify it and determine how it acted. This line of study was to lead to his best-known achievement.

After four years as professor at the University of Sheffield, Florey was appointed professor of pathology at Oxford in 1935. He consulted chemist **Frederick Gowland Hopkins** regarding a suitable person to lead the biochemistry work at Oxford. Hopkins recommended Chain. Beginning in 1938, Florey and Chain began to study antibacterial agents found in bacteria and molds. They decided first to study penicillin, described (but never isolated) by Fleming almost a decade earlier. By 1941, the two had produced concentrated penicillin and shown that it could successfully treat bacterial infections in laboratory animals without toxic effects. Florey and Chain began clinical trials on nine humans, all with dramatically successful results. The mass bloodshed of World War II created a desperate need for medications that could bring relief to thousands of victims of injury and sickness, so efforts to produce penicillin in large quantities were begun. Florey went to the United States to encourage production of the drug. He even traveled to battlefields to investigate the effectiveness of penicillin on wounded soldiers. Soon the drug was in common use.

After the war, Florey continued antibiotic research and later concentrated on experimental pathology. He also contributed research on the biology of mucus secretions, **electron** microscopy, and circulatory and pulmonary illnesses. Florey remained at Oxford as a professor of pathology until 1962, when he became provost of Queen's College, Oxford, and served as president of the Royal Society from 1960 to 1965. For his work with penicillin, Florey shared the 1945 Nobel Prize in Medicine with Fleming and Chain. Florey was knighted in 1944 and in 1965 was named Baron Florey of Adelaide.

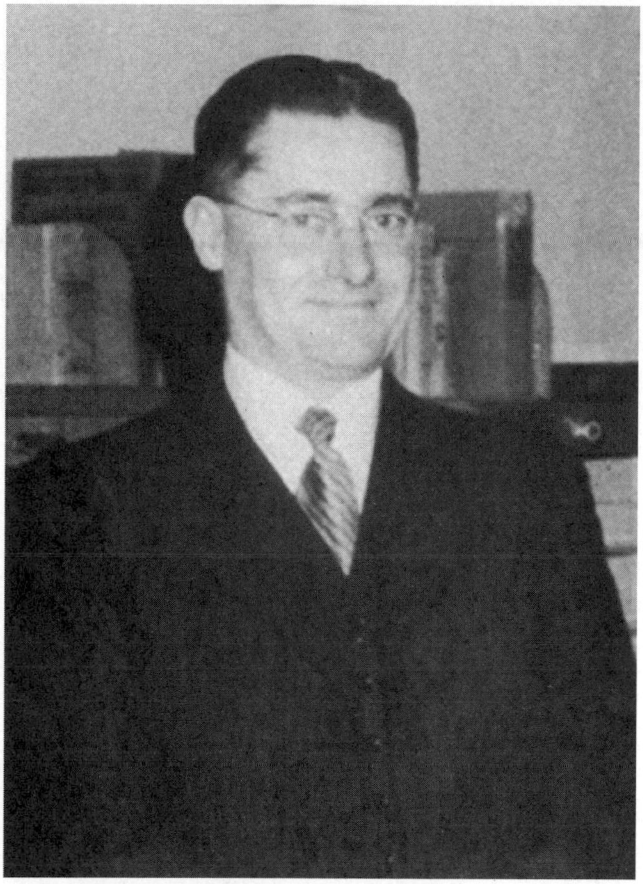
Howard Walter Florey

FLUKE INFECTIONS

Fluke infections are diseases of the digestive tract and other organ systems caused by parasitic flatworms (Trematodes) that involve hosts other than human beings. Trematode comes from a Greek word that means having holes and refers to the external suckers that adult flukes use to draw nourishment from their hosts. Fluke infections are contracted by eating uncooked fish, plants, or animals from fluke-infected waters. In humans, there are liver and lung flukes. Diseases caused by liver flukes include fascioliasis, opisthorchiasis, and clonorchiasis. Cases of liver fluke infection have been reported in Europe, the United States, the Middle East, China, Japan, and Africa. Diseases caused by lung flukes include paragonimiasis, a common infection in the Far East, Southeast Asia, Africa, Central and South America, Indonesia, and the Pacific Islands. It is estimated that between 40 million and 100 million people worldwide suffer from either liver or lung fluke infections. Liver and lung flukes enter through the mouth and can infect anyone. The symptoms differ according to the type of fluke involved but always include: Most people don't develop symptoms; the early symptoms are not unique to these diseases alone; infection does not confer immunity against re-infection by the same or other species of flukes; and infection is usually associated with eating uncooked fish, plants, or animals that live in fresh water.

Fascioliasis is caused by *Fasciola hepatica*, the sheep liver fluke. Humans become infected when they eat watercress, water chestnuts, or other plants covered with the encysted metacercariae. The metacercariae enter the liver, where they inflame and destroy tissue. After 10–15 weeks in the liver, the adult flukes move to the bile ducts and produce eggs. Acute fascioliasis is marked by abdominal **pain** with **headache**, loss of appetite, **anemia**, and vomiting. Some patients develop **hives**, muscle pains, or a yellow color to the skin and whites of the eyes (**jaundice**). Chronic disease may produce complications, including blockage of the bile ducts or the migration of adult flukes to other body parts.

Opisthorchiasis and clonorchiasis are caused by *Clonorchis sinensis*, the Chinese liver fluke, *Opisthorchis viverrini* or *O. felineus* and affect more than 20 million people in Japan, China, Southeast Asia, and India. The symptoms of opisthorchiasis and clonorchiasis are similar to those of fascioliasis and include acute and chronic forms. In acute infection, the patient may be tired, have a low-grade **fever**, pains in the joints, a swollen liver, abdominal pain, and a skin rash. The acute syndrome may be difficult to diagnose because the fluke eggs don't appear in the patient's stool for three to four weeks. Patients with chronic disease experience a loss of appetite, fatigue, low-grade fever, **diarrhea**, and an enlarged liver that feels sore when the abdomen is pressed.

Paragonimiasis is caused by a lung fluke, either *Paragonimus westermani* or *P. skrjabini*. These flukes are larger than liver flukes and also infect meat- or fish-eating animals. In humans, the metacercariae migrate to the lungs or the brain in 1% of cases. In the lungs, the flukes lay their eggs and form areas of inflammation covered with a thin layer of fibrous tissue. These areas may eventually rupture, causing the patient to **cough** up fluke eggs, blood, and inflamed tissue. It takes about six weeks for the eggs to appear. Patients with lung infections may have chest pain, fever, and rust-colored or bloody sputum. Lung infections can lead to lung **abscess**, **pneumonia**, or **bronchitis**. Patients with fluke infections of the brain may experience **seizures** or a fatal inflammation of brain tissue called **encephalitis**. Some patients also develop diarrhea and abdominal pain or lumps under the skin.

Diagnosis of fluke infections is based on the patient's history and identification of the fluke's eggs or adult forms. In the United States, stool specimens or body fluid samples may

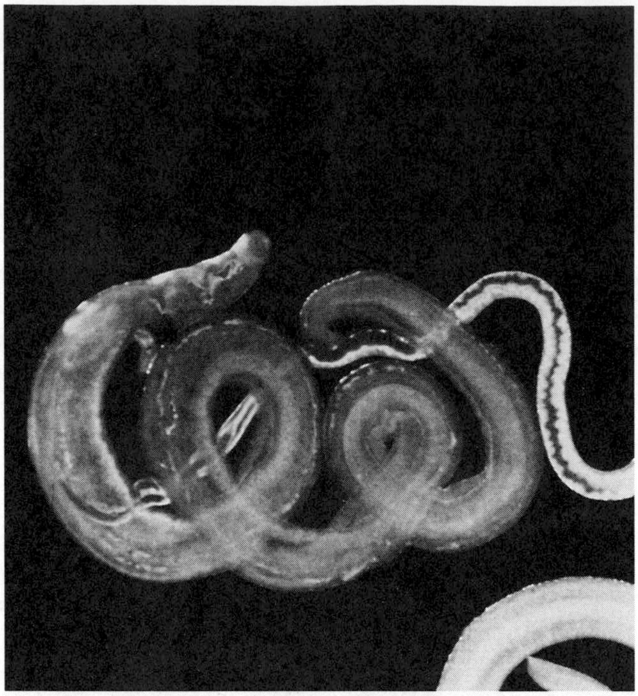

A micrograph of adult intestinal blood flukes, *Schistosoma mansoni*. Humans can become infected while bathing or working in contaminated water. *(Photo Researchers, Inc. Reproduced by permission.)*

be sent to a laboratory with experts in unusual diseases to identify the parasite. In some cases, adult flukes are found in the patient's stools, vomit, sputum, or skin lumps (for lung flukes). In lung flukes, it's important to rule out **tuberculosis** through a tuberculosis skin test and a **chest x ray**. Blood tests may be somewhat useful in diagnosing fluke infections. In some cases, **computed tomography scans** (CT scans) or **ultrasound** scans of the patient's chest or brain (for lung flukes) or abdomen (for liver flukes), are useful. Fluke infections are treated with medications such as triclabendazole, praziquantel, bithionol, albendazole, and mebendazole. Treatment varies from several days to several weeks. Cure rates range from 50–95%. Most patients experience mild side effects from these drugs. The prognosis for recovery from liver fluke infections is good, although patients with serious infections may be more vulnerable to other diseases. Most patients with lung fluke infections also recover, however, severe infections of the brain can cause **death**. There are no vaccines against fluke infections. Prevention includes: Boiling or purifying drinking water, avoiding raw or undercooked fish or salads made from fresh aquatic plants, thoroughly cooking all food eaten in areas with fluke infestations, and controlling or killing the snails that are the flukes' intermediate hosts.

FLUORIDE TREATMENT

Fluoride is a chemical found in many substances. In the human body, fluoride acts to prevent **tooth decay** by strengthening tooth enamel and inhibiting the growth of plaque-forming bacteria. After researchers discovered this characteristic of fluoride, *fluoridation*—the process of adding the fluoride to public water supplies—began. It all started with Frederick S. McKay, a Colorado Springs, Colorado, dentist, in the early 1900s. McKay noticed that many of his patients had brown stains, called ''mottled enamel,'' on their teeth. McKay set out to find the cause, helped by researcher Greene V. Black (1836-1915) of Northwestern University and other dentists. By 1916, McKay believed the mottling was caused by something in the patients' drinking water. By 1928, he concluded that mottling was linked to reduced tooth decay. In 1931, at the suggestion of an Alcoa chemist in Bauxite, Arkansas, McKay verified that drinking water from places with a high degree of tooth mottling contained unusually high levels of naturally occurring fluoride. H. Trendley Dean, a dentist with the United States Public Health Service, also studied the connection between mottling and fluoride in the 1930s. By the early 1940s, Dean and his research team had established that one part per million was the ideal level of fluoride in drinking water, substantially reducing decay while not causing mottling. Following safety tests on animals, the Public Health Service conducted field tests. In 1945 the public water systems of Newburgh, New York, and Grand Rapids, Michigan, became the first ever to be artificially fluoridated with sodium fluoride. Simultaneously, a group of Wisconsin dentists led by John G. Frisch inaugurated fluoridation in their state. Results of these tests seemed to show that fluoridation reduced dental cavities by as much as two thirds. Based on those results, the United States Public Health Service recommended in 1950 that all United States communities with public water systems fluoridate. Later that year the American Dental Association (ADA) followed suit, and the American Medical Association added its endorsement in 1951. Even though virtually the entire dental, medical, and public health establishment favored fluoridation, the recommendation was immediately controversial and has remained so. Opponents objected to fluoridation because of possible health risks (fluoride is toxic in large amounts) and concerns about being deprived of the choice whether or not to consume a chemical. While referenda have blocked fluoridation in a number of communities, nearly 60 percent of people in the United States now drink fluoridated water. Fluoridation is also practiced in about thirty other countries. The initial claims that fluoridation of drinking water produced two-thirds less tooth decay have been modified to about 20 to 25 percent reduction. Other ways of applying fluoride have been developed. In the 1950s Procter and Gamble had the idea of adding the chemical to toothpaste. First, researchers at Indiana University had to find a way to keep stannous fluoride from bonding with toothpaste abrasives. Once this problem was overcome, Procter & Gamble introduced its new ''Crest—with Fluoristan'' in 1956, launched with an advertising blitz that included the popular line ''Look, Mom—no cavities!'' Four years later, P&G scored a coup when the ADA Council on Dental Therapeutic gave Crest its seal of approval as ''an effective decay-preventive dentifrice.'' The ADA now estimates that brushing with fluoride-containing toothpaste reduces tooth decay by as much as 20 or 30 percent. In addition to toothpaste, fluoride can also be taken in tablet form and as a solution either ''painted'' directly onto the teeth or swished around as a mouthwash. Recently, a team of British scientists have been working on developing a vaccine to prevent tooth decay, which could one day serve as an alternative to fluoridation. A plant-based substance, the vaccine is ''painted'' on the teeth and prevents tooth decay by eliminating bacteria from the mouth.

See also Toothbrush and toothpaste

FOOD AND DRUG ADMINISTRATION

The Food and Drug Administration (FDA), one of the oldest consumer protection agencies in the United States (formed in 1927), ensures that foods are safe and wholesome, that medicines and medical devices are safe and effective, that cosmetics and products which emit radiation are harmless, and that products are honestly labeled and packaged. FDA is also responsible for feed and drugs for pets and farm animals.

Each year, the agency monitors the manufacture, import, transport, storage, and sale of $1 trillion worth of goods. It regulates almost 95,000 businesses in the United States. Headquartered in Rockville, Maryland, it is part of the United States Department of Health and Human Services, Public Health Service division. FDA has more than 9,000 employees working in district and local offices in 157 cities nationwide. Agency staff include 2,100 scientists working in 40 laboratories nationwide, and 1,100 investigators and inspectors who visit 15,000 facilities each year.

FDA enforces the Federal Food, Drug, and Cosmetic Act and related public health laws. If the agency finds a company in violation of any of the laws which it enforces, FDA can encourage the firm to voluntarily correct the problem or to recall the faulty product. If the company cannot or will not correct the problem voluntarily, FDA can go to court to force the company to stop selling the product and have products seized and destroyed, and seek criminal penalties against manufacturers and distributors. Each year, FDA finds about 3,000 products unfit for consumers and withdrawals them from the market, and 30,000 import products are detained from entering the United States.

Agency scientists prepare evidence for legal cases, and review test results submitted by companies seeking agency approval for drugs, vaccines, food additives, coloring agents, and medical devices. In reviewing new drug approvals, the agency determines whether the new drug's benefits outweigh risks.

To protect food, agency scientists test food samples to make sure that substances such as pesticide residues are not present in unacceptable amounts. If they are, FDA takes corrective action.

The agency sets labeling standards so people know what the food they buy contains and ensures that medicated feeds and drugs given to animals raised for food do not threaten public health. The agency also protects the nation's blood supply by examining blood bank operations and ensures that biologicals (medical preparations made from living organisms and their products), such as insulin and vaccines, are pure and effective. Medical devices that are life supporting, life sustaining, or implanted in the body must be approved by the agency before they can be marketed. FDA continues to monitor drugs and devices after they have been approved for marketing. Each year, the agency collects and analyzes tens of thousands of reports to monitor unexpected adverse reactions.

The agency can also have unsafe cosmetics taken off of the market. Dyes and others additives used in drugs, food, and cosmetics must be reviewed and approved before they can be sold.

The FDA Modernization Act of 1997 focused on reforming the way food, medical products, and cosmetics are regulated. The act's most important provisions: re-authorized the prescription drug user fees for five more years, modernized the regulation of biological products, increased patient access to experimental drugs and medical devices and accelerated agency review of important new medications, allowed drug manufacturers to distribute certain information on off-label use and drug economics, created an exemption to allow pharmacists to prepare individualized therapies not commercially available, focused resources on the riskiest medical devices, eliminated the requirement for food packaging and other substances that come in contact with food to be approved before being marketed, and simplified regulatory obligations while maintaining high standards for medical products.

FDA is comprised of: Office of the Commissioner, Office of Operations, Office of Policy, Office of External Affairs, and Office of Management and Systems. Within the Office of Operations, the Center for Biologics Evaluation and Review reviews the safety and efficacy of vaccines, blood and blood products, certain diagnostic products, and other biological and biotechnically-derived human products. The Center for Devices and Radiological Health ensures the safety and effectiveness of medical devices and eliminates unnecessary human exposure to man-made radiation. The Center for Drug Evaluation and Research ensures that marketed drugs are safe and effective. The Center for Food Safety and Applied Nutrition ensures that the nation's food supply is safe, sanitary, wholesome, and honestly labeled; and that cosmetic products are safe and properly labeled. The Center for Veterinary Medicine ensures animal health and the safety of food derived from animals. The National Center for Toxicological Research conducts research to define what makes some products regulated by FDA poisonous. The Office of Orphan Products Development promotes the development of products to treat rare diseases or conditions.

FOOD GROUPS AND NUTRIENTS

Millions of Americans take vitamin and mineral supplements every day. Most experts agree, however, that if one eats a healthy diet, there is probably no need to take daily supplements. Mineral and vitamin supplements cannot, completely make up for an unhealthy diet, such as one high in fat or low in fiber. Certain groups of people with special needs may benefit from taking supplements, however. These groups include pregnant women, frequent **aspirin** takers, heavy drinkers, and smokers.

Persons with special nutritional needs are advised to include in their **dietary supplements** the following **vitamins** and minerals: vitamin A (promotes good vision, healthy skin and mucous membranes and acts as an antioxidant), vitamin C (promotes healthy gums and teeth, aids in iron absorption, maintains normal connective tissue), vitamin E (aids the formation of red blood cells, acts as an antioxidant), folic acid (reduces the risk of certain birth defects, important in normal growth and **metabolism**), calcium (builds bone and teeth, helps regulate heartbeat), and iron (essential to formation of hemoglobin).

Fortunately, there are several federal guidelines available to help an individual plan a balanced **diet**. They include the United States **Food and Drug Administration**'s (FDA) Recommended Dietary Allowances (RDA), and the United States Department of Agriculture's (USDA) Food Guide Pyramid and Dietary Guidelines. Both guides assert that to achieve a balanced diet, one must consume a variety of foods from each of four basic food groups each day. In the RDA formulation, these four food groups consist of a milk group (including milk products such as cheese and yogurt); a meat group (including meat, chicken, fish, beef, pork, lamb, and vegetable sources of protein such as beans, peas, nuts, and seeds); a fruit and vegetable group; and a grain group (breads and cereals such as whole grain breads, enriched breads, rice, and pasta). In 1992, the United Stated Department of Agriculture (USDA) announced its Food Guide Pyramid and Dietary Guidelines, which were intended to shift the eating habits of Americans to diets that are low in fat, low in calories, high in fiber, with an emphasis on five servings of fruits and vegetables a day. The Food Guide Pyramid includes the RDA's four food groups, but the Food Guide Pyramid also identifies specific amounts of these foods to be eaten daily. What is also novel in the Food Guide Pyramid is that grains form the foundation of the diet pyramid, followed by an abundance of fruits and vegetables.

The RDA guidelines include eating at least three meals each day, not skipping breakfast, and above all, eating foods from each of the four food groups at every meal in order to achieve a balanced diet. (The term balanced simply means that a diet adequately meets one's nutritional needs while not providing any nutrients in excess. A balanced diet provides optimal protein and complex carbohydrates while supplying only moderate amounts of sodium, fats, and simple sugars. An unbalanced diet is one that can cause problems with maintenance of body tissues, growth and development, brain and **nervous system** function, as well as problems with bone and muscle systems.)

The USDA also recommends the consumption of small amounts of fish and poultry, with only occasional inclusion of red meat in the diet to reduce the amount of saturated fat and cholesterol consumed. Along with the Food Guide Pyramid, the USDA promotes the following dietary guidelines for maintaining good health: Eat a variety of foods; maintain healthy weight; choose a diet low in fat, saturated fat, and cholesterol; choose a diet with plenty of vegetables, fruits, and grain products; use sugars, salt, and sodium in moderation; and drink alcohol in moderation (if consumed at all). In 1993, the FDA mandated that all food packages show how much fat, saturated fat, cholesterol, dietary fiber, and sodium they contain, making it easier for the health-conscious consumer to abide by federal dietary guidelines.

See also Calcium imbalance; Cholesterol test; Iron deficiency anemia; Nutrition; Vitamin A deficiency; Vitamin E deficiency

FOOD LABELING

Federal law requires that food manufacturers place labels on most foods. The food label must provide complete, useful and accurate **nutrition** information. The requirement that packaged food be labeled has the effect of raising the quality of foods sold; it also gives the consumer a basis for making healthy food choices. Food labels appear in a consistent format to facilitate direct comparisons of the nutritional contents of various foods. These labels always appear on a package under the title *Nutrition Facts.*

Near the top of the label are the *Serving Size* and *Amounts per Serving* indications. Serving size is based on an average portion size. To make comparison between products easier, similar food products have similar serving sizes. Calories and the Calories from Fat are listed under *Amounts per Serving*. Besides providing valuable data about fat intake, this label also lists amounts of total fat, saturated fat, cholesterol, sodium, total carbohydrate, dietary fiber, sugars, and protein on a per serving basis.

The regulations require that only two **vitamins**, Vitamins A and C, and two **minerals**, calcium and iron, appear on the food label. Food manufacturers may, however, voluntarily list other vitamins and minerals in the food. And any added vitamins or minerals must be listed on the nutrition label.

The Percent Daily Value for vitamins and minerals provides a general idea of how much of a vitamin or mineral a single serving contributes to the total daily diet. The Percent Daily Value evaluates the food's nutritional content based on a 2,000-calorie diet. You can use the percent daily value to quickly compare foods and see how the amount of a nutrient in a serving of food fits into a 2,000 calorie diet.

Near the bottom of the label, there may be a list of six nutrients and the recommended daily intakes. Daily values are listed for 2000- and for 2500-calorie daily intakes. The amounts listed for the first four nutrients, i.e., total fat, saturated fat, cholesterol, and sodium, are maximum values. The amounts of total carbohydrate and dietary fiber are minimum amounts. This list is exactly the same on all food labels that carry it.

The terms most commonly used in nutritional labeling carry precise definitions; these terms include low calorie (40 calories or less per serving); reduced calorie (at least 25% fewer calories per serving when compared with a similar food

; light or lite (one-third fewer calories or 50% less fat per serving); sugar free (less than 0.5 grams of sugar per serving); reduced sugar (at least 25% less sugar per serving when compared with a similar food); fat free (less than 0.5 gram of fat per serving); 100% fat free (meets requirements for fat free); low fat (3 grams or less per serving); reduced fat (at least 25% less fat when compared with a similar food); cholesterol free (less than 2 milligrams cholesterol per serving and 2 grams or less saturated fat per serving); low cholesterol (20 milligrams of less cholesterol per serving and 2 grams or less saturated fat per serving); sodium free (less than 5 milligrams sodium per serving); salt free (meets requirements for sodium free).

Finally, the food label may contain a message that describes the relationship between a food or food component, such as fat, calcium or fiber and a disease or health-related condition. This message is known as a health claim. Federal law, backed by extensive scientific evidence, recognizes health claims for seven diet and health relationships: calcium and **osteoporosis**; fiber containing grain products, fruits, vegetables and **cancer**; fruits, vegetables and cancer; fruits, vegetables, and grain products that contain fiber and coronary heart disease; fat and cancer; saturated fat and cholesterol and coronary heart disease; and sodium and **hypertension**.

Food manufacturers must list ingredients in descending order by weight. The ingredient list must include FDA-approved color additives; sources of protein hydrolysates; and caseinate as a milk derivative in foods that claim to be non-dairy.

Many foods are exempt from the requirement of food labeling. These include restaurant foods; hospital cafeteria foods; airline foods; food from service vendors; ready-to-eat foods prepared primarily on site; bulk food that is not resold; food produced by small businesses; medical foods; plain coffee and tea; flavor extracts; food colors; spices; and any foods that contain no significant nutrients.

See also Food groups and nutrients

Food poisoning

Food poisoning means health problems from eating food contaminated by bacteria, viruses, environmental toxins, or toxins within the food. The Centers for Disease Control and Prevention (CDC) estimates that there are 6–33 million cases of food poisoning in the United States each year. Many are mild and pass rapidly. Common bacterial causes are *Salmonella*, *Staphylococcus aureus*, *Escherichia coli* O157:H7, *Shigella*, and *Clostridium botulinum*. Food and water can also be contaminated by viruses (**cholera**), environmental toxins (heavy metals), and poisons within the food (**mushroom poisoning** or **fish and shellfish poisoning**). Careless food handling enables bacteria to grow. Vegetables that are eaten raw may be contaminated by bacteria in soil, water, and dust during washing and packing. Home and commercially canned food may be improperly processed at too low a temperature or for too short a time. Raw meats carry many foodborne bacterial diseases. Thorough cooking kills the bacteria, but properly cooked food can be re-contaminated if it touches unclean objects used with raw meat, by food handlers, or by the environment. Anyone can get food poisoning but serious outbreaks are rare and most likely to affect the very young, the very old, those with immune system weaknesses, some travelers outside the United States, and people living in institutions. Sometimes food poisoning is called bacterial **gastroenteritis** or infectious **diarrhea**.

Symptoms of food poisoning are abdominal muscle cramping, vomiting, diarrhea, **fever**, and possibly **dehydration**. The severity depends on the type of bacteria, the amount consumed, and the individual. *Salmonella* is found in some egg yolks, raw and undercooked poultry, and other meats, dairy products, fish, and shrimp. Traditional food poisoning symptoms begin 12–72 hours after eating contaminated food and last two to five days. Dehydration can be a complication. People generally recover without treatment. *Staphylococcus aureus*, found in dust, air, and sewage, is spread by food handlers using poor sanitary practices. Salad dressings, milk products, cream pastries, and food kept at room temperature are most likely to be contaminated. Symptoms usually appear two to eight hours after eating contaminated food and usually last three to six hours. Most people recover without medical assistance.

E. coli O157:H7 causes most severe food poisoning. *E. coli* is found mainly in dairy products and beef, especially ground beef. Symptoms appear one to three days after eating contaminated food, when the victim begins to have severe abdominal cramps and watery diarrhea that usually becomes bloody and lasts one to eight days. According to the U.S. **Food and Drug Administration**, *Campylobacter jejuni (C. jejuni)* is the leading cause of bacterial diarrhea in the United States. Children under five and people ages 15–29 are most frequently infected. *C. jejuni* is carried by healthy cattle, chickens, birds, and flies and is found in ponds and streams. Symptoms begin two to five days after eating contaminated food and include fever, abdominal pain, **nausea**, **headache**, muscle pain, and watery or sticky diarrhea which may contain blood. Symptoms last 7–10 days. Dehydration is common.

Shigella, associated with contaminated food and water, crowded living conditions, and poor sanitation, commonly causes diarrhea in travelers to developing countries. The toxins affect the small intestine. Symptoms appear 36–72 hours after eating contaminated food. In addition to watery diarrhea, nausea, vomiting, abdominal cramps, and fever, up to 40% of children show neurological symptoms. The disease lasts two to three days. Dehydration is common. Most people recover on their own, but children who are malnourished or have weakened **immune systems** may die. Adult and infant *C. botulinum* **botulism** poisons the **nervous system**, causing **paralysis**. *C. botulinum* is an anaerobic bacterium that lives in an airless environment. Botulism is likely to be fatal. Adult botulism is usually associated with home canned food, and occasionally commercially canned or vacuum packed foods. Symptoms appear about 18–36 hours after eating contaminated food. They start with weakness and **dizziness**, followed by double vision, difficulty speaking and swallowing, and paralysis of the body.

When the respiratory muscles are paralyzed, **death** results. People with signs of botulism need immediate emergency medical care. Infant botulism occurs when a child under the age of one year ingests the spores of *C. botulinum* from soil or honey. Symptoms start gradually, with constipation followed by poor feeding, lethargy, weakness, drooling, and a wailing cry, and finally, paralysis of head muscles and the rest of the body.

The diagnosis of food poisoning is confirmed by finding the suspected bacteria in a **stool culture** or a fecal smear. Laboratory tests can isolate bacteria from a food sample. Botulism is usually diagnosed from its neurological symptoms. Many cases of food poisoning go undiagnosed. Treatment of food poisoning, except that caused by *C. botulinum,* focuses on preventing dehydration by replacing fluids and electrolytes lost through vomiting and diarrhea. Intravenous fluids may be used. In very serious cases, medications may be given to stop abdominal cramping and vomiting. People with food poisoning should not eat and drink only clear liquids during the period of vomiting and diarrhea, and then eat bland, soft, easy to digest foods for a few days. Severe bacterial food poisonings are sometimes treated with **antibiotics** such as Trimethoprim and sulfamethoxazole (Septra, Bactrim), ampicillin (Amcill, Polycill) or ciprofloxacin (Ciloxan, Cipro). Botulism requires hospitalization, often in the intensive care unit. Antitoxin is given to adults if it can be administered within 72 hours after symptoms start. If breathing is impaired, patients are put on a mechanical ventilator and fed intravenously. Alternative practitioners offer the same advice as traditional practitioners on diet and recommend taking charcoal tablets, *Lactobacillus acidophilus*, *Lactobacillus bulgaricus*, citrus seed extract, and electrolyte replacement fluid, and *Arsenicum album* or *Nux vomica*. Most cases of food poisoning (except botulism) clear up on their own within one week without medical assistance. Deaths are rare and usually occur in the very young, the very old and people whose immune systems are already weakened. Food poisoning is preventable through good sanitation and food handling techniques.

FOOD SAFETY

In the United States, agencies exist on the federal, state, and local levels to ensure a safe food supply and, in general, the food supply is very safe. However, as many as 81 million people experience foodborne illness annually, and an estimated 9,000 people die as a result. Most of these illnesses result from bacterial or viral contamination of food.

Producers, distributors, and consumers all share responsibility in ensuring safe food. Improper handling at any stage, from production and processing at a factory to preparation and storage at home, can cause food that was safe to become unsafe. Modern production and distribution systems open the door for problems that were not anticipated when congress passed the first food safety laws in 1906. In the last 20 years or so, individual food processing facilities have become very large and a single instance of contamination can result in tons of food being affected. New infectious diseases have emerged and old ones have turned up in new places or have adapted to **antibiotics**. Changes in dietary habits also affect the amount of risks consumers face. More people than ever are eating out on a regular basis, giving them little control over food preparation. Also, higher demand for fresh fruits and vegetables has increased the amount of food imports coming into the country. If safety standards are not followed in the countries of origin, these foods carry the risk of contamination. Since distribution systems reach over the entire globe, tracing illnesses back to the source of contamination can be very difficult.

Food safety concerns are generally biological, chemical, or physical in nature. The vast majority of foodborne illnesses are due to biological contaminants, primarily bacteria and viruses. Common ones include *Campylobacter jejuni* in raw or undercooked meats, unpasteurized milk, and untreated water; *Salmonella* in undercooked meats and eggs or in dairy products, seafood, fruits, and vegetables; hepatitis A virus from foods contaminated by human feces; and *Shigella* from dairy products, poultry, and raw vegetables. Less common are *Clostridium botulinum* (botulism) from improperly canned foods, sausages, meat products, and seafood; *Escherichia coli* O157:H7 from undercooked hamburgers or unpasteurized milk; *Listeria monocytogenes* in unpasteurized milk, soft cheeses and ice cream, raw vegetables, undercooked meats, and seafood; *Staphylococcus aureus* in cooked foods that contain a lot of protein; and *Vibrio vulnificus* in raw or undercooked seafood.

Chemicals are routinely added to processed foods to preserve them and to enhance flavor and appearance. These chemicals have been tested and are believed to be safe. However, some additives, such as artificial sweeteners or fat substitutes, carry warnings about potential bad effects of eating them. Many consumers worry about artificial chemicals, but naturally occurring chemicals can be more dangerous. Allergy-producing substances, called allergens, are a major concern. Some people have dangerous, potentially fatal allergic reactions to chemicals found in peanuts, tree nuts (e.g., walnuts, pecans, and almonds), shellfish, eggs, milk, soy, fish, and wheat. Other naturally occurring chemicals are added to foods as dietary supplements, but there may not be proof that these are either effective or safe. In rare cases, chemicals get into food accidentally and the potential exists for pesticides, animal drug residues, or cleaning substances to show up in foods. Other chemical hazards may arise from environmental pollution.

Foreign objects in food are the biggest concern with regard to physical hazards. During production and processing, small stones or fragments of glass, metal, wood, or other materials may appear in food due to accident, equipment failure, or negligence.

Hazard identification and prevention are the best means of making sure that food is safe. Producers and processors are required to handle food under sanitary conditions to prevent biological contamination. They must also use precautions to prevent chemical and physical contaminants from getting into food.

Food processors often use a set of instructions called the Hazard Analysis Critical Control Point (HACCP) program.

Through HACCP programs, processors identify everything that can go wrong and then take specific steps to prevent these problems. At the processing level, there also needs to be proper attention to labeling. Labeling is meant to inform consumers of nutritional aspects of the food as well as to alert them to potential allergens. Food has to be transported and stored properly using refrigeration to prevent spoiling and the growth of microorganisms.

Consumers need to be just as careful at home. To prevent foodborne illness, consumers should thoroughly cook meats, prepare food on clean surfaces, refrigerate foods, and cool prepared foods in a refrigerator. Fresh fruits and vegetables should be thoroughly washed even if the package indicates that the product has already been washed. Bulging cans, mold, discoloration, and bad flavor or odor are indications that a food is spoiled. If a consumer has any doubts about a food, it should not be eaten.

See also Botulism; Food and Drug Administration; Food poisoning

Foot care

Foot care involves all aspects of preventative and corrective care of the foot and ankle. Doctors specializing in foot care are called podiatrists. Three-quarters of people have foot problems during their lives from wearing ill-fitting shoes, general wear and tear, an injury, or as a complication of disease. People with **diabetes mellitus** or circulatory diseases are 20 times more likely to have foot problems than the general public. Foot problems include: foot **pain**, joint inflammation, plantar **warts**, fungal infections (like athlete's foot), nerve disorders, torn ligaments, broken bones, bacterial infections, and tissue injuries (like frostbite). People with diabetes or circulatory disorders should be alert to even small foot problems. In these people, a break in the skin can lead to infection, **gangrene**, and **amputation**.

Daily foot care for people likely to develop foot problems includes washing the feet in tepid water with mild soap and oiling the feet with vegetable oil or a lanolin-based lotion. Toenails should be cut straight across above the level of the skin after soaking the feet in tepid water. Corns and calluses, athletes foot and plantar warts in high risk patients should only be treated by a doctor. Many people with diabetes or circulatory disorders have problems with cold feet. These problems can be reduced by not **smoking**, wearing warm socks, not crossing the legs while sitting or not sitting in one position too long, and avoiding constricting stockings. People with circulatory problems should not use heating pads or hot water bottles on their feet. No special preparation other than an understanding of the nature of foot problems is necessary to begin routine foot care. With regular care, foot disorders such as infections, skin ulcers, and gangrene can be prevented.

Foot disorders

A variety of disorders can affect the feet. A bunion is an abnormal enlargement of the joint (the first metatarsophalangeal joint, or MTPJ) at the base of the great or big toe (hallux). It is caused by inflammation and usually results from chronic irritation and pressure from poorly fitting footwear.

A corn is a small, painful, raised bump on the outer skin layer. A callus is a rough, thickened patch of skin.

Hammertoe is a condition in which the toe is bent in a claw-like position. It can be present in more than one toe but is most common in the second toe.

A heel spur is a bony projection on the sole (plantar) region of the heel bone (also known as the calcaneous). This condition may accompany or result from severe cases of inflammation to the structure called plantar fascia. This associated plantar fascia is a fibrous band of connective tissue on the sole of the foot, extending from the heel to the toes.

A displacement of two major bones of the foot (hallux valgus) causes bunions, although not everyone with this displacement will develop the joint swelling and bone overgrowth that characterize a bunion. One of the bones involved is called the first metatarsal bone. This bone is long and slender, with the big toe attached on one end and the other end connected to foot bones closer to the ankle. This foot bone is displaced in the direction of the four other metatarsals connected with the toes. The other bone involved is the big toe itself, which is displaced toward the smaller toes. As the big toe continues to move toward the smaller toes, it may become displaced under or over the second toe. The displacement of these two foot bones causes a projection of bone on the inside portion of the forefoot. The skin over this projection often becomes inflamed from rubbing against the shoe, and a callus may form.

The joint contains a small sac (bursa) filled with fluid that cushions the bones and helps the joint to move smoothly. When a bunion forms, this sac becomes inflamed and thickened. The swelling in the joint causes additional **pain** and pressure in the toe.

Bunions may form as a result of abnormal motion of the foot during walking or running. One common example of an abnormal movement is an excessive amount of stress placed upon the inside of the foot. This leads to friction and irritation of the involved structures. Age has also been noted as a factor in developing bunions, in part because the underlying bone displacement worsens over time unless corrective measures are taken.

Wearing improperly fitting shoes, especially those with a narrow toe box and excessive heel height, often causes the formation of a bunion. This forefoot deformity is seen more often in women than men. The higher frequency in females may be related to the strong link between footwear fashion and bunions. In fact, in a recent survey of more than 350 women, nearly 90% wore shoes that were at least one size too small or too narrow.

Because genetic factors can predispose people to the hallux valgus bone displacement, a strong family history of bunions can increase the likelihood of developing this foot disorder. Various arthritic conditions and several genetic and neuromuscular diseases, such as **Down syndrome** and **Marfan syndrome**, cause muscle imbalances that can create bunions from displacement of the first metatarsal and big toe. Other possible causes of bunions are leg-length discrepancies, with the bunion present on the longer leg, and trauma occurring to the joint of the big toe.

Symptoms of bunions include the common signs of inflammation such as redness, swelling, and pain. The discomfort is primarily located along the inside of the foot just behind the big toe. Because of friction, a callus may develop over the bunion. If an overlapping of the toes is allowed, additional rubbing and pain occurs. Inflammation of this area causes a decrease in motion with associated discomfort in the joint between the big toe and the first metatarsal. If allowed to worsen, the skin over the bunion may break down causing an ulcer, which also presents a problem of potential infection. (Foot ulcers can be particularly dangerous for people with diabetes, who may have trouble feeling the ulcer forming and healing if it becomes infected.)

A thorough medical history and physical exam by a physician is always necessary for the proper diagnosis of bunions and other foot conditions. X rays can help confirm the diagnosis by showing the bone displacement, joint swelling, and, in some cases, the overgrowth of bone that characterizes bunions. Doctors will also consider the possibility that the joint pain is caused by or complicated by arthritis (which causes destruction of the cartilage of the joint), **gout** (which causes the accumulation of uric acid crystals in the joint), tiny **fractures** of a bone in the foot (stress fractures), or infection and may order additional tests to rule out these possibilities.

The first step in treating a bunion is to remove as much pressure from the area as possible. People with bunions should wear shoes that have enough room in the toe box to accommodate the bunion and avoid high-heeled shoes and tight-fitting socks or stockings. Dressings and pads help protect the bunion from additional shoe pressure. The application of splints or customized shoe inserts (orthotics) to correct the alignment of the big toe joint is effective for many bunions. Most patients are instructed to rest or choose **exercise**s that put less stress on their feet, at least until the misalignment is corrected. In some cases, physicians also use steroid injections with local anesthetic around the bunion to reduce inflammation.

If conservative treatment is not successful, surgical removal of the bunion may be necessary to correct the deformity. This procedure is called a bunionectomy, and there are many variations on the operation, which is usually performed by a surgeon who specializes in treating bone conditions (orthopedics) or by one who specializes in treating the foot (podiatry). Surgeons consider the angle of the bone misalignment, the condition of the bursa, and the strength of the bones when they choose which procedure to use. Most bunionectomies involve the removal of a section of bone and the insertion of pins to rejoin the bone. Sometimes the surgeons may move ligaments (which connect bone to bone in the joint) or tendons (which connect bone to muscle) in order to realign the bones. After this procedure, the bones and other tissues are held in place while they heal by compression dressings or a short cast. The individual must refrain from vigorous exercise for six weeks.

Often, modifications in footwear allow a good prognosis without surgery. If surgery is necessary, complete healing without complications requires approximately four to six weeks. Even after surgery corrects the bone misalignment, patients are usually instructed to continue wearing low-heeled, roomy shoes to prevent the bunion from reforming.

Corns and calluses are one of the three major foot problems in the United States. The other two are foot infections and toenail problems. Corns and calluses affect about 5% of the population.

Corns usually appear on non-weight-bearing areas like the outside of the little toe or the tops of other toes. Women have corns more often than men, probably because women wear high-heeled shoes and other shoes that do not fit properly. Corns have hard cores shaped like inverted pyramids. Sharp pain occurs whenever downward pressure is applied, and a dull ache may be felt at other times.

A hard corn is a compact lump with a thick core. Hard corns usually form on the tops of the toes, on the outside of the little toe, or on the sole of the foot.

A soft corn is a small, inflamed patch of skin with a smooth center. Soft corns usually appear between the toes.

A seed corn is the least common type of corn. Occurring only on the heel or ball of the foot, a seed corn consists of a circle of stiff skin surrounding a plug of cholesterol.

Calluses occur most often on the heels and balls of the feet, the knees, and the palms of the hands. However, they can develop on any part of the body that is subject to repeated pressure or irritation. Calluses are usually more than an inch wide—larger than corns. They generally don't hurt unless pressure is applied.

A plantar callus, a callus that occurs on the sole of the foot, has a white center. Hereditary calluses develop where there is no apparent friction, run in families, and occur most often in children.

Corns and calluses form to prevent injury to skin that is repeatedly pinched, rubbed, or irritated. The most common causes are:

- Shoes that are too tight or too loose, or have very high heels
- Tight socks or stockings
- Deformed toes
- Walking down a long hill, or standing or walking on a hard surface for a long time.

Jobs or hobbies that cause steady or recurring pressure on the same spot can also cause calluses.

Corns can be recognized on sight. A family physician or podiatrist may scrape skin off what seems to be a callus, but may actually be a wart. If the lesion is a wart, it will bleed. A callus will not bleed, but will reveal another layer of dead skin.

Corns and calluses do not usually require medical attention, unless the person who has them has diabetes mellitus, poor circulation, or other problems that make self-care difficult.

Treatment should begin as soon as an abnormality appears. The first step is to identify and eliminate the source of pressure. Placing moleskin pads over corns can relieve pressure, and large wads of cotton, lamb's wool, or moleskin can cushion calluses.

Using hydrocortisone creams or soaking feet in a solution of Epsom salts and very warm water for at least five minutes a day before rubbing the area with a pumice stone will remove part or all of some calluses. Rubbing corns just makes them hurt more.

Applying petroleum jelly or lanolin-enriched hand lotion helps keep skin soft, but corn-removing ointments that contain acid can damage healthy skin. They should never be used by pregnant women or by people who are diabetic or who have poor circulation.

It is important to see a doctor if the skin of a corn or callus is cut, because it may become infected. If a corn discharges pus or clear fluid, it is infected. A family physician, podiatrist, or orthopedist may:

- Remove (debride) affected layers of skin
- Prescribe oral **antibiotics** to eliminate infection
- Drain pus from infected corns
- Inject cortisone into the affected area to decrease pain or inflammation
- Perform surgery to correct toe deformities or remove bits of bone.

Most corns and calluses disappear about three weeks after the pressure that caused them is eliminated. They are apt to recur if the pressure returns.

Bursitis, a painful, inflamed fluid-filled sac, can develop beneath a corn. An ulcer or broken area within a corn can reach to the bone. Infection can have serious consequences for people who have diabetes or poor circulation.

Hammertoe is described as a deformity in which the toesbend downward with the toe joint usually enlarged. Over time, the joint enlarges and stiffens as it rubs against shoes. Other foot structures involved include the overlying skin and blood vessels and nerves connected to the involved toes.

The shortening of tendons responsible for the control and movement of the affected toe or toes cause hammertoe. Top portions of the toes become callused from the friction produced against the inside of shoes. This common foot problem often results from improper fit of footwear. This is especially the case with high-heeled shoes placing pressure on the front part of the foot that compresses the smaller toes tightly together. The condition frequently stems from muscle imbalance, and usually leaves the affected individual with impaired balance.

A thorough medical history and physical exam by a physician is always necessary for the proper diagnosis of hammertoe. X rays can help to confirm the diagnosis.

Wearing proper footwear and stockings with plenty of room in the toe region can provide treatment for hammertoe. Stretching exercises may be helpful in lengthening the excessively tight tendons.

In advanced hammertoe cases, where conservative treatment is unsuccessful, surgery may be recommended. The tendons that attach to the involved toes are located and an incision is made to free the connective tissue to the foot bones. Additional incisions are made so the toes no longer bend in a downward fashion. The middle joints of the affected toes are connected together permanently with surgical hardware such as pins and wire sutures. The incision is then closed with fine sutures. These sutures are removed approximately seven to ten days after surgery.

Heel spurs are a common foot problem resulting from excess bone growth on the heel bone. The bone growth is usually located on the underside of the heel bone, extending forward to the toes. One explanation for this excess production of bone is a painful tearing of the plantar fascia connected between the toes and heel. This can result in either a heel spur or an inflammation of the plantar fascia, medically termed plantar fascitis. Because this condition is often correlated to a decrease in the arch of the foot, it is more prevalent after the age of six to eight years, when the arch is fully developed.

One frequent cause of heel spurs is an abnormal motion and mal-alignment of the foot called pronation. For the foot to function properly, a certain degree of pronation is required. This motion is defined as an inward action of the foot, with dropping of the inside arch as one plants the heel and advances the weight distribution to the toes during walking. When foot pronation becomes extreme from the foot turning in and dropping beyond the normal limit, a condition known as excessive pronation creates a mechanical problem in the foot. In some cases the sole or bottom of the foot flattens and becomes unstable because of this excess pronation, especially during critical times of walking and athletic activities. The portion of the plantar fascia attached into the heel bone or calcaneous begins to stretch and pull away from the heel bone.

At the onset of this condition, pain and swelling become present, with discomfort particularly noted as pushing off with the toes occurs during walking. This movement of the foot stretches the fascia that is already irritated and inflamed. If this condition is allowed to continue, pain is noticed around the heel region because of the newly formed bone, in response to the stress. This results in the development of the heel spur. It is common among athletes and others who run and jump a significant amount.

An individual with the lower legs angulating inward, a condition called genu valgus or ''knock knees,'' can have a tendency toward excessive pronation. As a result, this too can lead to a fallen arch resulting in plantar fascitis and heel spurs. Women tend to have more genu valgus than men do. Heel spurs can also result from an abnormally high arch.

Other factors leading to heel spurs include a sudden increase in daily activities, an increase in weight, or a change of shoes. Dramatic increase in training intensity or duration may cause plantar fascitis. Shoes that are too flexible in the middle of the arch or shoes that bend before the toe joints will cause an increase in tension in the plantar fascia and possibly lead to heel spurs.

The pain this condition causes forces an individual to attempt walking on his or her toes or ball of the foot to avoid pressure on the heel spur. This can lead to other compensations during walking or running that in turn cause additional problems to the ankle, knee, hip, or back.

Heel spurs and plantar fascitis are usually controlled with conservative treatment. Early intervention includes stretching the calf muscles while avoiding re-injuring the plantar fascia. Decreasing or changing activities, losing excess weight, and improving the proper fitting of shoes are all important measures to decrease this common source of foot pain. Modification of footwear includes shoes with a raised heel and better arch support. Shoe orthotics recommended by a health-care professional are often very helpful in conjunction with **exercises** to increase strength of the foot muscles and arch. The orthotic prevents excess pronation and lengthening of the plantar fascia and continued tearing of this structure. To aid in this reduction of inflammation, applying ice for 10 to 15 minutes after activities and use of anti-inflammatory medication can be helpful. Physical therapy can be beneficial with the use of heat modalities, such as ultrasound, that create a deep heat and reduce inflammation. If the pain caused by inflammation is constant, keeping the foot raised above the heart and/or compressed by wrapping with an ace bandage will help.

Corticosteroid injections are also frequently used to reduce pain and inflammation. Taping can help speed the healing process by protecting the fascia from reinjury, especially during stretching and walking.

When chronic heel pain fails to respond to conservative treatment, surgical treatment may be necessary. Heel surgery can provide relief of pain and restore mobility. The type of procedure used is based on examination and usually consists of releasing the excessive tightness of the plantar fascia, called a plantar fascia release. Depending on the presence of excess bony build up, the procedure may or may not include removal of heel spurs. Similar to other surgical interventions, there are various modifications and surgical enhancements regarding surgery of the heel.

Usually, heel spurs are curable with conservative treatment. If not, heel spurs are curable with surgery. About 10% of those that continue to see a physician for plantar fascitis have it for more than a year. If there is limited success after approximately one year of conservative treatment, patients are often advised to have surgery.

FOREIGN OBJECTS

''Foreign'' means ''originating elsewhere'' or ''outside the body.'' Foreign bodies usually get stuck in the eyes, ears, nose, airways, and rectum of children and adults. Young children may intentionally put shiny objects into their mouths and stick things in their ears and up their noses. Adults may accidentally swallow a non-food object or inhale a foreign body that gets stuck in the throat. Airborne particles can get stuck in the eyes of anyone. Foreign bodies can be in hollow organs (like swallowed batteries) or in tissues (like bullets). They can be inert or irritating. If they irritate they will cause inflammation and scarring. They can bring infection with them or acquire it and protect it from the body's immune defenses. They can block passageways either by their size or by the scarring they cause. Some can be toxic.

Dust, dirt, sand, or other airborne material can lodge in the eyes, causing minor irritation and redness. More serious damage can be caused by hard or sharp objects that become embedded in the cornea or inner eyelid. Children will sometimes put things into their noses, ears, and other openings and, on occasion, insects may also fly into the ears and nose. At a certain age children will eat anything. Some items can get stuck and cause trouble. Batteries are corrosive and must be removed immediately. The most commonly inhaled item is probably a peanut. Inhaled items always cause symptoms and may be hard to detect. Adults commonly swallow dental devices, and adults with **mental illness** or subversive motives may swallow inappropriate objects. Sometimes a foreign object will get stuck between the rectum and the anal canal, or is self-introduced to enhance sexual stimulation and then get stuck.

The symptoms are as diverse as the objects and their locations. The most common symptom is infection. Blockage of passageways—breathing, digestive or excretory—is another result. **Pain** is common. Treatment varies depending on where the foreign object is. In the eyes, small particles like sand may be removable without medical help, but if the object is not visible or cannot be retrieved, emergency treatment is necessary. Eye trauma can lead to vision loss and should never be ignored. In a well-lighted area, use clean hands and materials to touch the eyes. If the particle is small, it can be dislodged by blinking or pulling the upper lid over the lower lid and flushing out the speck, or by picking it out with a clean cloth. Rinse the eye with clean, lukewarm water. If the foreign object cannot be removed at home, cover the eye lightly with sterile gauze. A physician will use surgical tweezers to remove it and may prescribe an antibiotic sterile ointment and a patch. If the foreign body is stuck in the deeper layers of the eye, an ophthalmic surgeon will be consulted. Many methods have been devised for removing foreign objects from the nose and ears. A bead in a nostril, for example, can be popped out by blowing into the mouth while holding the other nostril closed. Skilled practitioners have removed peas from the ears by tiny improvised corkscrews; marbles by q-tips with super glue. Tweezers often work well, too. Insects can be floated out of the ear by pouring warm (not hot) oil into the ear canal. Items that are stuck deep in the ear canal require emergency treatment. Mechanical obstruction of the airways, common when food gets stuck in the throat, can be treated with the **Heimlich maneuver**. If the object is lodged lower in the airway, a bronchoscope (an instrument to view the airway and remove obstructions) can be inserted. When the object is blocking the entrance to the stomach, a fiberoptic endoscope (an instrument to views the interior of a body cavity) may be used. After giving the patient a sedative and anesthetizing the throat, the physician either pulls the foreign object out or pushes it into the stomach. Objects in the digestive tract that aren't irritating, sharp, or large may be followed as they continue on through. Sterile objects that are causing no symptoms may be left in place. Surgical removal of the offending object is necessary if it is causing symptoms. A rectal retractor can remove objects that a physician can feel during **physical examination**. Surgery may be required for objects deeply stuck within the recturm.

Using common sense and following safety precautions are the best ways to prevent foreign objects from entering the body. For instance, parents and grandparents should toddler-proof their homes, storing batteries in a locked cabinet and properly disposing of used batteries, so curious preschoolers can't fish them out of a wastebasket. To minimize the chance of youngsters inhaling food, parents should not allow children to eat while walking or playing. Adults should chew food thoroughly and not talk while chewing. Many eye injuries can be prevented by wearing safety glasses while using tools.

Forssmann, Werner (1904-1979)

German physician

Werner Theodor Otto Forssmann, a surgeon and urologist, was born on August 29, 1904, in Berlin, the only child of Julius Forssmann, a lawyer employed by a life insurance company, and Emmy Hindenberg. Forssmann's father died in World War I while young Forssmann was still a student in the Askanische Gymnasium. His mother worked as an office clerk and his grandmother took over the role of running the household. Forssmann's uncle, a doctor just outside of Berlin, became an influential force in his nephew's life, ultimately convincing Forssmann to pursue a career in medicine. In 1922, after graduating from the Gymnasium, Forssmann entered the Friedrich Wilhelm University in Berlin, passing the state examination in 1928. Forssmann's doctoral thesis on the effects of concentrated liver on **pernicious anemia**, a blood deficiency, marked the way for his later experiments. Together with a small group of fellow students, Forssmann experimented on himself, taking large doses of liver concentrate daily and demonstrating its healthful effects on blood. After receiving his doctor's diploma in early 1929 and being frustrated in his efforts to obtain a post as an internist, Forssmann worked for a short time in a private women's clinic in Spandau. Then, through family connections, he secured an internship at the August Viktoria Home in Eberswalde, a small town northeast of Berlin.

Training as a surgeon, Forssmann nevertheless gave thought to an earlier passion of his: heart diagnosis. He was dissatisfied with the inaccuracy and uncertainty of diagnostic techniques such as percussion, auscultation, x ray, and even **electrocardiography**. He became convinced that there was an internal diagnostic method that would not involve major risks, trigger automatic reflex actions, or disturb the balance of pressure in the thorax. As early as the mid-nineteenth century, there had been a procedure known as cardiac catheterization in animal experiments. Doctors had performed the procedure in the late nineteenth century to determine blood pressure in the right and left chambers of the heart. Some of these procedures employed the use of a catheter inserted through the jugular vein of a horse. Forssmann believed that he could do this on humans through a vein at the elbow traditionally used for intravenous injections. His research on cadavers supported his idea, and by the summer of 1929 Forssmann approached his supervisor, Dr. Richard Schneider, with a plan to catheterize his own heart with a ureteric catheter. Schneider, however, would not allow such a dangerous experiment in his hospital.

Undaunted, Forssmann set out to convince a surgical nurse in his section of his experiment's feasibility so he could gain access to the sterilized instruments he needed. Eventually, the nurse agreed to aid him. He gave himself a local anesthetic in the left elbow and then made an incision. Once he had opened his vein, he inserted the catheter about a foot up his arm and had the nurse accompany him to the x-ray lab. There, Forssmann stood behind a fluoroscope screen with a mirror placed so that he could see the image of the catheter, which he pushed up until it was in the right ventricle of his heart. Then he calmly ordered that photographs be made of this momentous achievement.

The results of this experiment were published in a short paper in the prestigious *Klinische Wochenschrift* and won Forssmann a position at the Charité Hospital in Berlin. But the reception to his article by other physicians was cool and his superior at the Charité did not approve of his unorthodox techniques, so Forssmann was soon back in Eberswalde. He continued his experiments for the next two years, during which time he proved that the insertion of a catheter in the heart was painless and caused no damage to the blood vessels. He also pioneered techniques for measuring pressure inside the heart and for injecting opaque material for x-ray studies of the heart. Still, his work was reviled by most physicians, who called it unethical and considered his experiments stunts. By 1931, Forssmann, discouraged by the response to his work, gave up experimental medicine. He returned to the Charité Hospital in Berlin and soon moved on to the Mainz City Hospital. It was there, in 1932, that he met the woman who would become his wife, Dr. Elsbet Engel, a resident in internal medicine. Though their marriage was happy, it also necessitated another change of hospitals for Forssmann, for it was against the hospital's policy for a married couple to work together. Forssmann trained as a urologist in Berlin at the Rudolph Virchow Hospital, then took a position as a surgeon and urologist at the City Hospital of Dresden-Friedrichstadt for two years. Later, he became a senior surgeon at the Robert Koch Hospital in Berlin.

During World War II, Forssmann served as an army surgeon, surviving six years spent in Germany, Norway, Russia, and in a prisoner of war (POW) camp. Back in Germany after the War, he practiced as a country doctor in the Black Forest village of Wambach for three years before returning to the practice of urology in 1950 at Bad Kreuznach. It was only after the war that Forssmann discovered that others had continued working with his cardiac catheterization experiment of 1929. The most notable implementation was by two Americans, **Dickinson Woodruff Richards, Jr.**, and **André F. Cournand**, who developed it into a tool for diagnosis and research. In 1954, Forssmann received the Leibniz Medal from the German Academy of Science in Berlin, yet he was refused a professorship at the University of Mainz. He had resigned himself to being a little-known doctor in Bad Kreuznach when, on October 18, 1956, he was notified that he had won, along with Richards and Cournand, the Nobel Prize for Physiology or Medicine for his contribution to the knowledge of heart catheterization and pathological changes in the circulatory system.

The Nobel Prize finally earned Forssmann renown and respect; in *Clinical Cardiology,* H. W. Heiss called him "one of the great fathers of cardiology." In 1958, he became the chief of the surgical division of the Evangelical Hospital of Düsseldorf, and 10 years later he was awarded the gold medal of the Society of Surgical Medicine of Ferrara. He died of a heart attack in Schopfheim, West Germany, on June 1, 1979.

Foster care

Foster care is an arrangement by which children live temporarily with people other than their own families, who for various reasons are unable to care for them; often, the reason for foster care is abuse or neglect by the child's parent.

There are more than half a million children living in foster homes in the United States at any given time. Neglect, physical abuse, **sexual abuse**, and emotional abuse are the primary reasons that children are removed from their homes and placed in foster care. **Substance abuse** by one or both parents is a factor in more than 75% of all foster home placements.

There always has been an informal system of foster care in the United States. Earlier in this country's history, neighbors or relatives would come forward to care for children whose parents (for whatever reasons) were unable to do so. However, there was little government effort to care for children before 1912, when the U.S Children's Bureau was established to protect the health and welfare of children. In the early days of government-run foster care, children were usually placed in foster families because their own parents were sick, unable to care for them, or dead.

Since the turn of the century, changing circumstances and an increase in the need for foster parents has made it necessary for foster care programs to become better organized and regulated. Today there are both government programs that regulate foster care, and programs set up and run by private agencies.

Foster children can be any age, but about 25% of children entering foster care for the first time are infants, and 60% are under 4. Youngsters between the ages of 13 and 18 account for about a third of all children in foster care.

Because children placed in foster care often have special physical, emotional, behavioral, educational, or social needs, it can be very challenging to serve as a foster parent. It's estimated that more than one-third of all licensed foster parents are without foster children at any given time, either because they're either unwilling or unable to care for children with difficult problems.

As a result, children who could be living with foster parents are sent instead to group homes, or shuttled from one foster home to another for unsuccessful, short-term stays. To combat this problem, child welfare workers today turn more often to relatives of the children in need of foster care, appealing to them to take over the care of the child. This form of foster care is called ''kinship care.''

People who want to become foster parents are first screened to determine whether they're eligible. Those best qualified to be a foster parent are patient and empathetic, attentive, and determined to succeed. They should have an ability to love and then let go, and a willingness to grow and learn from the fostering experience. Applicants don't need to be married or live in a single-family home—or even be stay-at-home parents. Foster parents include retired persons, working parents, apartment dwellers, and single or divorced persons.

Qualified applicants receive training in how to be good foster parents. They are reimbursed for the cost of caring for their foster children, and they receive extra funds if there are special needs that must be met or unusual health problems that require treatment. Social workers oversee and supervise foster parents' work. In most cases, **counseling** and support are available to foster parents.

Fractures

Fractures, or broken bones, are one of the most common medical problems. It is estimated that 6.8 million fractures occur in the United States each year alone, with approximately 900,000 of them requiring hospitalization. To treat a fracture so that the patient regains full use of an injured arm or leg the bone ends must first be brought back into alignment; then, the fracture must be held together until the bone ends grow back together. Closed or simple fractures, in which the bone ends do not penetrate the skin, have always been relatively easy to treat. Open or compound fractures were usually fatal prior to the advent of **antiseptics** in the 1860s because infection would set in. The earliest method of holding a reduced fracture in place was to use splints—rigid strips laid parallel to each other alongside the bone. Ancient Egyptians used wood splints made of bark wrapped in linen to hold broken bones in place. Ancient Hindus treated fractures with bamboo splints. The writings of **Hippocrates** discuss management of fractures in some detail, recommending wooden splints plus exercise to prevent muscle atrophy during the **immobilization**. Next, medical practitioners thought of stiffening the **bandages** that held the splints in place. The ancient Greeks used waxes and resins for this purpose. The Roman **Celsus**, writing in A.D. 30, describes how to use splints and bandages stiffened with starch. Arabian doctors used lime derived from sea shells. The Italian School of Salerno in the twelfth century recommended bandages hardened with a flour and egg mixture. Medieval European bonesetters used casts made of egg white, flour, and animal fat. In the sixteenth century the famous French surgeon **Ambroise Paré** (1517-1590) made casts of wax, cardboard, cloth, and parchment that hardened as they dried. Splints remained the basic method of immobilization until 1852, when a Dutch army surgeon, Antonius Mathijsen, introduced *roller bandages* impregnated with quick-drying plaster of paris (gypsum). Broken bones could be held in place while the wet bandages were applied; when dry, the bandages became a rigid cast that held the bones perfectly in place during healing. As Mathijsen himself pointed out, Arab physicians had used plaster casts for centuries, but knowledge of the technique hadn't reached the West until the end of the eighteenth century. Plaster of paris casts have remained standard treatment for fractures. Beginning in the early 1980s, casts made of fiberglass plaster have also come into use and are favored for their light weight and water resistance. In addition to splints and casts, fractures have been treated with *extension* and **traction**. The ancient Greeks used traction—pulling on a broken limb with weights and pulleys—but that practice died out until after the Middle Ages. Traction was revived by the eminent French surgeon **Guy de Chauliac** (1300-1368) during the fourteenth century. The gifted orthopedist Hugh Owen Thomas (1833-1891) of England devised improved methods of traction as well as the Thomas splint, still used today, which allowed for extension of the limb. Hugh Arbuthnot Lane (1856-1943) of Great Britain devised a way to hold broken bone ends together mechanically when they would not heal together naturally. In 1893 he introduced the use of steel screws to rejoin bones and then improved the technique around 1905 by using steel plates screwed into the bone ends. Lane's method, of course, could only succeed after **Joseph Lister** (1827-1912) had introduced antisepsics to surgery, and successful treatment of compound fractures also depended on Lister's innovation. Compound fractures meant heavy contamination of the wound, which almost always led to severe infection and usually resulted in death. Since infection could not be avoided in pre-antiseptic days, the usual method of treating compound fractures until the late nineteenth century was amputation—which, in the case of removal of the thigh, also often resulted in fatal infection. Once Lister began the era of antiseptic surgery in 1865, infection in compound fractures could be controlled and these injuries could at last be treated successfully with surgery, casts, and plates.

FRANK, JOHANN PETER (1745-1821)

German physician

At a time when the **plague** and excrement dumped on streets was a common sight in Europe's cities, Johann Peter Frank began to stress the importance of proper hygiene for the masses. With a cry for the state to be responsible for the public's health at all times, Frank guided his career as a writer, teacher, and physician through prominent positions which preached his life-altering improvements in cities throughout several countries. His determination to make these changes led him to be known as the founder of modern **public health**.

Born into a large family of German and French descent in Rotalben near Zweibucken in 1745, Frank attended catholic schools including the Piarist Latin School in Rastadt and the Jesuit School in Bockenheim, Lorraine. While in school, he was leaning towards music and song as a career with his soprano voice both of which he could not follow due to **malaria** in his youth and gouty arthritis in later years.

In 1761, Frank began studying at Metz, then in Pont-a-Mousson the following year where he decided to focus on physics. The 18-year-old Frank then journeyed to Heidelberg to begin his studies in medicine. He spent two years there at Heidelberg, but concluded his training at the University of Strassburg. During medical school, Frank showed a strong interest in the basic issues of clinical medicine, such as the promotion of the **smallpox** inoculation that would be a precursor to his life's work.

Well versed in numerous languages, including Italian, English, Dutch, Latin, German, and French, Frank could fulfill his needs of restlessness that took him throughout Europe with each career move. After practicing for two years at Bitsch, Lorraine, he returned to practice in Baden, Germany. The events that would follow this move would forever strengthen his resolve to prepare an encyclopedic treatise of public health. After puerperal fever caused complications during a difficult labor that ended the life of his young wife, with his child's death occurring a few months later, Frank immediately focused on the study of obstetrics and **midwifery** in relation to public health. This focus lead him to the position of director of the Midwives Association in Baden, and an investigator of a typhus fever epidemic in Gernsbach by the court at Rastadt. Subsequent positions included court and garrison physician, and town and country physician in Bruschal. The next year, 1773, he began his position of physician to the Prince-Bishop of Speyer who commended his ideas on health reform. This support led to the founding of an obstetrics school where Frank served actively as a faculty member.

During 1779, Frank would unveil what would be the most important principles of public hygiene during this time in his *System einer vollständigen medizinischen Polizey*. With proposals for strict legislation that would ensure a legitimate way of life ''from womb to tomb,'' Frank's recommendations included chapters on conjugal hygiene, the protection of women engaged in manual labor, education of children, and proper hygiene in schools. While an immediate call to attention was needed on issues presented in his encyclopedic work, Frank proved to be ahead of his time his ideas of public and private health measures were only partly accomplished by public officials two centuries later.

When the fourth volume of *System* was published seven years later, Frank became well known throughout Europe. At this time he received offers from the University of Mainz as professor of physiology and preventive medicine, and a chance at a professorship of clinical medicine from Göttingen and Pavia. He chose Göttingen, and beginning in 1784 his days consisted of ward rounds, and lecturing on physiology, pathology, and therapeutics. After one year at Göttingen, Frank yearned for a position that would allow him more time to write and promote his national health reform: he then decided to immediately move to Pavia to begin his position in clinical medicine.

For nine years, Frank called Pavia home and brought a vast amount of change to the university. He upgraded the medical faculty, established new professional chairs, improved the guidelines of the practice of midwifery, and founded a museum of pathological anatomy, a surgical clinic, and an **apothecary** school. Also at this time, Frank presented the first volume of his treatment of diseases of man, *De curandis hominum morbis pitome*. This was expanded to six volumes and translated into numerous languages. He also published a series of clinical lectures and case reports a total of 12 volumes were resented between 1785 and 1793.

A need for change brought Frank to Vienna to begin his position as director of the Allgemeines Krankenhaus and a professorship at the University. His energy brought a variety of transformations, including a new postmortem room, a museum of pathological anatomy, and increased the number of available beds. With the emergence of a smallpox epidemic in 1800, Frank was able to vaccinate with **Edward Jenner**'s cowpox derived immunization. his event led to a government order that recommended vaccination for the entire population taking Frank's efforts one step closer to his ultimate goal. Following this time, he left Vienna for Russia. After one year at the University of Vilna, he went to serve the Czar as physician-in-ordinary and director of the Medico-Surgical Academy for three years.

As he aged, Frank dealt with **gout** and decreasing energy, and this led to his decision to reject Napoleon's request to be his personal physician, and instead retire to Freiburg to finalize the fifth volume of his encyclopedic work, *System*. Frank returned to Vienna in 1811 to continue a large clinical practice and write his sixth volume. He stayed there until his death in 1821.

Delivering the message of sound health and hygiene guided Frank throughout his life. With topics such as premarital sex education, suitable clothing for women, and protection and care of illegitimate children, all to be the responsibility of the State, his *System* and Frank's relentless efforts marked the beginning of public health reformation.

See also Apothecary; Community Health; Edward Jenner; Midwifery; Pathology; Smallpox; Vaccination

Franklin, Rosalind Elsie (1920-1958)

British chemist

Deoxyribonucleic acid (DNA) carries the genetic instructions for life. Johann Miescher (1844-1895), a Swiss physician, discovered DNA in 1869 while studying the composition of white blood cells. Nearly one hundred years passed before **James Watson** and **Francis Crick** were credited with the discovery of the actual structure of DNA. Many scientists contributed to this discovery—not the least of whom was Rosalind Franklin.

Franklin was born in London on July 25, 1920. She graduated from Cambridge University in 1941. She conducted experiments using chromatographic techniques and later worked at a laboratory in Paris, France, where she learned to develop x-ray diffraction photographs. In 1951, she used these skills to carefully construct x-ray diffraction photos of DNA under varying degrees of humidity. Together with her colleague, **Maurice Wilkins**, she noted that the pictures showed the molecule to be a helical shape. She remained skeptical, however, that DNA would actually take up a helical form under all conditions.

James Watson was later shown the photographs by Wilkins, apparently without the consent of Franklin. The photographs strongly supported Watson and Crick's hypothesis of a double-stranded helical DNA molecule. In 1953, this model was publicly presented by Watson and Crick. The double-helix, or twisted ladder shape, is made of sugar-phosphate units of nucleotides. These nucleotides form the sides of the ladder. The rungs are formed by four nitrogenous bases, including adenine and guanine (the purines) and thymine and cytosine (the pyrimidines). Each rung consists of two bases. Knowledge of the distances between the atoms, as determined by x-ray diffraction, was crucial in establishing the structure of the DNA model.

Francis Crick admitted in a *Nature* article that "Rosalind Franklin was only two steps away from the solution. She needed to realize that the two chains must run in opposite directions and that the bases, in their correct tautomeric forms, were paired together." Although Franklin was on the verge of solving the mystery of DNA structure, it was during this time that she chose to leave King's College and DNA to study the tobacco mosaic virus. She was instrumental in showing how the nucleic acid molecules of the virus existed in a helical array of repeated protein units.

Perhaps Rosalind Franklin's most amazing accomplishment is the relatively short period of time in which she contributed such valuable scientific information. She died in London of **cancer** on April 16, 1958, at the early age of 37. This was four years before Watson, Crick, and Wilkins received the Nobel Prize in physiology or medicine. Many people believe that Franklin's work has been underestimated due to her untimely death and the female prejudices of the English scientific establishment in the 1950s.

Frerichs, Friedrich Theodor von (1819-1885)

German pathologist

Frerichs is generally recognized as the founder of experimental **pathology**. As a professor of medicine for many years, his insistence on teaching medical biochemistry and pathology as part of the regular curriculum was instrumental in establishing a scientific foundation for clinical medicine.

Born in Aurich, Hanover, Germany, Frerichs received a medical education in his homeland and went on to become a professor of therapeutics and pathology at the illustrious University of Breslau in 1851. During his eight years there, he was known for his strict requirement that all his students' work be based on well designed experiments and precise laboratory analysis. One of the students whose medical career Frerichs helped shape was **Paul Ehrlich**, who would later win a Nobel Prize in Medicine for his research.

While he was working at Breslau, Frerichs also performed his own research on the biochemistry of diseased organisms. Through this work, he became the first scientist to observe the amino acids tyrosine and leucine in urine from **hepatitis** patients with acute yellow liver atrophy. He did extensive work on the pathologies of **nephritis** and liver **cirrhosis**, leading to better diagnostic and treatment methods for liver ailments. His *Treatise on Diseases of the Liver* was published in 1858. Frerichs's other research of note was on the pathology of **diabetes**.

Beginning in 1859, Frerichs served as director of the University of Berlin's Charity Hospital. He remained in that post until his death in 1885.

See also Pathology

FREUD, SIGMUND (1856-1939)

Austrian neurologist

Sigmund Freud was born in Moravia. When he was three years old, his family moved to Vienna, the city where he was to live until the last year of his life. At the age of 17, Freud entered the University of Vienna's medical school, where he pursued a variety of research interests. Although primarily interested in physiological research, Freud was forced to enter into clinical practice due to the difficulty of obtaining a university appointment—aggravated, in his case, by anti-Semitic attitudes and policies. After additional independent research and clinical work at the General Hospital of Vienna, Freud entered private practice, specializing in the treatment of patients with neurological and hysterical disorders.

During this period, Freud learned about his colleague Josef Breuer's "cathartic" treatment of hysterical symptoms, which disappeared when a patient recalled traumatic experiences while under **hypnosis** and was able to express original emotions that had been repressed and forgotten. Pursuing this idea further, Freud spent several months in France studying **Jean-Martin Charcot**'s method of treating hysteria by hypnosis. Upon his return to Vienna, Freud began the task of finding a similar method of treatment that did not require hypnosis, the limitations of which he found unsatisfactory. In addition to learning by observing the symptoms and experiences of his patients, Freud also engaged in a rigorous self-analysis based on his own dreams. In 1895, he and Breuer published *Studies on Hysteria,* a landmark text in the history of **psychoanalysis**, and in 1900 Freud's own groundbreaking work, *The Interpretation of Dreams,* appeared.

By this time, Freud had worked out the essential components of his system of psychoanalysis, including the use of free association and catharsis as a method of exploring the unconscious, identifying repressed memories and the reasons for their repression, and enabling patients to know themselves more fully. The patient, relaxed on a couch in his office, was directed to engage in a free association of ideas that could yield useful insights; the patient was asked to reveal frankly whatever came to mind. Through both his work with patients and his own self-analysis, Freud came to believe that mental disorders that have no apparent physiological cause are symbolic reactions to psychological shocks, usually of a sexual nature, and that the memories associated with these shocks, although repressed in the unconscious, indirectly affect the content not only of dreams but of conscious activity.

Freud published *The Psychopathology of Everyday Life* in 1904 and three more works the following year, including *Three Essays on the Theory of Sexuality,* which set forth his ideas about the development of the human sex instinct, or libido, including his theory of childhood sexuality and the Oedipus complex. While recognition from the scientific community and the general public was slow in coming, by the early 1900s Freud had attracted a circle of followers, including **Carl Jung**, Alfred Adler, and Otto Rank (1884-1939), who held weekly discussion meetings at his home and later became known as the Vienna Psychological Society. Although Jung and Adler were eventually to break with Freud, forming their own theories and schools of analysis, their early support helped establish psychoanalysis as a movement of international importance. In 1909, Freud was invited to speak at Clark University in Worcester, Massachusetts, by its president, the distinguished psychologist G. Stanley Hall (1844-1924), and was awarded an honorary doctorate. After World War I, Freud gained increasing fame as psychoanalysis became fashionable in intellectual circles and was popularized by the media.

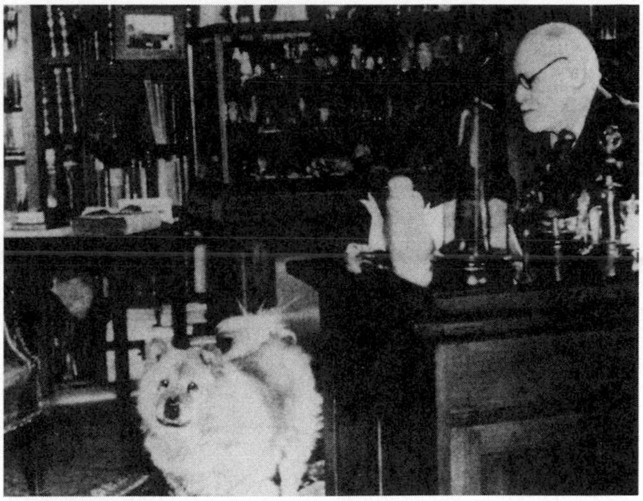

Sigmund Freud

Freud contended that the human personality is governed by forces called "instincts" or "drives." Later, he came to believe in the existence of a death instinct, or death wish (Thanatos), directed either outward as aggression or inward as self-destructive behavior (noted mainly as repetition compulsions). He constructed a comprehensive theory on the structure of the psyche, which he viewed as divided into three parts. The id, corresponding to the unconscious, is concerned with the satisfaction of primitive desires and with self-preservation. It operates according to the pleasure principle and outside the realm of social rules or moral dictates. The ego, associated with reason, controls the forces of the id to bring it into line with the reality principle and make socialization possible, and it channels the forces of the id into acceptable activities. The critical, moral superego—or conscience—developed in early childhood, monitors and censors the ego, turning external values into internalized, self-imposed rules with which to inhibit the id. Freud viewed individual behavior as the result of the interaction among these three components of the psyche.

At the core of Freud's psychological structure is the repression of unfulfilled instinctual demands. An unconscious process, repression is accomplished through a series of defense mechanisms. Those most commonly named by Freud include denial (failure to perceive the source of anxiety); rationalization (justification of an action by an acceptable motive); displacement (directing repressed feelings toward an acceptable substitute); projection (attributing one's own unacceptable impulse to others); and sublimation (transforming an unacceptable instinctual demand into a socially acceptable activity).

Freud continued modifying his theories in the 1920s and changed a number of his fundamental views, including his theories of motivation and **anxiety**. In 1923, he developed **cancer** of the jaw (he had been a heavy cigar smoker throughout his life) and underwent numerous operations for this disease over the next 16 years. Life in Vienna became increasingly precarious for Freud with the rise of Nazism in the 1930s, and he emigrated to London in 1938, only to die of his illness the following year. Many of the concepts and theories Freud introduced—such as the role of the unconscious, the effect of childhood experiences on adult behavior, and the operation of defense mechanisms—continue to be a source of both controversy and inspiration. His books include *Totem and Taboo* (1913), *General Introduction to Psychoanalysis* (1916), *The Ego and the Id* (1923), and *Civilization and Its Discontents* (1930).

See also Carl Jung; Psychoanalysis; Psychosis

FRISCH, KARL VON (1886-1982)

Austrian zoologist

Karl von Frisch won the Nobel Prize in 1973 for his pioneering work in the field of animal physiology and behavior. Frisch was a leading researcher in the study of insect behavior, and his studies proved that fish have acute hearing and that bees communicate effectively through a ritual dance. Frisch's discoveries and subsequent Nobel Prize were also significant because this was the first major acknowledgement of advances made in the study of ethology.

Frisch was born in Vienna in 1886 into a family dedicated to science. His father, Anton Ritter von Frisch, was a physician, and his mother, Marie Exner, came from a long line of distinguished scientists and scholars. From his earliest years, Frisch was exposed to the natural world, in large part due to a country house that his family retreated to every summer. There, the young Frisch spent his time collecting various species of animals. ''Even before I went to school,'' he wrote in his autobiography, *A Biologist Remembers,* ''I had a little zoo in my room.'' But Frisch was not simply a collector; he was also a keen observer. ''I discovered that miraculous worlds may reveal themselves to a patient observer where the casual passer-by sees nothing at all,'' he said in his autobiography. A few early observations—most notably that the sea animals he collected in an aquarium in his room waved their tentacles when he turned on the lights—piqued an interest in the sensory systems of animals that would last his lifetime.

By the time Frisch reached college age, it was clear that his interests were focused on zoology. Nevertheless, his father thought medicine a more practical field than zoology, and in 1905 Frisch enrolled as a student of medicine at the University of Vienna. Medical school, Frisch later wrote, proved invaluable in providing a background in histology, anatomy and human physiology. He studied with his uncle, Sigmund Exner, who was a renowned physiologist and lecturer at the university. Though Exner taught human physiology, he encouraged his nephew to pursue his interest in animals by aiding him in a research project on the position of pigments in the compound eyes of certain beetles, butterflies and crustaceans. According to Frisch, his uncle's openness toward the study of animals in a course limited to human physiology was unheard of at the time. Comparing the physiology of humans and animals would only later be seen as so invaluable that it was made into a separate discipline. In the middle of his third year as a medical student, Frisch found himself increasingly frustrated by the ''medical character'' of the curriculum. He finally decided to drop his medical studies to pursue the field of ethology, or the study of animal behavior. He transferred to the Zoological Institute at the University of Munich, where he studied under Richard von Hertwig. He continued to cultivate the interests he had developed under his uncle's leadership, researching light perception and color changes in minnows. It was at this time that he discovered minnows had an area on the forehead filled with sensory cells—a ''third, very primitive eye,'' he called it in *A Biologist Remembers.* This explained why blind minnows reacted to light by changing color in the same way as minnows with sight. Frisch wrote his doctoral thesis on this subject and received his degree in 1910.

Frisch also began to question the common assumption of the time that fish and all invertebrates were color blind. He successfully trained minnows to respond to colored objects, proving that they could perceive color. These findings, however, were not kindly received by members of the scientific community, and Frisch's most notable opponent was Karl von Hess, the director of Munich Eye Clinic. The debate arose partly because of the theoretical connection between Frisch and the views of the famous naturalist Charles Darwin. Frisch believed in Darwinism, which theorized that the survival of certain species of animals depended on the development of their senses. Frisch hypothesized that animal behavior, rather than simply being a fixed mechanism, had an ''adaptive biological significance,'' assumptions that were still a source of disagreement among scientists at the time. Despite the arguments about his research, Frisch was offered a teaching job at the University of Munich in 1921.

While teaching at the University of Munich, Frisch continued to study color perception in animals on vacations spent at his family's summer home. Having proved that **color-blindness** in fish was a fallacy, he turned to prove the same for bees. He conjectured that the adaptive purpose of the bright coloration of flowers was to guide bees to nectar. The bees, in turn, aided the flowers through pollination. That bees would be color-blind seemed untenable to Frisch. To test his hypothesis, he used research strategies similar to the ones he had used with fish. He conditioned their behavior by placing drops of sugar water on squares of blue-colored cardboard. He then placed these blue squares among plain gray squares. Eventually, he placed blue squares without sugar water among the gray squares. He found that the bees continued to go to the blue squares for their food, proving that they could differentiate color.

In 1914 Frisch's research was interrupted by the outbreak of World War I. He was excused from military duty because of poor eyesight but accepted a plea from his brother, who was a physician, to volunteer at a Red Cross hospital in dire need of help. His background in medical school qualified him to establish a bacteriologic laboratory at the hospital, enabling rapid diagnosis of diseases such as **cholera**, dysentery and **typhoid**. While at the hospital, he met a nurse, Margarethe Mohr, whom he married in 1917. Eventually they had three daughters and a son.

Meanwhile his research on bees continued to deepen. During the war, he would take a few weeks' leave from the hospital every summer, returning to his country house to research the bees. As the war came to an end, his work at the hospital lessened and his students returned to the Zoological Institute. After a 4-year hiatus, he began teaching again and in January 1919 became an assistant professor.

Eventually Frisch became interested in scout bees—those that left the hive to explore a region for food. He set out dishes of sugar water and observed their behavior. When the dish was empty a scout bee occasionally came to the dish. When the food dish was full the scout would return in a matter of minutes with a whole company of bees. "It was clear to me that the bee community possessed an excellent intelligence function," Frisch wrote in his autobiography, "but how it functioned I did not know."

In the spring of 1919 Frisch developed a glass cage in which he placed a single honeycomb that could be observed from all sides. Through continuous observation and experimentation, Frisch concluded that scout bees, who foraged for food for the whole honeycomb, conveyed this information to the other bees by performing a kind of dance on the honeycomb. This dance excited the forager bees, who then flew directly to the food. In retrospect, Frisch called his first discovery of the bees' dance "the most far-reaching observation of my life." It would be another 20 years before Frisch fully understood the complexity of this dance.

In the fall of 1921, Frisch was appointed professor of zoology and director of the Zoologic Institute at Rostock University and began investigating whether fish could hear. The physiology of fish indicated that they could not. They did not have any of the characteristics thought to be necessary for the sense of hearing, like ear lobes, auditory canals, middle ears, or a cochlea in the inner ear, which was thought to be the center of hearing in humans. Frisch used his proven methods of behavior conditioning to test hearing in fish. He whistled to blind catfish before feeding them. Eventually he whistled but did not feed them and the catfish continued to respond. The answer seemed simple—or, as one skeptical scientist put it, "There is no doubt. The fish comes when you whistle." Frisch eventually refined his early research in this area with the help of his students and discovered other facts that supported his initial findings.

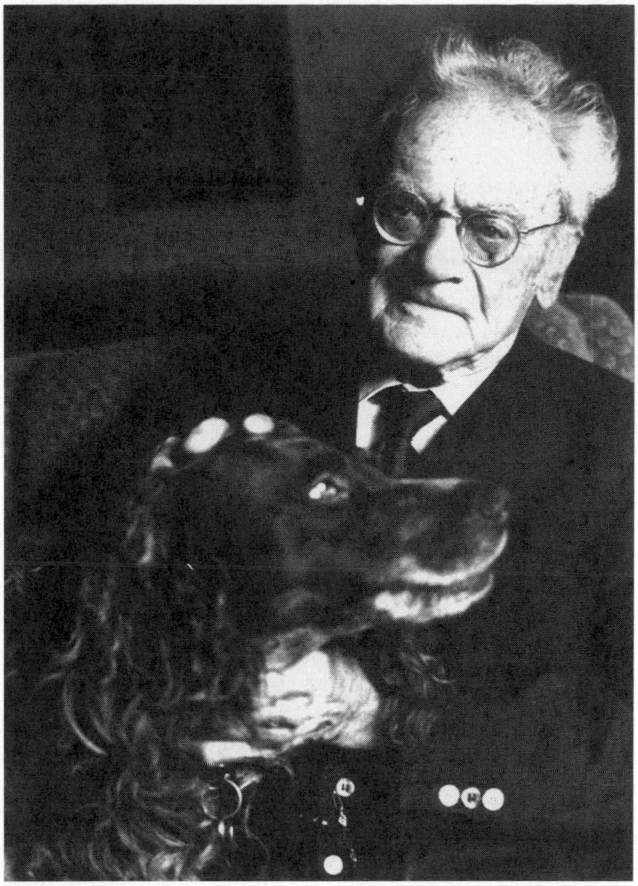
Karl von Frisch

In 1925 Frisch began working at the Zoological Institute of the University of Munich. However, during World War II, the Zoological Institute at the University was destroyed, and Frisch spent those years in his country home and at the University of Graz. In 1950 he returned to Munich to rebuild the Institute as its director. During this time, he wrote many books for the general public as well as for the scientific community. Frisch retired in 1958 and died in 1982.

About his life's work, Frisch wrote philosophically in *A Biologist Remembers:* "The layman may wonder why a biologist is content to devote 50 years of his life to the study of bees and minnows without ever branching out into research on, say, elephants, or at any rate the lice of elephants or the fleas of moles. The answer to any such question must be that every single species of the animal kingdom challenges us with all, or nearly all, the mysteries of life."

This attitude was shared by the Nobel committee, who rewarded him with the prize in medicine and physiology in 1973. The prize, which Frisch shared with two other animal behaviorists, **Konrad Lorenz** and **Nikolaas Tinbergen**, was a departure for the Nobel Committee. Never before had there been such public recognition of the interactive study of animals and humans. In an article in *Science* magazine regarding the Nobel Prize, Frisch was praised for teaching the world that "human behavior [is not] something... outside nature" but something that is "subject to the principles that mold the biology, adaptability and the survival of other organisms."

FROSTBITE AND FROSTNIP

Frostbite is damage to the skin and other tissues caused by freezing. Frostnip is a mild form of cold injury. In North America, frostbite is largely confined to Alaska, Canada, and the northern states. Recently, there has been a substantial decline in the number of cases and a change in the type of people at-risk, as outdoor winter activities have grown more popular and there are more homeless people. Exposure to temperatures a little below the freezing mark can take hours for skin to freeze, but very cold skin can freeze in minutes or seconds. Air temperature, wind speed, and moisture all affect how cold the skin becomes. The extent of permanent injury depends upon how long the skin and tissues remain frozen. Homeless people and others lacking strong self-preservation instincts face a greater risk of frostbite-related **amputation** because they are more likely to stay out in the cold when they should seek shelter or medical attention. Alcohol and **smoking** can increase the severity of injury. Other risk factors include inadequate clothing, previous cold injury, fatigue, wound infection, **atherosclerosis** (an arterial disease), and **diabetes**. Driving in poor weather can also be dangerous.

Frostbite injury is due to tissue freezing, tissue hypoxia, and the release of inflammatory mediators. Tissue freezing causes ice crystal formation and other changes that damage and kill cells. Tissue hypoxia (oxygen deficiency) occurs when the blood vessels in the hands, feet, and other extremities narrow in response to cold. Hypoxia, blood clots, and endothelial damage lead to the release of inflammatory mediators (substances that act as links in the inflammatory process), which cause further endothelial damage, hypoxia, and cell destruction. Frostbite is classified by degree of injury (first, second, third, or fourth), or type (superficial and deep). Ninety percent of frostbite injuries affect the feet or hands. The remainder involve the ears, nose, cheeks, or penis. Once frostbite sets in, the affected part begins to feel cold and numb; this is followed by clumsiness. The skin turns white or yellowish. As the skin begins to thaw, **edema** (excess tissue fluid) often accumulates, causing swelling. In second- and higher-degree frostbite, blisters appear. Third-degree cases produce deep, blood-filled blisters and, later, a hard black scab. Fourth-degree frostbite penetrates below the skin to the muscles, tendons, nerves, and bones. In severe cases the dead tissue can drop off. Infection is possible. Like frostbite, frostnip is associated with ice crystal formation in the tissues, but the tissues aren't destroyed and the crystals dissolve when skin is warmed. Frostnip generally affects the earlobes, cheeks, nose, fingers, and toes. The skin turns pale and feels numb or tingly until warming begins.

Frostbite is diagnosed by a **physical examination** and may include x rays, **angiography** (x ray examination of the blood vessels using an injected dye), thermography (a heat-sensitive device to measure blood flow), and other tests. Diagnostic tests are only useful 3–5 days after rewarming, once the blood vessels have stabilized. Emergency medical help is necessary when frostbite is suspected. While waiting for help to arrive, remove wet or tight clothing and put on dry, loose clothing or wraps. Use a splint and padding to protect the injured area. Never rub the area with snow or anything else. Avoid partial thawing and refreezing, which makes the injury worse. Keep the affected part away from heat sources such as campfires and car heaters. Rewarm in the field only when emergency help will take more than two hours to arrive and refreezing can be prevented. Hospital treatment begins by rapidly rewarming the affected part to stop ice crystal formation and dilate narrowed blood vessels. Aloe vera is applied, and the affected part is splinted, elevated, and wrapped in a dressing. Blisters may be cleaned. A **tetanus** shot and, possibly, penicillin, are used to prevent infection, and ibuprofen is given to fight inflammation. Narcotics are usually needed to reduce pain. Treatment generally requires a hospital stay of several days, during which **hydrotherapy** and physical therapy restore the affected part to health. Experts recommend that 22–45 days must pass before a decision on amputation can safely be made. For frostnip in fingers, blow air on them or hold them under the armpits; cover other frostnipped areas with the hands. Never rub the injured areas. To speed recovery after leaving the hospital, alternative practitioners suggest: bathing the affected part in warm water or using contrast hydrotherapy (a series of hot and cold water applications), nutritional therapy, homeopathic and botanical therapies, **acupuncture**, and **oxygen therapy**.

Prolonged frostbite symptoms include throbbing pain, tingling, a burning sensation, or a sensation resembling electric shocks. Possible consequences of frostbite include skin—color changes, nail deformation or loss, joint stiffness and pain, hyperhidrosis (excessive sweating), and heightened sensitivity to cold. A degree of sensory loss lasts at least four years—and sometimes a lifetime. Frostbite can be prevented. Appropriate clothing and footwear are essential. Clothing should be worn loosely and in layers. The hands, feet, and head should be covered. Outer garments should be wind and water resistant, and wet clothing and footwear must be replaced quickly. Avoid alcohol, drugs, and smoking. Pay close attention to the weather and avoid unnecessary risks such as driving in isolated areas during a blizzard.

FULLER, SOLOMON (1872-1953)

Liberian African American neurologist and psychiatrist

Solomon Fuller, the first black psychiatrist in the United States, played a key role in the development of psychiatry in the 1900s. Known for his research on **dementia,** Fuller helped make the United States the leader in psychiatry that it is today. In addition, as a professor at Boston University School of Medicine for more than 30 years, Fuller helped train the next generation of psychiatrists.

Solomon Carter Fuller was born on August 11, 1872 in Monrovia, Liberia. His family, however, had American roots;

his grandfather, John Lewis Fuller, had been a slave in Virginia who had been able to buy his freedom and move his family to Liberia. Solomon's father, also named Solomon, was a coffee planter and an official in the Liberian government. His mother, Anna Ursala James, whose parents were physicians and missionaries, set up a school to teach Carter and other area children. Fuller's early education also included six years—from age 10 to 16—at the College Preparatory School of Monrovia.

In 1889, at the age of 17, Fuller left Liberia to attend Livingstone College in North Carolina. He graduated in 1893, began studying medicine at Long Island College Hospital, and later transferred to Boston University School of Medicine. Fuller received his M.D. degree in 1897. Upon graduation, Fuller accepted a position as intern and official helper in the pathology lab at Westborough State Hospital in Massachusetts. After two years he was promoted to pathologist, a position in which he remained for 22 years. Fuller was also a consultant to the hospital for an additional 23 years.

At the same time that he was beginning his career in medicine, Fuller also became a member of the medical faculty at Boston University School of Medicine. He taught at BUSM for 34 years, becoming, in turn, an instructor, lecturer, associate professor, and emeritus professor of neurology.

According to Robert H. Sharpley in George E. Gifford, Jr.'s *Psychoanalysis, Psychotherapy, and the New England Medical Scene, 1844–1944,* Fuller's decision to pursue a career in neurology and psychiatry was influenced by a lecture at the American Medico-Psychological Association given by neurologist S. Weir Mitchell. According to Sharpley, Mitchell, in his lecture, criticized hospitals for not studying mental illness. In addition, he called for hospitals to study both the pathology and psychology of their patients. Fuller followed Mitchell's advice by collecting and analyzing data on patients with various mental disorders, Sharpley says. To further his knowledge, in 1900 Fuller took advanced courses at the Carnegie Laboratory in New York. He then went to Europe in 1904, studying under Emil Kraepelin and Alois Alzheimer, professors at the University of Munich's psychiatric clinic. Once back in the United States, Fuller continued his work at Westborough and BUSM. Fuller became known for his work on **Alzheimer's disease,** a degenerative neurological disorder in which memory, judgment, and the ability to reason progressively deteriorate. He also focused his research on the organic causes of disorders such as **schizophrenia** and manic-depressive psychosis (now called **bipolar disorder**). Finally, Fuller practiced psychiatry, which he continued past his retirement.

Fuller helped develop the neuropsychiatric unit at the Veterans Administration Hospital in Tuskegee, Alabama, personally training the doctors who went on to head the department. According to Sharpley, Fuller's knowledge of the venereal disease, syphilis later helped these doctors diagnose syphilis in black World War II veterans who had been misdiagnosed with behavioral disorders.

In 1909 Fuller married Meta Vaux Warrick, a sculptor who had at one point studied under Rodin. Fuller and his wife had three sons. In his personal life, Fuller enjoyed photography, gardening, and book binding. Though he became blind in his later years, by all reports he continued to work, seeing patients and reading via "talking books." Fuller died on January 16, 1953. Though Fuller hated being called "an excellent black psychiatrist," he is remembered to this day both for his work and for his pioneering role as the first black psychiatrist. The mental health facility at Boston University is now officially known as the Dr. Solomon Carter Fuller Mental Health Center. And in 1972, the American Psychiatric Association and the Black Psychiatrists of America established the Solomon Carter Fuller Institute.

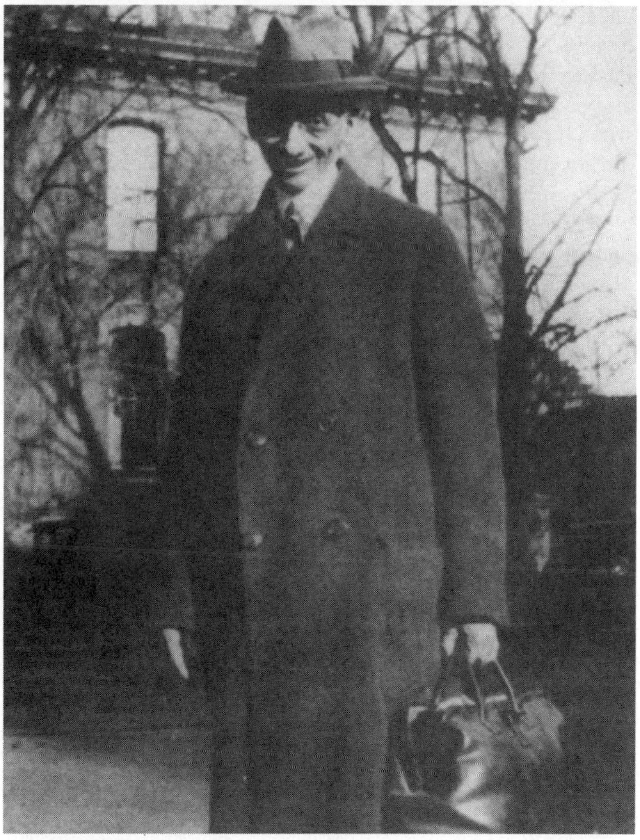

Solomon Fuller

FUNK, CASIMIR (1884-1967)

Polish-American biochemist

A biochemist and a forerunner in the field of nutritional science, Funk discovered that many human diseases are caused by a lack of certain nutrients that are readily available in some foods. He found cures for such devastating illnesses as **beriberi**, **pellagra**, ricketts, and **scurvy** based on this finding. Funk later did extensive research on hormones.

Funk was born in Warsaw, Poland, the son of a renowned dermatologist. As a young man, he studied organic chemistry at Switzerland's University of Berne, from which he received his Ph.D. in 1904. Afterward, Funk worked at the Pasteur Institute in Paris until 1906, then sporadically at the University of Berlin as an assistant. It was not until 1910, when he accepted an offer to work at London's Lister Institute of Preventative Medicine, that Funk's career as a scientist truly began. In this position, he was assigned to research beriberi, a common illness in the Far East that causes peripheral nerve damage and eventually heart failure. Scientists thought that the disease might be due to insufficient dietary protein, but Funk disregarded this notion and began experiments to determine what was absent in the typical Far Eastern diet of polished rice.

Funk discovered in 1911 that the bran, the partly ground husk of the rice grain that was usually thrown out in Far Eastern cultures, contained a vital substance called thiamine that prevents beriberi. Later that year, he isolated a substance now known as niacin (vitamin B_1), but he stopped researching it when he realized it did not prevent beriberi. He named thiamine and niacin "vitamines" after the Latin word for "life" and "amine" because he believed (incorrectly) that all these vital ingredients contained nitrogen. The word later became "**vitamins.**" When he published his findings in 1912, Funk immediately became well known in the scientific world, while people around the world soon began asking about these seemingly miraculous substances. Funk's famous book *The Vitamin* was published in 1913.

Funk left the Lister Institute later in 1913 to become head of the Biochemistry Department at the Cancer Hospital Research Institute in London. He remained there for two years, then moving to the United States after accepting a better paying job at New York's Cornell Medical College as a chemical researcher in **cancer**. In 1917, Funk became head of research at H. A. Metz and Company, where he remained until 1921. While at Metz, Funk developed Oscodol (a vitamin A and D concentrate) and Salvarsan (an arsenic-based treatment for **syphilis**).

After working as a biochemistry associate at Columbia University's College of Physicians and Surgeons from 1921 to 1923, Funk decided to return to his native country. He took a post in Warsaw as director of the State Institute of Hygiene's Biochemical Department, where he became interested in the function of hormones. In 1924 he showed that the pituitary gland's posterior portion produces hormones that regulate water balance and affect muscles.

Funk left Poland again in 1927 as the country's political climate worsened. At his own private laboratory called Casa Biochemica in Paris, he soon discovered that the sex hormones estrogen and testosterone are effective in treating some diseases. He also managed to extract the male hormone androsterone from human urine in 1929. Despite the progress he was making, Funk returned permanently to the United States when World War II started. He began a job in New York as a consulting scientist for the U.S. Vitamin Corporation, and in 1940 he became president of the Funk Foundation for Medical Research. He died in 1967.

See also Vitamins

FURCHGOTT, ROBERT (1916-)

American pharmacologist

Furchgott was one of three American pharmacologists who received the 1998 Nobel Prize in Physiology or Medicine for discoveries related to the role of nitric oxide as a signaling molecule in the **cardiovascular system.** His co-recipients were **Ferid Murad** and **Louis Ignarro.**

Not to be confused with **nitrous oxide** (a gas used in **anesthesia**), nitric oxide is a colorless, odorless gas that, thanks to initial work by these three Nobel laureates and a flurry of subsequent research by others, now has widespread potential including the treatment of heart disease, **shock, cancer, impotence,** and pulmonary **hypertension**—a potentially fatal condition in premature infants. In 1994, the respected journal *Science* declared nitric oxide as its "molecule of the year."

Born in Charleston, South Carolina, Furchgott moved with his parents to Orangeburg in the same state, where his maternal grandparents lived and his father set up a clothing store. There, the youthful Furchgott is best remembered for his scrappy play in Orangeburg High School's 14-6 win over Rock Hill High School to win the 1931 state football championship.

He studied chemistry at the University of North Carolina and biochemistry at Northwestern University, before accepting a professorship in pharmacology in 1956 at State University of New York (SUNY), where he became department chair and performed most of the research which earned him the Nobel Prize. Since 1988, he has been a distinguished professor at SUNY.

During the 1950s, Furchgott developed a method for determining how blood vessels respond to medications, neurotransmitters and hormones, using a piece of rabbit aorta cut in the form of a helix. This allowed him to study the effects of drugs on vascular smooth muscle. Another early contribution was his discovery that such muscle relaxes when exposed to ultraviolet light, a phenomenon known as photo-relaxation.

Furchgott's major research advance came in 1980, when he discovered a substance in the endothelium (a thin layer of flattened cells lining the inner surface of blood vessels) that caused relaxation in smooth muscle. He called this substance endothelium-derived relaxing factor (EDRF).

Earlier, Ferid Murad had postulated that nitric oxide and other nitrogen-containing compounds might be produced by one cell, travel through membranes, and then regulate the function other cells. At the time, this was an entirely new concept for signaling in biological systems. After six year years of further work, Furchgott discovered that his EDRF was, in reality, nitric oxide operating as Murid had suggested. Furchgott announced this important development in 1986 at a scientific conference at the Mayo Clinic in Rochester, Minnesota. At the same meeting, Louis Ignarro announced he had independently confirmed that EDRF was nitric oxide, using spectral analysis.

Nitric oxide is now known to play a key role in many biological functions including inflammation, blood flow regulation, cell growth, smooth muscle relaxation, and preserving memory.

G

GAJDUSEK, D. CARLETON (1923-)

American virologist

Gajdusek was born in Yonkers, New York, on September 9, 1923, the son of Hungarian immigrants. His parents provided a rich intellectual environment at home, and Gajdusek became interested in science at an early age. While still in high school, he spent summers working at the Boyce Thompson Institute for Plant Research in Yonkers. Gajdusek entered the University of Rochester in 1940 at the age of 16. He graduated with a bachelor of science degree in biophysics three years later. In 1946, he also received an M.D. from Harvard Medical School.

In the eight years following graduation from Harvard, Gajdusek completed residencies in Boston, Massachusetts, and New York City, New York, worked for two years at the California Institute of Technology with Linus Pauling, did research in virology at Harvard with John Enders, served in the United States Army at the Walter Reed Medical Center, and continued his studies in Iran at the Pasteur Institute. Finally, in 1954, he moved to the Walter and Eliza Hall Institute of Medical Research in Melbourne, Australia, to carry out additional research in virology.

During his tenure at the Hall Institute, Gajdusek learned about an unusual disease that infected members of the Fore tribe in New Guinea. The disease—called kuru—caused a slow, but ultimately fatal, degeneration of the brain and had never been studied by medical scientists. Gajdusek decided to travel to New Guinea, where he spent a year learning more about kuru.

Gajdusek spent much of the next decade trying to discover the causative agent for kuru. He felt sure that the disease was caused by a virus. An important clue was that the Fore, in a ritualistic practice, honored their dead by eating their brains. Gajdusek reasoned that this practice would be an ideal mechanism by which a viral infection could be transmitted from one person to another.

However, standard techniques for identifying viruses produced no results in this case. For a while, Gajdusek considered the possibility that kuru might be a hereditary disorder rather than an infectious disease.

In 1963 another possibility occurred to him. He realized that kuru was similar in some ways to scrapie, a neurological disorder that affects sheep. Scrapie begins to appear in sheep long after they have been infected. The incubation period can be many years. Scientists believed that scrapie was caused by an unusual type of virus that acts extremely slowly.

Gajdusek considered the possibility that kuru is also caused by a slow-acting virus. To test this hypothesis, he implanted pieces taken from the brains of kuru victims into apes. More than two years later, the disease began to appear in the apes. Evidence for the existence of a scrapie-like, slow-moving viral infection appeared to exist.

Gajdusek's success with his kuru research prompted him to attack other unexplained brain diseases. In 1971, he found that a slow-moving virus might also be responsible for **Creutzfeldt-Jacob disease**, a degenerative brain disorder that occurs throughout the world. For his work on slow-moving viruses, Gajdusek received a share of the 1976 Nobel Prize for physiology or medicine.

Some scientists now believe that the slow-moving virus responsible for scrapie, kuru, and Creutzfeldt-Jacob disease is actually a new type of infectious particle called a prion. First suggested in 1982 by American neurologist **Stanley Prusiner** (1942-), the prion is thought to be a naked piece of protein that has the ability to cause certain types of viral-like diseases.

In 1997, Gajdusek admitted in a Maryland circuit court that he had sexually molested a 17-year-old boy. The boy was one of more than 50 children he had brought back to the United States since the 1960s from the South Pacific. These children often lived with Gajdusek, who financed their educations. As a part of his plea bargain, Gajdusek received a one-year prison sentence and five years probation. While he has been sued in civil court for $2.2 million by one of the boys he took in, others he adopted rallied around Gajdusek and supported him during his trial. He retired from his position as chief of the Laboratory

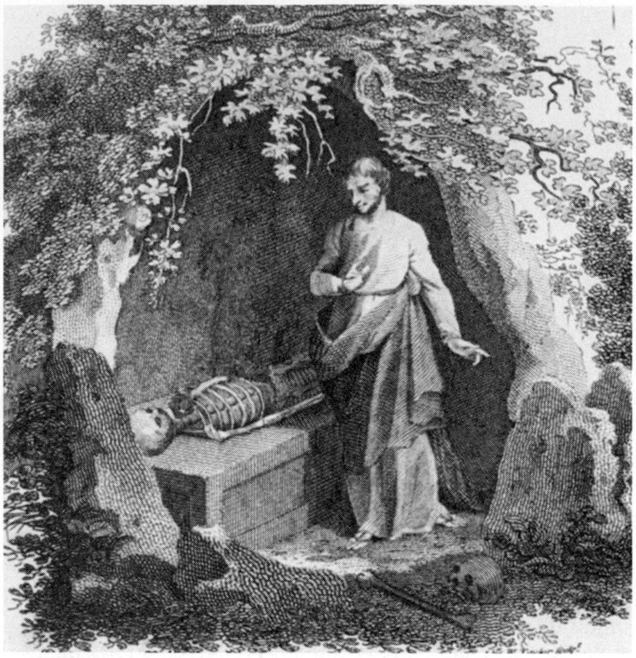

Galen

of Central Nervous Systems at the National Institutes of Health in 1997.

GALEN (130-200)

Greek physician

Galen, the last and most influential of the great ancient medical practitioners, was born in Pergamum, Asia Minor. His father, the architect Nicon, is supposed to have prepared Galen for a career in medicine following the instructions given him in a dream by the god of medicine, Asclepius. Accordingly, Galen studied philosophy, mathematics, and logic in his youth and then began his medical training at age sixteen at the medical school of Pergamum attached to the local shrine of Asclepius. At age twenty, Galen embarked on extensive travels, broadening his medical knowledge with studies at Smyrna, Corinth, and Alexandria. At Alexandria, the preeminent research and teaching center of the time, Galen was able to study skeletons (although not actual bodies).

Returning to Pergamum at age twenty-eight, Galen became physician to the gladiators, which gave him great opportunities for observations about human anatomy and physiology. In 161 A.D., Galen moved to Rome and quickly established a successful practice after curing several eminent people, including the philosopher Eudemus. Galen also conducted public lectures and demonstrations, began writing some of his major works on anatomy and physiology, and frequently engaged in polemics with fellow physicians. In A.D. 174, Galen was summoned to treat Marcus Aurelius and became the emperor's personal physician.

Galen once again returned to Pergamum in A.D. 166, perhaps to escape the quarreling, perhaps to avoid an outbreak of **plague** in Rome. After a few years, Galen was summoned back to Rome by Marcus Aurelius. He became physician to two subsequent emperors, Commodus and Septimius Severvs, and seems to have stayed in Rome for the rest of his career, probably dying there in about A.D. 199.

Galen was an astonishingly prolific writer, producing hundreds of works, of which about 120 have survived. His most important contributions were in anatomy. Galen expertly dissected and accurately observed all kinds of animals, but sometimes mistakenly—because human dissection was forbidden—applied what he saw to the human body. Nevertheless, his descriptions of bones and muscle were notable; he was the first to observe that muscles work in contracting pairs. He described the heart valves and the structural differences between arteries and veins. He used experiments to demonstrate paralysis resulting from spinal cord severing, control of the larynx through the laryngeal nerve, and passage of urine from kidneys to bladder. An excellent clinician, Galen pioneered diagnostic use of the pulse rate and described cardiac arrhythmias. Galen also collected therapeutic plants in his extensive travels and explained their uses.

In his observations about the heart and blood vessels, however, Galen made critical errors that remained virtually unchallenged for 1,400 years. He correctly recognized that blood passes from the right to the left side of the heart, but decided this was accomplished through minute pores in the septum, rather than through the pulmonary circulation. Like **Erasistratus**, Galen believed that blood formed in the liver and was circulated from there throughout the body in the veins. He did show that arteries contain blood, but thought they also contained and distributed *pneuma*, a vital spirit. In a related idea, Galen believed that the brain generated and transmitted another vital spirit through the (hollow) nerves to the muscles, allowing movement and sensation.

After Galen, experimental physiology and anatomical research ceased for many centuries. Galen's teachings became the ultimate medical authority, approved by the newly ascendant Christian church because of Galen's belief in a divine purpose for all things, even the structure and functioning of the human body. The medical world moved on from Galenism only with the appearance of **Andreas Vesalius**'s work on anatomy in 1543 and **William Harvey**'s work on blood circulation in 1628.

GALL BLADDER DISORDERS

There are various disorders that affect the gall bladder, and they usually involve gallstones.

A gallstone is a solid crystal deposit that forms in the gallbladder, which is a pear-shaped organ that stores bile salts until they are needed to help digest fatty foods. Gallstones can migrate to other parts of the digestive tract and cause severe **pain** with life-threatening complications.

Gallstones vary in size and chemical structure. A gallstone may be as tiny as a grain of sand or as large as a golf ball. 80 percent of gallstones are composed of cholesterol. They are formed when the liver produces more cholesterol than digestive juices can liquefy. The remaining 20% of gallstones are composed of calcium and an orange-yellow waste product called bilirubin. Bilirubin gives urine its characteristic color and sometimes causes **jaundice**.

Gallstones are the most common of all gallbladder problems. They are responsible for 90% of gallbladder and bile duct disease, and are the fifth most common reason for hospitalization of adults in the United States. Gallstones usually develop in adults between the ages of 20 and 50; about 20% of patients with gallstones are over 40. The risk of developing gallstones increases with age—at least 20% of people over 60 have a single large stone or as many as several thousand smaller ones. The gender ratio of gallstone patients changes with age. Young women are between two and six times more likely to develop gallstones than men in the same age group. In patients over 50, the condition affects men and women with equal frequency. Native Americans develop gallstones more often than any other segment of the population; Mexican-Americans have the second-highest incidence of this disease.

Gallstones can cause several different disorders. Cholelithiasis is defined as the presence of gallstones within the gallbladder itself. Choledocholithiasis is the presence of gallstones within the common bile duct that leads into the first portion of the small intestine (the duodenum). The stones in the duct may have been formed inside it or carried there from the gallbladder. These gallstones prevent bile from flowing into the duodenum. Ten percent of patients with gallstones have choledocholithiasis, which is sometimes called common-duct stones. Patients who don't develop infection usually recover completely from this disorder.

Cholecystitis is a disorder marked by inflammation of the gallbladder. It is usually caused by the passage of a stone from the gallbladder into the cystic duct, which is a tube that connects the gallbladder to the common bile duct. In 5–10% of cases, however, cholecystitis develops in the absence of gallstones. This form of the disorder is called acalculous cholecystitis. Cholecystitis causes painful enlargement of the gallbladder and is responsible for 10–25% of all gallbladder surgery. Chronic cholecystitis is most common in the elderly. The acute form is most likely to occur in middle-aged adults.

Cholesterolosis or cholesterol polyps is characterized by deposits of cholesterol crystals in the lining of the gallbladder. This condition may be caused by high levels of cholesterol or inadequate quantities of bile salts, and is usually treated by surgery.

Gallstone ileus, which results from a gallstone's blocking the entrance to the large intestine, is most common in elderly people. Surgery usually cures this condition.

Narrowing (stricture) of the common bile duct develops in as many as 5% of patients whose gallbladders have been surgically removed. This condition is characterized by inability to digest fatty foods and by abdominal pain, which sometimes occurs in spasms. Patients with stricture of the common bile duct are likely to recover after appropriate surgical treatment.

Gallstones are caused by an alteration in the chemical composition of bile. Bile is a digestive fluid that helps the body absorb fat. Gallstones tend to run in families. In addition, high levels of estrogen, insulin, or cholesterol can increase a person's risk of developing them.

Pregnancy or the use of birth control pills can slow down gallbladder activity and increase the risk of gallstones. So can diabetes, **pancreatitis**, and **celiac disease**. Other factors influencing gallstone formation are:

- Infection
- **Obesity**
- Intestinal disorders
- **Coronary artery disease** or other recent illness
- **Multiple pregnancies**
- A high-fat, low-fiber diet
- **Smoking**
- Heavy drinking
- Rapid weight loss.

Gallbladder attacks usually follow a meal of rich, high-fat foods. The attacks often occur in the middle of the night, sometimes waking the patient with intense pain that ends in a visit to the emergency room. The pain of a gallbladder attack begins in the abdomen and may radiate to the chest, back, or the area between the shoulders. Other symptoms of gallstones include:

- Inability to digest fatty foods
- Low-grade **fever**
- Chills and sweating
- **Nausea and vomiting**
- **Indigestion**
- Gas
- Belching
- Clay-colored bowel movements.

Gallstones may be diagnosed by a family doctor, a specialist in digestive problems (a gastroenterologist), or a specialist in internal medicine. The doctor will first examine the patient's skin for signs of jaundice and feel (palpate) the abdomen for soreness or swelling. After the basic **physical examination**, the doctor will order **blood count**s or blood chemistry tests to detect evidence of bile duct obstruction and to rule out other illnesses that cause fever and pain, including stomach **ulcers**, **appendicitis**, and **heart attack**s.

More sophisticated procedures used to diagnose gallstones include:

- **Ultrasound** imaging. Ultrasound has an accuracy rate of 96%.
- Cholecystography (cholecystogram, gallbladder series, gallbladder x ray). This type of study shows how the gallbladder contracts after the patient has eaten a high-fat meal.
- Fluoroscopy. This imaging technique allows the doctor to distinguish between jaundice caused by **pancreatic cancer** and jaundice caused by gallbladder or bile duct disorders.
- Endoscopy (ERCP). ERCP uses a special dye to outline the pancreatic and common bile ducts and locate the position of the gallstones.
- Radioisotopic scan. This technique reveals blockage of the cystic duct.

One-third of all patients with gallstones never experience a second attack. For this reason many doctors advise watchful waiting after the first episode. Reducing the amount of fat in the diet or following a sensible plan of gradual weight loss may be the only treatments required for occasional mild attacks. A patient diagnosed with gallstones may be able to manage more troublesome episodes by:

- Applying heat to the affected area.
- Resting and taking occasional sips of water.
- Using non-prescription forms of **acetaminophen** (Tylenol or Anacin-3).

A doctor should be notified if pain intensifies or lasts for more than three hours; if the patient's fever rises above 101°F (38.3°C); or if the skin or whites of the eyes turn yellow.

Surgical removal of the gallbladder (cholecystectomy) is the most common conventional treatment for recurrent attacks. Laparoscopic surgery, the technique most widely used, is a safe, effective procedure that involves less pain and a shorter recovery period than traditional open surgery. In this technique, the doctor makes a small cut (incision) in the patient's abdomen and removes the gallbladder through a long tube called a laparoscope.

If a stone is lodged in the bile ducts, additional surgery must be done to remove it. After surgery, the surgeon will ordinarily leave in a drain to collect bile until the system is healed. The drain can also be used to inject contrast material and take x rays during or after surgery.

A procedure called endoscopic retrograde cholangiopancreatoscopy (ERCP) allows the removal of some bile duct stones through the mouth, throat, esophagus, stomach, duodenum, and biliary system without the need for surgical incisions. ERCP can also be used to inject contrast agents into the biliary system, providing superbly detailed pictures.

Rare circumstances require different techniques. Patients too ill for a complete cholecystectomy (removal of the gallbladder), sometimes only the stones are removed, a procedure called cholelithotomy. But that does not cure the problem. The liver will go on making faulty bile, and stones will reform, unless the composition of the bile is altered.

For patients who cannot receive the laparoscopic procedure, there is also a nonsurgical treatment in which ursodeoxycholic acid is used to dissolve the gallstones. Extracorporeal shock-wave **lithotripsy** has also been successfully used to break up gallstones. During the procedure, high-amplitude sound waves target the stones, slowly breaking them up.

There are a number of imaging studies that identify gallbladder disease, but most gallstones will not show up on conventional x rays. That requires contrast agents given by mouth that are excreted into the bile. Ultrasound is very useful and can be enhanced by doing it through an endoscope in the stomach. CT (**computed tomography scans**) and MRI (**magnetic resonance imaging**) scanning are not used routinely but are helpful in detecting common duct stones and complications.

Without a gallbladder, stones rarely reform. Patients who have continued symptoms after their gallbladder is removed may need an ERCP to detect residual stones or damage to the bile ducts caused by the stones before they were removed. Once in a while the Ampulla of Vater is too tight for bile to flow through and causes symptoms until it is opened up.

The best way to prevent gallstones is to minimize risk factors. In addition, a 1998 study suggests that vigorous **exercise** may lower a man's risk of developing gallstones by as much as 28%. The researchers have not yet determined whether physical activity benefits women to the same extent.

Gallo, Robert C. (1937-)

American virologist

Robert C. Gallo, one of the best-known biomedical researchers in the United States, is considered the codiscoverer, along with **Luc Montagnier** at the Pasteur Institute, of the human **immunodeficiency** virus (HIV). Gallo established that the virus causes acquired immunodeficiency syndrome (**AIDS**), something which Montagnier had not been able to do, and he developed the blood test for HIV, which remains a central tool in efforts to control the disease. Gallo also discovered the human T-cell **leukemia** virus (HTLV) and the human T-cell growth factor interleukin–2.

Gallo's initial work on the isolation and identification of the AIDS virus has been the subject of a number of allegations, resulting in a lengthy investigation and official charges of scientific misconduct which were overturned on appeal. Although he has now been exonerated, the ferocity of the controversy has tended to obscure the importance of his contributions both to AIDS research and biomedical research in general. As Malcolm Gladwell observed in 1990 in the *Washington Post:* "Gallo is easily one of the country's most famous scientists, frequently mentioned as a Nobel Prize contender, and a man whose research publications were cited by other researchers publishing their own work during the last decade more often than those of any other scientist in the world."

Gallo was born in Waterbury, Connecticut, on March 23, 1937, to Francis Anton and Louise Mary (Ciancuilli) Gallo. He grew up in the house that his Italian grandparents bought after they came to the United States. His father worked long hours at the welding company which he owned. The dominant memory of Gallo's youth was of the illness and death of his only sibling, Judy, from childhood leukemia. The disease brought Gallo into contact with the nonfamily member who most influenced his life, Dr. Marcus Cox, the pathologist who diagnosed her disease in 1948. During his senior year in high school, an injury kept Gallo off the high school basketball team and forced him to think about his future. He began to spend time with Cox, visiting him at the hospital, even assisting in postmortem examinations. When Gallo entered college, he knew he wanted a career in biomedical research.

Gallo attended Providence College, where he majored in biology, graduating with a bachelor's degree in 1959. He continued his schooling at Jefferson Medical College in Philadelphia, where he got an introduction to medical research. In 1961 he worked as a summer research fellow in Alan Erslev's laboratory at Jefferson. His work studying the **pathology** of oxygen deprivation in coal miners led to his first scientific publication in 1962, while he was still a medical student.

In 1961 Gallo married Mary Jane Hayes, a woman he knew from his hometown whom he had begun dating in his first year of college. Together they had two children. Gallo graduated from medical school in 1963; on the advice of Erslev, he went to the University of Chicago because it had a reputation as a major center for blood-cell biology, Gallo's research interest. From 1963 to 1965 he did research on the biosynthesis of hemoglobin, the protein that carries oxygen in the blood.

In 1965 Gallo was appointed to the position of clinical associate at the **National Institutes of Health** (NIH) in Bethesda, Maryland. He spent much of his first year at NIH caring for cancer patients. Despite the often depressing work environment, he observed some early successes at treating **cancer** patients with chemotherapy. Children were being cured of the very form of childhood leukemia that killed his sister almost twenty years before. In 1966, Gallo was appointed to his first full-time research position, as an associate of Seymour Perry, who was head of the medicine department. Perry was studying how white blood cells grow in various forms of leukemia. In his laboratory Gallo studied the enzymes involved in the synthesis of the components of deoxyribonucleic acid (DNA), the carrier of genetic information.

The expansion of the NIH and the passage of the National Cancer Act in 1971 led to the creation of the Laboratory of Tumor Cell Biology at the National Cancer Institute (NCI), a part of the NIH. Gallo was appointed head of the new laboratory. He had become intrigued with the possibility that certain kinds of cancer had viral origins, and he set up his new laboratory to study human retroviruses. Retroviruses are types of viruses which possess the ability to penetrate other cells and splice their own genetic material into the genes of their hosts, eventually taking over all of their reproductive functions. At the time Gallo began his work, retroviruses had been found in animals; the question was whether they existed in humans. His research involved efforts to isolate a virus from victims of certain kinds of leukemia, and he and his colleagues were able to view a retrovirus through electron microscopes. In 1975, Gallo and Robert E. Gallagher announced that they had discovered a human leukemia virus, but other laboratories were unable to replicate their results. Scientists to whom they had sent samples for independent confirmation had found two different retroviruses not from humans, but from animals. The samples had been contaminated by viruses from a monkey or a chimp and the idea that a virus could cause cancer was publicly ridiculed.

Despite the humiliation Gallo suffered and the damage this premature announcement did to his reputation, he continued his efforts to isolate a human retrovirus. He turned his attention to T-cells, white blood cells which are an important part of the body's **immune system**, and developed a substance called T-cell growth factor (later called interleukin–2), which would sustain them outside the human body. The importance of this growth factor was that it enabled Gallo and his team to sustain cancerous T-cells long enough to discover whether a retrovirus existed within them. These techniques allowed Gallo and his team to isolate a previously unknown virus from a leukemia patient. He named the virus human T-cell leukemia virus, or HTLV, and he published this finding in *Science* in 1981. This time his findings were confirmed, and as Michael Specter noted in the *New York Review of Books,* Gallo was "transformed from a loser to a star."

It was Gallo's experience with viral research that made him so important in the effort to identify the cause of AIDS, after that disease had first been characterized by doctors in the United States. In further studies of HTLV, Gallo had established that it could be transmitted by **breast-feeding**, sexual intercourse, and blood **transfusions**. He also observed that the incidence of cancers caused by this virus was concentrated in Africa and the Caribbean. HTLV had these and other characteristics in common with what was then known about AIDS, and Gallo was one of the first scientists to hypothesize that the disease was caused by a virus. In 1982, the National Cancer Institute formed an AIDS task force with Gallo as its head. In this capacity he made available to the scientific community the research methods he had developed for HTLV, and among those whom he provided with some early technical assistance was Luc Montagnier at the Pasteur Institute in Paris.

Gallo tried throughout 1983 to get the AIDS virus to grow in culture, using the same growth factor that had worked in growing HTLV, but he was not successful. Finally, a member of Gallo's group named Mikulas Popovic developed a method to grow the virus in a line of T-cells. The method consisted, in effect, of mixing samples from various patients into a kind of a cocktail, using perhaps ten different strains of the virus at a time, so there was a higher chance that one would survive. This innovation allowed the virus to be studied, and observing the similarities to the retroviruses he had previously discovered, Gallo called it HTLV–3. In 1984, he and his colleagues published their findings in *Science.* Gallo and the other scientists in his laboratory were able to establish that this virus caused AIDS, and they developed a blood test for the virus. In a 1993 issue of *New York Times Magazine,* Nicholas Wade writes: "After twelve grim years, Gallo's blood test is still the only weapon of real value that scientists have yet managed to devise against this baffling disease."

Almost a year before Gallo announced his findings, Montagnier at the Pasteur Institute had identified a virus he called LAV, though he was not able to prove that it caused AIDS. The two laboratories were cooperating with each other in the race to find the cause of AIDS and several samples of this virus had been sent to Gallo at the National Cancer Institute. The controversy which would embroil the American scientist's career for almost the next decade began when the United States government denied the French scientists a patent for the AIDS test and awarded one to his team instead. The Pasteur Institute believed their contribution was not recognized in this decision, and they challenged it in court. Gallo did not deny that they had preceded him in isolating the virus, but he argued that it was proof of the causal relationship and the development of the blood test which were most important, and he maintained that these advances had been accomplished using a virus which had been independently isolated in his laboratory.

This first stage of the controversy ended in a legal settlement that was highly unusual for the scientific community:

Gallo and Montagnier agreed out of court to share equal credit for their discovery. This settlement followed a review of records from Gallo's laboratory and rested on the assumption that the virus Gallo had discovered was different from the one Montagnier had sent him. An international committee renamed the virus HIV, and in what Specter calls "the first such negotiated history of a scientific enterprise ever published," the American and French groups published an agreement about their contributions in *Nature* in 1987. In 1988, Gallo and Montagnier jointly related the story of the discoveries in *Scientific American.*

Questions about the isolation of the AIDS virus were revived in 1989 by a long article in the *Chicago Tribune.* The journalist, a Pulitzer Prize winner named John Crewdson, had spent three years investigating Gallo's laboratory, making over one hundred requests under the Freedom of Information Act. He directly questioned Gallo's integrity and implied he had stolen Montagnier's virus. The controversy intensified when it was established that the LAV virus which the French had isolated and the HTLV–3 virus were virtually identical. The genetic sequencing in the two were in fact so close that some believed they actually came from the same AIDS patient, and Gallo was accused of simply renaming the virus Montagnier had sent him. Gallo's claim to have independently isolated the virus was further damaged when it was discovered that in the 1984 *Science* article announcing his discovery of HTLV–3 he had accidently published a photograph of Montagnier's virus.

In 1990, pressure from a congressional committee forced the NIH to undertake an investigation. In the *Washington Post,* Malcolm Gladwell observed of this inquiry: "No other investigation has taken so long, dealt with a scientific discovery of such importance or directly implicated so distinguished a researcher." The NIH investigation found Popovic guilty of scientific misconduct but Gallo guilty only of misjudgment. A committee of scientists which oversaw the investigation was strongly critical of these conclusions, and the group expressed concern that Popovic had been assigned more than a fair share of the blame. In June 1992, the NIH investigation was superseded by the Office of Research Integrity (ORI) at the **U.S. Department of Health and Human Services**, and in December of that year ORI found both Gallo and Popovic guilty of scientific misconduct. Based largely on a single sentence in the 1984 *Science* article that described the isolation of the virus, the ORI report found Gallo guilty of misconduct for "falsely reporting that LAV had not been transmitted to a permanently growing cell line." This decision renewed the legal threat from the Pasteur Institute, whose lawyers moved to claim all the back royalties from the AIDS blood test, which then amounted to approximately $20 million.

Gallo strongly objected to the findings of the ORI, pointing to the fact that the finding of misconduct turned on a single sentence in a single paper. Other scientists objected to the panel's priorities, believing that the charge of misconduct concerned a misrepresentation of a relatively minor issue which did not negate the scientific validity of Gallo's conclusions. Lawyers representing both Gallo and Popovic brought their cases before an appeals board at the Department of Health and Human Services. Popovic's case was heard first, and in December 1993 the board announced that he had been cleared of all charges. As quoted in *Time,* the panel declared: "One might anticipate... after all the sound and fury, there would be at least a residue of palpable wrongdoing. This is not the case." The ORI immediately withdrew all charges against Gallo for lack of proof.

According to *Time,* in December 1993 Gallo considered himself "completely vindicated" of all the allegations that had been made against him. He has established that before 1984 his laboratory had succeeded in isolating other strains of the virus which were not similar to LAV. Many scientists now believe that the problem was simply one of contamination, a mistake which may have been a consequence of the intense pressure for results in many laboratories during the early years of the AIDS **epidemic**. It has been hypothesized that the LAV sample from the Pasteur Institute contaminated the mixture of AIDS viruses which Popovic concocted to find one strain that would survive in culture; it is believed that this strain was strong enough to survive and be identified by Gallo and Popovic for a second time.

In 1990, when the controversy was still at its height, Gallo published a book about his career called *Virus Hunting,* which seemed intended to refute the charges against him, particularly the *Tribune* article by Crewdson. Gallo made many of the claims that were later supported by the appeals board, and in the *New York Times Book Review,* Natalie Angier called him "a formidable gladiator who firmly believes in the importance of his scientific contributions." Angier wrote of the book: "His description of the key experiments in 1983 and 1984 that led to the final isolation of the AIDS virus are intelligent and persuasive, particularly to a reader who was heard the other side of the story. Although the reviews of *Virus Hunting* were not entirely sympathetic, many felt the controversy was misplaced. A number of reviewers commented on how this controversy had virtually paralyzed one of the most important AIDS research laboratories in the world. In the *Washington Post,* J. D. Robinson observed that "thousands of hours and untold psychic energy which could have been devoted to seeking a cure for AIDS have been spent responding to inquiries and accusations."

The many allegations and the long series of investigations have distracted many people from the accomplishments of a man whose name appears on hundreds of scientific papers and who has won most major awards in biomedical research except the Nobel Prize. Gallo has actually received the coveted Albert Lasker Award twice, once in 1982 for his work on the viral origins of cancer, and again in 1986 for his research on AIDS. He has also been awarded the American Cancer Society Medal of Honor in 1983, the Lucy Wortham Prize from the Society for Surgical Oncology in 1984, the Armand Hammer Cancer Research Award in 1985, and the Gairdner Foundation International Award for Biomedical Research in 1987. He has received eleven honorary degrees.

GALTON, FRANCIS (1822-1911)

English scientist

Francis Galton was born near Birmingham, England, in 1822. His impressive talents appeared early. At the age of three, he was already reading, and at four, he was studying Latin. His I.Q. at adulthood was estimated at 200. But as a young man of 22, a fresh graduate of Cambridge, Galton did not continue his training as a physician. His wealthy father had died and left Galton a large inheritance, so the young Galton was free to do whatever he fancied.

For a time he chose to travel, exploring virtually unknown parts of Sudan, Syria, and southwest Africa. Upon his return, Galton published two books about his travels. He was even recognized by the Geographical Society and the Royal Society with various medals and honors. He was also knighted in 1909.

Galton never held any academic or professional post. Instead, he did his experimenting at home or during his travels. His earliest researches had to do with meteorology. In his 1863 book *Meteorgraphica*, Galton presented the modern technique of weather-mapping and coined the term anticyclone to describe the high pressure systems that bring fair, calm weather. Because of these studies, Galton was instrumental in establishing the Meteorological Office and the National Physical Laboratory.

Galton's natural curiosity about nature and mankind soon led him to explore a new frontier: heredity. He felt that the study of heredity was not progressing as quickly or accurately as possible because of a lack in quantitative research. Galton strongly believed that virtually everything could be proven mathematically—everything was quantifiable. He even went so far as to develop a system to measure beauty and the effectiveness of prayer. These researches established him as the founder of the biometric school. (Followers of the biometric school use statistics to prove hypotheses in **genetics**.)

In 1859, Charles Darwin, who was Galton's relative, published *The Origin of Species*. In that book, Darwin asserted that certain characteristics from two different individuals blend together to create variations in their offspring. Darwin also believed that these characteristics are "copied" within the parents' bodies and carried to the reproductive organs, where they wait to pass on the traits to the offspring.

Galton, seeing that this theory could be tested statistically, set out to support Darwin's "pangene" theory. It made sense to him that these "copied" characteristics were probably floating around in the bloodstream. So he chose to transfuse or switch the blood of a purebred silver-gray rabbit with a common lop-eared rabbit. After breeding the silver-gray rabbits that had the blood of lop-eared rabbits, Galton found no difference in the rabbits' offspring. Silver-gray rabbits still produced silver-gray offspring. He thought this revealed the weakness of the inheritance aspect of Darwin's theory.

Several years later, Galton came up with his own theory to explain inheritance: the theory of ancestral heredity. According to Galton's theory, each parent contributes half of the traits to the offspring, each grandparent one-fourth, and so on.

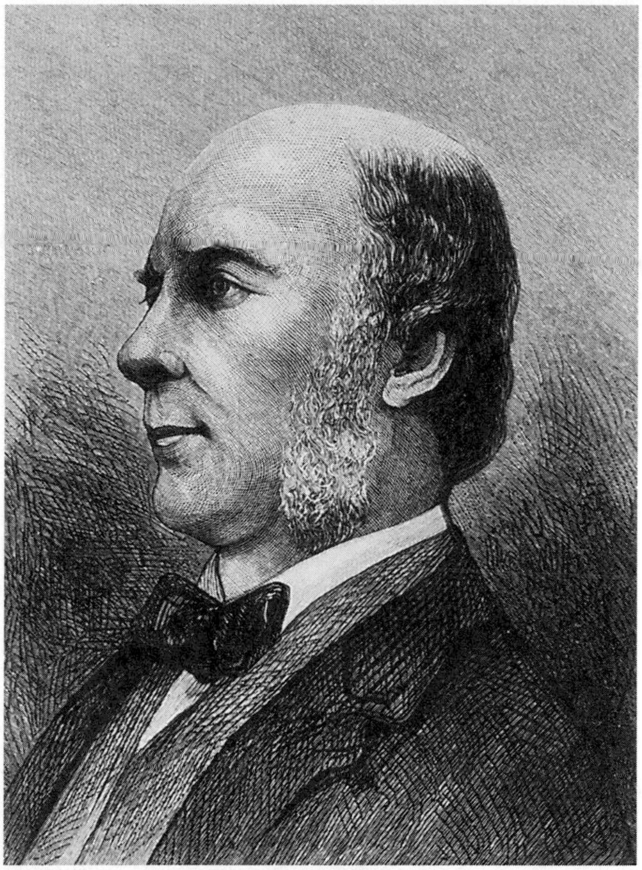

Francis Galton

With each generation, the traits become more diluted and the offspring begin exhibiting the average of race, not the average of the parents. Unfortunately, Galton's theory was still too similar to Darwin's "blending." It did not survive the rediscovery and eventual acceptance of Gregor Mendel's work, which stressed particulate heredity—or the notion of traits being inherited individually rather than being blended. Nevertheless, Galton's theory turns out to be mathematically sound in that one-half of any individual's genes come from each parent, one-fourth from each grandparent, and so forth.

Galton pioneered studies of identical twins, whose differences can be attributed to environmental factors since they are genetically identical. He also studied talented families to determine how artistic, intellectual, or athletic skill might be inherited. Galton's heredity studies led him to believe that scientific breeding could be applied to human populations. Galton called this science **eugenics**. Eugenics entails "breeding in" desirable traits of the human population, such as talent and healthiness, and "breeding out" undesirable traits, such as stupidity and weakness. Galton suspected that getting such a concept accepted would be difficult, but he devoted significant time and energy to ensure that the topic was not forgotten. He even donated a large amount of his inheritance money to establish a Chair of Eugenics at University College in London.

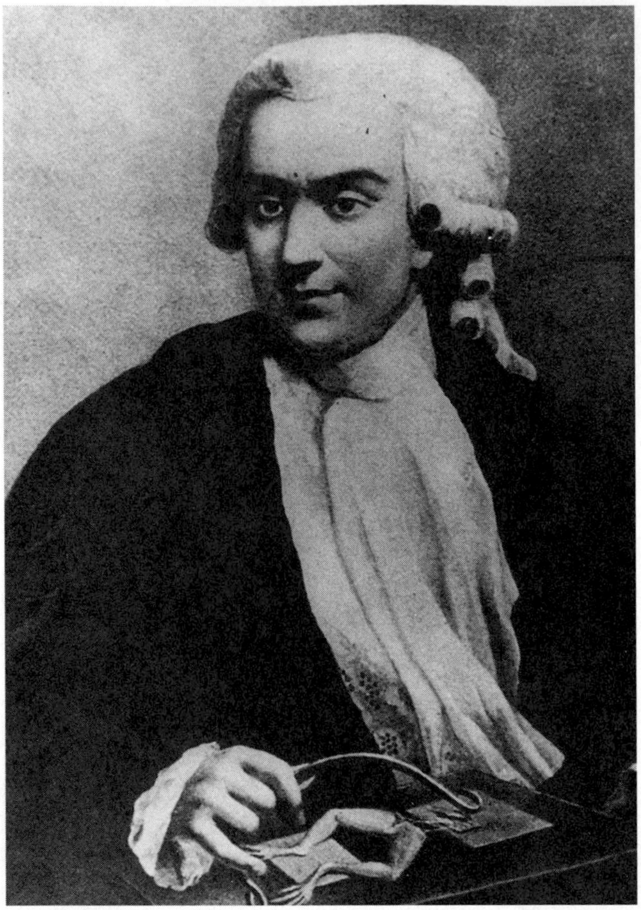

Luigi Galvani

Later in his life, Galton became interested in fingerprinting. He thought it might be a way to track differences in families, race, morals, and intellect. Although Galton never found any correlations to support this assumption, he did establish fingerprinting as an easy and almost infallible means of human identification. The fingerprinting methods he developed are essentially the same methods used today.

Among Galton's other books were *Hereditary Genius* (1869), *Inquiries into Human Faculty* (1883), *Natural Inheritance* (1889), and *Finger Prints* (1892). He was knighted in 1909, two years before his death in 1911.

Galvani, Luigi (1737-1798)

Italian anatomist

Luigi Galvani was not especially interested in electricity. At least, not at first. Born on September 9, 1737, at Bologna, Italy, Galvani was initially a student of theology; but he switched to the study of medicine, receiving his degree in 1762. In 1775 he was appointed Professor of Anatomy and Gynecology at the University of Bologna, the school from which he graduated.

In 1771, Galvani happened to observe the **dissection** of a frog and noticed the dead frog's legs would twitch when a spark touched them. This was no big surprise; it was known that live muscle tissue twitched when touched with a spark, so dead tissue ought to react the same way.

At first Galvani had no further interest in the incident, but later he recalled that a generation earlier Benjamin Franklin had shown lightning was an electrical phenomena. Galvani reasoned that if Franklin was right, lightning should have the same effect on a frog's legs as the spark. He set out to confirm Franklin's findings.

Galvani found that twitching did indeed occur during a thunderstorm. In fact, muscles could be made to twitch every time they came into contact with two different types of metal. Electricity was obviously involved, but was it coming from the muscle or the metal?

Keep in mind that Galvani was an anatomist. He decided that an "animal electricity" was responsible, and he published his findings in 1791. His paper, suggesting a different type of electric phenomena, received general acceptance; however, there were a few exceptions. Alessandro Volta was among those who disagreed with Galvani's conclusion. A spirited controversy erupted between the two. Volta ultimately prevailed, showing that the twitching was caused by the combination of the two different metals and the fluid within the muscle tissue.

Galvani was extremely disappointed. Worse, when he refused to swear allegiance to Napoleon Bonaparte's government in 1797, he lost his position at the university. He died in poverty on December 4, 1798.

Galvani is nonetheless remembered in a number of ways. A person who abruptly jumps into action is said to be galvanized. Iron that has had a layer of zinc crystals applied with electric current is known as galvanized iron. The steady flow of electricity that is created by the contact of two metals is known as galvanic electricity. Perhaps the best tribute to Galvani's memory came from André Ampère, who invênted a device to measure current in 1820, the galvanometer.

Gangrene

Gangrene is the destruction of body tissue by a bacteria called *Clostridium perfringens*, or a combination of *streptococci* and *staphylococci* bacteria. C. perfringens is wide-spread in soil and the intestinal tracts of humans and animals. It becomes dangerous only when its spores germinate, producing toxins and destructive enzymes, and germination occurs only in an *anaerobic* environment (one almost totally devoid of oxygen). While gangrene can develop in any part of the body, it is most common in fingers, toes, hands, feet, arms, and legs, the parts of the body most susceptible to restricted blood flow. Even a slight injury in such an area is at high risk of causing gangrene. Early treatment with antibiotics such as penicillin, and surgery to remove the dead tissue, will often reduce the need for amputation. Left untreated, gangrene results in amputation of the affected limb and/or death of the patient. Many wounded soldiers lost life and limb to gangrene before sterilization of surgical instruments and the development of antibiotics.

Because blood carries oxygen to all tissues of the body, diseases or injuries which interrupt that blood flow increase the risk of gangrene. **Diabetes**, arteriosclerosis, severe **frost bite**, blood clots, crushing injuries, and burns are common causes of restricted blood flow. Gangrene is classified into two types: dry and wet. Gas gangrene, the most deadly apart from gangrene in the abdominal organs, falls in the category of wet gangrene. Dry gangrene, in which the skin becomes painful, dark, dries up, and drops off, is less aggressive than moist gangrene, as some healing can occur where the living and dead skin meet. Moist gangrene, on the other hand, spreads quickly and can be fatal. Dying cells leak fluid and the moist environment encourages bacteria to grow and spread rapidly. Symptoms often begin with pain and loss of feeling followed by swelling of the skin and blisters which turn black and ooze a foul-smelling discharge. Infection can be accompanied by a fever up to 101° F (38.3°C).

Gas gangrene usually develops from infection following surgery, or when contaminated soil or other foreign matter enters a deep puncture wound, open wounds with muscle damage, or a compound fracture. Bacteria flourish in the moist, oxygen-reduced environment, producing gaseous bubbles which release poison into the body. Infection spreads rapidly through the dying skin, underlying muscle, and bone, which excrete a brown, foul-smelling puss. Ruptured appendix or gallbladder are the most common cause of abdominal gangrene, which is indicated by severe abdominal pain.

Risk factors associated with poor circulation and therefore gangrene are diabetes mellitus, **smoking**, excessive consumption of alcohol, poor circulation commonly experienced in old age, **Raynaud's disease**, and Buerger's disease. Individuals in these categories should take precautions such as close examination of extremities for signs of swelling, redness, warmth, or **pain** of the skin; avoid foot injuries by wearing comfortable shoes and keeping toe nails clipped; adhering strictly to dietary and medical regimes recommended for diabetes, and stop drinking alcohol and smoking tobacco. If infection is suspected, a doctor's advice should be sought immediately.

In 1994, physicians from Cornell University and New York Hospital reported considerable success with **angioplasty** to improve blood flow to lower extremities. In 1997, Jeffrey Isner, M.D. and his team at St. Elizabeth's Medical Center in Boston developed a gene therapy called "therapeutic angiogenesis," which encourages the growth of new blood vessels around restricted vessels. Success was achieved in the legs of eight out of 10 people treated, avoiding the need for amputation.

In 1994, seven people in England died of a "flesh-eating virus," or "galloping gangrene," caused by a*group A streptococcus* infection bringing about *necrotizing fasciitis*, the death of subcutaneous and adjacent tissue. These instances of necrosis were unusual because it usually involves an anaerobic bacteria.

See also Flesh-eating disease

Garrod, Archibald (1857-1936)

English physician and chemist

Archibald Garrod was a physician whose innovative work in clinical medicine and chemistry led him to discover a new class of human disease based on hereditary factors. A pioneer in biochemistry, Garrod stressed the chemical uniqueness of each person. For his work on inborn errors of **metabolism**, Garrod was elected to the Royal Society and received a knighthood.

Archibald Edward Garrod was born in London on November 25, 1857, the fourth and youngest son of Sir Alfred Baring Garrod and Elisabeth Ann Colchester. Garrod's father, a distinguished professor of medicine at University College in London, was the first physician to note the presence of uric acid in patients suffering from gout. In later years, Garrod would cite his father's discovery as the first quantitative biochemical investigation performed on living humans.

As a child, Garrod demonstrated an early talent for illustration and a lasting interest in color. He studied physical geography at Marlborough and astronomy at Oxford, where he graduated with first-class honors in natural science. Deciding to follow in his father's footsteps, Garrod began the study of medicine at St. Bartholomew's Hospital in London. He received a number of scholarships and spent a year attending medical clinics in Vienna, resulting in the publication of a book on the laryngoscope, a device used to examine the interior of the throat. A tall, handsome man, Garrod became a skilled clinician whose reassuring manner enabled him to gather detailed medical histories from his patients. In 1884, Garrod joined the staff of St. Bartholomew's Hospital, but promotion was slow and for nearly three decades he had ample time to pursue his interest in chemistry and disease. He wrote a number of papers on joint disorders, his father's specialty, pointing out the difference between rheumatism and **rheumatoid arthritis** as diseases.

Garrod's interest in joint disease led him to study the chemistry of pigments in urine. While working as a visiting physician at the Great Osmond Street Hospital for Sick Children, he examined a three-month old boy, Thomas P., whose urine was stained a deep reddish-brown. Garrod's diagnosis was alkaptonuria, which is caused by an abnormal build-up of homogentisic acid, or alkapton. In a normal person, the acid is broken down through a series of chemical reactions into carbon dioxide and water. But in rare cases, the metabolic process is interrupted and the acid is excreted in the urine, where it turns black on contact with the air. According to the **germ theory** of disease, which had transformed the study of medicine in Garrod's time, alkaptonuria was thought to be a bacterial infection of the intestine. The disorder was almost always diagnosed in infancy, lasted throughout life and was thought to be contagious. Garrod's training in physical science, however, led him to investigate the disease as a series of chemical reactions. He reviewed 31 cases of alkaptonuria from his own practice and from the medical literature, and presented his findings to the Royal Medical and Chirurgical (Surgical) Society of London in 1899. Alkaptonuria, he noted, although rare, tended to appear among children of healthy parents. It was not contagious and seemed to be a harmless error in metabolism.

When a third child with alkaptonuria was born to the parents of Thomas P., Garrod suspected that something more than mere chance was involved. When he learned that Thomas P.'s parents were blood relations—their mothers were sisters—he inquired into the backgrounds of other families with one or more children with alkaptonuria. In every instance, their parents were also first cousins. It was while walking home from the hospital one afternoon that Garrod conceived of the possibility that alkaptonuria might be a disease caused by heredity (**genetics**). Gregor Mendel's work on the principles of heredity, newly discovered in England, offered a simple explanation. The mating of first cousins apparently created conditions under which a rare, recessive Mendelian factor (or gene) appeared in the offspring. Garrod's classic paper on alkaptonuria was published in *Lancet* in 1902.

Garrod went on to study other metabolic disorders, including the pigment disorders **porphyria**, the cause of George III's madness, and **albinism**. Like alkaptonurics, albinos tended to be children of parents who were first cousins. In a series of lectures delivered before the Royal College of Physicians in 1908, Garrod described such disorders as "inborn errors of metabolism." In each instance, he claimed, a genetic factor caused a deficiency in a certain enzyme which led to a premature block in the chemistry of normal metabolism. In his book, *Inborn Errors of Metabolism* (1909), Garrod described an important new class of diseases which were genetic, not bacteriological in origin.

In recognition of his contributions to science, Garrod was made a fellow of the Royal Society in 1910, and was knighted in 1918. He spent World War I in the Army Medical Service on the island of Malta as consulting physician to the British forces in the Mediterranean. Two of his sons were killed in combat, a third died of the Spanish **influenza** following the armistice.

After the War, Garrod returned briefly to St. Bartholomew's, but was soon summoned to Oxford to become Regius Professor of Medicine. In his lectures, Garrod urged students to think of disease in terms of biochemistry. Clinicians, he argued, were uniquely placed to observe anomalies of nature which they could then investigate in the laboratory. In his later writings, Garrod hypothesized that there might be a molecular (genetic) basis for all variations in life functions, including physical appearance, susceptibility to disease, even behavior.

Garrod retired in 1927. He and his wife, Laura Elizabeth, whom he married in 1886, moved to Cambridge to be near their daughter, Dorothy, a noted archaeologist and teacher at Newnham College. Archibald Edward Garrod died at home on March 28, 1936. He was 78.

The significance of Garrod's contribution to the science of genetics was not appreciated in his lifetime; he was an elderly physician when most young geneticists were botanists and zoologists. It was not until the 1940s that Garrod's pathbreaking work in human genetics was rediscovered and applied to gene theory.

Gasser, Herbert Spencer (1888-1963)

American neurophysiologist and physician

Herbert Gasser was born in Platteville, Wisconsin, on July 5, 1888. His mother, Jane Griswold, who descended from an early Connecticut family, was a teacher trained in Wisconsin's first State Normal School in Platteville. Gasser's father, Herman, was born in the Tyrol and came to the United States as a boy. Herman was a self-educated man who eventually qualified in medicine and became a country doctor.

After attending State Normal School, Gasser received two degrees in science at the University of Wisconsin, a bachelor's degree in zoology in 1910 and a master's in anatomy in 1911. However, Gasser's future interests were determined by a physiology course in the University's newly organized medical school. The young lecturer who emphasized the new spirit of research in medicine was **Joseph Erlanger**, the man with whom Gasser would share the Nobel Prize 33 years later. In 1915, he earned his medical degree from Johns Hopkins University, where he conducted research on blood coagulation in his spare time. After another year of research in Wisconsin, Gasser joined Erlanger at Washington University in St. Louis, in 1916.

Earlier scientists had provided painstaking microscopic slides of neurons and general theories of nerve networks in the body. Gasser's contributions made it possible to trace pathways while keeping the **nervous system** intact. Physiologists knew that impulses (action potentials) travel along nerves to convey sensation and to stimulate muscles, and that these impulses could be recorded by electrical instruments. A hypothesis existed that impulses moved faster along thick fibers than they did thin ones. Gasser's dramatic new method involved stimulating a given region of nerves and then reading the transmitted signal as it reached its destination, much like a physician tests a patient's knee jerk response with a rubber mallet. His problem was in finding recording devices capable of measuring, in fractions of a second, impulses that were small in quantity and short in duration. The available devices were inadequate. The string galvanometer and the capillary electrometer were slow and insensitive. The cathode-ray oscillograph, although quick, was insensitive to small currents.

The first breakthrough for Gasser came with the same vacuum tube amplifier that made radio possible. The three-stage amplifier had been brought to St. Louis by H. Sidney Newcomer, one of Gasser's classmates at Hopkins, who had built the device with the help of friends at the Western Electric Company. Nerve impulses could now be recorded, though the instrument's inertia caused distortions in timing the impulses. Their report describing this apparatus and experiments on nerves in the diaphragm appeared in 1921. This article was less important for its new knowledge about nerves than for its description of how sensations could at last be signalized.

A new technology, again from Western Electric, allowed Gasser and Joseph Erlanger to conduct the pioneering studies that eventually led to their Nobel Prize. It had been believed for over a decade that, should a means be discovered to test the Braun tube, the nerve impulse might accurately be recorded. But the tube, invented in 1897, used a cold-cathode technology, wherein the emission of electrons from the cathode's electrode is triggered by an outside force—this proved to be its downfall. Western Electric had, on the other hand, developed an oscillograph tube fitted with a hot cathode. This permitted the instrument to operate at a low voltage, which made it more sensitive to the small currents of the nerve action potentials. The instrument could record both the time elapsed between impulses and the change in nerve reactions. Though the tube was a breakthrough for Gasser and Erlanger, they still had to devise auxiliary apparatus to coordinate their induction shocks with the action potentials that were displayed on the screen. This work was reported in 1922.

Using the cathode-ray oscilloscope, Gasser and Erlanger almost immediately made two discoveries about the unexpected complexity they found in nerve trunks. In one, they determined that the sequence of events of nerve impulse transmission consists of two parts. There is an initial, large, rapid deviation in electric potential, called the spike, which ascends then descends during the actual transmission. The spike is followed by a sequence of small, slow potential changes, called the after-potential, that first has a negative and then a positive deviation.

In their other discovery, Gasser and Erlanger found that the composite action potential of a nerve has a range of velocities. They eventually identified three distinct patterns based on the length of spikes and their after potentials, and classified the fibers into three main groups. The fastest and thickest are A fibers, the intermediate size are B fibers, while the thinnest and slowest are C fibers. Their findings thus confirmed the hypothesis that thick fibers conduct impulses faster than thin ones.

Erlanger and Gasser next showed how these three types of fibers are distributed over the incoming and outgoing fibers of the spinal cord, the sensory and motor roots. The perception of **pain** is carried by the thin, slow fibers, while muscle sense and touch and muscle movement are conducted by the fast fibers. Gasser subsequently explored the excitability of nerve fibers in relation to after-potentials. He also continued to refine the oscilloscope, first using x-ray film and eventually a camera to record the impulses.

Gasser served as professor of pharmacology at Washington University from 1921 to 1931. During a two-year leave of absence between 1923 and 1925, he worked with **Archibald V. Hill** and **Henry Hallett Dale** in London, Walter Straub in Munich, and Louis Lapicque at the Sorbonne, on investigations involving muscle contractions and excitation of nerves. In 1931, Gasser became professor of physiology at Cornell University Medical College in New York City. In 1935, at age 47, Gasser became the second scientific director of the Rockefeller Institute for Medical Research, succeeding Simon Flexner. Gasser's medical training and his grasp of mathematical and physical sciences equipped him well to lead and to comprehend the expanding field of scientific medicine. His tenure bridged the economic depression of the 1930s, World War II, and the unsettling changes in the funding of scientific research after the war. Despite these trying times, Gasser, nevertheless,

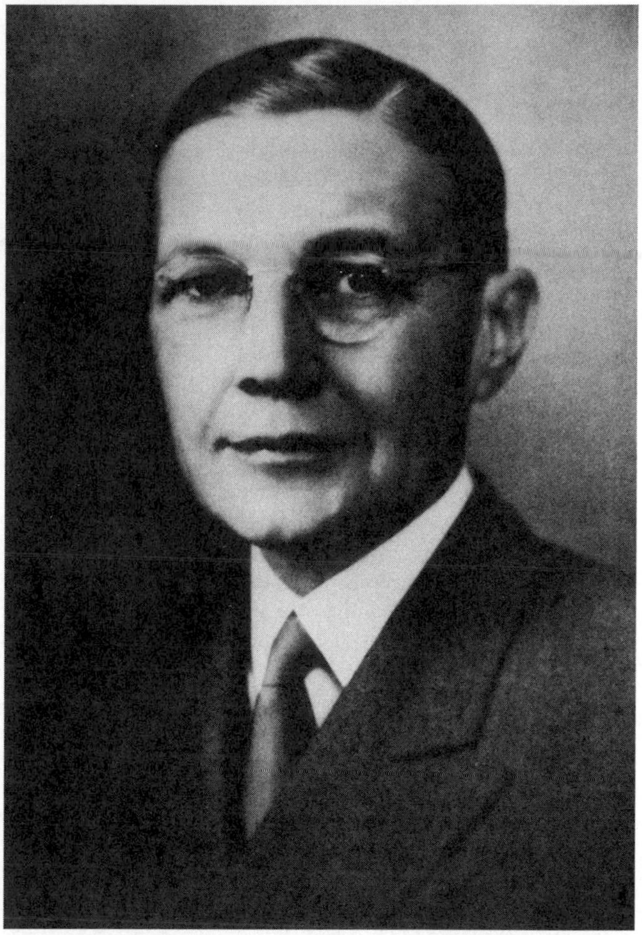

Herbert Spencer Gasser

led the institute's transition from its original emphasis on pathology and infectious diseases to a broader biological approach to human diseases. From 1936 to 1957, he also served as editor of *The Journal of Experimental Medicine.*

During World War II, many Rockefeller Institute laboratories closed and their facilities and staff were organized to support war efforts. Gasser returned to work he had done on chemical warfare during the first world war, chairing a civilian committee on research development in that field. So it was a great surprise for Gasser when a cable arrived in 1944 from Stockholm, announcing that he had won a Nobel prize. Gasser retired from the institute in 1953 and was succeeded by Detlev W. Bronk. With a change to emeritus status came the opportunity for Gasser to return to the laboratory. Instead of plunging into new areas of nerve physiology, he returned to unfinished work on differentiation of the thin C fibers. The introduction of electron microscopy helped him confirm many of his earlier findings. Gasser's scientific contributions were recognized by honorary degrees from twelve universities. He was elected to the National Academy of Sciences in 1934, the American Philosophical Society in 1937, and was a member of more than twenty other scientific societies in the United States, Europe, and South America. He received the Kober Medal in 1954, from the American Association of Physicians.

Following a second stroke, Gasser died in New York Hospital on May 11, 1963.

GASTRITIS

Gastritis is an inflammation of the lining of the stomach. There are several forms, including chronic gastritis (symptoms are usually indefinite or nonexistent) and acute erosive gastritis (symptoms may include vomiting, vomiting blood, black, tarry feces, anorexia nervosa, and **nausea**).

In the 1990s, scientists discovered that the main cause of chronic gastritis is infection from a bacterium called *Helicobacter pylori* (*H. pylori*). This micro-organism has an outer layer that is resistant to the normal effects of stomach acid in breaking down bacteria, so it may rest in the stomach for long periods, even years, causing symptoms of gastritis or ulcers when other factors are introduced, such as the presence of specific genes or ingestion of **nonsteroidal anti-inflammatory drugs** (NSAIDS). Study of the role of *H. pylori* in gastritis and peptic **ulcers** has disproved the former belief that stress led to most stomach and duodenal ulcers. *H. pylori* is most likely transmitted between humans, although the specific routes of transmission are not fully understood. As the millennium closed, studies were also underway to determine the role of *H. pylori* and resulting chronic gastritis in gastric **cancer**.

After *H. pylori*, the second most common cause of gastritis is nonsteroidal anti-inflammatory drugs. These commonly used pain killers, including aspirin, fenoprofen, ibuprofen and naproxen, can lead to acute erosive gastritis and peptic ulcers. Other forms of erosive gastritis can be caused by alcohol and corrosive agents or due to trauma such as ingesting foreign bodies. Patients with erosive gastritis sometimes show no symptoms.

Other types of gastritis include:

- Acute stress gastritis—this most serious form of gastritis usually occurs in critically ill patients.
- Atrophic gastritis results from chronic gastritis that is leading to wasting away of the stomach's lining. Gastric atrophy is the final stage of chronic gastritis and may be a forerunner to gastric cancer.
- Superficial gastritis is a term used to describe the initial stages of chronic gastritis.
- Uncommon specific forms of gastritis include granulomatous, eosiniphilic and lymphocytic gastritis.

Less common forms of gastritis may result from a number of generalized diseases or from complications of chronic gastritis.

Chronic gastritis is easily diagnosed with the urea breath test, which detects *H. pylori* infection, or through blood tests or endoscopy (examining the stomach area using a hollow tube inserted through the mouth). A **biopsy** of the stomach lining may also be ordered.

Diagnosis of acute erosive gastritis involves careful questioning of the patient, since this type of gastritis is most often the result of chronic use of NSAIDS, alcoholism, or other substances.

The discovery of *H. pylori's* role in gastritis and ulcers has led to improved treatment of chronic gastritis. Since the infection can be treated with **antibiotics**, the bacterium can be completely eliminated up to 90% of the time. Although *H. pylori* can be successfully treated, the treatment may be uncomfortable for patients and relies heavily on patient compliance. No single antibiotic has been found to eliminate *H. pylori* on its own, so a combination of antibiotics is usually prescribed.

In acute erosive gastritis, few patients show symptoms, so treatment may depend on severity of symptoms. When symptoms do occur, patients may be treated with therapy similar to that for *H. pylori*, especially since some studies have demonstrated a link between *H. pylori* and NSAIDS in causing ulcers. Avoidance of NSAIDS will most likely be recommended.

For other forms of gastritis, specific treatments will depend on the cause and type of gastritis, and may include prednisone or antibiotics. Critically ill patients at high risk for **bleeding** may be treated with preventive drugs to reduce risk of acute stress gastritis. If stress gastritis does occur, the patient is treated with a drug to stop bleeding. Sometimes surgery is recommended, but is weighed with the possibility of surgical complications or **death**. Once torrential bleeding occurs in acute stress gastritis, the death rate can be greater than 60%.

Alternative forms of treatment for gastritis and ulcers should be used cautiously and in conjunction with conventional medical care, particularly now that scientists have confirmed the role of *H. pylori* in gastritis and ulcers. Alternative treatments address gastritis symptoms with diet and nutritional supplements, herbal medicine and **ayurvedic medicine**. It is believed that zinc, vitamin A and beta-carotene aid the stomach lining's ability to repair itself. Herbs thought to stimulate the **immune system** and reduce inflammation include echinacea (*Echinacea* spp.) and goldenseal (*Hydrastis canadensis*).

The discovery of *H. pylori* has improved the prospects of recovery for patients with gastritis and ulcers. Research is continuing into the most effective treatment of *H. pylori*, especially in light of the bacterium's resistance to certain antibiotics. It is believed that *H. pylori* plays a role in the eventual development of serious gastritis complications and cancer. Detection and treatment of *H. pylori* infection may help reduce occurrence of these diseases. The prospects for patients with acute stress gastritis are much poorer, with a 60 percent or higher death rate among those bleeding heavily.

GASTROENTERITIS

Gastroenteritis is a catchall term for infection or irritation of the digestive tract, particularly the stomach and intestine. It is frequently called stomach or intestinal flu, although the influenza virus is not associated with this illness. Major symptoms include **nausea and vomiting**, **diarrhea**, and abdominal cramps. These symptoms are sometimes also accompanied by fever and overall weakness. Gastroenteritis typically lasts about three days. Adults usually recover without problems, but children, the elderly, and people with underlying disease are more vulnerable to complications such as **dehydration**.

Gastroenteritis is rarely life-threatening in the United States and other developed nations. However, an estimated 220,000 children younger than age five are hospitalized with gastroenteritis symptoms in the United States annually. Of these, 300 die as a result of severe diarrhea and dehydration. In developing nations, diarrheal illnesses are a major cause of death. In 1990, approximately three million deaths occurred worldwide as a result of diarrheal illness.

Gastroenteritis commonly arises from consuming food or beverages containing viruses, bacteria, or parasites. Certain medications and excessive alcohol can also irritate the digestive tract to the point of inducing gastroenteritis.

The most common cause of gastroenteritis is viral infection. Exposure often occurs by consuming materials contaminated by excrement (fecal-oral route). Viruses involved in gastroenteritis include rotavirus, **adenovirus**, astrovirus, and calicivirus and small round-structured viruses (SRSVs).

Bacterial gastroenteritis frequently results from unsanitary drinking water or food—common in developing nations. Natural or man-made disasters can make underlying **sanitation** and food-safety problems worse. In developed nations, modern food production can expose millions of people to disease-causing bacteria through its intensive production and distribution methods. Common types of bacterial gastroenteritis are linked to *Salmonella* and *Campylobacter* bacteria; however, *Escherichia coli* (**E. coli**) 0157 and *Listeria monocytogenes* are creating increased concern in developed nations. In developing countries, **cholera** and shigella remain of great concern, and research to develop long-term vaccines is underway.

Gastroenteritis usually shouldn't require a visit to the doctor. However, medical treatment is essential if symptoms worsen or if complications develop. Infants, young children, the elderly, and persons with underlying disease require special attention in this regard.

The greatest danger presented by gastroenteritis is dehydration. Fluid loss through diarrhea and vomiting can upset the body's electrolyte balance, leading to potentially life-threatening problems such as heartbeat abnormalities. Dehydration should be suspected if dry mouth, increased or excessive thirst, or scanty urination is experienced.

If symptoms do not clear up within a week, an infection or disorder more serious than gastroenteritis may be involved. Symptoms requiring prompt medical attention include high fever (102° F [38.9°C] or above), blood or mucus in the diarrhea, blood in the vomit, and severe abdominal pain or swelling.

Unless there is an outbreak affecting several people or complications are encountered in a particular case, identifying the specific cause of the illness is not a priority. However, if identification of the infectious agent is required, a stool sample will be collected and analyzed for the presence of viruses, disease-causing bacteria, or parasites.

For comfort and convenience, **over-the-counter** medications such as Pepto Bismol may be used to relieve symptoms. A doctor may prescribe a more powerful **antidiarrheal drug** such as motofen or lomotil. Should disease-causing bacteria or parasites be identified in the patient's stool sample, e, an antibiotic may be prescribed.

It is important to stay hydrated and nourished during a bout of gastroenteritis. If you are not dehydrated, it should be enough to drink generous amounts of nonalcoholic fluids such as water or juice. **Caffeine** should be avoided, since it increases urine output. The traditional BRAT diet—bananas, rice, applesauce, and toast—is tolerated by the tender gastrointestinal system, but it is not particularly nutritious. Many, but not all, medical researchers recommend a diet that includes complex carbohydrates (e.g., rice, wheat, potatoes, bread, and cereal), lean meats, yogurt, fruit, and vegetables. Milk and other dairy products shouldn't create problems if they are part of the normal diet. Fatty foods or foods with a lot of sugar should be avoided.

Minimal to moderate dehydration is treated with oral rehydrating solutions that contain glucose and electrolytes. These are commercially available under names such as Naturalyte, Pedialyte, Infalyte, and Rehydralyte. Oral rehydrating solutions are specially formulated. Fluids that are not so formulated—such as cola, apple juice, broth, and sports beverages—are not recommended to treat dehydration. If vomiting makes drinking difficult, small, frequent amounts of fluid may be better tolerated. Should oral rehydration fail or severe dehydration occur, medical treatment in the form of intravenous therapy is required.

Alternative treatments for uncomplicated gastroenteritis include meadowsweet (*Filipendula ulmaria*) slippery elm, (*Ulmus fulva*) or homeopathic remedies including *Arsenicum album*, ipecac, or *Nux vomica*. Live cultures of *Lactobacillus acidophilus* are said to soothe the digestive tract and return the intestinal flora to normal. *L. acidophilus* is found in live-culture yogurt, as well as in capsule or powder form at health food stores. Castor oil packs to the abdomen can reduce inflammation and also reduce spasms or discomfort.

There are few steps that can be taken to avoid gastroenteritis. Hand-washing, and ensuring that food is well-cooked and unspoiled can prevent bacterial gastroenteritis, but may not be effective against viral gastroenteritis.

GAYLE, HELENE DORIS (1955-)

African American epidemiologist and pediatrician

Helene Doris Gayle is a specialist in the epidemiology of acquired immune deficiency syndrome (**AIDS**) and the human **immunodeficiency** virus (HIV) in children and teenagers. She is the coordinator of the AIDS Agency and chief of the HIV/AIDS Division at the U.S. Agency for International Development, Office of Health. In her position she has travelled to Africa and Asia to investigate the ways the disease effects different societies and to help coordinate international efforts to study it.

Born the third of five children on August 16, 1955, in Buffalo, New York. Her father, Jacob Sr., was an entrepreneur and her mother, Marietta, was a psychiatric social worker. Gayle was influenced by her parents from an early age, for her parents impressed upon their children the importance of making a contribution to the world. Gayle was also affected by growing up during the Civil Rights movement, and served as head of the black student union in her high school.

Gayle pursued a bachelor of arts degree in psychology in 1976 at Barnard University, followed by a medical degree from the University of Pennsylvania in 1981. Medical school opened the door for Gayle to the "social and political aspects of medicine," she told *Ebony* writer Renee D. Turner. After hearing a noted researcher speak on the efforts to eradicate the deadly **smallpox** virus, Gayle decided to seek a masters of public health, which she received from Johns Hopkins University in 1981. She then began a residency and internship in pediatrics at Children's Hospital Medical Center in Washington, D.C., where she worked for three years.

In 1984, Gayle was accepted to the epidemiology training program at the **Centers for Disease Control** and Prevention (CDC) in Atlanta, where she focused on the AIDS virus. She held various positions at the CDC, concentrating her efforts on the effect of AIDS on children, adolescents and their families, both in the United States and worldwide. Gayle has found that the U.S. black community, especially its women, is at high risk of contracting the fatal disease. In the late 1980s, black women made up 52 percent of the female AIDS population nationwide even though they only constituted 11 percent of the entire population. Gayle is an advocate for education as an important tool for the prevention of HIV/AIDS; as she told Turner, "Learning more about the spread of the disease also will provide some ammunition" in combating it. Gayle has traveled extensively studying the risk factors which contribute to the spread of HIV/AIDS in her position with the AIDS division for the Agency for International Development. The author of many articles and studies on HIV/AIDS risk factors, Gayle has received numerous awards, including the Henrietta and Jacob Lowenburg Prize, the Gordon Miller Award, and the U.S. Public Health Service achievement medal. She taught at various universities and is on the editorial board of the *Annual Review of Public Health.* Gayle is unmarried and has no children. As she told Turner, "I don't regret having placed a high priority on a career that enables me to make a contribution to mankind." Besides, she added, "we have no choice but to try to make an impact."

GENDER IDENTITY DISORDER

The psychological diagnosis gender identity disorder (GID) is used to describe a male or female who feels a strong identification with the opposite sex and experiences considerable distress because of their actual sex.

Gender identity disorder can affect children, adolescents, and adults. Individuals with gender identity disorder have strong cross-gender identification. They believe that they are, or should be, the opposite sex. They are uncomfortable with their sexual role and organs and may express a desire to alter their bodies. While not all persons with GID are labeled as transsexuals, there are those who are determined to undergo sex change procedures or have done so, and, therefore, are classified as transsexual. They often attempt to pass socially as the opposite sex. Transsexuals alter their physical appearance cosmetically and hormonally, and may eventually undergo a sex-change operation.

Children with gender identity disorder refuse to dress and act in sex-stereotypical ways. It is important to remember that many emotionally healthy children experience fantasies about being a member of the opposite sex. The distinction between these children and gender identity disordered children is that the latter experience significant interference in functioning because of their cross-gender identification. They may become severely depressed, anxious, or socially withdrawn.

The cause of gender identity disorder is not known. It has been theorized that a prenatal hormonal imbalance may predispose individuals to the disorder. Problems in the individual's family interactions or family dynamics have also been postulated as having some causal impact.

The *Diagnostic and Statistical Manual of Mental Disorders*, Fourth Edition (*DSM-IV*), the diagnostic reference standard for United States mental health professionals, describes the criteria for gender identity disorder as an individual's strong and lasting cross-gender identification and their persistent discomfort with their biological gender role. This discomfort must cause a significant amount of distress or impairment in the functioning of the individual.

DSM-IV specifies that children must display at least four of the following symptoms of cross-gender identification for a diagnosis of gender identity disorder:

- A repeatedly stated desire to be, or insistence that he or she is, the opposite sex.
- A preference for cross-dressing.
- A strong and lasting preference to play make-believe and role-playing games as a member of the opposite sex or persistent fantasies that he or she is the opposite sex.
- A strong desire to participate in the stereotypical games of the opposite sex.
- A strong preference for friends and playmates of the opposite sex.

Gender identity disorder is typically diagnosed by a psychiatrist or psychologist, who conducts an interview with the patient and takes a detailed social history. Family members may also be interviewed during the assessment process. This evaluation usually takes place in an outpatient setting.

Treatment for children with gender identity disorder focuses on treating secondary problems such as depression and **anxiety**, and improving **self-esteem**. Treatment may also work on instilling positive identifications with the child's biological gender. Children typically undergo psychosocial therapy sessions; their parents may also be referred for family or individual therapy.

Transsexual adults often request hormone and surgical treatments to suppress their biological sex characteristics and acquire those of the opposite sex. A team of health professionals, including the treating psychologist or psychiatrist, medical doctors, and several surgical specialists, oversee this transitioning process. Because of the irreversible nature of the surgery, candidates for sex-change surgery are evaluated extensively and are often required to spend a period of time integrating themselves into the cross-gender role before the procedure begins. **Counseling** and peer support are also invaluable to transsexual individuals.

Long-term follow up studies have shown positive results for many transsexuals who have undergone sex-change surgery. However, significant social, personal, and occupational issues may result from surgical sex changes, and the patient may require psychotherapy or counseling.

See also Sexual orientation

GENE THERAPY

Gene therapy is the use of genes engineered for treating disease. The first human gene therapy was approved for clinical trial in the United States in May 1989. Because this powerful technique is still in the experimental stages, each country has its own approval process, designed to protect the patient, the health workers, and the public. In the United States, each procedure must be approved by the **National Institutes of Health**'s Recombinant DNA Advisory Committee, by the Food and Drug Administration, and by the director of the National Institutes of Health.

Gene therapy begins with the isolation of a gene that can have a therapeutic effect, such as producing a protein in patients who lack the protein-producing gene or who have defective genes. In the laboratory, the desired gene is cut out of a cell's deoxyribonucleic acid (DNA) with enzymes. It is then inserted into somatic (functional) cells removed from the patient, and the treated cells are returned to the patient's body. An alternative approach is to insert the gene into disabled (harmless) viral or bacterial genetic material, which serve as vectors. These molecular delivery trucks carrying the attached gene are then injected directly into the patient, where they seek and enter somatic cells. In some cases, the virus itself is altered to make many copies of the gene. Ideally the gene should be targeted to an exact location in the cell's DNA. Viral vectors are primarily retroviruses, whose genetic material is ribonucleic acid (RNA) instead of DNA. These viruses have the potential to be permanently integrated into host cells' DNA. Techniques also exist for altering the individual's germ (reproductive) cells, which not only treat the individual but are inherited by the next generation. Such techniques are already used in plants and animals. However, this approach raises ethical dilemmas when applied to humans because permanent genetic changes (eugenics) have been attempted to harm people or eliminate groups considered inferior or undesirable. Two early extensive gene therapy trials focused on **severe combined immunodeficiency** (SCID) and malignant melanoma.

This rare disease (SCID) inhibits **immune system** functioning. In a well-publicized case, a teenager named David lived for several years in a plastic bubble to protect him from infection. Some instances of SCID result from a genetic mutation that prevents production of the protein adenosine deaminase (ADA), which protects immune system white cells called *lymphocytes*. In September 1990, Drs. R. Michael Blaese and W. French Anderson at the U.S. National Institutes of Health performed the world's first gene therapy on a four-year-old with this condition. A normal gene for ADA was inserted into a virus and allowed to enter lymphocytes that were withdrawn from her body. Then she was injected with the altered cells. During the next year-and-a-half, she had several series of injections, along with conventional treatment. In continued studies of young SCID patients, the cells appeared to induce production of ADA, reducing infections and allowing the children to have normal lives. There were no side effects. However, because most of these children were also given a standard enzyme treatment (due to ethical considerations), scientists could not conclusively say that it was the gene therapy that caused the improvements.

Melanoma is a type of often-fatal **skin cancer**. Since 1991, the National Cancer Institute's Dr. Steven A. Rosenberg has been studying treatment of the disease using TIL (tumor-infiltrating lymphocytes) cells taken from the patient's cancerous tumor. These cells normally enter a tumor and produce the protein called *tumor necrosis factor*. But often the tumor isn't destroyed. Scientists insert a gene into the TIL cells that boosts production of tumor necrosis factor. The cells are injected into the patients, and the genes function for a short period of time. Then, as a safety feature, the injected cells die.

Cystic fibrosis. A genetic treatment for this lung disease was approved in 1992. Dr. Ronald Crystal, of the National Institutes of Health inserted a needed gene into an inactive cold virus that the patients inhale. The gene then entered the lung and functioned to prevent the production of the mucus that blocks a patient's breathing. In follow-up studies, liposomes—hollow spheres of fat molecules formed in solution—were used as vectors to prevent side effects possibly caused by the viral vectors, like inflamed lungs and swollen nostrils. Familial hypercholesterolemia. Patients with this condition lack a gene for disposing of harmful low-density lipoprotein cholesterol, allowing it to build up in their bodies. People lacking both copies of the gene usually die from a heart attack in their early teens. Someone with only one copy suffers from severe coronary disease. Scientists at several medical centers are studying insertion of the needed gene into cells from a patient's liver, then injecting the cells into the person's body.

Studies are under way on genetic therapies for a host of illnesses, including **Hemophilia** B, **AIDS**, liver failure, **leukemia**, **brain tumors**, several **cancers**, arthritis, and **sickle-cell anemia**.

Despite ongoing advances, gene therapy remains a highly experimental procedure. Geneticists must overcome the dilemma of ensuring that a sufficient number of the therapeutic genes reach the proper cells to become functional. Most likely, viral vectors will play a key role in accomplishing this goal. Although viruses are extremely efficient at entering cells, the difficulty has been to get them to enter the proper cells. In 1998, scientists from Harvard Medical School announced a technique that can essentially build a bridge with two proteins. The bridge enables the virus to bind to and enter a specific cell. If proven effective, this approach would allow gene therapists to pinpoint cells for therapy. In addition to retroviruses as vectors, scientists have been studying adenoviruses vectors to target nondividing cells, which retroviruses cannot do. However, viruses and liposomes, which adhere to cells like tumors and insert genes into them, have drawbacks as vectors. Viruses can infect many types of cells and cause immune responses or become inserted in the wrong cell. Liposomes also have a slight possibility of infecting germ cells, producing heritable changes. As a result, researchers continue to look for new vectors like plasmids (circular DNA packages) and human artificial chromosomes (HACs). These chromosomes are less likely to trigger an immune response like viruses and are not able to seep into and affect other tissues because they can only be inserted into cells that have been removed from the body. Although it is still too early to tell, HACs may be viable vectors for gene therapies in blood diseases, like hemophilia and sickle-cell anemia.

An alternative approach for delivery genes has been developed by two scientists at Northwestern University. The gene "gun" is powered by pressurized helium that injects microscopic gold "bullets" coated with genes. In animal studies focusing on skin cells around tumors, they found that the surrounding cells began producing immune cells, called cytokines, which are what the genes are encoded for. The therapy shrunk tumors and lengthened the lives of the mice. Unlike viral vectors, this approach does not seek to permanently integrate the gene into the cell's DNA. This would be a disadvantage for inherited disease because the "mutant" genes that cause the disease would eventually become dominant again. However, the gene gun may be useful in disease such as cancer because of the reduced likelihood of prolonged or permanent side effects like those associated with traditional **chemotherapy**.

Although many obstacles must be overcome, gene therapy has shown much promise in animal studies. In 1998 researchers from Stanford University announced a gene therapy that provides proteins to inhibit inflammation in **multiple sclerosis** in mice. Gene therapy may also prove to be especially effective in many types of cancer, which often has a strong genetic basis, such as gene mutations that cause cancers to grow and spread. One approach uses gene-modified cancer cells as vaccines. Cancer cells are extracted from tumors removed from the body, then scientists insert the corrective genes and reinsert them into the patients' tumors, essentially immunizing them with their own tumor cells. Although good result have been obtained in animals, the therapy has yet to be proven effective in humans.

GENETIC ELEMENTS, TRANSPOSABLE •

See McClintock, Barbara

GENETIC ENGINEERING

Genetic engineering is the altering of the genetic material of living cells in order to make them capable of producing new substances or performing new functions, like getting a microorganism to produce human insulin or a sheep to produce a human blood-clotting protein in its milk. The technique became possible during the 1950s when scientists discovered the structure of deoxyribonucleic acid (DNA) molecules and how DNA stores and transmit genetic information. Largely as the result of the pioneering work of **James Watson** (1928-) and **Francis Crick** (1916-), scientists found that the sequence of nitrogen bases that make up any specific DNA molecule codes for the manufacture of specific chemical compounds. That sequence acts, therefore, as an "instruction manual" that directs all cell functions. Certain practical consequences of that discovery became almost immediately apparent. Suppose that the base sequence T-G-G-C-T-A-C-T on a DNA molecule carries the instruction "make insulin." (The actual sequence for such a message would in reality be very much longer.) DNA in the cells of the islets of Langerhans in the pancreas would normally contain that base sequence since the islets are the region in which insulin is produced in mammals. But that base sequence carries the same message no matter where it is found. If a way could be found to insert the base sequence into the DNA of bacteria, for example, then those bacteria would be capable of manufacturing insulin.

Although the concept of gene transfer is relatively simple, its actual execution presents a number of difficult technical challenges. In 1973, American biochemist Paul Berg, often referred to as the father of genetic engineering, developed a method for joining the DNA from two different organisms, a monkey virus known as SV40 and a second virus known as lambda phage. The accomplishment was significant, but Berg's method was slow and laborious. A turning point came later the same year when Stanley Cohn at Stanford and Hubert Boyer at the University of California at San Francisco discovered an enzyme that greatly increased the efficiency of the Berg process. The technique of gene transfer developed by Berg, Boyer, and Cohen is fundamentally that used in most animal genetic engineering today. This technique requires three elements: the gene to be transferred, a host cell in which the gene is to be inserted, and a vector for transferring the gene to the body. Suppose, for example, that one wishes to insert the insulin gene into a bacterial cell. The first step is to obtain a copy of the insulin gene. This copy can be obtained from a natural source (like DNA in islets of Langerhans cells), or it can be manufactured artificially in the laboratory. The second step is to insert the insulin gene into the vector. Viruses, liposomes (hollow spheres of fat molecules formed in solution), and plasmids (circular forms of DNA) are common vectors. Scientists have discovered enzymes that can "recognize" certain base sequences in a DNA molecule and cut the molecule open at these locations. In this case, the plasmid vector can, therefore, be cleaved at almost any point chosen by the scientist. Once the plasmid has been cleaved, it is mixed with the insulin gene and another enzyme that has the ability to glue the DNA molecule back together. In this case, however, the insulin gene attaches itself to the plasmid before the plasmid is re-closed. The hybrid plasmid now contains the gene whose product (insulin) is desired. It can be inserted into the host cell where it begins to function as all bacterial genes function. In this case, however, in addition to normal bacterial functions, the host cell is also producing insulin as directed by the inserted gene. This method is sometimes referred to as gene splicing. Since genes from two different sources have been combined with each other, the technique is also called recombinant DNA (rDNA) research.

The possible applications of genetic engineering are nearly limitless. For example, rDNA methods now make it possible to produce a number of natural products that were previously available in only very limited amounts. Until the 1980s, for example, the only supply of insulin available to diabetics was animals slaughtered for meat or other purposes. That supply was never adequate to treat all diabetics at moderate cost. In 1982, however, the United States Food and Drug Administration approved insulin produced by genetically altered organisms, the first such product to become available. Since 1982, a number of additional products, including human growth hormone, alpha interferon, interleukin-2, erythropoietin, tumor necrosis factor, and tissue plasminogen activator have been produced by rDNA techniques. In addition to the production of insulin, this technique has been used to create recombinant factor VIII for the treatment of **hemophilia**, a hereditary blood defect that inhibits blood clotting and makes it difficult for the body to naturally control bleeding. This genetically engineered blood factor protein can help induce clotting. Available since 1993, factor VIII can, for example, be produced in hamster cell lines using Bovine serum proteins. It is considered safer than similar blood-derived factors which have the potential to pass on blood viruses, such as AIDS or hepatitis. Several other similar blood factor products are under development.

The potential commercial value of genetically engineered products was not lost on entrepreneurs in the 1970s. In many cases, the founders of the first genetic engineering firms were scientists themselves, often those involved in basic research in the field. Boyer, for example, joined with venture capitalist Robert Swanson in 1976 to form Genentech (Genetic Engineering Technology). Other early firms like Cetus, Biogen, and Genex were formed similarly through the collaboration of scientists and business people. The structure of genetic engineering (or, more generally, biotechnology) firms has been a source of controversy, with concerns about individual scientists making a profit by opening their own companies that are based on research carried out at public universities and paid for with federal funds. By the early 1990s, working relationships had, in many cases, been formalized among universities, individual researchers, and the corporations they establish. But not everyone is satisfied that the ethical issues involved in such arrangements are settled.

One of the most exciting potential applications of genetic engineering involves the treatment of genetic disorders. Medical scientists now know of more 3,000 disorders that arise because of errors in an individual's DNA and are continuously finding new links among genes and diseases. Conditions such as **sickle-cell anemia**, **Tay-Sachs disease**, Duchenne **muscular dystrophy**, **Huntington's** chorea, **cystic fibrosis**, and Lesch-Nyhan syndrome are the result of the loss, mistaken insertion, or change of a single nitrogen base in a DNA molecule. Genetic engineering makes it possible for scientists to provide individuals who lack a certain gene with correct copies of that gene. If and when that correct gene begins to function, the genetic disorder may be cured. This procedure is known as human **gene therapy**. The first approved trials of gene therapy with human patients were begun in 1989. One of the most promising sets of experiments involved a condition known as **severe combined immune deficiency** (SCID) or ADA deficiency. Children born with this disorder have no **immune system** because of the lack of a single gene. In 1990, a research team at the National Institutes of Health led by W. French Anderson attempted gene therapy with a four-year old patient with SCID. The patient received about a billion cells containing a genetically engineered copy of the ADA gene that the child's body lacked. Human gene therapy is the source of great controversy among scientists and non-scientists alike. Few individuals would say that the technique should never be used, especially for battling life threatening diseases, like **AIDS** and **cancer**. But many critics worry about where gene therapy might lead, such as genetically engineered humans.

Genetic engineering also promises a revolution in agriculture. Recombinant DNA techniques make it possible to produce plants that are resistant to herbicides, that will survive freezing temperatures, that will take longer to ripen, that will convert atmospheric nitrogen to a form they can use, that will manufacture their own resistance to pests, and so on. Scientists have tested a multitude of plants engineered to have special properties such as these. In 1994, a tomato was the first genetically engineered food to appear in American supermarkets. The genetically engineered tomato was created with an ''antisense'' gene that allows the tomato to ripen on the vine but remain firm for shipping. As with every other aspect of genetic engineering, however, these advances have been controversial. The development of herbicide-resistant plants, for example, only means that farmers will use still larger quantities of herbicides, critics say, not an especially desirable trend. How sure can we be, others ask, about the potential risk to the environment posed by the introduction of ''unnatural'' engineered plants? For example, in the case of the tomato, some people are concerned genes from the plant could spread into soil bacteria and then infect humans or animals. Many other applications of genetic engineering have already been developed or are likely to be realized in the future. In every case, however, the glowing promises of each new technique is somewhat tempered by the social, economic and ethical questions it raises.

Genetically engineered clones (exact genetic copies of an individual), for example, became a major issue in 1997 when scientists from Scotland announced that they had successfully created the first clone of an adult mammal. The genes used to clone Dolly the sheep came from the frozen mammary tissue of a six-year-old dead sheep. The cloning was accomplished by taking the cell nucleus from a Finn Dorset sheep and then substituting it with the egg from the dead Poll Dorset sheep. The nucleus with the egg was then implanted into a third Scottish Blackface sheep. Because of the three different breeds used, the researchers had ready evidence that Dolly was truly a clone. While Dolly was a major advance scientifically, she became more famous among the public because of the ethical furor that has surrounded her "creation." Using genetic engineering to clone humans could be abused to create certain "types" of people, bringing forth the specter of humans as objects instead of individuals. Both the United States and Great Britain have banned human cloning. Still, the cloning of animals has many potential benefits, including raising animals that could be genetically engineered to produce more meat or, perhaps, to produce a human gene protein that could then be used in gene therapy.

Genetic fingerprinting

Fingerprints are unique to each individual. Methods of recording and matching fingerprints have allowed police to correctly identify many criminals. Genetic scientists have recently developed another tool for identification based on the uniqueness of each person's genes. Genetic differences account for the large variations we see among individuals. This genetic variability is expressed in obvious traits like hair color and genetic disorders such as **hemophilia**. However, more genetic variability is hidden from view and can only be detected by directly studying the deoxyribonucleic acid (DNA). Each human has approximately 100,000 genes in the chemical form of DNA. The genetic information coded in the genes varies greatly between individuals. Thus, no two humans, except for identical twins, have exactly the same genetic code. A description of a person's DNA that is detailed enough to distinguish it from another person's DNA is called a DNA or genetic "fingerprint." In 1985, an English researcher named Alec Jeffreys developed a technique to visualize a person's genetic code. This direct DNA analysis revealed so much variation in the genetic code between different people that even a small section of the entire genetic code could identify an individual's special combination of traits. Jeffreys knew that human DNA had many multi-repeated segments called minisatellites, and that the number and length of minisatellite DNA varied widely from person to person. He used a special detergent to break open the human cells and release the DNA code into solution. Then a restriction enzyme called HinfI broke the chain of DNA codes at sites close to each minisatellite DNA. The fragments of DNA were then attached to a membrane and allowed to combine with a radioactive minisatellite probe. After several hours, these probe molecules located and attached to certain predefined areas of the DNA fragments. X-rays were taken of the membrane to show where the radioactive probes attached. These pictures were then used to compare bands of DNA just as fingerprints are compared. Three years later, Henry Erlich developed a method of DNA fingerprinting so sensitive that it could be used to identify an individual from an extremely small sample of hair, blood, semen, or skin. Erlich's technique used Jeffreys' traditional method and combined it with a technique called polymerase chain reaction (PCR). First discovered by Kary Mullis, PCR was used to duplicate DNA and thus copy the genetic code. Erlich was able to duplicate and heat-separate the DNA fragments from a single human hair root many times using PCR. Ultimately, PCR multiplied the DNA from one single hair to an amount equivalent to that found in a million identical strands of hair. The amplified DNA was then used to obtain a DNA fingerprint. Genetic fingerprinting has already proved to be a very useful tool. Initially, it was used exclusively in forensic science and law. This technique has helped to link suspects to crimes where a single drop of blood was the only clue. Maternity and paternity matters have also been settled using genetic fingerprinting. This technology's impact in the study of genetic disorders and evolutionary relationships between different animal groups is also extremely important. While genetic fingerprinting has attained a high public profile through several sensational criminal trials, the process is not accepted by all as definitive proof of guilt. Critics argue that DNA experts may overestimate the odds of having matching DNA fingerprints; they also say that DNA samples can be contaminated when collected and that poor lab procedures can result in mistakes. These problems have been used successfully by defense attorneys to negate some DNA fingerprinting evidence presented in criminal trials. However, most courts in the U.S. allow DNA evidence, and some states have passed specific laws allowing its use.

Genetics

All living things pass on traits from one generation to the next according to a systematic set of "blueprints." These blueprints are contained in the long, thread-like chromosomes that lie inside the cell nucleus of all living things. On these chromosomes are genes that determine the hereditary traits of the offspring.

Egg and sperm cells, or sex cells, are specially formed to carry only one set of the 23 different chromosomes that are normally found in the human body. (Regular body cells have *two* sets of the 23 chromosomes.) When a mother's egg is fertilized by the father's sperm, the egg inherits one set of chromosomes from each parent, for a total of 46 chromosomes.

Some characteristics can only be inherited through genes and chromosomes: blood type, eye color, maleness or femaleness, etc. These are called hereditary traits. Most characteristics, however, are a result of both heredity and environment. For instance, a person can inherit a general body type, but environmental factors such as diet and **exercise** may change that body type.

The study of heredity—the science called genetics—started in the 1800s, when scientists first began trying to explain the existence of different species and variations within the same species. At that time, French biologist Jean Baptiste de Lamarck strongly believed that acquired characteristics would improve when routinely used over time. Those characteristics that were not used simply faded away. Lamarck also maintained that acquired characteristics were inherited from one generation to the next. In other words, Lamarck believed that if a giraffe continuously stretched its neck to reach for food, it would develop a longer neck. And the longer neck would be passed on to the next giraffe generation. Although his belief that acquired characteristics were inherited was incorrect, Lamarck was on the right track. He implied that traits can be inherited from generation to generation—that species undergo long-term evolutionary changes.

In 1859, Charles Darwin published his landmark book *The Origin of Species*, in which he outlined his theory of evolution through natural selection. Darwin believed that members of a particular species have slightly different characteristics. In the competition for space, food, and shelter, some of these characteristics would make a particular plant or animal better able to survive and produce offspring than others of its species. Therefore, these advantageous characteristics would persist in future generations, while those less advantageous ones would disappear as their carriers died out. After centuries or millennia of competition or natural selection, recent members of a species might be quite different from their ancestors. This theory gained advocates like the revered English physician Thomas Huxley (1825-1895), who, as ''Darwin's Bulldog,'' did more than anyone else to overcome opposition to Darwinian theory. But even with all the support, Darwin's theory still lacked an explanation for how the differences in species occurred.

Darwin, realizing that he needed to explain the mechanics of variation, asserted that tiny particles floating in an individual's bloodstream entered the eggs and sperm to determine hereditary characteristics. But **Francis Galton** proved him wrong with a simple blood transfusion experiment between two different types of rabbits. The transfusion didn't change the offspring of the rabbits as it should have if Darwin were correct.

In 1884, August Weissmann proposed that a special hereditary substance existed in the egg nucleus, which he termed ''germ plasm.'' His theories concerning the behavior of this substance—later identified as chromosomes—were eventually proved correct. However, he mistakenly believed that the germ plasm passed intact from generation to generation, unchanged by any environmental factors. Weissmann's theory, therefore, could not adequately account for the changes that occurred between generations and drove Darwin's theory of evolution.

It wasn't until 1900 that the second important theory concerning heredity was discovered, although it had been formulated some forty-five years earlier. Gregor Mendel, an Austrian monk, had begun experimenting with pea plants at about the same time that Darwin set forth his ideas on natural selection. Through his efforts, Mendel demonstrated that actual physical ''hereditary factors'' could be transmitted independently. Mendel ultimately established the basic laws of heredity—the missing key to Darwin's natural selection theory—and set the standard for the field of genetics. His revolutionary theories, however, were met with disinterest during his lifetime and remained largely unknown until 1900, when they were independently rediscovered by Hugo de Vries, Karl Correns (1864-1933), and Erich Tschermak (1871-1962).

De Vries took Mendel's theories further. Unlike the Austrian monk, he believed that variations, rather than arising from gradual or transitional steps, occurred in jumps he called mutations. This formed the cornerstone of de Vries's mutation theory, which he proposed in 1901.

Despite these theories, no biological mechanism for heredity had yet been found. Walther Flemming had discovered chromosomes during the 1870s but, unaware of Mendel's work, did not understand their genetic significance. In 1903, a young graduate student, Walter S. Sutton, at last made the connection. He had observed that during cell division in regular cells, chromosomes were present in pairs. But in the cell division of reproductive cells, only one member of each pair entered a sperm or egg. The chromosomes became pairs again when the egg joined the sperm in the fertilization process. Sutton saw that this pairing, unpairing, and pairing again paralleled the movement of Mendel's ''hereditary units.'' Theodor Boveri independently came to the same conclusion, and together their hypothesis came to be known as the chromosomal theory of inheritance.

By 1909, when Wilhelm Johannsen coined the term *gene* to describe the ''hereditary units'' on the chromosome, Mendelian theory and chromosomal theory had been widely accepted by scientists. American geneticist **Thomas Hunt Morgan**, however, remained unconvinced and set out to empirically prove or disprove Mendel's theory of inheritance. Following his many experiments with the fruit fly, Morgan was won over, convinced that genes were the trait-determiners and that they are arranged in a certain order on each chromosome. He also noticed that all the genes on the same chromosome were usually inherited together. Morgan referred to these as *linked genes*.

Further experiments showed that traits did not always follow Mendel's basic laws of heredity. Morgan showed that offspring don't always inherit all of the genes on a chromosome. He called this occurrence *crossing over*. By 1915, Morgan, along with **Hermann Muller**, Calvin Bridges (1889-1938), and Alfred Sturtevant (1891-1970), had fully developed the concepts of linkage and crossing over.

Yet some still refused to acknowledge the great strides made by biologists. The Ukrainian biologist Trofirm Denisovich Lysenko (1898-1976) gained control of Soviet biological research between 1928 and 1965, and, with the backing of Joseph Stalin (1879-1953), imposed his erroneous view that acquired characteristics could be inherited. Although his influence waned with the rise of Nikita Khrushchev (1894-1971), Lysenko severely damaged the Soviet Union's reputation in the international scientific community. His legacy would not be erased until the launching of *Sputnik I* in 1957.

By 1953, **James Watson** and **Francis Crick** had developed a model of deoxyribonucleic acid (DNA), the building blocks of genes, thus deciphering the genetic code and providing a key to the chemical basis of heredity. In recent decades, most research on heredity has focused on the function of DNA, its regulatory processes, and its evolution.

GENETIC TESTING AND COUNSELING

Genetic testing examines the genetic information contained inside a person's cells to determine if that person has or will develop a certain disease or could pass a disease to his or her offspring.

Some families or ethnic groups have a higher incidence of a certain disease than does the population as a whole. Before having a child, a couple from such a family or ethnic group may want to know if their child would be at risk of having that disease.

Early in **pregnancy**, the baby's cells can be studied for certain defects that could result in physical abnormalities or **mental retardation**. This testing is most common when the mother is over the age of 35 or there is a family history of physical or mental abnormalities.

A genetic disease may be apparent when the child is born or may appear later as the child develops. Genetic testing can help diagnose these diseases. Couples who are having difficulty conceiving a child or who have suffered multiple miscarriages may be tested to see if a genetic cause can be identified.

Huntington's disease is an example of a genetic disease that doesn't appear until adulthood. If this disease or another late-onset disease is in a person's family, genetic testing may be able to predict if that person will develop the disease.

Some genetic defects may make a person more susceptible to certain types of **cancer**. Testing for these defects can help predict a person's risk. Other types of genetic tests help diagnose and predict and monitor the course of certain kinds of cancer, particularly **leukemia** and **lymphoma**.

Genetic counseling aims to facilitate the exchange of information regarding a person's genetic legacy. It attempts to:

- Accurately diagnose a disorder
- Assess the risk of recurrence in the concerned family members and their relatives
- Provide alternatives for decision-making
- Provide **support groups** that will help family members cope with the recurrence of a disorder.

With approximately 2,000 genes identified and approximately 5,000 disorders caused by genetic defects, genetic counseling is important in the medical discipline of obstetrics. Genetic counselors, educated in the medical and the psychosocial aspects of genetic diseases, convey complex information to help people make life decisions. There are limitations to the power of genetic counseling, though, since many of the diseases that have been shown to have a genetic basis currently offer no cure (for example, **Down syndrome** or Huntington's disease). Although a genetic counselor cannot predict the future unequivocally, he or she can discuss the occurrence of a disease in terms of probability.

A genetic counselor, with the aid of the patient or family, creates a detailed family pedigree that includes the incidence of disease in first-degree (parents, siblings, and children) and second-degree (aunts, uncles, and grandparents) relatives. Before or after this pedigree is completed, certain genetic tests are performed using DNA analysis, x ray, **ultrasound**, **urinalysis**, skin **biopsy**, and physical evaluation. For a pregnant woman, prenatal diagnosis can be made using amniocentesis or chorionic villus sampling.

An important aspect of the genetic counseling session is the compilation of a family pedigree or medical history. To accurately assess the risk of inherited diseases, information on three generations, including health status and/or cause of **death**, is usually needed. If the family history is complicated information from more distant relatives may be helpful, and medical records may be requested for any family members who have had a genetic disorder. Through an examination of the family history a counselor may be able to discuss the probability of future occurrence of genetic disorders. In all cases, the counselor provides information in a non-directive way that leaves the decision-making up to the client.

Genetic disease results from a change, or mutation, in a chromosome or in one or several base pairs in a gene. Several types of genetic tests are available to look for the mutations in genes and chromosomes associated with certain diseases. The cost of genetic tests vary: chromosome studies can cost hundreds of dollars and certain gene studies, thousands. Insurance coverage also varies with the company and the policy. It may take several days or weeks to complete a test.

Direct DNA mutation analysis examines DNA for specific gene mutations. Some genes contain more than 100,000 bases and a mutation of any one base can make the gene nonfunctional and cause disease. The more mutations possible, the less likely it is for a test to detect all of them. This test is usually done on white blood cells from a person's blood. The test begins by using chemicals to separate DNA from the rest of the cell. Next, the two strands of DNA are separated by heating. Special enzymes (called restriction enzymes) are added to the single strands of DNA and then act like scissors and cut the strands in specific places. The DNA fragments are then sorted by size through a process called electrophoresis. A special piece of DNA, called a probe, is added to the fragments. The probe is designed to bind to specific mutated portions of the gene. When bound to the probe, the mutated portions appear on x-ray film with a distinct banding pattern.

Family linkage studies are done to study a disease when a mutated gene's general location on a chromosome is known but its identity is not. These studies are possible when a chromosome marker has been found associated with a disease. Chromosomes contain certain regions that vary in appearance between individuals. These regions are called polymorphisms. If a polymorphism is always present in family members with the same genetic disease, and absent in family members without the disease, it is likely that the gene responsible for the disease is near that polymorphism. The gene mutation can be indirectly detected in family members by looking for the polymorphism.

To look for the polymorphism, DNA is isolated from cells in the same way it is for direct DNA mutation analysis. A probe is added that will detect the large polymorphism on the chromosome. When bound to the probe, this region will appear on x-ray film with a distinct banding pattern. The pattern of banding of a person being tested for the disease is compared to the pattern from a family member affected by the disease.

Linkage studies have disadvantages not found in direct DNA mutation analysis. These studies require multiple family members to participate in the testing. If key family members choose not to participate, the incomplete family history may make testing other members useless. The indirect method of detecting a mutated gene also causes more opportunity for error.

Many genetic diseases and syndromes are caused by structural chromosome abnormalities. To analyze a person's chromosomes, his or her cells are allowed to grow and multiply in the laboratory until they reach a certain stage of growth. The length of growing time varies with the type of cells. Cells from blood and bone marrow take 1–2 days; fetal cells from amniotic fluid take 7–10 days.

When the cells are ready, they are placed on a microscope slide using a technique to make them burst open, spreading their chromosomes. The slides are stained: the stain creates a banding pattern unique to each chromosome. Under a microscope, the chromosomes are counted, identified, and analyzed based on their size, shape, and stained appearance.

Karyotypes of the chromosomes are prepared for further study and to document the results. First, a photograph is taken of the chromosomes from one or more cells as seen through the microscope. Then the chromosomes are cut out and arranged side-by-side with their partner in ascending numerical order, from largest to smallest. The karyotype is done either manually or using a computer attached to the microscope. Chromosome analysis is also called cytogenetics.

A person who has a mutated gene associated with a disease is called a carrier. A carrier is a person who is not affected by the mutated gene he or she possesses, but can pass the gene to an offspring. Genetic tests have been developed that tell prospective parents whether or not they are carriers of certain diseases. If one or both of the parents is a carrier, the risk of passing the disease to a child can be predicted.

To predict the risk, it is necessary to know if the gene in question is autosomal or sex-linked. If the gene is carried on any one of chromosomes 1–22, the resulting disease is called an autosomal disease. If the gene is carried on the X or Y chromosome, it is called a sex-linked disease.

Sex-linked diseases, such as the bleeding condition **hemophilia**, are usually carried on the X (or female) chromosome. A woman who carries a disease-associated mutated gene on one of her X chromosomes, has a 50% chance of passing that gene to her son. A son who inherits that gene will develop the disease because he does not have another normal copy of the gene on a second X chromosome to compensate for the mutated copy.

The risk of passing an autosomal disease to a child depends on whether the gene is dominant or recessive. A prospective parent carrying a dominant gene, has a 50% chance of passing the gene to a child. A child needs to receive only one copy of the mutated gene to be affected by the disease.

If the gene is recessive, a child needs to receive two copies of the mutated gene, one from each parent, to be affected by the disease. When both prospective parents are carriers, their child has a 25% chance of inheriting two copies of the mutated gene and being affected by the disease; a 50% chance of inheriting one copy of the mutated gene, and being a carrier of the disease but not affected; and a 25% chance of inheriting two normal genes. When only one prospective parent is a carrier, a child has a 50% chance of inheriting one mutated gene and being an unaffected carrier of the disease, and a 50% chance of inheriting two normal genes.

Not all genetic diseases show their effect immediately at birth or early in childhood. Although the gene mutation is present at birth, some diseases don't appear until adulthood. If a specific mutated gene responsible for a late-onset disease, like Huntington's disease, has been identified, a person from an affected family can be tested before symptoms appear.

Cancer can result from an inherited mutated gene or a gene that mutated sometime during a person's lifetime. Some genes, called tumor suppressor genes, produce proteins that protect the body from cancer. If one of these genes develops a mutation, it can't produce the protective protein. If the second copy of the gene is normal, its action may be sufficient to continue production, but if that gene later also develops a mutation, the person is vulnerable to cancer. Other genes, called oncogenes, are involved in the normal growth of cells. A mutation in an oncogene can cause too much growth, the beginning of cancer.

Direct DNA tests are currently available to look for gene mutations identified and linked to several kinds of cancer. People with a family history of these cancers are those most likely to be tested. If one of these mutated genes is found, the person is more susceptible to developing the cancer. The likelihood that the person will develop the cancer, even with the mutated gene, is not always known because other genetic and environmental factors are also involved in the development of cancer.

Chromosome analysis is done on fetal cells primarily when the mother is over the age of 35, has had multiple miscarriages, or a family history of a genetic abnormality. Prenatal testing is done on the fetal cells in amniotic fluid (the fluid surrounding the baby) at 14–16 weeks of pregnancy or from a chorionic villus sampling (from the baby's placenta) at 8–12 weeks. Cells from amniotic fluid grow for 7–10 days before they are ready to be analyzed. Biopsy cells grow faster and can be analyzed sooner.

Chromosome analysis using blood cells is done on a child who is born with or later develops signs of mental retardation or physical malformation. In the older child, chromosome analysis may be done to investigate developmental delays.

Extra or missing chromosomes cause mental and physical abnormalities. A child born with an extra chromosome 21 (trisomy 21) has Down syndrome. An extra chromosome 13 or 18 also produce well known syndromes. A missing X chromosome causes Turner syndrome and an extra X in a male causes Klinefelter syndrome. Other abnormalities are caused by extra or missing pieces of chromosomes. Fragile X syndrome is a sex-linked disease, causing mental retardation in males. The abnormality is recognized by a fragile-looking area at the bottom of the X chromosome.

Chromosome material may also be rearranged, such as the end of chromosome 1 moved to the end of chromosome 3. If no material is added or deleted in the exchange, the person may not be affected. Such an exchange, however, can cause **infertility** or abnormalities if passed to children.

Evaluation of a man and woman's infertility or repeated miscarriages will include blood studies of both to check for a chromosome structural rearrangement. Many chromosome abnormalities are incompatible with life; babies with these abnormalities often miscarrry during the first trimester. Cells from a baby that died before birth can be studied to look for chromosome abnormalities that may have caused the **death**.

Certain cancers, particularly leukemia and lymphoma, are associated with changes in chromosomes: extra or missing complete chromosomes, extra or missing portions of chromosomes, or exchanges of material (called translocations) between chromosomes. Studies show that the locations of the chromosome breaks are at locations of tumor suppressor genes or oncogenes.

Chromosome analysis on cells from blood, bone marrow, or solid tumor helps diagnose certain kinds of leukemia and lymphoma and often helps predict how well the person will respond to treatment. After treatment has begun, periodic monitoring of these chromosome changes in the blood and bone marrow gives the physician information as to the effectiveness of the treatment.

A well-known chromosome rearrangement is found in chronic myelogenous leukemia. This leukemia is associated with an exchange of material between chromosomes 9 and 22. The resulting smaller chromosome 22 is called the Philadelphia chromosome.

Most tests for genetic diseases of children and adults are done on blood. To collect the 5–10 mL of blood needed, a healthcare worker draws blood from a vein in the inner elbow region. Collection of the sample takes only a few minutes.

Prenatal testing is done either on amniotic fluid or a chorionic villus biopsy. To collect amniotic fluid, a physician performs a procedure called amniocentesis. An ultrasound is done to find the baby's position and an area filled with amniotic fluid. The physician inserts a needle through the woman's skin and the wall of her uterus and withdraws 5–10 mL of amniotic fluid. Placental tissue for a chorionic villus biopsy is taken through the cervix. Each procedures take approximately 30 minutes.

Bone marrow is used for chromosome analysis in a person with leukemia or lymphoma. The person is given local **anesthesia**. Then the physician inserts a needle through the skin and into the bone (usually the sternum or hip bone). One-half to 2 mL of bone marrow is withdrawn. This procedure takes approximately 30 minutes.

Genital herpes

Genital herpes is a **sexually transmitted disease** caused by a herpes virus. The disease is characterized by painful blisters on the genital areas of men and women. It is spread person-to-person by sexual contact. It is not spread by toilet seats, doorknobs, swimming pools, hot tubs, or through the air.

There are eight kinds of human herpes viruses. Only two of these, herpes simplex types 1 and 2, cause genital herpes. Although it is commonly believed that herpes simplex virus type 1 causes only cold sores and herpes simplex virus type 2 causes only genital sores, this is not completely true. Both herpes virus type 1 and type 2 can cause herpes sores on either the lips or genitals.

Sometimes an active infection occurs without visible sores. An infected person can therefore spread herpes virus to other people without knowing it. The initial infection, known as the "primary" infection, can be followed by later "recurrent" infections.

The first symptoms of herpes usually occur within two to seven days after contact with an infected person but may take up to two weeks. For up to 70% of patients, the symptoms may affect the whole body (called "constitutional symptoms") including tiredness, **headache**, **fever**, chills, muscle aches, loss of appetite, as well as painful, swollen lymph nodes in the groin.

Most patients with genital herpes experience a prodrome (symptoms of oncoming disease) of **pain**, burning, **itching**, or tingling at the site where blisters will form. This stage may last anywhere from a few hours, to one to two days. The prodrome can occur for both primary and recurrent infections. The prodrome for recurrent infections may be severe and cause a severe burning or stabbing pain in the genital area, legs, or buttocks.

Following the prodrome come the herpes blisters. In dry areas, the blisters become covered with a scab and heal within two to three weeks. In moist areas, the blisters burst and form painful **ulcers** that heal by three to four weeks. In men, herpes blisters usually form on the penis but can also appear on the scrotum, thighs, and buttocks. In women, they most often appear on the labia and entrance to the vagina, but can also form on the buttocks, thighs, breasts, fingers, eyes, and around the urinary and anal openings.

Thirty percent to 40% of men have a discharge from the urinary tube. Men may also experience painful or difficult urination (44%), swelling of the urinary tube (27%), **meningitis** (13%), and throat infection (7%).

Women can experience a very severe and painful primary infection. Herpes blisters first appear on the labia and vaginal area, causing a watery discharge. Other symptoms may include painful or difficult urination (83%), swelling of the urinary tube (85%), meningitis (36%), and throat infection (13%). One in ten women also gets a vaginal yeast infection.

After the primary infection, the virus is latent, hiding in the cells. At some point, latent viruses may become activated again and cause a "recurrent" infection.

Newborn babies infected with herpes virus experience a very severe, possibly fatal disease called "neonatal herpes infection." Doctors will perform **Cesarean section**s on women who go into labor with active genital herpes.

Risk factors for genital herpes include: early age at first sexual activity, multiple sexual partners, and a medical history of other sexually transmitted diseases.

About 40% of the persons infected with herpes simplex virus type 2 will experience six or more outbreaks each year. Genital herpes recurrences are less severe than the primary infection; however, women still experience more severe symptoms and pain than men. Blisters will appear at the same sites during each outbreak.

Genital herpes is diagnosed primarily by symptoms, although laboratory tests may be performed to look for the virus.

Because genital sores can be symptoms of many other diseases, the doctor must determine the exact cause of the sores.

Certain **antiviral drugs** can lessen symptoms and decrease length of herpes outbreaks. Some may also prevent future outbreaks. These drugs are most effective when taken as early in the infection process as possible, preferably during the prodrome stage. Acyclovir (Zovirax) is the drug of choice for herpes infection. Other drugs that may be used include famciclovir (Famvir), valacyclovir (Valtrex), vidarabine (Vira-A), idoxuridine (Herplex Liquifilm, Stoxil), trifluorothymidine (Viroptic), and penciclovir (Denavir). Patients with frequent outbreaks (greater than six to eight per year) may benefit from long-term use of acyclovir which is called ''suppressive therapy.'' Alternatively, patients may use short-term suppressive therapy to lessen the chance of developing an active infection during special occasions such as weddings or holidays.

There are several things that a patient may do to lessen the pain of genital sores. Wearing loose fitting clothing and cotton underwear is helpful as is soaking in a tub of warm water and using a blow dryer on the ''cool'' setting to dry the infected area. Putting an ice pack on the affected area for 10 minutes, followed by 5 minutes off and then repeating this procedure may relieve pain. A zinc sulfate ointment may help to heal the sores. Application of a baking soda compress to sores may be soothing.

Newborn babies with herpes virus infections are treated with intravenous acyclovir or vidarabine, which have greatly reduced deaths and increased the number of babies who appear normal at one year of age. However, because neonatal herpes infection is so serious, even with treatment babies may not survive, or may suffer nervous system damage. Infected babies may be treated with long-term suppressive therapy.

Alternative treatments to avoid recurrences of genital herpes include a diet that is rich in lysine (found in most vegetables, legumes, fish, turkey, beef, lamb, cheese, chicken, and lysine supplements). Other remedies include herbs such as echinacea and garlic, and red marine algae. Ointments containing zinc sulphate, lithium succinate, glycyrrhizinic acid, vitamin E or tea tree oil may also be recommended. In addition, homeopathic remedies are available.

The only way to prevent genital herpes is to avoid contact with infected persons. This is not easy because many people are not aware that they are infected. Avoid all sexual contact with known infected persons during a herpes outbreak. Because herpes can spread at any time, **condom** use is recommended. As of mid-1999 no herpes vaccines had been approved, although new vaccines are being tested in humans.

GENITAL WARTS

Genital warts, also called condylomata acuminata or venereal warts, are growths in the genital area caused by a sexually transmitted virus.

Genital warts are the most common **sexually transmitted disease**. It is estimated that 1% of sexually active people between the ages of 18 and 45 have genital warts; however, as many as 40% of sexually active adults are believed to carry the human papillomavirus (HPV) that causes genital warts.

Genital warts vary somewhat in appearance. They may be either flat or resemble raspberries or cauliflowers. The warts begin as small red or pink growths and grow as large as four inches across, interfering with intercourse and childbirth. The warts grow in the moist tissues of the genital areas. In women, they occur on the external genitals and on the walls of the vagina and cervix; in men, they develop in the urethra and on the shaft of the penis. The warts then spread to the area behind the genitals surrounding the anus.

Risk factors for genital warts include:

- Multiple sexual partners
- Infection with another STD
- **Pregnancy**
- Anal intercourse
- Poor **personal hygiene**
- Heavy perspiration

There are about 80 types of human papillomavirus. Genital warts are caused by HPV types 1, 2, 6, 11, 16, and 18. HPV is transmitted by sexual contact. The time between infection and appearance of the first symptoms varies from one to six months.

Symptoms include bleeding, **pain**, and odor as well as the visible warts.

Diagnosis is usually made by examining scrapings from the warts under a darkfield microscope. If the warts are caused by HPV, they will turn white when a 5% solution of white vinegar is added. If the warts reappear, the doctor may order that tissue samples be examined to rule out **cancer**.

No treatment for genital warts is completely effective because therapy depends on destroying skin infected by the virus. There are no drugs that kill the virus directly.

Genital warts were treated until recently with applications of podophyllum resin, a corrosive substance that cannot be given to pregnant patients. A milder form of podophyllum, podofilox (Condylox), has been introduced. Women are also treated with 5-fluorouracil cream, bichloroacetic acid, or trichloroacetic acid. All of these substances irritate the skin and require weeks of treatment.

Genital warts can also be treated with injections of interferon. Interferon works best in combination with podofilox applications.

Surgery may be necessary to remove warts blocking the patient's vagina, urethra, or anus. Surgical techniques include the use of liquid nitrogen, electrosurgery, and **laser surgery**.

Genital warts are non-threatening growths and are not cancerous by themselves. Repeated HPV infection in women, however, appears to increase the risk of later **cervical cancer**. Women infected with HPV types 16 and 18 should have yearly cervical smears. It is not unusual for genital warts to return after all present methods of treatment—including surgery—because HPV can hide in apparently normal surrounding skin.

The only reliable method of prevention is sexual **abstinence**. The use of **condoms** minimizes but does not eliminate the risk of HPV transmission. The patient's sexual contacts should be notified and examined.

GERM THEORY

The Germ Theory of disease, which states that illness is caused by germlike substances, was first suggested in the fourth century B.C. by the Greek philosopher Democritus. More than two millennia later, in the latter half of the nineteenth century, the French chemist and microbiologist **Louis Pasteur** and the German physician **Robert Koch** were finally able to establish the theory, based on microscopic observation and experimental evidence. For most of the intervening centuries, the concept of Germ Theory was doubted and other ideas about the origin of disease prevailed. Predominant among these was the notion that illness was caused by lethal emanations in the atmosphere, also known as ''miasmas.'' Miasmas might be generated from swamps, from the decomposition of plant and animal matter, from sewage, or from various climatic events. As late as the 1840s, the mainstream medical profession in England was espousing the view that poisonous vapors released during decomposition would mix with the surrounding air, penetrate the air cells of the lungs, and spread diseases as varied as **cholera**, **typhoid fever**, and **plague** throughout the human body.

Then, in the 1860s, Louis Pasteur was commissioned by the French government to study the cause of a disease that had been ravishing silkworm populations and threatening the economically powerful silk industry. By 1868 he had determined that a tiny parasite was responsible, and he recommended that to curb its spread the infected silkworms had to be destroyed. Once the silkworms were destroyed the source of the parasite was eliminated and the disease was halted. Pasteur's demonstration of a link between the silkworm disease and a specific pathogen or disease-causing substance provided the first clear evidence in support of Germ Theory. Pasteur went on to develop techniques for reducing the virulence of disease-causing organisms, most notably developing the **sanitation** technique we know today as pasteurization.

Meanwhile, in the 1870s Robert Koch identified the bacterium responsible for **anthrax**, a disease of cattle. He developed a method for growing the bacteria ''in culture,'' that is, outside of the diseased animal. Placing a drop of his anthrax culture under the microscope, he observed that as the bacteria multiplied they produced spores. While the bacteria themselves were short-lived, the spores seemed to be resilient. Koch then injected healthy cattle with these spores and saw that they developed anthrax. This was the first demonstration that a disease could be caused by a pathogen that grew outside of a living organism. In 1882 Koch announced the discovery of the bacterium responsible for **tuberculosis**. In 1883 he isolated and identified the bacterium that caused cholera. Koch developed a four-step method, known today as Koch's postulates, for demonstrating that a particular pathogen is the cause of a disease. First, the pathogen must be found in every individual who has the disease. Second, the pathogen must be isolated from a diseased individual and grown separately in a pure culture. Third, the disease must be induced in an experimental animal by transferring the pathogen from the pure culture. And fourth, the same pathogen must be isolated from the experimental animal after it has contracted the disease.

While Pasteur and Koch demonstrated the connection between specific microorganisms and the occurrence of particular diseases, they did not attempt to explain all disease through Germ Theory. Although we know today that half of all human diseases are caused by bacteria, illness can be attributed to many other sources, including genetic mutation, environmental contaminants, malnutrition, prions, and a host of viruses, fungi, protozoans, and parasitic worms.

GESTALT THERAPY

Gestalt therapy seeks to treat psychological problems and mental disorders by gaining awareness of emotions and behaviors in the present rather than in the past. The therapist does not interpret experiences for the patient. Instead, the therapist and patient work together to help the patient understand him/herself. Patients are encouraged to become aware of immediate needs, meet them, and let them recede into the background. The well-adjusted person is seen as someone who has a constant flow of needs and is able to satisfy those needs.

In Gestalt therapy (from the German word meaning *form*), the major goal is self-awareness. Patients work on uncovering and resolving interpersonal issues during therapy. Unresolved issues are unable to fade into the background of consciousness because the needs they represent are never met. In Gestalt therapy, the goal is to discover people connected with a patient's unresolved issues and try to engage those people (or images of those people) in interactions that can lead to a resolution. Gestalt therapy is most useful for patients open to working on self-awareness.

The choice of a therapist is crucial. Some people who call themselves ''therapists'' have limited training in Gestalt therapy. It is important that the therapist be a licensed mental health professional. Additionally, some individuals may not be able to tolerate the intensity of this type of psychotherapy.

Gestalt therapy tends to emphasize medium to large groups, although many Gestalt techniques can be used in one-on-one therapy. Gestalt therapy probably has a greater range of formats than any other therapeutic technique. It is practiced in individual, couples, and family therapies, as well as in therapy with children.

Ideally, the patient identifies current sensations and emotions, particularly ones that are painful or disruptive. Patients are confronted with their unconscious feelings and needs, and are helped to accept and assert those repressed parts of themselves.

The most powerful techniques involve role-playing. For example, the patient talks to an empty chair, imagining that a person associated with an unresolved issue is sitting in the chair. As the patient talks to the ''person'' in the chair, the patient imagines that the person responds to the expressed feelings. Although this technique may sound artificial and might make some people feel self-conscious, it can be a powerful way to approach buried feelings and gain new insight into them.

Sometimes patients use battacca bats, padded sticks that can be used to hit chairs or sofas. Using a battacca bat can help a patient safely express anger. A patient may also experience a Gestalt therapy marathon, where the participants and one or more facilitators have nonstop **group therapy** over a weekend. The effects of the intense emotion and the lack of sleep can eliminate many psychological defenses and allow significant progress to be made in a short time. This is true only if the patient has adequate psychological strength for a marathon and is carefully monitored by the therapist.

Gestalt therapy begins with the first contact. There is no separate diagnostic or assessment period. Instead, assessment and screening are done as part of the ongoing relationship between patient and therapist. This assessment includes determining the patient's willingness and support for work using Gestalt methods, as well as determining the compatibility between the patient and the therapist. Unfortunately, some ''encounter groups'' led by poorly trained individuals do not provide adequate pre-therapy screening and assessment.

Sessions are usually held once a week. Frequency of sessions is based on how long the patient can go between sessions without losing momentum from the previous session. Patients and therapists discuss when to start sessions, when to stop, and what kind of activities to use. However, the patient is encouraged and required to make choices.

Disturbed people with severe mental illness may not be suitable candidates for Gestalt therapy. Facilities that provide Gestalt therapy and train Gestalt therapists vary widely.

Scientific documentation on the effectiveness of Gestalt therapy is limited. Some evidence suggests that this type of therapy may not be reliably effective.

The approach can be anti-intellectual and can discount thoughts, thought patterns, and beliefs. In the hands of an ineffective therapist, Gestalt procedures can become a series of mechanical exercises. Moreover, there is a potential for the therapist to manipulate the patient with powerful techniques, especially in therapy marathons where fatigue may make a patient vulnerable.

GESTATIONAL DIABETES

Gestational diabetes is a condition that occurs during **pregnancy**. Like other forms of **diabetes**, it involves a defect in the way the body processes and uses dietary sugars (glucose).

In gestational diabetes, the problem is in the placenta, an organ inside the womb that attaches the embryo to the womb's wall. During a normal pregnancy, the placenta provides the baby with nourishment. In addition, it produces hormones that interfere with the body's response to insulin, a hormone involved in regulating glucose levels in the blood. In most pregnant women, the pancreas (the gland that produces insulin), simply makes extra insulin during pregnancy to counteract the effect of these hormones. However, when a woman's pancreas cannot produce enough extra insulin, blood glucose levels stay abnormally high, and she is considered to have gestational diabetes

Most women with gestational diabetes have no recognizable symptoms. However, leaving this form of diabetes undiagnosed and untreated is risky to the developing fetus. Left untreated, a diabetic mother's blood sugar levels will be consistently high. This sugar will cross the placenta and pour into the baby's system through the umbilical cord. The unborn baby's pancreas will respond to this high level of sugar by constantly putting out large amounts of insulin, allowing the fetus's cells to take in glucose, where it will be converted to fat and stored. A baby who has been exposed to constantly high levels of sugar throughout pregnancy will be abnormally large, often so large that he or she cannot be born through the vagina, but will instead need to be born through a surgical procedure, a **cesarean section**.

Furthermore, after the baby is born, it will still have an abnormally large amount of insulin. When the mother and baby are no longer attached to each other via the placenta and umbilical cord, the baby will no longer receive the mother's high level of sugar. The baby's high level of insulin, however, will very quickly use up the glucose circulating in the baby's bloodstream. The baby is then at risk for having a dangerously low level of blood glucose (a condition called **hypoglycemia**). This is easily resolved by giving the baby glucose. It is important to monitor the baby's blood glucose levels.

About 1–3% of all pregnant women develop gestational diabetes. Women at risk for gestational diabetes include those who:

- Are overweight
- Have a family history of diabetes
- Have previously given birth to a very large, heavy baby
- Have previously had a baby who was stillborn, or born with a birth defect
- Have an excess amount of amniotic fluid (the cushioning fluid within the womb that surrounds the developing fetus)
- Are over 25 years of age
- Belong to an ethnic group known to experience higher rates of gestational diabetes (in the United States, these include Mexican-Americans, American Indians, African-Americans, as well as individuals from Asia, India, or the Pacific Islands)
- Have a previous history of gestational diabetes during a pregnancy.

Screening for gestational diabetes is a routine part of pregnancy care, usually done between the 24th and 28th week of pregnancy. Screening involves drinking a glucose solution, followed by a blood test that determines the glucose level.

When the screening level exceeds a certain amount, a further three-hour glucose tolerance test is performed. This involves following a special diet for three days prior to the test. Then, for 10–14 hours just before the test, the patient is instructed to eat and drink nothing except water. A blood sample is then taken to determine the fasting glucose level, after which the patient drinks a glucose solution and has her blood tested every hour for the next three hours. If two or more of these levels are elevated over normal, then the patient is considered to have gestational diabetes.

Treatment will depend on the severity of the diabetes. Mild forms can be treated with diet (decreasing the intake of sugars and fats, in particular). Many women are put on strict, detailed **diets**, and are asked to stay within a certain range of calorie intake. **Exercise** is sometimes used to lower blood sugar levels. Patients are often asked to regularly measure their blood sugar. This is done by poking a finger with a needle called a lancet, putting a drop of blood on a special type of paper, and feeding the paper into a meter which determines the blood sugar level. When diet and exercise do not keep blood glucose levels within an acceptable range, a patient may need regular shots of insulin.

The prospects for women with gestational diabetes, and their babies, is generally good. Almost all such women stop being diabetic after delivering. However, some research suggests that nearly 50% of these women will develop a permanent form of diabetes within 15 years. The child of a mother with gestational diabetes has a greater-than-normal chance of developing diabetes sometime in adulthood. A woman who has had gestational diabetes during one pregnancy has about a 66% chance of having it again during any subsequent pregnancies. Women who had gestational diabetes usually are tested for diabetes at the post-partum checkup or after stopping **breastfeeding**.

GI EXAMS

There are various kinds of GI exams. A barium **enema**, also known as a lower GI (gastrointestinal) exam, is a test that uses x-ray examination to view the large intestine. There are two types of this test: the single-contrast technique where barium sulfate is injected into the rectum in order to gain a profile view of the large intestine; and the double-contrast (or ''air contrast'') technique where air is inserted into the rectum. A barium enema may be performed for a variety of reasons, including to aid in the diagnosis of colon and rectal **cancer** (or **colorectal cancer**), and inflammatory disease. Detection of **polyps** (a benign growth in the tissue lining of the colon and rectum), diverticula (a pouch pushing out from the colon), and structural changes in the large intestine can also be established with this test. The double-contrast barium enema is the best method for detecting small tumors (such as polyps), early inflammatory disease, and bleeding caused by **ulcers**.

Colonoscopy is a medical procedure in which a long, flexible, tubular instrument called the colonoscope is used to view the entire inner lining of the colon (large intestine) and the rectum. It is generally recommended when the patient complains of rectal bleeding or has a change in bowel habits and other unexplained abdominal symptoms. The test is frequently used to test for colorectal cancer, especially when polyps or tumor-like growths have been detected using the barium enema and other diagnostic tests. Polyps can be removed through the colonoscope and samples of tissue (biopsies) can be taken to test for the presence of cancerous cells. The test also enables the physician to check for bowel diseases such as ulcerative colitis and Crohn's disease. It is a necessary tool in monitoring patients who have a past history of polyps or colon cancer.

An upper GI examination is a fluoroscopic examination (a type of x-ray imaging) of the upper gastrointestinal tract, including the esophagus, stomach, and upper small intestine (duodenum). It is frequently requested when a patient experiences unexplained symptoms of abdominal **pain**, difficulty in swallowing (dysphagia), regurgitation, **diarrhea**, or weight loss. It is used to help diagnose disorders and diseases of or related to the upper gastrointestinal tract, including cases of hiatal **hernia**, diverticuli, ulcers, tumors, obstruction, enteritis, gastroesophageal reflux disease, Crohn's disease, and pulmonary aspiration.

To begin a barium enema, the patient will lie with their back down on a tilting radiographic table in order to have x rays of the abdomen taken. After being assisted to a different position, a well-lubricated rectal tube is inserted through the anus. This tube allows the physician or assistant to slowly administer the barium into the intestine. While this filling process is closely monitored, it is important for the patient to keep the anus tightly contracted against the rectal tube to help maintain its position and prevent the barium from leaking. This step is emphasized to the patient due to the inaccuracy that may be caused if the barium leaks. A rectal balloon may also be inflated to help retain the barium. The table may be tilted or the patient moved to a different position to aid in the filling process.

As the barium fills the intestine, x rays of the abdomen are taken to distinguish significant findings.There are many ways to perform a barium enema. One way is that shortly after filling, the rectal tube is removed and the patient expels as much of the barium as possible. Upon completing this, an additional x ray is taken, and a double-contrast enema may follow. If this is done immediately, a thin film of barium will remain in the intestine, and air is then slowly injected to expand the bowel lumen. Sometimes no x rays will be taken until after the air is injected.

In order to conduct the most accurate barium enema test, the patient must follow a prescribed diet and bowel preparation instructions prior to the test. This preparation commonly includes restricted intake of diary products and a liquid diet for 24 hours prior to the test, in addition to drinking large amounts of water or clear liquids 12–24 hours before the test. Patients may also be given **laxatives**, and asked to give themselves a cleansing enema.

In addition to the prescribed diet and bowel preparation prior to the test, the patient can expect the following during a barium enema:

- They will be well draped with a gown as they are secured to a tilting x-ray table.
- As the barium or air is injected into the intestine, they may experience cramping pains or the urge to defecate.
- The patient will be instructed to take slow, deep breaths through the mouth to ease any discomfort.

A colonoscopy can be done either in the doctor's office or in a special procedure room of a local hospital. An intravenous (IV) line will be started in a vein in the arm. The patient is generally given a sedative and a pain-killer through the IV line.

During the procedure, the patient will be asked to lie on his or her left side with the knees drawn up toward the abdomen. The doctor begins the procedure by inserting a lubricated, gloved finger into the anus to check for any abnormal masses or blockage. A thin, well-lubricated colonoscope will then be inserted into the anus and it will be gently advanced through the colon. The lining of the intestine will be examined through the scope. Occasionally air may be pumped through the colonoscope to help clear the path or open the colon. If there are excessive secretions, stool, or blood that obstruct the viewing, they will be suctioned out through the scope. The doctor may press on the abdomen or ask the patient to change position in order to advance the scope through the colon.

The entire length of the large intestine can be examined in this manner. If suspicious growths are observed, tiny biopsy forceps or brushes can be inserted through the colon and tissue samples can be obtained. Small polyps can also be removed through the colonoscope. After the procedure, the colonoscope is slowly withdrawn and the instilled air is allowed to escape. The anal area is then cleansed with tissues.

The procedure may take anywhere from 30 minutes to 2 hours depending on how easy it is to advance the scope through the colon. Colonoscopy can be a long and uncomfortable procedure, and the bowel cleaning preparation may be tiring and can produce diarrhea and cramping. During the colonoscopy, the sedative and the pain medications will keep the patient very drowsy and relaxed. Most patients complain of minor discomfort and pressure from the colonoscope moving inside. However, the procedure is not painful.

The doctor should be notified if the patient has **allergies** to any medications or anesthetics; any bleeding problems; or if the woman is pregnant. The doctor should also be informed of all the medications that the person is currently on and if he or she has had a barium x-ray examination recently. If the patient has had heart valves replaced, the doctor should be informed, so that appropriate **antibiotics** can be administered to prevent any chance of infection. The risks of the procedure will be explained to the patient before performing the procedure and the patient will be asked to sign a consent form.

It is important that the colon be thoroughly cleaned before performing the examination. Hence, before the examination, considerable preparation is necessary to clear the colon of all stool. The patient will be asked to refrain from eating any solid food for 24 to 48 hours before the test. Only clear liquids such as juices, broth, and Jello are recommended. The patient is advised to drink plenty of water to avoid **dehydration**. The evening before the test, the patient will have to take a strong laxative that the doctor has prescribed. Several 1 qt enemas of warm tap water may have to be taken on the morning of the exam. Commercial enemas (e.g. Fleet) may be used.

The patient will be given specific instructions on how to use the enema and how many such enemas are necessary. Generally, the procedure has to be repeated until the return from the enema is clear of stool particles. On the morning of the examination, the patient is instructed not to eat or drink anything. The preparatory procedures are extremely important since, if the colon is not thoroughly clean, the exam cannot be done.

An upper GI series takes place in a hospital or clinic setting and is performed by an x-ray technician and a radiologist. A radiologist typically is in attendance to oversee the procedure, and view and interpret the fluoroscopic pictures. Before the test begins, the patient is sometimes administered an injection of glucagon, a medication which slows stomach and bowel activity, to allow the radiologist to get a clearer picture of the gastrointestinal tract. In order to further improve the clarity of the upper GI pictures, the patient may be given a cup of baking soda crystals to swallow, which distend the stomach by producing gas.

Once these preparatory steps are complete, the patient stands against an upright x-ray table, and a fluoroscopic screen is placed in front of him. The patient will be asked to drink from a cup of flavored barium sulfate, a thick and chalky-tasting liquid that allows the radiologist to see the digestive tract, while the radiologist views the esophagus, stomach, and duodenum on the fluoroscopic screen. The patient will be asked to change positions frequently in order to coat the entire surface of the gastrointestinal tract with barium. The technician or radiologist may press on the patient's abdomen in order to spread the barium. The x-ray table will also be moved several times throughout the procedure. The radiologist will ask the patient to hold his breath periodically while exposures are being taken. The entire procedure takes approximately 30 minutes.

In some cases, in addition to the standard upper GI series, a doctor may request a detailed intestine, or small bowel, radiography and fluoroscopy series; it is also called a small bowel follow-through (SBFT). Once the preliminary upper GI series is complete, the patient will be escorted to a waiting area while the barium travels down through the rest of the small intestinal path. Every 15–30 minutes, the patient will return to the x-ray suite for additional x rays, or films. Once the barium has completed its trip down the small bowel tract, the test is completed. This procedure can take anywhere from one to four hours.

Esophageal radiography, also called a barium esophagram or a barium swallow, is a study of the esophagus only, and is usually performed as part of the upper GI series. It is commonly used to diagnose the cause of difficulty in swallowing (dysphagia) and for detecting hiatal hernia. A barium sulfate liquid, and sometimes pieces of food covered in barium, are given to the patient to drink and eat while a radiologist examines the swallowing mechanism on a fluoroscopic screen. The test takes approximately 30 minutes.

Patients must not eat, drink, or smoke for eight hours prior to undergoing an upper GI examination. Longer dietary restrictions may be required, depending on the type and diagnostic purpose of the test. Patients undergoing a small bowel follow-through exam may be asked to take laxatives the day prior to the test. Upper GI patients are typically required to wear a hospital gown, or similar attire, and to remove all jewelry, so the camera has an unobstructed view of the abdomen.

GILMAN, ALFRED GOODMAN (1941-)

American biochemist and pharmacologist

Alfred Goodman Gilman was born in 1941 in New Haven, Connecticut, to Alfred Gilman Sr. and Mabel Schmidt Gilman.

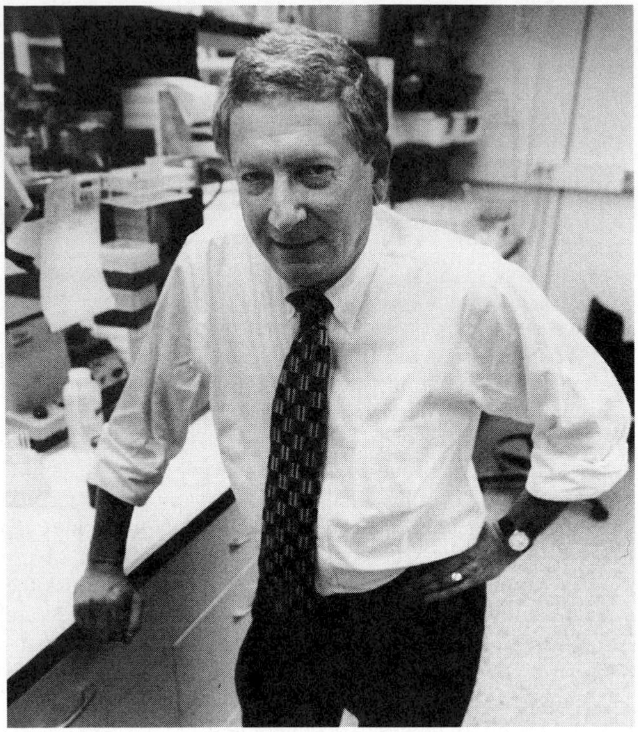

Alfred G. Gilman

Gilman grew up in White Plains, New York, where his father was on the faculty of The College of Physicians and Surgeons of Columbia University and then later a founding chairman of the Pharmacology Department at the new Albert Einstein College of Medicine. Visits to his father's laboratory peaked his interest in biology. Gilman was also able to observe intricate pharmacological experiments designed for medical students.

In 1955 Gilman was sent to the Taft School in Watertown, Connecticut, a prep school for boys. Gilman was not happy about being sent away, nor did he enjoy the rigid structure of the boys' school. From there, he went on to Yale where he majored in biochemisty. Gilman describes his first laboratory project, to test Francis Crick's adapter hypothesis, as "wildly overambitious." The experience was rewarding for him though, because of the encouragement he received from his lab instructor Melvin Simpson.

After receiving his B.A. from Yale in 1962, Gilman worked for Burroughs Wellcome in New York and published his first papers. He knew he wanted to go into research when he entered a unique M.D.-Ph.D. program at Case Western Reserve University in the fall of 1962. Gilman conducted research on the thyroid gland and was also interested in studying cells and **genetics**. He earned an M.D. and Ph.D. in pharmacology in 1969. His interest in genetics led him to the Pharmacology Research Associate Training Program at the National Institute of General Medical Sciences, where he researched cyclic adenosine monophosphate (AMP), a genetic regulator that moderates hormone actions. His work with Nobel laureate **Earl Sutherland** was the beginning of his interest in cell communication.

In 1971 Gilman accepted a position as an assistant professor of pharmacology at the University of Virginia in Charlottesville. It was here that Gilman began his Nobel Prize-winning work. He and his colleagues knew about **Martin Rodbell**'s work at the **National Institutes of Health** with guanine nucleotides (components of deoxyribonucleic acid [DNA] and ribonucleic acid [RNA]). Rodbell and his research associates at the NIH ascertained that the guanine nucleotides were somehow related to cell communication, but could not prove it. Gilman's research began where Rodbell left off, and in the late 1970s, he and his colleagues started looking for the chemicals that would confirm Rodbell's work. Gilman used genetically altered **leukemia** cells to detect the presence of G-proteins. He found that without the G-protein, the cells did not respond to outside stimulation the way a normal cell would. In 1980 they found the G-proteins, named because they bind to the guanine nucleotides.

G-proteins are instrumental in the fundamental workings of a cell. They allow us to see and smell by changing light and odors to chemical messages that travel to the brain. Understanding how G-proteins malfunction could lead to understanding serious diseases like **cholera** or **cancer**. Scientists have linked improperly working G-proteins to everything from alcoholism to **diabetes**. Pharmaceutical companies are developing drugs that would focus on G-proteins.

In 1979 Gilman was asked to chair the department of pharmacology at the University of Texas Southwestern Medical Center in Dallas. He eventually accepted the postion and his time at Southwestern was filled with many other awards. Among the awards are the Poul Edvard Poulson Award from the Norwegian Pharmacological Society in 1982 and the Gairdner Foundation International Award in 1984. In 1987 he shared the Richard Lounsbery Award from the National Academy of Sciences with Martin Rodbell in 1987, foreshadowing the Nobel. In 1989 he won the Albert Lasker Basic Medical Research Award. Finally, Gilman and Rodbell were awarded the 1994 Nobel Prize in Medicine for their collaborative work. Since his discovery, Gilman has been in the forefront of G-protein research. He predicts that eventually scientists will be able to map cell communication in a way that will allow scientists to predict how cells will respond to a variety of signals, leading the way to major advances in the treatment of disease.

GLAUCOMA

Glaucoma is a condition in which the optic nerve is subject to damage—usually, but not always, because of excessive pressure within the **eye**. If untreated, optic nerve damage results in progressive, permanent vision loss, starting with unnoticeable blind spots at the edge of the field of vision, progressing to tunnel vision, then to blindness.

More than two million people in the United States have glaucoma, 80,000 of whom are legally blind as a result. It is the leading cause of preventable blindness in the United States and the most frequent cause of blindness in African-Americans, who are at about a three-fold higher risk of glaucoma than the rest of the population. The risk of glaucoma increases dramatically with age, but it can strike any age group, even newborn infants and fetuses.

Glaucoma is actually a class of diseases—there are at least twenty different forms. It is a secondary condition of over 60 widely diverse diseases. It can also result from injury. Most glaucoma is probably inherited. At least ten defective genes causing glaucoma have been identified.

Glaucoma occurs when the aqueous humor (a watery fluid bathing the iris, cornea and lens of the eye) is not removed rapidly enough or when the body produces it too rapidly, causing pressure to build up. The pressure distorts the shape of the optic nerve and destroys it. This causes blind spots in places where the image from the eye is not being transmitted to the brain.

Open-angle glaucoma accounts for over 90% of all cases. It is called ''open-angle'' because the corner where the aqueous fluid drains is open, allowing drainage. Pressure usually builds slowly. At first, chronic open-angle glaucoma has no noticeable symptoms. The vision loss is too gradual to be noticed and each eye fills in the image where its partner has a blind spot. If not treated, however, vision loss becomes evident, and the condition can be very painful.

In narrow-angle glaucoma, the corner is narrow and may therefore drain slowly or may be at risk of closing.

A closed-angle glaucoma attack usually occurs suddenly, when the drainage area is blocked. Such an attack is obvious from the beginning. The symptoms are blurred vision, severe pain, sensitivity to light, **nausea**, and halos around lights. Normally clear corneas may be hazy. This is an emergency and needs to be treated immediately.

Similarly, congenital glaucoma is evident at birth. Symptoms are bulging eyes, cloudy corneas, excessive tearing, and sensitivity to light.

To diagnose glaucoma, pressure within the eye is measured with an instrument known as a tonometer. One type of tonometer involves numbing the eye with an eyedrop and touching it with a small probe. This quick test is a routine part of an eye examination.

Ophthalmoscopes, hand-held instruments with a light source, are used to detect optic nerve damage by looking through the pupil. Visual field tests (perimetry) can detect blind spots before the patient is aware of them.

Pressure within the eye can vary throughout the day, so several visits may be needed to measure pressure at different times.

When glaucoma is diagnosed, drugs, typically given as eye drops, are usually tried before surgery. **Beta blockers** (such as Timoptic), carbonic anhydrase inhibitors (acetazolamide), and alpha-2 agonists (Alphagan) inhibit the production of aqueous humor. Miotics (pilocarpine) and prostaglandin analogues (Xalatan) increase the outflow of aqueous humor.

It is important for patients to tell their doctors about any conditions they have or medications they are taking. Certain drugs used to treat glaucoma would not be prescribed for patients with pre-existing conditions. All of the drugs mentioned above have side effects, some of which are rare but serious and potentially life-threatening, so patients should be monitored closely, especially for cardiovascular, pulmonary, and behavioral symptoms.

Attacks of acute closed-angle glaucoma are medical emergencies. Pressure can be rapidly lowered by acetazolamide, hyperosmotic agents, a topical beta-blocker, and pilocarpine.

Laser surgery or microsurgery to open the drainage canals or make an opening in the iris can also increase the outflow of aqueous humor. These surgeries are usually successful, but the effects often last less than a year. Nevertheless, they are an effective treatment for patients whose pressure is not sufficiently lowered by drugs and for those who can't tolerate the drugs.

Sight lost due to glaucoma cannot be restored.

Vitamin C, vitamin B_1 (thiamine), chromium, zinc, and rutin may reduce pressure within the eye. There is evidence that marijuana lowers pressure, but it has serious side effects and contains substances linked to **cancer**. Although the U.S. **Food and Drug Administration** and **National Institutes of Health** currently recommend against treating glaucoma with marijuana, they are supporting research to learn more about it.

Any glaucoma patient using alternative methods to prevent optic nerve damage should also be under the care of a traditionally trained ophthalmologist or optometrist licensed to treat glaucoma.

About half of the people stricken by glaucoma are not aware of it. Many will become blind. On the other hand, the prospects for patients whose glaucoma is treated are excellent.

The best form of prevention is to have regular **eye exams**. Any person who is glaucoma-susceptible should read warning labels on over-the-counter medicines and inform their physician of products they are considering taking. Steroids may also raise pressure within the eye, so patients taking them may need to be monitored more frequently.

As more is learned about the genes that cause glaucoma, it will become possible to test DNA and identify potential glaucoma victims, so they can be treated before their pressure becomes elevated.

See also Visual impairment and blindness

GOLDSTEIN, JOSEPH L. (1940-)

American molecular geneticist and physician

Joseph Leonard Goldstein, the only son of Isadore E. and Fannie (Albert) Goldstein, was born on April 18, 1940, in Sumter, South Carolina. He graduated from Washington & Lee University in 1962 with a B.S. degree in chemistry, and attended Southwestern Medical School of the University of Texas Health Science Center in Dallas. There, Donald Seldin, chairman of the Health Science Center's department of internal medicine, offered him a future faculty appointment, provided he would specialize in **genetics** and then return to Dallas to establish a division of medical genetics there. He received his M.D. degree in 1966.

Goldstein's internship and residency at Massachusetts General Hospital brought him to Michael Brown, who had arrived from the University of Pennsylvania, having also obtained his M.D. degree in 1966. The two served in the same internship and residency program, and both were interested in research. After finishing their training in 1968, they joined the **National Institutes of Health** (NIH) in Bethesda, Maryland.

At the NIH biochemical genetics laboratory, Goldstein studied under the leadership of **Marshall Warren Nirenberg**, who was awarded the 1968 Nobel Prize in physiology or medicine for unraveling the way in which the genetic code determines the structure of proteins. Here, he learned about the excitement and efficiency of biology on a molecular level. At the same time he worked under Dr. Donald S. Fredrickson, clinical director of the National Heart Institute, who was investigating people with hypercholesterolemia, or abnormally high cholesterol levels. In particular, Goldstein was interested in those patients with homozygous familial hypercholesterolemia. Familial hypercholesterolemia, identified as a genetically acquired disease by Carl Müller of Oslo, Norway, involved a genetic defect which caused a metabolic error resulting in high blood cholesterol levels and heart attacks. But it was Fredrickson and Avedis K. Khachadurian of the American University of Beirut, who identified two forms of the disease: a heterozygous form, involving a single defective gene found in one in 500 people; and a homozygous form, in which two defective genes are present and which strikes about one in a million. Blood cholesterol levels reach four to eight times the normal amount with symptoms of **atherosclerosis**, or hardening of the arteries, beginning in childhood. Nearly every sufferer from the homozygous form dies from a heart attack before the age of 30.

In 1972 Goldstein left the National Institutes of Health for Seattle under a two-year NIH fellowship in medical genetics. During this time he worked with Arno G. Motulsky, an internationally recognized expert in the field of genetic aspects of heart disease, and devoted himself to a study investigating the frequency of various hereditary hyperlipidemias (diseases of high blood-fat levels) in a random sampling of **heart attack** survivors. The samples were taken from 885 patients (who survived three months or more) out of 1,166 coronary victims admitted in an eleven-month period to thirteen Seattle hospitals from 1970 to 1971. Studying 500 of those survivors and 2,520 members of their families revealed that thirty-one percent of the survivors had high blood-fat levels, either high cholesterol, high triglycerides, or a mixture of both. Eleven percent had an inherited combination of high cholesterol and high triglycerides. Goldstein and his associates defined this disease as familial combined hyperlipidemia. He knew that due to its complexity, combined hyperlipidemia would be an arduous area in which to begin research. Patients with homozygous hypercholesterolemia—having no normal genes at the area of the unknown defect—might be easier to study regarding gene functioning and cholesterol level.

Returning to the University of Texas Health Science Center in 1972 as head of the medical school's first division of medical genetics, and assistant professor in the department of internal medicine which was still directed by Donald Seldin, Goldstein addressed the task of identifying the fundamental genetic defect in familial hypercholesterolemia (FHC). Brown had joined the staff the previous year.

The idea of cell receptors was known, but it had never been studied in relationship to fat and cholesterol in the blood. Over 93% of the cholesterol in the human body is found inside cells. There, it participates in functions critical to cell development and cell membrane formation. Cholesterol also contributes to the essential production of sex hormones, **corticosteroid**s and bile acids. The remaining seven percent is dangerous, however, if it is not absorbed into the cells as it courses through the circulatory system, and sticks instead to the walls of blood vessels disrupting the flow of blood to the heart and brain.

Dietary cholesterol, found only in animal foods, is not necessary to the human body since the body produces its own cholesterol in the liver. If no cholesterol is available in the bloodstream, individual cells will produce their own. The human liver excretes that cholesterol which is not used by cells or deposited on artery walls. Cholesterol is fat-soluble, but attaches itself to water-soluble proteins, or lipoproteins, manufactured in the liver, as a means of moving through the bloodstream. The lipoproteins most favored by cholesterol are low-density ones, called LDLs, which are composed of much more fat than protein. Thus, high levels of LDLs are equated with the threat of heart disease.

Goldstein and Brown started their study by observing tissue cultures of the human skin cells known as fibroblasts, harvested from six FHC homozygotes, sixteen FHC heterozygotes and forty normal people. The cultured fibroblasts, like other animal cells, need cholesterol for the formation of the cell membrane. During this process, Goldstein and Brown were able to follow the manner in which the cells obtained cholesterol, and identify the process of cholesterol extraction from the lipoproteins in the serum of the culture medium, specifically LDLs. This discovery was made in 1973 with their demonstration of the presence of receptor molecules on the cells, which function to adhere LDLs and carry them into the cell. Goldstein and Brown noted that each individual cell normally has 250,000 receptors that bind low-density lipoproteins, and further located LDL receptors on circulating human blood cells as well as cell membranes from assorted animal tissues.

The cells of individuals with the heterozygous form of FHC have forty to fifty percent of the LDL receptors that are typically present on normal cells. Cells of individuals with the homozygous form of FHC have no LDL receptors or a very small number. Cholesterol, manufactured by the liver and attached to LDLs, is passed into the blood, but is removed from the circulatory system rather slowly. Under normal circumstances an LDL molecule spends a day and a half in the bloodstream, but in FHC heterozygotes this length of time is extended to three days, and in FHC homozygotes to five days, providing increased opportunity for cholesterol to accumulate in the walls of the blood vessels.

Cholestyramine, a drug used to treat high cholesterol levels, had been synthesized over 20 years before Goldstein's and Brown's study, but had never been fully understood. Goldstein and Brown discovered that cholestyramine works by multiplying LDL receptors in the liver, which then converts cholesterol into bile acids and passes them into the intestines. However, in spite of this action, cholestyramine had only limited effect on levels of serum cholesterol. Goldstein and Brown determined the reason for this: The increased numbers of LDL receptors in the liver signaled the need for more cholesterol and the liver responded by increasing cholesterol production. This increase in cholesterol level then shut down the production of LDL receptors in the liver. These findings indicated the need for a drug to impede the liver's synthesis of cholesterol that could be administered in tandem with cholestyramine. In 1976 Akiro Endo, a Japanese scientist, isolated compactin, an anticholesterol enzyme, from **penicillin** mold, and in the same year Alfred W. Alberts of Merck, Sharp and Dohme research laboratories isolated a structurally similar enzyme, mevinolin, from a different mold. Goldstein and Brown combined mevinolin and cholestyramine in animal experiments with good results, and in 1987 the **Food and Drug Administration** approved mevinolin, now called lovastatin, for marketing. The FDA made the recommendation with the stipulation that the drug should be used only when diet and exercise proved inadequate in treating high cholesterol. Goldstein anticipated a lapse of five to ten years before use of the drug would affect the nation's coronary death rate.

For revolutionizing scientific knowledge about the regulation of cholesterol metabolism and the treatment of diseases caused by abnormally elevated cholesterol levels in the blood, Goldstein and Brown received the 1985 Nobel Prize in physiology or medicine. They also have received awards from the National Academy of Sciences, the American Chemical Society, the Roche Institute of Molecular Biology, the American Heart Association and the American Society for Human Genetics.

Goldstein's and Brown's research illuminating the activity of LDL receptors and their function in the management of cholesterol levels has had far-reaching effects. Not only has their work increased understanding of an important aspect of human physiology, but it has also had a practical impact on the prevention and treatment of heart disease. The National Institutes of Health, in part because of Goldstein's and Brown's work, recommended the lowering of fat intake in the U.S. diet.

Golgi, Camillo (1843-1926)

Italian histologist

Golgi was born in Corteno, Italy, on July 7, 1843, the son of a physician. His home town was later renamed Corteno-Golgi in his honor. Golgi studied medicine at the University of Pavia, where he received his M.D. in 1865. After graduation, he worked briefly in a psychiatric clinic, but eventually decided to pursue a career in histological research.

Financial difficulties forced him in 1872 to accept a position as chief medical officer at the Hospital for the Chronically Ill in Abbiategrasso, Italy. No research facilities were available there, however, and he was able to continue his studies only by converting an unused kitchen into a laboratory. By 1875, Golgi had earned sufficient fame to receive an appointment as lecturer in histology at the University of Pavia. Four years later he was appointed Professor of Anatomy at the University of Siena, but he stayed only a year there before returning to Pavia as Professor of Histology. There he married Donna Lina Aletti, the niece of one of his former professors.

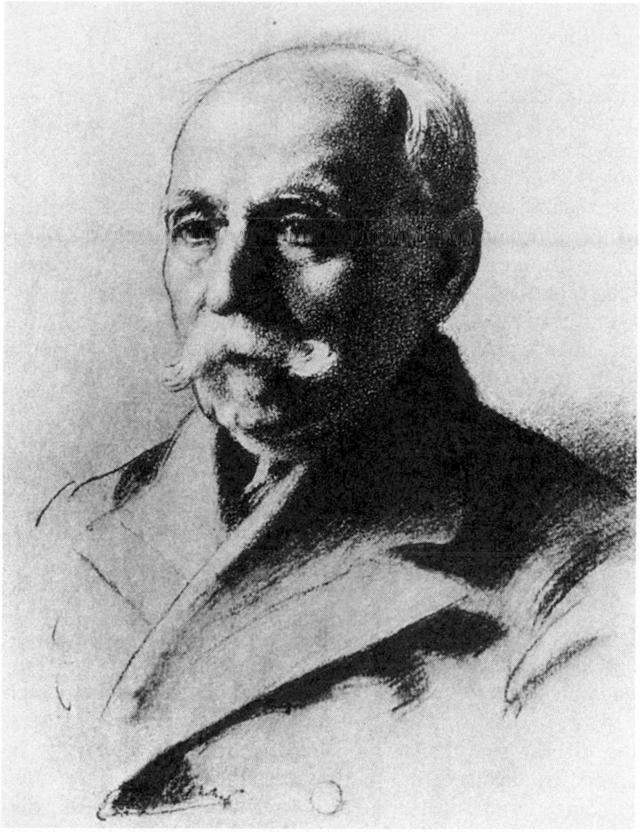

Camillo Golgi

Golgi's earliest research involved the study of neurons, or nerve cells. Neurons present a number of problems for researchers that other cells do not. While most cells are compact and have a relatively fixed shape, neurons are commonly very long and thin with structures that are difficult to see clearly. In the 1860s, techniques used to stain and study non-nerve cells were well developed, but they were largely useless with neurons. As a result, a great deal of uncertainty surrounded the structure and function of neurons and neuron networks.

In 1873, Golgi found that silver salts could be used to dye neurons. The neurons turned black and stood out clearly from surrounding tissue. Golgi perfected his technique so that the addition of just the right amount of dye for just the right period of time would highlight one or another part of the neuron, a single complete neuron, or a group of neurons.

Golgi's new technique resolved some questions about the **nervous system**, but not all. He was able, for example, to confirm the view of Wilhelm von Waldeyer-Hartz that neurons are separated by narrow gaps—synapses—and are not physically connected to each other. He was unable to completely explain, however, the complex, overlapping network of dendrites.

While studying the brain of a barn owl in 1896, Golgi made a second important discovery. He found previously undetected bodies near the nuclear membrane. Those bodies, now known as *Golgi bodies* or *Golgi complexes*, seem to be involved in the manufacture of proteins and carbohydrates. For his research on the nervous system, Golgi was awarded a share of the 1906 Nobel Prize for physiology or medicine.

Between 1885 and 1893, Golgi was also involved in research on **malaria**. He made one especially interesting discovery in this field; namely, that all the malarial parasites in an organism reproduce at the same time, a time that corresponds to the recurrence of **fever**.

In addition to his scientific work, Golgi was active in Italian politics. He was elected a Senator in 1900 and served in a number of administrative posts at Pavia. He died in Pavia on January 21, 1926.

GONORRHEA

Gonorrhea is a common sexually transmitted disease (STD) and the most common bacterial infection in adults. In the United States, approximately 1 million cases are reported each year, most occurring in people under age 30. In its early stages, the disease may cause no symptoms and therefore can be spread by unsuspecting victims. In females, gonorrhea often remains asymptomatic but can lead to vaginal itching, discharge, or uterine bleeding and other serious complications. An infected woman who gives birth can transmit the disease to her infant, most often resulting in childhood blindness. As a precaution, silver nitrate is administered to the eyes of newborns to prevent this condition. In males, gonorrhea causes infection of the urethra and painful urination. Though not deadly, the disease if untreated can infect other genital organs or the throat. If the infection spreads throughout the blood stream, it can cause an arthritis-**dermatitis** syndrome.

Gonorrhea was described in early writings from Egypt, China, and Japan. Warnings against ''unclean discharge from the body'' appear in the Bible. A diagnostic description of the disease was written in the Middle Ages. In the late fifteenth century, a **syphilis** epidemic raged throughout Europe, though at that time syphilis was often confused with gonorrhea, and some believed that gonorrhea was the first stage of syphilis. The gram-negative bacteria that causes gonorrhea was discovered in 1879 by Albert Neisser (1855-1916), a German physician who went on to identify the bacterial cause for **leprosy**. German immunologist **Paul Ehrlich** named the bacterium *gonococcus*. Since then, five types of the gonococcus organism have been identified.

A test for the presence of gonococcus bacterium serves as the diagnostic tool. The first effective treatment for gonorrhea were the **sulfonamides** which became available in 1937. During World War II, **penicillin** became widely available for the treatment of gonorrhea and other bacterial disease. However, while penicillin and related antibiotics are effective in about 90 percent of cases, some strains of the gonococcus are becoming resistant to these standard treatments.

While reported cases of gonorrhea in the United States have decreased annually since 1987, the disease and its complications still cost an estimated $1.1 million a year. Found mostly in high-density urban areas, the highest incidence is among people 24 years of age and under who have multiple sex partners and do not use **condoms** or other safe-sex measures. Interestingly, while the incidence of **AIDS** has gone down in the homosexual male population, epidemiologists have noted an increase in gonorrhea among homosexual men. The best way to prevent gonorrhea is to practice sexual **abstinence** or through the use of male condoms during sexual activity. Due to the dramatic rise of **antibiotic**-resistant strains of the disease, scientists are working on new approaches for the prevention, diagnosis, and treatment of gonorrhea.

GORGAS, WILLIAM CRAWFORD (1854-1920)

American physician and Surgeon General, U.S. Army

United States military man and physician, William Crawford Gorgas, first gained recognition for eradicating **yellow fever** and **malaria** in Havana, Cuba. Due to this amazing feat, in 1902, United States Surgeon General Dr. George M. Sternberg recommended Gorgas be placed in charge of solving the same problem in Panama. When the U.S. government assumed control of Panama from the French and took over construction of the Panama Canal, they were forced to abandon the project because of yellow fever. Gorgas was appointed chief sanitary officer of the zone in 1904, receiving commission to implement mosquito-control methods along the entire canal zone. By late 1907, his efforts had totally eliminated the disease from the area, enabling continued construction and successful completion of the canal. Gorgas was elected to the Alabama Hall of Fame in 1953.

Gorgas was born near Mobile, Alabama, the first child of General Josiah Gorgas who, originally from Pennsylvania, was a chief ordnance officer in the Confederate Army; and Amelia Gayle, the daughter of a governor of Alabama. Gorgas first attended Sewanee University, ultimately becoming a gold medal student. From 1876 to 1879, he attended Bellevue Medical College in New York City where he studied medicine and accepted an internship. His dream of entering the military was fulfilled in June 1880 when he was commissioned as second lieutenant in the U.S. Army Medical Corps.

When Dr. Ronald Reed discovered that mosquitoes carried the dreaded malaria and yellow fever, not everyone believed his findings. Gorgas did, however, and it was he who implemented the huge mosquito control program in Havana, Cuba, where, in the early 1900s, 500 people were dying each year from the diseases. By 1902, Gorgas' efforts had yellow fever entirely eradicated. When the United States assumed control of Panama, **tuberculosis**, **cholera**, **smallpox**, bubonic **plague**, and **diphtheria** were all troublesome; however, yellow fever and malaria alone had killed an estimated ten to twenty thousand people there between 1882 and 1888. When Gorgas was commissioned to take on the daunting task of eradicating those diseases, he found an abundance of open sewage drains and shallow trenches dug by the French and filled with water as protection from ferocious umbrella ants. These pools became stagnant and putrid in the hot climate—perfect breeding grounds for the disease-carrying mosquito.

Amazingly, Gorgas' work was greatly hampered by U.S. government officials in the zone who refused to accept the mosquito theory. They not only denied him authority to implement his plans and hindered shipment of supplies from the United States, they tried desperately to have him dismissed from the project—until, in 1905, several top officials died from yellow fever. Fortunately for the entire project, President Theodore Roosevelt knew of Gorgas' success in Havana and, encouraged by John F. Stevens, the newly appointed chief engineer of the canal project, gave Gorgas his full support. Stevens immediately assigned 4,000 workers to the **sanitation** effort and approved an unlimited budget for supplies.

The crews set to work, first covering the stagnant waterways with an oil and pesticide combination, then fumigating every house. Infected people were quarantined in screened-in tents, running water was supplied to the homes, streets were paved, and entirely new communities emerged. Within two years, 24,000 workers lived in a disease-free zone. When Gorgas wrote his book *Sanitation in Panama* in 1915, he said, "...it is now more than eight years, and not a case of yellow fever has originated in the Isthmus." He also wrote, with amazing perception, "No doubt the great centers of civilization will remain for centuries much as they are at present. The white settlers will go to the valleys of the Amazon and Congo, building up large agricultural communities which will supply the European and American centers...I believe that the peoples of that day will look back upon the sanitary work done at the Canal Zone as the first great demonstration that the white man could live as well in the tropics as in the temperate zone. I am inclined to think that at this time the sanitary phase of the work will be considered more important than the actual construction of the canal itself, as important to the world as this great waterway now is, and will be for generations to come."

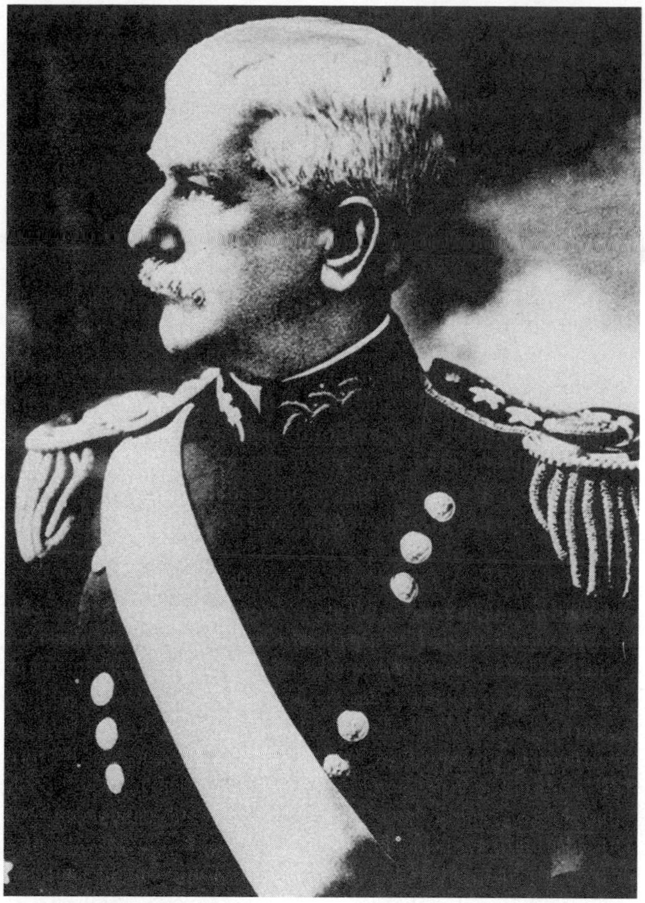

William Crawford Gorgas

Gout

Gout is a form of arthritis that causes severe **pain** and swelling in the joints. It most commonly affects the big toe, but may also affect the heel, ankle, hand, wrist, or elbow. Gout usually comes on suddenly, goes away after 5–10 days, and can keep recurring. It is different from other forms of arthritis because it occurs when there are high levels of uric acid circulating in the blood, which can cause urate crystals to settle in the tissues of the joints.

Normally the kidneys filter uric acid out of the blood and excrete it in the urine. Sometimes, however, the body produces too much uric acid or the kidneys aren't efficient enough at filtering it, and it builds up in the bloodstream. A person's susceptibility to gout may be inherited, or result from being overweight and eating a rich diet. In some cases, another disease (such as **lymphoma**, **leukemia**, or hemolytic **anemia**) may be the underlying cause.

An excess of uric acid doesn't always cause gout. However, over years, sharp urate crystals build up in the joints. Often, an infection, surgery, a stubbed toe, a heavy drinking binge, or some other event can lead to inflammation—the redness, swelling, and pain that are the hallmarks of a gout attack.

Often, the attack begins in the middle of the night. The pain can be so excruciating that the sufferer cannot bear weight on the joint or tolerate the pressure of bedcovers. The inflamed skin over the joint may be red, shiny, and dry, and there may be mild fever. These symptoms may go away in about a week and disappear for months or years. However, over time, attacks of gout recur more and more frequently, last longer, and affect more joints. Eventually, stone-like deposits may build up in the joints, ligaments, and tendons, leading to permanent joint deformity and decreased motion. An excess of uric acid can also cause **kidney stones**.

Gout affects an estimated one million Americans. It most commonly afflicts men (800,000 men versus 200,000 women). Uric acid levels tend to increase in men at **puberty**, and, because it takes 20 years of high levels to cause gout symptoms, men commonly develop gout in their late 30s or early 40s. Women tend to develop gout later in life, starting in their 60s. According to some medical experts, estrogen protects against gout, and when estrogen levels fall during **meno-**

pause, urate crystals can begin to build. Excess body weight, regular excessive alcohol intake, the use of blood pressure medications called **diuretics**, and high levels of certain fatty substances in the blood can all increase risk of gout.

Usually, doctors can diagnose gout based on the **physical examination** and medical history. They can also administer a test that measures the level of uric acid in the blood. The most definitive way to diagnose gout is to take a sample of fluid from the joint and test it for urate crystals.

Temporary attacks of gout can be treated with **nonsteroidal anti-inflammatory drugs** (NSAIDs) such as naproxen sodium (Aleve), ibuprofen (Advil), or indomethacin (Indocin). In some cases, these drugs can aggravate a peptic **ulcer** or existing kidney disease and cannot be used. Doctors sometimes also use colchicine (Colbenemid). **Corticosteroids** such as prednisone (Deltasone) and adrenocorticotropic hormone (Acthar) may be given orally or may be injected directly into the joint for more concentrated effect. While all of these drugs have potential side effects, they are used for only about 48 hours and are not likely to cause major problems. Aspirin and closely related drugs (salicylates) should be avoided because they can worsen gout.

Once an acute attack has been successfully treated, doctors try to prevent future attacks and long-term joint damage by lowering uric acid levels in the blood. Uricosuric drugs, such as probenecid (Benemid) and sulfinpyrazone (Anturane), lower the levels of urate in the blood by increasing its removal from the body (excretion) through the urine. These drugs may promote formation of kidney stones and may not work for all patients, especially those with kidney disease. Allopurinol (Zyloprim), blocks the production of urate in the body, and can also dissolve kidney stones. Once people begin taking these medications they must take them for life or the gout will continue to return.

Gout cannot be cured but usually it can be managed successfully. In some cases, however, medicines alone do not dissolve the uric acid deposits and they must be removed surgically. In addition to taking pain medications as prescribed by their doctors, people having gout attacks are encouraged to rest and to increase the amount of fluids that they drink.

For centuries, gout has been known as a ''rich man's disease,'' implying overindulgence in food and drink. While this is perhaps a little oversimplified, lifestyle factors clearly influence a person's risk of developing gout. Since **obesity** and excessive alcohol intake are associated with gout, losing weight and limiting alcohol intake can help reduce risk. **Dehydration** may also promote the formation of urate crystals, so people taking diuretics or ''water pills'' may be better off switching to another blood pressure medication, and everyone should be sure to drink at least six to eight glasses of water each day. It may also be helpful to avoid foods high in purine, such as organ meats, sardines, anchovies, red meat, gravies, beans, beer, and wine.

Graefe, Albrecht Friederich Wilhelm Ernst von (1828-1870)

German eye surgeon

Albrecht von Graefe is best known as the founder of modern ophthalmology. Von Graefe, whose full name was Friederich Wilhelm Ernst Albrecht von Graefe, dedicated his life to becoming an excellent teacher, surgeon, and clinician in the field of ophthalmology. Although born into a privileged life as the son of Carl Ferdinand von Graefe the Director of the Surgical Clinic for 30 years, author of the *Encyclopedic Dictionary of Medical Sciences*, a pioneer in plastic surgery, and general in the Prussian army Albrecht based his short life on utilizing his talent to benefit those who were in need.

Orphaned at the age of 12, von Graefe focused on his studies. As an extremely gifted student, he decided to follow in his father's footsteps and began by enrolling at the University of Berlin in 1843. At the age of 15, he was the youngest student on record to begin studies at the university. With instructors who were revered in the world of nineteenth-century Berlin medicine, such as **Schönlein**, Romberg, Dieffenbach, **Virchow**, Schlemm, von **Brücke**, Du Bouis-Reymond, and Johannes Müller, von Graefe left an impression on his teachers of being an intense student who would strive for great accomplishments. Four years later he graduated from medical school, and began to plan his *Wanderjahre* a trip through Europe that would allow him to study some of his day's leading ophthalmologists. Beginning in December of 1847, von Graefe made several stops along his journey, including the eye clinic of Ferdinand Arlt in Prague, and a 20-month stay in Paris with Sichel, Desmarres, Louis, and **Claude Bernard**. He then headed to Vienna to observe Eduard Jaeger, followed by a brief trip back to Berlin, then to London to stay with **William Bowman** and George Critchett. His voyage concluded with stays in Glasgow with William Mackenzie and Dublin with William Wilde.

Rich with experience from working with Europe's leading ophthalmologists for nearly three years, von Graefe returned to Berlin to open his first clinic in Behrenstrasse on November 1, 1850. Consisting of three small rooms and little equipment, von Graefe welcomed his first patients with a famous advertisement that ran in all Berlin papers for six weeks, stating that he would treat poor patients free of charge. Von Graefe's surgical cases were performed in two rooms he rented from a tailor. It is there that he completed a successful **cataract** extraction on a blind man and an artificial pupil on the scarred cornea of an organ grinder. While his treatment was successful for his first two surgical cases, the blind man developed delirium tremens during the evening while in recovery, fell out of bed and attacked the organ grinder with his fists.

Eager to deliver the best care for his patients, von Graefe searched for ways to properly examine the eyes. He pioneered the design and use of instruments for clinical perimetry, and in 1862, he developed the development of one of the first tonometers, which are instruments used to measure intraocular pressure. His talent as a doctor became apparent as the number of his patients grew. At the end of the first two months, his clinic saw 230 patients, and at the end of the first year von Graefe treated over 1,900 patients. To accommodate the recent growth in patients, the clinic was moved to a three-story building at 46 Karlstrasse, which became the most famous eye clinic in nineteenth-century Europe. Shortly after this move, von Graeffe would see over 10,000 patients a year in his clinic.

Recognition of von Graefe's achievements was also given by the students who came to observe and learn from him as he examined patients, operated and explained pathology and treatment. He lectured to many, and hundreds of students were trained at von Graefe's side. At the young age of 26, he published his own journal of materials in the first of many *Archiv fur Augenheilkunde*. Consisting of 480 pages written by himself, the first *Archiv* would be followed by journals containing articles from contributing experts, including Arlt and Donders, and the studies of Helmholtz on accomodation.

In 1857, von Graefe reached the peak of his career by reporting the cure of **glaucoma** with iridectomy at the first International Congress of Ophthalmology. He referred to glaucoma in three forms: the acute inflammatory, the chronic and amaurosis with advanced cupping of the disc. Von Graefe's work on glaucoma set a standard in the world of ophthalmology. It was at this time he also became engaged to Anna, Countess Knuth in 1861. While traveling that year, he was struck with acute tuberculous pleurisy. After resting on the Riviera that winter, he returned to Berlin and married Anna in 1862. The couple had five children throughout their eight years of marriage, two of whom died.

In 1864, von Graefe embarked on modifying the corneal flap procedure. By using a thin pointed knife (created by himself), a peripheral linear incision was made to avoid the large gap of the typically used semicircular corneal incision. This procedure was commended by von Graefe's peers as it reduced infection and the failure rate of the extraction of a cataract from 10-5%, and was soon used internationally by countless ophthalmic surgeons.

As von Graefe's clinic grew, so did his passion for his patients and work. Even as he dealt with an increasing pain caused by his heightened **tuberculosis**, he continued to perform an enormous amount of surgery, with up to 50 cataracts and 15 iridectomies in one week. Von Graefe was also influential in the founding of the Heidelberg Ophthalmological Society, which in 1864 joined together 80 ophthalmologists from around the world.

As the tuberculosis spread to von Graefe's lungs and throat, he began to work harder and was able to do so after injecting himself with **morphine**, a drug that he had become addicted to due to his continual pain. He died on July 20, 1870 at the age of 42, and his wife passed on two years later at the age of 30. After von Graefe's death, he was memorialized by fellow ophthalmologists who published an encyclopedia in his memory. His image also lives on in a statue that was erected by the Berlin Medical Society in 1882 in front of the Charité Hospital, and a Graefe Museum in the Heidelberg eye clinic by the Heidelberg Society. It was von Graefe's final wishes that his clinic be closed immediately after his death, ending 20 years of historical happenings in the world of ophthalmology.

See also Cataract; Claude Bernard; William Bowman; Eye; Glaucoma; Johann Lukas Schonlein; Rudolf Carl Virchow; Visual impairment and blindness

GRANIT, RAGNAR ARTHUR (1900-1991)

Finnish neurophysiologist

Ragnar Arthur Granit was born in Helsinki, Finland, on October 30, 1900, the eldest son of Arthur W. Granit, a government forester, and Albertina Helena Malmberg Granit. Since both his parents were of Swedish origin, Granit attended the Swedish Normal School there. In 1918, Granit fought in Finland's war for independence from the Soviet Union, for which he received the Finnish Cross of Freedom.

The following year Granit entered the University of Helsinki with the intention of studying experimental psychology. However, he decided that a medical education would provide the best foundation for this field. So he went on to complete a master's degree in 1923 and then an M.D. in 1927. It was while completing his medical studies that Granit became interested in studying the **nervous system**, particularly the **eye**. The English physiologist **Edgar Douglas Adrian** had just made the first recordings of electrical impulses in single nerve fibers, and Granit realized that Adrian's technique could be used to provide useful information about the nervous system as well as the retina. Thus, in 1928 Granit traveled to Oxford University to work with Adrian and another English physiologist, **Charles Scott Sherrington**, and learn the techniques of neurophysiology. Soon thereafter, Granit accepted a fellowship in medical physics at the University of Pennsylvania. It was here, while working at the university's Johnson Foundation for Medical Physics, that Granit first met **Haldan Keffer Hartline**, who along with **George Wald** would eventually share the Nobel Prize with Granit.

In 1935 Granit returned to the University of Helsinki as a professor of physiology, but he also continued his research into neurophysics. At this time, it was still unclear whether light could inhibit, as well as elicit, impulses in the optic nerve. During the early 1930s, Granit produced the first experimental evidence of this inhibition, a finding that remains fundamental to visual physiology. In early work, Granit employed such indirect measures as the sensitivity reported by human subjects to flickering lights. He showed that illumination focused on the retina would suppress the response of adjacent regions. This served to enhance the perception of visual contrasts. Granit soon confirmed these findings using an electroretinogram, a graphic record of electrical activity in the retina, similar to the record of heart activity known as an electrocardiogram.

The 1939 invasion of Finland by the Soviet Union interrupted Granit's work. During the war Granit served as a physician on three Swedish-speaking islands, including Korpo in the Baltic Sea. After the war, he was offered positions at both Harvard University in the United States as well as the Karolinksa Institute in Stockholm. He chose the latter, where he directed the Nobel Institute for Neurophysiology until his retirement in 1967.

While working at the Nobel Institute, Granit and his colleagues became the first scientists to use microelectrodes, tiny electrical conductors, for sensory research. By using microelectrodes to study individual cells in the retina, Granit now demonstrated that certain cells, called modulators, are color-specific, while others, called dominators, respond to a broad range of the spectrum. Although subsequent research has modified his views, Granit's studies were the earliest serious effort to investigate color vision by electrophysiological methods.

Beginning in 1945, Granit shifted the focus of his research to the study of muscle spindles, sensory end organs that are sensitive to muscle tension. Ultimately, the structure of muscle spindles and their function in motor control became one of the best-studied areas in neurophysiology, and Granit was at the forefront of the field. Throughout this period of his career, Granit maintained a hands-on presence in the laboratory and continued to take part in experimental operations on animals there. The procedures he most enjoyed performing were the meticulous dissection of nerves and the careful preparation of nerve roots for electrode placement.

Granit's dual contributions to neurophysiology were honored on numerous occasions. In addition to the Nobel he was awarded such prizes as the 1947 Jubilee Medal of the Swedish Society of Physicians, the 1957 Anders Retzius Gold Medal of the University of Utrecht, and the 1961 Jahre Prize of Oslo University. He was once president of the Royal Swedish Academy of Sciences, and a member of such learned societies as the American Academy of Arts and Sciences, the American National Academy of Sciences, and the Royal Society of London. Active even after his retirement, Granit was appointed a resident scholar at the Fogarty International Center in Bethesda, Maryland, during part of the 1970s. He also accepted a visiting professorship at St. Catherine's College in Oxford, England.

Granit had married Baroness Marguerite Emma ''Daisy'' Bruun on October 2, 1929, just before leaving for the Johnson Foundation fellowship in the United States. They had one son, Michael, who became a Stockholm architect. Granit died of a heart attack at his home in Stockholm on March 12, 1991.

GRAVE ROBBERY

Up until the late 14th century, **Galen**'s writings (A.D. 129-216) were an unchallenged source of information on **human anatomy**. In the late medieval period, however, the field of medicine began to change. Doctors and their students sought information that was drawn from their own observation and experience. They believed that a better understanding of the human body would allow them to practice medicine more effectively. Accordingly, **dissection** of cadavers for information and instruction became a part of medicine. The practice was not widespread until the 15th century and didn't reach the British Isles until the mid-16th century.

Initially, lecturers dissected a body while students observed, and the demand for cadavers was low. Later, as schools became more numerous and students began conducting dissections themselves, the need for cadavers grew. Countries on continental Europe met the challenge by passing anatomy laws on how anatomists could acquire bodies. In Great Britain, Ireland, and the United States, however, such laws did not exist until nearly the mid-19th century.

Previously, the laws that did exist were very restrictive. For example, the town council in Edinburgh, Scotland granted a charter to the city's surgeons allowing them one body per year.

In desperation, anatomists turned to grave robbery as a means of acquiring bodies for dissection. Initially, these thefts were conducted by anatomists and their students, but by the mid-18th century, there arose a class of thieves who made their living from this gruesome practice. These so-called resurrectionists or resurrection men entered graveyards on the night following a funeral. Working silently, with as little light as possible, they unburied the upper part of the coffin in the new grave. After breaking through the lid, they slipped a noose around the corpse's neck and dragged the body from the grave. The grave was returned to its original appearance, and the resurrectionists brought the body to an anatomy school. At the anatomy school, they received money for the body, generally with no questions asked.

Thousands of graves were robbed in the late 18th century and early 19th century, primarily in and around Dublin, Edinburgh, Glasgow, and London.

Descriptions of grave robbery turn up frequently in the literature of the time. For example, the character Jerry Cruncher in Charles Dickens's *A Tale of Two Cities* described his line of work as a ''tradesman'' dealing in ''a branch of scientific goods'' in answer to his son's questions about what a resurrection man did. Naturally, the public was disgusted and angry about the resurrectionists' activities and the anatomists' indirect involvement. It was not uncommon for people to sit guard by the grave of a friend or relative for several days following a burial. Some people installed heavy iron gates over the graves of their loved ones in order to discourage grave robbers. Locked gates, traps, and other devices were also used. The resurrectionists ran the risk of being attacked by guards defending a graveyard, and there are reports of some being shot and killed. Violence sometimes led to riots, and more than one anatomy school was destroyed by angry mobs both in Britain and the United States.

Laws regarding the practice were not changed until the British 1832 Anatomy Act. American laws were passed on a state by state basis and most had laws in place by the 1840s.

These laws were inspired in large part by the actions of resurrectionists who turned to murder to supply the anatomists with cadavers. The most notorious of these men were William Hare and William Burke who committed their crimes in Edinburgh in 1828. Burke and Hare first sold the body of a man who had died in Hare's boarding house. Afterward, they and two female associates allegedly planned and committed 16 murders within nine months and sold the bodies to an anatomy school. Friends of their last victim discovered what they were doing and reported them to the police. Only Burke was convicted of the crimes and was executed at the end of 1828. (Ironically, his body was turned over to an anatomist for public dissection.) Similar crimes were reported in London and in several American cities, and public outrage forced legislators to pass laws permitting anatomists a legal source of cadavers. Once these laws were in place, grave robbery quickly declined.

Grief

Grief refers to the feelings and associated behaviors accompanying loss, usually through **death**. It is a major component of our emotional repertoire, and has been captured unforgettably in numerous literary works through the ages; two notable examples are *The Confessions of St. Augustine* and *The Sorrows of Young Werther* by Johann Wolfgang von Goethe.

Grieving affects how people feel both mentally and physically, how they cope, interact with others, and see the world.

Because everyone is different, people feel grief in a range of intensities, but professionals agree that it typically follows three stages that may occur in sequence or that may overlap. The first phase is one of denial, in which the shock and numbness a person feels may disguise the full pain of their loss. These feelings may occur even when death is expected, but they are likely to last longer and to be more intense if death is unexpected.

The second phase is one of acute anguish once the realization begins to set in that the loss is forever. A person may have physical symptoms, for example, feelings of choking or emptiness in the abdomen. The bereaved may have no desire to see anyone, or may become forgetful or angry. People sometimes doubt themselves or even God. Parents of a murdered child may not be able to bring themselves to clean out the child's room. The process of grieving is so overwhelmingly intense that even well adjusted people can feel as though they are going insane. Acute anguish may last weeks or months, though gradually people find they are able to go on. For some people this is a period of oscillating between focusing on the pain of the loss and trying to divert themselves through work or planning for the future.

In a final phase called restitution, the bereaved is able to recognize the loss, but also sees that it is possible to have a life apart from the deceased, that is, to return to work, experience pleasure, and seek companionship and love.

Mourning is the public expression of grief. Since earliest history, every culture has recorded its own beliefs, customs, and behavior related to mourning. The purpose of mourning is to help the bereaved to acknowledge the reality of the death, to provide support for the bereaved, to pay tribute to the dead, and to offer the community an avenue for expressing sorrow. For example, in contemporary North America, the funeral and burial service provide these functions, though the exact practices vary depending on religion and culture. Mass public grieving, like the kind that accompanied the death of Diana, Princess of Wales, allows people to express private feelings in a public way; conversely, people may also use such public mourning as a way of expressing private losses.

Mourning in children can be expressed in different ways.

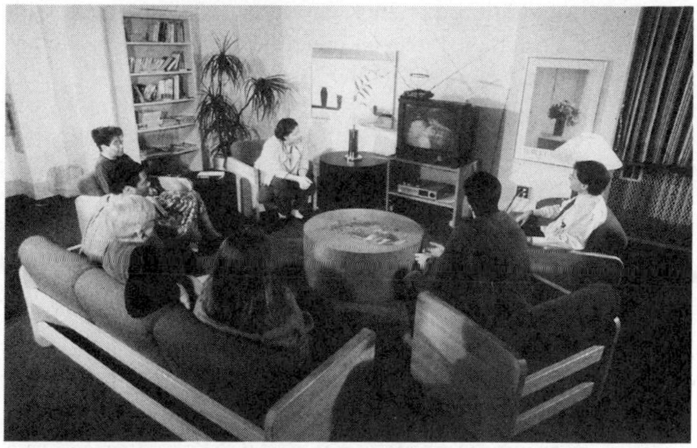

Group therapy is practiced in a variety of settings, including both inpatient and outpatient facilities, and is used to treat anxiety, mood, and personality disorders as well as psychoses. ***(Photo Researchers, Inc. Reproduced by permission.)***

Very young children may express grief in bodily functions, such as bed wetting, difficulty eating, and disturbed sleep, just as they may do in the absence of an adult on whom they depend. Most children five and older, however, understand the difference between separation and death, and their reactions are more complex. Children who have lost a parent may fear the death of the remaining parent; those who have lost a sibling may worry that any feelings of jealousy or resentment they felt toward their sibling actually caused the person's death. Some children develop behavioral problems.

People also experience losses other than death of a person for which they might grieve. Such losses include the death of a cherished pet, or material losses (for instance, a home) due to conflict or natural disaster. Unresolved grief refers to ambiguous loss, and it stems from the inability to mourn someone who is not properly gone. For example, a person might be still physically present but emotionally absent, as in the case of loved ones suffering from **Alzheimer's disease**, debilitating **stroke**, or a serious **mental illness**. Alternatively, a person might be physically absent but still emotionally present, as when a person is missing in military action, or a child disappears and is not found.

The symptoms of grief are the same as those for clinical depression, but expected in the wake of an intense loss. If they persist, they are then regarded as a clinical disorder rather than normal grief.

See also Sleep disorders

Group Therapy

Group therapy gives individuals a safe and comfortable place where they can work out problems and emotional issues with others. It takes place in small groups of patients that meet regularly to talk, interact, and discuss problems with each other and the group leader (therapist). Patients gain insight into their own thoughts and behavior, and offer suggestions and support to others. In addition, patients who have a difficult time with interpersonal relationships can benefit from the social interactions that are a basic part of the therapy.

Patients are typically referred for group therapy by a psychologist or psychiatrist. Some patients may need individual therapy first. Group therapy sessions are usually arranged and conducted by a psychologist, psychiatrist, social worker, or other healthcare professional. In some groups, two co-therapists share the leadership responsibility. Patients are selected based on what they might gain from group interaction and what they can contribute.

Therapy group members may have similar diagnostic backgrounds (for example, they may all suffer from depression), or they may be dealing with a variety of issues. The number of group members varies widely, but is typically no more than 12. Groups may be time-limited (with a predetermined number of sessions) or indefinite (where the group determines when therapy ends). Membership may be closed or open to new members once sessions begin.

The therapeutic approach depends on the focus of the group and the psychological training of the therapist. Some common techniques include psychodynamic, cognitive-behavioral, and **Gestalt therapy**.

In a group session, members are encouraged to openly and honestly discuss the issues that brought them to therapy. There are no definite rules for group therapy, only that members participate to the best of their ability. However, most therapy groups do have basic ground rules that are usually discussed during the first session. Patients are asked not to share what goes on in therapy sessions with anyone outside of the group. This protects the confidentiality of the other members. They may also be asked not to see other group members socially outside of therapy, because of the harmful effect it might have on the dynamics of the group.

The therapist's main task is to guide the group in self-discovery. He or she may lead the group interaction or allow the group to take its own direction. Typically, the leader does some of both, providing direction when the group gets off track while letting members set their own agenda. The therapist may simply reinforce positive behavior (such as empathy or constructive suggestions) within the group. In almost all group therapy situations, the therapist will emphasize the common traits among members so they gain a sense of group identity.

The main benefit group therapy may have over individual psychotherapy is that some patients behave and react more like themselves in a group setting than they would one-on-one with a therapist. The patient gains a sense of identity and social acceptance from membership in the group. Seeing how others deal with these issues may suggest new solutions to their problems. Feedback from group members offers unique insights into one's own behavior, and the group provides a safe forum in which to practice new behaviors. By helping others work through their problems, members can gain **self-esteem**. Group therapy may also simulate family experiences, allowing family dynamic issues to emerge.

The end of long-term group therapy may cause feelings of grief, loss, abandonment, anger, or rejection in some members. The group therapist will try to create a sense of closure by encouraging members to explore their feelings and use newly acquired coping techniques to deal with them. Working through this termination phase of group therapy is an important part of the treatment process.

Patients who have trouble communicating in group situations may be at risk for dropping out of group therapy. If no one comments on their silence or makes an attempt to interact with them, they may begin to feel even more isolated and alone instead of identifying with the group. Therefore, the therapist usually attempts to encourage silent members to participate early on in treatment.

Patients who are suicidal, homicidal, psychotic, or in the midst of a major crisis are typically not referred for group therapy until their behavior and emotional state have stabilized. Depending on their level of functioning, cognitively impaired patients (such as patients with organic brain disease or a traumatic brain injury) may also be unsuitable for group therapy. Some very fragile patients may not be able to tolerate aggressive or hostile comments from group members. Some patients with sociopathic traits are not suitable for most groups.

Both group and individual psychotherapy benefit about 85% of the patients who participate in them. Optimally, patients gain a better understanding of themselves, and perhaps a stronger set of interpersonal and coping skills. Some patients may continue therapy after group therapy ends, either individually or in another group setting.

Self-help groups like Alcoholics Anonymous and Weight Watchers offer many of the same benefits of social support, identity, and belonging, but are considered outside of the psychotherapy realm. These self-help groups meet to discuss a common area of concern (such as alcoholism, eating disorders, bereavement, parenting). Group sessions are not run by a therapist, but by a nonprofessional leader, group member, or the group as a whole. Self-help groups are sometimes used in addition to psychotherapy or regular group therapy.

GUIDED IMAGERY

The technique of guided imagery focuses the power of the mind on some aspect of the workings of the body, in order to cause a real, positive physical response.

Once learned, this self-help technique is used to relieve stress, explore psychological conflicts, and manage **pain**. Used either in a medical setting or as an effective means of self-care, it can be applied to any situation in which relaxation, symptom relief, and a feeling of personal empowerment is useful.

Guided imagery has been described as a kind of ''directed daydreaming.'' It is based on the generally accepted idea that the mind can influence the body. For example, if you relax and think about a juicy, fresh lemon, then imagine slicing it and slowly raising the dripping, pale yellow sections to your waiting lips and sucking on them, chances are you will experience a standard physical response: you will salivate. Advocates of this technique argue that people possess a remarkable degree of self-regulation that generally goes unknown, unexplored, and unused.

Thoughts or ''images'' can affect heart and breathing rate, as well as other involuntary functions such as hormone levels, gastrointestinal secretions, and brain wave patterns. Advocates of guided imagery therefore stress the importance of the image (thought) which, they say, does not have to be real to have a actual, physical effect. Guided imagery takes the next step and asks why the mind can't be used to cause good things to happen within the body. Also called visualization, creative visualization, or creative imagery, this technique teaches how to consciously create positive images to accomplish a desired goal. One neurological explanation of what might go on in the brain during guided imagery is that the image or message is sent from the higher centers of the brain (cerebral cortex) to the lower or more primitive centers that regulate a person's involuntary functions, like breathing and heart rate. Whether or not these images are real, the lower part of the brain apparently responds accordingly as long as there is no contradictory information.

In a typical guided imagery session, the patient or client is placed in a relaxed state by the verbal guidance of the practitioner. This calm, receptive state is deepened through breathing exercises. This allows the patient to give real focus and direction to his or her imagination. Once truly deep relaxation is achieved, the practitioner encourages the patient to choose a safe place, a very personal, truly serene site that may or may not actually exist, in which the patient feels perfect emotional security. It is at this point that the practitioner begins to work on the particular goal of therapy, whether it is to reduce stress or anxiety, manage the constant pain of a chronic condition, or assist in the healing process. Following several successful sessions with a practitioner, patients are usually able to use the technique on their own, often using written instructions or special tapes.

Guided imagery should not be used in place of conventional medicine or surgery in cases of a serious disease or condition. It is not recommended for psychotic patients who often cannot distinguish the difference between suggested images and reality. The only risk in guided imagery would be in viewing it as a cure-all rather than as an complement to conventional medicine.

Guillain-Barré syndrome

Guillain-Barré syndrome (GBS) causes progressive muscle weakness and **paralysis** (complete inability to use a particular muscle or muscle group), which develops over days or up to four weeks, and lasts several weeks or even months.

GBS typically occurs in a patient who has just recovered from a seemingly uncomplicated viral infection, most commonly cytomegalovirus, herpes, Epstein-Barr virus, or viral hepatitis. GBS may also follow a gastrointestinal infection with the bacteria *Campylobacter jejuni,* in which case the GBS is particularly severe. About 5% of GBS cases follow a surgical procedure. Individuals with **lymphoma**, **systemic lupus erythematosus**, or **AIDS** have a higher-than-normal risk of GBS. Other GBS patients may have recently received an immunization, while still others have no known preceding event. In 1976–77, there was a vastly increased number of GBS cases among people recently vaccinated against Swine flu. The reason for this has never been identified, and no other flu vaccine has caused such an increase in GBS cases.

The first symptoms of GBS start one to four weeks after the individual has recovered from the initial infection. They consist of muscle weakness (legs first, then arms, then face), accompanied by prickly, tingling sensations. Symptoms affect both sides of the body simultaneously, a fact that helps distinguish GBS from other causes of weakness and tingling. Normal reflexes are first diminished, then lost. The weakness eventually affects all the voluntary muscles, resulting in paralysis. When those muscles necessary for breathing become paralyzed, the patient must be placed on a mechanical ventilator which takes over the function of breathing. This occurs about 30% of the time. Severely ill GBS patients may also have problems with fluid balance, severely fluctuating blood pressure, and heart rhythm irregularities.

Diagnosis of GBS involves examining the fluid that bathes the brain and spinal canal through a spinal tap. This involves inserting a needle into the lower back.

There is no direct treatment for GBS. Instead, treatments are aimed at the disabilities caused by the disease. The progress of paralysis must be carefully monitored, in case mechanical breathing assistance becomes necessary. Careful attention must also be paid to the amount of fluid the patient is drinking and eliminating. Blood pressure, heart rate, and heart rhythm also must be monitored.

A procedure called plasmapheresis, performed early in the course of GBS, has been shown to shorten the course and severity of the disease. Plasmapheresis consists of withdrawing the patient's blood, passing it through an instrument that separates the different types of blood cells, and returning all the cellular components (red and white blood cells and platelets) along with either donor plasma or a manufactured replacement solution. This is thought to rid the blood of substances that cause GBS symptoms.

It has also been shown that high doses of immunoglobulin, a substance naturally manufactured by the body's immune system in response to various threats, given intravenously (by drip through a needle in a vein), may be just as helpful as plasmapheresis.

About 85% of GBS patients make reasonably good recoveries. However, 30% of adult patients, and a greater percentage of children, never fully regain their previous level of muscle strength. Some of these patients suffer from ongoing weakness, others from permanent paralysis. About 10% of GBS patients begin to improve, then suffer a relapse. These patients suffer chronic GBS symptoms. About 5% of all GBS patients die, most from cardiac rhythm disturbances.

Patients with certain characteristics tend to have a worse outcome. These include people of older age, those who required breathing support with a mechanical ventilator, and those who had their worst symptoms within the first seven days.

Guillemin, Roger (1924-)

French American endocrinologist

Roger Guillemin is one of the founders of the field of neuroendocrinology, the study of the interaction between the central **nervous system** (such as the brain) and endocrine glands (such as the pituitary, thyroid, and pancreas). Guillemin focused his research on hormones produced by the brain, and their subsequent effect on body processes. He proved the correctness of a hypothesis first proposed by English anatomist Geoffrey W. Harris that the hypothalamus releases hormones to regulate the pituitary gland. For discoveries which led to an understanding of hypothalamic hormone productions of the brain, Guillemin and fellow endocrinologist **Andrew V. Schally** shared the 1977 Nobel prize for physiology or medicine with physicist **Rosalyn Sussman Yalow**. Guillemin and Schally were pioneers in isolating, identifying, and determining the chemical nature of such hormones as TRF (thyrotropin-releasing factor which regulates the thyroid gland), LRF (luteinizing-releasing factor which controls male and female reproductive functions), somatostatin (which regulates the production of growth hormones and insulin), and endorphins (which may be involved in the onset of mental illness). Guillemin's work led to scientific advances including an understanding of thyroid diseases, infertility, juvenile diabetes, and the physiology of the brain. According to Guillemin, the determination of the chemical structure of TRF marked an end to the pioneering era in neuroendocrinology and the beginning of a major new science.

Roger Charles Louis Guillemin was born on January 11, 1924, and raised in Dijon, France, the son of Raymond Guillemin, a machine toolmaker, and Blanche Rigollot Guillemin. He attended the University of Dijon where he received a Bachelor's degree in 1942, and then entered the University of Lyons medical school, graduating with a medical degree in 1949. However, Guillemin interrupted his studies during World War II in order to join the French underground during the Nazi occupation, becoming part of an operation helping refugees escape to Switzerland over the Jura Mountains. During and after the war Guillemin received three years of clinical training and briefly practiced medicine before joining a well-known Canadian physiologist, Hans Selye, as a research assistant. To work with Selye, Guillemin moved to the Institute of Experimental Medicine and Surgery at the University of Montreal in Canada. In 1950, he suffered a near-fatal attack of tubercular **meningitis**. After his recovery in 1951, Guillemin married Lucienne Jeanne Billard, who had been his nurse during his illness. They had six children, five daughters—Chantal, Claire, Helene, Elizabeth, and Cecile, and a son François.

Guillemin received his Ph.D. from the University of Montreal in 1953, and accepted an assistant professorship at Baylor University Medical School in Houston, Texas. His research involved endocrinology, the study of the hormones that circulate in the blood. The **endocrine system** is a hierarchical one in which hormones from the pituitary gland regulate other endocrine glands. It was thought that the head of the entire system was the hypothalamus, located at the base of the brain just above the pituitary gland. However, the way in which hypothalamic hormonal regulation occurred was unclear. The theory of regulation by nerve impulses was marred by the anatomical fact that there are few nerves that extend from the hypothalamus to the pituitary. Anatomist Geoffrey W. Harris theorized that hypothalamic regulation occurred by means of hormones, which are transported by the blood. Harris's experiments supported his hypothesis, proving altered pituitary function when the blood vessels were cut between the hypothalamus and the pituitary. The problem was that no one had yet been successful in isolating and identifying a hormone from the hypothalamus.

Guillemin began an investigation to find the missing evidence, a task of extraordinary difficulty because very minute amounts of hypothalamic substances are involved. At Baylor, Guillemin worked together with Schally using a technique called mass spectroscopy and a new tool developed by physicists Solomon Berson and Rosalyn Sussman Yalow called **radioimmunoassays** (RIAs) which enabled scientists to isolate and identify the chemical structure of hormones. In the early 1960s Guillemin considered continuing his research in France, and obtained a concurrent appointment at both Baylor and the Collège de France in Paris. However, he left the Collège de France in 1963, and was appointed director of the Laboratory for Neuroendocrinology at Baylor University. By this time he and Schally had ended their scientific cooperation and had become fiercely competitive in a race to identify hypothalamic hormones.

Guillemin worked with sheep hypothalami which he obtained from slaughterhouses. Obtaining the specimens was a large-scale, difficult operation. Only very minute amounts of substance existed in each sheep hypothalamus and it had to be extracted very soon after death. Guillemin and Roger Burgus, a chemist who worked with Guillemin, reported that their laboratory collected about five million hypothalamic fragments from sheep brains, which involved handling about five hundred tons of brain tissue. Finally in 1968, Guillemin and his coworkers isolated the hypothalamic hormone that effects the release of thyrotropin. The following year Guillemin, as well as Schally, who had been working independently, revealed the structure of TRF (a hypothalamic hormone which today is called thyrotropin-releasing hormone or TRH). When TRF is secreted by the hypothalamus, it causes the pituitary gland to secrete another hormone that in turn causes the thyroid gland to secrete its own hormones. Shortly thereafter Guillemin and his colleagues isolated and determined the chemical structure of GRH (growth-releasing-hormone), a hypothalamic hormone that causes the pituitary to release gonadotropin which in turn influences the release of hormones in the testicles or ovaries. This discovery led to advancements in the medical treatment of infertility.

In 1970 Guillemin moved to the Salk Institute in La Jolla, California. There he isolated a third hypothalamic hormone which he named somatostatin. This hormone acts by inhibiting the release of growth hormone from the pituitary gland. In 1977 Guillemin and Schally were awarded the Nobel Prize for their research on hypothalamic hormones. Guillemin wrote on the importance of their discoveries in an autobiography, published in *Pioneers in Neuroendocrinology II,* stating that: "I consider the isolation and characterization of TRF as the major event in modern neuroendocrinology, the inflection point that separated confusion and a great deal of doubt from real knowledge. Modern neuroendocrinology was born of that event. Isolations of LRF, somatostatin, and the recent endorphins were all extensions (as there will be still more, I am sure) of that major event—the isolation of TRF, a novel molecule in hypothalamic extracts, with hypophysiotropic activity, the first so characterized.... The event was the vindication of 14 years of hard work."

Guillemin soon turned his attention to another class of substances, known as neuropeptides. Produced by the hypothalamus and other parts of the brain, neuropeptides act at the synapses of the nerves (the area where the nerve impulse passes from one neuron or nerve cell to another). One group of neuropeptides, for example, called endorphins, seem to affect moods and the perception of pain. Guillemin's recent research includes neurochemistry of the brain and growth factors.

Guillemin is known as an urbane conversationalist who is interested in the arts and enjoys painting. He and his wife have a collection of contemporary French and American paintings, pre-Columbian art objects, and artifacts from around the world. Guillemin is also a connoisseur of fine food and wine.

Gulf War Syndrome

Gulf War Syndrome (GWS), or Gulf War Illness (GWI), refers to an array of physical and emotional symptoms reported by thousands of United States veterans following their participation in the Persian Gulf War in 1990 and 1991. Considerable confusion and controversy surround GWS because symptoms are not only varied but often vary among individuals and may mimic symptoms of other diseases. Also, many vets remain symptom-free, and some researchers claim symptoms are no more prevalent among Gulf War vets than in the general population. Some are of the opinion GWS is related to **Post-Traumatic Stress Syndrome**. Regardless of the controversy, many vets who left for the war in perfect health now experience illnesses ranging from mild to incapacitating and which, in some cases, has resulted in **death**.

During the Gulf War, many service people were exposed to dense smoke from oil well fires, infectious diseases, pesticides, depleted uranium, chemical and biological weapons, pyridostigmine bromide—a pretreatment against potential exposure to poisonous gas, **anthrax** and botulinum toxin vaccines, and psychological and physiological stress. GWS symptoms include aches and pains and fatigue closely resembling **fibromyalgia** (FM) and **Chronic Fatigue Syndrome** (CFS), migraine **headaches**, depression, weight gain, **rashes** unresponsive to treatment, asthma, difficulty with concentration and memory, gastrointestinal upset, **sore throat** and swollen glands, fevers, and lowered **immune system**. Studies reported in the *Journal of the American Medical Association (JAMA)* in 1997 by Haley, et al determined 70 percent of 249 members of a battalion which served in the gulf had "serious health concerns." Researchers concluded neuropsychologic difficulties may have been caused by exposure to pesticides, chemical weapons, and/or pyridostigmine bromide. Also reported in *JAMA* in 1997 by Schwarts, et al was a study of service personnel from all branches of the armed services representing more than 800 military units. When compared to service personnel not sent to the Gulf, Gulf vets were much more likely to experience GWS and, of those, symptoms were significantly greater when contact with solvents, smoke, pesticides, pyridostigmine, and agents of chemical warfare were reported.

It was not until 1996 that the U.S. Department of Defense acknowledged the escape of neurotoxic chemicals following post-war destruction of Iraqi ammunition bunkers. The Gulf War Illness office established by the Pentagon is now conducting investigations, including studies done on Czechoslovakian and French troops, analysis of a theory of an Iraqi terrorist attack with chemical weapons at Al Jubayl, claims of biological weapon use, hazards from exposure to depleted uranium dust, and insecticide/pesticide use and exposure. These investigations and epidemiological studies have thus far failed to identify the cause of GWS, and medical research has failed to find clinical parameters by which it can be defined. A January 1997 article in *JAMA* concluded that these illnesses are real, not simply psychosomatic, and that treatment of symptoms, **counselling**, and emotional support are critical.

In an open trial conducted by Drs. Pietr Hitzig and Dan Malone, complete remission of GWS was reported in up to 90 percent of patients on the FEN/PHEN protocol, which is a combination of phentermine and fenfluramine. Fatigue and body aches experienced in GWS, FM, and CFS appear to be linked to low or unbalanced levels of serotonin and dopamine. The FEN/PHEN combination—which must be highly individualized and monitored because of potential adverse side affects—appears to balance the levels of these neurotransmitters. Results must now be tested in rigorous controlled trials.

Gullstrand, Allvar (1862-1930)

Swedish physician

Gullstrand conducted studies in ophthalmology and optics that contributed greatly to our understanding of the mechanisms of vision and disorders of the **eye**. The son of a prominent physician, Gullstrand was born in Landskrona, Sweden, and studied medicine in Uppsala, Vienna, and in Stockholm. He earned his medical degree in 1884 and his doctorate in 1890.

In 1892 Gullstrand became a lecturer at the Royal Caroline Institute and worked as head of the ophthalmological clinic in Stockholm. Two years later, he became professor at the University of Uppsala and in 1913, the university created a chair in his honor so that he could concentrate on his research in ophthalmological optics, the study of the optical system of the human eye.

Gullstrand's first contribution to the field was his study of astigmatism of the cornea. His findings on **astigmatism** led to the design of more effective corrective lenses for the condition. He then turned his attention to the role of the lens in accommodation. His detailed mathematical approach went beyond the findings of **Hermann von Helmholtz**, the German physicist who had published the *Handbook of Physiological Optics*, which Gullstrand edited. Gullstrand wrote many of his own papers on mathematical optics and, with his typical mathematical rigor, discovered inaccuracies in the traditional treatment of optical disorders.

Gullstrand also invented a slit lamp, which was used with a microscope to locate a foreign body in the eye with complete accuracy, and designed aspheric lenses that gave vision to patients whose lenses had been removed because of **cataracts**. In addition, he devised several other optical instruments including an ophthalmoscope, used to examine the interior of the eye.

Gullstrand received honorary degrees from the University of Uppsala, the University of Jena, and the University of Dublin. In 1911 he was awarded the Nobel Prize in physiology and medicine. Highly respected for his integrity and his exacting research, he was later appointed president of the Nobel Prize committee. He died in 1930 in Uppsala, Sweden.

GUY DE CHAULIAC (ca. 1300-1368)

French Surgeon

Medieval Frenchman Guy de Chauliac is known as one of the most influential surgeons of the fourteenth century. Born into a peasant-class family in 1290, he was guided in his studies by the lords of Mercoeur. One of the most scholarly individuals of his time, Chauliac studied medicine first at Toulouse, then at Montpellier, and concluded his education at Bologna. With direction from his master Nicolaus Bertrucius (Bertrucio) at Bologna, Chauliac's knowlege of anatomy excelled his teacher's methods left such an impression on Chauliac that he often quoted him throughout his life. He left Bologna for Paris, then to Lyons where Chauliac was appointed canon (clergyman) of St. Just. Later appointments included canon of Rheims and of Mende. With Avignon being home of the popes at this time, Chauliac became private physician to several bishops, including: Clement VI (1342-1352); Innocent VI (1352-1362); and Urban V (1362-1370). As a valued part of the church, he was appointed a papal clerk of the Roman Catholic Church. Chauliac also became acquainted with the Italian lyric poet and scholar Francesco Petrarch while serving at Avignon.

Upon receiving his master's degree in medicine from Montpellier a title equal to the M.D. of Bologna Chauliac began to refer to himself in his works as "cyrurgicus magister in medicine." In 1363, he created what would be considered the medical standard on surgery until the seventeenth century with the *Inventorium sive collectorium in parte chirurgiciali medicine*, commonly known as *Chirurgia*. Even after undergoing several editions and translations from Latin into Provencal, French, English, Italian, Dutch, and Hebrew, the seven parts of *Chirurgia* spanned three centuries as the guiding force in surgical medicine. Key information is found in the prologue ("Capitulum singulare") with topics ranging from liberal arts, diet, **surgical instruments**, and the process of performing an operation. Chauliac also describes a brief history of medicine and surgery as it evolved through earlier physicians and surgeons, in addition to personal information.

While Chauliac's book was highly regarded, noone admired it more than the writer himself, and he thought *Chirurgia* to be the best medical ideas of his time. In the book, he quotes 3,300 acknowledged writers and authors to reinforce his ideas. These include **Galen**, **Hippocrates**, **Aristotle**, **Razi** (Rhazes), Abul Kasim (Albucasis), Ign Sina (**Avicenna**), Ibn Rushd (Averroës), in addition to references to his own colleagues.

Great emphasis was placed on anatomy in the seven-volume text, and Chauliac indicates that a surgeon who was ignorant of anatomy carved the human body in the same way a blind man carved wood. In the section on anatomy (Tractatus I), Chauliac shows little understanding of his topic. While experienced at actual surgical procedures, this part of *Chirurgia* shows the limited amount of medical knowledge available to Chauliac and his peers at this time.

The plague epidemics of 1348 and 1360 are both described by Chauliac in the textbook, and he is the first to distinguish the difference between bubonic (also known as black death) and pneumonic (a result of bubonic that affects the lungs) **plague**. In addition to recording the prevalence of plague in Asia and Europe, Chauliac falsely blames the disease on the Jewish population. The plague is also recognized as being contagious, and Chauliac recommends the air to be purified, venesection (opening of a vein to remove blood), and having the sick maintain a healthy diet to combat the disease.

Chauliac's ideas on infection have caused continued controversy. According to the surgeon, wounds should not be permitted to heal as nature allows, but should be aggressively treated. His treatments included antidotal salves and plasters. Chauliac also believed that pus (laudable pus) from an infection was required in the healing process.

Three other works were written by Chauliac: *Practica astrolabii (De astronomia)*, an essay on astrology; *De ruptura*, which describes a **hernia**; and *De subtilianti diaeta*, explaining **cataracts** and treatments for the patient.

See also Aristotle; Cataracts; Diets and weight management; Galen; Hernia; Hippocrates of Cos; Infection control; Plague

GYNECOMASTIA

Gyne refers to female, and mastia refers to the breast. Gynecomastia is strictly a male disease and is any growth of the adipose (fatty) and glandular tissue in a male breast. Not all breast growth in men is considered abnormal, just excess growth.

Breast growth is directed exclusively by female hormones—estrogens. Although men have some estrogen in their system, it is usually insufficient to cause much breast enlargement because it is counterbalanced by male hormones—**androgens**. Upsetting the balance, either by more of one or less of the other, results in the male developing female characteristics, breast growth being foremost.

At birth both male and female infants will have little breast buds from their mother's hormones. These recede until adolescence, when girls always, and boys sometimes, have breast growth. At this time, the boy's breast growth is minimal, often one-sided and temporary.

Extra or altered sex chromosomes can produce **intersex** problems of several kinds. Breast growth along with male genital development is seen in Klinefelter syndrome—the condition of having an extra X (female) chromosome—and a few other chromosomal anomalies. One of the several glands that produce hormones can malfunction for reasons other than chromosomes. Failure of androgen production is as likely to produce gynecomastia as overabundant estrogen production. Testicular failure and castration can also be a cause. Some **cancers** and some benign tumors can make estrogens. **Lung cancer** is known to increase estrogens.

If the hormone manufacturing organs are functioning properly, problems can still arise elsewhere. The liver is the principle chemical factory in the body. Other organs like the thyroid and kidneys also effect chemical processes. If any of these organs are diseased, a chemical imbalance can result that alters the manufacturing process. Men with **cirrhosis** of the liver will often develop gynecomastia from increased production of estrogens.

Finally, drugs can also cause breast enlargement. Estrogens are given to men to treat **prostate cancer** and a few other diseases. Marijuana and heroin, along with some prescription drugs, have estrogen effects in some men. On the list are methyldopa (for blood pressure), cimetidine (for peptic **ulcers**), diazepam (Valium), antidepressants, and spironolactone (a diuretic).

Carefully feeling the area beneath the nipple of an adolescent boy with breast enlargement will reveal a discreet and sometimes tender lump the size of a fat nickel or quarter. For more serious gynecomastia, the underlying disease will require evaluation, if it is not already well understood.

This condition is usually not treated. If it is the result of endocrine disease, hormone manipulations may reduce the effects of the imbalance. There are a number of medical and surgical interventions possible. Radiation of misbehaving organs and cancers is considered an effective treatment.

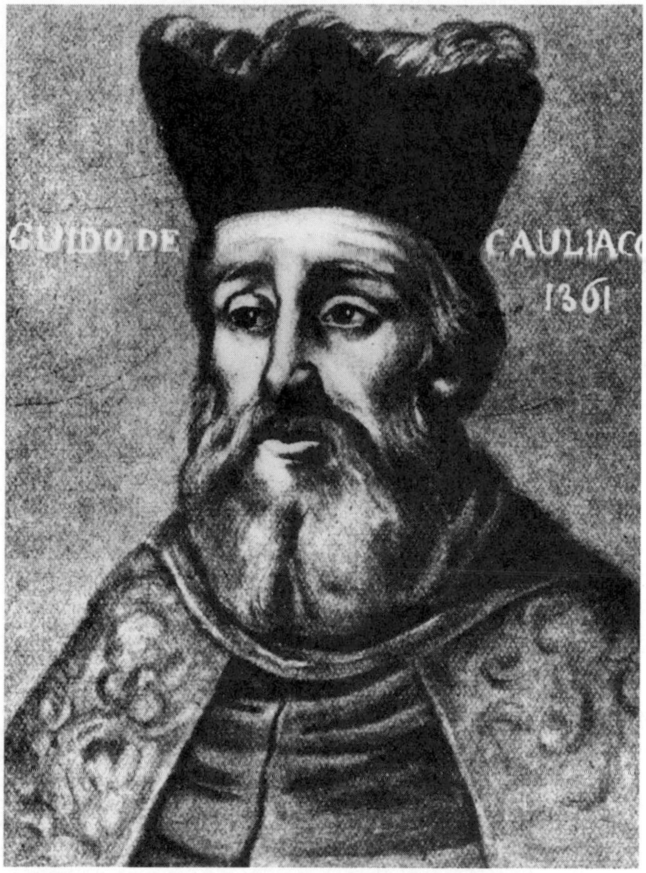

Guy de Chauliac

H

HAHNEMANN, SAMUEL (1755-1843)

German physician

Samuel Hahnemann is the founder of homeopathy, the concept that a disease can be cured by infinitesimal doses of a substance that in larger quantities mimics disease symptoms. During Hahnemann's life time, physicians routinely used **bleeding** and purging to treat disease, and many medicines were more likely to poison than to cure. Hahnemann was horrified by the toll such treatment took on patients and developed **homeopathic medicine** as an alternative.

Hahnemann was born on April 10, 1755, to Christian Gottfried and Johanna Christian Hahnemann, in Meissen, Germany. Hahnemann was highly intelligent but not physically strong as a child. His early schooling was often interrupted so he could help to support his family. Even when in school, his family also had trouble affording his tuition. When he was 15, his teachers proposed giving this bright student lessons for free. He was especially gifted in languages and later turned to translation for part of his income. After finishing school in Meissen in 1775, Hahnemann enrolled in the University of Leipzig to study medicine. However, he was frustrated with the quality of the teaching and left in late 1776 for Vienna. In Vienna, Hahnemann received medical training but was only able to remain a short time, again due to lack of funds. Nearly two years later, once he had saved up enough money, he entered the University of Erlangen and completed his medical studies. He was awarded his degree in August 1779 and began to practice medicine in 1780.

His first position was in Hettstedt, a small German mining town. While there, he witnessed an outbreak of a fever which intensified his disgust with current medical practices. He next moved to Dessau, where he focused his energy on chemistry. In Dessau, he met his future wife, Johanna Küchler, whom he married on November 17, 1782. The first of their 10 children was born the following year. Hahnemann and his young family initially lived in Gommern, where he continued to study chemistry and wrote extensively on the topic. In 1785, Hahnemann and his family moved to Dresden where the opportunities to study chemistry and medicine were greater.

The first hints of homeopathic medicine appeared in a 1788 paper authored by Hahnemann in which he recommended a highly diluted solution of silver nitrate to treat chronic sores. In 1789, he and his family moved back to Leipzig where he devoted himself to research, translations, and writing about chemistry and medicine. While living in a rural suburb of the city, Hahnemann came across a reference to cinchona bark, which was used to treat **malaria**. Hahnemann was curious about how the medicine worked and tried it on himself. He felt that cinchona caused the same symptoms as malaria: **fever**, chills, and exhaustion. Hahnemann conducted many experiments, which he called provings, to determine the precise effects that a substance would have on a healthy person. In 1810, he published *Organon der rationellen Heilkunde* (Handbook of Rational Healing), the book in which he set out the principles of homeopathic medicine.

The first principle was the law of similars, and the second principle was the law of infinitesimals. These two laws reflected Hahnemann's theory that provoking symptoms similar to those caused by a disease could help the body fight off the disease. He used herbs and plants, minerals, and other materials and proposed that they were most effective when they were highly diluted (present in infinitesimal amounts). The third principle had to do with prescribing homeopathic medicines. Hahnemann based prescriptions on the whole person with regard to his or her lifestyle and temperament, rather than just the symptoms of a disease. After publication of the book, Hahnemann began publicizing homeopathic medicine and giving lectures. He later published *Materia medica pura* (Pure Materia Medica) which included details about his provings and treatments of specific complaints.

Hahnemann's theories were met with scorn by the medical community, arguing that homeopathy was ineffective and science was on their side. A major argument against homeopathy is that substances are diluted so much that they no longer

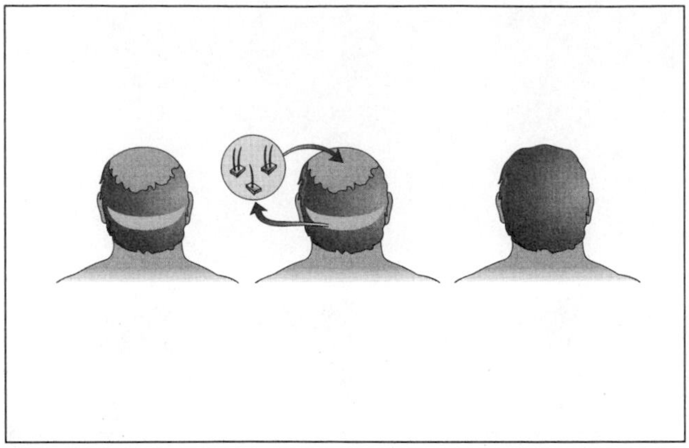

The most common hair transplant procedure involves taking small strips of scalp containing hair follicles from the donor area, usually at the sides or back of the head. These strips are then divided into several hundred smaller grafts. The surgeon relocates these grafts containing skin, follicle, and hair to tiny holes in the balding area by using microsurgical instruments or lasers. *(Illustration by Electronic Illustrators Group.)*

exist in a solution. In several places, laws against homeopathy were passed. To avoid prosecution and to continue his studies, Hahnemann and his family moved frequently. In 1830, Hahnemann's wife died, and five years later, at the age of 80, Hahnemann remarried. His new wife was Melanie D'Hervilly, a Frenchwoman. Shortly after they married, they moved to Paris where Hahnemann died in July 1843.

In the last decades of his life, Hahnemann witnessed a widespread acceptance of homeopathic medicine. A driving force behind its acceptance was the fact that homeopaths, the practitioners of homeopathic medicine, did not use bleeding, purging, and other brutal medical treatments. Acceptance of homeopathy has continued intermittently ever since. In the late 19th century and early 20th century, it was virtually replaced by medicines such as **antibiotics**. Towards the end of the 20th century, however, there has been renewed interest in homeopathy. Modern medicine considers homeopathic treatments as placebos at best and **quackery** at worst, but such criticism doesn't detract from Hahnemann's commitment to improve the practice of medicine. In rejecting standard medical practices of the day and promoting health measures such as **exercise** and a sensible diet, he showed himself to be a doctor ahead of his time.

See also Alternative medicine; homeopathic medicine

HAIR TRANSPLANTATION

Hair transplantation is a surgical procedure used to treat **baldness** or hair loss. Typically, tiny patches of scalp are removed from the back and sides of the head and implanted in the bald spots in the front and top of the head.

Hair transplantation is a cosmetic procedure performed on men (and occasionally on women) who have significant hair loss, thinning hair, or bald spots where hair no longer grows. In men, hair loss and baldness are most commonly due to genetic factors (a tendency passed on in families) and age. Male pattern baldness, in which the hairline gradually recedes to expose more and more of the forehead, is the most common form. Men may also experience a gradual thinning of hair at the crown or very top of the skull. For women, hair loss is more commonly due to hormonal changes and is more likely to be a thinning of hair from the entire head. Transplants can also be done to replace hair lost due to **burns**, injury, or diseases of the scalp.

Although hair transplantation is a fairly simple procedure, some risks are associated with any surgery. It is important to inform the physician about any medications currently being used and about previous allergic reactions to drugs or anesthetic agents. Patients with blood clotting disorders also need to inform their physician before the procedure is performed.

The surgery is performed by a physician in an office, clinic, or hospital setting. Each surgery lasts 2–3 hours, during which approximately 250 grafts will be transplanted. A moderately balding man may require up to 1,000 grafts to get good coverage of a bald area, so a series of surgeries scheduled 3–4 months apart is usually required. The patient may be completely awake during the procedure with just a local anesthetic applied to numb the areas of the scalp. Some patients may be given a drug to help them relax or to put them to sleep.

The most common transplant procedure uses a thin strip of hair and scalp from the back of the head. This strip is cut into smaller clumps of five or six hairs. Tiny cuts are made in the balding area of the scalp and a clump is implanted into each slit. The doctor performing the surgery will attempt to recreate a natural looking hairline along the forehead. Minigrafts, micrografts, or implants of single hair follicles can be used to fill in between larger implant sites and can provide a more natural-looking hairline. The implants will also be arranged so that thick and thin hairs are interspersed and the hair will grow in the same direction.

Another type of hair replacement surgery is called scalp reduction. This involves removing some of the skin from the hairless area and "stretching" some of the nearby hair-covered scalp over the cut-away area.

Health insurance will not pay for hair transplants that are done for cosmetic reasons. Insurance may pay for hair replacement surgery to correct hair loss due to accident, burn, or disease.

It is important to be realistic about what a hair transplant will finally look like. This procedure does not create new hair, it simply redistributes the hair that the patient already has. Some research has been conducted where chest hair has been transplanted to the balding scalp, but this procedure is not widely practiced.

It is important to find a respected, well-established, experienced surgeon and discuss the expected results prior to the surgery. The patient may need blood tests to check for bleeding or clotting problems and may be asked not to take Aspirin-type products before the surgery. The type of **anesthesia** used will depend on how extensive the surgery will be and where it will be performed.

The area may need to be bandaged overnight. The patient can return to normal activities; however, strenuous activities should be avoided in the first few days after the surgery. On rare occasions, the implants can be "ejected" from the scalp during vigorous **exercise**. There may be some swelling, bruising, **headache**, and discomfort around the graft areas and around the eyes. These symptoms can usually be controlled with a mild **pain** reliever like Aspirin. Scabs may form at the graft sites and should not be scraped off. There may be some numbness at the sites, but it will diminish within 2–3 months.

The transplanted hair will fall out within a few weeks, however, new hair will start to grow in the graft sites within about 3 months. A normal rate of hair growth is about 0.25–0.5 in (6–13 mm) per month.

Although there are rare cases of infection or scarring, the major risk is probably that the grafted area does not look the way the patient expected it to look.

Major complications as a result of hair transplantation are extremely rare. Occasionally, a patient may have problems with delayed healing, infection, scarring, or rejection of the graft; but this is uncommon.

HALDANE, JOHN SCOTT (1860-1936)

Scottish physiologist

John Scott Haldane is revered for his key advancements in respiratory physiology. Born into an affluent Scottish family, Haldane's father, Robert, worked as a lawyer and writer to the signet of Edinburgh, and his older brother Richard Burdon was the Viscount Haldane of Cloan. His advanced education took place at Edinburgh Academy and Edinburgh University, where he received a degree in medicine in 1884. Further education took place at Jena and Berlin.

Research became Haldane's passion as he began his first work on the composition of air in homes and schools at Dundee a piece that would be published in 1887. In the same year, he made his final professional move as he established a position at Oxford as demonstrator in physiology alongside his uncle. As Haldane refused to accept unproven distinctions between applied science and that based on speculation, he launched into his work on the relation between the carbon dioxide content of inhaled air and respiratory volume. Using information that was obtained in previous laboratory studies, he started his study of the hazards coal miners were exposed to. This report became a basis for the cause of death in mine disasters with an emphasis on carbon monoxide's lethal effects. Determined to establish the exact reason for carbon monoxide's toxicity, Haldane went back to the lab and by experimenting on mice in a hyperbaric environment, he developed facts that demonstrated carbon monoxide binds hemoglobin (the iron containing pigment of red blood cells), which prevents its crucial role in carrying oxygen throughout the body. This discovery was ahead of Haldane's time, as carbon monoxide poisoning's clinical connection would not be appreciated for over a half a century.

Determined to establish a logical method for his research, Haldane created the infamous Haldane gas analysis apparatus in 1898. Shortly after, along with Joseph Barcroft, he devised a method for determining blood gas content from small amounts of blood. As his work progressed, Haldane produced his most influential paper in 1905. Written with J. G. Priestly, he expressed that pulmonary ventilation is controlled by the limited pressure of carbon dioxide in blood throughout the arteries that reaches the respiratory center of the midbrain. While his research of chemical control of ventilation was changed several times, his basic premise clearly showed that, except under extreme conditions, the regulation of breathing depends much more on the amount of carbon dioxide in air that is inhaled than on the amount of oxygen. This crucial finding was not applied clinically until after World War II.

Haldane continued to show his interest in the human body's tolerance of stressful conditions as he looked further into work in the mines and deep-sea diving. His work presented the cause and cure for heatstroke and caisson disease, which is also known as bends, or the painful condition in limbs and abdomen as a result of rapid reduction of air pressure. His method for stage decompression to prevent the development of nitrogen bubbles in tissue spaces upon ascent is common among deep-sea diving operations and in underwater construction.

In 1911, Haldane led several physiologists from around the world to begin their study on the physiological effects of high altitude at the summit of Pike's Peak, Colorado. During this expedition Haldane persisted in the belief that oxygen could not pass across the lining of the tiniest air sacs (alveoli) in the lung only due to passive dispersion along a gradient of partial pressure. Instead, he believed in the oxygen secretion theory, which stated that oxygen travel was due to active secretion by the cells lining alveoli sacs. This thought held true only to Haldane, and has since been discarded.

Haldane's work also consists of studies on hemoglobin dissociation which presented the manner in which the degree of oxygenation of hemoglobin affects the uptake of carbon dioxide in the tissues and its release in the lung. The reaction of the kidney to water content in the blood and the physiology of **sweating** were also topics of study for Haldane. He was also in great demand by engineers who relied on his knowledge and counsel when planning safety measures for construction of tunnels and diving and mining operations, and for solutions to ventilation problems in buildings, ships, and submarines.

Most of Haldane's findings were summarized at his greatest academic accolade, the Silliman lectures at Yale in 1916. This lecture was published into a book in 1922, and after a revision in 1935, became the standard guide in respiratory physiology. Haldane was also known for his resounding interest in philosophical topics which show in his writings regarding the connection between science and philosophy. It is in these works that Haldane assumed "the mechanism of reproduction and heredity" by the "division from a pre-existing nuclear mechanism... that is capable of dividing itself to an absolute indefinite extent and yet retaining its original structure" all well before transfer of individual characteristics through genetic chains was known. Haldane's son, J. B. S. Haldane, is known for his work as a geneticist and philosopher.

Appointments to several royal commissions and as fellow of the Royal Society in 1897 were fulfilled by Haldane. Accolades include the Royal Medal in 1916, the Copley Medal in 1934, and for his work in industrial hygiene, he was created Companion of Honour in 1928. His career included a position as fellow of New College, Oxford that spanned from 1901 until his death. His interests in coal mining led him to the directorship of a research laboratory created by the coal mining industry, near Doncaster and later in Birmingham where he spent most of his time after 1921.

Haldane's ability to look beyond the laboratory and investigate theory brought crucial findings in respiratory physiology, including: the process by which oxygen in surrounding air of various environments enters the human body and arrives at the capillary (microscopic blood vessels); the reverse passage of carbon dioxide from capillary to exhaled air; the role of the vagus nerve (10th cranial nerve); and devising a method for estimating cardiac output. While he received honorary degrees from several institutions, Haldane never achieved full academic honors.

See also Blood gas analysis; Carbon monoxide poisoning; Respiratory system; Sweating

HALLUCINATIONS

Hallucinations are false or distorted sensory experiences that seem real and may be seen, heard, felt, and even smelled or tasted, yet are generated only by the mind.

A hallucination occurs when a misfire occurs within the mechanism of the brain that helps to distinguish conscious perceptions from internal, memory-based perceptions. This can be caused by stress, medication, extreme fatigue, **mental illness**, or other environmental, emotional, or physical factors. Hallucinations occur during periods of consciousness. They can take the form of visions, voices or sounds, tactile feelings (touch), smells, or tastes.

Patients suffering from **dementia** and psychotic disorders such as **schizophrenia** frequently experience hallucinations. Hallucinations can also occur in patients who are not mentally ill as a result of stress overload or exhaustion, or may be intentionally induced through the use of drugs, **meditation**, or sensory deprivation. Almost 40% of people are known to experience hallucinations as they are falling asleep. About 12% of people have experienced hallucinations upon waking.

Common causes of hallucinations include:

- Drugs. Hallucinogenics such as ecstasy (3,4-methylenedioxymethamphetamine, or MDMA), LSD (lysergic acid diethylamide, or acid), mescaline (3,4,5-trimethoxyphenethylamine, or peyote), and psilocybin (4-phosphoryloxy-N, N-dimethyltryptamine, or mushrooms) trigger hallucinations. Other drugs such as marijuana and PCP have hallucinatory effects. Certain prescription medications may also cause hallucinations. In addition, drug withdrawal may induce hallucinations of sight or touch; as in an alcoholic suffering from delirium tremens (DTs).
- Stress. Prolonged or extreme stress can impede thought processes and trigger hallucinations.
- Sleep deprivation and/or exhaustion. Physical and emotional exhaustion can induce hallucinations by blurring the line between sleep and wakefulness.
- Meditation and/or sensory deprivation. When the brain lacks external stimulation to form perceptions, it may form hallucinatory perceptions. This condition is commonly found in blind and deaf people.
- Electrical or neurochemical activity in the brain. A hallucinatory sensation (frequently visual) called an aura often appears before a migraine. Also, auras involving smell and touch are known to warn of an upcoming epileptic attack.
- Mental illness. Up to 75% of schizophrenic patients admitted for treatment report hallucinations.
- Brain damage or disease. Injuries to the brain may alter brain function and produce hallucinations.

Aside from hallucinations related to waking or falling asleep, more than one experience of hallucination suggests a person should see a general physician, psychologist, or psychiatrist to rule out organic, environmental, or psychological causes. If a psychological cause such as schizophrenia is suspected, a psychologist will typically conduct an interview with the patient and the patient's family, and administer one of several clinical inventories, or tests, to evaluate the mental status of the patient.

Occasionally, people who are in good mental health will experience a hallucination. If hallucinations are short-lasting and not frequent, and can be explained by short-term environmental factors such as sleep deprivation or meditation, no treatment may be necessary. However, if hallucinations are hampering an individual's ability to function, a general physician, psychologist, or psychiatrist should be consulted to pinpoint the source and recommend a treatment plan.

Hallucinations related to a mental illness such as schizophrenia should be treated by a psychologist or psychiatrist. In many cases, chronic hallucinations caused by schizophrenia or some other mental illness can be controlled by medication such as thioridazine (Mellaril), haloperidol (Haldol), chlorpromazine (Thorazine), clozapine (Clozaril), or risperidone (Risperdal). If hallucinations persist, psychosocial therapy can be helpful in teaching the patient the coping skills to deal with them. Hallucinations due to sleep deprivation or extreme stress generally stop after the cause is removed.

HALLUCINOGENS

Hallucinogens are a class of drugs that affects the brain and alters perceptions and mood. Human beings have used hallucinogens for centuries, primarily in ancient cultural and religious ceremonies. As a part of their religion, for example, certain American Indian tribes used the hallucinogen peyote to experience ''spiritual visions.''

Unlike most other drug classifications, hallucinogens are grouped primarily by causing hallucinations (which comes from Latin meaning "to wander in the mind"). Hallucinogens may be synthetic (man made) or organic (occurring in nature, such as certain plants). Organic hallucinogens include mescaline, peyote, and various fungi (certain mushrooms). Synthetic hallucinogens first appeared in 1938 when German chemist Albert Hoffman created a derivative of lysergic acid (LSD) in the laboratory. Scientists largely ignored the discovery until medical researchers in the 1950s began investigating LSD's possible therapeutic use for treating some psychiatric disorders.

In the 1960s, with the youth counterculture movement, the "hippie" movement, more and more people began experimenting with LSD to experience its mind altering effects. Sometimes referred to as "psychedelics," both natural and synthetic hallucinogens went on to influence many aspects of American pop culture, including clothing, music, art, and language.

As the use of LSD and other hallucinogens became more widespread and some of their dangers known, the United States and other countries made hallucinogens illegal.

Although not considered psychologically or physically addictive like heroin, alcohol, and tobacco, hallucinogens have many unexpected and serious effects. For example, although hallucinogens are often taken to feel good, some people can have unpleasant experiences, sometimes referred to as "bad trips." These psychological experiences are largely associated with moods and can include fear, paranoia, confusion, and behavior similar to **schizophrenia**. Depending on the hallucinogen and the amount taken, immediate physical effects can include an elevated heart rate and increased blood pressure. Some long-time users have shown damage to the brain resulting in impaired memory, inability to concentrate, mental confusion, and difficulty with abstract thinking. Some users also experience "flashbacks," in which they may re-experience some hallucinogenic effects days or months after taking the drug.

Another danger associated with synthetic hallucinogens is that it is impossible to know what ingredients have been used to make them because they are not regulated or distributed by a pharmacist. As a result, more serious side effects may occur, such as convulsions, **coma**, and heart or lung failure. Since hallucinogens affect the senses and impair motor skills, they can also result in serious and even fatal **accidents**, like car accidents, drownings, **burns**, and falls.

Hallucinogens work by disrupting the brain's chemical communication system. The brain controls thoughts and sends messages throughout the body by transmitting chemicals from nerve cell to nerve cell, both in the brain and the body. Called neurons, these nerve cells communicate with each other through chemical messengers called neurotransmitters. Exactly how hallucinogens affect neurons and neurotransmitters has not been clearly defined. Many hallucinogens, however, are believed to affect a neurotransmitter called serotonin, which plays a large role in sensory information and emotions. The synthetic hallucinogen MDMA (methylenedioxymethamphetamine), for example, can damage or destroy neurons that contain serotonin.

The illegal use of hallucinogens peaked in the United States in the late 1970s, and their use declined throughout the 1980s. However, surveys showed that hallucinogen use rose again during the 1990s, especially among young adults. Many of these hallucinogens are relatively new synthetics and are referred to as "designer" drugs, such as MDMA, sometimes called Ecstasy. Since these drugs are often made by combining an hallucinogen with some other drug, such as methamphetamine (or "speed"), they can have dangerous side effects, sometimes even resulting in death. People caught using and/or selling hallucinogens can be arrested and sent to prison. Certain religious groups, however, especially among American Indians, may still use hallucinogens in their ceremonies.

See also Schizophrenia

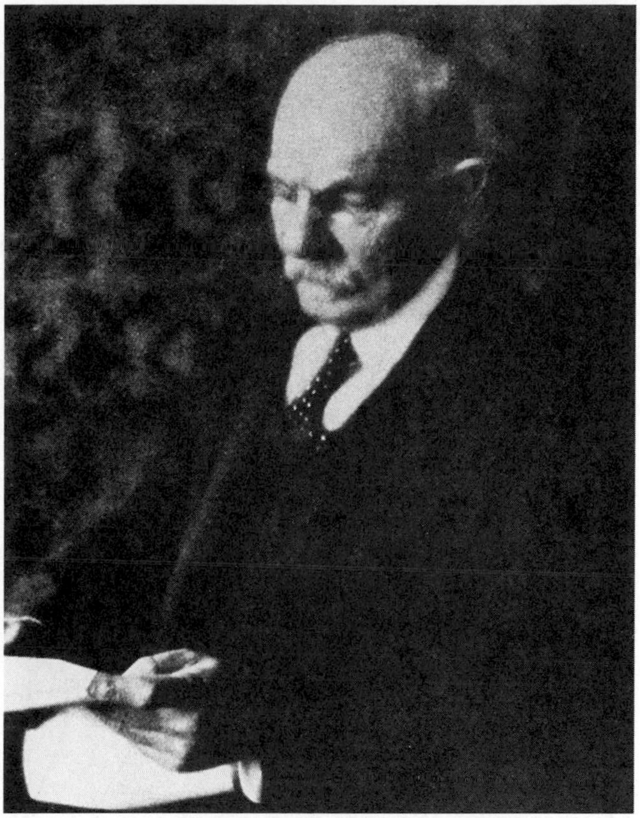
William Stewart Halsted

HALSTED, WILLIAM STEWART (1852-1922)

American surgeon

William Halsted was born in New York, New York, to a family of successful merchants. While at Yale University he was an indifferent student who became interested in medicine only during his senior year. Halsted received his M.D. from Columbia in 1877 as one of the top ten students in his class. He then studied in Europe and returned to New York as a surgeon in 1880.

In the early 1880s Halsted began experimenting with "conduction **anesthesia**"—injections of cocaine into nerves in the area to be operated on. While Halsted successfully established neuroregional anesthesia—anesthetization of only parts of the body rather than all of it—he became addicted to cocaine in the process and struggled for several years to free himself of the **addiction**.

Halsted then moved to Baltimore, Maryland, where in 1890 he became head of surgery at the recently established Johns Hopkins Hospital and Medical School. At Hopkins, Halsted became renowned as a meticulous, studious surgeon. He operated painstakingly slowly and spent many hours in the laboratory studying healing processes. His insistence on operating room cleanliness led to the development of *aseptic* procedures in surgery—keeping germs out rather than killing those that are present. When an antiseptic irritated the hands of his operating room nurse, Halsted ordered rubber gloves for her, and then began wearing sterilized gloves himself. (The nurse, Caroline Hampton, married Halsted.)

Halsted also improved radical operations for hernia and breast cancer and operating techniques for the thyroid gland and blood vessels. His laboratory studies and careful operating methods resulted in much improved healing of surgical **wounds**. Halsted died in 1922 the day after he underwent surgery for jaundice.

HAMILTON, ALICE (1869-1970)

American pathologist

Alice Hamilton was a pioneer in correcting the medical problems caused by industrialization, awakening the country in the early twentieth century to the dangers of industrial poisons and hazardous working conditions. Through her untiring efforts, toxic substances in the lead, mining, painting, pottery, and rayon industries were exposed and legislation passed to protect workers. She was also a champion of worker's compensation laws, and was instrumental in bringing about this type of legislation in the state of Illinois. A medical doctor and researcher, she was the first woman of faculty status at Harvard University, and was a consultant on governmental commissions, both domestic and foreign.

Alice Hamilton was born on February 27, 1869, in New York City, the second of five children born to Montgomery Hamilton, a wholesale grocer, and Gertrude (Pond) Hamilton. Alice Hamilton grew up in secure material surroundings. Her mother encouraged the children to follow their minds and inclinations, and this approach proved beneficial. Her sister, Edith, later became a noted Greek scholar and the editor of well-known books on Greek myths and literature. Alice was educated at home and for a few years at a private school.

Hamilton's decision to pursue a career in medicine came, in part, because it was one of the few professional fields open to women of her day. She earned a medical degree from the University of Michigan in 1893, without having completed an undergraduate degree and taking surprisingly few science courses. Realizing that she wanted to pursue research rather than medical practice, Hamilton went on to do further studies both in the United States and abroad: from 1895–1896 at Leipzig and Munich; 1896–1897 at Johns Hopkins; and 1902 in Paris at the Pasteur Institute. In 1897 she accepted a post as professor of pathology at the Women's Medical College at Northwestern University in Chicago, and when it closed in 1902, she became a professor of pathology at the Memorial Institute for Infectious Diseases, a position which she held until 1909.

In Chicago Hamilton became a resident of Hull House, the pioneering settlement designed to give care and advice to the poor of Chicago. Here, under the influence of Jane Addams, the founder of Hull House, Hamilton saw the effects of poverty up close. Investigating a **typhoid** epidemic in Chicago, she was instrumental in reorganizing the city's health department and in drawing attention to the role flies played in spreading the **epidemic**. After reading *Dangerous Trades* by Sir Thomas Oliver, Hamilton began her life-long mission to treat the excesses of industrialization. Unlike other countries such as Germany and England, the United States had no industrial safety laws at the time. During her time at Hull House, Hamilton investigated the steel industry and others for occupationally caused **lead poisoning**.

In 1910 Hamilton was chosen by the governor of Illinois to head up his Commission on Occupational Diseases, and her research and investigation into the dangers of lead and phosphorous paved the way to the state's first worker's compensation laws. In 1911 she took up similar, non-salaried, duties for the federal government, becoming an investigator of industrial poisons for the fledgling Department of Labor. During World War I, Hamilton investigated the high explosives industry, discovering that nitrous fumes were responsible for a great number of supposedly natural deaths.

In 1919 she became the first female faculty member of Harvard University as assistant professor of industrial medicine, but was denied access to the male bastion of the Harvard Club and to participation in graduation ceremonies. Hamilton kept up her international contacts, serving as the only woman delegate on the League of Nations Health Commission to the U.S.S.R. in 1924, as well as acting as a consultant to the International Labor Office in Geneva, Switzerland. In 1925, she published her *Industrial Poisons in the United States,* the first text on the subject, and became one of the few worldwide authorities in the area of industrial toxins. At this same time, she was also instrumental in influencing the surgeon general to investigate the dangerous effects of tetraethyl lead and radium.

Hamilton retired from Harvard in 1935, but not from active public life. She became a consultant in the U.S. Labor Department's Division of Labor Standards and from 1937–1938 conducted an investigation of the viscose rayon industry. Hamilton demonstrated the toxicity involved in rayon processes, and these findings that led to Pennsylvania's first compensation law for occupational diseases. In her later years, Hamilton, who never married, wrote an autobiography and continued to be active politically, advancing causes of social justice and pacifism. She died of a stroke at her home in Hadlyme, Connecticut, in 1970. Hamilton was 101 at the time of her death, and had been the recipient of honorary degrees from around the world for her work in revealing the dangers of industrial poisons.

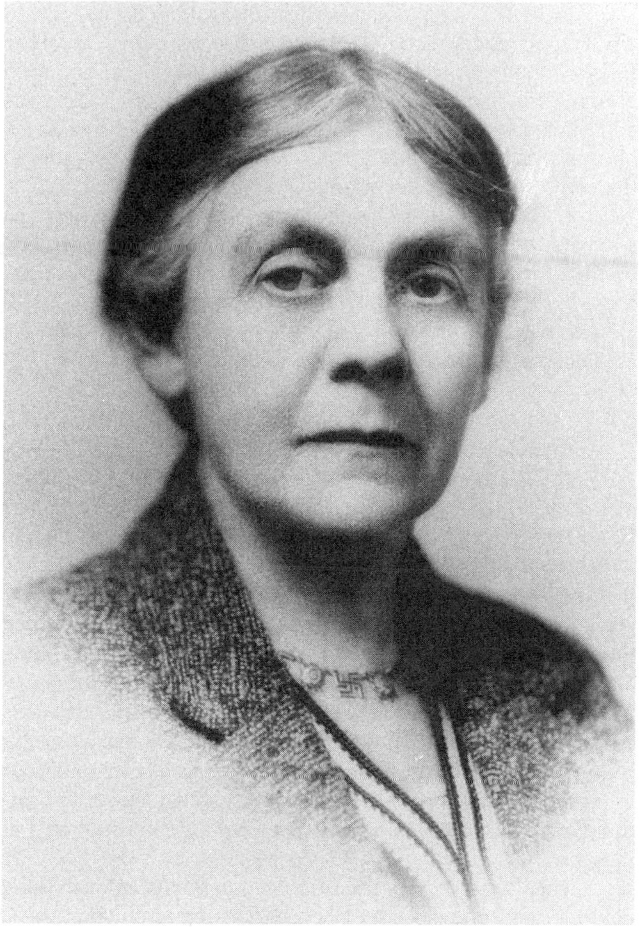

Alice Hamilton

HANAFUSA, HIDESABURO (1929-)

Japanese virologist and molecular oncologist

Hidesaburo Hanafusa is a prominent researcher in the **genetics** of cancerous viruses. As explained by Fulvio Bardossi and Judith N. Schwartz in a *Research Profile* distributed by the Rockefeller University, Hanafusa ''has used his training as a biochemist, combined with new insights and new technologies from molecular biology and genetics, to observe, isolate, control, and explain the events that occur and the elements that interact when virus meets cell.'' Hanafusa's early work with the Rous sarcoma virus (RSV), a virus that causes **cancer** in birds, has laid the foundation for a new hypothesis on how cancer may be caused by damaged genes—so-called ''oncogenes''—within an organism's own cells. The oncogene theory proposes that genes have the potential to cause a normal cell to become cancerous. Hanafusa's current investigations at the Rockefeller University in New York City focuses on oncogenes and explores how they induce cellular transformation from a normal to a cancerous state.

Hanafusa was born on December 1, 1929 in Nishinomiya, Japan. He is the son of Kamehachi and Tomi Hanafusa. He majored in biochemistry, and received his bachelor's degree in 1953, and his doctorate in 1960, both from Osaka University. On May 11, 1958, Hanafusa married Teruko Inoue, a fellow student at Osaka who has become one of his principal scientific colleagues. The couple have one daughter, Kei. In 1961, Hanafusa left his homeland in Japan and accepted a position in the laboratory of Harry Rubin, a pioneer in tumor virus research at the University of California in Berkeley.

When Nobel Prize-winning pathologist **Peyton Rous** made the pioneering discovery in 1910 that a virus causes cancer in chickens, the basic mechanisms of cancer were as yet poorly understood. A half century later, Hanafusa continued the research into the causes of viral cancer. Hanafusa's initial project with Rubin at the University of California produced a major discovery. While trying to isolate pure RSV, the researchers found that the virus could transform normal cells into cancerous ones. Interestingly, however, the virus could not replicate itself without a protein from a helper virus. This virus became a tool for future experiments. By changing the properties and activities of the altered RSV, Hanafusa could analyze key reactions that are responsible for bringing about a cancerous state. Hanafusa pursued these studies as a visiting scientist at the College de France in Paris from 1964 to 1966 and then as head of a laboratory of viral oncology at the Public Health Research Institute in New York City.

In 1973 Hanafusa became professor of viral oncology at the Rockefeller University. In a new set of experiments, he injected chickens with RSV that had been altered to remove most of the genetic information specifically responsible for tumor formation. To his surprise, the chickens developed tumors anyway. On examination, he found the viruses had reacquired the missing tumor gene—the oncogene—from the chicken cell's own genetic information. These experiments showed that inappropriate activation of normal cellular genes causes tumors. Since then, more than twenty such oncogenes have been identified as being responsible for various kinds of cancers.

While exploring the nature of the RSV sarcoma gene (an oncogene), Hanafusa learned that the RSV mutants which he had isolated were temperature sensitive. This proved to be an important clue that the substance produced was a protein. Subsequent speculations presume that oncogenes may have an important role in normal cell life—to manufacture a protein required by the cell. It is only when the protein is overproduced that cancer occurs. Hanafusa later learned that the RSV sarcoma gene induces the protein tyrosine kinase, which can, by itself, trigger a cell division. Further investigations by Hanafusa have explored the role of this protein in the cell's signaling apparatus, a complicated sequence of intracellular communication known as phosphorylation. Hanafusa found that when infected with RSV, many cellular proteins become phosphorylated on tyrosine, and this process is associated with changes in cell growth.

In 1988, Hanafusa identified a novel oncogene, *crk,* in an avian sarcoma virus. Although it has no known catalytic function, its overproduction induces tyrosine phosphorylation of some cellular proteins and causes cancer. This finding has contributed to a surge of interest in the interaction between the phosphotyrosine-containing proteins and peptide domains in the cell's signaling network.

For his contributions in cancer virus studies, Hanafusa received the Howard Taylor Ricketts Award in 1981, the Albert Lasker Basic Medical Research Award in 1982, the Asahi Press Prize in 1984, and the Alfred P. Sloan, Jr. Prize in 1993. He was elected a Foreign Associate of the National Academy of Sciences in 1985.

HAND-FOOT-MOUTH DISEASE

Hand-foot-mouth disease is an infection of young children in which characteristic fluid-filled blisters appear on the hands, feet, and inside the mouth.

Coxsackie viruses belong to a family of viruses called **Enteroviruses**. These viruses live in the gastrointestinal tract, and are therefore present in feces. They can be spread easily from one person to another when poor hygiene allows the virus within the feces to be passed from person to person. After exposure to the virus, development of symptoms takes only four to six days. Hand-foot-mouth disease can occur year-round, although the largest number of cases are in summer and fall months.

Hand-foot-mouth disease is very common among young children, and often occurs in clusters of children who are in daycare together. It is spread when poor hand-washing after a diaper change or contact with saliva (drool) allows the virus to be passed from one child to another.

Within about four to six days of acquiring the virus, an infected child may develop a relatively low-grade **fever**, ranging from 99–102°F (37.2–38.9°C). Other symptoms include fatigue, loss of energy, decreased appetite, and a sore sensation in the mouth, which may interfere with feeding. After one to two days, fluid-filled bumps (vesicles) appear on the inside of the mouth, along the surface of the tongue, on the roof of the mouth, and on the insides of the cheeks. These are tiny blisters, about 3–7 mm in diameter. Eventually, they may appear on the palms of the hands and on the soles of the feet. Occasionally, these vesicles may occur in the diaper region.

The vesicles in the mouth cause the majority of discomfort, and the child may refuse to eat or drink due to **pain**. This phase usually lasts for an average of a week. As long as the bumps have clear fluid within them, the disease is at its most contagious. The fluid within the vesicles contains large quantities of the causative viruses. Extra care should be taken to avoid contact with this fluid.

Diagnosis is made by most practitioners solely on the basis of the unique appearance of blisters of the mouth, hands, and feet, in a child not appearing very ill.

There are no treatments available to cure or decrease the duration of the disease. Medications like **acetaminophen** or ibuprofen may be helpful for decreasing pain, and allowing the child to eat and drink. It is important to try to encourage the child to take in adequate amounts of fluids, in the form of ice chips or popsicles if other foods or liquids are too uncomfortable.

The prognosis for a child with hand-foot-mouth disease is excellent. The child is usually completely better within about a week of the start of the illness.

Prevention involves careful attention to hygiene. Thorough, consistent hand-washing practices, and discouraging the sharing of clothes, towels, and stuffed toys are all helpful. Virus continues to be passed in the feces for several weeks after infection, so good hygiene should be practiced long after all signs of infection have passed.

HANTAVIRUS DISEASE

Hantavirus Disease, otherwise known as Hantavirus Pulmonary Syndrome (HPS) manifests as flu-like symptoms which rapidly progresses into **shortness of breath**, difficulty breathing, internal bleeding, **respiratory failure**, and **death**. Hantaviruses (HTV) are distantly related to the ebola virus and have been recognized as causes of disease in China and Asia for many years. They first came to the attention of health authorities in the United States in 1993 when several healthy young adults developed flu-like symptoms and more than half of them died. HTV is carried by rodents and transmitted to humans through urine, feces, and dust contaminated with feces of infected rodents. While HPS is rare—only 110 cases have been reported in the U.S. since 1993—there is no effective treatment.

On May 1993, several people became ill and five died of an ''unexplained illness'' on an Indian Reservation in ''Four Corners'' in the southwest United States, an area where the borders of Utah, Colorado, New Mexico and Arizona meet. Immediately, departments of health from the four states, aided by the Navajo Nation Division of Health, embarked on intensive investigations to determine the cause of these illnesses and deaths. They soon linked the disease outbreak to the hantavirus and now believe this form of hantavirus has been present in the U.S. since at least as early as 1959. Since the 1993 outbreak, HPS has been identified in more than half the states in the nation. Rodents carrying HTV have been found in at least 20 national parks, and may exist in all. Although authorities believe outdoor campers may be at a higher risk of infection from HTV, only two cases have been reported following camping trips.

Hantavirus originates from the *Hantaan Virus,* (HTN), found in the Asian striped field mouse. Once transmitted to humans, it causes a severe disease known as **hemorrhagic fever** with renal syndrome (HFRS) and which is estimated to infect more than 100,000 people in China each year. HTN was first identified in the western world in 1951 when many U.S. troops stationed in Korea became ill. Several and somewhat less severe illnesses are caused by related viruses, all of which are found in rodents indigenous to the Old World. Hantaviruses found in New World rodents appear to originate from the *Prospect Hill* (PH) virus carried by the meadow vole. This virus has not been implicated in human disease, but is believed to be the parent of the hantavirus, carried by deer mice and other rodents, which causes HPS. While carrier rodents do not manifest the disease, humans are at risk of developing HPS when they come into contact with infected rodent urine, feces, or dust contaminated with feces. The virus may enter the body with contaminated dirt or dust through a cut or wound, the eyes, by ingestion of contaminated water or food, or inhalation of contaminated dust. It does not seem to be passed from one human to another, nor to be transmitted by bites from fleas, ticks, mosquitos, or other biting insects. Although cats and dogs are not know to be carriers, they may bring infected rodents into contact with humans.

Symptoms of hantavirus infection, including fatigue, fever and chills, severe muscle aches, headaches, **dizziness**, vomiting **diarrhea**, abdominal **pain**, and a dry **cough**, may not develop for several weeks following infection. Because so few cases of HPS are found, determining its incubation period is difficult. Sometimes, symptoms will alleviate for one or two days, only to return with increased difficulty breathing caused by fluid seeping into the lungs and internal bleeding. Even treatment with **oxygen therapy** and respiratory support is only successful in 50 percent of severe cases. Experimental treatment with intravenous ribavirin—an **antiviral drug**—is undergoing clinical trials.

Hardy, Harriet (1905-1993)

American pathologist

Harriet Hardy intended to be a simple general practitioner, but fortuitous events changed that plan. Through the investigation of a respiratory illness that was common among factory workers in two towns in Massachusetts, she discovered the often-fatal respiratory disease berylliosis—a discovery that led to her becoming one of the world's foremost authorities in the field of occupational medicine. In the course of her long career she battled against numerous diseases caused by dangerous substances to which workers are exposed, including silicosis and asbestosis.

Born on September 23, 1905 in Arlington, Massachusetts, Harriet Louise Hardy set her course early on for a career in medicine. In 1928 she graduated from Wellesley College, and four years later earned her M.D. from Cornell University. After interning and spending her residency at Philadelphia General Hospital, she started her practice at Northfield Seminary in Massachusetts as a school doctor. This simple practice, however, did not last long, and by 1939 she had accepted a post as college doctor and director of health education at Cambridge's Radcliffe College. It was here, while researching the fields of **women's health** and fitness, that Hardy's interests expanded to include industrial diseases.

In the early 1940s, Hardy began a collaboration with Joseph Aubt to study the effects of lead poisoning. Like Alice Hamilton and other pioneering pathologists of the time, Hardy began to recognize the dangers inherent in the modern factory, with workers coming into contact with all manner of toxic substances. There soon came word of a strange respiratory disease among the workers in the Sylvania and General Electric fluorescent lamp factories in nearby Lynn and Salem, Massachusetts. The sufferers all complained of **shortness of breath**, **cough**ing, and loss of weight; in some cases, the disease was fatal. Hardy and her colleagues were initially baffled as to the cause of the disease, but it occurred to Hardy that the disease had to be occupationally related. Referring to research from Europe and Russia, Hardy finally found the connection to beryllium; a light metal used in the manufacture of fluorescent lamps, beryllium dust or vapor could be easily inhaled by factory workers. Hardy showed that this outbreak was indeed berylliosis, a condition whose symptoms sometimes are not manifested for up to 20 years after exposure to beryllium dust. Hardy subsequently became an expert in beryllium poisoning, writing papers which educated and alerted the medical community to its dangers. She also established a registry of berylliosis cases at the Massachusetts General Hospital (where she had been on staff since 1940); this registry later served as a model for the tracking of other occupation-related disorders.

Hardy went on to establish a clinic of occupational medicine at Massachusetts General Hospital in 1947, directing it for the next 24 years. She continued to explore the disease-producing properties of work-related substances, and in 1954 she was among the first scientists to identify a link between asbestos and cancer. Hardy was also concerned with the effects of radiation on the human body; she worked with the Atomic Energy Commission in Los Alamos, New Mexico, to study radiation poisoning, making a number of suggestions toward better working conditions in nuclear power plants. In 1949 she teamed up with **Alice Hamilton** to write the second edition of *Industrial Toxicology,* which has become a standard text on the subject. Other areas of Hardy's research and investigation included mercury poisoning and treatments for lead poisoning. She also researched the harmful effects of benzene, and as a result of her findings the highest permissible concentration of the hydrocarbon used in industry was reduced by fifty per cent.

In 1955 she was named Woman of the Year by the American Medical Women's Association. An outspoken and forceful critic for change, Hardy was appointed clinical professor at Harvard Medical School in 1971, and during the course of her long career authored over 100 scientific articles. She died of an **immune system** cancer, **lymphoma**, on October 13, 1993 at Massachusetts General Hospital.

Hartline, Haldan Keffer (1903-1983)

American physiologist and biophysicist

Haldan Keffer Hartline was born on December 22, 1903, in Bloomsburg, Pennsylvania, to Daniel Schollenberger Hartline and Harriet Franklin Hartline. He attended college at Lafayette College in Easton, Pennsylvania, graduating with a B.S. in 1923. He went on to study retinal electrophysiology as a graduate student at Johns Hopkins University, obtaining his M.D. in 1927. Hartline spent the next two years at Johns Hopkins University as a National Research Council fellow in medical sciences.

Between 1929 and 1931, Hartline was a Johnson Traveling Research Scholar from the University of Pennsylvania to the universities of Leipzig and Munich. He travelled extensively in Germany during those years before returning to the United States, where he joined the Eldridge Reeves Johnson Research Foundation for Medical Physics as an assistant professor of biophysics at the University of Pennsylvania. Hartline married Mary Elizabeth Kraus on April 11, 1936. They had three sons: Daniel Keffer, Peter Haldan, and Frederick Flanders.

From the early days of his career, Hartline was fascinated by the **metabolism** of nerve cells, and he eventually focused his attention on the workings of individual cells in the retina of the **eye**. During the late 1920s and early 1930s, Hartline used recently developed methods of fiber isolation to record the activity of single nerve fibers in the retina. He began by experimenting with *Limulus Polyphemus,* the horseshoe crab. He chose this primitive creature because it possessed a feature that was ideal for his research: a compound eye with a long optic nerve and large individual photoreceptors. It seemed to Hartline that working with the horseshoe crab might allow him to record the electrical behavior of single nerve fibers. He succeeded in 1932, while working at the Eldridge Reeves Johnson Foundation. Hartline and Columbia University psychophysiologist Clarence H. Graham managed to isolate single nerve fibers from the optic nerve, placed electrodes on those single fibers, stimulated them with light, and recorded the nerve impulses that occurred. This was the first record of the activity of a single optic nerve fiber, and it proved to Hartline and Graham that their theories had been correct: information is relayed through individual optic nerve fibers by a series of uniform nerve impulses.

Hartline moved into another field of vision in 1938, when he began to study the vertebrate eye, using microdissection techniques to record the activity of individual fibers in the optic nerve of frogs. While recording the nerve impulses from the single nerve fibers lying behind the rods and cones of the eye, he found that the fibers making up the nerve did not all behave in the same way. Some were stimulated by steady light, others were stimulated by the light when it first hit the retina, and still others were stimulated only as the light was shut off. Hartline demonstrated that visual information begins to be differentiated in the retina and in the receptors themselves, as soon as the stimulation occurs, before the information can be conducted more deeply into the central **nervous system**. This research afforded new insights into the working of the retina. It also provided a new understanding of how the mechanisms of vision were integrated with, and how they affected, the nervous system as a whole. For this discovery, Hartline was awarded the Howard Crosby Warren Medal of the Society of Experimental Psychologists in 1948.

Hartline continued his teaching and research at the University of Pennsylvania, becoming professor of biophysics and chair of the department at Johns Hopkins in 1949. In 1953, Hartline joined the faculty of Rockefeller University in New York as professor of neurophysiology. There, Hartline began investigating the phenomenon of inhibition in the retina of the compound eye, using the horseshoe crab as a subject once again. He and his colleague, Floyd Ratliff, demonstrated the electrical response of nerve fibers and cells to light hitting the retina, and the mechanism by which this response allows the eye to differentiate shapes. He found that the receptor cells in the eye are interconnected in such a way that when one is stimulated, others nearby are depressed, thus sharpening the contrast in light patterns. In the 1960s, Hartline extended these studies to the dynamics of the receptors and their interactions, with a view to understanding visual phenomena such as motion detection. Hartline's findings eventually led to the development of a set of mathematical equations expressing the interrelationship of the receptor units of the compound eye; this information has been key to understanding brightness and contrast in the retinal image.

For his work on electrical activity on the cellular level within the eye, Hartline shared the 1967 Nobel Prize for physiology or medicine with the American biologist **George Wald** and the Swedish neurophysiologist **Ragnar Granit**. This was not the only award received by Hartline during this period; he also received the A. A. Michelson Award of Case Institute, 1964, and the Lighthouse Award in 1969. In addition to the Nobel Prize and the other awards and honors received during his lifetime, Hartline was also presented with a number of honorary degrees. He was awarded doctorates from Lafayette College in 1959, the University of Pennsylvania in 1971, Rockefeller University in 1976, the University of Maryland in 1978, and Syracuse University in 1979; an LL.D. from Johns Hopkins University in 1971; and an M.D. from the University of Freiburg in 1971.

Hartline was a member of many important scientific organizations, many of them elective. He was elected to the National Academy of Sciences in 1948, and to the American Academy of Arts and Sciences in 1957. Hartline also held memberships in the American Philosophical Society and the Biophysics Society, and in 1966 was elected a foreign member of the Royal Society, London. The Optical Society of America made him an honorary member, as did the Physiology Society (U.K.).

Hartline died on March 17, 1983, in Fallston, Maryland.

HARVEY, WILLIAM (1578-1657)

English physician

William Harvey, the father of modern physiology, was born in Folkestone, Kent, England, in 1578, the eldest of seven sons of a yeoman farmer. While five of the other Harvey brothers became London merchants, William studied arts and medicine at Cambridge University, where he received a bachelor of arts degree in 1597, and then earned his medical degree in 1602 from the renowned medical school at Padua (Italy), where he studied under Girolamo Fabrici. Returning to London, Harvey began what became a very successful medical practice while also engaging extensively in medical research. In 1604 he married Elizabeth Browne, daughter of a prominent London doctor; they had no children.

In 1609 Harvey was appointed to the staff of St. Bartholomew's Hospital. He was elected a fellow of the Royal College of Physicians in 1607 and was Lumleian lecturer on anatomy and surgery for the College from 1615 to 1656. His ideas about circulation of the blood were first publicly expressed in these lectures in 1616. Harvey became court physician to King James I in 1618 and then to Charles I in 1625, a post he held until Charles was beheaded in 1649. Charles provided Harvey with deer from the royal parks for his medical research, and Harvey remained loyal to Charles even during the Cromwellian Civil War, which led to the sacking of Harvey's rooms in 1642 and the destruction of many of his medical notes and papers. Harvey retired at the end of the Civil War, a widower, and lived with his various brothers. He died of a stroke in 1657 in Roehampton and was buried in the family vault at Hempstead Church in Essex.

Harvey's great contribution to medicine was his revolutionary discovery of the circulation of blood. His many experimental **dissections** and **vivisections** convinced Harvey that **Galen**'s ideas about blood movement must be wrong, particularly the concepts that blood was formed in the liver and absorbed by the body, and that blood flowed through the septum (dividing wall) of the heart. Harvey first studied the heartbeat, establishing the existence of the *pulmonary* (heart-lung-heart) circulation and noting the one-way flow of blood. When he also comprehended how much blood was pumped by the heart, he realized there must be a constant amount of blood flowing through the arteries and returning through the veins of the heart, a continuing circular flow.

Harvey published this radical new concept of blood circulation in 1628. It provoked immediate controversy and hostility, contradicting as it did the usually unquestioned teachings of Galen, the basis of medical knowledge at the time. The most virulent critic, Jean Riolan, scorned Harvey as a "circulator"—a derisive term for a traveling quack. Harvey calmly and quietly defended his work, and although his medical practice declined for a time, his ideas had become widely accepted at the time of his death. The discovery of capillaries by **Marcello Malpighi** in 1661 provided the factual evidence to confirm Harvey's theory of blood circulation. Harvey's method of drawing reasoned conclusions from meticulous observation formed the basis of an entirely new approach to medicine—modern physiology.

Harvey's other important contribution to medicine was in the field of embryology. He was one of the first to study the development of the chick in the egg and performed many dissections of mammal embryos at various stages of formation. From these experiments Harvey was able to formulate the first new theory of generation since antiquity, emphasizing the primacy of the egg, even in mammals. His findings on generation were published in 1651 and became the foundation of the new science of embryology.

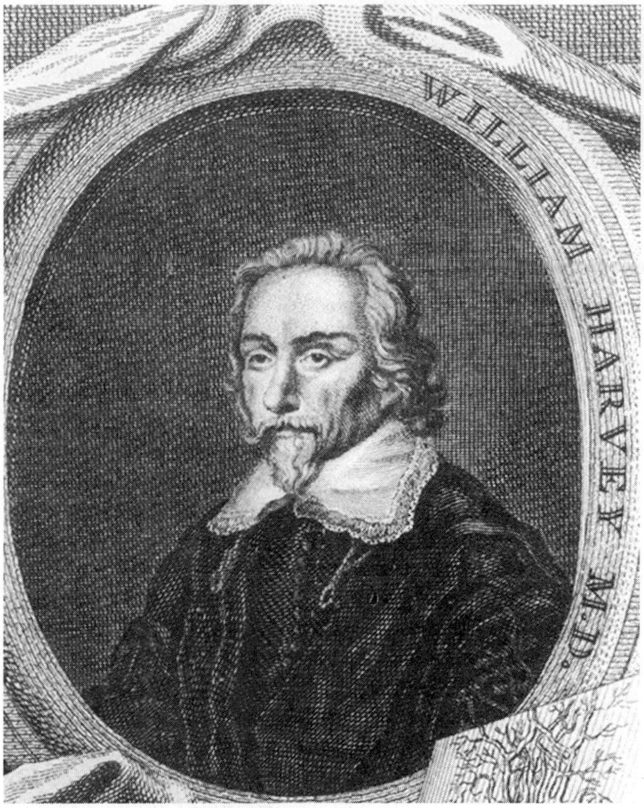

William Harvey

HAY FEVER

Allergic rhinitis (AR), more commonly known as hay fever, is an inflammation of the nasal passages caused by allergic reaction to airborne substances.

Allergic rhinitis is the most common allergic condition and one of the most common of all minor afflictions. It affects between 10-20% of all people in the United States, and is responsible for 2.5% of all doctor visits. **Antihistamines** and other drugs used to treat allergic rhinitis make up a significant fraction of both prescription and **over-the-counter drug** sales each year.

There are two types of allergic rhinitis: seasonal and perennial. Seasonal AR occurs in the spring, summer, and early fall, when airborne plant pollens are at their highest levels. Perennial AR can occur at any time of year and is usually caused by home or workplace airborne pollutants. A person can be affected by one or both types. Symptoms of seasonal AR are worst after being outdoors, while symptoms of perennial AR are worst after spending time indoors.

Both types of **allergies** can develop at any age, although onset in childhood through early adulthood is most common. Although allergy to a particular substance is not inherited, increased allergic sensitivity may "run in the family." While allergies can improve on their own over time, they can also become worse over time.

Allergic rhinitis is a type of immune reaction, in which immune proteins called antibodies react with otherwise harmless substances. Such substances are known as allergens.

AR involves a special set of cells in the **immune system** known as mast cells, which are found in the lining of the nasal passages and eyelids. Mast cells display on their surface a special type of antibody, called immunoglobulin type E (IgE). When these antibodies encounter allergens, they trigger release of a variety of chemicals onto neighboring cells, including blood vessels and nerve cells. One of these chemicals, histamine, binds to the surfaces of these other cells, through special proteins called histamine receptors. Interaction of histamine with receptors on blood vessels causes neighboring cells to become leaky, leading to the fluid collection, swelling, and increased redness characteristic of a runny nose and red, irritated eyes. Histamine also stimulates **pain** receptors, causing the itchy, scratchy nose, eyes, and throat common in allergic rhinitis. Because of the central role of histamine in the allergic response, antihistamine drugs are the primary weapon against allergies.

The number of possible airborne allergens is enormous. Seasonal AR is most commonly caused by grass and tree pollens. Different plants release their pollen at different times of the year, so seasonal AR sufferers may be most affected in spring, summer, or fall, depending on which plants they are most sensitive to. The amount of pollen in the air is reflected in the pollen count, often broadcast on the daily news during allergy season. Pollen counts tend to be lower after a good rain that washes the pollen out of the air and higher on warm, dry, windy days.

Virtually any type of tree or grass may cause AR. A few types of weeds that tend to cause the most trouble for people include the following:

- Ragweed
- Sagebrush
- Lamb's-quarters
- Plantain
- Pigweed
- Dock/sorrel
- Tumbleweed.

Perennial AR is often triggered by house dust, a complicated mixture of airborne particles, many of which are potent allergens. House dust contains some or all of the following:

- House mite body parts. All houses contain large numbers of microscopic insects called house mites. These harmless insects feed on fibers, fur, and skin shed by the house's larger occupants. Their tiny body parts easily become airborne.
- Animal dander. Animals constantly shed fur, skin flakes, and dried saliva. Carried in the air, or transferred from pet to owner by direct contact, dander can cause allergy in many sensitive people.
- Mold spores. Molds live in damp spots throughout the house, including basements, bathrooms, air ducts, air conditioners, refrigerator drains, damp windowsills, mattresses, and stuffed furniture. Mildew and other molds release airborne spores which circulate throughout the house.

Other potential causes of perennial allergic rhinitis include the following:

- Cigarette smoke
- Perfume
- Cosmetics
- Cleansers
- Copier chemicals
- Industrial chemicals
- Construction material gases.

Inflammation of the nose, or **rhinitis**, is the major symptom of AR. Inflammation causes **itching**, sneezing, runny nose, redness, and tenderness. AR usually also causes reddened, itching, and watery eyes.

Diagnosing seasonal AR is usually easy and can often be done without a medical specialist. When symptoms appear in spring or summer and disappear with the onset of cold weather, seasonal AR is almost certainly the culprit.

Allergy tests, including skin testing and provocation testing, can help identify the precise culprit, but may not be done unless a single source is suspected and subsequent avoidance is possible. Skin testing involves placing a small amount of a specific allergen under the skin to observe whether redness and swelling occurs.

Perennial AR can also usually be diagnosed by careful questioning about the timing of exposure and the onset of symptoms. Specific allergens can be identified through allergy skin testing.

Avoidance of the allergens is the best treatment, but this is often not possible. When it is not possible to avoid one or more allergens, there are two major forms of medical treatment, drugs and immunotherapy.

The most common drugs for treating AR are called antihistamines. Antihistamines block the histamine receptors on nasal tissue, decreasing the effect of histamine release by mast cells. They may be used after symptoms appear, though they may be even more effective when used preventively, before symptoms appear. A wide variety of antihistamines are available.

Most over-the-counter antihistamines may produce drowsiness as a major side effect. Newer antihistamines that do not cause drowsiness are available by prescription.

Other drugs used to treat AR include decongestants, corticosteroids, and mast cell stabilizers.

Immunotherapy, also known as desensitization or allergy shots, is also available for treatment of allergies. Immunotherapy alters the balance of antibody types in the body, thereby reducing the ability of IgE to cause allergic reactions. Immunotherapy is preceded by allergy testing to determine the precise allergens responsible. Injections involve very small but gradually increasing amounts of allergen, over several weeks or months, with periodic boosters. Full benefits may take up to several years to achieve and are not seen at all in about one in five patients.

Most people with AR can achieve adequate relief with a combination of preventive strategies and treatment. While allergies may improve over time, they may also get worse or expand to include new allergens. Early treatment can help prevent an increased sensitization to other allergens.

Reducing exposure to pollen may improve symptoms of seasonal AR. Strategies include the following:

- Stay indoors with windows closed during the morning hours, when pollen levels are highest.
- Keep car windows up while driving.
- Use a surgical face mask when outside.
- Wash clothes and hair after being outside.
- Clean air conditioner filters in the home regularly.

Preventing perennial AR requires identification of the responsible allergens.

Mold spores:

- Keep the house dry through ventilation and use of dehumidifiers.
- Use a disinfectant such as dilute bleach to clean surfaces such as bathroom floors and walls.
- Clean and disinfect air conditioners and coolers.

House dust:

- Vacuum frequently, and change the bag regularly. Use a bag with small pores to catch extra-fine particles.
- Clean floors and walls with a damp mop.

Animal dander:

- Avoid contact if possible.
- Wash hands after contact.
- Vacuum frequently.
- Keep pets out of the bedroom, and off furniture, rugs, and other dander-catching surfaces.
- Have your pets bathed and groomed frequently.

See also Allergies

HEADACHES

A headache involves **pain** in the head which can arise from many disorders or may be a disorder itself.

There are three types of primary headaches: tension-type (muscular contraction headache), migraine (vascular headaches), and cluster. Virtually everyone experiences a tension-type headache at some point. An estimated 18% of American women suffer migraines, compared to 6% of men. Cluster headaches affect fewer than 0.5% of the population, and men account for approximately 80% of all cases. Headaches caused by illness are secondary headaches and are not included in these numbers.

Approximately 40–45 million people in the United States suffer chronic headaches. Headaches have an enormous impact on society due to missed workdays and productivity losses.

Traditional theories about headaches link tension-type headaches to muscle contraction, and migraine and cluster headaches to blood vessel dilation (swelling). Pain-sensitive structures in the head include blood vessel walls, membranous coverings of the brain, and scalp and neck muscles. Brain tissue itself has no sensitivity to pain. Therefore, headaches may result from contraction of the muscles of the scalp, face or neck; dilation of the blood vessels in the head; or brain swelling that stretches the brain's coverings. Specific nerves of the face and head may also cause headaches. Sinus inflammation is a common cause of headache. Keeping a headache diary may help link headaches to stressful occurrences, menstrual phases, food triggers, or medication.

Tension-type headaches are often brought on by stress, overexertion, loud noise, and other external factors. The typical tension-type headache is described as a tightening around the head and neck, and an accompanying dull ache.

Migraines are intense throbbing headaches occurring on one or both sides of the head. The pain is accompanied by other symptoms such as **nausea**, vomiting, blurred vision, and aversion to light, sound, and movement. Migraines are often triggered by food items, such as red wine, chocolate, and aged cheeses. For women, a hormonal connection is likely, since headaches occur at specific points in the menstrual cycle, with use of **oral contraceptives**, or the use of **hormone replacement therapy** after **menopause**.

Cluster headaches cause excruciating pain. The severe, stabbing pain centers around one eye, and eye tearing and nasal congestion occur on the same side. The headache lasts from 15 minutes to four hours and may recur several times in a day. Heavy smokers are more likely to suffer cluster headaches, which are also associated with alcohol consumption.

Since headaches arise from many causes, a physical examination assesses general health and a neurological exam evaluates the possibility of disease causing the headache. If headache is the primary illness, a doctor asks about its frequency and duration, when it occurs, pain intensity and location, possible triggers, and any prior symptoms. This information helps in classifying the headache.

Warning signs indicating a need for prompt medical intervention include:

- ''Worst headache of my life.'' This may indicate a ruptured **aneurysm** (swollen blood vessel) in the head or other neurological emergency.
- Headache accompanied by one-sided weakness, numbness, visual loss, speech difficulty, or other signs. This may indicate a **stroke**. Migraines may include neurological symptoms.
- Headache that becomes worse over a period of six months, especially if most prominent in the morning or if accompanied by neurological symptoms. This may indicate a **brain tumor**.
- Sudden onset of headache. If accompanied by **fever** and stiff neck, this can indicate **meningitis**.

Headache diagnosis may include neurological imaging tests such as **computed tomography scan** (CT scan) or **magnetic resonance imaging** (MRI).

Headache treatment is divided into two forms: one aimed at stopping a headache in progress, the other at trying to prevent the headache.

Tension-type and migraine headaches can be treated with **aspirin**, **acetaminophen**, ibuprofen, naproxen, or Extra-strength Excedrin, which includes **caffeine**. Prescription medications such as **antidepressants** and **muscle relaxants** can address tension-type headaches, and ergotamine tartrate or sumatriptan can relieve or prevent migraines. Cluster headaches may also be treated with ergotamine and sumatriptan, as well as by inhaling pure oxygen. Prophylactic treatments include prednisone, calcium channel blockers, and methysergide.

Alternative headache treatments include:

- **Acupuncture or acupressure**
- **Biofeedback**
- **Chiropractic**
- Herbal remedies using feverfew (*Chrysanthemum parthenium*), valerian (*Valeriana officinalis*), white willow (*Salix alba*), or skullcap (*Scutellaria lateriflora*), among others
- **Homeopathic** remedies
- **Hydrotherapy**
- **Massage**
- Magnesium supplements
- Regular physical **exercise**
- Relaxation techniques, such as **meditation** and **yoga**
- Transcutaneous electrical nerve stimulation (TENS). A test that electrically stimulates nerves and blocks the signals of pain transmission.

Some headaches may be prevented by avoiding triggering substances and situations, or by employing alternative therapies, such as yoga and regular exercise. Since foods are often linked to headaches, especially cluster headaches and migraines, identification and elimination of the allergy-causing food(s) from the diet can be an important preventive measure.

Head and neck cancer

The term head and neck cancers refers to a group of **cancer**s found in the head and neck region. This includes tumors found in the oral cavity (mouth), the oropharynx (which includes the back one-third of the tongue, the back of the throat and the tonsils); the nasopharynx (which includes the area behind the nose); the hypopharynx (lower part of the throat), and the larynx (voice box, located in front of the neck, in the region of the Adam's apple). The most frequently occurring cancers of the head and neck area are oral cancers and laryngeal cancers. Almost half of all the head and neck cancers occur in the oral cavity, and a third of the cancers are found in the larynx. By definition, the term ''head and neck cancers'' usually excludes tumors that occur in the brain.

Although the exact cause for these cancers is unknown, tobacco is regarded as the single greatest risk factor: 75–80% of the oral and laryngeal cancer cases occur among smokers. Heavy alcohol use has also been included as a risk factor. In rare cases, irritation to the lining of the mouth, due to jagged teeth or ill-fitting dentures, has been known to cause oral cancer. Exposure to asbestos appears to increase the risk of developing laryngeal cancer.

In the case of lip cancer, just like **skin cancer**, exposure to sun over a prolonged period has been shown to increase the risk. In the Southeast Asian countries (India and Sri Lanka), chewing of betel nut has been associated with cancer of the lining of the cheek. An increased incidence of nasal cavity cancer has been observed among furniture workers, probably due to the inhalation of wood dust. A virus (Epstein-Barr) has been shown to cause nasopharyngeal cancer.

Head and neck cancers are one of the easiest to detect. The early signs can be both seen and felt. The signs and symptoms depend on the location of the cancer:

- Mouth and oral cavity: a sore that does not heal within two weeks, unusual bleeding from the teeth or gums, a white or red patch in the mouth, a lump or thickening in the mouth, throat, or tongue.
- Larynx: persistent hoarseness or **sore throat**, difficulty breathing, or **pain**.
- Hypopharynx and oropharynx: difficulty in swallowing or chewing food, ear pain.
- Nose, sinuses, and nasopharyngeal cavity: pain, bloody discharges from the nose, blocked nose, and frequent sinus infections that do not respond to standard **antibiotics**.

Specific diagnostic tests used depend on the location of the cancer. The first step in diagnosis is a complete and thorough examination of the oral and nasal cavity, using mirrors and other visual aids. The tongue and the back of the throat are examined as well. Any suspicious looking lumps or lesions are examined with fingers (palpation). In order to look inside the larynx, the doctor may sometimes perform a procedure known as **laryngoscopy**. The doctor may order blood or other immunological tests. These tests are aimed at detecting antibodies to the Epstein-Barr virus, which has been known to cause cancer of the nasopharynx.

X rays of the mouth, the sinuses, the skull, and the chest region may be required. Imaging techniques such as a **computed tomography scan** (CT scan); Ultrasonograms or an MRI (**magnetic resonance imaging**) may be used to get detailed pictures of the areas inside the body.

When a sore does not heal or a suspicious patch or lump is seen in the mouth, larynx, nasopharynx, or throat, a **biopsy** may be performed to rule out the possibility of cancer. The biopsy is the most definitive diagnostic tool for detecting the cancer. If cancerous cells are detected in the biopsied sample, the doctor may perform more extensive tests in order to find whether, and to where, the cancer may have spread.

The cancers can be treated successfully if diagnosed early. The choice of treatment depends on the size of the tumor, its location, and whether it has spread to other parts of the body. Surgery, radiation and **chemotherapy**, are the most common mods of treatment. Surgery is generally recommended for small tumors. If the cancer cannot be removed by surgery, radiotherapy is used alone. After aggressive surgery and radiation, rehabilitation is often necessary and is an essential part of the treatment. The patient may experience difficulties with swallowing, chewing, and speech and may require a team of health care workers, including speech therapists, prosthodontists, occupational therapists etc.

With early detection and immediate treatment, survival rates can be dramatically improved. For lip and oral cancer, if detected at its early stages, almost 80% of the patients survive five years or more. Cancers of the nasal cavity often go undetected until they reach an advanced stage. If diagnosed at the early stages, the five-year survival rates are 60–70%. In cancer of the oropharynx, 60–80% of the patients survive five years or more if the cancer is detected in the early stages. Patients who are diagnosed with early stage cancers that have originated in the nasopharynx have an excellent chance of a complete cure (almost 95%). Similarly, small cancers of the larynx have an excellent five-year survival rate of 75–95%. However, in all of the head and neck cancers, the survival rates drop dramatically as the cancer advances.

Refraining from the use of all tobacco products (**cigarettes**, cigars, pipe tobacco, chewing tobacco), consuming alcohol in moderation, and practicing good **oral hygiene** are some of the measures that one can take to prevent head and neck cancers. Since there is an association between excessive exposure to the sun and lip cancer, people who spend a lot of time outdoors in the sun should protect themselves from the sun's harmful rays. Regular **physical examinations**, or mouth examination by the patient himself, or by the patient's doctor or dentist, can help detect oral cancer in its very early stages.

HEAD INJURY

Injury to the head may damage the scalp, skull or brain, with results ranging from mild to fatal. Head injuries can be caused by traffic **accidents**, **sports injuries**, falls, workplace accidents, assaults, or firearms. About 70% of all accidental deaths are due to head injuries, as are most injury-related disabilities.

The brain can be damaged even if there is no external evidence of damage. A person who has had a head injury and who is experiencing the following symptoms should seek medical care immediately:

- Serious bleeding from the head or face
- Loss of consciousness, however brief
- Confusion and lethargy
- Lack of pulse or breathing
- Clear fluid drainage from the nose or ear.

A head injury may cause damage both from the direct physical injury and from secondary factors such as lack of oxygen, brain swelling, and disturbance of blood flow. It can cause swirling movements throughout the brain, tearing nerve fibers and causing widespread bleeding or a blood clot. Swelling may raise pressure within the skull and can block the flow of oxygen to the brain.

Head injury may involve **concussion**, in which there is a brief loss of consciousness without visible structural damage to the brain. Initial symptoms of brain injury may also include: memory loss and confusion, vomiting, **dizziness**, partial **paralysis** or numbness, **shock**, and **anxiety**.

After a head injury, there may be a period of impaired consciousness followed by confusion and impaired memory with disorientation and a breakdown in the ability to store and retrieve new information. Others experience temporary **amnesia** involving loss of memory of the weeks, months, or years before the injury. As the patient recovers, memory slowly returns. Post-traumatic amnesia refers to loss of memory for events during and after the accident. Epilepsy occurs in 2–5% of those who have had a head injury.

Closed head injury refers to brain injury without any penetrating injury to the brain. It may be the result of a direct blow to the head; of the moving head being rapidly stopped (as when it hits a windshield), or by the sudden deceleration of the head without striking anything. A moving head will cause a "contrecoup injury" where damage occurs on the side of the brain opposite the point of impact, as a result of the brain slamming into that side of the skull. Even when no object contacts the head, sudden deceleration can result in whiplash, causing delicate brain tissues to hit against the rough, jagged inner surface of the skull.

If the skull is fractured, bone fragments may be driven into the brain. Any object that penetrates the skull may implant foreign material and dirt into the brain, leading to infection.

A skull fracture is a medical emergency that must be treated promptly to prevent possible brain damage. Such an injury may be obvious if blood or bone fragments are visible, but there may also be no apparent damage. A fracture should be suspected if there is: blood or clear fluid leaking from nose or ears, unequal pupil size, bruises or discoloration around the eyes or behind the ears, swelling or depression of the part of the head.

If a blood vessel between the skull and the brain ruptures; leaking blood can form a clot, which can press against brain tissue. If the blood flow is not stopped, it can lead to unconsciousness and death. Symptoms of bleeding within the skull include: **nausea and vomiting**, **headache**, loss of consciousness, unequal pupil size, and lethargy.

If the head injury is mild, there may be no symptoms other than slight headache, or confusion, dizziness, and blurred vision. Up to 60% of patients who sustain a mild brain injury continue to experience a range of symptoms called "post-concussion syndrome," for as long as a year. This syndrome can involve a puzzling interplay of difficult-to-diagnose complaints, including: headache, dizziness, mental confusion, behavior changes, memory loss, depression, emotional outbursts, and cognitive deficits that impair functions such as awareness.

Damage in a severe head injury can be assessed with **computed tomography scan** (CT scan), **magnetic resonance imaging** (MRI), **positron emission tomography** (PET) scans, electroencephalograms (EEG), and routine neurological and neuropsychological evaluations.

A penetrating wound (such as caused by a bullet) may require surgery. If there is bleeding inside the skull, the blood may need to be surgically drained; if a clot has formed, it may need to be removed. Severe skull **fractures** also require surgery.

In the event of long-term disability, there are a variety of treatment programs, including long-term **rehabilitation**, coma treatment centers, transitional living programs, behavior management programs, life-long residential or day treatment programs and independent living programs.

Patients with a mild head injury who experience symptoms are advised to seek out a specialist. A local chapter of a head-injury foundation can provide names of nearby experts.

Prompt diagnosis and treatment can alleviate some of the problems after a head injury. However, a patient's prospects for recovery may not be known for many months or even years. The outlook for a minor head injury is generally good, although symptoms can persist for a year or longer. This can limit ability to work and cause strain in personal relationships.

Serious head injuries can be devastating, producing permanent mental and physical disability. Full healing may take five years or longer.

Many severe injuries could be prevented by wearing protective helmets during certain sports and occupations, and when riding bikes or motorcycles. Seat belts and airbags can prevent injuries.

HEALTH CARE ADMINISTRATION

Health care administration, also called health services administration, is the planning, organizing, and coordinating of the delivery of health care. Health care administrators help all types of health care organizations effectively deliver health care. They are responsible for facilities, services, programs, staff, budgets, and relations with other organizations.

Health care administrators can work in a variety of settings. More than half of all health care administrators work in hospitals. In the hospital setting, they work in executive management, day-to-day management, or specialized departments such as finance, systems analysis, or marketing. **Health maintenance organizations** and other managed care organizations are another major employer of health care administrators. Health care administrators in HMOs or other managed care organizations perform the same functions as administrators in large medical practices, and also establish and manage medical benefits packages that will attract enrollees and help the organization succeed.

Health care administrators also work in **nursing homes**, hospices, **home health care** agencies, **rehabilitation** centers, community mental health centers, urgent care centers, diagnostic imaging centers, and in offices of doctors, dentists, and other health care practitioners.

As the United States health care system continues to expand and diversify, the demand for skilled health care administrators is expected to grow through the year 2006. Although hospitals will continue to employ the majority of health care administrators, other types of organizations (long term care facilities, home health care agencies, and doctors' offices and clinics) will begin to use more health care administrators.

Most health care administrators have at least a bachelor's degree in a field such as finance, public administration, or personnel administration. Many also have a graduate degree in health services administration, nursing administration, or business administration, as well as work experience in a health care setting. Larger organizations generally require more specialized education than smaller ones do. Most health care administrators do not need to be licensed. Nursing home administrators in most states and the District of Columbia, however, must have a bachelor's degree, pass a licensing examination, finish a state training program, and enroll in continuing education.

HEALTH CARE SYSTEM

A health care system is an assemblage of institutions, agencies, and individuals whose primary goal is to deliver medical service for the benefit of society at large. The key elements of our nation's health care system are wide ranging in function. Public and private **hospitals** provide emergency care, surgical treatment, and clinical services to patients. **Hospices** and **nursing homes** care for individuals at the end of their lives. Medical schools and other training institutions educate and prepare health professionals to serve the public. State and municipal health boards conduct sanitation inspections, set public health standards, and, along with federal organizations like the **Centers for Disease Control**, investigate outbreaks of illness. Public medical insurance programs, such as **Medicare and Medicaid**, provide assistance to the poor and the elderly. Municipal, state, and federal agencies provide disaster and emergency response services. Government organizations such as the **National Institutes of Health** conduct and sponsor research and monitor the nation's health status. Millions of individuals who are doctors, nurses, therapists, and other medical providers, are most directly linked to the delivery of health care.

Today's complex, costly, and highly regulated health care industry has evolved in response to the public expectation that the enjoyment of a high standard of health is a fundamental right. This expectation has, in turn, arisen as the result of the extraordinary increase in medical knowledge, unique to our era. An improved understanding of the mechanisms and causes of illness, coupled with the development of vaccines and pharmaceutical treatments, has enabled health providers to manage or cure vast numbers of disease conditions that only a century ago were untreatable. Advances in technology now allow for early and rapid detection of many illnesses, as well as more accurate diagnosis. The availability of safe and effective **anesthesia**, the development of complex surgical procedures, and the invention of sophisticated prosthetic devices have helped extend the human lifespan and have greatly reduced the suffering from disease and disability. With these enormous improvements in our ability to care for the ill and disabled, comes the unfortunate drawback that health care is increasingly costly. As medical knowledge continues to improve in the coming decades and as health care technology continues to develop, the growing challenge will be to ensure that all members of society have access to cost effective care of the highest standard.

HEALTH INSURANCE

Health insurance is a form of insurance that helps pay for medical services, such as doctor visits, tests, and hospitalization. Private insurance companies and government agencies, like the **Medicare and Medicaid** programs in the United States, are the primary providers of health insurance. Health insurance assures that people can afford medical care and protects the individual from being overburdened with enormous health care bills. Private companies charge a monthly fee, or premium, for health care coverage. Government-based health insurance is usually free and sometimes based on certain criteria, such as age (Medicare) or income (Medicaid).

Health insurance is a relatively recent phenomenon, having emerged primarily during the course of the twentieth century. As early as 1883, Germany had established a government-sponsored health services system to provide care for low income people who could not afford it. Still, as recently as 1929, no insurance was available to cover the costs of hospitalization in the United States. In the 1930s, individual hospitals began to initiate health insurance plans to subscribing members in the community, often an individual company or group, such as teachers, who could receive care in the hospital providing the insurance. The ''free-choice'' approach to hospital care coverage (in which the insured can seek medical attention from a health care provider of his or her own choice) soon evolved through a consortium of area hospitals as well as through private insurance companies.

After World War II, Great Britain initiated the first comprehensive compulsory governmental health plan, which provided free medical care to any patient seeing a doctor within the system. Known today as socialized medicine, this approach has been adopted by many countries. However, in the United States, employer-based and individual purchases of private health insurance became the primary source of health coverage, although governmental programs do exist. One advantage associated with the private insurance approach is that it offers patients a greater freedom of choice since most physicians and hospitals provide services covered by the major medical insurers, such as Blue Cross. However, relying on private insurance also has a major drawback. People who can not afford to pay for health insurance traditionally have much more limited access to services. In 1965, the U.S. government took efforts to address the problem of people who could not afford insurance when it enacted the Medicare and Medicaid programs. These programs provide care to people over the age of 65 and the poor, respectively. Other programs, such as workers' compensation and disability, also evolved to provide for health care services and are primarily run by the individual states.

In the early 1990s, a growing debate over health care and insurance in the United States began, focusing primarily on the growing costs of health care and the ever-expanding population base unable to afford health care insurance. The U.S. is the only Western industrialized nation without a government-sponsored comprehensive health insurance plan for its citizens. As a result, by the mid-1990s, the U.S. spent 40 percent of its Gross National Product (GNP) on health care and nearly 40 million people were uninsured. Statistics such as these led to a proposal by President Clinton to establish a federal program that would ensure coverage for nearly all U.S. citizens. This proposal was opposed by many in the health care industry, including the medical and insurance professions, who viewed government interference as an encroachment of ''free-choice'' for both patients and health care providers. No legislation was enacted, and the health care insurance debate continued.

On the one hand, socialized medicine reduces health care costs and provides insurance for all. But many argue that the approach erodes the quality of health care and stifles new approaches and quality improvement in health care services. However, in 1997, ten million children in the United States had no health insurance. As a result, they either went without care or sought services in hospital emergency rooms, which represents a costly and in-effective use of health care resources.

As a result of the debate over health care and health insurance, new approaches seek to contain costs. **Health Maintenance Organizations** (HMOs), for example, offer treatment through their own network of doctors organized to lower costs. By the late 1990s, **managed care,** which incorporates HMOs and other similar health services organizations and insurances, had become the dominant mode of providing health care services and insurance in the U.S. Ideally, this approach allows consumer to pick and choose insurance plans while avoiding government price controls and rationing of health care services. However, it has resulted in less freedom of choice in health care because people must seek care from physicians and hospitals associated with their particular managed care plan. It has also failed to addresss successfully the issue of the uninsured.

See also Managed care; Medicare and Medicaid

Health maintenance organization

Traditionally in the United States, if you got sick, you went to the doctor, who examined you, treated you, and sent you a bill. This was called ''fee-for-service'' medicine, and it was the way medical care was given for decades. But as medical costs spiraled upwards (sometimes reaching hundred of thousands of dollars for care), insurers began looking for a way that patients could get their care and keep costs in control. The Health Maintenance Organization (HMO) was the proposed solution to the problem. Most people join HMOs through their workplace. In fact, according to NBC News, 87% of adults who receive health coverage through their employer are members of an HMO. These members, or subscribers, receive comprehensive medical care through paying a fixed monthly fee, or premium. There are several types of HMOs. Network HMOs contract with two or more group practices of physicians to provide care to members. Group HMOs contract with independent physician groups; some HMOs contract with individual practices, which makes them an independent practitioner association, or IPA. Or, HMOs may hire physicians as staff doctors at their own clinic or hospital (the staff model). In an HMO, each member has a primary care physician, or a ''gatekeeper.'' This PCP sees the patient for all his or her health needs. The PCP can be a family practitioner, a pediatrician, an internist, a general practitioner, or a obstetrician-gynecologist (OB-GYN). In many ways, the PCP serves the same function as the old-time family doctor did. The PCP can prescribe medicines, give physicals, answer questions, and diagnose ailments—and in the case of the OB-GYN, deliver babies. But in the HMO, the primary care physician has an extra responsibility: he or she is the one who decides whether a patient needs to see a specialist (such as a dermatologist), is admitted to the hospital, or needs special tests or procedures. Usually, subscribers choose their primary care physician from the HMO's list of member doctors; in some cases, the PCP is the choice of the HMO. In many cases, subscribers may find that the doctor they have already been seeing is a member of the HMO; physicians can be part of several HMOs at once. However, it is not guaranteed that a person's physician will be part of a plan, so before switching from a traditional health insurance plan to an HMO, he or she should check with the physician to be sure. HMO subscribers are not discouraged from seeing their primary care doctor. Preventive care is emphasized by HMOs, and so patients are not limited in the number of visits they can make. In fact, the more often a doctor sees a patient, the better, because the doctor will get to know the patient and be able to judge when there is something out of the ordinary going on. HMOs have been criticized for affecting the quality of care that patients receive, and for taking the decision-making about health care out of the hands of the physicians. It is true that HMOs have sometimes balked at providing patients with expensive or experimental treatments. However, the laws governing HMOs vary from state to state, and the insurer may be required by law to pay for a procedure. For example, Massachusetts law requires that HMOs pay for infertility treatment and for the birth and newborn care of the baby that results, even in the case of a multiple birth. Such procedures can easily exceed $150,000 total, making it unlikely that a couple outside of an HMO, who would be paying almost of quarter of that amount themselves under traditional insurance, would pursue infertility treatments. HMO subscribes generally do not have significant out-of-pocket expenses. They must pay a small amount at each visit to the doctor (a "co-pay"), which usually amounts to five or ten dollars. In some cases, such as for obstetric care, the co-pay is waived. Coverage varies from HMO to HMO. Some, as mentioned, will pay for infertility treatments. Others cover vision care and **eyeglasses** or contact lenses (or at least some part of their cost), and even dental care. Some will also offer discounts on wellness programs to their members, such as fitness center memberships and even discounts of child car seats. Being a member of an HMO has its advantages and disadvantages. Patients who are on traditional plans can choose any doctor and go to any hospital without pre-approval from anyone. They will pay about 20% of the doctor's or hospital's fees out of their own pockets, which may make them less likely to visit the doctor with an apparently minor ailment or a health concern. Patients on an HMO may face limited choices and curtailment of certain tests and procedures, but can enjoy many benefits that will go toward keeping them healthy. It is a decision that needs to be made with care and consideration.

See also Health insurance; Managed care

HEALTH SCREENING

A health screening is a test to determine the possible presence of a disease or other health problem. Health screenings often are conducted routinely as a preventive measure, or may be done when there is reason to suspect a particular health problem exists.

It should be noted that there is not universal agreement as to which tests should be performed and when they should be performed. Individual doctors and insurers may have their own philosophies about health screening tests. What follows, then, are common recommendations; individuals should consult their doctors and insurers for information specific to their needs.

Children's health screenings normally include height, weight and blood pressure checks, together with possible hearing, vision or dental problems.

Other screenings might include tests to measure learning progress, a check to make sure the spine is straight and developing properly, and skin screenings to check for the presence of unusual **moles** or **birthmarks**. Tests normally are done to detect the possibility of **diabetes**, **tuberculosis** and **anemia**.

It is recommended that children get dental check-ups at least once a year as soon as they have several teeth; an initial vision screening by age 3; and a blood pressure check by age 10. Some pediatricians also give cholesterol checks to children if family history and circumstances warrant.

Beginning with adulthood, health care providers have established a set of recommended health screens for men and women depending on the age of the patient. (In addition, the frequency of some health screenings depends on risk factors of the patient.) **Eye** (every three years) and dental exams (twice a year) and hearing checks are recommended for everyone.

For women between the ages of 20 and 39, the following screenings are recommended:

- **Pelvic exam**: every year.
- **Pap test**: every year until three satisfactory tests have been completed, and then at the doctor's discretion.
- Breast: at least every three years.
- Skin: at least every three years.

For women between the ages of 40 and 49, the following health screenings are recommended:

- Blood pressure: at least every two years
- **Cholesterol test**: every five years
- Skin exam: every year
- Breast exam: every year
- Pelvic exam: every year
- Pap test: every year (or at the doctor's discretion)
- **Mammography**: every one to two years (depending on risk)
- Fasting plasma glucose test: to check for the possibility of diabetes, every three years after age 45

After age 50, women should have the following screenings:

- Blood pressure: at least every two years
- Cholesterol: every five years (or every three years starting at age 65
- Skin exam: every year
- Breast exam: every year
- Mammogram: every year
- **Fecal occult blood test**: every year

- Pelvic exam: every year
- Pap test: yearly (or at the doctor's discretion)
- Bone mineral density test: once as a baseline
- Fasting plasma glucose test: for diabetes, every three years
- Thyroid-stimulating hormone test: every 3-5 years starting at age 65
- **Colorectal cancer** test: every five to ten years

For men between the ages of 20 an 39, the following screenings are recommended:

- Blood pressure: at least every two years
- Cholesterol: every five years
- Skin exam: every three years

Men between the ages of 40 and 49 should have screenings for:

- Blood pressure: at least every two years
- Cholesterol: every five years
- Skin exam: every year
- Fasting plasma glucose test: to check for the possibility of diabetes, every three years after age 45

Men who are 50 years or older should have the following screenings:

- Blood pressure: at least every two years
- Cholesterol: every five years (or every three years starting at age 65)
- Skin exam: every year
- Digital rectal exam: (to check for the possibility of **prostate cancer**) every year
- Prostate specific antigen (PSA) test: every year
- Fasting plasma glucose test: (for diabetes) every three years
- Colorectal cancer test: every five to ten years

Health screenings are important for early detection of diseases or other possible health problems. Any suspected problems should be reported to a health care provider immediately.

See also Colorectal cancer; Prostate cancer; Thyroid function tests

HEALY, BERNADINE (1944-)

American cardiologist

Bernadine Healy is a cardiologist and health administrator who was the first woman to head the **National Institutes of Health** (NIH) from 1991 to 1993. Known for her outspokenness, innovative policy making, and sometimes controversial leadership in medical and research institutions, Healy has been particularly effective in addressing medical policy and research pertaining to women. She spent the early part of her career at Johns Hopkins University where she rose to full professor on the medical school faculty while also undertaking significant administrative responsibilities. She served as deputy science advisor to President Ronald Reagan from 1984–1985. In 1985 she was appointed Head of the Research Institute of the Cleveland Clinic Foundation where she remained until her appointment as director of the NIH in 1991. Healy was also president of the American Heart Association from 1988–1989 and has served on numerous national advisory committees. Healy was named dean of the College of Medicine and Public Health at Ohio State University in 1995. And in the fall of 1999 she became president of the American Red Cross.

The second of Michael J. and Violet (McGrath) Healy's four daughters, Bernadine Patricia Healy was born August 2, 1944, in New York City and grew up in Long Island City, Queens, New York. Her parents, second generation Irish-Americans, operated a small perfume business from the basement of their home. Healy attended Hunter College High School, a prestigious public school in Manhattan and graduated first in her class. At Vassar College she majored in chemistry and minored in philosophy, graduating summa cum laude in 1965. One of ten women in a class of 120 at Harvard Medical School, she received her M.D. cum laude in 1970.

Healy completed her internship and residency at Johns Hopkins Hospital in Baltimore and spent two years at the National Heart, Lung, and Blood Institute at NIH before returning to Johns Hopkins and working her way up the academic ranks to professor of medicine. During these years, she also served as director of the coronary care unit (1977–1984) and assistant dean for post-doctoral programs and faculty development (1979–1984). From there, Healy served the Reagan Administration as deputy director of the White House Office of Science and Technology Policy. President George Bush nominated her for director of NIH in September 1990 and she was later confirmed by the U.S. Senate. Her tenure with NIH ended when incoming President Clinton appointed a new director in 1993. Healy has been married to cardiologist Floyd D. Loop since 1985. With Loop she has a daughter, Marie McGrath Loop; her other daughter, Bartlett Ann Bulkley, is from her previous marriage to surgeon George Bulkley, whom she divorced in 1981.

Healy has manifested her talent and interest in shaping research policy through her many appointments to federal advisory panels, editorial boards of scientific journals, and other decision-making bodies. As the president of the American Heart Association she initiated pioneering research into women's heart disease and demonstrated that medical progress depends on the public and medical community's perception that there is a problem to be solved. Previously, heart disease was perceived as a male affliction despite the fact that it kills more women than men. Medical practitioners for years treated women's heart disease far less aggressively than men's, and most research on coronary heart disease (like most other medical research) used male subjects either predominantly or exclusively. Healy has set out to ''convince both the lay and medical sectors that coronary heart disease is also a woman's disease, not a man's disease in disguise,'' she wrote in *New England Journal of Medicine.*

At the time that Healy was appointed director of the National Institutes of Health in 1991, the agency included thirteen research institutes, sixteen thousand employees, a research budget of over nine billion dollars, and was a world leader in bio-medical research. Yet when Healy assumed control, the agency was beset with problems, its effectiveness was in decline, and it had been without a permanent director for twenty months. Scientists were leaving in record numbers because of non-competitive salaries, politicization of scientific agendas (a prime example was the ban on fetal-tissue research because the Republican administration believed it encouraged **abortion**), and congressional investigations into alleged cases of scientific misconduct. The agency had been accused of sexism and racism in hiring and promotion. Low morale and bureaucratization added to the institute's problematic image. Healy brought an aggressive and visible management style to the NIH. Her appointment was viewed positively by many because of her outstanding experience in dealing with science policy issues. In addition, because she had been a member of a panel that advised continuation of fetal-tissue research, her appointment was also seen as a move away from politicized science. She also held a series of ''town meetings'' with NIH scientists to pinpoint problems and form committees to make recommendations concerning NIH research priorities. Furthermore, she initiated a large scale study of the effects of vitamin supplementation, **hormone replacement therapy**, and dietary modification on women between the ages of forty-five and seventy-nine. She established a policy whereby the NIH would fund only those **clinical trials** that included both men and women when the condition being studied affected both genders.

Healy's policy decisions at times proved controversial. For example, Healy charged the NIH Office of Scientific Integrity (OSI), whose job it was to investigate ethical matters, with improper conduct, including leaking confidential information and failing to protect the rights of scientists being investigated. In response, the head of OSI accused Healy of mishandling a scientific misconduct case at the Cleveland Clinic Foundation. The allegations led to a hearing in 1991 in which Healy vigorously defended herself, as well as the changes that she had implemented at OSI.

Another controversy involved gene patenting. Despite the objections of Nobel laureate **James Watson,** head of NIH's human genome project, Healy approved patent applications for 347 genes. She believed that patenting genes would promote, not hinder, the ability to access information about them and also spark much-needed international debate on the subject. A third controversy strained her relationship with the Congressional Caucus for Women's Issues. Healy lobbied against provisions in a congressional bill concerning the NIH that would make the inclusion of women and minorities in clinical studies a legal requirement, arguing that it represented ''micro-management'' of NIH. Attempting to negotiate a political compromise on another issue, she lobbied against overturning the Bush administration's ban on fetal tissue research, despite her previous support for such research.

Dr. Healy has received several awards, including the Charles A. Dana Foundation Award for exceptional leadership in the strategic direction of NIH; the *Glamour* magazine ''Woman of the Year'' Award; the Sara Lee Frontrunner Award for unprecedented dedication, vision, and commitment to the government; and the Golden Heart Award of the national American Heart Association. She has been awarded a distinguished service award from the Greater Cleveland Hospital Association; the Excellence in Leadership Award from the National Women's Economic Alliance Foundation; the McDonough Center Distinguished Leadership Award; the Health Advocacy Award of the Friends of the National Institute of Nursing Research; and in October 1996 she was inducted into the Ohio Women's Hall of Fame. Dr. Healy was named a Women's Health Hero by *American Health for Women* magazine in October 1997; and in November 1997, with her husband, was named Humanitarian of the Year by the American Red Cross. In April 1998 she received the Democracy in Action Award from the League of Women Voters, and in September of that year the National Museum of Women's History presented her with its Women Making History Award. Dr. Healy received the YWCA Women of Achievement Award in April 1999. She has received numerous honorary degrees.

HEARING AIDS AND COCHLEAR IMPLANTS

Hearing aids are devices that amplify sound so a person who has a hearing impairment can enjoy sounds from a musical symphony to a lively conversation to the rustle of leaves. Two types of hearing aids either conduct sound through the air or through bone. Usually a person who is hearing impaired can use an *air-conduction* hearing aid, as it amplifies sound and brings it directly to the **ear**. The *bone-conduction* hearing aid brings sound waves to the bony part of the head behind the ear and uses the bone to transmit sound waves to the nerves of the ear. A typical hearing aid contains a microphone that picks up sounds and converts them into electric signals, an amplifier, which increases the strength of the electric signals, and the receiver, which converts the signals back into sound waves that can be heard by the wearer. There are three main styles of hearing aids: those that fit behind the ear, those that fit into the ear, and those which slip into the ear canal. Power is provided by a small battery.

Devices to aid hearing have a long history. The idea of bone conduction was known in the early seventeenth century and the ear trumpet was used even before that time. The ear trumpet was shaped to gather sound and funnel it into the ear. In seventeenth century Germany, Marcus Banzer used a piece of swine bladder connected to a tube made of elk hoof to make an artificial ear drum. Later in that century the audiphone or dentiphone was invented. Made of a flexible material, the device was shaped like a fan and held at its end between the teeth as the fan was bent toward the sound. The sound vibrations captured by the fan were carried to the teeth, the jaw bones, the skull, and finally to the auditory nerve. Perhaps the largest hearing aid ever made was an imposing throne built for King John VI of Portugal in 1819. Hollow carved arms of the chair terminated with the wooden mouths of lions through which people would speak and have their voices carried by tubes to the king's ear. An artificial ear drum was devised in 1852 when an English physician, Joseph Toynbee, used a disk of vulcanized rubber attached to a rod. The Victorian era was known for some of its more elaborate concealed hearing devices, in urns, top-hats, even tiaras. In the 1870s, Alexander Graham Bell began experimenting with the conduction of sound through electrical devices originally intending to help deaf children hear. His experiments led to the invention of the telephone instead, but his work did bring public awareness to the needs of the hearing impaired. The first electrical hearing aid was made in 1901 by Miller Reese Hutchinson and he called it the Telephone-Transmitter. During the era of vacuum tubes, like those used in early radio, new hearing aids were developed starting in 1920 with Earl Charles Hanson's Vactuphone. A 1923 model produced by the Marconi Company was the Otophone, consisting of an amplifier placed in a large case weighing 16 pounds (7 kg) making it rather bulky to use. The first "wearable" hearing aid weighed 2.5 pounds (1.1 kg) and was made by A. Edwin Steven in 1935. During the 1950s transistors revolutionized electronics and Microtone introduced its compact and powerful transistor hearing aid in 1953.

For individuals whose hearing cannot be aided with a hearing aid, there is the possibility of having a cochlear implant, the first of which were done in 1973 and which involved the implantation of an electrical device which stimulated the remaining nerves in the inner ear in people suffering from nerve deafness. Although the implant did not restore normal hearing, it helped the recipient hear and interpret environmental sound. Today, multichannel electrical cochlear implants are more sophisticated and contain speech processors which allow some patients to understand speech without reading lips. Implants consist of tiny electrodes inserted in the ear and connected to a receiver implanted under the skin by an implanted wire. Robert V. Shannon of the House Ear Institute of Los Angeles has developed an auditory brainstem implant for people whose auditory nerve has been severed. The implant consists of a tiny microphone, sound processor, and transmitter all outside the ear, and an electrode that is implanted inside the head and connected to the auditory brain stem. When the microphone picks up sound, the unit converts sound energy into electric signals that are sent directly to the brain where they are interpreted as sound. Although the implant is not enough to restore hearing, it upgrades the level of environmental sound heard by the user and, in a trial situation, at least one recipient could understand limited human speech.

Computer microchips are now being used in programmable hearing aids, allowing the device to be adjusted by computer. Through programming based on the needs of the individual, signal amplification is automatically adjusted, which means softer sounds can amplified more than louder sounds. Multi-channel capability allows for programmable reception of high- and low-frequency ranges, and some devices have multi-microphone capability, which means one microphone picks up broad-range sound and the other, narrow-range sound, improving the capability of distinguishing conversation from background noise. Digital hearing aids in which a computer- controlled sound processor is contained, are also available.

Hearing loss

Hearing loss is any degree of impairment of the ability to understand sound. A drop of more than 10 decibels (a unit measuring the loudness of sound) in what a person can hear is significant.

Hearing can be interrupted at many stages as sound waves pass through the air of the external **ear**, the bones of the middle ear, and the liquid of the inner ear. Hearing loss can also occur as hearing-related impulses are transmitted along the nerves to the brain, or within the brain, where the impulses may be misinterpreted.

The external ear canal can be blocked by ear wax, **foreign objects**, infection, and tumors. Overgrowth of bone, which occurs when the ear canal has been flushed with cold water repeatedly for years, can also narrow the passageway, making blockage and infection more likely. This condition occurs often in Northern California surfers and is therefore called "surfer's ear."

The ear drum is so thin a physician can see through it into the middle ear. Sharp objects, pressure from an infection in the middle ear, even a firm cuffing or slapping of the ear, can rupture it. It is also susceptible to pressure changes during scuba diving.

Otitis media (an infection in the middle ear) occurs when fluid cannot escape into the throat because of blockage of the Eustachian tube. The pus or mucus accumulates, dampening the motion of the small bones in the middle ear. A disease called otosclerosis can bind the bones, causing deafness.

Sensory hearing loss involves damage to the acoustic nerve, or to the Organ of Corti in the inner ear. The leading cause of sensory hearing loss is prolonged exposure to loud noise, often rock music or job-related noise. A third of people over 65 have presbycusis—sensory hearing loss due to aging. Whether induced by noise or age, these conditions involve primarily the loss of high-frequency hearing. In most languages, it is the high-frequency sounds that define speech, so these people have trouble understanding speech over background noise. Brain infections like **meningitis**, drugs such as the aminoglycoside **antibiotics** (streptomycin, gentamycin, kanamycin, tobramycin), and **Meniere's disease** also cause permanent sensory hearing loss. Meniere's disease combines attacks of hearing loss with attacks of vertigo, a condition in which the person's surroundings seem to spin dizzily. These symptoms may occur together or separately. High doses of salicylates like **aspirin** and quinine can cause a temporary high-frequency loss. Prolonged high doses can lead to permanent deafness. Sensory deafness can also be caused by **rubella** (German **measles**). Sudden hearing loss—at least 30 decibels in less than three days—is most commonly caused by cochleitis, a viral infection.

Another category of hearing loss is neural. Damage to the acoustic nerve and the parts of the brain involved in hearing are the most likely to produce permanent hearing loss. **Strokes**, **multiple sclerosis**, and tumors on the acoustic nerve are all possible causes of neural hearing loss.

Hearing can also be diminished by extra sounds generated by the ear, most of them from the same kinds of disorders that cause diminished hearing. These sounds are referred to as tinnitus and can be ringing, blowing, clicking, or anything else that no one but the patient hears.

An examination of the ears and nose combined with simple hearing tests done in the physician's office can detect many common causes of hearing loss. If the defect is in the brain or the acoustic nerve, further neurological testing and imaging will be needed.

Conductive hearing loss, involving an interruption in the transmission of sound waves, can almost always be restored to some degree, if not completely. Matter in the ear canal can be easily removed. Surfer's ear gradually improves if cold water is avoided or a special ear plug is used. In advanced cases, surgeons can grind away the excess bone. Middle ear infection with fluid is also simple to treat. If medications do not work, surgical drainage of the ear is accomplished through the ear drum, which heals completely. Damaged ear drums can be repaired with a tiny skin graft. Surgical repair of otosclerosis through an operating microscope can substitute tiny artificial parts for original bones in the inner ear.

Sensory and neural hearing loss, on the other hand, cannot readily be cured. Fortunately it is not often complete, so that hearing aids can help correct the problem. In-the-ear hearing aids can boost sound volume by up to 70 decibels. (Normal speech is about 60 decibels.) Also available are bone-conduction hearing aids and devices that can be surgically implanted in the inner ear.

Tinnitus can sometimes be relieved by adding white noise (like the sound of wind or waves crashing on the shore) to the environment.

Decreased hearing is such a common problem that there are legions of organizations to provide assistance. Special language training, both in lip reading and signing, special schools and camps for children are widely available.

Hearing loss may be helped by homeopathic therapies, and oral doses of essential fatty acids such as flax oil and omega 3 oil can help alleviate the accumulation of wax in the ear.

Prompt treatment and attentive follow-up of middle-ear infections in children will prevent this cause of hearing loss. Control of infectious childhood diseases such as measles has greatly reduced sensory hearing loss as a complication of epidemic diseases. Laws that require protection from loud noise in the workplace have achieved substantial reduction in noise induced hearing loss. Surfers should use the right kind of ear plugs.

HEARING TESTS

The testing of a person's ability to hear various sound frequencies is known as audiometry. The test is performed using electronic equipment called an audiometer and is usually administered by an audiologist, a trained technician.

Audiometry is used to identify and diagnose hearing loss. The equipment is used in health screening programs, for example in grade schools, to detect hearing problems in children. It is also used in the doctor's office or hospital audiology department to diagnose hearing problems in children, adults, and the elderly. With correct diagnosis of a person's specific pattern of hearing impairment, the right type of therapy can be prescribed. It might include hearing aids, corrective surgery, or **speech therapy**.

Testing with audiometry equipment is simple and painless. The equipment emits sounds or tones, like musical notes, at various frequencies, or pitches, and at differing volumes or levels of loudness. Testing is usually done in a soundproof testing room.

The person being tested wears a set of headphones that blocks out other distracting sounds and delivers a test tone to one ear at a time. At the sound of a tone, the patient holds up a hand or finger to indicate that the sound is detected. The audiologist lowers the volume and repeats the sound until the patient can no longer detect it. This process is repeated over a wide range of tones or frequencies from very deep, low sounds, like the lowest note played on a tuba, to very high sounds, like the pinging of a triangle. Each ear is tested separately. It is not unusual for levels of sound sensitivity to differ from one ear to the other.

A second type of audiometry testing uses a headband rather than headphones. The headband is worn with small plastic rectangles that fit behind the ears to conduct sound through the bones of the skull. The patient being tested senses the tones that are transmitted as vibrations through the bones to the inner ear. As with the headphones, the tones are repeated at various frequencies and volumes.

The results of the audiometry test may be recorded on a grid or graph called an audiogram. This graph is generally set up with low frequencies or tones at one end and high ones at the other end, much like a piano keyboard. Low notes are graphed on the left and high notes on the right. The graph also charts the volume of the tones used; from soft, quiet sounds at the top of the chart to loud sounds at the bottom. Hearing is measured in units called decibels. Most of the sounds associated with normal speech patterns are in the range of 20-50 decibels. An adult with normal hearing can detect tones between 0-20 decibels.

Speech audiometry is another type of testing that uses a series of simple recorded words spoken at various volumes into headphones worn by the patient. The patient repeats each word back to the audiologist as it is heard. An adult with normal hearing will be able to recognize and repeat 90-100% of the words.

The ears may be examined with an otoscope prior to audiometry testing to determine if there are any blockages in the ear canal due to ear wax or other material.

Audiometry test results are considered abnormal if there is a significant or unexplained difference between the levels of sound heard between the two ears, or if the person being tested is unable to hear in the normal range of frequencies and volume. The pattern of responses displayed on the audiogram can be used by the audiologist to identify if a significant hearing loss is present and if the patient might benefit from hearing aids or corrective surgery.

A vibrating tuning fork held next to the ear or placed against the skull will stimulate the inner ear to vibrate, and can help determine if there is hearing loss.

Two types of tests with tuning forks are typically conducted. In the Rinne test, the vibrating tuning fork is held against the skull, usually on the bone behind the ear (mastoid process) to cause vibrations through the bones of the skull and inner ear. It is also held next to, but not touching, the ear, to cause vibrations in the air next to the ear. The patient is asked to determine which sound is louder, the sound heard through the bone or through the air. A second tuning-fork test is the Weber test, which places the stem or handle of the vibrating tuning fork at various points along the midline of the skull and face. The patient is then asked to identify which ear hears the sound created by the vibrations. Tuning forks of different sizes produce different frequencies of vibrations and can be used to establish the range of hearing.

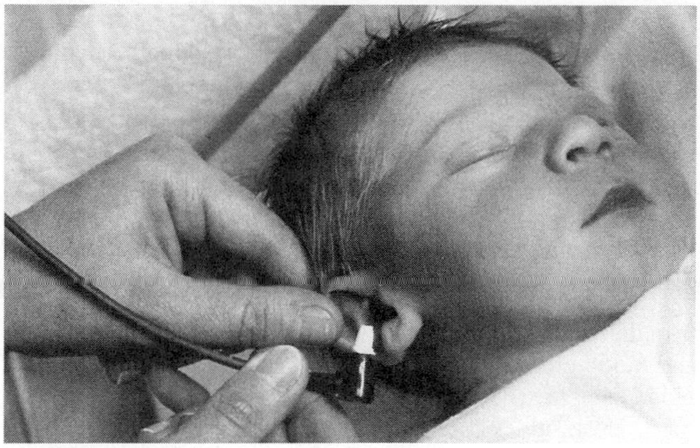

A technician is testing little girl's hearing with an audiometer.

HEART ATTACK

A heart attack is the death of, or damage to, part of the heart muscle because the supply of blood to the heart muscle is severely reduced or stopped.

Also called myocardial infarctions, heart attacks are the leading cause of death in the United States. Each year, more than 1.5 million Americans suffer an attack, and almost half a million die. Most heart attacks follow years of silent but progressive **coronary artery disease**, which can be prevented in many people. A heart attack is often the first symptom of coronary artery disease. According to the American Heart Association, 63% of women and 48% of men who die suddenly of coronary artery disease had no previous symptoms.

A heart attack occurs when one or more of the coronary arteries that supply blood to the heart is completely blocked, cutting off blood to the heart muscle. The blockage is usually caused by **atherosclerosis**, the build-up of plaque in the artery walls, and/or by a blood clot in a coronary artery. Sometimes, a healthy or atherosclerotic coronary artery has a spasm and the blood flow to part of the heart decreases or stops. Why this happens is unclear, but it can result in a heart attack.

About half of all heart attack victims wait at least two hours before seeking help. This increases their chance of sudden death or being disabled. It is important to recognize the signs of a heart attack and seek prompt medical attention at the nearest hospital with 24-hour emergency cardiac care.

About one fifth of all heart attacks are silent, that is, the patient does not know one has occurred. Although the patient feels no **pain**, silent heart attacks can still damage the heart.

Major risk factors significantly increase the risk of coronary artery disease. Those which cannot be changed are:

- Heredity. People whose parents have coronary artery disease are more likely to develop it. African Americans are also at increased risk, due to their higher rate of severe high blood pressure.
- Sex. Men under the age of 60 years of age are more likely to have heart attacks than women of the same age.
- Age. Men over the age of 45 and women over the age of 55 are considered at risk. Older people (those over 65) are more likely to die of a heart attack. Older women are twice as likely to die within a few weeks of a heart attack as a man.

Major risk factors which can be changed are:

- **Smoking**. It greatly increases both the chance of developing coronary artery disease and the chance of dying from it. Second-hand smoke may also increase risk.
- High cholesterol from eating foods such as meat, eggs, and other animal products.
- High blood pressure. High blood pressure makes the heart work harder, and over time, weakens it, increasing the risk of heart attack, **stroke**, **kidney failure**, and congestive **heart failure**. When combined with **obesity**, smoking, high cholesterol, or **diabetes**, the risk of heart attack or stroke increases several times.
- Lack of physical activity. Even modest physical activity is beneficial if done regularly.

Contributing risk factors have been linked to coronary artery disease, but their significance and prevalence are not known yet. Contributing risk factors are:

- Diabetes mellitus. More than 80% of diabetics die of some type of heart or blood vessel disease.
- Obesity. Excess weight increases the strain on the heart and increases the risk of developing coronary artery disease, even if no other risk factors are present. Obesity increases both blood pressure and blood cholesterol, and can lead to diabetes.
- **Stress** and anger. Stress, the mental and physical reaction to life's irritations and challenges, increases the heart rate and blood pressure, and can injure the lining of the arteries. Evidence shows that anger increases the risk of dying from heart disease and more than doubles the risk of having a heart attack right after an episode of anger.

More than 60% of heart attack victims experience symptoms before the attack, sometimes days or weeks before. Sometimes people do not recognize the symptoms of a heart attack or are in denial that they are having one. Symptoms are:

- Uncomfortable pressure, fullness, squeezing, or pain in the center of the chest. This lasts more than a few minutes, or may go away and return.

- Pain that spreads to the shoulders, neck, or arms.
- Chest discomfort accompanied by lightheadedness, **fainting**, **sweating**, **nausea**, or **shortness of breath**.

All of these symptoms do not occur with every heart attack. Sometimes, symptoms disappear and then reappear. A person with any of these symptoms should immediately call an emergency rescue service or be driven to the nearest hospital with a 24-hour cardiac care unit, whichever is quicker.

Experienced emergency care personnel can usually diagnose a heart attack simply by looking at the patient. To confirm this diagnosis, they talk with the patient, check heart rate and blood pressure, perform an electrocardiogram, and take a blood sample.

Heart attacks are treated with **cardiopulmonary resuscitation** (CPR) when necessary to start and keep the patient breathing and his heart beating. Additional treatment can include close monitoring, electric shock, drug therapy, revascularization procedures, **coronary artery bypass surgery**, or repair of blood vessels using a tiny plastic tube tipped with a balloon that compresses the plaque and opens the blocked artery (**angioplasty**).

The aftermath of a heart attack is often severe. Two-thirds of heart attack patients never recover fully. Within one year, 27% of men and 44% of women die. Within six years, 23% of men and 31% of women have another heart attack, 13% of men and 6% of women experience sudden death, and about 20% have heart failure. People who survive a heart attack have a chance of sudden death four to six times greater than others and a chance of illness and death two to nine times greater. Older women are more likely than men to die within a few weeks of a heart attack.

Many heart attacks can be prevented through a healthy lifestyle including eating right (foods that are low in fat, especially saturated fat; low in cholesterol; and high in fiber; plenty of fruits and vegetables; and limited sodium), regular exercise, maintaining a healthy weight, no smoking, moderate drinking, no illegal drugs, controlling **hypertension**, and managing stress.

Daily **aspirin** therapy may help prevent blood clots associated with atherosclerosis. It can also prevent heart attacks from recurring, prevent heart attacks from being fatal, and lower the risk of strokes.

HEART CATHETERIZATION

Heart catheterization (also called cardiac catheterization) is a diagnostic procedure that carefully examines how the heart and its blood vessels function. One or more catheters (tubes designed to enter small openings) are inserted into the organ through a blood vessel in the arm or leg. The procedure gathers information about the pressure, flow, and supply of blood, as well as supplying blood samples and x rays of the heart and surrounding blood vessels.

The primary reason for conducting a heart catheterization is to diagnose and manage suspected cases of heart disease, a frequently fatal condition that leads to 1.5 million **heart attacks** annually in the United States.

To understand how heart catheterization is able to diagnose and manage heart disease, the basic workings of the heart muscle must be understood. Just as the body relies on a constant supply of blood, so does the heart. The organ possesses an intricate web of blood vessels (coronary arteries) that ensure an adequate supply of blood rich in oxygen and nutrients. An abnormality in any of these arteries can cause the heart's blood flow to decrease, resulting in **coronary artery disease**.

Typically performed along with **angiography** (injecting dye into the bloodstream to outline the heart and blood vessels), catheterization can help identify blockages, narrowing, or abnormalities in the coronary arteries. If these signs are visible, the patient may need coronary bypass surgery or other treatment.

Symptoms and diagnoses that can lead to performing a heart catherization include:

- Chest **pain**, characterized by prolonged heavy pressure or a squeezing pain
- An abnormal treadmill stress test
- A heart attack
- Heart problems originating from birth
- Valvular heart disease
- A need to measure the heart's ability to pump blood.

Becasue heart catheterization is considered an "invasive" procedure, it is important to consider the following conditions:

- A bleeding disorder, poor kidney function, or weakness. These typically increase risk and may be reason to cancel the procedure.
- Heart valve disease. If this is detected, **antibiotics** may be given to prevent inflammation of the membrane lining the heart (**endocarditis**).

Like all surgical procedures, cardiac catheterization involves some risk of complications. These may include:

- Cardiac **arrhythmias** (an irregular heartbeat)
- Pericardial tamponade (a condition causing excess pressure in the membrane surrounding the heart)
- In rare cases, a heart attack or stroke may develop due to clotting or rupture of one or more of the heart or brain arteries.

The risk of catheterization increases in patients over the age of 60, those who have severe **heart failure**, or persons with serious valvular heart disease.

Prior to cardiac catheterization, it is important to relay information to the doctor or nurse regarding **allergies** to shellfish (such as shrimp or scallops) that contain iodine or dyes commonly used in other diagnostic tests.

The patient must not eat or drink anything for at least six hours prior to the test. Just before the procedure, the patient will urinate and change into a hospital gown, then lie flat on a padded table that may be tilted to allow the heart to be examined from a variety of angles.

Catheterization typically lasts two to three hours. A patient should expect the following:

- A mild sedative may be given to allow the patient to relax but remain conscious during the procedure.
- An intravenous needle will be inserted into the arm to administer medication. Electrodes will be attached to

the chest to enable the painless procedure known as **electrocardiography**.

- Prior to inserting a catheter into the arm or leg, the point of entry will be made numb by injecting a local anesthetic. Pressure may also be experienced as the catheter travels through the blood vessel.
- After the catheter is guided into the coronary-artery system, a dye is injected to help identify abnormalities of the heart. During this time, the patient may experience a hot, flushed feeling or a quickly passing nausea. Coughing or breathing deeply may alleviate discomfort.
- Medication may be given if chest pain occurs, and nitroglycerin may also be administered to allow expansion of the heart's blood vessels.
- When the test is complete, the physician will remove the catheter and close the skin with sutures or tape.

While cardiac catheterization may be performed on an out-patient basis, patients may require close monitoring afterward, remaining in hospital for at least 24 hours. The patient will be instructed to rest in bed for at least eight hours. If the catheter was inserted in the leg or groin area, the leg will be kept extended for four to six hours. If a vein or artery in the arm was used, the arm will need to remain extended for a minimum of three hours.

The patient should expect a hard ridge to form over the incision site that diminishes as it heals. Bluish discoloration under the skin at the point of insertion should also be expected but fades in two weeks. It is not uncommon for the incision site to bleed during the first 24 hours following surgery. If this should happen, the patient should apply pressure to the site with a clean tissue or cloth for 10-15 minutes.

HEART FAILURE

Heart failure is a condition in which the heart has lost ability to pump enough blood to the body's tissues. With too little blood, the organs and other tissues do not receive enough oxygen and nutrients to function properly.

Heart failure happens when disease affects the heart's ability to deliver blood. Often, a person with heart failure may have a buildup of fluid in the tissues, called **edema**. Heart failure with this kind of fluid buildup is called congestive heart failure. According to the American Heart Association, about 4.9 million Americans are living with congestive heart failure. Ten out of every 1,000 people over age 65 have this condition.

Where edema occurs in the body depends on the part of the heart affected. Heart failure caused by abnormality of the lower left chamber of the heart (left ventricle) means that the ventricle cannot pump blood to the body as fast as it returns from the lungs. Because blood cannot get back to the heart, it begins to back up in the lungs. Some of the fluid in the blood is forced into the breathing space of the lungs, causing **pulmonary edema**. A person with pulmonary edema has shortness of breath, which may be severe and life threatening. A patient with congestive heart failure feels tired.

In right-sided heart failure, the lower right chamber of the heart (right ventricle) cannot pump blood to the lungs as fast as it returns from the body through the veins. Blood then engorges the right side of the heart and the veins. Fluid backed up in the veins is forced out into the tissues, causing swelling, usually in the feet and legs.

When the heart cannot pump enough blood, it tries to make up for this by becoming larger. Enlarged, the ventricle can contract more strongly and pump more blood. The heart also compensates by pumping more often to improve blood output and circulation. The kidneys try to compensate for a failing heart by retaining more salt and water to increase the volume of blood. This extra fluid can also cause edema. Eventually, as the condition worsens, these measures are not enough to keep the heart pumping enough blood. Kidneys often weaken under these circumstances, further aggravating the situation.

The most common causes of heart failure are **coronary artery disease** and **heart attack** (which may be ''silent''), disease of th the heart muscle (**cardiomyopathy**), high blood pressure (**hypertension**), heart valve disease, congenital heart disease (present at birth), alcoholism and drug abuse.

A person with heart failure may experience the following: **shortness of breath**; frequent **coughing** (especially when lying down); swollen feet, ankles, and legs; abdominal swelling and **pain**; fatigue, **dizziness** or **fainting**; or sudden **death**. Pulmonary edema may cause the person to cough up bubbly phlegm that contains blood.

To diagnose heart failure, a doctor may use a **chest x ray**, electrocardiogram (ECG; also called EKG) or other imaging tests, or heart catheterization.

Shortness of breath while engaging in activities or that wakes a person from sleep are classic symptoms of heart failure. Rapid breathing or other changes in breathing may also be present. Patients with heart failure may also have a rapid pulse The skin of the fingers and toes may have a bluish tint and feel cool.

Heart failure usually is initially treated with lifestyle changes and medicines. Dietary changes may be needed to maintain proper weight and reduce salt intake. Appropriate exercise may also be recommended, but it is important that heart failure patients only begin an **exercise** program with the advice of their doctors. Walking, bicycling, swimming, or low-impact aerobic exercises may be recommended. There are good heart **rehabilitation** programs at most larger hospitals.

Other lifestyle changes that may reduce the symptoms of heart failure include stopping **smoking** or other tobacco use, eliminating or reducing alcohol consumption, and not using harmful drugs.

Medicines that may be prescribed for heart failure include **diuretics**, **digitalis**, **vasodilators**, **beta blockers**, angiotensin converting enzyme inhibitors (ACE inhibitors), angiotensin receptor blockers (ARBs), and calcium channel blockers.

Surgery is used to correct certain heart conditions that cause heart failure. Congenital heart defects and abnormal heart valves can be surgically repaired. Blocked coronary arteries can usually be treated with **angioplasty** or **coronary artery bypass surgery**.

With severe heart failure, the heart muscle may become so damaged that available treatments do not help. Patients with this end-stage heart failure may be considered for heart transplantation when all other treatments have stopped working.

Most patients with mild or moderate heart failure can be successfully treated with dietary and exercise programs and the right medications. Many people are able to participate in normal daily activities and lead relatively active lives.

Patients with severe heart failure may eventually have to consider transplantation. Approximately 50% of patients diagnosed with congestive heart failure live for five years with the condition. Women with heart failure usually live longer than men with heart failure.

The best way to try to prevent heart failure is to eat a healthy diet and get regular exercise, but many causes of heart failure cannot be prevented. People with risk factors for coronary disease (such as high blood pressure and high cholesterol levels) should work closely with their doctor to reduce their likelihood of heart attack and heart failure.

Finally, diagnosing and treating heart failure before the heart becomes severely damaged can improve the prognosis. With proper treatment, many patients may continue to lead active lives for a number of years.

Heart-lung machine

The heart-lung machine is an essential component in **open-heart surgery**. Blood from the veins is shunted via catheter to the machine, which introduces oxygen into the blood and then pumps the blood back into the patient's arteries. With the machine thus performing all the functions of the heart and lungs, the heart itself can be stopped while surgery is performed. Before the heart-lung machine, heart surgeons operated blindly, either with the heart still pumping, by slowly chilling the patient's body until circulation nearly stopped, or by connecting the patient's circulatory system to a second person's system during the operation. All of these methods were extremely risky.

While the idea of a heart-lung machine had been proposed as long ago as 1812, the device was not developed until American surgeon, John H. Gibbon, Jr. (1903-1974), decided in 1931 to build a heart-lung machine after a young female patient died of blocked lung circulation. At the time, experimental devices existed for pumping and oxygenating blood during perfusion (artificial circulation). Gibbon, who received his medical degree in 1927 from Jefferson Medical College, began his heart-lung work in 1934 at Massachusetts General Hospital during a research fellowship with the assistance of research technician Mary Hopkinson, who later became his wife. They found the action of roller pumps gentle enough to minimize both clotting and damage to blood cells, and they employed centrifugal force to spread the blood in a layer thin enough to absorb the required amounts of oxygen. In 1935 the Gibbons went to the University of Pennsylvania School of Medicine and continued their experiments, reporting successful results with animals by 1939. In 1946 John Gibbon became head of the surgical department at his alma mater and soon secured the backing of Thomas J. Watson, chairman of IBM. With the use of IBM laboratories and engineers, Gibbon's heart-lung machine was perfected after the introduction of wire-mesh screens to enhance oxygenation, filters to block air bubbles or clots, and monitoring devices. By 1952, the heart-lung bypass surgery had a ninety percent success rate on animals, and Gibbon decided to use the machine on a human patient. The first attempt failed, although the pump-oxygenator worked as required. On May 6, 1953, the second surgery using the heart-lung machine was successfully performed on Cecilia Bavolek. Despite the deaths of two subsequent patients, the era of open-heart surgery had begun. The heart-lung machine was rapidly improved: oxygenation, for example, was accomplished by more sophisticated methods. Once patients could be kept alive during heart surgery, a whole new range of operations became possible. Congenital heart defects could be repaired, diseased or damaged valves could be replaced, and **coronary bypass surgery** became possible through sewing in a replacement blood vessel to carry blood flow around a blocked section of artery. Thanks to Gibbon's heart-lung machine, open-heart surgery—especially coronary bypass—has become routine throughout the world.

By the late 1990s, a laser system being used in many protocols across the United States, allowed traditional bypass surgery without the heart-lung machine. This surgery requires only a small incision between the ribs (no cutting of the chest bone as with traditional bypass surgery) to expose the heart muscle. The laser is aimed at the portion of the heart starved for oxygen and, synchronized with the heartbeat, fires automatically when the ventricle is full of blood until about 20 to 40 new channels are created through the wall of the heart muscle. The outside of these channel heals almost immediately while the inside remains open. As the heart pumps, blood is forced from the left ventricle into these new channels, providing oxygenated blood to the previously starved section. This surgery takes one-to-two hours as opposed to the four-to-six required for traditional bypass surgery.

Heart murmurs

A heart murmur is an abnormal, extra sound during the heartbeat cycle made by blood moving through the heart and its valves. It is detected by the doctor's examination using a **stethoscope**.

A heart beating normally makes two sounds: ''lubb'' when the valves in one part of the heart close, and ''dupp'' when other valves close. A heart murmur is a series of vibratory sounds made by turbulent blood flow. The sounds last longer than normal heart sounds and can be heard between the normal sounds of the heart.

Heart murmurs are common in children, but they can also result from heart or valve defects. Nearly two thirds of heart murmurs in children are produced by a normal heart and are harmless. This type of heart murmur is usually called an ''innocent'' murmur. Innocent heart murmurs are typically very faint, intermittent, and occur in a small area of the chest. ''Pathologic'' heart murmurs involve disease and may indicate the presence of a serious heart defect. They are louder, continual, and may be accompanied by a click or gallop.

Some heart murmurs are continually present; others happen only when the heart is working harder than usual, including during **exercise** or certain types of illness.

Innocent heart murmurs are caused by blood flowing through the chambers and valves of the heart or the blood vessels near the heart. Sometimes **anxiety**, **stress**, **fever**, **anemia**, overactive thyroid, and **pregnancy** will cause innocent murmurs that can be heard by a physician using a stethoscope. Pathologic heart murmurs, however, are caused by structural problems of the heart. These include defective heart valves or holes in the walls of the heart. Valve problems are more common. Valves that do not open completely cause blood to flow through a smaller opening than normal, while those that do not close properly may cause blood to go back through the valve. A hole in the wall between the left and right sides of the heart, called a septal defect, can cause heart murmurs. Some septal defects close on their own; others require surgery to prevent progressive damage to the heart.

Symptoms of heart murmurs differ depending on the cause. Innocent heart murmurs and those which do not impair the function of the heart have no symptoms. Murmurs due to severe abnormalities of a heart valve may cause **shortness of breath**, **dizziness**, chest **pain**s, **palpitations**, and lung congestion.

Heart murmurs can be heard when a physician listens to the heart through a stethoscope during a regular check-up. Very loud heart murmurs and those with clicks or extra heart sounds should be evaluated further. Infants with heart murmurs who do not thrive, eat, or breath properly and older children who lose consciousness suddenly or are intolerant to exercise should also be evaluated further. If the murmur sounds suspicious, the physician may order a **chest x ray**, an **electrocardiogram**, and an **echocardiogram**.

An electrocardiogram (ECG) shows the heart's activity and may reveal muscle thickening, damage, or a lack of oxygen. Electrodes covered with conducting jelly are placed on the patient's chest, arms, and legs. They send impulses of the heart's activity to a recorder which traces them on paper. The test takes about 10 minutes and is commonly performed in the doctor's office. An exercise ECG (a stress test conducted on a treadmill or stationary bicycle) can reveal additional information.

An echocardiogram (cardiac ultrasound), may be ordered to identify a structural problem that is causing the heart murmur. An echocardiogram uses sound waves to create an image of the heart's chambers and valves. The technician applies gel to a hand-held transducer, then presses it against the patient's chest. The sound waves are converted into an image that can be displayed on a monitor. Performed in a cardiology outpatient diagnostic laboratory, the test takes 30 minutes to an hour.

Innocent heart murmurs do not affect the patient's health and require no treatment. Heart murmurs due to septal defects may require surgery. Those due to valvular defects may require **antibiotics** to prevent infection during certain surgical or dental procedures. Severely damaged or diseased valves can be repaired or replaced through surgery.

Most children with innocent heart murmurs grow out of them by the time they reach adulthood. Severe causes of heart murmurs may progress to severe symptoms and **death**.

If the heart murmur is innocent, heart activity can be supported using the herb hawthorn (*Crataegus laevigata* or *C. oxyacantha*) or coenzyme Q10. These remedies improve heart contractility and the heart's ability to use oxygen. If the murmur originates in the valves, herbs that act like antibiotics may be considered, as well as options that build resistance to infection.

HEART SURGERY FOR CONGENITAL DEFECTS

A variety of surgical procedures can be performed to repair the many types of heart defects that may be present at birth (congenital defects). Heart surgery is done to correct such defects to the greatest extent possible and to improve the flow of blood and oxygen to the body. While congenital heart defects vary in their severity, most require surgery.

Surgery is recommended for defects that result in a lack of oxygen, a poor quality of life, or a child who does not gain sufficient weight. Some types of congenital heart defects that cause no symptoms are nonetheless treated surgically because they can lead to serious complications.

There are many types of congenital heart defects. Most obstruct the flow of blood in the heart, or the vessels near it, or cause abnormal blood flow through the heart. Rarer types include newborns born with one ventricle, one side of the heart that is not completely formed, or the pulmonary artery and the aorta coming out of the same ventricle. Most congenital heart defects require surgery during infancy or childhood. Sometimes, multiple surgical procedures are necessary.

These procedures are performed under general **anesthesia**. Some require the use of a **heart-lung machine**, which cools the body to reduce the need for oxygen and takes over for the heart and lungs during the procedure.

Before surgery for congenital heart defects, the patient will receive a complete evaluation, which includes a **physical exam**, a detailed family history, a **chest x ray**, an **electrocardiogram**, an **echocardiogram**, and usually cardiac catheterization. For six to eight hours before the surgery, the patient cannot eat or drink anything. An electrocardiogram shows the heart's activity and may reveal a lack of oxygen. Electrodes covered with conducting jelly are placed on the patient's chest, arms, and legs and the heart's impulses are traced on paper. An echocardiogram uses sound waves to create an image of the heart's chambers and valves. Gel is applied to a hand-held transducer and then pressed against the patient's chest. Cardiac catheterization is an invasive diagnostic technique used to evaluate the heart, in which a long tube is inserted into a blood vessel and guided into the heart. A contrast solution is injected to make the heart visible on x rays.

After heart surgery for congenital defects, the patient goes to an intensive care ward where he or she is connected to a variety of tubes and monitors, including a ventilator. Patients are monitored every 15 minutes until vital signs (pulse and breathing rate, for example) are stable. Heart sounds, oxygenation of the blood, and the electrocardiogram are monitored. Chest tubes will be checked to ensure that they are draining properly and there is no bleeding. **Pain** medications will be administered. Complications such as stroke, lung blood clots, and reduced blood flow to the kidneys will be watched for. After the ventilator and breathing tube are removed, chest physical therapy and exercises to improve circulation will be started.

Complications from heart surgery for congenital defects can be severe. They include shock, congestive heart failure, lack of oxygen or too much carbon dioxide in the blood, irregular heartbeat, **stroke**, infection, kidney damage, lung blood clot, low blood pressure, hemorrhage, cardiac arrest, and **death**.

Smaller congenital heart defects can now be repaired in a cardiac catheterization lab instead of an operating room. Cardiac catheterization procedures can save the lives of critically ill newborns and in some cases eliminate or delay more invasive surgical procedures. It is expected that catheterization procedures will continue to replace more types of surgery for congenital heart defects in the future. A thin tube called a catheter is inserted into an artery or vein in the leg, groin, or arm and threaded into the area of the heart which needs repair. The patient receives a local anesthetic at the insertion site and is awake but sedated during the procedure.

HEART VALVE DISORDERS

There are various kinds of heart valve disorders. Five major ones are mitral valve insufficiency, mitral valve prolapse, mitral valve stenosis, tricuspid valve insufficiency, and tricuspid valve stenosis.

Mitral valve insufficiency is a term used when the valve between the upper left chamber of the heart (atrium) and the lower left chamber (ventricle) doesn't close well enough to prevent back flow of blood when the ventricle contracts. Mitral valve insufficiency is also known as mitral valve regurgitation or mitral valve incompetence.

Mitral valve prolapse (MVP) is a ballooning of the support structures of the mitral heart valve into the left upper collection chamber of the heart.

The term stenosis means an abnormal narrowing of an opening. Mitral valve stenosis refers to a condition in the heart in which one of the valve openings has become narrow and restricts the flow of blood from the upper left chamber (left atrium) to the lower left chamber (left ventricle).

Tricuspid valve insufficiency occurs when a tricuspid valve does not close tightly enough to prevent leakage. This condition is also called tricuspid valve regurgitation and tricuspid incompetence.

Tricuspid valve stenosis is a narrowing or stiffening of the opening in the valve. This stenosis causes increased resistance to blood flow through the valve.

Normally, blood enters the left atrium of the heart from the lungs and is pumped through the mitral valve into the left ventricle. The left ventricle contracts to pump the blood forward into the aorta. The aorta is a large artery that sends oxygenated blood through the circulatory system to all of the tissues in the body. If the mitral valve is leaky due to mitral valve insufficiency, it allows some blood to get pushed back into the atrium. This extra blood creates an increase in pressure in the atrium, which then increases blood pressure in the vessels that bring the blood from the lungs to the heart. Increased pressure in these vessels can result in increased fluid buildup in the lungs.

When these structures weaken or lengthen abnormally, the valve may balloon into the left atrium. Sometimes this can cause the mitral valve to leak blood backward.

This condition may be inherited and occurs in approximately 10% of the population. It affects more women than men and often peaks after the age of 40.

If the mitral valve is abnormally narrow, due to disease or birth defect, blood flow from the atrium to the ventricle is restricted. This restricted flow leads to an increase in the pressure of blood in the left atrium. Over a period of time, this back pressure causes fluid to leak into the lungs. It can also lead to an abnormal heart rhythm (atrial fibrillation), which further decreases the efficiency of the pumping action of the heart.

The tricuspid valve is located between the right atrium and the right ventricle of the heart. When the right ventricle contracts, it is supposed to pump blood forward into the lungs. If the tricuspid valve does not close tightly, some of that blood leaks back into the right atrium. When the atrium receives its usual quantity of blood from veins leading to the heart, plus the leaking blood, the pressure inside the atrium increases. This higher pressure creates resistance to the flow of blood in the veins that enter the atrium from the body. In addition, this increase in pressure causes the right atrium to enlarge over time. Congestion from fluid buildup occurs, particularly in the liver and legs.

The tricuspid valve is the largest of the four valves in the heart. When it is narrowed or stiffened, it decreases the amount of blood that can flow through it. This decrease raises the pressure in the right atrium and causes the atrium to enlarge. It also causes the right ventricle to shrink, and lowers the cardiac output.

In the past, **rheumatic fever** was the most common cause of mitral valve insufficiency. However, the increased use of **antibiotics** for **strep throat** has made rheumatic fever rare in developed countries. In these countries, mitral valve insufficiency caused by rheumatic fever is seen mostly in the elderly. In countries with less developed health care, rheumatic fever is still common and is often a cause of mitral valve insufficiency.

Heart attacks that damage the structures that support the mitral valve are a common cause of mitral valve insufficiency. Myxomatous degeneration can cause a ''floppy'' mitral valve that leaks. In other cases, the valve simply deteriorates with age and becomes less efficient.

People with mitral valve insufficiency may not have any symptoms at all. It is often discovered during a doctor's visit when the doctor listens to the heart sounds.

Both the left atrium and left ventricle tend to get a little bigger when the mitral valve does not work properly. The ventricle has to pump more blood so it gets bigger to increase the force of each beat. The atrium gets bigger to hold the extra blood. An enlarged ventricle can cause **palpitations**. An enlarged atrium can develop an erratic rhythm (atrial fibrillation), which reduces its efficiency and can lead to blood clots forming in the atrium.

MVP may occur due to rheumatic heart disease but is usually found in healthy people. Changes that occur in the valve are caused by rapid multiplication of cells in the middle layer that presses on the outer layer. The outer layer weakens, causing a prolapse of the valve toward the left atrium.

Most persons do not have symptoms. Those that do may experience sharp, left-sided chest **pain**. Some complain of fatigue, or a pounding feeling in the chest. Others can have an irregular heart beat and even pass out. Some persons may experience difficulty breathing, ankle swelling, and fluid in the lungs. Other symptoms may include **anxiety**, **headache**s, morning tiredness, and constantly cold hands and feet. **Death** from this condition is rare.

Mitral valve stenosis is also almost always caused by rheumatic fever. As a result of rheumatic fever, the leaflets that form the opening of the valve are partially fused together. Mitral valve stenosis can also be present at birth. Babies born with this problem usually require surgery if they are to survive. Sometimes, growths or tumors can block the mitral valve, mimicking mitral valve stenosis.

If the restriction is severe, the increased blood pressure can lead to **heart failure**. The first symptoms of heart failure, which are fatigue and **shortness of breath**, usually appear only during physical activity. As the condition gets worse, symptoms may also be felt even during rest. A person may also develop a deep red coloring in the cheeks.

Tricuspid valve insufficiency usually produces vague symptoms, such as general weakness and fatigue. As the conditions worsens, a person experiences pain in the upper right part of the abdomen, caused by a congested and enlarged liver. The legs may also swell (**edema**).

Tricuspid valve stenosis, again, is most often the result of rheumatic fever. On rare occasions, it is caused by a tumor or disease of the connective tissue. The rarest cause is a **birth defect**.

A person with tricuspid valve stenosis may experience generalized weakness and fatigue. Many people have palpitations and can feel fluttering in their neck. Over time, there may be pain in the upper right abdomen, due to increased congestion and enlargement of the liver.

When the doctor listens to the heart sounds, mitral valve insufficiency is generally recognized by the sound the blood makes as it leaks backward. It sounds like a regurgitant murmur. The next step is generally a **chest x ray** and an electrocardiogram (ECG) to see if the heart is enlarged. The most definitive noninvasive test is **echocardiography**, a test that uses sound waves to make an image of the heart. This test gives a picture of the valve in action and shows the severity of the problem.

The diagnosis of MVP is based on symptoms and physical exam. During the exam, the physician may hear a click and/or heart murmur with a stethoscope. The best diagnostic test for MVP is the echocardiogram.

Mitral valve stenosis is usually detected by a physician listening to heart sounds. Normal heart valves open silently to permit the flow of blood. A stenotic valve makes a snapping sound followed by a ''rumbling'' murmur. The condition can be confirmed with a chest x ray and an electrocardiogram, both of which will show an enlarged atrium. If surgery is necessary, cardiac catheterization may be done to fully evaluate the heart before the operation.

A severely impaired valve needs to be repaired or replaced. Either option will require surgery. Repairing the valve can fix the problem completely or reduce it enough to make it bearable and prevent damage to the heart. Valves can be replaced with either a mechanical valve or one that is partly mechanical and partly from a pig's heart.

Mechanical valves are effective but can increase the incidence of blood clots. To prevent blood clots from forming, the patient will need to take drugs that prevent abnormal blood clotting (**anticoagulants**). The valves made partly from a pigs heart don't have as great a risk of blood clots, but they don't last as long as fully mechanical valves. If a valve wears out, it must be replaced again.

Repair can be accomplished in two ways. In the first method, balloon valvuloplasty, the doctor will try to stretch the valve opening by threading a thin tube (catheter) with a balloon tip through a vein and into the heart. Once the catheter is positioned in the valve, the balloon is inflated, separating the fused areas. The second method involves opening the heart and surgically separating the fused areas.

Damaged heart valves are easily infected. Anytime a procedure is contemplated that might allow infectious organisms to enter the blood, the person with mitral valve insufficiency should take antibiotics to prevent possible infection.

Persons who experience certain types of an irregular heartbeat with MVP should be treated. Propranolol (Inderal) or other **beta blockers** or digoxin (Lanoxin) are often helpful. Persons who develop moderate to severe symptoms with a leaky mitral valve may require repair or replacement of the mitral valve with an artificial heart valve. Persons with MVP and a leaky valve need to protect themselves from heart or heart valve infections. Antibiotics should be taken before any surgical, dental or oral procedures according to the American Heart Association recommendations.

Tricuspid valve insufficiency itself usually does not require treatment, since a tiny leakage occurs in most normal people. In certain cases, however, if there is underlying pulmonary valve disease or lung disease, those conditions should be treated.

If irregular heart rhythms or heart failure are present, they are usually treated independently of the valve insufficiency.

Since a person with known tricuspid valve insufficiency is at risk for infections of the heart, antibiotics should be taken before and after oral or dental surgery, or urologic procedures.

Tricuspid valve stenosis itself usually doesn't require treatment. However, if there is damage to other valves in the heart as well, then surgical repair or replacement must be considered.

The only possible way to prevent mitral valve insufficiency and stenosis, as well as tricuspid valve stenosis, is to prevent rheumatic fever. This can be done by evaluating sore throats for the presence of the bacteria that causes strep throat. Strep throat is easily treated with antibiotics.

In general, tricuspid valve insufficiency cannot be prevented.

Heat disorders

Heat disorders are a group of related illnesses caused by prolonged exposure to hot temperatures, restricted fluid intake, or failure of the body's temperature regulation mechanisms. Disorders related to heat exposure include heat cramps, heat exhaustion, and heat **stroke** (also called sunstroke). Heat stroke is especially dangerous and requires immediate medical attention.

As perspiration evaporates from the skin during hot weather, the body is cooled. Salt helps the cells retain water. If the body loses too much salt and fluids, the symptoms of **dehydration** can occur. In hot weather, a healthy body loses enough water to cool itself while creating the lowest level of chemical imbalance. The healthy body maintains a temperature of approximately 98.6°F (37°C) regardless of surrounding conditions.

Heat cramps are the least severe of the heat-related illnesses. They are often the first signal that the body is having difficulty with increased temperature. Think of heat cramps as a warning sign to a potential heat-related emergency. They are painful muscle spasms caused by excessive loss of salts (electrolytes) due to heavy perspiration. They occur more often in the legs and abdomen than in other areas of the body. Individuals at higher risk are those working in extreme heat, elderly people, young children, people with health problems, and those who are unable to naturally and properly cool their bodies. Individuals with poor circulation and who take medications to reduce excess body fluids can be at risk when conditions are hot and humid.

The care of heat cramps includes placing the individual at rest in a cool environment, while giving cool water with a teaspoon of salt per quart, or a commercial sports drink. Usually rest and liquids are all that is needed. Mild stretching and massaging of the muscle area can follow once the condition improves. The individual should not take salt tablets, since this may actually worsen the condition. When the cramps stop, activity can usually be started again if there are no other signs of illness. The individual needs to continue drinking fluids and should be watched carefully for further signs.

Heat exhaustion, more serious and complex than heat cramps, often affects athletes, firefighters, construction workers, factory workers, and anyone who wears heavy clothing in hot humid weather. The skin may appear cool, moist, and pale. The individual may complain of **headache** and **nausea** with a feeling of overall weakness and exhaustion. **Dizziness**, faintness, and mental confusion are often present, as is rapid and weak pulse. Breathing becomes fast and shallow. Fluid loss reduces blood volume and lowers blood pressure. Yellow or orange urine often is a result of inadequate fluid intake, along with associated intense thirst.

Individuals suffering from heat exhaustion should stop all physical activity and move immediately to a cool place out of the sun, preferably an air-conditioned location. They should then lay down with feet slightly elevated, remove or loosen clothing, and drink cold (but not iced), slightly salty water or commercial sports drink. This is often all the treatment that is needed, and the person usually recovers within one or two days.

Heat exhaustion can develop rapidly into heat stroke, which can be life threatening. Because the percentage of victims dying from heat stroke is very high, immediate medical attention is critical when problems first begin. The body's temperature reaches a dangerous level, higher than 104°F (40°C) and as high as 106°F (41.1°C). Other symptoms include mental confusion with possible combativeness and bizarre behavior, staggering, and faintness. The pulse becomes strong and rapid (160–180 beats per minute) with the skin taking on a dry and flushed appearance. There is often very little perspiration. The individual can quickly lose consciousness or have convulsions.

Simply moving the individual afflicted with heat stroke to a cooler place is not enough to reverse the internal overheating. Emergency medical assistance should be called immediately. While waiting for help to arrive, quick action to lower body temperature must take place. Clothes should be loosened or removed, allowing air to circulate around the body. Next, the individual should be wrapped in wet towels or clothing, with ice packs placed in areas with the greatest blood supply. These areas include the neck, under the arm and knees, and in the groin. Once the patient is under medical care, **cooling treatments** may continue as appropriate. Body temperature should be monitored constantly to guard against overcooling. Breathing and heart rate should also be monitored closely, and a health professional may replace fluids and electrolytes intravenously. **Anti-convulsant drugs** may be given. After severe heat stroke, bed rest may be recommended for several days. Heat stroke is a very serious condition and its outcome depends upon general health and age. Due to the high internal temperature of heat stroke, permanent damage to internal organs is possible.

Because heat cramps, heat exhaustion, and heat stroke have a cascade effect on each other, the prevention of the onset of all heat disorders is similar. Avoid strenuous exercise when it is very hot. Individuals exposed to extreme heat conditions should drink plenty of fluids. It is important to wear light and loose-fitting clothing, and to consume water often without waiting until thirst develops. Eating lightly salted foods can help replace salts lost through perspiration. Ventilation in working areas can be improved by opening a window or using an electric fan. Sunblocks and **sunscreens** with a protection factor of 15 (SPF 15) can be very helpful in extreme direct sunlight.

Heat disorders are harmful to people of all ages, but their severity is likely to increase as people age. Heat cramps in a 16-year-old may be heat exhaustion in a 45-year-old and heat stroke in a 65-year-old.

HEAT TREATMENTS

Heat treatments are applied to body areas that are injured or functioning in an abnormal way.

The general purposes of a heat treatment are to improve the flexibility of soft tissues, remove toxic substances, enhance blood flow, increase function of tissue cells, encourage muscle relaxation, and help relieve **pain**. There are two types of heat treatments: superficial and deep. Superficial treatments apply heat to the outside of the body. Deep heat treatments direct it toward specific inner tissues through **ultrasound** or electric current. Heat treatments are beneficial prior to exercise, providing a warm-up effect.

Hot packs are a very common form of heat treatment. Moist heat packs are readily available in most hospitals, physical therapy centers, and athletic training rooms. Treatment temperature should not exceed 131°F (55°C). The pack is used over multiple layers of toweling to achieve a comfortable warming effect for approximately 30 minutes.

Hot-water bottles are another form of superficial heat treatment. The bottles are filled half-way with hot water between 115–125°F (46.1–52°C). Covered by a protective toweling, the bottle is placed on the treatment area and left until the water has cooled.

Electrical heating pads continue to be used, however because of the need for an electrical outlet, safety and convenience become issues.

Paraffin is often used for heating uneven surfaces of the body such as the hands. It consists of melted paraffin wax and mineral oil. While solid at room temperature, parrafin is used as a liquid heat treatment when heated to 126–127.4°F (52–53°C). The most common form of paraffin application is called the dip-and-wax method. In this technique, the patient will dip 8–12 times and then the extremity will be covered with a plastic bag and a towel for insulation. Most treatment sessions are about 20 minutes.

Hydrotherapy tanks or pools are used to treat many musculoskeletal disorders. The water is generally set at warm temperatures, never exceeding 150°F (65.6°C). Because the patient often performs resistance exercises while in the water, higher temperatures become a concern as the treatment becomes more physically draining. Because of this, many hydrotherapy baths are now set at 95–110°F (35–43.3°C). There are also units available with moveable turbine jets, which provide a light massage effect.

Fluidotherapy is a form of heat treatment developed in the 1970s. It uses dry heat in the form of cellulose particles suspended in air. Temperatures in this treatment range from 110–123°F (43.3–50.5°C). Fluidotherapy allows the patient to exercise the limb during the treatment, and also provides massage, increasing blood flow.

Ultrasound heat treatments penetrate the body, providing relief to inner tissue. Ultrasound energy comes from the acoustic or sound spectrum, but is not detected by the human ear. Using conducting agents such as gel or mineral oil, the ultrasound transducer warms muscle tissue and other connective tissue such as ligaments and tendons. Fat, however, absorbs the energy to a much lesser degree. Ultrasound has a relatively longlasting effect, continuing up to one hour.

Diathermy is another deep-heat treatment. An electrode drum is used to apply heat to an affected area. It consists of a wire coil surrounded by an insulating plastic housing. Plenty of toweling must be layered between the unit and the patient. This device is helpful with chronic **low back pain** and muscle spasms. Prior to ultrasound technology, diathermy was a popular heat therapy of the 1940s–1960s.

Once heat treatment has been completed, any symptoms of **dizziness** and **nausea** should be noted and documented along with any skin irritations or discoloring not previously present. A one-hour interval between treatments is needed to avoid restriction of blood flow.

Supervision should be present during any form of heat treatment, especially hydrotherapy. All heat treatments can potentially damage tissue, if temperatures are excessive. In all cases, proper insulation and length of treatment should be carefully administered. Overexposure during a superficial heat treatment may result in redness, blisters, **burns**, or reduced blood circulation. During ultrasound therapy, excessive treatment over bony areas with little soft tissue (such as hand, feet, and elbow) can cause excessive heat resulting in pain and possible tissue damage. Exposure to the electrode drum during diathermy may produce hot spots.

Heat treatments should not be used on individuals with circulation problems, heat intolerance, or lack of sensation in the affected area. Low blood circulation may contribute to heat-related injuries. Heat treatments also should not be used on individuals afflicted with heart, lung, or kidney diseases. Deep heat treatments should not be used on areas above the eye, heart, or on a pregnant patient. Deep heat treatments over areas with metal surgical implants should be avoided in case of rapid temperature increase and subsequent injury.

HEAVY METAL POISONING

Heavy metal poisoning is the toxic accumulation of heavy metals in the soft tissues of the body.

Heavy metals are chemical elements that have a specific gravity (a measure of density) at least five times that of water. The heavy metals most often involved in human poisoning are lead, mercury, arsenic, and cadmium. Some heavy metals, such as zinc, copper, chromium, iron, and manganese, are required by the body in small amounts, but these same elements can be toxic in larger quantities.

Heavy metals may enter the body in food, water, or air, or by absorption through the skin. Once in the body, they compete with essential **minerals** such as zinc, copper, magnesium, and calcium, and interfere with the function of the organs. People may come in contact with heavy metals in industrial work, pharmaceutical manufacturing, and agriculture. Children may be poisoned as a result of playing in contaminated soil.

Symptoms will vary, depending on the nature and the quantity of the heavy metal ingested. Patients may complain of **nausea**, vomiting, **diarrhea**, stomach **pain**, **headache**, **sweating**, and a metallic taste in the mouth. Depending on the metal, there may be blue-black lines in the gums. In severe cases, patients exhibit obvious impairment of awareness, judgment, language, and motor skills. The expression ''mad as a hatter'' comes from the mercury **poisoning** prevalent in 17th-century France among hatmakers who soaked animal hides in a solution of mercuric nitrate to soften the hair.

Heavy metal poisoning may be detected using blood and urine tests, hair and tissue analysis, or x ray. If acute arsenic poisoning is suspected, an x ray may reveal arsenic in the abdomen (since arsenic is opaque to x rays).

The treatment for most heavy metal poisoning is **chelation therapy**. A chelating agent specific to the metal involved is given either by mouth, injection or intravenously. The three most common chelating agents are calcium disodium edetate, dimercaprol, and penicillamine. The chelating agent binds to the metal in the body's tissues, forming a complex; which is then released to the bloodstream. The complex is filtered out of the blood by the kidneys and excreted in the urine. This process may be lengthy and painful, and typically requires hospitalization. Chelation therapy is effective in treating lead, mercury, and arsenic poisoning, but is not useful in cadmium poisoning. To date, no treatment has been proven effective for cadmium poisoning.

In cases of acute mercury or arsenic ingestion, vomiting may be induced. A health professional may decide to wash out the stomach (gastric lavage). The patient may also require treatment such as intravenous fluids for complications of poisoning such as **shock**, **anemia**, and **kidney failure**.

The chelation process can only halt further effects of the poisoning; it cannot reverse neurological damage already sustained.

Because exposure to heavy metals is often an occupational hazard, protective clothing and respirators should be provided and worn on the job. Protective clothing should then be left at the work site and not worn home, where it could carry toxic dust to family members. Industries are urged to reduce or replace the heavy metals in their processes wherever possible. Exposure to environmental sources of lead, including lead-based paints, plumbing fixtures, vehicle exhaust, and contaminated soil, should be reduced or eliminated.

HEIMLICH MANEUVER

The Heimlich maneuver is an emergency procedure for removing a foreign object lodged in the airway that is preventing a person from breathing.

Every year about 3,000 adults die because they accidentally inhale rather than swallow food. The food blocks their windpipe (trachea), making breathing impossible. Death follows rapidly unless the food or other foreign material can be displaced from the airway.

The Heimlich maneuver, or abdominal thrusts, is simple enough that it can be performed immediately by anyone trained in the maneuver. By compressing the abdomen, air is forced out of the lungs, dislodging the obstruction and bringing the foreign material up into the mouth.

The maneuver is used mainly when solid material like food, coins, vomit, or small toys are blocking the airway. There has been some controversy about whether it is appropriate to use routinely on near-drowning victims. The American Red Cross and American Heart Association both recommend that the Heimlich maneuver be used only as a last resort, after traditional airway clearance techniques and **cardiopulmonary resuscitation** (CPR) have been tried repeatedly and failed, or if it is clear that a solid foreign object is blocking the airway.

The Heimlich maneuver can be performed on all people, but modifications are necessary if the **choking** victim is very obese, pregnant, a child, or an infant.

Indications that a person's airway is blocked include:

- The person can not speak or cry out.
- The face turns blue from lack of oxygen.
- The person desperately grabs at his or her throat.
- The person has a weak **cough**, and labored breathing produces a high-pitched noise.
- The person does all of the above, then becomes unconscious.

To perform the Heimlich maneuver on a conscious adult, the rescuer stands behind the victim, who may either be sitting or standing. The rescuer makes a fist with one hand, and places it, thumb toward the victim, below the rib cage and above the waist. The rescuer encircles the victim's waist, placing his other hand on top of the fist.

In a series of 6–10 sharp and distinct thrusts upward and inward, the rescuer attempts to develop enough pressure to force the foreign object back up the trachea. If the maneuver fails, it is repeated. It is important not to give up if the first attempt fails. As the victim is deprived of oxygen, the muscles of the trachea relax slightly. Because of this loosening, it is possible that the foreign object may be expelled on a second or third attempt.

Unconscious victims should be laid on the floor. Bend the chin forward, make sure the tongue is not blocking the airway, and feel in the mouth for **foreign objects**, being careful not to push any farther into the airway. The rescuer kneels astride the victim's thighs and places his or her fists between the bottom of the victim's breastbone and the navel. The rescuer then executes a series of 6–10 sharp compressions by pushing inward and upward.

After the abdominal thrusts, the rescuer repeats the process of lifting the chin, moving the tongue, feeling for and possibly removing the foreign material. If the airway is not clear, the rescuer repeats the abdominal thrusts as often as necessary. If the foreign object has been removed, but the victim is not breathing, the rescuer starts CPR.

In pregnant or very obese people, the main difference in performing the Heimlich maneuver is in the placement of the fists. Instead of abdominal thrusts, chest thrusts are used. The fists are placed against the middle of the breastbone, and the motion of the thrust is in and downward, rather than upward. If the victim is unconscious, the thrusts are similar to those used in CPR.

The technique in children over one year of age is the same as in adults, except that the force used is less than used with adults, to avoid damaging the child's ribs, breastbone, and internal organs.

With infants less than one year old, the rescuer sits down and lays the infant along his or her forearm with the face pointed toward the floor. The rescuer's hand supports the infant's head, and with the rescuer's forearm resting on his or her own thigh for additional support. Using the heel of the other hand, the rescuer administers four or five rapid blows to the infant's back between the shoulder blades.

After the back blows, the rescuer sandwiches the infant between his or her arms, and turns the infant over so that the child is lying face up supported by the opposite arm. Using the free hand, the rescuer places the index and middle finger on the center of the breastbone and makes four sharp chest thrusts. This series of back blows and chest thrusts is alternated until the foreign object is expelled.

To apply the Heimlich maneuver to yourself, make a fist with one hand and place it in the middle of the body at a spot above the navel but below the breastbone, then grasp the fist with the other hand and push sharply inward and upward. If this fails, press the upper abdomen over the back of a chair, edge of a table, porch railing or something similar, and thrust up and inward until the object is dislodged.

Before doing the maneuver on anyone, it is important to determine if the airway is completely blocked. If the person choking can talk or cry, Heimlich maneuver is not appropriate. If the airway is not completely blocked, the choking victim should be allowed to try to cough up the foreign object on his or her own.

Many people vomit after being treated with the Heimlich maneuver. Depending on the length and severity of the choking episode, the choking victim may need to be taken to a hospital emergency room.

Incorrectly applied, the Heimlich maneuver can break bones or damage internal organs. In infants, the rescuer should never attempt to sweep the baby's mouth without looking to remove foreign material. This is likely to push the material farther down the trachea.

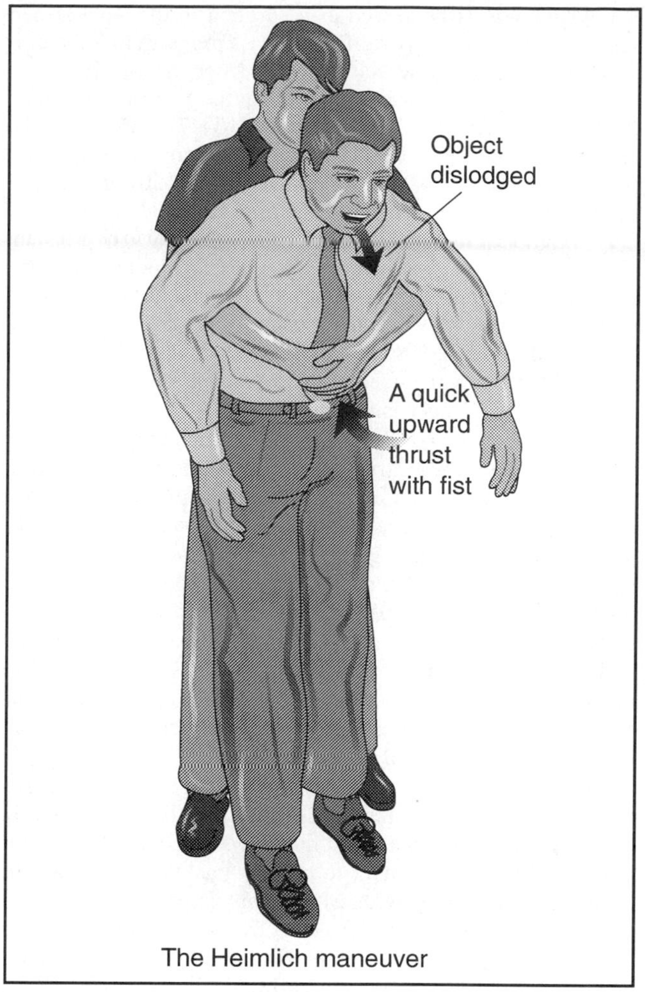

To perform the Heimlich maneuver on a conscious adult (as illustrated above), the rescuer stands behind the victim and encircles his waist. The rescuer makes a fist with one hand and places the other hand on top, positioned below the rib cage and above the waist. The rescuer then applies pressure by a series of upward and inward thrusts to force the foreign object back up the victim's trachea. ***(Illustration by Electronic Illustrators Group.)***

HEIMLICH, HENRY JAY (1920-)

American surgeon and inventor

Henry Jay Heimlich has achieved wide recognition for the **Heimlich maneuver**, a lifesaving squeeze that has replaced the backslap as a remedy for choking and is responsible for the saving of thousands of lives. Among his other innovations are a surgical procedure for replacing a damaged esophagus by using a flap from the patient's stomach, a simple emergency chest drainage device for victims of chest wounds, and a long-lasting portable oxygen tank to enhance mobility for victims of chronic lung disease. His publications include a home guidebook to emergency medicine, and he is a frequent and popular lecturer on medical topics. His public visibility, which began with his development of the Heimlich maneuver, has been heightened by his television appearances and an award-winning television series in which a cartoon Dr. Heimlich teaches first aid to children. He has also produced instructional videos. Heimlich directs the Heimlich Research Institute in Cincinnati, Ohio, where a staff of volunteers aids him in a range of activities, including work on malariotherapy and promotion of Computers for Peace, an international program aimed at preventing war.

Heimlich was born in Wilmington, Delaware, on February 3, 1920, to Philip and Mary Epstein Heimlich. The elder Heimlich was a prison social worker, and as a child Henry accompanied his father on visits to all of New York State's prisons. Heimlich received a bachelor's degree in 1941 from Cornell University, and an M.D. degree in 1943 from Cornell's medical school. His internship at Boston City Hospital was interrupted in 1944 by his entry into the U.S. Navy. During World War II he served as a surgeon in the Gobi Desert of Inner Mongolia, as part of America's program to forge alliances with the Chinese Nationalists. After the war Heimlich spent four years as a surgical resident at the Veterans Administration Hospital in the Bronx (1946–47), Mount Sinai (1947–48) and Bellevue (1948–49) hospitals in New York City, and Triboro Hospital in Jamaica (1949–50). In 1950 he became attending surgeon at Montefiore Hospital in New York City, where he remained through 1969, acting also as assistant clinical professor of surgery at New York Medical College. Heimlich served on the board of the National Cancer Foundation from 1960 to 1970, and was president for five of those years. In the mid–1960s he was also president of Cancer Care, and in 1965 was a member of the President's Commission on Heart Disease, Cancer, and Stroke.

Heimlich's first medical innovation, devised in 1950, was a procedure for gastric tube esophagoplasty, constructing a new esophagus from a section of the patient's stomach. Having first proposed the idea to the chief of surgery at Montefiore to no effect, Heimlich negotiated a small grant and laboratory space at New York Medical College, and tried the procedure on dogs. Although interest in the procedure lagged in the United States, Heimlich's work came to the attention of a surgeon in Bucharest, Romania, who had been performing a similar procedure on humans. Heimlich conferred with the Romanian surgeon and tried the operation on U.S. patients in 1956. It has since become a standard surgical practice.

Heimlich's emergency chest drainage device for use with victims of chest injury was inspired by his World War II experiences. Heimlich's small unit used a flutter valve from a "Bronx cheer" noisemaker to prevent backflow of fluids. He tested it successfully with a hospital patient who was also hooked up to the conventional electrical suction device. The Heimlich chest drainage valve was widely used in Vietnam and is common in emergency facilities.

In 1969 Heimlich became director of surgery at the Jewish Hospital of Cincinnati, Ohio. At about that time he began thinking about a treatment for **choking**, which was the sixth most common cause of accidental deaths in the United States, responsible for about four thousand deaths annually. Heimlich was aware that a hard slap on the back meant to aid a choking victim could easily lodge an obstruction more firmly. As a chest surgeon, Heimlich was also aware of the reserve volume of air that stays in the lungs after exhalation, and he reasoned that this reserve could be used to help expel an object. He tested his ideas on laboratory dogs. He closed off the upper end of an endotracheal tube and put it down the throat of an anesthetized dog; when he compressed the air in the dog's chest, the tube was forced out of the dog's airway. Heimlich found the best results were obtained by a subdiaphragmatic thrust, pushing up suddenly on the soft tissue under the diaphragm. When the technique is applied to humans, a rescuer stands behind the choking victim, wraps his arms around the victim's waist, makes a fist with one hand (thumb side in) and grasps it with the other hand, then gives a quick upward thrust. If a choking victim is lying unconscious, the diaphragm may be compressed by the heel of the rescuer's hand.

In 1974 Heimlich published his study in *Emergency Medicine.* He also brought the article to the attention of the press, and references to it began to appear in newspapers nationwide. A week later, the *Seattle Times* reported that a seventy-year-old restaurateur had saved the life of his neighbor's wife using Heimlich's technique. Many similar stories followed, including cases of children successfully performing the maneuver, and Heimlich was thrust into the national limelight. Heimlich has also defined the symptoms of choking—inability to speak or breathe, pallor followed by bluish skin color, and finally, loss of consciousness and collapse. He has publicized the fact that choking is often mistaken for a **heart attack**—the so-called café coronary. In 1975 the Heimlich maneuver was endorsed by the emergency medical services division of the **American Medical Association**. It was later recommended by the American Red Cross and the American Heart Association, who in addition advised its use with drowning victims. Deaths from choking declined dramatically following widespread publicity about the Heimlich maneuver, and in 1984 Heimlich was recognized with the Albert Lasker Public Service Award.

In 1977 Heimlich became professor of advanced clinical sciences at Xavier University in Cincinnati. There he established the Heimlich Institute to continue work on innovations such as a portable oxygen system, the Micro-Trach. He is the founder and president of the Dysphagia Foundation, and has developed techniques for teaching stroke victims how to swallow. With the philosophy that elimination of war will promote the well-being of the largest number of people, Heimlich has developed Computers for Peace, a program that uses computer projections to show that the benefits of trade among hostile nations are so great it is against the self-interest of nations to go to war.

In 1985 he received a research grant from the Fannie L. Rippel Foundation to study the effects of malariotherapy, a new treatment against **cancer**. Heat was known to kill cancer cells, and Heimlich reasoned that the fevers of **malaria** may be useful in the treatment of cancer. When a cancer patient is deliberately infected with malaria, the resulting fever combats the cancer cells. Once the cancer is under control, drugs can be used to eradicate the malaria organism. The idea is not new; a similar procedure was used in the 1920s against **syphilis**. Heimlich has also advocated malariotherapy for treatment of **Lyme disease**, which like syphilis, is caused by a spirochete and has similar clinical manifestations.

Heimlich's projects are diverse, some are deceptively simple, and many have been controversial. "You're not being original if all your peers agree with what you're doing," he told an *Omni* interviewer in 1983. Heimlich is the author of many scientific and popular articles, and has used television to increase his audience. "I can do more toward saving lives in three minutes on television than I could do all my life in the operating room," he told *Omni.* Heimlich's television series for children, "Dr. Henry's Emergency Lessons for People," won an Emmy Award in 1980. Also in 1980, Heimlich published *Dr. Heimlich's Home Guide to Emergency Medical Situations,* and was named as one of the top ten speakers in the country by the International Platform Association. In 1984 he was honored by the Chinese ministry of health for his World War II service.

He married Jane Murray, daughter of dance studio personalities Arthur and Katherine Murray, on June 3, 1951; they

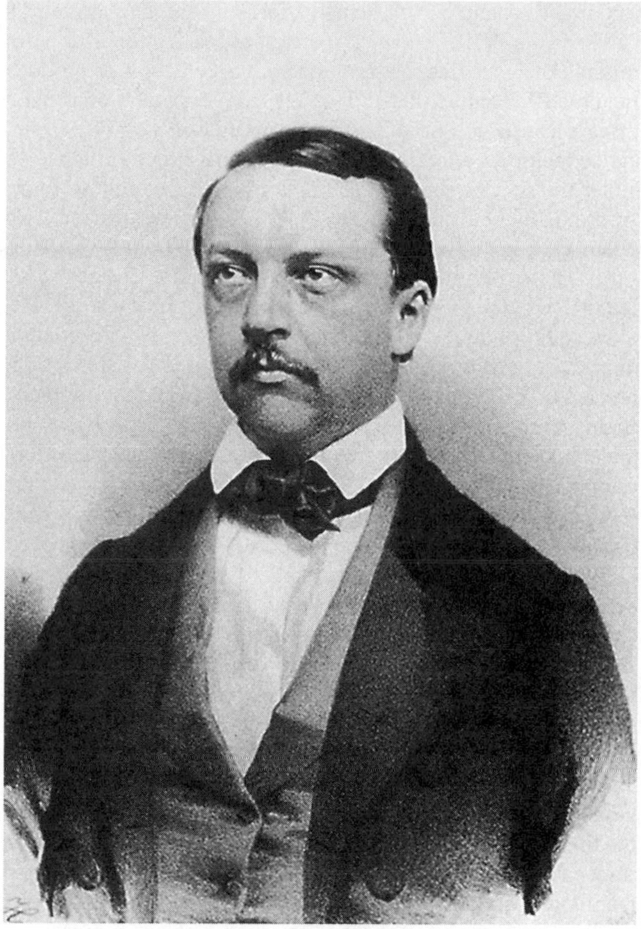

Hermann Ludwig Ferdinand von Helmholtz

have four children: Philip, Peter, and Janet and Elizabeth (twins).

HELMHOLTZ, HERMANN VON (1821-1894)

German physiologist and physicist

Hermann Helmholtz was one of the few scientists to master two disciplines: medicine and physics. He conducted breakthrough research on the **nervous system**, as well as the functions of the **eye** and **ear**. In physics, he is recognized (along with two other scientists) as the author of the concept of conservation of energy.

Helmholtz was born into a poor but scholarly family; his father was an instructor of philosophy and literature at a gymnasium in his hometown of Potsdam, Germany. At home, his father taught him Latin, Greek, French, Italian, Hebrew, and Arabic, as well as the philosophical ideas of Immanuel Kant and J. G. Fichte (who was a friend of the family). With this background, Helmholtz entered school with a wide perspective. Though he expressed an interest in the sciences, his father could not afford to send him to a university; instead, he was persuaded to study medicine, an area that would provide him with government aid. In return, Helmholtz was expected to use his medical skills for the good of the government—particularly in army hospitals.

Helmholtz entered the Friedrich Wilhelm Institute in Berlin in 1898, receiving his M.D. four years later. Upon graduation he was immediately assigned to military duty, practicing as a surgeon for the Prussian army. After several years of active duty he was discharged, free to pursue a career in academia. In 1848 he secured a position as lecturer at the Berlin Academy of Arts. Just a year later he was offered a professorship at the University of Konigsberg, teaching physiology. Over the next twenty-two years he moved to the universities at Bonn and Heidelberg, and it was during this time that he conducted his major works in the field of medicine.

Helmholtz began to study the human eye, a task that was all the more difficult for the lack of precise medical equipment. In order to better understand the function of the eye he invented the ophthalmoscope, a device used to observe the retina. Invented in 1851, the ophthalmoscope—in a slightly modified form—is still used by modern eye specialists. Helmholtz also designed a device used to measure the curvature of the eye called an ophthalmometer. Using these devices he advanced the theory of three-color vision first proposed by Thomas Young. This theory, now called the Young-Helmholtz theory, helps ophthalmologists to understand the nature of **color blindness** and other afflictions.

Intrigued by the inner workings of the sense organs, Helmholtz went on to study the human ear. Being an expert pianist, he was particularly concerned with the way the ear distinguished pitch and tone. He suggested that the inner ear is structured in such a way as to cause resonations at certain frequencies. This allowed the ear to discern similar tones, overtones, and timbres, such as an identical note played by two different instruments.

In 1852 Helmholtz conducted what was probably his most important work as a physician: the measurement of the speed of a nerve impulse. It had been assumed that such a measurement could never be obtained by science, since the speed was far too great for instruments to catch. Some physicians even used this as proof that living organisms were powered by an innate ''vital force'' rather than energy. Helmholtz disproved this by stimulating a frog's nerve first near a muscle and then farther away; when the stimulus was farther from the muscle, it contracted just a little slower. After a few simple calculations Helmholtz announced the impulse velocity within the nervous system to be about one-tenth the speed of sound.

After completing much of the work on sensory physiology that had interested him, Helmholtz found himself bored with medicine. In 1868 he decided to return to his first love—physical science. However, it was not until 1870 that he was offered the physics chair at the University of Berlin and only after it had been turned down by Gustav Kirchhoff. By that time, Helmholtz had already completed his groundbreaking research on energetics.

The concept of conservation of energy was introduced by Julius Mayer in 1842, but Helmholtz was unaware of

Mayer's work. Helmholtz conducted his own research on energy, basing his theories upon his previous experience with muscles. It could be observed that animal heat was generated by muscle action, as well as chemical reactions within a working muscle. Helmholtz believed that this energy was derived from food and that food got its energy from the sun. He proposed that energy could not be created spontaneously, nor could it vanish—it was either used or released as heat. This explanation was much clearer and more detailed than the one offered by Mayer, and Helmholtz is often considered the true originator of the concept of conservation of energy.

While this was undoubtedly Helmholtz's greatest legacy, he also began several projects that were later completed by other scientists. He advanced a number of hypotheses on electromagnetic radiation, speculating that it lay far into the invisible ranges of the spectrum. This line of research was later resumed, very successfully, by one of Helmholtz's students, Heinrich Rudolph Hertz, the discoverer of radio waves. Helmholtz's theories on electrolysis were also the basis for future work conducted by Svante August Arrhenius.

Helmholtz had been a sickly child; even throughout his adult life he was plagued by migraine **headaches** and dizzy spells. In 1894, shortly after a lecture tour of the United States, he fainted and fell, suffering a **concussion**. He never completely recovered, dying of complications several months later.

HEMOPHILIA

Suffering an occasional cut, scratch, or bruise is a normal consequence of life. When there is damage to the skin and a blood vessel ruptures, bleeding occurs. The human body is then able to initiate a series of reactions which cause the bleeding to stop. First, platelet cells in the blood move toward and attach to the site of the wound. The platelets are further held in place by strands of *fibrin*. The formation of the strands is the key event in a complex series of enzymatic reactions that are still somewhat of a mystery today. Without this cascade clotting process, people would be in danger of bleeding to death from very minor injuries.

However, the scenario described above could be fatal for a person afflicted with hemophilia. The term *hemophiliac,* coined by the German physician **Johann Schönlein** (1793-1864) in 1828, is made up of Greek and Latin terms which refer to ''one who loves to hemorrhage or bleed.'' First described by the Islamic surgeon Abu al-Qasim in the tenth century, this genetic disease has existed for several hundred years and has directly influenced history. Queen Victoria (1819-1901) had several hemophilic sons that died before they had the opportunity to become King of England. As early as the nineteenth century, scientists suspected that hemophilia may be passed from parents to offspring, or inherited. They also noticed that generally only males showed the uncontrolled bleeding that is a major symptom of the disease.

Today we know that hemophilia is caused by a small defect in a single human gene. When this particular defect occurs, as in classic or type A hemophilia, the body lacks an important protein which helps to form fibrin. This protein is called factor VIII. About 85 percent of all hemophiliacs are missing the gene that instructs the body's cells how to produce factor VIII. Hemophilia B is a less common type of genetic disease caused by a deficiency in another necessary protein, called factor IX. In each type of bleeding disorder, proteins are either missing or deficient and thus fibrin is not able to form. Approximately 2 out of every 10,000 males are afflicted with either type A or type B hemophilia.

Hemophilia is a sex-linked trait because the genes for factor VIII and IX are located on the X sex chromosome. Female cells contain two X chromosomes and male cells contain one X chromosome and one Y chromosome. All males inherit one factor VIII gene on the X chromosome from their mothers. If this gene is defective, the male will be hemophilic. A female, in contrast, has two factor VIII genes, one inherited from each parent. If one gene is defective but the other is not, the female will not be affected by this disease. The normal gene on the second X chromosome protects her. She will, however, carry the defective gene and may pass this gene on to her children. Generally, carrier females will pass their defective gene on to half their daughters, who will be carriers, and to half their sons, who will be hemophilic. For example, Queen Victoria was a carrier, and the genetic profile of her offspring supports this fact. Only in a very rare situation would a female acquire two defective genes and be hemophilic.

Fortunately, hemophiliacs can be treated with **transfusions** of concentrated factor VIII protein. This has increased the life expectancy of some hemophiliacs. The protein concentrate can be prepared by combining volumes of blood donated from many humans with normal clotting blood. However, this method usually spreads viral diseases which were present in the original donated blood. Many hemophiliacs are chronically infected with these viruses which include the virus that causes **AIDS** and **hepatitis**. In fact, in the early to mid-1980s, over 90% of the people with severe hemophilia contracted the AIDS virus through contaminated human blood plasma. Only recently has a process been invented where certain viruses, including the AIDS virus, can be detected in the blood supply. Cow and pig blood have also been concentrated and used as a therapy, since these animals have higher concentrations of factor VIII than humans. Transfusion reactions and other problems have caused a decline in the use of animal-derived factor VIII.

In the early 1980s, a completely new way of making factor VIII was discovered. Scientists from several research companies have been able to make the factor VIII protein by isolating the normal gene and inserting this human gene into hamster cells. The hamster cells then produce large amounts of pure factor VIII protein. The protein is then harvested and used as a therapy for hemophiliacs. This process is called **genetic engineering**. In addition to eliminating many of the side effects associated with previous factor VIII therapies (for example, complications from bleeding and from transfused blood and blood products that may be contaminated with a virus), a gene therapy approach promises to provide a permanent programming of cells to make clotting factor. Studies in mice has shown the process to be effective, and clinical trials in humans are on the horizon. According to the World Federation of Hemophilia, the cure for hemophilia using gene therapy is imminent.

Hemorrhagic fevers

Hemorrhagic fevers are caused by viruses that exist throughout the world but are most common in tropical areas. Early symptoms, such as muscle aches and fever, can progress either to mild illness or to a more serious, potentially fatal disease. In severe cases, a prominent symptom is **bleeding** (hemorrhaging) from orifices, such as the nose or vagina, and from internal organs.

These viruses also exist in insects, spiders and other animals that become infected but do not die and often have no symptoms. The viruses are transmitted to humans either directly by one of these infected animals or by an intervening species such as mosquitoes.

Hemorrhagic fevers are generally linked to specific locations. If many people reside in one of these areas, the number of cases may be high. Fatality rates are variable. In cases of dengue hemorrhagic fever-dengue shock syndrome, 1–5% of those afflicted die. On the other end of the spectrum is Ebola, an African hemorrhagic fever that kills 30–90% of those infected.

The onset of hemorrhagic fevers may be sudden or gradual. Not all cases progress to the very serious symptom of bleeding. The severity of bleeding ranges from pinpoint hemorrhages under the skin surface to distinct bleeding from body orifices. Depending on the particular virus, a wide range of other symptoms may occur, including abdominal **pain**, apathy, appetite loss, blurry vision, chills, **coma**, convulsions, **coughing**, **delirium**, **diarrhea**, disorientation, **dizziness**, **fever**, gastrointestinal upset, **headache**, **jaundice**, joint pain, **low back pain**, malaise, muscle aches, **nausea**, **rash**, runny nose, **seizures**, **sore throat**, stupor, swelling or flushing of the face, or vomiting.

The viruses that cause hemorrhagic fevers are found most commonly in tropical locations; however, some are found in cooler climates. The disease is typically harbored by rodents, ticks, or mosquitoes, but person-to-person transmission can also occur in health care settings or through sexual contact.

Ebola, caused by a member of the Filoviridae family of viruses, is most commonly found in Africa, particularly the Republic of the Congo and Sudan. Ebola is fatal in 30–90% of cases. Another, rarer filovirus, the Marburg virus, is found in sub-Saharan Africa. It is not known which animals harbor filoviruses.

Argentinian, Brazilian, Bolivian, and Venezuelan hemorrhagic fevers are caused by viruses of the Arenaviridae family. Lassa fever, which occurs in west Africa, also arises from an arenavirus. Infected rodents shed virus particles in their urine and saliva, which humans may inhale or otherwise contact. Untreated, South American hemorrhagic fevers have a 10–30% fatality rate. Lassa fever has an overall fatality rate lower than 2%, but hospitals may encounter 20% fatality rates, treating typically the most serious of cases.

Yellow fever and dengue fever are caused by the Flaviviridae family of viruses. Yellow fever occurs in tropical areas of the Americas and Africa and is transmitted from monkeys to humans by mosquitoes. Mosquitoes also transmit the dengue virus. Dengue fever is most common in southeast Asia and areas of the Americas.

Rift Valley fever is caused by the phlebovirus, a member of the Bunyaviridae family found in sub-Saharan Africa and the Nile delta. Natural reservoirs are wild and domestic animals, and transmission occurs through contact with infected animals or through mosquito bites. **Death**, which occurs in fewer than 3% of cases, is attributable to massive liver damage.

Crimean-Congo hemorrhagic fever is caused by nairovirus (another member of the Bunyaviridae family) and occurs in central and southern Africa, Asia, Eurasia, and the Middle East. The virus is found in hares, birds, ticks, and domestic animals and may be transmitted by ticks or by contact with infected animals. Death rates range from 10% in southern Russia to 50% in parts of Asia.

Hemorrhagic fever with renal (kidney) syndrome is caused by other members of the Bunyaviridae family: the **hantaviruses**: Hantaan, Seoul, Puumala, and Dobrava. Hantaan virus occurs in northern Asia, the Far East, and the Balkans; Seoul virus is found worldwide; Puumala virus is found in Scandinavia and northern Europe; while Dobrava virus occurs in the Balkans. Wild rodents transmit the virus via their excrement or body fluids or through direct contact. Death rates range from 0–10%.

Since the hemorrhagic fevers share symptoms with many other diseases, positive identification relies on evidence of the viruses in the bloodstream—such as detection of antigens and antibodies, or finding the virus itself in the body.

Lassa fever, and possibly other hemorrhagic fevers, respond to ribavirin, an antiviral medication. However, most of the hemorrhagic fever viruses can only be treated with supportive care. Such care centers around maintaining correct fluid and electrolyte balances in the body and protecting the patient against secondary infections. Heparin and vitamin K administration, coagulation factor replacement, and blood transfusions may lessen or stop bleeding in some cases.

Permanent disability can occur with some types of hemorrhagic fever. About 10% of severely ill Rift Valley fever victims suffer retina damage and may be permanently blind, and 25% of South American hemorrhagic fever victims suffer potentially permanent deafness.

Proper treatment is vital. For individuals who survive hemorrhagic fevers, prolonged convalescence is usually inevitable. However, survivors seem to gain lifelong immunity against the virus that made them ill.

To prevent hemorrhagic fevers, attempts have been made in urban and settled areas to destroy mosquito and rodent populations. In places where such measures are impossible, individuals can use insect repellents, mosquito netting, and other methods to minimize exposure.

Vaccines have been developed against yellow fever, Argentinean hemorrhagic fever, and Crimean-Congo hemorrhagic fever. Vaccines against other hemorrhagic fevers are being researched.

HEMORRHOIDS

Hemorrhoids are enlarged veins in the anus or lower rectum. They often go unnoticed and usually clear up after a few days, but can cause long-lasting discomfort, bleeding and be excruciatingly painful. However, effective medical treatments are available.

Hemorrhoids (also called piles) can be divided into two kinds, internal and external. Internal hemorrhoids lie inside the anus or lower rectum. External hemorrhoids lie outside the anal opening. Both kinds can be present at the same time.

More than 75% of Americans have hemorrhoids at some point in their lives, typically after age 30. Pregnant women often develop hemorrhoids, but the condition usually clears up after childbirth. Men are more likely than women to suffer from hemorrhoids that require professional medical treatment.

Precisely why hemorrhoids develop is unknown. Researchers have identified a number of explanations for hemorrhoidal swelling, including the simple fact that people's upright posture places a lot of pressure on the anal and rectal veins. **Aging**, **obesity**, **pregnancy**, chronic **constipation** or **diarrhea**, excessive use of **enemas** or **laxatives**, straining during bowel movements, and spending too much time on the toilet are considered contributing factors. Heredity may also play a part in some cases. There is no reason to believe that hemorrhoids are caused by jobs requiring, for instance, heavy lifting or long hours of sitting, although activities of that kind may make existing hemorrhoids worse.

The most common symptom of internal hemorrhoids is bright red blood in the toilet bowl or on one's feces or toilet paper. When hemorrhoids remain inside the anus they are almost never painful, but they can prolapse (protrude outside the anus) and become irritated and sore. Sometimes, prolapsed hemorrhoids move back into the anal canal on their own or can be pushed back in, but at other times they remain permanently outside the anus until treated by a doctor.

Small external hemorrhoids usually do not produce symptoms. Larger ones, however, can be painful and interfere with cleaning the anal area after a bowel movement. When, as sometimes happens, a blood clot forms in an external hemorrhoid (creating what is called a thrombosed hemorrhoid), the skin around the anus becomes inflamed and a very painful lump develops. On rare occasions the clot will begin to bleed after a few days and leave blood on the underwear. A thrombosed hemorrhoid will not obstruct blood flow.

Hemorrhoids can often be effectively dealt with by dietary and lifestyle changes. Softening the feces and avoiding constipation by adding fiber to one's diet is important, because hard feces lead to straining during defecation. Fruit, leafy vegetables, and whole-grain breads and cereals are good sources of fiber, as are bulk laxatives and fiber supplements such as Metamucil or Citrucel. Exercising, losing excess weight, and drinking six to eight glasses a day of water or another liquid (not alcohol) also helps. Soap or toilet paper that is perfumed may irritate the anal area and should be avoided, as should excessive cleaning, rubbing, or wiping of that area. Reading in the bathroom is also a bad idea, because it adds to the time one spends on the toilet and may increase the strain placed on the anal and rectal veins. After each bowel movement, wiping with a moistened tissue or pad sold for that purpose helps lessen irritation. Hemorrhoid pain is often eased by sitting in a tub of warm water for about 10 or 15 minutes two to four times a day (sitz bath). A cool compress or ice pack to reduce swelling is also recommended (it should be wrapped in a cloth or towel to prevent direct contact with the skin). Many people find that over-the-counter hemorrhoid creams and foams bring relief, but these medications do not make hemorrhoids disappear.

When painful hemorrhoids do not respond to home-based remedies, professional medical treatment is necessary. Rubber-band ligation is probably the most widely used of the many treatments for internal hemorrhoids, and the least costly. This procedure is performed in the office of a family doctor or specialist, or in hospital on an outpatient basis. An applicator is used to place one or two small rubber bands around the base of the hemorrhoid, cutting off its blood supply. After 3 to 10 days with the bands, the hemorrhoid falls off, leaving a sore that heals in a week or two. Because internal hemorrhoids are located in a part of the anus that does not sense pain, anesthetic is unnecessary. Although there can be minor discomfort and bleeding for a few days after the bands are applied, complications are rare and most people are soon able to return to work and other activities. If more than one hemorrhoid exists or if banding is not entirely effective the first time (as occasionally happens), the procedure may need to be repeated a few weeks later. After five years, 15–20% of patients experience a recurrence of internal hemorrhoids, but in most cases all that is needed is another banding.

External hemorrhoids, and some prolapsed internal hemorrhoids, are removed by conventional surgery in a hospital. Depending on the circumstances, this requires a local, regional, or general anesthetic. Surgery does cause a fair amount of discomfort, but an overnight hospital stay is usually not necessary. Full healing takes two to four weeks, but most people are able to resume normal activities at the end of a week. Hemorrhoids rarely return after surgery.

Hemorrhoids do not cause **cancer** and are rarely dangerous or life-threatening. However, because **colorectal cancer** and other **digestive system** diseases can cause anal bleeding and other hemorrhoid-like symptoms, people should always consult a doctor when those symptoms occur.

HENCH, PHILIP SHOWALTER (1896-1965)

American medical researcher

Philip Hench made important advances in the understanding and hormonal treatment of arthritis and other rheumatic diseases. For his accomplishments, he received part of the 1950 Nobel prize for physiology or medicine, which he shared with his co-worker **Edward Kendall** and **Tadeus Reichstein**, who had isolated cortisone in 1936.

Hench was born in Pittsburgh, Pennsylvania, where his father was a teacher. He graduated from Lafayette College in 1912 and received his medical degree in 1920 from the University of Pittsburgh Medical School. He was affiliated with the Mayo Clinic in Rochester, Minnesota in 1921, specializing in such rheumatic diseases as **rheumatoid arthritis**, which is characterized by swelling of the joints.

In the 1930s, Hench's Mayo Clinic colleague Edward Kendall was studying the pituitary gland hormone ACTH (adrenocorticotropic hormone) and the adrenal gland hormones scortisol and cortisone. ACTH signals the adrenal gland to produce cortisol, and both cortisone and cortisol block the body's ability to inflame the joints and other tissues.

Hench and Kendall studied the hormones' possible use in treating arthritis. During World War II, Hench headed the first program to mass-produce ACTH for medical use. In 1948 and 1949, he and another colleague became the first to use cortisone and ACTH to successfully treat arthritis.

It was soon discovered, however, that the benefits lasted only while the hormones were being administered. Also, they produced dangerous side effects such as high blood pressure, high blood sugar, and **obesity**, and the use of hormones for these purposes was discontinued.

In addition to his Nobel prize, Hench was honored with such awards as the Heberden Medal, the Lasker Award in 1949, the Passano Foundation Award and the Criss Award. He was also a founder of the American Rheumatism Association and a member of the Royal Society of Medicine.

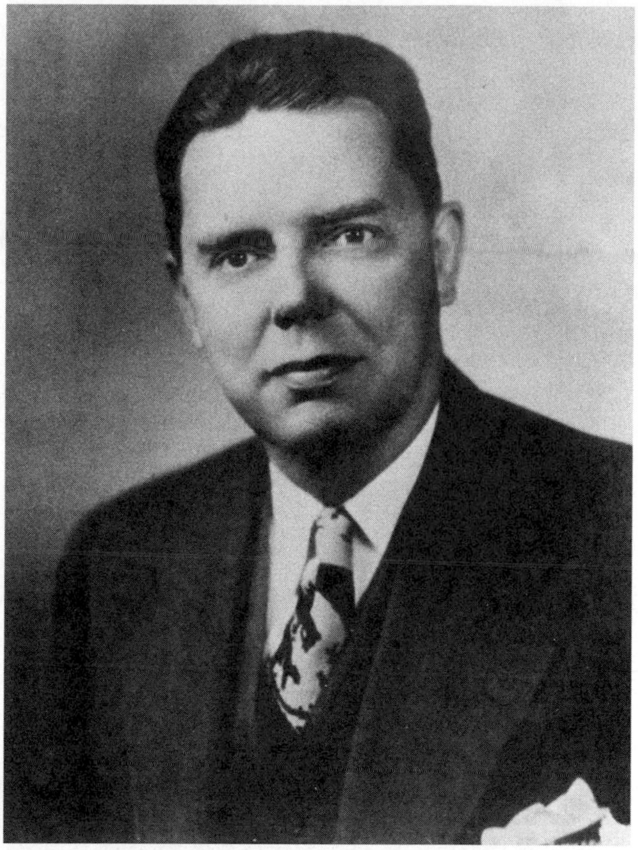

Philip Showalter Hench

HEPATITIS

Perhaps the first account of hepatitis occurred in the second century B.C., when Greek physicians described a mysterious and often fatal disease that caused inflammation of the liver. They noted that the skin of afflicted patients had a distinguishing yellow appearance, later called **jaundice**. A thousand years later, St. Zacharias (d.752) described a similar disease; and, between the seventeenth and nineteenth centuries, about 80 epidemics of jaundice occurred throughout the world. Today, it is known that hepatitis can cause a variety of other symptoms, including malaise, liver disease, gastrointestinal upset, **liver cancer**, and scarring of the liver (**cirrhosis**). When the liver becomes infected and inflamed, it is unable to perform its vital functions. This causes a reduction in the blood flow to the liver and subsequent cell death. Cirrhosis may follow.

Many types of hepatitis can be prevented, however. Alcoholic hepatitis is caused by an increase in the fat deposits within the liver. This non-infectious type of hepatitis is common among heavy drinkers. There are also several types of hepatitis caused by viruses. These include hepatitis types A, B, C, and D.

Hepatitis A, also known as *epidemic* or infectious hepatitis, is spread by the intestinal-oral route. Infection occurs in conditions of poor **sanitation** and overcrowding. Once the virus has been contracted, it usually takes about 20-40 days before symptoms appear. This is known as the incubation period.

Hepatitis B, or serum hepatitis, is transmitted mainly by blood transfusion. Sexual transmission of hepatitis B has also been reported. The incubation period takes between 60 and 180 days. Type B viral hepatitis (HBV) has a higher fatality rate than type A.

Hepatitis C, also referred to as non-A, non-B hepatitis (NANB), is also transmitted through blood transfusion. Researchers believe that the causative agent may actually be several viruses. A 1998 study from Scotland has found that hepatitis C might also be spread through saliva, which may account for the fifty percent of cases in which there is no history of blood transfusions or intravenous drug use. People infected with hepatitis C usually show relatively mild symptoms which may become chronic.

In 1977, hepatitis D was discovered and found to be present only in the liver cells of people who had been exposed to HBV. Scientists strongly believe that this virus requires HBV to survive. Hepatitis D is an important factor in the development of chronic liver disease.

Many other viruses can cause hepatitis, including Epstein-Barr, herpes simplex, **measles**, **mumps**, and **chicken pox** viruses.

Many methods are available to help prevent transmission of viral hepatitis. Maintaining clean living conditions, designing adequate sewage facilities, and testing blood supplies for contamination are obvious approaches. **Baruch S. Blumberg** (1925-) and Irving Millman (1923-) developed a test to identify hepatitis B in blood samples, which helped blood banks screen out carriers of hepatitis B after they began using the test in 1971. The test was based on Blumberg's discovery of an antigen that detected hepatitis B in blood samples.

One of the best modes of prevention is **vaccination**. Safe and effective vaccines are now available for protection against hepatitis B, including one developed by Blumberg and Millman. In 1986, a new type of vaccine that used genetic engineering was developed. Scientists were able to make the vaccine by inserting part of the HBV gene into baker's yeast cells. The yeast cells then produced large amounts of viral protein. This protein resembled the infectious hepatitis virus but lacked certain parts that would cause the disease in humans. The viral protein was then injected into the human body, causing the **immune system** to produce antibodies against the virus, thus creating an immunity against hepatitis B. This yeast-derived hepatitis B vaccine is the first recombinantly produced vaccine approved for human use.

Studies continue into the treatment of hepatitis. Injections of interferon alfa has been approved for treatment of hepatitis B and C; and a number of new drugs, called nucleoside analogues, are also be developed for treating hepatitis B.

HERBAL REMEDIES, WESTERN

Herbal remedies involve the use of plants as medicines to restore and maintain health. The origins of western herbal remedies are found in the ancient civilizations of Egypt, Greece, Rome, and the Middle East. After the arrival of Columbus, many New World plants became available to Europeans, and by the time of Henry VIII in England (1491-1547), a European medical system that blended plant use and **astrology** had developed.

For centuries, medicine in the West meant herbal remedies. During the late 20th century, modern medicine with its synthetic drugs and high technology became so dominant that herbal cures were almost totally eclipsed. However, at the turn of the millennium, herbal remedies were beginning to be accepted as being at least complementary to conventional medicine. Much of this renewed popularity is attributable not only to a belief in the effectiveness of herbals, but also because of herbal medicine's holistic emphasis, its respect for the individual, and its emphasis on self-help.

Herbal medicine expresses great concern for the uniqueness of the individual. As a result, two people with the same medical condition may receive two very different herbal prescriptions. Another difference from modern medicine is the makeup of herbal remedies: they are not just a single, chemical ingredient, but the entire plant, made up of hundreds, if not thousands, of different chemicals.

Herbal remedies must be treated with care, especially if combinations are taken. A qualified professional herbalist or naturopathic physician should consulted, since mainstream physicians only rarely prescribe herbal remedies. Certain insurance companies cover the cost of herbals, but only when prescribed by a healthcare professional.

Herbal remedies can be dangerous and must be treated with respect. Some of the most potent and toxic chemicals come from plants. Simply because something is described as ''natural'' does not mean that it cannot have serious side effects. While most commonly used herbal remedies are safe, it is best to obtain the advice of a well-trained practitioner before using any plant-based medication that is not well known, especially since herbals may interact with conventional drugs. Further, it is important to use herbal remedies correctly and stick to the prescribed doses. It should also be recognized that the sale of herbals in the United States is largely unregulated, and consumers cannot be certain of their quality.

The improper use of herbal remedies can bring unwanted and sometimes dangerous results. Some remedies are toxic when taken in high doses, or if taken by pregnant women or small children. Herbal remedies should never be substituted in cases of severe, acute illness when rapid and strong-acting medicines are required, nor in cases of major physical injury when n surgery is necessary. Self-prescribing without consulting an herbal expert can be dangerous.

Many of modern medicine's standard pharmaceuticals were derived from plants. **Aspirin**, for example, came from the bark of the willow tree. **Morphine** and codeine are derived from the opium poppy. Chamomile and peppermint are recognized relaxants, and aloe effectively soothes skin problems. The heart drug digoxin comes from the common flower called foxglove. Tubocurarine, a powerful **muscle relaxant**, is derived from a South American plant containing curare. Cocaine comes from the cocoa plant, and the anti-malarial quinine is derived from the cinchona tree. Valerian has been helpful for **insomnia**, garlic has reduced blood pressure and cholesterol levels, and St. John's wort has been shown to have powerful antiviral and antidepressive qualities. Herbal remedies are indeed chemicals in their natural state and should be regarded as dilute forms of drugs that can produce a biological effect.

Plant or herb remedies have shown to be particularly effective for skin conditions, such as eczema, for problems of digestion, such as **irritable bowel syndrome**, and for urinary conditions, like **cystitis**. What should not be expected, however, is for conditions to respond immediately as is sometimes the case with modern synthetic drugs. Since herbal remedies attempt to treat the underlying condition or problem rather than the symptoms, individuals who take these natural remedies should not expect the symptoms to disappear until the basic underlying physical problem has responded to the herbal and been resolved.

The **World Health Organization** (WHO) of the United Nations estimates that as much as 80% of the world population relies on the use of various forms of traditional (herbal) medicine for its primary healthcare.

While herbal remedies in the United States demonstrated the beginnings of a real renaissance in the late 1990s, no such resurgence was necessary in Europe. There, herbal remedies have never really gone out of fashion. Still, even in countries with a strong herbal tradition, interest and actual use of herbal remedies has increased.

Despite this increase in attention, research, and use, herbal products sold in the United States remain largely unregulated, since they are considered to be dietary supplements, and, therefore, are regarded as "food" rather than "drugs." For drugs to be sold, the **Food and Drug Administration** (FDA) requires manufacturers to conduct lengthy studies to prove the safety and efficiency of both prescription and over-the-counter drugs. However, manufacturers of herbal remedies are held to no such rigorous standard. By placing herbal remedies in the same category as **dietary supplements**, like **vitamins** and **minerals**, the FDA effectively exempts them from having to be rigorously tested. Further, the 1994 Dietary Supplement Health and Education Act allows herbal manufacturers to make "limited claims" on their labels as long as they do not claim to "diagnose, prevent, mitigate, treat or cure a specific disease."

See also Chinese traditional herbal medicine; Dietary supplements

HERNIA

A hernia is a bulge or protrusion of an organ through the structure or muscle that contains it. There are many different types of hernias.

The most familiar are those in which part of the intestines protrude through the abdominal wall. An inguinal hernia appears as a bulge in the groin. It can occur with or without **pain**. Inguinal hernias account for 80% of all hernias and are more common in men, in whom they may descend into the scrotum.

Most hernias result from a weakness in the abdominal wall that either develops or is present at birth. Any increase in pressure in the abdomen, such as coughing, straining, heavy lifting, or **pregnancy**, can help cause an abdominal hernia. **Obesity** or recent excessive weight loss, as well as aging and previous surgery, are also risk factors.

Most abdominal hernias appear suddenly when the abdominal muscles are strained. The person may feel tenderness, a slight burning sensation, or a feeling of heaviness in the bulge. It may be possible to push the hernia back into place with gentle pressure, or it may disappear by itself when the person reclines.

Generally, abdominal hernias need to be seen and felt to be diagnosed. The doctor may ask the person to **cough** while he or she feels the area. Once a diagnosis of abdominal hernia is made, the doctor will usually send the person to a surgeon for a consultation. Surgery provides the only cure for a hernia through the abdominal wall.

Once an abdominal hernia occurs it tends to increase in size. Some patients with abdominal hernias wait for a while prior to choosing surgery. In these cases, they must avoid strenuous physical activity such as heavy lifting or straining with **constipation**. They may also wear a truss, which is a support worn like a belt to keep a small hernia from protruding. People can tell if their hernia is getting worse if they develop severe constant pain, **nausea and vomiting**, or if the bulge does not return to normal when lying down or when they try to gently push it back in place. In these cases they should consult with their doctor immediately. But, ultimately, surgery is the treatment in almost all cases.

There are risks to not repairing a hernia surgically. Left untreated, a hernia may become trapped outside the abdomen, causing a blockage in the intestine. If severe enough, it may cut off the blood supply to the intestine and part of the intestine might die. When the blood supply is cut off, the hernia is termed "strangulated." A strangulated hernia is a medical emergency requiring immediate surgery. Repairing a hernia before it becomes strangulated is much safer than waiting until complications develop. The surgeon will push the bulging part of the intestine back into place and sew the overlying muscle back together. When the muscle is not strong enough, the surgeon may reinforce it with a synthetic mesh.

Surgery can be done on an outpatient basis, under either local or general **anesthesia**, and is frequently done with a laparoscope. In this case, a tube that allows visualization of the abdominal cavity is inserted through a small puncture wound. Several small punctures are made to allow surgical instruments to be inserted. This type of surgery avoids a larger incision. The prospect of recovery is excellent if the hernia is corrected before it becomes strangulated. Abdominal hernias generally do not recur in children but can recur in up to 10% of adult patients.

Some hernias can be prevented by maintaining a reasonable weight, avoiding heavy lifting and constipation, and following a moderate **exercise** program to maintain good abdominal muscle tone.

A hiatal or diaphragmatic hernia is not visible on the outside of the body. In hiatal hernia, the stomach bulges upward through the muscle that separates the chest from the abdomen (the diaphragm). This occurs more often in women than in men.

About 50% of people with hiatal hernias have no symptoms. If symptoms exist they will include heartburn, usually 30–60 minutes following a meal. There may be some mid-chest pain due to gastric acid from the stomach being pushed up into the esophagus. The pain and heartburn are usually worse when lying down. Frequent belching and feelings of abdominal fullness may also be present.

With a hiatal hernia, the diagnosis is based on the symptoms reported by the patient. The doctor may then order tests to confirm the diagnosis. If a barium swallow is ordered, the person drinks a chalky white barium solution, which will help any protrusion through the diaphragm show up on the x ray that follows. Currently, a diagnosis of hiatal hernia is often made by endoscopy. This procedure is done by a gastroenterologist (a specialist in digestive diseases). The person is given an intravenous sedative and a small tube is inserted through the mouth, then into the esophagus and stomach where the doctor can visualize the hernia. The procedure usually causes no discomfort. It is done on an outpatient basis.

Treatments for hiatal hernia include: avoiding reclining after meals; avoiding spicy foods, acidic foods, alcohol, and tobacco; eating small, frequent, bland meals; and a high-fiber diet.

Medications can also help to manage the symptoms of a hiatal hernia. **Antacids** are used to neutralize gastric acid and decrease heartburn. Drugs that reduce the amount of acid produced in the stomach (H2 blockers) are also used. This class of drugs includes famotidine (sold under the name Pepcid), cimetidine (Tagamet), and ranitidine (Zantac). Omeprazole (Prilosec) is not an H2 blocker, but is another drug that suppresses gastric acid secretion and is used for hiatal hernias. Metoclopramide (Reglan), a drug that increases the tone of the muscle around the esophagus and causes the stomach to empty more quickly.

Hiatal hernias are treated successfully with medication and diet modifications 85% of the time and the prospect of recovery is excellent.

HERNIATED DISK

Disk herniation is a rupture of fibrous material surrounding the disks that separate the vertebrae of the spine. Each disk is made up of a jelly-like center surrounded by a tough ring of fibres arranged in concentric layers like those of an onion. Any forceful vertical pressure on the disks can cause them to push their fluid contents outward, placing pressure on a spinal nerve that can cause both nerve damage and considerable **pain**. Herniation may occur suddenly from lifting, twisting, or direct injury, or gradually from degenerative changes. The condition most frequently occurs in the low back region and is also called herniated nucleus pulposus, prolapsed disk, ruptured intervertebral disk, or slipped disk. Disk herniation can also occur in the neck, and less commonly, in the chest area.

Depending on the location, the ruptured material may press directly on nerve roots or on the spinal cord, causing a shock-like pain (sciatica) down the legs, weakness, numbness, or problems with bowels, bladder, or sexual function.

The peak age for occurrence of disk herniation is between 20–45 years of age. Males are more commonly affected than females by low-back disk herniation by a 3:2 ratio. A prolonged, bent-forward work posture is linked to increased cases of disk herniation.

X rays, **computed tomography scans** (CT or CAT scans), and **magnetic resonance imaging** (MRI) are useful for confirming disk herniation. Myelography is a special x ray in which a dye or air is injected into the patient's spinal canal. The patient lies strapped to a table as the table tilts in various directions and spot x rays are taken of the spine. Electomyograms (EMGs), measuring the electrical activity of muscle contractions, assess muscle fatigue associated with **low back pain**.

Unless serious symptoms occur, herniated disks can initially be treated with pain medication and up to 48 hours of bed rest. There is no proven benefit from resting more than 48 hours. Patients are then encouraged to gradually increase their activity. Medications including antiinflammatories, muscle relaxers, or in severe cases, narcotics, may be continued if needed.

Physical therapists can use therapies such as ultrasound or diathermy to project heat deep into the tissues of the back. They can also administer manual therapy, if mobility of the spine is impaired. Physical therapy may also help improve posture and develop an exercise program for recovery and long-term protection. Traction can be used to try to decrease pressure on the disk. A lumbar support can be helpful as a temporary measure to reduce pain and improve posture.

Surgery is often appropriate for conditions that do not improve with the usual treatment. A strong, flexible spine is important for a quick recovery after surgery. There are several surgical approaches to treating a herniated disk, including the classic discectomy, microdiscectomy, or percutanteous discectomy. The basic differences among these procedures are the size of the incision, how the disk is reached surgically, and how much of the disk is removed.

Discectomy is the surgical removal of the portion of the disk that is putting pressure on a nerve causing the back pain. The surgeon first enters through the skin and then removes a bony portion of the vertebra called the lamina, hence the term laminectomy. The disk material that is pressing on a nerve is removed. Rarely is the entire lamina or disk removed.

In microdiscectomy, the offending bone or disk tissue is removed with the surgeon using an operating microscope. This procedure can be done under local **anesthesia**. Advantages include a smaller incision, less injury to the muscles and nerves, and easier identification of structures.

Percutaneous disk excision is performed on an outpatient basis, is less expensive than other surgical procedures, and does not require general anesthesia. The purpose is partial removal of the disk's soft center, leaving all the structures important to stability practically unaffected. In this procedure, large incisions are avoided by inserting devices that have cutting and suction capability.

Athroscopic microdiscectomy is similar to percutaneous discectomy. A video scope is introduced through one entry site and surgical instruments through another site. The surgeon is able to search and extract material while directly observing what he is doing.

Laser disk decompression is also similar to percutaneous excision and arthroscopic microdiscectomy, however laser energy, introduced through a needle, vaporizes a small portion of the disk's center.

It is important to realize that only a very small percentage of people with herniated low-back disks require surgery. Further, surgery should be followed by appropriate **rehabilitation** to decrease the chance of reinjury.

Spinal fusion is the process by which bone grafts harvested from the pelvis are placed between the vertebrae after the disk material is removed. In the low back, spinal fusion can help prevent further disk herniation.

Chemonucleolysis is an alternative to surgery. Chymopapain, a purified enzyme derived from the papaya plant, is injected into the disk space to relieve pressure on the nerve root.

Acupuncture is an alternative therapy involving the use of fine needles inserted along the pathway of the pain to relieve pain. Massage therapists may also provide short-term relief from a herniated disk. **Chiropractic** treatment usually includes manipulation to correct muscle and joint malfunctions.

Many patients with herniated disks in the low back respond well to conservative treatment. Only 5–10% of patients with unrelenting sciatica and chronic low-back pain need to have a surgical procedure performed. For those patients who do require surgery, success rates for the above-mentioned procedures varies from 60–90%. Disk surgery has progressively become less invasive, but each procedure has possible complications that can lead to chronic low back pain and restricted lifestyle.

Proper exercises to strengthen the lower back and abdominal muscles are key in preventing excess stress on the disks. Good posture, a flexibility program, losing weight, and proper lifting of heavy objects are all important. Proper footwear may reduce impact forces while walking on hard surfaces. Special back-support devices may help if heavy lifting is required with combinations of twisting.

HEROPHILUS (335 B.C.-280 B.C.)

Greek anatomist and physiologist

Sometimes called the father of anatomy, Herophilus was born in Chalcedon, Asia Minor. Little is known about his life; the date and place of his death have been completely lost, as have all his writings. Herophilus studied medicine under **Praxagoras** of Cos and then at Alexandria, where he later taught and practiced medicine. In Alexandria, Herophilus had the unique opportunity to practice human dissection, a research technique not allowed elsewhere. Herophilus even performed public dissections. His work was highly regarded, and the medical school he founded at Alexandria attracted scores of students.

Herophilus made many anatomical studies of the brain. He distinguished the *cerebrum* (larger portion) from the *cerebellum* (smaller portion), pronounced the brain to be the seat of intelligence, and identified several structures of the brain, several of which still carry his name. He discovered that the nerves originate in the brain, was the first to distinguish nerves from tendons, and noted the difference between *motor nerves* (those concerned with motion) and *sensory nerves* (those related to sensation). He traced the optic nerve and described the retina. He studied the liver extensively and described and named the duodenum, the first part of the small intestine.

Drawing a distinction between arteries and veins, Herophilus noted the arterial pulse and developed standards for its measurement and use in diagnosis. He thought that arterial pulsation was involuntary, rising from dilation and contraction of arteries due to impulses sent from the heart. He corrected the idea that arteries carry air rather than blood. Herophilus also wrote a treatise on midwifery and accurately described the ovaries, the uterus, and the tubes leading from the ovaries to the uterus (later named the Fallopian tubes). In the field of medical treatment, Herophilus sensibly recommended good diet and exercise, but was also an enthusiastic advocate of bleeding and frequent drug therapy.

Although his medical school languished after his death, Herophilus (and his younger successor **Erasistratus**) established the disciplines of anatomy and physiology, which did not significantly advance before **Galen** in the second century and then the early modern anatomists of the thirteenth century.

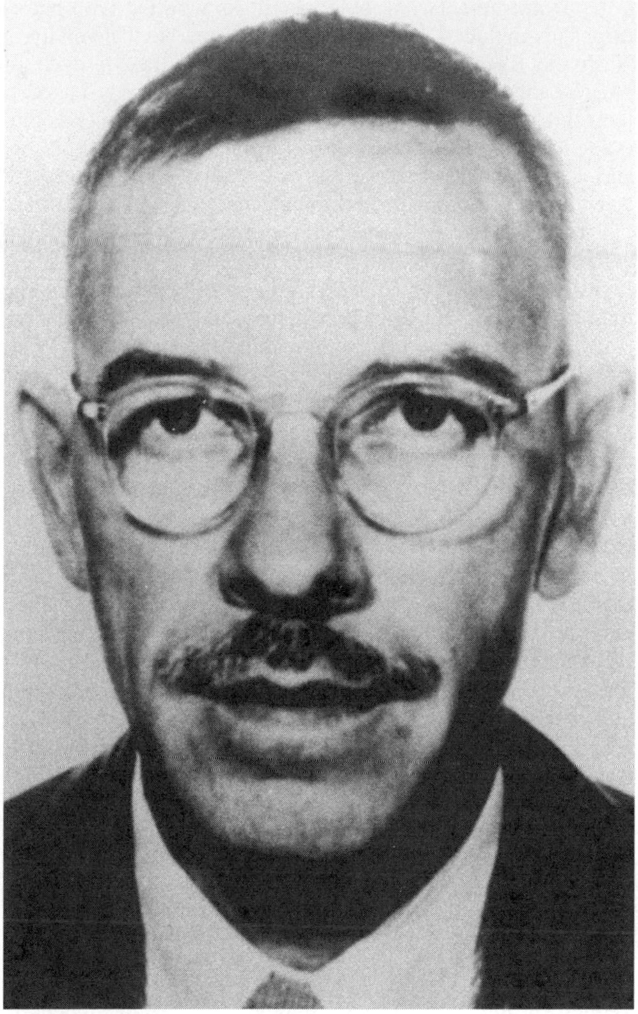

Alfred Day Hershey

HERSHEY, ALFRED DAY (1908-1997)

American virologist

Alfred Day Hershey was born on December 4, 1908, in Owosso, Michigan. He received his Ph.D. in bacteriology from Michigan State in 1934. He was appointed to the staff of the Department of Bacteriology at Washington University in St. Louis, Missouri. There he worked under J. J. Bronfenbrenner, who had been studying bacteriophages. A bacteriophage, or simply phage, is a type of virus that infects bacteria cells. It consists of only nucleic acid and protein. Nucleic acids, notably DNA and RNA, contain genetic material inherited by every cell. The basic structure of a bacteriophage includes a head and a tail; the head is made of protein encasing a core of nucleic acid, and the tail is protein.

During the 1940s, other scientists working with bacteriophages included **Max Delbruck** at Vanderbilt University in Nashville, Tennessee, who was working on the life cycle of phages, and **Salvador Luria** of Columbia University. Together they showed that bacterial cells can undergo spontaneous mutation in order to resist destruction by phages. Delbruck, Luria, and Hershey formed the core of the Phage Group, a group of scientists dedicated to bacteriophage research, especially those phages that infect the bacillus ***E. coli*** strain B.

In 1946, both Hershey and Delbruck, working separately, found that different strains of phage will exchange genetic material if both have infected the same bacterial cell. Hershey called this phenomenon genetic recombination. Then in 1952, at Cold Spring Harbor Laboratory in New York with Martha Chase, a geneticist, the pair discovered how phages infect bacteria. First the phage attaches itself to the bacterial cell membrane by its tail, and then the nucleic acid core is injected into the bacterial cell. The phage DNA enters the bacterial cell and then directs the cell to produce more bacteriophages. This experiment helped to prove that DNA is the genetic material of bacteriophages as well as other organisms. Throughout the remainder of the 1950s and 1960s, Hershey investigated the nucleic acid of bacteriophages, establishing that bacteriophage DNA is single-stranded, unlike the double-stranded DNA that exists in higher life forms. For their work on the replication and genetic structure of viruses, the 1969 Nobel Prize for physiology or medicine was awarded to Hershey, Luria, and Delbruck.

Hershey married Harriet Davidson in 1945. They had one son. Hershey died in 1997.

HESS, WALTER RUDOLF (1881-1973)

Swiss physiologist

Walter Rudolf Hess was born in the Swiss town of Frauenfeld to Clemens and Gertrud (Fischer Saxon) Hess on March 17, 1881. He inherited a strong interest in science from his father, a physics teacher. After finishing high school, Hess began his college career, changing universities frequently and taking every opportunity to travel. He eventually received a medical degree from the University of Zurich in 1905, and took a hospital residency under the famous surgeon Dr. Konrad Brunner.

While working for Brunner, Hess designed an improved blood viscometer (to measure blood's thickness and consistency) and began thinking about research in earnest. He took a second residency in Zurich and specialized in ophthalmology (the physiology and diseases of the **eye**) under the mistaken impression that the discipline would allow him time to continue his circulatory system investigations. He indeed developed a successful ophthalmology practice with a good income, but it took up all of his time. In 1912 Hess gave up his practice and moved to the Institute of Physiology in Zurich. Eventually he was named chair of the Physiology department, and began traveling to conferences and meetings throughout Europe. The stresses inherent in administrative work and World War I cut into his research time again, but he still managed to publish two important monographs, *The Regulation of the Circulatory System* in 1930, and *The Regulation of Respiration* in 1931.

Hess brought an unusual variety of tools and skills to his research. He had learned the basic principles of physics from his father, he knew a great deal about optics and hand-eye coordination from his days as an ophthalmologist, and he was a skilled surgeon. These all proved useful when he began conducting brain research on experimental animals. Hess's work on the circulatory and **respiratory systems** had included investigations of their interrelationship with other parts of animal physiology, including how blood flow and breathing were affected by the **nervous system**. Gradually this led to research on the areas of the brain responsible for regulating internal organs.

Of particular interest to Hess was the diencephalon, which is located under the cerebellum and is thus very difficult to access without damaging the rest of the brain. Hess designed very small electrodes and a mechanical guidance system that could implant the electrodes in experimental animals (cats) with the least possible disruption of their normal behavior. He also designed a method of delivering electrical stimulus pulses swiftly and accurately. On at least one occasion there was a public outcry about the use of animals for experimentation. Hess was instrumental in convincing the activists that, if properly regulated and humanely conducted, animal experiments were important for human welfare.

Using the electrodes to stimulate different areas of the brain, Hess observed the results on other areas of bodily function, such as blood pressure, respiration, and body temperature. He recorded his observations not only on paper, but also on film, and maintained meticulous records of **dissections** and cell studies. He also compared the results of electrical stimulation with behaviors resulting from naturally occurring brain lesions. He found that the diencephalon, and particularly the hypothalamus, controlled many of the body's responses, such as fear and hunger, and he was able to map out some of these responses in detail. Partly due to the isolation imposed by World War II, and partly because his papers were written entirely in German, the outside world knew little of his work until he had accumulated about 25 years worth of experiments. This may have been fortunate, because, as he wrote in his sketch, "The vast number of experiments turned out to be decisive; for generalization concerning symptoms, syndromes, and localizations could be supported only by such a large body of data."

In 1949, Hess won a share of the Nobel Prize for physiology or medicine for his work in analyzing the function of the diencephalon, part of the interbrain, and its role in coordinating the body's internal organs; Portuguese neurosurgeon **Antonio Egas Moniz** shared the award for his work on white brain matter. Other recognitions he received included Switzerland's Marcel Benorst Prize in 1933 and the German Society for Circulation Research's Ludwig Medal in 1938.

Hess married the former Louise Sandmeyer in 1908; the couple had two children, Rudolf and Gertrud. He retired in 1951, although he continued his work and was instrumental in the establishment of an institute for brain research. He died in Locarno, Switzerland, on August 12, 1973.

HEYMANS, CORNEILLE JEAN-FRANÇOIS (1892-1968)

Belgian physiologist and pharmacologist

Born in Ghent, Belgium on March 28, 1892, Corneille Jean François Heymans was the eldest of six sons of Jan-Frans Heymans, a noted pharmacologist who founded the J. F. Heymans Institute of Pharmacology and Therapeutics at the University of Ghent. He and his father were to become a scientific team of considerable reputation—one of the few father-son scientific teams in history.

Heymans' career was delayed by four years of service as a field artillery officer in the Belgian Army during World War I. His performance won him the Belgian War Cross and the Order of the Crown of Leopold, among other decorations for valor.

After the war, Heymans received his medical degree from the University of Ghent in 1920. His father was his principal teacher and later would become his primary co-researcher in the experiments that ultimately led to the Nobel Prize in 1938. Had his father not died in 1932, he most likely would have shared the award with his son.

The year following his graduation from the university, Heymans married Berthe May, an ophthalmologist. The young couple studied abroad for several years, permitting Heymans to establish valuable contacts with some of the leading scientists of the day in his field, among them Eugène Gley at the Collège de France, Maurice Arthus at the University of Lausanne in Switzerland, Ernest H. Starling at University College in London, and Carl Wiggers at Western Reserve University's medical school in Cleveland, Ohio.

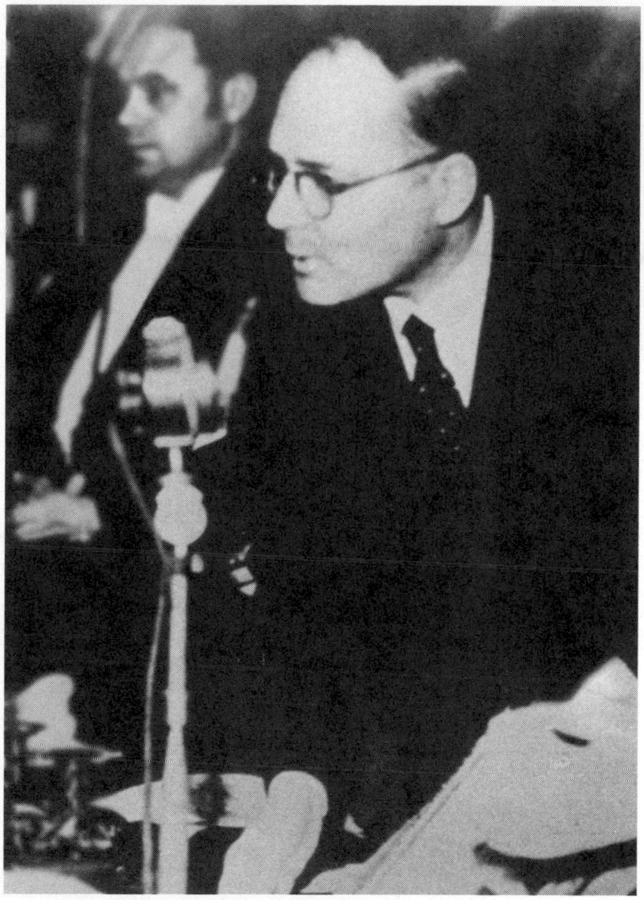

Corneille Jean-Francois Heymans

Heymans returned to the University of Ghent in 1922 to become a lecturer in pharmacodynamics, the study of the action of drugs in the body. He succeeded his father as professor of pharmacology and director of the Institute in 1930, but father and son continued to collaborate on many projects, including respiratory experiments that revealed previously unknown facts about how breathing is regulated in human beings and animals.

At that time, it had been well known for half a century that changes in blood pressure were associated with changes in the rate and the depth of breathing. The mechanism enforcing these changes in respiration was not known. It was believed, however, that alterations of breathing rates were the result of the direct action of blood pressure on the brain's respiratory center, the medulla. It was assumed that the medulla was able to detect changes in the blood circulating through it and regulate the rate of breathing accordingly.

Another scientist, Heinrich E. Hering, however, had noted a reflex action in the carotid artery (two major arteries on each side of the neck) that appeared to influence the heart beat. Through a series of experiments originally intended to refute Hering's contention, Heymans instead demonstrated that the reflex in the artery also exerted control over breathing.

The effort to determine this fact involved what became known as the ''isolated head'' technique. The head of an anesthetized dog, attached to its body only by the vagus aortic nerves, was kept alive by the shared circulation of blood of a second anesthetized dog. The Heymans found that when they induced **hypertension** (increased blood pressure) in the isolated body of the first dog its medullary respiratory center was stimulated or inhibited appropriately. But when the aortic nerves were severed, all respiratory response to changes in the blood pressure ceased. This experiment enabled the Heymans team to demonstrate conclusively that the aortic nerves were the reflex mechanism's sole sensory pathway.

The experiment thus disproved the classical theory of the blood's direct action on the brain and provided the evidence for an alternative explanation. The Heymans later determined the sites at which changes in the blood were detected. They discovered that the reflex in the carotid artery contains pressure-sensitive areas, or presso-receptors, that can detect even slight changes in blood pressure. They also found small structures on the inside walls of the carotid artery and the aorta. These chemoreceptors responded to changes in the chemical composition of the blood. By making clear why certain drugs affected respiration and circulation, Heymans' discovery opened the way for improvements in the treatment of many diseases.

Heymans' colleagues appreciated the thoroughness and accuracy of his work, which he documented in over eight hundred articles and papers published during his career. Heymans also won great recognition as a gifted teacher.

Many scientific honors came to him. In addition to the Nobel Prize, he was awarded the Alvarenga Prize of the (Belgian) Académie Royale de Medécine, the Prix Quinquennal de Medécine of the Belgian government, the Pius XI Prize of the Pontificia Academia Scientiarum and the Monthyon Prize of the Institut de France. Heymans held sixteen honorary degrees and belonged to more than forty scientific and medical societies.

Throughout his career, he traveled widely both as a lecturer and a tourist. He lectured at several major American universities, including Harvard and the University of Chicago. He was fluent in many languages and conducted seminars in Montevideo, Chile, to help organize scientific exchange programs between that country and his own. He visited India on behalf of the World Health organization. During World War II, he helped organize relief efforts to provide food for Belgian children. In so doing, he made several trips to Berlin to obtain the cooperation of German officials in getting Red Cross food shipments into Belgium.

Heymans and his wife had four children: Marie-Henriette, Pierre, Joan and Berthe. In 1963, upon his retirement from the Heymans Institute, he was designated professor emeritus. He continued to visit the institute several times a week until his death following a stroke in Knokke, Belgium, on July 18, 1968.

Hiccups

Hiccups are the result of an involuntary, spasmodic contraction of the diaphragm followed by the closing of the throat.

Hiccups are one of the most common, but thankfully mildest, disorders to which humans are prey. Virtually everyone experiences them at some point, but they rarely last long or require a doctor's care. Occasionally, a bout of hiccups will last longer than two days, earning it the name ''persistent hiccups.'' Very few people will experience intractable hiccups, in which hiccups last longer than one month.

A hiccup involves the coordinated action of the diaphragm and the muscles which close off the windpipe (trachea). The diaphragm is a dome-shaped muscle separating the chest and abdomen, normally responsible for expanding the chest cavity for inhalation. Sensation from the diaphragm travels to the spinal cord through the phrenic nerve and the vagus nerve, which pass through the chest cavity and the neck. Within the spinal cord, nerve fibers from the brain monitor sensory information and adjust the outgoing messages that control contraction. These messages travel along the phrenic nerve.

Irritation of any of the nerves involved in this loop can cause the diaphragm to undergo involuntary contraction, or spasm, pulling air into the lungs. When this occurs, it triggers a reflex in the throat muscles. Less than a tenth of a second afterward, the trachea is closed off, making the characteristic ''hic'' sound.

Hiccups can be caused by central **nervous system** disorders, injury or irritation to the phrenic and vagus nerves, and toxic or metabolic disorders affecting the central or peripheral nervous systems. They may be of unknown cause or may be a symptom of psychological **stress**. Hiccups often occur after drinking carbonated beverages or alcohol. They may also follow overeating or rapid temperature changes. Persistent or intractable hiccups may be caused by any condition which irritates or damages the relevant nerves, including:

- Overstretching of the neck
- **Laryngitis**
- Heartburn (gastroesophageal reflux)
- Irritation of the eardrum (which is innervated by the vagus nerve)
- General anesthesia
- Surgery
- Bloating
- Tumor
- Infection
- **Diabetes**.

Hiccups are diagnosed by observation, and by hearing the characteristic sound. Diagnosing the cause of intractable hiccups may require imaging studies, blood tests, pH monitoring in the esophagus, and other tests.

Most cases of hiccups will disappear on their own. Home remedies which interrupt or override the spasmodic nerve circuitry are often effective. Such remedies include:

- Holding one's breath for as long as possible
- Breathing into a paper bag
- Swallowing a spoonful of sugar
- Bending forward from the waist and drinking water from the wrong side of a glass.

Treating any underlying disorder will usually cure the associated hiccups. Chlorpromazine (Thorazine) relieves intractable hiccups in 80% of cases. Metoclopramide (Reglan), carbamazepam, valproic acid (Depakene), and phenobarbital are also used. As a last resort, surgery to block the phrenic nerve may be performed, although it may lead to significant impairment of respiration.

Most cases of hiccups last no longer than several hours, with or without treatment.

Some cases of hiccups can be avoided by drinking in moderation, avoiding very hot or very cold food, and avoiding cold showers. Carbonated beverages when drunk through a straw deliver more gas to the stomach than when sipped from a container; therefore, avoid using straws.

High-risk pregnancy

A **pregnancy** can be considered high-risk for a variety of reasons. Twins, triplets, and other **multiple pregnancies** are always considered high-risk because of the increased chance of **premature labor**. A pregnancy is also considered high-risk when **prenatal tests** indicate that the baby has a serious health problem (for example, a heart defect). In such cases, the mother will need special tests and possibly medication, to carry the baby safely through to delivery. Complications caused by pregnancy itself, such as preeclampsia or **gestational diabetes** can also turn a normal pregnancy into a high-risk pregnancy.

Finally, many women who have chronic illnesses require special attention when they become pregnant. Thousands of women live successfully with diseases like **asthma**, epilepsy, and ulcerative colitis, but when these women become pregnant they are often considered to have high-risk pregnancies. It is difficult to predict what will happen to various medical conditions during pregnancy. Of the women who have asthma, for example, 25% will get worse during pregnancy, 50% will have no change due to pregnancy, and 25% will actually get better during pregnancy. No one understands why this is so, and no one can predict the experience a woman might have.

Most women will see one healthcare provider during pregnancy, either an obstetrician, a midwife, or a nurse practitioner. Women who have a medical problem may also need the expert advice and care of a perinatologist, a medical doctor (obstetrician) specializing in the care of women at high risk for having problems during pregnancy. Perinatologists care for women who have pre-existing medical problems as well as women who develop complications during pregnancy.

A woman who has a medical problem will have more tests than the average pregnant woman. These might include tests to monitor the medical problem or blood tests to check the levels of medication. In most medical conditions, pregnancy changes the amount of medication needed.

Some medical conditions can increase the risk of birth defects. The doctor may suggest an **ultrasound** to check the baby early in the second trimester (16–18 weeks of pregnancy). At that point, the fetus is large enough that the doctor can see the organs and structures clearly. The caregiver may request ultrasound exams every few weeks to make sure the medical condition is not interfering with the baby's growth and health. Treatment varies widely with type of disease. Additional tests may help determine the need for changes in medication or additional treatment.

The prospects for successful childbirth depend in large part on the specific medical condition. Some conditions make it difficult to get pregnant and lead to a higher risk of problems in the baby. An example is thyroid disease, in which the thyroid gland (located in the neck) may produce too much or too little thyroid hormone. Abnormal levels of thyroid hormone can cause problems in pregnancy and affect the health of the baby. Fortunately, thyroid disease can be treated with medication. As long as the level of thyroid hormone is controlled throughout pregnancy, there should be no problems for mother or baby.

There is a large group of medical conditions that usually do not interfere with pregnancy, but are affected by pregnancy. This group includes asthma, epilepsy, and ulcerative colitis. For example, some women with ulcerative colitis experience a worsening of their symptoms during pregnancy, while others will have no change or may get better during pregnancy. Each of these women should be monitored very carefully throughout pregnancy.

A further group of medical conditions may have a major impact on pregnancy. Women with lupus (disease caused by alterations in the **immune system** that result in inflammation of connective tissue and organs) or kidney disease face real risks during pregnancy. Pregnancy can cause their symptoms to worsen significantly and can lead to serious illness. Because these diseases can affect the mother's ability to supply oxygen and nutrients to the baby through the placenta, they can cause problems for the baby as well. These babies may not be able to grow and gain weight properly (intrauterine growth retardation). There is also an increased risk of the birth of a dead fetus.

Diabetes is a condition that is both affected by pregnancy and affects pregnancy. It can lead to miscarriages, **birth defects**, and stillbirths. When a woman monitors her blood sugar carefully and treats high levels with insulin, the risk of these negative outcomes drops considerably. Unfortunately, pregnancy makes diabetes much harder to control. In general, blood sugar and the need for insulin to control it rise throughout pregnancy.

Most medical conditions do not lead to complications in pregnancy. With frequent visits to healthcare providers, and careful attention to medication, women with medical problems usually enjoy healthy, successful pregnancies. Women with medical problems that cause health risks during pregnancy should consider those risks before deciding to become pregnant. Only rarely (in the case of severe heart disease, for example) are the risks to the mother so high that she should not consider pregnancy at all.

A pre-pregnancy visit with a healthcare provider is especially important for a woman who has a medical problem. A woman who has not had a pre-pregnancy visit should contact a healthcare provider as soon as she learns she is pregnant. Often, the provider will schedule the first prenatal visit within a day or two, instead of waiting until 8–10 weeks of pregnancy. This is because certain medical conditions can increase the risk of miscarriage. The provider will want to be sure that any medication is adjusted properly to increase the chance of having a successful pregnancy.

HILL, ARCHIBALD VIVIAN (1886-1977)

English physiologist

Hill was born in Bristol, England, on September 26, 1886. His father, a timber merchant, abandoned the family when Hill was three, leaving his mother to educate the boy and his younger sister. After completing his primary education, Hill earned a scholarship to Trinity College, Cambridge, which he entered in 1905. At Trinity, Hill majored in mathematics and completed the usual three-year course in two years. In the process, however, he found that he was more interested in physiology than in mathematics.

After graduating in 1909 with a degree in natural sciences, Hill began research on frog muscle at the Cambridge Physiological Laboratory. At the time, muscle research was proceeding in a number of directions. Walter Fletcher (1873-1934) and **Frederick Gowland Hopkins**, for example, had earlier studied the chemical changes that occur in muscles during contraction, discovering the role of lactic acid in that process.

Hill, however, decided to forego the study of the chemical process to concentrate instead on the heat changes that

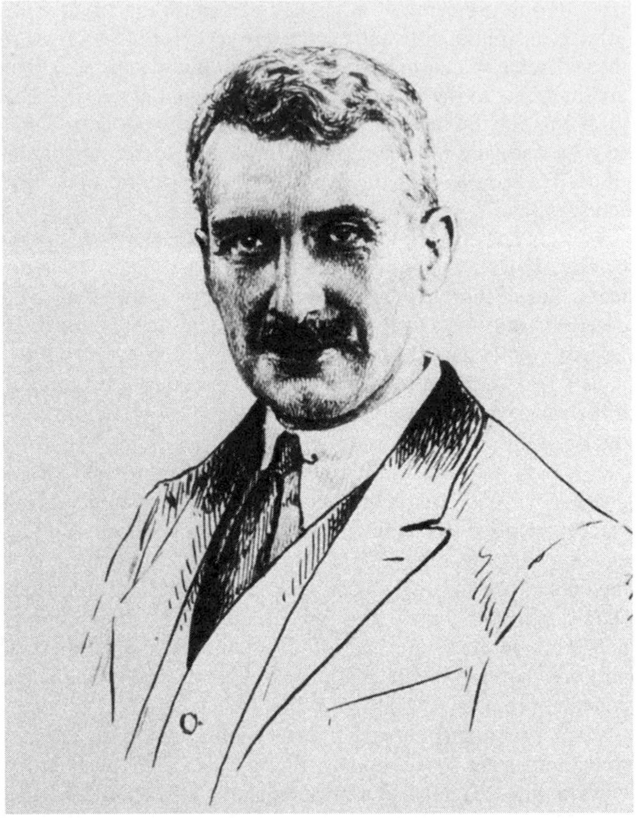

Archibald Vivian Hill

occur during muscular activity. Scientists had already found that a small amount of heat is produced during muscular contraction. Hill's goal was to analyze that process in greater detail. The task was a challenging one. Only very small amounts of heat are produced during muscular activity and for only very short periods of time. To deal with these problems, Hill used a thermocouple to measure heat changes. A thermocouple is a very sensitive kind of thermometer that converts heat changes into electrical currents that are more easily read and recorded.

With the thermocouple, Hill was able to find that heat is formed twice during muscular activity, once during the contraction itself and once following the contraction. In the former case, heat is evolved rapidly, and in the second case, more slowly, but often in larger quantities. Hill also demonstrated that oxygen is consumed during the second phase rather than during the contraction. His techniques were so precise in this research that he was able to detect temperature changes as small as 0.003° C in a few hundredths of a second. For his accomplishments, Hill was awarded a share of the 1922 Nobel Prize for physiology or medicine.

After serving with distinction in World War I, Hill did research on anti-aircraft artillery at King's College, Cambridge, work for which he was knighted in 1918. He became Professor of Physiology at Manchester University in 1920 and then moved to University College, London, in 1923. From 1926 to 1951, he was professor at the Royal Society, serving also as Secretary of the organization from 1935 to 1946. He continued his research in physiology after his retirement in 1952.

Hill married Margaret Neville Keynes in 1913. They had two sons and two daughters. Hill died in Cambridge on June 3, 1977.

Hinton, William Augustus (1883-1959)

African American medical researcher

William Augustus Hinton was the first black professor at Harvard Medical School, where he taught **preventative medicine** and hygiene, as well as bacteriology and immunology. He earned an international reputation as a medical researcher with his work on the detection and treatment of **syphilis** and other **sexually transmitted diseases**. He was integral in developing two common diagnostic procedures for syphilis, the Hinton test and the Davies-Hinton test.

Hinton was born on December 15, 1883, in Chicago, Illinois. His parents were Augustus Hinton and Maria Clark, both former slaves. Hinton grew up in Kansas and became the youngest student to ever graduate from Kansas City High School. After high school, he studied at the University of Kansas, completing the three-year premed program in two years. Hinton did some additional undergraduate work at Harvard University and received his B.S. there in 1905.

After graduation, Hinton spent some time working in a law office, but, as he reported in *Twenty-fifth Anniversary Report—Harvard Class of 1905,* he ''discovered that legal appetite can't always be cultivated.'' Instead of pursuing work in law, Hinton turned to education, teaching science at Waldo University in Tennessee from 1905 to 1906 and at State School in Langston, Oklahoma, from 1906 to 1909. It was during this time—in Langston—that Hinton met and married Ada Hawes, a teacher, in 1909. They subsequently had two daughters, Ann and Jane.

In 1909, Hinton entered Harvard Medical School. Though offered a scholarship reserved for African American students, Hinton instead chose to compete for a scholarship offered to all students. He won the Wigglesworth scholarship two years in a row . By skipping the second year of school and finishing the Harvard medical program in only three years, Hinton received his M.D. in 1912.

After graduating, Hinton's first job was as a serologist at the Wassermann Laboratory of the Harvard Medical School. By 1915, he was named the director of the lab, which at the time had become the official lab for the Massachusetts State Department of Public Health. In 1916, Hinton also became chief of the laboratory department at the Boston Dispensary. One of his accomplishments there was developing a program to train women as lab technicians, a profession that at the time was not generally open to women.

From the start of his career until his retirement, his attention was directed toward ''syphilis and the laboratory tests used in connection with its diagnosis and treatment,'' Hinton reported in *Fiftieth Anniversary Report—Harvard Class of 1905.* In 1927, Hinton developed a test—subsequently known as the Hinton test—to diagnose syphilis. Because it was easier, less expensive, and more accurate than previously used tests, the Hinton test was adopted as standard procedure for diagnosing syphilis. Later, with Dr. J. A. V. Davies, Hinton developed another diagnostic test for syphilis, know as the Davies-Hinton test.

Hinton began teaching at Harvard Medical School in 1923, as assistant lecturer in preventive medicine and hygiene. He continued teaching for 27 years. Hinton wrote one book during his career—*Syphilis and Its Treatment,* published in 1936. At the time, the book was considered controversial. In *Fiftieth Anniversary Report—Harvard Class of 1905,* Hinton wrote that the book contained ''specific ways in which laboratory tests for syphilis should be used correctly.'' Though the book had ''little support'' at first, by 1955 Hinton noted that ''except where new and superior drugs have replaced those then in use, most of it has been recognized.'' The *Harvard Medical Alumni Bulletin* of July 1959, in fact, described the book as ''widely acclaimed.'' In an interview with the *Boston Daily Globe* in 1952, Hinton told reporter Frances Burns that he considered the book his most important contribution because it summed up both his research and the experience he gained through patients in clinics who had syphilis. ''I had learned that race was not the determining factor but that it was, rather, the socioeconomic condition of the patient,'' he told Burns. ''It is a disease of the underprivileged.''

In addition to his work as a researcher, Hinton was a special consultant to the U.S. Public Health Service and, beginning in 1936, chief of the labs of the Boston Floating Hospital. He also taught at both Tufts University and Simmons College. In 1940, Hinton lost a leg in a car accident. This disability, however, did not keep him from teaching. In fact, in 1949, Harvard appointed Hinton clinical professor of bacteriology and immunology. He was the school's first black professor. Hinton retired one year later, in 1950. According to the *Boston Daily Globe,* however, he continued to teach without a salary. Hinton retired from the Massachusetts Department of Public Health Wassermann Laboratory in 1953.

At home, Hinton's hobbies were gardening and making furniture. He died at the age of 75 on August 8, 1959, in Canton, Massachusetts.

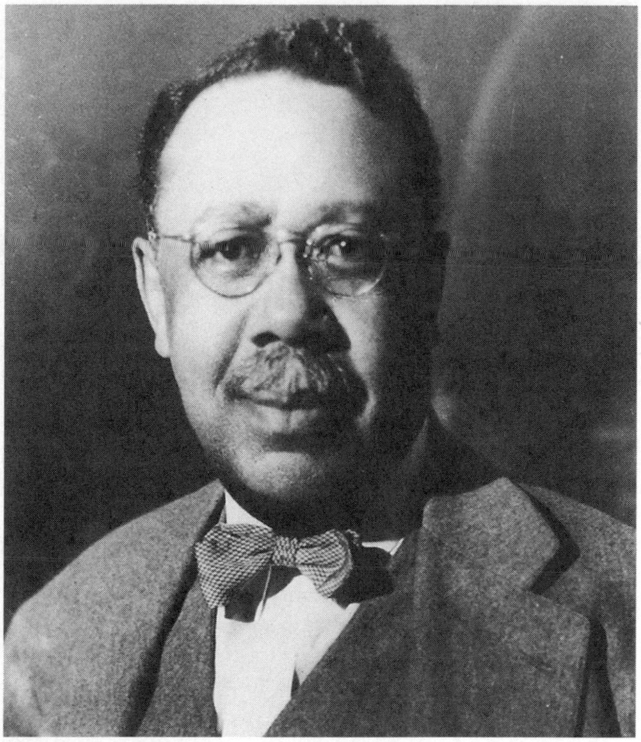

William Augustus Hinton

HIPPOCRATES OF COS (460 B.C.-377 B.C.)

Greek physician

Hippocrates was a famous Greek physician who is widely known as the ''Father of Medicine.'' Although little is known about his life, a few facts are considered accurate.

Hippocrates was born on the Greek island of Cos around 460 B.C. to a family of physicians. Cos was the site of one of the great medical schools of ancient Greece, and Hippocrates taught there for many years. He also traveled widely, lecturing in Greece and probably throughout the ancient Mideast. He was well known in his lifetime and died around 377 B.C. in Larissa.

Hippocrates is considered the father of medicine because, through his school, he separated medical knowledge and practice from myth and superstition basing them instead on fact, observation, and clinical experience. Our knowledge of Hippocrates' methods and teachings comes from the *Corpus Hippocraticum*, the Hippocratic Collection. This is a series of about 60 books that seem to have been collected in the great Library of Alexandria after about 200 B.C. While Hippocrates may have written only a few and possibly none of these books, they are considered to be an expression of his medical teachings and philosophy, which became an important basis of Western medicine.

The Hippocratic approach to medicine, expressed in the books, emphasized that disease arose from natural causes, not from whims of the gods. Hippocrates insisted on careful observation of medical conditions; the books contain dozens of detailed clinical descriptions of diseases. He recommended as little interference as possible with the body's own ability to heal. Treatment focused on diet, rest, and cleanliness. He advanced the doctrine of the four **humors**, whereby disease was supposed to result from an imbalance among the body's four important fluids.

Hippocrates also emphasized a high ethical standard for physicians. The Hippocratic Oath is a statement of medical ethics. Developed over 2,000 years ago, it probably reflects the views of Hippocrates while not actually having been written

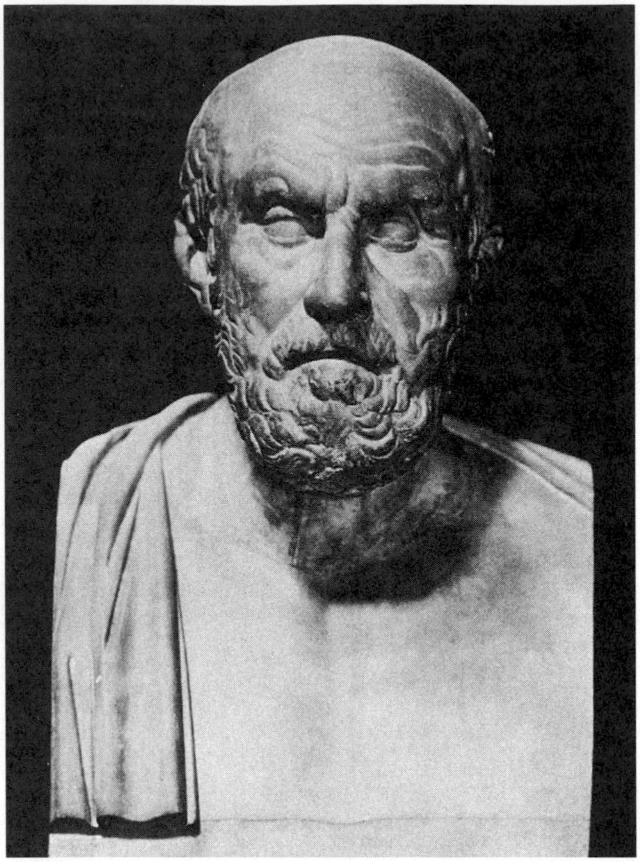

Hippocrates

by him. The oath pledges a physician to serve only the benefit of the patient, and to keep confidential anything he or she sees or hears in the course of treatment. Many medical students today still take a form of the Hippocratic Oath when they receive their medical degrees.

Hirschsprung's disease / Congenital megacolon

Hirschsprung's disease, also known as congenital megacolon, is an abnormality in which certain nerve fibers are absent in segments of the bowel, resulting in severe bowel obstruction.

The disease occurs approximately once in every 5,000 births, and is about four times more common in males than females. Hirschsprung's disease affects varying lengths of bowel segment, most often involving the region near the rectum. In 10% of affected children, the entire colon and part of the small intestine are involved.

Hirschsprung's disease is caused when cells in the wall of the colon (parasympathetic ganglion cells, which help control the movement of bowel contents) do not develop before birth. The affected segment of the intestine is prevented from relaxing and moving the bowel contents. As a result of this constriction, portions of the bowel above the affected segment are enlarged.

Hirschsprung's disease develops in the fetus early in **pregnancy**. There may be a genetic basis to the disease, since 4–50% of brothers and sisters are also afflicted and about 10% of children with the disease have a genetic condition, such as **Down's syndrome**.

The initial symptom is usually severe, continuous **constipation**. A newborn may fail to pass the first stool within 24 hours of birth, may repeatedly vomit yellow or green colored bile, and may have a swollen, uncomfortable abdomen. Occasionally, infants may have only mild or intermittent constipation, often with **diarrhea**.

While two thirds of cases are diagnosed in the first three months of life, Hirschsprung's disease may also be diagnosed later in infancy or childhood. Occasionally, even adults are found to have a variation of the disease. In older infants, symptoms and signs may include anorexia (lack of appetite or inability to eat), lack of the urge to move the bowels, empty rectum during a doctor's **physical examination**, swollen abdomen, and a lump in the colon that can be felt by the doctor. It should be suspected in older children with abnormal bowel habits, especially a history of constipation dating back to infancy and ribbon-like stools.

Occasionally, a child may have a severe intestinal infection called enterocolitis, which is life threatening. The symptoms are usually explosive, watery stools and fever in a very ill-appearing infant. It is very important to get medical attention before the intestinal obstruction causes an overgrowth of bacteria that evolves into a medical emergency. Enterocolitis can lead to severe diarrhea and massive fluid loss, which can cause death from **dehydration** unless surgery is done immediately to relieve the obstruction.

Hirschsprung's disease must be treated surgically. The goal is to remove the diseased, nonfunctioning segment of the bowel and restore bowel function. This is often done in two stages. The first stage relieves the intestinal obstruction by performing a **colostomy**. This is the creation of a stoma, an opening in the abdomen, through which bowel contents can be discharged into a waste bag. When the child's weight, age, or condition is deemed appropriate, surgeons close the stoma, remove the diseased portion of bowel, and perform a "pull-through" procedure, which connects the working part of the bowel to the anus. This usually establishes fairly normal bowel function.

Most infants with Hirschsprung's disease achieve good bowel control after surgery, but a small percentage of children may have lingering problems with soilage or constipation. These infants are also at higher risk for an overgrowth of bacteria in the intestines, including subsequent episodes of enterocolitis, and should be closely followed by a doctor.

Hirsutism

Hirsutism is excessive growth of facial or body hair in women. It is not a disease. The condition usually develops during **pu-**

berty and becomes more pronounced as the years go by. However, an inherited tendency, over-production of male hormones (**androgens**), medication, or disease, can cause it to appear at any age.

Women who have hirsutism usually have irregular menstrual cycles. They sometimes have small breasts and deep voices, and their muscles and genitals may become larger than women without the condition.

In those cases in which the cause is not clear, hirsutism is probably hereditary, because there is often a family history of the disorder.

''Secondary'' hirsutism is most often associated with polycystic ovary syndrome, an inherited hormonal disorder characterized by menstrual irregularities, biochemical abnormalities, and **obesity**. This type of hirsutism may also be caused by malfunctions of the pituitary or adrenal glands, use of male hormones or minoxidil (Loniten), a drug used to widen blood vessels, or adrenal or ovarian tumors.

Hirsutism is rarely caused by a serious underlying disorder. **Pregnancy** occasionally stimulates its development. Hirsutism triggered by tumors is very unusual.

In hirsutism, hair follicles usually become enlarged and the hairs themselves become larger and darker. A woman whose hirsutism is caused by an increase in male hormones has a pattern of hair growth similar to that of a man. Patients whose hirsutism is not hormone-related have long, fine hairs on their faces, arms, chests, and backs.

Diagnosis is based on a family history of hirsutism, a personal history of menstrual irregularities, and masculine traits. Laboratory tests are not needed to assess the status of patients whose menstrual cycles are normal and who have mild, gradually progressing hirsutism.

A family physician or endocrinologist may order blood tests to measure hormone levels in women with long-standing menstrual problems or more severe hirsutism. **Computed tomography scans** (CT scans) are sometimes performed to evaluate diseases of the adrenal glands. Additional diagnostic procedures may be used to confirm or rule out underlying diseases or disorders.

Primary hirsutism can be treated mechanically, which involves bleaching or physically removing unwanted hair by cutting, electrolysis, shaving, tweezing, waxing, or using hair-removing creams (depilatories).

Low-dose dexamethasone (a synthetic adrenocortical steroid), birth-control pills, or medications that suppress male hormones (for example, spironolactone) may be prescribed for patients whose condition stems from high androgen levels.

Treatment of secondary hirsutism is determined by the underlying cause of the condition.

Birth-control pills alone cause this condition to stabilize in one of every two patients and to improve in one of every 10.

When spironolactone (Aldactone) is prescribed to suppress hair growth, 70% of patients experience improvement within six months. When women also take birth-control pills, menstrual cycles become regular and hair growth is suppressed even more.

HISTOPLASMOSIS

Histoplasmosis is an infectious disease caused by inhaling themicroscopic spores of the fungus *Histoplasma capsulatum.* The disease exists in three forms. Acute or primary histoplasmosis causes flu-like symptoms. Most people who are infected recover without medical intervention. Chronic histoplasmosis affects the lungs and can be fatal. Disseminated histoplasmosis affects many organ systems in the body and is often fatal, especially to people with acquired immunodeficiency syndrome (**AIDS**).

Histoplasmosis is an airborne infection. The spores that cause it are found in soil contaminated with bird or bat droppings. Sometimes histoplasmosis is called Ohio Valley disease, Central Mississippi River Valley disease, Appalachian Mountain disease, Darling's disease, or *Histoplasma capsulatum* infection.

Anyone can get histoplasmosis, but people who come into contact with bird and bat droppings are more likely to be infected. This includes farmers, gardeners, demolition and construction workers, bridge inspectors, painters, people installing or servicing heating and air conditioning units, roofers, building renovators, and cave explorers. Dust suppression measures may help limit exposure. Individuals at risk of developing the more severe forms of the disease should avoid situations where they will be exposed to bat and bird droppings.

The very young and the elderly are more likely to develop severe symptoms, especially if they have a pre-existing lung disease or are heavy smokers. People who have a weakened **immune system**, either from diseases such as AIDS or **leukemia**, or as the result of medications they take (**corticosteroids** or **chemotherapy** drugs) are more likely to develop chronic or disseminated histoplasmosis.

A simple skin test similar to that given for tuberculosis will tell if a person has previously been infected by the fungus *H. capsulatum.* **Chest x rays** often show lung damage caused by the fungus, but do not lead to a definitive diagnosis because the damage caused by other diseases has a similar appearance. Diagnosis of chronic or disseminated histoplasmosis can be made by culturing a sample of sputum or other body fluids in the laboratory to isolate the fungus. The urine, blood serum, washings from the lungs, or cerebrospinal fluid can all be tested for a substance that the body produces in response to the infection.

When the spores of *H. capsulatum* are inhaled, they lodge in the lungs where they divide and cause injury. This is known as acute or primary histoplasmosis. It is not contagious. Many otherwise healthy people show no symptoms of infection at all. When symptoms do occur, they appear 3–17 days after exposure (average time is 10 days). The symptoms are usually mild and resemble those of a cold or flu: **fever**, dry **cough**, enlarged lymph glands, tiredness, and a general feeling of ill health. A small number of people develop bronchopneumonia. About 95% of people who are infected either experience no symptoms or have symptoms that clear up on their own. This creates partial immunity to re-infection. Acute histoplasmosis generally requires no treatment other than rest.

Non-prescription drugs such as **acetaminophen** (Tylenol) may be used against pain and fever. Avoiding smoke and using a cool air humidifier may ease chest pain.

In some people, spores that cause the disease continue to live in the lungs. In about 5% of infected people, (usually those with chronic lung disease, **diabetes mellitus**, or weakened immune systems), the disease progresses to chronic histoplasmosis. This can take months or years. Symptoms of chronic histoplasmosis resemble those of tuberculosis. Cavities form in the lung tissue, parts of the lung may collapse, and the lungs fill with fluid. Chronic histoplasmosis is a serious disease that can result in **death**. Patients with an intact immune system who develop chronic histoplasmosis are treated with the drug ketoconazole (Nizoral) or amphotericin B (Fungizone). In patients with healthy immune systems, alternative therapies can be very successful. These focus on creating an environment where the fungus cannot survive, by maintaining good health and eating a diet low in dairy products, sugars (including honey and fruit juice) and foods like beer that contain yeast. This is complemented by a diet high in raw food. Supplements of antioxidant **vitamins** C, E, and A, along with B complex, may also be added to the diet. *Lactobacillus acidophilus* and *Bifidobacteria* will replenish the good bacteria in the intestines. Antifungal herbs, like garlic, can be consumed in relatively large doses and for an extended time.

In patients with suppressed immune systems, chronic histoplasmosis is treated with amphotericin B, which is given intravenously. Because of its potentially toxic side effects, hospitalization is often required. The patient may also receive other drugs to minimize the side effects of the amphotericin B. Patients with AIDS must continue to take the drug itraconazole (Sporonox) orally for the rest of their lives in order to prevent a relapse. If the patient can not tolerate itraconazole, the drug fluconazole (Diflucan) can be substituted. Patients with chronic histoplasmosis who are treated with antifungal drugs generally recover rapidly if they do not have underlying illness.

The rarest form of histoplasmosis is disseminated histoplasmosis. Disseminated histoplasmosis is seen almost exclusively in patients with AIDS or other immune defects. In disseminated histoplasmosis the infection may move to the spleen, liver, bone marrow, or adrenal glands. Symptoms include a worsening of those found in chronic histoplasmosis, as well as weight loss, **diarrhea**, the development of open sores in the mouth and nose, and enlargement of the spleen, liver, and adrenal gland. Little is known about the prospects of recovery from disseminated histoplasmosis, because AIDS patients typically have other infections that complicate the issue.

HITCHINGS, GEORGE H. (1905-1998)

American pharmacologist

George H. Hitchings was among the most prolific of modern pharmaceutical scientists. He worked at Burroughs Wellcome Company, a British pharmaceutical company with research facilities in the United States, for more than thirty years before his retirement in 1975. Hitchings produced many important pharmaceuticals for treating diseases such as **cancer**, **gout**, and **malaria**, and for preventing rejection of transplanted organs. His contributions were based on the premise that an understanding of what makes diseased cells different from normal cells makes it possible to exploit those differences to destroy cancer cells or foreign invaders such as bacteria or viruses with drugs. For his work in finding treatments for serious diseases, Hitchings and his long-time Burroughs Wellcome collaborator **Gertrude Elion** shared the 1988 Nobel Prize in physiology or medicine with British pharmaceutical scientist Sir **James Black**. It was the first time since 1957 that pharmaceutical scientists had been awarded the prize.

George Herbert Hitchings was born to George Herbert Hitchings, Sr., a naval architect, and Lillian H. Belle Hitchings on April 18, 1905, in Hoquiam, Washington, on the Olympic Peninsula. His father's death when he was twelve and his admiration for **Louis Pasteur**, a preeminent scientist-philanthropist who became his role model, aimed Hitchings toward a career in medicine. As the salutatorian of his high school class, Hitchings gave an address to the graduating class on the **germ theory** and Pasteur's life.

Hitchings attended the University of Washington, where he received a bachelor's degree in chemistry in 1927 and a master's degree in chemistry in 1928. He also showed a fondness for many scholarly subjects, studying the arts and history in college. He began his career in scientific research at an early age. ''The Chemistry of the Waters of Argyle Lagoon,'' the first of his more than three hundred scientific publications, appeared in the publications of the Puget Sound Biological Station in 1928, when he had just entered graduate school. He continued his graduate work in biological chemistry at Harvard College, where he received his Ph.D. in 1933. Hitchings' doctoral dissertation concerned the **metabolism** of nucleic acids, the chemicals that make up DNA, the carrier of genetic information. Hitchings did his work on nucleic acids before **James Watson** and **Francis Crick** discovered the structure of DNA, and at that time no one was interested in nucleic acids. Hitchings couldn't find a job. Finally, after working for nine years as a teaching fellow at Harvard (1933–39) and Western Reserve University (1939–42), he was hired by Burroughs Wellcome in 1942 and resumed his work on nucleic acids. He became vice president of research in 1967 and held the position until 1975, when he became scientist emeritus.

Until Hitchings and the pharmacologist Gertrude Elion came along, drug researchers sought new drugs by modifying natural products. The two pioneered a method that has come to be known as ''rational'' drug design. They reasoned that if they understood the differences between normal and diseased or infected cells, these differences could serve as a entry point to selectively kill diseased tissue without harming surrounding normal tissue. They implemented these ideas by investigating the chemical pathways of nucleic acid synthesis, which is crucial to cell metabolism. Hitchings synthesized chemicals similar in structure to natural nucleic acids, the purines and pyrimidines. These related compounds interfered with DNA synthesis. Because cancer cells divide quickly, the compounds are particularly disruptive to them, killing them as they try to divide. This form of **chemotherapy** is just one instance of the rational drug design that helped Hitchings accumulate eighty-five patents over his thirty-year career.

One compound in particular, 6-mercaptopurine (6MP), a purine analog synthesized in 1951, proved to be particularly effective. Working with scientists at Sloan-Kettering Institute, Hitchings and Elion perfected the drug, which was used to combat childhood leukemia. 6MP and thioguanine, also produced by Hitchings and Elion, are still used to treat acute **leukemias**.

In 1959 Hitchings discovered that 6MP inhibited production of antibodies in rabbits. A less toxic form called azathioprine, marketed under the trade name Imuran, was developed in 1957 to control rejection of transplanted organs and treat autoimmune diseases. In the nearly nine thousand kidney transplants performed each year, Imuran remains the drug most commonly used to prevent organ rejection. 6MP is broken down in the body by xanthine oxydase, the same enzyme that converts purines into uric acid, the cause of the painful joint disease gout. Further investigation of purine analogs led to the development of allopurinol in the 1960s. It blocks uric acid production by competing for xanthine oxydase, an enzyme that converts purines to uric acid. Hitchings was also active in the development of other drugs, including pyrimethamine, which is used to treat malaria, and trimethoprim, which is used to treat urinary tract infections and other bacterial infections.

Philanthropy had always been a part of Hitchings' life, and he has said that when he was baptized his father dedicated his life to the service of mankind. He served as president of the Burroughs Wellcome fund, a charitable organization, from 1971 to 1990. In addition, he has served as director of a dozen local chapters of philanthropic organizations.

Hitchings married Beverly Reimer in 1933. The couple had two children, Laramie Ruth and Thomas Eldridge. Beverly died in 1985. In 1989, Hitchings was remarried to Joyce Shaver. He died on February 27, 1998 in Chapel Hill, North Carolina.

Besides the Nobel Prize, Hitchings received numerous awards, including the Gregor Mendel Medal from the Czechoslovakian Academy of Science in 1968 and the Albert Schweitzer International Prize for Medicine in 1989. He was awarded eleven honorary degrees and was a member of the National Academy of Sciences. In addition, he traveled widely, lecturing in Africa, Asia, Europe and South America.

HIVES

Hives is an allergic skin reaction causing localized redness, swelling, and **itching**.

Hives is a reaction of the body's **immune system** that causes areas of the skin to swell, itch, and become reddened (wheals). When the reaction is limited to small areas of the skin, it is called ''urticaria.'' Involvement of larger areas, such as whole sections of a limb, is called ''angioedema.''

Hives is an allergic reaction. The body's immune system is normally responsible for protection from foreign invaders. When it becomes sensitized to normally harmless substances, the resulting reaction is called an allergy. An attack of hives is set off when such a substance, called an allergen, is ingested, inhaled, or otherwise contacted. It interacts with immune cells called mast cells, which reside in the skin, airways, and **digestive system**. When mast cells encounter an allergen, they release histamine and other chemicals, both locally and into the bloodstream. These chemicals cause blood vessels to become more porous, allowing fluid to accumulate in tissue and leading to the swollen and reddish appearance of hives. Some of the chemicals released sensitize **pain** nerve endings, causing the affected area to become itchy and sensitive.

A wide variety of substances may cause hives in sensitive people, including foods, drugs, and insect **bites or stings**. Common culprits include:

- Nuts, especially peanuts, walnuts, and Brazil nuts
- Fish, mollusks, and shellfish
- Eggs
- Wheat
- Milk
- Strawberries
- Food additives and preservatives
- **Penicillin** or other **antibiotics**
- Flu vaccines
- **Tetanus** toxoid vaccine
- Gamma globulin
- Bee, wasp, and hornet stings
- Bites of mosquitoes, fleas, and **scabies**.

Urticaria is characterized by redness, swelling, and itching of small areas of the skin. These patches usually grow and recede in less than a day, but may be replaced by others in other locations. Angioedema is characterized by more diffuse swelling. Swelling of the airways may cause **wheezing** and respiratory distress. In severe cases, airway obstruction may occur.

Hives are easily diagnosed by visual inspection. The cause of hives is usually apparent, but may require a careful medical history in some cases.

Mild cases of hives are treated with **antihistamines**, such as diphenhydramine (Benadryl). An oatmeal bath may also relieve itching. More severe cases may require oral **corticosteroids**, such as prednisone. Topical corticosteroids are not effective. Airway swelling may require emergency injection of epinephrine (adrenaline).

Most cases of hives clear up within one to seven days without treatment, providing the cause (allergen) is found and avoided.

Preventing hives depends on avoiding the allergen causing them. Analysis of new items in the diet or new drugs taken may reveal the likely source of the reaction. Chronic hives may be aggravated by **stress**, **caffeine**, alcohol, or tobacco; avoiding these may reduce the frequency of reactions.

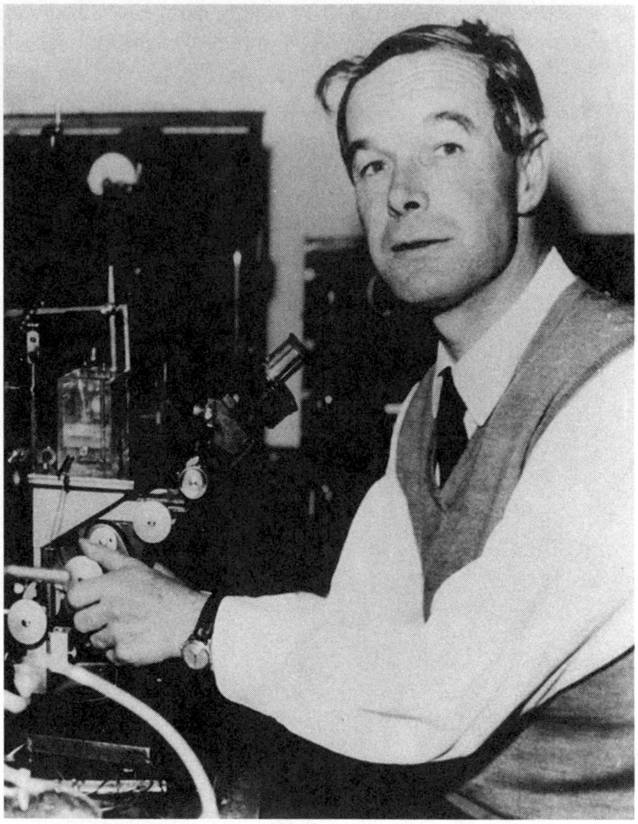

Alan Lloyd Hodgkin

HODGKIN, ALAN LLOYD (1914-1998)

English biophysicist

Alan Lloyd Hodgkin was best known for his work in defining the electrical and chemical characteristics of nerve impulses. Along with **Andrew F. Huxley** he performed experiments on the nerve fibers of squid and described the nerve impulses with a series of mathematical equations. For their research in this area, which resulted in the ionic theory of nerve impulses, the two men shared the 1963 Nobel Prize in physiology or medicine with **John C. Eccles**.

Hodgkin was born on February 5, 1914, in Banbury, Oxfordshire, England, to George L. and Mary Wilson Hodgkin. Hodgkin's father died in Baghdad during World War I, only a few years after his birth. Hodgkin was educated at the Downs School in Malvern and the Gresham School in Holt. In 1932, he entered Trinity College, Cambridge, where he first became interested in physiology. Hodgkin became a fellow at Trinity in 1936, serving as lecturer and later as assistant director of research at the physiological laboratory.

Hodgkin began studying the electrical properties of the nerve fibers in the shore crab while at Cambridge. He spent a year at the Rockefeller Institute in New York City between 1937 and 1938, and while there he met scientists who had developed new methods for studying nerve fibers. Hodgkin brought these ideas back to Cambridge, where with Andrew Huxley he devised an experiment to test an hypothesis about nerve impulses first proposed by German physiologist Julius Bernstein.

Bernstein had hypothesized that nerve cells possess a resting or unstimulated potential and an action or stimulated potential. During the resting potential, he believed, the nerve cell membrane had an unequal distribution of positively and negatively charged ions, with more negative ones on the inside. During resting potential, the membrane was permeable to the positively charged ions, but the negatively charged ions could not permeate the cell membrane. When the cell was stimulated, Bernstein argued, the membrane ''gates'' were temporarily opened, allowing ions to pass in both directions. By using the nerve cells of the shore crab, Hodgkin was able to establish that the resting potential was due to an outward movement of potassium ions; during the action potential the cell membrane's gates allowed in the more concentrated sodium ions. He also discovered that the action potential was usually much larger than the resting potential.

Some of the researchers Hodgkin had met in the United States were working with squid, whose nerve fibers are larger than those of most organisms. Hodgkin and Huxley were able to develop a method to study these fibers using microelectrodes, and they were able to confirm the results of their earlier experiment. Their progress, however, came to a halt during World War II, when Hodgkin worked on radar systems for aircraft for the Air Ministry. Hodgkin and Huxley were back in Cambridge in 1945, and they formed a small research group to pursue their pre-war investigations into nerve fibers.

In 1951, Hodgkin and his colleagues published the results of their research. They found that the membrane is permeable only to specific ions during the resting potential, because of the differing concentrations of potassium and sodium. The concentration of the positively charged sodium ions is greater on the outside of the membrane and the concentration of negative potassium ions higher on the inside during resting potential. During the action potential, the negative and positive ions travel through the membrane, so that the interior charge becomes positive and the exterior negative. This is followed by an equilibrium charge, then a return to the resting potential charge state. All this happens in milliseconds.

The work done by Hodgkin and Huxley which was most responsible for bringing them to the attention of the Nobel Prize committee was the development of a series of mathematical formulae they published in 1952. The purpose of these equations was to synthesize the experimental information then available about the electrical and chemical nature of nerve transmissions. Their goal was to analyze and predict each stage in the passage of the nerve cell membrane from resting to action potential. They were awarded the 1963 Nobel Prize in physiology or medicine, which they shared with John C. Eccles, an Australian who advanced the British team's findings by showing what happens to nerve impulses transmitted across the synapses, or intersections, between nerve cells.

Hodgkin was appointed Foulerton Research Professor of the Royal Society in 1952, and was awarded the Royal Medal in 1958. He was John Humphrey Plummer Professor of Biophysics at Cambridge from 1970 to 1981, president of the Marine Biological Association from 1966 to 1976, and a master of Trinity College.

Hodgkin was married in 1944 to Marion Rous, the daughter of American Nobel Laureate **Peyton Rous**. The couple met during Hodgkin's year at the Rockefeller Institute in New York. They had four children. Hodgkin died December 20, 1998.

HODGKIN'S DISEASE

Hodgkin's disease is a cancerous enlargement of the lymph nodes, spleen, and other lymphoid tissue. Examples of the syndrome were first recorded by the Italian physician **Marcello Malpighi** in 1666, but it was an English physician, Thomas Hodgkin (1798-1866), who first described the disease in detail in 1832.

Born in London in 1798, Hodgkin received his medical degree in 1821 from the University of Edinburgh and served as lecturer on morbid anatomy at Guy's Hospital in London from 1825 to 1837. Hodgkin introduced the use of the newly invented **stethoscope** to Great Britain from the Continent and promoted the importance of postmortem examination. Passed over for an appointment as assistant physician at Guy's, Hodgkin, a Quaker, devoted increasing amounts of time in his later years to philanthropic and humanitarian concerns. He died of dysentery in Jaffa on a mission to Palestine in 1866.

Hodgkin's interest in postmortem investigations led to the presentation of a paper in 1832 titled "On Some Morbid Appearances of the Absorbent Glands and Spleen" describing a particular type of lymphoma characterized by swollen lymph tissue. The importance of this paper wasn't recognized until 1856, when the English doctor Samuel Wilks redescribed the condition and named it Hodgkin's disease.

Hodgkin's disease is distinguished from other conditions that cause lymphatic tissue swelling by the presence of giant, mostly multi-nuclear, cells. These Sternberg-Reed cells were first recorded by pathologists Carl Sternberg (Germany) in 1898 and Dorothy Reed (U.S.) in 1902.

Hodgkin's disease occurs primarily between the ages of 15 and 35 and after the age of 55. Once almost certainly fatal, Hodgkin's disease can now, for the most part, be successfully treated, especially if it is discovered in the early stages. The standard therapy combines radiation and **chemotherapy**. Clinical trials are also being conducted using bone marrow transplants as an adjuvant therapy. The transplants are designed to replace bone marrow which may have been destroyed by chemotherapy, thus compromising the patient's **immune system**. Ironically, immune deficiency may be a risk factor for acquiring Hodgkin's disease. As a result, it is often found in patients with the acquired immunodeficiency syndrome, or **AIDS**.

HOLISTIC MEDICINE

Holistic (also spelled "wholistic") medicine is the ancient art and science of healing that addresses the whole person and emphasizes the inseparable connection of mind, body, and spirit in promoting health and treating illness. Holistic medical care adheres to three basic tenets: recognizing the psychological, environmental, and social contributions to disease; actively involving the patient in the treatment process; and emphasizing **preventive medicine**, alternative therapies, and a lifestyle that lessens the probability of developing disease.

Over 5,000 years ago, ancient healing traditions in India and China stressed living a healthy life that was in harmony with nature. Socrates (4th century B.C.) also advocating treating the whole person, stating that "the part can never be well unless the whole is well."

The term *holism* was introduced by Jan Christiaan Smuts in 1926 as a way of viewing living things as "entities greater than and different from the sum of their parts." The holistic movement, however, gathered impetus in the late 1960s as a reaction to what some observers viewed as the increasing role of costly and depersonalizing medical technology, and a nearly universal dependence on drugs in the diagnosis and treatment of disease. Although the older, nineteenth-century concept of a physician had been basically humanistic, critics of more recent developments charged that advanced medical technology had led **physicians** to treat organs rather than whole persons. In addition, many chronic conditions did not respond to standard medical treatments.

Several publications that provided the groundwork for this movement include *Man, Medicine, and Environment* (1958) and *Health and Disease* (1965). In both books, the author, microbiologist René Dubos, emphasized the role played by social change in conquering infectious diseases. In addition, social critic Ivan Illich, in *Medical Nemesis* (1975), and health-care policy expert, Rick Carlson, in *The End of Medicine* (1975), addressed the dehumanizing aspect of technological medicine and predicted its replacement by a more individualized medical system.

By the 1970s, the word "holistic" was commonly used in the field of health and medicine, and in 1978 the American Holistic Medical Association was founded in the United States.

In addition to the belief that the whole is more than the sum of its parts, the principles of holistic medicine state that health is more than the absence of disease. A common explanation is to view wellness as line on a continuum. The line represents all possible degrees of health. The left end of the line represents premature death. On the right end is the highest possible level of wellness and maximum well being. The midpoint of the line represents an apparent lack of disease, thus placing all levels of illness on the left side of the wellness continuum. The right half indicates that even when no illness seems to be present, there is still much room for improvement. Holistic health, therefore, is looked at as an ongoing process.

Holistic medicine maintains that the majority of illnesses and premature death can be traced back to lifestyle choices. While the dangers connected with drugs, alcohol, nicotine, and unprotected sexual activity are well known, the impact of excesses in such things as sugar, **caffeine**, and negative attitudes are considerably less publicized. Combined with deficiencies in exercise, nutritious foods, and **self-esteem**, these excesses gradually accumulate harmful effects. With time, they diminish the quality of life within that human being and can set the stage for illness.

According to the ideas of holistic medicine, quality of life, in the present and in the future, is being determined by a multitude of seemingly insignificant choices made every day.

While preventing illness is important, holistic medicine focuses on reaching higher levels of wellness. However, when disease and chronic conditions occur, the principles of holistic medicine can also be applied. Holistic health care professionals (physicians, nurses, acupuncturists, herbalists, for example) use the holistic approach in partnership with their patients and recommend treatments that support the body's natural healing system.

A holistic approach to healing means more than eliminating symptoms. In holistic medicine, a symptom is considered the body's message that something needs attention. The symptom is used as a guide to look beneath the surface for the root cause.

See also Herbal remedies, Western; Physician; Preventive medicine

Holley, Robert William (1922-1993)

American biochemist

Robert William Holley is best known for his 1962-1965 work in chemically isolating pure strands of transfer ribonucleic acid (tRNA), which retrieves specific amino acids for assembly by the cell's ribosomes into proteins. He also determined the complete sequence of one RNA strand. For this work, he shared the 1968 Nobel Prize for physiology or medicine with **Har Gobind Khorana** and **Marshall Nirenberg**.

Holley was born in Urbana, Illinois, where his parents were teachers, and received his bachelor's degree from the University of Illinois. He obtained his Ph.D. from Cornell University and spent almost his entire career there, in 1964 becoming professor of biochemistry and molecular biology.

Working with yeast RNA, Holley used techniques developed for proteins by Frederick Sanger, including chemical fragmenting, cutting with restriction enzymes, and separating by ion-exchange chromatography and paper electrophoresis. He used snake venom for the first cuts on long strands. After deciphering the base sequences on the fragments, he reconstructed the sequence of the entire strand.

Following this, Holley studied the relationship between messenger RNA (mRNA), the first copy of a DNA instruction, and tRNA. He also partially identified the three-dimensional structure of RNA and showed that tRNA was a cloverleaf, rather than a helix as deoxyribonucleic acid (DNA) is.

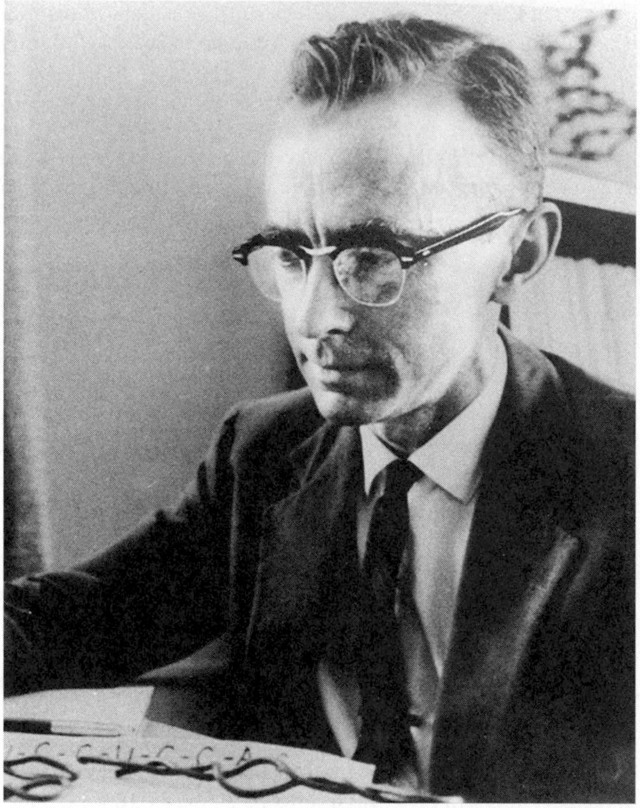

Robert William Holley

Holmes, Oliver Wendell (1809-1894)

American physician and author

Best known as a poet and essayist, Oliver Wendell Holmes was also a renowned physician. Born in Cambridge, Massachusetts, Holmes came from an old New England family. He earned both his undergraduate and medical degrees from Harvard, then served as professor of anatomy at Dartmouth from 1838-1840 and at Harvard from 1847 until his retirement in 1882. His ability to hold his students' attention was legendary. During these years, he wrote medical papers, literary essays, and poems, including the famous ''Old Ironsides'' and ''The Deacon's Masterpiece.'' He also suggested the name **anesthesia** for the use of ether in surgery when it began in 1846.

During 1842 and 1843 the medical community of Boston was especially concerned about puerperal **fever**, or childbed fever. This dreaded and usually fatal contagion regularly swept through maternity wards of hospitals, striking women who had just given birth. Holmes did a study of cases of the fever and presented his findings in *The Contagiousness of Puerperal Fever*, published in 1843 and reprinted with additions in 1855. He deduced that the disease was a contagious infection carried from dead or infected patients to new victims by the doctors who examined them. Holmes recommended hand washing and other sanitary precautions by physicians to pre-

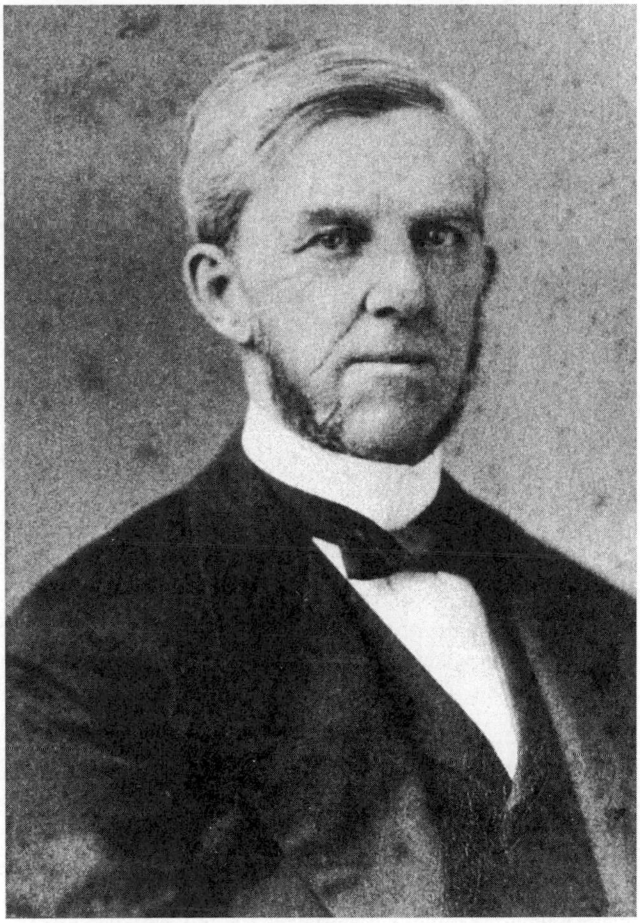

Oliver Wendell Holmes

vent the spread of the disease. This discovery preceded similar findings by **Ignaz Semmelweiss** four years later.

Unfortunately, Holmes's advice was largely ignored or attacked by his colleagues, especially since microbiological proof of the theory was unavailable. But Holmes, unlike Semmelweiss, did live to see his conclusions proven and put into practice.

HOME HEALTH CARE

Home health care can include many different services. While the services may differ, they all have in common the fact that they are delivered to the patient at his or her home. The patient may be recovering from recent surgery or illness and need medical checkups or **wound** care, or may be a disabled patient who received physical or occupational therapy at home. In general, the care needed is more skilled than can be provided by the family or friends of the patient, and the patient prefers to stay home rather than enter a nursing facility.

Home care suppliers vary depending on the kind of services they provide.

Home health agencies provide skilled care from physicians, nurses and trained therapists. For instance, a home health agency nurse might visit a woman who has just given birth and her new baby to do a well-baby check and answer any of the mother's questions. A physical therapist working for a home health agency might visit an accident victim who is trying to regain the use of his leg. Because they often provide more than just one medical specialty, a home health agency can meet the varying needs of the same patient.

Sometimes home health agencies will also provide **hospice** care (which can also be provided by independent hospice care organizations). Hospice care professionals (such as nurses) and volunteers provide not only medical care but also emotional and psychological care to people who are terminally ill. Hospice care workers also help support the family in caring for the patient and dealing with their own emotional health. They also help keep the patient as comfortable and pain-free as possible.

A homemaker or home care aide agency supplies trained personnel who can assist clients with housekeeping, bathing, dressing and preparing meals. These personnel are sometimes called ''companions.''

Some home care agencies assist patients not by delivering medical care but by providing essential equipment and supplies. Suppliers of durable medical equipment (equipment that can be used and reused after it is thoroughly decontaminated and cleaned) can provide, deliver and set up a variety of medical equipment and teach patients their proper use. Examples of durable medical equipment include wheelchairs, breast pumps, and walkers. These firms may also provide home oxygen services, delivering and maintaining an oxygen tank in the patient's home if such an arrangement is necessary.

Similarly, other companies can provide in-home delivery of medication and equipment for patients who need intravenous drug delivery or **tube feeding**.

Other health care professionals that can provide their services in the home health care setting include social workers, occupational therapists, speech-language pathologists, and dietitians.

Home health care can be paid for directly by the patient. However, many services (if provided by a qualified individual or agency) will be paid for under the federal **Medicare** program (which covers most people over age 65), Medicaid (which is joint federal-state funded program), the Veterans Administration (available only to veterans who are at least 50% disabled by a service-related injury), and the Older Americans Act.

Commercial insurance carriers and managed care companies will also sometimes pay for home health care services. Paying for home care can actually be a bargain for an insurer, because treating a patient at home with home health care can cost thousands of dollars less than treating the patient in the hospital.

Like **hospitals** and **nursing homes**, home care providers must meet strict standards for the quality of services and the delivery of care. Meeting these standards results in a provider being accredited, a sign of quality that persons seeking home care should look for. The major accrediting organizations for home care include the National Committee for Quality Assurance (NCQA) (202-955-3510), the Joint Commission on Accreditation of Healthcare Organization (JCAHO) (630-792-5600), the Community Health Accreditation Council (212-989-9393) and the National Home Caring Council (202-547-6586).

For more information about home health care, contact the National Association for Home Care, 228 Seventh St. SE, Washington, DC, 20003 (202-547-7424).

HOMEOPATHIC MEDICINE

Homeopathic medicine, or homeopathy, is a holistic system of treatment that originated in the late eighteenth century. The name homeopathy is derived from two Greek words that mean ''like disease'' because the system is based on the notion that a medicine capable of curing a disease will mimic or imitate its symptoms. **Samuel Hahnemann** (1755-1843), the founder of homeopathic medicine, used the Latin phrase *similia similibus curentur*, or ''let like be cured with like,'' to summarize the underlying principle of his system. Homeopaths use the term allopathy, or ''other disease,'' to describe the use of drugs in conventional medicine to oppose or counteract the symptom being treated.

Hahnemann was trained in the standard medical practice of his day and licensed as a physician in 1779. In 1796, he gave up his practice because he was disturbed by the poor results of orthodox medical treatment. He supported himself by working as a translator of medical texts. While translating an English physician's research on a treatment for **malaria**, Hahnemann experimented on himself with small doses of the drug until he developed symptoms resembling malaria. He concluded that the substance's curative powers came from its ability to produce symptoms resembling those of its target disease. Hahnemann's reasoning was similar to that of **Edward Jenner**, who discovered the principle of **vaccination** in 1798 by observing that exposure to a mild form of pox conferred immunity against **smallpox**, a deadly disease with similar symptoms.

Hahnemann followed up his experiment by studying local records of accidental **poisoning**s from commonly used medications. He found that when these substances were taken in overdose, they produced symptoms similar to those of the diseases for which they were given. For example, mercury was used to treat **syphilis**, but could cause syphilis-like ulcers in high doses. Hahnemann referred to his discovery as ''the law of similars.'' By this, he meant that substances producing specific symptoms when given to healthy people in sufficient quantity could heal sick people of similar symptoms when given in highly diluted forms.

The purpose of homeopathy is the restoration of the body to homeostasis, or healthy balance, which is considered its natural state. The symptoms of a disease are regarded as the body's own defensive attempt to correct its imbalance, rather than as enemies to be defeated. Because a homeopath regards symptoms as evidence of the body's inner intelligence, he or she will prescribe a remedy designed to stimulate this internal curative process rather than suppress the symptoms.

The holistic nature of homeopathic treatment means that practitioners do not focus on isolated symptoms when treating patients. Even if the patient seeks help for only one illness, such as a cold or a skin rash, the homeopath will evaluate the disorder in the context of the patient's overall physical and psychological characteristics. It is thought that a careful assessment of all the patient's symptoms over the course of years will reflect a basic weakness specific to that person's constitution. In acute treatment, which is given for colds, vomiting, **fever**, and similar problems, the homeopath selects a remedy on the basis of the patient's symptomatic reactions to recent stresses in his or her life.

The first stage in homeopathic treatment is the practitioner's detailed notation of the patient's symptoms. Homeopathic case-taking includes not only the symptoms directly associated with the illness but other physical complaints that the patient may have and his or her psychological reactions. Homeopathy uses the word symptom in a broader sense than mainstream medicine. In homeopathy, symptoms include any physical or emotional change observed during the course of an illness. In addition to noting the location and severity of the symptoms, the homeopath will ask about the circumstances or factors (e.g., weather, time of day, behavior or activity, etc.) that make the symptom either better or worse.

The practitioner will choose the medication by matching the patient's symptom profile with the symptoms that the remedy has been proved to cause in healthy people. Dose repetition or change of medication is based on observation of the patient's response.

A homeopathic medication is formulated by preparing what is called a mother tincture, which is made by soaking plant, animal, or mineral materials in a solution of alcohol. The mother tincture is then diluted with either 10 or 100 parts of alcohol. The process of dilution is repeated many times in order to achieve the desired potency.

There are few risks associated with homeopathic treatment in the United States. In terms of training, some homeopaths are licensed graduates of conventional medical schools in many fields. Others are naturopaths and registered nurses. In addition, there are lay practitioners of homeopathy whose practice should be more limited than licensed professionals.

The heavily diluted remedies used in homeopathy are safe in terms of their chemical composition and have fewer side effects than conventional medications. However, symptoms may briefly worsen when a remedy is first used. A number of practitioners have written books emphasizing the limitations of homeopathic home treatment. The complexity of the case-taking process and determining the appropriate prescriptions persuade most patients to consult practitioners for serious illnesses rather than attempting to treat themselves.

HOMICIDE

Homicide is the formal term for one person killing another person, whether the act was criminal or not. There are four legal categories of homicide, which vary in their definitions and associated punishments from country to country.

The main categories of homicide are murder, which denotes a crime committed with malicious or clear intent; manslaughter, which includes acts committed in a moment of passion or recklessness without malice aforethought; noncriminal homicide; and excusable, negligent, or accidental homicide, such as when someone dies during surgery due to unforeseen complications.

In the United States, the categories of murder and manslaughter are subdivided into levels of seriousness, or ''degrees.''

Homicides generally not regarded as criminal are those committed in self-defense, to aid a police officer or other representative of the law (for instance, during a sanctioned execution), or to stop someone from committing a serious crime. In addition, the legal systems of some countries consider the ''mercy killing'' or **euthanasia** of a terminally ill or grievously injured person to be noncriminal.

Penalties for homicide can vary to the same degree as the definition of the crime, but usually murder is punishable by death or life imprisonment, while a conviction for manslaughter may bring a certain maximum jail term.

HOOKWORM DISEASE

Hookworm disease is an illness caused by one of two types of S-shaped worms that infect the intestine of humans (the worm's host): *Necator americanus* and *Ancylostoma duodenale*. The two species cause illness by attaching themselves to the lining of the small intestine and sucking a person's blood.

Both types of hookworm are similar. The adult worm of both is about 10 mm long, pinkish-white in color, and curved into an S-shape or double hook. The females produce about 10,000–20,000 eggs per day. These eggs are passed out of the host's body in feces. The eggs enter the soil, where they incubate. After about 48 hours, the immature larval form hatches out of the eggs. These larvae take about six weeks to develop into the mature larval form that is capable of causing human infection. If exposed to human skin at this point (usually bare feet walking in the dirt or bare hands digging in the dirt), the larvae will bore through the skin and ride through the lymph circulation to the right side of the heart.

An itchy, slightly raised rash called ''ground itch'' may appear around the area where the larvae first bored through the skin. The skin in this area may become red and swollen. This lasts for several days and commonly occurs between the toes.

The larvae are then pumped into the lungs. There, they bore into the tiny air sacs (alveoli) of the lungs. Their presence within the lungs usually causes enough irritation to produce **cough**ing, **fever**, and **wheezing**. However, some people have none of these symptoms.

The larvae are coughed up into the throat and mouth, and are then swallowed and passed into the small intestine. Within the intestine that they develop into the adult worm. Hookworms cause trouble for their human host when they attach their mouths to the lining of the small intestine and suck the person's blood.

Once established within the intestine, the adult worms can cause **pain**, decreased appetite, **diarrhea**, and weight loss. The worms suck between 0.03–0.2 ml of blood per day. When a worm moves from one area of the intestine to another, it detaches its mouth from the intestinal lining, leaving an irritated area that may continue to bleed for some time. This results in even further blood loss. A single adult worm can live for up to 14 years in a patient's intestine. Over time, the patient's blood loss may be significant. **Anemia** is the most serious complication of hookworm disease, progressing over months or years. Children are particularly harmed by such anemia and can suffer from heart problems, **mental retardation**, slowed growth, and delayed sexual development. In infants, hookworm disease can be deadly.

To diagnose hookworm disease, a stool sample is examined under a microscope for hookworm eggs. Counting the eggs in a specific amount of feces allows the healthcare provider to estimate the severity of the infection. Minor infections are often left untreated, especially in areas where hookworm is very common. If treatment is required, the doctor will prescribe a three-day dose of medication. One to two weeks later, another stool sample will be taken to see if the infection is still present. Anemia is treated with iron supplements. In severe cases, blood transfusion may be necessary. Two medications, pyrantel pamoate and mebendazole, are frequently used with good results.

The prognosis for patients with hookworm disease is generally good. However, reinfection rates are extremely high in countries with poor **sanitation**. Preventing hookworm disease involves improving sanitation and avoiding contact with soil in areas with high rates of hookworm infection. Children should be required to wear shoes when playing outside in such areas, and people who are gardening should wear gloves.

Ancylostoma duodenale is found primarily in the Mediterranean, the Middle East, and throughout Asia. *Necator americanus* is common in tropical areas including Asia, parts of the Americas, and throughout Africa. Research suggests that at least 25% of all people in the world have hookworm disease. In the United States, 700,000 people are believed to be infected with hookworms at any given time.

HOPKINS, FREDERICK GOWLAND (1861-1947)

English biochemist

Born in Sussex, England, Hopkins had a lonely and unhappy childhood. He was brought up by his widowed mother and an unmarried uncle who tended to ignore him. When Hopkins was seventeen, his uncle chose a career in insurance for him and for several years he dutifully gave in to his uncle's wishes. At the same time, however, he also took part-time courses in chemistry at the University of London, eventually getting his degree. In 1888, already twenty-seven years old, Hopkins received the small inheritance that finally enabled him to enter medical school at Guy's Hospital in London.

After getting his doctoral degree in 1894, Hopkins joined the staff of Guy's Hospital and taught for several years. In 1898, he was invited to teach physiology and anatomy at

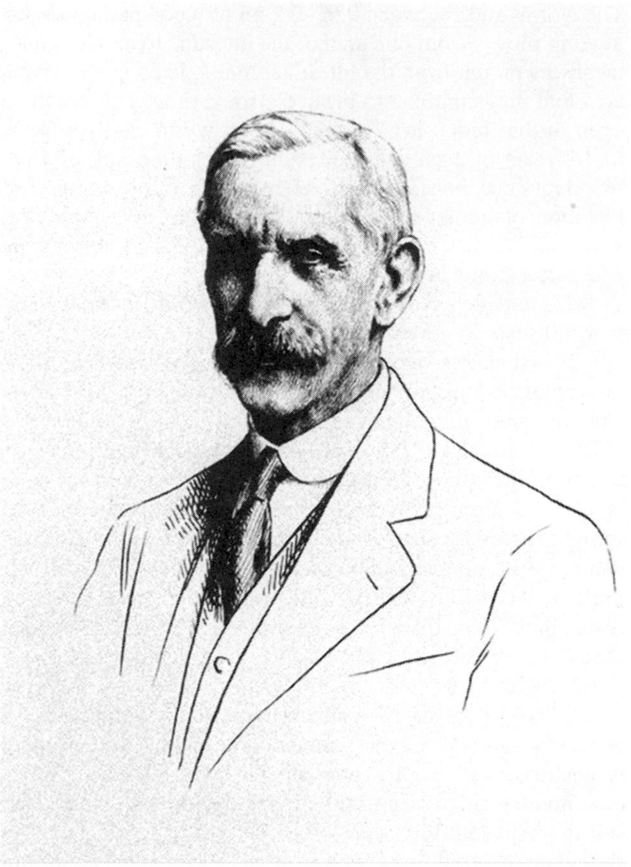

Frederick Gowland Hopkins

Cambridge University and it was at Cambridge—when Hopkins was well into his thirties—that his long, distinguished career really began.

Hopkins' early research was in uric acid and his studies of the effects of various diets on uric acid excretion first aroused his interest in proteins. In 1901, working with S.W. Cole, a student at Cambridge, Hopkins discovered tryptophan, an important amino acid, and was able to isolate it from protein. A few years later, he demonstrated that tryptophan, and certain other amino acids, could not be manufactured in the body from other nutrients but had to be supplied as such in the diet. (By so doing, he laid the foundation for the concept of the essential amino acid outlined by William Rose a generation later.)

After his work with tryptophan, Hopkins' primary interest became the study of diet and its effect on **metabolism**. At the time, nutritional science was in a fairly primitive stage. Most researchers confidently believed that a well-rounded diet consisted of the proper mixture of fats, proteins, carbohydrates, mineral salts, and water, and that the so-called diet-linked illnesses—such as **beriberi** or **scurvy**—were caused by some toxic substance in certain foodstuffs. Hopkins, studying the literature—including reports by **Christiaan Eijkman** that polished rice seemed to cause beriberi, while unpolished rice effected a cure—began to have serious doubts.

Hopkins had already noticed that his laboratory rats failed to grow on a diet of artificial nutrients, but grew rapidly when he added tiny amounts of cow's milk to their daily rations. He suspected, therefore, that normal food must contain substances missing from the pure fats, proteins and carbohydrates routinely used—for consistency—in nutritional studies. Terming these substances ''accessory food factors,'' he pointed out that they appeared to be necessary for growth. His two papers on the subject, in 1906 and 1912, are considered the first explanations of the concept of **vitamins**.

In 1907, Hopkins and Sir Walter Fletcher conducted pioneering research in another area of biochemistry when they demonstrated that working muscles accumulate lactic acid. And in 1922, Hopkins isolated the tripeptide (triple-linked) enzyme, glutathione, from living tissue and demonstrated its importance to the utilization of oxygen by tissue cells.

For his pioneering work in vitamin research, Hopkins received the 1929 Nobel Prize in medicine or physiology (sharing the prize with Eijkman). He was knighted in 1925 and received numerous other awards, including the Royal Medal of the Royal Society of London in 1918 and the Copley Medal in 1926.

HOPPE-SELYER, ERNST FELIX (1825-1895)

German biochemist

Ernst Hoppe-Selyer was one of the leaders in making biochemistry (or physiological chemistry, as it was called then) a scientific field distinct from medical physiology. He performed the first study of the nucleic acids, gave the name hemoglobin to the red blood cells, and discovered the enzyme invertase.

Ernst Hoppe was born in Freiburg-an-der-Unstrut, Germany. His father, a minister, and his mother died when he was a child. After he was adopted by his brother-in-law, he added Selyer to his name. He received his medical degree from the University of Berlin in 1851, then combined a medical practice with scientific research. Hoppe-Selyer's interest shifted gradually from physiology to chemistry. After serving on the faculties of the Universities of Berlin and Tubingen, in 1872 he became professor of physiological chemistry at the University of Strasbourg (then part of Germany). He established the first independent biochemistry laboratory in 1877 and the first biochemical journal.

Hoppe-Selyer's first important discovery came in 1862, when he used the newly invented spectrograph to determine the structure of the red blood cells, which he called hemoglobin. He later showed how hemoglobin binds and releases oxygen and how carbon monoxide can take oxygen's place in the blood cell. He also demonstrated some of the chemical similarities of hemoglobin and chlorophyll.

Hoppe-Selyer began studying the nucleic acids after they were discovered in 1869 by one of his students, the Swiss biochemist Johann Friedrich Miescher. Hoppe-Selyer showed that nucleic acids were present in yeast, and his work was extended by his one-time assistant, **Albrecht Kossel**.

Hoppe-Selyer's other research included the discovery in 1871 of invertase, the enzyme that converts sucrose (table sugar) into the simpler sugars glucose and fructose. He helped determine that lecithin is composed of nitrogen, phosphorus, fat, and choline (one of the B vitamins). And he demonstrated that lecithin and the steroid cholesterol are found in every cell.

HORMONE REPLACEMENT THERAPY

Hormone replacement therapy (HRT) is the use of synthetic or natural female hormones to make up for the decline or lack of natural hormones produced in a woman's body. HRT is sometimes referred to as estrogen replacement therapy (ERT), because the first medications that were used in the 1960s for female hormone replacement were estrogen compounds.

These drugs are given in a variety of prescription strengths and methods of administration. HRT has two primary purposes: preventive treatment against **osteoporosis** and heart disease; and relief of physical symptoms associated with **menopause**.

Women in midlife enter a stage of development called menopause, when their menstrual periods become irregular and finally stop. The early phase of this transition is called the perimenopause. In the United States, the average age at menopause is presently 50 or 51, but some women begin menopause as early as 40 and others as late as 55. It can take as long as 10 years for a woman to complete the process. Women who have had their ovaries removed surgically are said to have undergone surgical menopause.

During the menopausal transition, the levels of estrogen in the woman's body drop. The lowered estrogen level is responsible for a group of symptoms that include hot flashes (or flushes), weight gain, changes in skin texture, mood swings, heart **palpitations**, sleep disturbances, a need to urinate more frequently, and loss of sexual desire. The estrogen that is given in HRT can eliminate hot flashes, night sweats, lack of vaginal lubrication, and urinary tract problems. HRT will *not* prevent weight gain or wrinkles. It also does not cure depression in most women.

HRT is recommended by many doctors on the grounds that estrogen replacement helps to protect women against two serious midlife health problems.

Osteoporosis is a disorder in which the bones become more brittle and more easily fractured. It is a particular problem for postmenopausal women because the lower levels of estrogen in the blood lead to weakening of the bone. About 25% of Caucasian women will develop severe osteoporosis; Asian women have a slightly lower risk level; Latina and African American women are least at risk.

In addition to race, there are other factors that put some women at higher risk of developing osteoporosis. Women in any of the following groups should take bone loss into account when considering HRT.

- Family history of osteoporosis
- Menopause before age 40
- Kidney disease and dialysis
- Thin body build or being underweight
- History of colitis, Crohn's disease, or chronic **diarrhea**
- Thyroid medications
- Childlessness
- Chronic use of **antacids**
- Lack of **exercise**
- Poor food choices, including high salt intake, lack of vitamin D, high **caffeine** consumption, and low calcium intake
- **Smoking** and alcohol abuse
- Cortisone therapy.

Heart disease is a major health concern of women in midlife. It is the leading cause of **death** in women over 60. The primary disorders of the circulatory system in postmenopausal women are **stroke**, **hypertension**, and **coronary artery disease**. Current studies of women on HRT do not yield a completely clear picture. In particular, although estrogen given without progestins has been shown to offer some protection against heart disease, the effect of progestins in offsetting the benefits of estrogen complicates the research findings. It seems likely that estrogen levels are only part of the picture in evaluating a woman's risk of heart disease.

The major factors that are known to increase the risk of heart disease include:

- History of smoking
- Being overweight
- High-fat **diets**
- Alcohol abuse
- Family history of heart disease
- High blood pressure
- High blood cholesterol levels
- **Diabetes**.

Less important risk factors include being African American, having a sedentary lifestyle, undergoing menopause before age 45, and having high levels of family- or job-related **stress**.

HRT medications come in several different forms, including tablets, stick-on patches, injections, and creams or rings that are worn inside the vagina. The form prescribed depends on the purpose of the hormone replacement therapy. All HRT medications used in the United States are available only with a doctor's prescription.

It is important to know that there is still considerable disagreement over the advantages and disadvantages of HRT. As of June 1998, a major American research team was urging further research into other strategies for health care in menopausal women. In the United Kingdom, the so-called ''Million Women'' study is being conducted to evaluate different types of HRT and the long-term health risks of this treatment.

The most important controversy over HRT is whether it increases a woman's risk of developing **breast cancer**. Some studies not only indicate a connection, but suggest that the risk of breast cancer rises with the length of time that a woman has been taking HRT. According to an American study published in June 1998, the risk of breast cancer increases by 2.3% for each year that a woman takes HRT. A Swedish study found that the risk of breast cancer doubled after six years of HRT, which agrees with American findings that risk is connected to length of treatment.

Horsley, Victor Alexander Haden (1857-1916)

English physiologist

Sir Victor Horsley earned recognition as the father of neurosurgery because of his experiments in physiology, the study of living organisms. While a medical student at University College in London, Horsley served as clinical clerk to Henry Charlton Bastian and developed a lifelong interest in the nervous system. While still in medical school, Horsley assisted Bastian with the text *The Brain as an Organ of the Mind*, and he illustrated a lecture by neurologist Sir William Gowers on spinal nerves and their relationship to the vertebral column.

While a house surgeon at University College Hospital, Horsley was reported to have used himself as a research subject. After earning his medical degree with a gold medal in surgery, Horsley joined the medical service at University College Hospital and National Hospital, Queen Square. He was also appointed assistant professor of pathology at University College and became superintendent of the Brown Institution. Horsley's affiliation with Brown laid the groundwork for his career in neurosurgery.

Horsley's pioneering work would not have been possible without the discoveries of **anesthesia** (1846), antiseptic principles (1865) (see **Lister**), and cerebral localization, the process which matched brain function with anatomy.

In 1886, Horsley performed 10 operations to remove brain tumors and was named a Fellow of the Royal Society. In 1887, Horsley and his former professor, Sir William Gowers, performed the first surgery to remove a spinal tumor. Although the surgery was successful and the patient was able to walk again, the medical community was outraged. Cranial surgeries of blood clots, **abscess**es, tumors and cranial nerves were within acceptable ethical limits, but no one had operated on the spinal column before. Gowers influenced Horsley to carry out anatomical experiments which Gowers used in his text *Diagnosis of Diseases of the Spinal Cord*.

The American brain surgeon Harvey W. Cushing traveled to London in 1900 and wrote of his meetings with Horsley. To Cushing, Horsley appeared to lead a frenetic life. At the breakfast table, Horsley ate while dictating letters to a secretary and petting the family dog. When Horsley took Cushing on a case that involved drilling into a patient's skull, manipulating the temporal lobe and closing the wound in less than an hour, Cushing abruptly left the city. As far as he was concerned, Horsley's practice of surgery in London was too primitive for him to learn anything.

Horsley always managed to combine a large practice with ongoing research. Most of his practice was devoted to the treatment of nervous disorders, while his research interests lay in neurophysiology and neurological surgery. His wide ranging scientific curiosity led him to study woodpeckers, ducks and armadillos in a search for anatomical clues that would help with surgery on humans. He carried out research on canine chorea, cortical localization, thyroid function, and **Pasteur**'s antirabies vaccine.

Throughout his career, Horsley was controversial. One of his former medical professors called him an amateur, and a colleague referred to him as an intellectual hormone. Horsley tried to advance science by carrying out research and antivivisectionists (who opposed animal experimentation) bitterly criticized him. Horsley was often able to see only one side of a question and he spoke out on social issues such as temperance, female suffrage, and a National Insurance Bill.

Horsley's achievements relied on his willingness to be the first to try something new. He developed the use of wax, muscle and deep **anesthesia** to control bleeding. He invented many **surgical instruments**, including a device to hold the patient's head. He was the first to expose the pituitary gland and the first to try to remove a tumor of the pineal gland. In consultation with his mentor Gowers, Horsley was the first to perform a root section for trigeminal **neuralgia**, a painful nerve disease which had no known cure. He also promoted the idea of surgical treatment for intracranial expanding lesions.

Horsley received knighthood in 1902. He went on to draft a new constitution for the British Medical Association and was first chairman of its representative body. In 1911, he was the first recipient of the Lannelongue Prize, given to the person who had made the greatest contribution to surgery over the past 10 years, and in 1912 he was elected to Royal Society of Uppsalla, filling the vacancy created by Lister's death.During World War I, Horsley improved conditions in military hospitals in Egypt and Mesopotamia (now Iraq) and was promoted to colonel. He died of typhoid in the Middle East.

Horstmann, Dorothy Millicent (1911-)

American virologist

Dorothy Millicent Horstmann played a significant yet often unacknowledged role in the development of the **polio** vaccine. In the late 1940s and early 1950s, before polio immunizations were considered feasible, she conducted groundbreaking animal studies which proved that the polio virus reaches the nervous system through the bloodstream. In 1952, while working at the Yale School of Medicine, she set up an experiment to determine whether polio first appeared in the blood before moving on to the brain. She fed monkeys and chimpanzees small quantities of polio virus, then examined the blood for traces of the it. The animals did not immediately develop symptoms of polio, yet small traces of virus were observable in their blood. Many of the animals later developed **paralysis**, one of polio's debilitating symptoms.

Horstmann was born July 2, 1911, in Spokane, Washington, to Henry and Anna (Humold) Horstmann. She received her B.A. in 1936 and her M.D. in 1940 from the University of California. After holding an internship at the San Francisco City and County Hospital from 1939 to 1940, she did her medical residency at Vanderbilt University. In 1942, she began her long affiliation with the Yale University School of Medicine. In 1945, Horstmann was appointed associate professor of medicine at Yale; from 1947 to 1948, she held a National Institutes of Health postdoctoral research fellowship there. In 1961,

Horstmann rose to professor of epidemiology and pediatrics, and in 1969 she was named John Rodman Paul Professor of Epidemiology and Pediatrics. Since 1982, she has held the titles of emeritus professor and senior research scientist at Yale. Horstmann was led to her experiments by the work of William McDowell Hammon, who showed that injections of gamma globulin, an antibody-rich serum extracted from plasma, could produce temporary immunity to polio. From this lead, Horstmann hypothesized that the polio virus first travelled through the bloodstream before finally settling in the nervous system. The discoveries she made during her experiments with monkeys and chimpanzees were initially dismissed by some virologists as inconclusive, because in most patients who had developed polio, no virus had been found in their blood. It was subsequently established, however, that by the time the symptoms of polio became clinically evident, the virus had already left the bloodstream and established itself in the nervous system. Horstmann's work and the parallel studies of David Bodian at Johns Hopkins University proved that polio is an intestinal infection which can enter the nervous system through the bloodstream.

Throughout the 1950s and 1960s, Horstmann participated in field trials to establish the effectiveness and safety of polio vaccines. During her distinguished career, Horstmann also studied maternal rubella and the rubella syndrome in infants. She holds four honorary doctorates and has received numerous honors and awards, including the James D. Bruce Award of the American College of Physicians, 1975, Denmark's Thorvold Madsen Award, 1977, and the Maxwell Finland Award of the Infectious Diseases Society of America, 1978. She is a member of the National Academy of Sciences, the American Society of Clinical Investigations, the American College of Physicians, and the Royal Society of Medicine.

HOSPICES

Hospice care is comprehensive palliative medical care (treatment aimed at reducing or abating **pain** and other symptoms, rather than treatment aimed at cure) and supportive social, emotional, and spiritual services to the terminally ill and their families, primarily in the patient's home but also in a hospice in-patient facility. Hospice reaffirms the right of every person and family to participate fully in this final stage of life's journey.

The word ''hospice'' is derived from the Latin *hospe*, meaning both host and guest. The idea of hospice is rooted in the centuries old idea of offering hospitality to those on a long journey. This concept of providing care, comfort, and aid to travelers can be traced back to Syria in the year 475 A.D.. It was during the Middle Ages, however, that the concept of hospices as way stations for pilgrims and travelers proliferated. By early medieval times, there were more than 750 hospices in England alone. Not only offering hospitality to injured travelers, hungry wayfarers, orphans, and the poor, hospices also sheltered the sick and dying.

The modern hospice movement began in England in the 1940s when Cicely Saunders, a British **physician**, founded St. Christopher's Hospital, a place where the terminally ill were cared for and could die with dignity. St. Christopher's Hospital continued to be a model for hospices worldwide and was recognized as an innovator in the area of **pain management** and treatment of the terminally ill.

When Saunders visited Yale University in the late 1960s, her vision of a peaceful place where the dying could find comfort in their final weeks or months found enthusiastic support. She ignited a fire that would lead to the establishment of Hospice, Inc., of New Haven, Connecticut, the first home care hospice in the United States. Soon thereafter the Connecticut Hospice of Branford was established, a residential facility designed exclusively for the care of the terminally ill. Based on the hospice principles established at St. Christopher's, these two organizations became the prototypes for hospices throughout the United States.

Elisabeth Kübler-Ross, a Swiss-American psychiatrist and renowned authority in the field of **death** and dying, also provided an impetus to the hospice movement in the United States. In a book based on more than 500 interviews with dying patients entitled *On Death and Dying* (1969), Kübler-Ross identified the five stages through which many terminally ill patients progress. The book became an internationally known best seller. In it, Kübler-Ross made a plea for home care as opposed to treatment in an institutional setting and argued that patients should be able to participate in the decisions that affect their destiny.

It is significant that the hospice movement found sustenance in the social and moral climate of the late 1960s and early 1970s a time when great strides were made in the care of those with life threatening illnesses, extending their life expectancies. As medical costs continued to escalate, a great burden was placed on hospitals focusing on acute care. The option of the more humane, compassionate, cost-effective method of care offered by hospices provided an attractive alternative. For a populace enlightened by a growing awareness of the needs of the dying by the work of Elisabeth Kübler-Ross, the hospice movement's time had come.

A person is considered terminally ill when he or she has received the maximum treatment for a disease without achieving remission or eradication of the disease. To be admitted to a hospice program, a patient must be declared by his or her doctor to have six months to live and not be seeking active medical treatment. Hospice focuses on maximizing the quality of life when the quantity of life cannot be extended with the emphasis on the individual rather than the disease.

In order to die with dignity, the hospice philosophy is that one must be in relative comfort. Thus, medications are used to prevent pain from occurring rather than to control it once it is present. For this reason, medication is given on a 24 hour basis to maintain maximum levels of comfort. Frequently, family members are taught how to administer the medications, decreasing their sense of helplessness and bolstering faltering and fragile **self-esteem**. Informed consent and active participation in all aspects of care return control to patients and their families whenever possible and appropriate.

In hospice, the patient and family are the unit of care. Total care requires providing services for all those affected by terminal illness or death. Families are supported before and during the illness and bereavement period. They are given help in coping with their feelings, maintaining a fulfilling relationship with the patient and planning for the future. This support, provided by an interdisciplinary team the physician and primary care nurse, who is the case manager, social workers, home health aides, clergy, volunteers, and other medical personnel as needed both enhances the quality of the patient's life and offers comfort to family members.

Most hospices provide services without charge if patients have limited or no financial resources. Insurance coverage for hospice care, however, is available through **Medicare**, Medicaid, and most private insurance plans.

See also Death; Kübler-Ross, Elisabeth; Living will; Pain; Pain management

HOSPITAL-ACQUIRED INFECTIONS

A hospital-acquired infection is usually one that first appears three days after a patient is admitted to a hospital or other health-care facility. Such infections are also called nosocomial infections.

About 5–10% of patients admitted to hospitals in the United States develop one of these infections, which are usually related to a procedure or treatment used to treat the patient.

Hospital-acquired infections can be caused by bacteria, viruses, fungi, or parasites. These microorganisms may already be present in the patient's body or may come from the environment, contaminated hospital equipment, healthcare workers, or other patients. An infection may start in any part of the body. A localized infection, such as at an abdominal surgery site, is limited to a specific part of the body and has local symptoms. A generalized infection enters the bloodstream and causes general systemic symptoms such as **fever**, chills, low blood pressure, or mental confusion.

Hospital-acquired infections may develop from surgical procedures, catheters placed in the urinary tract or blood vessels, or from material from the nose or mouth that is inhaled into the lungs. The most common types of hospital-acquired infections are urinary tract infections (UTIs), **pneumonia**, and surgical wound infections. **Ulcers** can also become infected.

All hospitalized patients are susceptible to contracting a nosocomial infection. Some patients are at greater risk than others, such as young children, the elderly, and persons with compromised **immune systems**. Other risk factors for getting a hospital-acquired infection are a long hospital stay, the use of indwelling catheters, failure of healthcare workers to wash their hands, and overuse of **antibiotics**.

Other hospital procedures that put patients at risk for nosocomial infection are gastrointestinal procedures, obstetric procedures, and **kidney dialysis**.

Fever is often the first sign of infection. Other symptoms and signs of infection are rapid breathing, mental confusion, low blood pressure, reduced urine output, and a high white blood cell count.

An infection is suspected any time a hospitalized patient develops a fever that cannot be explained by a known illness. Some patients, especially the elderly, may not develop a fever. In these patients, the first signs of infection may be rapid breathing or mental confusion.

Hospital-acquired infections are serious illnesses that cause death in about 1% of cases. Rapid diagnosis and identification of the responsible microorganism is necessary, so treatment can be started as soon as possible.

Hospitals and other healthcare facilities have developed extensive **infection control** programs to prevent nosocomial infections. These programs focus on identifying high risk procedures and other possible sources of infection. High risk procedures such as urinary catheterization should be performed only when necessary and catheters should be left in for as little time as possible. Medical instruments and equipment must be properly sterilized to ensure they are not contaminated. Frequent handwashing by healthcare workers and visitors is necessary to avoid passing infectious microorganisms to hospitalized patients.

Antibiotics should only be used when necessary. Use of antibiotics creates favorable conditions for infection with the fungal organism *Candida*. Overuse of antibiotics is also responsible for the development of bacteria that are resistant to antibiotics.

HOSPITALS

There are various types of hospitals, but all are places in which people who need medical treatment are looked after and cared for.

The Hindus built the first known hospitals during the 5th century BC in what is now known as Sri Lanka. Hospitals didn't reach the western hemisphere until about 1500, however. when the first institution dedicated to medical care was constructed on the island of Hispaniola. Soon after, a hospital was erected in Mexico City, where it stands today.

The first hospital in the United States was called the Pennsylvania Hospital, built in Philadelphia in 1751. Today there are more than 6,600 hospitals throughout the United States available to people who require medical care. Those that treat a wide variety of minor and serious illnesses are called general hospitals. If the facility cares for those living around it, it is referred to as a community hospital.

Larger, more sophisticated hospitals which specialize in very serious or hard-to-treat illnesses by providing state-of-the-art medical care are known as "medical centers." Most provide tertiary (referral-based) care and are linked to medical schools. They may be known for a particular type of treatment, such as burn care, emergency medicine, open heart surgery or organ transplants. These university- or medical school-affiliated medical centers provide valuable teaching experiences for their students. These institutions are also known as "teaching hospitals."

In addition, there are a number of specialty hospitals including comprehensive cancer centers, children's hospitals, maternity hospitals, geriatric hospitals for the aged, and veterans hospitals (for members of the armed forces).

Most hospitals are designed to treat patients only for short periods of time, and most must follow **health insurance** guidelines limiting the number of days a patient can stay in the hospital. However, some hospitals deal with more chronic problems where patients with ongoing health problems are cared for.

Hospitals are regularly inspected by a national group known as the Joint Commission for the Accreditation of Healthcare Organizations (JCAHO) to assure they meet basic requirements of good medical care. In order to work in hospitals, doctors must apply for "hospital privileges" which allows them to admit their patients to that hospital.

Most hospitals in the United States are non-profit institutions. Those that are run with the intention of making a profit are called proprietary facilities. About a fourth of American hospitals are operated by a government agency, such as the Veterans Administration, or a city or state. Other hospitals are administered by religious groups.

No matter what type of hospital it may be, most are separated into departments in which certain kinds of medical services are available. Major departments in most hospitals include nursing, surgery, anesthesiology, obstetrics and gynecology, pediatrics, emergency department, radiology, nutrition and physical therapy.

Some larger hospitals contain specialized medical departments, such as **pathology** (where diseases are diagnosed and cause of death determined), dermatology, cardiology, neurology, and psychiatry.

HOTLINES

There are a multitude of hotlines available that can be a source of crisis intervention, support, referrals, and information for specific problems. Many hotlines may be reached toll-free from all 50 states, 24 hours a day, seven days each week. Finding a hotline in a nearby area can be accomplished by calling the social work department of the local hospital, or by looking in the telephone book, in the yellow pages under Social Service Organizations. The hotline may match the caller with a survivor with a similar history, or link survivors' family members with veteran family members who've coped with similar issues. The practical advice and/or emotional support given can provide a new lifeline for the caller.

One example of a nationally available hotline is that for **domestic violence**. In addition to having a toll-free line at 1-800-799-SAFE (7233), there is line for the hearing impaired (TTY) at 1-800-787-3224. Callers can converse in either English or Spanish, with interpreters available to translate an additional 139 languages. The National Domestic Violence Hotline links individuals to help in their area using a nationwide database that includes detailed information on domestic violence shelters, other emergency shelters, legal advocacy and assistance programs, and social service programs.

Some other national crisis hotlines include **Child Abuse** and Neglect Reporting Line (1-800-292-9582), Poison Information (1-800-722-7112), **Rape** Crisis (1-800-262-9800), Runaways Hotline (1-800-621-4000), Narcotics Anonymous (1-800-229-7244), and **Suicide** Hotline (1-800-345-6785).

See also Child abuse; Domestic violence; Rape; Suicide

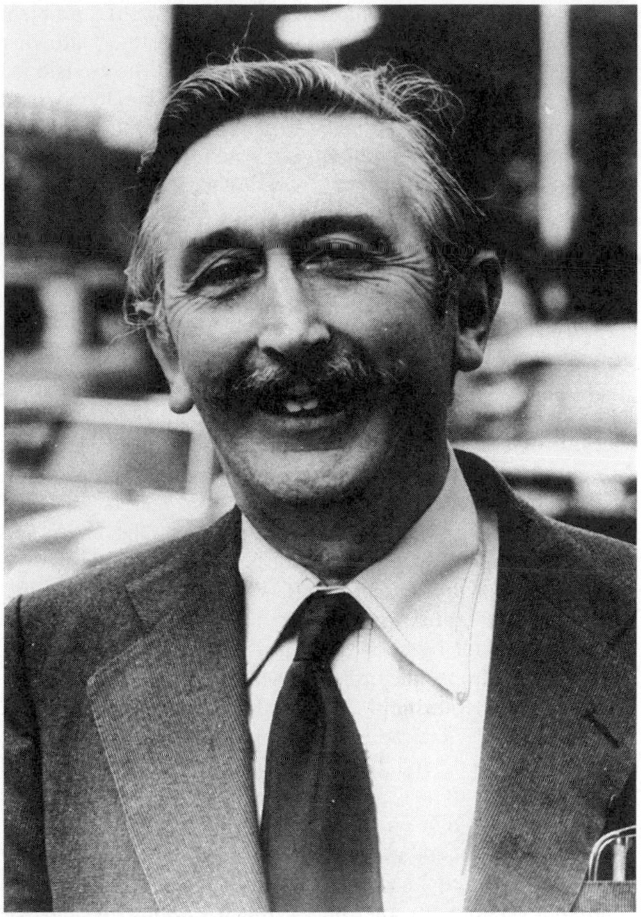

Godfrey Newbold Hounsfield

HOUNSFIELD, GODFREY N. (1919-)

English biomedical engineer

Godfrey Newbold Hounsfield was born August 28, 1919, in Newark, England, the youngest of five children of a steel-industry engineer turned farmer. He graduated from London's City and Guilds College in 1938 after studying radio communication. When World War II erupted, Hounsfield volunteered for the Royal Air Force (RAF), where he studied and later lectured on the new and vital technology of radar at the RAF's Cranwell Radar School. After the war he resumed his education, and received a degree in electrical and mechanical engineering from Faraday House Electrical Engineering College in 1951. Upon graduation, Hounsfield joined Thorn EMI (Electrical and Musical Industries) Ltd., an employer he has remained with his entire professional life.

At Thorn EMI, Hounsfield worked on improving radar systems and then on computers. In 1959, a design team led by Hounsfield finished production of Britain's first large all-transistor computer, the EMIDEC 1100. Hounsfield moved on to work on high-capacity computer memory devices, and was granted a British patent in 1967 titled "Magnetic Films for Information Storage."

Hounsfield's work in this period included the problem of enabling computers to recognize patterns, thus allowing them to "read" letters and numbers. In 1967, he envisioned a medical diagnostic system in which an **x-ray machine** would image thin "slices" through the patient's body and a computer would process the slices into an accurate representation which would display the tissues, organs, and other structures in much greater detail than a single x ray could produce. Computers available in 1967 were not sophisticated enough to make such a machine practical, but Hounsfield continued to refine his idea and began working on a prototype scanner. He enlisted two radiologists, James Ambrose and Louis Kreel, who assisted him with their practical knowledge of radiology and also provided tissue samples and test animals for scans. The project attracted support from the British Department of Health and Social Services, and in 1971 a test machine was installed at Atkinson Morely's Hospital in Wimbledon. It was highly successful, and the first production model followed a year later. These original scanners were designed for imaging the brain, and were hailed by neurosurgeons as a great advance. Before the computerized axial tomography (CAT) scanner, doctors wanting a detailed brain x ray had to help their equipment see through the skull by such dangerous techniques as pumping chemicals or air into the brain. As head of EMI's Medical Systems section, Hounsfield continued to improve the device, working to lower the radiation exposure required, sharpen the images produced, and develop larger models which could image any part of the body, not just the head. This "whole body scanner" went on the market in 1975.

CAT scanners generated some resistance because of their expense: even the earliest models cost over $300,000, and improved versions several times as much. Despite this, the machines were so useful they quickly became standard equipment at larger hospitals around the world. The scanner won Hounsfield and his company more than thirty awards, including the MacRobert Award, Britain's highest honor for engineering. In 1979, Hounsfield's collection of scientific tributes was topped off with the Nobel Prize. That year's Nobel was shared with **Allan M. Cormack**, an American nuclear physicist who had separately developed the equations involved in reconstructing an image via computer. A surprising feature of the selection was that neither man had a degree in medicine or biology, or a doctorate in any field.

Hounsfield moved on to positions as chief staff scientist and then senior staff scientist for Thorn EMI. He continued to improve the CAT scanner, working to develop a version which could take an accurate "snapshot" of the heart between beats. He has also contributed to the next step in diagnostic technology, nuclear magnetic resonance imaging. In 1986, he became a consultant to Thorn EMI's Central Research Laboratories in Middlesex, near his longtime home in Twickenham.

HOUSSAY, BERNARDO A. (1887-1971)

Argentine physiologist

Bernardo Alberto Houssay was born in Buenos Aires, Argentina, on April 10, 1887; his parents had emigrated from France before his birth. His father was Albert Houssay, a lawyer who also taught literature at the National College of Buenos Aires, and his mother was the former Clara Laffont.

Houssay completed his secondary education at the Colegio Británico at the age of 14. Three years later he earned his degree in pharmaceutical chemistry from the University of Buenos Aires, receiving the highest honors in his class. He then enrolled in the school of medicine at the university and was granted his M.D. at the age of 23. Houssay's medical studies took somewhat longer to complete than might have been expected, given his previous academic record, because he simultaneously worked as a hospital pharmacist in order to help pay for his expenses.

Having completed his studies, Houssay was appointed provisional professor, and, in 1912, full professor of physiology at the university's school of veterinary science. In 1913, he became chief physician at Alvear Hospital as well as a laboratory director in the newly created National Public Health Laboratories. Houssay's 1919 return to the university as chair of physiology marked the beginning of his greatest impact in the field. It was at the university that he established and became director of the Institute of Physiology, a research center that was to attain worldwide distinction. At its peak, the Institute was home to 135 graduate students from every part of the world, extending Houssay's influence far beyond the borders of Argentina. In 1920 Houssay married María Angélica Catán, a chemist. All three of their children, Alberto Bernardo, Héctor Emilio José, and Raúl Horacio, earned medical degrees.

In spite of his many administrative responsibilities, Houssay continued to be very active in research throughout his life. He was intensely interested in every aspect of physiology, from the cardiovascular to the respiratory to the gastrointestinal systems. But his major accomplishments resulted from his studies of the endocrine system, studies that dated to research begun while he was still a medical student. That research received an important impetus in 1921 when Canadians **Frederick Banting** and **Charles Best** and Scottish physiologist **John Macleod** discovered the role of insulin in the development of **diabetes**.

From 1923 to 1937, Houssay studied the interaction between the pancreas and insulin, on the one hand, and the pituitary gland (then called the hypophysis) and its secretions, on the other. One of his first major discoveries was the role of the anterior lobe of the pituitary gland in the **metabolism** of carbohydrates. A more important discovery was that the oxidation of sugars in the body depends not simply on the presence or absence of insulin, but on a complex interaction between insulin and other hormones, such as prolactin and somatotropin, produced in the pituitary gland. For his unraveling of this process, Houssay received a share of the 1947 Nobel Prize for physiology.

The political turmoil that swept Argentina in the 1940s altered Houssay's career. During the uprisings of 1943, he signed a petition calling for the democratization of the Argentine government. As a result, he was dismissed from his post at the university. Two years later, the dismissal was voided, and Houssay returned to the university. He was there only briefly, however, before he was asked to retire, which he did in 1946. In the meantime, he and some colleagues had founded the independent Institute of Biology and Experimental Medicine in order to continue with their research. Even when Houssay was yet again reinstated to his old post at the university in 1955, he continued to serve as director of the Institute.

Houssay was a major leader of Argentine science for many years. He founded, assisted in the establishment of, or served as head of nearly every major scientific organization in the country between 1920 and 1970. He was honored not only by his own nation, but by scientific societies all over the world. He was given honorary doctorates by more than 25 universities and was elected to membership in scientific societies in Great Britain, Germany, France, Italy, Spain, and the United States. Houssay died in Buenos Aires on September 21, 1971.

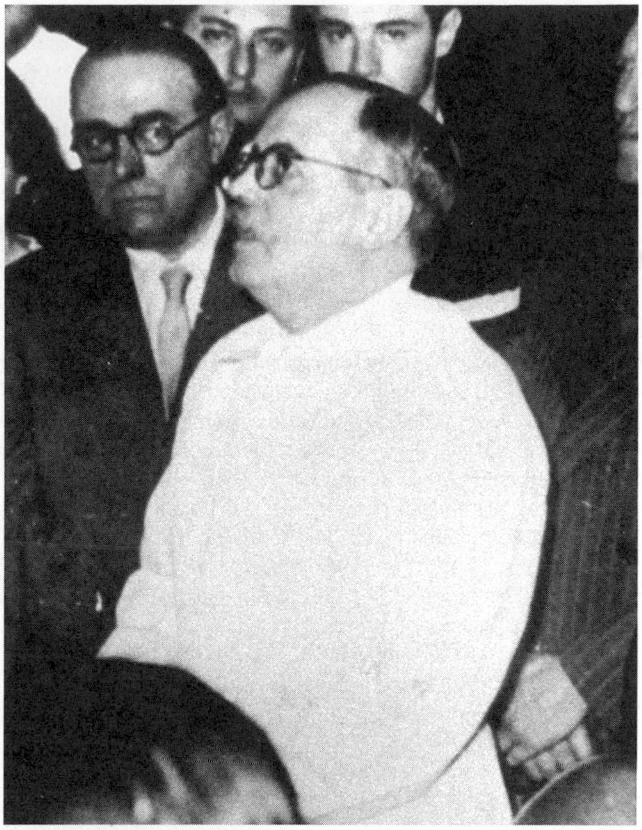
Bernardo Alberto Houssay

HUBEL, DAVID H. (1926-)

Canadian American neurobiologist

Born February 27, 1926, in Windsor, Ontario, of American parents, Elsie M. Hunter Hubel (pronounced hyü-ble) and Jesse H. Hubel, David Hunter Hubel grew up in Montreal. From his father, who was a chemical engineer, Hubel developed an interest in science, especially chemistry and electronics.

From 1932 to 1944, Hubel attended the Strathcona Academy in Outremont, Ontario. He began his college studies at McGill University in 1944. Although he received his B.S. with honors in mathematics and physics, he decided to enter McGill University Medical School in 1947—a decision which he appears to have made almost on the spur of the moment, since he had not taken any college course in biology. He also worked summers at the Montreal Neurological Institute, where he began his studies of the **nervous system**. He received his medical degree in 1951 and spent the next four years studying clinical neurology, first at the Montreal Neurological Institute and then at Johns Hopkins University in Baltimore, Maryland.

In 1955, Hubel was drafted into the United States Army, which sent him to the Neurophysiology Division of the **Walter Reed** Army Institute of Research in Washington, D.C. At Walter Reed, Hubel discovered a stimulating group of physiologists who encouraged him to do original research for the first time in his life. Determined to study **sleep**, he developed a device, known as a tungsten microelectrode, to record the electrical impulses of nerve cells. He used this device on cats to measure the activity of nerve cells in sleep.

During his research on sleep, Hubel became more interested in the reactions of his subjects to the firing responses recorded by the microelectrodes during waking states. He had placed the microelectrodes in the visual cortex area of the brain for his sleep experiments, and he began to realize that it was possible to understand how the brain operates in the visual process. In reading the work of other scientists on this subject, Hubel discovered the research papers of Stephen Kuffler, who was then a leading figure in the neurophysiology of vision.

After his army service ended in 1958, Hubel went to Johns Hopkins University where he did further research on the surface of the brain, the gray matter of the cerebral cortex, in the laboratory of Vernon Mountcastle. But shortly afterwards he moved to the Wilmer Institute, also at Johns Hopkins, and joined Stephen Kuffler's research team. There he met **Torsten Wiesel**, and under the direction of Kuffler the two of them began to make discoveries about the relationship of the retina to the visual cortex as part of the general physiology of the brain.

In 1959, Hubel and Wiesel, along with the rest of Kuffler's research team, followed Kuffler to the Harvard Medical School in Boston. By 1964, Harvard had formed a new department of neurobiology, naming Kuffler as its chairman. Hubel became chairman of this department in 1967, and in 1968 he was named the George Packer Berry Professor of Physiology.

Much of the work done by Hubel and Wiesel, using microelectrodes and electronic equipment, centered around a section of the visual cortex in the brain known as area 17. The cells in this section of the visual cortex form several thin layers that are arranged in columns running through the cortex. Hubel and Weisel discovered that certain cells of area 17 in the brain respond to the stimulation of specific retinal cells in the eye. In particular, they found that cells in the cortex are specialized to respond to different types of stimulation. There are types of cortical cells that respond to light spots and others that respond specifically to the different angles of a tilted line. They discovered that some respond only to definite directions of movement, while others respond only to definite colors.

Hubel and Wiesel's research has made the visual cortex the most mapped-out section of the brain, and it has deepened the scientific understanding of how the visual system works. In addition, their work has led to practical ophthalmological applications for the treatment of congenital **cataracts**, as well as a condition occurring in childhood known as **strabismus**, where one eye is unable to focus with the other because of a muscle imbalance. Hubel and Wiesel discovered that at birth the visual cortex begins to develop its structures from the stimulation of the newborn's retina. The development of the brain is shaped by the activity of the eye, and the sooner childhood eye disorders are corrected, therefore, the better the chances of avoiding serious **visual impairments** in the future. Before their research, the customary medical practice had been to delay operating on these conditions, but today doctors recognize the importance of the early removal of cataracts and the prompt treatment of strabismus.

For their work on how the retinal image is read and interpreted by the cells of the visual cortex, Hubel and Wiesel shared the first half of the 1981 Nobel Prize for physiology or medicine. For his work on split-brain physiology, **Roger W. Sperry** won the second half.

Hubel has been married to Shirley Ruth Izzard Hubel since 1953, and they have three sons.

HUGGINS, CHARLES B. (1901-1997)

American surgeon

Charles Brenton Huggins was born on September 22, 1901, in Halifax, Nova Scotia, to pharmacist Charles Edward and Bessie Marie (Spencer) Huggins. He earned his B.A. from Acadia University, Wolfville, Nova Scotia, in 1920. That same year, he moved to the United States to attend Harvard Medical School, graduating in four years with both an M.A. and M.D. He did his internship at the University of Michigan Hospital and was appointed instructor in surgery at the University's Medical School in 1926. The following year, he became instructor of surgery on the original faculty of the University of Chicago Medical School, and in that same year, he married Margaret Wellman. The couple had a son, Charles Edward, and daughter, Emily Wellman. In 1933, Huggins became an American citizen. He attained the rank of full professor of surgery in 1936. In 1946, he spent a brief period with the Johns Hopkins University as professor of urological surgery and director of the department of urology. He was director of the University of Chicago's Ben May Laboratory for Cancer Research from 1951 to 1969, continuing his research at the university until 1972, when he returned to Acadia University to become chancellor. He retired from the post in 1979 and moved to Chicago.

Huggins' initial specialty was urology, but his interest in **cancer** was actually sparked in 1930, when he met German Nobel Prize-winning cancer researcher **Otto Warburg**. Upon his return to the University of Chicago in the early 1930s, Huggins and his colleagues experimented with changing normal connective tissue elements into bone, using cells from the male urinary tract and bladder. His interest soon turned to the male urogenital system, particularly the role played by chemicals and hormones in the prostate gland, the male accessory reproductive gland located at the base of the urethra. In 1939, he and his colleagues developed a surgical procedure which isolated the prostate gland of dogs from the urinary tract. This procedure allowed the analysis and measurement of secretions of the gland which form much of the ejaculatory fluid. The research was at times frustrated by the formation of prostate tumors in some of the dogs. He turned his energy to studying the development and growth of **prostate cancer**.

Huggins discovered high levels of testosterone, a male sex hormone, in secretions from a cancerous prostate. He also discovered that reducing male hormone secretions by either orchiectomy (castration) or estrogen (a female hormone) therapy, or both, drastically reduced testosterone levels and inhibited the growth of advanced metastatic (spreading) prostate cancer. He also developed a blood test to measure acid phosphatase, which is secreted by the prostate, and alkaline phosphatase, which is secreted by bone-forming cells in bone tissue, both of which showed increased levels in patients with metastasized prostate cancer. Using these measurements, he could determine the extent of the cancer and the effect of the hormone treatments.

Huggins found that although the level of **androgens** (male sex hormones) dropped drastically after orchiectomy, in some cases they rose again, often to a level higher than before the surgery. Investigations led him to believe that the adrenal glands were producing androgens of their own, apparently compensating for the lowered levels induced by the hormone therapy, and encouraging the growth of the cancer. In 1944, he performed the first bilateral adrenalectomy, (removal of the two adrenal glands located above the kidneys), producing some positive results, even before cortisone was readily available for replacement therapy. In 1953, Huggins reported that, when used in combination, adrenalectomy and cortisone replacement had a beneficial effect on 50% of patients suffering from either prostate or **breast cancer**, but had no effect on other types of cancer.

In the 1950s, Huggins left the clinical environment to return to the laboratory where he began focusing on breast cancer. Huggins and two students, D. M. Bergenstal and Thomas Dao, developed a treatment for cancer that entailed removal of both ovaries and both adrenal glands. Combined with cortisone replacement therapy, the treatment brought about improvement in 30% to 40% of the patients with advanced breast cancer, sometimes with quite definite and prolonged improvement.

Breast cancer research was being hampered, however, because of the long delay between stimulation and growth of artificially induced mammary tumors in animals. In 1956, Huggins discovered that a single dose of 7,12-dimethylbens(a)anthracene (DMBA) would quickly induce mammary tumors in certain types of female rats and that many of these tumors were, like some in humans, hormone dependent and responded to regulation of the hormonal environment.

In the mid-1960s, a major scientific controversy developed around whether birth control pills encourage cancer of the breast and other reproductive organs. Huggins, who by that time had spent more than 30 years researching the relationship between hormones and cancer, studied data collected from thousands of women taking birth control pills. He believed that ''the pill'' did not encourage such cancers in women.

For his research on hormones and cancer, Huggins shared the 1966 Nobel Prize with **Peyton Rous**, who was honored for his work 55 years earlier on viral causes of cancer. In addition to the Nobel Prize, Huggins was awarded one of the highest honors to be bestowed by American medicine, the Lasker Clinical Research Award, in 1963. He was also the first recipient of the Charles L. Mayer Award in cancer research from the National Academy of Sciences in 1943. Huggins also was awarded two gold medals for research from the American Medical Association, the Order of Merit from Germany, and the Order of the Sun from Peru. He was made honorary fellow of the Royal College of Surgeons in both Edinburgh and London, and is the recipient of numerous honorary degrees.

He died at his home in Chicago in 1997.

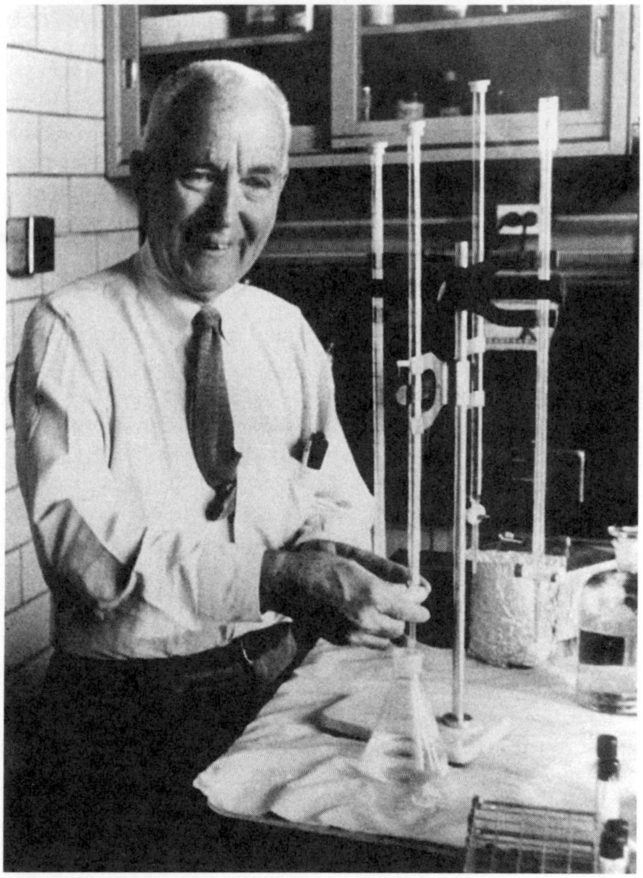

Charles Brenton Huggins

Human anatomy

Based on the same structure found in other mammals, human anatomy is characterized by bilateral symmetry. However, unlike other mammals, humans walk upright. This difference has caused significant evolutionary adaptations that set humans apart anatomically from the rest of the animal world. These changes mainly concern the pelvis, which has to bear more of the organs' weight and serve as the trunk's center of balance; the feet, which have a greater load to carry; the arms, which no longer have to bear the upper body's weight; the skull, which has grown to accommodate a larger brain that has also moved more toward the body's center line; and the femur and its associated musculature.

The building blocks of human anatomy, like those of the other mammals, are four kinds of tissues, each of which serves a specific purpose. Nerve tissues comprise the nervous system and send and receive the brain's electrical messages; connective tissues, which hold together the body's different structures (i.e, the ligaments that connect muscle to bone); epithelial tissues, including the skin, that line cavities and cover organs; and muscle tissues, which make up the body's musculature.

These building blocks all come together in the organs, discrete structures that perform certain specialized functions. The human body has nine major organ systems: the **respiratory system** (lungs and airways); the **digestive system** (stomach, intestines, esophagus); the **musculoskeletal system** (bones and skeletal muscles); the **reproductive system** (ovaries or testes, female or male genital); the **integumentary system** (skin); the circulatory system (blood vessels, heart, blood); the excretory system (kidneys, bladder, urethra, ureters); the **nervous system** (brain, spinal cord, nerves); and the **endocrine system** (hormone producing glands and tissues).

Certain terms exist that allow **physicians**, surgeons, and others to discuss human anatomy in a way that eliminates misunderstanding and ambiguity. For instance, the words ''trunk'' (neck, chest, and upper abdomen), ''pelvis'' (lower abdomen), ''perineum'' (below the abdomen), and ''vertebral column'' (spine) describe the main regions of the body. These and all of the more specific terms rely on the body always being in the same position so that they mean the same thing to everyone at all times. Even if a particular body is not in this position, the words medical professional use to describe it will correspond to the ''anatomical position.'' This consists of a body standing upright with its arms at its side, palms facing out, feet together, and head facing forward. From there, the body is divided by the median plane and two subplanes (sagittal or coronal); four directions (superior or inferior, posterior or anterior), and two directions relative to the medial plan (medial and lateral). In addition, the terms ''superficial'' and ''deep'' refer to location relative to the skin surface, while ''proximal'' and ''distal'' indicate location relative to the structure's root. The hands and feet each have their own descriptors as well (i.e., palmar/dorsal, dorsal/plantar, respectively).

Human bite infections

Human bite infections are potentially serious infections caused by rapid growth of bacteria in broken skin.

Bites—animal and human—are responsible for about 1% of visits to emergency rooms. Bite injuries are more common during the summer months.

In adults, the most common form of human bite is the closed-fist injury, sometimes called the "fight bite." These injuries result from the breaking of the skin over the knuckle joint when a person's fist strikes someone's teeth during a fight.

In children, bite infections result either from accidents during play or from fighting. Most infected bites in adults result from fighting.

The infection itself can be caused by a number of bacteria that live in the human mouth. These include streptococci and staphylococci. Infections that begin less than 24 hours after the injury are usually produced by a mixture of organisms and can cause an infection that will cause the death of a specific area of tissue, in which tissue is rapidly destroyed. If a bite is infected, the skin will be sore, red, swollen, and warm to the touch.

In most cases the diagnosis is made by an emergency room doctor on the basis of the patient's history. Because the human mouth contains a variety of bacteria, the doctor will order a laboratory culture in order to choose the most effective antibiotic.

Treatment involves surgical attention as well as medications. Because bites cause puncturing and tearing of skin rather than clean-edged cuts, they must be carefully cleansed. The doctor will wash the wound with water under high pressure and remove the dead tissue and foreign objects from the wound to prevent infection. If the bite is a closed-fist injury, the doctor will look for torn tendons or damage to the spaces between the joints. Examination includes x rays to check for bone fractures or foreign objects in the wound.

Doctors do not usually suture a bite wound because the connective tissues and other structures in the hand form many small closed spaces that make it easy for infection to spread. Emergency room doctors often consult surgical specialists if a patient has a deep closed-fist injury or one that appears already infected.

The doctor will make sure that the patient is immunized against **tetanus**, which is routine procedure for any open **wound**. Because of risk of infection, all patients with human bite should be given **antibiotics**. Patients with closed-fist injuries may need inpatient treatment in addition to an intravenous antibiotic.

The prognosis depends on the location of the bite and whether it was caused by a child or an adult. Bites caused by children rarely become infected because they are usually shallow. Between 15–30% of bites caused by adults become infected, with a higher rate for closed-fist injuries.

HUMAN EXPERIMENTATION

Human experimentation refers to the use of human beings as experimental subjects. A subject is defined as an individual who is observed or experimented with by an investigator; an investigator is a qualified individual who conducts research. Humans have long been used as subjects for a variety of experiments. However, the most publicized are those that are medical in nature, for medical science has an impact on human health and life in crucial ways. Although most medical experimentation is carried out using laboratory animals, the results cannot be extrapolated to humans with certainty. Some human diseases are known to occur spontaneously in certain animal species or can even be induced; however, most human diseases do not have animal models. Further, the functioning of an animal is not identical to that of humans. Therefore, the final tests need to be done on human subjects; for certain tests (e.g., drug tests) human testing is required by federal regulations.

Experiments on people have contributed in great measure to medical progress; human life span has increased significantly, **infant mortality** has decreased by more than 75%, and many human diseases that were once fatal or widespread have become curable or disappeared.

Two kinds of experimentation have contributed to this progress: self-experimentation by the investigator (in rare cases) and experiments using patient volunteers with the objective of their benefit. Of the variety of tests conducted in humans, the testing of clinically useful drugs is most common. A number of drugs that are preventive, curative, or palliative (pain reducer) in nature have been developed this way. The procedure for testing drug compounds involves multiple steps; the favorable outcome of the preceding step determines the next step in the study. Drug testing is divided into at least three phases. Phase I determines the safety of the compound under study when administered to human beings. It is carried out in normal healthy individuals under controlled conditions of diet, exercise, rest, etc. Once the drug is determined to be tolerated well by the human body, it is tried out on a limited number of patients suffering from the disease that the drug is meant to cure. This forms the second phase (Phase II). In Phase III, the drug is given to a large number of patients suffering from the particular disease to further assess the safety and effectiveness of the drug and determine optimal dosage schedules. This step is popularly known as **clinical trials**. The results from the clinical trials of a drug are evaluated statistically and medically; they are then reported to various health authorities around the world and are usually published in a scientific review.

Despite the compelling need for tests on human subjects and the resulting benefits for mankind, this issue has drawn considerable attention. Particularly controversial has been the use of human subjects for research that does not specifically entail the benefit of the subject. This is termed nontherapeutic experimentation. Its most grotesque form occurred during the second world war in the well-documented "experiments" conducted by the Nazis on prisoners in concentration camps. At least 26 different types of experiments were conducted for the explicit purpose of gaining medical and scientific information, with the larger goal of benefiting the German people and race. The Nazis' "experimentation" was in fact torture—it was characterized by coercion and lack of consent; the use of men, women, and children in blatant disregard of their health and humanity; a sadistic avoidance of **anesthesia**; dehumanizing conditions; and the murder of the subjects as part of the experimental design. These and other nontherapeutic experiments carried out since (in other parts of the world), have attracted public criticism and led people to question the ethics and morality of the whole endeavor and raise a fundamental question: is medical and scientific progress, though beneficial to mankind, above human rights and the individual or vice versa? What emerged from the concentration camp experience was a landmark document, the Nuremberg Code, which contains propositions for the ethical conduct of experiments in human beings. Over the years, several regulatory bodies all over the world (Declaration of Helsinki I and II, National Health and Medical Research Council, American Psychological Association, Transplantation and Anatomy Act, etc.) have refined existing regulations and expanded the scope for the enforcement of ethical conduct in various aspects of human experimentation. At the root of these guidelines lie the values of human freedom and the inviolability of the human person, regardless of the therapeutic or nontherapeutic nature of human experimentation. All codes share the principle of consent as their first commandment. This means that every effort should be made by the investigator to inform the potential subject about all aspects of the experiment, and an individual can be used as an experimental subject only upon receipt of his or her informed consent. Besides the issue of consent, there are numerous other aspects of human experimentation that merit ethical consideration and have been dealt with in the above mentioned codes. In contrast, the issue of limits on scientific enquiry—what kind of scientific questions one is permitted to ask and pursue in order to gain knowledge, and how far can one go in this pursuit—is not clearly addressed. The application of these principles is a continuously evolving process, and it is propelled by present day experimentation in, for example, **gene therapy**, human genome project, human fetal research, and human cloning.

See also Medical ethics

HUMAN PHYSIOLOGY

Physiology is the science of the functioning of living organisms. Like other animals, humans move, respond to environmental stimuli, breathe, eat and digest food, excrete wastes, reproduce, and grow. Multiple organ systems in the body perform these various functions. Each organ system is characterized by a specialized function and thus, division of labor is a basic principle underlying physiology. Another striking feature is the complex organization of an organ system. Several structurally and functionally distinct organs make up an organ system, and each organ contributes to the specialized function of the system as a whole. An organ is further made up of two or more related tissues that determine the specific function of the organ. Based on function, tissues in the human body have been classified into four primary types: epithelial, connective, muscle, and nervous tissues. A tissue is composed of functionally similar cells. Cells are the smallest living (distinct and functional) unit of an organism. Regardless of their differences, all cells are capable of synthesizing carbohydrates, proteins, lipids, and nucleic acids (the building blocks of the cell), producing chemical energy by breakdown of nutrients, secreting wastes, reproduction, and growth. It is the proper functioning of the individual cells that underlies the normal functioning of the organ system as a whole. Thus, within an organ system, there is both structural and functional hierarchy.

The human body consists of 11 organ systems: The **integumentary system** (skin, hair) covers the body externally and acts primarily as a boundary between the internal and external environments. The **musculoskeletal system** is really two systems: the skeletal system (bones, cartilage, joints) and the muscular systems (skeletal muscles); these provide support and control movement, respectively. The **nervous system** (brain, sensory receptors, spinal cord, nerves) is the fast-acting response system of the human body; it responds to changes within and outside the body. The function of the **respiratory system** (nasal cavity, pharynx, larynx, trachea, bronchus, lungs) is to exchange oxygen for carbon dioxide from the atmosphere. Food is digested by the **digestive system** (oral cavity, esophagus, stomach, small and large intestines, rectum, anus). Nutrients, oxygen, and wastes are transported within the body by the **cardiovascular system** (heart, arteries, veins). Nitrogen-containing wastes are excreted by the **urinary system** (kidneys, ureter, urinary bladder, urethra). The **lymphatic system** (lymph nodes, thoracic duct, lymphatic vessels) houses the white blood cells involved in immunity. Reproduction is carried out by the **reproductive systems** of males (seminal vesicles, prostate gland, vas deferens, testis, scrotum, penis) and females (ovary, fallopian tube, uterus, vagina), which primarily contribute the sperm and egg, respectively; fusion of the egg and sperm and subsequent development of the resulting embryo occurs in the female reproductive system. A number of processes such as growth, development, etc. are regulated by chemicals called hormones that are produced by a variety of glands that constitute the **endocrine system** (pineal, pituitary, thyroid, parathyroid, thymus, adrenal, pancreas, testis, ovary); hormones are transported through out the body by the blood and affect target cell function by binding to receptors present in the target tissue.

Although each organ system has a specific role to play, a number of human functions involve the interaction of more than one organ system—e.g., movement requires both the muscular and the skeletal systems. Given this level of complexity in the functioning of the human body, the tight regulation of the various organ systems is crucial for maintaining relatively stable internal conditions. Such a state is referred to as homeostasis. Homeostasis in the human body is sustained by both the nervous and endocrine systems, as they are able to access all parts of the body. These two systems act via electrical impulses (quick acting) and hormones (slow acting), respectively, to control the activity of all the organ systems (including themselves). Disruption of homeostatic control mechanisms in the body lead to altered physiology and, thus, disease.

See also Cardiovascular system; Digestive system; Endocrine system; Integumentary system; Lymphatic system; Musculoskeletal system; Nervous system; Reproductive system, female; Reproductive system, male; Respiratory system; Urinary system

Humors

The doctrine of humors (from the Latin for liquid or fluid) refers to the ancient Greek theory of the four bodily fluids: blood, phlegm, choler (yellow bile) and melancholy (black bile) that determined health and temperament. Humoral theory formed the basis of western medicine and had tremendous influence up to the 19th century. The common practice of blood letting, for example, was intended to rid the body of excess humors. Even such innovators as Franciscus Sylvius (1614-1672), who examined the chemical basis of disease, still kept their systems within the general framework of a humoral explanation. **William Harvey** (1578-1657), who proved that blood circulated in the body, was attacked by many of his contemporaries for trying to demolish established ideas.

Humoral theory was an extension of the earlier writings of Empedocles (504 to 443 B.C.), who proposed the universe and everything in it was composed of four cosmic elements, fire, air, earth, and water. These elements in turn were each associated with warm, cold, dry, and moist qualities. It was **Hippocrates of Cos** (c.460-c.377 B.C.) who proposed that an imbalance of the bodily humors resulted in pain and disease, and that, conversely, maintaining a balance of the fluids was the key to good health. For example, according to humoral theory, **epilepsy** was caused by phlegm blocking the airways, and seizures were the result of the body trying to free itself. Humors could be influenced by many factors in the environment: congenital (present from birth), accidental, or the result of natural phenomena. Hippocrates also believed the humors were essentially glandular secretions, that is, they originated in the heart, brain, liver, and spleen. The trick was to keep the bodily fluids in balance both with one another and with influences from outside.

Galen (c.130-c.200), the Greek-born court physician to Marcus Aurelius, enhanced the doctrine of the humors with another aspect, that of the four temperaments. These were features of personality that reflected the influence of particular humors: sanguine (from blood), or buoyant; phlegmatic, or sluggish; choleric, or quick-tempered, and melancholic, or dejected. Thus, not only general health but emotional stability depended on an appropriate balance among the four bodily humors. An excess of any one could produce illness or an exaggerated personality trait. Over time, ''humor'' came to mean any personality quirk. Elizabethen and Renaissance literature often featured humor characters whose monomaniacal passions served to point out human weaknesses.

Even in its heyday, humoral theory was not universally accepted. In 300 B.C., the Greek anatomist and physiologist **Erasistratus** held that health and disease were intimately connected with the pneuma, a subtle vapor permeating the air people breathe. Asclepiades of Bithynia (124 B.C.-c.40 B.C.) taught that disease results from physical states of the solid particles he believed made up the body, a concept derived from the atomic theory of the 5th-century philosopher Democritus.

Other medical traditions also embraced a kind of humoral theory. The ancient Chinese believed the body to be composed of five elements (earth, fire, water, wood, and metal) and they understood health to be a balance between these various elements. In India, the theory of tridosha (three humors) was the basis of the **Ayurvedic** system of medicine. Wind, bile, and phlegm were substances held to be present in all living creatures. Imbalance or derangement of these humors, or doshas, owing to diet, wrong conduct, or environmental conditions resulted in ill health and disease. Correcting the imbalance brought about a cure. The Hindu concept of doshas as a fundamental principle in Ayurveda shares many similar features with Galen's concept of humors in Greek medicine. Nevertheless, each system defines the terms by referring to their own philosophies and histories, and with that in mind some scholars of Ayurveda emphasize the differences rather than the similarities.

In 1858 with publication of Rudolf Virchow's (1821-1902) work showing that the basis of human disease is to be found in the cells, humoral theory fell out of favor. But humoral ideas remain pervasive as folk traditions among many people in the way they experience and describe their illness. Moreover, traditional medical systems such as Ayurveda and Unani continue to emphasize the role of humors in the course of their routine clinical practice.

See also Alternative medicine; Ayurvedic medicine; Chinese traditional medicine

Huntington, George Sumner (1850-1916)

American physician

Huntington was no academic or medical researcher, just a simple family doctor who wrote a landmark description of the fatal hereditary disease now known as **Huntington's disease**.

Neither was he the first to recognize the malady that now bears his name. In fact, his father, George Lee Huntington, and grandfather, Abel Huntington, were both family physicians who were aware of the disease. The original manuscript of Huntington's classic paper, presented in 1872 to a local medical society in Middleport, Ohio, and published later that year in the Philadelphia-based *Medical and Surgical Reporter*, contains penciled annotations from his father, offering advice incorporated into the final draft. In Huntington's birthplace—East Hampton, New York—the disease had been prevalent for several generations in families that had emigrated from Suffolk, England. It had also previously been reported by other doctors in Westchester County, New York, and Wyoming County, Pennsylvania.

But Huntington's paper is considered a classic of the literature of neurology. ''In the history of medicine, there are few instances in which a disease has been more accurately, more graphically or more briefly described,'' wrote the esteemed medical educator **William Osler**, referring to the three-paragraph description of the disease contained in Huntington's landmark paper. It was one of just two papers written by Huntington during his career. The second was an honorary essay requested 30 years later by the New York Neurological Society.

"The hereditary chorea, as I shall call it, is confined to certain and unfortunately a *few* families, and has been transmitted to them, an heirloom from generations away back in the dim past," wrote Huntington. "It is spoken of by those in whose veins the seeds of the disease are known to exist, with a kind of horror, and not at all alluded to except through dire necessity, when it is mentioned as *'that disorder.'*"

"...It begins as an ordinary chorea might begin, by the irregular and spasmodic action of certain muscles, as of the face, arms, etc. These movements gradually increase when muscles hitherto unaffected take on the spasmodic action, until every muscle in the body becomes affected (excepting the involuntary ones), and the poor patient presents a spectacle which is anything but pleasant to witness."

Huntington also recognized the effects of the disease on the mind: "The tendency to insanity, and sometimes that form of insanity which leads to suicide, is marked...."

The paper was written within one year of Huntington's graduation from the College of Physicians and Surgeons at Columbia University. After practicing briefly with his father on New York's Long Island, he had moved to Palmyra, Ohio. But he found Ohio did not agree with him and he returned in 1874 to Duchess County, New York, where he practiced medicine and enjoyed hunting, music, and his family until his death in 1916 at the age of 66.

HUNTINGTON'S CHOREA/DISEASE

The term chorea comes from the Greek word *choreia*, which means "to dance." The term aptly describes the fitful, jerking movements associated with the condition. One form of chorea was first described by the English physician, **Thomas Sydenham**, in 1685, at which time the disorder was known as St. Vitus' Dance. This condition is now called **Sydenham's chorea**.

A second form of chorea has also been known for centuries, although it was first described in detail only in 1872 by the American physician, **George Huntington** (1850-1916). Huntington was born and lived in East Hampton, Long Island, a community where chorea was widespread. His father and grandfather, also physicians, had both treated sufferers from chorea for many years. It was well known that the condition had been transmitted from Suffolk, England, to Connecticut in the seventeenth century by way of a single family, known as the Bures family group. Members of the Bures family group had been frequently accused of witchcraft and were among those convicted of this crime during the Salem witch trials.

Huntington, upon obtaining his medical degree from Columbia University, worked with his father in East Hampton, then moved to Palmyra, Ohio, before finally settling in Duchess County, New York. His paper on chorea was apparently his only published work, but was considered so exemplary that the disease he reported was eventually named for him.

Unlike Sydenham's chorea, which occurs most often in children and lasts only a few weeks or months, Huntington's chorea does not strike until middle age and is always fatal. The disorder first appears as irregular and spasmodic movements of the muscles. Eventually these movements become so severe that a person is disabled. In his paper, Huntington wrote that in the final stages of the disease "the hapless sufferer is but a quivering wreck of his former self." Mental deterioration often accompanies these physical symptoms. The patient becomes progressively worse until **death** occurs.

Huntington well described the terrifying outlook within families that had a history of chorea. Both the families and physicians knew that the disorder was hereditary, but had no means of finding out who would be afflicted until late in life. Huntington reported that the outcome of the disease "is so well known to the sufferer and his friends, that medical advice is seldom sought."

The disorder became well known to the American public in the late 1950s and early 1960s when the popular folk singer, Woody Guthrie (1912-1967), developed the condition. Guthrie's wife, Marjorie, and his son, Arlo Guthrie (b.1947), wrote and spoke about the agony they faced in dealing with Woody's illness as well as their uncertainties about Arlo's future as a father.

In 1993, after ten years of intensive research, scientists discovered the gene that causes Huntington's chorea. Even more important, four years later researchers uncovered how the mutated gene causes the devastating disorder. Investigators at the University of California at Los Angeles (UCLA) discovered that a genetic mutation results in the formation of 30 to 150 copies of glutamine (an amino acid) into certain proteins. As a result, the proteins clump together and then migrate into the nucleus of brain cells. This finding indicates that a single neurological mechanism may be responsible for inhibiting the production of neurotransmitters (substances that transmit nerve impulses) that would normally be produced by certain brain cells, resulting in the loss of muscular control characteristic of chorea. Scientists also know that the more severely the gene is mutated, the earlier the onset of the disease. Discovery of the genetic component and its functioning in Huntington's chorea has spurred research into drugs that would prevent the proteins from forming masses. Such drugs would, at the very least, delay the onset of symptoms.

The use of fetal cell transplants into the brain is regarded by some scientists as a promising treatment approach. In 1996, investigators at the Good Samaritan Hospital in Arizona announced the first successful use of fetal transplants to treat Huntington's chorea. Animal studies indicate that the transplanted cells are integrated into the brain's structure and then function normally to restore neural circuitry. In further patients studies, the scientists found some improvement in motor capacity and increased functioning lasting from six to nine months in some patients. However, outcomes have varied greatly among patients who have received transplants, and it is still not know whether the positive effects will persist over time. Other intriguing research currently under way includes using growth chemicals to stimulate brain stem cells to produce new neurons and studies of brain implants using a cell that secretes a substance that may prevent nerve cell death.

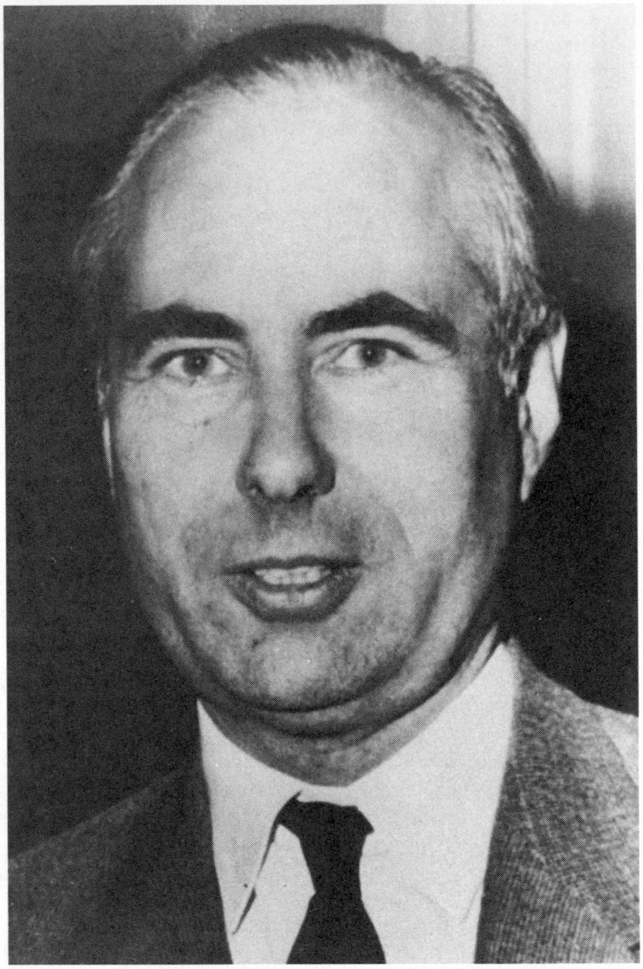

Andrew Fielding Huxley

Huxley, Andrew Fielding (1917-)

English physiologist

Andrew Fielding Huxley is an English physiologist whose research on nerve impulse transmission earned him the 1963 Nobel Prize for medicine and physiology, which he shared with his colleague **Alan Lloyd Hodgkin** and the Australian physiologist **John Carew Eccles**. Huxley and Hodgkin confirmed scientists' earlier discovery that nerve impulse transmission involves a momentary change in the nerve fiber's membrane, affecting the ability of particles to pass through it.

Huxley was born in London, England, on November 22, 1917, to a prominent and successful family. His grandfather was the nineteenth-century biologist Thomas Henry Huxley. Julian Sorel Huxley, also a noted biologist, was Andrew's half-brother, as was the author Aldous Huxley. Andrew's father, Leonard, was also a writer. His mother was Rosalind (Bruce) Huxley. Huxley was educated at Trinity College, Cambridge, where he received his B.A. in 1938 and his M.A. in 1941. He began studying the physical sciences but switched to physiology in his last year.

In 1939, Huxley joined Alan Hodgkin at the Plymouth Marine Biological Laboratory to study the transmission of nerve impulses. There, Huxley and Hodgkin attempted to verify the work of other scientists, including Julius Bernstein, **Joseph Erlanger**, and **Herbert Spencer Gasser**. These scientists had hypothesized that a nerve impulse produces an electrical current between the active and resting regions of a nerve, and that this impulse causes a fleeting change in the permeability of the nerve fiber membrane. Hodgkin and Huxley went about their research by experimenting on squid, which have giant axons, or nerve fibers, and therefore were known to be particularly useful in studying nerve systems. They inserted a small electrode into the squid's axon, and connected it to a system that would measure the electrical currents produced when the nerve was stimulated.

Huxley's work was interrupted during World War II, when he spent two years doing operational research for the Anti-Aircraft Command and later worked for the Admiralty. In 1946, he returned to his alma mater, serving in a variety of positions—fellow, assistant director of research, director of studies, and reader in experimental biophysics—while he carried out and perfected his research with Hodgkin. He was married to Jocelyn Richenda Gammell Pease in 1947; they had five daughters and one son.

In the course of their research, Huxley and Hodgkin were surprised to learn that, contrary to earlier hypotheses, the outer layer of a nerve fiber is not equally permeable to all ions (charged particles). While a resting cell has low sodium- and high potassium-permeability, Huxley and Hodgkin found that, during excitation, sodium ions flood into the axon, which instantaneously changes from a negative to a positive charge. It is this sudden change that constitutes a nerve impulse. The sodium ions then continue to flow through the membrane until the axon is so highly charged that the sodium becomes electrically repelled. The stream of sodium then stops, which causes the membrane to become permeable once again to potassium ions.

Huxley and Hodgkin first announced their findings in 1951 and published a series of highly regarded papers in 1952. In 1955, Huxley was named to the Royal Society, and in 1960 he became the Jodrell Professor of Physiology at University College, London, where, according to Ronald Clark's history of the Huxley family, *The Huxleys,* he occupied the desk of his grandfather, T. H. Huxley. He remained professor at University College until 1983. In 1974 he was knighted.

When he received the Nobel Prize in 1963, Huxley described the often laborious research and computations involved in his work. While crediting those scientists whose findings he built upon, he also allowed that there was much more work to be done in this field. One of the many applications of the methods and findings of Huxley and Hodgkin was discovered by John Carew Eccles, who shared the Nobel Prize with the two Englishmen. Eccles studied motor neurons in the spinal cord and synapses using microelectrodes similar to those used by Huxley and Hodgkin. Huxley himself devoted much of his later research to studying muscle contraction. His findings have increased the understanding of diseases of the nervous system, as well as similar ionic mechanisms in the kidney and heart.

Hydrocephalus

Hydrocephalus is an abnormal expansion of cavities (ventricles) within the brain caused by the accumulation of cerebrospinal fluid.

Hydrocephalus is the result of an imbalance between the formation and drainage of cerebrospinal fluid (CSF). Approximately 500 milliliters (about a pint) of CSF is formed within the brain each day, by structures called choroid plexus, with epidermal cells lining chambers called ventricles. Once formed, CSF usually circulates among all the ventricles before it is absorbed and returned to the circulatory system. The normal adult volume of circulating CSF is 150 ml, so that the CSF turn-over rate is more than three times per day. Production is independent of absorption, and reduced absorption causes CSF to accumulate within the ventricles.

Reduced absorption most often occurs when one or more passages connecting the ventricles become blocked, preventing movement of CSF to its drainage sites in the subarachnoid space just inside the skull. This type of hydrocephalus is called ''noncommunicating.'' Reduction in absorption rate can also be caused by damage to the absorptive tissue. This type is called ''communicating hydrocephalus.''

Both of these types lead to an elevation of the CSF pressure within the brain. This increased pressure squeezes the soft tissues of the brain, distorting and damaging them. In infants whose skull bones have not yet fused, the intracranial pressure is partly relieved by expansion of the skull, so that symptoms may not be as dramatic. Both types of elevated-pressure hydrocephalus may occur from infancy to adulthood.

A third type of hydrocephalus, called ''normal pressure hydrocephalus,'' is marked by ventricle enlargement without an apparent increase in CSF pressure. This type affects mainly the elderly.

Hydrocephalus may be caused by:

- Congenital brain defects
- Hemorrhage, either in the ventricles or the subarachnoid space
- Infection of the central **nervous system** (**syphilis**, herpes, **meningitis**, **encephalitis**, or **mumps**)
- Tumor.

Symptoms of elevated-pressure hydrocephalus include:

- **Headache**
- **Nausea and vomiting**, especially in the morning
- Lethargy
- Gait disturbance
- Double vision
- Subtle difficulties in learning and memory
- Delay in achievement of developmental milestones in children.

Irritability is the most common sign of hydrocephalus in infants and, if untreated, this may lead to lethargy. Bulging of the fontanelle, the soft spot between the skull bones, may also be an early sign. Hydrocephalus in infants prevents fusion of the skull bones, and causes expansion of the skull.

Symptoms of normal pressure hydrocephalus include **dementia**, gait abnormalities, and **incontinence** (involuntary urination or bowel movements).

Imaging studies—x ray, **computed tomography scan** (CT scan), **ultrasound**, and especially **magnetic resonance imaging** (MRI)—are used to assess the presence and location of obstructions, as well as changes in brain tissue that have occurred as a result of the hydrocephalus. Lumbar puncture (spinal tap) may be performed to aid in determining the cause.

The primary method of treatment for both elevated- and normal-pressure hydrocephalus is surgical installation of a shunt. The shunt is a tube connecting the ventricles to an alternative drainage site, usually the abdomen. The shunt contains a one-way valve to prevent reverse flow. In some cases of noncommunicating hydrocephalus, a direct connection can be made between one of the ventricles and the subarachnoid space, allowing drainage without a shunt.

Installation of a shunt requires lifelong monitoring by the patient or family members for signs of recurring hydrocephalus due to obstruction or failure of the shunt.

Some drugs may postpone the need for surgery by inhibiting the production of CSF. These include acetazolamide and furosemide. Other drugs used to delay surgery include glycerol, digoxin, and isosorbide.

Prognosis for elevated-pressure hydrocephalus depends on a wide variety of factors, including the cause, age of onset, and the timing of surgery. Studies indicate that about half of all children who receive appropriate treatment and follow-up will develop IQs greater than 85. Those with hydrocephalus at birth do better than those with later onset due to meningitis. For patients with normal pressure hydrocephalus, shunt installation may lead to improvement in approximately half.

Some cases of elevated pressure hydrocephalus may be preventable by preventing or treating the infectious diseases which precede them. Prenatal diagnosis of congenital brain malformation is often possible, offering the option of family planning.

Hydrotherapy

Hydrotherapy is a general term for a group of alternative treatments that use water for the relief of various diseases or injuries, or for cleansing the digestive tract. The use of hydrotherapy has a long history as a form of medical treatment. For example, in classical times the Romans and Greeks found sources of water that were considered to have healing properties.

Hydrotherapy is used to treat a wide range of conditions, often in conjunction with conventional medical treatment.

Some forms of hydrotherapy are not suitable for certain patients. Cold baths should not be given to young children or the elderly. Sauna baths should be avoided by people with heart conditions.

External hydrotherapy involves the immersion of the body in water or the application of water or ice to the body, while temperature-based treatments involve the different effects of hot or cold water on the skin and underlying tissues. Hot water (around 100°F/37.8°C) relaxes muscles and causes sweating. It is used to treat arthritis, rheumatism, poor circulation, and sore muscles. Hot water hydrotherapy can be used in combination with **aromatherapy** by adding scented oils to the water. Cold water (60°F/15.6°C) treatments are used to stimulate blood flow in the skin and underlying muscles.

Temperature-based treatments include the application of moist heat or cold to specific parts of the body. The application of moist heat is called fomentation, and is used for chest colds, influenza, or arthritis. Cold compresses or ice packs are used in the treatment of sprains, headaches, or dental surgery. Body packs, which consist of wet cloth wrapped around the patient, are sometimes used to calm psychiatric patients and for detoxification.

A sitz bath is a form of treatment in which the patient sits in a specially constructed tub that allows the lower abdomen to be submerged in water of a different temperature from the water around the feet. Sitz baths are recommended for hemorrhoids, prostate swelling, menstrual cramps, and other genitourinary disorders.

Motion-based hydrotherapy uses water under pressure in the form of jets, whirlpools, or aerated bubbles to massage the body. It is used to treat joint and muscle injuries as well as stress and anxiety.

Internal hydrotherapy includes colonic irrigations and enemas. Steam baths or inhalation of steam to relieve respiratory congestion is also a form of internal hydrotherapy, as is drinking mineral water to restore the body's electrolyte balance or cleanse the system.

Normal results for hydrotherapy are symptomatic relief of the condition for which it was recommended. Additionally, hydrotherapy can strengthen both the individually focused area and the entire body.

HYPERCOAGULATION DISORDERS

Hypercoagulation disorders (or hypercoagulable states or disorders) have the opposite effect of the more common coagulation disorders. In hypercoagulation, there is an increased tendency for clotting of the blood, which may put a patient at risk for obstruction of veins and arteries (phlebitis or pulmonary embolism).

In normal hemostasis, or the stoppage of bleeding, clots form at the site of the blood vessel's injury. However, in hypercoagulation, clots develop in circulating blood. This disorder can cause clots throughout the body's blood vessels, sometimes creating a condition known as thrombosis. Thrombosis can lead to infarction, or death of tissue, as a result of blocked blood supply to the tissue. However, hypercoagulability does not always lead to thrombosis. In **pregnancy**, and other hypercoagulable states, the incidence of thrombosis is higher than that of the general population, but is still under 10%. However, in association with certain genetic disorders, hypercoagulation disorders may be more likely to lead to thrombosis.

Hypercoagulation disorders may be acquired or hereditary. Some of the genetic disorders that lead to hypercoagulation are abnormal clotting factor V, variations in fibrinogen, and deficiencies in proteins C and S. Other body system diseases may also lead to these disorders, including **diabetes**, sickle-cell anemia, congenital heart disease, lupus, and others. Antithrombin III deficiency is a hereditary hypercoagulation disorder that affects both sexes. Symptoms include obstruction of a blood vessel by a clot (thromboembolic disease), vein inflammation (phlebitis), and ulcers of the lower parts of the legs. The role of proteins C and S is a complex one. In order for coagulation to occur, platelets (small, round fragments in the blood) help contract blood vessels to lessen blood loss and also to help plug damaged blood vessels. However, the conversion of platelets into actual clots is a complicated web involving proteins that are identified clotting factors. The factors are carried in the plasma, or liquid portion of the blood. Proteins C and S are two of the clotting factors that are present in the plasma to help regulate or activate parts of the clotting process. Protein C is considered an anticoagulant. Mutation defects in the proteins may decrease their concentrations in the blood, and may or may not affect their resulting anticoagulant activity. Factor V is an unstable clotting factor also present in plasma. Abnormal factor V resists the changes that normally occur through the influence of protein C, which can also lead to hypercoagulability. Prothrombin, a glycoprotein which converts to thrombin in the early stage of the clotting process, is affected by the presence of these proteins, as well as other clotting factors.

The diagnosis of hypercoagulation disorders is completed with a combination of physical examination, medical history, and blood tests. An accurate medical history is important to determine possible symptoms and causes of hypercoagulation disorders. There are a number of blood tests that can determine the presence or absence of proteins, clotting factors, and platelet counts in the blood. Among the tests used to detect hypercoagulation is the Antithrombin III assay. Protein C and protein S concentrations can be diagnosed with immunoassay or plasma antigen level tests.

Coumadin and heparin **anticoagulants** may be administered to reduce the clotting effects and maintain fluidity in the blood. Heparin is an anticoagulant that prevents thrombus formation and is used primarily for liver and lung clots.

The prognosis for patients with hypercoagulation disorders varies depending on the severity of the clotting and thrombosis. If undetected and untreated, thrombosis could lead to recurrent thrombosis and **pulmonary embolism**, a potentially fatal problem.

Hereditary hypercoagulation disorders may not be prevented. Genetic and blood testing may help determine a person's tendency to develop these disorders.

HYPERPIGMENTATION

Hyperpigmentation is the increase in the natural color of the skin. Melanin, a brown pigment manufactured by certain cells in the skin called melanocytes, is responsible for skin color. Melanin production is stimulated by a pituitary hormone called melanocyte stimulating hormone (MSH). Other pigments appear in the skin much less often. Melanin gives skin its natural color.

Darkened spots on the skin come in several varieties. The most ominous is malignant melanoma, a very aggressive **cancer** that begins as an innocent mole. Most **moles** (nevus), however, are and remain benign (harmless). The average person has several dozen, and certain people with a hereditary excess may have hundreds. Freckles, age spots, and cafe au lait spots, known as ephelides, are always flat and not as dark. Cafe au lait spots are seen mostly in people with another hereditary disorder called neurofibromatosis. ''Port wine stains'' are congenital dark red blotches on the skin. Other common dark colorations on the skin are called keratosis and consist of locally overgrown layers of skin that are dark primarily because there is more tissue than normal. A few of these turn into **skin cancers** of a much less dangerous kind than melanoma.

Darkened regions of the skin occur as a result of abnormal tanning when the skin is sensitive to sunlight. Several diseases and many drugs can cause **photosensitivity**. Among the common drugs responsible for this uncommon reaction are birth control pills, **antibiotics** and **diuretics**, **nonsteroidal anti-inflammatory drugs** (NSAID), pain relievers, and a couple psychoactive medications. Some of the same drugs may also cause patches of discolored skin known as localized drug reactions and representing an allergy to that drug. Sunlight darkens an abnormal chemical in the skin of patients with porphyria cutanea tarda. Several endocrine diseases, some cancers, and several drugs abnormally stimulate melanocytes, usually through an overproduction of MSH. Arsenic poisoning and Addison's disease are among these causes. A condition known as acanthosis nigricans is a velvety darkening of skin in folded areas (armpits, groin, and neck) that can signal a cancer or hormone imbalance.

Of particular note is a condition called melasma (dark pigmentation of the skin), caused by the female hormone estrogen. Normal in **pregnancy**, this brownish discoloration of the face can also happen with birth control pills that contain estrogen.

Overall darkening of the skin may be due to pigmented chemicals in the skin. Silver, gold, and iron each have a characteristic color when visible in the skin. Several drugs and body chemicals, like bilirubin, can end up as deposits in the skin and discolor it.

There are a number of other rare entities that color the skin, each in its own peculiar way. Among these are strange syndromes that seem to be birth defects and vitamin and nutritional deficiencies.

The pattern of discoloration is immediately visible to the trained dermatologist, a physician specializing in skin diseases, and may be all that is required to name and characterize the discoloration. Many of these pigment changes are signs of internal disease that must be identified. Because pigmentation changes may also be caused by medication, the drug responsible for the reaction must be identified and removed.

Skin sensitive to sunlight must be protected by shade or sunscreens with an SPF of 15 or greater. Skin cancers must be, and unsightly benign lesions may be, surgically removed. **Laser surgery** is an effective removal technique for many localized lesions. Because it spreads so rapidly, melanoma should be immediately removed, as well as some of the surrounding tissue to prevent regrowth.

Sunlight is the leading cause of dark spots on the skin, so shade and sunscreens are necessary preventive strategies, especially in people who burn easily.

Hypersplenism

Hypersplenism is a disorder that causes the spleen to rapidly and prematurely destroy blood cells.

The spleen is located in the upper left area of the abdomen. One of its major functions is to remove blood cells from the body's bloodstream. In hypersplenism, the spleen's normal function accelerates, and it begins to remove cells that may still be normal in function. Sometimes, the spleen will temporarily hold onto up to 90% of the body's platelets and 45% of the red blood cells. Hypersplenism may occur as a primary disease, leading to other complications, or as a secondary disease, resulting from an underlying disease or disorder. Hypersplenism is sometimes referred to as enlarged spleen (splenomegaly). An enlarged spleen is one of the symptoms of hypersplenism. What differentiates hypersplenism is its premature destruction of blood cells.

Hypersplenism may be caused by a variety of disorders. Sometimes, it is brought on by a problem within the spleen itself and is referred to as primary hypersplenism. Secondary hypersplenism results from another disease such as chronic **malaria**, **rheumatoid arthritis**, **tuberculosis**, or polycythemia vera, a blood disorder. Spleen disorders in general are almost always secondary in nature. Hypersplenism may also be caused by tumors.

Symptoms of hypersplenism include easy bruising, easy contracting of bacterial diseases, **fever**, weakness, heart **palpitations**, and ulcerations of the mouth, legs and feet. Individuals may also bleed unexpectedly and heavily from the nose or other mucous membranes, and from the gastrointestinal or urinary tracts. Most patients will develop an enlarged spleen, **anemia**, leukopenia, or abnormally low white blood cell counts, or **thrombocytopenia**, a deficiency of circulating platelets in the blood. Other symptoms may be present.

An enlarged spleen can be caused by a variety of diseases, including hemolytic anemia, **cirrhosis** of the liver, **leukemia**, malignant **lymphoma** and other infections and inflammatory diseases. Splenomegaly occurs in about 10% of patients with **systemic lupus erythematosus**. Sometimes, it is caused by recent viral infection, such as mononucleosis. An enlarged spleen may cause in the upper left side of the abdomen and a premature feeling of fullness at meals.

Diagnosis of hypersplenism begins with review of symptoms and patient history, and careful feeling (palpation) of the spleen. Sometimes, a physician can feel an enlarged spleen. **X-ray studies**, such as **ultrasound**, may help diagnose an enlarged spleen and possible underlying causes, such as tumors. Blood tests indicate decreases in white blood cells, red blood cells, or platelets. Another test measures red blood cells in the liver and spleen after injection of a radioactive substance, and indicates areas where the spleen is holding on to large numbers of red cells or is destroying them.

Enlarged spleens are diagnosed using a combination of patient history, physical examination, including palpation of the spleen, if possible, and diagnostic tests. A history of fever and systemic symptoms may be present because of infection, malaria, or an inflammatory disorder. A complete **blood count** is taken to check counts of young red blood cells. Liver function tests, CT scans, and ultrasound exams can also help to detect an enlarged spleen.

In secondary hypersplenism, the underlying disease must be treated to prevent further destruction of blood cells, and possible spleen enlargement. Those therapies will be tried prior to removal of the spleen, which is avoided if possible. In severe cases, the spleen must be removed. Splenectomy will correct the effects of low blood cell concentrations in the blood.

Prognosis depends on the underlying cause and progression of the disease. Left untreated, spleen enlargement can lead to serious complications. Hypersplenism can also lead to complications due to decreased blood cell counts.

Some of the underlying causes of hypersplenism or enlarged spleen can be prevented, such as certain forms of anemia and cirrhosis of the liver due to alcohol. In other cases, the hypersplenism may not be preventable, as it is a complication to an underlying disorder.

HYPERTENSION

Blood pressure is the force exerted by blood on the walls of the arteries. When the pressure is too high, the heart is working harder than it should, and the blood vessels are overstressed. High blood pressure, or hypertension, can range from mild to severe. Physicians knew for a long time that very high blood pressure was harmful, but it took the results of a long-term study of the residents of Framingham, Massachusetts, to convince doctors in the early 1960s that *all* hypertension was dangerous. It can lead to **heart attack**, **stroke**, and **kidney failure**. Researchers also announced in 1998 that high blood pressure could mean a higher risk of developing **dementia**. Hypertension affects sixty million, or nearly one out of four, Americans.

Attempts to find effective ways to treat hypertension led researchers to uncover the methods by which the body regulates blood pressure; knowledge of that process is still evolving. In 1898 R. Tigerstedt and P. G. Bergman found that an enzyme produced by the kidneys affected blood pressure. Henry Goldblatt and colleagues confirmed the role of the kidneys in 1934, producing hypertension in dogs by constricting the kidney arteries. In 1940 Braun-Menendez in Argentina and Irvine Page and Oscar Helmer at the Cleveland Clinic in Ohio found that renin, the kidney enzyme, catalyzed the formation of angiotensin, a very potent vasoconstrictor (a substance that causes blood vessels to contract). In the 1950s researchers discovered that renin causes the production of angiotensin I, which has little physiological effect but is stimulated by angiotensin converting enzyme to produce the vessel-constricting angiotensin II. In the 1960s Gross and others further found that angiotensin stimulates production of the hormone aldosterone by the adrenal glands, which in turn promotes retention of sodium and water, boosting the fluid content of the circulatory system and thus the pressure on blood vessel walls. Angiotensins were also shown to act on the **nervous system**, stimulating release of the neurotransmitter norepinephrine, which signals the arterioles to constrict. This complex is called the renin-angiotensin-aldosterone system. Exactly why the system malfunctions to produce hypertension is not yet known, except in the approximately 10 percent of cases in which high blood pressure is the result of specific, known physical disorders, particularly of the kidneys and adrenal glands.

Effective drug treatments to control high blood pressure were not developed until after World War II, although some early attempts at drug treatment were made. The French surgeon Mathieu Jaboulay (1860-1913) in 1900 reported on his drastic approach to alleviate severe hypertension: sympathectomy, or the cutting of the nerves that stimulate blood vessel constriction. Two American doctors took a dietary approach; Frederick Allen promoted salt and water restriction in 1920, and Walter Kempner (1903-1997) put patients on a no-salt rice diet in the 1940s.

The modern era of drug treatment for hypertension began with the introduction of reserpine in 1953. Reserpine was first derived from the snakeroot plant, *Rauwolfia serpentina*, long used by medical practitioners in India, both to lower blood pressure and induce relaxation. *Rauwolfia* was first mentioned in Western medical literature in a 1563 Portuguese work, but it was not studied seriously by Western-trained Indian physicians until 1931. The results of a clinical trial published by Dr. Rustom Jal Vakil in 1949 caught the attention Dr. Robert Wilkins, director of the hypertension clinic at Massachusetts General Hospital. Wilkins confirmed the hypotensive (anti-hypertensive) effect of *Rauwolfia* in 1952. The active ingredient was soon isolated and named reserpine; it was synthesized in 1956 by Robert Burns Woodward of Harvard. Reserpine was the first antihypertensive drug to achieve wide clinical use because of its nearly universal effectiveness. (It acts by interfering with transmission of norepinephrine.) It was also widely sold as a tranquilizer.

Other drugs took the place of reserpine as manufacturers and researchers focused their attention on **antihypertensive**s beginning in the 1950s. The discovery of the first thiazide diuretic, benzothiadiazine, was reported in 1957 by the drug company Merck, Sharp and Dohme. Thiazide diuretics, which increase excretion of sodium chloride and water by stimulating the flow of urine, are widely used today to lower blood pressure. They may be taken in combination with methyldopa, an antihypertensive introduced in 1963, or with the **beta-blockers**, a new class of drugs that came on the market in 1964. James Black, senior pharmacologist at Imperial Chemical Industries of Great Britain, was responsible for the development of the first beta blocker, propranolol. The American biochemist Raymond Ahlquist had suggested that epinephrine and norepinephrine transmit their signals—which cause an increase in heart rate and stronger contractions of the heart and blood vessels—to beta receptor sites on the heart muscle. In 1957, Black noted reports of a drug that blocked the stimulating effects of adrenaline on the heart, and set about creating a new chemical compound that would block the effects of epinephrine and norepinephrine at the beta receptor sites. This was accomplished by 1960, with the improved beta-blocker propranolol appearing in 1964. Beta blockers are now widely used to treat both **angina** and high blood pressure.

Two other antihypertensives were introduced in the 1980s. Calcium channel blockers work by blocking the channel that carries calcium to muscle cells; since calcium is required for contraction of the muscles in artery walls and affects the rate at which the heart beats, lowering calcium levels in muscle also lowers blood pressure. ACE (angiotensin converting enzyme) inhibitors interfere with the effect of an enzyme that stimulates angiotensin I to convert to the powerful vasoconstrictor angiotensin II and that also promotes the destruction of bradykinin, a powerful vasodilator (a substance that promotes the relaxation of blood vessels). Ferreira and his coworkers first found BPFs, factors that intensify the body's reaction to bradykinin, in the venom of pit vipers in the 1960s. The BPFs inhibited the action of an enzyme that Erdos and associates showed was identical to angiotensin converting enzyme. BPFs were then synthesized, and in 1977 Cushman and his colleagues developed the first orally effective ACE inhibitor, captopril. Recently, it has been discovered that ACE inhibitors also reduce the rate of heart failure and progress of heart disease following heart attack.

Other drug treatments include sympathetic (adrenergic) nervous system blockers, which inhibit the sympathetic nervous system; vasodilators, which lower vascular resistance by dilating the blood vessels; and HMG-CoA reductase inhibitors, which are used with dietary modifications to reduce cholesterol levels. However, drug therapy, which usually includes side effects, isn't the only way to treat hypertension. From the 1970s on, doctors have recommended **exercise**, weight loss, eliminating **smoking**, **stress** reduction, and a diet low in sodium, **caffeine**, alcohol, and cholesterol as a means of lowering blood pressure.

Advances are also being made in discovering the biological roots of hypertension. For example, in 1998 researchers reported that glucocorticoid (a specific group of corticoids, or adrenal cortex steroids) abnormalities may play a role in familial disposition to hypertension. Investigators also identified two oncogenes that may be related to sodium-related hypertension by affecting how sodium is released or retained by sodium channels in the kidneys. Variations of an ACE (angiotensin converting enzyme) gene, which encodes for an enzyme that helps regulate blood volume and controls salt and water balance, have also been linked to hypertension in men but not women.

Hypnosis

Hypnosis is a state described as sleeplike. It is usually induced by another individual for the purpose of tapping into the unconscious mind. As a result of the hypnosis, the subject may experience forgotten or suppressed memories. Hypnosis has also been described as a way to use a person's inherent healing capabilities that usually remain inaccessible to him and outside of his control.

Hypnosis can be helpful in relaxation and **pain** reduction by decreasing muscle tension. Hypnosis can also reduce pain by helping the subject visualize and create an alternate reality perceived as being safe and comfortable. Many doctors now use hypnosis to overcome the pain of **headaches**, backaches, childbirth, **cancer**, and pain and fear resulting from dental procedures. In some cases, surgeons use hypnosis in the operating room, not only to reduce the amount of **anesthesia** needed by the patient, but also to lessen **anxiety** and postoperative bleeding and swelling.

Psychologists use hypnosis in treating patients to overcome negative habits, anxiety, fear and depression. Also, it is commonly used to help patients recall past events, which is useful in psychotherapy. Family physicians have recently begun to use hypnosis to treat psychosomatic illness (physical illnesses or complaints that are largely caused by psychological factors). Professionals in the field of psychotherapy have also found positive results in helping patients control appetite and reduce the levels of drugs necessary in the treatment chronic illness.

Because hypnosis can sometimes completely remove or distract people from feeling pain, it is important that a doctor or other appropriate medical specialist assess the underlying medical or psychological condition prior to hypnosis. Another important precaution when dealing with hypnosis is that, despite potential medical benefits of hypnosis, misinterpretation is possible because of the questionable reliability of the memories recalled during hypnosis. Because there is no medical degree required for the practice of hypnotherapy, persons wishing to undergo hypnosis should be sure that the therapist is well trained. It may be helpful to find a therapist who is a licensed professional in a field where hypnotherapy is part of normal practice, such as social workers and psychologists. It is important to check credentials and background when choosing a hypnotherapist.

Hypnosis is not to be considered a form of psychotherapy, nor a treatment capable of solving problems immediately or on its own. Problems and habits take time to get implanted in one's life, and it takes considerable amount of time to remove them.

A hypnotic state results from gradually entering a state of consciousness unlike that of awareness or sleep. During this time, the attention of subjects is withdrawn from his or her surroundings. Most individuals can easily be hypnotized, but the depth and extent of the hypnotic state varies.

Hypnotherapy requires that the patient desire to change a certain type of behavior. Success is greater the more committed the subject is to change. If the patient is reluctant, hypnotherapy may be unsuccessful.

Hypochondriasis

Hypochondriasis is a mental disorder characterized by excessive fear of or preoccupation with a serious illness, despite medical testing and reassurance to the contrary. It was formerly called hypochondriacal neurosis.

Although hypochondriasis is often considered a disorder that primarily affects adults, it is now increasingly recognized in children and adolescents. In addition, hypochondriasis may develop in elderly people without previous histories of health-related fears. The disorder accounts for about 5% of psychiatric patients and is equally common in men and women.

The causes of hypochondriasis are not precisely known. Children may have physical symptoms that resemble or mimic those of other family members. In adults, hypochondriasis may sometimes reflect a self-centered character structure or a wish to be taken care of by others; it may also have been copied from a parent's behavior. In elderly people, hypochondriasis may be associated with depression or **grief**. It may also involve biologically based hypersensitivity to internal stimuli.

Most hypochondriacs are worried about being physically sick, although some express fear of insanity. The symptoms reported can range from general descriptions of a specific illness to unusual complaints. In many instances the symptoms reflect intensified awareness of ordinary body functions, such as heartbeat, breathing, or stomach noises. It is important to understand that a hypochondriac's symptoms are not ''in the head'' in the sense of being delusional. The symptoms are real, but the patient misinterprets bodily functions and attributes them to a serious or even lethal cause.

Diagnosis is often complicated by the patient's detailed understanding of symptoms and medical terminology from previous contacts with doctors. If a new doctor suspects hypochondriasis, he or she will usually order a complete medical workup in order to rule out physical disease.

- The patient is not psychotic (out of touch with reality or hallucinating).
- The patient gets upset or blames the doctor when told there is ''nothing wrong,'' or that there is a psychological basis for the problem.
- There is a correlation between episodes of hypochondriacal behavior and stressful periods in the patient's life.
- The behavior has lasted at least six months.

The goal of therapy is to help the patient (and family) live with the symptoms and to modify thinking and behavior that reinforces hypochondriacal symptoms. This treatment orientation is called supportive, as distinct from insight-oriented, because hypochondriacs usually resist psychological interpretations of their symptoms. Supportive treatment may include medications to relieve anxiety. Some clinicians look carefully for ''masked'' depression and treat with antidepressants.

Follow-up care includes regular physical checkups, because about 30% of patients with hypochondriasis will eventually develop a serious physical illness. The physician also tries to prevent unnecessary medical testing and ''doctor shopping'' on the patient's part.

From 33–50% of patients with hypochondriasis can expect significant improvement from the current methods of treatment.

HYPOGLYCEMIA

The condition called hypoglycemia is literally translated as low blood sugar. Hypoglycemia occurs when blood sugar (or blood glucose) concentrations fall below a level necessary to properly support the body's need for energy and stability throughout its cells.

Carbohydrates are the main dietary source of the glucose that is manufactured in the liver and absorbed into the bloodstream to fuel the body's cells and organs. Glucose concentration is controlled by hormones, primarily insulin and glucagon. Glucose concentration is also controlled by epinephrine (adrenalin) and norepinephrine, as well as growth hormone. If these regulators are not working properly, levels of blood sugar can become either excessive (as in hyperglycemia) or inadequate (as in hypoglycemia). If a person has a blood sugar level of 50 mg/dl or less, he or she is considered hypoglycemic, although glucose levels vary widely from one person to another.

Drug-induced hypoglycemia, a complication of **diabetes**, is the most commonly seen and most dangerous form of hypoglycemia. It occurs most often in diabetics who must inject insulin periodically to lower their blood sugar. While other diabetics are also vulnerable to low blood sugar episodes, they have a lower risk of a serious outcome than do insulin-dependent diabetics. Unless recognized and treated immediately, severe hypoglycemia in the insulin-dependent diabetic can lead to generalized convulsions followed by amnesia and unconsciousness. Death, though rare, is a possible outcome.

In insulin-dependent diabetics, hypoglycemia is known as an insulin reaction.

Ideopathic or reactive hypoglycemia (also called postprandial hypoglycemia) occurs when some people eat. A number of reasons for this reaction have been proposed, but no single cause has been identified. In some cases, this form of hypoglycemia appears to be associated with malfunctions or diseases of the liver, pituitary, adrenals, liver, or pancreas. These conditions are unrelated to diabetes.

HYPOGONADISM

Hypogonadism is the condition in which the production of sex hormones and germ cells are inadequate. It is more prevalent in males than in females.

The gonads are the organs of sexual differentiation—in the female, they are ovaries; in the male, the testes. Along with producing eggs and sperm, they produce sex hormones that generate all the differences between men and women. If they produce too little sex hormone, then either the growth or the function of the sexual organs is impaired.

The gonads are not independent in their function, however. They are loosely controlled by the pituitary gland. The pituitary hormones are the same for males and females, but the gonadal hormones are different. Men produce mostly **androgens**, and women produce mostly estrogens. These two kinds of hormones regulate the development of the embryo and direct the adolescent maturation of sex organs into their adult form. Further, they sustain those organs and their function throughout the reproductive years. The effects of estrogen reach beyond that to sustain bone strength and protect the **cardiovascular system** from degenerative disease.

Hormones can be inadequate during or after each stage of development—embryonic and adolescent. During each stage, inadequate hormone stimulation will prevent normal development. After each stage, a decrease in hormone stimulation will result in failed function and perhaps some shrinkage. The organs affected principally by sex hormones are the male and female genitals, and the female breasts. Body hair, fat deposition, bone and muscle growth, and some brain functions are also influenced.

Sex is determined at the moment of conception by the sex chromosomes, one of each of which is provided by the parent. A female receives two X chromosomes, one from her mother and one from her father. A male receives an X from his mother (the only kind she has to give) and a Y chromosome from his father. Genetic defects sometimes result in changes in the chromosomes. If sex chromosomes are involved, there is a change in the development of sexual characteristics.

Female is the default sex of the embryo, so most of the sex organ deficits at birth occur in boys. Some, but not all, are due to inadequate androgen stimulation. The penis may be small, the testicles undescended (cryptorchidism) or various degrees of "feminization" of the genitals may be present.

After birth, sexual development does not occur until **puberty**. Hypogonadism most often shows up as an abnormality in boys during puberty. Again, not every defect is due to inadequate hormones. Some are due to too much of the wrong hormone. Kallmann's syndrome is a birth defect in the brain that prevents release of hormones and appears as failure of male puberty. Some boys have an adequate amount of androgen in their system but fail to respond to it, a condition known as androgen resistance.

Female problems in puberty or with the **reproductive system** are rarely related to a lack of hormones, but rather to complex rhythms gone wrong. Women's problems with too little hormone happen during **menopause**, which is a normal hypogonadism.

A number of adverse events can damage the gonads and result in decreased hormone levels. The childhood **mumps**, if acquired after puberty, can infect and destroy the testicles—a disease called viral orchitis. Ionizing radiation and **chemotherapy**, trauma, several drugs (spironolactone, a **diuretic** and ketoconazole, an antifungal agent), alcohol, marijuana, heroin, methadone, and environmental toxins can all damage testicles and decrease their hormone production. Severe diseases in the liver or kidneys, certain infections, **sickle-cell anemia**, and some **cancers** also affect gonads. To treat some male cancers, it is necessary to remove the testicles, thereby preventing the androgens from stimulating cancer growth. This procedure, still called castration or *orchiectomy*, removes androgen stimulation from the whole body.

For several reasons the pituitary can fail. It happens rarely after **pregnancy**. It used to be removed to treat advanced breast or prostate cancer. Sometimes the pituitary develops a tumor that destroys it. Failure of the pituitary is called hypopituitarism and, of course, leaves the gonads with no stimulation to produce hormones.

Besides the tissue changes generated by hormone stimulation, the only other symptoms relate to sexual desire and function. Libido is enhanced by testosterone, and male sexual performance requires androgens. The role of female hormones in female sexual activity is less clear, although hormones strengthen tissues and promote healthy secretions, facilitating sexual activity.

Currently, there are accurate blood tests for most of the hormones in the body, including those from the pituitary and even some from the hypothalamus. Chromosomes can be analyzed, and gonads can be, but rarely are, biopsied.

Replacing missing body chemicals is much easier than suppressing excesses. Estrogen replacement is recommended for nearly all women after menopause for its many beneficial effects. Estrogen can be taken by mouth, injection, or skin patch. It is strongly recommended that the other female hormone, progesterone, be taken as well, because it prevents overgrowth of uterine lining and **uterine cancer**. Testosterone replacement is available for males who are deficient.

Hypopituitarism

Hypopituitarism is loss of function in an endocrine gland due to failure of the pituitary gland to secrete hormones that stimulate that gland's function. The pituitary gland is located at the base of the brain. Patients diagnosed with hypopituitarism may be deficient in one single hormone, several hormones, or have complete pituitary failure.

The pituitary is a pea-sized gland located at the base of the brain, and surrounded by bone. The hypothalamus, another endocrine organ in the brain, controls the function of the pituitary gland by providing "hormonal orders." In turn, the pituitary gland regulates the many hormones that control various functions and organs within the body. The posterior pituitary acts as a sort of storage area for the hypothalamus and passes on hormones that control function of the muscles and kidneys. The anterior pituitary produces its own hormones which help to regulate several endocrine functions.

In hypopituitarism, something interferes with the production and release of these hormones, thus affecting the function of the target gland. Commonly affected hormones may include:

Gonadotropin deficiency, which involves two distinct hormones affecting the **reproductive system**. Luteinizing hormone (LH) stimulates the testes in men and the ovaries in women. This deficiency can affect fertility in men and women and **menstruation** in women. Follicle-stimulating hormone (FSH) has similar effects to LH.

Thyroid stimulating hormone (TSH) is involved in stimulation of the thyroid gland. A lack of stimulation in the gland leads to hypothyroidism.

Also known as corticotropin, adrenocorticotopic hormone (ACTH) stimulates the adrenal gland to produce a hormone similar to cortisone, called cortisol. The loss of this hormone can lead to serious problems.

Growth hormone (GH) regulates the body's growth. Patients who lose supply of this hormone before physical maturity will suffer impaired growth. Loss of the hormone can also affect adults.

Other important hormones include prolactin, which stimulates the female breast to produce milk; antidiuretic hormone (ADH), which controls the function of the kidneys and, when deficient, can lead to **diabetes** insipidus. However, patients with hypopituitarism rarely suffer ADH deficiency, unless the hypopituitarism is the result of hypothalamus disease.

However, deficiency of a single pituitary hormone occurs less commonly than deficiency of more than one hormone. Sometimes referred to as progressive pituitary hormone deficiency or partial hypopituitarism, there is usually a predictable order of hormone loss. Generally, growth hormone is lost first, then luteinizing hormone deficiency follows. The loss of follicle-stimulating hormone, thyroid stimulating hormone and adrenocorticotopic hormones follow much later. The progressive loss of pituitary hormone secretion is usually a slow process, which can occur over a period of months or years. Hypopituitarism does occasionally start suddenly with rapid onset of symptoms.

Sometimes, all hormones released by the anterior pituitary will be lost, a condition called panhypopituitarism, or complete pituitary failure.

Hypopituitarism can result from the decreased release of hypothalmic hormones that stimulated pituitary function, from the interference of tumors, inflammation, infection, or interrupted blood supply, or from the damage to the pituitary stalk or destruction of the pituitary cells themselves by tumor or disease.

Symptoms of hypopituitarism vary with the affected hormones and severity of deficiency. Frequently, patients have had years of symptoms that were nonspecific until a major illness occurred. Overall symptoms may include fatigue, sensitivity to cold, weakness, decreased appetite, weight loss and abdominal pain. Low blood pressure, **headache** and visual disturbances are other associated symptoms.

Gonadotrophin deficiency may show up as infertility in women and men. Women may also have decreased interest in sex, premature cessation of menstruation, hot flashes, vaginal dryness and pain during intercourse. Men may also suffer sexual dysfunction.

A deficiency of TSH may first be indicated by intolerance to cold, fatigue, weight gain, constipation and pale, waxy, dry skin.

Symptoms of ACTH deficiency include fatigue, weakness, weight loss and low blood pressure.

In children, growth hormone deficiency will result in short stature and growth retardation.

Once the diagnosis of a single hormone deficiency is made, it is strongly recommended that tests for other hormone deficiencies be conducted.

Treatment varies, depending on the age and sex of the patient, severity of the deficiency, the number of hormones involved, and even the underlying cause of the hypopituitarism. Immediate hormone replacement is generally administered to replace the specific deficient hormone. Patients need to be tauch about how to manage the impact of their hormone deficiency on daily life. For instance, certain illnesses, accidents or surgical procedures may have adverse complications due to hypopituitarism.

The treatment of hypopituitarism is usually very straightforward, but must normally continue for the remainder of the patient's life. If the cause of the disorder is a tumor or lesion, radiation or surgical removal are treatment options. Successful removal may reverse the hypopituitarism. However, even after removal of the mass, **hormone replacement therapy** may still be necessary.

Most patients with hypopituitarism live normal lives as long as therapy is continued. However, hypopituitarism is usually a permanent condition and prognosis depends on the primary cause of the disorder. It can be potentially life threatening, particularly when acute hypopituitarism occurs as a result of a large pituitary tumor. The number of people who die from this disease has increased, and, although the cause is not known, may be due to overtreatment with hormones. Recovery of pituitary function is preferred to lifelong hormone therapy.

There is no known prevention of hypopituitarism, except for prevention of damage to the pituitary/hypothalamic area from injury.

Hypotension

Hypotension is the medical term for low blood pressure.

The pressure of the blood in the arteries rises and falls as the heart and muscles handle demands of daily living, such exercise, sleep and stress. Some healthy people have blood pressure well below the average for their age, even though they have a completely normal heart and blood vessels. This is often true of athletes who are in superior shape. The term ''hypotension'' is usually used only when blood pressure has fallen so far that enough blood can no longer reach the brain, causing **dizziness** and **fainting.**

Postural hypotension is the most common type of low blood pressure. In this condition, symptoms appear after a person sits up or stands quickly. In normal people, the **cardiovascular system** must make a quick adjustment to raise blood pressure slightly to account for the change in position. For those with postural hypotension, the blood pressure adjustment is inadequate or doesn't happen. Postural hypotension may occur if someone is taking certain drugs or medicine for high blood pressure. It also happens to diabetics when nerve damage has disrupted the reflexes that control blood pressure.

Many people have a chronic problem with low blood pressure that is not particularly serious. This may include people who require certain medications, who are pregnant, have bad veins, or have arteriosclerosis (hardening of the arteries).

The most serious problem with low blood pressure occurs when there is a sudden drop, which can be life-threatening due to widespread ischemia (insufficient supply of blood to an organ due to blockage in an artery). This type of low blood pressure may be due to a wide variety of causes, including:

- Trauma with extensive blood loss
- Serious **burns**
- **Shock** from various causes
- **Heart attack**
- Adrenal failure

- **Cancer**
- Severe **fever**
- Serious infection (septicemia).

Blood pressure is a measure of the pressure in the arteries created by the heart contracting. During the day, a normal person's blood pressure changes constantly, depending on activity. Low blood pressure can be diagnosed by taking the blood pressure with a sphygmomanometer. This is a device with a soft rubber cuff that is inflated around the upper arm until it's tight enough to stop blood flow. The cuff is then slowly deflated until the health care worker, listening to the artery in the arm with a stethoscope, can hear the blood first as a beat forcing its way along the artery. This is the systolic pressure. The cuff is then deflated more until the beat disappears and the blood flows steadily through the open artery; this gives the diastolic pressure.

Blood pressure is recorded as systolic (higher) and diastolic (lower) pressures. A healthy young adult has a blood pressure of about 110/75, which typically rises with age to about 140/90 by age 60 (a reading now considered mildly elevated).

Treatment of low blood pressure depends on the underlying cause, which can usually be resolved. For those people with postural hypotension, a medication adjustment may help prevent the problem. These individuals may find that rising more slowly, or getting out of bed in slow stages, helps the problem. Low blood pressure with no other symptoms does not need to be treated.

Low blood pressure as a result of injury or other underlying condition can usually be successfully treated if the trauma is not too extensive or is treated in time. Less serious forms of chronic low blood pressure have a good prognosis and do not require treatment.

HYPOTHERMIA

Hypothermia, a potentially fatal condition, occurs when body temperature falls below 95°F (35°C). Although it is an obvious danger for people living in cold climates, many cases have occurred when the air temperature is well above freezing. Elderly people, for instance, have succumbed to hypothermia after prolonged exposure to indoor air temperatures of 50–65°F (10–18.3°C).

Measured orally, a healthy person's body temperature can fluctuate between 97°F (36.1°C) and 100°F (37.8°C). Survival depends on maintaining temperature stability within this range by balancing the heat produced by **metabolism** with the heat lost to the environment through (for the most part) the skin and lungs. When environmental or other changes cause heat loss to outpace heat production, the brain triggers physiological and behavioral responses to restore the balance. Shivering, for example, aids heat production by accelerating metabolism. But if the cold stress is too great and the body's defenses are overwhelmed, body temperature begins to fall. Hypothermia is considered to begin once body temperature reaches 95°F (35°C), though even smaller drops in temperature can have an adverse effect.

Hypothermia is divided into two types: primary and secondary. Primary hypothermia occurs when the body's heat-balancing mechanisms are working properly but are subjected to extreme cold, such as exposure to cold air or cold water. Hypothermia due to cold air usually takes at least several hours to develop, but immersion hypothermia will occur within about an hour of entering the water because water draws heat away from the body much faster than air does. Secondary hypothermia affects people whose heat-balancing mechanisms are impaired in some way and cannot respond adequately to moderate or perhaps even mild cold. Among the reasons for the failure of the body's heat-balancing are **diabetes**, **malnutrition**, bacterial infection, thyroid disease, and the use of medications and other substances that affect the brain or spinal cord, such as alcohol.

Secondary hypothermia is often a threat to the elderly, who may be on medications or suffering from illnesses that affect their ability to conserve heat. Malnutrition and immobility can also put the elderly at risk. Some medical research also suggests that shivering and blood vessel narrowing (two of the body's defenses against cold) may not be triggered as quickly in older people. For these and other reasons, the elderly can, over a period of days or even weeks, fall victim to hypothermia in poorly insulated homes or other surroundings. In addition, hypothermia can easily be misdiagnosed as a **stroke** or some other common illness of old age.

The signs and symptoms of hypothermia follow a typical course. The impact of hypothermia on the nervous system becomes apparent quite early. Coordination, for instance, may begin to suffer as soon as body temperature reaches 95°F (35°C). Other early signs include cold and pale skin and intense shivering; the latter stops between 90°F (32.2°C) and 86°F (30°C). As body temperature continues to fall, speech becomes slurred, the muscles go rigid, and the victim becomes disoriented and has trouble seeing. Other harmful consequences include dehydration as well as liver and **kidney failure**. Heart rate, respiratory rate, and blood pressure rise during the first stages of hypothermia, but fall once the 90°F (32.2°C) mark is passed. Below 86°F (30°C), most victims are **comatose**, and below 82°F (27.8°C) the heart's rhythm becomes dangerously disordered. Yet even at very low body temperatures, people can survive for several hours and be successfully revived, though they may appear to be dead.

Emergency medical help should be summoned whenever a person appears hypothermic, exhibiting the danger signs described above. Until emergency help arrives, a victim of outdoor hypothermia should be brought to shelter and warmed by removing wet clothing and footwear, drying the skin, and wrapping him or her in warm blankets or a sleeping bag. Gentle handling is necessary when moving the victim to avoid disturbing the heart. Rubbing the skin or giving the victim alcohol can be harmful, though warm drinks such as clear soup and tea are recommended for those who can swallow.

Rewarming is the essence of hospital treatment for hypothermia. Mild hypothermia (in which the patient's body temperature is 90–95°F [32.2–35°C]) is reversed with passive rewarming, using the patient's own metabolism to rewarm the body. Moderate hypothermia (86–90°F [30–32.2°C]) is often treated first with active external rewarming and then with passive rewarming. Active external rewarming involves applying heat to the skin, for instance by placing the patient in a warm bath or wrapping the patient in electric blankets.

Severe hypothermia (a body temperature of less than 86°F [30°C]) requires active internal rewarming, such as cardiopulmonary bypass, in which the patient's blood is circulated through a rewarming device and then returned to the body. The alternative is to introduce warm oxygen or fluids into the body.

People who spend time outdoors in cold weather can reduce heat loss by wearing their clothing loosely and in layers and by keeping their hands, feet, and head well covered (30–50% of body heat is lost through the head). Because water draws heat away from the body so easily, staying dry is important, and wet clothing and footwear should be replaced as quickly as possible. Wind- and water-resistant outer garments are also crucial. Alcohol should be avoided because it promotes heat loss by expanding the blood vessels that carry body heat to the skin.

Preventing hypothermia among the elderly requires vigilance on the part of family, friends, and caregivers. An elderly person's home should be properly insulated and heated, with living areas kept at a temperature of 70°F (21.1°C). Warm clothing and bedding are essential, as are adequate food, rest, and exercise. Older people who live alone should be visited regularly—at least once a day during very cold weather—to ensure that their health remains sound and that they are taking good care of themselves. For help and advice, family members and others can turn to government and social service agencies. Meals on Wheels and visiting nurse programs, for instance, may be available, and it may be possible to obtain financial aid to winterize and heat homes.

Hyrtl, Joseph (1810-1894)

Austrian anatomist

Joseph Hyrtl earned an international reputation as a technical anatomist. In the mid-nineteenth century, the field of medicine depended heavily on anatomical discoveries, and Hyrtl's work was key to medical progress. Hyrtl was a lifelong academic, but the money he earned from producing anatomical supplies made him rich.

Hyrtl was born in Kismarton, Hungary, which is now part of Austria, and studied medicine in Vienna, serving as prosector (one who performs **dissections** for anatomical demonstrations) for the anatomist Joseph Berres. While he was still a student, Hyrtl taught anatomy to practitioners in the community. When he completed his doctorate in 1835, his dissertation advocated the study of anatomy and clinical instruction, seeing no value in conducting physiological experiments on animals. Hyrtl continued as prosector for another two years before accepting an anatomy professorship in Prague. In 1845, Hyrtl returned to teach anatomy at his alma mater in Vienna. He was awarded the teaching position that became vacant on the death of his old teacher, Berres. Hyrtl added to the demonstration collections, published frequently on his areas of research and taught applied anatomy to physicians.

Hyrtl published his first book, *Handbook of Human Anatomy*, in 1846, and well received being translated into all of the major languages and eventually went to 20 editions. Hyrtl reasoned that he had already provided his students with sketches and drawings at every lecture, so the book had no illustrations. The text focused on anatomical structure and function, which were most important to the practitioner.

In 1847, Hyrtl published the widely read *Handbook of Topographical Anatomy*, which organized the study of anatomy by region of the body. This text introduced topographical anatomy in Germany and established it as a separate discipline.

Hyrtl produced and sold specialized anatomical preparations that were used by scientists and all major anatomical museums. To better study anatomical structure, he used a preparation to inject vessels and bone cavities with a material that made them stiff. He then destroyed the adjacent bones or soft tissue. The technique enabled Hyrtl to study comparative anatomy across different species. Hyrtl's primary interest was anatomy, so he left the study of tissues to others. In 1860, Hyrtl published a manual on dissection and his text on corrosive anatomy came out in 1873. In his academic career, Hyrtl also improved and expanded the Anatomical Museum although the work was interrupted by political unrest in the 1850s.

During his tenure in Vienna, Hyrtl grew distant from his colleagues, who complained about his strong ambition and irritability. During the 30 years Hyrtl spent on the Viennese medical faculty, he was never chosen to serve as dean, a reflection on his strained relations with colleagues. In the lecture hall, Hyrtl had a flair for drama and liked to draw together concepts from history, scientific terminology, surgery and physiology. His students enjoyed the unusual approach and Hyrtl's lectures were always well attended. In the academic year 1864-1865, the year of the university's 500th anniversary, Hyrtl was asked to serve as rector.

Hyrtl was primarily interested in bone structure and the circulation of blood. He wrote about the characteristics of blood vessels in birds and amphibians and how these differed from human veins and arteries. In his comparative anatomy research, Hyrtl looked at patterns in veins, and the structure of the portal vein of the adrenal gland. He was interested in the role of cartilage in the knee, and the design of the hip joint.

When Hyrtl examined nonvascular hearts, his theories about coronary arteries conflicted with those of physiology professor Ernst von Brücke, leading to a bitter dispute. Although Hyrtl's hypotheses were later verified, the conflict wore him down. Hyrtl's comparative anatomy research of the ear led him to a previously unreported muscle of the incus which lay in an area which came to be known as Hyrtl's recess.

Hyrtl left the university in 1874, a little ahead of the customary retirement age, and spent the next 20 years writing about the history of anatomical terminology. Through the sale of his anatomic preparations, Hyrtl accumulated a substantial amount of money. After his death in Austria, Hyrtl's fortune was given to deserving medical students, an orphanage, a boarding school, and a church.

HYSTERECTOMY

Hysterectomy is the surgical removal of the uterus. In a total hysterectomy, the uterus and cervix are removed, and, in some cases, so are the fallopian tubes and ovaries. In a subtotal hysterectomy, only the uterus is removed. In a radical hysterectomy, the uterus, cervix, ovaries, oviducts, lymph nodes, and lymph channels are removed. The type of hysterectomy performed depends on the reason for the procedure. In all cases, **menstruation** stops and a woman can no longer bear children.

In the United States, about 600,000 hysterectomies are done every year, making it the second most common operation. By age 60, roughly one out of every three American women will have had a hysterectomy.

Most (30%) of all hysterectomies in the United States are done to remove fibroid tumors. Fibroid tumors, or "fibroids" are non-cancerous (benign) growths in the uterus. They can cause pelvic and **lower-back pain** and heavy or lengthy menstrual periods. Treatment of **endometriosis** is the reason for 20% of hysterectomies. In endometriosis, the cells of the uterine lining (the endometrium) begin growing outside the uterus. These outlying cells still respond to the hormones that control the menstrual cycle and bleed each month, just as they would if they were inside the uterus. This irritates the surrounding tissue, leading to **pain** and scarring.

Another 20% percent of hysterectomies are done because of heavy or abnormal vaginal bleeding that cannot be linked to any cause and cannot be controlled by other means. A further 20% of hysterectomies are performed to treat prolapsed uterus, **pelvic inflammatory disease**, and endometrial hyperplasia, a potentially precancerous condition.

About 10% of hysterectomies are performed to treat **cancer** of the cervix, ovaries, or uterus. Women with cancer in one or more of these organs almost always have the organ(s) removed as one part of their cancer treatment.

A total hysterectomy, sometimes called a simple hysterectomy, removes the entire uterus and the cervix. The ovaries are not removed and continue to secrete hormones. Total hysterectomies are always performed in the case of uterine and **cervical cancer**. The total hysterectomy is the most common kind of hysterectomy.

If the reason for the hysterectomy is to remove **uterine fibroids**, treat abnormal bleeding, or relieve pelvic pain, it may be possible to remove only the uterus and leave the cervix. This procedure, called a subtotal or partial hysterectomy), removes the least amount of tissue.

Radical hysterectomies are performed on women with cervical cancer or endometrial cancer that has spread to the cervix. A radical hysterectomy removes the uterus, cervix, top part of the vagina, ovaries, fallopian tubes, lymph nodes, lymph channels, and tissue in the pelvic cavity that surrounds the cervix. This type of hysterectomy removes the most tissue and requires the longest hospital stay and recovery period.

The frequency with which hysterectomies are performed in the United States has been questioned in recent years. It has been suggested that many hysterectomies are unnecessary. The United States has the highest rate of hysterectomies (number

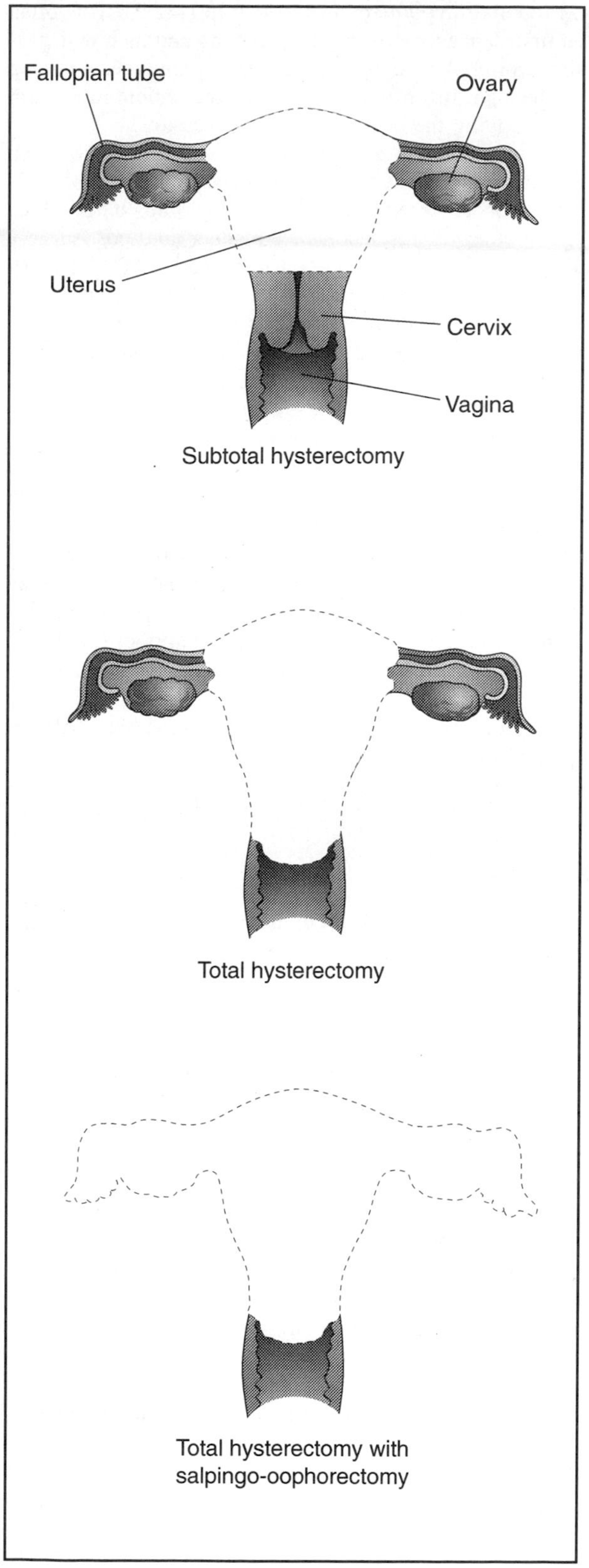

Three types of hysterectomy and the organs removed in each type.

body. Moderate hypothermia (86–90°F [30–32.2°C]) is often treated first with active external rewarming and then with passive rewarming. Active external rewarming involves applying heat to the skin, for instance by placing the patient in a warm bath or wrapping the patient in electric blankets.

Hysterectomy is a relatively safe operation, although like all major surgery it carries risks. These include unanticipated reaction to **anesthesia**, internal bleeding, blood clots, damage to other organs such as the bladder, and post-surgery infection. The risk of death is about 1 in every 1,000 (1/1,000) women having the operation.

Other complications sometimes reported after a hysterectomy include changes in sex drive, weight gain, **constipation**, and pelvic pain. Hot flashes and other symptoms of menopause can occur if the ovaries are removed. Women who have both ovaries removed and who do not take estrogen replacement therapy run an increased risk for heart disease and **osteoporosis**. Women with a history of psychological and emotional problems before the hysterectomy are more likely to experience psychological difficulties after the operation.

Although there is some concern that hysterectomies may be performed unnecessarily, there are many conditions for which the operation improves a woman's quality of life. In the Maine Woman's Health Study, 71% of women who had hysterectomies to correct moderate or severe painful symptoms reported feeling better mentally, physically, and sexually after the operation.

HYSTERIA

The term ''hysteria'' has been in use for more 2000 years and its definition has become broader and more diffuse over time. In modern psychology and psychiatry, hysteria is a feature of hysterical disorders in which a patient experiences physical symptoms that have a psychological, rather than an organic, cause; and histrionic personality disorder characterized by excessive emotions, dramatics, and attention-seeking behavior.

Patients with hysterical disorders experience physical symptoms that have no organic cause. These patients are not ''faking'' their ailments, as the symptoms are very real to them. Disorders with hysteric features typically begin in adolescence or early adulthood.

Histrionic **personality disorder** is found in approximately 2–3% of the general population. It begins in early adulthood and has been diagnosed more frequently in women than in men. Histrionic personalities are typically self-centered and attention seeking. They operate on emotion rather than fact or logic, and their conversation is full of generalizations and dramatic appeals. While the patient's enthusiasm, flirtatious behavior, and trusting nature may make them appear charming, their need for immediate gratification, mercurial displays of emotion, and constant demand for attention often alienates them from others.

Hysteria may be a defense mechanism to avoid painful emotions by unconsciously transferring this distress to the body. Symptoms may mimic a number of physical and neurological disorders which must be ruled out before a diagnosis of hysteria is made.

According to the *Diagnostic and Statistical Manual of Mental Disorders,* Fourth Edition (*DSM-IV*), individuals with histrionic personality possess at least five of the following symptoms or personality features:

- A need to be the center of attention
- Inappropriate, sexually seductive, or provocative behavior while interacting with others
- Rapidly changing emotions and superficial expression of emotions
- Vague and impressionistic speech (gives opinions without any supporting details)
- Easily influenced by others
- Believes relationships are more intimate than they are.

Hysterical disorders frequently prove to be actual medical or neurological disorders, which makes it important to rule these disorders out before diagnosing a patient with hysterical disorders. In addition to a patient interview, several clinical inventories may be used to assess the patient for hysterical tendencies, such as the Minnesota Multiphasic Personality Inventory-2 (MMPI-2) or the Millon Clinical Multiaxial Inventory-III (MCMI-III). These tests may be administered in an outpatient or hospital setting by a psychiatrist or psychologist.

For people with hysterical disorders, a supportive healthcare environment is critical. Regular appointments with a physician who acknowledges the patient's physical discomfort are important. Psychotherapy may be attempted to help the patient gain insight into the cause of their distress. Use of behavioral therapy can help to avoid re-enforcing symptoms.

Psychotherapy is generally the treatment of choice for histrionic personality disorder. It focuses on supporting the patient and on helping them develop the skills needed to create meaningful relationships with others.

The outcome for hysterical disorders varies by type. Some may last a lifetime, others for only a few months. Symptoms of hysterical disorders may suddenly disappear, only to reappear in another form later.

Individuals with histrionic personality disorder may be at a higher risk for suicidal gestures, attempts, or threats in an effort to gain attention. Providing a supportive environment for patients with both hysterical disorders and histrionic personality disorder is key to helping these patients.

I

IGNARRO, LOUIS J. (1941-)

American pharmacologist

Ignarro, together with fellow American pharmacologists **Robert Furchgott** and **Ferid Murad**, received the 1998 Nobel Prize in Physiology or Medicine for discoveries related to the role of nitric oxide as a signaling molecule in the **cardiovascular system**.

Not to be confused with **nitrous oxide** (a gas used in **anesthesia**), nitric oxide is a colorless, odorless gas that, thanks to initial work by these three Nobel laureates and a flurry of subsequent research by others, now has widespread potential including the treatment of heart disease, **shock**, **cancer**, **impotence**, and **pulmonary hypertension**—a potentially fatal condition in premature infants. In 1994, the respected journal *Science* declared nitric oxide as its ''molecule of the year.''

Born in Brooklyn, New York, Ignarro studied pharmacy at Columbia University and then obtained a Ph.D. in Pharmacology from the University of Minnesota. He served as professor of pharmacology at Tulane University in New Orleans from 1979 to 1985, when he joined the University of California at Los Angeles (UCLA).

There, Ignarro is known as an extraordinary teacher. By 1998, he had received 10 consecutive Golden Apple Awards, given by UCLA medical students annually to the best teacher in the basic sciences.

Ignarro started his research into nitric oxide in 1978. Earlier, Ferid Murad had postulated that nitric oxide and other nitrogen-containing compounds might be produced by one cell, travel through membranes, and then regulate the function of other cells. At the time, this was an entirely new concept for signaling in biological systems.

Then, in 1980. Robert Furchgott discovered a substance in the endothelium (a thin layer of flattened cells lining the inner surface of blood vessels) that caused relaxation in smooth muscle. Furchgott called this substance endothelium-derived relaxing factor (EDRF).

After several years of research, Ignarro discovered that Furchgott's EDRF was, in reality, nitric oxide operating as Murid had suggested. Ignarro announced this important development in 1986 at a scientific conference at the Mayo Clinic in Rochester, Minnesota. At the same meeting, Furchgott announced he had independently confirmed that EDRF was nitric oxide. This was the first time anyone had demonstrated that a gas could act as a signal molecule in the body, and it prompted a flood of research into nitric oxide worldwide.

Nitric oxide is now known to play a key role in many biological functions including inflammation, blood flow regulation, cell growth, smooth muscle relaxation, and preserving memory. Each year, thousands of research papers are written about the molecule, compared to just a dozen papers in published in 1980. Ignarro is editor-in-chief of the journal *Nitric Oxide, Biology and Chemistry*, and a founder of the Nitric Oxide Society.

IMHOTEP (ca. 27th century B.C.)

Egyptian physician, architect, and vizier

Imhotep was a priest/physician and wise man in ancient Egypt who was credited with many miraculous healings. Although he achieved great fame during his lifetime, Imhotep's renown continued to grow after his death. He eventually achieved status as a god among the Egyptians, who prayed to him about matters of health. He is best known today as the architect who began the ''age of pyramids'' in Egypt. He designed and supervised the building of the step pyramid complex at Saqqara (sometimes spelled Sakkara), which is believed to be the first colossal stone edifice ever built.

Because he was born a commoner, Imhotep's early life is largely unknown. He most likely was born in a suburb of Memphis, Egypt. Imhotep probably received a liberal education as a youth and, as a result, had wide ranging interests. Imhotep's superior intellect served him well, and he eventually

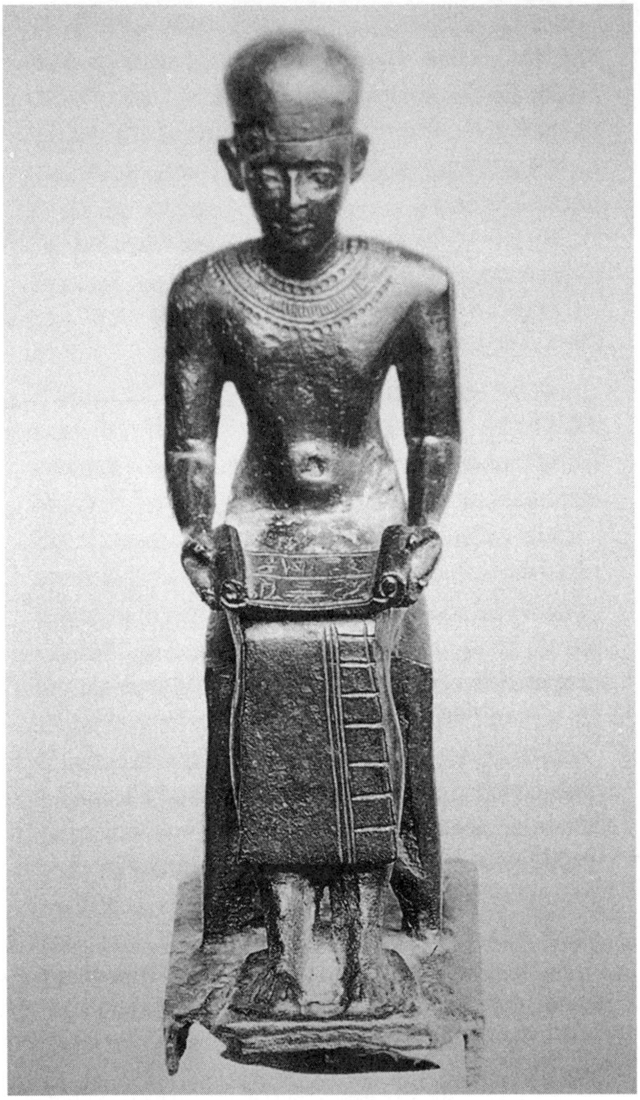

Imhotep

became chief vizier during Egypt's Third Dynasty for King Djoser (2630-2611 B.C.), or Zoser. As vizier, he was the king's chief advisor on nearly every aspect of Egyptian life, from law and finances to the military and agriculture. In this role, his reputation grew as a wise man. Many of his sayings were alleged to have become Egyptian proverbs, although none survive today.

Imhotep was a renowned as a physician and, because of his duties as vizier, he undoubtedly advised on medical matters. Scholars hypothesize, however, that his role as a physician may have been glorified after his death. Nevertheless, many legends of miraculous healings surround Imhotep. It was said that Imhotep often appeared in the dreams of those who were ill and provided them with remedies. Another legend relates that infertile couples would pray at Imhotep's temple and subsequently could conceive a child.

The deification of Imhotep began as a medical demi-god for the sick. Around 525 B.C., when Egypt was under Persian rule, Imhotep achieved full deity status, meaning that his birth was attributed to the direct intervention of one of Egypt's gods. As the son of Ptah, creator god of Memphis and of craftsmen, Imhotep had many shrines and small temples dedicated to him. A vigorous cult following grew during the New Kingdom (about 1580 B.C.) and lasted well into the Roman period of rule over Egypt. One of the temples built in his honor at Memphis became a renowned hospital and medical school. Imhotep is believed to be the only non-royal ever elevated to god status by the Egyptians. The Roman emperors Claudius and Tiberius also had inscriptions in praise of Imhotep on the walls of their Egyptian temples. Festivals were held in honor of Imhotep and the events of his life, such as his birthday and death, although there is not record of these exact dates.

Under the reign of King Djoser, Imhotep undertook the building of the step pyramid at Saqqara, south of Cairo. The pyramid and its compound were unique for several reasons. Imhotep decided not to use the then standard sun-dried mud bricks but rather would build the King's funerary complex using stone as a more permanent building material. The complex encompassed a towering six tiered step-like structure standing approximately 200 feet high and was the world's first large stone structure. When completed, the entire site, once surrounded by a single massive stone wall, was nearly 2,000 feet long and 1,000 feet wide. It included a 40 column colonnade, exquisite courtyard, and many shrines, temples, and outbuildings. The pyramid's burial chambers are an especially remarkable feat of design and engineering, with a series of shafts, tunnels and chambers that are more complex than any pyramid that followed. It is the oldest surviving Egyptian pyramid.

Although Imhotep's renown lasted for more than 3,000 years, many scholars believed him to be a mythological figure. In fact, the tomb or mummy of Imhotep has never been discovered. As a medical man, architect, scientist, faith healer, and god, Imhotep was not only one of the most influential people of his times but maintained a lasting influence for centuries after his death. In the words of famous English physician and scientist **Sir William Osler** (1849-1919), Imhotep was "the first figure of a physician to stand out clearly from the mists of antiquity."

IMMOBILIZATION

Immobilization refers to the process of holding a joint or bone in place with a splint, cast, or brace. This is done to prevent an injured area from moving while it heals.

When an arm, hand, leg, or foot requires immobilization, the cast, splint, or brace will generally extend from the joint above the injury to the joint below the injury. For example, an injury to the mid-calf requires immobilization from the knee to the ankle and foot. Injuries of the hip and upper thigh or shoulder and upper arm require a cast that encircles the body and extends down the injured leg or arm.

Casts are generally used for immobilization of a broken bone. Once the doctor makes sure the two broken ends of the bone are aligned, a cast is put on to keep them in place until they rejoin through natural healing. Casts are applied by a physician, a nurse, or an assistant. They are custom-made to fit each person, and are usually made of plaster or fiberglass. Fiberglass weighs less than plaster, is more durable, and allows the skin more adequate airflow than plaster. A layer of cotton or synthetic padding is first wrapped around the skin to cover the injured area and protect the skin. The plaster or fiberglass is then applied over this.

Most casts should not be gotten wet. However, some types of fiberglass casts use Gortex padding that is waterproof and allows the person to completely immerse the cast in water when taking a shower or bath. There are some circumstances when this type of cast material can not be used.

A splint is often used to immobilize a dislocated joint while it heals. Splints are also often used for finger injuries, such as **fractures** or baseball finger, an injury in which the tendon at the end of the finger is separated from the bone as a result of trauma. Splinting also is used to immobilize an injured arm or leg immediately after an injury. Before moving a person who has injured an arm or leg some type of temporary splint should be applied to prevent further injury to the area. Splints may be made of acrylic, polyethylene foam, plaster, or aluminum. In an emergency, a splint can be made from a piece of wood or rolled magazine.

Slings are often used to support the arm after a fracture or other injury. They are generally used along with a cast or splint, but sometimes are used alone as a means of immobilization. They can be used in an emergency to immobilize the arm until the person can be seen by a doctor. A triangular bandage is placed under the injured arm and then tied around the neck.

Braces are used to support, align, or hold a body part in the correct position. Braces are sometimes used after a surgical procedure is performed on an arm or leg. They can also be used for an injury. Since some braces can be easily taken off and put back on, they are often used when the person must have physical therapy or exercise the limb during the healing process. Many braces can also be adjusted to allow for a certain amount of movement.

Both braces and splints offer less support and protection than a cast and may not be a treatment option in all circumstances.

A collar is generally used for neck injuries. A soft collar can relieve pain by restricting movement of the head and neck. Collars also transfer some of the weight of the head from the neck to the chest. Stiff collars are generally used to support the neck when there has been a fracture in one of the bones of the neck. Cervical collars are widely used by emergency personnel at the scene of injuries when there is a potential neck or head injury.

Immobilization may also be secured by **traction**. Traction involves using a method for applying tension to correct the alignment of two structures (such as two bones) and hold them in the correct position. For example, if the bone in the thigh breaks, the broken ends may have a tendency to overlap. Use of traction will hold them in the correct position for healing to occur. The strongest form of traction involves inserting

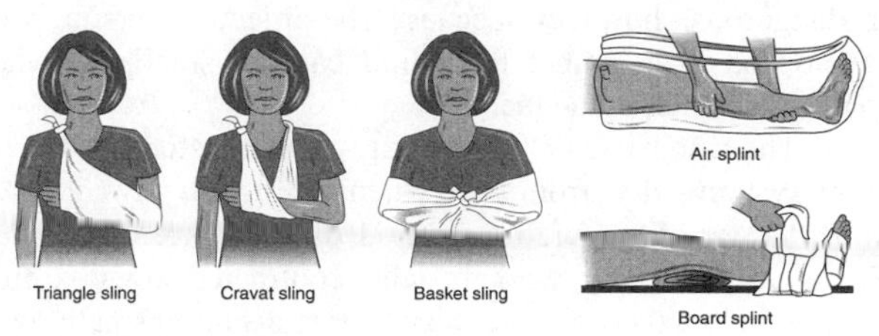

Several types of immobilization.

a stainless steel pin through a bony prominence attached by a horse shoe shaped bow and rope to a pulley and weights suspended over the end of the patient's bed.

After a cast or splint has been put on, the injured arm or leg should be elevated for 24 to 72 hours. It is recommended that the person lie or sit with the injured arm or leg raised above the level of the heart. Rest combined with elevation will reduce pain and speed the healing process by minimizing swelling.

After the cast, splint, or brace is removed, gradual exercise is usually performed to regain muscle strength and motion. The doctor may also recommend **hydrotherapy, heat treatments,** and other forms of **physical therapy**.

For some people, such as those in traction, immobilization will require long periods of bed rest. Lying in one position in bed for an extended period of time can result in sores on the skin and skin infection. Long periods of bed rest can also cause a build up of fluid in the lungs or **pneumonia**. **Urinary tract infections** can result from extended bed rest.

People who have casts, splints, or braces on their arms or legs will generally spend several weeks not using the injured arm or leg. This lack of use can result in decreased muscle tone and shrinkage of the muscle (atrophy). Much of this loss can usually be regained, however, through rehabilitation after the injury has healed.

IMMUNE SYSTEM

The immune system is the body's biological defense mechanism that protects against foreign invaders. Only in the last century have the components of that system and the ways in which they work been discovered, and more remains to be clarified.

Since ancient times medical observers had noticed that the body seemed to have powers to protect itself and resist disease. In particular, people who survived some infectious diseases did not suffer from those diseases again during their lifetime. This led to the practice of variolation in Asia, whereby people were injected with a mild case of **smallpox** to prevent the later development of a severe case of the disease. Lady Mary Wortley-Montague introduced variolation to Britain from the Ottoman Empire in 1720. The procedure was rather dangerous, however, because the injected person could develop an acute rather than mild case of smallpox, which could lead to an **epidemic**.

The true roots of immunology—or the study of the immune system—date from 1796 when an English physician, **Edward Jenner**, discovered a method of smallpox **vaccination**. He noted that dairy workers who contracted cowpox from milking infected cows were thereafter resistant to smallpox. In 1796 Jenner injected a young boy with material from a milkmaid who had an active case of cowpox. After the boy recovered from his own resulting cowpox, Jenner inoculated him with smallpox; the boy was immune. After Jenner published the results of this and other cases in 1798, the practice of Jennerian vaccination spread rapidly.

It was **Louis Pasteur** who established the cause of infectious diseases and the medical basis for immunization. First, Pasteur formulated his **germ theory** of disease—the concept that disease is caused by communicable microorganisms. In 1880 Pasteur discovered that aged cultures of fowl **cholera** bacteria lost their power to induce disease in chickens but still conferred immunity to the disease when injected. He went on to use *attenuated* (weakened) cultures of **anthrax** and **rabies** to vaccinate against those diseases. The American scientists Theobald Smith (1859-1934) and Daniel Salmon (1850-1914) showed in 1886 that bacteria killed by heat could also confer immunity.

Why vaccination imparted immunity was not yet known. In 1888 Pierre-Paul-Emile Roux (1853-1933) and Alexandre Yersin (1863-1943) showed that **diphtheria** bacillus produced a toxin that the body responded to by producing an antitoxin. **Emil von Behring** and Shibasaburo Kitasato found a similar toxin-antitoxin reaction in **tetanus** in 1890. He discovered that small doses of tetanus or diphtheria toxin produced immunity, and that this immunity could be transferred from animal to animal via serum. Von Behring concluded that the immunity was conferred by substances in the blood, which he called antitoxins, or antibodies. In 1894, Richard Pfeiffer (1858-1945) found that antibodies killed cholera bacteria (bacterioloysis). Hans Buchner (1850-1902) in 1893 discovered another important blood substance called complement (Buchner's term was *alexin*), and **Jules Bordet** in 1898 found that it enabled the antibodies to combine with antigens (foreign substances) and destroy or eliminate them. It became clear that each antibody acted only against a specific antigen. **Karl Landsteiner** was able to use this specific antigen-antibody reaction to distinguish the different blood groups.

A new element was introduced into the growing body of immune system knowledge during the 1880s by the Russian microbiologist **Elie Metchnikoff**. He discovered cell-based immunity: white blood cells (leucocytes), which Metchnikoff called phagocytes, ingested and destroyed foreign particles. Considerable controversy flourished between the proponents of cell-based and blood-based immunity until 1903, when Almroth Edward Wright brought them together by showing that certain blood substances were necessary for phagocytes to function as bacteria destroyers. A unifying theory of immunity was posited by **Paul Ehrlich** in the 1890s; his ''side-chain'' theory explained that antigens and antibodies combine chemically in fixed ways, like a key fits into a lock. Until now, immune responses were seen as purely beneficial. In 1902, however, **Charles Richet** and Paul Portier demonstrated extreme immune reactions in test animals that had become sensitive to antigens by previous exposure. This phenomenon of hypersensitivity, called **anaphylaxis**, showed that immune responses could cause the body to damage itself. Hypersensitivity to antigens also explained **allergies**, a term coined by Pirquet in 1906.

By the early 1900s immunology had become an established medical field with its own journals, first in Germany in 1909 and then in the United States in 1916 (the latter published by the world's first immunology society, founded in 1913).

Much more was learned about antibodies in the mid-twentieth century, including the fact that they are proteins of the gamma globulin portion of plasma and are produced by plasma cells; their molecular structure was also worked out. An important advance in immunochemistry came in 1935 when Michael Heidelberger and **Edward Kendall** (1886-1972) developed a method to detect and measure amounts of different antigens and antibodies in serum. Immunobiology also advanced. **Frank Macfarlane Burnet** suggested that animals did not produce antibodies to substances they had encountered very early in life; **Peter Medawar** proved this idea in 1953 through experiments on mouse embryos.

In 1957 Burnet put forth his clonal selection theory to explain the biology of immune responses. On meeting an antigen, an immunologically responsive cell (shown by C. S. Gowans (1923-) in the 1960s to be a lymphocyte) responds by multiplying and producing an identical set of plasma cells, which in turn manufacture the specific antibody for that antigen. Further cellular research has shown that there are two types of lymphocytes (nondescript lymph cells): B-lymphocytes, which secrete antibody, and T-lymphocytes, which regulate the B-lymphocytes and also either kill foreign substances directly (killer T cells) or stimulate macrophages to do so (helper T cells). Lymphocytes recognize antigens by characteristics on the surface of the antigen-carrying molecules. Researchers in the 1980s uncovered many more intricate biological and chemical details of the immune system components and the ways in which they interact.

Knowledge about the immune system's role in rejection of transplanted tissue became extremely important as organ transplantation became surgically feasible. Peter Medawar's work in the 1940s showed that such rejection was an immune reaction to antigens on the foreign tissue. Donald Calne (1936-) showed in 1960 that **immunosuppressant drugs**—drugs that suppress immune responses—reduced transplant rejection, and these drugs were first used on human patients in 1962. In the 1940s George Snell (1903-) discovered in mice a group of tissue-compatibility genes, MHC that played an important role in controlling acceptance or resistance to tissue grafts. **Jean Dausset** found human MHC, a set of antigens to human leucocytes (white blood cells), called HLA. Matching of HLA in donor and recipient tissue is an important technique to predict compatibility in transplants. **Baruj Benacerraf** in 1969 showed that an animal's ability to respond to an antigen was controlled by genes in the MHC complex.

Exciting new discoveries in immunology are on the horizon. Researchers are investigating the relation of HLA to disease; certain types of HLA molecules may predispose people to particular diseases. This promises to lead to more effective treatments and, in the long run, possible prevention. Autoimmune reaction—in which the body has an immune response to its own substances—may also be a cause of a number of diseases, like **multiple sclerosis**, and research proceeds on that front. Approaches to cancer treatment also involve the immune system. Some researchers, including Burnet, speculate that a failure of the immune system may be implicated in **cancer**. In the late 1960s Ion Gresser (1928-) discovered that the protein **interferon** acts against cancerous tumors. After the development of genetically engineered interferon in the mid-1980s finally made the substance available in practical amounts, research into its use against cancer accelerated. The invention of monoclonal antibodies in the mid-1970s was a major breakthrough. Increasingly sophisticated knowledge about the workings of the immune system holds out the hope of finding an effective method to combat one of the most serious immune system disorders, **AIDS**.

Avenues of research to treat AIDS includes a focus on supporting and strengthening the immune system. (However, much research has to be done in this area to determine whether strengthening the immune system is beneficial or whether it may cause an increase in the number of infected cells.) One area of interest is cytokines, proteins produced by the body that help the immune system cells communicate with each other and activate them to fight infection. Some individuals infected with the AIDS virus HIV (human immunodeficiency virus) have higher levels of certain cytokines and lower levels of others. A possible approach to controlling infection would be to boost deficient levels of cytokines while depressing levels of cytokines that may be too abundant. Other research has found that HIV may also turn the immune system against itself by producing antibodies against its own cells.

For many years it was believed that the immune system responded only to invading antigens and was not influenced by psychological events. However, building on research that began in the mid-1960s, scientists have determined that the immune system is also affected by a person's psychological health, or state of mind. This branch of research is referred to as pscyhoimmunology, or psychoneuroimmunology (the study of the relationship among psychology, neurology, and immunology). A complex network of nerves, hormones, and neuropeptides appear to link the immune system and an individual's psyche. For example, extreme psychological stress has been shown to suppress the immune system and accelerate disease in people with HIV. (Short-term stress is believed to have certain benefits to the body.) Other psychosocial factors—such as a fixation on dying, clinical depression, a lack of purpose in life, inability to be assertive, and lack of a supportive network of friends and family—may also affect the immune system. Research into pscyhoimmunology focuses on treatments that can impact stress levels and other psychological factors.

Advances in immunological research indicate that the immune system may be made of more than 100 million highly specialized cells designed to combat specific antigens. While the task of identifying these cells and their functions may be daunting, headway is being made. By identifying these specific cells, researchers may be able to further advance another promising area of immunological research—the use of recombinant DNA technology, in which specific proteins can be mass produced. This approach has led to new cancer treatments that can stimulate the immune system by using synthetic versions of proteins released by interferons.

IMMUNODEFICIENCY

In immunodeficiency disorders, part of the body's **immune system** is missing or defective, thus impairing the body's ability to fight infections. As a result, the person with an immunodeficiency disorder will have frequent infections that are generally more severe and last longer than usual.

The immune system is the body's main system to fight infections. The normal immune system involves a complex interaction of certain types of cells that can recognize and attack "foreign" invaders, such as bacteria, viruses, and fungi. It also plays a role in fighting **cancer**. People are born with certain parts of the immune system; such parts are called innate immunity. Other parts of the immune system people develop over time, which is called adaptive immunity.

The innate immune system is made up of the skin (which acts as a barrier to prevent organisms from entering the body), white blood cells called phagocytes, a system of proteins called the complement system, and chemicals called interferon. When phagocytes encounter an invading organism, they surround and engulf it to destroy it. The complement system also attacks bacteria. The elements in the complement system create a hole in the bacterium's outer layer of the target cell, which leads to its death.

The adaptive component of the immune system is extremely complex and still not entirely understood. Basically, it has the ability to recognize an organism or tumor cell as not being a normal part of the body, and to develop a response to attempt to eliminate it.

Defects can occur in any component of the immune system or in more than one component (combined immunodeficiency). Different immunodeficiency diseases involve different components of the immune system. The defects can be inherited and/or present at birth (congenital) or acquired.

Congenital immunodeficiency is present at birth, and is the result of genetic defects. Even though more than 70 different types of congenital immunodeficiency disorders have been identified, they rarely occur.

Disorders of innate immunity affect phagocytes or the complement system. These disorders also result in recurrent infections.

Acquired immunodeficiency is more common than congenital immunodeficiency. It is the result of an infectious process or other disease. For example, the human immunodeficiency virus (HIV) is the virus that causes acquired immunodeficiency syndrome (**AIDS**). However, this is not the most common cause of acquired immunodeficiency.

Acquired immunodeficiency often occurs as a complication of other conditions and diseases. For example, the most common causes of acquired immunodeficiency are malnutrition, some types of cancer, and infections. People who weigh less than 70% of the average weight of persons of the same age and gender are considered to be malnourished. Examples of infections that can lead to immunodeficiency are **chicken pox**, German measles, **measles**, **tuberculosis**, chronic **hepatitis**, lupus, and bacterial and fungal infections.

Sometimes, acquired immunodeficiency is brought on by drugs used to treat another condition. For example, patients who have an **organ transplant** are given drugs to suppress the immune system so the body will not reject the organ. During the period of time that these drugs are being taken, the risk of infection increases. It usually returns to normal after the person stops taking the drugs.

People with an immunodeficiency disorder tend to become infected by organisms that don't usually cause disease in healthy persons. The major symptoms of most immunodeficiency disorders are repeated infections that heal slowly. These chronic infections cause symptoms that persist for long periods of time. People with chronic infection tend to be pale and thin. They may have skin rashes. Broken blood vessels, especially near the surface of the skin, may be visible, resulting in black-and-blue marks in the skin.

There is no cure for immunodeficiency disorders. Therapy is aimed at controlling infections and, for some disorders, replacing defective or absent components.

Common variable immunodeficiency also is treated with periodic injections of gamma globulin throughout life. Additionally, **antibiotics** are given when necessary to treat infections.

In most cases, immunodeficiency caused by **malnutrition** is reversible. The health of the immune system is directly linked to the nutritional health of the patient. Among the essential nutrients required by the immune system are proteins, **vitamins**, iron, and zinc.

For people being treated for cancer, periodic relief from **chemotherapy** drugs can restore the function of the immune system.

In general, people with immunodeficiency disorders should maintain a healthy diet because malnutrition can aggravate immunodeficiencies. They should also avoid being near people who have colds or are sick because they can easily acquire new infections. For the same reason, they should practice good **personal hygiene**, especially dental care. People with immunodeficiency disorders should also avoid eating undercooked food because it might contain bacteria that could cause infection. This food would not cause infection in normal persons, but in someone with an immunodeficiency, food is a potential source of infectious organisms. People with immunodeficiency should be given antibiotics at the first indication of an infection.

There is no way to prevent a congenital immunodeficiency disorder. However, someone with a congenital immunodeficiency disorder might want to consider getting genetic counseling before having children to find out if there is a chance they will pass the defect on to their children.

Some of the infections associated with acquired immunodeficiency can be prevented or treated before they cause problems. For example, there are effective treatments for tuberculosis and most bacterial and fungal infections. HIV infection can be prevented by practicing ''safe sex'' and not using illegal intravenous drugs. These are the primary routes of transmitting the virus. For people who don't know the HIV status of the person with whom they are having sex, safe sex involves using a **condom**.

IMMUNOGLOBULIN DEFICIENCY SYNDROMES

Immunoglobulin deficiency syndromes are a group of **immunodeficiency** disorders in which the patient has reduced number of or lack of antibodies.

Immunoglobulins (Ig) are antibodies. There are five major classes of antibodies: IgG, IgM, IgA, IgD, and IgE.

- IgG is the most abundant of the classes of immunoglobulins. It is the antibody for viruses, bacteria, and antitoxins. It is found in most tissues and plasma.
- IgM is the first antibody present in an immune response.
- IgA is an early antibody for bacteria and viruses. It is found in saliva, tears, and all other mucous secretions.
- IgD's activity is unknown.
- IgE is present in the respiratory secretions. It is an antibody for parasitic diseases, hay fever, and allergic asthma.

All antibodies are made by B-cells. Any disease that harms the development or function of these cells will cause a decrease in the amount of antibodies produced. Since antibodies are essential in fighting infectious diseases, people with immunoglobulin deficiency syndromes become ill more often. However, the cellular **immune system** is still functional, so these patients are more prone to infection caused by organisms usually controlled by antibodies.

There are two types of immunodeficiency diseases: primary and secondary. Secondary disorders occur in normally healthy bodies that are suffering from an underlying disease. Once the disease is treated, the immunodeficiency is reversed. Immunoglobulin deficiency syndromes are primary immunodeficiency diseases, occurring because of defective B lymphocytes or antibodies. They account for 50% of all primary immunodeficiencies, and they are, therefore, the most prevalent type of immunodeficiency disorders.

Immunoglobulin deficiencies are the result of congenital defects affecting the development and function of B lymphocytes (B-cells). There are two main points in the development of B-cells when defects can occur. First, B-cells can fail to develop into antibody-producing cells. Second, B-cells can fail to make a particular type of antibody or fail to switch classes during maturation. Initially, when B-cells start making antibodies for the first time, they make IgM. As they mature and develop memory, they switch to one of the other four classes of antibodies. Failures in switching or failure to make a subclass of antibody leads to immunoglobulin deficiency diseases.

Symptoms are persistent and frequent infections, **diarrhea**, **failure to thrive**, and **malabsorption** (of nutrients).

An immunodeficiency disease is suspected when children become ill frequently, especially from the same organisms. Laboratory tests are performed to verify the diagnosis. Antibodies can be found in the blood. Depending on the type of immunoglobulin deficiency the laboratory tests will show a decrease or absence of antibodies or specific antibody subclasses.

Immunodeficiency diseases can not be cured. Patients are treated with antibiotics and immune serum. Immune serum is a source of antibodies. Antibiotics are useful for fighting bacteria infections. There are some drugs that are effective against fungi, but very few drugs that are effective against viral diseases.

Bone marrow transplantation can, in most cases, completely correct the immunodefiency.

Patients with immunoglobulin defiency syndromes must practice impeccable health maintenance and care, paying particular attention to optimal dental care, in order to stay in good health.

IMMUNOLOGIC THERAPIES

Immunologic therapy is the treatment of disease using medicines that boost the body's natural immune response.

It is used to improve the **immune system**'s natural ability to fight diseases such as **cancer**, **hepatitis**, and **AIDS**. These drugs also may be used to help the body recover from the harmful side effects of treatments such as **chemotherapy**.

Most drugs in this category are manufactured versions of substances the body produces naturally. In their natural forms, these substances help defend the body against disease. For example, aldesleukin (Proleukin) is an artificially made form of interleukin-2, which helps white blood cells work. Another type of drug, epoetin (Epogen, Procrit), stimulates the bone marrow to make new red blood cells. It is an artificially made version of human erythropoietin, which is made naturally in the body and has the same effect on bone marrow.

Most of these drugs come in an injectable form, and the recommended dosage depends on the type of immunologic therapy. For some medicines, the physician will decide the dosage for each patient, taking into account the patient's weight and whether he or she is taking other medicines. Some drugs used in immunologic therapy are given only in a hospital, under a physician's supervision. Some, the patients may give themselves under the guidance of a doctor or pharmacist.

IMMUNOSUPPRESSANT DRUGS

Immunosuppressant drugs are medicines that reduce the body's natural defenses against foreign invaders or materials. Used in transplant patients, these drugs help prevent their bodies from rejecting transplanted organs.

When an organ, such as a liver, a heart or a kidney, is transplanted from one person (the donor) into another (the recipient), the recipient's **immune system** has the same response it has to any foreign material: It attacks and tries to destroy the organ. Immunosuppressant drugs help prevent this from happening by subduing the natural immune response. However, the drugs' action also makes the body more vulnerable to infection. For that reason, people who take these kinds of medicine need to be especially careful to avoid infections.

In addition to being used to prevent organ rejection, immunosuppressant drugs sometimes are used to treat severe skin disorders such as **psoriasis** and other diseases such as **rheumatoid arthritis**, Crohn's disease (chronic inflammation of the digestive tract) and patchy hair loss (alopecia areata).

Immunosuppressant drugs are available only with a physician's prescription and come in tablet, capsule, liquid and injectable forms. Commonly used immunosuppressant drugs include azathioprine (Imuran), cyclosporine (Sandimmune) and tacrolimus (Prograf).

The physician will decide exactly how much of the medicine each patient needs. It is vital that the patient take this medicine exactly as directed. Never take smaller, larger or more frequent doses, and do not take the drug for longer than directed. Taking too much may increase the risk of side effects, while taking too little may not do any good. Nor should a patient stop taking the drug without checking with the physician who prescribed it.

Seeing a physician regularly while taking immunosuppressant drugs is important. These regular check-ups will allow the physician to make sure the medicine is working as it should and to watch for unwanted effects. These medicines are very powerful and can cause serious side effects, such as high blood pressure, kidney problems and liver problems. Some side effects may not show up until years after the medicine is used. However, the good these drugs can do may outweigh the possible harm. Anyone who has been advised to take immunosuppressant drugs should thoroughly discuss the risks and benefits with his or her physician

Immunosuppressant drugs lower a person's resistance to infection and can make infections harder to treat. The drugs can also increase the chance of uncontrolled bleeding. Anyone who has a serious infection or injury while taking immunosuppressant drugs should get prompt medical attention and should make sure that the physician in charge knows about the medicine.

Immunosuppressant drugs may cause the gums to become tender and swollen or to bleed. If this happens, check with a physician or dentist right away. Regular brushing, flossing, cleaning and gum massage may help prevent this problem. Ask the dentist for advice on how to clean the teeth and mouth without causing injury.

People who have certain medical conditions or who are taking certain other medicines may have problems if they take immunosuppressant drugs. Before taking these drugs, be sure to let the physician know about **allergies**, whether you are pregnant or on oral birth control pills, or who have **shingles** or **chicken pox**.

Taking immunosuppressant drugs with certain other drugs may affect the way the drugs work or may increase the chance of side effects.

People who take immunosuppressant drugs may be at higher than normal risk of developing certain kinds of **cancer** later in life. However, the drugs may be necessary to prevent the failure of a life-saving transplant. The possible harm must be carefully weighed against the drugs' benefits. Discussing the medicine's good and bad points with a physician will help a patient decide about whether to take immunosuppressant drugs.

Some side effects of immunosuppressant drugs are minor and usually go away as the body adjusts to the medicine. These include loss of appetite, **nausea or vomiting**, increased hair growth, and trembling or shaking of the hands. Medical attention is not necessary unless these side effects continue or cause problems.

The risk of cancer or infection may be greater when immunosuppressant drugs are combined with certain other drugs which also lower the body's ability to fight disease and infection. Anyone who takes immunosuppressant drugs should let the physician know all other medicines he or she is taking and should ask whether the possible interactions can interfere with treatment.

IMPETIGO

Impetigo refers to a very localized bacterial infection of the skin. It tends to afflict primarily children. Impetigo caused by the bacteria *Staphylococcus aureus* (or staph) affects children of all ages, while impetigo caused by the bacteria called group A. streptococci (or strep) are most common in children ages two to five.

The bacteria that cause impetigo are very contagious. They can be spread by scratching, or contact with a towel, clothing, or stuffed animal.

Impetigo tends to develop in areas of the skin that have already been damaged through some other mechanism (a cut, scrape, **burn**, insect **bite**, or pock from **chicken pox**).

There are two types of impetigo, bullous and **epidemic**. The first sign of bullous impetigo is a large bump on the skin, with a clear, fluid-filled top (called a vesicle). The bump develops a scab-like, honey-colored crust. There is usually no redness or pain, although the area may be quite itchy. Ultimately, the skin in this area will become dry, and flake away. Bullous impetigo is usually caused by staph bacteria.

Epidemic impetigo can be caused by staph or strep bacteria, and (as the name implies) is very easily passed between children. Certain factors, such as heat and humidity, crowded conditions, and poor hygiene increase the chance that this type of impetigo will spread rapidly among large groups of children. Epidemic impetigo involves the formation of a small vesicle surrounded by a circle of reddened skin. The vesicles appear first on the face and legs. When a child has several of these vesicles close together, they may spread to each other. The skin surface may become eaten away (ulcerated), leaving irritated pits. When there are many of these deep, pitting ulcers, with pus in the center and brownish-black scabs, the condition is called ecthyma. If left untreated, the type of bacteria causing this type of impetigo has the potential to cause a serious kidney disease. Even when impetigo is initially caused by strep bacteria, the vesicles are frequently secondarily infected with staph bacteria.

Impetigo is usually an uncomplicated skin condition. Left untreated, however, there is a chance of developing a serious disease, including bone infection, joint infection, or **pneumonia**. If large quantities of bacteria are present and begin circulating in the bloodstream, the child is in danger of developing an overwhelming systemic infection known as **sepsis**.

Characteristic appearance of the skin is the usual method of diagnosis, although fluid from the vesicles can be cultured and then examined in an attempt to identify the causative bacteria.

Uncomplicated impetigo is usually treated with a topical antibiotic cream called mupirocin. In more serious, widespread cases of impetigo, or when the child has a fever or swollen glands, oral or intravenous **antibiotics** may be given. The vast majority of children recover quickly, completely, and uneventfully.

Prevention involves good hygiene. Handwashing, never sharing towels, clothing, or stuffed animals, and keeping fingernails well-trimmed are easy precautions to take to avoid spreading the infection from one person to another.

IMPOTENCE

Impotence, or erectile dysfunction, is the inability to achieve or maintain an erection long enough to engage in sexual intercourse.

Under normal circumstances, when a man is sexually stimulated, his brain sends a message down the spinal cord and into the nerves of the penis. The nerve endings in the penis release chemical messengers, called neurotransmitters, which signal the corpora cavernosa (the two spongy rods of tissue that run the length of the penis) to relax and fill with blood. As they expand, the corpora cavernosa close off other veins that would normally drain blood from the penis. As the penis becomes engorged with blood, it enlarges and stiffens, causing an erection. Problems with blood vessels, nerves, or tissues of the penis can interfere with an erection.

It is estimated that 10-20 million American men frequently suffer from impotence and that it strikes up to half of all men between the ages of 40 and 70. Doctors used to think that most cases of impotence were psychological in origin, but they now recognize that, at least in older men, physical causes may play a primary role in 60% or more of all cases. In men over 60, the leading cause is **atherosclerosis**, or narrowing of the arteries, which can restrict the flow of blood to the penis. Injury or disease of the connective tissue, such as may prevent the corpora cavernosa from completely expanding, and damage to the nerves of the penis, from certain types of surgery or neurological conditions such as **Parkinson's disease** may also cause impotence. Men with diabetes are especially at risk for impotence because of their high risk of both atherosclerosis and a nerve disease called diabetic neuropathy.

Some drugs, including certain types of blood pressure medications, **antihistamines**, tranquilizers, and **antidepressants** can interfere with erections. **Smoking**, excessive alcohol consumption, and illicit drug use may also contribute. In rare cases, low levels of the male hormone testosterone may contribute to erectile failure. Finally, psychological factors, such as **stress**, guilt, or **anxiety**, may also play a role, even when the impotence is primarily due to organic causes.

Years ago, the standard treatment for impotence was an implantable penile prosthesis or long-term psychotherapy. Although physical causes are now more readily diagnosed and treated, individual or marital **counseling** is still an effective treatment for impotence when emotional factors play a role.

Injection therapy involves injecting a substance into the penis to enhance blood flow and cause an erection. The **Food and Drug Administration** (FDA) approved a drug called alprostadil (Caverject) for this purpose in July of 1995. Alprostadil, which relaxes smooth muscle tissue to enhance blood flow into the penis, must be injected shortly before intercourse. Another, similar drug that is sometimes used is papaverine, which has not yet been approved by the FDA for this use.

In a long-awaited breakthrough, a pill for combating impotence was cleared for marketing by the FDA in March 1998. Called sildenafil citrate (brand name Viagra), the drug boosts levels of a substance called cyclic GMP, which is responsible for widening the blood vessels of the penis. Viagra has been shown to be effective in about 70-80% of men who take it, and it can even work in men with some psychological component to their impotence. Unlike drugs that are injected into the penis, Viagra causes an erection only when the man is sexually aroused.

Implantable **penile prostheses** are usually considered a last resort for treating impotence. They are implanted in the corpora cavernosa to make the penis rigid without the need for blood flow. The semirigid type of prosthesis consists of a pair of flexible silicone rods that can be bent up or down. This type of device has a low failure rate but, unfortunately, it causes the penis to always be erect, which can be difficult to conceal under clothing.

The inflatable type of device consists of cylinders that are implanted in the corpora cavernosa, a fluid reservoir implanted in the abdomen, and a pump placed in the scrotum. The man squeezes the pump to move fluid into the cylinders and cause them to become rigid. (He reverses the process by squeezing the pump again.) While these devices allow for intermittent erections, they have a slightly higher malfunction rate than the silicon rods.

Men can return to sexual activity six to eight weeks after implantation surgery. Since implants affect the corpora cavernosa, they permanently take away a man's ability to have a natural erection.

A number of herbs have been promoted for treating impotence. The most widely touted herbs for this purpose are *Coryanthe yohimbe* (available by prescription as yohimbine, with the trade name Yocon) and gingko (*Gingko biloba*), although neither has been conclusively shown to help the condition in controlled studies. In addition, gingko carries some risk of abnormal blood clotting and should be avoided by men taking blood thinners such as coumadin.

There is no specific treatment to prevent impotence. Perhaps the most important measure is to maintain general good health and avoid atherosclerosis—by exercising regularly, controlling weight, controlling **hypertension** and high cholesterol levels, and avoiding smoking. Avoiding excessive alcohol intake may also help.

INCEST

There are two basic definitions of incest, psychological and legal. From a psychological perspective, incest is any overtly sexual contact between people who are either closely related or perceive themselves to be closely related. Legally, incest is prohibited sexual relations between members of the same kinship group. Incest is almost universally forbidden between unmarried members of the same family (between siblings or between parents and children). In many cultures the definition of incest includes other relatives, such as sexual contact between uncles or aunts and nieces or nephews, or between first cousins.

Most social scientists believe that the primary purpose of the prohibition, often called the incest taboo, is to protect the nuclear family from the consequences of sexual rivalry and jealousy. The taboo is linked with the rule of exogamy (marriage outside of one's kinship group, usually for the purpose of social alliance between groups). Besides reinforcing the incest prohibition, this rule prevents families from becoming culturally ingrown through continuous endogamy (marriage within a kinship group). Highly inbred populations have diminished reproductive capacity and have higher risks for hereditary disorders. Marriage to relatives outside the nuclear family is common in a number of cultures, however, and it is no longer widely believed that the incest taboo serves principally to guard against inbreeding as a negative biological result of incest.

Another theory, emphasizing socialization, argues that the incest taboo is an important method of regulating the erotic impulse in children, preparing them to function with mature restraint in adult society. The psychoanalytic explanation of **Sigmund Freud** speculated that the horror of incest resulted from the combination of ambivalent emotions toward one's immediate family, and repressed forbidden desires to commit sexual acts with family members.

The question has also been raised whether various categories of incest exist, suggesting that brother-sister, mother-son, and father-daughter sexual unions might be better understood as theoretically distinct.

Some societies permit exceptions to the incest prohibition for cultural reasons. Such exceptions have included the mandatory marital union of royal siblings in ancient Egypt, among the Inca, and in traditional Hawaiian society. Unsanctioned violations occur with varying frequency in all societies, with varying degrees of repercussion. As the immediacy of biological relationship decreases, sanctions against sexual intimacy may be relaxed or disappear.

However, incest in the form of **child abuse** is a major social concern worldwide. In the United States, every state has a statute punishing incest. In those states that have recodified laws dealing with sexual behavior, the victim must be a minor. Incest in which the victim is an adult reportedly occurs extremely rarely.

Retrospective case studies list many incest-promoting factors in modern society: a failure to desexualize family affection; family isolation; ignorance of incest prohibitions; family disintegration; **substance abuse**; unemployment; physical contiguity (sleeping in the same bed); and psychiatric problems such as pedophilia, retardation, and psychotic illness.

Aggressors rarely commit acts of incest because of sexual needs. Just as rape is not a sexual act but one of power, control, degradation, and hostility against women, it is known that incest is motivated by similar impulses. It is thought that two powerful forces operate in the majority of aggressors. The first is an almost insatiable need for unconditional love and adoration. Children tend to love totally and unconditionally. This kind of love may prove a powerful aphrodisiac to an individual who suffers from feelings of inadequacy.

Another type of aggressor attempts to overcome feelings of inadequacy by gaining power and control over a helpless child. At the same time, whether the aggressor is pursuing power or validation, he may also be unconsciously seeking revenge against either his wife, his mother, or other women for what he considers a variety of emotional (or perhaps physical) crimes against him.

Since some definitions list only sexual intercourse as behaviors involved in incest, while others include other types of sexual contact, it is difficult to estimate the incidence of incest, however defined. In addition, many victims of incest may fail to report the act, a tendency that incest shares with **rape**. However, various studies place the percentage of incest victims in the general population of America at about 10 to 20 million. Among the reported victims of incest, girls outnumber boys approximately ten to one. It has been estimated that the average age of an incest victim is seven years.

It has been suggested that brother-sister incest occurs far more often than father-daughter, which has been traditionally regarded as the most common form. Research also indicates that incest is somewhat more likely to occur in upper- and middle-class communities.

The impact of incest on the incest victim, especially its long-term effects, is often devastating. The incest victim's need for self-punishment often leads to self-abusive behaviors such as drug abuse, sexual promiscuity, **suicide** attempts, and a variety of other physical and psychological problems.

In social terms, instead of focusing on the psychological damage of incest, modern society tends to dwell on the violation of the taboo because of the tendency to view the act of incest with such horror, disdain, and often disbelief. This preoccupation often causes both victims and perpetrators to be too intimidated by the possibility of exposure to seek treatment, and the cycle is perpetuated.

See also Freud, Sigmund; Rape; Sexual abuse; Suicide

INCONTINENCE

Incontinence is the unintentional passage of urine, stool, or gas through the anus or urinary tract. For some people, incontinence is a relatively minor problem, as when it is limited to a slight occasional soiling of underwear, but for others it involves considerable physical and/or emotional distress.

Approximately 13 million Americans suffer from urinary incontinence. Women are affected by the disorder more frequently than are men; one in 10 women under age 65 suffer from urinary incontinence. Older Americans, too, are more prone to the condition. Twenty percent of Americans over age 65 are incontinent.

Fecal incontinence, also called bowel incontinence, can occur at any age, but is most common among people over the age of 65.

Incontinence sufferers often hesitate to ask their doctors for help because they are embarrassed or ashamed.

Incontinence can result from a wide variety of medical conditions, including **nervous system** problems, **Parkinson's disease**, and bladder dysfunction. **Childbirth** can also lead to incontinence. It can weaken the pelvic muscles and cause the bladder to lose some support from surrounding muscles, resulting in stress incontinence. Vaginal-delivery childbirth can result in damage to the anal sphincter, the ring of muscle that closes the anus. Childbirth-related incontinence is usually restricted to gas, but for some women involves the passing of liquid or solid stools.

Surgery can also result in incontinence. For example, **hysterectomy** or other gynecological surgery can damage or weaken the pelvic muscles that control the flow of urine. The removal of **hemorrhoids** by surgery or other techniques can also cause anal damage and fecal incontinence, as can more complex operations affecting the anus and surrounding areas. Anal and rectal infections as well Crohn's disease can lead to incontinence by damaging the muscles that control defecation. For some people, incontinence becomes a problem when the anal muscles begin to weaken in midlife or old age.

Dementia, **mental retardation**, **strokes**, **brain tumors**, and other conditions that affect the nervous system can cause incontinence by interfering with muscle function or the normal sensations that trigger bladder and bowel control. One study of **multiple sclerosis** patients discovered that about half were incontinent. Nerve damage caused by long-lasting **diabetes mellitus** (diabetic neuropathy) is another condition that can give rise to incontinence.

Medical assessments in cases of incontinence typically involve asking questions about the patient's past and current health. For women who have given birth, a detailed obstetric history is also necessary. A **physical examination** is typically performed, along with specific diagnostic testing to determine the cause of the incontinence. Diagnostic testing may include x rays, **ultrasound**, urine tests, and a physical examination of the pelvis and perianal area.

Incontinence arising from an underlying condition such as diabetic neuropathy can sometimes be helped by treating the underlying condition. When that does not work, or no underlying condition can be discovered, medication may be used, such as loperamide (Imodium), anticholinergics (i.e., propantheline, or Pro-Banthine) and **antispasmodics** (i.e., oxybutynin, or Ditropan). Other **over-the-counter** medications such as pseudoephedrine (i.e., Actifed, Benadryl, Dimetapp) and phenylpropanolamine (i.e., Dexatrim, Acutrim) may be prescribed to tighten the urethral sphincter.

In addition, the doctor may have the incontinent patient establish regularly toileting habits, either by creating a schedule or by using a suppository or **enema** to stimulate defecation at the same time every day or every other day.

Dietary changes and exercises done at home to strengthen the muscles may also help.

Incontinence usually responds well to professional medical treatment, even among elderly and institutionalized patients. If complete control cannot be restored, the impact of incontinence on everyday life can still be lessened considerably in most cases. When incontinence remains a problem despite medical treatment, disposable underwear and other commercial incontinence products are available to make life easier. Doctors and nurses can offer advice on coping with incontinence, and people should never be embarrassed about seeking their assistance. **Counseling** and information are also available from **support groups**.

Independent living

Surveys conducted by the American Association of Retired Persons (AARP) and others indicate that retired people, given the choice, prefer to live in the homes in which they had been living prior to retirement. One's own home tends to represent security and independence to most retired Americans. But because most housing in this country is designed for young, active and mobile people, individuals wishing to live in their own homes upon retiring must, at the very least, be able to drive, shop, cook, and perform household chores. Because most elderly persons lose one or more of these abilities as they grow older, the percentage of elderly persons living alone in the 1990s is currently only about 28% according to the AARP.

Not everyone, however, is in complete agreement about the meaning of living independently. Some elderly persons think living independently means being able to take care of oneself in general or to be able to manage on one's own, while others think living independently means living in one's own home. But mostly everyone agrees that the key to independent living is being able to take care of oneself. Studies have shown that the problems most seniors identify as impediments to living independently are physical health problems, and, to a lesser extent, mental health problems.

In terms of the types of assistance that seniors feel they need to enable them to continue living independently, most seniors point first to financial support, and secondly to transportation assistance. Turning to the need for information, many elderly persons feel they need help with finances, budgeting, and paying bills if they are to continue living independently; they also point to their need for help getting health information. One alternate to living alone that has worked for many retired persons is to move into an independent living retirement community where meals, housekeeping, activities, transportation and security are provided as part of a comprehensive service package. Yet another alternative is homesharing, in which two or more unrelated persons share a house or apartment. Everyone in the homesharing arrangement is free to use the common areas of the house, such as the kitchen and living room. However, each homesharer also has some personal space, usually a bedroom, where he or she can have privacy.

Homesharing has helped elderly people remain independent and at the same time reduce their housing costs. Not surprisingly, weighing the advantages of service-oriented housing or homesharing against the independence offered by a single family home can prove a complicated task for many seniors. Studies have shown that those persons who are most successful in maintaining an independent lifestyle in old age are those who continue to maintain a positive outlook on life, pay close attention to their diets, remain physically active, take precautions to eliminate causes of accidents and prepare for emergencies in the home, keep mentally alert, and plan carefully for their financial needs.

See also Aging; Diets and weight management; Exercise; Nursing homes; Retirement; Medicare and Medicaid

Indigestion

Indigestion, sometimes called dyspepsia, is a general term covering a group of nonspecific symptoms in the digestive tract. It is often described as a feeling of fullness, bloating, **nausea**, heartburn, or gassy discomfort in the chest or abdomen. The symptoms develop during meals or shortly afterward. In most cases, indigestion is a minor problem that often clears up without professional treatment.

Indigestion is a widespread condition, estimated to occur in 25% of the adult population of the United States.

The symptoms associated with indigestion have a variety of possible physical causes, ranging from commonplace food items to serious systemic disorders:

- Diet. Milk, milk products, alcoholic beverages, tea, and coffee cause indigestion in some people because they stimulate the stomach's production of acid.
- Medications. Certain prescription drugs as well as **over-the-counter** medications can irritate the stomach lining. These medications include **aspirin**, **non-steroidal anti-inflammatory drugs**, some **antibiotics**, and **oral contraceptives**.
- Disorders of the pancreas and gallbladder, including inflammation of the gallbladder or pancreas, **cancer** of the pancreas, and
- Intestinal parasites, such as fluke and tapeworm infections, giardiasis, and strongyloidiasis.

- Systemic disorders, including **diabetes**, thyroid disease, collagen vascular disease.
- Cancers of the digestive tract.
- Conditions associated with women's **reproductive system**, including menstrual cramps, **pregnancy**, and **pelvic inflammatory disease**.

Indigestion often accompanies an emotional upset because the part of the **nervous system** involved in the so-called "fight-or-flight" response also affects the digestive tract. Many people in the general population will experience heartburn, "butterflies in the stomach," or stomach cramps when they are in upsetting situations—such as school examinations, arguments with family members, crises in their workplace, and so on. Some people's **digestive systems** appear to react more intensely to emotional stress due to hypersensitive nerve endings in their intestinal tract.

In some cases, the patient's description of the symptoms suggests a specific digestive disorder as the cause of the indigestion. Some doctors classify these cases into three groups:

Esophagitis is an inflammation of the tube that carries food from the throat to the stomach (the esophagus). The tissues of the esophagus can become irritated by the flow (reflux) of stomach acid backward into the lower part of the esophagus. If the patient describes the indigestion in terms of frequent or intense heartburn, the doctor will consider gastroesophageal reflux disease (GERD) as a possible cause. GERD is a common disorder in the general population, affecting about 30% of adults.

Patients who smoke and are over 45 are more likely to have indigestion of the peptic ulcer type. This group also includes people who find that their indigestion is relieved by taking **antacids** or eating a small amount of food.

Most cases of chronic indigestion—as many as 65%—fall into this category. Nonulcer dyspepsia is sometimes called functional dyspepsia because it appears to be related to abnormalities in the way that the stomach empties its contents into the intestine. In some people, the stomach empties either too slowly or too rapidly. In others, the stomach's muscular contractions are irregular and uncoordinated. These disorders of stomach movement (motility) may be caused by hypersensitive nerve endings in the stomach tissues. Patients in this group are likely to be younger than 45 and have a history of taking medications for **anxiety** or depression.

Because indigestion is a nonspecific set of symptoms, patients who feel sick enough to seek medical attention are likely to go to their primary care doctor. The history does not always point to an obvious diagnosis. The doctor can, however, use the process of history-taking to evaluate the patient's mood or emotional state in order to assess the possibility of a psychiatric disturbance. In addition, asking about the location, intensity, timing, and recurrence of the indigestion can help the doctor weigh the different diagnostic possibilities.

Since most cases of indigestion are not caused by serious disorders, many doctors prefer to try medications and other treatment measures before ordering an endoscopy. During this procedure, the doctor uses an endoscope, a slender tube-shaped instrument, to look at the lining of the patient's stomach. If the patient has indigestion of the esophagitis type or nonulcer type, the stomach lining will appear normal. If the patient has PUD, the doctor will be able to see breaks or ulcerated areas in the tissue. He or she may also order other imaging tests, such as ultrasound, or blood tests, especially if the patient is over 45.

Many patients benefit from the doctor's reassurance that they do not have a serious or fatal disorder. Cutting out alcoholic beverages and drinks containing **caffeine** often helps. The patient may also be asked to keep a record of food intake, daily schedule, and symptom severity. Food diaries sometimes reveal psychologic or dietary factors that influence indigestion.

Patients with the esophagitis type of indigestion are often treated with drugs that block the secretion of stomach acid, such as ranitidine (Zantac) and famotidine (Pepcid).

Patients with motility disorders may be given prokinetic drugs, which speed up the emptying of the stomach and increase intestinal motility. They include metoclopramide (Reglan) and cisapride (Propulsid).

Most cases of mild indigestion do not need medical treatment. For patients who consult a doctor and are given an endoscopic examination, 5-15% are diagnosed with GERD and 15-25% with PUD. About 1% of patients who are endoscoped have **stomach cancer**. Most patients with functional dyspepsia do well on medication.

Indigestion can often be prevented by attention to one's diet, general stress level, and ways of managing stress. Specific preventive measures include:

- Quitting **smoking**.
- Cutting down on or eliminating alcohol, tea, or coffee.
- Avoiding fatty and spicy foods.
- Eating slowly and keeping mealtimes relaxed.
- Practicing **yoga** or **meditation**.
- Not taking aspirin or other medications on an empty stomach.
- Keeping one's weight within normal limits.

INDOOR AIR QUALITY

Indoor air quality is an area of increasing concern in the United States. While most people are aware of the threat posed by outdoor air pollution (such as smog), few realize that inside homes, schools and offices one can be exposed to two to five times as many pollutants as outdoors, according to the U.S. Environmental Protection Agency. Indoor air pollution has been ranked as one of the top five environmental risks to public health by the EPA and its Science Advisory Board. In addition, the U.S. Occupational Safety and Health Administration has estimated that 30 percent of Americans who work in nonindustrial buildings are exposed to indoor air pollution.

During the 1970s energy crisis, buildings were designed to be airtight, conserving as much warm air during the winter and cooled air during the summer as was possible. Windows that could not be opened became a common part of building design. Ventilation systems were altered from past practice as well. Rather than drawing in large amounts of fresh air from the outside and put in the effort and expense of heating or cooling it, the new systems drew in relatively little outside air and instead recirculated indoor air. These energy-conserving features became widely used in the designs of office buildings, shopping centers, schools and homes.

It is now clear that such airtight buildings create problems. Because of inadequate ventilation to the outside, the air pollutants inside the buildings are neither diluted or removed. The results can range from nose, eye and throat irritation and aggravation of **asthma** to an increased risk of **lung cancer**.

Where do these pollutants come from?

- Some pollutants come from outside sources. These include pesticides, outdoor pollution, and radon. Radon is a naturally occurring gas that is given off as a byproduct of the decay of the element uranium. Uranium is present is many types of soil and rock, especially phosphate, granite and shale. If rock or exposed soil is present in the basement of a building, radon can leach into the air inside the basement. If inhaled, its radioactive particles can become trapped in lung tissue and lead, possibly, to lung cancer.
- Building materials and furnishings can add to indoor air pollution. Among these products are asbestos-based insulation, carpet adhesives, and furniture or cabinets made from pressed wood that uses certain types of adhesives.
- Combustion sources are also sources of indoor air pollution. These include oil, gas, coal and wood burned for heat or used in cooking, and also tobacco products. As they burn, these materials release carbon monoxide (CO), a colorless and odorless gas that can be fatal in high concentrations. People are often exposed to CO by improperly adjusted gas stoves, cars left idling inside a closed, attached garage, and from tobacco smoke. Tobacco smoke, in addition to carrying CO, carries more than 4,000 substances, of which more than 40 have been known to cause **cancer**.
- Biological sources of indoor air pollution include mold, mildew, fungi and bacteria (which are found in areas with high moisture levels such as bathrooms), dust mites and animal dander.
- Common household products add to the problem of indoor air pollution. Cleaning products and air fresheners, personal care products such as hair sprays, paint strippers and paints, and glues can all linger in the air long after they have been used.

Exposure to small amounts of indoor air pollutants can cause minor irritations, such as dry, scratchy eyes and throats, or **headaches**. However, in large concentrations pollutants can lead to **dizziness**, tiredness, and **nausea**, and **rashes**. Each year there are news reports of buildings being evacuated because of ''sick building syndrome,'' a group of health symptoms listed above that stem from poor air quality inside a building and usually subside after leaving the building. Long-term exposure to some indoor air pollutants can lead to damage of the central **nervous system**, kidneys and liver.

Although anyone can have problems because of indoor air pollution, most susceptible are children, the elderly, and people who have respiratory ailments such as **bronchitis**, asthma or emphysema.

Adequate ventilation goes a long way in eliminating problems with indoor air pollution, as does controlling the humidity in a building. Other steps to take to maintain the quality of air inside your home, office or school include:

- Do not allow anyone to smoke inside the building, whether cigarettes, pipes or cigars.
- Be sure that gas stoves and other gas appliances are properly adjusted and in proper working condition.
- Do not idle your car in the garage.
- Have a professional inspect, clean and tune up home heating systems each year.
- Test your home for radon with a radon test kit, which can be purchased at hardware stores and home centers.
- Regularly clean air conditioners, humidifiers and dehumidifiers to control the growth and spread of mold and milder spores.
- Vacuum often to control pet dander and dust mites (it's best to use a vacuum cleaner equipped with a high-efficiency particulate air filter for the job).
- Keep indoor moisture between 30 and 50 percent to control the growth of mold and mildew.

If you feel consistently better after you leave a certain building, whether your home, school or office, you might have reason to suspect a problem with the air quality.

For more information, you can contact the EPA's Indoor Air Quality Information Clearinghouse, which is available Monday through Friday, 9 a.m. to 5 p.m. Eastern time, at 800-438-4318. Other sources of information include the National Radon Information Hotline (1-800-644-6999) and the National Hispanic Indoor Air Quality Hotline (1-800-725-8312).

INFANT MORTALITY

A statistical term referring to the number of infants per 1,000 births who die before they reach one year of age, infant mortality occurs for many reasons. More than 60% of infant deaths happen in the first month after birth, known formally as the neonatal period, and are most often attributed to premature birth (before the 30th week) or serious **birth defects**.

Infant mortality rates are sometimes used as indicators of a particular area's sociological or economic status. For instance, an industrialized country such as France has a lower infant mortality rate than a less developed country such as Mozambique because there is generally more access to advanced medical technology, adequate **sanitation**, **contraception**, good **nutrition** for prenatal and postnatal care, and other advantages in Europe. Likewise, the rate can highlight discrepancies in the care available to a single country's different racial groups. In the early 1980s in the United States, for instance, more black babies died in infancy than white babies.

In a typical population, the mortality rate is higher among male infants than female infants, mainly because males' birth rate is also higher.

From a global perspective as of 1999, the mortality rate was about 80 infants per 1,000 (8%), whereas in developed countries the rate was below 10 per 1,000 (1%) and in undeveloped nations it neared 200 per 1,000 (20%).

Some of the most common reasons for infant mortality are **low birth weight**, caused by premature birth or any of a variety of problems with the mother's health during pregnancy; **respiratory distress syndrome**, which may involve **atelectasis** (collapsed lung or lungs), hypoxemia (low oxygen), and high carbon dioxide levels; and lack of the essentials of life, i.e., adequate food, warmth, shelter, and water.

Infectious arthritis

Infectious arthritis, which is sometimes called septic arthritis or pyogenic arthritis, is a serious infection of the joints characterized by **pain**, **fever**, occasional chills, inflammation and swelling in one or more joints, and loss of function in the affected joints. It is considered a medical emergency.

Infectious arthritis can occur in any age group, including newborns and children. In adults, it usually affects the wrists or one of the patient's weight-bearing joints—most often the knee—although about 20% of adult patients have symptoms in more than one joint. Multiple joint infection is common in children and typically involves the shoulders, knees, and hips.

Some groups of patients are at greater risk for developing infectious arthritis. These high-risk groups include:

- Patients with chronic **rheumatoid arthritis**.
- Patients with certain systemic infections, including **gonorrhea** and HIV infection. Women and male homosexuals are at greater risk for gonorrheal arthritis than are male heterosexuals.
- Patients with certain types of **cancer**.
- IV drug abusers and alcoholics.
- Patients with artificial (prosthetic) joints.
- Patients with **diabetes**, **sickle-cell anemia**, or **systemic lupus erythematosus** (SLE).
- Patients with recent joint injuries or surgery, or patients receiving medications injected directly into a joint.

In general, infectious arthritis is caused by the spread of a bacterial, viral, or fungal infection through the bloodstream to the joint. The disease agents may enter the joint directly from the outside as a result of an injury or a surgical procedure, or they may be carried to the joint by the blood from infections elsewhere in the body. The specific organisms vary somewhat according to age group. Newborns are most likely to acquire gonococcal infections of the joints from a mother with gonorrhea. Children may also acquire infectious arthritis from a hospital environment, often as a result of catheter placement. The organisms involved are usually either *Haemophilus influenzae* (in children under two years of age) or *Staphylococcus aureus*. In older children or adults, the infectious organisms include *Streptococcus pyogenes* and *Streptococcus viridans* as well as *Staphylococcus aureus*. *Staphylococcus epidermidis* is usually involved in joint infections related to surgery. Sexually active teenagers and adults frequently develop infectious arthritis from *Neisseria gonorrhoeae* infections. Older adults are often vulnerable to joint infections caused by gram-negative bacilli, including *Salmonella* and *Pseudomonas*.

Infectious arthritis often has a sudden onset, but symptoms sometimes develop over a period of three to 14 days. The symptoms include swelling in the infected joint and pain when the joint is moved. Infectious arthritis in the hip may be experienced as pain in the groin area that becomes much worse if the patient tries to walk. In 90% of cases, there is some leakage of tissue fluid into the affected joint. The joint is sore to the touch; it may or may not be warm to the touch, depending on how deep the infection lies within the joint. In most cases the patient will have fever and chills, although the fever may be only low-grade. Children sometimes develop **nausea and vomiting**.

Septic arthritis is considered a medical emergency because of the damage it causes to bone as well as cartilage, and its potential for creating septic shock, which is a potentially fatal condition. *Staphylococcus aureus* is capable of destroying cartilage in one or two days. Destruction of cartilage and bone in turn leads to dislocations of the joints and bones. If the infection is caused by bacteria, it can spread to the blood and surrounding tissues, causing **abscess**es or even blood poisoning. The most common complication of infectious arthritis is osteoarthritis.

The diagnosis of infectious arthritis depends on a combination of laboratory testing with careful history-taking and physical examination of the affected joint. Infectious arthritis can coexist with other forms of arthritis, **gout**, **rheumatic fever**, **Lyme disease**, or other disorders that can cause a combination of joint pain and fever. In some cases, the doctor may consult a specialist in orthopedics or rheumatology to avoid misdiagnosis.

Infectious arthritis requires usually requires several days of treatment in a hospital, with follow-up medication and physical therapy lasting several weeks or months. Because of the possibility of serious damage to the joint or other complications if treatment is delayed, the patient will be started on intravenous **antibiotics** before the specific organism is identified. After the disease organism has been identified, the doctor may give the patient a drug that targets the specific bacterium or virus. Nonsteroidal anti-inflammatory drugs are usually given for viral infections. Intravenous antibiotics are given for about two weeks, or until the inflammation has disappeared. The patient may then be given a two- to four-week course of oral antibiotics.

In some cases, surgery is necessary to drain fluid from the infected joint.

Patients with severe damage to bone or cartilage may need reconstructive surgery, but it cannot be performed until the infection is completely gone.

Infectious arthritis requires careful monitoring while the patient is in the hospital. The doctor will drain the joint on a daily basis and remove a small sample of fluid for culture to check the patient's response to the antibiotic.

About 70% of patients will recover without permanent joint damage. However, many patients will develop osteoarthritis or deformed joints. Children with infected hip joints sometimes suffer damage to the growth plate of the bone. If treatment is delayed, infectious arthritis has a mortality rate between 5% and 30% due to septic **shock** and **respiratory failure**.

Some cases of infectious arthritis are preventable by lifestyle choices. These include avoidance of self-injected drugs; sexual **abstinence** or monogamous relationships; and prompt testing and treatment for suspected cases of gonorrhea.

INFECTION CONTROL

Infection control refers to policies and procedures used to minimize the risk of spreading infections, especially in hospitals and health care facilities.

The purpose of infection control is to reduce the occurrence of infectious diseases. These diseases are usually caused by bacteria or viruses and can be spread by human to human contact, animal to human contact, human contact with an infected surface, airborne transmission through tiny droplets of infectious agents suspended in the air, and, finally, by a common vehicle such as food or water.

Infections obtained in hospitals are also called nosocomial infections. They occur in approximately 5% of all hospital patients. This results in increased time spent in the hospital and, in some cases, **death**. There are many reasons nosocomial infections are common, one of which is that many hospital patients have a weakened **immune system** which makes them more susceptible to infections. This weakened immune system can be caused either by the patient's diseases or by treatments given to the patient. Second, many medical procedures can increase the risk of infection by introducing infectious agents into the patient. Thirdly, many patients are admitted to hospitals because of infectious disease. These infectious agents can then be transferred from patient to patient by hospital workers or visitors.

Infection control has become a formal discipline in the United States since the 1950s, due to the spread of **staphylococcal infections** in hospitals. Because there is both the risk of health care providers acquiring infections themselves, and of them passing infections on to patients, the **Centers for Disease Control** and Prevention have established guidelines for infection control procedures. In addition to **hospitals**, infection control is important in **nursing homes**, clinics, child care centers, and restaurants, as well as in the home.

Due to constant changes in our lifestyles and environments, there are constantly new diseases that people are susceptible to, making protection from the threat of infectious disease urgent. Many new contagious diseases have been identified in the past 30 years, such as **AIDS**, Ebola, and **hantavirus**. Increased travel between continents makes the worldwide spread of disease a bigger concern than it once was. Additionally, many common infectious diseases have become resistant to known treatments.

Because of the overuse of **antibiotics**, many bacteria have developed a resistance to common antibiotics. This means that newer antibiotics must continually be developed in order to treat an infection. However, further resistance seems to come about almost simultaneously. This indicates to many scientists that it might become more and more difficult to treat infectious diseases. The use of antibiotics outside of medicine also contributes to increased antibiotic resistance. One example of this is the use of antibiotics in animal husbandry. These negative trends can only be reversed by establishing a more rational use of antibiotics through treatment guidelines.

The goals of infection control programs are: immunizing against preventable diseases, defining precautions that can prevent exposure to infectious agents, and restricting the exposure of health care workers to an infectious agent. An infection control practitioner is a specially trained professional, often a nurse, who oversees infection control programs.

Commonly recommended precautions to avoid and control the spread of infections include:

- Vaccinate against diseases for which a vaccine is available.
- Wash hands often.
- Cook food thoroughly.
- Use antibiotics only as directed.
- See a doctor for infections that do not heal.
- Avoid areas with a lot of insects.
- Be cautious around unfamiliar animals.
- Do not engage in unprotected sex or in intravenous drug use.
- Inquire about infectious diseases when you travel.

Because of the higher risk of spreading infectious disease in a hospital setting, higher levels of precautions are taken there. Typically, health care workers wear gloves with all patients, since it is difficult to know whether a transmittable disease is present or not. Patients who have a known transmittable infectious disease are isolated to decrease the risk of transmitting the infectious agent to another person. Hospital workers who come in contact with infected patients must wear gloves and gowns to decrease the risk of carrying the infectious agent to other patients. All articles of equipment that are used in an **isolation** room are decontaminated before reuse. Patients who are immunocompromised may be put in protective isolation to decrease the risk of infectious agents being brought into their room. Any hospital worker with infections, including colds, are restricted from that room.

Hospital infections can also be transmitted through the air. Thus care must be taken when handling infected materials so as to decrease the numbers of infectious agents that become airborne. Special care should also taken with hospital ventilation systems to prevent recirculation of contaminated air.

INFECTIOUS MONONUCLEOSIS

Infectious mononucleosis is a contagious illness caused by the Epstein-Barr virus that can affect the liver, lymph nodes, and oral cavity. While mononucleosis is not usually a serious disease, its primary symptoms of fatigue and lack of energy can linger for several months.

Infectious mononucleosis, frequently called ''mono'' or the ''kissing disease,'' is caused by the Epstein-Barr virus (EBV) found in saliva and mucus. The virus affects a type of white blood cell called the B lymphocyte, producing characteristic atypical lymphocytes that may be useful in the diagnosis of the disease.

While anyone, even young children, can develop mononucleosis, it occurs most often in young adults between the ages of 15 and 35 and is especially common in teenagers. The mononucleosis infection rate among college students who have not previously been exposed to EBV has been estimated to be about 15%. In younger children, the illness may not be recognized.

The disease typically runs its course in four to six weeks in people with normally functioning **immune systems**. People with weakened or suppressed immune systems are particularly vulnerable to the potentially serious complications of infectious mononucleosis.

The EBV that causes mononucleosis is related to a group of herpes viruses, including those that cause cold sores and **chicken pox**. Most people are exposed to EBV at some point during their lives. Mononucleosis is most commonly spread by contact with virus-infected saliva through coughing, sneezing, kissing, or sharing drinking glasses or eating utensils.

In addition to general weakness and fatigue, symptoms of mononucleosis may include any or all of the following:

- **Sore throat** and/or swollen tonsils
- **Fever** and chills
- **Nausea and vomiting**, or decreased appetite
- Swollen lymph nodes in the neck and armpits
- **Headaches** or joint **pain**
- Enlarged spleen
- **Jaundice**
- Skin **rash**.

Complications that can occur with mononucleosis include a temporarily enlarged spleen or inflamed liver. In rare instances, the spleen may rupture, producing sharp pain on the left side of the abdomen, a symptom that warrants immediate medical attention. Additional symptoms of a ruptured spleen include light-headedness, rapidly beating heart, and difficulty breathing. Other rare, but potentially life-threatening, complications may involve the heart or brain. The infection may also cause significant destruction of the body's red blood cells or platelets.

Symptoms do not usually appear until four to seven weeks after exposure to EBV. An infected person can be contagious during this incubation time period and for as many as five months after the disappearance of symptoms. Also, the virus will be excreted in the saliva intermittently for the rest of their lives, although the individual will experience no symptoms. Contrary to popular belief, the EBV is not highly contagious. As a result, individuals living in a household or college dormitory with someone who has mononucleosis have a very small risk of being infected unless they have direct contact with the person's saliva.

If symptoms associated with a cold persist longer than two weeks, mononucleosis is a possibility; however, a variety of other conditions can produce similar symptoms. If mononucleosis is suspected, a physician will typically conduct a physical examination, including a ''Monospot'' antibody blood test that can indicate the presence of proteins or antibodies produced in response to infection with the EBV. These antibodies may not be detectable, however, until the second or third weeks of the illness. Occasionally, when this test is inconclusive, other blood tests may be conducted.

The most effective treatment for infectious mononucleosis is rest and a gradual return to regular activities. Individuals with mild cases may not require bed rest but should limit their activities. Any strenuous activity, athletic endeavors, or heavy lifting should be avoided until the symptoms completely subside, since excessive activity may cause the spleen to rupture.

The sore throat and dehydration that usually accompany mononucleosis may be relieved by drinking water and fruit juices. Gargling salt water or taking throat lozenges may also relieve discomfort. In addition, taking **over-the-counter** medications, such as **acetaminophen** or ibuprofen, may relieve symptoms, but **aspirin** should be avoided because mononucleosis has been associated with **Reye's syndrome**, a serious illness aggravated by aspirin.

While **antibiotics** do not affect EBV, the sore throat accompanying mononucleosis can be complicated by a streptococcal infection, which can be treated with antibiotics. Cortisone anti-inflammatory medications are also occasionally prescribed for the treatment of severely swollen tonsils or throat tissues.

While the severity and length of illness varies, most people diagnosed with mononucleosis will be able to return to their normal daily routines within two to three weeks, particularly if they rest during this time period. It may take two to three months before a person's usual energy levels return. One of the most common problems in treating mononucleosis, particularly in teenagers, is that people return to their usual activities too quickly and then experience a relapse of symptoms. Once the disease has completely run its course, the person cannot be re-infected.

Although there is no way to avoid becoming infected with EBV, paying general attention to good hygiene and avoiding sharing beverage glasses or having close contact with people who have mononucleosis or cold symptoms can help prevent infection.

INFERTILITY

Infertility is the failure of a couple to conceive a child after trying to do so for at least one full year. In primary infertility, pregnancy has never occurred. In secondary infertility, one or both members of the couple have previously conceived, but are unable to conceive again after a full year of trying.

Currently, in the United States, about 20% of couples struggle with infertility at any given time. Infertility has increased as a problem over the last 30 years.

Unlike most medical problems, infertility is an issue requiring the careful evaluation of two separate individuals, as well as an evaluation of their interactions with each other. In about 3-4% of couples, no cause for their infertility will be discovered. About 40% of the time, the root of the couple's infertility is due to a problem with the male partner; about 40% of the time, the root of the infertility is due to the female partner; and about 20% of the time, there are fertility problems with both the man and the woman.

Male infertility can be caused problems with the sperm. A semen sample is examined under the microscope for four basic characteristics:

- The number of sperm present in a semen sample (the sperm count). (The normal number of sperm present in one milliliter (ml) of semen is over 20 million. An individual with only 5-20 million sperm per ml of semen is considered subfertile; an individual with less than 5 million sperm per ml of semen is considered infertile.)
- Sperm motility (how well the sperm swim).
- The sperm's physical structure (Not all sperm within a specimen of semen will be perfectly normal. Some may be immature, and some may have abnormalities of the head or tail. A normal semen sample will contain no more than 25% abnormal forms of sperm.)
- Volume of the semen sample (An abnormal amount of semen could affect the ability of the sperm to successfully fertilize an ovum.)

Treatment of male infertility includes addressing known reversible factors first; for example, discontinuing any medication known to have an effect on spermatogenesis or ejaculation, as well as decreasing alcohol intake, and treating thyroid or other endocrine disease. Abnormally large veins in the testicles (varicoceles) can be treated surgically. Testosterone in low doses can improve sperm motility.

The first step in diagnosing a woman's fertility problems is to make sure that she is producing an ovum each month. A woman's morning body temperature is slightly higher around the time of ovulation. A woman can measure and record her temperatures daily and a chart can be drawn to show whether or not ovulation has occurred. Luteinizing hormone (LH) is released just before ovulation. A simple urine test can be done to check if LH has been released around the time that ovulation is expected.

Treatment of ovulatory problems depends on the cause. If a thyroid or pituitary problem is responsible, simply treating that problem can restore fertility. (The thyroid and pituitary glands release hormones that also are involved in regulating a woman's menstrual cycle.) Medication can also be used to stimulate fertility. The most commonly used of these are called Clomid and Pergonal. These drugs increase the risk of multiple births (twins, triplets, etc.).

Pelvic adhesions and endometriosis can cause infertility by preventing the sperm from reaching the egg or interfering with fertilization. However, both these conditions can be treated.

Some couple who are having trouble conceiving turn to assisted reproductive techniques, which include in vitro fertilization (IVF), gamete intrafallopian transfer (GIFT), and zygote intrafallopian tube transfer (ZIFT). These are usually used after other techniques to treat infertility have failed.

In vitro fertilization involves the use of a drug to induce the simultaneous release of many eggs from the female's ovaries, which are retrieved surgically. Meanwhile, several semen samples are obtained from the male partner, and the ova and sperm are then combined in a laboratory, where several of the ova may be fertilized. Cell division is allowed to take place up to the embryo stage. Three or four of the embryos are transferred to the female's uterus, and the wait begins to see if any or all of them implant and result in an actual pregnancy.

GIFT involves retrieval of both multiple ova and semen, and the mechanical placement of both within the female partner's fallopian tubes, where one hopes that fertilization will occur. ZIFT involves the same retrieval of ova and semen, and fertilization and growth in the laboratory up to the zygote stage, at which point the zygotes are placed in the fallopian tubes. Both GIFT and ZIFT seem to have higher success rates than IVF.

In general, it is believed that of all couples who undergo a complete evaluation of infertility followed by treatment, about half will ultimately have a successful pregnancy. Of those couples who do not choose to undergo evaluation or treatment, about 5% will go on to conceive after a year or more of infertility.

INFERTILITY DRUGS

Infertility drugs are medicines that help bring about **pregnancy**.

Infertility is the inability of a man and woman to achieve pregnancy after at least a year of having regular sexual intercourse without any type of birth control. There are many possible reasons for infertility, and finding the most effective treatment for a couple may involve many tests to find the problem. For pregnancy to occur, the woman's **reproductive system** must release eggs regularly—a process called ovulation. The man must produce healthy sperm that are able to reach and unite with an egg. And once an egg is fertilized, it must travel to the woman's uterus (womb), become implanted and remain there to be nourished.

If a couple is infertile because the woman is not ovulating, infertility drugs may be prescribed to stimulate ovulation. The first step usually is to try a drug such as clomiphene. If that doesn't work, human chorionic gonadotropin (HCG) may be tried, usually in combination with other infertility drugs.

Clompiphene and HCG may also be used to treat other conditions in both males and females.

Clomiphene (Clomid, Serophene) comes in tablet form and is available only with a physician's prescription. Human chorionic gonadotropin is given as an injection, only under a physician's supervision.

The dosage may be different for different patients. Check with the physician who prescribed the drug or the pharmacist who filled the prescription for the correct dosage.

Clomiphene must be taken at certain times during the menstrual cycle. Be sure to follow directions exactly.

Seeing a physician regularly while taking infertility drugs is important.

Treatment with infertility drugs increases the chance of multiple births. Although this may seem like a good thing to couples who want children very badly, multiple fetuses can cause problems during pregnancy and delivery and can even threaten the babies' survival.

Having intercourse at the proper time in the woman's menstrual cycle helps increase the chance of pregnancy. The physician may recommend using an ovulation prediction test kit to help determine the best times for intercourse.

Some people feel dizzy or lightheaded, or less alert when using clomiphene. The medicine may also cause blurred vision and other vision changes. Anyone who takes clomiphene should not drive, use machines or do anything else that might be dangerous until they have found out how the drugs affect them.

Questions remain about the safety of long-term treatment with clomiphene. Women should not have more than 6 courses of treatment with this drug and should ask their physicians for the most up-to-date information about its use.

People who have certain medical conditions or who are taking certain other medicines may have problems if they take infertility drugs. Before taking these drugs, be sure to let the physician know about any of these conditions:

Anyone who has had unusual reactions to infertility drugs in the past should let his or her physician know before taking the drugs again. The physician should also be told about any **allergies** to foods, dyes, preservatives, or other substances.

Clomiphene may cause **birth defects** if taken during pregnancy. Women who think they have become pregnant while taking clomiphene should stop taking the medicine immediately and check with their physicians.

Infertility drugs may make some medical conditions worse. Before using infertility drugs, people with any of these medical problems should make sure their physicians are aware of their conditions:

- **Endometriosis**
- Fibroid tumors of the uterus
- Unusual vaginal bleeding
- Ovarian cyst
- Enlarged ovaries
- Inflamed veins caused by blood clots
- Liver disease, now or in the past
- Depression.

Taking infertility drugs with certain other medicines may affect the way the drugs work or may increase the chance of side effects.

When used in low doses for a short time, clomiphene and HCG rarely cause side effects. However, anyone who has stomach or pelvic **pain** or bloating while taking either medicine should check with a physician immediately. Infertility drugs may also cause less serious symptoms such as hot flashes, breast tenderness or swelling, heavy menstrual periods, bleeding between menstrual periods, **nausea or vomiting**, **dizziness**, lightheadedness, irritability, nervousness, restlessness, **headache**, tiredness, sleep problems, or depression. These problems usually go away as the body adjusts to the drug and do not require medical treatment unless they continue or they interfere with normal activities.

Other side effects are possible. Anyone who has unusual symptoms after taking infertility drugs should get in touch with a physician.

Infertility drugs may interact with other medicines. When this happens, the effects of one or both of the drugs may change or the risk of side effects may be greater. Anyone who takes infertility drugs should let the physician know all other medicines she is taking.

INFERTILITY THERAPIES

Infertility is the inability of a man and a woman to conceive a child through sexual intercourse. There are many possible reasons for the problem, which can involve the man, the woman, or both. Various treatments are available that enable a woman to become pregnant; the correct one will depend on the specific cause of the infertility.

Infertility treatment is aimed at enabling a woman to have a baby by treating the man, the woman, or both partners. During normal conception of a child, the man's sperm will travel to the woman's fallopian tubes, where, if conditions are right, it will encounter an egg that has been released from the ovary. The sperm will fertilize the egg, which will enter the uterus where it implants and begins to divide, forming what's called an embryo. The embryo will develop during **pregnancy** into a baby.

Infertility treatment attempts to correct or compensate for any abnormalities in this process that prevent the fertilization of an egg or development of an embryo.

It's important for a couple contemplating infertility treatment to examine their own ideas and feelings about the process and consider ethical objections before the woman becomes pregnant from such treatment.

About 90% of women who are trying to get pregnant and use no birth control will do so within one year. If, after one year of having frequent sexual intercourse with no **contraception** a couple has not conceived, they should seek the advice of a physician. Tests can be performed to look for possible infertility problems.

Treating an underlying infection or illness is the first step in infertility treatment. The physician may also suggest improving general health, dietary changes, reducing **stress**, and **counseling**.

The most common cause of male infertility is failure to produce enough healthy sperm. For fertilization to happen, the number of sperm cells in the man's semen (the fluid ejected during sexual intercourse) must be sufficient, and the sperm cells must have the right shape, appearance, and activity (motility).

Defects in the sperm can be caused by an infection resulting from a **sexually transmitted disease**, a blockage caused by a varicose vein in the scrotum (varicocele), an endocrine imbalance, or problems with other male reproductive organs (such as the testicles, prostate gland, or seminal vesicles).

If a low sperm count is the problem, it's possible to restore fertility by:

- Treating underlying infections.
- Timing sex to coincide with the time the woman is ovulating, which means that the egg is released from the ovary and is beginning to travel down the fallopian tube (the site of fertilization).
- Having sex less often to build up the number of sperm in the semen.

- Treating any endocrine imbalance with drugs.
- Having a surgical procedure to remove a varicocele (varicocelectomy).

If infertility is due to a woman's failure to release eggs from the ovary (ovulate), fertility drugs can help bring hormone levels into balance, stimulating the ovaries and triggering egg production.

In some women, infertility is due to blocked fallopian tubes. The egg is released from the ovary, but the sperm is prevented from reaching it because of a physical obstruction in the fallopian tube. If this is the case, surgery may help repair the damage. Microsurgery can sometimes repair the damage to scarred fallopian tubes if it is not too severe. Not all tube damage can be repaired, however, and most tubal problems are more successfully treated with in vitro fertilization.

Fibroid tumors in the uterus also may cause infertility, and they can be surgically treated. **Endometriosis**, a condition in which parts of the lining of the uterus become imbedded on other internal organs (such as the ovaries or fallopian tubes) may contribute to infertility. It may be necessary to surgically remove the endometrial tissue to improve fertility.

Artificial insemination may be tried if sperm count is low, the man is impotent, or the woman's vagina creates a hostile environment for the sperm. The procedure is not always successful. In this procedure, the semen is collected and placed into the woman's cervix with a small syringe at the time of ovulation. From the cervix, it can travel to the fallopian tube where fertilization takes place. If the partner's sperm count is low, it can be mixed with donor sperm before being transferred into the uterus.

If there is no sperm in the male partner's semen, then artificial insemination can be performed using a donor's sperm obtained from a sperm bank.

Some fertility treatments require removal of the eggs and/or sperm and manipulation of them in certain ways in a laboratory to assist fertilization. These techniques are called assisted reproductive technologies.

When infertility can't be treated by other means or when the cause is not known, it's still possible to become pregnant through in vitro fertilization (IVF), a costly, complex procedure that achieves pregnancy 20% of the time.

In this procedure, a woman's eggs are removed by withdrawing them with a special needle. Attempts are then made to fertilize the eggs with sperm from her partner or a donor. This fertilization takes place in a petri dish in a laboratory. The fertilized egg (embryo) is then returned to the woman's uterus.

Often, three to six fertilized eggs are returned at the same time into the uterus. Usually one or two of the embryos survive and grow into fetuses, but sometimes three or more fetuses result.

A child born in this method is popularly known as a "test tube baby," but in fact the child actually develops inside the mother. Only the fertilization of the egg takes place in the laboratory.

In a variation of IVF called intracytoplasmic sperm injection (ICSI), single sperm cells are injected directly into each egg. This may be helpful for men with severe infertility.

In this technique, sperm and eggs are placed directly into the woman's fallopian tubes to encourage fertilization to occur naturally. This procedure is done with the help of **laparoscopy**. In laparoscopy, a small tube with a viewing lens at one end is inserted into the abdomen through a small incision. The lens allows the physician to see inside the patient on a video monitor.

If infertility is caused by a low sperm count, zygote intrafallopian transfer (ZIFT) can be tried. This technique combines GIFT and IVF. This procedure is also called a "tubal embryo transfer."

In this technique, in-vitro fertilization is first performed, so that the actual fertilization takes place and is confirmed in the laboratory. Two days later, instead of placing the embryo in the uterus, the physician performs laparoscopy to place the embryos in the fallopian tube, much like the GIFT procedure.

A woman must have at least one functioning fallopian tube in order to participate in ZIFT.

Couples who are having fertility problems may want to limit or avoid:

- Tobacco
- Alcohol
- **Caffeine**
- Stress
- Tight-fitting undershorts (men)
- Hot tubs, saunas and steam rooms (high temperatures can kill sperm).

Women who take fertility drugs have a higher likelihood of getting pregnant with more than one child at once. There are also rare but serious side effects to fertility drugs.

INFLAMMATORY BOWEL DISEASE

Inflammatory bowel disease (IBD), the major example of which is Crohn's disease, involves inflammation of the intestine, especially the small intestine. Inflammation refers to swelling, redness, and loss of normal function. There is evidence that the inflammation is caused by various products of the immune system, which attack the body itself instead of helpfully attacking a foreign invader (a virus or bacteria, for example). The inflammation of Crohn's disease most commonly affects the last part of the ileum (a section of the small intestine), and often includes the large intestine (the colon). However, inflammation may also occur in other areas of the gastrointestinal tract, affecting the mouth, esophagus, or stomach. Crohn's disease differs from ulcerative colitis, the other major type of IBD, in two important ways:

- The inflammation of Crohn's disease may be discontinuous, meaning that areas of involvement in the intestine may be separated by normal, unaffected segments of intestine. The affected areas are called "regional enteritis," while the normal areas are called "skip areas."
- The inflammation of Crohn's disease affects all the layers of the intestinal wall, while ulcerative colitis affects only the lining of the intestine.

Also, ulcerative colitis does not usually involve the small intestine; in rare cases it involves the terminal ileum (so-called "backwash" ileitis).

In addition to inflammation, Crohn's disease causes ulcerations, or irritated pits in the intestinal wall. These pits occur because the inflammation has made areas of tissue shed.

Crohn's disease may be diagnosed at any age, although most diagnoses are made between the ages 15-35. About .02-.04% of the population suffers from this disorder, with men and women having an equal chance of being stricken. Whites are more frequently affected than other racial groups, and people of Jewish origin are between three and six times more likely to suffer from IBD. IBD runs in families; an IBD patient has a 20% chance of having other relatives who are fellow sufferers.

The cause of Crohn's disease is unknown. No infectious agent (virus, bacteria, or fungi) has been identified as the cause of Crohn's disease. Still, some researchers have theorized that some type of infection may have originally been responsible for triggering the **immune system**, resulting in the continuing and out-of-control cycle of inflammation that occurs in Crohn's disease. Other evidence for a disorder of the immune system includes the high incidence of other immune disorders that may occur along with Crohn's disease.

The first symptoms of Crohn's disease include **diarrhea**, **fever**, abdominal **pain**, inability to eat, weight loss, and fatigue. Some patients have severe pain that mimics **appendicitis**. It is rare, however, for patients to notice blood in their bowel movements. Because Crohn's disease severely limits the ability of the affected intestine to absorb the nutrients from food, a patient with Crohn's disease can have signs of **malnutrition**, depending on the amount of intestine affected and the duration of the disease.

The combination of severe inflammation, ulceration, and scarring that occurs in Crohn's disease can result in serious complications, including obstruction, **abscess** formation, and fistula formation.

An obstruction is a blockage in the intestine. This obstruction prevents the intestinal contents from passing beyond the point of the blockage. The intestinal contents ''back up,'' resulting in **constipation**, vomiting, and intense pain. Although rare in Crohn's disease (because of the increased thickness of the intestinal wall due to swelling and scarring), a severe bowel obstruction can result in an intestinal wall perforation (a hole in the intestine). Such a hole in the intestinal wall would allow the intestinal contents, usually containing bacteria, to enter the abdomen. This complication could result in a severe, life-threatening infection.

Abcess formation is the development of a walled-off pocket of infection. A patient with an abscess will have bouts of fever, increased abdominal pain, and may have a lump or mass that can be felt through the wall of the abdomen.

Fistula formation is the formation of abnormal channels. These channels may connect one area of the intestine to another neighboring section of intestine. Fistuals may join an area of the intestine to the vagina or bladder, or they may drain an area of the intestine through the skin. Abscesses and fistulas commonly affect the area around the anus and rectum (the very last portions of the colon allowing waste to leave the body). These abnormal connections allow the bacteria that normally live in the intestine to enter other areas of the body, causing potentially serious infections.

Patients suffering from Crohn's disease also have a significant chance of experiencing other disorders. Some of these may relate specifically to the intestinal disease, and others appear to have some relationship to the imbalanced immune system. The faulty absorption state of the bowel can result in gallstones and **kidney stones**. Inflamed areas in the abdomen may press on the tube that drains urine from the kidney to the bladder (the ureter). Ureter compression can make urine back up into the kidney, enlarge the ureter and kidney, and can potentially lead to kidney damage. Patients with Crohn's disease also frequently suffer from:

- Arthritis (inflammation of the joints)
- Spondylitis (inflammation of the vertebrae, the bones of the spine)
- Ulcers of the mouth and skin
- Painful, red bumps on the skin
- Inflammation of several eye areas; and
- Inflammation of the liver, gallbladder, and/or the channels (ducts) that carry bile between and within the liver, gallbladder, and intestine.

The chance of developing **cancer** of the intestine is greater than normal among patients with Crohn's disease, although this chance is not as high as among those patients with ulcerative colitis.

Diagnosis is first suspected based on a patient's symptoms. Blood tests may reveal an increase in certain types of white blood cells, an indication that some type of inflammation is occurring in the body. The blood tests may also reveal anemia and other signs of malnutrition due to malabsorption (low blood protein; variations in the amount of calcium, potassium, and magnesium present in the blood; changes in certain markers of liver function). Stool samples may be examined to make sure that no infectious agent is causing the diarrhea, and to see if the waste contains blood.

During an endoscopic exam, a doctor passes a flexible tube with a tiny, fiber-optic camera device through the rectum and into the colon. The doctor can then carefully examine the lining of the intestine for signs of inflammation and ulceration that might suggest Crohn's disease. A tiny sample (a **biopsy**) of the intestine can also be taken through the endoscope, and the tissue will be examined under a microscope for evidence of Crohn's disease.

X rays can be helpful for diagnosis, and also for determining how much of the intestine is involved in the disease. For these x rays, the patient must either drink a chalky solution containing barium, or receive a barium enema (a solution that is administered through the rectum). Barium helps to ''light up'' the intestine, allowing more detail to be seen on the resulting x rays.

Treatments for Crohn's disease try to reduce the underlying inflammation, the resulting **malabsorption/malnutrition**, the uncomfortable symptoms of crampy abdominal pain and diarrhea, and the possible complications (obstructions, abscesses, and fistulas).

Inflammation can be treated with a drug called sulfasalazine. Sulfasalazine is made up of two parts. One part is related to the sulfa **antibiotics**; the other part is a form of the anti-inflammatory chemical, salicylic acid (related to **aspirin**). Sulfasalazine is not well-absorbed from the intestine, so it stays mostly within the intestine, where it is broken down into its components. It is believed that the salicylic acid component actively treats Crohn's disease by fighting inflammation. Some patients do not respond to sulfasalazine, and require steroid medications (such as prednisone). Steroids, however, must be used carefully to avoid the complications of these drugs, including increased risk of infection and weakening of bones (**osteoporosis**). Some very potent immunosuppressive drugs, which interfere with the products of the immune system and can hopefully decrease inflammation, may be used for those patients who do not improve on steroids.

Serious cases of malabsorption/malnutrition may need to be treated by providing nutritional supplements. These supplements must be in a form that can be absorbed from the damaged, inflamed intestine. Some patients find that certain foods are hard to digest, including milk, large quantities of fiber, and spicy foods. When patients are suffering from an obstruction, or during periods of time when symptoms of the disease are at their worst, they may need to drink specially formulated, high-calorie liquid supplements. Those patients who are severely ill may need to receive their nutrition through a needle inserted in a vein (intravenously), or even by a tiny tube (a catheter) inserted directly into a major vein in the chest.

A number of medications are available to help decrease the cramping and pain associated with Crohn's disease. These include loperamide, tincture of opium, and codeine. Some fiber preparations (methylcellulose or psyllium) may be helpful, although some patients do not tolerate them well.

Crohn's disease is a life-long illness. The severity of the disease can vary, and a patient can experience periods of time when the disease is not active and he or she is symptom free. However, the complications and risks of Crohn's disease tend to increase over time. Well over 60% of all patients with Crohn's disease will require surgery, and about half of these patients will require more than one operation over time. About 5-10% of all Crohn's patients will die of their disease, primarily due to massive infection.

INFLUENZA

Influenza is an infectious disease caused by the influenza virus. The term *influenza* is used to describe influenza and other similar illnesses. The general symptoms of influenza, also known as the flu or grippe, are chills, **headache**, **fever**, weakness and aching of the joints. The incubation period is short—between one and three days—and the first symptom is a fever that may reach 103° F. Cough and gastrointestinal discomfort may also accompany the disease. Usually, the viral infection runs its course in about a week. However, the virus weakens the **immune system**, making the human body subject to secondary infections such as bacterial **pneumonia**. Fatalities associated with influenza usually result from such secondary complications. The presence of viral pneumonia was probably the cause of many deaths during the great influenza **epidemics** of the past.

Historically, influenza has been known for centuries and may have been what **Hippocrates** of Cos described as the cause of an epidemic as early as 412 B.C. In the sixteenth century, John Keys (1510-1573), also known by his Latinized name, Johannes **Caius**, was a well-educated English physician who wrote a treatise on the "Sweatyng Sickness." In this curious book he describes a highly contagious illness in which death frequently occurred within a few days or even hours after symptoms began to show. The symptoms he described included fever, **delirium** and labored breathing—not very different from influenza symptoms. At that time the cause was sometimes attributed to the English diet—but nobody really knew how the sweating sickness was transmitted. Treatment included bed rest and doing anything that would promote sweating.

Even at the beginning of the twentieth century, doctors had difficulty determining how influenza spread. They knew it was not spread by bacteria from unsanitary conditions, nor by insects. But what doctors did know was that the disease could be fatal. Between 1918 and 1919, influenza killed about 20 million people all over the globe. In the United States more than 550,000 people died of the flu—ten times more Americans than were killed in action during World War I. There were emergency hospitals set up to treat flu patients. Soldiers were made to gargle with salt water to prevent the disease.

Scientists and physicians searched for the cause of influenza but could not find one. Not until the 1930s with the invention of more powerful microscopes did scientists began to see pathogens much smaller than bacteria—viruses. During that decade the nature of viruses was discovered. Wendell Stanley, an American biochemist, prepared large quantities of viruses, and found that they could be crystallized. Viruses are very simple structures made of only proteins and nucleic acids which could be crystallized in much the same way as other nonliving chemicals. However, when a virus is inside a living cell it uses the cell's genetic machinery to make more copies of itself. Stanley had discovered that viruses are on the borderline between living and nonliving things because they grow only when inside living cells. During World War II, Stanley worked on culturing the influenza virus. Today influenza is grouped with other viruses known as **adenoviruses**.

Because viruses are so tiny, vast numbers are found in human body fluids like mucus and saliva. Coughing or sneezing releases an aerosol spray filled with viruses. The pathogen easily travels from one person to another, making influenza very contagious. The viruses usually enter the upper respiratory tract and begin reproducing. The body's immune system, including antibodies and T lymphocytes, work to kill the viruses, but may be not be enough to stop the disease from running its course.

Scientists are still puzzled by the influenza outbreak that occurred around the time of the First World War. Originating in the American Midwest, the epidemic spread world wide, possibly carried abroad by American soldiers during World War I. Incredibly, lung tissue from an Army private who died from the flu was preserved in paraffin and stored in Washington, DC. In 1997, scientists used polymerase chain reaction—which amplifies minute genetic material—to extract the virus.

Genetic studies found the flu contained a pig virus. The study further proved that pigs, which are susceptible to both bird and human viruses, can serve as a cauldron where new and dangerous viral strains can intermingle and form other strains. The finding also dispelled a long-time belief that the epidemic may have developed from an avian, or bird, virus.

In 1997 a three-year-old boy in Hong Kong died from a virus previously thought to occur only in birds. Investigators believe that the transmission was direct from bird to human without the usual intermediary pig. Prior to the boy's infection, thousands of chickens in Hong Kong died from the virus. By the end of 1997, 15 additional cases had occurred in the city.

Research has shown that viruses have a phenomenal ability to change, or mutate, very quickly. A treatment that may have worked on one flu virus may not work on another. Each year different strains develop and are named for places where they first occur. The Asian flu caused a worldwide epidemic in 1957-1958 and the Hong Kong flu in 1968-1969. Fewer deaths resulted because antibiotics were used to treat secondary infections.

The best treatment for influenza is prevention; and flu vaccines (both killed and live virus) are recommended, especially for the very young and the very old. In addition the antiviral drug known as amantadine has been used to treat certain strains of influenza.

Influenza pandemic of 1918

Pandemics are **epidemics** that occur on a global scale. They generally result from the emergence of an influenza A virus that is novel for the human population. The hallmark of pandemic **influenza** is excess mortality—the number of deaths observed during an epidemic of influenza-like illness in excess of the number expected. During this century, pandemics occurred in 1918, 1957 (Asian flu), and 1968 (Hong Kong flu). The 1918 influenza outbreak is regarded as the worst in human history—it killed up to 40 million people world wide.

The outbreak started in the United States at an army base in the Midwest and then spread to Europe and other parts of the world. This epidemic was different from most others because it preyed heavily upon the 20 to 40 year old age group, which was normally the most healthy and resistant to disease.

It all started on March 11, 1918 at an army camp in Kansas. A company cook named Albert Mitchell reported to the infirmary with typical flu-like symptoms—a low grade **fever**, mild **sore throat**, a light **headache**, and muscle aches. Bed rest was recommended. By noon, 107 soldiers were sick. Within 2 days, 522 people were sick. Many were gravely ill with severe **pneumonia**. Then reports started coming in from other military bases around the country. Thousands of soldiers docked off the East Coast were sick. Within a week, the influenza was hitting isolated places, such as the island of Alcatraz. Every state in the United States had been infected. The death toll in United States was 850,000 people. The actual killer was the pneumonia that accompanied the infection.

A subset of patients died extremely quickly, within two or three days of symptoms. Massive amounts of fluid accumulated in the lungs of these people; in a sense these patients drowned. Other people died of secondary infections with bacterial pneumonia. **Antibiotics** did not exist in 1918 and hence there was no way to treat those secondary infections.

In order to curtail the spread of the disease, the Health Department adopted many measures. Theaters, lodges, dance halls, and places of amusement were closed for several weeks. Fresh air and adequate heat were counseled. People were advised to get 9 hours of sleep. **Smoking** was prohibited on streetcars in order to prevent spitting.

The infection, which was airborne, spread across the Atlantic. By April, French troops and civilians were infected. By mid-April, the disease had spread to China and Japan. By May, the virus had spread throughout Africa and South America. 60% of the Eskimo population was wiped out in Alaska. 80 to 90% of the Samoan population was infected. In the end, 25 million people had died. Some estimates put that number as high as 37 million. 18 months after the disease appeared, the flu bug vanished and has never shown up again. Even with a death toll of 850,000, the United States was the area that was the least devastated by the virus.

No one at the time was really sure what had happened. Viruses were not known then. However, while conducting autopsies in 1918, some army doctors had preserved specimens in formaldehyde. One of these jars contained the lungs of a 21 year old soldier that died on September 26, 1918. The researchers at Armed Forces Institute of Pathology in Washington, D.C., managed to isolate genetic material from the virus and were successful in gathering a wealth of information.

The virus had apparently passed from birds to pigs and then to humans. Viruses tend to remain stable in birds, but occasionally when they infect pigs, the pig's immune system kicks into action and produces antibodies. In order to survive, the virus is forced to mutate. And it was this mutated swine virus that caused the most deadly pandemic on Earth.

At present a lot of work is being done to figure out whether there is a genetic basis for why this particular virus was so virulent. Influenza viruses often mutate and new strains arise continually, which is why vaccines have to be made every year to match the current strain. It is possible that such a pandemic could occur again. If scientists are able to unravel the mystery of how the genetic structure of the virus is related to its lethal ability, future epidemics could perhaps be prevented.

See also Influenza

Inhalation therapies

Inhalation therapies are a group of respiratory, or breathing, treatments designed to help restore or improve breathing function in patients with a variety of diseases, conditions, or injuries. The treatments range from at-home **oxygen therapy** for patients with **chronic obstructive pulmonary disease** to mechanical ventilation for patients with acute **respiratory failure**. Inhalation therapies usually include the following categories:

- Oxygen therapy

- Incentive spirometry
- Continuous positive airway pressure (CPAP)
- Oxygen chamber therapy
- Mechanical ventilation
- Newborn life support.

Inhalation therapies are ordered for various stages of diseases that are causing progressive or sudden respiratory failure.

Oxygen therapy is most commonly ordered to support patients with emphysema and other chronic obstructive pulmonary disease (COPD). The oxygen therapy is usually ordered once decreased oxygen saturation in the blood or tissues is shown. Oxygen therapy may also be used in the hospital setting to help return a patient's breathing and oxygen levels to normal.

Once a patient shows hypoxemia, or decreased oxygen in arterial blood, supplemental oxygen may be ordered. The main purpose of the oxygen is to prevent damage to vital organs resulting from inadequate oxygen supply. The lowest possible saturation will be given to keep the patient's measurements at a minimum acceptable level. The oxygen is administered through a mask or nasal tube, or sometimes directly into the trachea. The amount of oxygen prescribed is measured in liters of flow per minute.

In the case of respiratory distress in newborns or adults, oxygen therapy may be attempted before mechanical ventilation since it is a noninvasive and less expensive choice.

Incentive spirometry may be ordered to help patients practice and improve controlled breathing. It may be ordered after surgery to the abdomen, lungs, neck, or head. It is designed to mimic natural sighs and yawns. A device provides positive feedback when a patient inhales at a predetermined rate and sustains the breath for a specific period of time. This helps teach the patient to take long, slow, and deep breaths. A spirometer, or equipment that measures pulmonary function, is provided to the patient and a respiratory therapist will work with the patient to demonstrate and explain the technique. Once patients show mastery of the technique, they are instructed to practice the exercises frequently on their own.

Common uses of continuous positive airway pressure include the treatment of **sleep apnea** and **respiratory distress syndrome** in both adults and infants. Patients with sleep apnea will receive continuous positive airway pressure to prevent upper airway collapse. It is usually administered through a tight-fitting mask as humidified oxygen. The pressure of flow is constant during both exhaling and inhaling and the level of pressure is determined based on each individual. Most patients undergoing CPAP in a hospital setting will receive continuous monitoring of some vital signs and periodic sampling of blood gas values.

Oxygen chamber therapy is ordered for various causes that indicate immediate need for oxygen saturation in the blood. Divers with **decompression** illness, climbers in high altitude, patients suffering from severe carbon dioxide poisoning, and children or adults in acute respiratory distress may require oxygen chamber therapy. In recent years, physicians have also used the forced pressure of oxygen chambers to help heal burns and other wounds because the pressure under which the oxygen is delivered can reach areas that are blocked off or suffering from poor circulation.

Also known as hyperbaric oxygen chamber or hyperbaric oxygen therapy (HBO), this treatment delivers pure oxygen under pressure equal to that of 2-3 times normal atmospheric pressure.

Mechanical ventilation is ordered for patients in acute respiratory distress, and is often used in intensive care situations. In some cases, mechanical ventilation is a final attempt to continue the breathing function in a patient and may be considered "life-sustaining."

In general, mechanical ventilation replaces or supports the normal lung function of a patient. Although normally delivered in a hospital, often to treat serious illness, mechanical ventilation may be performed at home under the order and supervision of a physician and home health agency. The patient will usually be intubated and the ventilator machine "takes over" the breathing function.

Newborn babies, particularly those who were premature, may require inhalation therapies immediately upon birth because the lungs are among the last organs to fully develop. Some newborns suffer from serious respiratory problems or birth complications, such as respiratory distress syndrome, neonatal wet lung syndrome, apnea of prematurity or persistent fetal circulation, which may require inhalation therapies.

Premature infants, especially those born before the 28th week of gestation, have underdeveloped breathing muscles and immature structures within the lungs. These infants will require breathing support, often in the form of mechanical ventilation. The support delivers warm, humidified, oxygen-enriched gases either by oxygen hood or through mechanical ventilation. In serious cases, the infant may require mechanical ventilation with CPAP or positive-end expiratory pressure (PEEP) through a tightly fitting face mask or even by endotracheal intubation.

Need for continued resuscitation for newborns depends not only on gestational age, but on signs indicating ineffective breathing, including color, heart rate, and respiratory effort. CPAP will be delivered through nasal or endotracheal tubes with a continuous-flow ventilator specifically designed for infants. An alarm system alerts the neonatal staff to problems and monitoring of breathing and other vital functions will accompany the therapy. As respiratory distress syndrome begins to resolve, usually in four or five days, the type of support will be reduced accordingly and the infant may be weaned from the ventilator and moved to only CPAP or an oxygen hood.

INSOMNIA

Insomnia is the inability to obtain an adequate amount or quality of **sleep**. The difficulty can be in falling asleep, remaining asleep, or both. People with insomnia do not feel refreshed when they wake up. Insomnia is a common symptom affecting millions of people that may be caused by many conditions, diseases, or circumstances.

Sleep is essential for mental and physical restoration. It is a cycle with two separate states: rapid eye movement

(REM), the stage in which most dreaming occurs; and non-REM (NREM). Four stages of sleep take place during NREM: stage I, when the person passes from relaxed wakefulness; stage II, an early stage of light sleep; stages III and IV, which are increasing degrees of deep sleep. Most stage IV sleep (also called delta sleep), occurs in the first several hours of sleep. A period of REM sleep normally follows a period of NREM sleep.

Insomnia is more common in women and older adults. People who are **divorced**, widowed, or separated are more likely to have the problem than those who are married, and it is more frequently reported by those with lower socioeconomic status. Short-term, or transient, insomnia is a common occurrence and usually lasts only a few days. Long-term, or chronic, insomnia lasts more than three weeks and increases the risk for injuries in the home, at the workplace, and while driving because of daytime sleepiness and decreased concentration. Chronic insomnia can also lead to **mood disorders** like depression.

Transient insomnia is often caused by a temporary situation in a person's life, such as an argument with a loved one, a brief medical illness, or **jet lag**. When the situation is resolved or the precipitating factor disappears, the condition goes away, usually without medical treatment.

Chronic insomnia usually has different causes, and there may be more than one. These include medical conditions or treatment; use of **caffeine**, alcohol, and nicotine; psychiatric conditions such as mood or **anxiety disorders**; **stress**; disturbed sleep cycles caused by a change in work shift; sleep-disordered breathing, such as snoring; periodic jerky leg movements (*nocturnal myoclonus*), which happen just as the individual is falling asleep; and repeated nightmares or **panic** attacks during sleep.

If a person worries whether he will be able to sleep, that too can cause insomia. The more one worries about falling asleep, the harder it becomes. This is called psychophysiological insomnia.

People who have insomnia do not start the day refreshed from a good night's sleep. They are tired. They may have difficulty falling asleep, and commonly lie in bed tossing and turning for hours. Or the individual may go to sleep without a problem but wakes in the early hours of the morning and is either unable to go back to sleep, or drifts into a restless, unsatisfying sleep. This is common in the elderly and in those suffering from depression.

The diagnosis of insomnia is made by a physician based on the patient's reported signs and symptoms. It can be useful for the patient to keep a daily record for two weeks of sleep patterns, food intake, use of alcohol, medications, and any other information recommended by the physician. If the patient has a bed partner, information can be obtained about whether the patient snores or is restless during sleep. This, together with a medical history and physical examination, can help confirm the doctor's assessment.

A wide variety of healthcare professionals can recognize and treat insomnia, but when a patient with chronic insomnia does not respond to treatment, or the condition is not adequately explained by the patient's physical, emotional, or mental circumstances, then more extensive testing by a specialist in sleep disorders may be warranted.

Treatment of insomnia includes alleviating any physical and emotional problems that are contributing to the condition and exploring changes in lifestyle that will improve the situation.

Patients can make changes in their daily routine that are simple and effective in treating their insomnia. If they are unable to go to sleep, they should go into another room and do something that relaxing, like reading. The patients should return to bed only when they feel sleepy. Patients should set the alarm and get up every morning at the same time, no matter how much they have slept, to establish a regular sleep-wake pattern. Naps during the day should be avoided, but if absolutely necessary, than a 30 minute nap early in the afternoon may not interfere with sleep at night.

Another successful technique is called sleep-restriction therapy, which restricts the amount of time spent in bed to the actual time spent sleeping. This approach allows a slight sleep debt to build up, which increases the individual's ability to fall asleep and stay asleep. If a patient is sleeping five hours a night, the time in bed is limited to 5-5 1/2 hours. The time in bed is gradually increased in small segments,with the individual rising at the same time each morning; at least 85% of the time in bed must be spent sleeping.

Medications given for insomnia include sedatives, tranquilizers, and **antianxiety drugs**. All require a doctor's prescription and may become habit-forming. They can lose effectiveness over time and can reduce alertness during the day. **Over-the-counter drugs** such as **antihistamines** are not very effective in bringing about sleep and can affect the quality of sleep.

INTEGUMENTARY SYSTEM

The human integumentary system is made up of the skin, hair, nails, and glands, and it serves many protective functions for the body. It prevents excessive water loss, keeps out microorganisms that could cause illness, and protects the underlying tissues from mechanical damage. Pigments in the skin called melanin absorb and reflect the sun's harmful ultraviolet radiation. The skin also helps to regulate body temperature. If heat builds up in the body, sweat glands in the skin produce sweat, which evaporates and cools the skin. In addition, when the body overheats, blood vessels in the skin expand and bring more blood to the surface, which allows body heat to be lost. If the body is too cold, on the other hand, the blood vessels in the skin contract, resulting in less blood at the body surface; heat is, thus, conserved. In addition to temperature regulation, the skin serves as a minor excretory organ, because sweat removes small amounts of nitrogenous wastes produced by the body. The skin also functions as a sense organ in that it contains millions of nerve endings that detect **touch**, heat, cold, **pain**, and pressure. Finally, the skin produces vitamin D in the presence of sunlight, and renews and repairs damage to itself.

In an adult, the skin covers about 21.5 sq ft (2 sq m) and weighs about 11 lb (5 kg). Depending on location, the skin ranges from 0.02-0.16 in (0.5-4.0 mm) thick. Its two principal parts are the outer layer, or epidermis, and a thicker inner layer, the dermis. A subcutaneous layer of fatty or adipose tissue is found below the dermis. Fibers from the dermis attach the skin to the subcutaneous layer, and the underlying tissues and organs also connect to the subcutaneous layer.

Ninety percent of the epidermis, including the outer layers, contains keratinocytes—cells that produce keratin, a protein that helps waterproof and protect the skin. Melanocytes are pigment cells that produce melanin, a brown-black pigment that adds to skin color and absorbs ultraviolet light, thereby shielding the genetic material in skin cells from damage. Merkel's cells are touch-sensitive cells found in the deepest layer of the epidermis of hairless skin.

In most areas of the body, the epidermis consists of four layers. On the soles of the feet and palms of the hands, where there is a lot of friction, the epidermis has five layers. In addition, calluses, abnormal thickenings of the epidermis, occur on skin subject to constant friction. At the skin surface, the outer layer of the epidermis constantly sheds the dead cells containing keratin. The uppermost layer consists of about 25 rows of flat dead cells that contain keratin.

The dermis is made up of connective tissue that contains protein, collagen, and elastic fibers. It also contains blood and lymph vessels, sensory receptors, related nerves, and glands. The outer part of the dermis has fingerlike projections, called dermal papillae, that indent the lower layer of the epidermis. Dermal papillae cause ridges in the epidermis above it, which in the digits give rise to fingerprints. The ridge pattern of fingerprints is inherited, and is unique to each individual. The dermis is thick in the palms and soles, but very thin in other places, such as the eyelids. If a part of the body, such as a working muscle, needs more blood, blood vessels in the dermis constrict, causing blood to leave the skin and enter the circulation that leads to muscles and other body parts. Sweat glands, the ducts of which pass through the epidermis to the outside and open on the skin surface through pores, are embedded in the deep layers of the dermis. Hair follicles and hair roots also originate in the dermis, and the hair shafts extend from the hair root through the skin layers to the surface. Also in the dermis are sebaceous glands associated with hair follicles that produce an oily substance called sebum. Sebum softens the hair and prevents it from drying; if sebum blocks up a sebaceous gland, a whitehead appears on the skin. A blackhead results if the material oxidizes and dries. **Acne** is caused by infections of the sebaceous glands. When this occurs, the skin breaks out in pimples and can become scarred.

The skin is an important sense organ, and as such it includes a number of nerves, which are mainly in the dermis (a few reach the epidermis). Nerves carry impulses to and from hair muscles, sweat glands, and blood vessels, and receive messages from touch, temperature, and pain receptors. Some nerve endings are specialized, such as sensory receptors that detect external stimuli. The nerve endings in the dermal papillae are known as Meissner's corpuscles, which detect light touch, such as a pat, or the feel of clothing on the skin. Pacinian corpuscles, located in the deeper dermis, are stimulated by stronger pressure on the skin. Receptors near hair roots detect displacement of the skin hairs by stimuli such as touch or wind. Bare nerve endings throughout the skin report information to the brain about temperature change, texture, pressure, and trauma.

Some skin disorders result from overexposure to the ultraviolet (UV) rays in sunlight. At first, overexposure to sunlight results in injury known as **sunburn**. UV rays damage skin cells, blood vessels, and other dermal structures. Continual overexposure leads to leathery skin, wrinkles, and discoloration and can also lead to **skin cancer**. Anyone excessively exposed to UV rays runs a risk of skin cancer, regardless of the amount of pigmentation normally in the skin. Seventy-five percent of all skin cancers are basal cell carcinomas that arise in the epidermis and rarely spread (metastasize) to other parts of the body. Physicians can surgically remove basal cell cancers. Squamous cell carcinomas also occur in the epidermis, but these tend to metastasize. Malignant melanomas are life-threatening skin cancers that metastasize rapidly. There can be a 10-20 year delay between exposure to sunlight and the development of skin cancers.

See also Acne; Skin cancer; Skin grafting; Skin lesions; Skin resurfacing

Intelligence tests

The Stanford-Binet Intelligence Scale and the Wechsler Intelligence Scales are standardized tests that assesses intelligence and cognitive abilities in children and adults.

The Stanford-Binet Intelligence Scale, the Wechsler Intelligence Scales for Children (regular, revised, and third edition), and the Wechsler Preschool and Primary Scale of Intelligence are used as tools in school placement, in determining the presence of a learning disability or a developmental delay, and in tracking intellectual development.

The Wechsler Adult Intelligence Scales (regular and revised) are used to determine vocational ability, to assess adult intellectual ability in the classroom, and to determine organic deficits. Both adult and children's Wechsler scales, as well as Stanford-Binet, are often included in neuropsychological testing to assess the brain function of individuals with neurological impairments.

Although the Stanford-Binet was developed for children as young as two, examiners should be cautious in using the test to screen very young children for developmental delays or disabilities. The test cannot be used to diagnose **mental retardation** in children aged three and under, and the scoring design may not detect developmental problems in preschool-age children.

Intelligence testing requires a clinically trained examiner. These should be administered and interpreted by a trained professional, preferably a psychologist or psychiatrist.

The fourth edition of the Stanford-Binet Intelligence Scale is a direct descendent of the Binet-Simon scale, the first intelligence scale created in 1905 by psychologist **Alfred Binet** and Dr. Theophilus Simon. This revised edition, released in

1986, was designed with a larger, more diverse, representative sample to minimize the gender and racial inequities that had been criticized in earlier versions of the test.

The Stanford-Binet scale tests intelligence across four areas: verbal reasoning, quantitative reasoning, abstract/visual reasoning, and short-term memory. The areas are covered by 15 subtests, including vocabulary, comprehension, verbal absurdities, pattern analysis, matrices, paper folding and cutting, copying, quantitative, number series, equation building, memory for sentences, memory for digits, memory for objects, and bead memory.

All test subjects take an initial vocabulary test, which along with the subject's age, determines the number and level of subtests to be administered. Total testing time is 45-90 minutes, depending on the subject's age and the number of subtests given. Raw scores are based on the number of items answered, and are converted into a standard age score corresponding to age group, similar to an IQ measure.

All of the Wechsler scales are divided into six verbal and five performance subtests. The complete test takes 60-90 minutes to administer. Verbal and Performance IQs are scored based on the results of the testing, and then a composite Full Scale IQ score is computed. Although earlier editions of some of the Wechsler Scales are still available, the latest revisions are described below:

Wechsler Adult Intelligence Scale-Revised (WAIS-R). The WAIS-R, the 1981 revision of the original Wechsler Adult Intelligence Scale, is designed for adults, age 16-74. The 11 subtests of the WAIS-R include information, digit span, vocabulary, arithmetic, comprehension, similarities, picture completion, picture arrangement, block design, object assembly, and digit symbol. An example of questions on the subtest of similarities might be: "Describe how the following pair of words are alike or the same—hamburger and pizza." A correct response would be "Both are things to eat."

Wechsler Intelligence Scale for Children, Third Edition (WISC-III). The WISC-III subtests includes many of the same categories of subtests as the WAIS-R. In addition, there are two optional performance subtests: symbol search and mazes.

Wechsler Preschool and Primary Scale of Intelligence (WPPSI). The WPPSI is designed for children age 4-6½ years. The test is divided into six verbal and five performance subtests. The eleven subtests are presented in the following order: information, animal house and animal house retest, vocabulary, picture completion, arithmetic, mazes, geometric design, similarities, block design, comprehension, and sentences.

The 1997 **Medicare** reimbursement rate for psychological and neuropsychological testing, including intelligence testing, is \$58.35 an hour. Billing time typically includes test administration, scoring and interpretation, and reporting. Many insurance plans cover all or a portion of diagnostic psychological testing.

The Stanford-Binet is a standardized test, meaning that norms were established during the design phase of the test by administering the test to a large, representative sample of the test population. The test has a mean, or average, standard score of 100 and a standard deviation of 16 (subtests have a mean of 50 and a standard deviation of 8). The standard deviation indicates how far above or below the norm the subject's score is. For example, an eight-year-old is assessed with the Stanford-Binet scale and achieves a standard age score of 116. The mean score of 100 is the average level at which all eight-year-olds in the representative sample performed. This child's score would be one standard deviation above that norm.

The Wechsler Intelligence Scales are standardized tests, meaning that as part of the test design, they were administered to a large representative sample of the target population, and norms were determined from the results. The scales have a mean, or average, standard score of 100 and a standard deviation of 15. The standard deviation indicates how far above or below the norm the subject's score is. For example, a ten-year-old is assessed with the WISC-III scale and achieves a full-scale IQ score of 85. The mean score of 100 is the average level at which all 10-year-olds in the representative sample performed. This child's score would be one standard deviation below that norm.

While the full-scale IQ scores provide a reference point for evaluation, they are only an average of a variety of skill areas. A trained psychologist will evaluate and interpret an individual's performance on the scale's subtests to discover their strengths and weaknesses and offer recommendations based upon these findings.

Interferon

While the middle years of the twentieth century saw the development of **antibiotics**, potent new weapons against bacterial diseases, no such chemical defenses against viral diseases had yet emerged other than a few anti-viral vaccines. This was and continues to be a significant gap, since more than half of the communicable diseases that affect human beings are caused by ribonucleic acid (RNA) viruses. The first step was to find out how the body protected itself against viruses; it was known that antibodies acted only against bacteria. That step was taken by Alick Isaacs, a Scottish virologist, in 1957.

Isaacs was born in Glasgow, Scotland, in 1921, to a Russian Jewish family. He studied medicine at Glasgow University but found he preferred research to the actual practice of medicine. Accordingly, he pursued graduate studies in bacteriology at Glasgow and secured fellowships to research **influenza** with eminent microbiologists Stuart Harris of England and **Frank MacFarlane Burnet** in Australia. Returning to England, Isaacs joined the World Influenza Centre at the National Institute for Medical Research in 1951. There, he carried out his continuing studies of viral influenza until his untimely death in 1967.

Early in his studies of influenza, Isaacs became interested in the viral interference phenomenon—the fact that an RNA virus in a cell inhibits the growth of any other viruses in that cell. He found that this interference seemed to be caused by something inside the cell. In 1957, while working with the visiting Swiss scientist Jean Lindenmann, Isaacs found that chick embryos injected with influenza virus released very small amounts of a protein that destroyed the virus and also inhibited the growth of any other viruses in the embryos. Isaacs and Lindenmann named the interfering protein *interferon.*

Further research showed that interferon was produced within hours of a viral invasion (antibodies take several days to form), and that most living things, including plants, can make the protective protein. Interferon was seen as the cell's first line of defense against viral infections, and its discovery was expected to pave the way for successful treatment of viral diseases.

Because interferon was thought to be species-specific (meaning only human interferon will work in human beings) and the body produces it in only minute amounts, interferon research inched forward at a snail's pace.

Interest in interferon was revived in the late 1960s when Ion Gresser (1928-), an American researcher in Paris, discovered that the protein stopped or slowed the growth of tumors in mice and also stimulated the production of tumor-killing lymphocytes. Gresser and the Finnish virologist Kari Cantell then developed a way to make interferon in useful amounts from human blood cells. Monoclonal antibodies, first produced in 1975, made large-scale purification of interferon possible, and the mid-1980s saw the advent of genetically engineered interferon, the first example of which was produced from bacteria by Swiss scientist Charles Weissmann in 1980. Scientists now know that there are three major types of interferon: alpha, beta, and gamma. They have also learned that interferons are not species specific but can have activity in other species.

Research of interferon's ability to kill **cancer** cells is active. It has been used successfully against **leukemia**, osteogenic sarcoma (a **bone cancer**), and as a therapy for delaying disease recurrence and prolonging survival in patients with melanoma (**skin cancer**). Research also continues on the use of interferon to treat viral diseases like **rabies**, hepatitis, and herpes infections. In December 1997, researchers from the Duke University Medical Center also announced study results that indicate interferon may be a way to preserve donor livers longer prior to transplantation.

International Red Cross

The International Red Cross works to alleviate human suffering and promote public health. In 1986, its name was changed to the International Red Cross and Red Crescent Movement. It is one of the largest humanitarian networks in the world. Based in Geneva, Switzerland, the movement has a presence and activities in nearly every country in the world. The Red Cross or Red Crescent flag is known worldwide as a symbol of mercy and neutrality. The International Red Cross and Red Crescent Movement is guided by seven fundamental principles: humanity, impartiality, neutrality, independence, voluntary service, unity, and universality.

The International Red Cross was established in 1863, after a book by Swiss businessman **Jean Henry Dunant**, *A Memory of Solferino*, raised awareness about the lack of medical services on the battlefield of Solferino in northern Italy. The book appealed for the establishment of peacetime volunteer societies with nurses who could care for the wounded in wartime and for those societies to be recognized and protected through an international agreement. Dunant's ideas led to the formation of the International Committee for Relief of the Wounded. This committee convinced the Swiss government to convene a diplomatic conference in Geneva in 1864 to adopt the first international humanitarian law: the Geneva Convention for the Amelioration of the Condition of the Wounded in Armies in the Field. The International Committee for Relief of the Wounded later became the International Committee of the Red Cross.

Today, the International Red Cross and Red Crescent Movement is made up of National Red Cross and Red Crescent Societies; the International Committee of the Red Cross; and the International Federation of Red Cross and Red Crescent Societies. The International Committee of the Red Cross, from which the movement began, was established in 1863. It is an independent humanitarian institution which serves as a neutral intermediary in armed conflict or unrest to protect and assist victims. The International Federation of Red Cross and Red Crescent Societies, established in 1919, promotes the humanitarian activities of the National Societies among vulnerable people, coordinating disaster relief and encouraging development support.

As of March 1999, there were 175 National Red Cross and Red Crescent Societies throughout the world. After World War II, the movement expanded the scope of its activities, and began working extensively with refugees. In 1949, another diplomatic conference was held and the four Geneva Conventions of 1949, which protected civilians in wartime, were adopted. In 1977, two additional protocols were added to the conventions.

The American Red Cross, headquartered in Washington, D.C., was established by **Clara Barton** in 1881 and received its first Federal charter in 1900. The American Red Cross is led by volunteers and guided by its Congressional Charter and the principals of the International Red Cross and Red Crescent Movement. Its mission is to provide relief to disaster victims and help people prevent, prepare for, and respond to emergency. It focuses on disaster relief, services to the armed forces and veterans, and **public health** and safety programs. One of its best known programs is the nationwide Red Cross blood program, which collects, stores, treats, and distributes blood and blood products to people who are ill and injured throughout the United States. The President of the United States serves as the honorary chairman.

Intersex states

Intersex states are conditions where a newborn's sex organs (genitals) look unusual, making it impossible to identify the sex of the baby from its outward appearance.

All developing babies start out with external sex organs that look female. If the baby is male, the internal sex organs

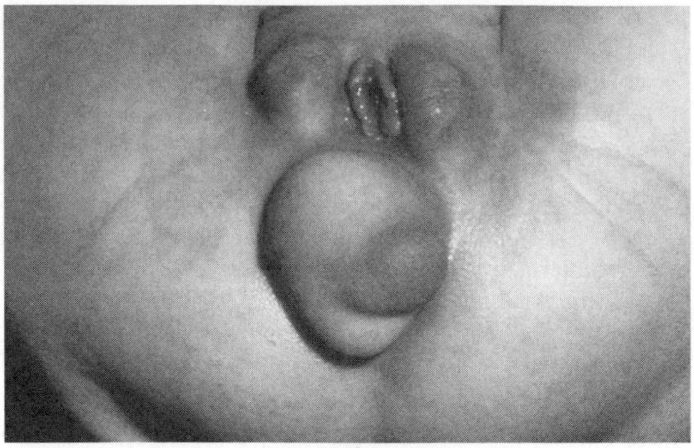

Photo of an infant with female and male genitalia.

mature and begin to produce the male hormone testosterone. If the hormones reach the tissues correctly, the external genitals that looked female change into the scrotum and penis. Sometimes, the genetic sex (as indicated by chromosomes) may not match the appearance of the external sex organs. About 1 in every 2,000 births results in a baby whose sex organs look unusual.

Patients with intersex states can be classified as a true hermaphrodite, a female pseudohermaphrodite, or a male pseudohermaphrodite. This is determined by examining the internal and external structures of the child.

A true hermaphrodite is born with both ovaries and testicles. They also have mixed male and female external genitals. This condition is extremely rare.

A female pseudohermaphrodite is a genetic female. However, the external sex organs have been masculinized and look like a penis. This may occur if the mother takes the hormone progesterone to prevent a miscarriage, but more often it is caused by an overproduction of certain hormones.

A male pseudohermaphrodite is a genetic male. However, the external sex organs fail to develop normally. Intersex males may have testes and a female-like vulva, or a very small penis.

Any abnormality in chromosomes or sex hormones, or in the unborn baby's response to the hormones, can lead to an intersex state in a newborn.

Intersex states may also be caused by a condition called congenital adrenal hyperplasia, which occurs in about 1 out of every 5,000 newborns. This disease blocks the baby's metabolism and can cause a range of symptoms, including abnormal genitals.

When doctors are uncertain about a newborn's sex, a specialist in infant hormonal problems is consulted as soon as possible. **Ultrasound** can locate a uterus behind the bladder and can determine if there is a cervix or uterine canal. Blood tests can check the levels of sex hormones in the baby's blood, and chromosome analysis (called karyotyping) can determine sex. Explorative surgery or a **biopsy** of reproductive tissue may be necessary. Only after thorough testing can a correct diagnosis and determination of sex be made.

Treatment of intersex states is controversial. Traditional treatment assigns sex according to test results, the potential for the child to identify with a sex, and the ease of genital surgery to make the organs look more normal. Treatment may then include reconstructive surgery followed by hormone therapy. Babies born with congenital adrenal hyperplasia can be treated with cortisone-type drugs and sometimes surgery.

Counseling should be given to the entire family of an intersex newborn. Families should explore all available medical and surgical options. Counseling should also be provided to the child when he or she is old enough.

Since the mid-1950s, doctors have typically assigned a sex to an intersex infant based on how easy reconstructive surgery would be. The American Academy of Pediatrics states that children with these types of genitals can be raised successfully as members of either sex, and recommends surgery within the first 15 months of life.

Some people are critical of this approach, including intersex adults who were operated on as children. The remolded genitals do not function sexually and can be the source of lifelong pain. They suggest that surgery be delayed until the patient can make informed choices about surgery and intervention.

Iron deficiency anemia

Iron deficiency anemia is the most common type of **anemia** throughout the world. In the United States, iron deficiency anemia occurs to a lesser extent than in developing countries because of the higher consumption of red meat and the practice of food fortification (addition of iron to foods by the manufacturer). Anemia in the United States is caused by a variety of sources, including excessive losses of iron in menstrual fluids and excessive bleeding in the gastrointestinal tract. In developing countries located in tropical climates, the most common cause of iron deficiency anemia is infestation with hookworm.

Infants are at increased risk for iron deficiency. They are born with a built-in supply of iron, which can be tapped during periods of drinking low-iron milk or formula. Both human milk and cow milk contain rather low levels of iron (0.5-1.0 mg iron/liter). However, the iron in human milk is about 50% absorbed by the infant, while the iron of cow milk is only 10% absorbed. During the first six months of life, a baby's growth is made possible by the milk in the diet and by the infant's built-in supply. However, premature infants have a lower supply of iron and, for this reason, it is recommended that preterm infants (beginning at 2 months of age) be given oral supplements of 7 mg iron/day, as ferrous sulfate. Iron deficiency can result if an infant is fed a formula based on unfortified cow milk.

Blood is lost from the body every day through the feces. The normal rate of this loss is 0.5-1.0 ml per day. However, more blood can be lost if colon or rectal cancer is present. About 60% of **colorectal cancers** result in further blood losses, where the extent of blood loss is 2-10 ml/day, and can lead to iron deficiency anemia.

Infection with hookworm can provoke iron deficiency and iron deficiency anemia. The hookworm is a parasitic worm that thrives in warm climates, including in the southern United States. It enters the body through the skin, as through bare feet. The hookworm then migrates to the small intestines where it attaches itself to the villi, the small sausage-shaped structures in the intestines that absorb nutrients. The hookworms damage the villi, resulting in blood loss, and they produce anti-coagulants that cause continued bleeding. Each worm can cause the loss of up to 0.25 ml of blood per day.

Bleeding and blood losses through gastrointestinal tract can also be caused by **hemorrhoids**, anal fissures, **irritable bowel syndrome**, and blood clotting disorders.

Symptoms of iron deficiency anemia include weakness and fatigue. These symptoms result because the red blood cells do not function properly and cannot carry oxygen to the muscles. Iron deficiency can also affect other tissues, including the tongue and fingernails. Prolonged iron deficiency can make the tongue smooth, shiny, and reddened, a condition called glossitis. The fingernails may grow abnormally and acquire a spoon-shaped appearance.

Decreased iron intake contributes to iron deficiency. The iron content of food varies widely; cabbage, for example, contains about 1.6 mg of iron per kg, spinach contains 33 mg/kg. Apples, tomatoes, and vegetable oil are relatively low in iron, while whole wheat bread and beef are relatively high in iron. Whether a food is low or high in iron can also be determined by comparing its iron content with the recommended dietary allowance (RDA) for iron. The RDA for iron for the adult male is 10 mg/day, while that for the adult woman is 15 mg/day. The RDA during pregnancy is 30 mg/day. The RDA for infants of up to six months years of age is 6 mg/day, while that for infants of between six months and one year is 10 mg/day. The RDA values are based on the assumption that the person eats a mixture of plant and animal foods.

Oral iron supplements (pills) can be used to treat iron deficiency anemia. They may contain various iron salts, such as ferrous sulfate, ferrous gluconate, or ferrous fumarate. Injections and infusions of iron (which may be necessary if oral supplements fail) involve iron dextran. In patients with poor iron absorption (by the gut), therapy with injection or infusion is preferable over oral supplements. Treatment of iron deficiency anemia sometimes requires more than therapy with iron. If the deficiency was provoked by hemorrhoids, surgery may prove essential to prevent recurrent iron deficiency anemia. Likewise, a deficiency caused by hookworm infestations should involve eliminating the parasite. The prognosis for treating and curing iron deficiency anemia is excellent. As long as the patient takes the iron supplements as directed. Iron deficiency anemia in infants and young children can be prevented by the use of fortified foods, such as formula and cereal.

IRON LUNG AND OTHER RESPIRATORS

The iron lung is a mechanical respiratory device used to force air into and out of the lungs of a person unable to breathe for themselves. Invented in 1929 by Philip Drinker (1893-1977), a professor at the School of Public Health at Harvard University, the iron lung was one of the first of several inventions designed for this purpose. During the 1920s, people with **respiratory failure** were aided by a pulmotor, a contraption similar to fireplace bellows, which inflated and deflated the lungs by forcing air in and sucking it out. This process worked; however patients experienced chest **pain** because the amount of air forced into the lungs was not adjustable to the individual patient's lung capacity. Many people suffering from poliomyelitis—which often paralyzes muscles of the diaphragm, the large, dome-shaped muscle above the stomach which rises and falls to draw air into and push it out of the lungs—required the aid of these devices to keep them alive.

Drinker's idea for a breathing device came from a Swedish physician named Thunberg who had been experimenting with a vacuum to help patients breathe. Enlisting the help of his brother, Cecil, and Louis Shaw (1886-1940) Drinker, built a prototype, tested it on cats, and designed a device large enough for humans. The patient's body was positioned inside an airtight metal box while the head remained outside. The box was connected to a pump which reduced the air pressure inside the box, causing a negative change in pressure in the chest cavity similar to that which occurs when the diaphragm moves downward allowing air to rush into the lungs. With this decrease in air pressure inside the box, the weight of the atmosphere outside the box forced air through the nose and mouth of the patient into the lungs. In October 1928 an eight-year-old girl unable to breathe as a result of polio was the first person to be put into the iron lung. Drinker's invention was initially known as the ''Drinker tank respirator,'' but was soon earned the nickname *iron lung*. Drinker and Shaw received numerous awards for their invention, which allowed many polio patients to be kept alive, and it remained the standard treatment for this purpose well into the 1950s.

Since Drinker's invention, a class of breathing machines called *ventilators* and *respirators* has been developed. A modern ventilator consists of an electrical pump connected to an air supply, a humidifier which adds moisture to the air, and a tube which is inserted into the patient's nose or mouth. Ventilators, unlike the iron lung, use positive air pressure from the pump to force air into the lungs and the patient exhales the air naturally. To adjust the oxygen-carbon dioxide ratio supplied by the ventilator, blood samples from the patient are analyzed to determine the metabolic rate. The volume of air required and the number of times per minute the patient needs to breathe in order to maintain the desired metabolic rate, is also calculated, and positive air pressure administers the correct mix and volume into the lungs, which deflate passively. Today's sophisticated hospital respiratory care units may utilize up to 15 different kinds of respirators. Ventilators assist patients unable to breathe for themselves, who suffer from degenerative muscle disease, or **burns** to the nose and throat. Some patients may be connected to a ventilator for months at a time, in which case a breathing tube is surgically inserted directly into the trachea (windpipe). Today, in such places as Stanford University Hospital in California, the iron lung of the 1950s is making a comeback due to it's non-invasive, negative air pressure which eliminates the possibility of infections or scarring prevalent with respirators which require a **tracheotomy**. The iron lung can also be used at home to help a patient rest respiratory muscles either during the day or night.

Miniature ventilators are also used to help premature babies breathe and provide temporary breathing assistance to patients undergoing surgery requiring anesthesia. At University Hospital in Stony Brook, New York, mini-iron lungs are used for some patients. Nicknamed *turtles* because of their green color and shell-like shape, these miniature iron lungs can be strapped onto a patient's chest. For treating **sleep apnea**, a **sleep disorder** in which breath becomes obstructed, a small ventilator about the size of a vanity case is connected to a tiny mask placed over the nose. Intermittent positive air pressure is delivered through the nostrils and the timing can be preset to correspond with the patient's natural breathing rate.

IRRITABLE BOWEL SYNDROME

Irritable bowel syndrome (IBS) is a common intestinal condition characterized by abdominal **pain** and cramps; changes in bowel movements (**diarrhea**, **constipation**, or both); gassiness; bloating; **nausea**; and other symptoms. There is no cure for IBS. Much about the condition remains unknown or poorly understood; however, dietary changes, drugs, and psychological treatment are often able to eliminate or substantially cureduce its symptoms.

IBS was once called—among other things—colitis, spastic colon, nervous colon, and spastic bowel. Some of these names reflected the now outdated belief that IBS is a purely psychological disorder, a product of the patient's imagination. Although modern medicine recognizes that **stress** can trigger IBS attacks, medical specialists agree that IBS is a genuine physical disorder—or group of disorders—with specific identifiable characteristics.

The symptoms of IBS tend to rise and fall in intensity rather than growing steadily worse over time. They always include abdominal pain, which may be relieved by defecation; diarrhea or constipation; or diarrhea alternating with constipation. Other symptoms—which vary from person to person—include cramps; gassiness; bloating; nausea; a powerful and uncontrollable urge to defecate (urgency); passage of a sticky fluid (mucus) during bowel movements; or the feeling after finishing a bowel movement that the bowels are still not completely empty. The accepted diagnostic criteria—known as the Rome criteria—require at least three months of continuous or recurrent symptoms before IBS can be confirmed.

Researchers remain unsure about the cause or causes of IBS. It is called a functional disorder because it is thought to result from changes in the activity of the major part of the large intestine (the colon). After food is digested by the stomach and small intestine, the undigested material passes in liquid form into the colon, which absorbs water and salts. This process may take several days. In a healthy person the colon is quiet during most of that period except after meals, when its muscles contract in a series of wavelike movements called peristalsis. Peristalsis helps absorption by bringing the undigested material into contact with the colon wall. It also pushes undigested material that has been converted into solid or semisolid feces toward the rectum, where it remains until defecation. In IBS, however, the normal rhythm and intensity of peristalsis is disrupted. Sometimes there is too little peristalsis, which can slow the passage of undigested material through the colon and cause constipation. Sometimes there is too much, which has the opposite effect and causes diarrhea.

Some kinds of food and drink appear to play a key role in triggering IBS attacks. Food and drink that healthy people can ingest without any trouble may disrupt peristalsis in IBS patients, which probably explains why IBS attacks often occur shortly after meals. Chocolate, milk products, **caffeine** (in coffee, tea, colas, and other drinks), and large quantities of alcohol are some of the chief culprits. Other kinds of food have also been identified as problems, however, and the pattern of what can and cannot be tolerated is different for each person. Characteristically, IBS symptoms rarely occur at night and disrupt the patient's sleep.

Stress is an important factor in IBS because of the close nervous system connections between the brain and the intestines. Although researchers do not yet understand all of the links between changes in the **nervous system** and IBS, they point out the similarities between mild digestive upsets and IBS. Just as healthy people can feel nauseated or have an upset stomach when under stress, people with IBS react the same way, but to a greater degree. Finally, IBS symptoms sometimes intensify during **menstruation**, which suggests that female reproductive hormones are another trigger.

Diagnosing IBS is a fairly complex task because the disorder does not produce changes that can be identified during a physical examination or by laboratory tests. When IBS is suspected, the doctor (who can be either a family doctor or a specialist) needs to determine whether the patient's symptoms satisfy the Rome criteria. The doctor must rule out other conditions that resemble IBS by questioning the patient about his or her physical and mental health (the medical history), performing a **physical examination**, and ordering laboratory tests.

Dietary changes, sometimes supplemented by drugs or psychotherapy, are considered the key to successful treatment. A low-fat, high-fiber diet free of problem-causing substances such as lactose, caffeine, beans, cabbage, cucumbers, broccoli, fatty foods, alcohol, and medications should be followed. Bran or 15-25 grams a day of an over-the-counter psyllium laxative (Metamucil or Fiberall) may also help both constipation and diarrhea. The patient can still have milk or milk products if lactose intolerance is not a problem. People with irregular bowel habits—particularly constipated patients—may be helped by establishing set times for meals and bathroom visits.

Although a high-fiber diet remains the standard treatment for constipated patients, **laxatives** may be prescribed. Loperamide (Imodium) and cholestyramine (Questran) are suggested for diarrhea. Abdominal pain after meals can be reduced by taking **antispasmodic drugs** such as hyoscyamine (Anaspaz, Cystospaz, or Levsin) or dicyclomine (Bemote, Bentyl, or Di-Spaz) before eating.

Psychological counseling or behavioral therapy may be suggested for some patients to reduce anxiety and to learn to cope with the pain and other symptoms of IBS.

IBS is not a life-threatening condition. It does not cause intestinal bleeding or inflammation, nor does it cause other bowel diseases or **cancer**. Although IBS can last a lifetime, in up to 30% of cases the symptoms eventually disappear. Even if the symptoms cannot be eliminated, with appropriate treatment they can usually be brought under control to the point where IBS becomes merely an occasional inconvenience. Treatment requires a long-term commitment, however; six months or more may be needed before the patient notices substantial improvement.

Isolation

Isolation refers to the precautions that are taken in the hospital to prevent the spread of an infectious agent from an infected or colonized patient to susceptible persons. Isolation practices are designed to minimize the transmission of infection in the hospital, using current understanding of the way infections can transmit. Isolation should be done in a user friendly, well-accepted, inexpensive way that interferes as little as possible with patient care, minimizes patient discomfort, and avoids unnecessary use.

The type of precautions used should be viewed as a flexible scale that may range from the least to the most demanding methods of prevention. These methods should always take into account that differences exist in the way that diseases are spread. Recognition and understanding of these differences will avoid use of insufficient or unnecessary interventions.

Isolation practices can include placement in a private room or with a select roommate, the use of protective barriers such as masks, gowns and gloves, a special emphasis on handwashing (which is always very important), and special handling of contaminated articles. Because of the differences among infectious diseases, more than one of these precautions may be necessary to prevent spread of some diseases but may not be necessary for others.

The **Centers for Disease Control** and Prevention (CDC) and the Hospital Infection Control Practice Advisory Committee (HICPAC) have led the way in defining the guidelines for hospital-based infection precautions. The most current system recommended for use in hospitals consists of two levels of precautions. The first level is Standard Precautions which apply to all patients at all times because signs and symptoms of infection are not always obvious and therefore may unknowingly pose a risk for a susceptible person. The second level is known as Transmission-Based Precautions which are intended for individuals who have a known or suspected infection with certain organisms.

Frequently, patients are admitted to the hospital without a definite diagnosis, but with clues to suggest an infection. These patients should be isolated with the appropriate precautions until a definite diagnosis is made.

Standard Precautions define all the steps that should be taken to prevent spread of infection from person to person when there is an anticipated contact with:

- Blood
- Body fluids
- Secretions, such as phlegm
- Excretions, such as urine and feces (not including sweat) whether or not they contain visible blood
- Nonintact skin, such as an open wound
- Mucous membranes, such as the mouth cavity.

Standard Precautions includes the use of one or combinations of the following practices. The level of use will always depend on the anticipated contact with the patient:

- Handwashing, the most important infection control method
- Use of latex or other protective gloves
- Masks, eye protection and/or face shield
- Gowns
- Proper handling of soiled patient care equipment
- Proper environmental cleaning
- Minimal handling of soiled linen
- Proper disposal of needles and other sharp equipment such as scalpels
- Placement in a private room for patients who cannot maintain appropriate cleanliness or contain body fluids.

Transmission Based Precautions may be needed in addition to Standard Precautions for selected patients who are known or suspected to harbor certain infections. These precautions are divided into three categories that reflect the differences in the way infections are transmitted. Some diseases may require more than one isolation category.

Airborne Precautions prevent diseases that are transmitted by minute particles called droplet nuclei or contaminated dust particles. These particles, because of their size, can remain suspended in the air for long periods of time; even after the infected person has left the room. Some examples of diseases requiring these precautions are **tuberculosis**, **measles**, and **chickenpox**.

A patient needing Airborne Precautions should be assigned to a private room with special ventilation requirements. The door to this room must be closed at all possible times. If a patient must move from the isolation room to another area of the hospital, the patient should be wearing a mask during the transport. Anyone entering the isolation room to provide care to the patient must wear a special mask called a respirator.

Droplet Precautions prevent the spread of organisms that travel on particles much larger than the droplet nuclei. These particles do not spend much time suspended in the air, and usually do not travel beyond a several foot range from the patient. These particles are produced when a patient **cough**s, talks, or sneezes. Examples of disease requiring droplet precautions are meningococcal **meningitis** (a serious bacterial infection of the lining of the brain), **influenza**, **mumps**, and German measles (**rubella**).

Patients who require Droplet Precautions should be placed in a private room or with a roommate who is infected with the same organism. The door to the room may remain open. Health care workers will need to wear masks within three feet of the patient. Patients moving about the hospital away from the isolation room should wear a mask.

Contact Precautions prevent spread of organisms from an infected patient through direct (touching the patient) or indirect (touching surfaces or objects that that been in contact with the patient) contact. Examples of patients who might be placed in Contact Precautions are those infected with:

- **Antibiotic**-resistant bacteria
- **Hepatitis** A
- **Scabies**
- **Impetigo**
- Lice.

This type of precaution requires the patient to be placed in a private room or with a roommate who has the same infection. Health care workers should wear gloves when entering the room. They should change their gloves if they touch material that contains large volumes of organisms such as soiled dressings. Prior to leaving the room, health care workers should remove the gloves and wash their hands with medicated soap. In addition, they may need to wear protective gowns if there is a chance of contact with potentially infective materials such as **diarrhea** or wound drainage that cannot be contained or if there is likely to be extensive contact with the patient or environment.

Patient care items, such as a stethoscope, that are used for a patient in Contact Precautions should not be shared with other patients unless they are properly cleaned and disinfected before reuse. Patients should leave the isolation room infrequently.

Itching

Itching is an intense, distracting irritation or tickling sensation that may be felt all over the skin's surface, or confined to just one area. The medical term for itching is ''pruritus.''

Itching instinctively leads most people to scratch the affected area. Different people can tolerate different amounts of itching, and anyone's threshold of tolerance can be changed due to **stress**, emotions, and other factors. In general, itching is more severe if the skin is warm, and if there are few distractions. This is why people tend to notice itching more at night.

The reason for the sensation of itching is not well understood. While itching is the most noticeable symptom in many skin diseases, it doesn't necessarily mean that a person who feels itchy has a disease.

Stress and emotional upset can make itching worse, no matter what the underlying cause. If emotional problems are the primary reason for the itch, the condition is known as psychogenic itching. Some people become convinced that their itch is caused by a parasite; this conviction is often linked to burning sensations in the tongue, and may be caused by a major psychiatric disorder.

Generalized itching is a condition that occurs all over the body that may indicate a medical condition such as **diabetes mellitus**, **liver disease**, **kidney failure**, **jaundice**, **thyroid disorders** (and rarely, **cancer**). Blood disorders such as **leukemia**, and lymphatic conditions such as **Hodgkin's disease** may sometimes cause itching as well.

Some people may develop an itch without a rash when they take certain drugs (such as **aspirin**, codeine, cocaine); others may develop an itchy red ''drug rash'' or **hives** because of an allergy to a specific drug.

Itching also may be caused when any of the family of hookworm larvae penetrate the skin. This includes swimmer's itch and creeping eruption caused by cat or dog hookworm, and ground itch caused by the ''true'' hookworm.

Many skin conditions cause an itchy rash. These include:

- Atopic dermatitis
- **Chickenpox**
- Contact dermatitis
- **Dermatitis** herpetiformis (occasionally)
- Eczema
- Fungus infections (such as **athlete's foot**)
- Hives (urticaria)
- Insect bites
- Lice
- **Lichen planus**
- Neurodermatitis (lichen simplex chronicus)
- **Psoriasis** (occasionally)
- **Scabies**.

On the other hand, itching all over the body can be caused by something as simple as bathing too often, which removes the skins natural oils and may make the skin too dry and scaly.

Localized itching refers to specific itchy areas that may occur if a person comes in contact with soap, detergents, and wool or other rough-textured, scratchy material. Adults who have **hemorrhoids**, anal fissure, or persistent **diarrhea** may notice itching around the anus (called ''pruritus ani''). In children, itching in this area is most likely due to worms.

Intense itching in the external genitalia in women (''pruritus vulvae'') may be due to **candidiasis**, hormonal changes, or the use of certain spermicides or vaginal suppositories, ointments, or deodorants.

It's also common for older people to suffer from dry, itchy skin (especially on the back) for no obvious reason. Younger people also may notice dry, itchy skin in cold weather. Itching is also a common complaint during **pregnancy**.

Itching is a symptom that is quite obvious to its victim. Someone who itches all over should seek medical care. Because itching can be caused by such a wide variety of triggers, a complete **physical exam** and medical history will help diagnose the underlying problem. A variety of blood and stool tests may help determine the underlying cause.

Antihistamines such as diphenhydramine (Benadryl) can help relieve itching caused by hives, but won't affect itching from other causes. Most antihistamines also make people sleepy, which can help patients sleep who would otherwise be awake from the itch.

Specific treatment of itching depends on the underlying condition that causes it. In general, itchy skin should be treated very gently. While scratching may temporarily ease the itch, in the long run scratching just makes it worse. In addition, scratching can lead to an endless cycle of itch—scratch—more itching.

To avoid the urge to scratch, a person can apply a cooling or soothing lotion or cold compress when the urge to scratch occurs. Soaps are often irritating to the skin, and can make an itch worse; they should be avoided, or used only when necessary.

Creams or ointments containing cortisone may help control the itch from insect bites, contact dermatitis or eczema. Cortisone cream should not be applied to the face unless a doctor prescribes it.

Probably the most common cause of itching is dry skin. There are a number of simple things a person can do to ease the annoying itch:

- Don't wear tight clothes
- Avoid synthetic fabrics
- Don't take long baths
- Wash the area in lukewarm water with a little baking soda
- For generalized itching, take a lukewarm shower
- Try a lukewarm oatmeal (or Aveeno) bath for generalized itching
- Apply bath oil or lotion (without added colors or scents) right after bathing.

While most cases of itching go away when the underlying cause is treated successfully, people who itch as a result of mental problems or stress should seek help from a mental health expert.

There are certain things people can do to avoid itchy skin. Patients who tend toward itchy skin should:

- Avoid a daily bath
- Use only lukewarm water when bathing
- Use only gentle soap
- Pat dry, not rub dry, after bathing, leaving a bit of water on the skin
- Apply a moisture-holding ointment or cream after the bath
- Use a humidifier in the home.

Patients who are allergic to certain substances, medications, and so on can avoid the resulting itch if they avoid contact with the allergen. Avoiding insect bites, bee stings, poison ivy and so on can prevent the resulting itch. Treating sensitive skin carefully, avoiding overdrying of the skin, and protecting against diseases that cause itchy **rashes** are all good ways to avoid itching.

IUD

An IUD is an intrauterine device made of plastic and/or copper that is inserted into the womb (uterus) by way of the vaginal canal. One type releases a hormone (progesterone), and is replaced each year. The second type is made of copper and can be left in place for five years. The most common shape in current use is a plastic ''T'' which is wrapped with copper wire.

IUDs are used to prevent **pregnancy** and are considered to be 95-98% effective. It should be noted that IUDs offer no protection against the acquired immunodeficiency syndrome (**AIDS**) virus or other **sexually transmitted diseases** (STDs).

IUDs are placed in the uterus by physicians. Prior to placement the doctor will take a medical history, do a **physical examination**, and take a **Pap test**. Women who have had tubal pregnancies, an abnormal Pap smear, or abnormal vaginal bleeding are generally disqualified from using this form of **contraception**. Also, women who have STDs, an allergy to copper, severe **pain** with periods (**menstruation**), sex with multiple partners, or who are currently pregnant are not eligible for an IUD. There are no age restrictions.

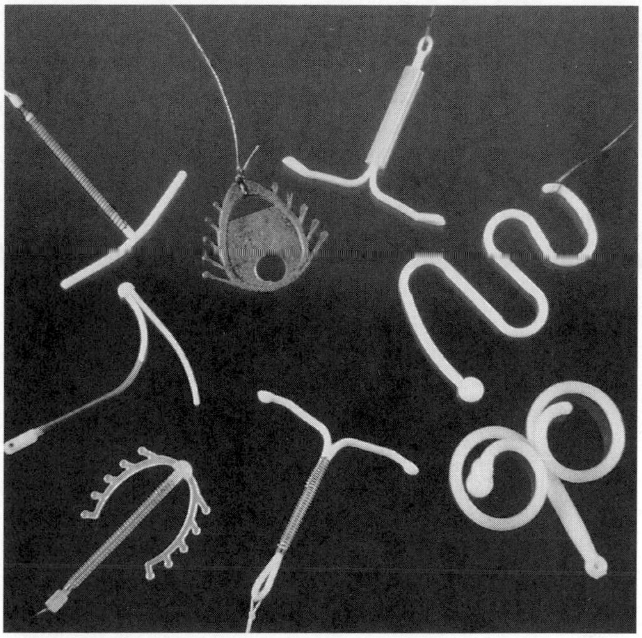

Various kinds of IUDs.

There is continuing controversy over exactly how IUDs prevent pregnancy. Some researchers think pregnancy is controlled by preventing conception (fertilization), while others believe that the devices prevent embryo attachment to the uterine wall (implantation).

IUDs which release a hormone may prevent pregnancy in several ways. Since one hormonal response is a thickening of the mucous at the entrance to the uterus, it is more difficult for the sperm to gain entry. This prevents the sperm from reaching an ovum. At the same time, the lining of the uterus becomes thinner, making it more difficult for a fertilized egg to implant itself in the uterus. The copper device slowly releases copper which is believed to weaken and perhaps kill sperm. An alternate explanation is that these objects ''sweep'' the uterus, dislodging any fertilized egg that attempts to implant itself. In addition, both devices tend to cause a mild inflammatory reaction in the lining of the uterus which also has an adverse impact on implantation.

After the physician approves the use of an IUD, the woman's genital area is washed thoroughly with soap and water in preparation of IUD insertion. The opening into the uterus (cervix) will also be cleaned with an antiseptic such as an iodine solution. Actual IUD insertion takes about five minutes, during which a local **anesthesia** is used to reduce any discomfort associated with the procedure. A plastic string connected to the IUD will hang out of the uterus into the vagina. The string is used to periodically check the position of the IUD.

The woman will be taught to watch for the signs and symptoms of potential complications and how to check the string, which should be done at least once a week. To check the string, the woman should first wash her hands with soap and water. From a squatting position, or with one foot elevated (such as on a chair), she should gently insert her finger into the vagina until she locates the cervix. If she cannot feel the string, if the string feels longer than it should, or if she can feel part of the IUD, she should notify her physician immediately. Additional information that needs to be reported includes painful intercourse and unusual discharge from the vagina.

Serious risks from IUDs are rare, but include heavy bleeding, pain, infection, cramps, **pelvic inflammatory disease**, perforation of the uterus, and **ectopic pregnancy**.

J

Jacob, François (1920-)

French biologist

François Jacob was born in June 1920 in Nancy, Meurthe-et-Moselle, France. He intended to be a surgeon, but injuries he sustained during World War II prevented this, and he switched to research. He received his M.D. in 1947 from the University of Paris and his Doctor of Science in 1954 from the Sorbonne. He then joined the faculty of the Pasteur Institute, becoming head of the Department of Cellular Genetics in 1960. He became a professor of cellular **genetics** at the College de France in 1964.

Jacob's experiments with ***E. coli*** showed that the medium in which the bacteria are grown affects the type and amount of enzymes the bacteria produce (induction). From this, the three scientists proposed that the bacteria regulate enzyme production. If grown in the sugar glucose, the bacteria produce very little of the enzyme β-galactosidase, because they do not require it for metabolizing glucose. But if they grow in lactose, *E. coli* bacteria produce much more β-galactosidase, which they need to metabolize lactose.

To explain how the bacteria regulate enzyme production, Jacob (with Andre Lwoff and Jacques Monod) theorized that there are three types of genes, a gene being a deoxyribonucleic acid (DNA) triplet or triplet cluster. An operon is a gene cluster composed of two types of genes: Z (structural) genes, which carry the instructions for protein production, such as for the β-galactosidase, and O (operator) genes, which control whether the Z genes' instructions are carried to the cell's ribosomes for protein production. The third type, called R (regulator) genes, instruct production of proteins that control the activity of other genes. In *E. coli*, when lactose is not present, an R gene instructs production of a repressor protein that binds to the O gene, turning the gene ''off'' by preventing it from being copied by ribonucleic acid (RNA). When lactose is present, the repressor binds to it rather than the O gene. This allows the O gene to turn the Z gene ''on.'' Research showed the theory to be correct.

Jacobi, Abraham (1830-1919)

German-American physician

The father of American pediatrics, Abraham Jacobi championed children's care in both academic and medical spheres. During his life, every medical school in the United States established a department of pediatrics.

Jacobi earned his medical degree at the University of Bonn in 1851. When he traveled to Berlin to take his state medical exams, he was arrested and held in prison for nearly two years on a charge of promoting political and social reform in the German revolution of 1848. Though he viewed his imprisonment as a badge of honor, he left Germany in 1853 to avoid being arrested again.

Jacobi arrived in New York later in 1853, where he practiced general medicine, surgery, and obstetrics, as was the custom of most of his contemporaries. Medical specialization was frowned on as being degrading, making physicians too much like tradesmen.

Jacobi wrote prolifically, publishing 200 articles and books during his career. His early contributions to the *New York Medical Journal* helped establish the field of pediatrics. In 1857, Jacobi lectured on childhood diseases of the larynx at the College of Physicians and Surgeons, his first formal pediatric lecture.

In 1860, Jacobi accepted a position as professor of infantile pathology and therapeutics at New York Medical College (not connected with the modern medical school of the same name). This appointment signaled a turning point as it was the first pediatric medical position and launched pediatrics as a medical and academic discipline in the United States.

In his first year at New York Medical College, Jacobi established a method of bedside clinical teaching, a landmark in medical education. Up to that point, physicians did not conduct teaching rounds on medical wards. In the same year, Jacobi also founded the first pediatric free clinic.

Jacobi accepted the position of clinical professor of diseases of children at New York University Medical College in

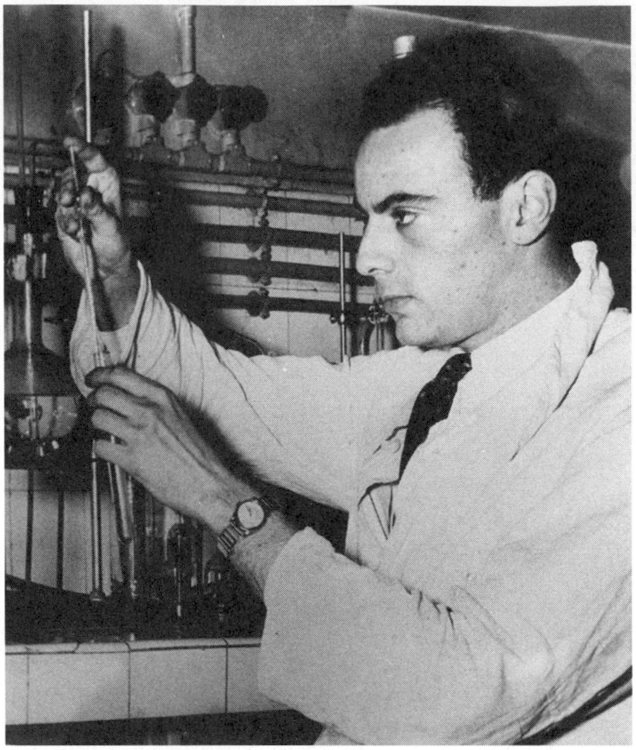

François Jacob

1865. The College of Physicians and Surgeons (Columbia University) appointed Jacobi as professor of clinical pediatrics in 1870. Jacobi worked at almost every hospital in New York, but he concentrated on the Jews Hospital (later Mount Sinai Hospital), where he set up the first outpatient pediatric clinic in 1874. By 1878, the Jews Hospital had the first department of pediatrics in a US general hospital. Jacobi declined several invitations to accept prestigious medical appointments in Germany.

Throughout his career, Jacobi took care to balance professional success with social commitment, and he advocated medical care for children on the basis of social justice. Though he tempered his socialist views later in life, he corresponded with Karl Marx through the 1860s. Jacobi is best recognized for his achievements in infant **nutrition**. He studied **breast feeding** and safe breast milk substitutes. After the safety of pasteurization (**Louis Pasteur**) was proven, he fought to dispel the old belief that raw milk was beneficial. He advised parents to boil milk until bubbles appeared and advocated diluting milk. His support of boiled milk was thought to have saved more lives than any measure besides **antibiotics**.

Jacobi also studied **diphtheria**, gastrointestinal disorders, dental disease, and treatment of pediatric diseases. He invented the first laryngoscope but never patented it. He was one of the early advocates of birth control. Jacobi wrote about medical history and specialized in topics of pediatrics in the era of 1800, **meningitis**, **tracheotomy** and **nursing**. Jacobi's best known text is *Intestinal Diseases of Infants and Children*, published in 1887.

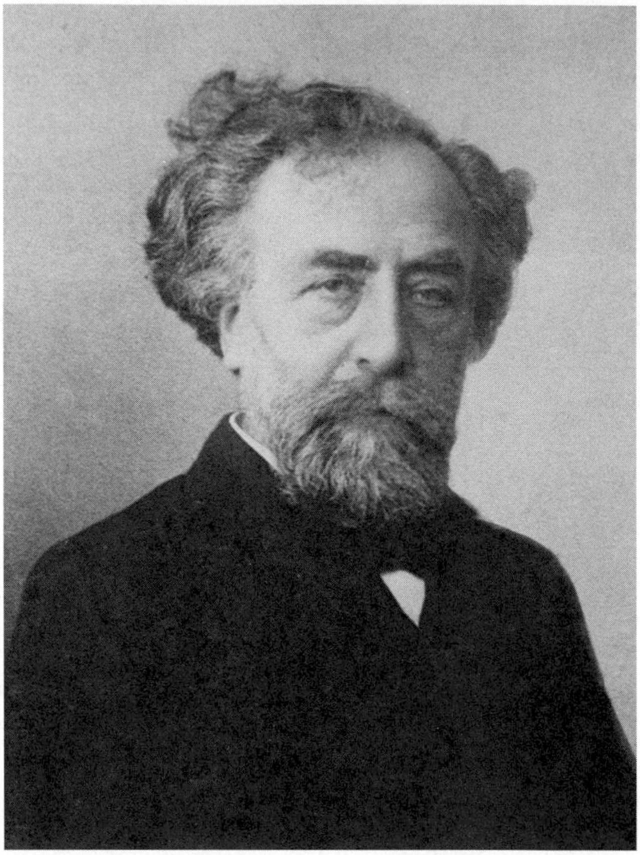

Abraham Jacobi

Jacobi was one of the first to treat diphtheric **croup** with intubation, the passage of a tube down the throat to help the patient breathe. Previously, physicians had been treating diphtheric croup by cutting into the larynx to establish an airway. Jacobi used diphtheria antitoxin as soon as it was available and advocated its use. In 1880, he published monograph on diphtheria.

Jacobi, who had been widowed twice, married the physician Mary Corinna Putnam in 1873. Mary Putnam Jacobi worked tirelessly with her husband on issues of child welfare and aid for the needy. They coauthored an article on infant feeding and Mary Putnam Jacobi published nearly 100 articles on her own, in addition to receiving the Boyleston Prize from Harvard. In 1883, the Jacobis were devastated to lose their 7-year-old son to diphtheria.

Professional recognition of pediatrics took another leap forward when Jacobi established the Pediatric Section of the American Medical Association in 1880, and the Pediatric Section of the New York Academy of Medicine followed in 1885. With the founding of the American Pediatric Society in 1888, Jacobi set up the first independent medical specialty society in the United States. Jacobi also served as president of the American Medical Association in 1912. Throughout his career, he pressed for regular attendance at medical society meetings. He wrote for numerous medical journals and lobbied Congress to publish the *Index Catalogue of the Library of the Surgeon General's Office,*

Jacobi had nearly completed his autobiography when a 1918 fire destroyed his only manuscript, along with his personal papers, letters and notes. He died within a year. Jacobi was honored with pediatric divisions named after him at Lenox Hill and Roosevelt hospitals in New York City. The Albert Einstein College of Medicine established the Abraham Jacobi Hospital as a memorial

JARVIK, ROBERT K. (1946-)

American physician, biomedical engineer, and inventor

Physician Robert K. Jarvik is designer and biomedical engineer of the first **artificial heart** used as a permanent implant in a human being. The device, named Jarvik–7, was implanted in Barney Clark on December 2, 1982, at the University of Utah Medical Center. Mr. Clark lived 112 days with the artificial heart. Jarvik has also performed research on other artificial organs and is author of more than 60 technical articles. He holds a number of patents on medical devices and has received numerous awards, including two citations of "Inventor of the Year"—from Intellectual Property Owners in 1982 and from National Inventors Hall of Fame in 1983. Jarvik also holds honorary doctorates from Syracuse University and Hahnemann University, presented in 1983 and 1985 respectively.

Robert Koffler Jarvik was born May 11, 1946, in Midland, Michigan, son of physician Norman Eugene Jarvik and Edythe Koffler Jarvik, and was raised in Stamford, Connecticut. As a teenager, Jarvik was a tinkerer and inventor. He watched his father in surgery and before he graduated from high school had invented an automatic stapler for use during surgery, which would replace the process of manually sewing up living body parts. He entered Syracuse University in 1964 and took courses in mechanical drawing and architecture, but his father's heart disease prompted him to change his course of study. Jarvik began premedical course work and graduated in 1968 with a bachelor's degree in zoology. His immediate plans were stalled when mediocre grades prevented him from acceptance into an American medical school. As an alternative, he attended medical school at the University of Bologna in Italy. After two years he returned to the United States to pursue a degree in occupational biomechanics at New York University, receiving an M.A. in 1971.

Shortly following graduation, Jarvik was hired as an assistant design engineer at the University of Utah by Willem Kolff, a leading expert in the development of artificial organs. Dr. Kolff had been working on inventing an artificial heart since the mid–1950s. In 1967 he had been appointed head of a new division at the University of Utah, which became known as the Institute of Biomedical Engineering. Its primary project was to develop an artificial heart.

Jarvik's achievements in biomedical engineering are closely tied to his employment at the institute, as it was headed by a world expert on man-made organs who had been working on developing an artificial heart for more than fifteen years, and had the full institutional support of the University of Utah, an essential condition for such a large-scale and complex medical project. Jarvik's inventive genius soon solved several problems associated with the devices. By the early 1980s, Jarvik developed an artificial heart that could be implanted in a human being. While working at the institute, Jarvik received his M.D. from the University of Utah in 1976.

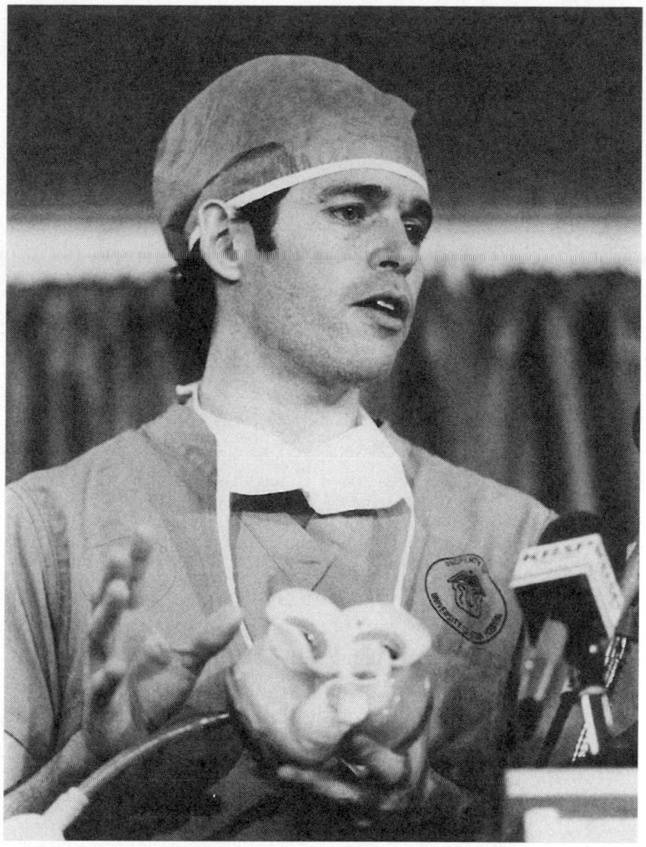

Robert K. Jarvik

The artificial heart program at the Utah institute aimed to re-create the lower two chambers or ventricles of the heart, which comprise the pumping portion of the organ. Creating the pump with a suitable power-source was the major obstacle facing the project. The ideal solution was considered a single unit containing both the pump and the power source that would be completely encased in the recipient's body. Before Jarvik arrived, Kolff had worked hard to create an electrical power source and, after failing at that, a nuclear one. When this strategy also failed, Kolff decided to concentrate on the pump and to rely on power from compressed air from a machine outside the body connected by tubes to the artificial heart. Scientifically, the decision was sound, as it divided a complex problem into two simpler parts. In practicality, however, it meant that recipients of the artificial heart would be permanently attached by tubes to a machine.

When Jarvik arrived at the institute, he immediately began working on the "Kwann-Gett heart," which was designed in 1971 by a member of Kolff's team, Clifford S. Kwann-Gett. This device used a rubber diaphragm as the pumping element that forced blood in and out of the artificial heart. The diaphragm represented an improvement in that it lowered the possibility of mechanical failure. However, it also caused blood to clot on its surface, which could cause death. Jarvik's improved version, called the "Jarvik–3," was shaped to better fit the anatomy of the experimental animals. In addition, the rubber of the diaphragm had been replaced by three highly flexible layers of a smooth polyurethane called 'biomer,' which eliminated the clotting problem. By the mid–1970s, Jarvik was working on a version intended for the human body. The plastic and aluminum device would replace the lower pumping chambers, known as the ventricles, and would be attached to the two upper chambers of the heart known as the atria, which receive blood from the veins. Such a device, called the "Jarvik–7," was implanted into Barney Clark on December 2, 1982.

Clark was a 61-year-old retired dentist suffering from **cardiomyopathy**, a degenerative disease of the heart muscles. He was a terminally ill man who believed that the experimental surgery would give him hope and would also contribute to the progress of medical science. In a seven and a half hour operation performed by surgeon William C. DeVries with assistance from Jarvik, Clark's ventricles were replaced by the Jarvik–7 which was driven by an outside air-compressor connected to the artificial heart by tubes. The surgery received world-wide publicity. Shortly after the operation, Clark suffered from disabling brain seizures. He died less than four months later. The artificial heart itself (except for a malfunctioning valve, which was replaced) functioned throughout, and was still pumping when Clark died of multiple organ failure. The surgery performed on Clark has provoked debate concerning various issues of medical ethics.

In 1976, Jarvik became a vice-president of Symbion, Inc., (originally known as Kolff Associates) an artificial organs research firm founded by Dr. Kolff. Jarvik was an aggressive officer of the company, and was appointed president in 1981. Seeking venture capital, Jarvik arranged a deal with an outside investment firm in which Kolff was to be deliberately excluded from direct management of the company. The move became the source of friction between Kolff and Jarvik, but has since been resolved. Under Jarvik's direction, the company branched out to include development and manufacturing of other organs, including an artificial ear.

After Barney Clark's surgery, a number of other modified Jarvik hearts were implanted but none of the recipients lived more than 620 days. The Jarvik–7 was also frequently and more successfully used as a temporary measure for patients awaiting a natural heart transplant. After Jarvik's own departure from the University of Utah and Symbion in 1987, the Jarvik–7 artificial heart did not fare well. Federal funding for the Jarvik project stopped in 1988, and artificial heart implantation was restricted to temporary implantation only. In 1990, the **Food and Drug Administration** (FDA) withdrew approval for the experimental use of the Jarvik–7, citing Symbion's poor quality control in the manufacturing process and inadequate service of equipment.

In 1987, Jarvik moved to New York City where he became president of his own company, Jarvik Research, Inc. In the same year, he married Marilyn vos Savant, a writer who is reported by the *Guinness Book of World Records* to have the highest IQ score in the world and whose writings include a well-known column in *Parade* magazine. Jarvik had been previously married to journalist Elaine Levin, with whom he had two children, Tyler and Kate. Jarvik continued artificial heart research, concentrating on the Jarvik 2000, described by Julie Baumgard in *New York* as a "rotary hydrodynamic axial-flow pump" in which "the valves have been eliminated and the whole device miniaturized." Based on principles quite different from the Jarvik–7, both the pump and its power source would be implanted entirely inside the heart. In an article in *After Barney Clark,* contributor Renée C. Fox described Jarvik as the "boyishly glamorous culture hero of bioengineering in whom the values of the 1960s and of the 1980s seem to be joined." Jarvik's interests are skiing, weight-lifting, poetry, art, sculpting, and physics.

JASON, ROBERT S. (1901-1984)

African American physician and pathologist

Robert S. Jason was the first African American to earn a Ph.D. in pathology. Jason had a medical degree as well and served as head of the department of **pathology** at Howard University and later as dean of its college of medicine. During his last years at Howard, he was coordinator for design and planning of its new University Hospital. In recognition of his many contributions to the university, the department of pathology at Howard's College of Medicine established in 1967 the Robert S. Jason Award in Pathology.

Robert Stewart Jason was born in Santurce, Puerto Rico on November 29, 1901. He was the son of Reverend Howard Talbot Jason, a Presbyterian missionary who was originally from Maryland, and his missionary wife, Lena B. (Wright) Jason. After attending local schools in Corozal, Puerto Rico and graduating from the Polytechnic Institute of San German, Puerto Rico, Jason entered Lincoln University in Pennsylvania and received his B.A. degree in 1924. He then attended the Howard University College of Medicine in Washington, D.C., and was awarded his M.D. degree in 1928. From the local schools of Puerto Rico through college and medical school, Jason was regularly ranked first in his class. In 1929 he completed his internship at Freedman's Hospital in Washington, D.C., and chose to continue his studies at the University of Chicago, where he was awarded his Ph.D. in pathology in 1932.

During that time, Jason joined the medical faculty at Howard's College of Medicine as an assistant professor of pathology. In 1934 he became associate professor and acting head of the department of pathology, and, by 1937, he was the department head and a full professor as well. He then served as vice dean of the college of medicine from 1946 to 1953, and as dean from 1955 to 1965. In that year he took on a new position as coordinator for the design and planning stages of a new facility to replace Howard's old Freedman's Hospital. He retired as professor emeritus in 1970 and lived in San Diego, California, before moving to New York City in 1979. As a pathologist, he was concerned with the structural and functional changes in cells, tissues, and organs caused by disease, and he focused specifically during his research career on the pathology of **syphilis** and **tuberculosis**. As department head and dean, he ran an extremely efficient operation, and these same skills were used to plan and organize Howard's new hospital.

Besides research, teaching, and administration, Jason held many professional appointments. He was a consultant in pathology to the National Institutes of Health from 1955 to 1970, consultant to the Veterans Administration Hospital from 1960 to 1970, member of the International Committee on Health of the Agency for International Development, and member of the National Advisory Council on Education for the Health Professions from 1964 to 1968. Jason also received several honors and awards during his long career. Besides two honorary doctorates and several awards from Howard University, he received the Professional Achievement Award given by the University of Chicago Alumni Association in 1970 and the Distinguished Service Award of the National Medical Association in 1969. Jason considered the most significant honor he received to be Howard University's College of Medicine naming an award after him in 1967. According to the *Journal of the National Medical Association,* "it is presented to a graduating student chosen on the basis of distinguished scholastic achievements, demonstrated interest in fundamental aspects of disease, integrity, self-discipline, and compassion, attributes common to the recipient and Dr. Robert S. Jason."

Jason was a volunteer with the American Cancer Society as well as a member of the American Medical Association, the American Association of Pathologists and Bacteriologists, and the International Academy of Pathologists. He was also a fellow of the College of American Pathologists and belonged to Alpha Omega Alpha (a national medical honor society), Alpha Phi Alpha Fraternity, and the Alpha Pi Boule of Sigma Pi Phi Fraternity.

Jason died of **Alzheimer's disease** at his home in New York City on April 6, 1984. He was survived by his wife, the former Elizabeth Gaddis, a daughter, Mrs. Jean Elizabeth Wright, a son, Robert S. Jason, Jr. M.D., and one brother and four sisters.

JAUNDICE

Jaundice is a condition in which a person's skin and the whites of the eyes are discolored yellow due to an increased level of bile pigments in the blood resulting from **liver disease**. Jaundice is sometimes called icterus, from a Greek word for the condition.

In order to understand jaundice, it is useful to know about the role of the liver in producing bile. The most important function of the liver is the processing of chemical waste products like cholesterol and excreting them into the intestines as bile. The liver is the premier chemical factory in the body—most incoming and outgoing chemicals pass through it. It is the first stop for all nutrients, toxins, and drugs absorbed by the digestive tract. The liver also collects chemicals from the blood for processing. Many of these outward-bound chemicals are excreted into the bile. One particular substance, bilirubin, is yellow. Bilirubin is a product of the breakdown of hemoglobin, which is the protein inside red blood cells. If bilirubin cannot leave the body, it accumulates and discolors other tissues. The normal total level of bilirubin in blood serum is between 0.2 mg/dL and 1.2 mg/dL. When it rises to 3 mg/dL or higher, the person's skin and the whites of the eyes become noticeably yellow.

Bile is formed in the liver. It then passes into the network of hepatic bile ducts, which join to form a single tube. A branch of this tube carries bile to the gallbladder, where it is stored, concentrated, and released on a signal from the stomach. Food entering the stomach is the signal that stimulates the gallbladder to release the bile. The tube, which is now called the common bile duct, continues to the intestines. Before the common bile duct reaches the intestines, it is joined by another duct from the pancreas. The bile and the pancreatic juice enter the intestine through a valve called the ampulla of Vater. After entering the intestine, the bile and pancreatic secretions together help in the process of digestion.

There are many different causes for jaundice, but they can be divided into three categories based on where they start—before, in, or after the liver (pre-hepatic, hepatic, and post-hepatic). When bilirubin begins its life cycle, it cannot be dissolved in water. The liver changes it so that it is soluble in water. These two types of bilirubin are called unconjugated (insoluble) and conjugated (soluble). Blood tests can easily distinguish between these two types of bilirubin.

Bilirubin begins as hemoglobin in the blood-forming organs, primarily the bone marrow. If the production of red blood cells (RBCs) falls below normal, the extra hemoglobin finds its way into the bilirubin cycle and adds to the pool.

Once hemoglobin is in the red cells of the blood, it circulates for the life span of those cells. The hemoglobin that is released when the cells die is turned into bilirubin. If for any reason the RBCs die at a faster rate than usual, bilirubin can accumulate in the blood and cause jaundice.

Many disorders speed up the death of red blood cells. The process of red blood cell destruction is called hemolysis, and the diseases that cause it are called hemolytic disorders. If red blood cells are destroyed faster than they can be produced, the patient develops **anemia**. Hemolysis can occur in a number of diseases, disorders, conditions, and medical procedures, including **malaria**; as a side effects of certain drugs, including some antibiotic and anti-**tuberculosis** medicines, drugs that regulate the heartbeat, and levodopa, a drug used to treat **Parkinson's disease**); certain drugs in combination with a hereditary enzyme deficiency known as glucose-6-phosphate dehydrogenase (G6PD); poisons (snake and spider venom, certain bacterial toxins, copper, and some organic industrial chemicals directly attack the membranes of red blood cells); artificial heart valves; hereditary RBC disorders; enlargement of the spleen; diseases of the small blood vessels; immune reactions to RBCs; **transfusions**; **kidney failure** and other serious diseases; **erythroblastosis fetalis**, a disease of newborns marked by the presence of too many immature red blood cells in the baby's blood; and high bilirubin levels in newborns.

Normal newborn jaundice is the result of two conditions occurring at the same time—a pre-hepatic and a hepatic source of excess bilirubin. First of all, the baby at birth immediately begins converting hemoglobin from a fetal type to an adult type. The fetal type of hemoglobin was able to extract oxygen from the lower levels of oxygen in the mother's blood. At birth the infant can extract oxygen directly from his or her own lungs and does not need the fetal hemoglobin any more. So fetal hemoglobin is removed from the system and replaced with adult hemoglobin. The resulting bilirubin loads the system and places demands on the liver to clear it. But the liver is not quite ready for the task, so there is a period of a week or so when the liver has to catch up. During that time the baby is jaundiced.

Liver diseases of all kinds threaten the organ's ability to keep up with bilirubin processing. **Starvation**, circulating infections, certain medications, **hepatitis**, and **cirrhosis** can all cause hepatic jaundice, as can certain hereditary defects of liver chemistry, including Gilbert's syndrome and Crigler-Najjar syndrome.

Post-hepatic forms of jaundice include the jaundices caused by failure of soluble bilirubin to reach the intestines after it has left the liver. These disorders are called obstructive jaundices. The most common cause of obstructive jaundice is the presence of gallstones in the ducts of the biliary system. Other causes have to do with **birth defects** and infections that damage the bile ducts; drugs; infections; cancers; and physical injury. Some drugs—and **pregnancy** on rare occasions—simply cause the bile in the ducts to stop flowing.

Certain chemicals in bile may cause **itching** when too much of them ends up in the skin. In newborns, insoluble bilirubin may get into the brain and do permanent damage. Longstanding jaundice may upset the balance of chemicals in the bile and cause stones to form. Apart from these potential complications and the discoloration of skin and eyes, jaundice by itself is inoffensive. Other symptoms are determined by the disease producing the jaundice.

In many cases the diagnosis of jaundice is suggested by the appearance of the patient's eyes and complexion. The doctor will ask the patient to lie flat on the examining table in order to feel (palpate) the liver and spleen for enlargement and to evaluate any abdominal **pain**. The location and severity of abdominal pain and the presence or absence of fever help the doctor to distinguish between hepatic and obstructive jaundice.

Disorders of blood formation can be diagnosed by more thorough examination of the blood or the bone marrow, where blood is made. Occasionally a bone marrow biopsy is required, but usually the blood itself will reveal the diagnosis. The spleen can be evaluated by an ultrasound examination or a nuclear scan if the **physical examination** has not yielded enough information.

Liver disease is usually assessed from blood studies alone, but again a biopsy may be necessary to clarify less obvious conditions. A liver **biopsy** is performed at the bedside. The doctor uses a thin needle to take a tiny core of tissue from the liver. The tissue sample is sent to the laboratory for examination under a microscope.

Newborns are more likely to have problems with jaundice if:

- They are premature.
- They are Asian or Native Americans.
- They have been bruised during the birth process.
- They have lost too much weight during the first few days.
- They are born at high altitude.
- The mother has diabetes.
- Labor had to be induced.

Disease in the biliary system can be identified by imaging techniques, of which there are many. X rays are taken a day after swallowing a contrast agent that is secreted into the bile. This study gives functional as well as anatomical information. There are several ways of injecting x ray dye directly into the bile ducts. It can be done through a thin needle pushed straight into the liver or through a scope passed through the stomach that can inject dye into the Ampulla of Vater. CT and MRI scans are very useful for imaging certain conditions like cancers in and around the liver or gall stones in the common bile duct.

Newborns are the only major category of patients in whom the jaundice itself requires attention. Because the insoluble bilirubin can get into the brain, the amount in the blood must not go over certain levels. If there is reason to suspect increased hemolysis in the newborn, the bilirubin level must be measured repeatedly during the first few days of life. If the level of bilirubin shortly after birth threatens to go too high, treatment must begin immediately. Exchanging most of the baby's blood was the only way to reduce the amount of bilirubin until a few decades ago. Then it was discovered that bright blue light will render the bilirubin harmless. Now jaundiced babies are fitted with eye protection and placed under bright fluorescent lights. The light chemically alters the bilirubin in the blood as it passes through the baby's skin.

Hemolytic diseases are treated, if at all, with medications and blood transfusions, except in the case of a large spleen. Surgical removal of the spleen (splenectomy) can sometimes cure hemolytic anemia. Drugs that cause hemolysis or arrest the flow of bile must be stopped immediately.

Most liver diseases have no specific cure, but the liver is so robust that it can heal from severe damage and regenerate itself from a small remnant of its original tissue.

JAW WIRING

Jaw wiring (also known as maxillomandibular fixation) is a surgical procedure where metal pins and wires are anchored into the jaw bones and surrounding tissues to keep an injured jaw from moving.

Jaw wiring keeps the bones aligned and stable while the jaw heals. Wiring the jaw may also be used if it's necessary to remove or reconstruct the jaw as a result of **cancer** or disease. Wiring the jaws shut also has been used in the past as a weight loss aid in cases of extreme **obesity** where other treatments had failed, although this procedure is rarely used for that purpose today.

Jaw wiring surgery can be performed by an oral surgeon or specially trained dentist called a maxillofacial surgeon, or by a doctor specializing in surgeries of the head and neck (otolaryngologist). The procedure may be done in a medical or dental office if the office is staffed and equipped to handle this type of surgery. More often, this surgery is performed in a hospital or medical center surgical area.

Depending on the extent of the facial injury or condition to be corrected, the patient may receive a sedative for relaxation, a local anesthetic drug to numb the area, or general **anesthesia** before surgery.

During surgery, the surgeon realigns the fractured bones. Every effort is made to restore the shape and appearance of the original jaw line. If any teeth were damaged, repair or replacement may be done at the same time. Small incisions may be made through the skin and surrounding tissue so the pins and wires can be set into the jawbone to hold the fracture together. To prevent the lower jaw from moving during healing, pins and wires may be inserted into the top jaw, as well. The upper and lower jaws are then wired together in order to stabilize the fracture.

As with other types of bone **fractures**, the jaw may take several weeks to heal. Another type of jaw **immobilization** that has been developed more recently is called rigid fixation. This method uses small metal plates and screws rather than pins and wires to secure the jaw bones. The main benefit of this technique is that the jaws don't have to be wired shut, allowing the patient to more quickly return to a normal lifestyle.

A patient whose jaw has been wired will not be able to eat solid foods for several weeks, but good nutrition is vital for the bone and surrounding tissues to heal. A liquid diet that can be consumed through a straw will be required. Soft, precooked foods can be liquefied in a blender, but liquid diet formulas may be a good alternative. The patient will also have to be taught how to care for the mouth, teeth, and injured area while the wires are in place.

There may be some scars from the small incisions used to insert the wires. With any surgical procedure, there are risks associated with the anesthetic drugs and the possibility of infection. If there is a risk that the patient may vomit, the jaw wiring may pose a **choking** hazard. It may be recommended that wire cutters be kept available in case the wires need to be cut in an emergency situation.

JENNER, EDWARD (1749-1823)

English physician

Jenner was born in Berkeley, England, the third son and youngest of six children of Stephen Jenner, a clergyman of the Church of England. He was orphaned at age five and was raised by his older brother, also a clergyman. When Jenner was

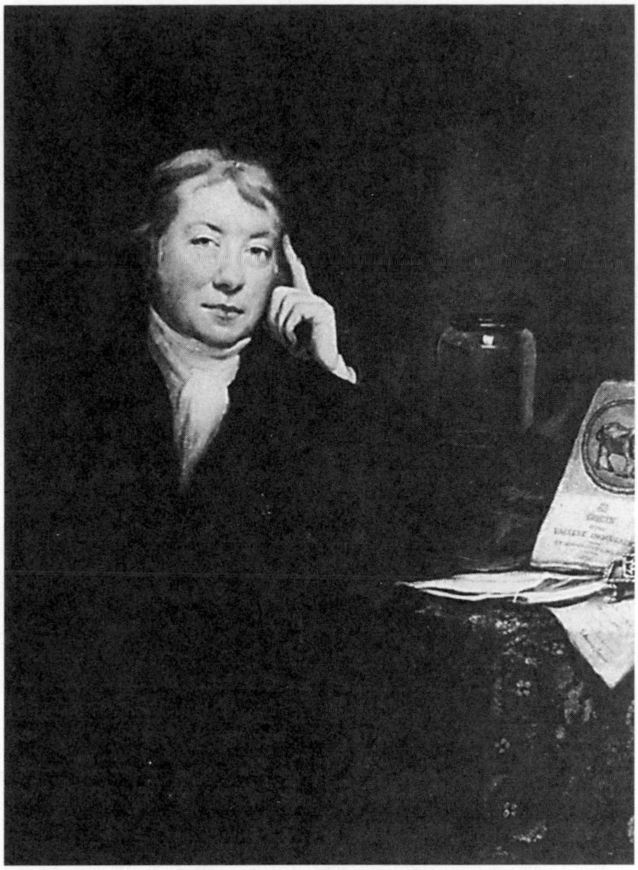

Edward Jenner

thirteen years old, he was apprenticed to a surgeon. Then in 1770, he moved to London, England, to work with John Hunter (1728-1798), an eminent Scottish anatomist and surgeon who encouraged Jenner to be inquisitive and experimental in his approach to medicine. Jenner returned to Berkeley in 1773, and set up practice as a country doctor. His curiosity about natural phenomena and dedication to medicine ultimately earned him status as a pioneer of virology and immunology, as well as the founder of the practice of **vaccination**.

During and prior to Jenner's lifetime, **smallpox** was a common and often fatal disease worldwide. Many centuries before Jenner's time, the Chinese had begun the practice of blowing flakes from smallpox scabs up the nostrils of healthy persons to confer immunity to the disease. By the seventeenth century, the Turks and Greeks had discovered that, when injected into the skin of healthy individuals, the serum from the smallpox pustule induced a mild case of the disease and subsequent immunity. This practice of inoculation reached England by the eighteenth century. However, it was quite risky as those who were inoculated frequently suffered a severe or fatal case of smallpox. Despite the risk, people willingly agreed to inoculation because of the widespread incidence of smallpox and the fear of suffering from terribly disfiguring pockmarks that resulted from the disease.

As a young physician, Jenner noted that dairy workers who had been exposed to cowpox, a disease like smallpox only milder, seemed immune to the more severe infection. He continually put forth his theory that cowpox could be used to prevent smallpox, but his contemporaries shunned his ideas. They maintained that they had seen smallpox victims who claimed to have had earlier cases of cowpox.

It became Jenner's task to transform a country superstition into an accepted medical practice. For up until the mid-1770s, the only documented cases of vaccinations using cowpox came from farmers such as Benjamin Jesty of Dorsetshire who vaccinated his family with cowpox using a darning needle.

After observing cases of cowpox and smallpox for a quarter century, Jenner took a step that could have branded him a criminal, just as easily as a hero. On May 14, 1796 he removed the fluid of a cowpox from dairymaid Sarah Nelmes, and inoculated James Phipps, an eight-year-old boy, who soon came down with cowpox. Six weeks later, he inoculated the boy with smallpox. The boy remained healthy. Jenner had proved his theory. He called his method *vaccination*, using the Latin word *vacca*, meaning cow, and *vaccinia*, meaning cowpox. He also introduced the word virus.

The publication of Jenner's *An Inquiry into the Causes and Effects of the Variolae Vaccinae* set off an enthusiastic demand for vaccination throughout Europe. Within 18 months, the number of deaths from smallpox had dropped by two-thirds in England after 12,000 people were vaccinated. By 1800, 100,000 people had been vaccinated worldwide. As the demand for the vaccine rapidly increased, Jenner discovered that he could take lymph from a smallpox pustule and dry it in a glass tube for use up to three months later. The vaccine could then be transported.

Jenner was honored and respected throughout Europe and the United States. At his request, Napoleon released several Englishmen who had been jailed in France in 1804 while France and Great Britain were at war. Across the Atlantic Ocean, Thomas Jefferson received the vaccine from Jenner and proceeded to vaccinate his family and neighbors at Monticello. However, in his native England, Jenner's medical colleagues refused to allow him entry into the College of Physicians in London, insisting that he first pass a test on the theories of **Hippocrates** and **Galen**. Jenner refused to bow to their demands, saying his accomplishments in conquering smallpox should have qualified him for election. He was never elected to the college.

Nearly two centuries after Jenner's experimental vaccination of young James, the **World Health Organization** (WHO) declared smallpox to be eradicated. However, when WHO announced its plan to destroy the last remaining stocks of the smallpox virus (which was used for research) on June 30, 1999, not everyone was pleased with the decision. Some scientists believe the stockpiled virus could still prove beneficial in terms of research to help fight other deadly viruses, including the human immunodeficiency virus (HIV), which causes **AIDS**.

See also Immune system

JERNE, NIELS K. (1911-1994)

Danish immunologist

Niels Kaj (sometimes transliterated Kai) Jerne was born on 23 December 1911, in London, England, to Danish parents Else Marie Lindberg and Hans Jessen Jerne. The family moved to the Netherlands at the beginning of World War I. Jerne earned his baccalaureate in Rotterdam in 1928 and studied physics for two years at the University of Leiden. Twelve years later, he entered the University of Copenhagen to study medicine, receiving his doctorate in 1951 at the age of 40. From 1943 until 1956 he worked at the Danish State Serum Institute, conducting research in immunology.

In 1955, Jerne traveled to the United States with noted molecular biologist **Max Delbrück** to become a research fellow at the California Institute of Technology at Pasadena. The two worked closely together, and it was not until his final two weeks at the Institute that Jerne completed work on his first major theory—on selective antibody formation. At this time, scientists believed that specific antibodies (molecules that defend the body from infection) do not exist until an antigen (any substance originating outside the body such as a virus) is introduced and acts as a template from which cells in the **immune system** create the appropriate antibody to eliminate it. Jerne's theory postulated instead that the immune system inherently contains all the specific antibodies it needs to fight specific antigens; the appropriate antibody, one of millions that are already present in the body, attaches to the antigen, thus neutralizing or destroying the antigen and its threat to the body.

In 1960, Jerne left his research in immunology to became chief medical officer with the World Health Organization in Geneva, Switzerland, where he oversaw the departments of biological standards and immunology. From 1960 to 1962, he served on the faculty at the University of Geneva's biophysics department.

From 1962 to 1966, Jerne was professor of microbiology at the University of Pittsburgh in Pennsylvania. During this period he developed a method, now known as the Jerne plaque assay, to count antibody-producing cells by first mixing them with other cells containing antigen material, causing the cells to produce an antibody that combines with red blood cells. Once combined, the blood cells are then destroyed, leaving a substance called plaque surrounding the original antibody-producing cells, which can then be counted. Jerne became director of the **Paul Ehrlich** Institute, in Frankfurt, Germany, in 1966, and, in 1969, established the Basel Institute for Immunology in Switzerland, where he remained until taking emeritus status in 1980.

In 1971, Jerne unveiled his second major theory, which deals with how the immune system identifies and differentiates between self molecules (belonging to its host) and nonself molecules (invaders). Noting that the immune system is specific to each individual, immunologists had concluded that the body's self-tolerance cannot be inherited and is therefore learned. Jerne postulated that such immune system "learning" occurs in the thymus, an organ in the upper chest cavity where the cells that recognize and attack antigens multiply, while those that could attack the body's own cells are suppressed. Over time, mutations among cells that recognize antigens increase the number of different antibodies the body has at hand, thereby increasing the immune system's arsenal against disease.

Jerne introduced what is considered his most significant work in 1974—the network theory, wherein he proposed that the immune system is a dynamic self-regulating network that activates itself when necessary and shuts down when not needed. At that time, scientists knew that the immune system contains two types of immune system cells, or lymphocytes: B cells, which produce antibodies, and T cells, which function as "helpers" to the B cells by killing foreign cells, or by regulating the B cells either by suppressing or stimulating their antibody producing activity. Further, antibody molecules produced by the B cells also contain antigen-like components (idiotypes) which can attract another antibody (anti-idiotype), allowing one antibody to recognize another antibody as well as an antigen. Jerne's theory expanded on this knowledge, speculating that a delicate balance of lymphocytes and antibodies and their idiotypes and anti-idiotypes exists in the immune system until an antigen is introduced. The antigen, he believed, replaces the anti-idiotype attached to the antibody. The immune system then senses the displacement and, in an attempt to find the anti-idiotype a "mate," produces more of the original antibody. This chain-reaction strengthens the body's immunity to the invading antigen.

Jerne shared the 1984 Nobel Prize for medicine or physiology with **Cesar Milstein** and **Georges J. F. Köhler** for his body of work that explained the function of the immune system

Jerne retired to southern France with his wife, Ursula Alexandra Kohl, whom he married in 1964; the couple had two sons. A citizen of both Denmark and Great Britain, Jerne received honorary degrees from American and European universities, was a foreign honorary member of the American Academy of Arts and Sciences, a member of the Royal Danish Academy of Sciences, and won, among other honors, the Marcel Benorst Prize in 1979 and the Paul Ehrlich Prize in 1982. Jerne died on 7 October 1994 at his home in Pont du Gard, southern France.

Jet lag

Jet lag is a condition marked by fatigue and irritability as a result of air travel across several time zones.

Living organisms are accustomed to periods of night and day alternating at set intervals. Most of the body's regulating hormones follow this cycle, known as circadian rhythm. Body temperature, sleepiness, thyroid function, metabolic processes, and the **sleep** hormone melatonin all cycle with daylight. There is a direct connection between the retina (where light hits the back of the **eye**) and the part of the brain that controls all these hormones.

When people are without clocks in a compartment that is completely closed to sunlight, most of them fall into a circadian cycle of about 25 hours. Every morning the sunlight resets the cycle, stimulating the leading chemicals and thus compensating for the difference between the 24 hour day and the 25 hour innate rhythm.

Today, technology has surpassed adaptability, at least momentarily. In a single day, we can completely reverse the night-day rhythm by flying to the other side of the earth. The chemicals are thrown into confusion. Most people reset their rhythms within a few days, demonstrating the adaptability of the human species; some, however, have trouble resetting their rhythms.

Traveling through a few time zones at a time is not as disruptive to circadian rhythms as traveling around the world, and people who travel west are less likely to experience jet lag than those who travel east.

The main symptom of jet lag is an altered sleep pattern—sleepiness during the day and trouble getting to sleep at night, together with **indigestion** and trouble concentrating. Individuals afflicted by jet lag will alternate in and out of a normal day-night cycle.

Exposure to bright morning sunlight in most cases will cure jet lag after a few days, although a few people will continue to have problems with sleep patterns.

Jet lag can be prevented in a number of ways. Eating a high-protein, low-calorie diet before taking off may help reduce the effects of jet lag. Drinking a lot of water to prevent **dehydration** can prevent jet lag. Moving around as much as possible during an airline flight also helps by maintaining circulation and moving nutrients and waste through the body. Extra doses of **vitamins** A, C, and E, as well as zinc and selenium, two days before and two days after a flight help to ease jet lag. People who don't have enough melatonin may avoid jet lag by taking this hormone, although its use is controversial due to concerns about its safety.

Jet lag usually lasts from 24-48 hours after air travel. In that short time period, the body adjusts to the time changes, and with enough rest, it returns to normal circadian rhythm.

Johnson, Jr., John B. (1908-1972)

African American physician and cardiologist

John B. Johnson, Jr. was one of the first African American physicians to assume a leadership position as department chairman of the Howard University Medical College. A pioneer in the diagnostic use of angiocardiography and cardiac catheterization, he also was one of two African American physicians appointed to Georgetown University Hospital's staff in 1954 as part of a successful effort to offer District of Columbia physicians equal opportunity.

John Beauregard Johnson, Jr., was born in Bessemer, Alabama, on April 29, 1908. He was the eldest of three sons of John B., Sr., a postman, and his wife Leona Duff Johnson. After completing high school at Tuskegee Institute, Alabama, he attended Oberlin College in Ohio, and earned a letter in track as well as his B.A. degree in 1931. From there, he went directly to medical school at Western Reserve University in

Cleveland and earned his M.D. there in 1935. After serving his internship at Cleveland City Hospital, he went to Howard University in 1936 as a laboratory assistant in physiology and spent his entire career in that institution. The following year he joined the Department of Medicine as an assistant and became an instructor in 1938.

When Johnson first joined Howard, its Dean, Numa P. G. Adams, was beginning to search for well-trained young physicians to staff the medical school's full-time clinical faculty. Adams selected Johnson as a promising potential candidate for leadership in the medical school, and sent him to the University of Rochester in 1939 for two years of postgraduate study in internal medicine. Johnson was given a General Education Board Fellowship. Upon returning to Howard, Johnson became director of Clinical Laboratories in 1941 and was made acting chair of the Department of Medicine from 1944 to 1949. During those years, Johnson spent one year at the Columbia University Division of Bellevue Hospital in New York under another General Education Board fellowship. In 1954, Johnson and another African American physician, Dr. R. Frank Jones, were appointed to the staff of Georgetown University Hospital. This marked a major breakthrough in the long campaign to secure parity of opportunity for minority physicians in the District of Columbia. At Howard, Johnson ended his career as the director of its Division of Cardiology.

As a cardiologist, or specialist in the treatment of heart disease, Johnson was an early proponent of angiocardiography, which is a diagnostic procedure that X rays the heart and its vessels after an intravenous injection of dye has been administered. The resulting picture shows blockages and abnormalities in the circulatory system. He also pioneered the technique of cardiac catheterization, in which a catheter—a thin, flexible tube—is inserted into the heart itself through a major vein in the arm. Johnson employed this technique to obtain samples of blood in the heart, to discover its abnormalities, and to determine the pressure of the heart itself. In addition, the physician studied **hypertension**—high blood pressure—and its disproportionate effects on African Americans. Johnson excelled in his field and published 64 papers during his career. One of these was awarded a citation from the journal *Angiology Research* for the Outstanding Publication of 1966.

As an educator, Johnson was described as an excellent teacher with infectious energy and enthusiasm whose lectures were both dramatic and exciting, as well as an individual who drove himself hard. He served on the board of directors of the American Heart Association from 1958 to 1961, and was awarded the Distinguished Service Medal of the National Medical Association. Twice he received the Susan B. and Theodore Cummings Humanitarian Award of the American College of Cardiology, in 1964 and 1965. After his retirement, the Howard University College of Medicine voted unanimously to name a chair after him. Its incumbent has the title of John Beauregard Johnson Professor of Medicine. When Johnson died in Freedman's Hospital on December 16, 1972, after a cerebral hemorrhage, he was survived by his third wife, Audrey Ingram Johnson, a stepdaughter, Adrienne, and a daughter from his second marriage, Linda.

Johnson, Joseph Lealand (1895-1991)

African American physiologist and physician

Joseph Lealand Johnson was the second African American to earn both a Ph.D. and an M.D. degree. Although his parents had been born into slavery in North Carolina, Johnson was able to secure an education and eventually became dean of the Howard University Medical School and chairman of its Department of Physiology. It was through his efforts that this department became a fully modernized place of research.

Johnson was born in Philadelphia, Pennsylvania, on January 14, 1895. His parents had moved there from North Carolina and eventually had fourteen children. Johnson was the youngest of the ten that survived infancy. His father was a laborer who died when Johnson was two, and his mother supported the family as a midwife. Although the ten-year-old Johnson was so interested in the law that he would regularly cut school to attend trials at City Hall, he took the advice of his high school principal and applied for a scholarship in agronomy at Pennsylvania State University. "I knew I first had to get to college if I wanted to study law," Johnson recalled later in an interview with Allen B. Weisse in *Conversations in Medicine,* "and this was the first step."

Upon admission, Johnson found himself to be the only black on the entire campus. His education was interrupted by World War I, and when Johnson discovered there were no officer training camps available to him as there were for his white classmates, he wrote directly to the Secretary of War. The Secretary responded that a special camp was being formed at Fort Des Moines, Iowa. Johnson joined up, was commissioned second lieutenant, and was assigned to the 350th Field Artillery at Fort Dix, New Jersey. After being honorably discharged in January, 1919, he returned to Penn State and received his B.S. degree in June of that year.

That autumn, Johnson began teaching at the Kansas Vocational and Industrial Institute in Topeka, Kansas, where he also was an assistant coach of the men's basketball team as well as coach of the women's basketball team. The next year he moved to Kansas City to teach general science and zoology at Lincoln High School. It was while attending a summer education course at the University of Chicago that Johnson first became interested in medicine as a way of helping the people of his poor Kansas City neighborhood called West Bottoms. "I got the feeling that those people were not getting the medical care that they should have because they couldn't afford it," Johnson explained to Weisse. "The idea struck me that I would go away and prepare myself thoroughly in medicine, and then come back to Kansas City and serve the people in the West Bottoms." With the help of the Lincoln High School principal who secured the backing of a wealthy friend, Johnson was able to resign from teaching and to dedicate himself to medical school.

By 1931, Johnson had earned his combined M. D. and Ph.D. degree in medicine and physiology at the University of Chicago. He was offered a physiology professorship at Howard University in Washington, D.C., by Dr. Numa P. G. Adams who had just become the first black dean of its medical school. Johnson accepted the offer, and it was under his guidance and direction that Howard's physiology department was completely revamped, renovated, and redirected into a modern facility where meaningful research could take place. When Dr. Adams died suddenly in 1940, Johnson became acting dean of Howard's medical school. In 1947 he became dean and remained in that position until 1955 when he returned to full-time teaching and research in physiology. He retired in 1971.

Johnson was a member of the board of directors of the National Medical Association and a member of the Medico Chirurgical Society of the District of Columbia. He also held memberships in the AAAS, NAACP, AMA, Foundation for Tropical Medicine, International College of Surgeons, Walter Reed Society, American Physiology Society, and was a fellow of the New York Academy of Sciences. He was a member of the honorary medical society, Alpha Omega Alpha, and Alpha Phi Alpha fraternity. He also served as the 1960–61 Imhotep Conference Chairman. Johnson died of cancer in Silver Spring, Maryland, in 1991.

JOHNSON, VIRGINIA E. (1925-)

American psychologist and sex therapist

In collaboration with Dr. **William Howell Masters**, psychologist and sex therapist Virginia E. Johnson pioneered the study of human sexuality under laboratory conditions. She and Masters published the results of their study as a book entitled *Human Sexual Response* in 1966, causing an immediate sensation. As part of her work at the Reproductive Biology Research Foundation in St. Louis and later at the Masters and Johnson Institute, she counseled many clients and taught **sex therapy** to many professional practitioners.

Johnson was born Virginia Eshelman on February 11, 1925, in Springfield, Missouri, to Hershel Eshelman, a farmer, and Edna (Evans) Eshelman. The elder of two children, she began school in Palo Alto, California, where her family had moved in 1930. When they returned to Missouri three years later, she was ahead of her school peers and skipped several grades. She studied piano and voice, and read extensively. She entered Drury College in Springfield in 1941. After her freshman year, she was hired to work in the state insurance office, a job she held for four years. Her mother, a republican state committeewoman, introduced her to many elected officials, and Johnson often sang for them at meetings. These performances led to a job as a country music singer for radio station KWTO in Springfield, where her stage name was Virginia Gibson. She studied at the University of Missouri and later at the Kansas City Conservatory of Music. In 1947, she became a business writer for the St. Louis *Daily Record.* She also worked briefly on the marketing staff of KMOX-TV, leaving that position in 1951.

In the early 1940s she married a Missouri politician, but the marriage lasted only two days. Her marriage to an attorney many years her senior also ended in divorce. On June 13, 1950, she married George V. Johnson, an engineering student and leader of a dance band. She sang with the band until the birth of her two children, Scott Forstall and Lisa Evans. In 1956, the Johnsons divorced.

In 1956, contemplating a return to college for a degree in sociology, Johnson applied for a job at the Washington University employment office. William Howell Masters, associate professor of clinical obstetrics and gynecology, had requested an assistant to interview volunteers for a research project. He personally chose Johnson, who fitted the need for an outgoing, intelligent, mature woman who was preferably a mother. Johnson began work on January 2, 1957, as a research associate, but soon advanced to research instructor.

Gathering scientific data by means of **electroencephalography**, **electrocardiography**, and the use of color monitors, Masters and Johnson measured and analyzed 694 volunteers. They were careful to protect the privacy of their subjects, who were photographed in various modes of sexual stimulation. In addition to a description of the four stages of sexual arousal, other valuable information was gained from the photographs, including evidence of the failure of some contraceptives, the discovery of a vaginal secretion in some women that prevents conception, and the observation that sexual enjoyment need not decrease with age. In 1964, Masters and Johnson created the non-profit Reproductive Biology Research Foundation in St. Louis and began treating couples for sexual problems. Originally listed as a research associate, Johnson became assistant director of the Foundation in 1969 and co-director in 1973.

In 1966, Masters and Johnson released their book *Human Sexual Response,* in which they detailed the results of their studies. Although the book was written in dry, clinical terms and intended for medical professionals, its titillating subject matter made it front-page news and a runaway best seller, with over 300,000 volumes distributed by 1970. While some reviewers accused the team of dehumanizing and scientizing sex, overall professional and critical response was positive.

At Johnson's suggestion, the two researchers went on the lecture circuit to discuss their findings and appeared on such television programs as NBC's *Today* show and ABC's *Stage '67.* Their book and their public appearances heightened public interest in sex therapy, and a long list of clients developed. Couples referred to their clinic would spend two weeks in intensive therapy and have periodic follow-ups for five years. In a second book, *Human Sexual Inadequacy,* published in 1970, Masters and Johnson discuss the possibility that sex problems are more cultural than physiological or psychological. In 1975, they wrote *The Pleasure Bond: A New Look at Sexuality and Commitment,* which differs from previous volumes in that it was written for the average reader. This book describes total commitment and fidelity to the partner as the basis for an enduring sexual bond. To expand **counseling**, Masters and Johnson trained dual-sex therapy teams and conducted regular workshops for college teachers, marriage counselors, and other professionals.

After the release of this second book, Masters divorced his first wife and married Johnson on January 7, 1971, in Fayetteville, Arkansas. They continued their work at the Reproductive Biology Research Foundation, and in 1973 founded the Masters and Johnson Institute. Johnson was co-director of the institute, running the everyday business, and Masters concentrated on scientific work. Johnson, who never received a college degree, was widely recognized along with Masters for her contributions to human sexuality research. Together they received several awards, including the Sex Education and Therapists Award in 1978 and Biomedical Research Award of the World Sexology Association in 1979.

In 1981, the team sold their lab and moved to another location in St. Louis, where they had a staff of twenty-five and a long waiting list of clients. Their book *Homosexuality in Perspective,* released shortly before the move, documents their research on gay and lesbian sexual practice and homosexual sexual problems and their work with "gender-confused" individuals who sought a "cure" for their homosexuality. One of their most controversial conclusions from their ten-year study of eighty-four men and women was their conviction that homosexuality is primarily not physical, emotional, or genetic, but a learned behavior. Some reviewers hailed the team's claims of success in "converting" homosexuals. Others, however, observed that the handpicked individuals who participated in the study were not a representative sample; moreover, they challenged the team's assumption that heterosexual performance alone was an accurate indicator of a changed sexual preference.

The institute had many associates who assisted in research and writing. Robert Kolodny, an M.D. interested in sexually transmitted diseases, coauthored the book *Crisis: Heterosexual Behavior in the Age of AIDS* with Masters and Johnson in 1988. The book, commented Stephen Fried in *Vanity Fair,* "was politically incorrect in the extreme": it predicted a large-scale outbreak of the virus in the heterosexual community and, in a chapter meant to document how little was known of the **AIDS** virus, suggested that it might be possible to catch it from a toilet seat. Several prominent members of the medical community questioned the study, and many accused the authors of sowing **hysteria**. Adverse publicity hurt the team, who were distressed because they felt the medical community had turned against them. The number of therapy clients at the institute declined.

The board of the institute was quietly dissolved and William Young, Johnson's son-in-law, became acting director. Johnson went into semi-retirement. On February 19, 1992, Young announced that after twenty-one years of marriage, Masters and Johnson were filing for divorce because of differences about goals relating to work and retirement. Following the divorce, Johnson took most of the institute's records with her and is continuing her work independently.

JOINT REPLACEMENT

Great advances have been made in joint replacement in the United States since the first hip was replaced in 1969. Improvements have been made in the materials and the surgical techniques used to install artificial joints.

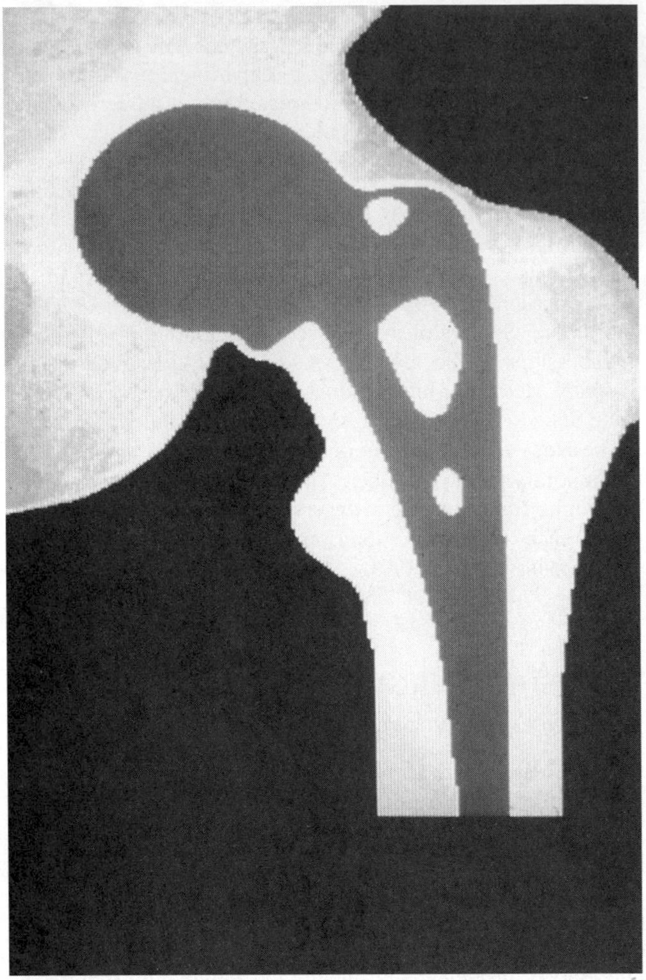

X-ray image of a human pelvis with a prosthetic hip joint.

Custom joints can be made using a mold that duplicates the original with a very high degree of accuracy.

The most common joints to be replaced are hips and knees. There is ongoing work on elbow and shoulder replacement, but some joint problems are still treated by surgically removing the joint in question or by reassembling the joint from smaller parts.

Seventy percent of replacements are performed because arthritis has caused the joint to stiffen and become painful to the point where normal daily activities are no longer possible. Joint replacement is appropriate if the joint doesn't respond to conservative treatment such as medication, weight loss, restricting activity and canes.

Patients with **rheumatoid arthritis** or other connective tissue diseases may also be candidates for joint replacement, but the results are usually not as good. Elderly people who fall and break a hip often undergo hip replacement when the probability of successful bone healing is low.

More than 170,000 hip replacements are performed in the United States each year. Since the lifetime of the artificial joint is limited, the best candidates for joint replacement are

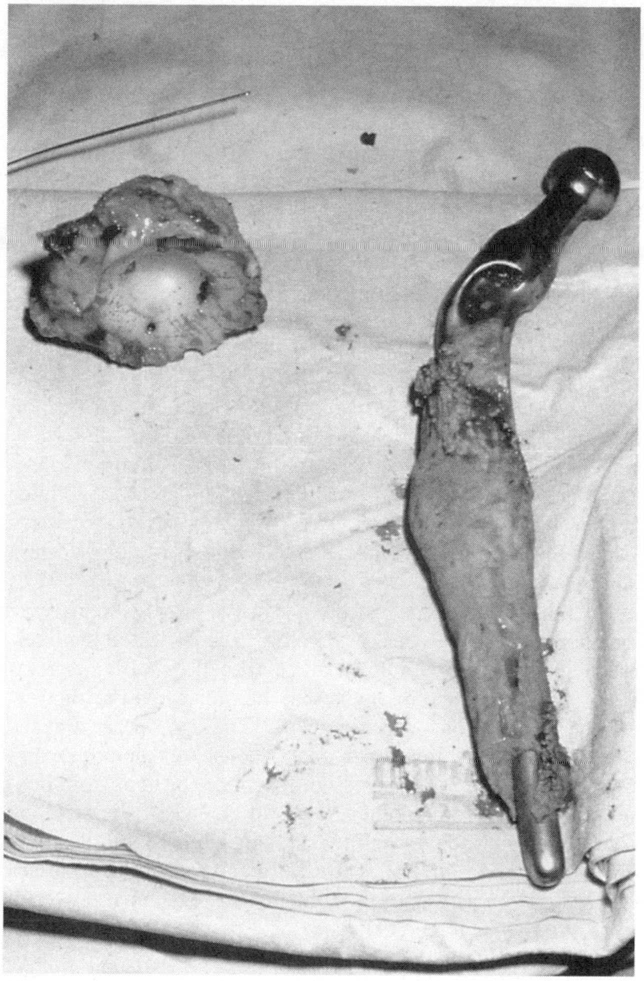

The components of a prosthetic hip joint: a plastic socket (left) and a steel rod encased in the cement that secures it inside the femur.

over age 60. In fact, joint replacements are performed successfully on an older-than-average group of patients. People with diseases that interfere with blood clotting are not good candidates, nor would anyone with any heart, kidney or lung problems that would make it risky to undergo general **anesthesia**.

Joint replacements are performed under general or regional anesthesia in a hospital by an orthopedic surgeon. Some medical centers specialize in joint replacement, and these centers generally have a higher success rate than less specialized facilities. The specific techniques of joint replacement vary depending on the joint involved.

In a hip replacement, the surgeon makes an incision along the top of the thigh bone and pulls it away from the socket of the hip bone. Next, the doctor inserts an artificial socket made of metal coated with plastic to reduce friction. After cutting the top of the thigh bone, the doctor fits a piece of artificial thigh made of metal into the lower thigh bone on one end and the new socket on the other. The artificial hip can either be held in place by a synthetic cement or by natural bone ingrowth.

While the cement is good at locking the prosthesis to the remaining bone, bubbles left in the cement after it cures may act as weak spots, causing cracks to develop. This promotes loosening of the prosthesis later in life. If more surgery is needed, all the cement must be removed before surgery can be performed.

On the other hand, an artificial hip fixed by natural bone in-growth requires more precise surgical techniques to assure maximum contact between the remaining natural bone and the prosthesis. The prosthesis is made so that it contains small pores that encourage the natural bone to grow into it. Growth begins 6 to 12 weeks after surgery. The short-term outcome with non-cemented hips is less satisfactory (patients report more thigh **pain**) but the long-term outlook is better with this technique. In both methods, hospital stays last from four to eight days.

In a knee replacement, the doctor makes a cut to expose the knee joint and then loosens the ligaments surrounding the knee. Next, the surgeon cuts the shin and thigh bone, and removes the knee. The artificial knee is cemented into place on the remaining stubs of those bones, the excess cement is removed and the knee is closed. Hospital stays range from three to six days.

In both types of surgery, preventing infection is very important. **Antibiotics** are given intravenously and continued in pill form after the surgery. Fluid and blood loss can be great, and sometimes blood **transfusion**s are needed. Many patients choose to donate their own blood for transfusion during the surgery. This prevents any blood incompatibility problems or the transmission of bloodbourne diseases.

Immediately after the operation the patient will be catheterized and monitored for infection. Antibiotics are continued and pain medication is prescribed. **Physical therapy** begins (first passive **exercise**s, then active ones) as soon as possible using a walker, cane, or crutches for additional support.

The immediate risks during and after surgery include infection, the development of blood clots that may block the arteries, and loss of too much blood. Infection caused by the operation can occur as long as a year later and can be difficult to treat. Some doctors add antibiotics directly to the cement used to fix the replacement joint in place. Blood-thinning medication is usually given to reduce the risk of clots. Loosening of the joint is the most common cause of failure in hip joints that are not infected. This may require another joint replacement surgery in about 12% of patients within a 15-year period following the first procedure.

Some elderly people experience short-term confusion and disorientation from the anesthesia. Although joint replacement surgery is highly successful, there is a risk of nerve injury. Dislocation or fracture of the hip joint is also a possibility.

More than 90% of patients receiving hip replacements have no more relief and much better joint function. The success rate is slightly lower in knee replacements, and drops still more for other joint replacement operations.

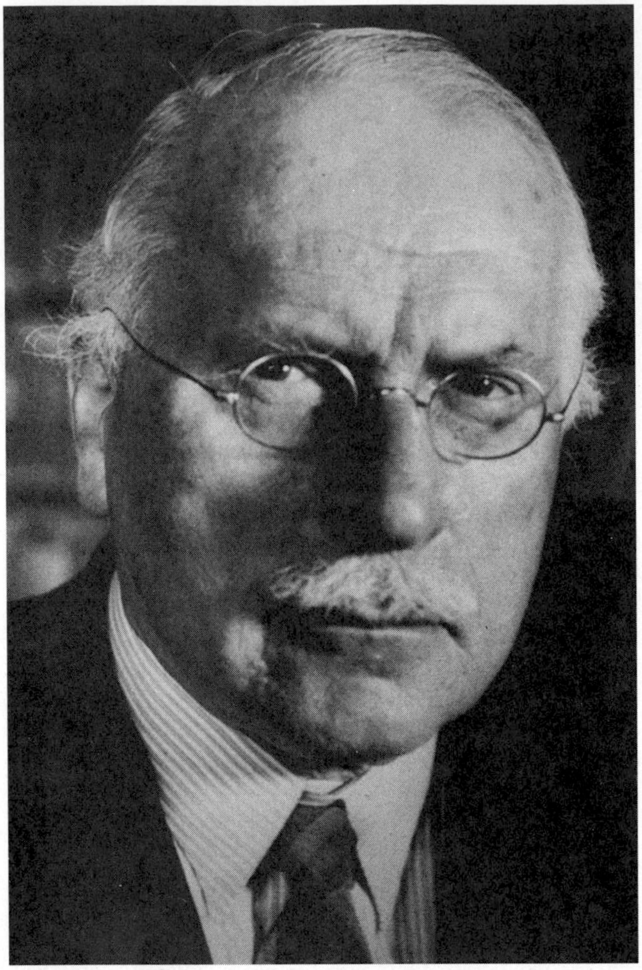

Carl Jung

JUNG, CARL GUSTAV (1875-1961)
Swiss psychiatrist

Carl Jung was born in Switzerland, the son of a Swiss Reform pastor. Having decided to become a psychiatrist, he enrolled in medical school at the University of Basel, from which he received his degree in 1900. Serving as an assistant at the University of Zurich Psychiatric Clinic, Jung worked under psychiatrist Eugen Bleuler (1857-1939), a psychiatrist renowned for his work on schizophrenia. Jung also traveled to France to study with the well-known psychiatrist Pierre Janet (1859-1947) as well. In 1905, he was appointed to a faculty position in psychiatry at the University of Zurich and became a senior physician at its clinic. Eventually, a growing private practice forced him to resign his university position. Jung's early published studies on **schizophrenia** established his reputation, and he also won recognition for developing a word association test.

Jung had read **Sigmund Freud**'s *The Interpretation of Dreams* shortly after its publication in 1900 and entered into a correspondence with its author. The two men met in 1907 and began a close association that was to last for over six years. In 1909, they both traveled to the United States to participate in the 20th-anniversary commemoration at Clark University in Worcester, Massachusetts, at the invitation of American psychologist, G. Stanley Hall (1844-1924). Jung became part of a weekly discussion group that met at Freud's house and included, among others, Alfred Adler and Otto Rank (1884-1939). This group evolved into the Vienna Psychoanalytic Society, and Jung became its first president in 1911. By this time, however, Jung had begun to develop concepts about **psychoanalysis** and the nature of the unconscious that differed from those of Freud, especially Freud's insistence on the sexual basis of neurosis. After the publication of Jung's *Psychology of the Unconscious* in 1912, the disagreement between the two men grew, and their relationship ended in 1914. At this period, Jung underwent a period of personal turmoil and, like Freud at a similar juncture in his own life, undertook a thorough self-analysis based on his dreams. Jung also explored myths and symbols, an interest he was to investigate further in the 1920s with trips to Africa and the southwestern United States to study the myths and religions of non-Western cultures.

Jung developed his own system of psychoanalysis, which he called analytical psychology, that reflected his interest in symbolism, mythology, and spirituality. A major premise of analytical psychology is that the individual personality, or psyche, functions on three levels. The ego operates at the conscious level, while the personal unconscious includes experiences that have been repressed, forgotten, or kept from consciousness in some other way. It is also the site of complexes—groups of feelings, thoughts, and memories, usually organized around a significant person (such as a parent) or object (such as money). At the deepest and most powerful level, Jung posited the existence of a racial or collective unconscious, which gathers together the experiences of previous generations and even animal ancestors, preserving traces of humanity's evolutionary development over time. The collective unconscious is a repository of shared images and symbols, called archetypes, that emerge in dreams, myths, and other forms. These include such common themes as birth, rebirth, death, the hero, the earth mother, and the demon. Certain archetypes form separate systems within the personality, including the persona, or public image; the anima and animus, or gender characteristics; the shadow, or animal instincts; and the self, which strives for unity and wholeness. In Jung's view, a thorough analysis of both the personal and collective unconscious is necessary to fully understand the individual personality.

Perhaps Jung's best-known contribution is his theory that individuals can be categorized according to general attitudinal types, as either introverted (inward-looking) or extroverted (outward-looking). The psychic wholeness, or individuation, for which human beings strive depends on reconciling these tendencies as well as the four functional aspects of the mind that are split into opposing pairs: sensing versus intuiting as ways of knowing, and thinking versus feeling as ways of evaluating. If any of these personality characteristics is overly dominant in the conscious mind, its opposite will be exaggerated in the unconscious. These pairs of functions have been widely adapted in vocational and other types of testing.

From 1932 to 1942, Jung was a professor at the Federal Polytechnical University of Zurich. Although his health forced him to resign, he continued writing about analytical psychology for the rest of his life and promoting the attainment of psychic wholeness through personal transformation and self-discovery. Jung's work has been influential in disciplines other than psychology, and his own writing includes works on religion, the arts, literature, and occult topics including alchemy, astrology, yoga, fortune telling, and flying saucers. Jung's autobiography, *Memories, Dreams, Reflections,* was published in 1961, the year of his death. Institutes of analytical psychology have been established throughout the world, although its international center remains the C. G. Jung Institute in Zurich, founded in 1948. Jung was a prolific writer; his collected works fill 19 volumes, but many of his writings were not published in English until after 1965. Shortly before his death, Jung completed work on *Man and His Symbols,* which has served as a popular introduction to his ideas on symbols and dreams.

See also Sigmund Freud; Psychoanalysis; Psychosis

"JUMPING" GENE • See McClintock, Barbara

JUVENILE ARTHRITIS

Juvenile arthritis (JA) refers to a number of different conditions, all of which strike children, and all of which have joint inflammation as their major manifestation.

The skeletal system of the body is made up of different types of the strong, fibrous tissue known as connective tissue. Bone, cartilage, ligaments, and tendons are all forms of connective tissue which have different compositions, and thus different characteristics.

The joints are structures that hold two or more bones together. Some joints (synovial joints) allow for movement between the bones being joined (called articulating bones). The simplest model of a synovial joint involves two bones, separated by a slight gap called the joint cavity. The ends of each articular bone are covered by a layer of cartilage. Both articular bones and the joint cavity are surrounded by a tough tissue called the articular capsule. The articular capsule has two components: the fibrous membrane on the outside, and the synovial membrane (or synovium) on the inside. The fibrous membrane may include tough bands of fibrous tissue called ligaments, which are responsible for providing support to the joints. The synovial membrane has special cells and many capillaries (tiny blood vessels). This membrane produces a supply of synovial fluid which fills the joint cavity, lubricates it, and helps the articular bones move smoothly about the joint.

In JA, the synovial membrane becomes intensely inflamed. Usually thin and delicate, the synovium becomes thick and stiff, with numerous infoldings on its surface. The membrane becomes invaded by white blood cells, which produce a variety of destructive chemicals. The cartilage along the articular surfaces of the bones may be attacked and destroyed, and the bone, articular capsule, and ligaments may begin to be worn away (eroded). These processes severely interfere with movement in the joint.

JA specifically refers to chronic arthritic conditions which affect a child under the age of 16 years, and which last for a minimum of three to six months. JA is often characterized by a waxing and waning course, with flares separated by periods of time during which no symptoms are noted (remission). Some literature refers to JA as juvenile **rheumatoid arthritis**, although most types of JA differ significantly from the adult disease called rheumatoid arthritis, in terms of symptoms, progression, and prognosis.

A number of different causes have been sought to explain the onset of JA. There seems to be some genetic link, based on the fact that the tendency to develop JA sometimes runs in a particular family, and based on the fact that certain genetic markers are more frequently found in patients with JA and other related diseases. Many researchers have looked for some infectious cause for JA, but no clear connection to a particular organism has ever been made. JA is considered by some to be an autoimmune disorder. **Autoimmune disorders** occur when the body's **immune system** mistakenly identifies the body's own tissue as foreign, and goes about attacking those tissues, as if trying to rid the body of an invader (such as a bacteria, virus, or fungi). While an autoimmune mechanism is strongly suspected, certain markers of such a mechanism (such as rheumatoid factor, often present in adults with such disorders) are rarely present in children with JA.

Joint symptoms of arthritis may include stiffness, **pain**, redness and warmth of the joint, and swelling. Bone in the area of an affected joint may grow too quickly, or too slowly, resulting in limbs which are of different lengths. When the child tries to avoid moving a painful joint, the muscle may begin to shorten from disuse. This is called a contracture.

Symptoms of JA depend on the particular subtype. JA is classified by the symptoms which appear within the first six months of the disorder:

- Pauciarticular JA: This is the most common and the least severe type of JA, affecting about 40-60% of all JA patients. This type of JA affects fewer than four joints, usually the knee, ankle, wrist, and/or elbow. Other more general (systemic) symptoms are usually absent, and the child's growth usually remains normal. Very few children (less than 15%) with pauciarticular JA end up with deformed joints. Some children with this form of JA experience painless swelling of the joint. Some children with JA have a serious inflammation of structures within the eye, which if left undiagnosed and untreated could even lead to blindness. While many children have cycles of flares and remissions, in some children the disease completely and permanently resolves within a few years of diagnosis.
- Polyarticular JA: About 40% of all cases of JA are of this type. More girls than boys are diagnosed with this form of JA. This type of JA is most common in children up to age three, or after the age of 10. Polyarticular JA

affects five or more joints simultaneously. This type of JA usually affects the small joints of both hands and both feet, although other large joints may be affected as well. Some patients with arthritis in their knees will experience a different rate of growth in each leg. Ultimately, one leg will grow longer than the other. About half of all patients with polyarticular JA have arthritis of the spine and/or hip. Some patients with polyarticular JA will have other symptoms of a systemic illness, including anemia (low red blood cell count), decreased growth rate, low appetite, low-grade **fever**, and a slight rash. The disease is most severe in those children who are diagnosed in early adolescence. Some of these children will test positive for a marker present in other autoimmune disorders, called rheumatoid factor (RF). RF is found in adults who have rheumatoid arthritis. Children who are positive for RF tend to have a more severe course, with a disabling form of arthritis which destroys and deforms the joints. This type of arthritis is thought to be the adult form of rheumatoid arthritis occurring at a very early age.

- Systemic onset JA: Sometimes called Still disease (after a physician who originally described it), this type of JA occurs in about 10-20% off all patients with JA. Boys and girls are equally affected, and diagnosis is usually made between the ages of 5-10 years. The initial symptoms are not usually related to the joints. Instead, these children have high fevers; a rash; decreased appetite and weight loss; severe joint and muscle pain; swollen lymph nodes, spleen, and liver; and serious **anemia**. Some children experience other complications, including inflammation of the sac containing the heart (**pericarditis**); inflammation of the tissue lining the chest cavity and lungs (pleuritis); and inflammation of the heart muscle (**myocarditis**). The eye inflammation often seen in pauciarticular JA is uncommon in systemic onset JA. Symptoms of actual arthritis begin later in the course of systemic onset JA, and they often involve the wrists and ankles. Many of these children continue to have periodic flares of fever and systemic symptoms throughout childhood. Some children will go on to develop a polyarticular type of JA.
- Spondyloarthropathy: This type of JA most commonly affects boys older than eight years of age. The arthritis occurs in the knees and ankles, moving over time to include the hips and lower spine. Inflammation of the eye may occur occasionally, but usually resolves without permanent damage.
- Psoriatic JA: This type of arthritis usually shows up in fewer than four joints, but goes on to include multiple joints (appearing similar to polyarticular JA). Hips, back, fingers, and toes are frequently affected. A skin condition called **psoriasis** accompanies this type of arthritis. Children with this type of JA often have pits or ridges in their fingernails. The arthritis usually progresses to become a serious, disabling problem.

Diagnosis of JA is often made on the basis of the child's collection of symptoms. Laboratory tests often show normal results. Some nonspecific indicators of inflammation may be elevated, including white blood cell count, erythrocyte sedimentation rate, and a marker called C-reactive protein. As with any chronic disease, anemia may be noted. Children with an extraordinarily early onset of the adult type of rheumatoid arthritis will have a positive test for rheumatoid factor.

Treating JA involves efforts to decrease the amount of inflammation, in order to preserve movement. Medications which can be used for this include **nonsteroidal anti-inflammatory drugs** (such as ibuprofen and naproxen). Oral (by mouth) steroid medications are effective, but have many serious side effects with long-term use. Injections of steroids into an affected joint can be helpful. Steroid eye drops are used to treat eye inflammation. Other drugs which have been used to treat JA include methotrexate, sulfasalazine, penicillamine, and hydroxychloroquine. **Physical therapy** and **exercise**s are often recommended in order to improve joint mobility and to strengthen supporting muscles. Occasionally, splints are used to rest painful joints and to try to prevent or improve deformities.

The prognosis for pauciarticular JA is quite good, as is the prognosis for spondyloarthropathy. Polyarticular JA carries a slightly worse prognosis. RF-positive polyarticular JA carries a difficult prognosis, often with progressive, destructive arthritis and joint deformities. Systemic onset JA has a variable prognosis, depending on the organ systems affected, and the progression to polyarticular JA. About 1-5% of all JA patients die of such complications as infection, inflammation of the heart, or kidney disease.

Because so little is known about what causes JA, there are no recommendations available for how to avoid developing it.

K

Kaposi, Moriz (1837-1902)

Hungarian physician

Moriz Kaposi, a Hungarian who devoted his professional life to the study of dermatology at the University of Vienna, was first to document nine previously unknown skin diseases. He educated a generation of distinguished academic dermatologists and laid the groundwork for subsequent researchers to study conditions such as **Kaposi's sarcoma** and lupus erythematosus.

Kaposi earned a medical degree in 1861 at the University of Vienna, where he studied with the dermatologist Ferdinand von Hebra. Kaposi went to work in Hebra's clinic and qualified as a privatdocent (lecturer) with a dissertation on the effect of **syphilis** on the mucous membranes. Eventually, Kaposi married Hebra's daughter. Hebra's death left Kaposi the heir apparent to the role of the most respected dermatologist in Vienna.

Kaposi's reputation brought students and patients from many countries. He trained dermatologists who went on to serve as chairmen of academic dermatology departments throughout Europe. With Hebra, Kaposi coauthored the *Handbook of Diseases of the Skin*, then Kaposi went on to write *Pathology and Treatment of Diseases of the Skin* on his own. Both texts were successful and were promptly translated into English, as were many of Kaposi's scholarly articles.

Kaposi was the first to observe nine previously undocumented skin conditions between 1872 and 1887. He is best known for his discovery in 1872 of Kaposi's sarcoma, a malignant disease of the skin and lymph nodes, marked by purplish blotches. Until the 1980s, Kaposi's sarcoma was rarely seen in the United States. When the US **Centers for Disease Control** recorded 26 cases of Kaposi's sarcoma in 1981, it was an important clue that helped scientists put together the first clinical description of the acquired immunodeficiency syndrome (**AIDS**). As of 1997, Kaposi's sarcoma was the most common tumor in patients with AIDS.

Kaposi was also first to document lupus erythematosus in 1872. This **autoimmune disorder** was considered rare in the nineteenth century, when Kaposi and several British and American dermatologists studied it as a skin disease. After the turn of the century, dermatologists traced internal symptoms to lupus and it gradually came to be seen as an illness with symptoms that might involve the skin alone or might involve the whole body. By 1999, about two million Americans were affected by the disease, which still has no definitive cure.

Kaposi's discoveries of lesser-known conditions include **impetigo** herpetiformis, a rare skin infection that affects pregnant women in the third trimester, often killing the fetus. In 1876, he documented diabetic **dermatitis**. In one gruesome disease first noted by Kaposi, lymphodermia perniciosa, the patient's symptoms began with skin rash and swelling, then the skin became knobby with open sores. The disease spread to the glands and spleen. On **autopsy**, the patient's spleen was enlarged fourfold, the bone marrow was filled with abnormal cells, and lungs contained nodules. Kaposi's meticulous clinical observations enabled him to identify many unusual conditions and set the standard for subsequent research in dermatology.

Kaposi's sarcoma

Kaposi's sarcoma produces pink, purple, or brown tumors on the skin, mucous membranes, or internal organs. It was a very rare form of **cancer**, primarily affecting elderly men of Mediterranean and eastern European background, until the 1980s, when it began to appear among **AIDS** patients. Milder forms of the disease can be managed successfully with topical agents and therapies; widespread disease requires **chemotherapy**.

Investigators recognize four distinct forms of Kaposi's sarcoma (KS). The first form, called classic KS, was described by the Austrian dermatologist **Moriz Kaposi** more than a century ago. Classic KS usually affects older men of Mediterranean or eastern European backgrounds by producing tumors on the lower legs. Though at times **pain**ful and disfiguring, they are not generally life-threatening. The second form of the disease, African endemic KS, primarily affects boys and men. It can appear as classic KS, or in a more deadly form that quickly spreads to tissues below the skin, the bones and lymph system, leading to **death** within a few years of diagnosis. Another form of KS, iatrogenic KS, is observed in kidney and liver transplant patients who take immunosuppressive drugs to prevent rejection of their organ transplant. Iatrogenic KS usually reverses after the immunosuppressive drug is stopped. The fourth form of KS, AIDS-related KS, emerged as one of the first illnesses observed among those with AIDS. Unlike classic KS, AIDS-related KS tumors generally appear on the upper body, including the head, neck, and back. The tumors also can appear on the soft palate and gum areas of the mouth, and in more advanced cases, they can be found in the stomach and intestines, the lymph nodes, and the lungs.

A variety of factors appear to contribute to the development of KS:

- Genetic predisposition. People with classic KS, and those who develop the tumors after transplantation, are more likely than others to possess a genetically determined immune factor called HLA-DR. Cases of KS that run in families, however, are rare.
- Sex hormones. The fact that the disease is more likely to afflict men than women suggests sex hormones, such as testosterone in men, may stimulate the growth of KS tumors, and that estrogen in women may retard their growth.
- Immune suppression. Liver, kidney, and bone marrow patients who take immunosuppressive drugs to prevent transplant rejection frequently develop KS lesions. Similarly, KS has been observed in patients receiving systemic treatment with high-dose **corticosteroids**, which also suppresses the **immune system**. Immune suppression is the hallmark of AIDS.
- Infectious, sexually transmitted agent. AIDS-related KS is ten times more likely to appear in homosexual or bisexual men with AIDS than it is to appear in IV drug users, **hemophilia**cs, or women. In addition, the proportion of AIDS patients who develop KS has decreased markedly as safer-sex practices have become more widespread. A number of viruses have been proposed as possible causes. They include cytomegalovirus and human papilloma virus, fragments of which have been found in KS tumor specimens. A more likely candidate, however, is a new herpes virus that has been called human herpes virus 8 (HHV-8) or KS-associated herpes virus (KSHV). Since fragments of the virus were first disclosed in KS samples in 1994, they have since been found in KS samples taken from patients with classic KS, African endemic KS, and KS in transplant patients. Fragments of HHV-8, however, have also been found in patients who have other skin diseases but who do not have KS.

Many physicians will diagnose KS based on the appearance of the skin tumors and the patient's medical history. Unexplained **cough** or chest pain, as well as unexplained stomach or intestinal pain or bleeding, could suggest that the disease has moved beyond the skin. The most certain diagnosis can be achieved by taking a **biopsy** sample of a suspected KS lesion and examining it under high-power magnification. For suspected involvement of internal organs, physicians will use a bronchoscope to examine the lungs or an endoscope to view the stomach and intestinal tract.

There is no single best treatment for KS. Treatments range from topical agents for mild disease with few tumors to more aggressive systemic chemotherapy for more serious KS that has spread to large areas of skin or the internal organs. Physicians will frequently combine topical, radiation, and various systemic chemotherapy drugs, depending on the sites of the body affected, the speed at which it is progressing, and the patient's overall health, among other considerations.

When the number of KS tumors is small and the disease appears to be progressing slowly, physicians will consider destroying the lesions with **cryotherapy** (using a liquid nitrogen spray or probe to freeze the tumor); injections directly into the tumor of vinblastine (a drug also used for systemic chemotherapy); or **radiation therapy** targeted at the tumor sites.

With widespread KS lesions over the body surface, or evidence of spread to other parts of the body, physicians will consider systemic chemotherapy drugs, either alone or in a variety of combinations. Combination therapy generally produces a better response, with fewer toxic side effects associated with large doses of any single drug. Among the chemotherapy agents that physicians will consider using are vinblastine, bleomycin, and doxorubicin. A new class of chemotherapy drugs, called liposomally encapsulated drugs, appears to produce good results with fewer toxic side effects than do more conventional chemotherapy drugs.

Evidence suggests that for some individuals, the class of AIDS drugs called **protease inhibitors**, in combination with other anti-HIV drugs, can reduce the levels of detectable HIV in the blood to nearly zero, and in some patients stabilize or reverse KS tumors. More research is needed in this area. Since the discovery of HHV-8, interest in an antiviral approach to KS has increased. There is no evidence, however, that two **antiviral drugs** commonly prescribed for herpes, acyclovir and ganciclovir, have any effect on the disease. One study of 20,000 patients with HIV and AIDS found that those who took foscarnet, another antiviral medication that works in a different way than acyclovir and ganciclovir, were less likely to develop KS tumors.

A number of other treatments for KS are under investigation, including:

- **Interferon**-alpha. Interferon-alpha is made by the body and has powerful effects on the immune system. Investigators have tried injecting it directly into lesions, and also in combination with other anti-HIV drugs such as zidovudine, with some success.
- Retinoids. These derivatives of vitamin A have long been used to treat **acne** and other skin diseases. Investigators are evaluating both topical preparations of these drugs as well as systemic versions.
- Laser therapy. In patients with small tumors, some investigators report success using lasers to destroy KS le-

sions. The reappearance of new tumors, may be high, however.

The prognosis for patients with classic KS is good. Tumors can frequently be controlled and patients frequently die of other causes before any serious spread. African endemic KS can progress rapidly and lead to premature death, despite treatment. In AIDS-related KS, milder cases can frequently be controlled; the prognosis for more advanced and rapidly progressing cases is less certain and dependent on the patient's overall medical condition. There are indications that KS can be stabilized or reversed in patients whose level of HIV in the blood is reduced to undetectable levels via antiretroviral therapy.

Safer sex practices may help to prevent AIDS-related KS by decreasing the risk of transmission of HHV-8. Treatment with antiretrovirals and protease inhibitors may help to preserve the function of the immune system in HIV patients and delay the appearance and progression of KS lesions.

KATZ, BERNARD (1911-)

German English physiologist

Katz was born in Leipzig, Germany, on March 26, 1911. He received his M.D. from the University of Leipzig in 1934, just as Adolf Hitler (1889-1945) was gaining power in Germany. Katz, who was Jewish, left his homeland for England where he pursued his post-graduate studies at the University of London. He eventually earned a Ph.D. in 1938 and a Sc.D. in 1934 from London.

During his years in London and (briefly, during World War II) Sydney, Australia, Katz worked with other scientists on the transmission of nerve impulses along a neuron and across the synaptic gap between neurons and muscles. With **Alan Hodgkin** and **Andrew Huxley**, he found that the movement of a nerve impulse along a single neuron can be described in terms of the diffusion of potassium and sodium ions across the cell membrane. This diffusion of ions creates a small electric potential that corresponds to the movement of the electrical impulse in the neuron.

In the 1950s, Katz concentrated on the transfer of the nerve message across synapses, the spaces between neurons or between neurons and muscle cells. Earlier research by **Henry Dale** (1875-1968) and **Otto Loewi** (1873-1961) had indicated that the neural message is carried across the synaptic gap by means of a chemical substance, a neurotransmitter, later identified as acetylcholine.

Katz eventually found that molecules of acetylcholine are apparently "packaged" in tiny vesicles stored at the end of a neuron. Upon stimulation, the neuron releases packages of acetylcholine that travel across the synapse and stimulate the adjacent muscle cell or second neuron. For this discovery, Katz was awarded a share of the 1970 Nobel Prize for physiology or medicine. He was also knighted by Queen Elizabeth II (1926) in 1969.

KAWASAKI SYNDROME

Kawasaki syndrome is a potentially fatal inflammatory disease that affects several organ systems in the body, including the heart, circulatory system, mucous membranes, skin, and **immune system**. Infants and children are at highest risk (80% are children under 4), but adults have also been diagnosed with the condition. Its cause is unknown.

Nearly twice as common among men, the disease affects Asians more often than either blacks or whites, but it doesn't seem to be found in any one particular part of the world. Although the disease usually occurs in single cases, it sometimes affects several members of the same family and occasionally occurs in small **epidemics**.

The specific cause of Kawasaki syndrome is unknown, although the disease resembles infections in many ways. Kawasaki syndrome may represent an allergic reaction or another unusual response to certain infections. Some researchers think that the syndrome may be caused by the interaction of an immune cell (called the T cell) with certain poisons produced by bacteria.

The symptoms of Kawasaki disease include a **fever** and a rash that spreads over the patient's chest and genital area. The fever is followed by peeling of the skin beginning at the fingertips and toenails. In addition to the body rash, the patient's lips become very red and the tongue takes on a "strawberry" appearance. The palms, soles, and mucous membranes that line the eyelids and cover the exposed portion of the eyeball become purplish-red and swollen. The lymph nodes in the patient's neck may also become swollen. These symptoms may last from two weeks to three months, with relapses in some patients.

In addition to the major symptoms, about 30% of patients develop joint **pain**s or arthritis, usually in the large joints of the body. Others develop **pneumonia**, **diarrhea**, dry or cracked lips, **jaundice**, or an inflammation of the membranes covering the brain and spinal cord (**meningitis**). A few patients develop symptoms of inflammation in the liver, gallbladder, lungs, or tonsils. About 20% of patients with Kawasaki syndrome develop complications of the **cardiovascular system**. These complications include inflammation of the heart tissue (**myocarditis**), disturbances in heartbeat rhythm (**arrhythmias**), and areas of blood vessel dilation (**aneurysms**). Other patients may develop inflammation of an artery in their arms or legs. Complications of the heart or arteries begin to develop around the tenth day after infection. The specific causes of these complications are not yet known.

Because Kawasaki syndrome is primarily a disease of infants and young children, the disease is most likely to be diagnosed by a pediatrician. The doctor will first rule out other diseases that cause fever and skin **rashes**, including **scarlet fever**, **measles**, Rocky Mountain spotted fever, **toxoplasmosis** (a disease carried by cats), juvenile **rheumatoid arthritis**, and a blistering and inflammation of the skin caused by reactions to certain medications.

Chest x ray may show enlargement of the heart (cardiomegaly). Urine may show the presence of pus or an abnormally high level of protein. An electrocardiogram may show changes in the heartbeat rhythm. In addition to these tests, it is important to take a series of echocardiograms during the course of the illness because 20% of Kawasaki patients will develop coronary aneurysms or arteritis that will not appear during the first examination.

Kawasaki syndrome is usually treated with a combination of **aspirin** to control the patient's fever and skin inflammation, and high doses of intravenous immune globulin to reduce the possibility of coronary artery complications. Some patients with heart complications may be treated with drugs that reduce blood clotting or may receive corrective surgery. Follow-up care includes two to three months of monitoring with chest x rays, **electrocardiography**, and **echocardiography**. Treatment with aspirin is often continued for several months.

Most patients with Kawasaki syndrome will recover completely, but about 1-2% will die as a result of blood clots forming in the coronary arteries or as a result of a **heart attack**. Deaths are sudden and unpredictable. Almost 95% of fatalities occur within six months of infection, but some have been reported as long as 10 years after.

KEEN, WILLIAM WILLIAMS (1837-1932)

American surgeon

William Williams Keen was internationally known as an innovative surgeon, prolific writer, and outstanding teacher of surgery and anatomy. He was class valedictorian at Brown University and earned his MD at Jefferson Medical College in 1862.

Soon after graduation from medical school, he served as acting surgeon in the US Army during the Civil War. He served near the front before being called to Turner's Lane Hospital in Philadelphia. The military was organizing hospitals that offered specialized treatment and in 1863, Union soldiers with neurological injuries and illnesses were sent to Turner's Lane Hospital. Physicians S. Weir Mitchell and George R. Morehouse had requested Keen's transfer and the three doctors observed the neurological patients closely, keeping detailed notes. They were the first to document and name causalgia, a severe burning sensation which can follow partial injury of the nerves. The doctors also studied the exaggeration of symptoms in **malingering** patients, primary and secondary **shock**, and reflex **paralysis**. They noted that when an important nerve is severed, there can be a paradoxical reaction where the patient suffers increased sensitivity to pain and touch. In 1864, the three physicians published a monograph on injuries to the nerves from gunshot wounds and other causes. They had gathered other materials in the expectation of publishing much more on nerve injuries, but the papers were ruined in a fire.

Keen pursued additional studies in Paris, Berlin, and Vienna between 1864 and 1866, when he returned to Philadelphia to begin private practice. In 1866, Keen began lecturing at the Philadelphia School of Anatomy and at Jefferson Medical College, his alma mater. In addition, he held academic appointments at the Pennsylvania Academy of Fine Arts and Women's Medical College.

Keen was one of the first physicians in the world to adopt antiseptic surgical technique, which probably accounted for some of his success as a surgeon. The prompt adoption of antiseptic practice was unusual because there had been very little understanding of infection. During the Civil War, the appearance of pus in a wound was interpreted as a sign of healing. In his account of his work as a military surgeon during the second battle of Bull Run, Keen mentioned pus being a positive sign. However, as soon as antisepsis was scientifically proven, Keen taught his students to maintain a sterile environment during every step of medical care. During his career, Keen estimated that he taught 6,000 to 7,000 medical students.

In 1886, after the death of his wife Emma, Keen revised the American edition of Gray's *Anatomy* and expanded the section on the **nervous system**. He was interested in the surgical treatment of disorders such as epilepsy and trigeminal neuralgia, a severe pain that often begins in the area of the mouth. One of Keen's triumphs in the newly recognized field of neurosurgery involved removing a **brain tumor** in a patient who went on to live another 30 years.

Keen participated in a clandestine surgery in 1893, performed on the presidential yacht in Long Island Sound. The patient was President Grover Cleveland, who suffered from a malignant tumor of the upper jaw. Keen assisted Joseph Bryant in the operation, which was carried out through the mouth and involved no external incisions. Cleveland lived another 15 years with no recurrence of the tumor, and the surgery was not made public until 1917.

Keen published more than 650 articles, books and editorials. He wrote about the first clinical use of X-rays in 1896. In 1892, he published *An American Text-book of Surgery* with J. W. White, which went to four editions and developed an international audience. His eight-volume *Principles and Practice of Surgery* was released between 1906 and 1921.

Keen was 80 years old when the United States entered World War I. He rejoined the service, this time as a major in the US Army Medical Corps, and edited *Principles and Practice of Surgery.*

Keen's achievements were widely recognized by the international medical community. He received honorary degrees from 12 universities in six countries and was an honorary fellow of three royal colleges of surgeons. He was president of the American Surgical Association in 1899 and president of the **American Medical Association** in 1900.

In addition to his significant role as surgeon and neurosurgeon, Keen was recognized for his many contributions to medical education. Over and above his writing and lecturing, he was active in numerous medical organizations and corresponded with surgeons and physicians around the world. On his ninetieth birthday, Keen announced that his only regret was having so little time to accomplish everything he still wanted to do. He died at home five years later.

Keller, Helen Adams (1880-1968)

American author, lecturer

Helen Adams Keller was born in Tuscumbia, Alabama, on June 27, 1880. She developed normally until the age of nineteen months, when she was stricken by a severe **fever**. In Keller's writings, she describes her parents' relief that she recovered from the fever, touching on the irony that, in their early rejoicing, they were unaware that she could no longer see or hear.

Keller spent the next five or so years locked into her isolated, dark world. Unable to see or hear, she also became mute. Her frustrations frequently boiled to the surface, and her behavior was described as angry, wild, and animal-like. She struck out at others, scratched, and hurled herself to the ground in fury at being unable to communicate with the people around her. Finally, when Keller was six, her parents reached the end of their rope. The consulted Alexander Graham Bell (inventor of the telephone and an expert on the deaf). He was able to make referrals which ended up in a young teacher, Annie Sullivan (**Anne Sullivan Macy**), being sent to the Keller family from the Perkins Institute for the Blind in Boston. Sullivan had herself been blind for a time, only to regain partial sight through surgery. Annie Sullivan proved to be the key to unlock Keller's world.

Using an alphabet of hand shapes which can be spelled into another person's hand, Sullivan followed Keller everywhere. As Keller experienced the world, Sullivan would spell pertinent words into Keller's hand. Finally, as Keller felt water from a pump gushing out over one of her hands, Sullivan formed the letters for the word ''water'' into Keller's other hand. At that moment, Keller suddenly underwent an epiphany, and she understood that Sullivan's fingers were communicating with her to identify the cold, liquid substance her other hand was experiencing.

From this point on, Keller was ravenous for knowledge. Sullivan taught her finger spelling, and Keller went on to learn a technique for ''hearing'' what people were saying by placing her hands on their nose, mouth and larynx. Keller quickly learned to read Braille, and a specialized typewriter allowed Keller to communicate in writing.

At age 10, Keller became determined to learn to speak, and attended the Horace Mann School for the Deaf, where she began the process. She also attended the Wright-Humason School for the Deaf, and the Cambridge School for Young Ladies. She was an excellent student, and was admitted to Radcliffe College at age 20. Annie Sullivan attended classes with Keller, patiently spelling the lectures into Keller's hand. Keller read material for her courses in Braille textbooks. By 1904, she had graduated with honors.

Keller and Sullivan traveled and lectured widely in the United States and overseas to raise money for the blind and deaf. Together, they helped put a stop to the practice of placing all disabled children permanently in institutions. As a living example, Keller was able to convince the public of the importance and value of appropriate education for even disabled children. During World War II, Keller championed the cause of veterans who had been blinded in battle.

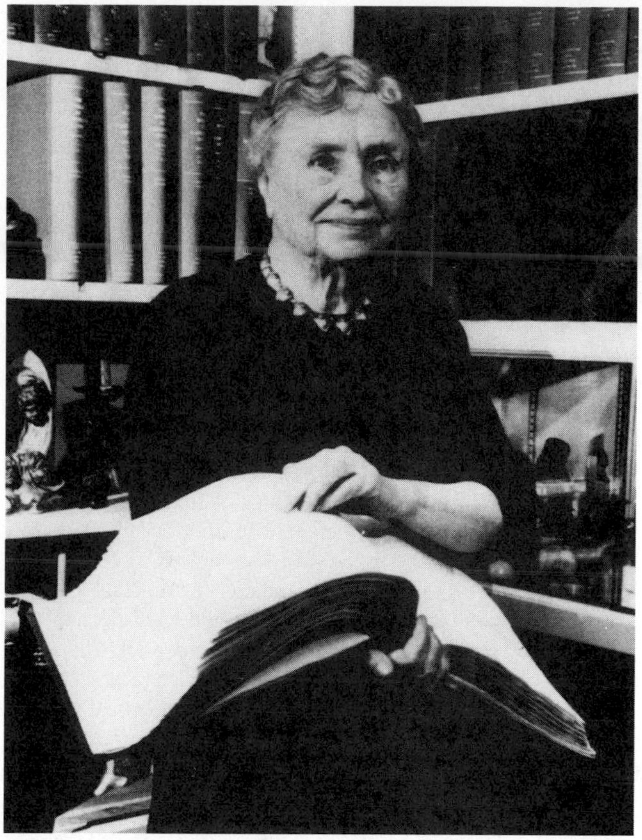

Helen Keller

In 1930, Annie Sullivan's eyes failed again, and she became blind. Polly Thompson, Sullivan and Keller's housekeeper/secretary since 1914, stepped into the role that Sullivan could no longer fill, caring for both Sullivan and Keller, and helping Keller travel and lecture. In 1936, Sullivan died. Thompson stayed with Keller until Thompson's death in 1960.

Keller wrote a number of very well-received books, including *The Story of My life* (1902); *Optimism* (1903); *The World I Live In* (1908); *The Song of the Stone Wall* (1910); *Out of the Dark* (1913); *My Religion* (1929); *Midstream: My Later Life* (1930); and *Teacher* (1930). Numerous biographies have been written about Helen Keller. William Gibson wrote the Pulitzer prize-winning play *The Miracle Worker* about Annie Sullivan's teaching of Helen Keller. *The Miracle Worker* was made into a 1962 film which garnered Academy Awards for Anne Bancroft (as Sullivan) and Patty Duke (as the young Helen Keller).

On June 1, 1968, Helen Keller died at the age of 87. Her own words make a fitting eulogy for the turning point in her life: ''Once I knew only darkness and stillness.... My life was without past or future.... But a little word from the fingers of another fell into my hand that clutched at emptiness, and my heart leaped to the rapture of living.''

See also Hearing loss; Macy, Anne Sullivan; Visual impairment and blindness

KELLY, HOWARD ATWOOD (1858-1943)

American physician

Howard A. Kelly served as one of the four original medical professors when Johns Hopkins Medical School was formed. He developed new techniques in abdominal surgery, particularly gynecologic surgery, and was one of the first to recognize the potential for treating **cancer** with radium.

Kelly received his MD from the University of Pennsylvania in 1882 and traveled to Europe to learn more about advanced gynecologic techniques. He founded Kensington Hospital in Philadelphia in 1888 and served as assistant professor of obstetrics at the University of Philadelphia.

Kelly moved to Baltimore in 1889 to work as gynecologist-in-chief at the new Johns Hopkins Hospital. At age 31, Kelly was one of four original faculty of Johns Hopkins University Medical School. He served as professor of gynecology for 30 years before becoming professor emeritus. Johns Hopkins was founded to raise the standards for medical schools. Admissions standards were very high, and each hospital department led a corresponding section at the school. The Johns Hopkins philosophy was to combine knowledge and clinical teaching for the benefit of the patient and the medical student. Kelly developed new surgical methods and diagnostic techniques to help make Baltimore a leading center of gynecology.

Kelly realized only a few of his medical students would go on to become gynecologists. His goal was to give every student a one-year foundation in gynecology for general purposes. All gynecologists had to first show proficiency in abdominal surgery. Kelly refused to teach gynecology by performing surgery before students in a large classroom. He reasoned that the students couldn't see very much and the exposure posed a risk to the patient. Students were permitted to observe many surgeries in the operating room, but they could not assist. Only students who finished medical school and were accepted for specialty training in gynecology could eventually assist in surgeries.

While still on staff at Johns Hopkins, Kelly founded the Howard A. Kelly Hospital in Baltimore in 1892. It was a **sanatorium** first founded because Johns Hopkins had few facilities for private patients. Kelly took over the sanitorium from a colleague who was moving away and added three adjacent houses which retained their original elegant architecture.

The discovery of radium in 1903 by **Pierre** and **Marie Curie** was exciting to doctors as they looked for ways to employ radium for new cures. Kelly bought a small tube of radium in 1904, keeping it at his private clinic, and began using it to treat external lesions. His aunt was his first radium patient. By 1907, Kelly had bought $12,000 worth of radium and in 1913, he traveled to Colorado to see if radium could be mined economically. He formed a partnership with other investors, including the US Bureau of Mines, to begin a $400,000 project. Kelly also developed a partnership with the federal government when he and another doctor founded the National Radium Institute. Eventually the government bowed out of both ventures in the wake of pressure from private interests.

Kelly wrote more than 500 scientific articles and 18 books. His medical textbooks on gynecology, the appendix, and topics such as the kidneys and bladder were valued for their comprehensive descriptions and detailed illustrations. Kelly wrote several medical biographies and a religious tract, *A Scientific Man and the Bible*. He held membership in professional societies throughout the world, including dozens of honorary fellowships and doctorates. Kelly is best known for his leadership in three areas: as a founding faculty member of Johns Hopkins University Medical School, as a physician who established high standards in gynecology, and as one of the first clinicians to see the medical potential of radium.

KELSEY, FRANCES OLDHAM (1914-)

Canadian American pharmacologist and physician

Frances Oldham Kelsey became nationally famous in 1962 when she prevented the sedative drug thalidomide from entering the United States. Thalidomide was found to have caused **birth defects** in 10,000 European children in the late 1950s and early 1960s. For preventing an American thalidomide tragedy, Kelsey was awarded the government's highest civilian award, the President's Distinguished Federal Civilian Service Award. Kelsey's vigilance led to the strengthening of investigational drug regulations, greater attention to the safety of drugs in **pregnancy**, and increased interest in research on teratology, the biological study of congenital deformities and abnormal development.

Kelsey was born in Cobble Hill, British Columbia, on July 24, 1914. In 1934, she received a bachelor's degree in science from McGill University in Montreal and attained a master's degree in science there in 1935. Kelsey received her professional degrees, a doctorate in pharmacology in 1938 and an M.D. in 1950, from the University of Chicago. She completed an internship at Sacred Heart Hospital in Yankton, South Dakota, in 1954 and was associate professor of pharmacology at the University of South Dakota from 1954 to 1957. She remained in South Dakota until 1960, and was in private practice there between 1957 and 1960. In 1955, Kelsey became a naturalized U.S. citizen. She had married F. Ellis Kelsey in 1943, and they had two children.

Early in her career, Kelsey investigated the cause of 107 deaths, most of them in children, from a new sulfa drug. In the 1940s, she coauthored several papers with her husband on the **metabolism** of antimalarial drugs. In 1943, they published a study in the *Journal of Pharmacy and Experimental Therapy* about the effects of antimalarial drugs on the embryo. They found that the drug could be broken down by the liver of adult rabbits, but fetal livers could not break it down, and the drug could have deleterious effects. This research laid the groundwork for Kelsey's continuing interest in the safety of drugs during pregnancy.

Kelsey's civil service career began in August, 1960, when she became a medical officer for the **Food and Drug Administration** (FDA). After one month on the job, Kelsey was asked to review what was expected to be a simple and routine marketing application for thalidomide. Thalidomide, a sleep inducer, had been developed in West Germany in the 1950s, and was widely marketed in Europe; belief in its safety was so widespread that the drug was available without prescription.

Kelsey soon became suspicious of the safety of thalidomide. In February, 1961, she read a letter from a doctor in the *British Medical Journal* suggesting an association between thalidomide and peripheral neuritis, a tingling sensation in the arms and legs of adult users. Kelsey promptly asked Richardson-Merrill, distributor of thalidomide, for additional animal study data and reports of all clinical trials of thalidomide to supplement the company's application for American approval. She later notified the company that she suspected thalidomide might have some effect on unborn children, although she did not yet suspect it as a cause of deformity. Throughout her review, Kelsey remained concerned that the company had failed to provide adequate data to demonstrate the safety of thalidomide.

In November, 1961, a German scientist alleged a strong association between use of the drug by pregnant women and an increase in deformed babies born in Germany. Finally, in December, 1961, the company acknowledged the German reports and requested that women of childbearing age discontinue its use. More than 10,000 cases of phocomelia, a condition causing underdevelopment or absence of arms and legs, in European children were eventually attributed to use of thalidomide. Seventeen cases of thalidomide embryopathy resulting from a then-legal experimental distribution of the drug were later documented in the United States.

On July 15, 1962, the *Washington Post* ran an article about Kelsey that began, "This is the story of how the skepticism and stubbornness of a government physician prevented what could have been an appalling American tragedy...." A wave of publicity and acclaim swept the world. Only a month later, Congress voted to award a gold medal to Kelsey "in recognition of the distinguished service to mankind... by withholding, despite the great pressures brought to bear upon her, approval of the horror-drug thalidomide which has caused thousands of babies to be deformed." In October, 1962, with Kelsey present at the ceremony, President Kennedy signed a landmark drug law, the Kefauver-Harris Amendments. The law required drug manufacturers to register with the Food and Drug Administration proof that new drugs were both effective and safe, and provided for more rapid recall of new drugs deemed hazardous. In 1963, Kelsey became chief of the Investigational Drug Branch of the FDA, and in 1968 was appointed to her current position as director of the Office of Scientific Investigations.

KENDALL, EDWARD CALVIN (1886-1972)

American biochemist

Edward Kendall is known for two major contributions to biochemical knowledge. The first of these was his isolation of the

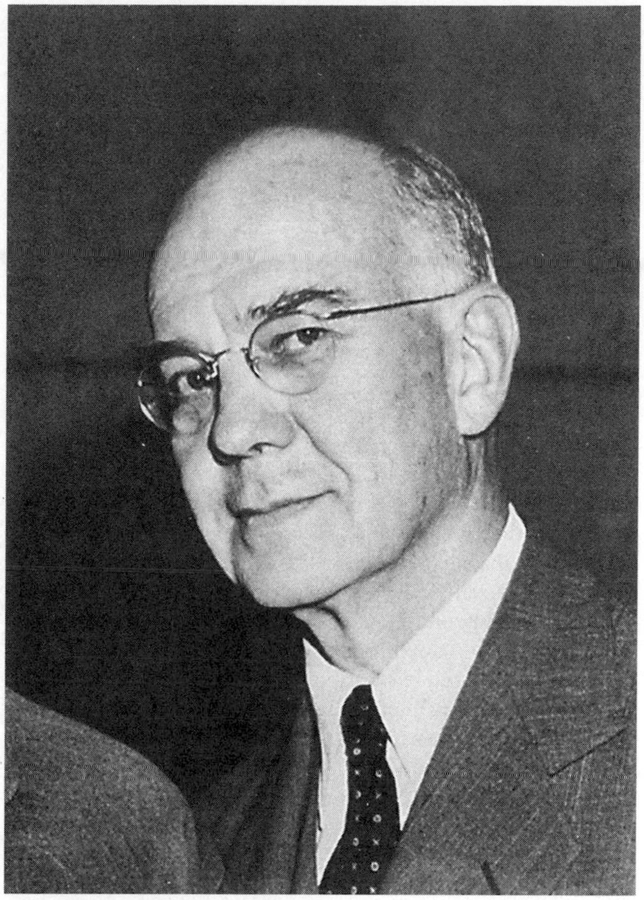

Edward Calvin Kendall

thyroid hormone thyroxine. In addition, he isolated several steroid hormones produced by the cortex (outer covering) of the adrenal gland, one of which is cortisone, playing a major role in demonstrating its medical use. For his work with cortisone, Kendall shared part of the 1950 Nobel Prize in physiology or medicine with his colleague **Philip Hench**.

Throughout his career, Kendall often relied on intuition rather than strict laboratory procedure in performing his research. After retiring from the Mayo Clinic in 1951, he continued his research at Princeton University. Kendall was born in South Norwalk, Connecticut, where his father was a dentist. He received both his bachelor's degree (1908) and his doctorate (1910) from Columbia University. The theory of hormones had been developed in the early years of the century by the British physiologists Ernest Starling and William Bayliss (1860-1924), describing glandular secretions that control body functions. In 1910, Kendall began working to isolate a thyroid hormone, first at a pharmaceutical company (Parke Davis and Co.) and then at St. Luke's Hospital in New York. By 1913, he had made a much more pure thyroid gland extract than previously was available, showing its activity in both experimental dogs and human patients.

In 1914, he joined the staff of the Mayo Clinic, in Rochester, Minnesota, where the founders were interested in studying and treating thyroid diseases. By the end of the year, Kendall had isolated the crystalline form of the hormone, later named thyroxine, and shown its activity in successful treatment of patients with underactive thyroid glands. In studying how thyroxine affects oxidation processes in the body, he needed the coenzyme glutathione, a peptide formed from the amino acids cysteine, glutamic acid, and glycine. Since it was not available in pure form, Kendall and his associates independently isolated and synthesized it.

During the 1930s, Kendall turned his attention to the hormones of the adrenal cortex after an adrenal extract had been successfully used to treat Addison's disease, which results from atrophy of the gland. In 1933, he isolated a crystalline substance, which he called "the" hormone, because it was then believed that the cortex secreted only a single hormone. However, further research showed that several substances were present in his crystals, none of them necessarily a hormone. The next year, Kendall and others independently suggested that the adrenal cortex secretes more than one hormone.

Over the next two years, Kendall isolated a series of crystalline substances, to which he gave alphabetical titles. Kendall's Compound E, later named cortisone, was independently isolated by three groups of scientists, but only Kendall converted it to a related compound, a diketone, which had already been demonstrated to be active. Kendall deduced that Compound E is a steroid. During World War II Kendall directed a program to synthesize and produce quantities of Compound E, because some medical authorities thought it might help prevent injury-related stress and surgical shock in wounded military personnel. Hench, who was working on treatment methods for rheumatoid arthritis, and Kendall determined to try using Compound E on arthritic patients. In 1948, after a supply of it was available, they used it as a treatment for the first time. In 1949, they named Compound E cortisone. Kendall's Compounds B and F were later identified by other scientists as the hormones corticosterone and cortisol (hydrocortisone).

KENNY, ELIZABETH (1886-1952)

Australian nurse

Also known as Sister Kenny, Elizabeth Kenny was born 1886 in Warialda, New South Wales. Without formal **nursing** training, she worked initially as a bush country nurse, treating the first stages of **polio** and in 1933, established a clinic at Townsville, Queensland. She became best known for her treatment of poliomyelitis. In the acute phase of the disease, the patient's back and limbs are wrapped in woolen clothes, wrung out after soaking in hot water. After the painful phase has passed, the paralyzed muscles are slowly stimulated and reeducated with passive **exercise**. In the early 1940s, Kenny lectured in the United States and often found opposition from those accustomed to the old methods of immobilization of patients using splints and casts. She soon gained the support of the **American Medical Association**. In 1943, the Elizabeth Kenny Institute of Minneapolis, Minnesota was set up to train nurses and **physical therapy** staff in Kenny's treatment methods.

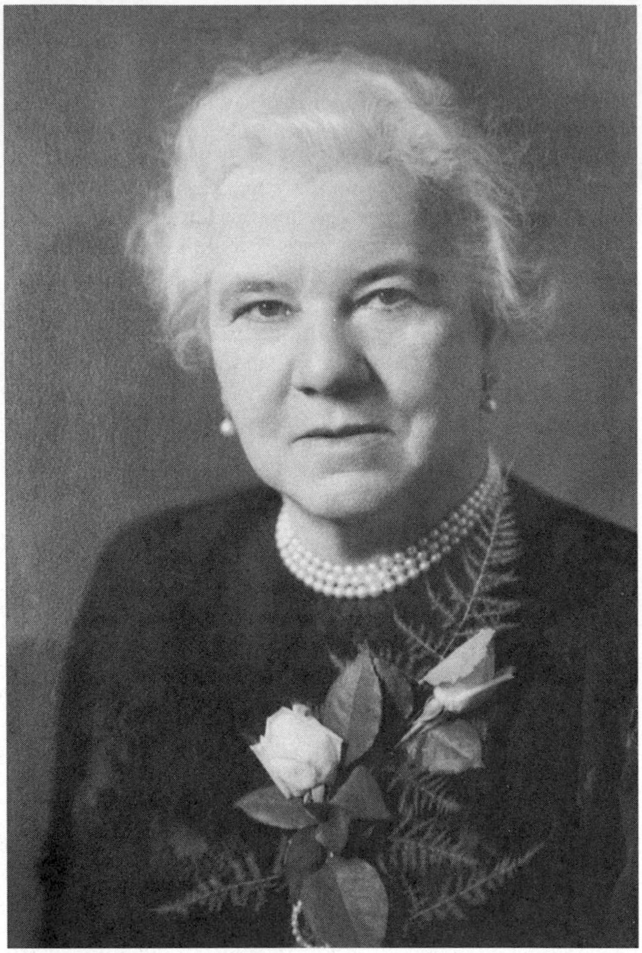

Elizabeth Kenny

KERATITIS

Keratitis is an inflammation of the cornea, the transparent membrane that covers the colored part of the **eye** (iris) and pupil of the eye.

There are many types and causes of keratitis, which can occur in both children and adults. Germs can't usually invade a healthy cornea, but certain conditions can allow an infection to occur, such as a scratch or a very dry eye can decrease the cornea's ability to protect itself.

Illnesses or other factors that reduces the body's ability to overcome infection, including **cold sore**s; **genital herpes**; crowded, dirty living conditions; poor hygiene poor **nutrition** (especially a deficiency of vitamin A, which is essential for normal vision).

Herpes simplex keratitis is a major cause of adult eye disease, and may lead to chronic inflammation of the cornea, development of tiny blood vessels in the eye, scarring, blindness, or **glaucoma**.

The infection generally begins with inflammation of the membrane lining the eyelid and the portion of the eyeball that comes into contact with it. It usually occurs in one eye. Subsequent infections are characterized by a pattern of lesions that resemble the veins of a leaf. These infections, called dendritic keratitis, can aid in the diagnosis. Recurrences may be brought on by **stress**, fatigue, or ultraviolet light (UV) exposure.

It is very important not to use topical **corticosteroids** with herpes simplex keratitis as it can make the condition much worse, possibly leading to blindness.

People who have bacterial keratitis wake up with their eyelids stuck together. There can be **pain**, sensitivity to light, redness, tearing, and a decrease in vision. Bacterial keratitis makes the cornea cloudy and may cause **abscess**es. This condition can be caused by wearing soft contact lenses overnight. One study found that overnight wear can increase risk by 10-15 times more than daily-wear contact lenses. Improper lens care is also a factor. Contaminated makeup can also contain bacteria.

Fungal keratitis, which often develops slowly, usually occurs if the cornea is injured in a farm-like setting or in a place where plant material is present. This condition usually affects people with weakened **immune systems**, often causes infection within the eyeball, and may cause abscesses.

Peripheral ulcerative keratitis is often associated with active or chronic: **Rheumatoid arthritis**, Wegener's granulomatosis, a rare condition characterized by kidney disease and development of nodules in the respiratory tract.

Superficial punctate keratitis is often associated with the type of viruses that cause the common cold; it's characterized by the destruction of pinpoint areas in the outer layer of the cornea. One or both eyes may be affected.

Acanthamoeba keratitis is a very painful, pus-producing condition commonly found in people who wear soft or rigid contact lenses. The bacteria can be found in tap water, soil, and swimming pools.

Photokeratitis (snowblindness) is caused by too much exposure to UV light such as in sunlight, suntanning lamps, or a welding arc. The condition is very painful and may occur several hours after exposure, and may last one to two days.

Interstitial keratitis is a chronic inflammation of tissue deep within the cornea that affects both eyes and usually occurs as a complication of congenital or acquired **syphilis**. It is rare in the United States. It also may occur in people with **tuberculosis**, **leprosy**, or other fungal infections.

Symptoms of keratitis include, but are not limited to:

- Tearing
- Pain
- Sensitivity to light
- Inflammation of the eyelid
- Decrease in vision
- Redness.

A doctor will test the patient's vision and then examine the eyes with a slit lamp. The cornea can be examined with fluorescein, a yellow dye which will highlight defects in the cornea. Deeper layers of the cornea can also be examined with the slit lamp. Samples of infectious matter removed from the eye will be sent for laboratory analysis.

Antibiotics, antifungals, and antiviral medication will be used to treat the appropriate organism. Broad spectrum antibiotics sterile, cotton-tipped applicator may be used to gently remove infected tissue and allow the eye to heal more rapidly. **Laser surgery** is sometimes performed to destroy unhealthy cells, and some severe infections require corneal transplants.

Antifungal, antibiotic, or antiviral eyedrops or ointments are usually prescribed to cure keratitis, but they should be used only by patients under a doctor's care. Inappropriate prescriptions or over-the-counter preparations can make symptoms more severe and cause tissue deterioration. Topical corticosteroids can cause great harm to the cornea in patient's with herpes simplex keratitis.

A patient with keratitis may wear a patch to protect the healing eye from bright light, **foreign objects**, the lid rubbing against the cornea, and other irritants. Sometimes a patch can make it worse, so again, the patient must discuss with the doctor whether or not a patch is necessary. The patient will probably return every day to the eye doctor to check on the progress.

Although early detection and treatment can cure most forms of keratitis, the infection can cause glaucoma, permanent scarring, ulceration of the cornea, or blindness.

Children and adults who wear contact lenses should always use sterile lens-cleaning and disinfecting solutions. Tap water is not sterile and should not be used to clean contact lenses. Contact lenses should be removed if the eyes become red or irritated, and replaced every three months.

Eating a well-balanced **diet** and wearing protective glasses when working or playing in potentially dangerous situations can reduce anyone's risk of developing keratitis. Protective goggles can even be worn mowing the lawn so that if twigs are tossed up they can't hurt the eye. Goggles or sunglasses with UV coatings can help protect against damage from UV light.

KHORANA, HAR GOBIND (1922-)

Indian American biochemist

Har Gobind Khorana is best known for developing chemical methods to determine the nucleotide sequence of ribonucleic acid (RNA) and for deciphering the genetic code. For this he shared the 1968 Nobel Prize for physiology or medicine with **Marshall Nirenberg** and **Robert Holley**.

Khorana was born in the small village of Raipur, India, where his father was a clerk in the British colonial service. Encouraged by his parents to obtain an education, he received a master's degree in 1945 from the University of Punjab, Lahore (now part of Pakistan). He then went to the United Kingdom, where he earned a doctorate in 1948 from the University of Liverpool. After brief visits to Switzerland and India, he returned to the United Kingdom to do research at Cambridge University during 1950-52, becoming interested in the nucleic acid investigations there. After further study in Switzerland, Khorana took a research position with the British Columbia (Canada) Research Council in Vancouver. In 1960 he joined the faculty of the University of Wisconsin.

Khorana's genetic code work involved using chemical methods and the enzymes deoxyribonucleic acid (DNA)

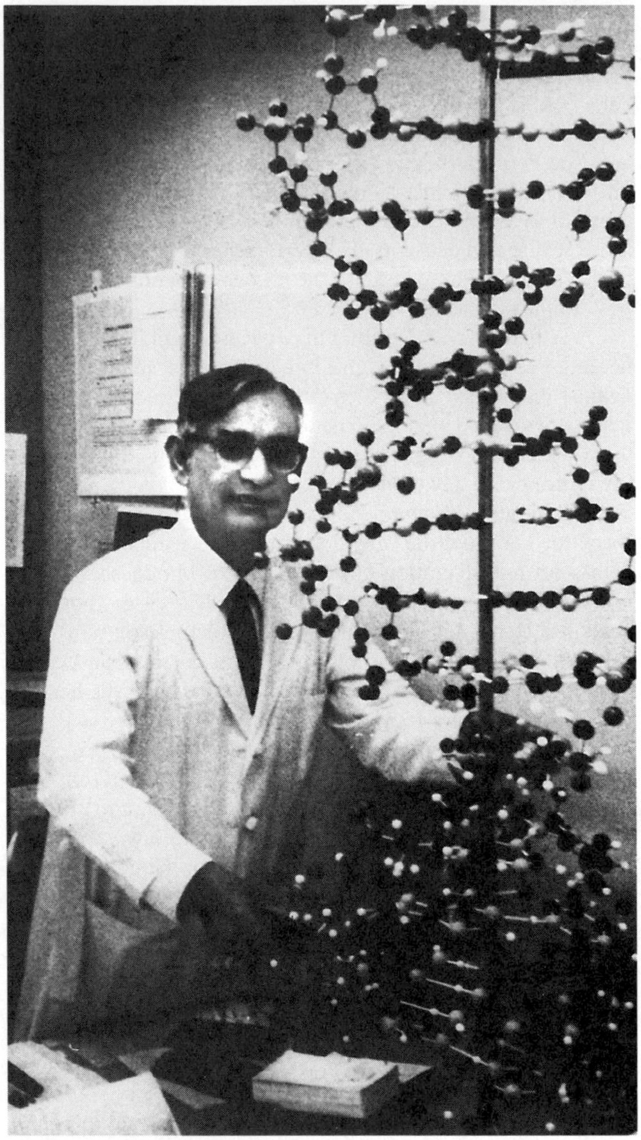

Har Gobind Khorana

polymerase and RNA polymerase, which he called ''beautifully precise copying machines,'' to produce long strands of nucleic acids with known base sequences. This allowed him to compare the information-bearing DNA with the corresponding transfer RNA (tRNA) that retrieved specific amino acids for assembly into proteins. Building on Nirenberg's work, Khorana precisely spelled out all sixty-four genetic code triplets (three-base information units) and related them to specific amino acids or terminating functions.

Two years after receiving the Nobel Prize for this work, he made pioneering progress in the construction of yeast and bacteria genes in the laboratory. Khorana also advanced knowledge of the way a cell's protein synthesizing bodies recognize a triplet and correctly assemble the amino acids, as well as how RNA and amino acids recognize each other.

Kidney cancer

Kidney cancer is a disease in which the cells in certain tissues of the kidney start to grow uncontrollably and form tumors. Renal cell carcinoma, which occurs in the cells lining the kidneys (epithelial cells), is the most common type of kidney cancer. Eighty-five percent of all kidney tumors are renal cell carcinomas.

The kidneys are a pair of organs shaped like kidney beans that lie on either side of the spine just above the waist. Inside each kidney are tiny tubes (tubules) that filter and clean the blood, taking out the waste products and making urine. The urine that is made by the kidney passes through a tube called the ureter into the bladder. Urine is held in the bladder until it is discharged from the body. Renal cell carcinoma generally develops in the lining of the tubules that filter and clean the blood.

The causes of kidney cancer are unknown, but men seem to have twice the risk of contracting the disease. There is a strong association between cigarette smoking and kidney cancer. Working around coke ovens has been shown to increase people's risk of developing this cancer. Certain types of painkillers that contain the chemical phenacetin are associated with kidney cancer. **Obesity** may be yet another risk factor for kidney cancer.

The most common symptom of kidney cancer is blood in the urine (hematuria). Other symptoms include painful urination, pain in the lower back or on the sides, abdominal pain, a lump or hard mass that can be felt in the kidney area, unexplained weight loss, **fever**, weakness, fatigue, and high blood pressure.

A diagnostic examination for kidney cancer includes taking a thorough medical history and making a complete **physical examination** in which the doctor will probe (palpate) the abdomen for lumps. Blood tests will be ordered to check for changes in blood chemistry caused by substances released by the tumor. Laboratory tests may show abnormal levels of iron in the blood. Either a low red blood cell count (**anemia**) or a high red blood cell count (erythrocytosis) may accompany kidney cancer. Occasionally, patients will have high calcium levels.

If the doctor suspects kidney cancer, an intravenous pyelogram (IVP) may be ordered. An IVP is an x-ray test in which a dye in injected into a vein in the arm. The dye travels through the body, and it outlines the kidneys, ureters, and the urinary bladder. On an x-ray image, the dye will reveal any abnormalities of the urinary tract. The IVP may miss small kidney cancers.

Renal ultrasound is a diagnostic test in which sound waves are used to form an image of the kidneys. Imaging tests such as **computed tomography scans** (CT scans) and **magnetic resonance imaging** (MRI) can be used to check whether the tumor has spread outside the kidney to other organs in the abdomen. A kidney **biopsy** is used to positively confirm the diagnosis of kidney cancer. During this procedure, a small piece of tissue is removed from the tumor and examined under a microscope. The biopsy will give information about the type of tumor, the cells that are involved, and the aggressiveness of the tumor (tumor stage).

Each person's treatment is different and depends on several factors. The location, size, and extent of the tumor have to be considered in addition to the patient's age, general health, and medical history. The primary treatment for kidney cancer that has not spread to other parts of the body is surgical removal of the diseased kidney (nephrectomy). Because most cancers affect only one kidney, the patient can function well on the one remaining. **Radiation therapy**, which consists of exposing the cancer cells to high-energy gamma rays from an external source, generally destroys cancer cells with minimal damage to the normal tissue. Side effects are **nausea**, tiredness, and stomach upsets. These symptoms disappear when the treatment is over. In kidney cancer, radiation therapy has been shown to alleviate pain and bleeding, especially when the cancer is inoperable. However, it has not proven to be of much use in destroying the kidney cancer cells. Therefore radiation therapy is not used very often.

Treatment of kidney cancer with **anticancer drugs** (**chemotherapy**) has not produced good results. However, new drugs and new combinations of drugs continue to be tested in clinical trials.

Because kidney cancer is often caught early and sometimes progresses slowly, the chances of a surgical cure are good. It is also one of the few cancers for which there are well-documented cases of spontaneous remission without therapy.

The exact cause of kidney cancer is not known, so it is not possible to prevent all cases. However, because a strong association between kidney cancer and tobacco has been shown, avoiding tobacco is the best way to lower one's risk of developing this cancer. Using care when working with cancer-causing agents such as asbestos and cadmium and eating a well-balanced **diet** may also help prevent kidney cancer.

KIDNEY FAILURE

Kidney failure is described in two ways: acute or chronic. Acute kidney failure occurs when illness, infection, or injury damages the kidneys. Temporarily, the kidneys cannot adequately remove fluids and wastes from the body or maintain the proper level of certain kidney-regulated chemicals in the bloodstream. Similarly, chronic kidney failure occurs when a number of diseases or inherited disorders injure the kidneys, but this form leads to irreversible damage, and eventually total kidney failure or end-stage renal disease (ESRD). Without proper treatment intervention to remove wastes and fluids from the bloodstream, ESRD is fatal.

The kidneys are the body's natural filtration system. They perform the critical task of processing approximately 200 quarts of fluid in the bloodstream every 24 hours. Waste products like urea and toxins, along with excess fluids, are removed from the bloodstream in the form of urine. Kidney (or renal) failure occurs when kidney functioning becomes impaired. Fluids and toxins begin to accumulate in the bloodstream. As fluids build up in the bloodstream, the patient with acute kidney failure may become puffy and swollen (edematous) in the face, hands, and feet. Their blood pressure typically begins to rise, and they may experience fatigue and **nausea**.

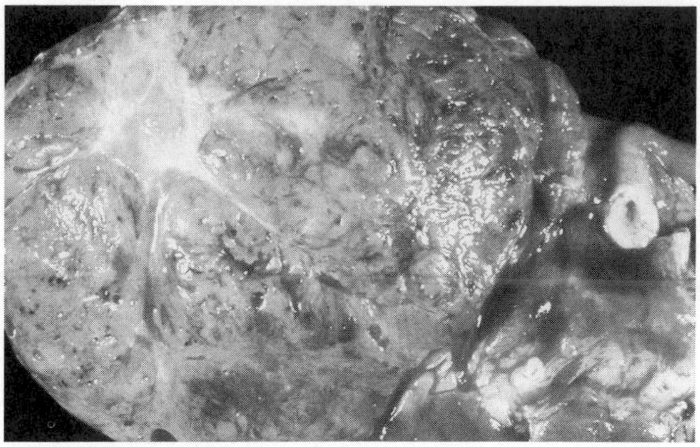

An extracted cancerous kidney. ***(Custom Medical Stock Photo. Reproduced by permission.)***

Unlike chronic kidney failure, which is long term and irreversible, acute kidney failure is a temporary condition. With proper and timely treatment, it can typically be reversed. Often there is no permanent damage to the kidneys. Acute kidney failure appears most frequently as a complication of serious illness, like **heart failure**, liver failure, **dehydration**, severe **burns**, and excessive bleeding (hemorrhage). It may also be caused by an obstruction to the urinary tract or as a direct result of kidney disease, injury, or an adverse reaction to a medicine.

Acute kidney failure can be caused by many different illnesses, injuries, and infections. These conditions fall into three main categories: *prerenal*, *postrenal*, and *intrarenal* conditions.

Prerenal conditions do not damage the kidney, but can cause diminished kidney function. They are the most common cause of acute renal failure, and include: dehydration; hemorrhage, or excessive bleeding; septicemia, or **sepsis** (a poisoning of the blood); heart failure; liver failure; and burns.

Postrenal conditions cause kidney failure by obstructing the urinary tract. These conditions include: inflammation of the prostate gland in men (**prostatitis**); enlargement of the prostate gland (benign prostatic hypertrophy); bladder or pelvic tumors; and kidney stones(calculi).

Intrarenal conditions involve kidney disease or direct injury to the kidneys. These conditions include: lack of blood supply to the kidneys (ischemia); the use of radiocontrast agents during diagnostic tests in patients with kidney problems; drug abuse or overdose; long-term use of nephrotoxic medications, like certain **pain** medicines; acute inflammation of the glomeruli, or filters, of the kidney; and kidney infections

Kidney failure is triggered by disease or a hereditary disorder in the kidneys. Both kidneys are typically affected. The four most common causes of chronic kidney failure include: diabetes, which consists of **diabetes mellitus** (DM), both insulin dependant (IDDM) and non-insulin dependant (NIDDM), a condition that occurs when the body cannot produce and/or use insulin, the hormone necessary for the body to process glucose; glomerulonephritis, or the chronic inflammation of the glomeruli, or filtering units of the kidney. Certain types of glomerulonephritis are treatable, and may only cause a temporary disruption of kidney functioning; **hypertension**, or high blood pressure is unique to chronic kidney failure in that it is both a cause and a major symptom of the condition.

Other possible causes of chronic kidney failure include **kidney cancer**, obstructions such as **kidney stones**, pyelonephritis (inflammation within kidney and of the surrounding pelvis), reflux nephropathy, **systemic lupus erythematosus**, amyloidosis, **sickle-cell anemia**, Alport syndrome, and oxalosis.

Initially, symtpoms of chronic kidney failure develop slowly. Even individuals with mild to moderate kidney failure may show few symtpoms in spite of increased urea in their blood. Among the symptoms that may be present at this point are frequent urination during the night and high blood pressure.

There are several symptoms of acute and chronic kidney failure, but most symptoms of chronic kidney failure are not apparent until kidney disease has progressed significantly. Common symptoms for both acute and chronic conditions include:

- **Anemia**. The kidneys are responsible for the production of erythropoietin (EPO), a hormone which stimulates red cell production. If kidney disease causes shrinking of the kidney, this red cell production is hampered.
- **Bad breath** or a bad taste in mouth. Urea, or waste products, in the saliva may cause an ammonia-like taste in the mouth.
- Bone and joint problems. The kidneys produce vitamin D, which aids in the absorption of calcium and keeps bones strong. For patients with kidney failure, bones may become brittle, and in the case of children, normal growth may be stunted. Joint **pain** may also occur as a result of unchecked phosphate levels in the blood.
- **Edema**. Puffiness or swelling around the eyes, arms, hands, and feet.
- Frequent urination.
- Foamy or bloody urine. Protein in the urine may cause it to foam significantly. Blood in the urine may indicate bleeding from diseased or obstructed kidneys, bladder, or ureters.
- **Headache**s. High blood pressure may trigger headaches.
- Hypertension, or high blood pressure. The retention of fluids and wastes causes blood volume to increase, which in turn, causes blood pressure to rise.
- Increased fatigue. Toxic substances in the blood and the presence of anemia may cause feelings of exhaustion.
- **Itching**. Phosphorus, which is typically eliminated in the urine, accumulates in the blood of patients with kidney failure. This heightened phosphorus level may cause itching of the skin.
- Lower back pain. Pain where the kidneys are located, in the small of the back below the ribs.
- Nausea, loss of appetite, and vomiting. Urea in the gastric juices may cause upset stomach. This can lead to malnutrition and weight loss.

Kidney failure is typically diagnosed and treated by a nephrologist, a doctor that specializes in treating the kidneys. The patient that is suspected of having kidney failure will undergo an extensive blood work-up. A blood test will assess the levels of creatinine, blood urea nitrogen (BUN), uric acid, phosphate, sodium, and potassium in the blood. Urine samples will also be collected, usually over a 24-hour period, to assess protein loss and/or creatinine clearance.

Determining the cause of kidney failure is critical to proper treatment. A full assessment of the kidneys is necessary to determine if the underlying disease is treatable and if the kidney failure is chronic or acute. X rays, **magnetic resonance imaging** (MRI), **computed tomography scan** (CT), **ultrasound**, renal **biopsy**, and/or arteriogram of the kidneys may be used to determine the cause of kidney failure and level of remaining kidney function. X rays and ultrasound of the bladder and/or ureters may also be needed.

Treatment for acute kidney failure varies. Treatment is directed to the underlying, primary medical condition that has triggered kidney failure. Prerenal conditions may be treated with replacement fluids given through a vein, **diuretics**, blood **transfusion**, or medications. Postrenal conditions and intrarenal conditions may require surgery and/or medication.

Frequently, patients in acute or chronic kidney failure require *hemodialysis*, *hemofiltration*, or *peritoneal dialysis* to filter fluids and wastes from the bloodstream until the primary medical condition can be controlled.

A primary type of treatment for both acute and chronic kidney failure is hemodialysis which involves circulating the patient's blood outside of the body through an extracorporeal circuit (ECC), or dialysis circuit. The ECC is made up of plastic blood tubing, a filter known as a dialyzer (or artificial kidney), and a dialysis machine that monitors and maintains blood flow and administers dialysate. Dialysate is a sterile chemical solution that is used to draw waste products out of the blood. The patient's blood leaves the body through the vein and travels through the ECC and the dialyzer, where fluid removal takes place.

During dialysis, waste products in the bloodstream are carried out of the body. At the same time, electrolytes and other chemicals are added to the blood. The purified, chemically-balanced blood is then returned to the body.

A dialysis ''run'' typically lasts three to four hours, depending on the type of dialyzer used and the physical condition of the patient. Dialysis is used several times a week until acute kidney failure is reversed.

Blood pressure changes associated with hemodialysis may pose a risk for patients with heart problems. Peritoneal dialysis may be the preferred treatment option in these cases.

Another type of treatment is hemofiltration, also known as continuous renal replacement therapy (CRRT). This procedure is a slow, continuous blood filtration therapy used to control acute kidney failure in critically ill patients. These patients are typically very sick and may have heart problems or circulatory problems. They cannot handle the rapid filtration rates of hemodialysis. They also frequently need **antibiotics**, nutrition, vasopressors, and other fluids given through a vein to treat their primary condition. Because hemofiltration is continuous, prescription fluids can be given to patients in kidney failure without the risk of fluid overload.

Like hemodialysis, hemofiltration uses an ECC. A hollow fiber hemofilter is used instead of a dialyzer to remove fluids and toxins. Instead of a dialysis machine, a blood pump makes the blood flow through the ECC. The volume of blood circulating through the ECC in hemofiltration is less than that in hemodialysis. Filtration rates are slower and gentler on the circulatory system. Hemofiltration treatment will generally be used until kidney failure is reversed.

If an acute kidney failure patient is stable and not in immediate crisis, peritoneal dialysis may be used. In peritoneal dialysis (PD), which is also used as a treatment for chronic kidney failure, the lining of the patient's abdomen, the peritoneum, acts as a blood filter. A flexible tube-like instrument (catheter) is surgically inserted into the patient's abdomen. During treatment, the catheter is used to fill the abdominal cavity with dialysate. Waste products and excess fluids move from the patient's bloodstream into the dialysate solution. After a certain time period, the waste-filled dialysate is drained from the abdomen, and replaced with clean dialysate. There are three type of peritoneal dialysis, which vary according to treatment time and administration method.

Peritoneal dialysis is often the best treatment option for infants and children. Their small size can make vein access difficult to maintain. It is not recommended for patients with abdominal adhesions or other abdominal defects (like a **hernia**) that might reduce the efficiency of the treatment. It is also not recommended for patients who suffer frequent bouts of an inflammation of the small pouches in the intestinal tract (diverticulitis).

Kidney transplantation involves surgically attaching a functioning kidney, or graft, from a brain dead organ donor (a cadaver transplant), or from a living donor, to a patient with ESRD. Patients with chronic renal disease who need a transplant and don't have a living donor register with UNOS (United Network for Organ Sharing), the federal organ procurement agency, to be placed on a waiting list for a cadaver kidney transplant. Kidney availability is based on the patient's health status. When the new kidney is transplanted, the patient's existing, diseased kidneys may or may not be removed, depending on the circumstances surrounding the kidney failure. A regimen of immunosuppressive, or anti-rejection medication, is required after transplantation surgery.

A diet low in sodium, potassium, and phosphorous, three substances that the kidneys regulate, is critical in managing kidney disease Other dietary restrictions, such as a reduction in protein, may be prescribed depending on the cause of kidney failure and the type of dialysis treatment employed. Patients with chronic kidney failure also need to limit their fluid intake.

Kidney failure patients with hypertension typically take medication to control their high blood pressure. Epoetin alfa, or EPO (Epogen), a hormone therapy, and intravenous or oral iron supplements are used to manage anemia. A multivitamin may be prescribed to replace **vitamins** lost during dialysis treatments. Vitamin D, which promotes the absorption of calcium, along with calcium supplements, may also be prescribed.

Since 1973, Medicare has picked up 80% of ESRD treatment costs, including the costs of dialysis and transplantation and of some medications. To qualify for benefits, a patient must be insured or eligible for benefits under Social Security, or be a spouse or child of an eligible American. Private insurance and state Medicaid programs often cover the remaining 20% of treatment costs.

Early diagnosis and treatment of kidney failure is critical to improving length and quality of life in chronic kidney failure patients. Patient outcome varies by the cause of chronic kidney failure and the method chosen to treat it. Overall, patients with chronic kidney disease leading to ESRD have a shortened life span. According to the United States Renal Data System (USRDS), the life span of an ESRD patient is 18-47% of the life span of the age-sex-race matched general population. ESRD patients on dialysis have a life span that is 16-37% of the general population

The demand for kidneys to transplant continues to exceed supply. In 1996, over 34,000 Americans were on the UNOS waiting list for a kidney transplant, but only 11,330 living donor and cadaver transplants were actually performed. Cadaver kidney transplants have a 50% chance of functioning 9 years, and living donor kidneys that have two matching antigen pairs have a 50% chance of functioning for 24 years. However, some transplant grafts have functioned for over 30 years.

Because many of the illnesses and underlying conditions that often trigger acute kidney failure are critical, the prognosis for these patients many times is not good. Studies have estimated overall **death** rates for acute kidney failure at 42-88%. Many people, however, die because of the primary disease that has caused the kidney failure. These figures may also be misleading because patients who experience kidney failure as a result of less serious illnesses (like kidney stones or dehydration) have an excellent chance of complete recovery. Early recognition and prompt, appropriate treatment are key to patient recovery.

Up to 10% of patients who experience acute kidney failure will suffer irreversible kidney damage. They will eventually go on to develop chronic kidney failure or end-stage renal disease. These patients will require long-term dialysis or kidney transplantation to replace their lost renal functioning.

Since acute kidney failure can be caused by many things, prevention is difficult. Medications that may impair kidney function should be given cautiously. Patients with pre-existing kidney conditions who are hospitalized for other illnesses or injuries should be carefully monitored for kidney failure complications. Treatments and procedures that may put them at risk for kidney failure (like diagnostic tests requiring radiocontrast agents or dyes) should be used with extreme caution.

KIDNEY FUNCTION TESTS

Kidney function tests is a collective term for a variety of individual tests and procedures that can be done to evaluate how well the kidneys are functioning.

The kidneys, the body's natural filtration system, perform many vital functions, including removing metabolic waste products from the bloodstream, regulating the body's water balance, and maintaining the pH (acidity/alkalinity) of the body's fluids. Approximately one and a half quarts of blood per minute are circulated through the kidneys, where waste chemicals are filtered out and eliminated from the body (along with excess water) in the form of urine. Kidney function tests help to determine if the kidneys are performing their tasks adequately.

Many conditions can affect the ability of the kidneys to carry out their vital functions. Some lead to a rapid (acute) decline in kidney function; others lead to a gradual (chronic) decline in function. Both result in a build-up of toxic waste substances in the blood. A number of clinical laboratory tests that measure the levels of substances normally regulated by the kidneys can help determine the cause and extent of kidney dysfunction. These tests are done on urine samples, as well as on blood samples.

There are a variety of urine tests that assess kidney function. A simple, inexpensive screening test, called a routine **urinalysis**, is often the first test administered if kidney problems are suspected. A small, randomly collected urine sample is examined physically for things like color, odor, appearance, and concentration (specific gravity); chemically for substances such a protein, glucose, and pH (acidity/ alkalinity); and microscopically for the presence of cellular elements (red blood cells, white blood cells, and epithelial cells), bacteria, crystals, and casts (structures formed by the deposit of protein, cells, and other substances in the kidneys' tubules). If results indicate a possibility of disease or impaired kidney function, one or more of the following additional tests is usually performed to more specifically diagnose the cause and the level of decline in kidney function.

- Creatinine clearance test. This test evaluates how efficiently the kidneys clear a substance called creatinine from the blood. Creatinine, a waste product of muscle energy metabolism, is produced at a constant rate that is proportional to the muscle mass of the individual. Because the body does not recycle it, all of the creatinine filtered by the kidneys in a given amount of time is excreted in the urine, making creatinine clearance a very specific measurement of kidney function.The test is performed on a timed urine specimen—a cumulative sample collected over a two to twenty-four hour period. Determination of the blood creatinine level is also required to calculate the urine clearance.
- Urea clearance test. Urea is a waste product that is created by protein **metabolism** and excreted in the urine. The urea clearance test requires a blood sample to measure the amount of urea in the bloodstream and two urine specimens, collected one hour apart, to determine the amount of urea that is filtered, or cleared, by the kidneys into the urine.
- Urine osmolality test. Urine osmolality is a measurement of the number of dissolved particles in urine. It is a more precise measurement than specific gravity for evaluating the ability of the kidneys to concentrate or dilute the urine. Kidneys that are functioning normally will excrete more water into the urine as fluid intake is increased, diluting the urine. If fluid intake is decreased, the kidneys excrete less water and the urine becomes more concentrated. The test may be done on a urine sample collected first thing in the morning, on multiple timed samples, or on a cumulative sample collected over a twenty-four hour period. The patient will typically be prescribed a high-protein diet for several days before the test and asked to drink no fluids the night before the test.
- Urine protein test. Healthy kidneys filter all proteins from the bloodstream and then reabsorb them, allowing no protein, or only slight amounts of protein, into the urine. The persistent presence of significant amounts of protein in the urine, then, is an important indicator of kidney disease. A positive screening test for protein (included in a routine urinalysis) on a random urine sample is usually followed-up with a test on a 24-hour urine sample that more precisely measures the quantity of protein.

There are also several blood tests that can aid in evaluating kidney function. These include:

- Blood urea nitrogen test (BUN). Urea is a by-product of protein metabolism. This waste product is formed in the liver, then filtered from the blood and excreted in the urine by the kidneys. The BUN test measures the amount of nitrogen contained in the urea. High BUN levels can indicate kidney dysfunction, but because blood urea nitrogen is also affected by protein intake and liver function, the test is usually done in conjunction with a blood creatinine, a more specific indicator of kidney function.
- Creatinine test. This test measures blood levels of creatinine, a by-product of muscle energy metabolism that, like urea, is filtered from the blood by the kidneys and excreted into the urine. Production of creatinine depends on an individual's muscle mass, which usually fluctuates very little. With normal kidney function, then, the amount of creatinine in the blood remains relatively constant and normal. For this reason, and because creatinine is affected very little by liver function, an elevated blood creatinine is a more sensitive indication of impaired kidney function than the BUN.
- Other blood tests. Measurement of the blood levels of other elements regulated in part by the kidneys can also be useful in evaluating kidney function. These include sodium, potassium, chloride, bicarbonate, calcium, magnesium, phosphorus, protein, uric acid, and glucose.

Patients will be given specific instructions for collection of urine samples, depending on the test to be performed. Some timed urine tests require an extended collection period of up to 24 hours, during which time the patient collects all urine voided and transfers it to a specimen container. Refrigeration and/or preservatives are typically required to maintain the integrity of such urine specimens. Certain dietary and/or medication restrictions may be imposed for some of the blood and urine tests. The patient may also be instructed to avoid **exercise** for a period of time before a test.

Normal values for many tests are determined by the patient's age and sex. Reference values can also vary by laboratory, but are generally within the ranges that follow.

- Creatinine clearance. For a 24-hour urine collection, normal results are 90-139 ml/min for adult males less than 40 years old, and 80-125 ml/min for adult females less than 40 years old. For people over 40, values decrease by 6.5 ml/min for each decade of life.
- Urea clearance. With maximum clearance, normal is 64-99 ml/min.
- Urine osmolality. With restricted fluid intake (concentration testing), osmolality should be greater than 800 mOsm/kg of water. With increased fluid intake (dilution testing), osmolality should be less than 100 mOSm/kg in at least one of the specimens collected.
- Urine protein. A 24-hour urine collection should contain no more than 150 mg of protein.

- Blood urea nitrogen (BUN). 8-20 mg/dl.
- Creatinine. 0.8-1.2 mg/dl for males, and 0.6-0.9 mg/dl for females.

Low clearance values for creatinine and urea indicate diminished ability of the kidneys to filter these waste products from the blood and excrete them in the urine. As clearance levels decrease, blood levels of creatinine and urea nitrogen increase. Since it can be affected by other factors, an elevated BUN, by itself, is suggestive, but not diagnostic, for kidney dysfunction. An abnormally elevated blood creatinine, a more specific and sensitive indicator of kidney disease than the BUN, is diagnostic of impaired kidney function.

Inability of the kidneys to concentrate the urine in response to restricted fluid intake, or to dilute the urine in response to increased fluid intake during osmolality testing may indicate decreased kidney function. Because the kidneys normally excrete almost no protein in the urine, its persistent presence, in amounts that exceed the normal 24-hour urine value, usually indicates some type of kidney disease as well.

KIDNEY STONES

Kidney stones are solid accumulations of material that form in the tubal system of the kidney. They cause painful problems when they block the flow of urine through or out of the kidney.

Urine is formed by the kidneys. As blood flows into the kidneys, specialized tubes within the kidneys extract a certain amount of fluid and other substances from the blood, which then flows out of the body as urine. Sometimes, a problem in the kidneys makes these dissolved substances become solid again. Sometimes, tiny crystals called ''silent stones'' may form in the urine that never cause any pain.

Kidney stones cause problems when they interfere with the normal flow of urine. They can block the flow down the ureter—the tube that carries urine from the kidney to the bladder. Because the kidney isn't used to feeling any pressure, when pressure builds from backed-up urine the kidney may swell. If the kidney is subjected to this pressure for some time, it may damage delicate kidney structures. If a kidney stone is lodged further down the ureter, the backed-up urine may also cause the ureter to swell. Because the ureters are muscular tubes, the presence of a stone will make these muscular tubes spasm, causing severe pain.

About 10% of all people will have a kidney stone at some point in life. Kidney stones are most common among:

- Caucasians
- Males
- People over the age of 30
- People who have had other kidney stones
- Relatives of kidney stone patients.

Kidney stones can be made up of a variety of substances, but the most common types are calcium stones; about 80% of all kidney stones fall into this category. People with calcium stones may have other diseases that cause them to have higher blood levels of calcium. These diseases include primary parathyroidism, sarcoidosis, hyperthyroidism, **multiple myeloma**, and some types of **cancer**. A diet heavy in meat, fish, and poultry also can cause calcium oxalate stones.

About 10% of all kidney stones are struvite stones (also called ''staghorn kidney stones''), made up of magnesium ammonium phosphate. These stones occur most often in patients who have had repeated urinary tract infections caused by certain types of bacteria. These bacteria produce a substance that makes the urine less acidic, which allows struvite to settle out of the urine and form stones.

About 5% of all kidney stones are uric acid stones, which occur when higher amounts of uric acid circulate in the blood. When the uric acid content becomes very high, solid bits of uric acid settle out of the urine. A kidney stone is formed when these bits of uric acid begin to cling to each other within the kidney, slowly growing into a solid mass. About half of all patients with this type of stone also have deposits of uric acid elsewhere in their body, commonly in the joint of the big toe. This painful disorder is called **gout**. Uric acid stones also may be caused by **chemotherapy**, certain bone marrow disorders, and an inherited disorder called Lesch-Nyhan syndrome.

About 2% of all kidney stones are stones made of cystine, a type of amino acid. People with this type of kidney stone don't process amino acids normally.

If a kidney stone is present, some people may notice blood in their urine, but patients don't usually notice symptoms until the stones pass into the ureter. At this point, most people will experience bouts of very severe crampy and spasmodic pain known as **colic**. The pain usually begins in the area between the lower ribs and the hip bone. As the stone moves closer to the bladder, a patient will often feel the pain radiating along the inner thigh. Women may feel pain in the vulva. Men may notice pain in the testicles. **Nausea**, vomiting, extremely frequent and painful urination, and obvious blood in the urine are common signs of kidney stones. **Fever** and chills usually mean that the ureter has become obstructed, trapping bacteria in the kidney and causing an infection (pyelonephritis).

Diagnosing kidney stones is based on a patient's history of very severe, distinctive pain together with an X-ray and a urine test. During the passage of a stone, there is almost always blood in the urine. A number of x-ray tests are used to diagnose kidney stones. X-ray of the kidneys, ureters, and bladder may or may not reveal the stone; a series of x-rays taken after injecting iodine dye into a vein is usually a more reliable way of seeing a stone. This procedure is called an intravenous pyelogram (IVP). The dye ''lights up'' the **urinary system** as it travels. In the case of an obstruction, the dye will be stopped by the stone or will only be able to get past the stone at a slow trickle.

When a patient is passing a kidney stone, it is important that all urine is strained so that they stone can be analyzed to determine its chemical composition. Collecting urine for 24 hours, followed by careful analysis of its chemical makeup, can often determine a number of reasons for stone formation.

Because the pain of passing a kidney stone is so severe, narcotic pain medications such as morphine are usually needed. Stones may pass more quickly if the patient is encouraged to drink large amounts of water (2-3 quarts per day). If the patient is vomiting or unable to drink because of the pain, it may be necessary to provide fluids through a vein. If there is infection, **antibiotics** will be needed.

Although most kidney stones will pass on their own, some will not. Surgical removal of a stone may become necessary when a stone appears too large to pass. Surgery may also be required if the stone is causing serious obstructions, pain that cannot be treated, heavy bleeding, or infection.

There are several surgical alternatives. In one method, the surgeon inserts a tube into the bladder and up into the ureter. A tiny basket is then passed through the tube, and the surgeon tries to snare the stone and pull it out. Open surgery to remove an obstructing kidney stone was relatively common in the past, but current methods allow the stone to be crushed with shock waves (called **lithotripsy**). These shock waves may be aimed at the stone from outside of the body; the stone fragments may then pass on their own or may be removed through an incision. All of these methods reduce the patient's recovery time considerably when compared to the traditional open operation.

Alternative treatments for kidney stones include the use of herbal medicine, **acupuncture**, **acupressure**, **hypnosis**, or **guided imagery** to relieve pain. Starfruit may relieve pain and increase the amount of urine a patient passes. Dietary changes may reduce the risk of future stones and to help absorb existing stones. Supplements of magnesium (a smooth muscle relaxant), can help ease pain and help the stone to pass.

How easily a patient recovers depends on the underlying disorder that caused the kidney stone in the first place. In most cases, patients with simple calcium stones will recover very well. However, about 60% of these patients will have other kidney stones. Struvite (''staghorn'') stones are particularly dangerous because they may grow extremely large, filling the tubes within the kidney. These won't pass out in the urine, and require surgical removal. Uric acid stones may also become staghorn tones.

Patients may be able to prevent certain types of kidney stones. Drinking several quarts of water every day is an important way to head off the problem. Patients with calcium stones may benefit from taking a medication called a **diuretic**, which decreases the amount of calcium passed in the urine. Eating less meat, fish, and chicken may help patients with calcium oxalate stones. Other items in the diet that may encourage calcium oxalate stone formation include beer, black pepper, berries, broccoli, chocolate, spinach, and tea. When a disease is identified as the cause of stone formation, treatment for that disease may lessen the likelihood of repeated stones.

KINESIOLOGY

Kinesiology is a series of tests that locate weaknesses in specific muscles that cause imbalances throughout the body. Once the weaknesses are found, specific **massage** or **acupressure** techniques are used in an attempt to rebalance what has been revealed by the kinesiology tests. Thus, kinesiology is used both to asses a problem and as a way to help treat the problem.

Kinesiology is a healing system that proponents believe can help find and correct imbalances in the body before they develop into a disease, and can restore overall balance and harmony. It is used to treat muscle, bone, and joint problems, all types of aches and **pain**s, and correct many areas of imbalance and discomfort.

Since interpretation of the muscle tests is complex, it should only be performed by a licensed health professional trained to look for subtle symptoms which have not yet become a major problem. Kinesiology itself is more of a diagnostic technique and should not be thought of as a cure for any particular problem.

Traditionally, the word ''kinesiology'' refers simply to the study of muscles and body movement. In 1964, however, American chiropractor George J. Goodheart founded what has become known as applied kinesiology when he linked eastern ideas about energy flow in the body with western techniques of muscle testing. Because Goodheart noted that one muscle contracts while another one relaxes, when he was presented with a painful, overly-tight muscle, he would observe and treat the opposite (weaker) muscle to restore balance. At the time, this was a novel technique. Further, Goodheart argued that there is a definite connection between muscles, glands, and organs, and that by testing the strength of certain muscles he could uncover the condition of the gland or organ to which it was related.

Applied kinesiology is based on the idea that the body is an interactive unit of different parts that affect each other. Everything a person does affects the body as a whole, so that a problem in one area can cause trouble in another area. According to kinesiology, the muscles eventually register and reflect anything that is wrong with any part of the body, whether physical or mental. Thus, a particular digestive problem might show up in the related muscles of the legs. By testing the strength of certain muscles, a kinesiologist claims to be able to gain access to the body's communication system, and, thus, to read the health status of each of the body's major components.

The manual testing of muscles was used in the late 1940s to evaluate muscle function and strength and to assess the extent of an injury. Applied kinesiology measures whether a muscle is tense or weak and flaccid. Done without instruments, the technique uses only the kinesiologist's fingertip pressure. During the first and longest appointment which lasts about an hour, the kinesiologist conducts a complete consultation, asking about the patient's history and background. During the physical exam, the patient sits or lies down as the kinesiologist holds the patient's leg or arm to isolate a particular muscle. The practitioner then touches a point on the body which he believes is related to that muscle, and, with quick, gentle, and painless pressure, pushes down on the limb. Patients are asked to resist this pressure, and, if they can't, an imbalance is suspected in the related organ, gland, or body part. This diagnostic technique is based on traditional Chinese medicine's belief that the body has common energy meridians for both organs and muscles. Kinesiologists also claim they can locate muscle weaknesses that stem from a variety of causes such as **allergies**, mineral and vitamin deficiencies, as well as from problems with the lymph system.

Once the exact cause is determined, the kinesiologist uses his fingertips to work the appropriate corresponding acupressure points in order to rebalance the flow of energy and restore health and recommend a nutrition therapy.

There are no major risks associated with this gentle, noninvasive therapy; it is generally safe for people of all ages and has no side effects.

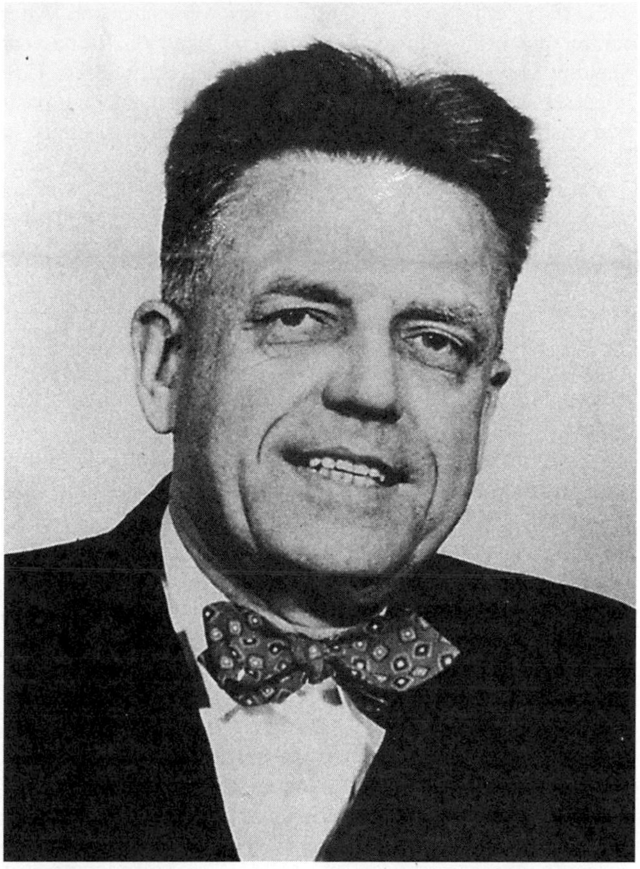

Alfred Kinsey

KINSEY, ALFRED (1894-1956)

American zoologist and sex researcher

Alfred Kinsey became a household name in the 1950s for his research on the sexual mores of American women and men. His two major texts, *Sexual Behavior in the Human Male* (1948) and *Sexual Behavior in the Human Female* (1953), broke new ground in the field of sex research and led to more open and honest investigations of sexual practices. Before he achieved international fame as a sex researcher, Kinsey had already established himself in the world of science as a leading zoologist and entomologist, becoming the world's foremost authority on the American gall wasp. Throughout his career, regardless of the subject, Kinsey remained inquisitive and scientifically high-minded.

Kinsey was born in Hoboken, New Jersey, on June 23, 1894. His father, Alfred, taught at the Stevens Institute of Technology, despite having only an eighth-grade education. His mother, Sarah Ann (Charles), the daughter of a carpenter, had completed only four years of schooling. Kinsey was a sickly child, plagued by **rheumatic fever**, rickets, and **typhoid**. His parents were strict and deeply religious, rejecting many of life's aesthetic pleasures. In spite of this puritanical upbringing, Kinsey acquired a life-long appreciation of music and poetry. Starting in the seventh grade, he began collecting botanical specimens. He undertook rigorous nature expeditions, which seemed to improve his poor health. He joined the Boy Scouts of America shortly after the organization was founded in 1910, earned the prestigious designation of Eagle Scout, and became a scout leader during high school. His early botanical studies were encouraged by his high school biology teacher, Natalie Roeth, with whom he would correspond throughout his life. During high school, inspired by Roeth, he wrote a paper entitled "What Do Birds Do When It Rains?"

After high school, Kinsey considered a career in the natural sciences, but his father wanted him to train as an engineer. He obligingly enrolled at the Stevens Institute and studied mechanical engineering for two years. His interest in engineering was limited, however, and, after reaching a compromise with his father, he enrolled as a junior at Bowdoin College in Brunswick, Maine, to study biology. During his two years at Bowdoin, he earned a reputation as a deadly serious student and a first-rate pianist. He received his B.S. from Bowdoin magna cum laude in 1916 and gave the commencement address at graduation.

In 1916, Kinsey received a scholarship from Harvard University and began his postgraduate work at the Bussey Institution. He was immediately drawn to the study of gall wasps (American Cynipidae), a small, ant-sized insect which lays its eggs inside growths (or galls) in large plants. The gall wasp can stay in its pupal state for years, and its life-span is extremely short, often less than a few hours. During his time at the Bussey Institution, Kinsey wrote his first text, *Edible Wild Plants of Eastern North America,* which was not published until 1943, when survivalist concerns were stronger. After completing his graduate work, he embarked on a one-year Sheldon Traveling Fellowship, touring the southwestern U.S. in pursuit of gall wasps. In 1920, he accepted a teaching position in the department of zoology at Indiana University in Bloomington.

Kinsey, a well-respected teacher and lecturer, was an easily identifiable figure on Indiana University's campus due to his trademark bow tie, white shirt, and crew cut. He often took undergraduates outdoors for hands-on nature studies. In the summer of 1921, he married Clara Brachen McMillen, a Phi Beta Kappa chemistry scholar. In typical Kinsey fashion, the couple spent their honeymoon on a camping expedition in the White Mountains of New Hampshire. The Kinsey's four children were all born between 1922 and 1928.

During the late 1920s, Kinsey continued his entomological research, contributing numerous articles on the gall wasp to scientific journals. His high school textbook, *An Introduction to Biology,* appeared in 1926, to enthusiastic reviews. The next year a companion text, *Field and Laboratory Manual in Biology,* was published. Soon after the appearance of this text, Kinsey's oldest child, Donald, died, succumbing to complications from **diabetes**.

Kinsey's first major text, *The Gall Wasp Genus Cynips: A Study in the Origin of the Species,* was published in 1930. In 1936, *The Origin of Higher Categories of Cynips,* appeared and bolstered Kinsey's reputation as the leading authority on the gall wasp and as one of the most original thinkers in the field of genetic theory. At this point, his firmly established career took an unusual twist. In the summer of 1938, Kinsey, then age 44, began teaching a noncredit marriage course for seniors at Indiana University. The course was the result of a petition sent to the Board of Trustees by a group of students the previous spring.

Before the course began, Kinsey, always the scientist, decided to study the subject of sex and marriage in detail. He read every known reference on the subject and was appalled by the inaccuracies and lack of scientific detail and honesty. The course he designed took a more biological approach. As part of the course, students were asked to complete detailed questionnaires, which constituted the first of Kinsey's case histories. Finding the questionnaires inappropriate and open to errors of interpretation, he began conducting face-to-face interviews, using a corner of his busy laboratory. By 1940, Kinsey's marriage course was opened to freshman and sophomores and grew so popular that enrollment soon reached 400 students per semester.

Around this time, Kinsey realized he needed a more general human sample in order to conduct meaningful research. He began to travel out of town to conduct interviews with additional subjects. At first, his trips were relegated to the weekends but, as his interest grew, his time away from the campus increased. Kinsey's growing involvement with sex research did not go unnoticed by his college's administration nor by the local clergy, the medical community, and, strangely enough, the University's department of sociology, all of whom wanted the course and Kinsey stopped. In 1940, he was called before Indiana University's president, Herman Wells, who demanded that Kinsey make a choice between his marriage course and sexual research. Kinsey resigned from the course. He then increased his number of out-of-town interviews and spent long hours interpreting data and training interviewers. David Halberstam, writing in *American Heritage,* reported that Mrs. Kinsey often said of her husband at this time, "I hardly see him at night any more since he took up sex."

During the 1940s, Kinsey embarked on a large-scale study of the sexual habits of men and women. Initially, his resources were limited, and he used his own money to hire staff and pay expenses. In 1943, he received a $23,000 grant from the Rockefeller Foundation, which enabled him to hire more staff and expand his efforts. Chief among his staff were colleagues W. B. Pomeroy, who also conducted thousands of sex interviews, Paul Gebhard, and Clyde Martin. The funding briefly legitimized his undertaking, which became known as the Institute for Sex Research of Indiana University.

By 1948 Kinsey and his colleagues were ready to release their initial findings. He chose a well-established medical publications firm, W. B. Saunders of Philadelphia, to publish the book, attempting to stress the scientific nature of the text rather than its potentially more lurid aspects. To avoid possible financial retribution against Indiana University, the book was published while the Indiana legislature was in recess in December 1948. The 804 page book, *Sexual Behavior in the Human Male,* sold 185,000 copies in its first year in print and made the *New York Times* bestseller list. The book employed frank descriptions of biological functions and was nonjudgmental of its subject's activities. Kinsey reported his findings simply and directly, pointing out a number of falsely held assumptions. In particular, the book reported that extramarital and premarital sex were more prevalent than generally believed; that nearly all males, especially teenagers, masturbated and that **masturbation** did not cause **mental illness**; and that one in three men reported having at least one homosexual encounter in their lifetimes.

Early polls indicated that most Americans agreed with Kinsey's findings. The most vehement criticism came later from the expected sources: conservative and religious organizations. Most of these attacks were emotionally rather than scientifically based, but few of Kinsey's colleagues came to his defense. The growing criticism jeopardized Kinsey's relationship with the Rockefeller Foundation. One of his chief critics, Henry Pitney Van Dusen, head of the Union Theological Seminary, was a member of the Rockefeller Board. And the new head of the foundation, Dean Rusk—who would later serve as secretary of state during John F. Kennedy's presidential administration—was growing weary of the foundation's well-publicized relationship with the Institute for Sex Research. The final break with the Rockefeller Foundation would come after Kinsey and his colleagues published their next book, *Sexual Behavior in the Human Female.*

The second sex book, as Kinsey expected, caused an even greater uproar than the first. Some of the book's more controversial findings concerned the low rate of frigidity, high rates of premarital and extramarital sex, the rapidness of erotic response, and a detailed discussion of clitoral versus vaginal orgasm. The book soared up the best-seller charts, eventually reaching sales of 250,000 in the U.S. alone. Criticism was harsh, and Kinsey's methods and motives were once again questioned. Evangelist Billy Graham was quoted by Halberstam in *American Heritage* as stating: "It is impossible to estimate the damage this book will do to the already deteriorating morals of America."

In August 1954, the Rockefeller Foundation, under increasing political pressure, announced its decision to cease funding for Kinsey's Institute. The nonpolitical Kinsey was now branded a subversive and accused of furthering the Communist cause by undermining American morals. He responded to these attacks by working even more diligently. The Institute turned its focus to a large-scale study of sex offenders, and Kinsey seemed determined to carry on. But the incessant criticism and lack of support took their toll. He wrote a scathing letter to Rusk, excerpted in *American Heritage,* pointing out that, "to have fifteen years of accumulated data in this area fail to reach publication would constitute an indictment of the Institute, its sponsors, and all others who have contributed time and material resources to this work."

Kinsey searched in vain for new sources of funding. He was troubled by insomnia and began taking sleeping pills and other medications. In 1955, he traveled to England and Europe, where he lectured on various topics and studied local sexual morés. Upon his return, he developed heart trouble and was hospitalized several times. In the spring of 1956, despite his poor health, he traveled to Chicago to conduct his final interviews, subjects 7,934 and 7,935. On August 25, 1956, at the age of 62, Kinsey died of **pneumonia** and heart complications.

KITTRELL, FLEMMIE PANSY (1904-1980)

African American nutritionist and educator

Flemmie Pansy Kittrell was an internationally-known **nutritionist** whose emphasis on child development and family welfare drew much-needed attention to the importance of the early home environment. During her more than forty years as an educator, she traveled abroad extensively, helping to improve home-life conditions in many developing nations. She was a founder of Howard University's school of human ecology and the recipient of several major awards which acknowledged her unique accomplishments. As the first African American woman to earn a Ph.D. in nutrition, she strove constantly to focus attention on the important role that women could play in the world and to push for their higher education.

Kittrell was born in Henderson, North Carolina, on Christmas Day, 1904. She was the youngest daughter of Alice (Mills) and James Lee Kittrell, both of whom were descended from African American and Cherokee forebears. Learning was of central importance to Kittrell's parents, and her father often read stories and poetry to her and her eight brothers and sisters. Her parents knew the importance of encouragement and the children frequently received praise for their perseverance and achievements.

After graduating from high school in North Carolina, Kittrell attended Hampton Institute in Virginia, receiving her Bachelor of Science degree in 1928. With the encouragement of her professors she enrolled at Cornell University, although there were not many black women during that era who became graduate students. In 1930 Kittrell received her M.A. from Cornell and in 1938, from the same institution, she accepted her Ph.D. in nutrition with honors.

Kittrell was offered her first job teaching home economics in 1928 by Bennett College in Greensboro, North Carolina, and it was to Bennett she returned after obtaining her Ph.D. She then became dean of women and the head of the home economics department at Hampton Institute in 1940, where she remained until 1944. In that year Kittrell accepted the personal offer of Howard University president Mordecai Johnson to preside over the home economics department at Howard University in Washington, D.C. At Howard, Kittrell developed a curriculum that broadened the common perception of home economics so that it included such fields as child development research.

In 1947 Kittrell embarked upon a lifetime of international activism, carrying out a nutrition al survey of Liberia sponsored by the United States government. Her findings concerning "hidden hunger," a type of **malnutrition** which occurred in ninety percent of the African nation's population, led to important changes in Liberian agricultural and fishing industries. Kittrell then received a 1950 Fulbright award which led to her work with Baroda University in India, where she developed an educational plan for nutritional research. In 1953, Kittrell went back to India as a teacher of home economics classes and nutritional seminars. Then, in 1957, Kittrell headed a team which traveled to Japan and Hawaii to research activities in those countries related to the science of home economics. Between 1957 and 1961, Kittrell was the leader of three more tours, to West Africa, Central Africa, and Guinea.

During this period Kittrell remained at Howard University. In 1963, her fifteen-year struggle to obtain a building for the school of human ecology resulted in the dedication of a new facility. This innovative building attracted national attention as it provided a working example for the nation's Head Start program, which was just getting off the ground. Retiring from Howard University in 1972, Kittrell was named Emeritus Professor of Nutrition.

Kittrell's achievements were regularly recognized by awards and honors. For instance, she was chosen by Hampton University as its outstanding alumna for 1955. In 1961 she received the Scroll of Honor by the National Council of Negro Women in recognition of her special services. Cornell University gave her an achievement award in 1968 and the University of North Carolina at Greensboro conferred on her an honorary degree in 1974. Also, a scholarship fund was founded in honor of Kittrell's career by the American Home Economics Association.

Kittrell continued to work despite her retirement from teaching in 1972. From 1974 to 1976 she was a Cornell Visiting Senior Fellow, and she served as a Moton Center Senior Research Fellow in 1977 and a Fulbright lecturer in India in

1978. Kittrell died unexpectedly of cardiac arrest on October 3, 1980, in Washington, D.C. During her life she had credited much of her success not only to her education, but also to the strength, love, and family unity she enjoyed in her parents' home, where learning was a very important aspect of family life.

Kocher, Theodor (1841-1917)

Swiss surgeon

Emil Theodor Kocher was born August 25, 1841, the son of Jacob Alexander and Maria (Wermuth) Kocher, in Bern, Switzerland. Schooled in Berlin, Germany; London, England; Paris, France; and Vienna, Austria, Kocher received his M.D. from the University of Bern in 1869. That same year he married Marie Witschi-Courant—the couple would have three sons. Newly married and newly graduated from medical school, Kocher visited various European clinics, including one in Vienna, where he studied under the most famous European surgeon of the day, **Theodor Billroth**. In 1872 Kocher, who was only 31 years old at the time, was named professor of clinical surgery at Bern University, a post he would hold for the next 45 years.

Kocher first gained recognition for developing a method for treating a dislocated shoulder, a technique now known by his name. Subsequently, he also created new methods or improvements in existing methods for operations upon the lungs, stomach, gall bladder, intestine, cranial nerves, and hernia. He also developed a special pair of surgical forceps, now known as "Kocher's forceps."

Kocher further contributed to medicine with his *Textbook of Operative Surgery*, his pioneering of ovariotomy and, especially, his application of the antiseptic techniques of the English researcher and doctor Joseph Lister.

Kocher himself credited his success with thyroidectomy operations in part to Lister's method of antisepsis. However, despite his mastery over the operation, Kocher himself considered the increased knowledge about the *physiological* function of the thyroid gland an even greater advancement in medical science. In 1883, at the congress of the German Surgical Society, Kocher reported that out of his first 100 thyroidectomies, 30 had resulted in a serious disorder. This ailment was apparently a result of the whole, rather than partial, removal of the goiter. The symptoms Kocher described were called operative myxedema, and were akin to naturally occurring myxedema. Patients suffering from myxedema usually reported weight gain, slowing of intellect and speech, hair loss, tongue thickening, and abnormal heart rates, as well as developing blood-related problems of **anemia** and altered white blood-cell counts. Kocher further related that myxedema symptoms were similar to problems experienced by patients suffering from sporadic cretinism and cachexia strumipriva, diseases that resulted in mental retardation and dwarfism. Because of Kocher's postulations, it was discovered that a lack of thyroid secretions was the cause of all these diseases. Kocher further pointed out that hypothyroidism can be traced not only to absence of the gland, whether congenital or surgical, but also to a goiter which has caused the gland to stop working.

Kocher's observations opened the way for future treatment of thyroid disorders. Although initial attempts to rectify the condition by administering thyroid hormone were not particularly successful, researchers recognized the importance of iodine, and in 1914 the effective part of the hormone, thyroxin, was isolated for effective treatment. Meanwhile, Kocher helped perfect the surgical technique for thyroidectomy, and his surgical mortality rates dropped by a great margin over the years.

During his long surgical career Kocher performed more than 2,000 thyroidectomies. In time the need for the operation declined as iodine-deprived regions incorporated supplements into their diets. Nevertheless, Kocher's contributions to combatting endemic goiter continue to be recognized in a world where nearly 5% of the population still continues to suffer this disorder.

For his many contributions to medicine, and especially the treatment of goiter, Kocher received the Nobel Prize in medicine in 1909. He died in Bern eight years after receiving the award.

Koch, Robert (1843-1910)

German bacteriologist

Robert Koch is considered to be one of the founders of the field of bacteriology. He pioneered principles and techniques in studying bacteria and discovered the specific agents that cause **tuberculosis**, **cholera**, and **anthrax**. For this he is also regarded as a founder of **public health**, aiding legislation and changing prevailing attitudes about hygiene to prevent the spread of various infectious diseases. For his work on tuberculosis, he was awarded the Nobel Prize in 1905.

Robert Heinrich Hermann Koch was born in a small town near Klausthal, Hanover, Germany, on December 11, 1843, to Hermann Koch, an administrator in the local mines, and Mathilde Julie Henriette Biewend, a daughter of a mine inspector. The Koch's had a total of thirteen children, two of whom died in infancy. Robert was the third son. Both parents were industrious and ambitious. Robert's father rose in the ranks of the mining industry, becoming the overseer of all the local mines. His mother passed her love of nature on to Robert who, at an early age, collected various plants and insects.

Before starting primary school in 1848, Robert taught himself to read and write. At the top of his class during his early school years, he had to repeat his final year. Nevertheless, he graduated in 1862 with good marks in the sciences and mathematics. A university education became available to Robert when his father was once again promoted and the family's finances improved. Robert decided to study natural sciences at Gottingen University, close to his home.

After two semesters, Koch transferred his field of study to medicine. He had dreams of becoming a physician on a ship. His father had traveled widely in Europe and passed a desire for travel on to his son. Although bacteriology was not taught then at the University, Koch would later credit his interest in that field to Jacob Henle, an anatomist who had published a theory of contagion in 1840. Many ideas about contagious diseases, particularly those of chemist and microbiologist Louis Pasteur, who was challenging the prevailing myth of spontaneous generation, were still being debated in universities in the 1860s.

During Koch's fifth semester at medical school, Henle recruited him to participate in a research project on the structure of uterine nerves. The resulting essay won first prize. It was dedicated to his father and bore the Latin motto, Nunquam Otiosus, or Never idle. During his sixth semester, he assisted Georg Meissner at the Physiological Institute. There he studied the secretion of succinic acid in animals fed only on fat. Koch decided to experiment on himself, eating a half pound of butter each day. After five days, however, he was so sick that he limited his study to animals. The findings of this study eventually became Koch's dissertation. In January 1866, he finished the final exams for medical school and graduated with highest distinction.

After finishing medical school, Koch held various positions; he worked as an assistant at a hospital in Hamburg, where he became familiar with cholera, and also as an assistant at a hospital for retarded children. In addition, he made several attempts to establish a private practice. In July, 1867, he married Emmy Adolfine Josephine Fraatz, a daughter of an official in his hometown. Their only child, Gertrude, was born in 1868. Koch finally succeeded in establishing a practice in the small town of Rakwitz where he settled with his family.

Shortly after moving to Rakwitz, the Franco-Prussian War broke out and Koch volunteered as a field hospital physician. In 1871, the citizens of Rakwitz petitioned Koch to return to their town. He responded, leaving the army to resume his practice, but he didn't stay long. He soon took the exams to qualify for district medical officer and in August 1872 was appointed to a vacant position at Wollstein, a small town near the Polish border.

It was here that Koch's ambitions were finally able to flourish. Though he continued to see patients, Koch converted part of his office into a laboratory. He obtained a microscope and observed, at close range, the diseases his patients confronted him with.

One such disease was anthrax, which is spread from animals to humans through contaminated wool, by eating uncooked meat, or by breathing in airborne spores emanating from contaminated products. Koch examined under the microscope the blood of infected sheep and saw specific microorganisms that confirmed a thesis put forth ten years earlier by biologist C. J. Davaine (1812-1882) that anthrax was caused by a bacillus. But Koch was not content to simply verify the work of another. He attempted to culture, or grow, these bacilli in cattle blood so he could observe their life cycle, including their formation into spores and their germination. Koch performed scrupulous research both in vitro and in animals before showing his work to **Ferdinand Cohn**, a botanist at the University of Breslau. Cohn was impressed with the work and replicated the findings in his own laboratory. He published Koch's paper in 1876.

In 1877, Koch published another paper that elucidated the techniques he had used to isolate *Bacillus anthracis*. He

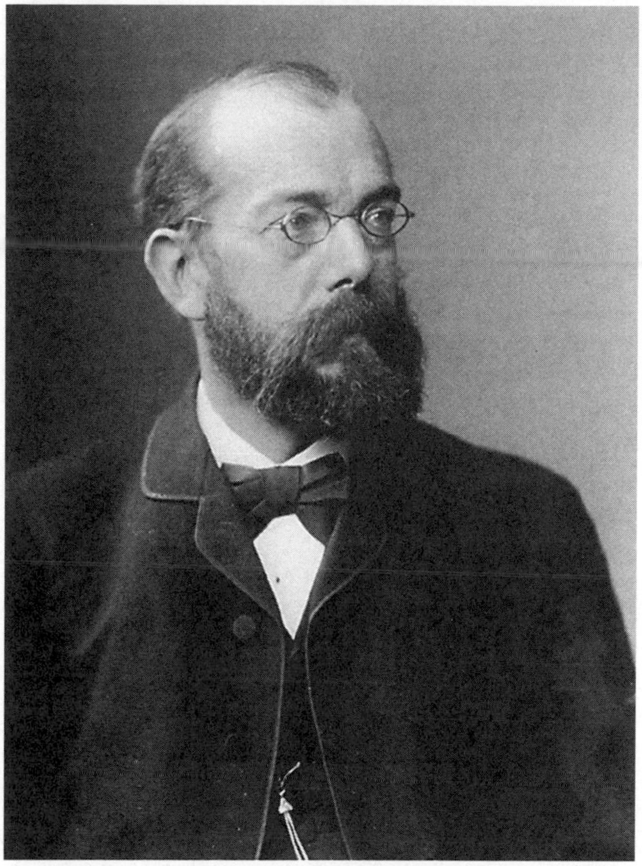

Robert Koch

had dry-fixed bacterial cultures onto glass slides, then stained the cultures with dyes to better observe them, and photographed them through the microscope.

It was only a matter of time that Koch's research eclipsed his practice. In 1880, he accepted an appointment as a government advisor with the Imperial Department of Health in Berlin. His task was to develop methods of isolating and cultivating disease-producing bacteria and to formulate strategies for preventing their spread. In 1881 he published a report advocating the importance of pure cultures in isolating disease-causing organisms and describing in detail how to obtain them. The methods and theory espoused in this paper are still considered fundamental to the field of modern bacteriology. Four basic criteria, now known as Koch's postulates, are essential for an organism to be identified as pathogenic, or disease-causing. First, the organism must be found in the tissues of animals with the disease and not in disease-free animals. Second, the organism must be isolated from the diseased animal and grown in a pure culture outside the body, or in vitro. Third, the cultured organism must be able to be transferred to a healthy animal, who will subsequently show signs of infection. And fourth, the organisms must be able to be isolated from the infected animal.

While in Berlin, Koch became interested in **tuberculosis**, which he was convinced was infectious, and, therefore, caused by a bacterium. Several scientists had made similar claims but none had been verified. Many other scientists persisted in believing that tuberculosis was an inherited disease. In six months, Koch succeeded in isolating a bacillus from tissues of humans and animals infected with tuberculosis. In 1882, he published a paper declaring that this bacillus met his four conditions—that is, it was isolated from diseased animals, it was grown in a pure culture, it was transferred to a healthy animal who then developed the disease, and it was isolated from the animal infected by the cultured organism. When he presented his findings before the Physiological Society in Berlin on March 24, he held the audience spellbound, so logical and thorough was his delivery of this important finding. This day has come to be known as the day modern bacteriology was born.

In 1883, Koch's work on tuberculosis was interrupted by the Hygiene Exhibition in Berlin, which, as part of his duties with the health department, he helped organize. Later that year, he finally realized his dreams of travel when he was invited to head a delegation to Egypt where an outbreak of **cholera** had occurred. **Louis Pasteur** had hypothesized that cholera was caused by a microorganism; within three weeks, Koch had identified a comma-shaped organism in the intestines of people who had died of cholera. However, when testing this organism against his four postulates, he found that the disease did not spread when injected into other animals. Undeterred, Koch proceeded to India where cholera was also a growing problem. There, he succeeded in finding the same organism in the intestines of the victims of cholera, and although he was still unable to induce the disease in experimental animals, he did identify the bacillus when he examined, under the microscope, water from the ponds used for drinking water. He remained convinced that this bacillus was the cause of cholera and that the key to prevention lay in improving hygiene and **sanitation**.

Koch returned to Germany and from 1885–1890 was administrator and professor at Berlin University. He was highly praised for his work, though some high-ranking scientists and doctors continued to disagree with his conclusions. But Koch was an adept researcher, able to support each claim with his exacting methodology. In 1890, however, Koch faltered from his usual perfectionism and announced at the International Medical Congress in Berlin that he had found an inoculum that could prevent tuberculosis. He called this agent tuberculin. People flocked to Berlin in hopes of a cure and Koch was persuaded to keep the exact formulation of tuberculin a secret, in order to discourage imitations. Although optimistic reports had come out of the clinical trials Koch had set up, it soon became clear from autopsies that tuberculin was causing severe inflammation in many patients. In January 1891, under pressure from other scientists, Koch finally published the nature of the substance, but it was an uncharacteristically vague and misleading report which came under immediate criticism from his peers.

Koch left Berlin for a time after this incident to recover from the professional setback. He also suffered from a personal scandal during this time, divorcing his wife in 1893 and immediately marrying an actress, Hedwig Freiberg, thirty years his junior. But the German government continued to support him throughout this time. An Institute for Infectious Diseases was established and Koch was named director. With a team of researchers, he continued his work with tuberculin, attempting to determine the ideal dose at which the agent could be the safest and most effective. The discovery that tuberculin was a valuable diagnostic tool (causing a reaction in those infected but none in those not infected), rather than a cure, helped restore Koch's reputation. In 1892 there was a cholera outbreak in Hamburg. Thousands of people died. Koch advocated strict sanitary conditions and isolation of those found to be infected with the bacillus. Germany's senior hygienist, Max von Pettenkofer, was unconvinced that the bacillus alone could cause cholera. He sneered at Koch's ideas, going so far as to drink a freshly isolated culture. Several of his colleagues joined him in this demonstration. Two developed symptoms of cholera, Pettenkofer suffered from diarrhea, but no one died; Pettenkofer felt vindicated in his opposition to Koch. Nevertheless, Koch focused much of his energy on testing the water supply of Hamburg and Berlin and perfecting techniques for filtering drinking water to prevent the spread of the bacillus.

In the following years, he gave the directorship of the Institute over to one of his students so he could travel again. He went to India, New Guinea, Africa, and Italy, where he studied diseases such as the **plague**, **malaria**, **rabies**, and various unexplained **fevers**. In 1905, after returning to Berlin from Africa, he was awarded the Nobel Prize for physiology and medicine for his work on tuberculosis. Subsequently, many other honors were awarded him recognizing not only his work on tuberculosis, but his more recent research on tropical diseases, including the Prussian Order Pour le Merits in 1906 and the Robert Koch medal in 1908. The Robert Koch Medal was established to honor the greatest living physicians, and the Robert Koch Foundation, established with generous grants from the German government and from the American philanthropist, Andrew Carnegie (1835-1919), was founded to work toward the eradication of tuberculosis.

Meanwhile, Koch settled back into the Institute where he supervised clinical trials and production of new tuberculins. He attempted to answer, once and for all, the question of whether tuberculosis in cattle was the same disease as it was in humans. Between 1882 and 1901 he had changed his mind on this question, coming to believe that bovine tuberculosis was not a danger to humans, as he had previously thought. He espoused his beliefs at conferences in the United States and Britain during a time when many governments were attempting large-scale efforts to minimize the transmission of tuberculosis through meat and milk.

Koch did not live to see this question answered. On April 9, 1910, three days after lecturing on tuberculosis at the Berlin Academy of Sciences, he suffered a heart attack from which he never fully recovered. He died at Baeden Baeden on May 27 at the age of 67. He was honored after death by the naming of the Institute after him.

Koch's obituaries are full of admiration for his perseverance and his scrupulous scientific process. Yet underneath the praise there is an acceptance that these same qualities—so useful to science—produced in the man a stubborn arrogance and an inability to give credit to the work of others or to admit his own mistakes. His early work with tuberculin and his defense that bovine tuberculosis was not harmful to humans are examples of his mistakes. Nevertheless, his strong will proved to be remarkably productive for science. He never left laboratory findings in the laboratory. Rather, he insisted, albeit stubbornly at times, that what he found in the laboratory should make a difference in the world. In the first paper he wrote on tuberculosis, he stated his lifelong goal, which he clearly achieved: ''I have undertaken my investigations in the interests of public health and I hope the greatest benefits will accrue therefrom.''

KÖHLER, GEORGES (1946-1995)

German immunologist

Born in Munich, in what was then occupied Germany, on April 17, 1946, Georges Jean Franz Köhler attended the University of Freiburg, where he obtained his Ph.D. in biology in 1974. From there he set off to Cambridge University in England, to work as a postdoctoral fellow for two years at the British Medical Research Council's laboratories. At Cambridge, Köhler worked under Dr. **César Milstein**, an Argentinean-born researcher with whom Köhler would eventually share the Nobel Prize. At the time, Milstein, who was Köhler's senior by 19 years, was a distinguished immunologist, and he actively encouraged Köhler in his research interests. Eventually, it was while working in the Cambridge laboratory that Köhler discovered the hybridoma technique.

Antibodies are produced by human plasma cells in response to any threatening and harmful bacterium, or tumor cell. The body forms a specific antibody against each antigen; and César Milstein has told the *New York Times* that the potential number of different antigens may reach ''well over a million.'' Therefore, for researchers working to combat diseases like **cancer**, an understanding of how antibodies could be harnessed for a possible cure was of great interest. And although scientists knew the benefits of producing antibodies, until Köhler and Milstein published their findings, there was no known technique for maintaining the long-term culture of antibody-forming plasma cells.

Köhler's interest in the subject had been aroused years earlier, when he had become intrigued by the work of Dr. Michael Potter (1924-) of the National Cancer Institute in Bethesda, Maryland. In 1962 Potter had induced myelomas, or plasma-cell tumors in mice, and others had discovered how to keep those tumors growing indefinitely in culture. Potter showed that plasma tumor cells were both immortal and able to create an unlimited number of identical antibodies. The only drawback was that there seemed no way to make the cells produce a certain *type* of antibody. Because of this, Köhler wanted to initiate a cloning experiment that would fuse plasma cells able to produce the desired antibodies with the ''immortal'' myeloma cells. With Milstein's blessing, Köhler began his experiment.

For several weeks after he made the hybrid cells, Köhler put off testing the outcome of his experiment for fear of failure. But disappointment turned to joy when Köhler discovered his test had been a success: Astoundingly, his hybrid cells were making pure antibodies against the test antigen. The result was dubbed ''monoclonal antibodies.'' For his contribution to medical science, Köhler—who in 1977 had relocated to Switzerland to do research at the Basel Institute for Immunology—was awarded the Nobel Prize in Medicine in 1984.

The implications of Köhler's discovery were immense. In the early 1980s Köhler's discovery had led scientists to identify various lymphocytes, or white blood cells. Among the kinds discovered were the T-4 lymphocytes, the cells destroyed by **AIDS**. Monoclonal antibodies have also improved tests for **hepatitis** B and **streptococcal infections** by providing guidance in selecting appropriate **antibiotics**, and they have aided in the research on **thyroid disorders**, lupus, **rheumatoid arthritis**, and inherited brain disorders. More significantly, Köhler's work has led to advances in research that can harness monoclonal antibodies into certain drugs and toxins that fight cancer, but would cause damage in their own right. Researchers are also using monoclonal antibodies to identify antigens specific to the surface of cancer cells so as to develop tests to detect the spread of cancerous cells in the body.

Despite the significance of the discovery, which has also resulted in vast amounts of research funds for many research laboratories, for Köhler and Milstein—who never patented their discovery—there was little remuneration. In fact, during the years following the discovery until they won the Nobel Prize, Köhler received only a single honorary doctorate. Following the award, however, he and Milstein, together with Michael Potter, were named winners of the Lasker Medical Research Award.

In 1985, Köhler moved back to his hometown of Freiburg, Germany, to assume the directorship of the Max Planck Institute for Immune Biology. He died on March 1, 1995.

KOLFF, WILLEM JOHAN (1911-)

Dutch American physician and biomedical engineer

Willem Johan Kolff was born in Leiden, the Netherlands, on February 14, 1911, the son of Adriana (de Jonge) and Jacob Kolff, a doctor who ran a **tuberculosis** sanatorium. After graduating from medical school at the University of Leiden in 1938, Kolff accepted a teaching post at the University of Groningen. There he was influenced by a professor who introduced Kolff to the basic concepts of dialysis—the principle whereby a solution of a high concentration passes through a semipermeable membrane to a solution with a lower concentration. He was affected as well by patients who were dying of **kidney failure**.

The kidneys are vital organs in the body; among other duties, the pair of organs is responsible for eliminating liquid wastes from the body, filtering over 400 gallons of blood daily. When the kidneys are not functioning correctly, uremia—a pathological condition caused by the accumulation of waste products normally removed in the urine—develops. The body swells, and if there is no intervention, death results. By the early twentieth century, doctors knew that they needed to create an external "kidney" to replace the function of damaged kidneys. As early as 1913 in the United States, doctors had managed a crude blood dialysis, or blood filtering, of dogs using celloidin as the filtering membrane. A major problem that they could not overcome, however, was preventing the coagulation of the blood once it was outside the animal. During and just after World War I, a German doctor, Georg Haas, using a new anticoagulant, heparin, successfully managed the first human dialysis, but still there were problems: Haas's apparatus could not filter enough blood quickly, and the supply of the anticoagulant was minimal.

At Groningen, Kolff was able to capitalize on these ground-breaking achievements and completed his own dialysis research with a simple sausage packing made of cellophane. He discovered that when the sausage casing was filled with a liquid, such as blood, then agitated in saline solution, the casing made a perfect membrane for filtering wastes. With the German takeover of Holland in 1940, Kolff, an outspoken anti-Nazi, left Groningen for the country town of Kampen, where he became the internist at the local hospital. There, in addition to carrying out his hospital duties and helping the resistance whenever possible, Kolff continued work on his dialysis machine. The anticoagulant heparin had become commercially available by that time. To solve the problem of adequate blood supply he created large rotating drums, adopting an idea automotive magnate Henry Ford had used to design water pumps in his engines. Kolff's attempts with humans initially were unsuccessful, and it was not until just after the end of the war, in September of 1945, that he successfully treated a patient, saving her life.

While still a medical student in 1937, Kolff had married Janke C. Huidekoper, and they already had four children, with another on the way, by 1950, when Kolff accepted a position in the United States at Ohio's Cleveland Clinic. Meanwhile, Kolff's dialysis machine was being improved upon by others around the world. Kolff then moved on to other medical endeavors: he was intent on creating a **heart-lung machine** that could be used to keep bodily functions operating and thus enable **open-heart surgery** to take place. In the 17 years he spent at the Cleveland Clinic Foundation as professor of clinical investigation, Kolff, working with C. P. Dubbelman, designed an artificial heart-lung device known as a pump-oxygenator. By 1961 another of Kolff's designs was in service: the intra-aortic balloon pump to be used in cases of circulation failure. In addition, his attention increasingly turned to designing and implanting an **artificial heart**. In December of 1957, Kolff and his Cleveland team removed the heart from a dog and replaced it with a pneumatic pump which kept the dog alive for 90 minutes, proving the viability of the artificial heart.

In 1967 Kolff moved from Cleveland to accept a position at the University of Utah as the head of both the Division of Artificial Organs and the Institute of Biomedical Engineering. As such, he led a team of surgeons, physicists, and cardiologists in designing an implantable artificial heart for humans. It was this team, using a heart designed by one of Kolff's students, Robert K. Jarvik, that implanted the first artificial heart in a human on December 2, 1982. The patient, Barney Clark, lived for 112 days, proving the viability of such a procedure. Kolff also designed an artificial **ear** and **eye**, though the latter, with its numerous devices necessary for operation, is far from a practical stage. Kolff has gone on to develop a portable kidney dialysis machine, introducing, as early as 1975, the Wearable Artificial Kidney (or WAK), which allows for home dialysis.

Kolff became a naturalized U.S. citizen in 1956 and is the author of close to 700 articles and papers on the kidney, heart, and artificial organs. Recognized worldwide for his efforts in bionics, Kolff is the recipient of more than 100 awards and honors, including the Landsteiner Silver Medal in 1942 from the Red Cross of the Netherlands, the Frances Amory Award in 1948 from the American Academy of Arts and Science, the Gairdner Prize in 1966, the Leo Harvey Prize in 1972, and the Japan Prize in 1986. He was named one of the one hundred most important Americans of the twentieth century by *Life* magazine in 1990.

KOOP, CHARLES EVERETT (1916-)

American pediatric surgeon; former U.S. Surgeon General

Charles Everett Koop (known as C. Everett Koop) was born in Brooklyn, New York, on October 14, 1916. As a pun on his last name (Koop/coop), Koop was nicknamed Chick. Koop displayed an early interest in medicine, sneaking into Columbia Presbyterian Hospital at the age of 15 in order to observe abdominal surgery. He was also known to anesthetize neighborhood cats with ether in order to perform surgery on them and practice stitching them up.

At only 16 years of age, Koop began classes at Dartmouth College, graduating with a B.A. degree in 1937. By 1941, Koop had received his M.D. from Cornell Medical College. He trained in pediatrics at Pennsylvania Hospital, continuing on in pediatric surgery at University of Pennsylvania School of medicine, Boston Children's Hospital, and the Graduate School of Medicine at the University of Pennsylvania. Koop earned an Sc.D degree in medicine from the University of Pennsylvania in 1947.

In 1948, when Koop became surgeon-in-chief at Children's Hospital in Philadelphia, pediatric surgery was still a relatively new field. Koop was one of the first physicians in the country to commit his entire practice to pediatric surgery. He worked hard to improve the then-dismal mortality rates associated with surgery on children. Koop established excellent practices of pre- and post-surgical care, which greatly reduced post-operative mortality rates. He also established a number of innovative surgical and diagnostic procedures. He worked to refine **anesthesia** practices for pediatric patients, improving both its safety and its efficacy. Some of his more well-known surgeries included the reconstruction of the chest of a baby whose heart had been outside its body at birth, and the separation of several different sets of Siamese (conjoined) twins.

Koop's career followed a very successful trajectory, and he moved quickly through the faculty ranks at the University

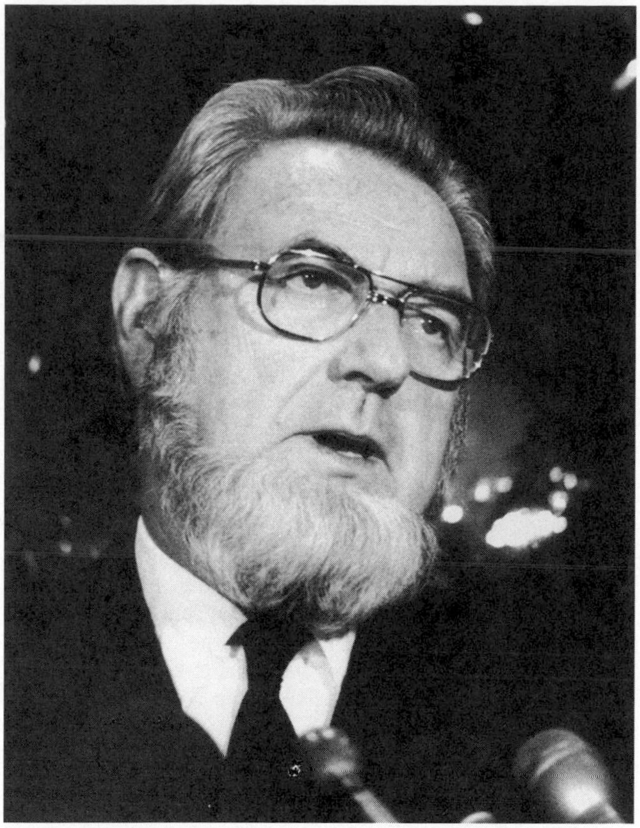

C. Everett Koop

of Pennsylvania School of Medicine, becoming professor of pediatric surgery at the School of Medicine in 1959 and at the Graduate School of Medicine in 1960. In 1971, he was appointed professor of pediatrics.

Koop's entree into a very visible public life came in 1981, when President Ronald Reagan chose him as surgeon general. Confirmation hearings were controversial, as liberals opposed his unmoving stance against **abortion**. He was perceived as dangerously conservative. Still, he was confirmed in November of 1981, and sworn in on January 21, 1982.

In Koop's tenure as surgeon general, he proved himself to be an outspoken advocate of **public health**. He lectured the nation about the medical dangers associated with tobacco (an unpopular issue with his conservative supporters). Koop compared nicotine addiciton with addiction to cocaine and heroine. He supported a ban on **smoking** in the workplace, and spoke out frankly against the practice of exporting tobacco products to developing nations. He supported bans on alcohol advertising. He tried to encourage Americans to become more mindful of their diet, decreasing fat and sugar and increasing fiber and complex carbohydrates.

Koop also continued to draw some liberal fire, by supporting the ''squeal rule,'' which mandated that health officials were obligated to contact parents if their children wanted to acquire contraceptives.

Koop had an important role in moving the nation out of silence about the **AIDS** epidemic. In 1996, he wrote a long re-

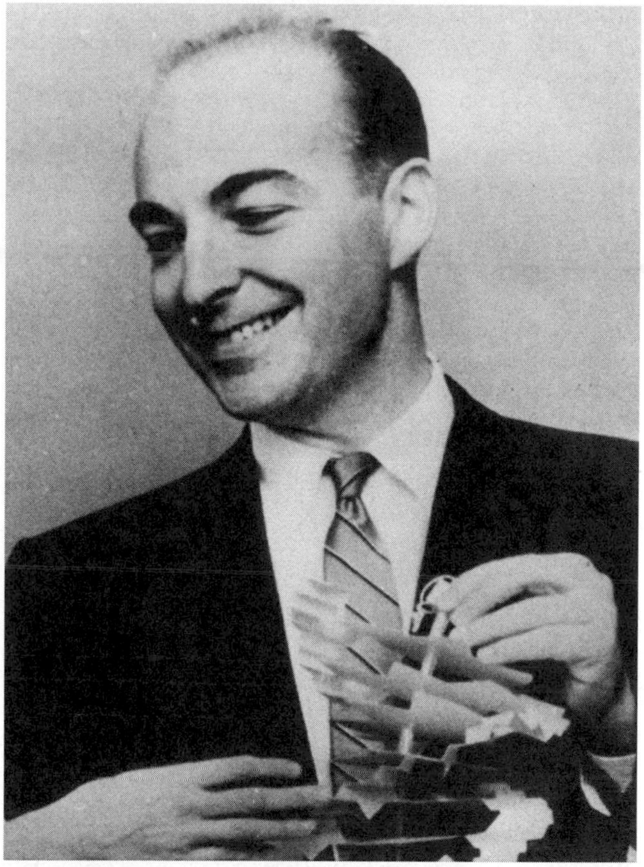

Arthur Kornberg

port, in which he advocated educating children about the dangers of AIDS, supplying adults with **condoms**, allowing pregnant women with AIDS to obtain abortions, and speaking out against requiring AIDS testing. Again, his conservative backers were disappointed in him, but his previous liberal opponents were pleased. Koop tried to explain himself to both groups, saying ''We are fighting a disease, not a people'' and ''You may hate the sin, but love the sinner.''

Koop decided not to serve a second term as surgeon general, resigning as of October 1989. Some believe that his resignation stemmed from pressure from various friends who felt that Koop had strayed too far from conservative ideals.

Koop went to Dartmouth College, this time as a faculty member. He helped to establish the C. Everett Koop Institute, where he serves as Senior Scholar. Koop continues to travel around the nation speaking on issues of public health.

See also Elders, Jocelyn

KORNBERG, ARTHUR (1918-)

American biochemist

Arthur Kornberg was the first to synthesize deoxyribonucleic acid (DNA) outside the cell. He also isolated and purified one of the enzymes necessary for successful synthesis. His results showed that a chromosome is composed of a continuous strand of DNA. For his success, he received half of the 1959 Nobel Prize in physiology or medicine.

Kornberg was born in Brooklyn, NY. He graduated from the City College of New York in 1937, and received his M.D. from the University of Rochester in 1941. After serving in the Coast Guard during World War II, he began his career in biochemical research. He headed the biochemistry department at Stanford University for many years.

After American biochemist **Severo Ochoa** synthesized ribonucleic acid (RNA) nucleotides in 1955, Kornberg began attempting to synthesize DNA. As a starting point, Kornberg isolated a pure form of the *E. coli* bacterial enzyme now known as DNA polymerase I, which plays a role in copying DNA within the cell. He then used as a synthesizing template a circular, single-stranded DNA from a bacteriophage (virus which parasitizes bacteria) called ϕX174, which was isolated by Robert Sinsheimer (1920-) at the California Institute of Technology. In nature, ϕX174 reproduces inside *E. coli*, forming a complementary second DNA circle that acts as a template for its new copy. Kornberg, Sinsheimer, and Mehran Goulian (1929-) (Stanford University) isolated this second DNA circle to use as their template. Then they added the enzyme and the four DNA nucleosides (base-sugar groups) with three-phosphate groups attached—ATP (adenosine triphosphate), GTP (guanosine triphosphate), CTP (cytidine triphosphate), and TTP (thymidine triphosphate). Finally, DNA nucleotides were formed. The scientists also showed that their synthetic DNA was biologically active. Since Sinsheimer's group had already found that even a single copying error would make the virus inactive, the activity proved that error-free DNA could be synthesized.

Later research by other scientists revealed details of the natural DNA-copying process. It is now known that DNA polymerase I's main task is examining copied DNA for errors, removing incorrect nucleotides, and repairing damaged ones. Both DNA polymerase I and polymerase III—the main synthesizing enzyme in many species—are needed for this replication.

Kornberg's current research focus at Stanford has changed from DNA replication to inorganic polyphosphate (poly P), a linear polymer with many functions, including phosphate and energy reservoirs, buffering against alkali, bacteria capsule formation, and regulation of growth and development especially under stress or deprivation.

KOSSEL, ALBRECHT (1853-1927)

German biochemist

Albrecht Kossel isolated several major structural parts of the nucleic acids and discovered histidine, an essential amino acid. He received the 1910 Nobel prize in physiology or medicine for his work with the nucleic acids and cellular proteins.

Kossel was born in Rostock, Germany, where his father was a merchant. Kossel's first scientific love was botany, but he was convinced by his father to study medicine and received his medical license in 1877. He next went to the University of Strasbourg (then part of Germany), where he became interested in physiological chemistry and worked with **Ernst Hoppe-Seyler** on the nucleic acids. After serving on university faculties in Berlin and Marburg, in 1901 he became head of the physiology department at the University of Heidelberg.

Between 1877 and 1881 he served as Ernst Hoppe-Selyer's assistant and began his studies of the nucleic acids, which had been discovered ten years earlier by one of Hoppe-Selyer's pupils, the Swiss biochemist Johann Miescher (1844-1895). Miescher had called his substance nuclein because it was found in a cell's nucleus, and it was thought to be a phosphorus-rich protein. Kossel showed that nuclein was actually composed of a protein portion and a non-protein portion, which was the nucleic acid.

Over the next 20 years, Kossel and his own research team made important discoveries about the structure of both the nucleic acids and cellular proteins. He showed that nucleic acid is made up in part of purines and pyrimidines. He identified their structures, showing that a pyrimidine has a single six-sided ring, while a purine has a six-sided ring that shares one side with a five-sided ring. He isolated the two purines, adenine and guanine, which are now known to exist in both ribonucleic acid (RNA) and deoxyribonucleic acid (DNA). He also isolated the three pyrimidines— thymine and cytosine, found in DNA, and uracil, which RNA contains instead of thymine. Adenine is composed of carbon, hydrogen, and nitrogen; the others also contain oxygen. In addition, he identified carbohydrates in the nucleic acids and made preliminary predictions about the types of sugars involved. His work was continued by the American biochemist Phoebus Levene (1869-1940), who had once studied with him. In addition to these findings, Kossel was the first to isolate the protein histone—a component of chromatin, the structural material of the chromosomes that supports the DNA.

Kossel was always motivated to find the biological functions of the chemicals he studied and isolated. In a famous 1912 lecture, he expressed his conviction about the importance of nucleic acids and cellular proteins as the chemical basis for **genetics**. He published many papers detailing his work and held honorary doctorates at six universities. He was also a member of the Royal Swedish Academy of Sciences and the Royal Society of Sciences of Uppsala.

KREBS, EDWIN G. (1918-)

American biochemist

Edwin Gerhard Krebs was born to William Carl Krebs and Louisa Helena Stegeman Krebs in Lansing, Iowa, on June 6, 1918. He was the third of four children. His father, a Presbyterian minister, died while Krebs was in his first year of high school. In order to keep Krebs's two older brothers enrolled at the University of Illinois in Urbana, Louisa Krebs moved the family from Greenville, where Edwin Krebs grew up, to the university town.

In 1940, after completing his high-school and undergraduate work in Urbana, Krebs entered medical school at

Washington University School of Medicine in St. Louis, Missouri. He had the opportunity to work under Arda A. Green, who was associated with **Carl Ferdinand Cori and Gerty T. Cori**. The Coris were a husband-and-wife team who had won the Nobel Prize in 1947 for research on carbohydrate **metabolism** and the enzyme phosphorylase. Krebs's later collaboration with **Edmond Fischer** at the University of Washington in Seattle had its beginning in the research conducted by the Coris.

After receiving his medical degree in 1943 and completing an eight-month residency in internal medicine at Barnes Hospital in St. Louis, Krebs became a medical officer in the navy, serving in that capacity until 1946. Due to the unavailability of a resident position, and on the advice of one of his professors, Krebs began studying science. Because of his background in chemistry, Krebs chose to work in biochemistry and was accepted by the Coris as a postdoctoral fellow in their laboratory. For two years, while working for the Coris, Krebs studied the interaction of protamine (a basic protein) with rabbit muscle phosphorylase. This work seemed so rewarding to him that he decided to continue his efforts in the field of research, and when in 1948 he was invited by Hans Neurath to join the faculty as an assistant professor in the department of biochemistry at the University of Washington.

At this time Neurath's department greatly emphasized protein chemistry and enzymology (enzymes are proteins that act as catalysts in biochemical reactions). Work in the Coris' laboratory had established that the enzyme phosphorylase existed in active and inactive forms, but what controlled its activity was unknown. Combining his experience on mammalian skeletal muscle phosphorylase with Edmond Fischer's experience with potato phosphorylase after Fischer joined the department, Krebs and Fischer teamed up to uncover the molecular mechanism by which phosphorylase makes energy available to a contracting muscle. What they discovered was reversible protein phosphorylation. An enzyme called protein kinase takes phosphate from adenosine triphosphate (ATP), the supplier of energy to cells, and adds it to inactive phosphorylase, changing the shape of the phosphorylase and consequently switching it on. Another enzyme, called protein phosphatase, reverses this process by removing the phosphate from phosphorylase, thus deactivating it. Protein kinases are present in all cells.

Once it became evident that reversible protein phosphorylation was a general process, the impact of Krebs and Fischer's work was immeasurable. Their collaboration opened the field of biochemical research and paved the way to much of the work done in the area of biotechnology and genetic engineering. Protein phosphorylation has even been posited as the basis of learning and memory. Medical applications have included development of the drug cyclosporin, which blocks the body's immune response by interfering with phosphorylation to prevent rejection of transplants. As important as what happens when the process functions normally is what happens when it goes awry: protein kinases are involved in almost 50 percent of cancer-causing oncogenes.

Recognition for Krebs's work came through various awards besides the Nobel Prize. In 1988 Krebs and Fischer shared the Passano Award for their research, and Krebs was one of four scientists to share the Lasker Award for Basic Medical Research in 1989. He was co-recipient of the Robert A. Welch Award in Chemistry in 1991, followed by the Nobel Prize in physiology or medicine a year later. Besides concentrating his research on protein phosphorylation, Krebs has investigated signal transduction and carbohydrate **metabolism**.

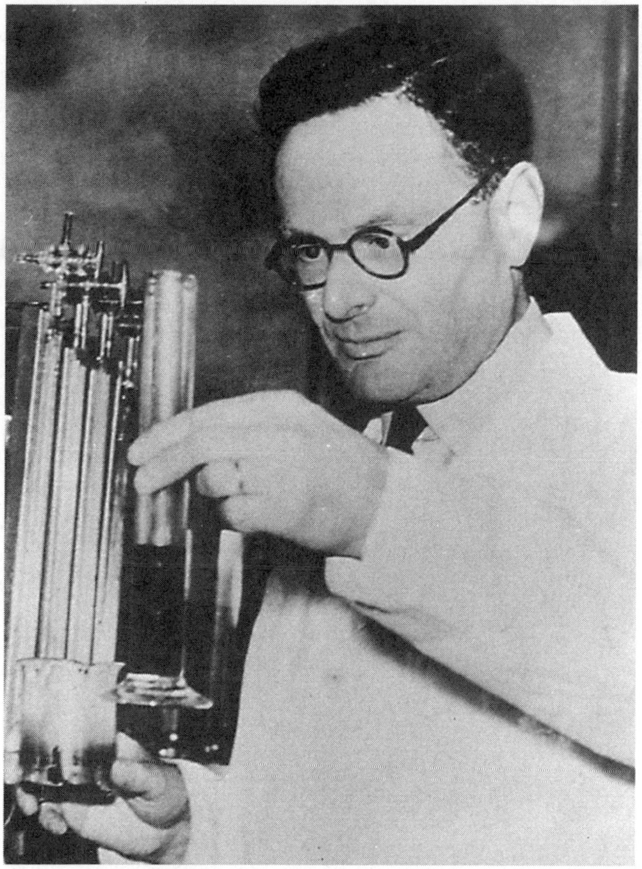

Hans Adolf Krebs

In 1968 Krebs had left the University of Washington to accept the position of founding chairman of the department of biological chemistry at the University of California in Davis. When he returned to Washington in 1977 he became chairman of the department of pharmacology. From 1977 until 1983, Krebs was associated with the Howard Hughes Medical Institute as well.

Krebs was married on March 10, 1945, to Virginia Deedy French, and they have three children, Sally, Robert, and Martha.

KREBS, HANS ADOLF (1900-1981)

German British biochemist

The son of a physician, Hans Krebs attended several German universities before receiving his medical degree from the University of Hamburg in 1925. Although he set up practice as an ear, nose and throat specialist (his father's occupation), he soon realized he preferred doing research and, a year later, became an assistant to the noted biochemist **Otto Warburg** at the Kaiser Wilhelm Institute in Berlin, Germany. While there, Krebs became interested in amino acids, the building blocks of protein. He particularly wanted to know more about the then-unknown process by which the body, under certain circumstances, breaks down the amino acids instead of using them for constructive purposes.

In the course of several years of research, Krebs discovered that when amino acids were broken down (or degraded), their nitrogen atoms were the first to be stripped away. After this deamination process, the nitrogen atoms were excreted from the body in the form of urea, a major component in urine. By 1932, Krebs was able to describe several of the basic steps in urea formation and to discuss what happened to the remainder of the amino acids. His ''urea cycle'' won Krebs some fame but by then the Nazi movement was becoming more powerful and, like almost all of Germany's Jewish scientists, Krebs decided to leave the country.

In 1933, Krebs went to England, where he studied for a while at Cambridge University, working under Frederick Gowland Hopkins. In 1935, he joined the faculty of Sheffield University, where he remained until 1954, then moved on to Oxford University, finally retiring in 1967. While at Sheffield, Krebs concentrated much of his attention on carbohydrate **metabolism** and discovered the process for which he is best known: the citric acid cycle (also called the tricarboxylic acid cycle or, more simply, the Krebs cycle). Several other biochemists—in particular, **Otto Meyerhof** and **Carl and Gerty Cori**—had already shown that glycogen, the carbohydrate stored in the liver and muscles, was broken down to lactic acid by a process that required no oxygen and that released very little energy. Krebs was interested in discovering how the lactic acid was then broken down into carbon dioxide and water—and was now somehow able to release a comparatively great deal of energy.

From the work of **Albert Szent-Györgyi**, Krebs knew that several four-carbon compounds were able to increase the consumption of oxygen by cellular tissues. Krebs then located two six-carbon acids with similar oxygen-increasing powers, (one of them the citric acid that gave the cycle its original name). All these various compounds, Krebs felt, must be involved in the chain that led from carbohydrates to carbon dioxide, water and energy. And, by performing countless studies—most of them on pigeon breast muscles—by 1937, he was able to work out most of the long, complicated chain.

The chain is, in fact, a cycle—a series of chemical changes that begins when lactic acid (a three-carbon compound) is broken down into a mysterious two-carbon compound (determined by **Fritz Lipmann** to be acetyl coenzyme A). The two-carbon compound, when combined with the four-carbon oxaloacetic acid, becomes the six-carbon citric acid. The citric acid then undergoes a complicated series of chemical changes, during which hydrogen atoms occasionally break off (and combine with atmospheric oxygen to produce energy), and two-carbon fragments either attach themselves to the chain to regenerate certain compounds or break off (to be broken down into carbon dioxide and water, liberating more energy in the process).

The Krebs cycle, it soon became clear, not only helped explain the metabolic pathways followed by carbohydrates but by fats and proteins as well. The cycle, in fact, appears to play a fundamental role in virtually all cell metabolism and Krebs' discovery is therefore considered a major contribution to biochemistry. For his work, Krebs shared the 1953 Nobel Prize in physiology or medicine with Lipmann. He was also knighted by Queen Elizabeth II (1926-) in 1958.

KRETSCHMER, ERNST (1888-1964)

German psychiatrist

Ernst Kretschmer was a prominent German psychiatrist best known for his studies showing a correlation between body type and personality. He earned a doctorate in medicine at the University of Tübingen in 1913 and began a residency in psychiatry. In 1914 he completed a dissertation on the role of delusion in manic depression (**bipolar disorder**).

At the beginning of World War I, Kretschmer joined the medical corps of the German Wehrmacht and served at a field hospital, then at a rehabilitation center for emotionally disturbed soldiers. He observed soldiers who suffered shell shock which led to conversion reactions, in which emotional problems took a physical form. He also recorded paranoid reactions that were linked with brain trauma. Based on his observations, he published the monograph *Hysteria, Reflex and Instinct* in 1923. Kretschmer devised a treatment for military victims of **hysteria** which involved lying quiet in a dark room and receiving electrical impulses.

Kretschmer continued his investigation into **paranoia** as it was influenced by the meeting of body, environment and personality and published this multidimensional theory in 1918 in *Ideas of Reference in Oversensitive Personalities, a Contribution to the Theory of Paranoia*. While some of the psychiatric community debated Kretschmer's research over the years, the book went into three editions and the ideas were well accepted.

In 1921 Kretschmer published his famous book, *Body Structure and Character*, which quickly drew international attention. He claimed that physical properties of the face, skull, and body structure were linked to character and psychiatric illness. Although this hypothesis was eventually discredited, Kretschmer's writing style was very persuasive and his book went into 20 editions. Kretschmer refined his theories of body structure and character throughout his career and never abandoned his original hypothesis. He carefully measured and photographed patients and thought of his research as a marriage of psychiatry and anthropology. Although he mentioned correlation in his text, he never applied any statistical analysis and relied on intuition. However, others in the psychological community used Kretschmer's findings as a starting point for new research.

All of Kretschmer's books were translated into English and Columbia University invited Kretschmer as a guest of honor at the opening of the New York State Psychiatric Institute in 1929.

Kretschmer went on to link his classification of physical properties to a theory of genius which was designed to appeal to psychiatrists and the lay public. He published *Psychology of Men of Genius* in 1931. Kretschmer believed genius could be cultivated by mixing ethnic groups and classes, a belief which contradicted the Nazi doctrine of a superior Aryan race. When the Nazis took over the German government in 1933, Kretschmer protested by resigning his position as president of the German Society of Psychotherapy. Surprisingly, Kretschmer worked in Germany throughout the period of Nazi domination without being persecuted. Many of his German colleagues in psychiatry and psychology left the country.

From 1926 to 1946, Kretschmer served as chairman of the department of neuropsychiatry at Marburg and director of the neurologic clinic. After World War II, he returned to the neurologic clinic at Tübingen and published *Psychotherapeutic Studies* in 1949. In Kretschmer's estimation, Germany was a generation behind other Western countries in using psychotherapy, and he developed new guidelines for using psychotherapy and **hypnosis**. Criminal behavior of the mentally ill was another research interest of Kretschmer, and he advocated psychiatric treatment for prisoners. Kretschmer retired from the University of Tübingen in 1959.

KROGH, AUGUST (1874-1949)

Danish physiologist

Schack August Steenberg Krogh (pronounced Krawg) was born on November 15, 1874, in Grenaa, Jutland. Throughout his life Krogh was active in both zoology and human physiology, accomplishing his major discoveries in the physiology of respiration.

Krogh attended school at the Gymnasium at Aarhus, and then went on to the University of Copenhagen in 1893. He first entered Copenhagen with the intention of studying physics and medicine, but under the influence of zoologist William Sorensen, he changed to the study of zoology and physiology. So slash rensen had advised Krogh to attend the lectures of Christian Bohr, an expert in circulatory and respiratory physiology. After attending Bohr's lectures at Copenhagen, Krogh began to work in Bohr's laboratory in 1897, and after receiving his master of science degree in 1899, he became Bohr's laboratory assistant.

One of Krogh's earliest achievements was his invention of a microtonometer—an instrument that measures gas pressure in fluids—which he developed to help in his research with a marine organism named *Corethra.* As a student Krogh had done research on the larvae of *Corethra* to determine how its air bladders operated (he found that they worked like the diving tanks of submarines). Traveling in 1902 to Greenland, Krogh studied the amounts of oxygen and carbon dioxide dissolved in fresh and sea water. His research cast a new understanding on the role of the oceans in carbon dioxide regulation and at the same time he was able to improve his techniques for measuring gas pressures in fluids.

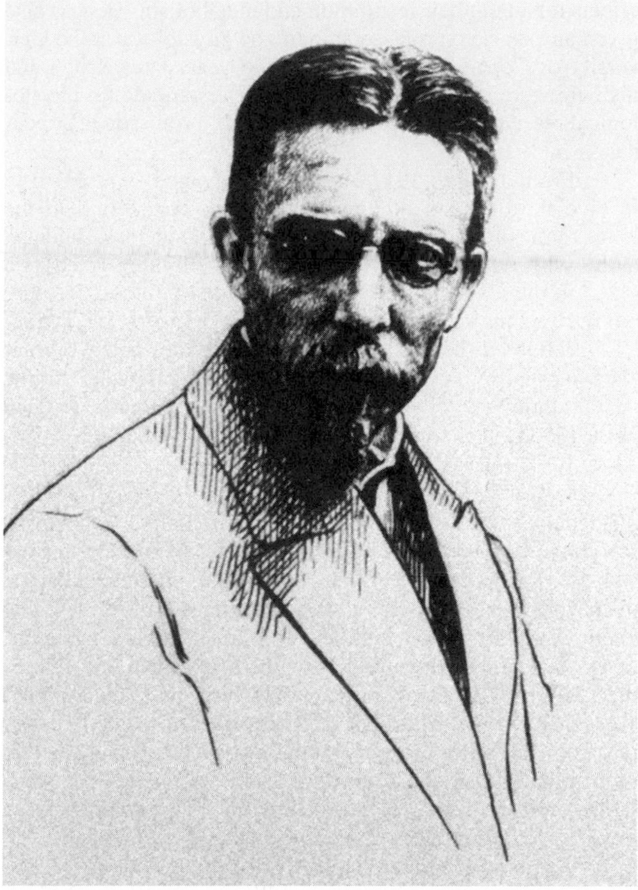

August Krogh

In 1903 Krogh received a Ph.D. in zoology from the University of Copenhagen, where, in his doctoral dissertation, he demonstrated the difference between the skin and lung respiration of the frog. Whereas the frog's skin respiration was constant and regular, Krogh found that the frog's lung respiration varied and was controlled by the autonomic system through the mechanism of the vagus nerve. Oxygen passed from the air sacs (alveoli) of the lung through a membrane to the capillaries and then to the blood stream where it formed carbon dioxide after it was used by the different tissues in the body. The process then reversed when the blood carried carbon dioxide to the alveoli of the lungs, where it was exhaled.

Krogh was married in 1905 to Marie Jorgensen, a physiologist who also worked in Bohr's laboratory. (The couple would eventually have three daughters and one son.) In 1906 the first of Krogh's papers to receive international recognition, a work which showed that nitrogen is not involved in animal **metabolism**, was awarded the Seegen Prize from the Vienna Academy of Sciences. In 1907 Krogh received further international attention at Heidelberg, Germany, when he discussed his findings on the diffusion of pulmonary gases at the International Congress of Physiology.

In 1908 Krogh made another trip to Greenland with his wife to study the Eskimo's meat-eating dietary habits and the effects it had on their respiration and metabolism. He was also given an associate professorship of zoo physiology at the University of Copenhagen that year. Two years later Krogh and his wife were given a laboratory at Ny Vestergade for physiological research. Krogh then became a full professor at Copenhagen in 1916.

From 1908 to 1912 Krogh was engaged in research to resolve the question of how oxygen was transferred in the lungs to the blood. Bohr and John Burdon Sanderson Haldane, along with other scientists, believed that the lung acted as a gland in the alveolar transfer of oxygen to the blood; in other words, the lung secreted the oxygen. Krogh, in 1912, convincingly delivered the fatal blow to the secretion theory by first showing that in fishes there is no secretion of oxygen into the air sacs, and then by demonstrating that the amount of oxygen in the blood always equalled the amount that should be provided by his diffusion theory.

It was not until 1916, however, that Krogh accomplished the work that would, in 1920, earn him the Nobel Prize for physiology or medicine. He showed that muscle tension was always slightly lower than the tensions in the capillaries, even when the muscle was at work. Noting that there were few open capillaries when a muscle was at rest, Krogh demonstrated that as soon as the muscle became active many capillaries began to open up. He was also able to show that blood did not enter the capillaries through the pressure of the blood vessels but from the relaxed tonus (partial contraction) of the active muscle. The relaxation of the muscle allowed the field of capillaries to open and the blood to flow in, thus providing more oxygen to the muscle, organ, or tissue.

Krogh's discoveries relating to gas exchanges in the lung and to the operation of the capillary system helped to develop medical techniques for breathing through the trachea. His work also improved surgical methods for open heart surgery, such as the procedure for reducing body temperature to below normal levels to slow down the rate of gaseous exchange.

In 1922 Krogh became interested in insulin (which had been discovered by **Frederick G. Banting** and **John James Rickard Macleod** the year before), partly because his own wife had **diabetes**. Besides being active in insulin research, Krogh helped to promote manufacturing facilities in Denmark for its production. Krogh also maintained his interest in zoology, writing about insects and becoming particularly attentive to theories about the way honey bees communicate.

Krogh died on September 13, 1949, in Copenhagen.

KÜBLER-ROSS, ELISABETH (1926-)

Swiss-American psychiatrist and researcher

Elisabeth Kübler-Ross, internationally renown psychiatrist, researcher, and writer in the field of thanatology (the study of death), is known primarily for her theory of the five stages in the dying process. Her revolutionary approach to **death** and dying was both compassionate and humane; it defied taboos and laid the groundwork for further study. Kübler-Ross is often given credit for having imported the **hospice** concept to the United States from its origins in England.

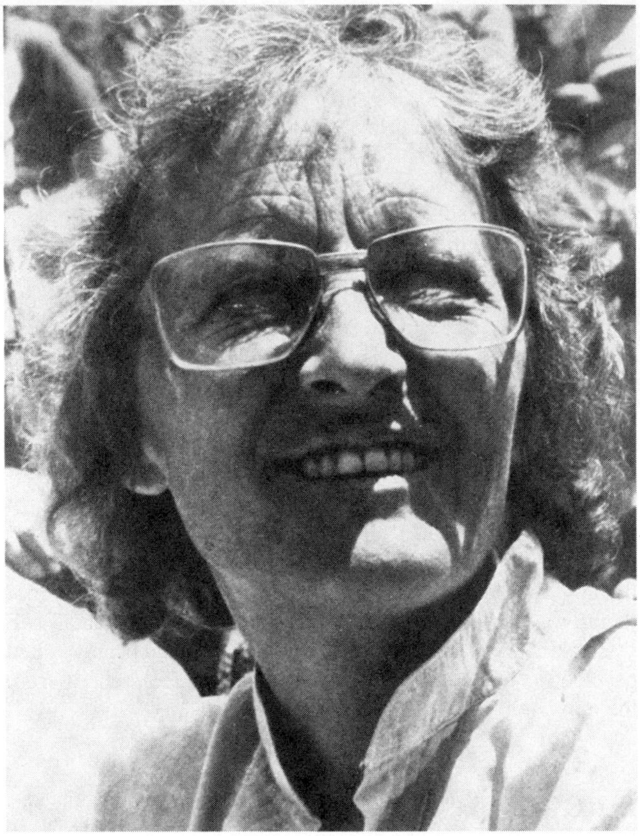

Elisabeth Kübler-Ross

The daughter of Ernst and Emmy (Villiger) Kübler, Elisabeth was the first-born of triplet girls. At birth Elisabeth and one of her sisters barely weighed two pounds, yet the triplets survived. Ernst Kübler, although conservative and a strict disciplinarian, enjoyed singing to his children and took them hiking in the mountains surrounding the family's retreat in Furlegi. These trips inspired in Elisabeth a deep reverence for nature and for all living things.

Although their brother's education was intended to prepare him to enter the business world, the girls were sent to local schools to prepare them for marriage. When Elisabeth developed a passion for science, however, she received no support her parents and pursued a post-secondary education on her own.

In Elisabeth's youth, the deaths of several individuals were instrumental in determining the direction of her personal and professional life. These experiences with death intensified the belief that later became the focus of her philosophy that death is only a stage of life, and that the terminally ill should be allowed to confront death with dignity.

When Elisabeth learned that the Germans had invaded Poland in 1939, she longed to assist the Polish people in any way she could. To that end, she became involved with refugees sent to Swiss hospitals; joined the International Volunteers for Peace in 1945; and worked on the French-Swiss border and in Sweden before she was finally sent to Poland in 1948. In Poland, she worked at numerous jobs, including camp cook, gardener, carpenter, and nurse.

Elisabeth Kübler graduated from the University of Zurich in 1957 and began working as a rural doctor in Switzerland. In 1958 she married Emanuel Robert Ross, a native New Yorker and fellow medical student to whom she remained married for 11 years.

Kübler-Ross traveled to the United States with her new husband, and they both obtained internships at Community Hospital in Glen Cove, Long Island. Elisabeth then secured a three-year residency in psychiatry at Manhattan State Hospital in Ward's Island while spending a year at Montefiore Hospital in the Bronx. Patients with even the most severe illnesses seemed to respond to Kübler-Ross's compassionate approach. The indifferent and even inhumane treatment of patients in psychiatric hospitals appalled the young doctor, and the more freedom she was allowed in treating patients, the more successful results she achieved.

After the birth of their first child, the couple left New York City, and in 1962 they accepted positions at the University of Colorado School of Medicine in Denver. Elisabeth Kübler-Ross was given a fellowship in psychiatry and the following year became an instructor at Colorado General Hospital. In 1965, the family, with their new daughter, moved to Chicago, where Kübler-Ross was appointed an assistant professor of psychiatry and assistant director of psychiatric consultation and liaison services at the University of Chicago Medical School.

Throughout her career, Kübler-Ross had been troubled by the widespread attitude of avoidance that prevailed in the care of terminally ill patients. Consequently, she began developing her own techniques for dealing with the dying and for allowing them to express their feelings. It was in Chicago that fame for her work in thanatology began. Although there were administrative pressures to suppress the attention her work received, she continued to work with nurses, sympathetic doctors, and priests to better counsel the dying. She held weekly seminars eventually canceled by the administration that attracted huge crowds. The administrative focus was on treating patients rather than on discussing death.

In her ground-breaking seminars, Kübler-Ross interviewed dying patients behind a one-way glass through which attendees could observe. Viewing death as the final stage of life, Kübler-Ross began to identify five stages in the death process. These stages, universal to all patients she encountered, were: denial, anger, bargaining, depression, and acceptance. Her research and findings were set forth in her best-selling book *On Death and Dying* (1969), a book that became a standard resource for counselors, physicians, and lay persons.

Life magazine published an article on November 21, 1969, that exposed to the public for the first time the openness with which Kübler-Ross approached the issue of death with patients and described their open conversations with her. The public response was overwhelming and was a turning point in Kübler-Ross's career. She decided to work exclusively with dying patients and their families.

In 1977 she founded ''Shanti Nilaya'' (Home of Peace), a healing center for the dying and their families in Escondido, California. She moved there from Chicago, and profits from her lectures and books funded the center. In 1990 she moved the Elisabeth Kübler-Ross Center to her own 200-acre farm in Headwater, Virginia, where she succeeded in training professionals and laypersons to deal with the terminally ill until 1994. In 1986 Kübler-Ross attempted to establish a hospice for babies with **acquired immunodeficiency syndrome (AIDS)**, but after strong community opposition, she abandoned the idea.

In addition to her most influential work, *On Death and Dying*, Kübler-Ross is the author of 19 books on dealing with the dying process. Throughout her career, Kübler-Ross received numerous awards and recognitions for her selfless devotion to the cause of the terminally ill. She also co-founded the American Holistic Medical Association.

See also Death; Holistic medicine; Hospices; Hospitals

L

LAENNEC, RENÉ THÉOPHILE HYACINTHE (1781-1826)

French physician

René Théophile Hyacinthe Laennec, known as the father of modern knowledge of pulmonary disease, is considered by many as one of the greatest clinicians of all time. He made a major contribution to medical science by introducing a method of diagnosing diseases called auscultation. Auscultation involves listening to and identifying various sounds made by different body structures. Laennec's specialty was chest diseases. Initially, his diagnostic method involved placing his **ear** to the chest of his patient. Ultimately, it led him to inventing the **stethoscope**, which he called the ''chest examiner.''

Although he is most famous for this work, he was the first person to describe the rare disease **tuberculosis** verrucosa cutis (tuberculosis of the skin), and gave **cirrhosis** its name from the Greek word *kirrhos*, meaning tawny. The term ''Laennec's cirrhosis'' is still used to describe alcoholic liver cirrhosis. He was also a pioneer in matching postmortem (**autopsy**) findings with physical signs of disease.

Laennec was born in Brittany, France. His father was a lawyer and writer of poetry. His mother died when he was six years old and he went to live with his grand-uncle, the Abbé Laennec. At the age of 12, he went to Nantes where his uncle was a professor at the university. An excellent student, the young Laennec soon became fluent in English and German, won many academic prizes, and began studying medicine under his uncle's direction. In 1800, at the age of 19, he entered the university in Paris, gaining first prize in both medicine and surgery in less than a year. He became a student of medicine under the personal physician to Napoleon Bonaparte's (1769-1821), Jean-Nicolas Corvisart (1755-1821), who used percussion (tapping with the fingers) to diagnose chest disorders. Laennec improved upon this method by placing his ear directly on the patient's chest to identify and differentiate between healthy and unhealthy sounds of the heart and respiratory system.

By performing autopsies, he identified precise causes of unhealthy sounds, enabling him to better diagnose and treat future patients. He named dozens of different sounds, coining the terms rale, used to define any abnormal sound in the chest, and rhonchi which described a loud, low-pitched crackles during exhalation. These terms are still used by medical professionals.

In 1819, Laennec wrote his famous treatise, *De l'auscultation médiate (On mediate auscultation)*, in which he described in unprecedented detail the sounds of chest disease and how he came to invent the chest examiner. This treatise, which laid the groundwork for modern pulmonary medicine, has been ranked in importance and insight with works of **Hippocrates** (c. 460-c. 377 B.C.) Laennec wrote ''the most important part of an art is to be able to observe properly.''

Ironically, his observation of children playing led to his inventing the stethoscope. He noticed children holding the end of a long piece of wood to their ears, listening to the tapping sounds made by a pin at the other end, the sound of which was transmitted through the wood. Laennec wrote about a young woman who came to him with symptoms of heart disease. Examination by percussion was ineffective ''...on the account of the great degree of fatness...the other method (placing the ear to the chest) being rendered inadmissible by the age and sex of the patient.'' Recalling the children and the stick, he rolled several sheets of paper into a cylinder, placing one end on the woman's chest and the other to his ear. ''I was not a little surprised and pleased to find that I could thereby perceive the action of the heart in a manner much more clear and distinct than I had ever been able to do by the immediate application of the ear,'' he wrote.

Experimenting with materials of different types, densities, lengths, and thicknesses, he settled on a ''...cylinder of wood, an inch and a half (3.8 cm) in diameter, and a foot (30.48 cm) long, perforated longitudinally by a bore three lines wide, and hollowed out into a funnel shape, to the depth of an inch and a half (3.8 cm) at one of its extremities.'' He then made his instrument available for purchase through the publishers of the treatise.

In 1822, Laennec succeeded Corvisart as chair of medicine at the Collège de France. Four years later, while studying tuberculosis (the contagious properties of which were not yet understood), he contracted the disease and died. Laennec was an intensely religious man and devout Catholic, well known for his charity to the poor, highly respected for his extreme kindness, beloved by students and colleagues. It is said that, near the end of his life, his primary goal was to "keep as far as possible from giving trouble to others."

See also Stethoscope

Lancefield, Rebecca Craighill (1895-1981)

American bacteriologist

Rebecca Craighill Lancefield is known throughout the world for the system she developed to classify the bacterium streptococcus. Her colleagues called her laboratory at the Rockefeller Institute for Medical Research (now Rockefeller University) "the Scotland Yard of streptococcal mysteries." During a research career that spanned six decades, she meticulously identified over fifty types of this bacteria. She used her knowledge of this large, diverse bacterial family to learn about pathogenesis and immunity of its afflictions, ranging from **sore throats**, **rheumatic fever** and **scarlet fever** to heart and kidney disease. The Lancefield system remains a key to the medical understanding of streptococcal diseases.

Born Rebecca Craighill on January 5, 1895, in Fort Wadsworth on Staten Island in New York on January 5, 1895, she was the third of six daughters. Her mother, Mary Montague Byram, married William Edward Craighill, a career army officer in the Army Corps of Engineers who had graduated from West Point. Lancefield received a bachelor's degree in 1916 from Wellesley College, after changing her major from English to zoology. Two years later, she earned a master's degree from Columbia University, where she pursued bacteriology in the laboratory of **Hans Zinsser**. Immediately on graduating from Columbia, she formed two lifelong partnerships. She married Donald Lancefield, who had been a classmate of hers in a genetics class. And she was hired by the Rockefeller Institute to help bacteriologists Oswald Avery and Alphonse Dochez, whose expertise on pneumococcus was then being applied to a different bacterium. This was during World War I, and the project at Rockefeller was to discover whether distinct types of streptococci could be isolated from soldiers in a Texas **epidemic** so that a serum might be produced to prevent infection. The scientists employed the same serological techniques that Avery had used to distinguish types of pneumococci. Within a year, Avery, Dochez, and Lancefield had published a major report which described four types of streptococci. This was Lancefield's first paper.

Lancefield and her husband took a short hiatus to teach in his home state at the University of Oregon, then returned to New York. Lancefield worked simultaneously on a Ph.D. at Columbia and on rheumatic fever studies at the Rockefeller Institute in the laboratory of Homer Swift, and her husband joined the Columbia University faculty in biology. Before World War I, physicians had suspected that a streptococcus caused rheumatic fever. But scientists, including Swift, had not been able to recover a specific organism from patients. Nor could they reproduce the disease in animals using patient cultures. Lancefield's first project with Swift, which was also her doctoral work, showed that the alpha-hemolytic class of streptococcus, also called green or viridans, was not the cause of rheumatic fever.

As a result of her work with Swift, Lancefield decided that a more basic approach to rheumatic fever was needed. So she began sorting out types among the disease-causing class, the beta-hemolytic streptococci. She used serological techniques while continuing to benefit from Avery's advice. Her major tool for classifying the bacteria was the precipitin test. This involved mixing soluble type-specific antigens, or substances used to stimulate immune responses, with antisera (types of serum containing antibodies) to give visible precipitates. Precipitates are the separations of a substance, in this case bacteria, from liquid in a solution—the serum—in order to make it possible to study the bacteria on its own.

Lancefield soon recovered two surface antigens from these streptococci. One was a polysaccharide, or carbohydrate, called the C substance. This complex sugar molecule is a major component of the cell wall in all streptococci. She could further subdivide its dissimilar compositions into groups and she designated the groups by the letters A through O. The most common species causing human disease, *Streptococcus pyogenes,* were placed in group A. Among the group A streptococci, Lancefield found another antigen and determined it was a protein, called M for its matt appearance in colony formations. Because of differences in M protein composition, Lancefield was able to subdivide group A streptococci into types. During her career, she identified over fifty types, and since her death in 1981 bacteriologists have identified thirty more.

Lancefield's classification converged with another typing system devised by Frederick Griffith in England. His typing was based on a slide agglutination method, in which the bacteria in the serum collects into clumps when an antibody is introduced. For five years the two scientists exchanged samples and information across the Atlantic Ocean, verifying each other's types, until Griffith's tragic death during the bombing of London in 1940. Ultimately, Lancefield's system, based on the M types, was chosen as the standard for classifying group A streptococci.

In further studies on the M protein, Lancefield revealed this antigen is responsible for the bacteria's virulence because it inhibits phagocytosis, thus keeping the white blood cells from engulfing the streptococci. This finding came as a surprise, because Avery had discovered that virulence in the pneumococcus was due to a polysaccharide, not a protein. Lancefield went on to show the M antigen is also the one that elicits protective immune reactions.

Lancefield continued to group and type strep organisms sent from laboratories around the world. Until the end of her life, her painstaking investigations helped unravel the complexity and diversity of these bacteria. Lancefield's colleague Maclyn McCarty, told contributor Carol L. Moberg that Lancefield was "never satisfied with quick answers," and her success came from a determination to stick with scientific problems for a long time. Her thoroughness, he added, was a significant factor in her small but substantial bibliography of nearly sixty papers.

Once her system of classification was in place, however, Lancefield returned to her original quest to elucidate connections between the bacteria's constituents and the baffling nature of streptococcal diseases. She found that a single serotype of group A can cause a variety of streptococcal diseases. This evidence reversed a long-standing belief that every disease must be caused by a specific microbe. Also, because the M protein is type-specific, she found that acquired immunity to one group A serotype could not protect against infections caused by others in group A.

From her laboratory at Rockefeller Hospital, Lancefield could follow patient records for very long periods. She conducted a study which determined that once immunity is acquired to a serotype, it can last up to thirty years. This particular study revealed the unusual finding that high titers, or concentrations, of antibody persist in the absence of antigen. In the case of rheumatic fever, Lancefield illustrated how someone can suffer recurrent attacks, because each one is caused by a different serotype.

In other studies, Lancefield focused on antigens. She and Gertrude Perlmann purified the M protein in the 1950s. Twenty years later she developed a more conservative test for typing it and continued characterizing other group A protein antigens designated T and R. Ten years after her official retirement, she made a vital contribution on the group B streptococci. She clarified the role of their polysaccharides in virulence and showed how protein antigens on their surface also played a protective role. During the 1970s, an increasingly high-rate of infants were being born with group B **meningitis**, and her work laid the basis for the medical response to this problem.

During World War II, Lancefield had performed special duties on the Streptococcal Diseases Commission of the Armed Forces Epidemiological Board. Her task involved identifying strains and providing antisera for epidemics of scarlet and rheumatic fever among soldiers in military camps. After the commission dissolved, her colleagues in the "Strep Club" created the Lancefield Society in 1977, which continues to hold regular international meetings on advances in streptococcal research.

An associate member at Rockefeller when Maclyn McCarty took over Swift's laboratory in 1946, Lancefield became a full member and professor in 1958 and emeritus professor in 1965. While her career and achievements took place in a field dominated by men, Lewis Wannamaker in *American Society for Microbiology News* quotes Lancefield as being "annoyed by any special feeling about women in science." In *Profiles of Pioneer Women Scientists,* Elizabeth O'Hern cites Lancefield as saying that women "sometimes expect too much." Nevertheless, most recognition for Lancefield came near her retirement. In 1961, she was the first woman elected president of the American Association of Immunologists, and in 1970 she was one of few women elected to the National Academy of Sciences. Other honors included the T. Duckett Jones Memorial Award in 1960, the American Heart Association Achievement Award in 1964, the New York Academy of Medicine Medal in 1973, and honorary degrees from Rockefeller University in 1973 and Wellesley College in 1976.

In addition to her career as a scientist, Lancefield had one daughter. Lancefield was devoted to research and preferred not to go on lecture tours or attend scientific meetings. Rockefeller's laboratories were not air-conditioned and her main diversion was leaving them during the summer and spending the entire season in Woods Hole, Massachusetts. There she enjoyed tennis and swimming with her family, which eventually included two grandsons. Official retirement did not change her lifestyle. She drove to her Rockefeller laboratory from her home in Douglaston, Long Island, every working day until she broke her hip in November 1980. She died of complications from this injury on March 3, 1981, at the age of eighty-six. Her husband Donald died the following August.

The pathogenesis of rheumatic fever still eludes scientists, and antibiotics have not eliminated streptococcal diseases. Yet the legacy of Lancefield's system and its fundamental links to disease remain and a vaccine against several group A streptococci is being developed in her former laboratory at Rockefeller University by Vincent A. Fischetti.

LANDSTEINER, KARL (1868-1943)

Austrian American chemist

Karl Landsteiner, who has been called the father of immunology, was the only child of Leopold Landsteiner, a prominent Austrian journalist and editor, and Fanny Hess Landsteiner. Landsteiner was educated at the University of Vienna, where he received his medical degree in 1891. While in medical school, Landsteiner began experimental work in chemistry, as he was greatly inspired by Ernst Ludwig, one of his professors. After receiving his medical degree, Landsteiner spent the next five years doing advanced research in organic chemistry for Emil Fischer, although medicine remained his chief interest. During 1886-1897, he combined these interests at the Institute of Hygiene at the University of Vienna where he researched immunology and serology. These fields were developing rapidly in the late 1800s as scientists explored numerous physiological changes associated with bacterial infection. Immunology and serology then became Landsteiner's lifelong focus. Landsteiner was primarily interested in the lack of safety and effectiveness of blood **transfusions**. Prior to his work, blood transfusions were dangerous and underutilized because the donor's blood frequently clotted in the patient. Landsteiner was intrigued by the fact that when blood from different subjects was mixed, the blood did not always clot. He believed there were intrinsic biochemical similarities and dissimilarities in blood. He was unsure, however, whether clotting was primarily a function of disease or a result of individual differences.

By 1901 Landsteiner discovered the answer. Using blood samples from his colleagues, he separated the blood's

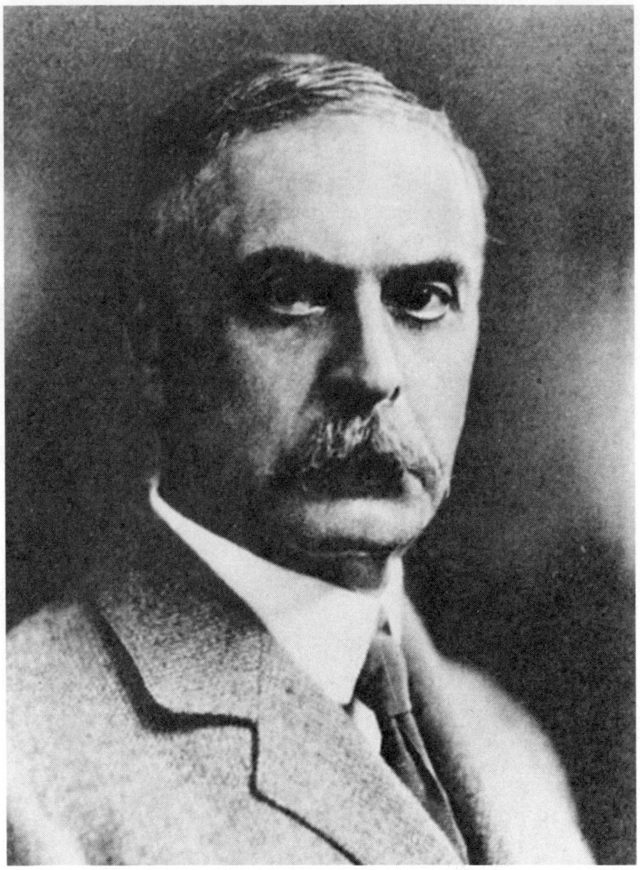

Karl Landsteiner

cells from its serum, and suspended the red blood cells in a saline solution. He then mixed each individual's serum with a sample from every cell suspension. Clotting occurred in some cases; in others there was no clotting. Landsteiner determined that human beings could be separated into blood groups according to the capacity of their red cells to clot in the presence of different serums. He named his blood classification groups A, B, and O. A fourth group AB, was discovered the following year. The result of this work was that patient and donor could be blood-typed beforehand, making blood transfusion a safe and routine medical practice. This discovery ultimately earned Landsteiner the 1930 Nobel Prize in physiology or medicine.

In 1927, Landsteiner and Philip Levine (1900-1987) also discovered two other inheritable factors, M and N, which do not affect transfusions. There exist two other practical applications of Landsteiner's blood classification work. The first is the significance of blood grouping in cases of disputed paternity. Today, most paternity questions are settled by very exact serological (**blood typing**) means. Second, Landsteiner's work provided the foundation for the field of forensic serology. Blood stains became serological ''fingerprints'' used to distinguish one person from another due to blood types being inheritable. Due to Landsteiner's outstanding achievements, in 1908 he was appointed chief of pathology at the University of Vienna. During the same year he became the first to isolate the poliomyelitis virus and was also the first to use monkeys as an experimental animal in **polio** research.

Landsteiner left the University of Vienna in 1919 and accepted a position in Holland due to the civil disorders in Vienna caused by World War I, as well as the lack of funding and facilities for research. In 1922 he accepted an offer to join the staff of the Rockefeller Institute for Medical Research in New York. He became an American citizen in 1929, and remained at the Institute for the rest of his life. Landsteiner continued his blood group research with Levine and Alexander Weiner and in 1940 discovered the Rhesus (Rh) factor during studies with the Rhesus monkey. The Rh factor is important in both blood transfusions and in pregnancy. If Rh-positive blood is introduced into the circulation of an Rh-negative person, it is recognized as foreign and the recipient may form antibodies capable of destroying the Rh-positive red blood cells. **Erythroblastosis fetalis**, a blood disease in newborn infants, is linked to this factor. Knowledge of the Rh factor led to ways of preventing brain damage, severe **jaundice** and **death** caused by the disease. Landsteiner retired from his post at the Rockefeller Institute in 1939, but continued his laboratory research. In 1943 he suffered a fatal heart attack while at his laboratory bench.

LANGUAGE DEVELOPMENT

Human infants are acutely attuned to the human voice and prefer it above all other sounds. In fact, they prefer the higher pitch ranges characteristic of female voices. They are also attentive to the human face, particularly the eyes, which they stare at even more if the face is talking. These preferences are present at birth, and some research indicates that babies even listen to their mother's voice during the last few months of pregnancy.

Since the early 1970s, it has been known that babies can detect very subtle differences between English phonemes (the functional units of speech sound). For example, they can detect the difference between ''pa'' and ''ba,'' or between ''da'' and ''ga.'' Of course, they do not attach meaning to the differences for 12 months or more.

At the beginning of infancy, vegetative noises and crying predominate. Observers note that by the age of four months, the baby's repertoire has expanded in more interesting ways. By this point babies are smiling at caregivers and making cooing and gurgling noises that are irresistible to most parents. It is common for the caregiver to respond by echoing these noises, thereby creating an elaborate interchange that can last many minutes.

At some point between four and 10 months, the infant begins producing more speech-like syllables, with a full resonant vowel and an appropriate ''closure'' of the stream of sound, approaching a true consonant. This stage is called ''canonical babbling.''

At about six to eight months, the range of vocalizations grows dramatically. Not all of these are human phonemes, and not all of them are found in the language around them. Research has shown that Japanese and American infants sound alike at this stage, and even congenitally deaf infants babble, though less frequently. These facts suggest that the infant is ''exercising'' her speech organs but is not being guided very much, if at all, by what she has heard.

By age 10 or 12 months, however, the range of sounds being produced has somewhat narrowed, and now babies' babbling in different cultures begin to take on sound characteristics of the language that surrounds them. The babbling at this stage often consists of repeated syllables like ''bababa'' or ''dadada'' or ''mamama.'' It is no accident that most of the world's languages have chosen some variant of ''papa,'' ''mama,'' ''dada,'' and ''nana'' as names for parents.

The first words make their appearance any time between 9 and 15 months or so, depending on the child's precocity and the parent's enthusiasm in noticing. What the baby ''means'' by these sounds is questionable at first. But before long the baby uses the sounds to draw a caregiver's attention, and persists until she gets it, or uses a sound to demand an object, and persists until it is given to her. There is a fairly protracted period for most babies in which their first words come and go, as if there is a ''word of the week.'' After several months of slow growth, there is an explosion of new words, often called the ''word spurt.'' This usually coincides with an interest in what things are called. Vocabulary climbs precipitously from then on, with an estimated nine new words a day from ages two to 18 years. These developments are noted in all the cultures that have been studied to date.

The nature of the child's first 50 words is quite similar across cultures: the child often names foods, pets, animals, family members, toys, vehicles, and clothing that the child can manipulate; she generally omits words for furniture, geographical features, buildings, weather, and so forth. Researchers agree that the child learns most effectively from social and interactive routines with an accomplished talker (who may be an older child), and not, at least at the start, from passive observations of adults talking or from radio or TV shows. Experiments and observations show that children pick up words at this stage most rapidly when the caregiver uses them to name or comment on what the child is already focused on.

The meanings of the child's first words are not necessarily the same as those of the adults around her. For instance, children may ''overgeneralize'' their first words to refer to items beyond their usual scope of application. A child might call all men ''Daddy,'' or all animals ''doggie,'' or all round objects ''ball.'' Others have pointed out that ''undergeneralization'' also occurs, though it is less likely to be noticed. For instance, a child might call only her own striped ball ''ball,'' and stay silent about all the rest, or refer to the family dog and others of the same type as ''doggie'' but not name any others. The child may also use a word to refer to a wide variety of objects that hold no single property in common except a shifting form of resemblance to the named object. It has been argued that children's first word meanings have only a family resemblance rather than a common thread. In fact, there are philosophers who argue that such is the nature of many adult words as well.

Most toddlers produce their first spontaneous two-word sentence at 18 to 24 months, usually once they have acquired between 50 and 500 words. At the start, the child combines the single words into two-word strings that usually preserve the common order of parents' sentences in English. At the time the English-speaking child is producing many two-word utterances, comprehension tests show he can also distinguish between sentences that contrast in word order and hence meaning:

The dog licks the cat
The cat licks the dog.

Most studies on early child language conclude that the child at the two-word stage is concerned with the expression of a small set of semantic relationships. All over the world, children apparently talk about the same meanings or ideas in their first sentences, despite the variety of forms in those languages. For example, the children refer to possession (Mommy dish, my coat), action-object sequences (hit ball, drop fork), attribute of an object (big truck, wet pants), or an object's location (cup shelf, teddy bed).

In the next stage of development of English, the extra little function words and inflections that modulate the meaning of the major syntactic relations make their appearance, though it is years until they are fully mastered. A classic error noticed in the acquisition of English inflections is the overgeneralization of plurals and past tenses. In each case, when the regular inflection begins to be mastered, it is overgeneralized to irregular forms, resulting in errors like foots, sheeps, goed, and eated. Two kinds of overgeneralizations occur: one in which the -ed ending is attached to the root form of the irregular verb (e.g. sing/singed) and the other in which the ending is attached to the irregular past form (e.g. broke/broked).

Children's first sentences lack any auxiliaries or tense markers: ''Me go home''; ''Daddy have tea.'' They also lack auxiliary-inversion for questions at this stage: ''I ride train?'' ''Sit chair?''

They also lack a system for assigning nominative case to the subject, that is, adult sentences mark the subject as nominative: ''I want that book''; but children at this stage frequently use the accusative case: ''Me want that book.''

LAPAROSCOPY

Laparoscopy is a type of surgical procedure that allows a doctor to observe a woman's uterus, ovaries and fallopian tube. It is often used to detect **ovarian cysts**, scar tissue, and diagnose pelvic or abdominal **pain**, **endometriosis**, **ectopic pregnancy**, or blocked fallopian tubes.

Laparoscopies are usually done as an outpatient procedure under general anesthesia. The viewing tube (called the laparoscope) — which is equipped with a small camera on the eyepiece — is inserted through a small incision in the navel. The doctor can then examine the abdominal and pelvic organs on a video monitor connected to the tube. Other small incisions can be made to insert instruments to perform a variety of procedures. Laparoscopy is less invasive than regular open abdominal surgery (laparotomy).

Laparoscopy was first used by gynecologists to diagnose and treat conditions relating to the female reproductive organs:

uterus, fallopian tubes, and ovaries. It is now used for a wider range of procedures, including operations that in the past required open surgery, such as removal of the appendix (appendectomy) or as an important tool in trying to find out the cause of **infertility**. Laparoscopy can also be used to examine the appendix, gallbladder, or liver.

Laparoscopy is also used during surgery for female sterilization (**tubal ligation**), some vaginal hysterectomies, for the treatment of ectopic pregnancy or endometriosis, and to collect eggs for in vitro fertilization. It also is a useful technique for taking a biopsy, aspirating a cyst, or locating and removing an intrauterine device (**IUD**) that has perforated the uterus.

Laparoscopy also can be used as an alternative to surgery for some non-gynecologic operations, such as removal of the appendix, gallstones, or gallbladder.

While many of these procedures can be done using regular open surgery, laparoscopy usually involves less pain, less risk, less scarring, and faster recovery. Because laparoscopy is so much less invasive than traditional abdominal surgery, patients can leave the hospital sooner.

Laparoscopy is a surgical procedure that is usually done in the hospital on an outpatient basis. After the patient is anesthetized, a hollow needle is inserted into the abdomen in or near the navel so that carbon dioxide gas can be pumped through the needle to expand the abdomen. This allows the surgeon a better view of the internal organs. The laparoscope is then inserted through this incision. The image from the camera attached to the end of laparoscope can be seen on a video monitor.

Sometimes, other small incisions are made to insert other instruments which are used to lift internal organs for examination or to perform surgical procedures.

One of the most common reasons for having diagnostic laparoscopy is to discover the cause of infertility. A laparoscopy can be used to uncover the reasons for infertility, such as physical problems or disease. Laparoscopy is also often used to discover the source of pelvic pain. There are many possible causes of pelvic pain that can be diagnosed with this technique, such as endometriosis, ovarian cysts, ectopic pregnancy, **pelvic inflammatory disease** (PID), and uterine abnormalities.

Patients should not eat or drink after midnight on the night before the procedure; afterwards, patients may leave the hospital within four to eight hours. (Traditional abdominal surgery requires a hospital stay of four days).

There may be some slight pain or throbbing at the incision sites in the first day or so after the procedure. The gas that is used to expand the abdomen may cause discomfort under the ribs or in the shoulder for a few days. Depending on the reason for the laparoscopy in gynecological procedures, some women may experience some vaginal bleeding.

Many patients can return to work within a day or so after having this type of procedure. The risk of complications is less than 0.5%. The procedure carries a slight risk of puncturing an organ, which could cause blood to seep into the abdominal cavity. Puncturing the intestines could allow intestinal contents to seep into the cavity. These are serious complications and major surgery may be required to correct the problem.

In rare cases, one of the following complications may occur:

- Hemorrhage
- Inflammation of the abdominal cavity lining
- **Abscess**
- Problems related to general anesthesia.

Laryngitis

Laryngitis is caused by an inflammation of the voice box (larynx). As the area around the vocal cords swells, they can't vibrate normally, so the voice sounds hoarse and painful; in some cases, the patient can't speak at all.

Laryngitis is a very common problem, and often occurs during a cold. It is almost always caused by the same viruses which cause most colds. Very rarely, bacteria such as Group A streptococcus may cause laryngitis. In people with faulty immune systems (particularly people with **AIDS**), fungal infections may be responsible for laryngitis.

Symptoms usually appear at the same time as cold symptoms, and include sore, scratchy throat, **fever**, runny nose, achiness, and tiredness. Problems in swallowing sometimes occur with **streptococcal infections**. The patient may **cough** and wheeze. Most often, the patient's voice will sound strained and hoarse. This is most common in infants, because the diameter of their airways is so small. In that case, the baby may breathe much faster and with a loud high-pitched sound (called stridor).

A doctor can diagnose laryngitis from a patient history of a cold followed by hoarseness. The throat usually appears red and somewhat swollen. Listening to the chest and back with a stethoscope may reveal some harsh **wheezing** sounds as the patient inhales.

If the laryngitis lingers for a long time, the doctor may suspect tuberculosis. Examining the airway will reveal redness, swelling, small bumps of tissue called nodules, and irritated pits in the tissue called ulcerations.

Simple viral laryngitis is treated by easing symptoms. Patients can gargle with warm salt water, take **pain** relievers such as **acetaminophen**, use vaporizers to create moist air, and rest. Rarely, an infant who is clearly struggling for air may need to have an artificial airway for a short period.

A patient with tubercular laryngitis is treated with a combination of drugs used to treat classic TB. Patients with fungal laryngitis may need a variety of anti-fungal medications.

Alternative treatments include decoctions (extracts made by boiling an herb in water) or infusions (extracts made by steeping an herb in boiling water) can be made with red sage and yarrow or with licorice. These are used for gargling, and are said to reduce pain. Echinacea tincture taken in water every hour for 48 hours is recommended to boost the immune system. Antiviral herbs, including lomatium and ligusticum, may help hasten recovery from laryngitis. Some people may get relief from placing cold compresses on the throat. Most patients recover from laryngitis within a week.

A person can prevent laryngitis in the same way as any common cold, by washing hands often, avoiding touching the face and nose as much as possible, and by disinfecting household surfaces commonly touched by others such as door handles and telephone receivers. However, even with relatively good hygiene practices, most people will get about five to six colds per year. It's hard to tell which of these may lead to laryngitis.

LARYNGOSCOPY

Laryngoscopy is a diagnostic method that allows the larynx to be seen directly during an examination. In one method, a flexible tube with a fiber-optic device is threaded through the nasal passage and down into the throat. The other method uses a rigid viewing tube passed directly from the mouth through the throat and into the larynx.

Both methods make use of a light source and a lens that are attached to a viewing tube. The endoscopic viewing tube may also be equipped to suction debris or remove material for biopsy.

Laryngoscopy procedures are performed in a hospital, using a local anesthetic spray to ease pain and suppress the gag reflex. Patients should not eat for several hours before the test. After the procedure is over, soothing liquids or lozenges can ease any temporary sore throat.

This procedure carries no serious risks, although the patient may have a sore throat or cough up small amounts of blood until the irritation subsides.

If a tumor or an object lodged in the tissue is discovered during the laryngoscopy, it would either be removed or described for further medical attention.

LASER SURGERY

Laser (light amplification by stimulated emission of radiation) surgery uses an intensely hot, precisely focused beam of light to remove or vaporize tissue and control bleeding in a wide variety of non-invasive and minimally invasive procedures. It is generally used to cut or destroy tissue that is abnormal or diseased without harming healthy, normal tissue; shrink or destroy tumors and lesions; or cauterize (seal) blood vessels to prevent excessive bleeding.

Because some lasers can temporarily or permanently discolor the skin of Blacks, Asians, and Hispanics, a dark-skinned patient should make sure that his surgeon has successfully performed laser procedures on people of color.

Some types of laser surgery should not be performed on pregnant women or on patients with severe cardiopulmonary disease or other serious health problems.

The first working laser was introduced in 1960. The device was initially used to treat diseases and disorders of the eye, whose transparent tissues gave ophthalmic surgeons a clear view of how the narrow, concentrated beam was being directed. Dermatologic surgeons also helped pioneer laser surgery, and developed and improved upon many early techniques and more refined surgical procedures.

The three types of lasers most often used in medical treatment are the:

- Carbon dioxide (CO_2) laser. Primarily a surgical tool, this device converts light energy to heat strong enough to minimize bleeding while it cuts through or vaporizes tissue.
- Neodymium:yttrium-aluminum-garnet (Nd:YAG) laser. Capable of penetrating tissue more deeply than other lasers, the Nd:YAG makes blood clot quickly and can enable surgeons to see and work on parts of the body that could otherwise be reached only through open (invasive) surgery.
- Argon laser. This laser provides the limited penetration needed for eye surgery and superficial skin disorders. In a special procedure known as photodynamic therapy (PDT), this laser uses light-sensitive dyes to shrink or dissolve tumors.

Sometimes described as "scalpels of light," lasers are used alone or with conventional surgical instruments in a diverse array of procedures that:

- Improve appearance
- Relieve **pain**
- Restore function
- Save lives.

Laser surgery is often standard operating procedure for specialists in:

- Cardiology
- Dentistry
- Dermatology
- Gastroenterology (treatment of disorders of the stomach and intestines)
- Gynecology
- Neurosurgery
- Oncology (**cancer** treatment)
- Ophthalmology (treatment of disorders of the eye)
- Orthopedics (treatment of disorders of bones, joints, muscles, ligaments, and tendons)
- Otolaryngology (treatment of disorders of the ears, nose, and throat)
- Pulmonary care (treatment of disorders of the respiratory system
- Urology (treatment of disorders of the urinary tract and of the male reproductive system).

Routine uses of lasers include erasing **birthmarks**, skin discoloration, and skin changes due to aging, and removing benign, precancerous, or cancerous tissues or tumors. Lasers are used to stop snoring, remove tonsils, remove or transplant hair, and relieve pain and restore function in patients who are too weak to undergo major surgery. Lasers are also used to treat:

- **Angina** (chest pain)
- Cancerous or non-cancerous tumors that cannot be removed or destroyed
- Cold and **canker sores**, gum disease, and tooth sensitivity or decay
- **Ectopic pregnancy** (development of a fertilized egg outside the uterus)
- **Endometriosis**
- Fibroid tumors

- Gallstones
- **Glaucoma**, mild-to-moderate nearsightedness and **astigmatism**, and other conditions that impair sight
- Migraine headaches
- Non-cancerous enlargement of the prostate gland
- **Nosebleeds**
- **Ovarian cysts**
- **Ulcers**
- **Varicose veins**
- **Warts**
- And numerous other conditions, diseases, and disorders.

Often referred to as "bloodless surgery," laser procedures usually involve less bleeding than conventional surgery. The heat generated by the laser keeps the surgical site free of germs and reduces the risk of infection. Because a smaller incision is required, laser procedures often take less time (and cost less money) than traditional surgery. Sealing off blood vessels and nerves reduces bleeding, swelling, scarring, pain, and the length of the recovery period.

Although many laser surgeries can be performed in a doctor's office rather than in a hospital, the person guiding the laser must be at least as thoroughly trained and highly skilled as someone performing the same procedure in a hospital setting. The American Society for Laser Medicine and Surgery, Inc. urges that:

- All operative areas be equipped with oxygen and other drugs and equipment required for **cardiopulmonary resuscitation (CPR)**
- Non-physicians performing laser procedures be properly trained, licensed, and insured
- A qualified and experienced supervising physician be able to respond to and manage unanticipated events or other emergencies within five minutes of the time they occur
- Emergency transportation to a hospital or other acute-care facility be available whenever laser surgery is performed in a non-hospital setting.

Because laser surgery is used to treat so many dissimilar conditions, the patient should ask his physician for detailed instructions about how to prepare for a specific procedure. Diet, activities, and medications may not have to be limited prior to surgery, but some procedures require a **physical examination** and a medical history that:

- Determines the patient's general health and current medical status
- Describes how the patient has responded to other illnesses, hospital stays, and diagnostic or therapeutic procedures
- Clarifies what the patient expects the outcome of the procedure to be.

Laser surgery can involve risks that are not associated with traditional surgical procedures. Being careless or not practicing safe surgical techniques can severely burn the patient's lungs or even cause them to explode. Patients must wear protective eye shields while undergoing laser surgery on any part of the face near the eyes or eyelids, and the United States Food and Drug Administration (FDA) has said that both doctors and patients must use special protective eyewear whenever a CO_2 laser is used.

Laser beams can burn or destroy healthy tissue, cause injuries that are painful and sometimes permanent, and actually compound problems they are supposed to solve. Errors or inaccuracies in laser surgery can worsen a patient's vision, for example, and lasers can scar and even change the skin color of some patients.

LAVERAN, ALPHONSE (1845-1922)

French biologist

Charles Louis Alphonse Laveran was born on June 18, 1845, into a military family in Paris. He was the second child and only son of Louis-Theodore Laveran, a career military physician, and Marie-Louise Anselme Guénard de la Tour Laveran. Laveran received his secondary education at the College Sainte-Barbe and the Lycée Louis-le-Grand. In 1863, he entered the military medical school at Strasbourg, which his father had also attended; Laveran graduated in 1867. He joined the military medical service following graduation and saw active duty during the Franco-Prussian War of 1870–1871. In 1874, he won by competitive examination an appointment to a professorship earlier held by his father at the École du Val-de-Grace, a military medical school in Paris. This was a temporary appointment, and at its conclusion in 1878 he was sent to the military hospital at Bône (now Annaba) in Algeria.

It was while at Bône that Laveran began a careful study of **malaria**, common in many parts of Algeria, in an effort to learn its cause. He set up a small laboratory and with the primitive, low-powered microscope available to him, he spent much time examining blood samples from malaria patients both living and deceased. His studies were briefly interrupted when he was transferred to Biskra, Algeria, where malaria was rare, but they were resumed when he moved on to Constantine, also in Algeria. There, on November 6, 1880, he first observed under the microscope circular and cylindrical bodies which had moving filaments, or flagella. This confirmed his earlier suspicion that malaria was caused by living animal cells, minute single-celled creatures called protozoa, which acted as parasites in the human body. The particular protozoan which Laveran had discovered to be the cause of malaria later came to be called plasmodium.

Laveran's discovery was presented to the Academy of Medicine in Paris on November 23, 1880. A second paper, based upon further research, was published by the Société Médicale des Hopitaux on December 24 of that year. In 1881, Laveran published a brief monograph, *Nature parasitaire des accidents de l'impaludisme,* which provided more details of his findings. Laveran's conclusions were not immediately accepted by other scientists studying malaria.

Laveran, however, continued his research, examining the blood of hundreds of malaria patients, both in Algeria and in Italy. By 1884, in a personal microscopic demonstration, he was able to persuade Louis Pasteur that his theory was correct.

Other noted scientists such as **William Osler** were convinced during the course of the 1880s. Also in 1884, Laveran published a book, *Traité des fièvres palustres avec la description des microbes du paludisme,* which summarized all of his research on malaria. In this work, he revealed his suspicion that the malaria protozoa were nurtured and transmitted to human beings by some species of mosquito. It remained for the British physician, **Ronald Ross**, working in India in the late 1890s, to prove that the malaria parasite was indeed transmitted by the Anopheles mosquito.

Laveran returned to Paris from Algeria in 1883 and became professor of military hygiene at the École du Val-de-Grace in 1884. He married Sophie Marie Pidancet in 1885. He resigned from the military medical service in December of 1896 and accepted a position at the Pasteur Institute in Paris. There he pursued his research for the rest of his life.

Laveran's demonstration that protozoa, as well as bacteria, could be the causes of disease in both human beings and animals led many other researchers into the field. Laveran himself did much significant work on disease-causing parasites. He was especially concerned with the trypanosome family of protozoa, one of which is the cause of the disease trypanosomiasis, or African sleeping sickness, transmitted by the tsetse fly. He also studied the trypanosome responsible for another tropical disease, kala azar, or dumdum fever. He was awarded the Nobel Prize in medicine in 1907 for his work on all disease-causing protozoa. He used half of the prize money to establish a laboratory for research on tropical diseases at the Pasteur Institute.

Laveran was honored with membership in the French Academy of Sciences in 1901. The French government made him a Commander of the Legion of Honor in 1912. During World War I he served on several committees concerned with preserving the health of French soldiers, and he served as president of the Academy of Medicine in 1920. He died after a short illness on May 18, 1922.

LAUGHING GAS • See Nitrous oxide

LAXATIVES

Laxatives are products that promote bowel movements, and are used to treat **constipation** (the passage of hard, dry stools). People who are constipated may find it difficult and even painful to have bowel movements. They may also feel bloated, sluggish, and generally uncomfortable and may have other symptoms such as a dull **headache** and **low back pain**. However, these symptoms don't always mean that laxatives are necessary. A great deal of misunderstanding exists about their use. A range of normal bowel habits exist, depending on the individual and the person's diet. Some people have bowel movements as often as three times a day, some only three times a week; anything within this range is considered normal. In addition, some people's stools are naturally firmer than others.

Occasional constipation can often be treated without laxatives. Increasing the amount of fiber in the diet, drinking plenty of water and other liquids (such as fruit and vegetable juices), exercising regularly, and setting aside time every day to have a bowel movement are the first steps. These measures will also help prevent constipation from occurring again.

If these methods don't relieve the problem, a doctor may suggest using a laxative for a limited time. A doctor should always be the one to decide when a laxative is needed and which type of laxative should be used.

Laxatives come in various forms liquids, tablets, suppositories, powders, granules, capsules, chewing gum, chocolate-flavored wafers, and caramels. The basic types include bulk-forming products, lubricants, stool softeners (also called emollient laxatives), and stimulant laxatives.

Bulk-forming laxatives contain materials like cellulose and psyllium that pass through the digestive tract without being digested. In the intestines, these materials absorb liquid and swell, making the stool soft, bulky, and easier to pass. The bulky stool then stimulates the bowel to move. Laxatives in this group include such brands as FiberCon, Fiberall, and Metamucil.

Mineral oil is the mostly widely used lubricant laxative. Taken by mouth, the oil coats the stool. This keeps the stool moist and soft and makes it easier to pass. Lubricant laxatives are often used for patients who need to avoid straining, such as after abdominal surgery.

Stool softeners such as docusate (Colace, Sof-Lax) make stools softer and easier to pass by increasing their moisture content. This type of laxative doesn't really stimulate a bowel movement, but makes it possible to have bowel movements without straining. Stool softeners are best used to prevent constipation in people who need to avoid straining. However, they are not very effective at treating existing constipation.

Ingredients in stimulant laxatives (Correctol or Senokot) trigger the action of muscles and nerves in the intestines to help move stool along. Although these laxatives are popular and effective, they should be used with care, as they are more likely than other types to cause side effects. They may also work more quickly and powerfully than other laxatives.

Laxatives are among the most widely misused over-the-counter medicines. The overuse of laxatives can lead the body to depend on them. When used regularly over a long time, laxatives can damage nerve cells in the colon, causing the colon to lose its natural ability to contract. This makes constipation worse. In addition, overuse of certain laxatives can weaken the bones and cause other serious problems. Because of these possible problems, patients should not use laxatives unless told to do so by a doctor. If a laxative is prescribed, it should be used only as directed.

Occasional, temporary constipation is usually caused by an improper diet, too little **exercise**, changes in daily routines, or the use of certain medicines such as pain relievers, antidepressant drugs, or **diuretics** (water pills). Constipation also can be caused by a number of diseases. A doctor should be consulted for any of the following symptoms:

- Persistent constipation in a person who has always had regular bowel movements

- Constipation that doesn't get better with the proper use of laxatives
- Rectal bleeding or blood in the stool
- Pain when having a bowel movement
- Loss of appetite or unexplained weight loss
- Bloating that continues or gets worse
- Nausea
- Vomiting
- Continuing abdominal pain or cramps
- Sores or irritation in the anal area.

Patients should not combine stool softeners (such as Colace) and lubricant laxatives (such as mineral oil) at the same time; this may cause unwanted side effects, such as watery **diarrhea**.

People whose gag reflexes don't work properly (such as those who have had **strokes**) should not use mineral oil laxatives. They may inhale small amounts of mineral oil, which could lead to inflammation of the lungs and possible **pneumonia**.

Some types of laxatives contain large amounts of sugar. People who have diabetes or who must limit their intake of sugar or other carbohydrates should read package labels carefully or check with a pharmacist before using laxatives. Bulk-forming laxatives must be taken with at least 8 oz. of water or other liquid; otherwise, it may form a mass that can block the throat, esophagus, or bowel. Anyone who develops a skin rash while taking a laxative should stop taking it immediately and call a physician.

Older people are especially likely to have constipation, and need to be careful not to overuse laxatives. Instead, older individuals should manage their constipation with proper diet and exercise. When laxatives are necessary, the bulk-forming types (such as FiberCon and Metamucil) are best for older people. Stimulants and lubricants should be avoided.

Bowel habits vary in children, as they do in adults, but in general children should not be given laxatives unless a doctor has directed it.

People with certain medical conditions or who are taking certain other medicines can have problems if they take laxatives. People who are sensitive to psyllium or who have respiratory disorders may have severe reactions if they inhale dry particles of psyllium (found in some bulk-forming laxatives, such as Metamucil). The risk of this problem can be reduced by using a spoon to add the powder to liquid in a glass, rather than pouring the powder directly from the container. Anyone who has had unusual reactions to laxatives in the past should tell the doctor before taking the drugs again. Pregnant women should also be careful about taking laxatives; bulk-forming products (such as Metamucil and FiberCon) and stool softeners (such as Colace) are the only kinds recommended for pregnant women. Stimulants and lubricants should be avoided. Because some kinds of laxatives may pass into breast milk, breastfeeding mothers should check with their doctors before using laxatives.

Before using laxatives, people with any of these medical problems should make sure their physicians are aware of their conditions:

- Kidney disease
- Past or present gastrointestinal surgery or disease
- Abnormally high amount of calcium in the blood (hypercalcemia)
- Throat problems
- Swallowing problems
- Partial bowel obstruction.

Taking laxatives with other drugs may affect the way the medicine works or may increase the chance of side effects. Recommended dosage depends on the type of laxative, but patients should always take laxatives exactly as the doctor directs or as the package label directs. Patients should never take larger or more frequent doses, or take the drug for longer than directed.

Serious side effects aren't common, but may occur. Patients should check with a doctor if any of the following side effects occur:

- Skin rash
- Confusion
- Unusual tiredness or weakness
- Irregular heartbeat
- Muscle cramps

Less common side effects, such as cramping, diarrhea, nausea, belching, throat irritation, or skin irritation around the rectal area also may occur and don't need medical attention unless they don't go away or they interfere with normal activities. Other rare side effects are possible. Anyone who has unusual symptoms after taking laxatives should get in touch with a doctor.

Some laxatives may make it more difficult for the body to absorb other medicines taken by mouth. For example, bulk-forming laxatives may interfere with the absorption of **aspirin**, the blood-thinning anticoagulant drug warfarin (Coumadin), digitalis drugs, and other drugs. Other types of laxatives such as Colace boost the absorption of other drugs taken by mouth. The stimulant laxative Correctol should not be taken with drugs that reduce stomach acid, such as cimetidine (Tagamet), ranitidine (Zantac), or omeprazole (Prilosec). This drug also should not be taken within one hour of drinking milk. Anyone who is taking any other medicines should check with a doctor or pharmacist before using a laxative.

LEAD POISONING

Lead poisoning occurs when a person swallows or inhales lead in any form, damaging the brain, nerves, and many other parts of the body. Acute lead poisoning, which is relatively rare, occurs when a large amount of lead is taken into the body all at once. Chronic lead poisoning, which is a common problem in children, occurs when small amounts of lead are taken in over a longer period.

Lead can damage almost every system in the human body, and it can also cause high blood pressure. It is particularly harmful to the developing brain of unborn babies and young children. The higher the level of lead in a child's body, the more serious the problems, which can include slowed reflexes, learning problems and even **mental retardation**. At very high levels, lead poisoning can cause seizures, **coma**, and **death**.

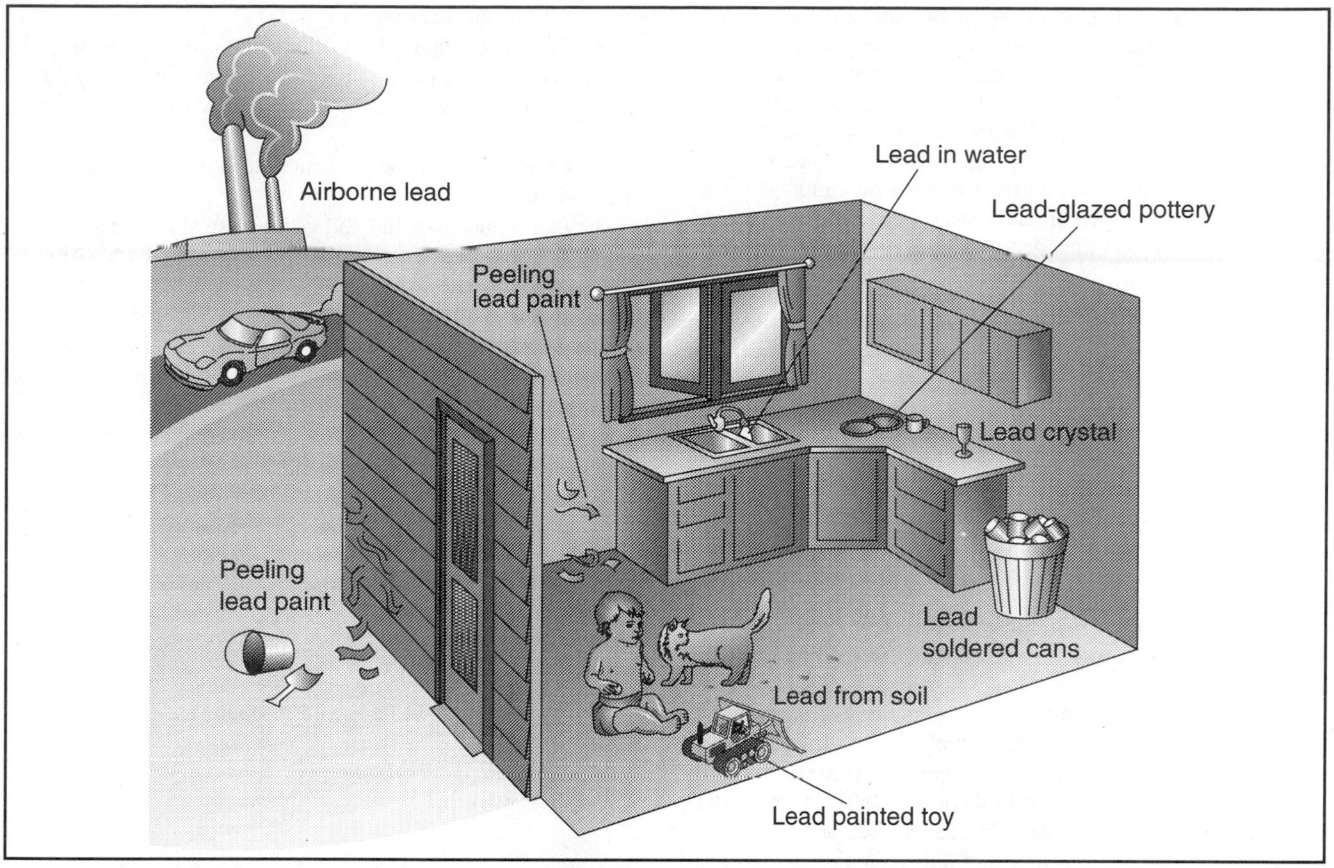

Common sources of lead exposure.

About one out of every six children in the United States has a high level of lead in the blood, according to the Agency for Toxic Substances and Disease Registry. Many of these children are exposed to lead through peeling paint in older homes. Others are exposed through dust or soil that has been contaminated by old paint or past emissions of leaded gasoline. Since children between the ages of 12-36 months tend to put things in their mouths, they are more likely than older children to take in lead. Pregnant women who come into contact with lead can pass it along to their unborn babies.

More than 80% of American homes built before 1978 have lead-based paint. The older the home, the more likely it is to contain lead paint, and the higher the concentration of lead in the paint is apt to be. Some homes also have lead in the water pipes or plumbing. In addition, people may have lead in the paint, dust, or soil around their homes or in their drinking water without knowing it, since lead can't be seen, smelled, or tasted. Because lead doesn't break down naturally, it can continue to cause problems until it is removed. Lead-based paint is the most common source of exposure among preschoolers. Children may eat paint chips from older homes that have fallen into disrepair or chew on painted surfaces. In addition, paint may be disturbed during remodeling. Pollution from operating or abandoned industrial sites can find its way into the soil.

Other sources of lead poisoning include:

- Drinking water. Exposure may come from lead water pipes, found in many homes built before 1930. Even newer copper pipes may have lead solder, and some new homes have brass faucets and fittings that can leach lead.
- Jobs and hobbies. A number of activities can expose participants to lead, such as making pottery or stained glass, refinishing furniture, doing home repairs, or using indoor firing ranges. When adults take part in such activities, they may inadvertently expose children to lead residue that is on their clothing or on scrap materials.
- Food. Imported food cans often have lead solder, and lead is found in leaded crystal glassware and some imported or old ceramic dishes. In addition, food may be contaminated by lead in the water or soil.
- Folk medicines. Certain folk medicines (for example, alarcon, alkohl, azarcon, bali goli, coral, ghasard, greta, liga, pay-loo-ah, and rueda) and traditional cosmetics (such as kohl) contain large amounts of lead.

Chronic lead poisoning may lead to learning disabilities, hyperactivity, mental retardation, slowed growth, **hearing loss**, or **headache**s. In adults, lead poisoning can cause high blood pressure, digestive problems, nerve disorders, severe abdominal pain, **diarrhea**, nausea and vomiting, weakness, seizures and coma.

A high level of lead in the blood can be detected with a simple blood test. In fact, testing is the only way to know for sure if children without symptoms have been exposed to lead, since they can appear healthy even after long-term damage occurs. The Centers for Disease Control recommends testing all children at 12 months of age and, if possible, again at 24 months. Testing should start at 6 months for children at risk for lead poisoning. Based on these test results and a child's risk factors, the doctor will then decide whether and how often further testing is needed. In some states, more frequent testing is required by law.

Children are at risk if they:

- Live in or regularly visit a house built before 1978 in which chipped or peeling paint is present or where remodeling is underway.
- Have a brother or sister, housemate, or playmate who has been diagnosed with lead poisoning.
- Live with an adult whose job or hobby involves exposure to lead.
- Live near an active lead smelter, battery-recycling plant, or other industry that can create lead pollution.

Adults may be at risk if they own glazed pottery or make stained glass, or are involved in renovating an old house which may be contaminated with lead.

The first step in treating lead poisoning is to avoid further contact with lead. For adults, this usually means making changes at work or in hobbies. For children, it means finding and removing sources of lead in the home. In most states, the public health department can help identify lead sources in the home. A professional with special training should remove lead paint. Scraping or sanding lead paint creates large amounts of dust that can poison people in the home and that may linger long after the work is completed. In addition, heating lead paint can release lead into the air. For these reasons, lead paint should only be removed by someone who knows how to do the job safely and has the equipment to clean up thoroughly. Occupants (especially children and pregnant women) should leave the home until the cleanup is finished.

If blood levels of lead are high enough, the doctor may also prescribe **chelation therapy**, a type of treatment using chemicals that bind to the lead and help the body pass it in urine at a faster rate. There are four chemical agents that may be used for this purpose, either alone or in combination: Edetate calcium disodium, dimercaprol, succimer, and penicillamine. (Although many doctors prescribe penicillamine for lead poisoning, this use of the drug has not been approved by the Food and Drug Administration.)

Changes in diet are no substitute for medical treatment. However, getting enough calcium, zinc, and protein may help reduce the amount of lead the body absorbs. Iron is also important.

If acute lead poisoning reaches the stage of seizures and coma, there is a high risk of death. Even if the person survives, there is a good chance of permanent brain damage. The long-term effects of lower levels of lead can also be permanent and severe. However, if chronic lead poisoning is caught early, these negative effects can be limited by reducing future exposure to lead and getting proper medical treatment.

To prevent lead poisoning:

- Play areas should be as clean and dust-free as possible.
- Pacifiers and bottles should be washed after they fall on the floor; stuffed animals and toys should be washed often.
- Children should wash hands before meals and at bedtime.
- Floors, windowsills and other chewable surfaces (such as cribs) should be washed twice a week with a solution of powdered dishwasher detergent in warm water.
- Bushes should be planted next to an older home with painted exterior walls to keep children at a distance.
- Grass or another ground cover should be planted in soil that is likely to be contaminated, such as soil around a home built before 1960 or located near a major highway.
- Household tap water should be tested for lead.
- Water from the cold-water tap only should be used for drinking, cooking, and making baby formula, since hot water is likely to contain higher levels of lead. The more time water has been sitting in the pipes, the more lead it may contain.
- People who work with lead should change clothes before going home.
- Food should not be stored in open cans (especially imported cans).
- Food should not be stored or served in pottery meant for decorative use.

LEARNING DISABILITY

A learning disability is a disorder that inhibits or interferes with the skills of learning, including speaking, listening, reading, writing, or mathematical ability. Legally, a learning-disabled child is one whose level of academic achievement is two or more years below the standard for his age and IQ level. It is estimated that anywhere from five to 20% of school-age children in the United States, mostly boys, suffer from learning disabilities (currently, most sources place this figure at 20%). Often, learning disabilities appear together with other disorders, such as attention deficit/hyperactivity disorder (ADHD). They are thought to be caused by irregularities in the functioning of certain parts of the brain. Evidence suggests that these irregularities are often inherited (a child is more likely to develop a learning disability if other family members have them). However, learning disabilities are also associated with certain conditions occurring during fetal development or birth, including maternal use of alcohol, drugs, and tobacco, exposure to infection, injury during birth, **low birthweight**, and sensory deprivation.Aside from underachievement, other warning signs t a child may have a learning disability include overall lack of organization, forgetfulness, taking unusually long amounts of time to complete assignments, and a negative attitude toward school and schoolwork. In the classroom, the child's teacher may observe one or more of the following characteristics: difficulty paying attention, unusual sloppiness and disorganization, social withdrawal, difficulty working independently, and trouble switching from one activity to another. In addition to the preceding signs, which relate directly to school and schoolwork, certain general behavioral and emotional features often accompany learning disabilities. These include impulsiveness, restlessness, distractibility, poor physical coordination, low tolerance for frustration, low **self-esteem**, daydreaming, inattentiveness, and anger or sadness.

Learning disabilities are associated with brain dysfunctions that affect a number of basic skills. Perhaps the most fundamental is sensory-perceptual ability—the capacity to take in and process information through the senses. Difficulties involving vision, hearing, and touch will have an adverse effect on learning. Although learning is usually considered a mental rather than a physical pursuit, it involves motor skills, and it can also be impaired by problems with **motor development**. Other basic skills fundamental to learning include memory, attention, and language abilities.

The three most common academic skill areas affected by learning disabilities are reading, writing, and arithmetic. Some sources estimate that between 60 and 80% of children diagnosed with learning disabilities have reading as their only or main problem area. Learning disabilities involving reading have traditionally been known as **dyslexia**; currently the preferred term is developmental reading disorder. A wide array of problems is associated with reading disorders, including difficulty identifying groups of letters, problems relating letters to sounds, reversals and other errors involving letter position, chaotic spelling, trouble with syllabication, failure to recognize words, hesitant oral reading, and word-by-word rather than contextual reading. Writing disabilities, known as dysgraphia, include problems with letter formation and writing layout on the page, repetitions and omissions, punctuation and capitalization errors, "mirror writing," and a variety of spelling problems. Children with dysgraphia typically labor at written work much longer than their classmates, only to produce large, uneven writing that would be appropriate for a much younger child. Learning abilities involving math skills, generally referred to as dyscalcula (or dyscalculia), usually become apparent later than reading and writing problems—often at about the age of eight. Children with dyscalcula may have trouble counting, reading and writing numbers, understanding basic math concepts, mastering calculations, and measuring. This type of disability may also involve problems with nonverbal learning, including spatial organization.

The first step in dealing with a learning disability is assessment by one or more qualified professionals, such as a learning specialist with a master's or doctoral degree, a psychologist, or a psychiatrist. The person performing the assessment gathers comprehensive background information about the child and the family and administers several types of testing. Psychological testing consists of IQ tests to assess a child's verbal and nonverbal intelligence and projective tests to evaluate his emotional state. Educational tests evaluate academic skills in basic areas including reading, writing, and arithmetic. Neuropsychological tests determine possible deficiencies in brain functioning by assessing motor skills, perception, memory, and language. After the testing is completed, referral may be made to other professionals, such as a speech-language pathologist, audiologist, ophthalmologist, or psychiatrist.

The principal forms of treatment for learning disabilities are remedial education and psychotherapy. Schools are required by law to provide specialized instruction for children with learning disabilities. A remediator works with the child individually, often devising strategies to circumvent the barriers caused by the disability. The earlier remediation is begun, the more effective it will be. At the same time that they are receiving remedial help, children with learning disabilities spend as much time as possible in the regular classroom.

While remediation addresses the obstacles created by the learning disability itself, psychotherapy deals with the emotional and behavioral problems associated with the condition. The inability to succeed at tasks that pose no unusual problems for one's peers creates a variety of unpleasant feelings. These feelings pose several dangers if they are allowed to persist. First, they may aggravate the disability: excessive stress can interfere with the performance of many tasks, especially those that are difficult to begin with. In addition, previously developed abilities may suffer as well, further eroding the child's self-confidence. Finally, destructive emotional and behavioral patterns that begin in response to a learning disability may become entrenched and extend to other areas of a child's life. Both psychoanalytic and behaviorally oriented methods are used in therapy for children with learning disabilities.

The sensitivity developed over the past two decades to the needs of students with learning disabilities has extended to college campuses, virtually all of which have special resource and advocacy centers for students with disabilities, including learning disabilities. Many learning-disabled students have been accommodated by special measures such as extra time on exams and classroom note takers. However, this trend has recently produced a backlash at some colleges by persons who are concerned with declining academic standards and who question whether the increasing claims of learning disabilities among college students—which have doubled since 1988—are all justified.

See also Attention-deficit disorder and Attention deficient hyperactivity disorder; Dyslexia

LEDERBERG, JOSHUA (1925-)

American geneticist

Joshua Lederberg is a Nobel Prize-winning American geneticist whose pioneering work on genetic recombination in bacteria helped propel the field of molecular genetics into the forefront of biological and medical research. In 1946, Lederberg, working with **Edward Lawrie Tatum**, showed that bacteria may reproduce sexually, disproving the widely held theory that bacteria were asexual. The two scientists' discovery also

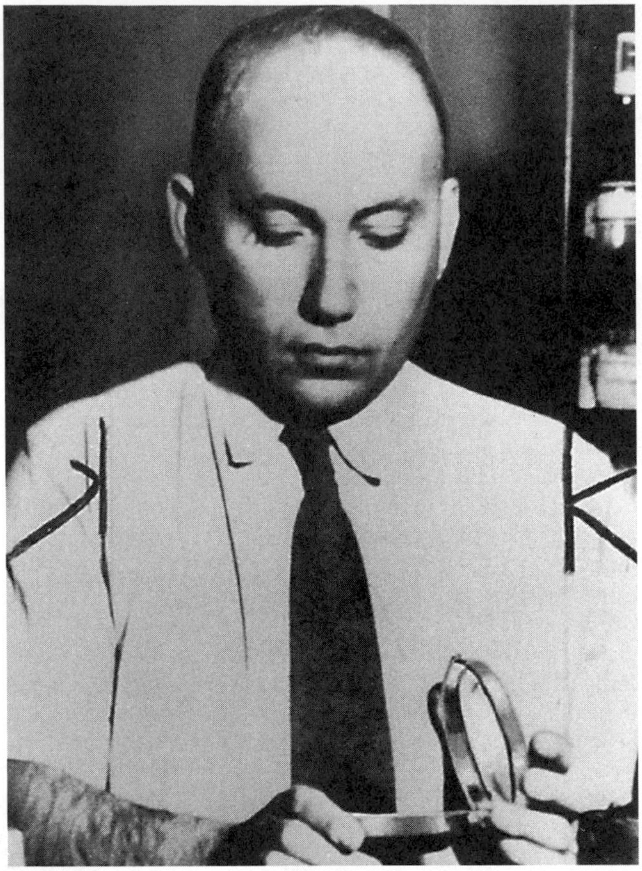

Joshua Lederberg

substantiated that bacteria possess genetic systems comparable to those of higher organisms, thus providing a new repertoire for scientists to study the genetic basis of life.

Continuing with his work in bacteria, Lederberg also discovered the phenomena of genetic conjugation and transduction—or the transfer of either the entire complement of chromosomes or chromosome fragments, respectively—from cell to cell. In his work on conjugation and transduction, Lederberg became the first scientist to manipulate genetic material, which had far-reaching implications for subsequent efforts in genetic engineering and gene therapy. In addition to his laboratory research, Lederberg lectured widely on the complex relationship between science and society and served as a scientific adviser on biological warfare to the World Health Organization.

Lederberg was born in Montclair, New Jersey, on May 23, 1925. His father, Zwi Hirsch Lederberg, was a rabbi; his mother, Esther Goldenbaum, had emigrated from Palestine two years before Lederberg was born. Lederberg's parents moved to New York City, eventually settling in the Washington Heights district. Lederberg attended the city's public schools, where, as he wrote in the book *The Excitement and Fascination of Science: Reflections of Eminent Scientists,* he was a precocious youth whose inquiring mind was nurtured by "a cadre of devoted and sympathetic teachers." At Stuyvesant High School (which specialized in science education), Lederberg first encountered other youths who could compete with him intellectually. Through a program known as the American Institute Science Laboratory, Lederberg was given the opportunity to conduct original research in a laboratory after school hours and on weekends. Here he pursued his interest in biology, working in cytochemistry, or the chemistry of cells. A voracious reader, Lederberg was influenced early on by science-oriented writers such as Bernard Jaffe, Paul de Kruif, and H. G. Wells. For a Bar Mitzvah present he received Meyer Bodansky's *Introduction to Physiological Chemistry,* and on his sixteenth birthday, E. B. Wilson's *The Cell in Development and Heredity.*

After graduating from high school in 1941, Lederberg entered Columbia University as a premedical student. He received a tuition scholarship from the Hayden Trust, which, coupled with his living at home and commuting to school, made it financially possible for him to attend college. Although his undergraduate studies focused on zoology, Lederberg also received a foundation in humanistic studies under Lionel Trilling, James Gutman, and others. Lederberg's work in zoology was fostered by H. Burr Steinbach, who helped Lederberg get space in a histology lab to pursue his own research. This early undergraduate research included an interest in the cytophysiology of mitosis in plants and the uses of genetic analysis in cell biology. In 1942, Lederberg met Francis Ryan, whose work in the biochemical genetics of *Neurospora* was Lederberg's first opportunity to see significant scientific research as it occurred. Lederberg graduated with a B.A. with honors in 1944 at the age of nineteen.

At the age of seventeen, Lederberg had enlisted in the United States Navy V–12 college training program, which featured a condensed pre-med and medical curriculum to produce medical officers for the armed services during World War II. While an undergraduate he also was assigned duty at the U.S. Naval Hospital at St. Albans in Long Island. He began his medical courses at the Columbia College of Physicians and Surgeons in 1944, but left after two years to study under Edward L. Tatum in the microbiology department at Yale University.

In spring of 1945 Ryan had suggested that Lederberg ask Tatum—who had made substantial contributions to biochemical genetics—if Lederberg could work in Tatum's lab at Yale. Lederberg was interested in natural recombination; and Tatum, working with **George W. Beadle**, had done pioneering investigations proving that the DNA (deoxyribonucleic acid) of *Neurospora* (a genus of fungi) played a fundamental role in many of the chemical reactions in *Neurospora* cells. While Lederberg helped Tatum continue his studies of *Neurospora,* the two proceeded to embark on a more tenuous line of research, studying *Escherichia coli* (a bacterium that lives in the gastrointestinal tract) for evidence of genetic inheritance. At the international Cold Spring Harbor Symposium of 1946, Lederberg and Tatum were graciously granted additional time to talk about their *E. Coli* research in addition to the *Neurospora* studies. The scientists' announcement that they had discovered sexual or genetic recombination in the bacterium was met with keen interest by an audience that included the leading molecular biologists and geneticists in the world. The prevailing theory among biologists of the time was that bacteria reproduced asexually by cells essentially splitting, creating two cells with a complete set of chromosomes (threadlike structures in the cell nucleus that carry genetic information). Lederberg and Tatum had found evidence that some strains of *E. coli* pass on hereditary material cell to cell. They found that a conjugation of two cells produced a cell that subsequently began dividing into offspring cells. These offspring showed that they inherited traits from each of the parent strains.

In *The Excitement and Fascination of Science,* Lederberg recalled the intense scrutiny this discovery came under at the Cold Spring Harbor Symposium. **André Lwoff** suggested that perhaps what they had found was a cross-feeding of nutrients between the cells. But in general at that meeting and a second one the following year, Lederberg found the giants of genetics, such as **Jacques Monod**, **Salvador E. Luria**, and Lwoff, to be supportive of and interested in his research. Lederberg also received requests for *E. coli* cultures by others who wanted to investigate his findings.

Lederberg's interest in basic research began to draw him further and further away from pursuing a medical career. In 1947 while at Yale he received an offer from the University of Wisconsin to become an assistant professor of genetics with a focus on the new field of microbial genetics. Although only two years away from receiving his M.D. degree, Lederberg viewed his return to medical school in *The Excitement and Fascination of Science* as a ''grave (if not total) interruption of research at its most exciting stage.'' His prospective appointment at Wisconsin was met with some skepticism concerning his youth (he was only twenty-two) and his yet-to-be fully-accepted research. More troubling personally were references to his character and his Jewish heritage. But the strong support of senior colleagues at Wisconsin and Yale prevailed. Lederberg accepted the position at Wisconsin (receiving his Ph.D. degree from Yale in 1948) and spent a fruitful and satisfying decade there. He never regretted abandoning his medical training, although he noted his later honorary medical degrees from Tufts University and the University of Turin as being among his most valued.

Lederberg continued to make groundbreaking discoveries at Wisconsin and firmly established himself as one of the most promising young intellects in the burgeoning field of genetics. By perfecting a method to isolate mutant bacteria species using ultraviolet light, Lederberg was able to prove the long-held theory that genetic mutations occurred spontaneously. He found he could ''mate'' two strains of bacteria—one resistant to penicillin and the other to streptomycin—and produce a bacteria resistant to both antibiotics. He also found that he could manipulate a virus's virulence.

Working with graduate student Norton Zinder, Lederberg discovered genetic transduction, which involves the transfer only of hereditary fragments of information between cells as opposed to complete chromosomal replication (conjugation). Lederberg went on to breed unique strains of viruses. Although these strains promised to reveal much about the nature of viruses in hopes of one day controlling them, they also posed a clear threat in terms of creating harmful biochemical substances. At the time, the practical aspect of Lederberg's work was hard to evaluate. The Nobel Prize Committee, however recognized the significance of his contributions to genetics and, in 1958, awarded him the Nobel Prize in physiology or medicine for the bacterial and viral research that provided a new line of investigations of viral diseases and cancer. Lederberg shared the prize with Beadle and Tatum. Lederberg's work in genetics eventually proved to be one of the foundations of gene mapping, which eventually led to efforts to genetically treat disease and identify those at risk of developing certain diseases.

A brilliant laboratory scientist and technician, Lederberg was also concerned with the role of science in society and the far-reaching effects of scientific discoveries, particularly in genetics. In a Pan American Health Organization/World Health Organization lecture in biomedical sciences called ''Health in the World Tomorrow,'' Lederberg acknowledged concerns of the public, and even some scientists, over the newfound ability to tamper with the genetic code of life. But he was more concerned with the many ethical questions that would arise over the inevitable successes the advancing fields of microbiology and genetics were ushering in. Lederberg saw the biological revolution as ''a philosophical one'' that was to bring a ''new depth of scientific understanding about the nature of life.'' He foresaw advancements in the treatment of cancer, organ transplants, and geriatric medicine as presenting a whole new set of ethical and social problems, such as the availability and allocation of expensive health-care resources.

Although Lederberg had a profound faith in science, he was not so confident of scientists' ability to rationally communicate the ramifications of their work. In *Man and His Future,* he lamented the ''archaic clumsiness of our basic mechanisms of communication. Man's dilemma,'' he said, ''is the discrepancy between the size of his population and the complexity of his institutions, on one hand, and his individual feebleness, measured as a data input rate of no more than fifty bits per second.''

Lederberg was also interested in the study of biochemical life outside of earth and coined the term *exobiology* to refer to such studies. Along with physicist Dean B. Cowie, he expressed concern in *Science* over the possible contamination of biological life on other planets from microbes carried by human spacecraft. He was also a consultant to the U.S. Viking space missions to the planet Mars.

Lederberg's career included an appointment as chairman of the new genetics department at Stanford University in 1958. In 1978 he was appointed president of Rockefeller University. Working with his first wife, Esther Zimmer, a former student of Tatum's whom Lederberg married in 1946, Lederberg investigated the role of bacterial enzymes in sugar metabolism. He also discovered that penicillin's ability to kill bacteria was due to its preventing synthesis of the bacteria's cell walls. Among Lederberg's many honors were the Eli Lilly Award for outstanding work by a scientist under thirty-five years of age and the Alexander Hamilton Medal of Columbia

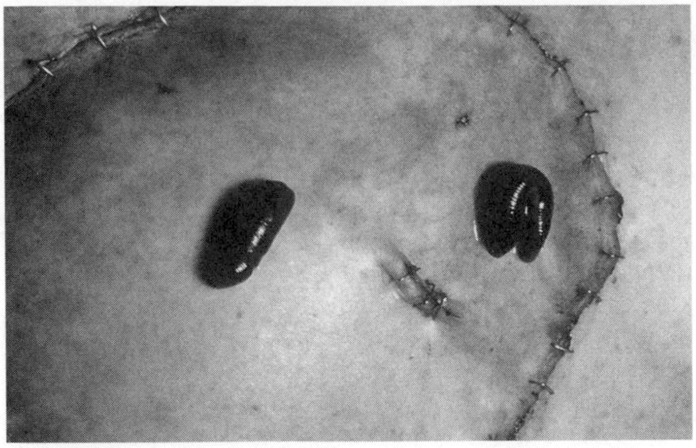

These leeches are being used to reduce venous congestion, or excessive amounts of blood in the blood vessels. *(Photograph by Michael English, M.D., Custom Medical Stock Photo. Reproduced by permission.)*

University. After divorcing his first wife, Lederberg married Marguerite Stein Kirsch in 1968, with whom he had two children, a daughter and a son.

While Lederberg recognized the intense competition that sometimes arises among modern-era scientists, he described his own personal scientific dealings as congenial. ''The shared interests of scientists in the pursuit of a universal truth,'' said Lederberg in *The Excitement and Fascination of Science,* ''remain among the rare bonds that can transcend bitter personal, national, ethnic, and sectarian rivalries.''

Leeches

Leeches are bloodsucking worms with segmented bodies. They belong to the same large classification of worms as earthworms and certain oceanic worms.

Leeches can primarily be found in freshwater lakes, ponds, or rivers. They range in size from 0.2 in (5 mm) to nearly 18 in (45 cm) and have two characteristic suckers located at either end of their bodies. Leeches consume the blood of a wide variety of animal hosts, ranging from fish to humans. To feed, a leech first attaches itself to the host using the suckers. One of these suckers surrounds the leech's mouth, which contains three sets of jaws that bite into the host's flesh, making a Y-shaped incision. As the leech begins to feed, its saliva releases chemicals that dilate blood vessels, thin the blood, and deaden the pain of the bite. Because of the saliva's effects, a person bitten by a leech may not even be aware of it until afterwards, when he or she sees the incision and the trickle of blood that is difficult to stop.

For centuries, leeches were a common tool of doctors, who believed that many diseases were the result of ''imbalances'' in the body that could be stabilized by releasing blood. For example, leeches were sometimes attached to veins in the temples to treat headaches. Advances in medical knowledge led doctors to abandon bloodletting and the use of leeches in the mid-nineteenth century. In recent years, however, doctors have found a new purpose for leeches—helping to restore blood circulation to grafted or severely injured tissue.

There are many occasions in medicine, mostly in surgery and trauma care, when blood accumulates and causes trouble. Leeches can be used to reduce the swelling of any tissue that is holding too much blood. This problem is most likely to occur in two situations:

- Trauma. Large blood clots resulting from trauma can threaten tissue survival by their size and pressure. Blood clots can also obstruct the patient's airway.
- Surgical procedures involving reattachment of severed body parts or tissue reconstruction following **burns**. In these situations it is difficult for the surgeon to make a route for blood to leave the affected part and return to the circulation. The hardest part of reattaching severed extremities like fingers, toes and ears is to reconnect the tiny veins. If the veins are not reconnected, blood will accumulate in the injured area. A similar situation occurs when plastic surgeons move large flaps of skin to replace skin lost to burns, trauma or radical surgery. The skin flaps often drain blood poorly, get congested, and begin to die. Leeches have come to the rescue in both situations.

It is important to use only leeches that have been raised in the laboratory under sterile conditions in order to protect patients from infection. Therapeutic leeches belong to one of two species—*Hirudo michaelseni* or *Hirudo medicinalis.*

One or more leeches are applied to the swollen area, depending on the size of the graft or injury, and left on for several hours. The benefits of the treatment lie not in the amount of blood that the leeches ingest, but in the anti-bloodclotting (anticoagulant) enzymes in the saliva that allow blood to flow from the bite for up to six hours after the animal is detached, effectively draining away blood that could otherwise accumulate and cause tissue death. Leech saliva has been described as a better anticoagulant than many currently available to treat **stroke**s and **heart attack**s. Active investigation of the chemicals in leech saliva is currently under way, and one anticoagulant drug, hirudin, is derived from the tissues of *Hirudo medicinalis.*

The leeches are removed by pulling them off or by loosening their grip with cocaine, heat, or acid. The used leeches are then killed by being placed in an alcohol solution and disposed of as a biohazard. Proper care of the patient's sore is important, as is monitoring the rate at which it bleeds after the leech is removed. Any clots that form at the wound site during treatment should be removed to ensure effective blood flow.

Infection is a constant possibility until the sore heals. It is also necessary to monitor the amount of blood that the leeches have removed from the patient, since a drop in red blood cell counts could occur in rare cases of prolonged bleeding.

Leeuwenhoek, Antoni van (1632-1723)

Dutch biologist and microscopist

Antoni van Leeuwenhoek is best remembered as the first person to study **bacteria** and "animalcules," or one-celled animals, now known as *protozoa.* Unlike his contemporaries **Robert Hooke** and **Marcello Malpighi**, Leeuwenhoek did not use the more advanced compound microscope; instead, he strove to manufacture magnifying lenses of unsurpassed power and clarity that would allow him to study the microcosm in far greater detail than any other scientist of his time.

Leeuwenhoek was born on October 24, 1632, in Delft, Holland. Although his family was relatively prosperous, he received little formal education. After completing grammar school in Delft, he moved to Amsterdam to work as a draper's apprentice. In 1654, he returned to Delft to establish his own shop, and he worked as a draper for the rest of his life. In addition to his business, Leeuwenhoek was appointed to several positions within the city government, which afforded him the financial security to spend a great deal of time and money in pursuit of his hobby—lens grinding. Lenses were an important tool in Leeuwenhoek's profession, since cloth merchants often used small lenses to inspect their products. His hobby soon turned to obsession, however, as he searched for more and more powerful lenses.

In 1671, Leeuwenhoek constructed his first simple microscope. It consisted of a tiny lens that he had ground by hand from a globule of glass and placed within a brass holder. To this, he had attached a series of pins designed to hold the specimen. It was the first of nearly six hundred lenses ranging from 50 to 500 times magnifications that he would grind during his lifetime. Through his microscope, Leeuwenhoek examined such substances as skin, hair, and his own blood. He studied the structure of ivory as well as the physical composition of the flea, discovering that fleas, too, harbored parasites.

Leeuwenhoek began writing to the British Royal Society in 1673. At first, the Society gave his letters little notice, thinking that such magnification from a single lens microscope could only be a hoax. However, in 1676, when he sent the Society the news that he had discovered tiny one-celled animals in rainwater, the interest of member scientists was piqued. Following Leeuwenhoek's specifications, they built microscopes of comparable magnitude and confirmed his findings. In 1680, the Society unanimously elected Leeuwenhoek as a member.

Until this time, Leeuwenhoek had been operating in an informational vacuum; he read only Dutch and, consequently, was unable to learn from the published works of Hooke and Malpighi (though he often gleaned what he could from the illustrations within their texts). As a member of the Society, he was finally able to interact with other scientists. In fact, the news of his discoveries spread worldwide, and he was often visited by royalty from England, Prussia, and Russia. The traffic through his laboratory was so persistent that he eventually allowed visitors by appointment only. Near the end of his life, he had reached near-legendary status and was often referred to by the local townsfolk as a magician.

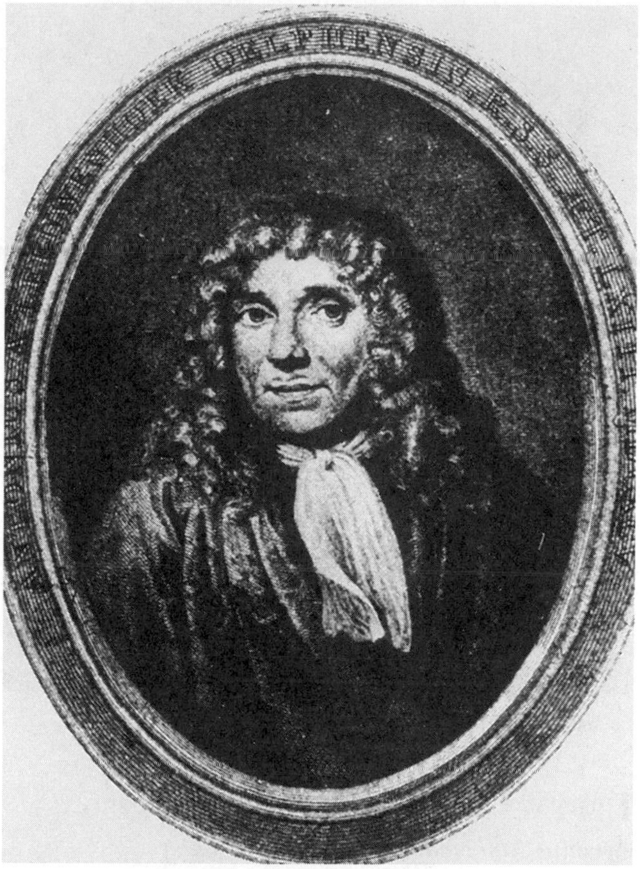

Antoni van Leeuwenhoek

Amid all the attention, Leeuwenhoek remained focused upon his scientific research. Specifically, he was interested in disproving the common belief in spontaneous generation, a theory proposing that certain inanimate objects could generate life. For example, it was believed that mold and maggots were created spontaneously from decaying food. He succeeded in disproving spontaneous generation in 1683, when he discovered bacteria cells. These tiny organisms were nearly beyond the resolving power of even Leeuwenhoek's remarkable equipment and would not be seen again for more than a century.

Leeuwenhoek created and improved upon new lenses for most of his long life. For the forty-three years that he was a member of the Royal Society, he wrote nearly 200 letters that described his progress. However, he never divulged the method by which he illuminated his specimens for viewing, and the nature of that illumination is still a mystery. Upon his death on August 30, 1723, Leeuwenhoek willed twenty-six of his microscopes—a few of which survive in museums—to the British Royal Society.

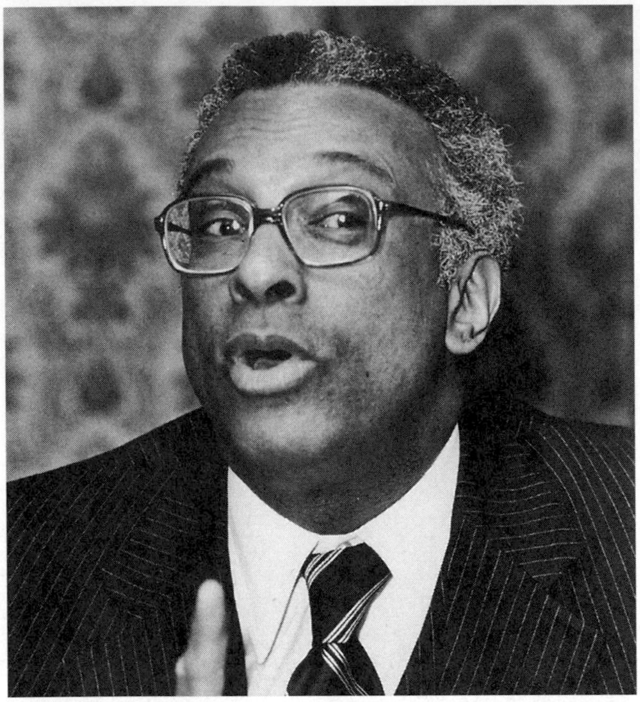

LaSalle D. Leffall, Jr

LEFFALL, JR., LASALLE D. (1930-)

African American surgical oncologist

Surgical oncologist LaSalle D. Leffall, Jr. has worked to focus attention on the problem of high cancer death rates among minorities, especially African Americans. As the first black president of the American Cancer Society and as an educator at Howard University, Leffall has dedicated his career to educating both the medical profession and the lay public about cancer risks for minorities.

Leffall, the son of Martha (Jordan) Lefall and LaSalle Leffall, Sr., was born in Tallahassee, Florida, on May 22, 1930. He attended public school and was the valedictorian of his high school class, graduating in 1945. In 1948, he received a B.S., summa cum laude, from Florida A & M University. From there, Leffall enrolled in Howard University College of Medicine. Again, he achieved academic excellence, graduating first in his class and receiving his M.D. degree in 1952. Leffall's formal medical education continued for the next seven years. He was an intern at Homer G. Phillips Hospital in St. Louis and assistant resident in surgery at both D.C. General Hospital and Freedmen's Hospital, both in Washington, D.C. From 1957 to 1959, Leffall was a senior fellow in cancer surgery at Memorial Sloan-Kettering Cancer Center in New York. He decided to study at Sloan-Kettering because of the new frontiers posed by cancer surgery, Leffall stated in an interview with Devera Pine for *Notable Twentieth-Century Scientists.* "I thought surgery was the most dynamic field," he recalled. "Memorial Sloan-Kettering was using some of the most exciting techniques."

After one year as Chief of General Surgery in the U.S. Army Hospital in Munich (1960 to 1961), Leffall turned to a career in education, becoming an assistant professor at Howard University in 1962. Leffall continued at Howard, serving as assistant dean of the College of Medicine from 1964 to 1970. In 1970, he was appointed professor and chair of the Department of Surgery. "I have a very strong feeling for Howard University. If I had not been accepted there, I wouldn't be a physician and surgeon today," he said in his interview. "When I came along in 1948, predominantly white medical schools rarely accepted blacks." As a researcher, Leffall has focused on clinical studies of cancer of the breast, colorectum, head and neck. He has published more than 116 articles in various professional journals and forums.

In addition to his careers in medicine and education, Leffall has led an active professional life. Leffall became a diplomate of the American Board of Surgery in 1958 and a fellow of the American College of Surgeons in 1964. He was a consultant to the National Cancer Institute beginning in 1972 and a consultant to Walter Reed Army Medical Center beginning in 1971. In 1978 he became the first black president of the American Cancer Society. He used this national forum to emphasize the problems of cancer in minorities, holding the first conference on cancer among black Americans in February of 1979. "I have tried to point out the problems of lack of access to care and the increased death rate," he told Pine. In 1980, President Carter appointed him to a six-year term as a member of the National Cancer Advisory Board.

Leffall has lectured extensively and has served as visiting professor at more than 200 medical institutions. He has received many awards, including the St. George Medal and Citation, the highest divisional award of the American Cancer Society, and the Distinguished Volunteer Service Award from the Secretary of the U.S. Department of Health and Human Services. In 1987, M.D. Anderson Hospital and Tumor Institute in Houston established the Biennial LaSalle D. Leffall Jr. Award. Though Leffall told Pine that he was grateful for all the awards, he said he considers the ones he received from his students over the years "first among equals." In fact, along with his medical career, Leffall considers his teaching one of his most important accomplishments. The role of a teacher, he said, is "to inspire, to instruct, to stimulate, to stretch the imagination and to expand the aspirations of others. It's an honor to be a teacher."

Leffall married Ruth McWilliams in 1956; the couple had one son.

LEGIONNAIRE'S DISEASE

Legionnaire's Disease is an infection caused by the *Legionella pneumophilia* bacterium which manifests as a severe type of pneumonia. The disease was first identified in the United States in 1976—and was subsequently named—when more than 200 Legionnaires participating in America's bicentennial celebrations in Philadelphia became ill. Thirty-four of those infected died. Authorities were at a loss to identify the cause.

Only after prolonged and intense investigations did researchers discover a previously unidentified bacteria which they believe was introduced into the air conditioning system through contaminated water supply. The disease is contracted through airborne transmission of the bacteria and progresses rapidly. Because it proves fatal in approximately 15-25% of reported cases, hospitalization is recommended in almost all instances.

Following identification of the Legionella bacterium, it is now known that the outbreak of a disease in Pontiac, Michigan in 1968, named "Pontiac Fever," was caused by the same species, as were outbreaks elsewhere which had previously gone unidentified. It is also believed to be the primary cause of atypical pneumonia in hospitalized patients and the second largest cause of bacterial pneumonia in the general public. The Center for Disease Control (CDC) recorded 1,241 cases in 1995, or an incidence of 0.48 in every 100,000 people. However, authorities believe more than 20,000 cases may occur in the United States annually. Reports of the disease have come from Africa, Australia, Europe, and North and South America and, while it is no respecter of race or sex, the mortality rate increases with the age of the patient and appears higher in males. Cases reported in people younger than 35 are 0.1 of 100,000, the mean age of reported cases is 52.7 years, and there is an increased frequency to the age of 79. People at high risk are people who use ventilators, the middle-aged, those with **diabetes**, **cancer**, **AIDS**, end-stage kidney disease, or other immunosuppressing factors such as alcoholism or those receiving chemotherapeutic or steroidal medications.

Legionella pneumophilia bacteria survive, thrive, and multiply in the warm, moist conditions found in air conditioning cooling towers, showers, decorative fountains, humidifiers, respiratory therapy equipment, and whirlpool spas. Legionnaire's disease appears more prevalent in the summer, and more so in August, and is slightly more common in the Northern United States than elsewhere. The incubation period ranges from two to 10 days. Symptoms usually begin with one or two days of mild head and body aches, joint pain, and loss of energy, followed by high fever—up to 104°F—chills, rigors, shortness of breath, chest pain, diarrhea, lack of coordination, a dry cough which often progresses to coughing up sputum and/or blood, and—on occasion— seizures. Inflammation of the upper respiratory tract is uncommon, which is a helpful indicator in diagnosis. Treatment consists of antibiotics, which should begin as soon as the disease is suspected, and supportive inpatient treatment with fluids, electrolyte replacement, and oxygen administered by mask or, in sever cases, mechanical ventilator. The disease is not transmitted through person-to-person contact, and recovery usually leaves no chronic complications.

See also Diabetes

LEISHMANIASIS

Leishmaniasis refers to several different illnesses caused by infection with an organism called a protozoan.

Protozoa are considered to be the most simple organisms in the animal kingdom. They are all single-celled. The types of protozoa which cause leishmaniasis are carried by the blood-sucking sandfly. The sandfly is referred to as the disease vector, simply meaning that the infectious agent (the protozoan) is carried by the sandfly and passed on to other animals or humans in whom the protozoan will set up residence and cause disease. The animal or human in which the protozoan then resides is referred to as the host.

Once the protozoan is within the human host, the human's **immune system** is activated to try to combat the invader. Specialized immune cells called macrophages work to swallow up the protozoa. Usually, this technique kills a foreign invader, but these protozoa can survive and flourish within macrophages. The protozoa multiply within the macrophages, ultimately causing the macrophage to burst open. The protozoa are released, and take up residence within other neighboring cells.

At this point, the course of the disease caused by the protozoa is dependent on the specific type of protozoa, and on the type of reaction the protozoa elicits from the immune system. There are several types of protozoa which cause leishmaniasis, and they cause different patterns of disease progression.

At any one time, about 20 million people throughout the world are infected with leishmaniasis. While leishmaniasis exists as a disease in 88 countries around the globe, some countries are hit harder than others. These include Bangladesh, India, Nepal, Sudan, Afghanistan, Brazil, Iran, Peru, Saudi Arabia, and Syria. Other areas which harbor the causative protozoa include China, many countries throughout Africa, Mexico, Central and South America, Turkey, and Greece. Although less frequent, cases have occurred in the United States, in Texas.

In some areas of southern Europe, leishmaniasis is becoming an important disease which infects people with weakened immune systems. In particular, individuals with acquired immunodeficiency syndrome (**AIDS**) are at great risk of this infection.

There are a number of types of protozoa which can cause leishmaniasis. Each type exists in specific locations, and there are different patterns to the kind of disease each causes. The overall species name is Leishmania (commonly abbreviated L.). The specific types include: *L. Donovani, L. Infantum, L. Chagasi, L. Mexicana, L. Amazonensis, L. Tropica, L. Major, L. Aethiopica, L. Brasiliensis, L. Guyaensis, L. Panamensis, L. Peruviana.* Some of the names are reflective of the locale in which the specific protozoa is most commonly found, or in which it was first discovered.

Localized cutaneous leishmaniasis occurs most commonly in China, India, Asia Minor, Africa, the Mediterranean Basin, and Central America. It has occurred in an area ranging from northern Argentina all the way up to southern Texas. It is called different names in different locations, including chiclero ulcer, bush **yaws**, uta, oriental sore, Aleppo boil, and Baghdad sore.

This is perhaps the least drastic type of disease caused by any of the Leishmania. Several weeks or months after being bitten by an infected sandfly, the host may notice an itchy bump (lesion) on an arm, leg, or face. Lymph nodes in the area of this bump may be swollen. Within several months, the bump develops a crater (ulceration) in the center, with a raised, reddened ridge around it. There may be several of these lesions near each other, and they may spread into each other to form one large lesion. Although localized cutaneous leishmaniasis usually heals on its own, it may take as long as a year. A depressed, light-colored scar usually remains behind. Some lesions never heal, and may invade and destroy the tissue below. For example, lesions on the ears may slowly, but surely, invade and destroy the cartilage which supports the outer ear.

Diffuse cutaneous leichmaniasis occurs most often in Ethiopia, Brazil, Dominican Republic, and Venezuela.

The lesions of diffuse cutaneous leishmaniasis are very similar to those of localized cutaneous leishmaniasis, except they are spread all over the body. The body's immune system apparently fails to battle the protozoa, which are free to spread throughout. The characteristic lesions resemble those of the dread biblical disease, **leprosy**.

Mucocutaneous leishmaniasis occurs primarily in the tropics of South America. The disease begins with the same sores noted in localized cutaneous leishmaniasis. Sometimes these primary lesions heal, other times they spread and become larger. Some years after the first lesion is noted (and sometimes several years after that lesion has totally healed), new lesions appear in the mouth and nose, and occasionally in the area between the genitalia and the anus (the perineum). These new lesions are particularly destructive and painful. They erode underlying tissue and cartilage, frequently eating through the septum (the cartilage which separates the two nostrils). If the lesions spread to the roof of the mouth and the larynx (the part of the wind pipe which contains the vocal cords), they may prevent speech. Other symptoms include **fever**, weight loss, **anemia** (low red blood cell count). There is always a large danger of bacteria infecting the already open sores.

Visceral leishmaniasis occurs in India, China, the southern region of Russia, and throughout Africa, the Mediterranean, and South and Central America. It is frequently called Kala-Azar or Dumdum fever.

In this disease, the protozoa uses the bloodstream to travel to the liver, spleen, lymph nodes, and bone marrow. Fever may last for as long as eight weeks, disappear, and then reappear again. The lymph nodes, spleen, and liver are often quite enlarged. Weakness, fatigue, loss of appetite, **diarrhea**, and weight loss are common. Kala-azar translates to mean "black fever." The name kala-azar comes from a characteristic of this form of leishmaniasis. Individuals with light-colored skin take on a darker, grayish skin tone, particularly of their face and hands. A variety of lesions appear on the skin.

Diagnosis for each of these types of leishmaniasis involves taking a scraping from a lesion, preparing it in a laboratory, and examining it under a microscope to demonstrate the causative protozoan. Other methods that have been used include culturing a sample piece of tissue in a laboratory to allow the protozoa to multiply for easier microscopic identification; injecting a mouse or hamster with a solution made of scrapings from a patient's lesion to see if the animal develops a leishmaniasis-like disease; and demonstrating the presence in macrophages of the characteristic-appearing protozoan, called Leishman-Donovan bodies.

In some forms of leishmaniasis, a skin test (similar to that given for TB) may be used. In this test, a solution containing a small bit of the protozoan antigen (cell markers which cause the human immune system to react) is injected or scratched into a patient's skin. In a positive reaction, cells from the immune system will race to this spot, causing a characteristic skin lesion. Not all forms of leishmaniasis cause a positive skin test, however.

The treatment of choice for all forms of leishmaniasis is a type of drug containing the element antimony. These include sodium sitogluconate, and meglumin antimonate. When these types of drugs do not work, other medications with anti-protozoal activity are utilized, including amphotericin B, pentamidine, flagyl, and allopurinol.

The prognosis for leishmaniasis is quite variable, and depends on the specific strain of infecting protozoan, as well as the individual patient's immune system response to infection. Localized cutaneous leishmaniasis may require no treatment. Although it may take many months, these lesions usually heal themselves completely. Only rarely do these lesions fail to heal and become more destructive.

Disseminated cutaneous leishmaniasis may smolder on for years without treatment, ultimately causing **death** when the large, open lesions become infected with bacteria.

Mucocutaneous leishmaniasis is often relatively resistant to treatment. Untreated visceral leishmaniasis has a 90% death rate, but only a 10% death rate with treatment.

Prevention involves protecting against sandfly bites. Insect repellents used around homes, on clothing, on skin, and on bednets (to protect people while sleeping) are effective measures.

Reducing the population of sandflies is also an important preventive measure. In areas where leishmaniasis is very common, recommendations include clearing the land of trees and brush for at least 984 ft (300 m) around all villages, and regularly spraying the area with insecticides. Because rodents often carry the protozoan which causes leishmaniasis, careful rodent control should be practiced. Dogs, which also carry the protozoan, can be given a simple blood test and then either treated or put to sleep.

LEPROSY

The disease now known as Hansen's disease was for centuries called leprosy. It was once among the most feared of all medical disorders. Patients were commonly isolated from the general community in leper colonies, such as the one founded in the Hawaiian Islands by Father Damien. In fact, the term leper long ago became synonymous with the person who was outcast by society.

Until the mid-nineteenth century, Hansen's disease was thought to be a hereditary condition or a disease of the blood. Researchers had unsuccessfully attempted to induce the disease in animals by injecting them with cells from Hansen's patients. Some scientists had even tried to infect themselves in this way, without success. As a result, most authorities were convinced that the disease was not infectious.

The correct explanation for the disease was provided in about 1869 by the Norwegian physician, Gerhard Henrik Armauer Hansen. Hansen was born in Bergen, Norway, on July 29, 1841. He received his medical degree from the University of Christiana (now Oslo) and two years later joined the medical staff at the Lungegard Hospital for Leprosy in Bergen. He spent most of his life working on the cause and treatment of the disease that ultimately received his name.

In the early 1870s, Hansen began to report his observations on the epidemiology and etiology of leprosy. He was fortunate to discover a number of communities in which the disease was very common, occurring as frequently as one in a thousand. Through extensive interviewing, he was able to demonstrate that the disease was almost certainly not transmitted genetically. He wrote that although he had ''not been able to furnish any decisive proof in any direction,'' he was convinced that leprosy fell in the ''category of specific diseases which are contagious.''

An important element in this conclusion was the discovery of ''small staff-like bodies, much resembling bacteria, lying within the cells [of leprosy patients].'' He suspected that the ''large brown elements'' he found in patients' cells were involved in the transmission of the disease. In 1880, Hansen named these infectious particles Bacillus leprae.

The identity of the ''large brown elements'' was finally determined when the German physician, Albert Neisser (1855-1916), visited Hansen in 1879. As a result of Neisser's work, the infectious agent was identified as the organism, Mycobacterium leprae.

Hansen's career at the Lungegard Hospital came to an end in 1880 when he inoculated one of his patients with live leprosy bacilli without obtaining her permission. Despite this setback, he continued working to improve the conditions of leprosy patients until his death in Fluro, Norway, on February 12, 1912. In 1997, there were an estimated 1.2 million cases of leprosy worldwide, with an estimated half a million new cases occurring each year.

As of 1998, India, Indonesia, and Myanmar account for 70% of all leprosy cases. The World Health Organization has recommended combinations of rifampicin, clofazimine, and dapsone for the treatment of leprosy. Thalidomide has also been approved by the U.S. Food and Drug Administration for use against ENL (type II lepra reaction), a severe complication of leprosy.

An important breakthrough in leprosy research occurred in 1985. A research team at Stanford University cloned five genes from *M. leprae*. This accomplishment is of considerable significance since it provides a basis on which an anti-leprosy vaccine can be developed. In fact, the development of such a vaccine is now well under way, providing hope that this disease may some day be controlled.

LEPTOSPIROSIS

Leptospirosis is a febrile disease (**fever**) caused by infection with the bacteria *Leptospira interrogans*. The disease can range from very mild and symptomless to a more serious, even life threatening form, that may be associated with kidney (renal) failure.

An infection by the bacterium *Leptospira interrogans* goes by different names in different regions. Alternate names for leptospirosis include mud fever, swamp fever, sugar cane fever, and Fort Bragg fever. More severe cases of leptospirosis are called Weil's syndrome or icterohemorrhagic fever. This disease is commonly found in tropical and subtropical climates but occurs worldwide.

As of the mid 1980s, there were 35-60 cases of leptospirosis reported in the United States each year. Most cases occur in Hawaii, followed by the south Atlantic, Gulf, and Pacific coastal states. However, because of the nonspecific symptoms of leptospirosis, it is believed that the occurrence in the United States is actually much higher. Leptospirosis occurs year-round in the United States, but about half of the cases occur between July and October.

Leptospirosis is a disease of animals and can be a very serious problem in the livestock industry. *Leptospira* bacteria have been found in dogs, rats, livestock, mice, voles, rabbits, hedgehogs, skunks, possums, frogs, fish, snakes, and certain birds and insects. Infected animals will pass the bacteria in their urine for months, or even years. In the United States, rats and dogs are more commonly linked with human leptospirosis than other animals.

Humans are considered ''accidental hosts'' and become infected with *Leptospira interrogans* by coming into contact with urine from infected animals. This is either through direct contact with urine, or through contact with soil, water, or plants that have been contaminated by animal urine. *Leptospira interrogans* can survive for as long as six months outdoors under favorable conditions. Leptospira bacteria can enter the body through cuts or other skin damage or through mucous membranes (such as the inside of the mouth and nose). It is believed that the bacteria may be able to pass through intact skin, but this is not known.

Once past the skin barrier, the bacteria enter the blood stream and rapidly spread throughout the body. The infection causes damage to the inner lining of blood vessels. The liver, kidneys, heart, lungs, central nervous system, and eyes may be affected.

There are two stages in the disease process. The first stage is during the active Leptospira infection and is called the ''bacteremic,'' or ''septicemic,'' phase. The bacteremic phase lasts from three to seven days and presents as typical flu-like symptoms. During this phase, bacteria can be found in the patient's blood and cerebrospinal fluid. The second stage, or ''immune phase,'' occurs either immediately after the bacteremic stage or after a one to three day symptom-free period. The immune phase can last up to one month. During the immune phase, symptoms are milder but **meningitis** (inflammation of spinal cord and brain tissues) is common. Bacteria can be isolated only from the urine during this second phase.

Leptospirosis is caused by an infection with the bacterium *Leptospira interrogans*. The bacteria are spread through contact with urine from infected animals. Persons at an increased risk for leptospirosis include farmers, miners, animal health care workers, fish farmers and processors, sewage and canal workers, cane harvesters, and soldiers. High risk activities include care of pets, hunting, trail biking, freshwater swimming, rafting, canoeing, kayaking, and participating in sports in muddy fields.

Symptoms of *Leptospira* infection occur within seven to 12 days following exposure to the bacteria. Because the symptoms can be nonspecific, most people who have antibodies to *Leptospira* do not remember having had an illness. Eighty-five to 90% of the cases are not serious and clear up on their own. Symptoms of the first stage of leptospirosis last three to seven days and are: fever (100-105°F [37.8-40.6°C]), severe **headache**, muscle **pain**, stomach pain, chills, nausea, vomiting, back pain, joint pain, neck stiffness, and extreme exhaustion. **Cough** and body rash sometimes occur.

Following the first stage of disease, a brief symptom-free period occurs for most patients. The symptoms of the second stage vary in each patient. Most patients have a low grade fever, headache, vomiting, and rash. Aseptic meningitis is common in the second stage, symptoms of which include headache and **photosensitivity** (sensitivity of the eye to light). *Leptospira* can affect the eyes and make them cloudy and yellow to orange colored. Vision may be blurred.

Ten percent of the persons infected with *Leptospira* develop a serious disease called Weil's syndrome. The symptoms of Weil's syndrome are more severe than those described above and there is no distinction between the first and second stages of disease. The hallmark of Weil's syndrome is liver, kidney, and blood vessel disease. The signs of severe disease are apparent after three to seven days of illness. In addition to those listed above, symptoms of Weil's syndrome include **jaundice** (yellow skin and eyes), decreased or no urine output, **hypotension** (low blood pressure), rash, anemia (decreased number of red blood cells), **shock**, and severe mental status changes. Red spots on the skin, ''blood shot'' eyes, and bloody sputum signal that blood vessel damage and hemorrhage have occurred.

Leptospirosis can be diagnosed and treated by doctors who specialize in infectious diseases. During the bacteremic phase of the disease, the symptoms are relatively nonspecific. This often causes an initial misdiagnosis because many diseases have similar symptoms to leptospirosis. The later symptoms of jaundice and kidney failure together with the bacteremic phase symptoms suggest leptospirosis. Blood samples will be tested to look for antibodies to *Leptospira interrogans*. Blood samples taken over a period of a few days would show an increase in the number of antibodies. Isolating *Leptospira* bacteria from blood, cerebrospinal fluid (performed by spinal tap), and urine samples is diagnostic of leptospirosis. It make take six weeks for *Leptospira* to grow in laboratory media. Most insurance companies would cover the diagnosis and treatment of this infection.

Leptospirosis is treated with **antibiotics**, penicillin (Bicillin, Wycillin), doxycycline (Monodox), ibramycin, or erythromycin (E-mycin, Ery-Tab). As of early 1998, the timing of antibiotic treatment is controversial. It is generally agreed that antibiotic treatment during the first few days of illness is helpful. However, leptospirosis is often not diagnosed until the later stages of illness. The benefit of antibiotic treatment in the later stages of disease is controversial. A rare complication of antibiotic therapy for leptospirosis is the occurrence of the Jarisch-Herxheimer reaction, which is characterized by fever, chills, headache, and muscle pain.

Patients with severe illness will require hospitalization for treatment and monitoring. Medication or other treatment for pain, fever, vomiting, fluid loss, bleeding, mental changes, and low blood pressure may be provided. Patients with kidney failure will require hemodialysis to remove waste products from the blood.

The majority of patients infected with *Leptospira interrogans* experience a complete recovery. Ten percent of the patients will develop eye inflammation (uveitis) up to one year after the illness. In the United States, about one out of every 100 patients will die from leptospirosis. **Death** is usually caused by kidney failure, but has also been caused by **myocarditis** (inflammation of heart tissue), septic shock (reduced blood flow to the organs because of the bacterial infection), organ failure, and/or poorly functioning lungs.

Persons who are at an extremely high risk (such as soldiers who are training in wetlands) can be pretreated with 200 mg of doxycycline once a week. As of early 1998, there were no vaccines available to prevent leptospirosis.

There are many ways to decrease the chances of being infected by *Leptospira*. These include:

- Avoid swimming or wading in freshwater ponds and slowly moving streams, especially those located near farms.
- Do not conduct canoe or kayak capsizing drills in freshwater ponds. Use a swimming pool instead.
- Boil or chemically treat pond or stream water before drinking it or cooking with it.
- Control rats and mice around the home.
- Have pets and farm animals vaccinated against *Leptospira*.
- Wear protective clothing (gloves, boots, long pants, and long-sleeved shirts) when working with wet soil or plants.

LEUKEMIAS

Leukemia is a **cancer** that starts in the organs that make blood, namely the bone marrow and the lymph system. Depending on their characteristics, leukemias can be divided into two broad types. Acute leukemias are the rapidly progressing leukemias, while the chronic leukemias progress more slowly. The vast majority of the childhood leukemias are of the acute form.

The cells that make up blood are produced in the bone marrow and the lymph system. The bone marrow is the spongy tissue found in the large bones of the body. The lymph system includes the spleen (an organ in the upper abdomen), the thymus (a small organ beneath the breastbone), and the tonsils (an organ in the throat). In addition, the lymph vessels (tiny tubes that branch like blood vessels into all parts of the body) and lymph nodes (pea-shaped organs that are found along the network of lymph vessels) are also part of the lymph system. The lymph is a milky fluid that contains cells. Clusters of lymph nodes are found in the neck, underarm, pelvis, abdomen, and chest.

The cells found in the blood are the red blood cells (RBCs), which carry oxygen and other materials to all tissues of the body; white blood cells (WBCs) that fight infection; and the platelets, which play a part in the clotting of the blood. The white blood cells can be further subdivided into three main types: granulocytes, monocytes, and lymphocytes.

The granulocytes, as their name suggests, have particles (granules) inside them. These granules contain special proteins (enzymes) and several other substances that can break down chemicals and destroy microorganisms, such as bacteria. Monocytes are the second type of white blood cell. They are also important in defending the body against pathogens.

The lymphocytes form the third type of white blood cell. There are two main types of lymphocytes: T lymphocytes and B lymphocytes. They have different functions within the immune system. The B cells protect the body by making ''antibodies.'' Antibodies are proteins that can attach to the surfaces of bacteria and viruses. This ''attachment'' sends signals to many other cell types to come and destroy the antibody-coated organism. The T cells protect the body against viruses. When a virus enters a cell, it produces certain proteins that are projected onto the surface of the infected cell. The T cells recognize these proteins and make certain chemicals that are capable of destroying the virus-infected cells. In addition, the T cells can destroy some types of cancer cells.

The bone marrow makes stem cells, which are the precursors of the different blood cells. These stem cells mature through stages into either RBCs, WBCs, or platelets. In acute leukemias, the maturation process of the white blood cells is interrupted. The immature cells (or ''blasts'') proliferate rapidly and begin to accumulate in various organs and tissues, thereby affecting their normal function. This uncontrolled proliferation of the immature cells in the bone marrow affects the production of the normal red blood cells and platelets as well.

Unlike acute leukemias, in which the process of maturation of the blast cells is interrupted, in chronic leukemias, the cells do mature and only a few remain as immature cells. However, even though the cells appear normal, they do not function as normal cells.

Acute leukemias are of two types: acute lymphocytic leukemia and acute myelogenous leukemia. Different types of white blood cells are involved in the two leukemias. In acute lymphocytic leukemia (ALL), it is the T or the B lymphocytes that become cancerous. The B cell leukemias are more common than T cell leukemias. Acute myelogenous leukemia, also known as acute nonlymphocytic leukemia (ANLL), is a cancer of the monocytes and/or granulocytes.

Chronic leukemias develop very gradually. The abnormal lymphocytes multiply slowly, but in a poorly regulated manner. They live much longer and thus their numbers build up in the body. The two types of chronic leukemias can be easily distinguished under the microscope. Chronic lymphocytic leukemia (CLL) involves the T or B lymphocytes. B cell abnormalities are more common than T cell abnormalities. T cells are affected in only 5% of the patients. The T and B lymphocytes can be differentiated from the other types of white blood cells based on their size and by the absence of granules inside them. In chronic myelogenous leukemia (CML), the cells that are affected are the granulocytes.

Chronic lymphocytic leukemia (CLL) often has no symptoms at first and may remain undetected for a long time. Chronic myelogenous leukemia (CML), on the other hand, may progress to a more acute form.

Chronic leukemias account for 1.2% of all cancers. Because leukemia is the most common form of childhood cancer, it is often regarded as a disease of childhood. However, leukemias affect nine times as many adults as children. In chronic lymphoid leukemia, 90% of the cases are seen in people who are 50 years or older, with the average age at diagnosis being 65. The incidence of the disease increases with age. It is almost never seen in children. Chronic myeloid leukemias are generally seen in people in their mid-40s. It accounts for about 4% of childhood leukemia cases. According to the estimates of the American Cancer Society (ACS), approximately 29,000 new cases of leukemia will be diagnosed in 1998.

Leukemia strikes both sexes and all ages. The human T-cell leukemia virus (HTLV-I) is believed to be the causative agent for some kinds of leukemias. However, the cause of most leukemias is not known. Acute lymphoid leukemia (ALL) is more common among Caucasians than among African-Americans, while acute myeloid leukemia (AML) affects both races equally. The incidence of acute leukemia is slightly higher among men than women. People with Jewish ancestry have a higher likelihood of getting leukemia. A higher incidence of leukemia has also been observed among persons with **Down syndrome** and some other genetic abnormalities.

Exposure to ionizing radiation and to certain organic chemicals, such as benzene, is believed to increase the risk of getting leukemia. Having a history of diseases that damage the bone marrow, such as aplastic anemia, or a history of cancers of the lymphatic system puts people at a high risk for developing acute leukemias. Similarly, the use of anticancer medications, immunosuppressants, and the antibiotic chloramphenicol are also considered risk factors for developing acute leukemias.

The symptoms of leukemia are generally vague and non-specific. A patient may experience all or some of the following symptoms:

- Weakness or chronic fatigue
- **Fever** of unknown origin
- Weight loss that is not due to dieting or **exercise**
- Frequent bacterial or viral infections
- **Headache**s
- Skin rash
- Non-specific bone **pain**
- Easy bruising
- Bleeding from gums or nose
- Blood in urine or stools
- Enlarged lymph nodes and/or spleen

- Abdominal fullness.

Like all cancers, acute and chronic leukemias are best treated when found early. There are no screening tests available.

If the doctor has reason to suspect leukemia, he or she will conduct a very thorough **physical examination** to look for enlarged lymph nodes in the neck, underarm, and pelvic region. Swollen gums, enlarged liver or spleen, **bruises**, or pinpoint red **rashes** all over the body are some of the signs of leukemia. Urine and blood tests may be ordered to check for microscopic amounts of blood in the urine and to obtain a complete differential **blood count**. This count will give the numbers and percentages of the different cells found in the blood. An abnormal blood test might suggest leukemia; however, the diagnosis has to be confirmed by more specific tests.

The doctor may perform a bone marrow **biopsy** to confirm the diagnosis of leukemia. During the biopsy, a cylindrical piece of bone and marrow is removed. The tissue is generally taken out of the hipbone. These samples are sent to the laboratory for examination. In addition to diagnosis, the biopsy is also repeated during the treatment phase of the disease to see if the leukemia is responding to therapy.

A spinal tap (lumbar puncture) is another procedure that the doctor may order to diagnose leukemia. In this procedure, a small needle is inserted into the spinal cavity in the lower back to withdraw some cerebrospinal fluid and to look for leukemic cells.

Standard imaging tests, such as x rays, **computed tomography scans** (CT scans), and **magnetic resonance imaging** (MRI) may be used to check whether the leukemic cells have invaded other areas of the body, such as the bones, chest, kidneys, abdomen, or brain. A gallium scan or bone scan is a test in which a radioactive chemical is injected into the body. This chemical accumulates in the areas of cancer or infection, allowing them to be viewed with a special camera.

There are two phases of treatment for leukemia. The first phase is called "induction therapy." As the name suggests, during this phase, the main aim of the treatment is to reduce the number of leukemic cells as far as possible and induce a remission in the patient. Once the patient shows no obvious signs of leukemia (no leukemic cells are detected in blood tests and bone marrow biopsies), the patient is said to be in remission. The second phase of treatment is then initiated. This is called continuation or maintenance therapy, and the aim in this case is to kill any remaining cells and to maintain the remission for as long as possible.

Chemotherapy is the use of drugs to kill cancer cells. It is usually the treatment of choice and is used to relieve symptoms and achieve long-term remission of the disease. Generally, combination chemotherapy, in which multiple drugs are used, is more efficient than using a single drug for the treatment. Some drugs may be administered intravenously through a vein in the arm; others may be given by mouth in the form of pills. If the cancer cells have invaded the brain, then chemotherapeutic drugs may be put into the fluid that surrounds the brain through a needle in the brain or back. This is known as intrathecal chemotherapy.

Because leukemia cells can spread to all the organs via the blood stream and the lymph vessels, surgery is not considered an option for treating leukemias.

Radiation therapy, which involves the use of x rays or other high-energy rays to kill cancer cells and shrink tumors, may be used in some cases. For acute leukemias, the source of radiation is usually outside the body (external radiation therapy). If the leukemic cells have spread to the brain, radiation therapy can be given to the brain.

Bone marrow transplantation is a process in which the patient's diseased bone marrow is replaced with healthy marrow. There are two ways of doing a bone marrow transplant. In an allogeneic bone marrow transplant, healthy marrow is taken from a donor whose tissue is either the same as or very closely resembles the patient's tissues. The donor may be a twin, a brother or sister (sibling), or a person who is not related at all. First, the patient's bone marrow is destroyed with very high doses of chemotherapy and radiation therapy. Healthy marrow from the donor is then given to the patient through a needle in a vein to replace the destroyed marrow.

In the second type of bone marrow transplant, called an autologous bone marrow transplant, some of the patient's own marrow is taken out and treated with a combination of **anticancer drugs** to kill all the abnormal cells. This marrow is then frozen to save it. The marrow remaining in the patient's body is destroyed with high-dose chemotherapy and radiation therapy. The marrow that was frozen is then thawed and given back to the patient through a needle in a vein. This mode of bone marrow transplant is currently being investigated in clinical trials.

Biological therapy or immunotherapy is a mode of treatment in which the body's own immune system is harnessed to fight the cancer. Substances that are routinely made by the immune system (such as growth factors, hormones, and disease-fighting proteins) are either synthetically made in a laboratory or their effectiveness is boosted and they are then put back into the patient's body. This treatment mode is also being investigated in clinical trials all over the country at major cancer centers.

Like all cancers, the prognosis for leukemia depends on the patient's age and general health. According to statistics, more than 60% of the patients with leukemia survive for at least a year after diagnosis. Acute myelocytic leukemia (AML) has a poorer prognosis rate than acute lymphocytic leukemias (ALL) and the chronic leukemias. In the last 15 to 20 years, the five-year survival rate for patients with ALL has increased from 38% to 57%.

In CML, if bone marrow transplantation is performed within one to three years of diagnosis, 50-60% of the patients survive three years or more. If the disease progresses to the acute phase, the prognosis is poor. Less than 20% of these patients go into remission.

Interestingly enough, since most childhood leukemias are of the ALL type, chemotherapy has been highly successful in their treatment. This is because chemotherapeutic drugs are most effective against actively growing cells. Due to the new combinations of anticancer drugs being used, the survival rates among children with ALL have improved dramatically. Eighty percent of the children diagnosed with ALL now survive for five years or more, as compared to 50% in the late 1970s.

Most cancers can be prevented by changes in lifestyle or diet, which will reduce the risk factors. However, in leukemias, there are no such known risk factors. Therefore, at the present time, no way is known to prevent leukemias from developing. People who are at an increased risk for developing leukemia because of proven exposure to ionizing radiation or exposure to the toxic liquid benzene, and people with Down syndrome, should undergo periodic medical checkups.

LEVI-MONTALCINI, RITA (1909-1989)

Italian American biochemist

Rita Levi-Montalcini revealed a fundamental process for cell growth and differentiation by discovering the hormone-like protein nerve growth factor (NGF). For this work, she received part of the 1986 Nobel prize in physiology or medicine.

Levi-Montalcini was born in Turin, Italy, where her father was an electrical engineer and mathematician, and her mother an artist. Despite the objections of her father, who did not approve of education for women, she earned two medical degrees in 1936 and 1940 from the University of Turin, specializing in neurology and psychiatry. She was particularly interested in embryo nervous systems, inspired by an article on limb growth in chick embryos published in 1934 by the nerve development specialist Viktor Hamburger. During World War II Levi-Montalcini, who was Jewish, lived and worked underground to avoid the Italian government's anti-Semitic practices, developing a theory that many immature nerve cells are normally programmed to die. After Italy was liberated in 1944, she worked as a physician in a refugee camp. In 1947, Hamburger invited Levi-Montalcini to Washington University in St. Louis, Missouri, to pursue her nerve theory, which their research confirmed in 1949. Intending to stay there just one year, she remained for thirty years, becoming a United States citizen in 1956.

After 1962, she divided her research time between St. Louis and Rome. Levi-Montalcini's discovery of NGF began when she observed that mouse tumors grafted to chick embryos stimulated the development of embryo nerves. Furthermore, rapid growth occurred whether the tumors were in direct contact with the embryo or not. In searching for a chemical that accounted for the growth, she went to Brazil (with one of her research mice in her purse) to use the latest procedures for the then-new technique of tissue culture-the mixing of tumor slices with chick blood and embryo extract. During twenty-four hours of incubation, a dense halo of nerve axons grew near the tumor. Further research conducted in St. Louis with her assistant **Stanley Cohen** identified a substance she named nerve growth factor.

Her work showed how target cells produce NGF and determine the direction axons grow. It also showed that nerve cells die when antibodies block NGF. After 1977, when she retired from Washington University, she lived in Rome with her twin sister Paola Levi-Montalcini, a well-known painter, where she published her autobiography, *In Praise of Imperfection* in 1988, one year before she died.

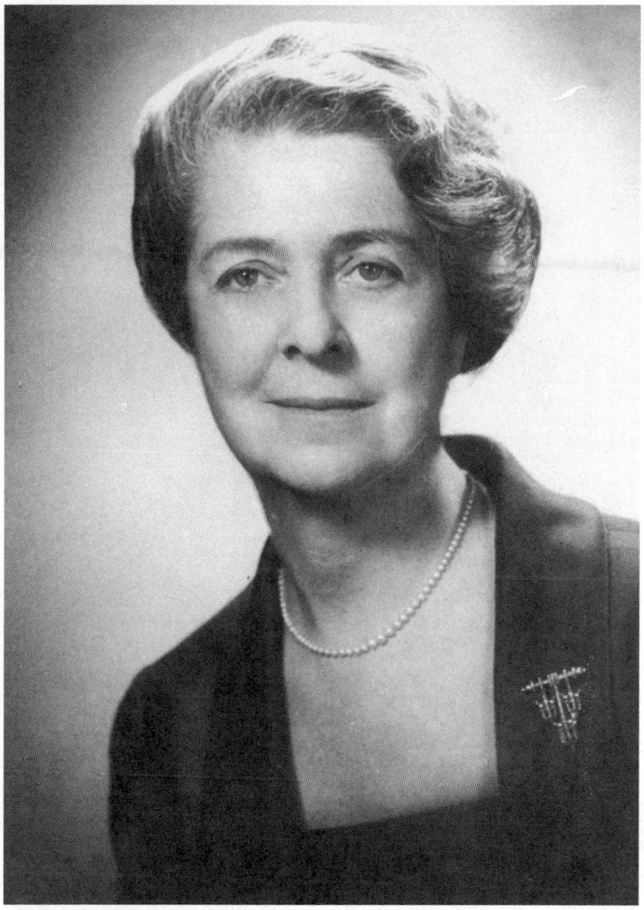

Rita Levi-Montalcini

LEWIS, EDWARD B. (1918-)

American developmental geneticist

Edward B. Lewis, sometimes called the father of developmental genetics, has dedicated a lifetime of research to the study of gene clusters responsible for early embryonic development. His tenacity resulted in important discoveries and led to formal recognition of his work. In 1995, Lewis was awarded the Nobel Prize in Physiology or Medicine for his groundbreaking genetic research. He shared the prize with two other scientists, **Eric Wieschaus** of Princeton University and **Christiane Nüsslein-Volhard** of the Max Planck Institute for Developmental Biology in Germany. Working independently of his corecipients, Lewis studied ''master control'' gene clusters in fruit flies and subsequently discovered their corresponding human counterparts. Such a discovery promises to explain and eventually prevent congenital human malformations (about 40% of all human birth defects). It may also lead to improved

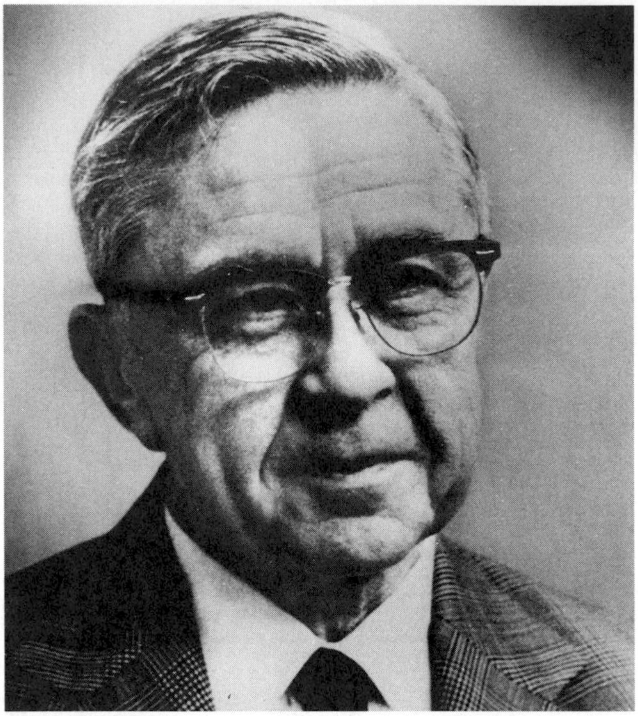

Edward B. Lewis

in-vitro fertilization techniques, as well as a better understanding of substances harmful to early pregnancy.

Edward B. Lewis was born May 20, 1918, in Wilkes-Barre, Pennsylvania, to Edward B. Lewis and Laura (Histed) Lewis. His early years were spent trying to satiate his thirst for scientific knowledge in an environment that did not lend itself to learning. Books were not commonplace at home and as he remembered, "the high school library had nothing at all on genetics." Lewis found solace in playing the flute. He practiced daily, and during high school played with the local symphony orchestra. His musical abilities led to a scholarship at Bucknell University; however, Lewis transferred to the University of Minnesota, which offered course work in genetics. In 1939, Lewis received a B.A. degree in biostatistics from the University of Minnesota. He went on to earn a Ph.D. in genetics at the California Institute of Technology (Caltech) in 1942 and a M.S. in meteorology the following year. After serving as a weatherman in the Army during World War II, Lewis returned to Caltech to reestablish his affiliation with his alma mater.

Since the 1940s, Lewis has been a pioneer in the field of developmental genetics. The direction of his research was already set as a sophomore in high school: with the encouragement of a biology teacher, Lewis and a friend, Edward Novitski, purchased 100 fruit flies from Purdue University for one dollar. Lewis and Novitski let the flies breed, checking each day for any unusual new hatchlings. Their eagerness to learn something from a living specimen sparked careers in biology for both boys. In Lewis it created a lifelong obsession with the genetic workings of the fruit fly. In fact, it was a mutated fruit fly discovered by Novitski that led to Lewis's first postulations about the genetic factors causing mutations in the flies. Like Lewis, Novitski spent his professional life immersed in genetics research. Now retired, he resides in Eugene, Oregon.

Continuing his work with fruit fly specimens, Lewis was able to collect, crossbreed, and ultimately study an enormous amount of mutant flies. By mutating fly embryos so that the flies developed extra pairs of wings, Lewis was able to discern that it was not only the wings that were duplicated but the whole body segment that contained the wings. Because the fruit fly has only eight chromosomes (humans have 23 sets), Lewis was able to pinpoint the gene sequence responsible for the development and order of each fly-body segment. His findings were published in a 1978 *Nature* paper entitled "A Gene Complex Controlling Segmentation in Drosophila." Since then, geneticists have discovered that the gene sequences are almost identical for all other animal species as well.

Lewis has often received recognition for his contributions to developmental genetics. In 1981, he was honored with a Ph.D. from the University of Umeå in Sweden. He received the Thomas Hunt Morgan Medal from the Genetics Society of America in 1983. He was awarded the Canadian Gairdner Foundation International Award in 1987 and Israel's Wolf Prize in Medicine in 1989. In 1990, he received three separate awards: the Lewis S. Rosenstiel Award in basic medical research, the National Medal of Science, and an honorary membership in the Genetical Society in Great Britain. Lewis won the prestigious Albert Lasker Basic Medical Research Award in 1991, the Louisa Gross Horwitz Prize in 1992, and was given an honorary Doctor of Science degree from the University of Minnesota in 1993.

LICE INFESTATION

Lice infestations (pediculosis) are infections of the skin, hair, or genital region caused by lice living directly on the body or in hats or other garments. Lice are small wingless insect-like parasites with sucking mouthparts that feed on human blood and lay their eggs on body hairs or in clothing. The name pediculosis comes from the Latin word *pediculosus* (lousy).

Lice infestations are not dangerous infections by themselves. It is, however a serious public health problem because some lice can carry organisms that cause other diseases, including **relapsing fever**, trench fever, and epidemic **typhus**. Although trench fever is self-limiting, the other two diseases have mortality rates of 5%-10%. Pubic lice are often associated with other **sexually transmitted diseases** (STDs) but do not spread them.

Lice infestations are frequent occurrences in areas of overcrowding or inadequate facilities for bathing and laundry. They are often associated with homelessness in the general population or with military, refugee, or prisoner camps in war-torn areas. All humans are equally susceptible to louse infestation; the elderly, however, are more vulnerable to typhus and other diseases carried by lice.

The symptoms of lice infestations vary somewhat according to body location, although all are characterized by intense **itching**, usually with injury to the skin caused by scratching or scraping. The itching is an allergic reaction to a toxin in the saliva of the lice. Repeated bites can lead to a generalized skin eruption or inflammation.

Head lice is caused by *Pediculosis humanus capitis*, the head louse. Head lice can be transmitted from one person to another by the sharing of hats, combs, or hair brushes. Epidemics of head lice are common among school-age children from all class backgrounds in all parts of the United States. The head louse is about 1/16 of an inch in length. The adult form may be visible on the patient's scalp, especially around the ears; or its grayish-white nits (eggs) may be visible at the base of the hairs close to the scalp. It takes between three and 14 days for the nits to hatch. After the nits hatch, the louse must feed on blood within a day or die.

Head lice can spread from the scalp to the eyebrows, eyelashes, and beard in adults, although they are more often limited to the scalp in children. The itching may be intense, and may be followed by bacterial infection of skin that has been scratched open. Another common complication is swelling or inflammation of the neck glands. Head lice do not spread typhus or other systemic diseases.

Infestations of body lice are caused by *Pediculosis humanus corporis*, an organism that is similar in size to head lice. Body lice, however, are rarely seen on the skin itself because they come to the skin only to feed. They should be looked for in the seams of the patient's clothing. This type of infestation is associated by wearing the same clothing for long periods of time without laundering, as may happen in wartime or in cold climates; or with poor personal hygiene. It can be spread by close personal contact or shared bedding.

Patients with body lice often have intense itching with deep scratches around the upper shoulders, flanks, or neck. The bites first appear as small red pimples but may cause a generalized skin rash. If the infestation is not treated, the patient may develop complications that include **headache**, **fever**, and bacterial infection with scarring. Body lice can spread systemic typhus or other infections.

Pubic lice are sometimes called ''crabs.'' This type of infestation is caused by *Phthirus pubis* and is commonly spread by intimate contact. People can also get public lice from using the bedding, towels, or clothes of an infected person.

Pubic lice usually appear first on pubic hair, but may spread to other parts of the body, particularly if the patient is very hairy. Pubic lice are also sometimes seen on the eyelashes of children born to infected mothers. It is usually easier for the doctor to see marks from the patient's scratching than the bites from the lice, but pubic lice sometimes produce small bluish spots called maculae ceruleae on the patient's trunk or thighs. Pubic lice also sometimes leave small dark brown specks from their own excreted matter on the parts of the patient's underwear that cover the anal or genital areas.

Doctors can diagnose lice infestations from looking closely at the parts of the body where the patient has been scratching. Lice are large enough to be easily seen with the naked eye or a magnifying glass. The eggs of pubic lice as well as head lice can often be found by looking at the base of the patient's hairs. Pediatricians are most likely to diagnose lice in school-age children.

It is important for doctors to rule out other diseases that can cause scratching and skin inflammation because the medications used to kill lice are very strong and can have bothersome side effects. The doctor will need to distinguish between head lice and dandruff; between body lice and **scabies** (a disease caused by skin mites); and between pubic lice and eczema. Blood tests or other laboratory tests are not useful in diagnosing lice infestations.

Lice infestations are treated with externally applied medications that either kill the lice or prevent them from feeding. Cases of head lice are usually treated with shampoos or rinses containing either lindane (Kwell) or permethrin (Nix). Because lindane is absorbed through the skin, the person giving the application should wear rubber gloves and rinse the patient's hair or body completely after use. Following the treatment, nits should be removed from the hair with a fine-toothed comb or tweezers. Lindane is also effective for treating infestations of body or pubic lice, but it should not be used by pregnant women. In most cases one treatment is sufficient, but the medication can be reapplied a week later if living lice have reappeared.

Infestations of body lice can also be treated by washing the patient's clothes or bedding in boiling water, ironing seams with an iron on a high setting, or treating the clothes with 1% malathion powder or 10% DDT powder.

If the patient's eyelashes have been infested, the only safe treatments are either a thick coating of petroleum jelly (Vaseline) applied twice daily for eight days, or 1% yellow oxide of mercury applied four times a day for two weeks. Any remaining nits should be removed with tweezers.

Patients with pubic lice should be examined and tested for other STDs.

For pubic lice, some practitioners of holistic medicine recommend a mixture of 25% oil of pennyroyal (*Mentha pulegium*), 25% garlic (*Allium sativum*) oil, and 50% distilled water applied three times in a three-day period, followed by removal of dormant eggs to prevent reinfestation.

Lice can be successfully eradicated in almost all cases, although some cases of lindane-resistant lice have been reported. In general, patients are more at risk from typhus and other diseases spread by lice than from the lice themselves.

There are no vaccines or skin treatments that will protect a person against lice prior to contact. In addition, lice infestation does not provide immunity against reinfection; recurrences are in fact quite common. Prevention depends on adequate personal hygiene at the individual level and the following public health measures:

- Teaching school-age children the basics of good personal hygiene, including the importance of not lending or borrowing combs, brushes, or hats.
- Notifying and treating an adult patient's close personal and sexual contacts.
- Examining homeless people, elderly patients incapable of self-care, and other high-risk individuals prior to hospital admission for signs of louse infestation. This measure is necessary to protect other hospitalized people from the spread of lice.

LICHEN PLANUS

Lichen planus is a skin condition of unknown origin that produces small, shiny, flat-topped, itchy pink or purple raised spots on the wrists, forearms or lower legs, especially in middle-aged patients.

Lichen planus affects between 1-2% of the population, most of whom are middle-aged women. The condition is less common in the very young and the very old. The lesions are found on the skin, genitals, and in the mouth. Most cases resolve spontaneously within two years. Lichen planus is found throughout the world and is equally distributed among races.

No one knows what causes lichen planus, although some experts suspect that it is an abnormal immune reaction following a viral infection, probably aggravated by **stress**. The condition is similar to symptoms caused by exposure to arsenic, bismuth, gold, or developers used in color photography. Occasionally, lichen planus in the mouth appears to be an allergic reaction to medications, filling material, dental hygiene products, chewing gum or candy.

Symptoms can appear suddenly, or they may gradually develop, usually on the arms or legs. The lesions on the skin may be preceded by a dryness and metallic taste or burning in the mouth.

Once the lesions appear, they change over time into flat, glistening, purple lesions marked with white lines or spots. Mild to severe **itching** is common. White, lacy lesions are usually painless, but eroded lesions often burn and can be painful. As the lesions clear up, they usually leave a brown discoloration behind, especially in dark skinned people.

Lichen planus in the mouth occurs in six different forms with a variety of symptoms, appearing as lacy-white streaks, white plaques, or eroded ulcers. Often the gums are affected, so that the surface of the gum peels off, leaving the gums red and raw.

A doctor can probably diagnose the condition simply from looking at the characteristic lesions, but a skin biopsy may be needed to confirm the diagnosis.

Treatment for lichen planus is aimed at easing symptoms. Itching can be treated with steroid creams and oral **antihistamines**. Severe lesions can be treated with **corticosteroids** by mouth, or combinations of photochemotherapy (PUVA) and griseofulvin.

Patients with lesions in the mouth may find that regular professional cleaning of the teeth and conscientious dental care improve the condition. Using milder toothpastes instead of tartar control products also seems to lessen the number of ulcers and makes them less sensitive.

While lichen planus can be annoying, it is usually fairly benign and clears up on its own. It may take months to reach its peak, but it usually clears up within 18 months.

LIND, JAMES (1716-1794)

English physician

James Lind, an English physician, proved through his experimentation that citrus fruits like oranges and limes could prevent scurvy, a deadly disease caused by a vitamin C deficiency.

Lind was born on October 4, 1716, in Edinburgh, Scotland, to Margaret (Smelum) and James Lind, a prosperous merchant. He attended grammar school in his youth, and then was apprenticed to the Edinburgh physician George Langlands in 1731. He became a surgeon's mate in the British navy in 1739, and in 1747, was promoted to surgeon.

Lind performed one of his most important experiments on curing scurvy in 1747. Many people knew that far more sailors on British warships died from scurvy than from battle. In retrospect, if sailors did not get vitamin C in their food, especially from fruits like oranges, lemons, or limes, then they developed the symptoms of scurvy: bleeding gums, loosened teeth, stiff or swollen joints, and bleeding under the skin. Infections often resulted, and if infections did not kill the sailors, then they soon died from convulsions or coma if they were left untreated. On long voyages, entire crews could be decimated by scurvy. Before Lind's work, others had noticed that citrus fruits were good for health. The Spanish physician, **Michael Servetus**, said in 1537 that citrus fruits were good for digestion. Admiral Sir Richard Hawkins of the British Navy noticed in 1593 that feeding his men citrus fruit each day seem to eliminate scurvy.

Lind set out in 1747 to prove experimentally that citrus fruits cured scurvy. While he was aboard the H.M.S. *Salisbury* from August to October 1747, Lind created an experiment in which he tested the effectiveness of dietary supplements on scurvy patients. He administered cider, vinegar, seawater, garlic, oranges and lemons, and other foods to patients with scurvy. He noticed that the most rapid and visible improvements came to his patients who received the citrus fruits.

In 1748, Lind left the navy and returned to Scotland, where he enrolled at the University of Edinburgh to obtain his M.D. degree. Because of his long training and experience in medicine, he received his M.D. that same year. He then practiced medicine in Edinburgh and married Isobel Dickie. In 1754, Lind published *A Treatise of the Scurvy*. In 1757, Lind published a second book, *On the Most Effectual Means of Preserving the Health of Seamen*, which also recommended giving sailors citrus fruits on long voyages. In 1758, Lind was appointed the chief physician of the Royal Naval Hospital at Gosport in the south of England.

In 1768, Lind published *An Essay on Diseases Incidental to Europeans in Hot Climates*, which was a leading source of information about tropical medicine for 50 years. Lind retired as chief physician of the Royal Naval Hospital in 1783. His son, John, replaced him. Lind died in Gosport on July 13, 1794. In spite of Lind's works, his advice about giving sailors citrus fruits to prevent scurvy was not taken seriously by the British Navy until after his death. Some physicians of the time simply did not believe that scurvy was caused by dietary problems. Others refused to believe that any disease as bad as scurvy could be cured so easily with an orange a day. In the next year, 1795, the Royal Navy adopted the practice of giving seamen citrus fruits and juices as part of their diets. Scurvy promptly vanished from the Royal Navy.

See also Michael Servetus

LIPID DISORDERS

Lipid disorders, like hyperlipoproteinemia, occur when there is too much lipid (fat) in the blood. Shorter terms that mean the same thing are hyperlipidemia and hyperlipemia. Dyslipidemia refers to a redistribution of cholesterol from one place to another that increases the risk of vascular disease without increasing the total amount of cholesterol. When more precise terms are needed, hypercholesterolemia and hypertriglycericemia are used.

It is commonly known that oil and water do not mix unless another substance like a detergent is added. Yet the body needs to transport both lipids (fats) and water-based blood within a single circulatory system. There must be a way to mix the two, so that essential fatty nutrients can be transported in the blood and so that fatty waste products can be carried away from tissues. The solution is to combine the lipids with protein to form water-soluble packages that can be transported in the blood.

These packages of fats are called lipoproteins. They are a complex mixture of triglycerides, cholesterol, phospholipids and special proteins. Some of these chemicals are fatty nutrients absorbed from the intestines on their way to being made part of the body. Cholesterol is a waste product on its way out of the body through the liver, the bile, and ultimately the bowel for excretion. The proteins and phospholipids make the packages water-soluble.

There are five different sizes of these chemical packages. Each package needs all four chemicals in it to hold everything in solution. They differ in how much of each they contain. If blood serum is spun very rapidly in an ultracentrifuge, these five packages will layer out according to their density. They have, therefore, been named according to their densities—high-density lipoproteins (HDL), low-density lipoproteins (LDL), intermediate-density lipoproteins (IDL), very low density lipoproteins (VLDL), and chylomicrons. Only the HDLs and the LDLs will be discussed in the rest of this article.

If there is not enough detergent in the laundry, the oily stains will remain in the clothes. In the same way, if the balance of chemicals in these packages is not right, cholesterol will stay in tissues rather than being excreted from the body. What is even worse, if the chemical composition of these packages changes, the cholesterol can fall out of the blood and stay where it lands. On the other hand, a different change in the balance can remove cholesterol from tissues where there is too much. This appears to be exactly what is going on in **atherosclerosis**. The lesions contain lots of cholesterol.

The LDLs are overloaded with cholesterol. A minor change in the other chemicals in this package will leave cholesterol behind. The HDLs have a third to a half as much cholesterol. They seem to be able to pick up cholesterol left behind by the LDLs. It seems that atherosclerosis begins with tiny tears at stressed places in the walls of the arteries. Low density lipoproteins from the blood enter these tears, where their chemistry changes enough to leave cholesterol behind. The cholesterol causes irritation; the body responds with inflammation; damage and scarring follow. Eventually the artery gets so diseased blood cannot flow through it. Strokes and **heart attacks** are the result.

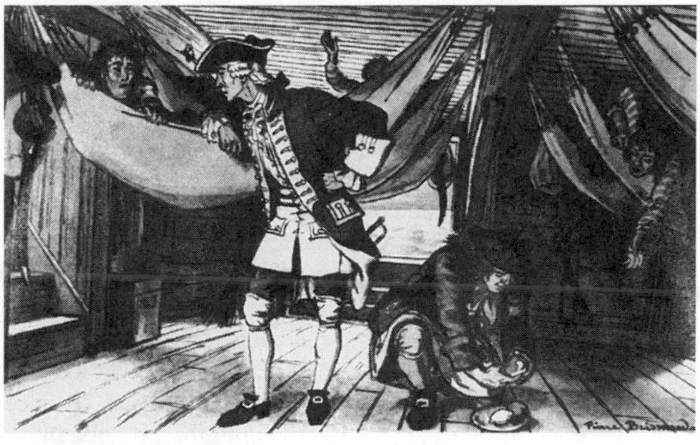

James Lind

But if there are lots of HDLs in the blood, the cholesterol is rapidly picked up and not allowed to cause problems. Women before **menopause** have estrogen (the female hormone), which encourages the formation of HDLs. This is the reason they have so little vascular disease, and why they rapidly catch up to men after menopause, when estrogen levels fall. Replacement of estrogen after menopause sustains the protection through the later years.

Cholesterol is the root of the problem, but like any other root it cannot just be eliminated. Ninety percent of the cholesterol in the body is created there as a waste product of necessary processes. The solution lies in getting it out to the body without clogging the arteries.

Of course the story is much more complex. The body has dozens of chemical processes that make up, break down, and reconfigure all these chemicals. It is these processes that are the targets of intervention in the effort to cure vascular disease.

Near the dawn of concern over cholesterol and vascular disease a family of hereditary diseases was identified, all of which produced abnormal quantities of blood fats. These diseases were called dyslipoproteinemias and came in both too much and too little varieties. The hyperlipoproteinemias found their way into five categories, depending on which chemical was in excess.

- Type 1 has a pure elevation of triglycerides in the chylomicron fraction. These people sometimes get **pancreatitis** and abdominal **pain**s, but they do not seem to have an increase in vascular disease.
- Type 2 appears in two distinct genetic patterns and a third category, which is by far the most important kind, because everyone is at risk for it. All Type 2s have elevated cholesterol. Some have elevated triglycerides also. The familial (genetic) versions of Type 2 often develop xanthomas, which are yellow fatty deposits under the skin of the knuckles, elbows, buttocks or heels. They may also have xanthelasmas, smaller yellow patches on the eyelids.
- Type 3 appears in one in 10,000 people and elevates both triglycerides and cholesterol with consequent vascular disease.

- Type 4 elevates only triglycerides and does not increase the risk of vascular disease.
- Type 5 is similar to Type 1.
- Dyslipidemia refers to a normal amount of cholesterol that is mostly in LDLs, where it causes problems.

All but Type 2 are rare and of interest primarily because they give insight into the chemistry of blood fats.

In addition to the above genetic causes of blood fat disorders, a number of acquired conditions can raise lipoprotein levels.

- **Diabetes mellitus**, because it alters the way the body handles its energy needs, also affects the way it handles fats. The result is elevated triglycerides and reduced HDL cholesterol. This effect is amplified by **obesity**.
- Hypothyroidism is a common cause of lipid abnormalities. The thyroid hormone affects the rate of many chemical processes in the body, including the clearing of fats from the blood. The consequence is usually an elevation of cholesterol.
- Kidney disease affects the blood's proteins and consequently the composition of the fat packages. It usually raises the LDLs.
- Liver disease, depending on its stage and severity, can raise or lower any of the blood fats.
- Alcohol raises triglycerides. In moderate amounts (if they are very moderate) it raises HDLs and can be beneficial.
- Cigarette smoking lowers HDL cholesterol, as does **malnutrition** and obesity.

Certain medications elevate blood fat levels. Because some of these medications are used to treat heart disease, it has been necessary to reevaluate their usefulness:

- Thiazides, water pills used to treat high blood pressure, can raise both cholesterol and triglycerides.
- Beta-blockers, another class of medication used to treat high blood pressure, cortisone-like drugs, and estrogen can raise triglycerides.
- Progesterone, the **pregnancy** hormone, raises cholesterol.

Not all of these effects are necessarily bad, nor are they necessarily even significant. For instance, estrogen is clearly beneficial. Each effect must be considered in the overall goal of treatment.

A combination of heredity and diet is responsible for the majority of fat disorders. It is not so much the cholesterol in the diet that is the problem, because that accounts for only 10% of the body's store. It is the other fats in the diet that alter the way the body handles its cholesterol. There is a convincing relation between fats in the diet and the incidence of atherosclerosis. The guilty fats are mostly the animal fats, but palm and coconut oil are also harmful. These fats are called saturated fats for the chemical reason that most of their carbon atoms have as many hydrogen atoms attached as they can accommodate. More important than the kind of fat is the amount of fat. For many people, fat is half of their diet. A quarter to a fifth is a much healthier fraction, the rest of the diet being made up of complex carbohydrates and protein.

This disease is silent for decades, until the first episode of heart disease or stroke.

It would be easier if simple cholesterol and triglyceride tests were all it took to assess the risk of atherosclerosis. But the important information is which package the cholesterol is in—the LDLs or the HDLs. That takes a more elaborate testing process. To complicate matters further, the amount of fats in the blood varies greatly in relation to the last meal—how long ago it was and what kind of food was eaten. A true estimate of the risk comes from several tests several weeks apart all done after at least twelve hours of **fasting**.

Diet and lifestyle change are the primary focus for most cholesterol problems. It is a mistake to think that a pill will reverse the effects of a bad diet, obesity, smoking, excess alcohol, stress, and inactivity. Reducing the amount of fat in the diet by at least half is the most important move to make. Much of the food eaten to satisfy a "sweet tooth" is higher in fat than in sugar. A switch away from saturated fats is the next step, but the rush to polyunsaturated fats was ill-conceived. These, and particularly the hydrogenated fats in margarine, have problems of their own. They raise the risk of **cancer** and are considered more dangerous than animal fat by many experts. Theory supports population studies that suggest monounsaturated olive oil may be the healthiest of all.

There is a tremendous push at the end of the twentieth century to use lipid-lowering medications. The most popular and most expensive agents, the "statins," hinder the body's production of cholesterol and sometimes damage the liver as a side effect. Their full name is 3-hydroxy-3-methylglutaryl-coemzyme A *(HMG-CoA)* reductase inhibitors. Their generic names are cervistatin, fluvastatin, lovastatin, pravastatin, and simvastatin. Studies show that these do lower cholesterol. Only recently, though, has any evidence appeared that this affects health and longevity. Earlier studies showed, in fact, an increased death rate among users of the first class of lipid-altering agents—the fibric acid derivatives. The chain of events connecting raised HDL and lowered LDL cholesterol to longer, healthier lives is still to be forged.

High-tech methods of rapidly reducing very high blood fat levels are performed for those rare disorders that require it. There are resins that bind cholesterol in the intestines. They taste awful, feel like glue and routinely cause gas, bloating, and **constipation**. For acute cases, there is a filtering system that takes fats directly out of the blood.

Niacin (nicotinic acid) lowers cholesterol very effectively and was the first medication proven to improve overall life expectancy. It can also be liver toxic, and the usual formulation causes a hot flash in many people. This can be overcome by taking a couple of **aspirin**s half-an-hour before the niacin, or by taking a special preparation called "flush free," "inositol-bound" or inositol hexanicotinate. Omega-3 oil is a special kind found mostly in certain kinds of fish. It is beneficial in lowering cholesterol. An herbal alternative called gugulipid, *Commiphora mukul*, an extract of an Indian plant, is supposed to work the same way as the expensive and liver toxic cholesterol-lowering medications.

The prognosis is good for Type 1 hyperlipoproteinemia with treatment; without treatment, death may result. For Type

2 the prognosis is poor even with treatment. The prognosis for type 3 is good when the prescribed diet is strictly followed. For types 4 and 5 the prognosis is uncertain, due to the risk of developing premature coronary artery disease and pancreatitis, respectively.

Genetic inheritance cannot be changed, but its effects may be modified with proper treatment. Family members of an individual with hyperlipoproteinemia should consider having their blood lipids assessed. The sooner any problems are identified, the better the chances of limiting or preventing the associated health risks. Anyone with a family history of disorders leading to hyperlipoproteinemia also may benefit from genetic testing and counseling to assist them in making reproductive decisions.

LIPIDOSES

Lipidoses are heredity disorders, passed from parents to their children, characterized by defects of the digestive system that impair the way the body uses fat from the diet. When the body is unable to properly digest fats, lipids accumulate in body tissues in abnormal amounts.

The digestion, storage, and use of fats from foods is a complex process that involves hundreds of chemical reactions in the body. In most people, the body is already programmed by its genetic code to produce all of the enzymes and chemicals necessary to carry out these functions. These genetic instructions are passed from parents to their offspring during reproduction.

People with lipidoses are born without the genetic codes needed to tell their bodies how to complete a particular part of the fat digestion process. In most of these disorders, the body does not produce a certain enzyme or chemical. Over 30 different disorders of fat metabolism are related to genetic defects. Although the defects are passed from parents to children, the parents often do not have the disorders themselves.

The symptoms, available treatments, and long-term consequences of these conditions vary greatly. Some of the conditions become apparent shortly after the infant is born; in others, symptoms may not develop until adulthood. For most of the lipidoses, diagnosis is suspected based on the symptoms and family history. Blood tests, urine tests, and tissue tests can be used to confirm the diagnosis. **Genetic testing** can be used, in some cases, to identify the defective gene. Some of these disorders can be controlled with changes in the diet, medications, or enzyme supplements. For many, no treatment is available. Some may cause **death** in childhood or contribute to a shortened life expectancy. Some of the most common or most serious lipidoses are discussed below.

Approximately 1 in every 40,000 males is born with Fabry's disease. This condition has an X-linked, recessive pattern of inheritance, meaning that the defective gene is carried on the X chromosome. A female who carries a defective recessive gene on one of her two X chromosomes has a 50% chance of passing the defective gene to her sons who will develop the disorder associated with the defective gene (a male receives one X chromosome from his mother and one Y chromosome from his father). She also has a 50% chance of passing the defective recessive gene to her daughters who will be carries of the disorder (like their mother). Some female carries of Fabry's disease show mild signs of the disorder, especially cloudiness of the cornea.

The gene that is defective in Fabry's disease causes a deficiency of the enzyme alpha-galactosidase A. Without this enzyme, fatty compounds starts to line the blood vessels. The collection of fatty deposits eventually affects blood vessels in the skin, heart, kidneys, and nervous system. The first symptoms in childhood are **pain** and discomfort in the hands and feet brought on by **exercise**, **fever**, **stress**, or changes in the weather. A raised rash of dark red-purple spots is common, especially on skin between the waistline and the knees. Other symptoms include a decreased ability to sweat and changes in the cornea or outer layer of the eye. Although the disease begins in childhood, it progresses very slowly. Kidney and heart problems develop in adulthood.

The diagnosis of Fabry's disease can be confirmed by a blood test to measure for alpha-galactosidase A. Women who are carries of the defective gene can also be identified by a blood test.

Treatment of Fabry's disease focuses on prevention of symptoms and long-term complications. Daily doses of diphenylhydantoin (Dilantin) or carbamazapine (Tegretol) can prevent or reduce the severity of pain in the hands and feet associated with the condition. A low sodium, low protein diet may be beneficial to those patients who have some kidney complications. If kidney problems progress, kidney dialysis or kidney transplantation may be required. Enzyme replacement therapy is currently being explored.

Although patients with Fabry's disease usually survive to adulthood, they are at increased risk for **stroke**, **heart attack**s, and kidney damage.

Gaucher (pronounced go-shay) disease is the most common of the lipid storage disorders. It is found in populations all over the world (20,00 to 40,000 people have a type of the disease), and it occurs with equal frequency in males and females. Gaucher disease has a recessive pattern of inheritance, meaning that a person must inherit a copy of the defective gene from both parents in order to have the disease. The genetic defect causes a deficiency of the enzyme glucocerebrosidase that is responsible for breaking down a certain type of fat and releasing it from fat cells. These fat cells begin to crowd out healthy cells in the liver, spleen, bones, and nervous system. Symptoms of Gaucher disease can start in infancy, childhood, or adulthood.

Three types of Gaucher disease have been identified, but there are many variations in how symptoms develop. Type 1 is the most common and affects both children and adults. It occurs much more often in people of Eastern European and Russian Jewish (Ashkenazi) ancestry, affecting one out of every 450 live births. The first signs of the disease include an enlarged liver and spleen, causing the abdomen to swell. Children with this condition may be shorter than normal. Other symptoms include tiredness, pain, bone deterioration, broken bones, anemia, and increased bruising. Type 2 Gaucher disease is more serious, beginning within the first few months after birth. Symptoms, which are similar to those in Type 1, progress rapidly, but also include nervous system damage. Symptoms of Type 3 Gaucher disease begin during early childhood with symptoms like Type 1. Unlike Type 2, the progress of the disease is slower, although it also includes nervous system damage.

Gaucher disease may be suspected based on symptoms and is confirmed with a blood test for levels of the enzyme. Samples of tissue from an affected area may also be used to confirm a diagnosis of the disease.

The symptoms of Gaucher disease can be stopped and even reversed by treatment with injections of enzyme replacements. Two enzyme drugs currently available are alglucerase (Ceredase) and imiglucerase (Cerezyme). Other treatments address specific symptoms such as anemia, broken bones, or pain.

The pain and deformities associated with symptoms can make coping with this illness very challenging for individuals and families. With treatment and control of symptoms, people with Type 1 Gaucher disease may lead fairly long and normal lives. Most infants with Type 2 die before the age of two. Children with Type 3 Gaucher disease may survive to adolescence and early adulthood.

Krabbe's disease is caused by a deficiency of the enzyme galactoside beta-galactosidase. It has a recessive pattern of inheritance and is believed to occur in one of 40,000 births in the United States. This condition, which is also called globoid cell leukodystrophy or Krabbe leukodystrophy, is characterized by acute nervous system degeneration. It develops in early infancy with initial symptoms of irritability, vomiting and episodes of partial unconsciousness. Symptoms progress rapidly to seizures, difficulty swallowing, blindness, deafness, **mental retardation**, and **paralysis**. No treatment is available for Krabbe's disease, and children born with the disease die in infancy.

At least five different forms of Niemann-Pick disease (NPD) have been identified. The different types seem to be related to the activity level of the enzyme sphingomyelinase. In patients with Types A and B NPD, there is a build up of sphingomyelin in cells of the brain, liver, spleen, kidney and lung. Type A is the most common form of NPD and the most serious, with death usually occurring by the age of 18 months. Symptoms develop within the first few months of life and include poor appetite, failure to grow, enlarged liver and spleen, and the appearance of cherry red spots in the retina of the eye. Type B develops in infancy or childhood with symptoms of mild liver or spleen enlargement and lung problems. Some adults with this form (Type E) may also show a loss of muscle coordination. Types C or D NPD are related to cholesterol transfer out of cells. Children with Types C or D grow normally in early childhood, but eventually develop difficulty in walking and loss of muscle coordination. Ultimately, the nervous system becomes severely damaged and these patients die. Type C occurs in any population, while Type D has been identified only in patients from Nova Scotia, Canada.

Diagnosis is confirmed by analyzing a sample of tissue. Prenatal diagnosis of Types A and B of NPD can be done with amniocentesis or chorionic villus sampling.

Treatment consists of supportive care to deal with symptoms and the development of complications. **Bone marrow transplantation** is being investigated as a possible treatment. Low-cholesterol **diets** may be helpful for patients with Types C and D.

Patients with Type A NPD usually die within the first year and a half of life. Type B patients generally live to adulthood but suffer from significant liver and lung problems. With Types C and D NPD, there is significant nervous system damage leading to severe muscle spasms, seizures, and eventually, to **coma** and death. Some patients with Types C and D die in childhood, while less severely affected patients may survive to adulthood.

Refsum's disease has a recessive pattern of inheritance and affects populations from Northern Europe, particularly Scandinavians most frequently. It is due to a deficiency of phytanic acid hydroxylase, an enzyme that breaks down a fatty acid called phytanic acid. This condition affects the nervous system, eyes, bones, and skin. Symptoms, which usually appear by age 20, include vision problems [**retinitis pigmentosa** and rhythmic eye movements (nystagmus)], loss of muscle coordination, loss of sense of smell (anosmia), pain, numbness, and elevated protein in the cerebrospinal fluid.

A diet free of phytanic acid (found in dairy products, tuna, cod, haddock, lamb, stewed beef, white bread, white rice, boiled potatoes, and egg yolk) can reduce some of the symptoms o. Plasmapheresis, a process where whole blood is removed from the body, processed through a filtering system, and then return to the body, may be used to filter phytanic acid from the blood.

Tay-Sachs disease (TSD) is a fatal condition caused by a deficiency of the enzyme hexosaminidase A (Hex-A). The defective gene that causes this disorder is found in roughly 1 in 250 people in the general population. However, certain populations have significantly higher rates of TSD. French-Canadians living near the St. Lawrence River and in the Cajun regions of Louisiana are at higher risk of having a child with TSD. The highest risk seems to be in people of Eastern European and Russian Jewish (Ashkenazi) descent. Tay-Sachs disease has a recessive pattern of inheritance, and approximately 1 in every 27 people of Jewish ancestry in the United States carries the TSD gene. Symptoms develop in infancy and are due to the accumulation of a fatty acid compound in the nervous system. Early symptoms include loss of vision and physical coordination, seizures, and mental retardation. Eventually, the child develops problems with breathing and swallowing. Blindness, paralysis, and death follow.

Carriers of the Tay-Sachs related gene can be identified with a blood test. Amniocentesis or chorionic villi sampling can be used to determine if the fetus has Tay-Sachs disease.

There is no treatment for Tay-Sachs disease. Parents who are identified as carriers may want to seek **genetic counseling**. If a fetus is identified as having TSD, parents may consider termination of the **pregnancy**.

Children born with Tay-Sachs disease become increasingly debilitated; most die by about age four.

Wolman's disease is caused by a genetic defect (with a recessive pattern of inheritance) that results in deficiency of an enzyme that breaks down cholesterol. This causes large amounts of fat to accumulate in body tissues. Symptoms begin in the first few weeks of life and include an enlarged liver and spleen, adrenal calcification (hardening of adrenal tissue due to deposits of calcium salts), and fatty stools. No treatment is currently available for Wolman's disease, and death generally occurs before six months of age.

Couples who have family histories of genetic defects can undergo genetic testing and counseling to see if they are at risk for having a child with one of the lipidoses disorders. During pregnancy, cell samples can be collected from the fetus using amniocentesis or chorionic villi sampling. The results of these test can indicate if the developing fetus has a lipidosis disorder. Termination of the pregnancy may be considered in some cases.

LIPMANN, FRITZ ALBERT (1899-1986)

German American biochemist

Born in Königsberg, Germany, Fritz Lipmann earned his medical degree at the University of Berlin in 1922 and, five years later, received his Ph.D. there as well. For the next several years, Lipmann conducted research at **Otto Meyerhof**'s laboratory in Heidelberg, Germany, and taught at the Kaiser Wilhelm Institute in Berlin. In 1932, when the Nazi movement in Germany made life increasingly uncomfortable, he accepted a position with the Carlsberg Foundation in Copenhagen, Denmark. In 1939, Lipmann immigrated to the United States, settling first at the Cornell Medical School and then, two years later, moving on to Harvard (1941-49) and then the staff of Massachusetts General Hospital (1949-57). In 1957, he became Professor of Biochemistry at the Rockefeller Institute in New York.

For a long time, most of Lipmann's research at these institutions centered around carbohydrate **metabolism**, especially the role played by phosphates. In 1937, Lipmann had discovered, almost by accident, that phosphates were somehow important to the metabolic process. He was not certain exactly what role they played, but believed it had something to do with the delivery of energy to the body's cells. In 1941, he finally came up with some of the answers he had been seeking. He found a molecule that released low-energy phosphate—*adenosine monophosphate*—and discovered that, during the course of carbohydrate metabolism, the molecule picked up two energy-rich phosphate bonds, and became adenosine triphosphate (ATP), a high-energy configuration that was able to release small traces of energy, when needed, to cells throughout the body.

In 1947, Lipmann made an even more important discovery. Working with pigeon liver extracts, he found a catalytically-active, heat-stable compound that appeared able to control the transfer of acetyl groups from one molecule to another. After isolating the compound and determining its structure (it was composed largely of pantothenic acid, or vitamin B2) he named it coenzyme A (CoA), with the ''A'' standing for acetylation. Lipmann speculated that CoA probably played an important role in the Krebs cycle, a complicated cycle of fatty acid, carbohydrate and protein oxidation.

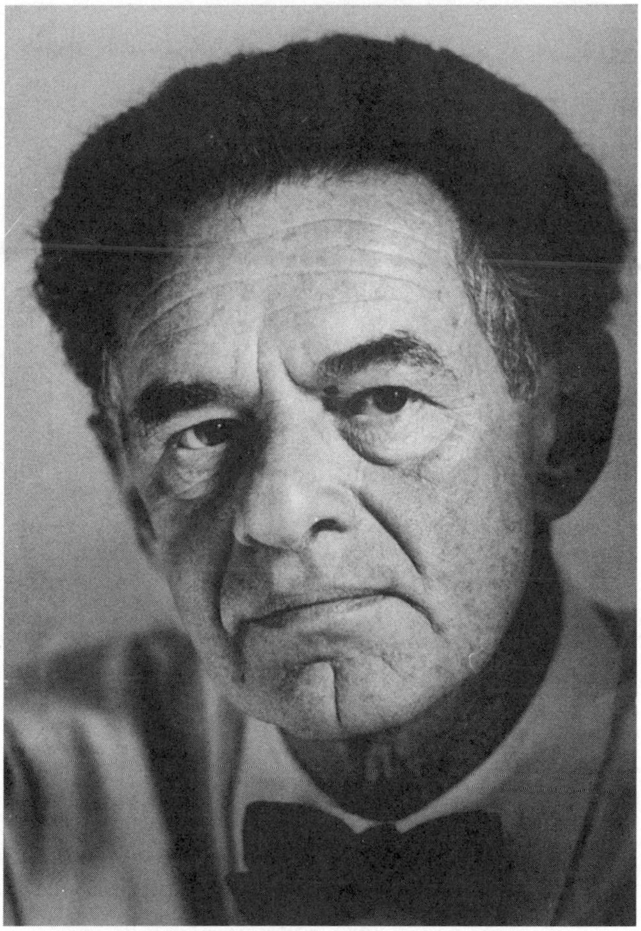

Fritz Albert Lipmann

Hans Krebs had already shown that lactic acid was broken down to carbon dioxide by way of a two-carbon compound that was part of his cycle. Lipmann believed that Krebs' two-carbon compound needed the help of CoA in order to enter the cycle and, by 1951, proved this to be the case. The two-carbon compound in the Krebs' cycle combined with CoA to form acetylcoenzyme A, a kind of super coenzyme that served as the hub of numerous biochemical reactions. For instance, in 1950, the coenzyme was found by Feodor Lynen (1911-1979) to play a key role in the metabolism of fats.

For his work on coenzyme A, Lipmann received the 1953 Nobel Prize in physiology or medicine, sharing the prize with Krebs. He also received several other honors including membership in the Faraday Society, the Danish Royal Academy of Sciences and the Royal Society of England.

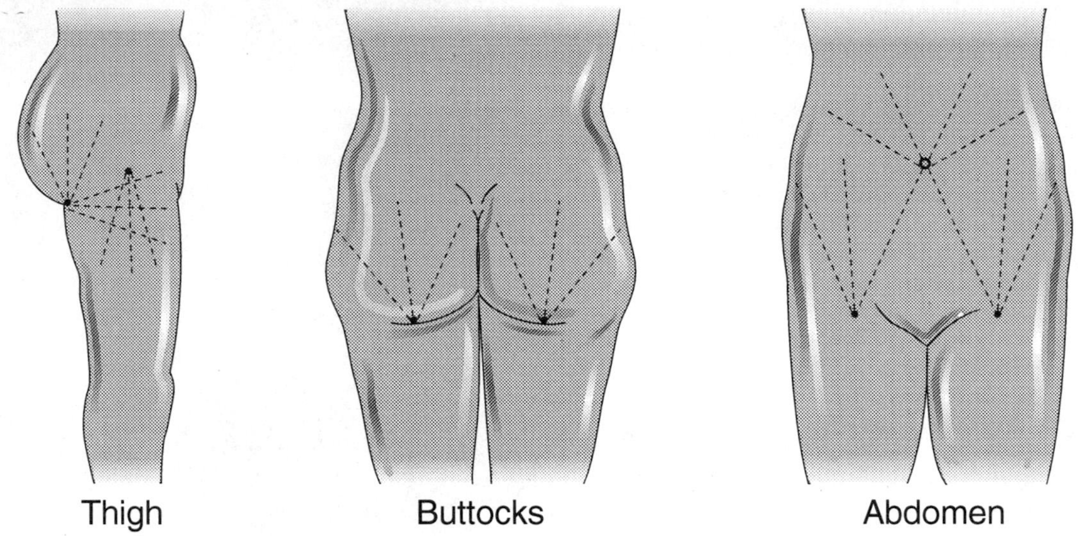

Common entry sites for liposuction procedures. ***(Illustration by Electronic Illustrators Group.)***

LIPOSUCTION

Liposuction, also known as lipoplasty or suction-assisted lipectomy, is cosmetic surgery performed to remove unwanted deposits of fat from under the skin. The doctor sculpts and recontours the patient's body by removing excess fat deposits that have been resistant to reduction by diet or **exercise**. The fat is permanently removed from under the skin with a suction device.

Liposuction is intended to reduce and smooth the contours of the body and improve the patient's appearance. Its goal is cosmetic improvement. It is the most commonly performed cosmetic procedure in the United States.

Liposuction does not remove large quantities of fat and is not intended as a weight reduction technique. The average amount of fat removed is about a liter, or a quart. Although liposuction is not intended to remove cellulite (lumpy fat), some doctors believe that it improves the appearance of cellulite areas (thighs, hips, buttocks, abdomen, and chin).

A new technique called liposhaving shows more promise at reducing cellulite.

Liposuction is most successful on patients who have firm, elastic skin and concentrated pockets of fat in cellultite areas. To get good results after fat removal, the skin must contract to conform to the new contours without sagging. Older patients have less elastic skin and therefore may not be good candidates for this procedure. Patients with generalized fat distribution, rather than localized pockets, are not good candidates.

Patients should be in good general health and free of heart or lung disease. Patients with poor circulation or who have had recent surgery at the intended site of fat reduction are not good candidates.

Most liposuction procedures are performed under local anesthesia (loss of sensation without loss of consciousness) by the tumescent or wet technique. In this technique, large volumes of very dilute local anesthetic (a substance that produces anesthesia) are injected under the patient's skin, making the tissue swollen and firm. Epinephrine is added to the solution to reduce bleeding, and make possible the removal of larger amounts of fat.

The doctor first numbs the skin with an injection of local anesthetic. After the skin is desensitized, the doctor makes a series of tiny incisions, usually 0.12-0.25 in (3-6 mm) in length. The area is then flooded with a larger amount of local anesthetic. Fat is then extracted with suction through a long, blunt hollow tube called a cannula. The doctor repeatedly pushes the cannula through the fat layers in a radiating pattern creating tunnels, removing fat, and recontouring the area. Large quantities of intravenous fluid (IV) is given during the procedure to replace lost body fluid. Blood **transfusions** are possible.

Some newer modifications to the procedure involve the use of a cutting cannula called a liposhaver, or the use of ultrasound to help break up the fat deposits. The patient is awake and comfortable during these procedures.

The length of time required to perform the procedure varies with the amount of fat that is to be removed and the number of areas to be treated. Most operations take from 30 minutes to 2 hours, but extensive procedures can take longer. The length of time required also varies with the manner in which the anesthetic is injected.

The cost of liposuction can vary depending upon the standardized fees in the region of the country where it is performed, the extent of the area being treated, and the person performing the procedure. Generally, small areas, such as the chin or knees, can be done for as little as $500, while more extensive treatment, such as when hips, thighs, and abdomen are done simultaneously, can cost as much as $10,000. These procedures are cosmetic and are not covered by most insurance policies.

The doctor will do a physical exam and may order blood work to determine clotting time and hemoglobin level for transfusions should the need arise. The patient may be placed on **antibiotics** immediately prior to surgery to ward off infection.

After the surgery, the patient will need to wear a support garment continuously for 2-3 weeks. If ankles or calves were treated, support hose will need to be worn for up to 6 weeks. The support garments can be removed during bathing 24 hours after surgery. A drainage tube, under the skin in the area of the procedure, may be inserted to prevent fluid build-up.

Mild side effects can include a burning sensation at the site of the surgery for up to one month. The patient should be prepared for swelling of the tissues below the operated site for 6-8 weeks after surgery. Wearing the special elastic garments will help reduce this swelling and help to achieve the desired final results.

The incisions involved in this procedure are tiny, but the surgeon may close them with stitches or staples. These will be removed the day after surgery. However, three out of eight doctors use no sutures. Minor bleeding or seepage through the incision site is common after this procedure. Wearing the elastic bandage or support garment helps reduce fluid loss.

This operation is virtually painless. However, for the first postoperative day, there may be some discomfort which will require light pain medication. Soreness or aching may persist for several days. The patient can usually return to normal activity within a week. Postoperative bruising will go away by itself within 10-14 days. Postoperative swelling begins to go down after a week. It may take 3-6 months for the final contour to be reached.

Liposuction under local anesthesia using the tumescent technique is exceptionally safe. A 1995 study of 15,336 patients showed no serious complications or **deaths**. Another study showed a 1% risk factor. However, as with any surgery, there are some risks and serious complications. Death is possible.

The main hazards associated with this surgery involve migration of a blood clot or fat globule to the heart, brain, or lungs. Such an event can cause a **heart attack**, **stroke**, or serious lung damage. However, this complication is rare and did not occur even once in the study of 15,336 patients. The risk of blood clot formation is reduced with the wearing of special girdle-like compression garments after the surgery, and with the resumption of normal mild activity soon after surgery.

Staying in bed increases the risk of clot formation, but not getting enough rest can result in increased swelling of the surgical area. Such swelling is a result of excess fluid and blood accumulation, and generally comes from not wearing the compression garments. If necessary, this excess fluid can be drained off with a needle in the doctor's office.

Infection is another complication, but this rarely occurs. If the physician is skilled and works in a sterile environment, infection should not be a concern.

If too much fat is removed, the skin may peel in that area. Smokers are at increased risk for shedding skin because their circulation is impaired. Another and more serious hazard of removing too much fat is that the patient may go into **shock**. Fat tissue has an abundant blood supply and removing too much of it at once can cause shock if the fluid is not replaced.

A rare complication is perforation or puncture of an organ. The procedure involves pushing a cannula vigorously through the fat layer. If the doctor pushes too hard or if the tissue gives way too easily under the force, the blunt hollow tube can go too far and injure internal organs.

Liposuction can damage superficial nerves. Some patients lose sensation in the area that has been suctioned, but feeling usually returns with time.

The loss of fat cells is permanent, and the patient should have smoother, more pleasing body contours without excessive bulges. However, if the patient overeats, the remaining fat cells will grow in size. Although the patient may gain weight back, the body should retain the new proportions and the suctioned area should remain proportionally smaller.

Tiny scars about 0.25-0.5 in (6-12 mm) long at the site of incision are normal. The doctor usually makes the incisions in places where the scars are not likely to show.

In some instances, the skin may appear rippled, wavy, or baggy after surgery. Pigmentation spots may develop. The recontoured area may be uneven. This unevenness is common, occurring in 5-20% of the cases, and can be corrected with a second procedure that is less extensive than the first.

Listeriosis

Listeriosis is an illness caused by the bacterium *Listeria monocytogenes* that is acquired by eating contaminated food. The organism can spread to the blood stream and central nervous system. During **pregnancy**, listeriosis often causes miscarriage or **stillbirth**.

Listeriosis is caused by an infection with the bacterium *Listeria monocytogenes*. This bacteria can be carried by many animals and birds, and it has been found in soil, water, sewage, and animal feed. Five out of every 100 people carry *Listeria monocytogenes* in their intestines. Listeriosis is considered a ''food-borne illness'' because most people are probably infected after eating food contaminated with *Listeria monocytogenes*. However, a woman can pass the bacteria to her baby during pregnancy. In addition, there have been a few cases where workers have developed *Listeria* skin infections by touching infected calves or poultry.

In the 1980s, the United States government began taking measures to decrease the occurrence of listeriosis. Processed meats and dairy products are now tested for the presence of *Listeria monocytogenes*. The Food and Drug Administration (FDA) and the Food Safety and Inspection Service (FSIS) can legally prevent food from being shipped, or order food recalls, if they detect any *Listeria* bacteria. These inspections, in combination with the public education regarding the proper handling of uncooked foods, appear to be working. In 1989, there were 1,965 cases of listeriosis with 481 **death**s. In 1993, the numbers fell to 1,092 cases with 248 deaths.

In 1996, the Centers for Disease Control and Prevention (CDC) began a nationwide food-borne disease surveillance program called ''FoodNet,'' in which seven states were participating by January 1997. Results from the program indicated that, in 1996, one person out of every 200,000 people got listeriosis. FoodNet also revealed that the hospitalization rate was higher for listeriosis (94%) than for any other food-borne illness. In addition, FoodNet found that the *Listeria* bacteria reached the blood and cerebrospinal fluid in 89% of cases, a higher percentage than in any other food-borne illness.

Persons at particular risk for listeriosis include the elderly, pregnant women, newborns, and those with a weakened immune system (called ''immunocompromised''). Risk is increased when a person suffers from diseases such as **AIDS**, **cancer**, kidney disease, diabetes mellitus, or by the use of certain medications. Infection is most common in babies younger than one month old and adults over 60 years of age. Pregnant women account for 27% of the cases and immunocompromised persons account for almost 70%. Persons with AIDS are 280 times more likely to get listeriosis than others.

As noted, persons become infected with *Listeria monocytogenes* by eating contaminated food. *Listeria* has been found on raw vegetables, fish, poultry, raw (unpasteurized) milk, fresh meat, processed meat (such as deli meat, hot dogs, and canned meat), and certain soft cheeses. Listeriosis outbreaks in the United States since the 1980s have been linked to cole slaw, milk, Mexican-style cheese, undercooked hot dogs, undercooked chicken, and delicatessen foods. Unlike most other bacteria, *Listeria monocytogenes* does not stop growing when food is in the refrigerator — its growth is merely slowed. Fortunately, typical cooking temperatures and the pasteurization process do kill this bacteria.

Listeria bacteria can pass through the wall of the intestines, and from there they can get into the blood stream. Once in the blood stream, they can be transported anywhere in the body, but are commonly found the central nervous system (brain and spinal cord); and in pregnant women they are often found in the placenta (the organ which connects the baby's umbilical cord to the uterus). *Listeria monocytogenes* live inside specific white blood cells called macrophages. Inside macrophages, the bacteria can hide from immune responses and become inaccessible to certain **antibiotics**. *Listeria* bacteria are capable of multiplying within macrophages, and then may spread to other macrophages.

After consuming food contaminated with this bacteria, symptoms of infection may appear anywhere from 11-70 days later. Most people do not get any noticeable symptoms. Scientists are unsure, but they believe that *Listeria monocytogenes* can cause upset stomach and intestinal problems just like other food-borne illnesses. Persons with listeriosis may develop flu-like symptoms such as **fever**, **headache**, nausea and vomiting, tiredness, and **diarrhea**.

Pregnant women experience a mild, flu-like illness with fever, muscle aches, upset stomach, and intestinal problems. They recover, but the infection can cause miscarriage, **premature labor**, early rupture of the birth sac, and stillbirth. Unfortunately, half of the newborns infected with *Listeria* will die from the illness.

There are two types of listeriosis in the newborn baby: early-onset disease and late-onset disease. Early-onset disease refers to a serious illness that is present at birth and usually causes the baby to be born prematurely. Babies infected during the pregnancy usually have a blood infection (**sepsis**) and may have a serious, whole body infection called granulomatosis infantisepticum. When a full-term baby becomes infected with *Listeria* during **childbirth**, that situation is called late-onset disease. Commonly, symptoms of late-onset listeriosis appear about two weeks after birth. Babies with late-term disease typically have **meningitis** (inflammation of the brain and spinal tissues); yet they have a better chance of surviving than those with early-onset disease.

Immunocompromised adults are at risk for a serious infection of the blood stream and central nervous system (brain and spinal cord). Meningitis occurs in about half of the cases of adult listeriosis. Symptoms of listerial meningitis occur about four days after the flu-like symptoms and include fever, personality change, uncoordinated muscle movement, **tremors**, muscle contractions, seizures, and slipping in and out of consciousness.

Listeria monocytogenes causes **endocarditis** in about 7.5% of the cases. Endocarditis is an inflammation of heart tissue due to the bacterial infection. Listerial endocarditis causes death in about half of the patients. Other diseases which have been caused by *Listeria monocytogenes* include brain abscess, eye infection, hepatitis (liver disease), **peritonitis** (abdominal infection), lung infection, joint infection, arthritis, heart disease, bone infection, and gallbladder infection.

Listeriosis may be diagnosed and treated by infectious disease specialists and internal medicine specialists. The diagnosis and treatment of this infection should be covered by most insurance providers.

The only way to diagnose listeriosis is to isolate *Listeria monocytogenes* from blood, cerebrospinal fluid, or stool. A sample of cerebrospinal fluid is removed from the spinal cord using a needle and syringe. This procedure is commonly called a spinal tap. The amniotic fluid (the fluid which bathes the unborn baby) may be tested in pregnant women with listeriosis. This sample is obtained by inserting a needle through the abdomen into the uterus and withdrawing fluid. *Listeria* grows well in laboratory media and test results can be available within a few days.

Listeriosis is treated with the antibiotics ampicillin (Omnipen) or sulfamethoxazole-trimethoprim (Bactrim, Septra). Because the bacteria live within macrophage cells, treatment may be difficult and the treatment periods may vary. Usually, pregnant women are treated for two weeks; newborns, two to three weeks; adults with mild disease, two to four weeks; persons with meningitis, three weeks; persons with brain abscesses, six weeks; and persons with endocarditis, four to six weeks.

Patients are often hospitalized for treatment and monitoring. Other drugs may be provided to relieve **pain** and fever and to treat other reactions to the infection.

The overall death rate for listeriosis is 26%. This high death rate is due to the serious illness suffered by newborns, the elderly, and immunocompromised persons. Healthy adults and older children have a low death rate. Complications of *Listeria* infection include: meningitis, sepsis, miscarriage, stillbirth, **pneumonia**, **shock**, endocarditis, **abscess** (localized infection) formation, and eye inflammation.

The United States government has already done much to prevent listeriosis. Persons at extremely high risk (pregnant women, immunocompromised persons, etc.) must use extra caution. High risk persons should: avoid soft cheeses, such as Mexican cheese, feta, Brie, Camembert, and blue cheese (cottage cheese is safe), thoroughly cook leftovers and ready-to-eat foods (such as hot-dogs), and avoid foods from the deli.

For all people, the risk of listeriosis can be reduced by taking these precautions:

- Completely cook all meats and eggs.
- Carefully wash raw vegetables before eating.
- Keep raw meat away from raw vegetables and prepared foods. After cutting raw meat, wash the cutting board with detergent before using it for vegetables.
- Avoid drinking unpasteurized milk or foods made from such milk.
- Wash hands thoroughly after handling raw meat.
- Follow the instructions on food labels. Observe food expiration dates and storage conditions.

LISTER, JOSEPH (1827-1912)

English surgeon

Joseph Lister, born in Upton, Essex, the son of a London wine merchant, developed antiseptic surgery, saving innumerable patients from the dreadful pain and death of post-surgical infection.

Lister's father invented the achromatic lens which created the modern microscope and encouraged the boy's interest in microbiology. After receiving his medical degree from University College Hospital in London in 1852, Lister practiced and taught surgery first in Edinburgh and then, from 1860, in Glasgow, Scotland.

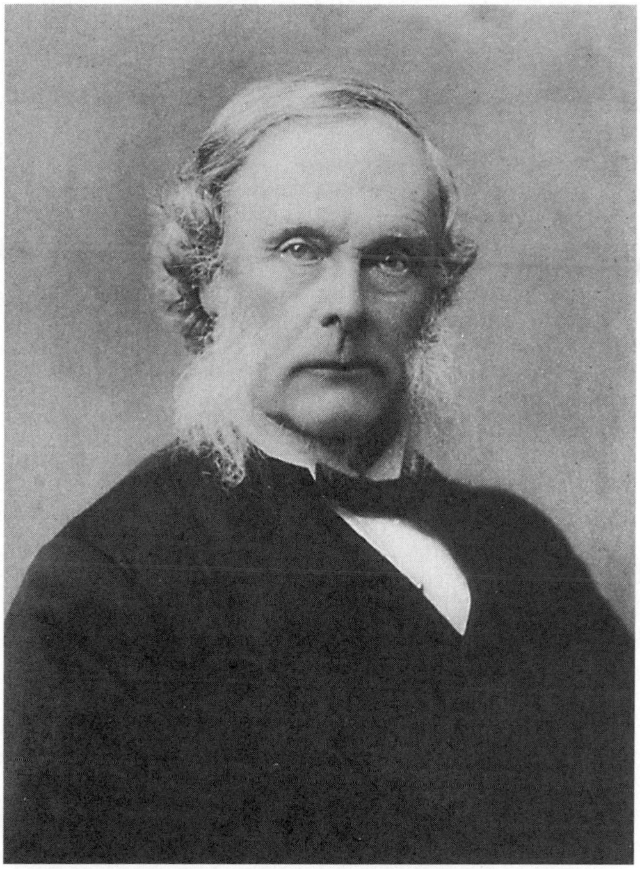

Joseph Lister

As a surgeon, Lister became increasingly disturbed by the high rate of the often fatal infection that developed in his patients after surgery. A professor of chemistry, Thomas Anderson (1819-1874), drew Lister's attention to the ideas of **Louis Pasteur**. Lister immediately concluded that the microorganisms described by Pasteur and carried in the air caused wound infections. He developed a method to destroy these organisms using carbolic acid as an antiseptic.

Lister first used his new antiseptic surgical technique in March 1865. Although this and many subsequent operations proved the effectiveness of Lister's method to prevent infection, Lister's ideas were vigorously opposed by many of his fellow physicians, who thought the antiseptic procedures ridiculously complicated and superfluous.

In 1877 Lister became a professor at London's King's College Hospital, where he continued to promote antisepsis. As the significance of his innovation became widely recognized in the late 1870s and 1880s, Lister gained many honors, including elevation to the peerage in 1897, and was a greatly venerated figure by the time of his death in 1912. His other contributions to surgery include the use of absorbable sutures and the introduction of wound drainage.

LITHOTRIPSY

Lithotripsy is the use of high-energy shock waves to fragment and disintegrate **kidney stones**. The shock wave, created by using a high-voltage spark or an electromagnetic impulse, is focused on the stone. This shock wave shatters the stone and this allows the fragments to pass through the urinary system. Since the shock wave is generated outside the body, the procedure is termed extracorporeal shock wave lithotripsy, or ESWL.

ESWL is used when a kidney stone is too large to pass on its own, or when a stone becomes stuck in a ureter (a tube which carries urine from the kidney to the bladder) and will not pass. Kidney stones are extremely painful and can cause serious medical complications if not removed.

ESWL should not be considered for patients with severe skeletal deformities, patients weighing over 300 lbs (136 kg), patients with abdominal aortic aneurysms, or patients with uncontrollable bleeding disorders. Patients who are pregnant should not be treated with ESWL. Patients with cardiac **pacemakers** should be evaluated by a cardiologist familiar with ESWL. The cardiologist should be present during the ESWL procedure in the event the pacemaker needs to be overridden.

Lithotripsy uses the technique of focused shock waves to fragment a stone in the kidney or the ureter. The patient is placed in a tub of water or in contact with a water-filled cushion, and a shock wave is created which is focused on the stone. The wave shatters and fragments the stone. The resulting debris, called gravel, then passes through the remainder of the ureter, through the bladder, and through the urethra during urination. There is minimal chance of damage to skin or internal organs because biologic tissues are resilient, not brittle, and because the the shock waves are not focused on them.

Prior to the lithotripsy procedure, a complete **physical examination** is done, followed by tests to determine the number, location, and size of the stone or stones. A test called an intravenous pyelogram, or IVP, is used to locate the stones. An IVP involves injecting a dye into a vein in the arm. This dye, which shows up on x ray, travels through the bloodstream and is excreted by the kidneys. The dye then flows down the ureters and into the bladder. The dye surrounds the stones, and x rays are then used to evaluate the stones and the anatomy of the urinary system. (Some people are allergic to the dye material, so it cannot be used. For these people, focused sound waves, called ultrasound, can be used to see where the stones are located.) Blood tests are done to determine if any potential bleeding problems exist. For women of childbearing age, a **pregnancy** test is done to make sure the patient isn't pregnant; and elderly patients have an EKG done to make sure no potential heart problems exist. Some patients may have a stent placed prior to the lithotripsy procedure. A stent is a plastic tube placed in the ureter which allows the passage of gravel and urine after the ESWL procedure is completed.

Most patients have a lot of blood in their urine after the ESWL procedure. This is normal and should clear after several days to a week or so. Lots of fluids should be taken to encourage the flushing of any gravel remaining in the urinary system. The patient should follow up with the urologist in about two weeks to make sure that everything is going as planned. If a stent has been inserted, it is normally removed at this time. Patients may return to work whenever they feel able.

Abdominal pain is not uncommon after ESWL, but it is usually not cause to worry. However, persistent or severe abdominal pain may imply unexpected internal injury. Colicky renal pain is very common as gravel is still passing. Other problems may include perirenal hematomas (blood clots near the kidneys) in 66% of the cases; nerve palsies; **pancreatitis** (inflammation of the pancreas); and obstruction by stone fragments. Occasionally, stones may not be completely fragmented during the first ESWL treatment and further ESWL procedures may be required.

LIVER CANCER

Liver cancer is a form of **cancer** with a high mortality rate. Liver cancers can be classified into two types. They are either primary, when the cancer starts in the liver itself; or metastatic, when the cancer has spread to the liver from some other part of the body.

Primary liver cancer is a relatively rare disease in the United States, representing about 2% of all malignancies. It is, however, much more common in other parts of the world, representing from 10-50% of malignancies in Africa and parts of Asia. The American Cancer Society estimates that in 1998, at least 14,000 new cases of liver cancer will be diagnosed. It will also cause roughly 13,000 **death**s in the United States in 1998.

In adults, most primary liver cancers belong to one of two types: hepatomas, or hepatocellular carcinomas, which start in the liver tissue itself; and cholangiomas, or cholangiocarcinomas, which are cancers that develop in the bile ducts inside the liver. About 90% of primary liver cancers are hepatomas. In the United States, about five persons in every 200,000 will develop a hepatoma; in Africa and Asia, over 40 persons in 200,000 will develop this form of cancer. Two rare types of primary liver cancer are mixed-cell tumors and Kupffer cell sarcomas.

There is one type of primary liver cancer that usually occurs in children younger than four years of age and between the ages of 12-15. This type of childhood liver cancer is called a hepatoblastoma. Unlike liver cancers in adults, hepatoblastomas have a good chance of being treated successfully. Approximately 70% of children with hepatoblastomas experience complete cures. If the tumor is detected early, the survival rate is over 90%.

The second major category of liver cancer, metastatic liver cancer, is about 20 times as common in the United States as primary liver cancer. Because blood from all parts of the body must pass through the liver for filtration, cancer cells from other organs and tissues easily reach the liver, where they can lodge and grow into secondary tumors. Primary cancers in the colon, stomach, pancreas, rectum, esophagus, breast, lung, or skin are the most likely to spread (metastasize) to the liver. It is not unusual for the metastatic cancer in the liver to be the first noticeable sign of a cancer that started in another organ. After **cirrhosis**, metastatic liver cancer is the most common cause of fatal liver disease.

The exact cause of primary liver cancer is still unknown. In adults, however, certain factors are known to place some individuals at higher risk of developing liver cancer. These factors include:

- Male sex. The male/female ratio for hepatoma is 4:1.
- Age over 60 years
- Exposure to substances in the environment that tend to cause cancer (carcinogens). These include a substance produced by a mold that grows on rice and peanuts (aflatoxin); thorium dioxide, which was used at one time as a contrast dye for x rays of the liver; and vinyl chloride, used in manufacturing plastics.
- Use of oral estrogens for birth control
- Hereditary hemochromatosis. Hemochromatosis is a disorder characterized by abnormally high levels of iron storage in the body. It often develops into cirrhosis.
- Cirrhosis. Hepatomas appear to be a frequent complication of cirrhosis of the liver. Between 30-70% of hepatoma patients also have cirrhosis. It is estimated that a patient with cirrhosis has 40 times the chance of developing a hepatoma than a person with a healthy liver.
- Exposure to hepatitis B (HBV) or hepatitis C (HBC) viruses. In Africa and most of Asia, exposure to hepatitis B is an important factor; in Japan and some Western countries, exposure to hepatitis C is connected with a higher risk of developing liver cancer. In the United States, nearly 25% of patients with liver cancer show evidence of HBV infection. Hepatitis is commonly found among intravenous drug abusers.

The early symptoms of primary, as well as metastatic, liver cancer are often vague and not unique to liver disorders. The long lagtime between the beginning of the tumor's growth and signs of illness is the major reason why the disease has such a high mortality rate. At the time of diagnosis, patients are often tired, with **fever**, abdominal **pain**, and loss of appetite. They may look emaciated and generally ill. As the tumor grows bigger, it stretches the membrane surrounding the liver (the capsule), causing pain in the upper abdomen on the right side. The pain may extend into the back and shoulder. Some patients develop a collection of fluid, known as ascites, in the abdominal cavity. Others may show signs of bleeding into the digestive tract. In addition, the tumor may block the ducts of the liver or the gall bladder, leading to **jaundice**. In patients with jaundice, the whites of the eyes and the skin may turn yellow, and the urine becomes dark-colored.

If the doctor suspects a diagnosis of liver cancer, he or she will check the patient's history for risk factors and pay close attention to the condition of the patient's abdomen during the **physical examination**. Masses or lumps in the liver and ascites can often be felt while the patient is lying flat on the examination table. The liver is usually swollen and hard in patients with liver cancer; it may be sore when the doctor presses on it. In some cases, the patient's spleen is also enlarged. The doctor may be able to hear an abnormal sound (bruit) or rubbing noise (friction rub) if he or she uses a stethoscope to listen to the blood vessels that lie near the liver. The noises are caused by the pressure of the tumor on the blood vessels.

Blood tests may be used to test liver function or to evaluate risk factors in the patient's history. Between 50-75% of primary liver cancer patients have abnormally high blood serum levels of a particular protein (alpha-fetoprotein or AFP). The AFP test, however, cannot be used by itself to confirm a diagnosis of liver cancer, because cirrhosis or chronic hepatitis can also produce high alpha-fetoprotein levels. Tests for alkaline phosphatase, bilirubin, lactic dehydrogenase, and other chemicals indicate that the liver is not functioning normally. About 75% of patients with liver cancer show evidence of hepatitis infection. Again, however, abnormal liver function test results are not specific for liver cancer.

Imaging studies are useful in locating specific areas of abnormal tissue in the liver. Liver tumors as small as an inch across can now be detected by ultrasound or computed tomography scan (CT scan). Imaging studies, however, cannot tell the difference between a hepatoma and other abnormal masses or lumps of tissue (nodules) in the liver. A sample of liver tissue for biopsy is needed to make the definitive diagnosis of a primary liver cancer. CT or ultrasound can be used to guide the doctor in selecting the best location for obtaining the biopsy sample.

Chest x rays may be used to see whether the liver tumor is primary or has metastasized from a primary tumor in the lungs.

Liver biopsy is considered to provide the definite diagnosis of liver cancer. A sample of the liver or tissue fluid is removed with a fine needle and is checked under a microscope for the presence of cancer cells. In about 70% of cases, the biopsy is positive for cancer. In most cases, there is little risk to the patient from the biopsy procedure. In about 0.4% of cases, however, the patient develops a fatal hemorrhage from the biopsy because some tumors are supplied with a large number of blood vessels and bleed very easily.

The doctor may also perform a **laparoscopy** to help in the diagnosis of liver cancer. A laparoscope is a small tube-shaped instrument with a light at one end. The doctor makes a small cut in the patient's abdomen and inserts the laparoscope. A small piece of liver tissue is removed and examined under a microscope for the presence of cancer cells.

Treatment of liver cancer is based on several factors, including the type of cancer (primary or metastatic); stage (early or advanced); the location of other primary cancers or metastases in the patient's body; the patient's age; and other coexisting diseases, including cirrhosis. For many patients, treatment of liver cancer is primarily intended to relieve the pain caused by the cancer but cannot cure it.

Few liver cancers in adults can be cured by surgery because they are usually too advanced by the time they are discovered. If the cancer is contained within one lobe of the liver, and if the patient does not have either cirrhosis, jaundice, or ascites, surgery is the best treatment option. Patients who can have their entire tumor removed have the best chance for survival. Unfortunately, only about 5% of patients with metastatic cancer (from primary tumors in the colon or rectum) fall into this group. If the entire visible tumor can be removed, about 25% of patients will be cured. The operation that is performed is called a partial hepatectomy, or partial removal of the liver. The surgeon will remove either an entire lobe of the liver (a lobectomy) or cut out the area around the tumor (a wedge resection).

Some patients with metastatic cancer of the liver can have their lives prolonged for a few months by **chemotherapy**, although cure is not possible. If the tumor cannot be removed by surgery, a tube (catheter) can be placed in the main artery of the liver and an implantable infusion pump can be installed. The pump allows much higher concentrations of the cancer drug to be carried to the tumor than is possible with chemotherapy carried through the bloodstream. The drug that is used for infusion pump therapy is usually floxuridine (FUDR), given for 14-day periods alternating with 14-day rests. Systemic chemotherapy can also be used to treat liver cancer. The medications usually used are 5-fluorouracil (Adrucil, Efudex) or methotrexate (MTX, Mexate). Systemic chemotherapy does not, however, significantly lengthen the patient's survival time.

Radiation therapy is the use of high-energy rays or x rays to kill cancer cells or to shrink tumors. Its use in liver cancer, however, is only to give brief relief from some of the symptoms. Liver cancers are not sensitive to radiation, and radiation therapy will not prolong the patient's life.

Removal of the entire liver (total hepatectomy) and liver transplantation are used very rarely in treating liver cancer as of 1998. This is because very few patients are eligible for this procedure, either because the cancer has spread beyond the liver or because there are no suitable donors. Further research in the field of transplant immunology may make liver transplantation a possible treatment method for more patients in the future.

Liver cancer has a very poor prognosis because it is often not diagnosed until it has metastasized. Fewer than 10% of patients survive three years after the initial diagnosis; the overall five-year survival rate for patients with hepatomas is around 4%. Most patients with primary liver cancer die within several months of diagnosis. Patients with liver cancers that metastasized from cancers in the colon live slightly longer than those whose cancers spread from cancers in the stomach or pancreas.

There are no useful strategies at present for preventing metastatic cancers of the liver. Primary liver cancers, however, are 75-80% preventable. Current strategies focus on widespread **vaccination** for hepatitis B; early treatment of hereditary hemochromatosis; and screening of high-risk patients with alpha-fetoprotein testing and ultrasound examinations.

Lifestyle factors that can be modified in order to prevent liver cancer include avoidance of exposure to toxic chemicals and foods harboring molds that produce aflatoxin. Most important, however, is avoidance of alcohol and drug abuse. Alcohol abuse is responsible for 60-75% of cases of cirrhosis, which is a major risk factor for eventual development of primary liver cancer. Hepatitis is a widespread disease among persons who abuse intravenous drugs.

LIVER DISEASE

More than 25 million people in the United States suffer from liver disease, and more than 43,000 of those people die every year. The only remedy for advanced disease is a liver transplant. The liver, an essential organ, is located behind the lower ribs on the right side of the chest. The largest organ in the body, it processes food and most medications. As the blood leaves the stomach and intestines, it passes through the liver, picking up and carrying nutrients throughout the body. The liver also cleanses the blood, discharges waste products, maintains hormone balance, produces immune factors, stores iron, synthesizes blood clotting factors, and manufactures bile which is stored in the gallbladder and excreted into the intestines to aid digestion. Howard J. Worman, M.D. at Columbia University, lists more than 30 different liver diseases on a World Wide Web page entitled ''Diseases of the Liver.'' Perhaps the most common and critical of these are viral **hepatitis**, **cirrhosis**, gallstones, alcohol-related disorders, and **cancer**.

Hepatitis, or ''inflammation of the liver,'' is primarily caused by different strains of virus and affects more than five million Americans. Hepatitis A virus is a milder form which may last around six weeks. Hepatitis B and C, severe and often fatal, result in permanent liver damage—such as cancer and cirrhosis—in 50% of cases.

Cirrhosis, the seventh leading cause of death in the United States, can result from any injury or disease of the liver—including certain chemicals and poisons, severe reaction to certain drugs, a build up of copper or iron, and obstruction in the bile duct. However, hepatitis, alcohol abuse, and other viruses cause more than half the cirrhosis fatalities. Cirrhosis develops when damaged tissue forms scars, which obstruct blood flow, which, in turn, kills more cells. Symptoms can include enlarged liver and spleen, accumulation of fluid in the abdomen and body tissue, **jaundice** (yellowing of the skin and eyes), and vomiting large amounts of blood. Because the liver can no longer purify the blood, toxins are carried to the brain causing anything from poor concentration to **coma**, brain swelling, and **death**. Certain types of cirrhosis can be treated but never reversed.

Gallstones develop when cholesterol and/or bile pigment crystalize creating ''stones'' which, when passing through the bile duct, cause extreme abdominal pain. If stones become lodged, bile backs up, spills into the blood stream, causing jaundice. Ultimately, cirrhosis can develop. Approximately 500,000 people undergo surgery each year to remove gall stones, and dissolving drugs have some success.

Alcoholic liver diseases include steatosis (fatty liver), acute and chronic hepatitis—both of which can be reversible if patients stop drinking—cancer, and cirrhosis. Alcoholic cirrhosis is the tenth leading cause of death in the United States.

Liver cancer develops most often as a result of cancer spreading from other organs. Little is known about *primary liver cancers*, except that it is often associated with other liver diseases. Although only about 1,000 people die each year in the United States from primary liver cancer, the death rate is almost at epidemic proportions in Africa and the Orient. Researcher Brian Carr at the Starzel Transplant Institute at the University of Pittsburgh believes dietary **carcinogens** may be a culprit and, in particular, a mold called *Aspergillus flavus*, which grows on unrefrigerated cooked rice.

The incidence of liver disease is on the rise, perhaps because of increased use of medications and exposure to environmental chemicals. While liver diseases are still poorly understood, researchers believe almost half could be prevented through application of knowledge already available.

Living will

A living will is a legal document that lets a person decide in advance what kind of medical treatment he/she does and does not want if he/she become physically or mentally unable to make decisions or communicate his/her wishes. Also called a Directive to Physicians or Healthcare Directive, it is a type of advance directive. Although a living will is typically used to reject heroic lifesaving measures to prolong life, such as intravenous feeding and mechanical respirators when the patient is dying, it can also be used to request that all available medical treatment be used. A living will can be general or specific, but it is limited because the manner of death cannot be anticipated and medical technology changes rapidly. It is called a living will because it is a will that is used while the person is still alive.

In 1990, the U.S. Supreme Court affirmed the use of living wills. A living will creates a contract with the attending doctor. When the doctor receives the living will, he/she must honor its instructions or turn the patient's care over to another doctor who will do so. A person who has drafted a living will should make sure that his/her family, lawyer, and doctor know about it. A living will relieves family and friends from having to make tough decisions about actions to prolong a loved one's life. It can be changed or canceled at any time. Every state recognizes a patient's right to make choices about health care and treatment, but state laws about living wills are different. A living will can be drafted without an attorney, but it is important to make sure that it conforms with the state's requirements, including the proper signatures and witnesses. Some states require that certain forms be used for a living will.

A living will does not let a person name someone to make medical decisions for him/her. Many people combine a living will with a durable power of attorney for health care. A **durable power of attorney for health care** lets the person select someone to make health care decisions for him/her if he/she becomes incapacitated and gives that person the legal authority to make those decisions. Depending on what state a person lives in, it may be better to have a living will, a durable power of attorney for health care, or both. Having both documents provides maximum protection for the many medical situations which could arise and require difficult decisions. Decisions on medical care for a person who does not have a living will or durable power of attorney for health care are made by doctors. If there are questions, the doctors will ask a close relative for consent. If relatives disagree about the decision, the case would wind up in court and be decided by a judge.

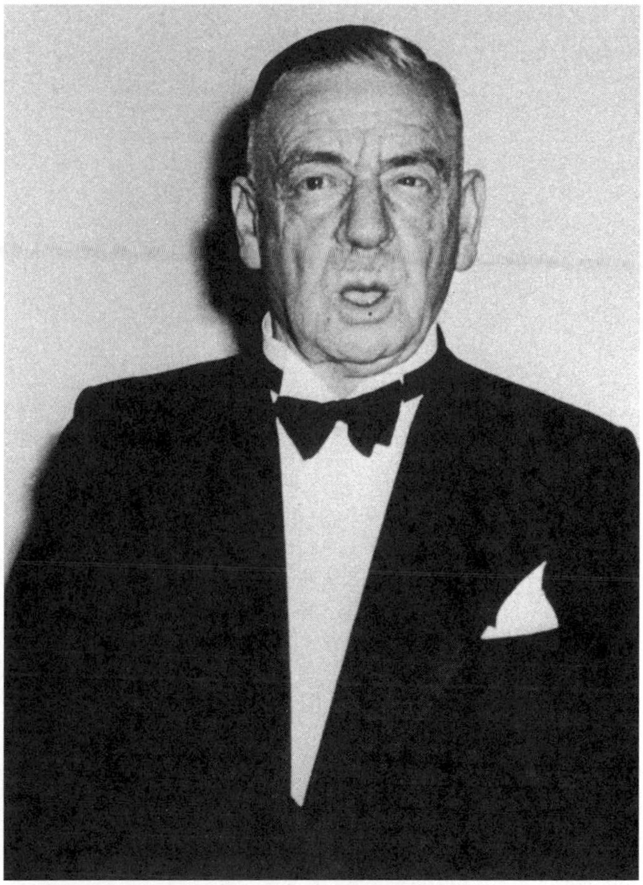

Otto Loewi

See also Durable power of attorney for health care

Loewi, Otto (1873-1961)

German American pharmacologist and physiologist

Otto Loewi (pronounced *lō–ee*) was born in Frankfurt am Main, Germany, on June 3, 1873. On the advice of his parents, Loewi entered the University of Strasbourg to study medicine, and received his medical degree in 1896. After graduation, he briefly visited Italy, and then returned to Germany for more training in chemistry and experimental methods. During this period, he also worked in the **tuberculosis** and **pneumonia** wards at the City Hospital of Frankfurt, where he was discouraged from continuing with clinical medicine because of high death rates. Instead, he turned his attention to an academic career in scientific research, and in 1898 he joined the department of pharmacology at the University of Marburg, first with an assistantship and then as a lecturer.

By 1902, Loewi had published the results of his scientific research at Marburg. His work dealt with the functioning of the kidneys and the effects on these organs of substances that increase the production of urine, known as **diuretics**. In 1903, along with other researchers including **Henry Hallett Dale**, Loewi began to consider the chemical transmission of nerve impulses. The hormone adrenaline and the chemical muscarine had already been identified as possible nerve transmitters by several English physiologists. In 1905, Loewi followed Hans Meyer, under whom he had worked at Marburg, to the University of Vienna. The same year, he met Gulda Goldschmiedt, the daughter of a chemistry professor, in Switzerland, and he married her the following year. They would have four children.

At the University of Vienna, Loewi concentrated on the effects of adrenaline and noradrenaline on **diabetes** and blood pressure. He also studied the response of the heart to the stimulation of the vagus nerve, one of the main cranial nerves in the autonomic system. In 1909, he was appointed to the University of Graz as a professor of pharmacology, where he remained until the German occupation of Austria in 1938.

By 1921, fifteen years after the idea of chemical transmission of nerve impulses had first been proposed by the English physiologists, scientists had still not discovered definite evidence of the existence of a chemical transmitter within the **nervous system**. One night Loewi had a dream that would help; he dreamed the design of an experiment that would determine the existence of a chemical transmitter. He jotted down some notes from the dream, still half asleep, but when he awoke the next morning he could not read his scrawl. The next night at three o'clock the idea returned to him; this time he immediately went to his laboratory.

For this pathbreaking experiment, Loewi used two hearts from frogs. He removed the vagus nerve from the first heart, and he stimulated the same nerve in the second one. After stimulating the nerve in the second heart, he removed some fluid and injected it into the heart without the vagus nerve. He observed that the rate of this heart slowed as if the vagus nerve had been stimulated. Then he stimulated the heart with the vagus nerve so it would beat faster. He again removed fluid and injected it into the heart without the vagus nerve. Its rate increased as if it had been stimulated directly by the missing nerve.

Loewi had established the role chemicals play in the transmission of nerve impulses, but he was not sure at first what these chemicals were. He called one "vagus substance" and the other "accelerator substance." Over the next fifteen years, Loewi, along with his colleagues, published a number of papers on the results of his initial experiment. What he had called vagus substance was identified as acetylcholine in 1926; other transmitters were later identified. In 1936, Loewi identified adrenaline as one of the sympathetic nervous system transmitters and noradrenaline as the most important one. Henry Hallett Dale shared the 1936 Nobel Prize with Loewi for his discovery of chemical transmitters in the voluntary nervous system.

After the German occupation of Austria in 1938, Loewi was only allowed to leave because he turned over his Nobel Prize money to the Nazis. His family was also able to escape, and they joined him in New York City in 1940. He became a United States citizen in 1946. He spent the rest of his life writing articles, delivering lectures, and writing his memoirs. He died on December 25, 1961, at the age of 88 in New York City.

LOGAN, MYRA A. (1908-1977)

African American physician and surgeon

Myra A. Logan fulfilled the image of the selfless, humanitarian doctor, practicing medicine to serve the community rather than simply to earn money. An urbane, modest person who never lost sight of her civic responsibilities, she is thought to be the first African American woman elected a fellow of the American College of Surgeons, and was the first woman to perform open heart surgery. Additionally, her research on **antibiotics** and **breast cancer** saved countless lives.

Myra Adele Logan was born in 1908 in Tuskegee, Alabama, the eighth child of Warren and Adella Hunt Logan. She enjoyed a relatively privileged upbringing, for her father was a trustee and treasurer of the prestigious Tuskegee Institute and her mother was a noted activist in health care and the suffrage movement. Booker T. Washington was a neighbor. Education and optimism were in the air of the Logan household, as was an interest in health care: in addition to her mother, Logan also had an aunt and sister who were or became involved in health matters, and her brother, Arthur, as well as a brother-in-law, was a physician. Logan attended Atlanta University in Georgia, graduating with a B.A. in 1927 as valedictorian of her class. She went north for graduate studies, taking her M.S. in psychology from Columbia University in New York. After working for a time on a YWCA staff in Connecticut, Logan finally made up her mind to study medicine, winning the first Walter Gray Crump $10,000 four-year scholarship to New York Medical College. She graduated in 1933 and interned as well as served her residency at Harlem Hospital in New York.

Her years at Harlem Hospital in the emergency room and riding ambulance as a young internee prepared Logan well for her future career in surgery. She not only delivered babies on the way to the hospital, but also repaired numerous stab wounds to the heart. Remaining at Harlem Hospital, she became an associate surgeon there, and was also a visiting surgeon at Sydenham Hospital. In 1943 she became the first woman to perform open heart surgery, in the ninth operation of its kind anywhere in the world. She also became interested in the then-new antibiotic drugs, researching aureomycin and other drugs and publishing her results in *Archives of Surgery* and *Journal of American Medical Surgery.* In the 1960s, Logan began to work on breast cancer, developing a slower x-ray process that could detect more accurately differences in the density of tissue and thus help discover tumors much earlier. In addition to maintaining a private practice, she was also a charter member of one of the first group practices in the nation, the Upper Manhattan Medical Group of the Health Insurance Plan, a concept that houses physicians of various specialties under one roof and that is the norm today.

Logan found time in her busy schedule to stay committed to social issues. Early in her career, she was a member of the New York State Committee on Discrimination, but resigned in protest in 1944 when Governor Dewey ignored the anti-discrimination legislation the committee had proposed. She was also active in Planned Parenthood as well as the National Association for the Advancement of Colored People (NAACP), and after her retirement in 1970 she served on the New York State Workmen's Compensation Board. Her myriad medical and civic achievements led to her election to the American College of Surgeons.

Logan married the well known painter Charles Alston in 1943. The couple had no children, devoting their lives to professional pursuits. She was a lover of music and a fine classical pianist. She also enjoyed the theater and reading. Myra Adele Logan died at Mount Sinai Hospital in New York on January 13, 1977, of lung cancer at the age of 68. Her husband, Charles Alston, died only a few months later.

LONG, CRAWFORD WILLIAMSON (1815-1878)

American physician

Long was the first physician to use ether to anesthetize a patient in surgery. Long performed his ground-breaking surgery in 1842, but the credit for the first public demonstration of the anesthetic effects of ether went to **William Thomas Green Morton**, who demonstrated its use in 1846.

Long was born November 1, 1815, in Danielsville, Georgia, to James and Elizabeth Long. He received his bachelor's degree from the University of Georgia in Athens, Georgia, in1835, and his Doctor of Medicine degree from the University of Pennsylvania School of Medicine in 1839. After a year and a half practicing medicine in several hospitals in New York City, he returned to Jefferson, Georgia, a small, country town, where he became a general practitioner. In August, 1842, he married Caroline Swain. They had six children.

Long performed his famous surgery a few months before he was married. For years, people had known that nitrous oxide (laughing gas) and ether made people feel exhilarated and intoxicated. Some people even held "ether frolics," or parties in which they inhaled ether for fun. Long had been to such parties, and had noticed that people suffered no pain if they fell down. One of Long's acquaintances, James M. Venables had used ether himself at social events, and wanted some cysts removed from his neck. In his office on the evening of March 30, 1842, Long soaked a towel with ether and had Venables inhale it. While Venables was unconscious, Long surgically removed his cysts. When Venables woke up, he was surprised that he had no cysts and no pain. Long charged Venables $2 for the surgery and anesthesia. Long continued to use ether in minor surgical procedures and obstetrics for years to come, but he did not publish his discovery until 1849, three years after William Thomas Green Morton had created a huge stir in Boston, Massachusetts, with his public demonstration of the powers of ether.

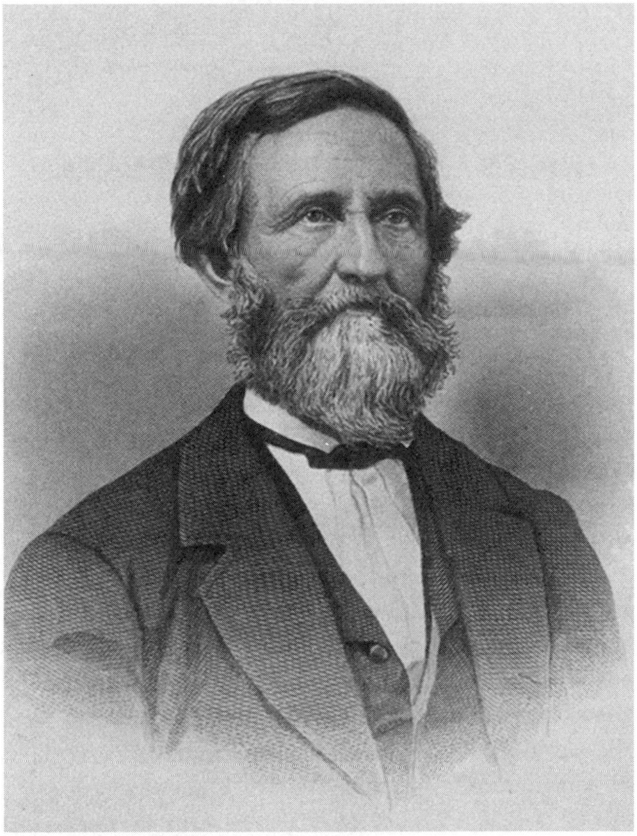

Crawford Williamson Long

In 1850, Long moved back to Athens, Georgia. There he spent the rest of his life, practicing medicine. He died in Athens on June 16, 1878.

See also William Thomas Green Morton

LONG-TERM CARE

About one out of eight Americans is over the age of 65. While Americans are remaining active longer and living longer than in the past, **aging** and its attendant illness can make it difficult for a person to manage without help. The system of health care that takes care of the many varied needs of older Americans is long-term care.

In the past, long-term care meant simply a nursing home. As people remain vital longer and as the health care needs of the elderly change, however, new alternatives have sprung up in the field of long-term care.

Long-term care can mean a **nursing home**. Nursing homes provide various levels of care. Some facilities provide skilled nursing care, with care delivered by nurses (both registered nurses and licensed practical nurses), following the orders of a physician. Skilled nursing facilities are not limited to helping elderly patients. Younger persons who have suffered debilitating illness or accidents may be placed in a skilled nursing facility for a short period of rehabilitation. Other nursing homes provide intermediate care (for patients who are more mobile but still need medical care from professionals), or custodial care (for patients who do not need constant medical care but who can no longer live on their own).

Long-term care, however, includes more than just nursing homes. Elderly people have varying degrees of independence, which long-term care professional describe as their activities of daily living (ADLs). ADLs include bathing, preparing and eating meals, using the toilet, dressing and getting around.

Some elderly people may still be able to manage their ADLs on their own, but may be finding a house too much to take care of. A person like this may find an ideal living situation in an independent living facility, where people live in their own apartments in a secure building.

A person who is able to live independently but needs nursing care may find home care to be the ideal solution. In home care, a nurse will visit every day or every other day and provide medical care, such as changing the dressing on wounds.

A person who cannot quite manage his or her ADLs but doesn't need the constant nursing care that would be found in a nursing home can move into a relatively new kind of long-term care, an assisted living facility. Assisted living facilities provide residents with their own apartments and usually provide daily maid service and meals, which may be served in a communal dining room. Assisted living residents often have access to on-site medical care if they need it.

Other levels of care also exist. If an elderly person lives with an adult child who is uncomfortable with leaving Mom or Dad home alone during the day, adult day care can be the answer. At an adult day care facility, the elderly person can enjoy social activities and meals and return home at night. This is also a good alternative for an older person who wants to live independently but needs some help during the day.

Continuing care retirement communities are seniors-only communities that provide a spectrum of care options from independent living to nursing home care.

Another form of long-term care is hospice care. Hospice care provides care and compassion to people who are dying, such as terminally ill cancer patients. The goal of hospice is to make patients as comfortable as possible, either in a home or a nursing-facility setting.

Paying for these many levels of care is a growing issue. In 1995,the U.S. General Accounting Office estimated that spending for long-term care totaled almost $91 billion. Of that amount, 60% was paid for by Medicaid, but 40% (over $36 billion) came out of the pockets of the elderly and their families, particularly their adult children. About 48% of people have done little or no planning for long-term care, and 80% of the post-World War II generation have little idea how long-term care is paid for. It is no wonder, then, that long-term care insurance is an area of increasing interest to both the elderly and their children.

However, a survey of Baby Boomers also indicated that a quarter of them were not willing to pay for extra insurance to cover the expense of long-term care.

See also Aging; Health insurance; Nursing homes

LORENZ, KONRAD (1903-1989)

Austrian zoologist and ethologist

Konrad Lorenz was born on November 7, 1903, in Vienna, Austria, as the younger of two sons born to Adolf Lorenz and his wife and assistant, Emma Lecher. Lorenz's love of animals began outside of school, primarily at the family's summer home in Altenberg, Austria, and his interests became more grounded in science when he read about Charles Darwin's evolutionary theory at the age of 10. In 1922, Lorenz began premedical training at Columbia University in New York but returned early to Austria to continue the program at the University of Vienna. Despite his medical studies, Lorenz found time to informally study animals. He also kept a detailed diary of the activities of his pet bird Jock, a jackdaw. In 1927, his career as an animal behaviorist was launched when an ornithological journal printed his jackdaw diary. During the following year, he received an M.D. degree from the University of Vienna and became an assistant to a professor at the anatomical institute there. His interests led him to study zoology at the University of Vienna, and in 1933, Lorenz earned his Ph.D. in that field.

Lorenz developed the theories for which he is best known during the years 1935 to 1938. He spent what he called his "goose summers" at the Altenberg home, concentrating on the behavior of greylag geese and confirming many hypotheses that he had formed while observing his pet birds. While working with the geese, Lorenz developed the concept of imprinting. Imprinting occurs in many species, most noticeably in geese and ducks, when—within a short, genetically set time frame—an animal will accept a foster mother in the place of its biological mother, even if that foster mother is a different species.

In addition, he and **Nikolaas Tinbergen**, future Nobel Prize cowinner, developed the concept of the innate releasing mechanism. Lorenz found that animals have instinctive behavior patterns, or fixed-action patterns, that remain dormant until a specific event triggers the animal to exhibit this behavior for the first time. The fixed-action pattern is a specific, ordered series of behaviors, such as the fighting and surrender postures used by many animals. He emphasized that these fixed-action patterns are not learned but are genetically programmed. The stimulus is called the "releaser," and the nervous system structure that responds to the stimulus and prompts the instinctive behavior is the innate releasing mechanism. Lorenz later devised a hydraulic model to explain an animal's motivation to perform fixed-action patterns.

While the research continued, Lorenz accepted an appointment in 1937 as lecturer in comparative anatomy and animal psychology at the University of Vienna. In 1940, he became professor of psychology at the University of Konigsberg in Germany but a year later answered the call to serve in the German Army. In 1944, Lorenz was captured by the Russians and sent to a prison camp. It was not until 1948 that he was released. Upon his return, Lorenz went back to the University of Vienna before accepting a small stipend from the Max Planck Society for the Advancement of Science to resume his studies at Altenberg. By 1952, Lorenz had published a popular book *King Solomon's Ring,* an account of animal behavior presented in easily understood terminology. Included in the book are many of his often-humorous experiences with his study subjects. The book also includes a collection of his illustrations.

In 1955, with the increased support of the Max Planck Society, Lorenz, ethologist Gustav Kramer, and physiologist Erich von Holst established and then codirected the Institute for Behavioral Physiology in Seewiesen, Bavaria, near Munich. During the ensuing years at Seewiesen, Lorenz again drew attention, this time for the analogies he drew between human and animal behavior—which many scientists felt were improper—and his continuing work on instinct. Following the deaths of codirectors von Holst and Kramer, Lorenz became the sole director of the Seewiesen Institute in 1961.

In 1966, Lorenz again faced some controversy with his book *On Aggression,* an example of his shift from solely studying animal behavior to including human social behavior. In the book, Lorenz describes aggression as ''the fighting instinct in beast and man which is directed against members of same species.'' He writes that this instinct aids the survival of both the individual and the species, in the latter case by giving the stronger males the better mating opportunities and territories. The book goes on to state that animals will use rank, territory, or evolved instinctual behavior patterns to avoid actual violence and fatalities. Lorenz says only humans purposefully kill each other—a fact that he attributes to the development of artificial weapons outpacing the human evolution of killing inhibitions.

In 1973, Lorenz, Tinbergen, and Karl Frisch, who studied bee communication, jointly accepted the Nobel Prize for their behavioral research. In the same year, Lorenz retired from his position as director of the Seewiesen institute. He then returned to Altenberg where he continued writing and began directing the department of animal sociology at the Austrian Academy of Science. In addition, the Max Planck Society for the Promotion of Science set up a research station for him at his ancestral home in Altenberg.

In 1927, the same year his career-launching diary was published, Lorenz married childhood friend Margarethe ''Gretl'' Gebhardt, a gynecologist. They had two daughters, Agnes and Dagmar, and a son, Thomas. Lorenz died February 27, 1989, of kidney failure at his home in Altenburg, Austria, at age 85.

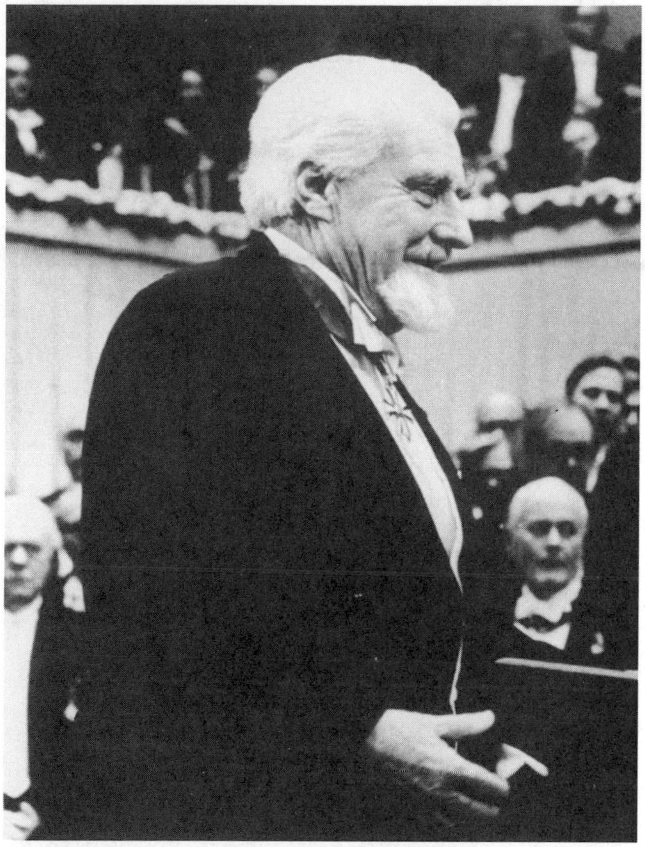

Konrad Lorenz

Lou Gehrig's disease

Amyotrophic lateral sclerosis (ALS) is a disease that breaks down tissues in the nervous system (a neurodegenerative disease) of unknown cause that affects the nerves responsible for movement. It is also known as motor neuron disease and Lou Gehrig's disease, after the baseball player whose career it ended.

ALS is a disease of the motor neurons, those nerve cells reaching from the brain to the spinal cord (upper motor neurons) and the spinal cord to the peripheral nerves (lower motor neurons) that control muscle movement. In ALS, for unknown reasons, these neurons die, leading to a progressive loss of the ability to move virtually any of the muscles in the body. ALS affects ''voluntary'' muscles, those controlled by conscious thought, such as the arm, leg, and trunk muscles. ALS, in and of itself, does not affect sensation, thought processes, the heart muscle, or the ''smooth'' muscle of the digestive system, bladder, and other internal organs. Most people with ALS retain function of their eye muscles as well. However, various forms of ALS may be associated with a loss of intellectual function (**dementia**) or sensory symptoms.

''Amyotrophic'' refers to the loss of muscle bulk, a cardinal sign of ALS. ''Lateral'' indicates one of the regions of the spinal cord affected, and ''sclerosis'' describes the hardened tissue that develops in place of healthy nerves. ALS affects approximately 30,000 people in the United States, with about 5,000 new cases each year. It usually begins between the ages of 40 and 70, although younger onset is possible. Men are slightly more likely to develop ALS than women.

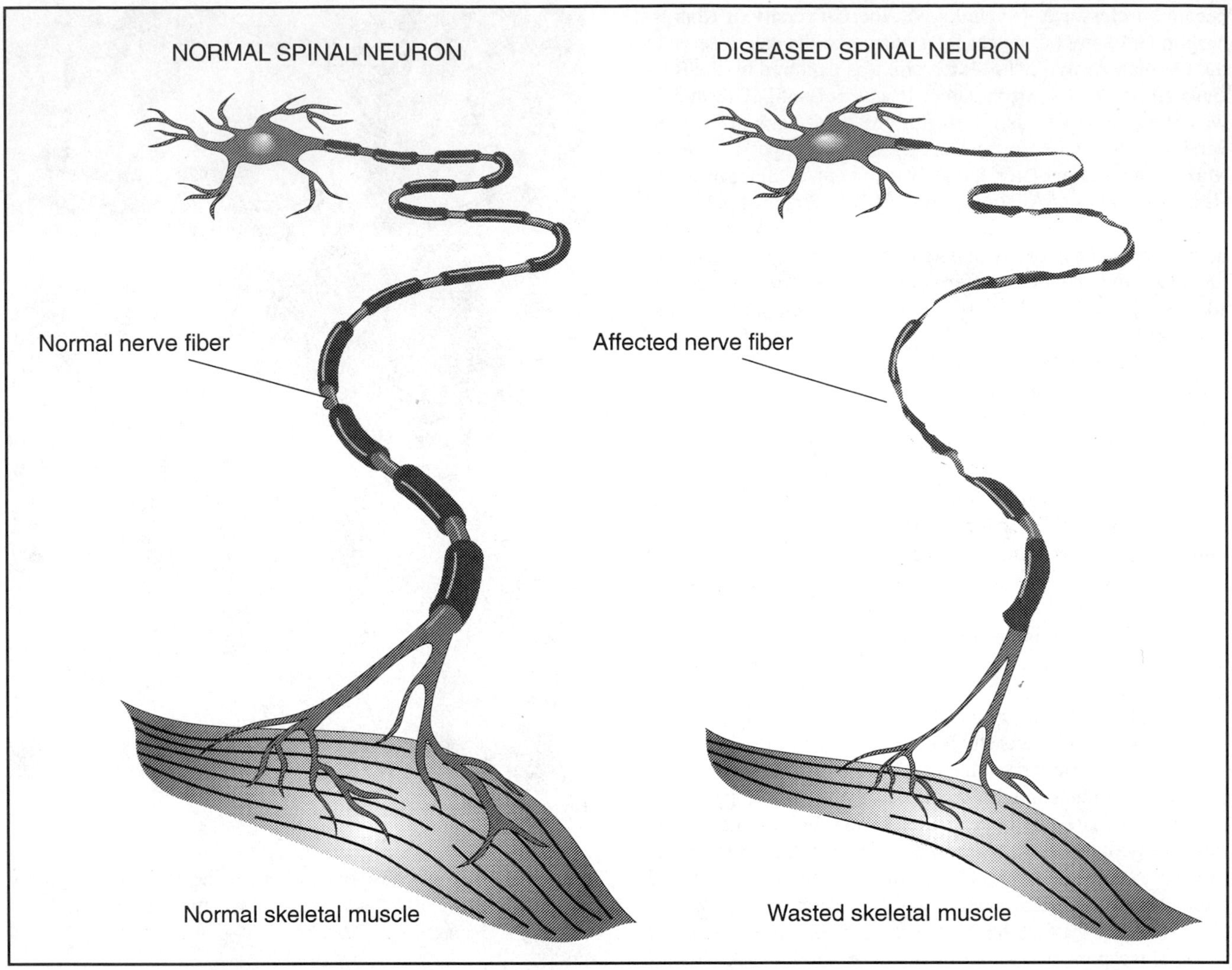

Amyotrophic lateral sclerosis (ALS) is caused by the degeneration and death of motor neurons in the spinal cord and brain. These neurons convey electrical messages from the brain to the muscles to stimulate movement in the arms, legs, trunk, neck, and head. As motor neurons degenerate, the muscles are weakened and cannot move as effectively, leading to muscle wasting. ***(Illustration by Electronic Illustrators Group.)***

ALS progresses rapidly in most cases. It is fatal within three years for 50% of all people affected, and within five years for 80%. Ten percent of people with ALS live beyond eight years.

The symptoms of ALS are caused by the death of motor neurons in the spinal cord and brain. Normally, these neurons convey electrical messages from the brain to the muscles to stimulate movement in the arms, legs, trunk, neck, and head. As motor neurons die, the muscles cannot be moved as effectively, and weakness results. In addition, lack of stimulation leads to muscle wasting, or loss of bulk. Involvement of the upper motor neurons causes spasms and increased tone in the limbs, and abnormal reflexes. Involvement of the lower motor neurons causes muscle wasting and twitching (fasciculations).

Two major forms of ALS are known: familial and sporadic. Familial ALS accounts for about 10% of all ALS cases. As the name suggests, familial ALS is believed to be caused by the inheritance of one or more faulty genes. About 15% of families with this type of ALS have mutations in the gene for SOD-1. SOD-1 gene defects are dominant, meaning only one gene copy is needed to develop the disease. Therefore, a parent with the faulty gene has a 50% chance of passing the gene along to a child.

Sporadic ALS has no known cause. While many environmental toxins have been suggested as causes, to date no research has confirmed any of the candidates investigated, including aluminum and metal dental fillings. As research progresses, it is likely that many cases of sporadic ALS will be shown to have a genetic basis as well.

A third type, called Western Pacific ALS, occurs in Guam and other Pacific islands. This form combines symptoms of both ALS and **Parkinson's disease**.

The earliest sign of ALS is most often weakness in the arms or legs, usually more pronounced on one side than the other at first. Loss of function is usually more rapid in the legs among people with familial ALS and in the arms among those with sporadic ALS. Leg weakness may first become apparent by an increased frequency of stumbling on uneven pavement, or an unexplained difficulty climbing stairs. Arm weakness may lead to difficulty grasping and holding a cup, for instance, or loss of dexterity in the fingers.

Less often, the earliest sign of ALS is weakness in the *bulbar* muscles, those muscles in the mouth and throat that control chewing, swallowing, and speaking. A person with bulbar weakness may become hoarse or tired after speaking at length, or speech may become slurred.

In addition to weakness, the other cardinal signs of ALS are muscle wasting and persistent twitching (fasciculation). These are usually seen after weakness becomes obvious. Fasciculation is quite common in people without the disease, and is virtually never the first sign of ALS.

While initial weakness may be limited to one region, ALS almost always progresses rapidly to involve virtually all the voluntary muscle groups in the body. Later symptoms include loss of the ability to walk, to use the arms and hands, to speak clearly or at all, to swallow, and to hold the head up. Weakness of the respiratory muscles makes breathing and coughing difficult, and poor swallowing control increases the likelihood of inhalation of food or saliva (aspiration). Aspiration increases the likelihood of lung infection, which is often the cause of death. With a ventilator and scrupulous bronchial hygiene, a person with ALS may live much longer than the average, although weakness and wasting will continue to erode any remaining functional abilities. Most people with ALS continue to retain function of the extraocular muscles that move the eyes, allowing some communication to take place with simple blinks or through use of a computer-assisted device.

The diagnosis of ALS begins with a complete medical history and physical exam, plus a neurological exam to determine the distribution and extent of weakness. An electrical test of muscle function, called an electromyogram, or EMG, is an important part of the diagnostic process. Various other tests, including blood and urine tests, x rays, and CT scans, may be done to rule out other possible causes of the symptoms, such as tumors of the skull base or high cervical spinal cord, thyroid disease, spinal arthritis, **lead poisoning**, or severe vitamin deficiency. ALS is rarely misdiagnosed following a careful review of all these factors.

There is no cure for ALS, and no treatment that can significantly alter its course. There are many things which can be done, however, to help maintain quality of life and to retain functional ability even in the face of progressive weakness.

As of early 1998, only one drug had been approved for treatment of ALS. Riluzole (Rilutek) appears to provide on average a three-month increase in life expectancy when taken regularly early in the disease, and shows a significant slowing of the loss of muscle strength. Riluzole acts by decreasing glutamate release from nerve terminals. Experimental trials of nerve growth factor have not demonstrated any benefit. No other drug or vitamin currently available has been shown to have any effect on the course of ALS.

A physical therapist works with the patient and family to implement **exercise** and stretching programs to maintain

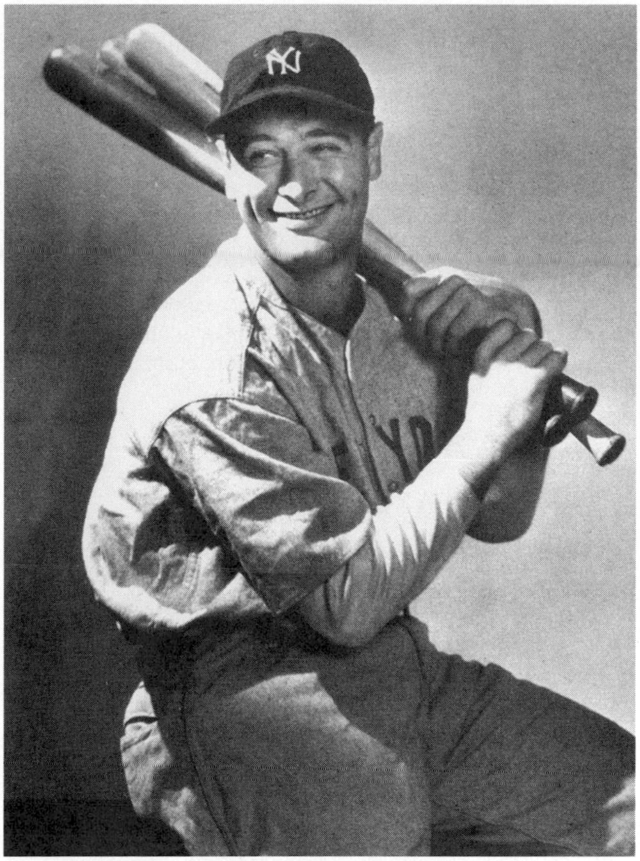

Lou Gehrig

strength and range of motion, and to promote general health. Swimming may be a good choice for people with ALS, as it provides a low-impact workout to most muscle groups. One result of chronic inactivity is contracture, or muscle shortening. Contractures limit a person's range of motion, and are often painful. Regular stretching can prevent contracture. Several drugs are available to reduce cramping, a common complaint in ALS.

An occupational therapist can help design solutions to movement and coordination problems, and provide advice on adaptive devices and home modifications.

Speech and swallowing difficulties can be minimized or delayed through training provided by a speech-language pathologist. This specialist can also provide advice on communication aids, including computer-assisted devices and simpler word boards.

Nutritional advice can be provided by a nutritionist. A person with ALS often needs softer foods to prevent jaw exhaustion or **choking**. Later in the disease, nutrition may be provided by a gastrostomy tube inserted into the stomach.

Mechanical ventilation may be used when breathing becomes too difficult. Modern mechanical ventilators are small and portable, allowing a person with ALS to maintain the maximum level of function and mobility. Ventilation may be administered through a mouth or nose piece, or through a tracheostomy tube. This tube is inserted through a small hole made in the windpipe. In addition to providing direct access to the airway, the tube also decreases aspiration. While many people with rapidly progressing ALS choose not to use ventilators for lengthy periods, they are increasingly used to prolong life for a short time.

The progressive nature of ALS means that most patients will eventually require full-time nursing care. This care is often provided by the spouse or other family member. While the skills involved are not difficult to learn, the physical and emotional burden of care can be overwhelming. Caregivers need to recognize and provide for their own needs as well as those of the patient, to prevent depression, burnout, and bitterness.

Low back pain

Low back pain is a common musculoskeletal symptom that may be either acute or chronic. It may be caused by a variety of diseases and disorders that affect the lumbar spine. Low back pain is often accompanied by sciatica, which is **pain** that involves the sciatic nerve and is felt in the lower back, the buttocks, and the backs of the thighs.

Low back pain is a symptom that affects 80% of the general United States population at some point in life with sufficient severity to cause absence from work. It is the second most common reason for visits to primary care doctors, and is estimated to cost the American economy $75 billion every year.

Low back pain may be experienced in several different ways:

- Localized. In localized pain the patient will feel soreness or discomfort when the doctor palpates, or presses on, a specific surface area of the lower back.
- Diffuse. Diffuse pain is spread over a larger area and comes from deep tissue layers.
- Radicular. The pain is caused by irritation of a nerve root. Sciatica is an example of radicular pain.
- Referred. The pain is perceived in the lower back but is caused by inflammation elsewhere—often in the kidneys or lower abdomen.

Acute pain in the lower back that does not extend to the leg is most commonly caused by a sprain or muscle tear, usually occurring within 24 hours of heavy lifting or overuse of the back muscles. The pain is usually localized, and there may be muscle spasms or soreness when the doctor touches the area. The patient usually feels better when resting.

Chronic low back pain has several different possible causes:

Mechanical reasons. Chronic strain on the muscles of the lower back may be caused by **obesity**; **pregnancy**; or job-related stooping, bending, or other stressful postures.

Malignancy. Low back pain at night that is not relieved by lying down may be caused by a tumor in the cauda equina (the roots of the spinal nerves controlling sensation in and movement of the legs), or a **cancer** that has spread to the spine from the prostate, breasts, or lungs. The risk factors for the spread of cancer to the lower back include a history of smoking, sudden weight loss, and age over 50.

Ankylosing spondylitis is a form of arthritis that causes chronic pain in the lower back. The pain is made worse by sitting or lying down and improves when the patient gets up. It is most commonly seen in males between 16 and 35. Ankylosing spondylitis is often confused with mechanical back pain in its early stages.

Disk herniation is a disorder in which a spinal disk begins to bulge outward between the vertebrae. Herniated or ruptured disks are a common cause of chronic low back pain in adults.

Back pain that is out of proportion to a minor injury, or that is unusually prolonged, may be associated with a somatoform disorder or other psychiatric disturbance.

Low back pain that radiates down the leg usually indicates involvement of the sciatic nerve. The nerve can be pinched or irritated by **herniated disk**s, tumors of the cauda equina, **abscess**es in the space between the spinal cord and its covering, spinal stenosis, and compression **fractures**. Some patients experience numbness or weakness of the legs as well as pain.

The diagnosis of low back pain can be complicated. Most cases are initially evaluated by primary care physicians rather than by specialists.

When beginning an initial workup of the patient's history, the doctor will ask the patient specific questions about the location of the pain, its characteristics, its onset, and the body positions or activities that make it better or worse. If the doctor suspects that the pain is referred from other organs, he or she will ask about a history of diabetes, peptic **ulcers**, **kidney stones**, urinary tract infections, or **heart murmurs**.

During the physical examination, the doctor will examine the patient's back and hips to check for conditions that require surgery or emergency treatment. The examination includes several tests that involve moving the patient's legs in specific positions to test for nerve root irritation or disk herniation. The flexibility of the lumbar vertebrae may be measured to rule out ankylosing spondylitis.

Imaging studies are not usually performed on patients whose history and **physical examination** suggest routine muscle strain or overuse. X rays are ordered for patients whose symptoms suggest cancer, infection, inflammation, pelvic or abdominal disease, or bone fractures. MRIs are usually ordered only for patients with certain types of masses or tumors.

It is important to know that the appearance of some abnormalities on imaging studies of the lower back does not necessarily indicate that they cause the pain. Many patients have minor deformities that do not create symptoms. The doctor must compare the results of imaging studies very carefully with information from the patient's history and physical examination.

All forms of treatment of low back pain are aimed either at symptom relief or to prevent interference with the processes of healing. None of these methods appear to speed up healing.

Acute back pain is treated with nonsteroidal anti-inflammatory drugs (NSAIDs), such as ibuprofen, **muscle re-**

laxants, or **aspirin**. Applications of heat or cold compresses are also helpful to most patients. If the patient has not experienced some improvement after several weeks of treatment, the doctor will reinvestigate the cause of the pain.

Patients with chronic back pain are treated with a combination of medications, physical therapy, and occupational or lifestyle modification. The medications given are usually NSAIDs, although patients with **hypertension**, kidney problems, or stomach ulcers should not take these drugs. Patients who take NSAIDs for longer than six weeks should be monitored periodically for complications.

Physical therapy for chronic low back pain usually includes regular **exercise** for fitness and flexibility, and **massage** or application of heat if necessary. Lifestyle modifications include giving up smoking, weight reduction (if necessary), and evaluation of the patient's occupation or other customary activities. Patients with herniated disks are treated surgically if the pain does not respond to medication. Patients with chronic low back pain sometimes benefit from **pain management** techniques, including **biofeedback**, **acupuncture**, and **chiropractic** manipulation of the spine.

Psychotherapy is recommended for patients whose back pain is associated with a somatoform, **anxiety**, or depressive disorder.

Treatment of sciatica and other disorders that involve the legs may include NSAIDs. Patients with long-standing sciatica or spinal stenosis that do not respond to NSAIDs are treated surgically. Although some doctors use cortisone injections to relieve the pain, this form of treatment is still debated.

A thorough differential diagnosis is important before any treatment is considered. There are times when alternative therapies are the most beneficial, and other times when more invasive treatments are needed.

Chiropractic treats patients by manipulating or adjusting sections of the spine. It is one of the most popular forms of alternative treatment in the United States for relief of back pain caused by straining or lifting injuries. Some osteopathic physicians, physical therapists, and naturopathic physicians also use spinal manipulation to treat patients with low back pain.

Practitioners of traditional Chinese medicine treat low back pain with acupuncture, *tui na* (push-and-rub) massage, and the application of herbal poultices.

Herbal medicine can utilize a variety of antispasmodic herbs in combination to help relieve low back pain due to spasm. Lobelia (*Lobelia inflata*) and myrrh (*Commiphora molmol*) are two examples of antispasmodic herbs.

Homeopathic treatment for acute back pain consists of applications of *Arnica* oil to the sore area or oral doses of *Arnica* or *Rhus toxicodendron*. *Bellis perennis* is recommended for deep muscle injuries. Other remedies may be recommended based on the symptoms presented by the patient.

Massage and the numerous other body work techniques can be very effective in treating low back pain. Yoga, practiced regularly and done properly, can be most useful in preventing future episodes of low back pain.

The prognosis for most patients with acute low back pain is excellent. About 80% of patients recover completely in 4-6 weeks. The prognosis for recovery from chronic pain depends on the underlying cause.

Low back pain due to muscle strain can be prevented by lifestyle choices, including regular physical exercise and weight control, avoiding smoking, and learning the proper techniques for lifting and moving heavy objects. Exercises designed to strengthen the muscles of the lower back, and chairs or car seats with lumbar supports are also recommended.

LOW BIRTHWEIGHT

Low birthweight is defined as being less than 2500 grams (or 5.5 pounds) at birth, with premature birth being a common cause of such low birthweight babies.

Birthweight is one of the key indicators of the health and viability of a newborn infant. It is one of the leading causes of infant mortality. Low birthweight infants are 40 times more likely to die in their first month of life than normal birthweight infants. They are also twice as likely as other infants to exhibit health problems and serious developmental delays during childhood.

Several factors contribute to low birthweight. These include teenage pregnancies, unwanted or unintended pregnancies, lack of prenatal care, poor nutrition during pregnancy leading to poor maternal weight gain, maternal smoking, and the use of alcohol and other drugs during pregnancy. All of these factors are preventable, and are called ''preventable risk factors.''

Maternal age, maternal health, fetal infection, ethnicity, multiple births, socio-economic status, genetic makeup, obstetric history, and a variety of genetic and metabolic disorders can also contribute to low birthweight. Women over 45 years and under 20 years of age are more likely to have a low birthweight baby. African American infants are twice as likely as infants of all other racial groups in American to be born low birthweight. Poor families are at a higher risk of having low birthweight babies. Multiple births also pose an increased risk of low birthweight. Despite that, the rate of triplets and other multiple births are on an increase because of the usage of fertility drugs.

The belief that a mother's psychological state can influence her unborn baby exists in many cultures all around the world. By the same token, it has been shown that mothers who live in high risk neighborhoods and encounter crime, poverty, and violence on a daily basis are very likely to have low birth weight babies. This may be because of the stress in their lives. Stress has been shown to reduce blood flow to the uterus and that could possibly slow fetal growth.

The problems of being low birthweight do not resolve even if the infant survives the first year after birth. As a group, these infants have higher rates of developmental problems, subnormal growth, and health problems than other children. By school age, these children are more likely to have **learning disabilities**, **attention deficit disorder**, developmental impairments, and breathing problems. Research has shown that low birthweight babies also have higher rates of psychosocial disabilities at adolescence.

There have been some studies which show that prematurity leading to low birthweight is associated with developmental speech and language difficulties as well as an increased risk for diabetes as adults. Researchers speculate that this may be because of some biochemical modifications being made in the body of the undernourished infant before birth.

The factors that contribute to low birthweight are complex, and hence low birthweight prevention is not an easy issue to address. Without doubt, however, it is problem worthy of a national effort. The overall social environment has to considered and a community wide approach has to be adopted.

Life style behaviors such as cigarette **smoking**, weight gain during pregnancy and the use of alcohol and other drugs play an important role in determining fetal growth. Cigarette smoking is one of the biggest known risk factors for low birthweight. About 20% of all low birthweights can be avoided if women did not smoke during pregnancy. Reducing heavy use of alcohol and other drugs could also significantly reduce the rate of low birthweight babies.

Pregnancy and the prospect of motherhood provide an important window of opportunity in a woman's life to improve her health and bring about some life style changes. Adoption of healthy lifestyle behaviors such as ceasing to smoke, giving up drug and alcohol use, eating an adequate diet, and gaining enough weight during pregnancy could positively affect the health of the woman and the health of her children.

For expectant mothers of all age groups and income levels, the same advice holds true. Early and good prenatal care increases the chances of a healthy baby and provides an array of medical, nutritional and educational interventions. These should reduce the incidence of low birthweight and other adverse outcomes.

Lower, Richard (1631-1691)

English physician and physiologist

Richard Lower was a pioneer in seventeenth century medicine because of his studies in experimental physiology. His observations about the circulation and **transfusion** of blood led to some of the most significant discoveries in the history of medicine. He is still regarded as one of Oxford's finest doctors.

Lower studied at Westminster School and Christ Church College, Oxford, where he earned an M.A. in 1655 and an M.D. in 1665. He was named Sedleian professor of natural philosophy in 1660. Lower was a medical student under Thomas Willis and then collaborated with him to investigate the nervous system. Simultaneously, Lower began his own research on the heart. He traced the circulation of blood as it passes through the lungs and learned that it changes when exposed to air. Lower was the first to observe the difference in arterial and venous blood.

Lower showed it was possible for blood to be transfused from animal to animal and from animal to man intravenously. In November 1667, Lower worked with Sir William King, another student of Willis, to transfuse sheep's blood into a man who was mentally ill. Lower was interested in advancing science but also believed the man could be helped, either by the infusion of fresh blood or by the removal of old blood. It was difficult to find people who would agree to be transfused, but an eccentric scholar, Arthur Coga, consented and the procedure was carried out by Lower and King before the Royal Society on November 23, 1667. Transfusion gathered some popularity in France and Italy, but medical and theological debates arose, resulting in transfusion being prohibited in France.

Lower studied the arterial circle at the base of the brain, named the circle of Willis after his teacher. He wanted to see if blood would continue to flow through the head if three of the four arteries supplying blood to the head were tied.

Lower also investigated to see how **cerebrospinal fluid** was formed and how it circulated. These experiments led to a study of **hydrocephalus**, a disease in which fluid collects in the cavities of the brain. In Lower's time, it was thought that catarrh, an inflammation of the mucous membranes, might be caused by seepage of fluid from the brain to the nose. *De Catarrhis*, Lower's book, is of historical significance because it was the first scholarly attempt by an English physician to take a classical doctrine (the theory that nasal secretions are an overspill from the brain) and to disprove it by scientific experiment.

Lower wrote *Diatribae T. Willisii de Febribus Vindicatio*, an eight-volume defense of Dr. Willis and his doctrine of fevers. In keeping with his interest in the circulatory system, Lower went on to write *Tractatus de Corde*, which described the muscular fibers of the heart, a method of ligaturing veins to produce dropsy, blood coagulation in the heart, the motion of digestive fluids, and other physiologic topics. Lower presented his *Tractatus de Corde* to the Royal Society in 1669.

Willis died in 1675 and Lower became busy with the demands of his medical practice and didn't have time to conduct experiments.

Lower took care of Charles II during his last illness in 1685. When James II took the throne, Lower did not continue as court physician because of the unpopularity of his anti-Catholic and Whiggish sentiments. Lower died in London from a fever.

Ludwig, Karl Friedrich Wilhelm (1816-1895)

German physiologist

Karl Friedrich Wilhelm Ludwig was one of the greatest researchers and teachers in the history of physiology. Born in Witzenhausen, Germany, he was the son of a former cavalry officer in the Napoleonic wars who became a civilian official at Hanau. After finishing his schooling at the Hanau gymnasium in 1834, Ludwig studied medicine at the University of Marburg, where he was expelled for dueling and political activities. He later returned to the university and earned his medical degree in 1840 after writing a dissertation on renal secretion. He then progressed through a series of anatomy and physiology professorships combined with research in Marburg in 1846; Zurich in 1849; Vienna, at the Josephinum (1855);

and finally Leipzig (1865), where he remained until his death thirty years later.

Ludwig had based his investigation and teaching of physiology on chemical and physical laws, explaining all physiological processes on the basis of measurable and experimentally demonstrable phenomena—not on some speculative "vital force." He invented a number of devices and methods to carry out his scientific approach to physiology, many of them related to his interest in circulation and respiration. In 1847 he devised the kymograph to prove that blood is moved by mechanical forces, not the invisible "vital force." Ludwig's kymograph used a mercury manometer tube and a revolving drum to graphically record blood pressure variations and other vital signs. With later modifications, the kymograph became a standard tool for recording results of experiments.

In 1859 Ludwig and a student designed a mercury pump that separated and measured quantities of gases—oxygen and carbon dioxide—in the blood. Ludwig's *stromuhr*, or stream gauge, of 1867 measured the flow of blood. Ludwig also discovered that he could keep organs alive outside an animal by pumping blood or a saline solution through the excised part, a process called perfusion.

In addition to his important inventions, Ludwig produced a long list of major physiological observations and findings, including discoveries about salivary secretions, the mechanism of cardiac activity, respiration, blood, and blood circulation. Ludwig used his appointment in 1864 to the newly created chair of physiology at Leipzig to create a model teaching center for physiology, which became a world center for physiological study. Ludwig's textbooks of 1852 and 1856 (the first modern one on physiology), his hundreds of students, and his numerous scientific contributions have made him perhaps the most influential physiologist of the second half of the nineteenth century.

LUMPECTOMY

A lumpectomy is one type of surgery for **breast cancer**. The malignant tumor and a surrounding margin of normal breast tissue are removed. Lymph nodes in the armpit (axilla) may also be removed.

Lumpectomy is a surgical treatment for newly diagnosed breast cancer. It is estimated that at least 50% of women with breast cancer are good candidates for this procedure. The location, size, and type of tumor are of primary importance when considering breast cancer surgery options. The size of the breast is another variable. The patient's psychological outlook, as well as her lifestyle choices, should also be taken into account when treatment decisions are made.

The severity of a **cancer** is evaluated or "staged" according to a fairly complex system. This considers the size of the tumor and whether the cancer has spread directly to adjacent tissues, such as the chest wall, the lymph nodes, and/or to distant parts of the body. Women with early stage breast cancers are usually better candidates for lumpectomy. In most cases, a course of **radiation therapy** after surgery is part of the treatment. **Chemotherapy** or hormone treatment may also be prescribed.

Many studies have compared the survival rates of women who have had removal of a breast (**mastectomy**) with those who have undergone lumpectomy and radiation therapy. The data is clear that for women with comparable stages of breast cancer, survival rates are equal between the two groups.

In some circumstances, a woman with later stage breast cancer may be able to have a lumpectomy. Chemotherapy can be administered before surgery to decrease tumor size and the chance of spread in selected cases.

There are a number of factors that may prohibit a breast cancer patient from having a lumpectomy. The tumor itself may be too large or located in an area, such as near the nipple, where it would be difficult to remove with good cosmetic results. Sometimes several areas of cancer are found in one breast, so the tumor cannot be removed in a single mass of tissue. Tumors known to grow very rapidly would most likely not be treated with lumpectomy. A cancer which has already attached itself to nearby structures, such as the skin or the chest wall, needs more extensive surgery.

Certain medical or physical circumstances may also eliminate lumpectomy as a treatment option. Sometimes lumpectomy may be attempted, but the surgeon is unable to remove the tumor with a sufficient amount of normal tissue surrounding it. This may be termed "persistently positive margins," or "lack of clear margins," referring to the margin of unaffected tissue around the tumor. Lumpectomy is not used for women who have had a previous lumpectomy and have a recurrence of the breast cancer.

Because of the need for radiation therapy after lumpectomy, this surgery may be medically unacceptable. A breast cancer discovered during **pregnancy** is not amenable to lumpectomy, due to the need for radiation therapy as part of the treatment. Radiation therapy cannot be administered to pregnant women, for fear of injuring the fetus. Women with collagen vascular disease, such as lupus erythematosus, or **scleroderma**, would experience scarring and damage to their connective tissue if exposed to radiation treatments. A woman who has already had therapeutic radiation to the chest area for other reasons cannot have additional exposure for breast cancer therapy.

Some women may choose not to have a lumpectomy for other reasons. They may strongly fear a recurrence of breast cancer, and may consider a lumpectomy too risky. Other women feel uncomfortable with a breast that has had a cancer, and they experience more peace of mind with the entire breast removed.

The need for radiation therapy may also be a barrier due to non-medical concerns. Some women simply fear this type of treatment and chose more extensive surgery so radiation will not be required. The commitment of time, usually five days a week for six weeks, may not be acceptable for others. This may be due to financial, personal, or job-related constraints. Finally, in geographically isolated areas, a course of radiation therapy may require lengthy travel, and perhaps unacceptable amounts of time away from the family and other responsibilities.

Lumpectomy is an imprecise term. Any amount of tissue, from 1-50% of the breast, may be removed and called a lumpectomy. Other names are no more definite in their meaning, although some idea of the scope of tissue removal may be implied. Breast conservation surgery is a frequently used synonym for lumpectomy. Partial mastectomy, quadrantectomy, segmental excision, wide excision, and tylectomy are other names for this procedure.

A lumpectomy is typically done in a hospital setting, but specialized outpatient facilities are sometimes preferred. The surgery is usually done while the patient is under general anesthetic. Local anesthetic with additional sedation may be used for some patients. The tumor and surrounding margin of tissue is removed and sent to the pathologist. The surgical site is closed. If axillary lymph nodes were not removed before, a second incision is made in the armpit. The fat pad which contains lymph nodes is removed from this area and is also sent to the pathologist for analysis. This portion of the procedure is called an axillary node dissection; it is critical for determining the stage of the cancer. Typically, 10-15 nodes are removed, but the number may vary. Surgical drains may be left in place in either location to prevent fluid accumulation. The surgery may last from one to three hours.

The patient may stay in the hospital one or two days, or return home the same day. This generally depends on the extent of the surgery, the medical condition of the patient, and physician and patient preferences. A woman usually goes home with a small bandage. The inner part of the surgical site usually has dissolvable stitches. The skin may be sutured or stitched; or the skin edges may be held together with steristrips, which are special thin, clear pieces of tape.

Routine preoperative preparations, such as taking nothing to eat or drink the night before surgery, are typically ordered for a lumpectomy. Information regarding expected outcomes and potential complications should also be part of preparation for lumpectomy, as for any surgical procedure. It is especially important that women know about sensations they might experience after the operation, so the sensations are not misinterpreted as signs of further cancer or poor healing.

If the tumor is not able to be felt (not palpable), a preoperative localization procedure is needed. A fine wire, or other device, is placed at the tumor site, using x ray or ultrasound for guidance. This is usually done in the radiology department of a hospital. The woman is most often sitting up and awake, although some sedation may be administered.

After a lumpectomy, patients are usually cautioned against lifting anything which weighs over five pounds for several days. Other activities may be restricted, according to individual needs. **Pain** is often enough to limit inappropriate motion. Women are often instructed to wear a well-fitting support bra both day and night for approximately one week after surgery.

Pain is usually well controlled with prescribed medication. If it is not, the patient should contact the surgeon, as severe pain may be a sign of a complication which needs medical attention. A return visit to the surgeon is normally scheduled approximately ten days to two weeks after the operation.

Radiation therapy is usually started as soon as feasible after lumpectomy. Other additional treatments, such as chemotherapy or hormone therapy, may also be prescribed. The timing of these is specific to each individual patient.

The risks are those which are common to any surgical procedure, including bleeding, infection, **anesthesia** reaction, or unexpected scarring. A lumpectomy may also cause loss of sensation in the breast. The size and shape of the breast will be affected by the operation. Fluid can accumulate in the area where tissue was removed, requiring drainage.

If lymph node dissection is performed, there are several potential complications. A woman may experience decreased feeling in the back of her armpit; or experience other sensations, including numbness, tingling, or increased skin sensitivity. An inflammation of the arm vein, called phlebitis, can occur. There may be injury to the nerves controlling arm motion.

Approximately 2-10% of patients develop **lymphedema** after axillary lymph node dissection. This swelling of the arm can range from mild to very severe. It can be treated with elastic bandages and specialized physical therapy, but it is a chronic condition, requiring continuing care. Lymphedema can arise at any time, even years after surgery.

A new technique that may eliminate the need for removing many axillary lymph nodes is being tested. The term ''sentinel node biopsy'' is most frequently used to refer to this method. It is based on the idea that the condition of the first lymph node in the network, which drains the affected area, can predict whether the cancer may have spread to the rest of the nodes. If this first, or sentinel, node is cancer-free, it is thought there is no need to look further. Many patients with early-stage breast cancers may be spared the risks and complications of axillary node dissection as the use of this approach continues to increase.

When lumpectomy is performed, it is anticipated that it will be the definitive surgical treatment for breast cancer. Other forms of therapy, especially radiation, are often prescribed as part of the total treatment plan. The expected outcome is no recurrence of the breast cancer.

Lung cancer

Lung cancer is a disease in which the cells of the lung tissues grow uncontrollably and form tumors. There are two kinds of lung cancers, primary and secondary. Primary lung cancer starts in the lung itself. Primary lung cancer is divided into small cell lung cancer and non-small cell lung cancer, depending on how the cells look under the microscope. Secondary lung cancer is cancer that starts somewhere else in the body (for example, the breast or colon) and spreads to the lungs.

Small cell cancer was formerly called oat cell cancer, because the cells resemble oats in their shape. About a fourth of all lung cancers are small cell cancers. It is a very aggressive cancer and spreads to other organs within a short time. It is generally found in people who are heavy smokers. Non-small cell cancers account for the remaining 75% of lung cancers.

Tobacco **smoking** is the leading cause of lung cancer. Exposure to asbestos fibers, either at home or in the workplace, is also considered a risk factor for lung cancer. Besides asbestos, mining industry workers who are exposed to coal products

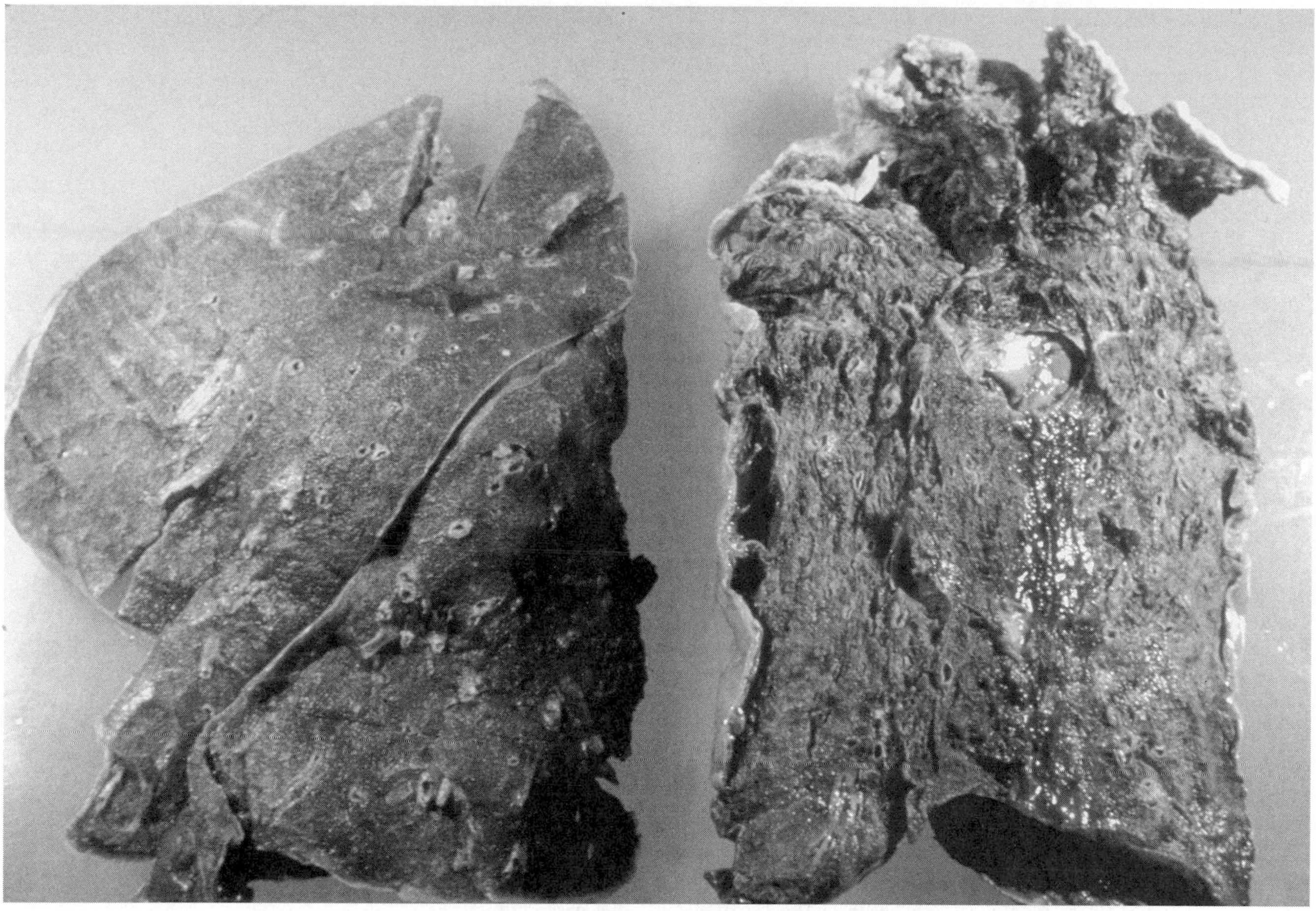

A normal lung (left) and the lung of a cigarette smoker (right). ***(Photograph by A. Glauberman, Photo Researchers, Inc. Reproduced by permission.)***

or radioactive substances such as uranium, and workers exposed to chemicals such as arsenic, vinyl chloride, mustard gas, and other **carcinogens** also have a higher than average risk of contracting lung cancer. High levels of a radioactive gas (radon) that cannot be seen or smelled also pose a risk for lung cancer.

Inflammation and scar tissue produced in the lung due to certain diseases such as **tuberculosis**; and certain types of **pneumonia** may increase the risk of developing lung cancer. Although the exact cause of lung cancer is not known, people with a family history of lung cancer appear to have a slightly higher risk of contracting the disease.

The early symptoms of lung cancer are:

- A **cough** that does not go away
- Chest **pain**
- **Shortness of breath**
- Persistent hoarseness
- Swelling of the neck and face
- Significant weight loss that is not due to dieting or vigorous **exercise**; fatigue and loss of appetite
- Bloody or brown-colored spit or phlegm (sputum)
- Unexplained **fever**
- Recurrent lung infections, such as **bronchitis** or pneumonia.

These symptoms may be caused by diseases other than lung cancer. It is vital, however, to consult a doctor to rule out the possibility that they are the first symptoms of lung cancer.

If the patient's doctor suspects lung cancer, he or she will take a detailed medical history to check all the symptoms and assess the risk factors. This will be followed by a complete **physical examination**. If the doctor has reason to suspect lung cancer—particularly if the patient has a history of heavy smoking or occupational exposure to substances that are known to irritate the lungs— he or she may order a chest x ray to see if there are any masses in the lungs. Special imaging techniques, such as CT scans or MRIs, may provide more precise information about the size, shape, and location of any tumors.

Sputum analysis involves microscopic examination of the cells that are either coughed up from the lungs, or are collected through a special instrument called a bronchoscope. Sputum analyses can diagnose at least 30% of lung cancers. Lung **biopsy** is the most definitive diagnostic tool for cancer. After obtaining samples of the lung tissue or a sample of tissue from the tumor, it is sent to the laboratory. A pathologist examines the tumor samples to identify the cancer's type and stage.

Treatment for lung cancer depends on the type of cancer, its location, and its stage. The most commonly used modes of treatment are surgery, **radiation therapy**, and **chemotherapy**.

Surgery is not usually an option for small cell lung cancers, because they have usually spread beyond the lung by the time they are diagnosed. Because non-small cell lung cancers are less aggressive, however, surgery can be used to treat them. Surgery may be the primary method of treatment, or radiation therapy and/or chemotherapy may be used to shrink the tumor before surgery is attempted.

Radiotherapy involves the use of high-energy rays to kill cancer cells. It is used either by itself or in combination with surgery or chemotherapy. The amount of radiation used depends on the size and the location of the tumor. Radiation therapy may produce some side effects which may disappear either during the course of the treatment or after the treatment is over. The side effects should be discussed with the doctor.

Chemotherapy uses anti-cancer medications that are either given intravenously or taken by mouth. These drugs enter the bloodstream and travel to all parts of the body, killing cancer cells that have spread to different organs. Chemotherapy is used as the primary treatment for cancers that have spread beyond the lung and cannot be removed by surgery. It can also be used in addition to surgery or radiation therapy.

If the lung cancer is detected before it has had a chance to spread to other organs, and if it is treated appropriately, at least 49% of patients can survive five years or longer after the initial diagnosis. Only 15% of lung cancers, however, are found at this early stage. Due to improvements in surgical technique and the development of new approaches to treatment, the one-year survival rate for lung cancer has improved considerably.

The best way to prevent lung cancer is not to smoke or to quit smoking if one has already started. Secondhand smoke from other people's tobacco should also be avoided. Appropriate precautions should be taken when working with cancer-causing substances (carcinogens). Eating well-balanced meals, testing houses for the presence of radon gas, and removing asbestos from buildings are also useful preventive strategies.

Luria, Salvador Edward (1912-1991)

Italian American biologist

Salvador Luria was born on August 13, 1912, in Turin, Italy. In 1929, he entered medical school there and soon developed a technical facility for culturing cells; that is, he was able to grow cells in artificial media inside culture dishes. He received a medical degree in 1935 and then served in the Italian Army for three years. After this service, he studied at the Curie Institute in Paris, where he became curious about bacteriophages, viruses that attack bacteria. He was especially interested in how X-ray radiation affects bacteriophages by causing mutations. Luria emigrated to the United States in 1940 and accepted an appointment to Columbia University. He met **Max Delbrück** shortly thereafter, and the latter invited Luria to carry on research at Vanderbilt University in Nashville, where Delbruck was teaching.

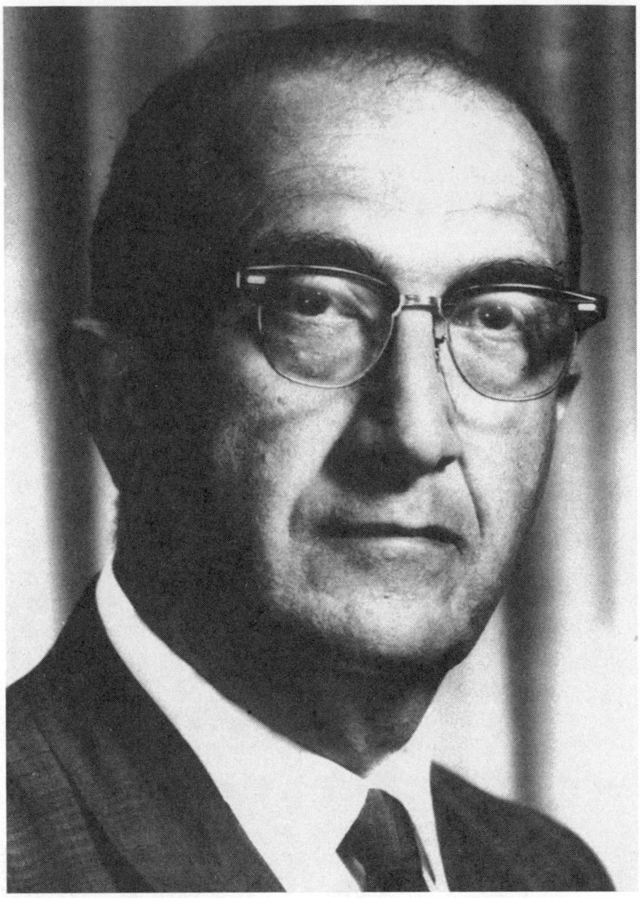

Salvador Luria

Together, Luria and Delbrück planned a series of experiments to study bacteria that had developed resistance to bacteriophages. They wanted to see if the resistance was the result of some action by bacteriophages on normal cells, or if the bacteria had become resistant because of mutation. Luria's ideas about random mutation were inspired by an unlikely source—watching people play slot machines at a country club dance during Luria's tenure at Indiana University in Bloomington. He observed how the payoff from a slot machine varied from just a few coins to a big pile of coins, a rather rare occurrence. Luria likened the bacteria to slot machines. Sometimes there were small clusters and sometimes large clusters, probably the descendants of a mutation. Luria's idea led to the development of the fluctuation test, which, with Delbrück's mathematical analysis, demonstrated that the bacterial resistance was an adaptive response caused by spontaneous, random mutation.

Luria and Delbrück began to collaborate with **Alfred Hershey**, a biologist also conducting bacteriophage research. The three became members of the "Phage Group," an informal assembly of scientists who worked exclusively with seven strains of bacteriophage so that their experimental results could be compared. Luria's research contributed a great deal to the understanding of the structure of viruses. This work was recognized in 1969, when Luria, Delbrück, and Hershey shared the Nobel Prize in physiology or medicine.

Luria had married Zella Hurwitz, a psychology professor, in 1945. They had one son. Luria died at home in Lexington, Massachusetts, after suffering a heart attack in 1991.

LWOFF, ANDRÉ (1902-1994)

French microbiologist

André Lwoff was a French microbiologist whose seminal work in the genetic control of virus synthesis helped guide successive generations of scientists toward a new outlook on cell physiology. Lwoff's primary contributions have come from his study of the biology of viruses, including the genetics of bacteria and the mechanisms of viral infection and replication. An erudite man who painted and was well versed in philosophy and literature, Lwoff was one of the foremost teachers and mentors to guide a generation of scientists who would move biology to a new frontier. Lwoff, who was Jewish, actively participated in the French Resistance during World War II.

André Michel Lwoff was born in Ainay-le-Château, in central France, on May 8, 1902. His parents were Russian immigrants who had come to France in the late nineteenth century. His father, Solomon Lwoff, was a physician in a psychiatric hospital; his mother, Marie Siminovitch, was a sculptor. Although Lwoff—who early on loved to paint, listen to music, and read—inherited his mother's artistic temperament, his interest in science was cultivated by his father, who often took the boy with him on his daily rounds. Lwoff spent most of his younger years in a rural community near Paris.

On the advice of his father, Lwoff attended the University of Paris (the Sorbonne) to study medicine, a field in which he could earn a comfortable living. But his real interest lay in his other major field of study, biology. Lwoff spent his summers at the Marine Biology Laboratory at Roscoff, in Britanny. He graduated with a bachelor's degree in the natural sciences in 1921 and, at the age of nineteen, became an assistant at the Pasteur Institute in Paris, working under microbiologists Édouard Chatton and Félix Mesnil. While conducting research part-time at the Institute, Lwoff continued to work toward his medical degree, which he received in 1927. He received his doctorate in natural science in 1932.

Lwoff's keen intellect was first applied to morphological studies of protozoa, one-celled animals that often live as parasites on other animals. Lwoff focused specifically on ciliates, which are covered with cilia (hair-like structures), and discovered a new species of ciliated protozoa. These studies eventually culminated in the discovery of the extranuclear inheritance characteristic of these organisms and earned Lwoff recognition as a leader in protozoology. Lwoff next turned his attention to an even simpler form of life, bacteria. The scientific community at that time primarily studied bacteria in terms

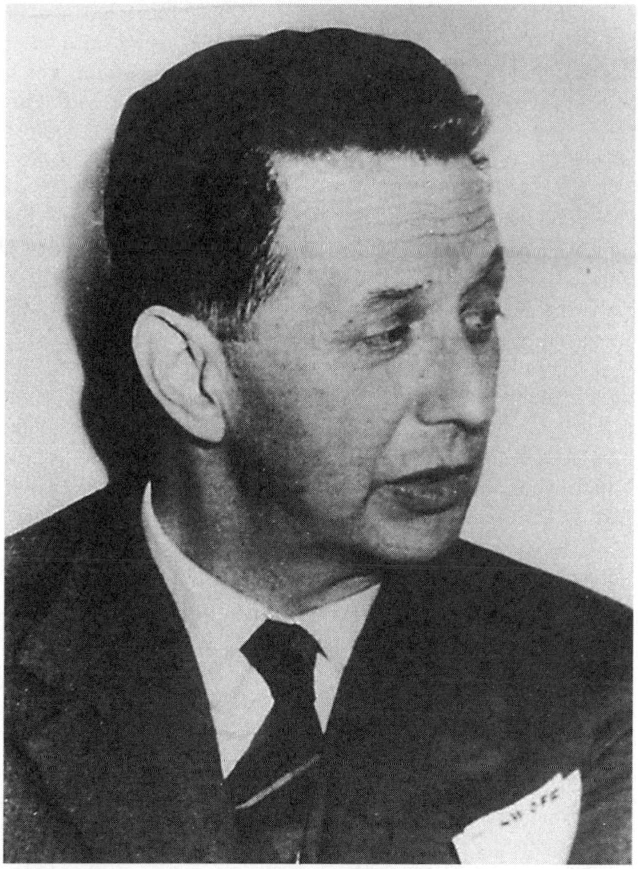
André Lwoff

of their role in putrefaction, fermentation, and the biological factors involved in disease. Lwoff, however, was more interested in the general biological properties of bacteria. Focusing on the ways such simple organisms get nutrition, he discovered how to produce chemically defined media for their growth—a discovery that led him to identify specific growth factors identified as **vitamins**.

Lwoff's discovery astounded the scientific community because it pointed to the bacterium as an organism much like higher organisms that need nutritional factors to grow and survive. Lwoff continued his research on vitamins, analyzing how vitamin deficiencies cause interruptions at certain points during metabolic processes. In 1936, in collaboration with his wife, Marguerite, whom he had married in 1925 and with whom he worked throughout his life, Lwoff published what was to become an extremely influential paper on how vitamins function as coenzymes, small molecules that help the larger enzyme molecules perform their catalytic functions. These discoveries revealed Lwoff's remarkable intuitive approach to research and demonstrated the unity of biochemical action in all living things. In 1938, the Pasteur Institute made Lwoff the chief of a new program focusing on the emerging field of microbial physiology.

During the 1930s, Lwoff developed a friendship with Eugène Wollman, a pioneer researcher of lysogenic bacteria, which have the hereditary power to produce bacteriophage, or bacterial viruses. In effect, these bacteriophage parasitize other bacteria and can cause bacterial lysis or cell destruction, which releases a host of bacteriophage particles, or phages. Initial interest in bacteriophages stemmed from scientists who thought it might be possible to use bacteriophages to fight specific diseases. Although this approach was, for the most part, ineffective, scientists were intrigued by the phenomenon since the appearance and disappearance of phages was highly unpredictable. Wollman, working with his wife, Elisabeth, had theorized that bacteriophages may be types of "lethal genes" that were reintroduced into the genetic makeup of an organism.

By the early 1940s, however, lysogeny had become an area that was considered of little importance by the young school of American bacterial virologists and many others, who now focused their work on T strains of *Escherichia coli,* in which lysogeny did not occur. The advance of World War II further disrupted the study of lysogeny. The Wollmans, who were Jewish, were captured by the Gestapo in Paris in 1943 and sent to the notorious Auschwitz concentration camp in Poland, never to be heard from again. Lwoff, meanwhile, had joined a resistance group in France that focused primarily on gathering intelligence for the Allies. He managed to escape capture when his underground network was destroyed by the Gestapo, who arrested many of Lwoff's compatriots. But Lwoff was soon involved in another underground network. He also hid American airmen in his apartment as they tried to make their way to unoccupied France after having being shot down over Nazi territory. After the war, Lwoff was awarded the Médaille de la Résistance, and was made Commander of the Légion d'Honneur for his efforts in resisting the Nazi occupation of France.

At war's end, Lwoff chose to continue the work of his friends the Wollmans. At the time, scientists who still worked in the field of bacterial lysogeny maintained that the haphazard release of phages probably occurred because of one of two reasons: the release of phages either resulted from bacteria mutation that spontaneously created phages (virus particles), or that the lysogenic bacteria leaked the phages without bursting. Furthermore, Félix Hérelle had hypothesized that bacteria are resistant to phages released by other bacteria and only absorb the phage from like bacteria. He also theorized that cells in cultured lysogenic bacteria carry "free" phages on their surface, which further strengthen the phage-host association that render bacteria resistant to later viral destruction. He believed that the increase of phages in a lysogenic bacterial culture was due to a few susceptible, or phage-sensitive, bacteria.

Lwoff began working with a lysogenic strain of soil bacteria called *Bacillus megaterium* and a second strain of bacteria susceptible to phage infection. Lwoff exhibited remarkable dexterity and skill in the extremely difficult procedure of growing individual bacteria in a microdrop and then fishing out the newly divided bacteria with a capillary pipette—only a few microns in diameter—without contaminating the specimen. He would then transfer the bacteria to a new noncontaminated medium. Although the approach was time-consuming and cumbersome, Lwoff was able to show that, contrary to D'Hérelle's theory, lysogenic bacteria could multiply for nineteen successive generations without the intervention of exogenous, or cell surface, phages. These successive generations were also lysogenic, which proved that lysogeny was a genetic trait. Lwoff's discoveries once again made lysogeny a viable area of study. Lwoff had also dispelled the notion that the host-virus relationship was one that always ended in morbidity, showing that the two could coexist.

Through his experiments, Lwoff also determined that lysogenic bacteria release the phages they produce by lysing, or breaking down, the cell. Still, Lwoff had not explained what actually took place during lysogeny. He did, however, go on to confirm Wollman's earlier finding that when the enzyme lysozyme was used to artificially break open lysogenic bacteria without affecting the phages, no phage particles could be found. He soon discovered what he called "prophages," which, unlike normal bacteriophages, were noninfectious. Furthermore, Lwoff discovered that the prophages acted as "bacterial genes" that integrated themselves into the chromosome of the host, where the genes are located. Reproduction of the phage particle was halted by a regulatory gene in the phage DNA.

Lwoff next theorized that some external environmental stimulus could interfere with the dormant merger of phage particles and host DNA and thus cause the production of bacteriophage. After months and months of experiments, Lwoff and his colleagues at the Pasteur Institute decided to irradiate the bacteria with ultraviolet light, which normally kills bacteria and bacteriophages. To their surprise, they found that ultraviolet light caused the phage to multiply and eventually destroy the bacterial cell. Lwoff would later note this discovery as one of the most thrilling of his scientific career. Further research showed that other stimuli, including chemicals that were known to cause cancers, could produce the same effect.

Lwoff's studies of lysogeny provided a viable model for a viral theory of cancer; and, in 1953, Lwoff proposed that "inducible lysogenic bacteria" might serve as a way of testing cancerous and noncancerous activity in cells. Although this proved difficult and engendered much debate over the possible viral origins of some **cancers**, Lwoff was correct in postulating that viruses' protein coats contain carcinogenic properties that can be activated by outside factors such as ultraviolet light. His research on lysogeny also led Lwoff to study poliomyelitis virus. He demonstrated that, unlike vaccine strains of the virus, some strains of the **polio** virus were not affected by temperature fluctuations.

Lwoff was awarded the Nobel Prize for physiology or medicine in 1965 for his lysogeny studies. He shared the award with fellow Pasteur Institute scientists **Jacques Lucien Monod** and **François Jacob**. These three were the first French scientists to win the Nobel Prize in thirty years, and Lwoff and his fellow Nobel Prize winners were largely unknown in France until they received the award. But this was not the case in the United States, where Lwoff had traveled and conducted some of his most important scientific dialogues. Soon, many young scientists came from the U.S. to visit Lwoff and learn as much about his expertise in the field of microbiology as possible.

They were also drawn to Lwoff because his line of research was fundamentally similar to that used in studying the genetic manipulation of microorganisms. Lwoff's influence was also enhanced because he spoke fluent English.

Unfortunately for many of his devotees, Lwoff was in no position to take them under his wing. His quarters in the attic of the Pasteur Institute were cramped and crowded with equipment. At the Institute, Lwoff was not obligated to teach and preferred to dedicate his time to his research. Even François Jacob had to plead with Lwoff on several occasions to work with him at the Institute. Despite this obstacle, many students and fellow scientists formed close relationships with Lwoff over the years. Lwoff had also helped Monod early in his career by allowing Monod to work with him in his laboratory at the Institute. In one series of studies, scientist Alice Audureau isolated a genus of bacterium taken from the gut of Lwoff; Monod eventually named the genus *Moraxella lwoffii* in Lwoff's honor.

In the book *Of Microbes and Life,* many of Lwoff's former students and colleagues contributed essays in celebration of the ''fiftieth anniversary of [Lwoff's] immersion in biology.'' In the book, **Salvador Edward Luria** aptly described Lwoff's Renaissance nature, which made him so interesting to so many of his fellow scientists. ''André Lwoff—scientist, painter, master of language, leader of one of the great schools of biology—is a prototype scientist-humanist, in whom the 'two cultures,' supposedly divergent and losing touch of each other, remain happily married.'' Lwoff was also noted for his marvelous sense of humor and enthusiasm, which, to the careful reader, would often shine through in even his most scientific papers. Lwoff retired from the Pasteur Institute in 1968 and became director of the Cancer Research Institute at Villejuif, near Paris, a position he held until 1972. He died in October 1994.

Lyme disease

Though it has probably been in existence for a long time, Lyme disease was only recently identified as a distinct illness. The disease is caused by the spirochete *Borrelia burgdorferi*, a corkscrew-shaped microorganism which is spread by ticks that thrive in wooded areas and tall grasses and infect deer, mice, and domestic animals as well as humans. Most common in New England, the upper Midwest, and northern California, it has been diagnosed in more than 40 states. Although Lyme disease is not fatal, it can cause lasting debilitation.

A Lyme disease infection progresses through three stages. The first stage includes a bull's-eye-like rash that can appear at the site of the tick bite in a few days to a few weeks. There can also be symptoms similar to **influenza**, **headaches**, and soreness in the neck. The second stage includes irregular heartbeat, joint pains, disturbances of vision and memory, and facial-nerve **paralysis**. The disease can then progress to a third stage which includes joint inflammation and **arthritis**. While it can be easily treated with **antibiotic**s, especially oral *tetracycline*, in the early stages, Lyme disease is often misdiagnosed until it has progressed to the second or third stage, during which the damage can become permanent. Antibiotics are also being developed for chronic Lyme disease which is characterized by chronic or intermittent symptoms.

The disease was first reported in Lyme, Connecticut, in 1974 by rheumatologist Allen Steere (1943-), who noticed that certain patients were exhibiting a distinct set of symptoms that could not be attributed to other known illnesses. Symptoms resembling those of Lyme disease had been reported in parts of Europe since the turn of the century, but clinicians were not sure whether the European syndrome had a similar origin to Lyme disease.

Then, in 1981, a survey of microorganisms in ticks revealed that a tick-borne spirochete was responsible for both the European and American syndromes. Because many people in the United States and Europe contract the disease without apparent exposure to the tick, many experts believe that mosquitoes, biting flies, and birds may also spread the organism.

Despite a full understanding of the disease, researchers have been developing a vaccine. At Yale University, scientists isolated the gene in the Lyme disease spirochete that leads to the production of the protein OspA, a protein common to many bacteria. Using **genetic engineering**, the researchers induced another bacterium to produce large quantities of OspA. When they injected laboratory mice with the protein and exposed the mice to the Lyme disease organism, none of them developed the disease. Furthermore, antibodies could be extracted from the mice and injected into uninfected mice, affording them protection from the disease as well.

While vaccines are undergoing testing in humans, scientists have recently discovered the DNA sequence for the causative agent, *Borrelia burgdorferi.* This advance will help researchers develop new diagnostic tests and vaccines, as well as determine individual susceptibility to chronic symptoms. Until then, education and proper early diagnosis appear to be the best means to control the disease. Experts advise campers and hikers to cover exposed skin, especially on the legs, when walking in the woods or tall grasses. People should also check themselves and their children thoroughly for ticks (particularly deer ticks roughly the size of a pinhead), and gently remove any ticks they find with tweezers to insure that the mouthparts of the tick are not left in the bite. Because the Lyme disease spirochete resides in the midguts of ticks, crushing the ticks could inject the contents of the midgut into the bite wound.

Lymphatic system

The lymphatic system is the body's network of organs, ducts, and tissues that filter harmful substances out of the fluid that surrounds body tissues. Lymphatic organs include the bone marrow, thymus, spleen, appendix, tonsils, adenoids, lymph nodes, and Peyer's patches (in the small intestine). The thymus and bone marrow are called primary lymphatic organs, because lymphocytes are produced in them. The other lymphatic organs are called secondary lymphatic organs.

Lymphocytes are a type of white blood cell (WBC), which is highly concentrated in lymphatic fluid. This clear fluid, also called lymph, travels through the lymphatic vessels, which connect the lymphatic organs. The terminal lymphatic vessels feed into the thoracic duct that returns body fluids to the heart prior to blood reoxygenation. The reincorporated fluid originates in the bloodstream, bathes organs and tissues, and is returned to the bloodstream after passing through lymphatic filters that function as part of the body's defense system against infection and **cancer**.

Lymph nodes, primarily clustered in the neck, armpits, and pelvic area, are the system's battle stations against infection. Lymph nodes are connected to one another by lymphatic vessels. It is in the nodes and other secondary organs where WBCs engulf and destroy debris to prevent them from reentering the bloodstream. Of the other two major secondary lymphatic organs, the spleen removes dead red blood cells (RBCs), and Peyer's patches remove intestinal antigens (foreign or harmful substances in the body).

Lymphocytes are the lymphatic system's foot soldiers. These cells identify enemy particles and attempt to destroy them. Lymphocytes fall into two general categories: T lymphocytes (T cells) and B lymphocytes (B cells). T cells form in the thymus (in the chest), and B cells form in the bone marrow of the long, thick bones of the thigh, arm, spine, or pelvis. While T cells primarily attack viral antigens, B cells attack bacterial antigens. Both T and B cells travel in lymph, through lymphatic vessels, and into lymph nodes.

T cells are further divided into three primary classes: helper T cells (T-H cells), cytotoxic T cells (ctx T cells), and T suppressor T cells. T-H cells augment B cell responses to bacterial antigens. Ctx T cells attack viral antigens and some early cancer cells. And suppressor T cells halt immune cell functions, allowing the body to rest.

B cells produce antibodies. According to their basic immunoglobulin type, antibodies are subdivided into five classes (IgM, IgD, IgG, IgE, and IgA). B cell antibodies recognize specific bacterial invaders and destroy them. Certain antibodies are more concentrated in areas of the body where they are most needed. For example, IgA-producing B cells are most concentrated in the Peyer's patches where they sample intestinal contents for potential antigens that could signal an infectious invasion of food-born bacteria.

Lymph nodes are pockets of lymph that orchestrate the removal of foreign material (including bacteria, viruses, and cancerous cells) from the lymph. They vary in size from microscopic to about 1 in (.394 cm) in diameter. Some nodes cluster at key sites where the limbs join the torso. Lymph nodes are named after their locations in the body. The nodes at the arm are called axial and brachial, those under the jaw are called subclavian, and those in the groin are called inguinal. Fibrous connective tissue covers the lymphatic tissue inside the lymph node.

Each node, also called a lymph gland, has both arterial blood supply and venous drainage. Lymphocytes drain out of the arteries into the node interior, usually through a high endothelial venule that facilitates their entry. This venule (small vein) derives its name from the higher-than-usual tightly joined endothelial cells that line it.

Before they can enter the lymph node, lymphocytes are carefully selected from other blood cells. They are recognized and distinguished by a lymphocyte-cellsurface protein called E-selectin. Receptors on the endothelial cells bind the E-selectin positive lymphocytes and slowly roll them toward a gap between adjacent cells. Then the lymphocyte is fed through this area much the way film is fed into a camera. The lymphocytes emerge on the interior of the node.

The internal lymph node tissue is separated into lobes. The lobe end at the center of the node is called the medulla, whereas the wider lobe end toward the perimeter of the node is called the cortex. The lobe area just next to the cortex is called the paracortex. Surrounding the lobes is an area called the medullary sinus. T cells are concentrated in the paracortex, whereas B cells primarily are concentrated in the cortex in structures called primary follicles. Lymphocytes first travel to the medullary sinus before migrating to the cortical and paracortical regions.

In addition to lymphocytes, several other kinds of antigen-fighting WBCs are contained within the nodes. Macrophages destroy and devour foreign antigens under direction from lymphocytes. Within the cortex, a large WBC called an interdigitating dendritic cell actually gathers the foreign antigen and presents it to the T cells that, in turn, trigger the antigen's destruction. This system is carefully controlled to avoid destroying host cells. Within the paracortex, follicular dendritic cells present antigens to B cells in a region of the follicles called the germinal centers. Within germinal centers, memory B cells are formed that are specifically primed to launch an attack against an antigen if it is encountered again. Like seasoned soldiers who know how to fight a particular enemy, memory B cells are molecularly armed to combat a known antigen.

Foreign antigens are constantly being destroyed; however, when a particularly strong infection occurs, the lymph nodes will sometimes swell with the influx of backup troops (more WBCs) sent in to help fight a particular molecular attacker. Eventually, the lymphocytes leave the node through the efferent lymphatic vessel.

Lymphatic vessels infiltrate tissues that are bathed in fluid released from blood into those tissues. Pockets of fluid collect in the tissues, and increased pressure allows the fluid to seep into the lymphatic vessels. Whereas blood vessels return deoxygenated blood to the heart to be pumped to the lungs for oxygen, lymphatic vessels return fluid that has leaked out of the capillaries into various tissues. However, before this lymphatic fluid is rejoined with venous fluid at the thoracic duct, it is filtered through the lymph nodes to remove infectious agents.

Lymphatic vessels are made up of single-cell epithelial layers that drain fluid away from tissue. Smooth muscles controlled by the autonomic nervous system direct the fluid away from tissues toward the lymph nodes and, eventually, the heart. The vessels contain one-way valves that close behind fluid traveling back to the heart so that lymphatic fluid cannot go backward. Lymphatic fluid is usually returned to circulation within 24 hours. When the lymphatic vessels become clogged, stopped up, or blocked, severe **edema** (bloating due to water retention) can result in a condition known as **lymphedema**.

Of the remaining lymphatic system components, the thymus, bone marrow, spleen, and Peyer's patches have fairly unique roles. Both the bone marrow and thymus introduce "virgin" lymphocyte to the lymphatic system. The spleen filters old RBCs from the blood and fights infections with lymphocytes and monocytes (cells that engulf and devour antigens). And the Peyer's patches are lymph tissue pockets under raised intestinal projections that examine intestinal contents for foreign antigens. Although the spleen's role is important, the human body is capable of functioning without it if it becomes injured or diseased.

Although the thymus is critical for T cell development in children, it begins to shrink as they progress toward adulthood and thereafter plays an increasingly reduced role. T cells are "educated" in the thymus to recognize "self" versus "nonself" (foreign) antigens. Without the ability to recognize self-antigens, T cells would target a person's own tissues in a very destructive manner. The thymus is also responsible for fostering maturation of T cells into their various subclasses. T cells function in a cell-mediated way such that they only recognize antigens presented to them by other cells; hence, T cell immunity is called cell-mediated immunity.

Both T cells (before branching off to develop in the thymus) and B cells originate in the pluripotential stem cells of the bone marrow or the fetal liver. Pluripotential stem cells are the body's cellular sculpting clay. They can be shaped into any cell—including lymphocytes, RBCs, macrophages, and numerous other blood constituents—and become increasingly specialized as they reach maturity. The B cells can generate an infinite number of antibodies in response to a multitude of foreign antigens. This amazing diversity arises from the many combinations of antibody components that can be rearranged to recognize individual antigens. Once a B cell identifies a particular enemy, it undergoes a process called clonal expansion. During this process, it makes many clones (copies) of itself in order to fight several invaders of a single type. This highly sophisticated molecular process destroys infections wherever they arise in the body.

One specialized form of antibody, IgA, detects antigens in the gastrointestinal tract at Peyer's patches. IgA contained within small projections, called lamina propriae, that extend into the small intestine test the intestinal lining for pathogens. The IgA binds to the foreign antigen, returns to exit the patch at its efferent lymphatic vessel, and travels to a mesenteric lymph node that gears up to fight the invader. IgA antibodies are also passed to nursing babies in their mothers' milk, because newborns do not synthesize IgAs until later.

See also Hodgkin's disease; Lymphomas, malignant

LYMPHEDEMA

Lymphedema is the swelling of tissues (**edema**), usually in the feet and legs, due to lymphatic obstruction.

Lymphatic fluid seeps out of the blood circulation into the tissues. It returns to the heart through separate channels called lymphatics, carrying waste products and germs. On its way to the heart, it passes through lymph nodes, where infecting germs (including some **cancer**s) are attacked by the body's defense mechanisms.

If lymphatic channels are obstructed or inadequate, fluid backs up and causes edema. Tissue fluid can also return to the circulation through tissues, without using the lymphatics, but gravity hinders this flow. So lymphedema is usually confined to the feet and legs.

There are several types of congenital abnormalities associated with other **birth defects** of the lymphatics, which cause this condition. One in 10,000 people have this type of lymphedema.

Lymphatics can be damaged or obstructed by many different agents. Repeated bouts of blood poisoning can scar the vessels. Surgery to remove cancerous lymph nodes or **radiation therapy** can damage them. Cancer itself, as it invades the lymph system, as well as several other infectious and inflammatory conditions, can result in blockage of lymph flow. The most common worldwide cause of lymphedema is a group of worms known as filaria. Filaria can be found in most of the developing regions of the world. They enter humans through insect bites, mostly mosquitoes, and take up residence in lymphatic channels, irritating them enough to scar them and impair their ability to carry lymph. Long-standing lymphatic **filariasis** can cause massive swelling of the legs, earning the name **elephantiasis**.

Since other types of swelling may look similar to lymphedema, precise diagnostic tools must be used. Ultrasound, **computed tomography scans** (CT), and **magnetic resonance imaging** (MRI) scans may help with diagnosis. Lymphangiography may be needed to clarify the cause.

Physical activity can pump some of the fluid out of the tissues. Compression stockings are of some value, as are devices that actively squeeze fluid out of tissues. **Diuretics** may alleviate some of the edema. Because the ability of the skin to defend itself is hampered by the swelling, infections are more common. It is therefore important to care for **wounds** and to treat infections early.

When caused by infection, lymphedema can be treated by eliminating the underlying infection with **antibiotics**.

Reconstructing lymphatic channels using microvascular surgery has recently achieved some success.

If congenital, lymphedema is a progressive and lifelong condition. If secondary or caused by an underlying disease or infection, lymphedema can be treated by treating the disease.

When traveling in regions known to have filaria, avoidance of insect bites is crucial. Prompt and effective treatment of the infection will prevent the consequences.

LYMPHOMAS, MALIGNANT

Lymphomas are a group of **cancer**s in which cells of the **lymphatic system** become abnormal and start to grow uncontrollably. Because there is lymph tissue in many parts of the body, lymphomas can start in almost any organ of the body.

The lymphatic system is made up of ducts or tubules that carry a milky fluid (lymph) to all parts of the body. Lymph contains the lymphocytes or white blood cells, which are the infection- fighting cells of the body. Small pea-shaped organs are found along the network of lymph vessels. These are called the lymph nodes, and their main function is to make and store the lymphocytes. Clusters of lymph nodes are found in the pelvis region, underarm, neck, chest, and abdomen. The spleen (an organ in the upper abdomen), the tonsils, and the thymus (a small organ found beneath the breastbone) are part of the lymphatic system.

The lymphocyte is the main cell of the lymphoid tissue. There are two main types of lymphocytes: the T lymphocyte and the B lymphocyte. These two types of cells perform different jobs within the immune system. B cell lymphomas are more common among adults, while among children, the incidence of T and B cell lymphomas are almost equal.

Lymphomas can be divided into two main types: Hodgkin's lymphoma and non-Hodgkin's lymphomas. A majority of non-Hodgkin's lymphomas begin in the lymph nodes. Malignant lymphocytes multiply uncontrollably and do not perform their normal functions. Hence, the body's ability to fight infections is affected. In addition, these malignant cells may crowd the bone marrow, and, prevent the production of normal blood cells.

The exact cause of non-Hodgkin's lymphomas is not known. However, the incidence has increased significantly in the recent years. Part of the increase is due to the **AIDS** epidemic. Individuals infected with the AIDS virus have a higher likelihood of developing non-Hodgkin's lymphomas. In general, males are at a higher risk for having non-Hodgkin's lymphomas than are females. The risk increases with age.

The symptoms of lymphomas are often vague and non-specific. Patients may experience loss of appetite, weight loss, nausea, vomiting, abdominal discomfort, and **indigestion**. The patient may complain of a feeling of fullness, which is a result of enlarged lymph nodes in the abdomen. Pressure or **pain** in the lower back is another symptom. In the advanced stages, the patient may have bone pain, **headache**s, constant coughing, and abnormal pressure and congestion in the face, neck, and upper chest. Some may have **fever**s and night sweats. In most cases, patients go to the doctor because of the presence of swollen glands in the neck, armpits, or groin area.

Like all cancers, lymphomas are best treated when found early. However, it is often difficult to diagnose lymphomas. There are no screening tests available, and, since the symptoms are non-specific, lymphomas are rarely recognized in their early stages. Detection often occurs by chance during a routine **physical examination**.

When the doctor suspects lymphoma, a complete medical history is taken, and a thorough physical examination is performed. Enlargement of the lymph nodes, liver, or spleen may suggest lymphomas. Blood tests will determine the cell counts and obtain information on how well the organs, such as the kidney and liver, are functioning. A biopsy of the enlarged lymph node is the most definitive diagnostic tool for staging purposes.

Conventional imaging tests, such as x rays, **computed tomography scans** (CT scans), **magnetic resonance imaging**, and abdominal sonograms, are used to determine the extent of spread of the disease.

Treatment options for lymphomas depend on the type of lymphoma and its present stage. In most cases, treatment consists of **chemotherapy**, radiotherapy, or a combination of the two methods.

Chemotherapy is the use of **anticancer drugs** to kill cancer cells. In non-Hodgkin's lymphomas, combination therapy, which involves the use of multiple drugs, has been found more effective than single drug use. The treatment may last about six months, but in some cases may last as long as a year. The drugs may either be administered intravenously (through a vein) in the arm or given orally in the form of pills. **Radiation therapy**, where high-energy ionizing rays are directed at specific portions of the body, such as the upper chest, abdomen, pelvis, or neck, is often used for treatment of lymphomas.

Like all cancers, the prognosis for lymphoma depends on the stage of the cancer, and the patient's age and general health. The survival rate among children is definitely better than among older people. About 90% of the children diagnosed with early stage disease survive 5 years or more.

Although many cancers may be prevented by making diet and life style changes which reduce risk factors, there is currently no known way to prevent lymphomas. Protecting oneself from developing AIDS, which may be a risk factor for lymphomas, is the only preventive measure that can be practiced.

LYNEN, FEODOR (1911-1979)

German biochemist

Feodor Felix Konrad Lynen was born in Munich, Germany, on April 6, 1911, the seventh of eight children, to Wilhelm and Frieda (Prym) Lynen. Lynen showed an early interest in his older brother's chemistry an eventually, enrolled in the Department of Chemistry at the University of Munich in 1930. There he studied with German chemist and Nobel laureate Heinrich Wieland (1877-1957), who was Lynen's principal teacher both as an undergraduate and graduate student. On February 12, 1937, Lynen received his doctorate degree. Three months later, on May 17, he married Wieland's daughter, Eva, with whom he would have five children: Peter, Annemarie, Susanne, Eva-Marie, and Heinrich.

Upon his graduation, Lynen stayed at the University of Munich in a postdoctoral research position. In 1942, he was appointed a lecturer, and eventually was made a full professor in 1953. A year later, he was named director of the newly established Max Planck Institute for Cell Chemistry. Throughout his years with the University, where he stayed until his death, Lynen supervised the research of nearly ninety students, many of whom reached leading positions in academia or industry.

In the first years after World War II, German scientists were spurned by their European and American colleagues. Only four German biochemists were invited to attend the First International Congress of Biochemistry held in Cambridge, England, in July of 1949. Lynen, one of the four, made an ideal good-will ambassador for Germany because of his good sense of humor and the fondness he had for parties. His cheery nature and solid research drew many foreign scientists to Munich. His magnetic personality was formally recognized years

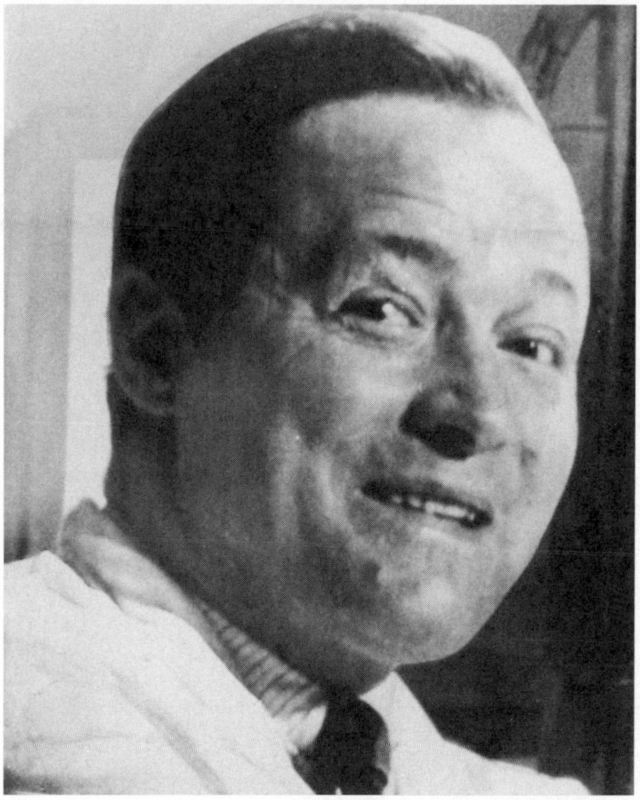

Feodor Lynen

later when, in 1975, he was chosen to serve as president of the Alexander von Humboldt Foundation, an institution devoted to fostering relations between Germany and the international scientific community.

During the 1940s, Lynen began studying how the living cell changes simple chemical compounds into sterols and lipids, complex molecules that the body needs to sustain life. The long sequence of steps and the roles various enzymes and **vitamins** played in this complicated metabolic process were not well understood. After the war, Lynen began to publish his early findings. At the same time, he became aware of similar work being conducted in the United States by **Konrad Bloch**. Eventually, Lynen and Bloch began to correspond, sharing their preliminary discoveries with each other. By working in this manner, the scientists determined the sequence of thirty-six steps by which animal cells produce cholesterol.

One of the breakthroughs in the cholesterol synthesis work came in 1951 when Lynen published a paper describing the first step in the chain of reactions that resulted in the production of cholesterol. He had discovered that a compound known as acetyl-coenzyme A, which is formed when an acetate radical reacts with coenzyme A, was needed to begin the chemical chain reaction. For the first time, the chemical structure of acetyl-coenzyme A was described in accurate detail. By solving this complex biochemical problem, Lynen established his international reputation and created a new set of challenging biochemical problems. Determining the structure of acetyl-coenzyme A supplied Lynen with the discovery he needed to advance his research.

During his rehabilitation from a serious ski injury at the end of 1951, Lynen contemplated how the structure and action of acetyl-coenzyme A made it a likely participant in other biochemical processes. Upon his return to the lab, Lynen began investigating the role of acetyl-coenzyme A in the biosynthesis of fatty acids and discovered that, as with cholesterol, this substance was the necessary first step. Lynen also investigated the catabolism of fatty acids, the chemical reactions that produce energy when fatty acids in foods are burned up to form carbon dioxide and water.

In addition to elucidating the role of acetyl-coenzyme A, Lynen's research revealed the importance of many other chemicals in the body. One of the most significant of these was his work with the vitamin biotin. In the late 1950s, Lynen demonstrated that biotin was needed for the production of fat.

Lynen and Bloch shared the Nobel Prize in medicine or physiology in 1964, largely because the Nobel Committee recognized the medical importance of their work. Medical authorities knew that an accumulation of cholesterol in the walls of arteries and in blood contributed to diseases of the circulatory system, including arteriosclerosis, **heart attacks**, and **strokes**. In its tribute to Lynen and Bloch, the Nobel Committee noted that a more complete understanding of the **metabolism** of sterols and fatty acids promised to reveal the possible role of cholesterol in heart disease. Any future research into the link between cholesterol and heart disease, the Nobel committee observed, would have to be based on the findings of Lynen and Bloch.

In 1972, Lynen moved to the Max Planck Institute for Biochemistry, which had just recently been founded. Between 1974 and 1976, Lynen was acting director of the Institute. He continued to oversee a lab at the University of Munich, however.

At the end of his life, Lynen was a renowned scientist, and a proud Bavarian. The author of over three hundred scholarly pieces, Lynen was also praised as a hard-working man who expected much of himself and his students. Six weeks after an aneurism operation, Lynen died on August 6, 1979, at the age of 68.

M

MACLEOD, JOHN JAMES RICKARD (1876-1935)

Scottish physiologist

John James Rickard Macleod was born in Cluny, near Dunkeld, Scotland, on September 6, 1876, the son of the Reverend Robert Macleod. Soon after his birth, the family moved to Aberdeen. Macleod attended Aberdeen Grammar School and Aberdeen University. He went on to study medicine at Marischal College, where he graduated with honors in 1898. With an Anderson traveling scholarship, Macleod continued his education at Leipzig's Physiology Institute where he studied biochemistry for a year. In 1900 he returned to London to become a demonstrator in physiology at the London Hospital Medical College, and the following year became a biochemistry lecturer there. The same year he was named a Mackinnon research scholar by the Royal Society. During this period, Macleod published his experiments on intracranial circulation and caisson's disease. In 1902 he attended Cambridge University and obtained a diploma in public health. He married Mary Watson in 1903, and journeyed to America to become professor of physiology at Western Reserve University in Cleveland, where he stayed for 15 years. The same year he arrived at Western Reserve, his text, *Practical Physiology,* was published.

Macleod began his investigations into the human body's carbohydrate **metabolism** during his early years at Western Reserve, studying salt and urea metabolism. Studies of the breakdown of liver glycogen followed, and in 1913, he published *Diabetes: Its Physiological Pathology.* In 1918, Macleod went to the University of Toronto to become a professor of physiology and associate dean of the faculty of medicine. Macleod's major areas of interest at this time were the effects of oxygen excess and deprivation. He also studied respiration in animals whose brains had been removed or spines cut. During this period, he wrote *Physiology and Biochemistry in Modern Medicine.* The 1,000-page book went through seven editions and became a standard text in the field.

In 1921 Macleod returned to his work on carbohydrate **metabolism**, comparing the blood-sugar level in normal animals with that of animals with their pancreas removed. At the time it was known that **diabetes** was caused by the failure of the pancreas to secrete a substance that regulates sugar metabolism, causing an abnormally high concentration of glucose in the blood and an excretion of sugar into the urine. It was also understood that the unidentified substance sped the passage of sugar in the form of glucose through the body to be oxidized as a source of energy or converted the sugar into glycogen for storage for later use as glucose. Macleod appointed **Frederick Grant Banting**, a Canadian orthopedic surgeon, to specifically investigate the function of a cluster of cells in the pancreas known as the islet of Langerhans. Macleod chose Charles Herbert Best, one of his senior medical students, to be Banting's chief laboratory assistant. Together the three men planned how they would separate the islet from the pancreas to isolate the substance secreted by the cell cluster. This substance, Macleod believed, was the sugar regulator they were seeking.

When Banting and Best tied the ducts of the pancreas so that it would atrophy, they were able to isolate a residue in the islet. They injected this extract into dogs and found that it did indeed lower blood glucose. The problem of how to obtain larger quantities of the extract, named **insulin**, remained. For help, Banting turned to James Bertram Collip, a young Canadian biochemist. Collip used pancreas glands bought from a butcher as a source of insulin. To demonstrate how safe the extract was, Banting and Best injected themselves with insulin. By January, 1922, they had begun clinical trials. A youngster named Leonard Thompson was the first diabetic to receive insulin injections. The results proved that the new treatment controlled the debilitating disease. Solving the final problem of making insulin therapy available to the general public, an American biochemist, John Jacob Abel, converted insulin into a crystalline form in 1926, so that it could be given in precise dosages. Today insulin is prepared from the pancreatic tissue of domestic animals.

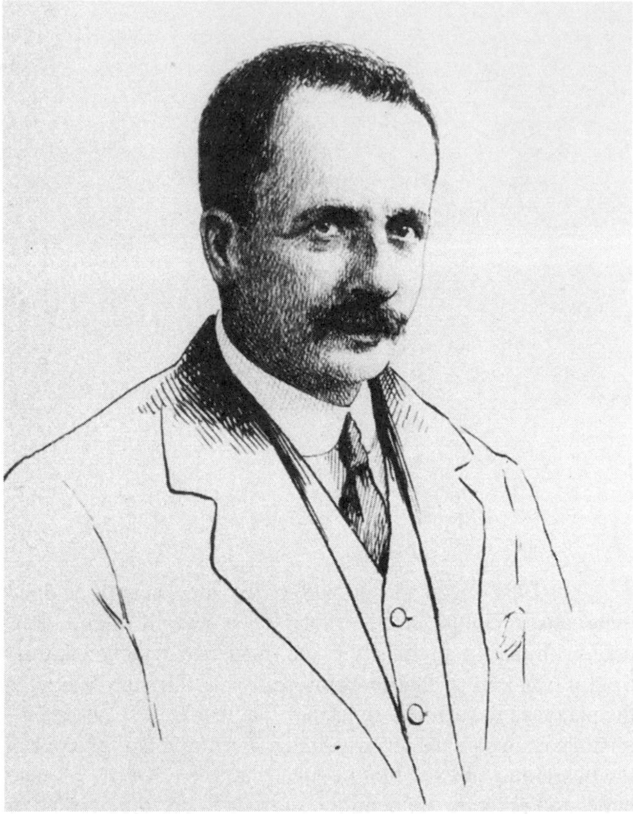

John James Rickard Macleod

The Nobel Prize committee acted with remarkable swiftness to recognize the achievement. Macleod and Banting were given the Nobel Prize in 1923, only a year after their discovery. Collip later noted that Macleod's outstanding position in the field of carbohydrate metabolism had made it appropriate and fortunate that the discovery of insulin had been made in his laboratory. Macleod, for his part, maintained that it was only through team work that insulin could be isolated. He shared his prize money with Collip, while Banting divided his with Best.

In 1928 Macleod returned to Scotland to become chairman of the physiology department at the University of Aberdeen. He continued his research into carbohydrate metabolism there and at the Rowett Institute, publishing numerous papers on insulin, experimental glycosuria—the presence of sugar in the urine—respiration and lactic acid metabolism. Arthritis forced him to discontinue his laboratory work, but he continued supervising the work of the physiology department. He died on March 16, 1935, at the age of 58.

MACULAR DEGENERATION

Macular degeneration is the progressive deterioration of a critical region of the retina called the macula. The macula is a 3-5 mm area in the retina that is responsible for central vision. This disorder leads to irreversible loss of central vision, although peripheral vision is retained. In the early stages, vision may be gray, hazy, or distorted.

Macular degeneration is the most common cause of legal blindness in people over 60, and accounts for approximately 11.7% of blindness in the United States. About 28% of the population over age 74 is affected by this disease.

Age-related macular degeneration (ARMD) is the most common form of macular degeneration. It is also known as age-related maculopathy (ARM), aged macular degeneration, and senile macular degeneration. Approximately 10 million Americans have some vision loss that is due to ARMD.

ARMD is subdivided into a dry (atrophic) and a wet (exudative) form. The dry form is more common and accounts for 70-90% of cases of ARMD. It progresses more slowly than the wet form and vision loss is less severe. In the dry form, the macula thins over time as part of the aging process and the pigmented retinal epithelium (a dark-colored cell layer at the back of the eye) is gradually lost. Words may appear blurred or hazy and colors may appear dim or gray.

In the wet form of ARMD, new blood vessels grow underneath the retina and distort the retina. These blood vessels can leak, causing scar tissue to form on the retina. The wet form may cause visual distortion and make straight lines appear wavy. A central blind spot develops. The wet type progresses more rapidly and vision loss is more pronounced. Treatments are available for some, but not most, cases of the wet form.

Other less common forms of macular degeneration include

- Cystoid macular degeneration. Loss of vision in the macula due to fluid-filled areas (cysts) in the macular region. This may be a result of other disorders, such as aging, inflammation, or high myopia.
- Diabetic macular degeneration. Deterioration of the macula due to diabetes.
- Senile disciform degeneration (also known as Kuhnt-Junius macular degeneration). A specific and severe type of the wet form of ARMD that involves leaking blood vessels (hemorrhaging) in the macular region. It usually occurs in people over 40 years old.

Age-related macular degeneration is part of the aging process. There may be a hereditary component. Having a family member with ARMD increases a person's risk for developing it. There is a slightly higher incidence in females. Whites and Asians are more susceptible to developing ARMD than blacks, in whom the disorder is rare.

ARMD is thought to be caused by hardening and blocking of the arteries (arteriosclerosis) in the blood vessels supplying the retina. Some of the same things that are bad for the heart are thought to contribute to the development of macular degeneration. These risk factors include smoking and a diet that is rich in saturated fat. Smokers have a risk of developing ARMD that is approximately 2.4-3 times that of non-smokers. Smoking increases the risk of developing wet-type ARMD, and may increase the risk of developing dry-type as well. Dietary fat also increase the risk. In one study of older (age 45-

84) Americans, signs of early ARMD were 80% more common in the group who ate the most saturated fat compared to those who ate the least. Low consumption of antioxidants, such as foods rich in vitamin A, is associated with a higher risk for developing ARMD. Consumption of moderate amounts of red wine and foods rich in vitamin A is associated with a lower risk. It is generally believed that exposure to ultraviolet (UV) light may contribute to disease development, but this has not been proven.

The main symptom of macular degeneration is a change in central vision. The patient may notice blurred central vision or a blank spot on the page when reading. The patient may notice visual distortion such as bending of straight lines. Images may appear smaller. Some patients notice a change in color perception and some experience abnormal light sensations. These symptoms may come on suddenly and become progressively more troublesome. Sudden onset of symptoms, particularly vision distortion, is an indication for immediate evaluation by an ophthalmologist.

To make the diagnosis of macular degeneration, the doctor dilates the pupil with eye drops and examines the interior of the eye, looking at the retina for the presence of yellow bumps called drusen and for gross changes in the macula such as thinning. The doctor also administers a visual field test, looking for blank spots in the central vision. The doctor may call for fluorescein **angiography** (intravenous injection of fluorescent dye followed by visual examination and photography of the back of the eye) to determine if blood vessels in the retina are leaking.

A central visual field test called an Amsler grid is usually given to patients who are suspected of having ARMD. It is a grid printed on a sheet of paper (so it is easy to take home). When looking at a central dot on the page, the patient should call the doctor right away if any of the lines appear to be wavy or missing. This may be an indication of fluid and the onset of wet ARMD. Patients may also be asked to come in for more frequent checkups.

While loss of vision cannot be reversed, early detection is important because treatments are available that may halt or slow the progression of the wet form of ARMD. Treatment for the dry form is not available as of 1998, but cell transplantation studies are under study.

In wet-type ARMD and in senile disciform macular degeneration, new capillaries grow in the macular region and leak. This leaking of blood and fluid causes a portion of the retina to detach. Blood vessel growth, called neovascularization, can be treated with laser photocoagulation in some cases, depending upon the location and extent of the growth. Argon or krypton lasers can destroy the new tissue and flatten the retina. This treatment is effective in about half the cases but results may be temporary. A concern with laser therapy is that the laser also destroys the photoreceptors in the treated area. If the blood vessels have grown into the fovea (a region of the macula responsible for fine vision), treatment may not be possible. Because capillaries can grow very quickly, this form of macular degeneration should be handled as an emergency and treated quickly. Patients who are experiencing visual distortion should seek help immediately.

Another form of treatment for the wet form of ARMD is **radiation therapy** with either x rays or a proton beam. Blood vessels that are proliferating (growing) are sensitive to treatment with low doses of ionizing radiation. Nerve cells in the retina are not growing and are insensitive, so they are not harmed by this treatment. External beam radiation treatment has shown promising results at slowing progression in limited, early trials. An alternative treatment is internal beam radiation therapy. For this treatment, the patient is given a local anesthetic and an applicator containing strontium 90 is inserted into the affected eye. This brief and localized radiation therapy prevents the growth of blood vessels.

Other therapies that are under study include treatment with alpha-interferon, thalidomide, and other drugs that slow the growth of blood vessels. Subretinal surgery also has shown promise in rapid-onset cases of wet ARMD. This surgery carries the risk of **retinal detachment**, hemorrhage, and acceleration of cataract formation. Other experimental treatments include photodynamic therapy (PDT). For this treatment, a photosensitizing dye is injected, followed by irradiation of the area of new blood vessel growth with a special, low-intensity diode laser. This treatment damages the cells in the blood vessel walls and causes them to stop growing.

A controversial treatment called rheotherapy involves pumping the patient's blood through a device that removes some proteins and fats. As of 1998, this had not been proven to be safe or effective.

Consumption of a diet rich in antioxidants (beta carotene and the mixed carotenoids that are precursors of vitamin A, **vitamins** C and E, selenium, and zinc), or taking antioxidant nutritional supplements, may help prevent macular degeneration, particularly if started early in life. Good dietary sources of antioxidants include citrus fruits, cauliflower, broccoli, nuts, seeds, orange and yellow vegetables, cherries, blackberries, and blueberries. Research has shown that nutritional therapy can prevent ARMD or slow its progression once established. Some doctors recommend taking beta carotene and zinc as a precautionary measure. Some vitamins are marketed specifically for the eyes.

The dry form of ARMD is self-limiting and eventually stabilizes. The loss of vision is permanent. The vision of patients with the wet form of ARMD often stabilizes or improves even without treatment, at least temporarily. However, after a few years, patients with the wet form of ARMD are usually left with only coarse peripheral vision remaining.

Many patients with macular degeneration lose their central vision permanently and may become legally blind. However, macular degeneration rarely causes total loss of vision. Peripheral vision is retained. The patient can compensate, to some extent, for the loss of central vision, even though macular degeneration may render them legally blind. Improved lighting and special low-vision aids may help even if sharpness of vision (visual acuity) is poor. Vision aids include special magnifiers that allow the patient to read and telescopic aids for long-distance vision. The use of these visual aids plus the retained peripheral vision usually allow the patient to remain independent. Registration as a legally blind person will enable a patient to obtain special services and considerations.

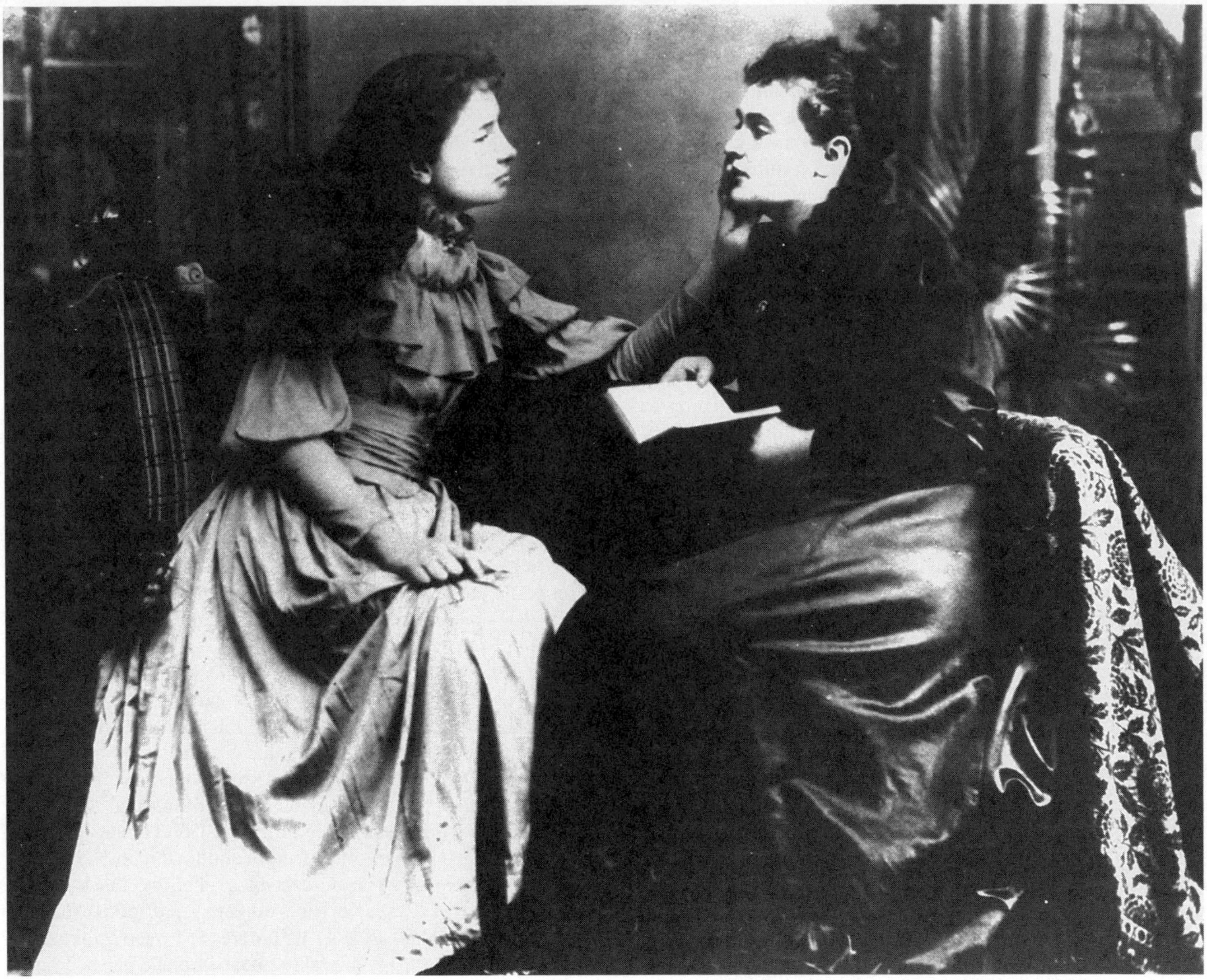

Anne Sullivan Macy (right), with Helen Keller.

Avoiding the risk factors for macular degeneration may help prevent it. This includes avoiding tobacco smoke and eating a diet low in saturated fat. Some other behaviors that may help reduce the risk of wet-type ARMD are eating a diet rich in green, leafy vegetables and yellow vegetables such as carrots, sweet potatoes, and winter squash; drinking moderate amounts of alcohol, such as one or two glasses of red wine a day; and taking an antioxidant vitamin supplement, especially vitamin A. Some vitamins may be toxic in large doses, so patients should speak with their doctors. Vitamins C and E have not been shown to reduce risk, nor did selenium in one large study. The use of zinc is controversial: some studies showed a benefit, others showed no benefit, and one actually showed an increased risk of ARMD with increased levels of zinc in the blood. Some doctors suggest that wearing UV-blocking sunglasses reduces risk. Use of estrogen in postmenopausal women is associated with a lower risk of developing ARMD.

See also Visual impairment and blindness

Macy, Anne Sullivan (1866-1936)

American Teacher

Anne Sullivan Macy was an American educator, best known for her work as Helen Keller's teacher. Born in Feeding Hills, Massachusetts, on April 14, 1866, she was named Joanna Mansfield Sullivan, but was always called Anne or Annie.

Sullivan's youth was not a happy one. As a child, an infection damaged her eyes, causing them to weaken throughout her early life until she was nearly blind. Her mother died of **tuberculosis** when she was 8, and her father deserted Sullivan and her siblings three years later. At age 11, Sullivan and her lame brother were sent to the state poorhouse in Tewksbury.

She lived in the almshouse for four years. One day, during a visit by the State Board of Charities, Sullivan asked a board member if she could go to school. The board agreed, and in 1880 Sullivan was assigned to the Perkins Institute for the Blind in Watertown, Massachusetts. While a student there, she had several surgeries that partially restored her sight. Sullivan graduated from Perkins in 1886 as class valedictorian.

While at Perkins, Sullivan learned the manual alphabet, a kind of language that uses a series of hand motions to represent letters and is used mostly by people who are both blind and deaf. Sullivan learned this alphabet in order to communicate with Laura Bridgman, a fellow student and the first deaf-blind person to be educated in the United States.

A year after graduating from Perkins, Sullivan took the train from Boston to Tuscumbia, Alabama, to meet Helen Keller, an undisciplined, angry child she had been hired to teach. Helen had been left blind, deaf, and mute as the result of an illness during infancy and had no means of communicating with others.

After an extremely difficult adjustment period, Sullivan worked to calm Helen down and gain her trust. She began trying to communicate with Helen through the manual alphabet she had learned at the Perkins School. She taught Helen by using her finger to spell the names of objects into Helen's palm, while allowing the child to feel or hold the objects at the same time. One day, while spelling w-a-t-e-r into Helen's palm as running water poured over their hands, Helen suddenly made the connection between the letters in her hand and the water she could feel running through her fingers. From then on, she was able to learn rapidly.

From that moment on, Sullivan became Keller's trusted constant companion. She accompanied Helen to the Perkins Institute where the child was educated, and later to the Wright-Humason School in New York City. They both went to the Cambridge School for Young Ladies. Eventually, Sullivan accompanied Helen to Radcliffe College in Boston. Sullivan served as Helen's translator, spelling out the lectures into her palm, and reading to her through the use of the manual alphabet for long periods every day. While Helen has been praised as an excellent student, Sullivan's role as her teacher and friend has been widely recognized as vital to Helen's success.

When Helen graduated from Radcliffe in 1904, she and Sullivan moved to a farm in Wrentham, Massachusetts, that had been donated to them by a benefactor. While living there, Helen wrote her famous autobiography, *The Story of My Life*. A Harvard instructor, John Albert Macy, worked with Helen to edit the book. Eventually, he and Sullivan fell in love and were married in the living room of the Wrentham home. However, Sullivan found it difficult to spend time away from Helen, and John Macy grew discouraged at having to share his wife with her blind student. The couple stayed together for eight years, separating in 1913. While they did not live together after that time, the couple remained married.

Meanwhile, Sullivan remained the constant companion of Helen, who had become a celebrated socialist commentator and advocate for the educational rights of handicapped persons. They traveled together on lecture tours that took them all over the world. In 1917, the two moved from Wrentham, and in 1924 they began working as fundraisers and advocates for the American Foundation for the Blind. In 1927, Nella Braddy began writing Sullivan's biography, *Anne Sullivan Macy*. The book was published in 1933.

Sullivan's health began declining rapidly at about this time, and her eyesight, which had never been good, continued to deteriorate. By 1935 she was completely blind, and she died October 20, 1936 in Forest Hills, New York, at 70 years of age.

See also Hearing loss; Keller, Helen; Mutism; Visual impairment and blindness

Magnetic resonance imaging (MRI)

Magnetic resonance imaging (MRI) allows physicians to examine tissues and organs inside the body by observing the response of atoms exposed to a strong magnetic field. In a closed MRI, the patient lies inside a machine in a 48-inch tube; in an open—or ''accessible''—MRI the patient lies on a table. More sensitive than X-ray spectroscopy, MRI does not rely upon potentially harmful radiation. Instead, a powerful electromagnet creates radio waves that cause hydrogen atoms in the body to release energy. The magnet can map this energy from almost 360 degrees, projecting images to a computer which gives an extremely high-resolution picture. Because MRI can scan through bone, it can probe the brain in search of a tumor, to assess stroke damage, or identify degeneration. It also ''sees'' under nerve coverings to help diagnose multiple sclerosis; reports joint injuries in muscle and ligaments; identifies blocked blood vessels; helps diagnose heart, liver and kidney disease; and is among the most powerful tools for detecting tissue abnormalities such as cancer.The series of scientific developments leading to the invention of MRI actually began in the late 1930s. Isidor Isaac Rabi (1898-1988), an American scientist, designed a process by which the magnetic strengths of atomic nuclei could be recorded. Firing a vaporized beam of silver through a magnetic field, he noted that the nuclei behaved like spinning tops, and that they wobbled at very precise frequencies; when radio signals that matched the frequencies of the wobble were applied, the nuclei reversed their spin. This phenomenon, called magnetic resonance, was very easy to observe, and much could be learned about the structure of the atom by knowing the resonance frequency. After World War II, two other American scientists, working independently, devised improvements upon Rabi's process, making it more precise and eliminating the need to vaporize (and thus destroy) the sample. Scientists Felix Bloch (1905-1983) and Edward Purcell (1912-1997) shared the 1952 Nobel Prize for Physics for *nuclear magnetic resonance (NMR) spectroscopy*, which gained an immediate place in nuclear laboratories as the most precise tool for studying molecules. Chemists had earlier discovered that a nucleus' wobble revealed information about surrounding molecules, and that each atom and molecule carried a ''signature wobble.'' By recognizing these signatures, researchers could use NMR to identify the composition of unknown chemical samples.

The most important application was forthcoming, however. Raymond V. Damadian (1916-) was the first to realize that NMR could be used on living tissue. He tested first on animals and then on humans, finding that the process was excellent for detecting areas of disease inside the body—areas that had previously required exploratory surgery to locate. NMR was especially useful for detecting cancer, since cancer cells carry their own signature resonance frequency. About this same time, the Swiss physical chemist, Richard R. Ernst (1933-), was working upon improving the NMR process yet again. By changing the radio signals, Ernst succeeded in making the technology more sensitive and easier to interpret—improvements that paved the way for the development of MRI, for which Ernst was awarded the 1991 Nobel Prize for Chemistry. MRI enables physicians to create three-dimensional images of large sections of molecules. It can define areas of soft tissue too thin to be picked up by X-rays. Using the radio signals, the computer will search for the frequencies of specific types of atoms (such as cancer cells). Once the radio waves are turned off, the atoms emit pulses of absorbed energy; the computer reads these pulses, creating a three-dimensional image of the scanned area. MRI scanners are generally found only in large medical research centers: the equipment is extremely expensive, and a trained radiologist must be present to supervise the procedure. The technology required to perform NMR scanning is much more affordable and easier to use; NMR units can be found in a variety of sizes at most hospitals. Both inventions have become important diagnostic tools. In fact, the Royal Swedish Academy (while announcing Ernst's Nobel Prize) described NMR spectroscopy as "perhaps the most important instrumental measuring technique within chemistry."

MAINSTREAMING

Mainstreaming is an inclusive form of education where students are taught in a comprehensive school system. Special education is available for students with special needs, but the goal is for the majority of students and those with special needs to learn in the same classroom whenever possible.

From the 1920s until the 1970s, the trend in Western countries was to set up special schools to educate students with special needs. With the passage of the Individuals with Disabilities Education Act (IDEA), Section 504 of the Rehabilitation Act in 1973, schools tried to bring all students under the same roof and provide services as needed. In 1975, PL 94-142 (Education for All Handicapped Children Act) was passed, giving every child the right to education in the least restrictive environment. In effect, all schoolchildren were given the right to a free public education.

With the advent of IDEA in the 1970s, educators and advocates for students with disabilities began pushing for all students to be taught among their peers in regular neighborhood schools. Mildly and moderately handicapped students began to be placed in regular classes, at least part time. Students with more profound handicaps began attending regular schools. Even when students had handicaps severe enough to prevent placement in regular classes, the reasoning was that all students would benefit from interacting in the hallway, homeroom, bus, and playground. The goal was to provide common meeting places so students could form friendships and share a feeling of community in their neighborhood school.

By the late 1980s, after additional observation and research, many educators and parents favored the merging of special and regular education into a comprehensive school system. Advocates pointed out that a dual system did not meet students' needs, was inefficient to administer, and promoted inappropriate attitudes toward students with disabilities.

Advocates were more interested in increasing the ability of mainstream education to meet the needs of all students, rather than spending time classifying students to see who should be in the mainstream. A federal system of definitions, however, was already in place, though it was not used consistently. School districts found themselves on shifting ground. They had to understand and accommodate students with special needs, without creating a counterproductive separate-but-equal atmosphere.

In a 1991 modification to IDEA, the federal government defined 13 categories of disability: **autism**, deaf-blindness, deafness, hearing impairment, **mental retardation**, multiple disabilities, orthopedic impairment, other health impairment, serious emotional disturbance, special learning disability, speech or language impairment, traumatic brain injury, and visual impairment. States and school districts were free, however, to use their own definitions, and there is wide variety in classification.

National statistics show that enrollment in special education is highest in the elementary school years. By high school, typically 4 to 5 percent of special education students are returned to general education classrooms.

Until the 1990s, boys were referred for special education more frequently than girls, but some 1996 statistics show boys and girls being referred in equal numbers. Research in the 1960s suggested a pattern of minority children being placed in special education in disproportionate numbers, spurring federal lawsuits. Some 1990s findings, however, suggest that overrepresentation of minorities is decreasing. Statistics on incidence of disability among African American, Native American, Hispanic, and other racial groups now show a closer match with population figures. Analysts point out, however, that it is very difficult to measure the individual effects of socioeconomic status, poverty, race, and ethnicity.

An overview of the guidelines shows that for a student to be eligible for special education, he or she must have a disability that can only be helped by special education. Special education can be used only when education in a regular classroom does not work. For example, a school district would need to make other arrangements if a special needs student was disruptive and prevented the students in a standard classroom from learning, or if the standard classroom wasn't providing a sufficient education for a special needs student.

The trend is for school districts to appoint support facilitators who help regular teachers with resources and equipment. Ideally, support facilitators work in the classroom with all students who need help, rather than focusing exclusively on the special needs student and drawing undue attention to him or her.

Students with medical and physical disabilities are protected by Section 504 and may still receive special accommodations at school, such as adaptive equipment, but they do not receive special education unless they show educational need.

The various trends in mainstreaming come to a head at the end of high school, when districts award diplomas differently. Some high schools grant diplomas with the same set of standards, exams, and course work applied to all students. Other schools offer a different credential or certificate of completion for special education students. The diploma, therefore, may not always mean the same thing. A 1990 congressional study showed about 30 percent of disabled students dropping out of school between grades 9 and 12.

To address some of these problems, Congress passed the Goals 2000: Educate America Act in 1994. The act calls for standards-based reform that would reorganize educational standards. The ultimate goal would be to devise a fair way of developing one system of accountability that applies to all students. Special education students would still have an individualized educational program (IEP) and achievable goals, and there would be more of an effort to tailor goals to every student's abilities and needs. Advocates would like to see school districts break away from evaluating students chiefly on norms that are based on peer performance. Ideally, all graduates would have a credential that accurately reflected their skills and achievements.

The Committee on Goals 2000 recognized that not enough is known about special education and standards-based reform and recommended long-term research in search of new information. Education studies have either omitted special education students or have measured them inconsistently. There is very little data on how special education students compare with general education students. There isn't enough information on funding special education and there is no information on how standards-based reform would be paid for. While educators acknowledge that schools classify disabled students in many different ways, there is little information on how these local decisions are actually made. In addition, families of disabled students are often overlooked and more models are needed for using families in educational planning.

Inclusive education is of great interest internationally, and as of 1997, some 24 countries of the Organization for Economic Cooperation and Development were conducting studies on restructuring special education.

MALABSORPTION SYNDROME

Malabsorption syndrome is an alteration in the ability of the intestine to absorb nutrients adequately into the bloodstream.

Protein, fats, and carbohydrates (macronutrients) normally are absorbed in the small intestine; the small bowel also absorbs about 80% of the eight to ten liters of fluid ingested daily. There are many different conditions that affect fluid and nutrient absorption by the intestine. A fault in the digestive process may result from failure of the body to produce the enzymes needed to digest certain foods. Congenital structural defects or diseases of the pancreas, gall bladder, or liver may alter the digestive process. Inflammation, infection, injury, or surgical removal of portions of the intestine may also result in absorption problems; reduced length or surface area of intestine available for fluid and nutrient absorption can result in malabsorption. **Radiation therapy** may injure the mucosal lining of the intestine, resulting in **diarrhea** that may not become evident until several years later. The use of some **antibiotics** can also affect the bacteria that normally live in the intestine and affect intestinal function.

Risk factors for malabsorption syndrome include:

- Family history of malabsorption or **cystic fibrosis**
- Use of certain drugs, such as mineral oil or other **laxatives**
- Travel to foreign countries
- Intestinal surgery
- Excess alcohol consumption.

The most common symptoms of malabsorption include:

- Anemia, with weakness and fatigue due to inadequate absorption of vitamin B_{12}, iron, and folic acid
- Diarrhea, steatorrhea (excessive amount of fat in the stool), and abdominal distention with cramps, bloating, and gas due to impaired water and carbohydrate absorption, and irritation from unabsorbed fatty acids. The individual may also report explosive diarrhea with greasy, foul-smelling stools.
- **Edema** (fluid retention in the body's tissues) due to decreased protein absorption
- **Malnutrition** and weight loss due to decreased fat, carbohydrate, and protein absorption. Weight may be 80-90% of usual weight despite increased oral intake of nutrients.
- Muscle cramping due to decreased vitamin D, calcium, and potassium levels
- Muscle wasting and atrophy due to decreased protein absorption and metabolism
- Perianal skin burning, **itching**, or soreness due to frequent loose stools.

Irregular heart rhythms may also result from inadequate levels of potassium and other electrolytes. Blood clotting disorders may occur due to a **vitamin K deficiency**. Children with malabsorption syndrome often exhibit a failure to grow and thrive.

Several disorders can lead to malabsorption syndrome, including cystic fibrosis, chronic **pancreatitis**, lactose intolerance, and gluten enteropathy (non-tropical sprue.)

Tropical sprue is a malabsorptive disorder that is uncommon in the United States, but seen more often in people from the Caribbean, India, or southeast Asia. Although its cause is unknown, it is thought to be related to environmental factors, including infection, intestinal parasites, or possibly the consumption of certain food toxins. Symptoms often include a sore tongue, anemia, weight loss, along with diarrhea and passage of fatty stools.

Whipple's disease is a relatively rare malabsorptive disorder, affecting mostly middle-aged men. The cause is thought to be related to bacterial infection, resulting in nutritional deficiencies, chronic low-grade **fever**, diarrhea, joint **pain**, weight loss, and darkening of the skin's pigmentation. Other organs of the body may be affected, including the brain, heart, lungs, and eyes.

Short bowel syndromes—which may be present at birth (congenital) or the result of surgery—reduce the surface area of the bowel available to absorb nutrients and can also result in malabsorption syndrome.

The diagnosis of malabsorption syndrome and identification of the underlying cause can require extensive diagnostic testing. The first phase involves a thorough medical history and **physical examination** by a physician, who will then determine the appropriate laboratory studies and x rays to assist in diagnosis. A 72-hour stool collection may be ordered for fecal fat measurement; increased fecal fat in the stool collected indicates malabsorption. A biopsy of the small intestine may be done to assist in differentiating between malabsorption syndrome and small bowel disease. Ultrasound, computed tomography scan (CT scan), **magnetic resonance imaging** (MRI), barium enema, or other x rays to identify abnormalities of the gastrointestinal tract and pancreas may also be ordered.

Laboratory studies of the blood may include:

- Serum cholesterol. May be low due to decreased fat absorption and digestion.
- Serum sodium, potassium, and chloride. May be low due to electrolyte losses with diarrhea.
- Serum calcium. May be low due to vitamin D and amino acid malabsorption.
- Serum protein and albumin. May be low due to protein losses.
- Serum vitamin A and carotene. May be low due to bile salt deficiency and impaired fat absorption.
- D-xylose test. Decreased excretion may indicate malabsorption.
- Schilling test. May indicate malabsorption of vitamin B_{12}.

Fluid and nutrient monitoring and replacement is essential for any individual with malabsorption syndrome. Hospitalization may be required when severe fluid and electrolyte imbalances occur. Consultation with a dietitian to assist with nutritional support and meal planning is helpful. If the patient is able to eat, the diet and supplements should provide bulk and be rich in carbohydrates, proteins, fats, **minerals**, and **vitamins**. The patient should be encouraged to eat several small, frequent meals throughout the day, avoiding fluids and foods that promote diarrhea. Intake and output should be monitored, along with the number, color, and consistency of stools.

The individual with malabsorption syndrome must be monitored for **dehydration**, including dry tongue, mouth and skin; increased thirst; low, concentrated urine output; or feeling weak or dizzy when standing. Pulse and blood pressure should be monitored, observing for increased or irregular pulse rate, or **hypotension** (low blood pressure). The individual should also be alert for signs of nutrient, vitamin, and mineral depletion, including nausea or vomiting; fissures at corner of mouth; fatigue or weakness; dry, pluckable hair; easy bruising; tingling in fingers or toes; and numbness or burning sensation in legs or feet. Fluid volume excess, as a result of diminished protein stores, may require fluid intake restrictions. The physician should also be notified of any **shortness of breath**.

Other specific medical management for malabsorption syndrome is dependent upon the cause. Treatment for tropical sprue consists of folic acid supplements and long-term antibiotics. Depending on the severity of the disorder, this treatment may be continued for six months or longer. Whipple's disease also may require long-term use of antibiotics, such as tetracycline. Management of some individuals with malabsorption syndrome may require injections of vitamin B_{12} and oral iron supplements. The doctor may also prescribe enzymes to replace missing intestinal enzymes, or antispasmodics to reduce abdominal cramping and associated diarrhea. People with cystic fibrosis and chronic pancreatitis require pancreatic supplements. Those with lactose intolerance or gluten enteropathy (non-tropical sprue) will have to modify their **diets** to avoid foods that they cannot properly digest.

The expected course for the individual with malabsorption syndrome varies depending on the cause. The onset of symptoms may be slow and difficult to diagnose. Treatment may be long, complicated, and changed often for optimal effectiveness. Patience and a positive attitude are important in controlling or curing the disorder. Careful monitoring is necessary to prevent additional illnesses cause by nutritional deficiencies.

MALARIA

Malaria is a group of parasitic diseases common in tropical and subtropical areas. Approximately 300 million cases occur annually worldwide, and one to nearly three million people die of malaria each year with about 90 percent of these deaths occurring in sub-Saharan Africa, with the majority being children. Malaria has been known for centuries, having been described in ancient Greek, Hebrew, and Roman writings and in Chinese and Indian medical chronicles. Efforts to eradicate malaria by draining the swamps around ancient Rome were some of the first successful public health measures recorded. Like most diseases, malaria was originally thought a result of poisonous vapors in the air, and the name of the disease comes form two Italian words, *mal* (meaning bad) and *aria* (meaning air).

One of the most predominant health problems in the world, malaria is a much-researched disease. The use of cinchona bark extracts (**quinine**) as treatment in the early seventeenth century by Peruvian Indians marked the first recognition of malarial fevers as a specific disease, and the clinical observations of malaria made by F. Torti and **Thomas Sydenham** in the later seventeenth century gave the disease a scientific basis. Malaria is caused by blood **parasite**s of the genus *Plasmodium*, which are transmitted to humans by the bite of the female *Anopheles* mosquito. When an *Anopheles* mosquito bites a human already infected with malaria, *Plasmodia* in the human's blood enter the mosquito's body and reproduce in her stomach. The offspring travel to her salivary glands and are transmitted to another human by her bite. In a human, the parasites travel to the liver, reproduce, and form clumps. Several days later, the clumps burst and new *Plasmodia* are released. Each parasite then invades a red blood cell and reproduces again. The infected cells rupture, releasing parasites which then invade other cells.

Charles Louis Alphonse Laveran (1845-1922) first discovered parasites in a malaria patient's blood in 1880, demonstrating its parasitic origin to those doubtful scientists who expected **Louis Pasteur**'s discovery of **bacteria** to explain all illnesses. Laveran's theory was validated in 1886 by the renowned histologist **Camillo Golgi**, who identified two distinct human malaria parasites (*Plasmodium vivax* and *P. malariae*) by examining the blood of malaria patients. Golgi discovered the life cycle of these parasites and correctly concluded that they divide at regular intervals. Each division causes a corresponding attack of fever in the human host.

Patrick Manson (1844-1922) suggested the mosquito as the mode of transmission among humans in 1894, and **Ronald Ross** and Giovanni Grassi (1854-1925) provided an explanation of the parasite's life cycle in 1897, also confirming that the mosquito is the vector. *Plasmodium* 's life cycle was further clarified by H. E. Shortt and P. C. C. Garnham in 1948. Malaria is characterized by a 10-40 day incubation period preceding a brief stage of chills, followed by a rapid rise in body temperature ranging as high as 107° F (41.7° C) accompanied by a severe headache, and finally a sweating stage during which the patient begins to feel well.

When the next batch of red blood cells ruptures, the cycle begins again. The cycle's periodicity, ranging from 48 to 72 hours, is determined by which of four species of *Plasmodium* (*P. vivax, P. malariae, P. falciparum* or *P. ovale*) is present. When more than one species of parasite is present, the cycles of symptoms can overlap.

The rate of death in untreated patients is greater than ten percent, and from the time of its introduction into Western medicine in the late seventeenth century until 1920, quinine was the only specific drug available to combat malaria's symptoms. Today, the synthetic drugs chloroquine, mefloquine, and doxycycline are commonly used in the prevention of malaria.

Because preventive drugs and vaccines are costly and *Plasmodium* tends to develop resistance to them, the prevention of malaria largely depends upon the eradication of the *Anopheles* mosquito. In 1905, construction on the Panama Canal was interrupted by **epidemic**s of malaria and **yellow fever**. The Isthmanian Canal Commission depended on **William Crawford Gorgas** (1854-1920) as chief sanitary officer to eliminate the diseases. With mosquito eradication supplies and 4000 men, Gorgas eliminated yellow fever and reduced malaria to a prevalence of less than ten percent among the workers by 1906 using public health measures.

During the 1950s and 1960s, the **World Health Organization** launched a worldwide campaign to eradicate malaria using the insecticide DDT to kill *Anopheles*. The disease disappeared in several countries where it had been endemic and was greatly reduced in others, but it began to return as *Anopheles* developed resistance to DDT. Other areas—particularly tropical areas where mosquitos inhabit large spaces, making control by insecticide inefficient—were relatively unaffected by these measures, and research was begun into biological or genetic means of control. DDT was banned in the United States in 1972 following the publication of Rachel Carson's *Silent Spring*, in which she demonstrated the harmful effects of DDT in ecosystems and on vertebrates. Canada has also banned the use of DDT, but this insecticide continues to be used in Mexico, India, and the republics of the former Soviet Union.

Malaria remains a serious public health problem in Central and South America, North and Central Africa, East Asia, the Middle East, and along the borders of the Mediterranean. In parts of Africa and South Asia, virtually the entire population is infected. Resistance to attacks of malaria develops with age, making children the most vulnerable to this disease. (Every 30 seconds a child dies of malaria.)

A promising new weapon in the war on malaria is a vaccine developed by Dr. Manuel Elkin Patarroyo and his colleagues at the Immunology Institute of Colombia's National University in Bogota. While Dr. Patarroyo's vaccine is not the first attempt at triggering the body's natural defense system to fight the parasites, it is the first malaria vaccine to be tested and shown safe and effective in extensive field trials. (It has been tested in Brazil, Colombia, Ecuador, Venezuela, and Africa. This vaccine is only effective against parasites of the species *P. falciparum* (responsible for 95 percent of malaria cases worldwide), and seems to confer immunity in only two-thirds of vaccinated people. Nonetheless, scientists believe it may prove an invaluable tool in a comprehensive attack on the disease when used in conjunction with mosquito control and treatment of victims with antimalarial drugs. The two other main types of vaccine under development are anti-sporozoite vaccines, which are designed to prevent infection, and anti-asexual blood stage vaccines, which reduce severe manifestations of the disease. Any effective vaccine against malaria will most likely have to induce a immune response to the various stages of malaria infection. In terms of prevention, the World Health Organization conducted a study which showed that bed nets impregnated with mosquito pesticides could lower childhood mortality due to malaria by 15 to 35 percent in certain situations.

See also Immune system

MALINGERING

In the context of medicine, malingering is the act of intentionally feigning or exaggerating physical or psychological symptoms for personal gain.

People may feign physical or psychological illness for any number of reasons. Faked illness can get them out of work, military duty, or criminal prosecution. It can also help them obtain financial compensation through insurance claims, lawsuits, or workers' compensation. Feigned symptoms may also be a way of getting the doctor to prescribe certain drugs.

According to the American Psychiatric Association, patients who malinger are different from people who invent symptoms for sympathy (**factitious diseases**). Patients who malinger clearly have something tangible to gain. People with factitious diseases appear to have a need to play the ''sick'' role. They may feign illness for attention or sympathy.

Malingering may take the form of complaints of chronic whiplash pain from automobile accidents. Whiplash claims are controversial. Although some people clearly do suffer from whiplash injury, others may be exaggerating the pain for insurance claims or lawsuits. Some intriguing scientific studies have shown that chronic whiplash pain after automobile accidents is almost nonexistent in Lithuania and Greece. In these countries, the legal systems do not encourage personal injury lawsuits or financial settlements. The psychological symptoms experienced by survivors of disaster (**post-traumatic stress disorder**) are also faked by malingerers.

People malinger for personal gain. The symptoms may vary. Generally malingerers complain of psychological disorders such as **anxiety**. They may also complain of chronic pain for which objective tests such as x rays can find no physical cause. Because it is often impossible to determine who is malingering and who is not, it is impossible to know how frequently malingering occurs.

Malingering may be suspected:

- When a patient is referred for examination by an attorney
- When the onset of illness coincides with a large financial incentive, such as a new disability policy
- When objective medical tests do not confirm the patient's complaints
- When the patient does not cooperate with the diagnostic work-up or prescribed treatment
- When the patient has antisocial attitudes and behaviors (antisocial personality).

The diagnosis of malingering is a challenge for doctors. On the one hand, the doctor does not want to overlook a treatable disease. On the other hand, he or she does not want to continue ordering tests and treatments if the symptoms are faked. Malingering is difficult to distinguish from certain legitimate **personality disorders**, such as factitious diseases or post-traumatic distress syndrome. In legal cases, malingering patients may be referred to a psychiatrist. Psychiatrists use certain written tests to try to determine whether the patient is faking the symptoms.

In a sense, malingering cannot be treated because the American Psychiatric Association does not recognize it as a personality disorder. Patients who are purposefully faking symptoms for gain do not want to be cured. Often, the malingering patient fails to report any improvement with treatment, and the doctor may try many treatments without success.

MALLON, MARY (1869-1938)

Irish Cook, Typhoid Carrier

An Irish immigrant cook, Mallon became the focus of one of the best-known episodes in the history of communicable disease when U.S. health officials identified her as a healthy carrier of the organism causing **typhoid fever**. Mallon, who refused to acknowledge her role in spreading the disease as a cook, is known to have infected at least 53 people, resulting in three deaths. Unable to stop her from cooking for others, New York City authorities confined her for 26 years on North Brother Island in the East River.

Prior to Mallon, authorities including Robert Koch and Walter Reed had speculated that the disease might be spread by carriers who transmitted typhoid bacteria even though they looked and felt perfectly well. Mallon became the first healthy carrier to be positively identified by U.S. health officials, when she was tracked down by George Soper, an epidemiologist and sanitary engineer from the New York City Department of Health.

Soper was hired by the owner of a summer retreat at Oyster Bay, Long Island, to investigate a typhoid outbreak there during the summer of 1906. Six cases of typhoid had developed among 11 members of the household of a visiting New York banker, and the retreat owner was concerned his property might not be rented again unless the source was exposed and eliminated.

Soper's investigation led to Mallon, who had been hired as cook 23 days before the first typhoid case materialized at Oyster Bay. She had left shortly after the outbreak began. Tracing Mallon through her employment agency, Soper found that she had cooked for seven other wealthy families, six of whom were afflicted by typhoid around the time of her employment.

Soper finally caught up with Mallon in an affluent household on Manhattan's Park Avenue, where an only daughter was critically ill with typhoid and a laundress had been hospitalized with the disease. Encountering Mallon in the kitchen, Soper explained his investigation and asked for samples of her urine, blood, and feces. Mallon responded with a sharp kitchen instrument.

When a subsequent visit by Soper and a medical colleague only pushed Mallon into another rage, the City Department of Health dispatched **Sara Josephine Baker**, a female physician who visited with a group of New York City policemen. Mallon lunged at the visitors with a long kitchen fork and fled to a nearby shed, where she was arrested and taken to hospital in an ambulance, kicking, screaming, and biting, with Baker sitting on her chest.

Mallon's feces repeatedly tested positive for typhoid bacteria and various medical treatments did not eliminate them. Soper tried unsuccessfully to persuade the cook to have her gallbladder removed, an operation that sometimes halted production of the bacteria but was considered a high risk at the time.

Mallon subsequently was sent to the Riverside Hospital for communicable diseases on North Brother Island. The New

York press learned of her case and dubbed her "Typhoid Mary" in sensational articles, one of which was accompanied by a drawing showing her cracking human skulls onto a grill.

After two years at North Brother Island, Mallon applied to a judge to be released, describing her involuntary confinement as "unjust, outrageous, uncivilized," and complaining that she was "treated like an outcast a criminal" even though she was charged with no crime.

The fact that Mallon was healthy was a new twist on existing quarantine practices, but the judge ruled in 1909 that she was a menace to public health and that health officials had a right to confine her. However, the following year, a New York health commissioner agreed to release Mallon on her promise to refrain from cooking or handling food for others. The terms of release required her to report to health officials every three months, but Mallon disappeared.

She was finally located in 1915 at New York's Sloane Hospital for Women, where she was working in the kitchen under the assumed name of Mary Brown. An outbreak of typhoid cases had occurred among the nursing staff there and co-workers had jokingly taken to calling her "Typhoid Mary," never suspecting that she was the infamous Mary Mallon they had read about in the newspapers.

She returned to the hospital on North Brother Island, where a special cottage was built for her in 1923. In her long years of life quarantine there, Mallon never admitted her status as a typhoid carrier. She did, however, become more compliant and was allowed to work at Riverside Hospital as a laboratory technician and even to visit friends in Manhattan and Queens.

On Christmas Day, 1932, Mallon suffered a stroke, which left her paralyzed until her death from bronchopneumonia six years later. Her funeral, held in a spacious church in the Bronx, was attended by nine people. Apparently still doubtful that a typhoid carrier could be free of symptoms, the doctor who filled out her death certificate wrongly listed typhoid as a contributing factor in her death.

See also Typhoid Fever

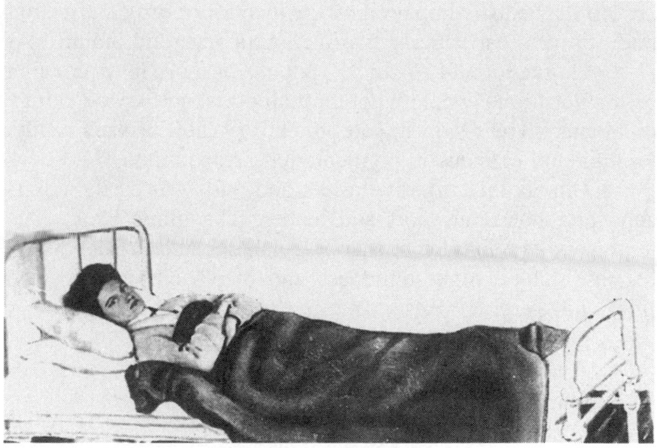

Mary Mallon, "Typhoid Mary."

MALNUTRITION

Malnutrition occurs when the body does not get enough **vitamins**, **minerals**, and other nutrients it needs to maintain healthy tissues and organ function. Both undernourished or overnourished people can suffer from malnutrition.

Undernutrition is a consequence of consuming too few essential nutrients or using or excreting them more rapidly than they can be replaced.

Infants, young children, and teenagers need additional nutrients. So do women who are pregnant or breastfeeding. Nutrient loss can be accelerated by **diarrhea**, excessive sweating, heavy **bleeding** (hemorrhage), or **kidney failure**. Nutrient intake can be restricted by age-related illnesses and conditions, excessive dieting, severe injury, serious illness, a lengthy hospitalization, or substance abuse.

The leading cause of death in children in developing countries is protein-energy malnutrition. This type of malnutrition results from inadequate intake of calories from proteins, vitamins, and minerals. Children who are already undernourished can suffer from protein-energy malnutrition when rapid growth, infection, or disease increases the need for protein and essential minerals.

In the United States, nutritional deficiencies generally have been replaced by dietary imbalances or excesses associated with many of the leading causes of **death** and disability. Overnutrition results from eating too much, eating too many of the wrong things, not exercising enough, or taking too many vitamins or other dietary replacements.

Risk of overnutrition is also increased by being more than 20% overweight, consuming a diet high in fat and salt, and taking high doses of:

- Nicotinic acid (niacin) to lower elevated cholesterol levels
- Vitamin B_6 to relieve **premenstrual syndrome**
- Vitamin A to clear up skin problems
- Iron or other trace minerals not prescribed by a doctor.

Nutritional disorders can affect any system in the body and the senses of sight, taste, and smell. Malnutrition begins with changes in nutrient levels in blood and tissues. Alterations in enzyme levels, tissue abnormalities, and organ malfunction may be followed by illness and death.

Poverty and lack of food are the primary reasons why malnutrition occurs in the United States. Ten percent of all low income households members do not always have enough healthful food to eat, and malnutrition affects one in four elderly Americans. Protein-energy malnutrition occurs in 50% of surgical patients and in 48% of all other hospital patients.

There is an increased risk of malnutrition associated with chronic diseases, especially disease of the intestinal tract, kidneys, and liver. Patients with chronic diseases like cancer, AIDS, and intestinal disorders may lose weight rapidly and become susceptible to undernourishment because they cannot absorb valuable vitamins, calories, and iron.

People with drug or alcohol dependencies are also at increased risk of malnurtrition. These people tend to maintain inadequate diets for long periods of time, and their ability to absorb nutrients is impaired by the alcohol or drug's affect on body tissues, particularly the liver, pancreas, and brain.

Unintentionally losing 10 pounds or more may be a sign of malnutrition. People who are malnourished may be skinny or bloated. Their skin is pale, thick, dry, and **bruises** easily. **Rashes** and changes in pigmentation are common.

Hair is thin, tightly curled, and pulls out easily. Joints ache and bones are soft and tender. The gums bleed. The tongue may be swollen or shriveled and cracked. Visual disturbances include night blindness and increased sensitivity to light and glare.

Other symptoms of malnutrition include:

- Anemia
- Diarrhea
- Disorientation
- **Goiter** (enlarged thyroid gland)
- Loss of reflexes and lack of coordination
- Muscle twitches
- Scaling and cracking of the lips and mouth.

Malnourished children may be short for their age, thin, listless, and have weakened immune systems.

Overall appearance, behavior, body-fat distribution, and organ function can alert a family physician, internist, or nutrition specialist to the presence of malnutrition. Patients may be asked to record what they eat during a specific period. X rays can determine bone density and reveal gastrointestinal disturbances, and heart and lung damage.

Blood and urine tests are used to measure levels of vitamins, minerals, and waste products. Nutritional status can also be determined by:

- Comparing a patient's weight to standardized charts
- Calculating body mass index (BMI) according to a formula that divides height into weight
- Measuring skin-fold thickness or the circumference of the upper arm.

Normalizing nutritional status starts with a nutritional assessment. This process enables a clinical nutritionist or registered dietician to confirm the presence of malnutrition, assess the effects of the disorder, and formulate **diets** that will restore adequate nutrition.

Patients who cannot or will not eat, or who are unable to absorb nutrients taken by mouth, may be fed intravenously (parenteral nutrition) or through a tube inserted into the gastrointestinal (GI) tract (enteral nutrition).

Tube feeding is often used to provide nutrients to patients who have suffered **burns** or who have **inflammatory bowel disease**. In this procedure,a thin tube is inserted through the nose and carefully guiding along the throat until it reaches the stomach or small intestine. If long-term tube feeding is necessary, the tube may be placed directly into the stomach or small intestine through an incision in the abdomen.

Tube feeding cannot always deliver adequate nutrients to patients who:

- Are severely malnourished
- Require surgery
- Are undergoing **chemotherapy** or radiation treatments
- Have been seriously burned
- Have persistent diarrhea or vomiting
- Whose gastrointestinal tract is paralyzed.

Intravenous feeding can supply some or all of the nutrients these patients need.

Up to 10% of a person's body weight can be lost without side effects, but if more than 40% is lost, the situation is almost always fatal. Death usually results from heart failure, electrolyte imbalance, or low body temperature. Patients with semiconsciousness, persistent diarrhea, **jaundice**, or low blood sodium levels have a poorer prognosis.

Some children with protein-energy malnutrition recover completely. Others have many health problems throughout life, including mental retardation and the inability to absorb nutrients through the intestinal tract. Prognosis for patients with malnutrition seems to be dependent on the the patient's age and the length and severity of the malnutrition, with young children and the elderly having the highest rate of long-term complications and death.

Breastfeeding a baby for at least six months is considered the best way to prevent early-childhood malnutrition. The United States Department of Agriculture and Health and Human Service recommend that all Americans over the age of two:

- Consume plenty of fruits, grains, and vegetables
- Eat a variety of foods that are low in fats and cholesterols and contain only moderate amounts of salt, sugars, and sodium
- Engage in moderate physical activity for at least 30 minutes, at least several times a week
- Achieve or maintain their ideal weight
- Use alcohol sparingly or avoid it altogether.

Every patient admitted to a hospital should be screened for the presence of illnesses and conditions that could lead to protein-energy malnutrition. Patients with higher-than-average risk for malnutrition should be more closely assessed and reevaluated often during long-term hospitalization or nursing-home care.

See also Inflammatory Bowel Disease; Jaundice

MALOCCLUSION

Malocclusion is a problem in the way the upper and lower teeth fit together in biting or chewing. Malocclusion literally means ''bad bite.'' The condition may also be referred to as an irregular bite, crossbite, or overbite.

Malocclusion may be seen as crooked, crowded, or protruding teeth. It may affect a person's appearance, speech, or ability to eat.

Malocclusions are most often inherited, but may be acquired. Inherited conditions include too many or too few teeth, too much or too little space between teeth, irregular mouth and jaw size and shape, and atypical formations of the jaws and face, such as a **cleft palate**. Malocclusions may be acquired from habits like finger or thumb sucking, tongue thrusting, premature loss of teeth from an accident or dental disease, and medical conditions such as enlarged tonsils and adenoids that lead to mouth breathing.

Malocclusions may be symptomless or they may produce **pain** from increased stress on the oral structures. Abnormal signs of wear on the teeth's chewing surfaces or tooth decay may occur in areas of tight overlap. Chewing may be difficult.

Malocclusion is most often found during a routine dental examination. A dentist will check a patient's occlusion by watching how the teeth make contact when the patient bites down normally. The dentist may ask the patient to bite down with a piece of coated paper between the upper and lower teeth; this paper will leave colored marks at the points of contact. When malocclusion is suspected, photographs and x rays of the face and mouth may be taken for further study. To confirm the presence and extent of malocclusion, the dentist makes plaster, plastic, or artificial stone models of the patient's teeth from impressions. These models duplicate the fit of the teeth and are very useful in treatment planning.

Malocclusion may be remedied by orthodontic treatment; **orthodontics** is a specialty of dentistry that manages the growth and correction of dental and facial structures. **Braces** are the most commonly used orthodontic appliances in the treatment of malocclusion. At any given time, approximately 4 million people in the United States are wearing braces, including 800,000 adults.

Braces apply constant gentle force to slowly change the position of the teeth, straightening them and properly aligning them with the opposing teeth. Braces consist of brackets cemented to the surface of each tooth and wires of stainless steel or nickel titanium alloy. When the wires are threaded through the brackets, they exert pressure against the teeth, causing them to gradually move.

Braces are not removable for daily tooth brushing, so the patient must be especially diligent about keeping the mouth clean and removing food particles which become easily trapped, to prevent **tooth decay**. Foods that are crunchy should be avoided to minimize the risk of breaking the appliance. Hard fruits, vegetables, and breads must be cut into bite-sized pieces before eating. Foods that are sticky, including chewing gum, should be avoided because they may pull off the brackets or weaken the cement. Carbonated beverages may also weaken the cement, as well as contribute to tooth decay. Teeth should be brushed immediately after eating sweet foods. Special floss threaders are available to make flossing easier.

If overcrowding is creating malocclusion, one or more teeth may be extracted (surgically removed), giving the others room to move. If a tooth has not yet erupted or is prematurely lost, the orthodontist may insert an appliance called a space maintainer to keep the other teeth from moving out of their natural position. In severe cases of malocclusion, surgery may be necessary and the patient would be referred to yet another specialist, an oral or maxillofacial surgeon.

Once the teeth have been moved into their new position, the braces are removed and a retainer is worn until the teeth stabilize in that position. Retainers do not move teeth, they only hold them in place.

Orthodontic treatment is the only effective treatment for malocclusion not requiring surgery. However, depending on the cause and severity of the condition, an orthodontist may be able to suggest other appliances as alternatives to braces.

There are some techniques of craniosacral therapy that can alter structure. This therapy may allow correction of some cases of malocclusion. If surgery is required, pre- and post-surgical care with homeopathic remedies, as well as vitamin and mineral **dietary supplements**, can enhance recovery. Night guards are sometimes recommended to ease the strain on the jaw and to limit teeth grinding.

Depending on the cause and severity of the malocclusion and the appliance used in treatment, a patient may expect correction of the condition to take two or more years. Patients typically wear braces 18-24 months and a retainer for another year. Treatment is faster and more successful in children and teens whose teeth and bones are still developing. The length of treatment time is also affected by how well the patient follows orthodontic instructions.

In general, malocclusion is not preventable. It may be minimized by controlling habits such as finger or thumb sucking. An initial consultation with an orthodontist before a child is seven years old may lead to appropriate management of the growth and development of the child's dental and facial structures, circumventing many of the factors contributing to malocclusion.

See also Cleft lip and palate; Orthodontics

MALONEY, ARNOLD HAMILTON (1888-1955)

Trinidadian African American physician and pharmacologist

Arnold Hamilton Maloney began his career planning to be a druggist in his native Trinidad, but his ultimate influence in the field of pharmacology was to be far greater than the local level. Maloney immigrated to the United States in 1909 where he completed his education and eventually became the first black professor of pharmacology in the nation. He had a varied career as ordained minister in the Episcopal Church, professor, researcher, consultant, and author. Through his research, he is perhaps most known for discovering an antidote for barbiturate poisoning (or an overdose of sedatives). He was also the second person of African descent to obtain both a medical degree and a doctorate of philosophy in the United States.

Maloney, the oldest male of ten children, was born July 4, 1888, in Cocoye Village, Trinidad, British West Indies. His father, Lewis Albert Maloney, was a building contractor and grocery chain operator, and his mother, Estelle Evetta (Bonas) Maloney, taught needlework to young women and later operated a general store. As a student, Maloney excelled and won numerous awards. He had a love of learning that led him to pursue many different interests as an adult. He studied at Naparima College in Trinidad, which is affiliated with Cambridge University, England, earning his bachelor's degree in 1909. That same year, he immigrated to the United States where he attended Lincoln University in Pennsylvania. In 1910, he received his master's degree from Columbia University. Maloney then received a bachelor of science degree in theology from the General Theological Seminary, New York, in 1912. He began his ministry at age 23 with the distinction of being the youngest minister in the Protestant Episcopal Church.

After practicing for several years, Maloney felt that the Episcopal Church was neglecting young black men. A suggestion he made prompted the church to establish St. Augustine in Raleigh, North Carolina, as a college for black youth. Although there were aspects of the ministry that Maloney enjoyed, he became disillusioned and left the church in 1922. He published a book outlining his views, *The Essentials of Race Leadership,* in 1924. On leaving the ministry, Maloney turned to teaching, accepting a professorship of psychology at Wilberforce University in Ohio. While he was very enthusiastic about teaching and found it rewarding, he decided to continue his own education.

Maloney entered Indiana University School of Medicine in 1925, graduating with a medical degree in 1929. He then attended the University of Wisconsin, where he engaged in research in pharmacology, earning a doctorate in this field in 1931. Maloney has the distinction of being the second man of African descent to earn both the M.D. and the Ph.D. degrees. Upon accepting a position at Howard University in the same year, he also became the first black professor of pharmacology in the United States.

From 1931 until 1953, Maloney worked in the department of pharmacology at Howard University School of Medicine in Washington, D.C. He began as an associate professor of pharmacology, becoming a full professor, and then head of the department. During these years, he also worked as a consultant in pharmacology for Freedmen's Hospital. Maloney's research involved several areas of pharmacology, but his most important work was the discovery of an antidote for barbiturate overdose. High levels of barbiturates (drugs used as sedatives) cause potentially deadly symptoms such as shallow respiration, central nervous system depression, and deep anesthesia. Maloney determined that administering picrotoxin (a potentially lethal poison) quickly reversed these symptoms. His first paper on this subject was published in 1931.

Maloney was hugely affected by the written word. He devoted two chapters of his autobiography, *Amber Gold: An Adventure in Autobiography,* to books he had been influenced by or enjoyed. He also wrote more than 50 articles during his career before retiring in 1953. Maloney was a member of many learned societies and several medical associations, including the American Negro Academy, American Academy of Political Sciences and the National Medical Association. In 1916, he married Beatrice Pocahontas Johnston; they had two children: Arnold Maloney, Jr. and Louise Beatrice. Maloney died in Washington, D.C., on August 8, 1955.

MALPIGHI, MARCELLO (1628-1694)

Italian physiologist

In the second half of the seventeenth century, Marcello Malpighi used the newly invented microscope to make a number of important discoveries about living **tissues** and structures, earning himself enduring recognition as a founder of scientific microscopy, histology (the study of tissues), embryology, and the science of plant anatomy.

Malpighi was born at Crevalcore, just outside Bologna, Italy, on March 10, 1628. The son of small landowners, Malpighi studied medicine and philosophy at the University of Bologna. While at Bologna, Malpighi was part of a small anatomical society headed by the teacher Bartolomeo Massari, in whose home the group met to conduct **dissection**s and **vivisection**s. Malpighi later married Massari's sister.

In 1655, Malpighi became a lecturer in logic at the University of Bologna; in 1656, he assumed the chair of theoretical medicine at the University of Pisa; in 1659, he returned to Bologna as lecturer in theoretical, then practical, medicine; from 1662 to 1666, he held the principal chair in medicine at the University of Messina; finally in 1666, he returned again to Bologna, where he remained for the rest of his teaching and research career. In 1691, at the age of sixty-three, Malpighi was called by his friend Pope Innocent XII to serve as the pontiff's personal physician. Reluctantly, Malpighi agreed and moved to Rome, where he died on November 29, 1694, in his room in the Quirinal Palace.

Early in his medical career, Malpighi became absorbed in using the microscope to study a wide range of living tissue—animal, insect, and plant. At the time, this was an entirely new field of scientific investigation. Malpighi soon made a profoundly important discovery. Microscopically examining a frog's lungs, he was able for the first time to describe the lung's structure accurately—thin air sacs surrounded by a network of tiny **blood** vessels. This explained how air (**oxygen**) is able to diffuse into the blood vessels, a key to understanding the process of respiration. It also provided the one missing piece of evidence to confirm **William Harvey**'s revolutionary theory of the **blood circulation**: Malpighi had discovered the capillaries, the microscopic connecting link between the veins and arteries that Harvey—with no microscope available—had only been able to postulate. Malpighi published his findings about the lungs in 1661.

Malpighi used the microscope to make an impressive number of other important observations, all "firsts." He observed a "host of red atoms" in the blood—the red blood corpuscles. He described the papillae of the tongue and skin—the receptors of the senses of taste and touch. He identified the rete mucosum, the Malpighian layer, of the skin. He found that the nerves and spinal column both consisted of bundles of fibers. He clearly described the structure of the kidney and suggested its function as a urine producer. He identified the spleen as an organ, not a gland; structures in both the kidney and spleen are named after him. He demonstrated that bile is secreted in the liver, not the gall bladder. In showing bile to be a uniform color, he disproved a 2,000-year-old idea that the bile was yellow and black. He described glandular adenopathy, a syndrome rediscovered by Thomas Hodgkin (1798-1866) and given that man's name 200 years later.

As if this catalog of human-tissue discovery weren't enough, Malpighi also conducted groundbreaking research in plant and insect microscopy. His extensive studies of the silkworm were the first full examination of insect structure. His detailed observations of chick embryos laid the foundation for microscopic embryology. His botanical investigations established the science of plant anatomy. The amazing variety of Malpighi's microscopic discoveries piqued the interest of countless other researchers and firmly established microscopy as a science.

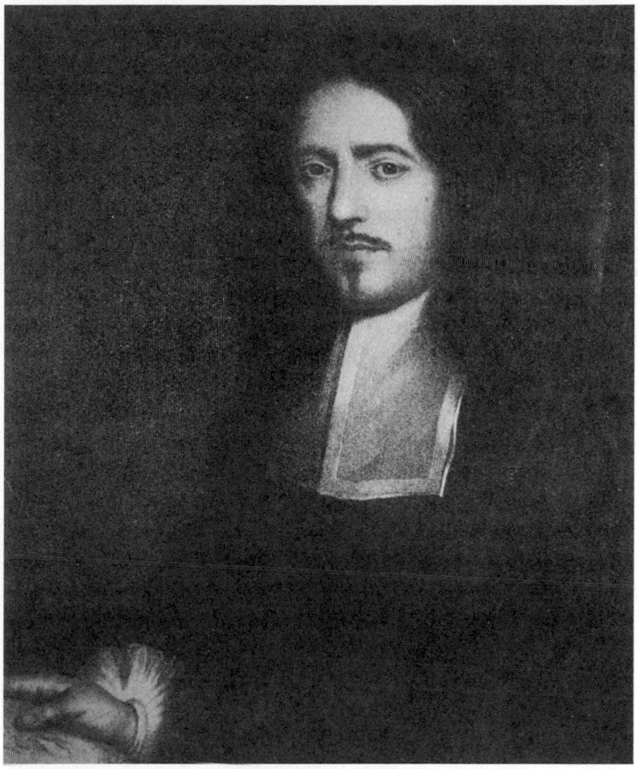

Marcello Malpighi

Mammography

Over the past century, mammography, or X-ray imaging of the breast, has become an accepted, although controversial, tool in the diagnosis of breast cancer. Breast cancer remains one of the deadliest diseases that strikes women; an estimated one out of every nine women will develop the disease in her lifetime. Mammography is considered an important screening and diagnostic tool because it can detect tumors while still small and most easily treated. In one study, women whose breast cancers were found early through mammograms had a five-year survival rate of 82 percent, while a group of women whose cancers were not found by mammograms had a five-year survival rate of just 60 percent. The American Cancer Institute guidelines recommend women aged 40 to 49 be screened every one to two years, and that women aged 50 and older be screened annually because the incidence of breast cancer increases with age.

Researchers began experimenting with X-ray technology in detecting cancer in the late nineteenth century. German surgeon, Albert Salomon, became the first person to use the X-ray to study breast cancer. Working with breast tissue that had been removed during surgery, he used the X-ray to determine the difference between cancerous and noncancerous tumors and found that the technique could successfully be used to detect breast cancer. He also discovered, based upon the differing X-ray images he obtained, that a number of different types of breast cancer existed. Salomon, who published his findings in 1913, is considered the inventor of breast radiology. However, he never used the technique in his own practice. In the 1920s, other German scientists continued Salomon's research. Out of these experiments came a study written by Leipzig researcher W. Vogel that fully described how X-rays could detect the difference between cancerous and noncancerous tissues. The detailed information is still considered useful to scientists who diagnose cancer.

Stafford L. Warren, a Rochester, New York, physician, became the first to experiment with the new technology in the United States. Using a fluoroscope, he discovered images similar to those found by Salomon in breast tissue. Warren used his technique for detailed examinations prior to breast cancer surgery. Using radiology, he also discovered changes in breast tissue as a result of pregnancy, menstruation, lactation, and the beginning of breast disease. His findings were published in 1930. The first physician to advocate the wide use of X-rays to screen women for breast cancer was Jacob Gershon-Cohen. In the mid-1950s, he and his colleagues began a five-year study of more than 1,300 women, screening each woman every six months. As a result, 92 were diagnosed with nonmalignant tumors and 23 with malignant tumors. A similar study conducted in Houston, Texas, found that women diagnosed early through mammography had a better recovery rate than those whose disease was discovered at a later stage by breast biopsy. By the 1960s, mammography was becoming a widely used diagnostic tool, although some critics alleged that the procedure exposed women to unnecessary levels of X-radiation. Through the development of more sensitive film, the amount of radiation needed to produce clear pictures of breast tissue was reduced significantly. By 1971, a quarter-million women over age thirty-five had been screened for breast cancer with mammography. The National Cancer Institute conducted a four-year study (1973-1977) of some 270,000 women throughout the United States. Some women were found to have very small benign growths, yet large numbers of these women had surgery, which some researchers felt was unnecessary. As a result of the study, the National Cancer Institute issued a set of guidelines regarding which groups of women will benefit from regularly scheduled mammograms. For women under age forty, the procedure was recommended only to those at risk of developing the disease because of family history other indicators such as palpable breast lumps.

See also X-ray machine; X-ray studies

Managed Care

Managed care is a method of health care delivery that shifts some of the financial risk involved to those providing care. Arising out efforts to control health care costs in the early 1980s, this risk shifting, in theory, creates incentives for the plan to provide appropriate levels of medical care and preventive health care with a focus on maintaining wellness. The key features of this concept include: service for defined population voluntarily enrolled in the managed care plan; assumption of contractual responsibility and financial risk by the managed care plan to provide a stated range of services; and, payment of a fixed annual or monthly fee by the enrollee(the insured member), independent of the actual services used. One type of managed care is the **health maintenance organization** (HMO). The enrollee selects a primary care provider (for example, a family practice or internal medicine physician) to manage their overall health care within the HMO; often a referral is required for the enrollee to consult with a specialist (such as a dermatologist, a podiatrist, or a surgeon). This method of providing health care is in contrast to the old traditional fee-for-service plans.

Most significant in a managed care plan is the control of what is deemed by the insurer as inappropriate medical care. Many studies have documented the wide variation in medical practice patterns, many of which resulted in costly and sometimes inappropriate medical testing and treatments. Some estimate that up to 30 percent of all health care costs result from unnecessary medical care. Selected aspects of managed care programs that have significantly reduced health care spending include requirements for preauthorization for selected **hospital** medical and surgical admissions, review of lengths of hospital stays, second surgical opinions, and requirements for outpatient surgery and diagnostic testing.

Although HMOs and other managed care plans have been effective in reducing inappropriate and unnecessary health-care measures and procedures, there is considerable concern from many quarters that they may overstep their prerogative in this area by cutting back or eliminating certain activities that may be necessary for the patient's care; their goal in cutting costs may jeopardize patients' well-being.

See also Health Maintenance Organization

Manson, Patrick (1884-1922)

Scottish Parasitologist

Born in Aberdeen, Scotland, Patrick Manson worked in China for 23 years. His interest in tropical parasites made him a pioneer in the founding of the specialty of **tropical medicine**. Manson earned his MD from Aberdeen Medical School in 1865. His first medical appointment, as assistant medical officer at Durham County Mental Asylum, lasted one year. Manson's older brother was working in Shanghai and persuaded him to travel.

Manson was posted to Formosa (Taiwan) as medical officer for the Chinese Imperial Maritime Customs in the southwestern port of Takao (Kaohsiung). It was Manson's responsibility to inspect ships and treat crews, which gave him ample opportunity to observe tropical diseases. He kept a careful diary and described elephantiasis, **leprosy** (Hansen's disease) and what he thought was heart disease but later learned was **beriberi**.

At end of 1870, Manson was caught in between a political dispute between Japan and China and on the advice of the British consul, he left Formosa in early 1871 to settle at Amoy (Xiamen), a port on the Chinese mainland. At Amoy, Manson had a post with the Baptist Missionary Hospital and a private practice, giving him experience with a large number of cases. He continued to see many cases of elephantiasis and developed a surgical method for removing the copious extra tissue that is part of the disease. His records show that he removed one ton of tissue over a three-year period.

Manson returned to Great Britain for a one-year leave at the end of 1874 and he scoured the libraries for more information on elephantiasis. In the British Museum, Manson found material from surgeon Timothy Lewis speculating that the parasite *Filaria sanguinis hominis* (FSH) was the immature form of a larger worm discovered by Thomas Lane Bancroft. Lewis suspected FSH embryos somehow caused elephantiasis, but he could not identify the method. Manson pored over these studies and developed his own theory of mosquito transmission.

When he returned to Amoy, Manson was so caught up in this scientific problem that he spent all of his spare time on it. He asked two medical students to look for FSH in blood samples. One of the students could only work at night, and he observed many more positive samples than the day observer. From this phenomenon, Manson suspected that there was a recurring pattern in the FSH life cycle. In the next phase of his research, Manson trained two men whose blood contained FSH to examine one another at three-hour intervals over a period of six weeks. This proved the embryos were present in the blood in higher numbers at night than during the day. Manson also showed that the embryos were enclosed in a sheath and they could escape the sheath when the blood was cooled in ice. From this step, Manson theorized that the embryos or embryonic worms could develop outside the human body, perhaps in the body of the common brown mosquito of Amoy. Again, Manson sought a human model and asked his gardener, whose blood was infected with FSH, to allow mosquitos to feed on him. Manson dissected a newly fed mosquito and was able to find parts of the FSH worm inside the mosquito.

During this period, 1877 through 1878, there was no scientific literature on the life cycle of mosquitos and Manson's work was held back by several mistaken assumptions. He thought mosquitos ate only one blood meal before dying, and he thought humans caught FSH by drinking water contaminated with larvae.

Despite these setbacks, Manson's work was significant because it was the first time anyone had proven the role of an arthropod (essentially, an insect with feet) in the life cycle of a parasite. This preliminary research eventually led to the discovery of vast numbers of parasites that require an arthropod as part of the life cycle. However, when Manson presented his work to the Linnean Society of London in 1878, no one understood the significance of his work. Manson continued his research and clinical work in Asia until the depreciation of the Chinese dollar in 1890, when he returned to London to work at the Seamen's Hospital.

There were many examples of tropical diseases at the Seamen's Hospital and Manson looked at the relationship between mosquitos and **malaria**, publishing a paper in 1894. With colleague Ronald Ross, he further examined the mosquito-malaria theory. Through the India Office, Manson arranged for Ross to investigate this theory in India. Ross and Manson were in close communication during this research, and their correspondence has been published. In August of 1897, Ross dissected a mosquito that had bitten a malaria patient and found evidence of malaria in the wall of the mosquito's stomach. Ross sent specimens to Manson, who confirmed the findings.

At this point, Ross was sent to an area where there was no human malaria, but that actually benefited his research. He studied a malaria parasite in sparrows and this helped Ross and Manson reconstruct the complete life cycle of the mosquito. These findings were presented to the British Medical Association. In 1898, an Italian scientist was able to replicate the discovery. Manson was credited with publicizing the research, explaining its significance and eventually helping to control malaria. One portion of his research showed that sleeping in a mosquito-proof hut could save lives while unsheltered people were dying of malaria.

Manson was involved in many aspects of tropical medicine, studying parasites such as flukes, ringworms, and guinea worms, and tracing their life cycles. He helped found the College of Medicine at Hong Kong and served as its first dean. He advocated specialized training for doctors planning to work in the tropics. Manson helped set up the world's first school of tropical medicine in Liverpool and was an organizer in the founding of the London School of Tropical Medicine in 1899, at a time when some practitioners thought medical specialization cheapened the profession. Manson helped found the Royal Society of Tropical Medicine in 1907 and served as its first president. He advised the Colonial Office for 20 years. Manson published his best known work, *Tropical Diseases: A Manual of the Diseases of Warm Climates*, in 1898 and it became a classic textbook, running to 17 editions. The Royal Society elected Manson a fellow in 1900 and he received a knighthood in 1903. He taught at the London School of Tropical Medicine until 1914. After retiring, Manson frequently traveled to Ceylon (Sri Lanka), Rhodesia (Zambia and Zimbabwe), and South Africa. He last addressed the London School two weeks before his death at age 77.

Marfan's syndrome

Antoine Marfan (1858-1942) was a French physician who became interested in pediatrics when he deputized for a colleague at Paris's Hospital for Sick Children in the late 1800s. Marfan believed medicine should be based on methodical and vigorous observation of the patient. It was in the course of his clinical studies in 1896 that he described the main features of a syndrome that later was given his name. Marfan's patient, a five-year-old girl, was thin, and had long limbs and abnormally long fingers and toes. Marfan compared the girl's long digits to the legs of a spider, which gave the condition its medical name, arachnodacryly, from the Greek word for ''spider,'' *arachne*.

Marfan's findings had been suggested 20 years earlier by an eye doctor in Cincinnati, Ohio, who described a tremor in the irises of a brother and sister with long limbs and exceptionally flexible joints—all subsequently shown to be characteristic symptoms of Marfan's syndrome. Later observers noted that Marfan's patients also are often tall and thin, with a long and narrow face, and may have a curved spine and a protruding or sunken breastbone. Most serious, it was found that the heart valves in Marfan's patients tend to leak, and the aorta—the body's largest artery—tends to enlarge and develop aneurysms, weak spots that may suddenly and fatally burst.

The cause of Marfan's is a (usually inherited) disorder of the body's connective tissue. In 1991, researchers discovered that a defective gene on chromosome 15 causes the syndrome. The severity of the disease will vary depending on the type of mutation, which affects the production of a protein call fibrillin. As a result, individuals with the syndrome apparently have insufficient amounts tiny fibers, which provide strength and elasticity to normal connective tissue. Research is under way to identify the various mutations that cause the disorder. Marfan's patients must be regularly monitored via echocardiography to check the size of the aorta and may need to be medicated with beta blockers, which reduce stress on the aorta by lowering the heart rate and contraction strength. The results of undiagnosed or unmonitored Marfan's can be tragic, as in the case of Flo Hyman, a 6-foot-5-inch Olympic volleyball star who died of an aorta rupture while on tour; her Marfan's was discovered only by autopsy. Another famous figure who may have had Marfan's was Abraham Lincoln (1809-1865), whose physical appearance suggests that conclusion to many observers. It is estimated that one in 10,000 people have Marfan's syndrome.

Marriage counseling

Marriage counseling is a type of psychotherapy for a married couple or established partners that tries to resolve problems in the relationship. Typically, two people attend counseling sessions together to discuss specific issues.

Marriage counseling is based on research that shows that individuals and their problems are best handled within the context of their relationships. Marriage counselors are trained in psychotherapy and family systems, and focus on understanding their clients' symptoms and the way their interactions contribute to problems in the relationship.

Marriage counseling is usually a short-term therapy that may take only a few sessions to work out problems in the relationship. Typically, marriage counselors ask questions about the couple's roles, patterns, rules, goals, and beliefs. Therapy often begins as the couple analyzes the good and bad aspects of the relationship. The marriage counselor then works with the couple to help them understand that, in most cases, both partners are contributing to problems in the relationship. When this is understood, the two can then learn to change how they interact with each other to solve problems. The partners may be encouraged to draw up a contract in which each partner describes the behavior he or she will be trying to maintain.

Marriage is not a requirement for two people to get help from a marriage counselor. Anyone person wishing to improve his or her relationships can get help with behavioral problems, relationship issues, or with mental or emotional disorders. Marriage counselors also offer treatment for couples before they get married to help them understand potential problem areas. A third type of marriage counseling involves postmarital therapy, in which divorcing couples who share children seek help in working out their differences. Couples in the midst of a divorce find that marriage therapy during separation can help them find a common ground as they negotiate interpersonal issues and child custody.

A marriage counselor is trained to use different types of therapy in work with individuals, couples, and groups. American Association of Marriage and Family Therapy (AAMFT) training includes supervision by experienced therapists, a minimum of a master's degree (including specific training in marriage and family therapy), and specific graduate training in marriage and family therapy.

When looking for a marriage counselor, a couple should find out the counselor's training and educational background, professional associations, such as AAMFT, and state licensure, and whether the person has experience in treating particular kinds of problem. Also, questions should be asked concerning fees, insurance coverage, the average length of therapy, and so on.

Marriage counseling helps couples learn to deal more effectively with problems, and can help prevent small problems from becoming serious. Research shows that marriage counseling, when effective, tends to improve a person's physical as well as mental health, in addition to improving the relationship.

MASSAGE

Massage is the manual rubbing and kneading of the body's soft tissues to stimulate circulation and promote relaxation of muscles. Many forms of massage are usedin use throughout the world, including Swedish, deep tissue, Tui Na, Hawaiian, and others. Massage helps the muscles relax by stimulating a reflex response of the nervous system. The application of smooth, steady, rhythmical massage can relieve tension and soothe sore muscles. This decrease in muscle tension causes the muscle to become more relaxed and elastic. Also, massage's effect on the circulatory system is beneficial for the healing of soft tissue injuries.

Massage's ability to aid in the recovery from soft tissue injuries, such as **sprains and strains**, is an important use of massage. Many soft tissue injuries are not serious enough for doctor or hospital for treatment; but they still may cause some discomfort and disability long after the initial injury. Massage can speed and improve the rate of recovery and reduce discomfort.

To understand how massage helps healing in cases of soft tissue injury, it is important to understand the inflammatory process. Inflammation begins because blood circulates to the injured area to bring important chemicals essential for healing. After a period of time, the initial inflammation stops. If applied at this point, massage will help increase circulation and promote healing as the increased blood flow brings additional oxygen and nutrients to the injured area. In this way, massage helps bridge the gap between common neglect of injury and major expensive medical intervention. Massage can also help stimulate the flow of lymph, the fluid that helps the body remove waste products.

Massage can stimulate inactive muscles whose inactivity is due to illness or injury. Deep continuous massage can relieve muscle tension and help prevent painful muscle spasms, which are common following injury. Also, massage can stretch and break down fibrous scar tissue that is not healing properly because it is not aligned to the adjoining muscle fibers.

Massage affects pain through the central **nervous system**. In one theory of pain called the ''gate theory,'' messages of pain which normally travel from the injury to the brain are blocked before reaching the centers responsible for interpreting pain. Massage helps stimulate and close the so-called gate of pain messages. As a result, the intensity of pain perceived by the brain is decreased.

Psychosomatic studies show how **stress** factors can cause migraines, **hypertension**, depression, some peptic **ulcers**, etc. Some researchers have estimated that 80% of disease is stress related. Soothing and relaxing massage therapy can help reduce illness by counteracting stress effects.

Massage usually is not recommended for individuals with a circulatory problem; it could produce complications in individuals with high blood pressure or a history of heart trouble. Injury to bone can occur if massage is performed too soon after injury over an area of advanced **osteoporosis** or bone fracture. Also, in cases of **cancer**, massage is not used because an increase in circulation might help the cancer spread more rapidly. Severe diabetes, skin infection, tubercular joints, **burns**, or abrasions may also be indications to avoid massage.

When selecting a massage therapist, it is important to check credentials, including whether the therapist has graduated from a school approved by a credible accrediting agency, such as the Commission for Massage Training Accreditation (COMTA) and the American Massage Therapy Association (AMTA).

Massage is a valuable tool in the management of many musculoskeletal disorders. While there are many forms of massage in use around the world, Swedish type massage is the type most commonly used in sports medicine in the United States. Sports medicine massage can be separated into five basic categories.

Massage can have adverse effects if not used properly, or if used over inappropriate areas. Massage will also have a

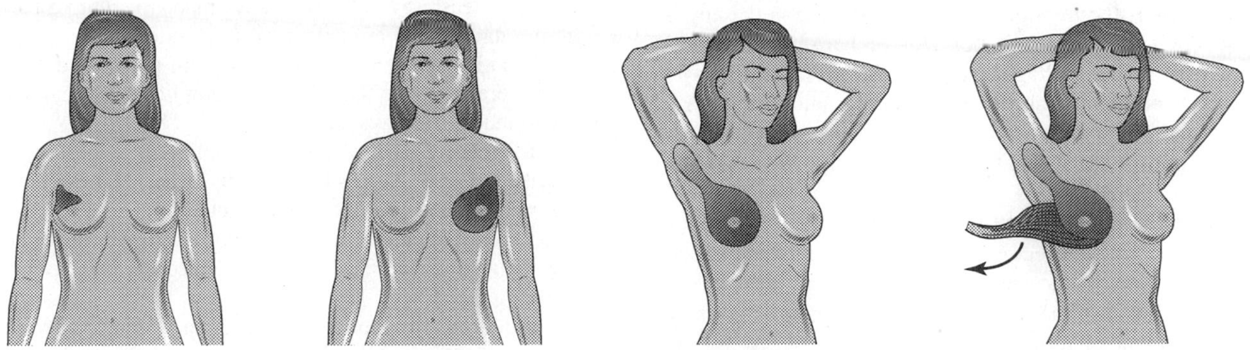

There are four types of mastectomies: partial mastectomy, or lumpectomy, in which the tumor and surrounding tissue is removed; simple mastectomy, where the entire breast and some axillary lymph nodes are removed; modified radical mastectomy, in which the entire breast and all axillary lymph nodes are removed; and the radical mastectomy, where the entire breast, axillary lymph nodes, and chest muscles are removed. *(Illustration by Electronic Illustrators Group.)*

negative effect if applied over an area that is infected. Massage over a recent injury may increase the inflammation and cause additional soft tissue injury. If an individual has poor circulation, a decrease or unwanted fluctuation in blood supply to critical areas of the body may occur. As noted, massage can produce abnormal blood flow in individuals with high blood pressure or a history of heart trouble. Injury to bone can occur if massage is performed too soon over a bone fracture, or over an area of advanced osteoporosis.

However, if applied properly and under the correct conditions, massage enhances muscle relaxation and increases circulation, resulting in the enhancement of the healing process.

See also Central nervous system; Osteoporosis; Sprains and strains; Stress and stress management

Mastectomy

Mastectomy is the surgical removal of all or part of the breast for the treatment or prevention of **breast cancer**. The size, location, and type of tumor are very important when choosing the best surgery to treat a woman's breast cancer. The size of the breast is also an important factor. A woman's psychological concerns, and her lifestyle choices should also be considered when decisions are made.

The severity of a **cancer** is evaluated according to a complex system called staging. This takes into account the size of the tumor, and whether it has spread to the lymph nodes, adjacent tissues, and/or distant parts of the body. A mastectomy is usually recommended for more advanced breast cancers. Women with earlier stage breast cancers, who could have breast conserving surgery, in which only the tumor and surrounding tissue are removed (called a **lumpectomy**), may decide to have a mastectomy.

There are many factors that make a mastectomy the treatment of choice. A large tumor is indicates a later stage of breast cancer, when the removal of the entire breast is recommended. In addition, large tumors are difficult to remove with good cosmetic results, especially if the woman has small breasts. Very rapidly growing breast cancers are usually treated with a mastectomy. Sometimes multiple areas of cancer are found in one breast, making removal of the whole breast necessary. A cancer that has already attached itself to nearby tissues, such as the skin or chest wall, is most likely to be removed with a mastectomy. Breast conserving may also prove unsuccessful. The surgeon is sometimes unable to remove the tumor with a sufficient amount, or margin, of normal tissue surrounding it. The entire breast needs to be removed in this situation. Recurrence of breast cancer after a lumpectomy is another indication for mastectomy.

Radiation therapy is almost always recommended following a lumpectomy. If a woman is unable to have radiation, a mastectomy is the treatment of choice. Radiation therapy is not used in regnant women for fear of harming the fetus; women with certain collagen vascular diseases, such as **systemic lupus erythematosus** or **scleroderma**; and any woman who has had therapeutic radiation to the chest area for other reasons cannot tolerate additional exposure for breast cancer therapy.

The need for radiation therapy after breast conserving surgery may make mastectomy more appealing for nonmedical reasons. Some women fear radiation, and choose the more extensive surgery, so radiation treatment will not be required. The commitment of time, usually five days a week, for six weeks, may not be acceptable for other women.

Some women choose mastectomy because they strongly fear recurrence of the breast cancer, and lumpectomy seems too risky. The issue of prophylactic mastectomy, or removal of the breast to prevent future breast cancer, is controversial. Women with a strong family history of breast cancer and/or who test positive for a known cancer-causing gene may choose this option. Patients who have had certain types of breast cancers that are more likely to recur may elect to have the unaffected breast removed. Evidence suggests that this procedure can decrease the chances of developing breast cancer, but it is not a guarantee that all breast tissue has been removed. Breast cancers have occurred after both breasts have been removed.

There are several types of mastectomies. The radical mastectomy, also called the Halsted mastectomy, is rarely performed today. It was developed in the late 1800s, when it was thought that more extensive surgery was most likely to cure cancer. A radical mastectomy involves removal of the breast, all surrounding lymph nodes up to the collarbone, and the underlying chest muscle. Women were often left disfigured and disabled, with a large defect in the chest wall and significantly decreased arm sensation and motion. Unfortunately, it is still the operation many women inaccurately picture, when the word mastectomy is mentioned.

Surgery that removes breast tissue and some axillary or underarm lymph nodes and leaves the chest muscle intact is usually called a modified radical mastectomy. The most common type of mastectomy performed in the 1990s, the surgery leaves a woman with a more normal chest shape than the older radical mastectomy procedure and a scar which is not visible in most clothing. It also allows for immediate or delayed breast reconstruction.

In a simple mastectomy, only the breast itself is removed. If a few of the axillary lymph nodes closest to the breast are also taken out, the surgery may be called an extended simple mastectomy.

There are other variations on the term mastectomy. A skin-sparing mastectomy uses special techniques that preserve the patient's breast skin for use in reconstruction. Total mastectomy is a confusing expression, as it may be used to refer to a modified radical mastectomy or a simple mastectomy.

A mastectomy is typically performed in a hospital setting, but specialized outpatient facilities are sometimes used. The surgery is done under general anesthesia and may take from two to five hours. In the past, women often stayed in the hospital at least several days. Now many patients go home within a day or two after their mastectomies.

Pain is usually well controlled with prescribed medication. Severe pain may be a sign of complications, and should be reported to the physician.

Exercises to maintain shoulder and arm mobility may be prescribed as early as 24 hours after surgery. These help restore strength and promote good circulation.

Emotional care is another important aspect of recovery. Patients are often advised to seek counseling and/or support groups.

Additional treatment for breast cancer may be necessary after a mastectomy. Depending on the type of tumor, lymph node status, and other factors, **chemotherapy**, radiation therapy, and/or hormone therapy may be prescribed.

After mastectomy and axillary lymph node dissection, a number of complications are possible. A woman may experience decreased feeling in the back of her armpit, or other sensations including numbness, tingling, or increased skin sensitivity. Some women report phantom breast symptoms, experiencing **itching**, aching, or other sensations in the breast that has been removed. There may be injury to the nerves controlling arm motion, resulting in decreased arm mobility.

Approximately 2-10% of patients develop **lymphedema** after axillary lymph node removal. This swelling of the arm, caused by faulty lymph drainage, can range from mild to very severe. It can be treated with elevation, elastic bandages, and specialized physical therapy. A new technique called sentinel node biopsy, which may eliminate the need for removing many lymph nodes, is being tested.

Although mastectomy remains the definitive surgical treatment for breast cancer, research continues into nonsurgical interventions, such as drug therapy. The most important research, however, may be the investigations into how to avoid or prevent breast cancer, which eliminates the need for a disfiguring mastectomy.

See also Breast cancer and care; Lumpectomy; Radiation therapy

MASTERS, WILLIAM HOWELL (1915-)

American obstetrician and gynecologist

William Howell Masters was the first to study the anatomy and physiology of human sexuality in the laboratory, and the publication of the reports on his findings created much interest and criticism. Since then, Masters and his colleague, **Virginia E. Johnson**, have become well-known as researchers and therapists in the field of human sexuality, and together they have established the Reproduction Biology Center and later the Masters and Johnson Institute in St. Louis, Missouri.

Masters was born on December 27, 1915, in Cleveland, Ohio, to Francis Wynne and Estabrooks (Taylor) Masters. He attended public school in Kansas City through the eighth grade and then went to the Lawrenceville School in Lawrenceville, New Jersey. In 1938 he received a B.S. degree from Hamilton College, where he divided his time between science courses and sports such as baseball, football, and basketball. He was also active in campus debate. He entered the University of Rochester School of Medicine and started working in the laboratory of Dr. George Corner, who was comparing and studying the reproductive tracts of animals and humans.

During his junior year in medical school, Masters became interested in sexuality because it was the last scientifically unexplored physiological function. After briefly serving in the navy, he received his M.D. degree in 1943. Masters became interested in the work of Dr. Alfred Kinsey, a University of Indiana zoology professor who had interviewed thousands of men and women about their sexual experiences. Choosing a field that would help him prepare himself for human sexuality research, Masters became an intern and later a resident in obstetrics and gynecology at St. Louis Hospital and Barnes Hospital in St. Louis. He also did an internship in pathology at the Washington University School of Medicine. In 1947 he joined the faculty at Washington and advanced from instructor to associate professor of clinical obstetrics and gynecology. Masters conducted research in the field and contributed dozens of papers to scientific journals. One of his areas of interest was hormone treatment and replacement in post-menopausal women.

By 1954 Masters decided that he was ready to undertake research on the physiology of sex. He was concerned that the medical profession had too little information on sexuality to understand clients' problems. Kinsey had depended on case histories, interviews, and secondhand data. Masters took the next step, which was to study human sexual stimulation using measuring technology in a laboratory situation.

Masters launched his project at Washington University, assisted by a grant from the United States Institute of Health. At first he recruited prostitutes for study, but found them unsuitable for his studies of "normal" sexuality. In 1956 he hired Virginia Eshelman Johnson, a sociology student, to help in the interviewing and screening of volunteers. The study was conducted over an eleven-year period with 382 women and 312 men participating. Subjects ranged in age from eighteen to eighty-nine and were paid for their time. Masters found a four-phased cycle relating to male and female sexual responses. To measure physiological changes, he used electroencephalographs, electrocardiographs, color cinematography, and biochemical studies.

Masters was very cautious and meticulous about protecting the identity of his volunteers. In 1959 he sent some results to medical journals, but continued to work in relative secrecy. After the content of the studies leaked out, the team had difficulty procuring grant money, so in 1964 Masters became director of the Reproductive Biology Foundation, a non-profit group, to obtain private funds. In November of that same year, Dr. Leslie H. Farber, a respected Washington D.C. psychiatrist, wrote an article in *Commentary* entitled "I'm sorry, Dear," in which he attacked the "scientizing" of sex. This attack was only the beginning of the criticism the research would receive.

In 1966 Masters and Johnson published *Human Sexual Response.* In this book, the researchers used highly technical terminology and had their publisher, Little, Brown and Co., promote the book only to medical professionals and journals. Nevertheless, the book became a popular sensation and the team embarked on a speaking and lecture tour, winning immediate fame. As early as 1959 Masters and Johnson had begun counseling couples as a dual-sex team. Believing that partners would be more comfortable talking with a same-sex therapist, the team began working with couples' sexual problems. In their second book, *Human Sexual Inadequacy* (1970), they discuss problems such as impotence.

Masters divorced his first wife, Elisabeth Ellis, not long after the publication of *Human Sexual Inadequacy* and married Johnson on January 1, 1971, in Fayetteville, Arkansas. In 1973 they became codirectors of the Masters and Johnson Institute. In 1979 Masters and Johnson studied and described the sexual responses of homosexuals and lesbians in *Homosexuality in Perspective.* They also claimed to be able to change the sexual preferences of homosexuals who wanted it. Masters also maintained a biochemistry lab and continued to receive fees from a gynecology practice. He retired from practice in 1975 at the age of sixty. In 1981 Masters and Johnson sold their lab and moved to another location in St. Louis. At this time they had a staff of twenty-five and a long list of therapy clients.

Further controversy over their work developed when in 1988 Masters and Johnson coauthored a book with an associate, Dr. Robert Kolodny. The book, *Crisis: Heterosexual Behavior in the Age of AIDS* predicted an epidemic of AIDS among the heterosexual population. Some members of the medical community severely condemned the study, and **C. Everett Koop**, then surgeon general of the United States, called Masters and Johnson irresponsible. Perhaps as a result of the negative publicity, the number of clients seeking sex therapy at the institute decreased. In early 1992, Bill Walters, acting director of the institute, announced that Masters and Johnson were divorcing after twenty-one years of marriage—conflict in their ideas about retirement was cited as the reason for the breakup. Masters vowed he would never retire and continued speaking and lecturing at the institute, in addition to working on another book. The divorce ended their work together at the clinic.

For his pioneering efforts in making human sexuality a subject of scientific study, Masters received the Paul H. Hoch Award from the American Psychopathic Association in 1971, the Sex Information and Education Council of the United States (SIECUS) award in 1972, and three other prestigious awards. He belongs to the American Association for the Advancement of Science (AAAS), the American Fertility Society, and several other medical associations.

Masturbation

Although the mere mention of the word masturbation still makes many people uncomfortable, attitudes toward the activity have become slightly more liberal because of its frequent discussion in the fields of psychology, psychiatry, and sociology, among others. However, despite evidence that masturbation is a healthy, normal part of human sexual development, the act is still regarded as unwholesome and shameful in some quarters. Indeed, the Roman Catholic Church still officially considers masturbation a mortal sin.

Masturbation is the self-stimulation of the genitals, usually with the aim of sexual pleasure and orgasm. It is generally performed alone and in private, but sometimes it occurs between people as part of a sexual relationship apart from sexual intercourse. The practice was taboo in most premodern societies—particularly those that espoused Christianity—and there were frightening myths and superstitions built up around it. These included that self stimulation would cause blindness, insanity, and other illnesses, some that would plainly mark the person as a masturbator. Many of these fears were based on observations of unwell people masturbating in public, but the observers were often unaware that such ailments as severe **mental retardation**, **dementia**, and **schizophrenia** can produce this behavior, not vice versa. Such myths still have the power to produce extreme guilt and fear in people who venture to explore self-pleasure, while others regard masturbation only as a nonemotional release or as a physical pleasure to be enjoyed for its own sake.

According to literature on the topic, as of the late 1990s, more people of all ages and both sexes are practicing masturbation, whether alone or with a partner, perhaps because of the fear of **AIDS** and the desire to have safe sex. However, the act remains most common among young adults and teenagers (particularly males), while it is also not infrequent among infants and children as a form of self-gratification similar to thumb-sucking. The practice is widely agreed to be a normal part of the sexual development process.

It is estimated that more than 90% of men and roughly 60% of women masturbate at least once during their lives. The act can bring about relaxation, pleasure, tension release, and physical satisfaction. Some sources indicate that masturbation in older children and teenagers can produce better control over sexual urges. Researchers generally agree that since masturbation does not usually bring the same psychological satisfaction as sexual interaction with another person, the activity declines or ceases altogether (especially in females) once an individual becomes involved in a sexual relationship with a partner.

Most people fantasize during masturbation, although studies have indicated that these scenarios and images many times involve situations or people that the subject would actually avoid if he or she encountered them in real life. Masturbation can much more effectively lead to orgasm than sexual activity with a partner, since there is sole control over what and how stimulation occurs. The practice is frequently recommended in **sex therapy**.

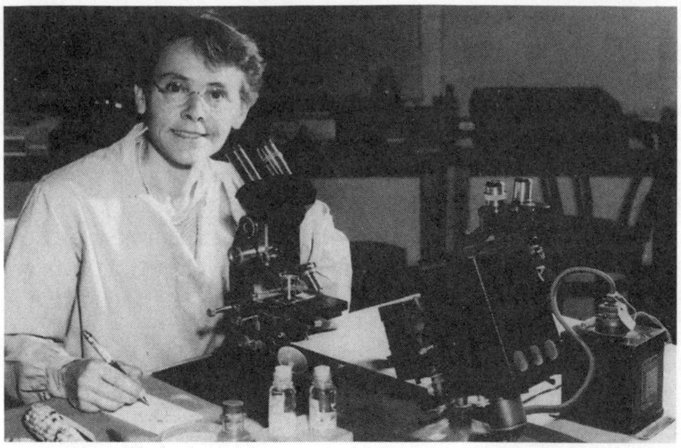

Barbara McClintock.

McClintock, Barbara (1902-1992)

American geneticist

Barbara McClintock was born on June 16, 1902, in Connecticut. The daughter of a physician, she grew up in the Flatbush section of Brooklyn, New York—a rural area during that time. During high school, McClintock's interests turned from sandlot baseball to science. Despite her parents' misgivings, she persuaded them to let her study at Cornell University, an agricultural college in Ithaca, New York. McClintock was fascinated with a genetics course she took in her junior year. However, in the plant breeding department where most of the genetics courses were taught, women were not permitted as graduate students. So McClintock signed up in the botany department and became assistant to a cytology professor who encouraged her interest in plant genetics.

After McClintock completed her graduate work at Cornell, she stayed on as an instructor and researcher, associating herself with Rollins Emerson's famous maize (corn) genetics group. During this time, she discovered the function of each chromosome in corn. Cultivating her own crops on university grounds, she spent summers recording changes in each plant, then returned to the lab after the harvest. By observing cell divisions at various stages of a corn plant's development, she was able to tell what each chromosome did in the process. Between 1929 and 1931, she published nine papers on the subject of genetics.

In 1931, McClintock assigned graduate student Harriet Creighton a problem in genetic crossover in corn. With McClintock's guidance, Creighton was able to show that genetic information is transferred after chromosomes cross over during the formation of sex cells. While on a visit to Cornell, Thomas Hunt Morgan, one of the pioneers in the study of genetics, urged McClintock and Creighton to publish their findings on genetic crossover in corn. They did, receiving favorable reviews for their work.

McClintock's major contribution to genetics came after she left Cornell, which at the time had no women above the level of professor outside the home economics department. It was difficult at first, because she had gained a reputation as being a difficult, independent loner. She worked briefly at the University of Missouri, but felt isolated from the administration and constrained by its bureaucratic rules (she often ignored building hours and would break into her lab on Sundays). In 1941, she found a permanent position at Cold Spring Harbor Laboratory on Long Island, a residential research site run by the Carnegie Institution of Washington, where she could conduct her experiments free of administrative interference.

Over the years, McClintock had developed an interest in the mutations caused by x-rays. She was so familiar with maize plants and their chromosomes that she instantly recognized anything unusual. One season, some of her corn seedlings had developed odd streaks and spots on the leaves. There appeared to be a pattern, but it was unlike any pattern made from the x-rays. Something in the plant itself seemed to be controlling the appearance of the patterns. She studied more closely and found that many color patches showed up in opposite pairs. For instance, if part of a leaf contained more green streaks than usual, a nearby portion would contain fewer than usual.

To McClintock, these were not signs of disorder, but of a larger and different system of order. She set out to make that difference understandable. For six years, she researched her unusual observations, and in 1951, she presented her theory of genetic transposition (also called genetic mobility or gene jumping). According to her theory, genes in a chromosome could actually move from one position to another within that same chromosome. McClintock saw transposition as a way that individual organisms regulate their development, and even their survival, in times of stress. McClintock's discovery, however, was met with derision. The majority of geneticists believed that genes were preprogrammed, and, like beads on a string, occupied a fixed place on chromosomes. Any changes, therefore, occurred only as a result of random accidents. When McClintock presented her findings at a symposium, her colleagues dismissed her as "an old bag who'd been hanging around Cold Spring Harbor for years."

By the 1970s, McClintock had expanded her theory, arguing that genes could not only change their positions on a chromosome, but that they could also serve different purposes in those different positions. Slowly, her ideas gained acceptance, as scientists began to witness transposition in other life forms. But it wasn't until 1983, some 30 years after her discovery, that McClintock received the Nobel Prize in physiology or medicine. She was also the recipient of the National Medal of Science (1970) and the first MacArthur Laureate Award (1981), a lifetime annual prize of $60,000.

When asked about the long delay in recognition for her discovery, McClintock observed, "If you know you're right, you don't care. You know that sooner or later, it will come out in the wash." McClintock died on September 2, 1992.

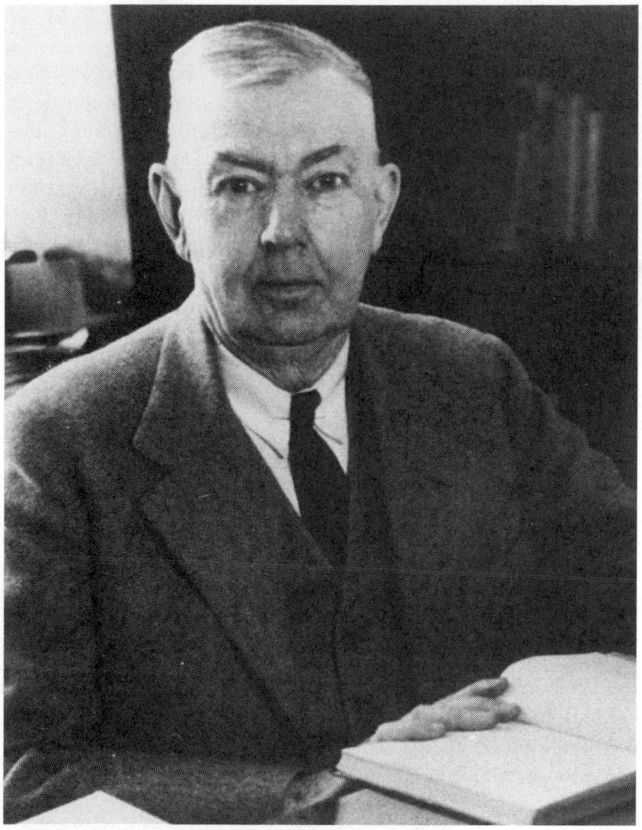

Elmer McCollum.

McCollum, Elmer Verner (1879-1967)

American biochemist

Elmer McCollum was born on a farm near Fort Scott, Kansas, where he spent his first seventeen years. Money was scarce and the rural community's single school was rarely in operation. But the young Kansan was bright, energetic, and determined to get an education. By moonlighting at numerous jobs, he worked his way, first through high school, then through the University of Kansas, graduating in 1903, and finally through Yale University, where he earned his doctorate in 1906.

Throughout his academic career, McCollum's first love was always organic chemistry. Shortly after graduation, however, he was offered a position at the University of Wisconsin as an instructor in biochemistry (then known as agricultural chemistry). With no better job offers in sight, he decided to accept—a decision that was to alter his life. In 1907, when McCollum arrived at the University's Agricultural Experiment Station, a research study was already in progress. The study was designed to examine the dietary effects of three widely used grains on the health and reproductive capacity of dairy cattle. Because the three grains were chemically similar, the researchers expected similar results. To everyone's intense surprise, however, only one grain—corn—kept the cattle healthy and strong. McCollum immediately resolved to try some nutritional experiments of his own.

Before long, McCollum had set up own laboratory and established the country's first colony of albino laboratory rats devoted to nutritional research. With the help of a young biochemist-in-training named Marguerite Davis, McCullum began the studies that were to lead to the discovery of vitamin A. By 1913, McCollum was able to report that the laboratory rats failed to grow when fed diets in which lard or olive oil was the only source of fat. These same rats, however, quickly resumed normal growth when ether-soluble extracts of butter or eggs were added to the diet. He concluded that butterfat and egg yolks contained some ''growth-promoting factor'' missing in other fats—a factor he soon isolated and termed *fat-soluble A* (to distinguish it from a water-soluble factor previously discovered by Christiaan Eijkman), eventually to be named vitamin A.

In the years that followed, McCollum contributed to the discovery of other fat-soluble **vitamin**s, such as vitamin D in 1922, and did important work in the field of trace minerals. In 1917, he went to Johns Hopkins University as professor of biochemistry, remaining there until 1944. In his later years, he lectured widely on nutritional topics, wrote several outstanding textbooks, and received numerous awards. Shortly before he died, at the age of 88, McCollum mused on his accomplishments and concluded: ''I have had an exceptionally pleasant life and am thankful.''

MEASLES

Measles is an infectious disease that is caused by a virus and primarily infects children. The symptoms of measles include high fever, headache, hacking cough, conjunctivitis and a rash which usually begins inside the mouth as white spots, (called Koplik's spots) and progresses to a red rash that spreads to face, neck, trunk and extremities. The incubation period varies but is usually 10–12 days until symptoms appear. Measles are sometimes called rubeola or the nine-day measles. Normally recovery is full. However, complications can arise if a secondary bacterial infection occurs, such as **pneumonia** or ear infection.

Measles was described as long ago as the ninth century when a Persian physician, Rhazes, first differentiated between measles and **smallpox**. He also made the observation that fever is a defense the body has against a disease, not a disease itself. His writings on the subject were translated into English and published in 1847.

The measles virus was first discovered in the 1930s; **John F. Enders** of Children's Hospital in Boston eventually isolated the measles virus in 1954 and began looking for an attenuated strain to be suitable for a live-virus vaccine. A successful immunization program for measles was begun soon after. Today measles is controlled in the United States with a vaccination that confers immunity against measles, **mumps** and **rubella** and is commonly called the MMR vaccine. Since a series of measles epidemics occurred in the teenage population, a second MMR shot is now required of many school-age children as it was found that only one vaccination appeared not to confer lifelong immunity.

MECHNIKOV, ILYA • See Metchnikoff, Elie

MEDAWAR, PETER BRIAN (1915-1987)

English biologist

Peter Brian Medawar was a renowned biologist who made major contributions to the study of immunology. Working extensively with skin grafts, he and his collaborators proved that one's immune system ''learns'' to distinguish between ''self'' and ''non-self''—that is, such distinctions are not inherent. During his career, Medawar also became a prolific author, penning books such as *The Uniqueness of the Individual* and *Advice to a Young Scientist.* Winner of the Nobel Prize in physiology or medicine in 1960, he was also knighted in 1965.

Medawar was born on February 28, 1915, in Rio de Janeiro, Brazil, to businessperson Nicholas Medawar and the former Edith Muriel Dowling. When he was a young boy, his family moved to England, which he thereafter called home. Medawar attended secondary school at Marlborough College, where he first became interested in biology. He once described his biology master at Marlborough as a rough individual whose selection for the position was meant to discourage the students from taking up science. However, Medawar acknowledged his teacher's devotion to biology, while the educator, in turn, recognized the pupil's interest. The biology master encouraged Medawar to pursue the science under the tutelage of one of his former students, John Young, at Magdalen College. Medawar followed this advice and enrolled at Magdalen in 1932 as a zoology student. He found Young to be an excellent teacher.

Medawar earned his bachelor's degree from Magdalen in 1935, the same year he accepted an appointment as Christopher Welch Scholar and Senior Demonstrator at Magdalen College. He followed Young's recommendation that he work with pathologist Howard Florey, who was undertaking a study of penicillin, work for which he would later become well-known. Medawar leaned toward experimental embryology and tissue cultures. While at Magdalen, he met zoology student Jean Shinglewood Taylor, who also joined Florey's lab. They married in 1937. In a 1984 interview with *New Scientist,* she recalled her impressions of Medawar at Magdalen: ''Nobody could forget him, because he was very tall, very untidy, obviously extremely clever, and very dominant.'' She spent less than a year in Florey's lab. The couple had their first child in 1938. In all they had four children, sons Charles and Alexander, and daughters Caroline and Louise.

In 1938, Medawar, by examination, became a fellow of Magdalen College and received the Edward Chapman Research Prize. A year later, he received his master's from Oxford. When World War II broke out in Europe, the Medical Research Council asked Medawar to concentrate his research on tissue transplants, primarily skin grafts. While this took him away from his initial research studies into embryology, his work with the military would come to drive his future research and eventually lead to a Nobel Prize. During the war, Medawar developed a concentrated form of fibrinogen, a component of the blood. This substance acted as a glue to reattach severed nerves, and found a place in the treatment of skin grafts and in other operations. More importantly to Medawar's future research, however, were his studies at the Burns Unit of the Glasgow Royal Infirmary in Scotland. His task was to determine why patients rejected donor skin grafts. He observed that the rejection time for donor grafts was noticeably longer for initial grafts, compared to those grafts that were transplanted for a second time. Medawar noted the similarity between this reaction and the body's reaction to an invading virus or bacteria. He formed the opinion that the body's rejection of skin grafts was immunological in nature; the body built up an immunity to the first graft and then called on that already-built-up immunity to quickly reject a second graft.

Upon his return from the Burns Unit to Oxford, he began his studies of immunology in the laboratory. In 1944 he became a senior research fellow of St. John's College, Oxford, and university demonstrator in zoology and comparative anatomy. Although he qualified for and passed his examinations for a doctorate in philosophy while at Oxford, Medawar opted against accepting it because it would cost more than he could afford. In his autobiography, *Memoir of a Thinking Radish,* he wrote, "The degree served no useful purpose and cost, I learned, as much as it cost in those days to have an appendectomy. Having just had the latter as a matter of urgency, I thought that to have both would border on self-indulgence, so I remained a plain mister until I became a prof." He continued as researcher at Oxford University through 1947.

During that year Medawar accepted an appointment as Mason professor of zoology at the University of Birmingham. He brought with him one of his best graduate students at Oxford, Rupert Everett "Bill" Billingham. Another graduate student, Leslie Brent, soon joined them and the three began what was to become a very productive collaboration that spanned several years. Their research progressed through Medawar's appointment as dean of science, through his several-month-long trip to the Rockefeller Institute in New York in 1949—the same year he received the prestigious title of fellow from the Royal Society—and even a relocation to another college. In 1951 Medawar accepted a position as Jodrell Professor of Zoology and Comparative Anatomy at University College, London. Billingham and Brent followed him.

Their most important discovery had its experimental root in a promise Medawar made at the International Congress of Genetics at Stockholm in 1948. He told another investigator, Hugh Donald, that he could formulate a foolproof method for distinguishing identical from fraternal twin calves. He and Billingham felt they could easily tell the twins apart by transplanting a skin graft from one twin to the other. They reasoned that a calf of an identical pair would accept a skin graft from its twin because the two originated from the same egg, whereas a calf would reject a graft from its fraternal twin because they

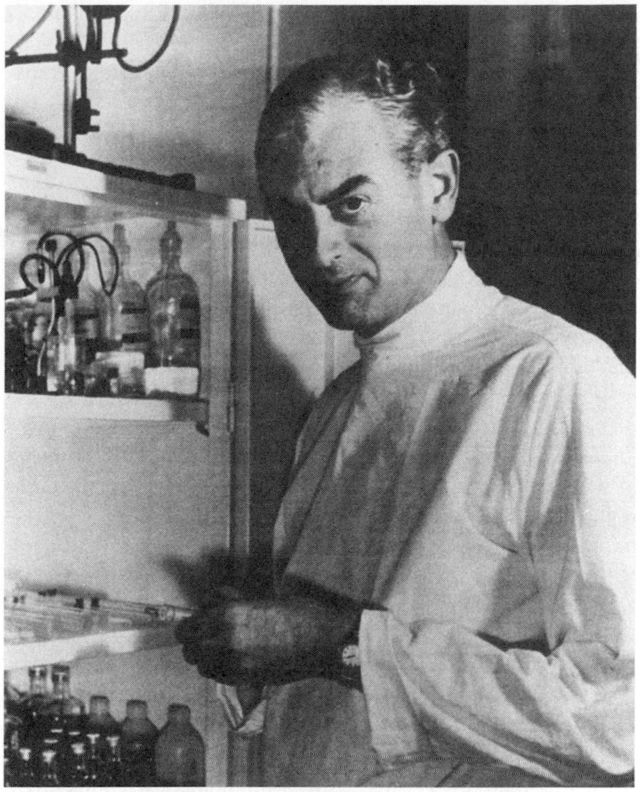

Peter Brian Medawar.

came from two separate eggs. The results did not bear this out, however. The calves accepted skin grafts from their twins regardless of their status as identical or fraternal. Puzzled, they repeated the experiment, but received the same results.

They found their error when they became aware of work done by Dr. Frank Macfarlane Burnet of the University of Melbourne, and Ray D. Owen of the California Institute of Technology. Owen found that blood transfuses between twin calves, both fraternal and identical. Burnet believed that an individual's immunological framework developed before birth, and felt Owen's finding demonstrated this by showing that the immune system tolerates those tissues that are made known to it before a certain age. In other words, the body does not recognize donated tissue as alien if it has had some exposure to it at an early age. Burnet predicted that this immunological tolerance for non-native tissue could be reproduced in a lab. Medawar, Billingham, and Brent set out to test Burnet's hypothesis.

The three-scientist team worked closely together, inoculating embryos from mice of one strain with tissue cells from donor mice of another strain. When the mice had matured, the trio grafted skin from the donor mice to the inoculated mice. Normally, mice reject skin grafts from other mice, but the inoculated mice in their experiment accepted the donor skin grafts. They did not develop an immunological reaction. The prenatal encounter had given the inoculated mice an acquired immunological tolerance. They had proven Burnet's hypothesis. They published their findings in a 1953 article in *Nature.*

Although their research had no applications to transplants among humans, it showed that transplants were possible. The scientific world previously held no hope for successful transplants. In *Memoir of a Thinking Radish,* Medawar explained: "Thus the ultimate importance of the discovery of tolerance turned out to be not practical, but moral. It put new heart into the many biologists and surgeons who were working to make it possible to graft, for example, kidneys from one person to another."

In the years following publication of the research, Medawar accepted several honors, including the Royal Medal from the Royal Society in 1959. A year later he and Burnet accepted the Nobel Prize for Physiology or Medicine for their discovery of acquired immunological tolerance: Burnet developed the theory and Medawar proved it. Medawar shared the prize money with Billingham and Brent.

Medawar's scientific concerns extended beyond immunology, even during the years of his work toward acquired immunological tolerance. While at Birmingham, he and Billingham also investigated pigment spread, a phenomenon seen in some guinea pigs and cattle where the dark spots spread into the light areas of the skin. "Thus if a dark skin graft were transplanted into the middle of a pale area of skin it would soon come to be surrounded by a progressively widening ring of dark skin," Medawar asserted in his autobiography. The team conducted a variety of experiments, hoping to show that the dark pigment cells were somehow "infecting" the pale pigment cells. The tests never panned out. "It was a weary and disheartening business representing a loss of about two years' work, at the end of which I had to admit that the hypothesis on which I had been working was mistaken."

Medawar also delved into animal behavior at Birmingham. He edited a book on the subject by noted scientist **Nikolaas Tinbergen**, who ultimately netted a Nobel Prize in 1973. Medawar felt Tinbergen's work was important enough that he went beyond his literary assistance, and wrote to a granting agency to assure that Tinbergen's work was funded. In 1957, Medawar also became a book author with his first offering, *The Uniqueness of the Individual,* which was actually a collection of essays. In 1959, his second book, *The Future of Man,* was issued, containing a compilation of a series of broadcasts he read for British Broadcasting Corporation (BBC) radio. The series examined the impacts of evolution on man.

Medawar remained at University College until 1962 when he took the post of director of the National Institute for Medical Research in London, where he continued his study of transplants and immunology. While there, he continued writing with mainly philosophical themes. *The Art of the Soluble,* published in 1967, is an assembly of essays, while his 1969 book, *Induction and Intuition in Scientific Thought,* is a sequence of lectures examining the thought processes of scientists. In 1969 Medawar, then president of the British Association for the Advancement of Science, experienced the first of a series of strokes while speaking at the group's annual meeting. As soon as possible, he returned to work, sometimes relying on research assistants to conduct the laboratory bench work. He finally retired from his position as director of the National Institute for Medical Research in 1971. In spite of his physical limitations, he went ahead with scientific research in his lab at the clinical research center of the Medical Research Council. There he began studying cancer. In the 1984 interview with *New Scientist,* he said, "I believe that vaccination is possible against a wide range of cancers, in principle. This is now our principal line of research."

Through the 1970s and 1980s, Medawar produced several other books—some with his wife as co-author—in addition to his many essays on growth, aging, immunity, and cellular transformations. In one of his most well-known books, *Advice to a Young Scientist,* he states that scientists are not geniuses, but people who have the combined characters of common sense and curiosity. He writes, "Like any other human being, a young scientist growing up will probably say to himself at the end of each decade, 'Ah well, that's it then. It has all been great fun, but nothing now remains except to play out time with dignity and composure and hope that some of my work will last a bit longer than I do.'" Medawar died on October 2, 1987, at the age of seventy-two.

Medical ethics

From the beginning of the history of medicine, healers have had to deal with questions of ethics. However, the separate discipline of medical ethics has existed for less than 50 years, largely prompted by 20th-century advances in life-support technology. Today, medical ethics has become a multidisciplinary endeavor, often involving teams that may include clergy, philosophers, scientists, and lawyers, as well as physicians and nurses.

The Hippocratic Oath, attributed to the ancient Greek physician **Hippocrates**, is one of the best-known statements of ethical practice. It required physicians to "abstain from whatever is deleterious and mischievous," seeking only the benefit of their patients. Doctors taking the oath swore: "I will give no deadly medicine to anyone if asked, nor suggest any such counsel; and in like manner I will not give to a woman a pessary (a device worn in the vagina) to produce abortion. With purity and with holiness I will pass my life and practice my art. I will not cut persons laboring under the stone, but will leave this to be done by men who are practitioners of this work." Furthermore, the Hippocratic Oath prohibited sexual relations with patients, and established the principle of medical confidentiality: "Whatever, in connection with my professional practice or not in connection with it, I see or hear, in the life of men, which ought not to be spoken of abroad, I will not divulge, as reckoning that all such should be kept secret."

Another landmark work was the Code of Ethics of the **American Medical Association**, created at the AMA's first meeting in 1847. At that gathering, 268 doctors from 22 U.S. states agreed to be bound by a uniform code of ethics, which added humanistic elements not present in the Hippocratic Oath. For example, the 5,298-word AMA document required physicians to treat their patients with "attention, steadiness, and humanity" and to be "vigilant for the welfare of the community.'' In cases when ''pestilence prevails,'' doctors were expected to ''face the danger and to continue their labors for the alleviation of suffering, even at the jeopardy of their own lives.'' The 1847 code required AMA members to respect patient confidentiality, avoid overcharging for their services, provide free services in cases of poverty, and to never abandon a patient if a case was considered incurable. Since 1847, the AMA code has been revised extensively. The current version begins with seven basic principles that serve as an introduction to medical ethics:

- ''A physician shall be dedicated to providing competent medical service with compassion and respect for human dignity.''
- ''A physician shall deal honestly with patients and colleagues, and strive to expose those physicians deficient in character or competence, or who engage in fraud or deception.''
- ''A physician shall respect the law and recognize a responsibility to seek changes in those requirements which are contrary to the best interests of the patient.''
- ''A physician shall respect the rights of patients, of colleagues, and of other health professionals, and shall safeguard patient confidences within the constraints of the law.''
- ''A physician shall continue to study, apply, and advance scientific knowledge, make relevant information available to patients, colleagues, and the public, obtain consultation, and use the talent of other health professionals when indicated.''
- ''A physician shall, in the provision of appropriate patient care, except in emergencies, be free to choose whom to serve, with whom to associate, and the environment in which to provide medical services.''
- ''A physician shall recognize a responsibility to participate in activities contributing to an improved community.''

In addition to these fundamental principles, the AMA code also includes a statement about the doctor-patient relationship, and dozens of opinions released by the AMA's Council on Ethical and Judicial Affairs. These opinions, released at an average rate of about eight per year, cover a wide range of ethical issues. Medical ethics is far from being a static field.

Developments in life-support technology during the 1960s, and more recent advances in reproductive technology and genetics, have prompted intense interest in medical ethics. Many current issues in medical ethics revolve around definitions of human life or the value placed upon it. Such issues include **abortion**, defining death, **eugenics**, **euthanasia** and physician-assisted suicide, **human experimentation**, in-vitro fertilization, and **organ transplantation**.

The growing need to contain health care costs has given rise to economic issues related to distribution of resources. For example, should governments spend more on approaches such as preventative medicine, homeopathy or **naturopathic medicine**? Should resources be concentrated on the young at the expense of the elderly? Will the introduction of **managed care** result in the dehumanization of medicine?

As advances in genetic technology and other fields continue at a revolutionary pace, medical ethics will undoubtedly remain a important discipline for many years to come.

See also Religion and medicine

Medical malpractice

Most physicians are competent, ethical, and highly skilled. However, medical doctors are human. Medical malpractice occurs when a doctor or other health care provider is negligent or fails to follow accepted standards of practice, causing harm to a patient.

Medicine is not without risk. Doctors cannot reasonably guarantee that their treatments will be successful, but they are expected to do what a reasonably qualified and prudent colleague would do under the same circumstances.

The law of medical malpractice varies from nation to nation, and in the United States, from state to state. Generally, however, a successful malpractice claim must first establish that the caregiver had a legal duty to the affected patient. Inhumane as it might seem, a doctor walking down a street or eating at a restaurant in most U.S. states has no legal responsibility to help an injured person. However, a doctor who offers voluntary aid becomes liable for any injury resulting from malpractice. Clearly, a legal duty exists when a patient visits a doctor's office seeking treatment and the doctor agrees to provide it. In certain cases, physicians may also have a duty to non-patients. For example, a jury might determine that a doctor who failed to diagnose epilepsy in a patient has a legal responsibility to others injured in an automobile accident caused by an epileptic seizure suffered by the patient.

A valid malpractice lawsuit must establish that the caregiver's duty to the patient was breached, failing to meet accepted standards of care. For this reason, medical malpractice suits often involve testimony from expert witnesses, who sometimes provide conflicting opinions about what constitutes a reasonable standard of care. Often, such standards are established by medical specialty associations. Doctors are expected to keep themselves informed about current treatment methods, but in many cases more than one treatment option exists and a physician is free to select from those options that would be considered reasonable by a substantial number of medical colleagues. In some cases, doctors try to perform procedures that are beyond their capabilities. It can be useful to check the credentials of your doctor. Physicians who claim to be specialists but are not certified by the appropriate specialty board may lack the training or skills to provide appropriate treatment.

Finally, a valid malpractice suit must establish that the doctor's breach of duty caused real damage to the patient. Depending on the jurisdiction, such harm may include physical and mental suffering, lost income, and other financial losses. However, some states (California and Indiana, for instance) significantly limit compensation available in cases of medical negligence.

How common is medical malpractice? One landmark study, based on case records from New York State, found that among 31,429 records from the year 1984, there were 1,278 cases of injury likely caused by medical management (as opposed to disease) that either lengthened the hospital stay or was responsible for a disability at the time of release from hospital. Of those cases, 306 were attributed to negligence. The researchers found that more than half of the injuries reported were minor, with complete recovery reported within one month. However, 14% of the injuries lasted between one and six months, 2.6% involved permanent disability, and 13.6% resulted in death.

Based on those findings, the researchers concluded that negligence was involved in the care of about one percent of all New York State hospital inpatients. Individual hospitals were found to have widely varying rates of negligence, and university hospitals had less than half the rates of negligence attributed to non-teaching hospitals.

The study also found that lawsuits are not filed in most cases of medical malpractice. On the other hand, the researchers were unable to find any evidence of negligence in 39 of the 47 cases in which malpractice suits were actually filed. Furthermore, they found that payments were made in 40% of those malpractice suits, even though most appeared to be without merit.

Other researchers have reported that as few as two percent of patients affected by doctor negligence ever file lawsuits, that less than 10% of medical malpractice claims ever go to trial, and only five percent proceed to a verdict. Most malpractice cases—more than 70%—are won by the caregivers sued.

Many malpractice suits involve not just doctors, but numerous codefendants including nurses, hospital staff, pharmacists, therapists, even manufacturers of drugs or medical equipment.

A doctor's violation of patient confidentiality could be grounds for a malpractice suit, if the breach caused harm to the patient. An example might be an AIDS patient written out of an inheritance after a doctor gossiped about his condition and word got to the patient's family.

Malpractice may also be present if a patient has not given informed consent before undergoing treatment. Your doctor should discuss the nature, risks and benefits of any proposed treatment, as well as other reasonable options. Many hospitals and doctors require patients to sign a consent form indicating that they assume any risks from the procedure. However, such forms may not shield a caregiver from a malpractice suit if negligence has occurred or the risks were not fully explained to the patient. In the case of needed emergency treatment, a doctor is not required to obtain informed consent. When patients are considered unable to make an informed decision because of age or other factors, consent is required from the patient's legal guardian.

A misdiagnosis by your doctor is not necessarily grounds for a malpractice suit, unless the doctor was negligent in failing to take a proper medical history, ordering appropriate tests, or recognizing obvious symptoms. Critics of the health care system argue that the threat of malpractice suits forces doctors to practice "defensive" medicine, ordering costly tests that would otherwise be unnecessary. Many doctors, however, argue that "defensive" medicine is good medicine.

Medicare and Medicaid

Although private health insurance in the United States dates back to the 1860s, the modern era of health insurance in this country did not begin until 1929 when a group of schoolteachers contracted with Baylor Hospital in Dallas, Texas, to provide room, board and specified medical services at a predetermined monthly rate. Congress' establishment of government-financed healthcare for elderly Americans (Medicare) in 1965 spurred tremendous growth in geriatric, or elderly, care efforts and its associated costs. Medicare now provides hospital and medical benefits to persons age 65 and older and to some others. The original Medicare Plan has two parts, Part A for hospital services and Part B for physician services, with certain eligibility restrictions. Medicare pays its share of the bill and the subscriber pays the balance. The plan participant may choose to go to any doctor, hospital, or other health care provider that accepts Medicare payment.

In the 1980s, Medicare **Health Maintenance Organizations** (HMOs) became available in some parts of the country, and beginning in 1999, **Preferred Provider Organizations** (PPOs) and Provider Sponsored Organizations, and other insurance options like Private-Fee-For Service Plans and Medicare Medical Savings Accounts became available in selected parts of the country. Medicare, which covers short-term acute medical conditions, rather than long-term, chronic conditions requiring custodial care is administered by the Social Security Administration.

In 1965, Congress established health coverage known as Medicaid for the poor of all ages whose income and resources are insufficient to pay for healthcare. Medicaid is state-administered and financed by both the states and federal government through the Social Security Administration. Thus, the Medicaid program varies considerably from state to state, as well as within each state over time. In 1995, Medicaid served the following populations: 18.7 million children; 7.6 million adults who care for these children; 4.4 million elderly; and 5.9 million blind and disabled. When family financial resources are exhausted, it is often Medicaid rather than Medicare that covers the costs of caring for patients who require long-term nursing services, for example those diagnosed with **Alzheimer's disease**.

Surveys have shown that most Americans believe that some type of Medicare reform is necessary, even though they do not always agree on the nature of the changes. One concern that many Americans share is that Medicare may face bankruptcy in the twenty-first century. Noting that the number of elderly U.S. citizens in the year 2040 will range anywhere from 288 million to 458 million people, a variance of nearly 200 million (based on U.S. Census Bureau projections), it is questioned whether the working population will be able to support a federally assisted medical program for the elderly. Some analysts believe, however, that Medicare will survive: their conclusion is based on the observation that although the population over 65 has doubled since 1960 and is expected to do so again over the next 35 years, the nation's income more than tripled since 1960. They also point out that between 1980 and

1998, almost as many babies were born in the U.S. (72 million) as were born between 1946 and 1964 (76 million). In 1999, the U.S. government's annual bill for healthcare spending was $3,925 per person, which is much higher than in other nations. This is thought to be largely due to the fact that physicians' salaries and hospital costs are higher here, and advanced medical technology is more widely used.

See also Aging; Retirement

MEDITATION

Meditation is a discipline or practice of contemplation or awareness found in most of the world's major religions and not a medical treatment in the usual sense. Meditation is, however, frequently recommended by mainstream medical practitioners as well as alternative therapists because of its demonstrated healing effects on the central nervous system, heart rate, and level of muscular tension.

Meditation is reputed to have benefits for the entire person: physical, mental, emotional, and spiritual. Persons who practice meditation on a regular basis may experience lowered blood pressure, more restful sleep, and relief from such physical effects of **stress** as **ulcers**, **headaches**, chronic muscle **pain**, and skin **rashes**. Therapeutic visualization has also been shown to extend the survival time and quality of life of terminally ill patients.

The purposes of meditation have been variously defined as increased awareness, greater ability to live in the moment, freedom from the ego, spiritual growth, or union with God or the universe. It is important to understand that although better health is a frequent side effect of meditation, it is not the goal or focus of meditation practice. The paradox of meditation as an approach to treatment of diseases and disorders is that it asks the patient to put aside immediate concerns with health or wellness.

Meditation is suitable for most people who are not vulnerable to psychotic episodes. Some people may experience **hallucinations** or dissociative episodes. The other major precaution concerns the patient's expectations. Most persons beginning a meditation practice will not find it easy; they are often disturbed by the distractions of their mental processes or the physical discomfort of sitting still for a period of time.

The form of meditation with which most Westerners are familiar involves sitting quietly in a chair or on the floor with eyes closed in order to concentrate or focus the mind. There are, however, a variety of approaches to meditation practice. But the goal of all forms of meditation is single-mindedness—to let go of all distractions and focus on one object of attention or devotion. There are several techniques that meditators use to achieve this level of concentration. Some techniques work better for individuals than others. Beginners should use the approach that they find the most comfortable.

Breathing exercises are often recommended to beginners. Meditation on the breath does not require changing one's breathing in any way, but only paying attention to it. This narrowness of focus helps to develop the ability to concentration. When the person becomes aware that his or her attention has wandered, he or she simply returns to focusing on the breath again. A variation of this approach is focusing on body sensations, sometimes called body scanning. The meditator simply focuses attention on the sensations in each part of his or her body in turn. Sometimes body scanning is combined with a breathing exercise; the meditator imagines breathing into and out of each part of the body as he or she attends to its sensations.

Meditation is a holistic practice that regards the body's positioning or activity as an important dimension of concentration. If the meditator is sitting, he or she is usually instructed to sit upright and wear loose or comfortable clothing in order to be alert as well as relaxed. Some forms of meditation, however, use body motion or postures as an intentional technique of concentration.

In this form of meditation, the person slows down the pace of walking in order to focus on each movement of his or her legs or feet. Walking meditation is often done inside in a large room or without a particular destination. Sufi walking (or dancing) is a form of moving meditation that developed in medieval Islam. The person walks in a rhythmic fashion, usually chanting, in order to focus the mind on a specific quality of God.

A mantra is a name of God or other sacred phrase that the meditator repeats over and over in order to focus the mind. Mantra repetition is the basic technique of transcendental meditation, or TM. TM was introduced to the West in the 1960s by the Maharishi Mahesh Yogi and helped to make meditation acceptable to mainstream medical doctors. There is some disagreement as to the importance of the mantra's content. Some think that any word or phrase is as effective as any other in focusing the mind. Others, however, maintain that the mantra must have some connection to the sacred. Examples of religious mantras include the Jesus prayer of Christian tradition, the holy Name of God in Judaism, or the Om mantra of Tibetan Buddhism.

Devotional meditation has an interpersonal quality in that the meditator focuses on a being who represents the divine or some quality of holiness to him or her. This approach also allows the meditator to integrate feelings of love or gratitude. It can take the form of chanting hymns that use the names of God, or visualizing the person or being that represents God to the meditator. Meditation in the Christian tradition sometimes includes visualizing Jesus or certain events in his life. Visualization is a useful approach to meditation for people who are sensitive to visual stimuli. Visualization meditation has also been used in the treatment of **cancer**, **AIDS** and other disease processes. In visualization therapy, the patient visualizes the inner workings of the body, with healthy cells fighting off the cancer or AIDS virus or rebalancing what is out of alignment with health. The patient can combine visualizations with breathing exercises by imagining that the breath is sending healing energy to the body. Patients with any illness can use devotional visualization as a way of integrating religious beliefs with visualization therapy.

People can learn to meditate in a variety of ways, including self-help books and from experienced teachers. The following guidelines are recommended for beginners in meditation:

- Regularity of practice. A minimum of 10-20 minutes daily is recommended for beginners, at the same time each day if at all possible.
- Quiet and privacy. Meditators should select a room or other location where they will not be disturbed by other people or the telephone. Setting aside a specific place as well as time for regular practice is ideal.
- Posture. The meditator should sit upright in a chair or on the floor with eyes closed. Good posture helps to maintain the flow of energy during breathing exercises.
- Proper breathing. Meditators should breathe deeply from the diaphragm rather than from the upper chest.

The major risk associated with meditation is the emergence of **hallucinations**, energy states or spiritual phenomena that are startling or worrisome to most Westerners. In most cases these experiences are byproducts of the attitudinal or behavioral changes that result from regular meditation practice. They do not indicate that the meditator is psychotic. One advantage of practicing under the guidance of a teacher is his or her experience in dealing with these phenomena.

MENDENHALL, DOROTHY REED (1874-1964)

American obstetrician and medical researcher

Dorothy Reed Mendenhall was a well-respected researcher, obstetrician, and pioneer in methods of childbirth. She was the first to discover that **Hodgkin's disease** was not a form of **tuberculosis**, as had been thought. This finding received international acclaim. As a result of her work, the cell type characteristic of Hodgkin's disease bears her name. The loss of her first child due to poor obstetrics changed her research career to a lifelong effort to reduce **infant mortality** rates. Mendenhall's efforts paid off with standards being set for weight and height for children ages birth to six, and also in programs that stressed the health of both the mother and child in the birthing process.

Dorothy Reed Mendenhall, the last of three children, was born September 22, 1874, in Columbus, Ohio, to William Pratt Reed, a shoe manufacturer, and Grace Kimball Reed, both of whom had descended from English settlers who came to America in the seventeenth century. Mendenhall attended Smith College and obtained a baccalaureate degree. Although she initially contemplated a career in journalism, Mendenhall's interest in medicine was inspired by a biology course she attended.

When they opened the school up to women, Mendenhall applied to Johns Hopkins Medical School in Baltimore, Maryland. In 1900, she was one of the first women to graduate from this school with a doctorate of medicine degree. The next year she received a fellowship in pathology at Johns Hopkins. While there, she taught bacteriology and performed research on Hodgkin's disease, which physicians then believed was a form of tuberculosis. She disproved this theory when she discovered a common link between diagnosed patients. She found that the blood of these patients carried a specific type of cell. The presence of these giant cells, now known as the Reed cell, distinctly identifies the disease. Mendenhall's work produced the first thorough descriptions, both verbal and illustrated, of the tissue changes that occur with Hodgkin's. She was the first to describe the disease's growth through several progressive states. Mendenhall determined that a patient's prognosis worsened with each successive stage. She incorrectly speculated, however, that the disease was a chronic inflammatory process. Her finding of the distinctive cell had world-wide importance and was a significant step forward in the understanding and treatment of Hodgkin's disease. Today, researchers know that Hodgkin's is a type of cancer characterized by a progressive enlargement of the lymph nodes.

Because she felt that there were few opportunities for advancement at Johns Hopkins, Mendenhall transferred her work to Babies Hospital of New York, becoming the first resident physician there. In 1906, she married Charles Elwood Mendenhall and began to raise a family. She had four children, one who died a few hours after birth. This loss was to shape the rest of her career. Mendenhall undertook a study of infant mortality, that, when released, brought government attention to the problems of maternal and child health. To determine the extent of infant mortality in the United States, she obtained epidemiological data for the Wisconsin State Board of Health. A major problem she identified was the prevalence of **malnutrition** among children. In her efforts to remedy the problems of childbearing and childrearing, Mendenhall developed correspondence courses for new and prospective mothers. She also lectured to groups across Wisconsin and wrote bulletins on nutrition for the United States Department of Agriculture. Mendenhall's efforts helped create some of Wisconsin's first infant welfare clinics, particularly in Madison. In 1937, she was gratified when Madison had the lowest infant mortality rate in the United States.

While employed as a field lecturer for the Department of Home Economics at the University of Wisconsin, in 1918, Mendenhall initiated a nationwide effort in which all children under six years of age were weighed and measured. This project helped establish standards for that normal, healthy children of these ages should weigh and how tall they should be. In 1926, Mendenhall undertook a study of birthing methods in Denmark, which had one of the lowest rates of childbirth complications. She later travelled to the country to gain firsthand information on their techniques, which included the utilization of specialized midwives and a reduced role of medical procedures. Through this, Mendenhall determined that there was too much medical intervention in normal childbirth, and that this intervention is often the source of health problems for the mother and child. She helped institute natural childbirth in the U.S. and also suggested that obstetrics become a specialty profession. From 1917 to 1936, Mendenhall also worked intermittently as a medical officer for the United States Children's Bureau. After her husband's death, she withdrew from public life. In her spare time she loved to read Marcus Aurelius. As a tribute to her dedication as a researcher, teacher, and physician, Smith College dedicated Sabin-Reed Hall in 1965. The hall honors Mendenhall and Florence Sabin, a fellow student at both Smith and Johns Hopkins. Mendenhall died July 31, 1964, in Chester, Connecticut, from heart disease.

Meniere's disease

Named for the French physician Prosper Meniere who first described the illness in 1861, Meniere's disease is an abnormality within the inner ear characterized by recurring vertigo (**dizziness**), **hearing loss**, and **tinnitus** (a roaring, buzzing or ringing sound in the ears). A fluid called endolymph moves in the membranous labyrinth or semicircular canals within the bony labyrinth inside the inner ear. When the head or body moves, the endolymph moves, causing nerve receptors in the membranous labyrinth to send signals to the brain about the body's motion. A change in the volume of the endolymph fluid, or swelling or rupture of the membranous labyrinth, is thought to result in Meniere's disease symptoms.

The cause of Meniere's disease is unknown. However, scientists are studying several possible causes including noise pollution, viral infections, and other biological factors. Symptoms include severe dizziness or vertigo, tinnitus, hearing loss, and the sensation of **pain** or pressure in the affected ear. Symptoms appear suddenly, last up to several hours, and can occur as often as daily to as infrequently as once a year. A typical attack includes vertigo, tinnitus and hearing loss; however, some individuals with Meniere's disease may experience a single symptom, like an occasional bout of slight dizziness or periodic, intense ringing in the ear. Attacks of severe vertigo can force the sufferer to have to sit or lie down, and may be accompanied by **headache**, nausea, vomiting, or **diarrhea**. Hearing tends to recover between attacks, but becomes progressively worse over time.

Meniere's disease usually starts between the ages of 20 and 50 years and affects men and women in equal numbers. In most patients, only one ear is affected; but both ears are involved in about 15% of patients.

An estimated 3 to 5 million people in the United States have Meniere's disease, and almost 100,000 new cases are diagnosed each year. Diagnosis is based on medical history, **physical examination**, hearing and balance tests, and medical imaging with **magnetic resonance imaging** (MRI).

Several types of tests are used to diagnose the disease and to evaluate the extent of hearing loss. In patients with Meniere's disease, audiometric tests (hearing tests) usually indicate a sensory type of hearing loss in the affected ear. Speech discrimination or the ability to distinguish between words that sound alike is often diminished. In about 50% of patients, the balance function is reduced in the affected ear. An electronystagnograph (ENG) may be used to evaluate balance. Since the eyes and ears work together through the nervous system to coordinate balance, measurement of eye movements can be used to test the balance system. For this test, the patient is seated in a darkened room and recording electrodes, similar to those used with a heart monitor, are placed near the eyes. Warm and cool water or air are gently introduced into each ear canal, and eye movements are recorded.

Another test that may be used is an electrocochleograph (EcoG), which can measure increased inner ear fluid pressure.

There is no cure for Meniere's disease, but medication, surgery, and dietary and behavioral changes, can help control or improve the symptoms. Symptoms may be treated with a variety of oral or injectable medications. Antihistamines, like diphenhydramine, meclizine, and cyclizine can be prescribed to sedate the vestibular system. A barbiturate medication like pentobarbital may be used to completely sedate the patient and relieve the vertigo. Anticholinergic drugs, like atropine or scopolamine, can help minimize **nausea and vomiting**. Diazepam has been found to be particularly effective for relief of vertigo and nausea in Meniere's disease.

There have been some reports of successful control of vertigo after **antibiotics** (gentamicin or streptomycin) or a steroid medication (dexamethasone) are injected directly into the inner ear. This procedure is done in the doctor's office and is less expensive and less invasive than a surgical procedure.

Surgical procedures may be recommended if the vertigo attacks are frequent, severe, or disabling and cannot be controlled by other treatments. The most common surgical treatment is insertion of a small tube, or shunt, to drain some of the fluid from the canal. This treatment usually preserves hearing and controls vertigo in about one-half to two-thirds of cases, but it is not a permanent cure in all patients.

The vestibular nerve leads from the inner ear to the brain and is responsible for conducting nerve impulses related to balance. A vestibular neurectomy is a procedure where this nerve is cut so the distorted impulses causing dizziness no longer reach the brain. This procedure permanently cures the majority of patients, and hearing is preserved in most cases. There is a slight risk that hearing or facial muscle control will be affected.

A labyrinthectomy is a surgical procedure in which the balance and hearing mechanism in the inner ear are destroyed on one side. This procedure is considered when the patient has poor hearing in the affected ear. Labyrinthectomy results in the highest rates of control of vertigo attacks; however, it also causes complete deafness in the affected ear.

Changes in diet and behavior are sometimes recommended. Eliminating **caffeine**, alcohol, and salt may relieve the frequency and intensity of attacks in some people with Meniere's disease. Reducing **stress** levels and eliminating tobacco use may also help.

Since the cause of Meniere's disease is unknown, there are no current strategies for its prevention. Research continues on the environmental and biological factors that may cause Meniere's disease or induce an attack, as well as on the physiological components of the fluid and labyrinth system involved in hearing and balance. Preventive strategies and more effective treatment should become evident once these mechanisms are better understood.

See also Dizziness; Hearing loss; Tinnitus

MENINGITIS

Meningitis is an inflammation of the *meninges*—the three layers of protective membranes that line the spinal cord and the brain. Meningitis can occur when there is an infection near the brain or spinal cord, such as a respiratory infection in the sinuses, the mastoids, or the cavities around the ear. Disease organisms can also travel to the meninges through the bloodstream. The first signs may be a severe headache and neck stiffness followed by fever, vomiting, a rash, then convulsions leading to loss of consciousness.

To diagnose meningitis, a sample of spinal fluid must be drawn from the lumbar region of the spine, a procedure known as a spinal tap. The spinal fluid is examined to reveal the microorganisms present in it. A diagnosis of bacterial meningitis requires immediate treatment with antibiotics.

The meningococcus bacteria, *Neisseria meningitides*, is a diplococcus that cannot move on its own. The bacteria spread from person to person in droplets in the air. Untreated, the disease advances quickly. It is fatal in about 15% of cases—significantly higher in infants and adults over sixty. In the United States, it affects between 2,000 and 5,000 young people each year, 70% of whom are under five years of age. Those who recover may suffer from some brain damage. Another type of bacterial meningitis, tuberculous meningitis, affects young children in third world countries where **tuberculosis** is common. Meningitis can also be caused by a virus. Viral meningitis usually requires little treatment and subsides within a week or two. It occurs most often in winter time. While data indicate that between 9,000 and 12,000 young people each year in the United States are affected with viral meningitis, many more cases may actually occur because people with mild forms of viral meningitis often do not see a physician.

Before antibiotics were available, bacterial meningitis was a dreaded disease, taking a toll on the young and leaving those who survived blind, deaf, or mentally retarded. A pioneer in the research of this disease and its cure was Dr. Sara Elizabeth Branham (1888-1962), who worked at the National Institute of Health in the early part of the twentieth century. Initially she did some research on bacterially caused food poisoning; but after the epidemic years of World War I she worked on the specific antiserum to combat meningitis. During World War I, cases of the disease ran rampant among soldiers, often leading to lengthy quarantines to prevent its further spread. Knowing that many strains of infectious bacteria could be responsible, Dr. Branham developed laboratory procedures that enabled technicians to determine which type of infection was present. At that time, the only treatment for meningitis was an antiserum (developed from horses) which had been losing its power over the years. Branham substituted a more effective serum extracted from rabbits. In 1937, Dr. Branham and a coworker discovered that the newly developed sulfonamide drugs (**sulfonamide**s) were effective in treating meningitis. Sulfadiazine was then used along with antiserum as an effective treatment and was responsible for keeping meningitis at bay during World War II. Dr. Branham wrote widely about the disease and was recognized for her dedicated work with awards and honorary degrees.

Today bacterial meningitis is curable if treated promptly with **antibiotics**, usually administered intravenously. Vaccines against meningitis are sometimes administered during epidemics. A vaccine against haemophilus influenzae type b (Hib), which was a major cause of bacterial meningitis, has reduced Hib meningitis cases by as much as 95 percent. However, because of the variety of disease organisms that can cause meningitis, this vaccine is not effective against other types of meningitis, and vaccines are generally of limited use for prevention.

MENOPAUSE

Menopause represents the end of **menstruation**. Although it refers to the final period, it is not an abrupt event, but a gradual process. Menopause is not a disease that needs to be cured, but a natural life-stage transition. However, women have to make important decisions about "treatment," including the use of **hormone replacement therapy** (HRT).

Many women have irregular periods and other problems of "pre-menopause" for years. It's not easy to predict when menopause begins, although doctors agree it is complete when a woman has not had a period for a year. Eight out of every 100 women stop menstruating before age 40. At the other end of the spectrum, five out of every 100 continue to have periods until they are almost 60. The average age of menopause is 51.

There is no mathematical formula to predict when menopause will begin, but a woman can get a general idea based on her family history, body type, and lifestyle. Women who began menstruating early will not necessarily stop having periods early as well. Many women will likely enter menopause at about the same age as their mothers. Menopause may occur later than average among smokers.

Once a woman enters **puberty**, each month her body releases one of the more than 400,000 eggs that are stored in her ovaries, and the lining of the womb (uterus) thickens in anticipation of receiving a fertilized egg. If the egg is not fertilized, progesterone hormone levels drop and the uterine lining sheds and bleeds.

By the time a woman reaches her late 30s or 40s, her ovaries begin to shut down, producing less of the hormones estrogen and progesterone and releasing eggs less often. The gradual decline of estrogen causes a wide variety of changes in tissues that respond to estrogen—including the vagina, vulva, uterus, bladder, urethra, breasts, bones, heart, blood vessels, brain, skin, hair, and mucous membranes. Over the long run, the lack of estrogen can make a woman more vulnerable to **osteoporosis** (which can begin in the 40s) and heart disease.

As hormone levels fluctuate, the menstrual cycle begins to change. Some women may have longer periods with heavy flow followed by shorter cycles and hardly any bleeding. Others will begin to miss periods completely. During this time, a woman also becomes less able to get pregnant.

The most common symptom of menopause is a change in the menstrual cycle, but there are a variety of other symptoms as well, including:

- Hot flashes
- Night sweats
- **Insomnia**
- Mood swings/irritability
- Memory or concentration problems
- Vaginal dryness
- Heavy bleeding
- Fatigue
- Depression
- Hair changes
- **Headache**s
- Heart **palpitations**
- Sexual disinterest
- Urinary changes
- Weight gain.

The clearest indication of menopause is the absence of a period for one year. It is also possible to diagnose menopause by testing hormone levels. One important test measures the levels of follicle-stimulating hormone (FSH), which rise steadily as a woman ages.

However, as a woman first enters menopause, her hormones often fluctuate wildly from day to day. For example, if a woman's estrogen levels are high and progesterone is low, she may have mood swings, irritability, and other symptoms similar to **premenstrual syndrome** (PMS). As hormone levels shift and estrogen level falls, hot flashes occur. Because of these fluctuations, a normal hormone level when the blood is tested may not necessarily mean the levels were normal the day before or will be the day after.

If it has been at least three months since a woman's last period, an FSH test might help determine whether menopause has occurred. Most doctors believe that the FSH test alone can't be used as proof that a woman has entered early menopause. A better measure of menopause is a test that checks the levels of estrogen, progesterone, testosterone and other hormones at mid-cycle, in addition to FSH.

When a woman enters menopause, her levels of estrogen drop and annoying symptoms (such as hot flashes and vaginal dryness) begin. Hormone replacement therapy can treat these symptoms by boosting the estrogen levels enough to suppress symptoms while also providing protection against heart disease and osteoporosis, which causes the bones to weaken. Experts disagree on whether HRT increases or decreases the risk of developing **breast cancer**. A Harvard study concluded that short-term use of hormones carries little risk, while HRT used for more than five years among women 55 and over seems to increase the risk of breast cancer.

Many women find that **yoga** (the ancient **meditation/exercise** developed in India 5,000 years ago) can ease menopausal symptoms. Because yoga has been shown to balance the endocrine system, some experts believe it may affect hormone-related problems. Studies have found that yoga can reduce **stress**, improve mood, boost a sluggish metabolism, and slow the heart rate. Specific yoga positions deal with particular problems, such as hot flashes, mood swings, vaginal and urinary problems, and other **pain**s.

Exercise helps ease hot flashes by lowering the amount of circulating FSH and LH and by raising endorphin levels (which drop while you're having a hot flash). Even exercising 20 minutes three times a week can significantly reduce hot flashes.

Regular, daily bowel movements to eliminate waste products from the body can be crucial in maintaining balance through menopause. The bowels are where circulating hormones are gathered and eliminated, keeping the body from recycling them and causing an imbalance.

Acupuncture is an ancient Asian art that involves placing very thin needles into different parts of the body to stimulate the system and unblock energy. It is has also been used for many menopausal symptoms, including insomnia, hot flashes, and irregular periods. Therapeutic **massage** involving **acupressure** can bring relief from a wide range of menopause symptoms by placing finger pressure at the same meridian points on the body that are used in acupuncture. Some women have been able to control hot flashes through **biofeedback**, a painless technique that helps a person train the mind to control the body.

See also Hormone replacement therapy; Hysterectomy; Premenstrual syndrome

MEN'S HEALTH

The field of men's health is concerned with health issues and aging changes peculiar to post-pubescent males. Growth in adolescent boys (**puberty** to 19) occurs in spurts, usually over 4-5 years, with the first growth spurt occurring between ages 10 and 14. Puberty is accompanied by an increase in height; the appearance of body hair; an enlargement of the testicles, penis, and scrotum; growth of the larynx, or voice box; and development of sweat glands.

Health problems potentially affecting adolescent males include the abuse of (tobacco, (alcohol and illicit drugs; overexposure to the sun; unhealthy eating habits; and **sexually transmitted diseases**.

Most men between the ages of 20 and 39 enjoy relatively good health. Their bodies do not change much physiologically, and their health concerns are often focused on sexuality, reproduction, and preventing **accidents**. Additional health concerns may include weight gain due to excessive calorie consumption, **skin cancer**, and **testicular cancer**.

The onset and increased rate of hair loss in men between the ages of 40 and 65 is often the first sign of aging. It is almost entirely genetically determined and nearly impossible to prevent. In the same way, a man in this age group has little ability to control changes in his eyesight and hearing. Other aspects of aging, however, respond to lifestyle, with the consequences of diet and other health-related habits becoming increasingly evident as a man enters his 50s. Examples of aging changes that respond to lifestyle include loss of skin elasticity and muscle strength, increase in body fat, narrowing and hardening of the arteries, rise in blood pressure, increase in cholesterol levels and bone loss. Many men experience a gradual lessening of sexual desire at this time, a result of the body secreting less testosterone and decreased nerve conduction. The risk of heart disease starts to increase significantly in men older than 45, and the incidence of colon cancer, skin cancer, and **cataracts** and **glaucoma** increases in this age group. Enlargement of the prostate is also common in men over 40. For men over 50, cancer of the prostrate is the most common type of **cancer** and the second leading cause of cancer death, following **lung cancer**. These changes continue gradually for most men into old age.

It is not uncommon for men over 65 to experience a gradual decline in height, continued decline in eyesight and hearing, loss of flexibility due to **osteoarthritis**, loss of aerobic capacity, increase in cholesterol levels, changes in sleeping patterns, further decline in the intensity of sexual interest, and memory loss. In addition, men over 65 are especially prone to chronic diseases such as heart disease, certain cancers, and diabetes; falls; flu and **pneumonia**; gastrointestinal ailments; physiological intolerance of heat and cold; and **incontinence**.

See also Adolescent health; Nutrition; Food groups and nutrients; Cardiovascular system

MENSTRUATION

Menstruation is one of the signs of **puberty**. The purpose of menstruation is to prepare the women's bodies for **pregnancy** and **childbirth**. Every month, the lining of the uterus thickens to receive and nourish a fertilized egg (if a woman becomes pregnant). If, however, the egg does not become fertilized, the uterus lining is shed. This process of shedding the lining is called menstruation.

A woman's first menstrual period generally occurs between the ages of 9 and 16. The first period is called menarche. There is no way to predict when a girl will have her first period; the age at which her mother started menstruating can give a rough estimate. There is a theory that when the amount fat in the girl's body reaches a certain level, it gives the body the permission to proceed menstruating. Women who lose a lot of their body fat through athletic training may therefore, start menstruating late or menstruate infrequently. In addition, women who lose most of their body fat through starvation, like women with anorexia, stop menstruating. Girls who are undernourished start their periods later than girls who are well fed. The length of each period varies. Some girls menstruate for only 3 days and some for as long as 7 or 8 days. However, the average menstrual period is 5 days. For the first year or two, periods are often irregular. For women in their 40s or 50s, the periods become irregular again and eventually stop. This process is known as **menopause**.

The biological cycle that leads to menstruation starts in the hypothalamus, a gland in the brain. It releases a special hormone called Follicle Stimulating Hormone Releasing Factor (FSH-RF) that stimulates the pituitary, another gland in the brain. In response to this chemical signal, the pituitary secretes two different hormones called Follicle Stimulating Hormone (FSH) and Luteinizing Hormone (LH) into the blood. These two hormones cause the follicles to begin to mature. The follicles are little sacs in the ovaries that carry the woman's eggs. The follicles ripen over a period of seven days, and while doing so, they secrete another hormone, estrogen into the blood. Estrogen causes the lining of the uterus to thicken. When the estrogen reaches a certain level in the blood, it signals the hypothalamus in the brain to release yet another hormone called the Luteinizing Hormone Releasing Factor (LH-RF). This hormone, in turn stimulates the pituitary to secrete the Luteinizing Hormone (LH). The surge of LH triggers the mature follicles to burst open and release an egg. This process is called ovulation. Ovulation takes place midway in a woman's monthly cycle.

Midway between ovulation and menstruation, the follicle from which the egg burst becomes the corpeus luteum (yellow body). It produces the hormone estrogen and another hormone progesterone that is necessary for the maintenance of a pregnancy. Progesterone causes the surface lining of the uterus, the endometrium, to thicken and become covered with mucus. The uterus is now well prepared to receive the fertilized egg and maintain a healthy pregnancy. If however, fertilization (the process where an egg and a sperm unite) does not occur, the blood flow to the uterus lining is stopped. The shedding of this blood along with the endometrial lining forms the menstrual flow.

Women can experience a variety of symptoms before, during, or after the monthly period. Common complaints include backache, stomach cramps, bloating, nausea, **diarrhea**, **constipation**, **headaches**, breast tenderness, irritability, and other mood changes. Some women experience positive sensations such as relief, release, euphoria, invigoration, creative energy, and increased sex drive. The symptoms that occur before or during menstruation are collectively called the "**Premenstrual syndrome** (PMS)." The hormones in our body are extremely sensitive to diet and nutrition. Hence, the negative symptoms of PMS are often attributed to poor nutrition. PMS does not affect every woman. Some women are not affected at all or only occasionally. In some women, the symptoms are mild and in others they can be severe and require medical intervention.

It is common to experience problems with menstruation from time to time. The problems can be related to the length of the period, its frequency, the amount of flow, or other symptoms related to the monthly cycle. The normal amount of fluid during one menstrual period varies from several ounces to less than one ounce. Most women have monthly cycles that are around 28 days. However, even if a woman has only three or four cycles a year, she can still be healthy, normal, and capable of producing a baby. Factors like significant weight loss can alter the monthly cycle. In addition, it can also be affected by emotions or changes in routine and stress levels.

Menstrual blood generally clots in the uterus and these clots dissolve before passing to the vagina. Sometimes, however, the clots will pass through the cervical opening before dissolving. It is also normal for the flow to change color from bright red to a dark brown. When menstrual fluid is exposed to air, menstrual odor occurs. Women use a variety of things to absorb their menstrual flow. Disposable pads or sanitary napkins and tampons are the most commonly used products.

Menstruation is neither a curse nor an illness, nor is it shameful or dirty. It is, in fact, a sign of good health, a sign that the body is functioning normally. In the United States, there is no official celebration, like a birthday party for the first period. However, several other cultures around the world have big celebrations for a girl's first period—she is congratulated on becoming a woman.

See also Puberty; Menstrual disorders; Menopause

MENSTRUAL DISORDERS

The menstrual cycle, while normally a smooth, regular process, is a complex phenomenon whose usual operation can break down at any point along the way. Menstrual disorders can be roughly divided into four categories: amenorrhea, dysfunctional uterine bleeding, dysmenorrhea, and oligomenorrhea.

The complete absence of menstrual periods is *amenorrhea.* There are two categories within this disorder: (1) primary amenorrhea, the relatively rare failure to start having a period by age 16 (the average age is 12), and (2) secondary amenorrhea, which is more common and refers to the temporary or permanent ending of periods in a woman who has menstruated normally in the past. Many women miss a period occasionally, but missing three or more periods in a row is considered amenorrhea. Prolonged amenorrhea can lead to **infertility** and other medical problems such as **osteoporosis** (thinning of the bones).

The absence of menstrual periods is a symptom, not a disease. Primary amenorrhea can result from hormonal imbalances, psychiatric disorders, **malnutrition**, excessive thinness or heaviness, and rapid weight loss. Drugs such as antidepressants, tranquilizers, steroids, and heroin can induce amenorrhea, as can chronic illness and **stress**. However, the main reason for amenorrhea is a delay in the beginning of **puberty**—either from natural reasons (such as heredity, intense physical training, or poor nutrition) or because of a problem in the **endocrine system**, such as a pituitary tumor or hypothyroidism.

The most common cause of secondary amenorrhea is **pregnancy**. Also, a woman's periods may end temporarily after she stops taking birth control pills. Secondary amenorrhea may also result from hormonal problems related to stress, depression, anorexia nervosa, or drugs; any condition affecting the ovaries, such as a tumor; or polycystic ovary syndrome (PCOS), which involves cysts in the egg-producing ovaries. The cessation of menstruation also occurs permanently after **menopause** or a **hysterectomy**.

Dysfunctional uterine bleeding (DUB) is irregular, abnormal uterine bleeding not caused by a tumor, infection, or pregnancy. It often occurs when the endometrium, the lining of the uterus, receives too much stimulation from the hormone estrogen, overgrows, and then must be shed from the uterus more frequently than usual. DUB occurs most often in women at the beginning and end of their reproductive lives.

DUB is suspected after other causes of uterine bleeding have been eliminated. Some of DUB's causes are **pelvic inflammatory disease** (PID), adenomyosis (a benign condition involving endometrial growths), **cancer**, fibroid tumors, and hypothyroidism. DUB is common in women with PCOS, while women who are on kidney **dialysis** or who use an intrauterine device (**IUD**) for birth control may also have heavy or prolonged periods.

Generally, the first approach to controlling DUB is to use **oral contraceptives** that provide a balance between estrogen and progesterone. NSAIDs (**nonsteroidal anti-inflammatory drugs**) can also be helpful. When bleeding cannot be controlled by hormone treatment, surgery may be necessary. Iron supplements, vitamin C, bioflavonoids, and stiptic (blood vessel-tightening) herbs may also be beneficial, while phytoestrogens and phytoprogesterone (from plant-based substances such as soy) can address hormonal imbalances.

Dysmenorrhea is the occurrence of painful cramps during menstruation. More than half of all girls and women suffer from this dull or throbbing pain that usually centers in the lower mid-abdomen, radiating toward the lower back or thighs. Menstruating women of any age can experience cramps. The first year or two of a girl's periods are not usually very painful. However, once ovulation begins, blood levels of prostaglandins (hormone-like substances that trigger strong muscle contractions in the uterus) rise, leading to stronger contractions. While the pain may be mild for some women, others suffer severe discomfort that can significantly interfere with everyday activities for several days each month. Some women may even experience **nausea and vomiting**, **diarrhea**, irritability, sweating, or **dizziness**. Dysmenorrhea often disappears after a woman's first childbirth, probably due to the stretching of the uterine opening or because the birth improves the uterine blood supply and muscle activity.

Dysmenorrhea is called "primary" when there is no specific abnormality and "secondary" when the pain is caused by an underlying gynecological problem. Experts believe that the presence and/or severity of cramps is also strongly influenced by genetics, whether a woman has PID, **stress**, higher **caffeine** intake, too little exercise, and certain body types. Secondary dysmenorrhea may be caused by **endometriosis**, fibroid tumors, or a pelvic infection.

If an NSAID is not available, **acetaminophen** and applying heat may help. While birth control pills ease the pain of dysmenorrhea because they lead to lower hormone levels, they are not usually prescribed for **pain management** unless the woman also wants to use them for birth control, because these pills may carry other, more significant side effects and risks. Likewise, several **yoga** postures and lying in the fetal position may bring relief. Dietary recommendations to ease cramps include increasing fiber, calcium, and complex carbohydrates and reducing or eliminating **smoking**, fat, red meat, dairy products, caffeine, salt, and sugar. Recent research suggests that vitamin B supplements, magnesium, and fish oil supplements (omega-3 fatty acids) may be beneficial.

Oligomenorrhea is a disorder characterized by light, infrequent menstrual periods in women whose periods were regularly established before they developed problems. Periods occur at intervals of greater than 35 days, with only four to nine periods in a year. Women who have oligomenorrhea often have difficulty conceiving children and may receive fertility drugs for this reason. The absence of adequate estrogen increases risk for bone loss, **uterine cancer**, and cardiovascular disease.

Women with PCOS are likely to suffer from oligomenorrhea, but other factors can also bring on the condition, including emotional stress, chronic illness, poor nutrition, **eating disorders**, excessive exercise, estrogen-secreting tumors, and using anabolic steriods to enhance athletic performance. Oligomenorrhea in adolescents is often caused by physical immaturity or lack of synchronization between the hypothalamus, pituitary gland, and ovaries. Adequate nutrition and moderate exercise usually prevent oligomenorrhea in healthy women.

In adolescents and women near menopause, oligomenorrhea usually needs no treatment. Most patients are treated with birth control pills. Other women, including those with PCOS, are treated with hormones. Glandular therapy can assist in bringing about the crucial balance involved in the normal reproductive cycle. **Homeopathy** and **acupuncture** may also be helpful, along with Western and **Chinese traditional herbal medicines**.

MENTAL HEALTH CARE

Just as medical health care addresses a person's physical condition, mental health care addresses a person's psychological condition. There are many kinds of emotional and mental health problems, most of which can be successfully treated and controlled.

Unfortunately, however, only one in five people suffering from mental or emotional disorders will seek help. The treatment rate is even lower among children suffering from mental disorders. It is estimated that only four to fifteen percent of children who have mental illnesses receive appropriate treatment.

A wide range of mental health conditions can be effectively treated with a combination of psychotherapy and medication, including **depressive disorders**, **schizophrenia**, **personality disorders**, and a wide variety of **anxiety disorders** (**panic disorder**, **obsessive-compulsive disorder**, **post-traumatic stress disorder**, **phobias**, social phobia, and generalized anxiety disorder). With proper treatment, as many as eight in 10 people suffering from mental disorders can effectively lead productive lives.

Mental health care is provided by different types of mental health professionals, including psychiatrists, psychologists, social workers, pastoral counselors, nurse-psychotherapists, and psychiatric nurses.

Psychiatrists are medical doctors with a specialty in mental health problems. Licensed by the state, they can prescribe drugs and typically treat more seriously ill clients (other mental health professionals have specific training in therapy but can't prescribe drugs). In many states, nurse-psychotherapists may be licensed to prescribe medications in collaboration with a doctor. Psychologists are licensed mental health professionals with an advanced degree (usually a Ph.D.) and many years of training in therapy techniques. Social workers are also trained in therapy and usually hold a master's degree in social work. Pastoral counselors are religious leaders who are also trained in therapeutic techniques.

There are three primary ways of treating mental health disorders: therapy (**counseling**), medication, and self-help techniques. Likewise, there are many different kinds of therapy, including cognitive therapy, behavioral therapy, interpersonal therapy (including **marriage counseling**), psychodynamic therapy, and **psychoanalysis**.

Cognitive therapy is based on the idea that a mental health problem is caused by a distortion in thinking, that how you feel is the direct result of how you think. Developed specifically to treat depression and anxiety by psychiatrist Aaron T. Beck, M.D., at the University of Pennsylvania, this type of counseling can pinpoint problem patterns of thinking. Clients learn how to recognize and label these distortions and understand why they are being used.

Behavioral therapy is similar to cognitive therapy in that it teaches clients how to alter thought distortions, but it also seeks to alter behavior as well. Based on the idea that a troubled person is not getting enough positive feedback, this type of therapy offers practical suggestions on how to reinforce healthy behavior with a system of self-rewards. This type of counseling is especially helpful for people with phobias or panic attacks.

Interpersonal counseling focuses on the development and improvement of relationships. This type of therapy helps people identify and solve their problems with others. The client is helped to understand how important positive relationships are to mental health, to assess current relationships, and to develop treatment goals.

Psychodynamic counseling, much like classical psychoanalysis, explores the past for the seeds of unresolved emotional conflicts with a counselor who actively directs the treatment and offers suggestions and interpretations.

Many specific mental health conditions are not just psychological in nature, but are also caused or at least influenced by physical problems in the brain. As a result, medications can treat many of these conditions. Research has found that the best way to treat these problems, including depression, anxiety, and phobias, are with a combination of therapy and medication.

There are a wide range of drugs that are used to treat mental and emotional disorders, including **antianxiety drugs**, **antipsychotic drugs**, **antidepressant drugs**, sedatives, mood-stabilizing drugs, stimulants, and side-effect control medications, which decrease the unpleasant effects of some drugs.

Other treatment methods are more controversial. **Electroconvulsive therapy** (ECT), also known as shock treatment, has a frightening reputation but is still used for some problems, such as very serious depressions that don't respond to drugs. The modern practice of ECT is less than 65 years old. By the 1950s it was the primary method of treating depression until the discovery of antidepressants led to its substantial decline. Today, patients undergoing ECT are given an anesthetic and a muscle relaxant. Afterwards, some patients may have a period of confusion and memory problems, but some patients have longer-term memory problems. It remains unclear whether ECT affects permanent memory, and it remains a controversial treatment.

Mental health care has improved dramatically over the last several decades, as the public has become more aware of, and more accepting of, emotional and mental health problems. In addition, the discovery of more and better medications (especially antidepressants) has made a dramatic improvement over mental health care. It is estimated that more than five million Americans suffer from an acute episode of mental illness each year, and that one in every five families will be affected at some point by a severe mental illness. Nearly 21 percent of all hospital admissions nationwide are due to mental disorders.

See also Counseling; Depressive disorders; Psychosis; Psychoanalysis; Family therapy

Mental Illness

Mental illnesses are biologically-based disorders which interfere with an individual's ability to think, feel, act, and relate within the standard norms of society. The American Psychiatric Association identifies hundreds of mental disorders ranging from **Attention Deficit Hyperactivity Disorder** to Violent/Self-Destructive Behaviors. Mental illness can be physical as well as psychological and emotional, and some are classified as "major mental illnesses" because of their propensity to seriously impair an individual's ability to function. Severe mental illnesses are more common than cancer, diabetes, or heart disease. Mental illness can strike any person at any time (one in five Americans and Australians, and one in six Canadians, will be affected some time in their life), account for more hospital admissions than any other single disease, and cost U.S. society more than $150 billion annually.

Mental illness afflicts people of every age, race, creed, and socioeconomic background. It can be extremely frightening and confusing to the sufferer, their families and their friends. It was not until the 1950s that mental illness became part of mainstream medicine. For centuries, it was so misunderstood and feared that sufferers were confined to insane asylums where they were shackled and treated as mere animals. In 1953, metal from such shackles was melted down and formed into a 300-pound Mental Health Bell and placed at the headquarters of the National Mental Health Association in Alexandria, Virginia, as a symbol of hope and liberty for people with mental illnesses. Yet even today, mental illness brings about feelings of shame, disapproval, discrimination, and rejection.

There is no clear understanding of what causes mental illness. Biochemical imbalances may be triggered by environmental and emotional stresses, and genetic predisposition is a factor. Symptoms are usually behavioral, such as confused thinking, prolonged depression, high anxiety/panic attacks, delusions of grandeur and hallucinations, suicidal thoughts, social withdrawal, dramatic swings between highs (mania) and lows (depression). Depression in the elderly is common and commonly unrecognized. Mental illness is often unrecognized in children; warning signs include poor grades despite strong efforts, excessive worry or anxiety, hyperactivity, persistent nightmares, frequent temper tantrums, substance abuse, excessive complaints of physical ailments, inability to cope with daily activities, and frequent outbursts of anger.

Major mental illnesses include **schizophrenia**, mood or affective disorders (depression/manic-depression), panic/anxiety disorders, **eating disorders** (anorexia nervosa and bulimia nervosa), personality disorders, posttraumatic stress syndrome, obsessive-compulsive disorder, and organic brain disorders. Treatment aims at reducing symptoms, improving social and personal functioning, and strengthening coping skills. Many types of therapies and medications are available and can be grouped in categories of psychosocial rehabilitation, biomedical therapy, psychotherapy, and behavioral therapy. These can be used alone or in combination.

Mental illness is not mental retardation. While it cannot be cured, most can be treated effectively. The first step in the road to recovery is awareness that something is wrong followed by accurate diagnosis and treatment from well-informed specialists. Appropriately licensed psychiatrists, psychologists, psychiatric nurses and social workers, mental health counsellors, case managers, and outreach workers are all available to treat and rehabilitate people suffering from mental illness.

See also Depressive disorders; Eating disorders; Obsessive-compulsive disorder; Schizophrenia

Mental retardation

Mental retardation is a developmental disability that first appears in children under the age of 18 and, in most cases, persists throughout adulthood. A person is considered mentally retarded if he or she has an intellectual functioning level well below average and significant limitations in two or more adaptive skill areas. Intellectual functioning level is defined by standardized tests that measure the ability to reason in terms of mental age (intelligence quotient or IQ). Mental retardation is defined as IQ score below 70-75. Adaptive skills are the skills needed for daily life and include the ability to produce and understand language (communication); home-living skills; use of community resources; health, safety, leisure, self-care, and social skills; self-direction; functional academic skills (reading, writing, and arithmetic); and work skills. Mental retardation occurs in 2.5-3% of the general population, and about 6-7.5 million mentally retarded individuals live in the United States alone.

In general, mentally retarded children reach developmental milestones such as walking and talking much later than the general population. Symptoms may appear at birth or later in childhood, depending on the cause. Some cases of mild mental retardation are not diagnosed before the child enters preschool. These children typically have difficulties with social, communication, and functional academic skills. Children who have a neurological disorder or illness such as **encephali-**

tis or **meningitis** may suddenly show signs of cognitive impairment and adaptive difficulties.

The Diagnostic and Statistical Manual of Mental Disorders, Fourth Edition (*DSM-IV*) classifies four different degrees of mental retardation: *mild, moderate, severe*, and *profound.* These categories are based on the individual's functioning level.

Approximately 85% of the mentally retarded population is in the mildly retarded category. Their IQ score ranges from 50-75, and they can often acquire academic skills up to the 6th grade level. They can become fairly self-sufficient and, in some cases, live independently with community and social support.

About 10% of the mentally retarded population is considered moderately retarded with IQ scores ranging from 35-55. They can carry out work and self-care tasks with moderate supervision. They typically acquire communication skills in childhood and are able to live and function successfully within the community in a supervised environment such as a group home.

About 3-4% of the mentally retarded population is severely retarded with IQ scores of 20-40. They may master very basic self-care skills and some communication skills. Many are able to live in a group home.

Only 1-2% of the mentally retarded population is classified as profoundly retarded with IQ scores under 20-25. They may be able to develop basic self-care and communication skills with appropriate support and training and need a high level of structure and supervision. Their retardation is often caused by an accompanying neurological disorder.

The American Association on Mental Retardation (AAMR) has developed another widely accepted diagnostic classification system for mental retardation that focuses on the capabilities of the retarded individual rather than on the limitations. The categories describe the level of support required. They are: *intermittent support, limited support, extensive support*, and *pervasive support.* Intermittent support, for example, is support needed only occasionally, perhaps during times of **stress** or crisis. It is the type of support typically required for most mildly retarded individuals. At the other end of the spectrum, pervasive support, or life-long, daily support for most adaptive areas, would be required for profoundly retarded individuals.

Aggression, self-injury, and **mood disorders** are sometimes associated with the disability. The severity of the symptoms and the age at which they first appear depend on the cause. If retardation is caused by **genetics** in the form of an inherited disorder, it is often apparent from infancy. If retardation is caused by childhood illnesses or injuries, learning and adaptive skills that were once easy may suddenly become difficult or impossible to master.

In about 35% of cases, the cause of mental retardation cannot be found. Biological and environmental factors include inherited abnormality of the genes, such as fragile X syndrome; single gene defects such as **phenylketonuria** (PKU); and accidents or mutations in genetic development such as the development of an extra chromosome 18 (trisomy 18) and **Down syndrome**. Environmental factors include cigarette smoking and drug abuse during pregnancy and **fetal alcohol syndrome** (which affects one in 600 children in the United States and is caused by excessive alcohol intake in the first twelve weeks (trimester) of **pregnancy**. Some studies have shown that even mo! derate alcohol use during pregnancy may cause learning disabilities in children.

Maternal infections and illnesses such as glandular disorders, **rubella**, **toxoplasmosis**, and cytomegalovirus infection may cause mental retardation. When the mother has high blood pressure (**hypertension**) or blood poisoning (toxemia), the flow of oxygen to the fetus may be reduced, causing brain damage and mental retardation.

Birth defects that cause physical deformities of the head, brain, and central nervous system frequently cause mental retardation. Neural tube defect, for example, is a birth defect in which the neural tube that forms the spinal cord does not close completely. This defect may cause children to develop an accumulation of cerebrospinal fluid on the brain (**hydrocephalus**). Hydrocephalus can cause learning impairment by putting pressure on the brain.

Hyperthyroidism, **whooping cough**, chickenpox, **measles**, and Hib disease (a bacterial infection) may cause mental retardation if they are not treated adequately. An infection of the membrane covering the brain (meningitis) or an inflammation of the brain itself (encephalitis) cause swelling that, in turn, may cause brain damage and mental retardation. Traumatic brain injury caused by a blow or a violent shake to the head may also cause brain damage and mental retardation in children.

Ignored or neglected infants who are not provided the mental and physical stimulation required for normal development may suffer irreversible learning impairments. Children who live in poverty and suffer from **malnutrition**, unhealthy living conditions, and improper or inadequate medical care are at a higher risk. Exposure to lead can also cause mental retardation. Many children have developed **lead poisoning** by eating the flaking lead-based paint often found in older buildings.

Federal legislation entitles mentally retarded children to free testing and appropriate, individualized education and skills training within the school system from ages 3-21. For children under the age of three, many states have established early intervention programs that assess, recommend, and begin treatment programs. Many day schools are available to help train retarded children in basic skills such as bathing and feeding themselves. Extracurricular activities and social programs are also important in helping retarded children and adolescents gain self-esteem.

Training in independent living and job skills is often begun in early adulthood. The level of training depends on the degree of retardation. Mildly retarded individuals can often acquire the skills needed to live independently and hold an outside job. Moderate to profoundly retarded individuals usually require supervised community living.

Family therapy can help relatives of the mentally retarded develop coping skills. It can also help parents deal with feelings of guilt or anger. A supportive, warm home environment is essential to help the mentally retarded reach their full potential.

Individuals with mild to moderate mental retardation are frequently able to achieve some self-sufficiency and to lead happy and fulfilling lives. To reach these goals, they need appropriate and consistent educational, community, social, family, and vocational supports. The outlook is less promising for those with severe to profound retardation. Studies have shown that these individuals have a shortened life expectancy. The diseases that are usually associated with severe retardation may cause the shorter life span. People with Down syndrome will develop the brain changes that characterize **Alzheimer's disease** in later life and may develop the clinical symptoms of this disease as well.

See also Birth defects; Down Syndrome; Genetics

Metabolic acidosis

Metabolic acidosis is a pH imbalance that occurs when the body has accumulated too much acid and does not have enough bicarbonate (an acid neutralizer) to effectively neutralize the acid's effects. This disruption of the body's acid/base balance can be a mild symptom brought on by a lack of insulin (an **antidiabetic drug**), a **starvation** diet, or a gastrointestinal disorder like vomiting and **diarrhea**. Metabolic acidosis can indicate a more serious problem with a major organ like the liver, heart, or kidneys. It can also be one of the first signs of **drug overdose** or **poisoning**.

Metabolic acidosis occurs when the body has more acid than base in it. Chemists use the term ''pH'' to describe how acidic or basic a substance is. Based on a scale of 14, a pH of 7.0 is neutral. A pH below 7.0 is an acid; the lower the number, the stronger the acid. A pH above 7.0 is a base; the higher the number, the stronger the base. Blood pH is slightly basic (alkaline), with a normal range of 7.36-7.44. Although metabolic acidosis is suspected based on symptoms, it is usually confirmed by laboratory tests on blood and urine samples. Blood pH below 7.35 confirms the condition. Levels of other blood components, including potassium, glucose, ketones, or lactic acid, may also be above normal ranges. The level of bicarbonate in the blood will be low, usually less than 22 mEq/L. Urine pH may fall below 4.5 in metabolic acidosis.

Acid is a natural by-product of the breakdown of fats and other processes in the body; however, in some conditions, the body does not have enough bicarbonate to balance the acids produced. This can occur when the body uses fats for energy instead of carbohydrates. Conditions where metabolic acidosis can occur include chronic **alcoholism**, **malnutrition**, and diabetic ketoacidosis. Consuming a diet low in carbohydrates and high in fats can also produce metabolic acidosis. The disorder may also be a symptom of another condition like kidney failure, liver failure, or severe diarrhea. The build up of lactic acid in the blood, due to such conditions as **heart failure**, **shock**, or **cancer**, induces metabolic acidosis. Some poisonings and overdoses (**aspirin**, methanol, or ethylene glycol) also produce symptoms of metabolic acidosis.

In mild cases of metabolic acidosis, symptoms include **headache**, lack of energy, and sleepiness. Breathing may become fast and shallow. Nausea, vomiting, diarrhea, **dehydration**, and loss of appetite are also associated with metabolic acidosis. Diabetic patients with symptoms of metabolic acidosis may also have breath that smells fruity. The patient may lose consciousness or become disoriented. Severe cases can produce **coma** and **death**.

Treatment focuses first on correcting the acid imbalance. Usually, sodium bicarbonate and fluids are injected into the blood through a vein. An intravenous line may be started to administer fluids and allow for the quick injection of other drugs that may be needed. If the patient is diabetic, insulin may be administered. Drugs to regulate blood pressure or heart rate, to prevent seizures, or to control **nausea and vomiting** might be given. Vital signs like pulse, respiration, blood pressure, and body temperature will be monitored. The underlying cause of the metabolic acidosis must also be diagnosed and corrected.

If metabolic acidosis is recognized and treated promptly, the patient may have no long-term complications; however, the underlying condition that caused the acidosis needs to be corrected or managed. Severe metabolic acidosis that is left untreated will lead to coma and death.

Diabetic patients especially need to routinely test their urine for sugar and acetone, strictly follow their appropriate diet, and take any medications or insulin to prevent metabolic acidosis. Patients receiving **tube feedings** or intravenous feedings must be monitored to prevent dehydration or the accumulation of ketones or lactic acid.

Metabolic alkalosis

Metabolic alkalosis is a pH imbalance that occurs when the body accumulates too much of an alkaline substance, such as bicarbonate, and does not have enough acid to effectively neutralize the effects of the alkali. This disturbance of the body's acid/base balance, can be a mild condition, brought on by vomiting, the use of steroids or diuretic drugs, or the overuse of **antacids** or **laxatives**. Metabolic alkalosis can also indicate a more serious problem with a major organ such as the kidneys.

Metabolic alkalosis results from the body having more base than acid in the system. Chemists use the term ''pH'' to decribe how acidic or alkaline (also called basic) a substance is. Based on a scale of 14, a pH of 7.0 is neutral. A pH below 7.0 is an acid; the lower the number, the stronger the acid. A pH above 7.0 is alkaline; the higher the number, the stronger the alkali. Blood pH is slightly alkaline, with a normal range of 7.36-7.44.

Conditions that lead to a reduced amount of fluid in the body, like vomiting or excessive urination due to use of diuretic drugs, change the balance of fluids and salts. The blood levels of potassium and sodium can decrease dramatically, causing symptoms of metabolic alkalosis. Slowed breathing may be an initial symptom. The patient may also have episodes of apnea (not breathing) that may go on 15 seconds or longer. **Cyanosis**, a bluish or purplish discoloration of the skin, may also develop as a sign of inadequate oxygen intake. Nausea, vomiting, and **diarrhea** may also occur. Other symptoms can include irritability, twitching, confusion, and picking at bedclothes. Rapid heart rate, irregular heart beats, and a drop in blood pressure are also symptoms. Severe cases can lead to convulsions and **coma**.

Although metabolic alkalosis may be suspected based on symptoms, they are often not noticeable. The condition is usually confirmed by laboratory tests on blood and urine samples. Blood pH above 7.45 confirms the condition. Levels of other blood components, including salts like potassium, sodium, and chloride, fall below normal ranges. The level of bicarbonate in the blood will be high, usually greater than 29 mEq/L. Urine pH may rise to about 7.0 in metabolic alkalosis.

Treatment focuses first on correcting the imbalance. An intravenous line may be started to administer fluids (generally normal saline, a salt water solution) and allow for the quick injection of other drugs that may be needed. Potassium chloride will be administered. Drugs to regulate blood pressure or heart rate, or to control **nausea and vomiting** might be given. Vital signs like pulse, respiration, blood pressure, and body temperature will be monitored. The underlying cause of the metabolic alkalosis must also be diagnosed and corrected.

If metabolic alkalosis is recognized and treated promptly, the patient may have no long-term complications; however, the underlying condition that caused the alkalosis needs to be corrected or managed. Severe metabolic alkalosis that is left untreated will lead to convulsions, **heart failure**, and coma.

Patients receiving **tube feedings** or intravenous feedings must be monitored to prevent an imbalance of fluids and salts, particularly potassium, sodium, and chloride. Overuse of some drugs, including **diuretics**, laxatives, and antacids, should be avoided.

METABOLISM

Metabolism refers to the highly integrated network of chemical reactions by which living cells grow and sustain themselves. This network is composed of two major types of pathways: anabolism and catabolism. Anabolism uses energy stored in the form of adenosine triphosphate (ATP) to build larger molecules from smaller molecules. Catabolic reactions degrade larger molecules in order to produce ATP and raw materials for anabolic reactions.

Together, these two general metabolic networks have three major functions: (1) to extract energy from nutrients or solar energy; (2) to synthesize the building blocks that make up the large molecules of life: proteins, fats, carbohydrates, nucleic acids, and combinations of these substances; and (3) to synthesize and degrade molecules required for special functions in the cell.

These reactions are controlled by enzymes, protein catalysts that increase the speed of chemical reactions in the cell without themselves being changed. Each enzyme catalyzes a specific chemical reaction by acting on a specific substrate, or raw material. Each reaction is just one in a sequence of catalytic steps known as metabolic pathways. These sequences may be composed of up to 20 enzymes, each one creating a product that becomes the substrate—or raw material—for the subsequent enzyme. Often, an additional molecule called a coenzyme is required for the enzyme to function. For example, some coenzymes accept an electron that is released from the substrate during the enzymatic reaction. Most of the water-soluble **vitamins** of the B complex serve as coenzymes; riboflavin (Vitamin B_2) for example, is a precursor of the coenzyme flavine adenine dinucleotide, while pantothenate is a component of coenzyme A, an important intermediate metabolite.

The series of products created by the sequential enzymatic steps of anabolism or catabolism are called metabolic intermediates, or metabolites. Each step represents a small change in the molecule, usually the removal, transfer, or addition of a specific atom, molecule, or group of atoms that serves as a functional group, such as the amino groups ($-NH_2$) of proteins.

Most such metabolic pathways are linear, that is, they begin with a specific substrate and end with a specific product. However, some pathways, such as the Krebs cycle, are cyclic. Often, metabolic pathways also have branches that feed into or out of them. The specific sequences of intermediates in the pathways of cell metabolism are called intermediary metabolism.

Among the many hundreds of chemical reactions there are only a few that are central to the activity of the cell, and these pathways are identical in most forms of life.

All reactions of metabolism, however, are part of the overall goal of the organism to maintain its internal orderliness, whether that organism is a single celled protozoan or a human. Organisms maintain this orderliness by removing energy from nutrients or sunlight and returning to their environment an equal amount of energy in a less useful form, mostly heat. This heat becomes dissipated throughout the rest of the organism's environment.

According to the first law of thermodynamics, in any physical or chemical change, the total amount of energy in the universe remains constant, that is, energy cannot be created or destroyed. Thus, when the energy stored in nutrient molecules is released and captured in the form of ATP, some energy is lost as heat. But the total amount of energy is unchanged.

The second law of thermodynamics states that physical and chemical changes proceed in such a direction that useful energy undergoes irreversible degradation into a randomized form—entropy. The dissipation of energy during metabolism represents an increase in the randomness, or disorder, of the organism's environment. Because this disorder is irreversible, it provides the driving force and direction to all metabolic enzymatic reactions.

Even in the simplest cells, such as bacteria, there are at least a thousand such reactions. Regardless of the number, all cellular reactions can be classified as one of two types of metabolism: anabolism and catabolism. These reactions, while opposite in nature, are linked through the common bond of energy. Anabolism, or biosynthesis, is the synthetic phase of metabolism during which small building block molecules, or precursors, are built into large molecular components of cells, such as carbohydrates and proteins.

Catabolic reactions are used to capture and save energy from nutrients, as well as to degrade larger molecules into smaller, molecular raw materials for reuse by the cell. The energy is stored in the form of energy-rich ATP, which powers the reactions of anabolism. The useful energy of ATP is stored in the form of a high-energy bond between the second and third phosphate groups of ATP. The cell makes ATP by adding a phosphate group to the molecule adenosine diphosphate (ADP). Therefore, ATP is the major chemical link between the energy-yielding reactions of catabolism, and the energy-requiring reactions of anabolism.

In some cases, energy is also conserved as energy-rich hydrogen atoms in the coenzyme nicotinamide adenine dinucleotide phosphate in the reduced form of NADPH. The NADPH can then be used as a source of high-energy hydrogen atoms during certain biosynthetic reactions of anabolism.

In addition to the obvious difference in the direction of their metabolic goals, anabolism and catabolism differ in other significant ways. For example, the various degradative pathways of catabolism are convergent. That is, many hundreds of different proteins, polysaccharides, and lipids are broken down into relatively few catabolic end products. The hundreds of anabolic pathways, however, are divergent. That is, the cell uses relatively few biosynthetic precursor molecules to synthesize a vast number of different proteins, polysaccharides, and lipids.

The opposing pathways of anabolism and catabolism may also use different reaction intermediates or different enzymatic reactions in some of the steps. For example, there are 11 enzymatic steps in the breakdown of glucose into pyruvic acid in the liver. But the liver uses only nine of those same steps in the synthesis of glucose, replacing the other two steps with a different set of enzyme-catalyzed reactions. This occurs because the pathway to degradation of glucose releases energy, while the anabolic process of glucose synthesis requires energy. The two different reactions of anabolism are required to overcome the energy barrier that would otherwise prevent the synthesis of glucose.

Another reason for having slightly different pathways is that the corresponding anabolic and catabolic routes must be independently regulated. Otherwise, if the two phases of metabolism shared the exact pathway (only in reverse) a slowdown in the anabolic pathway would slow catabolism, and vice versa.

See also Vitamins

Metchnikoff, Elie (1845-1916)

Russian microbiologist

An important early researcher in immunology, Elie Metchnikoff was born in Kharkov, Russia, on May 16, 1845. His father was an officer of the Imperial Guard. His mother was the daughter of a Jewish writer, and she encouraged her son's interest in natural sciences. After graduating from the University of Kharkov in 1864, Metchnikoff continued his studies in Germany, then returned to Russia and earned his Ph.D. from the University of St. Petersburg in 1867. Metchnikoff's early career was difficult. His first faculty positions, at the University of Odessa beginning in 1862 and at St. Petersburg in 1868, were marred by difficult working conditions and severe eyestrain. After his first wife died in 1873, Metchnikoff attempted suicide. Thanks to a happy and financially successful second marriage, Metchnikoff became financially independent and moved to Messina, Italy, in 1882 to devote himself to research. There, he made his great discovery.

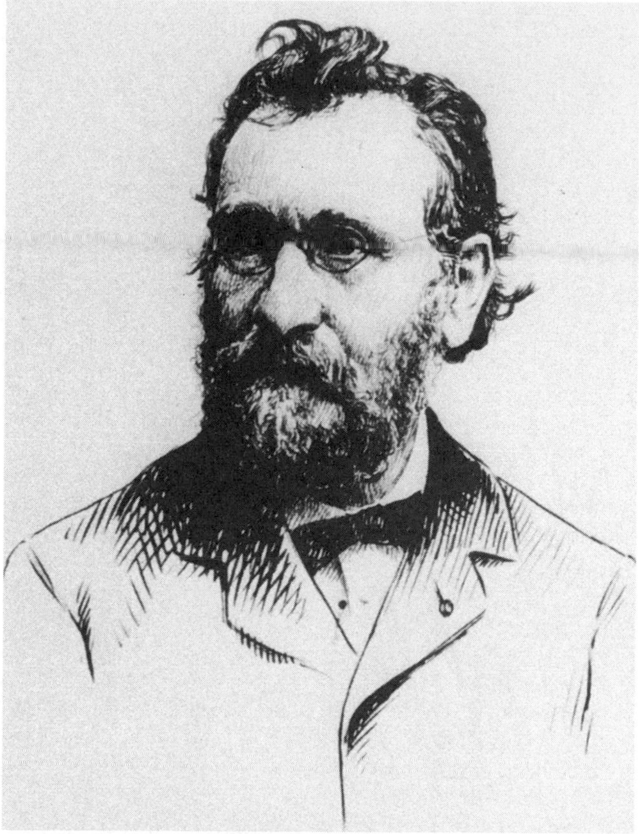

Elie Metchnikoff

In 1865, Metchnikoff had studied roundworms for the purpose of observing intracellular **digestion**. In Messina, he studied transparent starfish larvae and observed a similar process, whereby mobile cells surrounded and engulfed invading foreign particles. He called these bacteria-eating cells phagocytes and devoted the next twenty-five years of his life to developing and promoting his concept of phagocytosis. Continuing his research, he showed that white blood corpuscles in higher animals and humans are also phagocytes. Metchnikoff first published his ideas about phagocytes in 1883 and wrote a comprehensive book on immunity in 1901. This new concept met with serious objections: first, because it contradicted the prevalent idea that white blood cells aided rather

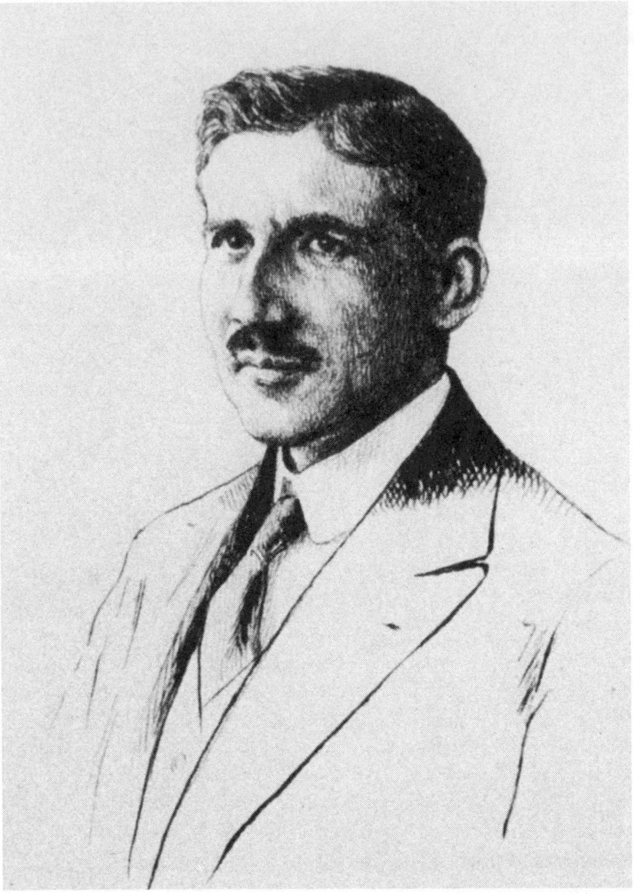

Otto Meyerhof

than attacked bacteria, and second, because it seemed to conflict with findings that antibody substances in the blood were responsible for immune responses. Metchnikoff worked, wrote, and spoke vigorously in support of his ideas, which became accepted as a component of the **immune system** in the early 1900s. He shared the 1908 Nobel Prize for medicine or physiology with **Paul Ehrlich** for his work on white blood corpuscles.

Metchnikoff returned to Russia to head Odessa's Bacteriological Institute from 1886-1887. After his work came to the attention of **Louis Pasteur**, Metchnikoff settled in Paris in 1888 as a member and then director of the Pasteur Institute. Late in his life, he became interested in longevity, which he linked to bacteria in the intestinal tract. He believed that regularly ingesting lactic-acid bacilli—found in sour milk and yogurt—would increase a person's life span. Metchnikoff died in Paris of cardiac failure on July 16, 1916.

MEYERHOF, OTTO (1884-1951)

German-American biochemist

The son of a merchant, Meyerhof received his medical degree from the University of Heidelberg in 1909. Although he was originally attracted to psychology, a meeting with Otto Warburg aroused his interest in cellular physiology and, in 1913, when he joined the faculty of Kiel, he began what was to be a lifelong investigation into the biochemistry of muscle.

At the time, it was already common knowledge that muscle contained glycogen and that—as **Frederick Gowland Hopkins** and his coworkers had shown a decade earlier—a working muscle accumulates lactic acid. With these facts as starting points, Meyerhof conducted a series of experiments and, in 1919, demonstrated how the glycogen-lactic acid cycle works. In phase one, when the muscle begins to contract, glycogen is converted to lactic acid. Oxygen is not consumed, but an oxygen debt is built up. In phase two, when the muscle rests after work, molecular oxygen is then consumed to pay off the ''debt'' and to oxidize about one-fifth of the lactic acid. The energy yielded from the oxidation process makes it possible for the remaining four-fifths of lactic acid to be reconverted to glycogen.

Meyerhof's discovery elaborated the observation of Archibald Vivian Hill, in 1913, that heat was emitted and oxygen consumed only during a muscle's contraction and its recovery. Hill and Meyerhof shared the 1922 Nobel Prize in physiology or medicine for their work on the biochemistry of muscular action. Meyerhof's work also laid the groundwork for **Carl and Gerty Cori**'s more detailed explanation, a few years later, of the steps by which glycogen is converted to lactic acid (a process thereafter often known as the Embden-Meyerhof pathway, after Meyerhof and a coworker)

Like many other Jewish scientists, Meyerhof left Germany in 1938 after the Nazis rose to power. Unfortunately, the biochemist settled in Paris, France, and was therefore forced to flee a second time when the Germans invaded France in 1940. Meyerhof then came to the United States and became a professor of physiological chemistry at the University of Pennsylvania, in Philadelphia, remaining there until his death.

MIDWIFERY

Midwifery, practiced around the world for thousands of years, is the act of assisting at childbirth and during pregnancy. Worldwide, midwives deliver more than two-thirds of all babies. In the United States, midwifes were replaced by **physicians** when advances in medical care shifted childbearing from the home to hospitals in the early 1900s. Since the 1960s, women interested in natural childbirth began turning to midwifes again.

Midwives focus on the physical, emotional, and social needs of women and their babies. They view childbirth as a normal event and encourage patients and their families to actively participate in decision making. They use medical technology only when necessary.

There are three types of midwifes in the United States today: certified nurse-midwives, certified midwives, and lay-midwives. Certified nurse-midwifes, also called nurse-midwives, are educated in nursing and midwifery, and certified by the American College of Nurse-Midwives Certification

Council. In some states, they also have to meet other requirements to practice. Certified nurse-midwifes provide routine women's health care as well as assistance with pregnancy and childbirth. Their services include: prenatal care, labor and delivery management, care after birth, newborn care, family planning, preconception care, managing menopause, birth-control advice, counseling on staying healthy and managing diseases. They are affiliated with physicians, who they can turn to when problems come up. Most work at hospitals, family planning clinics, or birthing centers affiliated with hospitals. Educating patients is an important role of certified nurse-midwifes. They counsel women about how to have a healthy pregnancy, labor and delivery techniques, breast feeding, parenting, sexually transmitted diseases, spousal and child abuse, and social support networks.

Certified midwives have formal midwifery education, including an apprenticeship, but they are not nurses. They usually help women deliver babies at home or in birthing centers. Certified midwives are legally recognized in 29 states. They perform most of the same services that certified nurse-midwives do and usually are affiliated with doctors, hospitals, and laboratories.

Lay-midwives are generally trained informally through apprenticeships with midwives; some do have formal education. They are not certified or licensed and typically assist only in home births. Many practice as part of a religious community or an ethnic group. In some states it is illegal for a lay midwife to charge for services.

Migrant Health

There are estimated to be as many as 4 million migratory, seasonal farmworkers in the United States, comprised of a variety of races and cultures. Often the migrant family is besieged and weakened by sporadic unemployment and loss of extended family support systems. Because income may be irregular and often falls below the national poverty level, a considerable amount of insecurity exists regarding food, clothing, shelter, transportation, health care and other essentials. Some have difficulty proving claims for Social Security benefits. Children may be forced or encouraged to contribute to the financial needs of the family, and may not remain in school beyond the minimum legal age.

Race and level of income and education contribute to differences in health care service utilization. Minority populations and those with lower levels of income and education utilize the **health care system** less frequently. Nonwhite populations spend fewer days in the **hospital**, see a physician less often, and are more often treated in outpatient or emergency departments. Exposure to pesticides and infectious diseases, and life in crowded, substandard housing place the migrant population at high risk for a multitude of complex health problems.

In an effort to address this problem, the Migrant Health Act of 1962 provided federally funded health care services in medically underserved areas throughout the United States and its territories. Grants were given to over 120 community based and state organizations to facilitate comprehensive medical care services with a culturally sensitive focus on migrant and seasonal farmworkers and their families.This program not only to serves this special needs population, but also protects farm community residents from prevalent communicable diseases and assists the often overburdened rural health care systems.

See also Minority health

Military Medicine

Traditionally, military medicine has progressed when war has forced doctors to devise better ways of caring for the wounded. Many advances in the treatment of shock, trauma, and infectious disease were developed under the pressure of war.

The Cold War (that period of indirect conflict and proxy wars between the United States and the Soviet Union that lasted from the end of World War II in 1946 until the disintegration of the Soviet Union in the early 1990s) forced military medicine into a period of self-examination and planning for new and varied demands.

Post-Cold War questions focus on how to balance a medical staff's combat readiness with other missions. In an environment where the military is highly mobile and fast-moving, and when it is deployed against considerably weaker forces, nonbattle injuries must be expected. For example, in 1991, in Operation Desert Storm (in which the US attacked Iraq after the latter invaded its oil-rich neighbor Kuwait), soldiers were far more likely to be evacuated for noncombat injuries than for combat injuries. Motor vehicle accidents were the most common cause of noncombat injuries.

Military medical staff must be prepared for disease and nonbattle injuries such as environmental and safety hazards. In military operations in Haiti and Somalia, about 10 percent of United States forces were seen for disease and nonbattle injuries, usually accidental injuries. Sports injuries are also persistent problems.

Military medical staff must make many special preparations based on the living conditions of the countries to which they will be traveling. More than one-fifth of the world lives in extreme poverty with little **sanitation**, where infectious diseases are the leading cause of death (17 million deaths per year). As a result of war, more than 50 million refugees and other displaced persons face additional risk for disease fostered by poor sanitation in camps. Under such conditions, United States military members have limited protection, because so many pathogens are resistant to **antibiotics** and insecticides. Diseases such as **cholera** and **malaria** were once thought to be under control but are now found in many countries. Malaria affected entire battalions during the wars in Korea and Vietnam. During the occupation of Somalia, 350 U.S. troops contracted malaria.

Poor sanitation also leads to **diarrheal** diseases, such as **dysentery**. During the Civil War, diarrheal diseases caused more deaths than battle wounds. Though diarrheal diseases rarely kill modern United States troops, they reduce combat capability. For example, when U.S. troops arrived in Saudi Arabia for Operation Desert Storm, more than half contracted diarrhea during the first month and of these, about 20 percent missed at least one day of work. Again, military medical personnel can offer very little, since the organisms that cause diarrhea quickly develop resistance to new drugs.

Troops exposed to rough living conditions are also at risk for incurable insect-borne diseases such as dengue fever, **yellow fever**, and Japanese **encephalitis**. Military medicine must be prepared to cope with **influenza**, **tuberculosis**, **hepatitis**, **meningitis**, biological weapons, **sexually transmitted diseases**, and heat casualties.

In addition to care of the troops, military medical personnel are responsible for the families of troops and for some military retirees. Retirees make up more than 50 percent of patients, up from 8 percent of patients in the early 1950s. Between 1986 and 1996, 35 percent of military hospitals closed. During the same decade, the number of people seeking help from the Military Health Services System has dropped only 9 percent. The trend is to accept fewer inpatients at military base hospitals.

Military medical personnel must be prepared to support large deployments, such as those in the Balkans, but must also prepare for expanding roles in treating victims of natural disasters and terrorism.

Military medical personnel have assisted in emergencies such as the bombing of the federal building in Oklahoma City and in major jet crashes. These outreach missions help military medical personnel hone their skills in addition to providing humanitarian aid. In the post-Cold War climate, military medical personnel are called upon to provide medical support for peacekeeping missions. Sometimes medical personnel are seen as less threatening than others in United States military uniforms, and their humanitarian efforts are more likely to be accepted.

The medical education of military physicians is changing to prepare for the military's new role. The military medical school curriculum includes training in casualty care research, **public health**, **preventive medicine**, humanitarian assistance, disaster medicine, medical simulation training, **tropical medicine**, specialized family care, and teleradiology (diagnostic images transmitted over telephone lines).

MILSTEIN, CÉSAR (1927-)

Argentine-English biochemist

César Milstein was born on October 8, 1927, in the eastern Argentine city of Bahía Blanca, one of three sons of Lázaro and Máxima Milstein. He studied biochemistry at the National University of Buenos Aires from 1945 to 1952, graduating with a degree in chemistry. Heavily involved in opposing the policies of President Juan Peron and working part-time as a chemical analyst for a laboratory, Milstein barely managed to pass with poor grades. Nonetheless, he pursued graduate studies at the Instituto de Biología Química of the University of Buenos Aires and completed his doctoral dissertation on the chemistry of aldehyde dehydrogenase, an alcohol enzyme used as a catalyst, in 1957.

With a British Council scholarship, he continued his studies at Cambridge University from 1958 to 1961 under the guidance of Frederick Sanger, a distinguished researcher in the field of enzymes. Sanger had determined that an enzyme's functions depend on the arrangement of amino acids inside it. In 1960 Milstein obtained a Ph.D. and joined the Department of Biochemistry at Cambridge, but in 1961, he decided to return to his native country to continue his investigations as head of a newly created Department of Molecular Biology at the National Institute of Microbiology in Buenos Aires.

A military coup in 1962 had a profound impact on the state of research and on academic life in Argentina. Milstein resigned his position in protest of the government's dismissal of the Institute's director, Ignacio Pirosky. In 1963 he returned to work with Sanger in Great Britain. During the 1960s and much of the 1970s, Milstein concentrated on the study of antibodies, the protein organisms generated by the immune system to combat and deactivate antigens. Milstein's efforts were aimed at analyzing myeloma proteins, and then DNA and RNA. Myeloma, which are tumors in cells that produce antibodies, had been the subject of previous studies by **Rodney R. Porter**, **MacFarlane Burnet**, and **Gerald M. Edelman**, among others.

Milstein's investigations in this field were fundamental for understanding how antibodies work. He searched for mutations in laboratory cells of myeloma but faced innumerable difficulties trying to find antigens to combine with their antibodies. He and Köhler produced a hybrid myeloma called hybridoma in 1974. This cell had the capacity to produce antibodies but kept growing like the cancerous cell from which it had originated. The production of monoclonal antibodies from these cells was one of the most relevant conclusions from Milstein and his colleague's research. The Milstein-Köhler paper was first published in 1975 and indicated the possibility of using monoclonal antibodies for testing antigens. The two scientists predicted that since it was possible to hybridize antibody-producing cells from different origins, such cells could be produced in massive cultures. They were, and the technique consisted of a fusion of antibodies with cells of the myeloma to produce cells that could perpetuate themselves, generating uniform and pure antibodies.

In 1983 Milstein assumed leadership of the Protein and Nucleic Acid Chemistry Division at the Medical Research Council's laboratory. In 1984 he shared the Nobel Prize with Köhler and Jerne for developing the technique that had revolutionized many diagnostic procedures by producing exceptionally pure antibodies. Upon receiving the prize, Milstein heralded the beginning of what he called "a new era of immunobiochemistry," which included production of molecules based on antibodies. He stated that his method was a by-product of basic research and a clear example of how an investment in research that was not initially considered commercially viable had "an enormous practical impact." By 1984 a thriving business was being done with monoclonal antibodies for diagnosis, and works on vaccines and cancer based on Milstein's breakthrough research were being rapidly developed.

In the early 1980s Milstein received a number of other scientific awards, including the Wolf Prize in Medicine from the Karl Wolf Foundation of Israel in 1980, the Royal Medal from the Royal Society of London in 1982, and the Dale Medal from the Society for Endocrinology in London in 1984. He is a member of numerous international scientific organizations, among them the U.S. National Academy of Sciences and the Royal College of Physicians in London. His hobbies include walking, outdoor cooking, and attending the theater. Milstein is married to biochemist Celia Prilleltensky; they have no children.

MINERAL DEFICIENCY

Mineral deficiency is a condition where the concentration of any one of the **minerals** essential to human health is abnormally low in the body. In some cases, an abnormally low mineral concentration is defined as that which leads to an impairment in a bodily function dependent on the mineral. In other cases, an abnormally low mineral concentration is defined as a level lower than that found in the healthy population.

Mineral nutrients are all the inorganic elements or inorganic molecules that are required for life. As far as human **nutrition** is concerned, inorganic nutrients include water, sodium, potassium, chloride, calcium, phosphate, sulfate, magnesium, iron, copper, zinc, manganese, iodine, selenium, and molybdenum. There is some evidence that other inorganic nutrients, such as chromium and boron, also play a part in human health, but their role is not well established. Fluoride has been proven to increase the strength of bones and teeth, but there is little or no reason to believe that it is needed for human life.

Severe deficiencies in any one of the inorganic nutrients can result in specific symptoms and sometimes in **death**, due to the failure of functions associated with that nutrient. A deficiency in one nutrient may occur less often than deficiency in several nutrients. A patient suffering from **malnutrition** is deficient in a variety of nutrients. In the United States, malnutrition is most often found among severe alcoholics. Deficiencies in one nutrient do occur, for example, in human populations living in iodine-poor regions of the world and in iron-deficient persons who lose excess iron by abnormal bleeding.

Inorganic nutrients have a wide variety of functions in the body. Water, sodium, and potassium deficiencies are most closely associated with abnormal nerve action and cardiac **arrhythmias**. Deficiencies in these nutrients tend to result not from a lack of content in the diet, but from excessive losses due to severe **diarrhea** and other causes. Iodine deficiency is a global public health problem. It occurs in parts of the world with iodine-deficient soils and results in goiter, which involves a relatively harmless swelling of the neck, and cretinism, a severe birth defect. The body uses iodine for making thyroid hormone. However, since thyroid hormone has a variety of roles in development of the embryo, iodine deficiency during **pregnancy** results in a number of **birth defects**.

Calcium deficiency due to lack of dietary calcium occurs only rarely. However, calcium deficiency due to **vitamin D deficiency** can be found among certain populations. Vitamin D is required for the efficient absorption of calcium from the diet, and vitamin D deficiency in growing infants and children can result in calcium deficiency.

Dietary phosphate deficiency is rare because phosphate is plentiful in plant and animal foods, but also because phosphate is efficiently absorbed from the diet into the body. Iron deficiency causes **anemia** (lack of red blood cells), which results in tiredness and shortness of breath.

Dietary deficiencies in the remaining inorganic nutrients tend to be rare. Magnesium deficiency tends to occur in chronic alcoholics, in persons taking diuretic drugs, and in those suffering from severe and prolonged diarrhea. Magnesium deficiency tends to occur with the same conditions that provoke deficiencies in sodium and potassium. Zinc deficiency has been found in poor Middle Eastern populations who rely on unleavened whole wheat bread as a major food source. Copper deficiency is also rare, but dramatic and health-threatening changes in copper metabolism occur in two genetic diseases, Wilson's disease and Menkes' disease.

Selenium deficiency may occur in regions of the world where the soils are poor in selenium, thus producing foods that are also low in this mineral. Premature infants may also be at risk for selenium deficiency. Manganese deficiency is extremely rare.

Sodium deficiency (hyponatremia) and water deficiency are the most serious and widespread deficiencies in the world. These deficiencies tend to arise from excessive losses from the body, as during prolonged and severe diarrhea or vomiting. Diarrheal diseases are a major world health problem and are responsible for about a quarter of the 10 million infant deaths that occur each year. Nearly all of these deaths occur in impoverished parts of Africa and Asia due to contamination of the water supply by animal and human feces. The main concern in treating diarrheal diseases is **dehydration**, that is, the losses of sodium and water which deplete the fluids of the circulatory system (the heart, veins, arteries, and capillaries). Severe losses of the fluids of the circulatory system result in **shock**, which is defined as inadequate supply of blood to the various tissues of the body resulting in a lack of oxygen to all of the body's cells. The main concern in avoiding shock is the replacement of sodium and water.

Sodium deficiency and potassium deficiency also frequently result during treatment with drugs called **diuretics**, which are used to treat high blood pressure (**hypertension**). However, diuretics can lead to sodium deficiency, excessive loss of potassium, and low plasma potassium (hypokalemia).

Iodine deficiency tends to occur in regions of the world where the soil is poor in iodine. Goiter, an enlargement of the thyroid gland (located in the neck), results from iodine deficiency. Goiter continues to be a problem in eastern Europe, parts of India and South America, and in Southeast Asia. Goiter has been eradicated in the United States because of the fortification of foods with iodine. Iodine deficiency during pregnancy results in cretinism in the newborn. Cretinism involves mental retardation, a large tongue, and sometimes deafness, muteness, and lameness.

Iron deficiency occurs due to periods of dietary deficiency, rapid growth, and excessive loss of the body's iron. Infants are at risk for acquiring iron deficiency because their rapid rate of growth needs a corresponding increased supply of dietary iron for use in making blood and muscles. Human milk is a better source of iron than cow milk, since about half of the iron in human breast milk is absorbed by the infant's digestive tract. In contrast, only 10% of the iron in cow milk is absorbed by the infant. Surveys of lower-income families in the United States have revealed that about 6% of the infants are anemic indicating a deficiency of iron in their diets. Blood loss that occurs with **menstruation** in women, as well as with a variety of causes of intestinal bleeding, is a major cause of iron deficiency. The symptoms of iron deficiency are generally limited to anemia and the resulting tiredness, weakness, and a reduced ability to perform physical work.

Calcium and phosphate are closely related nutrients. About 99% of the calcium and 85% of the phosphate in the body occur in the skeleton. Both of these nutrients occur in a great variety of foods, especially milk, eggs, and green, leafy vegetables are rich in calcium and phosphate. Dietary deficiencies in calcium (hypocalcemia) or phosphate are extremely rare throughout the world. Vitamin D deficiency can be found among young infants, the elderly, and others who may be shielded from sunshine for prolonged periods of time. Vitamin D deficiency impairs the absorption of calcium from the diet and, as a result, can provoke calcium deficiency even when the diet contains adequate calcium.

Zinc deficiency has been found among peasant populations in rural areas of the Middle East. Unleavened whole wheat bread can account for 75% of the energy intake in these areas. This diet, which does not contain meat, does contain zinc, but it also contains phytic acid, which naturally occurs in wheat and inhibits zinc absorption. The yeast used to leaven bread produces enzymes that inactivate the phytic acid. Unleavened bread does not contain yeast and, therefore, contains intact phytic acid. The symptoms of zinc deficiency include lack of sexual maturation, lack of pubic hair, and small stature. Zinc deficiency is relatively uncommon in the United States, but it may occur in adults with **alcoholism** or intestinal malabsorption problems. Low plasma zinc has been found in patients with alcoholic **cirrhosis**, Crohn's disease, and **celiac disease**. The signs of zinc deficiency include a rash on the face, groin, hands, and feet and diarrhea. These symptoms can easily be reversed by administering zinc. An emerging concern is that increased calcium intake can interfere with zinc absorption or retention. Hence, there is some interest in the question of whether persons taking calcium to prevent **osteoporosis** should also take zinc supplements.

Severe alterations in copper metabolism occur in two genetic diseases, Wilson's disease and Menkes' disease. Both of these diseases are rare and occur in about one in 100,000 births.

Selenium deficiency may occur in premature infants, since this population naturally tends to have low levels of plasma selenium. Selenium deficiency occurs in regions of the world containing low-selenium soils. These regions include Keshan Province in China, New Zealand, and Finland. In Keshan Province, a disease (Keshan disease) occurs which results in deterioration of regions of the heart and the development of fibers in these regions.

Minerals serve strikingly different functions in the body, and the tests for the corresponding deficiency are markedly different from each other. The mineral content of the body may be measured by testing samples of blood plasma, red blood cells, or urine. In the case of calcium and phosphate deficiency, the diagnosis may also involve taking x rays of the skeleton. In the case of iodine deficiency, the diagnosis may include examining the patient's neck with the eyes and hands. In the case of iron deficiency, the diagnosis may include the performance of a stair-stepping test by the patient.

In the healthy population, all mineral deficiencies can be prevented by the consumption of inorganic nutrients at levels defined by the RDA. Where a balanced diet is not available, government programs for treating individuals, or for fortifying the food supply, may be used. Ensuring an adequate intake of these minerals, by eating a balanced diet or by taking mineral supplements, is the best way to prevent deficiencies.

See also Malnutrition; Minerals; Vitamin D deficiency

Minerals

Minerals are inorganic substances that occur in nature. Many minerals are relevant to human nutrition, including water, sodium, potassium, chloride, calcium, phosphate, sulfate, magnesium, iron, copper, zinc, manganese, iodine, selenium, and molybdenum. Cobalt is a required mineral for human health, but it is supplied by vitamin B_{12}. Cobalt appears to have no other function, aside from being part of this vitamin. There is some evidence that chromium, boron, and other inorganic elements play some part in human nutrition, but the evidence is indirect and not yet convincing. Fluoride seems not to be required for human life, but its presence in the diet contributes to long-term dental health. Some of the minerals do not occur as single atoms, but occur as molecules, which are composed of one or more atoms. These include water, phosphate, sulfate, and selenite (a form of selenium). Sulfate contains an atom of sulfur, and the body can acquire all the sulfate it needs from protein.

Various minerals, or inorganic nutrients, are required for life, meaning that their continued supply in the diet is needed for growth, maintenance of body weight in adulthood, and for reproduction. The amount of each mineral that is needed to support growth during infancy and childhood, to maintain body weight and health, and to facilitate **pregnancy** and lactation, are listed in a table called the Recommended Dietary Allowances (RDA), which was compiled by the United States Food and Nutrition Board. All of the values listed in the RDA indicate the daily amounts that are expected to maintain health throughout most of the general population. However, studies on small groups of healthy human subjects indicate that the actual levels of each inorganic nutrient required by any given individual is likely to be less than that stated by the RDA, which set the standards in order to accommodate the variability expected among the general population.

The RDAs for adult males are 800 mg of calcium, 800 mg of phosphorus, 350 mg of magnesium, 10 mg of iron, 15 mg of zinc, 0.15 mg of iodine, and 0.07 mg of selenium. The RDA for sodium is expressed as a range (0.5-2.4 g/day). The minimal requirement for chloride is about 0.75 g/day, and the minimal requirement for potassium is 1.6-2.0 g/day, though RDA values have not been set for these nutrients. The RDAs for several other minerals has not been determined, and here the estimated safe and adequate daily dietary intake has been listed by the Food and Nutrition Board. These values are listed for copper (1.5-3.0 mg), manganese (2-5 mg), fluoride (1.5-4.0 mg), molybdenum (0.075-0.25 mg), and chromium (0.05-0.2 mg). (The function of chromium is essentially unknown, and evidence for its necessity exists only for animals.)

People are treated with minerals for several reasons. The primary reason is to relieve a **mineral deficiency** such as **iron deficiency anemia**. Chemical tests suitable for the detection of all mineral deficiencies are available. The diagnosis of the deficiency is also often aided by non-chemical tests such as the hematocrit test for the red blood cell content in blood for iron deficiency, the visual examination of the neck for iodine deficiency, or the examination of bones by densitometry for calcium deficiency.

Mineral treatment can also help prevent the development of a possible or expected deficiency. Examples include the practice of giving young infants iron supplements and the food industry's practice of supplementing infant formulas with iron. The purpose here is to reduce the risk for iron deficiency anemia. Another example is women taking calcium supplements with the hope of reducing the risk of **osteoporosis**.

There is reason to believe that the purchase and consumption of most, but not all, of these minerals is beneficial to health. Potassium supplements are useful for reducing blood pressure in cases of persons with high blood pressure. The effect of potassium varies from person to person. The consumption of calcium supplements is likely to have some effect on reducing the risk for osteoporosis. Selenium supplements are expected to be of value only for residents of Keshan Province, China, because of the established association of selenium deficiency and ''Keshan disease'' in this region.

Minerals are used in medical treatments by replacing a poor diet with a diet that supplies the RDA, by consuming oral supplements (commercially available in stores), or by injections or infusions. Injections are especially useful for infants, for mentally disabled persons, or where the physician wants to be totally sure of compliance. Infusions, as well as injections, are essential for medical emergencies, as during mineral deficiency situations like hyponatremia (sodium deficiency), hypokalemia (potassium deficiency), hypocalcemia (calcium deficiency), and hypomagnesemia (magnesium deficiency). Oral mineral supplements are especially useful for mentally alert persons who otherwise cannot or will not consume food that is a good mineral source, such as meat. For example, a vegetarian who! will not consume meat may be encouraged to consume oral supplements of iron, as well as supplements of vitamin B_{12}.

Calcium supplements, along with naturally occuring hormones estrogen and calcitonin therapy, are commonly used in the prevention and treatment of osteoporosis. Fluoride has been proven to reduce the rate of **tooth decay**. Magnesium is often used to treat eclampsia, which occasionally occurs during pregnancy. In this case, magnesium is used as a drug (magnesium sulfate) to prevent convulsions, and not to relieve a deficiency. Treatment with cobalt, in the form of vitamin B_{12}, is used for relieving the symptoms of **pernicious anemia**, a relatively common disease which tends to occur in persons older than 40 years. Free cobalt is never used for the treatment of disease. The response to mineral treatment can be monitored by chemical tests, by an examination of red blood cells or white blood cells, or by physiological tests, depe! nding on the exact mineral deficiency.

There are some risks associated with mineral treatment, and **mineral toxicity** can be life theatening in some instances. Selenium, for example, is distinguished among most of the nutrients in that dietary intakes at levels only ten times that of the RDA can be toxic. In treating emergency cases of hyponatremia, hypokalemia, or hypocalcemia by intravenous injections, too much sodium, potassium, or calcium, can result in hypernatremia, hyperkalemia, or hypercalcémia, respectively. Risk for toxicity is rare where treatment is by dietary means because the intestines act as a barrier, and absorption of any mineral supplement is gradual. The gradual passage of any mineral through the intestines, especially when the mineral supplement is taken with food, allows the various organs of the body to acquire the mineral. Gradual passage of the mineral into the bl! oodstream also allows the kidneys to excrete the mineral in the urine, should levels of the mineral rise to toxic levels in the blood.

See also Calcium imbalance; Iron deficiency anemia; Mineral deficiency; Mineral toxicity; Osteoporosis; Pernicious anemia; Potassium imbalance; Phosphorous imbalance; Sodium imbalance

Mineral toxicity

Mineral toxicity is a condition in which the concentration in the body of any one of the **minerals** is abnormally high and results in an adverse effect on health. Mineral nutrients are the inorganic elements or inorganic molecules that are required for life. The inorganic nutrients in human nutrition include water, sodium, potassium, chloride, calcium, phosphate, sulfate, magnesium, iron, copper, zinc, manganese, iodine, selenium, and molybdenum.

In general, mineral toxicity results when there is an accidental consumption of too much of a mineral, as with drinking ocean water (sodium toxicity); taking too much of a mineral supplement (available in most drug and health stores); or with overexposure to industrial pollutants, household chemicals, or certain drugs. Mineral toxicity may also apply to toxicity that can be the result of certain diseases or injuries. For example, hemochromatosis leads to iron toxicity; Wilson's disease results in copper toxicity; severe trauma can lead to hyperkalemia (potassium toxicity).

Depending on the mineral, the effects vary and toxicity occurs at different levels of the mineral in the body. An increase in the concentrations of sodium in the bloodstream can result in seizures and **death**. Increased plasma sodium, which is called hypernatremia, causes various cells of the body, including those of the brain, to shrink. Shrinkage of the brain cells results in confusion, **coma**, **paralysis** of the lung muscles, and death. Death has occurred where table salt (sodium chloride) was accidently used, instead of sugar, for feeding infants. Death due to sodium toxicity has also resulted when baking soda (sodium bicarbonate) was used during attempted therapy of excessive **diarrhea** or vomiting. Although a variety of processed foods contain high levels of sodium chloride, the levels used are not enough to result in sodium toxicity.

Excessive levels of potassium in the bloodstream (severe hyperkalemia) can result in cardiac **arrhythmias** or even death due to cardiac arrest. Potassium is potentially quite toxic, however toxicity or death due to potassium poisoning is usually prevented because of the vomiting reflex. The consumption of food results in mild increases in the concentration of potassium in the bloodstream, but levels of potassium do not become toxic because of the uptake of potassium by various cells of the body, as well as by the action of the kidneys transferring the potassium ions from the blood to the urine. The body's regulatory mechanisms can easily be overwhelmed, however, when potassium chloride is injected intravenously, and high doses of injected potassium can result in death.

Iodine toxicity results in impairment of the creation of thyroid hormone, resulting in lower levels of thyroid hormone in the bloodstream. The thyroid gland enlarges, as a consequence, and goiter is produced. This enlargement is also called hyperthyroidism. (Goiter is usually caused by iodine deficiency.) Iodine toxicity produces ulcers on the skin called ''kelp **acne**'' because of its association with eating kelp, an ocean plant which contains high levels of iodine. Iodine toxicity occurs in Japan, where large amounts of seaweed are consumed.

Iron toxicity is not uncommon, due to the wide distribution of iron pills. A lethal dose of iron is in the range of 200-250 mg iron/kg body weight. Hence, a child who accidently eats 20 or more iron tablets may die as a result of iron toxicity. Within six hours of ingestion, iron toxicity can result in vomiting, diarrhea, abdominal **pain**, seizures, and possibly coma. Although symptoms may appear to improve, this improvement can be followed by **shock**, low blood glucose, liver damage, convulsions, and death within 12-48 hours after toxic levels of iron are ingested.

Nitrite poisoning occurs during a reaction with the iron atom of hemoglobin, an iron-containing protein that resides within the red blood cells. This protein is responsible for the transport of nearly all of the oxygen from the lungs to various tissues and organs of the body. A very small fraction of hemoglobin spontaneously oxidizes per day, producing a protein of a slightly different structure, called methemoglobin. Normally, the amount of methemoglobin constitutes less than 1% of the total hemoglobin. Methemoglobin can accumulate in the blood as a result of nitrite poisoning. Infants are especially susceptible to poisoning by nitrite.

Nitrate, which is naturally present in green leafy vegetables and in water is rapidly converted to nitrite by the naturally occurring bacteria residing on the tongue, as well as in the intestines, and then absorbed into the bloodstream. Poisoning by nitrite, or nitrate after its conversion to nitrite, results in the inability of hemoglobin to carry oxygen throughout the body, identifited by a bluish skin color. Adverse symptoms occur when over 30% of the hemoglobin has been converted to methemoglobin, and these symptoms include cardiac arrhythmias, **headache**, **nausea and vomiting**, and in severe cases, **seizures**.

Calcium and phosphate are closely related nutrients. Calcium toxicity is rare, but overconsumption of calcium supplements may lead to deposits of calcium phosphate in the soft tissues of the body. Phosphate toxicity can occur with overuse of **laxatives** or **enemas** that contain phosphate. Severe phosphate toxicity can result in hypocalcemia, and in various symptoms resulting from low plasma calcium levels. Moderate phosphate toxicity, occurring over a period of months, can result in the deposit of calcium phosphate crystals in various tissues of the body.

Zinc toxicity is rare but can occur in metal workers who are exposed to fumes containing zinc. Excessive dietary supplements of zinc can result in nausea, vomiting, and diarrhea, and copper deficiency because zinc inhibits the absorption of copper.

Severe alterations in copper metabolism occur in two genetic diseases, Wilson's disease and Menkes' disease, both of which are rare and occur in about one in 100,000 births. Both diseases involve mutations in the proteins that transport copper, that is, in special channels that allow the passage of copper ions through cell membranes. Wilson's disease tends to occur in teenagers and in young adults and usually lasts throughout their lives. Copper accumulates in the liver, kidney, and brain, resulting in damage to the liver and nervous system. Wilson's disease can be successfully controlled by lifelong treatment with d-penicillamine. Treatment also involves avoiding foods that are high in copper, such as liver, nuts, chocolate, and mollusks. After an initial period of treatment with penicillamine, Wilson's disease may be treated with zinc supplements to inhibit the absorption of dietary copper.

Selenium toxicity occurs in regions of the world, including some parts of China, where soils contain high levels of selenium that are then found in foods and water. Early signs of selenium toxicity include nausea, weakness, and diarrhea. With continued intake of selenium, changes in fingernails and hair loss results, and damage to the nervous system occurs. The breath may acquire a garlic odor.

Manganese toxicity occurs in manganese mine workers, where men breath air containing dust bearing manganese. It has been documented in Chile, India, Japan, Mexico, and elsewhere. Symptoms of manganese poisoning can occur within several months or years of exposure and include a mental disorder resembling **schizophrenia**, as well as hyperirritability, violent acts, **hallucinations**, and difficulty in walking.

The prognosis for treating toxicity due to sodium, potassium, calcium, iodine and phosphate is usually excellent. Toxicity due to the deposit of calcium phosphate crystals is not usually reversible. For any mineral overdose that causes coma, seizures, or nerve damage the prognosis for recovery is often poor, and death results in a small fraction of patients.

See also Minerals; Mineral deficiency

MINORITY HEALTH

The United States is a nation of immigrants. By the year 2050, one-half of the country's population will be members of minority groups, defined as Native Americans and Alaska Natives, African Americans, Asian Americans and Pacific Islanders, and Hispanics. Because racial and ethnic minority populations have poorer health than the general population and suffer disproportionately from the added stresses of poverty, their health care needs are different from those of much of the majority population.

Racial division has been a feature of the American experience, and the **health care system** reflects the race and class divisions within society. Nonwhites have historically suffered from higher mortality rates, higher incidence of major diseases, and lower availability and use of medical services. Discrimination may be obvious, for example, in location and number of providers to serve minority groups, or subtle, for example, in the personal interactions among health care providers, patients, and their families. The special health care needs of minorities are also a concern in other countries with substantial mixed immigrant populations, such as Canada and the United Kingdom.

Disparities in health care that affect minorities negatively are reflected by higher rates of **infant mortality**; diabetes; cardiovascular diseases; HIV infection; breast and **cervical cancer** screening and management; and deficits in child or adult immunization rates. African Americans in particular have a higher death rate than whites for 12 of the 15 leading causes of death.

Infant mortality is an important measure of a nation's health and a worldwide indicator of health status. In the United States, the infant mortality rate for blacks is twice that of whites. Blacks have twice the mortality rate for cardiovascular disease as whites, and all racial and ethnic minorities have higher risk factors for cardiovascular disease, including **hypertension**, **obesity**, and higher levels of cholesterol. Although black women have a lower rate of breast cancer than white women, they are less likely to survive it. Minority women in general have low rates of screening and treatment for breast and cervical cancer, diseases for which early intervention can significantly reduce the risk of death.

Rates of diabetes and diabetic complications are higher among all minorities than among whites. Underimmunization in urban areas with traditionally underserved populations increases the likelihood of vaccine-preventable diseases among both children and adults. Racial and ethnic minorities constitute approximately 25% of the total U.S. population, yet they account for nearly 54% of all cases of AIDS.

In addition to perceptions of inadequate treatment related to race or ethnicity, other factors affect access to care. Minorities have higher rates of unemployment, and may not be covered by **health insurance**. Even among the working poor, employment benefits may not include health insurance, and salaries may be too low for workers to purchase their own. Minority groups are more likely to have to rely on mass transportation for access to health care, which restricts their mobility. Low rates of literacy make it difficult to identify and to take advantage of entitlements that do exist.

Not only do minorities have less access to the best care, but, though the situation has been improving in more recent years, researchers have sometimes failed to include them in studies and have not taken into account the role of ethnic differences and their distinctive needs in defining health. National databases lack useful information to improve services for minorities, although this is changing.

Cultural differences, such as language difficulties or use of alternative types of health care treatment, may also create obstacles to care. For some groups, there is a stigma attached to seeking care for a problem such as **depression**. Research efforts to include minorities may be hampered by suspicion of researchers' hidden agendas. These fears are grounded in experiences such as the Tuskegee **syphilis** study, in which patients were left untreated in ways that would not have been tolerated in the majority population.

Minorities comprise about 30% of the poor living in rural areas. The particular problems of rural minorities include chronic poverty in some areas, a lack of stable medical care for migrant workers, and language and other barriers, for example, clashes between Native American culture and mainstream medicine.

A 1985 landmark report by the **U.S. Department of Health and Human Services** Task Force on Black and Minority Health led to the institutionalization of minority-related health and service initiatives at the federal and state level, including President Clinton's 1998 racial and ethnic health disparities initiative. National, state, and local agencies have all improved their data collection methods, which makes it possible to measure the health problems of minorities with increasing sophistication. Serious study of class, race, ethnicity, and health has much to offer in the way of answers to major scientific and policy questions.

See also Alternative medicine; Breast cancer and care; Diabetes mellitus

MINOT, GEORGE RICHARDS (1885-1950)

American hematologist and physician

George Richards Minot was born on December 2, 1885, in Boston, Massachusetts, the eldest of three sons of a prominent Boston family. George's father was a physician, and several other men on both sides of the family had been distinguished medical practitioners as well. Minot graduated from Harvard College in 1908, and despite an apparent lack of ambition, entered Harvard medical school thereafter and did well in his courses. It was in medical school that he became interested in the study of human blood, and after he received his M.D. in 1912 he immediately began his internship at the Massachusetts General Hospital in Boston. In 1914 he became an assistant at the Johns Hopkins University medical school in Baltimore. There he continued his studies of blood in the laboratory and did some of the research that led to Dr. William H. Howell's discovery of the anticoagulant drug heparin.

In 1915 Minot began to focus his attention on various forms of **anemia**, but especially on **pernicious anemia**, a dis-

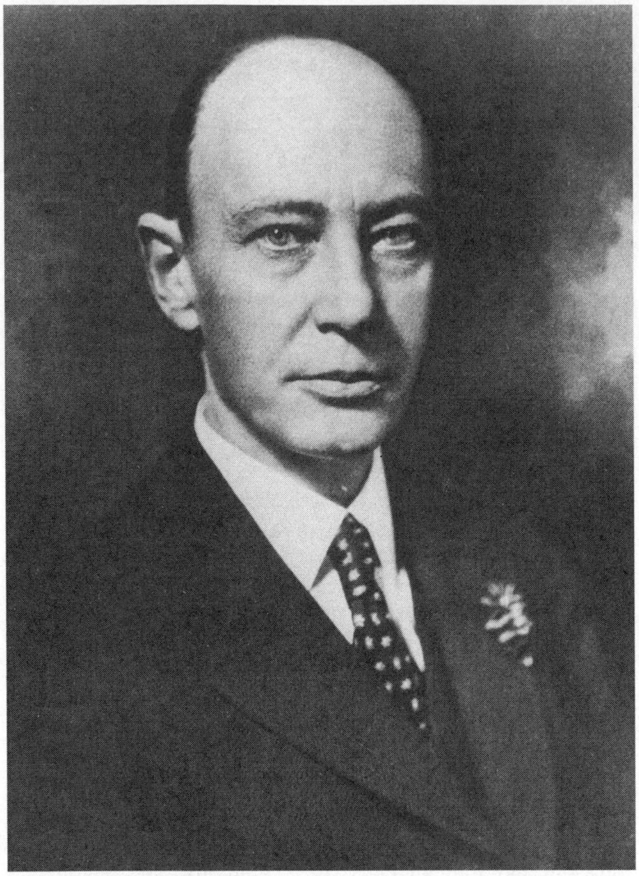

George Richards Minot

ease for which there was then no known cure and which was almost always fatal to the patient. In his prolonged study of blood smears under the microscope, Minot made the important discovery that the number of reticulocytes (young red blood cells) found in a sample provided a good index of the activity of the bone marrow, the part of the body which produces all red blood cells. He also began to suspect that the cause of pernicious anemia was some malfunction in the bone marrow, and that this in turn was somehow related to the diet of the patient. Around 1917 he turned his attention to **cancer** research and treatment. He did significant research on several forms of **leukemia**, a cancerous disease of the blood. In 1918 he became an assistant professor at the Harvard Medical School. In 1921 Minot was diagnosed with diabetes. The discovery of insulin in 1922 led to his rapid improvement and the resumption of his research.

In 1925 Minot returned to the problem of the treatment of pernicious anemia. He was partly inspired by reading reports of experiments by Dr. **George Hoyt Whipple** of Rochester, who had bled dogs to make them anemic and then restored their health by feeding them a diet rich in red meat, especially liver. Minot speculated that feeding liver to human patients with pernicious anemia might have a beneficial effect. Minot enlisted a young colleague, Dr. William P. Murphy, to assist him in the experiment, and together they began feeding up to half a pound of liver per day to as many patients with pernicious anemia as they could persuade to eat it. This simple treatment produced dramatic results: nearly all the patients showed striking improvement, many within only two weeks or so. More important, they continued to improve with further liver feeding rather than suffering relapses following temporary remission of symptoms, as victims of pernicious anemia often did.

In 1926 Minot and Murphy presented a report on the successful treatment of forty-five patients suffering from pernicious anemia. A year later, they reported favorable results in the treatment of 105 patients. The next step was to develop an extract of pure liver which would be less bulky and more palatable to the patient. Minot persuaded Dr. Edward J. Cohn, a professor of physical chemistry at the Harvard medical school, to work on this problem, and Cohn soon isolated what was called Fraction G from pure liver. The Eli Lilly Company then began to manufacture the substance as a commercial product. In 1929 Minot and others discovered that much smaller dosages of the extract, given intravenously, had the same effect as large doses taken by mouth. The discovery of a cure for pernicious anemia marked the culmination of Minot's career as a scientific researcher. He was appointed professor of medicine at the Harvard medical school and director of the Thorndike Memorial Laboratory at Boston City Hospital in 1928. Minot remained active as an administrator until 1947, when he suffered a severe stroke. He died three years later.

Moles

A mole (nevus) is a pigmented (colored) spot on the outer layer of the skin (epidermis)and can be round, oval, flat, or raised. Moles can occur singly or in clusters on any part of the body. Most moles are brown, but colors can range from pinkish flesh tones to yellow, dark blue, or black.

Everyone has at least a few moles. They generally appear by the time a person is 20 and look, at first, like freckles. A mole's color and shape don't usually change. Changes in hormone levels that occur during **puberty** and **pregnancy** can make moles larger and darker. New moles may also appear during this period.

A mole usually lasts about 50 years before beginning to fade. Some moles disappear completely, and some never lighten at all. Some moles develop stalks that raise them above the skin's surface; these moles eventually drop off.

About 1-3% of all babies have one or more moles when they are born. Moles that are present at birth are called congenital nevi.

Other types of moles include:

- Junctional moles, which are usually brown and may be flat or slightly raised.
- Compound moles, which are slightly raised, range in color from tan to dark brown, and involve pigment-producing cells (melanocytes) in both the upper and lower layers of the skin (epidermis and dermis).

- Dermal moles, which range from flesh-color to brown, are elevated, most common on the upper body, and may contain hairs.
- Sebaceous moles, which are produced by over-active oil glands and are yellow and rough-textured.
- Blue moles, which are slightly raised, colored by pigment deep within the skin, and most common on the head, neck, and arms of women.

Most moles are benign, but atypical moles (dysplastic nevi) may develop into malignant melanoma, a potentially fatal form of **skin cancer**. Most atypical moles are bigger than a pencil eraser, and the shape and pigmentation are irregular. They are more apt to become cancerous than moles that develop after birth, especially if they are more than eight inches in diameter. Lentigo maligna (melanotic freckle of Hutchinson), most common on the face and after the age of 50, first appears as a flat spot containing two or more shades of tan. It gradually becomes larger and darker. One in three of these moles develop into a form of skin cancer known as lentigo maligna melanoma.

The cause of moles is unknown, although atypical moles are hereditary and may also result from exposure to sunlight. Only a small percentage of moles require medical attention. A mole that has the following symptoms should be evaluated by a dermatologist (a physician spealizing in skin diseases).

- Appears after the age of 20
- Bleeds
- Itches
- Looks unusual or changes in any way.

A doctor who suspects skin cancer will remove all or part of the mole for microscopic examination. This procedure, which is usually performed in a doctor's office, is simple, relatively painless, and takes little more than a few minutes. It does leave a scar.

If laboratory analysis confirms that a mole is cancerous, the dermatologist will remove the rest of the mole. However, moles are rarely cancerous and, once removed, unlikely to recur. A dermatologist should be consulted if a mole reappears after being removed.

Wearing a sunscreen and limiting sun exposure may prevent some moles. Anyone who has moles should examine them every month and see a dermatologist if they change in size, shape, color, or texture or if new moles appear. Anyone with a family history of melanoma should also see a dermatologist for an annual skin examination. Everyone, especially people who spend large amounts of time with their skin directly exposed to the sun's rays, should know the ABCDs of melanoma:

- A: Asymmetry, which occurs when the two halves of the mole are not identical
- B: Borders that are irregular or indistinct
- C: Color that varies in a single mole
- D: Diameter, which should be no larger than the eraser on a pencil.

A mole exhibiting any of these characteristics should be evaluated by a dermatologist.

MONOAMINE OXIDASE INHIBITORS

Monoamine oxidase inhibitors (MAO inhibitors) are a type of antidepressant used to treat mental **depression**. Like other **antidepressant drugs**, MAO inhibitors help reduce the extreme sadness, hopelessness, and lack of interest in life that are typical in people with depression. MAO inhibitors are especially useful in treating people whose depression is combined with other problems such as **anxiety**, panic attacks, **phobias**, or the desire to sleep too much.

Discovered in the 1950s, MAO inhibitors work by correcting chemical imbalances in the brain. Normally, natural chemicals called neurotransmitters carry signals from one brain cell to another. Some neurotransmitters, such as serotonin and norepinephrine, play important roles in controlling mood. But other substances in the brain may interfere with mood control by breaking down these neurotransmitters. Researchers believe that MAO inhibitors work by blocking the chemicals that break down serotonin and norepinephrine. This gives the neurotransmitters more time to do their important work.

Because MAO inhibitors also affect other chemicals throughout the body, these drugs may produce many unwanted side effects. They can be especially dangerous when taken with certain foods, beverages and medicines. Anyone taking these drugs should ask his or her physician or pharmacist for a list of products to avoid.

MAO inhibitors are available only with a physician's prescription and are sold in tablet form. Some commonly used MAO inhibitors are isocarboxazid (Marplan), phenelzine (Nardil), and tranylcypromine (Parnate). The recommended dosage depends on the type of MAO inhibitor and the type of depression for which it is being taken.

MAO inhibitors can cause serious and possibly life-threatening reactions, such as sudden **hypertension**, when taken with certain foods, beverages, or medicines. The dangerous reactions may not begin until several hours after consuming these things. Aged cheeses, red wines, smoked or pickled meats, chocolate, caffeinated beverages, and foods containing monosodium glutamate (MSG) are among the foods and drinks to be avoided.

People who take MAO inhibitors should not drink alcoholic beverages or use any other medicine unless it has been approved or prescribed by a physician who knows that they are taking MAO inhibitors. This includes nonprescription (over-the-counter) medicines such as sleep aids; medicines for **common colds**, **cough**, **hay fever**, or **asthma** (including nose drops or sprays); medicines to increase alertness or keep from falling asleep; and appetite control products.

Because MAO inhibitors work on the central nervous system, they may add to the effects of alcohol and other drugs that slow down the central nervous system, such as **antihistamines**, cold medicine, allergy medicine, sleep aids, medicine for seizures, tranquilizers, some **pain** relievers, and **muscle relaxants**.

MAO inhibitors may also interact with medicines used during surgery, dental procedures, or emergency treatment. These interactions could increase the chance of side effects.

Some people feel drowsy, dizzy, lightheaded, or less alert when using MAO inhibitors. The drugs may also cause blurred vision. For these reasons, anyone who takes these drugs should not drive, use machines or do anything else that might be dangerous until they have found out how the drugs affect them. Older people may be especially sensitive to the side effects of MAO inhibitors, especially **dizziness** or lightheadedness.

Anyone who has had unusual reactions to MAO inhibitors in the past should let his or her physician know before taking the drugs again. The physician should also be told about any **allergies** to foods, dyes, preservatives, or other substances.

Studies suggest that taking MAO inhibitors during **pregnancy** may increase the risk of **birth defects** or problems in the newborn after birth. MAO inhibitors may pass into breast milk, but no problems have been reported in nursing babies whose mothers took the medicine.

MAO inhibitors may also affect blood sugar levels, and diabetics who take them must be cautious. Before using MAO inhibitors, people with any of these medical problems should make sure their physicians are aware of their conditions:

- Alcohol abuse
- High blood pressure
- Recent **heart attack** or **stroke**
- Heart or blood vessel disease
- Liver disease
- Kidney disease
- Frequent or severe **headache**s
- Epilepsy
- **Parkinson's disease**
- Current or past mental illness
- Asthma or **bronchitis**
- Overactive thyroid
- Pheochromocytoma (a tumor of the adrenal gland).

Taking MAO inhibitors with certain other drugs may affect the way the drugs work or may increase the chance of side effects. The most common side effects are dizziness, lightheadedness, drowsiness, tiredness, weakness, blurred vision, shakiness or trembling, restlessness, sleep problems or twitching during sleep, increased appetite (especially for sweets), weight gain, decreased sexual ability, decreased amount of urine, and mild headache. These problems usually go away as the body adjusts to the drug and do not require medical treatment unless they interfere with normal activities.

More serious side effects may include:

- Severe chest pain
- Severe headache
- Stiff, sore neck
- Enlarged pupils
- Increased sensitivity of eyes to light
- Fast or slow heartbeat
- Sweating, with or without fever or cold, clammy skin
- **Nausea and vomiting**.

Anyone who takes MAO inhibitors must check with his or her physician before taking any other prescription or nonprescription (over-the-counter) medicine. Among the drugs that may interact with MAO inhibitors are:

- Central nervous system (CNS) depressants such as medicine for allergies, colds, hay fever, and asthma; sedatives; tranquilizers; prescription pain medicine; muscle relaxants; medicine for seizures; sleep aids; **barbiturates**; and anesthetics.
- Medicine for high blood pressure
- Other antidepressants, including **tricyclic antidepressants** (such as Tofranil and Norpramin), antidepressants that raise serotonin levels (such as Prozac and Zoloft), and bupropion (Wellbutrin)
- Diabetes medicines taken by mouth
- Insulin
- Water pills (**diuretics**).

See also Antidepressant drugs; Depressive disorders

MONOD, JACQUES LUCIEN (1910-1976)

French biologist

The structure of all living matter is determined by the composition of its deoxyribonucleic acid, or DNA, molecule; the discovery in the early 1950s that the genetic code carried by DNA is responsible for the shape of all the proteins that make up skin, eyes, hair—all the tissues of life—astounded the scientific community at the time. But how this master plan is carried out, and how its instructions are read and followed by the body, were facts discovered much later by French biologist Jacques Lucien Monod and a small cadre of scientists working with him. Monod and his colleagues postulated, and later demonstrated, the process by which messenger ribonucleic acid (mRNA) carries instructions for protein synthesis from the DNA in a cell's nucleus to its cytoplasm, where the instructions are carried out. Monod and two fellow researchers, **Francois Jacob** and **André Lwoff**, won the 1965 Nobel Prize for physiology or medicine.

Monod was born in Paris, on February 9, 1910, to Lucien Hector Monod, a painter and intellectual of Swiss Huguenot descent, and Charlotte Todd (MacGregor) Monod, a Scottish-American from Milwaukee, Wisconsin. At the age of seven, Monod moved with his family to Cannes in the South of France. His parents were very influential in his education, and Monod later credited his father for his own passionate interest in music, and, later, biology. The young Monod learned to play the cello at an early age, and even during the years he was doing research in molecular biology, he played in and directed a string quartet and a Bach choir. Although Monod later confessed a serious inclination towards a career in conducting, he also showed an early interest in biology, collecting beetles and tadpoles in the woods around his southern France home. His interest developed further, and he entered the College de Cannes from where he graduated in the summer of 1928. Monod went on to receive a B.S. from the Faculte des Sciences at the University of Paris, Sorbonne, in 1931. Although he stayed on at the university for further studies, Monod felt that the academic curriculum at the Sorbonne was deficient and did not reflect contemporary biological research. Therefore, it was through the personal contacts he developed during excursions to the nearby Roscoff marine biology station that Monod received his true scientific grounding.

While working at the Roscoff station, Monod met Andre Lwoff, with whom he would establish a life-long collaboration. Lwoff introduced Monod to the potentials of microbiology and microbial nutrition, and these became the focus of Monod's early research. Boris Ephrussi, another scientist working at Roscoff, opened Monod to the importance of physiological and biochemical genetics. And Louis Rapkine, also a Roscoff contemporary, impressed upon Monod the importance of learning the chemical and molecular aspects of living organisms.

During the autumn of 1931 Monod took up a fellowship at the University of Strasbourg in the laboratory of Edouard Chatton, France's leading protistologist. Then, in October, 1932, he won a Commercy Scholarship that called him back to Paris to work at the Sorbonne once again. This time he was an assistant in the Laboratory of the Evolution of Organic Life, which was directed by the French biologist Maurice Caullery at the time. Moving to the zoology department in 1934, Monod became an assistant professor of zoology in less than a year. That summer, Monod also embarked on a natural history expedition to Greenland aboard the *Pourquoi pas?* This expedition was a great success and developed in Monod a life-long love for sailing. In 1936 Monod left for the United States with Ephrussi, where he spent time at the California Institute of Technology on a Rockefeller grant. His research centered on studying the fruit fly (*Drosophila melanogaster*) under the direction of Thomas Hunt Morgan, an American geneticist. Here Monod not only met with refreshingly new opinions, but he also got his first look at a new way of studying science—a research style based on collective effort and a free passage of critical discussion. This was in contrast to the rigid, sometimes sterile, attitude among the faculty at the Sorbonne. Returning to France, Monod completed his studies at the Institute of Physiochemical Biology. In this time he also worked with Georges Teissier, a scientist at the Roscoff station, who influenced Monod's interest in the study of bacterial growth. This later became the subject of Monod's doctoral thesis at the Sorbonne.

This was a time of war in Europe, and despite a medical exemption from military service which allowed him to retain his academic position, Monod joined the French resistance movement. His Sorbonne laboratory became an underground meeting place and propaganda print shop. Thereafter Monod also joined the Franc-Tireurs Partisans and was captured by the Gestapo. He managed to escape and continued his underground resistance efforts. Monod is also credited with helping to organize the general strike that led to Paris' ultimate liberation, and he was honored with several military commendations for his efforts.

During this period Monod also continued his pursuit of music, forming a Bach choir, La Cantate, which he would direct until 1948. In 1938, he met his future wife, Odette Bruhl, an archeologist and orientalist, through the choir. In the postwar period Monod served as the laboratory director of Lwoff's Department, and he also became an officer in the Free France Forces. As a member of General de Lattre de Tassigny's staff, he met a number of American scientists. They provided Monod with several scientific journals in which he read articles about the spontaneous mutations of bacteria. Monod later recalled the influence these articles had on the course of his career. He noted that these journals in particular, lead him to the study of genetics and later, his research into the structure of DNA.

Monod's work comprised four separate but interrelated phases beginning with his practical education at the Sorbonne. In the early years of his education, he concentrated on the kinetic aspects of biological systems, discovering that the growth rate of bacteria could be described in a simple, quantitative way. The size of the colony was solely dependent on the food supply; the more sugar Monod gave the bacteria to feed on, the more they grew. Although there was a direct correlation between the amount of food Monod fed the bacteria and their rate of growth, he also observed that in some colonies of bacteria, growth spread over two phases, sometimes with a period of slow or no growth in between. Monod termed this phenomenon "diauxy" (double growth), and guessed that the bacteria had to employ different enzymes to metabolize different kinds of sugars.

When Monod brought the finding to Lwoff's attention in the winter of 1940, Lwoff suggested that Monod investigate the possibility that he had discovered a form of "enzyme adaptation," in which the latency period represents a hiatus during which the colony is switching between enzymes. In the previous decade, a similar phenomenon had been recorded by the Finnish scientist, Henning Karstroem while working with protein synthesis. Although the outbreak of war and a conflict with his director took Monod away from his lab at the Sorbonne, Lwoff offered him a position in his laboratory at the Pasteur Institute where Monod would remain until 1976. Here he began working with Alice Audureau to investigate the genetic consequences of his kinetic findings, thus beginning the second phase of his work.

To explain his findings with bacteria, Monod shifted his focus to the study of enzyme induction. He theorized that certain colonies of bacteria spent time adapting and producing enzymes capable of processing new kinds of sugars. Although this slowed down the growth of the colony, Monod realized that it was a necessary process as the bacteria needed to adapt to varying environments and foods to survive. Therefore, in devising a mechanism that could be used to sense a change in the environment, and thereby enable the colony to take advantage of the new food, a valuable evolutionary step was taking place. In Darwinian terms, this colony of bacteria would now have a very good chance of surviving, by passing these changes on to future generations. Monod would summarize his research and views on relationship between the roles of random chance and adaptation in evolution in his 1970 book *Chance and Necessity.*

Between 1943 and 1945, working with Melvin Cohn, a specialist in immunology, Monod hit upon the theory that an "inducer" acted as an internal signal of the need to produce the required digestive enzyme. This hypothesis challenged the German biochemist Rudolf Schoenheimer's theory of the ''dynamic state'' of protein production, which stated that it was the mix of proteins that resulted in a large number of random combinations. Monod's theory, in contrast, projected a fairly stable and efficient process of protein production which seemed to be controlled by a master plan. In 1953, Monod and Cohn published their findings on the generalized theory of induction.

That year Monod also became the director of the department of cellular biology at the Pasteur Institute and began his collaboration with Francois Jacob and Jacob's team. In 1955, working with Jacob, he began the third phase of his work by investigating the relationship between the roles of heredity and environment in enzyme synthesis, that is, how the organism creates these vital elements in its metabolic pathway and how it knows when to create them.

It was this research that led Monod and Jacob to formulate their model of protein synthesis. They identified a gene cluster they called the operon, at the beginning of a strand of bacterial DNA. These genes, they postulated, send out messages signalling the beginning and end of the production of a specific protein in the cell, depending on what proteins are needed by the cell in its current environment. Within the operons, Monod and Jacob discovered two key genes, which they named the ''operator ''and ''structural'' genes. The scientists discovered that during protein synthesis, the operator gene sends the signal to begin building the protein. A large molecule then attaches itself to the structural gene to form a strand of messenger RNA (mRNA). In addition to the operon is the regulator gene, which codes for a repressor protein. The repressor protein either attaches to the operator gene and inactivates it, in turn, halting structural gene activity and protein synthesis; or the repressor protein binds to the regulator gene instead of the operator gene, thereby freeing the operator and permitting protein synthesis to occur. As a result of this process, the mRNA, when complete, acts as a template for the creation of a specific protein encoded by the DNA, carrying instructions for protein synthesis from the DNA in the cell's nucleus, to the ribosomes outside the nucleus, where proteins are manufactured. With such a system, a cell can adapt to changing environmental conditions, and produce the proteins it needs when it needs them.

Word of the importance of Monod's work began to spread, and in 1958 he was invited to become professor of biochemistry at the Sorbonne, a position he accepted conditional to his retaining his post at the Pasteur Institute. At the Sorbonne, Monod was the chair of chemistry of metabolism, but in April, 1966, his position was renamed the chair of molecular biology in recognition of his research in creating the new science. His Nobel prize in 1965 both increased his responsibilities and thrust him to the center of a growing limelight in the field of biochemistry.

Monod's life following the Nobel prize reveals a dramatic shift to the administrative side of scientific research. Elected to the College de France and named chair of molecular biology in 1967, Monod used his influence and fame to bolster the cause of the organized student movement against the academic establishment in France. In 1971 he was offered the directorship of the Pasteur Institute and, on April 15, 1971, he was named director general of the institute. At this time the institute was on the verge of financial collapse, and Monod set aside his research to devote all his efforts to modernize and revitalize the organization. As his administrative duties grew, his research activities rapidly slowed and finally stopped in 1972 after the death of his wife. Not long thereafter, Monod himself fell ill with aplastic anemia. Four years later, with his own death imminent, and having completed only the first phase of his intended sweeping changes at the institute, Monod returned to his home in Cannes. He died there on May 31, 1976.

His twin sons, Olivier and Philippe, followed him into scientific research, Olivier as a geologist and Philippe as physicist. Monod's list of awards and honors was impressive, and it included the Montyon Physiology Prize, the Louis Rapkine Medal, and the Charles Leopold Mayer Prize. He was made a Chevalier de l'Ordre des Palmes Academiques and later an officer in the Legion of Honor. He also received both the Croix de Guerre and the Bronze Star Medal.

MONTAGNIER, LUC (1932-)

French virologist

Luc Montagnier of the Institut Pasteur in Paris has devoted his career to the study of viruses. He is perhaps best known for his 1983 discovery of the human immunodeficiency virus (HIV), which has been identified as the cause of acquired immunodeficiency syndrome (**AIDS**). However, in the twenty years before the onset of the AIDS epidemic, Montagnier made many significant discoveries concerning the nature of viruses. He made major contributions to the understanding of how viruses can alter the genetic information of host organisms, and significantly advanced cancer research. His investigation of interferon, one of the body's defenses against viruses, also opened avenues for medical cures for viral diseases. Montagnier's ongoing research focuses on the search for an AIDS vaccine or cure.

Montagnier was born in Chabris (near Tours), France, the only child of Antoine Montagnier and Marianne Rousselet. He became interested in science in his early childhood through his father, an accountant by profession, who carried out experiments on Sundays in a makeshift laboratory in the basement of the family home. At age fourteen, Montagnier himself conducted nitroglycerine experiments in the basement laboratory. His desire to contribute to medical knowledge was also kindled by his grandfather's long illness and death from colon cancer.

Montagnier attended the Collège de Châtellerault, and then the University of Poitiers, where he received the equivalent of a bachelor's degree in the natural sciences in 1953. Continuing his studies at Poitiers and then at the University of Paris, he received his *licence ès sciences* in 1955. As an assistant to the science faculty at Paris, he taught physiology at the Sorbonne and in 1960 qualified there for his doctorate in medicine. He was appointed a researcher at the Centre National de la Recherche Scientifique (C.N.R.S.) in 1960, but then went to London for three and a half years to do research at the Medical Research Council at Carshalton.

Viruses are agents which consist of genetic material surrounded by a protective protein shell. They are completely dependent on the cells of a host animal or plant to multiply, a process which begins with the shedding of their own protein shell. The virus research group at Carshalton was investigating ribonucleic acid (RNA), a form of nucleic acid that normally is involved in taking genetic information from deoxyribonucleic acid (DNA) (the main carrier of genetic information) and translating it into proteins. Montagnier and F. K. Sanders, investigating viral RNA (a virus that carries its genetic material in RNA rather than DNA), discovered a double-stranded RNA virus that had been made by the replication of a single-stranded RNA. The double-stranded RNA could transfer its genetic information to DNA, allowing the virus to encode itself in the genetic make-up of the host organism. This discovery represented a significant advance in knowledge concerning viruses.

From 1963 to 1965, Montagnier did research at the Institute of Virology in Glasgow, Scotland. Working with Ian MacPherson, he discovered in 1964 that agar, a gelatinous extractive of a red alga, was an excellent substance for culturing **cancer** cells. Their technique became standard in laboratories investigating oncogenes (genes that have the potential to make normal cells turn cancerous) and cell transformations. Montagnier himself used the new technique to look for cancer-causing viruses in humans after his return to France in 1965.

From 1965 to 1972, Montagnier worked as laboratory director of the Institut de Radium (later called Institut Curie) at Orsay. In 1972, he founded and became director of the viral oncology unit of the Institut Pasteur. Motivated by his findings at Carshalton and the belief that some cancers are caused by viruses, Montagnier's basic research interest during those years was in retroviruses as a potential cause of cancer. Retroviruses possess an enzyme called reverse transcriptase. Montagnier established that reverse transcriptase translates the genetic instructions of the virus from the viral (RNA) form to DNA, allowing the genes of the virus to become permanently established in the cells of the host organism. Once established, the virus can begin to multiply, but it can do so only by multiplying cells of the host organism, forming malignant tumors. In addition, collaborating with Edward De Mayer and Jacqueline De Mayer, Montagnier isolated the messenger RNA of interferon, the cell's first defense against a virus. Ultimately, this research allowed the cloning of interferon genes in a quantity sufficient for research. However, despite widespread hopes for interferon as a broadly effective anti-cancer drug, it was initially found to be effective in only a few rare kinds of malignancies.

AIDS (acquired immunodeficiency syndrome), a tragic epidemic that emerged in the early 1980s, was first adequately characterized around 1982. Its chief feature is that it disables the immune system by which the body defends itself against numerous diseases. It is eventually fatal. By 1993, more than three million people had developed full-blown AIDS. Montagnier believed that a retrovirus might be responsible for AIDS. Researchers had noted that one pre-AIDS condition involved a persistent enlargement of the lymph nodes, called lymphadenopathy. Obtaining some tissue culture from the lymph nodes of an infected patient in 1983, Montagnier and two colleagues, Françoise Barré-Sinoussi and Jean-Claude Chermann, searched for and found reverse transcriptase, which constitutes evidence of a retrovirus. They isolated a virus they called LAV (lymphadenopathy-associated virus). Later, by international agreement, it was renamed HIV, human immunodeficiency virus. After the virus had been isolated, it was possible to develop a test for antibodies that had developed against it—the HIV test. Montagnier and his group also discovered that HIV attacks T4 cells which are crucial in the immune system. A second similar but not identical HIV virus called HIV–2 was discovered by Montagnier and colleagues in April 1986.

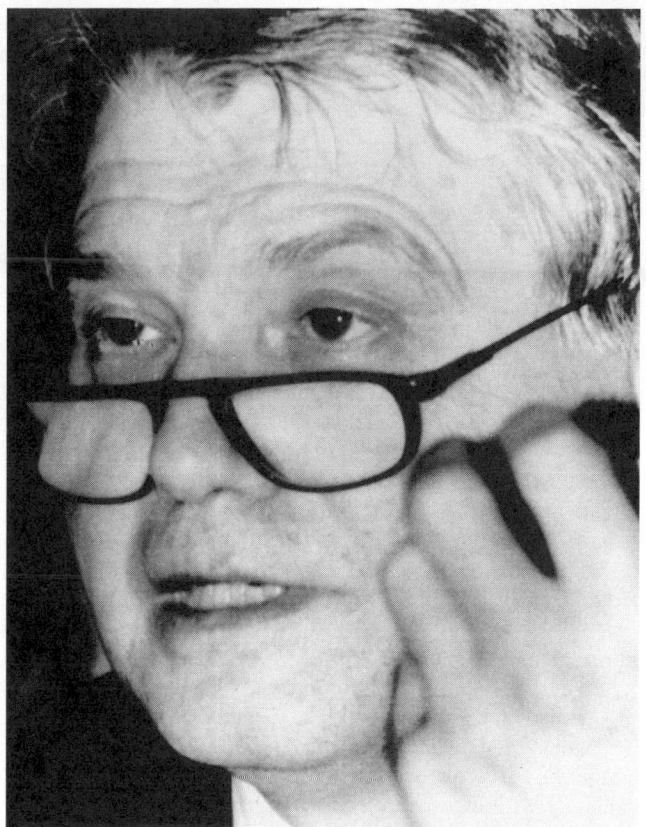

Luc Montagnier

A controversy developed over the patent on the HIV test in the mid–1980s. **Robert C. Gallo** of the National Cancer Institute in Bethesda, Maryland, announced his own discovery of the HIV virus in April 1984 and received the patent on the test. The Institut Pasteur claimed the patent (and the profits) on the basis of Montagnier's earlier discovery of HIV. Despite the controversy, Montagnier continued research and attended numerous scientific meetings with Gallo to share information. Intense mediation efforts by **Jonas Salk** (the scientist who developed the first polio vaccine) led to an international agreement signed by the scientists and their respective countries in 1987. Montagnier and Gallo agreed to be recognized as codiscoverers of the virus, and the two governments agreed that the profits of the HIV test be shared (most going to a foundation for AIDS research).

The scientific dispute continued to resurface, however. Most HIV viruses from different patients differ by six to twenty percent because of the remarkable ability of the virus to mutate. However, Gallo's virus was less than two percent different from Montagnier's, leading to the suspicion that both viruses were from the same source. The laboratories had exchanged samples in the early 1980s, which strengthened the suspicion. Charges of scientific misconduct on Gallo's part led to an investigation by the National Institutes of Health in 1991, which initially cleared Gallo. In 1992 the investigation was reviewed by the newly created Office of Research Integrity. The ORI report, issued in March of 1993, confirmed that Gallo had in fact "discovered" the virus sent to him by Montagnier. Whether or not Gallo had been aware of this fact in 1983 could not be established, but it was found that he had been guilty of misrepresentations in reporting his research and that his supervision of his research lab had been desultory. The Institut Pasteur immediately revived its claim to the exclusive right to the patent on the HIV test. Gallo objected to the decision by the ORI, however, and took his case before an appeals board at the Department of Health and Human Services. The board in December of 1993 cleared Gallo of all charges, and the ORI subsequently withdrew their charges for lack of proof.

Montagnier's continuing work includes investigation of the envelope proteins of the virus that link it to the T-cell. He is also extensively involved in research of possible drugs to combat AIDS. In 1990 Montagnier hypothesized that a second organism, called a mycoplasma, must be present with the HIV virus for the latter to become deadly. This suggestion, which has proved controversial among most AIDS researchers, is the subject of ongoing research.

Montagnier married Dorothea Ackerman in 1961. They have three children, Jean-Luc, Anne-Marie, and Francine. He has described himself as an aggressive researcher who spends much time either in the laboratory or traveling to scientific meetings. He enjoys swimming and classical music, and loves to play the piano, especially Mozart sonatas.

MOOD DISORDERS

Mood disorders are mental disorders characterized by periods of **depression**, sometimes alternating with periods of elevated mood. While many people go through sad or elated moods from time to time, people with mood disorders suffer from severe or prolonged mood states that disrupt their daily functioning. Among the general mood disorders classified in the fourth edition (1994) of the *Diagnostic and Statistical Manual of Mental Disorders* (*DSM-IV*) are major depressive disorder, **bipolar disorder**, and dysthymia.

In classifying and diagnosing mood disorders, doctors determine if the mood disorder is unipolar or bipolar. When only one extreme in mood (the depressed state) is experienced, the depression is called unipolar. Major depression refers to a single severe period of depression, marked by negative or hopeless thoughts and physical symptoms like fatigue. In major depressive disorder, some patients have isolated episodes of depression. In between these episodes, the patient does not feel depressed or have other symptoms associated with depression. Other patients have more frequent episodes.

Bipolar depression or bipolar disorder (sometimes called manic depression) refers to a condition in which people experience two extremes in mood. They alternate between depression (the "low" mood) and mania or hypomania (the "high" mood), which are abnormal elevations in mood. Mania and hypomania are similar, but mania is usually more severe and debilitating to the patient. The person may be excessively cheerful, have grandiose ideas, and may sleep less. They may talk nonstop for hours, have unending enthusiasm, and demonstrate poor judgement. Sometimes the elevation in mood is marked by irritability and hostility rather than cheerfulness. The patient may seem to be in a frenzy and will often make poor, bizarre, or dangerous choices in his/her personal and professional lives. Hypomania is not as severe as mania and does not cause the level of impairment in work and social activities that mania can.

Dysthymia is a recurrent or lengthy depression that may last a lifetime. It is similar to major depressive disorder, but dysthymia is chronic, long-lasting, persistent, and mild. Patients may have symptoms that are not as severe as major depression, but the symptoms last for many years. It seems that a mild form of the depression is always present. In some cases, people may also experience a major depressive episode on top of their dysthymia, a condition sometimes referred to as a "double depression."

Mood disorders tend to run in families. These disorders are associated with imbalances in certain chemicals that carry signals between brain cells (neurotransmitters). These chemicals include serotonin, norepinephrine, and dopamine. Women are more vulnerable to unipolar depression than are men. Major life **stress**ors (like divorce, serious financial problems, **death** of a family member, etc.) will often provoke the symptoms of depression in susceptible people.

Major depression is more serious than just feeling "sad" or "blue." The symptoms of major depression may include:

- Loss of appetite
- A change in the sleep pattern, like not sleeping (**insomnia**) or sleeping too much
- Feelings of worthlessness, hopelessness, or inappropriate guilt
- Fatigue
- Difficulty in concentrating or making decisions
- Overwhelming and intense feelings of sadness or grief
- Disturbed thinking. The person may also have physical symptoms like stomachaches or **headache**s.

Doctors diagnose mood disorders based on the patient's description of the symptoms and the patient's family history. The length of time the patient has had symptoms is also important. Generally patients are diagnosed with dysthymia if they feel depressed more days than not for at least two years. In major depressive disorder, the patient is depressed almost all day nearly every day of the week for at least two weeks. The depression is severe. Sometimes laboratory tests are performed to rule out other causes for the symptoms (like thyroid disease). The diagnosis may be confirmed when a patient responds well to medication.

The most effective treatment for mood disorders is a combination of medication and psychotherapy. The four different classes of drugs used in mood disorders are heterocyclic antidepressants (HCAs), selective serotonin reuptake inhibitors (SSRI inhibitors), **monoamine oxidase inhibitors** (MAOI inhibitors), and mood stabilizers such as lithium.

A number of psychotherapy approaches are useful as well. Interpersonal psychotherapy helps the patient recognize the interaction between the mood disorder and interpersonal relationships. Cognitive-behavioral therapy explores how the patient's view of the world may be affecting his or her mood and outlook.

When depression fails to respond to treatment or when there is a high risk of suicide, **electroconvulsive therapy** (ECT) is sometimes used. ECT is believed to affect neurotransmitters like the medications do. Patients are anesthetized and given **muscle relaxants** to minimize discomfort. Then low-level electric current is passed through the brain to cause a brief convulsion. The most common side effect of ECT is mild, short-term memory loss.

There are many alternative therapies that may help in the treatment of mood disorders, including **acupuncture**, botanical medicine, **homeopathy**, **aromatherapy**, constitutional **hydrotherapy**, and light therapy. Short-term clinical studies have shown that the herb St. John's wort (*Hypericum perforatum*) can effectively treat some types of depression. Though it appears very safe, the herb may have some side effects and its long-term effectiveness has not been proven. It has not been tested in patients with bipolar disorder. St. John's wort and antidepressant drugs should not be taken simultaneously.

Most cases of mood disorders can be successfully managed if properly diagnosed and treated. People can also take steps to improve mild depression and keep it from becoming a condition that needs medical attention. For example, stress management (like relaxation training or breathing exercises), **exercise**, and avoidance of drugs or alcohol may be beneficial in improving a mild depression or mood disorder.

See also Bipolar disorder; Depressive disorders; Psychoanalysis

MORGAGNI, GIOVANNI BATTISTA (1682-1771)

Italian Physician

Giovanni Battista Morgagni was born at Forli, Italy, on February 20, 1682; he died at Padua on December 6, 1771. He was educated at the University of Bologna, receiving a degree in philosophy and medicine there in 1701. He studied under A. M. Valsalva (1666–1723), whom he venerated for the rest of his life; when Valsalva left Bologna for Parma, Morgagni succeeded him as demonstrator in anatomy. He was made President of the *Accademia* at the age of 24, and he gained a reputation for his dislike of speculation as opposed to accurate observation. In 1706 he began publication of a series of anatomical works, which led to his becoming known in Europe as an anatomist. In 1712, he left Bologna for Padua, where, except for a short unsuccessful attempt at practicing medicine in Forli, he was to spend the rest of his life as Professor of Anatomy. Shortly after settling in Padua, he married Paola Vergieri of Forli, with whom he had 15 children. His eight daughters all entered convents, which is said to have caused him considerable sadness near the end of his life. After his wife died in 1770, the aged widower did not have much desire to continue living. Ironically, his life, which had contributed so much to the understanding of the pathological basis of **stroke**, came to an end on December 6, 1771, when he (like his teacher Valsalva before him) succumbed to the condition.

Morgagni taught at the renowned University of Padua for 56 years (1715 to 1771). His greatest professional achievement came in 1761 when, at the age of 79, he published his masterpiece, *De Sedibus et Causis Morborum* (translated into English as *On the Sites and Causes of Disease*). The book, consisting of five volumes of letters (for a total of 70 letters), described Morgagni's observations of some 700 autopsies, and it included his correlations between clinical symptoms and postmortem findings (lesions) for each of the cases studied. (Morgagni expressed his debt in *De Sedibus* to previously published work by Theophile Bonet, 1629-1689, although the latter's work, *Sepulcretum*, translated in English as *Graves*), is generally considered to be a poorly organized and inconclusive summary of autopsy findings up to 1679.) It was Morgagni's study that introduced the clinical principles and practices that are still used today. Morgagni also drew on the ideas of **Hippocrates**, whose methods of observation and reasoning formed the basis for many of Morgagni's own ideas. For example, whereas Hippocrates made systematic differentiations of diseases based on observed external symptoms, Morgagni went farther and related the external expressions of the particular disease to the internal conditions within the body. Morgagni thus focused on the internal damage within the body that gives rise to disease. In clinical practice, Morgagni carefully noted the symptoms during the course of a patient's illness, and then attempted to identify the organic or pathological causes of that disease during the postmortem examination.

Because Morgagni's studies were so extensive, it became possible for him to predict or visualize internal conditions based on symptomatic observations. Morgagni's work was also instrumental in debunking the ancient humoral theory of disease, according to which there is one cause for all diseases. Morgagni's *De Sedibus* clearly identifies the pathologies of a number of diseases, including hepatic **cirrhosis** (acute yellow atrophy), cerebral gummata, cardiac valvular lesions, renal **tuberculosis**, pneumonic solidification of the lungs, and syphilitic lesions (**aneurysms**) of the brain. Morgagni also proved,

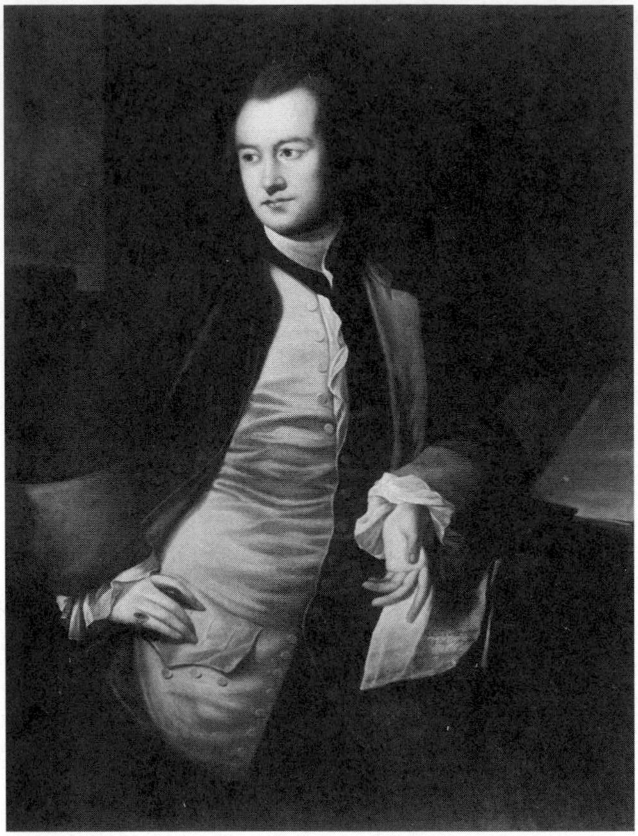
John Morgan

through many autopsies, that cerebral lesion in stroke occurs on the opposite side from the resulting **paralysis**. Morgagni has bequeathed his name to many anatomical part's and conditions of the human body, e.g., the Morgagnian cataract.

Morgagni was held in high esteem by his colleagues and students; he was the friend of many Venetian senators and several popes. His international reputation was attested to by his election to the *Academia Naturae Curiosorum* (1708); the Academy of Science, Paris (1731); the Imperial Academy of St. Petersburg (1735); and the Berlin Academy (1754).

Morgagni was largely responsible during the more than 50 years he spent as a professor at the University of Padua for that university's foremost reputation in Europe during the 18th century. Besides being recognized today as one of the leading figures in 18th-century medicine, he is considered the father of morbid anatomy, and a founder of modern anatomy and **pathology**.

See also Human anatomy

MORGAN, JOHN (1735-1789)

American Physician

John Morgan was born June 10, 1735 in Philadelphia, Pennsylvania; he died on October 15, 1789 in the same city. He was the son of Evan Morgan, a realtor and dealer in iron and hardware, and Joanna Biles Morgan. He married Mary Hopkinson in 1765 (they had no children). His education consisted of matriculation from Reverend Finley's Nottingham Academy; graduation with an A.B. degree from the College of Philadelphia in 1757; a medical apprenticeship with John Redman; studies in London and Edinburgh from 1760 through 1763, culminating with his taking the M.D. degree from the University of Edinburgh in 1763 (where he studied under William Hunter, the Munros, and William Cullen); and finally postgraduate studies in Paris and Italy from 1763 to 1765. In 1765 he returned to Philadelphia where he began his medical practice. In the same year he was appointed Professor of Theory and Practice of Physic at the College of Philadelphia. From 1775 on, he served as Director-General of Hospitals and Physician-in-Chief of the Continental Army, but the enmity of his subordinates and the nature of Revolutionary politics led to his being dismissed from his position by Congress in 1777 and to his replacement by William Shippen. From 1773 to 1783 he was senior medical officer at Pennsylvania Hospital. Following two years of deliberation, a court of inquiry honorably acquitted Morgan in 1779 of all charges that had led to his dismissal as Director-General of the Army. But these events had by then taken their toll on Morgan, and he returned to private practice, broken in spirit, poor, and in ill health. He died 12 years later.

John Morgan was a principal founder, with Shippen, of the first medical school in America and of the American Physical Society and the College of Physicians of Philadelphia. As Director General and Physician-in-Chief of the Continental Army, he attempted to improve the quality of medical care provided to members of the American army, and insisted on rigorous examinations for medical officers and on the subordination of regimental surgeons to the hospital chiefs. Morgan's library became the cornerstone for the Library of the College of Physicians. Among his writings were *A Discourse upon the Institution of Medical Schools in America* (1765), which files the first brief for adequate medical education in this country and commemorates the organization at the College of Philadelphia of the Medical Department of the University of Pennsylvania; *A Recommendation of Inoculation According to Baron Dimsdale's Method* (1776); *A Vindication of His Public Character in the Station of Director-General of the Military Hospitals* (1777), in which he ably defends his actions as Director-General of the Army and demands a court of inquiry to investigate the grounds for his dismissal.

See also Military medicine

MORGAN, THOMAS HUNT (1866-1945)

American geneticist

Thomas Hunt Morgan was born on September 25, 1866, in Lexington, Kentucky. As a child growing up in rural Kentucky, he was surrounded by nature and wildlife. Perhaps that environment contributed to his intense interest in biology, for

Morgan later majored in zoology at State College of Kentucky. After his graduation in 1886, he investigated chemistry and morphology (the study of organism development to better understand evolutionary relationships) at Johns Hopkins University, completing his doctorate in 1890. From his graduate days on, Morgan believed that heredity was in some way central to understanding all biological phenomena—especially development and evolution. His persistence in trying to prove and develop heredity theories led to his winning the Nobel Prize for physiology or medicine in 1933.

In 1903, there were several attempts to explain variations in plants and animal species. One was Charles Darwin's theory of natural selection, a process by which organisms best adapted to local environments leave more offspring that survive to spread their favorable traits throughout a population. But Morgan wondered how complex organisms such as humans could have evolved from such a process. To him, the theory seemed incomplete. Morgan viewed natural selection as a process that sorted out variations in an organism, not as one that created the variations. So what was it that determined whether a baby would be a boy or a girl, or whether it would have blue eyes or green eyes? The three widely known heredity theories of the time offered competing explanations: the Mendelian (or gene) theory, the chromosome theory, and the mutation theory.

Gregor Mendel, by cross-breeding pea plants, had first determined some of the rules of inheritable traits—those of sex determination, gene linkage (inheritance of characteristics together), and mimicry. Advocates of the chromosome theory maintained that genes located on chromosomes were responsible for specific inherited traits. Morgan was skeptical of the Mendelian and chromosome theories because the conclusions were speculative, based on nothing more than observation, inference, and analogy. Morgan wanted to be able to draw firm, rigorous, testable conclusions based on quantitative and analytical data. His strong belief in experimental analysis attracted Morgan to Hugo de Vries's mutation theory. De Vries, a Dutch botanist, had physical evidence that large-scale variations in one generation could produce offspring that were of a different species than their parent plants. Morgan set out to test de Vries's theory in animals and also to disprove the other heredity theories.

His first experiments using the fruit fly (*Drosophila melanogaster*) were unsuccessful; Morgan was not able to duplicate the magnitude of mutations that de Vries had claimed for plants. Then in 1910, Morgan noticed a natural mutation in one of the male fruit flies: it had white eyes instead of red. He began breeding the white-eyed male to its red-eyed sisters and found that all of the offspring had red eyes. When Morgan bred those offspring, he found that they produced a second generation of both red- and white-eyed fruit flies. Morgan was fascinated to find that all of the white-eyed flies were male. He traced the unusual finding to a difference between male and female chromosomes. The white-eye gene of the fruit fly was located on the male sex chromosome. By studying future generations of fruit flies, Morgan found that genes were linearly arranged on chromosomes. His work with the fruit fly strongly backed Mendel's gene concept and, moreover, established that chromosomes definitely carried genetic traits. For the first time, the association of one or more hereditary characteristics with specific chromosomes was clear, thereby unifying Mendelian ''trait'' theory and chromosome theory.

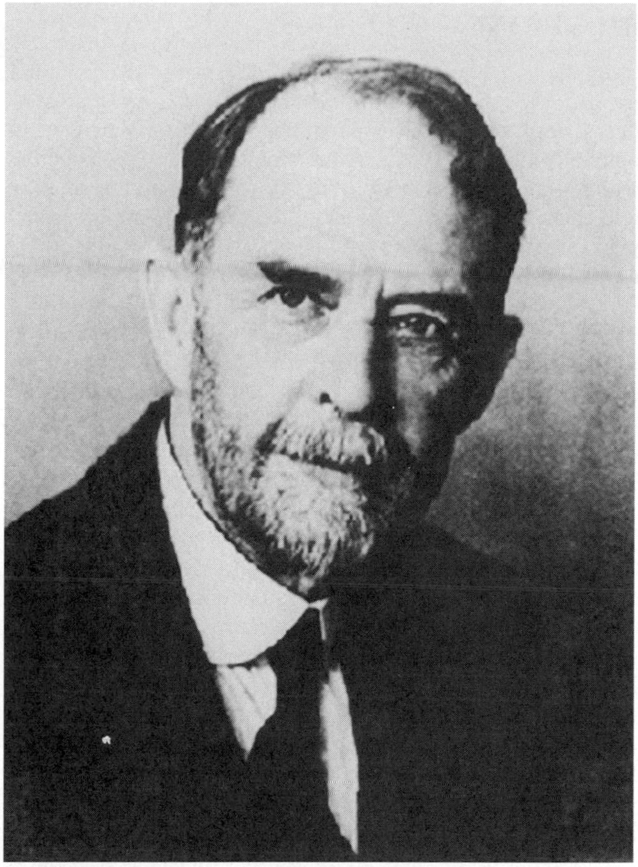

Thomas Hunt Morgan

That was only the first of Morgan's discoveries. Working with students **Hermann Muller**, Alfred H. Sturtevant, and Calvin Bridges, Morgan went on to develop and perfect his concepts of linkage by explaining why, for instance, he occasionally found a white-eyed female in his studies. Morgan concluded that traits found on the same chromosome were not always inherited together. This genetic ''mistake'' was called crossing over, because one chromosome actually exchanged material with (or crossed over to) another chromosome. This process was an important source of genetic diversity. In 1915, Morgan, along with his students, published the culmination of his work, *The Mechanism of Mendelian Heredity*. These results provided the key to all further work in the area of genetics and laid the groundwork for all genetically-based research.

In 1904, Morgan had married Lilian Vaughan Sampson, who assisted in his research. They had one son and three daughters. Morgan died in 1945.

See also Genetics

Morphine

Morphine is the most effective naturally occurring compound used for the relief of **pain** in medicine and surgery. It also induces sleep and produces euphoria. The active ingredient in opium, from which it is derived, morphine is highly addictive with repeated use. Its story is the story of the founding of alkaloid chemistry, which grew out of the study of plant bases and plays an essential role in medicine.

In 1805, opium was widely used for its euphoric effects, and a German pharmacist named Friedrich Sertürner (1783-1841) decided to investigate the components of poppy juice, from which opium is derived. He found an unknown acid, converted it into a crystalline precipitate, and named it principium somniferum. Having determined that this substance was the active ingredient in opium, in 1809 he recommended the cultivation of the poppy on a large scale as a way to further the national economy since morphine was used in the production of the popular drug and poppy seed oil.

In 1815, Sertürner and three young volunteers each took three 30 mg doses of principium somniferum over a period of 45 minutes, and were not fully themselves again until several days later. In 1817 he published a paper describing the drug, in which he changed its name to *morphium*, after Morpheus, the Greek god of dreams. The same year, the name was changed to ''morphine'' by the French chemist Joseph Gay-Lussac.

During the 1800s, the French physiologist François Magendie advanced the use of morphine in medicine, administering it both orally and by injection. Morphine's greatest medical advantage is its depressant action, which causes the threshold of pain to rise, relieving pain many other analgesics are unable to control. Its narcotic properties also produce a calming effect, protecting the body's system in traumatic shock. Its greatest disadvantage, however, is its addictiveness.

Morphine is an alkaloid, which means that it is an organic compound that contains carbon, hydrogen and nitrogen, and which forms a water-soluble salt. The chemistry of alkaloids is crucial in medicine; the analgesic properties of the opium alkaloids are a case in point, but other examples of important alkaloids include strychnine, which is a respiratory stimulant; codeine, which is a painkiller; and conine, which is the active ingredient in hemlock and was responsible for the poisoning of Socrates (469 B.C.-399 B.C.). Sertürner's groundbreaking research provided the foundations for the field of alkaloid chemistry and these contributions to medicine.

Morphine's popularity on the Civil War battlefields boosted its general use in the treatment of many kinds of discomfort, and a leading British doctor called morphine ''God's own medicine.'' However, thousands of people worldwide were tragically addicted. Many chronicles of **addiction** have been written, including Eugene O'Neill's (1888-1953) semi-autobiographical play *Long Day's Journey Into Night*. Once addicted, a person is likely to experience severe symptoms of withdrawal, including pain, hyperventilation, restlessness and confusion.

In 1898, the Bayer corporation synthesized heroin from morphine and marketed it as an antidote to morphine addiction, but the concurrent moral reform movements were beginning to give rise to anti-opiate sentiments, and morphine's popularity and acceptance began to decline. Today, morphine is often replaced in medicine by methadone, which also treats chronic pain and prevents morphine withdrawal symptoms.

Morton, William Thomas Green (1819-1868)

American Dental Surgeon

Morton was the first person to show publicly that ether could be used as an anesthetic during surgery. After his demonstration, the use of ether as an anesthetic spread rapidly to Europe.

Morton was born August 9, 1819, to James and Rebecca Morton. His father was a farmer. Though Morton wanted to be a physician, his father could not afford the tuition, so Morton settled for a diploma from the Baltimore College of Dental Surgery in 1840. He then practiced dentistry for several years. In 1844, he married Elizabeth Whitman. They had five children.

Several people had used ether as an anesthetic before Morton. Another dentist, Dr. Elijah Pope, extracted a patient's tooth using ether in January, 1842. Two months later, **Crawford Williamson Long**, a physician, used ether to remove cysts from a patient's neck. Neither Pope nor Long publicized their applications of ether, and so Morton was first given credit for using ether as an anesthetic. Like many people of his time, Morton knew that some gases could make a person insensible to pain. Scientific lecturers traveled America promoting the discoveries of new substances, among them, nitrous oxide (laughing gas), and ether. Typically, the lecturer would give one of these substances to a member of the audience, who would stagger around intoxicated or burst into fits of laughter. Hardly anyone thought that these chemicals could be anesthetics. In fact, **Oliver Wendell Holmes** did not invent the term ''anesthetic'' until November, 1846.

One person who made the connection was a dentist partner of Morton's, Horace Wells. Wells had one of his own teeth extracted while using nitrous oxide, and he felt nothing. He wanted to show others this new application of nitrous oxide. He persuaded Dr. John Collins Warren, a famous Boston surgeon, to let him demonstrate nitrous oxide to a class of medical students at the Massachusetts General Hospital. During the operation, someone prematurely removed the bag supplying the nitrous oxide to the young patient, who yelled out as though he were in pain. The assembled medical students thought the demonstration was a hoax, and they shouted insults at Wells. Though the patient later said he had felt no pain, Wells' career was doomed. He committed suicide in jail in January1848.

Morton had assisted Wells during the failed demonstration at Massachusetts General Hospital, and he refused to repeat Wells' mistake. Morton consulted with one of his teachers, Charles T. Jackson, who suggested that he use sulfuric ether. Morton then thoroughly studied the application of sulfuric ether in dental surgery. He even disguised its odor by blending it with aromatic chemicals. He called the resulting compound, "letheon." Morton tried his ether compound on one patient on September 30, 1846, and it successfully worked. One Boston newspaper, the *Journal*, reported his success the next day. Then Morton tried another demonstration with the same Dr. Warren at the Massachusetts General Hospital. On October 16, 1846, as a number of medical students watched, Morton applied ether to his patient, Gilbert Abbot. Then, with Abbot safely unconscious, Morton removed a tumor from his jaw. Abbot felt nothing. After his successful demonstration, Morton made a point of telling the assembled students that his "letheon" was no hoax. Before 1846 was over, ether was used in surgeries in London and Paris.

Having triumphed in the surgical auditorium, Morton promptly made a costly mistake. He tried to prevent others from using his ether anesthesia, and he became embroiled in a legal battle with Charles T. Jackson over who had first discovered the anesthetic properties of ether. Jackson claimed that Morton was acting as his agent, Morton claimed otherwise, and Morton eventually lost his practice and nearly all of his money fighting Jackson. Jackson eventually died in an insane asylum, and on July 15, 1868, Morton died in poverty in New York City. When Oliver Wendell Holmes was asked his opinion about who should get the credit for discovering the anesthetic properties of ether, he punned, "e(i)ther."

See also Crawford Williamson Long

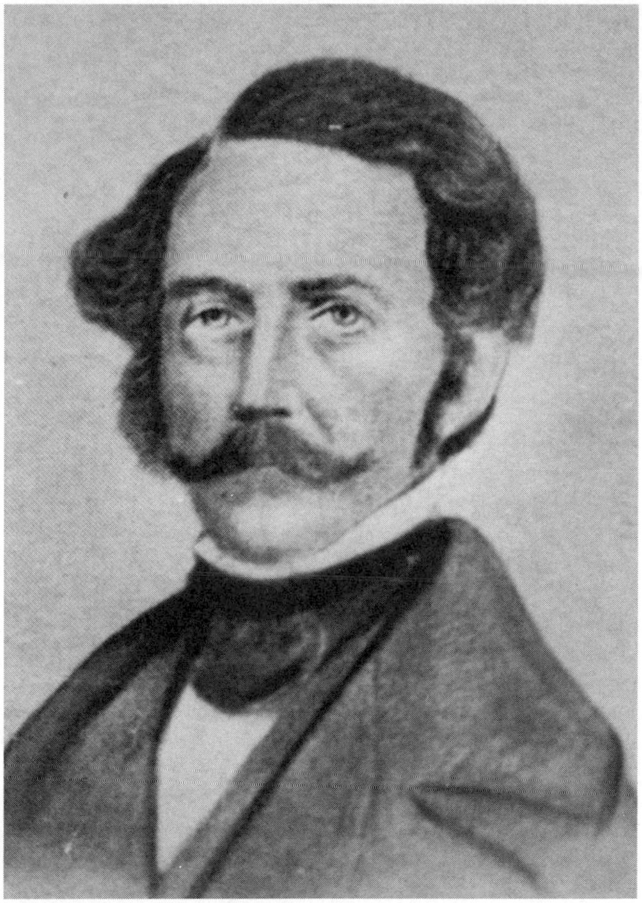

William Thomas Green Morton

MOTION SICKNESS

Motion sickness is the uncomfortable **dizziness**, nausea, and vomiting that people experience when their sense of balance and equilibrium are disturbed by constant motion. Motion sickness is a common problem, with nearly 80% of the population enduring its affects at one time in their lives. While it may occur at any age, motion sickness most often afflicts children over the age of two, with the majority outgrowing their susceptibility.

When looking at why motion sickness occurs, it is helpful to understand the role of the sensory organs. The sensory organs control a body's sense of balance by telling the brain what direction the body is pointing, the direction it is moving, and if it is standing still or turning. These messages are relayed by the inner ears, the eyes, the skin pressure receptors (such as in those in the feet), and the muscle and joint sensory receptors. The central nervous system (the brain and spinal cord) is responsible for processing all incoming sensory information.

Motion sickness and its symptoms surface when conflicting messages are sent to the central nervous system. An example of this is reading a book in the back seat of a moving car. The inner ears and skin receptors sense the motion, but the eyes register only the stationary pages of the book. This conflicting information may cause the usual motion sickness symptoms of dizziness, **nausea, and vomiting**.

While all five of the body's sensory organs contribute to motion sickness, excess stimulation to the vestibular system within the inner ear (the body's "balance center") is the primary reason for this condition. Balance problems or dizziness are caused by a conflict between what is seen and how the inner ear perceives it, leading to confusion in the brain. This confusion may result in higher heart rates, rapid breathing, nausea and sweating, dizziness, and vomiting.

Pure optokinetic motion sickness is caused solely by visual stimuli, or what is seen. The optokinetic system is the reflex that allow the eyes to move when an object moves. Many people suffer when what they view is rotating or swaying, even if they are standing still.

Additional factors that may contribute to the occurrence of motion sickness include: poor ventilation; **anxiety** or fear; a full stomach; alcohol; and a genetic predisposition to motion sickness.

Often viewed as a minor annoyance, some travelers are temporarily immobilized by motion sickness, and a few continue to feel its effects for hours and even days after a trip. Most cases of motion sickness are mild and self-treatable disorders. Severe cases of motion sickness symptoms, and those that become progressively worse, may require the attention of a doctor with specialized skills in diseases of the ear, nose, throat, equilibrium, and neurological system.

Medications that help ease the symptoms of motion sickness are available without a prescription (over-the-counter or OTC medicine). Alcohol should be avoided when taking any drug for motion sickness. Large doses of drugs for motion sickness may also cause dry mouth and occasional blurred vision. People with emphysema, chronic **bronchitis**, **glaucoma**, or difficulty urinating due to an **enlarged prostate** should not use OTC drugs for motion sickness unless directed to by their doctor.

Longer trips may require a prescription medication called scopolamine (Transderm Scop). Formerly used in the transdermal skin patch (now discontinued), it is now available in the form of a prescription gel. The gel is most effective when smeared on the arm or neck and covered with a bandage.

Alternative treatments for motion sickness have become widely accepted. Ginger (*Zingiber officinale*) in various forms is often used to calm the stomach. It is now known that the oils ginger contains to relax the intestinal tract and mildly depress the central nervous system. Some of the most effective forms of ginger include the powdered, encapsulated form; ginger tea prepared from sliced ginger root; or candied pieces. All forms of ginger should be taken on an empty stomach.

Placing manual pressure on the **acupuncture** point located about three finger-widths above the wrist on the inner arm, either by acupuncture, **acupressure**, or a mild, electrical pulse, has been shown to be effective against the symptoms of motion sickness. Elastic wristbands sold at most drugstores are also used to put pressure on this area.

Motion sickness is easier to prevent than to eliminate once it has begun. The following steps may help prevent the unpleasant symptoms of motion sickness:

- Avoid reading while traveling, and do not sit in a backward facing seat.
- Always ride where the eyes may see the same motion that the body and inner ears feel. Safe positions include the front seat of the car while looking at distant scenery; the deck of a ship where the horizon can be seen; and sitting by the window of an airplane. The least motion on an airplane is in a seat over the wings.
- Maintain a fairly straight-ahead view.
- Eat a light meal before traveling, or if already nauseated, avoid food altogether.
- Take motion sickness medicine at least 30-60 minutes before travel begins.

While there is no cure for motion sickness, its symptoms can be controlled or even prevented. Most people respond successfully to treatment, or avoid the unpleasant symptoms through prevention methods.

Motor development

Developing motor (muscular movement) skills is an essential part of normal child development. Muscles are controlled by the brain, which learns through experience how to send proper signals to muscles controlling such motor activities as walking, balancing, throwing, and writing. Even the simplest of motor skills may be far more complex than is readily apparent. For example, no fewer than 200 opposing muscles must coordinate just to allow an infant to stand.

In a newborn child, the first movements are random, involving the larger muscles. Through developmental experiences, the child progresses to intentional motions: grasping objects with the hands, rolling over, standing, walking, and then to complex activities such as catching a ball, which requires carefully co-ordinated use of the eyes and hands.

Gross motor skills are those that involve large muscles. Fine motor skills use the smaller muscles (such as those in the fingers) in conjunction with the eyes.

Some typical motor development milestones follow:

- Smiling, 1 month
- Rolling over, 5 months
- Sitting, 7 months
- Crawling, 8 months
- Creeping, 10 months
- Standing, 11 months
- Walking, 13 months
- Talking (words), 10 months
- Talking (sentences), 21 months

When considering the above list of development milestones, it is important to remember that all children learn at their own pace. Many perfectly normal children will progress faster or slower than their colleagues. For instance, the typical range for walking is between eight and 18 months, and for talking (words) is from six to 14 months.

Parents may encourage gross motor development by providing indoor and outdoor play environments that promote motor skills. These may include balls, swings, slides, jungle gyms, or an improvised obstacle course. Such equipment should be checked regularly to make sure it is safe. Watch for loose nuts or bolts, splinters, sharp edges, and other hazards. Fine motor skills may be encouraged by providing pegboards, shape sorters, building blocks, popbeads, ring stackers, puzzles, crayons, chalk, paint, and craft supplies.

When selecting age-appropriate motor activities for a child, it is important to choose those that encourage, not frustrate. Some children will try almost anything, while others may be 'motor cautious' and may choose to let others lead, observing them before attempting the activity themselves.

Motor vehicle safety

Considering the physical size of the United States, where people regularly travel over large distances for recreation and as a means of getting to work, it is not surprising that dependence on the automobile has become so prevalent. There is something fundamentally appealing about traveling in a vehicle that allows for sudden changes in plans and routine.

Driving is as likely to provide headaches as pleasure, however, depending on whether one happens to be speeding along on an the open-road or stuck in a traffic jam. But above all, driving can also be, and frequently is, fatal.

In 1997, 41,967 people died in highway accidents in this country, down slightly from the previous year. In addition, motor vehicle accidents cost more than $150 billion every year in medical, **rehabilitation** and long-term care costs, lost productivity, lost tax revenue, property damage, and police, judicial, and social service costs. In light of these facts, it is quite surprising that highway safety expenses account for only one percent of the budget of the U.S. Department of Transportation.

Alcohol impairment is the leading factor in automobile fatalities. In 1997, alcohol was a factor in 39 percent of all fatal traffic crashes. The second most important problem was excessive speed, which contributed to approximately one-third of all fatal crashes.

In an attempt to make driving safer, automobile manufacturers have added seatbelts, shoulder straps, headrests, airbags, padded dashes, safety glass, collapsible steering columns, controlled crush characteristics, anti-lock breaks, and many other improvements to new vehicles. In addition, improvements in highway construction have led to a decrease in the number accidents and deaths among drivers. Stricter enforcement of drunk-driving laws have removed many intoxicated drivers from the road.

The Advocates for Highway and Auto Safety organization suggests the following tips for safe driving. First, make sure you are clear-headed before you get behind the wheel. Alcohol and drugs (including prescription drugs), can severely impair your ability to drive. Pay attention to the labels on the bottles of any medications you are taking. If a label says the medication you are taking causes drowsiness, don't drive. Consult your doctor or pharmacist if you have any questions. Make sure you have had a good night's rest. Always designate another driver or select an alternate means of transportation if you are in doubt about your ability to drive safely. Try not to drive alone when you are tired. Driving when accompanied by a passenger can increase your alertness. Driving while sleep-deprived at night can increase your chances of a crash. Plan your trips ahead of time. Give yourself plenty of time to reach your destination, allowing for emergencies and traffic jams. By planning ahead, you will be more relaxed when operating your vehicle. You will also be less likely to experience road rage, or feel the need for excessive speeding, tailgating, or weaving between cars.

When you shop for a new car, research the safety performance of the vehicle you are thinking about buying. Find out how the vehicle performs in crash tests. Look for side-impact air bags. If you are shopping for a used vehicle, look for one with air bags. Buy a safe vehicle to protect you and your family in the event of a collision. When you are in the driver's seat, be relaxed. Be alert to signs of fatigue; if you start to feel tired while driving, pull over and let someone else drive. Always follow common sense safety rules, being sure to use seat belts and other restraints. Always keep your eyes on the road, and make sure any important items such as directions and maps, sunglasses, etc. are in easy reach before you set out, and be sure to pull over to a safe place before you attempt to use a cellular telephone.

Although there are 18.1 auto-related deaths per 100,000 people for all ages in this country, male drivers between 15 and 24 years of age have 48.2 auto-related deaths per 100,000 population, a rate that is 2 1/2 times the national average. The rate for female drivers between 15 and 24 years of age is 18.4 auto-related deaths per 100,000 population, or approximately the national average. These figures suggest that young male drivers stand to gain the most from adopting safer driving habits. According to automobile insurance companies, teenage driving deaths frequently occur after dark, in the presence of passengers other than family members, after using alcohol, and during recreational use of the automobile.

Experts point out a number of precautions that the male teenage driver can and should take to increase his safety on the road.

First, he should take a driver's education course; these courses have been demonstrated to decrease the frequency of accidents among those that have taken them. For the first 3 to 6 months after obtaining his driver's license, the teenager should not drive alone; he should not carry passengers; and he should avoid driving after dark. Above all, he should become knowledgeable about the effects of alcohol.

See also Accidents; Adolescent health; Alcohol use and abuse; Drunk driving

Movement disorders

Movement disorders are a group of diseases and syndromes affecting the ability to produce and control movement.

Though it seems simple and effortless, normal movement in fact requires an astonishingly complex system of control. Disruption of any portion of this system can cause a person to produce movements that are too weak, too forceful, too uncoordinated, or too poorly controlled for the task at hand. Unwanted movements may occur at rest. Intentional movement may become impossible. Such conditions are called movement disorders.

Abnormal movements themselves are symptoms of underlying disorders. In some cases, the abnormal movements are the only symptoms. Disorders causing abnormal movements include:

- **Parkinson's disease**
- Parkinsonism caused by drugs or poisons
- Parkinson-plus syndromes (progressive supranuclear palsy, multiple system atrophy, and cortical-basal ganglionic degeneration)
- **Huntington's disease**
- Wilson's disease
- Inherited ataxias (Friedreich's ataxia, Machado-Joseph disease, and spinocerebellar ataxias)
- **Tourette syndrome** and other tic disorders
- Essential tremor
- **Restless leg syndrome**
- Dystonia
- **Stroke**
- **Cerebral palsy**
- Encephalopathies
- Intoxication

- **Poisoning** by carbon monoxide, cyanide, methanol, or manganese.

Movement is produced and coordinated by several interacting brain centers, including the motor cortex, the cerebellum, and a group of structures in the inner portions of the brain called the basal ganglia.

Both the cerebellum and the motor cortex send information to a set of structures deep within the brain that help control involuntary components of movement (basal ganglia). The basal ganglia send output messages to the motor cortex, helping to initiate movements, regulate repetitive or patterned movements, and control muscle tone.

Motor cortex damage can cause weakness of paralysis, and may lead to spasticity. Cerebellar disorders cause inability to control the force, fine positioning, and speed of movements (ataxia). Disorders of the cerebellum may also impair the ability to judge distance so that a person under- or over-reaches the target (dysmetria). Tremor during voluntary movements can also result from cerebellar damage.

Basal ganglia damage causes a variety of movement disorders, depending on the portion of the basal ganglia that is damaged. Parkinson's disease, the most common basal ganglia disorder, is caused by cell death in the portion known as the substantia nigra. Disruptions in other portions of the basal ganglia are thought to cause tics, **tremors**, dystonia, and a variety of other movement disorders, although the exact mechanisms are not well understood.

Some movement disorders, including Huntington's disease and inherited ataxias, are caused by inherited genetic defects. Some disease that cause sustained muscle contraction limited to a particular muscle group (focal dystonia) are inherited, but others are caused by trauma. The cause of most cases of Parkinson's disease is unknown, although genes have been found for some familial forms.

Abnormal movements are broadly classified as either hyperkinetic—too much movement—and hypokinetic—too little movement. Hyperkinetic movements include:

- Dystonia. Sustained muscle contractions, often causing twisting or repetitive movements and abnormal postures. Dystonia may be limited to one area (focal) or may affect the whole body (general). Focal dystonias may affect the neck (cervical dystonia or **torticollis**), the face (one-sided or hemifacial spasm, contraction of the eyelid or blepharospasm, contraction of the mouth and jaw or oromandibular dystonia, simultaneous spasm of the chin and eyelid or Meige syndrome), the vocal cords (laryngeal dystonia), or the arms and legs (writer's cramp, occupational cramps). Dystonia may be painful as well as incapacitating.
- Tremor. Uncontrollable (involuntary) shaking of a body part. Tremor may occur only when muscles are relaxed or it may occur only during an action or holding an active posture.
- Tics. Involuntary, rapid, nonrhythmic movement or sound. Tics can be controlled briefly.
- Myoclonus. A sudden, shock-like muscle contraction. Myoclonic jerks may occur singly or repetitively. Unlike tics, myoclonus cannot be controlled even briefly.
- Chorea. Rapid, nonrhythmic, usually jerky movements, most often in the arms and legs.
- Ballism. Like chorea, but the movements are much larger, more explosive and involve more of the arm or leg. This condition, also called ballismus, can occur on both sides of the body or on one side only (hemiballismus).
- Akathisia. Restlessness and a desire to move to relieve uncomfortable sensations. Sensations may include a feeling of crawling, **itching**, stretching, or creeping, usually in the legs.
- Athetosis. Slow, writhing, continuous, uncontrollable movement of the arms and legs.

Hypokinetic movements include:

- Bradykinesia. Slowness of movement.
- Freezing. Inability to begin a movement or involuntary stopping of a movement before it is completed.
- Rigidity. An increase in muscle tension when an arm or leg is moved by an outside force.
- Postural instability. Loss of ability to maintain upright posture caused by slow or absent righting reflexes.

Treatment of a movement disorder begins with determining its cause. Physical and occupational therapy may help make up for lost control and strength. Drug therapy can help compensate for some imbalances of the basal ganglionic circuit. For instance, levodopa (L-dopa) or related compounds can substitute for lost dopamine-producing cells in Parkinson's disease. Conversely, blocking normal dopamine action is a possible treatment in some hyperkinetic disorders, including tics. Oral medications can also help reduce overall muscle tone. Local injections of botulinum toxin can selectively weaken overactive muscles in dystonia and spasticity. Destruction of peripheral nerves through injection of phenol can reduce spasticity. All of these treatments may have some side effects.

Surgical destruction or inactivation of basal ganglionic circuits has proven effective for Parkinson's disease and is being tested for other movement disorders. Transplantation of fetal cells into the basal ganglia has produced mixed results in Parkinson's disease.

MOVEMENT THERAPY

Movement therapy uses body movement to affect physiological functioning. It includes muscle and tissue manipulation, education and awareness, breathing and emotional expression, and specific movement patterns. Movement therapy is used to enhance an individual's mind/body awareness and promote a healthier lifestyle.

Movement therapies work on the premise that by repatterning muscle relationships, one can overcome discomfort and experience a heightened sense of the body and its relationship to the environment. Most therapies were developed by individuals who sought relief from chronic **pain** or saw others who needed therapeutic relief. Neuromuscular reeducation is integral to the process of movement therapy. Some therapies involve deep muscle massage which acts as a first step in releasing tension. The field of movement therapy can be broken down into specific theories and techniques.

Aston patterning is a deep muscle manipulation technique used in conjunction with neuromuscular reeducation. It is particularly beneficial for individuals with chronic pain such as **tennis elbow** and for people with postural problems. It differs from other techniques in that the patient receives long term relief. Reeducation is essential to the technique, for one must consciously change the movement patterns that caused the pain.

The Alexander technique was developed by F. Mathias Alexander, an Australian actor who suffered severe vocal difficulties and studied his own habits of movement to determine what might be causing them. He discovered a habit of tensing his neck muscles with the intake of each breath that resulted in distortion of the head-neck-spine relationship. He named this head-neck-spine relationship the "primary control" and promoted a system of movement reeducation to bring increased awareness of these anatomical relationships. This technique results in a sense of kinesthetic lightness where thinking becomes clearer, sensations livelier, and movement more pleasurable.

The Feldenkrais method deals with structural integration of the mind and the body using movement training, gentle touch, and verbal dialogue. Moshe Feldenkrais was a physicist who suffered a sports related injury which drove him to explore his own movement patterns. He succeeded in overcoming his handicap, and in the process he developed sequences of movements designed to replace old negative habits with new structurally integrated ones. He developed two approaches: *awareness through movement,* which uses group sessions, and *functional integration,* which specializes in individualized gentle touch. Results include improved posture, better flexibility, coordination, and less pain and tension.

Hellerwork combines deep tissue massage, guided verbal dialogue, and movement education. The purpose is to structurally realign the body, release tension, and enhance mind/body awareness. The technique involves deep massage along with dialogue on how to move properly and how to change habits and lifestyle in order to reduce tension. Results are improved posture, relief of common aches and pains, and increased awareness of emotional problems contributing to physical disabilities.

The Pilates method is a system of physical conditioning and **rehabilitation**. Pilates works from the inside out, beginning with pelvic stabilization, intense concentration, patience, body alignment, breathing, and intelligence. Joseph Pilates was a gymnast and bodybuilder born in 1880. During World War I, he devised a series of **exercise**s to aid rehabilitation of wounded soldiers using springs attached to a hospital bed. He moved to New York City in 1923 and began to use the wooden bed, now called the universal reformer, to recondition dancers and athletes. Pilates later added other apparatus to his system, such as the chair, the trapeze table, and the barrel, as well as an extensive series of mat exercises. Deep breathing and abdominal support are important ingredients in the technique. Results are strength, control, lengthening through the spine, and correction of imbalance and faulty neuromuscular patterning.

Trager work is a method of gentle, rhythmical touch combined with movement reeducation. As the individual lies on a table, a certified practitioner uses gentle, non-intrusive touch to loosen muscles and joints. These gentle movements trigger sensory motor feedback between the mind and body, which in turn produces psychophysical integration. After the manipulation session, the patient is introduced to a series of movements to maintain a sense of lightness and awareness called *mentastics*. Trager work is beneficial for severe neuromuscular disturbances and produces increased body awareness.

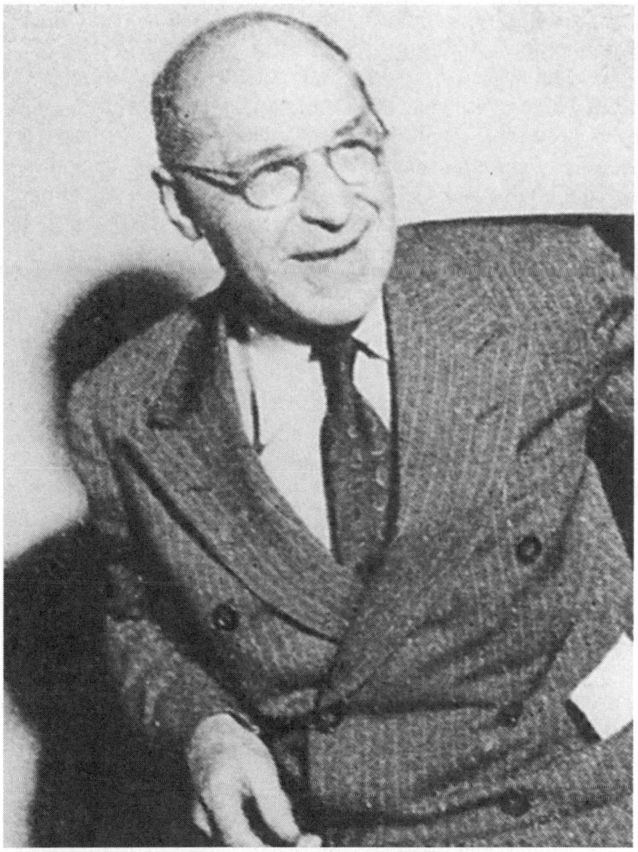

Hermann Joseph Muller

Movement therapy has proven beneficial for individuals who seek not only relief from chronic pain, but for those who want to enjoy movement as a part of daily life. When taught by a qualified teacher in the proper setting, there are no risks, and the patient feels a release of tension and relief from muscular pain, while experiencing a heightened awareness of his or her own body and its relationship to the environment.

Muller, Hermann Joseph (1890-1967)

American geneticist

In a career that took him through Hitler's Germany and Stalin's Russia, Muller achieved scientific distinction while spawning political controversy. He is best known for his discovery that x-rays could induce artificial mutations in genes, a finding that won him a Nobel Prize in 1946.

Muller was born in New York City on December 1, 1890. His studies began at Columbia University, where he was influenced by Edmund Beecher Wilson and his emphasis on the role of chromosomes in heredity. Perhaps more importantly, Muller also became an associate of **Thomas Hunt Morgan**, researching natural mutations in *Drosophilia* (fruit fly). In Morgan's fly lab, Muller first established himself as an untraditional thinker, proposing imaginative theories and designing creative experiments. He may have been too much of an iconoclast, though, for his relationships with others were fractious, and Morgan himself found Muller somewhat presumptuous and idealistic. Personal conflicts aside, Muller's research at Columbia established several fundamentals of genetics, including the crossing-over of genes and their linear linkage in heredity.

Muller earned his Ph.D. in 1916, and left New York to continue his research at Rice Institute in Texas. There, while analyzing mutations, he isolated and mapped the modifier genes that control inherited characteristics. From this, Muller concluded that heredity was determined by variations in individual genes, giving them a primacy not realized before. Muller returned to Columbia for a brief period in 1918. During this time, he formulated one of his most important theories: that since genes are the only parts of cells that can replicate the changes that occur in them, they must be the source of everything in the cell, and, by extension, of life itself.

Muller finally left Columbia for good two years later, when he landed a position at the University of Texas. During his twelve years there, he achieved his most important discovery: that x-rays induced mutations in *Drosophila* chromosomes by altering gene structure. This finding, published in 1927, established Muller as an international figure. It also formed the nucleus of a new discipline, radiation genetics.

Muller became a member of the American Academy of Sciences in 1931, but personal difficulties soon took over. His socialist views garnered suspicion at the university, his marriage dissolved, and a financial crisis loomed. The combined stress was overwhelming; he suffered a nervous breakdown and attempted suicide. Muller recovered, but found himself ostracized in the uncompromising political climate of the thirties. He spent 1933 in Berlin as a Guggenheim fellow, investigating genetic structure and mutations at the Kaiser Wilhelm Institute. Hitler's Germany, however, proved equally inhospitable to a socialist, and he soon departed for Moscow and the Soviet Institute of Genetics.

Muller believed that the Soviet Union was an enlightened society, where his work on genetics and its tangent, eugenics, would be supported. Unfortunately, there he ran afoul of Trofim Lysenko (1898-1976), a politically ambitious scientist who had rejected the Mendelian laws of heredity and adopted instead the fallacious belief that acquired characteristics could be inherited. Stalin was convinced of this pseudoscience as well, and Lysenko's useless theories were taught as gospel. Soviet scientists who dared to disagree were banished. Muller scoffed at these ideas and asserted his own by writing *Out of the Night*. He sent Stalin a copy of the book, but to no avail. His proposals were rejected, and the Institute was accused of racism and that gravest of socialist sins, class elitism. For the next four years, Muller contented himself with diatribes against Lysenko and a futile defense of genetics.

The situation gradually became intolerable, and Muller left to join the Spanish Civil War, another quixotic cause, in 1937. The year 1938 brought Muller an appointment to the University of Edinburgh. He spent three years at the Institute of Animal Genetics, analyzing radiation-induced lethal mutations in embryos. As the war loomed, he returned to the United States. He had remarried, and since both he and his new wife were part Jewish, they had begun to fear for their own safety. He went first to Amherst College. Then in 1945, he secured a professorship in zoology at Indiana University, a position he held until his death.

It was while working at Indiana University in 1946 that Muller finally received the Nobel Prize in physiology or medicine. He used the fame the award finally brought as an opportunity to champion various causes. Muller warned that the increasing medicinal and industrial use of radiation could wreak havoc on the human gene pool, affecting future generations. He continued his attacks on Lysenko, withdrawing from the Soviet Academy of Sciences in 1947. He urged educators to reform the teaching of biology, emphasizing genetics and evolution in science curricula.

His most controversial idea was a eugenics program in which the sperm of highly gifted and intelligent men would be frozen and stored for later use. In a nation still polarized by race and horrified by the Nazis' use of genocide and selective breeding, such a suggestion could only meet with resistance. Muller was motivated, though, by his genuine concern for the future of the human race, which he thought was threatened by technology and the loss of natural selection. He believed that it was possible to guide the evolution of mankind and create a better allotment of positive qualities than would naturally occur.

Müller, Paul (1899-1965)

Swiss chemist

Paul Müller was an industrial chemist who discovered that dichlorodiphenyltrichloroethane (DDT) could be used as an insecticide. This was the first insecticide that could actually target insects; in small doses it was not toxic to humans and yet it was stable enough to remain effective over a period of months. When DDT was introduced in 1942, the effects it would have on the environment were not well understood. It was widely hailed, in particular for its ability to reduce the incidence of tropical diseases by reducing insect populations. For his work with DDT and the role his discovery played in the fight against diseases such as typhus and malaria, Müller was awarded the 1948 Nobel Prize in medicine or physiology.

Paul Hermann Müller was born in Olten, Switzerland, on January 12, 1899, to Gottlieb and Fanny Leypoldt Müller. His father was an official on the Swiss Federal Railway, and the family moved to Lenzburg and then to Basel, where Müller was educated until the age of seventeen. After finishing his secondary education, Müller worked for several years in a succession of jobs with local chemical companies. In 1919, he entered the University of Basel to study chemistry. He did his doctoral work under F. Fichter and H. Rupe, and his dissertation examined the chemical and electrochemical reactions of m-xylidine and some related compounds. Xylidines are used in the manufacture of dyes, and when Müller received his Ph.D. in 1925 he went to work in the dye division of the J. R. Geigy Corporation, a very large Swiss chemical company. Müller married Friedel Rügsegger in 1927; they had two sons and a daughter. Müller initially conducted research on the natural products that could be derived from green plants, and the compounds he synthesized were used as pigments and tanning agents for leather. In 1935, he was assigned to develop an insecticide. At that time the only available insecticides were either expensive natural products or synthetics ineffective against insects; the only compounds that were both effective and inexpensive were the arsenic compounds, which were just as poisonous to human beings and other mammals. Müller noticed that insects absorbed and processed chemicals much differently than the higher animals, and he postulated that for this reason there must be some material that was toxic to insects alone. After testing the biological effects of hundreds of different chemicals, in 1939 he discovered that the compound DDT met most of his design criteria. First synthesized in 1873 by German chemist Othmar Zeidler, who had not known of its insecticide potential, DDT could be sprayed as an emulsion with water or could be mixed with talcum or chalk powder and dusted on target areas. It was first used against the Colorado potato beetle in Switzerland in 1939; it was patented in 1940 and went on the market in 1942.

Müller had set out to find a specific compound that would be cheap, odorless, long-lasting, fast in killing insects, and safe for plants and animals. He almost managed it. DDT in short term application is so non-toxic to human beings that it can be applied directly on the skin without ill effect. It is cheap and easy to make, and it usually needs to be applied only once during a growing season, unlike biodegradable pesticides which must often be applied several times, in larger amounts and at much higher cost. Typhus and malaria are very severe, often fatal illnesses, which are carried by body lice and mosquitoes respectively; in the 1940s several potentially severe epidemics of these diseases were averted by dusting the area and the human population with DDT. The insecticide saved many lives during World War II and increased the effectiveness of Allied forces. Soldiers fighting in both the Mediterranean and the tropics were dusted with DDT to kill lice, and entire islands were sprayed by air before invasions.

Despite these successes, environmentalists were concerned from the time DDT was introduced about the dangers of its indiscriminate use. DDT was so effective that all the insects in a dusted area were killed, even beneficial ones, eradicating the food source from many birds and other small creatures. Müller and other scientists were actually aware of these concerns, and as early as 1945 they had attempted to find some way to reduce DDT's toxicity to beneficial insects, but they were unsuccessful. Müller also believed that insecticides must be biodegradable.

Hailed as a miracle compound, DDT came into wide use, and the impact on beneficial insects was not the only problem. Because it was such a stable compound, DDT built up in the environment; this was a particular problem once it began to be used for agricultural purposes and applied over wide areas year after year. Higher animals, unharmed by individual small doses, began to accumulate large amounts of DDT in their tissues (called bio-accumulation). This had serious effects and several bird species, most notably the bald eagle, were almost wiped out because frequent exposure to the chemical caused the shells of their eggs to be thin and fragile. Many insects also developed resistances to DDT, and so larger and larger amounts of the compound needed to be applied yearly, increasing the rate of bio-accumulation. The substance was eventually banned in many countries; in 1972 it was banned in the United States.

In addition to the 1948 Nobel Prize in physiology or medicine, Müller received an honorary doctorate from the University of Thessalonica in Greece in recognition of DDT's impact on the Mediterranean region. He retired from Geigy in 1961, continuing his research in a home laboratory. He died on October 13, 1965.

Multiple chemical sensitivity

Multiple chemical sensitivity, also known as MCS syndrome is a disorder in which a person develops symptoms from exposure to chemicals in the environment. With each incidence of exposure, lower levels of the chemical trigger a reaction, and the person becomes increasingly vulnerable to reactions triggered by other chemicals.

Multiple chemical sensitivity typically begins with one high-dose exposure to a chemical, but it may also develop with long-term exposure to a low level of a chemical. Chemical exposure is often a result of indoor air pollution. Buildings that are tightly sealed for energy conservation may cause a related illness called sick building syndrome, in which people develop symptoms from chronic exposure to airborne environmental chemicals such as formaldehyde from the furniture, carpet glues, and latex caulking. A person moving into a newly constructed building that has not had time to degas may experience the initial high-dose exposure to chemicals that leads to MCS.

Chemicals most often connected with MCS include: formaldehyde; pesticides; solvents; petrochemical fuels such as diesel, gasoline, and kerosene; waxes, detergents, and cleaning products; latex; tobacco smoke; perfumes and fragrances; and artificial colors, flavors, and preservatives. People who develop MCS are commonly exposed in one of the following situations: on the job as an industrial worker; residing or working in a poorly ventilated building; or living in conditions of high air or water pollution. Others may be exposed in unique incidents.

Because MCS is difficult to diagnose, estimates vary as to what percentage of the population develops MCS. However, most MCS patients are female. The median age of MCS patients is 40 years old, and most sufferers experience symptoms before they are 30 years old.

The symptoms of MCS vary from person to person and are not chemical-specific. Symptoms are not limited to one physiological system, but primarily affect the respiratory and nervous systems. Commonly reported symptoms are **headache**, fatigue, weakness, difficulty concentrating, short-term memory loss, **dizziness**, irritability and depression, **itching**, numbness, burning sensation, congestion, **sore throat**, hoarseness, **shortness of breath**, **cough**, and stomach **pain**s.

Multiple chemical sensitivity is a modern disorder, becoming more prevalent as more man-made chemicals are introduced into the environment in greater quantities. It is especially difficult to diagnose because it presents no consistent or measurable set of symptoms and has no single diagnostic test or marker. Physicians are often unaware of MCS as a condition. They may be unable to diagnose it, or may misdiagnose it as another degenerative disease, or may label it as a psychosomatic illness (a physical illness that is caused by emotional problems). Their lack of understanding generates frustration, **anxiety**, and distrust in patients already struggling with MCS. However, a new specialty of medicine is evolving to address MCS and related illnesses: occupational and environmental medicine.

A physician looking for MCS takes a complete patient history and try to identify chemical exposures. Doctors may recommend **antihistamines**, **analgesics**, and other medications to combat the symptoms. The most effective treatment for MCS is to avoid chemicals that trigger symptoms. This becomes increasingly difficult as the number of offending chemicals increases and people with MCS often remain at home where they are able to control the chemicals in their environment. This **isolation** limits their abilities to work and socialize, so supportive counseling may also be appropriate.

Some MCS patients find relief with detoxification programs of **exercise** and sweating, and chelation of heavy metals. Others support their health with nutritional regimens and immunotherapy vaccines. Some undergo food-allergy testing and testing for accumulated pesticides in the body to learn more about their condition and what chemicals to avoid. **Homeopathy** and **acupuncture** can give added support to any treatment program for MCS patients. Botanical medicine can help to support the liver and other involved organs.

Multiple chemical sensitivity is difficult to prevent because even at high-dose exposures, different people react differently. Ensuring adequate ventilation in situations with potential for chemical exposure and wearing the proper protective equipment in industrial situations minimizes the risk. Once MCS sets in, sensitivity continues to increase and a person's health continues to deteriorate. Strictly avoiding exposure to triggering chemicals for a year or more may improve health.

MULTIPLE ENDOCRINE NEOPLASIA SYNDROMES

The multiple endocrine neoplasia (MEN) syndromes are three related disorders affecting the thyroid and other hormone producing (endocrine) glands of the body.

The three forms of MEN are MEN1 (Wermer's syndrome), MEN2A (Sipple syndrome), and MEN2B (previously known as MEN3). Each is a genetic condition that predisposes the carrier of the gene to excessive growth of cells (hyperplasia) and tumor formation in a number of endocrine glands.

MEN1 patients experience hyperplasia or tumors of several endocrine glands, including the parathyroids, the pancreas, and the pituitary. The most frequent symptom of MEN1 is overgrowth of the parathyroid glands. This leads to an excess secretion of parathyroid hormone causing elevated blood calcium levels, **kidney stones**, weakened bones, and nervous system depression. Almost all MEN1 patients show these symptoms by age 40.

Tumors of the pancreas are also common in MEN1. Excessive secretion of gastrin (a hormone secreted into the stomach to aid in digestion) by these tumors can cause upper gastrointestinal **ulcers**. The anterior pituitary and the adrenal glands can also be affected.

Patients with MEN2A and MEN2B experience two main symptoms, medullary **thyroid cancer** (MTC) and a tumor of the adrenal gland medulla known as pheochromocytoma. MTC is a slow-growing **cancer**, but one that can be cured in less than 50% of cases. Pheochromocytoma is usually a benign tumor that causes excessive secretion of adrenal hormones, which, in turn, can cause life-threatening **hypertension** and cardiac arrhythmia.

MEN2A patients have a tendency to develop tumors of the parathyroid gland. Although similar to MEN1, less than 20% of MEN2A patients will show parathyroid involvement. MEN2B patients show a variety of additional conditions: swollen lips; tumors of the mucous membranes of the eye, mouth, tongue, and nasal cavity; enlarged colon; and skeletal abnormalities. Symptoms develop early in life (often before five years of age) in cases of MEN2B and the tumors are more aggressive. MEN2A is about ten times more common than MEN2B.

All types of MEN are caused by inherited genetic defects in genes that control tumor suppression. A patient who inherits one defective copy of a tumor suppressor gene from either parent has a strong predisposition to the disease. For all types of MEN, the children of an affected individual have a 50% chance of inheriting the defective gene.

MEN is diagnosed from clinical symptoms and testing for elevated hormone levels. For MEN1, the relevant hormone is parathyroid hormone. For both types of MEN2, the greatest concern is development of medullary thyroid cancer. Numerous other hormone levels can be measured to assess the involvement of the various endocrine glands.

Before 1994, there was no way of definitively identifying which children or symptom-free adults who had inherited the MEN defective gene. Now genetic screening using DNA

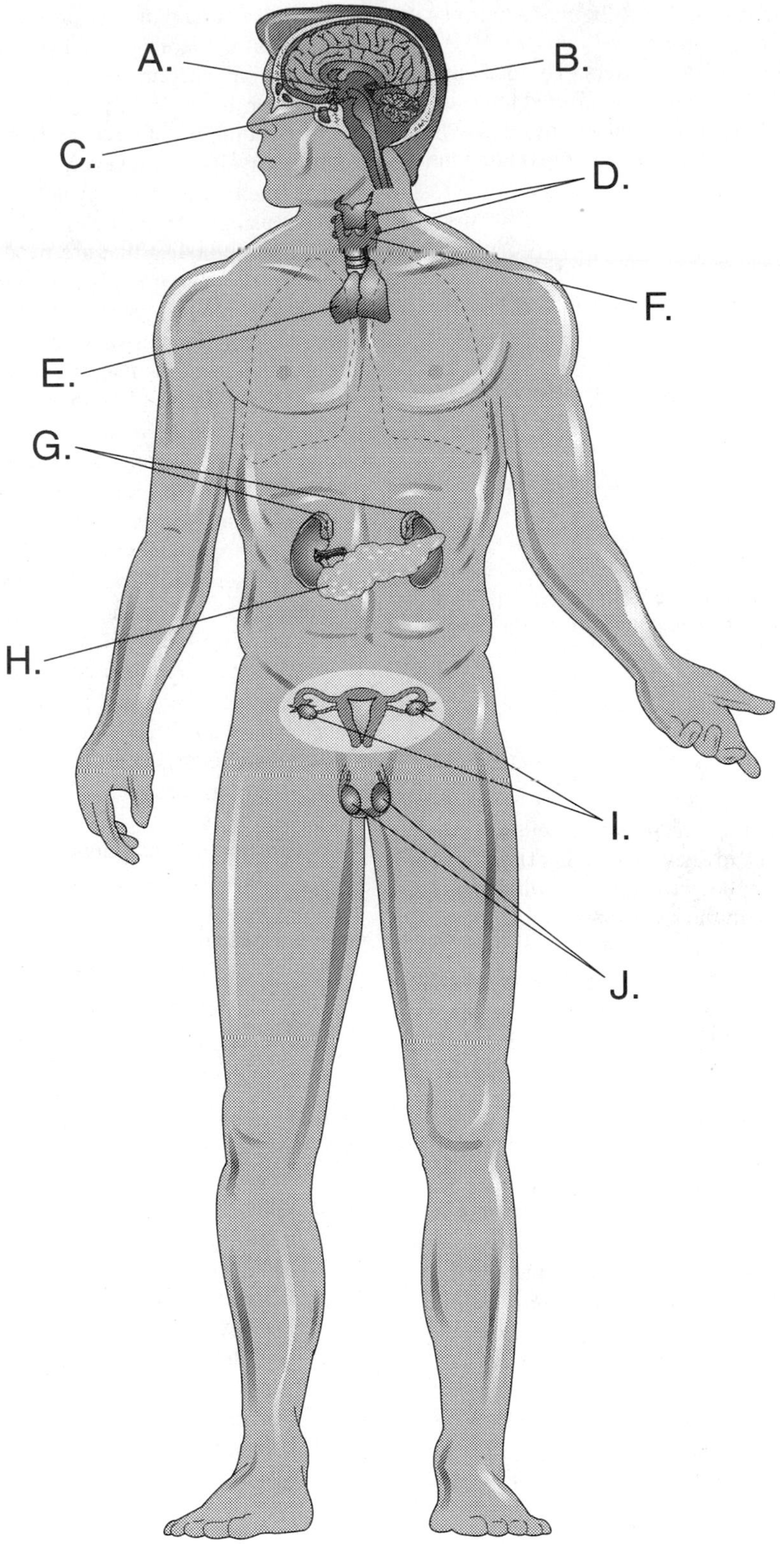

The human endocrine system: A. Hypothalamus. B. Pineal. C. Pituitary. D. Parathyroid. E. Thymus. F. Thyroid. G. Adrenals. H. Pancreas. I. Ovaries (female). J. Testes (male). *(Illustration by Electronic Illustrators Group.)*

technology allows a positive distinction to be made between children who are and who are not at risk.

Children who are identified as carriers. The defective genes that cause MEN2A or MEN2B can be offered total surgical removal of the thyroid gland (thyroidectomy) and synthetic thyroid hormone replacement as a way of preventing the development of thyroid cancer.

No single treatment is available for MEN. However, some of the symptoms caused by MEN can be treated. Surgical removal of some slow growing tumor is possible as is treatment of thyroid cancer by surgical removal of the thyroid. However, among doctors there is some disagreement about when thyroid removal should occur. After thyroidectomy, the patient receives replacement thyroid hormone either orally or by injection. Even when surgery is performed early, cancer may spread or metastasized to other parts of the body. **chemotherapy** and radiation therapy may not be effective in controlling its spread.

Diagnosed and treated early, patients with MEN may do very well. Untreated MEN may be fatal. Analysis of at-risk family members using genetic testing leads to earlier treatment and improved outcomes. There is no way to prevent the genetic mutations that cause MEN.

Multiple myeloma

Multiple myeloma is a disorder in which plasma cells are produced in an uncontrolled and invasive (malignant) fashion. Plasma cells develop from lymphocytes, a type of white blood cell. They are found primarily in the bone marrow and lymph nodes.

Plasma cells are responsible for helping the body fight infection. They produce antibodies that circulate in the blood and recognize markers, called antigens, on the cells of invading organisms like bacteria. These antibodies defend the body against foreign organisms.

Multiple myeloma occurs when the plasma cells in the bone marrow begin reproducing uncontrollably. While normal bone marrow contains less than 5% plasma cells, bone marrow in a patient with multiple myeloma contains over 10% plasma cells.

Multiple myeloma tends to be a disease of the elderly. The average patient is 68 years old when diagnosed. During the last 10 years, doctors have seen an increase in cases of multiple myeloma occurring at younger ages, but patients are usually over age 40. Men have a slightly increased chance of having multiple myeloma, and African-Americans are twice as likely as Caucasians to develop the disease.

Although the exact cause of multiple myeloma has not been determined, researchers believe that it may be linked to exposure to certain environmental substances such as radiation and chemicals.

Bone **pain** is an extremely common symptom among patients with multiple myeloma. About 70% of all patients report bone pain as their first symptom. This pain is caused by plasma cells growing in number within the bone marrow, replacing normal marrow and putting pressure on the bone. Plasma cells also produce chemicals called osteoclast activating factors (OAF). OAF encourage special cells called osteoclasts to break down bone. In healthy people this process is balanced by the building up of new bone by cells called osteoblasts. In multiple myeloma, however, excess OAF are produced and bone is eaten away by overly active osteoclasts. Bones become weak (causing **osteoporosis**) and may break.

The antibodies that are over-produced in multiple myeloma function abnormally. Furthermore, other types of antibodies are under produced. Destruction of circulating antibodies also increases. This results in an increased chance of developing serious bacterial infections. The most common types of infections include **pneumonia** and kidney infections.

Abnormalities in the structure and function of kidney cells are extremely common in multiple myeloma. About half of all patients have kidney problems. These problems occur because of high levels of calcium in the blood (due to bone breaking down), protein build-up, and increased circulating uric acid. Increased strain on the kidney to eliminate large amounts of the broken down products of antibodies and proteins may cause kidney damage or kidney failure.

Other problems are common in multiple myeloma. Because plasma cells take up space within the bone marrow, other cells normally produced there decrease and are sometimes defective in shape and function. Red blood cells decrease, resulting in anemia in about 80% of all people with multiple myeloma.

Circulating antibodies may interfere with clotting, resulting in an increased risk of bleeding. Abnormally thick blood may interfere with blood circulation anywhere in the body, but particularly in the fingers, toes, ears, and nose. Blood thickening may also cause **headache**, fatigue, and vision problems. Excess calcium in the blood may cause patients to feel weak, depressed, and confused. Sometimes, the plasma cells create a tumor called a plasmacytoma. Plasmacytomas may press on bone, causing fractures. Fractured bones may place unusual pressure on nearby nerves, resulting in nerve damage, pain, burning, tingling, and weakness of the affected muscle.

Diagnosis of multiple myeloma involves examination of blood, urine, bone marrow, and bones. Blood tests will reveal abnormalities, including anemia with abnormal red blood cells. Blood calcium will be high in about 33% of all patients. A specialized test called electrophoresis can be used to show an increased amount of antibodies in the blood and urine.

Examination of the bone marrow requires a test called a bone marrow aspiration. A long, thin needle is placed into the hip, and a sample of bone marrow is withdrawn. In multiple myeloma, the bone marrow has a significantly increased percentage of plasma cells, usually well over 10%.

Because the treatments for multiple myeloma can be very damaging, and because the disease often progresses slowly, many patients are not treated until measurements of antibodies in the blood reach a particularly high level. **Chemotherapy** agents used in multiple myeloma include melphalan, cyclophosphamide, chlorambucil, and prednisone. These may be given over four to seven days in four to six week intervals. Chemotherapy may be given for several years. The disease usually recurs within a year after treatment has stopped. Chemotherapy can be given again, but each time the disease reappears it is less responsive to treatment.

Bone pain is often treated with radiation directed at the problem area. High blood levels of calcium may respond to treatment with prednisone. High blood levels of uric acid may improve with allopurinol. When anemia causes symptoms, blood **transfusions** may be necessary.

One general recommendation for alternative **cancer** treatment includes dietary supplementation with beta-carotene, vitamin B_6, vitamin C, vitamin E, selenium, and zinc as antioxidant protection. Other recommendations include reducing **stress** through techniques such as **biofeedback** training, **guided imagery**, and **meditation**. These same techniques are useful for pain relief.

About 15% of patients with multiple myeloma die within three months of diagnosis. About 60% of all patients respond to treatment and live for an average of two and a half to three years after diagnosis. About 23% of all patients die of other illnesses associated with advanced age.

MULTIPLE PERSONALITY DISORDER

Multiple personality disorder (MPD) is a mental illness. It is classified as a dissociative disorder and has been renamed dissociative identity disorder (DID). MPD or DID is a condition in which two or more distinct identities or personality states alternate in controlling the patient's consciousness and behavior.

The precise nature of DID (MPD) is still a subject of debate. Some researchers think that DID may be a culture-specific syndrome found in western society, caused primarily by both childhood abuse and unspecified long-term societal changes. Unlike depression or **anxiety disorders**, which have been recognized for centuries, the earliest cases of persons reporting DID symptoms were not recorded until the 1790s. Most were considered medical oddities or curiosities until the late 1970s, when increasing numbers of cases were reported in the United States.

Psychiatrists are still debating whether DID was previously misdiagnosed and underreported, or whether it is currently over-diagnosed. Because childhood trauma is a factor in the development of DID, some doctors think it may be a variation of **post-traumatic stress disorder** (PTSD).

The most distinctive feature of DID is the formation and emergence of alternate personality states, or "alters." Patients with DID experience their alters as distinct individuals possessing different names, histories, and personality traits. It is not unusual for DID patients to have alters of different genders, sexual orientations, ages, or nationalities. The average DID patient has between two and 10 alters, but some have been reported to have over one hundred.

The severe dissociation that characterizes patients with DID is currently understood to result from a set of causes that include: an innate ability to dissociate easily; repeated episodes of severe physical or sexual abuse in childhood; and lack of a supportive or comforting person to counteract abusive relative(s).

The major dissociative symptoms experienced by DID patients are amnesia, depersonalization, derealization, and identity disturbances.

Amnesia in DID is marked by gaps in the patient's memory for long periods of their past, in some cases, their entire childhood. Most DID patients have amnesia, or "lose time," for periods when another personality is "out." They may report finding items in their house that they can't remember having purchased, finding notes written in different handwriting, or other evidence of unexplained activity.

Depersonalization is a dissociative symptom in which the patient feels that his or her body is unreal, is changing, or is dissolving. Some DID patients experience depersonalization as a feeling of being outside their body or as watching a movie of themselves.

With derealization the patient perceives the external environment as unreal. Patients may see walls, buildings, or other objects as changing in shape, size, or color. DID patients may fail to recognize relatives or close friends.

Identity disturbances in DID result from the patient's having split off entire personalities or characteristics as well as memories. When a stressful or traumatic experience triggers the reemergence of these dissociated parts, the patient switches — usually within seconds — into an alternate personality.

Diagnosis of DID is complex. Patients are often treated under a variety of other psychiatric diagnoses for a long time before being re-diagnosed with DID. Many DID patients are misdiagnosed as depressed because their primary personality is subdued and withdrawn.

Other misdiagnoses include schizophrenia, borderline personality disorder, somatization disorder, and panic disorder. DID patients are often frightened by their dissociative experiences and may go to emergency rooms or clinics because they fear they are going insane.

When a doctor evaluates a patient for DID, he first rules out physical conditions that sometimes produce amnesia, depersonalization, or derealization. If the patient appears physically normal, the doctor next rules out psychotic disturbances, including schizophrenia. Many patients with DID are misdiagnosed as schizophrenic because they may "hear" their alters "talking" inside their heads. If the doctor suspects DID, he or she can use a screening test called the Dissociative Experiences Scale (DES) followed by specific additional testing.

Treatment of DID may last for five to seven years in adults and usually requires several different treatment methods. Patients should be treated by a therapist with specialized training in dissociation. Psychotherapy for DID patients has several stages: an initial phase for uncovering and "mapping" the patient's alters; a phase of treating the traumatic memories and "fusing" the alters; and a phase of consolidating the patient's newly integrated personality. Many DID patients are helped by group as well as individual treatment, provided that the group is limited to people with dissociative disorders.

Some doctors prescribe tranquilizers or antidepressants for DID patients because their alter personalities may have

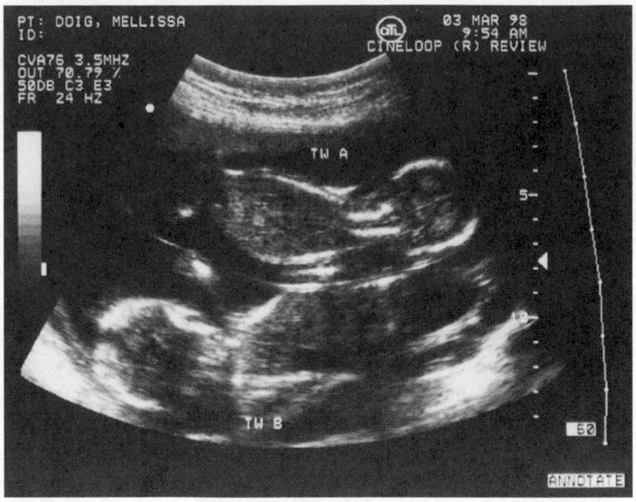

An ultrasound image of identical twin male fetuses. The distortion is due to "twin B" being closer to the transducer. *(Courtesy of Melissa Walsh Doig. Reproduced by permission.)*

anxiety or **mood disorders**. Other therapists prefer to keep medications to a minimum because DID patients can easily become psychologically dependent on drugs. In addition, many DID patients have at least one alter who abuses drugs or alcohol, substances which are dangerous in combination with many medications.

While not always necessary, **hypnosis** is a standard treatment to help patients recover repressed ideas and memories. Hypnosis can also be used to control problem behaviors that many DID patients exhibit, such as self-mutilation or eating disorders. In the later stages of treatment, the therapist may use hypnosis to "fuse" the alters.

Alternative treatments that help to relax the body are often recommended for DID patients as an adjunct to psychotherapy and/or medication. These include **hydrotherapy**, herbal medicine, therapeutic **massage**, and **yoga**. **Meditation** is usually discouraged until the patient's personality has been reintegrated.

Some therapists believe that the prognosis for recovery is excellent for children and good for most adults. Although treatment takes years, it is often ultimately effective. As a general rule, the earlier the patient is diagnosed and properly treated, the better the chances for improvement.

MULTIPLE PREGNANCY

Multiple pregnancy is a **pregnancy** where more than one fetus develops in the womb. Twins happen naturally about one in every 100 births. There are two types of twinning—identical and fraternal. Identical twins represent the splitting of a single fertilized zygote (union of a male sperm and a female egg that produce a developing fetus) into two separate individuals. They normally have identical genes. When they do not separate completely, the result is Siamese (or conjoined) twins.

Fraternal twins are three times more common than identical twins. They occur when two eggs are fertilized by separate sperm. Each has a different selection of its parents' genes. Fraternal twins and are genetically no more closely related than any siblings with the same parents.

The natural incidence of multiple pregnancy has been upset by advances in fertility treatments that may cause the simultaneous release of multiple eggs. The result is an increased rate of multiple births in the U.S. These children are fraternal; they each arise from a separate egg and a separate sperm. Cloning produces identical twins.

Women are designed to release one egg every menstrual cycle. A hormone called progesterone, released by the first egg to be produced, prevents any other egg from maturing during that cycle. When this control fails, release and fertilization of more than one egg is possible. Fertility drugs inhibit these hormonal controls, allowing multiple pregnancy to occur. Multiple pregnancy is more difficult and poses more health risks than single pregnancy. Premature birth is more likely with each additional fetus.

The problem with multiple births is that there is limited room in even the womb (uterus). Developing fetuses need to reach a certain size and gestational age before they can survive outside the uterus. **Prematurity** is the constant threat of multiple pregnancies. Twins have five times the **death** rate of single births. Triplets and larger multiples die even more often. The principle threat of prematurity is that the lungs are not fully developed. A condition called hyaline membrane disease afflicts premature infants. The lungs do not stay open after their first breath because they lack a chemical called surfactant that is present in full-term babies. Survival of premature infants was greatly improved when surfactant was finally synthesized in a form that could be used in premature babies. Tiny babies also have trouble regulating their body temperature.

Fertility drugs prevent the normal process of single ovulation by permitting more than one egg at a time to mature and be released for fertilization. The first drug to accomplish this was clomiphene. Subsequently, two natural hormones—follicle stimulating hormone (FSH) and chorionic gonadotrophin-have been used to treat infertility.

Multiple pregnancies cause the uterus to grow faster than usual. Obstetricians can detect this unusually rapid growth as the pregnancy progresses. Before birth, an **ultrasound** will also detect multiple fetuses in the uterus. After birth, physical appearance or a careful examination of the placenta and amniotic membranes will usually reveal whether the babies were in the same water bag or separate ones. One bag means identical twins.

Mothers generally do well with multiple births. Depending on whether they are greatly premature, babies may remain hospitalized, where their breathing can be assisted and their temperature controlled in an incubator. Extremely premature babies need artificial ventilation until their lungs mature. These babies are fragile in many other ways, but modern methods of intensive care have successfully stabilized babies as small as one pound.

There are no specific treatments to alleviate medical difficulties caused by multiple pregnancies, however supportive measures may help both mother and children recover from the birthing process. With modern medical advances and excellent prenatal care, many multiple pregnancies occur without difficulties. If the babies are born prematurely, immediate medical care increases the chance of survival without any complications.

Multiple sclerosis

Multiple sclerosis (MS) is a chronic autoimmune disorder affecting movement, sensation, and bodily functions. It is caused by destruction of the myelin insulation covering nerve fibers (neurons) in the central nervous system (brain and spinal cord). This insulation, called myelin, helps electrical signals pass quickly and smoothly between the brain and the rest of the body. When the myelin is destroyed, nerve messages are sent more slowly and less efficiently. Patches of scar tissue, called plaques, form over the affected areas, further disrupting nerve communication. The symptoms of MS occur when the brain and spinal cord nerves no longer communicate properly with other parts of the body. Because there appears to be no pattern in the appearance of new plaques, the progression of MS can be unpredictable.

Multiple sclerosis affects more than a quarter of a million people in the United States. Most people have their first symptoms between the ages of 20 and 40; symptoms rarely begin before 15 or after 60. Women are almost twice as likely to get MS as men, especially in their early years. Despite considerable research, the trigger for this autoimmune destruction is still unknown. At various times, evidence has pointed to genes, environmental factors, viruses, or a combination of these.

The symptoms of multiple sclerosis may occur in one of three patterns:

- The most common pattern is the ''relapsing-remitting'' pattern, in which there are clearly defined symptomatic attacks lasting 24 hours or more, followed by complete or almost complete improvement. The period between attacks may be a year or more at the beginning of the disease, but may shrink to several months later on. This pattern is especially common in younger people who develop MS.
- In the ''primary progressive'' pattern, the disease progresses without remission or with occasional plateaus or slight improvements. This pattern is more common in older people.
- In the ''secondary progressive'' pattern, the person with MS begins with relapses and remissions, followed by more steady progression of symptoms.

Between 10–20% of people have a benign type of MS, meaning their symptoms progress very little over the course of their lives.

Because plaques may form in any part of the central nervous system, the symptoms of MS vary widely from person-to-person and from stage-to-stage of the disease. Initial symptoms often include:

- Muscle weakness, causing difficulty walking
- Loss of coordination or balance
- Numbness, ''pins and needles,'' or other abnormal sensations
- Visual disturbances, including nystagmus (eye tremor), and blurred or double vision.

Later symptoms may include:

- Fatigue
- Muscle spasticity and stiffness
- **Tremors**
- **Paralysis**
- **Pain**
- Vertigo
- Speech or swallowing difficulty
- Loss of bowel and bladder control
- **Incontinence**, **constipation**
- **Sexual dysfunction**
- Cognitive changes, especially depression.

Symptoms of MS may be worsened by heat or increased body temperature, including **fever**, intense physical activity, or exposure to sun, hot baths, or showers.

As of 1997, there are three drugs approved for the treatment of multiple sclerosis which have been shown to affect the course of the disease. None of these drugs is a cure, but they can slow disease progression in many patients.

Avonex and Betaseron are forms of the immune system protein beta interferon, while Copaxone is glatiramer acetate (formerly called copolymer-1). All three have been shown to reduce the rate of relapses in the relapsing-remitting form of MS. Different measurements from tests of each have demonstrated other benefits as well: Avonex may slow the progress of physical impairment, Betaseron may reduce the severity of symptoms, and Copaxone may decrease disability. All three drugs are administered by injection—Copaxone daily, Betaseron every other day, and Avonex weekly. Betaseron, at least, has led to the development of neutralizing antibodies, which reduce the effectiveness of treatment.

Immunosuppressant drugs have been used for many years to treat acute exacerbations (relapses). Drugs used include **corticosteroids** such as prednisone and methylprednisone; the hormone adrenocorticotropic hormone (ACTH); and azathioprine. Recent studies indicate that several days of intravenous methylprednisone may be more effective than other immunosuppressant treatments for acute symptoms. This treatment may require hospitalization.

MS causes a large variety of symptoms, and the treatments for these are equally diverse. Most symptoms can be treated and complications avoided with good care and attention from medical professionals. Good health and nutrition remain important preventive measures. **Vaccination** against **influenza** can prevent respiratory complications, and contrary to earlier concerns, is not associated with worsening of symptoms. Preventing complications such as **pneumonia**, bed sores, injuries from falls, or urinary infection requires attention to the primary problems which may cause them. Shortened life spans with MS are almost always due to complications rather than primary symptoms themselves.

Physical therapy helps the person with MS to strengthen and retrain affected muscles; to maintain range of motion to prevent muscle stiffening; to learn to use assistive devices such as canes and walkers; and to learn safer and more energy-efficient ways of moving, sitting, and transferring. **Exercise** and stretching programs are usually designed by the physical therapist and taught to the patient and caregivers for use at home. Exercise is an important part of maintaining function for the person with MS. Swimming is often recommended, not only for its low-impact workout, but also because it allows strenuous activity without overheating.

Occupational therapy helps the person with MS adapt to her environment and adapt the environment to her. The occupational therapist suggests alternate strategies and assistive devices for activities of daily living, such as dressing, feeding, and washing, and evaluates the home and work environment for safety and efficiency improvements that may be made.

Training in bowel and bladder care may be needed to prevent or compensate for incontinence. If the urge to urinate becomes great before the bladder is full, some drugs may be helpful, including propantheline bromide (Probanthine), oxybutynin chloride (Ditropan), or imipramine (Tofranil). Baclofen (Lioresal) may relax the sphincter muscle, allowing full emptying. Intermittent catheterization is effective in controlling bladder dysfunction. In this technique, a catheter is used to periodically empty the bladder.

Spasticity can be treated with oral medications, including baclofen and diazepam (Valium), or by injection with botulinum toxin (Botox). Spasticity relief may also bring relief from chronic pain. Other more acute types of pain may respond to carbamazepine (Tegretol) or diphenylhydantoin (Dilantin). **Low back pain** is common from increased use of the back muscles to compensate for weakened legs. Physical therapy and over-the-counter pain relievers may help.

Fatigue may be partially avoidable with changes in the daily routine to allow more frequent rests. Amantadine (Symmetrel) and pemoline (Cylert) may improve alertness and lessen fatigue. Visual disturbances often respond to corticosteroids. Other symptoms that may be treated with drugs include seizures, vertigo, and tremor.

It is difficult to predict how multiple sclerosis will progress in any one person. Most people with MS will be able to continue to walk and function at their work for many years after their diagnosis. The factors associated with the mildest course of MS are being female, having the relapsing-remitting form, having the first symptoms at a younger age, having longer periods of remission between relapses, and initial symptoms of decreased sensation or vision rather than of weakness or incoordination.

Less than 5% of people with MS have a severe progressive form, leading to **death** from complications within five years. At the other extreme, 10-20% have a benign form, with a very slow or no progression of their symptoms. The most recent studies show that about seven out of 10 people with MS are still alive 25 years after their diagnosis, compared to about nine out of 10 people of similar age without disease. On average, MS shortens the lives of affected women by about six years, and men by 11 years. Suicide is a significant cause of death in MS, especially in younger patients.

The degree of disability a person experiences five years after onset is, on average, about three-quarters of the expected disability at 10–15 years. A benign course for the first five years usually indicates the disease will not cause marked disability.

Mumps

Mumps is a contagious viral disease that causes painful enlargement of the salivary glands, most commonly the parotids. For this reason, the scientific name for mumps is *Epidemic parotitis*.

The condition was first described by **Hippocrates** with a clarity and thoroughness that one historian says is "worthy of any modern medical textbook." Hippocrates observed that the diseases occurred most commonly in young men, a fact that he attributed to their congregating at sports grounds. Women, who were inclined to be isolated in their own homes, were seldom taken ill with the disease, he noted. Interestingly enough, Hippocrates did not given a name to the condition that he described so well.

Over the centuries, medical writers paid little attention to mumps. Occasionally, mention was made of a local epidemic of the disease, as was recorded for Paris, France, in the sixteenth century by **Guillaume de Baillou** (1538-1616). Most experts seemed to believe that the disease was contagious, but no studies were done to confirm this suspicion.

The first detailed scientific description of mumps was provided by the British physician Robert Hamilton (1721-1793) in 1790. Hamilton's paper in the *Transactions of the Royal Society of Edinburgh* finally made the disease well known among physicians.

Efforts to prove the contagious nature of mumps date to 1913. In that year, two French physicians, Charles-Jean-Henri Nicolle (1866-1936) and Ernest Alfred Conseil, attempted to transmit mumps from humans to monkeys, but were unable to obtain conclusive results. Eight years later, Martha Wollstein injected viruses taken from the saliva of a mumps patient into cats, producing inflammation of the parotid, testes, and brain tissue in the cats. Conclusive proof that mumps is transmitted by a filterable virus was finally obtained by two American researchers, Claude D. Johnson and Ernest William Goodpasture (1886-1960), in 1934.

A vaccine for mumps was developed by an American microbiologist, **John Enders**, in 1948. During World War II, Enders had developed a vaccine using a killed virus, but it was only moderately and temporarily successful. After the war, he began to investigate ways of growing mumps virus in a suspension of minced chick embryo and ox blood. The technique was successful and Enders' live virus vaccine is now routinely used to vaccinate children against this ancient disease.

Munchausen syndrome

Munchausen syndrome is a psychiatric disorder that causes an individual to self-inflict injury or illness or to fabricate symptoms of physical or mental illness in order to receive medical care or hospitalization. In a variation of the disorder, Munchausen syndrome by proxy (MSBP), the primary caretaker, typically the mother, intentionally causes or fabricates illness in a child or other person under her care.

Munchausen syndrome takes its name from Baron Karl Friederich von Munchausen, an 18th century German military man known for his tall tales. The disorder first appeared in psychiatric literature in the early 1950s when it was used to describe patients who sought hospitalization by inventing symptoms and complicated medical histories, and/or inducing illness and injury in themselves. Categorized as a factitious disorder (a disorder in which the physical or psychological symptoms are under voluntary control), Munchausen's syndrome seems to be motivated by a need to assume the role of a patient. Unlike **malingering**, there does not appear to be any clear secondary gain (e.g., money or relief from duty) in Munchausen syndrome.

Individuals with Munchausen syndrome by proxy use their child or other dependent person to fulfill their need to step into the patient role. The disorder most commonly victimizes children from birth to 8 years old. Parents with MSBP may exaggerate or fabricate their child's symptoms, or they may deliberately induce symptoms through various methods, including **poisoning**, suffocation, **starvation**, or infecting the child's bloodstream.

The exact cause of Munchausen syndrome is unknown. It has been theorized that Munchausen patients are motivated by a desire to be cared for, a need for attention, dependency, an ambivalence toward doctors, or a need to suffer. Factors that may predispose an individual to Munchausen's include a serious illness in childhood or an existing personality disorder.

The Munchausen patient presents a wide array of physical or psychiatric symptoms, usually limited only by their medical knowledge. Many Munchausen patients are very familiar with medical terminology and symptoms. Some common complaints include **fever**s, **rashes**, **abscess**es, bleeding, and vomiting. Common Munchausen syndrome by proxy symptoms include apnea (cessation of breathing), fever, vomiting, and **diarrhea**. In both Munchausen and MSBP, the suspected illness does not respond to a normal course of treatment. Patients or parents may push for invasive diagnostic procedures and display an extraordinary depth of knowledge of medical procedures.

Because Munchausen sufferers often go from doctor to doctor, gaining admission into many hospitals along the way, diagnosis can be difficult. They are typically detected rather than diagnosed. During a course of treatment, they may be discovered by a hospital employee who has encountered them during a previous hospitalization. Their caregivers may also notice that symptoms such as high fever occur only when the patient is left unattended. Occasionally, unprescribed medication used to induce symptoms is found with the patient's possession. When patients are confronted, they often react with outrage and check out of the hospital to seek treatment at another facility with a new caregiver.

There is no clearly effective treatment for Munchausen syndrome. Extensive psychotherapy may be helpful with some Munchausen patients. If Munchausen syndrome co-exists with other mental disorders, such as a personality disorder, the underlying disorder is typically treated first.

The infections and injuries Munchausen patients self-inflict can cause serious illness. Patients often undergo countless unnecessary surgeries throughout their lifetimes. In addition, because of their frequent hospitalizations, they have difficulty holding down a job. Further, their chronic health complaints may damage interpersonal relationships with family and friends. Children victimized by sufferers of MSBP are at a real risk for serious injury and possible **death**. Those who survive physically unscathed may suffer developmental problems later in life.

Because the cause of Munchausen syndrome is unknown, formulating a prevention strategy is difficult. Some medical facilities and healthcare practitioners have attempted to limit hospital admissions for Munchausen patients by sharing medical records. While these attempts may curb the number of hospital admissions, they do not treat the underlying disorder and may endanger Munchausen sufferers that have made themselves critically ill and require treatment. Children who are found to be victims of persons with Munchausen by proxy syndrome should be immediately removed from the care of the abusing parent or guardian.

MURAD, FERID (1936-)

American physician, pharmacologist

Together with fellow American pharmacologists **Robert Furchgott** and **Louis Ignarro**, Murad received the 1998 Nobel Prize in Physiology or Medicine for discoveries related to the role of nitric oxide as a signaling molecule in the cardiovascular system.

Not to be confused with **nitrous oxide** (a gas used in **anesthesia**), nitric oxide is a colorless, odorless gas that, thanks to initial work by these three Nobel laureates and a flurry of subsequent research by others, now has widespread potential including the treatment of heart disease, **shock**, **cancer**, **impotence**, and pulmonary **hypertension**—a potentially fatal condition in premature infants. In 1994, the respected journal *Science* declared nitric oxide as its ''molecule of the year.''

Born in Whiting, Indiana, Murad studied medicine and pharmacology simultaneously at Western Reserve University, receiving both his M.D. and Ph.D. in 1965. He was an intern and resident in internal medicine at Massachusetts General Hospital until 1967, and then worked until 1970 at the **National Institutes of Health**'s National Heart and Lung Institute as a clinical associate and staff fellow.

Then followed a series of academic, research, and administrative appointments at the University of Virginia (1975-1981), Stanford University and Palo Alto Veterans Administration Medical Center (1981-1988), and Northwestern University and the University of Texas (starting in 1996).

Murad has also worked in the pharmaceutical industry. From 1988 to 1992 he worked for Abbott Laboratories, becoming vice president of pharmaceutical research and development, and from 1993-1995 he was full-time president and chief executive officer of Molecular Geriatrics Corporation.

Murad's work with nitric oxide began when he was in graduate school. He set out to learn how nitroglycerin, used for more than 100 years to treat **angina**, affected blood vessels. He found that nitroglycerin was effective because it prompted release of nitric oxide, which relaxed smooth muscle cells. Prior to this, nitric oxide was best known as an air pollutant present in automobile exhaust fumes. The gas was known to be present in bacteria, but it was not thought to be important in higher animals such as mammals.

Based on this, Murad postulated that nitric oxide and other nitrogen-containing compounds (he coined the term nitrovasodilators to describe them) might be produced by one cell, travel through membranes, and then regulate the function other cells. At the time, this was an entirely new concept for signaling in biological systems, but it was independently confirmed by Furchgott and Ignarro, clearing the way for entirely new therapies and diagnostic methods.

Nitric oxide is now known to play a key role in many biological functions including inflammation, blood flow regulation, cell growth, smooth muscle relaxation, and preserving memory.

Murad's winning of the Nobel Prize for discovering that nitric oxide is nitroglycerin's secret weapon against angina had an odd coincidence noted by some after the Nobel awards presentation. Alfred Nobel, the Swedish chemist who founded the famous prizes named after him, made his fortune using nitroglycerin to invent dynamite. In fact, Nobel suffered from angina and his doctor once advised him to take nitroglycerin to ease his chest pain. The industrialist would not take the substance, saying that, in his case, it caused headaches.

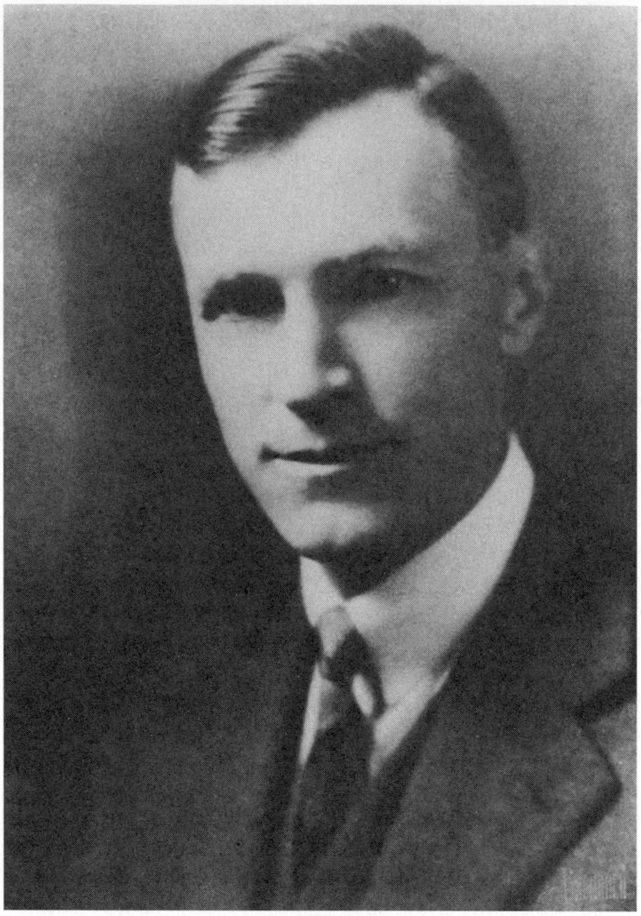

William Parry Murphy

Murphy, William Parry (1892-1987)

American physician and pathologist

William Parry Murphy was born 1892 in Wisconsin, to Congregational minister Thomas Francis Murphy and his wife, Rose Anna Parry. He attended public schools in Wisconsin and received his B.A. in 1914 from the University of Oregon. Murphy taught high school math and physics for two years in Oregon before entering the University of Oregon Medical School in Portland, where he also worked in the anatomy department as a laboratory assistant. He later received the William Stanislaus Murphy Fellowship award and entered Harvard Medical School in Boston, from which he graduated in 1922.

In 1925, Murphy began a collaboration with **George Richards Minot** that would ultimately earn them the Nobel Prize. Minot recruited Murphy to join his study, in which **pernicious anemia** patients were fed one-quarter to one-half pound of liver daily. Reputed for his diligence and dedication, Murphy assumed the painstaking, time-consuming responsibility of counting the microscopic reticulocytes (red blood cells) in the blood samples of pernicious anemia patients before and during the liver diet. The dramatic increase in reticulocytes in the samples following the patient's consumption of liver clearly identified the critical connection between liver ingestion and the production of mature red blood cells.

The liver diet therapy for pernicious anemia presented certain problems. Patients found it difficult to ingest such large quantities of liver every day. Also troublesome was the question of how to feed it to patients so ill they could no longer eat. Following a suggestion from one of his patients, Murphy partially solved the problem by feeding patients liquefied liver through stomach tubes. Murphy, however, was not satisfied. He and Minot enlisted the expertise of Edwin J. Cohn, a physical chemistry professor at Harvard Medical School. Cohn chemically reduced large amounts of liver to a concentrated extract fifty to one hundred times more potent than the liver itself. Ingestion of three vials a day of this extract, which cost $17.00 a month, proved just as effective as the cheaper but less palatable liver diet, which cost approximately $5.50 a month. Murphy felt the cost of the extract was prohibitive for many people and continued to search for a less expensive method of administering it. He sought the help of Guy W. Clark of the Lederle Laboratories; soon they developed an extremely concentrated extract. Injected into the muscle only once a month, the extract provided the same therapeutic effect as the liver diet or the oral extract. The monthly cost of this injection was $1.20.

Medical professionals, however, were skeptical of the results of the carefully documented study, which Murphy and Minot presented in 1926, because the treatment seemed too simple. Pernicious anemia had been thought to be caused by some type of poison, and patients were treated with arsenic, blood transfusions, or surgery, all to no avail. Worldwide treatment by the liver diet soon convinced the skeptics. Murphy's work was advanced by Harvard physician William Castle, who, in 1948, isolated the active ingredient in liver which promoted the development of fully mature red blood cells in patients suffering from pernicious anemia. That factor, named cyanocobalamin for its high concentration of cobalt, is commonly called Vitamin B_{12}, which is now used universally via intramuscular injection for the lifesaving treatment of pernicious anemia.

In addition to working with Minot on the liver diet study, Murphy became Minot's partner in private practice in Boston. In 1924, he was appointed assistant in medicine at Harvard Medical School, promoted to associate in medicine at the Brigham Hospital in 1935, and became a senior associate in medicine and consultant in hematology there. He married Pearl Harriet Adams in 1919; they had a son and a daughter. Murphy's honors include the Cameron Prize and Lectureship of the University of Edinburgh, the Bronze Medal of the American Medical Association, and the Gold Medal of the Massachusetts Humane Society. He died in 1987, in Massachusetts.

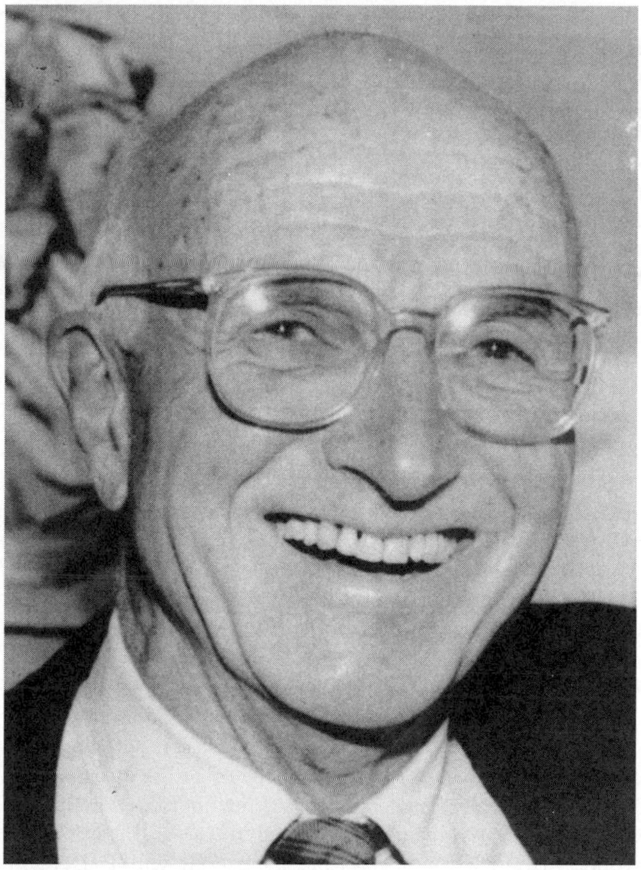

Joseph Edward Murray

MURRAY, JOSEPH E. (1919-)

American surgeon

Joseph Edward Murray was born 1919 in Massachusetts, the son of William Andrew Murray and Mary DePasquale Murray. He earned an A.B. in 1940 from Holy Cross College and then went on to Harvard University to earn his medical degree in 1943. His early work specialized in plastic surgery, in particular reconstructive surgery of the eye and hand. It was a training that would stand Murray in good stead with his later research, for one of the major problems plastic surgeons had to deal with was the rejection of skin grafts by the **immune system**. Murray and other plastic surgeons soon learned that grafts would take between identical twins.

In the late 1940s, Murray became drawn to the work of a team of doctors at Brigham Hospital who were studying end-stage renal disease, and one of the directions their researches was taking was transplantation. Research had been progressing over the past half century on kidney transplants in dogs, but there had never been a successful human transplant. These Harvard researchers, led by John Merrill and David Hume, had been doing experiments transplanting kidneys from cadavers onto the thigh of patients with kidney failure, grafting the third kidney to the femoral vessel of the recipient. One such thigh transplant functioned for about six months, enough time to allow the patient's own kidneys to heal and resume functioning. Kidney dialysis was also being perfected at this time, but Murray felt that it was only a temporary solution. He developed a surgical technique to connect the blood vessels of the donor kidney with those in the abdomen of the recipient, implanting the ureter directly into the urinary bladder.

The new procedure required the right patient; he or she would have to be one of a pair of identical twins with the other twin willing and able to donate a kidney, thus avoiding rejection by the immune system of the recipient. Such an opportunity came in 1954 when the Herrick brothers turned up at Brigham Hospital. The subsequent operation lasted five and one-half hours and was an immediate success. Richard Herrick lived another seven years on the transplanted kidney before dying of heart failure.

Murray continued to perform more successful operations on identical twins, including Edith Helm, who went on to have children and grandchildren, but the real problem now became how to suppress the immune reaction so that the operation would be more generally available. At first Murray and other researchers tried total body X rays and infusions of bone marrow from the donor to adapt the recipient's immune system. In most cases the transplants functioned for several weeks, but there were many failures. Finally in 1959, after a course of total body X rays, a non-identical twin survived a kidney transplant from his brother and went on to lead a normal life. Later in 1959 two Boston hematologists, William Dameshek and Robert Schwartz, demonstrated that the compound 6-mercaptopurine would prevent a host animal from rejecting a foreign protein. This was the opening Murray was looking for, and working with chemists and other researchers, Murray developed a drug regimen to suppress the immune system and thus allow an organ from a non-related donor to be accepted by the recipient's body. In 1962 Murray successfully completed the first organ transplant from a cadaver.

Murray's successes became known worldwide and inspired other surgeons to experiment with a variety of organ transplants. With the development of less toxic immune suppressants such as azathioprine, transplants became a growth industry with registries for organs documented worldwide. A related medical benefit was the increase in research into the rejection phenomenon, and thus into the functioning of the human immune system, research that has proved invaluable with the onset of Acquired Immunodeficiency Syndrome (**AIDS**).

After this work on renal transplants, Murray went back to his first love, plastic surgery, developing ways to repair inborn facial defects in children. He headed the plastic surgery divisions of Peter Bent Brigham Hospital from 1951–1986 and Children's Hospital Medical Center from 1972–1985, and he has also been a professor of surgery at Harvard Medical School since 1970. Murray was the recipient of the Gold Medal from the International Society of Surgeons in 1963. Four years after retiring from surgery, but not from administrative duties at Brigham Hospital, Murray was awarded the Nobel Prize for physiology or medicine along with E. Donnall Thomas, whose work in bone marrow transplants was closely related to Murray's research. By tackling the difficult problem of organ transplants, he provided a definitive solution to end-stage renal disease as well as stimulating worldwide research into immunology. His work in craniofacial reconstruction as a plastic surgeon has not only mended and saved lives, but also enlarged the scope and diversity of plastic surgery.

MUSCLE RELAXANTS

Strains, sprains, and other muscle injuries can result in **pain**, stiffness, and muscle spasms. Muscle relaxants do not heal the injuries, but they do relax muscles and help ease discomfort and stop muscle spasms. The muscle relaxant cyclobenzaprine (Flexeril) is also sometimes used to treat **fibromyalgia**, a condition that involves aches, stiffness, and fatigue.

Muscle relaxants work by acting on the central nervous system. In the United States, they are available only with a physician's prescription. Examples of muscle relaxants are carisoprodol (Soma), chlorzoxazone (Parafon Forte DSC), cyclobenzaprine (Flexeril), and methocarbamol (Robaxin). Most come only in tablet form. However, methocarbamol (Robaxin) is available in both tablet and injectable forms. Some muscle relaxants are available in Canada without a prescription.

Muscle relaxants are usually prescribed along with rest, **exercise**, physical therapy, or other treatments. Although the drugs may provide relief, they should never be considered a substitute for these other forms of treatment. These drugs may make the injury feel so much better that one is tempted to go back to normal activity, but doing too much too soon can actually make the injury worse.

Muscle relaxants work quite well for relieving muscle pain due to injuries, but are not effective for other types of pain. Some people feel drowsy, dizzy, confused, lightheaded, or less alert when using muscle relaxants drugs. These drugs may also cause blurred vision, clumsiness, or unsteadiness.

Because muscle relaxants work on the central nervous system, they may add to the effects of alcohol and other drugs that slow down the central nervous system. They may also add to the effects of anesthetics, including those used for dental procedures. For this reason, anyone who takes these drugs should not drive, operate machinery, or do anything else that might be dangerous until they have found out how the drugs affect them.

People with certain medical conditions or who are taking certain other medicines can have problems if they take muscle relaxants. Diabetes should be aware that the metaxalone (Skelaxin) may cause false test results on one type of test for sugar in the urine. People with epilepsy should be cautioned that taking the muscle relaxant methocarbamol may increase the likelihood of seizures.

Anyone who has allergies, who is breastfeeding has kidney disease, has suffered a recent **heart attack** or irregular heartbeat, has an overactive thyroid gland, hepatitis or liver disease, is a current or former drug or alcohol abuser, has **glaucoma**, or has problems with urination should discuss their condition with their doctor before taking muscle relaxants.

The most common side effects or muscle relaxants are vision changes, such as double vision or blurred vision; **dizziness**; lightheadedness; drowsiness; and dry mouth. These problems usually go away as the body adjusts to the drug and do not require medical treatment. Methocarbamol and chlorzoxazone may cause harmless color changes in urine—orange or reddish-purple with chlorzoxazone and purple, brown, or green with methocarbamol. The urine will return to its normal color when the patient stops taking the medicine.

Less common side effects, such as stomach cramps or pain, nausea and vomiting, **constipation**, **diarrhea**, **hiccups**, clumsiness or unsteadiness, confusion, nervousness, restlessness, irritability, flushed or red face, **headache**, heartburn, weakness, trembling, and sleep problems also may occur and do not need medical attention unless they do not go away or they interfere with normal activities.

More serious side effects are not common, but may occur. Anyone who experiences breathing problems, facial swelling, **fainting**, unusually fast or unusually slow heartbeat, **fever**, tightness in the chest, rash, **itching**, **hives**, burning, stinging, red, or bloodshot eyes, or unusual thoughts or dreams after taking muscle relaxants should seek medical help promptly

The muscle relaxant chlorzoxazone (Parafon Forte DSC) has caused serious, life-threatening liver problems in some people. The reaction is rare, but anyone taking the drug should stop taking it and notify his or her physician immediately if any of these symptoms occur: fever, rash, loss of appetite, nausea, vomiting, fatigue, pain in the upper right part of the abdomen, dark urine, or yellow skin or eyes.

Muscle relaxants may interact with some other medicines. When this happens, the effects of one or both of the drugs may change or the risk of side effects may be greater. Anyone who plans to take muscle relaxants should let the physician know all other medicines, including over-the-counter or nonprescription medicines, that he or she is taking.

MUSCLE SPASMS AND CRAMPS

Muscle spasms and cramps are spontaneous, often painful muscle contractions.

Most people are familiar with the sudden pain of a muscle cramp. The rapid, uncontrolled contraction, or spasm, happens unexpectedly, with either no stimulation or some trivially small one. The muscle contraction and pain last for several minutes, and then slowly ease. Cramps may affect any muscle, but are most common in the calves, feet, and hands. While painful, they are harmless, and in most cases, not related to any underlying disorder. Nonetheless, cramps and spasms can be manifestations of many neurological or muscular diseases.

The terms cramp and spasm can be somewhat vague, and they are sometimes used to include types of abnormal muscle activity other than sudden painful contraction. These include stiffness at rest, slow muscle relaxation, and spontaneous contractions of a muscle at rest (fasciculation). Fasciculation is a type of painless muscle spasm, marked by rapid, uncoordinated contraction of many small muscle fibers. A critical part of diagnosis is to distinguish these different meanings and to allow the patient to describe the problem as precisely as possible.

Normal voluntary muscle contraction begins when electrical signals are sent from the brain through the spinal cord along nerve cells called motor neurons. These include both the upper motor neurons within the brain and the lower motor neurons within the spinal cord and leading out to the muscle. At the muscle, chemicals released by the motor neuron stimulate the internal release of calcium ions from stores within the muscle cell. These calcium ions then interact with muscle proteins within the cell, causing the proteins (actin and myosin) to slide past one another. This motion pulls their fixed ends closer, thereby shortening the cell and, ultimately, the muscle itself. Recapture of calcium and unlinking of actin and myosin allows the muscle fiber to relax.

Abnormal contraction may be caused by abnormal activity at any stage in this process. Certain mechanisms within the brain and the rest of the central nervous system help regulate contraction. Interruption of these mechanisms can cause spasm. Motor neurons that are overly sensitive may fire below their normal thresholds. The muscle membrane itself may be over sensitive, causing contraction without stimulation. Calcium ions may not be recaptured quickly enough, causing prolonged contraction.

Interuption of brain mechanisms and overly sensitive motor neurons may result from damage to the nerve pathways. Possible causes include **stroke**, **multiple sclerosis**, **cerebral palsy**, neurodegenerative diseases, trauma, **spinal cord injury**, and nervous system poisons such as strychnine, **tetanus**, and certain insecticides. Nerve damage may lead to a prolonged or permanent muscle shortening called contracture.

Changes in muscle responsiveness may be due to or associated with:

- Prolonged **exercise**. Curiously, relaxation of a muscle actually requires energy to be expended. The energy is used to recapture calcium and to unlink actin and myosin. Normally, sensations of pain and fatigue signal that it is time to rest. Ignoring or overriding those warning signals can lead to such severe energy depletion that the muscle cannot be relaxed, causing a cramp. The familiar advice about not swimming after a heavy meal, when blood flow is directed away from the muscles, is intended to avoid this type of cramp. Rigor mortis, the stiffness of a corpse within the first 24 hours after **death**, is also due to this phenomenon.
- **Dehydration** and salt depletion. This may be brought on by protracted vomiting or **diarrhea**, or by copious sweating during prolonged exercise, especially in high temperatures. Loss of fluids and salts—especially sodium, potassium, magnesium, and calcium—can disrupt ion balances in both muscle and nerves. This can prevent them from responding and recovering normally, and can lead to cramp.
- Metabolic disorders that affect the energy supply in muscle. These are inherited diseases in which particular muscle enzymes are deficient. They include deficiencies of myophosphorylase (McArdle's disease), phosphorylase b kinase, phosphofructokinase, phosphoglycerate kinase, and lactate dehydrogenase.
- Myotonia. This causes stiffness due to delayed relaxation of the muscle, but does not cause the spontaneous contraction usually associated with cramps. However, many patients with myotonia do experience cramping from exercise. Symptoms of myotonia are often worse in the cold. Myotonias include myotonic dystrophy, myotonia congenita, paramyotonia congenita, and neuromyotonia.

Fasciculations may be due to fatigue, cold, medications, metabolic disorders, nerve damage, or neurodegenerative disease, including amyotrophic lateral sclerosis (**Lou Gehrig's Disease**). Most people experience brief, mild fasciculations from time to time, usually in the calves.

The pain of a muscle cramp is intense, localized, and often debilitating Coming on quickly, it may last for minutes and fade gradually. Contractures develop more slowly, over days or weeks, and may be permanent if untreated. Fasciculations may occur at rest or after muscle contraction, and may last several minutes.

Abnormal contractions are diagnosed through a careful medical history, physical and neurological examination, and electromyography of the affected muscles. Electromyography records electrical activity in the muscle during rest and movement.

Most cases of simple cramps require no treatment other than patience and stretching. Gently and gradually stretching and massaging the affected muscle may ease the pain and hasten recovery.

More prolonged or regular cramps may be treated with drugs such as carbamazepine, phenytoin, or quinine. Fluid and salt replacement, either orally or intravenously, is used to treat dehydration. Treatment of underlying metabolic or neurologic disease, where possible, may help relieve symptoms.

Cramps may be treated or prevented with Gingko (*Ginkgo biloba*) or Japanese quince (*Chaenomeles speciosa*). Supplements of vitamin E, niacin, calcium, and magnesium may also help. Taken at bedtime, they may help to reduce the likelihood of night cramps.

Occasional cramps are common, and have no special medical significance.

The likelihood of developing cramps may be reduced by eating a healthy diet with appropriate levels of **minerals**, and getting regular exercise to build up energy reserves in muscle. Avoiding exercising in extreme heat helps prevent heat cramps. Heat cramps can also be avoided by taking salt tablets and water before prolonged exercise in extreme heat. Taking a warm bath before bedtime may increase circulation to the legs and reduce the incidence of nighttime leg cramps.

Muscular dystrophy

The term *muscular dystrophy* refers to any condition in which healthy muscle cells die and are replaced by fat and connective tissue. The result of this change is a weakening and wasting of muscles that progress over time. Eventually a person with this condition loses all control over his or her muscles, is no longer able to walk, and eventually dies of respiratory failure. Most patients do not live beyond the age of 30.

At least seven distinct forms of muscular dystrophy are known: *Duchenne*, *facioscapulohumoral*, *limb-girdle*, *distal myopathy*, *ocular myopathy*, *myotonic*, and *Werdnig-Hoffman*. All are hereditary disorders, although the genetic mechanisms by which they are transmitted differ from type to type.

The most common and most severe form of muscular dystrophy is named for a French neurologist, **Guillaume B. A. Duchenne** (1806-1875), who first described the disorder in 1861. Our current understanding of Duchenne muscular dystrophy is due in large part on the work of the American geneticist, Elizabeth Shull Russell (b.1913). In 1951, Russell accidentally observed Duchenne muscular dystrophy symptoms in a colony of mice with which she was working. Over a period of years, she was able to show that this form of muscular dystrophy is inherited as an X-linked recessive trait.

An important step forward in understanding and possibly treating Duchenne muscular dystrophy occurred in 1986 when scientists at Harvard Medical School discovered that the defective gene responsible for Duchenne muscular dystrophy is located on the short arm of the X chromosome. They found that the protein produced by the normal gene, dystrophin, is absent from the cells of Duchenne muscular dystrophy patients. One consequence of this discovery was a 1989 research project in which mice with a defective Duchenne muscular dystrophy gene were treated with immature muscle cells. The new muscle cells apparently contained correct copies of the gene and began producing dystrophin in normal amounts.

More recently, gene therapy has come to the forefront as a therapeutic approach for muscular dystrophy, especially since scientists have identified the mutated genes that can cause myotonic, Duchenne, Becker, some forms of limb-girdle, a form of congenital, and Emery-Dreifuss muscular dystrophies. For example, researchers have developed an artificial dystrophin gene to replace the absent protein in Duchenne muscular dystrophy, and research is ongoing into how to best deliver copies of these genes into muscle cells so that they work efficiently and continue to function.

One approach set for human clinical trials will involve injections of genes into the biceps muscle. In 1998, researchers also showed that genes containing the muscle protein sarcoglycan can correct defects in limb-girdle muscular dystrophy when the genes are injected into the leg muscles of hamsters. Since these studies are using a naturally occurring sarcoglycan protein, it can be inserted with minimal use of immunosuppressive drugs. The use of these drugs during gene therapy research using artificial proteins has proven to be a major obstacle to gene therapy because suppressing the **immune system** can make the patient susceptible to other diseases and immunosuppressive drugs have many potentially serious side effects. In addition to opening up a window for new therapies, research into the genetics of muscular dystrophy are helping scientists to better understand the disease. For example, because of recent insights into the genetic components of muscular dystrophy, researchers now know that Duchenne and Becker dystrophies are really the same disease distinguished only by variations in severity. In other cases, some types of muscular dystrophy thought to be one disease are now known to be different diseases caused by various genetic defects.

Musculoskeletal system

The muscular system is the body's network of tissues for both conscious and unconscious movement. Movement is generated through the contraction and relaxation of specific muscles. Some muscles, like those in the arms and legs, are involved in voluntary movements such as raising a hand or flexing the foot. Other muscles are involuntary and function without conscious effort. Voluntary muscles include skeletal muscles and total about 650 in the whole human body. Skeletal muscles are controlled by the somatic **nervous system**; whereas the autonomic nervous system controls involuntary muscles. Involuntary muscles include muscles that line internal organs. These smooth muscles are called visceral muscles, and they perform tasks not generally associated with voluntary activity throughout the body even when it is asleep. Smooth muscles control several automatic physiological responses such as pupil constriction when iris muscles contract in bright light and blood vessel dilation when smooth muscles around them relax, or lengthen. In addition to skeletal and smooth muscle which are considered voluntary and involuntary, respectively, cardiac muscle exists which is considered neither. Cardiac muscle is not under conscious control, and it can also function without external nervous system regulation.

Smooth muscles derive their name from their appearance when viewed in polarized light microscopy; in contrast to cardiac and skeletal muscles which have striations (appearance of parallel bands or lines), smooth muscle is unstriated. Striations result from the pattern of the myofilaments, actin and myosin, which line the myofibrils within each muscle cell. When many myofilaments align along the length of a muscle cell, light and dark regions create the striated appearance. This microscopic view of muscle reveals some hint of how muscles alter their shape to induce movement. Because muscle cells tend to be elongated, they are often called muscle fibers. Muscle cells are distinct from other cells in the body in shape, protein composition, and in the fact that they are multi-nucleated (have more than one nucleus per cell).

Skeletal muscles are probably the must familiar type of muscle to people. Skeletal muscles are the ones that ache when someone goes for that first outdoor run in the spring after not running much during the winter. And skeletal muscles are heavily used when someone carries in the grocery bags. **Exercise** may increase muscle fiber size, but muscle fiber number generally remains constant. Skeletal muscles take up about 40% of the body's mass, or weight. They also use a great deal of oxygen and nutrients from the blood supply. Multiple levels of skeletal muscle tissue receive their own blood supplies.

Like all muscles, skeletal muscles can be studied at both a macroscopic and a microscopic level. At the macroscopic level, skeletal muscles usually originate at one point of attachment to a tendon and terminate at another tendon at the other end of an adjoining bone. Tendons are rich in the protein collagen which is arranged in a wavy way so that it can stretch out and provide additional length at the muscular-bone junction.

Skeletal muscles act in pairs where the flexing (shortening) of one muscle is balanced by a lengthening (relaxation) of its paired muscle or a group of muscles. These antagonistic (opposite) muscles can open and close joints such as the elbow or knee. Muscles which contract and cause a joint to close are called flexor muscles, and those which contract to cause a joint to stretch out are called extensors. Skeletal muscle which support the skull, backbone, and rib cage are called axial skeletal muscles; whereas, skeletal muscles of the limbs are called distal. These muscles attach to bones via strong, thick connective tissue called tendons. Several skeletal muscles work in a highly coordinated manner in activities such as locomotion, walking.

Skeletal muscles are organized into extrafusal and intrafusal fibers. Extrafusal fibers are the strong, outer layers of muscle. This type of muscle fiber is the most common. Intrafusal fibers which make up the central region of the muscle are weaker than extrafusal fibers. Skeletal muscles fibers are additionally characterized as "fast" or "slow" based on their activity patterns. Fast, also called "white," muscle fibers contract rapidly, have poor blood supply, operate anaerobically, and fatigue rapidly. Slow, also called "red," muscle fibers contract more slowly, have better blood supplies, operate aerobically, and do not fatigue as easily. Slow muscle fibers are used in movements which are sustained such as maintaining posture.

Skeletal muscles are enclosed in a dense sheath of connective tissue called the epimysium. Within the epimysium, muscles are sectioned into columns of muscle fiber bundles, called primary bundles or fasciculi, which are each covered by connective tissue called the perimysium. An average skeletal muscle may have 20 - 40 fasciculi which are further subdivided into several muscle fibers. Each muscle fiber (cell) is covered by connective tissue called endomysium. Both the epimysium and the perimysium contain blood and lymph vessels to supply the muscle with nutrients and oxygen and remove waste products, respectively. The endomysium has an extensive network of capillaries that supply individual muscle fibers. Individual muscle fibers vary in diameter from 10-60 micrometers and in length from a few millimeters to about 12 in (30 cm) in the sartorius muscle of the thigh.

Skeletal muscles function as the link between the somatic nervous system and the skeletal system. One does not move a skeletal muscle for the sake of moving the muscle unless one is a bodybuilder. Skeletal muscles are used to carry out instructions from the brain so that someone can accomplish something. For instance, someone decides that they would like a bite of cake. Unless the cake will come to the mouth by itself, the person needs to figure out some way to get that cake to their mouth. The brain tells the muscle to contract in the forearm allowing it to flex so that the hand is in position to get a forkful of cake. But the muscle alone cannot support the weight of a fork; it is the sturdy bones of the forearm that allow the muscles to complete the task of obtaining the cake. Hence, the skeletal and muscular systems work together as a lever system with joints acting as a fulcrum to carry out instructions from the nervous system.

The somatic nervous system controls skeletal muscle movement through motor neurons. Alpha motor neurons extend from the spinal cord and terminate on individual muscle fibers. The axon, or signal sending end, of the alpha neurons branch to innervate multiple muscle fibers. The nerve terminal forms a synapse, or junction, with the muscle to create a neuromuscular junction. The neurotransmitter, acetylcholine (Ach) is released from the axon terminal into the synapse. From the synapse, the Ach binds to receptors on the muscle surface which triggers events leading to muscle contraction. While alpha motor neurons innervate extrafusal fibers, intrafusal fibers are innervated by gamma motor neurons.

Voluntary skeletal muscle movements are initiated by the motor cortex in the brain. Then signals travel down the spinal cord to the alpha motor neuron to result in contraction. However, not all movement of skeletal muscles is voluntary. Certain reflexes occur in response to dangerous stimuli, such as extreme heat. Reflexive skeletal muscular movement is controlled at the level of the spinal cord and does not require higher brain initiation. Reflexive movements are processed at this level to minimize the amount of time necessary to implement a response.

In addition to motor neuron activity in skeletal muscular activity, a number of sensory nerves carry information to the brain to regulate muscle tension and contraction to optimize muscle action. Muscles function at peak performance when they are not overstretched or overcontracted. Sensory neurons within the muscle send feedback to the brain with regard to muscle length and state of contraction.

Cardiac muscles, as is evident from their name, make up the muscular portion of the heart. While almost all cardiac muscle is confined to the heart, some of these cells extend for a short distance into cardiac vessels before tapering off completely. The heart muscle is also called the myocardium. The heart muscle is responsible for more than two billion beats in a lifetime. The myocardium has some properties similar to skeletal muscle tissue, but it is also unique. Like skeletal muscles, myocardium is striated; however, the cardiac muscle fibers are smaller and shorter than skeletal muscle fibers averaging 5-15 micrometers in diameter and 20-30 micrometers in length. In addition, cardiac muscles align lengthwise more than side-by-side compared to skeletal muscle fibers. The microscopic structure of cardiac muscle is also unique in that these cells are branched such that they can simultaneously communicate with multiple cardiac muscle fibers.

Cardiac muscle cells are surrounded by an endomysium like the skeletal muscle cells. But innervation of autonomic nerves to the heart do not form any special junction like that found in skeletal muscle. Instead, the branching structure and extensive interconnectedness of cardiac muscle fibers allows for stimulation of the heart to spread into neighboring myocardial cells; this does not require the individual fibers to be stimulated. Although external nervous stimuli can enhance or diminish cardiac muscle contraction, heart muscles can also contract spontaneously making them myogenic. Like skeletal muscle cells, cardiac muscle fibers can increase in size with physical conditioning, but they rarely increase in number.

Smooth muscle falls into two general categories, visceral smooth muscle and multi-unit smooth muscle. Visceral smooth muscle fibers line internal organs such as the intestines, stomach, and uterus. They also facilitate the movement of substances through tubular areas such as blood vessels and the small intestines. Multi-unit smooth muscles function in a highly localized way in areas such as the iris of the eye. Contrary to contractions in visceral smooth muscle, contractions in multi-unit smooth muscle fibers do not readily spread to neighboring muscle cells.

Smooth muscle is unstriated with innervations from both sympathetic (flight or fight) and parasympathetic (more relaxed) nerves of the autonomic nervous system. Smooth muscle appears unstriated under a polarized light microscope, because the myofilaments inside are less organized. Smooth muscle fibers contain actin and myosin myofilaments which are more haphazardly arranged than they are in skeletal muscles. The sympathetic neurotransmitter, Ach, and parasympathetic neurotransmitter, norepinephrine, activate this type of muscle tissue.

The concentric arrangement of some smooth muscle fibers enables them to control dilation and constriction in the intestines, blood vessels, and other areas. While innervation of these cells is not individual, excitation from one cell can spread to adjacent cells through nexuses which join neighbor cells. Smooth muscle cells have a small diameter of about 5-15 micrometers and are long, typically 15-500 micrometers. They are also wider in the center than at their ends. Gap junctions connect small bundles of cells which are, in turn, arranged in sheets.

Within hollow organs, such as the uterus, smooth muscle cells are arranged into two layers. The outer layer is usually arranged in a longitudinal fashion surrounding the inner layer which is arranged in a circular orientation. Many smooth muscles are regulated by hormones in addition to the neurotransmitters of the autonomic nervous system. In addition, contraction of some smooth muscles are myogenic or triggered by stretching as in the uterus and gastrointestinal tract.

Smooth muscle differs from skeletal and cardiac muscle in its energy utilization as well. Smooth muscles are not as dependent on oxygen availability as cardiac and skeletal muscles are. Smooth muscle uses glycolysis to generate much of its metabolic energy.

MUSHROOM POISONING

Mushroom poisoning refers to the severe and often deadly effects of various toxins that are found in certain types of mushrooms. The toxins initially cause severe abdominal cramping, vomiting, and watery **diarrhea**, and then lead to liver and kidney failure.

The highest reported incidences of mushroom poisoning occur in western Europe, where a popular pastime is amateur mushroom hunting. Since the 1970s, the United States has seen an increase in mushroom poisoning due to an increase in the popularity of "natural" foods, the use of mushrooms as recreational hallucinogens, and an increasing awareness of the gourmet qualities of wild mushrooms.

About 90% of the deaths due to mushroom poisoning in the United States and western Europe result from eating *Amanita phalloides*. This mushroom is recognized by its metallic green cap (the color may vary from light yellow to greenish brown), white gills (located under the cap), white stem, and bulb-shaped structure at the base of the stem. A pure white variety of this species also occurs. **Poisoning** results from ingestion of as few as one to three mushrooms. Higher death rates occur with children less than 10 years old and with the elderly.

Poisonous mushrooms contain at least two different types of toxins, each of which can cause death if taken in large enough quantities. Some of the toxins found in poisonous mushrooms are among the most potent ever discovered. One group of poisons, known as amatoxins, blocks the production of DNA. This leads to the death of many cells, especially those that reproduce frequently such as in the liver, intestines, and kidney. Other mushroom poisons affect the proteins needed for muscle contraction, and therefore reduce the ability of muscles to function.

Symptoms of *Amanita* poisoning occur in different stages or phases. Abdominal cramping, nausea, vomiting, and severe watery diarrhea occur anywhere from 6-24 hours after eating the mushroom and last for about 24 hours. These intestinal symptoms can lead to **dehydration** and low blood pressure (**hypotension**).

A period of remission of symptoms that lasts 1-2 days occurs next. During this time, the patient feels better, but blood tests begin to show evidence of liver and kidney damage. Liver and kidney failure continue to develop and either lead to death within about a week or recovery within 2-3 weeks.

Other symptoms are due to either a decrease in blood clotting factors that leads to internal bleeding or reduced muscle function, with the development of weakness and **paralysis**.

In most cases, the fact that the patient has recently eaten wild mushrooms is the clue to the cause of symptoms. Moreover, the identification of any remaining mushrooms by a qualified mushroom specialist (mycologist) can be a key to diagnosis. When in doubt, the toxin known as alpha-amantin can be found in the blood, urine, or stomach contents of an individual who has ingested poisonous *Amanita* mushrooms.

There is no specific antidote for mushroom poisoning. However, several advances in therapy have decreased the death rate over the last several years. Early replacement of lost body fluids has been a major factor in improving survival rates.

Therapy is aimed at decreasing the amount of toxin in the body. Initially, attempts are made to remove toxins from the upper gastrointestinal tract by inducing vomiting or by gastric lavage (stomach pumping). After that, continuous aspiration of the upper portion of the small intestine through a nasogastric tube is done, and oral charcoal (every four hours for 48 hours) is given to prevent absorption of toxin. These measures work best if started within six hours of ingestion.

In the United States, early removal of mushroom poison by way of an artificial kidney machine (dialysis) has become part of the treatment program. This is combined with the correction of any imbalances of salts such as sodium or potassium (electrolytes) dissolved in the blood. An enzyme called thioctic acid and **corticosteroids** also appear to be beneficial, as well as high doses of penicillin. In Europe, a chemical taken from the milk thistle plant, *Silybum marianum*, is also part of treatment.

When liver failure develops, liver transplantation may be the only treatment option. Although the mortality rate has decreased with improved and rapid treatment, according to some medical reports death still occurs in 20-30% of cases, with a higher mortality rate in children.

The most important factor in preventing mushroom poisoning is to avoid eating wild mushrooms. For anyone not expert in mushroom identification, there are generally no easily recognizable differences between nonpoisonous and poisonous mushrooms. Some edible European mushrooms look very similar to poisonous mushrooms found in the United States, putting European immigrant mushroom hunters at special risk. Most mushroom poisons are not destroyed or deactivated by cooking, canning, freezing, drying, or other means of food preparation.

Music therapy

Music therapy is administered by a trained music therapist to individuals of all ages who require special services because of behavioral, social, learning, or physical disabilities. The controlled use of music helps people overcome problem conditions or behaviors. Music therapy can be found in hospitals, clinics, day care facilities, schools, community mental health centers, substance abuse facilities, nursing homes, hospices, **rehabilitation** centers, correctional facilities, and private practices.

Music therapy sessions can be conducted in a group setting or in an individual one-on-one setting. The length of the sessions can vary, but are on average 30-60 minutes.

A qualified music therapist first assesses the strengths and needs of each client and then provides the appropriate treatment, including creating, singing, moving to, and/or listening to music. A client's abilities are strengthened and then transferred to other areas of their lives through their musical involvement in a therapeutic context. Research supports the effectiveness of music therapy in improving communication, facilitating movement and overall physical rehabilitation, providing emotional support for clients and their families, motivating people to cope with treatment, and providing an outlet for the expression of feelings. Clients can develop their auditory, visual, motor, communication, social, academic (cognitive), and self-help skills through many different types of music activities.

A music therapist must prepare and carefully plan in order for music therapy treatment programs and intervention strategies to be effective. The four basic steps for a music therapist to prepare for a new client are: (1) define the client's problem or area of need (assessment); (2) set a therapeutic goal for the client; (3) devise music activities that are related to the goal and appropriate to the client's level of functioning and capacity to respond; and (4) implement the procedure and evaluate the client's responses.

Music therapy often elicits changes in non-target behaviors that may be just as significant as those initially sought. In the music therapy literature, positive "side effects" are almost always reported, as a result of the many influences of music. Frequently observed increases which often accompany musical experiences are: motivation to try new things, pride in self, and enhanced fine motor coordination.

Mutism

Mutism is a rare childhood condition characterized by a consistent failure to speak in situations where talking is expected. The child has the ability to converse normally, and does so, for example, in the home, but consistently fails to speak in specific situations such as at school or with strangers. It is estimated that one in every 1,000 school-age children are affected by mutism.

Experts believe that this problem is associated with **anxiety** and fear in social situations such as in school or in the company of adults. Therefore mutism is often considered a type of social phobia. This is not a communication disorder because the affected children can converse normally in some situations. It is not a developmental disorder because their ability to talk, when they choose to do so, is appropriate for their age level. This problem has been linked to anxiety, and one of the major ways in which both children and adults attempt to cope with anxiety is by avoiding whatever provokes the anxiety.

Affected children are typically shy, and are especially so in the presence of strangers and unfamiliar surroundings or situations. However, the behaviors of children with this condition go beyond shyness. Refusing to speak, or speaking in a whisper, spares the child from the possible humiliation or embarrassment of "saying the wrong thing." When asked a direct question by teachers, for example, the affected child may act as if they are unable to answer. Some children may communicate via gestures, nodding, or very brief utterances. Additional features may include excessive shyness, oppositional behavior, and impaired learning at school.

The diagnosis of mutism is fairly easy to make because the signs and symptoms are clear-cut and easily observable. However, other social disorders effecting social speech, such as **autism** or **schizophrenia**, must be considered when making the diagnosis.

There are two recommended treatments for mutism: behavior modification therapy and antidepressant medication. Treatment is most effective when individualized to each patient. It has been suggested that speech pathologists may also be able to help these children.

The prognosis for mutism is good. Sometimes it disappears suddenly on its own. The negative impact on learning and school activities may, however, persist into adult life. Mutism cannot be prevented because the cause is not known. However, family conflict or problems at school contribute to the seriousness of the symptoms.

Myasthenia gravis

Myasthenia gravis (MG) is an autoimmune disease that causes muscle weakness. MG affects the neuromuscular junction, interrupting the communication between nerve and muscle, and thereby causing weakness. A person with MG may have difficulty moving their eyes, walking, speaking clearly, swallowing, and even breathing, depending on the severity and distribution of weakness. Increased weakness with exertion, and improvement with rest, is a characteristic feature of MG. MG affects "voluntary" muscles, which are those muscles under conscious control responsible for movement. It does not affect heart muscle or the "smooth" muscle found in the digestive system and other internal organs.

About 30,000 people in the United States are affected by MG. It can occur at any age, but is most common in women who are in their late teens and early twenties, and in men in their sixties and seventies.

While the trigger for the autoimmune attack is unknown, about 10% of those with MG also have thymomas, or benign tumors of the thymus gland. The thymus is a principal organ of the immune system, and researchers speculate that thymic irregularities are involved in the progression of MG, even in many people without overt thymomas. Other possible factors that may contribute to MG are infections, genes, and abnormal immune system development.

The earliest symptoms of MG often result from weakness of the extraocular muscles, which control eye movements. Symptoms involving the eye (ocular symptoms) include double vision (diplopia), especially when not gazing straight ahead, and difficulty raising the eyelids (ptosis). A person with ptosis may need to tilt their head back to see. Eye-related symptoms remain the only symptoms for about 15% of MG patients. Another common early symptom is difficulty chewing and swallowing, due to weakness in the bulbar muscles, which are in the mouth and throat. **Choking** becomes more likely, especially with food that requires extensive chewing.

Weakness usually becomes more widespread within several months of the first symptoms, reaching their maximum within a year in two-thirds of patients. Weakness may involve muscles of the arms, legs, neck, trunk, and face, and affect the ability to lift objects, walk, hold the head up, and speak.

Symptoms of MG become worse upon exertion, and better with rest. Heat, including heat from the sun, hot showers, and hot drinks, may increase weakness. Infection and **stress** may worsen symptoms. Symptoms may vary from day to day and month to month, with intervals of no weakness interspersed with a progressive decline in strength.

While there is no cure for myasthenia gravis, there are a number of treatments that effectively control symptoms in most people.

Pyridostigmine (Mestinon) is usually the first drug tried. Like edrophonium, pyridostigmine blocks acetylcholinesterase. It is longer-acting, taken by mouth, and well-tolerated. Loss of responsiveness and disease progression combine to eventually make pyridostigmine ineffective in tolerable doses in many patients.

Thymectomy, or removal of the thymus gland, has increasingly become standard treatment for MG. Up to 85% of people with MG improve after thymectomy, with complete remission eventually seen in about 30%. The improvement may take months or even several years to fully develop. Thymectomy is not usually recommended for children with MG, since the thymus continues to play an important immune role throughout childhood.

Immune-suppressing drugs are used to treat MG if response to pyridostigmine and thymectomy are not adequate. Drugs include **corticosteroids** such as prednisone, and the nonsteroids azathioprine (Imuran) and cyclosporine (Sandimmune).

Plasma exchange may be performed to treat myasthenic crisis or to improve very weak patients before thymectomy. In this procedure, blood plasma is removed and replaced with purified plasma free of autoantibodies. It can produce a temporary improvement in symptoms, but is too expensive for long-term treatment. Another blood treatment, intravenous immunoglobulin therapy, is also used for myasthenic crisis. In this procedure, large quantities of purified immune proteins (immunoglobulins) are injected. For unknown reasons, this leads to symptomatic improvement in up to 85% of patients. It is also too expensive for long-term treatment.

People with weakness of the bulbar muscles may need to eat softer foods that are easier to chew and swallow. In more severe cases, it may be necessary to obtain nutrition through a feeding tube placed into the stomach (gastrostomy tube).

Most people with MG can be treated successfully enough to prevent their condition from becoming debilitating. In some cases, however, symptoms may worsen even with vigorous treatment, leading to generalized weakness and disability. MG rarely causes early **death** except when untreated.

MYCOPLASMA INFECTIONS

Mycoplasma are the smallest of the free-living organisms; unlike viruses, mycoplasma can reproduce outside of living cells. Many species within the genus *Mycoplasma* thrive as parasites in human, bird, and animal hosts. Some species can cause disease in humans.

Mycoplasma are found most often on the surfaces of mucous membranes. They can cause chronic inflammatory diseases of the respiratory system, urogenital tract, and joints. The most common human illnesses caused by mycoplasma are due to infection with *M. pneumoniae,* which is responsible for 10-20% of all **pneumonia**s.

Pneumonia caused by mycoplasma is also called atypical pneumonia, walking pneumonia, or community-acquired pneumonia. Infection moves easily among people in close contact because it is spread primarily when infected droplets from the respiratory system circulate in the air due to coughing, spitting, or sneezing.

Atypical pneumonias can affect otherwise healthy people who have close contact with one another. Pneumonia caused by *M.pneumoniae* may start out with symptoms of an upper respiratory infection, probably a **sore throat**, progressing to a dry cough within a few days. Gradually, **fever**, fatigue, muscle aches, and a cough that produces thin sputum (spit or phlegm) will emerge. Non-respiratory symptoms may occur too: abdominal **pain**, **headache**, and **diarrhea**. About 20% of patients may have ear pain.

Another mycoplasma species, *M. hominis*, is common in the mucous membranes of the genital area and can cause infection in both males and females. Its presence does not always cause symptoms.

Usually, mycoplasma pneumonia will be identified after other common diagnoses have been eliminated. For example, a common antibiotic might be prescribed for a respiratory infection producing fever and cough. If symptoms do not improve in 3-5 days, the organism causing the disease is not a typical one and not susceptible to this antibiotic.

If a Gram's stain (a common test done on sputum) does not indicate a gram-positive pathogen, the doctor will suspect a gram-negative organism, such as mycoplasma. The actual underlying organism may not be identified (it isn't in almost 50% of cases of atypical pneumonia). Although it is rare, a rash may appear along with pneumonia symptoms. This should trigger suspicion of mycoplasma pneumonia, even if laboratory tests are inconclusive.

Standard x rays may reveal a patchy material that has entered the lung tissue; this can be evident for months. Highly sophisticated and specific polymerase chain reaction methods (PCR) have been developed for many respiratory pathogens, including *M. pneumoniae*. They are not readily available and are very expensive.

A 2-3 week course of certain antibiotics (erythromycin, azithromycin, clarithromycin, dirithromycin, or doxycycline) is generally prescribed for atypical pneumonia. This disease is infectious for weeks, even after the patient starts antibiotics. A persistent cough may linger for 6 weeks.

Mycoplasma pneumonia may be involved in the onset of **asthma** in adults. Other rare complications include meningoencephalitis, **Guillain-Barré syndrome**, mononeuritis multiplex, **myocarditis**, or **pericarditis**. This may increase the risk of acute heart **arrhythmias** leading to **sudden cardiac death**. However, with proper treatment and rest, recovery should be complete.

At this time, there are no vaccines for mycoplasma infection. It is difficult to control its spread, especially in a group setting. The best measures are still the simplest ones. Avoid exposure to people with respiratory infections whenever possible, wash hands frequently, and cover the moth while coughing or sneezing.

MYOCARDITIS

Myocarditis is an inflammatory disease of the heart muscle (myocardium). Most cases of myocarditis in the United States originate from a virus, and the disease may remain undiagnosed by doctors due to lack of initial symptoms. The disease may also present itself as an acute, catastrophic illness that requires immediate treatment. Although the inflammation or degeneration of the heart muscle that myocarditis causes may be fatal, this disease often goes undetected. It may also disguise itself as ischemic, valvular, or hypertensive heart disease. Myocarditis is a rare but serious condition that affects both males and females of any age.

An inflammation of the heart muscle may occur as an isolated disorder or be the dominant feature of a systemic disease (one that affects the whole body).

While there are several contributing factors that may lead to myocarditis, the primary cause is viral. Myocarditis usually results from the Coxsackie B virus, and may also result from **measles**, **influenza**, chicken pox, hepatitis virus, or the adenovirus in children.

If an acute onset of severe myocarditis occurs, a patient may display the following symptoms: rhythm disturbances of the heart; rapid heartbeat (ventricular tachycardia); left or right ventricular enlargement; shortness of breath (dyspnea); **pulmonary edema** (the accumulation of fluid in the lungs); and swollen legs.

Additional causes of myocarditis include: bacterial infections, such as **tetanus**, **gonorrhea**, or **tuberculosis**; parasite infections; **rheumatic fever**; surgery on the heart; **radiation therapy** for **cancer** and certain medications.

As of 1996, research has shown that illegal drugs and toxic substances may also produce acute or chronic injury to the myocardium. These studies also indicate an increase in the incidence of myocarditis from the use of cocaine. Further studies conducted in 1996 indicate that **malnutrition** encourages the Coxsackie B virus to flourish, leading to the potential development of myocarditis. Human **immunodeficiency** virus (HIV) is also now recognized as a cause of myocarditis, although its prevalence is not known.

The best way to diagnose myocarditis may be through a person's observation of his or her own symptoms, followed by a thorough medical history and physical exam conducted by a doctor. Tests usually include laboratory blood studies and **echocardiography**. An electrocardiogram (ECG) is also routinely used due to its ability to detect a mild case of the disease. Cardiac catheterization and **angiography** are additional diagnostic tests used to determine the presence of myocarditis, or to rule out other possible heart diseases that may lead to heart failure.

Another measure used to diagnosis myocarditis is the endomyocardial biopsy procedure. This invasive catheterization procedure examines a piece of the endocardium (the lining membrane of the inner surface of the heart) to verify the presence of the disease.

While myocarditis is a serious condition, there is no medical treatment necessary if it results from a general viral infection. The only steps to recovery include rest and avoidance of physical exertion. Adequate rest becomes more important to recovery if the case or myocarditis is severe with signs of dilated cardiomyopathy (disease of the heart muscles). In this case, medical treatment for congestive heart failure may include medications such as angiotensin converting enzyme (ACE) inhibitors, **diuretics** to reduce fluid retention, digitalis to stimulate a stronger heartbeat, and/or low-dose beta-blockers.

If myocarditis is caused by a bacterial infection, the disease is treated with **antibiotics**. If severe rhythm disturbances are involved, cardiac assist devices, an ''**artificial heart**,'' or heart transplantation may be the only option for complete recovery.

The outlook for a diagnosed case of myocarditis caused by a viral infection is excellent, with many cases healing themselves spontaneously. Because this disease ranges from mild to severe, the disease resolution may vary from complete healing (with or without significant scarring), to severe congestive heart failure leading to death or requiring a heart transplant.

Inflammation of the myocardium may also cause acute **pericarditis** (inflammation of the outer lining of the heart). Due to the potential effects of the disease, including sudden death, it is imperative that proper medical attention be obtained.

MYOPATHIES

Myopathies are diseases of skeletal muscle which are not caused by nerve disorders. These diseases cause the skeletal or voluntary muscles to become weak or wasted. There are many different types of myopathies, some of which are inherited, some inflammatory, and some caused by endocrine problems. Myopathies are rare and not usually fatal. Typically, effects are mild, largely causing muscle weakness and movement problems, and many are transitory. Only rarely will patients become dependent on a wheelchair. However, **muscular dystrophy** (which is technically a form of myopathy) is far more severe. Some types of this disease are fatal in early adulthood.

Myopathies are usually degenerative, but they are sometimes caused by drug side effects, chemical **poisoning**, or a chronic disorder of the immune system. Among their many functions, genes are responsible for overseeing the production of proteins important in maintaining healthy cells. Muscle cells produce thousands of proteins. With each of the inherited myopathies, a genetic defect is linked to a lack of, or problem with, one of the proteins needed for normal muscle cell function. Different kinds of myopathy caused by different defective genes.

Most, but not all, of these genetic myopathies are dominant, which means that a child needs to inherit only one copy of the defective gene from one parent in order to show symptoms of the disease. Male and female children are equally at risk.

The major symptoms associated with the genetic myopathies include: weakness of voluntary muscles (affected muscles almost always lack reflexes); delays in reaching developmental motor milestones; problems with running, jumping, and climbing stairs that develop in childhood; muscle stiffness triggered by fatigue, **stress**, cold, or long rest periods, such as a night's sleep; attacks of temporary muscle weakness (muscles work normally between attacks); or multisystem problems primarily involving the brain and muscles.

In some cases, myopathies can be caused by a malfunctioning endocrine gland (or glands), which produces either too much or too little of the chemical messengers called hormones. Hormones are carried by the blood and one of their many functions is to regulate muscle activity. Problems in producing hormones can lead to muscle weakness.

Other myopathies are inflammatory, leading to inflamed, weakened muscles. Inflammation is a protective response of injured tissues characterized by redness, increased heat, swelling, and/or **pain** in the affected area. Examples of this type include polymyositis, dermatomyositis, and myositis ossificans.

Dermatomyositis is a disease of the connective tissue that also involves weak, tender, inflamed muscles. In fact, muscle tissue loss may be so severe that the person may be unable to walk. Skin inflammation is also present. The cause is unknown, but viral infection and **antibiotics** are associated with the condition. In some cases, dermatomyositis is associated with rheumatologic disease or **cancer**.

Polymyositis involves inflammation of many muscles usually accompanied by deformity, swelling, sleeplessness, pain, sweating, and tension. It, too, may be associated with cancer. Myositis ossificans is a rare inherited disease in which muscle tissue is replaced by bone, beginning in childhood.

While considered to be a separate group of diseases, the muscular dystrophies also technically involve muscle wasting and can be described as myopathies. These relatively rare diseases appear during childhood and adolescence, and are caused by muscle destruction or degeneration. They are genetic disorders caused by problems in the production of key proteins.

The forms of muscular dystrophy (MD) differ according to the way they are inherited, the age of onset, the muscles they affect, and how fast they progress. The most common type is Duchenne MD, affecting one or two in every 10,000 boys. Other types of MD include Becker's, myotonic dystrophy, limb-girdle MD, and facioscapulohumeral MD.

Early diagnosis of myopathy is important so that the best possible care can be provided as soon as possible. An experienced physician can diagnose a myopathy by evaluating a person's medical history and by performing a thorough physical exam. Diagnostic tests can help differentiate between the different types of myopathy, as well as between myopathy and other neuromuscular disorders. If the doctor suspects a genetic myopathy, a thorough family history will also be taken.

Treatment depends on the specific type of myopathy the person has and the prognosis for patients with myopathy depends on the type and severity. In most cases, the myopathy can be successfully treated and the patient returned to normal life. Muscular dystrophy, however, is a much more serious condition. Duchenne's MD is usually fatal by the late teens; Becker's MD is less serious and may not be fatal until the 50s.

MYRINGOTOMY AND EAR TUBES

Myringotomy is a surgical procedure in which a small incision is made in the eardrum (the tympanic membrane), usually in both ears. The word comes from *myringa,* modern Latin for drum membrane, and *tomē*, Greek for cutting. Fluid in the middle ear can be sucked out through the incision.

Ear tubes, or tympanostomy tubes, are small tubes, open at both ends, that are inserted into the incisions in the eardrums during myringotomy. They come in various shapes and sizes and are made of plastic, metal, or both.

Myringotomy with the insertion of ear tubes is an optional treatment for inflammation of the middle ear with fluid collection (effusion), also called glue ear, that lasts more than three months, and does not respond to drug treatment. It is the recommended treatment if the condition lasts four to six months. Effusion is the collection of fluid that escapes from blood vessels or the lymphatic system. In this case, the fluid collects in the middle ear.

Initially, acute inflammation of the middle ear with effusion is treated with one or two courses of **antibiotics**. **Antihistamines** and **decongestants** have been used, but they have not been proven effective unless there is also hay fever or some other allergic inflammation that contributes to the problem. Myringotomy with or without the insertion of ear tubes is NOT recommended for initial treatment of otherwise healthy children with middle ear inflammation with effusion.

In about 10% of children, the effusion lasts for three months or longer, when the disease is considered chronic. In children with chronic disease, systemic steroids may help, but the evidence is not clear, and there are risks.

When medical treatment doesn't stop the effusion after three months in a child who is one to three years old, is otherwise healthy, and has **hearing loss** in both ears, myringotomy with insertion of ear tubes becomes an option. If the effusion lasts for four to six months, myringotomy with insertion of ear tubes is recommended.

The purpose of myringotomy is to relieve symptoms, to restore hearing, to take a sample of the fluid to examine in the laboratory in order to identify any microorganisms present, or to insert ear tubes.

Ear tubes can be inserted into the incision during myringotomy and left there. The eardrum heals around them, securing them in place. They usually fall out on their own in 6-12 months or are removed by a doctor.

While ear tubes are in place they keep the incision from closing, keeping a channel open between the middle ear and the outer ear. This allows fresh air to reach the middle ear, allowing fluid to drain out, and preventing pressure from building up in the middle ear. The patient's hearing returns to normal immediately after the insertion and the risk of recurrence diminishes.

Parents often report that children talk better, hear better, are less irritable, sleep better, and behave better after myringotomy with the insertion of ear tubes.

The procedure is usually done in an ambulatory surgical unit under general anesthesia, although some physicians do it in the office with sedation and local anesthesia, especially in older children. The ear is washed, a small incision made in the eardrum, the fluid sucked out, a tube inserted, and the ear packed with cotton to control bleeding.

A child undergoing myringotomy with the insertion of ear tubes may not have food or water for four to six hours before anesthesia. Antibiotics are usually not needed.

After the insertion there are a few steps to take to insure that everything heals correctly. The use of antimicrobial drops is controversial. Water should be kept out of the ear canal until the eardrum is intact. A doctor should be notified if the tubes fall out. Many doctors also recommend that the child use ear plugs to keep water out of the ear during bathing or swimming, to reduce the risk of infection and discharge.

The risks of myringotomy with the insertion of ear tubes include: cutting the outer ear, formation at the myringotomy site of granular nodes due to inflammation, formation of a mass of skin cells and cholesterol in the middle ear that can grow and damage surrounding bone (cholesteatoma), and permanent perforation of the eardrum.

If the procedure is repeated, structural changes in the eardrum can occur, such as loss of tone (flaccidity), shrinkage or retraction, or hardening of a spot on the eardrum (tympanosclerosis).

It is possible that the incision won't heal properly, leaving a permanent hole in the eardrum, which increases the risk of infection and can cause some hearing loss.

It is also possible that the ear tube will move inward and get trapped in the middle ear, rather than move out into the external ear. The exact incidence of tubes moving inward is not known, but it could increase the risk of further episodes of middle-ear inflammation, inflammation of the eardrum or the part of the skull directly behind the ear, formation of a mass in the middle ear, or infection due to the presence of a foreign body.

The surgery may not be a permanent cure. As many as 30% of children undergoing myringotomy with insertion of ear tubes need to undergo another procedure within five years.

N

NARCISSISM

Narcissism is a **personality disorder** characterized by excessive love for and preoccupation with one's self.

Clinically, narcissism is considered a personality disorder and is listed in the *Diagnostic and Statistical Manual of Mental Disorders* (DSM IV). Individuals with this disorder display an exaggerated sense of their own importance and abilities, brag about their accomplishments, and downplay the achievements of others. They believe themselves to be uniquely gifted and commonly engage in fantasies of fabulous success, power, or fame. Arrogant and egotistical, narcissistics are often snobs, defining themselves by their ability to associate with (or purchase the services of) the ''best'' people, and display a sense of entitlement, expecting (and taking for granted) special treatment and concessions from others. Paradoxically, individuals with narcissistic personality disorder are generally very insecure and have low **self-esteem**. They require the continual attention and admiration of others and find it difficult to cope with adversity or criticism, which may result in either rage and counterattack or social withdrawal. Because narcissistics cannot handle failure, they will take great lengths to avoid risks and situations in which defeat is a possibility. Another common characteristic of narcissistic individuals is envy and the expectation that others are envious as well. The self-aggrandizement and self-absorption of narcissistic individuals is accompanied by a pronounced lack of interest in and empathy for others. They expect people to be devoted to them but have no impulse to reciprocate, being unable to identify with the feelings of others or anticipate their needs. Narcissistics are exploiters; their relationships are often based on what other people can do for them.

The first psychologist to address narcissism was Havelock Ellis (1859-1939) in a paper on autoeroticism published in 1898. **Sigmund Freud** claimed that sexual perversion is linked to the narcissistic substitution of the self for one's mother as the primacy love object in infancy. In 1933, psychoanalyst Wilhelm Reich (1897-1957) described the ''phallic-narcissistic'' personality type in terms that foreshadow the present-day definition: self-assured, arrogant, and disdainful. The social-learning-oriented criteria for narcissistic personality disorder drawn up by Theodore Milton in 1969 were included in the third edition of the *Diagnostic and Statistical Manual of Mental Disorders* (and are very similar to those found in the current edition of DSM): 1) inflated self-image; 2) exploitative; 3) cognitive expansiveness; 4) insouciant temperament; 5) deficient social conscience.

Secondary features of narcissism include feelings of shame or humiliation, depression, and mania. Narcissistic personality disorder has also been linked to anorexia nervosa, substance-related disorders (especially cocaine abuse), and other personality disorders. The incidence of the disorder in the American population is estimated at under 1%, and approximately 50 to 75% of those diagnosed are male.

See also Personality development; Personality disorders

NASAL IRRIGATION

Nasal irrigation is the practice of flushing the nasal cavity with a sterile solution. The solution may contain **antibiotics**. Nasal irrigation is used to clear infected sinuses or may be performed after surgery to the nose region. It may be performed by adding antibiotics to the solution to treat nasal polyps, nasal septal deviation, allergic nasal inflammation, chronic sinus infection, and swollen mucous membranes. Irrigation may also be used to treat long-term users of inhalants, such as illicit drugs (cocaine), or occupational toxins, like paint fumes, sawdust, pesticides, or coal dust.

Nasal irrigation should not be performed on people who have frequent nosebleeds; have recently had nasal surgery; or whose gag reflex is impaired, as fluid may enter the windpipe.

Nasal irrigation can be performed by the patient at home, or by a medical professional. A forced-flow instrument, such as a syringe, is filled with a warm saline solution. The so-

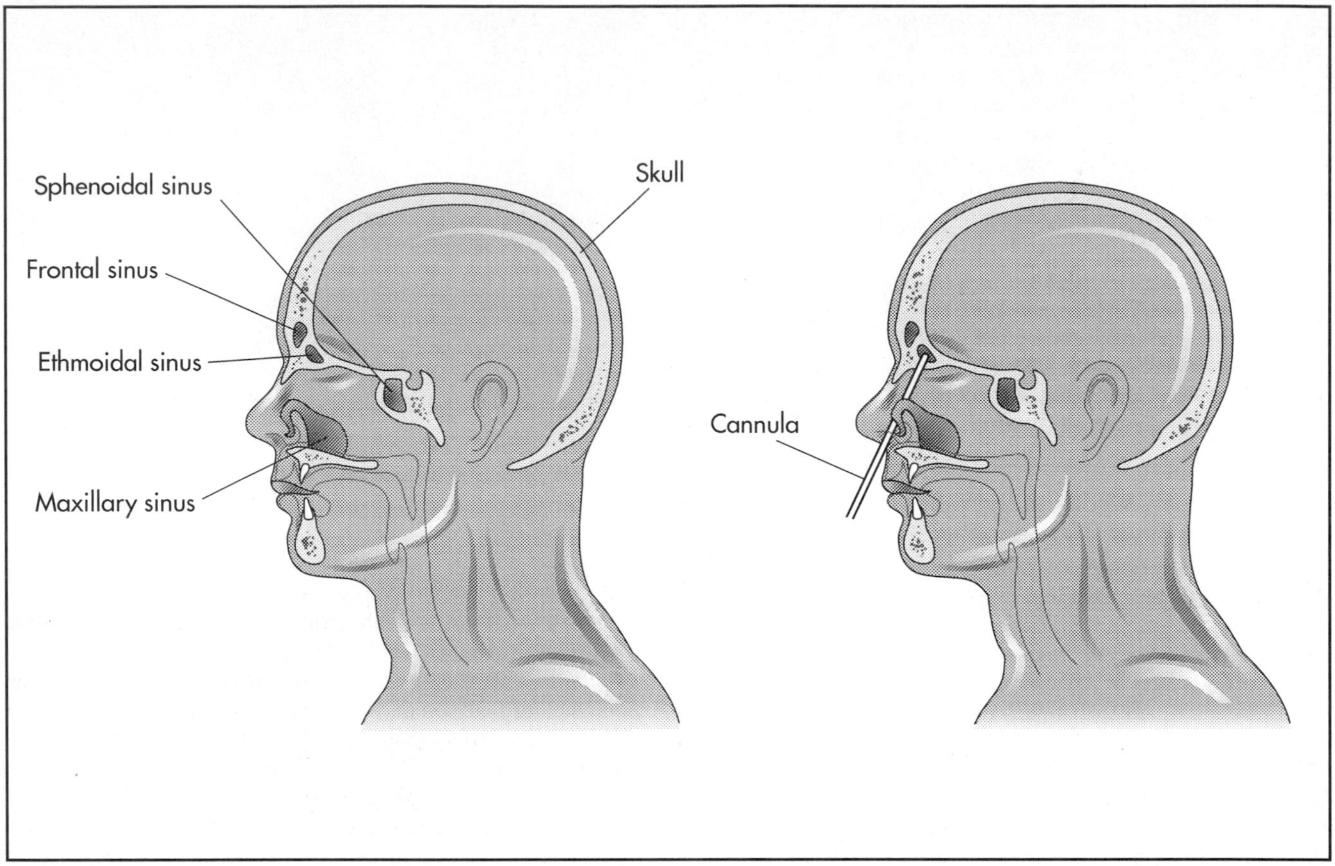

Because surgery in the nasal area has a high incidence rate for contamination with pathogenic bacteria, nasal irrigation is performed to remove loose tissue and prevent infection. The illustration (right) shows a cannula in place while the sinus passages are being flushed. ***(Illustration by Electronic Illustrators Group.)***

lution can be commercially prepared (Ayr, NaSal) or can be prepared by the patient, using one half teaspoon salt with each eight ounces of warm water. Occasionally, antibiotics are added to the solution, to kill bacteria and aid healing of irritated membrane. The syringe is then directed into the nostril. The irrigation solution loosens encrusted material in the nasal passage, and drainage takes place through the nose. The patient leans over a catch basin during irrigation, into which the debris flows. Irrigation continues until all debris is cleared from the passage. Nasal irrigation can be performed up to twice daily, unless the irrigation irritates the mucous membrane.

To help prevent complications, the patient is instructed not to open his or her mouth or swallow during the procedure. Opening the mouth or swallowing could cause infectious material to move from the nasal passage into the sinuses or the ear.

Complications of nasal irrigation include irritation of the nasal passage due to extreme temperature of the irrigation solution. Rarely, irrigation fluid may enter the windpipe. This most often occurs in people with a poor gag reflex.

Nasogastric Suction

Nasogastric suction is the process of removing solids, liquids, or gasses from the stomach or small intestine by inserting a tube through the nose and suctioning the material through the tube. This procedure may be done in the following situations:

- To relieve pressure on the stomach or small intestine when intestinal obstruction is suspected.
- Before operations on the stomach or intestines.
- To obtain a sample of the stomach contents for analysis.
- To remove toxic substances.
- To flush the stomach during gastrointestinal **bleeding** or **poisoning**s.

For this procedure, the patient sits upright while a lubricated tube is slipped through the nose and down the throat. The patient may be asked to sip water at a certain point in the procedure to help the tube slide in more easily. If the tube is to be placed into the small intestine, the doctor may use an endoscope (a thin, flexible instrument containing a camera and a light) to help see where the tube is going. Once the tube is in place, material can be removed from the stomach or intestines with gentle suction.

Different types of nasogastric tubes are used for different purposes. Tubes used for **stomach flushing** are called orogastric tubes and are the largest in diameter. Tubes that are threaded through the lower opening of the stomach (pylorus) and into the small intestine are stiffer and have a balloon tip.

Most patients tolerate nasogastric suctioning well. After the tube is removed, the patient's throat may feel irritated, but no special care is needed. The most serious risk from this procedure is that the patient will inhale some of the stomach contents into the lungs (aspiration). This may lead to bronchial infections and aspiration **pneumonia**. There is also the chance that the tube will be misplaced in the windpipe (trachea), causing violent **cough**ing. Irritation to the throat and esophagus can cause bleeding.

NATHANS, DANIEL (1928-)

American molecular biologist

Nathans was born in 1928 in Delaware. He was the last of nine children born to Samuel and Sarah Nathans, Russian Jewish immigrants. Nathans received his B.A. from the University of Delaware in 1950 and his M.D. from Washington University in St. Louis in 1954. It was during the summer after his first year of medical school that Nathans had his initial exposure to laboratory work.

After medical school, Nathans completed a one-year internship at Columbia-Presbyterian Medical Center. After this, he spent two years (1955–57) at the National Cancer Institute as a clinical associate studying protein synthesis. In 1956, Nathans married Joanne Gomberg, with whom he had three sons. Returning to Columbia-Presbyterian, Nathans completed his residency in 1959. That same year Nathans won a United States Public Health Service grant to do biochemical research at Rockefeller University in New York with Fritz Lipmann and Norton Zinder. It was at this point that Nathans fully committed to work in the laboratory rather than in a clinical practice. In New York, Nathans continued his work on protein synthesis and began viral research, mostly related to host-controlled variations in viruses.

In 1962, Nathans began his long relationship with Johns Hopkins University as assistant professor of microbiology and director of genetics. He was elevated to associate professor in 1965 and full professor in 1967. He was named director of the molecular biology and genetics department in 1972 and Boury Professor of Molecular Biology and Genetics in 1976, positions he retained for many years.

In 1962, when Nathans first arrived at Johns Hopkins, **Werner Arber**, at Basel University in Switzerland, predicted the existence of an enzyme capable of cutting DNA at specific sites. Deoxyribonucleic acid (DNA) is assumed to be the source of autoreproduction in many viruses. An ability to cut or cleave the DNA into specific and predictable fragments was important to greatly improving our capabilities for researching and understanding viruses. The necessity of ''specific'' and ''predictable'' fragments relates to the need of the scientist to know the fragment he or she is studying is identical to the fragment any other scientist would get following the same laboratory procedure.

In 1968, Arber got halfway to his goal, finding an enzyme (type I) capable of cleaving DNA, but in seemingly random patterns. In 1969, **Hamilton O. Smith**, a colleague of Nathans at Johns Hopkins, wrote to Nathans (who was in Israel at the time) to tell him he had developed a type II enzyme. This enzyme, named Hind II, was capable of cleaving DNA into specific and predictable fragments.

At this time, Nathans was working on a simian virus (SV40) which causes tumors in monkeys. SV40 was particularly impervious to then-current methods of study, so Nathans immediately saw an application of Smith's tool. Nathans, with Kathleen Danna, used Hind II to cut SV40 into eleven pieces and show its method of replication. One technique they employed in this process was radioactive labeling. The combined efforts of Arber, Smith, and Nathans over a period of more than a decade led to their receipt of the Nobel Prize in physiology or medicine in 1978. Their inter-laboratory cooperation greatly advanced the potential for consistent DNA and gene research.

Nathans continued his work with Hind II and cleared the path for much of the work that has been done since in research on DNA function and structure (such as restrictions maps, used to define DNA structure). This early work has also led to the area of recombinant DNA research, which involves the process of joining two DNA fragments from separate sources into one molecule. Since this field of research was uncharted territory and carried some risks, including the creation of new pathogens, Nathans was among an early group of scientists who, in 1974, encouraged the publication of research guidelines and some self-imposed limits on DNA research. Despite the risks, recombinant DNA research has been put to good use in creating supplies of heretofore scarce enzymes and **hormones**, including human-produced **insulin**. In the 1980s, Nathans's research continued to be linked closely to DNA and genetics. A good portion of his scientific work during this time related to the effect of growth factors on genes and **gene** regulation.

NATIONAL INSTITUTES OF HEALTH

The National Institutes of Health (NIH), which oversees one of the world's foremost biomedical research centers, is a federal agency administered by the **U.S. Department of Health and Human Services**. NIH's beginnings can be traced to 1887 and the establishment of a one-room Laboratory of Hygiene. NIH is one of eight **Public Health** Service agencies that fall under control of the U.S. Department of Health and Human Services. There are 24 separate institutes, centers, and divisions within NIH. By 1999, the NIH budget had grown to more than $15.6 billion (from about $300 in 1887).

NIH supports research whose goal is to provide better health for everyone. NIH seeks to acquire new knowledge to ''help prevent, detect, diagnose, and treat disease and disability, from the rarest genetic disorder to the common cold.''

Besides conducting research in its own laboratories, NIH supports the research of scientists in universities, medical schools, hospitals, and research institutions; helps train researchers; and facilitates the transfer of biomedical information to physicians, patients, and the general public.

NIH invests more than 81 percent of its budget in research and research training at more than 1,700 institutions in the United States and abroad. About 35,000 scientists receive NIH funding.

Only about 11 percent of NIH's budget funds projects conducted in the agency's own laboratories, mostly located at the main campus (consisting of 75 buildings on more than 300 acres) in Bethesda, Maryland. The Bethesda facilities include the Warren Grant Magnuson Clinical Center (a research hospital and laboratory to allow researchers at NIH access to patients); the Children's Inn at NIH (where chronically ill children and their families live while the children are being treated and studied at NIH); the Clinical Center's Ambulatory Care Research Facility (providing additional space for laboratories and for the Center's rapidly growing outpatient programs); the Fogarty International Center (promoting international cooperation and scholarship in science); the Mary Woodard Lasker Center for Health Research and Education (supporting a program for medical students); and the National Library of Medicine (the world's largest medical library with a collection of more than 5 million books, journals, pamphlets, rare historical volumes and manuscripts, films, and other items).

Other facilities in the NIH network include the National Institute of Environmental Health Sciences, located in Research Triangle Park, North Carolina, which studies the adverse effects of environmental factors on human health; the NIH Animal Center in Poolesville, Maryland; the Gerontology Research Center in Baltimore, Maryland; the Addiction Research Center of the National Institute on Drug Abuse also in Baltimore; Rocky Mountain Laboratories in Hamilton, Montana; and several smaller field stations.

To acquire NIH funding, the prospective grantee submits a research application to NIH. This application is reviewed for scientific merit by a panel of scientific experts (a process called peer review), primarily from outside the government, who are active in the biomedical sciences. A group of eminent scientists and members of the public who share an interest in health issues or the biomedical sciences then determine the application's overall merit and priority.

Ninety-seven scientists who have received NIH support have won Nobel Prizes for their scientific achievements. Five of these Nobelists were employed in NIH's own laboratories, Drs. Christian B. Anfinsen, **Julius Axelrod**, **D. Carleton Gajdusek**, **Marshall W. Nirenberg**, and **Martin Rodbell**.

NIH funding has played an important role in reducing deaths from coronary heart disease and from **stroke**; in improving the detection and treatment of **cancer**s; in reducing the extent of paralysis from **spinal cord injury**; in the development of vaccines that protect against infectious diseases; in developing new medications for **schizophrenia**; in increasing the chances for survival of infants with **respiratory distress syndrome**; in relieving suffering from **depressive disorders**; and in advancing the fields of molecular **genetics** and genomics.

Much of NIH-supported research focuses on such diseases and health concerns as mental disorders, infectious diseases, and chronic illnesses. Specific objectives are to improve the prevention and treatment of cancer, heart disease, stroke, blindness, arthritis, diabetes, kidney diseases, **Alzheimer's disease**, **communication disorders**, **mental illness**, drug abuse and alcoholism, **AIDS** and other unconquered diseases. Efforts continue to improve the health of infants and children, women, and minorities. Other studies seek a better understanding of the **aging** process, and of behavior and lifestyle practices that affect health.

NATUROPATHIC MEDICINE

Naturopathic medicine, or naturopathy, is an alternative approach to health care. It emphasizes preventive measures to maintain health; patient education and active participation in therapy; and noninterference with the body's natural healing processes. In most states of the United States, naturopaths (practitioners of naturopathy) do not prescribe synthetic drugs or practice major surgery. Naturopathy is not one particular approach to health care. Rather it is a collection of treatment methods that share a common philosophy.

The term naturopathy, or nature cure, was first used in 1895 by Dr. John Scheel, a physician practicing in New York City. Scheel combined natural healing techniques that dated back to **Hippocrates** (c. 400 BC) with more recent practices, such as the 19th century German custom of vacationing at hot springs or health spas. Bennedict Lust, who popularized naturopathy in the United States around the turn of the century, defined naturopathy as a discipline covering a range of natural healing techniques, including **hydrotherapy**, herbal medicine, and **homeopathy**. Lust maintained that disease could be cured naturally when patients adopted what he called corrective habits and new principles of living, as well as giving up the ''evil habits'' of overeating, the use of tea and coffee, and consumption of alcohol. In 1951, Dr. Paul Wendel published a book titled *Standardized Naturopathy*, which described nearly 300 different forms of naturopathic treatment. Naturopathy was popular in the United States until the mid-1930s, when legislation was passed that restricted the licensing and practice of naturopathic practitioners.

There has been a revival of interest in naturopathy in the United States and Canada since the 1970s. Most of today's naturopathic practitioners have been trained in family practice or general medicine. As of 1998, four accredited colleges in the United States and Canada that offered degrees in naturopathic medicine. Ten states (Alaska, Arizona, Connecticut, Hawaii, Montana, Oregon, Vermont, Maine, New Hampshire, and Washington) had licensing procedures for naturopathic practitioners.

Naturopathic treatments are holistic—intended to benefit all dimensions of the patient's being, rather than focused on a specific physical condition or organ—and as noninvasive as possible. Naturopaths define health as a condition of positive well-being, not as the absence of disease. The philosophy that underlies naturopathic medicine is called vitalism. Vitalism is the belief that life cannot be reduced to a collection of physical and chemical data, and that the human body has an innate wisdom or inner drive toward vitality and health. Following this belief, naturopaths expect patients to be active participants in recovering or maintaining their health, rather than passive recipients of medications or surgical procedures.

Naturopathic treatments are directed toward removal of the underlying causes of illness and not simply relief of symptoms. Symptoms are regarded as signs that the body is healing itself and showing "interior wisdom" in responding to disease agents. The naturopathic physician tries to assist the body in this process rather than suppressing or fighting the symptoms.

Naturopaths may use one or more types of therapy in treating patients. Most practitioners regard diet and nutrition as the core of naturopathic treatment, although some choose to specialize in specific approaches. Naturopathic diets emphasize beans, grains, vegetables and fruit. Patients are not required to be vegetarians, but are encouraged to substitute chicken and fish for red meat.

Naturopaths in the United States have borrowed elements of Native American, Ayurvedic, and Chinese herbal medicine in their treatments of specific diseases. Naturopathic practitioners receive training in traditional herbalism as well as standard medical pharmacology. Herbal medicines are frequently used in naturopathy to strengthen weakened immune systems, as tonics, and as nutritional supplements. Most naturopathic physicians also are trained in the philosophy of homeopathy.

Hydrotherapy (the use of water to treat diseases and injuries and to cleanse the digestive tract) has been an important part of naturopathic medicine since the 19th century, particularly in the German-speaking parts of Europe. Detoxification therapy is another key principle of naturopathic medicine. Naturopaths maintain that a person's basic level of health is largely determined by the body's ability to rid itself of toxic substances. **Fasting** is a commonly recommended feature of a naturopathic detoxification program. Many patients undertake periodic fasts of three to five days during which they are allowed only water or unsweetened herbal tea. Other features of naturopathic detoxification include the use of vitamin C, fiber and mineral supplements, and botanical preparations. **Exercise**, **massage**, joint manipulation and other physical techniques are used to treat patients with muscle, bone and joint problems.

The holistic orientation of naturopathy includes an emphasis on the psychological and spiritual dimensions of human life. The patient's general "life stance" is considered a major factor in the prevention and treatment of diseases, particularly those that affect the immune system. Naturopathic physicians receive formal training in psychology and **counseling** techniques, including the use of **hypnosis**, **guided imagery**, and **family therapy**.

NAUSEA AND VOMITING

Nausea is the sensation of feeling like you are about to vomit. Vomiting, or emesis, is the expelling of undigested food through the mouth.

Occasional nausea can have a number of causes, including overeating, drinking too much alcohol, infection, and **stress**. Morning sickness is a type of nausea caused by **pregnancy**-related hormone changes. Some people experience motion sickness when riding in a car or traveling by plane or boat. Certain medicines, including **cancer chemotherapy** drugs also cause nausea.

Mild nausea can often be relieved by getting some fresh air or eating bland crackers. Vomiting relieves nausea right away, but can cause dehydration. Sipping clear juices, weak tea, and some sports drinks help replace lost fluid and **minerals** without irritating the stomach. After a period of nausea and vomiting, food should be reintroduced gradually, beginning with small amounts of dry, bland food like crackers and toast.

Various medications are available for nausea. Meclizine (Bonine), a medication for motion sickness, also diminishes the feeling of queasiness in the stomach. Dimenhydrinate (Dramamine), another motion-sickness drug, is not effective on other types of nausea and may cause drowsiness.

Advocates of alternative treatments suggest **biofeedback**, **acupressure** and the use of herbs to calm the stomach. Biofeedback uses **exercise** and deep relaxation to control nausea. Acupressure (applying pressure to specific areas of the body) can be performed by wearing a special wristband or by applying firm pressure to the back of the jawbone; the webbing between the thumb and index finger; the top of the foot; the inside of the wrist; or the base of the rib cage.

Chamomile (*Matricaria recutita*) or lemon balm (*Melissa officinalis*) tea may relieve symptoms. Ginger (*Zingiber officinale*), another natural remedy, can be drunk as tea or taken as candy or powered capsules.

Persistent, unexplained, or recurring nausea and vomiting can be symptoms of serious illness and should be checked by a doctor. It is important to call a doctor if nausea and vomiting:

- Occur after eating rich or spoiled food or taking a new medication
- Is repeated or continues for 48 hours or longer
- Follows intense **dizziness**.
- Is accompanied by yellowing of the skin and whites of the eyes; **pain** in the chest or lower abdomen; trouble swallowing or urinating; **dehydration** or extreme thirst; drowsiness or confusion; or a fruity breath odor.

A doctor should also be notified if vomiting is heavy and/or bloody, if the vomited material looks like feces or if the patient has been unable to keep food down for 24 hours.

An ambulance or emergency response number should be called immediately if:

- Diabetic **shock** is suspected
- Nausea and vomiting continue after other symptoms of viral infection have subsided
- The patient has a severe headache.
- The patient is sweating and having chest pain and trouble breathing
- Nausea, vomiting, and breathing problems occur after exposure to a known allergen.

NEAR-DROWNING

Drowning is suffocation that results from being submerged in water or another fluid. Near-drowning is the term for surviving such suffocation.

The number of near-drownings in the United States is hard to estimate because not all incidents are reported, but estimates range from 15,000-70,000. Nearly half of all drownings and near-drownings involve children less than four years old, and 60-90% of drownings in this age group are in home swimming pools. Teenage boys also face a heightened risk of drowning and near-drowning, because of their tendency to behave recklessly and use drugs and alcohol (drugs and alcohol are implicated in 40-50% of teenage drownings). At all ages, males are more likely than females to drown, possibly because they are not supervised as closely.

Not all drownings and near-drownings occur because a nonswimmer accidentally ventures into deep water. Many are a result of some other event such as a **heart attack** that causes unconsciousness or a head or spinal injury that prevents a diver from resurfacing. Drownings can occur in shallow, as well as deep, water. Young children have drowned or almost drowned in bathtubs, toilets, large buckets, and washing machines. Bathtubs are especially dangerous for infants six months to one year old, who can sit up straight in a bathtub but may not be able to pull themselves out of the water if they slip under the surface.

Human life depends on a constant supply of oxygen-laden air reaching the blood by way of the lungs. When drowning begins, the larynx (an air passage) closes, preventing both water and air from entering the lungs. If the larynx stays closed, the concentration of oxygen in the blood drops. This is called "dry drowning." In "wet drowning," the larynx relaxes and water enters the lungs, also resulting in a drop in oxygen concentration. All of this happens very quickly: within three minutes of submersion most people are unconscious, and within five minutes the brain begins to suffer from lack of oxygen. Other problems that often occur in near-drowning cases are abnormal heart rhythms (cardiac dysrhythmias), cardiac arrest, an increase in blood acidity (acidosis), and a severe drop in body temperature (**hypothermia**).

The signs and symptoms of near-drowning can differ widely from person to person. Some victims are alert but agitated, while others are **coma**tose. Breathing may stop, or the victim may gasp for breath. Bluish skin (**cyanosis**), **cough**ing, and frothy pink sputum (material expelled from the respiratory tract by coughing) are often observed. Rapid breathing (tachypnea), a rapid heart rate (tachycardia), and a low-grade **fever** are common during the first few hours after rescue. Conscious victims may appear confused, lethargic, or irritable.

Treatment begins with removing the victim from the water and performing **cardiopulmonary resuscitation (CPR)**. One purpose of CPR—which should be attempted only by people trained in its use—is to bring oxygen to the lungs, heart, brain, and other organs by breathing into the victim's mouth. When the victim's heart has stopped, a person administering CPR also attempts to get the heart pumping again by pressing down on the victim's chest. After CPR has been performed and emergency medical help has arrived on the scene, the victim is given oxygen and intravenous fluids and is checked for injuries.

In the emergency department, victims continue receiving oxygen until blood tests show a return to normal. Patients who have experienced hypothermia are rewarmed. Comatose patients usually do not benefit from treatment. Patients who recover can be discharged from the emergency department after four to six hours if their blood oxygen level is normal and they have no other problems. But because lung problems can develop 12 or more hours after submersion, patients are dismissed only if the medical staff is convinced they will seek medical help if necessary. Patients who do not recover fully in the emergency department are admitted to the hospital for at least 24 hours for further observation and treatment.

Brain damage is the major long-term problem from near-drowning. However, most patients who are not comatose when they arrive at the hospital survive with brain function intact. Death or permanent brain damage are very likely when patients arrive comatose. Early rescue of near-drowning victims (within 5 minutes of submersion) and prompt CPR (within less than 10 minutes of submersion) seem to be the best guarantees of a complete recovery.

Prevention of drowning and near-drowning depends on educating people about water safety. Parents should never leave young children in or near water without supervision for even a short time. Everyone should follow the rules for safe swimming and boating, and adults and teenagers should learn CPR. Anyone who has a medical condition that can cause a seizure or otherwise threaten safety in the water should swim only with a partner. People also need to be aware that alcohol and drug use substantially increase the chances of an accident.

NEARSIGHTEDNESS AND FARSIGHTEDNESS

Nearsightedness (myopia) and farsightedness (hyperopia) are vision problems. People who are nearsighted see objects clearly when they are close to the eye, while distant objects appear blurred or fuzzy. Symptoms of hyperopia can vary from no visual problems at all, to clear distance vision combined with blurry near vision, to blurry distance and near vision.

To understand nearsightedness and farsightedness, it helps to know something about the main parts of the eye's focusing system: the cornea, lens, and retina. The cornea is a tough, transparent, dome-shaped tissue that covers the front of the eye, lying in front of the iris (the colored part of the eye). The lens is a transparent structure located behind the iris. The retina is a thin membrane that lines the rear of the eyeball. Light-sensitive cells in the retina convert incoming light rays into electrical signals that are sent to the brain, which then interprets the images. In people with normal vision, parallel light rays enter the eye and are bent by the cornea and lens to focus precisely on the retina, producing a crisp, clear image. In a nearsighted person, the cornea and lens bend the light rays too much for the length of the eye, and the rays converge in front of the retina. The resulting image that goes to the brain appears fuzzy. In farsightedness, the point of focus falls behind the retina.

Typical symptoms of nearsightedness are blurred distance vision, eye discomfort, squinting, and eye strain. People usually are diagnosed with this problem during the first several years of elementary school when a teacher notices a child having difficulty seeing the blackboard, reading, or concentrating.

Newborn babies usually are slightly farsighted, but their vision tends to improve over time. However, some people have hyperopia for life. If the condition is not too severe, the lens may be able to adjust enough to bring the image back onto the retina. When this happens, a person can see clearly at a distance, but the constant refocusing may cause **headaches** or eyestrain. Nearby objects may appear blurry because the eyes have to shift from focusing on something at a distance to focusing on something near. If the lens cannot adjust enough to bring images of distant objects onto the retina, those objects may appear blurry. This explains why symptoms of farsightedness are so variable.

The usual treatment for nearsightedness and farsightedness is corrective lenses, which may be worn in eyeglasses or as contact lenses. For people who find glasses and contact lenses inconvenient or uncomfortable, and who meet certain selection criteria, corrective eye surgery may be an option. Several types of surgery, including **radial keratotomy** (RK), photorefractive keratectomy (PRK), and laser-assisted in-situ keratomileusis (LASIK) are used to correct these vision problems.

Presbyopia is another type of vision problem that occurs as a part of normal aging and has symptoms similar to those of farsightedness. As people age, the lens becomes less flexible, and the muscles that adjust its curvature become less powerful. As a result, it loses its ability to focus the rays of light coming from nearby objects. People with presbyopia have trouble reading small print and doing close work. The problem may be worse early in the morning, in dim light, or when the person is tired.

Symptoms of presbyopia usually begin to appear between age 40-45 and continue to develop until the condition stabilizes 10-20 years later. Presbyopia cannot be cured, but the problem can be corrected with eyeglasses or contact lenses.

See also Visual impairment and blindness

NEHER, ERWIN (1944-)

German biophysicist

Erwin Neher was born in Landsberg, Germany, in 1944, the son of Franz Xavier Neher and Elisabeth Pfeiffer Neher. In 1967, he earned his master's degree from the University of Wisconsin under a Fulbright scholarship. He then went on to complete his doctorate at the Institute of Technology in Munich, Germany, in 1970.

While the existence of ion channels that transmit electrical charges was hypothesized as early as the 1950s, no one had been able to see these channels. As a doctoral student, Neher was drawn to the question of how electrically charged ions control such biological functions as the transmission of nerve impulses, the contraction of muscles, vision, and the process of conception. He realized that in order to get answers to these questions he would have to look for the ion channels.

It was in his doctoral thesis that Neher first developed the concept of the patch clamp technique as a way of discovering the ion channels. In 1974 he shared a laboratory space with Bert Sakmann at the Max Planck Institute in Göttingen. They both agreed that understanding the nature of ion channels was the most important problem in the biophysics of the cell membrane, and they set out to develop the techniques of patch clamping.

In 1976 Neher and Sakmann published their landmark paper on the use of glass recording electrodes with microscopic tips, called micropipettes, pressed against a cell membrane. With these devices, which they called patch clamp electrodes, they were able to electrically isolate a tiny patch of the cell membrane and to study the protein s in that area. They could then see how the individual proteins acted as channels or gates for specific ions, allowing certain ions to pass through the cell membrane one at a time, while preventing others from entering. Their work with patch clamps allowed them to remove a patch of the membrane and to enter the interior of the cell. They then were able to conduct various experiments to observe the intricate mechanism of ion channels. Several years later, Neher, Sakmann, and their colleagues refined the technique of patch clamping. Creating a better seal between the micropipette and the patch of cell membrane it pressed against was one of the refinements they sought. Without a tight seal there was interference by ''noise'' that overshadowed the smaller electrical currents.

Neher solved the problem of outside noise interference in 1980 when he was able to observe on his oscilloscope a marked drop in the noise level to almost zero. From this drop he was able to infer that he had produced a seal that was one hundred times better than previously attained. While other researchers had noticed an abatement of noise at times, Neher was the first to realize the significance of the drop in noise level.

Neher found that by using a light suction with a super clean pipette, he could create a high-resistance seal of 10–100 gigohms (a gigohm is a measure of electrical resistance equal to one billion ohms). He called this seal a ''gigaseal.'' With the gigaseal, background noise could be decreased, and a number of new ways could be used to control cells for patch clamp experimentation. Patches from the cell could now be torn away from the membrane to act as a membrane coating over the mouth of the pipette, thus allowing for more exact measurement of electrical ion movement. A strong suction could force the pipette into the cell while still maintaining a tight seal for the cell as a whole.

In 1976 Neher returned to the Max Planck Institute in Göttingen. In 1978, he married microbiologist Eva-Maria Ruhr; they have five children. He became director of the membrane biophysics department at the Max Planck Institute in 1983, and in 1987 he was made an honorary professor.

In 1991 Neher and Sakmann won the Nobel Prize for proving the existence of ion channels. The Nobel Committee also praised the work of Neher and Sakmann for helping in research on heart disease, **epilepsy**, and disorders affecting the nervous and muscle systems. Patch clamp research has helped in the development of new drugs for these conditions.

Neonatal Jaundice

Neonatal jaundice (hyperbilirubinemia) is a higher-than-normal level of bilirubin in the blood. Bilirubin, a by-product of the breakdown of hemoglobin (the oxygen-carrying substance in red blood cells), is produced when the body breaks down old red blood cells. Normally, the liver processes the bilirubin and excretes it in the stool. An excess of bilirubin in the blood leads to a yellow discoloration of the skin and the whites of the eyes called **jaundice**. This condition is particularly common in newborn infants. Before birth, an infant gets rid of bilirubin through the mother's blood and liver systems. After birth, the baby's liver has to take over processing bilirubin on its own. Almost all newborns have higher than normal levels of bilirubin. In most cases, the baby's systems continue to develop and can soon process bilirubin. This development can be encouraged by beginning breastfeeding or formula feeding as soon as possible after delivery and continuing to feed the baby frequently.

Most cases of newborn jaundice resolve without medical treatment within two to three weeks. However, infants with very high bilirubin levels may need medical treatment to prevent serious complications, such as **mental retardation**, **hearing loss**, behavior disorders, **cerebral palsy**, or **death**.

One type of treatment is **phototherapy**—exposure of the baby's skin to fluorescent light. The bilirubin in the baby's skin absorbs the light and is changed to a substance that can be excreted in the urine. This treatment can be done in the hospital or at home with special lights which parents can rent for the treatment. Treatment may be needed for several days before bilirubin levels in the blood return to normal. The baby's eyes are shielded to prevent the optic nerves from absorbing too much light. Another type of treatment uses a special fiber optic blanket. There is no need to shield the baby's eyes with this treatment, and it can be done at home. In rare cases, where bilirubin levels are extremely high, the baby may need to receive a blood **transfusion**.

All infants with jaundice should be evaluated by a health care provider to rule out more serious problems. Signs of severe hyperbilirubinemia include listlessness, high-pitched crying, apnea (periods of not breathing), arching of the back, and seizures.

Premature infants are especially likely to develop jaundice. The condition also is more common in some populations, such as Native American and Asian. But in general, there is no way to predict which infants will be affected by hyperbilirubinemia.

Hyperbilirubinemia and jaundice can also be the result of other diseases or conditions. Hepatitis, **cirrhosis** of the liver, and mononucleosis are diseases that can affect the liver. **Gallstones**, a blocked bile duct, or the use of drugs or alcohol can also cause jaundice.

Nephritis

Nephritis is inflammation of the kidney. The most common form, glomerulonephritis, affects children and teenagers far more often than adults. It is inflammation of the glomeruli, small round filters located in the kidney. Pyelonephritis affects adults more than children, and is recognized as inflammation of the kidney and upper urinary tract. A third type of nephritis is hereditary nephritis, a rare inherited condition.

Acute glomerulonephritis usually develops a few weeks after a strep infection of the throat or skin. Symptoms of glomerulonephritis include fatigue, high blood pressure, and swelling (especially in the hands, feet, ankles and face). Ninety percent of children with glomerulonephritis recover without complications. With proper medical treatment, symptoms usually subside within a few weeks, or at the most, a few months. Treatment normally includes drugs such as cortisone or cytotoxic drugs (drugs that destroy certain cells or antigens). **Diuretics** may be prescribed to increase urination. In patients with high blood pressure, drugs may be prescribed to lower blood pressure. Iron and vitamin supplements may be recommended if the patient becomes anemic.

Streptococcal infections that may lead to glomerulonephritis can be prevented by avoiding exposure to strep infection and obtaining prompt medical treatment for **scarlet fever** or other infection.

Pyelonephritis usually occurs suddenly, and the acute form of this disease is more common in adult women. It is commonly caused when bacteria are carried into the urinary tract by the backward flow of urine from the bladder. Symptoms include **fever** and chills, fatigue, burning or frequent urination, cloudy or bloody urine, and aching **pain** on one of both sides of the lower back or abdomen. It can be treated successfully if diagnosed early. Follow-up urinalysis studies will determine if the patient remains bacteria-free. If the infection is not cured or continues to recur, it can lead to serious complications such as bacteremia (bacterial invasion of the bloodstream), hypertension, chronic pyelonephritis and even permanent kidney damage. Patients who are severely ill with acute pyelonephritis may need to be hospitalized. **Antibiotics** will be prescribed, with the length of treatment based on the severity of the infection. In the case of chronic pyelonephritis, a six-month course of antibiotics may be necessary to rid the body of infection. Surgery is sometimes necessary. Pyelonephritis can best be avoided if those with a history of urinary tract infections drink plenty of fluids, urinate frequently, and practice good hygiene following urination.

Hereditary nephritis is present at birth. The rare disease appears in many different forms and can be responsible for up to 5% of end-stage renal disease in men. Although it cannot be prevented, early detection and treatment can prevent complications such as eye problems, deafness or kidney failure. Treatment of hereditary nephritis depends of the variety of the disease and its severity at the time of treatment.

For any type of nephritis, alternative treatment should be used as a complement to medical care and under the supervision of a licensed practitioner. Some herbs thought to relieve symptoms of nephritis include cleavers (*Galium* spp.) and wild hydrangea.

Diagnosis of nephritis is based on:

- The patient's symptoms and medical history
- **Physical examination**
- Laboratory tests
- **Kidney function tests**
- Imaging studies such as **ultrasound** or x rays to determine blockage and inflammation.

NEPHROTIC SYNDROME

Nephrotic syndrome is a collection of symptoms that occur because tiny filters (glomeruli) in the kidney become leaky. The glomeruli (a single one is called a glomerulus) are tufts of capillaries (the smallest type of blood vessels). They act as filters in the kidneys, allowing a certain amount of water and waste products to leave the blood and eventually pass out of the body in the form of urine. Normally, proteins are unable to pass through the glomerular filter. However, in people with nephrotic syndrome, this filter becomes defective, allowing large quantities of protein to leave the blood circulation and pass out of the body in the urine.

Patients with nephrotic syndrome are from all age groups, but children between 18 months and four years are at increased risk for the disorder. In children, boys are more frequently affected; in adults, the ratio of men to women is closer to equal.

Nephrotic syndrome can be caused by a number of different diseases. Generally, the damage that results is due to immune system changes. For some reason, the immune system becomes directed against the person's own kidney. The glomeruli become increasingly leaky as various substances from the immune system are deposited within the kidney.

A number of kidney disorders are associated with nephrotic syndrome, including:

- Minimal change disease or MCD (responsible for about 80% of nephrotic syndrome in children, and about 20% in adults). MCD is a disorder of the glomeruli.
- Focal glomerulosclerosis
- Membranous glomerulopathy
- Membranoproliferative glomerulonephropathy.

Other types of diseases can also result in nephrotic syndrome. These include diabetes, sickle-cell anemia, amyloidosis, **systemic lupus erythematosus**, sarcoidosis, leukemia, lymphoma, **cancer** of the breast, colon, and stomach, reactions to drugs (including nonsteroidal anti-inflammatory drugs, lithium, and street heroin), allergic reactions (to insect stings, snake venom, and poison ivy), infections (**malaria**, various bacteria, **hepatitis** B, herpes zoster, and the virus that causes **AIDS**), and severe high blood pressure.

The first symptom of nephrotic syndrome is often foamy urine. As the syndrome progresses, swelling (**edema**) develops in the eyelids, hands, feet, knees, scrotum, and abdomen. The patient feels increasingly weak and fatigued and loses appetite. Over time, the loss of protein causes the muscles to shrink and weaken (called muscle wasting). The patient may have abdominal **pain** and difficulty breathing. Because the kidneys are involved in blood pressure regulation, abnormally low or abnormally high blood pressure may develop.

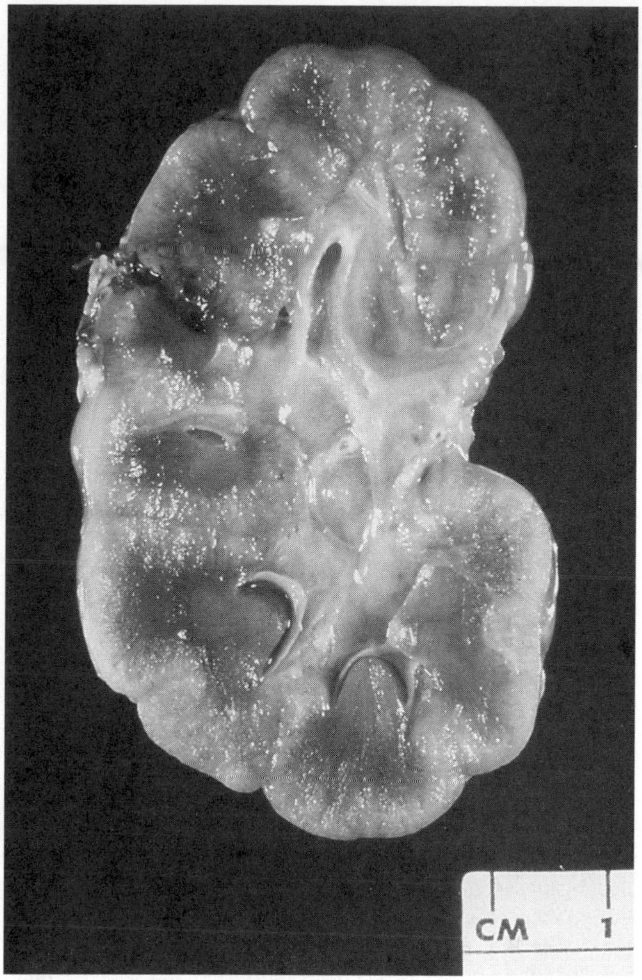

A specimen of a nephrotic human kidney. *(Custom Medical Stock Photo. Reproduced by permission.)*

Over time, the protein loss occurring in nephrotic syndrome results in general malnutrition. Hair and nails become brittle, and growth is stunted. Bones become weak, and the body begins to lose other important nutrients (sugar, potassium, calcium). Infection is a serious and frequent complication, as are disorders of blood clotting. Acute kidney failure may develop.

Diagnosis is based first on urine and blood tests. In people with nephrotic syndrome, the urine contains too much protein, while the blood has too little. Blood tests will also reveal a high level of cholesterol. In order to diagnose one of the kidney disorders that cause nephrotic syndrome, a small sample (biopsy) of the kidney is removed for examination. This biopsy can be done with a long, very thin needle which is inserted through the skin under the ribs.

The type of treatment for nephrotic syndrome depends on the type of disorder that caused it. Medications that suppress the immune system are commonly used. The first choice is usually a steroid drug (such as prednisone). Some conditions may require even more potent medications, such as cyclophosphamide or cyclosporine. Treating the underlying conditions (lymphoma, cancers, heroin use, infections) that have led to nephrotic syndrome often improves the symptoms of nephrotic syndrome as well. Some patients will need medications to control high blood pressure. Occasionally, patients are told to limit the amount of fluid they drink. Swelling can sometimes be relieved with the use of **diuretics**, which allow the kidney to produce more urine and thus remove excess fluid from the body.

The success of treatment depends on the underlying disorder. Of all the kidney disorders, minimal change disease has the best treatment success, with 90% of all patients responding to treatment. Other types of kidney diseases have less favorable outcomes, with high rates of progression to kidney failure. When nephrotic syndrome is caused by another, treatable disorder (infection, allergic or drug reaction), the likelihood of successful treatment is high.

Nephrotoxic Injury

Nephrotoxic injury is damage to one or both of the kidneys that results from exposure to a toxic material, usually something taken by mouth.

The kidneys are the primary organs of the urinary system, which removes waste from the blood and excretes them from the body in urine. Every day, the kidneys filter about 45 gal (180 l) of blood, about four times as much as the amount that passes through any other organ. Because of this high volume, the kidneys are more often exposed to toxic substances in the blood and are very vulnerable to injury from those materials.

Each kidney contains more than one million structures called nephrons. Each nephron consists of two parts: the renal corpuscle and the renal tubule. The renal corpuscle is where the blood is filtered. It is made up of a network of capillaries (the glomerulus) and the structure that surrounds these capillaries (Bowman's capsule). Blood flows into the glomerulus, where the liquid part of the blood (plasma) passes through the walls of the capillaries and into Bowman's capsule. The plasma, now called filtrate, contains substances that the body needs, such as water, glucose, and other nutrients, as well as wastes, excess salts, and excess water. When the filtrate moves from Bowman's capsule into the renal tubules, the beneficial substances are reabsorbed into the blood stream. The remaining filtrate is then passed to the bladder as urine.

When the kidneys are exposed to a toxic material, damage can occur in a number of ways. Some toxins directly kill cells in the glomerulus or the renal tubules. Other toxins create substances or conditions, such as allergic reactions, that cause cell death. Nephrotoxic injury can lead to acute renal failure, in which the kidneys suddenly lose their ability to function, or chronic renal failure, in which kidney function slowly deteriorates. Untreated, renal failure can result in seizures, coma, and death.

Several different substances can be toxic to the kidneys. These include **antibiotics**; pain relievers (**analgesics**); contrast agents used in some diagnostic tests, such as sodium iodide; heavy metals, such as lead, mercury, arsenic, and uranium; **anticancer drugs**; solvents and fuels, such as carbon tetrachloride, methanol, and ethylene glycol; herbicides and pesticides; and excess uric acid.

The elderly and people whose kidneys are already weakened by disease are especially susceptible to nephrotoxic injury. So are people who are exposed over long periods to heavy metals or solvents on the job or at home. Severe dehydration increases the risk of nephrotoxic injury, as do diseases that cause overproduction of uric acid.

Symptoms of nephrotoxic injury include excess urea in the blood (azotemia), anemia, increased acidity of the blood (acidosis), excess fluids in the body (**overhydration**), and high blood pressure (**hypertension**). Blood, pus, or uric acid crystals may be present in the urine, and urine output may decrease.

Physicians detect kidney damage through **physical examination**, blood tests, urine tests, and imaging procedures. To find out whether the damage is due to nephrotoxic injury, the physician will ask about the patient's medical history, current prescriptions and exposure to solvents and other toxins.

Nephrotoxic injury is treated in the hospital. The goal of treatment is to remove the toxin from the patient's system, while maintaining kidney function. The removal method depends on the type of toxin and may include the use of **diuretics** or chelates to enhance excretion of the toxin in urine, or, in extreme cases, the direct removal of toxins from the blood using an artificial filtering system.

If the damage has not caused acute renal failure, kidney function can be fully restored once the toxin is removed from the body. However, if permanent damage has resulted in chronic renal failure, lifelong dialysis or a kidney transplant may be necessary.

The risk of nephrotoxic injury can be reduced by taking no more than the recommended dosages of antibiotics or analgesics. Elderly patients who take analgesics daily (for heart problems or arthritis, for example) should be closely monitored to prevent accidental overdose. Patients should alert health care workers to any underlying conditions, such as diabetes or **allergies** to antibiotics, that may heighten the effect of a potential nephrotoxin. Safety recommendations for using solvents or handling heavy metals should be followed.

Nervous system

The nervous system coordinates behavior and helps to maintain the internal stability of animals. It may be as simple as the nerve net of Cnidarians or as complex as the centralized system of mammals. In all nervous systems the functional unit is the nerve cell or neuron, a cell specialized to transmit and receive a stimulus.

In humans, the brain and spinal cord are formed early in embryonic development. At the beginning of the third week of gestation, the embryo has already formed a neural plate on the dorsal surface that eventually folds together to form a hollow tube from which the brain and spinal cord develop. During this time the 100 billion neurons found in the brain are produced—the sum total of all the neurons that the brain will ever contain in an individual's lifetime. The brain is one of the largest organs in the body and consists of three main regions: the forebrain, midbrain, and hindbrain. The cerebrum, which is the most important area for neural processing, together with the thalamus and hypothalamus, forms the forebrain. In the midbrain are centers for the receipt and integration of several types of sensory information, such as seeing and hearing. The information is then sent on to specific areas in the cerebrum to be processed. The hindbrain consists of three parts: the medulla oblongata, the pons, and cerebellum, and it functions in maintaining homeostasis and coordinating movement. The pons and medulla of the hindbrain, together with the midbrain, form the brainstem, which is the location of reflex centers such as those that control heart beat rate and breathing rate. The other part of the central nervous system, the spinal cord, serves as a pathway for nerve tracts carrying impulses to and from the brain. It acts as the site for simple reflexes such as the familiar knee jerk. If a slice were made into the spinal cord, it would show a cord with a small central canal surrounded by an area of gray matter shaped like a butterfly surrounded by white matter. The gray matter is composed of large masses of cell bodies, dendrites and unmyelinated axons; the white matter is composed of bundles of axons that are called tracts, which send information to and from the brain.

The central nervous system operates through the peripheral nervous system, which is the ''roadway'' that links the central nervous system to the rest of the body. The nerves that carry information to the central nervous system from sensory receptors such as the **eye** are called sensory nerves or afferent nerves; those that carry impulses away from the central nervous system to effector organs such as the muscles are called motor nerves or efferent nerves. Commonly the fibers of sensory and motor neurons are bundled together to form mixed nerves. There are 12 pairs of cranial nerves that run to or from the brain, such as the optic and vagus nerves. There are 31 pairs of nerves called spinal nerves that originate from the spinal cord, such as the sciatic nerve and ulnar nerve, the nerve that is stimulated when you hit your elbow. Specific areas of the body are served by each of the spinal nerves. All sensory nerves enter the cord through a dorsal root, and all motor nerves exit through a ventral root. If the dorsal section of a root is destroyed, sensation from that area is also destroyed, but the muscles are still able to function. In the opposite situation, damage to the ventral root destroys muscle function, but sensory information is still processed.

There are two main divisions to the peripheral nervous system, the somatic and the autonomic. The somatic system involves the skeletal muscles and is considered voluntary since there is control over movement such as writing or throwing a ball. The autonomic nervous system (ANS) affects internal organs and is considered involuntary since the processes such as heart beat rate and glandular secretions occur with usually little control on the part of the individual. The autonomic nervous system, in turn, is divided into two divisions, the parasympathetic and sympathetic. The parasympathetic system is most active in normal, restful situations and is dominant during quiet, relaxed periods. It acts to decrease the heartbeat and to stimulate the motility and secretions necessary for digestion. The sympathetic nervous system is most active during times of stress and arousal and is dominant when energy is required, when it increases the rate and strength of the contractions of the heart and inhibits the motility of the intestine. Together with hormones, the autonomic system maintains homeostasis, the internal balance of the body.

The functional unit of the nervous system is the neuron, a cell specialized to receive and transmit impulses. Even though there are a variety of neurons, the essential structures are the same in each: a cell body containing the nucleus and two kinds of processes extending from it, the axon and dendrite. Axons transmit impulses away from the cell body to the dendrites of adjoining neurons. Some axons may be over 3 ft (1 m) in length, such as the sciatic nerve, which runs from the spinal cord to the lower leg. The axons of the peripheral nerves are enclosed in a fatty (myelin) sheath formed from specialized cells called Schwann cells. The myelin sheath acts to insulate the axon, which helps to accelerate the transmission of a nerve impulse. Gaps along the sheath expose the axon fiber and are important in allowing nerve impulses to jump from one section of the axon to another. The speed at which nerve impulses travel depends on the diameter of the axon and the presence of the myelin sheath; some impulses from the large motor nerves to the leg muscles travel as fast as 394 ft (120 m) per second. Damage to the sheath in **multiple sclerosis** patients causes impaired muscle control and other symptoms, an indication of the importance of the myelin sheath in the transmission of nerve impulses. Axons are bundled together and enclosed by connective tissue to form nerves. Dendrites are usually highly branched extensions of the cell body that receive impulses from axons. In some cases they may be very small, as seen in some of the neurons of the brain, or long, as is the sensory dendrite that runs from the foot to the spinal cord.

See also Human physiology

NEURALGIA

Neuralgia is an intense burning or stabbing **pain** caused by nerve irritation or damage. The pain is usually brief but may be severe. It is usually felt in the part of the body that is supplied by the irritated nerve and often feels as if it is shooting along the nerve.

Disease, infection, and inflammation can cause neuralgia, as can pressure on a nerve or irritation of a nerve. The problem can arise from **tooth decay**, eye strain, poor diet, nose infections, or exposure to damp and cold. Postherpetic neuralgia is an intense debilitating pain felt at the site of a previous attack of shingles. Trigeminal neuralgia (also called tic douloureux, the most common type of neuralgia), causes a brief, searing pain along the trigeminal nerve, which supplies sensation to the face. The facial pain of migraine neuralgia lasts between 30 minutes and an hour and occurs at the same time on successive days. The cause is not known.

Glossopharyngeal neuralgia is an intense pain felt at the back of the tongue, in the throat, and in the ear—all areas served by the glossopharyngeal nerve. The pain may occur spontaneously, or it can be triggered by talking, eating, or swallowing (especially cold foods such as ice cream). Its cause is not known.

Occipital neuralgia is caused by a pinched occipital nerve. There are two occipital nerves, each located at the back of the neck, each supplying feeling to the skin over half of the back of the head. These nerves can be pinched due to factors ranging from arthritis to injury, but the result is the same: numbness, pain, or tingling over half the base of the skull.

Neuralgia is a symptom of an underlying disorder; its diagnosis depends on finding the cause of the condition creating the pain.

Glossopharyngeal, trigeminal, and postherpetic neuralgias sometimes respond to **anticonvulsant drugs**, such as carbamazepine or phenytoin, or to painkillers, such as **acetaminophen**. Trigeminal neuralgia may also be relieved by surgery in which the nerve is cut or decompressed. In some cases, compression neuralgia (including occipital neuralgia) can be relieved by surgery.

People with shingles should see a doctor within three days of developing the rash, since aggressive treatment of the blisters that appear with the rash can ease the severity of the infection and minimize the risk of developing postherpetic neuralgia. However, it is not clear whether the treatment can prevent postherpetic neuralgia.

If postherpetic neuralgia develops, the physician may try a variety of treatments, as their effectiveness varies from person to person. These treatments may include:

- Antidepressants such as amitriptyline (Elavil)
- Anticonvulsants (phenytoin, valproate, or carbamazepine)
- Capsaicin (Xostrix), the only medication approved by the FDA for treatment of postherpetic neuralgia
- Topical painkillers
- Desensitization
- TENS (transcutaneous electrical nerve stimulation)
- Dorsal root zone (DREZ) surgery (a treatment of last resort).

Some alternative treatments also are used for neuralgia. B-complex **vitamins**, primarily given by intramuscular injection, can be effective. A whole foods diet with adequate protein, carbohydrates, and fats that also includes yeast, liver, wheat germ, and foods that are high in B vitamins may be helpful. Acupuncture is a very effective treatment, especially for postherpetic neuralgia. Some botanical medicines may also be useful. For example, black cohosh (*Cimicifuga racemosa*) appears to have anti-inflammatory properties.

The effectiveness of the any type of treatment depends on the cause of the neuralgia, but many cases respond to pain relief. Trigeminal neuralgia tends to come and go, but successive attacks may be disabling. Although neuralgia is not fatal, the patient's fear of being in pain can seriously interfere with daily life. Some people with postherpetic neuralgia respond completely to treatment. Most people, however, experience some pain after treatment, and a few receive no relief at all. Some people live with this type of neuralgia for the rest of their lives, but for most, the condition gradually fades away within five years.

Neuroblastoma

Neuroblastoma is a solid **cancer**ous tumor that develops in the nerve tissue of the neck, chest, abdomen, or pelvis. The tumor usually spreads from the adrenal gland, which is located in the abdomen near the kidneys.

Neuroblastoma affects mainly children. It is the fourth most common cancer that occurs in children, affecting one in 100,000 children in the United States each year. Approximately 60% of cases of neuroblastoma occur in children younger than two years old, and 70-90% occur in children under five. The disease is sometimes present at birth, but is usually not noticed until later. By the time the disease is diagnosed, it has often spread to the lymph nodes, liver, lungs, bones, or bone marrow.

Physicians classify neuroblastoma in stages, based on how far the disease has spread from its original site to other tissues in the body. The best treatment for the disease depends on its stage. Neuroblastoma that is confined to the site of origin, with no evidence that it has spread to other tissues, is called localized resectable (able to be cut out) neuroblastoma. At this stage, the cancer can be surgically removed. Localized unresectable neuroblastoma is confined to the site of origin, but the cancer cannot be completely removed surgically. Regional neuroblastoma has extended beyond its original site, to nearby lymph nodes, organs or tissues, but has not spread to distant sites in the body. Disseminated neuroblastoma has spread to distant lymph nodes, bone, liver, skin, bone marrow, and/or other organs. Stage IV's (or ''special'') neuroblastoma has spread only to liver, skin, and/or, to a very limited extent, bone marrow. Recurrent neuroblastoma is cancer that has come back or continued to spread after it has been treated. It may come back in the original site or in another part of the body.

The most common symptoms of neuroblastoma arise because of pressure caused by the tumor and bone **pain** from cancer that has spread to the bone. Cancer that has spread to the area behind the eye may cause bulging eyes and dark circles around the eyes. Pressure on the spinal cord may cause **paralysis**. **Fever**, anemia, and high blood pressure occur occasionally. Some children may have watery **diarrhea**, uncoordinated or jerky muscle movements, or uncontrollable eye movements, but these symptoms are rare.

Physicians use physical examination and imaging techniques, such as computed tomography scan (CT scan) and **magnetic resonance imaging** (MRI), to diagnose neuroblastoma.

The physician may also take a small tissue sample (biopsy) from the tumor or bone marrow and examine the cells under the microscope. Once neuroblastoma has been found, the physician will perform more tests to find out if the cancer has spread to other tissues in the body.

Treatments are available for children with all stages of neuroblastoma. More than one type of treatment may be used, depending on the stage of the disease. Surgery is used whenever possible, to remove as much of the cancer as possible, and can generally cure the disease if the cancer has not spread to other parts of the body. **Radiation therapy** is often used after surgery; high-energy rays (radiation) are used to kill as many of the remaining cancer cells as possible. **Chemotherapy** (using drugs to kill cancer cells) may also be used after surgery to kill remaining cells. Also, before surgery, chemotherapy is used to shrink the tumor so that it can be more easily removed during surgery. **Bone marrow transplantation** is used to replace bone marrow cells killed by radiation or chemotherapy. In some cases the patient's own bone marrow is removed before treatment and saved for transplantation later. Other times the bone marrow comes from a ''matched'' donor, such as a brother or sister.

The chances of recovery from neuroblastoma depend on the stage of the cancer, the age of the child, the location of the tumor, and other factors. Infants have a higher rate of cure than do children over one year of age, even when the disease has spread. In general, the prospects for a young child with neuroblastoma are good: about 85% of children who develop the disease as infants are still alive five years after treatment, as are 35% of children whose disease developed later.

Neurofibromatosis

Neurofibromatosis (NF), or von Recklinghausen disease, is a genetic disease in which patients develop many soft tumors (neurofibromas) under the skin and throughout the nervous system. The tumors develop from cells called neural crest cells, which are found in developing fetuses (unborn babies). Normally, neural crest cells turn into other types of cells that form nerves; bony structures of the head and neck; and pigment cells, which provide color to body structures. But in a person with neurofibromatosis, a genetic defect causes the neural crest cells to develop abnormally, producing tumors and malformations of the nerves, bones, and skin.

About one in every 4,000 babies born has neurofibromatosis (NF). Two types of NF exist, NF-1 (90% of all cases), and NF-2 (10% of all cases). The chance of a person with NF passing on the genetic defect to a child is 50%. However, not all cases of NF are inherited. About half are due to a spontaneous mutation (a permanent change in the structure of a specific gene) that occurs after birth.

NF-1 is suspected if any two of these signs are present:

- The presence of café-au-lait (French for coffee-with-milk) spots. These are patches of tan or light brown skin, usually about 5-15 mm in diameter. Nearly all patients with NF-1 have these spots.
- Multiple freckles in the armpit or groin.
- Tiny tumors called Lisch nodules in the iris (colored area) of the eye.
- Neurofibromas. These are soft, rubbery tumors that occur under the skin, along nerves or within the gastrointestinal tract. The skin over neurofibromas may be purplish.
- Skeletal deformities, such as a twisted spine (**scoliosis**), curved spine (humpback), or bowed legs.
- Tumors along the optic nerve, which cause vision problems in about 20% of patients.
- The presence of NF-1 in a patient's parent, child, brother or sister.

Children with NF-1 are very likely to have speech problems, learning disabilities, or attention deficit disorder. They may also develop **seizure disorder**s, or the abnormal accumulation of fluid within the brain (**hydrocephalus**). A number of **cancer**s are more common in patients with NF-1.

Patients with NF-2 do not necessarily have café-au-lait spots, freckling, and neurofibromas of the skin. They are more likely to have hearing loss, due to tumors along the acoustic nerve. These tumors may spread to neighboring nerves, causing weakness of the muscles of the face, **headache**, **dizziness**, poor balance, and uncoordinated walking. Cloudy areas on the lens of the eye (called **cataracts**) frequently develop at an unusually early age. As in NF-1, the chance of brain tumors developing is unusually high.

Monitoring the progression of neurofibromatosis involves careful testing of vision and hearing. X-ray studies of the bones are frequently done to watch for the development of deformities. CT scans and MRI scans are performed to track the development and progression of tumors in the brain and along the nerves.

There are no available treatments for the genetic disorders that underlie neurofibromatosis, but some of the symptoms can be treated. Skin tumors can be surgically removed. Some brain tumors and tumors along the nerves, can be surgically removed or treated with drugs (**chemotherapy**) or x-ray treatments (**radiation therapy**). Twisting or curving of the spine and bowed legs may require surgical treatment, or the wearing of a special brace.

The outlook for a person with NF depends on the type of tumors that develop. As tumors grow, they begin to destroy surrounding nerves and structures. This can cause blindness, deafness and problems with balance and coordination, making it difficult to walk. Deformities of the bones and spine can also interfere with walking and movement.

There is no known way to prevent NF cases which occur due to a spontaneous change in the genes (mutation). New cases of inherited NF can be prevented with careful **genetic counseling**. A person with NF can be made to understand that each of his or her offspring has a 50% chance of also having NF. When a parent has NF, and the specific genetic defect causing the parent's disease has been identified, tests can be performed on the fetus (developing baby) during **pregnancy**. The tissue can then be examined for the presence of the parent's genetic defect. Some families use this information to prepare for the arrival of a child with a serious medical problem. Other families choose not to continue the pregnancy.

Nicolle, Charles J. H. (1866-1936)

French bacteriologist

Born in 1866, in Rouen, France, Charles Jules Henri Nicolle was the son of physician Eugène Nicolle. Charles took his medical degree in 1893 in Paris, then returned to Rouen for a staff position in a hospital. Shortly thereafter, he married Alice Avice. Nicolle agreed in 1902 to assume the directorship of the Institute Pasteur in Tunis, Tunisia. Until his death in 1936, Nicolle lived and worked in Tunis with occasional lecturing in Paris.

Affiliated with the original Institute Pasteur (which was founded in Paris in 1888), the institute in Tunis was basically an organization in name only. Over the years to come, however, Nicolle improved a run-down antirabies vaccination unit into a leading center for the study of North African and tropical diseases. It was in Tunis where Nicolle accomplished his groundbreaking work on **typhus**. He became intrigued by the observation that an outbreak of typhus did not seem to take hold in hospital wards as it did among the general populace of the city. Although the contagion infected workers who admitted patients into the hospital, it did not affect other patients or attendants in the actual wards. Those who collected or laundered the dirty clothes of newly admitted patients typically came down with the disease.

Realizing that the washing, shaving, and providing of clean clothes to the new patient was possibly the key to the pattern of infection, Nicolle initiated a series of experiments in 1909 to confirm his suspicion of the arthropod-borne nature of typhus. He theorized that lice, which attached themselves to the bodies and clothes of human beings, transmitted the disease, so he began his investigation by infusing a chimpanzee with human blood infected with typhus, then transferred the chimpanzee's blood to a healthy macaque monkey. When the fever and rash of typhus was seen on the monkey, Nicolle placed twenty-nine human body lice obtained from healthy humans on the skin of the macaque. These lice were later placed on the skin of a number of healthy monkeys, which all contracted the disease.

For his research into the cause of typhus, Nicolle was awarded the 1928 Nobel Prize for physiology or medicine. Once Nicolle isolated the relationship between typhus and the louse, preventative measures were established to counter unsanitary conditions. The development of the insecticide DDT by Paul Müller in 1939 was the most effective prophylactic against typhus.

Nicolle is also responsible for other important contributions to the science of bacteriology. Stemming from his research into typhus was his recognition of a phenomenon known as ''inapparent infection,'' a state in which a carrier of a disease exhibits no symptoms. This theoretical discovery suggested how diseases survived from one epidemic to another.

Nicolle, along with a variety of other colleagues over time, also researched African infantile leishmaniasis, which affected humans, and a related disease in dogs. Another significant discovery concerned the role of flies in the transmission of the blinding disease trachoma. For these and other works, Nicolle received the French Commander of the Legion of Honor and was named to the French Academy of Medicine. In 1932 he became a professor in the College de France.

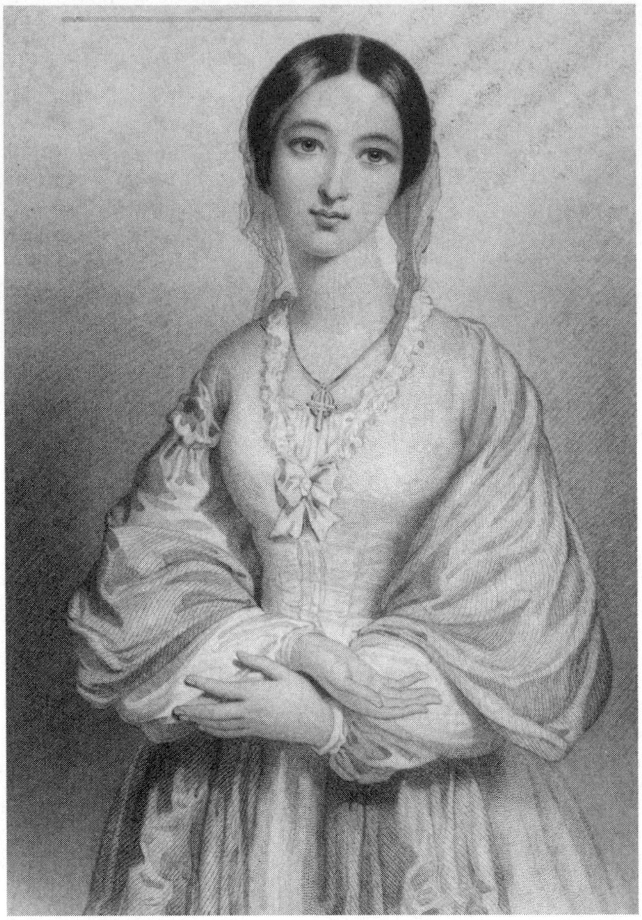

Florence Nightingale

Nightingale, Florence (1820-1910)

British Nurse, Public Health advocate

Florence Nightingale is generally regarded as having founded the modern profession of **nursing**. She was born in Florence, Italy, to very wealthy parents who were on an extended honeymoon (2 years) throughout Europe. Her family returned to their estate in England, where Nightingale's father taught her languages, history, and philosophy. It was expected that Nightingale would follow the conventions of the era, learning needlework and leisurely, lady's activities, eventually marrying as befitted her station in high society. At 16, however, Nightingale felt herself to be called to higher purpose by the voice of God.

Nightingale approached her parents about her desire to enter training to become a nurse, but they were horrified at the low-class nature of her interest, and tried to dissuade her. Ultimately, they forbade her, but within a few years she ignored their protests and enrolled in the Institution of Deaconesses in Germany. She returned to London at age 33 to become superintendent of a woman's hospital.

In 1854, reports were returning to England about the horrifying conditions in the Crimea, where Britain and France had battled Russia. Thousands of wounded British soldiers were dying of the suboptimal medical conditions in the makeshift hospitals that had been set up in Turkey. The British people were angered that their men, who had served their country so well, were now being neglected in their hour of need.

In October of 1854, Nightingale was tapped by the secretary of war to lead a contingent of nurses to the Crimea. Nightingale arrived in Scutari with 38 other nurses. Indeed, the reports had been understated. Wounded and ill soldiers lay in filth on straw pallets in crowded hallways. Rats and insects crawled the floors and walls, and the hospitals lacked basic supplies, such as cots, mattresses, bandages, washbasins, soap, towels. Water was rationed, and available in totally inadequate amounts. While Nightingale did not understand basic "**germ theory**," she still recognized that overcrowding, filth, and poor ventilation all contributed to the illness she saw before her. She immediately requisitioned 200 scrub brushes, and, enlisting the most well of the soldiers, set a team to work cleaning the filthy building. Nightingale worked tirelessly caring for the soldiers, day and night. By night, she carried a lamp through the corridors, stopping to help the suffering. For this, she was nicknamed "the lady of the lamp."

Nightingale tried to go to the Crimea to work, but was met with protests from officials, who said that her only area of authority was in Scutari. Furthermore, shortly after her arrival, she fell severely ill with Crimean fever. She returned to England in 1856, and remained a bedridden invalid for the rest of her life.

Despite her lifelong illness, Nightingale continued to have amazing influence. She also continued to write about appropriate medical practices for the military, prompting the establishment of the Royal Commission on the Health of the Army. Officials came to her residence to meet with her, and she read and stayed abreast of various **public health** issues around the world. In fact, she was considered an expert on health issues in India, although she had never traveled there. Nightingale wrote extensively about hospital planning and organization, and about educating health professionals, especially nurses. Nightingale died on August 13, 1910.

See also Nursing; Public health

NIRENBERG, MARSHALL WARREN (1927-)

American biochemist

Marshall Nirenberg is best known for first determining a relationship between a genetic code triplet (a *codon*) and its corresponding amino acid. He followed this by deciphering most of the entire genetic code, independent of the work of **Har Gobind Khorana**. For his work, Nirenberg shared the 1968 Nobel Prize for physiology and medicine with Khorana and **Robert Holley**.

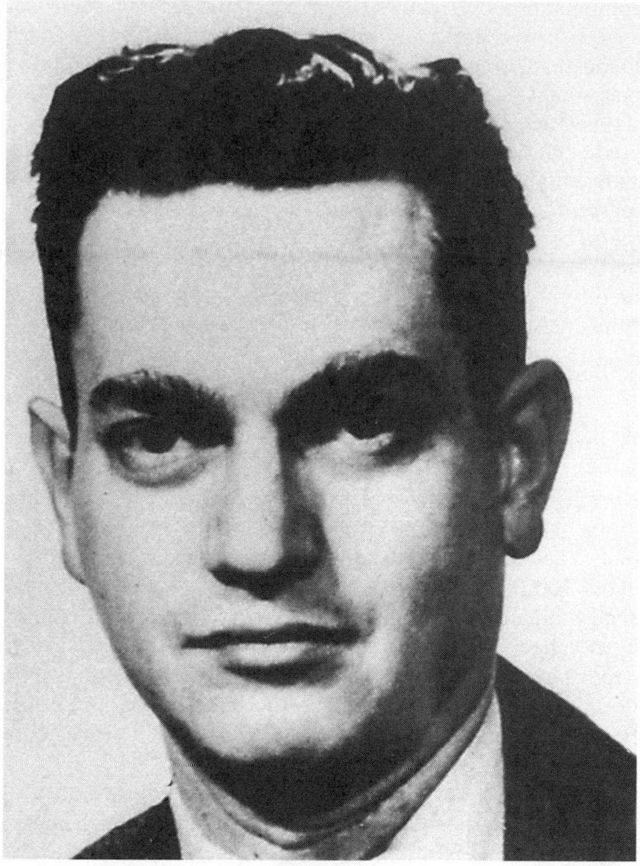

Marshall W. Nirenberg

Nirenberg was born in New York City, New York. After receiving bachelor's and master's degrees from the University of Florida, he earned his doctorate in biological chemistry from the University of Michigan in 1957. He then joined the U.S. National Institutes of Health, where he has spent his career.

When Nirenberg began his work, it was already known that a series of three nucleic acid nucleotides (or bases) carry the instruction that specifies a single amino acid. These three bases make up a codon. Messenger ribonucleic acid (mRNA), in the form of a triplet of bases complementary to the codon (called an *anticodon* carries the DNA information from the DNA to ribosomes in the cytoplasm. The mRNA then binds with the ribosome. Proteins begin to be constructed when transfer ribonucleic acid (tRNA) binds with mRNA.

Nirenberg and his colleague J. H. Matthaei set out to determine which codons coded for the twenty amino acids necessary for protein production. First they synthesized artificial RNA (first developed by **Severo Ochoa**) composed entirely of the RNA nucleotide uracil (U) so that the only possible codon was UUU. Then they introduced the artificial RNA into a solution of ground bacteria containing all components: DNA, amino acids, enzymes, etc. The mixture produced phenylalanine, leading Nirenberg to conclude that UUU coded for this amino acid. This experiment was repeated for all possible combinations of codons. Using a combination of statistical analysis and chemical processes, Nirenberg and his colleagues found that some codons produced the same amino acid and that some did not code any amino acid. Chemical analysis showed that almost all of the 50 codons whose amino acids he predicted were accurate. Nirenberg and Philip Leder also showed that the three bases which make up a codon of tRNA must be in a specific order to bring the correct amino acid to the ribosome.

Besides the Nobel Prize, Nirenberg has also been honored by the National Medal of Science in 1965 and membership in the National Academy of Sciences in 1967.

Nitrogen Narcosis

Nitrogen narcosis, also called ''rapture of the deep,'' is a condition that occurs in divers breathing compressed air from a tank. The condition becomes noticeable when divers go below about 100 ft. At that point, they experience an altered mental state similar to alcohol intoxication. Nitrogen narcosis has also been called ''the martini effect'' because for every 50 ft of depth beyond the initial 100 ft, the effect is something like drinking one martini on an empty stomach. At 300 ft, the effect becomes disabling, causing stupor, blindness, unconsciousness, and even **death**.

Nitrogen narcosis occurs because gases in the body behave according to Dalton's Law of partial pressures. The law states that the total pressure of a gas mixture is equal to the sum of the partial pressures of gases in the mixture. Partial pressure is the pressure exerted by any one of the gases in the mixture. The greater the concentration of a gas in the mixture, the greater its partial pressure. As a diver goes deeper into the water, total gas pressure increases. As total gas pressure increases, the partial pressure of each individual gas also increases, in proportion to its concentration in the mixture. As the partial pressure of nitrogen increases, more nitrogen becomes dissolved in the blood. This high nitrogen concentration slows the nervous system and mimics the effects of alcohol or narcotics.

Symptoms of nitrogen narcosis include: wooziness; giddiness; euphoria (an exaggerated feeling of happiness or well-being); disorientation; loss of balance; clumsiness; slowing of reaction time; and fuzzy thinking. Cold, **stress**, and rapid changes in depth make the effects worse.

Except for death, the effects of nitrogen narcosis are completely reversed as the gas pressure decreases. They are typically gone by the time the diver returns to a water depth of 60 ft. Nitrogen narcosis has no hangover or lasting effects requiring further treatment. However, a doctor should be consulted whenever a diver has lost consciousness.

Some experienced divers seem to become accustomed to the effects of increased nitrogen. The more often they dive, the less it affects them. Nitrogen narcosis can be prevented by using helium instead of nitrogen to mix with oxygen for deep water diving. Helium is colorless, odorless, and tasteless. However, it is more expensive than nitrogen, and it drains body heat from a diver. In some situations, the helium-oxygen mixture may produce nausea, **dizziness**, and trembling, but these reactions are not as severe than nitrogen narcosis. Another way to avoid nitrogen narcosis is by limiting the depth of dives. The risk may also be minimized by following safe diving practices, including proper equipment maintenance, low work effort, proper buoyancy, maintenance of visual cues, and focused thinking. In addition, no alcohol should be consumed within 24 hours of diving.

Nitrous oxide

The gas nitrous oxide was first identified by Joseph Priestley in 1772. Years later, in the late 1790s, the British chemist Humphry Davy began experimenting with the effects of inhaling nitrous oxide. He noted its exhilarating effects, and the way it made him want to laugh—which gave the gas its popular name of ''laughing gas.'' Davy published his findings in 1800, remarking that ''As nitrous oxide... appears capable of destroying pain, it may probably be used with advantage during surgical operations.''

Little attention was paid to Davy's observations, or to those of Henry Hill Hickman (1800-1830), a general practitioner from Shropshire, England, who in 1824 explored methods of painless surgery on animals using both carbon dioxide and nitrous oxide gas. Nevertheless, nitrous oxide became widely known in the first half of the nineteenth century. Davy repeatedly demonstrated the gas's exhilarating effects to gatherings of his friends, and inhalation parties became quite popular. Use spread to the United States as traveling lecturers spread knowledge about the new chemistry to the general public, usually including a demonstration of the effects of nitrous oxide inhalation on audience volunteers. One of these public lectures in Hartford, Connecticut, in December 1844, given by Gardner Quincy Colton (1814-1898), was attended by local dentist Dr. Horace Wells (1815-1848). Wells observed that a volunteer, Samuel Cooley, obviously hurt himself while under the influence of nitrous oxide but didn't notice the pain. Wells immediately thought of using the gas to banish pain during tooth extraction; the next day he took some of Colton's gas while a fellow dentist removed one of Wells's teeth. As he had expected, Wells felt no pain.

After confirming the anesthetic effect of nitrous oxide on other patients, Wells arranged through his former dental partner, William T. G. Morton (1819-1868), to demonstrate his discovery to a group of Morton's Harvard Medical School classmates in January 1845. Unfortunately, the nitrous oxide was applied incorrectly, and the patient yelped with pain when his tooth was pulled, embarrassing Wells before the group.

After Morton used ether successfully as an anesthetic in 1846, Wells pressed his claims for primacy as the discoverer of **anesthesia**. Frustrated in these attempts, Wells began to abuse chloroform. He committed suicide in 1848 after being arrested for throwing acid at two women in New York, New York.

Nitrous oxide was finally made a practical anesthetic by Colton in 1863. Edmund Andrews (1824-1904), a Chicago surgeon, began to use nitrous oxide in combination with oxygen in 1868, and as this method gained popularity, nitrous oxide became a staple in surgical as well as dental practice.

Nonsteroidal anti-inflammatory drugs

Nonsteroidal anti-inflammatory drugs (NSAIDs) are medicines that relieve **pain**, swelling, stiffness, and inflammation. They are prescribed for a variety of painful conditions, including arthritis, **bursitis**, **tendinitis**, **gout**, menstrual cramps, sprains, strains, and other injuries. Two drugs in this category, ibuprofen and naproxen, also reduce **fever**. While NSAIDs relieve symptoms, they do not cure the diseases or injuries responsible for these problems. Some nonsteroidal anti-inflammatory drugs can be bought over the counter; others are available only with a prescription from a physician or dentist.

Among the drugs in this group are diclofenac (Voltaren), etodolac (Lodine), flurbiprofen (Ansaid), ibuprofen (Motrin, Advil, Rufen), ketorolac (Toradol), nabumetone (Relafen), naproxen (Naprosyn); naproxen sodium (Aleve, Anaprox, Naprelan); and oxaprozin (Daypro). They are sold as tablets, capsules, caplets, liquids, and rectal suppositories and some are available in chewable, extended-release, or delayed-release forms.

NSAIDs should always be taken as directed. Patients who take this medicine for severe arthritis must take it regularly over a long time. Several weeks may be needed to feel the results, so it is important to keep taking the medicine, even if it does not seem to be working at first.

When taking NSAIDs in tablet, capsule, or caplet form, always take them with a full, 8-ounce glass of water or milk. Taking these drugs with food or an antacid will help prevent stomach irritation.

NSAIDs can cause a number of side effects, from indigestion, dizziness, drowsiness and heartburn to more serious problems such as fast heartbeat, tightness in the chest, convulsions, and unusual bleeding. Most minor symptoms go away as the patient's body adjusts to the medicine. If they do not, or if severe side effects occur, call a physician.

Side effects are more likely when the drugs are taken in large doses or for a long time or when two or more nonsteroidal anti-inflammatory drugs are taken together. Also, older people may be more likely than younger people to have side effects. Health care professionals can help patients weigh the risks of benefits of taking these medicines.

Some NSAIDs can increase the chance of bleeding after surgery (including dental surgery), so anyone who is taking the drugs should alert the physician or dentist before surgery. It may be necessary to stop taking the medicine or to switch to another type several days before surgery.

NSAIDs make some people more sensitive to sunlight. Even brief exposure to sunlight can cause severe **sunburn**, **rashes**, redness, **itching**, blisters, or discoloration. Vision changes also may occur. To reduce the chance of these problems, avoid direct sunlight, especially from mid-morning to mid-afternoon; wear protective clothing, a hat, and sunglasses; and use a sunscreen with a skin protection factor (SPF) rating of at least 15. Do not use sunlamps, tanning booths or tanning beds while taking these drugs.

NSAIDs may interact with a variety of other medicines. When this happens, the effects of the drugs may change, and the risk of side effects may be greater. Anyone who takes these drugs should let the physician know all other medicines he or she is taking. Among the drugs that may interact with NSAIDs are:

- Blood thinning drugs, such as warfarin (Coumadin)
- Other nonsteroidal anti-inflammatory drugs
- Heparin
- **Tetracyclines**
- Cyclosprorine
- **Digitalis drugs**
- Lithium
- Phenytoin (Dilantin)
- Zidovudine (AZT, Retrovir).

Nosebleed

A nosebleed, also called epistaxis, is bleeding from the nose. Often, nosebleeds are caused by blowing the nose too hard, picking the nose, or being hit in the nose. Nosebleeds are more common in people with hay fever, because the swollen membranes inside the nose are fragile. While most nosebleeds are not a sign of serious medical problems, persistent bleeding—from the nose or from any other part of the body—should be investigated, as it could be an early sign of **cancer**.

Nosebleeds most often come from the front of the septum, the wall of cartilage that separates the nostrils. The septum has a mass of blood vessels on either side called Kiesselbach's plexus that is easy to injure. Nosebleeds from areas farther inside the nose are less common and much harder to manage.

The first treatment for nosebleed is to pinch the nostrils together, bend forward at the waist and stay in that position for 5-10 minutes. Bleeding that continues is usually from the back of the nose and will flow down the throat. If that happens, emergency medical attention is needed.

For a nosebleed that won't stop, health care professionals may pack the nose with cotton cloth and a rubber balloon, which may cause some discomfort. Having no place to flow, the blood should clot. Then a physician can find the source of the bleed and permanently repair it. If the packing has to remain in place for some time, **antibiotics** and **pain** medication will be necessary. Nose packing may so interfere with breathing that the patient will need supplemental oxygen.

Many bleeds are from small exposed blood vessels. They can be sealed with cautery (burning with electricity or chemicals). Larger vessels may not respond to cautery. The surgeon may have to tie them off.

Estrogen cream, the same preparation used to revitalize vaginal tissue, can toughen fragile blood vessels in the front of the septum and delay the need for cauterization. Plant-based medicines known as stiptics, which slow down and can stop bleeding, may be taken internally or applied to the inside of the nose. Some of the plants used are achillea (yarrow), trillium, geranium, and shepherd's purse (*Capsella bursa-pastoris*).

To reduce the chance of getting a nosebleed, blow the nose gently and do not pick. Treatment of hay fever helps make the tissues inside the nose less fragile.

NOVOCAIN

Cocaine was widely used as a local anesthetic after Carl Koller (1857-1944) demonstrated its effectiveness in 1884. By the end of the 1800s, however, the addictive properties of cocaine had been recognized. Doctors, realizing they needed to develop substitutes for cocaine's active anesthetic ingredient, carefully studied the drug's exact chemical structure. Many of the initial synthetic cocaine products that were developed were too irritating to be of any practical use. The first successful substitute was Ernest Fourneau's (1872-1949) stovaine, discovered in 1904.

Fourneau's product was soon followed, in 1905, by procaine, the discovery of German Alfred Einhorn. Einhorn gave his substance the trade name Novocain, from the Latin *novus* (''new'') plus *cocaine*. Introduced by Heinrich Braun (1862-1934) in 1905, novocain soon showed that it had all the positive effects of cocaine with none of that drug's drawbacks. Guido Fisher popularized Novocain, or procaine, in the United States. Injected by needle, Novocain immediately became popular as a local anesthetic for both medical and dental purposes.

Other similar synthetic substitutes for cocaine produced after novocain include tropocaine, aucaine, monocaine, and lignocaine.

See also Anesthesia

NURSING

Throughout history nursing has played an essential role in society as a profession that embodies the preservation and restoration of health along with the care of the terminallly ill. With records from early in the first millennium A.D., ancient cultures referred to nurses as attendants who prepared and administered medicines, cared for the physical needs of patients, and knowingly followed physician's orders. While still focused on the same basic desire to provide wellness, comfort, care, and assurance to the sick, the role of the nurse has evolved into one of the most crucial support functions of modern medicine.

The influences of an everchanging society have promoted the radical developments in nursing throughout time. First seen as a role suitable only for uneducated women or slaves in ancient times, Christianity along with other religious orders soon helped the nurse gain respect as the role of caregiver to the sick became an increasingly prominent practice. The Christian Church brought the formation of the Order of the Deaconesses in the first century a group similar to public health or visiting nurses. This happened at a time when caring for the sick was a Christian duty, ''a sacred vocation based upon Christ's actual command.'' The love and brotherhood of Christianity also led to the establishment of the first nursing order by the Augustinian Sisters during the Middle Ages. With the approach of the Protestant Reformation in England, monastic medicine (care given by monasteries and the monks and nuns who live there) and the nursing orders of the sixteenth century were destroyed, leaving **hospitals** overcrowded with the only care for the sick provided by illiterate, indigent women. Chaos ruled until the early eighteenth century when voluntary hospitals offered some relief for England, and the continued presence of nursing orders in Europe aided those in need. Reformation of societal factors, including prisons and social welfare during this dark period led to the organization of new nursing orders to supply improved, humane services where none existed before.

While the first nursing order with a systematic educational program was established in the sixteenth century by the Sisters of Charity, continued growth of cities along with the emergence of **epidemic**s led to an increased need for formal training apart from the church to meet the demand for more nurses. To help meet this need, a special nursing school, La Source was founded by Countess Agénor de Gasparin in 1859 near Lausanne in Switzerland. The countess introduced nursing as a vocation that should be salaried all without the presence of religious vows.

The Crimean War (1854-1856) produced the founder of modern nursing, **Florence Nightingale**. Born into an affluent family, her stature helped structure nursing into an orderly work force during the war, and in 1860, Nightingale established her renowned school of nursing at St. Thomas' Hospital in London. Similar in thought to the countess, Nightingale observed nursing as a career and a calling, rather than a religious vocation. Her high expectations inducted thousands of students into a profession she thought demanded intelligence and impeccable morals and behavior. The Nightingale Training Schools infiltrated Britain, Canada, Australia, and New Zealand, in addition to influencing the education of nurses in the United States.

As Nightingale's values of nursing traveled overseas, the United States was in the midst of the Civil War (1861-1865). Bringing care to the soldiers on the battlefields was led by many nurses, but **Clara Barton** would ultimately stimulate the growth of nursing in this country due to her role as founder of the American Red Cross. Her cause was initiated by Swiss banker, **Jean Henri Dunant**, who after witnessing the Battle of Solferino on June 24, 1859, was determined that no soldier would go without medical support. His founding of the **International Red Cross** in 1864 instigated the development of nurses' training throughout the world. This catalyst also brought about the Women's Central Relief Committee. Led by Dr. **Elizabeth Blackwell**, a former associate of Nightingale's, this group of women was dedicated to serving several needs of the war, including, identifying the army's nursing needs, and creating ''a bureau for the examination and registration of nurses.'' Their persistence led to the organization of the National Sanitary Commission that would guide the government to oversee medical support for the army.

Although religious orders still dominated nursing in parts of Europe throughout the early nineteenth century, the United States placed proper education and training of lay nurses as a top priority. Hospitals became the accepted route for preparation and employment, and nursing schools throughout America and Canada began to follow the Nightingale vision of providing classroom instruction and clinical practice. Mary Agnes Snively established the Canadian Nurses' Association (CNA) in 1884, and the Nurses Associated Alumni of the United States, which later became the American Nurses' Association (ANA) was founded in part by Isabel Hampton Robb in 1886.

With the emergence of professional organizations and the Red Cross serving as the nursing profession's liasion to the world, a need to further prove their professional identity was provoked as oppposition surfaced from physicians and other rivalries within the vocation itself. In order to protect and define their status, high standards were set with strict entrance requirements, prescribed curricula, and licensing regulations for the profession. The United States became the touchstone of nursing as they moved into the twentieth century with national nursing organizations and state governments working together toward defining standards and educational requirements these efforts led to the first registry law in 1938 by New York State which established the difference between the registered nurse, who had met state requirements for a licensed professional nurse, and the less rigorous training requirements of the practical nurse.

Advancement in the world of medicine and public health launched the nursing profession into the twentieth century. The Goldmark Report, funded by the Rockefeller Foundation in the early 1900s, resulted in expansion of nursing programs at Yale University, Vanderbilt University, and the University of Toronto. Alternatives to the hospital diploma setting has become a reality as education in senior colleges and universities has became standard worldwide. Nursing programs include: the associate degree (ADN) program that lasts two years and is offered by junior or community colleges with a focus on the technical elements of nursing; and the four-year baccalaureate program with curriculum including liberal arts and sciences and clinical experience which leads to a bachelor or science degree in nursing (BSN). Although each program is unique, the interaction and collaboration of all three are reinforced by state mandates for articulation agreements in the United States. The practical nurse (LPN) or vocational nurse (LVN) is also an approved program that is offered by high schools, community colleges, vocational schools, and a variety of health care agencies throughout the country.

Opportunities continue to increase for the nurse as a need for their expertise escalates. The profession has met the demand for its changing role with an increasing number employed in long-term care, home health care, ambulatory and school-based clinics, health maintenance organizations, and community nursing centers. In addition to their presence on medical/surgical units or intensive care units, nurses teach in schools, serve in executive positions, conduct research, and work alongside physicians in joint practices. While historically a profession typically occupied by women, the twentieth century has seen the entrance of more men to nursing roles in the emergency room, critical care, and surgical settings. Trends in the United States also include the growth of graduate nursing education, which prepares nurse practitioners, nurse anesthetists, nurse-midwives, and clinicians for numerous specialties.

As science and technology continue to flourish, so will the demand for the advancement of nursing. With a abundance of organizations across the world to guide their efforts and shape policy, including the National League of Nursing in the United States, the incentives for a career in nursing will continue to proliferate and match the opportunities offered by other professions.

See also Barton, Clara; Dunant, Jean Henri; Epidemic and pandemic; Health maintenance organization; Nightingale, Florence

Nursing Homes

Nursing homes are institutions that provide living quarters and care for individuals who require assistance with their day to day activities. Most often the residents of nursing homes are elderly and have chronic, disabling or terminal health conditions. The activities for which they need assistance can range from very basic ones, such as bathing, eating, and dressing, to more instrumental ones such as shopping, preparing meals, taking medications, doing housework, and managing money.

Prior to the twentieth century, nursing homes were virtually non-existent. The elderly, the sick, and the disabled were cared for primarily by family members. Public poorhouses took in those who had no means or family to care for them. The need for long-term nursing care was less significant, since life expectancy was shorter and most mortality was the result of infectious diseases that took a relatively rapid course. Medication and technology that now enable people with chronic and debilitating conditions to sustain an acceptable quality of life over a longer period of time, were not available.

In 1935 the United States Congress passed the Social Security Act and established the Old Age Assistance (OAA) program. The OAA stimulated the development of the nursing home industry because it provided public funds to care for the elderly in non-public institutions. In 1950 an amendment to the Social Security Act required that states establish licensing procedures for nursing homes. While the amendment did not specify standards of care, it was the first legislative step toward providing some measure of quality assurance for residents. In 1956 a federal government commission on chronic health problems reported that most nursing homes had poor standards for service and employed vastly undertrained personnel. After a series of studies and hearings at both state and federal levels, the Nursing Homes Standards Guide was issued by the U.S. Public Health Service in 1963. Meanwhile, in 1960 the OAA was replaced by a far more extensive program, called Medical Assistance for the Aged (MAA). During the 1950s, federal spending for nursing home care had increased from approximately $35 million to nearly three hundred million. By 1965 the MAA was providing about $1.3 billion of assistance. That same year, the Medicaid and Medicare programs were inaugurated. Federal funding increased even more dramatically, and as a result government involvement in the regulation of the nursing home industry grew substantially. In 1974 certification and licensing regulation went into effect, establishing standards of quality that were more uniform across the country. Over the past few decades, quality of care has improved substantially, though regulation and enforcement continue to be important legislative issues. The rights of nursing home patients with respect to such issues as privacy, disclosure of medical information, and freedom from abuse have also arisen as important legal and societal issues.

Nursing homes are now classified as either ''intermediate care'' or ''skilled care,'' according to the degree of medical assistance they provide to their residents. Skilled nursing facilities provide extensive medical care, and their services are often covered by Medicare. Within many nursing homes both intermediate and skilled care are available, offered in different sections of the same facility so that residents may be moved easily from one level of care to another. Today well over two million elderly Americans live in nursing homes. It is expected that by the year 2040 that number will approach five million.

Nüsslein-Volhard, Christiane (1942-)

German genetic researcher

Christiane Nüsslein-Volhard was born on October 20, 1942, in Magdeburg, Germany. The daughter of Rolf Volhard, an architect, and Brigitte (Hass) Volhard, a musician and painter. And while few women of her generation chose scientific careers, Nüsslein-Volhard found that being female in a male-dominated field presented little in the way of an obstacle to her studies. She received degrees in biology, physics, and chemistry from Johann-Wolfgang-Goethe-University in 1964 and a diploma in biochemistry from Eberhard-Karls University in 1968. In 1973 she earned a Ph.D. in biology and genetics from the University of Tübingen. Nüsslein-Volhard was married for a short time as a young woman and never had any children. She decided to keep her husband's last name because it was already associated with her developing scientific career.

In the late 1970s Nüsslein-Volhard finished post-doctoral fellowships in Basel, Switzerland, and Freiburg, Germany, and accepted her first independent research position at the European Molecular Biology Laboratory (EMBL) in Heidelberg, Germany. She was joined there by **Eric F. Wieschaus** who was also finishing his training. Because of their common interest in *Drosophila*, or fruit flies, Nüsslein-Volhard and Wieschaus decided to work together to find out how a newly fertilized fruit fly egg develops into a fully segmented embryo.

Nüsslein-Volhard and Wieschaus chose the fruit fly because of its incredibly fast embryonic development. They began to pursue a strategy for isolating genes responsible for the embryos' initial growth. This was a bold decision by two scientists just beginning their scientific careers. No one had done anything like this before, and it wasn't certain whether they would be able to actually isolate specific genes.

Their experiments involved feeding male fruit flies sugar water laced with chemicals that damaged the flies' deoxyribonucleic acid (DNA). When the male fruit flies mated with females, the females often produced dead or mutated embryos. Nüsslein-Volhard and Wieschaus studied these embryos for over a year under a microscope which had two viewers, allowing them to examine an embryo at the same time. They were able to identify specific genes that basically told cells what they were going to be—part of the head or the tail, for example. Some of these genes, when mutated, resulted in damage to the formation of the embryo's body plan.

Nüsslein-Volhard and Wieschaus published the results of their research in the English scientific journal *Nature* in 1980. They received a great deal of attention because their studies showed that there were a limited number of genes that control development and that they could be identified. This was significant because similar genes existed in higher organisms and humans and, importantly, these genes performed similar functions during development. Nüsslein-Volhard and Wieschaus's breakthrough research could help other scientists find genes that could explain birth defects in humans. Their research could also help improve in-vitro fertilization and lead to an understanding of what causes miscarriages.

In 1991 she and Wieschaus received the Albert Lasker Medical Research Award, which is considered second only to the Nobel. During this time Nüsslein-Volhard had begun new research at the Max Planck Institute in Tübingen, Germany, similar to the work she did on the fruit flies. This time she wanted to understand the basic patterns of development of the zebra fish. She chose zebra fish as her subject because most of the developmental research on vertebrates in the past was on mice, frogs, or chickens, which have many technical difficulties, one of which was that one couldn't see the embryos developing. Zebra fish seemed like the perfect organism to study because they are small, they breed quickly, and the embryos develop outside of the mother's body. The most important consideration, however, was the fact that zebra fish embryos are transparent, which would allow Nüsslein-Volhard a clear view of development as it was happening.

Despite her prize-winning research on fruit flies, she received skeptical feedback on her zebra fish work. Other scientists claimed it was risky and foolish. When she submitted papers about her laboratory's work for publication, one reviewer even asked her why she was bothering. Nüsslein-Volhard was not one to be stopped by criticism or to rest on her laurels. Even though her reputation was built on her fruit fly research, her love of new challenges pushed her to take on this risky new project and set her sights to the future.

On October 9, 1995, in the midst of criticism about her new research, Nüsslein-Volhard (the first German woman to win in this category), Wieschaus, and Edward B. Lewis of the California Institute of Technology won the Nobel Prize in

Physiology or Medicine for their work on genetic development in *Drosophila*. Lewis had been analyzing genetic mutations in fruit flies since the forties and had published his results independently from Nüsslein-Volhard and Wieschaus.

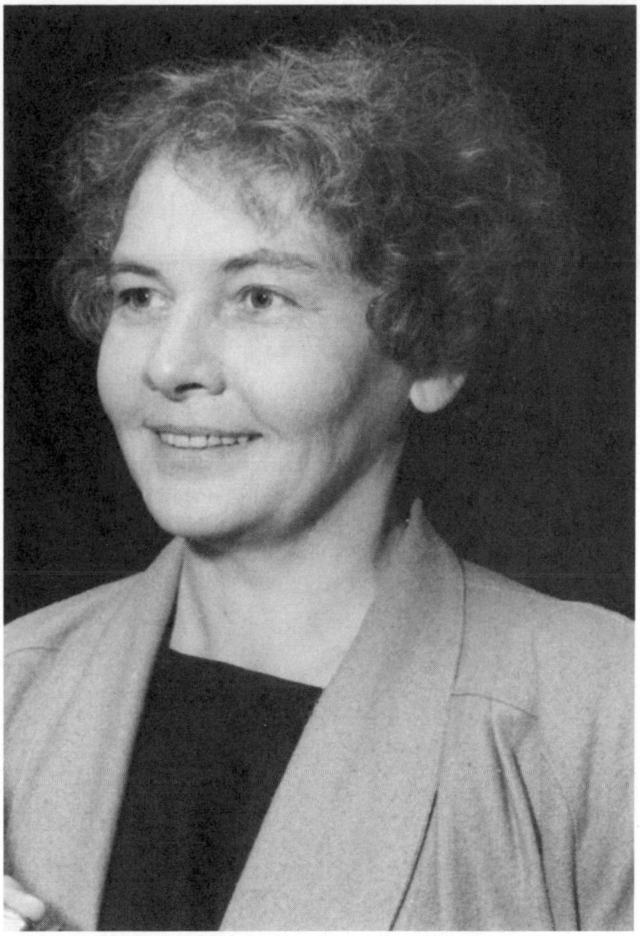

Christiane Nüsslein-Volhard

Nutrition

Nutrition is both the process by which humans take in and utilize food and the study of diet as it relates to health.

With the proliferation of fast food restaurants, the number of junk food commercials on television, and the increased trend toward eating out, it is more difficult than ever for parents to ensure that their children maintain a nutritious diet. In recent decades, increasing affluence and the widespread availability of vitamin-enriched foods have shifted the focus of nutritional concerns in the United States from obtaining minimum requirements to cutting down on harmful elements in one's diet. According to a 1988 report from the office of the U.S. Surgeon General, health problems are more likely to be caused by nutritional excesses and imbalances than by deficiencies. In other words, parents need to be as concerned about high levels of fat, cholesterol, sugar, and salt as about adequate intake of **vitamins**, **minerals**, and other nutrients.

The American Academy of Pediatrics, the National Academy of Sciences, the American Heart Association, and other nutrition-oriented organizations agree that fat should not account for more than 30% of the calorie intake of children over the age of two, and saturated fat should account for under 10%. The main dietary sources of saturated fat include whole milk, cheese, hot dogs, and luncheon meats. Recommendations for dietary change include switching to 1% or skim milk, low-fat cheese, and meats from which the fat can be trimmed. (Because fat is important for growth, experts also caution that fat intake should not be lowered to under 25% of daily calorie intake, and that parents of children under two should not restrict fat in their diets.) Hardening of the arteries and heart disease have been linked not only to the conversion of saturated fats into cholesterol but also to cholesterol that comes directly from food (dietary cholesterol), often found in the same foods that are high in saturated fat. Egg yolks are the primary source of dietary cholesterol, and their consumption should be monitored in children as in adults.

The amount of refined sugar in children's diets—typically accounting for 14% of calorie intake by adolescence—is another cause for concern. Although sugar is known to cause **tooth decay** and may be associated with behavior problems, the greatest danger in consuming foods high in added sugar is that these "empty calories" will replace the more nutritious foods that children need in order to maintain good health. (Soft drinks, perhaps the single greatest source of refined sugar in the diet of children and teenagers, get virtually all their calories from sugar and offer no nutrients whatsoever.)

Another element that needs to be restricted in children's diets is the intake of sodium through salted foods. Sodium has been closely linked to **hypertension** (high blood pressure), which increases a person's risk of heart disease and **strokes**. It has been determined that 18-year-olds need only 500 milligrams of sodium daily. However, the average two-year-old already consumes more than five times that amount (2,670 milligrams), and this figure rises to 3,670 milligrams by the age of 17. The National Academy of Sciences recommends limiting sodium intake to 2,400 milligrams daily (if possible, 1,800 milligrams). Contrary to what most people might think, the vast majority of sodium enters a person's diet through salt that is added in food preparation rather than table salt used when a person is eating.

In addition to limiting the amounts of fat, cholesterol, salt, and sugar in children's diets, health authorities also recommend that parents concerned about nutrition ensure that their children obtain a generous supply of complex carbohydrates (found in foods such as beans, potatoes, whole-grains, and pasta) and have at least five servings of fresh fruits and vegetables daily.

A special problem that may affect childhood nutrition is the presence of food **allergies**, which are more common in children than in adults. They are most likely to begin when a child is very young and the **immune system** is still sensitive—

most begin in infancy. Food allergies also tend to run in families: if one parent has food allergies, a child has a 40% likelihood of developing one. This figure rises to 75% if both parents have allergic sensitivities to food. Common symptoms of food allergies include hives, rashes, swelling of the eyes, lips, and mouth, respiratory symptoms, and digestive problems. Foods that most often produce allergic reactions in infants are cow's milk, soy products, and citrus fruits. Other common childhood allergens include wheat, nuts, chocolate, strawberries, tomatoes, corn, and seafood. A widely used method for detecting food allergies is to temporarily place children on diets free of known allergy-causing foods and then add one ''suspect'' food at a time for a week or so and observe the reaction. Once the causes of food allergies are known, the best treatment method is to remove those foods from the child's diet. If the causes of a food allergy cannot be determined, antihistamines can be used to reduce the symptoms of allergic reactions. In time, childhood food allergies are often outgrown.

Feeding a child with food allergies is a challenging but not impossible task for parents. A variety of foods can be substituted for those to which a child is allergic: soy products for milk and other dairy products; carob for chocolate; and, in the case of wheat allergies, products or flour made from grains such as rice or oats.

Many authorities, including the American Academy of Pediatrics, agree that healthy children receiving a well-balanced diet do not need to take nutritional supplements. Nevertheless, some pediatricians still recommend vitamins for children until they are eating solid foods. Special situations that may call for supplements include **vitamin K deficiencies** in **low birthweight** babies; iron deficiency in young children or adolescent girls; weight-reduction or allergy diets that may cause vitamin deficiencies; vitamin B12 deficiencies in children from strict vegetarian families who do not receive animal protein from dairy products; and various illnesses, including metabolic disorders. Recommendations for supplements are universally accompanied by the precaution that they should not be considered substitutes for an adequate diet.

See also Dietary supplements; Minerals; Vitamins

O

OBESITY

Obesity traditionally has been defined as a weight at least 20% above a person's ideal body weight. Twenty to forty percent over ideal weight is considered mildly obese; 40–100% over ideal weight is considered moderately obese; and more than 100% over ideal weight is considered severely, or morbidly, obese. According to some estimates, approximately one quarter of the U.S. population can be considered obese, 4 million of whom are morbidly obese.

Excessive weight can result in many serious, and potentially deadly, health problems, including high blood pressure, diabetes, infertility and increased risk for heart disease and heart attack.

The physical explanation for weight gain is simple: more calories are consumed than burned, and the body stores the excess calories as fat. However, the exact reasons why some people become obese while others do not is not clear. Genetic factors influence how the body regulates appetite and the rate at which it turns food into energy (metabolic rate). But a genetic tendency to gain weight does not automatically mean that a person will be obese. Eating habits and patterns of physical activity also are important. Recent studies have shown that the amount of fat in a person's diet may be more important than the number of calories. Carbohydrates like cereals, breads, fruits, and vegetables and protein (fish, lean meat, turkey breast, skim milk) are converted to fuel almost as soon as they are consumed. Most fat calories, however, are immediately stored in fat cells, which add to the body's weight and girth as they expand and multiply.

Obesity can also be a side-effect of certain disorders and conditions, including an underactive thyroid gland or damage to the part of the brain that helps regulate appetite. Certain medicines, such as steroids and antidepressants may cause weight gain.

The location of fat on a person's body is one clue to the risk of developing certain obesity-related conditions. ''Apple-shaped'' people who store most of their weight around the waist and abdomen are at greater risk for **cancer**, heart disease, **stroke**, and **diabetes** than ''pear-shaped'' people whose extra pounds settle primarily in their hips and thighs.

Successful treatment of obesity must involve life-long behavioral changes rather than short-term weight loss. Weight-loss programs that emphasize realistic goals, gradual progress, sensible eating, and **exercise** can be very helpful and are recommended by many doctors. Programs that promise instant weight loss or feature severely restricted diets are not effective and, in some cases, can be dangerous. Studies have shown that ''yo-yo'' dieting, in which weight is repeatedly lost and regained, increases a person's likelihood of developing fatal health problems more than losing weight gradually or not losing it at all.

For people who are severely obese, diet and lifestyle changes may be accompanied by surgery to reduce or bypass portions of the stomach or small intestine. Such surgery can be risky, and it is done only after other weight-loss strategies have failed, on patients whose obesity seriously threatens their health. Other surgical procedures, such as **liposuction** and **jaw wiring**, are not recommended.

Appetite-suppressant drugs are sometimes prescribed to aid in weight loss. These drugs work by increasing levels brain chemicals that control feelings of fullness and satisfaction. However, most of the weight lost while taken appetite suppressants is usually regained after stopping them. Also, suppressants containing amphetamines can be abused by patients. Two weight-loss drugs, dexfenfluramine hydrochloride (Redux) and fenfluramine (Pondimin) as well as a combination fenfluramine-phentermine (Fen/Phen) drug, were taken off the market when they were shown to cause potentially fatal heart defects. In November, 1997, the United States **Food and Drug Administration** (FDA) approved a new weight-loss drug, sibutramine, (Meridia). Available only with a doctor's prescription, Meridia can significantly elevate blood pressure and cause dry mouth, **headache**, **constipation**, and **insomnia**. This medication should not be used by patients with a history of congestive heart failure, heart disease, stroke, or uncontrolled high blood pressure.

The Chinese herb ephedra (*Ephedra sinica*), combined with **caffeine**, exercise, and a low-fat diet in physician-supervised weight-loss programs, is an alternative approach that can cause at least a temporary weight loss. However, the large doses of ephedra required to achieve the desired result can also cause serious medical problems including high blood pressure, heart attack, seizures, stroke, and death. Ephedra should not be used by anyone with a history of diabetes, heart disease, or thyroid problems.

Acupressure and acupuncture can also suppress food cravings. Visualization and **meditation** can create and reinforce a positive self-image that enhances the patient's determination to lose weight. By improving physical strength, mental concentration, and emotional serenity, **yoga** can provide the same benefits.

Diuretic herbs, which increase urine production, can cause short-term weight loss but cannot help patients achieve lasting weight control.

The best approach to achieving and maintaining weight loss is a life-long commitment to regular exercise and sensible eating habits. As many as 85% of dieters who do not exercise on a regular basis regain their lost weight within two years. In five years, the figure rises to 90%. Exercise increases the metabolic rate by creating muscle, which burns more calories than fat. When regular exercise is combined with regular, healthful meals, calories continue to burn at an accelerated rate for several hours.

Obsessive-Compulsive Disorder

Obsessive-compulsive disorder (OCD) is a type of **anxiety** disorder. People with anxiety disorders cannot stop worrying. In OCD, people have intense, repetitive thoughts, images, or impulses that are frightening, absurd, or unusual. These are called obsessions. Typical obsessions include fears of dirt, germs, contamination, and violent or aggressive impulses. People with obsessive-compulsive disorder may have an intense preoccupation with order and symmetry, or be unable to throw anything away. To reduce the anxiety caused by their irrational thoughts, people with OCD perform ritualized actions, known as compulsions, that also are usually bizarre and irrational. Examples are repeated hand-washing, constant counting or arranging of items, and checking over and over again to make sure an appliance is turned off. As the person performs these acts, he may feel temporarily better, but there is no long-lasting sense of satisfaction or completion after the act is performed. Often, a person with obsessive-compulsive disorder believes that something terrible will happen if the ritual isn't performed.

OCD is often described as the ''disease of doubt,'' because a person who has it usually knows the obsessive thoughts and compulsions are irrational but, on another level, fears they may be true. Because the symptoms are upsetting and embarrassing, people with the condition often hide their fears and rituals but cannot avoid acting on them.

Most people with OCD have both obsessions and compulsions, but a few have just one or the other. Some people are barely bothered by the condition, while others find the obsessions and compulsions to be profoundly traumatic and spend much time each day in compulsive actions.

While no one knows for sure, research suggests that the tendency to develop obsessive-compulsive disorder is inherited. If one person in a family has obsessive-compulsive disorder, there is a 25% chance that another immediate family member has the condition. Stress and psychological factors may worsen symptoms, which usually begin during adolescence or early adulthood.

There are several theories behind the cause of OCD. Some experts believe that OCD is related to a chemical imbalance within the brain that causes a communication problem between the front part of the brain (frontal lobe) and deeper parts of the brain responsible for the repetitive behavior. Research has shown that a particular part of the brain is overactive in OCD patients. This overactivity may cause brain cells to get ''stuck,'' much as a jammed transmission in a car damages the gears. This could lead to the development of rigid thinking and repetitive movements. Drugs that boost the levels of serotonin, a natural brain chemical linked to emotion and many different anxiety disorders can reduce OCD symptoms. This suggests that OCD may be related to levels of serotonin in the brain.

Out of shame, people with obsessive-compulsive often avoid seeking treatment. Because they are so good at hiding their problem, many people with OCD don't get the help they need until the behaviors are deeply ingrained habits and hard to change. More than a decade can pass between the onset of symptoms and proper diagnosis and treatment.

Obsessive-compulsive disorder can be effectively treated with a combination of cognitive-behavioral therapy and medication that regulates the brain's serotonin levels. Cognitive-behavioral therapy teaches patients how to confront their fears and obsessive thoughts by waiting out the urge to perform the calming rituals. Eventually their anxiety decreases, and they learn to focus their attention elsewhere. Drugs that are approved to treat obsessive-compulsive disorder include fluoxetine (Prozac), fluvoxamine (Luvox), paroxetine (Paxil), and sertraline (Zoloft). Drugs should be taken for at least 12 weeks before deciding whether or not they are effective.

Without treatment, obsessive-compulsive disorder can last for decades, fluctuating from mild to severe and worsening with age. Treatment with drugs and behavioral therapy is completely successful for some patients. Unfortunately, not all patients have such a good response, and hospitalization may be required in some cases.

Occupation Safety and Health

A relatively new concern that dates roughly to the post-Industrial Revolution era, occupation health and safety is a field that involves measures to prevent or minimize dangers to people in their places of work, i.e., the office, farm, building site, factory, or store. These hazards generally fall into two categories: those presented by toxic chemicals and those presented by physical factors.

In industrialized countries, job-related accidents kill more people every year than any diseases except cancer and heart disease. The National Safety Council (NSC) estimated in 1990 that some 100,000 new work-related illnesses occur every year in the United States and that people who work in the mining, agriculture, construction, and quarrying industries are three to four times more likely to die than their counterparts in other industries. The NSC also reported in 1990 that industrial accidents led to almost 2 million disabling injuries and approximately 11,000 deaths in the United States.

While it would seem practical to implement strong health and safety provisions in all workplaces, there are several factors that sometimes bar these provisions from going into effect. One of them, not surprisingly, is that company owners and operators perceive safety and health laws as expensive and unnecessary meddling by the government. Sometimes even the workers themselves resist health and safety regulations because they seem overcautious and may interfere with comfort. However, while bureaucracies can be frustrating to deal with, laws such as those imposed by the Occupational Safety and Health Administration (OSHA) and its subsidiary agencies can potentially save millions of dollars in worker compensation claims, sick time, and law suits every year.

The most effective ways to mitigate worker exposure to toxic chemicals are process or equipment modification, local exhaust ventilation, elimination or substitution of a substance, isolation or enclosure, and providing personal protective equipment and clothing if the substance's harmful effects cannot be minimized by the other means. To lessen the risk of accident or injury present by physical factors, employers can offer training, for instance, on how to operate machinery or lift heavy loads properly to avoid back strain.

The most common health risks that workers face are caused by inhaling dust from coal, grains, clay, quartz, asbestos, silica, fungal spores, and metals; by being exposed to radiation, whether from the sun or ionizing sources; and by coming into contact with such common industrial chemicals as lead, beryllium, cadmium, arsenic, benzene, or vinyl chloride, which all can cause severe damage to all organs of the body when inhaled, touched, or ingested. **Allergies** to or long-term contact with irritating chemicals can cause **dermatitis**, while exposure to serious diseases such as **AIDS**, **leptospirosis**, and **brucellosis**, among many others, are dangers for people who work with blood, rats, and livestock, respectively. Many people are also hurt every year by lifting heavy loads; running or working around machinery unsafely; working outdoors for too long or with too little protection in sunny, windy, or hot conditions; receiving electric shocks; and sustaining **carbon monoxide poisoning**. In the 1990s, doctors identified a new group of work-related disorders called **repetitive motion injuries**; these include **carpal tunnel syndrome**. In addition, many workers suffer from various levels of psychological stress induced by noise, repetition, and other job-related factors.

Since the Industrial Revolution, during which a period of rapid economic growth and the introduction of mechanical and technical inventions led to many thousands of injuries and deaths from poor working conditions and lack of safety provisions, there have emerged entire state and federal bureaucracies dedicated solely to health and safety in the workplace. However, it was not until 1970 that the Occupational Health and Safety Act was passed. This, in turn, established the National Institute for Occupational Safety and Health and the Department of Labor's powerful OSHA, which supports reduction of workplace hazards, establishes training programs, creates mandatory safety and health standards, and provides for occupational and health research.

In the 21st century, as in the 20th, the greatest challenge will be making sure that occupation health and safety measures keep pace with the rapid development of new technologies in the workplace.

Occupational Therapy

The American Occupational Therapy Association defines occupational therapy as ''the therapeutic use of self-care, work/productive activities, and play/leisure activities to increase independent function, enhance development, and prevent disability.'' As such, occupational therapy includes the adaptation of tasks and the environment to maximize independence and quality of life.

The term occupation refers not to employment per se, but to activities that are meaningful to the individual within the environments in which he or she lives and functions.

Occupational therapy involves assisting people who for one reason or another cannot function independently; increasing independence by assisting with activities of daily living; enhancing an individual's ability to work, play, and enjoy leisure; and helping others to help themselves. Occupational therapy is not, however, helping people find jobs (although occupational therapists may assist people in returning to work after a mishap, illness, or injury); or physical therapy (although occupational therapy students may attend many of the same classes as physical therapists).

Occupational therapists use daily activities to help people achieve independence. In the cases of individuals with physical disabilities, the occupational therapist first focuses on helping the individual perform essential daily activities, which may include dressing, grooming, bathing, and eating. After these skills have been mastered, the occupational therapist works on imparting the skills needed to meet daily responsibilities, such as caring for a home and family, going to school, or seeking and holding a job.

In the case of a client with a **mental illness**, the goal is also to help the individual function independently. In treating mental or emotional problems, the occupational therapist may work with the patient to help him or her manage time more effectively, work productively with others, and enjoy leisure time.

Occupational therapists work in public schools, **rehabilitation** hospitals, mental health centers, **nursing homes**, physician's offices, and home health agencies. They are primarily, however, employed in hospitals, skilled nursing facilities, and schools.

Occupational therapists may work with victims of neurodegenerative disease such as **multiple sclerosis**, transverse myelitis, and **Lou Gehrig's disease** (amyotrophic lateral sclerosis); **carpal tunnel syndrome**; **stroke**; traumatic brain injury; hip fracture/replacement; **spinal cord injury**; **low back pain**; poor vision; **schizophrenia**; **Alzheimer's disease**; **attention-deficit/hyperactivity disorders**; **cerebral palsy**; chronic **pain**; substance use disorders; and tendon injuries. They also work with young children with delayed development.

In addition, the occupational therapist may help with the growth and development of premature babies; work to establish learning environments for physically challenged school children; modify home environments for victims of stroke; analyze job requirements for an injured worker; or conduct research on the effectiveness of specific treatments.

In 1997, annual salaries for occupational therapists working full-time averaged $47,095, ranging from a low of $12,000 to a high of $130,000. To become an occupational therapist, a student must complete an education program accredited by the Accreditation Council for Occupational Therapy Education. The student may choose either to pursue a bachelor's degree, a post baccalaureate certificate, or a professional master's degree. All academic programs in occupational therapy include a period of supervised clinical experience.

See also Hospitals; Independent living; Physical therapy

Occupational lung diseases

There are various occupational lung diseases. Among them are: Asbestosis, a chronic, progressive inflammation of the lung; it is a consequence of prolonged exposure to large quantities of asbestos, a material once widely used in construction, insulation, and manufacturing. It is not contagious.

Black lung disease is the common name for coal workers' pneumoconiosis (CWP) or anthracosis, a lung disease of older workers in the coal industry, caused by inhalation, over many years, of small amounts of coal dust.

Silicosis is a progressive disease that belongs to a group of lung disorders called pneumoconioses. Silicosis is marked by the formation of lumps (nodules) and fibrous scar tissue in the lungs. It is the oldest known occupational lung disease, and is caused by exposure to inhaled particles of silica, mostly from quartz in rocks, sand, and similar substances.

When asbestos is inhaled, fibers penetrate the breathing passages and irritate, fill, inflame, and scar lung tissue. In advanced asbestosis, the lungs shrink, stiffen, and become honeycombed (riddled with tiny holes).

Legislation has reduced use of asbestos in the United States, but workers who handle automobile brake shoe linings, boiler insulation, ceiling acoustic tiles, electrical equipment, and fire-resistant materials are still exposed to the substance. Asbestos is used in the production of paints and plastics. Significant amounts can be released into the atmosphere when old buildings or boats are razed or remodeled.

Asbestosis is most common in men over 40 who have worked in asbestos-related occupations. Smokers or heavy drinkers have the greatest risk of developing this disease. Between 1968 and 1992, more than 10,000 Americans over the age of 15 died as a result of asbestosis. Nearly 25% of those who died lived in California or New Jersey, and most of them had worked in the construction or shipbuilding trades.

The risk of having black lung disease is directly related to the amount of dust inhaled over the years; the disease typically affects workers over age 50. Its common name comes from the fact that the inhalation of heavy deposits of coal dust makes miners lungs look black instead of a healthy pink. Although people who live in cities often have some black deposits in their lungs from polluted air, coal miners have much more extensive deposits.

In the years since the federal government has regulated dust levels in coal mines, the number of cases of black lung disease has fallen sharply. Since the Federal Coal Mine Health and Safety Act of 1969, average dust levels have fallen from 8.0 mg. per cubic meter to the current standard of 2.0 mg. per cubic meter. The 1969 law also set up a black lung disability benefits program to compensate coal miners who have been disabled by on-the-job dust exposure.

Despite the technology available to control the hazard, however, miners still run the risk of developing this lung disease. The risk is much lower today, however; fewer than 10% of coal miners have any x ray evidence of coal dust deposits. When there is such evidence, it often shows up as only small black spots less than 1 cm. in diameter, and may have been caused by smoking rather than coal dust. This condition is called ''simple CWP'' and does not lead to symptoms or disability.

It is estimated that there are 2 million workers in the United States employed in occupations at risk for the development of silicosis. These include miners, foundry workers, stonecutters, potters and ceramics workers, sandblasters, tunnel workers, and rock drillers. Silicosis is mostly found in adults over 40. It has four forms:

- Chronic silicosis may take 15 or more years of exposure to develop. There is only mild impairment of lung functioning. Chronic silicosis may progress to more advanced forms.
- Patients with complicated silicosis have noticeable **shortness of breath**, weight loss, and extensive formation of fibrous tissue (fibrosis) in the lungs. These patients are at risk for developing **tuberculosis** (TB).
- Accelerated silicosis appears after 5-10 years of intense exposure. The symptoms are similar to those of complicated silicosis. Patients in this group often develop **rheumatoid arthritis** and other **autoimmune disorders**.
- Acute silicosis develops within six months to two years of intense exposure to silica. The patient loses a great deal of weight and is constantly short of breath. These patients are at severe risk of TB.

Occupational exposure is the most common cause of asbestosis, but the condition also strikes people who inhale asbestos fiber or who are exposed to waste products from plants near their homes. Family members can develop the disease as a result of inhaling particles of asbestos dust that cling to workers' clothes.

It is rare for asbestosis to develop in anyone who hasn't been exposed to large amounts of asbestos on a regular basis for at least 10 years. Symptoms of the disease do not usually appear until 15–20 years after initial exposure to asbestos.

The first symptom of asbestosis is usually shortness of breath following **exercise** or other physical activity. The early stages of the disease are also characterized by a dry **cough** and a generalized feeling of illness.

As the disease progresses and lung damage increases, shortness of breath occurs even when the patient is at rest. Recurrent respiratory infections and coughing up blood are common. So is swelling of the feet, ankles, or hands. Other symptoms of advanced asbestosis include chest pain, hoarseness, and restless sleep. Patients who have asbestosis often have clubbed (widened and thickened) fingers. Other potential complications include **heart failure**, collapsed (deflated) lung, and **pleurisy** (inflammation of the membrane that protects the lung).

Since the particles of fine coal dust, which a miner breathes when he is in the mines, cannot be destroyed within the lungs or removed from them, builds up. Eventually, this build-up causes thickening and scarring, making the lungs less efficient in supplying oxygen to the blood.

The primary symptom of the disease is shortness of breath, which gradually gets worse as the disease progresses. In severe cases, the patient may develop **cor pulmonale**, an enlargement and strain of the right side of the heart caused by chronic lung disease. This may eventually cause right-sided heart failure.

Some patients develop emphysema (a disease in which the tiny air sacs in the lungs become damaged, leading to shortness of breath, and respiratory and heart failure) as a complication of black lung disease. Others develop a severe type of black lung disease called progressive massive fibrosis, in which damage continues in the upper parts of the lungs even after exposure to the dust has ended. Scientists aren't sure what causes this serious complication. Some think that it may be due to the breathing of a mixture of coal and silica dust that is found in certain mines. Silica is far more likely to lead to scarring than coal dust alone.

The precise mechanism that triggers the development of silicosis is still unclear. What is known is that particles of silica dust get trapped in the tiny sacs (alveoli) in the lungs where air exchange takes place. White blood cells called macrophages in the alveoli ingest the silica and die. The resulting inflammation attracts other macrophages to the region. The nodule forms when the immune system forms fibrous tissue to seal off the reactive area. The disease process may stop at this point, or speed up and destroy large areas of the lung. The fibrosis may continue even after the worker is no longer exposed to silica.

Early symptoms of silicosis include shortness of breath after exercising and a harsh, dry cough. Patients may have more trouble breathing and cough up blood as the disease progresses. Congestive heart failure can give their nails a bluish tint. Patients with advanced silicosis may have trouble sleeping and experience chest **pain**, hoarseness, and loss of appetite. Silicosis patients are at high risk for TB, and should be checked for the disease during the doctor's examination.

Screening of at-risk workers can reveal lung inflammation and lesions characteristic of asbestosis. Patients' medical histories can identify occupations, hobbies, or other situations likely to involve exposure to asbestos fibers.

X rays can show shadows or spots on the lungs or an indistinct or shaggy outline of the heart that suggests the presence of asbestosis. Blood tests are used to measure concentrations of oxygen and carbon dioxide. Pulmonary function tests can be used to assess a patient's ability to inhale and exhale, and a computed tomography scan (CT) of the lungs can show flat, raised patches associated with advanced asbestosis.

Black lung disease can be diagnosed by checking a patient's history for exposure to coal dust, followed by a chest x-ray to discover if the characteristic spots in the lungs caused by coal dust are present. A pulmonary function test may aid in diagnosis.

X rays can detect black lung disease before it causes any symptoms. If exposure to the dust is stopped at that point, progression of the disease may be prevented.

Diagnosis of silicosis is based on:

- A detailed occupational history.
- **Chest x ray**s will usually show small round opaque areas in chronic silicosis. The round areas are larger in complicated and accelerated silicosis.
- Bronchoscopy.
- Lung function tests.

It should be noted that the severity of the patient's symptoms does not always correlate with x-ray findings or lung function test results.

The goal of treatment is to help patients breathe more easily, prevent colds and other respiratory infections, and control complications associated with advanced disease. Ultrasonic, cool-mist humidifiers or controlled coughing can loosen bronchial secretions.

Regular exercise helps maintain and improve lung capacity. Although temporary bed rest may be recommended, patients are encouraged to resume their regular activities as soon as they can.

Antibiotics may be prescribed to combat infection. **Aspirin** or **acetominophen** (Tylenol) can relieve minor discomfort and **bronchodilators** that are swallowed or inhaled can relax and widen breathing passages.

Diuretics (drugs that increase urine production and excretion) or digitalis glycoside (*Digitalis purpurea*) are prescribed for some patients. Others may need to use supplemental oxygen or use less salt.

Anyone who develops symptoms of asbestosis should see a family physician or lung disease specialist. A doctor should be notified if someone who has been diagnosed with asbestosis:

- Coughs up blood
- Continues to lose weight
- Is short of breath
- Has chest pain
- Develops a sudden **fever** of 101°F (38.3°C) or higher
- Develops unfamiliar, unexplained symptoms.

There is no treatment or cure for black lung disease, although it is possible to treat complications such as lung infections and cor pulmonale. Further exposure to coal dust must be stopped.

Likewise, there is no cure for silicosis. Therapy is intended to relieve symptoms, treat complications, and prevent respiratory infections. It includes careful monitoring for signs of TB. Respiratory symptoms may be treated with bronchodilators, increased fluid intake, steam inhalation, and physical therapy. Patients with severe breathing difficulties may be given **oxygen therapy** or placed on a mechanical ventilator. Acute silicosis may progress to complete **respiratory failure**. Heart-lung transplants are the only hope for some patients.

Patients with silicosis should call their doctor for any of the following symptoms:

- Tiredness or mental confusion
- Continued weight loss
- Coughing up blood
- Fever, chest pain, breathlessness, or new unexplained symptoms.

Patients with silicosis should be advised to quit **smoking**, prevent infections by avoiding crowds and persons with colds or similar infections, and receive **vaccinations** against **influenza** and **pneumonia**. They should be encouraged to increase their exercise capacity by keeping up regular activity, and to learn to pace themselves with their daily routine.

Asbestosis can't be cured, but its symptoms can be controlled. Doctors don't know why the health of some patients deteriorates and the condition of others remain the same, but believe the difference may be due to varying exposures of asbestos. People with asbestosis who smoke, particularly those who smoke more than one pack of cigarettes each day, are at increased risk for developing lung cancer and should be strongly advised to quit smoking.

Those miners with simple CWP can lead a normal life. However, patients who develop black lung disease at an early age, or who have progressive massive fibrosis, have a higher risk of premature **death**.

Silicosis is currently incurable. The prognosis for patients with chronic silicosis is generally good. Acute silicosis, however, may progress rapidly to respiratory failure and death.

Workers in asbestosis-related industries should have regular x rays to determine whether their lungs are healthy. A person whose lung x ray shows a shadow should eliminate asbestos exposure even if no symptoms of the condition have appeared.

Anyone who works with asbestos should wear a protective mask or a hood with a clean-air supply and obey recommended procedures to control asbestos dust. Anyone who is at risk of developing asbestosis should:

- Not smoke
- Be vaccinated against influenza and pneumonia
- Exercise regularly to maintain cardiopulmonary fitness
- Avoid crowds and people who have respiratory infections.

A person who has asbestosis should exercise regularly, relax, and conserve energy whenever necessary.

The only way to prevent black lung disease is to avoid long-term exposure to coal dust. Coal mines may help prevent the condition by lowering coal dust levels and providing protective clothes to coal miners.

Silicosis is a preventable disease. Preventive occupational safety measures include:

- Controls to minimize workplace exposure to silica dust
- Substitution of substances—especially in sandblasting—that are less hazardous than silica
- Clear identification of dangerous areas in the workplace
- Informing workers about the dangers of overexposure to silica dust, training them in safety techniques, and giving them appropriate protective clothing and equipment.

Coworkers of anyone diagnosed with silicosis should be examined for symptoms of the disease. The state health department and the Occupational Safety and Health Administration (OSHA) or the Mine Safety and Health Administration (MSHA) must be notified whenever a diagnosis of silicosis is confirmed.

OCHOA, SEVERO (1905-1993)

American biochemist

Severo Ochoa is best known for being the first to synthesize ribonucleic acid (RNA) outside the cell. He has also discovered several important metabolic processes. For his work with RNA, he received half of the 1959 Nobel Prize in physiology or medicine.

Ochoa was born in Luarca, Spain, where his father was a lawyer, and graduated from the University of Malaga in 1921. He received a medical degree in 1928 from the University of Madrid. After further studies in experimental biology, in 1940 he joined the Medical School faculty of Washington University in St. Louis. In 1942, he moved to New York University's College of Medicine, becoming chairman of the biochemistry department in 1954. He became an American citizen in 1956.

Ochoa's synthesis in 1955 of RNA was pure serendipity—an unexpected byproduct of his study of the way cells use glucose that is stored as ATP (adenosine triphosphate). Ochoa and a French associate, Marianne Grunberg-Manago, had purified an enzyme (now called polynucleotide phosphorylase) from the bacteria *Azotobacter vinelandii*. They were trying to study its reactions with ATP and other base-sugar combinations (called nucleosides) with one or three phosphate groups attached. No reaction occurred. However, when they added the enzyme and some magnesium to a nucleoside with two phosphate groups (diphosphate), over half of the nucleoside disappeared and some phosphorus was freed.

Ochoa traced the nucleoside to a new molecule that ultraviolet chromatography identified as a nucleotide. He then repeated the reaction with other nucleoside-diphosphates, in each case finding a nucleotide. Further analysis showed that the sugar was ribose, meaning that the reaction produced ribonucleic acid (RNA). Since the reaction was also reversible, Ochoa concluded that adding and removing phosphorus groups is a major mechanism in the synthesis and breakdown of nucleotide chains. Ochoa and other scientists used this method to decipher the genetic code. Later studies by others showed that RNA polymerase, not Ochoa's enzyme, is the main RNA synthesizing enzyme.

Ochoa is also known for his work on how the body uses carbon dioxide, and he helped identify a key compound in the **metabolism** of carbon dioxide. He also identified Krebs cycle reactions leading to energy storage in phosphate bonds.

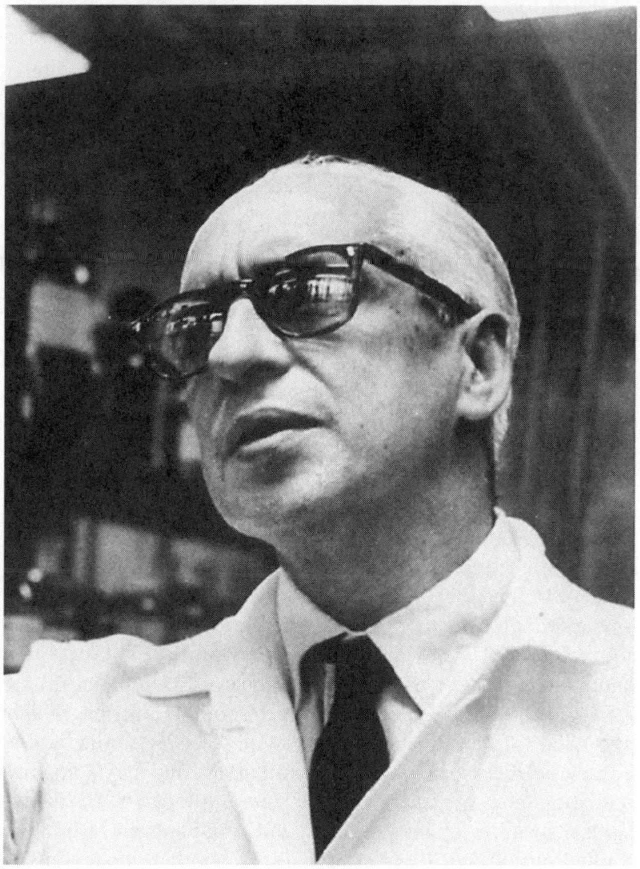

Severo Ochoa

OPEN-HEART SURGERY

For many years, major heart surgery—opening the chest to operate directly on an exposed heart—was considered outside the realm of possibility. The heart would cease beating during such operations. How could patients survive? A few pioneers did perform emergency surgery directly on the open heart, one of the first being African-American surgeon **Daniel Hale Williams**, who opened the chest of a stabbing victim and sewed up the pericardium (the sac surrounding the heart) in 1893. Both Ludwig Rehn (1849-1930) and Forina sutured heart wounds 1896. More lengthy and complicated heart operations, however, required a way to keep the blood oxygenated and circulating while a patient's heart was undergoing the operation. American surgeon, John H. Gibbon, Jr., devoted himself to solving this problem in the 1930s. Assisted by his wife Mary, Gibbon persisted until he had developed a workable pump-oxygenator, or **heart-lung machine**, that shunted blood from the veins through a catheter to a machine that supplied the blood with oxygen and then pumped the blood back into the arteries. On May 6, 1953, Gibbon connected Cecilia Bavolek, a patient suffering from **heart failure**, to the heart-lung machine and operated directly on her heart, closing an opening between her atria. This operation ushered in the era of open-heart surgery.

The methods and technical details of open cardiac surgery were refined throughout the 1950s by a number of surgeons and engineers, notably Owen Wangenstein at the University of Minnesota and John W. Kirklin at Minnesota's Mayo Clinic. By 1960 open-heart surgery was standard practice and began to be used not just for repair of cardiac malfunctions but also for replacement of defective heart parts—even the whole heart itself. Surgeons Albert Starr and M. L. Edwards of Portland, Oregon, designed a ball-and-cage **artificial heart valve** and successfully implanted it in a 52-year-old patient in 1961. Rene G. Favalaro introduced coronary artery bypass surgery in 1967. The heart gets its blood supply from coronary arteries that branch off from the aorta. These arteries can narrow from accumulations of plaque, which also promote clot formation, and can thereby become blocked, causing severe chest pain (angina) and, in some cases, heart attack. Favalaro and his surgical team at the Cleveland Clinic devised a technique of grafting a vein from the patient's leg around a blocked portion of a coronary artery, creating an alternate blood pathway. Favalaro's bypass surgery was made possible by the use of microsurgical techniques arteriography (direct images of the heart prior to open-heart surgery) and the heart-lung machine. Within three years of Favalaro's pioneering 1967 operation, coronary bypass surgery gained wide acceptance. Its use in cases of mildly clogged arteries dropped off in the late 1970s with the advent of balloon **angioplasty**.

The most dramatic development in open-heart surgery was the heart transplant, first successfully performed in Cape Town, South Africa, by Dr. **Christiaan Barnard** in 1967. Another dramatic step in open-heart surgery was revealled in 1996 when Randas Batista, an obscure cardiac surgeon from a country clinic in southern Brazil, hit the headlines in the United States. Batista cuts a triangular chunk from the left ventricular muscle of an enlarged heart in an effort to save the life of patient with chronic heart failure. Researchers do not yet understand why a weak heart thickens and grows—sometimes ballooning to twice it's normal size—but they do know it no longer pumps efficiently and eventually fails completely. Contrary to popular opinion, Batista believes it is the size of the heart, not the weakened muscle, that kills people. He has used his controversial technique on more than 400 people since 1994. In 1996, prominent U.S. surgeons travelled with the ABC news team from *20/20* to Brazil to see Batista's technique first-hand. Since May, 1996, Patrick McCarthy of the Cleveland Clinic has performed the surgery on more than 24 patients. All but one were still living four months later.

Ophthalmoscope

An ophthalmoscope enables a physician to examine the interior of the eye by directing a tiny beam of light through the pupil, the black ''window'' of the eye. Using the ophthalmoscope, the physician can look through the pupil to detect any abnormalities or pathological changes that could signal disease.

The first ophthalmoscope was invented by Charles Babbage, an English mathematician, in 1847. He gave the device to a physician for testing, but it was laid aside and forgotten. Four years later, German physician and physiologist **Hermann von Helmholtz** (1821-1894), unaware of Babbage's invention, developed his own version of the ophthalmoscope. Because he had better luck making his device known, Helmholtz is often credited as the sole inventor. Helmholtz's instrument operated by using a mirror to shine a beam of light into the eye. The observer would look through a tiny aperture attached to the mirror. Helmholtz eventually found that looking through the retina into the back of the eye only produced a red reflex; consequently, he attached a condenser lens to obtain an inverted image, which was then magnified five times. He called this combination of a mirror and condenser lens an indirect ophthalmoscope. It was used regularly for eye examinations until 1920. Helmholtz also invented the ophthalmometer, which was used to measure the curvature of the eye; studied color blindness; the speed of nervous impulses; and physiological acoustics; and wrote the classic *Handbook of Physiological Optics.* Swedish ophthalmologist, **Allvar Gullstrand**, who also studied physiological optics, developed another version of the ophthalmoscope and invented a slit lamp used with a microscope that enabled a physician to locate foreign bodies in the eye.

The modern ophthalmoscope is a hand-held instrument containing a small battery-powered lamp that directs the beam of light into the eye of a patient by way of a mirrored prism. The observer looks through a tiny hole in the prism and the instrument, which can be focused by a series of revolving lenses, magnifies the image. The lens needed to focus the image gives an approximation of the spectacle lenses needed to correct the patient's vision. A new type of ophthalmoscope that can project a laser beam is used in eye surgery to correct a detached retina. Another, larger type of ophthalmoscope, called the binocular ophthalmoscope, is used in clinical research and provides an image of the eye that is magnified fifteen times.

Opportunistic Infections

Opportunistic infections are so named because they occur in people whose immune systems are not working properly; they are ''opportunistic'' insofar as the infectious agents take advantage of their hosts' compromised **immune system**s and invade to cause disease.

The organisms that cause opportunistic infections are categorized as protozoa, fungi, viruses and bacteria. These organisms are found widely in nature and often live in the human body. When the immune system is working properly, it can control the germs. However, persons with defective immune systems are unable to fight off the growth and destructive action of these organisms within the body. Opportunistic infections are seldom spread to people who have normal healthy immune systems.

One of the ways the immune system can be damaged is when the person is infected by **HIV**. In addition, drugs used to treat **cancer**, and drugs used to facilitate **organ transplants** can also suppress the immune system.

A person infected with HIV can get an opportunistic infection, when the counts of a particular immune cell (T cell) in the blood falls below a certain critical number. The most common opportunistic infections that an HIV-infected person get are **Candidiasis** or Thrush, Cytomegalovirus, Herpes simplex virus, Mycobacterium avium complex, Pneumocystis carinii **pneumonia**, **Toxoplasmosis**, and **Tuberculosis**.

Most of the germs that cause opportunistic infections are quite common. One can reduce the risk of infection by keeping clean, having hygienic practices, and avoiding known sources of infection. Diagnosing an opportunistic infection can be very tricky. Generally, the symptoms are rather vague and nonspecific and could be due to a multitude of factors. Hence, the physician has to order blood culture and other laboratory tests to make a definitive diagnosis. Even if an immunocompromised person gets an opportunistic infection, there are medications that will prevent active disease. This is called prophylaxis. Getting vaccinated against pneumococci, a leading cause of bacterial pneumonia in the immuno-compromised people, is now recommended by the Ntaional Institutes of Health.

Because of the **AIDS** epidemic and the mortality associated with it, a lot of money and effort has been expended in the past decade on research aimed at the prevention and treatment of opportunistic infections. Much progress has been made and currently, there are specific drugs or combinations of drugs that seem to work best for each infection. Many researchers are also of the opinion that if a person's damaged immune system can be rebuilt, he will be better protected against opportunistic infections. When people use the newest drugs that fight HIV, its possible that their immune system can repair some of the damage done by HIV, and can do a better job of fighting opportunistic infections.

See also AIDS; Immune system

Oral Contraceptives

Oral contraceptives are medicines taken by mouth to help prevent **pregnancy**. Also known as birth control pills, they contain artificially made forms of two hormones produced naturally in the body. These hormones, estrogen and progestin, regulate a woman's menstrual cycle. When taken in the proper amounts, following a specific schedule, oral contraceptives are very effective in preventing pregnancy.

Oral contraceptives have several effects that help prevent pregnancy. For pregnancy to occur, an egg must ripen inside a woman's ovary, be released, and travel to the fallopian tube (the passageway from the ovary to the uterus). A man's sperm must also reach the fallopian tube, where it fertilizes the egg. Then the fertilized egg must travel to the woman's uterus (womb), where it lodges in the uterus lining and develops into a fetus. The main way that oral contraceptives prevent pregnancy is by keeping an egg from ripening fully. Eggs that do not ripen fully cannot be fertilized. In addition, birth control pills thicken mucus in the woman's body through which the sperm has to swim. This makes it more difficult for the sperm to reach the egg. Oral contraceptives also change the uterus lining so that a fertilized egg cannot lodge there to develop.

Birth control pills may cause good or bad side effects. For example, a woman's menstrual periods are regular and usually lighter when she is taking oral contraceptives, and the pills may reduce the risk of **ovarian cysts**, breast lumps, **pelvic inflammatory disease**, and other medical problems. However, taking birth control pills increases the risk of **heart attack**, **stroke**, and blood clots in certain women. Serious side effects such as these are more likely in women over 35 years of age who smoke cigarettes and in those with specific health problems such as high blood pressure, diabetes, or a history of breast or uterine **cancer**. A woman who wants to use oral contraceptives should ask her physician for the latest information on the risks and benefits of all types of birth control and should consider her age, health, and medical history when deciding what to use. No form of birth control (except not having sex) is 100% effective. However, oral contraceptives can be highly effective when used properly.

Oral contraceptives do not protect against **AIDS** or other **sexually transmitted diseases**. For protection against such diseases, it is necessary to use a latex **condom**.

Oral contraceptives come in a wide range of estrogen-progestin combinations. The pills in use today contain much lower doses of estrogen than those available in the past, and this change has made serious side effects less likely. Some pills contain only progestin. These are prescribed mainly for women who need to avoid estrogens and may not be as effective in preventing pregnancy as the estrogen-progestin combinations.

These medicines come in tablet form, in containers designed to help women keep track of which tablet to take each day. The tablets are different colors, indicating amounts of hormones they contain. Some may contain no hormones at all. These are included simply to help women stay in the habit of taking a pill every day, as the hormone combination needs to be taken only on certain days of the menstrual cycle. Keeping the tablets in their original container and taking them exactly on schedule is very important. They will not be as effective if they are taken in the wrong order or if doses are missed. Oral contraceptives are not effective immediately after a woman begins taking them. Physicians recommend using other forms of birth control for the first 1–3 weeks.

Oral contraceptives are available only with a physician's prescription. Some commonly used brands are Demulen, Desogen, Loestrin, Lo/Ovral, Nordette, Ortho-Novum, and Ovcon.

See also Contraception

Oral Hygiene

Oral hygiene is the practice of keeping the mouth clean and healthy by brushing and flossing to prevent **tooth decay** and gum disease. Brushing and flossing prevent the build-up of plaque, the sticky film of bacteria and food that forms on the teeth. Plaque sticks to grooves in the teeth and produces acids that can slowly eat away, or decay, the protective enamel surface of the teeth, causing holes (cavities) to form. Plaque also irritates gums and can lead to gum disease and tooth loss. In addition to brushing and flossing, antiseptic mouthwashes improve oral hygiene by killing some of the bacteria that help form plaque. Fluoride—in toothpaste, drinking water, or dental treatments—also helps to protect teeth by binding with enamel to make it stronger. Daily care is important in oral health, but so are regular visits to the dentist. At the dentist's office, the dentist or dental hygienist can perform preventive services such as fluoride treatments, sealant application, and scaling (scraping off the hardened plaque, called tartar). Diagnostic services, such as x-ray imaging and oral cancer screening, and treatment services, such as fillings, crowns, and bridges, can also be performed.

Maintaining oral hygiene should be a lifelong habit. An infant's gums and, later, teeth should be kept clean by wiping them with a moist cloth or a soft toothbrush. However, only a pea-sized amount of fluoride toothpaste should be used, as too much fluoride can be harmful to young children.

Even people with partial or full dentures should maintain good oral hygiene. Bridges and dentures must be kept clean to prevent gum disease. Dentures should be relined and adjusted by a dentist as necessary to maintain proper fit so the gums do not become red, swollen, and tender. Dentures should not be worn overnight.

Brushing should be performed with a toothbrush and a fluoride toothpaste at least twice a day and preferably after every meal and snack. Effective brushing must clean each outer tooth surface, inner tooth surface, and the flat chewing surfaces of the back teeth. To clean the outer and inner surfaces, the toothbrush should be held at a 45-degree angle against the gums and moved back and forth in short strokes (no more than one tooth width distance). To clean the inside surfaces of the front teeth, the toothbrush should be held vertically and the bristles at the tip (called the toe of the brush) moved gently up and down against each tooth. To clean the chewing surfaces of the large back teeth, the brush should be held flat and moved back and forth. Finally, the tongue should also be brushed using a back-to-front sweeping motion to remove food particles and bacteria that may sour the breath.

Toothbrushes wear out and should be replaced every three months. The best toothbrushes to use have soft, rounded, nylon bristles. The size and shape should allow for reaching all tooth surfaces easily.

Flossing once a day helps prevent gum disease by removing food particles and plaque at and below the gumline as well as between teeth. To begin, most of an 18-in (45-cm) strand of floss is wrapped around the third finger of one hand. A 1-in (2.5-cm) section is then grasped firmly between the thumb and forefinger of each hand. The floss is eased between two teeth and worked gently up and down several times with a rubbing motion. At the gumline, the floss is curved first around one tooth and then the other with gentle sliding into the space between the tooth and gum. After the space between each two teeth is cleaned, a fresh section of floss is unwrapped from one hand as the used section of floss is wrapped around the third finger of the opposite hand. Flossing should be done between all teeth and behind the back teeth.

Dental floss comes in many varieties (waxed, unwaxed, flavored, tape). The choice of dental floss is a matter of personal preference. People who have trouble handling floss can use floss holders and other types of cleaning aids, such as brushes and picks.

Brushing and flossing should not be done so vigorously as to irritate or damage sensitive tissues. When a person first starts flossing regularly, the gums may be sore and may bleed for a few days. Bleeding that continues for more than a week should be brought to a dentist's attention. As a general rule, any mouth sore or abnormal condition that does not disappear after 10 days should be examined by a dentist.

ORGAN DONATION

In recent decades, major advances have occurred in the field of **organ transplantation**. Success rates have improved, more patients are now considered eligible for organ grafts, and more and more cities have established transplant centers.

However, the demand for donor organs drastically exceeds the supply. In the United States, for example, 63,782 patients were on the National Transplant Waiting List on June 30, 1999. Despite this need, only 20,961 transplants were performed the previous year, because organs were available from just 9,913 donors.

This critical shortage of donor organs is considered the number-one issue in organ transplantation, because many more lives could have been saved. In 1998, 4,855 Americans died while awaiting organ transplants. Of those, 2,295 were awaiting kidney transplants and 1,319 were awaiting livers. Other patients died waiting for donor hearts (767), lungs (486), kidneys and pancreas (93), intestines (45), hearts and lungs (41), and pancreases (9).

During the 1990s, the number of people on U.S. transplant waiting lists tripled, while virtually no increase was recorded in the number of organs available for transplant. It is estimated that between one-third and one-half of people now on waiting lists will die.

Although surveys have indicated that a majority of people are willing to donate their organs when they die, most families refuse to grant permission when approached. Even if a donor card has been signed, doctors usually seek consent from the family before removing organs for transplant. Many bereaved families who do consent derive considerable comfort from the fact that several lives can be saved or improved by organs and tissue grafts from a single donor.

According to the U.S. United Network for Organ Sharing, many myths surround the subject of organ donations. For example, many people believe that their medical histories make their organs unusable for transplant purposes, although recent advances make it possible to use many previously unusable organs. If one wishes to donate one's organs, it is best to leave this decision to trained professionals who will determine it at the time of death.

The cost of removing organs will not be charged to either the family or the estate. Instead, it is charged to the transplant recipient, usually through health insurance or Medicare. Removal of organs will not disfigure the body nor alter its appearance (a concern of family members thinking of funeral arrangements).

Indicating your wish to donate organs for transplant will not reduce efforts to save your life. Organs will not be removed until all life-preserving efforts have failed, and the organ procurement team will not be the same doctors who have tried to save you.

Your age at time of death is not an issue. Even newborns can supply much-needed organs. In fact, 25% of patients awaiting livers are under the age of ten.

If you wish to donate your organs, it is important to advise your family and loved ones of this decision. Including this wish in your will is not enough, because the organs will be unusable by the time your will is read.

Organs are especially needed from members of ethnic and racial minorities, because the risk of rejection by the body's immune system is reduced when organs are genetically similar. In addition, some minorities are more vulnerable than the general population to certain heart, lung, kidney, liver, and pancreas conditions that make transplants necessary.

You may also wish to donate your entire body for scientific research, but this is not possible if you are to donate organs. To donate your whole body to science, contact the medical school or research institution of your choice to make the necessary arrangements.

See also Organ transplantation

ORGAN TRANSPLANTATION

Organ transplantation is surgery in which a diseased or damaged organ is removed from a patient and replaced with a healthy organ from an organ donor. A number of major organs, including the heart, lungs, liver, and kidneys, can be transplanted. Normally, organ transplantation is a last resort. It is performed only on patients who are in the last stages of organ failure and for whom other treatments have not been successful.

Because healthy donor organs are in short supply, strict rules dictate who should or should not receive a transplant. Patients who have conditions that might cause the new organ to fail should not receive transplants. Similarly, patients who may be too sick to survive the surgery or the side effects of the drugs they must take to keep their new organ working are not good transplant candidates.

Once a person has been approved for an organ transplant, he or she is placed on a waiting list at a transplant center.

All patients on waiting lists are registered with the United Network for Organ Sharing (UNOS). UNOS runs a national computer network that connects all the transplant centers and organ-donation organizations. When a donor organ becomes available, information about it is entered into the UNOS computer and compared to information from patients on the waiting list. The computer program then produces a ranked list of patients who are good candidates for that particular organ. Finding an organ that is a good match for the recipient's blood type is important, so the computer program takes that into account when producing the list. The ranking is also based on other factors, such as the size of the organ relative to the patient's size, and how badly the patient needs a transplant.

When a good match is found, the donor organ rushed to the transplant center where the patient is waiting, and the patient is prepared for surgery. Transplant patients usually are given drugs to prevent the body from rejecting the new organ. These drugs, called immunosuppressive drugs, are usually started before or during the transplant operation. **Immunosuppressive drugs** keep the body's immune system from recognizing and attacking the new organ as foreign tissue. Normally, immune system cells recognize and attack foreign or abnormal cells, such as bacteria, **cancer** cells, and the cells that make up a transplanted organ. Immunosuppressive drugs suppress the immune cells and allow the new organ to function properly. However, they can also allow the patient to get infections and can cause undesirable side effects. Because the chance of rejection is highest during the first few months after the transplantation, recipients are usually given a combination immunosuppressive drugs in high doses during this time. Afterward, they must take lower doses of immunosuppressive drugs for the rest of their lives.

Like all surgery, organ transplantation carries the risk of complications, such as infection and bleeding. In addition, certain other complications can develop from specific types of transplants. In kidney transplants, for example, the ureter, which carries urine from the kidney to the bladder, may be damaged, resulting in urine leakage. However, this problem usually can be corrected with follow-up surgery.

Patients are monitored closely after transplant surgery for any signs of infection, rejection of the new organ, or other complications. The likelihood of success depends on a number of factors, including the patient's age and health, the type of organ transplanted, the match between donor and recipient, and how well the patient follows the physician's instructions after surgery. For some types of organ transplantation, the results can be quite dramatic. For example, heart patients who could hardly get out of bed before the surgery begin feeling much better soon afterward. Most are able to go back to work and resume normal activities, and many are even able to participate in sports.

Orthodontics

Orthodontics is a specialized branch of dentistry dealing with ''malocclusions,'' or bad bite. The ''bandolet,'' created in 1723, was the first known orthodontic apparatus; the most common modern orthodontic appliances include braces, retainers, tooth guards, and splints, all used to correct tooth and jaw problems such as crossbite, protruding or misaligned teeth, protruding or retruding jaw, tooth grinding, speech difficulties, and temporomandibular joint dislocation. Teeth-straightening and extraction to improve alignment of remaining teeth has been practiced since early times (Leonardo Da Vinci perhaps made the first written observation regarding teeth and bite); today, approximately one in every 50 people (25% being adults), is being treated by an orthodontist.

Orthodontics as an independent science began developing in the l880s. The first comprehensive treatise on dentistry, *The Surgeon Dentist*, published in 1728 by Pierre Fauchard (1678-1761), devoted an entire chapter to tooth irregularities and ways to correct them. In 1757, French dentist Bourdet wrote *The Dentist's Art*, devoting a chapter to tooth alignment; in 1771, John Hunter wrote the first English text on the subject entitled*The Natural History of the Human Teeth* ; and the term *orthodontia* was coined in 1841 by Lafoulon and appeared in a book by J. M. Alexis Schange on malocclusion. In 1858, the first article on orthodontics was written by Norman W. Kingsley. His 1880 *Treatise on Oral Deformities* served as the catalyst for the new dental science, earning him the title of ''The Father of Orthodontics.'' J. N. Farrar who published the two volume, profusely illustrated *A Treatise on the Irregularities of the Teeth and Their Corrections* and was adept at designing orthodontic appliances, suggested the use of mild force at intervals to move teeth; he ultimately became known as ''The Father of Modern Orthodontics.'' The third influential figure in orthodontics, Edward H. Angle (1855-1930), devised the first simple and logical classification system for malocclusions which is still used as the basis for orthodontic diagnosis. He contributed significantly to the design of orthodontic appliances, founded the first school and college of orthodontia, organized the American Society of Orthodontia in 1901, and founded the first orthodontic journal in 1907. His highly praised reference book, *Malocclusion of the Teeth*, went through seven editions. Other innovations in orthodontics in the late 1800s and early 1900s included the first textbook on orthodontics for students, published by J. H. Guilford in 1889; Eugene Solomon Talbot's (1847-1924) suggestion to use X-rays for orthodontic diagnosis; and the use of rubber elastics, pioneered by Calvin S. Case (or perhaps H. A. Baker).

Developments in orthodontics include more convenient, comfortable and less noticeable appliances such as tiny brackets instead of bands; ''space age'' wires for braces and bands developed through NASA, which require fewer replacements; braces with clear, tooth-colored, or multi-colored brackets with matching or interchangeable colored elastics; retainers with a favorite logo or photo; tiny magnets attached to upper and lower molars instead of head gear to realign teeth; ''lingual'' braces connected to the back of teeth for completely invisible treatment; and computer technology to diagnose and plan treatment, and produce images of the end results.

For more extreme problems, such as a jaw too narrow to accommodate a full mouth of adult teeth, expanders—

devices used to widen upper and lower jaws—prevent overcrowding. Most effective when applied before puberty, upper expanders fit over the roof of the mouth and connect to the back teeth on either side exerting outward pressure. A tiny key turned periodically further expands the frame, opening the sutures (the juncture where the bones of the mouth roof meet) allowing new bone to grow into that opening. As there is no lower suture to open, lower expanders, which fit under the tongue, are designed to upright tipped teeth.

Disorders of the *temporomandibular joint* (TMJ), located immediately in front of the ears where the jaw bone connects to the skull, affect 60 million or more Americans and has many origins—from injury to high levels of stress. Symptoms include difficulty opening and closing the mouth—often the jaw will lock in one position; pain and noise when chewing; ear, temple, head, or face pain; debilitating headaches; loss of hearing or ringing in the ears; nausea; blurred vision; and dizziness. Diagnosis is difficult, as pain often emulates that caused by other problems. Treatments include reversible (splints, physical therapy, psychotherapy to relieve stress, chiropractic adjustments, and massage therapy), and non-reversible (crowns, surgery, and bite adjustment). Splints allow joints, muscles, and ligaments to rest, heal, and function more normally, and also reduce the damaging effects of clenching and grinding teeth, usually a stress-related activity.

ORTHOPEDIC SURGERY

Orthopedic (sometimes spelled orthopaedic) surgery corrects problems that arise in the skeleton and its attachments, the ligaments and tendons. It may also deal with some problems of the nervous system, such as those that arise from injury of the spine. These problems can occur at birth, through injury, or as the result of aging.

Medical doctors trained to deal with such problems are called orthopedic surgeons or orthopedists (the terms are used interchangeably). The word ''orthopedic''comes from two Greek words, *ortho*, meaning straight and *pais,* meaning child. Originally orthopedic surgeons dealt with bone deformities in children, using braces to straighten the child's bones. With the development modern surgical techniques, orthopedic surgeons expanded their role to include surgery involving the bones and related nerves and connective tissue.

Some orthopedic surgeons specialize in one particular aspect of orthopedics, such as hand surgery, **joint replacements**, or disorders of the spine. Others specialize in trauma medicine and can be found in emergency rooms and trauma centers treating injuries. The work of orthopedists can overlap with that of plastic surgeons, geriatric specialists, pediatricians, or podiatrists (foot care specialists). A rapidly growing area of orthopedics is sports medicine, and many sports medicine doctors are board certified orthopedists.

Choosing an orthopedist is an important step in seeking treatment. Patients looking for a qualified orthopedist should ask if the physician is ''board certified'' by his or her accrediting organization.

The kinds of treatments done by orthopedists range from **traction** to **amputation**, hand reconstruction to spinal fusion or joint replacements. They also treat broken bones, strains and sprains, and dislocations. Some specific procedures done by orthopedic surgeons are covered as separate entries in this book, including arthroscopic surgery, **bone grafting**, and traction.

Orthopedists usually are affiliated with hospitals, medical centers, trauma centers, or free-standing surgical centers where they work closely with surgical teams including anesthesiologists and surgical nurses. Orthopedic surgery can be performed under general, regional, or local anesthesia.

Much of the work of the surgeon involves adding foreign material to the body in the form of screws, wires, pins, tongs, and prosthetics to hold damaged bones in their proper places or to replace damaged bone or connective tissue. Great improvements have been made in the development of artificial limbs and joints, and in the materials available to repair damage to bones and connective tissue. As developments continue in the fields of materials science and tissue engineering, surgeons will be able to more nearly duplicate the natural functions of the bones, joints, and ligaments, and to more accurately restore damaged parts to their original range of motion.

As with any surgery, there is always a risk of excessive bleeding, infection, and allergic reaction to anesthesia. Risks specifically associated with orthopedic surgery include inflammation at the site where foreign material (pins, prosthesis) is introduced into the body, infection as the result of surgery, and damage to nerves or to the spinal cord.

Rehabilitation from orthopedic injuries or surgery can be a long, arduous task. The doctor will work closely with physical therapists to assure that the patient gets the proper treatment to enhance range of motion and return function to the affected part.

Thousands of people have successful orthopedic surgery each year to recover from injuries or restore lost function. The likelihood of success for depends on the age and general health of the patient, the medical problem being treated, and the patient's willingness to comply with rehabilitative therapy after the surgery.

OSLER, WILLIAM (1849-1919)

Canadian Medical educator

After Osler's death at the age of 70, the prestigious British medical journal *The Lancet* described him as the most significant medical personality of his day. Oddly, this giant of the healing profession was not known for any breakthrough discovery. Rather, through persistence and a powerful personality, Osler inspired doctors worldwide to adopt a more humanistic approach of medicine focused on patients rather than profits. He has been described as ''the model of a cultured, articulate, insatiably curious, highly principled physician.''

Born at Bond Head, Ontario, Osler was one of nine children fathered by an Anglican clergyman. His medical career is jokingly said to have started with a surgical procedure on his sister Chattie, conducted at a Sunday School picnic when he was just five. As Osler was trying to chop kindling wood, Chattie repeatedly put her finger on the chopping block to annoy him. After warning her, he proceeded to cut off the tip of her finger.

Osler's formal education also had a less-than-distinguished beginning. Starting a lifelong habit of practical jokes, he hid all the desks in the attic of the one-room schoolhouse. On another occasion he locked a gaggle of geese in the school. These pranks were rewarded by expulsion and Osler was sent to an Anglican boarding school in Weston, Ontario, where he managed to surpass his earlier mischief. There, he was involved in barricading an unpopular school matron in her room, which then was then filled with smoke from burning mustard, molasses, and pepper. The housekeeper was almost asphyxiated, causing a Toronto newspaper to report ''Pupils turn Outlaws.'' Osler was briefly jailed over that incident but was spared further punishment by the persuasive skills of his older brother Featherston, who was starting what would become a brilliant career as a criminal lawyer.

Despite his mischievous activities, Osler originally intended to follow his father into the clergy. He was diverted from that goal, however, by the founder of the Weston school, Father Johnson ''who delighted in the woods in springtime, and told us about the frog-spawn and the caddis worms, and who....showed us with the microscope the marvels in a drop of dirty pond water.''

''No more dry husks for me after such a diet,'' Osler wrote. ''From the study of nature to the study of man was an easy step.'' Also at Weston, Osler was profoundly moved reading Thomas Browne's *Religio Medici.* He later described Browne as a ''life-long mentor'' and commented that ''no book has had so enduring an influence on my life.''

Osler started his medical studies at the University of Toronto, later transferring to McGill University in Montreal. There, he performed more than 1,000 autopsies, carefully recording his findings and applying them to patient care. Osler graduated from McGill in 1872. After two years of further study in Europe, he returned to Canada and was appointed by McGill, first as a medical lecturer, and the following year as professor of medicine.

After 10 years in Montreal, Osler went to the University of Pennsylvania as professor of clinical medicine. Then, in 1888, he was appointed as physician-in-chief of the new Johns Hopkins Hospital, which grew into one of the world's most respected medical centers.

At Johns Hopkins, Osler trained more than 1,000 medical students who proudly dubbed themselves ''first-generation Oslerians.'' Over time, Osler and three other founders at Johns Hopkins transformed the way in which medicine is studied. Believing that the best learning occurs at bedsides, Osler opened the hospital wards to students and encouraged them to learn by doing. Assigned to wards as clinical clerks, students performed physical examinations, prepared extensive case histories, and presented them for criticism.

Using a term derived from his early interest in divinity, Osler taught that medicine is a ''calling.'' ''He once told a

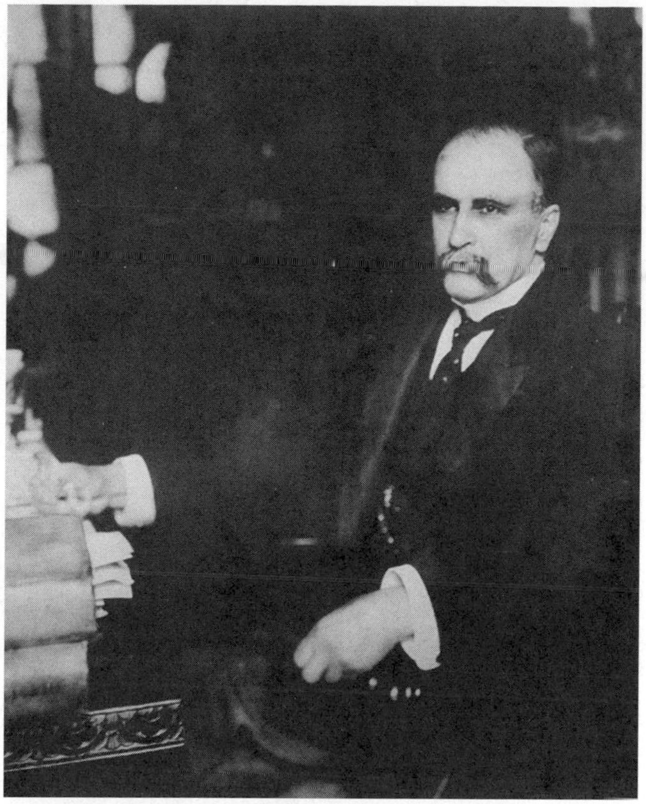

William Osler

group of medical students, ''You are in this profession as a calling, not as a business... Once you get down to a purely business level, your influence is gone and the true light of your life is dimmed. You must work in the missionary spirit, with a breadth of charity that raises you far above the petty jealousies of life.'' Osler also emphasized that medical school was just the beginning of a lifetime commitment to learning, and he continued using the term ''fellow students'' long after he had become an esteemed teacher.

Osler wrote one of the most successful textbooks in medical history. His 1892 *Principles and Practice of Medicine* was published in eight editions and translated into four other languages. After his death, it continued in print with numerous editions produced by other editors.

Although he is best known as a bedside teacher and for his efforts to marry medicine with the humanities, Osler was responsible for some scientific advances. In 1873 he identified blood platelets as a third type of blood corpuscle. He also did research on malaria, pneumonia, typhoid fever, tuberculosis, cardiovascular disease, and other medical conditions.

By 1903, Osler had suffered what is now known as burnout, and in 1905 he accepted the less-strenuous but equally prestigious position of Regius Professor of Medicine at England's Oxford University. His reduced duties at Oxford allowed him to pursue his interest in the humanities, especially the history of medicine. His *A Concise History of Medicine*

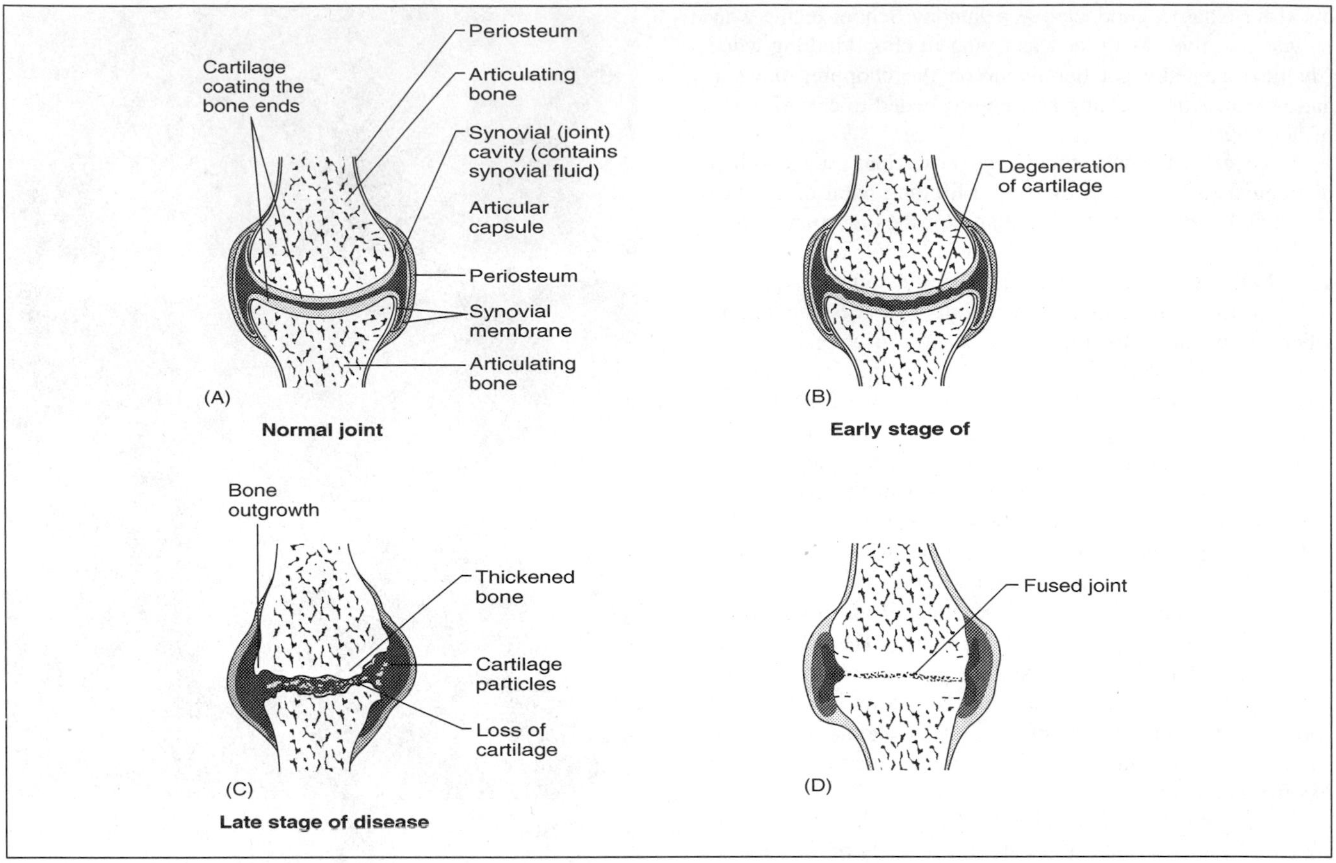

The progression of osteoarthritis. ***(Illustration by Hans & Cassady, Inc.)***

was published in 1919, the same year Osler died from complications of pneumonia.

Throughout his life, Osler was an avid collector of books, urging medical students to ''start at once a bed-side library and spend the last half-hour of the day in communion with the saints of humanity.'' After his death, his large collection was presented to McGill University in Montreal. There, it is specially housed in the Osler Library. Osler's ashes rest behind a wood panel in the library's central room, surrounded by floor-to-ceiling books.

Osler's love of books and his philosophy of medicine were both summarized in a speech he gave to dedicate a new section of the Boston Medical Library: ''To study the phenomena of disease without books is to sail an uncharted sea, while to study books without patients is not to go to sea at all.''

OSTEOARTHRITIS

Osteoarthritis (OA), which is also known as osteoarthrosis or degenerative joint disease (DJD), is a disorder of the joints that worsens over time. It results from deterioration or loss of the cartilage that acts as a protective cushion between bones, particularly in weight-bearing joints such as the knees and hips. As the cartilage wears away, the bone forms hardened areas called spurs and fluid-filled pockets in the marrow, known as subchondral cysts. The deformed bones and fluid accumulation in the joints cause pain, which is made worse by moving the joint or putting weight on it. Rest usually relieves the pain.

People with osteoarthritis may have joint **pain** on one or both sides of the body. It affects mainly the knees, hands, hips, feet, and spine.

Osteoarthritis usually appears after age 40. About 90% of Americans will show some signs of the disorder in their weight-bearing joints by that 40. In the early stages of osteoarthritis, the pain is minor and may take the form of mild stiffness in the morning. In later stages, inflammation develops. The patient may have pain even when the joint is not being used and may lose the ability to move the joint normally.

Until the late 1980s, osteoarthritis was thought to be a normal part of aging, caused by simple ''wear and tear'' on the joints. But recent research into cartilage formation has led to new understanding. Osteoarthritis is now considered to be the end result of several different factors contributing to cartilage damage, and is classified as either primary or secondary.

Primary osteoarthritis is caused by from abnormal stresses on weight-bearing joints or normal stresses on weak joints. Finger joints, hips, knees, the neck and back and big toe are most frequently affected. People with certain gene mutations appear to be more susceptible to primary osteoarthritis.

Obesity also contributes to the problem by increasing the pressure on the weight-bearing joints of the body. Age is a factor, too. As the body ages, cartilage loses its ability to repair itself. In addition to these factors, some researchers theorize that primary osteoarthritis may be triggered by enzyme disturbances, bone disease, or liver problems.

Secondary osteoarthritis results from repeated or sudden injury to a joint. It can occur in any joint. **Sports injuries**, gout, poor posture, metabolic disorders, and repetitive stress injuries associated with certain occupations (like the performing arts, construction or assembly line work, and computer keyboard operation) may lead to secondary osteoarthritis.

Physicians diagnose osteoarthritis using a combination of **physical examination** and imaging methods such as x rays, **magnetic resonance imaging** (MRI) and **computed tomography scans** (CT scans). In the physical examination, the doctor will touch and move the patient's joint, checking for swelling, pain, and cracking or grinding sounds. In patients with osteoarthritis, x rays may show narrowed joint spaces, unusually dense areas in the bone, and the presence of subchondral cysts or bone spurs.

Treatment for osteoarthritis usually involves a combination of medication and physical therapy. Most patients with are given **nonsteroidal anti-inflammatory drugs (NSAIDs)**, such as ibuprofen (Motrin, Advil), ketoprofen (Orudis), and flurbiprofen (Ansaid), which reduce inflammation as well as relieving pain. However, NSAIDs also may have undesirable side effects including stomach **ulcers**, sensitivity to sun exposure, kidney problems, and nervousness or depression. Some osteoarthritis patients are treated with **corticosteroids** injected directly into the joints to reduce inflammation. However, this should be done no more than two or three times a year.

Exercises that increase balance, flexibility, and range of motion are recommended for osteoarthritis patients. These may include walking, swimming and other water exercises, **yoga** and other stretching exercises, or isometric exercises. Physical therapy may also include **massage**, moist hot packs, or soaking in a hot tub.

In severe cases, surgery may be necessary to replace a damaged joint with an artificial one or to remove parts of bone.

Several new treatments are being investigated, including drugs that help the body repair damaged cartilage; injections of hyaluronic acid, which may help lubricate protect cartilage; and cartilage transplantation.

Some osteoarthritis patients say they get relief from taking supplements of glucosamine or a combination of glucosamine and chondroitin. These substances are believed to help the body maintain and repair cartilage, and studies conducted in Europe have shown some effectiveness.

While there is no permanent cure for osteoarthritis, many people are able to find relief and slow the progression of the condition with a combination of weight control, appropriate exercise and medication.

Osteochondroses

Osteochondroses refers to a group of diseases of children and adolescents in which bone tissue dies, and is usually replaced with healthy bone tissue. The singular term is osteochondrosis.

During the years of rapid bone growth, the growing ends of bones (epiphyses) may not receive enough blood supply to keep the bone tissue alive. Since bone is normally undergoing a continuous rebuilding process, the dead (necrotic) tissue usually repairs itself over a period of weeks or months.

Osteochondrosis can affect different areas of the body and is often categorized by its location as articular, non-articular, or physeal osteochondrosis. Physeal osteochondrosis is known as Scheuermann's disease. It occurs in the spine at the joints between vertebrae (known as physes), especially in the chest region. Articular disease occurs at the joints (articulations). One of the more common forms is Legg-Calvé-Perthes disease, occurring at the hip. Other forms include Köhler's disease (foot), Freiberg's disease (second toe), and Panner's disease (elbow). Freiberg's disease is the one type of osteochondrosis that is more common in females than in males. All others affect the sexes equally. Non-articular osteochondrosis occurs at any other skeletal location. For instance, Osgood-Schlatter disease of the tibia (the large inner bone of the leg between the knee and ankle) is relatively common.

No one knows exactly why osteochondrosis develops. Stress and ischemia (reduced blood supply) are two of the most commonly mentioned factors. Athletic young children are often affected when they overstress their developing limbs with a particular repetitive motion. In many cases, no specific cause can be found.

The most common symptom for most types of osteochondrosis is simply **pain** at the affected joint, especially when pressure is applied. Locking of a joint or limited range of motion at a joint can also occur.

Scheuermann's disease can lead to kyphosis (hunchback condition) due to the wearing down of the vertebrae. Usually, however, the kyphosis is mild, causing no further symptoms and requiring no special treatment.

In many cases, simply resting the affected body part for a period of days or weeks will bring relief from osteochondrosis. A cast may be applied if needed to prevent movement of a joint. Some patients heal with no treatment at all. Others heal with little treatment other than keeping weight or stress off the affected limb. The younger a person is when osteochondrosis occurs, the better the prospects for full recovery.

Osteogenesis imperfecta

Osteogenesis imperfecta (OI) is a term for a group of genetic diseases in which the bones are formed improperly, making them fragile and likely to break. This happens when collagen, the fibrous protein material that makes up skin, bone, cartilage, and ligaments, is faulty.

Osteogenesis imperfecta affects equal numbers of males and females. It occurs in about one of every 30,000 births.

Osteogenesis imperfecta is a genetic disorder, but not everyone who has it received a defective gene from his or her mother or father. Some cases are due to a spontaneous mutation (a permanent defect in a specific gene) that occurs after birth. A person who has osteogenesis imperfecta due to a spontaneous mutation can then pass on this defective gene to his or her future offspring.

There are four forms of osteogenesis imperfecta, called Types I through IV. Of these, Type II tends to be the most severe, and usually causes death shortly after birth. Types I, III, and IV have some symptoms in common, but each also has distinctive symptoms. Symptoms include:

- Weak bones which break (fracture) easily. In some forms of osteogenesis imperfecta, these **fractures** occur even before birth. People with Type I have about 20–40 fractures before **puberty**; people with Type III may have more than 100 fractures before puberty. Fractures usually occur less after puberty, but may increase again in women after **menopause**.
- Loose, unstable joints (due to abnormal structure of the ligaments), resulting in a high risk of dislocation.
- A bluish tinge to the white of the eye (the sclera).
- A curved and twisted spine (**scoliosis**).
- **Hearing loss** (due to malformation and fractures of the tiny bones in the middle ear which are necessary for hearing).
- Abnormally fragile, discolored (bluish-yellow) teeth.
- Shorter-than-normal final height, depending on the type of osteogenesis imperfecta. In Type I, height is slightly short or close to normal; in Type III, height is quite abnormal, with growth stopping around three feet; in Type IV, height is somewhat shorter than normal.
- Thin, fragile skin.
- A high risk of complications such as **hernia**s and heart valve abnormalities.

Other complications vary according to the type of osteogenesis imperfecta. In Type I, the face is often triangular in shape. In Type II, the rib cage may be abnormally formed, restricting the lungs and causing breathing difficulties. The arms and legs are often shorter than normal, and the bones are bowed.

Osteogenesis imperfecta is usually suspected when a baby has bone fractures for no obvious reason. The bluish sclera of the eye also is a clue to this condition. Unfortunately, because of the unusual nature of the fractures appearing in a baby who cannot yet move, some parents have been falsely accused of **child abuse** before osteogenesis imperfecta was diagnosed in the child.

Doctors confirm the diagnosis of osteogenesis imperfecta by taking a tiny sample of the patient's skin (a biopsy), and performing tests on this sample in a laboratory. However, it takes a long time to get results from this test, and it produces falsely negative results in about 15% of all people who have obvious symptoms of osteogenesis imperfecta.

There is no cure for osteogenesis imperfecta. Most treatments are aimed at repairing the fractures and bone deformities which the condition causes. Splints, casts, and braces are all used. When repeated fractures or bowed bones interfere with a child's ability to walk, surgeons may implant a metal rod in the bone.

Other treatments include **hearing aids** and early capping of teeth. Some patients need to use a walker or wheelchair. **Pain** may be treated with a variety of medications. Swimming is a good form of **exercise** for someone with osteogenesis imperfecta, because it increases muscle and joint strength without putting too much strain on bones and joints.

Acupuncture, **hypnosis**, relaxation training, visual imagery, and **biofeedback** have all been used to try to decrease the pain of fractures.

There is no known way to prevent osteogenesis imperfecta, but adults with the condition should have genetic counseling to understand the chance of passing it to their offspring.

OSTEOMYELITIS

Osteomyelitis is a bone infection, almost always caused by bacteria. Over time, the infection can destroy the bone.

Bone infections may occur at any age. Certain conditions increase the risk of developing such an infection, including **sickle-cell anemia**, injury, the presence of a foreign object (such as a bullet or a screw placed to hold together a broken bone), intravenous drug use (such as heroin), diabetes, kidney dialysis, surgical procedures to bony areas, and untreated infections of tissue near a bone (for example, extreme cases of untreated sinus infections have led to osteomyelitis of the bones of the skull).

Staphylococcus aureus is the type of bacterium usually involved in osteomyelitis. Others include the mycobacterium which causes **tuberculosis**, a type of Salmonella bacterium in patients with sickle cell anemia, and *Pseudomonas aeurginosa* in drug addicts. The viruses that cause **chickenpox** and **smallpox** can cause viral osteomyelitis, but this is very rare.

Infecting bacteria can find their way to the bone by traveling through the bloodstream or by spreading from nearby infected soft tissue. Children are most likely to be infected in the long bones of the arms and legs, because their growing bones are richly supplied with blood. Adults have different blood circulation patterns, so they are less likely to get osteomyelitis in the arms and legs, but more likely to develop the condition in the spine. People with diabetes are especially likely to develop osteomyelitis by the spread of infection from nearby soft tissue. This is because diabetes interferes with nerve sensation and good blood flow to the feet, making patients prone to developing poorly healing **wounds** to their feet. These wounds can become infected, and the infection can spread to bone.

Acute osteomyelitis refers to a bone infection that develops and peaks over a relatively short time. In children, symptoms of acute osteomyelitis usually include **pain** in the affected bone, tenderness to over the infected area, **fever** and chills. Patients who develop osteomyelitis due to the spread of infection from nearby soft tissue may only notice poor healing of the original wound or infection.

Adult patients with osteomyelitis of the spine usually have a longer period of dull, aching pain in the back, and no fever. Some patients notice pain in the chest, abdomen, arm, or leg. This occurs when the inflammation in the spine causes pressure on a nerve root serving one of these other areas.

Doctors use several tests to diagnose osteomyelitis. Blood tests or cultures, x rays and **magnetic resonance imaging** (MRI) all may be used.

Antibiotics (medications used to kill bacteria) are used to treat osteomyelitis. These medications are usually given through a needle in a vein (intravenously) for at least part of the time. In children, these antibiotics can be given by mouth after initial treatment by vein. In adults, four to six weeks of intravenous antibiotic treatment is usually recommended, along with bed rest for part or all of that time. Occasionally, a patient will have such extensive osteomyelitis that surgery will be required to clean the infected area.

When osteomyelitis is not properly treated, a chronic (long-term) type of infection may occur. However, with quick, appropriate treatment, only about 5% of all cases of acute osteomyelitis will eventually become chronic osteomyelitis. Patients with chronic osteomyelitis may require antibiotics periodically for the rest of their lives.

Carefully caring for any wounds or injuries will lessen the risk of developing osteomyelitis.

Osteopathy

Osteopathy is a system and philosophy of health care that separated from traditional (allopathic) medical practice about a century ago. Osteopathy shares many of the same goals as traditional medicine, but places greater emphasis on the relationship between the organs and the **musculoskeletal system**. Osteopaths strongly believe in the healing power of the body and try to take advantage of that strength. They believe in treating the whole individual rather than just the disease.

Osteopathy was founded in the 1890s by Dr. Andrew Taylor, who believed that the musculoskeletal system was central to health. **Chiropractic**, a related health discipline, also emphasizes the importance of the musculoskeletal system. The original theory behind both approaches presumed that energy flowing through the nervous system is influenced by the supporting structure that encases and protects it—the skull and vertebral column. A defect in the musculoskeletal system was believed to alter the flow of this energy and cause disease. Correcting the defect cured the disease. Defects were thought to be misalignments—parts out of place by tiny distances. Treating misalignments became a matter of restoring the parts to their natural arrangement by adjusting them.

As medical science advanced, defining causes of disease and discovering cures, schools of osteopathy adopted modern science, incorporated it into their curriculum, and redefined their original theory of disease in light of these discoveries. Since the middle of the 20th century, the Doctor of Osteopathy (D.O.) degree has been considered equivalent to the doctor of medicine (M.D.) degree. However, osteopaths have continued their emphasis on the musculoskeletal system and their traditional focus on ''whole person'' medicine. As of 1998, osteopaths constituted 5.5% of American physicians, approximately 45,000. From its origins in the United States, osteopathy has spread to countries all over the world.

Osteopaths, chiropractors, and physical therapists all practice manipulations (adjustments). Back and neck pain are the main reasons patients come to these specialists for manipulation. The place of manipulation in medical care is far from settled, but millions of patients find relief from it.

When a patient comes to an osteopath with pain, the first step is to determine the cause of the pain. It is important to rule out serious conditions such as cancer and brain or spinal cord disease. Once it is clear that the pain is originating in the musculoskeletal system, manipulation may be appropriate.

Techniques for manipulation vary among practitioners. Most try to get the muscles to relax first. This can be done with heat, medication, or gentle but persistent stretching. The manipulation is most often done by a short, fast motion called a thrust, precisely in the right direction. A satisfying ''pop'' is evidence of success. Others practitioners use steady force until relaxation permits movement.

Returning the joint to its normal position may be only the first step. If a misalignment is due to a short leg, for example, a patient may need a lift in one shoe. Longstanding pain may have caused muscle deterioration. In that case, additional methods of physical therapy may be necesssary to rebuild muscles, correct posture and change habits that the patient developed to compensate for the pain. Patients may also be given medicines to relieve muscle spasms and pain.

Manipulation has rarely caused problems. Once in a while too forceful a thrust has damaged structures in the neck and caused serious damage. The most common adverse event, though, is misdiagnosis. Cancers have been missed and serious back problems that could have been corrected by surgery have been ignored until spinal nerves have been permanently damaged.

Osteoporosis

The word osteoporosis literally means ''porous bones.'' It occurs when bones lose too much of their protein and mineral content, particularly calcium. Over time, bone mass, and therefore bone strength, is decreased. As a result, bones become fragile and break easily. Even a sneeze or a sudden movement may be enough to break a bone in someone with severe osteoporosis.

To understand osteoporosis, it is helpful to understand the basics of bone formation. Bone is living tissue that's constantly being renewed in a two-stage process (resorption and formation) that occurs throughout life. In the resorption stage, old bone is broken down and removed by cells called osteoclasts. In the formation stage, cells called osteoblasts build new bone to replace the old. During childhood and early adulthood, more bone is produced than removed. After the mid-30s, bone is lost faster than it's formed, so the amount of bone in the skeleton slowly declines. Osteoporosis that occurs as an acceleration of this normal aging process is called primary osteoporosis. Osteoporosis that occurs because of other diseases or prolonged use of certain medicines is called secondary osteoporosis.

Osteoporosis occurs most often in older people. Women, however, are five times more likely than men to develop the disease. They have smaller, thinner bones than men to begin with, and they lose bone mass more rapidly after menopause (usually around age 50), when they stop producing a bone-protecting hormone called estrogen. In the five to seven years following menopause, women can lose about 20% of their bone mass. By age 65 or 70, though, men and women lose bone mass at the same rate.

A number of factors increase the risk of developing osteoporosis. They include:

- Age.
- Gender.
- Race. Caucasian and Asian women are most at risk for the disease, but African American and Hispanic women can get it too.
- Figure type. Women who are thin with small bones are more liable to have osteoporosis.
- Early menopause. Women who stop menstruating early because of heredity, surgery or heavy physical **exercise** may lose large amounts of bone tissue early in life. Conditions such as anorexia and bulimia may also lead to early menopause and osteoporosis.
- Lifestyle. People who smoke or drink too much, or don't get enough exercise have an increased chance of getting osteoporosis.
- Diet. Those who don't get enough calcium or protein are more likely to have osteoporosis.

Before making a diagnosis of osteoporosis, the doctor usually takes a complete medical history, conducts a physical exam, and orders x rays, as well as blood and urine tests, to rule out other diseases that cause loss of bone mass. The doctor may also recommend a **bone density test**. This is the only way to know for certain if osteoporosis is present and far it has progressed.

Ordinary x rays don't reveal bone loss until the disease is advanced and most of the damage already has been done. Machines called densitometers, which are designed specifically to measure bone density, can catch the disease in earlier stages. The most accurate and advanced densitometers use a technique called DEXA (dual energy x-ray absorptiometry). People should talk to their doctors about their risk factors for osteoporosis and should discuss whether they should get the test.

For most women who've gone through menopause, **hormone replacement therapy** (HRT), also called estrogen replacement therapy, is an effective treatment for osteoporosis, as well as for relief of other menopause-related symptoms. HRT increases a woman's supply of estrogen, which helps build new bone, while preventing further bone loss. Some women, however, do not want to take hormones, because some studies show they are linked to an increased risk of **breast cancer** or **uterine cancer**. Whether or not a woman takes hormones is a decision she should make carefully with her doctor.

For people who can't or don't want to take estrogen, two other medications, alendronate and calcitonin, can be good choices. Both stop bone loss, help build bone, and decrease fracture risk by as much as 50%.

Unfortunately, much of the treatment for osteoporosis is for fractures that result from advanced stages of the disease. For complicated fractures, such as broken hips, hospitalization and a surgical procedure are required. Though the surgery itself is usually successful, complications of the hip fracture can be serious. People who have had the surgery have a 5–20% greater risk of dying within the first year following that injury than do others in their age group. A large percentage of those who survive are unable to return to their previous level of activity, and many end up moving from self-care to a supervised living situation or nursing home. That's why getting early treatment and taking steps to reduce bone loss are vital.

Building strong bones, especially before the age of 35, and maintaining a healthy lifestyle are the best ways of preventing osteoporosis. To build as much bone mass as early as possible in life, and to help slow the rate of bone loss later in life:

Experts recommend 1,500 milligrams (mg) of calcium per day for adolescents, pregnant or breast-feeding women, older adults (over 65), and postmenopausal women not using hormone replacement therapy. All others should get 1,000 mg per day. Good sources of calcium are milk, cheese, yogurt, green leafy vegetables, tofu, shellfish, Brazil nuts, sardines, and almonds.

Those with calcium carbonate have the greatest amount of useful calcium. Supplements should be taken with meals and accompanied by six to eight glasses of water a day.

Vitamin D helps the body absorb calcium. People can get vitamin D from sunshine with a quick (15–20 minute) walk each day or from foods such as liver, fish oil, and vitamin-D fortified milk.

Smoking and heavy drinking reduce bone mass. To reduce risk, do not smoke, and limit alcoholic drinks to no more than two per day. An alcoholic drink is one-and-a-half ounces of hard liquor, 12 ounces of beer, or five ounces of wine.

Weight-bearing exercises—where bones and muscles work against gravity—are best. These include aerobics, dancing, jogging, stair climbing, tennis, walking, and lifting weights. Try to exercise three to four times per week for 20–30 minutes each time.

Ovarian cancer

Ovarian cancer is a disease in which the cells in the ovaries become abnormal and start to grow uncontrollably, forming tumors. The ovaries are a pair of almond-shaped organs that lie in the pelvis on either side of the uterus. The ovaries produce and release an egg each month during the menstrual cycle. In addition, they also produce the female hormones estrogen and progesterone, which regulate and maintain the secondary female sexual characteristics.

Ovarian cancer can develop at any age, but more than half the cases are among women who are 65 years or older.

It is difficult to diagnose ovarian cancer early, because often there are no warning symptoms and the disease grows relatively quickly. In addition, the ovaries are situated deep in the pelvis and, therefore, small tumors cannot be detected easily during a routine **physical examination**.

The actual cause of ovarian cancer is not known, but several factors are known to increase one's chances of developing the disease. These are called risk factors. Age may be considered a risk factor for ovarian cancer, because the incidence of the disease increases with age. Half of all cases are diagnosed after age 65. Race may be another risk factor for the disease, since the incidence of the disease is noted to be the highest among white women and lowest among blacks. A high-fat diet may have something to do with an increased incidence of ovarian cancer, because when Asian women move to the more affluent western countries and adopt a diet that is rich in fat, the incidence of ovarian cancer among them rises.

A family history of ovarian cancer may also put a woman at an increased risk for developing the disease. It is believed that the longer a woman ovulates, the higher is her risk of ovarian cancer. Therefore, starting to menstruate at a very early age (before age 12) and late **menopause** seems to put women at a higher risk for ovarian cancer.

Ovarian cancer has no specific signs or symptoms in the early stages of the disease. The patient may complain of the following symptoms: pain or swelling in the abdomen, bloating, and general feeling of abdominal discomfort, constipation, nausea or vomiting loss of appetite, fatigue. There may be unexplained weight gain due to an accumulation of fluid in the abdomen and sometimes post-menopausal women may have vaginal bleeding.

If ovarian cancer is suspected, the physician typically begins the diagnosis by taking a complete medical history to assess all the risk factors. A thorough pelvic examination is conducted. Blood tests to determine the level of a particular blood protein, CA125, may be ordered. This protein is usually elevated when a woman has ovarian cancer. However, it is not a definitive test.

In order to determine if the tumor is benign or cancerous, minor surgery may be necessary. A piece of the tissue is removed and microscopically examined to determine whether the tumor was benign or malignant. Standard imaging techniques such as **computed tomography scans** (CT scans) and **magnetic resonance imaging** (MRI) may be used to determine if the disease has spread to other parts of the body.

The cornerstone of treatment for ovarian cancer is surgery. It is aimed at removing as much of the cancer as possible. **Chemotherapy**, which involves the use of **anticancer drugs** to kill the cancer cells, is usually administered after the surgery to destroy any remaining cancer. **Radiation therapy** is not routinely used for ovarian cancer.

The type of surgery depends on the extent of spread of the disease. In most procedures, the ovaries, uterus, and fallopian tubes are completely removed. In rare cases, if the cancer is not very aggressive and the woman is young and has not had children, a more conservative approach may be adopted. Only one ovary may be removed, and, if possible, the fallopian tubes and the uterus may be left intact.

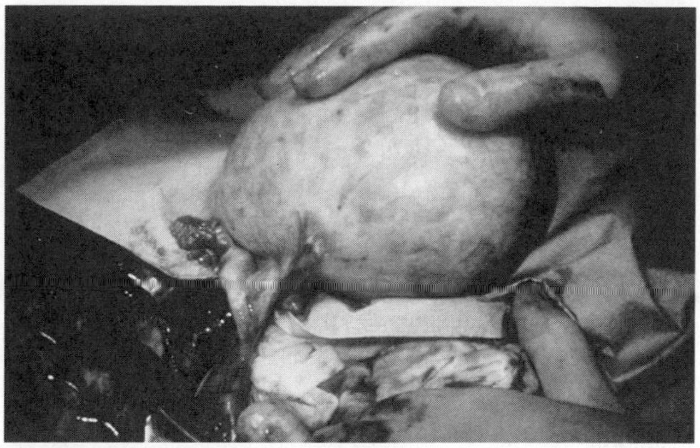

An ovarian cyst is being surgically removed from a 25-year-old female patient. ***(Photograph by Art Siegel, Custom Medical Stock Photo. Reproduced by permission.)***

Most often ovarian cancer is not diagnosed until it is in an advanced stage, making it the most deadly of all the female reproductive cancers. More than 50% of the women who are diagnosed with the disease die within five years.

Since there is no known cause for ovarian cancer, it is not possible to prevent the disease. Nevertheless, there are ways to reduce one's risks of developing the disease. Having one or more children, preferably having the first before age 30, and breastfeeding may decrease one's risk of developing the disease.

There are no simple tests or screening procedures to detect ovarian cancer in its early stages. High-risk women are therefore advised to undergo periodic screening with the transvaginal ultrasound or a blood test for CA125 protein. The American Cancer Society recommends annual pelvic examinations for all women after age 40, in order to increase the chances of early detection of ovarian cancer.

OVARIAN CYSTS

Ovarian cysts are sacs containing fluid or semisolid material that develop in or on the surface of an ovary. Most are harmless, but because they cause some of the same symptoms as ovarian tumors that may be **cancer**ous, ovarian cysts should always be checked out.

The most common types of ovarian cysts are follicular cysts and corpus luteum cysts, which are related to the menstrual cycle. Follicular cysts occur when the cyst-like follicle on the ovary in which the egg develops does not burst and release the egg. These cysts are usually small and harmless, disappearing within two to three menstrual cycles. Corpus luteum cysts occur when the corpus luteum—a small, yellow body that secretes hormones—doesn't dissolve after the egg is released. They usually disappear in a few weeks but can grow to more than 4 in (10 cm) in diameter and may twist the ovary.

Ovarian cysts can develop any time from **puberty** to **menopause**, including during **pregnancy**.

Many ovarian cysts have no symptoms. However, when the growth is large or there are multiple cysts, the patient may experience any of the following symptoms:

- Fullness or heaviness in the abdomen.
- Pressure on the rectum or bladder.
- A constant dull ache in the pelvic area that may spread to the lower back and thighs. The pain occurs shortly before the beginning or end of menstruation or may occur during intercourse.

A physician may find ovarian cysts during a routine pelvic exam. If a patient complains of symptoms typical of ovarian cysts, a doctor can confirm the diagnosis using a pelvic exam and ultrasound. For an ultrasound test, a technician uses a hand-held wand to send and receive sound waves to create images of the ovaries on a computer screen. The images are photographed for later analysis. This painless test takes about 15 minutes and is usually done in a hospital or a physician's office.

Many ovarian cysts require no treatment and disappear on their own. Often the physician will wait and re-examine the patient in four to six weeks before taking any action. Postmenopausal patients and patients who have not reached puberty and have an ovarian mass may need surgery. Surgery is also recommended for growths that are larger than 4 in (10 cm), and are complex, growing, persistent, solid and irregularly shaped and for growths that are on both ovaries or that cause pain or other symptoms.

More than 90% of noncancerous ovarian cysts can be removed using **laparoscopy**, a simple, outpatient procedure. The patient receives a general or local anesthetic, then a small incision is made in the abdomen. The laparoscope is inserted into the incision and the cyst or the entire ovary is removed. Usually, the patient can return to normal activities within two weeks.

For cysts that cannot be removed with laparoscopy, regular surgery may be necessary. The operation is performed under general anesthesia in a hospital and requires a stay of five to seven days. Recovery takes four weeks.

OVERHYDRATION

Overhydration, also called water excess or water intoxication, is a condition in which the body contains too much water. It occurs when the body takes in more water than it excretes, and its normal sodium level is diluted. This can result in digestive problems, behavioral changes, brain damage, seizures, or **coma**. An adult whose heart, kidneys, and pituitary gland are functioning properly would have to drink more than two gallons of water a day to develop water intoxication. The condition is most common in patients whose kidney function is impaired and may occur when health care professionals administer greater amounts of water-producing fluids and medications than the patient's body can handle.

Infants are especially likely to develop overhydration. The **Centers for Disease Control** and Prevention has cautioned that babies are particularly susceptible to the problem during the first month of life, when the kidneys' filtering mechanism is too immature to excrete fluid as rapidly as older infants do. Breast milk or formula provide all the fluids a healthy baby needs. Water should be given slowly, sparingly, and only during extremely hot weather.

For adults, drinking too much water rarely causes overhydration when the body's systems are working normally. People with heart, kidney, or liver disease are more likely to develop overhydration because their kidneys are unable to excrete water normally. It may be necessary for people with these disorders to restrict the amount of water they drink and/or adjust the amount of salt in their diets.

Overhydration can cause acidosis (a condition in which blood and body tissues have an abnormally high acid content), anemia, **cyanosis** (a condition that occurs when oxygen levels in the blood drop sharply), hemorrhage, and **shock**. The brain is the organ most vulnerable to the effects of overhydration. If excess fluid levels accumulate gradually, the brain may be able to adapt to them and the patient will have only a few symptoms. If the condition develops rapidly, confusion, seizures, and coma are likely to occur.

Since the brain particularly susceptible, behavior changes are the usually the first symptoms of water intoxication. The patient may become confused, drowsy, or inattentive. Shouting and **delirium** are common. Other symptoms of overhydration may include blurred vision, muscle cramps and twitching, **paralysis** on one side of the body, poor coordination, **nausea and vomiting**, rapid breathing, sudden weight gain, and weakness. Blood pressure is sometimes, but not always higher than normal.

Chronic illness, **malnutrition**, a tendency to retain water, and kidney diseases and disorders increase the likelihood of becoming overhydrated. Infants and the elderly are at increased risk for overhydration, as are people with certain mental disorders or alcoholism.

Before treatment can begin, a doctor must determine whether a patient's symptoms are due to overhydration, in which excess water is found inside and outside cells, or excess blood volume, in which high sodium levels prevent the body from storing excess water inside the cells.

Mild overhydration can generally be corrected by following a doctor's instructions to limit fluid intake. In more serious cases, **diuretics** may be prescribed to increase urination, although these drugs tend to be most effective in the treatment of excess blood volume. Identifying and treating any underlying condition (such as impaired heart or kidney function) is crucial.

In patients with severe symptoms, fluid imbalances must be corrected immediately. A powerful diuretic and fluids to restore normal sodium concentrations are given rapidly at first. When the patient has absorbed 50% of these substances, blood levels are measured. Treatment then continues at a more moderate pace in order to prevent brain damage that could occur from sudden changes in blood chemistry.

Untreated water intoxication can be fatal, but this outcome is quite rare.

Over-the-counter drugs

Over-the-Counter (OTC) drugs can be bought without a prescription and used by consumers to self-treat certain conditions. As Americans participate more in their own health care and more prescription drugs are converted to OTC drugs, the use of OTC drugs is growing. They are widely available in supermarkets, drug stores, and other types of stores. Common examples include aspirin, and many cough and cold medicines. Over-the-counter drugs can be safely used without the help of a doctor or another health care practitioner as long as the directions on the package and the label are followed. Pharmacists can help consumers determine which OTC drug to buy. A doctor should be consulted, however, before buying an OTC drug for children.

As of April 1999, there were more than 100,000 OTC drugs on the market, in more than 80 product classes. The **Food and Drug Administration** (FDA) regulates OTC drugs to ensure that their benefits outweigh their risks and that they are properly labeled. FDA must approve new OTC drugs and new ingredients in OTC drugs before they can be put on the market. Most OTC drugs were developed and marketed before the law required proof of their safety and effectiveness. FDA is evaluating the ingredients and labeling of these older OTC drugs as part of ''The OTC Drug Review Program.'' For each class of OTC drugs, FDA is developing a monograph (kind of like a recipe book) with information about acceptable ingredients, doses, formulations, and labeling. Products that follow the monographs can be marketed without going through a separate FDA review process. This will ensure that these products are safe and effective and help consumers understand how best to use them.

On March 27, 1999, FDA published a final rule to require a new label format on nearly all over-the-counter drug labels. The new format makes the main messages of the labeling more prominent, includes easier-to-read type, presents information in a standard order, and includes other requirements to make it easier to read labels. The new labels were required starting April 16, 1999.

See also Food and Drug Administration

Oxygen tent

A French physician, Charles Michel (1850-1935), first realized the importance of oxygen to aid the healing process. It was perhaps around 1900 that he first used an oxygen chamber to improve the health of some of his patients, probably those suffering from respiratory disorders. Later the oxygen chamber was expanded around a patient's entire bed and became known as the oxygen tent. Oxygen tents then began to appear in hospitals in Europe and North America.

Oxygen tents are most often used when a medical patient suffers from pneumonia or other respiratory disease, or carbon monoxide poisoning. They are also used following an event in which the patient's body tissues have been deprived of oxygen. The gas inside the tent has a higher percentage of oxygen than found in normal air and thus the patient breathes in more oxygen per breath. The tent is a framed ''envelope'' fitted completely around the patient's hospital bed. Air inside the tent is extracted with a fan and passes through a dust filter and cooling unit where moisture in the exhaled air is condensed and removed. Oxygen-enriched air is pumped into the tent and, if necessary, humidity inside the tent can be increased by an atomizer so the patient's lungs do not dry out. Access to the patient is through a large, zippered opening.

Oxygen therapy

Oxygen therapy is a form of treatment that uses oxygen to heal various disease conditions and strengthen the immune system. Hyperbaric oxygen therapy (HBO) is a mainstream treatment that involves placing the patient in a pressurized chamber with pure oxygen (O_2). Bio-oxidative therapies are alternative treatment approaches that emphasize increasing the oxygen content of the blood through proper breathing and diet, together with the use of ozone and/or hydrogen peroxide in the treatment of specific diseases or weakened immune systems. Ozone therapy is considered a mainstream form of medical treatment in Germany, Austria, Switzerland, France, and Russia.

HBO therapy is used to reverse conditions or processes caused by inadequate oxygen in the body (e. g., **asthma**, **carbon monoxide poisoning**, **smoke inhalation**, **decompression sickness**, and mountain sickness) or to speed up the healing of injuries or infections by increasing the amount of oxygen in body tissues.

For this type of treatment, the patient is placed in a pressurized chamber and breathes pure oxygen either circulating within the chamber itself or through a mask or tube. Patients being treated for carbon monoxide or smoke inhalation **poisoning** receive oxygen through a tight-fitting aviator or anesthesia mask. The length of time in the oxygen chamber, the degree of pressurization, and the number of treatments depend on the condition being treated. For example, decompression sickness from diving accidents may require up to two weeks of oxygen treatment. Patients with **osteomyelitis** may require as many as 40–60 treatments. Treatment sessions for most conditions are 90 minutes, with one or two five-minute ''air breaks'' at 20-minute or half-hour intervals.

Risks associated with hyperbaric oxygen treatment include seizures, irritation of the inner ear, numbness in the fingers, and temporary changes in the lens of the eye. In rare cases, HBO causes inflammation of the optic nerve that may lead to blindness.

Bio-oxidative therapies are used to treat conditions ranging from **AIDS**, **cancer**, and cardiovascular diseases to **acne**, dental surgery, **allergies**, arthritis, and herpes infections. Ozone therapy and hydrogen peroxide therapy are used to treat a variety of diseases. Ozone and hydrogen peroxide are thought to inhibit tumor growth, kill viruses, stimulate the production of disease-fighting white blood cells, and improve the efficiency of oxygen transfer from the blood to body tissues.

Ozone can be administered in various ways. Mixtures of ozone and oxygen may be injected into muscle or introduced into the rectum. Doctors in Germany and Russia inject ozonated water into patients' joints to treat arthritis, rheumatism, and other joint diseases. Ozonated water is also used to cleanse or disinfect wounds, burns and skin infections and to treat the mouth after dental surgery. Ozone-treated oils are used to treat fungal infections, insect **bites and stings**, acne, and similar skin problems. Slow-healing wounds are sometimes treated by pumping a mixture of ozone and oxygen into an airtight bag surrounding the area to be treated. The mixture is absorbed into body tissues through the skin. A method called autohemotherapy is used in Cuba to treat HIV infection, herpes, arthritis, and cancer. It involves removing 10–50 mL of a patient's blood, treating it with a mixture of ozone and oxygen, and then reinjecting or reinfusing it into the patient.

Hydrogen peroxide (H_2O_2) is a colorless liquid that mixes easily with water. Weak solutions of hydrogen peroxide are given intravenously for treatment of **pneumonia**, or **influenza**, and certain chronic diseases. Intravenous infusions of hydrogen peroxide also appear to help the immune system by stimulating production of white blood cells. Hydrogen peroxide solutions can also be injected directly into joints and soft-tissue to treat arthritis and other inflammatory conditions.

Patients should always check with a physician before trying any of these treatments.

P

PACEMAKER

The rhythmic, regular beating of the heart is controlled by a natural pacemaker—a small patch of cells at the top of the right atrium called the sinus node which sends rhythmic electric impulses along specific conducting fibers to the heart muscles, stimulating them to contract and relax in a regular sequence. When the heart muscles fail to receive the pacemaker's signals, the heart ceases pumping blood ceases. Within a few minutes, the patient faints, and within a few more minutes, dies—unless the heart muscles can be stimulated to resume contracting. An artificial pacemaker is designed to help a damaged heart beat normally, programmed to send an electrical impulse to stimulate the heart muscle if it does not sense a normal heart beat within a specific amount of time. Dual-chamber pacemakers, the most common type, sense and pace activity in both the atrium (upper chamber) and ventricle (lower chamber). Single-pass pacemakers use only one lead and sense only one chamber, usually the ventricle. Faster and more easily implanted than the dual lead type, this pacemaker is indicated only in certain instances.

The English surgeon W. H. Walshe first suggested using electric impulses to restart the heart in 1862. Nearly a century later, Harvard-educated American cardiologist, Paul Zoll, believed he could use the heart's responsiveness to electrical stimulation to treat cases of ''heart block.'' His first attempt, passing an electrode down the esophagus, failed, but in 1952 he developed an external pacemaker, passing an electric shock to the heart through electrodes placed on a patient's chest. In October 1952, Zoll's pacemaker was used to maintain a heartbeat in a man suffering from congestive heart failure; after two days, the patient's own heart took over again.

Zoll's machine, while effective, had inherent limitations: The shocks were painful to the chest muscles, and the machine—and thus the movement of the patient—were restricted to the nearest electrical outlet. Researchers envisioned an implantable pacemaker, and American inventor Wilson Greatbatch had dreamed of building one since he first heard of heart block in 1951. The restrictive size of vacuum tubes and storage batteries made it impossible, however. As transistors became widely available in the late 1950s, Greatbatch mentioned his idea to Dr. William Chardack of the Buffalo, New York, Veterans Administration Hospital and, with Chardack's encouragement, put together an implantable pacemaker in three weeks, working in the barn behind his home. After two years of animal testing, in 1960, Chardack and his associates implanted the first pacemakers in the chest wall of a human patient. Also in 1960, Ake Senning and his colleague, Elmqvist, also designed an implantable pacemaker with an external coil and internal receiver. Modern pacemakers are much improved over these designs. Lightweight and relatively easy to install, and their lithium batteries last up to ten years as opposed to the mercury-zinc battery's life of twenty months. The first generation of pacemakers sent signals at a preset rate; researchers Ken Anderson and Dennis Brumwell of Medtronic, Inc., in Minneapolis, Minnesota, advanced pacemaker technology immensely when they invented activity-responsive pacing in 1981 by using piezoelectric crystals that reacted to differing levels of body exertion. Medtronic's ''Activitrax,'' introduced in 1985, was the first pacemaker to adjust pacing rate to exercise level. Several even more advanced pacemakers became available in the late 1980s, among them Medtronic's ''Legend.'' These devices can be reprogrammed while they're still implanted, using radio-frequency signals to reset the pacemaker's microprocessor. They also store information about cardiac events, and some models can even transmit that information over the telephone, directly from the patient's chest to the doctor's office.

Two concerns surrounding the pacemaker are interference by digital wireless telephones and the ''Year 2000'' effect. Research indicates that some digital phones may interfere with some pacemakers but pose no more risk than metal detectors at airport security checkpoints or X-rays, and that interference is unlikely if the phone is held six in (15.24 cm) or more from the pacemaker. Research is underway to determine how this interference can be prevented. Medtronic, the world's largest supplier of implantable medical devices, issued a statement in March 1998 that the anticipated "Year 2000" computer problems will in no way affect their computer-aided pacemakers because therapy is based on internal counters which are unrelated to any specific calendar date.

PAGET'S DISEASE OF BONE

Paget's disease of bone (*osteitis deformans*) is the abnormal formation of bone tissue that results in weakened and deformed bones.

Named for Sir James Paget (1814-1899), this disease affects 1-3% of people over 50 years of age, but affects over 10% of people over 80 years of age. Paget's disease can affect one or more bones in the body. Most often, the pelvis, bones in the skull, the long bones (the large bones that make up the arms and legs), and the collarbones are affected by Paget's disease. In addition, the joints between bones (the knees or elbows, for example) can develop arthritis because of this condition.

Paget's disease is characterized by changes in the normal mechanism of bone formation. Bone is a living material made by the body through the continual processes of formation and breakdown (resorption). The combination of these two actions is called remodeling and is used by the body to build bone tissue that is strong and healthy. Strong bones are formed when bone tissue is made up of plate-shaped crystals of **minerals** called hydroxyapatite. Normal wear and tear on the skeletal system is repaired throughout life by the ongoing process of remodeling. In fact, the entire human skeleton is remodeled every five years.

Healthy bone tissue has an ordered structure that gives the bone its strength. Bones affected by Paget's disease, however, have a structure that is disorganized. This disorganized structure weakens the diseased bone and makes people suffering from this disease more likely to have **fractures**. These fractures are slow to heal.

Paget's disease of bone is most commonly found in Europe, England, Australia, New Zealand, and North America. In these areas, up to 3% of all people over 55 years of age are affected with the disease. It is interesting to note that Paget's disease is rare in Asia, possibly showing that this disease may affect some ethnic groups and geographic areas more than others.

The cause of Paget's disease is not known. Various viruses have been suggested to be involved in this disease, but the relationship between viral infections and Paget's disease remains uncertain.

Paget's disease usually begins without any symptoms. However, as the disease progresses, bone and joint **pain** develop. A unique feature of Paget's disease is the enlargement of areas of affected bone. This type of enlargement is clearly identifiable on an x ray.

If the bones of the skull are affected by Paget's disease, enlargement of the skull can occur and may result in a loss of hearing. When the long bones in the legs are affected, they can become bent under the body's weight because of their weakness. Little or no injury to a bone can cause fractures in the weakened bones. Fractures that occur when no traumatic injury is present are known as spontaneous fractures.

Although rare, bone **cancer** can occur in less than 1% of patients with Paget's disease. Such cancer is often accompanied by an abrupt increase in the intensity of pain at the diseased site. Unfortunately, this type of cancer has a poor prognosis; the survival time is within one to three years.

Paget's disease is often found when an individual is having x rays taken for medical reasons unrelated to this bone disease. A diagnosis of Paget's disease can also be made when higher than normal levels of a chemical called alkaline phosphatase are found in the blood. Alkaline phosphatase is a substance involved in the bone formation process, so if its levels are abnormally high this indicates that the balance between bone formation and resorption is upset.

Treatment, given only when symptoms are present, consists of the following types:

Drugs: Paget's disease is most often treated with drug therapy, with bone pain lessening within weeks of starting the treatment. While **nonsteroidal anti-inflammatory drugs** can reduce bone pain, two additional categories of drugs are used to treat this disease; they are described below.

Hormone Treatment: The hormone calcitonin, which is made naturally by the thyroid gland, is used to treat Paget's disease. This compound rapidly decreases the amount of bone breakdown or loss (resorption). After approximately two to three weeks of treatment with calcitonin, bone pain lessens and new bone tissue forms. Calcitonin is commonly given as daily injections for one month, followed by three injections each week for several additional months. The total dose of calcitonin given to an individual depends upon the amount of disease present and how well the individual's condition responds to the treatment.

Although calcitonin is effective in slowing the progression of Paget's disease, the favorable effects of the drug do not continue for very long once administration of the drug is stopped. In addition, some temporary side effects can occur with this drug. Nausea and flushing are the most common side effects and have been found in 20-30% of individuals taking calcitonin. Vomiting, **diarrhea**, and abdominal pain can also occur, but these effects are also temporary. A form of calcitonin taken nasally causes fewer side effects, but requires higher doses because less of the drug reaches the diseased bone.

Bisphosphonates: The bisphosphonate group of drugs are drugs that bind directly to bone minerals because of their specific chemical structure. Once bound to the bone, these drugs inhibit bone loss by reducing the action of bone cells that normally degrade bone during the remodeling process. Unlike treatment with calcitonin, the positive effects of increased bone formation and reduced pain can continue for many months or even years after bisphosphonate treatment is stopped. Bisphosphonates are considered the treatment of choice for Paget's disease and are usually given for 3-6 months at a time.

Bisphosphate drugs suitable for the treatment of Paget's disease are etidronate, pamidronate, alendronate, clodronate, and tiludronate. Other bisphosphonate drugs are under development as well. The main side effects of these drugs include a flu-like reaction (pamidronate), gastrointestinal disturbances (alendronate, clodronate), and abnormal bone formation (etidronate, when taken in high doses).

Surgery: Treatment of Paget's disease usually begins with drug therapy. However, various surgical treatments can also be used to treat skeletal conditions that occur in patients with Paget's disease.

In patients with severe arthritis of the hip or knee, a **joint replacement** operation can be beneficial. Notably, in addition to the malformation of bone tissue caused by this condition, there are greater numbers of blood vessels that also form in the diseased bone, making surgery to bones affected with Paget's disease more difficult.

There is no cure for Paget's disease. However, the development of potent bisphosphonate drugs like alendronate and pamidronate has resulted in the ability to slow the progress of the disease.

PAIN

Pain is an unpleasant feeling that is carried to the brain by the nervous system. Injury is a major cause, but pain may also arise from an illness. It may accompany a psychological condition, such as depression, or may even occur for no obvious reason.

Pain can be classified as acute or chronic (long-lasting) Acute pain often results from tissue damage, such as a skin burn or broken bone. Acute pain can also be associated with **headache**s or muscle cramps. This type of pain usually goes away as the injury heals or the cause of the pain is removed.

Chronic pain is pain that lingers after an injury heals, or is related to a disease, or has no known cause but will not go away. It is estimated that one in three people in the United States will experience chronic pain at some time in their lives.

Some types of pain are considered abnormal. For example, phantom limb pain occurs after part of the body is amputated. Although the person is missing a body part, the nervous system still perceives pain coming from that part. Another type of pain, allodynia, is unbearable discomfort in response to a normally harmless stimulus, such as the weight of one's clothing on the skin. A somewhat related condition, hyperalgesia, is a feeling of extreme pain from something that should be only mildly painful, such as a pin prick.

Because pain is the most common symptom of injury and disease, the first step in treating it is to try to find out what is causing it. Sometimes, there is an obvious injury, such as a broken bone. But finding the cause of internal pain can be more difficult. Other symptoms, such as **fever** or nausea, help narrow down the possibilities. In some cases, such as lower back pain, it may not be possible to find a specific cause. Finding the cause of a specific pain can be further complicated by the fact that pain sometimes originates in one part of the body but is felt in another part. For example, pain arising from fluid accumulating at the base of the lung may be felt in the shoulder.

Everyone experiences and describes pain in their own way, so it can be difficult to communicate precisely about its quality and intensity. There are no tests that can show what type of pain a person is having or how severe it is. This is why doctors ask patients a lot of questions about their pain, including where it is located and what type of pain it is—burning, shooting, stinging, stabbing, throbbing, or aching, for example. Doctors also ask what kinds of things increase or relieve the pain, how long it has lasted, and whether there are any variations in it. Sometimes patients are asked to rate their pain on a scale of 0 (no pain) to 10 (the worst pain ever experienced).

Many drugs are available for preventing or treating pain. Drugs from different classes may be combined to handle certain types of pain.

Nonopioid analgesics, such as **aspirin**, **acetaminophen** (Tylenol), and ibuprofen (Advil) are most often used for minor pain. These drugs are available without a doctor's prescription, but there are also some prescription-strength medications in this class.

Narcotic analgesics are available only with a doctor's prescription and are used for more severe pain, such as cancer pain. These drugs include codeine, morphine, and methadone. Contrary to earlier beliefs, **addiction** to these painkillers is not common; people who genuinely need these drugs for pain control typically do not become addicted.

Anticonvulsants as well as antidepressant drugs, initially developed to treat seizures and depression, respectively, also can be used as pain-killers. Furthermore, it is not unusual for people with chronic or extreme pain to experience some depression, so treatment with antidepressants may serve a dual role. Commonly prescribed anticonvulsants for pain include phenytoin, carbamazepine, and clonazepam. Antidepressants used for this purpose include doxepin, amitriptyline, and imipramine.

Pain that can't be relieved with the drugs discussed above may be treated by injections of local anesthetics directly into or near the nerve that is transmitting the pain signal. These root blocks may also be useful in determining the source of pain.

Drugs are not always effective in controlling pain. Surgical methods are used as a last resort if drugs and local anesthetics fail.

Alternative treatments are sometimes used to help patients deal with both the physical and psychological aspects of pain. Some of the most popular treatment options include **acupressure** and **acupuncture**, **massage**, **chiropractic**, and relaxation techniques, such as **yoga**, **hypnosis**, and **meditation**. Herbal therapies are gaining increased recognition as viable options. For example, capsaicin, the component that makes cayenne peppers spicy, is used in ointments to relieve the joint pain associated with arthritis. Contrast hydrotherapy can also be very beneficial for pain relief.

Lifestyles that incorporate a healthier diet and regular **exercise** can also be helpful. In addition to relieving **stress**, regular exercise has been shown to increase endorphins, the body's natural painkillers.

Pain management

Pain management is the use of medicines and other approaches to prevent, reduce, or stop **pain** sensations.

Pain has the important role of alerting the brain to potential or actual damage to the body, from injury, disease, or other causes. But after the brain receives and processes the message, further pain can be a nuisance and can actually interfere with recovery from illness or injury. Unrelieved pain can become a syndrome in its own right and cause a downward spiral in a person's health and outlook. Managing pain properly speeds recovery, prevents additional health complications, and improves a person's of life.

Finding and treating the cause of the pain is the first step in managing it. Injuries must be repaired and diseases must be diagnosed and treated. But treating the cause doesn't always relieve the pain. Pain-relieving drugs and other treatments are often necessary.

Pain-relieving drugs, otherwise called **analgesics**, include **nonsteroidal anti-inflammatory drugs** (NSAIDs), **acetaminophen**, narcotics, antidepressants, anticonvulsants, and others. NSAIDs and acetaminophen are available as **over-the-counter** and prescription medications, and are frequently the first treatment for pain. These drugs can also be used along with other drugs that may require a doctor's prescription.

NSAIDs include **aspirin**, ibuprofen (Motrin, Advil, Nuprin), naproxen sodium (Aleve), and ketoprofen (Orudis KT). These drugs are used to treat pain from inflammation. Acetaminophen is also effective against pain, but its ability to reduce inflammation is limited.

NSAIDs and acetaminophen are effective for most forms of acute (sharp, but not long-lasting) pain, but moderate and severe pain may require stronger medication. Narcotics handle intense pain effectively, and are used for cancer pain and acute pain that does not respond to milder drugs. This drug class includes drugs such as oxycodon, methadone, and meperidine (Demerol). Narcotics may be ineffective against some forms of chronic pain. In addition, they are not recommended for long-term use because the body develops a tolerance to the drugs, making them less effective over time.

Although antidepressant drugs were developed to treat depression, they are also effective in combating chronic **headaches**, **cancer** pain, and pain associated with nerve damage. **Antidepressants** that have been shown to have analgesic (pain reducing) properties include amitriptyline (Elavil), trazodone (Desyrel), and imipramine (Tofranil). **Anticonvulsant drugs** share a similar background with antidepressants. Developed to treat epilepsy, anticonvulsants were found to relieve pain as well. Drugs such as phenytoin (Dilantin) and carbamazepine (Tegretol) are prescribed to treat the pain associated with nerve damage.

Other prescription drugs are used to treat specific types of pain or specific pain syndromes. For example, **corticosteroids** are very effective against pain caused by inflammation and swelling, and sumatriptan (Imitrex) was developed to treat migraine headaches.

Some drugs for pain can be taken by mouth. Others are not absorbed very well from the stomach and must be injected into muscles or veins. Following surgery and other medical procedures, patients may have the option of controlling the pain medication themselves. By pressing a button, they can release a set dose of medication into a solution that flows into the body through a needle inserted in a vein. Another mode of administration involves implanted tubes that deliver pain medication directly to the spinal cord. Delivering drugs in this way can reduce side effects and increase the effectiveness of the drug.

Pain treatment options that do not use drugs are often used in addition to drug therapy. Non-drug therapies help some people gain a greater sense of control over their pain. Relaxation techniques, such as **yoga** and **meditation**, are used to decrease muscle tension and reduce **stress**. Tension and stress can also be reduced through **biofeedback**, in which a person consciously attempts to modify skin temperature, muscle tension, blood pressure, and heart rate.

Participating in normal activities and exercising can also help control pain. Through physical therapy, a person can learn **exercise**s for reducing stress, strengthening muscles, and staying fit. Regular exercise has been linked to production of endorphins, the body's natural pain killers.

Acupuncture involves the inserting of small needles into the skin at key points. **Acupressure** uses these same key points, but involves applying pressure rather than inserting needles. Both of these methods may work by prompting the body to release endorphins. Applying heat or being **massage**d are very relaxing and help reduce stress. Transcutaneous electrical nerve stimulation (TENS) applies a small electric current to certain parts of nerves, potentially interrupting pain signals and inducing release of endorphins. To be effective, use of TENS should be medically supervised.

If other treatment methods are not effective in reducing pain, surgery may be an option. Some types of surgery are designed to relieve pressure on a nerve. Another type of surgical procedure is neurolysis, also called a nerve block, which involves destroying a portion of a nerve that is transmitting a pain signal. A third approach is to electrically stimulate or directly apply drugs to nerves that are transmitting pain signals. Electrical stimulation works on the same principle as TENS. But instead of applying the current across the skin, electrodes are implanted to stimulate nerves. Finally, a surgeon may cut a nerve and disconnect it from the central nervous system. However, this does not always relieve the pain, so the technique is not widely used.

Palade, George (1912-)

Romanian American cell biologist

George Emil Palade was born in 1912, in northeastern Romania. One of three children, Palade came from a professional family and earned his medical degree from the University of Bucharest in 1940. In 1941, he married Irina Malaxa; they eventually had two children together.

In 1945, after being discharged from the army, Palade obtained a research position at New York University. While there he met the eminent cell biologist Albert Claude, who had pioneered both the use of the electron microscope in cell study and techniques of cell fractionation (the separation of the constituent parts of cells by centrifugal action). The older scientist invited Palade to join the staff at the Rockefeller Institute (now Rockefeller University), and in 1946 Palade accepted a two-year fellowship as visiting investigator. Political instability in Romania caused Palade to stay in the United States permanently. He became a U.S. citizen in 1952 and a full professor of cytology at Rockefeller in 1958.

At the Rockefeller Institute, Palade and his collaborators reported groundbreaking descriptions of the fine appearance of the cell and of its biochemical function. Concentrating on the cytoplasm—the living material in the cell outside the nucleus—Palade was first attracted to larger organelles (bodies of definite structure and function in the cytoplasm) which Claude had earlier called ''secretory granules.'' Palade showed that these tiny sausage-shaped structures, mitochondria, are the site where energy for the cell is generated. Animal cells typically contain a thousand such mitochondria, each creating adenosine triphosphate (ATP), a high-energy phosphate molecule—through enzymic (enzyme-catalyzed) oxidation or breakdown of fat and sugar. The ATP is then released into the cytoplasm where it powers energy-requiring mechanisms such as nerve impulse conduction, muscle contraction, or protein synthesis.

Using the high-power electron microscope (a device that utilizes electrons instead of light to form images of minute objects), Palade next revealed a delicate tracery, subsequently termed the endoplasmic reticulum. The endoplasmic reticulum is a series of double-layered membranes present throughout all cells except mature erythrocytes, or red blood cells. Its function is the formation and transport of fats and proteins. By far Palade's most significant work was with so-called microsomes, small bodies in the cytoplasm that Claude had earlier identified and shown to have a relatively high ribonucleic acid (RNA) content. RNA is the genetic messenger in protein synthesis. Palade observed these microsomes both as free bodies within the cytoplasm, and attached to the endoplasmic reticulum. In 1956, using a high-speed centrifuge, Palade and his colleague Philip Siekevitz were able to isolate microsomes and observe them under the electron microscope. They discovered that these microsomes were made of equal parts of RNA and protein.

Palade assumed that these RNA-rich microsomes were in fact the factories producing protein to sustain not only the cell but the entire organism. The microsome was renamed the ribosome, and Palade and his team went to work to investigate the pathway of protein synthesis in the cell. Palade and Siekevitz began a series of experiments on ribosomes of the liver and pancreas, employing autoradiographic tracing, a sophisticated process similar to X-ray photography in which a picture is produced by radiation. Investigating in particular exocrine cells (those that secrete externally) of the guinea pig pancreas, the team was able, by 1960, to show that ribosomes do in fact synthesize proteins that are then transported through the endoplasmic reticulum. Further research elucidated the function of the larger ribosomes attached to the endoplasmic reticulum, establishing them as the site where amino acids assemble into polypeptides (chains of amino acids).

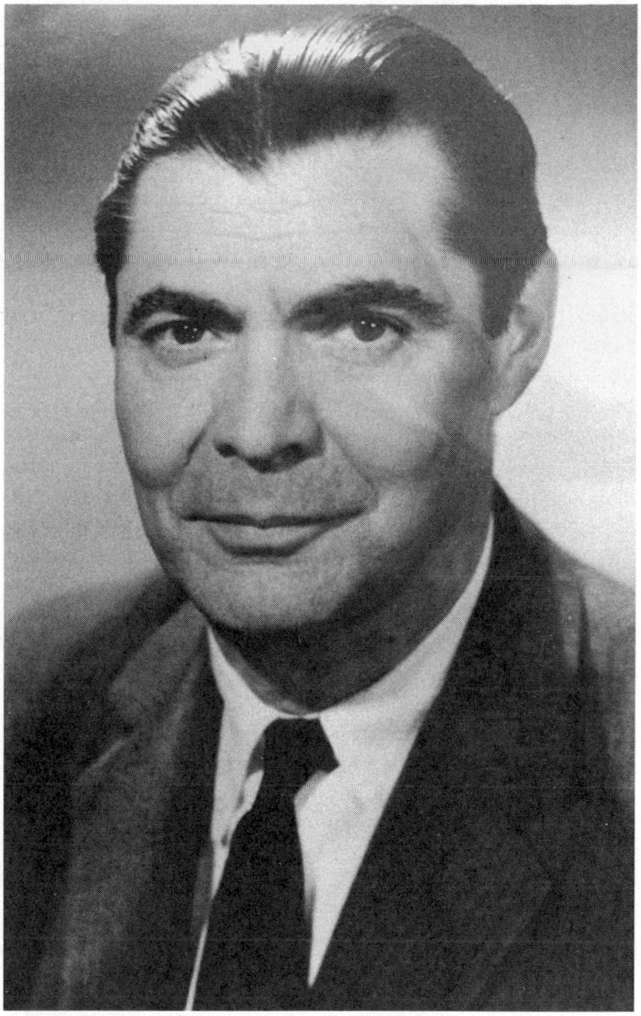

George Emil Palade

Having completed his work on protein synthesis, Palade turned his attention to cellular transport—the means by which substances move through cell membranes. Working with Marilyn G. Farquhar, Palade demonstrated by electron micrography (images formed using an electron microscope) that molecules and ions were engorged by sacs or vesicles that move to the surface from within the cell. These vesicles actually merge with the outer membrane for a time, and then swallow up and bring the substances inside the cell. This vesicular model was in distinct contrast to the then current pore model whereby it was thought that molecules simply entered the cell through pores in the membrane.

Palade's later work at Yale University has been an attempt to establish links between defects in cellular protein production and various illnesses. In 1974 Palade shared the Nobel Prize in Physiology or Medicine with his former mentor, Albert Claude, and with **Christian R. de Duvé**, for their descriptions of the detailed microscopic structure and functions of the cell. In 1990, Palade left Yale to become the dean for scientific affairs at the University of California, San Diego.

Palpitations

A sensation in which a person is aware of an irregular, hard, or rapid heartbeat.

Palpitations mean that the heart is not behaving normally. It can appear to skip beats, beat rapidly, beat irregularly, or thump in the chest. Although palpitations are very common and often harmless, they can be frightening to the person, who is usually unaware of his or her heartbeat.

Palpitations can also be a sign of serious heart trouble. Palpitations that are caused by certain types of abnormal heart rhythms (**arrhythmias**) can be serious, and even fatal if left untreated. Recognizable arrhythmias are present in a small number of patients who have palpitations. Immediate medical attention should be sought for palpitations that feel like a very fast series of heartbeats, last more than two or three minutes, and are unrelated to strenuous physical activity or obvious fright or anger. Medical attention should also be sought if palpitations are accompanied by chest **pain**, **dizziness**, **shortness of breath**, or an overall feeling of weakness.

Most people have experienced a skipped or missed heartbeat, which is really an early beat and not a skipped beat at all. After a premature heartbeat, the heart rests for an instant then beats with extra force, making the person feel as if the heart has skipped a beat. This type of palpitation is nothing to worry about unless it occurs frequently. Severe palpitations feel like a thudding or fluttering sensation in the chest. After chest pain, palpitations are the most common reason that people are referred for cardiology evaluation.

Palpitations can be caused by **anxiety**, arrhythmias, **caffeine**, certain medications, cocaine and other amphetamines, emotional stress, overeating, panic, somatization, and vigorous **exercise**. There may be no other symptoms. But, anxiety, dizziness, shortness of breath, and chest pain may be signs of more severe arrhythmias.

Palpitations are diagnosed through a medical history, a **physical examination**, an electrocardiogram (ECG), and screening for psychiatric disorders. It is often difficult to distinguish palpitations from **panic disorder**, a common problem in which the person experiences frequent and unexplained ''fight-or-flight'' responses, which is the body's natural physical reaction to extreme danger or physical exertion, but without the obvious external stimulus.

To accurately diagnose palpitations, one of the irregular heartbeats must be ''captured'' on an EKG, which shows the heart's activity. Electrodes covered with a type of gel that conducts electrical impulses are placed on the patient's chest, arms, and legs. These electrodes send impulses of the heart's activity to a recorder, which traces them on paper. This **electrocardiography** test takes about 10 minutes and is performed in a physician's office or hospital. Because the palpitations are unlikely to occur during a standard EKG, Holter monitoring is often performed. In this procedure, the patient wears a small, portable tape recorder that is attached to a belt or shoulder strap and connected to electrode disks on his or her chest. The Holter monitor records the heart's rhythm during normal activities. Some medical centers are now using ''event recorders'' that the patient can carry for weeks or months. When the palpitations occur, the patient presses a button on the device, which captures the information about the palpitations for physician evaluation. Later the recording can be transmitted over the telephone line for analysis.

Most palpitations require no treatment. Persistent palpitations can be treated with small doses of a beta blocker. **Beta blockers** are drugs that tend to lower blood pressure. They slow the heart rate and decrease the force with which the heart pumps. If the cause of the palpitations is determined to be an arrhythmia, medical, or surgical treatment may be prescribed, although surgery is rarely needed.

Most palpitations are harmless, but some can be a sign of heart trouble which could be fatal if left untreated.

Palpitations not caused by arrhythmias can be prevented by reducing or eliminating anxiety and emotional stress, and reducing or eliminating consumption of tea, cola, coffee, and chocolate. Exercise can also help, but a treadmill **stress test** performed by a physician should be considered first to make sure the exercise is safe.

Pancreatic cancer

Pancreatic cancer is a disease in which **cancer**ous cells are found within the tissues of the pancreas. The pancreas is a pear-shaped gland that lies behind the stomach, surrounded by other digestive organs, such as the liver, gallbladder, and small intestine. It has two main functions, to produce digestive juices that help break down food, and to produce hormones (like insulin) that control how the body stores and uses the food.

The part of the pancreas that produces the digestive juices is called the exocrine pancreas, and almost 95% of pancreatic cancers occur in the tissues of the exocrine pancreas.

Although the exact cause for pancreatic cancer remains unknown, several risk factors, such as smoking and diets rich in red meat and fat, have been shown to increase the susceptibility to this particular cancer. It has been observed that a third of pancreatic cancer cases occur among smokers. Therefore, smoking is regarded as the single greatest risk factor for this cancer. The disease is more common among diabetics. Conditions such as chronic **pancreatitis** (long-term inflammation of the pancreas) have also been associated with an increased risk for pancreatic cancer.

The most common signs and symptoms of the disease are abdominal **pain**; digestive problems, **diarrhea**, and **nausea**. Weight loss that is not due to drastic dieting or exercising is a common occurrence in pancreatic cancer patients. Gallbladder enlargement and **jaundice** (a yellowish discoloration of the whites of the eyes and the skin) may sometimes occur.

The first step in diagnosing pancreatic cancer is a thorough medical history and a complete **physical examination** to check for fluid accumulation, or any lumps, or masses, in the abdomen. The skin and the whites of the eyes will be checked for jaundice. Blood tests will be performed to rule out the possibility of liver diseases that can also contribute to jaundice. Imaging tests such as CT scans, MRI imaging, or ultrasonography may be ordered in order to get a detailed picture of the internal organs. This will also help to check whether the cancer has spread to other organs beyond the pancreas. The most definitive test for pancreatic cancer is a **biopsy**, where a sample of the tumor is removed and examined microscopically.

Pancreatic cancer can be treated by any of the three standard modalities: surgery, **radiation therapy**, or **chemotherapy**.

If the imaging studies show that the cancer is contained within the pancreas, the doctors will attempt surgery to remove all the cancer. Depending on the location of the tumor, different types of surgery can be performed, where either the whole pancreas or only parts of the pancreas are removed. If the tumor is too widespread to be removed by surgery, radiation therapy in combination with chemotherapy is used.

The disease is often fatal. Once diagnosed with this cancer, 95% of patients will die within five years. More than 80% of the patients will not survive the first year after initial diagnosis. The poor prognosis is because of late diagnosis; the pancreas is a small gland located deep within the abdominal cavity, and, hence, cannot be seen or felt during routine physical examination. There are no early symptoms, and by the time the symptoms are manifested, the cancer has already spread to other organs and is in an advanced stage.

Since the exact cause of pancreatic cancer is not known, there are no guidelines for prevention. The wisest approach would be to avoid all the risk factors for pancreatic cancer. Quitting cigarette **smoking** will certainly reduce the risk for many cancers, including pancreatic cancer. In countries where the diet is low in fat, the incidence of pancreatic cancer is much lower. The American Cancer Society recommends a diet rich in fruits, vegetables, and dietary fiber in order to reduce the risk of pancreatic cancer.

PANCREATITIS

Pancreatitis is inflammation of the pancreas, an organ that is important in digestion. Pancreatitis can be acute (beginning suddenly, usually with the patient recovering fully) or chronic (progressing slowly with continued, permanent injury to the pancreas).

The pancreas is located in the abdomen, near the liver, stomach, and duodenum (the first part of the small intestine). The pancreas is considered a gland. A gland is an organ whose main function is to produce chemicals that pass either into the main blood circulation (called an endocrine function), or pass into another organ (called an exocrine function). The pancreas is unusual because it has both endocrine and exocrine functions. Its endocrine function produces three hormones. Two of these hormones, insulin and glucagon, help the body process sugars in the diet. The third hormone, vasoactive intestinal polypeptide (VIP), affects the functioning of the stomach and intestines. In its exocrine function, the pancreas produces a variety of digestive enzymes that pass into the duodenum through a channel called the pancreatic duct. In the duodenum, the enzymes begin the process of breaking down proteins, fats, starches, and other components of food.

Acute pancreatitis occurs when the pancreas suddenly becomes inflamed but improves. Patients recover fully from the disease, and in almost 90% of cases the symptoms disappear within about a week after treatment. With chronic pancreatitis, damage to the pancreas occurs slowly over time. Symptoms may come and go, but the condition does not disappear, and the pancreas is permanently damaged.

Acute pancreatitis has a number of causes. The most common, gallbladder disease and alcoholism, account for more than 80% of all hospitalizations for acute pancreatitis. Other factors, including infections, injuries to the abdomen, and certain drugs, may also contribute to pancreatitis.

Pain in the upper right hand corner of the abdomen is a major symptom in pancreatitis. The pain is usually quite intense and steady and often feels as if it is boring through to the patient's back. Nausea, vomiting, abdominal swelling, increased heart rate, low blood pressure and slight **fever** also are common symptoms.

Patients who are seriously ill with pancreatitis may show classic signs of **shock**. Shock is a very serious syndrome that occurs when the volume (quantity) of fluid in the blood is very low. The patient's arms and legs become extremely cold, the blood pressure drops dangerously low, the heart rate is quite fast, and the patient may have changes in mental function. When shock occurs, all of body's major organs are deprived of blood (and, therefore, oxygen), resulting in damage. Kidney, respiratory, and **heart failure** are serious risks of shock.

In very severe cases of pancreatitis (called necrotizing pancreatitis), the pancreatic tissue begins to die. When this happens, the pancreas becomes extremely susceptible to serious infection. As the pancreatic tissue continues to be destroyed, many digestive functions are disturbed. The inability to digest and use proteins results in smaller muscles (wasting) and weakness. The inability to digest and use the nutrients in food leads to **malnutrition**, and a generally weakened condition. As the disease progresses, permanent injury to the pancreas can lead to diabetes.

Treatment of pancreatitis involves quickly replacing lost fluids through a needle inserted in a vein (intravenous or IV fluids). These IV solutions need to contain appropriate amounts of salts, sugars, and sometimes even proteins, in order to correct the patient's disturbances in blood chemistry. Pain is treated with a variety of medications. Until the gastrointestinal tract begins functioning normally, the patient is not allowed to eat. The patient is carefully monitored for any complications that may develop. If infections occur, **antibiotics** are given through the IV. Severe necrotizing pancreatitis may require surgery to remove part of the dying pancreas.

Patients who develop chronic pancreatitis because of alcohol consumption must stop drinking alcohol entirely.

PANIC DISORDER

A panic attack is a sudden, intense feeling of fear coupled with an overwhelming sense of danger, accompanied by physical symptoms of **anxiety**, such as pounding heart, sweating, and rapid breathing. A person with panic disorder may have repeated panic attacks (at least several a month) and feel severe anxiety about having another attack.

Almost everyone has occasional moments of anxiety, but panic attacks are sudden and unprovoked, having little to do with real danger. Panic disorder is a chronic (long-term) condition that can have a devastating impact on a person's family, work, and social life.

People with panic disorder usually have their first panic attack in their 20s. The first attack usually strikes without warning. A person might be walking down the street, driving a car, or riding an escalator when suddenly panic strikes. Pounding heart, sweating palms, and an overwhelming feeling of impending doom are common features. Some people feel an overwhelming urge to escape. Others are convinced they are about to have a **heart attack**, suffocate, lose control, or "go crazy." While the attack may last only seconds or minutes, the experience can be so disturbing that the person starts to worry that it might happen again any time.

As the fear of future panic attacks deepens, the person begins to avoid places or situations in which panic occurred in the past. People with severe panic disorder may even become afraid to leave home. This fear of being in exposed places is called agoraphobia.

People with untreated panic disorder may have problems getting to work or keeping their jobs. As the person's world narrows, untreated panic disorder can lead to depression, substance abuse, and in rare cases, suicide.

Scientists aren't sure what causes panic disorder, but they suspect the tendency to develop the condition can be inherited. Some experts think that people with panic disorder may have a hypersensitive nervous system that responds to nonthreatening situations as if they were dangerous. Research suggests that people with panic disorder may not be able to make proper use of their body's normal **stress**-reducing chemicals.

Because its physical symptoms are easily confused with other conditions, panic disorder often goes undiagnosed. A thorough physical examination is needed to rule out a medical condition. Because the physical symptoms are so pronounced and frightening, panic attacks can be mistaken for a heart problem. Some people experiencing a panic attack go to an emergency room and endure many tests before a diagnosis is made.

Once a medical condition is ruled out, a mental health professional is the best person to diagnose panic disorder, taking into account not just the actual episodes, but how the patient feels about the attacks and how the attacks affect everyday life. Most patients with panic disorder respond best to a combination of cognitive-behavioral therapy and medication. Cognitive-behavioral therapy usually runs from 12-15 sessions. It teaches patients:

- How to identify and alter thought patterns so as not to mistake the symptoms of panic disorder for true disasters.
- How to prepare for the situations and physical symptoms that trigger a panic attack.
- How to identify and change unrealistic self-talk (such as "I'm going to die!") that can worsen a panic attack.
- How to calm down and learn breathing exercises to counteract the physical symptoms of panic.
- How to gradually confront the frightening situation step by step until it becomes less terrifying.
- How to "desensitize" themselves to their own physical sensations, such as rapid heart rate.

In addition, some medications can help reduce or prevent panic attacks by changing the way certain chemicals interact in the brain. It may be necessary to take a drug for several months to determine whether it is working. With effective drugs, treatment usually continues for at least six months to a year.

Patients can make certain lifestyle changes to help keep panic at bay, such as reducing or eliminating **caffeine** and alcohol and avoiding cocaine, amphetamines, and marijuana.

A variety of alternative therapies may also be helpful in treating panic attacks. Nutritional supplementation (especially with B **vitamins**, magnesium, and antioxidant vitamins), creative visualization, **guided imagery**, and relaxation techniques may help some people suffering from panic attacks. Hydrotherapies, especially hot epsom salt baths or baths with essential oil of lavender (*Lavandula officinalis*), can help patients relax.

While there may be occasional periods of improvement, the episodes of panic rarely disappear on their own. Fortunately, panic disorder responds very well to treatment; panic attacks decrease in up to 90% of people after 6-8 weeks of a combination of cognitive-behavioral therapy and medication.

Unfortunately, many people with panic disorder never get the help they need. If untreated, panic disorder can last for years and may become so severe that normal life is impossible. Many people who struggle with untreated panic disorder and try to hide their symptoms end up losing their friends, family, and jobs.

Papanicolaou, George (1883-1962)

Greek-American physician and anatomist

George Papanicolaou was a physician and researcher who was associated with the Cornell University school of medicine for forty-eight years. While studying microscopic slides of cells that had been cast off (exfoliated) in body fluids of laboratory animals and humans, he recognized the presence of abnormal cancer cells. The discovery led to the famous test that bears the first syllable of his last name, the Pap test. He is recognized by his colleagues as the father of modern cytology.

George Nicholas Papanicolaou was born on May 13, 1883, in Coumi, Greece, to Nicholas (a physician) and Mary Critsutas Papanicolaou. He received an M.D. degree from the University of Athens in 1904 and a Ph.D. from the University of Munich in 1910. He married Mary A. Mavroyeni on September 15, 1910. His first position was as a physiologist for an expedition of the Oceanographic Institute of Monaco for one year. In 1912, during the Balkan War, he became an officer in the Greek army medical corps. He came to the United States in 1913, working initially as a salesman, but soon securing work in his field as an anatomy assistant at Cornell University, where he eventually became a full professor in 1924. He also served on the pathology staff of New York Hospital from 1913. Papanicolaou became a United States citizen in 1927.

In the pathology lab at Cornell, Papanicolaou began working with microscope slides of vaginal secretions of guinea pigs. He found that changes in forms of the epithelial cells (the outer layer of the skin or of an organ) correspond with the animal's estrus or menstrual cycle. Using the changes as a measuring device, he was able to study sex hormones and the menstrual cycles of other laboratory animals.

In 1923 Papanicolaou studied vaginal smears of women who had cervical cancer and found cancer cells present. Writing in the medical journal *Growth* in 1920, he outlined his theory that a microscopic smear of vaginal fluid could detect the presence of cancer cells in the uterus. At this time physicians relied on biopsy and curettage to diagnose and treat cancer and ignored the possibilities of a new test based on Papanicolaou's research.

Papanicolaou himself paid little attention to his research in this area for the next decade. At the encouragement of a colleague, Dr. Herbert F. Traut, and with the support of Dean Joseph C. Hinsey of Cornell medical college, he later continued his work in this field and was allowed to devote full time to his research. In 1943 he published conclusive findings that showed smears of vaginal fluid could indicate cervical and uterine cancer before symptoms appear. This time the medical community took notice, and the "new cancer diagnosis," the Pap smear test, won acceptance and became a routine screening technique.

During a Pap test, a scraping or smear is taken from the woman's cervix (the mouth of the uterus) or from the vagina, then is stained and examined under the microscope, where cells may appear normal, cancerous, or suspicious. It is a simple, painless, and effective means of early cancer detection.

Papanicolaou soon won international acclaim for his discovery. The American Cancer Society (ACS) launched massive education campaigns for the test, and Dr. Charles Cameron, a Philadelphia surgeon (who was director of the ACS), said that this test was the most significant and practical discovery in our time. Papanicolaou spent much of his time promoting the test and trained thousands of students in the microscopic detection techniques. Once the test had been accepted, he began to apply the same principle of exfoliate cytology to cancers of the lung, stomach, and bladder.

At Cornell Papanicolaou founded the Papanicolaou Research Center and worked six and a half days a week peering at slides and looking for malignant cells. He seldom took a vacation. When associates advised him to rest, he stated that the work was so interesting and that there was so much to be done. His wife worked as his research assistant and driver.

Papanicolaou was a member of many societies and won twelve prestigious awards including the Borden award of the Association of Medical Colleges in 1940, the Lasker award of the Public Health Association in 1950, and the honor medal from the American Cancer Society in 1952. The king of Greece gave him the medal of the Cross of the Grand Commander award, and his native town of Coumi renamed their town square in his honor. He was the author of four books and over one hundred articles.

At the age of seventy-eight, Papanicolaou ended his forty-eight year association with Cornell and took over the Papanicolaou Cancer Institute in Miami. He maintained a busy schedule and was planning for the further expansion of the institute when he suffered a heart attack and died on February 19, 1962. He was buried in Clinton, New Jersey.

In 1983, the hundredth anniversary of Papanicolaou's birth, several articles appeared in scientific journals honoring him and his persistent spirit of scientific discovery. In December, 1992, the *Journal of the Florida Medical Association* issued a thirty year commemorative of his death, which states that because of his persistence, there has been a seventy-percent decrease in cervical and uterine cancer. His techniques are also being applied to other organs and systems in the use of fine needle aspiration.

Pap test

The Pap test is a simple and painless procedure for the early detection of the two most common and fatal forms of cancer in women: cervical and uterine. It is considered one of the most effective and significant weapons in the modern fight against cancer.

The test, also known as Papanicolaou's Smear, is named for the Greek doctor who developed it, **George Nicholas Papanicolaou** (1883-1962), who received his M.D. from the University of Athens in 1904. He emigrated to the United States in 1913 and was affiliated with New York Hospital and Cornell Medical College throughout his career. In 1917, Papanicolaou began a microscopic study of vaginal discharge cells in pigs. After expanding his research to humans, he observed cell abnormalities in a woman with cervical cancer, which inspired him to develop a method of detecting cancer through microscopic cell examination, or cytology. This technique had first been suggested by English physician Lionel Smith Beale (1828-1906) in 1867. Papanicolaou began publishing reports on his cytologic method of uterine and cervical cancer detection in 1928, but most of his colleagues remained committed to the standard procedures of cervical biopsy and curettage. In 1939 Papanicolaou began collaborating with gynecologist Herbert Traut. Their 1943 monograph, *Diagnosis of Uterine Cancer by the Vaginal Smear*, won wide acceptance for the procedure, and Papanicolaou began teaching it to physicians from around the world.

The significance of the Pap smear is that it allows detection of cancer in its presymptomatic stage, when the disease can best be treated. Cancer of the cervix in its earliest stages is almost 100% curable, while 80% of uterine cancer cases detected by a Pap test can also be cured. The smear technique of abnormal cell detection has been expanded to early diagnosis of cancer of many other organs.

Paralysis

Paralysis is defined as complete loss of strength in an affected limb or muscle group.

The chain of nerve cells that runs from the brain through the spinal cord out to the muscle is called the motor pathway.

Normal muscle function requires intact connections all along this motor pathway. Damage at any point reduces the brain's ability to control the muscle's movements. This reduced efficiency causes weakness, also called paresis. Complete loss of communication prevents any willed movement at all. This lack of control is called paralysis. Certain inherited abnormalities in muscle cause periodic paralysis, in which the weakness comes and goes.

The line between weakness and paralysis is not absolute. A condition causing weakness may progress to paralysis. On the other hand, strength may be restored to a paralyzed limb. Nerve regeneration or regrowth is one way in which strength can return to a paralyzed muscle. Paralysis almost always causes a change in muscle tone. Paralyzed muscle may be flaccid, flabby, and without appreciable tone, or it may be spastic, tight, and with abnormally high tone that increases when the muscle is moved.

Paralysis may affect an individual muscle, but it usually affects an entire body region. The distribution of weakness is an important clue to the location of the nerve damage that is causing the paralysis. Words describing the distribution of paralysis use the suffix ''-plegia,'' from the Greek word for ''**stroke**.'' The types of paralysis are classified by region:

- Monoplegia, affecting only one limb
- Diplegia, affecting the same body region on both sides of the body (both arms, for example, or both sides of the face)
- Hemiplegia, affecting one side of the body
- Paraplegia, affecting both legs and the trunk
- Quadriplegia, affecting all four limbs and the trunk.

The nerve damage that causes paralysis may be in the brain or spinal cord (the central nervous system) or it may be in the nerves outside the spinal cord (the peripheral nervous system). The most common causes of damage to the brain are:

- Stroke
- Tumor
- Trauma (caused by a fall or a blow)
- **Multiple sclerosis** (a disease of that destroys the protective sheath that covers nerve cells)
- **Cerebral palsy** (a condition caused by a defect or injury to the brain that occurs at or shortly after birth)
- Metabolic disorder (a disorder that interferes with the body's ability to maintain itself).

Damage to the spinal cord or peripheral nerves is most often caused by trauma, such as a fall or a car crash.

The only treatment for paralysis is to treat its underlying cause. The loss of function caused by long-term paralysis can be treated through a comprehensive **rehabilitation** program. Rehabilitation includes:

- **Physical therapy**. The physical therapist focuses on mobility. Physical therapy helps develop strategies to compensate for paralysis by using those muscles that still have normal function, helps maintain and build any strength and control that remain in the affected muscles, and helps maintain range of motion in the affected limbs to prevent muscles from shortening (contracture) and becoming deformed. If nerve regrowth is expected, physical therapy is used to retrain affected limbs during recovery. A physical therapist also suggests adaptive equipment such as braces, canes, or wheelchairs.
- **Occupational therapy**. The occupational therapist focuses on daily activities such as eating and bathing. Occupational therapy develops special tools and techniques that permit self-care and suggests ways to modify the home and workplace so that a patient with an impairment may live a normal life.
- Other specialties. The nature of the impairment may mean that the patient needs the services of a respiratory therapist, vocational rehabilitation counselor, social worker, speech-language pathologist, nutritionist, special education teacher, recreation therapist, or clinical psychologist.

Paramedics

Literally meaning ''beside doctor,'' paramedics refers to two groups of health care workers, both of which assist physicians in treating patients and share direct responsibility for their care. Neither has training as extensive as that required for physicians.

One type of paramedic is specifically trained for emergency situations. These individuals, also known as emergency medical technicians, are often the first people at the scene of an accident or other event where people have been injured or need to be rescued. They provide patients with emergency care (i.e., resuscitation) to stabilize them, and then accompany them in an ambulance to a hospital emergency room to inform the attending **physician** of their status.

Also included in this category are nurse practitioners and physician's assistants, although these people usually deal with patients at the hospital or doctor's office rather than in the field. They perform much of the routine work required in patient care, such as drawing blood, giving injections, taking medical histories, and providing basic medical care and diagnosis.

The other type of paramedic comprises the general group of highly trained professionals who support physicians, including x-ray and laboratory technicians and physical therapists.

Paranoia

Paranoia is an unfounded or exaggerated distrust of others, sometimes reaching delusional proportions. Paranoid individuals constantly suspect the motives of those around them, and believe that certain individuals, or people in general, are ''out to get them.''

Paranoid perceptions and behavior may appear as features of a number of mental illnesses, including depression and **dementia**, but are most prominent in three types of psychological disorders: paranoid **schizophrenia**, delusional disorder (persecutory type), and paranoid personality disorder (PPD).

Individuals with paranoid schizophrenia and persecutory delusional disorder experience what is known as persecutory delusions: an irrational, yet unshakable, belief that someone is plotting against them. Persecutory delusions in paranoid schizophrenia are bizarre, sometimes grandiose, and often accompanied by auditory **hallucinations**. Delusions experienced by individuals with delusional disorder are more plausible than those experienced by paranoid schizophrenics; not bizarre, though still unjustified. Individuals with delusional disorder may seem offbeat or quirky rather than mentally ill, and, as such, may never seek treatment.

Persons with paranoid personality disorder tend to be self-centered, self-important, defensive, and emotionally distant.Their paranoia manifests itself in constant suspicions rather than full-blown delusions. The disorder often impedes social and personal relationships and career advancement. Some individuals with PPD are described as ''litigious,'' as they are constantly initiating frivolous law suits. PPD is more common in men than in women, and typically begins in early adulthood.

The exact cause of paranoia is unknown. Potential causal factors may be genetics, neurological abnormalities, changes in brain chemistry, and **stress**. Paranoia is also a possible side effect of drug use and abuse (for example, alcohol, marijuana, amphetamines, cocaine, PCP). Acute, or short term, paranoia may occur in some individuals overwhelmed by stress.

The diagnosis of patients with paranoid symptoms includes a thorough **physical examination** and patient history to rule out possible organic causes (such as dementia) or environmental causes (such as extreme stress). If a psychological cause is suspected, a psychologist will conduct an interview with the patient and may administer one of several tests to evaluate mental status.

Paranoia that is symptomatic of paranoid schizophrenia, delusional disorder, or paranoid personality disorder should be treated by a psychologist and/or psychiatrist. **Antipsychotic** medication such as thioridazine (Mellaril), haloperidol (Haldol), chlorpromazine (Thorazine), clozapine (Clozaril), or risperidone (Risperdal) may be prescribed, and cognitive therapy or psychotherapy may be employed to help the patient cope with their paranoia and/or persecutory delusions. It is uncertain whether antipsychotic medication benefit individuals with paranoid personality disorder and may even pose long-term risks.

If an underlying condition, such as depression or drug abuse, is found to be triggering the paranoia, an appropriate course of medication and/or psychosocial therapy is employed to treat the primary disorder.

Because of the inherent mistrust felt by paranoid individuals, they often must be coerced into entering treatment. As unwilling participants, their recovery may be hampered by efforts to sabotage treatment (for example, not taking medication or not being forthcoming with a therapist). They may also exhibit a lack of insight into their condition or the belief that the therapist is plotting against them. Although their lifestyles may be restricted, some patients with PPD or persecutory delusional disorder continue to function in society without treatment.

PARATHYROID DISORDERS

Parathyroid glands are four pea-sized glands located just behind the thyroid gland in the front of the neck. The function of parathyroid glands is to produce a hormone called parathyroid hormone (parathormone), which helps regulate calcium and phosphorous in the body. Hyperparathyroidism is the overproduction of this hormone. Hypoparathyroidism is the result of a decrease in production of parathyroid hormones; the result is a low level of calcium in the blood.

Thyroid glands and parathyroid glands, despite their similar name and proximity, are entirely separate, and each produces hormones with different functions. Hyperparathyroidism may be primary or secondary. It most often occurs in those over age 30, and most commonly in patients 50 to 60 years old. It rarely occurs in children or the elderly. Women are affected by the disease up to three times more often than men. It is estimated that 28 of every 100,000 people in the United States will develop hyperparathyroidism each year. Hypoparathyroidism affects both males and females of all ages.

Normally, parathyroid glands produce the parathormone as calcium levels drop and lower to meet the demands of a growing skeleton, **pregnancy**, or lactation. However, when one or more parathyroid glands malfunctions, it can lead to overproduction of the hormone and elevated calcium level in the blood. Therefore, a common result of hyperparathyroidism is hypercalcemia, or an abnormally high level of calcium in the blood. Primary hyperparathyroidism occurs as a malfunction of one of the glands, usually as a result of a benign tumor, called adenoma. Secondary hyperparathyroidism occurs as the result of a metabolic abnormality outside the parathyroid glands, which causes a resistance to the function of the parathyroid hormones. Primary hyperparathyroidism is one of the most common endocrine disorders, led only by diabetes and hyperthyroidism.

Often, there are no obvious symptoms or suspicion of hyperparathyroidism, and it is first diagnosed when a patient is discovered to be hypercalcemic during a routine blood chemistry profile. Patients may believe they have felt fine, but realize improvements in sleep, irritability, and memory following treatment. When symptoms are present, they may include development of gastric **ulcers** or **pancreatitis** because high calcium levels can cause inflammation and **pain** in the linings of the stomach and pancreas.

Most of the symptoms of hyperparathyroidism are those present as a result of hypercalcemia, such as **kidney stones**, **osteoporosis**, or bone degradation resulting from the bones giving up calcium. Muscle weakness, central nervous system disturbances such as depression, psychomotor and personality disturbances, and rarely, even **coma** can occur. Patients may also experience heartburn, **nausea**, **constipation**, or abdominal pain. In secondary hyperparathyroidism, patients may show signs of calcium imbalance such as deformities of the long bones. Symptoms of the underlying disease may also be present.

Most commonly, hyperparathyroidism occurs as the result of a single adenoma, or benign tumor, in one of the parathyroid glands. About 90% of all cases of hyperparathyroidism are caused by an adenoma. The tumors are seldom **cancer**ous. They will grow to a much larger size than the parathyroid glands, often to the size of a walnut. Genetic disorders or multiple endocrine tumors can also cause a parathyroid gland to enlarge and oversecrete hormone. In 10% or fewer of patients with primary hyperparathyroidism, there is enlargement of all four parathyroid glands. This condition is called parathyroid hyperplasia.

The accidental removal of the parathyroid glands during neck surgery is the most frequent cause of hypoparathyroidism. Complications of surgery on the parathyroid glands is another common cause of this disorder. There is the possibility of autoimmune genetic disorders causing hypoparathyroidism such as Hashimoto's thyroiditis, **pernicious anemia**, and Addison's disease. The destruction of the gland by radiation is a rare cause of hypoparathyroidism. Occasionally, the parathyroids are absent at birth causing low calcium levels and possible convulsions in the newborn. Symptoms in the advanced and continuous stages of hypoparathyroidism include splitting of the nails, inadequate tooth development and **mental retardation** in children, and seizures.

Abnormal low levels of calcium result in irritability of nerves, causing numbness and tingling of the hands and feet, with painful-cramp like muscle spasms known as tetany. Laryngeal spasms may also occur causing respiratory obstruction.

Diagnosis of hyperparathyroidism is most often made when a blood test (radioimmunoassay) reveals high levels of parathyroid hormone and calcium. A blood test that specifically measures the amount of parathyroid hormone has made diagnosis simpler. X-ray examinations may be performed to look for areas of diffuse bone demineralization, bone cysts, outer bone absorption and erosion of the long bones of the fingers and toes. Hypercalcemia is mild or intermittent in some patients, but is an excellent indicator of primary hyperparathyroidism. Dual energy x-ray absorptiometry (DEXA or DXA), a tool used to diagnose and measure osteoporosis, is used to show reduction in bone mass for primary hyperparathryroidism patients. Once a diagnosis of hyperparathyroidism is reached, the physician will probably order further tests to evaluate complications. For example, abdominal radiographs might reveal kidney stones.

For secondary hyperparathyroidism, normal or slightly decreased calcium levels in the blood and variable phosphorous levels may be visible. Patient history of familial kidney disease or convulsive disorders may suggest a diagnosis of secondary hyperparathyroidism. Other tests may reveal a disease or disorder, which is causing the secondary hyperparathyroidism.

Hyperparathyroidism cases will usually be referred to an endocrinologist, a physician specializing in hormonal problems, or a nephrologist, who specializes in kidney and mineral disorders.

Patients with mild cases of hyperparathyroidism may not need immediate treatment if they have only slight elevations in blood calcium level and normal kidneys and bones. These patients should be regularly checked, probably as often as every six months, by **physical examination** and measurement of kidney function and calcium levels. A bone densitometry measurement should be performed every one or two years. After several years with no worsened symptoms, the length of time between exams may be increased.

Patients with more advanced hyperparathyroidism will usually have all or half of the affected parathyroid gland or glands surgically removed. This surgery is relatively safe and effective. The primary risks are those associated with general anesthesia. There are some instances when the surgery can be performed with the patient under regional, or cervical block, anesthesia. Often studies such as ultrasonography prior to surgery help pinpoint the affected areas.

Removal of the enlarged parathyroid gland or glands cures the disease 95% of the time and relief of bone pain may occur in as few as three days. In up to 5% of patients undergoing surgery, chronically low calcium levels may result, and these patients will require calcium supplement or vitamin D treatment. Damage to the kidneys as a result of hyperparathyroidism is often irreversible. Prognosis is generally good, however complications of hyperparathyroidism such as osteoporosis, bone **fractures**, kidney stones, peptic ulcers, pancreatitis, and nervous system difficulties may worsen prognosis.

Presently hypoparathyroidism is considered incurable. The disorder requires lifelong replacement therapy to control symptoms. Medical research however, continues to search for a cure.

Secondary hyperparathyroidism may be prevented by early treatment of the disease causing it. Early recognition and treatment of hyperparathyroidism may prevent hypercalcemia. Since the cause of primary hyperparathyroidism, or the adenoma which causes parathyroid enlargement, is largely unknown, there are not prescribed prevention methods.

There are no specific preventive measures for hypoparathyroidism. However, careful surgical techniques are critical to reduce the risk of damage to the gland during surgery.

PARÉ, AMBROISE (1510-1590)

French surgeon

Ambroise Paré, the uneducated son of a country artisan, became the greatest surgeon of the sixteenth century. Renowned as much for his compassion as his surgical skill, Paré guided his life with a humble credo of patient care: ''I dressed him, God cured him.'' Paré was born in an era in which physicians considered surgery well beneath their dignity; they left all cutting to the lowly **barber-surgeons**. At an early age, he served an apprenticeship to a barber in the French provinces, travelling to Paris at age 19 where he became a surgical student at the Hôtel Dieu hospital. After attaining the rank of master barber-surgeon in 1536, he joined the army as a regimental surgeon. He served intermittently in the army for the next 30 years, during which time he developed a flourishing practice and gained fame through his writings and his considerate, democratic treatment of soldiers of all ranks. Before his career ended, he had served as surgeon to four French kings.

It was during the siege of Turin in 1536-37 that Paré made his first great medical discovery. Gunshot **wounds**, a new medical condition, were considered to be poisonous and were routinely treated by cauterization with boiling oil. When Paré ran out of oil during the siege, he turned instead to simple dressings and soothing ointment, and immediately noted the improved condition of his patients. Paré popularized this revolutionary treatment in his *Method of Treating Wounds* in 1545. Paré's second critical contribution to medicine was his promotion of ligature of blood vessels to prevent hemorrhage during amputations. Paré's classic *Treatise on Surgery*, written in 1564, disseminated knowledge of this life-saving technique. In this book, Paré also included large parts of **Andreas Vesalius**'s authoritative work on anatomy, translated from the original Latin into the vernacular French. This dramatically opened the doors of anatomical knowledge to the barber-surgeons of Paré's time who, like Paré, were unable to read Latin and were scorned and left untrained by establishment physicians.

Paré was an innovator, willing to depart from established practices. He advocated massage and designed a number of artificial limbs as well as an artificial eye. He advanced obstetrics by reintroducing podalic version (turning a fetus *in utero* into a position possible for birth) and inducing premature labor in cases of uterine hemorrhage. As always, he spread knowledge of these discoveries through his vernacular writings. Because of his dissemination of surgical knowledge among the barber-surgeons of his time and his efforts to elevate the status of surgery to a level of some prestige and professionalism, Paré is regarded as the "Father of Modern Surgery."

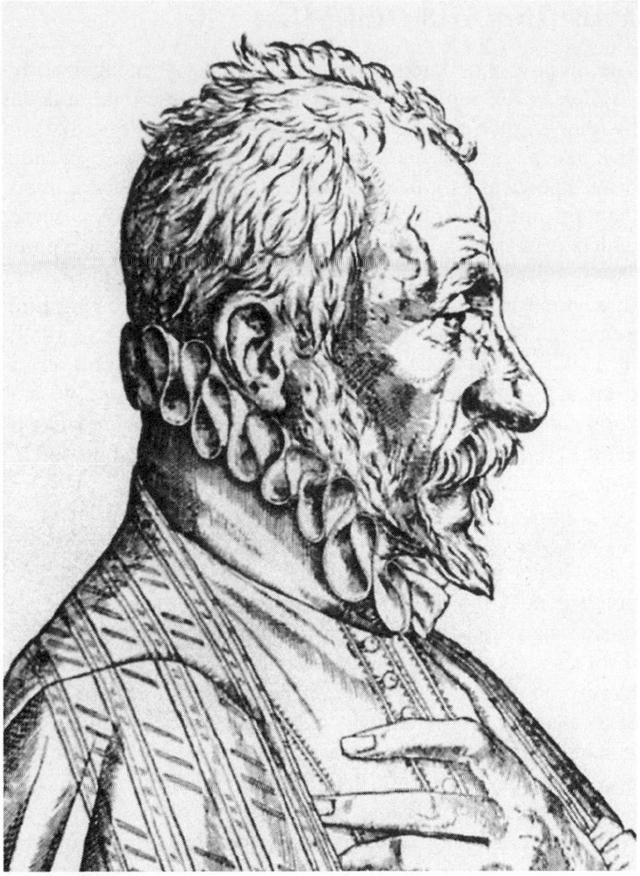

Ambroise Paré

PARKINSON, JAMES (1755-1824)

English Physician

Parkinson's disease is named after James Parkinson, who provided a detailed description of what he termed "shaking palsy" in an essay published in 1817. Parkinson was also the first to recognize a perforated appendix as a cause of death.

Parkinson was born in 1755, son of a surgeon and apothecary who ran his practice in London, England. Parkinson's early education included Latin, Greek, natural philosophy and shorthand—all subjects he considered indispensable to a doctor's basic training. It is believed that Parkinson took over the medical practice before his father died in 1784.

The following year, Parkinson attended a surgical lecture series by John Hunter, considered the founder of pathological anatomy in England and a researcher with wide interests in biology and medical science. Over his career, Parkinson developed similarly broad interests. In addition to his medical work, he wrote about chemistry, geology, sports, and with special influence, about paleontology (the science of fossils). Parkinson was also an aggressive social reformer. He is not known to have participated in riots or public demonstrations of the day, but he issued pamphlets calling for fair taxes, revolution without bloodshed, and civil rights for the disenfranchised, among many other reforms. On weekends, he established Sunday schools for the poor.

In 1805, Parkinson published a treatise about gout, observing that daily doses of soda provided considerable relief.

His best-know work is *Essay on the Shaking Palsy*, published in 1817. Describing what would later be known as Parkinson's disease, he observed: "The first symptoms perceived are, a slight sense of weakness, with a proneness to trembling in some particular part; ... but most importantly in one of the hands and arms." As the disorder progressed, Parkinson wrote, patients were forced to lean forward while walking, so much so that "... being at the same time, irresistibly impelled to take much quicker and shorter steps, and thereby to adopt unwillingly a running pace. In some cases it is found necessary to substitute running for walking." Still later, the tremors made even sleep difficult, Parkinson wrote. "It now seldom leaves him for a moment; but even when exhausted nature seizes a small portion of sleep, the motion becomes so violent as not only to shake the bed-hangings, but even the floor and sashes of the room."

Others had written previously about the so-called shaking palsy, including the ancient Greek doctor **Galen**, but Parkinson's description was so comprehensive that his name became synonymous with the disorder. He encouraged pathologists to take a greater interest in learning about shaking palsy.

PARKINSON'S DISEASE

The disease once known as "shaking palsy," recognized by physicians for hundreds of years, was first described in detail by the English physician James Parkinson (1755-1824) in 1817. As a result of his work, shaking palsy gradually became better known as *Parkinson's disease.* By some estimates, more than 1.5 million Americans suffer from Parkinson's Disease, which primarily afflicts older people and usually develops slowly over a period of years causing slowness of movement (bradykinesia), gradual loss of muscular control, resting limb tremors, and gait disturbance (difficulty walking). Eventually the condition becomes so severe that the person becomes incapacitated. The cause of Parkinson's disease is usually not known; however, symptoms can appear after a **stroke**, **encephalitis**, carbon monoxide or manganese **poisoning**, and **head injury**.

James Parkinson was born in London on April 11, 1755, the son of a surgeon. He studied under the famous physician John Hunter (1728-1793) and later opened a thriving medical practice. In 1817, Parkinson completed his exhaustive study of shaking palsy, describing in detail the characteristics of the disorder and outlining the stages by which it develops. Based largely on a single post-mortem examination, he also hinted at a cause for the condition—a swelling of the medulla. This line of investigation was largely abandoned, however, for well over a century. Not until the 1970s did scientists obtain evidence for a possible cause of Parkinson's disease. Then, researchers began to receive reports of Parkinson's disease among users of certain types of illegal synthetically manufactured drugs. Eventually it became clear that Parkinson's disease results from the death of brain cells in the substantia nigra, a small area deep within the brainstem that produce the neurotransmitter, dopamine. With this knowledge, scientists began to explore methods for controlling symptoms of Parkinson's disease.

One approach is to provide patients with a drug known as L-dopa, a compound that is converted into dopamine in the brain. This therapy has been fairly successful, although it decreases in efficiency as the disease develops. In 1985, the Israeli researcher, Joussa Youdim, found that a compound called deprenyl slows the progress of Parkinson's disease; this drug has been used with considerable success on patients. However, eventually, these drugs produce dyskinesia—uncontrollable movements of the head and limbs. Thus, without drugs, the patient becomes rigid and cannot move; with them, certain movements are uncontrollable.

One promising treatment involves the grafting of brain cells to replace the dopamine-producing ones that have died. This procedure was first attempted by scientists from the United States and Sweden in the late 1970s using cells from fetal rats because the cells were still immature and capable of developing into the type of cell needed in the brain of the patient. In recent years, the procedure has been modified by the use of human fetal tissue, tissue taken from another part of the patient's body, and tissue genetically engineered to produce the missing dopamine. Another promising treatment is surgery called "stereotactic pallidotomy," first introduced by Dr. Lars Leksell in 1952 and reintroduced in the 1980s by a Finnish surgeon working in Sweden, Dr. Lauri Laitinen, who had worked with Leksell. In this procedure, a needle-fine probe is inserted through a tiny hole in the skull, positioned in a small area within the globus pallidus, and an electrical current is applied to destroy cells. Of 38 patients Laitinen treated in January, 1992, 80-90% had long-term relief of symptoms.

In 1997, researchers identified a gene thought to produce defective proteins which accumulate in the brain killing dopamine neurons and causing early-onset Parkinson's disease. Current research also shows that people who smoke may have only half the risk of contracting Parkinson's disease as do nonsmokers because monoamine oxidase B (MAO B), which breaks down dopamine, was found to be 40% lower in smokers than in nonsmokers. Researchers therefore speculate they would have more available dopamine and thus be less prone to Parkinson's. Which ingredient in cigarettes lowers MAO B is not yet known.

PARROT FEVER

Parrot fever is a rare infectious disease that causes **pneumonia** in humans. It is transmitted from pet birds or poultry. The illness is caused by chlamydia, a parasitic type of microorganism closely related to bacteria. Parrot fever is also called chlamydiosis, psittacosis or ornithosis.

Parrot fever, which is referred to as avian psittacosis when it infects birds, is caused by a type of Chlamydia known as *Chlamydia psittaci*. Pet birds in the parrot family, including parakeets, macaws, and cockatiels, are the most common carriers of the infection. Other birds that may also spread *C. psittaci* include pigeons, doves, mynah birds, and turkeys. Birds carrying the organism may appear healthy but can expel the parasite in their feces.

The symptoms of avian psittacosis include inactivity, loss of appetite, and ruffled feathers, **diarrhea**, runny eyes, and nasal discharge, and green or yellow-green urine. Sick birds can be treated with **antibiotics** by a veterinarian.

C. psittaci is usually spread from birds to humans through exposure to infected bird feces during cage cleaning or by handling infected birds. In humans, parrot fever can range in severity from minor flu-like symptoms to severe and life-threatening pneumonia.

Although a rare occurrence, humans can also spread the disease by person-to-person contact. If infected, symptoms usually develop within 5-14 days of exposure and include **fever**, **headache**, chills, loss of appetite, **cough**, and fatigue. In severe cases, the patient develops pneumonia. People who work in pet shops or who keep pet birds are the most likely to become infected.

Only about 100-200 cases of parrot fever are reported each year in the United States. It is possible, however, that the illness is more common since it is easily confused with other types of **influenza** or pneumonia. Doctors are most likely to consider a diagnosis of parrot fever if the patient has a recent history of exposure to birds. The diagnosis can be confirmed by blood tests for antibodies. In addition, a chest x ray may also be used to diagnose the pneumonia caused by *C.psittaci.*

Psittacosis is treated with oral antibiotics, which are typically prescribed for at least 10-14 days. Severely ill patients may be given intravenous antibiotics for the first few days of therapy. There is no effective vaccine against parrot fever.

The prognosis for recovery is excellent; with antibiotic treatment, more than 99% of patients with parrot fever recover. Severe infections, however, may be fatal to the elderly, the untreated, and persons with weak immune systems.

Birds imported into the United States as pets should be quarantined to ensure that they are not infected. Health authorities recommend that breeders and importers feed imported birds a special blend of feed mixed with antibiotics for 45 days to ensure that any *C. psittaci* organisms are destroyed before the birds are sold. In addition, bird cages and food and water bowls should be cleaned daily.

PASTEUR, LOUIS (1822-1895)

French chemist and microbiologist

Louis Pasteur was one of the most extraordinary scientists in history, leaving a legacy of scientific contributions which include an understanding of how microorganisms carry on the biochemical process of fermentation, the establishment of the causal relationship between microorganisms and disease, and the concept of destroying microorganisms to halt the transmission of communicable disease. These achievements led him to be called the founder of microbiology.

After his early education Pasteur went to Paris, studied at the Sorbonne, then began teaching chemistry while still a student. After being appointed chemistry professor at a new university in Lille, France, Pasteur began work on yeast cells and showed how they produce alcohol and carbon dioxide from sugar during the process of fermentation. Fermentation is a form of cellular respiration carried on by yeast cells, a way of getting energy for cells when there is no oxygen present. He found that fermentation would take place only when living yeast cells were present.

Establishing himself as a serious, hard-working chemist, Pasteur was called upon to tackle some of the problems plaguing the French beverage industry at the time. Of special concern was the spoiling of wine and beer, which caused great economic loss and tarnished France's reputation for fine vintage wines. Vintners wanted to know the cause of l'amer, a condition that was destroying the best burgundies. Pasteur looked at wine under the microscope and noticed that when aged properly the liquid contained little spherical yeast cells. But when the wine turned sour, there was a proliferation of bacterial cells which were producing lactic acid. Pasteur suggested that heating the wine gently at about 120°F would kill the bacteria that produced lactic acid and let the wine age properly. Pasteur's book *Etudes sur le Vin*, published in 1866 was a testament to two of his great passions—the scientific method and his love of wine. It caused another French Revolution—

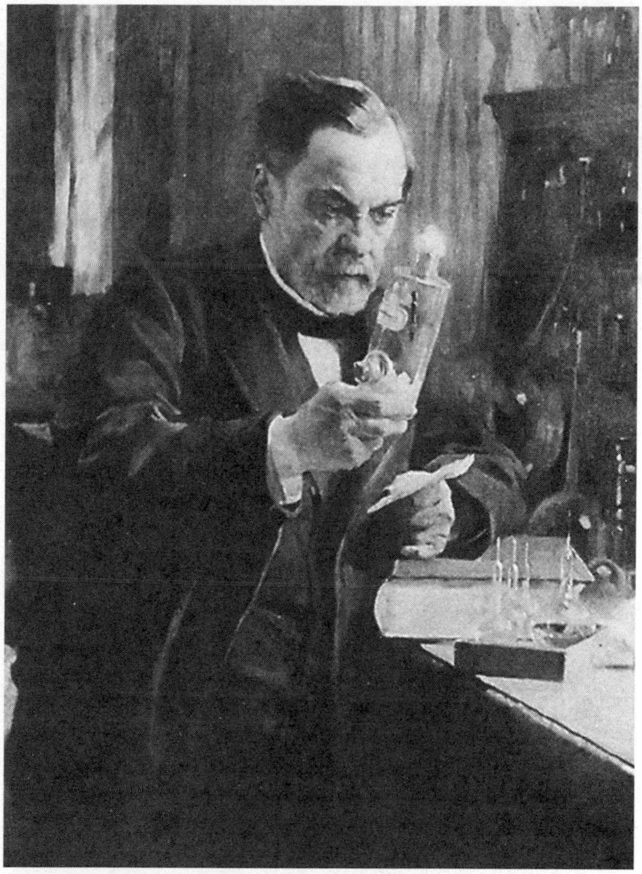

Louis Pasteur

one in wine-making, as Pasteur suggested that greater cleanliness was need to eliminate bacteria and that this could be done with heat. Some wine-makers were aghast at the thought but doing so solved the industry's problem.

The idea of heating to kill microorganisms was applied to other perishable fluids like milk and the idea of pasteurization was born. Several decades later in the United States the pasteurization of milk was championed by American bacteriologist **Alice Catherine Evans** who linked bacteria in milk with the disease **brucellosis**, a type of fever found in different variations in many countries.

In his work with yeast, Pasteur also found that air should be kept from fermenting wine, but was necessary for the production of vinegar. In the presence of oxygen, yeasts and bacteria break down alcohol into acetic acid—vinegar. Pasteur also informed the vinegar industry that vinegar production could be increased by adding more microorganisms to the fermenting mixture. Pasteur carried on many experiments with yeast. He showed that fermentation can take place without oxygen (*anaerobic* conditions), but that the process still involved living things such as yeast. He did several experiments to show (as **Lazzaro Spallanzani** had a century earlier) that living things do not arise spontaneously but rather come from other living things. To disprove the idea of spontaneous generation, Pasteur boiled meat extract and left it exposed to air in a flask with a long S-shaped neck. There was no decay observed because microorganisms from the air did not reach the extract. On the way to performing his experiment Pasteur had also invented what has come to be known as sterile technique, boiling or heating of instruments and food to prevent the proliferation of microorganisms.

In 1862 Pasteur was called upon to help solve a crisis in another ailing French industry. The silkworms that produced silk fabric were dying of an unknown disease. So armed with his microscope, Pasteur went to the south of France in 1865. He found the tiny parasites that were killing the silkworms and affecting their food, mulberry leaves. His solution seemed drastic at the time. He suggested destroying all the unhealthy worms and starting with new cultures. The solution worked and French silk scarves were back in the marketplace.

Pasteur then turned his attention to human and animal diseases. He had believed for some time that microscopic organisms cause disease and that these tiny microorganisms could travel from person to person spreading the disease. Other scientists had expressed this thought before, but Pasteur had more experience using the microscope and identifying different kinds of microorganisms such as bacteria and fungi.

In 1868, Pasteur suffered a stroke and much of his work thereafter was carried out by his wife Marie Laurent Pasteur. After seeing what military hospitals were like during the Franco-Prussian War, Pasteur impressed upon physicians that they should boil and sterilize their instruments. This was still not common practice in the nineteenth century.

Pasteur developed techniques for culturing and examining several disease-causing bacteria. He identified *Staphylococcus pyogenes*bacteria in boils and *Streptococcus pyogenes* in puerperal fever. He also cultured the bacteria that cause **cholera**. Once when injecting healthy chickens with cholera bacteria, he expected the chickens to get sick. Unknown to Pasteur, the bacteria were old and no longer virulent. The chickens failed to get the disease, but instead they received immunity against cholera. Thus Pasteur discovered that weakened microbes make a good vaccine by imparting immunity without actually producing the disease.

Pasteur then began work on a vaccine for **anthrax**, a disease that killed many animals and infected people who contracted it from their sheep and thus was known as ''woolsorters' disease.'' Anthrax causes sudden chills, high fever, pain, and can affect the brain. Pasteur experimented with weakening or attenuating the bacteria that cause anthrax, and in 1881 produced a vaccine that successfully prevented the deadly disease.

Pasteur's last great scientific achievement was developing a successful treatment for **rabies**, a deadly disease contracted from bites of an infected, rabid dog. Rabies, or hydrophobia, first causes terrible pain in the throat that prevents swallowing, then brings on spasms, fever, and finally death. Pasteur knew that rabies took weeks or even months to become active. He hypothesized that if people were given an injection after being bitten, it could prevent the disease from manifesting. After methodically producing a rabies vaccine from the spinal fluid of infected rabbits, Pasteur sought to test it. In 1885 nine-year-old Joseph Meister, who had been mauled and bitten by a rabid dog, was brought to Pasteur, and after a series of shots of the new rabies vaccine, the boy did not develop any of the deadly symptoms of rabies. Pasteur's triumphant success was a great relief to many worldwide.

To treat cases of rabies, the Pasteur Institute was established in 1888 with monetary donations coming from all over the world. It later became one of the most prestigious biological research institutions in the world. When Pasteur died in 1895 he was well-recognized for his outstanding achievements in science.

PASTEUR, MARIE LAURENT • See Pasteur, Louis

PATAU'S SYNDROME

Patau's syndrome, also called trisomy 13, occurs when a child is born with three copies of chromosome 13. Normally, two copies of the chromosome are inherited, one from each parent. The extra chromosome causes numerous physical and mental abnormalities. Owing mostly to heart defects, the lifespan of trisomy 13 babies is usually measured in days. Survivors have profound **mental retardation**.

Individuals normally inherit 23 chromosomes from each parent, for a total of 46 chromosomes. However, genetic errors can occur before or after conception. In the case of Patau's syndrome, a random error occurs, and the embryo has three copies of chromosome 13, rather than the normal two copies.

Trisomy 13 occurs in approximately 1 in 12,000 live births. In many cases, spontaneous abortion (miscarriage) occurs, and the fetus does not survive. The risks of trisomy 13 seem to increase with the mother's age, particularly if she is over 30. Male and female children are equally affected, and the syndrome occurs in all races.

Newborns with trisomy 13 have numerous internal and external abnormalities. Commonly, the front of the brain fails to divide into lobes or hemispheres, and the entire brain is unusually small. Children who survive infancy usually exhibit profound mental retardation.

Incomplete development of the optic (sight) and olfactory (**smell**) nerves often accompanies the brain defects, and the child may also be deaf. Frequently, a child with trisomy 13 has cleft lip, cleft palate, or both. Facial features are flattened and ears are malformed and lowset. Extra fingers or toes may be present in addition to other hand and foot malformations.

Patau's syndrome can be detected during **pregnancy** through the use of ultrasonography, amniocentesis, and other testing. In infants the abnormality can be confirmed by examining the infant's chromosomal pattern. However, Patau's syndrome cannot be cured. Although certain structural abnormalities can be treated through surgery, malformations are often numerous and severe. Decisions regarding measures to prolong life are best made on an individual basis by parents and doctors. Medical treatment may simply focus on ameliorating symptoms rather than prolonging life.

Approximately 82% of trisomy 13 babies die within their first month of life; only 5-10% survive to one year. Children who survive infancy require medical treatment to correct structural abnormalities and associated complications. Survival to adulthood is very rare. Only one adult is known to have survived to age 33.

PATENT MEDICINE

Patent medicines originated in 16th century England. These medicines were ready-made remedies and could be purchased to treat many conditions. Originally, the term referred to medicines that actually were patented. To receive a patent, however, the maker had to reveal all ingredients that went into the medicine. Inventors were often reluctant to reveal a formula and would just register the name of the medicine. In this way they could keep their ingredients secret while retaining exclusive use of a name. In time, all ready-made medicines whether they were patented or not became known as patent medicines.

The term patent medicine has a negative meaning today because of the amount of quackery tied to patent medicines in the 18th, 19th, and early 20th centuries. Some patent medicines actually did contain effective substances and worked as promised. Quinine, digitalis, ipecac, and other substances have genuine medical uses, and they were found in several patent medicines of the era. However, because patent medicine makers were not required to disclose ingredients, consumers bought medicines on faith. Unethical manufacturers took advantage of that faith. Some patent medicine makers heavily advertised cure-alls that contained nothing more than water, flavoring, and coloring. Other patent medicines supposedly contained exotic ingredients, such as snake oil, which inferred special curative powers. The patent medicines seemed to work because many conditions for which they were advertised simply went away by themselves. If a person were to take a patent medicine, he or she would naturally attribute a return to health to the medicine. Through this ploy, patent medicine makers had many people willing to write testimonials about the effectiveness of the medicine. These testimonials served as the best kind of advertising. In most cases, even if patent medicines didn't help, they didn't cause any harm either. However, some patent medicines were dangerous. Tonics for general health, bitters for stomach complaints, and medicines for ''female weakness'' often contained high percentages of alcohol. Patent medicines meant to soothe teething babies contained **morphine**. Cures for colds and congestion contained heroin or cocaine. Used indiscriminately, these medicines could be addictive, sickening, or even deadly.

At the beginning of the 20th century, the tide began to turn against patent medicines. The public had been defrauded too often and it was angry. In 1906, the United States Congress passed the Pure Food and Drug Act. This law required manufacturers to list the amounts of alcohol, opium, cocaine and other substances in their medicines if they were present. It did not prohibit these substances from being sold over the counter, however. Still, many patent medicines were forced off the shelf by this law and others had to change their content or advertising. There were high hopes that this law would mean the end of ineffective and dangerous patent medicines. However, the law had loopholes, and there was incomplete knowledge about some substances. One such substance was radium, a highly radioactive material. For a short time after the discovery of radioactivity, both the medical community and the public believed that it had special curative powers. Patent medicine makers picked up on this belief and produced medicines to meet the public demand. Radium could be taken by injection, tablet, suppository, or inhalation, and it was advertised as a cure for baldness, impotence, aging, rheumatism, and a variety of other ills. Radioactive patent medicines were sold into the early 1930s, demonstrating that the Pure Food and Drug Act and other laws passed in 1912 and 1914 weren't stringent enough. Progressively stricter regulation followed in the Federal Food, Drug and Cosmetic Act (1938), the Durham-Humphrey Act (1951), and the Kefauver-Harris Amendment (1962). These laws imposed strict controls on non-prescription medicines, but have not completely eliminated the production and sale of patent medicines.

See also Quackery

PATHOLOGY

Pathology is the science that studies the nature of diseases and the changes they produce in the body.

Since ancient times, physicians have concerned themselves with the distinguishing features of health and disease. Until the early 19th century, however, their ideas were based on a theory of **humors** (that is, elemental fluids in the body), rather than systematic examination of body parts and disease processes. Disease was believed to result from an imbalance of these humors. **Dissection** of dead bodies to learn about disease was not allowed by religious leaders and obstructed progress in the study of anatomy and pathology through the Middle Ages. By the Renaissance, however, reports from post-mortem dissections began to provide a new and important source of information contributing to medical knowledge. In his *Universa medicina,* **Jean François Fernel** (1497-1558) introduced the term pathology to describe the abnormalities detected by anatomists when they dissected cadavers. But Fernel still held to the ancient teachings of the humors.

In the 18th century, the anatomical basis of disease began to emerge. Public hospitals provided a seemingly endless supply of corpses for dissections after death, and hospitals became centers for teaching and practicing morbid anatomy (the abnormal structures in the body associated with disease). By the second half of the 18th century, in both America and Europe, surgeons and physicians had already begun to correlate signs and symptoms of patients with findings from autopsies after the patients died.

In 1761, **Giovanni Battista Morgagni** (1682-1771) published the first textbook to systematically detail morbid anatomy and to locate diseases within individual organs. But humoral theories remained firmly entrenched, and the study of anatomy was still limited to what pathologists could observe of organs, muscles, and bones with the naked eye. All the same, as a result of their investigations into corpses, pathologists in many different countries were beginning to ask questions about what made a tumor benign or malignant, the nature of pus, how wounds heal, and whether blood clots are beneficial or harmful.

Major progress was quick to follow. In France, **Marie François Xavier Bichat** (1771-1802) studied tissues rather than organs. One of his important contributions was the announcement that the disease of a tissue is the same no matter which organ the tissue is in. Bichat worked without the aid of a microscope. But the introduction of improved compound microscopes in the 1820s made it possible to study both normal and diseased tissue more extensively and more accurately than ever before. In 1858, **Rudolf Carl Virchow** (1821-1902) proved conclusively that diseases arose in the cells of organs and tissues, not in the organs and tissues generally. Not long after, the investigations of **Louis Pasteur** (1822-1895) and **Robert Koch** (1843-1910) into bacteria were a major step in rounding out understanding of how disease works.

By the end of the 19th century, pathology had come into its own as a separate medical specialty. Today, pathologists perform, evalute, or supervise diagnostic tests, using materials from living or dead patients. Their work is mostly carried in the laboratory, and they work closely with physicians who are directly in charge of patients. Among the materials a pathologist examines (in procedures generally known as biopsies) are surgically removed body parts, blood and other body fluids, urine, feces, and so on. Pathologists also practice **autopsy**, which allows them to reconstruct the end of the physical life of a dead person by providing information about the workings of disease they would not be able to get any other way. It is not possible for any one person to know all there is to know about pathology, so pathologists who specialize in one area or another frequently work together. For example, pediatric pathology studies disease processes in children. Forensic pathology is a subspecialty whose goal is to clarify crimes or legal issues.

Advances in laboratory techniques and increasingly fine-scaled instrumentation have greatly expanded the information available to the pathologist in determining the causes of disease. Research in **genetics** is also changing the study of pathology. More and more, pathologists are being called on to examine the molecular structure of DNA and to identify molecular markers of disease, as well as to study the impact of environmental factors on heredity.

Training in pathology requires a medical degree and roughly five years of postgraduate study.

Patient's Rights

The health care rights of patients have been the subject of much public debate and legislative action in the latter half of the 20th century. The fundamental right to quality medical care and compensation for **medical malpractice**, the right to informed consent, and the right to health care privacy, are all protected under United States congressional law. While these and other laws ensure many rights for medical patients, the changing nature of medical knowledge and care also ensures the continued need to regulate the relationships among patients, care-givers, and care-giving institutions.

One of the first comprehensive statements of a patient's rights was drafted by the American Hospital Association in 1973. Today it must be posted in the corridors of every hospital facility the association has accredited and includes twelve basic rights:

1. A patient has the right to considerate and respectful care.

2. A patient has the right to receive complete information from a physician about a patient's diagnosis, treatment plan, and prognosis.

3. To obtain information about the specific nature of a proposed treatment or procedure, a disclosure of the risks involved, and information about medical alternatives.

4. To be able to refuse treatment and to be informed of the medical consequences.

5. Privacy during discussion of one's medical condition and while undergoing medical care.

6. To expect all records related to medical care will be kept confidential.

7. Reasonable efforts are made to respond to a patient's request for services, and that a patient not be transferred to another medical facility without being advised of the need to be transferred and without insuring that the new facility will accept transfer of the patient.

7. To be able to obtain information about the relationships amongst care providers in the hospital and related medical and educational institutions. This is designed to protect patients from conflicting interests that might affect quality of care.

8. To be able to obtain information about human experimentation and research that might affect treatment or care, and to refuse to take part in such experimentation and research.

9. To expect reasonable continuity of care. This is meant to assure the patient that, for example, diagnoses will be followed up with continued treatment.

10. To be able to examine and receive an explanation of the hospital bill.

11. To be informed of hospital rules and regulations that apply to patient conduct. This one provides benefit to both patient and hospital.

12. Though the quality of resolution varies widely, most hospitals have grievance committees that will hear complaints and staff representatives that act as patient advocates when a right is called into question.

Since the Hospital Patients Bill of Rights was drafted in 1973, a number of important laws related to patient's rights have been enacted by state and federal government. The Nursing Home Reform Act, passed by Congress in 1987 and put into effect in 1990, guarantees the standard of care in nursing home facilities, regulating aspects of care such as the provision of nutritious food, the respectful and courteous treatment of patients, and the quality of rehabilitation services. The federal Emergency Medical Treatment and Active Labor Act of 1989, and similar state laws, protect patients who are in need of emergency care from being turned away from a hospital emergency room and or being denied treatment. In 1991, Congress passed the Patient Self-Determination Act, providing greater personal control over the medical care given at the end of life. The Federal Privacy Act of 1974 provided loose guarantees of protection for medical records. More recently additional laws have been passed to ensure the confidentiality of medical records. Bills to guarantee patients rights in Health Maintenance Organizations are currently under congressional review. As the 21st century is approached and medical procedures become more complex and costly, as infectious diseases and genetic conditions become easier to diagnose, and the ability to sustain and prolong life continues to improve, the need for new legislation will be even more prominent.

PAVLOV, IVAN PETROVITCH (1849-1936)

Russian physiologist

Born on September 14, 1849, in Ryazan, Russia, Pavlov was the son of a village priest. He planned to follow family tradition by becoming a priest himself. While at a theological seminary, however, Pavlov read Charles Darwin's *Origin of the Species* and found he really wanted a career in science instead. Soon afterward, in 1870, Pavlov transferred from the seminary to St. Petersburg University. There his professors included two renowned Russian chemists, Dmitri Mendeleev and Alexander Butlerov (1828-1886). Pavlov studied both chemistry and physiology. He obtained a medical degree from St. Petersburg Military Medical Academy in 1879, and a Ph.D. in 1883.

For the next few years, Pavlov studied cardiovascular and gastrointestinal physiology in Germany, then returned to the Medical Academy, where he was appointed Professor of Physiology and also conducted most of his research investigations. Pavlov's first major studies centered around the physiology of digestion. He was particularly interested in working out the nervous mechanism that controlled the secretion of the digestive tract's various glands.

In 1889, Pavlov designed one of his most important animal experiments: after severing a dog's gullet, he pulled the upper end out through an opening in the animal's neck. From then on, while the dog could be fed, his food would drop out through the open gullet rather than reach his stomach. Nevertheless, as Pavlov pointed out, after each feeding, the animal's gastric juices would flow, suggesting that nerves in his mouth must have been stimulated. These nerves must have then sent a message to the brain which, by way of other nerves, must have then stimulated the stomach's digestive glands, causing them secrete the juices. Pavlov performed a number of other experiments that not only helped demonstrate how digestion worked in a living animal, but also helped establish the importance of the autonomic **nervous system** in controlling the digestive process. For his work, Pavlov received the 1904 Nobel Prize in physiology or medicine.

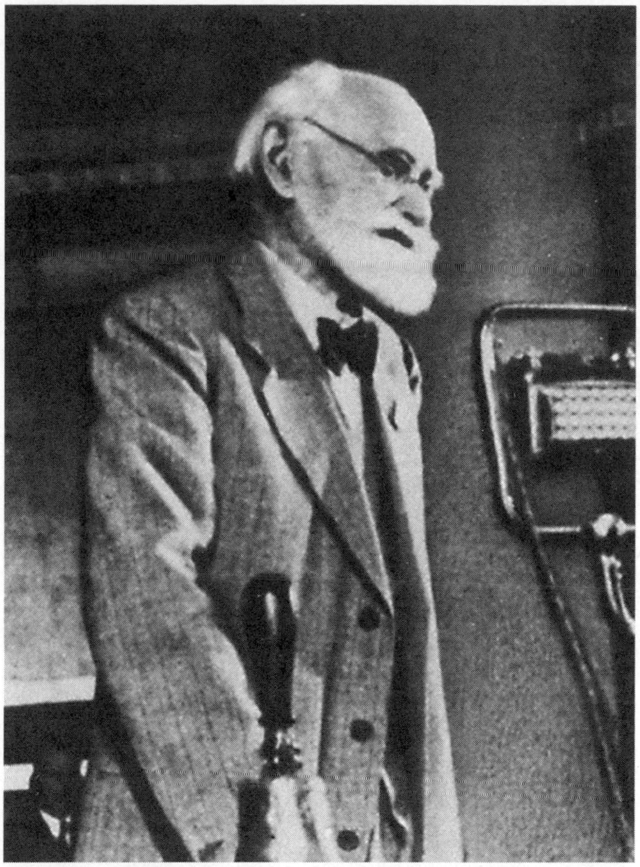

Ivan Petrovitch Pavlov

Ironically, Pavlov then went on to design the series of animal experiments for which he is most famous: the ''salivating dog'' studies. In these studies, Pavlov confined a laboratory dog in a room that was kept soundproof in order to eliminate distracting noises. The dog was held in place by a loose harness, was fed by an automatic apparatus that was operated from outside the room, and had a small measuring tube attached to his cheek to collect the flow of saliva from his parotid gland. The dog's saliva was measured under varying situations and, before long, Pavlov was able to report that the dog's salivation began, as expected, as soon as he saw his food (a natural and unconditioned reflex). However, if a neutral sound, such as a bell, always accompanied the offering of his food, the dog began to salivate as soon as he heard the bell—even if the food *did not* immediately appear. Pavlov termed this second reaction a conditioned reflex—a reaction that was not really instinctive but had been learned through a sequence of associations.

Pavlov's continuing investigation of the conditioned reflex—although it took place in a laboratory and was conducted on animals—clearly had implications for human learning behavior as well. Psychiatrists and psychologists around the world began incorporating the concept into a number of different doctrines, particularly those relating to behavioral psychology. Pavlov continued his own studies, even after the

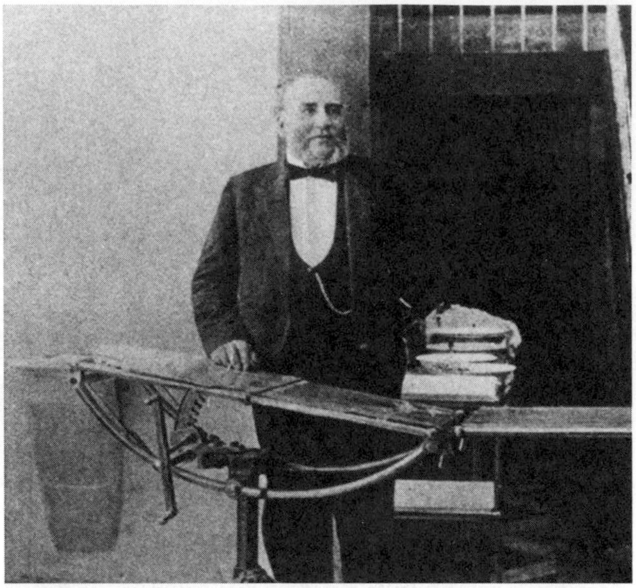

Jules-Émile Pean

Communist Revolution and, although he himself was an outspoken anti-Communist, he remained one of Russia's most highly treasured scientists until his death in Leningrad on February 27, 1936.

Pean, Jules Émile (1830-1898)

French Surgeon

Considered one of the founders of modern gynecology, Pean was so famous in his homeland for his advances in gynecological surgery and other innovations that Henri Toulouse-Lautrec (1864-1901) painted the surgeon's portrait.

Pean was born in Chateaudun, France and received his education from the College de Chartres. He began studying medicine at age 19 at the University of Paris, where he insisted on using aseptic surgical techniques throughout the 1850s despite his colleagues' general lack of concern about this crucial factor. Pean wrote the first of his many books, The Splenectomy, in 1860. He was instrumental in developing the arterial clamp in 1862, and by 1868, the gifted young man was chief surgeon of all hospitals in Paris.

In 1874, Pean was appointed chief of services at St. Louis Hospital. He wrote *The Elements of Pathological Surgery* the following year, *Lessons in Clinical Surgery* in 1876, and in 1877 a book on the use of hemostatic forceps, which he had invented in 1868.

In the realm of gynecology, which was in its infancy in the mid-1800s, Pean was a force of innovation and integrity. He invented effective ways to remove the ovaries and performed a vaginal **hysterectomy** for carcinoma in 1890. In addition, he devised a method for gastrectomy and is believed to have performed the first surgery to correct diverticula of the bladder in 1895. Late in the century, Pean also attempted the first known total joint arthroplasty, although unsuccessfully. He died in 1898.

Peer Pressure

Peers are the individuals with whom a child or adolescent identifies, who are usually but not always of the same age-group. Peer pressure occurs when the individual experiences implicit or explicit persuasion, sometimes amounting to coercion, to adopt similar values, beliefs, and goals, or to participate in the same activities as those in the peer group.

Although it is usually conceived of as primarily a negative influence acting on adolescents or teens, peer pressure can be a positive influence as well, and it can act on children at any age, depending on their level of contact with others. The influence of peer pressure is usually addressed in relation to the relative influence of the family on an individual. Some characteristics that peer groups offer and which families may be lacking are: (1) a strong belief structure; (2) a clear system of rules; and (3) communication and discussion about taboo subjects such as drugs, sex, and religion.

Peer pressure is strongly associated with level of academic success, drug and substance use, and gender role conformity. The level of peer influence increases with age, and resistance to peer influence often declines as the child gains independence from the family or caretakers, yet has not fully formed an autonomous identity. One study in particular confirms other research findings that the values of the peer group with whom the high schooler spends the most time are a stronger factor in the student's level of academic success than the values, attitudes, and support provided by the family. Compared to others who started high school with the same grades, students whose families were not especially supportive but who spent time with an academically oriented peer group were successful, while those students whose families stressed academics but who spent time with peers whose orientation was not academic performed less well.

The peer pressure study contradicts prevailing ideas about the influence of families on the success of racial and cultural minorities such as Asians and African Americans. While some Asian families were not especially involved in their children's education, the students, who found little social support of any type, tended to band together in academic study groups. Conversely, African American students, whose families tended to be highly involved in and supportive of education, were subjected to intense peer pressure not to perform academically. According to the study, the African American peer groups associated the activities of studying and spending time at the library with ''white'' behavior, and adopted the idea that the student who gets good grades, participates in school activities, or speaks standard English is betraying his racial heritage and community. Consequently, gifted students ''dumb-down'' as they make the choice between academics and ''fitting in.'' Research suggests that this type of peer pressure contributes to a decline in the grades of African American students (especially males) as early as the first through fourth grades.

Peer pressure similarly compels students of all ethnic backgrounds to engage in other at-risk behaviors such as cigarette **smoking**, truancy, drug use, sexual activity, fighting, theft, and daredevil stunts. Again, peer group values and attitudes influence, more strongly than do family values, the level of teenage alcohol use. Regardless of the parenting style, peer pressure also influences the degree to which children, especially girls, conform to expected gender roles. Up until about grade six, girls' performance in science and math are on par with that of boys, but during adolescence girls' test scores and level of expressed interest declines. The tendency is to abandon competition with boys in favor of placing more emphasis on relationships and on physical appearance.

Ideally the child, adolescent, or teen should make decisions based on a combination of values internalized from the family, values derived from thinking independently, and values derived from friends and other role models. In order to achieve this balance, rather than attempting to minimize peer influence, families and schools must provide strong alternative beliefs, patterns of behavior, and encourage formation of peer groups that engage in positive academic, athletic, artistic, and social activities.

In order to rival their children's peers, parents should convey a strong, clear (not necessarily rigid) value structure and open avenues of communication early in life, while the child is first being exposed to the group persuasions of preschoolers. In situations where decisions might be made about peer pressure, parents who are hesitant to discourage their children's independence and individuality often send vague messages or no message at all to the child about their perspective on the matter. Voicing parental opinion provides guidance, which the child can choose to accept or reject in future situations. In turn, the knowledge that the child is being guided on important matters gives parents a sense of confidence when the child succumbs to the numerous small, inconsequential peer pressures concerning interests, toys, and styles of dress throughout grade school.

Adults may vary in their level of independence from groups, the degree to which they follow the crowd, but even the most popular, independent teen feels the strong effect of peer pressure. Techniques of resisting teen peer pressure include:

1. Observe people and the groups with whom they socialize. Observe what they do and the consequences of their actions. When someone tries to argue ''everyone's doing it,'' you can prove otherwise. Make choices about who you spend time with, instead of joining a group just because it's there.

2. Avoid situations that present problems—parties with drugs, being alone with a boyfriend or girlfriend who might pressure you.

3. Communicate: Say ''No'' forcefully and with eye contact. (If you do not believe yourself, they will not either.) Talk about it. Find someone who feels the same way you do.

4. Anticipate what your friends will say or do and decide beforehand how you will react. Consider all the alternatives, including the consequences of doing it their way. Is it a matter of wearing something you do not like, or is it a matter of damaging your body?

5. If you find yourself anticipating conflict too often, seriously think about finding a new friend or set of friends. Start off gradually, spending less and less time with the person who is pressuring you.

6. Know yourself. Know what moods might make you more susceptible to negative peer influence. Know (or figure out) what activities build your **self-esteem**. Know why you are doing whatever you do everyday—be aware of your actions.

Two primary areas in which schools can discourage negative peer pressure and encourage formation of positive peer groups are in peer leader programs and in collaborative learning practices. Virtually every school trains student peer leaders to participate in **counseling**, **support groups**, drug or violence prevention programs, or peer mentoring and tutoring programs. For these programs, students are trained in cognitive awareness, goal setting, problem identification, decision-making, and communication skills in order to lead, coach, and support other students. Peer leader programs implicitly combat peer pressure as the students act as positive role models for other teens.

PELLAGRA

Pellagra, a niacin deficiency disease, begins unremarkably, usually with weakness, skin rash, mouth sores, and loss of appetite. Unless checked, however, it gradually worsens, producing severe inflammation of the skin, mental disturbances, and diarrhea—followed all too often by death. The word *pellagra* is Italian for ''rough skin,'' a description of the rough, scaly skin seen in most pellagra patients.

The disease was first noticed by scientists in Europe around 1720, just about the time that maize (or Indian corn) was beginning to be heavily imported from the Americas and planted in many countries. In 1735, the symptoms of pellagra were described by Spanish physician Gaspar Casal (1679-1759), who correctly observed that the disease seemed to be associated with maize-based diets. At the time, however, most scientists believed the disease was caused by a toxin somehow produced by maize, particularly by wet or spoiled maize, and spent many wasted years hunting for the elusive germ. Pellagra had always been troublesome in the American South where both corn and cornmeal were dietary staples. However, it was not until 1907 when a major epidemic began that the government launched a number of serious investigative studies. (The epidemic peaked in 1928, when close to 7,000 deaths were attributed to pellagra, and roughly 20,000 pellagra sufferers were seen in Georgia alone.) One of those investigating the problem was Joseph Goldberger (1874-1929), a doctor who from 1913 on devoted himself to finding a solution.

A few researchers, such as **Casimir Funk** (1884-1967), had already suggested that pellagra might be caused by an inadequate diet, and Goldberger and his associates agreed. Pellagra, they found, attacked people who, largely because of poverty, had diets that were often restricted to corn meal, salt pork, lard, and molasses. Milk, meat, and eggs were conspicuously absent but, when these were added to the diet, the patients' conditions dramatically improved. To test whether a limited diet could really cause pellagra, Goldberger conducted an experiment in 1915 in which volunteer prisoners in the study were placed on a typical meat-and milk-free cornmeal diet. Within six months, when virtually all prisoners developed pellagra—a pellagra that showed no signs of being infectious—Goldberger restored the meat and milk and promptly saw his patients restored to health. Goldberger concluded that pellagra was a dietary deficiency disease that could be cured by a "P-P factor" (pellagra preventive) that was clearly lacking in corn, but that could probably be found in meat or milk. Goldberger and his associates suspected that the high tryptophan, or amino acid, level in milk was involved in the cure of pellagra.

More than thirty years later, Conrad Arnold Elvehjem (1901-1962), an American biochemist, finally proved that the P-P factor was nicotinic acid, or niacin, one of the B **vitamin**s, which was indeed involved in tryptophan **metabolism**.

Pelvic examination

The pelvic examination is an important component of preventive health care. It is essential for early detection of genital cancers, infections, **sexually transmitted diseases**, or any other abnormalities. In addition to being valuable in preventing disease, the pelvic examination plays a very important part in the diagnosis and course of such diseases as uterine fibroids, pelvic inflammatory disease, status of pregnancy, etc.

It is recommended that women have an annual exam every year beginning at age 18, or within six months of the first sexual intercourse. During the exam, the vulva, vagina, and cervix are examined for any signs of diseases, infection, or abnormalities. The routine pelvic exam is done by a medical professional (gynecologist, general practitioner, or nurse practitioner).

When a woman first arrives for the pelvic exam, she will be asked for information regarding her medical background and **menstruation** and contraceptive history. During the pelvic exam, the woman will be asked to lie on her back on the examination table, with knees bent and feet in stirrups at the end of the table. This position makes it easier for the clinician to conduct the examination. First, the medical practitioner visually examines the vulvar (genital) area for any abnormalities.

After the external genitalia has been checked, a metal or plastic speculum will be inserted into the vagina. The speculum holds open the vaginal wall so that the practitioner can see the cervix (the opening to the uterus). With the help of a tiny cervical brush that is inserted through the speculum, the physician will lightly scrape the cervix and vagina in order to obtain some cells from it. These cells will be smeared on a glass slide and sent to the laboratory for examination. This procedure called a Pap smear allows for the early detection of precancerous cells. The physician may also take extra cell samples to test for sexually transmitted diseases or vaginal infections.

After this procedure, the speculum is gently removed, and the physician conducts a bi-manual examination. It is called bi-manual because both hands are used. The clinician places one hand on the abdomen and inserts a gloved finger into the vagina. While applying slight pressure on the abdomen with one hand, with the other hand the physician will feel the uterus, fallopian tubes, and ovaries. This helps the doctor to determine the size, mobility, shape, position, surface texture, and amount of tenderness of the uterus and ovaries. It also enables identification of any cysts or masses that may be present.

While the entire procedure may feel awkward and cause a small amount of pain and discomfort, this can be greatly minimized by relaxing the pelvic muscles. It is very important to avoid the use of douches and vaginal creams or medications for at least 48 hours prior to the pelvic exam because these substances can distort the appearance of the cells that will be studied in the Pap smear. For this reason, the test should not be scheduled when the woman is having her monthly period. It is also recommended that a woman not have sexual intercourse for 24 hours before the Pap smear is done

It is recommended that a woman have a pelvic exam and Pap smear once a year. If a woman has several sexual partners or has had an abnormal Pap smear in the past, her doctor may recommend that she be seen more often.

See also PAP test

Pelvic inflammatory disease

Pelvic inflammatory disease (PID) is a term used to describe any infection in the lower female reproductive tract that spreads upward to the upper female reproductive tract. The lower female genital tract consists of the vagina and the cervix. The upper female genital tract consists of the body of the uterus, the fallopian or uterine tubes, and the ovaries.

PID, also called salpingitis (inflammation of the fallopian tubes), endometritis (inflammation of the inside lining of the body of the uterus), or pelvic **peritonitis** (inflammation inside of the abdominal cavity surrounding the female reproductive organs), is the most common and most serious consequence of infection with **sexually transmitted diseases** (STDs) in women.

Over one million cases of PID are diagnosed annually in the United States, and it is the most common cause for hospitalization of reproductive-age women. Sexually active women aged 15-25 are at highest risk for developing PID. The disease can also occur, although less frequently, in women having monogamous sexual relationships.The most serious consequences of PID are increased risk of **infertility** and **ectopic pregnancy** (the fertilized ovum is implanted outside of the uterine cavity).

To understand PID, it is helpful to understand the basics of inflammation. Inflammation is the body's response to disease-causing microorganisms. The affected body part may swell due to accumulation of fluid in the tissue or may become reddened due to an excessive accumulation of blood. A discharge (pus) may be produced that consists of white blood cells and dead tissue. Following inflammation, scar tissue, called fibrosis, may form. Adhesions of fibrous tissue form and cause organs or parts of organs to stick together.

PID may be used synonymously with the following terms:

- Salpingitis (Inflammation of the fallopian tubes)
- Endometritis (Inflammation of the inside lining of the body of the uterus)
- Tubo-ovarian **abscess**es (Abscesses in the tubes and ovaries)
- Pelvic **peritonitis** (Inflammation inside of the abdominal cavity surrounding the female reproductive organs).

A number of factors affect the risk of developing PID. They include:

- Age. The incidence of PID is very high in younger women and decreases as a woman ages.
- Race. The incidence of PID is 8-10 times higher in non-whites than in whites.
- Socioeconomic status. The higher incidence of PID in women of lower socioeconomic status is due in part to a woman's lack of education and awareness of health and disease and her accessibility to medical care.
- **Contraception**. Induced abortion, use of an **IUD**, non-use of barrier contraceptives such as **condom**s, and frequent douching are all associated with a higher risk of developing PID.
- Lifestyle. High risk behaviors, such as drug and alcohol abuse, early age of first intercourse, number of sexual partners, and **smoking** all are associated with a higher risk of developing PID.
- Types of sexual practices. Intercourse during menses and frequent intercourse may offer more opportunities for the admission of pathogenic organisms to the inside of the uterus.
- Disease. 60-75% of cases of PID are associated with STDs. A prior episode of PID increases the chances of developing subsequent infections.

The two major causes of STDs are the organisms, *Neisseria gonorrhoeae* and *Chlamydia trachomatis*. The main symptom of *N. gonorrheae* infection (**gonorrhea**) is a vaginal discharge of mucus and pus. Sometimes bacteria from the colon normally in the vaginal cavity may travel upward to infect the upper female genital organs, facilitated by the infection with gonorrhea. Infections with *C. trachomatis* and other organisms are more likely to have mild or no symptoms.

Normally the cervix produces mucus which acts as a barrier to prevent disease-causing microorganisms, called pathogens, from entering the uterus and moving upward to the tubes and ovaries. This barrier may be breached in two ways. A sexually transmitted pathogen, usually a single organism, invades the lining cells, alters them, and gains entry. Another way for organisms to gain entry happens when trauma or alteration to the cervix occurs. **Childbirth**, spontaneous or induced abortion, or use of an intrauterine contraceptive device (IUD) are all conditions that may alter or weaken the normal lining cells, making them susceptible to infection, usually by several organisms. During **menstruation**, the cervix widens and may allow pathogens entry into the uterine cavity.

Recent evidence suggests that bacterial vaginosis (BV), a bacterial infection of the vagina, may be associated with PID. BV results from the alteration of the balance of normal organisms in the vagina, by douching, for example. While the balance is altered, conditions are formed that favor the overgrowth of anaerobic bacteria, which thrive in the absence of free oxygen. A copious discharge is usually present. Should some trauma occur in the presence of anaerobic bacteria, such as menses, abortion, intercourse, or childbirth, these organisms may gain entrance to the upper genital organs.

The most common symptom of PID is pelvic **pain**. However, many women with PID have symptoms so mild that they may be unaware that an infection exists.

In acute salpingitis, a common form of PID, swelling of the fallopian tubes may cause tenderness on **physical examination**. **Fever** may be present. Abscesses may develop in the tubes, ovaries, or in the surrounding pelvic cavity. Infectious discharge may leak into the peritoneal cavity and cause peritonitis, or abscesses may rupture causing a life-threatening surgical emergency.

Chronic salpingitis may follow an acute attack. Subsequent to inflammation, scarring and resulting adhesions may result in chronic pain and irregular menses. Due to blockage of the tubes by scar tissue, women with chronic salpingitis suffer a high risk of having an ectopic pregnancy. The fertilized ovum is unable to travel down the fallopian tube to the uterus and implants itself in the tube, on the ovary, or in the peritoneal cavity. This condition can also be a life-threatening surgical emergency.

IUD usage has been strongly associated with the development of PID. Bacteria may be introduced to the uterine cavity while the IUD is being inserted or may travel up the tail of the IUD from the cervix into the uterus. Uterine tissue in association with the IUD shows areas of inflammation that may increase its susceptibility to pathogens.

Susceptibility to STDs involves many factors, some of which are not known. The ability of the organism to produce disease and the circumstances that place the organism in the right place at a time when a trauma or alteration to the lining cells has occurred are factors. The individual's own immune response also helps to determine whether infection occurs.

If PID is suspected, the physician will take a complete medical history and perform an internal pelvic examination. Other diseases that may cause pelvic pain, such as **appendicitis** and **endometriosis**, must be ruled out. If pelvic examination reveals tenderness or pain in that region, or tenderness on movement of the cervix, these are good physical signs that PID is present.

Specific diagnosis of PID is difficult to make because the upper pelvic organs are hard to reach for samplings. The physician may take samples directly from the cervix to identify the organisms that may be responsible for infection. Two blood tests may help to establish the existence of an inflammatory process. A positive C-reactive protein (CRP) and an elevated erythrocyte sedimentation rate (ESR) indicate the presence of inflammation. The physician may take fluid from the cavity surrounding the ovaries called the *cul de sac*; this fluid may be examined directly for bacteria or may be used for culture. Diagnosis of PID may also be done using a laparoscope, but **laparoscopy** is expensive, and it is an invasive procedure which carries some risk for the patient.

The goals of treatment are to reduce or eliminate the clinical symptoms and abnormal physical findings, to get rid of the microorganisms, and to prevent long term consequences such as infertility and the possibility of ectopic pregnancy. If acute salpingitis is suspected, treatment with **antibiotics** should begin immediately. Early intervention is crucial to keep the fallopian tubes undamaged. The patient is usually treated with at least two broad spectrum antibiotics that can kill both *N. gonorrhoeae* and *C. trachomatis* plus other types of bacteria that may have the potential to cause infection. Hospitalization may be required to ensure compliance. Treatment for chronic PID may involve **hysterectomy**, which may be helpful in some cases. If a woman is diagnosed with PID, she should see that her sexual partner is also treated to prevent the possibility of reinfection.

Alternative therapy should be complementary to antibiotic therapy. For pain relief, an experienced practitioner may apply castor oil packs, or use **acupressure** or **acupuncture**. Some herbs, such as *Echinacea* (*Echinacea* spp.) and calendula (*Calendula officinalis*) are believed to have antimicrobial activity and may be taken to augment the action of prescribed antibiotics. General tonic herbs, as well as good nutrition and rest, are important in recovery and strengthening after an episode of PID. Blue cohosh (*Caulophyllum thalictroides*) and false unicorn root (*Chamaelirium luteum*) are recommended as tonics for the general well-being of the female genital tract.

PID can be cured if the initial infection is treated immediately. If infection is not recognized, as frequently happens, the process of tissue destruction and scarring that results from inflammation of the tubes results in irreversible changes in the tube structure that cannot be restored to normal. Subsequent bouts of PID increase a woman's risks manyfold. Thirty to forty percent of cases of female infertility are due to acute salpingitis.

With modern antibiotic therapy, **death** from PID is almost nonexistent. In rare instances, death may occur from the rupture of tubo-ovarian abscesses and the resulting infection in the abdominal cavity. One recent study has linked infertility, a consequence of PID, with a higher risk of **ovarian cancer**.

The prevention of PID is a direct result of the prevention and prompt recognition and treatment of STDs or of any suspected infection involving the female genital tract. The main symptom of infection is an abnormal discharge. To distinguish an abnormal discharge from the mild fluctuations of normal discharge associated with the menstrual cycle takes vigilance and self-awareness. Sexually active women must be able to detect symptoms of lower genital tract disease. Ideally these women will be able to have a frank dialogue regarding their sexual history, risks for PID, and treatment options with their physicians. Also, these women should have open discussions with their sexual partners regarding disclosure of significant symptoms of possible infection.

Lifestyle changes should be geared to preventing the transfer of organisms when the body's delicate lining cells are unprotected or compromised. Barrier contraceptives, such as condoms, diaphragms, and cervical caps should be used. Women in monogamous relationships should use barrier contraceptives during menses and take their physician's advice regarding intercourse following abortion, childbirth, or biopsy procedures.

PENICILLINS

Penicillins are one of a group of **antibiotics** that kill bacteria or prevent their growth. There are several types of penicillins, each used to treat different kinds of infections, such as skin, dental, ear, respiratory tract, urinary tract, and other bacterial infections. These drugs will *not* work for colds, flu, and other infections caused by viruses.

Examples of penicillins are penicillin V (Beepen-VK, Pen-Vee K, V-cillin K, Veetids) and amoxicillin (Amoxil, Polymox, Trimox, Wymox). Penicillins are sometimes combined with other ingredients called beta-lactamase inhibitors, which protect the penicillin from bacterial enzymes that may destroy it before it can do its work.

Penicillins are available only with a physician's prescription and are sold in capsule, tablet (regular and chewable), liquid, and injectable forms. The recommended dosage depends on the type of penicillin, the strength of the medication, and the medical problem for which it is being taken.

Penicillins must always be taken exactly as directed and should not be discontinued, even if symptoms improve. Following a physician's instructions carefully is important with all types of infections but is especially important with "strep" infections, which can lead to serious heart problems if the infection is not cleared up completely. In addition, different types of penicillins cannot be substituted for one another. Penicillins work best when they are at constant levels in the blood. To help keep levels constant, the medication should be taken in doses spaced evenly through the day and night. Doses should not be skipped. Some penicillins, notably penicillin V, are taken on an empty stomach; others may be taken with food. When taking penicillin, symptoms generally begin to improve within a few days after initiating treatment.

Penicillins may, however, cause problems such as **diarrhea**. Severe symptoms may indicate a potentially serious side effect. Penicillins may also alter the results of some medical tests or adversely interact with other medications. Also, people with hay fever, **asthma**, eczema, or other general **allergies** (or who have had such allergies in the past) may be more likely to have severe reactions to penicillins. Thus, it is important for the patient to inform his or her physician of any medications currently being used, of any medical conditions, or of any allergies to foods, dyes, preservatives, or other substances before taking penicillin.

The most common side effects of penicillin are mild diarrhea, **headache**, vaginal **itching** and discharge, sore mouth or tongue, or white patches in the mouth or on the tongue. These problems usually dissipate as the body adjusts to the drug and usually do not require medical treatment unless they continue or are bothersome.

More serious side effects are not common, but may occur. These include **shortness of breath** or rapid or irregular breathing; fever; sudden lightheadedness or faintness; joint **pain**; skin rash, **hives**, itching, or red, scaly skin; or swelling or facial puffiness.

Penile cancer

Penile cancer is the growth of malignant cells on the external skin and in the tissues of the penis. **Cancer** of the penis is a rare disease. It occurs most often in men who were not circumcised as infants.

The cause of penile cancer is unknown. There does, however, appear to be a connection between development of the disease and lack of personal hygiene. Failing to regularly and thoroughly cleanse the part of the penis covered by the foreskin increases the risk of developing the disease.

The most common symptom of penile cancer is a tender spot, an open sore, or a wart-like lump that originates at the tip of the penis, spreads slowly across the skin, and invades deeper layers of tissue. **Pain** and bleeding may develop as the cancer continues to grow. A urologist should be consulted about any growths on the penis or abnormal discharge from it. If left untreated penile, cancer infiltrates the lymph nodes. Through the lymphatic (infection-fighting) system, it spreads to the groin and other parts of the body.

The diagnosis of penile cancer is most commonly made by a doctor who specializes in the genitourinary tract (a urologist). The doctor examines the patient's penis for lumps or other abnormalities. A biopsy may be ordered to distinguish malignant changes from **syphilis** and penile **warts**. If the results confirm a diagnosis of cancer, additional tests are done to determine whether the disease has spread to other parts of the body. This process is called staging.

In Stage I of penile cancer, malignant cells are found only on the surface of the head (glans) of the penis. In Stage II, the penile cancer has spread to the surface of the glans, tissues beneath the surface, and the shaft of the penis. In Stage III, malignant cells have spread to lymph nodes in the groin, where they cause swelling. In Stage IV, the disease has spread throughout the penis and lymph nodes in the groin, or has traveled to other parts of the body.

Amputation of all or part of the penis (total or partial penectomy) is the most common and most effective treatment. If the disease is diagnosed early enough, surgeons are often able to preserve enough of the organ for urination and sexual activity.

Wide local excision is a form of surgery that removes only cancer cells and a small amount of normal tissue adjacent to them. Microsurgery removes cancerous tissue and the smallest possible amount of normal tissue. During microsurgery, the doctor uses a special instrument that provides a comprehensive view of the area where cancer cells are located and makes it possible to determine that all malignant cells have been removed. **Laser surgery** uses an intense precisely focused beam of light to dissolve or burn away cancer cells.

Radiation therapy may be administered to enhance the effects of surgery or as an alternative to surgery. External radiation is provided by a machine. Internal radiation involves implanting radioactive elements into the part of the body where malignant cells are located.

Superficial cancers that are limited to a small area can be treated with fluorouracil (Adrucil, Efudex), a medication that is applied as a cream directly to the skin of the penis.

More advanced disease requires systemic treatments with **chemotherapy** that is administered intravenously or taken by mouth. These drugs enter the bloodstream and kill cancer cells that have spread to any part of the body.

Biological therapy is a type of treatment that is sometimes called biological response modifier (BRM) therapy. It uses natural or artificial substances to boost, focus, or reinforce the body's disease-fighting resources.

Cure rates are high for cancers diagnosed in Stage I or II, but much lower for Stages III an IV, by which time cancer cells have spread to the lymph nodes.

Penile prostheses

Penile prostheses are semirigid or inflatable devices that are implanted into penises to alleviate **impotence**. The penis is composed of one channel for urine and semen and three compartments with tough, fibrous walls containing "erectile tissue." With appropriate stimulation, the blood vessels that lead out of these compartments constrict, trapping blood. Blood pressure fills and hardens the compartments producing an erection of sufficient firmness to perform sexual intercourse. Additional stimulation leads to ejaculation, where semen is pumped out of the urethra. When this system fails, impotence (failure to create and maintain an erection) occurs.

Impotence can be caused by a number of conditions, including diabetes, **spinal cord injury**, prolonged drug abuse, and removal of a prostate gland. If the medical condition is irreversible, a penile prosthesis may be considered. Patients whose impotence is caused by psychological problems are not recommended for implant surgery.

Penile implant surgery is conducted on patients who have exhausted all other areas of treatment. The semirigid device consists of two rods that are easier and less expensive to implant than the inflatable cylinders. Once implanted, the semirigid device needs no follow-up adjustments, however it produces a penis which constantly remains semi-erect. The inflatable cylinders produce a more natural effect. The patient is able to simulate an erection by using a pump located in the scrotum.

With the patient asleep under general **anesthesia**, the device is inserted into the erectile tissue of the penis through an incision in the fibrous wall. In order to implant the pump for the inflatable implant, incisions are made in the abdomen and the perineum (area between the anus and the genitals). A fluid reservoir is inserted into the groin and the pump is placed in the scrotum. The cylinders, reservoir, and pump are connected by tubes and tested before the incisions are closed.

Surgery always requires an adequately informed patient, both as to risks and benefits. In this case, the sexual partner

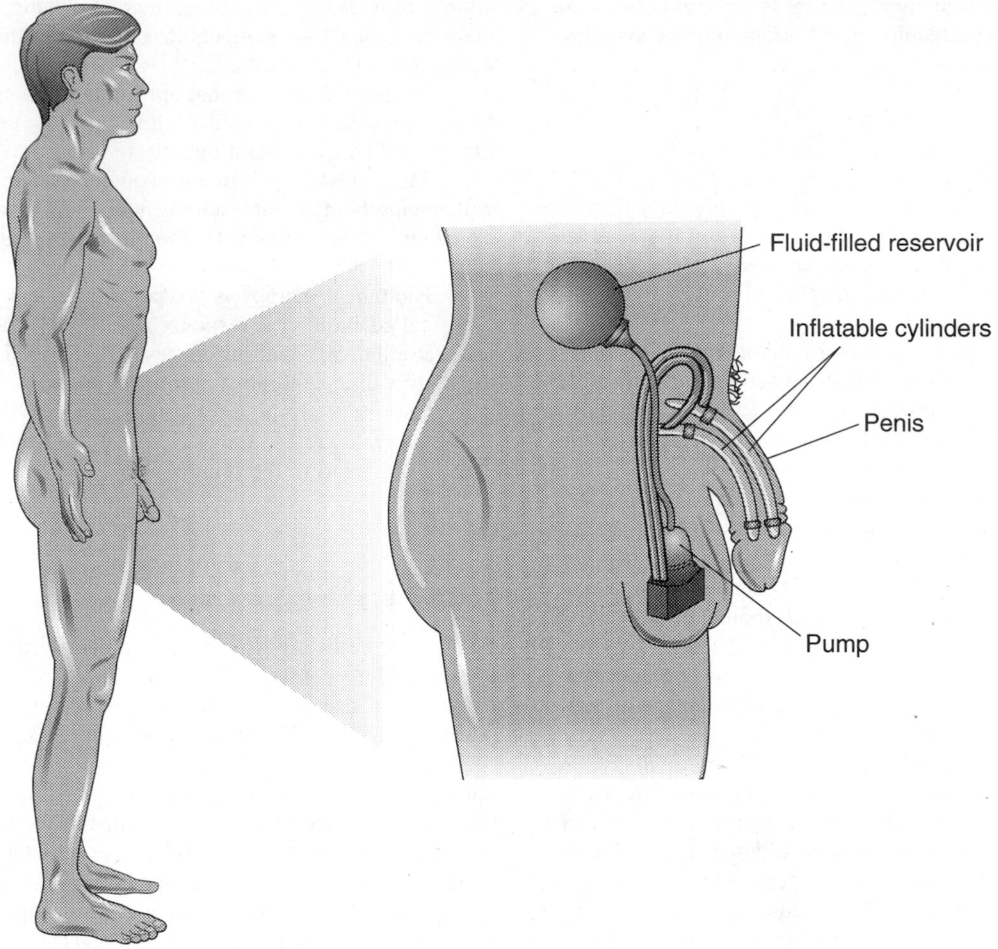

A diagram of the inflatable implant device.

should also be involved in the discussion. Prior to surgery, antibacterial cleansing occurs and the surrounding areas are shaved.

To minimize swelling, ice packs are applied to the penis for the first 24 hours following surgery. The incision sites are cleansed daily to prevent infection. **Pain** relievers may be taken.

With any implant, there is a slightly greater risk of infection. The implant may irritate the penis and cause continuous pain. The inflatable prosthesis may need follow-up surgery to repair leaks in the reservoir or to reconnect the tubing.

PERCEPTION

Perception refers to how the brain organizes and interprets sensory information. Until fairly recently, perception was considered by the school of psychology called behaviorism to be largely a passive and inevitable response to stimuli. Today's cognitive scientists, however, explain perception as an active process in which the brain treats external stimuli as raw material to be shaped, aided by our experience. Earlier in this century gestalt psychologists made a major contribution to the theory of perception by studying the ways people organize and select from the multitude of stimuli that are presented to them.

The brain receives information from the environment by way of specialized sensors called receptors. These receptors respond to physical stimuli such as light, sound, touch, taste, and smell. Nature has conveniently distributed these receptors in places on the body where they will be most useful, for example, in the retina, tongue, ears, nose, and skin—what we call our sensory apparatus. Environmental inputs are received by the senses and distributed to different parts of the brain for analysis. By a process that is not understood, the brain assembles the different elements into the perceptual experiences that make up our everyday lives.

Vision is our most important sense. If our brains had to process every bit of sensory stimulus we receive from the world, we would soon be overwhelmed. Selective attention helps us to focus only on stimuli that are needed or wanted at any instant, and to ignore less important ones. Perceptual constancy explains our tendency to interpret one object in the same way, no matter how near or far away it is, the angle we are viewing it from, or how bright it is. In other words, the world should look chaotic, but it doesn't.

Context—the setting in which something happens—is important to perception because we do not perceive objects in isolation. So how near one stimulus element (object in the environment) is to another, how similar the elements are, the human tendency to see complete figures, and our ability to distinguish important figures from the background will all contribute to the pattern that we perceive. Perception is also influenced by the intensity and physical dimensions of the stimulus, our own past experience, how ready we are to respond, and our motivation and emotional state.

Some perceptual abilities appear to be innate. For example, six-month-old infants are able to perceive depth. Similarly, experiments with young animals in the laboratory show that they are reluctant to step off the edge of what appears to be a steep cliff. But learning is also assumed to play a role in perception, since infants who are deprived of sensory experience show impaired perception.

Normally the brain is able to seamlessly integrate its mental equivalent of the world outside our bodies, based on an interplay between the physiological activity of the brain and external sensory stimuli. When the interplay breaks down, however, owing to a variety of causes, perceptual disturbances can result.

Sometimes these disturbances are benign, as in certain auditory or visual illusions. An illusion is a false impression of an object or event. For example, the sound of a siren drops as it moves away from the observer, which we call the Doppler effect. Another familiar illusion is the perception we have that we are moving when we are seated on a stationary train and the train on the next track begins to pull away.

Disordered perception is also associated with a range of diseases and conditions. **Hallucinations** are perceptions of objects and events in the absence of any external stimulus or situation. Auditory hallucinations are a cardinal feature of **schizophrenia**; patients suffering from alcoholic delerium tremens may feel insects crawling on their skin; and patients with temporal lobe **epilepsy** experience certain taste sensations even when they have not eaten anything. In phantom limb syndrome, patients who have had arms or legs amputated continue to feel the arm or leg as though it were still there. Neurological diseases also cause perceptual disturbances. For example, a lesion of the right parietal cortex results in a condition called hemispatial neglect: a patient can only perceive the right side of things. If you ask them to draw a clock, they will only draw the numbers 12 to 6. In somatoparaphrenia, patients deny possession of their own limbs.

PERFORATED EARDRUM

A perforated eardrum is caused by a hole or rupture in the eardrum, the thin membrane that separates the outer ear canal from the middle ear. A perforated eardrum may cause temporary **hearing loss** and occasional discharge.

The eardrum (tympanic membrane) is a thin wall that separates the outer ear from the middle ear, vibrating when sound waves strike the membrane. The middle ear is connected to the nose by the Eustachian tube. In addition to conducting sound, the eardrum also protects the middle ear from bacteria. When it is perforated, bacteria can more easily get into this part of the ear, causing ear infections.

In general, the larger the hole in the eardrum, the greater the temporary loss of hearing. The location of the perforation also affects the degree of hearing loss. Severe hearing loss may follow a skull fracture that disrupts the bones in the middle ear. Eardrum perforation caused by a loud noise may result in ringing in the ear (**tinnitus**), in addition to a temporary hearing loss. Over time, this hearing loss improves and the ringing usually fades in a few days.

The eardrum can become damaged by a direct injury. It is possible to perforate the eardrum in many ways, for example with a cotton-tipped swab or another foreign object, by hitting the ear with an open hand, ater a skull fracture, or after a loud explosion or other loud noise. In addition, an ear infection can rupture the eardrum as pressure within the middle ear rises when fluid builds up. If the eardrum is punctured by pressure from an ear infection, there may be infected or bloody drainage from the ear. Rarely, a small hole may remain in the eardrum after a pressure-equalizing tube falls out or is removed by a doctor.

Symptoms of a performated eardrum include an earache or pain in the ear, which may be severe, or a sudden decrease in ear **pain**, followed by ear drainage of clear, bloody, or pus-filled fluid, hearing loss, or ear noise/buzzing. A physician usually diagnoses perforated eardrum by direct inspection with an otoscope. Hearing tests may reveal a hearing loss.

A perforated eardrum usually heals on its own within two months, and any hearing loss that accompanies the perforation is usually temporary. **Antibiotics** may be given to prevent infection or to treat an existing ear infection. Painkillers may also be given to relieve any ear pain. Occasionally, a paper patch is placed over the eardrum until the membrane heals. Three or four patches may be needed before the perforation closes completely. If the eardrum does not heal on its own, surgical repair (tympanoplasty) may be necessary.

PERICARDITIS

Pericarditis is an inflammation of the two layers of the thin, sac-like membrane that surrounds the heart. This membrane is called the pericardium; thus the term pericarditis means inflammation of the pericardium.

Pericarditis is fairly common. It affects approximately one in 1,000 people. The most common form is caused by a viral infection. People in their 20s and 30s who have had a recent upper respiratory infection are most likely to be affected, along with men aged 20-50. One out of every four people who have had pericarditis will get it again, but after two years these relapses are less likely to occur.

The viruses that cause pericarditis include those that cause **influenza**, **polio**, and **rubella** (German **measles**). In children, the most common viruses that cause pericarditis are the adenovirus and the cocksackievirus (which is most likely to affect children during warmer weather).

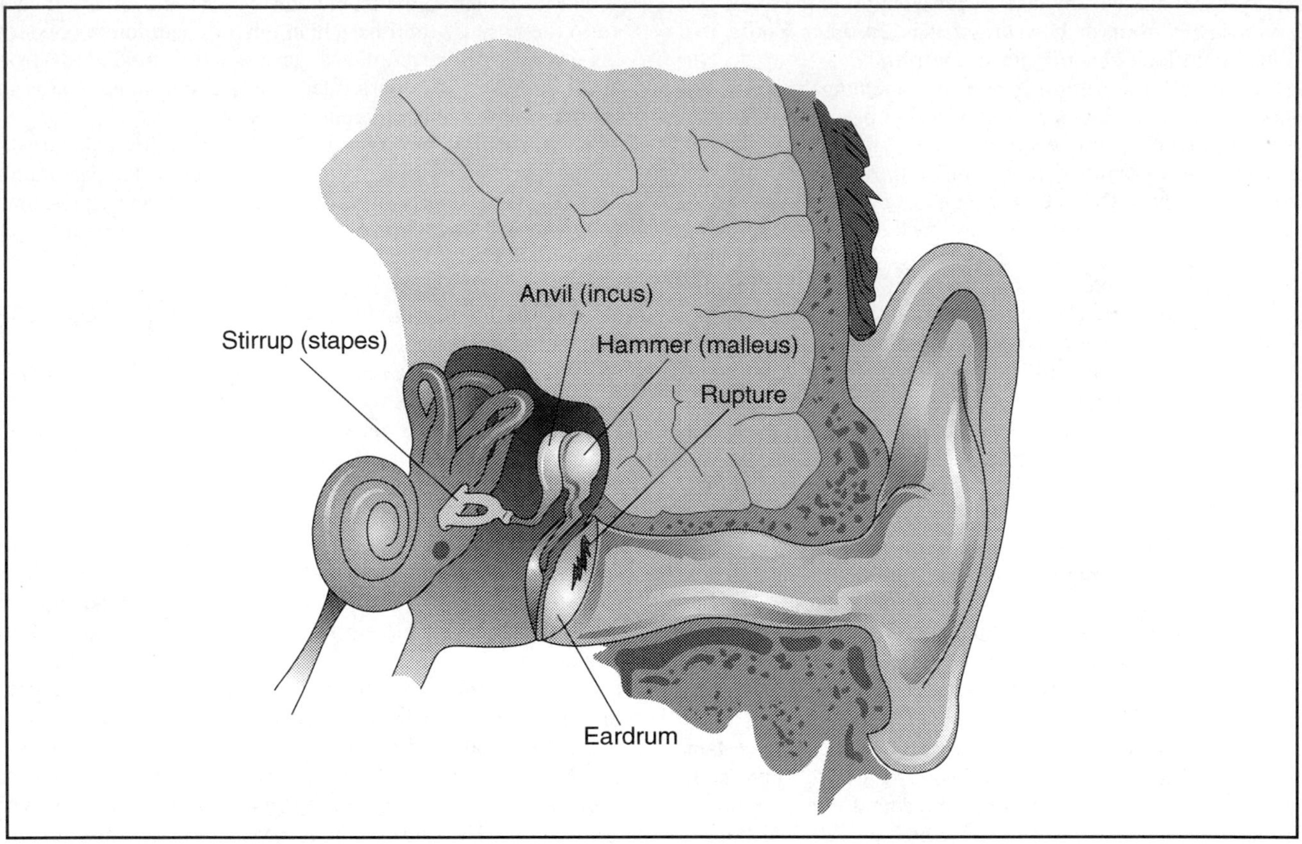

A diagram showing a perforated eardrum.

Although pericarditis is usually caused by a virus, it also can be caused by an injury to the heart or it can follow a **heart attack**. It may also be caused by certain inflammatory diseases such as **rheumatoid arthritis** or systemic lupus erythematosus. Bacteria, fungi, parasites, **tuberculosis**, **cancer**, or **kidney failure** may also affect the pericardium. Sometimes the cause is unknown.

There are several forms of pericarditis, depending on the cause. One type of pericarditis is caused by infection with a virus, bacteria, or fungus usually in the lungs and upper respiratory tract. This form of the disease causes a sharp, severe **pain** that starts in the region of the breastbone. If the pericarditis is caused by a bacteria, it is called bacterial or purulent pericarditis.

Sometimes fluid collects between the heart and the pericardium. This is called pericardial effusion, and may lead to a condition called **cardiac tamponade**. When the fluid accumulates, it can squeeze the heart and prevent it from filling with blood. This block of blood-flow keeps the rest of the body from getting its necessary supply of oxygen and can cause dangerously low blood pressure. A cardiac tamponade can occur when the chest is injured during surgery, **radiation therapy**, or an accident. Cardiac tamponade is a serious medical emergency and must be treated immediately.

When the pericardium is scarred or thickened, the heart has difficulty contracting. This is because the pericardium has shrunken or tightened around the heart, constricting the muscle's heart movement. This usually occurs as a result of tuberculosis, which now is rarely found in the United States, except in immigrant, **AIDS**, and prison populations.

Symptoms likely to be associated with pericarditis include:

- Rapid breathing
- Breathlessness
- Dry **cough**
- **Fever** and chills
- Weakness
- Broken blood vessels (hemorrhages) in the mucus membrane of the eyes, the back, the chest, fingers, and toes
- Feelings of **anxiety**
- A sharp or dull pain that starts in the front of the chest under the breastbone and radiates to the left side of the neck, upper abdomen, and left shoulder. The pain is less intense when the patient sits up or leans forward and worsens when lying down. The pain may worsen with a deep breath, like **pleurisy**, which may accompany pericarditis.

The heart of a person with pericarditis is likely to produce a grating sound (friction rub) when heard through a stethoscope. This sound occurs because the roughened pericardium surfaces are rubbing against each other.

The following tests will also help diagnose pericarditis and what is causing it:

- Electrocardiograph (ECG) and echocardiogram to distinguish between pericarditis and a heart attack.
- X-ray to show the traditional ''water bottle'' shadow around the heart that is often seen in pericarditis where there is a sufficient fluid build up.
- **Computed tomography scan** (CT scan) of the chest.
- Heart catheterization to view the heart's chambers and valves.
- Pericardiocentesis to test for viruses, bacteria, fungus, cancer, and tuberculosis.
- Blood tests such as LDH and CPK to measure cardiac enzymes and distinguish between a heart attack and pericarditis, as well as a complete **blood count** (CBC) to look for infection.

Since most pericarditis is caused by a virus and will heal naturally, there is no specific, curative treatment. Ordinarily **antibiotics** do not work against viruses. Pericarditis stemming from a virus usually clears up in 2 weeks to 3 months. Medications may be used to reduce inflammation, however. They include **nonsteroidal anti-inflammatory drugs** (NSAIDs), such as ibuprofen and **aspirin**. **Corticosteroids** are helpful if the pericarditis was caused by a heart attack or **systemic lupus erythematosus**. **Analgesics** (painkillers such as aspirin or **acetaminophen**) also may be given.

If the pericarditis recurs, removal of all or part of the pericardium (pericardiectomy) may be necessary. In the case of constrictive pericarditis, the pericardiectomy may be necessary to remove the stiffened parts of the pericardium that are preventing the heart from beating correctly. If a cardiac tamponade is present, it may be necessary to drain excess fluid from the pericardium. Pericardiocentesis, the same procedure used for testing, is used to withdraw the fluid.

For most people, home care with rest and medications to relieve pain are sufficient. A warm heating pad or compress also may help relieve pain. Sitting in an upright position and bending forward helps relieve discomfort. A person with pericarditis may also be kept in bed, with the head of the bed elevated to reduce the heart's need to work hard as it pumps blood. Along with painkillers and antibiotics, diuretic drugs (''water pills'') to reduce fluids may also be used judiciously.

The prognosis for those with pericarditis is good. Most people recover within three weeks to several months and do not require any additional treatment.

Although pericarditis cannot be prevented, a healthy lifestyle with proper nutrition and **exercise** will help keep the body's immune system strong and more likely to fight off invading microorganisms.

PERINATAL INFECTIONS

Perinatal infections include bacterial or viral illnesses that can be passed from a mother to her baby either while the baby is still in the uterus, during the delivery process, or shortly after birth. Maternal infection can, in some cases, cause complications at birth. The mother may or may not experience active symptoms of the infection during the **pregnancy**. The most serious and most common perinatal infections, and the impact of these diseases on the mother and infant, are discussed below in alphabetical order. It is important to note that men can become infected and can transmit many of these infections to other women. The sexual partners of women who have these infections should also seek medical treatment.

Chlamydia trachomatis is the most common bacterial sexually transmitted disease in the United States, causing more than 4 million infections each year. The majority of women with chlamydial infection experience no obvious symptoms. The infection affects the reproductive tract and causes **pelvic inflammatory disease**, **infertility**, and **ectopic pregnancy** (the fertilized egg implants somewhere other than in the uterus). This infection can cause premature rupture of the membranes and early labor. It can be passed to the infant during delivery and can cause ophthalmia neonatorum (an eye infection) within the first month of life and **pneumonia** within one to three months of age. Symptoms of chlamydial pneumonia are a repetitive **cough** and rapid breathing. **Wheezing** is rare and the infant does not develop a **fever**

Cytomegalovirus (CMV) is a very common virus in the herpes virus family. It is found in saliva, urine and other body fluids and can be spread through sexual contact or other more casual forms of physical contact like kissing. In adults, CMV may cause mild symptoms of swollen lymph glands, fever, and fatigue. Many people who carry the virus experience no symptoms at all. Infants can become infected with CMV while still in the uterus if the mother becomes infected or develops a recurrence of the infection during pregnancy. Most infants exposed to CMV before birth develop normally and do not show any symptoms. As many as 6,000 infants who were exposed to CMV before birth are born with serious complications each year. CMV interferes with normal fetal development and can cause **mental retardation**, blindness, deafness, or epilepsy in these infants.

Genital herpes, which is usually caused by Herpes simplex virus type 2 (HSV-2), is a sexually transmitted disease that causes painful sores on the genitals. Women who have their first outbreak of genital herpes during pregnancy are at high risk of **miscarriage** or delivering a low birth weight baby. The infection can be passed to the infant at the time of delivery if the mother has an active sore. The most serious risk to the infant is the possibility of developing HSV-2 **encephalitis**, an inflammation of the brain, with symptoms of irritability and poor feeding.

Hepatitis B is a contagious virus that causes liver damage and is a leading cause of chronic liver disease and **cirrhosis**. Approximately 20,000 infants are born each year to mothers who test positive for the hepatitis B virus. These infants are at high risk for developing hepatitis B infection through exposure to their mothers blood during delivery.

Human **immunodeficiency** virus (HIV) is a serious, contagious virus that causes acquired immunodeficiency syndrome (**AIDS**). About one-fourth of pregnant women with HIV pass the infection on to their newborn infants. An infant with HIV usually develops AIDS and dies before the age of two.

Human papillomavirus (HPV) is a sexually transmitted disease that causes **genital warts** and can increase the risk of developing some **cancer**s. HPV appears to be transferred from the mother to the infant during the birth process.

Rubella is a virus that causes German **measles**, an illness that includes rash, fever, and symptoms of an upper respiratory tract infection. Most people are exposed to rubella during childhood and develop antibodies to the virus so they will never get it again. Rubella infection during early pregnancy can pass through the placenta to the developing infant and cause serious **birth defects** including heart abnormalities, mental retardation, blindness, and deafness.

Group B streptococcus (GBS) infection is the most common bacterial cause of infection and **death** in newborn infants. In women, GBS can cause vaginitis and urinary tract infections. Both infections can cause premature birth and the bacteria can be transferred to the infant in the uterus or during delivery. GBS causes pneumonia, **meningitis**, and other serious infections in infants.

Syphilis is a sexually transmitted bacterial infection that can be transferred from a mother to an infant through the placenta before birth. Up to 50% of infants born to mothers with syphilis will be premature, stillborn, or will die shortly after birth. Infected infants may have severe birth defects. Those infants who survive infancy may develop symptoms of syphilis up to two years later.

Periodontal disease

Periodontal diseases are a group of diseases that affect the tissues that support and anchor the teeth. Left untreated, periodontal disease results in the destruction of the gums, alveolar bone (the part of the jaws where the teeth arise), and the outer layer of the tooth root.

Periodontal disease is usually seen as a chronic (long-term) inflammatory disease. An acute (short-term) infection of the periodontal tissue may occur, but is not usually reported to the dentist. The tissues that are involved in periodontal diseases are the gums, which include the gingiva, periodontal ligament, cementum, and alveolar bone. The gingiva is a pink-colored mucus membrane that covers parts of the teeth and the alveolar bone. The periodontal ligament is the main part of the gums. The cementum is a calcified structure that covers the lower parts of the teeth. The alveolar bone is a set of ridges from the jaw bones (maxillary and mandible) in which the teeth are embedded. The main area involved in periodontal disease is the gingival sulcus, a pocket between the teeth and the gums. Several distinct forms of periodontal disease are known. These are gingivitis, acute necrotizing ulcerative gingivitis, adult periodontitis, and localized juvenile periodontitis. Although periodontal disease is thought to be widespread, serious cases of periodontitis are not common. Gingivitis is also one of the early signs of leukemia in some children.

Gingivitis is an inflammation of the outermost soft tissue of the gums. The gingivae become red and inflamed, loose their normal shape, and bleed easily. Gingivitis may remain a chronic disease for years without affecting other periodontal tissues. Chronic gingivitis may lead to a deepening of the gingival sulcus. Acute necrotizing ulcerative gingivitis is mainly seen in young adults. This form of gingivitis is characterized by painful, bleeding gums, and death (necrosis) and erosion of gingival tissue between the teeth. It is thought that **stress**, **malnutrition**, fatigue, and poor **oral hygiene** are among the causes for acute necrotizing ulcerative gingivitis.

Adult periodontitis is the most serious form of the periodontal diseases. It involves the gingiva, periodontal ligament, and alveolar bone. A deep periodontal pocket forms between the teeth, and the cementum and the gums. Plaque, calculus, and debris from food and other sources collect in the pocket. Without treatment, the periodontal ligament can be destroyed and resorption of the alveolar bone occurs. This allows the teeth to move more freely and eventually results in the loss of teeth. Most cases of adult periodontitis are chronic, but some cases occur in episodes or periods of tissue destruction.

Localized juvenile periodontitis is a less common form of periodontal disease and is seen mainly in young people. Primarily, localized juvenile periodontitis affects the molars and incisors. Among the distinctions that separate this form of periodontitis are the low incidence of bacteria in the periodontal pocket, minimal plaque formation, and mild inflammation.

Herpes infection of the gums and other parts of the mouth is called herpetic gingivostomatitis and is frequently grouped with periodontal diseases. The infected areas of the gums turn red in color and have whitish herpetic lesions. There are two principal differences between this form of periodontal diseases and most other forms. Herpetic gingivostomatitis is caused by a virus, Herpes simplex, not by bacteria, and the viral infection tends to heal by itself in approximately two weeks. Also, herpetic gingivostomatitis is infectious to other people who come in contact with the herpes lesions or saliva that contains virus from the lesion.

Pericoronitis is a condition found in children who are in the process of producing molar teeth. The disease is seen more frequently in the lower molar teeth. As the molar emerges, a flap of gum still covers the tooth. The flap of gum traps bacteria and food, leading to a mild irritation. If the upper molar fully emerges before the lower one, it may bite down on the flap during chewing. This can increase the irritation of the flap and lead to an infection. In bad cases, the infection can spread to the neck and cheeks.

Trench mouth is an acute, necrotizing (causing tissue death), ulcerating (causing open sores) form of gingivitis. It causes pain in the affected gums. **Fever** and fatigue are usually present also. Trench mouth, also known as Vincent's disease, is a complication of mild cases of gingivitis. Frequently, poor oral hygiene is the main cause. Stress, an unbalanced diet, or lack of sleep are frequent cofactors in the development of trench mouth. This form of periodontal disease is more common in people who smoke. The term "trench mouth" was created in World War I, when the disease was common in soldiers who lived in the trenches. Symptoms of trench mouth appear suddenly. The initial symptoms include painful gums and foul breath. Gum tissue between teeth becomes infected and dies, and starts to disappear. Often, what appears to be remaining gum is dead tissue. Usually, the gums bleed easily, especially when chewing. The pain can increase to the point where eating and swallowing become difficult. Inflammation or infection from trench mouth can spread to nearby tissues of the face and neck.

Periodontitis is a condition in which gingivitis has extended down around the tooth and into the supporting bone structure. Periodontitis is also called pyorrhea. Plaque and tarter buildup sometimes lead to the formation of large pockets between the gums and teeth. When this happens, anaerobic bacteria grow in the pockets. The pockets eventually extend down around the roots of the teeth where the bacteria cause damage to the bone structure supporting the teeth. The teeth become loose and tooth loss can result. Some medical conditions are associated with an increased likelihood of developing periodontitis. These diseases include diabetes, **Down syndrome**, Cohn's disease, **AIDS**, and any disease that reduces the number of white blood cells in the body for extended periods of time.

Several factors play a role in the development of periodontal disease. The most important are age and oral hygiene. The number and type of bacteria present on the gingival tissues also play a role in the development of periodontal diseases. The presence of certain species of bacteria in large enough numbers in the gingival pocket and related areas correlates with the development of periodontal disease. Also, removal of the bacteria correlates with reduction or elimination of disease. In most cases of periodontal disease, the bacteria remain in the periodontal pocket and do not invade surrounding tissue.

The mechanisms by which bacteria in the periodontal pocket cause tissue destruction in the surrounding region are not fully understood. Several bacterial products that diffuse through tissue are thought to play a role in disease formation. Bacterial endotoxin is a toxin produced by some bacteria that can kill cells. Studies show that the amount of endotoxin present correlates with the severity of periodontal disease. Other bacterial products include proteolytic enzymes, molecules that digest protein found in cells, thereby causing cell destruction. The immune response has also been implicated in tissue destruction. As part of the normal immune response, white blood cells enter regions of inflammation to destroy bacteria. In the process of destroying bacteria, periodontal tissue is also destroyed.

Gingivitis usually results from inadequate oral hygiene. Proper brushing of the teeth and flossing decreases plaque buildup. The bacteria responsible for causing gingivitis reside in the plaque. Plaque is a sticky film that is largely made from bacteria. Tartar is plaque that has hardened. Plaque can turn into tartar in as little as three days if not brushed off. Tartar is difficult to remove by brushing. Gingivitis can be aggravated by hormones, and sometimes becomes temporarily worse during **pregnancy**, **puberty**, and when the patient is taking birth control pills. Interestingly, some drugs used to treat other conditions can cause an overgrowth of the gingival tissue that can result in gingivitis because plaque builds up more easily. Drugs associated with this condition are phenytoin, used to treat seizures; cyclosporin, given to organ transplant patients to reduce the likelihood of organ rejection; and calcium blockers, used to treat several different heart conditions. **Scurvy**, a vitamin C deficiency and **pellagra**, a niacin deficiency, can also lead to bleeding gums and gingivitis.

The initial symptoms of periodontitis are bleeding and inflamed gums, and **bad breath**. Periodontitis follows cases of gingivitis, which may not be severe enough to cause a patient to seek dental help. Although the symptoms of periodontitis are also seen in other forms of periodontal diseases, the key characteristic in periodontitis is a large pocket that forms between the teeth and gums. Another characteristic of periodontitis is that pain usually doesn't develop until late in the disease, when a tooth loosens or an **abscess** forms.

Diagnosis is made by observation of infected gums. Usually, a dentist is the person to diagnose and characterize the various types of periodontal disease. In cases such as acute herpetic gingivostomatitis, there are characteristic herpetic lesions. Many of the periodontal diseases are distinguished based on the severity of the infection and the number and type of tissues involved.

Diagnosis of periodontitis includes measuring the size of the pockets formed between the gums and teeth. Normal gingival pockets are shallow. If periodontal disease is severe, jaw bone loss will be detected in x-ray images of the teeth. If too much bone is lost, the teeth become loose and can change position. This will also be seen in x-ray images.

Tartar can only be removed by professional dental treatment. Following treatment, periodontal tissues usually heal quickly. Gingivitis caused by vitamin deficiencies is treated by administering the needed vitamin. There are no useful drugs to treat herpetic gingivostomatitis. Because of the pain associated with the herpes lesions, patients may not brush their teeth while the lesions are present. Herpes lesions heal by themselves without treatment. After the herpetic lesions have disappeared, the gums usually return to normal if good oral hygiene is resumed. Pericoronitis is treated by removing debris under the flap of gum covering the molar. This operation is usually performed by a dentist. Surgery is used to remove molars that are not likely to form properly.

Treatment for trench mouth starts with a complete cleaning of the teeth, removal of all plaque, tartar, and dead tissue on the gums. For the first few days after cleaning, the patient uses hydrogen peroxide mouth washes instead of brushing. After cleaning, the gum tissue will be very raw and rinsing minimizes damage to the gums that might be caused by the tooth brush. For the first few days, the patient should visit the dentist daily for checkups and then every second or third day for the next two weeks. Occasionally, antibiotic treatment is used to supplement dental cleaning of the teeth and gums. Surgery may be needed if the damage to the gums is extensive and they do not heal properly.

Treatment of periodontitis requires professional dental care. The pockets around the teeth must be cleaned, and all tartar and plaque removed. In periodontitis, tartar and plaque can extend far down the tooth root. Normal dental hygiene, brushing and flossing, cannot reach deep enough to be effective in treating periodontitis. In cases where pockets are very deep (more than one quarter inch deep), surgery is required to clean the pocket. This is performed in a dental office. Sections of gum that are not likely to reattach to the teeth may be removed to promote healing by healthy sections of gum. Abscesses are treated with a combination of **antibiotics** and surgery. The antibiotics may be delivered directly to the infected gum and bone tissues to ensure that high concentrations of the antibiotic reach the infected area. Abscess infections, especially of bone, are difficult to treat and require long term antibiotic treatments to prevent a reoccurrence of infection.

Periodontal diseases can be easily treated. The gums usually heal and resume their normal shape and function. In cases where they don't, prostheses or surgery can restore most of the support for proper functioning of the teeth.

Most forms of periodontal disease can be prevented with good dental hygiene. Daily use of a toothbrush and flossing is sufficient to prevent most cases of periodontal disease. Tartar control toothpastes help prevent tartar formation, but do not remove tartar once it has formed.

PERITONITIS

Peritonitis is an inflammation of the membrane which lines the inside of the abdomen and all of the internal organs. This membrane is called the peritoneum. Peritonitis may be primary (meaning that it occurs spontaneously, and not as the result of some other medical problem) or secondary (meaning that it results from some other condition). It is most often due to infection by bacteria, but may also be due to some kind of a chemical irritant (such as spillage of acid from the stomach, bile from the gall bladder and biliary tract, or enzymes from the pancreas during the illness called **pancreatitis**). Peritonitis has even been seen in patients who develop a reaction to the cornstarch which is used to powder gloves worn during surgery. Peritonitis with no evidence of bacteria, chemical irritant, or foreign body has occurred in such diseases as **systemic lupus erythematosus**, **porphyria**, and **familial Mediterranean fever**. When the peritoneum gets contaminated by blood, the blood can both irritate the peritoneum and serve as a source of bacteria to cause an infection. Blood may leak into the abdomen due to a burst tubal **pregnancy**, an injury, or bleeding after surgery.

Primary peritonitis usually occurs in people who have an accumulation of fluid in their abdomens. Ascites is a common complication of severe **cirrhosis** of the liver (a disease in which the liver grows increasingly scarred and dysfunctional). The fluid that accumulates creates a good environment for the growth of bacteria.

Secondary peritonitis most commonly occurs when some other medical condition causes bacteria to spill into the abdominal cavity. Bacteria are normal residents of a healthy intestine, but they should have no way to escape and enter the abdomen, where they could cause an infection. Bacteria can infect the peritoneum due to conditions in which a hole (perforation) develops in the stomach (due to an ulcer eating its way through the stomach wall) or intestine (due to a large number of causes, including a ruptured appendix or a ruptured diverticulum). Bacteria can infect the peritoneum due to a severe case of **pelvic inflammatory disease** (a massive infection of the female organs, including the uterus and fallopian tubes). Bacteria can also escape into the abdominal cavity due to an injury which causes the intestine to burst, or an injury to an internal organ which bleeds into the abdominal cavity.

Symptoms of peritonitis include **fever** and abdominal **pain**. An acutely ill patient usually tries to lie very still, because any amount of movement causes excruciating pain. Often, the patient lies with the knees bent, to decrease strain on the tender peritoneum. There is often **nausea and vomiting**. The usual sounds made by the active intestine and heard during examination with a stethoscope will be absent, because the intestine usually stops functioning. The abdomen may be rigid and boardlike. Accumulations of fluid will be notable in primary peritonitis due to ascites. Other signs and symptoms of the underlying cause of secondary peritonitis may be present.

A diagnosis of peritonitis is usually based on symptoms. Discovering the underlying reason for the peritonitis, however, may require some work. A blood sample will be drawn in order to determine the white blood cell count. Because white blood cells are produced by the body in an effort to combat foreign invaders, the white blood cell count will be elevated in the case of an infection. A long, thin needle can be used to take a sample of fluid from the abdomen in an effort to diagnose primary peritonitis. The types of immune cells present are usually characteristic in this form of peritonitis. X-ray films may be taken if there is some suspicion that a perforation exists. In the case of a perforation, air will have escaped into the abdomen and will be visible on the picture. When a cause for peritonitis cannot be found, an open exploratory operation on the abdomen (laparotomy) is considered to be a crucial diagnostic procedure, and at the same time provides the opportunity to begin treatment.

Treatment depends on the source of the peritonitis, but an emergency laparotomy is usually performed. Any perforated or damaged organ is usually repaired at this time. If a clear diagnosis of pelvic inflammatory disease or pancreatitis can be made, however, surgery is not usually performed. Peritonitis from any cause is treated with **antibiotics** given through a needle in the vein, along with fluids to prevent **dehydration**.

Prognosis for untreated peritonitis is likely to be **death**. With treatment, the prognosis is variable, dependent on the underlying cause.

There is no way to prevent peritonitis, since the diseases it accompanies are usually not under the voluntary control of an individual. However, prompt treatment can prevent complications.

PERNICIOUS ANEMIA

Pernicious anemia is a disease in which the red blood cells are abnormally formed, due to an inability to absorb vitamin B_{12}.

Vitamin B_{12}, or cobalamin, plays an important role in the development of red blood cells. It is found in significant quantities in liver, meats, milk and milk products, and legumes. During the course of the digestion of foods containing B_{12}, the B_{12} becomes attached to a substance called intrinsic factor. Intrinsic factor is produced by parietal cells which line the stomach. The B_{12}-intrinsic factor complex then enters the intestine, where the vitamin is absorbed into the bloodstream. In fact, B_{12} can only be absorbed when it is attached to intrinsic factor.

In pernicious anemia, the parietal cells stop producing intrinsic factor. The intestine is then completely unable to absorb B_{12}. So, the vitamin passes out of the body as waste. Although the body has significant amounts of stored B_{12}, this will eventually be used up. At this point, the symptoms of pernicious anemia will develop.

Pernicious anemia is most common among people from northern Europe and among African Americans. It is far less frequently seen among people from southern Europe and Asia. Pernicious anemia occurs in equal numbers in both men and women. Most patients with pernicious anemia are older, usually over 60. Occasionally, a child will have an inherited condition which results in defective intrinsic factor. Pernicious anemia seems to run in families, so that anyone with a relative suffering from the disease has a greater likelihood of developing it as well.

People with pernicious anemia seem to have a greater chance of having certain other conditions. These conditions include **autoimmune disorders**, particularly those affecting the thyroid, parathyroid, and adrenals. It is thought that the immune system, already out of control in these diseases, incorrectly becomes directed against the parietal cells. Ultimately, the parietal cells seem to be destroyed by the actions of the immune system.

True pernicious anemia refers specifically to a disorder of decayed parietal cells leading to absent intrinsic factor, resulting in an inability to absorb B_{12}. However, there are other related conditions which result in decreased absorption of B_{12}. These conditions cause the same types of symptoms as true pernicious anemia. Other conditions which interfere with either the production of intrinsic factor, or the body's use of B_{12}, include conditions that require surgical removal of the stomach, or **poisoning**s with corrosive substances which destroy the lining of the stomach. Certain structural defects of the intestinal system can result in an overgrowth of normal bacteria. These bacteria then absorb B_{12} themselves, for use in their own growth. Intestinal worms (especially one called fish tapeworm) may also use B_{12}, resulting in anemia. Various conditions that affect the first part of the intestine (the ileum), from which B_{12} is absorbed, can also cause anemia due to B_{12} deficiency. These ilium related disorders include tropical sprue, Whipple's disease, Crohn's disease, **tuberculosis**, and the Zollinger-Ellison syndrome.

Symptoms of pernicious anemia and decreased B_{12} affect three systems of the body: the system that is involved in the formation of blood cells (hematopoietic system); the gastrointestinal system; and the nervous system.

The hematopoietic system is harmed because B_{12} is required for the proper formation of red blood cells. Without B_{12}, red blood cell production is greatly reduced. Those red blood cells that are produced are abnormally large and defective in shape. Because red blood cells are responsible for carrying oxygen around the body, decreased numbers (termed anemia) result in a number of symptoms, including fatigue, **dizziness**, ringing in the ears, pale or yellowish skin, fast heart rate, enlarged heart with an abnormal heart sound (murmur) evident on examination, and chest **pain**.

Symptoms that affect the gastrointestinal system include a sore and brightly red tongue, loss of appetite, weight loss, **diarrhea**, and abdominal cramping.

The nervous system is severely affected when pernicious anemia goes untreated. Symptoms include numbness, tingling, or burning in the arms, legs, hands, and feet; muscle weakness; difficulty and loss of balance while walking; changes in reflexes; irritability, confusion, and depression.

Diagnosis of pernicious anemia is suggested when a blood test reveals abnormally large red blood cells. Many of these will also be abnormally shaped. The earliest, least mature forms of red blood cells (reticulocytes) also will be low in number. White blood cells and platelets may also be decreased in number. Measurements of the quantity of B_{12} circulating in the bloodstream will be low. Testing for true pernicious anemia is more complex.

Treatment of pernicious anemia requires the administration of lifelong injections of B_{12}. Vitamin B_{12} given by injection enters the bloodstream directly, and doesn't require intrinsic factor. At first, injections may need to be given several times a week, in order to build up adequate stores of the vitamin. After this, the injections can be given on a monthly basis. Other substances required for blood cell production may also need to be given; they may include iron and vitamin C.

Prognosis is generally good for patients with pernicious anemia. Many of the symptoms improve within just a few days of beginning treatment, although some of the nervous system symptoms may take up to 18 months to improve. Occasionally, when diagnosis and treatment have been delayed for a long time, some of the nervous system symptoms may be permanent.

Because an increased risk of **stomach cancer** has been noted in patients with pernicious anemia, careful monitoring is necessary, even when all the symptoms of the original disorder have improved.

Personality Development

The concept of personality refers to the profile of stable beliefs, moods, and behaviors that differentiate among children and adults who live in a particular society. The profiles that differentiate children across cultures of different historical times will not be the same because the most adaptive profiles vary with the values of the society and the historical era. For example, an essay on personality development written 300 years ago by a New England Puritan would have listed piety as a major psychological trait; but that would not be regarded as an important personality trait in contemporary America.

Contemporary theorists emphasize personality traits having to do with individualism, internalized conscience, sociability with strangers, the ability to control strong emotion and impulse, and personal achievement.

An important reason for the immaturity of our understanding of personality development is the heavy reliance on questionnaires that are filled out by parents of children or the responses of older children to questionnaires. Because there is less use of behavioral observations of children, our theories of personality development are not strong.

There are five different hypotheses regarding the early origins of personality. One assumes that the child's inherited biology, usually called a temperamental bias, is an important basis for the child's later personality. Alexander Thomas and Stella Chess suggested there were nine temperamental dimensions and three synthetic types, which they called the difficult child, the easy child, and the child who is slow to warm up to unfamiliarity. Studies of children suggest that a shy and fearful style of reacting to challenge and novelty predicts, to a modest degree, an adult personality that is passive to challenge and introverted in mood.

A second hypothesis regarding personality development comes from **Sigmund Freud**'s suggestion that variation in the sexual and aggressive aims of the id, which is biological in nature, combined with family experience, leads to the development of the ego and superego. Freud suggested that differences in parental socialization produced variation in anxiety, which, in turn, leads to different personalities.

A third set of hypotheses emphasizes direct social experiences with parents. After World War II, Americans and Europeans held the more benevolent idealistic conception of the child that described growth as motivated by affectionate ties to others rather than by the narcissism and hostility implied by Freud's writings. John Bowlby contributed to this new emphasis on the infant's relationships with parents in his books on attachment. Bowlby argued that the nature of the infant's relationship to the caretakers and especially the mother created a profile of emotional reactions toward adults that might last indefinitely.

A fourth source of ideas for personality centers on whether or not it is necessary to posit a self that monitors, integrates, and initiates reaction. This idea traces itself to the Judeo-Christian assumption that it is necessary to award children a will so that they could be held responsible for their actions. A second basis is the discovery that children who had the same objective experiences develop different personality profiles because they construct different conceptions about themselves and others from the same experiences. The notion that each child imposes a personal interpretation to their experiences makes the concept of self critical to the child's personality.

An advantage of awarding importance to a concept of self and personality development is that the process of identification with parents and others gains in significance. All children wish to possess the qualities that their culture regards as good. Some of these qualities are the product of identification with each parent.

A final source of hypotheses regarding the origins of personality comes from inferences based on direct observations of a child's behavior. This strategy, which relies on induction, focuses on different characteristics at different ages. Infants differ in irritability, three-year-olds differ in shyness, and six-year-olds differ in seriousness of mood. A major problem with this approach is that each class of behavior can have different historical antecedents. Children who prefer to play alone rather than with others do so for a variety of reasons. Some might be temperamentally shy and are uneasy with other children while others might prefer solitary activity.

The most important personality profiles in a particular culture stem from the challenges to which the children of that culture must accommodate. Most children must deal with three classes of external challenges: (1) unfamiliarity, especially unfamiliar people, tasks, and situations; (2) request by legitimate authority for conformity to and acceptance of their standards; and (3) domination by or attack by other children. In addition, all children must learn to control two important families of emotions: anxiety, fear, and guilt, on the one hand, and on the other, anger, jealousy, and resentment.

Of the four important influences on personality—identification, ordinal position, social class, and parental socialization—identification is the most important. By six years of age, children assume that some of the characteristics of their parents belong to them and they experience vicariously the emotion that is appropriate to the parent's experience. A six-year-old girl identified with her mother will experience pride should mother win a prize or be praised by a friend. However, she will experience shame or anxiety if her mother is criticized or is rejected by friends. The process of identification has great relevance to personalty development.

The child's ordinal position in the family has its most important influence on receptivity to accepting or rejecting the requests and ideas of legitimate authority. First-born children in most families are more willing than later-borns to conform to the requests of authority. They are more strongly motivated to achieve in school, more conscientious, and less aggressive.

The child's social class affects the preparation and motivation for academic achievement. Children from middle-class families typically obtain higher grades in school than children of working- or lower-class families because different value systems and practices are promoted by families from varied social-class backgrounds.

The patterns of socialization used by parents also influence the child's personality. Baumrind suggests that parents could be classified as authoritative, authoritarian, or permissive. More competent and mature preschool children usually have authoritative parents who were nurturant but made maturity demands. Moderately self-reliant children who were a bit withdrawn have authoritarian parents who more often relied on coercive discipline. The least mature children have overly permissive parents who are nurturant but lack discipline.

See also Child development

PERSONALITY DISORDERS

Personality disorders are a group of mental disturbances defined by the fourth (1994) edition of the *Diagnostic and Statis-*

tical Manual of Mental Disorders (*DSM-IV*) as ''enduring pattern[s] of inner experience and behavior'' that are sufficiently rigid and deep-seated to bring a person into repeated conflicts with his or her social and occupational environment. *DSM-IV* specifies that these dysfunctional patterns must be regarded as nonconforming or deviant by the person's culture, and cause significant emotional **pain** and/or difficulties in relationships and occupational performance. In addition, the patient usually sees the disorder as being consistent with his or her self image and may blame others.

To meet the diagnosis of personality disorder, which is sometimes called character disorder, the patient's problematic behaviors must appear in two or more of the following areas:

- **Perception** and interpretation of the self and other people
- Intensity and duration of feelings and their appropriateness to situations
- Relationships with others
- Ability to control impulses.

Personality disorders arise in late adolescence or early adulthood. Doctors rarely give a diagnosis of personality disorder to children on the grounds that children's personalities are still in the process of formation and may change considerably by the time they are in their late teens. But, in retrospect, many individuals with personality disorders could be judged to have shown evidence of the problems in childhood.

It is difficult to give close estimates of the percentage of the population that suffers from personality disorders. Patients with certain personality disorders, including antisocial and borderline disorders, are more likely to get into trouble with the law or otherwise attract attention than are patients whose disorders chiefly affect their capacity for intimacy. On the other hand, some patients, such as those with narcissistic or obsessive-compulsive personality disorders, may be outwardly successful because their symptoms are useful within their particular occupations. It has, however, been estimated that about 15% of the general population of the United States suffers from personality disorders, with higher rates in poor or troubled neighborhoods. The rate of personality disorders among patients in psychiatric treatment is between 30% and 50%. It is possible for patients to have a so-called dual diagnosis; for example, they may have more than one personality disorder, or a personality disorder together with a substance-abuse problem.

By contrast, *DSM-IV* classifies personality disorders into three clusters based on symptom similarities:

- Cluster A (paranoid, schizoid, schizotypal): Patients appear odd or eccentric to others.
- Cluster B (antisocial, borderline, histrionic, narcissistic): Patients appear overly emotional, unstable, or self-dramatizing to others.
- Cluster C (avoidant, dependent, obsessive-compulsive): Patients appear tense and **anxiety**-ridden to others.

The *DSM-IV* clustering system does not mean that all patients can be fitted neatly into one of the three clusters. It is possible for patients to have symptoms of more than one personality disorder or to have symptoms from different clusters.

Since the criteria for personality disorders include friction or conflict between the patient and his or her social environment, these syndromes are open to redefinition as societies change. One criticism that has been made of the general category of personality disorder is that it is based on Western notions of individual uniqueness. Its applicability to people from cultures with different definitions of human personhood is thus open to question. Furthermore, even within a culture, it can be difficult to define the limits of ''normalcy.''

The personality disorders defined by *DSM-IV* are as follows:

Patients with paranoid personality disorder are characterized by suspiciousness and a belief that others are out to harm or cheat them. They have problems with intimacy and may join cults or groups with paranoid belief systems. Some are litigious, bringing lawsuits against those they believe have wronged them. Although not ordinarily delusional, these patients may develop psychotic symptoms under severe **stress**. It is estimated that 0.5-2.5% of the general population meet the criteria for paranoid personality disorder.

Schizoid patients are perceived by others as ''loners'' without close family relationships or social contacts. Indeed, they are aloof and really do prefer to be alone. They may appear cold to others because they rarely display strong emotions. They may, however, be successful in occupations that do not require personal interaction. About 2% of the general population has this disorder. It is slightly more common in men than in women.

Patients diagnosed as schizotypal are often considered odd or eccentric because they pay little attention to their clothing and sometimes have peculiar speech mannerisms. They are socially isolated and uncomfortable in parties or other social gatherings. In addition, people with schizotypal personality disorder often have oddities of thought, including ''magical'' beliefs or peculiar ideas (for example, a belief in telepathy) that are outside of their cultural norms. It is thought that 3% of the general population has schizotypal personality disorder. It is slightly more common in males. Schizotypal disorder should not be confused with **schizophrenia**, although there is some evidence that the disorders are genetically related.

Patients with antisocial personality disorder are sometimes referred to as sociopaths or psychopaths. They are characterized by lying, manipulativeness, and a selfish disregard for the rights of others; some may act impulsively. People with antisocial personality disorder are frequently chemically dependent and sexually promiscuous. It is estimated that 3% of males in the general population and 1% of females have antisocial personality disorder.

Patients with borderline personality disorder (BPD) are highly unstable, with wide mood swings, a history of intense but stormy relationships, impulsive behavior, and confusion about career goals, personal values, or sexual orientation. These often highly conflictual ideas may correspond to an even deeper confusion about their sense of self (identity). People with BPD frequently cut or burn themselves, or threaten or attempt **suicide**. Many of these patients have histories of severe childhood abuse or neglect. About 2% of the general population have BPD; 75% of these patients are female.

Patients diagnosed with this disorder impress others as overly emotional, overly dramatic, and hungry for attention.

They may be flirtatious or seductive as a way of drawing attention to themselves, yet they are emotionally shallow. Histrionic patients often live in a romantic fantasy world and are easily bored with routine. About 2-3% of the population is thought to have this disorder. Although historically, in clinical settings, the disorder has been more associated with women, there may be bias toward diagnosing women with the histrionic personality disorder.

Narcissistic patients are characterized by self-importance, a craving for admiration, and exploitative attitudes toward others. They have unrealistically inflated views of their talents and accomplishments, and may become extremely angry if they are criticized or outshone by others. Narcissists may be professionally successful but rarely have long-lasting intimate relationships. Fewer than 1% of the population has this disorder; about 75% of those diagnosed with it are male.

Patients with avoidant personality disorder are fearful of rejection and shy away from situations or occupations that might expose their supposed inadequacy. They may reject opportunities to develop close relationships because of their fears of criticism or humiliation. Patients with this personality disorder are often diagnosed with dependent personality disorder as well. Many also fit the criteria for social phobia. Between 0.5-1.0% of the population have avoidant personality disorder.

Dependent patients are afraid of being on their own and typically develop submissive or compliant behaviors in order to avoid displeasing people. They are afraid to question authority and often ask others for guidance or direction. Dependent personality disorder is diagnosed more often in women, but it has been suggested that this finding reflects social pressures on women to conform to gender stereotyping or bias on the part of clinicians.

Patients diagnosed with this disorder are preoccupied with keeping order, attaining perfection, and maintaining mental and interpersonal control. They may spend a great deal of time adhering to plans, schedules, or rules from which they will not deviate, even at the expense of openness, flexibility, and efficiency. These patients are often unable to relax and may become ''workaholics.'' They may have problems in employment as well as in intimate relationships because they are very ''stiff'' and formal, and insist on doing everything their way. About 1% of the population has obsessive-compulsive personality disorder; the male/female ratio is about 2:1.

Personality disorders are thought to result from a bad interface between a child's temperament and character on one hand and his or her family environment on the other. Temperament can be defined as a person's innate or biologically shaped basic disposition. Human infants vary in their sensitivity to light or noise, their level of physical activity, their adaptability to schedules, and similar traits. Even traits such as ''shyness'' and ''novelty-seeking'' may be, at least in part, determined by the biology of the brain and the genes one inherits.

Character is defined as the set of attitudes and behavior patterns that the individual acquires or learns over time. It includes such personal qualities as work and study habits, moral convictions, neatness or cleanliness, and consideration of others. Since children must learn to adapt to their specific families, they may develop personality disorders in the course of struggling to survive psychologically in disturbed or stressful families. For example, nervous or high-strung parents might be unhappy with a baby who is very active and try to restrain him or her at every opportunity. The child might then develop an avoidant personality disorder as the outcome of coping with constant frustration and parental disapproval. As another example, **child abuse** is believed to play a role in shaping borderline personality disorder. One reason that some therapists use the term developmental damage instead of personality disorder is that it takes the presumed source of the person's problems into account.

Some patients with personality disorders come from families that appear to be stable and healthy. It has been suggested that these patients are biologically hypersensitive to normal family stress levels. Levels of the brain chemical (neurotransmitter) dopamine may influence a person's level of novelty-seeking, and serotonin levels may influence aggression.

Diagnosis of personality disorders is complicated by the fact that persons suffering from them rarely seek help until they are in serious trouble or until their families (or the law) pressure them to get treatment. The reason for this slowness is that the problematic traits are so deeply entrenched that they seem normal (ego-syntonic) to the patient. Diagnosis of a personality disorder depends in part on the patient's age. Although personality disorders originate during the childhood years, they are considered adult disorders. Some patients, in fact, are not diagnosed until late in life because their symptoms had been modified by the demands of their job or by marriage. After retirement or the spouse's **death**, however, these patients' personality disorders become fully apparent. In general, however, if the onset of the patient's problem is in mid- or late-life, the doctor will rule out **substance abuse** or personality change caused by medical or neurological problems before considering the diagnosis of a personality disorder. It is unusual for people to develop personality disorders ''out of the blue'' in mid-life.

There are no tests that can provide a definitive diagnosis of personality disorder. Most doctors will evaluate a patient on the basis of several sources of information collected over a period of time in order to determine how long the patient has been having difficulties, how many areas of life are affected, and how severe the dysfunction is.

The doctor may schedule two or three interviews with the patient, spaced over several weeks or months, in order to rule out an adjustment disorder caused by job loss, bereavement, or a similar problem. An office interview allows the doctor to form an impression of the patient's overall personality as well as obtaining information about his or her occupation and family. During the interview, the doctor will note the patient's appearance, tone of voice, body language, eye contact, and other important non-verbal signals, as well as the content of the conversation. In some cases, the doctor may contact other people (family members, employers, close friends) who know the patient well in order to assess the accuracy of the patient's perception of his or her difficulties. It is quite common for people with personality disorders to have distorted views of their situations, or to be unaware of the impact of their behavior on others.

Doctors use psychologic testing to help in the diagnosis of a personality disorder. Most of these tests require interpretation by a professional with specialized training. Doctors usually refer patients to a clinical psychologist for this type of test.

Personality inventories are tests with true/false or yes/no answers that can be used to compare the patient's scores with those of people with known personality distortions. The single most commonly used test of this type is the Minnesota Multiphasic Personality Inventory, or MMPI.

Projective tests are unstructured. Unstructured means that instead of giving one-word answers to questions, the patient is asked to talk at some length about a picture that the psychologist has shown him or her, or to supply an ending for the beginning of a story. Projective tests allow the clinician to assess the patient's patterns of thinking, fantasies, worries or anxieties, moral concerns, values, and habits. Common projective tests include the Rorschach, in which the patient responds to a set of ten inkblots; and the Thematic Apperception Test (TAT), in which the patient is shown drawings of people in different situations and then tells a story about the picture.

At one time psychiatrists thought that personality disorders did not respond very well to treatment. This opinion was derived from the notion that human personality is fixed for life once it has been molded in childhood, and from the belief among people with personality disorders that their own views and behaviors are correct, and that others are the ones at fault. More recently, however, doctors have recognized that humans can continue to grow and change throughout life. Most patients with personality disorders are now considered to be treatable, although the degree of improvement may vary. The type of treatment recommended depends on the personality characteristics associated with the specific disorder. Treatment options include inpatient treatment, insight-oriented approaches, group therapy, and family therapy, to name a few. Medications may be prescribed for patients with specific personality disorders. The type of medication depends on the disorder.

Treatment with medications is not recommended for patients with certain personality disorders, such as the avoidant, histrionic, dependent, or narcissistic personality types. The use of potentially addictive medications should be avoided in people with borderline or antisocial personality disorders. However, some avoidant patients who also have social phobia may benefit from **monoamine oxidase inhibitors** (MAO inhibitors), a particular class of antidepressant.

The prognosis for recovery depends in part on the specific disorder. Although some patients improve as they grow older and have positive experiences in life, personality disorders are generally life-long disturbances with periods of worsening and periods of improvement. Others, particularly schizoid patients, have better prognoses if they are given appropriate treatment. Patients with paranoid personality disorder are at some risk for developing delusional disorders or schizophrenia. The personality disorders with the poorest prognoses are the antisocial and the borderline. Borderline patients are at high risk for developing substance abuse disorders or bulimia. About 80% of hospitalized borderline patients attempt suicide at some point during treatment, and about 5% succeed in committing suicide.

The most effective preventive strategy for personality disorders is early identification and treatment of children at risk. High-risk groups include abused children, children from troubled families, children with close relatives diagnosed with personality disorders, children of substance abusers, and children who grow up in cults or political extremist groups.

PERSONAL HYGIENE

Attention to personal hygiene will help a person look their best, feel their best, and can even help in avoiding disease. People who are conscientious about personal hygiene take care of cleanliness, routine health care, and preventive health maintenance.

An overview of some of the most common preventable health problems illustrates the role of personal hygiene:

Mouth: Despite spending $1.5 billion on **oral hygiene** products each year, 98 percent of Americans have cavities or **tooth decay**. The combination of bacteria in the mouth, sugar in the diet, and susceptible teeth leads to decay, cavities, gum disease, and sometimes even the loss of teeth. These risks can be addressed by eating a variety of foods, limiting sugary foods, brushing and flossing regularly, and having regular dental checkups.

Eyes: Even people with normal vision need **eye examinations** to screen for disease, infection, and changes in vision. Protecting the eyes is a matter of following common sense measures such as guarding against poking the eyes or rubbing against them with dirty clothing, tissues, or fingers. It will also help to avoid exposure to strong light and avoid eyestrain.

Ears: Avoid poking at the inside of the ears. Have regular **hearing tests** and ear examinations to check for **hearing loss** or other disorders and illnesses.

Skin: Remove dirt, prevent odor, and make sure rough skin is moisturized. Breaks in the skin should be washed and bandaged. Pigment changes are usually not harmful, but too much sun can lead to **skin cancer**. A doctor should be consulted if there is a change in a **wart** or **mole**. Almost every teenager experiences some **acne**, and persistent cases can be treated by a family doctor or dermatologist. In cases of parasites such as head lice, body lice, and **scabies**, bedding and clothing must be treated in addition to the skin. The hair is part of the skin and it responds to good diet, exercise, good health habits, and regular shampooing.

Genitourinary: Conscientious patients can reduce the risk of cancer by performing the breast self-examination (women) and testicular self exam (men) at home and reporting any changes to a doctor. Prepubescent women need to learn special care of the body during **menstruation**. Adolescents face many pressures and decisions in the area of sexuality. Issues include **abstinence**, **contraception**, **pregnancy**, **abortion**, and **sexually transmitted diseases**, which can be incurable or fatal. Often parents and schools serve as resources on these topics.

Back: Care of the back requires correct procedures for lifting and bending. Many back problems can be prevented by keeping the muscles strong through **exercise** and good posture.

Feet: Most foot problems are preventable. Precautions include exposing the feet to fresh air, choosing shoes to promote healthy feet, rotating shoes on different days, and changing shoes when the feet are perspiring. Feet can also be protected by not sharing footwear, and by using footwear around pools and locker rooms. A routine **physical examination** should include a foot exam.

General: Many day-to-day complaints can be addressed with preventive health strategies such as eating a good diet, getting enough rest, taking care of emotional **stress**, and seeking help for large fluctuations in weight. The simple act of handwashing (at least 20 seconds according to Food and Drug Administration recommendations) can prevent the spread of many food-borne illnesses and upper respiratory infections. Staying home with a contagious illness will help keep it from spreading.

The medical profession has come to recognize violence as a **public health** issue. Teens need to learn about sexual assault, **domestic violence**, **conflict resolution**, and safety around weapons.

Sometimes lack of attention to personal health can be symptom of a deeper medical problem such as arthritis, poor eyesight, or **dementia**. Inattention to hygiene could also signal a depressive disorder or a substance abuse problem.

See also Adolescent health

Pharmacy

Pharmacy is the third largest health profession in the United States. In 1997, there were approximately 170,000 licensed pharmacists in the United States. Of these, some 43,000 worked in community pharmacies, with the others employed in all areas of health care and medical research. Pharmacists are employed in hospitals, **nursing homes**, home health care companies, **managed care** organizations, clinics, and physicians' offices. Other pharmacists work for federal agencies such as the **Food and Drug Administration** and the **National Institutes of Health**. Still others are faculty members at colleges and universities.

In the past, pharmacists were thought of as dispensers of medication, where their traditional role would be to count or pour medications. However, the role of the profession has evolved to include pharmaceutical care: the responsible provision of drug therapy to achieve specific outcomes that improve a patient's quality of life, and disease state management, and the systematic review of a disease process, the available treatment options, and the outcomes or drug interactions that those treatments may be expected to produce.

Pharmacists earn either a five-year bachelor of science (B.S.) degree, or a six-year doctor of pharmacy (PharmD.) degree, although some pharmacists earn master's or doctor of philosophy degrees in related fields. Before entering practice, pharmacy graduates must pass a national licensure examination and meet additional requirements in the states in which they intend to practice. The aging of the American population, and the on-going development of new medications coupled with the increasing complexity of drug therapies only bode well for the pharmaceutical profession in the twenty-first century.

There are many professional organizations that serve the needs of members of the pharmaceutical profession. These include the American Pharmaceutical Association (with offices in all 50 states and over 18,000 members), the National Pharmaceutical Association, the National Community Pharmacists Association, the American Association for Health System Pharmacists, and the American College of Apothecaries.

For the medical consumer, the most common source for obtaining prescription medicines is the local or community pharmacy. Medical consumers who belong to **Health Maintenance Organization**s (HMOs) may be required to use a pharmacy on site (at the location of the HMO) or the HMO may have contracted with certain pharmacies to take their business. Another avenue that some individuals and some insurance companies have chosen is mail-order pharmacy. With this arrangement, a prescription is normally sent to the mail-order pharmacy or phoned in by the physician. As it may take a week or more for the prescription to arrive at the home of the patient, mail order is best used for maintenance (long-term medications used to treat such chronic problems as high blood pressure and diabetes).

Since 1993, all pharmacists who practice in states receiving Medicaid funds have been required to provide counseling services on all matters pertaining to special directions for taking medications and to precautions about medication side effects, interactions, proper storage, techniques for self-monitoring, and other essential guidance. Once a community pharmacy has been chosen, it usually is in the medical consumer's best interest to stay with that pharmacy and not shop around for another pharmacy, especially if the selected pharmacy maintains patient drug histories. If the pharmacy maintains an accurate drug history on the patient, the pharmacist can more easily check for drug interactions that may be potentially harmful to the patient, or decrease the efficacy of medications prescribed by different physicians.

Phenylketonuria

Phenylketonuria (PKU) is a rare, inherited, metabolic disorder that can result in **mental retardation** and other neurological problems. People with this disease have difficulty breaking down and using (metabolizing) the amino acid phenylalanine. PKU is sometimes called Folling's disease in honor of Dr. Asbjorn Folling who first described it in 1934.

Phenylalanine is an essential amino acid. These substances are called ''essential'' because the body must get them from food to build the proteins that make up its tissues and keep them working. Therefore, phenylalanine is required for normal development. Phenylalanine is a common amino acid and is found in all natural foods. However, natural foods contain more phenylalanine than required for normal development. This level is too high for patients with PKU, making a special low-phenylalanine diet a requirement.

The incidence of PKU is approximately one in every 15,000 births (1/15,000). There are areas in the world where the incidence is much higher, particularly Ireland and western Scotland. In Ireland the incidence of PKU is 1/4,500 births. This is the highest incidence in the world and supports a theory that the genetic defect is very old and of Celtic origin. Countries with very little immigration from Ireland or western Scotland tend to have low rates of PKU. In Finland, the incidence is less than 1/100,000 births. Caucasians in the United States have a PKU incidence of 1/8,000, whereas Blacks have an incidence of 1/50,000.

There are a number of specific types of PKU. Maternal phenylketonuria is a condition in which a high level of phenylalanine in a mother's blood causes mental retardation in her child when in the uterus. A woman who has PKU and is not using a special low-phenylalanine diet will have high levels of phenylalanine in her blood. Her high phenylalanine levels will cross the placenta and affect the development of her child. The majority of children born from these pregnancies are mentally retarded and have physical problems, including small head size (microcephaly) and congenital heart disease. Most of these children do not have PKU. There is no treatment for maternal phenylketonuria. Control of maternal phenylalanine levels is thought to limit the effects of maternal phenylketonuria.

Hyperphenylalaninemia is a condition in which patients have high levels of phenylalanine in their blood, but not as high as seen in patients with classical PKU. There are two forms of hyperphenylalaninemia: mild and severe.

Tyrosinemia is characterized by a high levels of two amino acids in the blood, phenylalanine and tyrosine. Patients with this disease have many of the same symptoms as seen in classical PKU, including mental retardation. Treatment consists of a special diet similar to the diet for PKU. The main difference between the two **diets** is that patients with tyrosinemia must eat a diet that is low in both phenylalanine and tyrosine.

The underlying cause of PKU is mutation in the gene that tells the body to make the enzyme phenylalanine hydroxylase. This enzyme allows the body to break down phenylalanine and ultimately use it to build proteins. Normally, the first step in phenylalanine metabolism is conversion to tyrosine, another amino acid. The genetic mutations result in no enzyme or poor quality enzyme being made. As a consequence, phenylalanine is not converted and builds up in the body. The high levels of phenylalanine can be detected in the blood and urine.

PKU is a genetic disease. A child must inherit defective genes from both parents to develop PKU. A person with one defective gene and one good gene will develop normally because the good gene will make sufficient phenylalanine hydroxylase. People with one good gene are called carriers because they do not have the disease, but are capable of passing the defective gene on to their children.

If both parents are carriers of defective phenylalanine hydroxylase genes, then the chances of their child having PKU is one in four or 25%. The chances that their child will be a carrier is two in four, or 50%. These percentages hold for each **pregnancy**.

Children with PKU appear normal at birth, but develop irreversible mental retardation unless treated early. Treatment consists of a special diet that contains very little phenylalanine. This diet must be used throughout the patient's life. Untreated newborns develop disease symptoms at age three to five months. At first they appear to be less attentive and may have problems eating. By one year of age, they are mentally retarded.

Patients with PKU tend to have lighter colored skin, hair, and eyes than other family members. They are also likely to have eczema and seizures. PKU patients have a variety of neurologic symptoms. Approximately 75-90% of PKU patients have abnormal electrocardiograms (ECGs), which measure the activity of their heart. Their sweat and urine may have a ''mousy'' smell that is caused by phenylacetic acid, a byproduct of phenylalanine metabolism. Untreated PKU children tend to be hyperactive and demonstrate loss of contact with reality (**psychosis**).

PKU must be detected shortly after birth. Although children with PKU appear normal at birth, they already have high phenylalanine levels. Screening is the only way to detect PKU before symptoms start to develop. In many areas of the world, screening newborns for PKU is performed routinely. The test is typically performed between one and seven days after birth. Blood is obtained by pricking the heel of the newborn and analyzing it for phenylalanine concentration.

The only treatment for persons with PKU is to limit the amount of phenylalanine in their diet. PKU patients should eat a special diet that is low in phenylalanine. The diet has small amounts of phenylalanine because it is essential for normal growth and development. The diet should be started before the fourth week of life to prevent mental retardation. If started early enough, the diet is 75% effective in preventing severe mental retardation. Many natural foods, including breast milk, must be avoided because they contain more phenylalanine than PKU patients can tolerate. However, low protein, natural foods, including fruits, vegetables, and some cereals, are acceptable on the diet. Monitoring of blood phenylalanine levels must be done to ensure that normal levels are maintained.

Patients who make a small amount of phenylalanine hydroxylase can eat a limited amount of regular food if their phenylalanine levels remain within an acceptable range. Low-phenylalanine and phenylalanine-free foods are available commercially. The special diet must be used throughout the patient's life.

Phlebotomy

Phlebotomy is the act of drawing or removing blood from the circulatory system through a cut (incision) or puncture in order to obtain a sample for analysis and diagnosis. Phlebotomy is also done as part of the patient's treatment for certain blood disorders.

Phlebotomy is part of treatment (therapeutic phlebotomy) for several diseases such as polycythemia vera, a condition that causes an elevated red blood cell volume. Phlebotomy is also prescribed for patients with disorders that increase the amount of iron in their blood to dangerous levels, such as **hepatitis** B, and hepatitis C. Patients with **pulmonary edema** (fluid in the lungs) may undergo phlebotomy procedures to decrease their total blood volume. Phlebotomy is also used to remove blood from the body during blood donation and for analysis of the substances contained within it. Patients who are anemic or have a history of cardiovascular disease may not be good candidates for phlebotomy.

Phlebotomy, which is also known as venesection, is performed by a nurse or a technician known as a phlebotomist. Blood is usually taken from a vein on the back of the hand or inside of the elbow. Some blood tests, however, may require blood from an artery. The skin over the area is wiped with an antiseptic, and an elastic band is tied around the arm. The band acts as a tourniquet, slowing the blood flow in the arm and making the veins more visible. The patient is asked to make a fist, and the technician feels the veins in order to select an appropriate one. When a vein is selected, the technician inserts a needle into the vein and releases the elastic band. The appropriate amount of blood is drawn and the needle is withdrawn from the vein. The patient's pulse and blood pressure may be monitored during the procedure.

For some tests requiring very small amounts of blood for analysis, the technician uses a finger stick. A lance, or small needle, makes a small cut in the surface of the fingertip, and a small amount of blood is collected in a narrow glass tube. The fingertip may be squeezed to get additional blood to surface.

The amount of blood drawn depends on the purpose of the phlebotomy. Blood donors usually contribute a unit of blood (500 mL) in a session. The volume of blood needed for laboratory analysis varies widely with the type of test being conducted. Therapeutic phlebotomy removes a larger amount of blood than donation and blood analysis require.

Patients having their blood drawn for analysis may be asked to discontinue medications or to avoid food (to fast) for a period of time before the blood test. Patients donating blood will be asked for a brief medical history, have their blood pressure taken, and have their hematocrit checked with a finger stick test prior to donation.

After blood is drawn and the needle is removed, pressure is placed on the puncture site with a cotton ball to stop bleeding, and a bandage is applied. It is not uncommon for a patient to feel dizzy or nauseated during or after phlebotomy. The patient may be encouraged to rest for a short period once the procedure is completed. Patients are also instructed to drink plenty of fluids and eat regularly over the next 24 hours to replace lost blood volume. Patients who experience swelling of the puncture site or continued bleeding after phlebotomy should get medical help at once.

Most patients will have a small bruise or mild soreness at the puncture site for several days. Therapeutic phlebotomy may cause **thrombocytosis** (an increase in the number of blood platelets) and chronic iron deficiency (anemia) in some patients. As with any invasive procedure, infection is also a risk. This risk can be minimized by the use of prepackaged sterilized equipment and careful attention to proper technique.

PHOBIAS

A phobia is an intense, unrealistic fear, which can interfere with the ability to socialize, work, or go about everyday life, that is brought on by an object, event or situation.

Just about everyone is afraid of something—an upcoming job interview or being alone outside after dark. But about 18% of all Americans are tormented by irrational fears that interfere with their daily lives. They aren't ''crazy''—they know full well their fears are unreasonable—but they can't control the fear. These people suffer from phobias.

Phobias belong to a large group of mental problems known as ''anxiety disorders'' that include **obsessive-compulsive disorder** (OCD), panic disorder, and post-traumatic stress disorder. Phobias themselves can be divided into three specific types:

- Specific phobias (formerly called ''simple phobias'')
- Social phobia
- Agoraphobia.

As its name suggests, a specific phobia is the fear of a particular situation or object, including anything from airplane travel to dentists. Found in 1 out of every 10 Americans, specific phobias seem to run in families and are roughly twice as likely to appear in women. If the person doesn't often encounter the feared object, the phobia doesn't cause much harm. However, if the feared object or situation is common, it can seriously disrupt everyday life. Common examples of specific phobias, which can begin at any age, include fear of snakes, flying, dogs, escalators, elevators, high places, or open spaces.

People with social phobia have deep fears of being watched or judged by others and being embarrassed in public. This may extend to a general fear of social situations—or be more specific or ''circumscribed,'' such as a fear of giving speeches or of performing (''stage fright''). More rarely, people with social phobia may have trouble using a public restroom, eating in a restaurant, or signing their name in front of others.

Social phobia is not the same as shyness. Shy people may feel uncomfortable with others, but they don't experience severe **anxiety**, they don't worry excessively about social situations beforehand, and they don't avoid events that make them feel self-conscious. On the other hand, people with social phobia may not be shy—they may feel perfectly comfortable with people except in specific situations. Social phobias may be only mildly irritating, or they may significantly interfere with daily life. It is not unusual for people with social phobia to turn down job offers or avoid relationships because of their fears.

Agoraphobia is the intense fear of feeling trapped and having a panic attack in a public place. It usually begins between ages 15-35, and affects three times as many women as men—about 3% of the population.

An episode of spontaneous panic is usually the initial trigger for the development of agoraphobia. After an initial panic attack, the person becomes afraid of experiencing a second one. Sufferers literally ''fear the fear,'' and worry incessantly about when and where the next attack may occur. As they begin to avoid the places or situations in which the panic attack occurred, their fear generalizes. Eventually the person completely avoids public places. In severe cases, people with agoraphobia can no longer leave their homes for fear of experiencing a panic attack.

Experts don't really know why phobias develop, although research suggests the tendency to develop phobias may be a complex interaction between heredity and environment. Some hypersensitive people have unique chemical reactions in the brain that cause them to respond much more strongly to **stress**. These people also may be especially sensitive to **caffeine**, which triggers certain brain chemical responses.

While experts believe the tendency to develop phobias runs in families and may be hereditary, a specific stressful event usually triggers the development of a specific phobia or agoraphobia. For example, someone predisposed to develop phobias who experiences severe turbulence during a flight might go on to develop a phobia about flying. What scientists don't understand is why some people who experience a frightening or stressful event develop a phobia and others don't.

Social phobia typically appears in childhood or adolescence, sometimes following an upsetting or humiliating experience. Certain vulnerable children who have had unpleasant social experiences (such as being rejected) or who have poor social skills may develop social phobias. The condition also may be related to low self-esteem, unassertive personality, and feelings of inferiority.

A person with agoraphobia may have a panic attack at any time, for no apparent reason. While the attack may last only a minute or so, the person remembers the feelings of panic so strongly that the possibility of another attack becomes terrifying. For this reason, people with agoraphobia avoid places where they might not be able to escape if a panic attack occurs. As the fear of an attack escalates, the person's world narrows.

While the specific trigger may differ, the symptoms of different phobias are remarkably similar: e.g., feelings of terror and impending doom, rapid heartbeat and breathing, sweaty palms, and other features of a panic attack. Patients may experience severe anxiety symptoms in anticipating a phobic trigger. For example, someone who is afraid to fly may begin having episodes of pounding heart and sweating palms at the mere thought of getting on a plane in two weeks.

A mental health professional can diagnose phobias after a detailed interview and discussion of both mental and physical symptoms. Social phobia is often associated with other **anxiety disorders**, depression, or substance abuse.

People who have a specific phobia that is easy to avoid (such as snakes) and that doesn't interfere with their lives may not need to get help. When phobias do interfere with a person's daily life, a combination of psychotherapy and medication can be quite effective. While most health insurance covers some form of mental health care, most do not cover outpatient care completely, and most have a yearly or lifetime maximum.

Medication can block the feelings of panic, and when combined with cognitive-behavioral therapy, can be quite effective in reducing specific phobias and agoraphobia.

Cognitive-behavioral therapy adds a cognitive approach to more traditional behavioral therapy. It teaches patients how to change their thoughts, behavior, and attitudes, while providing techniques to lessen anxiety, such as deep breathing, muscle relaxation, and refocusing.

One cognitive-behavioral therapy is "desensitization" (also known as "exposure therapy"), in which people are gradually exposed to the frightening object or event until they become used to it and their physical symptoms decrease. For example, someone who is afraid of snakes might first be shown a photo of a snake. Once the person can look at a photo without anxiety, he might then be shown a video of a snake. Each step is repeated until the symptoms of fear (such as pounding heart and sweating palms) disappear. Eventually, the person might reach the point where he can actually touch a live snake. Three fourths of patients are significantly improved with this type of treatment.

Another more dramatic cognitive-behavioral approach is called "flooding," which exposes the person immediately to the feared object or situation. The person remains in the situation until the anxiety lessens.

Several drugs are used to treat specific phobias by controlling symptoms and helping to prevent panic attacks. These include anti-anxiety drugs (benzodiazepines) such as alprazolam (Xanax) or diazepam (Valium). Blood pressure medications called "**beta blockers**," such as propranolol (Inderal) and atenolol (Tenormin), appear to work well in the treatment of circumscribed social phobia, when anxiety gets in the way of performance, such as public speaking. These drugs reduce overstimulation, thereby controlling the physical symptoms of anxiety.

In addition, some antidepressants may be effective when used together with cognitive-behavioral therapy. These include the **monoamine oxidase inhibitors** (MAO inhibitors) phenelzine (Nardil) and tranylcypromine (Parnate), as well as selective serotonin reuptake inhibitors (SSRIs) like fluoxetine (Prozac), paroxetine (Paxil), sertraline (Zoloft) and fluvoxamine (Luvox).

In all types of phobias, symptoms may be eased by lifestyle changes, such as:

- Eliminating caffeine
- Cutting down on alcohol
- Eating a good diet
- Getting plenty of **exercise**
- Reducing stress.

Treating agoraphobia is more difficult than other phobias because there are often so many fears involved, such as open spaces, traffic, elevators, and escalators. Treatment includes cognitive-behavioral therapy with antidepressants or anti-anxiety drugs. Paxil and Zoloft are used to treat **panic disorder**s with or without agoraphobia.

Phobias are among the most treatable mental health problems; depending on the severity of the condition and the type of phobia, most properly treated patients can go on to lead normal lives. Research suggests that once a person overcomes the phobia, the problem may not return for many years—if at all.

Untreated phobias are another matter. Only about 20% of specific phobias will go away without treatment, and agoraphobia will get worse with time if untreated. Social phobias tend to be chronic, and without treatment, will not likely go away. Moreover, untreated phobias can lead to other problems, including depression, alcoholism, and feelings of shame and low self-esteem.

While most specific phobias appear in childhood and subsequently fade away, those that remain in adulthood often need to be treated. Unfortunately, most people never get the help they need; only about 25% of people with phobias ever seek help to deal with their condition.

There is no known way to prevent the development of phobias. Medication and cognitive-behavioral therapy may help prevent the recurrence of symptoms once they have been diagnosed.

PHOSPHORUS IMBALANCE

Phosphorus imbalance refers to conditions in which the element phosphorus is present in the body at too high a level (hyperphosphatemia) or too low a level (hypophosphatemia).

Almost all of the phosphorus in the body occurs as phosphate (phosphorus combined with four oxygen atoms), and most of the body's phosphate (85%) is located in the skeletal system, where it combines with calcium to give bones their hardness. The remaining amount (15%) exists in the cells of the body, where it plays an important role in the formation of key nucleic acids, such as DNA, and in the process by which the body turns food into energy (metabolism). The body regulates phosphate levels in the blood through the controlled release of parathyroid hormone (PTH) from the parathyroid gland and calcitonin from the thyroid gland. PTH keeps phosphate levels from becoming too high by stimulating the excretion of phosphate in urine and causing the release of calcium from bones (phosphate blood levels are inversely proportional to calcium blood levels). Calcitonin keeps phosphate blood levels in check by moving phosphates out of the blood and into the bone matrix to form a mineral salt with calcium.

Most phosphorus imbalances develop gradually and are the result of other conditions or disorders, such as malnutrition, poor kidney function, or a malfunctioning gland.

Hypophosphatemia (low blood phosphate) has various causes. Hyperparathyroidism, a condition in which the parathyroid gland produces too much PTH, is one primary cause. Poor kidney function, in which the renal tubules do not adequately reabsorb phosphorus, can result in hypophosphatemia, as can overuse of diuretics (water pills) and antacids containing aluminum hydroxide. Problems involving the intestinal absorption of phosphate, such as chronic diarrhea or a deficiency of Vitamin D (needed by the intestines to properly absorb phosphates) can cause the condition. **Malnutrition** due to chronic alcoholism can result in an inadequate intake of phosphorus. Recovery from various conditions such as severe burns can provoke hypophosphatemia, since the body must use larger-than-normal amounts of phosphate.

Symptoms generally occur only when phosphate levels have decreased profoundly. They include muscle weakness, tingling sensations, tremors, and bone weakness. Hypophosphatemia may also result in confusion and memory loss, seizures, and coma

Hyperphosphatemia (high blood phosphate) also has various causes. It is most often caused by a decline in the normal excretion of phosphate in urine as a result of kidney failure or impaired function. Hypoparathyroidism, a condition in which the parathyroid gland does not produce enough PTH, or pseudoparathyroidism, a condition in which the kidneys lose their ability to respond to PTH, can also contribute to decreased phosphate excretion. Hyperphosphatemia can also result from the overuse of **laxatives** or **enemas** that contain phosphate. Hypocalcemia (abnormally low blood calcium) can cause phosphate blood levels to increase abnormally. A side-effect of hyperphosphatemia is the formation of calcium-phosphate crystals in the blood and soft tissue.

Hyperphosphatemia is generally asymptomatic; however, it can occur in conjunction with hypocalcemia, the symptoms of which are numbness and tingling in the extemities, muscle cramps and spasms, depression, memory loss, and convulsions. When calcium-phosphate crystals build up in the blood vessels, they can cause arteriosclerosis, which can lead to heart attacks or strokes. When the crystals build up in the skin, they can cause severe itching.

Disorders of phosphate metabolism are assessed by measuring serum or plasma levels of phosphate and calcium. Hypophosphatemia is diagnosed if the blood phosphate level is less than 2.5 milligrams per deciliter of blood. Hyperphosphatemia is diagnosed if the blood phosphate level is above 4.5 milligrams per deciliter of blood. Appropriate tests are also used to determine if the underlying cause of the imbalance, including assessments of kidney function, dietary intake, and appropriate hormone levels.

Treatment of phosphorus imbalances focuses on correcting the underlying cause of the imbalance and restoring equilibrium. Treating the underlying condition may involve surgical removal of the parathyroid gland in the case of hypophosphatemia caused by hyperparathyroidism; initiating hormone therapy in cases of hyperphosphatemia caused by hypoparathyroidism; ceasing intake of drugs or medications that contribute to phosphorus imbalance; or instigating measures to restore proper kidney function.

Restoring phosphorus equilibrium in cases of mild hypophosphatemia may include drinking a prescribed solution that is rich in phosphorus; however, since this solution can cause diarrhea, many doctors recommend that patients drink 1 qt (.9 l) of skim milk per day instead, since milk and other diary products are significant sources of phosphate. Other phosphate-rich foods include green, leafy vegetables; peas and beans; nuts; chocolate; beef liver; turkey; and some cola drinks. Severe hypophosphatemia may be treated with the administration of an intravenous solution containing phosphate.

Restoring phosphorus equilibrium in cases of mild hyperphosphatemia involves restricting intake of phosphorus-rich foods and taking a calcium-based antacid that binds to the phosphate and blocks its absorption in the intestines. In cases of severe hyperphosphatemia, an intravenous infusion of calcium gluconate may be administered. Dialysis may also be required in severe cases to help remove excess phosphate from the blood. The prognosis for treating hyperphosphatemia and hypophosphatemia are excellent, though in cases where these problems are due to genetic disease, life-long hormone treatment may be necessary.

Phosphorus imbalances caused by hormonal disorders or other genetically determined conditions cannot be prevented. Hypophosphatemia resulting from poor dietary intake can be prevented by eating foods rich in phosphates, and hypophosphatemia caused by overuse of diuretics or antacids can be prevented by strictly following instructions concerning proper dosages, as can hyperphosphatemia due to excessive use of enemas or laxative. Finally, patients on dialysis or who are being fed intravenously should be monitored closely to prevent phosphorus imbalances.

Photorefractive keratectomy and laser-assisted in-situ keratomileusis

Photorefractive keratectomy (PRK) and laser-assisted in-situ keratomileusis (LASIK) are two similar surgical techniques that use an excimer laser to correct **nearsightedness** (myopia) by reshaping the cornea. The cornea is the clear outer structure of the eye that lies in front of the colored part of the **eye** (iris). PRK and LASIK are two forms of vision-correcting (refractive) surgery. The two techniques differ in how the surface layer of the cornea is treated. As of mid 1998, two eximer lasers (Summit and Visx) are approved for laser vision correction (refractive surgery using a laser) in the PRK procedure, but not yet approved by the **Food and Drug Administration** (FDA) for use in LASIK.

The purpose of both LASIK and PRK is to correct nearsightedness in persons who do not want to, or who cannot wear eye glasses or contact lenses. Most patients are able to see well enough to pass a driver's license exam without glasses or contact lenses after the operation. After approximately age 40, the lens in the eye stiffens making it harder to focus up close. Because laser vision correction only affects the cornea the procedures do not eliminate the need for reading glasses. Patients should be wary of any ads that ''guarantee'' 20/20 vision. Patients should also make sure that the laser being used is approved by the FDA.

Patients should be over 18 years of age, have healthy corneas, and have vision that has been stable for the past year. People who may not be good candidates for these procedures are pregnant women or women who are breastfeeding (vision may not be stable); people with scarred corneas or macular disease; people with autoimmune diseases or **rheumatoid arthritis**); or people with diabetes. Patients with **glaucoma** should not have LASIK because the intraocular pressure (IOP) of the eye is raised during the procedure. A patient with persistent lid infections may not be a good candidate because of an increased risk of infection. An ophthalmologist who specializes in laser vision correction can determine who would be likely to benefit from the operation and suggest which of the two operations might be more appropriate for any given patient.

If a patient is thinking of having **cataract** surgery, they should discuss it with the doctor. During cataract surgery an intracocular lens (IOL) will be inserted and that alone may correct distance vision.

PRK and LASIK are both performed with an excimer laser, which uses a cold beam of ultraviolet light to sculpt or reshape the cornea so that light will focus properly on the retina. The cornea is the major focusing structure of the eye. The retina sends the image focused on it to the brain. In myopia, the cornea is either too steep or the eye is too long for a clear image to be focused on the retina. PRK and LASIK flatten out the cornea so that the image will focus more precisely on the retina.

In PRK, the surface of the cornea is removed by the laser. In LASIK, the outer layer of the cornea is sliced, lifted, moved aside while the cornea is reshaped with the laser, then replaced to speed healing. Both procedures cause the cornea to become flatter, which corrects the nearsighted vision.

At least one laser has been approved to treat mild **astigmatism** (light spread over a diffuse area) as of 1998. Correcting farsightedness (hyperopia) may be possible in the future.

These laser vision-correcting procedures are rapidly replacing **radial keratotomy** (RK), an earlier form of refractive surgery that involved cutting the cornea with a scalpel in a pattern of radiating spokes. RK has declined in popularity since the approval of the excimer laser in 1995, falling from a high of 250,000 procedures performed per year in 1994 to 50,000 in 1997.

For both LASIK and PRK, the patient's eye is numbed with anesthetic drops. No injections are necessary. The patient is awake and relaxed during the procedure.

LASIK is sometimes referred to as a ''flap and zap'' procedure because a thin flap of tissue is temporarily removed from the surface of the cornea and the underlying cornea is then ''zapped'' with a laser. Prior to the surgery, the surface of the cornea is marked with a dye marker so that the flap of cornea can be precisely aligned when it is replaced. The doctor places a suction ring on the eye to hold it steady. During this part of the operation, which lasts only a few seconds, the patient is not able to see. A surgical instrument called a microkeratome is passed over the cornea to create a very thin flap of tissue. The IOP is increased at this time which is why it is contraindicated in patients with glaucoma. This thin tissue layer is folded back. The cornea is reshaped with the laser beam and the cell layer is replaced. Because the cell layer is not permanently removed, patients have a faster recovery time and experience far less discomfort than with PRK. An antibiotic drop is put in and the eye is patched until the following day's checkup.

In PRK, a small area of the surface layer of the cornea is vaporized. It takes about three days for the surface cells to grow back and vision will be blurred. Some patients describe it as ''looking through Vaseline.'' PRK is generally recommended for patients with mild to moderate myopia (usually under -5.00 diopters).

With both PRK and LASIK, there is a loud tapping sound from the laser and a burning smell as the cornea is reshaped. The surgery itself is painless and takes only a minute or two. Patients are usually able to return home immediately after surgery. Most patients wait (up to six months) before they have the second one done. This allows the first eye to heal and to see if there were complications from the surgery.

The cost of these procedures can vary with geographic area and the doctor. In general, the procedure costs $1,350-$2,500 per eye for PRK and about $500 more per eye for LASIK. PRK and LASIK are generally not covered by insurance. However, insurance may cover these procedures for people in certain occupations, such as police officers and firefighters.

Most patients return to work within one to three days after the procedure, although visual recovery from PRK may take as long as four weeks. An eye shield may be used for about one week at night and patients may be sensitive to bright light for a few days. Patients may be asked by their doctor to keep water out of their eye for a week and to avoid mascara or eyeliner during this period.

There is a risk of under- or over-correction with either of these procedures. If vision is under-corrected, a second procedure can be performed to achieve results that may be closer to 20/20 vision. About 5-10% of PRK patients return for an adjustment, as do 10-25% of LASIK patients. People with higher degrees of myopia have vision that is harder to correct and usually have LASIK surgery rather than PRK. This may account for the higher incidence of adjustments for LASIK patients. Patients with very high myopia (over -15.00 diopters) may experience improvement after LASIK, but they are not likely to achieve 20/40 vision without glasses. However, their glasses will not need to be as thick or heavy after the surgery. However, most patients, especially those with less extreme myopia, do not need glasses after the surgery.

Haze is another possible side effect. Although hazy vision is unlikely, it is more likely to occur after PRK than after LASIK. This haze usually clears up. Corneal scarring, halos, or glare at night, or an irritating bump on the cornea are other possible side effects. As with any eye surgery, infection is possible, but rare. Loss of vision is possible with these procedures, but this complication is extremely rare.

Most complications from LASIK are related to the creation and realignment of the flap. The microkeratome must be in good-working order and sharp. LASIK requires a great deal of skill on the part of the surgeon and the complication rate is related to the experience level of the surgeon. In one study, the rate of LASIK complications declined from 3% for surgeons during their first three months using this technique, to 1% after a year's experience in the technique, to 0% after 18 months experience.

Most patients experience improvement in their vision immediately after the operation and about half of LASIK patients are able to see 20/30 within one day of the surgery. Vision tends to become sharper over the next few days and then stabilizes; however, it is possible to have shifts in myopia for the next few months. Vision clears and stabilizes faster after LASIK than after PRK. Final vision is achieved within three to six months with LASIK and six to eight months with PRK. The vast majority of patients (95% for people with low to moderate myopia and 75% for people with high levels of myopia) are able to see 20/40 after either of these procedure and are able to pass a driver's license test without glasses or contact lenses.

LASIK is more complicated than PRK because of the addition of the microkeratome procedure. LASIK, as of mid 1998, is not approved by the FDA. However, LASIK generally has faster recovery time, less pain, and less chance of halos and scarring than PRK. LASIK can treat higher degrees of myopia (-5.00 to -25.00 diopters). LASIK also requires less use of steroids. Patients need to speak with qualified, experienced eye surgeons to help in choosing the procedure that is right for them.

Photosensitivity

Photosensitivity is any increase in the reactivity of the skin to sunlight. The skin is a carefully designed interface between the body and the outside world. It is infection-proof when intact, nearly waterproof, and filled with protective mechanisms. Sunlight threatens the health of the skin. Normal skin is highly variable in its ability to resist sun damage. Natural skin pigmentation is its main protection. The term photosensitivity refers to any increase beyond what is considered normal variation.

There are over three dozen diseases, two dozen drugs, and several perfume and cosmetic components that can cause photosensitivity. There are also several different types of reaction to sunlight phototoxicity, photoallergy, and polymorphous light eruption. In addition, prolonged exposure to sunlight, even in normal skin, leads to skin aging and **cancer**. These effects are accelerated in patients who have photosensitivity.

- Phototoxicity is a severely exaggerated reaction to sunlight caused by a new chemical in the skin. The primary symptom is **sunburn**, which is rapid and can be severe enough to blister (a second degree burn). The chemicals associated with phototoxicity are usually drugs. The list includes several common **antibiotics**—quinolones, **sulfonamides**, and **tetracyclines**; **diuretics** (water pills); major tranquilizers; oral diabetes medication; and cancer medicines. There are also some dermatologic drugs, both topical and oral, that can sensitize skin.
- Photoallergy produces an intense **itching** rash on exposure to sunlight. Patients develop chronic skin changes as a result of scratching. Some of the agents that cause phototoxicity can also cause photoallergy. Some cosmetic and perfume ingredients, including one of the most common **sunscreens**, para-amino benzoic acid (PABA), can do this.
- Polymorphous light eruption resembles photoallergy in its production of intensely itching **rashes** in sunlight. However, this condition lessens with continued light exposure, and so is seen mostly in the spring. Also, there does not seem to be an identifiable chemical involved. Diseases of several kinds increase skin sensitivity.

- A hereditary disease called xeroderma pigmentosum includes a defect in repair mechanisms that greatly accelerates skin damage from sunlight.
- A family of metabolic diseases called **porphyrias** produce chemicals (porphyrins) that absorb sunlight in the skin and thereby cause damage.
- Albinos lack skin pigment through a genetic defect and are thus very sensitive to light.
- **Malnutrition**, specifically a deficiency of niacin known as **pellagra**, sensitizes the skin.
- Several diseases like **acne**, systemic lupus erythematosus, and herpes simples (**fever** blisters) decrease the resistance of the skin to sun damage.

The pattern of appearance on the skin, a history of drug or chemical exposure, and the timing of the symptoms often suggests a diagnosis. A skin biopsy may be needed for further clarification.

Removal of the offending drug or chemical is primary. Direct sunlight exposure should be limited. Some people must avoid sunlight altogether, while others can tolerate some direct sunlight with the aid of sunscreens.

A sunscreen with an SPF of 15 or greater protects most skin from damage. Protective clothing such as hats are highly recommended in addition.

PHOTOTHERAPY

Phototherapy, or light therapy, is the administration of doses of bright light in order to normalize the body's internal clock and/or relieve depression. Phototherapy is prescribed primarily to treat **seasonal affective disorder** (SAD), a mood disorder characterized by depression in the winter months, and is occasionally employed to treat **insomnia** and **jet lag**.

The exact mechanisms by which the treatment works are not known, but the bright light employed in phototherapy may act to readjust the body's circadian (daily) rhythms, or internal clock. Other popular theories are that light triggers the production of serotonin, a neurotransmitter believed to be related to **depressive disorders**, or that it influences the body's production of melatonin, a hormone derived from serotonin that may be related to circadian rhythms.

Patients with eye problems should see an ophthalmologist regularly, both before and during phototherapy. Because some ultraviolet rays are emitted by the light boxes used in phototherapy, patients taking photosensitizing medications (medications making the skin more sensitive to light) and those who have sun-sensitive skin should consult with their physician before beginning treatment. Patients with medical conditions that make them sensitive to ultraviolet rays should also be seen by a physician before starting phototherapy. Patients who have a history of mood swings or mania should be monitored closely, since phototherapy may cause excessive mood elevation in some individuals.

Phototherapy is generally administered at home. The most commonly used phototherapy equipment is a portable lighting device known as a light box. The box may be mounted upright to a wall, or slanted downwards towards a table. The patient sits in front of the box for a prescribed period of time (anywhere from 15 minutes to several hours). Some patients with SAD undergo phototherapy sessions two or three times a day, others only once. The time of day and number of times treatment is administered depend on the physical needs and lifestyle of the individual patient. If phototherapy has been prescribed for the treatment of SAD, it typically begins in the fall months as the days begin to shorten, and continues throughout the winter and possibly the early spring.

The light from a slanted light box is designed to focus on the table it sits upon, so patients may look down to read or do other sedentary activities during therapy. Patients using an upright light box must face the light source (although they need not look directly into the light). The light sources in these light boxes typically range from 2,500-10,000 lux. (In contrast, average indoor lighting is 300-500 lux; a sunny summer day is about 100,000 lux).

Patients beginning light therapy for SAD may need to adjust the length, frequency, and timing of their phototherapy sessions to achieve the maximum benefit. These patients should keep their doctor informed of their progress and the status of their depressive symptoms. Occasionally, antidepressants and/or psychotherapy may be recommended as an adjunct to phototherapy.

An abnormally elevated or expansive mood (hypomania) may occur, but it is usually temporary. Some patients undergoing phototherapy treatment report side effects of eyestrain, **headache**s, insomnia, fatigue, **sunburn**, and dry eyes or nose. Most of these effects can be managed by adjusting the timing and duration of the phototherapy sessions. A strong sun block and eye and nose drops can alleviate the other problems. Long-term studies have shown no negative effects to the eye function of individuals undergoing phototherapy treatments. Patients with SAD typically report an alleviation of depressive symptoms within 2-14 days after beginning phototherapy.

PHYSICAL ALLERGY

Physical allergies are allergic reactions to cold, sunlight, heat, or minor injury. The **immune system** is designed to protect the body from harmful invaders such as germs. Occasionally, it goes awry and attacks harmless or mildly noxious agents, doing more harm than good. This event is termed allergy if the target is from the outside like pollen or bee venom and autoimmunity if it is caused by one of the body's own components.

The immune system usually responds only to certain kinds of chemicals, namely proteins. However, non-proteins can trigger the same sort of response, probably by altering a protein to make it look like a target. Physical allergy refers to reactions in which a protein is not the initial inciting agent.

Sometimes it takes a combination of elements to produce an allergic reaction. A classic example is drugs that are capable of sensitizing the skin to sunlight. The result is phototoxicity, which appears as an increased sensitivity to sunlight or as localized skin **rashes** on sun-exposed areas.

- Minor injury, such as scratching, causes itchy welts to develop in about 5% of people. The presence of itchy welts (urticaria) is a condition is called dermographism.
- Cold can change certain proteins in the blood so that they induce an immune reaction. This may indicate that there are abnormal proteins in the blood from a disease of the bone marrow. The reaction may also involve the lungs and circulation, producing **wheezing** and **fainting**
- Heat allergies can be caused by **exercise** or even strong emotions in sensitive people.
- Sunlight, even without drugs, causes immediate urticaria in some people. This may be a symptom of **porphyria**, a genetic metabolic defect.
- Elements like nickel and chromium, although not proteins, commonly cause skin rashes, and iodine allergy causes skin rashes and sores in the mouth in allergic individuals.
- Pressure or vibration can also cause urticaria.
- Water contact can cause aquagenic urticaria, presumably due to chlorine or some other trace chemical in the water, although distilled water has been known to cause this reaction.

When the inflammatory reaction involves deeper layers of the skin, urticaria becomes angioedema. The skin, especially the lips and eyelids, swells. The tongue, throat, and parts of the digestive tract may also be involved. Angioedema may be due to physical agents. Often the cause remains unknown.

Visual examination of the symptoms usually diagnoses the reaction. Further skin tests and review of the patient's photosensitivity may reveal a cause.

Removing the offending agent is the first step to treatment. If sun is involved, shade and sunscreens are necessary. The reaction can usually be controlled with epinephrine, **antihistamines**, or cortisone-like drugs. **Itching** can be controlled with cold packs or commercial topical agents that contain menthol, camphor, eucalyptus oil, aloe, antihistamines, or cortisone preparations.

If the causative agent has been diagnosed, avoidance of or protection against the allergen cures the allergy. Usually, allergies can be managed through treatment.

Physical Education

The history of physical education reflects people's attitudes about physical activity. From prehistoric times, because survival was related to physical stamina and to people's ability to find food, no separate physical fitness programs were needed. Gradually, ancient societies in China, Egypt, Greece, and Rome adopted physical education as part of military training. As the more developed societies came to value the scholarly life, physical education lost favor. Many developed countries have had to strike a balance between physical and intellectual interests.

The history of physical education frequently shows a pattern of military, social, and political influence.

In one high point of ancient history, Athenian Greeks came to the forefront in the era 700 to 600 B.C. with their quest for physical and intellectual perfection. In numerous festivals, Athenians celebrated the beauty of the human form in dance, art, religious rites, and athletics. Athenians honored the gods of Olympus, especially Zeus, with the first Olympic Games. The Olympic Games offered a civilizing influence, with social class disregarded and all citizens judged on athletic competition. If a war was being fought, it was halted during the Olympic Games. Many historians regard Athenian culture as the height of early physical education, but like their Chinese predecessors, the Athenians felt the competing influence of intellectualism.

The Middle Ages saw the fall of the Roman Empire and the rise of Christianity, and the Christian influence brought about a denial of physical activity for anything other than manual labor. Christians saw sports and physical play as immoral, and in 394 they halted the Olympic Games. This trend was not reversed until the medieval societies grew and sought power through military expansion.

During the Renaissance, the pendulum swung once again as artists showed the human body as an object of admiration. The humanist faction, centered in Italy, valued education in sports such as fencing, archery, swimming, running, and ball games. The moralist faction, influenced by the Protestant Reformation, saw physical activity only as a way for carrying out work. During this period, much of Europe was still Catholic, and Catholics favored recreational physical activity with the view that care should be taken of the body as the vessel that held the soul. The other major Renaissance faction was realism, which favored physical education as part of a sound mind in a sound body.

In 19th-century Europe, Sweden and Germany developed systems of gymnastics that were adopted internationally with Germany building the first indoor gymnasium. In Finland, which also built a gymnasium, exercise was for the first time seen as a way to achieve physical **rehabilitation**. Scholars began to study anatomy and physiology in relation to exercise. Denmark was among the first countries to require physical education in schools.

Physical education fulfilled a political role in early-20th-century Russia after the rise of communism. Physical fitness helped insure military strength, productivity, and nationalism. Sports were viewed as a way of achieving international fame.

The United States followed other countries in its approach to physical education. During the Colonial period, the sheer physical demands of survival made physical education unnecessary. War required physical training as a part of military preparation. Between the Revolution War and the Civil War, Americans followed some recreational activities such as riding, hunting, dancing, swimming, and early forms of golf and tennis. By the 1820s, some American schools offered gymnasia and physical education. Instruction included the development and care of the body, and training in hygiene. Students learned calisthenic exercises, gymnastics, and the performance and management of athletic games. Women's colleges offered exercise and dance classes. The Young Men's Christian Association (YMCA) opened its first American chapter in 1851. Many sports gained in popularity around this time, including baseball.

After the American Civil War, large school systems began to adopt physical education programs and many states passed laws requiring that physical education programs be taught. For the first time, specialized training was offered for physical education instructors. In another first, colleges offered intercollegiate sports such as rowing, football, and track and field. In keeping with this wave of interest in physical education, the Olympic Games were restored in 1896, after a 1,400-year interlude.

Surprisingly, many Americans were not physically fit for military service during World War I, and there were many postwar efforts to add physical education at all levels of schooling. During World War II, **physical fitness** was again required of soldiers—but it was also required of many others, particularly women, since the war effort required manual labor. Soldiers once again came up short in physical fitness requirements, so after the war, schools instituted more rigorous physical education requirements, and there was greater interest in the teaching of physical education.

By 1950, there were over 400 United States colleges and universities offering majors in physical education and there was increasing recognition of the scientific foundation of physical education. The fitness of the military in the Korean War again fell short of expectations, and the federal government set up the President's Council on Physical Fitness, which helped to raise fitness standards in schools across the country. A series of 1970s and 1980s recessions brought about cutbacks in many school programs, including physical education. By the 1970s, interest in the President's Council had waned and physical education courses began to emphasize lifetime sports such as golf, badminton, tennis, and bowling. In another swing of the pendulum, the American public spontaneously developed an intense interest in fitness in the late 1970s.

One of the most significant shifts of the 1970s was the Title IX amendment to the Federal Education Act, which stipulated that no federally funded education programs could discriminate on the basis of gender. Enforcement of Title IX opened up many new opportunities for women in competitive athletics, both at the high school and collegiate levels.

In a continuation of 1980s trends, during the 1990s many school districts have limited the amount of time students spend in physical education or have even dropped the program in response to economic problems or concerns about poor curriculum. Some reformers in the field are turning to **sports education** as a way of reengaging the students.

Physical examination

A physical examination is an evaluation of the body and its functions using inspection, palpation (feeling with the hands), percussion (tapping with the fingers), and auscultation (listening). A complete health assessment also includes gathering information about a person's medical history and lifestyle, doing laboratory tests, and screening for disease.

The annual physical examination has been replaced by the periodic health examination. How often this is done depends on the patient's age, sex, and risk factors for disease. The United States Preventative Services Task Force (USPSTF) has developed guidelines for preventive health examinations that health care professionals widely follow. Organizations that promote detection and prevention of specific diseases, like the American Cancer Society, generally recommend more intensive or frequent examinations.

A comprehensive physical examination provides an opportunity for the health care professional to obtain baseline information about the patient for future use, and to establish a relationship before problems happen. It provides an opportunity to answer questions and teach good health practices. Detecting a problem in its early stages can have good long-term results.

A complete physical examination usually starts at the head and proceeds all the way to the toes. However, the exact procedure will vary according to the needs of the patient and the preferences of the examiner. An average examination takes about 30 minutes. The cost of the examination will depend on the charge for the professional's time and any tests that are done. Most health plans cover routine physical examinations including some tests.

First, the examiner will observe the patient's appearance, general health, and behavior, along with measuring height and weight. The vital signs including pulse, breathing rate, body temperature, and blood pressure are recorded.

With the patient sitting up, the following systems are reviewed:

- Skin. The exposed areas of the skin are observed; the size and shape of any lesions are noted.
- Head. The hair, scalp, skull, and face are examined.
- Eyes. The external structures are observed. The internal structures can be observed using an ophthalmoscope (a lighted instrument) in a darkened room.
- Ears. The external structures are inspected. A lighted instrument called an otoscope may be used to inspect internal structures.
- Nose and sinuses. The external nose is examined. The nasal mucosa and internal structures can be observed with the use of a penlight and a nasal speculum.
- Mouth and pharynx. The lips, gums, teeth, roof of the mouth, tongue, and pharynx are inspected.
- Neck. The lymph nodes on both sides of the neck and the thyroid gland are palpated (examined by feeling with the fingers).
- Back. The spine and muscles of the back are palpated and checked for tenderness. The upper back, where the lungs are located, is palpated on the right and left sides and a stethoscope is used to listen for breath sounds.
- Breasts and armpits. A woman's breasts are inspected with the arms relaxed and then raised. In both men and women, the lymph nodes in the armpits are felt with the examiner's hands. While the patient is still sitting, movement of the joints in the hands, arms, shoulders, neck, and jaw can be checked.

Then while the patient is lying down on the examining table, the examination includes:

- Breasts. The breasts are palpated and inspected for lumps.
- Front of chest and lungs. The area is inspected with the fingers, using palpation and percussion. A stethoscope is used to listen to the internal breath sounds.

The head should be slightly raised for:

- Heart. A stethoscope is used to listen to the heart's rate and rhythm.The blood vessels in the neck are observed and palpated.

The patient should lie flat for:

- Abdomen. Light and deep palpation is used on the abdomen to feel the outlines of internal organs including the liver, spleen, kidneys, and aorta, a large blood vessel.
- Rectum and anus. With the patient lying on the left side, the outside areas are observed. An internal digital examination (using a finger), is usually done if the patient is over 40 years old. In men, the prostate gland is also palpated.
- Reproductive organs. The external sex organs are inspected and the area is examined for **hernia**s. In men, the scrotum is palpated. In women, a pelvic examination is done using a speculum and a Papanicolaou test (**PAP test**) may be taken.
- Legs. With the patient lying flat, the legs are inspected for swelling, and pulses in the knee, thigh, and foot area are found. The groin area is palpated for the presence of lymph nodes. The joints and muscles are observed.
- **Musculoskeletel system**. With the patient standing, the straightness of the spine and the alignment of the legs and feet is noted.
- Blood vessels. The presence of any abnormally enlarged veins (**varicose**), usually in the legs, is noted.

In addition to evaluating the patient's alertness and mental ability during the initial conversation, additional inspection of the nervous system may be indicated:

- Neurologic screen. The patient's ability to take a few steps, hop, and do deep knee bends is observed. The strength of the hand grip is felt. With the patient sitting down, the reflexes in the knees and feet can be tested with a small hammer. The sense of touch in the hands and feet can be evaluated by testing reaction to **pain** and vibration.
- Sometimes additional time is spent examining the 12 nerves in the head (cranial) that are connected directly to the brain. They control the sense of smell, strength of muscles in the head, reflexes in the eye, facial movements, gag reflex, and muscles in the jaw. General muscle tone and coordination, and the reaction of the abdominal area to stimulants like pain, temperature, and touch would also be evaluated.

Before visiting the health care professional, the patient should write down important facts and dates about his or her own medical history, as well as those of family members. He or she should have a list of all medications with their doses or bring the actual bottles of medicine along. If there are specific concerns about anything, writing them down is a good idea.

Before the physical examination begins, the bladder should be emptied, and a urine specimen can be collected in a small container. For some blood tests, the patient may be told ahead of time not to eat or drink after midnight.

The patient usually removes all clothing and puts on a loose-fitting hospital gown. An additional sheet is provided to keep the patient covered and comfortable during the examination.

Once the physical examination has been completed, the patient and the examiner should review what laboratory tests have been ordered and how the results will be shared with the patient. The medical professional should discuss any recommendations for treatment and follow-up visits. Special instructions should be put in writing. This is also an opportunity for the patient to ask any remaining questions about his or her own health concerns.

Normal results of a physical examination correspond to the healthy appearance and normal functioning of the body. For example, appropriate reflexes will be present, no suspicious lumps or lesions will be found, and vital signs will be normal.

Abnormal results of a physical examination include any findings that indicated the presence of a disorder, disease, or underlying condition. For example, the presence of lumps or lesions, fever, muscle weakness or lack of tone, poor reflex response, heart **arrhythmia**, or swelling of lymph nodes will point to a possible health problem.

Physical Fitness

Physical fitness is the ability to perform vigorous physical activity. It is not measured in terms of achieving specific motor skills, but rather it is assessed in terms of muscle strength, endurance, and flexibility. The circulatory and **respiratory systems** are also involved because of their role in supplying muscles with blood and oxygen.

In considering muscles, strength is the maximum force that can be exerted by a muscle, and endurance is the ability to perform a muscular activity at less than maximum force, for example, in doing a series of chin-ups. Flexibility is the ability of a joint to move through a normal range of motion. The components of physical fitness (strength, endurance, flexibility, and capacity of circulatory and respiratory systems) can only be maintained through regular **exercise**.

Although the percentage of body fat is not a main factor in physical fitness, it must be considered because of its effect on a person's ability to exercise. There is debate in the fitness community about whether an individual can be considered fit if he or she is overweight.

The body will adapt to a regular exercise program by improving the function of the cardiac and respiratory systems. The blood will have a greater capacity to carry oxygen, which in turn will improve the body's ability to work. The heart and respiratory systems will be more efficient during rest and exercise, and the resting heart rate is usually reduced. These changes take place when a person participates in a rhythmic endurance activity such as walking, running, and cycling, or continuous sports activities such as basketball or tennis.

In addition, an individual participating in a regular exercise program will notice the effects on the skeletal, muscular, and **nervous systems**. The body will show improved flexibility of the joints along with greater muscle strength and muscle endurance.

A regular exercise program also benefits the back. At least half of Americans are affected by **low back pain**, and about 80 percent of these problems are related to muscular problems rather than to the spine. Frequently back problems are linked to degenerative processes in which the abdominal muscles become too weak or the hamstring muscles at the back of the thighs become tight and inflexible. A consistent strengthening and conditioning program can alleviate symptoms of back pain.

The death rate from **coronary artery disease** in the United States is one of the highest in the world. Contrary to many popular ideas, **heart attacks** are caused by a degenerative process, not by individual instances of exercise, excitement, or heavy eating. Persons in sedentary occupations have a higher rate of coronary heart disease and related deaths than people who are more physically active. Regular physical activity will help reduce the risk of heart attack. If a person who engages in regular exercise does have a heart attack, it is likely to occur late in life and the individual is more likely to survive. Regular exercise helps lower blood triglyceride (fat) levels and cholesterol levels, both of which are related to heart disease.

The effectiveness of exercise depends on the demand on organs and body systems. Individuals participating in the same exercise may not all experience the same results. Moderation of intensity, duration, and frequency is recommended to prevent tissue damage.

While isolated attempts at strenuous exercise can cause discomfort, moderate regular exercise contributes to a sense of well-being. Studies of societies in which people commonly live for over 100 years show a common denominator of moderate physical activity. Growth and development studies show that active children have stronger muscles and sturdier frames than peers who do not exercise regularly.

Physical therapy

Physical therapists evaluate and treat people with health problems resulting from injury or disease. They assess joint motion, muscle strength and endurance, function of heart and lungs, and performance of activities required in daily living. Physical therapists employ a wide range of therapeutic **exercise** techniques, cardiovascular endurance training, and training in activities of daily living. Typical examples of persons who might benefit from physical therapy include an automobile mechanic with an injured back, an elderly person with arthritis; a newborn baby with a birth defect; a professional athlete in training; a stroke victim; a crippled child; a pregnant woman; and an overstressed business executive.

Physical therapy aids people who are recovering from injury or a disease by making them stronger, relieving their **pain**, and helping them to regain use of an affected limb or to relearn such daily activities as walking, dressing, and bathing. Some patients recovering from surgery require physical therapy as part of their recovery process. In these cases, the physical therapist attempts to achieve normal mobility through the relief of pain and the rehabilitation of impaired muscle function. The therapist may employ active or passive exercises designed to strengthen specific muscles or to coordinate muscle movement. In passive exercises, the therapist manipulates the affected parts until the patient is able to do so alone. In **hydrotherapy**, the patient exercises in water, which requires a smaller expenditure of energy than exercises out of water. Patients who are entirely immobilized may begin physical therapy in bed with **massage** and the application of heat.

Physical therapists also assist people in remaining well and safe from injury. Physical therapists teach people the importance of **physical fitness** and show them how to avoid injuries at work or play. They also design and supervise personalized exercise programs geared at helping people increase their overall fitness and muscular strength and endurance.

Physical therapy techniques may include therapeutic exercise, joint mobilization and range-of-motion exercises, cardiovascular endurance training, relaxation exercises, therapeutic massage, **biofeedback**, training in various activities of daily living, wound care, pulmonary physical therapy, and training in moving about. Specific therapies including **traction**, ultrasound, diathermy, electrotherapy, **cryotherapy**, hydrotherapy, and laser therapy may also be applied during treatment.

Although many physical therapists work in hospitals, more than 70 percent can be found in private physical therapy offices, community health centers, corporate or industrial health centers, sports facilities, research institutions, rehabilitation centers, **nursing homes**, home health agencies, schools, pediatric centers, and colleges and universities. As a specialist in rehabilitation, the physical therapist typically works with other health care personnel (including physicians, occupational therapists, rehabilitation nurses, and psychologists) to determine the patient's goals; evaluates patients and implements treatment programs; teaches patients to use prosthetic devices; and provides instruction to patients to continue the recovery when they are no longer under the direct care of the physical therapist. As a community health worker, the physical therapist may administer rehabilitative care in the home; teach prenatal and postnatal exercise classes; evaluate and treat children in public schools; and teach back-care classes to prevent back pain and injury. As an industrial therapist, the physical therapist may determine physical requirements for specific jobs; evaluate and treat an employee's job-related physical problems; identify potentially dangerous work conditions; modify job-related tasks to prevent injuries; and provide treatment to injured workers. As a sports therapist, the physical therapist may evaluate an athlete's performance abilities; condition athletes to improve their performance; recommend special equipment to reduce injuries; and develop fitness programs for the general public. As a researcher, the physical therapist may participate in scientific studies that will lead to new knowledge, new technologies, and more effective patient care. As an educator, the physical therapist may help prepare students for careers in physical therapy; teach entry-level and graduate-level physical therapy courses; participate in scholarly activities that contribute to the understanding of physical therapy; and participate in a variety of service activities in the university and community. As an administrator, the physical therapist may manage physical therapy departments and clinics and act as a consultant to colleagues and health care providers.

With Americans becoming more health- and exercise-conscious, participating in sports and fitness activities, more physical therapists will be needed to treat and help prevent knee, leg, back, shoulder, and other musculoskeletal injuries. The post War World II baby boom generation is now aging and beginning to experience conditions common to older people such as arthritis, **stroke**, heart disease, and other prolonged-care conditions. Physical therapists will be called on to care for them.

See also Low back pain; Musculoskeletal system; Occupational therapy; Sports injuries

PHYSICIAN

The term ''physician'' is often used as a more accurate version of ''doctor,'' since the latter can mean anyone who has completed a doctorate in any discipline. A physician, or doctor of medicine (MD), is a person who has graduated from an accredited medical school and passed the state licensing examinations required to become a professional provider of medical care, including surgery.

There are different categories of physician. A *resident* physician has completed an internship (now called PG1, post-graduate 1) and obtained a license to practice medicine, but works full- or part-time at a hospital to learn more about his or her chosen specialty. A *family* or *primary care* physician is a specialized medical professional who provides ongoing care for all ages and both sexes, planning and carrying out a thorough health care program for all members of a family over time; this is the physician people see before going on to a specialist and who coordinates patients' care if multiple health care professionals are involved. An *attending* physician visits a certain hospital at specified times to supervise his or her patients' treatment and give further instructions to **paramedics**. An *emergency* physician is an expert in the particular procedures and methods used in the emergency room.

PINCUS, GREGORY (1903-1967)

American endocrinologist

Gregory Pincus is best known for his central role in developing ''the pill''—the **oral contraceptive** or birth control pill. He also investigated the biochemistry of aging, arthritis, cancer, and the adrenal system's response to stress. Pincus was born in Woodbine, New Jersey. Both of his parents had interests in agriculture and the arts, and his father taught at an agricultural school. In 1924, Pincus graduated from Cornell University where he not only studied science but founded a literary magazine. In 1927 he received master's and doctoral degrees from Harvard University and, following further study in Europe, joined Harvard's biology faculty. In 1938 he joined the faculty at Clark University, in Worcester, Massachusetts, as an experimental zoologist and, in 1944, co-founded the independent Worcester Foundation for Experimental Biology where he continued his earlier research on the way the reproductive system and female hormones functioned.

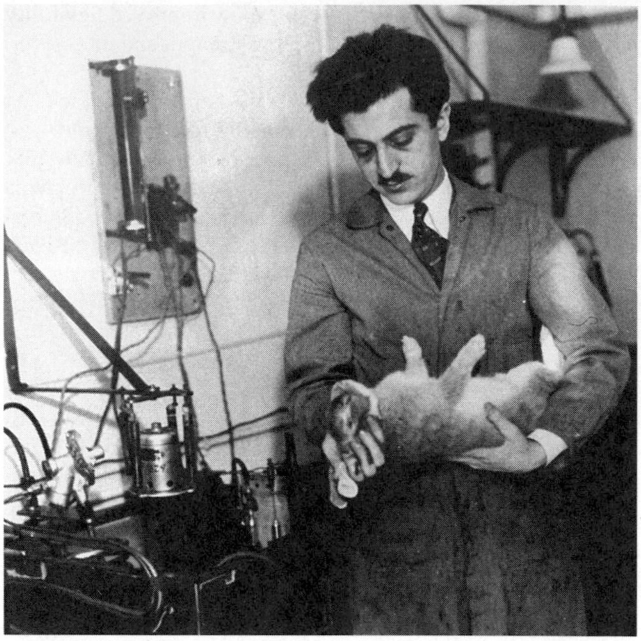

Gregory Pincus

Since the discovery of the sex hormones, scientists had searched for a natural, safe, and foolproof method of using female hormones to treat infertility and prevent pregnancy. Several scientists beginning in the 1920s showed that progesterone inhibited ovulation. In the 1940s, British chemist Robert Robinson tried unsuccessfully to synthesize various female hormones. Pincus's work attracted the attention of **Margaret Sanger** (1879-1966), the United States' best-known advocate of birth control. Financed by Sanger's friend, philanthropist Katherine Dexter McCormick (1875-1967), Pincus led a group of scientists in the early 1950s who began developing a hormone-based substance to make the body mimic pregnancy—the one time when a woman is almost certain not to become pregnant. The biologist Min-Chueh Chang carried out experiments on laboratory animals with various compounds of progestin, a synthetic progesterone developed in Mexico by the American chemist Carl Djerassi. Another collaborator, physician **John Rock**, had already been experimenting with progesterone to cure infertility. Tests of the new substance on women took place in Massachusetts, Puerto Rico, Haiti, Mexico, and California, supervised by Pincus, Rock, Celso-Ramon Garcia and Edris Rice-Wray. Because contraception was illegal in Massachusetts and due to objections from religious groups—principally the Roman Catholic Church—the initial tests were

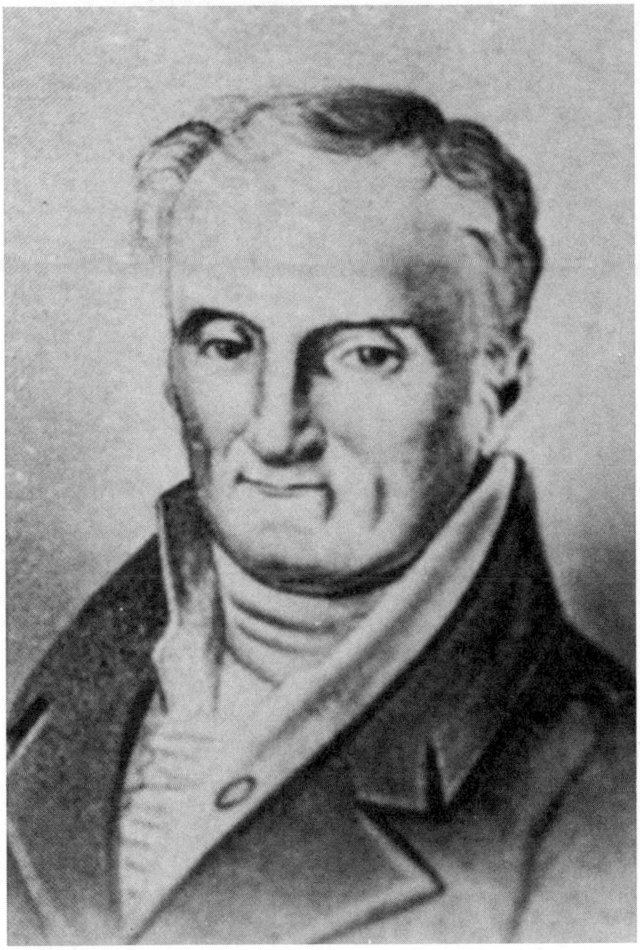

Phillippe Pinel.

to treat infertility rather than prevent pregnancy. However, these tests showed that the compound prevented ovulation and in 1960, progesterone was approved by the U.S. Food and Drug Administration as the first contraceptive pill.

Gregory Pincus continues to be hailed as the primary force behind the oral contraceptive. Among the many honors he received during his lifetime was membership in the National Academy of Sciences of the U.S.A.

PINEL, PHILIPPE (1745-1826)

French Physician

Pinel was one of the founders of modern psychiatry, as well as a distinguished teacher of internal medicine. His innovations in treating mentally ill patients were so stirring and profound that his ideas are still followed today.

Pinel was born on April 20, 1745 at Saint André, in southern France. His relatives on both sides of his family were physicians and surgeons. In college, he first studied literature before changing to religion. In April, 1770, he abandoned his religion classes at the University of Toulouse and enrolled in the college of medicine. He received his M.D. degree on December 21, 1773. In 1774, Pinel went to Montpellier, where he taught mathematics and anatomy, wrote theses for the lazy, rich students, and observed the practice of medicine. In 1778, he moved to Paris, where he edited a health journal, wrote articles for several publications, and translated English medical and scientific works into French.

A turning point in his life occurred in 1783, when a friend asked Pinel for help with his manic-depressive behavior. His friend was a law student in Paris, and his behavior alternated between depression and excitability. Finally, Pinel's friend ran away one night into the forest wearing only his shirt. He got lost and was discovered by a pack of wolves, killing him. Pinel was shocked by this incident and wondered what he could do to help such people. His interest in treating mentally ill people increased, and he began to publish articles on mental illness.

Powerful people noted Pinel's work on mental illness, and in 1793, with Paris controlled by the revolutionary government that had deposed King Louis XVI, he was appointed the director of the Bicêtre Insane Asylum, one of the most famous **asylums** in France. At Bicêtre, inmates were locked in dark cells, chained to walls, dunked in water, given drugs to make them vomit, and bled. The ruling theories of the time said that insane people were possessed by demons. Pinel thought that social and mental stress, heredity, and physical ailments caused insanity. He threw out the old treatments and recommended sunlight, friendly conversations with the doctor, discussing personal problems, exercise, cleanliness, and meaningful work. He especially wanted to unchain his patients.

Pinel's approach was revolutionary, but he did not implement it immediately. To unchain patients, he had to get permission from the revolutionary council controlling Paris. The council's president left the decision to Pinel and warned him that he could get killed by one of his patients. But Pinel had always been a careful observer and he knew his patients. Pinel quietly told one patient, an officer with a history of violence who had been at Bicêtre for 40 years, that he would like to take his chains off. Pinel asked the officer if he would be nonviolent. The officer promised, Pinel unchained him, and the officer went out into the sunlight for the first time in many years. He exclaimed how beautiful the light was. The officer remained calm, helped other inmates, and was released two years later. Pinel's methods also saved lives. Before Pinel, over half the people admitted to Bicêtre died in their first year of confinement. After Pinel began, only one person in eight died in the first year.

In 1795, Pinel became director of the Salp&ecircp;trière asylum for women, where he enforced the same changes with the same results. His assistants at the two asylums went on to administrative directorships of their own and spread his ideas around Europe.

Pinel married Jeanne Vincent in 1792. They had three sons, one of whom became a specialist in mental illnesses. In 1798, Pinel published a book on the classification of diseases, *Nosographie philosophique*, and in 1801, he published another book about mental illness, *Traité médico-philosophique sur l'aliénation mentale ou la manie*. His first wife died in 1811, and in 1815 he married Marie-Madeline Jacquelin-Lavallée.

Pinel died, much-loved and greatly honored, on October 25, 1826, in Paris. His funeral was attended by important state dignitaries, scientists, doctors, students, and former inhabitants of Bicêtre and Salpêtrière, the very patients whom Pinel had unchained and unleashed into the light.

See also Asylums

PITUITARY TUMORS

Pituitary tumors are abnormal growths on the pituitary gland. Some tumors secrete hormones normally made by the pituitary gland. Located in the center of the brain, the pituitary gland manufactures and secretes hormones that regulate growth, sexual development and functioning, and the fluid balance of the body. About 10% of all **cancer**s in the skull are pituitary tumors. Pituitary adenomas (adenomas are tumors that grow from gland tissues) and pituitary tumors in children and adolescencents (craniopharyngiomas) are the most common types of pituitary tumors. They are usually benign and grow slowly. Even malignant pituitary tumors rarely spread to other parts of the body.

Pituitary adenomas do not secrete hormones but are likely to be larger and more invasive than tumors that do. Craniopharyngiomas are benign tumors that are extremely difficult to remove. Radiation does not stop craniopharyngiomas from spreading throughout the pituitary gland. Craniopharyngiomas account for less than 5% of all **brain tumor**s. Pituitary tumors usually develop between the ages of 30 and 40, but half of all craniopharyngiomas occur in children, with symptoms most often appearing between the ages of five and ten.

The cause of pituitary tumors is not known, but may be genetic. Symptoms related to tumor location, size, and pressure on neighboring structures include:

- Persistent **headache** on one or both sides, or in the center of the forehead
- Blurred or double vision; loss of peripheral vision
- Drooping eyelid caused by pressure on nerves leading to the eye
- Seizures.

Symptoms related to hormonal imbalance include:

- Excessive sweating
- Loss of appetite
- Loss of interest in sex
- Inability to tolerate cold temperatures
- **Nausea**
- High levels of sodium in the blood
- Menstrual problems
- Excessive thirst
- Frequent urination
- Dry skin
- **Constipation**
- Premature or delayed **puberty**
- Delayed growth in children
- Galactorrea (milk secretion in the absence of **pregnancy** or breast feeding)
- Low blood pressure
- Low blood sugar.

As many as 40% of all pituitary tumors do not release excessive quantities of hormones into the blood. Known as clinically nonfunctioning, these tumors are difficult to distinguish from tumors that produce similar symptoms. They may grow to be quite large before they are diagnosed.

Endocrinologists and neuroendocrinologists base the diagnosis of pituitary tumors on:

- The patient's own observations and medical history
- **Physical examination**
- Laboratory studies of the patient's blood and cerebrospinal fluid
- X-rays of the skull and other studies that provide images of the inside of the brain (CT, MRI)
- Vision tests
- **Urinalysis.**

Some pituitary tumors stabilize without treatment, but a neurosurgeon will operate at once to remove the tumor (adenectomy) or pituitary gland (hypophysectomy) of a patient whose vision is deteriorating rapidly. Patients who have pituitary apoplexy may experience very severe headaches, have symptoms of stiff neck and sensitivity to light. This condition is considered an emergency. **Magnetic resonance imaging** (MRI) is the best imaging technique for patients with these symptoms. If the tumor is small, surgery may be done through the nose. If the tumor is large, it may require opening the skull for **tumor removal**. Selected patients do well with proton beam radiosurgery (the use of high energy particles in the form of a high energy beam to destroy an overactive gland).

Treatment is determined by the type of tumor and by whether it has invaded tissues adjacent to the pituitary gland. Hormone-secreting tumors can be successfully treated with surgery, radiation, or drugs. Surgery is usually used to remove all or part of a tumor within the gland or the area surrounding it, and may be combined with **radiation therapy** to treat tumors that extend beyond the pituitary gland. Removal of the pituitary gland requires life-long **hormone replacement therapy**.

Radiation therapy can provide long-term control of the disease if it recurs after surgery, and radioactive pellets can be implanted in the brain to treat craniopharyngiomas. CV205-502, a new dopamine agonist (a drug that increases the effect of another, in this instance dopamine) can control symptoms of patients who do not respond to bromocriptine.

Pituitary tumors are usually curable. Following surgery, adults may gradually resume their normal activities, and children may return to school when the effects of the operation have diminished, and appetite and sense of well-being have returned. Patients should wear medical identification tags identifying their condition and the hormonal replacement medicines they take.

PLACENTAL ABNORMALITIES

There are two major placental abnormalities. Placenta previa is a condition that occurs during **pregnancy** when the placenta is abnormally placed, and partially or totally covers the cervix.

Placental abruption occurs when the placenta separates from the wall of the uterus prior to the birth of the baby. This can result in severe, uncontrollable **bleeding** (hemorrhage).

The uterus is the muscular organ that contains the developing baby during pregnancy. The lowest segment of the uterus is a narrowed portion called the cervix. This cervix has an opening (the os) that leads into the vagina, or birth canal. The placenta is the organ that attaches to the wall of the uterus during pregnancy. The placenta allows nutrients and oxygen from the mother's blood circulation to pass into the developing baby (the fetus) via the umbilical cord.

During labor, the muscles of the uterus contract repeatedly. This allows the cervix to begin to grow thinner (called effacement) and more open (dilatation). Eventually, the cervix will become completely effaced and dilated, and the baby can leave the uterus and enter the birth canal. Under normal circumstances, the baby will emerge through the mother's vagina during birth.

In placenta previa, the placenta develops in an abnormal location. Normally, the placenta should develop relatively high up in the uterus, on the front or back wall. In about 1 in 200 births, the placenta will be located low in the uterus, partially or totally covering the os. This causes particular problems in late pregnancy, when the lower part of the uterus begins to take on a new formation in preparation for delivery. As the cervix begins to efface and dilate, the attachments of the placenta to the uterus are damaged, resulting in bleeding.

During a normal labor and delivery, the baby is born first. Several minutes to 30 minutes later, the placenta separates from the wall of the uterus and is delivered. This sequence is necessary because the baby relies on the placenta to provide oxygen until he or she begins to breathe independently.

Placental abruption occurs when the placenta separates from the uterus before the birth of the baby. Placental abruption occurs in about 1 out of every 200 deliveries. African-American and Latin-American women have a greater risk of this complication than do Caucasian women. It was once believed that the risk of placental abruption increased in women who gave birth to many children, but this association is still being researched.

While the actual cause of placenta previa is unknown, certain factors increase the risk of a woman developing the condition. These factors include:

- Having abnormalities of the uterus
- Being older in age
- Having had other babies
- Having a prior delivery by **cesarean section**
- **Smoking** cigarettes.

When a pregnancy involves more than one baby (twins, triplets, etc.), the placenta will be considerably larger than for a single pregnancy. This also increases the chance of placenta previa.

Placenta previa may cause a number of problems. It is thought to be responsible for about 5% of all miscarriages. It frequently causes very light bleeding (spotting) early in pregnancy. Sometime after 28 weeks of pregnancy (most pregnancies last about 40 weeks), placenta previa can cause episodes of significant bleeding. Usually, the bleeding occurs suddenly and is bright red. The woman rarely experiences any accompanying **pain**, although about 10% of the time the placenta may begin separating from the uterine wall (called abruptio placentae), resulting in pain. The bleeding usually stops on its own. About 25% of such patients will go into labor sometime in the next several days. Sometimes, placenta previa does not cause bleeding until labor has already begun.

Placenta previa puts both the mother and the fetus at high risk. The mother is at risk of severe and uncontrollable bleeding (hemorrhage), with dangerous blood loss. If the mother's bleeding is quite severe, this puts the fetus at risk of becoming oxygen deprived. The fetus' only source of oxygen is the mother's blood. The mother's blood loss, coupled with certain changes that take place in response to that blood loss, decreases the amount of blood going to the placenta, and ultimately to the fetus. Furthermore, placenta previa increases the risk of preterm labor, and the possibility that the baby will be delivered prematurely.

The cause of placental abruption is unknown. However, a number of risk factors have been identified. These factors include:

- Older age of the mother
- History of placental abruption during a previous pregnancy
- High blood pressure
- Certain disease states (**diabetes**, collagen vascular diseases)
- The presence of a type of uterine tumor called a leiomyoma
- Twins, triplets, or other **multiple pregnancies**
- Cigarette smoking
- Heavy alcohol use
- Cocaine use
- Malformations of the uterus
- Malformations of the placenta
- Injury to the abdomen (as might occur in a car accident).

Symptoms of placental abruption include bleeding from the vagina, severe pain in the abdomen or back, and tenderness of the uterus. Depending on the severity of the bleeding, the mother may experience a drop in blood pressure, followed by symptoms of organ failure as her organs are deprived of oxygen. Sometimes, there is no visible vaginal bleeding. Instead, the bleeding is said to be ''concealed.'' In this case, the bleeding is trapped behind the placenta, or there may be bleeding into the muscle of the uterus. Many patients will have abnormal contractions of the uterus, particularly extremely hard, prolonged contractions. Placental abruption can be total (in which case the fetus will almost always die in the uterus), or partial.

Placental abruption can also cause a very serious complication called consumptive coagulopathy. A series of reactions begin that involve the elements of the blood responsible for clotting. These clotting elements are bound together and used up by these reactions. This increases the risk of uncontrollable bleeding and may contribute to severe bleeding from the uterus, as well as causing bleeding from other locations (nose, urinary tract, etc.).

Placental abruption is risky for both the mother and the fetus. It is dangerous for the mother because of blood loss, loss of clotting ability, and oxygen deprivation to her organs (especially the kidneys and heart). This condition is dangerous for the fetus because of oxygen deprivation, too, since the mother's blood is the fetus' only source of oxygen. Because the abrupting placenta is attached to the umbilical cord, and the umbilical cord is an extension of the fetus' circulatory system, the fetus is also at risk of hemorrhaging. The fetus may die from these stresses, or may be born with damage due to oxygen deprivation. If the abruption occurs well before the baby was due to be delivered, early delivery may cause the baby to suffer complications of premature birth.

Diagnosis of placenta previa is suspected whenever bright red, painless vaginal bleeding occurs during the course of a pregnancy. The diagnosis can be confirmed by performing an **ultrasound** examination. This will allow the location of the placenta to be evaluated.

While many conditions during pregnancy require a **pelvic examination**, in which the healthcare provider's fingers are inserted into the patient's vagina, such an examination should never be performed if there is any suspicion of placenta previa. Such an examination can disturb the already susceptible placenta, resulting in hemorrhage.

Sometimes placenta previa is found early in a pregnancy, during an ultrasound examination performed for another reason. In these cases, it is wise to have a repeat ultrasound performed later in pregnancy (during the last third of the pregnancy, called the third trimester). A large percentage of these women will have a low-lying placenta, but not a true placenta previa where some or all of the os is covered.

Diagnosis of placental abruption relies heavily on the patient's report of her symptoms and a the **physical examination** performed by a healthcare provider. Ultrasound can sometimes be used to diagnose an abruption, but there is a high rate of missed or incorrect diagnoses associated with this tool when used for this purpose. Blood will be taken from the mother and tested to evaluate the possibility of life-threatening problems with the mother's clotting system.

Treatment of placenta previa depends on how far along in the pregnancy the bleeding occurs. When the pregnancy is less than 36 weeks along, the fetus is not sufficiently developed to allow delivery without a high risk of complications. Therefore, a woman with placenta previa is treated with bed rest, blood **transfusion**s as necessary, and medications to prevent labor. After 36 weeks, the baby can be delivered via cesarean section. This is almost always the preferred method of delivery in order to avoid further bleeding from the low-lying placenta.

The first line of treatment for placental abruption involves replacing the mother's lost blood with blood transfusions and fluids given through a needle in a vein. Oxygen will be administered, usually by a mask or through tubes leading to the nose. When the placental separation is severe, treatment may require prompt delivery of the baby. However, delivery may be delayed when the placental separation is not as severe, and when the fetus is too immature to insure a healthy baby if delivered. The baby is delivered vaginally when possible. However, a cesarean section may be performed to deliver the baby more quickly if the abruption is quite severe or if the baby is in distress.

In cases of placenta previa, the prognosis for the mother is very good. The baby, however, has a 15-20% chance of dying. This is 10 times the **death** rate associated with normal pregnancies. About 60% of these deaths occur because the baby delivered was too premature to survive.

The prognosis for cases of placental abruption varies, depending on the severity of the abruption. The risk of death for the mother ranges up to 5%, usually due to severe blood loss, **heart failure**, and kidney failure. In cases of severe abruption, 50-80% of all fetuses die. Among those who survive, nearly half will have lifelong problems due to oxygen deprivation in the uterus and premature birth.

There are no known ways to insure the appropriate placement of the placenta in the uterus. However, careful treatment of the problem can result in the best chance for a good outcome for both mother and baby.

Some of the causes of placental abruption are preventable. These include cigarette smoking, alcohol abuse, and cocaine use. Other causes of abruption may not be avoidable, like diabetes or high blood pressure. These diseases should be carefully treated. Patients with conditions known to increase the risk of placental abruption should be carefully monitored for signs and symptoms of this complication.

See also Childbirth; Pregnancy loss

Plague

Plague is a serious, infectious disease usually transmitted by the bites of rodent fleas. It was the scourge of our early history. There are three major forms of the disease: bubonic, septicemic, and pneumonic. Plague has been responsible for three great world pandemics, which caused millions of **death**s and significantly altered the course of history. A pandemic is a disease that occurs throughout the entire population of a country, a people, or the world. Although the cause of the plague was not identified until the third pandemic in 1894, scientists are virtually certain that the first two pandemics were plague because a number of the survivors wrote about their experiences and described the symptoms.

The first great pandemic appeared in 542 A.D. and lasted for 60 years. It killed millions of citizens, particularly along the Mediterranean Sea. This sea was the busiest, coastal trade route at that time and connected what is now southern Europe, northern Africa, and parts of coastal Asia.

The second pandemic occurred during the 14th century, and was called "the black death" because its main symptom

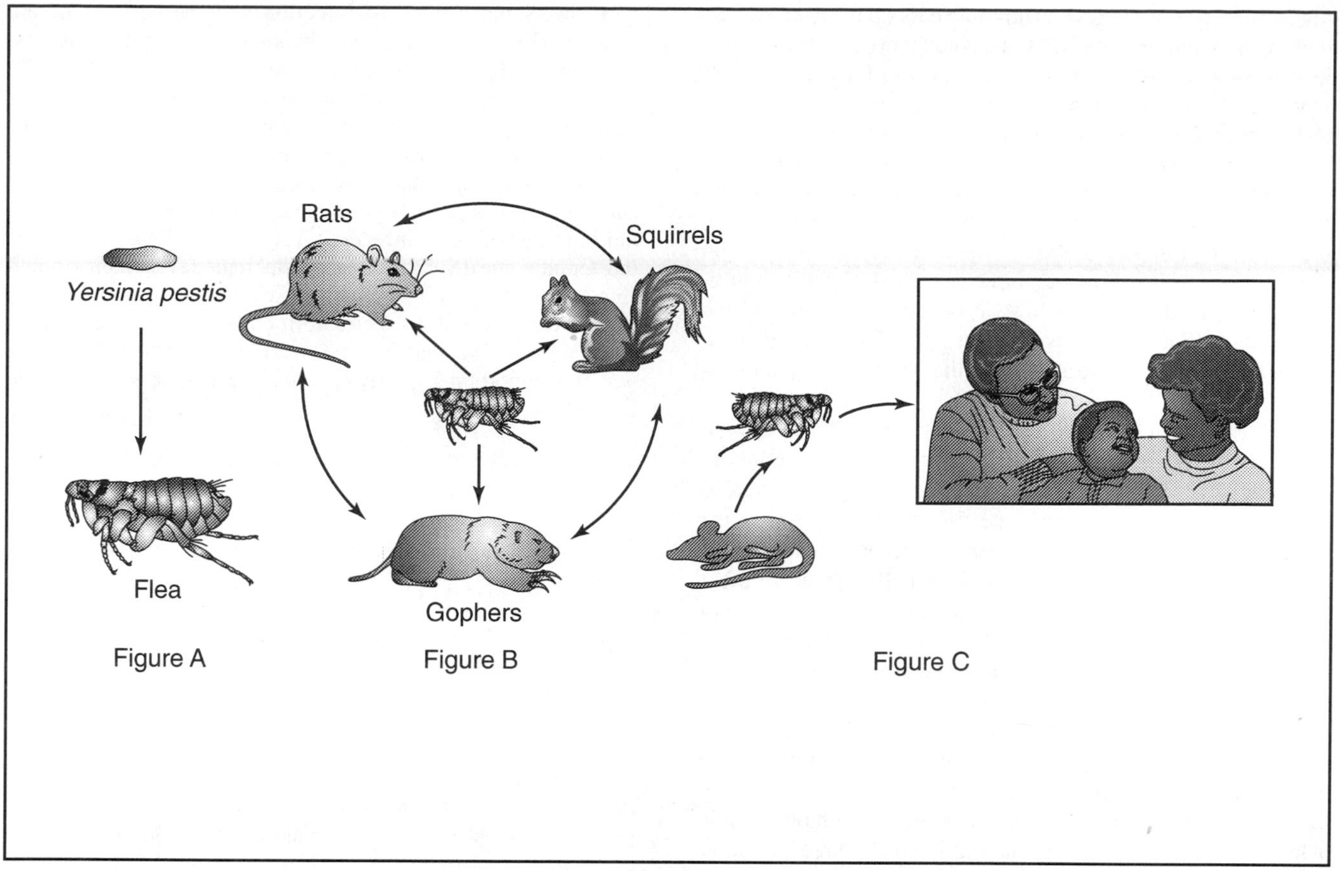

How plague spreads.

was the appearance of black patches on the skin. It was also a subject found in many European paintings, drawings, plays, and writings of that time. The connections between large, active trading ports, rats coming off the ships, and the severe outbreaks of the plague was known by the people. This was the most severe of the three, beginning in the mid 1300s with an origin in central Asia and lasting for 400 years. About a fourth of the entire European population died within a few years after plague was first introduced.

The final pandemic began in northern China, reaching Canton and Hong Kong by 1894. From here, it spread to all continents, killing millions.

The great pandemics of the past occurred when wild rodents spread the disease to rats in cities, and then to humans when the rats died. Another route for infection came from rats coming off ships that had traveled from heavily infected areas. Generally, these were busy, coastal or inland trade routes.

Curiously, between 10 and 50 Americans living in the southwestern United States contract plague each year during the spring and summer. The last rat-borne epidemic in the United States occurred in Los Angeles in 1924-25. Since then, all plague cases in this country have been sporadic, acquired from wild rodents or their fleas. Plague can also be acquired from ground squirrels and prairie dogs in parts of Arizona, New Mexico, California, Colorado, and Nevada. Around the world, there are between 1,000 and 2,000 cases of plague each year. Recent outbreaks in humans occurred in Africa, South America, and southeast Asia.

Some people and/or animals with bubonic plague go on to develop **pneumonia** (pneumonic plague). This can spread to others via infected droplets during coughing or sneezing.

Plague is one of three diseases still subject to international health regulations. These rules require that all confirmed cases be reported to the **World Health Organization** (WHO) within 24 hours of diagnosis. According to the 1998 regulations, passengers on an international voyage who have been to an area where there is an epidemic of pneumonic plague must be placed in **isolation** for six days before being allowed to leave.

Fleas carry the bacterium *Yersinia pestis*. When a flea bites an infected rodent, it swallows the plague bacteria. The bacteria is passed on when the fleas, in turn, bite a human. Humans also may become infected if they have a break or cut in the skin and come in direct contact with body fluids or tissues of infected animals.

More than 100 species of fleas have been reported to be naturally infected with plague; in the western United States, the most common source of plague is the ground squirrel flea.

Since 1924 there have been no documented cases in the United States of human-to-human spread of plague from droplets. All but one of the few pneumonic cases have been associated with handling infected cats. While dogs and cats can become infected, dogs rarely show signs of illness and are not believed to spread disease to humans. However, plague has been spread from infected coyotes (wild dogs) to humans.

Two to five days after infection, patients experience a sudden **fever**, chills, seizures, and severe **headache**s, followed by the appearance of swelling or ''buboes'' in armpits, groin, and neck. The most commonly affected sites are the lymph glands near the site of the first infection. As the bacteria multiply in the glands, the lymph node becomes swollen. As the nodes collect fluid, they become extremely tender. Occasionally, the bacteria will cause an ulcer at the point of the first infection.

Bacteria that invade the bloodstream directly (without involving the lymph nodes) causes septicemic plague. (Bubonic plague also can progress to septicemic plague if not treated appropriately.) Septicemic plague that does not involve the lymph glands is particularly dangerous because it can be hard to diagnose the disease. The bacteria usually spread to other sites, including the liver, kidneys, spleen, lungs, and sometimes the eyes, or the lining of the brain. Symptoms include fever, chills, prostration, abdominal pain, **shock**, and bleeding into the skin and organs.

Pneumonic plague may occur as a direct infection (primary) or as a result of untreated bubonic or septicemic plague (secondary). Primary pneumonic plague is caused by inhaling infective drops from another person or animal with pneumonic plague. Symptoms, which appear within one to three days after infection, include a severe, overwhelming pneumonia, with **shortness of breath**, high fever, and blood in the phlegm. If untreated, half the patients will die; if blood **poisoning** occurs as an early complication, patients may die even before the buboes appear.

Life-threatening complications of plague include shock, high fever, problems with blood clotting, and convulsions.

Plague should be suspected if there are painful buboes (inflamed lymph nodes), fever, exhaustion, and a history of possible exposure to rodents, rabbits, or fleas in the western states. The patient should be isolated. **Chest x-rays** are taken, as well as blood cultures, antigen testing, and examination of lymph node specimens. Blood cultures should be taken 30 minutes apart, before treatment.

As soon as plague is suspected, the patient should be isolated, and local and state departments notified. Drug treatment reduces the risk of death to less than 5%. The preferred treatment is with **antibiotics** such as streptomycin administered as soon as possible. Alternatives include gentamicin, chloramphenicol, tetracycline, or trimethoprim/sulfamethoxazole.

Plague can be treated successfully if it is caught early. Untreated pneumonic plague is almost always fatal, however, and the chances of survival are very low unless specific antibiotic treatment is started within 15-18 hours after symptoms appear. The presence of plague bacteria in a blood smear is a grave sign, and indicates septicemic plague.

Plague vaccines have been used with varying effectiveness since the late 19th century. Experts believe that **vaccination** lowers the chance of infection and the severity of the disease. However, the effectiveness of the vaccine against pneumonic plague is not clearly known.

Vaccinations against plague are not required to enter any country. Because immunization requires multiple doses over a 6-10 month period, plague vaccine is not recommended for quick protection during outbreaks. Moreover, its unpleasant side effects make it a poor choice unless there is a substantial long-term risk of infection. The safety of the vaccine for those under age 18 has not been established. Pregnant women should not be vaccinated unless the need for protection is greater than the risk to the unborn child. Even those who receive the vaccine may not be completely protected. This is why it is important to protect against rodents, fleas, and people with plague.

See also Black Death pandemics; Epidemic and pandemic

PLASTIC, COSMETIC, AND RECONSTRUCTIVE SURGERY

Plastic, cosmetic, and reconstructive surgery refers to a variety of operations performed in order to repair or restore body parts to look ''normal,'' or to change a body part to look better. These types of surgery are highly specialized. They are characterized by careful preparation of the patient's skin and tissues, by precise cutting and suturing techniques, and by care taken to minimize scarring. Recent advances in the development of miniaturized instruments, new materials for **artificial limbs** and body parts, and improved surgical techniques have expanded the range of plastic surgery operations that can be performed.

Although these three types of surgery share some common techniques and approaches, they have somewhat different emphases. Plastic surgery is usually performed to treat **birth defects** and to remove skin blemishes such as **warts**, **acne** scars, or **birthmarks**.

While cosmetic surgery procedures are performed to make the patient look younger or enhance his or her appearance in other ways, reconstructive surgery is used to reattach body parts severed in combat or accidents, to perform skin grafts after severe **burns**, or to reconstruct parts of the patient's body that were missing at birth or removed by surgery. Reconstructive surgery is the oldest form of plastic surgery, having developed out of the need to treat wounded soldiers in wartime.

Some patients should not have plastic surgery because of certain medical risks. These groups include:

- Patients recovering from a **heart attack**, severe infection (for example, **pneumonia**), or other serious illness
- Patients with infectious hepatitis or HIV infection
- **Cancer** patients whose cancer might spread (metastasize)
- Patients who are extremely overweight. Patients who are more than 30% overweight should not have **liposuction**
- Patients with blood clotting disorders.

Plastic, cosmetic, and reconstructive surgeries have an important psychological dimension because of the high value placed on outward appearance in Western society. Many people who are born with visible deformities or disfigured by accidents later in life develop emotional problems related to social rejection. Other people work in fields such as acting, modeling, media journalism, and even politics, where their employment depends on how they look. Some people have unrealistic expectations of cosmetic surgery and think that it will solve all their life problems. It is important for anyone considering nonemergency plastic or cosmetic surgery to be realistic about its results. One type of psychiatric disorder, called body dysmorphic disorder, is characterized by an excessive preoccupation with imaginary or minor flaws in appearance. Patients with this disorder frequently seek unnecessary plastic surgery.

Plastic surgery includes a number of different procedures that usually involve skin. Operations to remove excess fat from the abdomen (''tummy tucks''), dermabrasion to remove acne scars or tattoos, and reshaping the cartilage in children's ears (otoplasty) are common applications of plastic surgery.

Most cosmetic surgery is done on the face. The most common cosmetic procedure for children is correction of a cleft lip or palate. In adults, the most common procedures are remodeling of the nose (**rhinoplasty**), removal of baggy skin around the eyelids (blepharoplasty), **facelifts** (rhytidectomy), or changing the size of the breasts (mammoplasty). Although many people still think of cosmetic surgery as only for women, growing numbers of men are choosing to have facelifts and eyelid surgery, as well as hair transplants and ''tummy tucks.''

Reconstructive surgery is often performed on burn and accident victims. It may involve the rebuilding of severely fractured bones, as well as **skin grafting**. Reconstructive surgery includes such procedures as the reattachment of an amputated finger or toe, or implanting a prosthesis. Prostheses are artificial structures and materials that are used to replace missing limbs or teeth, or arthritic hip and knee joints.

Preparation for nonemergency plastic or reconstructive surgery includes patient education, as well as medical considerations. Some operations, such as nose reshaping or the removal of warts, small birthmarks, and tattoos can be done as outpatient procedures under local **anesthesia**. Most plastic and reconstructive surgery, however, involves a stay in the hospital and general anesthesia.

Preparation for plastic surgery includes the surgeon's detailed assessment of the parts of the patient's body that will be involved. Skin grafts require evaluating suitable areas of the patient's skin for the right color and texture to match the skin at the graft site. Facelifts and cosmetic surgery in the eye area require very close attention to the texture of the skin and the placement of surgical cuts (incisions).

Patients scheduled for plastic surgery under general anesthesia will be given a **physical examination**, blood and urine tests, and other tests to make sure that they do not have any previously undetected health problems or blood clotting disorders. The doctor will check the list of other prescription medications that the patient may be taking to make sure that none of them will interfere with normal blood clotting or interact with the anesthetic.

Patients are asked to avoid using **aspirin** or medications containing aspirin for a week to two weeks before surgery, because these drugs lengthen the time of blood clotting. Smokers are asked to stop **smoking** two weeks before surgery because smoking interferes with the healing process. For some types of plastic surgery, the patient may be asked to donate several units of his or her own blood before the procedure, in case a **transfusion** is needed during the operation. The patient will be asked to sign a consent form before the operation.

The doctor will meet with the patient before the operation is scheduled, in order to explain the procedure and to be sure that the patient is realistic about the expected results. This consideration is particularly important if the patient is having cosmetic surgery.

Medical aftercare following plastic surgery under general anesthesia includes bringing the patient to a recovery room, monitoring his or her vital signs, and giving medications to relieve **pain** as necessary. Patients who have had fat removed from the abdomen may be kept in bed for as long as two weeks. Patients who have had mammoplasties, breast reconstruction, and some types of facial surgery typically remain in the hospital for a week after the operation. Patients who have had liposuction or eyelid surgery are usually sent home in a day or two.

Patients who have had outpatient procedures are usually given **antibiotics** to prevent infection and are sent home as soon as their vital signs are normal.

The risks associated with plastic, cosmetic, and reconstructive surgery include the postoperative complications that can occur with any surgical operation under anesthesia. These complications include wound infection, internal bleeding, pneumonia, and reactions to the anesthesia.

In addition to these general risks, plastic, cosmetic, and reconstructive surgery carry specific risks:

- Formation of undesirable scar tissue
- Persistent pain, redness, or swelling in the area of the surgery
- Infection inside the body related to inserting a prosthesis. These infections can result from contamination at the time of surgery or from bacteria migrating into the area around the prosthesis at a later time.
- Anemia or fat **embolism**s from liposuction
- Rejection of skin grafts or tissue transplants
- Loss of normal feeling or function in the area of the operation. For example, it is not unusual for women who have had mammoplasties to lose sensation in their nipples.
- Complications resulting from unforeseen technological problems. The best-known example of this problem was the discovery in the mid-1990s that **breast implants** made with silicone gel could leak into the patient's body.

Platelet count

A platelet count is a diagnostic test that determines the number of platelets in the patient's blood. Platelets, which are also called thrombocytes, are small disk-shaped blood cells produced in the bone marrow and involved in the process of blood clotting. There are normally between 150,000-450,000 platelets in each microliter of blood. Low platelet counts or abnormally shaped platelets are associated with bleeding disorders. High platelet counts sometimes indicate disorders of the bone marrow.

The primary functions of a platelet count are to assist in the diagnosis of bleeding disorders and to monitor patients who are being treated for any disease involving bone marrow failure. Patients who have diseases such as leukemia, polycythemia vera, or aplastic anemia are given periodic platelet count tests to monitor their health.

Platelet counts use a freshly-collected blood specimen to which a chemical called EDTA has been added to prevent clotting before the test begins. About 5 mL of blood are drawn from a vein in the patient's inner elbow region. Blood drawn from a vein helps to produce a more accurate count than blood drawn from a fingertip. Collection of the sample takes only a few minutes.

After collection, the mean platelet volume of EDTA-blood will increase over time. This increase is caused by a change in the shape of the platelets after removal from the body. The changing volume is relatively stable for a period of one to three hours after collection. This period is the best time to count the sample when using electronic instruments, because the platelets will be within a standard size range.

Platelets can be observed in a direct blood smear for approximate quantity and shape. A direct smear is made by placing a drop of blood onto a microscope slide and spreading it into a thin layer. After staining to make the various blood cells easier to see and distinguish, a laboratory technician views the smear through a light microscope. Accurate assessment of the number of platelets requires other methods of counting. There are three methods used to count platelets; hemacytometer, voltage-pulse counting, and electro-optical counting.

The microscopic method uses a phase contrast microscope to view blood on a hemacytometer slide. A sample of the diluted blood mixture is placed in a hemacytometer, which is an instrument with a grid etched into its surface to guide the counting. For a proper count, the platelets should be evenly distributed in the hemacytometer. Counts made from samples with platelet clumping are considered unreliable. Clumping can be caused by several factors, such as clotting before addition of the anticoagulant and allowing the blood to remain in contact with a capillary blood vessel during collection. Errors in platelet counting are more common when blood is collected from capillaries than from veins.

Electronic counting of platelets is the most common method. There are two types of electronic counting, voltage-pulse and electro-optical counting systems. In both systems, the collected blood is diluted and counted by passing the blood through an electronic counter. The instruments are set to count only particles within the proper size range for platelets. The upper and lower levels of the size range are called size exclusion limits. Any cells or material larger or smaller than the size exclusion limits will not be counted. Any object in the proper size range is counted, however, even if it is not a platelet. For these instruments to work properly, the sample must not contain other material that might mistakenly be counted as platelets. Electronic counting instruments sometimes produce artificially low platelet counts. If a platelet and another blood cell pass through the counter at the same time, the instrument will not count the larger cell because of the size exclusion limits, which will cause the instrument to accidentally miss the platelet. Clumps of platelets will not be counted because clumps exceed the upper size exclusion limit for platelets. In addition, if the patient has a high white blood cell count, electronic counting may yield an unusually low platelet count because white blood cells may filter out some of the platelets before the sample is counted. On the other hand, if the red blood cells in the sample have burst, their fragments will be falsely counted as platelets.

Risks for a platelet count test are minimal in normal individuals. Patients with bleeding disorders, however, may have prolonged bleeding from the puncture wound or the formation of a bruise (hematoma) under the skin where the blood was withdrawn.

The normal range for a platelet count is 150,000-450,000 platelets per microliter of blood. An abnormally low platelet level (**thrombocytopenia**) is a condition that may result from increased destruction of platelets, decreased production, or increased usage of platelets. In idiopathic thrombocytopenic purpura (ITP), platelets are destroyed at abnormally high rates. **Hypersplenism** is characterized by the collection of platelets in the spleen. Disseminated intravascular coagulation (DIC) is a condition in which blood clots occur within blood vessels in a number of tissues. All of these diseases produce reduced platelet counts.

Abnormally high platelet levels (**thrombocytosis**) may indicate either a benign reaction to an infection, surgery, or certain medications; or a disease like polycythemia vera, in which the bone marrow produces too many platelets too quickly.

Platelet function disorders

Platelets are elements within the bloodstream that recognize and cling to damaged areas inside blood vessels. When they do this, the platelets trigger a series of chemical changes that result in the formation of a blood clot. There are certain hereditary disorders that affect platelet function and impair their ability to start the process of blood clot formation. One result is the possibility of excessive bleeding from minor injuries or menstrual flow.

Platelets are formed in the bone marrow a spongy tissue located inside the long bones of the body as fragments of a large precursor cell (a megakaryocyte). These fragments circulate in the bloodstream and form the first line of defense against blood escaping from injured blood vessels.

Damaged blood vessels release a chemical signal that increases the stickiness of platelets in the area of the injury. The sticky platelets adhere to the damaged area and gradually form a platelet plug. At the same time, the platelets release a series of chemical signals that prompt other factors in the blood to reinforce the platelet plug. Between the platelet and its reinforcements, a sturdy clot is created that acts as a patch while the damaged area heals.

There are several hereditary disorders characterized by some impairment of the platelet's action. Examples include von Willebrand's disease, Glanzmann's thrombasthenia, and Wiskott-Aldrich syndrome. Vulnerable aspects of platelet function include errors in the production of the platelets themselves or errors in the formation, storage, or release of their chemical signals. These defects can prevent platelets from responding to injuries or from prompting the action of other factors involved in clot formation.

Platelet function disorders can be inherited, but they may also occur as a symptom of acquired diseases or as a side effect of certain drugs, including **aspirin**. Common symptoms of platelet function disorders include bleeding from the nose, mouth, vagina, or anus; pinpoint **bruises** and purplish patches on the skin; and abnormally heavy menstrual bleeding.

In diagnosing platelet function disorders, specific tests are needed to determine whether the problem is caused by low numbers of platelets or impaired platelet function. A blood **platelet count** and **bleeding** time are common screening tests. If these tests confirm that the symptoms are due to impaired platelet function, further tests are done that pinpoint the exact nature of the defect.

Treatment is intended to prevent bleeding and stop it quickly when it occurs. For example, patients are advised to be careful when they brush their teeth to reduce damage to the gums. They are also warned against taking medications that interfere with platelet function. Some patients may require iron and folate supplements to counteract potential anemia. Platelet **transfusion**s may be necessary to prevent life-threatening hemorrhaging in some cases. **Bone marrow transplantation** can cure certain disorders but also carries some serious risks. Hormone therapy is useful in treating heavy menstrual bleeding. Von Willebrand's disease can be treated with desmopressin (DDAVP, Stimate). The outcome depends on the specific disorder and the severity of its symptoms. Platelet function disorders range from life-threatening conditions to easily treated or little-noticed problems.

Inherited platelet function disorders cannot be prevented except by **genetic counseling**; however, some acquired function disorders may be guarded against by avoiding substances that trigger the disorder.

PLEURISY

Pleurisy is an inflammation of the membrane that surrounds and protects the lungs (the pleura). Inflammation occurs when an infection or damaging agent irritates the pleural surface. As a consequence, sharp chest **pain**s are the primary symptom of pleurisy.

Pleurisy, also called pleuritis, is a condition that generally stems from an existing respiratory infection, disease, or injury. In people who have otherwise good health, respiratory infections or **pneumonia** are the main causes of pleurisy. This condition used to be more common, but with the advent of **antibiotics** and modern disease therapies, pleurisy has become less prevalent.

The pleura is a double-layered structure made up of an inner membrane, which surrounds the lungs, and an outer membrane, which lines the chest cavity. The pleural membranes are very thin, close together, and have a fluid coating in the narrow space between them. This liquid acts as a lubricant, so that when the lungs inflate and deflate during breathing, the pleural surfaces can easily glide over one another.

Pleurisy occurs when the pleural surfaces rub against one another, due to irritation and inflammation. Infection within the pleural space is the most common irritant, although the abnormal presence of air, blood, or cells can also initiate pleurisy. These disturbances all act to displace the normal pleural fluid, which forces the membranes to rub, rather than glide, against one another. This rubbing irritates nerve endings in the outer membrane and causes pain. Pleurisy also causes a chest noise that ranges from a faint squeak to a loud creak. This characteristic sound is called a ''friction rub.''

Pleurisy cases are classified either as having pleural effusion or as being ''dry.'' Pleural effusion is more common and refers to an accumulation of fluid within the pleural space; dry pleurisy is inflammation without fluid build-up. Less pain occurs with pleural effusion because the fluid forces the membrane surfaces apart. However, pleural effusion causes additional complications because it places pressure on the lungs. This leads to respiratory distress and possible lung collapse.

A variety of conditions can give rise to pleurisy. The following list represents the most common sources of pleural inflammation.

- Infections, including pneumonia, **tuberculosis**, and other bacterial or viral respiratory infections
- Immune disorders, including **systemic lupus erythematosus**, **rheumatoid arthritis**, and sarcoidosis
- Diseases, including **cancer**, **pancreatitis**, liver **cirrhosis**, and heart or kidney failure
- Injury, from a rib fracture, collapsed lung, esophagus rupture, blood clot, or material such as asbestos
- Drug reactions, from certain drugs used to treat tuberculosis (isoniazid), cancer (methotrexate, procarbazine), or the immune disorders mentioned above (hydralazine, procainamide, phenytoin, quinidine).

The hallmark symptom of pleurisy is sudden, intense chest pain that is usually located over the area of inflammation. Although the pain can be constant, it is usually most severe when the lungs move during breathing, coughing, sneezing, or even talking. The pain is usually described as shooting or stabbing, but in minor cases it resembles a mild cramp. When pleurisy occurs in certain locations, such as near the diaphragm, the pain may be felt in other areas such as the neck, shoulder, or abdomen (referred pain). Another indication of pleurisy is that holding one's breath or exerting pressure against the chest causes pain relief.

Pleurisy is also characterized by certain respiratory symptoms. In response to the pain, pleurisy patients commonly have a rapid, shallow breathing pattern. Pleural effusion can also cause **shortness of breath**, as excess fluid makes expanding the lungs difficult. If severe breathing difficulties persist, patients may experience a blue colored complexion (**cyanosis**).

Additional symptoms of pleurisy are specific to the illness that triggers the condition. Thus, if infection is the cause, then chills, **fever**, and fatigue will be likely pleurisy symptoms.

The distinctive pain of pleurisy is normally the first clue physicians use for diagnosis. Doctors usually feel the chest to find the most painful area, which is the likely site of inflammation. A stethoscope is also used to listen for abnormal chest sounds as the patient breathes. If the doctor hears the characteristic friction rub, the diagnosis of pleurisy can be confirmed, Sometimes, a friction rub is masked by the presence of pleural effusion and further examination is needed for an accurate diagnosis.

Identifying the actual illness that causes pleurisy is more difficult. To make this diagnosis, doctors must evaluate the patient's history, additional symptoms, and laboratory test results. A **chest x ray** may also be taken to look for signs of accumulated fluid and other abnormalities. Possible causes, such as pneumonia, fractured ribs, esophagus rupture, and lung tumors may be detected on an x ray. **Computed tomography scan** (CT scan) and ultrasound scans are more powerful diagnostic tools used to visualize the chest cavity. Images from these techniques more clearly pinpoint the location of excess fluid or other suspected problems.

The most helpful information in diagnosing the cause of pleurisy is a fluid analysis. Once the doctor knows the precise location of fluid accumulation, a sample is removed using a procedure called thoracentesis. In this technique, a fine needle is inserted into the chest to reach the pleural space and extract fluid. The fluid's appearance and composition is thoroughly examined to help doctors understand how the fluid was produced. Several laboratory tests are performed to analyze the chemical components of the fluid. These tests also determine whether infection-causing bacteria or viruses are present. In addition, cells within the fluid are identified and counted. Cancerous cells can also be detected to learn whether the pleurisy is caused by a malignancy.

In certain instances, such as dry pleurisy, or when a fluid analysis is not informative, a biopsy of the pleura may be needed for microscopic analysis. A sample of pleural tissue can be obtained several ways: with a biopsy needle, by making a small incision in the chest wall, or by using a thoracoscope (a video-assisted instrument for viewing the pleural space and collecting samples).

The pain of pleurisy is usually treated with analgesic and anti-inflammatory drugs, such as **acetaminophen**, ibuprofen, and indomethacin. People suffering from pleurisy may also receive relief from lying on the painful side. Sometimes, a painful cough will be controlled with codeine-based cough syrups. However, as the pain eases, a person with pleurisy should try to breathe deeply and cough to clear any congestion, otherwise pneumonia may occur. Rest is also important to aid in the recovery process.

The treatment used to cure pleurisy is ultimately defined by the underlying cause. Thus, pleurisy from a bacterial infection can be successfully treated with antibiotics, while no treatment is given for viral infections that must run their course. Specific therapies designed for more chronic illnesses can often cause pleurisy to subside. For example, tuberculosis pleurisy is treated with standard anti-tuberculosis drugs. With some illnesses, excess fluid continues to accumulate and causes severe respiratory distress. In these individuals, the fluid may be removed by thoracentesis, or the doctor may insert a chest tube to drain large amounts. If left untreated, a more serious infection may develop within the fluid, called empyema.

Alternative treatments can be used in conjunction with conventional treatment to help heal pleurisy. **Acupuncture** and botanical medicines are alternative approaches for alleviating pleural pain and breathing problems. An herbal remedy commonly recommended is pleurisy root (*Asclepias tuberosa*), so named because of its use by early American settlers who learned of this medicinal plant from Native Americans. Pleurisy root helps to ease pain, inflammation, and breathing difficulties brought on by pleurisy. This herb is often used in conjunction with mullein (*Verbascum thapsus*) or elecampane (*Inula helenium*), which serve as **expectorants** to clear excess mucus from the lungs. In addition, there are many other respiratory herbs that are used as expectorants or for other actions on the respiratory system. Herbs thought to combat infection, such as echinacea (*Echinacea* spp.) are also included in herbal pleurisy remedies. Anitviral herbs, such as *Lomatium dissectum* and *Ligusticum porteri*, can be used if the pleurisy is of viral origin. Traditional Chinese medicine uses the herb ephedra (*Ephedra sinica*), which acts to open air passages and alleviate respiratory difficulties in pleurisy patients. Dietary recommendations include eating fresh fruits and vegetables, adequate protein, and good quality fats (omega-3 fatty acids are anti-inflammatory and are found in fish and flax oil). Taking certain nutritional supplements, especially large doeses of vitamin C, may also provide health benefits to people with pleurisy. Contrast hydrotherapy applied to the chest and back, along with compresses (cloths soaked in an herbal solution) or poultices (crushed herbs applied directly to the skin) of respiratory herbs, can assist in the healing process. Homeopathic treatment, guided by a trained practitioner, can be effective in resolving pleurisy.

Preventing pleurisy is often a matter of providing early medical attention to conditions that can cause pleural inflammation. Along this line, appropriate antibiotic treatment of bacterial respiratory infections may successfully prevent some cases of pleurisy. Maintaining a healthy lifestyle and avoiding exposure to harmful substances (for example, asbestos) are more general preventive measures.

Pneumococcal pneumonia

Pneumococcal pneumonia is a common but serious infection and inflammation of the lungs. It is caused by the bacterium *Streptococcus pneumoniae*, which is the cause of many human diseases, including **pneumonia**.

Although the bacteria can normally be found in the nose and throat of healthy individuals, it can grow and cause infection when the immune system is weakened. Infection usually begins with the upper respiratory tract and then travels into the lungs. Pneumonia occurs when the bacteria find their way deep into the lungs, to the area called the alveoli, or air sacs. This is the functional part of the lungs where oxygen is absorbed into the blood. Once in the alveoli, *Streptococcus pneumoniae* begin to grow and multiply. White blood cells and immune proteins from the blood also accumulate at the site of infection in the alveoli. As the alveoli fill with these substances and fluid, they can no longer function in the exchange of oxygen. This fluid filling of the lungs is how pneumonia is defined.

Those people most at risk of developing pneumococcal pneumonia have a weakened immune system. This includes the elderly, infants, **cancer** patients, **AIDS** patients, post-operative patients, alcoholics, and those with diabetes. Pneumococcal pneumonia is a disease that has a high rate of hospital transmission, putting hospital patients at greater risk. Prior lung infections also makes someone more likely to develop pneumococcal pneumonia. The disease can be most severe in patients who have had their spleen removed. It is the spleen that is responsible for removing the bacteria from the blood. Cases of pneumonia, which is spread by close contact, seem to occur most often between November through April. If not treated, the disease can spread, causing continually decreasing lung function, heart problems, and arthritis.

Symptoms of bacterial pneumonia include a **cough**, sputum (mucus) production that may be puslike or bloody, shaking and chills, **fever**, and chest **pain**. Symptoms often have an abrupt beginning and occur after an upper respiratory infection such as a cold. Symptoms may differ somewhat in the elderly, with minimal cough, no sputum and no fever, but rather tiredness and confusion leading to **hypothermia** and **shock**.

The presence of symptoms and a physical exam which reveals abnormal lung sounds usually suggest the presence of pneumonia. Diagnosis is typically made from an x ray of the lungs, which indicates the accumulation of fluid. Additional tests that may be done include a complete **blood count**, a sputum sample for microscopic examination and culture for *Streptococcus pneumoniae*, as well as possibly **blood culture**s.

Depending on the severity of the disease, **antibiotics** are given either at home or in the hospital. Historically, the treatment for pneumococcal pneumonia has been penicillin. However, an increasing number of cases of pneumococcal pneumonia have become partially or completely resistant to penicillin, making it less effective in treating this disease. Other effective antibiotics include amoxicillin and erythromycin. If these antibiotics are not effective, vancomycin or cephalosporin may alternatively be used.

Being a serious, sometimes fatal disease, pneumococcal pneumonia is best treated as soon as possible with antibiotics. However, there are also alternative treatments that both support this conventional treatment and prevent recurrences. Maintaining a healthy immune system is important. One way to do this is by taking the herb, echinacea (*Echinacea* spp.). Getting plenty of rest and reducing **stress** can help the body heal. Some practitioners feel that mucus-producing foods (including dairy products, eggs, gluten-rich grains such as wheat, oats, rye, as well as sugar) can contribute to the lung congestion that accompanies pneumonia. Decreasing these foods and increasing the amount of fresh fruits and vegetables may help to decrease lung congestion.

Adequate protein in the diet is also essential for the body to produce antibodies. Contrast and constitutional hydrotherapy can be very helpful in treating cases of pneumonia. Other alternative therapies, including acupuncture, Chinese herbal medicine, and homeopathy, can be very useful during the recovery phase, helping the body to rebuild after the illness and contributing to the prevention of recurrences.

Simple, uncomplicated cases of pneumococcal pneumonia will begin to respond to antibiotics in 48-72 hours. Full recovery from pneumonia, however, is greatly dependent on the age and overall health of the individual. Normally healthy and younger patients can recover in only a few days, while the elderly or otherwise weakened individuals may not recover for several weeks. Complications may develop which give a poorer prognosis. Even when promptly and properly diagnosed, such weakened patients may die of their pneumonia.

Recently, a **vaccination** has become available for the prevention of pneumococcal pneumonia. This vaccination is generally recommended for people with a high likelihood of developing pneumococcal infection or for those in whom a serious complication of infection is likely to develop. This would include persons over the age of 65, as well as those with:

- Chronic pulmonary disease
- Advanced cardiovascular disease
- **Diabetes mellitus**
- Alcoholism
- **Cirrhosis**
- Chronic kidney disease
- Spleen dysfunction, or removal of spleen
- Iimmunosuppression (cancer, organ transplant or AIDS)
- **Sickle-cell anemia**.

Unfortunately, those people for whom the vaccination is most recommended are also those who are least likely to respond favorably to a vaccination. Therefore, there remains a question about the overall effectiveness of this vaccine.

The use of oral penicillin to prevent infection may be recommended for some patients at high risk, such as children with sickle cell disease and those with a spleen removed. This treatment, however, must be weighed with the increased likelihood of developing penicillin-resistant infections.

PNEUMOCYSTIS PNEUMONIA

Pneumocystis pneumonia is a lung infection that occurs primarily in people with weakened immune systems especially people who are HIV-positive. The disease agent is an organism whose biological classification is still uncertain. *Pneumocystis carinii* was originally thought to be a one-celled organism (a protozoan), but more recent research suggests that it is a fungus. Although its life cycle is known to have three stages, its method of reproduction is not yet completely understood. The complete name of the disease is *Pneumocystis carinii* **pneumonia** (PCP) and is also sometimes called pneumocystosis.

Pneumonia as a general term refers to a severe lung inflammation. In pneumocystis pneumonia, this inflammation is caused by the growth of *Pneumocystis carinii*, a fungus-like organism that is widespread in the environment. PCP is ordinarily a rare disease, affecting only people with weakened immune systems. Many of these people are patients receiving drugs for organ transplants or **cancer** treatment. With the rising incidence of **AIDS**, however, PCP has become primarily associated with AIDS patients. In fact, as many as 75% of AIDS patients have developed PCP. It has also been the leading cause of **death** in AIDS patients.

The organism that causes PCP is widely distributed in nature and is transmitted through the air. When the organism is inhaled, it enters the upper respiratory tract and infects the tiny air sacs at the ends of the smaller air tubes (bronchioles) in the lungs. These tiny air sacs are called alveoli. Under a microscope, alveoli look like groups of hollow spheres resembling grape clusters. The exchange of oxygen with the blood takes place in the alveoli. It appears that *P. carinii* lives in the fluid in the lining of the alveoli.

Person-to-person infection does not appear to be very common; however, clusters of PCP outbreaks in hospitals and groups of immunocompromised people indicate that patients with active PCP should not be exposed to others with weakened immune systems. It is thought that many people actually acquire mild *Pneumocystis carinii* infections from time to time, but are protected by their immune systems from developing a full-blown case of the disease.

P. carinii is an opportunistic organism. This means that it causes disease only under certain conditions, as when a person is immunocompromised. Under these circumstances, *P. carinii* can multiply and cause pneumonia. The mechanisms of the organism's growth within the alveoli are not fully understood. As the pneumocystis organism continues to replicate, it gradually fills the alveoli. As the pneumonia becomes more severe, fluid accumulates and tissue scarring occurs. These changes result in decreased respiratory function and lower levels of oxygen in the blood.

Some patients are at greater risk of developing PCP. These high-risk groups include:

- Premature infants
- Patients with **immunodeficiency** diseases, including severe combined immunodeficiency disease (SCID) and acquired immunodeficiency syndrome (AIDS).
- Patients receiving immunosuppressive drugs, especially cortisone-like drugs (**corticosteroids**)
- Patients suffering from protein **malnutrition**.

AIDS is currently the most common risk factor for PCP in the United States. PCP is, however, also found in countries with widespread hunger and poor hygiene.

The incubation period of PCP is not definitely known, but is thought to be between four and eight weeks. The major symptoms include **shortness of breath**, **fever**, and a nonproductive **cough**. Less common symptoms include production of sputum, blood in the sputum, difficulty breathing, and chest **pain**. Most patients will have symptoms for one to two weeks before seeing a physician. Occasionally, the disease will spread outside of the lung to other organs, including the lymph nodes, spleen, liver, or bone marrow.

The diagnosis of PCP begins with a thorough **physical examination** and blood tests. Although imaging studies are helpful in identifying abnormal areas in the lungs, the diagnosis of PCP must be confirmed by microscopic identification of the organism in the lung. Samples may be taken from the patient's sputum, or may be obtained via bronchoscopy or lung biopsy. Because of the severity of the disease, many physicians will proceed to treat patients with symptoms of pneumocystis pneumonia if they belong to a high-risk group, without the formality of an actual diagnosis. The severity of PCP can be measured by x-ray studies and by determining the amount of oxygen and carbon dioxide present in the patient's blood.

Treatment for PCP involves the use of **antibiotics**. These include trimethoprim-sulfamethoxazole (TMP-SMX, Bactrim, Septra) and pentamidine isoethionate (Nebupent, Pentam 300). Both of these anti-microbial drugs are equally effective. AIDS patients are typically treated for 21 days, whereas non-AIDS patients are treated for 14 days. TMP-SMX may be highly toxic in AIDS patients, causing severe side effects that include fever, rash, decreased numbers of white blood cells and platelets, and hepatitis. Pentamidine also causes side effects in immunocompromised patients. These side effects include decreased blood pressure, irregular heart beats, the accumulation of nitrogenous waste products in the blood, and electrolyte imbalances. Pentamidine can be given in aerosol form to minimize side effects. Alternative drugs can be used for patients experiencing these side effects.

P. carinii appears to be developing resistance to TMP-SMX. In addition, some patients are allergic to the standard antibiotics given for PCP. As a result, other antibiotics for the treatment of PCP are continually under investigation. Some drugs proven to be effective against *P. carinii* include dapsone (DDS) with trimethoprim (Trimpex), clindamycin (Cleocin) with primaquine, as well as atovaquone (Mepron). Paradoxically, corticosteroids have been found to improve the ability of TMP-SMX or pentamidine to treat PCP.

If left untreated, PCP will cause breathing difficulties that will eventually cause death. The prognosis for this disease depends on the amount of damage to the patient's lungs prior to treatment. Prognosis is usually better at a facility that specializes in caring for AIDS patients. Antibiotic treatment of PCP is about 80% effective.

Patients who have previously had PCP often experience a recurrence. Healthy lifestyle choices, including exercising, eating well, and giving up smoking may keep the disease at bay.

PNEUMONIA

It is the year 1900, and a young man falls ill, suffering from a shaking chill, sharp chest pain, cough, fever, and headache. These warning signs sound the alarm—he has pneumonia. At that time, in the days before **antibiotics**, it was often a fatal disease, killing thousands of people, especially during **epidemics**. Pneumonia—the two primary types being bacterial and viral—is acute infection of the air sacs inside the human lungs. It usually starts in the airways or bronchi and spreads to one or both lungs. Today, when treated properly, most people recover from bacterial pneumonia; however, it remains the sixth most common cause of death among older people in the United States. The very young and very old are especially likely to fall victim to pneumonia, the most common form of which is caused by *Streptococcus pneumoniae*—bacteria that are transmitted through the air and inhaled into the lungs. These bacteria cause pneumococcal disease, which results not only in pneumonia, but can also attack blood cells causing an infection called "**bacteremia**," and the brain, causing meningitis. An extremely safe and effective vaccine—one injection lasts most people a lifetime—protects against almost all bacteria which cause pneumococcal diseases. Staphylococcus bacteria will also cause pneumonia, as will certain viruses, protozoa, and even fungi. Only bacterial pneumonia can be effectively treated with antibiotics.

The treatment used to prevent pneumonia in the days before antibiotics is attributed to Almroth Edward Wright, an English bacteriologist and a pioneer in the infant field of immunology. Near the end of the nineteenth century, Wright became interested in developing inoculations using killed bacteria. These acted as vaccines, causing a mild infection that triggered future resistance to the bacteria. Wright first developed a vaccine against **typhoid fever** in the late 1890s. In 1911 he went to South Africa where he was asked to help prevent pneumonia among workers in the gold mines. There he developed an inoculation against pneumonia based on the same principles he had used to formulate the typhoid vaccine. His inoculation greatly reduced the number of pneumonia cases. Between 1926 and 1934, another Englishman, Frederick Griffith, developed laboratory techniques for classifying over thirty different strains of bacteria. At around the same time, Rebecca Craighill Lancefield, an American doctor, was working on a similar project identifying streptococcus bacteria. Finding out more about disease-causing bacteria was the focus of much medical research on both sides of the Atlantic. The race was on to come up with the cause and cure for many life-threatening diseases, including pneumonia.

By the 1930s other researchers were working on a new class of wonder drugs—antibiotics. Using Griffith's early classification work, Oswald T. Avery, a Canadian-American physician, as well as other bacteriologists such as Alphonse Dochez, made a discovery which would prove important to the science of genetics. As they studied two strains of the pneumococci bacteria, they recognized that one had a smooth coat—the S strain—and the other—the R strain—was without a coat, giving it a rough appearance. The R strain seemed to be missing an enzyme that would aid the bacteria in forming its carbohydrate coat. Avery and others found that when living R strain bacteria were added to extracts from the S strain, the R became S—that is, the R strain could replicate the coat and appear smooth. Most scientists thought that a protein from the S strain caused this reaction. However, in 1944, Avery and others demonstrated that the trigger was pure DNA (deoxyribonucleic acid). It became clear that DNA was the important compound in carrying traits in living things. This discovery opened the way for the exploration of the structure and behavior of DNA, a study which is fundamental to modern genetics. Around the time of Avery's discovery, the antibiotic **penicillin** was past the stage of trial usage and was being used to cure pneumonia among World War II soldiers as well as civilians. Today, penicillin is still the drug of choice in treating bacterial pneumonia. In severe cases, patients are placed on ventilators to aid breathing and clear the lungs of sputum.

Another form of pneumonia, **Legionnaire's disease**, is caused by *Legionella pneumophila* bacteria and is usually treated with the antibiotic erythromycin. Nonbacterial causes of pneumonia include viruses such as the **influenza** virus, adenovirus, and even the **chicken pox** virus. In viral cases, antibiotics are sometimes administered because the lungs are often infected by bacteria simultaneously. In recent years there has been an upsurge in the number of pneumonia cases caused by *Pneumocystis carinii*, a protozoan. This type of pneumonia is often associated with persons having an immunological deficiency such as that brought on by the **AIDS** virus. Treatment includes an aerosol misting of the lungs with antibiotics.

See also Immune system

PNEUMOTHORAX

Pneumothorax is a collection of air or gas in the chest or pleural space that causes part or all of a lung to collapse. Normally, the pressure in the lungs is greater than the pressure in the pleural space surrounding the lungs. However, if air enters the pleural space, the pressure in the pleura then becomes greater than the pressure in the lungs, causing the lung to collapse partially or completely. Pneumothorax can be either spontaneous or due to trauma.

If a pneumothorax occurs suddenly or for no known reason, it is called a spontaneous pneumothorax. This condition most often strikes tall, thin men between the ages of 20 to 40. In addition, people with lung disorders, such as emphysema, cystic fibrosis, and tuberculosis, are at higher risk for spontaneous pneumothorax. Traumatic pneumothorax is the result of accident or injury due to medical procedures performed to the chest cavity, such as thoracentesis or mechanical ventilation. Tension pneumothorax is a serious and potentially life-threatening condition that may be caused by traumatic injury, chronic lung disease, or as a complication of a medical procedure. In this type of pneumothorax, air enters the chest cavity, but cannot escape. This greatly increased pressure in the pleural space causes the lung to collapse completely, compresses the heart, and pushes the heart and associated blood vessels toward the unaffected side.

The symptoms of pneumothrax depend on how much air enters the chest, how much the lung collapses, and the extent of lung disease. Symptoms include the following, according to the cause of the pneumothorax:

- Spontaneous pneumothorax. Simple spontaneous pneumothorax is caused by a rupture of a small air sac or fluid-filled sac in the lung. It may be related to activity in otherwise healthy people or may occur during scuba diving or flying at high altitudes. Complicated spontaneous pneumothorax, also generally caused by rupture of a small sac in the lung, occurs in people with lung diseases. The symptoms of complicated spontaneous pneumothorax tend to be worse than those of simple pneumothorax, due to the underlying lung disease. Spontaneous pneumothorax is characterized by dull, sharp, or stabbing chest **pain** that begins suddenly and becomes worse with deep breathing or **cough**ing. Other symptoms are **shortness of breath**, rapid breathing, abnormal breathing movement (that is, little chest wall movement when breathing), and cough.

- Tension pneumothorax. Following trauma, air may enter the chest cavity. A penetrating chest wound allows outside air to enter the chest, causing the lung to collapse. Certain medical procedures performed in the chest cavity, such as thoracentesis, also may cause a lung to collapse. Tension pneumothorax may be the immediate result of an injury; the delayed complication of a hidden injury, such as a fractured rib, that punctures the lung; or the result of lung damage from **asthma**, chronic **bronchitis**, or emphysema. Symptoms of tension pneumothorax tend to be severe with sudden onset. There is marked **anxiety**, distended neck veins, weak pulse, decreased breath sounds on the affected side, and a shift of the mediastinum to the opposite side.

To diagnose pneumothorax, it is necessary for the healthcare provider to listen to the chest (auscultation) during a **physical examination**. By using a stethoscope, the physician may note that one part of the chest does not transmit the normal sounds of breathing. A chest x ray will show the air pocket and the collapsed lung. An electrocardiogram (ECG) will be performed to record the electrical impulses that control the heart's activity. Blood samples may be taken to check for the level of arterial blood gases.

A small pneumothorax may resolve on its own, but most require medical treatment. The object of treatment is to remove air from the chest and allow the lung to re-expand. This is done by inserting a needle and syringe (if the pneumothorax is small) or chest tube through the chest wall. This allows the air to escape without allowing any air back in. The lung will then re-expand itself within a few days. Surgery may be needed for repeat occurrences.

Most people recover fully from spontaneous pneumothorax. Up to half of patients with spontaneous pneumothorax experience recurrence. Recovery from a collapsed lung generally takes one to two weeks. Tension pneumothorax can cause death rapidly due to inadequate heart output or insufficient blood oxygen (hypoxemia), and must be treated as a medical emergency.

Preventive measures for a non-injury related pneumothorax include stopping smoking and seeking medical attention for respiratory problems. If the pneumothorax occurs in both lungs or more than once in the same lung, surgery may be needed to prevent it from occurring again.

Poisoning

Poisoning occurs when any substance interferes with normal body functions after it is swallowed, inhaled, injected, or absorbed. Poisonings are a common occurrence. About 10 million cases of poisoning occur in the United States each year. In 80% of the cases, the victim is a child under the age of five. About 50 children die each year from poisonings. Curiosity, inability to read warning labels, a desire to imitate adults, and inadequate supervision lead to childhood poisonings.

The elderly are the second most likely group to be poisoned. Mental confusion, poor eyesight, and the use of multiple drugs are the leading reasons why this group has a high rate of accidental poisoning. A substantial number of poisonings also occur as suicide attempts or **drug overdose**s.

Poisons are common in the home and workplace, yet there are basically two major types. One group consists of products that were never meant to be ingested or inhaled, such as shampoo, paint thinner, pesticides, houseplant leaves, and carbon monoxide. The other group contains products that can be ingested in small quantities, but which are harmful if taken in large amounts, such as pharmaceuticals, medicinal herbs, or alcohol. Other types of poisons include the bacterial toxins that cause **food poisoning**, such as *Escherichia coli*; heavy metals, such as the lead found in the paint on older houses; and the venom found in the bites and stings of some animals and insects. The staff at a poison control center and emergency room doctors have the most experience diagnosing and treating poisoning cases.

The effects of poisons are as varied as the poisons themselves; however, the exact mechanisms of only a few are understood. Some poisons interfere with the metabolism. Others destroy the liver or kidneys, such as heavy metals and some pain relief medications, including acetaminophen (Tylenol) and nonsteroidal anti-inflammatory drugs (Advil, Ibuprofen). A poison may severely depress the central nervous system, leading to coma and eventual respiratory and circulatory failure. Potential poisons in this category include anesthetics (for example, ether and chloroform), opiates (for example, morphine and codeine), and barbiturates. Some poisons directly affect the respiratory and circulatory system. Carbon monoxide causes death by binding with hemoglobin that would normally transport oxygen throughout the body. Certain corrosive vapors trigger the body to flood the lungs with fluids, effectively drowning the person. Cyanide interferes with respiration at the cellular level. Another group of poisons interferes with the electrochemical impulses that travel between neurons in the nervous system. Yet another group, including cocaine, ergot, strychnine, and some snake venoms, causes potentially fatal seizures.

Severity of symptoms can range from **headache** and **nausea** to convulsions and **death**. The type of poison, the amount and time of exposure, and the age, size, and health of the victim are all factors which determine the severity of symptoms and the chances for recovery.

There are more than 700 species of poisonous plants in the United States. Plants are second only to medicines in causing serious poisoning in children under age five. There is no way to tell by looking at a plant if it is poisonous. Some plants, such as the yew shrub, are almost entirely toxic: needles, bark, seeds, and berries. In other plants, only certain parts are poisonous. The bulb of the hyacinth and daffodil are toxic, but the flowers are not; while the flowers of the jasmine plant are the poisonous part. Moreover, some plants are confusing because portions of them are eaten as food while other parts are poisonous. For example, the fleshy stem (tuber) of the potato plant is nutritious; however, its roots, sprouts, and vines are poisonous. The leaves of tomatoes are poisonous, while the fruit is not. Rhubarb stalks are good to eat, but the leaves are poisonous. Apricots, cherries, peaches, and apples all produce healthful fruit, but their seeds contain a form of cyanide that can kill a child if chewed in sufficient quantities. One hundred mg of moist, crushed apricot seeds can produce 217 mg of cyanide.

Common houseplants that contain some poisonous parts include:

- Aloe
- Amaryllis
- Cyclamen
- Dumbcane (also called Diffenbachia)
- Philodendron

Common outdoor plants that contain some poisonous part include:

- Bird of paradise flower
- Buttercup
- Castor bean
- Chinaberry tree
- Daffodil
- English ivy
- Eucalyptus
- Foxglove
- Holly
- Horse chestnut
- Iris
- Jack-in-the-pulpit
- Jimsonweed (also called thornapple)
- Larkspur
- Lily-of-the-valley
- Morning glory
- Nightshade (several varieties)
- Oleander
- Potato
- Rhododendron
- Rhubarb
- Sweet pea
- Tomato
- Wisteria
- Yew

Symptoms of plant poisoning range from irritation of the skin or mucous membranes of the mouth and throat to nausea, vomiting, convulsions, irregular heartbeat, and even death. It is often difficult to tell if a person has eaten a poisonous plant because there are no tell-tale empty containers and no unusual lesions or odors around the mouth.

Many products used daily in the home are poisonous if swallowed. These products often contain strong acids or strong bases (alkalis). Toxic household cleaning products include:

- Ammonia
- Bleach
- Dishwashing liquids
- Drain openers
- Floor waxes and furniture polishes
- Laundry detergents, spot cleaners, and fabric softeners
- Mildew removers
- Oven cleaners
- Toilet bowl cleaners

Personal care products found in the home can also be poisonous. These include:

- Deodorant
- Hairspray
- Hair straighteners
- Nail polish and polish remover
- Perfume
- Shampoo

Signs that a person has swallowed one of these substances include evidence of an empty container nearby, nausea or vomiting, and **burns** on the lips and skin around the mouth if the substance was a strong acid or alkali. The chemicals in some of these products may leave a distinctive odor on the breath.

Both over-the-counter and prescription medicines can help the body heal if taken as directed. However, when taken in large quantities, or with other drugs where there may be an adverse interaction, they can act as poisons. Drug overdoses, both accidental and intentional, are the leading cause of poisoning in adults. Medicinal herbs should be treated like pharmaceuticals and taken only in designated quantities under the supervision of a knowledgeable person. Herbs that have healing qualities when taken in small doses can be toxic in larger doses.

Drug overdoses cause a range of symptoms, including excitability, sleepiness, confusion, unconsciousness, rapid heartbeat, convulsions, nausea, and changes in blood pressure. The best initial evidence of a drug overdose is the presence of an empty container near the victim.

People can be poisoned by fumes they inhale. Carbon monoxide is the most common form of inhaled poison. Other toxic substances that can be inhaled include:

- Farm and garden insecticides and herbicides
- Gasoline fumes
- Insect repellent
- Paint thinner fumes

Initially, poisoning is suspected if the victim shows changes in behavior and signs or symptoms previously described. Evidence of an empty container or information from the victim are helpful in determining exactly what substance has caused the poisoning. Some acids and alkalis leave burns on the mouth. Petroleum products, such as lighter fluid or kerosene, leave a distinctive odor on the breath. The vomit may be tested to determine the exact composition of the poison. Once hospitalized, blood and urine tests may be done on the patient to determine his metabolic condition.

Treatment for poisoning depends on the poison swallowed or inhaled. Contacting the poison control center or hospital emergency room is the first step in getting proper treatment. The poison control center's telephone number is often listed with emergency numbers on the inside cover of the telephone book, or it can be reached by dialing the operator. The poison control center will ask for specific information about the victim and the poison, then give appropriate first aid instructions. If the patient is to be taken to a hospital, a sample of vomit and the poison container should be taken along, if they are available.

Most cases of plant poisoning are treated by inducing vomiting, if the patient is fully conscious. Vomiting can be induced by taking syrup of ipecac, an over-the-counter product available at any pharmacy.

For acid, alkali, or a petroleum product poisonings, the patient should not vomit. Acids and alkalis can burn the esophagus if they are vomited, and petroleum products can be inhaled into the lungs during vomiting, resulting in **pneumonia**.

Once under medical care, doctors have the option of treating the patient with a specific remedy to counteract the poison (antidote) or with activated charcoal to absorb the substance inside the patient's digestive system. In some instances, pumping the stomach may be required. Medical personnel will also provide supportive care as needed, such as intravenous fluids or mechanical ventilation.

The outcome of poisoning varies from complete recovery to death, and depends on the type and amount of the poison, the health of the victim, and the speed with which medical care is obtained.

Most accidental poisonings are preventable. The number of deaths of children from poisoning has declined from about 450 per year in the 1960s to about 50 each year in the 1990s. This decline has occurred mainly because of better packaging of toxic materials and better public education.

Polio

Polio, or poliomyelitis, is a serious infectious disease caused by a virus that affects the central **nervous system**. Polio, sometimes called infantile paralysis, primarily affects children. When the virus first takes hold, symptoms begin with body aches and a stiff neck. As the disease progresses, it affects nerve tissue causing paralysis and the wasting of muscle tissue. Before inoculation was available, polio was a dread disease that killed many, because paralysis of the breathing muscles caused suffocation. Today, due to immunization programs and the **World Health Organization**'s Global Technical Consultative Group on Polio Eradication program, a total of only 4,116 polio cases were reported worldwide in 1997, a decline of 90 percent worldwide since the program began in the late 1980s. With the disease still widely found in Bangladesh, India, Nepal, Pakistan, South Asia, the Congo, Nigeria, West and Central Africa, Ethiopia, Somalia, Sudan, and the Horn of Africa, WHO is in the final stage of their push for the total eradication of polio.

There is evidence to suggest that polio was known more than 3,000 years ago in Egypt and continued to paralyze people well into this century. In the early part of the twentieth century in America, there were numerous outbreaks of the disease including the 1916 epidemic in which 27,000 people developed polio, almost 7,000 of whom died and many thousands more who were left paralyzed. The only treatment was physical therapy to ease the paralysis.

In 1929 a young man was the first polio patient to be aided by a new kind of therapy—the Drinker tank respirator, or iron lung, invented by Philip Drinker, a professor at the School of Public Health at Harvard University. Drinker placed his patient into an airtight metal box from the neck down. The patient's mouth and nose remained outside the box, which was connected to a pump which reduced air pressure inside the box, imitating the negative change in pressure in the chest cavity that occurs during an inhalation. The decreased air pressure inside the box drew air through the nose and mouth of the patient into the lungs. Use of the iron lung ushered in an era in which many polio patients could be kept alive. Still, there was no cure, and little was known of its causative agent.

An Austrian-American physician, **Karl Landsteiner** (who won a 1930 Nobel prize for discovering human blood groups) was the first to postulate that polio was caused by a virus. Between 1908 and 1919, while working at the Royal-Imperial Hospital in Vienna, he examined many patients who had died of polio. In experiments, he took spinal cord and brain tissue from a polio victim and injected it into monkeys. The animals developed polio symptoms, and when Landsteiner was unable to detect any bacteria, he believed the cause to be a virus.

After the discovery of the causative virus, the success of eradicating the disease is credited primarily to the work of two men, **Jonas Salk** and **Albert Sabin**. Salk began his immunology research in 1938 at New York University and participated in a program to identify the known strains of the polio virus at the University of Pittsburgh. His research was aided by the earlier work of Nobel Prize winners **John Enders**, Frederick C. Robbins, and **Thomas Weller**, who had perfected techniques of growing large quantities of polio virus on monkey kidney tissue. Salk grew the viruses and then killed them with formaldehyde. This killed-virus mixture proved to be an effective vaccine which was tested nationally starting in 1954. It is estimated that Salk's vaccine proved 60-90% effective against the disease.

During the time Salk was testing his vaccine, Sabin was developing a live-virus vaccine grown on monkey kidney tissue. In 1959, the Polish-American physician began testing his vaccine on millions of Russians. His vaccine proved more effective than Salk's and had two advantages: the live-virus vaccine conferred longer-lasting immunity, and could also be administered orally. After Great Britain began using the Sabin oral vaccine in 1962, the United States followed suite, and it is still the standard immunization practice today.

Although polio itself is almost conquered, many people who contracted the disease as long ago as thirty years are experiencing what some researchers believe to be ''post-polio syndrome,'' or PPS, which manifests as fatigue, pain, and muscle weakness. Some investigators have discovered viral fragments in the spinal fluid of PPS patients which closely resemble the poliovirus, indicating it may persist in the central nervous system in a mutated, nonvirulent, and nonreplicating form, prompting, however, immune system response.

POLYPS

The word polyp refers to any overgrowth of tissue from the surface of mucous membranes. Polyps come in a variety of shapes—round, droplet, and irregular being the most common; and they affect various parts of the body—the intestines, the nasal passages, the rectum, and the vocal cords.

Polyps are one of many forms of tissue overproduction that can occur in the body. Cells in many body tissues sometimes keep growing beyond their usual limits. Medical scientists call this process *neoplasia*, which means simply "new growth." An individual overgrowth is called a neoplasm. In most cases these growths are limited, and the result is a benign swelling or mass of cells called a tumor. If the new growth occurs on the surface of the tissue instead of inside an organ it is often called a polyp. **Cancer** is another type of neoplasm marked by unlimited tissue growth. The essential feature that distinguishes cancer from nonmalignant neoplasms is that it does not stop growing.

Intestinal polyps are a common form of neoplasm. All intestinal polyps arise from the inner lining of the intestinal wall. This layer of mucosal tissue does the work of digestion. About 30% of the general population will develop intestinal polyps at some point in life, with the likelihood increasing with age. Most of these polyps are never noticed during a person's lifetime because they cause no problems. They are often discovered accidentally at **autopsy**. The primary importance of intestinal polyps is that 1% of them become cancerous. Because the polyps that eventually turn malignant cannot be identified in advance, they are all suspect.

Nasal polyps tend to occur in people with respiratory **allergies**. Hay fever (**allergic rhinitis**) is an irritation of the membranes of the nose by airborne particles or chemicals. These membranes make mucus. When irritated, they can also grow polyps. The nose is not only a passageway for air to reach the lungs; it also provides the connection between the sinuses and the outside world. Sinuses are lined with mucus membranes, just like the nose. Polyps can easily obstruct the drainage of mucus from the sinuses. When any fluid in the body is trapped so it cannot flow freely, it becomes infected. The result, **sinusitis**, is a common complication of allergic rhinitis.

Rectal polyps are tissue growths that arise from the wall of the rectum and protrude into it. They may be either benign or malignant (cancerous). The rectum is the last segment of the large intestine, ending in the anus, the opening to the exterior of the body. Rectal polyps are quite common. They occur in 7-50% of all people, and in two thirds of people over age 60.

Vocal cord nodules and polyps are noncancerous growths on the vocal cords that affect the voice.

The vocal cords, located in the voice box in the middle of the neck, are two tough, fibrous bands that vibrate to produce sound. They are covered with a layer of tissue that is similar to skin. With use, this layer thickens. With heavy use, the thickening may localize, producing a nodule. Unlike skin, heavy usage over a short time may also produce polyps. A polyp is a soft, smooth lump containing mostly blood and blood vessels. A nodule is similar to a polyp, but tends to be firmer.

The chances of a polyp's becoming cancerous depend to some extent on its location within the digestive tract. 95 percent of all intestinal polyps develop inside the large bowel.

The stomach's lining is host to polyps of a similar appearance, but there is no agreement as to their potential for becoming **stomach cancer**.

Polyps in the small bowel do not seem to have malignant potential. Instead they can produce obstruction in either of two ways. A large polyp can obstruct the bowel by its sheer size. Smaller polyps can be picked up by the rhythmic contractions (peristalsis) of the intestines and pull the part of the bowel to which they are attached into the adjoining section. The result is a telescoping of one section of bowel into another, called intussusception.

Population studies of colon cancer suggest that diet plays an important role in the disease, and by implication in the formation of colon polyps. The most consistent interpretation of these data is that animal fats—though not vegetable fats—are the single most important dietary factor. Lack of fiber in the diet may also contribute to polyp formation. Other types of polyps are too rare to produce enough data for evaluation.

Most polyps cause no symptoms. Large ones eventually cause intestinal obstruction, which produces cramping abdominal **pain** with **nausea and vomiting**. As colon polyps evolve into cancers, they begin to produce symptoms that include bleeding and altered bowel habits.

Some people who are allergic to **aspirin** develop both **asthma** and nasal polyps.

Nasal polyps often plug the nose, usually one side at a time. People with allergic rhinitis are so used to having a stopped up nose they may not notice the difference when a polyp develops. Other polyps may be closer to a sinus opening, so airflow is not obstructed, but mucus becomes trapped in the sinus. In this case, there is a feeling of fullness in the head, no sense of smell, and perhaps a **headache**. The trapped mucus will eventually get infected, adding pain, fever, and perhaps bloody discharge from the nose.

The cause of most rectal polyps is unknown, however a diet high in animal fat and red meat, and low in fiber, is thought to encourage polyp formation. Some types of polyps are hereditary. In an inherited disease called familial polyposis, hundreds of small, malignant and pre-malignant polyps are produced before the age of 40. Also, inflammatory bowel disease may cause growth of polyps and pseudo-polyps. Juvenile polyps (polyps in children) are usually benign and often outgrow their blood supply and disappear at **puberty**.

Most rectal polyps produce no symptoms and are discovered on routine digital or endoscopic examination of the rectum. Rectal bleeding is the most common complaint when symptoms do occur. Abdominal cramps, pain, or obstruction of the intestine occur with some large polyps. Certain types of polyps cause mucous-filled or watery **diarrhea**.

Chronic infections caused by allergies and inhalation of irritants, such as cigarette smoke, may produce vocal nodules and polyps, but extensive use of the voice is their most common cause. Nodules and polyps are more common in male children, female adolescents, and female adults. This may be due in part to the faster speed at which the cords vibrate to produce higher-pitched voices.

Voice alterations are most apparent in singers, who may notice the higher registers are the first to change. Hoarseness causes others to seek medical attention.

Routine screening for bowel cancer is recommended for everyone over the age of 40. Screening may be as simple as testing the stool for blood or as elaborate as colonoscopy. Colonoscopy is a procedure in which the doctor threads an instrument called a colonoscope up through the entire large bowel. Most polyps are in the lower segment of the colon, called the sigmoid colon. These polyps can be seen with a shorter scope called a sigmoidoscope. X ray imaging can also used to look for polyps. For x rays, the colon is first filled with barium, which is a white substance that shows up as a shadowed area on the film. The colon can also be filled with barium and air, which is called a double contrast study.

Because polyps take about five years to turn into cancers, routine examinations are recommended every three years.

The head and neck surgeon (otorhinolaryngologist) is equipped to diagnose nasal polyps. In order to perform the exam, medicine must be applied to decongest the membranes. Cotton balls soaked with one of these agents and left in the nostrils for a few minutes provide adequate shrinkage.

Rectal polyps are commonly found by sigmoidoscopy (visual inspection with an instrument consisting of a tube and a light) or colonoscopy. If polyps are found in the rectum, a complete examination of the large intestine is done, as multiple polyps are common. Polyps do not show up on regular x rays, but they do appear on barium enema x rays.

The otorhinolaryngologist must see the vocal cords to diagnose vocal nodules and polyps. It is also important to confirm that there are not other problems instead of or in addition to these benign lumps. Other causes of hoarseness include throat cancers, vocal cord paralysis, and simple **laryngitis**. The cords can usually be seen using a mirror placed at the back of the tongue. More elaborate scopes, including a videostroboscope, allow better views while the cords are producing sounds.

A biopsy of a nodule or polyp will ensure they are not cancerous.

All intestinal polyps should be removed as preventive care. Most of them can be taken out through a colonoscope. Complications like obstruction and intussusception are surgical emergencies.

Most nasal polyps can be removed by the head and neck surgeon as an office procedure called a nasal polypectomy. Bleeding, the only complication, is usually easy to control. Nose and sinus infections can be treated with **antibiotics** and **decongestants**, but if airflow is restricted, the infection will recur.

Before the operation to remove rectal polyps, a colonoscopy (examination of the intestine with an endoscope) is performed, and standard pre-operative blood and urine studies are done. The patient is also given medicated **enemas** to cleanse the bowel.

The patient is given a sedative and a narcotic pain killer. A colonoscope is inserted into the rectum. The polyps are located and removed with a wire snare, ultrasound, or laser beam. After they are removed, the polyps are examined to determine if they are malignant or benign. When polyps are malignant, it may be necessary to remove a portion of the rectum or colon to completely remove cancerous tissue.

Voice rest is the first choice treatment for polyps. Polyps that appeared suddenly will resolve with a few days of complete silence. Nodules do not disappear with rest. Lesions that have been there longer may be slower to disappear and require voice training by a speech therapist.

Nodules and polyps may be surgically removed, using either conventional techniques or lasers.

Patients with hereditary disorders associated with polyps must undergo total colectomy early in adult life. All children of parents with these disorders should be screened early in adulthood, because half of them will have the same disease. For the bulk of the population, increased dietary fiber and decreased animal fat are the best preventives known at present. For the occasional intestinal polyp that arises in spite of good dietary habits, routine screening should prevent it from becoming cancerous.

Since most nasal polyps are the result of allergic rhinitis, they can be prevented by treating this condition. New treatments have greatly improved control of hay fever. There are now several spray medicines that are quite effective. Spray cortisone-like drugs are the most popular. Over-the-counter nasal decongestants have an irritating effect similar to the allergy they are supposed to be treating. Continued use can bring more trouble than relief and result in an **addiction** to nose sprays. The resulting disease, **rhinitis** medicamentosa, is more difficult to treat than allergic rhinitis.

Allergists and ENT surgeons both treat allergic rhinitis with a procedure called desensitization. After identifying suspect allergens using one of several methods, they will give the patient increasing doses of those allergens in order to produce blocking antibodies that will impede the allergic reaction. This is effective in a number of patients, but the treatment may take a period of months to years.

Eating a diet low in red meat and animal fat, and high in fiber, is thought to help prevent rectal polyps.

Careful use of the voice will prevent most vocal cord nodules and polyps. Avoiding inhaled irritants, may also prevent nodules and polyps from forming.

Porphyrias

The porphyrias are a group of rare disorders that affect heme biosynthesis (the formation of chemical compounds by living organisms). Heme is an essential component of hemoglobin (the iron-containing pigment of the blood that carries oxygen from the lungs to the tissues) as well as many enzymes throughout the body. Biosynthesis of heme is a process that starts with simple molecules and ends with a large, complex heme molecule. Each step of the biosynthesis pathway is directed by its own protein, called an enzyme. As a heme precursor molecule moves through each step, an enzyme modifies it in some way. If the precursor is not modified, it cannot proceed to the next step.

Due to a defect in one of the enzymes of the heme biosynthesis pathway, protoporphyrins or porphyrin (heme precursors) are prevented from proceeding further along the pathway. Instead, precursors accumulate at the stage of the enzyme defect and cause a variety of physical symptoms in the affected person. Specific symptoms depend on the point at which heme biosynthesis is blocked and which precursors accumulate. In general, the porphyrias primarily affect the skin and the nervous system. Symptoms can be debilitating or life threatening in some cases. Porphyria is an inherited condition, but it may be acquired after exposure to poisonous substances.

Heme is produced in several tissues in the body, but its main biosynthesis sites are the liver and the bone marrow. Although production is concentrated in the liver and bone marrow, heme is used in nearly every tissue in the body. In most cells, it is a key building block in the construction of factors that oversee metabolism as well as transport of oxygen and energy. In the liver, heme is used in several vital enzymes, particularly one that is involved in the metabolism of chemicals, **vitamins**, fatty acids, and hormones. It is very important in transforming toxic substances into easily excretable materials. In immature red blood cells, heme is a the major component of hemoglobin

The production of heme may be compared to a factory assembly line. At the start of the line, raw materials are fed into the process. At specific points along the line, an addition or adjustment is made to further development. Once additions and adjustments are complete, the final product roles off the end of the line.

The control of heme biosynthesis is complex. There are various chemical signals that can trigger increased or decreased production. These signals can affect the enzymes themselves or their production, starting at the genetic level. Under normal circumstances, when heme concentrations are at an appropriate level, precursor production decreases. However, a glitch in the biosynthesis pathway represented by a defective enzyme means that heme biosynthesis is incomplete. Because heme levels remain low, the synthesis pathway continues to churn out precursor molecules in an attempt to make up the deficit.

The net effect of this continued production is an abnormal accumulation of precursor molecules and development of some type of porphyria. Each type of porphyria corresponds with a specific enzyme defect and an accumulation of the associated precursor.

The porphyrias are divided into two general categories, depending on the location of the deficient enzyme. Porphyrias that affect heme biosynthesis in the liver are called hepatic porphyrias. The porphyrias that affect heme biosynthesis in immature red blood cells are called erythropoietic porphyrias (erythropoiesis is the process through which red blood cells are produced).

Enzymes involved in heme biosynthesis have subtle, tissue-specific variations; therefore, heme biosynthesis may be impeded in the liver, but normal in the immature red blood cells, or vice versa. Incidence of porphyria varies widely between types and occasionally by geographic location. Although certain porphyrias are more common than others, their greater frequency is only relative to other types. All porphyrias are considered rare disorders.

The underlying cause of all porphyrias is a defective enzyme somewhere along the heme biosynthesis pathway. In nearly all cases, the defective enzyme is a genetically linked factor. Therefore, porphyrias are inheritable conditions. However, an environmental trigger such as diet, drugs, or sun exposure may be necessary before any symptoms develop. In many cases, symptoms do not develop, and people may be completely unaware that they have a gene for porphyria.

Nearly all of the hepatic porphyrias follow a pattern of acute attacks interspersed among periods of complete symptom remission. For this reason, they are often referred to as the acute porphyrias. The erythropoietic porphyrias do not follow the same pattern and are considered chronic conditions.

The specific symptoms of each porphyria depend on the affected enzyme and whether it occurs in the liver or in the bone marrow. The severity of symptoms can vary widely, even within the same porphyria type. If the porphyria becomes symptomatic, the common factor between all types is an abnormal accumulation of protoporphyrins or porphyrin.

Depending on the symptoms presented, the possibility of porphyria may not immediately come to mind. In the absence of a family history of porphyria, some symptoms of porphyria, such as abdominal pain and vomiting, may be attributed to other disorders. Neurological symptoms, including confusion and hallucinations, can lead to an initial suspicion of psychiatric disease rather than a physical disorder. Diagnosis may be aided in cases in which these symptoms appear in combination with neuropathy (any disease of the nerves), sensitivity to sunlight, or other factors. Certain symptoms, such as urine the color of port wine, are hallmark signs of porphyria.

A common initial test measures protoporphyrins in the urine. However, if skin sensitivity to light is a symptom, a blood plasma test is indicated. If these tests reveal abnormal levels of protoporphyrins, further tests are done to measure heme precursor levels in the stool and in red blood cells. Whether heme precursors occur in the blood, urine, or stool gives some indication of the type of porphyria, but more detailed biochemical testing is required to determine their exact identity. Making this determination yields a strong indicator of which enzyme in the heme biosynthesis pathway is defective, which, in turn, allows a diagnosis of the particular type of porphyria.

Biochemical tests rely on the color, chemical properties, and other unique features of each heme precursor. Other biochemical tests rely on the fact that heme precursors become less water soluble (able to be dissolved in water) as they progress further through the heme biosynthesis pathway. As a final test, measuring specific enzymes and their activities may be done for some types of porphyrias.

Treatment for porphyria revolves around avoiding acute attacks, limiting potential effects, and treating symptoms. However, treatment options vary depending on the type of porphyria that has been diagnosed.

A person who has been diagnosed with, for example, intermittent porphyria, can prevent most attacks by avoiding precipitating factors, such as certain drugs that have been identified as triggers for acute porphyria attacks. Individuals must maintain adequate nutrition, particularly with respect to carbohydrates. In some cases, an attack can be stopped by increasing carbohydrate consumption or by receiving carbohydrates intravenously.

If an attack occurs, medical attention is needed. Pain is usually severe, and narcotic **analgesics** are the best option for relief. Medications can be used to counter nausea, vomiting, and **anxiety** as well as for sedation or to induce sleep. An intravenously administered drug called hematin may be used to curtail an attack. Women, who tend to develop symptoms more frequently than men owing to hormonal fluctuations, may find hormone therapy that inhibits ovulation to be helpful.

Acute porphyria attacks can be life-threatening events, so it is not advisable to try self-treatments in these situations. Alternative treatments can be useful adjuncts to conventional therapy. For example, some people may find relief for the pain associated with some porphyrias through **acupuncture** or **hypnosis**. Relaxation techniques, such as **yoga** or **meditation**, may also prove helpful in **pain management**.

Even in the presence of a genetic inheritance for a porphyria, symptom development depends on a variety of factors. In the majority of cases, a person remains asymptomatic throughout life. Porphyria symptoms are rarely fatal with proper medical treatment, but they may be associated with temporarily debilitating or permanently disfiguring consequences. Measures to avoid these consequences are not always successful, regardless of how diligently they are pursued. Although pregnancy has been known to trigger porphyria attacks, it is not as great a danger as was once thought.

If there is a family history of porphyria, a person should consider being tested to determine whether he or she carries the associated gene. Even if symptoms are absent, it is useful to know about the presence of the gene to assess the risks of developing the associated porphyria. This knowledge also reveals whether a person's offspring may be at risk. Theoretically, it is possible to do prenatal tests. However, these tests would not indicate whether the child would develop porphyria symptoms; only that they might have the potential to do so.

PORTER, RODNEY (1917-1985)

English biochemist

Rodney Robert Porter was born October 8, 1917, in Newton-le-Willows, near Liverpool in Lancashire, England. His mother was Isobel Reese Porter and his father, Joseph L. Porter, was a railroad clerk. He attended Liverpool University, where he earned a B.S. in biochemistry in 1939. During World War II he served in the Royal Artillery, the Royal Engineers, and the Royal Army Service Corps, and participated in the invasions of Algeria, Sicily, and Italy. After his discharge in 1946, he resumed his biochemistry studies at Cambridge University under the direction of Frederick Sanger.

Porter's doctoral research at Cambridge was influenced by Nobel laureate **Karl Landsteiner**'s book, *The Specificity of Serological Reactions,* which described the nature of antibodies and techniques for preparing some of them. Antibodies, at the time, were thought to be proteins that belonged to a class of blood-serum proteins called gamma globulins. From Sanger, who had succeeded in determining the chemical structure of insulin (a protein that metabolizes carbohydrates), Porter learned the techniques of protein chemistry. Sanger had also demonstrated tenacity in studying problems in protein chemistry involving amino acid sequencing that most believed impossible to solve, and he was a model for the persistence Porter would show in his later work on antibodies.

Fortunately, Porter chose rabbits to experiment on for his research. Although this was not known at the time, the antibody system is not as complex in this animal as it is in some. The most important antibody, or immunoglobulin, in the blood is called IgG, which contains more than 1,300 amino acids. The problem of discovering the active site of the antibody—the part that combines with the antigen—could be solved only by working with smaller pieces of the molecule. Porter discovered that an enzyme from papaya juice, called papain, could break up IgG into fragments that still contained the active sites but were small enough to work with. He received his Ph..D. for this work in 1948.

Porter remained at Cambridge for another year, then in 1949 he moved to the National Institute for Medical Research at Mill Hill, London. There, he improved methods for purifying protein mixtures and used some of these methods to show that there are variations in IgG molecules. He obtained a purer form of papaya enzyme than had been available at Cambridge and repeated his earlier experiments. This time the IgG molecules broke into thirds, and one of these thirds was obtained in a crystalline form which Porter called fragment crystallizable (Fc).

Obtaining the Fc crystal was a breakthrough; Porter now was able to show that this part of the antibody was the same in all IgG molecules, since a mixture of the different molecules would not have formed a crystal. He also discovered that the active site of the molecule (the part that binds the antigen) was in the other two-thirds of the antibody. These he called fragment antigen-binding (or FAB) pieces. After Porter's research was published in 1959, another research group, led by **Gerald M. Edelman** at Rockefeller University in New York, split the IgG in another way—by separating amino acid chains rather than breaking the proteins at right angles between the amino acids as Porter's papain had done.

In 1960 Porter was appointed professor of immunology at St. Mary's Hospital Medical School in London. There he repeated Edelman's experiments under different conditions. After two years, having combined his own results with those of Edelman, he proposed the first satisfactory structure of the IgG molecule. The model, which predicted that the FAB fragment consisted of two different amino acid chains, provided the basis for far-ranging biochemical research. Porter's continuing work contributed numerous studies of the structures of individual IgG molecules. In 1967 Porter was appointed Whitley Professor of Biochemistry and chairman of the biochemistry department at Oxford University. In his new position, Porter continued his work on the immune response, but his interest shifted from the structure of antibodies to their role as receptors on the surface of cells. To further this research, he developed ways of tagging and tracing receptors. He also became an authority on the structure and genetics of a group of blood proteins called the complement, which binds the Fc region of the immunoglobulin and is involved in many important immunological reactions.

Porter was killed in an automobile accident a few weeks before he was to retire from the Whitley Chair of Biochemistry. He had been planning to continue as director of the Medical Research Council's Immunochemistry Unit for another four years; he had also intended to continue his laboratory work, attempting to crystallize one of the proteins of the complement system.

Positron emission tomography (PET)

Positron emission tomography (PET) is a scanning technique used in conjunction with small amounts of radiolabeled compounds to visualize brain anatomy and function. PET was the first scanning method to provide information on brain function as well as anatomy. This information includes data on blood flow, oxygen consumption, glucose metabolism, and concentrations of various molecules in brain tissue.

PET has been used to study brain activity in various neurological diseases and disorders, including **stroke**, epilepsy; **Alzheimer's disease**, **Parkinson's disease**, and **Huntington's disease**; and in some psychiatric disorders, such as **schizophrenia**, depression, **obsessive-compulsive disorder**, **attention-deficit hyperactivity disorder**, and **Tourette syndrome**.

PET studies have helped to identify the brain mechanisms that operate in drug **addiction**, and to shed light on the mechanisms by which individual drugs work. PET is also proving to be more accurate than other methods in the diagnosis of many types of **cancer**. In the treatment of cancer, PET can be used to determine more quickly than conventional tests whether a given therapy is working. PET scans also give accurate and detailed information on heart disease, particularly in women, in whom breast tissue can interfere with other types of tests.

A very small amount of a radiolabeled compound is inhaled by or injected into the patient. The injected or inhaled compound accumulates in the tissue to be studied. As the radioactive atoms in the compound decay, they release smaller particles called positrons, which are positively charged. When a positron collides with an electron (negatively charged), they are both annihilated, and two photons (light particles) are emitted. The photons move in opposite directions and are picked up by the detector ring of the PET scanner. A computer uses this information to generate three-dimensional, cross-sectional images that represent the biological activity where the radiolabeled compound has accumulated.

A related technique is called single photon emission **computed tomography scan** (CT scan) (SPECT). SPECT is similar to PET, but the compounds used contain heavier, longer-lived radioactive atoms that emit high-energy photons, called gamma rays, instead of positrons. SPECT is used for many of the same applications as PET, and is less expensive than PET, but the resulting picture is usually less sharp than a PET image and reveals less information about the brain.

Some of radioactive compounds used for PET or SPECT scanning can persist for a long time in the body. Even though only a small amount is injected each time, the long half-lives of these compounds can limit the number of times a patient can be scanned.

Postpartum depression

Postpartum depression is a mood disorder that begins after **childbirth** and usually lasts beyond six weeks. The onset of postpartum depression tends to be gradual and may persist for many months, or develop into a second bout following a subsequent **pregnancy**. Postpartum depression affects approximately 15% of all childbearing women. Mild to moderate cases are sometimes unrecognized by women themselves. Many women feel ashamed if they are not coping and so may conceal their difficulties. This is a serious problem that disrupts women's lives and can have effects on the baby, other children, her partner, and other relationships. Levels of depression for fathers also increase significantly.

Postpartum depression is often divided into two types: early onset and late onset. An early onset most often seems like the "blues," a mild brief experience during the first days or weeks after birth. During the first week after the birth up to 80% of mothers will experience the "baby blues." This is usually a time of extra sensitivity and symptoms include tearfulness, irritability, **anxiety**, and mood changes, which tend to peak between three to five days after childbirth. The symptoms normally disappear within two weeks without requiring specific treatment apart from understanding, support, skills and practice. In short, some depression, tiredness, and anxiety may fall within the "normal" range of reactions to giving birth.

A late onset appears several weeks after the birth. This involves a slowly growing feeling of sadness, depression, lack of energy, chronic tiredness, inability to sleep, change in appetite, significant weight loss or gain, and difficulty caring for the baby.

At the present, experts cannot say what causes postpartum depression. Most likely, it is caused by many factors that vary from individual to individual. Mothers commonly experience some degree of depression during the first weeks after birth. Pregnancy and birth are accompanied by sudden hormonal changes that affect emotions. Additionally, the 24-hour responsibility for a newborn infant represents a major psychological and lifestyle adjustment for most mothers, even after the first child. These physical and emotional **stress**es are usually accompanied by inadequate rest until the baby's routine stabilizes, so fatigue and depression are not unusual.

Experiences vary considerably but usually include several symptoms.

Feelings:

- Persistent low mood
- Inadequacy, failure, hopelessness, helplessness
- Exhaustion, emptiness, sadness, tearfulness
- Guilt, shame, worthlessness
- Confusion, anxiety, and panic
- Fear for the baby and of the baby
- Fear of being alone or going out.

Behaviors:

- Lack of interest or pleasure in usual activities
- **Insomnia** or excessive sleep, nightmares
- Not eating or overeating
- Decreased energy and motivation
- Withdrawal from social contact
- Poor self-care
- Inability to cope with routine tasks.

Thoughts:

- Inability to think clearly and make decisions
- Lack of concentration and poor memory
- Running away from everything
- Fear of being rejected by partner
- Worry about harm or **death** to partner or baby
- Ideas about suicide.

Some symptoms may not indicate a severe problem. However, persistent low mood or loss of interest or pleasure in activities, along with four other symptoms occurring together for a period of at least two weeks, indicate clinical depression, and require adequate treatment.

There are several important risk factors for postpartum depression, including:

- Stress
- Lack of sleep
- Poor **nutrition**
- Lack of support from one's partner, family or friends
- Family history of depression
- Labor/delivery complications for mother or baby
- Premature or postmature delivery
- Problems with the baby's health
- Separation of mother and baby
- A difficult baby (temperament, feeding, sleeping, settling problems)
- Preexisting neurosis or **psychosis**.

Although there is no diagnostic test for post-partum depression, it is important to understand that it is, nonetheless, a real illness, and like a physical ailment, it has specific symptoms.

Several treatment options exist, including medication, psychotherapy, counseling, and group treatment and support strategies, depending on the woman's needs. One effective treatment combines antidepressant medication and psychotherapy. These types of medication are often effective when used for 3-4 weeks. Any medication use must be carefully considered if the woman are breast-feeding, but with some medications, continuing breast-feeding is safe. Nevertheless, medication alone is never sufficient and should always be accompanied by counseling or other support services.

Postpartum depression can be effectively alleviated through counseling and support groups, so that the mother does not feel she is alone in her feelings. Constitutional homeopathy can be the most effective treatment of the alternative therapies because it acts on the emotional level where postpartum depression is felt. **Acupuncture**, Chinese herbs, and Western herbs can all help the mother suffering from postpartum depression come back to a state of balance. Seeking help from a practitioner allows the new mother to feel supported and cared for and allows for more effective treatment.

A new mother also should remember that this time of stress does not last forever. In addition, there are useful things she can do for herself, including:

- Valuing her role as a mother and trusting her own judgment.
- Making each day as simple as possible.
- Avoiding extra pressures or unnecessary tasks.
- Trying to involve her partner more in the care of the baby from the beginning.
- Discussing with her partner how both can share the household chores and responsibilities.
- Scheduling frequent outings, such as walks and short visits with friends.
- Having the baby sleep in a separate room so she sleep more restfully.
- Sharing her feelings with her partner or a friend who is a good listener.
- Talking with other mothers to help keep problems in perspective.
- Trying to sleep or rest when the baby is sleeping.
- Taking care of her health and well-being.
- Not losing her sense of humor.

With support from friends and family, mild postpartum depression usually disappears quickly. If depression becomes severe, a mother cannot care for herself and the baby, and in rare cases, hospitalization may be necessary. Yet, medication, counseling, and support from others usually cure even severe depression in 3-6 months.

Exercise can help enhance a new mother's emotional well-being. New mothers should also try to cultivate good sleeping habits and learn to rest when they feel physically or emotionally tired. It is important for a woman to learn to recognize her own warning signs of fatigue respond to them by taking a break.

POST-TRAUMATIC STRESS DISORDER

Post-traumatic stress disorder (PTSD) is a debilitating condition that affects people who have been exposed to a major traumatic event. PTSD is characterized by upsetting memories or thoughts of the ordeal, "blunting" of emotions, increased arousal, and sometimes severe personality changes. Once called "shell shock" or battle fatigue, PTSD is most well known as a problem of war veterans returning from the battlefield. However, it can affect anyone who has experienced a traumatic event, such as rape, robbery, a natural disaster, or a serious accident. A diagnosis of a serious disease can trigger PTSD in some people. Considered to be one of a group of conditions known as "**anxiety disorders**," it can affect people of all ages who have experienced severe trauma. Children who have experienced severe trauma, such as war, a natural disaster, sexual or physical abuse, or the **death** of a parent, are also prone to PTSD.

PTSD is a response to a profoundly disturbing event. It isn not clear why some people develop PTSD following a trauma and others do not, although experts suspect it may be influenced both by the severity of the event, by the person's personality and genetic make-up, and by whether or not the trauma was expected. As the individual struggles to cope with life after the event, ordinary events or situations reminiscent of the trauma often trigger frightening and vivid memories or "flashbacks."

Symptoms usually begin within three months of the trauma, although sometimes PTSD does not develop until years after the initial trauma occurred. Once the symptoms begin, they may fade away again within six months. Others suffer with the symptoms for far longer and in some cases, the problem may become chronic. Some untreated Vietnam veterans with PTSD, for example, spent decades living alone in rural areas of the country, struggling to come to grips with the horror of war.

Among the most troubling symptoms of PTSD are flashbacks, which can be triggered by sounds, smells, feelings, or images. During a flashback, the person relives the traumatic event and may completely lose touch with reality, suffering through the trauma for minutes or hours at a time, believing that it is actually happening all over again.

For a diagnosis of PTSD, symptoms must include at least one of the following so-called "intrusive" symptoms:

- Flashbacks
- **Sleep disorders**: nightmares or night terrors
- Intense distress when exposed to events that are associated with the trauma.

In addition, the person must have at least three of the following "avoidance" symptoms that affect interactions with others:

- Trying to avoid thinking or feeling about the trauma
- Inability to remember the event
- Inability to experience emotion, as well as a loss of interest in former pleasures (psychic numbing or blunting)
- A sense of a shortened future.

Finally, there must be evidence of increased arousal, including at least two of the following:

- Problems falling asleep
- Startle reactions: hyper-alertness and strong reactions to unexpected noises
- Memory problems
- Concentration problems
- Moodiness
- Violence.

In addition to the above symptoms, children with PTSD may experience learning disabilities and memory or attention problems. They may become more dependent, anxious, or even self-abusing.

Not every person who experiences a traumatic event will experience PTSD. A mental health professional will diagnose the condition if the symptoms of **stress** last for more than a month after a traumatic event. While a formal diagnosis of PTSD is made only in the wake of a severe trauma, it is possible to have a mild PTSD-like reaction following less severe stress.

The most helpful treatment appears to be a combination of medication along with supportive and cognitive-behavioral therapies. Effective medications include **anxiety**-reducing medications and antidepressants, especially the selective serotonin reuptake inhibitors (SSRIs) such as fluoxetine (Prozac). Sleep problems can be lessened with brief treatment with an anti-anxiety drug, such as a benzodiazepine like alprazolam (Xanax), but long-term usage can lead to disturbing side-effects, such as increased anger.

Therapy can help reduce negative thought patterns and self talk. Cognitive-behavioral therapy focuses on changing specific actions and thoughts with the help of relaxation training and breathing techniques. **Group therapy** with other PTSD sufferers and family therapy can also be helpful.

The severity of the illness depends in part on whether the trauma was unexpected, the severity of the trauma, how chronic the trauma was (such as for victims of **sexual abuse**), and the person's inherent personality and genetic make-up.

With appropriate medication, emotional support, and counseling, most people show significant improvement. However, prolonged exposure to severe trauma such as experienced by victims of prolonged physical or sexual abuse and survivors of the Holocaust may cause permanent psychological scars.

POTASSIUM IMBALANCE

Potassium, a necessary electrolyte, facilitates nerve impulse conduction and the contraction of skeletal and smooth muscles, including the heart. It also facilitates cell membrane function and proper enzyme activity. Levels must be kept in a proper (homeostatic) balance for the maintenance of health. The normal concentration of potassium in the serum is in the range of 3.5 to 5.0 mM. Hyperkalemia refers to serum or plasma levels of potassium ions above 5.0 mM. Hypokalemia means serum or plasma levels of potassium ions that fall below 3.5 mM. The concentration of potassium is often expressed in units of milliequivalents per liter (mEq/L), rather than in units of millimolarity (mM). Both units mean the same thing when applied to concentrations of potassium ions.

A normal adult who weighs about 154 lbs (70 kg) contains a total of about 3.6 moles of potassium ions in the body. Most of this potassium (about 98%) occurs inside various cells and organs, where its concentration is about 150 mM. This level is in contrast to the much lower concentration found in the blood serum, where only about 0.4% of the body's potassium resides. Hyperkalemia can be caused by an overall excess of body potassium, or by a shift from inside to outside cells. For example, hyperkalemia can be caused by the sudden release of potassium ions from muscle into the surrounding fluids.

Hypokalemia can result from two general causes: either from an overall depletion in the body's potassium or from excessive uptake of potassium by muscle from surrounding fluids. Hypokalemia due to overall depletion tends to be a chronic phenomenon, while hypokalemia due to a shift in location tends to be a temporary disorder.

In a normal person, hyperkalemia from too much potassium in the diet is prevented by at least three types of regulatory processes. First, various cells and organs act to prevent hyperkalemia by taking up potassium from the blood. It is also prevented by the action of the kidneys, which excrete potassium into the urine. A third protective mechanism is vomiting. Consumption of a large dose of potassium ions, such as potassium chloride, induces a vomiting reflex to expel most of the potassium before it can be absorbed.

Hyperkalemia can occur from a variety of causes, including the consumption of too much of a potassium salt; the failure of the kidneys to normally excrete potassium ions into the urine; the leakage of potassium from cells and tissues into the bloodstream; and from acidosis. The most common cause of hyperkalemia is kidney (or renal) disease, which accounts for about three quarters of all cases.

Hyperkalemia can also be caused by a disease of the adrenal gland called Addison's disease. The adrenal gland produces the hormone aldosterone that promotes the excretion of potassium into the urine by the kidney.

Hyperkalemia can also result from injury to muscle or other tissues. Since most of the potassium in the body is contained in muscle, a severe trauma that crushes muscle cells results in an immediate increase in the concentration of potassium in the blood. Hyperkalemia may also result from severe **burns** or infections.

Acidic blood plasma, or acidosis, is an occasional cause of hyperkalemia. Acidosis, which occurs in a number of diseases, is defined as an increase in the concentration of hydrogen ions in the bloodstream. In the body's attempt to correct the situation, hydrogen is taken up by muscle cells out of the blood in an exchange mechanism involving the transfer of potassium ions into the bloodstream. This can abnormally elevate the plasma's concentration of potassium ions. When acidosis is the cause of hyperkalemia, treating the patient for acidosis has two benefits: a reversal of both the acidosis and the hyperkalemia.

Symptoms of hyperkalemia include abnormalities in the behavior of the heart. Heart abnormalities of mild hyperkalemia (5.0 to 6.5 mM potassium) can be detected by an electrocardiogram (ECG or EKG). With severe hyperkalemia (over 8.0 mM potassium), the heart may beat at a dangerously rapid rate (fibrillation) or stop beating entirely (cardiac arrest). Patients with moderate or severe hyperkalemia may also develop nervous symptoms such as tingling of the skin, numbness of the hands or feet, weakness, or a flaccid **paralysis**, which is characteristic of both hyperkalemia and hypokalemia (low plasma potassium).

Hypokalemia is most commonly caused by the use of **diuretics**. Diuretics are drugs that increase the excretion of water and salts in the urine. Diuretics are used to treat a number of medical conditions, including **hypertension** (high blood pressure), congestive **heart failure**, liver disease, and kidney disease. However, diuretic treatment can have the side effect of producing hypokalemia. In fact, the most common cause of hypokalemia in the elderly is the use of diuretics. The use of furosemide and thiazide, two commonly used diuretic drugs, can lead to hypokalemia. In contrast, spironolactone and triamterene are diuretics that do not provoke hypokalemia.

Other commons causes of hypokalemia are excessive **diarrhea** or vomiting. Diarrhea and vomiting can be produced by infections of the gastrointestinal tract. Due to a variety of organisms, including bacteria, protozoa, and viruses, diarrhea is a major world health problem. It is responsible for about a quarter of the 10 million infant **death**s that occur each year. Although nearly all of these deaths occur in the poorer parts of Asia and Africa, diarrheal diseases are a leading cause of infant death in the United States. Diarrhea results in various abnormalities, such as **dehydration** (loss in body water), hyponatremia (low sodium level in the blood), and hypokalemia.

Because of the need for potassium to control muscle action, hypokalemia can cause the heart to stop beating. Young infants are especially at risk for death from this cause, especially where severe diarrhea continues for two weeks or longer. Diarrhea due to laxative abuse is an occasional cause of hypokalemia in the adolescent or adult. Enema abuse is a related cause of hypokalemia. Laxative abuse is especially difficult to diagnose and treat, because patients usually deny the practice. Up to20% of persons complaining of chronic diarrhea practice laxative abuse. Laxative abuse is often part of **eating disorders**, such as anorexia nervosa or bulimia nervosa. Hypokalemia that occurs with these eating disorders may be life-threatening.

Alcoholism occasionally results in hypokalemia. About one half of alcoholics hospitalized for withdrawal symptoms experience hypokalemia. The hypokalemia of alcoholics occurs for a variety of reasons, usually poor nutrition, vomiting, and diarrhea. Hypokalemia can also be caused by hyperaldosteronism; Cushing's syndrome; hereditary kidney defects such as Liddle's syndrome, Bartter's syndrom, and Franconi's syndrome; and eating too much licorice.

Mild hypokalemia usually results in no symptoms, while moderate hypokalemia results in confusion, disorientation, weakness, and discomfort of muscles. On occasion, moderate hypokalemia causes cramps during **exercise**. Another symptom of moderate hypokalemia is a discomfort in the legs that is experienced while sitting still. The patient may experience an annoying feeling that can be relieved by shifting the positions of the legs or by stomping the feet on the floor. Severe hypokalemia results in extreme weakness of the body and, on occasion, in paralysis. The paralysis that occurs is ''flaccid paralysis,'' or limpness. Paralysis of the muscles of the lungs results in death. Another dangerous result of severe hypokalemia is abnormal heart beat (arrhythmia) that can lead to death from cardiac arrest (cessation of heart beat). Moderate hypokalemia may be defined as serum potassium between 2.5 and 3.0 mM, while severe hypokalemia is defined as serum potassium under 2.5 mM.

Insulin injections are used to treat hyperkalemia in emergency situations. Insulin is a hormone well known for its ability to stimulate the entry of sugar (glucose) into cells. It also provokes the uptake of potassium ions by cells, decreasing potassium ion concentration in the blood. When insulin is used to treat hyperkalemia, glucose is also injected. Serum potassium levels begin to decline within 30 to 60 minutes and remain low for several hours. In non-emergency situations, hyperkalemia can be treated with a low potassium diet. If this does not succeed, the patient can be given a special resin to bind potassium ions. One such resin, sodium polystyrene sulfonate (Kayexalate), remains in the intestines, where it absorbs potassium and forms a complex of resin and potassium. Eventually this complex is excreted in the feces. A typical dose of resin is 15 grams, taken one to four times per day. The correction of hyperkalemia with resin treatment takes at least 24 hours.

In emergency situations, when severe hypokalemia is suspected, the patient should be put on a cardiac monitor, and respiratory status should be assessed. If laboratory test results show potassium levels below 2.5 mM, intravenous potassium should be given. In less urgent cases, potassium can be given orally in the pill form. Potassium supplements take the form of pills containing potassium chloride (KCl), potassium bicarbonate ($KHCO_3$), and potassium acetate. Oral potassium chloride is the safest and most effective treatment for hypokalemia. Generally, the consumption of 40–80 mmoles of KCl per day is sufficient to correct the hypokalemia that results from diuretic therapy. For many people taking diuretics, potassium supplements are not necessary as long as they eat a balanced diet containing foods rich in potassium.

Pott, Percival (1714-1788)

English Surgeon

Percival Pott was a highly successful and influential 18th-century London surgeon. Pott, who was born in London, was one of the first physicians to describe many medical conditions, some of which now bear his name. Following an apprenticeship under surgeon Edward Nourse, Pott joined the staff at St. Bartholomew's Hospital, initially as an assistant, and later as a senior surgeon and professor, serving there from 1744 through 1787. Toward the end of the century, Pott had built up one of the most successful surgical practices in London. Those who knew him report that he had a kindly, charitable nature.

Disorders named after Pott include Pott's disease, which is a rare spinal condition caused by **tuberculosis** that eventually leads to bone disintegration and skeletal deformity (1779); Pott's puffy tumor (an **abscess** with associated localized headache, tenderness, and **edema** of the affected area (1768); and Pott's fracture (1750), which is a particular type of compound fracture of the ankle that Pott himself sustained after a fall in the street. Pott's lectures at St. Bartholomew's Hospital were well attended, not only by students but also by foreign visitors. Pott wrote extensively about his clinical observations. In 1765 he published *Fractures and Dislocations*, in which he identified the two conditions that now bear his name as well as many other conditions that relate to bone structure. Other writings treated various head injuries, **hernia**, *fistula-in-ano* (an abnormal channel between the lower bowel and the skin of the perineum), and hydrocele (a swelling of the scrotum). Pott also recognized a form of **cancer** located in the skin of the scrotum (epithelioma of the scrotum) as an occupational hazard peculiar to chimney sweeps. When one considers that Pott's contributions to medical knowledge came before the advent of **anesthesia**, at a time when surgeons were largely restricted to operating on the surface of the body (and avoided regions within the head, neck, or abdomen), one can begin to appreciate the genius of Pott's work. Pott was elected to the Royal Society in 1764. His published works include *That Kind of Palsy of the Lower Limbs which is Frequently Found to Accompany a Curvature of the Spine* (1779). His treatises on hernia (1756), head injuries (1760), hydrocele (1762), *fistula in ano* (1765), fractures and dislocations (1768), chimney sweep's cancer (1775), and spinal deformity (1779) are considered masterpieces.

Prader-Willi syndrome

Prader-Willi syndrome (PWS) is caused by a rare birth defect centered on chromosome 15. Characteristics of the syndrome include developmental delays, **mental retardation**, behavioral problems, and insatiable appetite leading to **obesity**. Affected individuals also experience incomplete sexual development, poor muscle tone, and short stature as adults.

PWS occurs in 1 in 12,000 to 15,000 births and is regarded as the most common genetic cause of obesity. It affects both genders and all races. Although PWS arises from a genetic defect, it is not an inherited condition—it is a birth defect. The defect occurs spontaneously and specifically involves chromosome 15.

A person normally inherits one copy of chromosome 15 from each parent. In PWS cases, the copy from the father either lacks a specific segment of DNA (70-75% of cases) or is missing altogether (25-30% of cases). If the father's chromosome 15 is absent, a person with PWS has two copies of the mother's chromosome 15. Although the individual has the proper number of chromosomes, inheriting two copies of a chromosome from one parent is an abnormal situation called uniparental disomy. If that parent is the mother, it is called maternal uniparental disomy.

Virtually all parents of individuals with PWS have normal chromosomes; fewer than 2% of cases are linked to an inherited genetic mutation. In most cases, an error occurs during embryo development. This error leads to deletion of part of the father's chromosome 15 or to maternal uniparental disomy for chromosome 15. In either case, genes that should have been inherited from the father are missing and PWS develops.

Newborns with PWS have low birth weight, poor muscle tone, are lethargic, do not feed well, and generally fail to thrive. Their genitalia are abnormally small, a condition that persists lifelong. At about two to four years of age, children with PWS develop an uncontrollable, insatiable appetite. Left to their own devices, they will eat themselves to extreme obesity.

Motor development is delayed 1-2 years, and speech and language problems are common. Mild mental retardation is present in about 63% of cases; moderate mental retardation occurs in 31% of cases. Severe mental retardation is seen in the remainder.

Individuals with PWS often develop behavior problems—ranging from stubbornness to temper tantrums—and are easily upset by unexpected changes. Other common characteristics include a high **pain** threshold, obsessive/compulsive behavior, dental problems, and breathing difficulties. About two-thirds of individuals cannot vomit even after consumption of spoiled food or other noxious substances.

Puberty may occur early or late, but it is usually incomplete. In addition to the effects on sexual development and fertility, individuals do not undergo the normal adolescent growth spurt and are short as adults. Muscles often remain underdeveloped.

Symptoms can lead to a diagnosis of PWS. This diagnosis can be confirmed through **genetic testing**. PWS cannot be cured. Treatment involves speech and language therapy and special education. Stringent control of food intake is vital to prevent obesity-related disease and **death**. A lifelong restricted-calorie diet accompanied by regular **exercise** is needed to control weight. Unfortunately, diet drugs do not work for individuals with PWS, but medications may be helpful in treating behavioral and psychological problems. Growth and development of secondary sexual characteristics can be achieved with hormone treatment, but decisions regarding such treatment are made on an individual basis.

Life expectancy for individuals with PWS may be normal if weight can be controlled. Individuals with PWS typically do best in settings that offer a stable routine and restricted access to food. PWS currently cannot be prevented.

Praxagoras (4th century B.C.-4th century B.C.)

Greek Physician

Praxagoras, a descendant of Asclepius, was a resident of Cos in Greece. He is believed to have been born around 340 BC, although some historians have placed his date of birth as late as the last third of the fourth century. His father, Nicharchus, was an eminent physician who, according to **Galen**, held the theory that the arteries contain only air, while the veins contain blood. This theory was later also expounded by Praxagoras.

Praxagoras, came to be regarded in antiquity as the most famous member (after **Hippocrates**, who was probably somewhat older than Praxagoras) of the Coan School. Galen ranked Praxagoras beside Hippocrates and Diocles among the famous physicians of the old school. Later medical historians classified Praxagoras as a follower of the *logical* or *dogmatic school*, which advocated rigid doctrine rather than investigation. (The dogmatists divided medical science into five branches: physiology, etiology, hygiene, semeiology, and therapeutics.) Praxagoras was the author of a book on the diseases of foreign lands, which suggests that he may have left his native country to travel abroad; this has led some scholars to conclude that Praxagoras had mainly a theoretical interest in medicine, though his reputation as a surgeon suggests that he could be rather daring in his medical procedures. He exerted tremendous influence on the development of Greek medical thinking, having been the teacher of some very illustrious physicians, including Plistonicus, Xenophon of Kos, and Herophilus (credited with differentiating the cerebrum and cerebellum, and with counting the pulse using a water clock). Praxagoras's work was widely known throughout antiquity. In the third century BC, the Stoic philosopher Chrysippus made reference to Praxagoras in discussing the origin of the nerves in the heart, suggesting that the latter was recognized as an outstanding authority on medical questions even in the third century BC. Yet another reference to Praxagoras appears in the first century BC by Krinagoras. Galen, who wrote a special book on the **humors** based on the theory of Praxagoras, attempted to show that Praxagoras's ideas were an extension of those of Hippocrates. Galen's opinion of Praxagoras is highly sympathetic, with Galen stating that one must praise those individuals who explain the truth once it is found and who make appropriate additions. References to Praxagoras also occur in the codex Crameri, the codex medicorum Laurentianus, and the codices Graeci Bonnonenses. One of Praxagoras's letters has also been preserved. Based on extant fragments of his writing, it is believed that Praxagoras authored at least 12 books, though the actual count is uncertain.

Precocious puberty

Sexual development before the age of eight in girls, and age 10 in boys is considered precocious puberty. Not every child reaches **puberty** at the same time, but in most cases it's safe to predict that sexual development will begin at about age 11 in girls and 12 or 13 in boys. However, occasionally a child begins to develop sexually much earlier. Between four to eight times more common in girls than boys, precocious puberty occurs in one out of every 5,000 to 10,000 American children.

Precocious puberty often begins before age 8 in girls, triggering the development of breasts and hair under the arms and in the genital region. The onset of ovulation and menstruation also may occur. In boys, the condition triggers the development of a large penis and testicles, with spontaneous erections and the production of sperm. Hair grows on the face, under arms and in the pubic area, and **acne** may become a problem.

While the early onset of puberty may seem fairly benign, in fact it can cause problems when hormones trigger changes in the growth pattern, essentially halting growth before the child has reached normal adult height. Girls may never grow above 5 ft (152 cm) and boys often stop growing by about 5 ft 2 in (157 cm).

The abnormal growth patterns are not the only problem, however. Children with this condition look noticeably different than their peers, and may feel rejected by their friends and socially isolated. Adults may expect these children to act more maturely simply because they look so much older. As a result, many of these children—especially boys—are noticeably more aggressive than others their own age, leading to behavior problems both at home and at school.

Puberty begins when the brain secretes a hormone that triggers the pituitary gland to release gonadotropins, which in turn stimulate the ovaries or testes to produce sex hormones. These sex hormones (especially estrogen in girls and testosterone in boys) cause the onset of sexual maturity.

The hormonal changes of precocious puberty are normal—it's just that the whole process begins a few years too soon. Especially in girls, there is not usually any underlying problem that causes the process to begin too soon. (However, some boys do inherit the condition; the responsible gene may be passed directly from father to son, or inherited indirectly from the maternal grandfather through the mother, who does not begin early puberty herself). This genetic condition in girls can be traced only in about 1% of cases.

In about 15% of cases, there is an underlying cause for the precocious puberty, and it is important to search for these causes. The condition may result from a benign tumor in the part of the brain that releases hormones. Less commonly, it may be caused by other types of **brain tumor**s, central nervous system disorders or adrenal gland problems.

Physical exams can reveal the development of sexual characteristics in a young child. Bone x-rays can reveal bone age, and pelvic ultrasound may show an enlarged uterus and rule out ovarian or adrenal tumors. Blood tests can highlight higher-than-normal levels of hormones. MRI or CAT scans should be considered to rule out intracranial tumors.

Treatment aims to halt or reverse sexual development so as to stop the accompanying rapid growth that will limit a child's height. There are two possible approaches: either treat the underlying condition (such as an ovarian or intracranial tumor) or change the hormonal balance to stop sexual development. It may not be possible to treat the underlying condition; for this reason, treatment is usually aimed at adjusting hormone levels.

There are several drugs which have been developed to do this including: histrelin (Supprelin), nafarelin (Synarel), synthetic gonadotropin-releasing hormone agonist, deslorelin, ethylamide, triptorelin, and leuprolide.

Drug treatments can slow growth to 2–3 in (5–7.5 cm) a year, allowing these children to reach normal adult height, although the long-term effects aren't known.

Preferred provider organization

A preferred provider organization (PPO) is a network of doctors and hospitals who form a corporation to provide medical services to self-insured businesses or for health insurance companies. A preferred provider organization negotiates with the business or insurance company to provide medical services at discounted rates in return for a large volume of patients. For members, a preferred provider organization is the least restrictive form of **managed care** organization. Many employers offer a preferred provider organization to help employees get used to managed care. Preferred provider organizations are the most popular type of employer-sponsored health plan in the United States. In 1999, Medicare added preferred provider organizations to its menu of health care insurance options.

A preferred provider organization is not like a **health maintenance organization**. Members choose from a large list of providers in private practice. They generally pay a small copayment to see a network provider and can see providers outside of the network by paying extra. They usually do not need a referral from their primary care doctor to see a specialist. The goal of a PPO is to lower costs for the insurance company, the employer, and the patient. A PPO uses a utilization review board to monitor the cost of health care by determining whether a patient should be hospitalized or not and whether services are medically necessary. This review can take place before, during, or after hospitalization. In some cases, a utilization review board monitors quality too.

See also Managed care; Health maintenance organization

Pregnancy-induced hypertension

Preeclampsia and eclampsia are complications of **pregnancy**. In preeclampsia, the woman has dangerously high blood pressure, swelling, and protein in the urine. If allowed to progress, this syndrome will lead to eclampsia.

High blood pressure in pregnancy (**hypertension**) is a very serious complication. It puts both the mother and the fetus at risk for a number of problems. Hypertension can exist in several different forms. One of these is the preeclampsia-eclampsia continuum (also called pregnancy-induced hypertension or PIH). In this type of hypertension, high blood pressure is first noted sometime after week 20 of pregnancy and is accompanied by protein in the urine and swelling. Chronic hypertension is another form of hypertension. It usually exists before pregnancy or may develop before week 20 of pregnancy. Chronic hypertension with superimposed preeclampsia is another form of chronic hypertension. This syndrome occurs when a woman with pre-existing chronic hypertension begins to have protein in the urine after week 20 of pregnancy. Late hypertension is another form of high blood pressure. It usually occurs after week 20 of pregnancy and is unaccompanied by protein in the urine and does not progress the way preeclampsia-eclampsia does.

Preeclampsia is most common among women who have never given birth. The disease is most common in mothers under the age of 20, or over the age of 35. African-American women have higher rates of preeclampsia than do Caucasian women. Other risk factors include poverty, multiple pregnancies (twins, triplets, etc.), pre-existing chronic hypertension, kidney disease, diabetes, excess amniotic fluid, and a condition of the fetus called nonimmune hydrops. The tendency to develop preeclampsia appears to run in families. The daughters and sisters of women who have had preeclampsia are more likely to develop the condition.

Experts are still trying to understand the exact causes of preeclampsia and eclampsia. It is generally accepted that preeclampsia and eclampsia are problematic because these conditions cause blood vessels to leak. The effects are seen throughout the body. When blood vessels leak they allow fluid to flow out into the tissues of the body. The result is swelling in the hands, feet, legs, arms, and face. While many pregnant women experience swelling in their feet, and sometimes in their hands, swelling of the upper limbs and face is a sign of a more serious problem. As fluid is retained in these tissues, the woman may experience significant weight gain (two or more pounds per week).

Blood vessels also sometimes leak in the brain. They can cause severe damage within the brain, resulting in seizures or coma. If the blood vessels in the eyes begin to leak the woman may experience problems seeing, and may have blurry vision or may see spots. Also, the retina may become detached. When blood vessels in the lungs leak fluid may leak into the tissues of the lungs, resulting in **shortness of breath**.

Leaky vessels within the liver may cause it to swell. The liver may be involved in a serious complication of preeclampsia, called the HELLP syndrome. In this syndrome, red blood cells are abnormally destroyed, chemicals called liver enzymes are abnormally high, and cells involved in the clotting of blood (platelets) are low. The small capillaries within the kidneys can leak. Normally, the filtration system within the kidney is too fine to allow protein (which is relatively large) to leave the bloodstream and enter the urine. In preeclampsia, however, the leaky capillaries allow protein to be dumped into the urine. The development of protein in the urine is very serious, and often results in a low birth weight baby.

In preeclampsia, the volume of circulating blood is lower than normal because fluid is leaking into other parts of the body. The heart tries to make up for this by pumping a larger quantity of blood with each contraction. Blood vessels usually expand in diameter (dilate) in this situation to decrease the work load on the heart. In preeclampsia, however, the blood vessels are abnormally constricted, causing the heart to work even harder to pump against the small diameters of the vessels. This causes an increase in blood pressure.

The most serious consequences of preeclampsia and eclampsia include brain damage in the mother due to brain swelling and oxygen deprivation during seizures. Mothers can also suffer from blindness, kidney failure, liver rupture, and placental abruption. Babies born to preeclamptic mothers are often smaller than normal, which makes them more susceptible to complications during labor, delivery, and in early infancy. Babies of preeclamptic mothers are also at risk of being born prematurely.

Diagnosing preeclampsia may be accomplished by noting painless swelling of the arms, legs, and/or face, in addition to abnormal weight gain. The patient's blood pressure is taken during every doctor's visit during pregnancy. An increase of 30 mm Hg in the systolic pressure, or 15 mm Hg in the diastolic pressure, or a blood pressure reading greater than 140/90 mm Hg is considered indicative of preeclampsia. A simple laboratory test in the doctor's office can indicate the presence of protein in a urine sample (a dipstick test).

With mild preeclampsia, treatment may be limited to bed rest, with careful daily monitoring of weight, blood pressure, and urine protein via dipstick. This careful monitoring will be required throughout pregnancy, labor, delivery, and even for 2–4 days after the baby has been born. If the diastolic pressure does not rise over 100 mm Hg prior to delivery, and no other symptoms develop, the woman can continue pregnancy until the fetus is mature enough to be delivered safely. Ultrasound tests can be performed to monitor the health and development of the fetus.

If the diastolic blood pressure continues to rise over 100 mm Hg, or if other symptoms like **headache**, vision problems, abdominal pain, or blood abnormalities develop, then the patient may require medications to prevent seizures. Magnesium sulfate is commonly given through a needle in a vein (intravenous, or IV). Medications that lower blood pressure (antihypertensive drugs) are reserved for patients with very high diastolic pressures (over 110 mm Hg), because lowering the blood pressure will decrease the amount of blood reaching the fetus. This places the fetus at risk for oxygen deprivation. If preeclampsia appears to be progressing toward true eclampsia, then medications may be given in order to start labor. Babies can usually be delivered vaginally. After the baby is delivered, the woman's blood pressure and other vital signs will usually begin to return to normal quickly.

The prognosis in preeeclampsia and eclampsia depends on how carefully a patient is monitored. Very careful, consistent monitoring allows quick decisions to be made, and improves the woman's prognosis. Still, the most common causes of death in pregnant women are related to high blood pressure.

About 33% of all patients with preeclampsia will have the condition again with later pregnancies. Eclampsia occurs in about 1 out of every 200 women with preeclampsia. If not treated, eclampsia is almost always fatal.

More information on how preeclampsia and eclampsia develop is needed before recommendations can be made on how to prevent these conditions. Research is being done with patients in high risk groups to see if calcium supplementation, **aspirin**, or fish oil supplementation may help prevent preeclampsia. Most importantly, it is clear that careful monitoring during pregnancy is necessary to diagnose preeclampsia early.

PREGNANCY

Pregnancy is the period from conception to birth. After the egg is fertilized by a sperm and then implanted in the lining of the uterus, it develops into the placenta and embryo, and later into

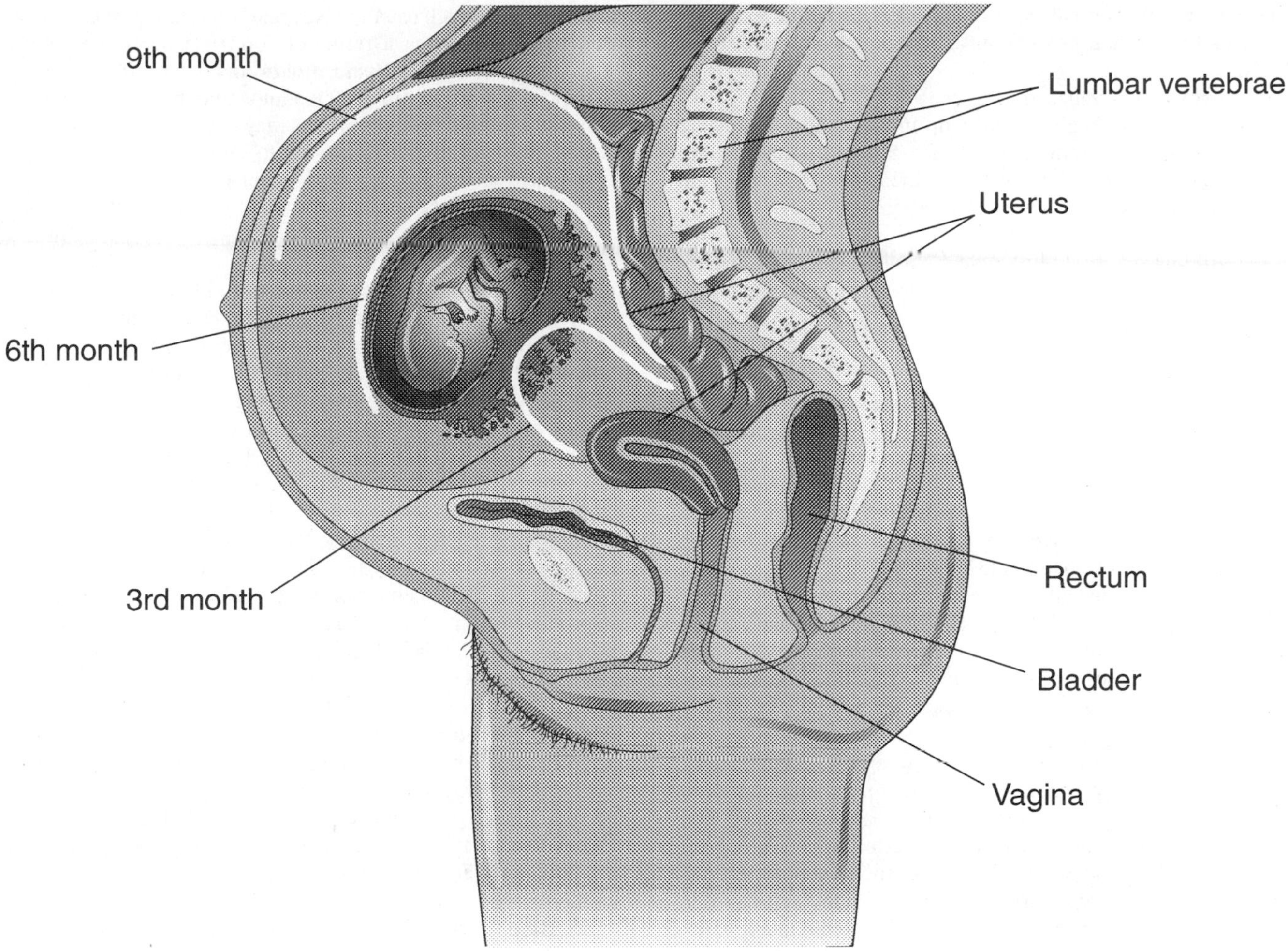

Pregnancy usually lasts 40 weeks in humans, beginning from the first day of the woman's last menstrual period, and is divided into three trimesters. The illustration above depicts the position of the developing fetus during each trimester. ***(Illustration by Electronic Illustrators Group.)***

a fetus. Pregnancy usually lasts 40 weeks, beginning from the first day of the woman's last menstrual period, and is divided into three trimesters, each lasting three months.

At the end of the first month, the embryo is about a third of an inch long, and its head and trunk—plus the beginnings of arms and legs—have started to develop. The embryo gets nutrients and eliminates waste through the umbilical cord and placenta. By the end of the first month, the liver and digestive system begin to develop, and the heart starts to beat.

In the second month, the heart starts to pump and the nervous system (including the brain and spinal cord) begins to develop. The 1 in (2.5 cm) long fetus has a complete cartilage skeleton, which is replaced by bone cells by month's end. Arms, legs and all of the major organs begin to appear. Facial features also begin to form.

By the third month the fetus has grown to 4 in (10 cm) and weighs a little more than an ounce (28 g). Now the major blood vessels and the roof of the mouth are almost completed, as the face starts to take on a more recognizably human appearance. Fingers and toes appear. All the major organs are now beginning to form; the kidneys are now functional and the four chambers of the heart are complete.

In the fourth month the fetus begins to kick and swallow, although most women still can't feel it move. Now 4 oz (112 g), the fetus can hear and urinate, and has established sleep-wake cycles. All organs are now fully formed, although they will continue to grow for the next five months. The fetus has skin, eyebrows and hair.

By the fifth month the fetus weighs up to a 1 lb (454 g) and measures 8-12 in (20-30 cm). The fetus experiences rapid growth as its internal organs continue to grow. At this point, the mother may feel the fetus move, and she can hear the heartbeat with a stethoscope.

Even though its lungs are not fully developed, a fetus born during the sixth month can survive with intensive care. Weighing 1-1.5 lbs (454-681 g), the fetus is red, wrinkly, and covered with fine hair all over its body. The fetus will grow very fast during this month as its organs continue to develop.

There is a better chance that a fetus born during the seventh month will survive. The fetus continues to grow rapidly, and may weigh as much as 3 lbs (1.3 kg). Now the fetus can suck its thumb and look around its watery womb with open eyes.

Growth continues during the eighth month but slows down as the baby begins to take up most of the room inside the uterus. Now weighing between 4-5 lbs (1.8-2.3 kg) and measuring 16-18 in (40-45 cm) long, the fetus may at this time prepare for delivery next month by moving into the head-down position.

Adding 0.5 lb (227 g) a week during the ninth month as the due date approaches, the fetus drops lower into the mother's abdomen and prepares for the onset of labor, which may begin any time between the 37th and 42nd week of gestation. Most healthy babies will weigh 6-9 lbs (2.7-4 kg) at birth, and will be about 20 inches long.

The first sign of pregnancy is usually a missed menstrual period, although some women bleed in the beginning. A woman's breasts swell and may become tender as the mammary glands prepare for eventual breastfeeding. Nipples begin to enlarge and the veins over the surface of the breasts become more noticeable. **Nausea and vomiting** are very common symptoms and are usually worse in the morning. Many women also feel extremely tired during the early weeks. Frequent urination is common, and there may be a creamy white discharge from the vagina. Some women crave certain foods, and an extreme sensitivity to smell may worsen the nausea. Weight begins to increase.

In the second trimester (13-28 weeks) a woman begins to look noticeably pregnant and the enlarged uterus is easy to feel. The nipples get bigger and darker, skin may darken, and some women may feel flushed and warm. Appetite may increase. By the 22nd week, most women have felt the fetus move. During the second trimester, nausea and vomiting often fade away, and the pregnant woman often feels much better and more energetic. Heart rate increases as does the volume of blood in the body.

By the third trimester (29-40 weeks), many women begin to experience a range of common symptoms. Stretch marks may develop on abdomen, breasts and thighs, and a dark line may appear from the navel to pubic hair. A thin fluid may be excreted from the nipples. Many women feel hot, sweat easily and often find it hard to get comfortable. Kicks from an active fetus may cause sharp **pain**s, and lower backaches are common. More rest is needed as the woman copes with the added **stress** of extra weight. Braxton Hicks contractions may get stronger.

At about the 36th week in a first pregnancy (later in repeat pregnancies), the baby's head drops down low into the pelvis. This may relieve pressure on the upper abdomen and the lungs, allowing a woman to breathe more easily. However, the new position places more pressure on the bladder.

The average woman gains 28 lbs (12.7 kg) during pregnancy, 70% of it during the last 20 weeks. An average, healthy full-term baby at birth weighs 7.5 lbs (3.4 kg), and the placenta and fluid together weigh another 3 lbs (1.3 kg). The remaining weight that a woman gains during pregnancy is mostly due to water retention and fat stores.

In addition to the typical, common symptoms of pregnancy, some women experience other problems that may be annoying but which usually disappear after delivery. **Constipation** may develop as a result of food passing more slowly through the intestine. **Hemorrhoids** and heartburn are fairly common during late pregnancy. Gums may become more sensitive and bleed more easily; eyes may dry out, making contact lenses feel painful. Pica (a craving to eat substances other than food) may occur. Swollen ankles and **varicose veins** may be a problem in the second half of pregnancy, and chloasma may appear on the face.

While the above symptoms are all considered to be normal, there are some symptoms that could be a sign of a more dangerous underlying problem. A pregnant woman with any of the following signs should contact her doctor immediately: abdominal pain, rupture of the amniotic sac or leaking of fluid from the vagina, bleeding from the vagina, no fetal movement for 24 hours (after the fifth month), continuous **headache**s, marked, sudden swelling of eyelids, hands or face during the last three months, dim or blurry vision during last 3 months, or persistent vomiting.

Many women first discover they are pregnant after a positive home pregnancy test. Pregnancy urine tests check for the presence of human chorionic gonadotropin (hCG), which is produced by a placenta. The newest home tests can detect pregnancy on the day of the missed menstrual period.

Home pregnancy tests are more than 97% accurate if the result is positive, and about 80% accurate if the result is negative. If the result is negative and there is no menstrual period within another week, the pregnancy test should be repeated. While home pregnancy tests are very accurate, they are less accurate than a pregnancy test conducted at a lab. For this reason, women may want to consider having a second pregnancy test conducted at their doctor's office to be sure of the accuracy of the result.

Blood tests to determine pregnancy are usually used only when a very early diagnosis of pregnancy is needed. This more expensive test, which also looks for hCG, can produce a result within 9-12 days after conception.

Once pregnancy has been confirmed, there are a range of screening tests that can be done to screen for **birth defects**, which affect about 3% of unborn children. Two tests are recommended for all pregnant women: alpha-fetoprotein (AFP) and the triple marker test.

Other tests are recommended for women at higher risk for having a child with a birth defect. This would include women over age 35, who had another child or a close relative with a birth defect, or who have been exposed to certain drugs or high levels of radiation. Women with any of these risk factors may want to consider amniocentesis, chorionic villus sampling (CVS) or **ultrasound**.

There are a range of other prenatal tests that are routinely performed, including: pap test, **gestational diabetes** screening test at 24-28 weeks, tests for sexually transmitted diseases, **urinalysis**, blood tests for anemia or blood type, and screening for immunity to various diseases, such as German **measles**.

Prenatal care is vitally important for the health of the unborn baby. A pregnant woman should be sure to eat a balanced, nutritious diet of frequent, small meals. Many doctors prescribe pregnancy **vitamins**, including folic acid and iron supplementation during pregnancy.

No medication (not even a nonprescription drug) should be taken except under medical supervision, since it could pass from the mother through the placenta to the developing baby. Some drugs have been proven harmful to a fetus, but no drug should be considered completely safe (especially during early pregnancy). Drugs taken during the first three months of a pregnancy may interfere with the normal formation of the baby's organs, leading to birth defects. Drugs taken later on in pregnancy may slow the baby's growth rate, or they may damage specific fetal tissue (such as the developing teeth).

To have the best chance of having a healthy baby, a pregnant woman should avoid: smoking, alcohol, street drugs, large amounts of **caffeine**, and artificial sweeteners. **Childbirth** education classes for the woman and her partner help prepare the couple for labor and delivery.

There are many ways to avoid pregnancy. A woman has a choice of many methods of **contraception** which will prevent pregnancy, including (in order of least to most effective): spermicide alone, natural (rhythm) method, diaphragm or cap alone, **condom** alone, diaphragm with spermicide, condom with spermicide, intrauterine device (**IUD**), contraceptive pill, sterilization (either a man or woman), and avoiding intercourse.

Pregnancy loss

There are various ways in which a **pregnancy** may be lost. Miscarriage means loss of an embryo or fetus before the 20th week of pregnancy. Most miscarriages occur during the first 14 weeks of pregnancy. The medical term for miscarriage is spontaneous abortion.

An abnormally weak cervix (the structure at the bottom of the uterus) is called "incompetent," and therefore it can gradually widen during pregnancy. Left untreated, this can result in repeated pregnancy losses or premature delivery.

A stillbirth is defined as the **death** of a fetus at any time after the 20th week of pregnancy. Stillbirth is also referred to as intrauterine fetal death (IUFD).

Miscarriages are very common. Approximately 20% of pregnancies (one in five) end in miscarriage. The most common cause is a genetic abnormality of the fetus. Not all women realize that they are miscarrying and others may not seek medical care when it occurs.

A miscarriage is often a traumatic event for both partners, and can cause feelings similar to the loss of a child or other member of the family. Fortunately, 90% of women who have had one miscarriage subsequently have a normal pregnancy and healthy baby; 60% are able to have a healthy baby after two miscarriages. Even a woman who has had three miscarriages in a row still has more than a 50% chance of having a successful pregnancy the fourth time.

Incompetent cervix is the result of an anatomical abnormality. Normally, the cervix remains closed throughout pregnancy until labor begins. An incompetent cervix gradually opens due to the pressure from the developing fetus after about the 13th week of pregnancy. The cervix begins to thin out and widen without any contractions or labor. The membranes surrounding the fetus bulge down into the opening of the cervix until they break, resulting in the loss of the baby or a very premature delivery.

It is important to distinguish between a stillbirth and other words that describe the unintentional end of a pregnancy. A pregnancy that ends before the 20th week is called a miscarriage rather than a stillbirth, even though the death of the fetus is a common cause of miscarriage. After the 20th week, the unintended end of a pregnancy is called a stillbirth if the infant is dead at birth and premature delivery if it is born alive.

Factors that increase a mother's risk of stillbirth include: age over 35; **malnutrition**; inadequate prenatal care; smoking; and alcohol or drug abuse.

There are many reasons why a woman's pregnancy ends in miscarriage. Often the cause is not clear. However, more than half the miscarriages that occur in the first eight weeks of pregnancy involve serious chromosomal abnormalities or **birth defects** that would make it impossible for the baby to survive. These are different from inherited genetic diseases. They probably occur during development of the specific egg or sperm, and therefore are not likely to occur again.

In about 17% of cases, miscarriage is caused by an abnormal hormonal imbalance that interferes with the ability of the uterus to support the growing embryo. This is known as luteal phase defect. In another 10% of cases, there is a problem with the structure of the uterus or cervix. This can especially occur in women whose mothers used diethylstilbestrol (DES) when pregnant with them.

The risk of miscarriage is increased by:

- **Smoking** (up to a 50% increased risk)
- Infection
- Exposure to toxins (such as arsenic, lead, formaldehyde, benzene, and ethylene oxide)
- **Multiple pregnancy**
- Poorly-controlled **diabetes**.

The most common symptom of miscarriage is bleeding from the vagina, which may be light or heavy. However, bleeding during early pregnancy is common and is not always serious. Many women have slight vaginal bleeding after the egg implants in the uterus (about 7-10 days after conception), which can be mistaken for a threatened miscarriage. A few women bleed at the time of their monthly periods through the pregnancy. However, any bleeding in the first three months of pregnancy (first trimester) is considered a threat of miscarriage.

Women should not ignore vaginal bleeding during early pregnancy. In addition to signaling a threatened miscarriage, it could also indicate a potentially life-threatening condition known as **ectopic pregnancy**. In an ectopic pregnancy, the fetus implants at a site other than the inside of the uterus. Most often this occurs in the fallopian tube.

Cramping is another common sign of a possible miscarriage. The cramping occurs because the uterus attempts to push out the pregnancy tissue. If a pregnant woman experiences both bleeding and cramping the possibility of miscarriage is more likely than if only one of these symptoms is present.

If a woman experiences any sign of impending miscarriage, she should be examined by a practitioner. The doctor or nurse will perform a pelvic exam to check if the cervix is closed as it should be. If the cervix is open, miscarriage is inevitable and nothing can preserve the pregnancy. Symptoms of an inevitable miscarriage may include dull relentless or sharp intermittent **pain** in the lower abdomen or back. Bleeding may be heavy. Clotted material and tissue (the placenta and embryo) may pass from the vagina.

A situation in which only some of the products in the uterus have been expelled is called an incomplete miscarriage. Pain and bleeding may continue and become severe. An incomplete miscarriage requires medical attention.

A "missed abortion" occurs when the fetus has died but neither the fetus nor placenta is expelled. There may not be any bleeding or pain, but the symptoms of pregnancy will disappear. The physician may suspect a missed abortion if the uterus does not continue to grow. The physician will diagnose a missed abortion with an **ultrasound** examination.

A woman should contact her doctor if she experiences any of the following:

- Any bleeding during pregnancy.
- Pain or cramps during pregnancy.
- Passing of tissue.
- **Fever** and chills during or after miscarriage.

Some factors that can contribute to the chance of a woman having an incompetent cervix include trauma to the cervix, physical abnormality of the cervix, or having been exposed to the drug diethylstilbestrol (DES) in the mother's womb. Some women have cervical incompetence for no obvious reason.

A number of different disorders can cause stillbirth. They include:

- Pre-eclampsia and eclampsia. These are disorders of late pregnancy characterized by high blood pressure, fluid retention, and protein in the urine.
- Diabetes in the mother.
- Hemorrhage.
- Abnormalities in the fetus caused by infectious diseases, including **syphilis**, **toxoplasmosis**, German **measles** (**rubella**), and **influenza**.
- Severe **birth defects**, including **spina bifida**. Birth defects are responsible for about 20% of stillbirths.
- Postmaturity. Postmaturity is a condition in which the pregnancy has lasted 41 weeks or longer.
- Unknown causes. These account for about a third of stillbirths.

In most cases the only symptom of stillbirth is that the mother notices that the baby has stopped moving. In some cases, the first sign of fetal death is **premature labor**. Premature labor is marked by a rush of fluid from the vagina, caused by the tearing of the membrane around the baby; and by abdominal cramps or contractions.

If a woman experiences any sign of impending miscarriage she should see a doctor or nurse for a pelvic examination to check if the cervix is closed, as it should be. If the cervix is open, miscarriage is inevitable.

An ultrasound examination can confirm a missed abortion if the uterus has shrunk and the patient has had continual spotting with no other symptoms.

Incompetent cervix is suspected when a woman has three consecutive spontaneous pregnancy losses during the second trimester (the fourth, fifth and sixth months of the pregnancy). The likelihood of this happening by random chance is less than 1%. Spontaneous losses due to incompetent cervix account for 20-25% of all second trimester losses. A spontaneous second trimester pregnancy loss is different from a miscarriage, which usually happens during the first three months of pregnancy.

The physician can check for abnormalities in the cervix by performing a manual examination or by an ultrasound test. The physician can also check to see if the cervix is prematurely widened (dilated). Because incompetent cervix is only one of several potential causes for this, the patient's past history of pregnancy losses must also be considered when making the diagnosis.

When the mother notices that fetal movement has stopped, the doctor can use several techniques to evaluate whether the baby has died. The doctor can listen for the fetal heartbeat with a stethoscope, use Doppler ultrasound to detect the heartbeat, or give the mother an electronic fetal nonstress test. In this test, the mother lies on her back with electronic monitors attached to her abdomen. The monitors record the baby's heart rate, movements, and contractions of the uterus.

For women who experience bleeding and cramping, bed rest is often ordered until symptoms disappear. Women should not have sex until the outcome of the threatened miscarriage is determined. If bleeding and cramping are severe, women should drink fluids only.

Although it may be psychologically difficult, if a woman has a miscarriage at home she should try to collect any material she passes in a clean container for analysis in a laboratory. This may help determine why the miscarriage occurred.

An incomplete miscarriage or missed abortion may require the removal of the fetus and placenta by a D&C (**dilatation and curettage**). In this procedure the contents of the uterus are scraped out. It is performed in the doctor's office or hospital.

After miscarriage, a doctor may prescribe rest or **antibiotics** for infection. There will be some bleeding from the vagina for several days to two weeks after miscarriage. To give the cervix time to close and avoid possible infection, women should not use tampons or have sex for at least two weeks. Couples should wait for one to three normal menstrual cycles before trying to get pregnant again.

Treatment for incompetent cervix is a surgical procedure called cervical cerclage. A stitch (suture) is used to tie the cervix shut to give it more support. It is most effective if it is performed somewhere between 14-16 weeks into the pregnancy. The stitch is removed near the end of pregnancy to allow for a normal birth.

Cervical cerclage can be performed under spinal, epidural, or general anesthesia. The patient will need to stay in the hospital for one or more days. The procedure to remove the suture is done without the need for anesthesia. The vagina is held open with an instrument called a speculum and the stitch is cut and removed. This may be slightly uncomfortable, but should not be painful.

Some possible risks of cerclage are premature rupture of the amniotic membranes, infection of the amniotic sac, and preterm labor. The risk of infection of the amniotic sac increases as the pregnancy progresses. For a cervix that is dilated 3 centimeters (cm), the risk is 30%.

After cerclage, a woman will be monitored for any preterm labor. The woman needs to consult her obstetrician immediately if there are any signs of contractions.

Cervical cerclage can not be performed if a woman is more than 4 cm dilated, if the fetus has already died in her uterus, or if her amniotic membranes are torn and her water has broken.

In most cases of intrauterine death, the mother will go into labor within two weeks of the baby's death. If the mother does not go into labor, the doctor will bring on (induce) labor in order to prevent the risk of hemorrhage. Labor is usually induced by giving the mother a drug (oxytocin) that cause the uterus to contract.

Emotional support from family and friends, self-help groups, and counseling by a mental health professional can help bereaved parents cope with their loss.

A miscarriage that is properly treated is not life-threatening, and usually does not affect a woman's ability to deliver a healthy baby in the future.

Feelings of grief and loss after a miscarriage are common. In fact, some women who experience a miscarriage suffer from major depression during the six months after the loss. This is especially true for women who don't have any children or who have had depression in the past. The emotional crisis can be similar to that of a woman whose baby has died after birth.

The success rate for cerclage correction of incompetent cervix is good. About 80-90% of the time women deliver healthy infants. The success rate is higher for cerclage done early in pregnancy.

With the exception of women with diabetes, women who have a stillbirth have as good a chance of carrying a future pregnancy to term as women who are pregnant for the first time.

The majority of miscarriages cannot be prevented because they are caused by severe genetic problems determined at conception. Some doctors advise women who have a threatened miscarriage to rest in bed for a day and avoid sex for a few weeks after the bleeding stops. Other experts believe that a healthy woman (especially early in the pregnancy) should continue normal activities instead of protecting a pregnancy that may end in miscarriage later on, causing even more profound distress.

If miscarriage was caused by a hormonal imbalance (luteal phase defect), this can be treated with a hormone called progesterone to help prevent subsequent miscarriages. If structural problems have led to repeated miscarriage, there are some possible procedures to treat these problems. Other possible ways to prevent miscarriage are to treat genital infections, eat a well-balanced diet, and refrain from smoking and using recreational drugs.

The risk of stillbirth can be lowered to some extent by good prenatal care and the mother's avoidance of exposure to infectious diseases, smoking, alcohol abuse, or drug consumption. Tests before delivery (antepartum testing), such as ultrasound, the alpha-fetoprotein blood test, and the electronic fetal nonstress test, can be used to evaluate the health of the fetus before there is a stillbirth.

PREMATURE EJACULATION

Premature ejaculation is male sexual climax (orgasm) prior to or immediately following penetration. In spite of the many theories and speculations about this disorder, the simple fact seems to be that sexual control is learned behavior. It can be learned correctly or incorrectly, and it can be relearned correctly. There is no definitive evidence that suggests disease or psychological conditions contribute to premature ejaculation.

In 1966, **William H. Masters** and **Virginia E. Johnson** published *Human Sexual Response,* in which they broke the first ground in approaching this topic from a new perspective. Their method was devised by Dr. James Seman and has been modified subsequently by Dr. Helen Singer Kaplan and others.

A competent and orthodox sex therapist will spend much more time focusing on the personal than the sexual relationship between the two people who come for treatment. Without emotional intimacy, sexual relations are superficial and sexual problems such as premature ejaculation are rarely overcome.

With that foremost in mind, a careful plan is outlined that requires dedication, patience and commitment by both partners. It necessarily begins by prohibiting intercourse for an extended period of time—at least a week, often a month. This is very important to the man because "performance **anxiety**" is the greatest enemy of performance. If he knows he cannot have intercourse he is able to relax and focus on the **exercise**s. The first stage is called "sensate focus" and involves his concentration on the process of sexual arousal and climax. He should learn to recognize each step in the process, most particularly the moment just before the "point of no return." Ideally, this stage of treatment requires the man's partner to be devoted to his sensations. In order to regain equality, he should in turn spend separate time stimulating and pleasing his mate, without intercourse.

At this point the techniques diverge. The original "squeeze technique" requires that the partner become expert at squeezing the head of the penis at intervals to prevent orgasm. The modified procedure, described by Dr. Ruth Westheimer, calls upon the man to instruct the partner when to stop stimulating him to give him a chance to draw back. A series of stages follows, each offering greater stimulation as the couple gains greater control over his arousal. This whole process has been called "outercourse." After a period of weeks, they will have together retrained his response and gained satisfactory control over it. In addition, they will each have learned much about the other's unique sexuality and ways to increase each other's pleasure.

With either technique, the emphasis is on the mutual goal of satisfactory sexual relations for both partners. Cures for premature ejaculation have had very high success rates. The ''squeeze technique'' has illicited a 95% success rate, whereby the patient is able to control ejaculation.

PREMATURE LABOR

The usual length of a human pregnancy is 38-42 weeks after the first day of the last menstrual period. Labor is a natural series of events that indicate that the birth process is starting. Premature labor is defined as contractions that occur after 20 weeks and before 37 weeks during the term of pregnancy. The baby is more likely to survive and be healthy if it remains in the uterus for the full term of the pregnancy. It is estimated that between 10% of births in the United States occur during the premature period. Premature birth is the greatest cause of newborn illness and **death**. In the U.S., **prematurity** has a greater impact on African-Americans.

The causes of premature labor cannot always be determined. Some research suggests that infection of the urinary or reproductive tract may stimulate premature labor and premature births. Multiple pregnancies (twins, triplets, etc.) are more likely to result in premature labor. Smoking, alcohol use, drug abuse and poor nutrition can increase the risk of premature labor and birth. Adolescent mothers are also at higher risk for premature delivery. Women whose mothers took diethylstilbestrol (DES) when they carried them are more likely to deliver prematurely, as are women who have had previous surgery on the cervix.

The symptoms of premature labor can include contractions of the uterus or tightening of the abdomen, which occur every ten minutes or more frequently. These contractions usually increase in frequency, duration, and intensity, and may or may not be painful. Other symptoms associated with premature labor can include menstrual-like cramps, abdominal cramping with or without **diarrhea**, pressure or pain in the pelvic region, low backache, or a change in the color or amount of vaginal discharge. As labor progresses, the cervix or opening of the uterus will open (dilate) and the tissue around it will become thinner (efface). Premature rupture of membranes (when the water breaks) may also occur.

An occasional contraction can occur anytime during the pregnancy and does not necessarily indicate that labor is starting. Premature contractions are sometimes confused with Braxton Hicks contractions, which can occur throughout the pregnancy. Braxton Hicks contractions do not cause the cervix to open or efface, and are considered ''false labor.''

To diagnose premature labor the health care provider will conduct a **physical examination** and ask about the timing and intensity of the contractions. A vaginal examination is the only way to determine if the cervix has started to dilate or efface. Urine and blood samples may be collected to screen for infection. A vaginal culture (a cotton-tipped swab is used to collect some fluid and cells from the vagina) may be done to look for a vaginal infection. A fetal heart monitor may be placed on the mother's abdomen to record the heartbeat of the fetus and to time the contractions. A fetal ultrasound may be performed to determine the age and weight of the fetus, the condition of the placenta, and to see if there is more than one fetus present.

The goal of treatment is to stop the premature labor and prevent the fetus from being delivered before it is full term. A first recommendation may be for the woman with premature contractions to lie down with feet elevated and to drink juice or other fluids. If contractions continue or increase, medical attention should be sought. In addition to bed rest, medical care may include intravenous fluids. Sometimes, this extra fluid is enough to stop contractions. In some cases, oral or injectable drugs like terbutaline sulfate, ritodrine, magnesium sulfate, or nifedipine must be given to stop the contractions. These are generally very effective; however, as with any drug therapy, there are risks of side effects. Some women may need to continue on medication for the duration of the pregnancy. **Antibiotics** may be prescribed if a vaginal or urinary tract infection is detected. If the membranes have already ruptured, it may be difficult or impossible to stop premature labor. If infection of the membranes that cover the fetus (chorioamnionitis) develops, the baby must be delivered.

If premature labor is managed successfully, the pregnancy may continue normally until the delivery of a healthy infant. Once symptoms of preterm labor occur during the pregnancy, the mother and fetus need to be monitored regularly since it is likely that premature labor will occur again. If the preterm labor cannot be stopped or controlled, the infant will be delivered prematurely. Infants that are born prematurely have an increased risk of health problems including **birth defects**, lung problems, **mental retardation**, blindness, deafness, and developmental disabilities. If the infant is born too early, its body systems may not be mature enough for it to survive. Evaluating the infant's lung maturity is one of the keys to determining its chance of survival. Fetuses delivered further into pregnancy and those with more mature lungs are more likely to survive.

Smoking, poor **nutrition**, and drug or alcohol abuse can increase the risk of premature labor and early delivery. A healthy diet and prenatal vitamin supplements (prescribed by the health care provider) are important for the growth of the fetus and the health of the mother. Pregnant women are advised to see a health care provider early in the pregnancy and receive regular prenatal examinations throughout the pregnancy.

PREMATURE MENOPAUSE

The average age American women go through **menopause** is age 51. If menopause (hormonal changes at the end of the female reproductive years) occurs before age 40, it is considered premature menopause. Possible causes include autoimmune problems and common **cancer** treatments.

About half of all women will go through menopause before age 51 and the rest will go through it after. Most women will finish menopause between the ages of 42 and 58. A small number of women will find that their periods stop prematurely, before age 40.

There are many possible causes of premature menopause. Women who have premature menopause often have **autoimmune disorders** like thyroid disease or diabetes mellitus. In these diseases, the body produces antibodies to one or more of its own organs. These antibodies interfere with the normal function of the organ. Just as antibodies might attack the thyroid or the pancreas (causing thyroid disease or diabetes), antibodies may attack the ovaries and stop the production of female hormones.

Cancer treatments like **chemotherapy** or radiation can cause premature menopause. The risk depends on the type and length of treatment and the age of the woman when she first begins radiation or chemotherapy. If the ovaries are surgically removed (during a **hysterectomy**, for example) menopause will occur within a few days, no matter how old the woman is.

The symptoms of premature menopause are similar to those of menopause at any time. Menstrual periods stop and women may notice hot flashes, vaginal dryness, mood swings, and sleep problems. Sometimes the first symptom of premature menopause is **infertility**. A woman may find that she cannot become pregnant because she is not ovulating (producing eggs) anymore.

When menopause occurs after the ovaries are surgically removed, the symptoms begin within several days after surgery and tend to be more severe. This happens because the drop in the level of estrogen is dramatic, unlike the gradual drop that usually occurs.

Premature menopause can be confirmed by blood tests to measure the levels of follicle stimulating hormone (FSH) and luteinizing hormone (LH). The levels of these hormones will be higher if menopause has occurred.

Because premature menopause is often associated with other hormonal problems, women who have premature menopause should be screened for diabetes, thyroid disease, and similar diseases.

There is no treatment to reverse premature menopause. **Hormone replacement therapy** (HRT) can prevent the common symptoms of menopause and lower the long-term risk of **osteoporosis**. Women who have premature menopause should take HRT. Estrogen relieves the unpleasant symptoms of menopause, including the hot flashes and the vaginal dryness. Estrogen is especially important for women who go through premature menopause. The long-term health risks of menopause (osteoporosis and increased risk of heart disease) are even more likely to occur after premature menopause. However, women who have certain medical conditions (like liver disease, uterine cancer, or **breast cancer**) may not be candidates for estrogen.

If a woman still has her uterus after premature menopause, she will need to take progesterone along with the estrogen. If her uterus has been removed, estrogen alone will be enough.

Women who wish to become pregnant after premature menopause now have the option of fertility treatments using donor eggs. This is similar to in vitro fertilization, but the eggs come from a donor instead of the woman who is trying to become pregnant. Premature menopause cannot be prevented.

Prematurity

The length of a normal **pregnancy** or gestation is considered to be 40 weeks (280 days) from the date of conception. Infants born before 37 weeks gestation are considered premature and may be at risk for complications.

More than one out of every ten infants born in the United States is born prematurely. Advances in medical technology have made it possible for infants born as young as 23 weeks gestational age (17 weeks premature) to survive. These premature infants, however, are at higher risk for **death** or serious complications, which include heart defects, respiratory problems, blindness, and brain damage.

The birth of a premature baby can be brought on by several different factors, including premature labor; placental abruption, in which the placenta detaches from the uterus; placenta previa, in which the placenta grows too low in the uterus; premature rupture of membranes, in which the amniotic sac is torn, causing the amniotic fluid to leak out; incompetent cervix, in which the opening to the uterus opens too soon; and maternal toxemia, or blood poisoning. While one of these conditions are often the immediate reason for a premature birth, its underlying cause is usually unknown. Prematurity is much more common in multiple pregnancy and for mothers who have a history of miscarriages or who have given birth to a premature infant in the past. One of the few, and most important, identifiable cause of prematurity is drug abuse, particularly cocaine, by the mother.

Infants born prematurely may experience major complications due to their low birth weight and the immaturity of their body systems. Some of the common problems among premature infants are **jaundice** (yellow discoloration of the skin and whites of the eyes), apnea (a long pause in breathing), and inability to breast or bottle feed. Body temperature, blood pressure, and heart rate may be difficult to regulate in premature infants. The lungs, digestive system, and nervous system (including the brain) are underdeveloped in premature babies, and are particularly vulnerable to complications. Some of the more common risks and complications of prematurity are described below.

Respiratory distress syndrome (RDS) is the most common problem seen in premature infants. Babies born too soon have immature lungs that have not developed surfactant, a protective film that helps air sacs in the lungs to stay open. With RDS, breathing is rapid and the center of the chest and rib cage pull inward with each breath. Sometimes the infant needs extra oxygen, and sometimes a surfactant drug can be given to coat the lung tissue. Bronchopulmonary dysplasia is the development of scar tissue in the lungs, and can occur in severe cases of RDS.

Necrotizing enterocolitis (NEC) is a further complication of prematurity. In this condition, part of the baby's intestines are destroyed as a result of bacterial infection. In cases where only the innermost lining of the bowel dies, the infant's body can regenerate it over time; however, if the full thickness of a portion dies, it must be removed surgically and an opening (ostemy) must be made for the passage of wastes until the infant is healthy enough for the remaining ends to be sewn together. Because NEC is potentially fatal, doctors are quick to respond to its symptoms, which include lethargy, vomiting, a swollen and/or red abdomen, fever, and blood in the stool. Measures include taking the infant off mouth feedings and feeding him or her intravenously; administering antibiotics; and removing air and fluids from the digestive tract via a nasal tube. Approximately 70% of NEC cases can be successfully treated without surgery.

Intraventricular hemorrhage (IVH) is another serious complication of prematurity. It is a condition in which immature and fragile blood vessels within the brain burst and bleed into the hollow chambers (ventricles) normally reserved for cerebrospinal fluid and into the tissue surrounding them. To drain fluid and relieve pressure on the brain, doctors will either perform lumbar punctures, a procedure in which a needle is inserted into the spinal canal to drain fluids; install a reservoir, a tube that drains fluid from a ventricle and into an artificial chamber under or on top of the scalp; or install a ventricular shunt, a tube that drains fluid from the ventricles and into the abdomen, where it is reabsorbed by the body. Infants who are at high risk for IVH usually have an ultrasound taken of their brain in the first week after birth, followed by others if bleeding is detected. IVH cannot be prevented; however, close monitoring can ensure that procedures to reduce fluid in the brain are implemented quickly to minimize possible damage.

Apnea of prematurity is a condition where the infant stops breathing for periods lasting up to 20 seconds. It is often associated with a slowing of the heart rate. The baby may become pale, or the skin color may change to a blue or purplish hue. Apnea occurs most commonly when the infant is asleep. Infants with serious apnea may need medications to stimulate breathing or oxygen through a tube inserted in the nose. Some infants may be placed on a ventilator or respirator with a breathing tube inserted into the airway. As the baby gets older, and the lungs and brain tissues mature, the breathing usually becomes more regular.

As the fetus develops, it gets the oxygen it needs from the mother's blood system. Most of the blood in the infant's system bypasses the lungs. Once the baby is born, its own blood must start pumping through the lungs to get oxygen. Normally, this bypass duct closes within the first few hours or days after birth. If it does not close, the baby may have trouble getting enough oxygen on its own. Patent ductus arteriosus is a condition where the duct that channels blood between two main arteries does not close after the baby is born. In some cases, a drug, indomethacin, can be given to close the duct. Surgery may be required, or the duct may close on its own as the baby develops.

Retinopathy of prematurity is a condition where the blood vessels in the baby's eyes do not develop normally, and can, in some cases, result in blindness. Premature infants are also more susceptible to infections because they are born with fewer antibodies.

Many of the problems associated with prematurity depend on how early the baby is born and how much it weighs at birth. The most accurate way of determining the gestational age of an infant in utero is calculating from a known date of conception or using **ultrasound** imaging to observe development. When a baby is born, doctors can use the Dubowitz exam to estimate gestational age. This standardized test scores responses to 33 specific neurological stimuli to estimate the infant's neural development. Once the baby's gestational age and weight are determined, further tests and electronic fetal monitoring may need to be used to diagnose problems or to track the baby's condition. A blood pressure monitor may be wrapped around the arm or leg. Several types of monitors can be taped to the skin. A heart monitor or cardiorespiratory monitor may be attached to the baby's chest, abdomen, arms, or legs with adhesive patches to monitor breathing and heart rate. A thermometer probe may be taped on the skin to monitor body temperature. Blood samples may be taken from a vein or artery. X rays or ultrasound imaging may be used to examine the heart, lungs, and other internal organs.

Treatment depends on the types of complications that are present. It is not unusual for a premature infant to be placed in a heat-controlled unit (an incubator) to maintain its body temperature. Infants that are having trouble breathing on their own may need oxygen either pumped into the incubator, administered through small tubes placed in their nostrils, or through a respirator or ventilator which pumps air into a breathing tube inserted into the airway. The infant may require fluids and nutrients to be administered through an intravenous line where a small needle is inserted into a vein in the hand, foot, arm, leg, or scalp. If the baby needs drugs or medications, they may also be administered through the intravenous line. Another type of line may be inserted into the baby's umbilical cord. This can be used to draw blood samples or to administered medications or nutrients. If heart rate is irregular, the baby may have heart monitor leads taped to the chest. Many premature infants require time and support with breathing and feeding until they mature enough to breath and eat unassisted.

Advances in medical care have made it possible for many premature infants to survive and develop normally. However, whether or not a premature infant will survive is still intimately tied to his or her gestational age. The longer the baby was able to develop in the womb the more likely it will be to survive outside it.

Physicians cannot predict long-term complications of prematurity and some consequences may not become evident until the child is school—aged. Minor disabilities like learning problems, poor coordination, or short attention span may be the result of premature birth, but can be overcome with early intervention. The risks of serious long term complications depend on many factors including how premature the infant was at birth, weight at birth, and the presence or absence of breathing problems. The development of infection or the presence of a birth defect can also effect long term prognosis. Severe disabilities like brain damage, blindness, and chronic lung problems are possible and may require ongoing care.

Some of the risks and complications of premature delivery can be reduced if the mother receives good prenatal care, follows a healthy diet, avoids alcohol consumption, and refrains from cigarette smoking. In some cases of premature labor, the mother may be placed on bed rest or given drugs that can stop labor contractions for days or weeks, giving the developing infant more time to develop before delivery. The physician may prescribe a steroid medication to be given to the mother before the delivery to help speed up the baby's lung development. The availability of a neonatal intensive care unit, a special hospital unit equipped and trained to deal with premature infants, can also increase the chances of survival.

Premenstrual syndrome

Premenstrual syndrome refers to symptoms that occur between ovulation and the onset of menstruation. The symptoms include both physical symptoms, such as breast tenderness, back **pain**, abdominal cramps, **headache**, and changes in appetite, as well as psychological symptoms of **anxiety**, depression, and unrest. Severe forms of this syndrome are referred to as premenstrual dysphoric disorder (PMDD). These symptoms may be related to hormones and emotional disorders.

Approximately 75% of all menstruating women experience some symptoms that occur before or during menstruation. PMS encompasses symptoms severe enough to interfere with daily life. About 3-7% of women experience the more severe premenstrual dysphoric disorder (PMDD). These symptoms can last 4-10 days and can have a substantial impact on a woman's life.

The reason some women get severe PMS while others have none is not understood. PMS symptoms usually begin between the ages of 20 and 30. The disease may run in families and is also more prone to occur in women with a history of psychological problems. Overall however, it is difficult to predict who is most at risk for PMS.

Because PMS is restricted to the second half of a woman's menstrual cycle, after ovulation, it is thought that hormones play a role. During a woman's monthly menstrual cycle, which lasts from 24-35 days, hormone levels change. The hormone estrogen gradually rises during the first half of a woman's cycle, the preovulatory phase, and falls dramatically at ovulation. After ovulation, the postovulatory phase, progesterone levels gradually increase until menstruation occurs. Both estrogen and progesterone are secreted by the ovaries, which are responsible for producing the eggs. The main role of these hormones is to cause thickening of the lining of the uterus (endometrium). However, estrogen and progesterone also affect other parts of the body, including the brain. In the brain and nervous system, estrogen can affect the levels of neurotransmitters, such as serotonin. Serotonin has long been known to have an effect on emotions, as well as eating behavior. It is thought that when estrogen levels go down during the postovulatory phase of the menstrual cycle, decreases in serotonin levels follow. Whether these changes in estrogen, progesterone, and serotonin are responsible for the emotional aspects of PMS is not known with certainty. However, most researchers agree that the chemical transmission of signals in the brain and nervous system is in some way related to PMS. This is supported by the fact that the times following **childbirth** and **menopause** are also associated with both depression and low estrogen levels.

Symptoms for PMS are varied and many, including both physical and emotional aspects that range from mild to severe. The physical symptoms include: bloating, headaches, food cravings, abdominal cramps, headaches, tension, and breast tenderness. Emotional aspects include mood swings, irritability, and depression.

The best way to diagnose PMS is to review a detailed diary of a woman's symptoms for several months. PMS is diagnosed by the presence of physical, psychological, and behavioral symptoms that are cyclic and occur in association with the premenstrual period of time. PMDD, which is far less common, was officially recognized as a disease in 1987. Its diagnosis depends on the presence of at least five symptoms related to mood that disappear within a few days of menstruation. These symptoms must interfere with normal functions and activities of the individual.

There are many treatments for PMS and PMDD depending on the symptoms and their severity. For mild cases, treatment includes **vitamins**, **diuretics**, and pain relievers. Vitamins E and B_6 may decrease breast tenderness and help with fatigue and mood swings in some women. Diuretics that remove excess fluid from the body seem to work for some women. For more severe cases and for PMDD, treatments available include **antidepressant drugs**, hormone treatment, or (only in extreme cases) surgery to remove the ovaries. Hormone treatment usually involves **oral contraceptives**. This treatment, as well as removal of the ovaries, is used to prevent ovulation and the changes in hormones that accompany it. Recent studies, however, indicate that hormone treatment has little effect over placebo.

The most progress in the treatment of PMS and PMDD has been through the use of antidepressant drugs. The most effective of these include sertraline (Zoloft), fluoxetine (Prozac), and paroxetine (Paxil). They are termed selective serotonin reuptake inhibitors (SSRIs) and act by indirectly increasing the brain serotonin levels, thus stabilizing emotions. Some doctors prescribe antidepressant treatment for PMS throughout the cycle, while others direct patients to take the drug only during the latter half of the cycle.

There are alternative treatments that can both affect serotonin and hormone responses, as well as affect some of the physical symptoms of PMS.

Some women find relief with the use of vitamin and mineral supplements. Magnesium can reduce the fluid retention that causes bloating, while calcium may decrease both irritability and bloating. Magnesium and calcium also help relax smooth muscles and this may reduce cramping. Vitamin E may reduce breast tenderness, nervous tension, fatigue, and **insomnia**. Vitamin B_6 may decrease fluid retention, fatigue, irritability, and mood swings. Vitamin B_5 supports the adrenal glands and may help reduce fatigue.

The most important way to alter hormone levels may be by eating more phytoestrogens. These plant-derived compounds have an effect similar to estrogen in the body. One of the richest sources of phytoestrogens is soy products, such as tofu. Additionally, many supplements can be found that contain black cohosh (*Cimicifugaracemosa*) or dong quai (*Angelica sinensis*), which are herbs high in phytoestrogens. Red clover (*Trifolium pratense*), alfalfa (*Medicago sativa*), licorice (*Glycyrrhiza glabra*), hops (*Humulus lupulus*), and legumes are also high in phytoestrogens. Increasing the consumption of phytoestrogens is also associated with decreased risks of **osteoporosis**, **cancer**, and heart disease.

Many antidepressants act by increasing serotonin levels. An alternative means of achieving this is to eat more carbohydrates. For instance, two cups of cereal or a cup of pasta has enough carbohydrate to effectively increase serotonin levels. An herb known as St. John's wort (*Hypericum perforatum*) has stood up to scientific trials as an effective antidepressant. As with the standard antidepressants, however, it must be taken continuously and does not show an effect until used for 4-6 weeks. There are also herbs, such as skullcap (*Scutellaria lateriflora*) and kava (*Piper methysticum*), that can relieve the anxiety and irritability that often accompany depression. An advantage of these herbs is that they can be taken when symptoms occur rather than continually. Chaste tree (*Vitex agnus-castus*) in addition to helping rebalance estrogen and progesterone in the body also may relieve the anxiety and depression associated with PMS.

The prognosis for women with both PMS and PMDD is good. Most women who are treated for these disorders do well.

Because the causes of PMS and PMDD are not completely understood prevention is difficult. Maintaining a good diet, one low in sugars and fats and high in phytoestrogens and complex carbohydrates, may prevent some of the symptoms of PMS. Women should try to **exercise** three times a week, keep in generally good health, and maintain a positive self image. Because PMS is often associated with **stress**, avoidance of stress or developing better means to deal with stress can be important.

PRENATAL CARE

Prenatal care is the comprehensive care that women receive throughout their **pregnancy**. It is an important part of making sure that the mother and baby are as healthy as possible. Regular prenatal visits gives the mother a chance to ask questions, be informed about the pregnancy, and also allows the doctor to keep a close watch on the progress of the fetus throughput the pregnancy. Women who begin prenatal care early in their pregnancies have better pregnancy outcomes.

Most pregnancies proceed normally, but there are some risks. Assessing these risks is an essential part of prenatal care. Prenatal care is not just medical care. It includes **childbirth** education, counseling, and providing support for the family. Prenatal care includes periodic regular visits to the doctor, good nutrition, regular physical activity, awareness and monitoring of the warning signs, and avoidance of unhealthy substances.

The first prenatal visit will be longer and more involved than later visits. During the first prenatal visit, the pregnancy is confirmed through a urine test and pelvic exam. The pelvic exam will help the doctor decide if the uterus is the right size and pinpoint the baby's due date, which is estimated from the date of the last missed period. The doctor will also be able to determine if there are any problems with the vagina and cervix and if the pelvis is large enough to get through a normal delivery. In addition to this, a thorough breast examination is conducted and height, weight, and blood pressure are recorded. A urine sample is collected which will be tested for sugar, protein, infection, and kidney problems. Blood is drawn in order to check the blood group, **anemia**, and the presence of **rubella** and **hepatitis** B antibodies. Laboratory tests for **gonorrhea**, chlamydia, and other **sexually transmitted diseases** will also be performed.

After the first visit, the pregnant woman will return once a month during the first 6 months of pregnancy. During the 7th and 8th months, visits will be scheduled every 2 weeks, and after that every week until delivery. During these visits weight, blood pressure, and urine will be checked. The abdomen will be examined for growth of the uterus, the baby's size, position, and heart beat. These examinations will help to ensure that the pregnancy is progressing normally. **Ultrasound** scans may be done to asses fetal growth and development, location of placenta, and amount of amniotic fluid.

In certain cases, a special test known as "chorionic villus sampling" may be performed in the first 12 weeks if there is any risk of certain genetic disorders being passed on to the fetus. Amniocentesis may be carried out on women over the age of 35 to detect any possible abnormalities such as **Down syndrome**, **spina bifida** in the fetus.

During pregnancy, women should certain substances that could harm the developing fetus. These substances are alcohol, cigarette smoking and other tobacco use, drug use, x-rays, lead, and common over the counter medications. Women should consult with their health care provider before taking any prescription or non-prescription medications.

Pregnant women should eat a balanced nutritional diet and increase their caloric intake to meet the needs of the developing fetus and their changing bodies. Good nutrition during pregnancy depends on eating a variety of wholesome foods, such as whole grains, vegetables, and fruit. It is recommended that pregnant women and women who wish to become pregnant should take a prenatal vitamin containing folic acid and other essential vitamins and minerals. Pregnant women should also eat foods that are rich in protein, calcium, iron, and folic acid. Eating healthfully during pregnancy is one of the most important things that women can do to ensure the normal development and growth of the developing fetus. It can also help to prevent **prematurity** and **low birthweight**. For the mother, good nutrition helps to prevent anemia, infection, difficult labor and poor post-partum healing.

A healthy woman with low risk pregnancy can exercise safely throughout their pregnancies. Moderate exercise is considered to be beneficial for most pregnant women as it helps to prevent **constipation**, **varicose veins**, relieves backaches, prepares the body for childbirth and maintains overall physical fitness.

For most women, pregnancy is a normal and happy event. The best thing a woman can do for herself is to eat a balance diet, cut out alcohol, smoking, drugs and get enough exercise. Most importantly, a complete prenatal program can help a woman to have the safest and healthiest pregnancy possible. Some women feel prenatal care costs too much and they cannot afford it. However, many programs are available for pregnant women who have little or no money for care. The county department can help the women find clinics if they need help finding affordable care.

See also Pregnancy; Prenatal diagnostic tests

Prenatal diagnostic tests

Amniocentesis is a procedure used to diagnose fetal defects in the early second trimester of **pregnancy**. A sample of the amniotic fluid which surrounds a fetus in the womb is collected through a pregnant woman's abdomen using a needle and syringe. Tests performed on fetal cells found in the sample can reveal the presence of many types of genetic disorders, thus allowing doctors and prospective parents to make important decisions about early treatment and intervention.

Since the mid-1970s, amniocentesis has been used routinely to test for **Down syndrome**, by far the most common genetic birth defect. By 1997, about 800 different diagnostic tests were available, most of them for hereditary genetic disorders such as **Tay-Sachs disease**, **muscular dystrophy** and **cystic fibrosis**.

Amniocentesis is recommended for women over age 35, or who have already borne children with **birth defects**, or when either of the parents has a family history of a birth defect for which a diagnostic test is available. Another reason for the procedure is to confirm indications of Down syndrome and certain other defects which may have shown up previously during routine blood tests.

The risk of bearing a child with a genetic defect such as Down syndrome is directly related to a woman's age (the older the woman, the greater the risk). At age 35, a woman's risk of carrying a fetus with Down syndrome roughly equals the risk of miscarriage caused by the procedure (about 1 in 200). In comparison, at age 25 the risk of this defect is about 1 in 1,400; by age 45 it increases to about 1 in 20. Nearly half of all pregnant women over 35 in the United States undergo amniocentesis and many younger women also decide to have the procedure.

One of the most common reasons for performing amniocentesis is an abnormal alpha-fetoprotein (AFP) test (see below). Alpha-fetoprotein is a protein produced by the fetus and present in the mother's blood. A simple blood screening, usually conducted around the 15th week of pregnancy, can determine the AFP levels in the mother's blood. Levels that are too high or too low may signal a problem with the fetus. Amniocentesis is recommended whenever the AFP levels fall outside the normal range.

The procedure is generally performed during the 16th week of pregnancy; results are usually available within three weeks. While it is possible to perform amniocentesis as early as the 11th week, there appears to be an increased risk of miscarriage when done at this time.

The advantage of an early test and speedy results lies in the extra time for decision making if a problem is detected. Potential treatment of the fetus can begin earlier. Important, also, is the fact that elective abortions are safer and less controversial the earlier they are performed.

As an invasive surgical procedure, amniocentesis poses a real, although small, risk to the health of a fetus. Parents must weigh the potential value of the knowledge or reassurance against the small risk of damaging what is probably a normal fetus. The serious emotional and ethical dilemmas that adverse test results can bring must also be considered. The decision to undergo amniocentesis is always a matter of personal choice. It is important for a woman to fully understand the procedure and to feel confident in the obstetrician performing it. Evidence suggests that a physician's experience with the procedure reduces the chance of problems. Almost all obstetricians are experienced in performing amniocentesis. The patient should feel free to ask questions and seek emotional support before, during and after the amnio is performed.

The word amniocentesis literally means "puncture of the amnion," the thin-walled sac of fluid in which a developing fetus is suspended during pregnancy. During the sampling procedure, the obstetrician inserts a very fine needle through the woman's abdomen into the uterus and amniotic sac and withdraws about an ounce of amniotic fluid for testing. The relatively painless procedure is performed on an outpatient basis, sometimes using local **anesthesia**.

The doctor uses ultrasound images to guide needle placement and collect the sample, lessening the risk of harming the fetus or having to insert the needle several times.

After the procedure, the woman should rest for the first 24 hours and avoid heavy lifting for two days.

The sample of amniotic fluid is sent to a laboratory where fetal cells contained in the fluid are isolated and grown in order to provide enough genetic material for testing. This takes about 7-14 days. The material is then examined under a microscope. For some disorders (like Tay-Sachs), the simple presence of a telltale chemical compound in the amniotic fluid is enough to confirm a diagnosis. Depending on the specific tests ordered and the skill of the lab conducting them, the results should be available between one and four weeks after the sample is taken.

Cost of the procedure depends on the doctor, the lab, and the tests ordered. Most insurers provide coverage for women over 35, as a follow-up to positive maternal blood screening results, and when genetic disorders run in the family.

An alternative to amniocentesis now widely used is chorionic villus sampling, or CVS, which can be performed as early as the eighth week of pregnancy. While this allows for the possibility of a first trimester abortion, if warranted, CVS is apparently also riskier and is more expensive.

The most promising area of new research in prenatal testing involves expanding the scope and accuracy of maternal blood screening, since this poses no risk to the fetus.

Once the procedure has been safely completed, the anxiety of waiting for the test results can prove to be the worst part of the process. A woman should seek emotional support from family and friends, as well as from her obstetrician and family doctor. Professional counseling may also prove necessary, particularly if a fetal defect is discovered.

There are several risks involved with the procedure. While slight bleeding (called ''spotting'') in pregnancy is fairly common, bleeding following amniocentesis should always be checked out. Rarely, infection can occur after the procedure. eaking of amniotic fluid or unusual vaginal discharge together with **fever** could signal the onset of infection. An unchecked infection can lead to severe complications. Unusual abdominal pain and/or cramping may indicate the onset of **Premature labor**, but mild cramping for the first day or two following the procedure is normal. There is a very slight risk of injury to the fetus resulting from contact with the needle. The rate of miscarriage occurring during amniocentesis appears to be about 0.5%, compared to a miscarriage rate of 1% for CVS. Many fetuses with severe genetic defects miscarry naturally during the first trimester.

Negative results from an amniocentesis indicate that everything about the fetus appears normal and the pregnancy can continue without undue concern. A negative result for Down syndrome means that it is 99% certain that the baby does not have the condition.

An overall ''normal'' result does not guarantee that the pregnancy will come to term, or that the fetus does not suffer from some other defect. Laboratory tests are not 100% accurate at detecting targeted conditions, nor is it possible to test for every fetal condition.

Positive results indicate the presence of a birth defect with an accuracy approaching 100%. Prospective parents are then faced with emotionally and ethically difficult choices regarding treatment options, the prospect of dealing with a severely affected newborn, and the option of elective abortion. At this point, the parents need expert medical advice and counseling.

The alpha fetoprotein (AFP) test is a measure of a substance called alpha fetoprotein in a pregnant woman's blood. Alpha fetoprotein (AFP) is produced by an unborn baby's liver and is found in both the amniotic fluid and the mother's blood. Abnormally high amounts of AFP in the mother's blood indicates the fetus may have one of several serious **birth defects**. This screening test cannot diagnose a specific condition; it only indicates a risk of several birth defects. The AFP test also can be used to detect liver disease, certain cancerous tumors, and to monitor the progress of cancer treatment.

The exact function of this protein is unknown. After birth, the infant's liver stops producing AFP, and an adult liver contains only trace amounts. During pregnancy, the fetus excretes AFP in urine and some of the protein crosses the fetal membranes to enter the mother's blood. The level of AFP can then be determined by analyzing a sample of the mother's blood. It is very important that the doctor know precisely how old the fetus is when the test is performed since the AFP level changes over the length of the pregnancy. Errors in determining the age of the fetus lead to errors when interpreting the test results. Since an AFP test is only a screening tool, more specific tests must follow to make an accurate diagnosis. An abnormal test result does not necessarily mean that the fetus has a birth defect. The test has a high rate of abnormal results (either high or low).

The AFP test is usually performed during the 16th week of pregnancy. AFP can be measured in a blood test or in the sample of amniotic fluid taken at the time of amniocentesis. Test results are usually available after about one week.

The most common and severe type of birth defect that the AFP test can detect are spinal column defects such as (**spina bifida**) and anencephaly (abasence of brain tissue). During pregnancy, if the neural tube (the structure that will become the brain and spinal cord) doesn't close correctly, AFP may leak through this abnormal opening and enter the amniotic fluid. This leakage creates abnormally high levels of AFP in amniotic fluid and in the mother's blood.

Other fetal conditions that can raise AFP levels above normal include:

- Cysts at the end of the spine
- Blockage in the esophagus or intestines
- Liver disease
- Defects in the abdominal wall
- Kidney or urinary tract defects or disease
- Brittle bone disease.
- Too little fluid in the amniotic sac around the fetus

Levels may also be high if there is more than one developing fetus, or a pregnancy that is farther along than estimated.

For unknown reasons, abnormally low AFP may indicate that the fetus has an increased risk of Down syndrome. Down syndrome is a condition that includes **mental retardation** and a distinctive physical appearance. If the screening test indicates an abnormally low AFP, amniocentesis is used to diagnose the problem. Abnormally low levels of AFP can also occur when the fetus has died.

Although AFP in human blood gradually disappears after birth, it never disappears entirely. It may reappear in liver disease, or in tumors of the liver, ovaries, or testicles. The AFP test is used to screen people at high risk for these conditions. After a cancerous tumor is removed, an AFP test can monitor the progress of treatment. Continued high AFP levels suggest the cancer is growing.

The risks associated with drawing blood are minimal, but may include bleeding from the puncture site, feeling faint or lightheaded after the blood is drawn, or blood accumulating under the puncture site (hematoma).

If results are abnormal, the doctor will inform the woman of her specific increased risk as compared to the ''normal'' risk of a standard case. If the risk of Down syndrome is greater than the standard risk for women who are 35 years old or older (1 in 270), then amniocentesis is recommended. This screening test only predicts risk; appropriate diagnostic testing will follow after an abnormal screening result. In tumor or liver disease testing, an AFP level greater than 50 ng/mL is considered abnormal.

Prenatal surgery

The first human fetal surgery, performed in the 1950s, were fetal blood transfusions for Rh-positive babies whose red blood cells were under attack by the Rh-negative mother's immune system. Attempts to improve this technique via direct access to the fetus through an open uterus were unsuccessful, and open-womb fetal surgery was abandoned. The development of real-time **ultrasound** imaging in 1977 made intrauterine fetal surgery feasible: visual imaging permitted surgeons to accurately guide needles similar to those used for amniocentesis without the risk of damage to placenta or fetus. In the early 1980s, surgeons at several medical centers attempted closed-womb surgery to relieve fetal hydrocephalus (abnormal accumulation of fluid around the brain) by draining excess fluid. Although fluid could be drained, most babies were born with severe neurological defects. In 1981, pediatric surgeon Michael Harrison of the University of California at San Francisco developed a closed-womb shunting procedure to correct a urinary tract obstruction which afflicts one in every 2,000 male fetuses. In this defect, a blocked bladder damages or destroys the unborn baby's kidneys and, because the presence of the baby's urine in the amniotic fluid is vital for its lung development, the absence of urine is fatal. Although this technique is now widely used, it remains high-risk.

Harrison performed the first successful major open-womb surgery on a fetus on June 15, 1989 when he repaired a hole in the diaphragm of a 24-week-old fetus. In this pioneering operation, the unborn baby's arm was lifted out of his mother's womb through an incision in her abdomen and uterus, exposing the left side. The baby's misplaced internal organs were repositioned and the diaphragm and abdominal incisions patched with Gortex. The baby was born seven weeks later, premature but healthy. Harrison and his team successfully performed the same operation on a second fetus soon after. These successes were preceded by minor surgery on fetuses either inside or partially removed from the womb, although six previous procedures on humans had failed. Harrison prepared for human prenatal surgery by performing more than a thousand intrauterine operations on animals—the first successful animal fetal operations being carried out in the 1920s.

Prenatal surgery is still in its earliest stages and the success rate is not yet high, even though it is higher for some closed-womb procedures such as the bladder shunt. Risk remains high for both fetus and mother, and prenatal surgery is recommended for only a few conditions. One technique that has exciting possibilities is fetal stem-cell transplantation in which stem cells, the source of all blood cells, from a dead fetus are injected into a living fetus, providing healthy genetic material in an effort to overcome defective genes in the recipient fetus.

Preventive Medicine

Preventive medicine seeks to reduce the incidence of disease by modifying the environmental or behavioral factors that caused the illness in the first place.

Originally, preventive medicine was largely concerned with understanding and preventing infectious disease. Today, however, its scope has widened. The aim of preventive medicine is to preserve good health; to prevent disease, injury, and disability; and to facilitate early diagnosis and treatment of illness.

Preventive medicine has become a very diverse and challenging medical specialty. Preventive medicine physicians are trained in the sciences of epidemiology, biostatistics, environmental and occupational health services, administration, as well as clinical prevention. They are uniquely qualified to work with both individuals and the community to promote health and prevent disease, initiating programs in infectious **disease prevention** and control, **sexually transmitted diseases**, and in chronic disease prevention. They use scientific methods to identify health hazards in the workplace and work to prevent occupational illness and injury.

Preventive services offered to infants and children, adolescents, pregnant women, and adults have three components. The first step is a thorough **health screening**. This is done to identify disease or discover risk factors for certain diseases. The screening includes taking an extensive medical history and assessing the lifestyle pattern for risk factors. A physical examination follows the screening, which may include laboratory tests.

The next step in preventive medicine involves **counseling**. If the person's lifestyle has too many risk factors—such as **smoking**, over use of alcohol or other drugs, sex with multiple partners, unprotected sex—the physician explains the relationship between the risk factors and disease. The preventive medicine specialist will then either assist the patient or will direct the patient toward somebody who will help him to acquire the knowledge, motivation, and skills needed to maintain healthful behavior.

Immunization against infectious diseases and chemoprophylaxis (medication to prevent future diseases) form the third step of preventive medicine.

Clinical prevention strategies have proved to be extremely successful. Certain diseases, which were once common and often debilitating, have declined following the introduction of preventive services. Infectious diseases such as **poliomyelitis**, which once occurred in regular epidemic waves, have become rare as a result of childhood immunization. Similar trends have been seen with **diphtheria**, pertussis, and other common childhood infections. As a result of newborn screening and treatment, children with metabolic disorders such as **phenylketonuria** can now lead normal lives. (If the disease were left unidentified and untreated, they would have suffered irreversible **mental retardation**.)

Similarly, implementation of the screening programs such as the **PAP test** has led to dramatic reductions in the incidence of **cervical cancer** and the mortality associated with it. Early detection and treatment of **hypertension** has significantly reduced the incidence of death from **stroke**.

Although immunizations and screening tests remain important preventive services, the most challenging role for preventive medicine specialists lies in altering the lifestyle patterns of patients long before clinical disease develops. Currently, some of the leading causes of death in the United States are **heart attacks**, **cancer**, cerebrovascular disease, **chronic obstructive pulmonary disease**, **accidents**, and human immunodeficiency virus infections. Almost all of these can be prevented (or the risks minimized) by changing lifestyle patterns. Smoking contributes to one out of every five deaths in the USA. It is responsible for a large number of deaths from cancer, **coronary artery disease**, cerebrovascular disease, and pulmonary diseases. Failure to use safety belts and **drunk driving** are the major contributors to motor vehicle fatalities. Physical inactivity and dietary factors contribute to heart disease, diabetes, cancer, **osteoporosis**, and other diseases. High-risk sexual practices increase the risk of sexually transmitted diseases and **AIDS**. Most of these deaths are potentially preventable by changes in personal health practices.

Environmental strategies for health protection, such as providing safe water for drinking, fluoridation, lead abatement, regulations on public smoking, seat-belt laws, and safer highways, require the commitment of the entire community. Once these changes are made, they can have a far-reaching impact.

Priapism

Priapism is a rare condition which causes a persistent, and often painful, penile erection. Priapism is drug induced, injury related, or caused by disease, not sexual desire. As in a normal erection, the penis fills with blood and becomes erect. However, unlike a normal erection that dissipates after sexual activity ends, the persistent erection caused by priapism is maintained because the blood in the penile shaft does not drain. The shaft remains hard, while the tip of the penis is soft. If it is not relieved promptly, priapism can lead to permanent scarring of the penis and inability to have a normal erection.

Priapism is caused by leukemia, sickle cell disease, or **spinal cord injury**. It has also been associated as a rare side effect to trazodone (Desyrel), a drug prescribed to treat depression. An overdose of self-injected chemicals to counteract **impotence** has also been responsible for priapism. The chemicals are directly injected into the penis, and at least a quarter of all men who have used this method of treatment for over three months develop priapism.

A **physical examination** is needed to diagnose priapism. Further testing, including nuclear scanning or Doppler ultrasound, will diagnose the underlying cause of the condition.

There are three methods of treatment. The most effective is the injection of medicines into the penis that allow the blood to escape. Cold packs may also be applied to alleviate the condition, but this method becomes ineffective after about eight hours. For the most serious cases and those that do not respond to the first two treatments, a needle can be used to remove the blood. The tissues may need to be flushed with saline or diluted medications by the same needle method. That failing, there are more extensive surgical procedures available. One of them shuts off much of the blood supply to the penis so that it can relax. If the problem is due to a sickle cell crisis, treatment of the crisis with oxygen or **transfusion** may suffice.

If priapism is relieved within the first 12-24 hours, there is usually no residual damage. After that, permanent impotence may result, since the high pressure in the penis compromises blood flow and leads to tissue death (infarction). For patients with priapism due to sickle cell disease, an antineoplastic drug (hydroxyurea) may prevent future episodes of priapism.

Pringle, John (1707-1782)

Scottish Physician

John Pringle was born in Roxburgh, Scotland. He was sent at an early age to receive a classical education at the University of St. Andrews, where he studied under his uncle, Francis Pringle. He entered the University of Edinburgh in 1727, intending to pursue a career in business. After one year, he left the university to work in Amsterdam, where he hoped to acquire practical experience in commerce. Upon visiting the University of Leyden, he happened to attend a lecture by the distinguished Dutch physician **Hermann Boerhaave**. Impressed by the lecture, Pringle decided to enroll in the University, where he subsequently studied anatomy and surgery under Boerhaave and Bernhard Siegfried Albinus. Pringle received his degree in 1730, and he later completed postgraduate medical training in Paris. In 1734 he returned to Scotland, where he established himself in private practice while serving as professor of metaphysics and moral philosophy at the University of Edinburgh. In 1741 Pringle was appointed attending physician at the British Army hospital in Flanders during the war of the Austrian succession. Pringle also served at the battle of Culloden in 1745. In 1748, with the signing of a peace accord, Pringle settled into civilian medical practice, but he retained his position as military physician and surgeon. In recognition of his distinguished career, the royal family honored him with medical appointments to the Duke of Cumberland, Queen Charlotte and King George III, as well as a baronetcy in 1766 (a baronetcy is a rank of honor below a baron and above a knight; the holder of that rank is a baronet). Pringle was a member of the Royal Society (and the first person to use the term antiseptic in a paper he read before that body), serving as its president from 1772 to 1778. In 1778 he succeeded the Swedish botanist Carl Linnaeus as one of eight foreign members of the Academie des Sciences in Paris.

Today, many historians recognize Pringle as the father of modern **military medicine**. Pringle's contributions to medicine included putting into place a set of guidelines aimed at protecting the health of army personnel and making efforts to improve the conditions of prisoners of war. Pringle was the author of *Observations of Disease of the Army* (1752), which became a classic reference work on military hygiene and contagious diseases. Through six editions over 25 years it covered the fundamental principles of **sanitation** and housing, and notably the need for latrines and ventilated barracks. (Pringle was instrumental in securing better ventilation for those confined in ships, jails, barracks, and mines.) *Observations* was based on extensive clinical studies conducted while he served as director of the British Army hospital in Flanders.

Within a year of assuming that position, he had seen combat duty in the battle of Dettingen in Germany. Noting the obstacles facing medical personnel in times of war, Pringle proposed an international convention that would protect all medical facilities from attack. It was not until more than 100 years later, with the establishment of the Red Cross (1863), that primary hospitals and medical personnel were finally granted neutrality status.

Observations looked at many of the infectious diseases associated with military life, including **typhus**, **malaria**, epidemic **meningitis**, and dysentery. In describing these diseases as they developed through stages, Pringle supplied clinical evidence in support of the theory of contagion occurring from the spread of *animalcules* (minute, usually microscopic, organisms). Pringle is also credited with naming **influenza**.

See also Military medicine; Morgan, John

Prolapse rectal

Rectal prolapse is protrusion of rectal tissue through the anus to the exterior of the body. The rectum is the final section of the large intestine.

Rectal prolapse can be either partial or complete. In partial prolapse, only the mucosa layer (mucous membrane) of the rectum extends outside the body. The projection is generally 0.75-1.5 inches (2-4 cm) long. In complete prolapse, called procidentia, the full thickness of the rectum protrudes for up to 4.5 inches (12 cm).

Rectal prolapse is most common in people over age 60, and occurs much more frequently in women than in men. It is also more common in psychiatric patients. Prolapse can occur in normal infants, where it is usually transient. In children it is often an early sign of **cystic fibrosis** or is due to neurological or anatomical abnormalities.

Although rectal prolapse in adults may initially reduce spontaneously after bowel movements, it eventually becomes permanent. Adults who have had prior rectal or vaginal surgery, who have chronic **constipation**, regularly depend on **laxatives**, have **multiple sclerosis** or other neurologic diseases, **stroke**, or **paralysis** are more likely to experience rectal prolapse.

Rectal prolapse in adults is caused by a weakening of the sphincter muscle or ligaments that hold the rectum in place. Weakening can occur because of aging, disease, or in rare cases, surgical trauma. Prolapse is brought on by straining to have bowel movements, chronic laxative use, or severe **diarrhea**.

Symptoms of rectal prolapse include discharge of mucus or blood, **pain** during bowel movements, and inability to control bowel movements (fecal incontinence). Patients may also feel the mass of tissue protruding from the anus. With large prolapses, the patient may lose the normal urge to have a bowel movement.

Prolapse is initially diagnosed by taking a patient history and giving a rectal examination while the patient is in a squatting position. It is confirmed by sigmoidoscopy (inspection of the colon with a viewing instrument called a endoscope) Barium **enema** x rays and other tests are done to rule out neurologic (nerve) disorders or disease as the primary cause of prolapse.

In infants, conservative treatment, consisting of strapping the buttocks together between bowel movements and eliminating any causes of bowel straining, usually produces a spontaneous resolution of prolapse. For partial prolapse in adults, excess tissue is surgically tied off with special bands causing the tissue to wither in a few days.

Complete prolapse requires surgery. Different surgical techniques are used, but all involve anchoring the rectum to other parts of the body, and using plastic mesh to reinforce and support the rectum. In patients too old, or ill, to tolerate surgery, a wire or plastic loop can be inserted to hold the sphincter closed and prevent prolapse. Treatment should be undertaken as soon as prolapse is diagnosed, since the longer the condition exists, the more difficult it is to reverse.

Successful resolution of rectal prolapse involves prompt treatment and the elimination of any underlying causes of prolapse. Infants and children usually recover completely without complications. Recovery in adults depends on age, general health, and the extent of the prolapse.

Reducing constipation by eating a diet high in fiber, drinking plenty of fluids, and avoiding straining during bowel movements help prevent the onset of prolapse. **Exercise**s that strengthen the anal sphincter may also be helpful.

Prophylaxis

A prophylaxis is a measure taken to maintain health and prevent the spread of disease. Antibiotic prophylaxis refers to the use of **antibiotics** to prevent infections.

Antibiotics are well known for their ability to treat infections. But some antibiotics also are prescribed to *prevent* infections. This usually is done only in certain situations or for people with particular medical problems. For example, people with abnormal heart valves have a high risk of developing heart valve infections after even minor surgery. This happens because bacteria from other parts of the body get into the bloodstream during surgery and travel to the heart valves. To prevent these infections, people with heart valve problems often take antibiotics before having any kind of surgery, including dental surgery.

Antibiotics also may be prescribed to prevent infections in people with weakened immune systems, such as people with **AIDS** or people who are having **chemotherapy** treatments for **cancer**. But even healthy people with strong immune systems may occasionally be given preventive antibiotics—if they are having certain kinds of surgery that carry a high risk of infection, or if they are traveling to parts of the world where they are likely to get an infection that causes **diarrhea**, for example.

In all of these situations, a physician should be the one to decide whether antibiotics are necessary. Unless a physician says to do so, it is not a good idea to take antibiotics to prevent ordinary infections.

Because the overuse of antibiotics can lead to resistance, drugs taken to prevent infection should be used only for a short time.

Among the drugs used for antibiotic prophylaxis are amoxicillin (a type of penicillin) and fluoroquinolones such as ciprofloxacin (Cipro) and trovafloxacin (Trovan). These drugs are available only with a physician's prescription and come in tablet, capsule, liquid, and injectable forms.

The recommended dosage depends on the type of antibiotic prescribed and the reason it is being used. For the correct dosage, check with the physician or dentist who prescribed the medicine or the pharmacist who filled the prescription. Be sure to take the medicine exactly as prescribed. Do not take more or less than directed, and take the medicine only for as long as the physician or dentist says to take it.

If the medicine causes **nausea**, vomiting, or diarrhea, check with the physician or dentist who prescribed it as soon as possible. Patients who are taking antibiotics before surgery should not wait until the day of the surgery to report problems with the medicine. The physician or dentist needs to know right away if problems occur.

For other specific precautions, see the entry on the type of drug prescribed such as **penicillins** or fluoroquinolones.

Antibiotics may cause a number of side effects. For details, see entries on specific types of antibiotics. Anyone who has unusual or disturbing symptoms after taking antibiotics should get in touch with his or her physician.

Whether used to treat or to prevent infection, antibiotics may interact with other medicines. When this happens, the effects of one or both of the drugs may change or the risk of side effects may be greater. Anyone who takes antibiotics for any reason should inform the physician about all the other medicines he or she is taking and should ask whether any possible interactions may interfere with drugs' effects. For details of drug interactions, see entries on specific types of antibiotics.

PROSTATE CANCER

Prostate cancer is a disease is which the cells of the prostate become abnormal and start to grow uncontrollably, forming tumors. It is the most common **cancer** among men in the United States,and is the second leading cause of cancer **death**s.

The prostate, testicles, and seminal vesicles are the major male sex glands. These three glands together secrete the fluid that makes up semen. The prostate is about the size of a walnut and lies just behind the urinary bladder. A tumor in the prostate interferes with proper control of the bladder and normal sexual functioning. Often, the first symptom of prostate cancer to develop is difficulty in urinating.

The cause of prostate cancer is not known, however, it is found mainly in men over the age of 55. 80% of the prostate cancer cases occur in men over the age of 65. Hence, age appears to be a risk factor for prostate cancer. Race may be another contributing factor, because African-Americans have the highest rate of prostate cancer in the world.

A family history of prostate cancer may put a man at a higher risk for getting this disease. In addition, there is some evidence to suggest that a diet high in fat increases the risk of prostate cancer.

Frequently, prostate cancer has no symptoms, and the disease is diagnosed when the patient goes for a routine screening examination. However, occasionally, when the tumor is big or the cancer has spread to the nearby tissues, the following symptoms may be seen:

- Weak or interrupted flow of the urine
- Frequent urination (especially at night)
- Difficulty starting urination
- Inability to urinate
- **Pain** or burning sensation when urinating
- Blood in the urine
- Persistent pain in lower back, hips, or thighs (bone pain)
- Painful ejaculation.

In order to diagnose the disease doctor may conduct a digital rectal examination (DRE) to feel for any lumps in the prostate. The rectum lies just behind the prostate gland, and a majority of prostate tumors begin in the posterior region of the prostate. If the doctor does detect an abnormality, he or she may order more tests in order to confirm these findings.

Blood tests are used to measure the amounts of certain protein markers, such as prostate-specific antigen (PSA), found circulating in the blood. A technique known as ''transrectal ultrasound'' can also be used to detect tumors. In this test, a small probe is placed in the rectum, and sound waves are released from the probe. These sound waves bounce off the prostate tissue and an image is created. Since normal prostate tissue and prostate tumors reflect the sound waves differently, the test can detect tumors quite efficiently. If cancer is suspected, the doctor will remove a small piece of prostate tissue with a hollow needle. This is then checked under the microscope for the presence of cancerous cells. Prostate **biopsy** is the most definitive diagnostic tool for prostate cancer.

The doctor and the patient will decide on the treatment mode after considering many factors. For example, the patient's age, the stage of the tumor, his general health, and the presence of any co-existing illnesses have to be considered. In addition, the patient's personal preferences and the risks and benefits of each treatment protocol are also taken into account before any decision is made.

For early stage prostate cancer, surgery is the best option and the most common one. Radical prostatectomy involves complete removal of the prostate. Because the seminal vesicles (the gland where the sperm is made) are removed along with the prostate, **infertility** is a side effect of this type of surgery. In a different surgical method, known as the transurethral resection procedure or TURP, only the cancerous portion of the prostate is removed, by using a small wire loop that is introduced into the prostate through the urethra. This technique is most often used in men who cannot have a radical prostatectomy due to age or other illness, and it is rarely recommended.

Radiation therapy involves the use of high-energy x rays to kill cancer cells or to shrink tumors. It can be used instead of surgery for early stage cancer. Hormone therapy is commonly used when the cancer is in an advanced stage and has spread to other parts of the body. Prostate cells need the male hormone testosterone to grow. Decreasing the levels of this hormone, or inhibiting its activity, will cause the cancer to shrink. Hormone levels can be decreased in several ways.

Drugs (such as LHRH agonists or anti-androgens) that bind to the male hormone testosterone and block its activity can be given. Another method tricks the body by administering the female hormone estrogen. When this is given, the body senses the presence of a sex hormone and stops making the male hormone testosterone. Alternatively, a surgical procedure which involves the complete removal of the testicles can be done. However, there are some unpleasant side effects to hormone therapy.

Chemotherapy is the use of drugs to kill cancer cells. The drugs can either be taken as a pill or injected into the body through a needle that is inserted into a blood vessel. Chemotherapy is sometimes used to treat prostate cancer that has recurred after other treatment.

Due to early detection and better screening methods, nearly 60% of the tumors are diagnosed while they are still confined to the prostate gland. The five-year survival rate for early stage cancers is almost 99%.

Because the cause of the cancer is not known, there is no definite way to prevent prostate cancer. However, the American Cancer Society (ACS) recommends that all men over age 40 have an annual rectal exam and that men have an annual PSA test beginning at age 50. African-American men and men with a family history of prostate cancer, who have a higher than average risk, should begin annual PSA testing even earlier, starting at age 45. A low fat diet may slow the progression of prostate cancer.

PROSTATITIS

Prostatitis is an inflammation of the prostate gland, a common condition in adult males. Often caused by infection, prostatitis may develop rapidly (*acute*) or slowly (*chronic*).

Prostatitis may be the symptom-producing disease of the genitourinary tract for which men most often seek medical help. About 40% of visits to a specialist in genitourinary problems (urologist) are for prostatitis. Forms of prostate inflammation include acute and chronic bacterial prostatitis and inflammation not caused by bacterial infection. A painful condition called *prostatodynia*, which may be caused by abnormal nerves or muscles in the region, is also thought to be a form of prostatitis. The chronic bacterial form is sometimes experienced by men whose sex partners have a bacterial infection of the vagina, making this a sexually transmitted disease. Other cases occur when small stones form within the prostate and become infected. Sometimes infection is caused by poor hygiene, surgical procedures, or even swimming in polluted water.

The sexually transmitted disease **gonorrhea** may sometimes cause prostatitis, and **tuberculosis** may spread to the prostate. Parasites and fungi may infect the prostate gland. Some men whose prostatitis is not caused by any microorganism have microscopic collections of cells called *granulomas* in their prostate tissue. Whether viruses also may cause prostatitis is debatable.

However the inflammation may begin, it causes blockages in the tiny glands within the prostate so that secretions build up, and the prostate swells. In acute cases, this swelling can occur very suddenly and cause considerable pain. When prostatitis develops gradually, trouble with the flow of urine may be the first symptom. Small stones may form, because the body attempts to neutralize bacteria by coating them with calcium. These stones may become infected themselves and make the condition worse.

Symptoms and signs that are typically experienced by men with prostatitis include:

- Difficulties in urinating. Most urinary problems are caused when the swollen prostate blocks the tube that carries urine from the bladder to the outside of the body (urethra). Patients feel the need to urinate more often than usual, often urgently. Urination is sometimes painful. It is hard to start the flow of urine and difficult to totally empty the bladder. Patients wake up at night to urinate. The stream may be weak or split. Dribbling after attempts to urinate may leave embarrassing wet spots on clothing. In severe prostatitis blood or sand-like particles (small calcium collections) may be passed in the urine.
- Pain. Besides pain when urinating, caused by prostate swelling, stimulation of nerves in the prostate gland may cause pain in the penis, one or both testicles, the lower stomach, the low back, and the area between the scrotum and the anus (perineum). Some patients experience pain during or after ejaculation, whenever they sit down or walk, or during bowel movements.
- Sex and fertility. The pain of prostatitis can make it impossible to enjoy sex. Men with prostatitis may be troubled by early release of sperm (**premature ejaculation**). Occasionally there is blood in the semen. Some of the drugs prescribed to ease the flow of the urine can dampen the desire to have sex. Because the normal prostate secretions make up part of the semen, prostatitis may lower fertility by severely lowering the number of sperm and making them less mobile.
- Psychological problems. A man with prostatitis who feels that nothing can be done and he ''just has to live with it'' may experience serious depression. Low sexual desire certainly contributes to depression.

A person with *acute prostatitis* may suddenly develop **fever** and chills, along with rapidly developing urinary symptoms and pain in the perineum or low back. This state is a medical emergency that demands immediate medical help.

Most often the symptoms and physical findings are enough to form a diagnosis of prostatitis. When the examiner inserts a finger in the rectum, the swollen prostate can be felt; it may be extremely tender when probed. Squeezing the gland slightly will produce a few drops of fluid that may be *cultured* to learn whether bacteria are present. The fluid typically contains a large number of white blood cells, especially the cells used to fight off infection (*macrophages*). Note: too much pressure on the prostate can force bacteria into the blood and cause a serious general infection. Many patients with chronic bacterial prostatitis also have recurring urinary tract infections (diagnosed by examining and culturing urine samples). These infections can be an important clue to the diagnosis. If doubt remains, the urologist may insert a special instrument called a *cystoscope* through the penis to directly view the prostate from inside and see whether it looks inflamed.

Acute prostatitis is first treated with **antibiotics**. Even though it may be difficult for drugs to actually get into the inflamed prostate, most patients do quickly get better. If intravenous antibiotics are needed or the bladder is retaining urine, a hospital stay may be necessary. Broad-spectrum antibiotics that work against most bacteria are used first. At the same time tests are done with samples of prostatic fluid to determine which bacterium is causing the infection, so that drugs can be prescribed to fight the specific germ. In chronic cases, the best results are obtained with a combination of the antibiotics trimethoprim and sulfamethoxazole. Oral antibiotics should be given for 1-3 months; longer, if necessary. If a fungus or some other organism is causing infection, special drugs are available. If chronic prostatitis continues despite all medical efforts and is seriously affecting the patient's life, the prostate may be removed surgically.

Nonbacterial prostatitis requires other measures to relieve urinary symptoms. These measures include drugs that fight inflammation (steroids or non-steroids) and a type of drug called an alpha-blocker that reduces muscle tension. Reduced muscle tension eases urine flow, allowing the bladder to empty. A narrowed urethra may be widened by placing a collapsed balloon at the site of obstruction and expanding it. This procedure is called *balloon dilation*. The effects of such dilation are usually temporary. Some physicians believe that stress is an important factor in prostatitis, and therefore prescribe diazepam (Valium) or another tranquilizer. The type of prostatitis known as prostatodynia is usually treated with a combination of muscle relaxing drugs, heat, special **exercise**s, and sometimes a tranquilizer.

There are a number of ''tips'' for relieving symptoms of prostatitis. They are especially helpful early on, before antibiotics have a chance to cure infection, or for patients with chronic or non-bacterial prostatitis:

- Hot sitz baths. Exposing the perineum to very hot water for 20 minutes or longer often relieves pain.
- Ice. When heat does not help, ice packs, or simply placing a small ice cube in the rectum, may relieve pain for hours.
- Water. A patient who has to urinate very often may want to cut back on his fluid intake but this will cause **dehydration** and increase the risk of bladder infection. Instead, it is best to drink plenty of water.
- Diet. Most doctors recommend cutting out—or cutting down on—**caffeine** (as in coffee or tea), alcohol, and spicy or acid foods. **Constipation** should be avoided because large, hard bowel movements may press on the swollen prostate and cause great pain. Bran cereals and whole-grain breads are helpful.
- Exercise. It is especially important for patients with chronic prostatitis to keep up their activity level. Simply walking often will help (unless walking happens to make the pain worse).
- Frequent ejaculation. Ejaculating two or three times a week often is recommended, especially when taking antibiotics.

A treatment popularized in the Philippines is called ''prostate drainage.'' At regular intervals, a finger is inserted into the rectum, to exert pressure on the prostate at the same time that an antibiotic treatment is given. Acupuncture and Chinese herbal medicine also can be effective in treating prostatitis. Nutritional supplements that support the prostate, including zinc, omega-3 fatty acids, several amino acids, and anti-inflammatory nutrients and herbs, can help reduce pain and promote healing. Western herbal medicine recommends saw palmetto *Serenoa repens* to support the prostate gland. Hot and cold contrast sitz baths can help reduce inflammation.

Most patients with acute bacterial prostatitis are cured if they receive proper antibiotic treatment. Every effort should be made to get a cure at the acute stage because chronic prostatitis can be much more difficult to eliminate. If the acute illness is *not* controlled, complications such as a localized infection (prostatic **abscess**), kidney infection, or infection of the blood (septicemia) may develop. When chronic prostatitis cannot be cured, it still is possible to keep urinary symptoms under control and keep the patient active by using low doses of antibiotics and other measures. If a man with any form of prostatitis develops serious psychological problems, he should be referred to a psychiatric specialist.

Potential sources of infection should be avoided. Good perineal hygiene should be maintained and sex should be avoided when one's partner has an active bacterial vaginal infection. If the kidneys, bladder, or other genitourinary organs are infected, prompt treatment may prevent the development of prostatitis. By far the best way of preventing chronic prostatitis is to treat an initial *acute* episode promptly and effectively.

PROTEASE INHIBITORS

A protease inhibitor is a type of drug that cripples the enzyme protease. An enzyme is a substance that triggers chemical reactions in the body. The human **immunodeficiency** virus (HIV) uses protease in the final stages of its reproduction (replication) process.

The drug is used to treat selected patients with HIV infection. Blocking protease interferes with HIV reproduction, causing it to make copies of itself that cannot infect new cells. The drug may improve symptoms and suppress the infection but does not cure it.

Patients should not discontinue this drug even if symptoms improve without consulting a doctor.

These drugs do not necessarily reduce the risk of transmitting HIV to others through sexual contact, so patients should avoid sexual activities or use **condom**s.

Protease inhibitors are considered one of the most potent medications for HIV developed so far.

This class of drugs includes indinavir (Crixivan), ritonavir (Norvir), nelfinavir (Viracept) and saquinavir (Invirase or Fortovase). Several weeks or months of drug therapy may be required before the full benefits are apparent.

The drug should be taken at the same time each day. Some types should be taken with a meal to help the body absorb them. Each of the types of protease inhibitor may have to be taken in a different way.

Common side effects include **diarrhea**, stomach discomfort, nausea, and mouth sores. Less often, patients may experience rash, muscle **pain**, **headache**, or weakness. Rarely, there may be confusion, severe skin reaction, or seizures. Some of these drugs can have interactions with other medication, and indinavir can be associated with **kidney stones**. Diabetes or high blood pressure may become worse when these drugs are taken.

Experts do not know whether the drugs pass into breast milk, so breastfeeding mothers should avoid them or should stop nursing until the treatment is completed.

PROTEIN-ENERGY MALNUTRITION

Protein-energy malnutrition (PEM) is a potentially fatal body-depletion disorder. It is the leading cause of death in children in developing countries.

PEM is also referred to as protein-calorie **malnutrition**. It develops in children and adults whose consumption of protein and energy (measured by calories) is insufficient to satisfy the body's nutritional needs. While pure protein deficiency can occur when a person's diet provides enough energy but lacks the protein minimum, in most cases the deficiency will be dual. PEM may also occur in persons who are unable to absorb vital nutrients or convert them to energy essential for healthy tissue formation and organ function.

Although PEM is not prevalent among the general population of the United States, it is often seen in elderly people who live in nursing homes and in children whose parents are poor. PEM occurs in one of every two surgical patients and in 48% of all other hospital patients.

Primary PEM results from a diet that lacks sufficient sources of protein and/or energy. Secondary PEM is more common in the United States, where it usually occurs as a complication of AIDS, cancer, chronic kidney failure, inflammatory bowel disease, and other illnesses that impair the body's ability to absorb or use nutrients or to compensate for nutrient losses. PEM can develop gradually in a patient who has a chronic illness or experiences chronic semi-**starvation**. It may appear suddenly in a patient who has an acute illness.

Kwashiorkor, also called wet protein-energy malnutrition, is a form of PEM characterized primarily by protein deficiency. This condition usually appears at the age of about 12 months when breastfeeding is discontinued, but it can develop at any time during a child's formative years. It causes fluid retention (edema); dry, peeling skin; and hair discoloration.

Primarily caused by energy deficiency, marasmus is characterized by stunted growth and wasting of muscle and tissue. Marasmus usually develops between the ages of six months and one year in children who have been weaned from breast milk or who suffer from weakening conditions like chronic **diarrhea**.

Secondary PEM symptoms range from mild to severe, and can alter the form or function of almost every organ in the body. The type and intensity of symptoms depends on the patient's prior nutritional status and on the nature of the underlying disease and the speed at which it is progressing.

Mild, moderate, and severe classifications have not been precisely defined, but patients who lose 10-20% of their body weight without trying are usually said to have moderate PEM. This condition is also characterized by a weakened grip and inability to perform high-energy tasks.

Losing 20% of body weight or more is generally classified as severe PEM. People with this condition can't eat normal-sized meals. They have slow heart rates and low blood pressure and body temperatures. Other symptoms of severe secondary PEM include baggy, wrinkled skin; **constipation**; dry, thin, brittle hair; lethargy; pressure sores and other **skin lesions**.

People who have kwashiorkor often have extremely thin arms and legs, but liver enlargement and ascites (abnormal accumulation of fluid) can distend the abdomen and disguise weight loss. Hair may turn red or yellow. Anemia, diarrhea, and fluid and electrolyte disorders are common. The body's immune system is often weakened, behavioral development is slow, and mental retardation may occur. Children may grow to normal height but are abnormally thin.

Kwashiorkor-like secondary PEM usually develops in patients who have been severely burned, suffered trauma, or had **sepsis** (tissue-destroying infection) or another life-threatening illness. The condition's onset is so sudden that body fat and muscle mass of normal-weight people may not change. Some obese patients even gain weight.

Profound weakness accompanies severe marasmus. Since the body breaks down its own tissue to use as calories, people with this condition lose all their body fat and muscle strength, and acquire a skeletal appearance most noticeable in the hands and in the temporal muscle in front of and above each ear. Children with marasmus are small for their age. Since their immune systems are weakened, they suffer from frequent infections. Other symptoms include loss of appetite, diarrhea, skin that is dry and baggy, sparse hair that is dull brown or reddish yellow, mental retardation, behavioral retardation, low body temperature (hypothermia), and slow pulse and breathing rates.

The absence of **edema** distinguishes marasmus-like secondary PEM, a gradual wasting process that begins with weight loss and progresses to mild, moderate, or severe malnutrition (cachexia). It is usually associated with cancer, **chronic obstructive pulmonary disease** (COPD), or another chronic disease that is inactive or progressing very slowly.

Some individuals have both kwashiorkor and marasmus at the same time. This most often occurs when a person who has a chronic, inactive condition develops symptoms of an acute illness.

Difficulty chewing, swallowing, and digesting food, **pain**, **nausea**, and lack of appetite are among the most common reasons that many hospital patients don't consume enough nutrients. Nutrient loss can be accelerated by bleeding, diarrhea, abnormally high sugar levels (glycosuria), kidney disease, malabsorption disorders, and other factors. **Fever**, infection, surgery, and benign or malignant tumors increase the amount of nutrients hospitalized patients need. So do trauma, **burns**, and some medications.

A thorough **physical examination** and a health history that probes eating habits and weight changes, focuses on body-fat composition and muscle strength, and assesses gastrointestinal symptoms, underlying illness, and nutritional status is often as accurate as blood tests and urinalyses used to detect and document abnormalities.

Some doctors further quantify a patient's nutritional status by:

- comparing height and weight to standardized norms
- calculating body mass index (BMI)
- measuring skinfold thickness or the circumference of the upper arm.

Treatment is designed to provide adequate nutrition, restore normal body composition, and cure the condition that caused the deficiency. Tube feeding or intravenous feeding is used to supply nutrients to patients who can't or won't eat protein-rich foods.

In patients with severe PEM, the first stage of treatment consists of correcting fluid and electrolyte imbalances, treating infection with **antibiotics** that don't affect protein synthesis, and addressing related medical problems. The second phase involves replenishing essential nutrients slowly to prevent taxing the patient's weakened system with more food than it can handle. Physical therapy may be beneficial to patients whose muscles have deteriorated significantly.

Most people can lose up to 10% of their body weight without side effects, but losing more than 40% is almost always fatal. Death usually results from heart failure, an electrolyte imbalance, or low body temperature. Patients with certain symptoms, including semiconsciousness, persistent diarrhea, jaundice, and low blood sodium levels, have a poorer prognosis than other patients. Recovery from marasmus usually takes longer than recovery from kwashiorkor. The long-term effects of childhood malnutrition are uncertain. Some children recover completely, while others may have a variety of lifelong impairments, including an inability to properly absorb nutrients in the intestines and mental retardation. The outcome appears to be related to the length and severity of the malnutrition, as well as to the age of the child when the malnutrition occurred.

Breastfeeding a baby for at least six months is considered the best way to prevent early-childhood malnutrition. Preventing malnutrition in developing countries is a complicated and challenging problem. Providing food directly during famine can help in the short-term, but more long-term solutions are needed, including agricultural development, public health programs (especially programs that monitor growth and development, as well as programs that provide nutritional information and supplements), and improved food distribution systems. Programs that distribute infant formula and discourage breast feeding should be discontinued, except in areas where many mothers are infected with HIV.

Every patient being admitted to a hospital should be screened for the presence of illnesses and conditions that could lead to PEM. The nutritional status of patients at higher-than-average risk should be more thoroughly assessed and periodically reevaluated during extended hospital stays or nursing home residence.

Prusiner, Stanley B. (1942-)

American neurologist

Prusiner won the 1997 Nobel Prize in Physiology or Medicine for his ground-breaking, yet controversial, work on a type of protein particle, a prion, that he hypothesized was responsible for a number of fatal neurodegenerative disorders, including **Creutzfeldt-Jakob disease** (CJD) and mad cow disease.

Prusiner was born on May 28, 1942, in Des Moines, Iowa. He earned his B.A., *cum laude*, at the University of Pennsylvania, in 1964, and then went on to receive an M.D. in 1968 from the same university. Prusiner then served his internship and residency at the prestigious University of California at San Francisco (UCSF) from 1968 to 1969, where he later served a residency in neurology. Prusiner soon became interested in neurodegenerative diseases. This interest was in part developed after one of his patients died of CJD, a disease of the cerebral cortex which leads to dementia and eventual death.

As a result of this experience, Prusiner learned that an entire category of diseases was yet to be elucidated. At the time, researchers thought many neurodegenerative diseases were caused by so-called slow viruses, which would take years and sometimes decades to incubate in the host. As early as 1967, a British team working at Hammersmith Hospital had proposed the existence of an infective agent that lacked nucleic acid in the sheep disease known as scrapie (so called because infected sheep tend to scrape the wool off their bodies). Their hypothesis grew out of the fact that when the genetic substance was destroyed in known infected material, extracts from the infected material were still able to spread the disease. This led to the conclusion that perhaps the infective agents in such animal diseases as scrapie and kuru (a disease of the cannibalistic Fore people of New Guinea which had been traced to the ritual eating of the brains of departed relatives) were non-viral.

Prusiner combined a zeal for research with a disarming political sense to win grants for the study of such diseases, including CJD, scrapie, kuru, fatal familial insomnia, and bovine spongiform encephalopathy (BSE), or mad cow disease. Over three decades, he managed to gain funding totaling 56 million dollars from the National Institutes of Health (NIH).

Expanding on work by British researchers as well as the NIH's Rocky Mountain Laboratories, which had shown similarities between kuru and scrapie, Prusiner set up a research team at UCSF employing ultimately a quarter million mice infected with diseased brain matter in an attempt to isolate the infective agent in neurodegenerative diseases. Such research was laborious and time-consuming, for the incubation period in mice took upwards of 200 days. Early breakthroughs occurred when Prusiner switched from mice to hamsters, as the onset of illness in those animals would occur twice as fast. By 1981, Prusiner was able to conclude that a protein was the causative agent in these brain diseases, and he dubbed this agent the prion. Such proteins were resistant to any modification of nucleic acids. When he and his team added enzymes that destroy nucleic acids in genes, they discovered that there was no reduction in the infective power of prions.

By 1992, Prusiner's research more clearly demonstrated the nature of the interaction between prion proteins. Prusiner showed that when the gene encoding for the prion protein in mice was destroyed, such mice (called prion knock-out mice) proved resistant to the diseases when injected with preparations of disease-causing prion protein. Later, when the prion gene was re-activated and the same mice were injected with diseased matter, they again became susceptible to infection. Though the role of prion proteins is unclear, what has become clear is the close causative effect of prions in a variety of neural diseases.

The diseases which Prusiner studied are life-threatening to only a tiny fraction of the world's population—the annual death toll of CJD in the United States annually, for example, is about 225, less than the number of traffic fatalities in two days. However, as the Nobel committee noted, Prusiner's research could lead to new therapies for a larger array of neurological disorders such as **Alzheimer's** and **Parkinson's disease**, which may or may not be caused by protein-based infective agents. In the case of prion-based diseases, Prusiner has suggested gene therapy to curtail the production of prion proteins and thus eliminate the spread of such diseases, as was done with his prion knock-out mice.

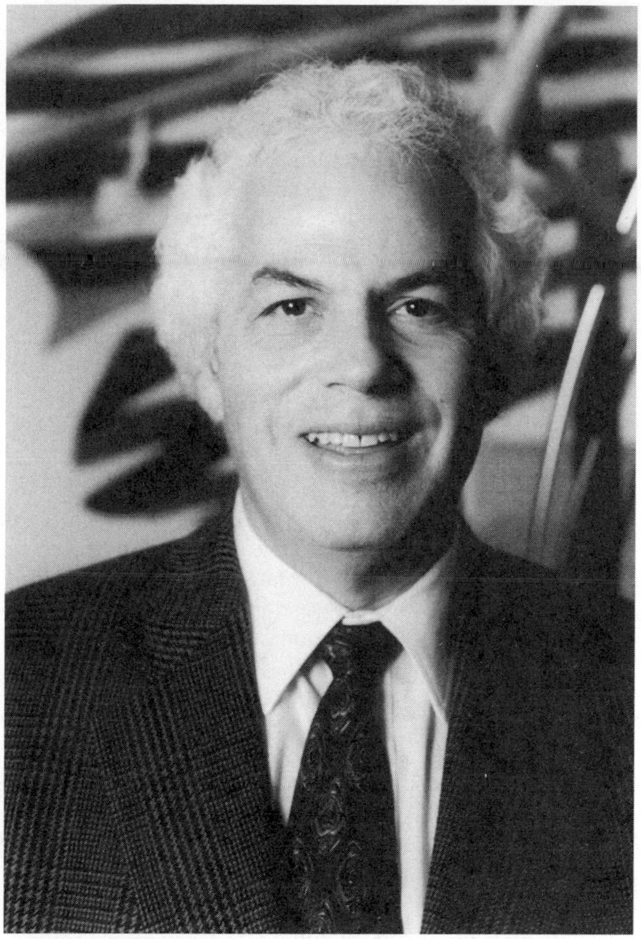

Stanley B. Prusiner

PSEUDOMONAS INFECTIONS

A pseudomonas infection is caused by a bacterium, *Pseudomonas aeruginosa*, and may affect any part of the body. In most cases, however, pseudomonas infections strike only persons who are very ill, usually hospitalized.

P. aeruginosa is a rod-shaped organism that can be found in soil, water, plants, and animals. Because it rarely causes disease in healthy persons, but infects those who are already sick or who have weakened immune systems, it is called an opportunistic pathogen. Opportunistic pathogens are organisms that do not ordinarily cause disease, but multiply freely in persons whose immune systems are weakened by illness or medication. Such persons are said to be immunocompromised. Patients with **AIDS** have an increased risk of developing serious pseudomonas infections. Hospitalized patients are another high-risk group, because *P. aeruginosa* is often found in hospitals. Infections that can be acquired in the hospital are sometimes called nosocomial diseases.

Of the 2 million nosocomial infections each year, 10% are caused by *P. aeruginosa*. The bacterium is the second most common cause of nosocomial **pneumonia** and the most common cause of intensive care unit (ICU) pneumonia. Pseudomonas infections can be spread within hospitals by health care workers, medical equipment, sinks, disinfectant solutions, and food. These infections are a very serious problem in hospitals for two reasons. First, patients who are critically ill can die from a pseudomonas infection. Second, many *Pseudomonas* bacteria are resistant to certain **antibiotics**, which makes them difficult to treat.

P. aeruginosa is able to infect many different parts of the body. Several factors make it a strong opponent. These factors include:

- The ability to stick to cells
- Minimal food requirements
- Resistance to many antibiotics
- Production of proteins that damage tissue
- A protective outer coat

Infections that can occur in specific body sites include:

- Heart and blood. *P. aeruginosa* is the fourth most common cause of bacterial infections of the blood (**bacteremia**). Bacteremia is common in patients with blood **cancer** and patients who have pseudomonas infections elsewhere in the body. *P. aeruginosa* infects the heart valves of intravenous drug abusers and persons with **artificial heart valves**.
- Bones and joints. Pseudomonas infections in these parts of the body can result from injury, the spread of infection from other body tissues, or bacteremia. Persons at risk for pseudomonas infections of the bones and joints include diabetics, intravenous drug abusers, and bone surgery patients.
- Central nervous system. *P. aeruginosa* can cause inflammation of the tissues covering the brain and spinal cord (**meningitis**) and brain **abscess**es. These infections may result from brain injury or surgery, the spread of infection from other parts of the body, or bacteremia.

- Eye and ear. *P. aeruginosa* can cause infections in the external ear canal—so-called ''swimmer's ear''—that usually disappear without treatment. The bacterium can cause a more serious ear infection in elderly patients, possibly leading to hearing problems, facial **paralysis**, or even **death**. Pseudomonas infections of the eye usually follow an injury. They can cause ulcers of the cornea that may cause rapid tissue destruction and eventual blindness. The risk factors for pseudomonas eye infections include: wearing soft extended-wear contact lenses; using topical corticosteroid eye medications; being in a **coma**; having extensive **burns**; undergoing treatment in an ICU; and having a tracheostomy or endotracheal tube.
- Urinary tract. Urinary tract infections can be caused by catheterization, medical instruments, and surgery.
- Lung. Risk factors for *P. aeruginosa* pneumonia include: **cystic fibrosis**; chronic lung disease; immunocompromised condition; being on antibiotic therapy or a respirator; and congestive **heart failure**. Cystic fibrosis patients often develop pseudomonas infections as children and suffer recurrent attacks of pneumonia.
- Skin and soft tissue. Even healthy persons can develop a pseudomonas skin rash following exposure to the bacterium in contaminated hot tubs, water parks, whirlpools, or spas. This skin disorder is called pseudomonas or ''hot tub'' folliculitis, and is often confused with **chickenpox**. Severe skin infection may occur in patients with *P. aeruginosa* bacteremia. The bacterium is the second most common cause of burn wound infections in hospitalized patients.

P. aeruginosa can be sudden and severe, or slow in onset and cause little **pain**. Risk factors for acquiring a pseudomonas infection include: having a serious illness; being hospitalized; undergoing an invasive procedure such as surgery; having a weakened immune system; and being treated with antibiotics that kill many different kinds of bacteria (broad-spectrum antibiotics).

Each of the infections listed above has its own set of symptoms. *Pseudomonas* bacteremia resembles other bacteremias, producing **fever**, tiredness, muscle pains, joint pains, and chills. Bone infections are marked by swelling, redness, and pain at the infected site and possibly fever. *Pseudomonas* meningitis causes fever, **headache**, irritability, and clouded consciousness. Ear infection is associated with pain, ear drainage, facial paralysis, and reduced hearing. Pseudomonas infections of the eye cause ulcers that may spread to cover the entire eye, pain, reduced vision, swelling of the eyelids, and pus accumulation within the eye.

P. aeruginosa pneumonia is marked by chills, fever, productive **cough**, difficult breathing, and blue-tinted skin. Cystic fibrosis patients with pseudomonas lung infections experience coughing, decreased appetite, weight loss, tiredness, **wheezing**, rapid breathing, fever, blue-tinted skin, and abdominal enlargement. Skin infections can cause a range of symptoms from a mild rash to large bleeding ulcers. Symptoms of pseudomonas folliculitis include a red itchy rash, headache, **dizziness**, earache, sore eyes, nose, and throat, breast tenderness, and stomach pain. Pseudomonas wound infections may secrete a blue-green colored fluid and have a fruity smell. Burn wound infections usually occur one to two weeks after the burn and cause discoloration of the burn scab, destruction of the tissue below the scab, early scab loss, bleeding, swelling, and a blue-green drainage.

Diagnosis and treatment of pseudomonas infections can be performed by specialists in infectious disease. Because *P. aeruginosa* is commonly found in hospitals, many patients carry the bacterium without having a full-blown infection. Consequently, the mere presence of *P. aeruginosa* in patients does not constitute a diagnostic finding. Cultures, however, can be easily done for test purposes. The organism grows readily in laboratory media; results are usually available in two to three days. Depending on the location of the infection, body fluids that can be tested for *P. aeruginosa* include blood, urine, cerebrospinal fluid, sputum, pus, and drainage from an infected ear or eye. X rays and other imaging techniques can be used to assess infections in deep organ tissues.

Because *P. aeruginosa* is commonly resistant to antibiotics, infections are usually treated with two antibiotics at once. Pseudomonas infections may be treated with combinations of ceftazidime (Ceftaz, Fortraz, Tazicef), ciprofloxacin (Cipro), imipenem (Primaxin), gentamicin (Garamycin), tobramycin (Nebcin), ticarcillin-clavulanate (Timentin), or piperacillin-tazobactam (Zosyn). Most antibiotics are administered intravenously or orally for two to six weeks. Treatment of an eye infection requires local application of antibiotic drops.

Surgical treatment of pseudomonas infections is sometimes necessary to remove infected and damaged tissue. Surgery may be required for brain abscesses, eye infections, bone and joint infections, ear infections, heart infections, and wound infections. Infected **wounds** and burns may cause permanent damage requiring arm or leg **amputation**.

Most pseudomonas infections can be successfully treated with antibiotics and surgery. In immunocompromised persons, however, *P. aeruginosa* infections have a high mortality rate, particularly following bacteremia or infections of the lower lung. Mortality rates range from 15-20% of patients with severe ear infections to 89% of patients with infections of the left side of the heart.

Most hospitals have programs for the prevention of nosocomial infections. Cystic fibrosis patients may be given periodic doses of antibiotics to prevent episodes of pseudomonas pneumonia.

Minor skin infections can be prevented by avoiding hot tubs with cloudy water; avoiding public swimming pools at the end of the day; removing wet swimsuits as soon as possible; bathing after sharing a hot tub or using a public pool; cleaning hot tub filters every six weeks; and using appropriate amounts of chlorine in the water.

Psoriasis

Named for the Greek word *psōra* meaning "itch," psoriasis is a chronic, non-contagious disease characterized by inflamed lesions covered with silvery-white scabs of dead skin.

Psoriasis, which affects at least four million Americans, is slightly more common in women than in men. Although the disease can develop at any time, and 10-15% of all cases are diagnosed in children under 10, and the average age at the onset of symptoms is 28. Psoriasis is most common in fair-skinned people and extremely rare in dark-skinned individuals.

Normal skin cells mature and replace dead skin every 28-30 days. Psoriasis causes skin cells to mature in less than a week. Because the body can't shed old skin as rapidly as new cells are rising to the surface, raised patches of dead skin develop on the arms, back, chest, elbows, legs, nails, folds between the buttocks, and scalp.

Psoriasis is considered mild if it affects less than 5% of the surface of the body; moderate, if 5-30% of the skin is involved, and severe, if the disease affects more than 30% of the body surface.

Dermatologists distinguish different forms of psoriasis according to what part of the body is affected, how severe symptoms are, how long they last, and the pattern formed by the scales.

Plaque psoriasis (psoriasis vulgaris), the most common form of the disease, is characterized by small, red bumps that enlarge, become inflamed, and form scales. The top scales flake off easily and often, but those beneath the surface of the skin clump together. Removing these scales exposes tender skin, which bleeds and causes the plaques (inflamed patches) to grow.

Plaque psoriasis can develop on any part of the body, but most often occurs on the elbows, knees, scalp, and trunk.

At least 50 of every 100 people who have any form of psoriasis have scalp psoriasis. This form of the disease is characterized by scale-capped plaques on the surface of the skull.

The first sign of nail psoriasis is usually pitting of the fingernails or toenails. Size, shape, and depth of the marks vary, and affected nails may thicken, yellow, or crumble. The skin around an affected nail is sometimes inflamed, and the nail may peel away from the nail bed.

Named for the Latin word *gutta,* which means "a drop," guttate psoriasis is characterized by small, red, drop-like dots that enlarge rapidly and may be somewhat scaly. Often found on the arms, legs, and trunk and sometimes in the scalp, guttate psoriasis can clear up without treatment or disappear and resurface in the form of plaque psoriasis.

Pustular psoriasis usually occurs in adults. It is characterized by blister-like lesions filled with non-infectious pus and surrounded by reddened skin. Pustular psoriasis, which can be limited to one part of the body (localized) or can be widespread, may be the first symptom of psoriasis or develop in a patient with chronic plaque psoriasis.

Generalized pustular psoriasis is also known as Von Zumbusch pustular psoriasis. Widespread, acutely painful patches of inflamed skin develop suddenly. Pustules appear within a few hours, then dry and peel within two days.

Generalized pustular psoriasis can make life-threatening demands on the heart and kidneys.

Palomar-plantar pustulosis (PPP) generally appears between the ages of 20 and 60. PPP causes large pustules to form at the base of the thumb or on the sides of the heel. In time, the pustules turn brown and peel. The disease usually becomes much less active for a while after peeling.

Acrodermatitis continua of Hallopeau is a form of PPP characterized by painful, often disabling, lesions on the fingertips or the tips of the toes. The nails may become deformed, and the disease can damage bone in the affected area.

Inverse psoriasis occurs in the armpits and groin, under the breasts, and in other areas where skin flexes or folds. This disease is characterized by smooth, inflamed lesions and can be debilitating.

Characterized by severe scaling, **itching**, and pain that affects most of the body, erythrodermic psoriasis disrupts the body's chemical balance and can cause severe illness. This particularly inflammatory form of psoriasis can be the first sign of the disease, but often develops in patients with a history of plaque psoriasis.

About 10% of partients with psoriasis develop a complication called **psoriatic arthritis**. This type of arthritis can be slow to develop and mild, or it can develop rapidly. Symptoms of psoriatic arthritis include:

- Joint discomfort, swelling, stiffness, or throbbing
- Swelling in the toes and ankles
- Pain in the digits, lower back, wrists, knees, and ankles
- Eye inflammation or pink eye (conjunctivitis)

The cause of psoriasis is unknown, but research suggests that an immune-system malfunction triggers the disease. Factors that increase the risk of developing psoriasis include:

- Family history
- **Stress**
- Exposure to cold temperatures
- Injury, illness, or infection
- Steroids and other medications
- Race

Trauma and certain bacteria may trigger psoriatic arthritis in patients with psoriasis.

A complete medical history and examination of the skin, nails, and scalp are the basis for a diagnosis of psoriasis. In some cases, a microscopic examination of skin cells is also performed.

Blood tests can distinguish psoriatic arthritis from other types of arthritis. Rheumatoid arthritis, in particular, is diagnosed by the presence of a particular antibody present in the blood. That antibody is not present in the blood of patients with psoriatic arthritis.

Age, general health, lifestyle, and the severity and location of symptoms influence the type of treatment used to reduce inflammation and decrease the rate at which new skin cells are produced. Because the course of this disease varies with each individual, doctors must experiment with or combine different treatments to find the most effective therapy for a particular patient.

Steroid creams and ointments are commonly used to treat mild or moderate psoriasis, and steroids are sometimes injected into the skin of patients with a limited number of lesions. In mid-1997, the United States **Food and Drug Administration** (FDA) approved the use of tazarotene (Tazorac) to treat mild-to-moderate plaque psoriasis. This water-based gel has chemical properties similar to Vitamin A.

Brief daily doses of natural sunlight can significantly relieve symptoms. **Sunburn** has the opposite effect.

Moisturizers and bath oils can loosen scales, soften skin, and may eliminate the itch. So can adding a cup of oatmeal to a tub of bath water. Salicylic acid (an ingredient in **aspirin**) can be used to remove dead skin or increase the effectiveness of other therapies.

Administered under medical supervision, ultraviolet light B (UVB) is used to control psoriasis that covers many areas of the body or that has not responded to topical preparations. Doctors combine UVB treatments with topical medications to treat some patients and sometimes prescribe home **phototherapy**, in which the patient administers his own UVB treatments.

Photochemotherapy (PUVA) is a medically supervised procedure that combines medication with exposure to ultraviolet light (UVA) to treat localized or widespread psoriasis. An individual with wide-spread psoriasis that has not responded to treatment may enroll in one of the day treatment programs conducted at special facilities throughout the United States. Psoriasis patients who participate in these intensive sessions are exposed to UVB and given other treatments for six to eight hours a day for two to four weeks.

Methotrexate (MTX) can be given as a pill or as an injection to alleviate symptoms of severe psoriasis or **psoriatic arthritis**. Patients who take MTX must be carefully monitored to prevent liver damage.

Psoriatic arthritis can also be treated with nonsteroidal anti-inflammatory drugs (NSAIDS), like **acetaminophen** (Tylenol) or aspirin. Hot compresses and warm water soaks may also provide some relief for painful joints.

Other medications used to treat severe psoriasis include etrentinate (Tegison) and isotretinoin (Accutane), whose chemical properties are similar to those of Vitamin A. Most effective in treating pustular or erythrodermic psoriasis, Tegison also relieves some symptoms of plaque psoriasis. Tegison can enhance the effectiveness of UVB or PUVA treatments and reduce the amount of exposure necessary.

Accutane is a less effective psoriasis treatment than Tegison, but can cause many of the same side effects, including **nosebleed**s, inflammation of the eyes and lips, bone spurs, hair loss, and **birth defects**. Tegison is stored in the body for an unknown length of time, and should not be taken by a woman who is pregnant or planning to become pregnant. A woman should use reliable birth control while taking Accutane and for at least one month before and after her course of treatment.

Cyclosporin emulsion (Neoral) is used to treat stubborn cases of severe psoriasis. Cyclosporin is also used to prevent rejection of transplanted organs, and Neoral, approved by the FDA in 1997, should be particularly beneficial to psoriasis patients who are young children or African-Americans, or those who have diabetes.

Other conventional treatments for psoriasis include:

- Capsaicin (*Capsicum frutecens*), an ointment that can stop production of the chemical that causes the skin to become inflamed and halts the runaway production of new skin cells. Capsaicin is available without a prescription, but should be used under a doctor's supervision to prevent **burns** and skin damage.
- Hydrocortisone creams, topical ointments containing a form of vitamin D called calcitriol, and coal-tar shampoos and ointments can relieve symptoms but may cause such side effects as folliculitis (inflammation of hair follicles) and heightened risk of **skin cancer**.

Most cases of psoriasis can be controlled, and most people who have psoriasis can live normal lives.

Some people who have psoriasis are so self-conscious and embarrassed about their appearance that they become depressed and withdrawn. The Social Security Administration grants disability benefits to about 400 psoriasis patients each year, and a comparable number die from complications of the disease.

A doctor should be notified if:

- Psoriasis symptoms appear or reappear after treatment
- Pustules erupt on the skin and the patient experiences fatigue, muscle aches, and **fever**
- Unfamiliar, unexplained symptoms appear.

PSORIATIC ARTHRITIS

Psoriatic arthritis is a form of arthritic joint disease associated with the chronic skin scaling and fingernail changes seen in **psoriasis**.

Physicians recognize a number of different forms of psoriatic arthritis. In some patients, the arthritic symptoms will affect the small joints at the ends of the fingers and toes. In others, symptoms will affect joints on one side of the body but not on the other. In addition, there are patients whose larger joints on both sides of the body simultaneously become affected, as in **rheumatoid arthritis**. Some people with psoriatic arthritis experience arthritis symptoms in the back and spine; in rare cases, called psoriatic arthritis mutilans, the disease destroys the joints and bones, leaving patients with gnarled and club-like hands and feet. In many patients, symptoms of psoriasis precede the arthritis symptoms; a clue to possible joint disease is pitting and other changes in the fingernails.

Most people develop psoriatic arthritis between ages 35-45, but it has been observed earlier in adults and children. Both the skin and joint symptoms will come and go; there is no clear relationship between the severity of the psoriasis symptoms and arthritis **pain** at any given time. It is unclear how common psoriatic arthritis is. Recent surveys suggest that between 1 in 5 people and 1 in 2 people with psoriasis may also have some arthritis symptoms.

The cause of psoriatic arthritis is unknown. As in psoriasis, genetic factors appear to be involved. People with psoriatic arthritis are more likely than others to have close relatives with the disease, but they are just as likely to have relatives with psoriasis but no joint disease. Researchers believe genes increasing the susceptibility to developing psoriasis may be located on chromosome 6p and chromosome 17, but the specific genetic abnormality has not been identified. Like psoriasis and other forms of arthritis, psoriatic arthritis also appears to be an autoimmune disorder, triggered by an attack of the body's own immune system on itself.

Symptoms of psoriatic arthritis include dry, scaly, silver patches of skin combined with joint pain and destructive changes in the feet, hands, knees, and spine. Tendon pain and nail deformities are other hallmarks of psoriatic arthritis.

Skin and nail changes characteristic of psoriasis with accompanying arthritic symptoms are the hallmarks of psoriatic arthritis. A blood test for rheumatoid factor, antibodies that suggest the presence of rheumatoid arthritis, is negative in nearly all patients with psoriatic arthritis. X rays may show characteristic damage to the larger joints on either side of the body as well as fusion of the joints at the ends of the fingers and toes.

Treatment for psoriatic arthritis is meant to control the **skin lesions** of psoriasis and the joint inflammation of arthritis. **Nonsteroidal anti-inflammatory drugs**, gold salts, and sulfasalazine are standard arthritis treatments, but have no effect on psoriasis. Antimalaria drugs and systemic **corticosteroids** should be avoided because they can cause **dermatitis** or exacerbate psoriasis when they are discontinued.

Several treatments are useful for both the skin lesions and the joint inflammation of psoriatic arthritis. Etretinate, a vitamin A derivative; methotrexate, a potent suppresser of the immune system; and ultraviolet light therapy have all been successfully used to treat psoriatic arthritis.

Food allergies/intolerances are believed to play a role in most autoimmune disorders, including psoriatic arthritis. Identification and elimination of food allergens from the diet can be helpful. Constitutional homeopathy can work deeply and effectively with this condition, if the proper prescription is given. Acupuncture, Chinese herbal medicine, and western herbal medicine can all be useful in managing the symptoms of psoriatic arthritis. Nutritional supplements can contribute added support to the healing process. Alternative treatments recommended for psoriasis and rheumatoid arthritis may also be helpful in treating psoriatic arthritis.

The prognosis for most patients with psoriatic arthritis is good. For many the joint and other arthritis symptoms are much milder than those experienced in rheumatoid arthritis. One in five people with psoriatic arthritis, however, face potentially crippling joint disease. In some cases, the course of the arthritis can be far more mutilating than in rheumatoid arthritis.

There are no preventive measures for psoriatic arthritis.

PSYCHOANALYSIS

Psychoanalysis is a form of psychotherapy used by qualified psychotherapists to treat patients who have a range of mild to moderate chronic life problems. It is related to a specific body of theories about the relationships between conscious and unconscious mental processes, and should not be used as a synonym for psychotherapy in general. Psychoanalysis is done one-on-one with the patient and the analyst; it is not appropriate for group work.

Psychoanalysis is the most intensive form of an approach to treatment called psychodynamic therapy. Psychodynamic refers to a view of human personality that results from interactions between conscious and unconscious factors. The purpose of all forms of psychodynamic treatment is to bring unconscious mental material and processes into full consciousness so that the patient can gain more control over his or her life.

Classical psychoanalysis has become the least commonly practiced form of psychodynamic therapy because of its demands on the patient's time, as well as on his or her emotional and financial resources. It is, however, the oldest form of psychodynamic treatment. The theories that underlie psychoanalysis were worked out by **Sigmund Freud** (1856-1939), a Viennese physician, during the early years of this century. Freud's discoveries were made in the context of his research into **hypnosis**. The goal of psychoanalysis is the uncovering and resolution of the patient's internal conflicts. The treatment focuses on the formation of an intense relationship between the therapist and patient, which is analyzed and discussed in order to deepen the patient's insight into his or her problems.

Psychoanalytic psychotherapy is a modified form of psychoanalysis that is much more widely practiced. It is based on the same theoretical principles as psychoanalysis, but is less intense and less concerned with major changes in the patient's character structure. The focus in treatment is usually the patient's current life situation and the way problems relate to early conflicts and feelings, rather than an exploration of the unconscious aspects of the relationship that has been formed with the therapist.

Not all patients benefit from psychoanalytic treatment. Potential patients should meet the following prerequisites:

- The capacity to relate well enough to form an effective working relationship with the analyst. This relationship is called a therapeutic alliance.
- At least average intelligence and a basic understanding of psychological theory.
- The ability to tolerate frustration, sadness, and other painful emotions.
- The capacity to distinguish between reality and fantasy.

People considered best suited to psychoanalytic treatment include those with depression, character disorders, neurotic conflicts, and chronic relationship problems. When the patient's conflicts are long-standing and deeply entrenched in his or her personality, psychoanalysis may be preferable to psychoanalytic psychotherapy, because of its greater depth.

Psychoanalysis is not suitable for patients suffering from severe depression or psychotic disorders such as **schizophrenia**. It is also not appropriate for people with **addiction**s or substance dependency, disorders of aggression or impulse control, or acute crises; some of these people may benefit from psychoanalysis after the crisis has been resolved.

In both psychoanalysis and psychoanalytic psychotherapy, the therapist does not tell the patient how to solve problems or offer moral judgments. The focus of treatment is exploration of the patient's mind and habitual thought patterns. Such therapy is termed "non-directed." It is also "insight-oriented," meaning that the goal of treatment is increased understanding of the sources of one's inner conflicts and emotional problems. The basic techniques of psychoanalytical treatment include:

Neutrality means that the analyst does not take sides in the patient's conflicts, express feelings about the patient, or talk about his or her own life. Therapist neutrality is intended to help the patient stay focused on issues rather than be concerned with the therapist's reactions. In psychoanalysis, the patient lies on a couch facing away from the therapist. In psychodynamic psychotherapy, however, the patient and therapist usually sit in comfortable chairs facing each other.

Free association means that the patient talks about whatever comes into mind without censoring or editing the flow of ideas or memories. Free association allows the patient to return to earlier or more childlike emotional states ("regress"). Regression is sometimes necessary in the formation of the therapeutic alliance. It also helps the analyst to understand the recurrent patterns of conflict in the patient's life.

Transference is the name that psychoanalysts use for the patient's repetition of childlike ways of relating that were learned in early life. If the therapeutic alliance has been well established, the patient will begin to transfer thoughts and feelings connected with siblings, parents, or other influential figures to the therapist. Discussing the transference helps the patient gain insight into the ways in which he or she misreads or misperceives other people in present life.

In psychoanalytic treatment, the analyst is silent as much as possible, in order to encourage the patient's free association. However, the analyst offers judiciously timed interpretations, in the form of verbal comments about the material that emerges in the sessions. The therapist uses interpretations in order to uncover the patient's resistance to treatment, to discuss the patient's transference feelings, or to confront the patient with inconsistencies. Interpretations may be either focused on present issues ("dynamic") or intended to draw connections between the patient's past and the present ("genetic"). The patient is also often encouraged to describe dreams and fantasies as sources of material for interpretation.

"Working through" occupies most of the work in psychoanalytic treatment after the transference has been formed and the patient has begun to acquire insights into his or her problems. Working through is a process in which the new awareness is repeatedly tested and "tried on for size" in other areas of the patient's life. It allows the patient to understand the influence of the past on his or her present situation, to accept it emotionally as well as intellectually, and to use the new understanding to make changes in present life. Working through thus helps the patient to gain some measure of control over inner conflicts and to resolve them or minimize their power.

Although psychoanalytic treatment is primarily verbal, medications are sometimes used to stabilize patients with severe **anxiety**, depression, or other **mood disorders** during the analysis.

The cost of either psychoanalysis or psychoanalytic psychotherapy is prohibitive for most patients without insurance coverage. A full course of psychoanalysis usually requires three to five weekly sessions with a psychoanalyst over a period of three to five years. A course of psychoanalytic psychotherapy involves one to three meetings per week with the therapist for two to five years. Each session or meeting typically costs between $80 and $200, depending on the locale and the experience of the therapist. The increasing reluctance of most HMOs and other managed care organizations to pay for long-term psychotherapy is one reason that these forms of treatment are losing ground to short-term methods of treatment and the use of medications to control the patient's emotions. It is also not clear that long-term psychoanalytically oriented approaches are more beneficial than briefer therapy methods for many patients.

Some patients may need evaluation for possible medical problems before entering psychoanalysis because numerous diseases—including virus infections and certain vitamin deficiencies—have emotional side effects or symptoms. The therapist will also want to know whether the patient is taking any prescription medications that may affect the patient's feelings or ability to concentrate. In addition, it is important to make sure that the patient is not abusing drugs or alcohol.

The primary risk to the patient is related to the emotional pain resulting from new insights and changes in long-standing behavior patterns. In some patients, psychoanalysis produces so much anxiety that they cannot continue with this treatment method. In other cases, the therapist's lack of skill may prevent the formation of a solid therapeutic alliance.

Psychoanalysis and psychoanalytic psychotherapy both have the goal of basic changes in the patient's personality structure and level of functioning, although psychoanalysis typically aims at more extensive and more profound change. In general, this approach to treatment is considered successful if the patient has shown:

- Reduction in intensity or number of symptoms
- Some resolution of basic emotional conflicts
- Increased independence and **self-esteem**
- Improved functioning and adaptation to life.

Attempts to compare the effectiveness of psychoanalytical treatment to other modes of therapy are difficult to evaluate. Some aspects of Freudian theory have been questioned since the 1970s on the grounds of their limited applicability to women and to people from non-Western cultures. There is, however, general agreement that psychoanalytic approaches work well for certain types of patients. In particular, these approaches are recommended for patients with neurotic conflicts.

Psychological tests

Psychological tests are written, visual, or verbal evaluations administered to assess the cognitive and emotional functioning of children and adults.

Psychological tests are used to assess a variety of mental abilities and attributes, including achievement and ability, personality, and neurological functioning.

For children, academic achievement, ability, and intelligence tests may be used as a tool in school placement, in determining the presence of a learning disability or a developmental delay, in identifying giftedness, or in tracking intellectual development. Intelligence testing may be used with adults to determine vocational ability (e.g., in career counseling) or to assess adult intellectual ability in the classroom.

Personality tests are administered for a wide variety of reasons, from diagnosing psychopathology (e.g., personality disorder, depressive disorder) to screening job candidates. They may be used in an educational or vocational setting to determine personality strengths and weaknesses, or in the legal system to evaluate parolees.

Patients who have experienced a traumatic brain injury, brain damage, or organic neurological problems (for example, **dementia**) are administered neuropsychological tests to assess their level of functioning and identify areas of mental impairment. They may also be used to evaluate the progress of a patient who has undergone treatment or **rehabilitation** for a neurological injury or illness. In addition, certain neuropsychological measures may be used to screen children for developmental delays and/or learning disabilities.

Psychological testing requires a clinically trained examiner. All psychological tests should be administered, scored, and interpreted by a trained professional, preferably a psychologist or psychiatrist with expertise in the appropriate area.

Psychological tests are only one element of a psychological assessment. They should never be used alone as the sole basis for a diagnosis. A detailed history of the test subject and a review of psychological, medical, educational, or other relevant records are required to lay the groundwork for interpreting the results of any psychological measurement.

Cultural and language differences in the test subject may affect test performance and may result in inaccurate test results. The test administrator should be informed before psychological testing begins if the test taker is not fluent in English and/or belongs to a minority culture. In addition, the subject's motivation and motives may also affect test results.

Psychological tests are formalized measures of mental functioning. Most are objective and quantifiable; however, certain projective tests may involve some level of subjective interpretation. Also known as inventories, measurements, questionnaires, and scales, psychological tests are administered in a variety of settings, including preschools, primary and secondary schools, colleges and universities, hospitals, outpatient healthcare settings, social agencies, prisons, and employment or human resource offices. They come in a variety of formats, including written, verbal, and computer administered.

Achievement and ability tests are designed to measure the level of an individual's intellectual functioning and cognitive ability. Most achievement and ability tests are standardized, meaning that norms were established during the design phase of the test by administering the test to a large representative sample of the test population. Achievement and ability tests follow a uniform testing protocol, or procedure (i.e., test instructions, test conditions, and scoring procedures) and their scores can be interpreted in relation to established norms. Common achievement and ability tests include the Wechsler **intelligence test** (WISC-III and WAIS) and the Stanford-Binet intelligence scales.

Personality tests and inventories evaluate the thoughts, emotions, attitudes, and behavioral traits that comprise personality. The results of these tests determine an individual's personality strengths and weaknesses, and may identify certain disturbances in personality, or psychopathology. Tests such as the Minnesota Multiphasic Personality Inventory-2 (MMPI-2) and the Millon Clinical Multiaxial Inventory III (MCMI-III), are used to screen individuals for specific psychopathologies or emotional problems.

Another type of personality test is the projective personality assessment. A projective test asks a subject to interpret some ambiguous stimuli, such as a series of inkblots. The subject's responses provide insight into his or her thought processes and personality traits. For example, the Rorschach Inkblot Test and the Holtzman ink blot test (HIT) use a series of inkblots that the test subject is asked to identify. Another projective assessment, the Thematic Apperception Test (TAT), asks the subject to tell a story about a series of pictures. Some consider projective tests to be less reliable than objective personality tests. If the examiner is not well-trained in psychometric evaluation, subjective interpretations may affect the evaluation of these tests.

Many insurance plans cover all or a portion of diagnostic neuropsychological or psychological testing. As of 1997, Medicare reimbursed for psychological and neuropsychological testing. Billing time typically includes test administration, scoring and interpretation, and reporting.

Prior to the administration of any psychological test, the administrator should provide the test subject with information on the nature of the test and its intended use, complete standardized instructions for taking the test (including any time limits and penalties for incorrect responses), and information on the confidentiality of the results. After these disclosures are made, informed consent should be obtained from the test subject before testing begins (except in cases of legally mandated testing, where consent is not required of the subject).

All psychological and neuropsychological assessments should be administered, scored, and interpreted by a trained professional. When interpreting test results for test subjects, the test administrator will review with subjects: what the test evaluates, its precision in evaluation, any margins of error involved in scoring, and what the individual scores mean in the context of overall test norms and the background of the test subject.

Psychosis

Psychosis is a symptom or feature of mental illness typically characterized by radical changes in personality, impaired functioning, and a distorted or non-existent sense of objective reality.

Patients suffering from psychosis have impaired reality testing; that is, they are unable to distinguish personal, subjective experience from the reality of the external world. They experience **hallucinations** and/or delusions that they believe are real, and may behave and communicate in an inappropriate and incoherent fashion. Psychosis may appear as a symptom of a number of mental disorders, including mood and **personality disorders**. It is also the defining feature of **schizophrenia**, schizophreniform disorder, schizoaffective disorder, delusional disorder, and the psychotic disorders (i.e., brief psychotic disorder, shared psychotic disorder, psychotic disorder due to a general medical condition, and substance-induced psychotic disorder).

Psychosis may be caused by the interaction of biological and psychosocial factors depending on the disorder it presents in; psychosis can also be caused by purely social factors, with no biological component.

Psychosis in schizophrenia and perhaps schizophreniform disorder appears to be related to abnormalities in the structure and chemistry of the brain, and appears to have strong genetic links; but its course and severity can be altered by social factors such as **stress** or a lack of support within the family. The cause of schizoaffective disorder is less clear cut, but biological factors are also suspected.

The exact cause of delusional disorder has not been conclusively determined, but potential causes include heredity, neurological abnormalities, and changes in brain chemistry. Some studies have indicated that delusions are generated by abnormalities in the limbic system, the portion of the brain on the inner edge of the cerebral cortex that is believed to regulate emotions.

Trauma and stress can cause a short-term psychosis (less than a month's duration) known as brief psychotic disorder. Major life-changing events such as the **death** of a family member or a natural disaster have been known to stimulate brief psychotic disorder in patients with no prior history of mental illness.

Psychosis may also be triggered by an organic cause, termed a psychotic disorder due to a general medical condition. Organic sources of psychosis include neurological conditions (for example, epilepsy and cerebrovascular disease), metabolic conditions (for example, porphyria), endocrine conditions (for example, hyper- or **hypothyroidism**), renal failure, electrolyte imbalance, or **autoimmune disorders**.

Psychosis is also a known side effect of the use, abuse, and withdrawal from certain drugs. So-called recreational drugs, such as hallucinogenics, PCP, amphetamines, cocaine, marijuana, and alcohol, may cause a psychotic reaction during use or withdrawal. Certain prescription medications such as steroids, anticonvulsants, chemotherapeutic agents, and antiparkinsonian medications may also induce psychotic symptoms. Toxic substances such as carbon monoxide have also been reported to cause substance-induced psychotic disorder.

Psychosis is characterized by the following symptoms:

- Delusions. Those delusions which occur in schizophrenia and its related forms are typically bizarre (i.e., they could not occur in real life). Delusions occurring in delusional disorder are more plausible, but still patently untrue. In some cases, delusions may be accompanied by feelings of **paranoia**.
- Hallucinations. Psychotic patients see, hear, smell, taste, or feel things that aren't there. Schizophrenic hallucinations are typically auditory or, less commonly, visual; but psychotic hallucinations can involve any of the five senses.
- Disorganized speech. Psychotic patients, especially those with schizophrenia, often ramble on in incoherent, nonsensical speech patterns.
- Disorganized or catatonic behavior. The catatonic patient reacts inappropriately to his environment by either remaining rigid and immobile or by engaging in excessive motor activity. Disorganized behavior is behavior or activity which is inappropriate for the situation, or unpredictable.

Patients with psychotic symptoms should undergo a thorough **physical examination** and history to rule out possible organic causes. If a psychiatric cause such as schizophrenia is suspected, a mental health professional will typically conduct an interview with the patient and administer one of several clinical inventories, or tests, to evaluate mental status. This assessment takes place in either an outpatient or hospital setting.

Psychosis that is symptomatic of schizophrenia or another psychiatric disorder should be treated by a psychologist and/or psychiatrist. An appropriate course of medication and/or psychosocial therapy is employed to treat the underlying primary disorder. If the patient is considered to be at risk for harming himself or others, inpatient treatment is usually recommended.

Antipsychotic medication such as thioridazine (Mellaril), haloperidol (Haldol), chlorpromazine (Thorazine), clozapine (Clozaril), sertindole (Serlect), olanzapine (Zyprexa), or risperidone (Risperdal) is usually prescribed to bring psychotic symptoms under control and into remission. Possible side effects of antipsychotics include dry mouth, drowsiness, muscle stiffness, and tardive dyskinesia (involuntary movements of the body). Agranulocytosis, a potentially serious but reversible health condition in which the white blood cells that fight infection in the body are destroyed, is a possible side effect of clozapine. Patients treated with this drug should undergo weekly blood tests to monitor white blood cell counts for the first six months, then every two weeks.

After an acute psychotic episode has subsided, antipsychotic drug maintenance treatment is typically employed and psychosocial therapy and living and vocational skills training may be attempted.

Prognosis for brief psychotic disorder is quite good; for schizophrenia, less so. Generally, the longer and more severe a psychotic episode, the poorer the prognosis is for the patient. Early diagnosis and treatment is critical to improving outcomes for the patient across all psychotic disorders.

Approximately 10% of America's permanently disabled population is comprised of schizophrenic individuals. The mortality rate of schizophrenic individuals is also high—approximately 10% of schizophrenics commit suicide, and 20% attempt it. However, early diagnosis and long-term follow up care can improve the outlook for these patients considerably. Roughly 60% of patients with schizophrenia will show substantial improvement with appropriate treatment.

Psychosurgery

Psychosurgery involves severing or otherwise disabling areas of the brain to treat a personality disorder, behavior disorder, or other mental illness. Modern psychosurgical techniques target the pathways between the limbic system (the portion of the brain on the inner edge of the cerebral cortex) that is believed to regulate emotions, and the frontal cortex, where thought processes are seated.

Lobotomy is a psychosurgical procedure involving selective destruction of connective nerve fibers or tissue. It is performed on the frontal lobe of the brain and its purpose is to alleviate mental illness and chronic **pain** symptoms. The bilateral cingulotomy, a modern psychosurgical technique which has replaced the lobotomy, is performed to alleviate mental disorders such as major depression, **bipolar disorder**, or **obsessive-compulsive disorder** (OCD), which have not responded to psychotherapy, behavioral therapy, electroshock, or pharmacologic treatment. Bilateral cingulotomies are also performed to treat chronic pain in **cancer** patients.

Psychosurgery should be considered only after all other non-surgical psychiatric therapies have been fully explored. Much is still unknown about the biology of the brain and how psychosurgery affects brain function.

Psychosurgery, and lobotomy in particular, reached the height of use just after World War II. Between 1946 and 1949, the use of the lobotomy grew from 500 to 5,000 annual procedures in the United States. At that time, the procedure was viewed as a possible solution to the overcrowded and understaffed conditions in state-run mental hospitals and asylums. Known as prefrontal or transorbital lobotomy, depending on the surgical technique used and area of the brain targeted, these early operations were performed with surgical knives, electrodes, suction, or ice picks, to cut or sweep out portions of the frontal lobe.

Today's psychosurgical techniques are much more refined. Instead of going in "blind" to remove large sections on the frontal lobe, as in these early operations, neurosurgeons use a computer-based process called stereotactic **magnetic resonance imaging** to guide a small electrode to the limbic system (brain structures involved in autonomic or automatic body functions and some emotion and behavior). There an electrical current burns in a small lesion (usually 1/2 in in size). In a bilateral cingulotomy, the cingulate gyrus, a small section of brain that connects the limbic region of the brain with the frontal lobes, is targeted. Another surgical technique uses a non-invasive tool known as a gamma knife to focus beams of radiation at the brain. A lesion forms at the spot where the beams converge in the brain.

Candidates for cingulotomies or other forms of psychosurgery undergo a rigorous screening process to ensure that all possible non-surgical psychiatric treatment options have been explored. Psychosurgery is only performed with the patient's informed consent.

Ongoing behavioral and medication therapy is often required in OCD patients who undergo cingulotomy. All psychosurgery patients should remain under a psychiatrist's care for follow-up evaluations and treatment.

As with any type of brain surgery, psychosurgery carries the risk of permanent brain damage, though the advent of non-invasive neurosurgical techniques, such as the gamma knife, has reduced the risk of brain damage significantly.

In a 1996 study at Massachusetts General Hospital, over one-third of patients undergoing cingulotomy demonstrated significant improvements after the surgery. And, in contrast to the bizarre behavior and personality changes reported with lobotomy patients in the 1940s and 50s, modern psychosurgery patients have demonstrated little post-surgical losses of memory or other high level thought processes.

Puberty

Puberty is the period of human development during which physical growth and sexual maturation occurs.

Beginning as early as age eight in girls—and two years later, on average, in boys—the hypothalamus (part of the brain) signals hormonal change that stimulates the pituitary. In turn, the pituitary releases its own hormones called gonadotrophins that stimulate the gonads and adrenals. From these glands comes a flood of sex hormones—**androgens** and testosterone in the male, estrogens and progestins in the female—that regulate the growth and function of the sex organs. It is interesting to note that the gonadotrophins are the same for males and females, but the sex hormones they induce are different.

In the United States, the first sign of puberty occurs on average at age 11 in girls, with menstruation and fertility following about two years later. Boys lag behind by about two years. Puberty may not begin until age 16 in boys and continue in a desultory fashion on past age 20. In contrast to puberty, adolescence is more of a social/cultural term referring to the interval between childhood and adulthood.

Puberty has been divided into five Sexual Maturity Rating (SMR) stages by two doctors, W. Marshall and J. M. Tanner. These ratings are often referred to as Tanner Stages 1-5. Staging is based on pubic hair growth, on male genital development, and female breast development. Staging helps determine whether development is normal for a given age. Both sexes also grow axillary (arm pit) hair and pimples. Males develop muscle mass, a deeper voice, and facial hair. Females redistribute body fat. Along with the maturing of the sex organs, there is a pronounced growth spurt averaging 3-4 in and culminating in full adult stature. Puberty can be precocious (early) or delayed. It all depends upon the sex hormones.

Puberty falling outside the age limits considered normal for any given population should prompt a search for the cause. As health and nutrition have improved over the past few generations, there has been a gradual decrease in the average age for the normal onset of puberty.

- Excess hormone stimulation is the cause for **precocious puberty**. It can come from the brain in the form of gonadotrophins or from the gonads and adrenals. Overproduction may be caused by functioning tumors or simple overactivity. Brain overproduction can also be the result of brain infections or injury.

- Likewise, delayed puberty is due to insufficient hormone. If the pituitary output is inadequate, so will be the output from the gonads and adrenals. On the other hand, a normal pituitary will overproduce if it senses there are not enough hormones in the circulation.
- There are several congenital disorders (polyglandular deficiency syndromes) that include failure of hormone output. These children do not experience normal puberty, but it may be induced by giving them the proper hormones at the proper time.
- Finally, there are in females abnormalities in hormone production that produce male characteristics—so called virilizing syndromes. Should one of these appear during adolescence, it will disturb the normal progress of puberty. Notice that virilizing requires abnormal hormones in the female, while feminizing results from absent hormones in the male. Each embryo starts out life as female. Male hormones transform it if they are present.

Delayed or precocious puberty requires measurement of the several hormones involved to determine which are lacking or which are in excess. There are blood tests for each one. If a tumor is suspected, imaging of the suspect organ needs to be done with x rays, **computed tomography scans** (CT scans), or **magnetic resonance imaging** (MRI).

Puberty is a period of great **stress**, both physically and emotionally. The psychological changes and challenges of puberty are made infinitely greater if its timing is off.

If early, the offending gland or tumor may require surgical attention, although there are several drugs now that counteract hormone effects. If delayed, puberty can be stimulated with the correct hormones. Treatment should not be delayed because necessary bone growth is also affected.

Properly administered hormones can restore the normal growth pattern.

PUBLIC HEALTH

The **Centers for Disease Control** and Prevention (CDC) define the role of public health as the active protection of the nation's health and safety, the distribution of credible information to enhance health decisions, and the establishment of partnerships with local communities and organizations to promote health. Public health comprises all activities that society does collectively to ensure conditions in which people can be healthy. This includes organized international (e.g., **World Health Organization**), national, state, and community efforts to prevent, identify, preempt, and counter threats to the public's health. Public health departments/districts include local (county or multicounty) health agencies, operated by local governments, with oversight and direction from a local board of health, which provides public health services throughout a defined geographic area.

Public health activities have increased the life expectancy of Americans in this century by 25 years, but few Americans are aware of their importance because most public health achievements involve prevention rather than cures. To cite an example, in 1900 **tuberculosis** (TB) was the primary cause of death in the United States and its cause was still under investigation. Once it became clear that TB was a contagious bacterial disease, public health control measures were implemented to stop the spread of this disease. Americans used to worry on a daily basis about infections, such as **polio**, diphtheria, **tetanus**, and **rubella**, that are now largely unheard of. Additionally there would still be a smoking rate in this country of nearly 60% of men and women, without its relation to health hazards and premature death, were it not for public health initiatives.

Examples of other activities that currently fall under public health control include the maintenance of clean air by monitoring radiation levels and developing strategies to keep them low, the maintenance of safe drinking water and its fluoridation, the inspection of dairy products to ensure consumer safety, the placement of doctors in rural areas, the assurance that children get proper nutrition to prevent sickness later in life, the demonstration of the efficacy on automobile seatbelt use in protecting human life, the licensing of child care centers, the provision of immunizations against life-threatening diseases, the demonstration of the role of exercise in reducing the risks of chronic disease, the promotion of cigarette-smoke-free environments for workers, the regulation of and the licensing of food service businesses, the protection of public water supplies from pollution, and overseeing the care provided by hospitals, nursing homes, and emergency medical services.

Other areas of interest among public health professionals include **alternative medicine**, **asthma**, bioethics, biological warfare, biometry, blindness, cardiology, **child abuse**, chronic disease, communicable **disease control**, communicable diseases, consumer health, **contraception**, dentistry, **diabetes**, disasters, **domestic violence**, drug resistance, emergencies, emergency medicine, environment, environmental exposure, **environmental health**, epidemiology, family planning, family practice, **food poisoning**, **genetics**, gynecology, health, health care reform, health education, health policy, health promotion, hearing disorders, heart diseases, **hepatitis**, history of medicine, HIV infections, **hospitals**, immunization, immunology, **influenza**, **leprosy**, **leptospirosis**, lung diseases, **lyme disease**, **malaria**, **measles**, medical indigency, medical informatics, medical oncology, medical societies, medical substance, medical technology, microbiology, **nursing**, **nutrition**, occupational health, ophthalmology, otolaryngology, parasitology, pediatrics, pharmacology, **plague**, **polio**myelitis, **preventive medicine**, primary health care, psychiatry, publishing, pulmonary disease, **rabies**, radiation, reproductive medicine, rheumatology, risk assessment, **rural health**, rural medicine, safety, schools, scientific sociology, **sexually transmitted diseases**, **smoking**, social medicine, standards, statistics, telemedicine, **tinnitus**, toxicology, traditional mental health, travel, **tropical medicine**, trypanosomiasis, **tuberculosis**, urban health, vaccines, veterinary medicine, **violence**, virology, virus diseases, vital statistics, **women's health**, world health, and **wounds** and injuries.

PULMONARY EDEMA

Pulmonary edema is a condition in which fluid accumulates in the lungs, usually because the heart's left ventricle does not pump adequately.

The build-up of fluid in the spaces outside the blood vessels of the lungs is called pulmonary edema. Pulmonary edema is a common complication of heart disorders, and most cases of the condition are associated with **heart failure**. Pulmonary edema can be a chronic condition, or it can develop suddenly and quickly become life threatening. The life-threatening type of pulmonary edema occurs when a large amount of fluid suddenly shifts from the pulmonary blood vessels into the lung, due to lung problems, **heart attack**, trauma, or toxic chemicals. It can also be the first sign of coronary heart disease.

In heart-related pulmonary edema, the heart's main chamber, the left ventricle, is weakened and does not function properly. The ventricle does not completely eject its contents, causing blood to back up and cardiac output to drop. The body responds by increasing blood pressure and fluid volume to compensate for the reduced cardiac output. This, in turn, increases the force against which the ventricle must expel blood. Blood backs up, forming a pool in the pulmonary blood vessels. Fluid leaks into the spaces between the tissues of the lungs and begins to accumulate. This process makes it more difficult for the lungs to expand. It also impedes the exchange of air and gases between the lungs and blood moving through lung blood vessels.

Most cases of pulmonary edema are caused by failure of the heart's main chamber, the left ventricle. It can be brought on by an acute heart attack, severe ischemia, volume overload of the heart's left ventricle, and mitral stenosis. Non-heart-related pulmonary edema is caused by lung problems like **pneumonia**, an excess of intravenous fluids, some types of kidney disease, bad **burns**, liver disease, nutritional problems, and **Hodgkin's disease**. Non-heart-related pulmonary edema can also be caused by other conditions where the lungs do not drain properly, and conditions where the respiratory veins are blocked.

Early symptoms of pulmonary edema include:

- **Shortness of breath** upon exertion
- Sudden respiratory distress after sleep
- Difficulty breathing, except when sitting upright
- **Cough**ing

In cases of severe pulmonary edema, these symptoms will worsen to:

- Labored and rapid breathing
- Frothy, bloody fluid containing pus coughed from the lungs (sputum)
- A fast pulse and possibly serious disturbances in the heart's rhythm (atrial fibrillation, for example)
- Cold, clammy, sweaty, and bluish skin
- A drop in blood pressure resulting in a thready pulse

A doctor can usually diagnose pulmonary edema based on the patient's symptoms and a physical exam. Patients with pulmonary edema will have a rapid pulse, rapid breathing, abnormal breath and heart sounds, and enlarged neck veins. A **chest x ray** is often used to confirm the diagnosis. Arterial blood gas testing may be done. Sometimes pulmonary artery catheterization is performed to confirm that the patient has pulmonary edema and not a disease with similar symptoms (called adult **respiratory distress syndrome** or "noncardiogenic pulmonary edema").

Pulmonary edema requires immediate emergency treatment. Treatment includes: placing the patient in a sitting position, oxygen, assisted or mechanical ventilation (in some cases), and drug therapy. The goal of treatment is to reduce the amount of fluid in the lungs, improve gas exchange and heart function, and, where possible, to correct the underlying disease.

To help the patient breath better, he/she is placed in a sitting position. High concentrations of oxygen are administered. In cases where respiratory distress is severe, a mechanical ventilator and a tube down the throat (tracheal intubation) will be used to improve the delivery of oxygen. Non-invasive pressure support ventilation is a new treatment for pulmonary edema in which the patient breaths against a continuous flow of positive airway pressure, delivered through a face or nasal mask. Non-invasive pressure support ventilation decreases the effort required to breath, enhances oxygen and carbon dioxide exchange, and increases cardiac output.

Drug therapy could include morphine, nitroglycerin, **diuretics**, angiotensin-converting enzyme (ACE) inhibitors, and **vasodilators**. Vasopressors are used for cardiogenic **shock**. Morphine is very effective in reducing the patient's **anxiety**, easing breathing, and improving blood flow. Nitroglycerin reduces pulmonary blood flow and decreases the volume of fluid entering the overloaded blood vessels. Diuretics, like furosemide (Lasix), promote the elimination of fluids through urination, helping to reduce pressure and fluids in the blood vessels. ACE inhibitors reduce the pressure against which the left ventricle must expel blood. In patients who have severe **hypertension**, a vasodilator such as nitroprusside sodium (Nipride) may be used. For cardiogenic shock, an adrenergic agent (like dopamine hydrochloride [Intropin], dobutamine hydrochloride [Dobutrex], or epinephrine) or a bipyridine (like amrinone lactate [Inocor] or milrinone lactate [Primacor]) are given.

Most patients with pulmonary edema who seek immediate treatment can be treated quickly and effectively.

Cardiogenic pulmonary edema can sometimes be prevented by treating the underlying heart disease. These treatments can including maintaining a healthy diet, taking appropriate medications correctly, and avoiding excess alcohol and salt.

PULMONARY EMBOLISM

Pulmonary embolism is an obstruction of a blood vessel in the lungs, usually due to a blood clot, which blocks a coronary artery.

Pulmonary embolism is a fairly common condition that can be fatal. According to the American Heart Association, an estimated 600,000 Americans develop pulmonary embolism annually; 60,000 die from it. As many as 25,000 Americans are hospitalized each year for pulmonary embolism, which is a relatively common complication in hospitalized patients. Even without warning symptoms, pulmonary embolism can cause sudden **death**. Treatment is not always successful.

Pulmonary embolism is difficult to diagnose. Less than 10% of patients who die from pulmonary embolism were diagnosed with the condition. It occurs when emboli block a pulmonary artery, usually due to a blood clot that breaks off from a large vein and travels to the lungs. More than 90% of cases of pulmonary embolism are complications of deep vein thrombosis, blood clots from the leg or pelvic veins. Emboli can also be comprised of fat, air, or tumor tissue. When emboli block the main pulmonary artery, pulmonary embolism can quickly become fatal.

Pulmonary embolism is caused by emboli that travel through the blood stream to the lungs and block a pulmonary artery. When this occurs, circulation and oxygenation of blood is compromised. The emboli are usually formed from blood clots but are occasionally comprised of air, fat, or tumor tissue. Risk factors include: prolonged bed rest, surgery, **childbirth**, **heart attack**, **stroke**, congestive **heart failure**, **cancer**, **obesity**, a broken hip or leg, **oral contraceptives**, **sickle-cell anemia**, congenital **coagulation disorders**, chest trauma, certain congenital heart defects, and old age.

Common symptoms of pulmonary embolism include:

- Labored breathing, sometimes accompanied by chest **pain**.
- A rapid pulse.
- A **cough** that produces bloody sputum.
- A low **fever**.
- Fluid build-up in the lungs.

Less common symptoms include:

- Coughing up a lot of blood.
- Pain caused by movement.
- Leg swelling.
- Bluish skin.
- **Fainting**.
- Swollen neck veins.

In some cases there are no symptoms.

Pulmonary embolism can be diagnosed through the patient's history, a physical exam, and diagnostic tests including **chest x ray**, lung scan, pulmonary **angiography**, **electrocardiography**, arterial blood gas measurements, and leg vein ultrasonography or venography.

A chest x ray can be normal or show fluid or other signs and rule out other diseases. The lung scan shows poor flow of blood in areas beyond blocked arteries. The patient inhales a small amount of radiopharmaceutical and pictures of airflow into the lungs are taken with a gamma camera. Then a different radiopharmaceutical is injected into an arm vein and lung blood flow is scanned. A normal result essentially rules out pulmonary embolism. A lung scan can be performed in a hospital or an outpatient facility and takes about 45 minutes.

Pulmonary angiography is the most reliable test for diagnosing pulmonary embolism but it is not used often, because it carries some risk and is expensive, invasive, and not readily available in many hospitals. Pulmonary angiography is a radiographic test which involves injection of a pharmaceutical "contrast agent" to show up the pulmonary arteries. A cinematic camera records the blood flow through the lungs of the patient, who lies on a table. Pulmonary angiography is usually performed in a hospital's radiology department and takes 30 minutes to one hour.

An electrocardiograph shows the heart's electrical activity and helps distinguish pulmonary embolism from a heart attack. Electrodes covered with conducting jelly are placed on the patient's chest, arms, and legs. Impulses of the heart's activity are traced on paper. The test takes about 10 minutes and can be performed in a physician's office or hospital lab.

Arterial blood gas measurements can be helpful, but they are rarely diagnostic for pulmonary embolism. Blood is taken from an artery instead of a vein, usually in the wrist and it is analyzed for oxygen, carbon dioxide and acid levels.

Venography is used to look for the most likely source of pulmonary embolism, deep vein thrombosis. It is very accurate, but it is not used often, because it is painful, expensive, exposes the patient to a fairly high dose of radiation, and can cause complications. Venography identifies the location, extent, and degree of attachment of the blood clots and enables the condition of the deep leg veins to be assessed. A contrast solution is injected into a foot vein through a catheter. The physician observes the movement of the solution through the vein with a fluoroscope while a series of x rays are taken. Venography takes between 30-45 minutes and can be done in a physician's office, a laboratory, or a hospital. Radionuclide venography, in which a radioactive isotope is injected, is occasionally used, especially if a patient has had reactions to contrast solutions. Most commonly performed are **ultrasound** and Doppler studies of leg veins.

Patients with pulmonary embolism are hospitalized and generally treated with clot-dissolving and clot-preventing drugs. **Oxygen therapy** is often needed to maintain normal oxygen concentrations. For people who can't take anticoagulants and in some other cases, surgery may be needed to insert a device that filters blood returning to the heart and lungs. The goal of treatment is to maintain the patient's cardiovascular and respiratory functions while the blockage resolves, which takes 10-14 days, and to prevent the formation of other emboli.

Thrombolytic therapy to dissolve blood clots is the aggressive treatment for very severe pulmonary embolism. Streptokinase, urokinase, and recombinant tissue plasminogen activator (TPA) are thrombolytic agents. Heparin is the injectable anticoagulant (clot-preventing) drug of choice for preventing formation of blood clots. Warfarin, an oral anticoagulant, is usually continued when the patient leaves the hospital and doesn't need heparin any longer.

About 10% of patients with pulmonary embolism die suddenly within the first hour of onset of the condition. The outcome for all other patients is generally good; only 3% of patients who are properly diagnosed and treated die. In cases of undiagnosed pulmonary embolism, about 30% of patients die.

Pulmonary embolism risk can be reduced in certain patients through judicious use of antithrombotic drugs such as heparin, venous interruption, gradient elastic stockings and/or intermittent pneumatic compression of the legs.

PULMONARY HYPERTENSION

Pulmonary hypertension is a rare lung disorder characterized by increased pressure in the pulmonary artery. The pulmonary artery carries oxygen-poor blood from the lower chamber on the right side of the heart (right ventricle) to the lungs where it picks up oxygen.

Pulmonary hypertension is present when the blood pressure in the circulation of the lungs is measured at greater than 25 mm of mercury (Hg) at rest or 30 mm Hg during **exercise**. Pulmonary hypertension can be either primary or secondary:

- Primary Pulmonary hypertension. The cause of pulmonary hypertension is unknown. It is rare, affecting 2 people per million. The illness most often occurs in young adults, especially women.
- Secondary Pulmonary Hypertension. Secondary pulmonary hypertension is increased pressure of the blood vessels of the lungs as a result of other medical conditions.

Regardless of whether pulmonary hypertension is primary or secondary, the disorder results in thickening of the pulmonary arteries and narrowing of these blood vessels. In response, the right side of the heart works harder to move the blood through these arteries and it becomes enlarged. Eventually overworking the right side of the heart may lead to right-sided **heart failure**, resulting in **death**.

While the cause of primary pulmonary hypertension is uncertain, researchers think that in most people who develop the disease, the blood vessels are sensitive to certain factors that cause them to narrow. Diet suppressants, cocaine, and **pregnancy** are some of the factors that are thought to trigger constriction or narrowing of the pulmonary artery. In about 6–10% of cases, primary pulmonary hypertension is inherited.

Secondary pulmonary hypertension can be associated with breathing disorders such as emphysema and **bronchitis**, or diseases such as **scleroderma**, **systemic lupus erythematosus** (SLE) or congenital heart disease involving heart valves, and pulmonary thromboembolism.

Symptoms of pulmonary hypertension include **shortness of breath** with minimal exertion, general fatigue, **dizziness**, and **fainting**. Swelling of the ankles, bluish lips and skin, and chest **pain** are among other symptoms of the disease.

Pulmonary hypertension is rarely detected during routine **physical examinations** and, therefore, often progresses to later stages before being diagnosed. In addition to listening to heart sounds with a stethoscope, physicians also use electrocardiogram, pulmonary function tests, perfusion lung scan, and/or right-heart cardiac catheterization to diagnose pulmonary hypertension.

The aim of treatment for pulmonary hypertension is to treat the underlying cause, if it is known. For example, thromboendarterectomy is a surgical procedure performed to remove a blood clot on the lung that is causing the pulmonary hypertension. Lung transplants are another surgical treatment.

Some patients are helped by taking medicines that make the work of the heart easier. Anticoagulants, drugs that thin the blood, decrease the tendency of the blood to clot and allow blood to flow more freely. **Diuretics** decrease the amount of fluid in the body and reduce the amount of work the heart has to do. Calcium channel blockers relax the smooth muscle in the walls of the heart and blood vessels and improve the ability of the heart to pump blood.

One effective medical treatment that dilates blood vessels and seems to help prevent blood clots from forming is epoprostenol (prostacyclin). Prostacyclin is given intravenously to improve survival, exercise duration, and well-being. It is sometimes used as a bridge to help people who are waiting for a lung transplant. In other cases it is used for long-term treatment.

Some people require supplemental oxygen through nasal prongs or a mask if breathing becomes difficult.

Pulmonary hypertension is chronic and incurable with an unpredictable survival rate. Length of survival has been improving, with some patients able to live 15–20 years or longer with the disorder.

Since the cause of primary pulmonary hypertension is still unknown, there is no way to prevent or cure this disease. A change in lifestyle may assist patients with daily activities. For example, relaxation exercises help to reduce stress. Good health habits such as a healthy diet, not smoking, and getting plenty of rest should be maintained.

Q

Quackery

The term quackery refers to promotion of a medical remedy that is false or unproven in order to earn a profit. The word derives from the term *quacksalver*, literally someone who boasts or quacks about his salves. Promoters of quackery, known as quacks, may not deliberately intend to deceive customers. In fact, they may genuinely believe that their products are worthwhile. However, good intentions don't make products effective for the purposes for which they are advertised, and Americans waste billions of dollars annually on false or unproven medical remedies.

Advertising and promotion are key ingredients of quackery. Quack remedies are available for virtually any condition from which a person may suffer, as well as a few that don't even exist. Promoters are expert at tapping into the normal concerns that people have about their health and their appearance. The products they offer range from the useless to the dangerous. Even graver are the quack remedies that offer false hope to desperate people who may be suffering from serious illness such as **cancer** or **AIDS**.

People who purchase quack remedies may be fooled, but they are not fools. Quackery succeeds because the promises are appealing, and they include impressive scientific language. A person might need a background in medicine, biochemistry, and physics in order to determine that certain promotions are based on misrepresented science. Promoters of quackery also misuse science by using preliminary studies to back up their claims and by selectively quoting from scientific sources. They may say they are ahead of their time and proclaim their product as a breakthrough. Genuine breakthroughs are rigorously studied and questioned by medical experts before they may be marketed. Promoters may complain that the medical establishment refuses to test their remedies. However, the burden of proof should rest with the person or company making the claim. The use of testimonials from satisfied customers contributes to the credibility of the advertising. However, the customer has no way of knowing whether the testimonial is real or not. Even if the testimonial is genuine, the results may or may not be due to the remedy being promoted.

Potential customers may believe that consumer protection laws prohibit quackery. Unfortunately, the laws are inadequate. The **Food and Drug Administration** (FDA) can take action when a food, drug, cosmetic, or medical device is promoted using false information. The FDA can also step in if a product is shown to be dangerous. The Federal Trade Commission can act in cases of false or misleading advertising. The U.S. Postal Service may be involved in cases in which the mail is used to defraud someone. The three agencies are hampered by small staffs and too many demands on their resources. Promoters can dodge charges by using vague wording in their advertising and by plainly stating that their products haven't been approved by the FDA. Customers who have been duped may be reluctant to complain, so it is difficult to build a case against promoters of quackery.

See also Patent medicine

R

Rabies

Rabies, a virus which affects the central nervous system, is found in saliva, brain tissue, and cerebral spinal fluid of animals and/or humans infected by it. Following years of decline in the United States, the number of reported rabies cases in animals is rising dramatically. Today, with improved vaccines and prompt treatment, human death from rabies is rare: six people died from the disease in 1994 and four in 1995.

Louis Pasteur's memories of witnessing—at the age of nine—a mad wolf snapping at animals and humans in his home town, and the cauterization of one of the nine victim's wounds by a blacksmith's red-hot poker, played a significant role in his decision to investigate the deadly rabies virus. Rabies was not very common in the eighteenth century, however victims eventually died due to destruction of nerve cells in the brain, but not before going through several days of intense suffering which included throat spasms, fevers, delirium, and paralysis. Since inability to swallow water is a symptom of rabies, it was also called hydrophobia, meaning *fear of water*.

Rabies is usually spread by saliva from the bite of an animal infected with the virus. François Magendie, a French neurophysiologist, also showed that saliva from infected humans could transmit the fatal disease to dogs. (The only reported case of human-to-human transmission was through a corneal transplant from an infected donor.) Pasteur and his coworkers, Charles-Edouard Chamberland (1851-1908) and Pierre-Paul-Emile Roux (1853-1933), failed to isolate the causative agent, which they believed to be a bacteria. Studying the tissue cultures from rabid and healthy animals, they soon discovered the heaviest concentrations of the pathogen in the spinal cords of rabid rabbits. Pasteur weakened the active rabies agents by hanging the spinal cords inside glass bottles with a drying agent and waiting two weeks for the viruses to become inactivated. Each day during that 14-day period, he made a broth suspension from the spinal cords. The 14-day-old suspension was not active, the seven-day-old suspension was more active, and the day-old suspension was very active. He began inoculating fifty dogs, using the inactive suspension first, working his way up to the most active. The inoculations had the same effect that the red-hot poker treatment had produced for the victim of the rabid wolf—it rendered the rabies virus inactive so that it could not enter the incubation stage for hydrophobia. By the time the final inoculation was given, the dogs were immune to the virus.

Pasteur was hesitant to test the vaccine on humans until July 1885 when a nine-year-old boy who had been bitten 14 times by a rabid dog was brought to him. The only chance this boy, Joseph Meister, had to stop the incubation and survive hydrophobia was from the vaccine Pasteur had developed. The treatment worked, and 23 days after being bitten, Joseph returned home, eventually returning to the Pasteur Institute in Paris where he became gate-porter. He committed suicide in 1940 after being ordered by the invading German troops to open Pasteur's crypt at the Institute. Pasteur scored another victory with a 14-year-old shepherd boy who battled a rabid dog to save his five friends from the fatal bites. Six days after Jean Baptiste Jupille was wounded, he was given vaccine treatment and survived. The vaccine's first failure was reported in 1885 when Louise Pelletier died eleven days after treatment was completed. Her death, however, was not surprising since she had been bitten on the head by a mountain dog and then waited 37 days to get treatment; the incubation had begun before she was vaccinated. Overall, the rabies vaccine proved to be a lifesaving treatment.

Rabies is still fatal unless the antirabies vaccine is started in time. Pasteur's method for diagnosing rabies could take 10-15 days before it became apparent that treatment was necessary. By the early twentieth century, American pathologist **Anna Wessels Williams** introduced a diagnostic procedure by which brain smears of the suspected rabid animal could be examined and diagnosis achieved in 30 minutes. Today, researchers believe a simple eye test may detect rabies faster than the blood, skin, or saliva tests currently used. Also available today is a ''preexposure'' vaccine for people exposed to high-risk situations, including veterinarians, researchers, forest rangers, and travellers to most third-world countries where rabid animals are prevalent.

Radial keratotomy

Radial keratotomy (RK) is a surgical procedure in which precisely placed micro incisions are made in a patient's cornea—the clear matter which covers the eyeball—to permanently correct near-sightedness, or myopia. In myopia, the curvature of the cornea causes light rays entering the eye to fall short of the *retina*. Radial keratotomy flattens the eyeball minutely, allowing light rays to focus at the retina. First performed in Japan in 1955 by T. Sato, Soviet ophthalmologist Svyatoslav Fyodorov developed the procedure in the 1970s after removing glass splinters from a patient whose vision actually improved once the eye healed. The procedure was brought to the United States in 1977 and further refined. Although once considered a risky procedure—and there are still risks involved—more than one million people worldwide have undergone treatment. In most instances, RK can improve myopic vision to 20/40 or better, even though some cases the patient still needs lenses due to under-correction and in others because of over-correction which causes far- sightedness.

Other permanent procedures as alternatives to RK include photorefractive keratectomy (PRK) which uses an excimer (ultraviolet) laser to vaporize corneal tissue; automated lamellar keratectomy (ALK), in which a microkeratome is used to remove portion of the cornea which is frozen, reshaped by grinding, and sewn back into the eye; laser-assisted intrastromal keratomileus (LASIK), which combines portions of ALK and LASIK to make a tiny flap on the cornea through which the inside layers are reshaped and the flap then closed; and orthokeratology—flattening the cornea by the rubbing of hard contact lenses which exert pressure on the eye.

Radiation injuries

Radio and television signals, radar, heat, infrared, ultraviolet, sunlight, starlight, cosmic rays, gamma rays, and x rays all belong to the electromagnetic spectrum and differ only in their relative energy, frequency, and wavelength. These waves all travel at the speed of light, and unlike sound they can all travel through empty space. The frequencies above visible light have enough energy to penetrate and cause damage to living tissue, damage that can be as minor as a **sunburn** caused by ultraviolet light or as extreme as the incineration of Hiroshima, Japan, during World War II. Lower frequencies do not penetrate, but can cause eye and skin damage, primarily due to the heat they transmit.

The energy of electromagnetic radiation is a direct function of its frequency. The high-energy, high-frequency waves, which can penetrate solids to various depths, cause damage by separating molecules into electrically charged pieces, a process known as ionization. Atomic particles, cosmic rays, gamma rays, x rays, and some ultraviolet are called ionizing radiation. The pieces they generate are called free radicals. They act like acid, but they last only fractions of a second before they revert to harmless forms. Adjusting the energy of therapeutic radiation can select a depth at which it will do the most damage. Ionizing radiation also does damage to chromosomes by breaking strands of DNA. DNA is so good at repairing itself that both strands of the double helix must be broken to produce genetic damage.

Because radiation is energy, it can be measured. There are a number of units used to quantify radiation energy. Some refer to effects on air, others to effects on living tissue. The roentgen, named after Wilhelm Conrad Roentgen, who discovered x rays in 1895, measures ionizing energy in air. A rad expresses the energy transferred to tissue. The rem measures tissue response. A roentgen generates about a rad of effect and produces about a rem of response. The gray and the sievert are international units equivalent to 100 rads and rems, respectively. A curie, named after French physicists who experimented with radiation, is a measure of actual radioactivity given off by a radioactive element, not a measure of its effect. The average annual human exposure to natural background radiation is roughly 3 milliSieverts (mSv).

It is reasonable to presume that any amount of ionizing radiation will produce some damage. However, there is radiation everywhere, from the sun (cosmic rays) and from traces of radioactive elements in the air (radon) and the ground (uranium, radium, carbon-14, potassium-40 and many others). Earth's atmosphere protects us from most of the sun's radiation. Living at 5,000 feet altitude in Denver, Colorado, doubles exposure to radiation, and flight in a commercial airliner increases it 150-fold by lifting us above 80% of that atmosphere. Because no amount of radiation is perfectly safe and because radiation is ever present, arbitrary limits have been established to provide some measure of safety for those exposed to unusual amounts. Less than 1% of them reach the current annual permissible maximum of 50 mSv.

It is therapeutic, accidental, and deliberate radiation that does the obvious damage. There has not been much in the way of deliberate radiation damage since Nagasaki, but accidental radiation exposure happens periodically. Between 1945 and 1987, there were 285 nuclear reactor accidents, injuring over 1,550 people and killing 64. The most striking example, and the only one to endanger the public, was the meltdown of the graphite core nuclear reactor at Chernobyl in 1986, which spread a cloud of radioactive particles across the entire continent of Europe. Information about radiation effects is still being gathered from that disaster. There have also been a few accidents with medical and industrial radioactivity.

Nevertheless, it is believed that radiation is responsible for less than 1% of all human disease and for about 3% of all cancers. This figure does not include **lung cancer** from environmental radon, because that information is unknown. The figure could be significant, but it is greatly confounded by the similar effects of tobacco.

Radiation can damage every tissue in the body. The particular manifestation will depend upon the amount of radiation, the time over which it is absorbed, and the susceptibility of the tissue. The fastest growing tissues are the most vulnerable, because radiation as much as triples its effects during the growth phase. Bone marrow cells that make blood are the fastest growing cells in the body. A fetus in the womb is equally sensitive. The germinal cells in the testes and ovaries are only slightly less sensitive. Both can be rendered useless with very small doses of radiation. More resistant are the lining cells of the body—skin and intestines. Most resistant are the brain cells, because they grow the slowest.

The relative sensitivity of various tissues gives a good idea of the wide range that presents itself. The numbers represent the minimum damaging doses; a gray and a sievert represent roughly the same amount of radiation:

- Fetus—2 grays (Gy).
- Bone marrow—2 Gy.
- Ovary—2-3 Gy.
- Testes—5-15 Gy.
- Lens of the eye—5 Gy.
- Child cartilage—10 Gy.
- Adult cartilage—60 Gy.
- Child bone—20 Gy.
- Adult bone—60 Gy.
- Kidney—23 Gy.
- Child muscle—20-30 Gy.
- Adult muscle—100+ Gy.
- Intestines—45-55 Gy.
- Brain—50 Gy.

Notice that the least of these doses is a thousand times greater than the background exposure and nearly 50 times greater than the maximum permissible annual dosage.

The length of exposure makes a big difference in what happens. Over time the accumulating damage, if not enough to kill cells outright, distorts their growth and causes scarring and/or cancers. In addition to leukemias, cancers of the thyroid, brain, bone, breast, skin, stomach, and lung all arise after radiation. Damage depends, too, on the ability of the tissue to repair itself. Some tissues and some types of damage produce much greater consequences than others.

Immediately after sudden irradiation, the fate of the patient depends mostly on the total dose absorbed. This information comes mostly from survivors of the atomic bomb blasts over Japan in 1945.

- Massive doses incinerate immediately and are not distinguishable from the heat of the source.
- A sudden whole body dose over 50 Sv produces such profound neurological, heart, and circulatory damage that patients die within the first two days.
- Doses in the 10-20 Sv range affect the intestines, stripping their lining and leading to **death** within three months from vomiting, diarrhea, **starvation**, and infection.
- Victims receiving 6-10 Sv all at once usually escape an intestinal death, facing instead bone marrow failure and death within two months from loss of blood coagulation factors and the protection against infection provided by white blood cells.
- Between 2-6 Sv gives a fighting chance for survival if victims are supported with blood **transfusion**s and **antibiotics**.
- One or two Sv produces a brief, non-lethal sickness with vomiting, loss of appetite, and generalized discomfort.

It is clearly important to have some idea of the dose received as early as possible, so that attention can be directed to those victims in the 2-10 Sv range that might survive with treatment. Blood transfusions, protection from infection in damaged organs, and possibly the use of newer stimulants to blood formation can save many victims in this category.

Local radiation exposures usually damage the skin and require careful wound care, removal of dead tissue, and **skin grafting** if the area is large. Again **infection control** is imperative.

There is considerable interest these days in benevolent chemicals called "free radical scavengers." How well they work is yet to be determined, but population studies strongly suggest that certain diets are better than others, and that those diets are full of free radical scavengers, otherwise known as antioxidants. The recommended ingredients are beta-carotene, **vitamins** E and C, and selenium, all available as commercial preparations. Beta-carotene is yellow-orange and is present in yellow and orange fruits and vegetables. Vitamin C can be found naturally in citrus fruits. Traditional Chinese medicine (TCM) and acupuncture, botanical medicine, and homeopathy all have contributions to make to recovery from the damage of radiation injuries. The level of recovery will depend on the exposure. Consulting practitioners trained in these modalities will result in the greatest benefit.

RADIATION THERAPY

Radiation therapy is the use of high energy, penetrating radiation (x rays, gamma rays, proton rays, and neutron rays) to kill **cancer** cells.

The primary purpose of radiation therapy is to eliminate or shrink localized cancers (as opposed to cancers that have spread to distant parts of the body). The aim is to kill as many cancer cells as possible, while doing as little damage as possible to healthy tissues. In some cases, the purpose is to kill all cancer cells and effect a cure. In other cases, when cures are not possible, the purpose is to alleviate **pain** by reducing the size of tumors that cause pain.

For some kinds of cancers (for example, **Hodgkin's disease**, non-Hodgkin's lymphoma, **prostate cancer**, and laryngeal cancer), radiation therapy alone is the preferred treatment. However, radiation is often used in conjunction with surgery, **chemotherapy**, or both, and survival rates for combination therapy in these cases are greater than for any single type of therapy. Radiation therapy is especially useful when surgical procedures cannot remove an entire tumor without damaging the function of surrounding organs. In these cases, surgeons remove as much of the tumor as possible, and the remainder is treated with radiation (irradiated).

Radiation therapy is also known as radiotherapy, radiation treatment, x ray therapy, cobalt therapy, and electron beam therapy. Recent advances have made it even more useful for patients and have cut down on some of the unpleasant side effects. **Radioactive implants** allow delivery of radiation to localized areas, with less injury to surrounding tissues than radiation from an external source that must pass through those tissues. Proton radiation also causes less injury to surrounding tissues than traditional photon radiation because proton rays can be more tightly focused. Current research with radioimmunotherapy and neutron capture therapy may provide ways to direct radiation exclusively at cancer cells, and in the case of radioimmunotherapy, to cancer cells that have spread to many sites throughout the body.

High energy radiation kills cells by damaging their DNA and thus blocking their ability to divide and proliferate. Radiation kills normal cells about as well as cancer cells, but cells that are growing and dividing quickly (such as cancer cells, skin cells, blood cells, immune system cells, and digestive system cells) are most susceptible to radiation. Fortunately, most normal cells are better able to repair radiation damage than are cancer cells. Accordingly, radiation treatments are parceled into component treatments that are spaced throughout a given time interval (usually about seven weeks). Thus, cells are given a chance to repair during the time between treatments. Since the repair rate of normal cells is greater than the repair rate of cancerous cells, a smaller fraction of the radiation-damaged cancerous cells will have been repaired by the time of the next treatment. This procedure is called ''fractionation'' because the total radiation dose is divided into fractions. Fractionation allows greater killing of cancer cells with less ultimate damage to the surrounding normal cells. Ideally all cancer cells will be dead after the last treatment session.

Before radiation therapy, the size and location of the patient's tumor and the nature of the surrounding tissue that may be in the path of the radiation beam must be determined as accurately as possible so that the radiation treatment can be designed to be maximally effective. **Magnetic resonance imaging** (MRI) and **computed tomography scan** (CT scan) are used to provide detailed images. The correct radiation dose, the number of sessions (fractions), the interval between sessions, and whether to give each fraction from the same direction or from different directions to lower the total dose imparted to any one nearby area, are calculated based on the tumor type, its size, and the sensitivity of the nearby tissues.

Shields are sometimes constructed for the patient to protect certain areas. The patient's skin may be marked with ink or tattoos to help achieve correct positioning for each treatment, or molds may be built to hold tissues in exactly the right place each time. When treatment may cause hair loss, some patients may want to purchase a wig, hat, or bandana in advance.

Follow-up is important for patients who have received radiation therapy. They should go to their radiation oncologist at least once within the first several weeks after their final treatment to see if their treatment was successful. They should also see an oncologist every six to twelve months for the rest of their lives so they can be checked to see if the tumor has reappeared or spread.

Treatment of symptoms following radiation therapy depends on which part of the body is being treated and the type of radiation. Nevertheless, many patients experience skin burn, fatigue, nausea, and vomiting regardless of the treatment area.

Affected skin should be kept clean and can be treated like a **sunburn**, with skin lotion or vitamin A and D ointment. Patients should avoid perfume and scented skin products and protect affected areas from the sun.

Nausea and vomiting are expected when the dose is high or if the abdomen or another part of the digestive tract is irradiated. Sometimes nausea and vomiting occur after radiation to other regions, but in these cases the symptoms usually disappear within a few hours after treatment. Nausea and vomiting can be treated with **antacids**, Compazine, Tigan, or Zofran.

Fatigue frequently starts after the second week of therapy and may continue until about two weeks after the therapy is finished. Patients may want to limit their activities, cut back their work hours, or take time off from work. They also may need to take naps and get extra sleep at night.

Patients who receive external beam therapy do not become radioactive and should be assured that they do not pose a danger to others. However, some patients who receive brachytherapy go home with low levels of radioactivity inside their bodies. These patients should be given instructions about any dangers they might pose to children and people of childbearing age and how long these dangers will last.

Emotional support is an important part of the care for patients undergoing any treatment for cancer.

Radioactive implants

Radioactive implants are devices that are placed directly within **cancer**ous tissue or tumors, in order to deliver **radiation therapy** intended to kill cancerous cells.

With the use of radioactive implants, the tumor is subjected to radioactive activity over a longer period of time, as compared to external beam therapy.

The patient is required to remain in his bed or room during the treatment. During the period of greatest radioactivity (24-72 hours), health care providers will limit the amount of time spent with the patient to that required for essential care.

Interstitial radiation therapy places the sources of radiation directly into the tumor and surrounding structures. Most commonly used in tumors of the head, neck, prostate, and breast, it may also be used in combination with external radiation therapy. The implant may be permanent or removable. A permanent implant of radioactive seeds, such as gold or iodine, is placed directly into the organ. Over several weeks or months, the seeds slowly deliver radiation to the tumor. More commonly used is the removable implant that requires an operation under general **anesthesia** to place narrow, hollow stainless steel needles through the tumor. Teflon tubes are inserted through the needles, and the needles are then removed. After the patient returns to his room, radioactive seeds are inserted into the tubes in a procedure called afterloading. Once the desired dosage is reached, the tubes and seeds are removed.

Intracavity radiation is often used for gynecologic cancers. Under general or spinal anesthesia, hollow applicators are placed directly inside the affected organ. Correct positioning is confirmed by x rays, and once the patient has returned to her room, a small plastic tube containing the radioactive isotope is inserted into the hollow applicator. The treatment is delivered over 48-72 hours, after which time the applicator and radioactive sources are removed. Very high doses of radiation can be delivered to the tumor, while the rapid removal of the radioactive dose limits damage to the surrounding structures.

Normal cells are subjected to the effects of radiation; any tissue near the radiation site may be damaged or destroyed. Some side effects are acute and temporary, while others develop over time and may be permanent. Skin reactions, such as redness, **itching**, flaking, or stripping of the top layer, are usually temporary; long-term effects can include scarring, and changes in texture. Radiation recall is a delayed skin side effect in which the area that had been exposed to radiation becomes irritated or blistered after the patient receives certain **chemotherapy**.

Following treatment for tumors of the head and neck region, the lining of the mouth and throat can become inflamed or irritated, resulting in a condition known as mucositis or **stomatitis**. Injury to the salivary glands can decrease saliva production, resulting in a condition known as xerostomia, or dry mouth. There also may be alteration in the patient's taste buds, resulting in decrease or loss of taste sensation (hypogeusia or ageusia), or the presence of unpleasant taste, sometimes described as metallic (dysgeusia). Patients may experience **nausea and vomiting** as a result of the effect of radiation on the brain. Hair loss (alopecia) may result from radiation's effect on hair follicles.

Radiation's effect on the rapidly growing cells of the gastrointestinal tract may result in **diarrhea** or abdominal cramping. Pelvic radiation can affect the bowel, bladder, or sexual function. Radiation can also affect production of blood cell components in the bone marrow.

RADIOIMMUNOASSAY (RIA)

Radioimmunoassay is an extremely sensitive method of measuring very small amounts of a substance in the blood. The isotopic method was developed in 1959 by the Americans, biophysicist **Rosalyn Yalow** and physician Solomon A. Berson (1918-1972) at the Bronx (New York) Veterans Administration Hospital.

Yalow had established the hospital's radioisotope laboratory in 1947. In 1950, she was joined by Berson, a resident in internal medicine who became interested in her work. Berson was born in New York City in 1918, and received his B.S. in 1938 from the City University of New York and his M.D. in 1945 from New York University.

Yalow and Berson developed their first radioisotopic technique to study blood volume and iodine metabolism, then adapted the method to study hormones. Working with very pure insulin, they became the first to discover that small molecules can induce production of antibodies. They were also able to show that, contrary to theory, Type II (adult onset) diabetes is caused by inefficient use of insulin, not by lack of it in the body.

In 1959 they perfected their method, naming it radioimmunoassay (RIA). Its extreme sensitivity—it measures one thousand billionths of a gram of material per milliliter of blood—quickly made it a standard laboratory tool. To measure insulin, the first step is mixing known amounts of radioisotope-tagged insulin and antibodies. These combine chemically. Next, a small amount of the patient's blood is added; the insulin it contains displaces some of the tagged insulin. The free tagged insulin is then measured with isotope detectors and the patient's insulin level is calculated.

RIA has been used for measuring peptide and steroid hormones, as well as other substances such as morphine, viruses, vitamins, cyclic adenosine monophosphate (cAMP), and messenger RNA (ribonucleic acid). It has been applied to narcotics detection, blood bank screening for hepatitis virus, early cancer detection, measurement of growth hormone levels in shorter-than-normal children, tracking of leukemia virus, diagnosis and treatment of peptic ulcers, and research with brain chemicals called neurotransmitters.

In 1968 Berson became chair of the Department of Medicine, Mt. Sinai School of Medicine, still continuing to work with Yalow. His death in 1972 made him ineligible to share the portion of the Nobel Prize in physiology or medicine that Yalow received in 1977 for their work.

RAMAZZINI, BERNARDINI (1633-1714)

Italian physician

Bernardini (or Bernardino) Ramazzini was born in Modena, Italy. He was a pioneer in the fields of epidemiology, trade diseases, and industrial hygiene. He taught at the university in Modena until the beginning of the eighteenth century, when he left Modena to join the faculty at the University of Padua. There he taught **pathology** up until three years before his death.

Ramazzini published the first treatise on occupational medicine in 1700. Entitled *De Morbis Aritificium Diatriba* (*On Artificially Caused Diseases*), this pioneering work systematically identified health hazards in more than forty occupations, including mining, **midwifery**, **pharmacy**, painting, printing and gilding. By recognizing the relationship between certain metals and the artisans who used them, Ramazzini effectively launched the science of industrial medicine. Ramazzini was the first person after Paracelsus to observe the prevalence of many other occupational disorders, including stone mason and miner's phthsis (pneumonoconiosis), the vertigo and sciatica of potters, and the eye troubles of gilders, printers and other occupations. He also investigated the presence of poisonous elements in some of the pigments used by painters. Besides his interest in the origins of occupational diseases, Ramazzini was also concerned with the possibilities of taking preventive measures. As a physician, Ramazzini made important epidemiological observations. He described and differentiated a number of disorders in various regions of the country where the disorders were endemic, including the outbreak of lathyrism in Modena in 1690 and the Paduan cattle plague of 1712. In keeping

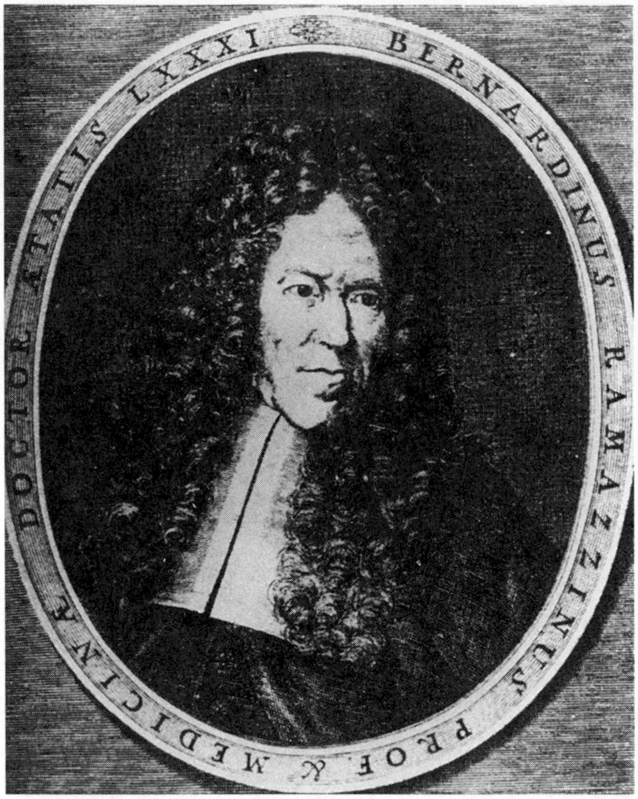

Bernardini Ramazzini

with the custom of clinicians of his time, he also recorded observations of the weather in (*Ephemerides barometricae*). He argued against the use of cinchona bark (the source of quinine) as a nonspecific treatment for disease, pointing out that the drug should only be used for cases of **malaria**. In modern times, Italian physicians have chosen to honor their compatriot Ramazzini by naming a medical journal after him.

Ramón y Cajal, Santiago (1852-1934)

Spanish histologist

Santiago Ramón y Cajal was born in Petilla, Aragón, Spain, on March 1, 1852. His father, a professor of applied anatomy, wanted young Santiago to pursue a medical career and enrolled his son first at the College of the Aesculpian Fathers and later at the Institute at Huesca. Young Ramón y Cajal was not really interested in medicine, however, and he left school to become apprenticed first to a barber, then to a shoemaker. At the age of 16, he returned to his formal education, entering the University of Saragossa. There he began studying the only medical subject in which he was really interested: anatomy. After graduation, Ramón y Cajal entered military service but, after contracting malaria in Cuba, he was discharged. He then returned to Saragossa, where he was made director of the museum in 1879. In 1883, he received a doctor of medicine degree from the University of Madrid.

Around this time, Ramón y Cajal became involved in a controversy then raging among anatomists. The question was how nerve messages are transmitted through the body. One theory—the reticular theory—held that nerve messages travel through a complex network of nerve fibers in physical contact with each other. Cell bodies observed within this network were thought to play primarily a structural and supportive role. Ramón y Cajal was able to provide new evidence about this issue by developing new cell-staining techniques. These stains showed more clearly than ever before the detailed structure of nerve tissue. With this technique, he was able to see that nerve cells are distinct units whose extensions—axons and dendrites—are *not* in contact with each other, but are separated by narrow gaps (synapses). For this discovery, Ramón y Cajal shared the 1906 Nobel Prize for physiology or medicine with **Camillo Golgi**.

Ramón y Cajal continued working on nerve structure and function for another three decades. In 1891, he found that nerve messages enter a neuron by way of the dendrites and leave by way of the axon. Later studies dealt with the growth and degeneration of neurons. He also developed new stains that made possible even more detailed studies of nerve tissue. For his many accomplishments in the field, Ramón y Cajal is often regarded as the father of modern neuroanatomy.

Ramón y Cajal's first academic appointment was as Professor of Descriptive and General Anatomy at the University of Valencia in 1883. He then went on to become Professor of Histology at the University of Barcelona in 1887 and Professor of Histology and Pathological Anatomy at the University of Madrid in 1892. He served at Madrid until 1921, when he became director of the Cajal Institute, founded in his honor by King Alfonso XIII. Ramón y Cajal died in Madrid on October 18, 1934.

See also Nervous system

Rape

Rape is a sexual assault on any unwilling victim. As with other violent crimes, sexual assaults are grossly under reported by victims due to feelings of embarrassment, fear of further injury and fear of court procedures. Rape can occur within the cycle of **domestic violence** in a marital relationship. It is estimated that only 20 percent of sexual assaults are committed by attackers unknown to the victim. Rape can be perpetrated upon individuals of both sexes, young or old, however some statistics suggest that the victims tend to be young women between the ages of 11 and 18.

One significant factor in date rape is the use of drugs and/or alcohol, leading to diminished judgment and self control on the part of either the victim and/or the assailant. In an effort to minimize chances of being raped, clear communication about sexual limits from the onset of a relationship will eliminate misinterpretation of nonverbal communication. Caution should be taken to avoid any places or situations that might lead to an especially vulnerable situation. Quick, assertive action in any forced attempt at sexual activity will have a higher chance of averting the assault. However, if the assailant is armed, passive resistance may be a safer option than fighting back.

Prompt medical attention is important following sexual assault. Before showering or cleansing the genital area, the victim should examined and treated for any injuries or possible venereal disease. Physical specimens will be collected as evidence for charges against the assailant. The rape should be reported to police, and the victim offered support. Most communities and college campuses offer rape or crisis **hotlines**. The victim who has **counseling** to assist them in dealing with the trauma of rape will have fewer lasting effects than those who get no help in dealing with the situation and their feelings.

See also Counseling; Domestic violence; Hotlines

Rashes

The popular term for a group of spots or red, inflamed skin that is usually a symptom of an underlying condition or disorder. Often temporary, a rash is only rarely a sign of a serious problem.

A rash may occur on only one area of the skin, or it could cover almost all of the body. Also, a rash may or may not be itchy. Depending on how it looks, a rash may be described as:

- Blistering (raised oval or round collections of fluid within or beneath the outer layer of skin)
- Macular (flat spots)
- Nodular (small, firm, knotty rounded mass)
- Papular (small solid slightly raised areas)
- Pustular (pus-containing skin blister).

There are many theories as to the development of skin rashes, but experts are not completely clear what causes some of them. Generally a skin rash is an intermittent symptom, fading and reappearing. Rashes may accompany a range of disorders and conditions, such as:

- Infectious illness. A rash is symptom of many different kinds of childhood infectious illnesses, including **chickenpox** and **scarlet fever**. It may be triggered by other infections, such as Rocky Mountain spotted fever or **ringworm**.
- Allergic reactions. One of the most common symptoms of an allergic reaction is an itchy rash. Contact dermatitis is a rash that appears after the skin is exposed to an allergen, such as metal, rubber, some cosmetics or lotions, or some types of plants (e.g. poison ivy). Drug reactions are another common allergic cause of rash; in this case, a rash is only one of a variety of possible symptoms, including **fever**, seizures, nausea and vomiting, **diarrhea**, heartbeat irregularities, and breathing problems. This rash usually appears soon after the first dose of the course of medicine is taken.

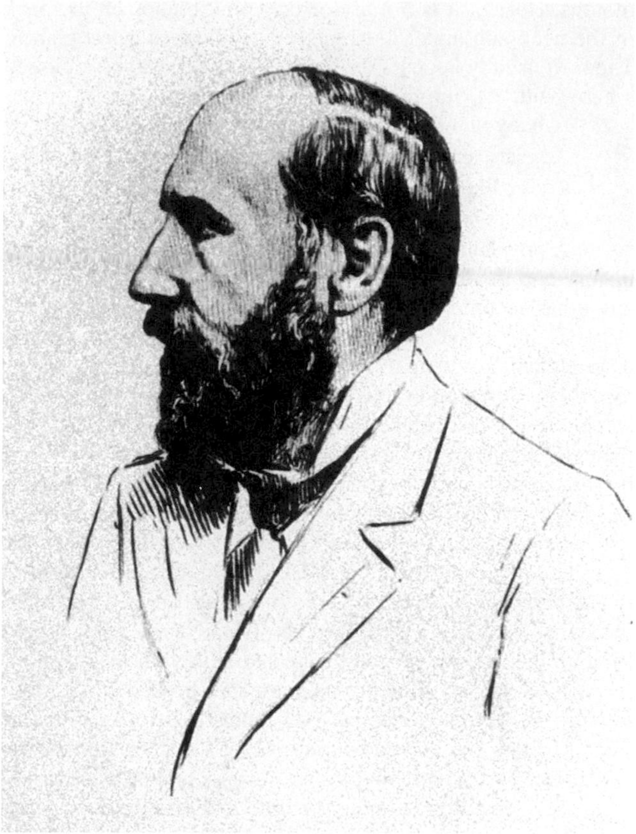

Santiago Ramón y Cajal

- Autoimmune disorders. Conditions in which the immune system turns on the body itself, such as systemic lupus erythematosus or purpura, often have a characteristic rash.
- Nutritional disorders. For example, scurvy, a disease caused by a lack of Vitamin C, has a rash as one of its symptoms.
- Cancer. A few types of cancer, such as chronic lymphocytic leukemia, can be the underlying cause of a rash.

Rashes are extremely common in infancy, and are usually not serious at all and can be treated at home.

Diaper rash is caused by prolonged skin contact with bacteria and the baby's waste products in a damp diaper. This rash has red, spotty sores and there may be an ammonia smell. In most cases the rash will respond within three days to drying efforts. A diaper rash that does not improve in this time may be a yeast infection requiring prescription medication. A doctor should be consulted if the rash is solid, bright red, causes fever, or the skin develops blisters, **boils**, or pus.

Infants also can get a rash on cheeks and chin caused by contact with food and stomach contents. This rash will come and go, but usually responds to a good cleaning after meals. About a third of all infants develop "acne" usually after the third week of life in response to their mothers' hormones before birth. This rash will disappear in a few weeks or a few months. Heat rash is a mass of tiny pink bumps on the back of the neck and upper back caused by blocked sweat glands. The rash usually appears during hot, humid weather, although a baby with a fever can also develop the rash.

A baby should see a doctor immediately if the rash:

- Appears suddenly and looks purple or blood-colored
- Looks like a burn
- Appears while the infant seems to be sick.

A physician can make a diagnosis based on the medical history and the appearance of the rash, where it appears, and any other accompanying symptoms.

Treatment of rashes focuses on resolving the underlying disorder and providing relief of the itching that often accompanies them. Soothing lotions or oral **antihistamines** can provide some relief, and topical antibiotics may be administered if the patient, particularly a child, has caused a secondary infection by scratching. The rash triggered by **allergies** should disappear as soon as the allergen is removed; drug rashes will fade when the patient stops taking the drug causing the allergy. For the treatment of diaper rash, the infant's skin should be exposed to the air as much as possible; ointments are not needed unless the skin is dry and cracked. Experts also recommend switching to cloth diapers and cleaning affected skin with plain water.

Most rashes that have an acute cause, such as an infection or an allergic reaction, will disappear as soon as the infection or irritant is removed from the body's system. Rashes that are caused by chronic conditions, such as autoimmune disorders, may remain indefinitely or fade and return periodically.

Some rashes can be prevented, depending on the triggering factor. A person known to be allergic to certain drugs or substances should avoid those things in order to prevent a rash. Diaper rash can be prevented by using cloth diapers and keeping the diaper area very clean, breast feeding, and changing diapers often.

RAT-BITE FEVER

Rat-bite fever refers to an infection which develops after having been bitten or scratched by an infected animal.

Rat-bite fever occurs most often among laboratory workers who handle lab rats in their jobs, and among people who live in poor conditions, with rodent infestation. Children are particularly likely to be bitten by rodents infesting their home, and are therefore most likely to contract rat-bite fever. Other animals that can carry the types of bacteria responsible for this illness include mice, squirrels, weasels, dogs, and cats. One of the causative bacteria can cause the same illness if it is ingested, for example in unpasteurized milk.

There are two variations of rat-bite fever, caused by two different organisms. In the United States, the bacteria *Streptobacillus moniliformis* is the most common cause (causing streptobacillary rat-bite fever). In other countries, especially Africa, *Spirillum minus* causes a different form of the infection (called spirillary rat-bite fever).

Streptobacillary rat-bite fever occurs up to 22 days after the initial bite or scratch. The patient becomes ill with fever, chills, nausea and vomiting, **headache**, and **pain** in the back and joints. A rash made up of tiny pink bumps develops, covering the palms of the hands and the soles of the feet. Without treatment, the patient is at risk of developing serious infections of the lining of the heart (**endocarditis**), the sac containing the heart (**pericarditis**), the coverings of the brain and spinal cord (**meningitis**), or lungs (**pneumonia**). Any tissue or organ throughout the body may develop a pocket of infection and pus, called an **abscess**.

Spirillary rat-bite fever occurs some time after the initial injury has already healed, up to about 28 days after the bite or scratch. Although the wound had appeared completely healed, it suddenly grows red and swollen again. The patient develops a fever. Lymph nodes in the area become swollen and tender, and the patient suffers from fever, chills, and headache. The skin in the area of the original wound sloughs off. Although rash is less common than with streptobacillary rat-bite fever, there may be a lightly rosy, itchy rash all over the body. Joint and muscle pain rarely occur. If left untreated, the fever usually subsides, only to return again in repeated two- to four-day cycles. This can go on for up to a year, although, even without treatment, the illness usually resolves within four to eight weeks.

In streptobacillary rat-bite fever, found in the United States, diagnosis can be made by taking a sample of blood or fluid from a painful joint. In a laboratory, the sample can be cultured, to allow the growth of organisms. Examination under a microscope will then allow identification of the bacteria *Streptobacillus moniliformis.* In spirillary rat-bite fever, diagnosis can be made by examining blood or a sample of tissue from the wound for evidence of *Spirillum minus.*

Shots of procaine penicillin G or penicillin V by mouth are effective against both streptobacillary and spirillary rat-bite fever. When a patient is allergic to the **penicillins**, erythromycin may be given by mouth for streptobacillary infection, or tetracycline by mouth for spirillary infection.

With treatment, prognosis is excellent for both types of rat-bite fever. Without treatment, the spirillary form usually resolves on its own, although it may take up to a year to do so.

The streptobacillary form, found in the United States, however, can progress to cause extremely serious, potentially fatal complications. In fact, before **antibiotics** were available to treat the infection, streptobacillary rat-bite fever frequently resulted in **death**.

Prevention involves avoiding contact with those animals capable of passing on the causative organisms. This can be an unfortunately difficult task for people whose economic situations do not allow them to move out of rat-infested buildings. Because streptobacillary rat-bite fever can occur after drinking contaminated milk or water, only pasteurized milk, and water from safe sources, should be ingested.

RAYNAUD'S DISEASE

Raynaud's disease refers to a disorder in which the fingers or toes (digits) suddenly experience decreased blood circulation.

Raynaud's disease can be classified as one of two types: primary (or idiopathic) and secondary (also called Raynaud's phenomenon).

Primary and idiopathic are words used to describe a condition which occurs by itself, with no other accompanying conditions that could be considered the cause. Primary Raynaud's disease is more mild, and causes fewer complications. About half of all cases of Raynaud's disease are of this type. Women are five times more likely than men to develop primary Raynaud's disease, and the average age of diagnosis is between 20 and 40 years. About 30% of all cases of primary Raynaud's disease progress after diagnosis, while 15% of cases actually improve.

Secondary Raynaud's disease is more complicated, severe, and more likely to progress. A number of medical conditions predispose a person to secondary Raynaud's disease, including:

- **Scleroderma**. Scleroderma is a serious disease of the connective tissue, in which tissues of the skin, heart, esophagus, kidney, and lung become thickened, hard, and constricted. About 30% of patients who develop scleroderma will first develop Raynaud's disease.
- Other connective tissue diseases, including **systemic lupus erythematosus**, **rheumatoid arthritis**, dermatomyositis, and polymyositis.
- Diseases which result in blockages of arteries (including **atherosclerosis** or hardening of the arteries).
- A severe form of high blood pressure which is caused by diseased arteries in the lung (called **pulmonary hypertension**).
- A number of nervous system disorders, including herniated discs in the spine, **stroke**s, tumors within the spinal cord, **polio**, and **carpal tunnel syndrome**.
- A variety of blood disorders.
- Injuries, including those due to exposure to constant vibration (workers who use chainsaws, jackhammers, or other vibrating equipment), repetitive movements (typists and piano players), electric shock, or extreme cold (frostbite).
- The use of certain medications, including drugs used for migraine **headache**s, high blood pressure, and some cancer **chemotherapy** agents.

Both primary and secondary types of Raynaud's symptoms are believed to be due to over-reactive arterioles (small arteries). While cold normally causes the muscle which makes up the walls of arteries to contract (squeeze down to become smaller), in Raynaud's disease the degree is extreme. Blood flow to the area is thus severely restricted. Some attacks may also be brought on or worsened by **anxiety** or emotional distress.

Classically, there are three distinct phases to an episode of Raynaud's symptoms. When first exposed to cold, the arteries respond by contracting intensely. The digits (fingers or toes) in question (or in rare instances, the tip of the nose or tongue) become pale and white as they are deprived of blood flow and, thus, oxygen. In response, the veins and capillaries dilate (expand). Because these vessels carry deoxygenated blood, the digit turns a bluish shade. The digit often feels cold, numb, and tingly. After the digit begins to warm up again, the arteries dilate. Blood flow increases significantly, and the digits turn a bright red. During this phase, the patient often describes the digits as feeling warm, and throbbing painfully.

Raynaud's disease may initially only affect the tips of the fingers or toes. When the disease progresses, it may eventually affect the entire finger or toe. Ultimately, all the fingers or toes may be affected. About 10% of the time, a complication called sclerodactyly may occur. In sclerodactyly, the skin over the affected digits becomes tight, white, thick, smooth, and shiny.

When the most serious complications of Raynaud's disease or phenomenon occur, the affected digits develop deep sores (ulcers) in the skin. The tissue may even die (**gangrene**), requiring **amputation**. This complication only occurs about 1% of the time in primary Raynaud's disease.

While the patient's symptoms will be the first clue pointing to Raynaud's disease, a number of tests may also be performed to confirm the diagnosis. Special blood tests called the antinuclear antibody test (ABA) and the erythrocyte sedimentation rate (ESR) are often abnormal when an individual has a connective tissue disease.

When a person has connective tissue disease, his or her capillaries are usually abnormal. A test called a nailfold capillary study can demonstrate such abnormalities. In this test, a drop of oil is placed on the skin at the base of the fingernail. This allows the capillaries in that area to be viewed more easily with a microscope.

A cold stimulation test may also be performed. In this test, specialized thermometers are taped to each of the digits that have experienced episodes of Raynaud's disease. The at-rest temperature of these digits is recorded. The hand or foot is then placed completely into a container of ice water for 20 seconds. After removing the hand or foot from this water, the temperature of the digits is recorded immediately. The temperature of the digits is recorded every five minutes until they reach the same temperature they were before being put into the ice water. A normal result occurs when this pre-test temperature is reached in 15 minutes or less. If it takes more than 20 minutes, the test is considered suspicious for Raynaud's disease or phenomenon.

The first type of treatment for Raynaud's symptoms is simple avoidance. Patients need to stay warm, and keep hands and feet well covered in cold weather. Patients who smoke cigarettes should stop, because nicotine will worsen the problem. Most people (especially those with primary Raynaud's) are able to deal with the disease by taking these basic measures.

People with more severe cases of Raynaud's disease may need to be treated with medications to attempt to keep the arterioles relaxed and dilated. Some medications which are more commonly used to treat high blood pressure (calcium-channel blockers, reserpine), are often effective for Raynaud's symptoms. Nitroglycerine paste can be used on the affected digits, and seems to be helpful in healing skin ulcers.

When a patient has secondary Raynaud's phenomenon, treatment of the coexisting condition may help control the Raynaud's as well. In the case of connective tissue disorders, this often involves treatment with corticosteroid medications.

Because episodes of Raynaud's disease have also been associated with **stress** and emotional upset, the disease may be improved by helping a patient learn to manage stress. Regular **exercise** is known to decrease stress and lower anxiety. **Hypnosis**, relaxation techniques, and visualization are also useful methods to help a patient gain control of his or her emotional responses. **Biofeedback** training is a technique during which a patient is given continuous information on the temperature of his or her digits, and then taught to voluntarily control this temperature.

Some alternative practitioners believe that certain dietary supplements and herbs may be helpful in decreasing the vessel spasm of Raynaud's disease. Suggested supplements include vitamin E (found in fruits, vegetables, seeds, and nuts), magnesium (found in seeds, nuts, fish, beans, and dark green vegetables), and fish oils. Several types of herbs have been suggested, including peony (*Paeonia lactiflora*) and dong quai (*Angelica sinensis*). The circulatory herbs cayenne (*Capsicum frutescens*), ginger (*Zingiber officinale*), and prickly ash (*Zanthoxylum americanum*) can help enhance circulation to the extremities.

The prognosis for most people with Raynaud's disease is very good. In general, primary Raynaud's disease has the best prognosis, with a relatively small chance for serious complications (1%). In fact, about 50% of all patients do well by taking simple precautions, and never even require medications. The prognosis for people with secondary Raynaud's disease (or phenomenon) is less predictable. This prognosis depends greatly on the severity of the patient's other associated condition (e.g. scleroderma or lupus).

There is no known way to prevent the development of Raynaud's disease. Once an individual realizes that he or she suffers from this disorder, however, steps can be taken to reduce the frequency and severity of episodes.

Razi, Abu Bakr Muhammad ibn Zakariya ar- (c. 850-c. 932)

Persian physician and philosopher

Abu Bakr Muhammad ibn Zakariya ar-Razi, also known as Rhazes, was born at Ray (near Tehran) in Persia. The actual years of his birth and death are uncertain. An Arabic physician and scientist, Rhazes is today recognized as one of the original portrayers of disease. Like many medieval scholars, Rhazes mastered a wide range of subjects, including philosophy, music (he wrote an encyclopedia on the subject), poetry, and logic. His interest in medicine apparently did not arise until he was in his thirties, when it is said that he was stimulated by a chance encounter with an apothecary. At various times he taught and practiced in Baghdad, where he also served as director and chief physician in that city's hospital. Very little is known of Rhazes' personal life, but it is believed that he was often persecuted for his open mindedness and beliefs in equality.

Rhazes rejected all forms of dogma as fanaticism, and argued that religious fanaticism breeds hatred and wars. He held that science is a continual and unlimited progression based on the accumulation of past knowledge and the pursuit of the unknown. This idea differed significantly from the Aristotelian view that there exists a point of intellectual perfection.

Rhazes' most celebrated work is a 25-volume Graeco-Arabic compendium of medical and surgical knowledge entitled *Al-Hawi*. Translated into Latin as *Liber continens* in 1279 (it was the largest and heaviest of all books published before 1501), this work contained information on many diseases. In this work, Rhazes listed medical theories for each disease entry from Greek, Syrian, Indian, Persian, and Arabic medicine; these theories were followed by then-current ideas and by his own observations and opinions. Following the tradition of Hippocrates, Rhazes supplied case histories, along with pragmatic suggestions for treatment. Rhazes advocated simple remedies, including **dietary supplements**, and warned against the dangers of complex preparations. He advocated medical receptivity as a means by which *all* observed phenomena could be given proper consideration.

Rhazes also made one of the first accurate descriptions of (and distinctions between) **smallpox** and **measles**. Although smallpox had been described by some of the church fathers in the sixth century, and again by the seventh century chronicler Aaron, Rhazes' description differs from the earlier ones by its greater completeness as well as by its close resemblance to modern descriptions. The ninth book of *Al-Hawi* remained the main source of therapeutic knowledge until long after the Renaissance.

Rhazes was familiar with a wide range of well defined chemicals, which he probably used in his medical work. Like many physicians of his time, Rhazes was also actively interested in alchemy; his *Book of the Secrets* contains a great deal of practical advice on chemical manipulations. He believed in the transmutation of metals, and believed that metals were derived primarily from two elements, sulfur and mercury. He attempted to classify all known substances, dividing them basically into animal, mineral, or vegetable categories.

Rhazes' views sometimes got him into political trouble, and he was obliged on more than one occasion to leave his native city. Although medical care was a luxury available mainly for wealthy and noble families during his lifetime, Rhazes treated poor patients at no charge out of compassion and dedication to clinical practice. When he was in his seventies, it is said that Rhazes was beaten and blinded by order of a caliph who objected to his views. Despite his achievements leading to distinction, honors, and acquired wealth, Rhazes is said to have died in poverty, his wealth having been distributed to those less fortunate than himself. Although this physician-philosopher was the author of over 200 treatises (and over half of them about medicine), it was finally his outspoken and antiauthoritarian views on religion, politics, and science that gained him distinction as a leading figure in the history of Islamic thought. He once said that all that is written in books is worth much less than the experience of one wise doctor.

Reed, Walter (1851-1902)

American physician

Walter Reed is best known for his research demonstrating that the mosquito is responsible for transmitting **yellow fever** from infected humans to uninfected humans. In its emphasis on sound scientific methodology, his work set the standards for twentieth-century experimental medicine.

Reed was born in Belroi, Virginia. He received an M.D. from the University of Virginia in 1869, and another from Bellevue Hospital Medical College in New York, New York in 1870. After briefly practicing medicine, he was commissioned in the United States Medical Corps in 1874, serving at frontier posts in the West. In 1898, Reed was appointed chair of a board to investigate **typhoid fever** in army camps. The board was able to show that typhoid is spread by flies and contact with fecal material, bringing an end to the epidemic.

In 1900, Reed was appointed head of the Commission of the United States Army on yellow fever in Havana, Cuba, of which James Carroll (1854-1907), Jesse William Lazear (1866-1900) and Aristides Agramonte (1869-1931) were also members. At this time, theories abounded on the mode of transmission, as well as the cause, of yellow fever—the sometimes fatal disease occurring in tropical and subtropical zones worldwide. In 1848 Josiah Nott (1804-1873), a physician in Alabama, proposed the mosquito as the vector of yellow fever between humans. In 1881, Carlos Juan Finlay (1833-1940) suggested that the *Aëdes* species specifically was involved.

Reed's commission was requested to investigate the bacterial basis of the disease, which the Italian physician, Giuseppe Sanarelli (1864-1940), had proposed in 1897, but in 18 cases they could not find one. Reed was skeptical of the bacterial origin theory because he knew of cases where no contact had occurred between infected individuals. The Commission decided to experiment with *Aëdes aegypti* mosquitos.

While conducting their research, Carroll and Lazear were accidentally infected with yellow fever. Lazear's case was fatal and, on November 20, 1900, Reed established an isolation camp called Camp Lazear where the three remaining scientists produced 22 cases of yellow fever in soldiers who had volunteered for the study, conclusively implicating *Aëdes* as the vector. In the process, they also disproved the bacterial theory, demonstrating that the causative organism is non-filterable—what we now know to be a virus. Harvard awarded Reed an honorary M.A. He died in 1902 of acute appendicitis.

The Commission's evidence made possible the eradication of yellow fever in areas where *Aëdes'* breeding grounds were destroyed. It also marked the first time a human viral disease had been thoroughly researched, and *Aëdes* was the first insect determined to be a vector of a human disease. The Commission's use of experimental controls and meticulous records served as a model for medical research through the early twentieth century.

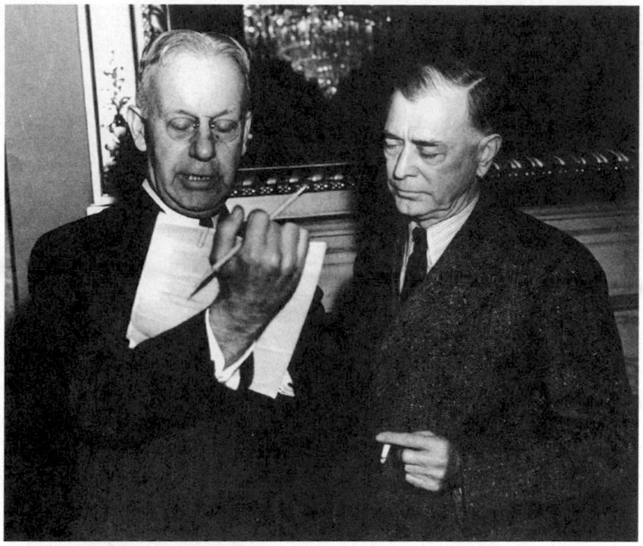

Walter Reed (right)

Reflexology

Based on the premise that there are reflex points in the hands and especially the feet that correspond to every part of the body, reflexology is the practice of applying pressure to these points in order to stimulate the body's natural healing powers.

Although reflexology does not treat specific diseases, its practitioners believe that stimulation of the proper reflex point in the foot will affect a particular organ, gland, or body part and can alleviate many health problems. Most use it to relieve stress and tension and to promote deep relaxation. Reflexologists also say that the overall health of a person benefits as the circulation is improved.

Reflexology employs no instruments or devices and involves only the application of pressure by hand on certain spots on the sides, soles, and tops of the feet. It is therefore safe for everyone when performed by a qualified therapist. There may be **pain** during the treatment when pressure is applied to specific points. It should, however, not be painful once the pressure is lifted.

Reflexology has its roots in the ancient civilizations of several different non-Western cultures. It first appeared in the West in the early 20th century as the ''zone therapy'' of American physician, William Fitzgerald, who divided the body into ten vertical zones. In the 1930s, the physiotherapist Eunice Ingham used this therapy on her patients and found that their feet were by far the most responsive areas to work, so she created a map of the entire body on the feet. Viewing the soles of the feet as a miniature representation of the body, she charted the toes as reflecting the head and neck; the soft balls of the feet, the shoulders and chest; the upper arch, the area from the diaphragm to the waist; the lower arch, the waist and pelvic area; and the heels, the sciatic nerve. The inside and outside curves of the feet as well as the ankles also corresponded to certain body areas.

Reflexology employs the principle that these ''reflex points'' on the feet, when worked by hand pressure, will reflexively stimulate energy to a related muscle or organ and promote healing. Although reflexology is medically unproven and no one really knows exactly how it works, it is known that

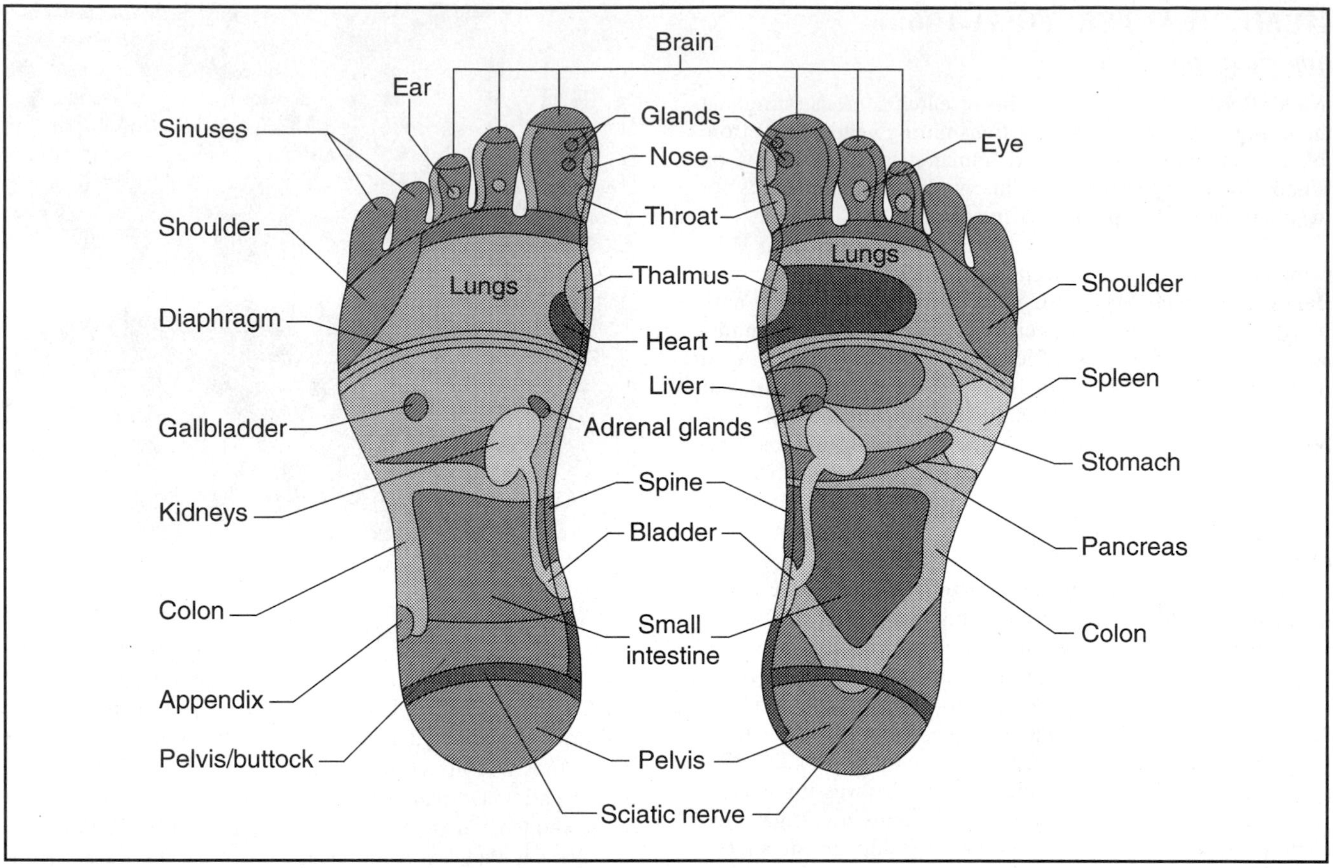

Reflex points on the feet.

the thousands of nerve endings in the feet have extensive interconnections through the spinal cord and can send messages via the brain to all areas of the body. Reflexologists claim that communication is essential to good health and that pressure on reflex points can release and clear blockages, improving the body's internal message-sending system. This, in turn, improves circulation and makes the body able to transport oxygen and nutrients more efficiently while eliminating toxins easily.

During the first session, the reflexologist will ask the patient about medical history and health conditions, as well as habits, work, and lifestyle. Patients need only to remove their shoes and socks, have their feet wiped, and cream or powder applied. The practitioner then ''works'' the reflex areas using several manual techniques, but always employing the thumbs or fingers. Blocked areas or blocked energy is often felt as deposits under the skin, and the practitioner will target these areas for breakup by manipulation and pressure. This can be slightly painful, although most people report feeling more relaxed after treatment. The number of treatments is variable, but most find that the best results are achieved over four to six sessions. As of 1993, there were nearly 25,000 certified practitioners around the world. In certain countries, like Thailand, people can get a reflexology treatment on the street, and in Denmark, it is the number one alternative health treatment.

When administered by a qualified therapist, there are virtually no risks involved in reflexology for people of all ages. However, it should not be used in cases of a serious illness or in place of traditional treatment for conditions that require medical attention.

Since the goal of reflexology is to normalize body functions rather than to cure any particular condition, it should be considered primarily a ''whole system'' kind of therapy. Many people do find however, that it works especially well on conditions that need to be regulated or cleared up, such as stress and fatigue, skin conditions, and menstrual or digestive irregularities. At a minimum, treatment is relaxing and can help relieve stress.

REHABILITATION

Rehabilitation is a treatment or treatments designed to facilitate the process of recovery from injury, illness, or disease to as normal a condition as possible.

The purpose of rehabilitation is to restore some or all of the patient's physical, sensory, and mental capabilities that were lost due to injury, illness, or disease. Rehabilitation includes assisting the patient to compensate for deficits that cannot be reversed medically. It is prescribed after many types of injury, illness, or disease, including **amputations**, arthritis, **cancer**, cardiac disease, neurological problems, orthopedic injuries, spinal cord injuries, **stroke**, and traumatic brain injuries.The Institute of Medicine has estimated that as many as 14% of all Americans may be disabled at any given time.

Rehabilitation should be carried out only by qualified therapists. **Exercises** and other physical interventions must take into account the patient's deficit. An example of a deficit is the loss of a limb.

A proper and adequate rehabilitation program can reverse many disabling conditions or can help patients cope with deficits that cannot be reversed by medical care. Rehabilitation addresses the patient's physical, psychological, and environmental needs. It is achieved by restoring the patient's physical functions and/or modifying the patient's physical and social environment. The main types of rehabilitation are physical, occupational, and speech therapy.

Each rehabilitation program is tailored to the individual patient's needs and can include one or more types of therapy. The patient's physician usually coordinates the efforts of the rehabilitation team, which can include physical, occupational, speech, or other therapists; nurses; engineers; physiatrists (physical medicine); psychologists; orthotists (makes devices such as braces to straighten out curved or poorly shaped bones); prosthetists (a therapist who makes artificial limbs or protheses); and vocational counselors. Family members are often actively involved in the patient's rehabilitation program.

Physical therapy helps the patient restore the use of muscles, bones, and the nervous system through the use of heat, cold, **massage**, whirlpool baths, ultrasound, exercise, and other techniques. It seeks to relieve **pain**, improve strength and mobility, and train the patient to perform important everyday tasks. Physical therapy may be prescribed to rehabilitate a patient after amputations, arthritis, **burns**, cancer, cardiac disease, cervical and lumbar dysfunction, neurological problems, orthopedic injuries, pulmonary disease, spinal cord injuries, stroke, traumatic brain injuries, and other injuries/illnesses. The duration of the physical therapy program varies depending on the injury/illness being treated and the patient's response to therapy.

Exercise is the most widely used and best known type of physical therapy. Depending on the patient's condition, exercises may be performed by the patient alone or with the therapist's help, or with the therapist moving the patient's limbs. Exercise equipment for physical therapy could include an exercise table or mat, a stationary bicycle, walking aids, a wheelchair, practice stairs, parallel bars, and pulleys and weights.

Heat treatment, applied with hot-water compresses, infrared lamps, short-wave radiation, high frequency electrical current, ultrasound, paraffin wax, or warm baths, is used to stimulate the patient's circulation, relax muscles, and relieve pain. Cold treatment is applied with ice packs or cold-water soaking. Soaking in a whirlpool can ease muscle spasm pain and help strengthen movements. Massage aids circulation, helps the patient relax, relieves pain and muscle spasms, and reduces swelling. Very low strength electrical currents applied through the skin stimulate muscles and make them contract, helping paralyzed or weakened muscles respond again.

Occupational therapy helps the patient regain the ability to do normal everyday tasks. This may be achieved by restoring old skills or teaching the patient new skills to adjust to disabilities through adaptive equipment, orthotics, and modification of the patient's home environment. Occupational therapy may be prescribed to rehabilitate a patient after amputation, arthritis, cancer, cardiac disease, head injuries, neurological injuries, orthopedic injuries, pulmonary disease, spinal cord disease, stroke, and other injuries/illnesses. The duration of the occupational therapy program varies depending on the injury/illness being treated and the patient's response to therapy.

Occupational therapy includes learning how to use devices to assist in walking (artificial limbs, canes, crutches, walkers), getting around without walking (wheelchairs or motorized scooters), or moving from one spot to another (boards, lifts, and bars). The therapist will visit the patient's home and analyze what the patient can and cannot do. Suggestions on modifications to the home, such as rearranging furniture or adding a wheelchair ramp, will be made. Health aids to bathing and grooming could also be recommended.

Speech therapy helps the patient correct speech disorders or restore speech. Speech therapy may be prescribed to rehabilitate a patient after a brain injury, cancer, neuromuscular diseases, stroke, and other injuries/illnesses. The duration of the speech therapy program varies depending on the injury/illness being treated and the patient's response to therapy.

Performed by a speech pathologist, speech therapy involves regular meetings with the therapist in an individual or group setting and home exercises. To strengthen muscles, the patient might be asked to say words, smile, close his mouth, or stick out his tongue. Picture cards may be used to help the patient remember everyday objects and increase his vocabulary. The patient might use picture boards of everyday activities or objects to communicate with others. Workbooks might be used to help the patient recall the names of objects and practice reading, writing, and listening. Computer programs are available to help sharpen speech, reading, recall, and listening skills.

Inhalation therapists, audiologists, and registered dietitians are other types of therapists. Inhalation therapists help the patient learn to use respirators and other breathing aids to restore or support breathing. Audiologists help diagnose the patient's **hearing loss** and recommend solutions. Dietitians provide dietary advice to help the patient recover from or avoid specific problems or diseases.

Rehabilitation services are provided in a variety of settings including clinical and office practices, hospitals, skilled-care nursing homes, sports medicine clinics, and some health maintenance organizations. Some therapists make home visits. Advice on choosing the appropriate type of therapy and therapist is provided by the patient's medical team.

REICHSTEIN, TADEUSZ (1897-1996)

Swiss chemist

Reichstein is best known for his work with the hormones produced by the adrenal gland cortex. He established that these corticoids were steroids, and in 1936 was the first to isolate cortisone. Reichstein shared the 1950 Nobel Prize in physiology or medicine for his work with cortisone.

Reichstein was born in Wloclawek, Poland. His father was an engineer and the family lived in various European countries; they became Swiss citizens in 1914. Reichstein received his Ph.D. in 1922 from the Swiss Technical Institute (ETH), Zurich. In 1931 he became the assistant of Leopold Ruzicka (1887-1976), the Swiss biochemist who was an expert on ring structures and was working to synthesize sex hormones. Reichstein also synthesized corticoids from a derivative of bile acid so they could be used to treat Addison's disease, which results from the adrenal glands' failure to produce a normal amount of hormones. Reichstein determined the locations of the oxygen molecules that characterize the individual, but closely related corticoids, permitting their synthesis. He also conducted research on other steroids including those derived from plants.

Another of Reichstein's interests was the structure of **vitamins**. In 1933, he independently synthesized ascorbic acid (vitamin C). In addition, he conducted research on pantothenic acid, one of the B vitamins.

Reichstein's many honors included honorary memberships in the U.S. National Academy of Sciences and the Royal Society (London). He also served as director of the Pharmaceutical Institute at the University of Basel. Reichstein retired in 1967 but he continued to conduct significant new research into his 90s. Reichstein died August 1, 1996.

Relapsing fever

Relapsing fever refers to two similar illnesses, both of which cause high **fever**s. The fevers resolve, only to recur again within about a week.

Relapsing fever is caused by spiral-shaped bacteria of the genus *Borrelia*. This bacterium lives in rodents and in insects, specifically ticks and body lice. The form of relapsing fever acquired from ticks is slightly different from that acquired from body lice.

In tick-borne relapsing fever (TBRF), rodents (rats, mice, chipmunks, and squirrels) which carry *Borrelia* are fed upon by ticks. The ticks then acquire the bacteria, and are able to pass it on to humans. TBRF is most common in sub-Saharan Africa, parts of the Mediterranean, areas in the Middle East, India, China, and the south of Russia. Also, *Borrelia* causing TBRF exist in the western regions of the United States, particularly in mountainous areas. The disease is said to be endemic to these areas, meaning that the causative agents occur naturally and consistently within these locations.

In louse-borne relapsing fever (LBRF), lice acquire *Borrelia* from humans who are already infected. These lice can then go on to infect other humans. LBRF is said to be epidemic, as opposed to endemic, meaning that it can occur suddenly in large numbers in specific communities of people. LBRF occurs in places where poverty and overcrowding predispose to human infestation with lice. LBRF has flared during wars, when conditions are crowded and good hygiene is next to impossible. At this time, LBRF is found in areas of east and central Africa, China, and in the Andes Mountains of Peru.

In TBRF, humans contract *Borrelia* when they are fed upon by ticks. Ticks often feed on humans at night, so many people who have been bitten are unaware that they have been. The bacteria is passed on to humans through the infected body fluids of the tick.

In LBRF, a louse must be crushed or smashed in order for *Borrelia* to be released. The bacteria then enter the human body through areas where the person may have scratched him or herself.

Both types of relapsing fever occur some days after having acquired the bacteria. About a week after becoming infected, symptoms begin. The patient spikes a very high fever, with chills, sweating, terrible **headache**, nausea, vomiting, severe **pain** in the muscles and joints, and extreme weakness. The patient may become dizzy and confused. The eyes may be bloodshot and very sensitive to light. A **cough** may develop. The heart rate is greatly increased, and the liver and spleen may be swollen. Because the substances responsible for blood clotting may be disturbed during the illness, tiny purple marks may appear on the skin, which are evidence of minor bleeding occurring under the skin. The patient may suffer from a **nosebleed**, or may cough up bloody sputum. All of these symptoms last for about three days in TBRF, and about five days in LBRF.

With or without treatment, a crisis may occur as the bacteria are cleared from the blood. This crisis, called a Jarisch-Herxheimer reaction, results in a new spike in fever, chills, and an initial rise in blood pressure. The blood pressure then falls drastically, which may deprive tissues and organs of appropriate blood flow (**shock**). This reaction usually lasts for about a day.

Recurrent episodes of fever with less severe symptoms occur after about a week. In untreated infections, fevers recur about three times in TBRF, and only once or twice in LBRF.

Diagnosis of relapsing fever is relatively easy, because the causative bacteria can be found by examining a sample of blood under the microscope. The characteristically spiral-shaped bacteria are easily identifiable. The blood is best drawn during the period of high fever, because the bacteria are present in the blood in great numbers at that time.

Either tetracycline or erythromycin is effective against both forms of relapsing fever. The medications are given for about a week for cases of TBRF; LBRF requires only a single dose. Children and pregnant women should receive either erythromycin or penicillin. Because of the risk of the Jarish-Herxheimer reaction, patients must be very carefully monitored during the initial administration of antibiotic medications. Solutions containing salts must be given through a needle in the vein (intravenously) to keep the blood pressure from dropping too drastically. Patients with extreme reactions may need medications to improve blood circulation until the reaction resolves.

In epidemics of LBRF, **death** rates among untreated victims have run as high as 30%. With treatment, and careful monitoring for the development of the Jarish-Herxheimer reaction, prognosis is good for both LBRF and TBRF.

Prevention of TBRF requires rodent control, especially in and near homes. Careful use of insecticides on skin and clothing is important for people who may be enjoying outdoor recreation in areas known to harbor the disease-carrying ticks.

Prevention of LBRF is possible, but probably more difficult. Good hygiene and decent living conditions would prevent the spread of LBRF, but these may be difficult for those people most at risk for the disease.

Religion and medicine

Throughout the history of human health, religion has had both beneficial and detrimental effects.

Consider, for example, the state of medicine during the Middle Ages. Then, as in much of history, the Church played a major role in providing health care. Priests were the principal caregivers. However, illness was viewed in those days as punishment from God, so treatment often involved tormenting the body to expel evil 'spirits.' Some Church teachings actively discouraged the advancement of medical science. For instance, priests were prohibited by papal decree from shedding blood, barring them from performing surgery. Also, the Church forbade dissections of human or animal cadavers, preventing any comprehensive knowledge of anatomy or physiology.

Religion and medicine are both concerned with making people whole. In fact, the words 'healing' and 'holiness' are both linguistically derived from the concept of wholeness.

Many health-care and teaching/research institutions have sprung from religious roots. The first hospitals were created by Christian and Islamic founders. Inspired by Christ's injunction to his followers to ''heal the sick'' and ''cleanse the lepers,'' Christian hospitals began appearing in Rome after Constantine declared Christianity as the state religion. This trend continued through the Medieval and Renaissance centuries, and was resurrected during the 19th century, when thousands of denominational hospitals, lunatic asylums and nursing homes were established throughout North America and Europe. Similar traditions of religious involvement in medical caregiving can be found in the histories of China and Hindu nations.

Just as there exists a wide range of religious traditions, there is also considerable difference of opinion on the overall health effects of religion. Sigmund Freud, the Austrian founder of psychoanalysis, considered religion to be a form of **mental illness**, needing to be replaced by ''rational operation of the intellect.'' (Oddly, Freud was himself deeply superstitious, especially about the number 17.) Others have argued that religious indoctrination is abusive and a cause of illness, intolerance and intellectual inflexibility.

Conversely, there are those who cite a large body of literature linking public and private religious activity with improved health. They cite benefits including reduced risk of **cancer**, stroke, heart attack, depression, and anxiety disorder; lower death rate from coronary artery disease; fewer cases of substance abuse; lower blood pressure; even faster recovery from a hip fracture. Numerous Christian traditions believe healing may result from intercessory prayer or a touch by a faith healer. In one telephone survey of almost 600 randomly selected adults, 14% reported they had experienced divine healing of a serious disease or condition. Another study associated intercessory prayer with a reduction in cardiovascular complications in patients in a coronary care unit.

On the other hand, some traditions have controversial beliefs that limit the medical interventions they are willing to accept. Christian Scientists, for example, reject use of medicine, trusting instead in prayer and counsel to invoke healing mental processes in the patient. Jehovah's Witnesses will not accept blood transfusions or blood products. Physicians sometimes seek court orders allowing treatment in such cases, especially if the life of a child is at risk because of the beliefs of the parents.

As to whether any particular religion has an overall positive or negative effect on human health, it is difficult to argue with the ancient advice: ''By their fruits ye shall know them.''

Remak, Robert (1815-1865)

German physician and physiologist

Robert Remak was born at Posen (Poznan), Poland on July 26, 1815; he died at Kissingen, Bavaria on August 29, 1865. He was a pioneer in neuroanatomy and neuro-embryology. Remak studied at the University of Berlin under Johannes Múller. He graduated in 1838, having written a very important thesis. He then became an unpaid assistant to Múller, supporting himself by general practice. From 1843 to 1847, he served as assistant to Johann Lukas Schonlein (1793 to 1864; founder of the Natural History School which proposed to study medicine as descriptive botany and zoology are studied), who was then physician at the Charité clinic in Berlin. In 1847, he became Privatdocent (an unsalaried professor paid directly by students) in the University of Berlin, and in 1859 was promoted to Associate Professor.

In 1836 Remak obtained a compound microscope, and subsequently published two papers on the **nervous system** based on work he did with it, even before he obtained his doctorate. His doctoral thesis (1838) dealt with his microscopical investigations of nervous tissue. Remak also showed in his thesis that the axon of a peripheral nerve arises from a nerve cell in the spinal cord, and that it runs continuously from the nerve cell to the terminal branching of the nerve. Although he earned a reputation as a microscopist, Remak also made significant contributions to several other areas of medicine. As a histologist, he is remembered for his discovery of the non-medullated nerve fibers (now known as the fibers of Remak) in 1838, as well as for his discovery of the ganglionic cells in the sinus venous of the frog's heart (1848), now considered to be the autonomous centers that cause the heart beat.

Remak was also the first to describe neurofibrils in nerve cells, the existence of six distinct layers of cells in the cerebral cortex, and the gangliated plexuses of sympathetic nerves in the stomach wall. In 1851, Remak simplified the conception of von Baer's classifications of germ-layers in embryology, showing the significance of three layers in the development of the organs and tissues of the body. He studied the development of the neural tube, and described the earliest development of vessels in the vascular area of the chick embryo. While working in Schonlein's clinic, he produced in his own person favus (a contagious disease affecting the skin and the scalp) experimentally, separating the fungus, which he named *Achorion Schonleini* after his chief, from the genus Oidium (1845). In 1852, he became one of the first scientists to point out that the proliferation of cells to form tissue is accompanied by cell division. (This was contrary to the opinions of Scheiden and Schwann who believed that tissue formation is accompanied by the endogenous formation of new cells.) Remak also wrote about lead **poisoning**, **paralysis** of the musculo-spinal nerve, and other nervous conditions. Along with Addison and Duchene of Boulogne, he pioneered the field of electrotherapy, substituting galvanic for induced current (1856). Remak was also the first person to describe ascending neuritis (1861).

REPETITIVE MOTION INJURY

Repetitive motion injury (RMI), sometimes called repetitive strain injury, cumulative trauma disorder, or overuse syndrome, is an umbrella term used to describe a variety of diagnostic conditions characterized by pain and discomfort that develop gradually in such soft-tissue structures as tendons, tendon sheaths, nerves, muscles, or blood vessels. Repetitive motion injuries may become progressively worse over time without treatment and may result in a complete loss of function in the affected area. Usually RMIs are associated with occupational causes, although nonoccupational activities, such as sports, hobbies, or driving may also contribute to the problem.

While the term ''repetitive motion injury'' is relatively new, gaining popularity in the final decades of the twentieth century, the occurrence of RMIs in industry is not new. In 1717, **Bernardino Ramazzini**, the father of occupational medicine, first introduced physicians to the common musculoskeletal disorders that arose from eighteenth-century occupations. As the Industrial Revolution gained momentum and assembly-line production, long hours, poor working conditions, and repetitive motions became the norm, the problem of work-related diseases and conditions was increasingly recognized. By the mid-1950s, automation contributed to a variety of physical and psychological problems.

When computers were introduced into the workplace during the 1980s, RMIs became a worldwide dilemma; the United States witnessed a gradual rise in RMIs from 1980 to 1986. The incidences then rose tremendously from 50,000 in 1985 to 281,800 in 1992, according to the Bureau of Labor Statistics. As the reported incidences of RMIs skyrocketed, researchers began documenting and examining the prevalence of RMIs in specific high-risk occupations.

Unlike sprains or strains, RMIs are not caused from a single incident. Each cycle of a work activity has the potential to cause microtears in the soft-tissue structures involved. One repetition may not produce inflammation or **pain**; however, if sufficient time is not allowed for tissue recovery, over time these microtears can accumulate to produce trauma to a specific area of the body. Thus, a worker on the job may be asymptomatic for years, while unknowingly accumulating job-related microtraumas.

Although they may develop anywhere in the body, RMIs are most common to the hand and wrist (such as **carpal tunnel syndrome**, hand-arm vibration syndrome), elbow and forearm (radial tunnel syndrome, cubital tunnel syndrome, tenosynovitis of the forearm extensor and flexor muscles), and shoulder and neck (tension neck syndrome, thoracic outlet syndrome).

The symptoms of an RMI may include one or more of the following: pain, stiffness, swelling, numbness or tingling in the hands, wrists, elbows, shoulders, back or neck; discomfort brought on by performing a particular task, and which then ceases or improves when no longer performing the task, such as on weekends or holidays. Often the discomfort begins in one area, for example neck and back, and then spreads to other parts of the body. Early warning signs may manifest as sore shoulders or neck pain, particularly when driving home after a day at work, or a loss of flexibility or strength. It is also possible that the effects of RMI may not manifest until the next morning as aches and stiffness in the arms or hands.

Repetitive motion injuries have long presented a problem to the health care professionals in that the injuries are notoriously difficult to diagnose and sometimes to treat, since they develop slowly and are characterized by pain that is not localized to one particular part of the body. Various criteria have been developed for detecting the presence of an RMI. These criteria vary depending on the specificity of physical symptoms, duration of time with symptoms, and the use of tests to determine specific diagnoses. The Occupational Safety and Health Administration (OSHA), for example, uses broad criteria to document the number of RMIs in industry. Once a condition is judged as an occupational illness, it must be recorded in the OSHA log.

It is of vital importance to understand why the RMI symptoms occurred in order eliminate the problem. Individuals who engage in repetitive tasks, according to ergonomics experts (ergonomics is the study of the relationship between the worker and the work environment), can prevent RMIs by following some simple guidelines such as varying tasks, avoiding awkward positions and posture, avoiding excessive force in operating equipment, and taking breaks as often as possible.

Most physicians began to accept and take seriously an RMI as a genuine physical problem in the late 1980s and early 1990s. They found that an RMI is very treatable in its early stages, but even a short delay in seeking rest and treatment can set recovery back by weeks, months or even years.

Treatment options for RMIs generally include: physical treatments (**physical therapists**, **chiropractors**, and **osteopaths**); **massage**; stretching; postural treatments aimed at correcting bad habits; relaxation (**yoga**, meditation); **exercise**; **acupuncture**; or pain clinics for those suffering from long-term pain. Medication such as **nonsteroidal anti-inflammatory drugs** may also play a valuable role in treating some individuals.

Future research into RMIs will continue to address the tolerances of human tissues and the body's means of adaptation. This information will help health care practitioners to develop training programs to improve and protect both the health and performance of workers. An additional area of research is the prevention of repetitive motion injuries through appropriate workplace engineering and ergonomic design.

See also Carpal tunnel syndrome; Occupation safety and health; Occupational therapy; Ramazzini, Bernardino; Tendinitis

REPRODUCTIVE SYSTEM

The reproductive system is the structural and physiological network whose purpose is the creation of a new life to continue the species. It is the only body system which is not concerned with supporting the life of its host. Human reproduction is sexual—meaning that both a male and a female are required to produce a life. Gender is determined at conception by the sex chromosome in the sperm that fertilizes an egg. The developing male or female has a reproductive system characteristic of its sex. However, boys and girls can not reproduce until sexual maturation occurs at puberty. The male reproductive system is designed specifically to produce and deliver sperm to the egg in the female. The female reproductive system is designed to develop ova (eggs) and prepare for egg fertilization by a sperm. The male and female systems are both anatomically and biochemically designed to join and make a new life. However, the reproductive system is unique among body systems in that a person may choose not to use it to its full capacity—to procreate. Individuals can decide not to reproduce.

The main tasks of the male reproductive system are to provide sex hormones, to produce sperm, and to transport sperm from the male to a female. The first two tasks are performed by the testes; while the third job is carried out by a series of ejaculatory ducts and the penis. The two testes are contained within the scrotum which hangs below the body between the legs. Each testis is attached at its top to an epididymis which contains numerous sperm ducts. The epidiymides (plural) send sperm through the vas deferens to the penis. However, the seminal vesicles, prostate, and bulbo-urethral glands each contribute to the seminal fluid which carries the sperm to the penis. The epididymides and part of the vas deferens are within the scrotum, but the glands creating the seminal fluid are in the abdomen.

Each of the testes is divided into lobes, or septae, containing coiled seminiferous tubules lined with spermatozoa-producing cells. Between the tubules are hormone-producing cells called interstitial cells, or cells of Leydig. Testosterone is produced by the interstitial cells. Since the testes-containing scrotum hangs below the body, it has a temperature around 89°F (32°C) which is ideal for sperm production which requires a low temperature. When the scrotum is held too close to the body by restrictive clothing, sterility can result.

The full maturation of a single sperm takes about 70-80 days. Hence, substances a male is exposed to during that period of time may effect the health of his sperm at the end of that time period. Sperm are always available in healthy males after puberty, because spermatogenesis is an ongoing process with cells in all stages of development existing in different layers of the seminiferous tubules. As many as several hundred million sperm can be produced each day. And one man has approximately a quarter mile of coiled seminiferous tubules which produce all these sperm.

The vas deferens carries concentrated sperm from the scrotum into the abdominal cavity to the ejaculatory duct. Sperm that remain in the ejaculatory duct longer than a couple of weeks degenerate and are disposed of. The prostate surrounds the ejaculatory duct and contains a sphincter that closes off the bladder during ejaculation. Seminal fluid from the seminal vesicles, the prostate, and the bulbo-urethral glands (or Cowper's glands) is added to the sperm. The seminal fluid plus the sperm is called semen.

Seminal fluid is designed to carry and nourish sperm. Seminal vesicles are located on either side of the bladder and contribute about 60% of the fluid. Seminal vesicle fluid is rich in essential sperm nutrients such as fructose which sustains sperm for up to 72 hours after ejaculation. Additional fluid is provided by the Cowper's glands (below the prostate) which secrete a pre-ejaculatory urethral lubricant that may contain some sperm. For this reason, withdrawal is not a foolproof contraceptive method. At ejaculation, additional Cowper secretions combine with the remaining seminal fluid and sperm. This semen is sent through the urethra in the penis.

The penis provides the route for transmitting sperm to an egg for reproduction. However, in its relaxed state, it can not effectively deliver sperm. In order for the sperm to have the best chance of fertilizing an egg, the penis must become erect and ejaculate semen close to an egg in the female reproductive tract.

The penis is part of the male's external reproductive system which becomes longer, thicker, and stiff during erection. It is comprised of a shaft region which is the cylindrical body of the penis and the glans, or head region. The glans and the shaft are separated at the coronal ridge which is a rim of tissue that is very sensitive to touch. The skin covering the penis is loose and allows for expansion during erection. Some males have a prepuce or foreskin which is a movable skin that covers the penile glans. Circumcised males have had this foreskin removed. Uncircumcised males must carefully clean the foreskin daily to prevent bacteria and foul-smelling secretions (called smegma) from accumulating.

Three cylinders of spongy erectile tissue make up the internal portion of the penis. Two cylinders run along the inner roof of the penis and are called the corpora cavernosa. The third cylinder runs along the lower side of the penis; it contains the urethra and is called the corpus spongiosum, or spongy body. The spongy body includes the penile tip and is more sensitive to touch than the rest of the penis. Several nerves and blood vessels run through the spongy body. An erection occurs when blood flow to the spongy tissue vessels increases. An average erect penis is 6.25 in (15.9 cm) long and 1.5 in (3.8 cm) wide at its base.

Sexual intercourse does not necessarily lead to reproduction, but the physiology of reproductive versus non-reproductive sexual arousal is indistinguishable. Sexual arousal has been divided into four stages by Masters and Johnson. These stages are the same whether the arousal results from physical stimulation (such as touch) or mental stimulation (such as reading an arousing book). Hence, arousal can be influenced by personal beliefs, desires, or values. The stages of arousal are: excitement, plateau, orgasm, and resolution.

The male stage of sexual excitement is marked by increased blood flow to the pelvic area and penis. Increased parasympathetic nerve activity causes the blood vessels in the penis to dilate, allowing for vasocongestion which leads to an erection. This may happen in a matter of seconds. Testes size also increases, and nipples become erect in some men.

The amount of time spent in the plateau phase varies considerably. In this stage, the head of the penis enlarges and darkens from blood pooling. Testes darken, enlarge from vasocongestion, and are lifted back away from the penis. At this point, pre-ejaculatory secretion from the bulbo-urethral gland occurs, and respiration, heart rate, and blood pressure increase.

Male orgasm results from both emission and ejaculation. Emission is the release of the ejaculatory fluid into the urethra. Emission is caused by increased sympathetic nerve stimulation in the ejaculatory ducts and glands which leads to rhythmic contractions that force the fluid out. For ejaculation, rhythmic contractions of the urethra expel the semen (usually 3-5 ml) while the prostate gland closes off the bladder.

In the resolution phase, blood exits the penis and testes, and the penis relaxes. Respiration, blood pressure, and heart rate return to normal, and sexual arousal enters a refractory period. During the refractory period, erection can not occur while the system "reloads." The length of refractory period varies from a couple of minutes to several hours and increases with fatigue and age.

The main tasks of the female reproductive system are to produce hormones, develop ova, receive sperm, and promote fertilization and the growth of a newly conceived life. These events occur internally. Ova mature in the ovaries. Sperm are received in the vagina and cervix. Fertilization takes place usually in the fallopian tubes and less often in the uterus, with the newly formed life developing in the endometrial lining of the uterus. The female reproductive tract can be pictured as a capital Y with the upper arms forming the fallopian tubes. The ovaries would be at the end of these arms. The uterus would be the upper half of the supporting stalk, and the vagina would be the lower half. External female genitals are involved in female sexual arousal.

The ovaries are oval-shaped and about 1-1.5 in (2.5-3.8 cm) long. They are connected to the body of the uterus by an ovarian ligament which tethers the ovaries in place. The ovaries parallel the testes in that they release sex hormones and develop gametes (ova or sperm). However, the job of the ovaries differs from that of the testes: while sperm are created daily through a man's life after puberty, all of a female fetus's eggs have been created by the sixth gestational month. Several million primordial follicles capable of forming ova are formed. About 1 million primordial follicles mature into primary follicles that still exist at birth. (The rest have degenerated.) When puberty begins, about 400,000 follicles remain. Mature eggs leave alternating ovaries monthly beginning in puberty in a process called ovulation. Unfertilized eggs are lost through menstruation, when the uterine lining is shed. Women typically menstruate for 30-40 years losing 360-480 eggs in a lifetime. Ovulation is hormonally suppressed during pregnancy and shortly after childbirth.

The formation of mature ova in the ovaries is called oogenesis. Unlike spermatogenesis, which occurs daily, oogenesis is on an average 28 day (or monthly) cycle. During embryonic development, primordial follicles are formed, each of which contains an oocyte surrounded by a layer of spindle-shaped cells. These spindle cells multiply during the mid-fetal stage of development and become granulosa cells which surround the egg. Granulosa cells function much like the Sertoli cells in men: they prevent destructive drugs from getting to the egg while also providing essential nutrients for its development. Granulosa cells also secrete a rich substance that forms a follicular coating called the zona pellucida. Before birth, the cellular layers surrounding the follicle differentiate into a layer of cells called the theca interna. At birth, a baby girl's ova are suspended at the first meiotic division inside the primary follicles. After the onset of puberty, a new follicle enters the next phase of follicular growth monthly.

The first two weeks of the menstrual cycle are called the follicular phase because of the follicular development that occurs during that time. Around day 14 of the cycle, LH and FSH surge to initiate ovulation. Ovulation entails the release of the mature oocyte from the ovarian follicle as it ruptures from the surface of the ovary into the abdominal cavity. Once released, the ovum is caught by the fimbria, which are finger-like projections off the ends of the fallopian tubes. The follicle which housed the growing egg remains in the ovary and is transformed into the corpus luteum. The corpus luteum secretes high levels of progesterone and some estrogen. The corpus luteum secures a position near the ovarian blood vessels to supply these hormones which prevent another follicle from beginning maturation. If the ovum is fertilized, then these hormone levels continue into pregnancy to prevent another cycle from beginning. However, if fertilization does not occur, then the corpus luteum degenerates allowing the next cycle to start. The second 14 days of the menstrual cycle are called the luteal phase because of the corpus luteum's hormonal control over this half of the cycle.

The optimal time for an oocyte to be fertilized is when it enters a fallopian tube. The fallopian tubes are fluid-filled, cilia-lined channels about 4-6 in (10-15 cm) long that carry the oocyte to the uterus. At ovulation, the primary oocyte completes its suspended meiosis and divides in two. A secondary oocyte and a small polar body result. If the secondary oocyte is fertilized, then it will go through another division which forms another polar body.

As the ripening egg travels along the fallopian tube, it is washed along by cilia which knock away residual nutrient cells on the outside of the egg. This array of cells leaving the cell forms a radiant cluster called the corona radiata. If sperm have made their way to the fallopian tube, then they have already been capacitated. Capacitation is the modification of a sperm's acrosomal tip which enables it to burrow into the egg. Fertilization blocks the ability of additional sperm to enter the egg. Once the nuclei of the egg and sperm cells have fused, the new cell is called a zygote. The zygote contains all the genetic information required to become a complete human being. This new life signifies the beginning of successful reproduction. As the zygotic cell divides into more cells, it travels from the fallopian tube to the uterus.

The uterus, or womb, is a muscular, inverted pear-shaped organ in the female pelvis which is specifically designed to protect and nurture a growing baby. It averages 3 in (7.6 cm) long by 2 in (5 cm) wide. However, during pregnancy, it expands with the growing embryo and fetus. Embryo is a term used to describe a human in the first eight weeks of development. After that, the human is called a fetus.

During the follicular phase of the menstrual cycle, the lining (or endometrium) of the uterus becomes thick and filled with many blood vessels in preparation for supporting an embryo. If fertilization does not occur within about eight days of ovulation, then this lining is shed in menstrual blood through the cervix. This cycle continues until menopause, when menstruation becomes less frequent and eventually stops altogether.

The cervix is the base of the uterus which extends into the vagina. The narrow passageway of the cervix is just large enough to allow sperm to enter and menstrual blood to exit. During childbirth, it becomes dilated (open) to allow the baby to move into the vagina, or birth canal. However, for most of the pregnancy, the cervix becomes plugged with thick mucous to isolate the developing baby from vaginal events. For this reason, non-reproductive, sexual intercourse is usually safe during pregnancy.

The vagina is a muscular tube about 5 in (12.7 cm) long. A thin layer of tissue called the hymen may cover the vaginal opening, but is usually gone in physically or sexually active females. A mucous membrane lines and moistens the vagina. During sexual intercourse, the vagina is lubricated further and functions to direct the penis toward the cervix to optimize fertilization. During childbirth, the vagina stretches to accommodate the passage of the baby. Both the uterus and the vagina contract to relatively original sizes some time after delivery.

External female genitals include the mons veneris, labia majora, labia minora, clitoris, and vestibule. They differ in size and color from female to female, but their location and function are consistent. The mons is a pad of fatty tissue filled with many nerve endings which becomes covered with pubic hair in puberty. The labia majora are two folds of skin which protect the opening to the urethra and internal genitals. Pubic hair grows on their outer surface in puberty. These fat padded folds of skin contain sweat glands, nerve endings, and numerous blood vessels. Inside these outer skin folds are the labia minora which are hairless. The labia minora form a spongy covering for the vaginal entrance. These smaller skin folds meet at the top of the genitals to form the clitoral hood. The hood houses the clitoris, a very sensitive organ which has a spongy shaft and a nerve-rich glans (tip). Between the labia minora and the vagina is the area called the vestibule. Within the vestibule are the two Bartholin's glands which lubricate the vagina.

Sexual arousal in females parallels the arousal stages in males. Female sexual arousal is not required to reproduce, but it does facilitate reproduction. In the excitement phase, blood flow to the vagina increases which, in turn, pushes fluid into the vaginal canal. This lubricating process is called transudation and allows for comfortable penile insertion. During this phase, blood infiltrates the spongy clitoris and labia, and the cervix and uterus are lifted up away from the vagina. Nipples often become erect, and respiration, heart rate, and blood pressure increase.

During the plateau stage, the vagina expands, forming a pocket near the cervix which is an ideal deposit site for sperm; this is called "tenting." The increased sensitivity of the clitoris causes it to retract in the clitoral hood, and breasts sometimes become flushed. In the orgasmic phase, the vaginal opening contracts rhythmically for about 15 seconds. Unlike the lengthy refractory period which males experience in the resolution stage, females are more likely to be multi-orgasmic and capable of more closely spaced orgasms. In the resolution stage, genital blood flow returns to normal. Respiration, heart rate, and blood pressure also return to normal. Within 72 hours of sexual intercourse reproduction will either have successfully begun or not succeeded.

RESPIRATORY ACIDOSIS

Respiratory acidosis is a condition in which a build-up of carbon dioxide in the blood produces a shift in the body's pH balance and causes the body's system to become more acidic. This condition is brought about by a problem either involving the lungs and respiratory system or signals from the brain that control breathing.

Respiratory acidosis is an acid imbalance in the body caused by a problem related to breathing. In the lungs, oxygen from inhaled air is exchanged for carbon dioxide from the blood. This process takes place between the alveoli (tiny air pockets in the lungs) and the blood vessels that connect to them. When this exchange of oxygen for carbon dioxide is impaired, the excess carbon dioxide forms an acid in the blood. The condition can be acute with a sudden onset, or it can develop gradually as lung function deteriorates.

Respiratory acidosis can be caused by diseases or conditions that effect the lungs themselves, such as emphysema, chronic **bronchitis**, **asthma**, or severe **pneumonia**. Blockage of the airway due to swelling, a foreign object, or vomit can induce respiratory acidosis. Drugs like anesthetics, sedatives, and narcotics can interfere with breathing by depressing the respiratory center in the brain. Head injuries or **brain tumor**s can also interfere with signals sent by the brain to the lungs. Such neuromuscular diseases as Guillain-Barré syndrome or **myasthenia gravis** can impair the muscles around the lungs making it more difficult to breath. Conditions that cause chronic **metabolic alkalosis** can also trigger respiratory acidosis.

The most notable symptom will be slowed or difficult breathing. **Headache**, drowsiness, restlessness, tremor, and confusion may also occur. A rapid heart rate, changes in blood pressure, and swelling of blood vessels in the eyes may be noted upon examination. This condition can trigger the body to respond with symptoms of metabolic alkalosis, which may include **cyanosis**, a bluish or purplish discoloration of the skin due to inadequate oxygen intake. Severe cases of respiratory acidosis can lead to **coma** and **death**.

Respiratory acidosis may be suspected based on symptoms. A blood sample to test for pH and arterial blood gases can be used to confirm the diagnosis. In this type of acidosis, the pH will be below 7.35. The pressure of carbon dioxide in the blood will be high, usually over 45 mmHg.

Treatment focuses on correcting the underlying condition that caused the acidosis. In patients with chronic lung diseases, this may include use of a bronchodilator or steroid drugs. Supplemental oxygen supplied through a mask or small tubes inserted into the nostrils may be used in some conditions, however, an oversupply of oxygen in patients with lung disease can make the acidosis worse. **Antibiotics** may be used to treat infections. If the acidosis is related to an overdose of narcotics, or a **drug overdose** is suspected, the patient may be given a dose of naloxone, a drug that will block the respiratory-depressing effects of narcotics. Use of mechanical ventilation like a respirator may be necessary. If the respiratory acidosis has triggered the body to compensate by developing metabolic alkalosis, symptoms of that condition may need to be treated as well.

If the underlying condition that caused the respiratory acidosis is treated and corrected, there may be no long term effects. Respiratory acidosis may occur chronically along with the development of lung disease or **respiratory failure**. In these severe conditions, the patient may require the assistance of a respirator or ventilator. In extreme cases, the patient may experience coma and death.

Patients with chronic lung diseases and those who receive sedatives and narcotics need to be monitored closely for development of respiratory acidosis.

Respiratory alkalosis

Respiratory alkalosis is a condition where the amount of carbon dioxide found in the blood drops to a level below normal range. This condition produces a shift in the body's pH balance and causes the body's system to become more alkaline (basic). This condition is brought on by rapid, deep breathing called *hyperventilation*.

Respiratory alkalosis is an alkali imbalance in the body caused by a lower-than-normal level of carbon dioxide in the blood. In the lungs, oxygen from inhaled air is exchanged for carbon dioxide from the blood. This process takes place between the alveoli (tiny air pockets in the lungs) and the blood vessels that connect to them. When a person hyperventilates, this exchange of oxygen for carbon dioxide is speeded up, and the person exhales too much carbon dioxide. This lowered level of carbon dioxide causes the pH of the blood to increase, leading to alkalosis.

The primary cause of respiratory alkalosis is hyperventilation. This rapid, deep breathing can be caused by conditions related to the lungs like **pneumonia**, lung disease, or **asthma**. More commonly, hyperventilation is associated with **anxiety**, **fever**, **drug overdose**, **carbon monoxide poisoning**, or serious infections. Tumors or swelling in the brain or nervous system can also cause this type of respiration. Other stresses to the body, including **pregnancy**, liver failure, high elevations, or **metabolic acidosis** can also trigger hyperventilation leading to respiratory alkalosis.

Hyperventilation, the primary cause of respiratory alkalosis, is also the primary symptom. This symptom is accompanied by **dizziness**, light headedness, agitation, and tingling or numbing around the mouth and in the fingers and hands. Muscle twitching, spasms, and weakness may be noted. **Seizures**, irregular heart beats, and tetany (muscle spasms so severe that the muscle locks in a rigid position) can result from severe respiratory alkalosis.

Respiratory alkalosis may be suspected based on symptoms. A blood sample to test for pH and arterial blood gas analysis can be used to confirm the diagnosis.

Treatment focuses on correcting the underlying condition that caused the alkalosis. Hyperventilation due to anxiety may be relieved by having the patient breath into a paper bag. By rebreathing the air that was exhaled, the patient will inhale a higher amount of carbon dioxide than he or she would normally. **Antibiotics** may be used to treat pneumonia or other infections. Other medications may be required to treat fever, seizures, or irregular heart beats. If the alkalosis is related to a drug overdose, the patient may require treatment for **poisoning**. Use of mechanical ventilation like a respirator may be necessary. If the respiratory alkalosis has triggered the body to compensate by developing metabolic acidosis, symptoms of that condition may need to be treated, as well. If the underlying condition is treated and corrected, there may be no long-term effects. In severe cases, the patient may experience seizures or heart beat irregularities that may be serious and life threatening.

Respiratory distress syndrome

Respiratory distress syndrome (RDS), also known as infant RDS and once known as hyaline membrane disease, is an acute lung disease present at birth, most frequently affecting premature babies. Abnormal layers of tissue called hyaline membranes keep oxygen breathed into the lungs from passing into the bloodstream. The lungs are said to be ''airless.'' Without treatment, the infant will die within a few days after birth, but if oxygen can be provided, and the infant receives modern treatment in a neonatal intensive care unit, complete recovery with no after-effects can be expected.

If a newborn infant is to breathe properly, the small air sacs (alveoli) at the ends of the breathing tubes must remain open so that oxygen can get into the tiny blood vessels that surround the alveoli. Normally, in the last months of **pregnancy**, cells in the alveoli produce a substance called surfactant, which allows these sacs to expand at the moment of birth so the infant can breathe normally. Surfactant is produced starting at about 34 weeks of pregnancy and, by the time the fetal lungs mature at 37 weeks, a normal amount is present.

If an infant is born prematurely, enough surfactant might not have formed, causing the lungs to collapse and making it very difficult for the baby to breathe. Sometimes, a layer of fibrous tissue, called a hyaline membrane, forms in the air sacs, making it even more difficult for oxygen to be absorbed into the blood vessels.

RDS nearly always occurs following premature births, and the more premature, the greater the chance that the infant will develop RDS. RDS is also seen in some infants whose mothers have **diabetes mellitus**; however, it is less likely to occur in the presence of certain conditions which themselves are harmful to the infant, such as abnormally slow growth of the fetus, high blood pressure in the mother causing a condition caused toxemia, and early rupture of the birth membranes.

Labored breathing (the ''respiratory distress'' of RDS) may begin as soon as the infant is born, or within a few hours. Breathing becomes very rapid, the nostrils flare, and the infant grunts with each breath. The ribs, which are very flexible in newborns, move inward each time a breath is taken. Soon, the muscles that move the ribs and diaphragm which draw air into the lungs become fatigued. When the blood oxygen level drops severely, the infant's skin turns bluish in color. Tiny, very premature infants may not even have signs of trouble breathing because their lungs may be so stiff they cannot even begin to breathe.

There are two major complications of RDS. One is **pneumothorax**, which means ''air in the chest.'' When the infant's own efforts to breathe, or a breathing machine, applies pressure on the lungs in an attempt to expand them, a lung may rupture, causing air to leak into the chest cavity. This air causes the lung to collapse further, making breathing even harder and interfering with blood flow in the lung arteries. The blood pressure can drop suddenly, cutting off the blood supply to the brain. Pneumothorax is an emergency that must be treated right away. Air may be removed from the chest using a needle and syringe. A tube is then inserted into the lung cavity and suction applied to remove the air. The other complication, intraventricular hemorrhage, is bleeding into the cavities (ventricles) of the brain, which may be fatal.

When a premature infant has obvious trouble breathing, RDS is a definite possibility. If premature birth is expected, or some condition calls for immediate delivery of the baby, the level of surfactant in the amniotic fluid which surrounds the baby in the uterus, will indicate how well the lungs have matured. If little surfactant is found in an amniotic fluid sample in a test called amniocentesis, which is taken by inserting a needle in the uterus and withdrawing fluid, there is a definite risk of RDS. Often this test is done at regular intervals so that the infant can be delivered as soon as the test indicates the lungs are mature. If the membranes have ruptured, surfactant can easily be measured in a sample of vaginal fluid.

The other major diagnostic test is a **chest x ray**. Collapsed lung tissue has a specific appearance; the more collapsed lung tissue, the more severe the RDS. An x ray can also determine if pneumothorax has occurred. Also, the oxygen level in the blood can be measured by taking an arterial blood gas analysis, or, more easily, by using a device called an oximeter, which is clipped to an earlobe. Pneumothorax may have occurred if the infant suddenly becomes worse while on mechanical ventilation—a machine that takes over the work of the lungs and delivers air under pressure.

If only a mild degree of RDS is present at birth, placing the infant in an oxygen hood may be sufficient. It is important, however, not to administer too much oxygen, as this may damage the retina and cause loss of vision. By using an oximeter to keep track of the blood oxygen level, repeated artery punctures, or pricking the heel to draw blood, RDS can be avoided. In more severe cases, a drug very like natural surfactant (Exosurf Neonatal or Survanta), can be dripped into the lungs through a fine tube (endotracheal tube) placed in the infant's windpipe (trachea). Typically the infant will be able to breathe more easily within a few days. The drug is continued until the infant starts producing its own surfactant. However, there is a risk of bleeding into the lungs from surfactant treatment; about 10% of the smallest infants are affected by this.

Infants with severe RDS may require treatment with a ventilator. In tiny infants, ventilation through a tracheal tube is an emergency procedure. Assisted ventilation must be closely supervised, as too much pressure can cause a collapsed lung. A gentler way to assist breathing, continuous positive airway pressure, or CPAP, delivers an oxygen mixture through nasal prongs or a tube placed through the nose rather than an endotracheal tube. CPAP may be tried before resorting to a ventilator, or after an infant placed on a ventilator begins to improve. Drugs that stimulate breathing may speed the recovery process.

If an infant born with RDS is not promptly treated, lack of an adequate oxygen supply will damage the body's organs and eventually cause them to stop functioning altogether. **Death** is the result. The central nervous system in particular—made up of the brain and spinal cord—is very dependent on a steady oxygen supply and is one of the first organ systems to feel the effects of RDS. On the other hand, if the infant's breathing is supported until the lungs mature and make their own surfactant, complete recovery within three to five days is the rule.

The best way of preventing RDS is to delay delivery until the fetal lungs have matured and are producing enough surfactant. If delivery cannot be delayed, the mother may be given a steroid hormone similar to a natural substance produced in the body. This steroid crosses the barrier of the placenta and helps the fetal lungs to produce surfactant. The steroid should be given at least 24 hours before the expected time of delivery. If the infant does develop RDS, the risk of bleeding into the brain will be much less if the mother has been given a dose of steroid.

If a very premature infant is born without symptoms of RDS, it may still be wise to deliver surfactant to its lungs. This may prevent RDS, or make it less severe if it does develop. An alternative is to wait until the first symptoms of RDS appear and then immediately give surfactant. Pneumothorax may be prevented by frequently checking the blood oxygen content, and limiting oxygen treatment under pressure to the minimum needed.

See also Pneumothorax

Respiratory failure

Respiratory failure is nearly any condition that affects breathing and ultimately results in failure of the lungs to function properly. The main tasks of the lungs and chest are to get oxygen into the bloodstream from air that is inhaled (breathed in) and, at the same to time, to eliminate carbon dioxide ($C0_2$) from the bloodstream through air that is exhaled (breathed out). In respiratory failure, either the level of oxygen in the blood becomes dangerously low, and/or the level of $C0_2$ becomes dangerously high.

Respiratory failure often is divided into two main types. One type is hypoxemic respiratory failure. This occurs when something interferes with normal gas exchange and too little oxygen gets into the blood (hypoxemia). All organs and tissues in the body suffer as a result. **Respiratory distress syndrome**, high altitudes (where there is less oxygen in the air), various forms of lung disease, severe **anemia**, and blood vessel disorders, can all prevent the lungs from extracting sufficient oxygen from the air.

The other type of respiratory failure is ventilatory failure. This occurs when breathing is not strong enough to rid the body of $C0_2$, which then builds up in the blood. This can happen when the respiratory center in the brainstem fails to drive breathing, when muscle disease keeps the chest wall from expanding when breathing in, or when **chronic obstructive pulmonary disease** is present, making it difficult to exhale. Many respiratory conditions cause both too little oxygen (hypoxemia) and too much $C0_2$ (ventilatory failure).

The major categories of respiratory failure, with specific examples of each, are:

- Obstruction of the airways. Examples are chronic **bronchitis** with heavy secretions; emphysema; **cystic fibrosis**; **asthma** (a condition in which it is very hard to get air in and out through narrowed breathing tubes).
- Weak breathing. This can be caused by drugs or alcohol, which depress the respiratory center; extreme **obesity**; or **sleep apnea**, where patients frequently stop breathing during sleep.
- Muscle weakness. This can be caused by **muscular dystrophy**; **polio**; a **stroke** that paralyzes the respiratory muscles; injury of the spinal cord; or **Lou Gehrig's disease**.
- Lung diseases. These include severe **pneumonia**; **pulmonary edema** (fluid in the lungs); heart disease; respiratory distress syndrome; pulmonary fibrosis and other scarring diseases of the lung; radiation exposure; smoke inhalation; and widespread **lung cancer**.
- An abnormal chest wall. This condition can be caused by scoliosis or severe injury to the chest wall.

Both low blood oxygen and high blood $C0_2$ can impair mental functions. Patients may become confused and disoriented and find it impossible to carry out their normal activities or do their work. Marked $C0_2$ excess can cause **headache**s and, in time, a semi-conscious state, or even **coma**. Low blood oxygen causes the skin to take on a bluish tinge. It also can cause an abnormal heart rhythm (**arrhythmia**). Lung disease may cause abnormal chest sounds upon examination with a **stethoscope** such as **wheezing** in asthma, and ''crackles'' in obstructive lung disease. Patients often breathe rapidly, are restless, and have a rapid pulse. A patient with ventilatory failure is prone to gasp for breath, and may use the neck muscles to help expand the chest.

The primary symptom of respiratory failure is shortness of breath. Other signs and symptoms are not specific but depend upon what is causing the failure. Good general health and some degree of ''reserve'' lung function will help a patient through an episode of respiratory failure. The key diagnostic method is to measure the amounts of oxygen, $C0_2$, and acid in the blood at regular intervals.

In treating respiratory failure, most patients are first given oxygen, then the underlying cause of respiratory failure must be treated. For example, **antibiotics** are used to fight a lung infection, or, for an asthmatic patient, a drug to open up the airways is commonly prescribed. A patient whose breathing remains very poor will require a mechanical ventilator to aid breathing. A plastic tube is placed through the nose or mouth into the windpipe and attached to a machine that forces air into the lungs. This can be a lifesaving treatment and should be continued until the patient's own lungs can take over the work of breathing. It is very important to use no more pressure than is necessary to provide sufficient oxygen, otherwise ventilation may cause further lung damage. Drugs are given to keep the patient calm, and the amount of fluid in the body is carefully adjusted so that the heart and lungs can function as normally as possible. Steroids, which combat inflammation, may sometimes be helpful but they can cause complications, including weakening the breathing muscles.

The respiratory therapist has a number of methods available to help patients overcome respiratory failure. They include:

- Suctioning the lungs through a small plastic tube passed through the nose, in order to remove secretions from the airways that the patient cannot **cough** up.
- Postural drainage, in which the patient is propped up at an angle or tilted to help secretions drain out of the lungs. The therapist may clap the patient on the chest or back to loosen the secretions, or a vibrator may be used for the same purpose.
- Breathing exercises after the patient recovers sufficiently to help strengthen the muscles that aid breathing.

The prognosis (outlook) for patients with respiratory failure depends chiefly on its cause. When respiratory failure develops slowly, pressure may build up in the lung's blood vessels, a condition called **pulmonary hypertension**. This condition may damage blood vessels and cause the heart to fail. If it is not possible to provide enough oxygen to the body, complications involving either the brain or the heart may also prove fatal. If the kidneys fail or the diseased lungs become infected, the prognosis is poor. In some cases, the primary disease causing respiratory failure is irreversible. Then, the patient, family, and physician together must decide whether to prolong life by ventilator support. Occasionally, lung transplantation is an option; however, this it is a highly complex procedure and availability of healthy lungs is small. If the underlying disease can be effectively treated, however, the outlook is usually good. Care is needed not to expose the patient to polluting substances in the atmosphere as it could tip the balance against recovery.

The best prevention of respiratory failure is early treatment of any lung disease or respiratory disease. Once serious respiratory failure is present, treatment in an intensive care unit with specialized personnel and equipment is desirable.

See also Cystic fibrosis; Emphysema; Mechanical ventilation; Pneumonia; Pulmonary edema; Respiratory distress syndrome; Stethoscope

RESPIRATORY SYNCYTIAL VIRUS INFECTION

Respiratory syncytial virus (RSV) is a virus that can cause severe lower respiratory infections in children under the age of two, and milder upper respiratory infections in older children and adults. RSV infection is also called bronchiolitis, because it is marked in young children by inflammation of the bronchioles. Bronchioles are the narrow airways that lead from the bronchi to the tiny air sacs (alveoli) in the lungs. The result is **wheezing**, difficulty breathing, and sometimes fatal **respiratory failure**.

RSV infection is caused by a group of viruses found worldwide. There are two different subtypes with numerous different strains. Taken together, these viruses account for a significant number of **death**s in infants.

RSV infection is primarily a disease of winter or early spring, with waves of illness sweeping through a community. The rate of RSV infection is estimated to be 11.4 cases in every 100 children during their first year of life. In the United States, RSV infection occurs most frequently in infants between the ages of two and six months.

RSV infection shows distinctly different symptoms, depending on the age of the infected person. In children under two, the virus causes a serious lower respiratory infection in the lungs. In older children and healthy adults, it causes a mild upper respiratory infection often mistaken for the **common cold**.

Although anyone can get this disease, infants suffer the most serious symptoms and complications. Breast feeding seems to provide partial protection from the virus. Conditions in infants that increase their risk of infection include:

- Premature birth
- Lower socio-economic environment
- Congenital heart disease
- Chronic lung diseases, such as **cystic fibrosis**
- **Immune system** deficiencies, including HIV infection
- Immunosuppressive therapy given to **organ transplant** patients.

Many older children and adults get RSV infection, but the symptoms are so similar to the common cold that the true cause often goes undiagnosed. People of any age with weakened immune systems, either from such diseases as **AIDS** or **leukemia**, or as the result of **chemotherapy** or **corticosteroid** medications, are more at risk for serious RSV infections. So are people with chronic lung disease.

RSV is spread through close contact with an infected person. It has been shown that if a person with RSV infection sneezes, the virus can be carried to others within a radius of six feet. This group of viruses is hardy. They can live on the hands for up to half an hour and on toys or other inanimate objects for several hours.

Scientists have yet to understand why RSV viruses attack the lower respiratory system in infants and the upper respiratory system in adults. In infants, RSV begins with such cold symptoms as a low **fever**, runny nose, and **sore throat**. Soon, other symptoms appear that suggest an infection which involves the lower airways. Some of these symptoms resemble those of **asthma**. RSV infection is suggested by:

- Wheezing and high-pitched, whistling breathing
- Rapid breathing (more than 40 breaths per minute)
- **Shortness of breath**
- Labored breathing out (exhalations)
- Bluish tinge to the skin (**cyanosis**)
- **Croup**y, seal-like, barking **cough**
- High fever.

Breathing problems occur in RSV infections because the bronchioles swell, making it difficult for air to get in and out of the lungs. If the child is having trouble breathing, immediate medical care is needed. Breathing problems are most common in infants under one year of age; they can develop rapidly.

RSV infection is usually diagnosed during a **physical examination** by the pediatrician or primary care doctor. The doctor listens with a **stethoscope** for wheezing and other abnormal lung sounds in the patient's chest. The doctor will also take into consideration whether there is a known outbreak of RSV infection in the area. **Chest x ray**s give some indication of whether the lungs are over-inflated from an effort to move air in and out. X rays may also show the presence of a secondary bacterial infection, such as **pneumonia**.

A blood test can also detect RSV infection. This test measures the level of antibodies (infection fighters) the body has formed against the virus. The blood test is less reliable in infants than in older children because antibodies in the infant's blood may have come from the mother during **pregnancy**. If infants are hospitalized, other tests such as an arterial **blood gas analysis** are done to determine if the child is receiving enough oxygen.

Home care for keeping a child with RSV comfortable and breathing more easily includes:

- Use a cool mist room humidifier to ease congestion and sore throat.
- Raise the baby's head by putting books under the head end of the crib.
- Give **acetaminophen** (Tylenol, Panadol, Tempra) for fever. **Aspirin** should not be given to children because of its association with **Reye's syndrome**, a serious disease.
- For babies too young to blow their noses, suction away any mucus with an infant nasal aspirator.

Dehydration can be a problem, so children should be encouraged to drink plenty of fluids. **Antibiotics** have no effect on viral illnesses, therefore, the body must make antibodies to fight the infection and return itself to health.

In the United States, RSV infections are responsible for more than 90,000 hospitalizations and 4,500 deaths each year. Children who are hospitalized receive oxygen and humidity through a mist tent or vaporizer. They also are given intravenous fluids to prevent dehydration. Mechanical ventilation may be necessary, and blood gases are monitored to assure that the child is receiving enough oxygen.

Bronchodilators, such as albuterol (Proventil, Ventilin), may be used to keep the airways open. Ribavirin (Virazole) is used for desperately ill children to stop the growth of the virus. Ribavirin is both expensive and has toxic side effects, so its use is restricted to the most severe cases.

Alternative medicine has little to say specifically about bronchiolitis, especially in very young children. However, practitioners emphasize that people get viral illnesses because their immune systems are weak. Prevention focuses on strengthening the immune system by eating a healthy diet low in sugars and high in fresh fruits and vegetables, reducing **stress**, and getting regular, moderate **exercise**. Like traditional practitioners, alternative practitioners recommend breast feeding infants so that the child may benefit from the positive state of health of the mother. Inhaling a steaming mixture of lemon oil, thyme oil, eucalyptus, and tea tree oil (**aromatherapy**) may make breathing easier.

RSV infection usually runs its course in 7-14 days. The cough may linger weeks longer. There are no medications that can speed the body's production of antibodies against the virus. Bacterial infections that take advantage of a weakened respiratory system may cause ear, sinus, and throat infections or pneumonia. These can be treated with antibiotics.

Hospitalization and death are much more likely to occur in children whose immune systems are weakened or who have underlying diseases of the lungs and heart. People do not gain permanent immunity to respiratory syncytial virus and can be infected many times. Children who suffer repeated infections seem to be more likely to develop asthma in later life.

As of 1998 there were no vaccines against RSV. The infection is so common that prevention is impossible. However, steps can be taken to reduce a child's contact with the disease. People with RSV symptoms should stay at least six feet away from young children; frequent hand washing, especially after contact with respiratory secretions, and the correct disposal of used tissues, help keep the disease from spreading; parents should try to keep their children under 18 months old away from crowded environments such as shopping malls during holiday seasons—where they are likely to come in contact with older people who have only mild symptoms of the disease; and child care centers should regularly disinfect surfaces that children touch.

See also Respiratory failure; Common cold

Respiratory system

The human respiratory system, working in conjunction with the **cardiovascular system**, supplies oxygen to, and removes carbon dioxide from, the cells of the body. The respiratory system conducts air to the respiratory surfaces of the lungs. There, the blood in the lung capillaries readily absorbs oxygen and gives off carbon dioxide gathered from the body cells. The circulatory system transports oxygen-laden blood to the body cells and picks up carbon dioxide. The term respiration describes the exchange of gases across cell membranes both in the lungs (external respiration) and in the body tissues (internal respiration). Pulmonary ventilation, or breathing, exchanges volumes of air with the external environment.

The human respiratory system consists of the respiratory tract and the lungs. The respiratory tract can be divided into an upper and a lower part. The upper part consists of the nose, nasal cavity, pharynx (throat), and larynx (voicebox). The lower part consists of the trachea (windpipe), bronchi, and bronchial tree. The respiratory tract cleans, warms, and moistens air during its trip to the lungs. The nose has openings to the outside that allow air to enter. Hairs inside the nose trap dirt and keep it out of the respiratory tract. The nose leads to a large cavity within the skull. This cavity and the space inside the nose make up the nasal cavity. A nasal septum, supported by cartilage and bone, divides the nasal cavity into a right and left side. Epithelium, a layer of cells that secrete mucus and cells equipped with cilia, lines the nasal passage. Mucus moistens the incoming air and traps dust. The cilia move pieces of the mucus with its trapped particles to the throat, where it is spit out or swallowed. Stomach acids destroy bacteria in swallowed mucus. Sinuses, epithelium-lined cavities in bone, surround the nasal cavity. Blood vessels in the nose and nasal cavity release heat and warm the entering air.

Air leaves the nasal cavity and enters the throat or pharynx. From there it passes into the larynx, which is located between the pharynx and the trachea or windpipe. A framework of cartilage pieces supports the larynx, which is covered by the epiglottis, a flap of elastic cartilage that moves up and down like a trap door. When we breathe, the epiglottis stays open, but when we swallow, it closes. This valve mechanism keeps solid particles and liquids out of the trachea. If we breathe in something other than air, we automatically cough and expel it. Should these protective mechanisms fail, allowing solid food to lodge in and block the trachea, the victim is in imminent danger of asphyxiation.

Air enters the trachea in the neck. Epithelium lines the trachea as well as all the other parts of the respiratory tract. C-shaped cartilage rings reinforce the wall of the trachea and all the passageways in the lower respiratory tract. Elastic fibers in the trachea walls allow the airways to expand and contract when we inhale and exhale, while the cartilage rings prevent them from collapsing. The trachea divides behind the sternum to form a left and right bronchus, each entering a lung. Inside the lungs, the bronchi subdivide repeatedly into smaller airways. Eventually they form tiny branches called terminal bronchioles. Terminal bronchioles have a diameter of about 0.02 in (0.5 mm). The branching air-conducting network within the lungs is called the bronchial tree.

The lungs are two cone-shaped organs located in the thoracic cavity, or chest, and are separated by the heart. The right lung is somewhat larger than the left. The pleural membrane surrounds and protects the lungs. One layer of the pleural membrane attaches to the wall of the thoracic cavity, and the other layer encloses the lungs. A fluid between the two membrane layers reduces friction and allows smooth movement of the lungs during breathing. The lungs are divided into lobes, each one of which receives its own bronchial branch. The bronchial branch subdivides and eventually leads to the terminal bronchi. These tiny airways lead into structures called respiratory bronchioles.

The respiratory bronchioles branch into alveolar ducts that lead into outpocketings called alveolar sacs. *Alveoli*, tiny expansions of the wall of the sacs, form clusters that resemble bunches of grapes. The average person has a total of about 300 million gas-filled alveoli in the lungs. These provide an enormous surface area for gas exchange. Spread flat, the average adult male's respiratory surface would be about 750 sq ft (70 m^2), approximately the size of a handball court. Arterioles and venules make up a capillary network that surrounds the alveoli. Gas diffusion occurs rapidly across the walls of the alveoli and nearby capillaries. The alveolar-capillary membrane together is extremely thin, about 0.5 in (6-37mm) thick.

The result of external respiration is that blood leaves the lungs laden with oxygen and cleared of carbon dioxide. When this blood reaches the cells of the body, internal respiration takes place. Under a higher partial pressure in the capillaries, oxygen breaks away from hemoglobin, diffuses into the tissue fluid, and then into the cells. Conversely, concentrated carbon dioxide under higher partial pressure in the cells diffuses into the tissue fluid and then into the capillaries. The deoxygenated blood carrying carbon dioxide then returns to the lungs for another cycle.

Pulmonary ventilation, or breathing, exchanges gases between the outside air and the alveoli of the lungs. Ventilation, which is mechanical in nature, depends on a difference between the atmospheric air pressure and the pressure in the alveoli. When we expand the lungs to inhale, we increase internal volume and reduce internal pressure. Lung expansion is brought about by two important muscles, the diaphragm and the intercostal muscles. The diaphragm is a dome-shaped sheet of muscle located below the lungs that separates the thoracic and abdominal cavities. When the diaphragm contracts, it moves down. The dome is flattened, and the size of the chest cavity is increased, lowering pressure on the lungs. When the intercostal muscles, which are located between the ribs, contract, the ribs move up and outward. Their action also increases the size of the chest cavity and lowers the pressure on the lungs. By contracting, the diaphragm and intercostal muscles reduce the internal pressure relative to the atmospheric pressure. As a consequence, air rushes into the lungs. When we exhale, the reverse occurs. The diaphragm relaxes, and its dome curves up into the chest cavity, while the intercostal muscles relax and bring the ribs down and inward. The diminished size of the chest cavity increases the pressure in the lungs, thereby forcing out the air.

Physicians use an instrument called a spirometer to measure the tidal volume, that is, the amount of air we exchange during a ventilation cycle. Under normal circumstances, we inhale and exhale about 500 ml, or about a pint, of air in each cycle. Only about 350 ml of the tidal volume reaches the alveoli. The rest of the air remains in the respiratory tract. With a deep breath, we can take in an additional 3,000 ml (3 liters or a little more than 6 pints) of air. The total lung capacity is about 6 liters on average. The largest volume of air that can be ventilated is referred to as the vital capacity. Trained athletes have a high vital capacity. Regardless of the volume of air ventilated, the lung always retains about 1200 ml (3 pints) of air. This residual volume of air keeps the alveoli and bronchioles partially filled at all times.

A healthy adult ventilates about 12 times per minute, but this rate changes with exercise and other factors. The basic breathing rate is controlled by breathing centers in the medulla and the pons in the brain. Nerves from the breathing centers conduct impulses to the diaphragm and intercostal muscles, stimulating them to contract or relax. There is an inspiratory center for inhaling and an expiratory center for exhaling in the medulla. Before we inhale, the inspiratory center becomes activated. It sends impulses to the breathing muscles. The muscles contract and we inhale. Impulses from a breathing center in the pons turn off the inspiratory center before the lungs get too full. A second breathing center in the pons stimulates the inspiratory center to prolong inhaling when needed. During normal quiet breathing, we exhale passively as the lungs recoil and the muscles relax. For rapid and deep breathing, however, the expiratory center becomes active and sends impulses to the muscles to bring on forced exhalations.

The normal breathing rate changes to match the body's needs. We can consciously control how fast and deeply we breathe. We can even stop breathing for a short while. This occurs because the cerebral cortex has connections to the breathing centers and can override their control. Voluntary control of breathing allows us to avoid breathing in water or harmful chemicals for brief periods of time. We cannot, however, consciously stop breathing for a prolonged period. A buildup of carbon dioxide and hydrogen ions in the bloodstream stimulates the breathing centers to become active no matter what we want to do. For this reason, people cannot kill themselves by holding their breath.

The respiratory system is open to airborne microbes and to outside pollution. It is not surprising that respiratory diseases occur, in spite of the body's defenses. Some respiratory disorders are relatively mild and, unfortunately, very familiar. We all experience the excess mucus, coughing, and sneezing of the common cold from time to time. The **common cold** is an example of **rhinitis**, an inflammation of the epithelium lining the nose and nasal cavity. Viruses, bacteria, and allergens are among the causes of rhinitis. Other respiratory disorders include **laryngitis**, **pneumonia**, **bronchitis**, **chronic obstructive pulmonary disease**, and **lung cancer**.

RESPITE CARE

Respite services provide a temporary break for the caregivers of the frail elderly or disabled, chronically ill individuals. The application of the concept to include **elder care** grew out of a combination of increasing interest in the role of the informal caregiver and the cost containment effort to reduce expenditure involved with institutionalization of the **aging** population. Services may be provided in or out of the person's home, with in-home services involving a temporary homemaker or **home health care**. Outside the home, help may include adult day care or temporary stays in **nursing homes**, group homes, or foster care homes. The type and scope of services, and eligibility for services, vary significantly from state to state.

Research has shown that the ability to free caregivers to care for the nondisabled family members, including themselves, reduced their level of stress, anxiety, and isolation. Time off, even for a few hours a week, can enable the caregiver to continue providing care. Brief periods of emergency relief or prescheduled respite from the physical and emotional strain can reenergize a caregiver and renew his or her dedication to the role. While the variety of respite care options available continues to expand, some caregivers are hesitant to arrange such services due to a fear that others may not provide adequate care. Caregivers should be encouraged to explore the various respite arrangements offered, recognizing that taking care of themselves is vital to their own well-being.

Relief from the emotional stress of caregiving can also prevent elder abuse. Family members and caretakers may express frustration in subtle ways, such as frequently reminding the patient that he is impaired and is a burden, talking to others about the patient as if he were not in the room, and arguing with the elder about unimportant issues. Potential for elder abuse is greatest when caregivers have no relief from the constant burden of care. The ability to visit with friends, attend church, or simply spend time alone will promote relaxation and leave the caregiver refreshed and better able to cope with the burdens of caregiving.

See also Elder Care; Home health care; Nursing homes; Foster care

Restless legs syndrome

Restless legs syndrome (RLS) is characterized by unpleasant sensations in the limbs, usually the legs, that occur at rest or before sleep and are relieved by activity such as walking. These sensations are felt deep within the legs and are described as creeping, crawling, aching, or fidgety.

Restless legs syndrome, also known as Ekbom syndrome, Wittmaack-Ekbom syndrome, *anxietas tibiarum*, or *anxietas tibialis*, affects up to 10-15% of the population. Some studies show that RLS is more common among elderly people. Almost half of patients over age 60 who complain of **insomnia** are diagnosed with RLS. In some cases, the patient has another medical condition with which RLS is associated. In idiopathic RLS, no cause can be found. In familial cases, RLS may be inherited from a close relative, most likely a parent.

Most people experience mild symptoms. They may lie down to rest at the end of the day and, just before sleep, will experience discomfort in their legs that prompts them to stand up, massage the leg, or walk briefly. Eighty-five percent of RLS patients either have difficulty falling asleep or wake several times during the night, and almost half experience daytime fatigue or sleepiness. It is common for the symptoms to be intermittent, disappearing for several months and then returning for no apparent reason. Two-thirds of patients report that their symptoms become worse with time. Some older patients claim to have had symptoms since they were in their early 20s, but were not diagnosed until their 50s. Suspected under-diagnosis of RLS may be attributed to the difficulty experienced by patients in describing their symptoms.

More than 80% of patients with RLS experience periodic limb movements in sleep (PLMS). These random movements of arms or legs may result in further sleep disturbance and daytime fatigue. Most patients have restless feelings in both legs, but only one leg may be affected. Arms may be affected in nearly half of patients.

There is no known cause for the disorder, but recent research has focused on several key areas. These include:

- Central nervous system (CNS) abnormalities. Several types of drugs have been found to reduce the symptoms of RLS. Based on an understanding of how these drugs work, theories have been developed to explain the cause of the disorder. Levodopa and other drugs that correct problems with signal transmission within the CNS can reduce the symptoms of RLS. It is therefore suspected that the source of RLS is a problem related to signal transmission systems in the CNS.
- **Iron deficiency anemia**. The body stores iron in the form of ferritin. There is a relationship between low levels of iron (as ferritin) stored in the body and the occurrence of RLS. Studies have shown that older people with RLS often have low levels of ferritin. Supplements of iron sulfate have been shown to significantly reduce RLS symptoms for these patients.

A careful history enables the physician to distinguish RLS from similar types of disorders that cause night time discomfort in the limbs, such as **muscle cramps**, burning feet syndrome, and damage to nerves that detect sensations or cause movement (polyneuropathy).

The most important tool the doctor has in diagnosis is the history obtained from the patient. There are several common medical conditions that are known to either cause or to be closely associated with RLS. The doctor may link the patient's symptoms to one of these conditions, which include **anemia**, **diabetes mellitus**, disease of the spinal nerve roots (lumbosacral radiculopathy), **Parkinson's disease**, late-stage **pregnancy**, **kidney failure** (uremia), and complications of stomach surgery. In order to identify or eliminate such a primary cause, blood tests may be performed to determine the presence of serum iron, ferritin, folate, vitamin B_{12}, creatinine, and **thyroid-stimulating hormones**. The physician may also ask if symptoms are present in any close family members, since it is common for RLS to run in families and this type is sometimes more difficult to treat.

In some cases, sleep studies such as a polysomnography are undertaken to identify the presence of PLMS that are reported to affect 70-80% of people who suffer from RLS. The patient is often unaware of these movements, since they may not cause him to wake. However, the presence of PLMS with RLS can leave the person more tired, because it interferes with deep sleep. A patient who also displays evidence of some neurologic disease may undergo electromyography (EMG). During EMG, a very small, thin needle is inserted into the muscle and electrical activity of the muscle is recorded. A doctor or technician usually performs this test at a hospital outpatient department.

The first step in treatment is to treat existing conditions that are known to be associated with RLS and that will be identified by blood tests. If the patient is anemic, iron (iron sulfate) or **vitamin** supplements—particularly folate or vitamin B_{12}—will be prescribed. If kidney disease is identified as a cause, treatment of the kidney problem will take priority.

In some people whose symptoms cannot be linked to a treatable associated condition, drug therapy may be necessary to provide relief and restore a normal sleep pattern. Prescription drugs that are normally used for RLS include:

- **Benzodiazepines** and low-potency opioids. These drugs are prescribed for use only on an ''as needed'' basis, for patients with mild RLS. Benzodiazepines appear to reduce nighttime awakenings due to PLMS. The benzodiazepine most commonly used to treat RLS is clonazepam (Klonopin, Rivotril). The main disadvantage of this drug type is that it causes daytime drowsiness. It also causes unsteadiness that may lead to accidents, especially for an elderly patient. **Opioid analgesics** are narcotic **pain** relievers. Those commonly used for mild RLS are low potency opioids, such as codeine (Tylenol #3) and propoxyphene (Darvocet). Studies have shown that these can be successfully used in the treatment of RLS on a long-term basis without risk of **addiction**. However, narcotics can cause **constipation** and difficulty urinating.
- Levodopa (L-dopa) and carbidopa (Sinemet). Levodopa is the drug most commonly used to treat moderate or severe RLS. It acts by supplying a chemical called dopamine to the brain. It is often taken in conjunction with carbidopa to prevent or decrease side effects. Although it is effective against RLS, levodopa may also causes a worsening of symptoms during the afternoon or early evening in 50-80% of patients. This phenomenon is known as ''restless legs augmentation,'' and if it occurs, the physician will probably discontinue Levodopa for a brief period while an alternate drug is used. Levodopa can often be reintroduced after a short break.
- Pergolide (Permax). Pergolide acts on the same part of the brain as Levodopa. It is less likely than Levodopa to cause daytime worsening of symptoms (occurs in about 25% of patients). However, it is not recommended as the first choice in drug therapy since it causes a high rate of minor side effects. Pergolide is often used only if Levodopa has been discontinued.
- High potency opioids. If the symptoms of RLS are difficult to treat with the above medication, higher dose opioids will be used. These include methadone (Dolophine), oxycodone, and clonidine (Catapres, Combipres, Dixarit). A significant disadvantage of these drugs is risk of addiction.
- Anticonvulsants. Some cases of RLS may be improved by **anticonvulsant drugs**, such as carbamazepine (Tegretol).
- Combination therapy. Some patients respond well to combinations of drugs such as a benzodiazepine and Levodopa.

Many drugs have been investigated for treatment of RLS, but it seems as though the perfect therapy has not yet been found. However, careful monitoring of side effects and good communication between patient and doctor can result in a flexible program of therapy that minimizes side effects and maximizes effectiveness.

It is likely that the best **alternative medicine** will combine both conventional and alternative therapies. Levodopa may be combined with a therapy that relieves pain, relaxes muscles, or focuses in general on the nervous system and the brain. Any such combined therapy that allows a reduction in dosage of levodopa is advantageous, since this will reduce the likelihood of unacceptable levels of drug side effects. Of course, the physician who prescribes the medication should monitor any combined therapy. Alternative methods may include:

- **Acupuncture**. Patients who also suffer from **rheumatoid arthritis** may especially benefit from acupuncture to relieve RLS symptoms. Acupuncture is believed to be effective in arthritis treatment and may also stimulate those parts of the brain that are involved in RLS.
- Homeopathy. Homeopaths believe that disorders of the nervous system are especially important because the brain controls so many other bodily functions. The remedy is tailored to the individual patient and is based on individual symptoms as well as the general symptoms of RLS.
- **Reflexology**. Reflexologists claim that the brain, head, and spine all respond to indirect massage of specific parts of the feet.
- Nutritional supplements. Supplementation of the diet with vitamin E, calcium, magnesium, and folic acid may be helpful for people with RLS.

Some alternative methods may treat the associated condition that is suspected to cause restless legs. These include:

- Anemia or low ferritin levels. Chinese medicine will emphasize stimulation of the spleen as a means of improving blood circulation and vitamin absorption. Other treatments may include acupuncture and herbal therapies, such as ginseng (*Panax ginseng*) for anemia-related fatigue.
- Late-stage pregnancy. There are few conventional therapies available to pregnant women, since most of the drugs prescribed are not recommended for use during pregnancy. Pregnant women may benefit from alternative techniques that focus on body work, including **yoga**, reflexology, and acupuncture.

RLS usually does not indicate the onset of other neurological disease. It may remain static, although two-thirds of patients get worse with time. The symptoms usually progress gradually. Treatment with Levodopa is effective in moderate to severe cases that may include significant PLMS. However, this drug produces significant side effects, and continued successful treatment may depend on carefully monitored use of combination drug therapy. The prognosis (expected outcome) is usually best if RLS symptoms are recent and can be traced to another treatable condition associated with RLS. Some associated conditions are not treatable, however. In these cases, such as for **rheumatoid arthritis**, alternative medicine such as acupuncture may be helpful.

Diet is key in preventing RLS. A preventive diet will include an adequate intake of iron and the B **vitamins**, especially B_{12} and folic acid. Strict vegetarians should take vitamin supplements to obtain sufficient vitamin B_{12}. Ferrous gluconate may be easier on the digestive system than ferrous sulfate, if iron supplements are prescribed. Some medications may cause symptoms of RLS. Patients should check with their doctor about these possible side effects, especially if symptoms first occur after starting a new medication. **Caffeine**, alcohol, and nicotine use should be minimized or eliminated. Even a hot bath before bed has been shown to prevent symptoms for some sufferers.

RETINAL DETACHMENT

Retinal detachment is movement of the transparent sensory part of the retina away from the outer pigmented layer of the retina. In other words, the portion of the retina pulls away from the outer wall of the eyeball.

There are three layers to the eyeball: The outermost layer is the tough, white sclera; the sclera is lined by the choroid, a thin membrane that supplies nutrients to part of the retina; and the innermost layer is the retina itself—the light-sensitive membrane that receives images through the pupil and transmits them to the brain. The retina is also made up of several layers. One layer contains the photoreceptors—the rods and cones—that send the visual message to the brain. Between this photoreceptor layer (also called the sensory layer) and the choroid is the pigmented epithelium.

Filling the inner space of the eyeball itself is the vitreous, a clear gel-like substance, which is in contact with the entire retina.

A retinal detachment occurs between the two outermost layers of the retina—the photoreceptor layer and the pigmented epithelium. Because the choroid supplies the photoreceptors with nutrients, retinal detachment can basically starve the photoreceptors. If a detachment is not repaired within 24-72 hours, permanent vision damage may occur.

Several conditions may cause retinal detachment:

- Scarring or shrinkage of the vitreous can pull the retina inward.
- Small tears in the retina allow liquid to seep behind it, forcing it forward.
- Injury to the eye can simply knock the retina loose.
- Bleeding behind the retina, most often due to diabetic retinopathy or injury, can force it forward.
- Retinal detachment may be spontaneous (without apparent cause). This occurs more often in the elderly or those with myopia (nearsightedness).
- **Cataract** surgery causes retinal detachment 2% of the time.
- Tumors.

Retinal detachment will cause a sudden defect in vision. It may look as if a curtain or shadow has just descended before the eye. If most of the retina is detached, there may be only a small hole of vision remaining. If just a part of the retina is involved, there will be a blind spot that may not even be noticed. It is often associated with *floaters*—little dark spots that float across the eye and can be mistaken for flies in the room. There may also be *flashes* of light. Anyone experiencing a sudden onset of flashes and/or floaters should contact their eye doctor immediately, as this may signal a detachment.

If the eye is clear—that is, if there is no clouding of the liquids inside the eye—the detachment can be seen by the ophthalmologist by looking into the eye with a hand-held instrument called an **ophthalmoscope**. Other lenses may also be used to examine the back of the eye. In binocular indirect ophthalmoscopy, the physician dilates the patient's pupil with eye drops and then examines the back of the eyes with a hand-held lens. In addition, to evaluate the blood vessels in the retina, a fluorescent dye (fluorescein) may be injected into a vein and photographed with ultraviolet light as it passes through the retina. Further studies may include computed tomography scan (CT scan), **magnetic resonance imaging** (MRI), or ultrasound study.

Reattaching the retina to the inner surface of the eye requires making a scar that will hold it in place and then bringing the retina close to the scarred area. The scar can be made from the outside, through the sclera, using either a laser or a freezing cold probe (cryopexy). Bringing the retina close to the scar can be done in two ways. In one method, a tiny belt tightened around the eyeball will bring the sclera in until it reaches the retina. This procedure is called scleral buckling and may be done under general **anesthesia**. Using this procedure permits the repair of retinal detachments without entering the eyeball. In the other method, air or gas must be pumped into the eye, forcing the retina outward against the sclera and its scar. This is called pneumatic retinopexy and can generally be done under local anesthesia.

If these methods fail, and especially if there is disease in the vitreous, the vitreous may have to be removed in a procedure called vitrectomy. This can be done through tiny holes in the eye, through which equally tiny instruments are placed to suck out the vitreous and replace it with saline, a salt walter solution. The procedure must maintain pressure inside the eye so that the eye does not collapse. Retinal reattachment has an 80-90% success rate.

In diseases such as **diabetes mellitus**, which have a high incidence of retinal disease, routine **eye examination**s can detect early changes. Early treatment can prevent progression to detachment and blindness from other events like hemorrhage. The most common problem is weakness of blood vessels that causes them to break down and bleed. When enough vessels have been damaged, new vessels grow to replace them. These new vessels may grow into the vitreous, producing blind spots and scarring. The scarring can in turn pull the retina loose. Other diseases can cause the tiny holes and tears in the retina through which fluid can leak. Preventive treatment uses a laser to cauterize (seal with heat) the blood vessels so that they do not bleed, and holes so they do not leak.

Good control of diabetes can help prevent diabetic eye disease. Blood pressure control can prevent **hypertension** from damaging the retinal blood vessels. Eye protection can prevent direct injury to the eyes. Regular eye exams can detect changes that the patient may not be aware of. This is important for patients with high myopia who may be more prone to detachment.

See also Cataracts; Ophthalmoscope; Retinopathies; Visual impairment and blindness

RETINITIS PIGMENTOSA

Retinitis pigmentosa (RP) refers to a group of inherited disorders that cannot be prevented and that slowly leads to the degeneration of part of the retina, primarily the photoreceptors. There is no known cure for RP, which will eventually lead to blindness.

The retina lines the interior surface of the back of the eye. The retina is made up of several layers. One layer contains two types of photoreceptor cells referred to as the rods and cones. The cones are responsible for sharp, central vision and color vision and are primarily located in a small area of the retina called the fovea. The area surrounding the fovea contains the rods, which are necessary for peripheral (side) vision and night vision (scotopic vision). The rod and cone photoreceptors convert light into electrical impulses and send the message to the brain via the optic nerve where the image of what we see is produced. Another layer of the retina, called the retinal pigmented epithelium (RPE), may also be affected in this disorder.

In RP, the photoreceptors (primarily the rods) begin to deteriorate and lose their ability to function. Because the rods are primarily affected, it becomes harder to see in dim light, thus producing a loss of night vision. As the condition progresses, peripheral vision disappears, resulting in tunnel vision. The ability to see color is eventually lost. In the late stages of the disease, there is only a small area of central vision remaining. Eventually, this too is lost.

The first symptom of RP is a loss of night vision followed by a loss of peripheral vision, usually begin in early adolescents or young adults. Occasionally, the loss of the ability to see color occurs before the loss of peripheral vision. Other symptoms can include seeing twinkling lights or small flashes of lights.

When a person complains of a loss of night vision, a doctor will examine the interior of the eye with an **ophthalmoscope** to determine if there are changes in the retina indicative of RP. However, the appearance of the retina is not enough for a diagnosis. There are other disorders that may give the retina a similar appearance to RP. There are also other reasons someone may have night blindness. For that reason, certain electrodiagnostic tests will be performed—either an electroretinogram (ERG) or an electro-oculogram (EOG); or a visual field examination, which can help determine if side vision is reduced.

There are no medications or surgery to treat this condition. Some doctors believe **vitamins** A and E will slightly slow the progression of the disease in some people. However, large doses of certain vitamins may be toxic and patients should speak to their doctors before taking certain supplements.

If a person with RP must be exposed to bright sunlight, some doctors recommend wearing dark glasses to reduce the effect on the retina. The glasses should protect against ultraviolet (UV) and infrared (IR) rays. Dark tint alone will not protect the eyes. Patients should talk to their eye doctors about the correct lenses to wear outdoors.

Because there is no cure for RP, the patient should be monitored for visual function and counselled about low-vision aids (for example, field-expansion devices). Also, when expectant parents—or couples who wish to become pregnant—are related to anyone who has had RP, they should receive **genetic counseling**.

See also Visual impairment and blindness

RETINOBLASTOMA

Retinoblastoma is a rare childhood **cancer** of the eye. It appears in infants or young children at a frequency of about one in every 15,000 births. In some cases, there is a family (familial) history of the disease. It is curable if detected early, but often requires surgical removal of the eye.

The genetic cause of retinoblastoma has been extensively studied. Normally, individuals have two good copies of the retinoblastoma gene (RB-1) on chromosome 13. This RB-1 gene carries the information for making a protein called pRB which regulates cell division. When pRB is absent or defective due to defective (mutated) copies of the gene, uncontrolled cell division occurs, and cancer results. These patients also have increased risk of developing other types of cancer because pRB appears to be involved in many types of cancer besides retinoblastoma.

Retinoblastoma develops in individuals in whom mutation (an abnormality) has occurred in both copies of RB-1. Retinoblastoma is described as a ''two-hit'' process. It appears that about 40% of patients are born with a defective copy on one gene (first ''hit''), inherited from one parent. The second copy is rendered defective by a separate mutation (second ''hit'') that occurs in the eye. Individuals with an inherited RB-1 defect have a high likelihood of developing retinoblastoma in both eyes. For individuals who do, diagnosis occurs at about age one.

The other 60% of patients inherit two normal copies of RB-1 and develop the disease only after each copy experiences an independent mutation. The likelihood of two independent ''hits'' is lower, and these individuals are less likely to develop retinoblastoma in both eyes. For these individuals, average age of diagnosis is 2.1 years.

Individuals with familial tumors in only one eye have a high incidence (70%) of recurrence in the other eye, and some patients experience secondary tumors in other non-ocular tissues of the body. Although chances of developing retinoblastoma decline sharply after age five, for those individuals who have had retinoblastoma in one eye, there is some possibility of the disease appearing in the other eye at any age into adulthood.

In cases with a family history of retinoblastoma, the child inherits a defective chromosome 13 from one parent. The tumor arises, however, only after a second, spontaneous mutation occurs in one of the cells of the retina; therefore, a situation then exists in which both copies of chromosome 13 carry defective genes. In the majority of cases, however, spontaneous mutations appear to occur in both copies of chromosome 13.

During diagnosis for retinoblastoma, a white reflection in the pupil of the eye is often the first sign of the disease. The presence of a tumor can be confirmed by an ophthalmologist directly examining the retina through the pupil.

Treatment depends upon the size and number of tumor locations in the eye, as well as whether the disease is found in one or both eyes. When only one eye is involved, the eye is surgically removed. If both eyes are involved, one eye can sometimes be saved by treating the tumor with **radiation therapy**, photocoagulation (use of intense laser light to destroy cancer cells), or **cryotherapy** (use of intense cold to kill cancer cells). **Chemotherapy** is increasingly used as a follow-up to one of these treatments. However, some forms of radiation therapy have been shown to promote other cancers, especially of the bone.

Because many patients have a strong predisposition to this disease, frequent **eye examination**s are recommended, especially after successful treatment for retinoblastoma in order to get the earliest possible warning if the disease recurs. Close monitoring is also important.

In a small percentage of cases, retinoblastoma is fatal because it has already spread through the optic nerve to the brain. However, if diagnosis occurs early, when the tumor is restricted to the eye, 90% of patients can be cured.

No preventative measures are possible for a genetic condition such as retinoblastoma. When expectant parents—or couples who wish to become pregnant—are related to anyone who has had retinoblastoma, they should receive **genetic counseling**. **Genetic testing** may be recommended to see if a defective gene has been inherited.

See also Cancer

RETINOPATHIES

Retinopathy is a noninflammatory disease of the retina, the thin membrane that lines the back of the eye and contains light-sensitive cells (photoreceptors). Light enters the eye and is focused onto the retina. The photoreceptors send a message to the brain via the optic nerve and the brain then ''interprets'' the electrical message sent to it, resulting in vision. The macula is a specific area of the retina responsible for central vision and the fovea is an tiny area about 1.5 mm located in the macula responsible for sharp vision. When looking at an object, the fovea should be directed right at it. Damage to the retina causes vision deficits and even blindness.

Retinopathy, or damage to the retina, has various causes. While each cause has its own specific effect on the retina, a general scenario for many of the retinopathies is as follows (note: not all retinopathies necessarily affect the blood vessels). Blood flow to the retina is disrupted, either by blockage or breakdown of the various vessels. This can lead to bleeding (hemorrhage) and fluids, cells, and proteins leaking into the area (exudates). There can be a lack of oxygen to surrounding tissues (hypoxia), or decreased blood flow (ischemia). Chemicals produced by the body then can cause new blood vessels to grow (neovascularization); however, these new vessels generally leak, cause the retina to swell, and vision will be affected.

Retinopathies are divided into two broad categories, *simple*—or *nonproliferative* retinopathies, and *proliferative* retinopathies. The simple retinopathies include the defects identified by bulging of the vessel walls, by bleeding into the eye, by small clumps of dead retinal cells called cotton wool exudates, and by closed vessels. This form of retinopathy is considered mild. The proliferative, or severe, forms include the defects caused by newly grown blood vessels, by scar tissue formed within the eye, by closed-off blood vessels that are badly damaged, and by the retina breaking away from its mesh of blood vessels that nourish it (**retinal detachment**).

There are many causes of retinopathy, and some of the more common ones are listed below.

Diabetic retinopathy—caused by **diabetes mellitus**—is the leading cause of blindness in people ages 20-74. Diabetes is a complex disorder characterized by an inability of the body to properly regulate the levels of sugar and insulin (a hormone made by the pancreas) in the blood. As diabetes progresses, the blood vessels that feed the retina become damaged in different ways. They can have bulges in their walls (**aneurysms**), they can leak blood into the jelly-like fluid that fills the eyeball (vitreous), they can become completely closed, or new vessels can begin to grow where there would not normally be blood vessels. However, these new blood vessels cannot nourish the retina and they bleed easily, releasing blood into the inner region of the eyeball, which can cause dark spots and cloudy vision. Diabetic retinopathy begins prior to any outward signs of the disease. Once symptoms are noticed, they include poorer than normal vision, fluctuating or distorted vision, cloudy vision, dark spots, episodes of temporary blindness, or permanent blindness. Diabetic retinopathy will occur in 90% of persons with type 1 diabetes (insulin-dependent, or insulin requiring) and 65% of persons with type 2 diabetes (non-insulin-dependent, or not requiring insulin) within about 10 years of diabetes onset. In the United States, new cases of blindness are most often caused by diabetic retinopathy. Among these new cases of blindness, 12% are people between the ages of 20-44 years, and 19% are people between the ages of 45-64 years.

Hypertensive retinopathy is caused by **hypertension** (high blood pressure). Some blood vessels can narrow, others can thicken and harden (arteriosclerosis). There will be flame-shaped hemorrhages and macular swelling (**edema**). This edema may cause distorted or decreased vision.

Sickle-cell anemia also affects blood vessels in the eye. This disease occurs mostly in American-African populations and is a hereditary disease that affects the red blood cells. The sickle-shaped blood cell reduces blood flow, which also includes blood flow in the retina. Vision problems will not appear early on in the disease; however, patients need to be followed closely in case neovascularization occurs.

Retinal vein occlusion generally occurs in the elderly. There is usually a history of other systemic disease, such as diabetes or high blood pressure. The central retinal vein (CRV), or the retinal veins branching off of the CRV, can become compressed, stopping the drainage of blood from the retina. This may occur if the central retinal artery hardens. Symptoms include a sudden, painless loss of vision or field of vision in one eye; there may be a sudden onset of floating spots (floaters) or flashing lights; or vision may decrease dramatically.

Retinal artery occlusion is generally the result of an **embolism** (blood clot) that dislodges from somewhere else in the body and travels to the eye. Temporary loss of vision may precede an occlusion. Symptoms include a sudden, painless loss of vision or decrease in visual field. Ten percent of the cases of a retinal artery occlusion occur because of giant cell arteritis (a chronic vascular disease).

Solar retinopathy can be caused by looking directly at the sun, as when watching an eclipse. This can cause loss of the central visual field or decreased vision. The symptoms can occur hours or days after the incident.

Certain medications can affect different areas of the retina. Doses of 20-40 mg a day of tamoxifen usually does not cause a problem, but much higher doses may cause irreversible damage. Patients taking chloroquine for lupus, **rheumatoid arthritis**, or other disorders may notice a decrease in vision. If so, discontinuing medication will stop, but not reverse, any damage. However, patients should never discontinue medication without the advise of their physician. Patients taking thioridazine may notice a decrease in vision or color vision. These drug-related retinopathies generally only affect patients taking large doses. However, patients need to be informed if medications will affect their eyes, and they also need to inform their doctors of any visual effects from medications.

Damaged retinal blood vessels and other retinal changes are visible to an eye doctor during an examination of the retina. This can be done using a hand-held instrument called an **ophthalmoscope**, or another instrument called a binocular indirect ophthalmoscope, that allow the doctor to see the back of the eye. Certain retinopathies have classic signs (for example, vascular ''sea fans'' in sickle cell, dot and blot hemorrhages in diabetes, flame-shaped hemorrhages in high blood pressure). Patients may then be referred for other tests to confirm the underlying cause of the retinopathy. These tests include blood tests and measurement of blood pressure. Also, fluorescein **angiography**, where a dye is injected into the patient and the back of the eyes are viewed and photographed, helps to locate leaky vessels.

Treatment for retinopathy usually begins with an ophthalmologist, a physician who specialize in eye disorders. Because retinopathy can result from underlying systemic causes, a general physician should be consulted as well. For drug-related retinopathies, the treatment is generally discontinuation of the drug (only under the care of a physician).

In some cases, **laser surgery** can help to prevent blindness or lessen vision loss. The high-energy light from a laser is aimed at the weakened blood vessels in the eye, destroying them. Scars will remain where the laser treatment was performed. For that reason, laser treatment cannot be performed in all sections of the retina. For example, laser photocoagulation at the fovea would destroy the area for sharp vision. Panretinal photocoagulation may be performed in which a larger area is treated at the periphery (edges) of the retina aimed at decreasing neovascularization. Prompt treatment of proliferative retinopathy may reduce the risk of severe vision loss by 50%. Patients with retinal artery occlusion should be referred to a cardiologist. Patients with retinal vein occlusion need to be referred to a physician, as they may have an underlying systemic disorder such as high blood pressure. Nonproliferative retinopathy has a better prognosis (expected outcome) than proliferative retinopathy. Prognosis depends upon the extent of the retinopathy, the cause, and promptness of treatment.

To help reduce the risk of retinopathy, complete **eye examinations** done regularly can help to detect early signs. Patients on certain medications should have more frequent eye exams, as well as a baseline eye exam when starting the drug. Persons with diabetes must take extra care to have thorough, periodic eye exams, especially if early signs of **visual impairment** are noticed. Anyone experiencing a sudden loss of vision, decrease in vision or visual field, flashes of light, or floating spots, should contact their eye doctor immediately.

Proper medical treatment for any of the systemic diseases known to cause retinal damage will help prevent retinopathy. For diabetics, maintaining proper blood sugar and blood pressure levels is important; however, some form of retinopathy will usually occur in diabetics, given enough time. A proper diet, particularly for those persons with diabetes, and stopping smoking, will also help delay retinopathy.

See also Diabetes mellitus; Laser surgery; Ophthalmoscope; Retinal detachment; Visual impairment and blindness

Retirement

Germany was the first country to provide workers with a comprehensive plan for social security. There, in 1881, Germany's imperial chancellor, Prince Otto von Bismarck, announced his plan to offer workers subsidized insurance against sickness, accident, and old age. In 1932, Franklin D. Roosevelt was elected President of the United States on a platform that promoted a social security program that would protect retirees against undue hardship, and that would provide them with an incentive to move out of the work force and make room for younger workers. After a 14-month fight in Congress, the Social Security Act was signed into law on August 14, 1935.

In over 60 years, there have been many additional government and private-sector agencies available to help meet the special needs of retired persons; these include **Public Health** Departments, Senior Centers, Social Service Agencies, the United Way and the American Association of Retired Persons (AARP). Although it appears that most retirees prefer to retire in a place specializing in retirement communities, such as Del Webb's pioneer Sun City (1960) in Arizona, many have sprung up near all major population centers. Most retired people obtain their retirement income from two or more of the following sources: social security retirement benefits, pensions and retirement plans (including IRAs and 401k plans), working part- or full-time, savings (especially amounts set aside after age 50), inheritances, gifts, early retirement bonuses, or withdrawal of equity form their homes.

In 1993, nine states had more than 1 million retired residents. California, with 3.3 million, led the way, followed by Florida, New York, Pennsylvania, Texas, Ohio, Illinois, Michigan, and New Jersey. During the 1980s, the largest increases in percentage of retired persons were mostly in western states and southeastern coastal states. According to the U.S. Census Bureau projections, the retired population will more than double between now and the year 2050 to 80 million. By that year, as many as one in five Americans could be retired. Most of this growth should occur between 2010 and 2030, when the baby boom generation enters their retirement years.

Poor health is not as prevalent among retired persons as many assume. In 1992, about 3 in every 4 noninstitutionalized persons aged 65-74 considered their health to be good. Two in three aged 75 or older felt similarly. On the other hand, as more people reach old age, there may also be more who face chronic, limiting illnesses such as arthritis, diabetes, **osteoporosis**, and senile dementia.

While 1% of those aged 65-74 years lived in a nursing home in 1990, nearly one in four aged 85 or older did. Among those who were not institutionalized in 1990-91, 9% aged 65-69 years, but 50% aged 85 or older, needed assistance performing everyday activities such as bathing, getting around inside the home, and preparing meals. Most people who require long-term care have suffered from physical problems such as heart attacks, **stroke**s or other debilitating problems, and not mental disabilities such as **Alzheimer's disease**.

Consequently, the ability to live independently and avoid long-term care facilities rests to a large extent in the hands of the retired person. Studies have shown that by exercising, the retired person increases his or her chances of staying out of a nursing home between the ages of 65 and 80. Many retirees in their 60s and 70s who are in reasonably good health manage their increased health care costs by supplementing their free Medicare coverage with a reasonably priced medi-gap insurance policy.

Reye's syndrome

Reye's syndrome is a serious medical condition associated with viral infection and aspirin intake. It usually strikes children under age 18, most commonly those between the ages of five and 12. Symptoms of Reye's syndrome develop after the patient appears to have recovered from the initial viral infection. Symptoms include fatigue, irritability, and severe vomiting. Eventually, neurological symptoms such as delirium and coma may appear. One third of all Reye's syndrome patients die, usually from heart failure, gastrointestinal bleeding, kidney failure, or cerebral edema (a condition in which fluid presses on the brain, causing severe pressure and compression).

Reye's syndrome is a particularly serious disease because it causes severe liver damage and swelling of the brain, a condition called encephalopathy. Recovery from the illness is possible if it is diagnosed early. Even with early diagnosis, some patients who survive Reye's syndrome may have permanent neurological damage, although this damage can be subtle.

Reye's syndrome was discovered in 1963 by Dr. Ralph D. Reye. However, the connection between aspirin and viral infection was not made until the 1980s. In a study conducted by the Centers for Disease Control, 25 out of 27 children who developed Reye's syndrome after a bout with **chicken pox** had taken aspirin during their illness. In 140 of the children with chicken pox who had not taken aspirin, only 53 developed Reye's syndrome. Researchers are still unsure about the exact mechanism that causes aspirin to damage the liver and brain during viral infections. Some researchers suspect that aspirin inhibits key enzymes in the liver, leading to liver malfunction. However, why the combination of aspirin intake and viral infection may lead to Rye's syndrome has never been fully explained.

Since the early 1980s, public health officials and physicians have warned parents about giving children aspirin to reduce pain during viral infections. As a result of these warnings, the numbers of cases of Reye's syndrome have dropped significantly: in 1977, 500 cases were reported; in 1989, only 25 cases were reported. Nonaspirin pain relievers, such as acetaminophen, are recommended for children and teenagers. Although children represent the majority of Reye's syndrome patients, adults can also develop Reye's syndrome. Therefore, pain relief for cold and flu symptoms, as well as for other viral infections such as chicken pox and **mumps**, should be restricted to nonaspirin medications in both children and adults.

Rheumatic fever

It is the end of summer vacation and a 10-year-old girl is outside playing when her mother notices the jerky and uncontrolled movements of her usually coordinated daughter. Earlier in the summer the girl had complained of a sore throat and later she had shown a skin rash for a day or two. When the girl said that her knee ached, her mother dismissed these complaints as "growing pains." Could these simple ailments be connected?

This young girl is showing symptoms of rheumatic fever, a disease that usually affects young people aged five to 15 and girls more frequently than boys. Symptoms often manifest themselves in late summer or early fall if a child has had a throat infection in the spring or early summer.

The disease begins as a bacterial infection such as strep throat caused by Group A streptococcus bacteria. To combat the infection, the human body produces antibodies which fight the bacteria. These antibodies then seem to turn on the body, attacking and inflaming healthy connective tissues of the joints, brain, and heart. What results may be a fever, inflammation of the joints (sometimes incorrectly called "growing pains"), and Sydenham's chorea—uncontrollable, spastic movements (traditionally called St. Vitus' Dance) caused by the immune system disorder's affect on the nervous system. By far the most dangerous and long-lasting effect of rheumatic fever can be permanent damage to the heart. Cardiac tissue, especially the heart valves, may become thickened and scarred, leading to the narrowing or leaking of heart valves, heart murmur, or even heart failure.

Much of what is known about the bacteria that cause rheumatic fever is from work done by Dr. Rebecca Craighill Lancefield of the Rockefeller Institute. Lancefield was a pioneer in classifying the chains of round bacteria known as streptococci. In her laboratory during the 1920s, she identified many types of streptococci and saw the connection between rheumatic fever and Group A streptococcus. However, she was frustrated in her efforts to discover how the bacteria cause the disease. Why they prompt such a destructive immune system response still remains a mystery.

After Lancefield's work, and with the coming of the age of **antibiotics**, penicillin was used to effectively treat rheumatic fever, and still is today. If the initial strep throat infection is treated with antibiotics, the disease cannot progress; however, without treatment, perhaps one percent of cases will develop into rheumatic fever. In conjunction with antibiotics, aspirin therapy is recommended to counteract joint pain and minimize heart damage. Sometimes a child with rheumatic fever continues to take **penicillin** over a long period of time to prevent recurrence.

Rheumatic fever had almost disappeared in the United States by the early 1980s—only 88 cases were recorded in 1983 as compared to 10,000 in 1961. However, in 1985, two hospitals in Utah alone reported 150 new cases, and outbreaks have since been reported in several other states. Also, the current strain appears to be more likely to cause heart damage because strep symptoms are much less severe, often being mistaken for a simple cold or other respiratory infection. In the developing countries of Asia and Africa, the disease is more common. There is no vaccine to prevent rheumatic fever, nor is there a cure once it develops.

Rheumatoid arthritis

Rheumatoid arthritis (RA) is a chronic disease causing inflammation and deformity of the joints. Other problems throughout the body (systemic problems) may also develop, including inflammation of blood vessels (**vasculitis**), the development of bumps (called rheumatoid nodules) in various parts of the body, lung disease, blood disorders, and weakening of the bones (**osteoporosis**).

The skeletal system of the body is made up of different types of strong, fibrous tissue called connective tissue. Bone, cartilage, ligaments, and tendons are all forms of connective tissue that have different compositions and different characteristics.

The joints are structures that hold two or more bones together. Some joints (synovial joints) allow for movement between the bones being joined (articulating bones). The simplest synovial joint involves two bones, separated by a slight gap called the joint cavity. The ends of each articular bone are covered by a layer of cartilage. Both articular bones and the joint cavity are surrounded by a tough tissue called the articular capsule. The articular capsule has two components, the fibrous membrane on the outside and the synovial membrane (or synovium) on the inside. The fibrous membrane may include tough bands of tissue called ligaments, which are responsible for providing support to the joints. The synovial membrane has special cells and many tiny blood vessels (capillaries). This membrane produces a supply of synovial fluid that fills the joint cavity, lubricates it, and helps the articular bones move smoothly about the joint.

In rheumatoid arthritis (RA), the synovial membrane becomes severely inflamed. Usually thin and delicate, the synovium becomes thick and stiff, with numerous infoldings on its surface. The membrane is invaded by white blood cells, which produce a variety of destructive chemicals. The cartilage along the articular surfaces of the bones may be attacked and destroyed, and the bone, articular capsule, and ligaments may begin to wear away (erode). These processes severely interfere with movement in the joint.

RA exists all over the world and affects men and women of all races. In the United States alone, about two million people suffer from the disease. Women are three times more likely than men to have RA. About 80% of people with RA are diagnosed between the ages of 35-50. RA appears to run in families, although certain factors in the environment may also influence the development of the disease.

The underlying event that promotes RA in a person is unknown. Given the known genetic factors involved in RA, some researchers have suggested that an outside event occurs that triggers the disease cycle in a person with a particular genetic makeup.

Many researchers are examining the possibility that exposure to an organism (like a bacteria or virus) may be the first event in the development of RA. The body's normal response to such an organism is to produce cells that can attack and kill the organism, protecting the body from the foreign invader. In an autoimmune disease like RA, this immune cycle spins out of control. The body produces misdirected immune cells, which accidentally identify parts of the person's body as foreign. These immune cells then produce a variety of chemicals that injure and destroy parts of the body.

RA can begin very gradually, or it can strike quickly. The first symptoms are **pain**, swelling, and stiffness in the joints. The most commonly involved joints include hands, feet, wrists, elbows, and ankles, although other joints may also be involved. The joints are affected in a symmetrical fashion. This means that if the right wrist is involved, the left wrist is also involved. Patients frequently experience painful joint stiffness when they first get up in the morning, lasting for perhaps an hour. Over time, the joints become deformed. The joints may be difficult to straighten, and affected fingers and toes may be permanently bent (flexed). The hands and feet may curve outward in an abnormal way.

Many patients also notice increased fatigue, loss of appetite, weight loss, and sometimes **fever**. Rheumatoid nodules are bumps that appear under the skin around the joints and on the top of the arms and legs. These nodules can also occur in the tissue covering the outside of the lungs and lining the chest cavity (pleura), and in the tissue covering the brain and spinal cord (meninges). Lung involvement may cause **shortness of breath** and is seen more in men. Vasculitis (inflammation of the blood vessels) may interfere with blood circulation. This can result in irritated pits (ulcers) in the skin, tissue death (**gangrene**), and interference with nerve functioning that causes numbness and tingling.

There are no tests available that can absolutely diagnose RA. Instead, a number of tests exist that can suggest the diagnosis of RA. Blood tests include a special test of red blood cells (called erythrocyte sedimentation rate), which is positive in nearly 100% of patients with RA. However, this test is also positive in a variety of other diseases. Tests for anemia are usually positive in patients with RA, but can also be positive in many other unrelated diseases. Rheumatoid factor is an autoantibody found in about 66% of patients with RA. However, it is also found in about 5% of all healthy people and in 10-20% of healthy people over the age of 65. Rheumatoid factor is also positive in a large number of other **autoimmune diseases** and other infectious diseases.

A long, thin needle can be inserted into a synovial joint to withdraw a sample of the synovial fluid for examination. In RA, this fluid has certain characteristics that indicate active inflammation. The fluid will be cloudy, relatively thinner than usual, with increased protein and decreased or normal glucose. It will also contain a higher than normal number of white blood cells. While these findings suggest inflammatory arthritis, they are not specific to RA.

There is no cure available for RA. However, treatment is available to combat the inflammation in order to prevent destruction of the joints, and to prevent other complications of the disease. Efforts are also made to maintain flexibility and mobility of the joints.

Nonsteroidal anti-inflammatory agents and **aspirin** are used to decrease inflammation and to treat pain. While these medications can be helpful, they do not interrupt the progress of the disease. Low-dose steroid medications can be helpful at both managing symptoms and slowing the progress of RA, as well as other drugs called disease-modifying antirheumatic drugs. These include gold compounds, D-penicillamine, antimalarial drugs, and sulfasalazine. Methotrexate, azathioprine, and cyclophosphamide are all drugs that suppress the immune system and can decrease inflammation. All of the drugs listed have significant toxic side effects, which require healthcare professionals to carefully compare the risks associated with these medications versus the benefits.

Total bed rest is sometimes prescribed during the very active, painful phases of RA. Splints may be used to support and rest painful joints. Later, after inflammation has somewhat subsided, physical therapists may provide a careful **exercise** regimen in an attempt to maintain the maximum degree of flexibility and mobility. **Joint replacement** surgery, particularly for the knee and the hip joints, is sometimes recommended when these joints have been severely damaged.

A variety of alternative therapies has been recommended. **Meditation**, **hypnosis**, **guided imagery**, and relaxation techniques; **acupressure** and **acupuncture** have all been used for pain relief. Body work can be soothing, decreasing **stress** and tension, and is thought to improve/restore chemical balance within the body.

A multitude of beneficial nutritional supplements include fish oils, the enzymes bromelain and pancreatin, and the antioxidants (**vitamins** A, C, and E, selenium, and zinc).

Anti-inflammatory herbs include tumeric (*Curcuma longa*), ginger (*Zingiber officinale*), feverfew (*Chrysanthemum parthenium*), devil's claw (*Harpagophytum procumbens*), Chinese thoroughwax (*Bupleuri falcatum*), and licorice (*Glycyrrhiza glabra*). Lobelia (*Lobelia inflata*) and cramp bark (*Vibernum opulus*) can be applied topically to the affected joints.

Homeopathic practitioners recommended *Rhus toxicondendron* and *Bryonia* (*Bryonia alba*) for acute prescriptions. **Yoga** promotes relaxation, relieves stress, and improves flexibility. Nutritionists suggest that a vegetarian diet low in animal products and sugar may help to decrease inflammation and pain. Beneficial foods include cold water fish (mackerel, herring, salmon, and sardines) and flavonoid-rich berries (cherries, blueberries, hawthorn berries, blackberries, etc.).

Because RA is often connected with food allergies/intolerances, an elimination/challenge diet can help to decrease symptoms as well as identify the foods that should be eliminated. **Hydrotherapy** can help to greatly reduce pain and inflammation. Moist heat is more effective than dry heat, and cold packs are useful during acute flare-ups.

About 15% of all RA patients will have symptoms for a short period of time and will ultimately get better, leaving them with no long-term problems. A number of factors are considered to suggest the likelihood of a worse prognosis. These include:

- Race and gender (female and Caucasian)
- More than 20 joints involved
- Extremely high erythrocyte sedimentation rate
- Extremely high levels of rheumatoid factor
- Consistent, lasting inflammation
- Evidence of erosion of bone, joint, or cartilage on x rays
- Poverty
- Older age at diagnosis
- Rheumatoid nodules
- Other coexisting diseases

- Certain genetic characteristics, diagnosable through testing.

Patients with RA have a shorter life span, averaging a decrease of three to seven years of life. Patients sometimes die when very severe disease, infection, and gastrointestinal bleeding occur. Complications due to the side effects of some of the more potent drugs used to treat RA are also factors in these **deaths**.

There is no known way to prevent the development of RA. The most that can be hoped for is to prevent or slow its progress.

See also Joint replacement; Osteoporosis

Rhinitis

Rhinitis, inflammation of the mucous lining of the nose, is a nonspecific term that covers infections, **allergies**, and other disorders whose common feature is the location of their symptoms. These symptoms include infected or irritated mucous membranes, producing a discharge, congestion, and swelling of the tissues of the nasal passages. The most widespread form of infectious rhinitis is the **common cold**.

The common cold is the most frequent viral infection in the general population, causing more absenteeism from school or work than any other illness. Colds are self-limited, lasting about 3-10 days, although they are sometimes followed by a bacterial infection. Children are more susceptible than adults; teenage boys than teenage girls; and adult women than adult men. In the United States, colds are most frequent during the late fall and winter.

Colds can be caused by as many as 200 different viruses which are transmitted by sneezing and coughing, contact with soiled tissues or handkerchiefs, or close contact with an infected person. Colds are easily spread in schools, offices, or any place where people live or work in groups. The incubation period ranges between 24 and 72 hours.

The onset of a cold is usually sudden. The virus causes the lining of the nose to become inflamed and produce large quantities of thin, watery mucus. Children sometimes run a **fever** with a cold. The inflammation spreads from the nasal passages to the throat and upper airway, producing a dry cough, **headache**, and watery eyes. Some people develop muscle or joint aches and feel generally tired or weak. After several days, the nose becomes less inflamed and the watery discharge is replaced by a thick, sticky mucus. This change in the appearance of the nasal discharge helps to distinguish rhinitis caused by a viral infection from rhinitis caused by an allergy.

There is no specific test for viral rhinitis, and diagnosis is based purely on symptoms. In children, the doctor will examine the child's throat and glands to rule out **measles** and other childhood illnesses that have similar early symptoms. Adults whose symptoms last longer than a week may require further testing to rule out a secondary bacterial infection or an allergy. Bacterial infections can usually be identified from a laboratory culture of the patient's nasal discharge. Allergies can be evaluated by blood tests, skin tests for reaction to specific substances, or nasal smears.

There is no cure for the common cold; treatment is given for symptom relief. Medications include **aspirin** or **nonsteroidal anti-inflammatory drugs** (NSAIDs) for headache and muscle **pain**, and **decongestants** to relieve stuffiness or runny nose. Patients should be warned against overusing decongestants, because they can cause a rebound effect. **Antibiotics** are not given for colds because they do not kill viruses. Supportive care includes bed rest and drinking plenty of fluid. Treatments under investigation include the use of ultraviolet light treatment and injections of **interferon**.

Any of ten different **homeopathic medicines** might be prescribed, depending on the appearance of the nasal discharge, the patient's emotional state, and the stage of infection. **Naturopaths** would recommend **vitamins** A and zinc supplements, together with botanical medicine made from echinacea (*Echinacea* spp.), goldenseal (*Hydrastis canadensis*), licorice (*Glycyrrhiza glabra*), or astragalus (*Astragalus membraneceus*) root.

Most colds resolve (cure themselves) completely in about a week. Complications are unusual but may include **sinusitis** (inflammation of the nasal sinuses), bacterial infections, or infections of the middle ear.

There is no vaccine effective against colds, and infection does not produce immunity against another cold. Prevention depends on:

- Washing hands often, especially before touching the face
- Minimizing contact with people already infected
- Not sharing hand towels or eating and drinking utensils.

See also Allergies; Common cold; Sinusitis

Rhinoplasty

The term rhinoplasty means ''nose molding'' or ''nose forming,'' a procedure in **plastic surgery** in which the structure of the nose is changed. The change can be made by adding or removing bone or cartilage, grafting tissue from another part of the body, or implanting synthetic material to alter the shape of the nose. This procedure is often called a ''nose job.''

Rhinoplasty is most often performed for cosmetic reasons. A nose that is too large, crooked, misshapen, malformed at birth, or deformed by an injury can be given a more pleasing appearance. If breathing is impaired due to the form of the nose or to an injury, it can often be improved with rhinoplasty.

The best candidates for rhinoplasty are those with relatively minor deformities. Nasal anatomy (structure) and proportions (size) are quite varied and the final look of any rhinoplasty will be a combination of the patient's anatomy and the surgeon's skill.

The quality of the patient's skin plays a major role in the outcome of rhinoplasty. Patients with extremely thick skin may not see a definite change in the underlying bone structure after surgery. On the other hand, thin skin provides almost no cushion to hide the most minor of bone irregularities or imperfections.

Rhinoplasty should not be performed until the pubertal growth spurt is complete—between ages 14 to 15 years for girls, and older for boys.

The cost of rhinoplasty depends on the difficulty of the work required and on the specialist chosen. Prices run from about $3,000 to more than $6,000. If the problem was caused by an injury, insurance will usually cover the cost. A rhinoplasty done only to change a person's appearance is not usually covered by insurance.

During the initial consultation, the patient and surgeon will determine what changes can be made in the shape of the nose. Most doctors take photographs at the same time. The surgeon will also explain the techniques and anesthesia options available to the patient.

The external nose is composed of a series of interrelated parts which include the skin, the bony pyramid, cartilage, and the tip of the nose, which is both cartilage and skin. The strip of skin separating the nostrils is called the columella.

Surgical approaches to nasal reconstruction are varied. Internal rhinoplasty involves making all incisions inside the nasal cavity. The external or ''open'' technique involves a skin incision across the base of the nasal columella. An external incision allows the surgeon to expose the bone and cartilage more fully and is most often used for complicated procedures. During surgery, the surgeon will separate the skin from the bone and cartilage support. The framework of the nose is then reshaped in the desired form by removing bone, cartilage, or skin. The remaining skin is then replaced over the new framework. If the procedure requires adding to the structure of the nose, the donated bone, cartilage, or skin can come from the patient or from a synthetic source. When the operation is over, the surgeon will apply a splint to help the bones maintain their new shape. The nose may also be packed, or stuffed with a dressing, to help stabilize the septum.

When a local anesthetic is used, light sedation is usually given first, after which the operative area is numbed. It will remain insensitive to **pain** for the length of the surgery. A general anesthetic is used for lengthy or complex procedures or if the doctor and patient agree that it is the best option.

Simple rhinoplasty is usually performed in an outpatient surgery center or in the surgeon's office. Most procedures take only an hour or two, and patients go home right away. Complex procedures may be done in the hospital and require a short stay.

Patients usually feel fine immediately after surgery; however, the first day there will be some swelling of the face, and patients should stay in bed with their heads elevated for at least a day. The nose may hurt, and a **headache** is not uncommon. The surgeon will prescribe medication to relieve these conditions. Swelling and bruising around the eyes will increase for a few days, but will begin to diminish after about the third day. Slight bleeding and stuffiness are normal, and vary according to the extensiveness of the surgery performed. Most people are up in two days, and back to school or work in a week. No strenuous activities are allowed for two to three weeks.

Patients are given a list of postoperative instructions, which include requirements for hygiene, **exercise**, eating, and follow-up visits to the doctor. Patients should not blow their noses for the first week to avoid disruption of healing. It is extremely important to keep the surgical dressing dry. Dressings, splints, and stitches are removed in one to two weeks, and patients should avoid **sunburn**.

Any type of surgery carries a degree of risk. There is always the possibility of unexpected events, such as an infection or a reaction to the **anesthesia**.

When the nose is reshaped or repaired from inside, the scars are not visible, but if the surgeon needs to make the incision on the outside of the nose, there will be some slight scarring. In addition, tiny blood vessels may burst, leaving small red spots on the skin. These spots are barely visible, but may be permanent.

About 10% of patients require a second procedure.

See also Plastic surgery

RIBOFLAVIN DEFICIENCY

Riboflavin deficiency is caused by a dietary lack of vitamin B_2. It occurs when the chronic (long-term) failure to eat sufficient amounts of foods that contain riboflavin produces **skin lesions**, lesions of smooth surfaces in the digestive tract, or nervous disorders.

Riboflavin, also called **vitamin** B_2, is a water-soluble vitamin. The recommended daily allowance (RDA) is 1.7 mg/day for an adult man and 1.3 mg/day for an adult woman. The best sources of this vitamin are meat, dairy products, and dark green vegetables, especially broccoli. Grains and legumes (beans and peas) also contribute riboflavin to the diet. Riboflavin is required for the processing of dietary fats, carbohydrates, and proteins to convert these nutrients to energy. It is also used for the continual process of renewal and regeneration of all cells and tissues in the body.

Riboflavin is sensitive to light. For this reason, commercially available milk is sometimes supplied in cartons rather than in clear bottles. Milk contains about 1.7 mg riboflavin/kg, cheese contains about 4.3 mg/kg, beef has 2.4 mg/kg, and broccoli has about 2.0 mg/kg. Riboflavin is not rapidly destroyed by cooking.

A deficiency in riboflavin alone has never occurred in the natural environment. Although poorer populations in the United States have a higher rate of riboflavin deficiency, the affected individuals are also deficient in a number of other nutrients, as well. In contrast, diseases where people are deficient in one vitamin only—such as thiamin, vitamin C, or vitamin D, for example—have been clearly documented. When riboflavin deficiency is actually detected, it is often associated with low consumption of milk, chronic **alcoholism**, or chronic **diarrhea**.

The symptoms of riboflavin deficiency include:

- Swelling and fissuring (breaking or cracking) of the lips (cheilosis)
- Ulceration and cracking of the angles of the mouth (angular **stomatitis**)

- Oily, scaly skin **rashes** on the scrotum, vulva, or area between the nose and lips
- Inflammation of the tongue
- Red, itchy eyes that are sensitive to light.

The nervous symptoms of riboflavin deficiency include:

- Numbness of the hands
- Decreased sensitivity to touch, temperature, and vibration.

Riboflavin status is diagnosed using a test conducted on red blood cells that measures the activity of an enzyme called glutathione reductase. An extract of the red blood cells is placed in two test tubes. One test tube contains no added riboflavin, while the second test tube contains a derivative of riboflavin, called flavin adenine dinucleotide. The added riboflavin derivative results in little or no stimulation of enzyme activity in patients with normal riboflavin levels. A stimulation of 20% or less is considered normal. A stimulation of more than 20% means the patient is deficient in riboflavin.

Riboflavin deficiency can be treated with supplemental riboflavin (0.5 mg/kg body weight per day) until the symptoms disappear. The prognosis (expected cure rate) for riboflavin deficiency is excellent, and it can be prevented by including milk, cheese, yogurt, meat, and/or certain vegetables in the daily diet. Of the vegetables, broccoli, asparagus, and spinach are highest in riboflavin, having a content ratio similar to that of milk, yogurt, or meat.

See also Alcoholism; Chronic diarrhea; Skin lesions; Stomatitis

Richardson, Benjamin Ward (1828-1896)

English physician

One of the most respected physicians of his day and an experimental pharmacologist who established precedents for the field's scientific integrity, Richardson was an active participant in some of the most popular reform movements of the 19th century. He was closely involved in the push for temperance and in the drives for improvements in **sanitation** and public hygiene. The physician was also one of the first scientists to advocate human treatment of laboratory animals.

Richardson was born in Somerby, Leicestershire, England. Some of his early medical education was as an apprentice to a surgeon in his hometown, after which he entered Anderson's University in 1847. He continued his medical studies in 1850 at the Faculty of Physicians and Surgeons in Glasgow, Scotland, and then received his medical degree from Scotland's University of St. Andrews in 1854.

In 1856, Richardson began working as a physician at the Royal Infirmary for Diseases of the Chest. The following year, he won a prestigious award for his discovery that ammonia maintains the fluidity of blood, yet volatizes to permit coagulation. He remained there for many years, during which he experimented with numerous organic compounds to determine their physiological effects. He described the chemical composition of amyl nitrate in 1863. From 1863 to 1871, Richardson concentrated on examining compounds in the amyl, ethyl, and methyl series and some hydrides, alcohols, chlorides, and iodides whose chemical composition he could determine. He then changed their molecular makeups by carefully substituting or adding different radicals in a process that he hoped would allow him to predict a particular compound's effects on the body.

Although Richardson was ultimately unable to establish a conclusive link between a compound's chemical makeup and its physiological effects, researchers later benefited from his assumption that only part of a molecule takes part in an actual physiological reaction, as well as his habit of experimenting with groups of like compounds. In addition, Richardson's research led to his introduction of 14 anesthetics, including methylene bichloride, and such useful medical tools as the disinfectant hydrogen peroxide and an ether spray for local **anesthesia**. He also invented some embalming methods and several medical devices.

In his role as reformer, Richardson wrote two books—*Diseases of Modern Life* (1876) and *National Health* (1890)—that warned about the dangers of poor sanitation, inadequate hygiene, and drinking alcoholic beverages. He began working at the London Temperance Hospital in 1892, and received a knighthood the following year for his contributions to the public health. Richardson died in London in 1896.

See also Anesthesia

Richards, Linda (1841-1930)

American nurse

The first professionally trained American nurse, Linda Richards is credited with establishing nurse training programs in various parts of the United States and in Japan. She also is recognized for creating the first system for keeping individual medical records for hospitalized patients.

Born on July 27, 1841, in West Potsdam, New York, Richards was the youngest of three daughters of Sanford and Betsy (Sinclair) Richards. Her father was a preacher who christened his youngest daughter Malinda Ann Judson Richards in hopes that she would follow in the footsteps of missionary Ann Judson Hasseltine.

When Richards was four years old, her family moved to the Wisconsin territory, where her father owned some land. Unfortunately, her father died from **tuberculosis** just six weeks after they arrived at their new home. Heartbroken, Richards returned with her mother and sisters to Newbury, Vermont, to stay with her grandfather. The family bought a small farm near Newbury where they lived until her mother also contracted tuberculosis. Linda, who was just 13, nursed her mother Betsy who also died from the infection.

The experience awakened young Linda's interest in **nursing**, and she received some informal training from a Doctor Currier, the local family practitioner who had cared for her mother. Despite her interest in nursing, however, she enrolled at the St. Johnsbury Academy when she was 15 to be trained as a teacher. Although she finished the one-year program and taught for several years, she was never happy teaching. At about the same time, she also worked for several years at the Union Straw Works in Foxboro, Massachusetts.

In 1860, Linda met George Poole, to whom she became engaged. Shortly after they met, Poole joined the Green Mountain Boys to fight in the U.S. Civil War; he was severely wounded in 1865. When he returned home, Richards cared for him until his death in 1869.

By this time, Richards had decided that she wanted to work as a nurse, and she moved to Boston to take a job at the Boston City Hospital. She received practically no training and was treated more like a maid than the nurse she wanted to be. She became ill and left the hospital after only three months. Undaunted by the experience, she was one of five women to sign up for a nurse-training program at the New England Hospital for Women and Children. She was the program's first graduate in 1873.

After her graduation, she traveled to New York City, where she was hired as night supervisor at Bellevue Hospital. It was there that she created a system for keeping individual records for each patient. Her system became widely used in this country and in England, where it was adopted by St. Thomas's Hospital, the institution founded by Florence Nightingale.

When she returned to Boston in 1874, she was named superintendent of the Boston Training School. The school's nurse-training program was only a year old at that time and was in danger of closing due to poor management. Richards, with her gift for organization and love of nursing, was able to turn the program around. Eventually, it became regarded as one of the best nursing programs in the country.

Longing for more skills, in 1877 Richards went to England to participate in an intensive, seven-month nurse training program. She studied at St. Thomas's Hospital in London, where she was able to spend some time with Florence Nightingale, widely regarded as the founder of modern nursing. At Nightingale's suggestion, she studied at King's College Hospital and the Edinburgh Royal Infirmary in Scotland.

Richards returned to America in 1878 to help set up a training school at Boston City Hospital. Named matron of the hospital and superintendent of the school, she stayed there until 1885 when she became ill. Later that year, she traveled to Japan to help establish that country's first nurse-training program. Richards supervised the school at Doshisha Hospital in Kyoto for five years before returning to the United States. Once home, she worked in the field of nursing for another 20 years, establishing and directing nurse-training programs in Philadelphia, Massachusetts, and Michigan. She was elected as the first president of the American Society of Superintendents of Training Schools and served as head of the Philadelphia Visiting Nurses Society. She also set up nurse-training schools in several hospitals for mentally ill patients.

Richards retired in 1911 to write her autobiography, *Reminiscences of Linda Richards.* Following a severe **stroke** in 1923, she returned to the New England Hospital for Women and Children where she remained until her death on April 16, 1930. Richards was named to the National Women's Hall of Fame in 1994.

See also Nursing

Richards, Jr., Dickinson Woodruff (1895-1973)

American physician

Dickinson Woodruff Richards, Jr. was born in 1895 in Orange, New Jersey to Sally (Lambert) and Dickinson Woodruff Richards. Richards received his A.B. from Yale University in 1917, and three months later enlisted in the United States Army, After serving in France with the American Expeditionary Force during World War I, Richards entered the College of Physicians and Surgeons at Columbia; there he completed his M.A. in physiology in 1922 and his M.D. in 1923. Richards immediately received his license to practice medicine. He spent his early career interning, conducting research, and studying experimental psychology. He then returned to Columbia University's Presbyterian Hospital to study pulmonary and circulatory physiology. In 1931 he married Constance Riley, a Wellesley College graduate who worked as a technician in his research lab at Presbyterian Hospital.

Richards' collaboration with André Cournand began in 1931 at Bellevue Hospital. Basing their research on Richards' concept ''that lungs, heart, and circulation should be thought of as one single apparatus for the transfer of respiratory gases between outside atmosphere and working tissues," these two physicians began a long and fruitful partnership. Their initial research involved the study of the physiological performance of the lungs and, in particular, a disorder known as chronic pulmonary insufficiency. Characterized by a malfunction in the heart's tricuspid and pulmonic valves, this defect causes blood to flow backward into the heart. Richards concluded, as had others before him, that it was necessary to be able to measure the amount of air in the lungs during different stages of pulmonary activity. Thus, he and Cournand unearthed studies done in 1929 by the German physician **Werner Forssmann**, wherein Forssmann had attempted to measure gases in the blood as it passed from the heart to the lungs.

Forssmann's technique was proven viable when he successfully inserted a narrow rubber catheter through a vein in his own arm and into the right atrium of his heart. This method gave access to blood as it entered the heart—blood that could then be examined in specific stages of pulmonary and cardiac activity and evaluated in terms of rate of flow, pressure relations, and gas contents. Catheterization would allow physicians to measure oxygen and carbon dioxide in blood returning from the right atrium, allowing for accurate measurement of blood flow through the lungs. Richards and Cournand sought to advance Forssmann's technique and to develop a safe procedure by first experimenting on animals. They began their research in 1936, and by 1941 they had successfully catheterized the right atrium of the human heart.

The measurements made possible through cardiac catheterization led Richards to other important assessments about functions of the heart and circulatory system. In 1941 he developed methods to measure the volume of blood pumped out of either ventricle (lower chamber) of the heart, and to measure blood pressure in the right atrium, the right ventricle, and the pulmonary artery, as well as total blood volume. More recent research has employed catheterization to diagnose abnormal exchange between the right and left sides of the heart, such as is present in some congenital cardiac defects. It has also contributed to the development of more sophisticated techniques such as angiocardiography (the X-ray examination of the heart after injection of dyes), which is used to determine whether normal circulation has resumed following a surgical procedure.

Richards and his colleagues also relied on their revolutionary research technique to study the effects of traumatic shock in heart failure and to identify congenital heart lesions. The most important result of this project was the discovery that whole blood, rather than just blood plasma, should be used in the treatment of shock to the cardiac system.

For their refinement of the catheterization procedure and the discoveries that followed, Richards, Cournand and Forssmann were awarded the Nobel Prize in physiology or medicine in 1956. Richards was passionate about health issues in the social arena as well as in the laboratory. For example, in 1957 he testified before the Joint Legislative Committee on Narcotics Study to suggest the construction of hospital clinics to legally distribute narcotics to recovering addicts.

Richards was elected to the National Academy of Sciences in 1958, and retired from practice in 1961, although he continued to lecture and publish frequent articles for several years. He died at his home in Lakeville, Connecticut on February 23, 1973, after suffering a heart attack.

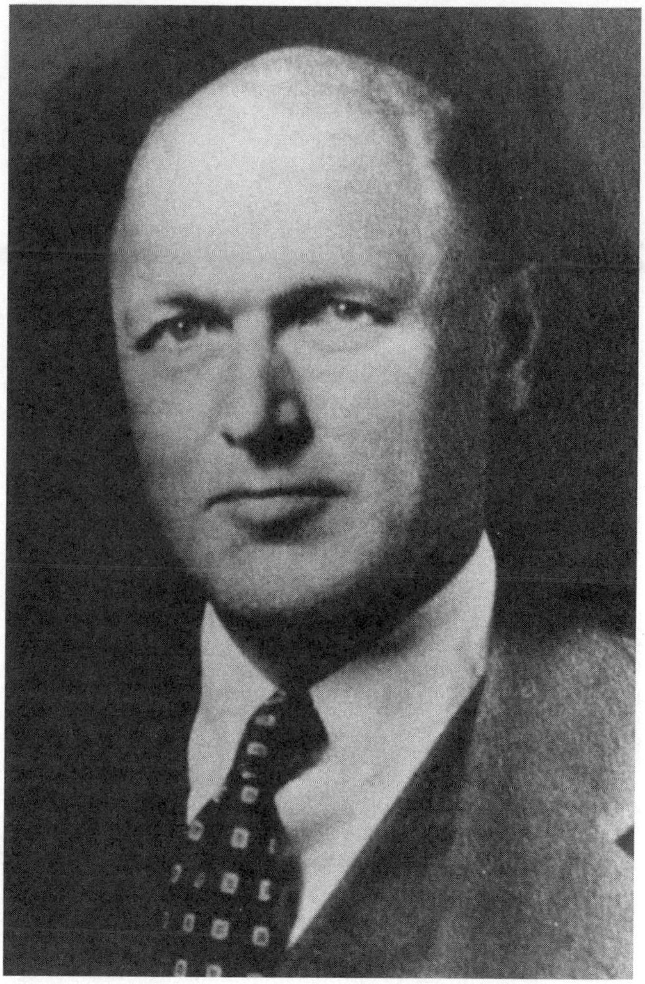

Dickinson Woodruff Richards, Jr.

RICHET, CHARLES ROBERT (1850-1935)

French physiologist

Charles Richet was born on August 25, 1850, in Paris, the son of a professor of clinical surgery. As a student, Richet found himself drawn to both the humanities and the sciences. Swayed perhaps by family influence, he entered medical school at the University of Paris, although he continued to write poetry and drama on the side. While at medical school, Richet became involved in studies of hypnotism, of the gastric juices involved in **digestion**, and of the phenomenon of pain. Deciding on a career in physiology rather than surgery, Richet, after receiving his medical degree in 1877, earned his doctor of science degree in 1878. Soon afterward, he was named a professor of the Faculty of Medicine at the University of Paris and immediately began research on muscle contraction. By 1883, he had turned to studies on how warm-blooded animals maintain their constant body temperature, demonstrating that the larger the animal, the less heat it produces per unit of weight.

In 1880, Richet began investigating microbiology, the field in which he would make his great contribution. He observed **Louis Pasteur** demonstrate the inoculation of chickens against the fatal fowl cholera with a weakened strain of the **cholera** bacteria. Richet was struck by the idea that microbes might cause disease by producing a toxin, and that immune animals might carry a substance in their blood that counteracts the toxin. Richet reasoned that, if blood from immune animals were injected into nonresistant animals, the transfused toxin-resistant substance might confer immunity on the blood recipient. His applications of this theory to produce an immune serum for **tuberculosis**, however, failed.

Nevertheless, Richet continued his studies of toxicity, and in 1900, at the request of Prince Albert of Monaco, he began investigating the toxicity of sea anemone poison. He discovered ''an extraordinary fact'' completely opposite to what he had expected: when dogs that had been previously injected with toxin were reinjected with small doses of that toxin, the animals quickly died. The initial dose, instead of conferring immunity, produced fatal hypersensitivity. Richet called this reaction **anaphylaxis**, and in subsequent investigations, he and others found that it could occur as the result of exposure to a number of substances. Richet summarized ana-

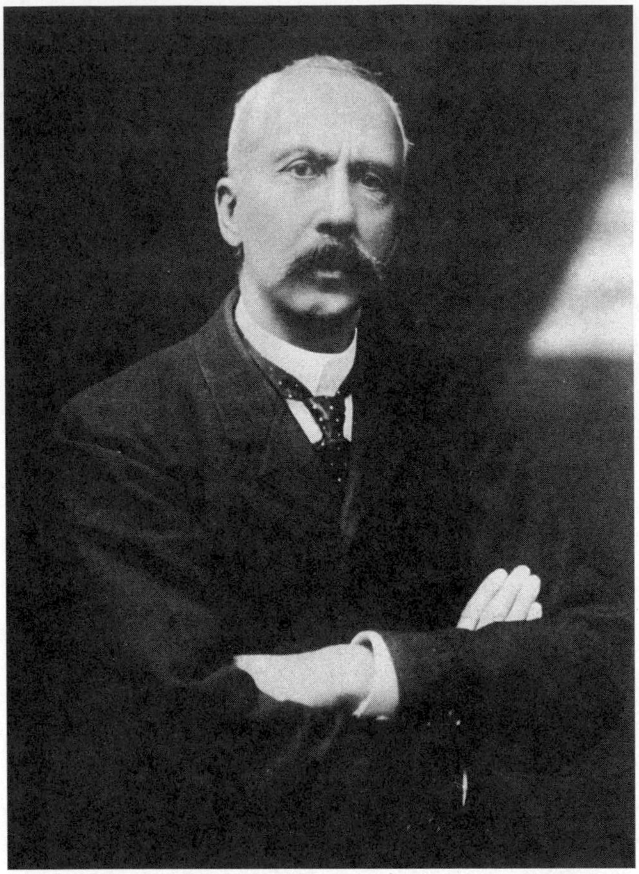

Charles Robert Richet

phylaxis research in a 1911 monograph. For his work on anaphylaxis, he earned the 1913 Nobel Prize.

During World War I, Richet investigated blood plasma transfusion. After the war, he continued research in a wide range of areas. During the 1890s, he took part in the design and construction of one of the early airplanes. He was deeply interested in psychic phenomena, and he was also a dedicated pacifist who wrote several histories showing the malevolent effects of war. In later life, Richet also continued writing poems, plays, and novels. He died in Paris on December 4, 1935.

Rickettsial infections

There are a number of rickettsial infections. Rickettsialpox is a relatively mild disease caused by a member of the bacterial family called Rickettsia. Rickettsialpox causes rash, **fever**, chills, heavy sweating, **headache**, eye **pain** (especially when exposed to light), weakness, and achy muscles. Rocky Mountain spotted fever (RMSF), a tick-borne illness, Q fever, and Trench fever are also caused by bacteria and result in high fevers and characteristic rashes.

Like other members of the family of Rickettsia, the bacteria causing rickettsialpox live in mice. Tiny mites feed on these infected mice, thus acquiring the organism. When these mites feed on humans, the bacteria can be transmitted.

Rickettsialpox occurs mostly within cities. In the United States, the disease has cropped up in such places as New York City, Boston, Philadelphia, Pittsburgh, and Cleveland. It has also been identified in Russia, Korea, and Africa.

The bacteria causing RMSF is passed to humans through the bite of an infected tick. The illness begins within about two weeks of such a bite. RMSF is the most widespread tick-borne illness in the United States, occurring in every state except Alaska and Hawaii. The states in the mid-Atlantic region, the Carolinas, and the Virginias have a great deal of tick activity during the spring and summer months, and the largest number of RMSF cases come from those states. About 5% of all ticks carry the causative bacteria. Children under the age of 15 years have the majority of RMSF infections.

C. burnetii, the bacteria that causes Q fever, lives in many different kinds of animals, including cattle, sheep, goats, tick, cats, rabbits, birds, and dogs. In sheep and cattle, for example, the bacteria tends to accumulate in large numbers in the female's uterus (the organ where lambs and calves develop) and udder. Other animals have similar patterns of bacterial accumulation within the females. As a result, *C. burnetii* can cause infection through contaminated milk, or when humans come into contact with the fluids or tissues produced when a cow or sheep gives birth. Also, the bacteria can survive in dry dust for months; therefore, if the female's fluids contaminate the ground, humans may become infected when they come in contact with the contaminated dust.

Persons most at risk for Q fever include anybody who works with cattle or sheep, or products produced from them. These include farm workers, slaughterhouse workers, workers in meat-packing plants, veterinarians, and wool workers.

Q fever has been found all over the world, except in some areas of Scandinavia, Antarctica, and New Zealand.

The term trench fever refers to the crowded conditions in which troops fought in during World War I and World War II. Because the causative bacteria is passed among humans through contact with body lice, overcrowding, and conditions which interfere with good hygiene (including regular washing of clothing) soldiers were predispose to this disease. Currently, homeless people in the United States are sometimes diagnosed with this illness. The bacteria is sometimes passed through the bite of an infected tick. This can cause the illness in people who participate in outdoor activity and encounter ticks in that particular area.

The specific bacteria responsible for rickettsialpox is called *Rickettsia akari*. A person contracts this bacteria through the bite of an infected mite. After a person has been bitten by an infected mite, there is a delay of about 10 days to three weeks prior to the onset of symptoms.

The first symptom is a bump which appears at the site of the original bite. The bump (papule) develops a tiny, fluid-filled head (vesicle). The vesicle sloughs away, leaving a crusty black scab in its place (eschar). In about a week, the patient develops a fever, chills, heavy sweating, headache, eye pain (especially when exposed to light), weakness, and achy muscles. The fever rises and falls over the course of about a weak. A bumpy rash spreads across the body. Each individual papule follows the same progression: papule, then vesicle, then eschar. The rash does not affect the palms of the hands or the soles of the feet.

The bacterial culprit in RMSF is called *Rickettsia rickettsii*. It causes no illness in the tick carrying it, and can be passed on to the tick's offspring. When a tick attaches to a human, the bacteria is passed. The tick must be attached to the human for about six hours for this passage to occur. Although prompt tick removal will cut down on the chance of contracting RMSF, removal requires great care. If the tick's head and body are squashed during the course of removal, the bacteria can be inadvertently rubbed into the tiny bite wound.

Symptoms of RMSF begin within two weeks of the bite of the infected tick. Symptoms usually begin suddenly, with high fever, chills, headache, severe weakness, and muscle pain. Pain in the large muscle of the calf is very common, and may be particularly severe. The patient may be somewhat confused and delirious. Without treatment, these symptoms may last two weeks or more.

The rash of RMSF is quite characteristic. It usually begins on the fourth day of the illness, and occurs in at least 90% of all patients with RMSF. It starts around the wrists and ankles, as flat pink marks (called macules). The rash spreads up the arms and legs, toward the chest, abdomen, and back. Unlike **rashes** which accompany various viral infections, the rash of RMSF does spread to the palms of the hands and the soles of the feet. Over a couple of days, the macules turn a reddish-purple color. They are now called petechiae, which are tiny areas of bleeding under the skin (pinpoint hemorrhages). This signifies a new phase of the illness. Over the next several days, the individual petechiae may spread into each other, resulting in larger patches of hemorrhage.

The most severe effects of RMSF occur due to damage to the blood vessels, which become leaky. This accounts for the production of petechiae. As blood and fluid leak out of the injured blood vessels, other tissues and organs may swell and become damaged, and:

- Breathing difficulties may arise as the lungs are affected.
- Heart rhythms may become abnormal.
- Kidney failure occurs in very ill patients.
- Liver function drops.
- The patient may experience nausea, vomiting, abdominal pain, and **diarrhea**.
- The brain may swell (**encephalitis**) in about 25% of all RMSF patients. Brain injury can result in seizures, changes in consciousness, actual **coma**, loss of coordination, imbalance on walking, muscle spasms, loss of bladder control, and various degrees of **paralysis**.
- The clotting system becomes impaired, and blood may be evident in the stools or vomit.

C. burnetii causes infection when a human breathes in tiny droplets, or drinks milk, containing the bacteria. After 3-30 days, symptoms of the illness appear.

The usual symptoms of Q fever include fever, chills, heavy sweating, headache, nausea and vomiting, **diarrhea**, fatigue, and **cough**. Also, a number of other problems may present themselves, including inflammation of the liver (hepatitis); inflammation of the sac containing the heart (**pericarditis**); inflammation of the heart muscle itself (**myocarditis**); inflammation of the coverings of the brain and spinal cord, or of the brain itself (meningoencephalitis); and **pneumonia**.

Chronic Q fever occurs most frequently in patients with other medical problems, including diseased heart valves, weakened immune systems, or kidney disease. Such patients usually have about a year's worth of vague symptoms, including a low fever, enlargement of the spleen and/or liver, and fatigue. Testing almost always reveals that these patients have inflammation of the lining of the heart (**endocarditis**).

Two different bacteria can cause trench fever: *Bartonella quintana* and *Bartonella henselae. B. quintana* is carried by body lice; *B. henselae* is carried by ticks.

Infection with *B. quintana* occurs when an infected louse defecates while feeding on a human. When the person scratches, the feces (which are full of bacteria) are rubbed into the tiny wound. Infection with *B. henselae* occurs when an infected tick bites a human, passing the bacteria along through the tiny bite wound.

Symptoms of trench fever begin about 2 weeks to a month after exposure to the bacteria. Sudden fever, loss of energy, **dizziness**, headache, weight loss, skin rash, severe muscle and bone pain can occur. Pain is particularly severe in the shins, leading to the nickname ''shin bone fever.'' The fever can reach 105°F (40.5°C) and stays high for five to six days at a time. The temperature then drops, and stays down for several days, usually recurring in five to six day cycles. An individual may experience as many as eight cycles of fever with the illness.

Most practitioners are able to diagnose rickettsial infections simply on the basis of their symptoms, their rising and falling fevers, and characteristic rashes. Occasionally, blood will be drawn and tests performed to demonstrate the presence of antibodies (immune cells directed against specific bacterial agents), which would confirm a diagnosis.

Because rickettsialpox is such a mild illness, some practitioners choose to simply treat the symptoms (giving **acetaminophen** for fever and achiness, pushing fluids to avoid **dehydration**). Others will give their patients a course of the antibiotic tetracycline, which will shorten the course of the illness to about one to two days.

It is essential to begin treatment absolutely as soon as RMSF is seriously suspected. Delaying treatment can result in death.

Antibiotics are used to treat RMSF. The first choice is a form of tetracycline; the second choice (used in young children and pregnant women) is chloramphenicol. If the patient is well enough, treatment by oral intake of medicine is perfectly effective. Sicker patients will need to be given the medication through a needle in the vein (intravenously). Penicillin and sulfa drugs are not suitable for treatment of RMSF, and their use may increase the death rate by delaying the use of truly effective medications.

Very ill patients will need to be hospitalized in an intensive care unit. Depending on the types of complications a particular patient experiences, a variety of treatments may be necessary, including intravenous fluids, blood **transfusions**, anti-seizure medications, **kidney dialysis**, and mechanical ventilation (a breathing machine).

Doxycycline and quinolone antibiotics are effective for treatment of Q fever. Treatment usually lasts for two weeks. Rifampin and doxycycline together are given for chronic Q fever. Chronic Q fever requires treatment for at least three years.

Erythromycin and azithromycin are both used to treat trench fever. Four weeks of treatment are usually necessary. Inadequate treatment often results in a relapse. In fact, relapses have been reported to occur as long as 10 years after the first episode.

Prognosis for full recovery from rickettsialpox is excellent. No **death**s have ever been reported from this illness, and even the skin rash heals without scarring.

Prior to the regular use of antibiotics to treat RMSF, the death rate was about 25%. Although the death rate from RMSF has improved greatly with an understanding of the importance of early use of antibiotics, there is still a 5% death rate. This rate is believed to be due to delays in the administration of appropriate medications.

Certain risk factors suggest a worse outcome in RMSF. Death rates are higher in males and increase as people age. It is considered a bad prognostic sign to develop symptoms of RMSF within only two to five days of a tick bite.

Death is rare from Q fever. Most people recover completely, although some patients with endocarditis will require surgery to replace their damaged heart valves.

Prognosis for patients with trench fever is excellent. Recovery may take a couple of months. Without treatment, there is always a risk of recurrence, even years after the original illness.

As with all mite- or tick-borne illnesses, prevention includes avoidance of areas known to harbor the insects, and/or careful application of insect repellents. Furthermore, because mice pass the bacteria on to the mites, it is important to keep mice from nesting in or around residences.

The mainstay of prevention involves avoiding areas known to harbor ticks. However, because many people enjoy recreational activities in just such areas, other steps can be taken:

- Wear light colored clothing (so that attached ticks are more easily noticed).
- Wear long sleeved shirts and long pants; tuck the pants legs into socks.
- Spray clothing with appropriate tick repellents.
- Examine. Anybody who has been outside for any amount of time in an area known to have a population of ticks should examine his or her body carefully for ticks. Parents should examine their children at the end of the day.
- Remove any ticks using tweezers, so that infection doesn't occur due to handling the tick. Grasp the tick's head with the tweezers, and pull gently but firmly so that the head and body are entirely removed.
- Keep areas around homes clear of brush, which may serve to harbor ticks.

Q fever can be prevented by the appropriate handling of potentially infective substances. For example, milk should always be pasteurized, and people who work with animals giving birth should carefully dispose of the tissues and fluids associated with birth. Industries which process animal materials (meat, wool) should take care to prevent the contamination of dust within the plant. Vaccines are available for workers at risk for Q fever.

Prevention of trench fever involves good hygiene and decent living conditions. When this is impossible, insecticide dusting powders are available to apply to clothing. Avoidance of areas known to harbor ticks or the use of insect repellents is necessary to avoid the type of infection passed by ticks.

Ringworm

Ringworm is a common fungal infection of the skin also be referred to as dermatophyte infection. The name ringworm is a misnomer since the disease is not caused by a worm. More common in males than in females, ringworm is characterized by patches of rough, reddened skin. Raised eruptions usually form the circular pattern that gives the condition its name. As lesions grow, the centers start to heal; however, the inflamed borders expand and spread the infection.

Ringworm is a term that is commonly used to encompass several types of fungal infection. Sometimes, however, only body ringworm is classified as true ringworm. Body ringworm (*tinea corporis*) can affect any part of the body except the scalp, feet, and facial area where a man's beard grows. The well-defined, flaky sores can be dry and scaly or moist and crusty.

Scalp ringworm (*tinea capitis*) is most common in children. It causes scaly, swollen blisters or a rash that looks like black dots. Sometimes inflamed and filled with pus, scalp ringworm lesions can cause crusting, flaking, and round bald patches, and can cause scarring and permanent hair loss.

Ringworm of the groin (*tinea cruris* or jock itch) produces raised red sores with well-marked edges. It can spread to the buttocks, inner thighs, and external genitals.

Ringworm of the nails (*tinea unguium*) generally starts at the tip of one or more toenails, which gradually thicken and discolor. The nail may deteriorate or pull away from the nail bed. Fingernail infection is far less common.

Ringworm can be transmitted by infected people or pets; or by towels, hairbrushes, or other objects contaminated by the fungi. **Diabetes mellitus** increases susceptibility, as do dampness, humidity, and dirty, crowded living areas. Tightly braided hair and using hair gel also raise the risk. Likelihood of infection can be lessened by avoiding contact with infected people, pets, or contaminated objects; and staying away from hot, damp places.

Symptoms include inflammation, scaling, and sometimes **itching**. Diagnosis is based on microscopic examination of scrapings taken from lesions. A dermatologist may also study the scalp of a patient with suspected tinea capitis under ultraviolet light. While some infections disappear without treatment, others respond to such topical antifungal medications as naftifine (Caldesene Medicated Powder) or tinactin (Desenex) or to griseofulvin (Fulvicin), which is taken by mouth. Medications should be continued for two weeks after lesions disappear.

A person with body ringworm should wear loose clothing and check daily for raw, open sores. Wet dressings applied to moist sores two or three times a day can lessen inflammation and loosen scales, and the doctor may suggest placing special pads between folds of infected skin. Anything the patient has touched or worn should be sterilized in boiling water. Infected nails should be cut short and straight and carefully cleared of dead cells with an emery board. Patients with jock itch should:

- Wear cotton underwear and change it more than once a day
- Keep the infected area dry
- Apply antifungal ointment over a thin film of antifungal powder.

Shampoo containing selenium sulfide can help prevent spread of scalp ringworm, but prescription shampoo or oral medication is usually needed to cure the infection.

Among the **homeopathic medicine** recommended includes:

- *Sepia* for brown, scaly patches
- *Tellurium* for prominent, well-defined, reddish sores
- *Graphites* for thick scales or heavy discharge
- *Sulphur* for excessive itching.

Topical applications of antifungal herbs and essential oils also can help resolve ringworm. Tea tree oil (*Melaleuca* spp.), thuja (*Thuja occidentalis*), and lavender (*Lavandula officinalis*) are the most common. Two drops of essential oil in 1/4 ounce of carrier oil is the dose recommended for topical application. Essential oils should not be applied to the skin undiluted. Botanical medicine can be taken internally to enhance the body's immune response. A person must be susceptible to exhibit this overgrowth of fungus on the skin. Echinacea (*Echinacea* spp.) and astragalus (*Astragalus membranaceus*) are the two most common immune-enhancing herbs. A well-balanced diet, including protein, complex carbohydrates, fresh fruits and vegetables, and good quality fats, is also important in maintaining optimal **immune system** function.

Ringworm can usually be cured, but recurrence is common. Chronic (recurring) infection develops in one patient in five.

It can take 6-12 months for new hair to cover bald patches, and 3-12 months to cure infected fingernails. Toenail infections do not always respond to treatment.

Robbins, Frederick (1916-)

American microbiologist

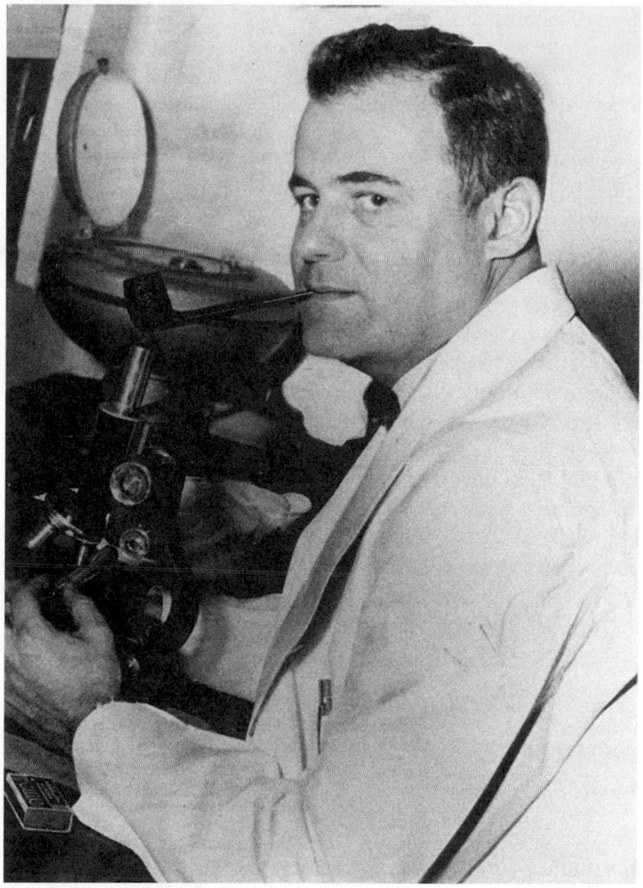

Frederick Chapman Robbins

Frederick Chapman Robbins was born in 1916, in Auburn, Alabama. He was the eldest of three boys born to Dr. William Jacob Robbins and Christine F. (Chapman) Robbins. His father was a noted plant physiologist and was director of the New York Botanical Garden. As a medical student at Harvard University, Robbins roomed with Thomas Weller and studied virology under **John F. Enders**, the men with whom he would later share the Nobel Prize. Service in World War II interrupted his residency at Children's Hospital in Boston, but it provided the opportunity to study viruses and bacterial diseases. In 1948, Robbins married Alice Havemeyer Northrop, who had been Weller's assistant in the Enders laboratory.

That year, Robbins went to work in Enders's lab. Concentrating on pediatrics, he and Weller attempted to grow poliomyelitis in embryonic and intestinal tissue. Prior to this time, polio had only been shown to grow in neural and brain tissue of men or monkeys. Vaccinations from this type of growth were potentially deadly because of something present in this tissue which could not be refined out, so there was no vaccine for polio. Growth of viruses in tissue culture, or in vitro, had historically been difficult because of the threat of bacterial invasion into the cell cultures. By the 1950s, however, antibiotics had been developed and introduced into the laboratory, such as **penicillin** and streptomycin, which enabled scientists to begin to grow tissue cultures of viruses without the threat of a bacterial invasion.

Robbins and Weller, in their polio experiments, were taking advantage of the new **antibiotics**. The human intestine cultures grew, which proved for the first time that polio could grow outside neural tissue. This made the feasibility of a polio vaccine far greater, both because it provided a non-deadly vaccine source and because the supply could be grown more cheaply in vitro than in a live animal. This work was a major breakthrough for scientific research and led to the awarding of the Nobel Prize to Enders, Weller, and Robbins in 1954. Their development provided the technology needed to produce a vaccination for polio, which was done in 1953 by virologist **Jonas Salk**.

Robbins's career then took a turn from laboratory work to the health policy arena. He served as president of the Society for Pediatric Research in 1961 and 1962 and in 1965 became dean of the school of medicine at Case Western Reserve. Robbins also began an intense involvement in national committees on a wide range of topics including human experimentation, Third World health policies, and public food and safety policy. His contribution to science in terms of laboratory research has been memorialized by the receipt of the Nobel Prize. For all his research work, however, it is possible his greater legacy will be in the area of health policy.

ROBERTS, RICHARD J. (1943-)

English biochemist

Richard John Roberts was born in 1943, in Derby, England. His father, John Roberts, was a motor mechanic, while his mother, Edna (Allsop) Roberts, took care of the family and served as Richard's first tutor. After graduating with honors in 1965, Roberts remained at Sheffield University to study for his doctoral degree under David Ollis, his undergraduate professor of organic chemistry. After becoming interested in molecular biology, he moved to Harvard University in 1969, where he spent the next four years deciphering the sequence of nucleotides in a form of ribonucleic acid known as tRNA. Using a new method devised by English biochemist Frederick Sanger at Cambridge, he was able to sequence the RNA molecule, while teaching other scientists Sanger's technique. His creative work with tRNA led an invitation by genetic pioneer and Nobel laureate, **James Watson**, to join his laboratory in Cold Spring Harbor, Long Island, New York.

In 1972, Roberts moved to Long Island to research ways to sequence DNA. American microbiologists Daniel Nathans and Hamilton Smith had shown that a restriction enzyme, Endonuclease R, could split DNA into specific segments. Roberts thought that such small segments could be used for DNA sequencing and began looking for other new restriction enzymes to expand the repertoire. (Enzymes are complex proteins that catalyze specific biochemical reactions.) In 1977, he developed a series of biological experiments to ''map'' the location of various genes in adenovirus and found that one end of a messenger ribonucleic acid (mRNA) did not react as expected. With the use of an electron microscope, Roberts and his colleagues observed that genes could be present in several, well-separated DNA segments.

In 1986, Roberts married his second wife, Jean. He moved back to Massachusetts in 1992 to join New England Biolabs, a small, private company involved in making research reagents, particularly restriction enzymes. In 1993, Roberts was awarded the Nobel Prize for his discovery of ''split genes.'' The Nobel Committee stated that, ''The discovery of split genes has been of fundamental importance for today's basic research in biology, as well as for more medically oriented research concerning the development of **cancer** and other diseases.''

ROCK, JOHN (1890-1984)

American gynecologist and obstetrician

John Rock was a gynecologist, obstetrician, and medical researcher who played a significant role in developing and promoting the use of oral contraceptives. As a leading authority on the reproductive system and embryology, he contributed to the understanding of infertility and reproductive problems and founded the Rock Reproductive Clinic in Brookline, Massachusetts. A devout Roman Catholic, he also challenged his church's opposition to the use of the birth control pill.

Rock, one of five children, was born March 24, 1890 in Marlborough, Massachusetts, to Frank Sylvester Rock and Ann Jane (Murphy) Rock. His father was an enterprising businessman who owned a liquor store, dealt in real estate, and promoted the local baseball team. The younger Rock graduated from Boston High School of Commerce and worked for a year and a half as an accountant for a fruit company in Guatemala and then with a construction firm in Rhode Island. Rock was fired from both jobs and decided to follow his father's advice to attend college.

Graduating with a baccalaureate degree from Harvard in 1915, he received the M.D. degree from Harvard Medical School in 1918. Rock interned at Massachusetts General Hospital, doing his residency in urology there and also at Boston Lying-in Hospital. After one year as a surgeon at Brookline Free Hospital for Women, he set up his own practice. His long professional relations with Harvard Medical School began in 1922 when he was appointed assistant professor of obstetrics.

Rock opened one of the first fertility and endocrine clinics at the Free Hospital for Women in the mid–1920s. At that time his main concern was solving reproductive problems rather than birth control. In 1944, along with Harvard scientist Miriam F. Menkin, Rock fertilized the first human egg in a test tube. He is also credited with the first recorded recovery of human embryos 2 to 17 days after fertilization as well as establishing the fact that ovulation occurs 14 days before menstruation.

In the early 1950s Rock began experimenting with progesterone, the female hormone that suppresses ovulation. Progesterone is secreted by the body during pregnancy so that no eggs are discharged—nature's way of preventing overlapping pregnancies. He surmised that giving the reproductive system a ''rest'' by injecting childless women with progesterone might increase fertility when the injections were stopped.

Though he was aware of the contraceptive possibilities of the hormone, he ignored those aspects for fear of the state's anti-birth control laws. At that time in Massachusetts, each instance of birth control advice would result in a fine of $1000 and a possible five-year prison sentence.

Rock corresponded with scientists Gregory Pincus, the world's foremost authority on the mammalian egg, and M. C. Chang, a specialist in the biology of sperm, about the possibility of developing a useful progestin, or synthetic progesterone, that could be given orally. With Pincus and Chang intent on investigating the hormones contraceptive properties, Rock's focus began to shift in that direction as well. Many pharmaceutical companies had developed progestins but none had been tried on humans. Chang and Pincus had methodically tested hundreds of variations of progestin and found two that could be safely tested on women. While Rock began the first tests for treatment of sterility on 50 females in 1954, simultaneous investigations into the effectiveness of progestin as a contraceptive were also undertaken. The researchers were amazed to discover that although 15 percent of the women on natural progesterone ovulated, none of those using the oral progestins did.

At this point Rock left the clinic at the Free Hospital for Women, having reached the mandatory retirement age of 65, and opened the Rock Reproductive Clinic. Realizing the need for more extensive tests, but aware of the legal and social complications involved, he chose to do field trials in Puerto Rico, Haiti, and Mexico, with a progestin manufactured by G. D. Searle Company. Of the women who followed directions, none became pregnant. The studies were now ready to present in the United States.

In 1959 Searle applied to license the ''Pill''—as the oral progestin became known—as a contraceptive, choosing Rock to present the findings of the experiences of 897 women before the Food and Drug Administration (FDA). The requirement at the time was that a drug must be proven safe and not necessarily effective. However, the young reviewer, who was aware of the implications of the Pill, was thorough in his examination, requiring further lab tests before approval. On May 11, 1960 the FDA approved Searle's Enovid, the first drug approved in order to prevent a medical happening. By 1964 some four million women were on the pill.

Rock was a devout member of the Roman Catholic church, whose traditional position was that no unnatural form of birth control be used. Believing in the right of choice, Rock became an outspoken activist for the use of contraceptives to control population explosion, in direct opposition to the teachings of the church. In 1931 he worked for the repeal of a Massachusetts law against the sale of birth control devices, and in 1945 he began teaching students at Harvard Medical School how to prescribe them. Rock took on the hierarchy of the Catholic church, arguing that the pill was a variant of the rhythm method. Using a strategy of logic, he showed that the pill of natural hormones extended the time when a woman was naturally sterile, hence increasing the rhythm method.

In 1963 he took his case through the mass media in a book, *The Time Has Come: A Catholic Doctor's Proposal to End the Battle Over Birth Control.* The book defended the morality of the pill and urged science and religion to unite on a system of population control. He was strongly criticized by conservative Catholic theologians but was described in the press as David taking on Goliath. As a result Pope Paul IV appointed a papal commission to study the issue. Although the commission recommended the pill, the hierarchy said no. With a clear conscience that he was right and the church leaders had made a mistake, Rock remained a devout Catholic, attending mass daily until his death on December 4, 1984.

Rock was a member of many societies, including Planned Parenthood, and was a founding fellow of the American College of Obstetricians and Gynecologists. Among the awards he received were the Lasker award from Planned Parenthood in 1940 and the Ortho award from the American Gynecological Society in 1949. He is credited not only with being the ''father'' of the first birth control pill but also popularizing and selling it to a skeptical world.

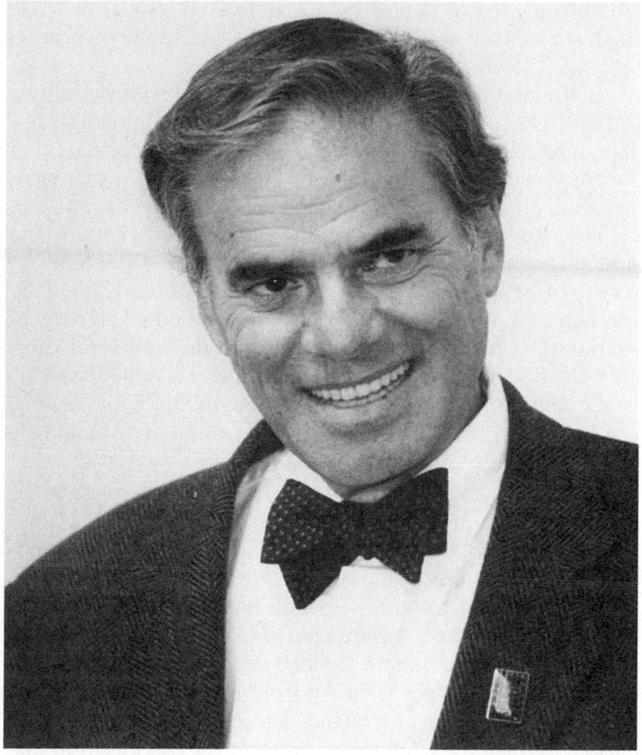

Martin Rodbell

RODBELL, MARTIN (1925-)

American biochemist

Rodbell was born on December 1, 1925 in Baltimore, Maryland. He attended a special Baltimore high school that accepted boys from all over the city and prepared them to enter college as sophomores. He entered Johns Hopkins University in 1943, pursuing his interest in chemistry. Not long after entering the university, Rodbell became bored with classes and felt (being Jewish) compelled to combat Hitler's armies. He spent the balance of World War II serving in the Navy, primarily in the South Pacific.

Rodbell returned to Johns Hopkins and received a B.A. in 1949. That same year he met his future wife, Barbara Lederman, a ballet dancer from Holland who had lost her family in the Auschwitz concentration camp. They married a year later, and Rodbell credits his wife for immersing him the world of the arts. Rodbell and his new wife traveled to Seattle, where Rodbell began his graduate studies in biochemistry at the University of Seattle. He studied the chemistry of lipids (the fatty substances in cells), and his thesis was on the biosynthesis of lecithin (fats found in cell membranes) in the rat liver. Unfortunately, his thesis was disproved by another scientist working on the same subject. This experience taught him not to assume that biological chemicials are pure, something that would help him later in his Nobel Prize-winning work.

Rodbell finished his Ph.D. in 1954 and then went to the University of Illinois for his post-doctoral fellowship. His research involved the biosynthesis of chloramphenicol, an antibiotic. When his fellowship advisor, Herbert Carter, asked him where he wanted to teach, Rodbell had to answer nowhere. After having taught a lecture course to freshman, only a few of whom passed his exams, Rodbell decided that teaching was not his calling. He accepted a position at the National Heart Institute in Bethesda, Maryland, and continued his research into fats, identifying important proteins that pertained to diseases concerning lipoproteins.

In the 1960s he returned to his original interest in cell biology and was awarded a fellowship to work at the University of Brussels, where he learned new lab techniques. He returned to the United States and accepted a postion at the NIH Institute of Arthritis and Metabolic Diseases in the Nutrition and Endocrinology lab. There he developed a simple procedure that would separate and purify fat cells. He was also able to remove the fat from a cell, conserving most of the structure of the cell. He named these cells ''ghosts.''

In several groundbreaking experiments, Rodbell and his colleagues at the NIH showed that cell communication involves three different working devices: (1) a chemical signal; (2) a ''second messenger'' like a hormone; and (3) a transducer, something that converts energy from one form to another. Rodbell's major contribution was in discovering that there was a transducer function. He and his colleagues also speculated that guanine nucleotides, components of deoxyribonucleic acid (DNA) and ribonucleic acid (RNA), were somehow involved in cell communication, something that would later be confirmed by Alfred Goodman, the biochemist with whom he would share the Nobel Prize. Gilman searched for the chemicals involved with guanine nucleotides and discovered the G-proteins.

G-proteins are instrumental in the fundamental workings of a cell. They allow us to see and smell by changing light and odors to chemical messages that travel to the brain. Understanding how G-proteins malfunction could lead to a better understanding of serious diseases like cholera or cancer. Scientists have already linked improperly working G-proteins to diseases like alcoholism and diabetes. Pharmaceutical companies are developing drugs that would focus on G-proteins.

Rodbell served as director of the National Institute of Environmental Health Sciences in Chapel Hill, North Carolina, from 1985 until his retirement in 1994. Ironically, only a few months before receiving the Nobel Award, Rodbell opted for early retirement, because there were no funds to support the research he wanted to do. Upon receiving the Nobel Prize, Rodbell was vocal in his criticism of the government because of its unwillingness to provide adequate support for fundamental research. He criticized them for favoring projects that yield obviously tangible and potentially profitable results, like drug treatments. Rodbell's other awards include the NIH Distinguished Service Award in 1973 and the Gairdner Award in 1984.

Röntgen, Wilhelm Konrad (1845-1923)

German physicist

Although Wilhelm Röntgen is credited with the discovery of x rays, he was almost certainly not the first to observe them, since they were readily produced using cathode ray devices. Many earlier scientists may have noticed but ignored such strange effects around their laboratories as glowing lights and foggy or overdeveloped photographic plates while experimenting with cathode rays, but probably dismissed or ignored them. It was Röntgen who recognized x rays as a new type of radiation.

Born in a small German village, Röntgen decided at an early age to study science, rather than follow his father as a cloth merchant. As a student, however, he preferred the outdoors to a classroom, and he was expelled from high school for assisting in a prank which had offended one of the instructors. Reputed to be insubordinate, Röntgen found the doors to the universities all but closed to him, and he was forced to apply to a local Technical School. Still, he completed his undergraduate studies in 1868, and in 1869 received his Ph.D. in philosophy. Röntgen then moved to Zurich, Switzerland, and became an assistant to German physicist August Kundt (1839-1894), who introduced him to the world of physics.

It was not until he was fifty years old that Röntgen began the work that made him internationally famous. While studying the effects of cathode rays emitted by luminescent chemicals, Röntgen noticed something very strange: when he turned on the power in his cathode ray tube, a sample of barium platinocyanide across the room glowed even though the tube was enclosed in black cardboard thick enough to prevent cathode rays from escaping. He deduced that the rays crossing the room must be of a completely new variety and many times more penetrating than cathode rays. He moved the barium platinocyanide sample away from the tube, finding that it glowed even when placed in the next room.

Röntgen, having discovered what was at that time the most powerful radiation known to science, was understandably excited. He knew that, in order to gain recognition, he must publish his findings before someone else discovered these rays. He spent the next seven weeks exhaustively researching and observing his new rays, which he named x rays, since ''x'' is the mathematical symbol for an unknown. During this period he found that x rays were completely invisible, traveled in a straight line, could be neither reflected nor refracted, and were unaffected by magnetic fields. Never before or since has there been a more dramatic reaction among the scientific community as well as the general populace as that which followed the publication of Röntgen's x-ray research in December, 1895. He delivered his first public lecture on x rays in January, 1896 and demonstrated therein the rays' ability to photograph the bones within living flesh. Less than twenty days later, an x-ray machine was used in the United States to locate a bullet within a patient's leg. Newspapers worldwide printed astounding photos of ''living skeletons.'' Physicians proclaimed it a modern miracle, while doomsayers predicted an end to privacy, envisioning devices that could peer through walls, doors, and clothing.

The repercussions of Röntgen's discovery spread exponentially. **Henri Becquerel** used x rays as the springboard for his own discovery of radioactivity, a discovery that ultimately led to a greater understanding of the atom and that opened the door to the nuclear age. Scientists today consider the discovery of x rays to be the beginning of the Second Scientific Revolution (just as Galileo's discoveries sparked the first).

Röntgen received numerous accolades for his discovery, including the very first Nobel Prize for physics, but he invariably declined or donated any monetary prizes that would accompany his awards. He strongly believed that science belonged to everyone, and that all nations should benefit from its advances; he also refused to patent any facet of x rays or their production. Thus, he was without substantial savings when the years following World War I brought hyperinflation to the German economy. He died in poverty in 1923 from intestinal **cancer**, probably caused by prolonged exposure to x rays.

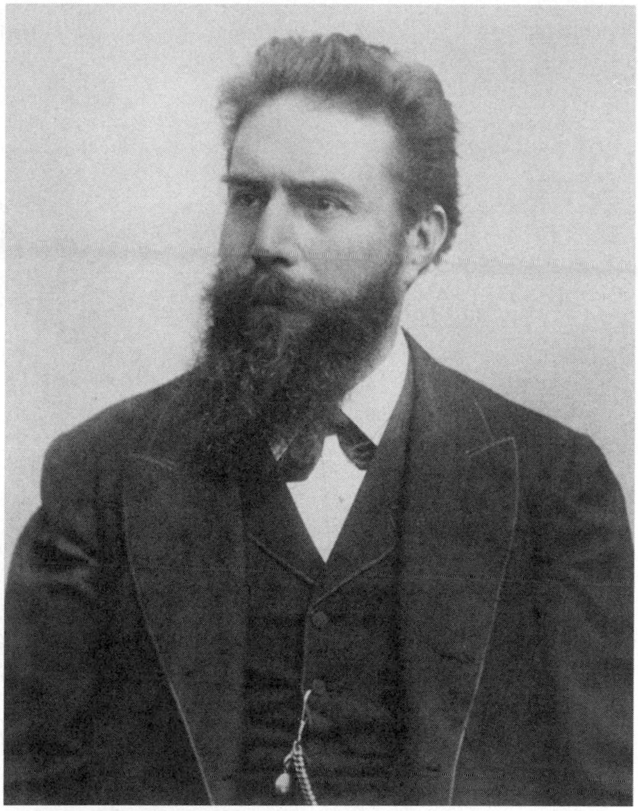

Wilhelm Konrad Röntgen

ROOT CANAL TREATMENT

Root canal treatment, also known as endodontic treatment, is a dental procedure in which the diseased or damaged pulp (core) of a tooth is removed and the inside areas (the pulp chamber and root canals) are filled and sealed.

Inflamed or infected pulp (pulpitis) most often causes a toothache. To relieve the **pain** and prevent further complications, the tooth may be extracted (surgically removed) or saved by root canal treatment. Root canal treatment has become a common dental procedure; more than 14 million are performed every year with a 95% success rate, according to the American Association of Endodontists.

Once root canal treatment is performed, the patient must have a crown placed over the tooth to protect it. The cost of the treatment and the crown may be expensive. However, replacing an extracted tooth with a fixed bridge, a removable partial denture, or an implant to maintain the space and restore the chewing function, is typically even more expensive.

Root canal treatment may be performed by a general dentist or by an endodontist, a dentist who specializes in endodontic (literally ''inside of the tooth'') procedures. Inside the tooth, the pulp's soft tissue contains the blood supply, by which the tooth gets its nutrients; and the nerve, by which the tooth senses hot and cold. This tissue is vulnerable to damage from deep dental decay, accidental injury, tooth fracture, or trauma from repeated dental procedures (such as multiple fillings over time). If a tooth becomes diseased or injured, bacteria build up inside the pulp, spreading infection from the natural crown of the tooth to the root tips in the jawbone. Pus accumulates at the ends of the roots, forming a painful **abscess** which can damage the bone supporting the teeth. Such an infection may produce pain that is severe, constant, or throbbing, as well as prolonged sensitivity to heat or cold, swelling and tenderness in the surrounding gums, facial swelling, and discoloration of the tooth. However, in some cases, the pulp may die so gradually that there is little noticeable pain.

Root canal treatment is performed under local **anesthesia**. A thin sheet of rubber, called a rubber dam, is placed in the mouth to isolate the tooth. The dentist removes any **tooth decay** and makes an opening through the natural crown of the tooth into the pulp chamber. Creating this access also relieves the pressure inside the tooth and can dramatically ease pain.

The dentist determines the length of the root canals, usually with a series of x rays. Small wire-like files are then used to clean the entire canal space of diseased pulp tissue and bacteria. The debris is flushed out with large amounts of water (irrigation). The canals are also slightly enlarged and shaped to

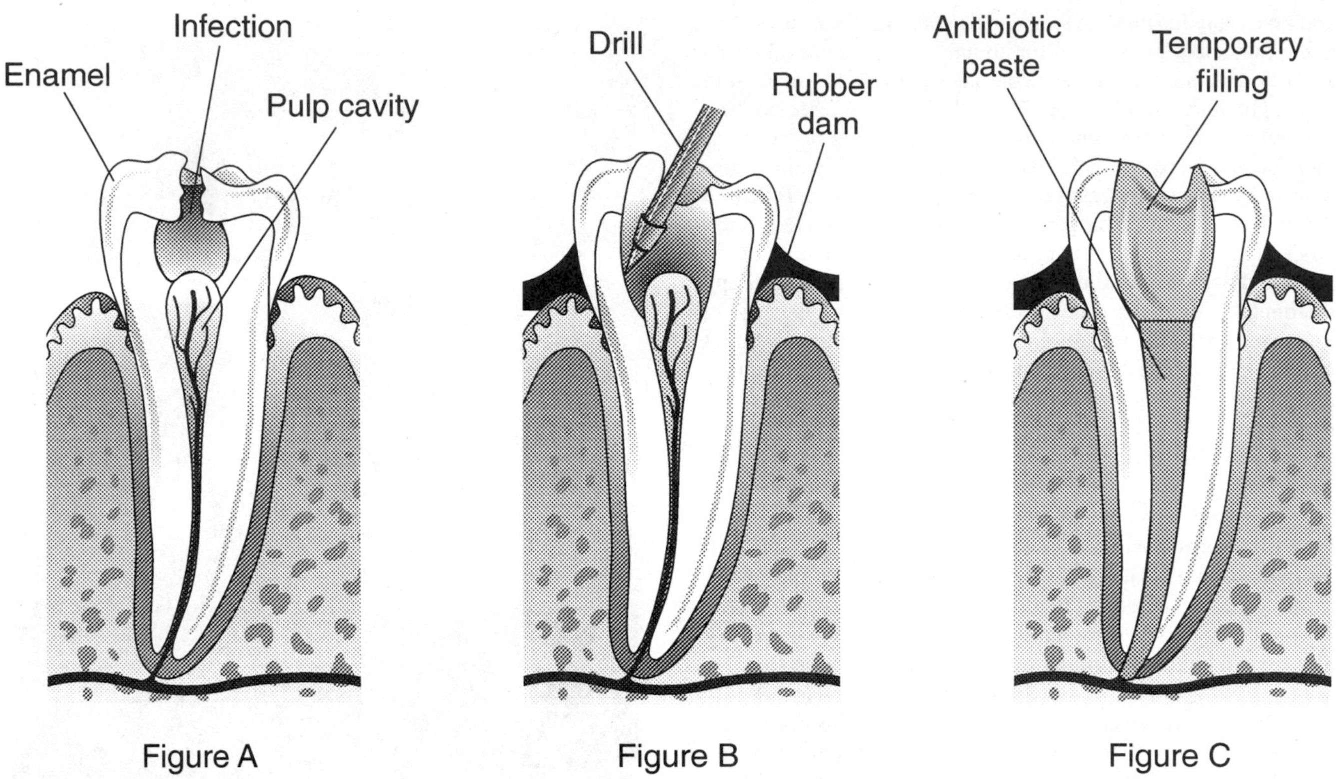

Root canal treatment is a dental procedure in which the diseased pulp of a tooth is removed and the inside areas are filled and sealed. In figure A, the infection can be seen above the pulp cavity. The dentist drills into the enamel and the pulp cavity is extracted (figure B). Finally, the dentist fills the pulp cavity with antibiotic paste and a temporary filling (figure C). ***(Illustration by Electronic Illustrators Group.)***

receive an inert (non-reactive) filling material called gutta percha. However, the tooth is not filled and permanently sealed until it is completely free of active infection. The dentist may place a temporary seal, or leave the tooth open to drain, and prescribe an **antibiotic** to counter any spread of infection from the tooth. This is why root canal treatment may require several visits to the dentist.

Once the canals are completely clean, they are filled with gutta percha and a sealer cement to prevent bacteria from entering the tooth in the future. A metal post may be placed in the pulp chamber for added structural support and better retention of the crown restoration. The tooth is protected by a temporary filling or crown until a permanent restoration may be made. This restoration is usually a gold or porcelain crown, although it may be a gold inlay, or an amalgam or composite filling (paste fillings that harden).

There is no typical preparation for root canal treatment. Once the tooth is opened to drain, the dentist may prescribe an antibiotic, then the patient should take the full prescribed course. With the infection under control, local anesthetic is more effective, so that the root canal procedure may be performed without discomfort.

The tooth may be sore for several days after filling. **Nonsteroidal anti-inflammatory drugs (NSAIDs)** to relieve pain—such as ibuprofen (Advil, Motrin)—may be taken to ease the soreness. The tissues around the tooth may also be irritated. Rinsing the mouth with hot salt water several times a day will help. Chewing on that side of the mouth should be avoided for the first few days following treatment. A follow-up appointment should be scheduled with the dentist for six months after treatment to make sure the tooth and surrounding structures are healthy.

There is a possibility that the root canal treatment will not be successful the first time. If infection and inflammation recur and an x ray indicates retreatment is feasible, the old filling material is removed and the canals are thoroughly cleaned out. The dentist will try to identify and correct problems with the first root canal treatment before filling and sealing the tooth a second time.

In cases where an x ray indicates that retreatment cannot correct the problem, endodontic (Surgery) surgery may be performed. In a procedure called an apicoectomy, or root resectioning, the root end of the tooth is accessed in the bone, and a small amount is shaved away. The area is cleaned of diseased tissue and a filling is placed to reseal the canal.

In some cases, despite root canal treatment and endodontic surgery, the tooth dies anyway and a **tooth extraction** must be performed.

With successful root canal treatment, the tooth will no longer cause pain. However, because it does not contain an internal nerve, it no longer has sensitivity to hot, cold, or sweets. These are signs of dental decay, so the patient must receive regular dental check-ups with periodic x rays to avoid further disease in the tooth. The restored tooth could last a lifetime;

however, with routine wear, the filling or crown may eventually need to be replaced.

See also Tooth decay; Tooth extraction

Roseola

Roseola is a common disease of babies or young children, in which several days of very high **fever** are followed by a **rash**. It is an extraordinarily common infection caused by a virus. About 90% of all children have been exposed to the virus, with about 33% actually demonstrating the syndrome of fever followed by rash. The most common age for a child to contract roseola is between six and twelve months. Roseola infection strikes boys and girls equally. The infection may occur at any time of year, although late spring and early summer seem to be peak times for it.

About 85% of the time, roseola is caused by a virus called Human Herpesvirus 6, or HHV-6. Although the virus is related to those herpesviruses known to cause sores on the lips or genitalia, HHV-6 causes a very different type of infection. HHV-6 is believed to be passed between people via infected saliva. A few other viruses (called **enteroviruses**) can produce a similar fever-then-rash illness, which is usually also called roseola.

Researchers believe that it takes about 5-15 days to develop illness after having been infected by HHV-6. Roseola strikes suddenly, when a previously-well child spikes an impressively high fever. The temperature may reach 106°F. As is always the case with sudden fever spikes, the extreme change in temperature may cause certain children to have **seizures**. About 5-35% of all children with roseola will have these "febrile seizures."

The most notable thing about this early phase of roseola is the absence of symptoms, other than the high fever. Although some children have a slightly reddened throat, or a slightly runny nose, most children have no symptoms whatsoever, other than the sudden development of high fever. This fever lasts for between three and five days.

Somewhere around the fifth day, a rash begins on the body. The rash is usually composed of flat pink patches or spots, although there may be some raised patches as well. The rash usually starts on the chest, back, and abdomen, and then spreads out to the arms and neck. It may or may not reach the legs and face. The rash lasts for about three days, then fades.

Very rarely, roseola will cause more serious disease. Patients so afflicted will experience significant swelling of the lymph nodes, the liver, and the spleen. The liver may become sufficiently inflamed to interfere with its functioning, resulting in a yellowish color to the whites of the eyes and the skin (**jaundice**). This syndrome (called a mononucleosis-like syndrome, after the disease called **infectious mononucleosis** that causes many of the same symptoms) has occurred in both infants and adults.

The diagnosis of roseola is often made by carefully examining the feverish child to make sure that other illnesses are not causing the temperature spike. Once it is clear that no

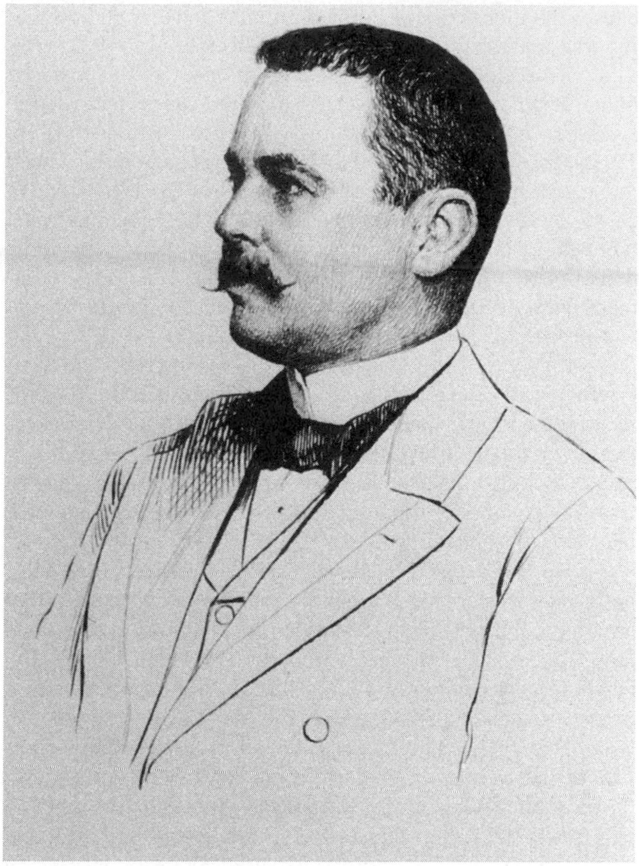

Ronald Ross

pneumonia, ear infection, **strep throat**, or other common childhood illness is present, the practitioner usually feels comfortable waiting to see if the characteristic rash of roseola begins.

There are no treatments available to stop the course of roseola. **Acetaminophen** or ibuprofen is usually given to try to lower the fever. Children who are susceptible to seizures may be given a sedative medication when the fever first spikes, in an attempt to prevent such a seizure. Children recover quickly and completely from roseola. The only complications are those associated with seizures, or the rare mononucleosis-like syndrome.

Other than the usual good hygiene practices always recommended to decrease the spread of viral illness, no methods are available to specifically prevent roseola.

See also Fever; Rash

Ross, Ronald (1857-1932)

English physician

Born in Almora, India, Ronald Ross spent much of his career in the Indian Medical Service. Because **malaria** was a devastating health problem in India, he began to study its cause in 1890. His research on the life-cycle of the parasite which causes the illness was instrumental in the modern understanding that malaria is a mosquito-borne disease.

It had long been thought that diseases were spread by odors, and that malaria was caused by the vapors produced in swamps. In 1880, Charles Louis Alphonse Laveran's (1845-1922) observations that the blood of malaria patients contained the pigmented bodies of parasites suggested an alternative cause. In 1894, Sir Patrick Manson (1844-1922) demonstrated the truth of this observation to Ross and suggested that mosquitos were responsible for transmitting these parasites to humans. Ross set out to investigate the life-history of the parasite and to test Manson's theory.

Progress was slow, but on August 16, 1897, Ross allowed ten *Anopheles* mosquitos—a species new to him—to feed on a malaria patient who had agreed to serve as a volunteer. Over the next few days, Ross dissected the mosquitos as usual, looking for some sign of malarial parasites acquired from the patient. He found nothing unusual, and by August 20 only two mosquitos were left.

He had decided to dissect one of these last *Anopheles*, but grew so discouraged when he found nothing unusual that he almost did not finish. But when he began to examine the mosquito's stomach tissue, he found several cells too small to be ordinary mosquito stomach cells. Inside each cell was a cluster of black granules just like those of Laveran's parasites.

Ross realized that if these were in fact the malarial parasites he had been seeking, they should continue to grow within the mosquito. When he dissected his last mosquito the next day and found still larger parasites in its stomach tissue, he knew he had discovered the parasite's stage of development which was the link between humans and mosquitos, and he named August 20 ''Mosquito Day.''

A published novelist, poet and playwright, he added a set of verses inspired by his discovery to his poem ''Exile'':

This day relenting God Hath placed within my hand A wondrous thing; and God Be praised. At his command, Seeking His secret deeds With tears and toiling breath, I find thy cunning seeds, O million-murdering Death. I know this little thing A myriad men will save. O Death, where is thy sting? Thy victory, O Grave?

The next step in his research was to demonstrate the mode of transmission of the parasite from mosquito to human. A transfer within the Service prevented further work with humans, but Ross was able to study avian malaria in caged birds. He followed the parasites from an infected bird into the stomach of a *Culex* (Aëdes) mosquito which had fed on the bird, and from there to the mosquito's salivary glands. The bite of this mosquito then transmitted the malarial parasite to another bird. The Italian scientist, Giovanni Grassi (1854-1925), demonstrated the same process between *Anopheles* and humans in 1898.

Devoting himself to the promotion of research into malaria and the stimulation of measures to control it, Ross published many reports based on the principle that, to eradicate malaria, mosquitos must be isolated from infected humans. He received the Nobel Prize in physiology or medicine in 1902, was knighted in 1911, served as a consultant in malaria to the War Office during World War I, and founded the Ross Institute of Tropical Hygiene in 1926.

ROUNDWORM INFECTIONS

Roundworm infections are diseases of the digestive tract and other organ systems caused by nematodes—parasitic worms with long, cylindrical bodies. Roundworm infections are widespread throughout the world, and humans acquire most types of roundworm infection from contaminated food or by touching the mouth with unwashed hands which have come into contact with the parasite larva. The severity of infection varies considerably from person to person. Children are more likely to have heavy infestations and are also more likely to suffer from **malabsorption** and **malnutrition** than adults.

The type and symptoms of roundworm infections vary according to the species of nematode which causes them. Anisakiasis infection is caused by anisakid roundworms. Humans are not the primary host for these parasites which infest whales, seals, and dolphins. However, crabs ingest roundworm eggs from the feces of these animals. In the crabs, the eggs hatch into larvae that can infect fish. The larvae enter the muscles of marine animals further up the food chain, including squid, mackerel, herring, cod, salmon, tuna, and halibut. Humans become accidental hosts when they eat raw or undercooked fish containing anisakid larvae. The larvae attach themselves to the tissues lining the stomach and intestines, and eventually die inside the inflamed tissue.

In humans, anisakiasis can produce either a severe syndrome that affects the stomach and intestines, or a mild chronic disease that may last for weeks or years. In acute anisakiasis, symptoms begin within one to seven hours after the individual eats infected seafood. Patients are often violently sick, with nausea, vomiting, **diarrhea**, and severe abdominal **pain** that may resemble **appendicitis**. In chronic anisakiasis, the patient has milder forms of stomach or intestinal irritation that resemble stomach **ulcers** or **irritable bowel syndrome**. In some cases, the acute form of the disease is followed by chronic infestation.

Ascariasis, which is caused by *Ascaris lumbricoides*, is one of the most widespread parasitic infections in humans, affecting over 1.3 billion people worldwide. Ascarid roundworms cause a larger burden on the human host than any other parasite; adult worms can grow as long as 12 or 14 inches, and release 200,000 eggs per day. The eggs infect people who eat unwashed vegetables from contaminated soil or touch their mouths with unwashed hands which have become contaminated. Once inside the digestive tract, the eggs release larvae that penetrate the intestinal wall and migrate (travel) to the lungs through the liver and the bloodstream. After about 10 days in the lungs, the larvae migrate further into the patient's upper lung passages and airway, where they are swallowed. When they return to the intestine, they mature into adults and reproduce. The time period from the beginning of the infection to egg production is 60-75 days.

The first symptoms of infection may occur when the larvae reach the lungs. The patient may develop chest **pain**, **cough**ing, difficulty breathing, and inflammation of the lungs. In some cases, the patient's sputum (phlegm) is streaked with blood. This phase of the disease is sometimes called Loeffler's syndrome. It is marked by an accumulation of parasites in the lung tissue and by eosinophilia (an abnormal increase in the number of a specific type of white blood cell). The intestinal phase of ascariasis is marked by stomach pain, cramping, nausea, and intestinal blockage in severe cases.

Toxocariasis is sometimes called visceral larva migrans (VLM) because the larval form of the organism hatches inside the intestines and migrates throughout the body to other organs (viscera). The disease is caused by *Toxocara canis* and *T. cati*, which live within the intestines of dogs and cats. Most human patients are children between the ages of two and four years, who become infected after playing in sandboxes or soil contaminated by pet feces, although adults are also susceptible. The eggs can survive in soil for as long as seven years.

The organism's eggs hatch inside the human intestine and release larvae that are carried in the bloodstream to all parts of the body, including the eyes, liver, lungs, heart, and brain. The patient usually has a **fever**, with coughing or **wheezing** and a swollen liver. Some patients develop skin **rashes** and inflammation of the lungs. The larvae may survive inside the body for months, producing allergic reactions and small granulomas (tissue swellings or growths produced in response to inflammation). Infection of the eye can produce ocular larva migrans (OLM), which is the first symptom of toxocariasis in some patients.

Trichuriasis, caused by *Trichuris trichiura*, is sometimes called whipworm because the organism has a long, slender, whiplike front end. The adult worm is slightly less than an inch long. Trichuriasis is most common in warm, humid climates, including the southeastern United States. The number of people with trichuriasis may be as high as 800 million worldwide.

Whipworm larvae hatch in the small intestine from swallowed eggs and move on to the upper part of the large intestine where they attach themselves to the lining. The adult worms produce eggs that are passed in the feces and mature in the soil. Patients with mild infections may have few or no symptoms. In cases of heavy infestation, the patient may have abdominal cramps and other symptoms resembling amebic dysentery. In children, severe trichuriasis may cause **anemia** and developmental retardation.

Roundworm infections are diagnosed by several different methods. Since the first symptoms of roundworm infection are common to a number of illnesses, a doctor is most likely to consider the possibility of a parasitic disease on the basis of the patient's history—especially in children. The definite diagnosis is based on the results of stool (feces) or tissue tests. In trichuriasis, adult worms may also be visible in the lining of the patient's rectum. In ascariasis, adult worms may appear in the patient's feces or vomit and can also be detected by x ray and **ultrasound tests**. In toxocariasis, larvae are sometimes found in tissue samples taken from a granuloma. If a patient with toxocariasis develops OLM, it is important to obtain a granuloma sample in order to distinguish between OLM and **retinoblastoma** (a type of cancerous eye tumor).

Anisakiasis is one of two roundworm infections that cannot be diagnosed from stool specimens. Instead, the diagnosis is made by x rays of the patient's stomach and small intestine. The larvae may appear as small threads when double contrast x rays are used. In acute cases, the doctor may use an endoscope (an instrument for examining the interior of a body cavity) to look for or remove larvae.

Blood tests cannot be used to differentiate among different types of roundworm infections, but the presence of eosinophilia can help to confirm the diagnosis.

Patients with trichuriasis or ascariasis should be examined for signs of infection by other roundworm species, as well, as many patients are infected by several parasites at the same time.

Treatment also depends upon the type being treated. Trichuriasis, ascariasis, and toxocariasis are treated with anthelminthic medications—drugs that destroy roundworms either by paralyzing them or by blocking them from feeding. Anthelminthic drugs include pyrantel pamoate, piperazine, albendazole, and mebendazole. Mebendazole cannot be given to pregnant women because it may harm the fetus. Treatment with anthelminthic drugs does not prevent reinfection. Patients with an intestinal obstruction caused by ascariasis may be given **nasogastric suction**, followed by anthelminthic drugs, in order to avoid surgery. If suction fails, the worms must be removed surgically to prevent intestinal rupture or blockage. There is no drug treatment for anisakiasis; however, symptoms usually resolve in one to two weeks when the larvae die. In some cases, the larvae are removed with an endoscope or by surgery.

The prognosis (expected outcome) for recovery from roundworm infections is good for most patients. Ascariasis is the only roundworm infection with a significant mortality rate. *A. lumbricoides* grows large enough to perforate the bile or pancreatic ducts; in addition, a mass of worms in the digestive tract can cause rupture or blockage of the intestines. It is estimated that 20,000 children die every year from intestinal ascariasis.

There are no effective **vaccines** against any of the soil-transmitted roundworms, nor does infection bring about immunity from reinfection. Prevention of infection or reinfection requires adequate hygiene and **sanitation** measures, including regular and careful handwashing before eating or touching the mouth with the hands.

With respect to specific infections, anisakiasis can be prevented by avoiding raw or improperly prepared fish or squid. Trichuriasis, ascariasis, and toxocariasis can be prevented by keeping children from playing in soil contaminated by human or animal feces, by teaching children to wash their hands before eating, and by having pets dewormed regularly by a veterinarian.

See also Malabsorption; Malnutrition

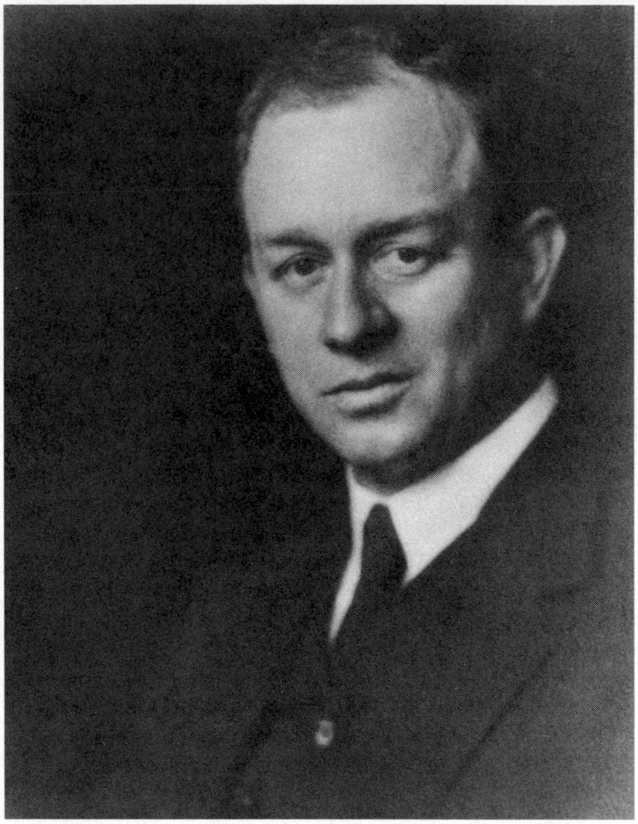

Peyton Rous

Rous, Peyton (1879-1970)

American physician and pathologist

Francis Peyton Rous was born in 1879, in Baltimore, Maryland, to Charles Rous, a grain exporter, and Frances Wood, the daughter of a Texas judge. He pursued his biological interests at Johns Hopkins University, receiving a B.A. in 1900 and an M.D. in 1905. After a medical internship at Johns Hopkins, however, he decided to concentrate on research and the natural history of disease. In 1909, Simon Flexner, director of the newly-founded Rockefeller Institute in New York City, asked Rous to take over **cancer** research in his laboratory.

A few months later, a poultry breeder brought a Plymouth Rock chicken with a large breast tumor to the Institute and Rous, after conducting numerous experiments, determined that the tumor was a spindle-cell sarcoma. When he transferred a cell-free filtrate from the tumor into healthy chickens of the same flock, they developed identical tumors. Moreover, after injecting a filtrate from the new tumors into other chickens, a malignancy exactly like the original formed. Further studies revealed that this filterable agent was a virus, although Rous carefully avoided this word. Now called the Rous sarcoma virus (RSV) and classed as an RNA retrovirus, it remains a prototype of animal tumor viruses and a favorite laboratory model for studying the role of genes in cancer.

Rous's discovery was received with considerable disbelief, both in the United States and in the rest of the world. His viral theory of cancer challenged all assumptions, going back to Hippocrates, that cancer was not infectious but rather a spontaneous, uncontrolled growth of cells and many scientists dismissed his finding as a disease peculiar to chickens. Discouraged by his failed attempts to cultivate viruses from mammal cancers, Rous abandoned work on the sarcoma in 1915. Nearly two decades passed before he returned to cancer research. During that time, Rous conducted breakthrough research on urgent medical problems such as emergency blood transfusions and culture-gathering techniques.

In 1933, a colleague's report stimulated Rous to renew his work on cancer. Richard Shope discovered a virus that caused warts on the skin of wild rabbits. Within a year, Rous established that this papilloma had characteristics of a true tumor. His work on mammalian cancer kept his viral theory of cancer alive. However, another twenty years passed before scientists identified viruses that cause human cancers and learned that viruses act by invading genes of normal cells. These findings finally advanced Rous's 1910 discovery to a dominant place in cancer research.

Meanwhile, Rous and his colleagues spent three decades studying the Shope papilloma to understand the role of viruses in causing cancer in mammals. Careful observations, over long periods of time, of the changing shapes, colors, and sizes of cells revealed that normal cells become malignant in progressive steps. Cell changes in tumors were observed as always evolving in a single direction toward malignancy.

The researchers demonstrated how viruses collaborate with carcinogens such as tar, radiation, or chemicals to elicit and enhance tumors. In a report co-authored by W. F. Friedewald, Rous proposed a two-stage mechanism of carcinogenesis, or the causing of cancer, called initiation and promotion. He further explained that a virus can be induced by carcinogens or it can hasten the growth and transform benign tumors into cancerous ones. For tumors having no apparent trace of virus, Rous cautiously postulated that these "spontaneous" growths might contain a virus that persists in a "masked" or latent state, causing no harm until its cellular environment is disturbed. Rous eventually ceased his research on this project due to the technical complexities involved with pursuing the interaction of viral and environmental factors. He then analyzed different types of cells and their nature in an attempt to understand why tumors go from bad to worse.

In 1915, Rous married Marion de Kay, daughter of a scholarly commentator on the arts, and they had three daughters. Rous was appointed a full member of the Rockefeller Institute in 1920 and member emeritus in 1945. Though officially retired, he remained active at his lab bench until the age of ninety, adding sixty papers to the nearly three hundred he published. In 1966 he was awarded the Nobel Prize in Medicine. He died of abdominal cancer in 1970, in New York City.

Rubella

Rubella, also known as German **measles**, is a fairly mild virus infection that generally affects children and young adults. The symptoms include slight fever, swollen lymph glands and a slight skin rash which may or may not be present. The relative mildness of the disease belies the fact that rubella in a pregnant woman can result in tragic consequences for the fetus. If a woman has the disease, especially in the early months of pregnancy, the virus travels through the placenta and affects development of the fetus. Spontaneous abortion occurs in 10 percent of cases, but if the pregnancy comes to term, the newborn infant is likely to be born with heart disease, eye defects, deafness, mental retardation or a combination of these.

The virus that causes rubella was first grown in laboratory culture by **Thomas Weller** of Harvard and Children's Hospital in Boston. However, an epidemic in the United States in 1964 prompted Paul D. Parkman, a physician who had isolated and propagated the virus, to work on developing an attenuated virus suitable for a vaccine. Working with associates Harry M. Meyer, Jr. and Theodore C. Panos, Parkman developed a vaccine made from attenuated viruses grown in monkey cells. Shortly thereafter, clinical trials were begun in children and women of child-bearing age.

By 1968, three other research groups had begun developing a vaccine for rubella. Stanley A. Plotkin obtained viruses from diploid human cells, while another doctor worked with rabbit cells. At the same time, Maurice R. Hilleman grew attenuated viruses in duck cells, knowing that mammalian cells sometimes contain other viruses that can infect human cells and cause **cancer**. All of these vaccines were tested and used throughout the 1970s leading to a reduction in cases of rubella, although the Parkman-Meyer vaccine was more virulent and caused more side effects in adults. Since that time, the MMR vaccine has been developed that offers protection against not only rubella, but also measles and **mumps**. MMR vaccinations are required for school-age children in many states.

Rufus of Ephesus (ca. 1st century B.C.-ca. 1st century)

Greek physician

Rufus of Ephesus was a renowned Greek physician who wrote numerous medical treatises in such areas as **pathology** and dietetics. Known primarily for his work in describing anatomy, Rufus's writings on anatomical nomenclature were of major importance to the advancement of medicine. Although not as well known in the annals of medicine as his predecessor Hippocrates (ca. 460-377 B.C.) or **Galen** (ca. 130-200 A.D.), who followed him, Rufus made important contributions to early medical knowledge and is rightly acclaimed as one of the great physicians of the ancient Greek era.

Little is known about Rufus's life. Although often depicted as living during the reign of Trajan (98-117 A.D.), he may well have lived during the earlier reigns of Nero (37-68 A.D.) and Vespasian (9-79 A.D.). Rufus was a common Roman name that meant "red-blond" in Latin and probably referred to his hair color. Rufus is believed to have been born in Ephesus, where he studied and practiced medicine. He may also have studied and worked in the ancient cultural center of Alexandria.

Although Rufus's personal life remains a mystery, his professional interests are well documented. His wide ranging treatises on medicine were preserved by chroniclers such as Paul of Aegina (625-690). At least 96 different medical works or sections are attributed to Rufus, who wrote in Greek and sometimes in traditional verse. Characterized by their precise clinical observations and the even-handed approach to evaluating his own and other physicians' (such as Hippocrates') beliefs and observations, Rufus's writings included *On the Naming of the Parts of the Human Body*, *On Kidney and Bladder Ailments*, and *On Joint-Diseases*.

Rufus gained most of his knowledge of anatomy by dissecting monkeys and pigs and reportedly was displeased that **dissection** of human corpses was outlawed. He described in detail the lens of the **eye** and its membrane and the optic chiasma. His work on pulse indicated he understood the difference between diastolic and systolic blood pressure. He accurately described **filariasis** (a tropical disease in which worms can be found in the blood) and accurately identified the cause of **gout** as an accumulation of poisons in the body. In one treatise, his keen powers of observation were applied to an epidemic of the **plague**, including environmental factors, disease symptoms, and treatment of the symptoms.

Rufus also wrote a famous treatise called *Questions of the Physician (to the Patients)*, which stressed the importance of the physician-patient interview as one of the foundations of good medical practice. He wrote: "One must put questions to the patient, for thereby certain aspects of the disease can be better understood, and the treatment rendered more effective." Although this approach is standard practice today, many ancient physicians believed that physical signs of disease alone were needed for diagnosis. Rufus also wrote extensively on sexual functioning, such as potency, and claimed that coitus was a remedy against melancholia and depression by helping to calm passions.

Although Rufus is not associated with any specific school of medical thought, he certainly adopted the Hippocratic approach. However, Rufus was often critical of the "father of medicine." Unlike many of his colleagues, who also wrote on philosophy, astronomy, and other disciplines, Rufus wrote solely on medical topics. His medical renown reached as far as Byzantium and Arabia, where he was especially esteemed. Galen also respected Rufus, who was said to have treated all patients with sympathy, whether they were noblemen or slaves. In the prologue to the *Canterbury Tales*, Geoffrey Chaucer (1342-1400) named Rufus among the great physicians of the past.

See also Hippocrates of Cos; Galen; Gout; Pathology

Rural health

One in five Americans live in rural areas. The definition of rural varies, but generally it is understood to be a sparsely populated nonurban area. Rural populations are very different one from the other, as is the geography of the regions they live in. For example, rural populations include seasonal farm workers,

Native American and Alaskan populations, and so-called frontier communities, those with fewer than six residents per square mile. The diversity of rural populations presents unique challenges in terms of health care. But all these communities have some things in common.

First, the decline of traditional rural occupations such as farming, mining, and timber has reduced employment opportunities for rural residents, contributing to poverty. Because poverty narrows the economic base from which health care delivery services are funded, rural residents have reduced access to essential health care services. Second, there is a higher concentration of elderly people in rural areas than in urban areas. And this number is increasing, as young adults move to urban areas to look for work. Third, the two most dangerous occupations are farming and mining, both of which are rural industries. Rural residents have higher rates of occupational injury. And finally, poverty and self-employment make it more likely that rural residents will be uninsured or underinsured. People without insurance are less likely to have money to spend on preventive health care, which means that when they do go to the doctor, their illnesses are usually more serious.

In rural areas, the ratio of primary care physicians to patients is 1 to 3,500, substantially under the ratio recommended by the **U.S. Department of Health and Human Services**. Because rural physicians do not make as much as physicians working in urban areas, work longer hours per week, and are professionally isolated, it is very difficult to hire and keep them. To offset this problem, nonphysician providers such as clinical nurse specialists, nurse practitioners, certified midwives, and physician assistants are increasingly taking on more of the primary care responsibilities for rural residents. Unfortunately, rural states have historically had the most restrictive laws governing the services of nonphysican providers. Over 50% of reimbursements to rural physicians for the care they provide to patients are made through public programs at rates substantially less than private payers. Limited opportunities to consult with colleagues and inadequate backup are additional difficulties that rural physicians and doctors for the poor must contend with. As **hospitals** merge or close to cut costs, such constraints worsen.

In response to these challenges, the federal government has set up a number of programs to address some of the health issues and problems facing rural America. Proposed measures include financial incentives to physicians and nonphysician providers who work in underserved areas, training opportunities for students, and grants and funds to develop innovative health care delivery models and to support rural health research centers. Information technology holds particular appeal for rural medicine. Telemedicine refers to the use of electronic commnication to provide clinical care, for example, 24-hour emergency consultation, medical support, and weekly instructional seminars and continuing medical education.

The proportion of inhabitants in other developed countries who live in rural, remote, and underserved communities is similar to that in the United States. The problems of these populations—the decline of traditional industries and an **aging** population owing to migration of the young to the cities—are also similar. Although fewer data are available in Europe, evidence indicates that, like their counterparts in the United States, rural physicians in Canada and across Europe suffer high workloads, limited access to training, isolation, poor morale, and a decline in recruitment. In countries long used to the particular demands of a vast geography such as Australia, New Zealand, and Canada, rural health has been better developed than in Europe. For example, since 1928, the Australian Royal Flying Doctor Service has provided a full range of medical services to rural residents for whom a visit to the doctor might otherwise entail a 400- to 600-mile (650 to 970 km) round trip.

Developing countries must cope with a chronic shortage of physicians and equipment, drugs, buildings, and nurses and other health staff. Those living in rural areas in developing areas are poor, and they cannot get medical attention unless it is paid for by the state. The quality of this medical care is often of low quality, and in remote regions it may be lacking completely. Poor infrastructure, for example, roads, telephones, emergency services, and per capita medical personnel, exacts a greater toll in developing than in developed countries. Rural health services in developing countries, of which India and Tanzania are typical examples, depend heavily on rural health centers and dispensaries, which are designed to provide comprehensive health services for the community. Staff are often nonphysician providers, and the emphasis is on diagnosis, treatment, and referral (to higher-level facilities), as well as a range of health promotion and disease prevention activities. These include maternal and child health, environmental health, and health education. Villages may be served by a village health post staffed by health workers supervised from centers in the primary health system. Because quality of infrastructure and ability to provide health services are directly related, the **World Health Organization** and the World Bank have increasingly linked improved health to development and alleviation of poverty.

See also Health care system; Health insurance; Medicare and Medicaid; Midwifery; Minority health; Physician

S

SABIN, ALBERT BRUCE (1906-1993)

Polish American virologist

Albert Sabin was born on August 26, 1906 in Bialystock, Poland (then Russia) and immigrated with his family to the United States in 1921. He attended New York University, received his medical degree in 1931, and began research on the virus that causes poliomyelitis or **polio**. Known at the time as infantile paralysis, it was a source of much fear because of its ability to cause paralysis and death, especially in infants and young children. By 1936, Sabin and his colleagues were able, for the first time, to grow the polio virus in human tissue cultures outside the body. In 1941, Sabin established that the human polio virus enters the body via the digestive tract and not the nose as was then thought. World War II interrupted his polio research and, while in the army, he studied several diseases affecting American troops such as sandfly fever, dengue fever, toxoplasmosis, and encephalitis lethargica. After the war, Sabin continued to engage in polio research.

By 1954, Sabin had developed a vaccine that gave protection against polio using a live virus rather than the killed virus used by **Dr. Jonas Salk**. Sabin believed that an attenuated (weakened and harmless) live virus would provide more rapid and longer-lasting protection than the Salk method. With some professional rivalry developing between Salk and Sabin, the latter persisted in bringing his vaccine to completion, and it became available to the public in 1961 following four years of worldwide tests. The Sabin vaccine has two advantages over the Salk vaccine: it can be administered orally rather than by injection, and offers protection with a single dose. Today, except for a few special cases, it is the preferred polio vaccine worldwide. The development of the Sabin vaccine was the result of 20 years of research on the nature, transmission, and epidemiology of three related virus types. Throughout his professional career, Sabin was known for his tireless and brilliant research. In his later years, Sabin's interests led him to research the possible connection between viruses and human **cancer**. Albert Sabin died March 3, 1993 at the age of 86.

SABIN, FLORENCE RENA (1871-1953)

American anatomist and biologist

Florence Sabin was born in the mining town of Central City, Colorado, to Vermont natives. Her paternal grandfather had been a Vermont country doctor; her father had studied medicine for two years before following the gold and silver rush West as a mining engineer. Her mother switched teaching posts from the South to Colorado during the Civil War. After her mother's death, when Florence was four, the girl attended boarding schools, first in Denver and then near relatives in Illinois and Vermont. She attended Smith College in Massachusetts with her sister, Mary, where she studied mathematics and zoology, graduating with a bachelor of science degree in 1893.

That same year, the Johns Hopkins Medical School opened, thanks to the funds raised by a group of Baltimore women who had stipulated that the school must admit women on an equal footing with men. After teaching for three years, Sabin could afford to enter the medical school in 1896. At Johns Hopkins, Sabin was greatly influenced by the prominent anatomy professor Franklin Mall, who encouraged her talent and inclination for research. While a student, Sabin constructed a three-dimensional model of a newborn infant's lower and mid brain, with an accompanying lab manual. Both became widely used in medical schools.

Sabin received her medical degree in 1900 and was appointed in 1901 to a fellowship at Hopkins created for her by the same group of Baltimore women. Thus began her twenty-five-year career of medical research and teaching at Hopkins, where she progressed from assistant to associate professor to first female full professor (of histology) in 1917. In her earlier years at Hopkins, Sabin investigated the structure and development of the **lymphatic system**, which was poorly understood at the time. Most scientists thought that the lymph vessels originated in tissue spaces and grew toward the veins. Using very small pig embryos she collected from a nearby slaughterhouse and injecting their lymph vessels with dye, Sabin convincingly

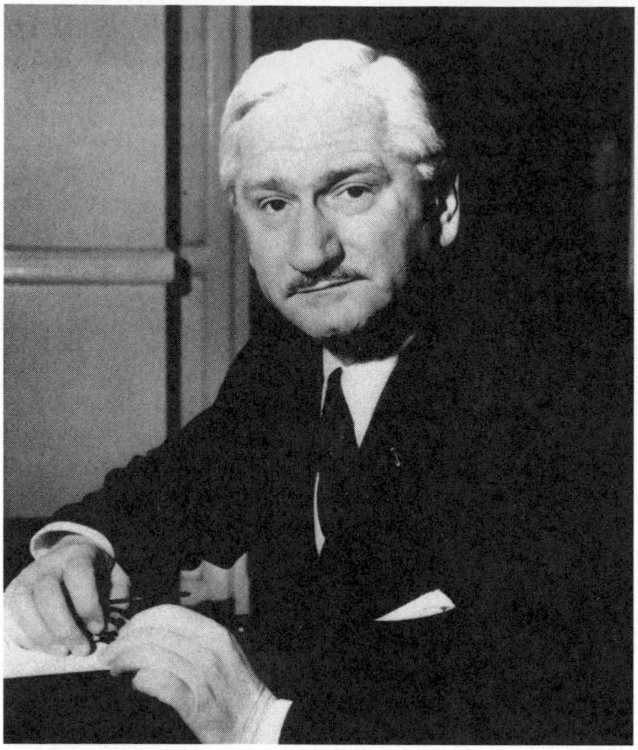

Albert Bruce Sabin

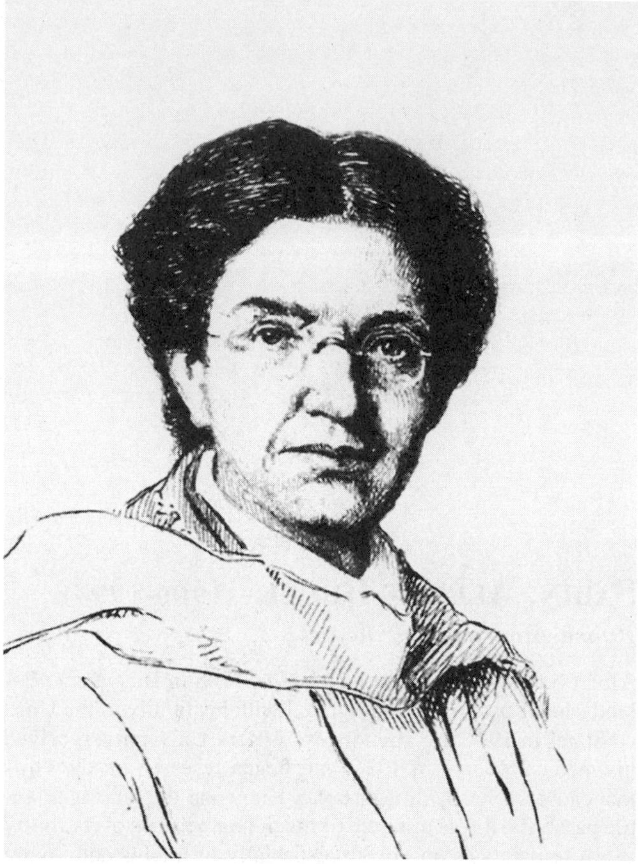

Florence Rena Sabin

demonstrated that the lymphatics start as buds from the veins and grow outward in a continuing series of buds. She also showed that the lymph system was one-way, the lymph vessels being closed at their ends. Sabin's series of published papers on her findings in 1916 established her scientific reputation.

Sabin's lymphatics investigations led her to a study of the origins of blood cells and vessels. Sabin observed in a live chick embryo under a microscope the actual formation of the blood vessels, followed by the red and white blood cells, and then the first heartbeat. Sabin also introduced, in the 1920s, the technique of ''supravital'' staining—staining of living cells with dyes, which made it possible to distinguish certain types of cells from others for the first time in living tissue. The supravital staining research, in turn, led Sabin to a study of cells (monocytes) involved in immune reactions, especially against the **tuberculosis** bacillus.

In 1925, Sabin left Johns Hopkins and continued her work at the Rockefeller Institute for Medical Research in New York City. There, she directed a laboratory dedicated to the investigation of cellular immune response, particularly in tuberculosis. While directing her staff's collaboration in an inter-institutional, inter-disciplinary effort to identify a tuberculin-resistant substance, Sabin continued her valuable original research on the formation of antibodies.

Required to retire in 1938 at the age of sixty-seven, Sabin moved back to Denver to live with her sister Mary. There, in the late 1940s, she applied her legendary enthusiasm and energy to reform Colorado's archaic public health laws. In October 1953, weakened by several years of caring for her failing sister, Sabin died of a heart attack in her living room chair.

Sakmann, Bert (1942-)

German physician and cell physiologist

Bert Sakmann, along with physicist Erwin Neher, was awarded the 1991 Nobel Prize in physiology or medicine for inventing the patch clamp technique. The technique made it possible to realize a goal that had eluded scientists since the 1950s: to be able to examine individual ion channels—pore-forming proteins found in the outer membranes of virtually all cells that serve as conduits for electrical signals. Introduced in 1976, the patch clamp technique opened new paths in the study of membrane physiology. Since then, researchers throughout the world have adapted and refined patch clamping, contributing significantly to research on problems in medicine and neuroscience. The Nobel Committee credited Sakmann and Neher with having revolutionized modern biology.

Sakmann was born in Stuttgart, Germany, on June 12, 1942. His later education involved much time around the laboratory. From 1969 to 1970, he was a research assistant in the department of neurophysiology at the Max Planck Institute for

Psychiatry in Munich. Between 1971 and 1973, Sakmann studied biophysics with Nobel Laureate Bernard Katz at University College in London as a British Council scholar. In 1974 he received his medical degree from the University ofGöttingen. From that year until 1979 he was a research associate inthe department of neurobiology at the Max Planck Institute for Biophysical Chemistry in Göttingen.

In the 1950s and 1960s, the existence of ion channels that allowfor the transmission of electrical charges from one cell to another was inferred from research since no one had been able to actually locate the sites of these channels. Cell physiologists were being drawn to thequestion of how electrically charged ions control such biological functions as the transmission of nerve impulses, the contraction of muscles, vision, and the process of conception. Sakmann's early interest in ion channels was stimulated by two papers published in 1969 and 1970 that gave strong evidence for the existence of ion channels. As stronger evidence began to accumulate for their existence, it became clear to Sakmann and Neher, who were sharing laboratory space at the Max Planck Institute, that they would have to develop a fine instrument to be able to locate the actual sites of the ion channels on the cell membrane.

Bedeviling efforts of researchers to that point was the electrical ''noise'' generated by the cell's membrane, which made it impossible todetect signals coming from individual channels. Sakmann and Neher set about to reduce the noise by shutting out most of the membrane. They applied a glass micropipette one micron wide and fitted with a recording electrode to a cell membrane and were able to measure the flow of current through a single channel. ''It worked the first time,'' Sakmann recalled in *Science* magazine. The biophysical community was exultant.

Over the next few years, Sakmann and Neher refined their patch clamp technique. The refinements made it possible to measure even very small currents, and established the patch clamp as a tremendously versatile tool in the field of cell biology. Patch clamping has been instrumental in studies of **cystic fibrosis**, hormone regulation, and insulin production in diabetes. The technique has also made possible the development of new drugs in the treatment of heart disease, epilepsy, and disorders affecting the nervous and muscle systems. In 1991 Sakmann and Neher won the 1991 Nobel Prize in physiology or medicine for their work on ion channels.

Sakmann has continued to work with other research teams, altering the genes for identified ion channels in order to trace the molecules in the channel responsible for opening and closing the ion pore. Even though Sakmann expressed surprise at receiving the Noble Prize, given all the other important work going on in cell physiology, the opinion of many of his colleagues was that the award was long overdue. Sakmann is married to Christianne, an ophthalmologist; they have three children.

SALK, JONAS (1914-1995)

American microbiologist

Jonas Salk was one of the United States's best known microbiologists, chiefly celebrated for his discovery of the polio vaccine. His greatest contribution to immunology was the insight that a ''killed virus'' is capable of serving as an antigen, prompting the body's immune system to produce antibodies that will attack invading organisms. This realization enabled Salk to develop a polio vaccine composed of killed polio viruses, producing the necessary antibodies to help the body to ward off the disease without itself inducing polio.

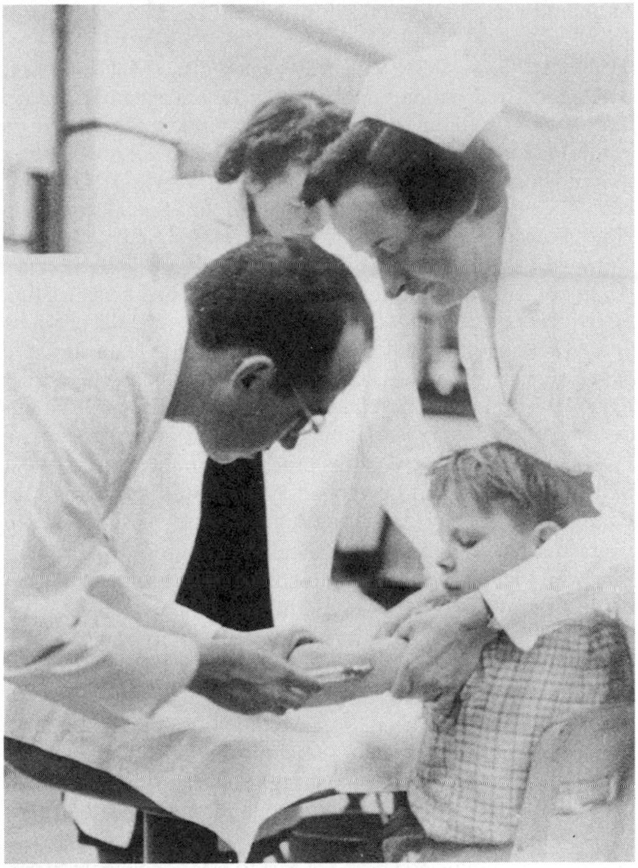

Jonas Salk

The eldest son of Orthodox Jewish-Polish immigrants, Jonas Edward Salk was born in East Harlem, New York, on 28 October 1914. His father, Daniel B. Salk, was a garment worker, who designed lace collars and cuffs and enjoyed sketching in his spare time. He and his wife, Dora Press, encouraged their son's academic talents, sending him to Townsend Harris High School for the gifted. There, young Salk was both highly motivated and high achieving, graduating at the age of fifteen and proceeding to enroll in the legal faculty of the City College of New York. Ever curious, however, he attended some science courses and quickly decided to switch fields. Salk graduated with a bachelor's degree in science in 1933, at the age of nineteen, and went on to New York University's School of Medicine. Initially he scraped by on money his parents had borrowed for him; after the first year, however, scholarships and fellowships paid his way. In his senior year, Salk met the man with whom he would collaborate on some of the most important work of his career, Dr. Thomas Francis, Jr.

On 7 June 1939, Salk was awarded his M.D. The next day, he married Donna Lindsay, a Phi Beta Kappa psychology major who was employed as a social worker. The marriage would produce three sons: Peter, Darrell, and Jonathan. After graduation, Salk continued working with Francis, and concurrently began a two-year internship at Mount Sinai Hospital in New York. Upon completing his internship, Salk accepted a National Research Council fellowship and moved to the University of Michigan to join Dr. Francis, who had been heading up Michigan's department of epidemiology since the previous year. Working on behalf of the U.S. Army, the team strove to develop a flu vaccine. Their goal was a ''killed-virus'' vaccine—able to kill the live flu viruses in the body, while simultaneously producing antibodies that could fight off future invaders of the same type, thus producing immunity. By 1943, Salk and Francis had developed a formalin-killed-virus vaccine, effective against both type A and B influenza viruses, and were in a position to begin clinical trials.

In 1946, Salk was appointed assistant professor of epidemiology at Michigan. Around this time he extended his research to cover not only viruses and the body's reaction to them but also their epidemic effects in populations. The following year he accepted an invitation to move to the University of Pittsburgh School of Medicine's Virus Research Laboratory as an associate research professor of bacteriology. When Salk arrived at the Pittsburgh laboratory, what he encountered was not encouraging. The laboratory had no experience with the kind of basic research he was accustomed to, and it took considerable effort on his part to bring the lab up to par. However, Salk was not shy about seeking financial support for the laboratory from outside benefactors, and soon his laboratory represented the cutting edge of viral research.

In addition to building a respectable laboratory, Salk also devoted a considerable amount of his energies to writing scientific papers on a number of topics, including the polio virus. Some of these came to the attention of Daniel Basil O'Connor, the director of the National Foundation for Infantile Paralysis—an organization that had long been involved with the treatment and rehabilitation of polio victims. O'Connor eyed Salk as a possible recruit for the polio vaccine research his organization sponsored. When the two finally met, O'Connor was much taken by Salk—so much so, in fact, that he put almost all of the National Foundation's money behind Salk's vaccine research efforts.

Poliomyelitis, traceable back to ancient Egypt, causes permanent paralysis in those it strikes, or chronic shortness of breath often leading to death. Children, in particular, are especially vulnerable to the polio virus. The University of Pittsburgh was one of four universities engaged in trying to sort and classify the more than one hundred known varieties of polio virus. By 1951, Salk was able to assert with certainty that all polio viruses fell into one of three types, each having various strains; some of these were highly infectious, others barely so. Once he had established this, Salk was in a position to start work on developing a vaccine.

Salk's first challenge was to obtain enough of the virus to be able to develop a vaccine in doses large enough to have an impact; this was particularly difficult since viruses, unlike culture-grown bacteria, need living cells to grow. The breakthrough came when the team of JohnF. Enders, Thomas Weller, and Frederick Robbins found that the polio virus could be grown in embryonic tissue—a discovery that earned them a Nobel Prize in 1954.

Salk subsequently grew samples of all three varieties of polio virus in cultures of monkey kidney tissue, then killed the virus with formaldehyde. Salk believed that it was essential to use a killed polio virus (rather than a live virus) in the vaccine, as the live-virus vaccine would have a much higher chance of accidentally inducing polio in inoculated children. He therefore exposed the viruses to formaldehyde for nearly 13 days. Though after only three days he could detect no virulence in the sample, Salk wanted to establish a wide safety margin; after an additional ten days of exposure to the formaldehyde, he reckoned that there was only a one-in-a-trillion chance of there being a live virus particle in a single dose of his vaccine. Salk tested it on monkeys with positive results before proceeding to human clinical trials.

Despite Salk's confidence, many of his colleagues were skeptical, believing that a killed-virus vaccine could not possibly be effective. His dubious standing was further compounded by the fact that he was relatively new to polio vaccine research; some of his chief competitors in the race to develop the vaccine—most notably Albert Sabin, the chief proponent for a live-virus vaccine—had been at it for years and were somewhat irked by the presence of this upstart with his unorthodox ideas.

As the field narrowed, the division between the killed-virus and the live-virus camps widened, and what had once been a polite difference of opinion became a serious ideological conflict. Salk and his chief backer, the National Foundation for Infantile Paralysis, were fairly lonely in their corner. But Salk failed to let his position in the scientific wilderness dissuade him and he continued, undeterred, with his research. To test his vaccine's strength, in early 1952 Salk administered a type I vaccine to children who had already been infected with the polio virus. Afterwards, he measured their antibody levels. His results clearly indicated that the vaccine produced large amounts of antibodies. Buoyed by this success, the clinical trial was then extended to include children who had never had polio.

In May 1952, Salk initiated preparations for a massive field trial in which over four hundred thousand children would be vaccinated. The largest medical experiment that had ever been carried out in the United States, the test finally got underway in April, 1954, under the direction of Dr. Francis and sponsored by the National Foundation for Infantile Paralysis. More than one million children between the ages of six and nine took part in the trial, each receiving a button that proclaimed them a ''Polio Pioneer.'' A third of the children were given doses of the vaccine consisting of three injections—one for each of the types of polio virus—plus a booster shot. A control group of the same number of children was given a placebo, and a third group was given nothing.

At the beginning of 1953, while the trial was still at an early stage, Salk's encouraging results were made public in the

Journal of the American Medical Association. Predictably, media and public interest were intense. Anxious to avoid sensationalized versions of his work, Salk agreed to comment on the results thus far during a scheduled radio and press appearance. However, this appearance did not mesh with accepted scientific protocol for making such announcements, and some of his fellow scientists accused him of being little more than a publicity hound. Salk, who claimed that he had been motivated only by the highest principles, was deeply hurt.

Despite the doomsayers, on 12 April 1955, the vaccine was officially pronounced effective, potent, and safe in almost 90% of cases. The meeting at which the announcement was made was attended by five hundred of the world's top scientists and doctors, 150 journalists, and sixteen television and movie crews.

The success of the trial catapulted Salk to instant stardom. He was inundated with offers from Hollywood and with pleas from top manufacturers for him to endorse their products. He received a citation from President Eisenhower and addressed the nation from the White House Rose Garden. He was awarded a congressional medal for great achievement in the field of medicine and was nominated for a Nobel Prize but, contrary to popular expectation, did not receive it. He was also turned down for membership in the National Academy of Sciences, most likely a reflection of the discomfort the scientific community still felt about the level of publicity he attracted and of continued disagreement with peers over his methods.

Wishing to escape from the glare of the limelight, Salk turned down the countless offers and tried to retreat into his laboratory. Unfortunately, a tragic mishap served to keep the attention of the world's media focused on him. Just two week after the announcement of the vaccine's discovery, eleven of the children who had received it developed polio; more cases soon followed. Altogether, about 200 children developed paralytic polio, eleven fatally. For a while, it appeared that the vaccination campaign would be railroaded. However, it was soon discovered that all of the rogue vaccines had originated from the same source, Cutter Laboratories in California. On May 7, the vaccination campaign was called to a halt by the Surgeon General. Following a thorough investigation, it was found that Cutter had used faulty batches of virus culture which were resistant to the formaldehyde. After furious debate and the adoption of standards that would prevent such a reoccurrence, the inoculation resumed. By the end of 1955, seven million children had received their shots, and over the course of the next two years more than 200 million doses of Salk's polio vaccine were administered, without a single instance of vaccine-induced paralysis. By the summer of 1961 there had been a 96 % reduction in the number of cases of polio in the United States, compared to the five-year period prior to the vaccination campaign.

After the initial inoculation period ended in 1958, Salk's killed-virus vaccine was replaced by a live-virus vaccine developed by Sabin; use of this new vaccine was advantageous because it could be administered orally rather than intravenously, and because it required fewer "booster" inoculations. To this day, though, Salk remains known as the man who defeated polio.

In 1954, Salk took up a new position as professor of preventative medicine at Pittsburgh, and in 1957 he became professor of experimental medicine. The following year he began work on a vaccine to immunize against all viral diseases of the central nervous system. As part of this research, Salk performed studies of normal and malignant cells, studies that had some bearing on the problems encountered in cancer research. In 1960, he founded the Salk Institute for Biological Studies in La Jolla, California; heavily funded by the National Foundation for Infantile Paralysis (by then known as the March of Dimes), the institute attracted some of the brightest scientists in the world, all drawn by Salk's promise of full-time, uninterrupted biological research.

When his new institute finally opened in 1963, Salk became its director and devoted himself to the study of multiple sclerosis and cancer. He remained a driven man, thinking nothing of working sixteen to eighteen hours a day, six days a week. In 1968, his marriage ended in divorce, and he made the headlines again in 1970 when he remarried, this time to Françoise Gilot, Pablo Picasso's first wife and mother of two of the artist's children. During the 1970s Salk turned to writing, producing books about the philosophy of science and its social role. In 1977, he received the Presidential Medal of Freedom.

Despite the sense of expectancy that he seemed to encourage, Jonas Salk took his successes and failures in stride. In the early 1990s, many people looked to him as the one would might finally develop a vaccine against the HIV virus. But Salk, though continuing to strive toward scientific breakthroughs, seems content simply to work at his chosen craft. "I don't want to go from one crest to another," he once said, as quoted by Sarah K. Bolton in *Famous Men of Science.* "To a scientist, fame is neither an end nor even a means to an end. Do you recall what Emerson said?—'The reward of a thing well done is the opportunity to do more'. "

Salk died on 23 June 1995, at a San Diego area hospital. His death, at the age of 80, was caused by heart failure.

SALMONELLA FOOD POISONING

Salmonella food poisoning is a bacterial **food poisoning** caused by the *Salmonella* bacterium. It results in the swelling of the lining of the stomach and intestines (**gastroenteritis**). While domestic and wild animals, including poultry, pigs, cattle and pets such as turtles, iguanas, chicks, dogs and cats can transmit this illness, most people become infected by ingesting foods contaminated with significant amounts of *Salmonella.*

Salmonella food poisoning occurs worldwide, however it is most frequently reported in North America and Europe. Only a small proportion of infected people are tested and diagnosed, and as few as 1% of cases are actually reported. While the infection rate may seem relatively low, even an attack rate of less than 0.5% in such a large number of exposures results in many infected individuals. The poisoning typically occurs in small, localized outbreaks in the general population or in large outbreaks in hospitals, restaurants, or institutions for children or the elderly. In the United States, *Salmonella* is responsible for about 15% of all cases of food poisoning.

Improperly handled or undercooked poultry and eggs are the foods which most frequently cause Salmonella food poisoning. Chickens are a major carrier of *Salmonella* bacteria, which accounts for its prominence in poultry products. However, identifying foods which may be contaminated with *Salmonella* is particularly difficult because infected chickens typically show no signs or symptoms. Since infected chickens have no identifying characteristics, these chickens go on to lay eggs or to be used as meat.

At one time, it was thought that *Salmonella* bacteria were only found in eggs which had cracked, thus allowing the bacteria to enter. Ultimately, it was learned that, because the egg shell has tiny pores, even uncracked eggs which sat for a time on a surface (nest) contaminated with *Salmonella* could themselves become contaminated. It is known also that the bacteria can be passed from the infected female chicken directly into the substance of the egg before the shell has formed around it.

Anyone may contract Salmonella food poisoning, but the disease is most serious in infants, the elderly, and individuals with weakened **immune systems**. In these individuals, the infection may spread from the intestines to the blood stream, and then to other body sites, causing **death** unless the person is treated promptly with **antibiotics**. In addition, people who have had part or all of their stomach or their spleens removed, or who have **sickle cell anemia**, **cirrhosis** of the liver, **leukemia**, **lymphoma**, **malaria**, louse-borne **relapsing fever**, or **Acquired Immunodeficiency Syndrome** (AIDS) are particularly susceptible to Salmonella food poisoning.

Salmonella food poisoning can occur when someone drinks unpasteurized milk or eats undercooked chicken or eggs, or salad dressings or desserts which contain raw eggs. Even if *Salmonella*-containing foods such as chicken are thoroughly cooked, any food can become contaminated during preparation if conditions and equipment for food preparation are unsanitary.

Other foods can then be accidentally contaminated if they come into contact with infected surfaces. In addition, children have become ill after playing with turtles or iguanas, and then eating without washing their hands. Because the bacteria are shed in the feces for weeks after infection with *Salmonella*, poor hygiene can allow such a carrier to spread the infection to others.

Symptoms appear about 1-2 days after infection, and include **fever** (in 50% of patients), nausea and vomiting, **diarrhea**, and abdominal cramps and **pain**. The diarrhea is usually very liquid, and rarely contains mucus or blood. Diarrhea usually lasts for about four days. The illness usually ends in about five to seven days.

Serious complications are rare, occurring most often in individuals with other medical illnesses. Complications occur when the *Salmonella* bacteria make their way into the bloodstream (**bacteremia**). Once in the blood stream, the bacteria can enter any organ system throughout the body, causing disease. Other infections which can be caused by *Salmonella* include:

- Bone infections (**osteomyelitis**)
- Joint infections (arthritis)
- Infection of the sac containing the heart (**pericarditis**)
- Infection of the tissues which cover the brain and spinal cord (**meningitis**)
- Infection of the liver (**hepatitis**)
- Lung infections (**pneumonia**)
- Infection of **aneurysms** (abnormal outpouchings which occur in weak areas of the walls of blood vessels)
- Infections in the center of existing tumors or cysts.

Under appropriate laboratory conditions, *Salmonella* can be grown and then viewed under a microscope for identification. Early in the infection, the blood is far more likely to positively show a presence of the *Salmonella* bacterium when a sample is grown on a nutrient substance (culture) for identification purposes. Eventually, however, positive cultures can be obtained from the stool (feces) and in some cases from a urine culture.

Even though Salmonella food poisoning is a bacterial infection, most practitioners do not treat simple cases with antibiotics. Studies have shown that using antibiotics does not usually reduce the length of time that the patient is ill. Paradoxically, it appears that antibiotics do, however, cause the patient to shed bacteria in their feces for a *longer* period of time. In order to decrease the length of time that a particular individual is a carrier who can spread the disease, antibiotics are generally not given.

In situations where an individual has a more severe type of infection with *Salmonella* bacteria, a number of antibiotics may be used. Chloramphenicol was the first antibiotic successfully used to treat Salmonella food poisoning. It is still a drug of choice in developing countries because it is so inexpensive, although some resistance has developed to it. Ampicillin and trimethoprim-sulfonamide have been used successfully in the treatment of infections caused by chloramphenicol-resistant strains. Newer types of antibiotics, such as **cephalosporin** or quinolone, are also effective. These drugs can be given by mouth or through a needle in the vein (intravenously) for very ill patients. With effective antibiotic therapy, patients feel better in 24-48 hours, the temperature returns to normal in three to five days, and the patient is generally recovered by 10-14 days.

A number of alternative treatments have been recommended for food poisoning. One very effective treatment that is strongly recommended is supplementation with *Lactobacillus acidophilus*, *L. bulgaricus*, and/or *Bifidobacterium* to restore essential bacteria in the digestive tract. These preparations are available as powders, tablets, or capsules from health food stores; yogurt with live *L. acidophilus* cultures can also be eaten. **Fasting** or a liquid-only diet is often used for food poisoning. **Homeopathic medicine** can work very effectively in the treatment of Salmonella food poisoning. The appropriate remedy for the individual and his/her symptoms must be used to get the desired results. Some examples of remedies commonly used are *Chamomilla*, *Nux vomica*, *Ipecac*, and *Colchicum*. Juice therapy, including carrot, beet, and garlic juices, is sometimes recommended, although it can cause discomfort for some people. Charcoal tablets can help absorb toxins and remove them from the digestive tract through bowel elimination. A variety of herbs with antibiotic action, including citrus seed extract, goldenseal (*Hydrastis canadensis*), and Oregon grape (*Mahonia aquifolium*), may also be effective in helping to resolve cases of food poisoning.

The prognosis (expected outcome) for uncomplicated cases of Salmonella food poisoning is excellent. Most people recover completely within a week's time. In cases where other medical problems complicate the illness, prognosis depends on the severity of the other medical conditions, as well as the specific organ system infected with *Salmonella.*

Prevention of Salmonella food poisoning involves the proper handling and cooking of foods likely to carry the bacteria. This means that recipes utilizing uncooked eggs (Caesar salad dressing, meringue toppings, mousses) need to be modified to eliminate the raw eggs. Not only should chicken be cooked thoroughly, until no pink juices flow, but all surfaces and utensils used on raw chicken must be carefully cleaned to prevent *Salmonella* from contaminating other foods. Careful handwashing is a must before, during, and after all food preparation involving eggs and poultry. Handwashing is also important after handling and playing with pets such as turtles, iguanas, chicks, dogs and cats.

See also Food poisoning; Gastroenteritis

Samuelsson, Bengt (1934-)

Swedish biochemist

Bengt Samuelsson shared the 1982 Nobel Prize for physiology or medicine with his compatriot **Sune K. Bergström** and British biochemist **John R. Vane** "for their discoveries concerningprostaglandins and related biologicallyactive substances." Because prostaglandins are involved in a diverserange of biochemical functions and processes, the research ofBergström, Samuelsson, and Vane opened up a new arena of medical research and pharmaceutical applications.

Bengt Ingemar Samuelsson was born on May 21, 1934, in Halmstad, Sweden, to Anders and Kristina Nilsson Samuelsson. Samuelsson entered medical school at the University of Lund, where he came under the mentorship of Sune K. Bergström. Called "the father of prostaglandin chemistry," Bergström was on the university faculty as professor of physiological chemistry. In 1958, Samuelsson followed Bergström tothe prestigious Karolinska Institute in Stockholm, which is associated with the Nobel Prize awards. There, Samuelsson received his doctorate in medical science in 1960 and his medical degree in 1961, and he was subsequently appointed as an assistant professor of medical chemistry. In1961, he served as a research fellow at Harvard University, and then in1962 he rejoined Bergström at the Karolinska Institute, where he remained until 1966.

At the Karolinska Institute, Samuelsson worked with a group of researchers who were trying to characterize the structures of prostaglandins. Prostaglandins are hormone-like substances found throughout the body, which were so named in the 1930s onthe erroneous assumption that they originated in the prostate. They play an important role in the circulatory system, and they help protect the body against sickness, infection, pain, and stress. Expanding on their earlier research, Bergström, Samuelsson, and other researchers discovered the role that arachidonic acid, an unsaturated fatty acid found in meats and vegetable oils, plays in the formation of prostaglandins. By developing synthetic methods of producing prostaglandins in the laboratory, this group made prostaglandins accessible for scientific research world wide. It was Samuelsson who discovered the process through which arachidonic acid is convert ed into compounds he named endoperoxides, which are in turn converted into prostaglandins.

Prostaglandins have many veterinary and livestock breeding applications, and Samuelsson joined the faculty of the Royal Veterinary College in Stockholm in 1967. He returned to the Karolinska Institute as professor of medicine and physiological chemistry in 1972. Samuelsson served as the chair of the department ofphysiological chemistry from 1973 to 1983, and as dean of the medical faculty from 1978 to 1983, combining administrative duties with a rigorous research schedule. During 1976 and 1977, Samuelsson also served as a visiting professor at Harvard University and the Massachusetts Institute of Technology.

During these years, Samuelsson continued his investigation of prostaglandins and related compounds. In 1973, he discovered the prostaglandins which are involved in the clotting of the blood; he called these thromboxanes. Samuelsson subsequently discovered the compounds he called leukotrienes, which are found in white blood cells (or leukocytes). Leukotrienes are involved in asthma and in **anaphylaxis**, the shock or hypersensitivity that follows exposure to certain foreign substances, such as the toxins in an insect sting. In the wake of such research, prostaglandins have been used totreat fertility problems, circulatory problems, asthma, arthritis, menstrual cramps, and ulcers. Prostaglandins have also been used medically to induce abortions.

The importance of Samuelsson's research has been recognized by numerous awards and honors in addition to the Nobel Prize. Such acknowledgments include the A. Jahres Award in medicine from Oslo University in 1970; the Albert Lasker Medical Research Award in 1977; the Ciba-Geigy Drew Award for biomedical research in 1980; the Gairdner Foundation Award in 1981; and the Abraham White Distinguished Scientist Award in 1991. Samuelsson has published widely on the biochemistry of prostaglandins, thromboxanes, and leukotrienes.

Sanatorium

A sanatorium is an institution where people suffering from physical or mental problems can go for treatment and recuperation. Often, the natural resources of the area in which a sanatorium is located, such as mineral springs, or clean mountain air, are used as part of the treatment or cure. In general, a sanatorium was designed to treat people suffering from a particular disease, such as **tuberculosis**.

Sanatoriums (also called sanitariums), were common in Europe for centuries, but they didn't become popular in the United States until the latter part of the 1800s.

American physician Edward Livingston Trudeau (1848-1915) is credited with popularizing the use of sanatoriums in the United States. Trudeau, who had contracted tuberculosis while nursing his brother through the disease, founded the first American tuberculosis sanatorium in 1885; he started what became known as the "sanatorium movement" in the United States.

After he became ill with his second bout of the deadly disease, and believed he would soon die, Trudeau traveled to upper New York State's Adirondack Mountains to live out his final days. Instead of dying, Trudeau recovered and his symptoms disappeared. He credited his cure to the fresh air of the surrounding mountains and decided to open a sanatorium on the site. Patients who came to his sanatorium were offered lots of fresh air, moderate exercise, and healthful diets.

The Trudeau Sanatorium at Saranac Lake was not the first sanatorium in the country, but it was the first one designed to treat people with tuberculosis. At that time, tuberculosis was a deadly illness, responsible for more than 10% of deaths caused by disease in the United States.

The Trudeau Sanatorium became the model for other tuberculosis treatment facilities, and by 1930, there were 600 such sanatoriums (or sanatoria) with a total of 84,000 beds.

Sanatoriums to treat tuberculosis were the most common type of these institutions, but others were established to help people suffering from other disorders. In 1879, American physician Leslie E. Keeley (1832-1900) established a sanatorium in Dwight, Illinois, designated for the treatment of alcoholics and drug addicts. John H. Kellog, an American physician best known for his development of dry breakfast cereals, started a sanatorium in Battle Creek, Michigan, in 1876. One of the first health food enthusiasts in this country, Kellog developed vegetable products for patients in order to add variation to their diets and improve their health.

Other sanatoriums are designed to treat patients suffering from mental problems. Once extremely popular in this country, the large mental health sanatoriums that warehoused hundreds of patients have been phased out and only partially replaced by smaller, community-based programs. However, large mental health sanatoriums are still popular in some other parts of the world.

Sanatoriums originally were favored by wealthy patients who had the time and money necessary to spend long periods away from home while recuperating from illness. Some sanatoriums later admitted middle-class and poor people as gestures of good-will and service.

See also Mental health care; Mental illness; Mental retardation

Sanger, Margaret Louise (1879-1966)

American nurse, birth control activist

Margaret Sanger was a pioneering feminist who advocated the right of women to control their bodies sexually and reproductively. She educated women about **contraception** and worked tirelessly for its legalization.

Born Margaret Higgins on September 11, 1879, in Corning, New York, Sanger was the sixth of eleven children. Her parents, Anne Purcell and Michael Hennessey Higgins, believed that it was every person's duty to help others and improve their lot. Her father was considered a freethinker who spoke out about labor reform and social equality. The Higgins home was a busy place where meetings were often held for like-minded progressives interested in social reform. The Higgins family was somewhat ostracized by their community for their outspoken activism. Margaret learned early in life to value controversy and to weather criticism.

Throughout Sanger's education, she displayed an interest and a passion for women's history and the push for equality. Sanger taught for a year after graduating from Claverick College and Hudson River Institute. After this year, her mother fell desperately ill with **tuberculosis** and Sanger returned home to nurse her. After her mother's death, Sanger recognized that **nursing** would be a profession that would allow her to help society in the way that she had always dreamed. Sanger went on to study nursing at White Plains Hospital and Manhattan Eye and Ear Clinic in New York. Shortly thereafter, she married her first husband, William Sanger.

After a hiatus in her career during which her three children were born, Sanger began her career as a visiting nurse in New York City. Serving women in the most desperate slums of the city, she was stricken by the specter of so many women dying in **childbirth** and dying of illegal attempts at **abortion**. Despite these desperate scenes, contraception remained illegal. Women told her of their agony: unable to prevent pregnancies, knowing that their health was compromised by many pregnancies, and bringing children into increasingly desperate poverty. Her female patients literally begged Sanger to teach them what they could do to change the cycle of poverty, childbirth, and death in which they were trapped.

Sanger became increasingly passionate about the topic of what she termed "birth control" (then called "voluntary motherhood"). She spent time researching such issues in the library, and even traveled with her family to Europe to learn more. She returned to New York in 1914, ready to champion the cause.

Sanger began publishing a magazine called *Woman Rebel.* She encouraged women to stand up and think for themselves. She published information on the right to vote and family planning. The Comstock Law, however, stated that the distribution of birth control information through the mail was illegal. The U.S. Postal Service, therefore, refused to deliver her magazine, terming its contents obscene. Eventually, Sanger was charged with breaking the law, and she fled to London for two years. She used this time to learn more about birth control and politics and returned to the United States in 1915, armed with more information and renewed passion.

Sanger began lecturing throughout the United States, gathering support for her political efforts to repeal the obscenity laws and anti-birth control laws that prevented activists from distributing both birth control information and birth control itself. She established the National Birth Control League, which over time became the Planned Parenthood Federation of American (still a vital advocate for safe contraception, family planning, and education about sexuality).

Sanger opened her own Brooklyn clinic in 1916, where she, her sister, and another nurse distributed pamphlets, collected histories to document the suffering of women, and provided health care. In short order, the police raided and closed down the clinic. Sanger was jailed and sentenced to labor in a workhouse. Upon her release, she simply reopened the clinic out of her own home. Her new publication, *The Birth Control Review,* debuted in 1921 and had a national mailing list. In 1928, Sanger collected 500 of the million letters she had received from women nationwide. These letters described the agony of poverty, their enslavement to uncontrollable pregnancies and childbirth, and the wrenching sadness of the many deaths of their own mothers, sisters, and daughters due to the lack of available contraception. Sanger published these letters in her 1928 book, *Mothers in Bondage.*

Throughout the 1920s and 1930s, Sanger traveled all over the world, lobbying and lecturing for appropriate birth control legislation. She published numerous articles, pamphlets, and books. She organized conferences on the subject of birth control, including the first International Birth Control Congress in Geneva, Switzerland. The Comstock Law was finally repealed in 1936, allowing information on birth control to be distributed through the mail. Shortly thereafter, the **American Medical Association** at last agreed that doctors could give their patients contraceptives.

In 1952 Sanger traveled to Bombay, India, for the founding of the International Planned Parenthood Federation, for which she served as the first president. Sanger helped fund research that led to Gregory Pincus's development of the birth control pill. Sanger died on September 6, 1966 in Tucson, Arizona.

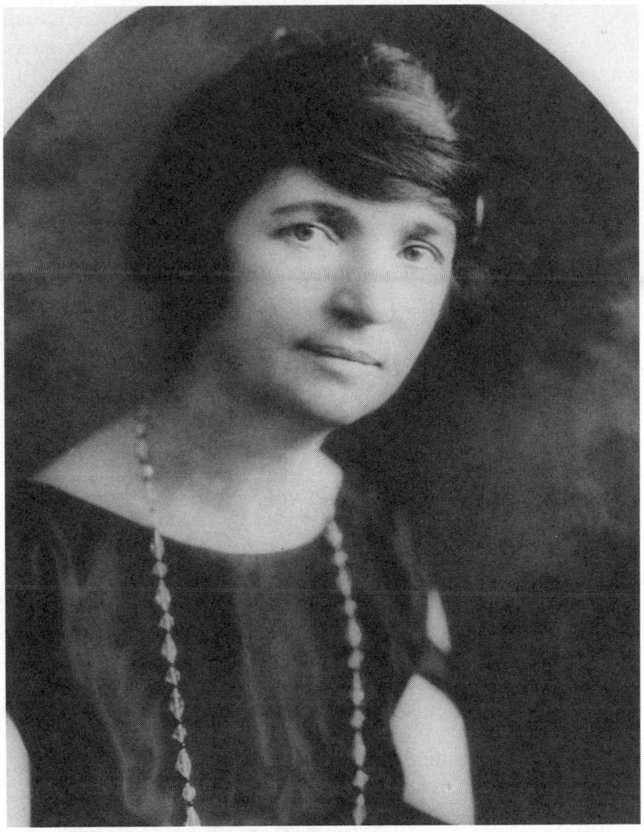

Margaret Sanger

SANITATION

Sanitation, or the use of measures that prevent disease and promote health, was practiced by civilization long before the origins of illness were understood. Underground systems designed to transport waste and surface water away from human dwellings date back as far as 1700 B.C., when the Minoan Kingdom thrived on the isle of Crete. The Palace at Knossos featured sinks, lavatories, a primitive flushing water closet, and four separate drainage systems that emptied into a sewer. Many of the homes in ancient Greece also included latrines that drained into subterranean sewers. In Rome, sewers designed to carry off surface water and provide drainage were built around 800 B.C.. Well-to-do citizens had water closets that drained into cesspools below their homes, and the Roman Empire assigned administrators to oversee the removal of rotting garbage and debris from city streets. Though today we equate such sanitary measures with an attempt to control disease, they were undertaken by the ancients primarily to reduce odor, increase human comfort, and improve the appearance of cities.

The link between good health and personal bathing was first suggested by the Greek physician Hippocrates (c. 460 - c.377 B.C.), who also believed that if water were boiled its impurities and poisons would be removed. In his day, most Greek cities had public hot and cold water baths. The Romans developed elaborate steam and hot water bathing facilities for pleasure and relaxation. With an ample water supply, transported by overhead aqueducts and underground channels, the first Roman baths were emptied and refilled each evening, after closing time. This practice undoubtedly reduced the incidence of bacterial contamination in the public waters, but as bathing became more popular, the pools became crowded and remained open all night. Water was replenished less frequently and the public baths eventually became a breeding ground for infection.

For centuries after the fall of the Roman Empire, sanitation measures such as personal bathing, the disposal of decaying plant and animal matter, and the use of indoor plumbing, were practiced only sporadically. During the medieval period in Europe, cities grew into crowded and unsanitary places. Homes were often infested with lice, fleas, and rats. Human and animal excrement frequently contaminated drinking water. Infectious diseases such as bubonic plague, typhus, typhoid fever, and smallpox took an extraordinary toll on human life. The prevailing view was that these illnesses arose from ''miasmas'', or deadly atmospheric vapors, and that such vapors could be created from foul smelling substances like human waste, rotting corpses, and decomposing food. Early European sanitation laws, dating back to the fourteenth century in France, were aimed at ridding cities of bad odors. In England, King Henry VIII passed an edict requiring homeowners to clear human waste and garbage from the system of open streams that flowed past their dwellings towards the Thames River. The 1348 ordinance of Philip VI of Valois established a street cleaning service in France. A century later King Charles IV created official waste dumping grounds outside of Paris.

The first comprehensive effort at improving sanitation in Europe did not occur till the nineteenth century. On the heels of a cholera epidemic in England, the civil servant Edwin Chadwick (1800-1890) started the Public Health movement. His Sanitary Report of 1842, in which he established the connections between overcrowding, squalor, and disease, led to the passage of the Public Health Act of 1848. The 1848 Act mandated that every dwelling have a human waste disposal arrangement, such as a toilet or ash pit, and it set aside five million British pounds for sanitation research. In 1875 a second Public Health Act, calling for a complete overhaul of London's water and sewer systems, was passed. At around the same time, sanitation efforts were beginning to take hold in America. The New York Board of Public Health was established in 1868, the first such health board of its time. In 1887, engineers devised a way to reverse the flow of the Chicago River, by creating the Sanitary and Ship Canal. The canal served as an efficient means of draining waste water from the city.

While these acts and engineering feats did much to improve public health, the biggest advances in sanitation were made as the result of scientific breakthroughs. In the 1860s, the British surgeon Joseph Lister (1827-1912), introduced the use of antiseptic solutions in hospitals. Two decades later considerable evidence began to emerge that disease could be caused by microscopic infectious agents, and the bacteria responsible for cholera, tuberculosis, anthrax and other deadly illnesses were discovered. Louis Pasteur (1822-1895), French chemist and microbiologist, created a technique for reducing th the virulence of disease-causing organisms, known today as pasteurization. The German physician Robert Koch (1843-1910) demonstrated the use of sterilization, employing steam to kill infectious microorganisms on surgical instruments. By the early twentieth century, it was learned that insects and arthropods could spread diseases such as malaria, yellow fever, and typhus.

Thoughout the past one hundred years, our understanding of the cause and spread of illnesses has increased dramatically. Modern sanitary techniques and public health laws are based on this understanding. Today, in most industrialized countries the use of sophisticated filtration devices and chemical treatment assures a clean water supply. Antiseptic hospital environments and sanitary food preparation facilities help to reduce the risk of disease transmission. Many formerly common illnesses can now be prevented, or their virulence reduced, because of the development of immunizations. The use of antibiotic treatments has also helped curb the spread of many diseases, though bacterial resistance to antibiotic agents is an ever-present threat to public health.

SANTORIO, SANTORIO (1561-1636)

Italian physician

Santorio Santorio, also known as Sanctorius, was born at Capodistria (now Italy) on March 29, 1561; he died in Venice on February 22, 1636. He was the founder of modern quantitative medical research. After graduating in medicine at the University of Padua in 1582, Sanctorius began practice in Venice. In 1587, he was appointed physician to the King of Poland, in which capacity he remained for 14 years. Upon returning from Poland, he re-established his practice in Venice. In 1611, he was called to the Chair of Theoretical Medicine at the University of Padua, where he remained until his resignation in 1629 and return to practice and research in Venice.

Sanctorius was largely responsible for the entry of clinical observation and experimental medicine into the physician's domain in the late sixteenth century. (His counterpart in England was William Harvey.) Sanctorius' introduction of the physical sciences into medical investigation has led to his being referred to as a principal architect of the *iatrophysical* school of medicine.

Sanctorius studied the process of metabolism by observing the weight fluctuations in his own body over the course of a day, and during various metabolic processes such as digestion, sleeping, and eating. To carry out these measurements, he used a set of specially constructed devices, including a balance scale, a pulse monitor (pulsilogium), a hydrometer to measure the moisture content in gas, and a chair suspended from a steelyard which was designed to measure what he referred to as *insensible perspiration* (which referred to the volatile substances that were supposed to leave the body). By weighing all the food and drink that he ingested and all the excreta that he passed, Sanctorius obtained numerical measurements for his insensible perspiration. Through these experiments, Sanctorius introduced the quantitative aspect into medical research, and at the same time founded the modern study of **metabolism**.

It is, however, for the invention of one of the first thermometers that Sanctorius is best known (described in his commentary on the first book of the Canon of Avicenna in 1625, which also gave a description of how the instrument was to be used in studying diseases). Sanctorius's thermometer, like the ones developed by Cornelius Drebbel, Robert Fludd, and Galileo at about the same time, consisted of an enclosed vessel containing air that contracted or expanded with the temperature, forcing water to move up or down a tube with arbitrary calibrations.

Other inventions for which Sanctorius is credited include an instrument for extracting bladder stones, a surgical device for the withdrawal of fluids from body cavities (i.e., trocar and cannula), an instrument for removing foreign bodies from the **ear**, a hygrometer to measure humidity, and a device for bathing patients in bed. In 1602, Sanctorius made reference to an instrument for comparing the rates of pulses that consisted of a pendulum attached to a string of variable length; the length of the string was adjusted until the beat of the pendulum coincided with that of the pulse. (Pulses were compared by comparing the lengths of string.)

Sanctorius's greatest inventions, i.e., his thermometer and pulse monitor, were eventually forgotten, only to be rediscovered 100 years later. Sanctorius authored *Ars de statica medicina* (*On Statistical Medicine*) in 1614, a work that reached its fifth edition in 1737. The frontispiece of this work shows Sanctorius seated in his chair suspended from a steelyard in the process of weighing himself after a meal; this plate has become a classic in the archives of medical illustration.

SATCHER, DAVID (1941-)

American physician and surgeon general

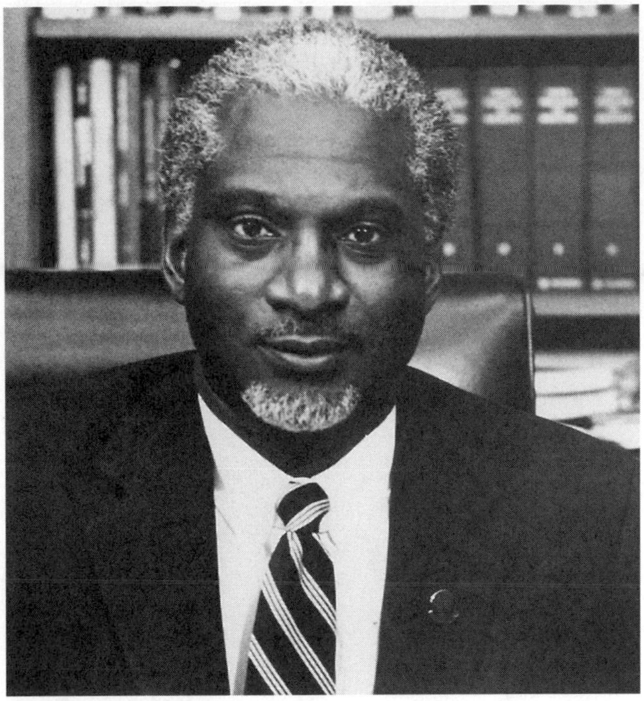

David Satcher

An African-American physician who grew up in the South at a time when white physicians would not treat black people, Satcher was sworn in as the 16th surgeon general of the United States and assistant secretary for health on February 13, 1998. In these posts, he has tried to make good on his youthful pledge to ''make the greatest difference to those with the greatest need.''

Satcher was born near Anniston, Alabama, on his parents' farm. His father worked at a local foundry, and neither parent had any formal education. Satcher graduated as valedictorian from his segregated high school and went on to the distinguished, all-black Morehouse College in Atlanta, Georgia, with a full scholarship. While there, he took an active part in the civil rights movement and was arrested several times for participating in sit-ins and other civil unrest. Satcher graduated magna cum laude from Morehouse in 1963, and enrolled at Case Western Reserve University's medical school as one of only two black students there. He earned his medical degree there and completed his Ph.D. in cytogenetics at the school in 1970, having won several coveted awards for academic work and quality of patient care.

After performing his internship from 1970 to 1971 at the University of Rochester School of Medicine, Satcher worked for a year as a resident physician at a migrant worker health center. In 1972 he left for California, where he took a position as director of the Community Hypertension Outreach Program at the Martin Luther King Jr. General Hospital, located in the crime- and poverty-plagued Watts section of Los Angeles. Satcher remained in that post until 1975, when he opened a free clinic in Watts in a church basement, serving as its medical director until 1979. In the meantime, Satcher had also become affiliated with the Drew Medical School in various capacities, eventually working there as interim dean from 1977 to 1979, and the University of California at Los Angeles School of Public Health, where he taught epidemiology as an assistant professor from 1974 to 1979.

Satcher returned to Morehouse in 1979 as a department chair in the medical school, but by 1982 he was on the move again—this time to Medharry Medical College in Nashville, Tennessee, to assume its presidency. His challenge was to rejuvenate the nearly bankrupt old predominantly black school and its associated teaching college, which he did by increasing federal grants and donations by millions of dollars. He also fought successfully to merge the Medharry teaching college with the ailing, white-controlled public hospital in Nashville in a controversial move that paid off with a stronger, integrated institution. In addition, Satcher worked hard to improve the outlook of many of Nashville's inner-city black youths, who were falling prey to drugs, teenage **pregnancy**, and violent crime at alarming rates.

Satcher remained at Medharry until 1993, when the federal government appointed him director of the **Centers for Disease Control** (CDC) and he became administrator of the Agency for Toxic Substances and Disease Registry. As CDC director, he mounted ambitious programs to educate people about ways to prevent early death from **AIDS**, lack of exercise, poor **nutrition**, and smoking. His advertising campaigns to encourage teens to use **condoms** caused outrage in some quarters, but Satcher responded with his characteristic composure that ''educating people about condoms does not increase sexual activity. It does increase the use of condoms by people who are sexually active.'' He has also sponsored programs to limit teenagers' access to guns, knives, alcohol, and areas in which violent crime often occur, such as abandoned buildings. These efforts, as well, have met with opposition from law-enforcement officials, who say Satcher's efforts infringe on their domain, but Satcher maintains that youth violence is a public-health issue, and so rightfully the province of the CDC.

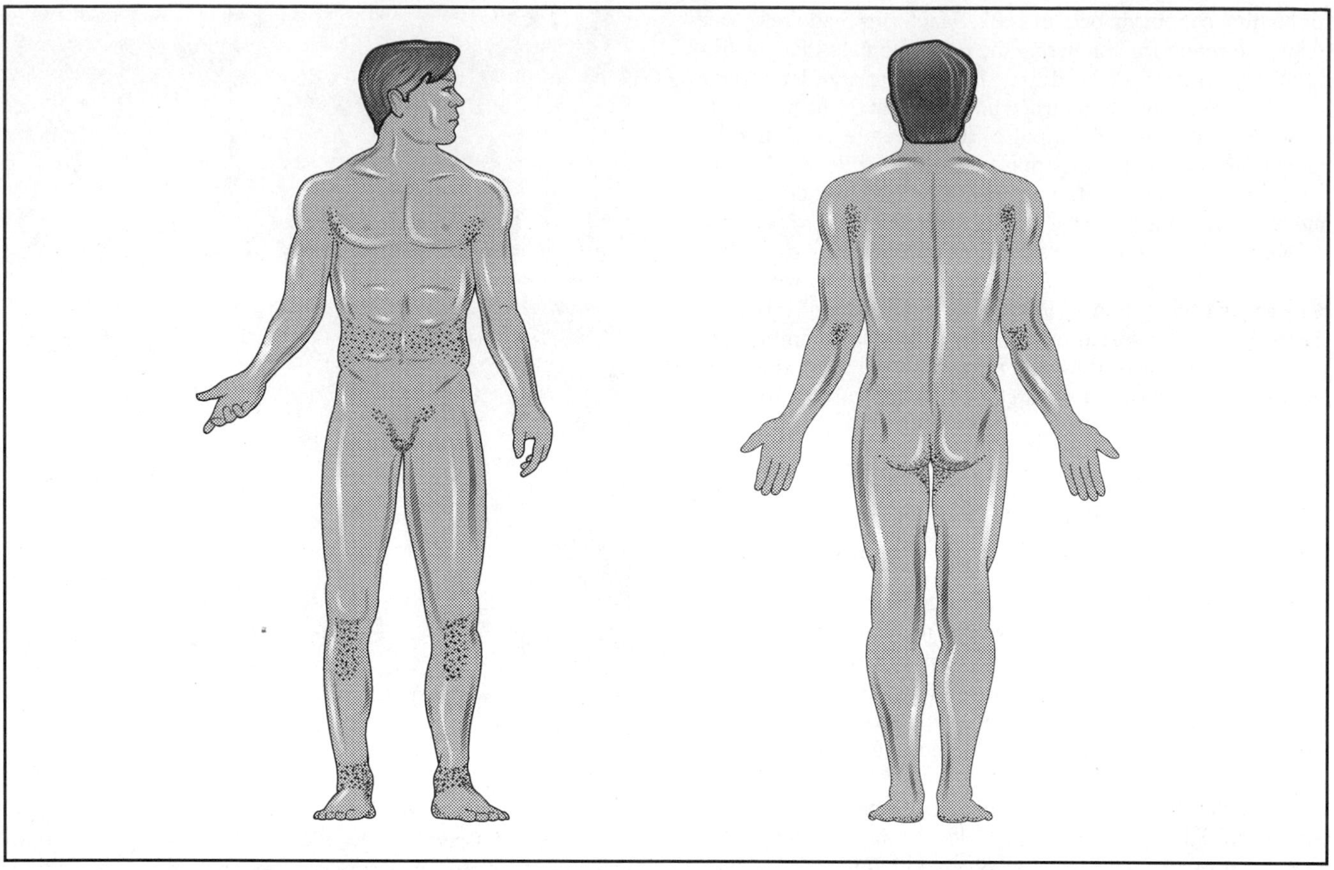

Scabies is a contagious skin infection common among people who live in overcrowded, less than ideal hygienic environments. It is caused by the infestation of female scab mites that, upon contact, burrows under the victim's skin and lays eggs along the lines of passage. Once the eggs hatch, the new mites rise to the skin's surface, mate, and repeat the infestation. Scabies can occur anywhere on the body, including the armpit, groin, buttocks, genital area, and ankles, as shown in the illustration above. ***(Illustration by Electronic Illustrators Group.)***

Under Satcher's direction, the CDC also expanded its **breast cancer**- and **cervical cancer** screening programs from only 18 states to 50.

President Bill Clinton nominated Satcher as surgeon general in 1997, praising the CDC and its director for declines in **infant mortality**, AIDS deaths, and teen pregnancy. Satcher accepted the nomination, saying that his goal would be to "take the best science in the world and place it firmly within the grasp of all Americans." He was sworn in as surgeon general for the Department of Health and Human Services (HHS) in early 1998, also assuming the position of assistant secretary for health for the organization. In the latter post, Satcher serves as director of the Office of Public Health and Science and as senior adviser to HHS Secretary Donna Shalala. As of 1999, he continued in both posts.

See also Centers for Disease Control

SCABIES

Scabies is a relatively contagious infection caused by a tiny, 0.3 mm long insect called a mite. When a human comes in contact with the female mite, the mite burrows under the skin, laying eggs along the line of its burrow. These eggs hatch, and the resulting offspring rise to the surface of the skin, mate, and repeat the cycle either within the skin of the original host, or within the skin of its next victim.

The intense **itching** almost always caused by scabies is due to a reaction within the skin to the feces of the mite. The first time someone is infected with scabies, he or she may not notice any itching for a number of weeks (four to six weeks). With subsequent infections, the itchiness will begin within hours of picking up the first mite. Scratching seems to serve some purpose in scabies, as the mites are apparently often inadvertently removed.

Scabies is most common among people who live in overcrowded conditions, and whose ability to practice good hygiene is limited. Scabies can be passed between people by close skin contact. Although the mites can only live away from human skin for about three days, sharing clothing or bedclothes can pass scabies among family members or close contacts.

The itching from scabies is worse after a hot shower and at night. Burrows are seen as winding, slightly raised gray lines along the skin. The female mite may be seen at one end of the burrow, as a tiny pearl-like bump underneath the skin. Because of the intense itching, burrows may be obscured by scratch marks left by the patient. The most common locations for burrows include the sides of the fingers, between the fingers, the top of the wrists, around the elbows and armpits, around the nipples of the breasts in women, in the genitalia of men, around the waist (beltline), and on the lower part of the buttocks. Babies may have burrows on the soles of their feet, palms of their hands, and faces.

Most infestations with scabies are caused by no more than 15 mites altogether. Infestation with huge numbers of mites (on the order of thousands to millions) occurs when an individual does not scratch, or when an individual has a weakened **immune system**. These patients include those who live in institutions; are mentally retarded, or physically infirm; have other diseases which affect the amount of sensation they have in their skin (**leprosy** or syringomyelia); have **leukemia** or **diabetes mellitus**; are taking medications which lower their immune response (**cancer chemotherapy**, drugs given after **organ transplantation**); or have other diseases which lower their immune response (such as acquired immunodeficiency syndrome or **AIDS**). This form of scabies, with its major infestation, is referred to as crusted scabies or Norwegian scabies. Infected patients have thickened, crusty areas all over their bodies, including over the scalp. Their skin is scaly. Their fingernails may be thickened and horny.

Diagnosis can be made simply by observing the characteristic burrows of the mites causing scabies. A sterilized needle can be used to explore the pearly bump at the end of a burrow, remove its contents, and place it on a slide to be examined. The mite itself may then be identified under a microscope.

Occasionally, a type of mite carried on dogs may infect humans. These mites cannot survive for very long on humans, and so the infection is very light.

Several types of lotions (1% lindane or 5% permethrin) can be applied to the body, and left on for 12-24 hours. This is usually sufficient, although it may be reapplied after a week if mites remain. Preparations containing lindane should not be used to treat pregnant women and infants. **Itching** can be lessened by the use of calamine lotion and **antihistamine** medications.

The prognosis (expected outcome) for complete recovery from scabies infestation is excellent. In patients with weak immune systems, the biggest danger is that the areas of skin involved with scabies will become secondarily infected with bacteria.

Good hygiene is essential in the prevention of scabies. When a member of a household is diagnosed with scabies, all that person's recently-worn clothing and bedding should be washed in very hot water.

SCARLET FEVER

Scarlet fever, caused by Group A streptococcal bacteria, was a common disease at one time, especially in children. Named for the flushing of the face that it causes, it is characterized by a sore throat, chills, fever, headache, vomiting, rapid pulse, red rash, and an inflamed or ''strawberry'' tongue. Scarlet fever (sometimes called *scarlatina*) was named by **Thomas Sydenham**, an English physician who was known as the ''English Hippocrates.'' From the time he began his medical career in 1656, Sydenham kept thorough records of patients. Astute observations led him to conclude that there were differences between **measles** and scarlet fever which up until that time were thought to be the same disease. He named scarlet fever for its most distinguishing characteristics.

In the early twentieth century, Alphonse Dochez, a pioneer in the field of respiratory diseases, studied many cases of scarlet fever as a doctor during World War I. When he returned to his professorship at Johns Hopkins Medical School, and later at Columbia University, he worked on the relationship between streptococcus bacteria and scarlet fever. Many doctors of the time did not believe that scarlet fever was caused by streptococci, but Dochez was convinced. Definitive proof was obtained when he inoculated a pig with the streptococcus bacteria. Late one night Dochez called an associate of his and asked him to come over to see ''his little pig, as rosy as a boiled lobster,'' thus showing that the bacteria did cause scarlet fever symptoms. He also used an *antitoxin* injection (called antiserum at the time) that whitened the rash of scarlet fever and had a therapeutic effect.

At the same time that Dochez was developing his scarlet fever antitoxin, another group of American researchers, George and Gladys Dick, were developing their diagnostic test for scarlet fever (the *Dick test*) and their antitoxin treatment. Although Dochez had obtained a British patent for his antitoxin in 1924 (earlier than the Dicks), his U.S. patent was dated 1926—later than those obtained by the Dicks. Thus, a court ruling forced Dochez to give up his work on the antitoxin in favor of the Dicks. From the mid 1920s, the Dick test was administered to thousands of children. For those without immunity to the disease, the antitoxin was prescribed.

In 1924, **Anna Wessels Williams**, an American doctor who isolated the **diphtheria** bacteria and developed lab procedures for detecting **typhoid fever** and **rabies**, also began working with scarlet fever. She published papers detailing the use of the Dick test to diagnose scarlet fever with more than 21,000 school children. Like Dochez, Williams performed laboratory experiments with the streptococci which cause scarlet fever. She helped discover that toxin-producing *hemolytic* (capable of destroying red blood cells) streptococci could be isolated not only from infected wounds but even from the throats of healthy people. She found that not all scarlet fever toxins were identical, which led to her explanation of why the disease could recur even after immunization.

During the 1930s and 1940s, the world was forever changed with the development of **antibiotic** drugs. Because scarlet fever is caused by streptococcus bacteria, it was a good candidate for treatment with antibiotics. **Penicillin** worked especially well, wiping out the streptococcus infection in individuals and, on a larger scale, preventing the kinds of epidemics which had been common in the past.

SCHALLY, ANDREW V. (1926-)

Polish American biochemist

Andrew V. Schally helped conduct pioneering research concerning hormones, identifying three brain hormones and greatly advancing scientists' understanding of the function and interaction of the brain with the rest of the body. His findings have proved useful in the treatment of diabetes and peptic ulcers, and in the diagnosis and treatment of hormone-deficiency diseases. Schally shared the 1977 Nobel Prize with French-born American endocrinologist Roger Guillemin and Rosalyn Yalow (an American scientist whose work in the discovery and development of radioimmunoassay, the use of radioactive substances to find and measure minute substances—especially hormones—in blood and tissue, helped Schally and Guillemin isolate and analyze peptide hormones).

Andrew Victor Schally was born on November 30, 1926, in Wilno, Poland, to Casimir Peter Schally and Maria Lacka Schally. His father served in the military on the side of the Allies during World War II, and Schally grew up during Nazi occupation of his homeland. The family later left Poland and immigrated to Scotland, where Schally entered the Bridge Allen School in Scotland. He studied chemistry at the University of London and obtained his first research position at London's highly regarded National Institute for Medical Research. Leaving London for Montreal, Canada, in 1952, Schally entered McGill University, where he studied endocrinology and conducted research on the adrenal and pituitary glands. He obtained his doctorate in biochemistry from McGill in 1957. Also in 1957, Schally became an assistant professor of physiology at Baylor University School of Medicine in Houston, Texas. There he was able to pursue his interest in the hormones produced by the hypothalamus.

Scientists had long thought that the hypothalamus, a part of the brain located just above the pituitary gland, regulated the endocrine system, which includes the pituitary, thyroid and adrenal glands, the pancreas, and the ovaries and testicles. They were, however, unsure of the way in which hypothalamic hormonal regulation occurred. In the 1930s British anatomist Geoffrey W. Harris theorized that hypothalamic regulation occurred by means of hormones, chemical substances secreted by glands and transported by the blood. Harris was able to support his hypothesis by conducting experiments that demonstrated altered pituitary function when the blood vessels between the hypothalamus and the pituitary were cut. Harris and others were unable to isolate or identify the hormones from the hypothalamus.

Schally devoted his work to identifying these hormones. He and Roger Guillemin, who also worked at Baylor University's School of Medicine, were engaged in research to unmask the chemical structure of corticotropin-releasing hormone (CRH). Their efforts, however, were unsuccessful—the structure was not determined until 1981. The two then focused their work, independently, on other hormones of the hypothalamus. Schally left Baylor in 1962, when he became director of the Endocrine and Polypeptide Laboratory at the Veterans Administration (VA) Hospital in New Orleans, Louisiana. Also that year, Schally became a U.S. citizen and took on the post of assistant professor of medicine at Tulane University Medical School.

Schally's first breakthrough came in 1966 when he and his research group isolated TRH, or thyrotropin-releasing hormone. In 1969 Schally and his VA team demonstrated that TRH is a peptide containing three amino acids. It was Guillemin, though, who first determined TRH's chemical structure. The success of this research made it possible to decipher the function of a second hormone, called luteinizing-hormone releasing factor (LHRH). Identified in 1971, LHRH is a decapeptide and controls reproductive functions in both males and females. The chemical makeup of the growth-releasing hormone (GRH) was also discovered by Schally's team in 1971. Schally was able to show that GRH, a peptide consisting of ten amino acids, causes the release of gonadotropins from the pituitary gland. These gonadotropins, in turn, cause male and female sex hormones to be released from the testicles and ovaries. In conjunction with this, Schally was able to identify a factor that inhibits the release of GRH in 1976. Guillemin, however, had determined its structure earlier and named it somatostatin. Subsequent studies by Schally showed that somatostatin serves multiple roles, some of which relate to insulin production and growth disorders. This led to speculation that the hormone could be useful for treating diabetes and acromegaly, a growth-disorder disease.

The hormone research done by Schally and his colleagues was tedious and expensive. Thousands of sheep and pig hypothalami were required to extract the smallest amount of hormone. These organs were solicited from many area slaughterhouses and required immediate dissection to prevent the hormones from degrading. Their accomplishment of isolating the first milligram of pure thyrotropin-releasing hormone, Guillemin stated, cost many times more than the NASA space mission that brought a kilogram of moon rock back to earth.

Schally's intense years of hard work and accomplishment were capped by the Nobel Prize, but he has also received many other awards and honors. In 1974 he was given the Charles Mickle Award of the University of Toronto, and the Gairdner Foundation International Award. He received the Borden Award in the Medical Sciences of the Association of American Medical Colleges in 1975 and, that same year, the Lasker Award and the Laude Award. He has held memberships in the National Academy of Sciences, the American Society of Biological Chemists, the American Physiology Society, the American Association for the Advancement of Science, and the Endocrine Society. In the years prior to receiving the Nobel Prize, Schally and his colleagues published more than 850 papers. Married to Brazilian endocrinologist, Ana Maria de Medeiros-Comaru, Schally often lectures in Latin America and Spain. He and his first wife, Margaret Rachel White, have two children.

SCHISTOSOMIASIS

Schistosomiasis, also known as bilharziasis, or snail **fever**, is a primarily tropical parasitic disease caused by the larvae of one or more of five types of flatworms or blood flukes known as schistosomes. The name bilharziasis comes from Theodor Bilharz, a German pathologist, who identified the worms in 1851.

Infections associated with worms present some of the most universal health problems in the world. In fact, only **malaria** accounts for more diseases than schistosomiasis. The World Health Organization (WHO) estimates that 200 million people are infected and 120 million display symptoms. Another 600 million people are at-risk of infection. Schistosomes are prevalent in rural and outlying city areas of 74 countries in Africa, Asia, and Latin America. In Central China and Egypt, the disease poses a major health risk.

There are five species of schistosomes that are prevalent in different areas of the world and produce somewhat different symptoms:

- *Schistosoma mansoni* is widespread in Africa, the Eastern-Mediterranean, the Caribbean, and South America and can only infect humans and rodents.
- *S. mekongi* is prevalent only in the Mekong river basin in Asia.
- *S. japonicum* is limited to China and the Philippines and can infect other mammals, in addition to humans, such as pigs, dogs, and water buffalos. As a result, it can be harder to control disease caused by this species.
- *S. intercalatum* is found in central Africa.
- *S. haematobium* occurs predominantly in Africa and the Eastern Mediterranean.

Intestinal schistosomiasis, caused by *Schistosoma japonicum, S. mekongi, mansoni*, and *S. intercalatum*, can lead to serious complications of the liver and spleen. Urinary schistosomiasis is caused by *S. haematobium*.

It is difficult to know how many individuals die of schistosomiasis each year because death certificates and patient records seldom identify schistosomiasis as the primary cause of death. Mortality estimates vary related to the type of schistosome infection but is generally low, for example, 2.4 of 100,000 die each year from infection with *S. mansoni*.

All five species are contracted in the same way, through direct contact with fresh water infested with the free-living form of the parasite known as cercariae. The building of dams, irrigation systems, and reservoirs, and the movements of refugee groups introduce and spread schistosomiasis.

Eggs are excreted in human urine and feces and, in areas with poor sanitation, contaminate freshwater sources. The eggs break open to release a form of the parasite called miracidium. Freshwater snails become infested with the miracidium, which multiply inside the snail and mature into multiple cercariae that the snail ejects into the water. The cercariae, which survive outside a host for 48 hours, quickly penetrate unbroken skin, the lining of the mouth, or the gastrointestinal tract. Once inside the human body, the worms penetrate the wall of the nearest vein and travel to the liver where they grow and sexually mature. Mature male and female worms pair and migrate either to the intestines or the bladder where egg production occurs. One female worm may lay an average of 200 to 2,000 eggs per day for up to twenty years. Most eggs leave the blood stream and body through the intestines. Some of the eggs are not excreted, however, and can lodge in the tissues. It is the presence of these eggs, rather than the worms themselves, that causes the disease.

Many individuals do not experience symptoms. If present, it usually takes four to six weeks for symptoms to appear. The first symptom of the disease may be a general ill feeling. Within twelve hours of infection, an individual may complain of a tingling sensation or light rash, commonly referred to as ''swimmer's itch,'' due to irritation at the point of entrance. The rash that may develop can mimic **scabies** and other types of **rashes**. Other symptoms can occur two to ten weeks later and can include fever, aching, **cough**, **diarrhea**, or gland enlargement. These symptoms can also be related to avian schistosomiasis which does not cause any further symptoms in humans.

Another primary condition, called Katayama fever, may also develop from infection with these worms, and it can be very difficult to recognize. Symptoms include fever, lethargy, the eruption of pale temporary bumps associated with severe **itching** (urticarial) rash, liver and spleen enlargement, and bronchospasm.

In intestinal schistosomiasis, eggs become lodged in the intestinal wall and cause an **immune system** reaction called a granulomatous reaction. This immune response can lead to obstruction of the colon and blood loss. The infected individual may have what appears to be a potbelly. Eggs can also become lodged in the liver, leading to high blood pressure through the liver, enlarged spleen, the build-up of fluid in the abdomen (ascites), and potentially life-threatening dilations or swollen areas in the esophagus or gastrointestinal tract that can tear and bleed profusely (esophageal varices). Rarely, the central **nervous system** may be affected. Individuals with chronic active schistosomiasis may not complain of typical symptoms.

Urinary tract schistosomiasis is characterized by blood in the urine, **pain** or difficulty urinating, and frequent urination and are associated with *S. haematobium*. The loss of blood can lead to **iron deficiency anemia**. A large percentage of persons, especially children, who are moderately to heavily infected experience urinary tract damage that can lead to blocking of the urinary tract and bladder cancer.

Proper diagnosis and treatment may require a tropical disease specialist because the disease can be confused with malaria or typhoid in the early stages. The healthcare provider should do a thorough history of travel in endemic areas. The rash, if present, can mimic scabies or other rashes, and the gastrointestinal symptoms may be confused with those caused by bacterial illnesses or other intestinal parasites. These other conditions will need to be excluded before an accurate diagnosis can be made. As a result, clinical evidence of exposure to infected water along with physical findings, a negative test for malaria, and an increased number of one type of immune cell, called an eosinophil, are necessary to diagnose acute schistosomiasis.

Eggs may be detected in the feces or urine. Repeated stool (feces) tests may be required to concentrate and identify the eggs. Blood tests may be used to detect a particular antigen or particle associated with the schistosome that induces an immune response. Persons infected with schistosomiasis may not test positive for six months, and as a result, tests may need to be repeated to obtain an accurate diagnosis. Blood can be detected visually in the urine or with chemical strips that react to small amounts of blood.

Sophisticated imaging techniques, such as **ultrasound**, computed tomography scan (CT scan), and **magnetic resonance imaging** (MRI), can detect damage to the blood vessels in the liver and visualize polyps and ulcers of the urinary tract, for example, that occur in the more advanced stages. *S. haematobium* is difficult to diagnose with ultrasound in pregnant women.

The use of medications against schistosomiasis, such as praziquantel (Biltricide), oxamniquine, and metrifonate, have been shown to be safe and effective. Praziquantel is effective against all forms of schistosomiasis and has few side effects. This drug is given in either two or three doses over the course of a single day. Oxamniquine is typically used in Africa and South America to treat intestinal schistosomiasis. Metrifonate has been found to be safe and effective in the treatment of urinary schistosomiasis. Patients are typically checked for the presence of living eggs three and six months after treatment. If the number of eggs excreted has not significantly decreased, the patient may require another course of medication.

If treated early, prognosis (expected outcome) is very good and complete recovery is expected. The illness is treatable, but people can die from the effects of untreated schistosomiasis. The severity of the disease depends on the number of worms, or worm load, in addition to how long the person has been infected. With treatment, the number of worms can be substantially reduced, and the secondary conditions can be treated. The goal of the World Health Organization is to reduce the severity of the disease rather than to completely stop transmission of the disease. There is, however, little natural immunity to reinfection. Treated individuals do not usually require retreatment for two to five years in areas of low transmission. The World Health Organization has made research to develop a vaccine against the disease one of its priorities.

Prevention of the disease involves several targets and requires long term community commitment. Infected patients require diagnosis, treatment, and education about how to avoid reinfecting themselves and others. Adequate healthcare facilities need to be available, water systems must be treated to kill the worms and control snail populations, and sanitation must be improved to prevent the spread of the disease.

To avoid schistosomiasis in endemic areas (areas where disease is highly prevalent):

- Contact the CDC for current health information on travel destinations.
- Upon arrival, ask an informed local authority about the infestation of schistosomiasis before being exposed to fresh water in countries that are likely to have the disease.
- Do not swim, stand, wade, or take baths in untreated water.
- Treat all water used for drinking or bathing. Water can be treated by letting it stand for three days, heating it for five minutes to around 122°F (50°C), or filtering or treating water chemically with chlorine or iodine, as with drinking water.
- Should accidental exposure occur, infection can be prevented by hastily drying off or applying rubbing alcohol to the exposed area.

See also Roundworm infections

SCHIZOPHRENIA

Schizophrenia, the most serious, complicated, and disabling of all **mental illnesses**, is a brain disorder which severely interferes with an individual's ability to think clearly, make decisions, and separate reality from what's happening in their mind. It affects one in every 100 people world-wide, males and females equally, has the highest suicide rate of all psychiatric disorders, and predominantly manifests in adolescence through the 30s. While there is still much controversy over the subject, many experts believe schizophrenia is a combination of a number of mental illnesses. Two studies by the National Institutes of Mental Health show that mood disorders (**bipolar disorder/depression**) are comorbid (present) in 80% of schizophrenics, prompting the belief that they are a fundamental part of the disease, not just a symptom of it. While schizophrenia cannot be cured, its symptoms are highly treatable with medication.

Schizophrenia, perhaps the most misunderstood mental illness, is not a split personality, a character floor, nor caused by poor parenting. It is a biological disorder due to very subtle abnormalities in the brain. Symptoms can be divided into three major categories: Positive, Negative, and Disorganized. *Positive* does not mean good in this sense, but ''something that should not be there.'' Positive symptoms are often referred to as psychotic because the individual experiences hallucinations- -hearing voices or seeing things which are not real, and delusions—believing people are reading their minds, controlling their thoughts, and plotting against them. *Negative* symptoms are things which ''should be there but are not.'' They interfere with the person's ability to function and include blunted emotions—laughing or crying is almost nonexistent, lack of motivation or energy—extreme cases need help even with simple tasks like taking a shower or changing clothes, lack of interest—even in the things that once brought pleasure, and limited speech—inability to say anything new or carry on a flowing conversation. *Disorganized* symptoms manifest in confused thought and speech, disjointed conversation, disorganized perceptions which cause everyday sights, sounds, and feelings to become terrifying, and disorganized behavior manifesting in repetitive movements which have no reason or purpose. In severe cases, the individual may become catatonic (resisting all attempts to be moved).

Discovery in the 1950s that schizophrenia responded dramatically to drugs settled the debate and determined its cause to be biological. Antipsychotic drugs, such as ''*atypical antipsychotics*'' because of fewer side effect—are either in use

might include **magnetic resonance imaging** (MRI) and **computed tomography scans** (CT scans). Other tests examine the conduction of electricity through nerve tissues, and include studies of the electrical activity generated as muscles contract (electromyography), nerve conduction velocity, and evoked potential testing. A more invasive test involves injecting a contrast substance into the space between the vertebrae and making x-ray images of the spinal cord (myelography), but this procedure is usually done only if surgery is being considered. All of these tests can reveal problems with the vertebrae, the disk, or the nerve itself.

Initial treatment for sciatica focuses on pain relief. For acute or very painful flare-ups, bed rest is advised for up to a week, along with medication for the pain. Pain medication includes **acetaminophen**, **nonsteroidal anti-inflammatory drugs** (NSAIDs), such as **aspirin**, or **muscle relaxants**. If the pain still does not cease, opioids (narcotic drugs) may be prescribed for short-term use or a local anesthetic will be injected directly into the lower back. **Massage** and heat application may be suggested as adjuncts (in addition).

If the pain is chronic, different pain relief medications are used to avoid long-term dosing of NSAIDs, muscle relaxants, and opioids. **Antidepressant drugs**, which have been shown to be effective in treating pain, may be prescribed alongside short-term use of muscle relaxants or NSAIDs. Local anesthetic injections or epidural steroids are used in selected cases.

As the pain allows, physical therapy is introduced into the treatment regime. Stretching **exercise**s that focus on the lower back, buttock, and hamstring muscles are suggested. The exercises also include finding comfortable, pain-reducing positions. Corsets and braces may be useful in some cases, but evidence for their general effectiveness is lacking. However, they may be helpful to prevent worsening of the condition related to certain activities.

With less pain and the success of early therapy, the individual is encouraged to follow a long-term program to maintain a healthy back and prevent re-injury. A physical therapist may suggest exercises and regular activity, such as water exercise or walking. Patients are instructed in proper body mechanics to minimize symptoms during light lifting or other activities.

If the pain is chronic and conservative treatment fails, surgery to repair a **herniated disk** or cut out part or all of the piriformis muscle may be suggested, particularly if there is evidence of nerve or nerve-root damage.

Massage is a recommended form of therapy, especially if the sciatic pain arises from muscle spasm. Symptoms may also be relieved by icing the painful area as soon as the pain occurs. Ice should be left on the area for 30-60 minutes several times a day. After two to three days, a hot water bottle or heating pad can replace the ice. **Chiropractic** or **osteopathy** may offer possible solutions for relieving pressure on the sciatic nerve and the accompanying pain. **Acupuncture** and **biofeedback** may also be useful as pain control methods. Body work, such as the Alexander technique, can assist an individual in improving posture and preventing further episodes of sciatic pain.

Most cases of sciatica are treatable with pain medication and physical therapy. After four to six weeks of treatment, an individual should be able to resume normal activities.

Some sources of sciatica are not preventable, such as disk degeneration, back strain due to **pregnancy**, or accidental falls. Other sources of back strain, such as poor posture, overexertion, being overweight, or wearing high heels, can be corrected or avoided. Cigarette smoking may also predispose (increase the chances of) people to pain, and should be discontinued.

General suggestions for avoiding sciatica, or preventing a repeat episode, include sleeping on a firm mattress, using chairs with firm back support, and sitting with both feet flat on the floor. Habitually crossing the legs while sitting can place excess pressure on the sciatic nerve. Sitting a lot can also place pressure on the sciatic nerves, so it's a good idea to take short breaks and move around during the work day, long trips, or any other situation that requires sitting for an extended length of time. If lifting is required, the back should be kept straight and the legs should provide the lift. Regular exercise, such as swimming and walking, can strengthen back muscles and improve posture. Exercise can also help maintain a healthy weight and lessen the likelihood of back strain.

SCLERODERMA

Scleroderma is a serious, progressive (worsening) disease thataffects the skin and connective tissue (including cartilage, bone, fat, and the tissue that supports the nerves and blood vessels throughout the body). Scleroderma is also frequently called systemic sclerosis.

Connective tissue is found throughout the body. It is a fibrous tissue produced by special cells called fibroblasts. Many cells of the **immune system** exist within the connective tissue. Connective tissue supports all of the structures of the body, including the skin, the organs, and all of the body's blood vessels and nerves. Collagen is a type of protein fiber present in connective tissue.

In scleroderma, collagen is over produced and is defective. Collagen then accumulates throughout the body, causing the hardening (sclerosis), scarring (fibrosis), and the damage characteristic of scleroderma. Because collagen is found so widely throughout the body, the effects of scleroderma are almost always widespread.

Scleroderma occurs in all races of people all over the world. Patients are most often diagnosed between the ages of 30-50 years old. Women are three to four times more likely to suffer from the disorder. Young Afro-American women and Choctaw Native Americans have particularly high rates of the disease. Although some cases of scleroderma clearly run in families, most cases of scleroderma occur without any known family tendency for the disease.

The cause of scleroderma remains puzzling. Although the accumulation of collagen appears to be a hallmark of the disease, doctors do not know why this happens. Some theories suggest that damage to blood vessels may occur prior to fibrosis. When blood vessels are damaged, the tissues of the body receive an inadequate amount of oxygen (a condition called ischemia). Some researchers believe that tissue ischemia and damage then causes the immune system to over react, creating an **autoimmune disorder**. The immune system is designed to produce antibodies—cells that fight foreign invaders like bacteria, viruses, and fungi. In this theory of scleroderma, the immune system gears up to fight an invader, but no invader is actually present. Instead, antibodies mistake the body's own tissues for foreign tissue. The immune system cells turn against the already damaged blood vessels and then the vessels' supporting tissues. These immune cells are designed to deliver potent chemicals in order to kill foreign invaders. Some of these cells dump these chemicals on the body's own tissues instead, causing inflammation, swelling, damage, and scarring.

Most cases of scleroderma occur with no recognizable initiating event. Some cases, however, have been traced to poisonous (toxic) exposures. For example, coal miners and gold miners (both of whom have a lot of exposure to silica dust) have higher than normal rates of scleroderma. Other types of chemicals that have been associated with scleroderma include polyvinyl chloride, benzine, toluene, and epoxy resins. In 1981, 20,000 people in Spain were stricken with a syndrome similar to scleroderma when a toxic substance accidentally contaminated cooking oil. Some claims of a scleroderma-like illness have been made by women with silicone breast implants.

About 95% of all patients with scleroderma have a condition called **Raynaud's disease** as their first symptom. In Raynaud's disease, the blood vessels of the fingers and/or toes (the digits) react abnormally to cold. The vessels clamp down, preventing blood flow to the end of the digit and, eventually, to the entire digit. The affected digit turns white, then blue, then red when it begins to get blood. Numbness, tingling, and **pain** are associated with this entire process. Over time, oxygen deprivation to these tissues may result in open, irritated pits (ulcers) in the surface of the skin. These ulcers can lead to tissue death (**gangrene**) and loss of the digit. These extreme symptoms of Raynaud's disease rarely occur, except when Raynaud's is associated with other conditions like scleroderma. When Raynaud's disease leads to scleroderma, the next symptoms are usually seen within two years of the first sign of Raynaud's.

Involvement of the skin leads to swelling underneath the skin of the hands, feet, legs, arms, and face. This is followed by thickening and tightening of the skin, which becomes taut and shiny. When this tightening is severe, it may cause deformity. For example, skin tightening on the hands may cause the fingers to become permanently curled (flexed), with no ability to straighten them. Structures within the skin are damaged (including those producing hair, oil, and sweat), and skin becomes dry and scaly. Ulcers may form, with the danger of infection. Calcium deposits often appear under the skin (calcinosis).

As the skin grows tight on the face, the mouth and nose become smaller. The small mouth may interfere with eating and caring for the teeth. Blood vessels under the skin may become enlarged and obvious through the skin, appearing as purplish marks (telangiectasis).

Muscle weakness, joint pain and stiffness, and **carpal tunnel syndrome** are common. Carpal tunnel syndrome involves scarring in the wrist, which puts pressure on the median nerve running through that area. This causes numbness, tingling, and weakness of some of the fingers.

The tube leading from the mouth to the stomach (the esophagus) becomes stiff and scarred. Patients may experience difficulty swallowing food. The acidic contents of the stomach may be allowed to flow backwards into the esophagus (esophageal reflux), causing severe symptoms of heartburn. Inflammation of the esophagus may occur (esophagitis).

The intestine becomes sluggish in processing food, causing bloating and pain. Foods are improperly processed, resulting in **diarrhea**, weight loss, and **anemia**. Telangiectasis developing in the stomach or intestine may cause rupture and bleeding.

The lungs are affected in about 66% of all patients with scleroderma. Complications include **shortness of breath**, coughing, difficulty breathing due to tightening of the tissue around the chest, inflammation of the air sacs of the lung (alveolitis), increased chance of **pneumonia**, and an increased risk of **cancer**. All of these have made lung disease the most likely cause of death in scleroderma.

The lining around the heart (pericardium) may become inflamed (**pericarditis**). The heart may have an increasing amount of difficulty pumping blood effectively (**heart failure**). Irregular heart rhythms and enlargement of the heart also occur in scleroderma.

Kidney disease is a common complication. Damage to blood vessels of the kidneys is often responsible for a huge spike in blood pressure, called malignant **hypertension**. The blood pressure may be so high that the patient suffers from swelling of the brain, with an extreme **headache**, damage to the retinas of the eyes, **seizures**, and failure of the heart to pump blood into the body's circulatory system. The kidneys may also stop filtering blood appropriately, leading to kidney failure. Treatments for high blood pressure and these kidney complications have greatly improved. Prior to these treatments, kidney problems were the most common cause of death for patients with scleroderma.

Other problems associated with scleroderma include painful dryness of the eyes and mouth, a low functioning thyroid gland (hypothyroidism), difficulty of male patients to achieve/sustain an erection of the penis, and enlargement and destruction of the liver.

Diagnosis involves recognizing the relatively unique characteristics of scleroderma symptoms. However, some of these symptoms can accompany other connective tissue diseases. Some nonspecific laboratory tests that may indicate an inflammatory disorder (but not specifically scleroderma) include:

- Elevated results from a special red blood cell test erythrocyte sedimentation rate)
- Decreased red blood cell count (anemia)

- Positive tests for certain antibodies (including rheumatoid factor, anti-Scl-70 antibodies, anticentrometre antibodies, and antinuclear antibodies).

Other tests can be performed to evaluate the extent of the disease. These can include:

- A test that reveals information about the electrical system of the heart (an electrocardiogram)
- Lung function tests
- X-ray studies of the gastrointestinal tract
- Various blood tests to study kidney functions.

There is no cure for scleroderma. A drug called D-penicillamine has been used to interfere with the defective collagen. It is believed to help decrease the degree of skin thickening and tightening, and to slow the progress of the disease in other organs. Steroid medications have been used to interfere with the inflammatory process in scleroderma. Other drugs have been studied that reduce the activity of the immune system (**immunosuppressants**), including azathioprine, colchicine, **interferon**, and 5-fluorouracil. Because they can have serious side effects, these medications are only used for the most severe cases of scleroderma.

The various complications of scleroderma are treated individually. Raynaud's disease requires that patients try to keep their hands and feet warm constantly, and avoid situations where they will be exposed to cold temperatures. Thick ointments and creams are used to treat dry skin. **Exercise** and **massage** may help joint involvement, and may help patients retain more movement despite skin tightening. Skin ulcers will need prompt attention and may require **antibiotics**. Patients with esophageal reflux will be advised to eat small meals more often. They should also avoid foods that may make the reflux worse, like spicy foods and **caffeine**-containing items like coffee, tea, and chocolate. Medications may be given to treat heartburn. Patients must be monitored for the development of high blood pressure, and promptly and aggressively treated with appropriate medications. When fluid accumulates due to heart failure, **diuretic** medications can be given to help get rid of the excess fluid.

The prognosis for patients with scleroderma varies. Some patients, in fact, have a very limited form of the disease and only their skin is affected. This is called morphea. These patients have a very good prognosis. Other patients with a cluster of symptoms called the CREST syndrome also have a relatively good prognosis. CREST stands for:

- C=Calcinosis
- R=Raynaud's disease
- E=Esophageal dysmotility (stiffness and malfunctioning of the esophagus)
- S=Sclerodactyly (thick, hard, rigid skin over the fingers)
- T=Telangiectasis.

In general, patients with very widespread skin involvement have the worse prognosis. This level of disease seems to be accompanied by involvement of other organs and the most severe complications. Although women are more commonly stricken with scleroderma, males more often die of the disease. The most common causes of death include heart, kidney, and lung diseases. About 65% of all patients survive 10 years or more following a diagnosis of scleroderma.

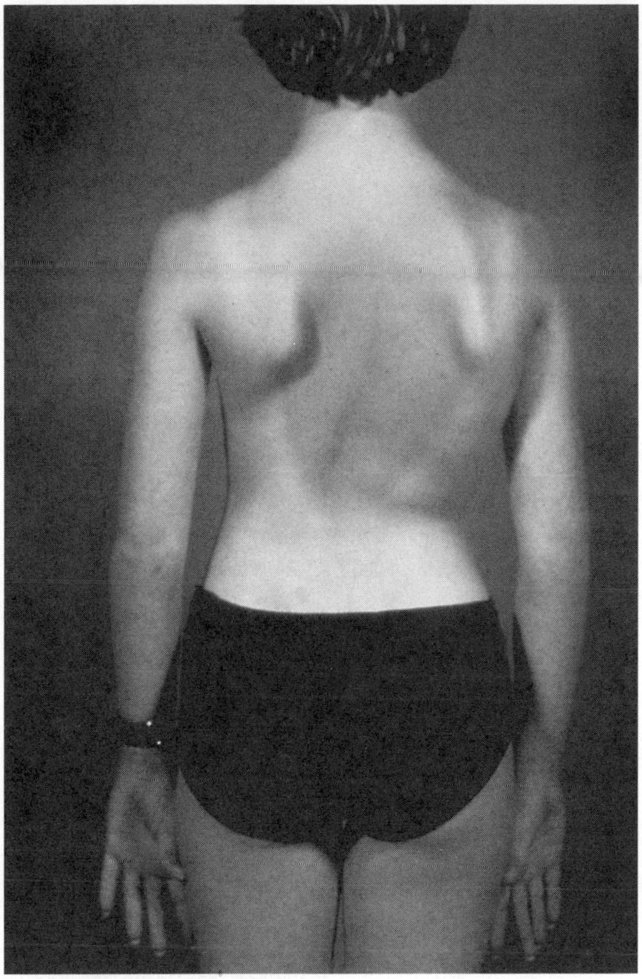

This woman suffers from scoliosis, or curvature of the spine. ***(Custom Medical Stock Photo. Reproduced by permission.)***

There are no known ways to prevent scleroderma. People can try to decrease exposure to those substances associated with high rates of the disease. These include silica dust, polyvinyl chloride, benzine, toluene, epoxy resins, and silicone breast implants.

See also Autoimmune disorders

Scoliosis

Scoliosis is a side-to-side curvature of the spine.

When viewed from the rear, the spine usually appears perfectly straight. Scoliosis is a lateral (side-to-side) curve in the spine, usually combined with a rotation of the vertebrae. (The lateral curvature of scoliosis should not be confused with the normal set of front-to-back spinal curves visible from the side.) While a small degree of lateral curvature does not cause any medical problems, larger curves can cause postural imbalance and lead to muscle fatigue and **pain**. More severe scoliosis can interfere with breathing and lead to arthritis of the spine (spondylosis).

Approximately 10% of all adolescents have some degree of scoliosis, though fewer than 1% have curves which require medical attention beyond monitoring. Scoliosis is found in both boys and girls, but a girl's spinal curve is much more likely to progress than a boy's. Girls require scoliosis treatment about five times as often. The reason for these differences is not known.

Four out of five cases of scoliosis are *idiopathic*, meaning the cause is unknown. While idiopathic scoliosis tends to run in families, no responsible genes had been identified as of 1997. Children with idiopathic scoliosis appear to be otherwise entirely healthy, and have not had any bone or joint disease early in life. Scoliosis is not caused by poor posture, diet, or carrying a heavy bookbag exclusively on one shoulder.

Idiopathic scoliosis is further classified according to age of onset:

- Infantile. Curvature appears before age three. This type is quite rare in the United States, but is more common in Europe.
- Juvenile. Curvature appears between ages 3 and 10. This type may be equivalent to the adolescent type, except for the age of onset.
- Adolescent. Curvature appears between ages of 10 and 13, near the beginning of **puberty**. This is the most common type of idiopathic scoliosis.
- Adult. Curvature begins after physical maturation is completed.

Causes are known for three other types of scoliosis:

- Congenital scoliosis is due to congenital **birth defects** in the spine, often associated with other organ defects.
- Neuromuscular scoliosis is due to loss of control of the nerves or muscles which support the spine. The most common causes of this type of scoliosis are **cerebral palsy** and **muscular dystrophy**.
- Degenerative scoliosis may be caused by degeneration of the discs which separate the vertebrae or arthritis in the joints that link them.

Scoliosis causes a noticeable asymmetry in the torso when viewed from the front or back. The first sign of scoliosis is often seen when a child is wearing a bathing suit or underwear. A child may appear to be standing with one shoulder higher than the other, or to have a tilt in the waistline. One shoulder blade may appear more prominent than the other due to rotation. In girls, one breast may appear higher than the other, or larger if rotation pushes that side forward.

Curve progression is greatest near the adolescent growth spurt. Scoliosis that begins early on is more likely to progress significantly than scoliosis that begins later in puberty.

More than 30 states have screening programs in schools for adolescent scoliosis, usually conducted by trained school nurses or gym teachers.

Treatment decisions for scoliosis are based on the degree of curvature, the likelihood of significant progression, and the presence of pain, if any.

Curves less than 20 degrees are not usually treated, except by regular follow-up for children who are still growing. Watchful waiting is usually all that is required in adolescents with curves of 20-30 degrees, or adults with curves up to 40 degrees or slightly more, as long as there is no pain.

For children or adolescents whose curves progress to 30 degrees, and who have a year or more of growth left, bracing may be required. Bracing cannot correct curvature, but may be effective in halting or slowing progression. Bracing is rarely used in adults, except where pain is significant and surgery is not an option, as in some elderly patients.

Surgery for idiopathic scoliosis is usually recommended if:

- The curve has progressed despite bracing
- The curve is greater than 40-50 degrees before growth has stopped in an adolescent
- The curve is greater than 50 degrees and continues to increase in an adult
- There is significant pain.

Orthopedic surgery for neuromuscular scoliosis is often done earlier. The goals of surgery are to correct the deformity as much as possible, to prevent further deformity, and to eliminate pain as much as possible. Surgery can usually correct 40-50% of the curve, and sometimes as much as 80%. Surgery cannot always completely remove pain.

The surgical procedure for scoliosis is called *spinal fusion*, because the goal is to straighten the spine as much as possible, and then to fuse the vertebrae together to prevent further curvature. To achieve fusion, the involved vertebra are first exposed, and then scraped to promote regrowth. Bone chips are usually used to splint together the vertebrae to increase the likelihood of fusion. To maintain the proper spinal posture before fusion occurs, metal rods are inserted alongside the spine, and are attached to the vertebrae by hooks, screws, or wires. Fusion of the spine makes it rigid and resistant to further curvature. The metal rods are no longer needed once fusion is complete, but are rarely removed unless their presence leads to complications.

Spinal fusion leaves the involved portion of the spine permanently stiff and inflexible. While this leads to some loss of normal motion, most functional activities are not strongly affected, unless the very lowest portion of the spine (the lumbar region) is fused. Normal mobility, exercise, and even contact sports are usually all possible after spinal fusion. Full recovery takes approximately six months.

Although important for general health and strength, exercise has not been shown to prevent or slow the development of scoliosis. It may help to relieve pain from scoliosis by helping to maintain range of motion. Good nutrition is also important for general health, but no specific dietary regimen has been shown to control scoliosis development. In particular, dietary calcium levels do not influence scoliosis progression. Most cases of mild adolescent idiopathic scoliosis need no treatment and do not progress.

Scurvy

Scurvy, now known to be caused by a lack of vitamin C, is one of the world's oldest and most devastating deficiency diseases.

Historians have been describing scurvy since ancient times primarily because the disease so often seemed to attack invading armies, sailors on long sea voyages, explorers, and even crusaders. For example, it was scurvy, rather than savage storms or hostile natives, that killed many of the crewmen who sailed with Vasco da Gama (1469-1524) in 1498 and with Ferdinand Magellan (1480-1521) in 1519.

Scurvy begins innocently enough, usually with mild fatigue, bleeding gums, and hemorrhagic bruises on the skin. However, after several months of a diet lacking any vegetables or fruits, worsening physical condition continues, resulting in weakened bones, loose teeth which ultimately fall out, severe joint pain, profuse bleeding from a simple cut, **anemia**, and eventually death.

Fortunately for later researchers, folk remedies for scurvy occasionally appeared in historical accounts. In 1536, for instance, Jacques Cartier (1491-1557) arrived in Newfoundland deeply concerned about the epidemic of scurvy among his crew members. Friendly Indians advised Cartier to give his men an extract of needles from a local tree (thought be white cedar or spruce). Cartier did so and found that almost all his men showed remarkable improvement. During that same century, several other writers reported similar dramatic cures from (among other foods) cloudberries, oranges, and lemons.

Nevertheless, Scottish naval surgeon, James Lind (1716-1794), is generally credited with being the first to discover the cure for scurvy. Shortly after the long sea voyage of Admiral George Anson (1697-1762), from 1740 to 1744 during which more than a thousand sailors out of a crew of 1,955 died primarily from scurvy, Lind began his own investigations into the disease.

From his readings of historical accounts, Lind realized that scurvy might be due to some dietary lack. In 1747, therefore, the physician began treating stricken sailors with various foods, and soon found that citrus fruits produced the fastest and most effective cures. Although Lind published his *Treatise on the Scurvy* in 1753, it was not until 1795 that the Admiralty prescribed a daily ration of lime juice for all British sailors (Lind's cure gave British sailors their nickname—''limeys''). Scurvy promptly diminished in the British navy; however, for the most part, the rest of the civilized world continued to ignore Lind's findings and to resist the idea that scurvy might be related to a dietary deficiency. During the American Civil War, then, scurvy was still killing soldiers in both the Union and Confederate armies. Ironically, even as late as 1912 when Robert Scott (1868-1912) explored the South Pole, he and his team succumbed not to the intense cold, but to the lack of fruits and vegetables in their diet.

In 1907, two Norwegian biochemists, Axel Holst (1861-1931) and Alfred Frohlich (1871-1953), proved conclusively that a scurvy-like condition could be produced in the guinea pig (one of the few animals unable to synthesize vitamin C from their intestinal bacteria) by restricting certain foods. Equally important, Holst and Frohlich then cured the lab animals by feeding them cabbage. The scientific community was finally convinced that the lack of a specific nutrient must be causing scurvy, and an intensive search began to find the nutrient. The antiscorbutic (or anti-scurvy) factor was not isolated until 1928, however. In that year, two teams of researchers, one headed by **Albert Szent-Györgyi** in Hungary, the second by Charles G. King in the United States, extracted an antiscorbutic substance from a variety of fruits. The substance was named vitamin C, or ascorbic acid which, in 1933, was synthesized by two other chemists, Norman Haworth (1883-1950) and **Tadeus Reichstein**. Soon afterward, vitamin C became the first vitamin to be artificially produced and, once marketed for medical purposes, marked the end of scurvy as a deadly disease. Today, those populations in the United States at high-risk for scurvy include alcoholics, drug abusers, and elderly men who live alone and who may experience extremely poor diets.

SEASONAL AFFECTIVE DISORDER

Seasonal affective disorder (SAD) is a **depressive disorder** most often associated with the lack of daylight in extreme northern and southern latitudes from the late fall to the early spring. Although researchers are not certain what causes seasonal affective disorder, they suspect that it has something to do with the hormone melatonin. Melatonin is thought to play an active role in regulating the body's circadian rhythm, or ''internal clock,'' which dictates when humans feel like going to bed at night and getting up in the morning. Although seasonal affective disorder is most common when light is low, it may occur in the spring, and it is then often called reverse SAD.

The body produces more melatonin at night than during the day, and scientists believe it helps people feel sleepy at nighttime. There is also more melatonin in the body during winter, when the days are shorter. Some researchers believe that excessive melatonin release during winter in people with SAD may account for their feelings of drowsiness or depression. One variation on this idea is that, during winter, people's internal clocks may become out of sync with the light-dark cycle, leading to a long-term disruption in melatonin release.

Seasonal affective disorder, while not an official category of **mental illness** listed by the American Psychiatric Association, is estimated to affect 10 million Americans, most of whom are women. Another 25 million Americans may have a mild form of SAD, sometimes called the ''winter blues'' or ''winter blahs.'' The risk of SAD increases the further from the equator a person lives.

The symptoms of SAD are similar to those of other forms of depression. People with SAD may feel sad, irritable, or tired, and may find themselves sleeping too much. They may also lose interest in normal or pleasurable activities (including sex), become withdrawn, crave carbohydrates, and gain weight.

Doctors usually diagnose seasonal affective disorder based on the patient's description of symptoms, including the time of year they occur. The first-line treatment for seasonal affective disorder is **phototherapy**, exposing the patient to bright artificial light to compensate for the gloominess of winter. Light therapy uses a device called a light box, which contains a set of fluorescent or incandescent lights in front of a reflector. Typically, the patient sits for 30 minutes next to a 10,000-lux box (which is about 50 times as bright as ordinary indoor light). Light therapy appears to be safe for most people. However, it may be harmful for those with eye diseases. The most common side effects are vision problems such as eye strain, **headache**s, irritability, and **insomnia**. In addition, hypomania (elevated or expansive mood, characterized by hyperactivity and inflated self esteem) may occasionally occur.

Recently, researchers have begun testing whether people who do not completely respond to light therapy can benefit from tiny doses of the hormone melatonin to reset the body's internal clock. Early results look promising, but the potential benefits must be confirmed in larger studies before this type of treatment becomes widely accepted.

Like other types of **mood disorders**, seasonal affective disorder may also respond to medication and **psychotherapy**. The four different classes of drugs used for mood disorders are:

- Heterocyclic **antidepressants** (HCAs), such as amitriptyline (Elavil).
- Selective serotonin reuptake inhibitors (SSRIs), such as fluoxetine (Prozac), paroxetine (Paxil), and sertraline (Zoloft).
- **Monoamine oxidase inhibitors** (MAO inhibitors), such as phenelzine sulfate (Nardil) and tranylcypromine sulfate (Parnate).
- Lithium salts, such as lithium carbonate (Eskalith), often used in people with bipolar mood disorders, are often useful with SAD patients. Many SAD patients also suffer from **bipolar disorder** (excessive mood swings; formerly known as manic depression).

A number of psychotherapy approaches are useful as well. Interpersonal psychotherapy helps patients recognize how their mood disorder and their interpersonal relationships interact. Cognitive-behavioral therapy explores how the patient's view of the world may be affecting mood and outlook.

Most patients with seasonal affective disorder respond to light therapy and/or antidepressant drugs.

See also Depressive disorder; Mood disorders; Phototherapy

Seborrheic dermatitis

Seborrheic dermatitis is a common inflammatory disease of the skin characterized by scaly lesions usually on the scalp, hairline, and face. It appears as red, inflamed skin covered by greasy or dry scales that may be white, yellowish, or gray. It can effect the scalp, eyebrows, forehead, face, folds around the nose and ears, the chest, armpits (axilla), and groin. Dandruff and cradle cap are mild forms of seborrheic dermatitis that appear as fine white scales without inflammation.

The cause of seborrheic dermatitis is unclear, although it is has been linked to **genetic** or environmental factors. *Pityrosporum ovale*, a species of yeast normally found in hair follicles, has been proposed as one possible causative factor. A high fat diet and alcohol ingestion are thought to play some role. Other possible risk factors include:

- **Stress** and fatigue
- Weather extremes (e. g. hot, humid weather or cold, dry weather)
- Oily skin
- Infrequent shampoos
- **Obesity**
- **Parkinson's disease**
- **acquired immunodeficiency syndrome** (AIDS)
- Use of drying lotions that contain alcohol
- Other skin disorders (for example **acne**, rosacea, or **psoriasis**)

Mild forms of the disorder may be asymptomatic (without symptoms). Symptoms also disappear and reappear, and vary in intensity over time. When scaling is present, it may be accompanied by **itching** that can lead to secondary infection.

The diagnosis of seborrheic dermatitis is based on assessment of symptoms, accompanied by consideration of medical history.

Treatment consists of vigorous shampoos with preparations that assist with softening and removing the scaly accumulations. For mild cases, a non-prescription shampoo with selenium sulfide or zinc pyrithione may be used. For more severe problems, the doctor may prescribe shampoos containing coal tar or scalp creams containing cortisone. The antiseborrheic shampoo should be left on the scalp for approximately five minutes before rinsing out. Hydrocortisone cream may also be ordered for application to the affected areas on the face and body. Application of the hydrocortisone should be discontinued when the condition clears and restarted with recurrence.

This chronic (ever-present) condition may be characterized by long periods of inactivity. Symptoms in the acute phase can be controlled with appropriate treatment. The condition cannot be prevented; however, severity and frequency of flare-ups may be minimized with frequent shampoos, thorough drying of skin folds after bathing, and wearing of loose, ventilating clothing. Foods that appear to worsen the condition should be avoided.

Sedgwick, William Thompson (1855-1921)

American biologist, educator, and sanitary engineer

William Thompson Sedgwick was born in West Hartford, Connecticut on December 29, 1855; he died in Boston, Massachusetts on January 26, 1921. Sedgwick was the son of William and Anne Louise Sedgwick, and the husband of Mary Katrine Rice, whom he married in 1881 (they had no children). A student of Newell Martin, Sedgwick obtained a Ph.B degree in 1877 from the Sheffield Scientific School (Yale); and a Ph.D. degree from Johns Hopkins University in 1881. From 1879 to 1883, he was a member of the physiological chemistry faculty at Johns Hopkins University; and from 1883 to 1921 of the biology faculty at the Massachusetts Institute of Technology (from 1911 to 1921 he belonged to the biology and **pub-**

lic health faculty). From 1888 to 1921, he served as consulting biologist for the Massachusetts State board of Health (from 1902 to 1921 he was a member of the advisory board of the Hygienic Laboratory of the U.S. Public Health Service); and from 1913 to 1922 he was the chairman of the administrative board of the Harvard-Massachusetts Institute of Technology School for Health Officers (the nation's first public health school). He was a member of the International Health Board of the Rockefeller Foundation; was president of the Society of American Bacteriologists in 1900; and belonged to the American Public Health Association from 1914 to 1915. Sedgwick is remembered as a biologist, educator, epidemiologist, and sanitary engineer, as well as one of the early advocates of the pasteurization of milk, and of the addition of chlorine to drinking water.

Sedgwick helped establish sanitary engineering as a profession in the United States, and he pioneered the use of bacteriology in sanitary science. In collaboration with William Ripley Nichols and Thomas M. Drown, Sedgwick did important work in the areas of sewage experimentation and water purification.

He made significant studies of sewage disposal at the Lawrence Experiment Station for the Massachusetts State Board of Health. Together with Hiram F. Mills, he proved that a severe typhoid epidemic (1890) in the Merrimac valley was the consequence of pollution in the Merrimac River, which supplied cities along its banks with drinking water; he published these findings in *Principles of Sanitary Science and the Public Health* (1902). Among his other contributions was the demonstration that chlorine can be used to disinfect water and sewage. He devised one of the first courses on **sanitation** and public health, and he trained many of the leading public health workers of his day, including Whipple, Winslow, Jordan, and Calkins. Among his writings are *General Biology* (1886, with E. B. Wilson); *A Report of the Biological Work of the Lawrence Experiment Station. Experimental Investigation by the State board of Health of Massachusetts upon Sewage, etc.* (1890); and *The Human Mechanism: Its Physiology and Hygiene and the Sanitation of its Surroundings* (1906, with Theodore Hough).

Seibert, Florence (1898-1991)

American biochemist

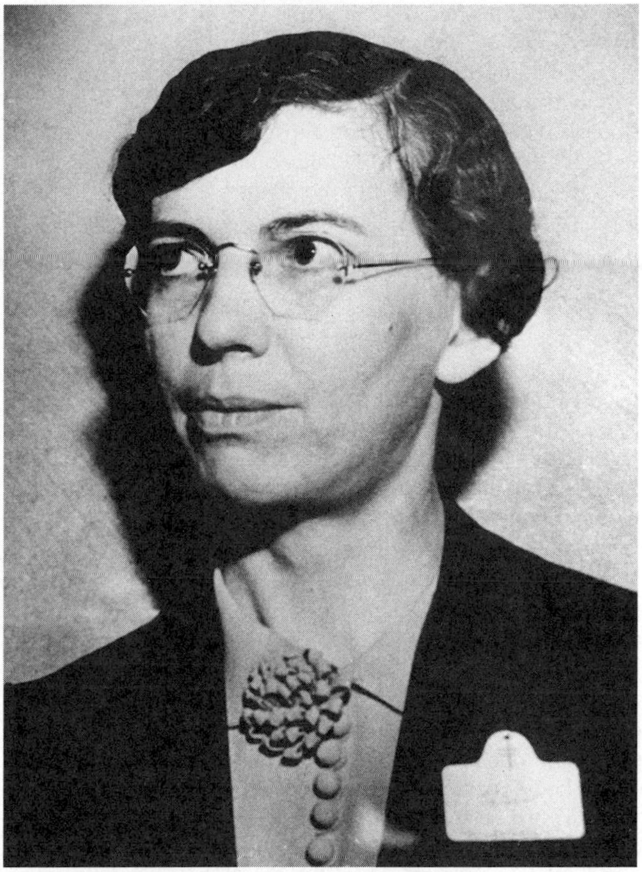

Florence B. Seibert

Florence B. Seibert was born in 1898 in Easton, Pennsylvania. At the age of three she was stricken with **polio** and her disability prompted her to pursue an academic career. She won a scholarship to Goucher College in Maryland and after graduation worked as a chemist during World War I. Dr. Seibert won a scholarship to earn her Ph.D. at Yale University. While there she became interested in why many people became ill with fever after receiving intravenous injections made with distilled water. During the 1920s she developed a distillation process that eliminated bacteria in distilled water and made intravenous injections safe.

Seibert's most well-known discovery was the development of a safe and accurate skin test for **tuberculosis**. Working on a Guggenheim Fellowship at Uppsala University in Sweden, she isolated the active substance in tuberculin—a derivative of purified bacterial protein and then used it to improve the accuracy of the skin test. In 1941, her improved TB skin test became the standard test in the United States and in 1952 it was adapted by the World Health Organization, and is still in use today.

Her other credits include teaching positions at the University of Chicago and University of Pennsylvania, serving with the United States Public Health Service, director of the Cancer Research Laboratory at the Mound Park Hospital in Florida, and induction into the National Women's Hall of Fame in 1990.

Seizures

A seizure is a sudden disruption of the brain's normal electrical activity accompanied by altered consciousness and/or other neurological and behavioral abnormalities. Epilepsy is a condition characterized by recurrent seizures that may include repetitive muscle jerking called convulsions.

There are more than 20 different seizure disorders. One in ten Americans will have a seizure at some time, and at least 200,000 have at least one seizure a month.

Epilepsy affects 1-2% of the population of the United States. Although epilepsy is as common in adults over 60 as in children under 10, 25% of all cases develop before the age of five. One in every two cases develops before the age of 25. About 125,000 new cases of epilepsy are diagnosed each year, and a significant number of children and adults that have not been diagnosed or treated have epilepsy.

Most seizures are benign (not life-threatening), but a seizure that lasts a long time can lead to status epilepticus, a life-threatening condition in which continuous seizures cause lengthy loss of consciousness and respiratory distress (severe breathing difficulties). Non-convulsive epilepsy can impair physical coordination, vision, and other senses. Undiagnosed seizures can lead to conditions that are more serious and more difficult to manage.

There are many different types of seizures: Generalized epileptic seizures occur when electrical abnormalities exist throughout the brain. A partial seizure does not involve the entire brain. A partial seizure begins in an area called an epileptic focus, but may spread to other parts of the brain and cause a generalized seizure. Some people who have epilepsy have more than one type of seizure.

Motor attacks cause parts of the body to jerk repeatedly. A motor attack usually lasts less than an hour and may last only a few minutes. Sensory seizures begin with numbness or tingling in one area. The sensation may move along one side of the body or the back before subsiding.

Visual seizures, which affect the area of the brain that controls sight, cause people to see things that are not there. Auditory seizures affect the part of the brain that controls hearing and cause the patient to imagine voices, music, and other sounds. Other types of seizures can cause confusion, upset stomach, or emotional distress.

A generalized tonic-clonic (grand-mal) seizure begins with a loud cry before the person having the seizure loses consciousness and falls to the ground. The muscles become rigid for about 30 seconds during the tonic phase of the seizure and alternately contract and relax during the clonic phase, which lasts 30-60 seconds. The skin sometimes acquires a bluish tint and the person may bite his tongue, lose bowel or bladder control, or have trouble breathing.

A grand mal seizure lasts between two and five minutes, and the person may be confused or have trouble talking when he regains consciousness (post-ictal state). He may complain of head or muscle aches, or weakness in his arms or legs before falling into a deep sleep.

A primary generalized seizure occurs when electrical discharges begin in both halves (hemispheres) of the brain at the same time. Primary generalized seizures are more likely to be major motor attacks than to be absence seizures.

Absence (petit mal) seizures generally begin at about the age of four and stop by the time the child becomes an adolescent. Absence seizures usually begin with a brief loss of consciousness and last between one and 10 seconds. A person having a petit mal seizure becomes very quiet and may blink, stare blankly, roll his eyes, or move his lips. A petit mal seizure lasts 15-20 seconds. When it ends, the person who had the seizure resumes whatever he was doing before the seizure began. He will not remember the seizure and may not realize that anything unusual has happened. Untreated, petit mal seizures can recur as many as 100 times a day and may progress to grand mal seizures.

Myoclonic seizures are characterized by brief, involuntary spasms of the tongue or muscles of the face, arms, or legs. Myoclonic seizures are most apt to occur when waking after a night's sleep.

A jacksonian seizure is a partial seizure characterized by tingling, stiffening, or jerking of an arm or leg and the seizure may progress along the limb. Loss of consciousness is rare.

Limp posture and a brief period of unconsciousness are features of akinetic seizures, which occur in young children. Akinetic seizures, which cause the child to fall, are also called drop attacks.

Simple partial seizures do not spread from the focal area where they arise. Symptoms are determined by what part of the brain is affected. The patient usually remains conscious during the seizure and can later describe it in detail.

A distinctive smell, taste, or other unusual sensation (aura) may signal the start of complex partial seizures that start as simple partial seizures, but move beyond the focal area and cause loss of consciousness. Complex partial seizures can become major motor seizures. Although a person having a complex partial seizure may not seem to be unconscious, he does not know what is happening and may behave inappropriately. He will not remember the seizure, but may seem confused or intoxicated for a few minutes after it ends.

The origin of 50-70% of all cases of epilepsy is unknown. Epilepsy is sometimes the result of trauma at the time of birth. Such causes include insufficient oxygen to the brain; **head injury**; heavy bleeding or incompatibility between a woman's blood and the blood of her newborn baby; and infection immediately before, after, or at the time of birth.

Other causes of epilepsy include:

- Head trauma resulting from a car accident, gunshot wound, or other injury.
- **Alcoholism**.
- Brain abscess or inflammation of membranes covering the brain or spinal cord.
- **Phenylketonuria** (PKU, a disease that is present at birth, is often characterized by seizures, and can result in **mental retardation**) and other inherited disorders.
- Infectious diseases like **measles**, **mumps**, and **diphtheria**.
- Degenerative disease.
- **Lead poisoning**, mercury **poisoning**, **carbon monoxide poisoning**, or ingestion of some other poisonous substance.
- Genetic factors.

Status epilepticus, a condition in which a person suffers from continuous seizures and may have trouble breathing, can be caused by:

- Suddenly discontinuing anti-seizure medication.
- Hypoxic or metabolic encephalopathy (brain disease resulting from lack of oxygen or malfunctioning of other physical or chemical processes).

- Acute **head injury**.
- Blood infection caused by inflammation of the brain or the membranes that cover it.

Diagnosis of seizures includes personal and family medical history, description of seizure activity, and physical and neurological examinations help primary care physicians, neurologists, and epileptologists diagnose this disorder. Doctors rule out conditions that cause symptoms that resemble epilepsy, including small **strokes** (transient ischemic attacks, or TIAs), **fainting** (syncope), pseudoseizures, and sleep attacks (narcolepsy).

Neuropsychological testing uncovers learning or memory problems. Neuro-imaging pr provides views of brain areas involved in seizure activity.

The **electroencephalography** (EEG) is the main test used to diagnose epilepsy. EEGs use electrodes placed on or within the skull to record the brain's electrical activity and pinpoint the exact location of abnormal discharges.

The patient may be asked to remain motionless during a short-term EEG or to go about his normal activities during extended monitoring. Some patients are deprived of sleep or exposed to seizure triggers, such as rapid, deep breathing (hyperventilation) or flashing lights (photic stimulation). In some cases, people may be hospitalized for EEG monitorings that can last as long as two weeks. Video EEGs also document what the patient was doing when the seizure occurred and how the seizure changed his behavior.

Other techniques used to diagnose epilepsy include:

- **Magnetic resonance imaging** (MRI), which provides clear, detailed images of the brain. Functional MRI (fMRI), performed while the patient does various tasks, can measure shifts in electrical intensity and blood flow and indicate which brain region each activity affects.
- **Positron emission tomography** (PET) and single photon emission tomography (SPECT) monitor blood flow and chemical activity in the brain area being tested. PET and SPECT are very effective in locating the brain region where metabolic changes take place between seizures.

The treatment goal for epilepsy is to eliminate seizures or make the symptoms less frequent and less severe. Long-term **anticonvulsant drug** therapy is the most common form of epilepsy treatment.

A combination of drugs may be needed to control some symptoms, but most patients who have epilepsy take one of the following medications:

- Dilantin (phenytoin)
- Tegretol (carbamazepine)
- Barbita (phenobarbital)
- Mysoline (primidone)
- Depakene (valproic acid, sodium valproate)
- Klonopin (clonazepam)
- Zarontin (ethosuximide).

Dilantin, Tegretol, Barbita, and Mysoline are used to manage or control generalized tonic-clonic and complex partial seizures. Depakene, Klonopin, and Zarontin are prescribed for patients who have absence seizures.

Neurontonin (gabapentin) and Lamictal (lamotrigine) are medications recently approved in the United States to treat adults who have partial seizures or partial and grand mal seizures.

Even a patient whose seizures are well controlled should have regular blood tests to measure levels of anti-seizure medication in his system and to check to see if the medication is causing any changes in his blood or liver. A doctor should be notified if any signs of drug toxicity appear, including uncontrolled eye movements; sluggishness, **dizziness**, or hyperactivity; inability to see clearly or speak distinctly; **nausea or vomiting**; or sleep problems.

Status epilepticus requires emergency treatment, usually with Valium (Ativan), Dilantin, or Barbita. An intravenous dextrose (sugar) solution is given to patients whose condition is due to low blood sugar, and a vitamin B_1 preparation is administered intravenously when status epilepticus results from chronic alcohol withdrawal. Because dextrose and thiamine are essentially harmless and because delay in treatment can be disastrous, these medications are given routinely, as it is usually difficult to obtain an adequate history from a patient suffering from status epilepticus.

Intractable seizures are seizures that cannot be controlled with medication or without sedation or other unacceptable side effects. Surgery may be used to eliminate or control intractable seizures.

Surgery can be used to treat patients whose intractable seizures stem from small focal lesions that can be removed without endangering the patient, changing the patient's personality, dulling the patient's senses, or reducing the patient's ability to function. Each year, as many as 5,000 new patients may become suitable candidates for surgery, which is most often performed at a comprehensive epilepsy center. Potential surgical candidates include patients with:

- Partial seizures and secondarily generalized seizures (attacks that begin in one area and spread to both sides of the brain).
- Seizures and childhood **paralysis** on one side of the body (hemiplegia).
- Complex partial seizures originating in the temporal lobe (the part of the brain associated with speech, hearing, and smell) or other focal seizures. However, the risk of surgery involving the speech centers is that the patient will lose speech function.
- Generalized myoclonic seizures or generalized seizures featuring temporary paralysis (akinetic) or loss of muscle tone (atonal).

A **physical examination** is conducted to verify that a patient's seizures are caused by epilepsy, and surgery is not used to treat patients with severe psychiatric disturbances or medical problems that raise risk factors to unacceptable levels. Surgery is never recommended unless:

- The best available anti-seizure medications have failed to control the patient's symptoms satisfactorily.
- The origin of the patient's seizures has been precisely located.
- There is good reason to believe that surgery will significantly improve the patient's health and quality of life.

Every patient considering epilepsy surgery is carefully evaluated by one or more neurologists, neurosurgeons, neuropsychologists, and/or social workers. A psychiatrist, chaplain, or other spiritual advisor may help the patient and his family cope with the **stress**es that occur during and after the selection process.

Surgical techniques used to treat intractable epilepsy include:

- Lesionectomy. Removing the lesion (diseased brain tissue) and some surrounding brain tissue is very effective in controlling seizures. Lesionectomy is generally more successful than surgery performed on patients whose seizures are not caused by clearly defined lesions, but removing only part of the lesion lessens the effectiveness of the procedure.
- Temporal resections. Removing part of the temporal lobe and the part of the brain associated with feelings, memory, and emotions (the hippocampus) provides good or excellent seizure control in 75-80% of properly selected patients with appropriate types of temporal lobe epilepsy. Some patients experience post-operative speech and memory problems.
- Extra-temporal resection. This procedure involves removing some or all of the frontal lobe, the part of the brain directly behind the forehead. The frontal lobe helps regulate movement, planning, judgment, and personality, and special care must be taken to prevent post-operative problems with movement and speech. Extra-temporal resection is most successful in patients whose seizures are not widespread.
- Hemispherectomy. This method of removing brain tissue is restricted to patients with severe epilepsy and abnormal discharges that often extend from one side of the brain to the other. Hemispherectomies are most often performed on infants or young children who have had an extensive brain disease or disorder since birth or from a very young age.
- Corpus callosotomy. This procedure, an alternative to hemispherectomy in patients with congenital (present at birth) hemiplegia, removes some or all of the white matter that separates the two halves of the brain. Corpus callosotomy is performed almost exclusively on children who are frequently injured during falls caused by seizures. If removing two-thirds of the corpus callosum doesn't produce lasting improvement in the patient's condition, the remaining one-third will be removed during another operation.
- Multiple subpial transection. This procedure is used to control the spread of seizures that originate in or affect the ''eloquent'' cortex, the area of the brain responsible for complex thought and reasoning.

Another form of treatment consists of a special high-fat, low-protein, low-carbohydrate diet is sometimes used to treat patients whose severe seizures have not responded to other treatment. Calculated according to age, height, and weight, the ketogenic diet induces mild **starvation** and **dehydration**. This forces the body to create an excessive supply of ketones, natural chemicals with seizure-suppressing properties.

The goal of this controversial approach is to maintain or improve seizure control while reducing medication. The ketogenic diet works best with children between the ages of one and 10. It is introduced over a period of several days, and most children are hospitalized during the early stages of treatment.

If a child following this diet remains seizure-free for at least six months, increased amounts of carbohydrates and protein are gradually added. If the child shows no improvement after three months, the diet is gradually discontinued.

Introduced in the 1920s, the ketogenic diet has had limited, short-term success in controlling seizure activity. Its use exposes patients to such potentially harmful side effects as:

- **Staphylococcal infections**
- Stunted or delayed growth
- Low blood sugar (**hypoglycemia**)
- Excess fat in the blood (hyperlipidemia)
- Disease resulting from calcium deposits in the urinary tract (urolithiasis)
- Disease of the optic nerve (optic neuropathy).

The United States Food and Drug Administration (FDA) has approved the use of vagus nerve stimulation (VNS) in patients over the age of 16 who have intractable partial seizures. This non-surgical procedure uses a **pacemaker**-like device implanted under the skin in the upper left chest, to provide intermittent stimulation to the vagus nerve. Stretching from the side of the neck into the brain, the vagus nerve affects swallowing, speech, breathing, and many other functions, and VNS may prevent or shorten some seizures.

A person having a seizure should not be restrained, but sharp or dangerous objects should be moved out of reach. Anyone having a complex partial seizure can be warned away from danger by someone calling his/her name in a clear, calm voice.

A person having a grand mal seizure should be helped to lie down. Tight clothing should be loosened. A soft, flat object like a towel or the palm of a hand should be placed under the person's head. Forcing a hard object into the mouth of someone having a grand mal seizure could cause injuries or breathing problems. If the person's mouth is open, placing a folded cloth or other soft object between his teeth will protect his tongue. Turning his head to the side will help him breathe. After a grand mal seizure has ended, the person who had the seizure should be told what has happened and reminded of where he is.

Alternative medicine can often be beneficial. Stress increases seizure activity in 30% of people who have epilepsy. Relaxation techniques can provide some sense of control over the disorder, but they should never be used instead of anti-seizure medication or used without the approval of the patient's doctor. **Yoga**, **meditation**, and favorite pastimes help some people relax and manage stress more successfully. **Biofeedback** can teach adults and older adolescents how to recognize an aura and what to do to stop its spread. Children under 14 are not usually able to understand and apply principles of biofeedback. **Acupuncture** treatments (acupuncture needles inserted for a few minutes or left in place for as long as half an hour) make some people feel pleasantly relaxed. **Acupressure** can have the same effect on children or on adults who dislike needles.

Aromatherapy involves mixing aromatic plant oils into water or other oils and massaging them into the skin or using a special burner to waft their fragrance throughout the room. Aromatherapy oils affect the body and the brain, and undiluted oils should never be applied directly to the skin. Ylang ylang, chamomile, or lavender can create a soothing mood. People who have epilepsy should not use rosemary, hyssop, sage or sweet fennel, which seem to make the brain more alert.

Dietary changes that emphasize whole foods and eliminate processed foods may be helpful. **Homeopathic** therapy also can work for people with seizures, especially constitution al homeopathic treatment that acts at the deepest levels to address the needs of the individual person.

The prognosis (expected outcome) for people suffering from seizures differs with the type of seizure. People who have epilepsy have a higher-than-average rate of **suicide**; sudden, unexplained **death**; and drowning and other accidental fatalities.

Benign focal epilepsy of childhood and some absence seizures may disappear in time, but remission is unlikely if seizures occur several times a day, several times in a 48-hour period, or more frequently than in the past.

Seizures that occur repeatedly over time and always involve the same symptoms are called stereotypic seizures. The probability that stereotypic seizures will abate is poor.

About 85% of all seizure disorders can be partially or completely controlled if the patient takes anti-seizure medication according to directions; avoids seizure-inducing sights, sounds, and other triggers; gets enough sleep; and eats regular, balanced meals.

Anyone who has epilepsy should wear a bracelet or necklace identifying his seizure disorder and listing the medication he takes.

Eating properly, getting enough sleep, and controlling stress and **fever**s can help prevent seizures. A person who has epilepsy should be careful not to hyperventilate. A person who experiences an aura should find a safe place to lie down and stay there until the seizure passes. Anticonvulsant medications should not be stopped suddenly and, if other medications are prescribed or discontinued, the doctor treating the seizures should be notified. In some conditions, such as severe head injury, brain surgery, or subarachnoid hemorrhage, anticonvulsant medications may be given to the patient to prevent seizures.

See also Anticonvulsant drugs; Electroencephalography (EEG); Head injury; Phenylketonuria; Positron emission tomography (PET)

SELF-ESTEEM

Considered an important component of emotional health, self-esteem encompasses both self-confidence and self-acceptance.

Experiences at home, at school, and with peers can all build or diminish a child's self-esteem. Psychologists and child-care authorities who write about self-esteem generally discuss it in terms of two key components: the feeling of being loved and accepted by others and a sense of competence and mastery in performing tasks and solving problems independently.

The value placed on self-esteem by the mental health profession over the past 30 years has been critiqued by psychologist Martin Seligman. Seligman claims that in order for children to feel good about themselves, they must feel that they are able to do things well. He claims that trying to shield children from feelings of sadness, frustration, and anxiety when they fail robs them of the motivation to persist in difficult tasks until they succeed. It is precisely such success in the face of difficulties that can truly make them feel good about themselves. Seligman believes that this attempt to cushion children against unpleasant emotions is in large part responsible for an increase in the prevalence of depression since the 1950s, an increase that he associates with a conditioned sense of helplessness.

Like Seligman, pediatrician and child-care expert **T. Berry Brazelton** emphasizes that children develop self-esteem through the sense of competence and mastery that comes from tackling and triumphing over challenges, even modest ones. He believes that parents can boost children's self-esteem even in infancy by giving them an active and autonomous role in casual play. As infants and toddlers advance to self-care activities, such as beginning to feed themselves, Brazelton encourages parents to let children complete tasks for themselves, however imperfectly, rather than jumping in and providing help. For example, he suggests allowing children to pick up small bits of food at the age of eight months even if they drop some, and letting them hold their own bottles at 12 months. Like Seligman, Brazelton emphasizes the value of leaving a child to work through a problem for herself, trying out different approaches to a task until she succeeds. For a child accustomed to learning by trial and error, frustration can serve as a source of motivation and energy rather than an obstacle. Brazelton also emphasizes the importance of encouraging the child in her endeavors and providing positive reinforcement when a goal is achieved.

In spite of his emphasis on the development of competence, Brazelton does advise parents to address their children in a positive way to reinforce feelings of love and acceptance. Among the harmful negative examples he points out are belittling comparisons with siblings (''Why can't you be more like your brother?'') and threats of abandonment (''If you don't stop that right now, I'm leaving you here!''). Various experts have noted that when parental communication is consistently delivered in a negative style it becomes internalized, and children start to practice negative ''self-talk,'' generating their own negative messages. In addition to their verbal communication style, parents also express acceptance and affirmation by showing physical affection and being good listeners, which make children feel important and cared about. Social critics have pointed out that it can be more difficult for children in the United States and other modern industrialized nations to achieve a sense of competence than it was for their counterparts in earlier historical periods. Children in the past, or in modern developing countries, participated actively in the economic life of the community, helping their families by doing some of the same jobs performed by adults. Today's children, especially in urban areas, perform little ''useful'' work and thus have few opportunities to master tasks that contribute to the welfare of their families and the community as a whole. In addition, their competence at the tasks that are demanded of them is continually challenged by competition in school, athletics, and other areas.

Self-esteem comes from different sources for children at different stages of development. The development of self-esteem in young children is heavily influenced by parental attitudes and behavior. Supportive parental behavior, including the encouragement and praise of mastery, as well as the child's internalization of the parents' own attitudes toward success and failure, are the most powerful factors in the development of self-esteem in early childhood. Later, older children's experiences outside the home—in school and with peers—become increasingly important in determining their self-esteem. Schools can influence their students' self-esteem through the attitudes they foster toward competition and diversity and their recognition of achievement in academics, sports, and the arts. By middle childhood, friendships have assumed a pivotal role in a child's life. Studies have shown that school-age youngsters spend more time with their friends than they spend doing homework, watching television, or playing alone. In addition, the amount of time they interact with their parents is greatly reduced from when they were younger. At this stage, social acceptance by a child's peer group plays a major role in developing and maintaining self-esteem.

See also Child development; Peer pressure

SELF-INJURY

Broadly speaking, self-injury (also called self-inflicted violence, self-harm, parasuicide, delicate cutting, self-abuse, and self-mutilation) is the act of attempting to alter a mood state by inflicting physical harm serious enough to cause tissue damage to the body. This harm may include cutting (with knives, razors, glass, pin, or any sharp object), burning, hitting the body with an object or fists, hitting a heavy object (like a wall), picking at skin until it bleeds, biting, pulling hair out. The most commonly observed forms are cutting, burning, and headbanging. It is not considered self-injury if the primary purpose is sexual pleasure, body decoration, or spiritual enlightenment through ritual.

The reasons why people engage in self-injurious behavior are numerous: biological predisposition, tension reduction, and lack of experience in dealing with intense emotions are some of the major factors. Studies have suggested that when people who self-injure get emotionally overwhelmed, an act of self-harm brings their level of psychological and physiological tension and arousal back to a bearable baseline level almost immediately. For this reason, self-injury is often addictive. However, eventually the negative consequences outweigh the immediate benefits, and the individual may feel trapped in a desperate cycle of self-harm.

People who inflict harm on themselves often indulge in the behavior as a way means of avoiding **suicide**. Although some individuals who self-injure do later attempt suicide, they almost always use a method different from their preferred method of self-harm.

One factor common to most individuals who self-injure is the feeling of invalidation. They are taught at an early age that their feelings are inconsequential or erroneous; they also learn that expressing certain feelings is forbidden. In homes in which these individuals are abused, they may have been severely punished for expressing these thoughts and feelings. Although sexual and physical abuse and neglect may precipitate self-injurious behavior and is often a predictor of the amount and severity of self-injury, many of those who harm themselves have no background of childhood abuse. In addition, those who self-injure usually have not been provided with adequate role models for learning how to deal with stress effectively.

Scientists believe that reduced levels of the brain chemical serotonin may predispose some individuals to self-injury by making them more aggressive and impulsive than most people. This tendency toward impulsive **aggression**, combined with a belief that their feelings are invalid, can lead to the agression being turned on the self. Once this behavior occurs, the individual harming him or herself learns that self-injury reduces the level of **stress**, and the cycle begins.

It has been estimated that about 1% of Americans self-injure, and women resort to this behavior more often than men. Although statistics vary, surveys of those who self-injure have found that about 85% of are women. The theory is that women are socialized to internalize anger and men to externalize it. It is also possible that because men are socialized to repress all emotion, they may have less trouble keeping things inside; or they may externalize it in seemingly unrelated violence.

A ''portrait'' of the self-injurer compiled by researchers found that the typical self-injurer is female, in her mid-20s to early 30s, and has been cutting herself since her teens. She tends to be middle- or upper-middle-class, intelligent, and from a background of physical and/or **sexual abuse** or from a home with at least one alcoholic parent. **Eating disorders** often coexist with self-injury. In addition, individuals who engage in repetitive self-injury have reported being diagnosed with other disorders, such as depression, **obsessive-compulsive disorder**, **dissociative disorders**, **anxiety and panic disorders**, and impuse-control disorders.

Self-injurers come from all races and socioeconomic levels. Some people who self-injure manage to function effectively in demanding jobs; others resort to disability compensation. They range in age from early teens to early 60s. The incidence of self-injury is reportedly similar to that of eating disorders, but because the disorder is so highly stigmatized even among health care professionals most people hide their scars, burns, and bruises carefully. Since self-injury is so socially unacceptable, it is not as understood or accepted by society as **alcoholism**, drug abuse, or other forms of addictive, compulsive, or avoidance behavior. Self-injurers are also adept at making excuses when questioned about their scars.

Research into medications that stabilize mood, ease depression, and calm anxiety have been found to be effective in treating individuals who self-injure. Hospitalization, it is thought, should only be used as a last resort when the patient is at risk for suicide or severe self-injury. According to experts, hospitals are artificially safe environments, and the necessary tasks of learning to identify the feelings behind the act and of choosing a less destructive method of coping need to be practiced and reinforced in the outside world.

Many therapeutic approaches have been developed to teach self-injurers effective ways of coping with stress. These approaches reflect a growing belief among mental health professionals that once a patient's pattern of self-inflicted **violence** stabilizes, real work can be done on the problems and issues underlying the disorder.

See also Anxiety disorders; Depression; Obsessive-compulsive disorder; Panic disorder; Suicide

Semen analysis

Semen analysis evaluates a man's sperm and semen to determine the cause of **infertility** or to confirm the success of a **vasectomy**. Semen is the thick yellow-white male ejaculate containing sperm; sperm are the male sex cells that fertilize the female egg (ovum) and contain the genetic information that the male will pass on to a child.

Abnormalities of sperm and semen can cause male infertility, and semen analysis is an initial step in investigating why a couple has been unable to conceive a child. Vasectomy is an operation done to sterilize a man by stopping the release of sperm into semen. Success of vasectomy is confirmed by the absence of sperm in semen.

The semen analysis test is usually done manually, though computerized test systems are available. Many laboratories base their procedures on standards published by the World Health Organization (WHO).

The volume of semen in the entire ejaculate is measured. The appearance, color, thickness, and pH is noted. A pH test looks at the range from a very acid solution to a very alkaline solution. Semen, like many other body fluids, has a standard pH range that would be considered optimal for fertilization of the egg to take place. The thick semen is then allowed to liquify; this usually takes 20-60 minutes.

Drops of semen are placed on a microscope slide and examined under the microscope. Motility, or movement, of 100 sperm are observed and graded in categories, such as rapid progressive or immotile.

The structure of sperm (sperm morphology) is assessed by carefully examining sperm for abnormalities in the size and shape in the head, tail, and neck regions. WHO standards define normal as a specimen with less than 30% abnormal forms. An alternative classification system (Kruger's) measures the dimensions of sperm parts. Normal specimens are allowed 14% or less abnormalities.

Sperm are counted by placing semen in a special counting chamber. The sperm within the chamber are counted under a microscope. White blood cells are recorded; these may indicate a reproductive tract infection. Laboratories may test for other biochemicals such as fructose, zinc, and citric acid. These are believed to contribute to sperm health and fertility.

Results of semen analysis for infertility must be confirmed by a second analysis seven days to three months after the first. Sperm counts may vary from day to day.

Semen analysis to confirm success of vasectomy is concerned only with discovering if sperm are still present. Semen is collected six weeks after surgery. If sperm are seen, another specimen is collected two to four weeks later. The test is repeated until two consecutive specimens are free of sperm.

A man should collect an entire ejaculate, by **masturbation**, into a container provided by his physician. To examine the best quality sperm, the specimen must be collected after two to three days of sexual abstinence, but not more than five to seven days. The specimen must not come into contact with any spermicidal agents used by a female partner for **birth control** purposes. The man should not have alcohol before the test.

A semen specimen to investigate infertility must be brought to the testing laboratory within one hour of obtaining it. Timing is not as critical for the postvasectomy test but the semen must be kept at body temperature. The most satisfactory sample is one obtained in the lab rather than at home.

WHO standards have established these normal values:

- Volume less than or equal to 2.0 mL
- Sperm count greater than or equal to 20 million per mL
- Motility (movement of the sperm) value is greater than or equal to 50% with forward progression, or greater than or equal to 25% with rapid progression within 60 minutes of ejaculation
- Morphology greater than or equal to 30% with normal forms
- White blood cell count less than 1 million per mL.

If infertility continues, despite normal semen analysis and female studies, further tests are done to evaluate sperm function.

Abnormalities of semen volume and liquidity, and sperm number and morphology decrease fertility. These abnormalities may be inherited or caused by a hormone imbalance, medications, or a recent infection. Further tests may be done to determine the cause of abnormalities.

See also Infertility; Vasectomy

Semmelweis, Ignaz Philipp (1818-1865)

Hungarian physician

Born in Budapest, Hungary, to a prosperous shopkeeping family of German origin, Semmelweis followed his undergraduate career at the University of Pest by earning his medical degree from the Vienna Medical School in 1844. After receiving his master's degree in midwifery, Semmelweis took a post as assistant in the Vienna General Hospital.

Semmelweis soon observed that the death rate among maternity patients in the ward treated by medical students was much higher (13%) than in the ward served by midwives (2%). When Semmelweis made a connection between the symptoms of a fatal dissection wound and puerperal fever, he concluded

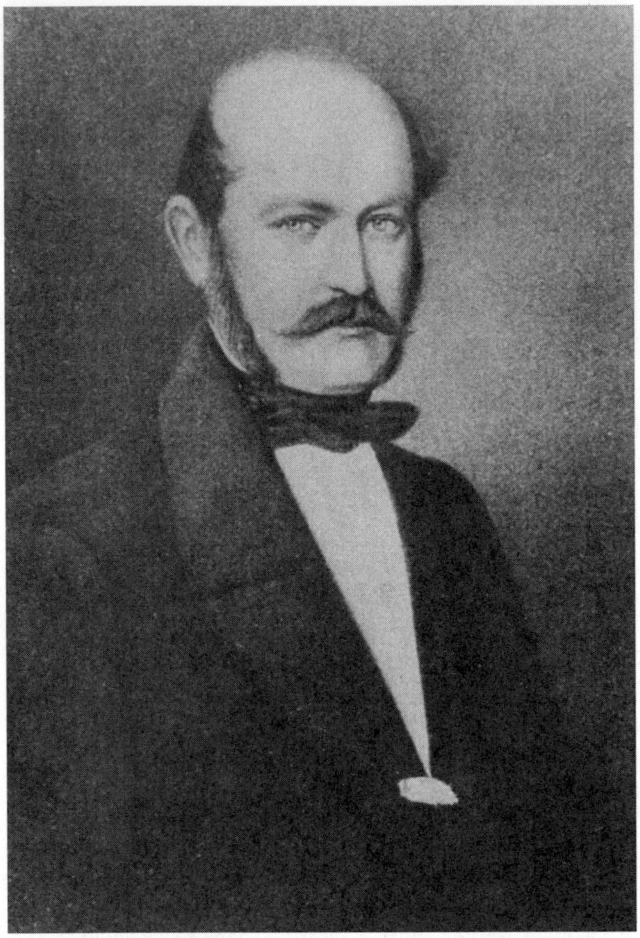

Ignaz Phillipp Semmelweis

that the fever was transmitted to the maternity patients by medical students carrying infectious materials on their fingers from dissected cadavers. Starting in May 1847 Semmelweis required his students to wash their hands in a solution of chlorinated lime before examining patients. Mortality rates from puerperal fever promptly plunged.

In spite of these dramatic results, Semmelweis's colleagues rejected the concept that they could be responsible for spreading disease. Forced out of his Viennese post, Semmelweis abruptly returned to Budapest, where he was head of maternity at St. Rochus Hospital from 1851 until 1857. Here again he introduced *antiseptic procedures* and nearly banished puerperal fever.

Semmelweis finally published his findings in 1861, but critics continued to attack him fiercely and he reacted with increasing anger and bitterness. Mental illness overtook him in 1865; he died after only two weeks in an asylum of, ironically, sepsis from a surgical wound. That same year, **Joseph Lister** performed his first antiseptic operation.

Sepsis

Sepsis refers to a bacterial infection in the bloodstream or body tissues. This is a very broad term covering the presence of many types of microscopic disease-causing organisms.

Sepsis is also called **bacteremia**. Closely related terms include septicemia and septic syndrome. In the general population, the incidence of sepsis is two people in 10,0000.

Sepsis can originate anywhere bacteria can gain entry to the body; common sites include the genitourinary tract, the liver and its bile ducts, the gastrointestinal tract, and the lungs. Broken or ulcerated skin can also provide access to bacteria commonly present in the environment. Invasive medical procedures, including dental work, can introduce bacteria or permit it to accumulate. Entry points and equipment left in place for any length of time present a particular risk. Heart valve replacement, catheters, ostomy sites, intravenous (IV) or arterial lines, surgical **wounds**, or surgical drains are examples. IV drug users are at high risk as well.

People with inefficient immune systems or blood disorders are at particular risk for sepsis and have a higher **death** rate (up to 60%); in people who have no underlying chronic disease, the death rate is far lower (about 5%). The growing problem of antibiotic resistance has increased the incidence of sepsis, partly because ordinary preventive measures (such as prophylactic **antibiotics**) are less effective.

The most common symptom of sepsis is **fever**, often accompanied by chills or shaking, or other flu-like symptoms. A history of any recent invasive procedure or dental work should raise the suspicion of sepsis and medical help should be sought.

The presence of sepsis is indicated by blood tests showing particularly high or low white blood cell counts. The causative agent is determined by blood culture.

Identifying the specific causative agent ultimately determines how sepsis is treated. However, time is of the essence, so a broad-spectrum antibiotic or multiple antibiotics will be administered until blood cultures reveal the culprit and treatment can be made specific to the organism. Intravenous antibiotic therapy is usually necessary and is administered in the hospital.

Septic shock is a potentially lethal drop in blood pressure due to the presence of bacteria in the blood.

Septic shock is a possible consequence of bacteremia, or bacteria in the bloodstream. Bacterial toxins, and the immune system response to them, cause a dramatic drop in blood pressure, preventing the delivery of blood to the organs. Septic shock can lead to multiple organ failure including **respiratory failure**, and may cause rapid **death**. **Toxic shock syndrome** is one type of septic shock.

During an infection, certain types of bacteria can produce and release complex molecules, called endotoxins, that may provoke a dramatic response by the body's immune system. Released in the bloodstream, endotoxins are particularly dangerous, because they become widely dispersed and affect the blood vessels themselves. Arteries and the smaller arterioles open wider, increasing the total volume of the circulatory system. At the same time, the walls of the blood vessels become leaky, allowing fluid to seep out into the tissues, lowering the amount of fluid left in circulation. This combination of increased system volume and decreased fluid causes a dramatic decrease in blood pressure and reduces the blood flow to the organs. Other changes brought on by immune response may cause coagulation of the blood in the extremities, which can further decrease circulation through the organs.

Septic shock is seen most often in patients with suppressed immune systems, and is usually due to bacteria acquired during treatment at the hospital. The immune system is suppressed by drugs used to treat **cancer**, autoimmune disorders, organ transplants, and diseases of immune deficiency such as **AIDS**. **Malnutrition**, chronic drug abuse, and long-term illness increase the likelihood of succumbing to bacterial infection. Bacteremia is more likely with preexisting infections such as urinary or gastrointestinal tract infections, or skin ulcers. Bacteria may be introduced to the blood stream by surgical procedures, catheters, or intravenous equipment.

Toxic shock syndrome most often occurs in menstruating women using highly absorbent tampons. Left in place longer than other types, these tampons provide the breeding ground for *Staphylococcus* bacteria, which may then enter the bloodstream through small tears in the vaginal lining. The incidence of toxic shock syndrome has declined markedly since this type of tampon was withdrawn from the market.

Septic shock is usually preceded by bacteremia, which is marked by **fever**, malaise, chills, and nausea. The first sign of **shock** is often confusion and decreased consciousness. In this beginning stage, the extremities are usually warm. Later, they become cool, pale, and bluish. Fever may give way to lower that normal temperatures later on in **sepsis**.

Other symptoms include:

- Rapid heartbeat
- Shallow, rapid breathing
- Decreased urination.
- Reddish patches in the skin.

Septic shock may progress to cause ''adult **respiratory distress syndrome**,'' in which fluid collects in the lungs, and breathing becomes very shallow and labored. This condition may lead to ventilatory collapse, in which the patient can no longer breathe adequately without assistance.

Diagnosis of septic shock is made by measuring blood pressure, heart rate, and respiration rate, as well as by a consideration of possible sources of infection. Blood pressure may be monitored with a catheter device inserted into the pulmonary artery supplying the lungs (Swan-Ganz catheter). Blood **culture**s are done to determine the type of bacteria responsible. The levels of oxygen, carbon dioxide, and acidity in the blood are also monitored to assess changes in respiratory function.

Septic shock is treated initially with a combination of **antibiotics** and fluid replacement. The antibiotic is chosen based on the bacteria present, although two or more types of antibiotics may be used initially until the organism is identified. Intravenous fluids, either blood or protein solutions, replace the fluid lost by leakage. Coagulation and hemorrhage may be treated with **transfusion**s of plasma or platelets. Dopamine may be given to increase blood pressure further if necessary.

Respiratory distress is treated with mechanical ventilation and supplemental oxygen, either using a nosepiece or a tube into the trachea through the throat.

Identification and treatment of the primary infection site is important to prevent ongoing proliferation of bacteria.

Septic shock is most likely to develop in the hospital, since it follows infections which are likely to be the objects of treatment. Because of this, careful monitoring and early, aggressive therapy can minimize the likelihood of progression. Nonetheless, death occurs in at least 25% of all cases.

The likelihood of recovery from septic shock depends on may factors, including the degree of immunosuppression of the patient, underlying disease, promptness of treatment, and type of bacteria responsible. Mortality is highest in the very young and the elderly, those with persistent or recurrent infection, and those with compromised immune systems.

The risk of developing septic shock can be minimized through treatment of underlying bacterial infections, and prompt attention to signs of bacteremia. In the hospital, scrupulous aseptic technique on the part of medical professionals lowers the risk of introducing bacteria into the bloodstream.

SERVETUS, MICHAEL (ca. 1511-1553)

Spanish physician and theologian

Servetus (also known as Miguel Serveto) was the first person to describe the circulation of blood from the heart into the lungs where it was oxygenated before going to the rest of the body.

Servetus' birthdate is uncertain, because he tried to mislead his accusers when he was on trial for his life in Geneva in 1553. Experts believe he was born on September 29, 1511, in Villanueva in northern Spain. Both of his parents, Antonio Serveto and Catalina Conesa, were nobles. He was educated at a church school, and then, at 15 years of age, he became an assistant to Juan de Quintana, a powerful Franciscan friar who later became the confessor to Charles V, the Holy Roman Emperor.

Servetus was very argumentative and stubborn, and he became involved in the bitter religious controversies that divided Europe. He went to Switzerland with Quintana, but then left in 1530 and moved to Strasbourg, France, where, at the age of 20, he published a book, *De trinitatis erroribus*, about the errors of believing in the Trinity of the father, son, and holy ghost. His book was condemned by Catholics and Protestants, and it was banned in Strasbourg.

Servetus returned to Switzerland, published a second scandalous book on the Trinity, and was forced to leave the country. He changed his name to Michel de Villeneuve, moved to France, and eventually settled in Lyons, where he worked as an editor and proofreader. He edited many books, including medical texts and several editions of the *Bible*.

Some time in 1535 or 1536, Servetus went to Paris to study medicine. There he associated with many important figures in medicine, and one of his teachers was **Jean Francois Fernel**. Another teacher wrote that Servetus was a fine assistant

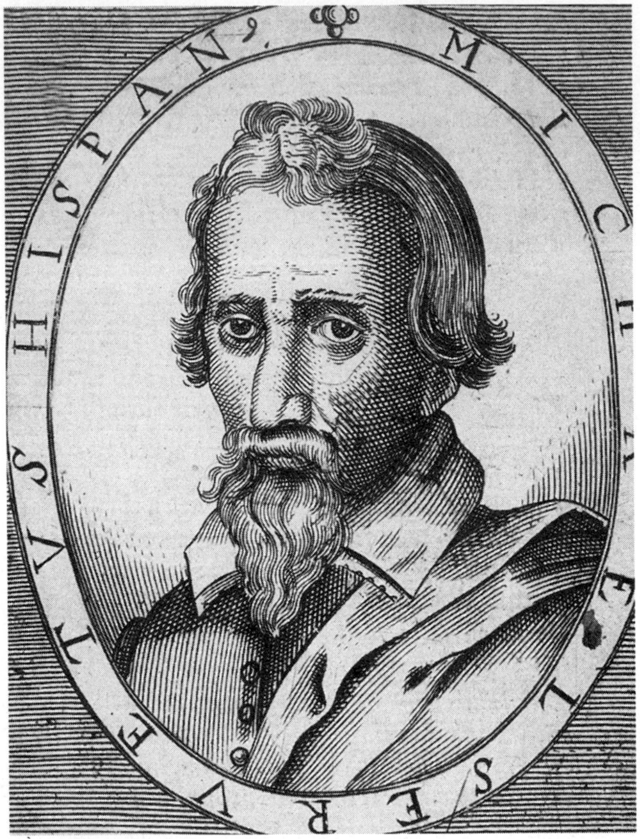

Miguel Serveto

in dissections. In 1537 Servetus published *Syruporum universa ratio*, a book about using syrups as a base for medicines. In his book, he mentioned that citrus fruits were good for digestion. Although there is no record that he was granted a diploma as a doctor of medicine, he left Paris in 1538 and began a career as a physician. One document of that time called him a medical doctor.

Although Servetus worked as a physician for years, his passion was still theology, and in January, 1553, he published yet another radical religious work, *Christianismi restitutio*. In this book, almost as an aside, Servetus made his most important contribution to medicine. He said that blood is pumped from the heart to the lungs, where it is oxygenated, then pumped back to the heart, from which it goes to the rest of the body. Prior to Servetus's description, medical experts, following **Galen**, believed that blood was oxygenated in the heart.

When Servetus published *Christianismi restitutio*, he was still living under the name Michel de Villeneuve. After the book came out, someone recognized who the author really was, and Servetus was arrested in Lyons. He escaped three days later and after hiding out for several months, he decided to go to Italy. Enroute to Italy, he traveled through Geneva, Switzerland, where he was known and recognized. He was arrested, but this time, he was unable to escape. He was accused and convicted of heresy, which carried the death penalty. On October 27, 1553, his executioners placed a crown of leaves and straw on his head, tied a copy of his last book to his arm, and burned him at the stake in Champel, Switzerland. In his last words, Servetus asked Jesus to have pity on him.

See also Galen; Fernel, Jean Francois

Severe combined immunodeficiency

Severe combined **immunodeficiency** (SCID) is the most serious human immunodeficiency disorder(s). It is a group of disorders existing from the time of birth (congenital) in which the patient's **immune system**, and the cells involved in immune responses fail to work properly. Children with SCID are vulnerable to recurrent severe infections, retarded growth, and early **death**. It is thought to affect between one in every 100,000 persons, and one in every 500,000 infants.

In order to understand why SCID is considered the most severe immunodeficiency disorder, it is helpful to have an outline of the human immune system which has three parts: cellular, humoral, and nonspecific. The cellular and humoral parts are both needed to fight infections—they recognize disease agents and attack them. The cellular system is composed of many classes of T-lymphocytes (white blood cells that detect foreign invaders called antigens). The humoral system is made up of B-cells, which are the only cells in the body that make antibodies. In SCID, neither the cellular nor the humoral part of the immune system is working properly.

Several different immune system disorders are currently grouped under SCID:

- Swiss-type agammaglobulinemia. This was the first type of SCID discovered, in Switzerland in the 1950s.
- Adenosine deaminase deficiency (ADA). About 50% of SCID cases are of this type. ADA deficiency leads to low levels of B and T cells in the child's immune system.
- Autosomal recessive. About 40% of SCID cases are inherited from the parents.
- Bare lymphocyte syndrome. In this form of SCID, the white blood cells (lymphocytes) in the baby's blood are missing certain proteins without which the lymphocytes cannot activate the T cells in the immune system.
- SCID with leukopenia. Children with this form of SCID are lacking a type of white blood cell called a granulocyte.

SCID is an inherited disorder. There are two ways in which a developing fetus' immune system can fail to develop normally. In the first type of genetic problem, both B and T cells are defective. In the second type, only the T cells are abnormal, but their defect affects the functioning of the B cells.

For the first few months of life, a child with SCID is protected by antibodies in the mother's blood. As early as three months of age, however, the SCID child begins to suffer from mouth infections (thrush), chronic **diarrhea**, otitis media (ear infections), and pulmonary (associated with the lungs) infections, including **pneumocystis pneumonia**. The child loses weight, becomes very weak, and eventually dies from an opportunistic infection—one which takes advantage of the patient's weakened state.

SCID is diagnosed by the typing of T and B cells in the child's blood. B cells can be detected by immunofluorescence tests for surface markers (unique proteins) on the cells. T cells can be identified in tissue sections (samples) using enzyme-labeled antibodies.

Patients with SCID can be treated with **antibiotics** and immune serum to protect them from infections, but these treatments cannot cure the disorder. **Bone marrow transplants** are currently regarded as one of the few effective standard treatments for SCID.

In 1990, the Food and Drug Administration (FDA) approved PEG-ADA, an orphan drug (not available in United States but available elsewhere), for the treatment of SCID. PEG-ADA, which is also called pegademase bovine, works by replacing the ADA deficiency in children with this form of SCID. Children who receive weekly injections of PEG-ADA appear to have normal immune functions restored. Another treatment that is still in the experimental stage is **gene therapy**.

As of 1998, there is no cure for SCID. Most untreated patients die before age two years. Genetic counseling is recommended for parents of a child with SCID.

See also Bone marrow transplantation; Gene therapy; Immune system; Immunodeficiency

SEX CHANGE SURGERY

Also known as sex reassignment surgery, sex change surgery is a procedure that changes genital organs from one gender to another.

There are two reasons to alter the genital organs from one sex to another.

- Newborns with intersex deformities must early on be assigned one sex or the other. These deformities represent intermediate stages between the primordial female genitals and the change into male caused by male hormone stimulation.
- Both men and women occasionally believe they are physically a different sex than they are mentally and emotionally. This dissonance is so profound they are willing to be surgically altered.

In both cases, technical considerations favor successful conversion to a female rather than a male. Newborns with ambiguous organs will almost always be assigned to the female sex, unless the penis is at least an inch long. Whatever their chromosomes, they are much more likely to be socially well adjusted as females, even if they cannot have children.

Sexual identity is probably the most profound characteristic humans have. Assigning it must take place immediately after birth, both for the child's and the parents' comfort. Changing sexual identity may be the most significant change one can experience. It therefore should be done with every care and caution. By the time most adults come to surgery, they have lived for many years with dissonant identity. The average in one study was 29 years. Nevertheless, even then they may not be fully aware of the implications of becoming the other sex.

Converting male to female anatomy requires removal of the penis, reshaping genital tissue to appear more female and constructing a vagina. A vagina can be successfully formed from a skin graft or an isolated loop of intestine. Following the surgery, female hormones (estrogen) will reshape the body's contours and grow satisfactory breasts.

Female to male surgery has achieved lesser success, due to the difficulty of building a functioning penis from the much smaller clitoral tissue available in the female genitals. Penis construction is not attempted less than a year after the preliminary surgery to remove the female organs. One study in Singapore found that a third of the patients would not undergo the surgery again. Nevertheless, they were all pleased with the change of sex. Besides the genital organs, the breasts need to be surgically altered for a more male appearance. This can be done quite successfully.

Orgasm, or at least "a reasonable degree of erogenous sensitivity," can be experienced by patients after surgery.

Social support, particularly from the family, is important for readjustment as a member of the opposite sex. If patients were socially or emotionally unstable before the operation, over 30, or had an unsuitable body build for the new sex, they tend to do poorly. In no case studied did the procedure diminish their ability to work.

All surgery runs the risk of infection, bleeding, and a need to return for repairs. This surgery is irreversible, so the patient must have no doubts about the results.

The most common complication of the male to female surgery is narrowing of the new vagina.

SEX CHROMOSOME ABNORMALITIES

Fragile X syndrome is caused by a mutated gene on the X chromosome. Affected individuals have developmental delays, variable levels of **mental retardation**, and behavioral and emotional problems. They may also have characteristic physical traits. Males are affected more severely than females.

Klinfelter syndrome is a genetic disorder affecting males. People with this syndrome are born with at least one extra X chromosome.

Turner syndrome is a disorder of the chromosomes affecting females, where one of the two X chromosomes is partially or completely absent.

Chromosomes are found in every cell in the body. Chromosomes contain genes, structures that direct the growth and functioning of all the cells and systems in the body. In other words, chromosomes are responsible for passing on hereditary traits from parents to child, like eye color, height, nose shape, etc. Chromosomes also determine whether the child will be male or female. Normally, a person has a total of 46 chromosomes in each cell, two of which are responsible for determining that individual's sex. These two sex chromosomes are called X and Y. The combination of these two types of chromosomes determines the sex of a child. Females have two X chromosomes (the XX combination); males have one X and one Y chromosome (the XY combination).

Fragile X syndrome is the most common form of inherited mental retardation. Estimates of the incidence of this syndrome vary, but it is thought to affect about one in 2,000 girls and one in 1,250 boys. The syndrome is caused by a mutation in the FMR-1 gene, located on the X chromosome. The role of the gene is unclear, but it is probably important in early development.

The mutation involves a short sequence of DNA in the gene. This sequence is designated CGG. Normally, there are fewer than 50 adjacent copies of the CGG sequence. If the CGG sequence repeats more than 200 times, the FMR-1 gene is disabled.

The inheritance pattern of fragile X syndrome is complex. A condition called premutation may exist through several generations of a family, and no symptoms of fragile X will appear. During this premutation phase, the CGG sequence repeats 50–200 times. The size of the premutation expands over succeeding generations. Once the premutation reaches more than 200 repetitions, it becomes a full mutation. Individuals who have the full mutation may have fragile X syndrome.

In Klinefelter syndrome, a problem very early in development results in an abnormal number and arrangement of chromosomes. Most commonly, a male with Klinefelter syndrome will be born with 47 chromosomes in each cell, rather than the normal number of 46. The extra chromosome is an X chromosome. This means that rather than having the normal XY combination, the male has an XXY combination. Some Klinefelter patients have more complex chromosomal errors, including the presence of 48, 49, or even 50 chromosomes. All of the extra chromosomes are Xs.

Klinefelter syndrome is one of the most common chromosomal abnormalities. About 1 in every 1,000 infant boy is born with some variation of this disorder.

In Turner syndrome, an error very early in development results in an abnormal number and arrangement of chromosomes. Most commonly, a patient with Turner syndrome will be born with 45 chromosomes in each cell rather than 46. The missing chromosome is an X chromosome.

About 1 in every 8,000 babies born has Turner syndrome.

Fragile X syndrome is caused by a full mutation in the FMR-1 gene on the X chromosome. Because boys have just one copy of the X chromosome, they are more likely to develop symptoms than girls are. Fragile X boys appear normal at birth but development is delayed and they may have behavioral problems as they get older. Common behavioral problems include hyperactivity and attention problems known as attention deficit disorder. Approximately 90% of fragile X boys are mentally retarded, although the severity of the retardation varies. Characteristic physical traits appear later in childhood. These traits include enlarged testes, prominent ears, and a long, narrow face.

A girl's normal X chromosome may compensate for her fragile X chromosome. Approximately 30–50% of girls with a full mutation develop symptoms. These symptoms include mental impairment, ranging from mild learning disability to mental retardation, and behavioral problems. Characteristic physical traits are less noticeable in girls than in boys. Girls may not have these traits at all.

Children with fragile X syndrome often have frequent ear and sinus infections. Nearsightedness and lazy eye are also common. Many children experience digestive disorders that cause frequent gagging, vomiting, and discomfort. A small percentage may also experience seizures.

The cause of Klinefelter syndrome is unknown, although it has been noted that the disorder is seen more frequently among the children of older mothers.

The presence of more than one X chromosome in a male results in a delay in **puberty**. The testicles and the penis tend to be smaller than normal, and **infertility** is common. The testicles may remain up in the abdomen, instead of descending into the scrotum as is normal. Body hair decreases and breast size increases. Sexual drive is often below normal. Boys with Klinefelter syndrome tend to be tall and thin.

While it was once believed that all boys with Klinefelter syndrome were mentally retarded, doctors now know that the disorder can exist without retardation. However, children with Klinefelter syndrome frequently have difficulty with language, including learning to speak, read, and write. Some children have difficulty with social skills and tend to be more shy, anxious, or immature than their peers. Overly aggressive behavior has also been noted.

The greater the number of X chromosomes present, the greater the disability. Boys with several extra X chromosomes have distinctive facial features, more severe retardation, deformities of bony structures, and even more disordered development of male features.

No cause has been identified for Turner syndrome. At birth, female babies with Turner syndrome are below average in weight and length. They have slightly swollen hands and feet, and sometimes have swelling at the nape of the neck. Girls with Turner syndrome are shorter than normal, and have short, webbed necks with extra, loose skin. The jaw is usually small and the ears are large. An extra fold of skin is often seen on either side of the nose, close to the eye (called an epicanthic fold). The chest is usually quite broad, with increased distance between the nipples.

Further examination of girls with Turner syndrome will reveal that the ovaries, normal at birth, begin to slowly disappear. Within about two years, the ovaries usually contain no eggs. By about 10 years of age, the ovaries themselves will be essentially gone, with only streaks of tissue remaining. Nearly all Turner syndrome patients have no eggs in their ovaries, and are unable to conceive. Various heart defects are more common in females with Turner syndrome, and about 33% of all patients will have kidney deformities.

Many patients have multiple middle ear infections, and **hearing loss** is a frequent problem. Coordination is often poor, and many babies with Turner syndrome learn to walk relatively late. Some language problems may exist, but testing usually reveals that patients have normal intelligence.

Some disorders occur more frequently in Turner syndrome patients. These include thyroid disorders, inflammatory bowel disease, and malformed blood vessels within the gastrointestinal tract.

Behavioral and developmental problems may indicate fragile X syndrome, particularly if there is a family history of mental retardation. Definitive identification is made by means of a genetic test for the mutation. Individuals with the premutation or mutation may also be identified through **genetic testing**. Amniocentesis, chorionic villus sampling, and percutaneous umbilical blood sampling can be used to identify a fragile X chromosome before birth.

Diagnosis of Klinefelter syndrome is made by examining chromosomes for evidence of more than one X chromosome present in a male. Other abnormalities of sex hormones are common, including a low level of the male hormone testosterone.

Diagnosis is made by studying the chromosomes. Patients with Turner syndrome will either lack all or a part of one X chromosome. The other X chromosome will be intact. It is important that careful analysis of the chromosomes be done in order to search for any pieces of Y chromosome present. Y chromosomes are usually present only in males. When Turner syndrome patients have pieces of a Y chromosome in their cells, they have a substantially increased risk of developing a type of tumor called a gonadoblastoma.

Once Turner syndrome has been diagnosed, it is important to perform careful ultrasound examination of the heart, kidneys, and ovaries to diagnose associated defects.

Fragile X syndrome cannot be cured. To reach his or her full potential, a child may require speech and language therapy, occupational therapy, and physical therapy. The expertise of psychologists, special education teachers, and genetic counselors may also be needed. Drugs are used to treat hyperactivity, seizures, and other problems. Establishing a regular routine, avoiding over stimulation, and using calming techniques can help reduce behavioral problems.

There is no treatment available to change chromosomal makeup. However, the delayed puberty and decreased sexual drive associated with Klinefelter syndrome can both be treated with injections of a testosterone preparation about every three weeks.

Similarly, there is no treatment available for Turner syndrome. However, girls are sometimes treated with growth hormones, which can help them reach a more normal height. Because the ovaries are normally responsible for producing the female hormone estrogen, replacement estrogen therapy will be necessary.

Early diagnosis and intensive intervention offer the best prognosis for fragile X individuals. They can learn and are often good at memorizing and imitation. Most behavioral problems decrease by adulthood. About 50% of fragile X individuals develop mitral valve prolapse, a heart condition, as adults. Life span is typically normal.

While many men with Klinefelter syndrome go on to live normal lives, nearly 100% of these men will be sterile (unable to produce a child). Because men with Klinefelter syndrome have enlarged breasts, they have nearly the same chance of developing **breast cancer** as do women. Lung disease and certain rare tumors are also increased in patients with Klinefelter syndrome.

The prognosis for a person with Turner syndrome is dependent on what (if any) other conditions are present. For example, heart or kidney defects, hearing loss, or the development of inflammatory bowel disease may significantly affect a person's quality of life. Without these types of conditions, however, a person with Turner syndrome can be expected to live a relatively normal life. Support will be necessary to help the adolescent girl cope with body image issues and to help some women accept the fact that they will never be able to have children.

SEX HORMONES TESTS

Sex hormones tests measure levels of the sex hormones, including estrogen, progesterone, and testosterone.The sex hormone tests are ordered to determine if secretion of these hormones is normal. Several different types of tests are used to evaluate the different sex hormones to help diagnose problems or disorders, and to monitor pregnancy.

Estrogen fraction test is done to evaluate sexual maturity, **menstrual disorders**, and fertility problems in females. This test may also be used to test for tumors that excrete estrogen. In pregnant women it aids in determining fetal-placental health. Estrogen fraction is also used to evaluate males who have enlargement of one or both breasts (**gynecomastia**), or who have feminization syndromes, where they display female sex characteristics.

Progesterone assay test is ordered to evaluate women who are having difficulty becoming pregnant or maintaining a **pregnancy**, and to monitor high-risk pregnancies.

Testosterone levels are ordered to evaluate:

- Ambiguous sex characteristics
- **Precocious puberty**
- Virilizing syndromes in the female
- **Infertility** in the male
- Rare tumors of the ovary and testicle.

The sex hormones control the development of primary and secondary sexual characteristics. They regulate the sex-related functions of the body, such as the menstrual cycle or the production of eggs or sperm. There are three main types of sex hormones:

- The female sex hormones (called the estrogen hormones)
- The progesterone hormones (which help the body prepare for and maintain pregnancy)
- The male sex hormones, or the androgen hormones.

Female sex hormones are responsible for normal menstruation and the development of secondary female characteristics. Testosterone is a hormone that induces **puberty** in the male and maintains male secondary sex characteristics. In females, the adrenal glands and the ovaries secrete small amounts of testosterone.

Estrogen is tested to evaluate menstrual status, sexual maturity, and gynecomastia (or feminization syndromes). It is a tumor marker for patients with certain ovarian tumors. E1, a type of estrogen, is the most active estrogen in the nonpregnant female.

E3 (estriol) is the major estrogen in the pregnant female. It is produced in the placenta. Excretion of estriol increases around the eighth week of gestation and continues to rise until shortly before delivery. Serial urine and blood studies of this hormone are used to assess placental function and fetal normality in high-risk pregnancies. Falling values during pregnancy suggest fetoplacental deterioration and require prompt reassessment of the pregnancy, including the possibility of early delivery.

Progesterone is essential for the healthy functioning of the female reproductive system. Produced in the ovaries during the second half of the menstrual cycle, and by the placenta during pregnancy, small amounts of progesterone are also produced in the adrenal glands and testes.

After ovulation, an increase of progesterone causes the uterine lining to thicken in preparation for the implantation of a fertilized egg. If this event does not take place, progesterone and estrogen levels fall, resulting in shedding of the uterine lining.

Progesterone is essential during pregnancy, not only ensuring normal functioning of the placenta, but passing into the developing baby's circulation, where it is converted in the adrenal glands to corticosteroid hormones.

Testosterone is the most important of the male sex hormones. It is responsible for stimulating bone and muscle growth, and sexual development. It is produced by the testes and in very small amounts by the ovaries. Most testosterone tests measure total testosterone.

Testosterone stimulates sperm production (spermatogenesis), and influences the development of male secondary sex characteristics. Overproduction of testosterone caused by testicular, adrenal, or **pituitary tumors** in the young male may result in precocious puberty.

Overproduction of testosterone in females, caused by ovarian and adrenal tumors, can result in masculinization, the symptoms of which include cessation of the menstrual cycle (amenorrhea) and excessive growth of body hair (**hirsutism**).

When reduced levels of testosterone in the male indicate underactivity of the testes (**hypogonadism**), testosterone stimulation tests may be ordered.

The progesterone and testosterone tests require a blood sample; it is not necessary for the patient to restrict food or fluids before the test. Testosterone specimens should be drawn in the morning, as testosterone levels are highest in the early morning hours. The estrogen fraction test can be performed on blood and/or urine. It is not necessary for the patient to restrict food or fluids for either test. If a 24-hour urine test has been requested, the patient should call the laboratory for instructions.

Risks for these blood tests are minimal, but may include slight bleeding from the puncture site, **fainting** or feeling lightheaded after having blood drawn, or blood accumulating under the puncture site (hematoma).

Estrogen levels vary in women, ranging from 24–149 picograms per milliliter of blood. In men, the normal range is between 12–34 picograms per milliliter of blood.

Progesterone levels vary from less than 150 nanograms per deciliter (ng/dL) of blood to 2,000 nanograms in menstruating women. During pregnancy, progesterone levels range from 1,500–20,000 ng/dL of blood.

Testosterone values vary from laboratory to laboratory, but can generally be found within the following levels:

- Men. 300-1,200 ng/dL
- Women. 30-95 ng/dL
- Prepubertal children. less than 100 ng/dL (boys), less than 40 ng/dL (girls).

Increased levels of estrogen are seen in feminization syndromes:

- When a male begins to develop female secondary sex characteristics
- During precocious puberty
- When children develop secondary sexual characteristics at an abnormally early age
- Because of ovarian, testicular, or adrenal tumor
- During normal pregnancy, **cirrhosis**, and increased thyroid levels (hyperthyroidism).

Decreased levels of estrogen are found in the following conditions:

- A failing pregnancy
- During **menopause**
- **Anorexia nervosa**
- Primary and secondary hypogonadism
- **Turner syndrome**, seen in females with one missing X chromosome.

Increased levels of progesterone are seen:

- During ovulation and pregnancy
- With certain types of **ovarian cysts**
- A tumor of the ovary known as a choriocarcinoma

Decreased levels of progesterone are seen:

- In toxemia of pregnancy
- With a threatened spontaneous abortion
- During placental failure
- After fetal **death**
- With amenorrhea
- Due to ovarian dysfunction.

Increased levels (male) of testosterone are found in:

- Sexual precocity
- The viral infection of **encephalitis**
- Tumors involving the adrenal glands
- Testicular tumor
- Excessive thyroid production (hyperthyroidism)
- Testosterone resistance syndromes.

Decreased levels (male) of testosterone are seen in:

- Klinefelter syndrome
- A chromosomal deficiency
- Primary and secondary hypogonadism
- **Down syndrome**
- Surgical removal of the testicles
- Cirrhosis.

Increased levels (females) of testosterone are found in ovarian and adrenal tumors and in the presence of excessive hair growth of unknown cause (hirsutism).

See also Amenorrhea; Hirsutism; Hypogonadism; Infertility; Menopause; Puberty

Sex therapy

Sex therapy is the treatment of **sexual dysfunction**. Sex therapy utilizes various techniques in order to relieve sexual dysfunction commonly caused by **premature ejaculation** or sexual **anxiety** and to improve the sexual health of the patient.

Sexual dysfunction conjures up feelings of guilt, anger, insecurity, frustration, and rejection. Therapy is slow and requires open communication and understanding between sexual partners. Therapy may inadvertently address interpersonal communication problems.

Sex therapy is conducted by a trained therapist, doctor, or psychologist. The initial sessions should cover a complete history not only of the sexual problem but of the entire relationship and each individual's background and personality. The sexual relationship should be discussed in the context of the entire relationship. In fact, sexual counseling may de-emphasize sex until other aspects of the relationship are better understood and communicated.

There are several techniques that combat sexual dysfunction and are used in sex therapy. They include:

- Semans' technique: helps to combat premature ejaculation with a ''start-stop'' approach to to penis stimulation. By stimulating the man up to the point of ejaculation and then stopping, the man will become more aware of his response. More awareness leads to greater control, and open stimulation of both partners leads to greater communication and less anxiety. The start-stop technique is conducted four times until the man is allowed to ejaculate.
- Sensate focus therapy: the practice of nongenital and genital touching between partners in order to decrease sexual anxiety and build communication. First, partners explore each other's bodies without touching the genitals or breasts. Once the couple is comfortable with nongenital touching, they can expand to genital stimulation. Intercourse is prohibited in order to allow the partners to expand their intimacy and communication.
- Squeeze technique: used to treat premature ejaculation. When the man feels the urge to ejaculate, his partner squeezes his penis just below the head. This stops ejaculation and gives the man more control over his response.

Habits change slowly. All the techniques must be practiced faithfully for long periods of time to relearn behaviors. Communication is imperative.

See also Sexual dysfunction

Sexual abuse

The National Victim Center reports that over 700,000 women are sexually abused annually, with an estimated 61% of these under the age of 18. Studies have shown that approximately 80% of sexual assaults are committed by friends, acquaintances, or family members of the victims.

Sexual assault, including **rape**, may also occur within marital relationships, often within the cycle of **domestic violence**. It is believed that less than half of marital sexual assaults and rapes are reported to authorities. Factors that contribute this under-reporting include embarrassment, fear of further injury, and fear of court procedures that often scrutinize and judge the victim's behavior and history. Myths that surround sexual abuse and **rape** include: ''no really doesn't mean no''; ''nice girls don't get raped''; and, ''she asked for it''. Each of these beliefs can allow the blame to be shifted from the abuser to the victim, leading to a lack of support for, and even condemnation with secondary victimization of the victim.

Use of drugs and alcohol has been found to contribute to the risk of sexual abuse. Rohypnol (Flunitrazepam) is a sleeping medication that, although not marketed in the United States, has been associated here with ''date rape'' due to the disinhibition it causes. Also known by the street names of Roachies, Rophies, Ruffies, or La Roche, it can impair memory and judgment for 8 to 24 hours. These side effects are greater when this medication is ingested in combination with alcohol.

Many victims of sexual assault experience symptoms of helplessness, guilt, humiliation, insomnia, impaired memory and sexual dysfunction. This post-traumatic stress syndrome, may also include flashbacks of the assault, avoidance of the place and circumstance in which the rape occurred, and avoidance of previously pleasurable activities. In a cross-sectional study of women who had been raped compared to women who had not experienced any criminal victimization, the victims rated themselves as significantly less healthy, visited the physician nearly twice as often, and incurred double the medical costs. Medical problems directly related to the assault may include acute injuries, acquired **sexually transmitted diseases**, and **preganancy**.

Research indicates that as many as one out of every four children will be a victim of sexual abuse. The abusers almost always are someone the child knows and trusts, including relatives, family friends, or caretakers. Sexual abuse of a child can be physical, verbal or emotional, often beginning gradually and increasing over time. Perpetrators of the abuse take advantage of the child's vulnerabilities, their trusting and dependent nature. Most children cannot or do not tell about their abuse. They may be too young to put the abuse into words, feel confused by the accompanying feelings, or be threatened or bribed by the abuser to keep the abuse a secret. They also may feel too ashamed or embarrassed to tell, be afraid no one will believe them or worry about getting in trouble or getting a loved one in trouble. Adults should be alert to symptoms of frequent abuse, including persistent sexual play with other children, toys or pets; unexplained pain, swelling, bleeding or irritation of the mouth, genital, or anal area; urinary tract infections; or displaying sexual knowledge, in language, or actions, beyond what is expected for their age. More subtle signs may include: fear or dislike of certain people or places; withdrawal from family friends, or usual activities; return to younger, more babyish behavior; and/or passive or overly pleasing behavior. There are many resources available to help victims and their families. Teaching children about sexual abuse with safety information appropriate to their developmental level, can help increase their awareness and coping skills.

See also Child abuse; Domestic violence; Rape

SEXUAL DYSFUNCTION

Sexual dysfunction is broadly defined as the inability to fully enjoy sexual intercourse. Specifically, sexual dysfunctions are disorders that interfere with a full sexual response cycle. These disorders make it difficult for a person to enjoy or to have sexual intercourse. While sexual dysfunction rarely threatens physical health, it can take a heavy psychological toll, bringing on depression, **anxiety**, and debilitating feelings of inadequacy.

Sexual dysfunction takes different forms in men and women. A dysfunction can be life-long and always present acquired, situational, or generalized (occurring despite the situation). A man may have a sexual problem if he:

- Ejaculates before he or his partner desires (**premature ejaculation**)
- Does not ejaculate, or experiences delayed ejaculation
- Is unable to have an erection sufficient for pleasurable intercourse
- Feels **pain** during intercourse
- Lacks or loses sexual desire.

A woman may have a sexual problem if she:

- Lacks or loses sexual desire
- Has difficulty achieving orgasm
- Feels anxiety during intercourse
- Feels pain during intercourse
- Feels vaginal or other muscles contract involuntarily before or during sex
- Has inadequate lubrication.

The most common sexual dysfunctions in men include:

- Erectile dysfunction: an impairment of the erectile reflex. The man is unable to have or maintain an erection that is firm enough for coitus or intercourse.
- Premature ejaculation, or rapid ejaculation with minimal sexual stimulation before, on, or shortly after penetration and before the person wishes it.
- Ejaculatory incompetence: the inability to ejaculate within the vagina despite a firm erection and relatively high levels of sexual arousal.
- Retarded ejaculation: a condition in which the bladder neck does not close off properly during orgasm so that the semen spurts backward into the bladder.

Until recently, it was presumed that women were less sexual than men. In the past two decades, traditional views of female sexuality were all but demolished, and women's sexual needs became accepted as legitimate in their own right.

Female sexual dysfunctions include:

- Sexual arousal disorder: the inhibition of the general arousal aspect of sexual response. A woman with this disorder does not lubricate, her vagina does not swell, and the muscle that surrounds the outer third of the vagina does not tighten—a series of changes that normally prepare the body for orgasm (''the orgasmic platform''). Also, in this disorder, the woman typically does not feel erotic sensations.
- Orgasmic disorder: the impairment of the orgasmic component of the female sexual response. The woman may be sexually aroused but never reach orgasm. Orgasmic capacity is less than would be reasonable for her age, sexual experience, and the adequacy of sexual stimulation she receives.
- Vaginismus: a condition in which the muscles around the outer third of the vagina have involuntary spasms in response to attempts at vaginal penetration.
- Painful intercourse: a condition that can occur at any age. Pain can appear at the start of intercourse, midway through coital activities, at the time of orgasm, or after intercourse is completed. The pain can be felt as burning, sharp searing, or cramping; it can be external, within the vagina, or deep in the pelvic region or abdomen.

Many factors, of both physical and psychological natures, can affect sexual response and performance. Injuries, ailments, and drugs are among the physical influences; in addition, there is increasing evidence that chemicals and other environmental pollutants depress sexual function. As for psychological factors, sexual dysfunction may have roots in traumatic events such as rape or incest, guilt feelings, a poor self-image, depression, chronic fatigue, certain religious beliefs, or marital problems. Dysfunction is often associated with anxiety. If a man operates under the misconception that all sexual activity must lead to intercourse and to orgasm by his partner, and if the expectation is not met, he may consider the act a failure.

With premature ejaculation, physical causes are rare, although the problem is sometimes linked to a neurological disorder, prostate infection, or urethritis. Possible psychological causes include anxiety (mainly performance anxiety), guilt feelings about sex, and ambivalence toward women. However, research has failed to show a direct link between premature ejaculation and anxiety. Rather, premature ejaculation seems more related to sexual inexperience in learning to modulate arousal.

When men experience painful intercourse, the cause is usually physical; an infection of the prostate, urethra, or testes, or an allergic reaction to spermicide or **condom**s. Painful erections may be caused by Peyronie's disease, fibrous plaques on the upper side of the penis that often produce a bend during erection. **Cancer** of the penis or testis and arthritis of the lower back can also cause pain.

Retrograde ejaculation occurs in men who have had prostate or urethral surgery, take medication that keeps the bladder open, or suffer from **diabetes mellitus**, a disease that can injure the nerves that normally close the bladder during ejaculation.

Erectile dysfunction is more likely than other dysfunctions to have a physical cause. Drugs, diabetes (the most common physical cause), **Parkinson's disease**, **multiple sclerosis**, and spinal cord lesions can all be causes of erectile dysfunction. When physical causes are ruled out, anxiety is the most likely psychological cause of erectile dysfunction.

Dysfunctions of arousal and orgasm in women also may be physical or psychological in origin. Among the most common causes are day-to-day discord with one's partner and inadequate stimulation by the partner. Finally, sexual desire can wane as one ages, although this varies greatly from person to person.

Pain during intercourse can occur for any number of reasons, and location is sometimes a clue to the cause. Pain in the vaginal area may be due to infection, such as urethritis; also, vaginal tissues may become thinner and more sensitive during breast-feeding and after **menopause**. Deeper pain may have a pelvic source, such as **endometriosis**, pelvic adhesions, or uterine abnormalities. Pain can also have a psychological cause, such as fear of injury, guilt feelings about sex, fear of **pregnancy** or injury to the fetus during pregnancy, or recollection of a previous painful experience.

Vaginismus may be provoked by these psychological causes as well, or it may begin as a response to pain, and continue after the pain is gone. Both partners should understand that the vaginal contraction is an involuntary response, outside the woman's control.

Similarly, insufficient lubrication is involuntary, and may be part of a complex cycle. Low sexual response may lead to inadequate lubrication, which may lead to discomfort, and so on.

In deciding when a sexual dysfunction is present, it is necessary to remember that while some people may be interested in sex at almost any time, others have low or seemingly nonexistent levels of sexual interest. Only when it is a source of personal or relationship distress, instead of voluntary choice, is it classified as a sexual dysfunction.

The first step in diagnosing a sexual dysfunction is usually discussing the problem with a doctor, who will need to ask further questions in an attempt to differentiate among the types of sexual dysfunction. The physician may also perform a **physical examination** of the genitals, and may order further medical tests, including measurement of hormone levels in the blood. Men may be referred to a specialist in diseases of the urinary and genital organs (urologist), and primary care physicians may refer women to a gynecologist.

Treatments break down into two main kinds: behavioral psychotherapy and physical. **Sex therapy**, which is ideally provided by a member of the American Association of Sexual Educators, Counselors, and Therapists (AASECT), universally emphasizes correcting sexual misinformation, the importance of improved partner communication and honesty, anxiety reduction, sensual experience and pleasure, and interpersonal tolerance and acceptance. Sex therapists believe that many sexual disorders are rooted in learned patterns and values. These are termed psychogenic. An underlying assumption of sex therapy is that relatively short-term outpatient therapy can alleviate learned patterns, restrict symptoms, and allow a greater satisfaction with sexual experiences.

In some cases, a specific technique may be used during intercourse to correct a dysfunction. One of the most common is the "squeeze technique" to prevent premature ejaculation. When a man feels that an orgasm is imminent, he withdraws from his partner. Then, the man or his partner gently squeezes the head of the penis to halt the orgasm. After 20-30 seconds, the couple may resume intercourse. The couple may do this several times before the man proceeds to ejaculation.

In cases where significant sexual dysfunction is linked to a broader emotional problem, such as depression or substance abuse, intensive psychotherapy and/or pharmaceutical intervention may be appropriate.

In many cases, doctors may prescribe medications to treat an underlying physical cause of sexual dysfunction. Possible medical treatments include:

- Clomipramine and fluoxetine for premature ejaculation
- Papaverine and prostaglandin for erectile difficulties
- **Hormone replacement therapy** for female dysfunctions
- Viagra, a pill approved in 1998 as a treatment for **impotence**.

A variety of alternative therapies can be useful in the treatment of sexual dysfunction. Counseling or psychotherapy is highly recommended to address any emotional or mental components of the disorder. Botanical medicine, either western, Chinese, or **ayurvedic**, as well as nutritional supplementation, can help resolve biochemical causes of sexual dysfunction. **Acupuncture** and homeopathic treatment can be helpful by focusing on the energetic aspects of the disorder.

Some problems with sexual function are normal. For example, women starting a new or first relationship may feel sore or bruised after intercourse and find that an over-the-counter lubricant makes sex more pleasurable. Simple techniques, such as soaking in a warm bath, may relax a person before intercourse and improve the experience. **Yoga** and **meditation** provide needed mental and physical relaxation for several conditions, such as vaginismus. Relaxation therapy eases and relieves anxiety about dysfunction. **Massage** is extremely effective at reducing **stress**, especially if performed by the partner.

There is no single cure for sexual dysfunctions, but almost all can be controlled. Most people who have a sexual dysfunction fare well once they get into a treatment program. For example, a high percentage of men with premature ejaculation can be successfully treated in two to three months. Furthermore, the gains made in sex therapy tend to be long-lasting rather than short-lived.

See also Impotence; Menopause; Pregnancy; Premature ejaculation; Sex therapy

SEXUAL ORIENTATION

The origins of sexual orientation have puzzled philosophers, theologians, and ordinary people for thousands of years. In a few cultures, homosexuality has been regarded as a normal part of life, or even as a gift from the gods. But in most cultures, homosexual behavior has been treated throughout history as a sin or even a crime. In the late 1800s, western medicine turned its attention on homosexuality and concluded it resulted from aberrant child-rearing practices. This disease model remained the prevailing paradigm in studies of homosexuality throughout most of the 20th century. Thus, the traditional attitude toward homosexuality in this country has been that homosexuality is a lifestyle that an individual chooses, and not something influenced by genes. This idea is consistent with the psychoanalytic theories of Sigmund Freud, who proposed that homosexuality arises either as a result of the castration complex that results when a boy realizes that his mother doesn't have a penis, or by a failure of a man to break the sexual bond with a smothering or domineering mother. In either case, Freud's ideas, which have not held up under scientific scrutiny, gave rise to the idea that homosexuality was a sickness that could be cured by treatment. The behaviorist school, on the other hand, argues that sexual orientation is a product of society and culture, but in a way more general than that proposed by Freud. According to behaviorist theory, if a boy is exposed to a homosexual role model, he may be swayed toward becoming gay. A variation in this idea has it that both heterosexual and homosexual orientation result from societal expectations. Unfortunately, this theory does not adequately explain how purely social factors could give rise to the propagation and survival of the human race. In 1993, Dr. Dean Hamer and his colleagues at the **National Institutes of Health** published the results of a study on the genetic origins of sexual orientation in the magazine *Science*. Hamer et al. reported that at least one subtype of sexual orientation, male homosexuality, appeared to be genetically influenced, and that it might be linked to a set of five DNA sequences located on the Xq28 region of the X chromosome, which is passed down by mothers to their offspring. Their study concluded that gay brothers tend to share these Xq28 sequences, which suggested a genetic origin for homosexuality passed through the female line. Hamer later cited twin and family studies as evidence that female sexual orientation is as likely to be inherited as male sexual orientation, but he felt it unlikely that the same version of Xq28 associated with male sexuality would be responsible for female homosexuality (lesbianism) in light of there being relatively few observations of families with large proportions of both gay men and women. Hamer's findings generated considerable interest, not the least because sexual orientation is at the center of fierce debates involving politics, the law, religion, ethics, and the very meaning of human behavior. The Pentagon was interested because of the potential effect the results might have on legislation about gays in the military. Observers have also pointed out that Supreme Court decisions could be influenced if it does indeed turn out that homosexuality is an immutable human characteristic. And there would also be ethical, medical, and economic issues to deal with if it turns out that there is indeed a gay gene. Since the publication of his 1993 article in *Science*, Hamer has stated that nature and nurture probably work together to determine sexual orientation. Using the analogy of the personal computer, Hamer says that sexual orientation could be the product of both genes and environment, in much the same way that the software in a computer is a mixture of what is installed in the factory and what the user adds later. It is significant, however, that the results of a 1999 study by Dr. George Rice of the University of Western Ontario have cast doubts on some of Hamer's findings. Specifically, Rice et al. failed to find a gene of large effect that influences sexual orientation, although they did not rule out the existence of such a gene elsewhere in the human genome. To this extent, the results of Rice et al. are not inconsistent with earlier studies in families and twins that have suggested that sexual orientation is at least partially linked to genetics.

This is, of course, a highly controversial issue, one that is far from settled at this time. The bulk of the evidence at present favors the concept that homosexuality is an immutable characteristic based on as yet undetermined mechanisms.

Sexual perversions

Sexual perversions are conditions in which sexual excitement or orgasm is associated with acts or imagery that are considered unusual within the culture. To avoid problems associated with the stigmatization of labels, the neutral term ''paraphilia,'' derived from Greek roots meaning ''alongside of'' and ''love,'' is used to describe what used to be called sexual perversions. A paraphilia is a condition in which a person's sexual arousal and gratification depend on a fantasy theme of an unusual situation or object that becomes the principal focus of sexual behavior.

Paraphilias can revolve around a particular sexual object or a particular act. They are defined by *DSM-IV* as ''sexual impulse disorders characterized by intensely arousing, recurrent sexual fantasies, urges and behaviors considered deviant with respect to cultural norms and that produce clinically significant distress or impairment in social, occupational or other important areas of psychosocial functioning.'' The nature of a paraphilia is generally specific and unchanging, and most of the paraphilias are far more common in men than in women.

Paraphilias differ from what some people might consider ''normal'' sexual activity in that these behaviors cause significant distress or impairment in areas of life functioning. They do not refer to the normal use of sexual fantasy, activity or objects to heighten sexual excitement where there is no distress or impairment. The most common signs of sexual activity that can be classified as paraphilia include: the inability to resist an impulse for the sexual act, the requirement of participation by non-consenting or under-aged individuals, legal consequences, resulting **sexual dysfunction**, and interference with normal social relationships.

Paraphilias include fantasies, behaviors, and/or urges which:

- Involve nonhuman sexual objects, such as shoes or undergarments
- Require the suffering or humiliation of oneself or partner
- Involve children or other non-consenting partners.

The most common paraphilias are:

- Exhibitionism, or exposure of the genitals
- Fetishism, or the use of nonliving objects
- Frotteurism, or touching and rubbing against a nonconsenting person
- Pedophilia, or the focus on prepubescent children

- Sexual masochism, or the receiving of humiliation or suffering
- Sexual sadism, or the inflicting of humiliation or suffering
- Transvestic fetishism, or cross-dressing
- Voyeurism, or watching others engage in undressing or sexual activity.

A paraphiliac often has more than one paraphilia. Paraphilias often result in a variety of associated problems, such as guilt, depression, shame, **isolation**, and impairment in the capacity for normal social and sexual relationships. A paraphilia can, and often does, become highly idiosyncratic and ritualized (excessively (habitual).

There is very little certainty about what causes a paraphilia. Psychoanalysts generally theorize that these conditions represent a regression to or a fixation at an earlier level of psychosexual development resulting in a repetitive pattern of sexual behavior that is not mature in its application and expression. In other words, an individual repeats or reverts to a sexual habit arising early in life. Another psychoanalytic theory holds that these conditions are all expressions of hostility in which sexual fantasies or unusual sexual acts become a means of obtaining revenge for a childhood trauma. The persistent, repetitive nature of the paraphilia is caused by an inability to erase the underlying trauma completely. Indeed, a history of childhood sexual abuse is sometimes seen in individuals with paraphilias.

However, behaviorists suggest, instead, that the paraphilia begins via a process of **conditioning** (when an act associated with one stimulus becomes associated with another). Nonsexual objects can become sexually arousing if they are frequently and repeatedly associated with a pleasurable sexual activity. The development of a paraphilia is not usually a matter of conditioning alone; there must usually be some predisposing (making susceptible) factor, such as difficulty forming person to person sexual relationships or poor self-esteem.

The following are situations or causes that might lead someone in a paraphiliac direction:

- Parents who humiliate and punish a small boy for strutting around with an erect penis
- A young boy who is sexually abused
- An individual who is dressed in a woman's clothes as a form of parental punishment
- Fear of sexual performance or intimacy
- Inadequate counseling
- Excessive alcohol intake
- Physiological problems
- Sociocultural factors
- Psychosexual trauma.

Whatever the cause, paraphiliacs apparently rarely seek treatment unless they are induced into it by an arrest or discovery by a family member. This makes diagnosis before a confrontation very difficult.

Paraphiliacs may select an occupation, or develop a hobby or volunteer work, that puts them in contact with the desired erotic stimuli, for example, selling women's shoes or lingerie in fetishism, or working with children in pedophilia. Other coexistent problems may be alcohol or drug abuse, intimacy problems, and personality disturbances especially emotional immaturity. Additionally, there may be sexual dysfunctions. Erectile dysfunction and an inability to ejaculate may be common in attempts at sexual activity without the paraphiliac theme.

Paraphilias may be mild, moderate, or severe. An individual with mild paraphilia is markedly distressed by the recurrent paraphiliac urges but has never acted on them. The moderate has occasionally acted on the paraphilic urge. A severe paraphiliac has repeatedly acted on the urge.

The literature describing treatment is fragmentary and incomplete. Traditional psychoanalysis has not been particularly effective with paraphilia and generally requires several years of treatment. Therapy with hypnosis has also had poor results. Current interests focus primarily on several behavioral techniques that include the following:

- Aversion imagery involves the pairing of a sexually arousing paraphilic stimulus with an unpleasant image, such as being arrested or having one's name appear in the newspaper.
- Desensitization procedures neutralize the **anxiety**-provoking aspects of nonparaphilic sexual situations and behavior by a process of gradual exposure. For example, a man afraid of having sexual contact with women his own age might be led through a series of relaxation procedures aimed at reducing his anxiety.
- Social skills training is used with either of the other approaches and is aimed at improving a person's ability to form interpersonal relationships.
- Orgasmic reconditioning may instruct a person to masturbate using his paraphilia fantasy and to switch to a more appropriate fantasy just at the moment of orgasm.

In addition to these therapies, drugs are sometimes prescribed to treat paraphilic behaviors. Drugs that drastically lower testosterone temporarily (antiandrogens) have been used for the control of repetitive deviant sexual behaviors and have been prescribed for paraphilia-related disorders as well. Cyproterone acetate inhibits testosterone directly at androgen receptor sites. In its oral form, the usual prescribed dosage range is 50-200 mg per day.

Serotonergics (drugs that boost levels of the brain chemical serotonin) are prescribed for anxious and depressive symptoms. Of the serotonergic agents reported, fluoxetine has received the most attention, although lithium, clomipramine, buspirone, and sertraline are reported as effective in case reports and open clinical trials with outpatients. Other alternative supplemental strategies that may be effective include adding a low dose of a secondary amine tricyclic antidepressant to the primary serotonergics, but these reports are only anecdotal (not scientifically proven).

Despite more than a decade of experience with **psychotherapy** treatment programs, most workers in the field are not convinced that they have a high degree of success. Furthermore, because some cases involve severe abuse, many in the general public would prefer to ''lock up'' the sex offender than to have him out in the community in a treatment program or on parole after the treatment program has been completed.

Paraphilia and paraphilia-related disorders are more prevalent than most clinicians suspect. Since these disorders are cloaked in shame and guilt, the presence of these conditions may not be adequately revealed until a therapeutic relationship is firmly established. Once a diagnosis is established, appropriate education about possible behavioral therapies and appropriate use of psychiatric medications can improve the outcome for these conditions.

See also Sex therapy

Sexually transmitted diseases

Sexually transmitted disease (STD) is a term used to describe more than 20 different infections that are transmitted through exchange of semen, blood, and other body fluids; or by direct contact with the affected body areas of people with STDs. Sexually transmitted diseases are also called venereal diseases.

The Centers for Disease Control and Prevention has reported that 85% of the most prevalent infectious diseases in the United States are sexually transmitted. The rate of STDs in this country is 50-100 times higher than that of any other industrialized nation. One in four sexually active Americans will be affected by an STD at some time in his or her life.

About 12 million new STD infections occur in the United States each year. One in four occurs in someone between the ages of 16 and 19. Almost 65% of all STD infections affect people under the age of 25.

STDs can have very **pain**ful long-term consequences as well as immediate health problems. They can cause:

- **Birth defects**
- Blindness
- Bone deformities
- Brain damage
- **Cancer**
- Heart disease
- **Infertility** and other abnormalities of the reproductive system
- **Mental retardation**
- **Death**.

Some of the most common and potentially serious STDs in the United States include:

- Chlamydial diseases— including lymphogranuloma venereum (LGV) and chlamydial urethritis—and **gonorrhea**. These STDs can cause sterility or potentially fatal infections of the upper genital tract. A chlamydia is a microscopic organism that lives as a parasite inside human cells.
- Human papillomavirus (HPV). HPV causes **genital warts**. It is the single most important risk factor for **cervical cancer** in women.
- **Genital herpes**. Herpes is an incurable viral infection thought to be one of the most common STDs in this country.
- **Syphilis**. Syphilis is a potentially life-threatening infection that increases the likelihood of acquiring or transmitting HIV. One type of syphilis is congenital syphilis, which causes irreversible health problems or death in as many as 40% of all live babies born to women with untreated syphilis.
- Human **immunodeficiency** virus (HIV) infection. As of 1998, there is no cure for this STD.

STDs affect certain population groups more severely than others. Women, young people, and members of minority groups are particularly affected. Women in any age bracket are more likely than men to develop medical complications related to STDs. With respect to racial and ethnic categories, the incidence of syphilis is 60 times higher among African Americans than among Caucasians, and four times higher in Hispanics than in Anglos. African Americans are 40 times more likely than Caucasians to develop gonorrhea, and as much as three times more likely to acquire genital herpes.

The symptoms of STDs vary somewhat according to the disease agent (whether a virus, a bacterium, or a chlamydia), the sex of the patient, and the body systems affected. The symptoms of some STDs are easy to identify; others produce infections that may either go unnoticed for some time or are easy to confuse with other diseases. Syphilis in particular can be confused with disorders ranging from **infectious mononucleosis** to allergic reactions to prescription medications. In addition, the incubation period of STDs varies. Some produce symptoms close enough to the time of sexual contact— often less than 48 hours later— for the patient to recognize the connection between the behavior and the symptoms. Others have a longer incubation period, so that the patient may not recognize the early symptoms as those of a sexually transmitted infection.

Some symptoms of STDs affect the genitals and reproductive organs:

- A woman who has an STD may bleed when she is not menstruating or have an abnormal vaginal discharge. Vaginal burning, **itching**, and odor are common, and she may experience pain in her pelvic area or while having sex.
- A discharge from the tip of the penis may be a sign that a man has an STD. Males may also have painful or burning sensations when they urinate.
- There may be swelling of the lymph nodes near the groin area.
- Both men and women may develop skin **rashes**, sores, bumps, or blisters near the mouth or genitals. Homosexual men frequently develop these symptoms in the area around the anus.

Other symptoms of STDs are systemic, which means that they affect the body as a whole. These symptoms may include:

- **Fever**, chills, and similar flu-like symptoms
- Skin rashes over large parts of the body
- Arthritis-like pains or aching in the joints
- Throat swelling and redness that lasts for three weeks or longer.

A sexually active person who has symptoms of an STD or who has had an STD or symptoms of infection should be examined without delay by a:

- Specialist in women's health (gynecologist)
- Specialist in disorders of the urinary tract and the male sexual organs (urologist)
- Family physician
- Nurse practitioner
- Specialist in skin disorders (dermatologist).

The diagnostic process begins with a thorough **physical examination** and a detailed medical history that documents the patient's sexual history and assesses the risk of infection.

The doctor or other healthcare professional will:

- Describe the testing process. This includes all blood tests and other tests that may be relevant to the specific infection.
- Explain the meaning of the test results.
- Provide the patient with information regarding high-risk behaviors and any necessary treatments or procedures.

The doctor may suggest that a patient diagnosed with one STD be tested for others. It's possible to have more than one STD at a time. One infection may hide the symptoms of another or create a climate that fosters its growth. At present, it is particularly important that persons who are HIV-positive be tested for syphilis as well.

The law in most parts of the United States requires public health officials to trace and contact the partners of persons with STDs. Minors, however, can get treatment without their parents' permission. Public health departments in most states can provide information about STD clinic locations; Planned Parenthood facilities provide testing and counseling. These agencies can also help with or assume the responsibility of notifying sexual partners who must be tested and may require treatment.

Although self-care can relieve some of the pain of genital herpes or genital warts that has recurred after being diagnosed and treated by a physician, other STD symptoms require immediate medical attention.

Antibiotics are prescribed to treat gonorrhea, chlamydia, syphilis, and other STDs caused by bacteria. Although prompt diagnosis and early treatment almost always cures these STDs, new infections can develop if exposure continues or is renewed.

The prognosis for recovery from STDs varies from disease to disease. The prognosis for recovery from gonorrhea, syphilis, and other STDs caused by bacteria is generally good, provided that the disease is diagnosed early and treated promptly. Untreated syphilis in particular can lead to long-term complications and disability. Viral STDs (genital herpes, genital warts, HIV) cannot be cured but must be treated on a long-term basis to relieve symptoms and prevent life-threatening complications.

Vaccines for the prevention of hepatitis A and hepatitis B are currently recommended for gay and bisexual men, users of illegal drugs, and others at risk of contracting these diseases. Vaccines to prevent other STDs are being tested and may be available within several years.

The risk of becoming infected with an STD can be reduced or eliminated by decisions about personal behavior. Abstinence from sexual relations or a monogamous relationship with a partner who is not having sex outside it are legitimate options. It is also wise to avoid sexual contact with partners who are known to be infected with an STD, whose health status is unknown, who abuse drugs, or who are involved in prostitution.

Men or women who have sex with an infected partner should make sure a new **condom** is used every time they have genital, oral, or anal contact. Used correctly and consistently, male condoms provide good protection against HIV and other STDs.

Female condoms (lubricated sheaths inserted into the vagina) have been shown to be effective in preventing HIV and other viral STDs. Researchers believe female condoms will substantially reduce the risk of developing other STDs; however, studies testing that theory have not yet been completed.

Spermicides and diaphragms can prevent transmission of some STDs. They do not protect women from contracting HIV. Birth-control pills, patches, or injections do not prevent STDs. Neither do surgical sterilization or **hysterectomy**.

Urinating and washing the genital area with soap and water immediately after having sex may eliminate some germs before they cause infection. Douching, however, can spread infection deeper into the womb. It may increase a woman's risk of developing **pelvic inflammatory disease** (PID).

Shaken baby syndrome

Shaken baby syndrome (SBS) is a collective term for the internal head injuries a baby or young child sustains from being violently shaken Shaken baby syndrome was first described in the medical literature in 1972. Physicians earlier labeled these injuries as accidental, but as more about **child abuse** became known, more cases of this syndrome were properly diagnosed.

Every year, nearly 50,000 children in the United States are forcefully shaken by their caretakers. More than 60% of these children are boys. The victims are on average six to eight months old, but may be as old as five years or as young as a few days.

Men are more likely than women to shake a child; typically, these men are in their early 20s and are the baby's father or the mother's boyfriend. Women who inflict SBS are more likely to be babysitters or child care providers than the baby's mother. The shaking may occur as a response of frustration to the baby's inconsolable crying or as an action of routine abuse.

Infants and small children are especially vulnerable to SBS because their neck muscles are still too weak to adequately support their disproportionately large heads, and their young brain tissue and blood vessels are extremely fragile. When an infant is vigorously shaken by the arms, legs, shoulders, or chest, the **whiplash** motion repeatedly jars the baby's brain with tremendous force, causing internal damage and bleeding. While there may be no obvious external signs of injury following shaking, the child may suffer internally from brain bleeding and bruising (called **subdural hemorrhage and hematoma**); brain swelling and damage (called cerebral **edema**); **mental re-**

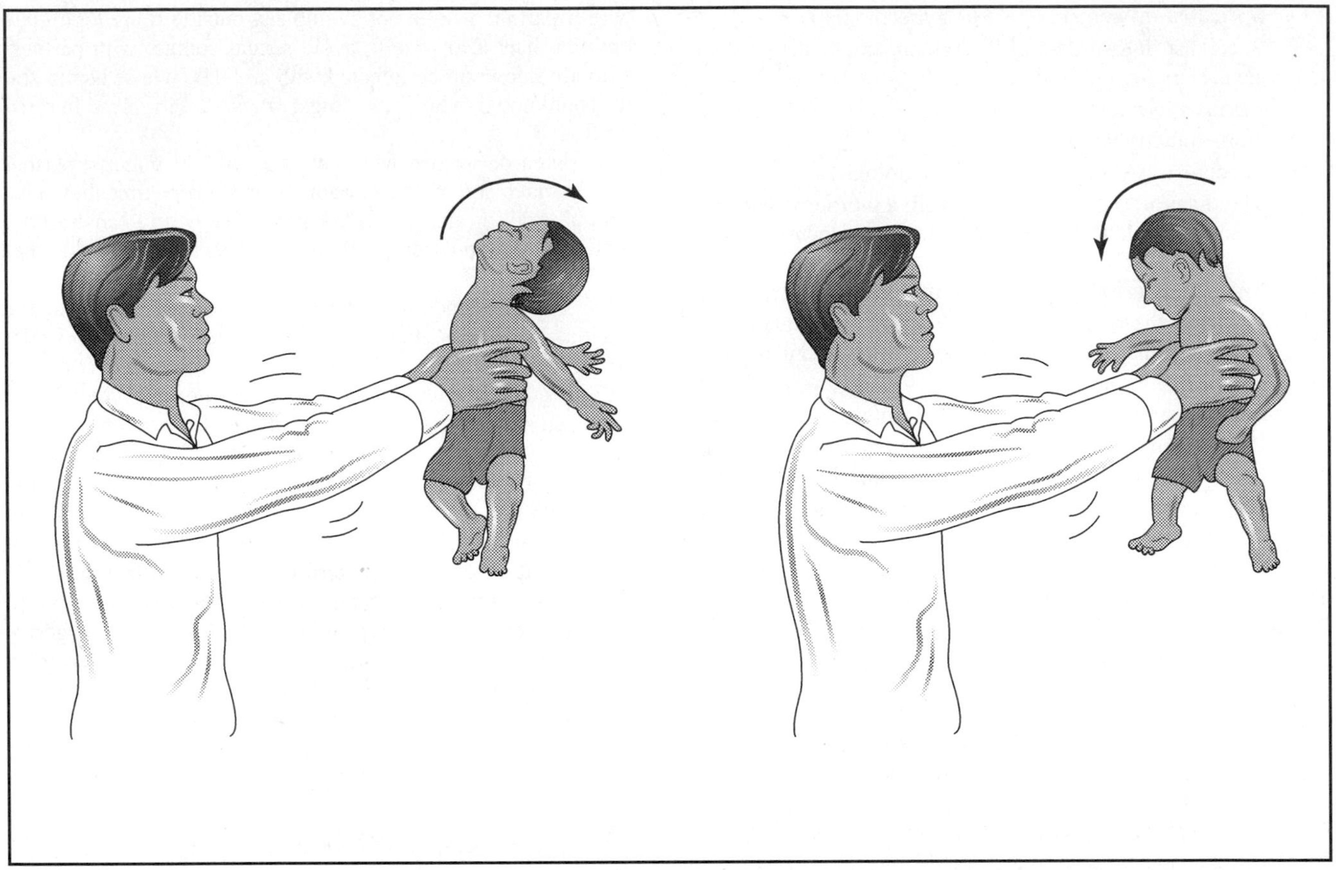

Shaken baby syndrome is a collective term for the internal head injuries a baby or young child sustains from being violently shaken. Because of the fragile state of an infant's brain tissue and blood vessels, when a baby is vigorously shaken by the chest, as shown in the illustration above, the whiplash motion repeatedly jars the baby's brain with extreme force, causing serious internal damage and bleeding. Nearly 2,000 American children die annually from this condition. ***(Illustration by Electronic Illustrators Group.)***

tardation; **blindness**, **hearing loss**, **paralysis**, speech impairment, and learning disabilities; and **death**. Nearly 2,000 children die every year as a result of being shaken.

Physicians may have difficulty initially diagnosing SBS because there are usually few witnesses to give a reliable account of the events leading to the trauma, few if any external injuries, and, upon close examination, the physical findings may not agree with the account given. A shaken baby may present one or more signs, including vomiting; difficulty breathing, sucking, swallowing, or making sounds; **seizures**; and altered consciousness.

To diagnose SBS, physicians look for at least one of three classic conditions: bleeding at the back of one or both eyes (retinal hemorrhage), subdural hematoma, and cerebral edema. The diagnosis is confirmed by the results of either a computed tomography scan (CT scan) or **magnetic resonance imaging** (MRI).

Appropriate treatment is determined by the type and severity of the trauma. Physicians may medically manage both internal and external injuries. Behavioral and educational impairments as a result of the injuries require the attention of additional specialists. Children with SBS may need physical therapy, speech therapy, vision therapy, and special education services.

There is no alternative to prompt medical treatment. An unresponsive child should never be put to bed, but must be taken to a hospital for immediate care.

Sadly, children who receive violent shaking have a poor prognosis for complete recovery. Those who do not die may experience permanent blindness, mental retardation, seizure disorders, or loss of motor control.

Shaken baby syndrome is preventable with public education. Adults must be actively taught that shaking a child is never acceptable and can cause severe injury or death.

When the frustration from an incessantly crying baby becomes too much, caregivers should have a strategy for coping that does not harm the baby. The first step is to place the baby in a crib or playpen and leave the room in order to calm down. Counting to 10 and taking deep breaths may help. A friend or relative may be called to come over and assist. A calm adult may then resume trying to comfort the baby. A warm bottle, a dry diaper, soft music, a bath, or a ride in a swing, stroller, or car may be offered to soothe a crying child. Crying may also indicate **pain** or illness, such as from abdominal cramps or an earache. If the crying persists, the child should be seen by a physician.

See also Child abuse; Seizures; Subdural hematoma

Sharp, Phillip A. (1944-)

American biologist

Phillip A. Sharp has conducted research into the structure of deoxyribonucleic acid (DNA —the chemical blueprint that synthesizes proteins) which has altered previous views on the mechanism of genetic change. For his work in this area, Sharp was presented with the 1977 Nobel Prize in medicine along with **Richard J. Roberts**. Sharp was born in Falmouth, Kentucky, on June 6, 1944 to Katherin Colvin and Joseph Walter Sharp. He attended Union College in Barbourville, Kentucky, where he received a B.A. degree in chemistry and mathematics in 1966. Sharp earned his Ph.D. degree from the University of Illinois in 1969.

Sharp and Richard J. Roberts discovered in 1977 that, in some higher organisms, genes may be comprised of more than one segment, separated by material which apparently plays no part in the creation of the proteins. Previously, most scientists believed that genes were continuous sections of DNA and that the string of coding information that makes up each gene was a single, linear unit. Sharp and Roberts, however, distinguished between the *exons,* the sequences that contain the vital information needed to create the protein, and the *introns,* incoherent biochemical information that interrupts the protein-manufacturing instructions. Each gene is apparently composed of fifteen to twenty exons, in between which introns may be located. During protein synthesis, exons are copied and spliced together, creating complete sequences, while the introns are ignored.

This discovery had not been made earlier largely because scientists had conducted most of their genetic research on prokaryotic organisms, such as bacteria, which do not have their genetic material located in clearly defined nuclei. Studies of bacteria had indicated that gene activity resulted in the transcription of double-stranded DNA into single-stranded messenger ribonucleic acid (mRNA); this is translated to the corresponding protein by ribosomes. Prokaryotic organisms have no introns, however, and therefore could not supply evidence for the existence, or the significance, of noncoding regions of DNA. Roberts and Sharp carried their research out on adenoviruses, the virus responsible for the common cold in humans. Although these are also prokaryotic organisms, Roberts and Sharp were able to take advantage of the fact that viruses reproduce themselves using the mechanisms of eukaryotic cells. Since their genome has some similarities to the genetic material in human cells, their protein synthesis was therefore relevant to the study of the cells of higher organisms.

In their experiments, Sharp's team created hybrid molecules in which they could observe mRNA strands binding to their complementary DNA strands. Electron micrographs allowed the scientists to identify which parts of the viral genomes had produced the mature mRNA molecules. What they discovered was that substantial sections of DNA were ignored in producing the final mRNA. This unexpected result gave evidence of a greater complexity of mRNA synthesis in eukaryotic organisms than in prokaryotic ones. Further research indicated that the mRNAs of eukaryotic organisms are synthesized as large mRNA precursor molecules; the introns are spliced out by means of enzyme activity to produce the mature mRNA that manufactures proteins. They found that a single gene could produce a variety of proteins—some defective as a result of different splicing patterns.

It is now believed that many hereditary diseases are caused by imperfect splicing of the genetic material, leading to the creation of faulty proteins. This may occur if the copying and splicing of the exons is not carried out accurately. One such disease is beta-thalassemia, a form of **anemia** prevalent in some Mediterranean areas that is caused by a faulty protein responsible for the formation of hemoglobin. Because of the insight Sharp's and Roberts's research has produced into the mechanisms of cell reproduction, it has important ramifications for research on malignant tumors and the viruses responsible for their development. It has also led to an investigation of methods for stopping the replication of the human immunodeficiency virus type 1 (HIV–1), with potential benefits in the search for a treatment for **AIDS**.

Sharp and Roberts's work has also led to new theories on the nature of evolutionary change; rather than being the cumulative effect of genetic mutation over time, it is now believed that it may be the result of the shuffling of large segments of DNA into new combinations to produce new proteins.

In 1990, before his earlier work had led to his Nobel Prize, Sharp was offered, and accepted, the presidency of the Massachusetts Institute of Technology. A short time later, he decided not to accept the position in order to devote his time exclusively to research. He has remained active in the field of academic administration, however, and has lobbied for research funding. He has also been active in industry; he was one of the founders of Biogen, a corporation started in Switzerland and now operating in Cambridge, Massachusetts, that has employed techniques developed in genetic engineering to produce the drug interferon.

Shattuck, Lemuel (1793-1859)

American public health innovator

Lemuel Shattuck was born on October 15, 1793 in Ashby, Massachusetts; he died on January 17, 1859 in Boston. He is remembered as a public health innovator, and for his work with vital statistics. Lemuel Shattuck was the son of John Shattuck, a farmer, and his wife Betsey. He married Clarissa Baxter in 1825; they had five children. Shattuck was almost entirely self-educated. From 1817 to 1822, he was a schoolteacher in Troy and Albany, New York, and in Detroit. From 1822 to 1833, he was a merchant in Concord, Massachusetts. He was a bookseller in Cambridge, Massachusetts in 1834. From 1840 to 1850, he was a self-employed bookseller, publisher, **public health** writer, and statistician in Boston. Intermittently, he served as a legislator for Boston and the state of Massachusetts.

Shattuck was one of the prime-movers of public hygiene in the United States. With his report to the Massachusetts Sanitary Commission in 1850, he accomplished for New England what such men as Chadwick, Rarr, and Simon had done for England. There had been in the United States few advances in public health aside from a few stray smallpox regulations until this report. Shattuck's report pointed out that much of the ill health and debility in the American cities at that time could be traced to unsanitary conditions, and stressed the need for local investigations and control of defects.

Shattuck was a prime mover in the adoption and expansion of public health measures at local and state levels. In 1850, he published a **Sanitation** Report that established a model for state boards of health in Massachusetts (1869) and other parts of the United States, including the District of Columbia (1870), California (1871), Virginia (1871), Minnesota (1872), Louisiana (1873), Alabama (1875), Georgia (1875), Maryland (1875), Colorado (1876), and Wisconsin (1876).

An early advocate of statistical surveys in mid-nineteenth century America, Shattuck helped establish the American Statistical Association (1839); in helping to reform the state vital statistics provisions for the state of Massachusetts (1840 to 1850), he established a prototype for other states. Shattuck expanded the scope of census reports in Boston (1845), and made suggestions for a federal census (1850). He was instrumental in improving and standardizing cause-of-death nomenclature (1842 to 1850) though his work on vital statistics registration in Massachusetts and through his **American Medical Association** (AMA) committee work. Shattuck sought improvements in genealogical records and local history sources (1830 to 1855), which fostered new interest in studies of heredity.

Shattuck also introduced measures to systemize and organize local and state government in Massachusetts.

He was the author of the following publications: *History of the Town of Concord* (1835); *Census of Boston for the Year 1845* (1846); *Report...Relating to a Sanitary Survey of the State* (1850); and *Memorials of the Descendants of William Shattuck* (1855).

Sherrington, Charles Scott (1857-1952)

English physiologist

Charles Scott Sherrington was born in London, England, on November 27, 1857. His father, who died while Sherrington was still young, was a physician, as was his step-father, who encouraged him to pursue a medical career. Sherrington studied at the Royal College of Surgeons, St. Thomas' Hospital in London, and Gonville and Caius College, Cambridge, before earning his medical degree from Cambridge in 1885. In the first years after receiving his degree, Sherrington traveled a number of times to Europe, investigating the effects of **cholera** epidemics and studying with **Rudolph Virchow**, Heinrich Hermann, and **Robert Koch** in Germany. While in Spain, he also became familiar with the work of **Santiago Ramón y Cajal**. As a result of these experiences, Sherrington became more interested in the study of pathology, physiology, and neurophysiology. Upon his return from Europe, Sherrington assumed the post of Professor of Physiology at the University of London and then, in 1895, at the University of Liverpool. He remained at Liverpool until 1913, when he accepted an appointment at Oxford.

Sherrington's accomplishments can be divided into three main areas: reflex action, decerebrate rigidity (changes that occur when part of the central **nervous system** is cut), and cortical localization (determining the function of various parts of the brain). Many of Sherrington's most important findings are summarized in his 1906 text, *The Integrative Action of the Nervous System*. That text is regarded as perhaps the most important single work establishing the basis of modern neurophysiology.

Sherrington's study of reflex action made clear that reflexes did not involve merely a few muscles, but that the brain integrated reactions to stimuli. For example, a dog's reaction to an itch involves 36 muscles performing two functions—scratching and maintaining balance.

Sherrington also made an important distinction among *exteroceptive* sensory nerves that detect stimuli from outside the body (such as smells, sounds, and light), *interoceptive* nerves that detect stimuli taken in to the body (foods), and *proprioceptive* nerves that detect states within the body such as the position of a muscle. The proprioceptive neurons carry out important functions such as maintaining balance and performing coordinated actions such as running. Sherrington was also the first to use the term neuron for the nerve cell and synapse for the junction between nerve cells.

Sherrington studied the effects on animals from which one or another part of the central nervous system had been removed, using his data to make detailed cortical maps of the brain. By cutting various parts of the cerebral cortex, he was able to determine with a high degree of accuracy where various motor functions are located in the brain. In 1919, he published a classic book, *Mammalian Physiology: A Course of Practical Exercises*. For his work in neurophysiology, Sherrington was knighted in 1922 and awarded a share of the 1932 Nobel Prize for physiology or medicine. Sherrington died of heart failure in Eastbourne on March 4, 1952, at the age of 95.

See also See also Neuron theory

Shingles

Shingles, also called herpes zoster, gets its name from both the Latin and French words for belt or girdle and refers to girdle-like skin eruptions that occur on the trunk of the body (although they occur elsewhere, as well). Shingles are caused by the virus that causes **chickenpox**, the varicella zoster virus (VSV), which can become dormant in nerve cells after an episode of chickenpox and later reemerge as shingles. Initially, red patches of **rash** develop into blisters. Because the virus travels along the nerve to the skin, it can damage the nerve and cause it to become inflamed. This condition can be very **painful**. If the pain persists long after the rash disappears, it is known as post-herpetic **neuralgia**.

Any individual who has had chickenpox can develop shingles. Approximately 300,000 cases of shingles occur every year in the United States. Overall, approximately 20% of those who had chickenpox as children develop shingles at some time in their lives. People of all ages, even children, can be affected, but the incidence increases with age. Newborn infants, bone marrow and other transplant recipients, as well as individuals with **immune systems** weakened by disease or drugs are also at increased risk. However, most individuals who develop shingles do not have any underlying malignancy or other immunosuppressive condition.

Shingles erupts along the course of the affected nerve, producing lesions anywhere on the body and may cause severe nerve pain. The most common areas to be affected are the face and trunk, which correspond to the areas where the chickenpox rash is most concentrated. The disease is caused by a reactivation of the chickenpox virus that has lain dormant in certain nerves following an episode of chickenpox. Exactly how or why this reactivation occurs is not clear, however, it is believed that the reactivation is triggered when the immune system becomes weakened, either as a result of **stress**, fatigue, certain medications, **chemotherapy**, or diseases, such as **cancer** or HIV infection. Further, it can be an early sign in persons with HIV that the immune system has deteriorated.

Early signs of shingles are often vague and can easily be mistaken for other illnesses. The condition may begin with **fever** and malaise (a vague feeling of weakness or discomfort). Within two to four days, severe pain, **itching**, and numbness/tingling (paresthesia) or extreme sensitivity to touch (hyperesthesia) can develop, usually on the trunk and occasionally on the arms and legs. Pain may be continuous or intermittent, usually lasting from one to four weeks. It may occur at the time of the eruption, but can precede the eruption by days, occasionally making the diagnosis difficult. Signs and symptoms may include the following:

- Itching, tingling, or severe burning pain
- Red patches that develop into blisters
- Grouped, dense, deep, small blisters that ooze and crust
- Swollen lymph nodes.

Diagnosis is usually not possible until the **skin lesions** develop. Once they develop, however, the pattern and location of the blisters and the type of cell damage displayed are very characteristic of the disease, allowing an accurate diagnosis primarily based upon the **physical examination**.

Although tests are rarely necessary, they may include the following:

- Viral culture of skin lesion.
- Microscopic examination using a Tzanck preparation. This involves staining a smear obtained from a blister. Cells infected with the herpes virus will appear very large and contain many dark cell centers or nuclei.

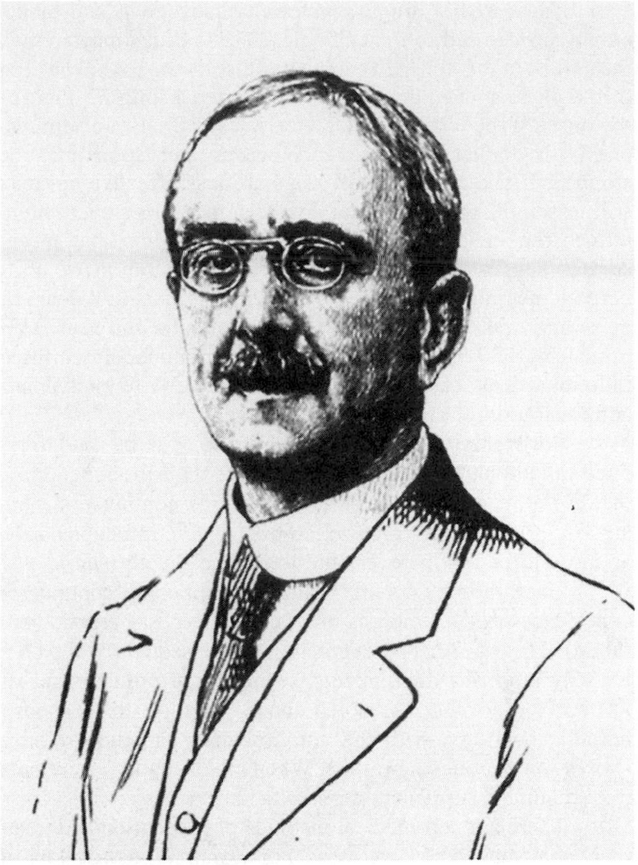

Charles Scott Sherrington

- Complete **blood count** (CBC) may show an elevated white blood cell count (WBC), a nonspecific sign of infection.
- Rise in antibody to the virus.

Shingles almost always resolves spontaneously (goes away) and may not require any treatment except for the relief of symptoms. In most people, the condition clears on its own in one or two weeks and seldom recurs.

Cool, wet compresses may help reduce pain. If there are blisters or crusting, applying compresses made with diluted vinegar will make the patient more comfortable. Mix one-quarter cup of white vinegar in two quarts of lukewarm water. Use the compress twice each day for 10 minutes. Stop using the compresses when the blisters have dried up.

Soothing baths and lotions such as colloidal oatmeal baths, starch baths or lotions, and calamine lotion may help to relieve itching and discomfort. Keep the skin clean, and do not re-use contaminated items. While the lesions continue to ooze, the person should be isolated to prevent infecting other susceptible individuals.

Later, when the crusts and scabs are separating, the skin may become dry, tight, and cracked. If that happens, rub on a small amount of plain petroleum jelly three or four times a day.

The **antiviral drugs acyclovir**, **valacyclovir**, and **famciclovir** can be used to treat shingles. These drugs may shorten the course of the illness. Their use results in more rapid healing of the blisters when drug therapy is started within 72 hours of the onset of the rash. In fact, the earlier the drugs are administered, the better, because early cases can sometimes be stopped. If taken later, these drugs are less effective but may still lessen the pain. Antiviral drug treatment does not seem to reduce the incidence of post-herpetic neuralgia, but recent studies suggest famciclovir may cut the duration of post-herpetic neuralgia in half. Side effects of typical oral doses of these antiviral drugs are minor with **headache** and nausea reported by 8-20 % of patients. Severely immunocompromised individuals, such as those with **AIDS**, may require intravenous administration of antiviral drugs.

Corticosteroids, such as prednisone, may be used to reduce inflammation but they do interfere with the functioning of the immune system. Corticosteroids, in combination with antiviral therapy, also are used to treat severe infections, such as those affecting the eyes, and to reduce severe pain.

Once the blisters are healed, some people continue to experience pain for months or even years (post-herpetic neuralgia). This pain can be excruciating. Consequently, the doctor may prescribe tranquilizers, sedatives, or **antidepressant**s to be taken at night. As noted above, attempts to treat post-herpetic neuralgia with the antiviral drug famciclovir have shown some promising results. When all else fails, severe pain may require a permanent nerve block.

There are non-medical methods of prevention and treatment that may speed recovery. For example, getting lots of rest, eating a healthy diet, regular **exercise** and minimizing stress are always helpful in preventing disease. Supplementation with vitamin B_{12} during the first one to two days and continued supplementation with vitamin B complex, high levels of vitamin C with bioflavenoids, and calcium, are recommended to boost the immune system. Herbal antivirals such as echinacea can be effective in fighting infection and boosting the immune system.

Although no single alternative approach, technique, or remedy has yet been proven to reduce the pain, there are a few options which may be helpful. For example, topical applications of lemon balm (*Melissa officinalis*) or licorice (*Glycyrrhiza glabra*) and peppermint (*Mentha piperita*) may reduce pain and blistering. **Homeopathic** remedies include *Rhus toxicodendron* for blisters, *Mezereum* and *Arsenicum album* for pain, and *Ranunculus* for itching. Practitioners of Eastern medicine recommend self-**hypnosis**, **acupressure**, and **acupuncture** to alleviate pain.

Shingles usually clears up in two to three weeks and rarely recurs. Involvement of the nerves that cause movement may cause a temporary or permanent nerve **paralysis** and/or **tremors**. The elderly or debilitated patient may have a prolonged and difficult course. For them, the eruption is typically more extensive and inflammatory, occasionally resulting in blisters that bleed, areas where the skin actually dies, secondary bacterial infection, or extensive and permanent scarring.

Similarly, an immunocompromised patient usually has a more severe course that is frequently prolonged for weeks to months. They develop shingles frequently and the infection can spread to the skin, lungs, liver, gastrointestinal tract, brain, or other vital organs. Cases of chronic shingles have been reported in patients infected with AIDS, especially when they have a decreased number of one particular kind of immune cell, called CD4 lymphocytes. Depletion of CD4 lymphocytes is associated with more severe, chronic, and recurrent varicella-zoster virus infections. These lesions are typical at the onset but may turn into ulcers that do not heal.

Potentially serious complications can result from herpes zoster. Many individuals continue to experience persistent pain long after the blisters heal. This pain can be severe and can persist for months or years after the lesions have disappeared. The incidence of post-herpetic neuralgia increases with age, and episodes in older individuals tend to be of longer duration. Most patients under 30 years of age experience no persistent pain. By age 40, the risk of prolonged pain lasting longer than one month increases to 33%. By age 70, the risk increases to 74%. The pain can adversely affect quality of life, but it does usually diminish over time.

Other complications include a secondary bacterial infection, and rarely, potentially fatal inflammation of the brain (**encephalitis**) and the spread of an infection throughout the body. These rare, but extremely serious, complications are more likely to occur in those individuals who have weakened immune systems.

Strengthening the immune system by making lifestyle changes is thought to help prevent the development of shingles. A lifestyle designed to strengthen the immune system and maintain good overall health includes eating a well-balanced diet rich in essential vitamins and **minerals**, getting enough sleep, exercising regularly, and reducing stress.

See also Chickenpox; Varicella

SHOCK

Shock is a medical emergency in which the organs and tissues of the body are not receiving an adequate flow of blood. This deprives the organs and tissues of oxygen (carried in the blood) and allows the buildup of waste products. Shock can result in serious damage or even **death**.

There are three stages of shock: Stage I (also called compensated, or nonprogressive), Stage II (also called decompensated or progressive), and Stage III (also called irreversible).

In Stage I of shock, when low blood flow (perfusion) is first detected, a number of systems are activated in order to maintain/restore perfusion. The result is that the heart beats faster, the blood vessels throughout the body become slightly smaller in diameter, and the kidney works to retain fluid in the circulatory system. All this serves to maximize blood flow to the most important organs and systems in the body. The patient in this stage of shock has very few symptoms, and treatment can completely halt any progression.

In Stage II of shock, these methods of compensation begin to fail. The systems of the body are unable to improve perfusion any longer, and the patient's symptoms reflect that fact. Oxygen deprivation in the brain causes the patient to become confused and disoriented, while oxygen deprivation in the heart may cause chest **pain**. With quick and appropriate treatment, this stage of shock can be reversed.

In Stage III of shock, the length of time that poor perfusion has existed begins to take a permanent toll on the body's organs and tissues. The heart's functioning continues to spiral downward, and the kidneys usually shut down completely. Cells in organs and tissues throughout the body are injured and dying. The endpoint of Stage III shock is the patient's death.

Shock is caused by three major categories of problems: cardiogenic (meaning problems associated with the heart's functioning); hypovolemic (meaning that the total volume of blood available to circulate is low); and **septic shock** (caused by overwhelming infection, usually by bacteria).

Cardiogenic shock can be caused by any disease, or event, which prevents the heart muscle from pumping strongly and consistently enough to circulate the blood normally. **Heart attack**, conditions which cause inflammation of the heart muscle (**myocarditis**), disturbances of the electrical rhythm of the heart, any kind of mass or fluid accumulation and/or blood clot which interferes with flow out of the heart can all significantly affect the heart's ability to adequately pump a normal quantity of blood.

Hypovolemic shock occurs when the total volume of blood in the body falls well below normal. This can occur when there is excess fluid loss, as in **dehydration** due to severe vomiting or **diarrhea**, diseases which cause excess urination (diabetes insipidus, **diabetes mellitus**, and **kidney failure**), extensive **burns**, blockage in the intestine, inflammation of the pancreas (**pancreatitis**), or severe bleeding of any kind.

Septic shock can occur when an untreated or inadequately treated infection (usually bacterial) is allowed to progress. Bacteria often produce poisonous chemicals (toxins) which can cause injury throughout the body. When large quantities of these bacteria, and their toxins, begin circulating in the bloodstream, every organ and tissue in the body is at risk of their damaging effects. The most damaging consequences of these bacteria and toxins include poor functioning of the heart muscle; widening of the diameter of the blood vessels; a drop in blood pressure; activation of the blood clotting system, causing blood clots, followed by a risk of uncontrollable bleeding; damage to the lungs, causing acute **respiratory distress syndrome**; liver failure; kidney failure; and **coma**.

Initial symptoms of shock include cold, clammy hands and feet; pale or blue-tinged skin tone; weak, fast pulse rate; fast rate of breathing; low blood pressure. A variety of other symptoms may be present, but they are dependent on the underlying cause of shock.

Diagnosis of shock is based on the patient's symptoms, as well as criteria including a significant drop in blood pressure, extremely low urine output, and blood tests that reveal overly acidic blood with a low circulating concentration of carbon dioxide. Other tests are performed, as appropriate, to try to determine the underlying condition responsible for the patient's state of shock.

The most important goals in the treatment of shock include: quickly diagnosing the patient's state of shock; quickly intervening to halt the underlying condition (stopping bleeding, re-starting the heart, giving **antibiotics** to combat an infection, etc.); treating the effects of shock (low oxygen, increased acid in the blood, activation of the blood clotting system); and supporting vital functions (blood pressure, urine flow, heart function).

Treatment includes keeping the patient warm, with legs raised and head down to improve blood flow to the brain, putting a needle in a vein in order to give fluids or blood **transfusions**, as necessary; giving the patient extra oxygen to breathe and medications to improve the heart's functioning; and treating the underlying condition which led to shock.

The prognosis of an individual patient in shock depends on the stage of shock when treatment was begun, the underlying condition causing shock, and the general medical state of the patient.

The most preventable type of shock is caused by dehydration during illnesses with severe vomiting or diarrhea. Shock can be avoided by recognizing that a patient who is unable to drink in order to replace lost fluids needs to be given fluids intravenously (through a needle in a vein). Other types of shock are only preventable insofar as one can prevent their underlying conditions, or can monitor and manage those conditions well enough so that they never progress to the point of shock.

See also Sepsis

Shockley, Dolores Cooper (1930-)

African American pharmacologist

Dolores Cooper Shockley is the first African American woman to earn a Ph.D. from Purdue University and the first African American woman in the United States to receive a Ph.D. in pharmacology. In 1977 she became chair of the department of microbiology at Meharry Medical College.

Shockley was born in Clarksdale, Mississippi, on April 21, 1930. She enrolled at Louisiana State University in 1947, intending to pursue a major in pharmacy with the goal of eventually opening her own drug store. During her college years, however, Shockley's interests shifted from retail business to research. When she earned her bachelor of science degree in 1951, she decided to continue her education in the field of pharmacology at Purdue University in Lafayette, Indiana. She was awarded her M.S. at Purdue in 1953 and then her Ph.D. in pharmacology two years later. After graduation, Shockley used a Fulbright Fellowship to do postdoctoral research at the University of Copenhagen.

When Shockley returned to the United States, she accepted an appointment as assistant professor of pharmacology at Meharry Medical College in Nashville, Tennessee. She was greeted in her new job with a certain amount of suspicion, she later told an interviewer for *Ebony,* because "some men thought that I was just working temporarily." She soon put those doubts to rest and became a valued and respected member of the faculty. In 1967 Shockley was promoted to associate professor, and ten years later she became head of the college's department of microbiology. She has since served also as Meharry's foreign student advisor and its liaison for international activities to the Association of American Medical Colleges. Shockley's research interests have focused on the consequences of drug action on stress, the effects of hormones on connective tissue, the relationships between drugs and nutrition, and the measurement of non-narcotic analgesics (pain killers). She was visiting assistant professor at the Einstein College of Medicine in New York City from 1959 to 1962 and was a recipient of the Lederle Faculty Award from 1963 to 1966. Shockley is married and the mother of four children.

SHORTNESS OF BREATH

Shortness of breath, or dyspnea, is a feeling of difficult or labored breathing that is out of proportion to the patient's level of physical activity. It is a symptom of a variety of different diseases or disorders and may be either acute or chronic.

The experience of dyspnea depends on its severity and underlying causes. The feeling itself results from a combination of impulses relayed to the brain from nerve endings in the lungs, rib cage, chest muscles, or diaphragm, combined with the patient's perception and interpretation of the sensation. In some cases, the patient's sensation of breathlessness is intensified by **anxiety** about its cause. Patients describe dyspnea variously as unpleasant shortness of breath, a feeling of increased effort or tiredness in moving the chest muscles, a panicky feeling of being smothered, or a sense of tightness or cramping in the chest wall.

Acute dyspnea with sudden onset is a frequent cause of emergency room visits. Most cases of acute dyspnea involve pulmonary (lung and breathing) disorders, cardiovascular disease, or chest trauma.

Pulmonary disorders that can cause dyspnea include airway obstruction by a foreign object, swelling due to infection, or **anaphylactic shock**; acute **pneumonia**; hemorrhage from the lungs; or severe bronchospasms associated with **asthma**.

Acute dyspnea can be caused by disturbances of the heart rhythm, failure of the left ventricle, mitral valve (a heart valve) dysfunction, or an embolus (a clump of tissue, fat, or gas) that is blocking the pulmonary circulation. Most pulmonary emboli (blood clots) originate in the deep veins of the lower legs and eventually migrate to the pulmonary artery.

Chest injuries, both closed injuries and penetrating **wounds**, can cause **pneumothorax** (the presence of air inside the chest cavity), **bruises**, or fractured ribs. **Pain** from these injuries results in dyspnea. The impact of the driver's chest against the steering wheel in auto accidents is a frequent cause of closed chest injuries.

Anxiety attacks sometimes cause acute dyspnea; they may or may not be associated with chest pain. Anxiety attacks are often accompanied by hyperventilation, which is a breathing pattern characterized by abnormally rapid and deep breaths. Hyperventilation raises the oxygen level in the blood, causing chest pain and **dizziness**.

Chronic dyspnea can be caused by asthma, **chronic obstructive pulmonary disease** (COPD), **bronchitis**, emphysema, inflammation of the lungs, **pulmonary hypertension**, tumors, or disorders of the vocal cords.

Disorders of the left side of the heart or inadequate supply of blood to the heart muscle can cause dyspnea. In some cases a tumor in the heart or inflammation of the membrane surrounding the heart may cause dyspnea.

Neuromuscular disorders cause dyspnea from progressive deterioration of the patient's chest muscles. They include **muscular dystrophy**, **myasthenia gravis**, and amyotrophic lateral sclerosis.

Patients who are severely anemic may develop dyspnea if they **exercise** vigorously. Hyperthyroidism or hypothyroidism may cause shortness of breath, and so may gastroesophageal reflux disease (GERD). Both chronic anxiety disorders, and a low level of physical fitness can also cause episodes of dyspnea. Deformities of the chest or **obesity** can cause dyspnea by limiting the movement of the chest wall and the ability of the lungs to fill completely.

The patient's history provides the doctor with such necessary information as a history of gastroesophageal reflux disease (GERD), asthma, or other allergic conditions; the presence of chest pain as well as difficulty breathing; recent accidents or recent surgery; information about smoking habits; the patient's baseline level of physical activity and exercise habits; and a psychiatric history of panic attacks or anxiety disorders.

How a person's body position affects his/her dyspnea symptoms sometimes gives hints as to the underlying cause of the disorder. Dyspnea that is worse when the patient is sitting up is called platypnea and indicates the possibility of liver disease. Dyspnea that is worse when the patient is lying down is called orthopnea, and is associated with heart disease or **paralysis** of the diaphragm. Paroxysmal nocturnal dyspnea (PND) refers to dyspnea that occurs during sleep and forces the patient to awake gasping for breath. It is usually relieved if the patient sits up or stands. PND may point to dysfunction of the left ventricle of the heart, **hypertension**, or narrowing of the mitral valve.

The doctor will examine the patient's chest in order to determine the rate and depth of breathing, the effort required, the condition of the patient's breathing muscles, and any evidence of chest deformities or trauma. He or she will listen for **wheezing**, stridor, or signs of fluid in the lungs. If the patient has a **fever**, the doctor will look for other signs of pneumonia. The doctor will check the patient's heart functions, including blood pressure, pulse rate, and the presence of **heart murmurs** or other abnormal heart sounds. If the doctor suspects a blood clot in one of the large veins leading to the heart, he or she will examine the patient's legs for signs of swelling.

Patients who are seen in emergency rooms are given a **chest x ray** and an **electrocardiography** (ECG) to assist the doctor in evaluating abnormalities of the chest wall, also to determine the position of the diaphragm, possible rib **fractures** or pneumothorax, irregular heartbeat, or the adequacy of the supply of blood to the heart muscle. Also, the patient may be given a breathing test on an instrument called a spirometer to screen for airway disorders.

The doctor may order blood tests and arterial blood gas tests to rule out **anemia**, hyperventilation from an anxiety attack, or thyroid dysfunction. A **sputum culture** can be used to test for pneumonia.

Specialized tests may be ordered for patients with normal results from basic diagnostic tests for dyspnea. High-resolution CT scans can be used for suspected airway obstruction or mild emphysema. Tissue biopsy performed with a bronchoscope can be used for patients with suspected lung disease.

If the doctor suspects a **pulmonary embolism**, he or she may order ventilation-perfusion scanning to inspect lung function, an angiogram of blood vessels, or ultrasound studies of the leg veins. **Echocardiography** can be used to test for pulmonary hypertension and heart disease.

Pulmonary function studies or **electromyography** (EMG) are used to assess neuromuscular diseases. Exercise testing is used to assess dyspnea related to COPD, anxiety attacks, poor physical fitness, and the severity of lung or heart disease. The level of acidity in the patient's esophagus may be monitored to rule out GERD.

Treatment of dyspnea depends on its underlying cause. Patients with acute dyspnea are given oxygen in the emergency room, with the following treatments for specific conditions:

- Asthma. Treatment with Alupent, epinephrine, or aminophylline.
- Anaphylactic shock. Treatment with Benadryl, steroids, or aminophylline, with hydrocortisone if necessary.
- heart failure. Treatment with oxygen, **diuretics**, and placing patient in upright position.
- Pneumonia. Treatment with **antibiotics** and removal of lung secretions.
- Anxiety attacks. Immediate treatment includes **antidepressant** medications. If the patient is hyperventilating, he or she may be asked to breathe into a paper bag to normalize breathing rhythm and the oxygen level of the blood.
- **Pneumothorax**. Surgical placement of a chest tube.

The treatment of chronic dyspnea depends on the underlying disorder. Asthma can often be managed with a combination of medications to reduce airway spasms and removal of allergens from the patient's environment. COPD requires both medication, lifestyle changes, and long-term physical **rehabilitation**. Anxiety disorders are usually treated with a combination of medication and **psychotherapy**. GERD can usually be managed with **antacids**, other medications, and dietary changes. There are no permanent cures for myasthenia gravis or muscular dystrophy.

Tumors and certain types of chest deformities can be treated surgically.

The appropriate alternative therapy for shortness of breath depends on the underlying cause of the condition. When dyspnea is acute and severe, **oxygen therapy** is used either in the doctor's office or in the emergency room. For shortness of breath with an underlying physical cause like asthma, anaphylactic shock, or pneumonia, the physical condition should be treated. Botanical and **homeopathic** remedies can be used for acute dyspnea, if the proper remedies and formulas are prescribed. If the dyspnea has a psychological basis (especially if it is caused by anxiety), **acupuncture**, botanical medicine, and homeopathy can help the patient heal at a deep level.

The prognosis (expected outcome) depends on the underlying cause of the dyspnea, its severity, and the type of treatment required.

Dyspnea caused by asthma can be minimized or prevented by removing dust and other triggers from the patient's environment. Long-term prevention of chronic dyspnea includes such lifestyle choices as regular aerobic exercise and avoidance of smoking.

See also Anxiety; Asthma; Anaphylactic shock; Bronchitis; Chronic obstructive pulmonary disease; Emphysema; Pneumonia; Pulmonary hypertension

SICKLE-CELL ANEMIA

Sickle-cell **anemia** is an inherited blood disorder that arises from a single amino acid substitution in one of the component proteins of hemoglobin. The component protein, or globin, that contains the substitution is defective. Hemoglobin molecules constructed with such proteins have a tendency to stick to one another, forming strands of hemoglobin within the red blood cells. The cells that contain these strands become stiff and elongated—that is, sickle shaped.

Sickle-shaped cells—also called sickle cells—die much more rapidly than normal red blood cells. Normal red blood cells survive for approximately 120 days in the bloodstream; sickle cells last only 10-12 days. The body cannot create replacements fast enough and anemia develops due to the chronic shortage of red blood cells. Further complications arise because sickle cells do not fit well through small blood vessels, and can become trapped. The trapped sickle cells form blockages that prevent oxygenated blood from reaching associated tissues and organs. Considerable **pain** results in addition to damage to the tissues and organs. This damage can lead to serious complications, including **stroke** and an impaired **immune system**. Sickle cell anemia primarily affects people with African, Mediterranean, Middle Eastern, and Indian ancestry. In the United States, African Americans are particularly affected.

Normal hemoglobin is composed of a heme molecule and two pairs of proteins called globins. Humans have the genes to create six different types of globins—alpha, beta, gamma, delta, epsilon, and zeta—but do not use all of them at once. Which genes are expressed depends on the stage of development: embryonic, fetal, or adult. Virtually all of the hemoglobin produced in humans from ages two to three months onward contains a pair of alpha-globin and beta-globin molecules.

A change, or mutation, in a gene can alter the formation or function of its product. In the case of sickle cell hemoglobin, the gene that carries the blueprint for beta-globin has a minute alteration that makes it different from the normal gene. This mutation affects a single nucleic acid along the entire DNA strand that makes up the beta-globin gene. (Nucleic acids are the chemicals that make up deoxyribonucleic acid, known more familiarly as DNA.) Specifically, the nucleic acid, adenine, is replaced by a different nucleic acid called thymine.

Because of this seemingly slight mutation, called a point mutation, the finished beta-globin molecule has an amino acid substitution: valine occupies the spot normally taken by glutamic acid. (Amino acids are the building blocks of all proteins.) This substitution creates a beta-globin molecule—and eventually a hemoglobin molecule—that does not function normally.

Normal hemoglobin, referred to as hemoglobin A, transports oxygen from the lungs to tissues throughout the body. In the smallest blood vessels, the hemoglobin exchanges the oxygen for carbon dioxide, which it carries back to the lungs for removal from the body. The defective hemoglobin, designated hemoglobin S, can also transport oxygen. However, once the oxygen is released, hemoglobin S molecules have an abnormal tendency to clump together. These aggregated hemoglobin molecules form strands within red blood cells, which then lose their usual shape and flexibility.

The rate at which hemoglobin S aggregation and cell sickling occur depends on many factors, such as the blood flow rate and the concentration of hemoglobin in the blood cells. If the blood flows at a normal rate, hemoglobin S is reoxygenated in the lungs before it has a chance to aggregate. The concentration of hemoglobin within red blood cells is influenced by an individual's hydration level—that is the amount water contained in the cells. If a person becomes **dehydrated**, hemoglobin becomes more concentrated in the red blood cells. In this situation, hemoglobin S has a greater tendency to clump together and induce sickle cell formation.

Genes are inherited in pairs, one copy from each parent. Therefore, each person has two copies of the gene that makes beta-globin. As long as a person inherits one normal beta-globin gene, the body can produce sufficient quantities of normal beta-globin. A person who inherits a copy each of the normal and abnormal beta-globin genes is referred to as a carrier of the sickle cell trait. Generally, carriers do not have symptoms, but their red blood cells contain some hemoglobin S. A child who inherits the sickle cell trait from both parents—a 25% possibility if both parents are carriers—will develop sickle cell anemia.

Worldwide, millions of people carry the sickle cell trait. Individuals whose ancestors lived in sub-Saharan Africa, the Middle East, India, or the Mediterranean region are the most likely to have the trait. The areas of the world associated with the sickle cell trait are also strongly affected by **malaria**, a disease caused by blood-borne parasites transmitted through mosquito bites. According to a widely accepted theory, the genetic mutation associated with the sickle cell trait occurred thousands of years ago. Coincidentally, this mutation increased the likelihood that carriers would survive malaria outbreaks. Survivors then passed the mutation on to their offspring, and the trait became established throughout areas where malaria was common.

Although modern medicine offers drug therapies for malaria, the sickle cell trait endures. Approximately 2 million Americans are carriers of the sickle cell trait. Individuals who have African ancestry are particularly affected; one in 12 African Americans are carriers. An additional 72,000 Americans have sickle-cell anemia, meaning they have inherited the trait from both parents. Among African Americans, approximately one in every 500 babies is diagnosed with sickle-cell anemia. Hispanic Americans are also heavily affected; sickle-cell anemia occurs in one of every 1,000-1,400 births. Worldwide, it has been estimated that 250,000 children are born each year with sickle-cell anemia.

The severity of the symptoms cannot be predicted based solely on the genetic inheritance. Some individuals develop health- or life-threatening problems in infancy, but others may have only mild symptoms throughout their lives. For example, genetic factors, such as the continued production of fetal hemoglobin after birth, can modify the course of the disease. Fetal hemoglobin contains gamma-globin in place of beta-globin; if enough of it is produced, the potential interactions between hemoglobin S molecules are reduced.

Common symptoms of anemia include fatigue, paleness, and a **shortness of breath**. A particularly severe form of anemia—aplastic anemia—occurs following infection with parvovirus. Parvovirus causes extensive destruction of the bone marrow, bringing production of new red blood cells to a halt. Bone marrow production resumes after 7-10 days; however, given the short lives of sickle cells, even a brief shut-down in red blood cell production can cause a precipitous decline in hemoglobin concentrations. This is called "aplastic crisis."

Painful crises, also known as vaso-occlusive crises, are a primary symptom of sickle-cell anemia in children and adults. The pain may be caused by small blood vessel blockages that prevent oxygen from reaching tissues. An alternate explanation, particularly with regard to bone pain, is that blood is shunted away from the bone marrow but through some other mechanism than blockage by sickle cells. These crises are unpredictable, and can affect any area of the body, although the chest, abdomen, and bones are frequently affected sites. There is some evidence that cold temperatures or infection can trigger a painful crisis, but most crises occur for unknown reasons. The frequency and duration of the pain can vary tremendously. Crises may be separated by more than a year or possibly only by weeks, and they can last from hours to weeks.

The hand-foot syndrome is a particular type of painful crisis, and is often the first sign of sickle-cell anemia in an infant. Common symptoms include pain and swelling in the hands and feet, possibly accompanied by a **fever**. Hand-foot syndrome typically occurs only during the first four years of life, with the greatest incidence at one year.

Sickle cells can impede blood flow through the spleen and cause organ damage. In infants and young children, the spleen is usually enlarged. After repeated incidence of blood vessel blockage, the spleen usually atrophies by late childhood. Damage to the spleen can have a negative impact on the immune system, leaving individuals with sickle-cell anemia more vulnerable to infections. Infants and young children are particularly prone to life-threatening infections.

Anemia can also impair the immune system, because stem cells—the precursors of all blood cells—are earmarked for red blood cell production rather than white blood cell production. White blood cells form the cornerstone of the immune system within the bloodstream.

The energy demands of the bone marrow for red blood cell production compete with the demands of a growing body. Children with sickle-cell anemia have delayed growth and reach **puberty** at a later age than normal. By early adulthood, they catch up on growth and attain normal height; however, weight typically remains below average.

Blockage of blood vessels in the brain can have particularly harsh consequences and can be fatal. When areas of the brain are deprived of oxygen, control of the associated functions may be lost. Sometimes this loss is permanent. Common stroke symptoms include weakness or numbness that affects one side of the body, sudden loss of vision, confusion, loss of speech or the ability to understand spoken words, and **dizziness**. Children between the ages of 1-15 are at the highest risk of suffering a stroke. Approximately two-thirds of the children who have a stroke will have at least one more.

Acute chest syndrome can occur at any age, and is caused by sickle cells blocking the small blood vessels of the lungs. This blockage is complicated by accompanying problems such as infection and pooling of blood in the lungs. Affected persons experience fever, **cough**, chest pain, and shortness of breath. Recurrent attacks can lead to permanent lung damage.

Males with sickle-cell anemia may experience a condition called **priapism**. (Priapism is characterized by a persistent and painful erection of the penis.) Due to blood vessel blockage by sickle cells, blood is trapped in the tissue of the penis. Damage to this tissue can result in permanent **impotence** in adults.

Both genders may experience kidney damage. The environment in the kidney is particularly conducive for sickle cell formation; even otherwise asymptomatic carriers may experience some level of kidney damage. Kidney damage is indicated by blood in the urine, incontinence, and enlarged kidneys.

Jaundice and an enlarged liver are also commonly associated with sickle-cell anemia. Jaundice, indicated by a yellow tone in the skin and eyes, may occur if bilirubin levels increase. Bilirubin is the final product of hemoglobin degradation, and is typically removed from the bloodstream by the liver. Bilirubin levels often increase with high levels of red blood cell destruction, but jaundice can also be a sign of a poorly functioning liver.

Some individuals with sickle-cell anemia may experience vision problems. The blood vessels that feed into the retina—the tissue at the back of the eyeball—may be blocked by sickle cells. New blood vessel can form around the blockages, but these vessels are typically weak or otherwise defective. Bleeding, scarring, and **retinal detachment** may eventually lead to blindness.

Sickle-cell anemia is suspected based on an individual's ethnic or racial background, and on the symptoms of anemia. A **blood count** reveals the anemia, and a sickle cell test reveals the presence of the sickle cell trait. The sickle cell test involves mixing equal amounts of blood and a two percent solution of sodium bisulfite. Under these circumstances, hemoglobin exists in its deoxygenated state. If hemoglobin S is present, the red blood cells are transformed into the characteristic sickle shape. This transformation is observed with a microscope, and quantified by expressing the number of sickle cells per 1,000 cells as a percentage. The sickle cell test confirms that an individual has the sickle cell trait, but it does not provide a definitive diagnosis for sickle-cell anemia.

To confirm a diagnosis of the sickle cell trait or sickle cell anemia, another laboratory test called gel electrophoresis is performed. This test uses an electric field applied across a slab of gel-like material to separate protein molecules based on their size, shape, or electrical charge. Although hemoglobin S (sickle) and hemoglobin A (normal) differ by only one amino acid, they can be clearly separated using gel electrophoresis. If both types of hemoglobin are identified, the individual is a carrier of the sickle cell trait; if only hemoglobin S is present, the person most likely has sickle-cell anemia. The gel electrophoresis test is also used as a screening method for identifying the sickle cell trait in newborns. More than 40 states screen newborns in order to identify carriers and individuals who have inherited the trait from both parents.

Early identification of sickle-cell anemia can prevent many problems. The highest **death** rates occur during the first year of life due to infection, aplastic anemia, and acute chest syndrome. If anticipated, steps can be taken to avert these crises. With regard to long-term treatment, prevention of complications remains a main goal. Sickle-cell anemia cannot be cured—other than through a risky **bone marrow transplantation**—but treatments are available for symptoms.

Pain is one of the primary symptoms of sickle-cell anemia, and controlling it is an important concern. The methods necessary for pain control are based on individual factors. Some people can gain adequate pain control through over-the-counter oral painkillers (**analgesics**), local application of heat, and rest. Others need stronger methods, which can include administration of narcotics.

Blood **transfusion**s are usually not given on a regular basis but are used to treat painful crises, severe anemia, and other emergencies. In some cases, such as treating spleen enlargement or preventing stroke from recurring, blood transfusions are given as a preventative measure. Regular blood transfusions have the potential to decrease formation of hemoglobin S, and reduce associated symptoms. However, regular blood transfusions introduce a set of complications, primarily iron loading, risk of infection, and sensitization to proteins in the transfused blood.

Infants are typically started on a course of **penicillin** that extends from infancy to age six. This treatment is meant to ward off potentially fatal infections. Infections at any age are treated aggressively with **antibiotics**. Vaccines for common infections, such as **pneumococcal pneumonia**, are administered when possible.

Emphasis is being placed on developing drugs that treat sickle cell anemia directly. The most promising of these drugs in the late 1990s is hydroxyurea, a drug that was originally designed for anticancer treatment. Hydroxyurea has been shown to reduce the frequency of painful crises and acute chest syndrome in adults, and to lessen the need for blood transfusions. Hydroxyurea seems to work by inducing a higher production of fetal hemoglobin. The major side effects of the drug include decreased production of platelets, red blood cells, and certain white blood cells. The effects of long-term hydroxyurea treatment are unknown.

Bone marrow transplantation has been shown to cure sickle cell anemia in severely affected children. Indications for a bone marrow transplant are stroke, recurrent acute chest syndrome, and chronic unrelieved pain. Bone marrow transplants tend to be the most successful in children; adults have a higher rate of transplant rejection and other complications.

The procedure requires a healthy donor whose marrow proteins match those of the recipient. Typically, siblings have the greatest likelihood of having matched marrow. Given this restriction, fewer than 20% of sickle-cell anemia individuals may be candidates. The percentage is reduced when factors such as general health and acceptable risk are considered. The procedure is risky for the recipient. There is approximately a 10% fatality rate associated with bone marrow transplants done for sickle-cell anemia treatment. Survivors face potential long-term complications, such as chronic graft versus host disease (an immune-mediated attack by the donor marrow against the recipient's tissues), **infertility**, and development of some forms of **cancer**.

In general, treatment of sickle-cell anemia relies on conventional medicine. However, **alternative** therapies may be useful in pain control. Relaxation, application of local warmth, and adequate hydration may supplement the conventional therapy. Further, maintaining good health through adequate nutrition, avoiding **stress**es and infection, and getting proper rest help prevent some complications.

Several factors aside from genetic inheritance determine the prognosis for affected individuals. Therefore, predicting the course of the disorder based solely on genes is not possible. In general, given proper medical care, individuals with sickle cell anemia are in fairly good health most of the time. The life expectancy for these individuals has increased over the last 30 years, and many survive well into their 40s or beyond. In the United States, the average life expectancy for men with sickle cell anemia is 42 years; for women, it is 48 years.

Inheritance cannot be prevented, but it may be predicted. Screening is recommended for individuals in high-risk populations; screening at birth offers the opportunity for early intervention; pregnant women and couples planning to have children may also wish to be screened to determine their carrier status; and carriers may consider genetic counseling to assess any risks to their offspring. The sickle cell trait can also be identified through prenatal testing; specifically through use of amniotic fluid sampling or chorionic villus sampling.

See also Blood count; Bone marrow transplantation; Transfusion

SIGN LANGUAGE

Sign language is a type of visual communication with the hands, body, and facial expressions used by deaf and hard-of-hearing people. American Sign Language (ASL) is the primary means of communication by a very large portion of the deaf population in the United States.

ASL has a unique grammar and syntax, unrelated to English (although it reflects English influences). American Sign Language also includes fingerspelling (also known as the manual alphabet) to spell out certain words that do not have a sign, including proper names and technical phrases.

In its true sense, ASL is the patterns used by deaf people when they communicate with sign in a non-English style. Neither articles nor speech are used. Only when American Sign Language differs completely from English is it properly considered true ASL; some people incorrectly use the term ''ASL'' to include a whole range of manual communication and types of sign languages.

Some deaf people use ASL exclusively, while others use ASL together with Signed English, a less complicated manual system of communication that is used to represent spoken English. Signed English includes gestures signed in the same word order as English and is often used with speech.

For many years, ASL was not considered a language; critics claimed it did not have grammatical structure, and warned that it isolated deaf people from the hearing world. Because it was considered ''grammatically incorrect'' by many educators, it was often forbidden in schools and programs for deaf children. For years, ASL was considered a suppressed language, despite its wide use by the deaf.

Today, linguists agree that ASL is indeed a separate and unique language complete unto itself, with its own grammar and syntax. Many schools and programs for deaf students advocate its use. However, there is still some resistance among educators about using ASL as a teaching tool. Some fear that it will interfere with the development of English skills, that English skills are imperative if the deaf person is to be able to survive in a hearing world.

In fact, deaf people themselves disagree about ASL. Some find it a source of pride and an example of cultural identity in the language, but others feel more ambivalent about its use in the wider hearing society.

ASL is not the only form of sign language. Fingerspelling is one method in which handshapes (representing letters) are used to spell out each word of the English language while speaking. It is an unpopular method of communication and is tiring to use and interpret.

Manually coded English systems use fingerspelling but also include signs and markers. The most common forms of this system include Signed English and Signing Exact English, which base their signs on ASL but include other aspects of the English language. Although this system is often used in schools, it is not used by deaf adults among themselves.

Pidgin Sign English is the system used most often by hearing people learning to communicate with deaf individuals. PSE combines the English language with the vocabulary and nonmanual features of ASL, and it is the preferred method of communication by many deaf people.

Other countries have their own sign languages; the best known is French Sign Language (known in France as "langue des signes Francaise," or LSF). It was first used with deaf students in the 19th century and was the first sign language to earn acceptance as a separate, complete language of its own. Research suggests that LSF is grammatically similar to ASL (handshapes, for example, are very much the same).

SIMON, JOHN (1816-1904)

English physician

Simon was a **physician** by training, but he is most famous for his dramatic reforms of London's **public health** system, which set the standard for 19th-century urban **sanitation** and health measures. Of the era's public health advocates, Simon is generally regarded as one of the most influential.

Born in London, Simon received his early medical education during his work as an apprentice to a well-known local surgeon at the St. Thomas Hospital. He completed his formal studies at the University of London's King's College, and from 1840 to 1847 served as a surgeon at the school's associated hospital.

Simon became the City of London's first medical officer of health in 1848, and in that capacity issued annual reports that led directly to the Sanitary Act of 1866. This landmark legislation formed the backdrop for industrial hygiene policy and created the first mandatory, universal, and science-based public health law. Simon's involvement here helped transform the issue of public health from a political platform to one rooted in scientific investigation and analysis. His reports also provided impetus for the Public Health Act of 1875, which established a comprehensive sanitary code that evolved and lasted for a century.

Simon remained in the city post until 1855, when he was appointed the first medical officer in the kingdom's central government. As such, Simon is credited with being a major force behind the 1858 Medical Reform Act. He used his office to establish a state medical department to oversee public health, solidify the concept of state scientific research, strengthen the existing public **vaccination** system, and supervise members of the medical profession.

Among Simon's other accomplishments while working for the central government were his implementation of building inspections, his development of methods to make the water supply cleaner and sewers more effective, his abolition of cesspools, and his creation of a set of procedures to follow for outbreaks of contagious diseases. He stepped down from his government post in 1876.

Aside from his considerable achievements as a government official, Simon was also a respected lecturer, researcher (particularly in the field of glandular phenomena), and surgeon. One of his most famous surgical feats was his development of a perineal urethra puncture method to correct urine retention caused by stricture. A chapter he wrote in *System of Surgery* (Holmes) on inflammation is now regarded as a classic on the subject. In his later years the physician wrote several books, including *English Sanitary Institutions* (1890) and *Personal Recollections* (1898). He received a knighthood in 1887 for his contributions to public health and welfare. Simon died in London in 1904.

SIMPSON, JAMES YOUNG (1811-1870)

Scottish physician

Sir James Young Simpson was born at Bathgate, West Lothian, Scotland on June 7, 1811; he died in London on May 6, 1870. He was one of the most prominent obstetricians of modern times. Simpson was the son of a village baker. At the age of 14, he entered Edinburgh Univeristy to study medicine, graduating in 1832. Seven years later, at the age of 29, Simpson was appointed Professor of **Midwifery** (obstetrics) at Edinburgh. He soon became Scotland's leading obstetrician, acquiring a sizable practice through demonstrated ability and remarkable personality. During his lifetime, Simpson received many honors, including a baronetcy (1866); the Freedom of the City of Edinburgh; and an honorary degree from Oxford University. Simpson is especially remembered for the wonderful influence he exerted on his patients, and for being one of the most noteworthy personalities of his time.

In November of 1847 (the same year he was appointed physician to the Queen in Scotland), Simpson began to employ chloroform in obstetrics and labor, but only after a preliminary test that involved inhaling it experimentally himself, as also did his assistants Matthews Duncan and George Keith. Simpson immediately found himself embroiled with Calvinists who were opposed to the use of any anaesthetic in childbirth. It was not until 1853, when Queen Victoria accepted the use of chloroform for the birth of her son that criticism of Simpson began to subside. In 1858, Simpson introduced iron wire sutures; between 1850 and 1864, he pioneered the use of long obstetric forceps. Other contributions in gynecology and obstetrics included the use of uterine sound (1843), the sponge tent, dilatation of the cervix uteri in diagnosis, *Simpson's pains* in uterine **cancer** (1863), and version in deformed pelves. He wrote important memoirs on fetal **pathology** and hermaphroditism, and made contributions to the fields of archeology and medical history (particularly on **leprosy** in Scotland; 1841 to 1842). He introduced village or pavilion **hospitals** in Scotland.

Simpson's statistical investigations of the results of major operations, published as *Hospitalism* in 1869, pointed out that in more than two thousand in-hospital extremity amputations in Britain, more than 41 percent of the patients died if their operation were done in hospitals with more than 300 beds, and that infection was by far the greatest cause of death. In the case of another 200 amputations done out-of-hospital in country practice, only 11 percent of the patients died. Postoperative mortality figures were also high in all of the hospitals of Europe (Paris: 60 percent, Zurich: 46 percent, Glasgow: 34 percent), and in America as well (Massachusetts General Hospital: 26 percent, Pennsylvania Hospital: 24 percent). Simpson warned "The man laid on the operating table in one of our hospitals, is exposed to more chances of death than the English soldier on the field of Waterloo.'' Simpson's article led to major improvements in hospital administration, and contributed to the tearing down of many of the most offending European hospitals.

Simpson fell into dispute with Joseph Lister over the latter's ideas for reasons that are not clearly understood, but which may have something had to do with Simpson's religious beliefs.

SIMS, JAMES MARION (1813-1883)

American physician

James Marion Sims, was born on January 25, 1813 in Lancaster, SC; he died on November 13, 1883 in New York, NY. Sims was the son of John and Mahala Sims, and the husband of Eliza Theresa Jones (parents of five surviving children). An American physician and surgeon, Sims was the first to establish gynecology as a separate branch of medicine, and as one of the first areas of surgical specialization. He is now recognized as the leading gynecologist of his time. Sims graduated from South Carolina College in 1832; a year later (1833), he entered Charleston Medical College. In 1834, he enrolled in Jefferson Medical School in Philadelphia, obtaining the M.D. degree from that school in 1835. He began practice in Lancaster, South Carolina, where his first two patients died. He subsequently lived in Mount Meigs, Alabama; Montgomery, Alabama (1840); New York City (where he practiced surgery; 1853); Europe (1861); New York (1868); France (1870-1872); and New York (1872). Sims was a member of the Board of Surgeons at Women's Hospital; president of the **American Medical Association** (1876), and president of the American Gynecological Society (1880). He established Women's Hospital in New York (1854) for the instruction of students and physicians in gynecological surgery. Sims is remembered as a kind-hearted but impulsive man, but more than that as one of the most gifted of American surgeons. A statue was erected to his memory in Bryant Park in New York City by his European and American admirers in 1894.

After settling in Alabama, Sims gained a reputation as a capable and inventive surgeon. He operated successfully for abscess of the liver in 1835, and successfully removed an upper and lower jaw in 1837. In 1845, he was called to examine a country woman who had sustained a displacement of the uterus as the result of a fall from a horse. Some accounts say that he hit upon the peculiar lateral examination position that now bears his name (*Sim's position*, still adopted in some gynecological procedures) while making a digital examination, others state that this discovery resulted from four years of experimentation on black slave women in Alabama. In any case, Sims did develop the first successful treatment of a vesticovaginal fistula (an abnormal opening between the vagina and the bladder), which most often occurs as the result of a mishap during childbirth. The success of Sim's procedure was largely due to his use of a special curved speculum and his positioning the patient semi-prone on her left side with her right knee drawn up to her chest. (It is important to note that, before Sims had developed his technique, many surgeons had attempted to treat this condition with no better results than to cause additional suffering and inconvenience to their patients). Sims published his results in 1852, creating a profound impression in the medical world. While visiting Europe in 1861, Sims performed his fistula operation before surgical leaders there. He was soon in request all over Europe as a specialist in the diseases of women.

Sims is also remembered as the inventor of two **surgical instruments** of his own design, Sim's catheter (to empty the bladder while the fistula was healing) and the afore-mentioned speculum (also known as a double-duck-billed vaginal speculum). He also experimented with silver sutures to avoid **sepsis**. Among his other contributions were his methods of amputating the cervix uteri (1861); his description of vaginismus (1861); his operation of cholecystotomy (1878); and his development of a careful method of aseptically invading the peritoneal cavity for the arrest of hemorrhage (1881).

Among Sim's writings are ''The Treatment of Epiethelioma of the Cevix Uterine,'' *Am. J. Obst.* (1879); ''Remarks on the Treatment of Gunshot Wounds of the Abdomen in Relation to Modern Peritonal Surgery,'' *British Med. J.* (1881); ''The Surgical Treatment of President Garfield,'' *North Am. Rev.* (1881).

SINUSITIS

Sinusitis is an inflammation of the sinuses (the paired air pockets within the bones of the face). Sinusitis is most often due to an infection within these spaces.

The sinuses, which are connected to the nose, are lined with the same kind of skin found elsewhere within the respiratory tract. This skin has tiny little hairs projecting from it called cilia. As the cilia beat constantly, they help move the mucus produced in the sinuses into the respiratory tract. As the mucus is swept along the respiratory tract, they help clear the respiratory tract of any debris or organisms.

When the lining of the sinuses is swollen, the mucus can't flow normally. Trapped mucus then fills the sinuses, causing an uncomfortable sensation of pressure and providing an excellent environment for the growth of infection-causing bacteria.

Sinusitis is almost always due to an infection, although swelling from **allergies** can mimic the symptoms of pressure, **pain**, and congestion; allergies also can set the stage for a bacterial infection. Bacteria are the most common cause of sinus infection. People with weakened immune systems (including patients with **AIDS**) or patients who are taking medications which lower their immune resistance may develop sinusitis caused by fungi.

Acute sinusitis usually follows some type of upper respiratory tract infection or cold. Instead of ending, the cold seems to linger on, with constant or even worsening congestion. Drainage from the nose often changes from a clear color to a thicker, yellowish-green. There may be **fever**, **headache** and pain over the affected sinuses, as well as pressure which may worsen when the patient bends over. There may be pain in the jaw or teeth. Some children, in particular, get upset stomachs from the infected mucus draining into the throat and stomach. Some patients develop a **cough**.

Chronic sinusitis occurs when the problem has existed for at least three months. There is rarely a fever with chronic sinusitis, but nasal congestion and sinus pain and pressure are frequent. Because of the nature of the swelling in the sinuses, mucus may drip constantly down the back of the throat, resulting in a constant **sore throat** and **bad breath**.

It can be hard to diagnose sinusitus because the symptoms so often resemble those of a common cold, but sinusitis should be strongly suspected when a cold lingers beyond a week. Doctors disagree about the value of certain basic office exams for sinusitis. For example, tapping over the sinuses may or may not cause pain in patients with sinusitis.

X-rays and CT scans of the sinuses are helpful for both acute and chronic sinusitis. People with chronic sinusitis also should be checked for allergies and the possibility of a physical obstruction that could be causing the illness. For example, the septum (the cartilage which separates the two nasal cavities from each other) may be slightly displaced. Called a **deviated septum**, this can cause chronic obstruction and constant infections.

Antibiotics are used to treat acute sinusitis. These may include sulfa drugs, amoxicillin, and a variety of **cephalosporins**. These medications are usually given for about two weeks, but may be given for even longer periods of time. **Decongestants**, or the short-term use of decongestant nose sprays, can be useful. **Acetaminophen** and ibuprofen can decrease the pain and headache, and a humidifier can prevent keep mucus moist, soothing any sore throat or cough.

Chronic sinusitis is often treated at first with antibiotics; steroid nasal sprays may be used to decrease swelling in the nasal passages. If an anatomic reason is found for chronic sinusitis, it may need to be corrected with surgery.

Fungal sinusitis requires surgery to clean out the sinuses followed by a relatively long course of a very strong antifungal medication called amphotericin B given through a needle in the vein.

Chronic sinusitis is often associated with food allergies, so identifying and eliminating the offending food can help. Irrigating the sinuses with a salt water solution or powdered goldenseal is often recommended for sinusitis and allergies in order to clear the nasal passages of mucus.

Acupuncture has been used to treat sinusitis, as have a variety of dietary supplements including **vitamins** A, C, and E, and the mineral zinc. Hot and cold compresses (3 minutes hot, 30 seconds cold, repeated 3 times always ending with cold) can be applied directly over the sinuses to relieve pressure and enhance healing. Inhalating essential oils (2 drops of oil to 2 cups of water) using thyme, rosemary, and lavender can help open the sinuses and kill bacteria that cause infection.

Prognosis for sinus infections is usually excellent, although some people may find that they are particularly prone to contracting such infections after a cold. Fungal sinusitis, however, has a relatively high **death** rate.

Prevention involves good hygiene to cut down on the number of colds an individual catches. Avoiding exposure to cigarette smoke, identifying and treating allergies, and avoiding deep dives in swimming pools may help prevent sinus infections. During the winter, it is a good idea to use a humidifier to prevent dry nasal passages from cracking and allowing bacteria to enter. When allergies are diagnosed, a number of nasal sprays are available to try to prevent inflammation within the nasal passageways, thus allowing the normal flow of mucus.

Sjögren's Syndrome

Sjögren's syndrome is a disorder in which the mouth and eyes become extremely dry. Sjögren's syndrome is often associated with other **autoimmune disorders** (a condition in which the body's immune system mistakenly begins treating parts of the body as foreign invaders). While the immune cells should attack and kill invaders like bacteria, viruses, and fungi, these cells should not attack the body itself.

There are three types of Sjögren's syndrome. Primary Sjögren's syndrome occurs by itself, with no other associated disorders. Secondary Sjögren's syndrome occurs along with other autoimmune disorders, like **systemic lupus erythematosus**, **rheumatoid arthritis**, **scleroderma**, **vasculitis**.

When the disorder is limited to involvement of the eyes, with no other organ or tissue involvement evident, it is called sicca complex.

Women are about nine times more likely to suffer from Sjögren's syndrome than are men. It affects all age groups, although most patients are diagnosed when they are between 40-55 years old. Sjögren's syndrome is commonly associated with other autoimmune disorders. In fact, 30% of patients with certain autoimmune disorders will also have Sjögren's syndrome.

The cause of Sjögren's syndrome has not been clearly defined, but several causes are suspected. The syndrome sometimes runs in families. Other potential causes include hormonal factors (since there are more women than men with the disease) and viral factors. The viral theory suggests that the immune system is activated in response to a viral invader, but then fails to turn itself off. Some other immune malfunction then causes the overly active immune system to begin attacking the body's own tissues.

The main problem in Sjögren's syndrome is dryness. The salivary glands are often attacked and slowly destroyed, leaving the mouth extremely dry and sticky feeling. Swallowing and talking become difficult. Normally, the saliva washes the teeth clean. Saliva cannot perform this function in Sjögren's syndrome, so the teeth develop many cavities and decay quickly. The parotid glands produce the majority of the mouth's saliva. They are located lying over the jaw bones behind the area of the cheeks and in front of the ears, and may become significantly enlarged in Sjögren's syndrome.

The eyes also become extremely dry as the tear glands (called glands of lacrimation) are slowly destroyed. Eye symptoms include **itching**, burning, redness, increased sensitivity to light, and thick secretions gathering at the eye corners closest to the nose. The cornea may have small irritated pits in its surface (ulcerations).

Destruction of glands in other areas of the body may cause a variety of symptoms. In the nose, dryness may result in **nosebleed**s. In the rest of the respiratory tract, the rates of ear infection, hoarseness, **bronchitis**, and **pneumonia** may increase. Vaginal dryness can be quite uncomfortable. Rarely, the pancreas may slow production of enzymes important for digestion. The kidney may malfunction. About 33% of all patients with Sjögren's syndrome have other symptoms unrelated to gland destruction. These symptoms include fatigue, decreased energy, **fever**s, muscle aches and **pain**s, and joint pain.

A patient with Sjögren's syndrome must have at least three consecutive months of bothersome eye and/or mouth dryness. A variety of tests can determine the quantity of tears produced, the quantity of saliva produced, and the presence or absence of antibodies that could be involved in the destruction of glands.

There is no cure for Sjögren's syndrome. Instead, treatment is aimed at easing discomfort and complications associated with dryness. Artificial tears may need to be used up to every 30 minutes in order to avoid complications. Dry mouth is treated by sipping fluids slowly but constantly throughout the day. Sugarless chewing gum also can be helpful. An artificial saliva is available for use as a mouthwash. Careful dental hygiene is important in order to avoid **tooth decay**. Vaginal dryness can be treated with gel preparations. Steroid medications may be required when other symptoms of autoimmune disorders complicate Sjögren's syndrome, but they carry risks of cornea damage.

The prognosis for patients with primary Sjögren's syndrome is good. Although the condition is annoying, serious complications rarely occur. The prognosis for patients with secondary Sjögren's syndrome varies since it depends on the prognosis for the accompanying autoimmune disorder.

No one knows how to prevent this syndrome.

SKIN CANCER

Skin cancer, malignant melanoma, is a type of skin tumor that is characterized by the **cancer**ous growth of melanocytes, which are cells that produce a dark pigment called melanin.

Cancer of the skin is the most common type of cancer and continues to grow in incidence. Skin cancer starts in the top layer of skin (the epidermis) but can grow down into the lower layers, the dermis and the subcutaneous layer. There are three main types of cells located in the epidermis, each of which can become cancerous. Melanocytes are the pigmented cells that are scattered throughout the skin, providing protection from ultraviolet (UV) light. Basal cells rest near the bottom of the epidermis and the layer of cells that continually grow to replace skin. The third type of epidermal cell is the squamous cells which make up most of the cells in human skin.

Malignant melanoma is the most serious type of skin cancer. It develops from the melanocytes. Although melanoma is the least common skin cancer, it is the most aggressive. It spreads (metastasizes) to other parts of the body—especially the lungs and liver—as well as invading surrounding tissues. Melanomas in their early stages resemble **moles**. In Caucasians, melanomas appear most often on the trunk, head, and neck in men and on the arms and legs in women. Melanomas in African Americans, however, occur primarily on the palms of the hand, soles of the feet, and under the nails. Melanomas appear only rarely in the eyes, mouth, vagina, or digestive tract. Although melanomas are associated with exposure to the sun, the greatest risk factor for developing melanoma may be genetic. People who have a first-degree relative with melanoma have an increased risk up to eight times greater of developing the disease.

Basal cell cancer is the most common type of skin cancer, accounting for about 75% of all skin cancers. It occurs primarily on the parts of the skin exposed to the sun and is most common in people living in equatorial regions or areas of high ozone depletion. Light-skinned people are more at risk of developing basal cell cancer than dark-skinned people. This form of skin cancer is primarily a disease of adults; it appears most often after age 30, peaking around age 70. Basal cell cancer grows very slowly; if it is not treated, however, it can invade deeper skin layers and cause disfigurement. This type of cancer can appear as a shiny, translucent nodule on the skin or as a red, wrinkled and scaly area.

Squamous cell cancer is the second most frequent type of skin cancer. It arises from the outer keratinizing layer of skin, so named because it contains a tough protein called keratin. Squamous cell cancer grows faster than basal cell cancer; it is more likely to metastasize to the lymph nodes as well as to distant sites. Squamous cell cancer most often appears on the arms, head, and neck. Fair-skinned people of Celtic descent are at high risk for developing squamous cell cancer. This type of cancer is rarely life-threatening but can cause serious problems if it spreads and can also cause disfigurement. Squamous cell cancer usually appears as a scaly, slightly elevated area of damaged skin.

Besides the three major types of skin cancer, there are a few other relatively rare forms. The most serious of these is **Kaposi's sarcoma** (KS), which occurs primarily in **AIDS** patients or older males of Mediterranean descent. When KS occurs with AIDS it is usually more aggressive. Other types of skin tumors are usually nonmalignant and grow slowly. These include:

- Bowen's disease. This is a type of skin inflammation (**dermatitis**) that sometimes looks like squamous cell cancer.
- Solar keratosis. This is a sunlight-damaged area of skin that sometimes develops into cancer.
- Keratoacanthoma. A keratoacanthoma is a dome-shaped tumor that can grow quickly and appear like squamous cell cancer. Although it is usually benign, it should be removed.

Most skin cancers are associated with the amount of time that a person spends in the sun and the number of **sunburn**s received, especially if they occurred at an early age. Skin cancer typically does not appear for 10-20 years after the sun damage has occurred. Because of this time lag, skin cancer rarely occurs before **puberty** and occurs more frequently with age.

The number of moles (nevi) on a person's skin is related to the likelihood of developing melanoma. There are three types of nevi: not cancerous (benign); atypical (dysplastic); or birthmark (congenital). All three types of nevi have been associated with a higher risk of developing melanoma. Sometimes the moles themselves can become cancerous; usually, however, the cancer is a new growth that occurs on normal skin.

The tendency to develop skin cancer also tends to run in families. As has already been mentioned, there appears to be a significant genetic factor in the development of melanoma.

Skin cancer begins to develop when a change or mutation occurs in one of the cells of the skin, causing it to grow without control. This mutation can be caused by ultraviolet (UV) light; most skin cancers are thought to be caused by overexposure to UV light from the sun. The incidence of severe, blistering sunburns is particularly closely related to skin cancer, more so when these **burns** occur during childhood. Exposure to ionizing radiation, arsenic, or polycyclic hydrocarbons in the workplace also appears to stimulate the development of skin cancers. The use of psoralen for treatment of **psoriasis** may be associated with the development of squamous cell cancer. Skin cancers are also more common in immunocompromised patients, such as AIDS patients or those who have undergone organ transplants.

The first sign of skin cancer is usually a change in an existing mole, the presence of a new mole, or a change in a specific area of skin. Any change in a mole or skin lesion, including changes in color, size, or shape, tenderness, scaliness, or **itching** should be suspected of being skin cancer. Areas that bleed or are ulcerated may be signs of more advanced skin cancer. By doing a monthly self-examination, a person can identify abnormal moles or areas of skin and seek evaluation from a qualified health professional. The ABCD rule provides an easy way to remember the important characteristics of moles when one is examining the skin:

- Asymmetry. A normal mole is round, whereas a suspicious mole is unevenly shaped.
- Border. A normal mole has a clear-cut border with the surrounding skin, whereas the edges of a suspect mole are often irregular.
- Color. Normal moles are uniformly tan or brown, but cancerous moles may appear as mixtures of red, white, blue, brown, purple, or black.
- Diameter. Normal moles are usually less than 5 millimeters in diameter. A skin lesion greater than 1/4 inch across may be suspected as cancerous.

A person who has a suspicious-looking mole or area of skin should consult a doctor. In many cases, the patient's primary care physician will refer him or her to a doctor who specializes in skin diseases (a dermatologist). The dermatologist will carefully examine the lesion for the characteristic features of skin cancer. If further testing seems necessary, the doctor will perform a skin **biopsy** by removing the lesion under local anesthesia. Because melanomas tend to grow in diameter, as well as downwards into the epidermis and fatty layers of skin, a biopsy sample that is larger than the mole will be taken. This tissue is then analyzed under a microscope by a specialist in diseased organs and tissues (a pathologist). The pathologist makes the diagnosis of cancer and determines how far the tumor has grown into the skin. The evaluation of the progression of the cancer is called staging. Staging refers to how advanced the cancer is and is determined by the thickness and size of the tumor. Additional tests will also be done to determine if the cancer has moved into the lymph nodes or other areas of the body. These tests might include chest x ray, computed tomography scan (CT scan), **magnetic resonance imaging** (MRI), and blood tests.

The primary treatment for skin cancer is to cut out (excise) the tumor or diseased area of skin. Surgery usually involves a simple excision using a scalpel to remove the lesion and a small amount of normal surrounding tissue. A procedure known as microscopically controlled excision can be used to examine each layer of skin as it is removed to ensure that the proper amount is taken. Depending on the amount of skin removed, the cut is either closed with stitches or covered with a skin graft. When surgical excision is performed on visible areas, such as the face, cosmetic surgery may also be performed to minimize the scar. Other techniques for removing skin tumors include burning, freezing with dry ice (cryosurgery), or **laser surgery**. For skin cancer that is localized and has not spread to other areas of the body, excision may be the only treatment needed.

Although **chemotherapy** is the normal course of therapy for most other types of advanced cancer, it is not usually effective and not usually used for advanced skin cancer. For advanced melanoma that has moved beyond the original tumor site, the local lymph nodes may be surgically removed. Immunotherapy in the form of interferon or interleukin is being used more often with success for advanced melanoma. There is growing evidence that **radiation therapy** may be useful for advanced melanoma. Other treatments under investigation for melanoma include **gene therapy** and **vaccination**. Recent studies have shown that the use of a vaccine prepared from the patient's own cancer cells may be useful in treating advanced melanoma. For people previously diagnosed with skin cancers, the chances of getting additional skin cancers are high. Therefore, regular monthly self-examination, as well as frequent examinations by a dermatologist, are essential.

The prognosis for skin cancer depends on several factors, the most important of which are the invasiveness of the tumor and its location. The prognosis is good for localized skin cancers that are diagnosed and treated early. For basal cell cancer and squamous cell cancer, the cure rate is close to 100%, although most of these patients will have recurrent skin cancer. For localized melanoma, the cure rate is approximately 95%. The prognosis worsens with larger tumors. Melanoma that has spread to the lymph nodes has a 5-year survival rate of 54%; advanced melanoma has a survival rate of only 13%. When melanoma has spread to other parts of the body, it is generally considered incurable; the median length of survival is six months.

Prevention is the best way to deal with skin cancer. Avoiding unnecessary sun exposure—including sun lamps and tanning salons— is relatively simple. Parents of small children should protect them against the risk of sunburn. Precautions include avoiding high sun, when the rays of the sun are most intense (between 11 A.M. and 1 P.M.) In addition, persons living at high elevations need to take extra precautions because the intensity of UV radiation increases by 4% with every 1000-foot rise above sea level.

There is presently some debate about the ability of sunscreen to protect against skin cancer. Some scientists believe that gradual exposure to the sun, in order to develop a mild tan, may offer the best protection from skin cancer. Skin cancer has also been related to diets that are high in fat. Decreasing the amount of fat consumed may also help to decrease the risk of skin cancer.

SKIN GRAFTING

Skin grafting is a surgical procedure in which skin or skin substitute is placed over a burn or wound to replace damaged skin or provide a temporary wound covering.

Wounds such as third-degree **burns** must be covered as quickly as possible to prevent infection and loss of fluid. Without a skin graft, wounds can contract, causing serious scars. Wounds that don't heal well, such as diabetic ulcers, or **bedsores**, can be treated with skin grafts to prevent infection. Skin grafting isn't necessary for first-or second-degree burns, which heal with little or no scarring.

Skin protects the body from fluid loss, helps to regulate temperature, and helps keep out germs. More than 50,000 people are hospitalized with burns each year in the United States, and 5,500 die. Approximately 4 million people suffer from non-healing wounds.

Skin for grafting can be obtained from another part of the patient's body if there is enough undamaged skin available and if the person is healthy enough to have extra surgery. Otherwise, skin can be obtained from another person (donor skin from cadavers is frozen, stored, and available for use), or from an animal (usually a pig). However, skin from these other sources are only used temporarily, since they are rejected by the patient's immune system within 7 to 10 days and must be replaced with a graft from the patient's own skin.

Several artificial skin products are available for burns or non-healing wounds. These products aren't rejected by the patient's body, and actually encourage the growth of new tissue. Artificial skin usually consists of a type of lattice which acts as a template for new skin to grow. This artificial lattice eventually breaks down as the new skin structure grows. A synthetic outer layer acts as a temporary barrier during this process, and is eventually replaced with a graft of the patient's own skin. The cost for the synthetic products in about $1,000 for a 40-inch square piece of artificial skin, in addition to the costs of the surgery. This procedure is covered by insurance.

Once a skin graft has been put in place (and even after it heals), it must be maintained carefully. Patients need to stay in bed for a few days and then wear special stockings or bandages to help support the new skin and keep it from contracting too much.

Since grafted skin doesn't contain sweat or oil glands, it should be lubricated daily for two to three months to prevent drying and cracking.

The risks of skin grafting include typical risks for any surgical procedure, including reactions to the drugs, breathing problems, bleeding, and infection. With a donor skin graft, there are also risks of getting an infectious diseases.

A skin graft should significantly improve the quality of the wound and may prevent serious complications. Sometimes grafts aren't successful, however, either because of poor blood flow, swelling, or infection.

SKIN LESIONS

A skin lesion is an abnormal growth or patch of skin that doesn't look like the area nearby. Skin lesions can be divided into two categories: primary and secondary.

Primary skin lesions are variations in color or texture that may be present at birth, such as **moles** or **birthmarks**. They also may appear during a person's lifetime, such as **warts**, **acne**, or **psoriasis**, allergic reactions such as **hives** or **sunburn**.

Secondary skin lesions include changes in the skin caused by primary skin lesions, either as a natural progression or because of scratching or picking at the skin.

The major types of primary lesions are:

- Macule. A small, circular, flat spot less than a quarter of an inch wide. The color of a macule is different from nearby skin, and are usually brown, white, or red. Freckles and flat moles are considered macules. Macules bigger than an inch are called patches.
- Vesicle. A raised lesion less than a a quarter of an inch across filled with clear fluid; vesicles bigger than this are called blisters. Vesicles may be caused by sunburn, insect bites, chemical irritation, or some viral infections, such as cold sores.
- Pustule. A raised lesion filled with pus usually caused by an infection, such as impetigo or **boils**.
- Papule. A solid, raised, rough lesion that may be red, pink or brown. A patch of closely-grouped papules is called a plaque. Papules are associated with conditions such as warts, **syphilis**, psoriasis, or **skin cancer**.
- Nodule. A solid lesion with distinct edges that is usually more deeply rooted than a papule. A nodule feels like a hard mass, distinct from the skin around it. A large nodule is called a tumor.
- Wheal. A raised skin lesion that can be itchy and usually disappears soon after it appears. Wheals are generally part of an allergic reaction.
- Telangiectasia. Small, dilated blood vessels that appear close to the surface of the skin. Telangiectasia is often a symptom of skin diseases such as rosacea or **scleroderma**.

The major types of secondary skin lesions are:

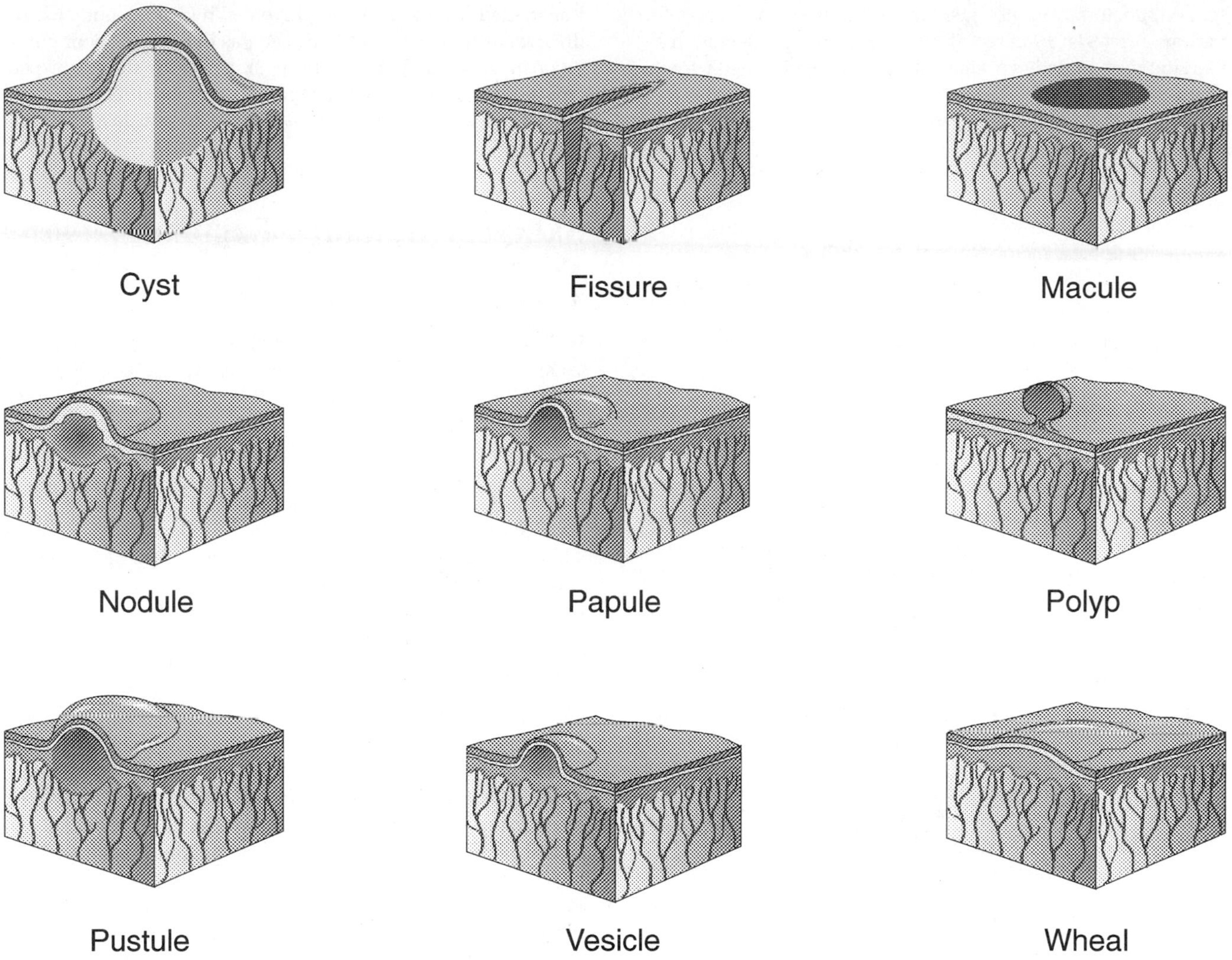

A skin lesion is an abnormal growth or an area of skin that doesn't look like the skin nearby. The illustrations above feature some of the different types of skin lesions. ***(Illustration by Electronic Illustrators Group.)***

- Ulcer. Lesion that erodes the upper portion of the skin and part of the lower portion beneath. Ulcers can be caused by conditions such as bacterial infection or injury, or from more long-lasting problems such as scleroderma. An ulcer that looks like a deep crack in the skin is called a fissure.
- Scale. A dry build-up of dead skin cells that often flakes off the surface of the skin. Diseases that cause scale include fungal infections and psoriasis.
- Crust. A dried collection of blood, serum, or pus. Also called a scab, a crust is often part of the normal healing process of many infectious lesions.
- Excoriation. A hollow, crusted area caused by scratching or picking at a skin sore.
- Scar. Discolored, fibrous tissue that permanently replaces normal skin after the tissue has been destroyed. A very thick and raised scar is called a keloid.
- Atrophy. An area of skin that has become very thin and wrinkled. Normally seen in older people and those who use very strong corticosteroid skin creams.

Skin lesions can be caused by a wide variety of conditions and diseases, and a tendency for developing moles, freckles, or birthmarks may be inherited. Infection of the skin itself by germs or parasites is the most common cause of skin lesions. Acne, **athlete's foot**, warts, and **scabies** are all examples of skin infections that cause lesions. Allergic reactions and sensitivity also can cause skin lesions. Underlying conditions can also trigger a skin lesion. For example, the decreased sensitivity and poor circulation that comes with **diabetes** can lead to the development of ulcers on the legs and feet. Infections of body's entire system can cause the sudden onset of skin lesions, such as witih chicken pox or herpes.

Diagnosis of the underlying cause of skin lesions is usually based on patient history, what the lesion looks like, and where it appears on the body. To determine the cause of an infection, doctors may also take scrapings or swab samples for various lab tests. In cases of suspected allergy, doctors may use skin tests to find out what substances are causing the reaction.

Doctors can determine if a skin lesion is cancerous by taking a sample of the skin and analyzing it under a microscope. Since early detection is a key to successful treatment of cancer, patients should examine their skin on a monthly basis for skin changes or the presence of new growths. When examining moles, factors to look for include:

- Asymmetry. A normal mole is round, but a suspicious mole is uneven.
- Border. A normal mole has a clear-cut border but the edges of a suspect mole may be irregular.
- Color. Normal moles are uniformly tan or brown, but cancerous moles may be mixtures of red, white, blue, brown, purple, or black.
- Diameter. Normal moles are usually less than 15 inches in diameter; anything bigger than that may be cancerous.

Treatment of skin lesions depends upon the cause, what type of lesions they are, and the patient's overall health. If the cause of the lesions is an allergic reaction, avoiding the allergy trigger is the most effective treatment. Skin preparations can be used to clean and protect irritated skin as well as to remove dead skin cells and scales. These may come in a variety of forms, including ointments, creams, lotions, and solutions. Topical **antibiotics**, fungicides, lice-killing and scabies-killing drugs can be applied to treat appropriate skin infections. Oral medications may be taken to treat body-wide infections or diseases. Deeply-infected lesions may require minor surgery to lance and drain pus. **Corticosteroids** are particularly effective in reducing inflammation and **itching** (puritis). Oatmeal baths, baking soda mixtures, and calamine lotion are also recommended to ease symptoms.

Sometimes surgical removal of a lesion may be recommended, especially when treating skin cancer. Surgical removal usually involves simply cutting away the growth under local anesthetic, but growths may be removed by freezing (**cryotherapy**) or **laser surgery**.

Skin lesions such as moles, freckles, and birthmarks are a normal part of skin and will not disappear unless deliberately removed by a surgical procedure. Lesions due to an allergic reaction often subside soon after the offending agent is removed. Healing of lesions due to infections or disorders depends upon the type of infection or disorder and the overall health of the individual. Prognosis for skin cancer mostly depends on whether or not the lesion has spread to other parts of the body.

Not all skin lesions are preventable; moles and freckles, for example, are common and unavoidable. However, others can be avoided or minimized by taking certain precautions. Skin lesions caused by an allergic reaction can be avoided by staying away from the offending agent, or figuring out how to safely handling it. Keeping the skin, nails, and scalp clean and moisturized, and not sharing personal care items such as combs and make-up with others, can help reduce or prevent infectious skin diseases. Skin lesions associated with **sexually transmitted diseases** can be prevented by using **condoms**. Individuals who have conditions such as diabetes or poor circulation that could lead to serious skin lesions should inspect their bodies regularly for changes in their skin. Staying out of the sun or using effective sunscreens can cut down on skin cancer.

Skinner, Burrhus Frederic (1904-1990)

American psychologist

B. F. Skinner was born in Susquehanna, Pennsylvania. As a youth, he showed talent for music and writing, as well as mechanical aptitude. He attended Hamilton College as an English major, with the goal of becoming a professional writer. After graduation, Skinner, discouraged over his literary prospects, became interested in behavioristic psychology after reading the works of John Watson and Ivan Pavlov. He entered Harvard University as a graduate student in psychology in 1928 and received his degree three years later. Skinner remained at Harvard through 1936, by which time he was a junior fellow of the prestigious Society of Fellows. While at Harvard, he laid the foundation for a new system of behavioral analysis through his research in the field of animal learning, utilizing unique experimental equipment of his own design.

His most successful and well-known apparatus, known as the Skinner Box, was a cage in which a laboratory rat could, by pressing on a bar, activate a mechanism that would drop a food pellet into the cage. Another device recorded each press of the bar, producing a permanent record of experimental results without the presence of a tester. Skinner analyzed the rats' bar-pressing behavior by varying his patterns of reinforcement (feeding) to learn their responses to different schedules (including random ones). Using this box to study how rats "operated on" their environment led Skinner to formulate the principle of operant **conditioning**—applicable to a wide range of both human and animal behaviors—through which an experimenter can gradually shape the behavior of a subject by manipulating its responses through reinforcement or lack of it. In contrast to Pavlovian, or response, conditioning, which depends on an outside stimulus, Skinner's operant conditioning depends on the subject's responses themselves. Skinner introduced the concept of operant conditioning to the public in his first book, *The Behavior of Organisms* (1938).

Between 1936 and 1948 Skinner held faculty positions at the University of Minnesota and the University of Indiana, after which he returned permanently to Harvard. His ideas eventually became so influential that the American Psychological Association created a separate division of studies related to them (Division 25: "The Experimental Analysis of Behavior"), and four journals of behaviorist research were established. In the 1940s Skinner began training animals to perform complex activities by first teaching them chains of simpler ones. He was quite successful in training laboratory animals to perform apparently remarkable and complex activities. One example of this involved pigeons that learned to play table tennis.

Skinner's observation of the effectiveness of incremental training of animals led him to formulate the principles of programmed instruction for human students, in which the concept of reward, or reinforcement, is fundamental, and complex subjects such as mathematics are broken down into simple components presented in order of increasing difficulty. Presented with a set of relatively simple questions, students receive immediate reinforcement—and thus incentive to continue—by being told that their answers were correct. The programmed learning movement became highly influential in the United States and abroad. Although this technique eventually came under criticism by educators advocating more holistic methods of instruction, it remains a valuable teaching tool. Courses and course materials based on it have been developed for many subjects, and at levels of difficulty ranging from kindergarten through graduate school.

Skinner's work was also influential in the clinical treatment of mental and emotional disorders. In the late 1940s he began to develop the behavior modification method, in which subjects receive a series of small rewards for desired behavior. Considered a useful technique for psychologists and psychiatrists with deeply disturbed patients, behavior modification has also been widely used by the general population in overcoming **obesity**, shyness, speech defects, **addiction** to **smoking**, and other problems. Extending his ideas to the realm of philosophy, Skinner concluded that all behavior was the result of either positive or negative reinforcement, and thus the existence of free will was merely an illusion. To explore the social ramifications of his behaviorist principles, he wrote the novel *Walden Two* (1948), which depicted a utopian society in which all reinforcement was positive. While detractors of this controversial work regarded its vision of social control through strict positive reinforcement as totalitarian, the 1967 founding of the Twin Oaks Community in Virginia was inspired by Skinner's ideas. Skinner elaborated further on his ideas about positive social control in his book *Beyond Freedom and Dignity* (1971), which critiques the notion of human autonomy, arguing that many actions ascribed to free will are performed due to necessity.

Skinner has been listed in *The 100 Most Important People in the World,* and in a 1975 survey he was identified as the best-known scientist in the United States. Skinner's other books include *Science and Human Behavior* (1953) and *Verbal Behavior* (1957).

See also Behavioral sciences; Ivan Petrovitch Pavlov; John Broadus Watson

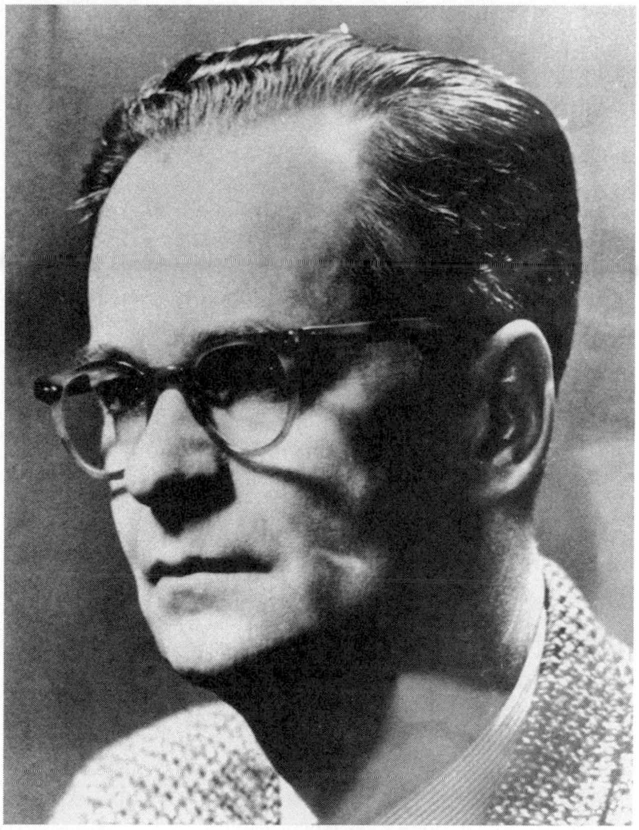

B. F. Skinner

SKIN RESURFACING

Skin resurfacing includes a variety of techniques to change the surface texture and appearance of the skin. Common skin resurfacing techniques include chemical peels, dermabrasion, and laser resurfacing.

Skin resurfacing may be used for cosmetic reasons, such as erasing wrinkles around the mouth or eyes. It also may be done as a medical treatment, such as removing precancerous lesions. Doctors sometimes combine techniques, using dermabrasion or laser resurfacing on some areas of the face, while performing a chemical peel on other areas.

In a chemical peel, the doctor paints on a variety of caustic chemicals to destroy several layers of skin, allowing new, fresh skin to grow. After the skin heals, discoloration, wrinkles, and other surface irregularities are often eliminated. Chemical peels are divided into three types: superficial, medium-depth, and deep. The type of peel depends on the strength of the chemical used, and on how deeply it penetrates.

Superficial peels are used for fine wrinkles, sun damage and acne. The medium-depth peel is used for more obvious wrinkles and sun damage, as well as for precancerous lesions. Deep peels are used for the most severe wrinkling and sun damage.

For dermabrasion, the doctor uses a sharp tool to selectively remove layers of skin. Some doctors use a hand-held motorized device with a small wire brush or grinding wheel. Others prefer to remove the skin by hand with an abrasive pad. Dermabrasion is often used to remove acne scars; it also can be used to treat wrinkling, surgical scars, and tattoos.

Laser resurfacing is the most recently developed technique for skin resurfacing. Specially designed, pulsing lasers can vaporize skin layer by layer without damaging nearby skin tissue. Special scanning devices move the laser light across the skin in predetermined patterns. Laser resurfacing can be used to remove wrinkles around the eyes, mouth, and cheeks, but smile lines tend to reappear after laser resurfacing. Laser resurfacing works best as a spot treatment; patients expecting complete removal of their wrinkles will not be satisfied.

Patients need to get ready for a chemical peel several weeks before the actual procedure. To promote turnover of skin cells, patients use a mild fruit acid lotion or cream in the morning, and an acne cream in the evening, together with a bleaching product that helps prevent later discoloration. To prevent reappearance of any herpes simplex virus infection, antiviral medicine is started a few days before the procedure and continues until the skin has healed.

Patients arrive for the procedure wearing no makeup. All peels cause some pain; for a superficial peel, a hand-held fan to cool the face during the procedure is often enough to ease discomfort. For medium-depth peels, the patient may take **aspirin** or a sedative. During the procedure, cold compresses and a hand-held fan reduce pain. Because deep peels can be extremely painful, some doctors prefer to use general **anesthesia**; however, local anesthetics with intravenous sedatives are often enough to control pain.

Dermabrasion doesn't require much preparation. It is usually performed under local anesthesia, although some doctors use intravenous sedation or general anesthesia. The doctor begins by marking the areas to be treated and then chilling them with ice packs. In order to stiffen the skin, a cold spray is applied, which also helps control pain. Some doctors prefer to inject the area with a saline solution and local anesthetic, which also leaves the skin's surface more solid.

Antiviral drugs are given several days before the procedure. Laser resurfacing is sometimes performed under local anesthesia or with an oral sedative. The patient's eyes must be shielded, and the area surrounding the face should be shielded with wet drapes or crumpled foil to catch stray beams of laser light. The doctor marks the areas to be treated before beginning the procedure.

Within a day or so following a superficial peel, the skin turns faint pink or brown. Over the next few days, dead skin will peel away. Patients should wash their skin often with a mild cleanser and cool water, and then apply an ointment to keep skin moist. After a medium-depth peel, the skin turns deep red or brown and crusts may form. Care is similar to that following a superficial peel. Redness may persist for a week or more. Deep-peeled skin will turn brown and crusty, and there may be swelling and some oozing. Frequent washing and ointments are better than bandages. The skin typically heals in about two weeks, but redness may persist.

Following dermabrasion, an ointment may be applied and the wound covered with a dressing and mask. Patients with a history of herpes infections will begin taking an antiviral medication to prevent a recurrence. After 24 hours, the dressing is removed, and ointment is reapplied to keep the wound moist. Patients are encouraged to wash their face with plain water and reapply ointment every few hours. This relieves **itching** and pain and helps removc oozing fluid and other matter. Patients may need pain medication, and steroids may be taken during the first few days to reduce swelling. The skin will take a week or more to heal, but may remain very red.

The skin should be kept moist after laser resurfacing to promote more rapid healing and reduce the risk of infection. Some doctors favor applying ointments only to the skin, but others prefer using dressings. In either case, care of the skin is similar to that given following a chemical peel. The face is washed with plain water to remove ooze, and an ointment is reapplied. Healing will take approximately two weeks. Pain medications and a steroid to reduce swelling may be taken.

All resurfacing procedures can lead to infection and scarring. It's also possible that skin color will be changed, or that redness will last for months. In addition, some of the peeling agents used in deep chemical peels can affect the function of the heart.

Depending on the resurfacing techniques selected, it's possible to improve the appearance of skin damaged by sun, age, or disease. Skin resurfacing techniques deal only the surface of the skin, however; procedures such as face-lift surgery or eyelid surgery may be needed to repair other age-related skin changes. All resurfacing procedures are accompanied by some pain, redness, and skin color changes which may last for several months following the procedure. Eventually, these problems usually fade away.

Complications of skin resurfacing techniques can be serious, including infection and scarring. Moreover, there are some people who don't make good candidates for the procedure. Patients who tend to scar easily may get poor results. Resurfacing procedures can reactivate herpes infections or lead to new, sometimes serious infections. All resurfacing techniques intentionally create skin **wounds**, which means that scarring is possible. These problems can be minimized by using antiviral drugs before the procedures and good wound care afterward. Selection of an experienced, reputable provider also is key.

As the popularity of skin resurfacing techniques has increased, unqualified or inexperienced providers have entered the field. Patients should choose their provider with the same degree of care they take for any other medical procedure.

Skoda, Josef (1805-1881)

Czech physician

Josef Skoda, a resident of Pilsen, Bohemia, became the leading clinician of the New Vienna School of medicine, and an exponent of the school's therapeutic nihilism, particularly in regard to the prevailing conservative ideas concerning disease causation then in vogue at the University of Vienna. In 1847, Skoda became the first medical teacher in Vienna to lecture in German. He taught for nearly his entire life at the Allegemeines Krankenhaus. Contemporaries remembered Skoda as a portly and rather cold and rigid bachelor who made few warm personal friendships. It is said he put up with a peculiar wardrobe for much of his life to avoid causing offense to his tailor, whom he considered a personal friend. He is also remembered for having once sued a clergyman to collect a debt.

In 1839, Skoda published his treatise on percussion and auscultation. In it he attempts to classify the sounds in the chest according to categories that take into account musical pitch and tonality, with alternations from full to hollow, clear to dull, tympanitic to muffled, and high to deep. The drum-like tympanic resonance heard on percussion above an area of **pneumonia** or lung fluid is known as Skodaic resonance. Although not much was known of the physics of sound during Skoda's lifetime, his acoustic categories, which were based more on the physical properties of the structures being investigated than their biological characteristics, were generally regarded as improvements on the descriptive terms used by the French clinicians of the period. Skoda's work has survived in elaborated form in the complicated instruments that some clinicians use to analyze the sounds of the chest for teaching purposes.

Skoda regarded his patients as objects for investigation only, and is said to have had no place for therapy in his medical practice. To his credit, however, he did not have much use for many of the ineffectual medical treatments of the time, which he dismissed as being ''all the same.'' He was also known for his practice of making snap diagnoses, which at that time were in vogue, and for looking askance at anyone who would think of using a post-mortem diagnosis to identify a disease.

Skoda was a proponent of **disease prevention**; he believed that the proper way to treat a disease was to stop it before it could begin its ravages; much of his time was devoted to the study of such epidemic diseases as typhoid and **cholera**.

Skoda is also remembered for his championing Ignac Semmelweis' at-the-time novel idea that the washing of the physician's hands in a disinfecting solution could reduce deaths due to puerperal fever in postpartum mothers. Skoda argued this point before the Austrian Academy of Sciences, as well as in print, at a time when there still existed tremendous resistance to prophylactic medical practices.

SLEEP

Sleep is a state of physical inactivity and mental rest in which conscious awareness, thought, and voluntary movement cease and intermittent dreaming takes place. This natural and regular phenomenon essential to all living creatures normally happens with the eyes closed and is divided into two basic types: REM (rapid eye movement) and NREM (non-rapid eye movement) sleep. As passive as sleep appears, it is actually a very active and deliberate process in which the brain busily turns off wakeful functions while turning on sleep mechanisms. No one knows exactly why we must sleep or how it happens, but the quality, quantity, and type of sleep affects the quality, quantity, and effectiveness of our wakeful mental and physical activities. These, in turn, influence the quality, quantity, and timing of sleep.

In the attempt to understand our need for sleep, experiments in sleep deprivation play an important role. Total sleep deprivation longer than 40 hours proves impossible, however, due to brief, totally unpreventable periods of ''microsleep,'' which will happen even during physical activity. These microsleeps barely last a few seconds, but they may explain performance lapses in waking activities. They demonstrate the body's obvious need for sleep and may even have some restorative function.

While sleep deprivation can eventually cause death, sleep deprivation lasting up to 10 days shows no serious, prolonged consequences and does not cause severe psychological problems or mental illness as once thought. Losing more than one night's sleep does produce a noticeable increase in irritability, lethargy, disinterest, and even paranoia. While not seriously impaired, psychomotor performance and concentration are adversely affected. While autonomic (involuntary) **nervous system** activity increases during sleep deprivation to keep heart rate, blood pressure, breathing, and body temperature normal, physical fitness cannot be maintained and immunological functions seem to suffer.

Another question that remains only partially answered is how sleep onset is determined and why. The factors involved include circadian rhythms (biological time clocks); the degree of stimulation in the wakeful state; the degree of personal sleepiness; the decrease in core body temperature; a quiet and comfortable sleep environment; conditioning arising from ''bedroom cues''; and homeostasis, the automatic attempt by the body to maintain balance and equilibrium (for example, the air temperature may fall to 50°F [10°C], but our body burns calories to maintain its normal temperature of 98.6°F [37°C]).

The fact that sleep deprivation increases the desire for sleep firmly points to a homeostatic element in sleep. This is intricately linked to highly influential circadian rhythms controlled by centers probably located in the hypothalamus, part of the brain primarily involved in autonomic nervous system functions. Circadian rhythms determine our approximate 24- to 25-hour sleep-wake pattern and a similar cycle in the rise and fall of core body temperature and other physiological functions.

Studies done on human circadian rhythms in situations totally devoid of time cues (such as sunrise, sunset, clocks, etc.) show that these rhythms are controlled completely internally and usually run on a cycle of almost 25 rather than 24 hours. In normal situations, factors called ''zeitgebers'' (from the German *zeit* for time and *geber* for giver) such as daylight, environmental noises, clocks, and work schedules virtually force us to maintain a 24-hour cycle. Therefore, our circadian rhythms must ''phase advance'' from their normal, approximate 25-hour cycle to an imposed 24-hour cycle.

The body has difficulty adapting to much more than an hour of phase-advance in one day. Drastic time changes—like those caused by rapid long-distance travel such as flying—require either phase-advancement or phase-delay. This is why travelers experience ''jet lag.'' Recovery from east-west travel requiring phase-delay adjustments is usually quicker than in phase-advancement resulting from west-east travel. Some people seem simply unable to phase-advance their biological clocks, which often results in sleep disorders.

The greatest contribution to sleep study was the development of the EEG, or electroencephalogram, by German psychiatrist Hans Berger in 1929. This electrode, attached to the scalp with glue, records electrical impulses in the brain called brain waves. The discovery triggered investigations into sleep in major centers around the world. Specific brain wave patterns became evident and sleep was generally classified into distinct stages.

In 1953, Professor Nathanial Kleitman and his graduate student Eugene Aserinsky reported their close observations of a sleep stage they called REM—rapid eye movement. An electro-oculogram, or EOG, taped close to the eyelids, recorded both vertical and horizontal eye movement, which became rapid and sporadic during REM sleep. The electromyogram, or EMG, recorded chin and neck muscle movement, which, for as yet undetermined reasons, completely relaxed during REM sleep. Kleitman and Aserinsky found that when subjects were awakened from REM sleep they almost always reported a dream, which was seldom the case when awakened from non-REM sleep.

Following the initial REM discoveries, sleep research greatly increased. One important discovery arising from this research was the high prevalence of **sleep disorders**, some of which now explain problems previously blamed on obscure physical or psychological disorders but which could not be effectively treated by medicine or psychiatry.

Non-REM sleep is generally believed to occur in four stages and is characterized by lack of dreaming. In the drowsy, light sleep of stage 1, which takes up about 5% of the sleep cycle, the sleeper is generally nonresponsive but is easily awakened. High chin muscle activity occurs and there is occasional slow, rolling eye movement.

Within a few minutes, the sleeper enters stage-2 sleep. Brain waves slow further and spindles (short bursts of electrical impulses) appear, along with K-complexes (sharp, high voltage wave groups, often followed by spindles). These phenomenon may be initiated by internal or external stimuli or by some as yet unknown source deep within the brain. This portion of sleep occupies about 45% of the sleep cycle.

Normally, stage-3 sleep follows stage 2 as a short (about 7% of total sleep) transition to stage-4 sleep. There is virtually no eye movement during stages 2, 3, and 4.

In stage-4 sleep, some sleep spindles may occur, but are difficult to record. This stage occupies about 13% of the sleep cycle, seems to be affected more than any other stage by the length of prior wakefulness, and reflects the most cerebral "shutdown." Accordingly, some researchers believe this stage to be the most necessary for brain tissue restoration. Usually grouped together, stages 3 and 4 are called delta, or slow wave sleep (SWS), and is normally followed by REM sleep.

The sleep cycle from stage 1 through REM occurs three to five times a night in a normal young adult. Stages 3 and 4 decrease with each cycle, while stage 2 and REM sleep occupy most of the last half of the night's sleep. Time spent in each stage varies with age, and age particularly influences the amount time spent in SWS. From infancy to young adult, SWS occupies about 20-25% of total sleep time and perhaps as little as 5% by the age of 60. This loss of time is made up in stage-1 sleep and wakeful periods.

The period comprised of the four stages between sleep onset and REM is known as REM latency. REM onset is indicated by a drop in amplitude and rise in frequency of brain waves. The subject's eyes flicker quickly under the eyelids, dream activity is high, and the body seems to become paralyzed because of the decrease in skeletal muscle tone. After REM, the subject usually returns to stage 2 sleep, sometimes after waking slightly. REM sleep occurs regularly during the night. The larger the brain, the longer the period between REM episodes—about 90 minutes for humans and 12 minutes in rats.

REM sleep is triggered by neural functions deep within the brain, which release one type of neurotransmitter (chemical agent) to turn REM sleep on and another to turn it off. Whereas autonomic activity (such as breathing and heart rate) slows and becomes more regular during non-REM sleep, it becomes highly irregular during REM sleep. Changes in blood pressure, heart rate, and breathing regularity take place, there is virtually no regulation of body temperature, and clitoral and penile erections are often reported. Most deaths, particularly of ill or aged individuals, happen early in the morning when body temperature is at its lowest and the likelihood of REM sleep is highest.

REM activity is seen in the fetus as early as six months after conception. By the time of birth, the fetus will spend 90% of its sleep time in REM but only about half that after birth. REM constitutes about 20-30% of a normal young adult's sleep, decreasing with age. These observations support one of several theories about our need for REM sleep which suggests that, to function properly, the central nervous system requires considerable stimulation, particularly during development. Because it receives no environmental stimulation during the long hours of sleep, it is possible that the high amount of brain wave activity in REM sleep provides the necessary stimulation.

Sleep apnea

Sleep apnea is a condition in which breathing stops for more than ten seconds during sleep. Sleep apnea is a major, though often unrecognized, cause of daytime sleepiness.

A sleeping person normally breathes continuously and uninterruptedly throughout the night. A person with sleep apnea, however, has frequent episodes (up to 400-500 per night) in which he or she stops breathing. This interruption of breathing is called "apnea." Breathing usually stops for about 30 seconds; then the person usually startles awake with a loud snort and begins to breathe again, gradually falling back to sleep.

There are two forms of sleep apnea. In *obstructive sleep apnea* (OSA), breathing stops because tissue in the throat closes off the airway. In *central sleep apnea,* (CSA), the brain centers responsible for breathing fail to send messages to the breathing muscles. OSA is much more common than CSA. It is thought that about 1-10% of adults are affected by OSA; only about one tenth of that number have CSA. OSA can affect people of any age and of either sex, but it is most common in middle-aged, somewhat overweight men, especially those who use alcohol.

A combination of the two forms is also possible, and is called "mixed sleep apnea."

Obstructive sleep apnea occurs when part of the airway is closed off (usually at the back of the throat) while a person is trying to inhale during sleep. People whose airways are slightly narrower than average are more likely to be affected by OSA. **Obesity**, especially obesity in the neck, can increase the risk of developing OSA, because the fat tissue tends to narrow the airway. In some people, the airway is blocked by enlarged tonsils, an enlarged tongue, jaw deformities, or growths in the neck that compress the airway. Blocked nasal passages may also play a part in some people.

People with OSA almost always snore heavily, because the same narrowing of the airway that causes snoring can also cause OSA. Snoring may actually help cause OSA as well, because the vibration of the throat tissues can cause them to swell. However, most people who snore do not go on to develop OSA.

OSA and CSA cause similar symptoms. The most common symptoms are:

- Daytime sleepiness
- Morning **headaches**
- A feeling that sleep is not restful
- Disorientation upon waking.

Sleepiness is caused not only by the frequent interruption of sleep, but by the inability to enter long periods of deep sleep, during which the body performs numerous restorative functions. OSA is one of the leading causes of daytime sleepiness, and is a major risk factor for motor vehicle accidents. Headaches and disorientation are caused by low oxygen levels during sleep, from the lack of regular breathing.

Sleep apnea can also cause serious changes in the cardiovascular system. Daytime **hypertension** (high blood pressure) is common. An increase in the number of red blood cells (polycythemia) is possible, as is an enlarged left ventricle of the heart (**cor pulmonale**), and left ventricular failure. In some people, sleep apnea causes life-threatening changes in the rhythm of the heart, including heartbeat slowing (bradycardia), racing (tachycardia), and other types of ''arrhythmias.'' Sudden **death** may occur from such arrhythmias. Patients with the Pickwickian syndrome (named after a Charles Dickens character) are obese and sleepy, with right **heart failure**, **pulmonary hypertension**, and chronic daytime low blood oxygen (hypoxemia) and increased blood CO_2 (hypercapnia).

Treatment of obstructive sleep apnea begins with reducing the use of alcohol or tranquilizers in the evening, if these have been contributing to the problem. Weight loss is also effective, but if the weight returns, as it often does, so does the apnea. Changing sleeping position may be effective: Snoring and sleep apnea are both most common when a person sleeps on his back. Turning to sleep on the side may be enough to clear up the symptoms. Raising the head of the bed may also help. Opening of the nasal passages can provide some relief. There are a variety of nasal devices such as clips, tapes, or holders which may help, though discomfort may limit their use. Nasal **decongestants** may be useful, but should not be taken for sleep apnea without the consent of the treating physician.

For moderate to severe sleep apnea, the most successful treatment is nighttime use of a ventilator, called a CPAP machine. CPAP (continuous positive airway pressure) blows air into the airway continuously, preventing its collapse. CPAP requires the use of a nasal mask. The appropriate pressure setting for the CPAP machine is determined by polysomnography in the sleep lab. Its effects are dramatic; daytime sleepiness usually disappears within one to two days after treatment begins. CPAP is used to treat both obstructive and central sleep apnea.

CPAP is tolerated well by about two-thirds of patients who try it. Bilevel positive airway pressure (BiPAP), is an alternative form of ventilation. With BIPAP, the ventilator reduces the air pressure when the person exhales. This is more comfortable for some.

Surgery can be used to correct the obstruction in the airways. The most common surgery is called UPPP, for uvulopalatopharngyoplasty. This surgery removes tissue from the rear of the mouth and top of the throat. The tissues removed include parts of the uvula (the flap of tissue that hangs down at the back of the mouth), the soft palate, and the pharynx. Tonsils and adenoids are usually removed in this operation. This operation significantly improves sleep apnea in slightly more than half of all cases.

Sleep disorders

Sleep disorders are a group of syndromes characterized by disturbance in a person's amount of sleep, quality or timing of sleep, or in behavior while sleeping. There are about 70 different sleep disorders.

Although sleep is a basic behavior in animals as well as humans, researchers still don't completely understand it. In the past 30 years, however, researchers have learned about the pattern of different types of sleep and its effects on breathing, heart rate, brain waves, and so on.

There are five stages of human sleep. Four stages occur during ''non-rapid eye movement (NREM) sleep,'' featuring unique brain wave patterns and body changes. Dreaming occurs in the fifth stage, known as ''rapid eye movement (REM)'' sleep. Stage 1 NREM sleep begins as a person falls asleep, progressing into Stage 2 NREM sleep, the beginning of ''true'' sleep. Experts can identify this stage by looking at a person's brain waves on a graph of brain activity. About 50% of sleep time is stage 2 REM sleep. Stages 3 and 4 (also called ''delta'' or ''slow-wave sleep'') are the deepest levels of human sleep and take up 10-20% of sleep time. Finally comes Stage 5 — REM sleep, which accounts for 20-25% of total sleep time. REM sleep, during which a person's eyes move rapidly back and forth behind closed eyelids, usually begins about 90 minutes after the person falls asleep. It alternates with NREM sleep about every hour and a half throughout the night. REM periods get longer during the night.

Sleep cycles vary with a person's age. Children and adolescents have longer periods of stage 3 and stage 4 NREM sleep than do middle aged or elderly adults. Total REM sleep also declines with age.

The average length of nighttime sleep varies among people. Most people sleep between seven and nine hours a night. In temperate climates, however, people often notice that sleep time varies with the seasons. It's not unusual for people in North America and Europe to sleep about 40 minutes longer per night during the winter.

Experts classify sleep disorders based on their cause. Most sleep disorders are ''secondary'' — that is, they are caused by other things such as mental disorders, prescription medications, substance abuse, or medical conditions. Sleep disorders that aren't caused by these things are considered to be ''primary'' disorders.

One of the best-known kinds of sleep disorders is **insomnia**— the inability to fall asleep. An occasional problem in falling asleep isn't considered to be insomnia; for a diagnosis, the person must have problems getting to sleep or staying asleep for at least one month. It's estimated that 35% of adults in the United States experience this problem during any given year, but the number of these adults who are experiencing true primary insomnia is unknown. Primary insomnia is usually caused by a traumatic event related to sleep or bedtime. People who experience primary insomnia are often anxious about not being able to sleep. They may then associate all sleep-related things (their bed, bedtime, and so on) with frustration, making the problem worse. The person then becomes more stressed about not sleeping. Insomnia usually begins when the person is a young adult or in middle age.

At the opposite end of the sleep disorder spectrum is the person who sleeps too much — this is called ''hypersomnia.'' The patient either sleeps a long time during the day, or takes quick naps each day with normal sleep at night. Sometimes, patients with hypersomnia have problems waking in the morning and may appear confused or angry. This condition is sometimes called sleep drunkenness and is more common in males. The number of people with hypersomnia is unknown, although 5-10% of patients in sleep disorder clinics have the disorder. Primary hypersomnia usually affects young adults between the ages of 15 and 30.

Restless legs syndrome (RLS) can cause either insomnia or hypersomnia in adults. Patients with RLS wake up because of cramps or twitches in their calves, and therefore they feel sleepy the next day. RLS patients have a crawly or aching feeling in their calves that can be relieved by moving or rubbing the legs. RLS often prevents the patient from falling asleep until the early hours of the morning, when the condition is less intense.

Kleine-Levin syndrome is a recurrent form of sleepiness that affects a person three or four times a year. Doctors don't know the cause of this syndrome, but it causes two to three days of excess sleeping 18 to 20 hours per day, extremely sexual behavior, compulsive eating, and irritability. Men are three times more likely than women to have the syndrome. There is no cure for this disorder.

Narcolepsy is a sleep problem in which a person has recurrent ''sleep attacks'' lasting between 10-20 minutes. Upon awakening, the patient feels refreshed but then feels sleepy again several hours later. Narcolepsy has three major symptoms in addition to sleep attacks: a sudden fall due to muscle tone loss, **hallucinations**, and sleep **paralysis**. Hallucinations may occur just before falling asleep or right after waking up and are associated with an episode of REM sleep. Sleep paralysis occurs during the transition from being asleep to waking up. About 40% of patients with narcolepsy have or have had another mental disorder. Although narcolepsy is often regarded as an adult disorder, it has been reported in children as young as 3 years old.

Breathing-related sleep disorders are syndromes in which the patient's sleep is interrupted by problems with breathing. There are three types of breathing-related sleep disorders:

- Obstructive **sleep apnea** syndrome is the most common form of breathing-related sleep disorder, marked by episodes of blockage in the upper airway during sleep. It's found primarily in obese people. Patients with this disorder typically alternate between periods of snoring or gasping (when their airway is partly open) and periods of silence (when their airway is blocked). Very loud snoring is a clue to this disorder.
- Central sleep apnea syndrome mostly occurs in elderly patients with heart or neurological conditions that affect their ability to breathe properly. It isn't associated with airway blockage, and it may be related to brain disease.
- Central alveolar hypoventilation syndrome is found most often in extremely obese people. While the patient's airway is clear, the oxygen level in the blood is too low.
- Mixed-type sleep apnea syndrome. This disorder combines symptoms of both the above sleep problems.

Circadian rhythm sleep disorders are caused by a difference between the person's daily sleep/wake patterns and demands of social activities, shift work, or travel. The term ''circadian'' comes from a Latin word meaning ''daily.''

There are three circadian rhythm sleep disorders: Delayed sleep phase, jet lag, and shift work type. In a ''delayed sleep phase,'' the sufferer goes to bed and gets up later than most people. **Jet lag** is caused by travel to a new time zone, temporarily throwing off a person's circadian rhythm. Shift work sleep disorder does the same thing, but this is more permanent, since the shift in schedule is caused by the person's job. People who are ordinarily early risers appear to be more vulnerable to jet lag and shift work-related circadian rhythm disorders than people who are ''night owls.''

In some sleep disorders, the patient's behavior is affected by specific sleep stages or transitions between sleeping and waking. Nightmare disorder is one version of this, in which the patient is awakened by frightening dreams and is fully alert on awakening. Between 10-50% of children between 3 and 5 have nightmares. The nightmares occur during REM sleep, usually in the second half of the night. The child is usually able to remember the content of the nightmare and may be afraid to go back to sleep. More females than males have this disorder, although some experts suspect it may be that women are more likely to report the problem. Nightmare disorder is most likely to occur in people under severe or traumatic stress.

Sleep terror (also called ''night terrors'') is a disorder of childhood in which the youngster seems to wake up screaming or crying, sweating or shaking — but in fact, the child is still asleep. It can be very difficult to awaken a child in this condition, and indeed, many experts recommend allowing the child to remain asleep. Sleep terror disorder affects about 3% of all children, usually between the ages of 4-12 years old; the problem is usually outgrown by adolescence. Fewer than 1% of adults have the disorder. Unlike nightmares, sleep terrors typically occur in stage 3 or stage 4 NREM sleep during the first third of the night. The patient may be confused or disoriented for several minutes, and not be able to remember the dream itself. Often, the child falls asleep again and doesn't remember the episode the next morning. In adults, it usually begins between the ages of 20 and 30. In children, more boys than girls have the disorder, but in adulthood the condition affects men and women equally.

Sleepwalking disorder (or somnambulism) occurs when a person is able to make complex movements during sleep, including walking. Like sleep terror disorder, sleepwalking occurs during stage 3 and stage 4 NREM sleep during the first part of the night. If the patient is awakened during a sleepwalking episode, he or she may be disoriented and have no memory of the behavior. In addition to walking around, patients with sleepwalking disorder have been reported to eat, use the bathroom, unlock doors, or talk to others. It is estimated that 10-30% of children have at least one episode of sleepwalking, but only 1-5% meet the criteria for sleepwalking disorder. The disorder is most common in children 8-12 years old. It is unusual for sleepwalking to occur for the first time in adults.

Unlike sleepwalking, REM sleep behavior disorder occurs later in the night and causes the patient to perform often violent physical movements. Unlike night terrors, the patients usually can remember what they were dreaming at the time.

In addition to the primary sleep disorders, there are also three categories of sleep disorders that are linked with other physical or mental disorders.

Many mental disorders, especially depression or one of the **anxiety disorders**, can cause sleep disturbances. They are the most common cause of chronic insomnia.

Some patients with chronic neurological conditions like Parkinson's disease or **Huntington's disease** may develop sleep disorders. Sleep disorders also have been associated with viral **encephalitis**, brain disease, and high or low levels of thyroid activity.

Sleeping sickness

Sleeping sickness refers to several related diseases that cause a deep sleep-like state and coma. Left untreated, it is fatal. The two most common types are East African and West African sleeping sickness with approximately 20,000 new cases reported each year. Few cases of the West African strain have ever been reported in the United States, with 17 cases of the East African strain reported since 1968. The technical name for the disease is *trypanosomiasis*, because it is caused by a thin, single-cell organism called a *trypanosome*. This parasite can be transmitted from infected animals to humans by the tsetse fly and, in extremely rare instances, by blood transfusion or organ transplant. The tsetse fly bite is painful, often developing into a red sore, or chancre.

Fever, headache, and chills are the first symptoms, followed by swollen lymph glands, aching muscles and joints, weight loss, skin rash, and extreme fatigue and general weakness. If the disease is not treated, it will progress to the **nervous system** causing confusion, personality changes, seizures and difficulty walking or talking. Once the parasites attack the brain, they cause deep sleep and coma. A physician can diagnose the disease with a microscopic examination of a patient's blood, spinal fluid, or fluid from a swollen gland. If the wiggling, long-tailed parasite is present, the disease is confirmed and can then be treated with arsenic-based drugs. Treatment is painful and dangerous (it has a five percent fatality rate), and only effective if begun before the nervous system is damaged. Once the deep sleep occurs, there is little chance for a cure and the patient usually dies.

More than one hundred years ago, several noted researchers contributed to the understanding of sleeping sickness. In the late nineteenth century, German bacteriologist **Robert Koch** went to Africa to do research on the disease. Koch was the first person to study the bacterium that caused **anthrax** in cattle by growing the organism outside the body in blood serum. He also helped develop the use of a gelatin medium for growing bacteria in Petri dishes so they could be more easily studied. Koch went on to isolate the **bacteria** that caused a number of important diseases, such as **cholera**, **tuberculosis**, and bubonic plague. After careful study, Koch established that sleeping sickness was transmitted by the tsetse fly, just as he had shown that the plague was transmitted by a flea that infested rats. He suggested that these diseases could be fought by attempting to control the insects that spread them.

David Bruce, an eminent Scottish microbiologist, made the next stride in the understanding of sleeping sickness. Bruce led the Royal Society's Sleeping Sickness Commission in Uganda in 1903. This team of scientists was able to prove that the disease was caused by trypanosomes and transmitted by tsetse flies. The final victory in the battle against sleeping sickness was provided by Louise Pearce (1855-1959). An American physician, Pearce joined a group of scientists at Rockefeller Institute charged with finding a drug that would kill the trypanosome organism. She and her partner, Wade Hampton Brown (1878-1942), decided to study chemicals related to Salvarsan—an arsenic-based cure for syphilis discovered by **Paul Ehrlich**. In 1919, they isolated a compound later called tryparsamide, which was effective against the disease. Pearce tested the chemical in the Belgian Congo (present-day Zaire), where its usefulness was convincingly demonstrated. Since that time, a number of effective drugs have been developed with the ability to destroy the trypanosomes.

Slye, Maud (1879-1954)

American pathologist

Maud Slye devoted her life to cancer research by investigating the inheritability of the disease in mice. Performing extensive

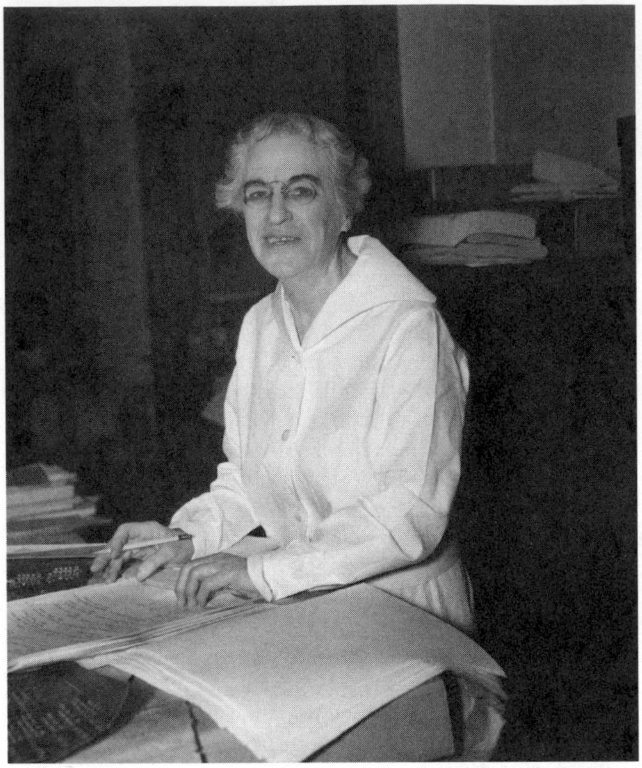

Maud Slye

breeding studies on the hereditary transmission of cancer, she kept meticulous pedigree records and autopsied thousands of mice during her lifetime. Her work was controversial, however; advocating the archiving of complete medical records for individuals, she believed that human beings could eradicate cancer by choosing mates with the appropriate genotype. Sometimes referred to as ''America's Curie,'' Slye received wide publicity for her work and was honored by many organizations.

Slye was born in Minneapolis, Minnesota, on February 8, 1879, the daughter of James Alvin and Florence Alden Wheeler Slye. Her family, though poor, traced their ancestry back to John Alden of the Plymouth colony. At age seventeen, Slye entered the University of Chicago with savings of forty dollars and the desire to become a scientist. Attending the university for three years, she supported herself by working as a secretary for university president William Harper. After a nervous breakdown, Slye convalesced in Woods Hole, Massachusetts, then completed her B.A. degree at Brown University in 1899. Hired as a teacher at the Rhode Island State Normal School, she stayed at the institution until 1905.

In 1908 Slye received a grant to do postgraduate work at the University of Chicago. Interested in the hereditary basis of disease, she began her work with six Japanese ''waltzing'' mice which were afflicted with a hereditary neurological disorder. Slye became intrigued by the inheritability of cancer when she heard of several heads of cattle at the Chicago stock yards—all with cancer of the eye—that had come from the same ranch. Inspired by this and other data, Slye went forward with her studies, breeding cancerous mice with one another as well as healthy mice with other healthy mice.

In 1911, Slye became a member of the university's newly created Sprague Memorial Institute, and in 1913 she presented her first paper on cancer before the American Society for Cancer Research. Becoming director of the Cancer Laboratory at the University of Chicago in 1919, she was promoted to assistant professor in 1922, then to associate professor in 1926. In 1936, Slye left her mice in the care of an assistant and took her first vacation in twenty-six years (earlier, when she had visited her ailing mother in California, she rented a boxcar and took her mice with her).

Although Slye discredited a prevailing theory that stated cancer was contagious, it became clear as her work proceeded that the appearance of cancer in an individual was not as simple as the presence of one gene. In later years, Slye posited that two conditions were necessary to produce cancer: inherited susceptibility, and prolonged irritation of the cancer-susceptible tissues. Nonetheless, further studies by other scientists have confirmed that while heredity can be a factor in certain types of cancer, it is much more complex than Slye had perceived.

Slye's work was recognized with several awards and honors, including the gold medal of the American Medical Association in 1914, and the Ricketts Prize in 1915. She also received the gold medal of the American Radiological Society in 1922. A member of the Association for Cancer Research, the American Medical Association, and the American Association for the Advancement of Science, Slye was the author of forty-two brochures on cancer and two volumes of poetry, *Songs and Solaces* and *I in the Wind.* At the time of her retirement in 1945 Slye was made professor emeritus of pathology, and she spent her retirement years analyzing data accumulated during her years of research. Slye never married. She died September 17, 1954, and was buried in Chicago's Oak Woods Cemetery.

Smallpox

Smallpox, or variola (from Latin *varus* meaning pimple), is a highly contagious viral disease, one of the very worst to afflict humankind since time immemorial. It is believed to have originated in northeastern Africa with the first agricultural settlements—around 10,000 B.C., spreading to India via Egyptian merchants, and was known in China in ancient times. Several early historians described plagues with the characteristic symptoms of smallpox (chills, headache, backache, nausea, vomiting, fever, and red spots on the skin that develop into pus-filled blisters). Greek historian Thucidydes (died c. 326 B.C.) chronicled a disease that broke out during the Peloponnesian War in the fifth century B.C., noting that a person who contracted this disease and survived was called ''fortunate and happy,'' since he could never get the disease again. The early Christian historian, Eusebius (died c. 379 B.C.), writing in the third century, referred to an epidemic (thought to be smallpox) in which "whole families were cut off very rapidly, so that two or three bodies of the dead were carried out from one house for burial at the same time. All places...overflowed with tears, sorrow and wailings."

Smallpox reached Europe from Arabia in the sixth century, and Crusaders returning to Europe from the Holy Land between 1094 and 1204 spread this disease across the continent. Smallpox probably arrived in the Western Hemisphere with the Spanish conquistadors in the sixteenth century, and slaves transported from Africa brought the disease to the American colonies. In 1721, nearly half the residents of Boston contracted the disease, establishing the record for the worst epidemic to hit the New England town.

Cotton Mather (1633-1728), a Puritan leader, tried to convince others that inoculation would deter the disease. Mather had learned about the art of inoculation from his slave, Onesimus, who was immune to smallpox because of the practices of the Garamanti in Africa. It had been 15 years earlier that Onesimus told Mather: "People take the Juice of the Small Pox, and Cut the Skin, and put in a drop; then by 'nd by a little sick; then few small pox; and no body dye of it; no body have small pox any more."

Mather tried to share his knowledge with medical practitioners, but he was chastised by those who believed inoculation was a "superstitious" African practice. Only Dr. Zabdiel Boylston (1679-1766) heeded Mather's pleadings. Boylston inoculated his own six-year-old son and two slaves, but his procedures appalled much of the community. At the time, Mather wrote: "The Destroyer, being enraged at the proposal of anything that may rescue the lives of our poor people from him, has taken a strange possession of the people on this occasion. They rave, they blaspheme, they talk not only like idiots, but also like Franticks, and not only the physician who began the experiment but I also am an object of their fury...."

Lady Mary Wortley Montagu (1689-1762) introduced smallpox inoculation into Europe in the early eighteenth century after she accompanied her husband, the British ambassador to Constantinople, to Turkey in 1717, there discovering a local practice called *ingrafting*. This procedure, nearly identical to the one performed by the Garamanti in Africa, also conferred immunity to smallpox. When Lady Montagu returned to England she had her own daughter inoculated and, with the support of Caroline, Princess of Wales, smallpox inoculation caught on despite vehement opposition from medical and religious leaders. However, inoculation was a double-edged sword. Because few people died from inoculated smallpox, they dropped their defenses and failed to take quarantine precautions; a mild case of inoculated smallpox was still contagious and could spawn a deadly natural epidemic. There were also side effects from these inoculations, such as blindness, **tuberculosis**, eye diseases, and disfiguring pock marks.

The first major step toward controlling smallpox came at the end of the eighteenth century when **Edward Jenner** heard stories from milkmaids who said they were immune to smallpox because they had contracted cowpox from cows' udders. Jenner heeded their folk wisdom, making it scientific fact when he performed his first vaccination on May 14, 1796, by scratching the arms of eight-year-old James Phipps with the lymph from a cowpox pustule on the hand of dairymaid Sarah Nelmes. On July 1, he introduced fresh smallpox lymph into young James, and waited for a reaction. There was none. This was the first scientific effort at controlling infectious diseases through deliberate vaccination. Jenner, envisioning the implications of his discovery, wrote in 1802, "it now becomes too manifest to admit of controversy, that the annihilation of the small pox, the most dreadful scourge of the human species, must be the final result of this practice." Over the next century and a half, vaccination against smallpox became a universally accepted public health practice.

At the end of World War II, smallpox was still reported in 95 countries. The World Health Organization of the United Nations believed global eradication of the virus was an attainable goal and, in 1966, appropriated $2.5 million for a program to promote mass vaccinations. The following year, 42 countries reported 10 million cases of smallpox. On October 22, 1977, the last known case of naturally acquired smallpox was reported in Somalia, and on December 9, 1979 in Geneva, Switzerland, a World Health Organization panel declared that smallpox had been eradicated from the world.

Stocks of the freeze-dried virus were maintained in several research labs to produce vaccine in the event that the disease reappeared. In 1978, medical photographer, Janet Parker, working at the University of Birmingham Medical School in Britain, contracted smallpox from an escaped laboratory virus and died. Public health officials worldwide realized that the real danger from smallpox no longer lay in nature but in the laboratory. The World Health Organization (WHO) encouraged all labs with stocks of the virus to destroy them or send them to two designated repositories: the Centers for Disease Control in Atlanta, Georgia, or the Research Institute of Viral Preparation in Moscow, Russia. The WHO, United States, and Russia subsequently agreed to destroy all remaining stock of the smallpox virus in December 1993. Because arguments remain against total destruction of the virus—one that no further studies of the virus will be possible, and another that complete eradication may not occur—total destruction of the stored virus has been postponed twice—once in 1993 and again in 1995. The current deadline for destruction of the variola strain of the smallpox virus is scheduled for June 31, 1999. If it does take place, it will be the first deliberate total elimination of any biological species.

SMELL

Smell is the ability of an organism to sense and identify a substance by detecting trace amounts of the substance that evaporate. Researchers have noted similarities in the sense of smell between widely differing species that reveal some of the details of how the chemical signal of an odor is detected and processed.

The sense of smell has been a topic of debate from humankind's earliest days. The Greek philosopher Democritus of Abdera (460-360 B.C.) speculated that we smell "atoms" of different size and shape that come from objects. His countryman **Aristotle** (384-322 B.C.), on the other hand, guessed that odors are detected when the ''cold'' sense of smell meets ''hot'' smoke or steam from the object being smelled. It was not until the late 18th century that most scientists and philosophers reached agreement that Democritus was basically right: the smell of an object is due to volatile, or easily evaporated, molecules that emanate from it.

Smell is the most important sense for most organisms. A wide variety of species use their sense of smell to locate prey, navigate, recognize and perhaps communicate with kin, and mark territory. The sense of smell differs from most other senses in its directness: we actually smell microscopic bits of a substance that have evaporated and made their way to the olfactory epithelium, a section of the mucus membrane in the roof of the olfactory cavity. The olfactory epithelium contains the smell-sensitive endings of the olfactory nerve cells, also known as the olfactory epithelial cells. These cells detect odors through receptor proteins on the cell surface that bind to odor-carrying molecules. A specific odorant docks with an olfactory receptor protein in much the same way as a key fits in a lock; this in turn excites the nerve cell, causing it to send a signal to the brain. This is known as the stereospecific theory of smell.

In the past few years molecular scientists have cloned the genes for the human olfactory receptor proteins. Although there are perhaps tens of thousands (or more) of odor-carrying molecules in the world, there are only hundreds, or at most about 1,000, kinds of specific receptors in any species of animal. Because of this, scientists do not believe that each receptor recognizes a unique odorant; rather, similar odorants can all bind to the same receptor. In other words, a few loose-fitting odorant ''keys'' of broadly similar shape can turn the same receptor ''lock.'' Researchers do not know how many specific receptor proteins each olfactory nerve cell carries, but recent work suggests that the cells specialize just as the receptors do, and any one olfactory nerve cell has only one or a few receptors rather than many.

It is the combined pattern of receptors that are tweaked by an odorant that allow the brain to identify it, much as yellow and red light together are intepreted by the brain as orange. (In fact, just as people can be color-blind to red or green, they can be ''odor-blind'' to certain simple molecules because they lack the receptor for that molecule.) In addition, real objects that we smell produce multiple odor-carrying molecules, so that the brain must analyze a complex mixture of odorants to recognize a smell.

Just as the sense of smell is direct in detecting fragments of the objects, it is also direct in the way the signal is transmitted to the brain. In most senses, such as vision, this task is accomplished in several steps: a receptor cell detects light and passes the signal to a nerve cell, which passes it on to another nerve cell in the central nervous system, which then relays it to the visual center of the brain. But in olfaction, all these jobs are performed by the olfactory nerve cell: in a very real sense, the olfactory epithelium is a direct outgrowth of the brain.

The olfactory nerve cell takes the scent message directly to the nerve cells of the olfactory bulb of the brain (or, in insects and other invertebrates that lack true brains, the olfactory ganglia), where multiple signals from different olfactory cells with different odor sensitivities are organized and processed. In higher species the signal then goes to the brain's olfactory cortex, where higher functions such as memory and emotion are coordinated with the sense of smell.

There is no doubt that many animals have a sense of smell far superior to that of humans. This is why, even today, humans use dogs to find lost persons, hidden drugs, and explosives, although research on ''artificial noses'' that can detect scent even more reliably than dogs continues. Humans are called microsmatic, rather than macrosmatic, because of their humble abilities of olfaction.

Still, the human nose is capable of detecting over 10,000 different odors, some in the range of parts per trillion of air; and many researchers are beginning to wonder whether smell does not play a greater role in human behavior and biology than has been thought. For instance, research has shown that human mothers can smell the difference between a vest worn by their baby and one worn by another baby only days after the child's birth.

Yet some olfactory abilities of animals are probably beyond humans. Most vertebrates have many more olfactory nerve cells in a proportionately larger olfactory epithelium than humans, which probably gives them much more sensitivity to odors. The olfactory bulb in these animals takes up a much larger proportion of the brain than humans, giving them more ability to process and analyze olfactory information.

In addition, most land vertebrates have a specialized scent organ in the roof of their mouth called the vomeronasal organ (also known as the Jacobson's organ or the accessory olfactory organ). This organ, believed to be vestigial in humans, is a pit lined by a layer of cells with a similar structure to the olfactory epithelium, which feeds into its own processing part of the brain, called the accessory olfactory bulb (an area of the brain absent in humans).

The vomeronasal sense appears to be sensitive to odor molecules with a less volatile, possibly more complex molecular structure than the odorants to which humans are sensitive. This sense is important in reproduction, allowing many animals to sense sexual attractant odors, or pheromones, thus governing mating behavior. It is also used by reptilian and mammalian predators in tracking prey.

Researchers have learned a lot about how the olfactory nerve cells detect odorants. However, they have not yet learned how this information is coded by the olfactory cell. Other topics of future research will be how olfactory cell signals are processed in the olfactory bulb, and how this information relates to higher brain functions and our awareness of smell.

Scientists are only beginning to understand the role that smell plays in animal and human behavior. The vomeronasal sense of animals is still largely not understood. Some researchers have even suggested that the human vomeronasal organ might retain some function, and that humans may have pheromones that play a role in sexual attraction and mating—although this hypothesis is very controversial.

In addition, detailed study of the biology of the olfactory system might yield gains in other fields. For instance, olfactory nerve cells are the only nerve cells that are derived from the central nervous system that can regenerate, possibly because the stress of their exposure to the outside world gives them a limited lifespan. Some researchers hope that studying regeneration in olfactory nerve cells or even transplanting them elsewhere in the body can lead to treatments for as yet irreversible damage to the spine and brain.

Smith, Hamilton O. (1931-)

American molecular biologist

Hamilton Othanel Smith shared the 1978 Nobel Prize in physiology or medicine with fellow biologists **Werner Arber** and Daniel Nathans for the set of linked discoveries that started off the boom in biotechnology. Because of these discoveries, researchers can more easily elucidate the structure and coding of deoxyribonucleic acid (DNA) molecules (the basic genetic map of an organism), and they hope to correct many genetic illnesses in the future. His research also made it possible to design new organisms, a controversial but potentially beneficial technology. Smith purified and explained the activity of the first restriction enzyme, which became the principal tool used by genetic engineers to selectively cut up DNA. (Arber had linked restriction and modification to DNA, and predicted the existence of restriction enzymes. Nathans, under Smith's encouragement at Johns Hopkins, developed techniques that enabled their practical use.)

Smith was born on August 23, 1931, in New York, New York, to Bunnie (Othanel) Smith and Tommie Harkey Smith. Smith graduated from University High School in three years, enrolling at a local university in 1948.

Smith came to the study of genetics by way of medicine. Initially a mathematics major at the University of Illinois, he transferred to the University of California at Berkeley in 1950 to study biology and graduated with a bachelor's degree in 1952. He obtained a medical degree from the Johns Hopkins School of Medicine in 1956. During the years 1956 to 1962, he held various posts, including an internship at Washington University in St. Louis, Missouri, a two-year Navy stint in San Diego, California, and a residency at Henry Ford Hospital in Detroit, Michigan. He gradually taught himself genetics and molecular biology in his spare time. In 1962 he began a research career at the University of Michigan on a postdoctoral fellowship from the National Institutes of Health, before finally returning to Johns Hopkins in 1965 as a research associate in the microbiology department. He was named a full professor of microbiology in 1973, and professor of molecular biology and genetics in 1981. In 1975, Smith was awarded a Guggenheim Fellowship for a year of study at the University of Zurich in Switzerland.

After his return to the United States, Smith purified the first Type II restriction endonuclease, which he obtained from the bacterium *Hemophilus influenzae,* and identified the nucleotide sequence which the enzyme would cut. He gave a supply of the enzyme to Daniel Nathans, who used it in his own work. The three men eventually won the 1978 Nobel Prize. The presenter of the prize noted that Smith proved Arbor's hypothesis about restriction enzymes, pointing the way for future research.

Smith's exacting specificity of Class II restriction enzymes makes them useful because biotechnologists can now cut DNA apart selectively. Then they can add and subtract specific nucleotides, and reproducibly weld (recombine) the links back together in a new order. This new piece of DNA now codes for a different protein. The current and potential uses of these procedures are enormous. Biotechnologists can genetically engineer bacteria that produce a particular chemical; human insulin for the treatment of **diabetes** is now made by such recombinant bacteria. Other bacteria have been designed to clean up oil slicks. One of the tasks that biotechnologists would like to accomplish is the eradication of genetic illness by correcting the mistaken DNA codes that cause it.

Smoke inhalation

Smoke inhalation is breathing in the harmful gases, vapors, and particulate matter contained in smoke.

Smoke inhalation typically occurs in victims or firefighters caught in a fire, but cigarette smoking also causes similar damage on a smaller scale over a longer period of time. People who are trapped in fires may suffer from smoke inhalation without having skin **burns**; however, the chance of smoke inhalation increases with the percentage of total body surface area burned. Smoke inhalation contributes to the total number of fire-related **death**s each year because the damage is serious, it may be hard to diagnose and patients may not show symptoms until a day or two after the fire. Children under age 11 and adults over age 70 are most vulnerable to the effects of smoke inhalation.

The harmful materials given off in a fire injure the airways and lungs by heat damage, irritation, and cutting off oxygen to body tissues. Signs of heat damage include singed nasal hairs, burns around and inside the nose and mouth, and a swollen throat. Tissue irritation of the throat and lungs may appear as noisy breathing, coughing, hoarseness, black or gray spittle, and fluid in the lungs. Oxygen starvation causes **shortness of breath** and blue-gray or cherry-red skin color. In some cases, the patient may be unconscious.

In addition to looking for the signs of heat damage, tissue irritation, and lack of oxygen, the doctor will check the patient's condition by evaluating breathing, pulse rate, and blood pressure. Blood tests indicate the oxygen level and byproducts of poisonous gases.

The doctor may visually examine the airways and lungs through a fiber optic tube inserted down the patient's windpipe. Other tests may be performed to measure how efficiently the lungs are working.

Treatment varies with the severity of damage. The primary focus of treatment is to keep the airway open with enough oxygen. If the airway is swelling shut, a tube may need to be inserted to keep an open airway.

Oxygen is often the only medication necessary. However, patients who are **wheezing** may be given medicine to relax the muscles and ease breathing. There are also antidotes for specific poisonous gases in the blood; dosage depends on the level indicated by blood tests. **Antibiotics** aren't given unless tests confirm there is a bacterial infection.

If available, hyperbaric **oxygen therapy** may be used to treat smoke inhalation. This treatment requires a special chamber in which the patient receives pure oxygen at high pressures much faster than normal.

Acupuncture can provide support to anyone who has suffered a traumatic injury such as smoke inhalation.

Although the outcome depends of the severity of the smoke inhalation and the severity of any accompanying burns or other injuries, with prompt medical treatment the prognosis for recovery is good. However, some patients may experience chronic breathing problems after smoke inhalation. People who already had **asthma** or other breathing problems may find their conditions have been worsened by the inhalation injury.

Smoke inhalation can be prevented by avoiding fires by using safe wiring, safely storing flammable liquids, and maintening clean, well-ventilated chimneys, wood stoves, and space heaters. Properly placed and working smoke detectors in combination with rapid evacuation plans will lessen a person's exposure to smoke in the event of a fire. When escaping a burning building, a person should move close to the floor where there is more cool, clear air to breathe because hot air rises, carrying gases and particulate matter upward. Finally, firefighters should wear proper protective gear.

SMOKING • See Cigarette smoking

SNELL, GEORGE DAVIS (1903-1996)

American immunogeneticist

One of three children, Snell was born on December 19, 1903, in Bradford, Massachusetts. By 1922, he had enrolled at Dartmouth pursuing studies in biology.

He obtained a B.S. degree in that subject in 1926 and enrolled at Harvard that same year to study genetics under the renowned biologist William Castle, who was among the first American scientists to delve into the biological laws of inheritance regarding mammals. Snell received a Ph.D. in 1930 after completing his dissertation on linkage (the means by which two or more genes on a chromosome are interrelated). That same year he became an instructor of zoology at Brown University, only to leave in 1931 to work at the University of Texas at Austin following receipt of a National Research Council Fellowship.

Snell's decision to accept the fellowship turned out to be a momentous one, as he began work for the famed geneticist Hermann Joseph Muller, whose research with fruit flies led to the discovery that x rays could produce mutations in genes. At the university, Snell experimented with mice, showing that x rays could produce mutations in rodents as well. Although Snell left the University of Texas in 1933 to serve as assistant professor at the University of Washington, he ventured to the Jackson Laboratory in Bar Harbor, Maine, in 1935 to return to research work. The laboratory, specializing in mammalian genetics, was well-known for its work in spite of its small size.

After continuing his work with x rays and mice, Snell decided to embark on a new study. Snell's project was concerned with the notion of transplants. Earlier scientific research had indicated that certain genes are responsible for whether a body would accept or reject a transplant. The precise genes responsible had not then been identified, however.

Snell began his experiments by performing transplants between mice with certain physical characteristics. He quickly discovered those mice with certain identical characteristics—in particular a twisted tail—tended to accept each other's skin grafts. In 1948 Peter Gorer came to Jackson Laboratory from London, England. Gorer, who had also conducted experiments on mice, developed an antiserum. He had discovered the existence of a certain antigen (foreign protein) in the blood of mice which induced an immune reaction when injected into other mice. Gorer had called this type of substance "Antigen II."

In collaboration, Snell and Gorer proved that Antigen II was present in mice with twisted tails, indicating that the genetics code for Gorer's antigen and the code found by Snell to be vital for tissue acceptance were identical. They called their discovery of this factor "H–2," for "Histocompatibility Two" (a term invented by Snell to describe whether a transplant would be accepted or rejected).

Later research revealed that instead of only a single gene being responsible for this factor, a number of closely related genes controlled histocompatibility. As a result, this was subsequently designated as the Major Histocompatibility Complex (MHC). The discovery of the MHC, and subsequent research by other scientists in the 1950s which proved it also existed in humans, made widespread organ transplantation possible. Donors and recipients could be matched (as had been done with blood types) to see if they were compatible.

Eventually Snell was able to produce what he called "congenic mice"—animals that are genetically identical except for one particular genetic characteristic. Unfortunately, the first strains of these mice were destroyed in a 1947 forest fire which burned down the laboratory. However, Snell's tenacity and dedication enabled him to rebound from this setback. Within three years he had created three strains of mice which differed genetically only in their ability to accept tissue grafts. The development of congenic strains of mice opened up a new field for experimental research, with Jackson Laboratory eventually being able to supply annually tens of thousands of these mice to other laboratories.

In 1952 Snell became staff scientific director and, in 1957, staff scientist at Jackson Laboratories. In those capacities he continued his research, particularly on the role that MHC plays in relation to cancer. Experiments he conducted with congenic mice found that on some occasions the mice rejected tumors which had been transplanted from their genetic twins. This "hybrid resistance" indicated that some tumors provoke an immune response, causing the body to produce antibodies to fight the tumor. This discovery could eventually be of great importance in developing weapons to fight **cancer**.

The success of Snell's work culminated in his winning the 1980 Nobel Prize in medicine or physiology for his work on histocompatibility. He shared this with two other immunogeneticists, **Jean Dausset** and **Baruj Benacerraf**. After being told of the Nobel committee's decision, Snell said there should have been a fourth recipient—his colleague Peter Gorer who died in 1962 and was thus ineligible to receive the prize.

Snow, John (1813-1858)

British physician

John Snow was a British physician of the Victorian era who helped introduce the use of **anesthesia** in surgery; he also attempted to show, in 1854, that **cholera** was a water-borne disease. His careful mapping of the distribution of cholera cases in London is the first known example of epidemiological research.

Snow was born in York, England, on March 15, 1813, the oldest of nine children. His father was an unskilled laborer and the family lived in one of the poorest sections of York, an industrial shipping area along the River Ouse. Snow was educated until the age of 14 at a common day school for the poor. In June of 1827 he arrived in Newcastle, 80 miles from his home, to begin a six year apprenticeship in medicine under William Hardcastle. Hardcastle taught him the day-to-day business of running a medical practice and dispensing medicine. During his apprenticeship, Snow also attended lectures at the Newcastle Infirmary.

In 1833 Snow became an assistant to a physician named Watson, not far from Newcastle. A year later he returned to York, where he joined the practice of Joseph Warburton. In October of 1836 he moved to London to begin advanced studies at the Hunterian School of Medicine. He became a Member of the Royal College of Surgeons of England in May of 1838, and in October of that year he qualified as a Licentiate of the Society of Apothecaries. Shortly afterward he set up his own practice in the Soho district of London. Although Snow was now fully qualified to practice medicine, he continued in his spare time to gain additional medical qualifications. He obtained a Bachelor of Medicine degree from the recently formed University of London in November 1843, and a year later received a Doctorate of Medicine from the same institution. In June 1850 he became a Licentiate of the Royal College of Physicians of London.

The use of anesthesia was first demonstrated in England in December 1846 by a dentist named James Robinson. Within days of its introduction, Snow had become sufficiently interested in its potential to investigate its scientific foundation. Soon he had designed his own inhaler for ether, and was using anesthesia in his hospital practice. In 1847 he published a small textbook on the proper administration and the effects of anesthetic vapors. He became widely acknowledged as the leading British expert on the subject and his medical practice was increasingly devoted to the use of anesthesia. His most famous patient was Queen Victoria, who called upon Snow to administer chloroform during the delivery of two of her nine children. His patients ranged widely in social position and wealth. Snow frequently practiced medicine in the poorest quarters of London.

In 1832, while still in his medical apprenticeship, Snow had treated cholera victims during an outbreak in the coal mining region near Newcastle. Cholera, which caused violent **diarrhea** and vomiting, was fatal to about half of its victims in the early 19th century. Between 1832 and 1854, a series of epidemics swept England and Snow had the occasion to witness its ravages many times. He observed that the disease tended to break out late in the summer, occurred most often amongst the poor, and seemed to arise in localized areas, often isolated geographically from one another. The prevailing belief at the time was that cholera was caused by "miasmas" or bad vapors, and that those of low moral character were more vulnerable. Snow, on the other hand, suspected the disease might be spread by a waterborne microorganism. In the first week of September 1854, over six hundred people died of cholera in a small area of Soho. Snow began to investigate the source of water that supplied this area, and traced the outbreak to a particular water pump on the now famous Broad Street. It had, for several weeks prior to the outbreak, been spewing forth a foamy brown water that smelled of raw sewage. Snow pleaded with the Board of Guardians of the local parish to remove the pump handle. By the time the handle was removed, the incidence of cholera had already begun to subside. Nonetheless, the publicity surrounding Snow's investigation drew attention to the general lack of **sanitation** efforts in London, and a complete overhaul of the city's water and sewage systems was begun. Cholera never returned. The data Snow collected and the maps he constructed showing the distribution of the disease in relation to source of water became the first known epidemiological survey of an illness. Because of this careful study, Snow is often referred to as the father of modern epidemiology.

Snow suffered from kidney disease and chronic poor health. He became incapacitated by a **stroke** shortly before he died, on June 16, 1858, at the age of 45.

Sodium imbalance

The normal concentration of sodium in the blood plasma is 136–145 mM. If the sodium level falls too late, it's called hyponatremia; if it gets too high, it's called hypernatremia.

A sodium level in the blood that is too low is dangerous and can cause seizures and **coma**. Very high sodium levels can lead to seizures and **death**.

Sodium is a mineral element and an important part of the human body. It controls the volume of fluid in the body and helps maintain the acid-base level. About 40% of the body's sodium is contained in bone, some is found within organs and cells and the remaining 55% is in blood plasma and other fluids outside cells. Sodium is important in proper nerve conduction, the passage of various nutrients into cells, and the maintenance of blood pressure.

The body continually regulates its handling of sodium. When a person eats too much or too little sodium, the intestines and kidneys respond to adjust concentrations to normal. During the course of a day, the intestines absorbs dietary sodium while the kidneys excrete a nearly equal amount of sodium into the urine.

The concentration of sodium in the blood depends on the total amount of sodium and water in arteries, veins, and capillaries (the circulatory system). The body regulates sodium and water in different ways, but uses both to help correct blood pressure when it is too high or too low.

If the body has too little sodium (called hyponatremia), the body can either increase sodium levels or decrease water in the body. Too high a concentration of sodium (hypernatremia), can be corrected either by decreasing sodium or by increasing body water.

There are many diseases that can cause abnormal salt levels, including diseases of the kidney, pituitary gland, and hypothalamus. This is especially a concern in elderly patients, who have a harder time regulating the concentrations of various nutrients in the bloodstream.

Low salt levels can be caused by eating too little salt or excreting too much sodium or water, and by diseases that impair the body's ability to regulate sodium and water. Keeping to a low-salt diet for many months or sweating too much during a race on a hot day, can make it hard to keep sodium levels high enough. While these conditions alone aren't likely to cause loss salt levels, it can occur under special circumstances. For example, patients taking diuretic drugs who eat a low-sodium diet may have hyponatremia. Diuretic drugs can correct high blood pressure by helping the body get rid of sodium into the urine — but excreting too much sodium can cause hyponatremia. Usually only mild hyponatremia occurs in patients taking diuretics. However, sodium levels can fall dangerously low in patients who eat a low-sodium diet and drinking too much water. Severe and prolonged **diarrhea** also can cause low sodium levels. A person with severe diarrhea can lose large amounts of water, sodium, and various nutrients. Some diarrheal diseases release especially large amounts of sodium and are most likely to cause hyponatremia. Drinking too much water may cause low sodium levels, because when the water is absorbed into the blood, it can dilute the sodium. This cause of hyponatremia is rare, but has been found in mentally ill patients who compulsively drink more than 20 liters of water a day. Excessive drinking of beer, which is mostly water without much sodium, can also produce hyponatremia when combined with a poor diet.

Marathon running under certain conditions can lead to hyponatremia, since sweat contains both sodium and water. Studies show that about 30% of marathon runners experience mild hyponatremia during a race. However, drinking water during a race isn't the answer — this can lead to severe hyponatremia because the drinking water dilutes the sodium in the bloodstream. Such runners may experience brain problems as a result of the severe hyponatremia and require emergency treatment.

Hyponatremia also develops from disorders in organs that control the body's regulation of sodium or water. The adrenal gland secretes a hormone that travels to the kidney, where it prompts the kidney to retain sodium by not excreting it into the urine. Addison's disease, which damages the adrenal gland, can therefore lead to low levels of sodium in the body.

The hypothalamus and pituitary gland are also involved in sodium regulation by making and releasing vasopressin, known as the anti-diuretic hormone, into the bloodstream. Vasopressin prompts the kidneys to reduce the amount of water released into urine. If the body produces too much vasopressin, it prompts the body to conserve water, causing a lower concentration of sodium in the blood. In addition, certain types of **cancer** cells produce vasopressin, which also can lead to hyponatremia. If the body produces too little vasopressin, the body doesn't conserve enough water and the level of sodium in the body rises.

High sodium levels may occur in diabetes insipidus, a disease that causes too much urine to be produced. In this type of diabetes, either the hypothalamus fails to make vasopressin, or the kidneys don't respond to vasopressin. In either case, the kidney is able to regulate the body's sodium levels, but can't retain water. High sodium levels don't occur in diabetes insipidus if the patient is able to drink enough water to keep up with urinary loss, which may be as high as 10 liters per day.

Sodium levels may rise in unconscious patients because they can't drink water. Water is continually lost by evaporation from the lungs and in the urine; if the patient isn't given water intravenously, the sodium concentration in the blood may increase and hypernatremia could develop. Hypernatremia can also occur in rare diseases in which the thirst impulse is impaired. Hypernatremia also can occur accidentally in the hospital when patients are given solutions containing sodium.

Symptoms of high sodium levels can include confusion, coma, **paralysis** of the lung muscles, and death. The severity of the symptoms is related to how quickly the high sodium levels developed. If the levels build up suddenly, the brain cells can't adapt to their new high-sodium environment. Hypernatremia is especially dangerous for children and the elderly. Moderately low sodium levels may trigger fatigue, confusion, **headache**, muscle cramps, and nausea. Severe hyponatremia can lead to seizures and coma.

Abnormal sodium levels are diagnosed by measuring the concentration of sodium in the blood. In low sodium levels, unless the cause is obvious, a variety of tests are needed to determine if sodium was lost from the urine, diarrhea, or from vomiting. Tests are also used to determine hormone problems. The patient's diet and use of diuretics must also be considered.

Severely low sodium levels can be treated by giving intravenous sodium and water into the blood. Moderate hyponatremia due to use of diuretics or high levels of vasopressin is often treated by drinking less water each day. Hyponatremia due to an abnormal adrenal gland is treated with hormone injections. High sodium level is treated with an intravenous solution of water a normal concentration of sodium. The infusion is performed over many hours or days to prevent abrupt and dangerous changes in brain cell volume. In emergencies, such as when a high sodium level is causing brain symptoms, infusions may be conducted with half the normal concentration of salt.

A low sodium level is just one manifestation of a variety of disorders. While it can easily be corrected, the prognosis for the underlying condition that causes it varies. The prognosis for treating a high sodium level is excellent, unless neurological symptoms are severe or if a doctor tries to reverse the condition too quickly.

It is not always easy to prevent abnormal salt levels. Patients who take diuretic medications must be checked regularly for the development of hyponatremia. High levels occur only in unusual circumstances that are not normally under a person's control.

Somatoform disorders

The somatoform disorders are a group of mental problems characterized by physical complaints that aren't caused by a physical disease or condition. Generally, the patient complains of uncomfortable physical sensations or the inability to walk or move the arms or legs. The physical symptoms must be serious enough to interfere with the patient's job or relationships, and must be symptoms that the patient can't control voluntarily.

As a group, the somatoform disorders are difficult to recognize and treat because patients often have long histories of medical or surgical treatment with several different doctors. In addition, the physical symptoms are not under the patient's conscious control, so that he or she isn't intentionally trying to confuse the doctor or complicate the process of diagnosis. Somatoform disorders are, however, a significant problem for the health care system because patients with these disturbances overuse medical services.

Somatization disorder was formerly called Briquet's syndrome, after the French physician who first recognized it. The distinguishing characteristic of this disorder is a pattern of symptoms in several different parts of the patient's body that can't be accounted for by medical illness. For a diagnosis, there must be complains of pain in the digestive system, sex organs, and the nervous system.

Somatization disorder usually begins before the age of 30. It is estimated that 0.2% of the United States population will develop this disorder sometime in their lives. Another researcher estimates that 1% of all women in the United States have symptoms of this disorder. The female-to-male ratio is estimated to range between 5:1 and 20:1.

Somatization disorder usually persists throughout the patient's life. It also tends to run in families. Some psychiatrists think that the high female-to-male ratio in this disorder reflects the cultural pressures on women in North American society and the social ''permission'' given to women to be physically weak or sickly.

Conversion disorder is a condition in which the patient's senses or ability to walk or move are impaired without a recognized medical or neurological disease. With this condition, psychological factors (such as **stress** or trauma) are temporarily related to the symptoms. The disorder gets its name from the notion that the patient is ''converting'' a psychological problem into an inability to move specific parts of the body or to use the senses normally. A patient who suddenly can't speak during a situation in which he or she is afraid to speak might be suffering from a conversion disorder. The symptom simultaneously contains the **anxiety** and serves to get the patient out of the threatening situation.

The specific physical symptoms of conversion disorder may include a loss of balance or **paralysis** of an arm or leg; the inability to swallow or speak; the loss of touch or pain sensation; going blind or deaf; seeing double; or having **hallucinations**, seizures, or convulsions.

Unlike somatization disorder, conversion disorder may begin at any age, and it does not appear to run in families. As many as 34% of the population experiences conversion symptoms over a lifetime, but the disorder is more likely to occur among less educated people; 90% of patients recover within a month, and most don't have recurrences. Male patients are likely to develop conversion disorders in occupational settings or military service.

Pain disorder is marked by the presence of severe pain. This category covers a range of patients with a variety of ailments, including chronic **headache**s, back problems, arthritis, muscle aches and cramps, or pelvic pain. In some cases the patient's pain appears to be largely due to psychological factors, but in other cases the pain is derived from a medical condition as well as the patient's mental problems.

Pain disorder is relatively common in the general population especially among older adults; the sex ratio is more nearly equal

Hypochondriasis is a somatoform disorder marked by excessive fear of or preoccupation with having a serious illness that doesn't get better in spite of medical testing and reassurance. It was formerly called hypochondriacal neurosis.

Although hypochondriasis is usually considered a disorder of young adults, it is now increasingly recognized in children and adolescents. It may also develop in elderly people without previous histories of health-related fears. The disorder accounts for about 5% of psychiatric patients, and is equally common in men and women. Hypochondriasis may persist over a number of years but usually occurs as a series of episodes rather than continuous treatment-seeking. The flare-ups of the disorder are often correlated with stressful events in the patient's life.

A patient with body dysmorphic disorder has a preoccupation with an imagined or exaggerated defect in appearance. Most cases involve features on the patient's face or head, but other body parts (especially those associated with sexual attractiveness, such as the breasts or genitals) may also be the focus of concern.

Body dysmorphic disorder is regarded as a chronic condition that usually begins in the patient's late teens and fluctuates over the course of time. It was initially considered to be a relatively unusual disorder, but may be more common than was formerly thought. It appears to affect men and women with equal frequency. Patients with body dysmorphic disorder often try to have plastic surgery or other procedures to repair or treat the supposed defect.

The most common somatoform disorders in children and adolescents are conversion disorders, although body dysmorphic disorders are being reported more frequently. Conversion reactions in this age group usually reflect stress in the family or problems with school rather than long-term mental health problems. Some mental health experts speculate that adolescents with conversion disorders often have overprotective or overinvolved parents with a subconscious need to see their child as sick; in many cases the son or daughter's symptoms become the center of family attention. The rise in body dysmorphic disorders in adolescents may reflect American society's preoccupation with physical perfection.

The somatoform disorders are grouped together on the basis of symptom patterns, so their causes include several different factors. Family stress is believed to be one of the most common causes of somatoform disorders in children and adolescents. Conversion disorders in this age group may also be connected with physical or sexual abuse within the family of origin.

Somatization disorder and hypochondriasis may result in part from the patient's unconscious imitation of their parents' behavior. This ''copycat'' behavior is particularly likely if the patient's parent benefitted in some way from symptoms.

Cultural influences appear to affect the somatoform disorders. Some cultures (for example, Greek and Puerto Rican) report higher rates of somatization disorder among men than is the case for the United States. In addition, somatization disorder is less common among people with higher levels of education. People in Asia and Africa are more likely to report certain types of physical sensations (for example, burning hands or feet, or the feeling of ants crawling under the skin) than are Westerners.

Genetic or biological factors may also play a role. For example, people who suffer from somatization disorder may also perceive pain differently.

Accurate diagnosis of somatoform disorders is important to prevent unnecessary surgery, lab tests, or other procedures. Diagnosis of somatoform disorders requires a thorough physical exam to rule out medical and brain conditions, or to assess their severity in patients with pain disorder. A detailed examination is especially necessary when conversion disorder is a possible diagnosis, because some neurological conditions (such as **multiple sclerosis** and **myasthenia gravis**) have sometimes been misdiagnosed as conversion disorder.

In addition to ruling out medical causes for the patient's symptoms, a doctor who is evaluating a patient for a somatization disorder will consider the possibility of other mental diagnoses. Patients with somatization disorder often develop panic attacks or **agoraphobia** (fear of going out in public) together with their physical symptoms. In addition to anxiety or personality disorders, the doctor will usually consider major depression as a possible diagnosis when evaluating a patient with symptoms of a somatoform disorder. Pain disorders may be associated with depression, and body dismorphic disorder may be associated with obsessive-compulsive disease.

Patients with somatoform disorders are sometimes given antianxiety drugs or antidepressant drugs if they have also been diagnosed with a mood or anxiety disorder. In general, however, it is considered better to avoid prescribing medications for these patients since they are likely to become psychologically dependent on them. (However, body dysmorphic disorder as been successfully treated with selective serotonin reuptake inhibitors (SSRI) antidepressants).

Patients with somatoform disorders can benefit from supportive approaches to treatment that are aimed at easing symptoms and stabilizing the patient's personality. Some patients with pain disorder benefit from **group therapy** or support groups, particularly if their social network has been limited by their pain symptoms.**Family therapy** is usually recommended for children or adolescents with somatoform disorders, particularly if the parents seem to be using the child as a focus to divert attention from other difficulties. Working with families of chronic pain patients also helps avoid reinforcing dependency within the family setting.

Hypnosis is a technique that is sometimes used to treat conversion disorder because it may allow patients to recover memories or thoughts connected with the onset of the physical symptoms.

Patients with somatization disorder or pain disorder may be helped by a variety of alternative therapies including **acupuncture**, **hydrotherapy**, therapeutic **massage**, or **meditation**.

The prognosis for somatoform disorders depends on the patient's age and whether the disorder is chronic or episodic. In general, somatization disorder and body dysmorphic disorder rarely disappear completely. Hypochondriasis and pain disorder may get better if there are great improvements in the patient's overall health and lifestyle. People with both disorders may go through periods when symptoms become less severe or become worse. Conversion disorder responds quickly to treatment, but may recur in about 25% of all cases.

Because these syndromes affect different age groups, have different symptom patterns and are caused by different problems of adjustment, it's hard to describe one way to prevent them all. In theory, allowing children to express emotional pain rather than regarding it as ''weak'' might reduce the attention that physical symptoms that bring from parents.

SORE THROAT

Sore throat (also called pharyngitis) is a painful inflammation of the mucous membranes lining the throat.It is a symptom of many conditions, but most often is associated with colds or **influenza**. Sore throat may be caused by either viral or bacterial infections or environmental conditions. Most sore throats heal without complications, but they shouldn't be ignored because some develop into serious illnesses.

Almost everyone gets a sore throat at one time or another, although children in child care or grade school have them more often than adolescents and adults. Sore throats are most common during the winter months when colds are more frequent.

Sore throats may appear suddenly and last from three to about seven days, or they may be chronic, lasting much longer. These chronic sore throats are often a symptom of an underlying condition or disease, such as a sinus infection.

Sore throats have many different causes, and may or may not be accompanied by cold symptoms, **fever**, or swollen lymph glands. Viruses cause 90% to 95% of all sore throats. Cold and flu viruses are the main culprits, inflaming the throat and occasionally the tonsils (**tonsillitis**). Cold symptoms almost always accompany a viral sore throat. These can include a runny nose, **cough**, congestion, hoarseness, **conjunctivitis** (eye inflammation), and fever. The level of throat pain varies from uncomfortable to excruciating, so that the patient can't eat, breathe, swallow, or speak without great discomfort.

Another group of viruses that cause sore throat are the adenoviruses, which also may cause infections of the lungs and ears. In addition to a sore throat, symptoms that accompany an adenovirus infection include cough, runny nose, white bumps on the tonsils and throat, mild **diarrhea**, vomiting, and a rash. The sore throat lasts about one week.

The coxsackie virus causes another type of severe sore throat linked to a disease called herpangina. Although anyone can get herpangina, it's most common in children up to age ten and is more prevalent in the summer or early autumn. Herpangina is sometimes called summer sore throat. Three to six days after being exposed to the coxsackie virus, an infected person develops a sudden sore throat with a fever between 102 and 104°F. Tiny grayish-white blisters form on the throat and in the mouth which turn into small ulcers. Throat pain is often severe, interfering with swallowing. Children may become dehydrated if they are reluctant to eat or drink because of the pain. In addition, people with herpangina may vomit, have abdominal pain, and generally feel ill and miserable.

Another common cause of a viral sore throat is mononucleosis, an infection caused by the Epstein-Barr virus that spreads to the lymphatic system, respiratory system, liver, spleen, and throat. Symptoms appear 30-50 days after exposure.

Mononucleosis, sometimes called the kissing disease, is extremely common; by the age of 40, as many as 95% of Americans will have had the infection. Often, symptoms are mild, especially in young children, and are diagnosed as a cold. Since symptoms are more severe in adolescents and adults, more cases are diagnosed as monomucleosis in this age group. One of the main symptoms of mononucleosis is a severe sore throat.

Although a runny nose and cough are much more likely to accompany a sore throat caused by a virus than one caused by a bacteria, there is no absolute way to tell what is causing the sore throat without a lab test. Viral sore throats are contagious and are passed directly from person to person by coughing and sneezing.

The other major cause of sore throats are bacterial infections, responsible for from 5% to 10% of painful throats. The most common bacterial sore throat results from an infection by group A streptococcus. This type of infection is commonly called **strep throat**. Anyone can get strep throat, but it is most common in school age children.

Pharyngeal **gonorrhea**, a sexually transmitted bacterial disease, causes a severe sore throat as a result of having oral sex with an infected person.

Not all sore throats are caused by infection, however. Postnasal drip (caused by hay fever and other **allergies**) can irritate the throat and make it sore. Heavy smoking or breathing secondhand smoke or dry air, abusing alcohol, breathing polluted air or chemical fumes, or swallowing substances that burn or scratch the throat can also cause sore throat. People who breathe through their mouths at night because of nasal congestion often get sore throats that improve as the day progresses.

It is easy for people to tell if they have a sore throat, but difficult to know what has caused it without lab tests. Most sore throats are minor and heal without any complications, but a few cases caused by bacterial infections can develop into serious diseases. Because of this, it's a good idea to see a doctor if a sore throat lasts more than a few days or is accompanied by fever, nausea, or abdominal pain.

Diagnosis of a sore throat by a doctor begins with a **physical examination** of the throat and chest. The doctor will also look for signs of other illness, such as a sinus infection or **bronchitis**. Since both bacterial and viral sore throat are contagious and pass easily from person to person, the doctor will ask whether the patient has been around other people with flu, sore throat, colds, or strep throat. If strep throat is a possibility, the doctor will do lab tests.

If mononucleosis is suspected, the doctor may do a mono spot test to look for antibodies indicating the presence of the Epstein-Barr virus. The test is cheap, takes only a few minutes, and can be done in a doctor's office. An inexpensive blood test can also determine the presence of antibodies to the mononucleosis virus.

Effective treatment varies depending on the cause of the sore throat. As frustrating as it may be to the patient, a viral sore throat is best left to run its course without drug treatment. **Antibiotics** have no effect on a viral sore throat. They don't shorten the length of the illness, nor do they lessen the symptoms.

Sore throat caused by bacteria must be treated with antibiotics. Patients need to take the full course of antibiotic prescribed, even if symptoms of the sore throat improve. Stopping the antibiotic early can lead to a return of the sore throat.

Because mononucleosis is caused by a virus, there is no specific drug treatment available. Rest, a healthy diet, plenty of fluids, limiting heavy **exercise** and competitive sports, and treatment of aches with **acetaminophen** (Datril, Tylenol, Panadol) or ibuprofen (Advil, Nuprin, Motrin, Medipren) will help ease symptoms. Nearly 90% of mononucleosis infections are mild, and one infection confers immunity.

In the case of chronic sore throat, it's important to treat the underlying disease to heal the sore throat. If a sore throat caused by environmental factors, the aggravating substance should be avoided.

Regardless of the cause of a sore throat, there are some home care steps that people can take to ease their discomfort. These include:

- Taking acetaminophen or ibuprofen for pain. **Aspirin** should not be given to children because of its association with **Reye's Syndrome**, a serious disease.
- Gargling with warm double strength tea or warm salt water made by adding one teaspoon of salt to eight ounces of water.

- Drinking plenty of fluids, but avoiding acid juices like orange juice, which can irritate the throat. Sucking on popsicles is a good way to get fluids into children.
- Eating soft, nutritious foods like noodle soup and avoiding spicy foods.
- Refraining from smoking.
- Resting until the fever is gone, then resuming strenuous activities gradually.
- A room humidifier may make sore throat sufferers more comfortable.
- Antiseptic lozenges and sprays may aggravate the sore throat rather than improve it.

There is no way to prevent a sore throat; however, the risk of getting one or passing one on to another person can be minimized by:

- Washing hands well and often
- Avoiding close contact with someone who has a sore throat
- Not sharing food and eating utensils with anyone
- Not smoking
- Staying out of polluted air

Spallanzani, Lazzaro (1729-1799)

Italian biologist and physiologist

Spallanzani was born on January 12, 1729, in Scandiano, Italy. He attended the University of Bologna and began his studies in law. However, his cousin, Laura Bassi, a professor of physics and mathematics, introduced him to a broad range of scientific studies. Spallanzani altered his educational course and, in 1754, he earned a Ph.D. in philosophy. He joined the priesthood to support himself while he studied natural phenomena, hoping to determine explanations for such events as a stone skipping on water, the regeneration of decapitated snail heads, and the electric discharge of torpedo fish. Over the course of his career, Spallanzani would examine the pits of spitting volcanoes, the world of reproduction, the waters of eels, the dark depths of the bat's home, and the intricacies of the vascular system.

Yet Spallanzani's greatest contribution was in the area of spontaneous generation of microorganisms. The theory of spontaneous generation held that living creatures could develop from lifeless matter, especially from decaying matter. For instance, **Aristotle** believed that animal life generated spontaneously from mud, dung, or decaying timber. Other scientists believed alligators arose from Nile River mud, worms came from Thames River mud, and mites came from cheese.

Francesco Redi, (1626-1697) an Italian physician and naturalist, conducted experiments in the seventeenth century that first dispelled the myths of spontaneous generation. Using the theory that decaying products only served as a nesting site for maggots to lay eggs, Redi showed that, in hot weather, maggots would appear on exposed meat or dead animals. If the fresh meat was placed in a jar covered with a fine gauze, no maggots appeared.

Spallanzani, meanwhile, set out in 1765 to prove that microorganisms existed because they were already present in some form in the solution, the container, or the air. He took solutions which he knew would ''breed'' organisms and boiled them for up to an hour. The flasks were hermetically sealed to keep out contaminated air. Nothing grew.

But proponents of the spontaneous generation theory dismissed Spallanzani's experiments, saying only that the boiling process had destroyed elements vital to the propagation of the organisms. It was not until **Louis Pasteur**'s experiments on bacteria a century later that Spallanzani was proved right. Spallanzani's work regarding spontaneous generation eventually led to means of food preservation through heat sterilization and canning.

Spallanzani also turned his attention to the circulatory system. Viewing the system of blood vessels within a hen's egg in 1771, he was able to determine that an arteriovenous network existed in a warm-blooded animal. With further study of the circulatory system, in which Spallanzani studied the changes that occur upon impending death as well as the effects of wounds on various parts of the system, he eventually developed a theory of **blood pressure**. He determined that the arterial pulse was not due simply to displacement of the cardiac muscle, but to an intentional and forceful push of blood against the vascular walls.

One of his next inquiries involved the fertilization of eggs. He began with the mating practices of frogs and toads. By 1785, when he was working with dogs, he induced the first case of artificial insemination. Spallanzani's curiosity surrounding natural phenomena took him on an expedition to the volcanoes of Vesuvius, Stromboli, Vulcano, and Etna. During his travels, he climbed to within five feet of red-hot lava in order to measure its flow. He suffered burned feet as he descended into the bowels of Vulcano. He was rendered unconscious by the gases at Etna. Spallanzani's volcanic studies earned him status as a pioneer in the volcanology.

One of Spallanzani's final investigations took him into the dark world of bats. He was fascinated by their ability to maneuver without light. Even blinded, the bats could travel and eat without interruption or hesitation. Spallanzani went through the senses one by one, trying to discover which one governed the habits of the bat. Through the process of elimination, he found that plugging up the bats' ears rendered them directionless. While Spallanzani accepted the theory of echolocation, this theory wasn't explained until 1941, when Donald R. Griffin described the bat's sensitivity to sound waves. Spallanzani died on February 11, 1799, in Pavia, Italy.

Speech Therapy

More than 6% of all adults in the United States have speech difficulties that involve articulation, language, voice, fluency, hearing, or swallowing. In addition, 5% of all children exhibit impaired speech, language, or hearing. Many of these individuals can be helped by speech therapy.

Speech and language disorders affect the way people speak to and understand each other. These disorders may range from problems with simple sounds to not being able to speak or use language at all. Speech and language disorders include stuttering, characterized by interruptions in the regular flow or rhythm of speech; articulation disorders, involving difficulties in forming or stringing sounds together; voice disorders, characterized by inappropriate voice pitch, loudness, or quality; **aphasia**, or the loss of speech and language abilities resulting from **stroke** or **head injury**; and delayed language disorder, characterized by slow development of the vocabulary and grammar required to express and understand thoughts and ideas.

Speech and language disorders are serious because the ability to communicate is in large part what makes us human. Without the ability to communicate, it is impossible to learn, work, or engage in social interactions.

Unfortunately, there is no single cause of speech and language disorders. These disorders may arise from **hearing loss**, **cerebral palsy** and other neuromuscular disorders, severe head injury, stroke, viral disease, **mental retardation**, certain drugs, physical impairments such as cleft lip or palate, vocal abuse or misuse, or inadequate speech and language models. The causes of a disorder may vary with the age and gender of the affected person. They may also depend on specific characteristics of the symptom. In some cases, it is not possible to determine the cause.

Indications that a person might be suffering from a speech and language disorder could include marked differences in that person's speech compared to that of others of the same age, sex, or ethnic group; difficulties on the part of others to understand that person's speech or language; that person becomes overly concerned with his or her own speech; or that person's avoidance of communication with others.

Speech-language pathologists, or speech therapists, specialize in human communication, its development, and its disorders. They are professionally trained to evaluate and treat persons with speech and language disorders.

The pathologist will have either a master's degree or doctoral degree in speech-language pathology, and he or she may also hold a Certificate of Clinical Competence from the American Speech-Language-Hearing Association. Some states also require licensing.

Methods of treating the disorder will depend upon the nature and severity of the problem, the age of the individual, and the individual's awareness of the problem. The speech-language pathologist typically employs specialized professional services that may include help with the production of speech sounds (articulation disorders); the development of proper voice production (voice disorders); the production of fluent speech and help coping with the inability to produce such speech (stuttering); and the compensation for lost language and speech skills and the relearning of language, speech skills, and sentence order (aphasia).

Speech therapists also help clients and their families come to understand the disorder and learn to communicate normally in educational, social, and work settings. They also provide advice on ways to help prevent speech and language disorders. Speech therapists may be found in a number of facilities, including public and private schools, **hospitals**, rehabilitation centers, **nursing homes**, community clinics, colleges and universities, private offices, state and local health departments, and state and federal government offices.

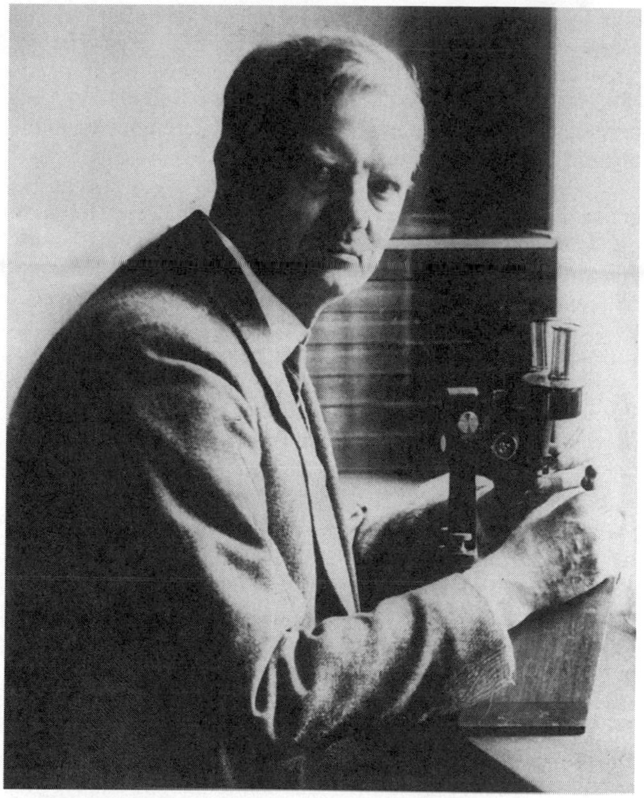

Hans Spemann

See also Communication disorders; Hearing loss

Spemann, Hans (1869-1941)

German embryologist

The son of a well known book publisher, Spemann was born on June 27, 1869, in Stuttgart, Germany. He was the eldest of four children in a family which was socially and culturally active, and lived in a large home that was well stocked with books (which helped shape the young Spemann's intellect). Upon entering the Eberhard Ludwig Gymnasium, Spemann first wished to study the classics. He later turned to embryology—the branch of biology that focuses on embryos and their development.

He entered the University of Heidelberg in 1891 to study medicine, however, his strict interest in medicine lasted only until he met German biologist and psychologist Gustav Wolff at the University of Heidelberg. Only a few years older than Spemann, Wolff had begun experiments on the embryological developments of newts and had shown how, if the lens of an embryological newt's eye is removed, it regenerates. Spemann remained interested and intrigued by both Wolff's finding and also in the newt, on which he based much of his future work. But more than the regeneration phenomenon, Spemann was interested in how the eye develops from the start. He devoted his scientific career to the study of how embryological cells become specialized and differentiated in the process of forming a complete organism.

Spemann left Heidelberg in the mid–1890s to continue his studies at the University of Munich; he then transferred to the University of Würzberg's Zoological Institute to study under the well-known embryologist Theodor Boveri. Spemann quickly became Boveri's prize student, and completed his doctorate in botany, zoology, and physics in 1895. Spemann stayed at Würzburg until 1908, when he accepted a post as professor at the University of Rostock. During World War I, he served as director of the Kaiser Wilhelm Institute of Biology (now the Max Planck Institute) in Berlin-Dahlem, and following the war, in 1919, he took a professorship at the University of Freiburg.

By the time Spemann began research at the Zoological Institute in Würzburg, he had already developed a keen facility and reputation for conducting well-designed experiments that centered on highly focused questions. His early research followed Wolff's closely. The eye of a newt is formed when an outgrowth of the brain, called the optic cup, reaches the surface layer of embryonic tissue (the ectoderm). The cells of the ectoderm then form into an eye. In removing the tissue over where the eye would form and replacing it with tissue from an entirely different region, Spemann found that the embryo still formed a normal eye, leading him to believe that the optic cup exerted an influence on the cells of the ectoderm, inducing them to form into an eye. To complete this experiment, as well as others, Spemann had to develop a precise experimental technique for operating on objects often less than two millimeters in diameter. In doing so, he is credited with founding the techniques of modern microsurgery, which is considered one of his greatest contributions in biology. Some of his methods and instruments are still used by embryologists and neurobiologists today.

In another series of experiments—conducted in the 1920s—Spemann was able to conclude that at a certain stage of development, the future roles of the different parts of the embryo have not been fixed, which supported his experiments with the newt's eye. In an experiment conducted on older eggs, however, Spemann found that the future role of some parts of the embryo had been decided, meaning that somewhere in between, a process he called ''determination'' must have taken place to fix the ''developmental fate'' of the cells.

One of Spemann's greatest contributions to embryology—and the one for which he won the 1935 Nobel Prize in physiology or medicine—was his discovery of what he called the ''organizer'' effect. In experimenting with transplanting tissue, Spemann found that when an area containing an organizer is transplanted into an undifferentiated host embryo, this transplanted area can induce the host embryo to develop in a certain way, or into an entirely new embryo. Spemann called these transplanted cells organizers, and they include the precursors to the central nervous system. In vertebrates, they are the first cells in a long series of differentiations of which the end product is a fully formed fetus.

Spemann remained at the University of Freiburg until his retirement in the mid–1930s. When not busy with his scientific endeavors, he cultivated his love of the liberal arts. He died at his home near Freiburg on September 12, 1941.

Sperry, Roger W. (1913-1994)

American psychobiologist

Roger Sperry was born on 20 August 1913, in Hartford, Connecticut. When Sperry was 11 years old, his father died and his mother returned to school and got a job as an assistant to a high school principal. Sperry attended local public schools through high school and then went to Oberlin College in Ohio on a scholarship. Although he majored in English, Sperry was especially interested in his undergraduate psychology courses with R. H. Stetson, an expert on the physiology of speech. Sperry earned his B.A. in English in 1935 and then worked as a graduate assistant to Stetson for two years. In 1937 he received an M.A. in psychology.

Thoroughly committed to research in the field of psychobiology by that time, Sperry went to the University of Chicago to conduct research on the organization of the central **nervous system** under the renowned biologist Paul Weiss. Before Weiss's research, scientists believed that the connections of the nervous system had to be very exact to work properly. Weiss disproved this theory by surgically crossing a subject's nerve connections. After the surgery was performed, the subject's behavior did not change. From this, Weiss concluded that the connections of the central nervous system were not predetermined, so that a nerve need not connect to any particular location to function correctly.

Sperry tested Weiss's research by surgically crossing the nerves that controlled the hind leg muscles of a rat. Under Weiss's theory, each nerve should eventually ''learn'' to control the leg muscle to which it was now connected. This did not happen. When the left hind foot was stimulated, the right foot responded instead. Sperry's experiments disproved Weiss's research and became the basis of his doctoral dissertation, ''Functional results of crossing nerves and transposing muscles in the fore and hind limbs of the rat.'' He received a Ph.D. in zoology from the University of Chicago in 1941.

Sperry did other related experiments that confirmed his findings and further contradicted Weiss's theory that ''function precedes form'' (that is, the brain and nervous system learn, through experience, to function properly). From these and other experiments, Sperry deduced that genetic mechanisms determine some basic behavioral patterns. According to his theory, nerves have highly specific functions based on genetically predetermined differences in the concentration of chemicals inside the nerve cells.

In 1941, Sperry moved to the laboratory of the renowned psychologist Karl S. Lashley. A year later, Lashley became director of the Yerkes Laboratories of Primate Biology in Orange Park, Florida. Sperry joined him there on a Harvard biology research fellowship. While there, he disproved some Gestalt psychology theories about brain mechanisms, as well as some theories of Lashley's.

After World War II, in 1946, Sperry accepted a position of assistant professor at the University of Chicago in the school's anatomy department. By 1954, he transferred to the California Institute of Technology (Caltech). At Caltech, Sperry conducted research on split-brain functions that he had first investigated when he worked at the Yerkes Laboratory. It had long been known that the cerebrum of the brain consists of two hemispheres. In most people the left hemisphere controls the right side of the body and vice versa. The two halves are connected by a bundle of millions of nerve fibers called the corpus callosum, or the great cerebral commissure.

Neurosurgeons had discovered that this connection could be cut into with little or no noticeable change in the patient's mental abilities. After experiments on animals proved the procedure to be harmless, surgeons began cutting completely through the commissure of epileptic patients in an attempt to prevent the spread of epileptic seizures from one hemisphere to the other. The procedure was generally successful, and beginning in the late 1930s, cutting through the forebrain commissure became an accepted treatment method for severe epilepsy. Observations of the split-brain patients indicated no loss of communication between the two hemispheres of the brain.

From these observations, scientists assumed that the corpus callosum had no function other than as a prop to prevent the two hemispheres from sagging. Scientists also believed that the left hemisphere was dominant and performed higher cognitive functions such as speech. This theory developed from observations of patients whose left cerebral hemisphere had been injured; these patients suffered impairment of various cognitive functions, including speech. Since these functions were not transferred over to the uninjured right hemisphere, scientists assumed that the right hemisphere was less developed.

Sperry's work shattered these views. He and his colleagues at Caltech discovered that the corpus callosum is more than a physical prop; it provides a means of communication between the two halves of the brain and integrates the knowledge acquired by each of them. They also learned that in many ways, the right hemisphere is superior to the left. Although the left half of the brain is superior in analytic, logical thought, the right half excels in intuitive processing of information. The right hemisphere also specializes in non-verbal functions, such as understanding music, interpreting visual patterns (such as recognizing faces), and sorting sizes and shapes.

Sperry started published technical papers on his split-brain findings in the late 1960s. The importance of his research was recognized relatively quickly, and in 1979 he was awarded the prestigious Albert Lasker Basic Medical Research Award, which included a $15,000 grant. The award was given in recognition of the potential medical benefits of Sperry's research, including possible treatments for mental or psychosomatic illnesses.

In 1981, Sperry was honored with the Nobel Prize in physiology or medicine. He shared it with two other scientists, Torsten N. Wieseland David H. Hubel, for research on the central nervous system and the brain. In describing Sperry's work, the Nobel Prize selection committee praised the researcher for demonstrating the difference between the two hemispheres of the brain and for outlining some of the specialized functions of the right brain.

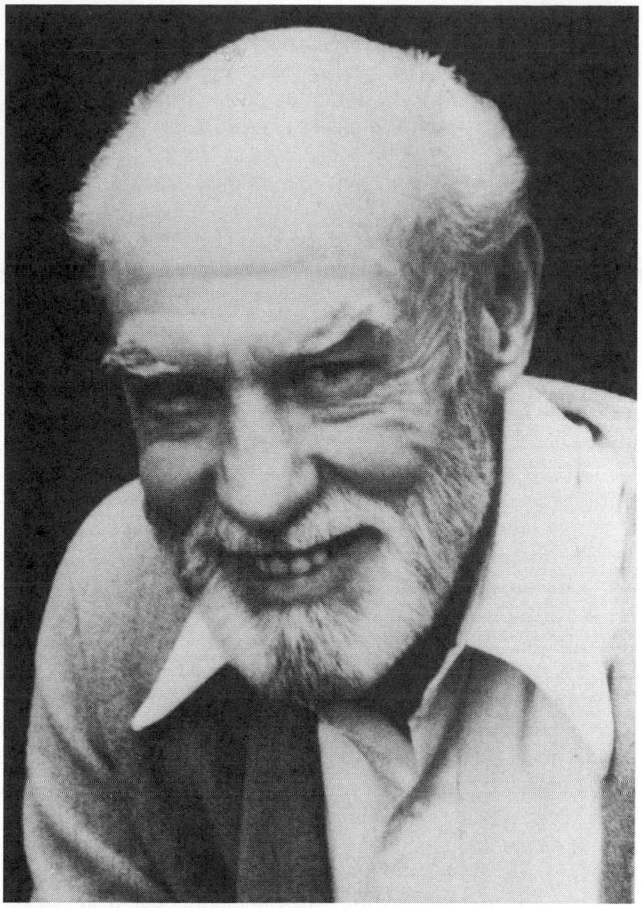

Roger W. Sperry

SPINA BIFIDA

Spina bifida is the common name for a range of **birth defects** caused by problems with the early development of the spine. The main defect of spina bifida is an abnormal opening in the spinal column through which the spinal cord passes. This leaves the spinal cord unprotected and vulnerable to either injury or infection.

Spina bifida occurs in one of every 700 births to whites in North America, but only one in every 3,000 births to blacks. In some areas of Great Britain, the occurrence of spina bifida is as high as one in every 100 births, leading to the hypothesis that some environmental factors must be at work.

The classic defect of spina bifida is an opening in the spine, obvious at birth, out of which protrudes a fluid-filled sac. This sac may include either just the membranes which cover the spinal cord or the membranes plus some part of the actual spinal cord. Often, the spinal cord itself has not developed properly. In spina bifida occulta, there may be some opening in the vertebrae, but no protruding sac. The entire defect may be covered with skin. The most severe form is called rachischisis, in which the entire length of the spine may be open.

The problems caused by spina bifida depend on a number of factors, including where along the spine the defect occurs and what other defects there are. The most severe types of spina bifida (raschischisis) is often fatal, either due to infection of the exposed tissues, or because of severe loss of function.

Spina bifida is one of a number of ''neural tube'' defects. The neural tube is the name for the very primitive structure which forms during fetal development, and which ultimately becomes the spinal cord and the brain. In spina bifida, the spinal column fails to wrap completely around the developing spinal cord. The abnormal development which causes in neural tube defects occurs very early in **pregnancy**, within the first three to four weeks.

Because different levels of the spinal cord are responsible for different functions, the location and the size of the defect in spina bifida will affect what kind of disabilities an individual will experience. Most patients with spina bifida have some degree of weakness in the legs ranging from slight to total **paralysis**, depending on the spinal cord condition. The higher up in the spine the defect occurs, the more severe the disabilities.

People with spina bifida frequently face severe problems with both bladder and bowel function, because complete emptying of both bladder and bowels requires an intact spinal cord. Difficulty in completely emptying the bladder can result in severe, repeated infections, ultimately causing kidney damage, which can be life threatening.

There are several types of defects which frequently accompany spina bifida. Arnold-Chiari malformations are changes in the brain structures that contribute to a condition called water on the brain (called **hydrocephalus**). Hydrocephalus is a condition in which there is too much cerebrospinal fluid (which protects the brain and spinal cord). If left to accumulate, this fluid puts damaging pressure on the brain.

Many children with spina bifida have other complications, including clubfeet and hip dislocations, as well as abnormal curves and bends in their spine causing a hunchbacked or twisted appearance.

Intelligence in children with spina bifida varies widely, and depends on the severity of the spinal defect and the presence of other conditions. Some children have normal intellectual potential, while others may operate at a slightly lower than normal capacity. Extreme intellectual deficits may occur in children with very severe spinal defects with associated Arnold-Chiari malformations and water on the brain.

It has recently been noted that children with spina bifida have a much higher risk of allergic sensitivity to latex causing anything from a minor skin **rash** to a more life-threatening reaction. This latex sensitivity is an important issue for these children, who have a much higher likelihood of coming into contact with latex surgical or exam gloves, as well as other medical supplies.

The protruding sac of severe spina bifida is quite apparent at birth, but other forms of spina bifida may be so subtle as to cause just the slightest dimple at the base of the spine. Clues that a baby has mild spina bifida include **birthmarks** located on the back along the area of the spine or areas of hair growth in the same general location. Other symptoms include muscle weakness and poor reflexes, as well as poor muscle tone of the ring of muscles that make up the anal opening (sphincter).

When spina bifida is suspected, spinal x rays, **computed tomography scans** (CT scans) of the spine, and ultrasound examinations of the area may help in diagnosis. Myelography is a procedure in which dye is injected into the area surrounding the spinal cord, followed by either x ray or CT scan. This allows the spinal cord to be examined more accurately. X ray, CT, and **magnetic resonance imaging** (MRI) exams are also needed in order to search for those problems which frequently accompany spina bifida, including hydrocephalus, Arnold-Chiari malformations, hip problems, and kidney damage.

Diagnosis prior to birth is an important area of concern. A particular substance, known as alpha-fetoprotein (AFP), is present at higher-than-normal levels in the blood of mothers who are carrying a fetus with a neural tube defect. AFP levels are tested during the 16 to 18 weeks of pregnancy. Abnormally high levels of AFP indicate that other tests should be done. These tests include withdrawing a sample of the fluid around the fetus (amniocentesis) to test for higher levels of AFP, and sophisticated ultrasound examination of the fetus. Results of amniocentesis, together with the results of careful ultrasound examination can diagnose more than 90% of all neural tube defects. Parents must then decide whether to terminate the pregnancy, or to use this information to prepare themselves to care for a child who will have significant medical needs.

Treatment of spina bifida is aimed first at closing the spinal defect in order to avoid complications which could be brought on by infection. Further operations are often necessary in order to repair the hip dislocations, clubfeet and spinal distortions which often go along with a spinal defect. Children with hydrocephalus will need drainage tubes to prevent brain damage. Many children who are able to learn to walk will require braces.

Many children with severe spina bifida are unable to completely empty their bladders, and can only do so with the insertion of a catheter tube. Such catheterization may be necessary at regular points throughout every day, in order to avoid the accumulation of urine which could back up, become infected, and damage the kidneys.

Children with significant bowel impairment may have severe **constipation**, which requires a high-fiber diet, laxative medications, **enemas**, or even removal of stool by hand to avoid bowel blockage.

Prognosis for a child with spina bifida has certainly improved, yet it still depends on the severity of the original spinal defect, as well as on other associated problems. The worst prognosis exists for those who are completely paralyzed, have a serious infection, or have hydrocephalus or other birth defects. Current care for children with spina bifida usually enables them to live into adulthood.

While doctors don't yet know how to prevent spina bifida or other neural tube defects, women who supplement their **diets** with folic acid prior to pregnancy and during the early weeks of pregnancy have a much lower risk of producing a baby with a neural tube defect. In fact, some studies indicate that taking 0.4 mg of folic acid decreases the risk of spina bifida by up to 75%. Because the defect which causes spina bifida occurs within the first 3 to 4 weeks of pregnancy, usually before a woman even realizes that she is pregnant, current recommendations state that any woman who is considering getting pregnant should immediately begin taking a folic acid supplement. Medications such as valproic acid, which increase the risk of neural tube defects if taken during pregnacy, should be avoided.

SPINAL CORD INJURY

Spinal cord injury is damage to the spinal cord that causes loss of sensation and motor control. Approximately 10,000 new spinal cord injuries (SCIs) occur each year in the United States. About 250,000 people are currently affected. Spinal cord injuries can happen to anyone at any time of life. The typical patient, however, is a man between the ages of 19 and 26, injured in a motor vehicle accident (about 50% of all SCIs), a fall (20%), an act of violence (15%), or a sporting accident (14%). Alcohol or other drug abuse plays an important role in a large percentage of all spinal cord injuries. Six percent of people who receive injuries to the lower spine die within a year, and 40% of people who receive the more frequent higher injuries die within a year.

Short-term costs for hospitalization, equipment, and home modifications are approximately $140,000 for an SCI patient capable of independent living. Lifetime costs may exceed one million dollars. Costs may be 3-4 times higher for the SCI patient who needs long-term institutional care. Overall costs to the American economy in direct payments and lost productivity are more than $10 billion per year.

The extent to which movement and sensation are damaged following spinal cord injury depends on the level of the injury, since nerves leaving the spinal cord at different levels control movement and sensation in diffferent parts of the body.

Damage below the base of the rib cage causes **paralysis** and loss of sensation in the legs and trunk below the injury. Injury at this level usually does no damage to the arms and hands. Paralysis of the legs is called paraplegia. Damage above this level involves the arms as well as the legs. Paralysis of all four limbs is called quadriplegia or tetraplegia. Cervical or neck injuries not only cause quadriplegia but also may cause difficulty in breathing. Damage in the lower part of the neck may leave enough diaphragm control to allow unassisted breathing. Patients with damage just below the base of the skull, require mechanical assistance to breathe.

Symptoms also depend on the extent of spinal cord injury. A completely severed cord causes paralysis and loss of sensation below the wound. If the cord is only partially severed, some function will remain below the injury. Damage limited to the front portion of the cord causes paralysis and loss of sensations of **pain** and temperature. Other sensation may be preserved. Damage to the center of the cord may spare the legs but paralyze the arms. Damage to the right or left half causes loss of position sense, paralysis on the side of the injury, and loss of pain and temperature sensation on the opposite side.

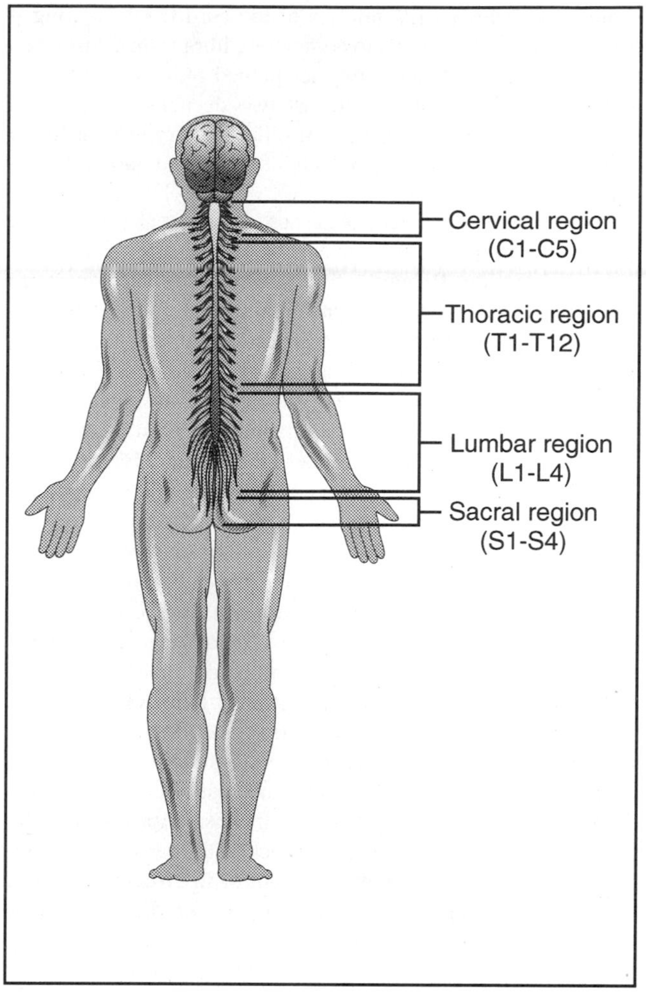

The extent of sensory and motor loss resulting from a spinal cord injury depends on the level of the injury because nerves at different levels control sensation and movement in different parts of the body. The distribution is as follows: C1-C4: head and neck; C3-C5: diaphragm; C5-T1: shoulders, arms, and hands; T2-T12: chest and abdomen (excluding internal organs); L1-L4: abdomen (excluding internal organs), buttocks, genitals, upper legs; L4-S3: legs; S2-S4: genitals, muscles of the perineum. *(Illustration by Electronic Illustrators Group.)*

Complications of spinal cord injury may include: •deep venous thrombosis, or blood clotting •pressure ulcers of the skin •spasticity and contracture of unused muscles •heterotopic ossification, or growth of bony tissue within muscle and tendons •autonomic dysreflexia, a lack of regulation of certain body systems •loss of bladder and bowel control •sexual dysfunction

A person who may have a spinal cord injury should not be moved. Treatment of SCI begins with **immobilization**. This strategy prevents partial injuries of the cord from severing it completely. Use of splints to completely immobilize suspected SCI at the scene of the injury has helped reduce the severity of spinal cord injuries in the last two decades. Intravenous methylprednisone, a steroidal anti-inflammatory drug, is given during the first 24 hours to reduce inflammation and tissue destruction.

Rehabilitation after spinal cord injury seeks to prevent complications, promote recovery, and make the most of remaining function. Rehabilitation is a complex and long-term process. It requires a team of professionals, including a neurologist, physiatrist or rehabilitation specialist, physical therapist, and occupational therapist. Other specialists who may be needed include a respiratory therapist, vocational rehabilitation counselor, social worker, speech-language pathologist, nutritionist, special education teacher, recreation therapist, and clinical psychologist. Support groups provide a critical source of information, advice, and support for SCI patients.

Some limited mobility and sensation may be recovered, but the extent and speed of this recovery cannot be predicted. Experimental electrical stimulation has been shown to allow some control of muscle contraction in paraplegia. This experimental technique offers the possibility of unaided walking. Further development of current control systems will be needed before useful movement is possible outside the laboratory.

The physical therapist focuses on mobility, to maintain range of motion of affected limbs and reduce contracture and deformity. Physical therapy helps compensate for lost skills by using those muscles that are still functional. It also helps to increase any residual strength and control in affected muscles. A physical therapist suggests adaptive equipment such as braces, canes, or wheelchairs.

An occupational therapist works to restore ability to perform the activities of daily living, such as eating and grooming, with tools and new techniques. The occupational therapist also designs modifications of the home and workplace to match the individual impairment.

A pulmonologist or respiratory therapist promotes airway hygiene through instruction in assisted coughing techniques and postural drainage. The respiratory professional also prescribes and provides instruction in the use of ventilators, facial or nasal masks, and tracheostomy equipment where necessary.

Pressure ulcers are prevented by turning in bed at least every two hours. The patient should be turned more frequently when redness begins to develop in sensitive areas. Special mattresses and chair cushions can distribute weight more evenly to reduce pressure. Electrical stimulation is sometimes used to promote muscle movement to prevent pressure ulcers.

Range of motion (ROM) **exercise**s help to prevent contracture. Chemicals can be used to prevent contractures from becoming fixed when ROM exercise is inadequate. Phenol or alcohol can be injected onto the nerve or botulinum toxin directly into the muscle. Botulinum toxin is associated with fewer complications, but it is more expensive than phenol and alcohol. Contractures can be released by cutting the shortened tendon or transferring it surgically to a different site on the bone where its pull will not cause as much deformity. Such tendon transfers may also be used to increase strength in partially functional extremities.

Normal bowel function is promoted through adequate fluid intake and a diet rich in fiber. Evacuation is stimulated by deliberately increasing the abdominal pressure, either voluntarily or by using an abdominal binder.

Bladder care involves continual or intermittent catheterization. The full bladder may be detected by feeling its bulge against the abdominal wall. Urinary tract infection is a significant complication of catheterization and requires frequent monitoring.

Counseling can help in adjusting to changes in sexual function after spinal cord injury. Erection may be enhanced through the same means used to treat erectile dysfunction in the general population.

The prognosis of SCI depends on the location and extent of injury. Injuries of the neck above C4 with significant involvement of the diaphragm hold the gravest prognosis. Respiratory infection is one of the leading causes of death in long-term SCI. Overall, 85% of SCI patients who survive the first 24 hours are alive 10 years after their injuries. Recovery of function is impossible to predict. Partial recovery is more likely after an incomplete wound than after the spinal cord has been completely severed.

Spinal cord tumors

A spinal cord tumor may be either a cancerous or noncancerous lesion in the spinal cord that grows between the membranes covering the spinal cord or in the spinal canal. A tumor here can compress the spinal cord or its nerve roots, so even a noncancerous growth may be disabling unless it's properly treated.

The spinal cord contains bundles of nerves that carry messages between the brain and the body. Because the spinal cord is encased in bone, any tumor that grows on or near it can press on the nerves, interfering with this brain-to-body communication. These tumors are fairly rare; about 10,000 Americans develop spinal cord growths each year, and about 40% of them are cancerous.

Newly-formed tumors that originate in the spinal cord are unusual, especially among children and the elderly. More typically, tumors start to grow elsewhere in the body and move through the bloodstream until they get to the spinal cord. Scientists don't know what causes these tumors, although the noncancerous growths may be either hereditary or present since birth.

When the tumor presses on the spinal cord, it causes a wide range of symptoms, including;

- Back **pain**
- Severe or burning pain in other parts of the body
- Numbness or cold
- Progressive loss of muscle strength or sensation in the legs
- Loss of bladder or bowel control.

A tumor at the top of the spinal column can cause pain radiating from the arms or neck; a tumor in the lower spine may cause leg or back pain. If there are several tumors in different areas of the spinal cord at the same time, it may cause symptoms in a variety of spots on the body.

Suspected spinal cord compression because of a tumor is a medical emergency. Prompt intervention may prevent **paralysis**. If basic nervous system tests and review of symptoms suggest a spinal cord tumor, a doctor may order some of these additional tests to diagnose the problem:

- MRI or CT scan
- Myelography
- Blood and spinal fluid tests
- X-rays of the spine
- Biopsy
- Bone scan

If the tumor is malignant and has spread into the spine from other parts of the body, treatment depends on the type of cancer it is. Surgery is usually the first step in treating cancerous and noncancerous tumors outside the spinal cord. Tumors inside the spinal cord may not be able to be completely removed with surgery. If they can't be removed, radiation and **chemotherapy** treatments may ease symptoms. Treatment also may include pain relievers and drugs to lessen swelling around the tumor, and relieve pressure on the spinal cord.

Early diagnosis and treatment can produce a higher success rate. Long-term survival depends on the tumor's type, location, and size. Surgery to remove the bone around the spinal cord can ease pressure on the spinal nerves and nerve pathways, which will usually ease pain and other symptoms; however, it may make walking more difficult. Physical therapy and **rehabilitation** may help.

Since spinal cord tumors usually are caused by spread of cancer that has first appeared elsewhere in the body, early detection of cancer in other organs may prevent spinal cord tumors. Lifestyle changes that may lower the risk of other types of cancer, may also help.

SPINAL INSTRUMENTATION

Spinal instrumentation is a method of straightening and stabilizing the spine after spinal fusion, by surgically attaching hooks, rods, and wire to the spine in a way that redistributes the stresses on the bones and keeps them in proper alignment.

Spinal instrumentation is used to treat instability and deformity of the spine. Instability occurs when the spine no longer maintains its normal shape during movement. Such instability results in nerve damage, spinal deformities, and disabling **pain**. Spinal deformities may be caused by:

- **Birth defects**.
- **Fractures**.
- Marfan syndrome.
- **Neurofibromatosis**.
- Neuromuscular diseases.
- Severe injuries.
- Tumors.

Curvature of the spine (**scoliosis**) is usually treated with spinal fusion and spinal instrumentation. Scoliosis is a disorder of unknown origin. It causes bending and twisting of the spine that eventually results in distortion of the chest and back. About 85% of cases occur in girls between the ages of 12-15, who are experiencing adolescent growth spurt.

Spinal instrumentation serves three purposes. It provides a stable, rigid column that encourages bones to fuse after spinal-fusion surgery. Second, it redirects the stresses over a wider area. Third, it restores the spine to its proper alignment.

Different types of spinal instrumentation are used to treat different spinal problems. Several common types of spinal instrumentation are explained below. Although the details of the insertion of rods, wires, and hooks varies, the purpose of all spinal instrumentation is the same—to correct and stabilize the backbone.

The Harrington Rod is one of the oldest and most proven forms of spinal instrumentation. It is used to straighten and stabilize the spine when curvature is greater than 60 degrees. It is an appropriate treatment for scoliosis.

Advantages of the Harrington rod are its relative simplicity of installation, the low rate of complications, and a proven record of reducing curvature of the spine. The main disadvantage is that the patient must remain in a body cast for about six months, then wear a brace for another three to six months while the bone fusion solidifies.

Luque rods are custom contoured metal rods that are fixed to each segment (vertebra) in the affected part of the spine. The main advantage is that the patient may not need to wear a cast or brace after the procedure. The main disadvantage is that the risk of injury to the nerves and spinal cord is higher than with a some other forms of instrumentation. This is because wires must be threaded through each vertebra near the spinal column, increasing the risk of such damage. Luque rods are sometimes used to treat scoliosis.

Drummond instrumentation, also called Harri-Drummond instrumentation, uses a Harrington rod on the concave side of the spine and a Luque rod on the convex side. The advantage is that each vertebra segment is fixed, with the risk of nerve injury decreased over Luque rod instrumentation. The disadvantage is that, like Harrington rod instrumentation, the patient must wear a cast and a brace after surgery.

Cotrel-Dubousset instrumentation uses hooks and rods in a cross-linked pattern to realign the spine and redistribute the biomechanical stress. The main advantage of Cotrel-Dubousset instrumentation is that, because of the extensive cross-linking, the patient may have to wear a cast or brace after surgery. The disadvantage is the complexity of the operation and the number of hooks and cross-links that may fail.

Zeilke instrumentation is similar to Cotrel-Dubousset instrumentation, but is used to treat double curvature of the spine. It requires wearing a brace for many months after surgery.

The Kaneda device is used to treat fractured thoracic or lumbar vertebrae when it is suspected that bone fragments are present in the spinal canal. Variations on the basic forms of spinal instrumentation, such as Wisconsin instrumentation, are being refined as technology improves. A physician chooses the proper type of instrumentation based on the type of disorder, the age and health of the patient, and on the physician's experience.

Since the hooks and rods of spinal instrumentation are anchored in the bones of the back, spinal instrumentation should not be performed on people with serious **osteoporosis**. To overcome this limitation, techniques are being explored that help anchor instrumentation in fragile bones.

Spinal instrumentation is performed by a neuro and/or orthopedic surgical team with special experience in spinal operations. The surgery is done in a hospital under **general anesthesia**. It is done at the same time as spinal fusion.

The surgeon strips the muscles away from the area to be fused. The surface of the bone is peeled away. A piece of bone is removed from the hip and placed along side the area to be fused. The stripping of the bone helps the bone graft to fuse.

After the fusion site is prepared, the rods, hooks, and wires are inserted. There is some variation in how this is done based on the spinal instrumentation chosen. In general, Harrington rods are the simplest instrumentation to install, and Cotrel-Dubousset instrumentation is the most complex and risky. Once the rods are in place, the incision is closed.

Spinal fusion with spinal instrumentation is major surgery. The patient will undergo many tests to determine that nature and exact location of the back problem. These tests are likely to include X-rays, **magnetic resonance imaging** (MRI), **computed tomography scans** (CT scans), and myleograms. In addition, the patient will undergo a battery of blood and urine tests, and possibly an electrocardiogram to provide the surgeon and anesthesiologist with information that will allow the operation to be performed safely. In Harrington rod instrumentation, the patient may be placed in **traction** or an upper body cast to stretch contracted muscles before surgery.

After surgery, the patient will be confined to bed. A catheter is inserted so that the patient can urinate without getting up. Vital signs are monitored, and the patient's position is changed frequently so that **bedsores** do not develop.

Recovery from spinal instrumentation can be a long, arduous process. Movement is severely limited for a period of time. In certain types of instrumentation, the patient is put in a cast to allow the realigned bones to stay in position until healing takes place. This can be as long as six to eight months. Many patients will need to wear a brace after the cast is removed.

During the recovery period, the patient is taught respiratory exercises to help maintain respiratory function during the time of limited mobility. Physical therapists assist the patient in learning self-care and in performing strengthening and range of motion exercises. Length of hospital stay depends on the age and health of the patient, as well as the specific problem that was corrected. The patient can expect to remain under a physician's care for many months.

Spinal instrumentation carries a significant risk of nerve damage and **paralysis**. The skill of the surgeon can affect the outcome of the operation, so patients should look for a hospital and surgical team that has a lot of experience doing spinal procedures.

After surgery there is a risk of infection or an inflammatory reaction due to the presence of the foreign material in the body. Serious infection of the membranes covering the spinal cord and brain can occur. In the long-term, the instrumentation may move or break, causing nerve damage and requiring a second surgery. Some bone grafts do not heal well, lengthening the time the patient must spend in a cast or brace, or necessitating additional surgery. Casting and wearing a brace may take an emotional toll, especially on young people. Patients who have had spinal instrumentation must avoid contact sports, and, for the rest of their lives, eliminate situations that will abnormally put stress on their spines.

Many young people with scoliosis heal with significantly improved alignment of the spine. Results of spinal instrumentation done for other conditions vary widely.

Spock, Benjamin McLane (1903-1998)

American pediatrician, psychiatrist, author

In a controversial book that sold more than 30 million copies in the three decades following its publication in 1946, pediatrician Benjamin Spock changed the way American parents raised their babies. *The Common Sense Book of Baby and Child Care,* based on Spock's 10 years of pediatric practice and psychoanalytic training, gave parents permission to use pacifiers, maintain flexible feeding schedules, and show ample affection to their babies. All were considered radical ideas at the time and, many believed, led to permissiveness that produced undisciplined, out-of- control behavior. The controversy created by the book catapulted Spock to fame, making him a worldwide child-rearing icon and prompting him to branch out in his career to include teaching and political activism.

Spock was born the eldest of six children in 1903 in New Haven, Connecticut. His father was a railroad lawyer whom Spock describes as ''grave'' and ''just,'' who commuted by trolley to his job and left most of the household and child-rearing duties to his wife. Spock's mother, the dominant influence in her son's life even many years later, rarely relied on any type of physical punishment for discipline. Rather, she controlled her children by instilling a strong sense of guilt. Spock credits his mother with encouraging him to read and inspiring him and his siblings to succeed later in life: ''She had a great sense of humor and delighted her children and her friends with stories about things she found amusing or ridiculous. She was a terrific mimic. She inspired her children with idealism and a drive to serve—five out of six of us became teachers or psychologists.''

After two years of schooling at the prestigious Andover Academy, Spock enrolled at Yale University where, as part of the school's varsity crew team, he won an Olympic gold medal in Paris in 1924. He earned an undergraduate degree in English literature and then, inspired by his summer job at a small home for crippled children, he began medical school. Two years at Yale's medical school were followed by a final two years at Columbia University, where he was at the top of his class both years. Now married—he and his wife Jane were married for 48 years before divorcing—Spock interned for two years at Presbyterian Hospital in New York. A subsequent one-year residency at New York Nursery and Child's Hospital led to what Spock has called "the most independent decision of my life": accepting a residency in psychiatry at New York Hospital.

As he started his own pediatric practice, Spock began psychoanalytic training and quickly saw a link between the medical and psychological aspects of treating children and helping their parents cope with their responsibilities. When he learned "that mothers were delighted to find a pediatrician interested in such common problems as thumb sucking and resistance to weaning or toilet training, I decided to stay in pediatrics. That was a momentous decision."

The publication of *The Common Sense Book of Baby and Child Care* led to teaching positions for Spock at Wayne State University in Detroit, Children's Hospital of the East Bay in Oakland, and the Mayo Clinic in Minnesota, and an administrative position at the University of Pittsburgh. Before he retired in 1967, Spock spent 12 years at Western Reserve University (now Case Western Reserve University) in Cleveland in the departments of psychiatry and pediatrics. Almost everywhere he went, he experienced some resistance from **physicians** uncomfortable with the psychoanalytic theories he used to supplement traditional medical norms.

In 1962 Spock joined the board of the National Committee for a Sane Nuclear Policy, prompted by his belief that the world's children were both physically and psychologically endangered by nuclear testing and the threat of nuclear war. It was just the beginning of Spock's life as a political activist. In 1968 he was convicted of conspiracy for his anti-Vietnam War activities, a conviction that later was overturned on appeal. In 1972, he ran for president, a candidate of the small People's Party. He received 80,000 votes in ten states.

Spock continued to write and speak, often about what he considered disturbing changes in society, such as increases in divorce, teen pregnancy, **suicide**, substance abuse, and violence. He remarried in 1976 to Mary Morgan, and she began to manage his speaking, writing, and consulting activities. Speaking with pride of his diverse career, all related to children's health, Spock said that people need to "realize that child care, the happiness of the family, the feelings of adults and children, and cultural and neighborhood activities are the most vital aspects of existence."

See also T. Berry Brazelton; Childcare; Child development

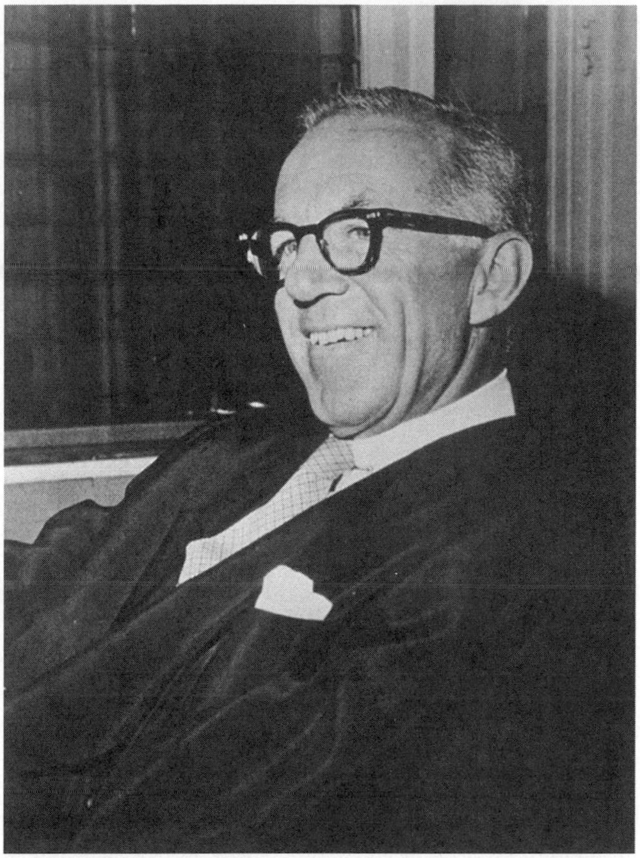

Benjamin Spock

SPORTS EDUCATION

Sports education is a form of **physical education** that emphasizes participation in sports as a way of developing skills, learning rules, practicing good sportsmanship, leading an active lifestyle, participating in a group, and learning leadership skills. Faced with cutbacks in physical education courses over the 1980s and 1990s, physical education teachers were often reduced to teaching sports skills apart from the actual game. Many teachers see sports education as a way of revitalizing physical education and making it more useful to students.

Sports education offers many features not present in standard physical education. By using seasons, teaching units that are two to three times longer than in physical education, sports education teachers have an opportunity to instruct in greater depth. Students are affiliated with a team throughout the semester, and all planning, practice, and competition is carried out in teams. Students find that sports are more meaningful in the context of the group effort and formal competition. Each season has a culminating event such as a championship, which gives students the opportunity to mark their progress. Record keeping is part of school sports as an effort to set standards, define goals, provide feedback, and set traditions. Teachers incorporate some sort of festivity into each season as an opportunity to celebrate effort, improvement, and fair play.

Sports education differs from institutionalized sports in many ways. Because of participation requirements, all students play at all times. Students are exposed to developmentally appropriate competition; adult forms of games are not used. Students learn the diverse roles inherent in sports competition, such as performer, referee, and scorekeeper. Depending on the season and the sport, they also have opportunities to serve as coach, manager, trainer, statistician, publicity officer, and sports board member. This gives students a better background to enjoy and participate in sports as adults. In addition, the teacher is relieved of some of the managerial responsibilities, enabling him or her to work more closely with students.

Sports education is set up so students can derive larger lessons in cooperation. A class may be divided into three teams, with two of the teams competing and members of the third team handling the diverse roles such as refereeing, then the teams rotate. Students benefit from peer teaching. Coaches lead skill practice, but because the students are organized in teams, they engage in peer teaching to help the team succeed. Because the season is longer than a physical education unit, teachers expect that conflicts will arise within teams and between teams; sportsmanship rules are enforced.

There are many advantages for students with low skills. They benefit from being part of the team and develop more confidence. In the longer season, they have more time to improve. At-risk students develop better social skills as a side benefit of learning sportsmanship and fair play. The ultimate goal of sports education is for students to become competent, literate, and enthusiastic in sports.

SPORTS INJURIES

Sports injuries are caused by sudden trauma or repetitive stress during athletic activities. Sports injuries can affect bones or ligaments, muscles, or tendons. Adults are less likely to suffer sports injuries than are children, who are more likely to hurt themselves because they:

- have immature reflexes
- can't recognize and judge risks
- aren't very coordinated

Each year, about 3.2 million children between the ages of 5 and 14 are injured while participating in athletic activities, accounting for 40% of all sports injuries. In fact, as many as 20% of children who play sports get hurt, and about one fourth of their injuries are considered to be serious. More than 775,000 boys and girls under age 14 are treated in hospital emergency rooms for sports-related injuries.

Injury rates are highest for athletes who play contact sports, but the most serious injuries are associated with individual activities. In any case, most of these childhood sports injuries occur during practice or during unorganized athletic activity.

The most common sports injury is a bruise caused when blood collects at the injured area and discolors the skin. Sprains account for a third of all sports injuries. A sprain is a partial or complete tear of a ligament (a strong band of tissue that connects bones to one another and steadies joints).

A strain is a partial or complete tear of a muscle or a tendon (strong connective tissue that links muscles to bones). Inflammation of a tendon (**tendinitis**) and inflammation of one of the fluid-filled sacs that allow tendons to move easily over bones (**bursitis**) is usually caused by minor stress that keeps bothering the same part of the body. These conditions often occur at the same time.

Fractures (usually the arm or leg) are another common sports-related injury. Sports activities rarely involve fractures of the spine or skull. The bones of the legs and feet are most susceptible to stress fractures, which occur when muscle strains make bones bend. Stress fractures are especially common in ballet dancers, long-distance runners, and in people whose bones are thin.

Shin splints are characterized by soreness and slight swelling of the front, inside, and back of the lower leg, and by sharp **pain** that develops and gradually gets stronger while exercising. Shin splints are caused by overuse or by stress fractures from repeated foot pounding associated with activities like aerobics, long-distance running, basketball, and volleyball.

A compartment syndrome is a potentially debilitating condition in which the muscles of the lower leg grow too large to be contained within membranes that enclose them. This condition is characterized by numbness and tingling. Untreated compartment syndrome can result in long-term disability.

Brain injury is the primary cause of fatal sports-related injuries. A **concussion**, which can occur even after a minor blow to the head, can cause loss of consciousness and may affect:

- Balance
- Comprehension
- Coordination
- Hearing
- Memory
- Vision.

Common causes of sports injuries include:

- Athletic equipment that malfunctions or is used incorrectly
- Falls
- Forceful high-speed collisions between players
- Wear and tear on areas of the body that are continually subjected to stress.

Symptoms include:

- Instability or obvious dislocation of a joint
- Pain
- Swelling
- Weakness.

Symptoms that persist, intensify, or reduce the athlete's ability to play without pain should be evaluated by an orthopedic surgeon. Prompt diagnosis can often prevent minor injuries from becoming major problems, or causing long-term or lasting damage.

An orthopedic surgeon should examine anyone:

- Who is prevented from playing by severe pain associated with acute injury
- Whose ability to play has declined due to chronic or long-term consequences of an injury
- Whose injury has caused visible deformities in an arm or leg.

The doctor will perform a **physical examination**, ask how the injury occurred, and what symptoms the patient has experienced. X rays and other tests may be ordered. Anyone who has suffered a blow to the head should be examined immediately, and at five-minute intervals afterwards until normal comprehension has returned. The initial examination measures the athlete's:

- Awareness
- Concentration

- Short-term memory

Follow-up evaluations of concussion test for:

- **Dizziness**
- **Headache**
- Nausea
- Visual disturbances.

Treatment for minor sports injuries generally consists of:

- Compressing the injured area with an elastic bandage.
- Elevation
- Ice
- Rest

Anti-inflammatory medications (such as ibuprofen) taken by mouth or as an injection into the swelling may be used to treat bursitis. Anti-inflammatory medications and **exercise**s to correct muscle imbalances are usually used to treat tendinitis. If the athlete keeps stressing inflamed tendons, they may rupture, and a cast or surgery is sometimes necessary to correct this condition. Orthopedic surgery may be needed to repair serious **sprains and strains**. Easing inflammation as well as restoring normal use and movement are the goals of treatment for overuse injuries.

Athletes who have been injured are usually advised to limit their activities until their injuries are healed. The doctor may suggest special exercises for athletes who have had several injuries. Athletes who have been severely injured may be advised to stop playing altogether.

Every child who plans to participate in organized athletic activity should have a pre-season sports physical. This special examination is performed by a pediatrician or family physician who:

- Carefully evaluates the site of any previous injury
- May recommend special stretching and strengthening exercises to help growing athletes create and preserve proper muscle and joint interaction
- Pays special attention to the cardiovascular and skeletal systems.

Telling the doctor which sport the athlete plays will help that physician determine which parts of the body will be subjected to the most stress. The doctor will then be able to suggest to the athlete steps to take to minimize the chance of getting hurt. Other injury-reducing game plans include:

- Being in shape
- Knowing and obeying the rules that regulate the activity
- Not playing when tired, ill, or in pain
- Not using steroids, which can improve athletic performance but cause life-threatening problems
- Taking good care of athletic equipment and using it properly
- Wearing appropriate protective equipment

SPORTS MEDICINE

Participation in sports can strengthen the body's **cardiovascular system**, improve stamina, and provide a sense of physical well-being. However, sports can also result in injury. Sports medicine concerns itself with preparing athletes to compete at an optimal level while avoiding injury, and with managing any injuries that do occur. Sports medicine practitioners can be both physicians and paramedical staff. In some cases, they are involved in developing helmets and other protective gear for athletes.

One of the earliest practitioners of sports medicine was the Greek physician Herodicus, who developed therapeutic diets and exercise regimes for athletes in the 5th century B.C. The first team physician was **Galen**, who in 157 trained and treated gladiators competing in public games. Despite these early examples, sports medicine did not come into its own until the 20th century. The first textbook on the subject was published in 1910, and the term ''sports medicine'' was coined in 1928, when 33 team physicians attending the Winter Olympics in St. Moritz, Switzerland, met to establish the International Assembly on Sports Medicine. The practice of ''doping''—trying to improve performance with drugs or other substances—was first reported in 1939, and the use of **anabolic steroids** to improve muscle mass and performance was first reported among Russian athletes in 1954. Athletes from numerous other nations quickly adopted the practice. The sports drink Gatorade was first used in 1965, in a test on the University of Florida football team, which achieved a winning season.

Performance in many sports has improved dramatically during the 20th century; however, the extent to which sports medicine has contributed to those improvements is subject to debate. In many cases, improved techniques and training methods were developed by the athletes themselves, with physiologists and other experts studying the developments after the fact. However, some improvements are directly attributable to sports medicine, including the benefits of carbohydrate-rich diets and proper fluid balance, which were discovered in basic research during the 1930s and 1940s.

Roger Bannister, the first human to run a sub-four-minute mile, was a medical student who studied the mechanics of running and developed a scientific training program. Bannister nonetheless seriously underestimated the capabilities of the human body. He believed that breaking the four-minute barrier would consume an athlete's oxygen reserve several yards before the finish line, and that he would have to complete the race in a semiconscious state. However, when Sebastian Coe ran the same distance in 3:49 in 1979, he was described as looking ''almost relaxed'' and ''hardly gasping.'' It is clear that the barriers to improved athletic performance are sometimes psychological.

Some of the principal advances made by sports medicine have been in the treatment of acute sports injuries. For example, techniques developed to treat shoulder problems including dislocations and problems with the rotator cuff and acromioclavicular joint proved so successful in athletes that they are now employed in mainstream medical practice.

Some injuries result from overuse and can be prevented by adjusting the athlete's training schedule or correcting bad technique. If no changes are made, permanent injury may follow, forcing retirement from the activity. Sometimes, rule changes can help. For example, junior baseball players in the United States may now make only a limited number of pitches per season, to prevent an overuse condition known as ''Little Leaguer's elbow.''

In recent years, there has been considerable interest in a variety of performance ''enhancers'' said to make athletes stronger, bigger, or faster.

Anabolic steroids, now disallowed in many sports, have been used by weight lifters and track-and-field athletes. They are similar to the natural hormone testosterone and can increase the size and strength of muscles. However, steroids also have serious side effects including heart disease, **liver cancer** or other liver damage, which far exceed any benefits obtained. It is worthwhile to observe that world records in the shot put were relatively stagnant during the late 1960s and 1970s, a period when many shot putters are believed to have used steroids. Similarly, growth hormone is believed both ineffective and dangerous, and is not permitted in many sports.

In 1999, Mark McGwire of the St. Louis Cardinals hit a record 70 home runs while using the supplements androstenedione and creatine. However, research results reported that same year found that androstenedione did not increase strength, but might instead promote heart disease, **cancer**, and enlarged breasts. Studies of athletes taking creatine have been inconclusive; some show minor improvements, others a detrimental effect. Long-term effects of the supplement are unknown.

Other so-called ''enhancers'' considered ineffective include ginseng, amino acids, coenzyme Q10, protein, and chromium picolinate.

One substance that may actually work is caffeine. Two cups of coffee taken before exercise has been shown to improve endurance. This effect does not occur during hot weather, and caffeine can be dangerous to persons who have heart disease.

Sprains and strains

Sprain refers to damage or tearing of ligaments or a joint. Strain refers to damage or tearing of a muscle.

When too much force is applied to a joint, the ligaments that hold the bones together may be torn or damaged. This causes a sprain, and its seriousness depends on how badly the ligaments are torn. Any joint can be sprained, but the most frequently injured joints are the ankle, knee, and finger.

Strains are tears in the muscle. Sometimes called ''pulled muscles,'' they usually occur because of overexertion or improper lifting techniques.

Children under age 8 are less likely to have sprains than are older people because their ligaments are tighter and their bones are more apt to break before a ligament tears. People who are active in sports suffer more strains and sprains than less active people. Repeated sprains in the same joint make the joint less stable and more prone to future sprains.

There are three types of sprains: Grade I sprains are mild injuries with no tearing of the ligament and no joint function is lost, although there may be tenderness and slight swelling.

Grade II sprains are caused by a partial tear in the ligament. These sprains have obvious swelling, extensive bruising, **pain**, problems bearing weight and in joint function.

Grade III sprains are caused by complete tearing of the ligament with severe pain, loss of joint function, widespread swelling and bruising, and the inability to bear weight. These symptoms are similar to those of bone **fractures**.

Strains can range from mild muscle stiffness to great soreness. Strains are caused by overusing or improperly using muscles, or by compensating for pain in another part of the body by changing the way it moves.

Patients don't need a doctor to diagnose Grade I sprains and mild strains, but Grade II and III sprains are often seen by a doctor to tell the difference between a sprain and a fracture.

Grade I sprains and mild strains can be treated at home. Basic first aid for sprains consists of RICE: Rest, Ice for 48 hours, Compression (wrapping in an elastic bandage), and Elevation of the sprain above the level of the heart. Over-the-counter pain medication such as **acetaminophen** (Tylenol) or ibuprofen (Motrin) will help.

In addition to RICE, people with grade II and grade III sprains in the ankle or knee usually need to use crutches until the sprains have healed enough to bear weight. Sometimes, physical therapy or home **exercise** is needed to restore the strength and flexibility of the joint.

Grade III sprains are usually immobilized in a cast for several weeks to see if the sprain heals. Pain medication is prescribed. Surgery may be necessary to relieve pain and restore function. Athletic people under age 40 are the most likely candidates for surgery, especially with grade III knee sprains. For complete healing, physical therapy usually will follow surgery.

Alternative practitioners endorse RICE and conventional treatments. In addition, nutritional therapists recommend vitamin C to supplement a diet high in whole grains, fresh fruits, and vegetables. If surgery is needed, alternative practitioners can recommend pre- and post-surgical therapies to enhance healing.

Moderate sprains heal within two to four weeks, but it can take months to recover from severe ligament tears. Until recently, tearing the ligaments of the knee meant the end to an athlete's career. Improved surgical and rehabilitation techniques now offer the possibility of complete recovery. However, once a joint has been sprained, it will never be as strong as it was before.

Sprains and strains can be prevented by warming up before exercising, using proper lifting techniques, wearing well-fit shoes, and taping or bracing the joint.

Sputum culture

Sputum is material coughed up from the lungs and spit out through the mouth. A sputum culture is done to find and identify the germ causing an infection such as **pneumonia** (an infection of the lung). If a specific germ is found, more testing is done to determine which antibiotic will best treat the infection.

A person with a **fever** and a continuing cough that produces pus-like material or blood may have an infection of the lungs and bronchial tubes. These infections are caused by several types of germs, including bacteria, fungi (molds and yeast), and viruses. A chest x ray helps a doctor see the infection; a culture can grow the germ causing the infection so it can be identified.

Based on the symptoms, the doctor decides what group of germ is probably causing the infection, and then orders one or more specific types of cultures: bacterial, viral, or fungal (for yeast and molds). For all culture types, the sputum must be carefully collected into a sterile container so that germs normally in the mouth don't contaminate the sample. Once in the laboratory, each culture type is handled differently.

A portion of the sputum is smeared on a microscope slide for a Gram stain. Another portion is spread over the surface of several different types of culture plates, and placed in an incubator at body temperature for one to two days.

To do a Gram stain test, the lab technician stains the slide with purple and red stain and examines it under a microscope. Gram staining makes sure the specimen doesn't contain saliva or material from the mouth. If there are many skin cells and few white blood cells, the specimen is not pure sputum and can't be cultured. The specimen may be rejected and a new specimen requested. If there are lots of white blood cells and bacteria of one type, this means there is an infection. The color of stain picked up by the bacteria (purple or red), the shape (such as round or rectangular), and the size provide valuable clues as to the bacteria's identity and helps the doctor predict what antibiotics might work best. Bacteria that stain purple are called gram-positive; those that stain red are called gram-negative.

During incubation, bacteria present in the sputum sample multiply and will appear on the plates as visible colonies. The bacteria are identified by their appearance, by the results of biochemical tests, and through a Gram stain of part of a colony.

A sensitivity test is also done to test which antibiotics will treat the infection by killing the bacteria.

The initial result of the Gram stain is available the same day, or in less than an hour if requested by the physician. An early report is usually available after one day, which will reveal if any bacteria have been found yet, and if so, their Gram stain appearance. The final report is usually available in one to three days, and includes complete identification and an estimate of the quantity of the bacteria and a list of the antibiotics to which they are sensitive.

A fungal culture is done to look for mold or yeast. The sputum sample is spread on special culture plates that will encourage the growth of mold and yeast. Different biochemical tests and stains are used to identify molds and yeast; cultures for fungi may take several weeks.

For a viral culture, sputum is mixed with commercially-prepared animal cells in a test tube. Characteristic changes to the cells caused by the growing virus help identify it. The time to complete a viral culture varies with the type of virus, but it may take from several days to several weeks.

Tuberculosis is caused by a slow-growing bacteria called *Mycobacterium tuberculosis*. Because it doesn't easily grow using routine culture methods, special procedures are used to grow and identify this bacteria. A small portion of the sputum is smeared on a microscope slide and stained with a special acid-fast stain. The stained sputum is examined under a microscope for tuberculosis organisms, which pick up the stain, making them visible. This smear can identify the bacteria within 24 hours.

To culture for tuberculosis, portions of the sputum are placed in tubes of broth that promote the growth of the organism; growth and identification may take two to four weeks.

Other microorganisms that cause various types of lower respiratory tract infections also require special culture procedures to grow and identify. *Mycoplasma pneumonia* causes a mild to moderate form of pneumonia, commonly called walking pneumonia; *Bordetella pertussis* causes **whooping cough**; *Legionella pneumophila*, Legionnaire's disease; *Chlamydia pneumoniae*, an atypical pneumonia; and *Chlamydia psittaci*, **parrot fever**.

*Pneumocystis carnii*causes pneumonia in people with weakened immune systems, such as people with **AIDS**. This organism does not grow in culture. Special stains are done on sputum for pneumonia caused by this organism. The diagnosis is based on the results of these stains, the patient's symptoms, and medical history.

The specimen for culture should be collected before antibiotics are started, since antibiotics may prevent germs in the sputum from growing in culture. The best time to collect a sputum sample is early in the morning, before the patient has anything to eat or drink. After rinsing the mouth with water to decrease mouth bacteria and dilute saliva, the patient must cough up sputum from within the chest. Taking deep breaths and lowering the head helps bring up the sputum. Sputum must not be held in the mouth but immediately spat into a sterile container. For tuberculosis, the doctor may want the patient to collect sputum samples on three consecutive mornings.

If coughing up sputum is difficult, a healthcare worker can have the patient breathe in sterile saline produced by a nebulizer. This nebulized saline coats the respiratory tract, loosening the sputum, and making it easier to cough up. Sputum may also be collected by a doctor.

If tuberculosis is suspected, collection of sputum should be carried out in an **isolation** room.

Sputum from a healthy person would have no growth on culture. A mixture of microorganisms, however, normally found in a person's mouth and saliva often contaminate the culture. If these microorganisms grow in the culture, they may be reported as normal flora contamination.

The presence of bacteria and white blood cells on the Gram stain and the isolation of a microorganism from culture is evidence of a lower respiratory tract infection.

Microorganisms commonly isolated from sputum include: *Streptococcus pneumoniae*, *Haemophilus influenzae*, *Staphylococcus aureus*, *Legionella pneumophila*, *Mycoplasma pneumonia*, *Klebsiella pneumoniae*, *Pseudomonas aeruginosa*, *Bordetella pertussis*, and *Escherichia coli*.

STAPHYLOCOCCAL INFECTIONS

Staphylococcal (staph) infections are communicable conditions caused by certain bacteria and generally characterized by the formation of **abscess**es. They are the leading cause of infections originating in hospitals in the United States.

Classified since the early 20th century as among the deadliest of all disease-causing organisms, staph exists on the skin or inside the nostrils of 20% to 30% of healthy people. The bacteria are sometimes found in breast tissue, the mouth, and the genital, urinary, and upper respiratory tracts.

Although staph bacteria are usually harmless, when injury or a break in the skin enables the organisms to invade the body and overcome the body's natural defenses, consequences can range from minor discomfort to **death**. Infection is most apt to occur in:

- Newborns
- Women who are breastfeeding
- Individuals whose immune systems have been impaired by radiation **chemotherapy**, or medication
- Intravenous drug users
- Those with surgical incisions, skin disorders, and serious illnesses such as **cancer**, diabetes, or lung disease.

Staph infections produce pus-filled pockets (abscesses) located just beneath the surface of the skin or deep within the body. The risk of infection is greatest among the very young and the very old.

A localized staph infection is confined to a ring of dead and dying white blood cells and bacteria. The skin above the infection feels warm to the touch. Most of these abscesses eventually burst, and the pus that leaks onto the skin can cause new infections.

A small fraction of localized staph infections enter the bloodstream and spread through the body. In children, these body-wide infections often affect the ends of the long bones of the arms or legs, causing a bone infection called **osteomyelitis**. When adults develop invasive staph infections, bacteria are most apt to cause abscesses of the brain, heart, kidneys, liver, lungs, or spleen.

Named for the golden color of the bacteria grown under laboratory conditions, *S. aureus* is a hardy organism that can survive in extreme temperatures or other inhospitable circumstances. About 70% to 90% of the population carry this strain of staph in the nostrils at some time. Although present on the skin of only 5% to 20% of healthy people, as many as 40% carry it elsewhere (such as in the throat, vagina, or rectum) for varying periods of time from hours to years without developing symptoms or becoming ill.

S. aureus flourishes in hospitals, where it infects staff and surgical patients; those who have skin irritations, insulin-dependent diabetes, kidney disease, or who receive frequent allergy-desensitization injections. Staph bacteria also can contaminate bedclothes, catheters, and other objects.

S. aureus causes a variety of infections. **Boils** and inflammation of the skin surrounding a hair shaft are the most common. Toxic shock (TSS) and scalded skin syndrome (SSSS) are among the most serious.

Toxic shock syndrome is a life-threatening infection characterized by severe **headache**, **sore throat**, **fever** as high as 105°F, and a **sunburn**-like rash that spreads from the face to the rest of the body. Symptoms appear suddenly; they also include **dehydration** and watery **diarrhea**.

Inadequate blood flow to peripheral parts of the body (shock) and loss of consciousness occur within the first 48 hours. Between the third and seventh day of illness, skin peels from the palms of the hands, soles of the feet, and other parts of the body. Kidney, liver, and muscle damage often occur.

Rare in adults and most common in newborns and other children under the age of five, scalded skin syndrome originates with a localized skin infection. A mild fever and/or an increase in the number of infection-fighting white blood cells may occur. A bright red rash spreads from the face to other parts of the body and eventually forms scales. Large, soft blisters develop at the site of infection and elsewhere. When they burst, they expose inflamed skin that looks as if it had been burned.

S. aureus can also cause:

- Arthritis
- Bacteria in the bloodstream
- Pockets of infection and pus under the skin
- Tissue inflammation that spreads below the skin, causing **pain** and swelling
- Inflammation of the valves and walls of the heart
- Inflammation of tissue that enclosed and protects the spinal cord and brain (**meningitis**)
- Inflammation of bone and bone marrow
- **Pneumonia**.

Capable of clinging to tubing (as in that used for intravenous feeding, etc.), prosthetic devices, and other non-living surfaces, *S. epidermidis* is the organism that most often contaminates devices that provide direct access to the bloodstream.

The primary cause of bacteremia in hospital patients, this strain of staph is most likely to infect cancer patients, whose immune systems have been compromised, and high-risk newborns receiving intravenous supplements.

S. epidermidis also accounts for two of every five cases of inflammation of prosthetic heart valves. This is a complication of the implantation of an artificial valve in the heart. Although contamination usually occurs during surgery, symptoms of infection may not become evident until a year after the operation. More than half of the patients who develop this condition die.

Existing within and around the urethra (the tube-like structure that carries urine from the bladder) of about 5% of healthy males and females, *S. saprophyticus* is the second most common cause of unobstructed urinary tract infections (UTIs) in sexually active young women. This strain of staph is responsible for 10% to 20% of infections affecting healthy outpatients.

Staph bacteria can spread through the air, but infection is almost always the result of direct contact with open sores or body fluids contaminated by these organisms. Staph bacteria often enter the body through inflamed hair follicles or oil glands. Or they penetrate skin damaged by **burns**, cuts and scrapes, infection, insect bites, or **wounds**.

Multiplying beneath the skin, bacteria infect and destroy tissue in the area where they entered the body. Staph infection of the blood develops when bacteria from a local infection infiltrate the lymph glands and bloodstream. These infections, which can usually be traced to contaminated catheters or intravenous devices, usually cause persistent high fever and sometimes shock. They also can cause death within a short time.

Common symptoms of staph infection include:

- Pain or swelling around a cut, or an area of skin that has been scraped
- Boils or other skin abscesses
- Blistering, peeling, or scaling of the skin. This is most common in infants and young children.
- Enlarged lymph nodes in the neck, armpits, or groin.

A family doctor should be notified whenever:

- Lymph nodes in the neck, armpits, or groin become swollen or tender
- An area of skin that has been cut or scraped becomes painful or swollen, feels hot, or produces pus. These symptoms may mean the infection has spread to the bloodstream.
- A boil or carbuncle appears on any part of the face or spine. Staph infections affecting these areas can spread to the brain or spinal cord.
- A boil becomes very sore. Usually a sign that infection has spread, this condition may be accompanied by fever, chills, and red streaks radiating from the site of the original infection.
- Boils which develop repeatedly. This type of recurrent infection could be a symptom of diabetes.

Blood tests that show very high concentrations of white blood cells can suggest a staph infection, but diagnosis is verified after lab analysis of material removed from pus-filled sores, and of normally-uninfected body fluids such as blood and urine. X-rays can help doctors find internal abscesses and estimate the severity of infection. Needle biopsy (removing tissue with a needle, then examining it under a microscope) may be used to find out if the bones are affected.

Mild staph infections can generally be cured by keeping the area clean, using soaps that leave a germ-killing film on the skin, and applying warm, moist compresses to the affected area for 20 to 30 minutes three or four times a day. Severe or recurrent infections may require a 7- to 10-day course of treatment with penicillin or other oral **antibiotics**. The precise antibiotic prescribed depends on the location of the infection and the type of bacteria involved

In case of a more serious infection, antibiotics may be administered intravenously for as long as six weeks. Intravenous antibiotics are also used to treat staph infections around the eyes or on other parts of the face. Surgery may be required to drain or remove abscesses that form on internal organs, or on shunts or other devices implanted inside the body.

Most healthy people who develop staph infections recover fully within a short time. Others develop repeated infections. Some become seriously ill, requiring long-term therapy or emergency care. A small percentage die.

Staphylococcal Scalded Skin Syndrome

Staphylococcal scalded skin syndrome (SSSS) is a disease caused by a type of bacteria in which large sheets of skin may peel away. It usually affects children under 5 (especially infants). Epidemics can occur in newborn nurseries when staff in those nurseries accidentally pass the causative bacteria between patients, but it also can strike others with weakened immune systems. This may include those with kidney disease, people undergoing **cancer chemotherapy**, organ transplant patients, and people with Acquired Immunodeficiency Syndrome (**AIDS**).

SSSS is caused by a type of bacteria called *Staphylococcus aureus* that produces a kind of chemical poison. While the bacteria itself doesn't spread throughout the body, it affects the skin by sending this toxin through the bloodstream.

SSSS begins with a small area of infection. In newborns, this may appear as a crusted area around the navel or the diaper area. In children between the ages of 1 and 6, a small red crusty bump appears near the nose or ear. The child may have no energy, and may have a **fever**. The skin becomes sensitive and uncomfortable, followed by a rash beginning as bright red patches around the original area of crusting. Blisters may appear, and the skin may look wrinkled. When the blisters pop, they leave pitted areas. Even gently touching these red patches of skin may cause them to peel away in jagged sheets. The skin below is shiny, moist, and bright pink. Within a day or two, the top layer of skin all over the body peels off in large sheets.

The danger of this illness lies in the fact that a different kind of bacteria may invade the raw areas of the skin and cause a serious bloodstream infection. A lot of body fluid is lost as the skin peels away, and the layer underneath dries out; **dehydration** is a danger at this point.

SSSS is usually diagnosed from the typical progression of symptoms in a child of this age. A sample of skin (skin **biopsy**) should be examined under a microscope, which will reveal a characteristic appearance.

Treatment involves applying a variety of lotions and creams to the skin to soothe the sensitive areas, and protect against drying and further moisture loss.

Most patients recover within 10 to 14 days without scarring in most patients. However, **death** may occur if severe dehydration or blood poisoning complicates the illness. About 3% of children die of these complications; about 50% of immunocompromised adults die of these complications.

As always, good hygiene can prevent the bacteria. In the event of an outbreak in a newborn nursery, staff members should have nasal smears taken to identify an adult who may be unknowingly carrying the bacteria and passing it on to the babies.

Starvation

Starvation is the result of a lack of nutrients needed for life to be maintained. Adequate nutrition includes two important parts — nutrients and calories. It's possible to eat what seems to be enough food without getting the required calories. For example, marasmus is the result of a diet that is deficient mainly in energy.

Starvation is caused by a number of factors. They include:

- Anorexia nervosa
- Fasting
- **Coma**
- **Stroke**
- Famine
- Poverty
- Severe gastrointestinal disease

Since the body will combat **malnutrition** by breaking down its own fat and eventually its own tissue, a whole host of symptoms can appear as starvation sets in.

Children who are chronically malnourished begin to grow much more slowly; anemia is the first sign to appear in an adult. Swelling of the legs is next as protein levels in the blood decrease. Loss of resistance to infection follows next, along with poor wound healing. There is also progressive weakness and difficulty swallowing, which may lead to inhaling food. At the same time, the signs of specific nutrient deficiencies may appear. Characteristic symptoms of starvation include:

- Shrinkage of vital organs, such as the heart, lungs, and ovaries or testes
- Chronic diarrhea
- Anemia
- Reduction in muscle mass
- Weakness
- Low body temperature
- Decreased ability to digest food
- Irritability
- Immune system problems
- Swelling
- Decreased sex drive

If the degree of malnutrition is severe, the intestines may not tolerate a fully balanced diet; in fact, they may not be able to absorb nutrients at all. Carefully prepared elemental diets or intravenous feeding is the first step in treatment. Gradually, solid foods are introduced and a daily diet of 5,000 calories or more is begun.

People can recover from severe degrees of starvation, but children may suffer from permanent **mental retardation** or growth defects if their lack of food was long and extreme.

Starzl, Thomas (1926-)

American surgeon

Thomas Starzl is a world-renowned transplant surgeon. He performed the first human liver transplant in 1963 and was a pioneer in kidney transplantation. He has continued his pioneering work by helping to develop better drugs to make human organ transplants safer and more successful. Starzl has also contributed to the fields of general and thoracic surgery and neurophysiology.

Thomas Earl Starzl was born on March 11, 1926, in Le Mars, Iowa, to Roman F. Starzl, the editor and publisher of the *Globe Post,* a local newspaper, and Anna Laura Fitzgerald Starzl. He was the second son and was followed by two younger sisters. He finished high school during World War II and enlisted in officers' training school at Westminster College in Fulton, Missouri, in 1944. After his discharge from military service, he entered the premedical program at Westminster College, graduating in 1947. After graduation he immediately returned home to care for his mother, who was suffering from breast cancer. She died less than two months later, on June 30.

In September 1947 he entered Northwestern University Medical School in Chicago. After completing three years of medical school, Starzl took a year off to do research with Dr. Horace W. Magoun, a professor of neuroanatomy. While in Magoun's laboratory, Starzl developed a recording technique to track deep brain responses to sensory stimuli. He and his advisor published the work, which continues to be cited, in 1951. His work in Magoun's laboratory earned him a Ph.D. degree in neurophysiology from Northwestern in 1952, the same year in which he received his M.D. Starzl also received an M.A. degree in anatomy from Northwestern.

Starzl enrolled in the prestigious surgical training program at Johns Hopkins University Hospital in Baltimore in 1952. During his time at Johns Hopkins he met and married Barbara J. Brothers of Hartville, Ohio. (The two had three children, Timothy, Rebecca and Thomas. The marriage ended in divorce in 1976, in part, Starzl admits, because of his nonstop work schedule.) Starzl stayed in the Johns Hopkins training program for four years, but left in anger when he learned he would not be offered the coveted position of chief resident. He went to Jackson Memorial Hospital in Miami for his fifth and final year as a resident. During this time he was attracted to the idea of liver transplantation. In an empty garage on the grounds of Jackson Memorial Hospital, Starzl set up a laboratory and began his research on the liver, doing experimental surgeries on dogs he obtained from the city pound. He developed a new technique for removing the liver, the first step in liver transplantation. He published his method, and it quickly became the worldwide standard.

In 1958 Starzl returned to Northwestern, where he had accepted a fellowship in thoracic surgery. He passed the thoracic surgery boards in 1959. More importantly, he received two awards to fund his experimental research. One was a five-year grant from the National Institutes of Health. The other was the prestigious Markle Scholarship, which persuaded him to remain in academic medicine. Starzl was a member of Northwestern's surgical faculty for four years. During that time, he further perfected techniques for liver transplantation.

Starzl accepted a position at the University of Colorado School of Medicine as an associate professor of surgery in 1962, believing it offered better opportunities to develop an active organ transplant program. In the late 1950s surgeons had begun to experiment with the first immune suppressive drugs to prevent the body from rejecting a transplanted organ. As a consequence, transplantations became possible for the first time. Despite his interest in liver transplantation, Starzl considered a human liver transplant to be too risky given current knowledge of immunosuppression. On March 27, 1962, Starzl performed his first kidney transplant operation in Denver. Starzl was to achieve considerable success in kidney transplantation, but his real target was the liver, and he soon turned to that challenge.

On March 1, 1963, five years before the surgeon Christiaan Neethling Barnard undertook the first human heart transplant, Starzl attempted the world's first liver transplant. His patient was a three-year-old boy named Bennie Solis born with an incomplete liver. The child did not survive the operation because of uncontrolled bleeding. Starzl was widely criticized because he failed in his attempt, but, undaunted, he tried again in May 1963. This time he gave his patient, a man with cancer of the liver, huge amounts of fibrinogen, a protein that forms blood clots. The operation appeared to be a success, but the patient died three weeks later from complications due to blood clotting.

During the next few years, Starzl worked to solve the problem of uncontrolled bleeding and tissue rejection. In 1964 he directed the first extensive trial of tissue matching ever attempted. In the early 1960s, the physician Paul Terasaki of the University of California at Los Angeles had developed a method for detection of tissue antigens, the agents responsible for organ rejection. This method began the field of human histocompatibility research, the search for compatible tissue types. These efforts made it possible to match organ donors and recipients. In addition, Starzl turned his attention to development of drugs that would block the immune system from rejecting a new organ.

In the late 1960s Starzl was ready to attempt liver transplantation once again. This time all the attempts were on infants and young children with severe liver disease, and a number of them were successful, although some of the patients who survived the operation died from unrelated illnesses not too long afterwards. By the late 1970s the survival rate for liver transplants had risen to 40 percent.

During the 1970s and early 1980s Starzl's career reputation skyrocketed. He was promoted to professor of surgery at the University of Colorado in 1964 and was made chairman of the department in 1972. During the late 1970s Starzl was wooed by the University of California at Los Angeles to move his transplantation program there. But he finally settled on the University of Pittsburgh and moved there in 1981. The same year he married Joy Conger, who had been a research technician working on a project with Starzl in Denver.

In the early 1980s the availability of cyclosporin, a new, superior drug to prevent organ rejection, was an encouraging sign to Starzl that the survivor rate for liver transplantation could be raised. However, bureaucratic roadblocks were in the way of using cyclosporin and other promising new drugs in organ transplant operations other than kidney transplantations because they were considered by the federal government to be experimental. Starzl took the problem to the then-acting U.S. Surgeon General C. Everett Koop. Koop suggested Starzl appear before a government committee at the National Institutes of Health that could approve the operation. Starzl assembled a group of children who had survived liver transplants performed in the 1970s and early 1980s. They served as witnesses to the value of the operation, and after much testimony the committee approved liver transplantation as a service to mankind.

What followed was a rush by surgeons to begin performing the operation. All came to learn from Starzl and the physicians he had trained, who were scattered across the country. At the same time it became clear that the country needed a national system of organ procurement and distribution. Starzl worked diligently to get a bill passed by Congress in 1984 that would set up such as system. Starzl designed the system at the University of Pittsburgh, which became the national standard.

Starzl also enhanced his fame by directing a series of multiple-organ transplants in these years. In 1984 a young child received a heart and liver in a single operation, while a young woman received a heart, liver and kidney in 1986. Starzl's attempts to transplant baboon livers into human patients remained controversial into the late 1980s, however. He had experimented with such transplantations since the early 1960s, performing the first successful one in 1989. The patient was dying from hepatitis B, to which baboon livers do not appear to be susceptible. Although the operation was initially successful, a surgical error caused a fatal infection some three weeks later. Although some people objected to the use of animals for "spare parts," a major controversy arose over the fact that the patient had been HIV positive. Virtually all medical centers take the position that organ transplants, which require a suppression of the immune system, are inappropriate for patients who have been infected with the virus that also attacks the immune system.

In 1990 Starzl underwent coronary bypass surgery himself, and shortly afterwards retired from active surgery. He now concentrates his efforts on research. He claims that the decision was motivated in part by his emotional involvement with patients, which made the surgeries particularly difficult and stressful for him.

Over the years, Starzl has won many awards and honors and has been awarded many honorary degrees, including a merit Award from Northwestern University in 1969, a Distinguished Achievement Award in Modern Medicine in 1969, Colorado Man of Year Award in 1967, David Hume Memorial Award from the National Kidney Foundation in 1978, and Pittsburgh Man of the Year Award in 1981. Starzl has written hundreds and hundreds of scientific papers, averaging fifty papers a year during the 1980s.

Stensen, Niels (1638-1686)

Danish geologist and anatomist

Niels Stenson, also known as Nicalaus Steno, was born in Copenhagen on January 1, 1638, and died in Schwerin, northern Germany in 1686. The son of a well-to-do goldsmith, Steno studied first in Copenhagen, where one of his teachers was the anatomist, Thomas Bartholin. In 1660, he began his travels and studies abroad; besides Copenhagen, he lived and studied in Paris, Amsterdam, Leyden, and Florence. While in Amsterdam, he discovered the parotid salivary duct (ductus Stenorzianus). After four years in Leyden, he returned to Copenhagen, but finding no post for him there, he went to Paris, where he made important observations on the anatomy of the brain. He arrived in Florence in 1665, where he became interested in geology after dissecting of the head of a shark and recognizing that the shark's teeth resembled certain unidentified fossils found from Tuscany (he concluded that the fossils were actually fossilized teeth). Steno went on to publish his findings in his treatise of 1669, entitled *De solido intra solidum*, which made significant contributions to the incipient field of geology. In 1672, Steno returned to Copenhagen, where he gave anatomical demonstrations for a while. In 1674, he returned to Florence. In the last decade of his life Steno completely abandoned science and devoted himself exclusively to missionary work, residing in various towns of northern Germany until his death. As a cleric he is remembered primarily for his conversion from Lutheranism in 1667 to become a priest (1675), and later vicar apostolic (1677). An international group of geologists erected a bust over his tomb in 1883.

As a scientist, Steno is remembered for his discoveries in geology, particularly for his observations of fossils, geologic strata, and crystallization; and in human anatomy, for his studies of the heart, muscles, brain and glands. Steno showed that a pineal gland like that found in man is also found in other animals, and used this observation plus other arguments to refute Descartes' claim that the pineal gland is the seat of the soul and uniquely human. He made a distinction between the glands and the lymph nodes, which are not part of the glandular system anatomically. He also confirmed Malpighi's theories on the incubation of the ovum in humans, and described the essential structure of the heart. He demonstrated that the long-held notion that tears arise in the brain was wrong, and in 1661, discovered (in sheep) the excretory duct of the parotid gland (one of two identical salivary glands), which is now known as the duct of Steno. In the same year he investigated the glands of the **eye**, and in 1664 he made observations on muscles and glands that contributed to recognition of the muscular nature of the heart. In 1667, Steno treated the physiology of muscles from a purely mechanical and mathematical point of view. His work with a microscope led him to describe the muscles as parallelepiped bundles of fascicles, subdivided into minute fibrils, with the tendon a tetragonal prism. He described contraction as a total response of a muscle to all of the tensile forces developed in each unit. His Paris discourse of 1669 argued that it is idle to speculate about the functions of the brain without knowing more about its structure.

Steptoe, Patrick (1913-1988)

English gynecologist

Patrick Steptoe, an English gynecologist and medical researcher, helped develop the technique of in vitro fertilization. In this process, a mature egg is removed from the female ovary and is fertilized in a test tube. After a short incubation period, the fertilized egg is implanted in the uterus, where it develops as in a typical pregnancy. This procedure gave women whose fallopian tubes were damaged or missing, and were thus unable to become pregnant, the hope that they too could conceive children. Steptoe and his colleague, English physiologist Robert G. Edwards, received international recognition—both positive and negative—when the first so-called test tube baby was born in 1978.

Patrick Christopher Steptoe was born on June 9, 1913 in Oxfordshire, England. His father was a church organist, while his mother served as a social worker. Steptoe studied medicine at the University of London's St. George Hospital Medical School and, after being licensed in 1939, became a member of the Royal College of Surgeons. His medical career, though, was interrupted by World War II. Steptoe volunteered as a naval surgeon, but he and his shipmates were captured by Italian forces in 1941 after their ship sank in the Battle of Crete. Initially granted special privileges in prison because he was a physician, Steptoe was placed in solitary confinement after officials detected his efforts to help fellow prisoners escape. Steptoe left the prison camp via a prisoner exchange in 1943. Following the war, Steptoe completed additional studies in obstetrics and gynecology. In 1948 he became a member of the Royal College of Obstetricians and Gynecologists and moved to Manchester to set up a private practice. In 1951 Steptoe began working at Oldham General and District Hospital in northeast England.

While at Oldham General and District Hospital, Steptoe pursued his interest in fertility problems. He developed a method of procuring human eggs from the ovaries by using a laparoscope, a long thin telescope replete with fiber optics light. After inserting the device—through a small incision in the navel—into the inflated abdominal cavity, Steptoe was able to observe the reproductive tract. Eventually the laparoscope would become widely used in various types of surgery, including those associated with sterility. But, at first, Steptoe had trouble convincing others in the medical profession of the merits of laparoscopy; observers from the Royal College of Obstetricians and Gynecologists considered the technique fraught with difficulties. Five years passed before Steptoe published his first paper on laparoscopic surgery.

In 1966 Steptoe teamed with Cambridge University physiologist Robert G. Edwards to propel his work with fertility problems. Utilizing ovaries removed for medical reasons, Edwards had pioneered the fertilization of eggs outside of the body. With his laparoscope, Steptoe added the dimension of being able to secure mature eggs at the appropriate moment in the monthly cycle when fertilization would normally occur. A breakthrough for the duo came in 1968 when Edwards successfully fertilized an egg that Steptoe had extracted. Not until 1970, however, was an egg able to reach the stage of cell division—into about 100 cells—when it generally moves to the uterus. In 1972 the pair attempted the first implantation, but the embryo failed to lodge in the uterus. Indeed, none of the women with implanted embryos carried them for a full trimester.

As their work progressed and word of it leaked out, the researchers faced criticism from scientific and religious circles concerning the ethical and moral issues relating to tampering with the creation of human life. Some opponents considered the duo's work akin to the scenario in Aldous Huxley's 1932 work, *Brave New World,* in which babies were conceived in the laboratory, cloned, and manipulated for society's use. Members of Parliament demanded an investigation and sources of funds were withdrawn. A *Time* reporter quoted Steptoe as saying, "All I am interested in is how to help women who are denied a baby because their tubes are incapable of doing their small part." Undaunted, Steptoe and Edwards continued their work at Kershaw's Cottage Hospital in Oldham, with Steptoe financing the research by performing legal abortions. Disturbed with the criticism, Steptoe and Edwards became more secretive, which made the speculation and criticism more intense.

In 1976 Steptoe met thirty-year-old Leslie Brown, who experienced problems with her fallopian tubes. Steptoe removed a mature egg from her ovary, and Edwards fertilized the egg using her husband Gilbert's sperm. The fertilized egg—implanted after two days—thrived, and on July 25, 1978, Joy Louise Brown, a healthy five pound twelve ounce girl was born in Oldham District and General Hospital. Even before the birth, reporters and cameramen congregated outside of the four story brick hospital, hoping for a glimpse of the expectant mother. After the birth, according to an article in *Time,* headlines in Britain heralded "OUR MIRACLE and BABY OF THE CENTURY."

Steptoe and Edwards were reluctant to discuss the procedures in press conferences and did not immediately publish their findings in a medical journal. In October of 1978, Steptoe was to receive an award from the Barren Foundation, a fertility research organization based in Chicago. The foundation suddenly cancelled the presentation because Steptoe and Edwards had not published an article on the event. As reported in a 1978 issue of *Time,* Steptoe called the foundation's action "the most utterly disgraceful exhibition of bad manners I've come across in the scientific world." In addition, rumors that the pair had sold their story to the tabloid the *National Enquirer* for a six figure amount were rampant. Steptoe declared that he rejected such offers and did not make any money on the highly publicized birth. Despite the furor, the New York Fertility Society subsequently presented Steptoe with an achievement award.

As to the claim of publishing, Steptoe answered that most scientists do not publish until several months after data is in and research complete. The procedures were fully presented at the January 26, 1979 meeting of the Royal College of Obstetricians and Gynecologists and at the conference of the American Fertility Society in San Francisco. Steptoe reported that with modified techniques, ten percent of the in vitro fertilization attempts could succeed. He further predicted that there could one day be a fifty percent success rate for the procedure.

In the aftermath of the first successful test tube baby, Steptoe received thousands of letters from couples seeking help in conception. He retired from the British National Health Service and constructed a new clinic near Cambridge. For their efforts, Steptoe and Edwards were both named Commanders of the British Empire, and in 1987 Steptoe was honored with fellowship in the Royal Society. Steptoe and his wife, a former actress, had one son and one daughter. His interests outside of medicine included piano and organ, cricket, plays, and opera. Steptoe died of cancer on March 21, 1988, in Canterbury. Yet, since the birth of baby Brown and the pioneering techniques of Steptoe, couples with various physiological problems have had children in clinics throughout the world.

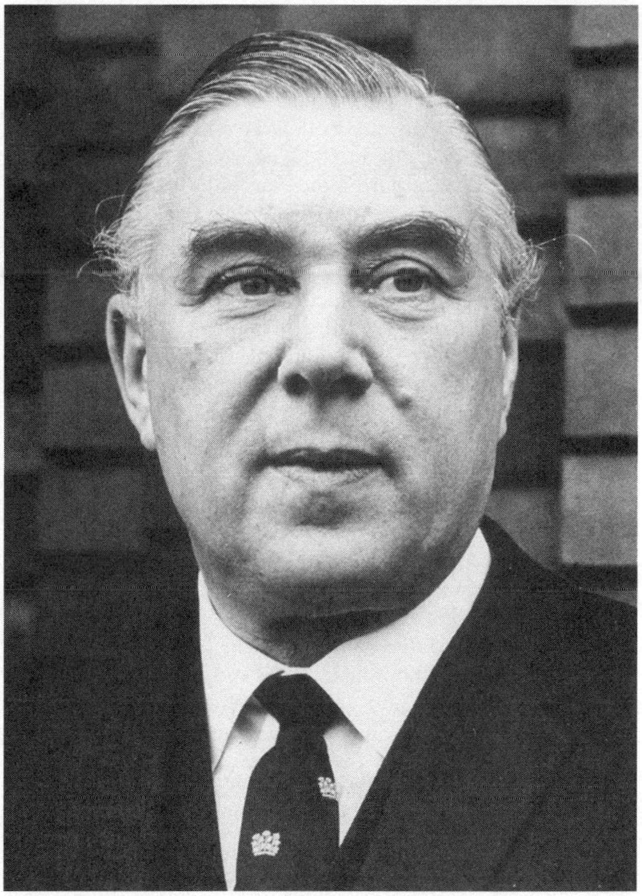

Patrick Steptoe

STERNBERG, GEORGE MILLER (1838-1915)

American physician and bacteriologist

George Miller Sternberg was born June 8, 1838 at Hartwick Seminary, Ostego County, New York. He died on November 3, 1915 in Washington, D.C. He was the son of Levi Sternberg, a Lutheran clergyman, and Margaret Levering Sternberg. In 1865, he married Louisa Russell, and in 1869, Martha L. Pattison (no children). He received his M.D. degree in 1860 from the College of Physicians and Surgeons at Columbia University. From 1860 to 1861, he practiced medicine in Elizabeth, New Jersey. From 1861 to 1902, he served with the U.S. Army Medical Corps (rising in rank from assistant surgeon to brigadier general). From 1861 to 1865 (during the Civil War), he assumed field and hospital duties. From 1865 to 1879, he served at various army posts during the Indian campaigns and **cholera** and **yellow fever** epidemics. In 1879, he was a member and secretary of the Havana Yellow Fever Commission of the National Board of Health. In 1898, he was placed in command of the medical service during the war with Spain. In 1885, he served as president of the American **Public Health** Association.

Sternberg is largely responsible for introducing Americans to the work of Louis Pasteur and Robert Koch; he also made pioneering bacteriological investigations of his own, publishing an important treatise in 1892. He announced the discovery of diplococcus of **pneumonia** in 1880, almost simultaneously with Pasteur. He was the first American researcher to demonstrate the protozoan responsible for **malaria** (1885), and the bacilli of **tuberculosis** and **typhoid fever** (1886). He and Koch began the scientific study of disinfection; he published a valuable treatise on the subject in 1900. He made advances in the field of photomicrography, and published a manual that became the authoritative American work on the subject. He started the Army Medical School in 1893. He organized the army's nurse and dental corps. In 1898, he established the Typhoid Fever Board, which demonstrated the importance of flies and contact infection in the spread of typhoid. He organized and supported Walter Reed's Yellow Fever Commission in Cuba (1900), which proved that the causative agent of yellow fever was transmitted by the *Aedes aegypti* mosquito. He was one of the first to show that viruses in people could be tracked by the antibodies they produced. Among Sternberg's writings are ''A Fatal Form of Septicemia in the Rabbit, Produced by the Subcutaneous Injection of Human Saliva,'' *Reports of the National Board of Health*, No. 3 (1881), 87-92; *Photomicrographs and How to Make Them* (1883); ''Disinfection and Individual prophylaxis Against Infectious Diseases,'' *The Lomb Prize Essays* (1886), 99-136; *A Manual of Bacteriology* (1892).

See also Military medicine

STETHOSCOPE

The stethoscope is an instrument for listening to sounds inside the human body for diagnostic purposes. Until the stethoscope was invented, clinical examination of patients was largely limited to external observations.

Medical knowledge about the inside of a patient's body took its first important step forward when Leopold Auenbrugger (1722-1809), a Viennese doctor, developed a technique he called percussion. Auenbrugger tapped on his patient's chest and then analyzed the different sounds to tell what conditions existed inside the chest. He published his findings in a 1761 pamphlet, which was ignored by the medical profession.

In the early 180Os, Jean Nicholas Covisart (1755-1821), Napoleon Bonaparte's personal physician, espoused Auenbrugger's percussion technique and translated the doctor's pamphlet into French. Covisart encouraged one of his students, Rene Theophile Laennec (1781-1826), to study acoustic diagnosis.

Laennec invented the stethoscope in 1816 during an examination of a young woman with a heart affliction. Due to both the patient's stoutness and prevailing standards of modesty, Laennec was unable to put his ear to the woman's chest. In a burst of inspiration, Laennec rolled a sheaf of paper tightly into a tube, placed one end of the tube over the patient's heart, and listened from the other end. The doctor later wrote, ''I was both surprised and gratified at being able to hear the beating of the heart with much greater clarity and distinctness than I had ever done before by direct application of my ear.''

Later, Laennec developed a wooden stethoscope. When his book describing his instrument and the diagnoses to be made with it appeared in 1819, the publisher gave a stethoscope to each purchaser of the book.

As the stethoscope came into standard use, promoted especially by the Austrian doctor Joseph Skoda (1805-1881), some modifications were made. Pliable tubing was introduced in 1850, the American doctor George P. Cammann developed a binaural stethoscope in 1852, and the electronic stethoscope appeared in 1980. Although advanced diagnostic tools such as CAT scans have reduced the importance of the stethoscope, it remains a valuable and widely used instrument.

STEVENS, NETTIE MARIA (1861-1912)

American cytogeneticist

Nettie Maria Stevens was born in Cavendish, Vermont, on July 7, 1861. She was an outstanding student, who finished high school during a time when most women never even reached that educational level. Still, her career opportunities were limited. Stevens earned her living as a school teacher and librarian, as did most unmarried women in the late 1800s. But unwilling to spend her whole life teaching high school, she sought further education. Since most universities did not admit women, she enrolled in Westfield Normal School, a teacher's college. After earning her certificate, she spent the next thirteen years working and saving in hopes of attending one of the country's few co-ed universities.

In 1896, she entered Stanford University in California, where Stevens received her master's degree in 1900. She was eventually attracted to Bryn Mawr College, where she conducted her postgraduate work under **Thomas Hunt Morgan**. (Another distinguished member of the faculty, Edmund Wilson, left the staff just before Stevens arrived.) Morgan, impressed with Stevens's brilliant work as a first-year student, helped her get a fellowship to study abroad. Her work in Germany with Thomas Boveri on the role of chromosomes in heredity helped prepare the way for her later contributions to science.

Upon her return to the United States in 1904, Stevens won a grant from the Carnegie Institute that allowed her to do original research. At this time, despite all the chromosome observations, experiments, and theories, no one knew for certain how the sex of a baby was determined. Stevens decided to find out. In her studies with mealworms, she observed that there were distinct differences in the chromosomes of a male versus the chromosomes of a female. Upon further study, she found a perfect correlation between sex and chromosome type. The females always carried two X chromosomes, but males produced either a large X chromosome or small Y chromosome. If an egg were fertilized with sperm carrying the male's X chromosome, it would produce a female. If it were fertilized with the male's Y chromosome, it would produce a male. Stevens published her findings on May 23, 1905. However, Wilson knew of Steven's work and was simultaneously conducting similar research. Wilson's paper, which essentially reached the same conclusions, was dated May 5, 1905, but was not published until August. Still, Wilson is usually given sole credit for the discovery, although he continued to acknowledge Stevens's work throughout his career.

Stevens remained at Bryn Mawr as a professor and researcher until her death of breast **cancer**. She died in Baltimore on May 4, 1912.

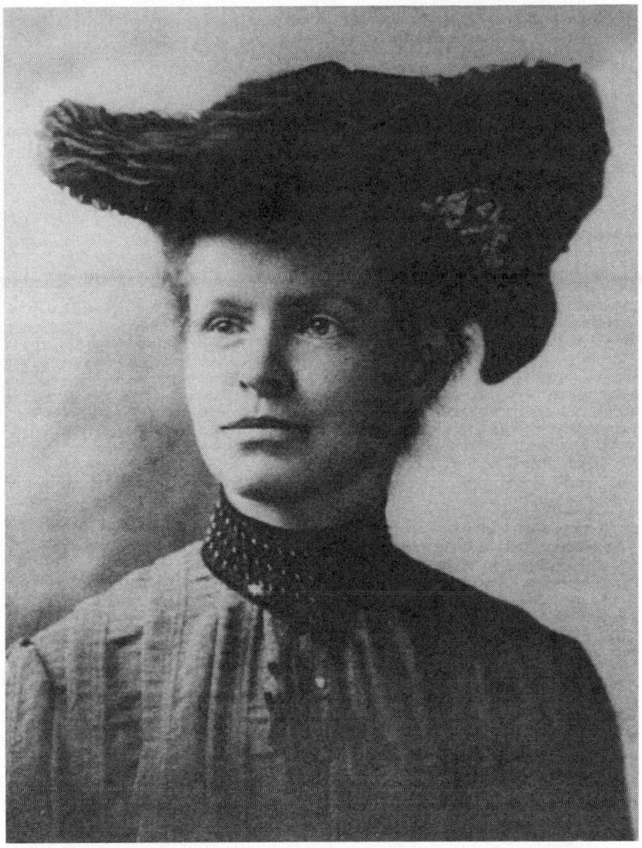

Nettie Maria Stevens

Stomach cancer

Stomach cancer is a disease in which the cells forming the inner lining of the stomach become abnormal and start to divide uncontrollably, forming a mass or a tumor. The stomach is a J-shaped organ that lies in the abdomen, on the left side. The esophagus (or the food pipe) carries the food from the mouth to the stomach. The stomach produces many digestive juices and acids that mix with the food and aid in the process of digestion. The stomach is divided into five sections. Cancer can develop in any of the five sections of the stomach.

While the exact cause for stomach cancer has not been identified, having poor nutritional habits, eating a lot of cured, pickled or smoked foods, eating foods high in starch and low in fiber, smoking, drinking alcohol, and **vitamin A deficiency** are believed to be risk factors for stomach cancer. Chronic (long-term) infection of the stomach with a bacterium (Helicobacter pylori) may lead to a particular type of cancer (lymphomas or mucosa-associated lymphoid tissue (MALT)) in the stomach. People who have had previous stomach surgery for ulcers or other conditions may have a higher likelihood of developing stomach cancers. Another risk factor is developing polyps (benign growths) in the lining of the stomach. Although polyps are not cancerous, some may have the potential to turn cancerous.

Stomach cancer is a slow-growing cancer and it can be years before it grows very large and produces distinct symptoms. In the early stages of the disease, the patient may only have mild discomfort, **indigestion**, heartburn, a bloated feeling after eating, and mild nausea. In the advanced stages, a patient will have loss of appetite and resultant weight loss, stomach **pain**s, vomiting, and blood in the stool. Stomach cancer often spreads (metastasizes) to adjoining organs such as the esophagus, adjacent lymph nodes, liver, or colon.

When a doctor suspects stomach cancer from the symptoms described by the patient, a thorough **physical examination** will be conducted to assess all the symptoms. Laboratory tests may be ordered to check for blood in the stool.

More specific tests such as a barium x ray of the upper gastrointestinal tract may be ordered. In this test, the patient is given a chalky, white solution of barium sulfate to drink. This solution coats the esophagus, the stomach, and the small intestine. Multiple x rays are then taken to identify any abnormalities in the lining of the stomach. In another test known as ''upper endoscopy,'' a thin, flexible, lighted tube (endoscope) is passed down the patient's throat. The doctor can view the lining of the esophagus and the stomach through the tube. If any suspicious-looking patches are seen, some of the tissue is collected for microscopic examination. This is known as a biopsy.

The three standard modes of treatment available for stomach cancer include surgery, **radiation therapy**, and **chemotherapy**. In the early stages of stomach cancer, surgery may be used to remove the cancer. If the cancer is too widespread and cannot be removed by surgery, an attempt will be made to remove blockage and control symptoms such as pain or bleeding. Depending on the location of the cancer, either the proximal portion or the distal part of the stomach may be removed. In a surgical procedure known as total gastrectomy, the entire stomach may be removed. Patients who have had parts of their stomachs removed can lead normal lives. Even when the entire stomach is removed, the patients quickly adjust to a different eating schedule. This involves eating small quantities of food more frequently. High protein foods are generally recommended.

Chemotherapy involves administering anti-cancer drugs either intravenously (through a vein in the arm) or orally (in the form of pills). This can either be used as the primary mode of treatment or after surgery to destroy any cancerous cells that may have migrated to distant sites. Radiation therapy is often used after surgery to destroy the cancer cells that may not have been completely removed during surgery.

By avoiding many of the risk factors associated with the disease, it is possible to prevent many stomach cancers. Excessive amounts of salted, smoked, and pickled foods should be avoided. A diet that is high in fiber and low in fats and starches is believed to lower the risk of several cancers. The American Cancer Society recommends eating at least five servings of fruits and vegetables daily and choosing six servings of food from other plant sources, such as grains, pasta, beans, cereals, and whole grain bread.

Stomach Flushing

Stomach flushing is a technique in which fluids are repeatedly pumped in and out of the stomach through a tube from the nose into the stomach. It's done to help control bleeding in the stomach or intestines, or to remove poisons from the stomach.

Bleeding from the esophagus from a ruptured vein, or from the stomach due to **ulcers** is a medical emergency. In an attempt to stop the bleeding, the stomach is flushed with lots of warm saline solution or ice water. This procedure is also known as gastric lavage or "stomach pumping."

Not all experts accept the use of stomach flushing to control bleeding becuase they believe it doesn't do much good and can create unnecessary risks. The procedure is usually done while giving drugs to constrict the blood vessels.

At one time, stomach flushing was a common way to remove certain poisons from the stomach, but today the American Academy of Clinical Toxicology advises against using stomach flushing routinely with poisoned patients. The technique is useful only if it can be done within an hour of swallowing a life-threatening quantity of poison. The stomach should not be flushed if the poison was a strong acid, alkali (such as lye or ammonia), or a substance such as gasoline. Anyone who is having convulsions should not have the stomach flushed.

Stomach flushing is performed in a hospital emergency room or intensive care unit by an emergency room doctor. After the tube is inserted through the nose into the stomach, small amounts of saline or ice water is pumped into the stomach and withdrawn. The procedure is repeated until the withdrawn fluid is clear.

Little preparation is needed for this procedure other than explaining the procedure to the patient.

After stomach flushing, the patient will be monitored. If necessary, additional treatment to prevent gastrointestinal bleeding or poisoning will be done.

There are a number of problems with the procedure. In poisoning cases, it delays the administration of activated charcoal, which may be more helpful. The procedure may speed up bleeding from the esophagus or stomach. The patient may inhale some of the stomach contents, which can cause a lung infection. Fluid and electrolyte imbalances are more likely to occur in older, sicker patients; damage to the throat is more likely in uncooperative patients.

Stomatitis

Stomatitis is an inflammation of the mucous lining of any of the parts of the mouth, including the cheeks, gums, tongue, lips, and roof or floor of the mouth. The word "stomatitis" literally means "inflammation of the mouth." This inflammation can be caused by conditions in the mouth itself, such as poor **oral hygiene**, poorly fitted dentures, mouth **burns** from hot food or drinks, or by conditions that affect the entire body, such as medications, allergic reactions, or infections.

Stomatitis is usually a painful condition, with redness, swelling, bleeding, or **bad breath**. Stomatitis affects all age groups, from the infant to the elderly.

A number of factors can cause stomatitis. Poorly fitted oral appliances, cheek biting, or jagged teeth can irritate the mouth. Chronic breathing through the mouth becuase of clogged nasal passages can dry the mouth, which can lead to irritation. Diseases such as cold sores, **gonorrhea**, **measles**, **AIDS**, and lack of vitamin C can cause stomatitis.

Canker sores are a specific type of stomatitis that causes shallow, painful ulcers usually located on the lips, cheeks, gums, or roof or floor of the mouth. These ulcers can range from pinpoint size to up to an inch or more. Though the cause of canker sores is unknown, nutritional deficiencies (especially vitamin B_{12}, folate, or iron) is suspected.

Generalized stomatitis can be caused by too much alcohol, spices, hot food, or tobacco products. Sensitivity to mouthwashes, toothpastes, and lipstick can irritate the lining of the mouth. Exposure to heavy metals, such as mercury, lead, or bismuth can cause stomatitis. Thrush (a type of fungal infection) is also a type of stomatitis.

It can be hard to diagnose stomatitis. A doctor will conduct a **physical examination** to evaluate the oral lesions and other skin problems. Blood tests or scrapings of the lining of the mouth may be evaluated in a culture or under a microscope to identify any infections.

The treatment of stomatitis is based on the problem causing it, but good oral hygiene is fundamental. Sharp-edged foods such as peanuts, tacos, and potato chips should be avoided. A soft-bristled toothbrush should be used to brush teeth and gums carefully without banging the toothbrush into the gums. Ill-fitting dental appliances or sharp-edged teeth can be corrected by a dentist. An infection can usually be treated with medication. Illnesses such as AIDS, leukemia, and anemia are treated by the appropriate medical specialist. Minor mouth burns from hot beverages or hot foods will usually get better on their own in a week or so. Chronic problems with canker sores are treated by first correcting any deficiencies of vitamin B_{12}, iron, or folate. If this is unsuccessful, a few patients may find relief with prescription medication applied to each ulcer with a cotton-tipped swab.

The herb calendula (*Calendula officinalis*), as an alcohol-based herbal extract and diluted for a mouth rinse can be quite effective in treating canker sores and other types of stomatitis.

The prognosis for stomatitis is based on the cause of the problem. Infectious causes of stomatitis can usually be managed with medication, or, if the problem is being caused by a certain drug, by changing the offending agent.

Stomatitis caused by local irritants can be prevented by good oral hygiene, regular dental checkups, and good dietary habits. Problems with stomatitis caused by disease can be minimized by good oral hygiene and closely following the medical therapy prescribed by the patients health care provider.

Stool Culture

Stool culture is a test to identify bacteria in patients with a suspected infection of the digestive tract. A sample of the patient's feces is placed in a special medium where bacteria is then grown. The bacteria that grow in the culture are identified using a microscope and biochemical tests.

Stool culture is used to identify bacteria or other germs in people with symptoms of stomach or intestinal infection, most often **diarrhea**. Identification of the organism is necessary to determine how to treat the patient's infection.

Stool culture is only performed if an infection of the digestive tract is suspected. The test has no harmful effects.

Stool culture also may be called fecal culture. To obtain a specimen for culture, the patient is asked to collect a stool sample into a special sterile container that may contain a solution. Specimens may need to be collected on three consecutive days. It is important to return the specimen to the doctor's office or the laboratory in the time specified by the doctor or nurse. Labs don't accept stool specimens contaminated with water, urine, or other materials.

The culture test involves placing a sample of the stool on a special substance called a medium that provides nutrients for certain organisms to grow and reproduce. The medium is usually a thick gel-like substance. The culture is done in a test tube (or on a flat round culture plate) which is kept at the proper temperature so bacteria can grow. After bacteria begin to grow in the medium, they are identified by observing physical characteristics and microscopic features. The bacteria may be dyed with special stains that make it easier to identify their features.

The length of time needed to perform a stool culture depends on the lab where it is done and the culture methods used. Stool culture usually takes 72 hours or longer to complete, but some organisms may take several weeks to grow in a culture.

An antibiotic sensitivity test may be done after a bacteria is identified to show which **antibiotics** will work the best in treating the infection.

Although most intestinal infections are caused by bacteria, in some cases a fungal or viral culture may be necessary.

Several intestinal parasites may cause gastrointestinal infection and diarrhea. Parasites are not cultured, but are identified microscopically in a test called ''Stool Ova and Parasites.''

Insurance coverage for stool culture may vary among different insurance plans. This common test usually is covered if ordered by an insurance-approved doctor at an approved lab.

The doctor or other healthcare provider will ask the patient for a complete medical history and perform a **physical examination** to determine possible causes of the problem. Information about the patient's diet, medications and recent travel may provide clues to the identity of possible infectious organisms.

Stool culture normally doesn't require any special preparation. Patients don't need to change their diet before collecting the specimen, but they should avoid castor oil, bismuth, and laxative preparations containing psyllium hydrophilic mucilloid that might contaminate the specimen.

Infection-causing bacteria that aren't normally found in the digestive tract include *Shigella*, *Salmonella*, *Campylobacter*, and *Yersinia*. *Clostridium difficile* produces a toxin that can cause severe diarrhea. Other bacteria that produce toxins are *Staphylococcus aureus*, *Bacillus cereus*, and *Escherichia coli*. Although *Escherichia coli* is a normal bacteria found in the intestines, one toxic type of this bacteria can be acquired from eating contaminated meat, juice, or fruits. It produces a toxin that causes severe inflammation and bleeding of the colon.

Strabismus

Strabismus is a condition in which the eyes don't point in the same direction, also called ''squint.'' It occurs in between 2% and 5% of all children, both boys and girls, and sometimes runs in families. About half of affected children are born with the condition, which causes one or both eyes to turn:

- Inward (crossed eyes)
- Outward (wall eyes)
- Upward (hypertropia)
- Downward (hypotropia).

Crossed eyes are the most common type of strabismus in infants. One type of this problem develops in children under age 2 who cross their eyes when focusing on nearby objects. This usually happens to children who are moderately to extremely farsighted. Another common form of strabismus (wall eyes), may only be noticeable when a child daydreams, looks at far-away objects, or is tired or sick.

Sometimes the eye turn is always in the same eye, but sometimes the turn alternates from one eye to the other. Most children with strabismus have an unchanging condition; no matter where they look, the degree of deviation doesn't change. In other forms of strabismus, the amount of misalignment depends upon which direction the eyes are pointed.

Sometimes a child may have ''false strabismus'' and seem to have a turned eye; in reality, this appearance may actually be due to:

- Extra skin that covers the inner corner of the eye
- A broad, flat nose
- Eyes set unusually close together or far apart. False strabismus usually disappears as the child's face grows.

In children with normal vision, both eyes send the brain the same message. It's necessary that both eyes look directly at the same object so that a child can see in three dimensions with good depth perception. When an eye is misaligned, the brain receives two different images. Young children learn to ignore distorted messages from a misaligned eye, but adults with strabismus often develop double vision.

Strabismus can be caused by a defect in muscles or the part of the brain that controls eye movement. It's especially common in children who have:

- **Brain tumors**
- **Cerebral palsy**
- **Down syndrome**
- **Hydrocephalus**

Diseases that cause partial or total blindness can cause strabismus. So can extreme farsightedness, **cataracts**, eye injury, or having much better vision in one eye than the other.

In adults, strabismus is usually caused by:

- Diabetes
- **Head injury**
- **Stroke**
- Brain tumor
- Other diseases affecting nerves that control eye muscles.

The most obvious symptom of strabismus is an eye that isn't always straight. The deviation can vary from day to day or during the day. People who have strabismus often squint in bright sunlight or tilt their heads to focus their eyes.

Every baby's eyes should be examined by the age of 6 months; a baby whose eyes haven't straightened by the age of 4 months should be examined to rule out serious disease.

A pediatrician, family doctor or eye specialist can check the health of the eye using drops that widen the pupils and temporarily paralyze eye-focusing muscles. Early diagnosis is important because some uneven eyes may be caused by a tumor, and untreated strabismus may damage vision in the unused eye and cause lazy eye (**amblyopia**).

Preserving or restoring vision and improving appearance may involve one or more of the following:

- Glasses to help focus and straighten the eye(s)
- Patching to force infants and young children to use and straighten the weaker eye
- Eye drops or ointments as a substitute for patching or glasses, or to make glasses more effective
- Surgery to tighten, relax, or reposition eye muscles
- Medication injected into an overactive eye muscle to allow the opposite muscle to straighten the eye
- **Vision training** (also called eye exercises).

Early consistent treatment usually improves vision and appearance. The best results are achieved if the condition is corrected before the age of 7.

STREP THROAT

Streptococcal sore throat (strep throat), is an infection of the mucous membranes lining the throat. Sometimes the tonsils are also infected (**tonsillitis**).

Caused by group A *Streptococcus* bacteria, untreated strep throat may develop into **rheumatic fever** or other serious conditions.

Strep throat accounts for between 5% and 10% of all sore throats. It occurs most often between November to April, and while anyone can get strep throat, it's most common among school children. People who smoke or who are tired, run down, or who live in damp, crowded conditions are more likely to become infected. Children under age 2 and adults who aren't around children are less likely to get the disease.

The disease passes directly from person to person by coughing or sneezing; rarely the bacteria is passed through food if a sick food handler accidentally contaminates food by coughing or sneezing. Statistically, if someone in the home is infected, one out of every four other household members may get strep throat within two to seven days.

A person with strep throat suddenly develops a **pain**ful sore throat one to five days after being exposed to the streptococcus bacteria. Unfortunately, it's impossible to tell the difference between a sore throat caused by strep or by other bacteria or viruses. The infected person usually feels tired and has a **fever**, sometimes accompanied by chills, **headache**, muscle aches, swollen lymph glands, and nausea. Young children may complain of abdominal pain. The tonsils look swollen and are bright red, with white or yellow patches of pus on them. Sometimes the roof of the mouth is red or has small red spots. Often a person with strep throat has **bad breath**.

Despite these common symptoms, strep throat can be deceptive. It's possible to have the disease and not show any of these symptoms. Many young children complain only of a headache and stomachache, without the characteristic sore throat.

There are complications. Occasionally, within a few days of developing the sore throat, a person may develop a fine, rough, **sunburn**-like rash over the face and upper body, together with a fever of between 101-104°F. The tongue becomes bright red, with a flecked, strawberry-like appearance. When a rash develops, this form of strep throat is called **scarlet fever**. The rash is a reaction to toxins released by the streptococcus bacteria. Scarlet fever is no more dangerous than strep throat, and is treated the same way. The rash disappears in about five days. One to three weeks later, patches of skin may peel off, especially on the fingers and toes.

Untreated strep throat can cause rheumatic fever. This is a serious illness, although it occurs rarely. The most recent outbreak appeared in the United States in the mid-1980s. Rheumatic fever occurs most often in children between the ages of five and 15, and may have a genetic component, since it seems to run in families. Although the strep throat that causes rheumatic fever is contagious, rheumatic fever itself is not.

Rheumatic fever begins one to six weeks after an untreated streptococcal infection. The joints, especially the wrists, elbows, knees, and ankles become red, sore, and swollen. The infected person develops a high fever, and possibly a rapid heartbeat when lying down, paleness, **shortness of breath**, and fluid retention. A red rash over the trunk may come and go for weeks or months. An acute attack of rheumatic fever lasts about three months. Rheumatic fever can cause permanent damage to the heart and heart valves. It can be prevented by promptly treating **streptococcal infections** with **antibiotics**. It does not occur if all the streptococcus bacteria are killed within the first 10-12 days after infection.

In the 1990s, outbreaks of a virulent strain of group A *Streptococcus* were reported to cause a toxic shock-like illness and a severe invasive infection called necrotizing fasciitis, which destroys skin and muscle tissue. Although these diseases are caused by group A *Streptococci*, they rarely begin with strep throat. Instead, in these cases the streptococcus bacteria enters the body through a skin wound. These complications are rare. However, since the **death** rate in necrotizing fasciitis is 30% to 50%, it's a good idea to seek prompt treatment for any streptococcal infection.

A doctor diagnoses strep throat by conducting a **physical examination** of the throat and chest. The doctor will also look for signs of other illness, such as a sinus infection or **bronchitis**, and ask if the patient has been around other people with strep throat. If it appears that the patient may have strep throat, the doctor will do laboratory tests.

There are two types of tests to determine if a person has strep throat: a rapid strep test or a throat culture. For both, a nurse will use a sterile swab to reach down into the throat and obtain a sample of material from the sore area. The procedure takes only a few seconds, but may cause gagging.

A rapid strep test can only determine the presence of streptococcal bacteria, but will not tell if the sore throat is caused by another kind of bacteria; these results are available in about 20 minutes. The advantage of this test is the speed with which a diagnosis can be made. However, in about 20% of cases where no strep is detected by the rapid test, the patient actually does have strep throat. Because of this, when the rapid strep test is negative, a doctor often does a **throat culture**.

For a throat culture, a sample of swabbed material is grown in the lab so that technicians can determine what kind of bacteria are present. Results take 24 to 48 hours. The test is very accurate and will show the presence of other kinds of bacteria besides *Streptococci*.

It's important not to take any antibiotics before having a throat culture, since even small amounts of antibiotics can mask the presence of the bacteria.

In the event that rheumatic fever is suspected, the doctor can do a blood test. This test, called an antistreptolysin-O test, will tell the doctor whether the person has recently been infected with strep bacteria. This helps the doctor distinguish between rheumatic fever and **rheumatoid arthritis**.

Strep throat is treated with antibiotics. Penicillin is the preferred medication. Oral penicillin must be taken for 10 days. Patients need to take the entire amount of antibiotic prescribed and not discontinue taking the medication when they feel better. Stopping the antibiotic early can lead to a return of the strep infection. Occasionally, a single injection of long-acting penicillin (Bicillin) is given instead of 10 days of oral treatment.

About 10% of the time, penicillin doesn't kill the strep bacteria. When this happens a doctor may prescribe other antibiotics such as amoxicillin (Amoxil), clindamycin (Cleocin), or a cephalosporin (such as Ceclor). Erythromycin, another relatively inexpensive antibiotic, is given to people who are allergic to penicillin. Scarlet fever is treated with the same antibiotics as strep throat.

Without treatment, the symptoms of strep throat begin subsiding in four or five days. However, because of the possibility of getting rheumatic fever, it's important to treat strep throat promptly. If rheumatic fever does occur, it's also treated with antibiotics. Anti-inflammatory drugs are used to treat joint swelling, and **diuretics** are used to reduce water retention. Once the rheumatic fever becomes inactive, children may continue on low doses of antibiotics to prevent a reoccurrence. Necrotizing fasciitis is treated with intravenous antibiotics.

There are some steps that people can take to ease the discomfort of their strep symptoms.

- Take **acetaminophen** or ibuprofen for pain. **Aspirin** should not be given to children because of its association with an increase in **Reye's syndrome**, a serious disease.
- Gargle with warm double strength tea or warm salt water (one teaspoon of salt to eight ounces of water) to relieve sore throat pain.
- Drink plenty of fluids, but avoid acidic juices like orange juice because they irritate the throat.
- Eat soft, nutritious foods like noodle soup. Avoid spicy foods.
- Avoid smoke and smoking.
- Rest until the fever is gone, then resume strenuous activities gradually.
- Use a room humidifier, as it may make sore throat sufferers more comfortable.
- Antiseptic lozenges and sprays may aggravate the sore throat rather than improve it.

It's possible also to ease the symptoms of strep throat by using various herbs and natural treatments. Some practitioners suggest using these treatments in addition to antibiotics, since they primarily address the comfort of the patient and not the underlying infection. Many practitioners recommend *Lactobacillus acidophilus* to offset the suppressive effects of antibiotics on the helpful bacteria of the intestines. Other suggested treatments include:

- Inhaling fragrances of the essential oils of lavender, thyme, eucalyptus, sage, or sandalwood
- Gargling with a mixture of water, salt, and tumeric powder or astringents, such as alum, sumac, sage, and bayberry
- Drinking tea made of sage or echinacea

Patients with strep throat begin feeling better — and are no longer contagious — 24 hours after starting antibiotics. Symptoms rarely last longer than five days. Children should not return to school or childcare until they are no longer contagious. Food handlers should not work for the first 24 hours after antibiotic treatment, because strep infections are occasionally passed through contaminated food. People who are not treated with antibiotics can continue to spread strep bacteria for several months.

About 10% of strep throat cases don't respond to penicillin. People who have even a mild sore throat after a 10-day treatment with antibiotics should return to their doctor. It's possible that the patient is just a carrier of strep, and that something else is causing the sore throat.

Taking antibiotics within the first week of a strep infection will prevent rheumatic fever and other complications. If rheumatic fever does occur, the outcomes vary considerably: Some people may be cured, but others may have permanent damage to the heart and heart valves. In rare cases, rheumatic fever can be fatal.

Necrotizing fasciitis has a death rate of 30% to 50%. Patients who survive often suffer a great deal of tissue and muscle loss. Fortunately, this complication of a streptococcus infection is very rare.

There is no way to prevent getting a strep throat. However, the risk of getting one or passing one on to another person can be minimized by:

- Washing hands often and well, especially after nose blowing or sneezing and before handling food
- Disposing of used tissues properly
- Avoiding close contact with someone who has a strep throat
- Not sharing food and eating utensils with anyone
- Not smoking.

STREPTOCOCCAL INFECTIONS

Streptococcal (strep) infections are communicable diseases that develop when Streptococcus bacteria normally found on the skin or in the intestines, mouth, nose, reproductive tract, or urinary tract invade other parts of the body and contaminate blood or tissue. Some strep infections don't produce symptoms, and some are fatal.

Most people have had some form of strep bacteria in their body at some point in their lives; people who host bacteria without showing signs of infection are considered to be carriers.

Primary strep infections invade healthy tissue (usually the throat). Secondary strep infections invade tissue already weakened by injury or illness, such as the bones, ears, eyes, joints, or intestines. Both primary and secondary strep infections can travel from affected tissues to the lymph glands, where they enter the bloodstream and spread throughout the body.

Numerous strains of strep bacteria have been identified. Types A, B, C, D, and G are most likely to make people sick. Group A strep (GAS) is the form of strep bacteria most apt to be associated with serious illness. Between 10,000 and 15,000 GAS infections occur in the United States every year. Most are mild inflammations of the throat or skin, where the bacteria are normally found; however, GAS infections can be deadly.

Two of the most severe invasive GAS infections are necrotizing fasciitis (flesh-eating bacteria) which destroys muscle tissue and fat, and **toxic shock syndrome** (a rapidly progressive disorder that causes **shock** and damages internal organs).

GAS is transmitted by direct contact with the saliva, nasal discharge, or open **wounds** of an infected person. Chronic illness, kidney disease treated by dialysis, and steroid use increase vulnerability to infection.

About one of five people with GAS infection develops a sore, inflamed throat, and pus on the tonsils. The majority of those infected by GAS either have no symptoms or develop enlarged lymph nodes, **fever**, **headache**, nausea, vomiting, weakness, and a rapid heartbeat.

Flesh-eating bacteria is characterized by fever, extreme **pain**, and swelling and redness at a site where skin is broken.

Symptoms of toxic shock include abdominal pain, confusion, **dizziness**, and widespread red skin rash.

Group B strep (GBS) most often affects pregnant women, infants, the elderly, and chronically ill adults. Since first emerging in the 1970s, GBS has been the primary cause of life-threatening illness and **death** in newborns. GBS exists in the reproductive tract of 20% to 25% of all pregnant women. Although no more than 2% of these women develop invasive infection, 40% to 73% transmit bacteria to their babies during delivery.

About 12,000 of the 3,500,000 babies born in this country each year develop GBS disease in infancy. About 75% of them develop early-onset infection. Sometimes evident within a few hours of birth and always apparent within the first week of life, this condition causes inflammation of the membranes covering the brain and spinal cord, (**meningitis**), **pneumonia**, blood infection, and other problems.

Late-onset GBS develops between the ages of seven days and three months, and often causes meningitis. About half of all cases of this rare condition can be traced to mothers who are GBS carriers. The cause of the others is unknown. GBS also has been linked to a history of **breast cancer**.

Group C strep (GCS) is a common source of infection in animals, but rarely causes human illness.

Group D strep (GDS) is a common cause of wound infections in hospital patients. GDS is also associated with:

- Abnormal growth of tissue in the gastrointestinal tract
- Urinary tract infection (UTI)
- Womb infections in women who have just given birth.

Group G strep (GGS) is normally present on the skin, in the mouth and throat, and in the intestines and genital tract, and is most likely to lead to infection in alcoholics and in people who have **cancer**, **diabetes mellitus**, **rheumatoid arthritis**, and other conditions that suppress immune-system activity. GGS can cause a variety of infections, including:

- Bacteria in the bloodstream
- **Bursitis** (Inflammation of the connective tissue structure surrounding a joint)
- **Endocarditis** (a condition that affects the lining of the heart chambers and the heart valves)
- Meningitis
- **Osteomyelitis**) (inflammation of bone and bone marrow)
- **Peritonitis** (inflammation of the lining of the abdomen).

A pregnant woman who has GBS infection can develop infections of the bladder, blood, and urinary tract, and deliver a baby who is infected or stillborn. The risk of transmitting GBS infection during birth is highest in a woman whose labor begins before the 37th week of **pregnancy** or lasts more than 18 hours or who:

- Becomes a GBS carrier during the final stages of pregnancy
- Has a GBS urinary-tract infection
- Has already given birth to a baby infected with GBS
- Develops a fever during labor.

More than 13% of babies who develop GBS infection during birth or within the first few months of life develop brain disorders. An equal number of them die.

Among men, and in women who are not pregnant, the most common consequences of GBS infection are pneumonia and infections of blood, skin, and soft tissue.

Other symptoms associated with strep infection include:

- Anemia
- Elevated white blood cell counts
- Inflammation of the epiglottis
- Heart murmur
- High blood pressure
- Infection of the heart muscle
- Kidney inflammation
- Swelling of the face and ankles.

To diagnose a strep infection, the doctor must obtain some bacteria by swabbing the back of the throat or the rectum with a piece of sterile cotton. Microscopic examination of the smear can identify which type of bacteria has been collected.

Penicillin and other **antibiotics** are used to treat strep infections. It takes less than 24 hours for antibiotics to stop an infected person's ability to transmit GAS. Guidelines developed by the American Academy of Obstetrics and Gynecology (AAOG), the American Academy of Pediatrics (AAP), and the Centers for Disease Control and Prevention (CDC) recommend giving intravenous antibiotics to a woman at high risk of passing GBS infection on to her child, and offering the medication to any pregnant woman who wants it.

Initiating antibiotic therapy at least four hours before birth allows medication to become concentrated enough to protect the baby during passage through the birth canal.

Babies infected with GBS during or shortly after birth may die. Those who survive often require lengthy hospital stays and develop vision or **hearing loss** and other permanent disabilities.

Conventional medicine is very successful in treating strep infections. However, several alternative therapies may relieve symptoms. For example, several herbs, including garlic, echinacea, and goldenseal are believed to strengthen the immune system, thus helping the body fight a current infection as well as helping prevent future infections.

GAS is responsible for more than 2,000 deaths a year. About 20% of people infected with flesh-eating bacteria die. So do three of every five who develop toxic shock syndrome.

Early-onset GBS kills 15% of the infants it affects. Late-onset disease claims the lives of 10% of babies who develop it. GBS infections are fatal in about 20% of the men and non-pregnant women who develop them.

About 10% to 15% of non-GAS strep infections are fatal. Antibiotic therapy, begun when symptoms first appear, may increase a patient's chance of survival.

Washing hands frequently (especially before eating and after using the toilet) and keeping wounds clean can help prevent strep infection. Exposure to infected people should be avoided, and a family physician should be notified by anyone who develops an extremely **sore throat** or pain, redness, swelling, or drainage at the site of a wound or break in the skin.

Until vaccines to prevent strep infection become available, 12 monthly doses of oral or injected antibiotics may prevent some types of recurrent infection.

Stress and stress management

Stress is the way a person responds to environmental demands or pressures. When stress was first studied in the 1950s, the term was used to explain both the causes and the effects of these pressures. More recently, however, the word ''stressor'' has been used to mean the trigger that provokes a stress response.

A certain degree of stress is a normal part of every day life; it is when stress becomes constant that it can lead to physical and mental problems. Stress-related disease is caused by excessive and prolonged demands on a person's coping resources.

The symptoms of stress can be either physical or psychological. Stress-related physical illnesses may be caused or at least influenced by stress-related overstimulation of a part of the nervous system that regulates the heart rate, blood pressure and digestive system. Some of these stress-related illnesses include **irritable bowel syndrome**, **heart attacks**, and chronic **headaches**.

Stress-related emotional illness may be influenced by stress resulting from major life changes, such as marriage, graduating, becoming a parent, getting fired, or retirement. In the workplace, stress-related illness often takes the form of burnout (a loss of interest in or ability to perform a job because of stress).

When a doctor suspects that a patient's illness is connected to stress, he or she will take a careful history of recent stress (family or job problems, other illnesses, and so on). Many doctors will evaluate the patient's personality as well, in order to judge how well the person copes with stress. There are a number of psychological tests that doctors can use to help diagnose the amount of stress that the patient experiences and the coping strategies used to deal with them.

Stress-related illness can be diagnosed by family doctors as well as by mental health specialists.

Recent advances in the understanding of the many complex connections between the mind and body have produced a variety of popular ways to treat stress-related illness:

- Medications. These may include drugs to control blood pressure or other physical symptoms of stress, as well as drugs that affect the patient's mood (tranquilizers or antidepressants).
- Stress management programs. These may be either individual or group treatments, and usually involve analysis of the stressors in the patient's life. They often focus on job or workplace related stress.
- Behavioral approaches. These strategies include relaxation techniques, breathing exercises, and physical exercise.

- **Massage**. Therapeutic massage relieves stress by relaxing the large groups of muscles in the back, neck, arms, and legs.
- Cognitive therapy. These approaches teach patients to reinterpret stress in order to alter the body's physical response.
- **Meditation** and spiritual practices. Relaxing, meditating and spiritual practices can help reduce stress.

Treatment of stress is one area in which the boundaries between traditional and alternative therapies have changed in recent years, in part because some forms of physical exercise (**yoga**, **tai chi**, aikido) that were once considered to be fads have become widely accepted as useful parts of mainstream stress reduction programs. Other alternative therapies for stress, which are occasionally recommended by mainstream medicine, include **aromatherapy**, dance therapy, nutrition-based treatments (including dietary guidelines and nutritional supplements), **acupuncture**, and herbal medicine.

The prognosis for recovery from a stress-related illness is related to a wide variety of factors in a person's life, many of which are inherited or beyond the individual's control (economic trends, cultural stereotypes and prejudices). It is possible, however, for humans to learn new responses to stress.

A person's ability to remain healthy in stressful situations is sometimes referred to as ''stress hardiness.'' Stress-hardy people have a cluster of personality traits that strengthen their ability to cope. These traits include believing in the importance of what they are doing; believing that they have some power to influence their situation; and viewing life's changes as positive opportunities rather than as threats.

It's not possible or desirable to totally prevent stress, which is an inevitable part of life. In addition, specific strategies for preventing stress vary widely from person to person, depending on the nature and number of the stressors in a person's life, and the amount of control he or she has over these factors. In general, a combination of attitude and behavior changes works well for most patients. The best way to prevent stress is for parents to teach healthy attitudes and behaviors within their family.

Stress test

Used to evaluate heart function, a stress test requires that a patient **exercise** on a treadmill or exercise bicycle so that the heart rate, breathing, blood pressure, and feeling of well being are monitored.

When the body is active, it requires more oxygen than when it is at rest, so the heart has to pump more blood. Because of the increased stress on the heart, exercise can reveal coronary problems that aren't obvious when the body is at rest. This is why the stress test (although not perfect) is the best noninvasive ''first step'' in assessing the health of the heart.

The stress test helps doctors determine how well the heart handles the stress imposed by exercise. It's especially helpful in detecting **coronary artery disease**, inadequate supply of oxygen-rich blood to the tissues of the heart muscle (ischemia), and determining safe levels of exercise in people with existing heart disease.

The exercise stress test carries a very slight risk (1 in 100,000) of causing a **heart attack**. For this reason, a doctor needs to stand by during the exercise stress test with emergency equipment on standby.

The patient must be aware of the symptoms of a heart attack and stop the test if any of the following symptoms appear:

- An unsteady gait
- Confusion
- Gray or cold, clammy skin
- **Dizziness** or **fainting**
- A drop in blood pressure
- Chest **pain** (**angina**)
- Irregular heart beat (cardiac **arrhythmias**).

Electrodes are attached to specific areas of the patient's chest with special adhesive patches and gel that conduct electrical impulses. Typically, electrodes are placed under each collarbone and each bottom rib, and six electrodes are placed across the chest in a rough outline of the heart. Then the technician attaches wires from the electrodes to a machine that records the heart's electrical activity picked up by the electrodes.

The heart is first tested while the patient is lying down, then standing up, and then breathing heavily for half a minute. These tests can later be compared with the tests performed while the patient is exercising. The patient's blood pressure is measured periodically throughout the test.

The patient begins riding a stationary bicycle or walking on a treadmill. Gradually the intensity of the exercise is increased. For example, if the patient is walking on a treadmill, the speed of the treadmill increases and the treadmill is tilted upward. If the patient is on an exercise bicycle, the resistance or ''drag'' is gradually increased. The patient continues exercising at higher intensities until he or she experiences severe fatigue, dizziness, chest pain, or until reaching target heart rate. (Target heart rate is usually 85% of the estimated top heart rate based on the patient's age). During this time, the patient's heart is continually monitored.

In some cases, other tests are also used together with the exercise stress test. For instance, recent studies suggest that women have a high rate of ''false negatives'' (results showing no problem when one exists) and ''false positives'' (results showing a problem when one does not exist) with the stress test.

Patients are usually instructed not to eat or smoke for several hours before the test. They should also tell the doctor about any medications they are taking. They should wear comfortable sneakers and exercise clothing.

After the test, the patient should rest until blood pressure and heart rate return to normal. If all goes well, and there are no signs of distress, the patient may return to his or her normal daily activities.

There is a very slight risk of a heart attack from the exercise, as well as cardiac arrhythmia (irregular heart beats), angina, or cardiac arrest (about 1 in 100,000).

A normal result of an exercise stress test shows normal heart rate, blood pressure and no angina, unusual dizziness, or **shortness of breath**.

A number of abnormalities may show up on an exercise stress test, indicating that not enough oxygen-rich blood is getting to the heart muscle, or that there are abnormal heart rhythms or structural problems, such as overgrowth of muscle (hypertrophy). If the blood pressure rises too high or the patient experiences distressing symptoms during the test, the heart may be unable to handle the increased workload. Stress test abnormalities usually require further evaluation and therapy.

STROKE

A stroke is the sudden death of brain cells in a localized area due to inadequate blood flow.A stroke occurs when blood flow is interrupted to part of the brain. Without blood to supply oxygen and nutrients and to remove waste products, brain cells quickly begin to die. Death of brain cells triggers a chain reaction in which toxic chemicals created by cell death affect other nearby cells. This is one reason why prompt treatment can have such a dramatic effect on final recovery.

Depending on the region of the brain affected, a stroke may cause **paralysis**, speech impairment, loss of memory and reasoning ability, **coma**, or death. A stroke is also sometimes called a brain attack or a cerebrovascular accident (CVA).

Some important stroke statistics:

- More than half a million people in the United States experience a new or recurrent stroke each year
- Stroke is the third leading cause of death in the United States and the leading cause of disability
- Stroke kills about 150,000 Americans each year, or almost one out of three stroke victims
- Three million Americans are currently permanently disabled from stroke
- In the United States, stroke costs about $30 billion per year in direct costs and loss of productivity
- Two-thirds of strokes occur in people over age 65
- Strokes affect men more often than women, although women are more likely to die from a stroke
- Strokes affect blacks more often than whites, and are more likely to be fatal among blacks.

Stroke is fatal for about 27% of white males, 52% of black males, 23% of white females, and 40% of black females. Stroke survivors may be left with significant deficits. Emergency treatment and comprehensive rehabilitation can significantly improve both survival and recovery.

- Other medical conditions. Stroke risk increases with **obesity**, high blood cholesterol level, or high red blood cell count.
- Lifestyle choices. Stroke risk increases with cigarette smoking (especially if combined with the use of **oral contraceptives**), low level of physical activity, alcohol consumption above two drinks per day, or use of cocaine or intravenous drugs.

There are four main types of stroke: cerebral thrombosis, cerebral embolism, subarachnoid hemorrhage, and intracerebral hemorrhage.

Cerebral thrombosis and cerebral **embolism** are caused by blood clots that block an artery supplying the brain, either in the brain itself or in the neck. These account for 70-80% of all strokes.

Clots most often form due to ''hardening'' (**atherosclerosis**) of brain arteries. Cerebral thrombosis is often preceded by a transient ischemic attack, or TIA, sometimes called a ''mini-stroke.'' In a TIA, blood flow is temporarily interrupted, causing short-lived stroke-like symptoms.

Cerebral embolism occurs when a blood clot from elsewhere in the circulatory system breaks free. If it becomes lodged in an artery supplying the brain, either in the brain or in the neck, it can cause a stroke. The most common cause of cerebral embolism is atrial fibrillation, a disorder of the heart beat.

Subarachnoid hemorrhage and intracerebral hemorrhage occur when a blood vessel bursts around or in the brain, either from trauma or excess internal pressure. The vessels most likely to break are those with preexisting defects such as an aneurysm. An aneurysm is a ''pouching out'' of a blood vessel caused by a weak arterial wall. Brain aneurysms are surprisingly common. According to **autopsy** studies, about 6% of all Americans have them. Aneurysms rarely cause symptoms until they burst.

Intracerebral hemorrhage affects vessels within the brain itself, while subarachnoid hemorrhage affects arteries at the brain's surface, just below the protective arachnoid membrane.

Symptoms of an embolic stroke usually come on quite suddenly and are at their most intense right from the start, while symptoms of a thrombotic stroke come on more gradually. Symptoms may include:

- Blurring or decreased vision in one or both eyes
- Severe **headache**, often described as ''the worst headache of my life''
- Weakness, numbness, or paralysis of the face, arm, or leg, usually confined to one side of the body
- **Dizziness**, loss of balance or coordination, especially when combined with other symptoms.

Stroke is a medical emergency requiring immediate treatment. Prompt treatment improves the chances of survival and increases the degree of recovery that may be expected. A person who may have suffered a stroke should be seen in a hospital emergency room without delay. Treatment to break up a blood clot, the major cause of stroke, must begin within three hours of the stroke to be effective. Improved medical treatment of all types of stroke has resulted in a dramatic decline in death rates in recent decades. In 1950, nine in ten died from stroke, compared to slightly less than one in three today.

Emergency treatment of stroke from a blood clot is aimed at dissolving the clot. This ''thrombolytic therapy'' is currently performed most often with tissue plasminogen activator, or t-PA. t-PA must be administered within three hours of the stroke event. Emergency treatment of hemorrhagic stroke is aimed at controlling intracranial pressure.

Surgery for hemorrhage due to aneurysm may be performed if the aneurysm is close enough to the cranial surface to allow access. Ruptured vessels are closed off to prevent rebleeding. For aneurysms that are difficult to reach surgically, endovascular treatment may be used. In this procedure, a catheter is guided from a larger artery up into the brain to reach the aneurysm. Small coils of wire are discharged into the aneurysm, which plug it up and block off blood flow from the main artery.

After the stroke has occurred and the brain has been damaged, treatment is aimed at **rehabilitation**. Rehabilitation refers to a comprehensive program designed to regain function as much as possible and compensate for permanent losses. Approximately 10% of stroke survivors are without any significant disability and able to function independently. Another 10% are so severely affected that they must remain institutionalized for severe disability. The remaining 80% can return home with appropriate therapy, training, support, and care services.

Rehabilitation is coordinated by a team of medical professionals and may include the services of a neurologist, a physician who specializes in rehabilitation medicine (physiatrist), a physical therapist, an occupational therapist, a speech-language pathologist, a nutritionist, a mental health professional, and a social worker. Rehabilitation services may be provided in an acute care hospital, rehabilitation hospital, long-term care facility, outpatient clinic, or at home.

The rehabilitation program is based on the patient's individual deficits and strengths. Strokes on the left side of the brain primarily affect the right half of the body, and vice versa. In addition, in left brain dominant people, who constitute a significant majority of the population, left brain strokes usually lead to speech and language deficits, while right brain strokes may affect spatial perception. Patients with right brain strokes may also deny their illness, neglect the affected side of their body, and behave impulsively.

Rehabilitation may be complicated by cognitive losses, including diminished ability to understand and follow directions. Poor results are more likely in patients with significant or prolonged cognitive changes, sensory losses, language deficits, or incontinence.

Damage from stroke may be significantly reduced through emergency treatment. Knowing the symptoms of stroke is as important as knowing those of a **heart attack**. Patients with stroke symptoms should seek emergency treatment without delay, which may mean dialing 911 rather than their family physician.

The risk of stroke can be reduced through lifestyle changes:

- Stop smoking
- Control blood pressure
- Get regular exercise
- Keep body weight down
- Avoid excessive alcohol consumption.
- Get regular checkups and follow the doctor's advice regarding diet and medicines.

Treatment of atrial fibrillation may significantly reduce the risk of stroke. Preventive anticoagulant therapy may benefit those with untreated atrial fibrillation. Warfarin (Coumadin) has proven to be more effective than aspirin for those with higher risk.

Screening for aneurysms may be an effective preventive measure in those with a family history of aneurysms or autosomal polycystic kidney disease, which tends to be associated with aneurysms.

Subdural Hematoma

A subdural hematoma is a collection of blood in the space between the outer and middle layers of the covering of the brain (the meninges). It is most often caused by torn, bleeding veins on the inside of the brain covering after a blow to the head.

A subdural hematoma most often affects people who are prone to falling. Only a slight bump on the head (or even a fall to the ground without hitting the head) may be enough to tear veins in the brain, often without fracturing the skull. There may be no external evidence of the bruising on the brain's surface.

Small subdural hematomas may not be very serious, and the blood that seeps out can be slowly absorbed over several weeks. Larger hematomas, like a big bruise, can gradually enlarge over several weeks even after the bleeding has stopped. This enlargement can compress the brain itself, and may lead to **death** if the blood isn't removed.

The time between the injury and the appearance of symptoms can vary from less than 48 hours to several weeks or more. Symptoms that appear in less than 48 hours indicate a serious subdural hematoma which may be fatal. However, if symptoms don't appear until at least two weeks after the accident, the condition is not so serious. The very young and the elderly are most likely to experience this type of chronic condition, which is less risky. Prompt medical care can reduce the probability of permanent brain damage in these cases.

Symptoms (which may come and go) include:

- **Headache**
- Episodes of confusion and drowsiness
- One-sided weakness or **paralysis**
- Lethargy
- Enlarged pupils
- Two different sizes of pupils
- Convulsions or loss of consciousness
- **Coma**.

A doctor should be contacted immediately if symptoms appear. Because these symptoms mimic the signs of a **stroke**, the patient should tell the doctor about any head injury within the previous few months. In an infant, symptoms may include increased pressure within the skull, growing head size, bulging soft spots on an infant's skull), vomiting, irritability, lethargy, and seizures.

A chronic subdural hematoma can be difficult to diagnose, but a slow loss of consciousness after a head injury is assumed to be a hematoma unless proven otherwise. The hematoma can be confirmed with **magnetic resonance imaging** (MRI) (a hematoma can be hard to see on a computed tomography scan (CT scan), depending on how long after the hemorrhage the scan is done).

If the hematoma is small and doesn't cause symptoms, no treatment is necessary. In more serious cases, hematomas

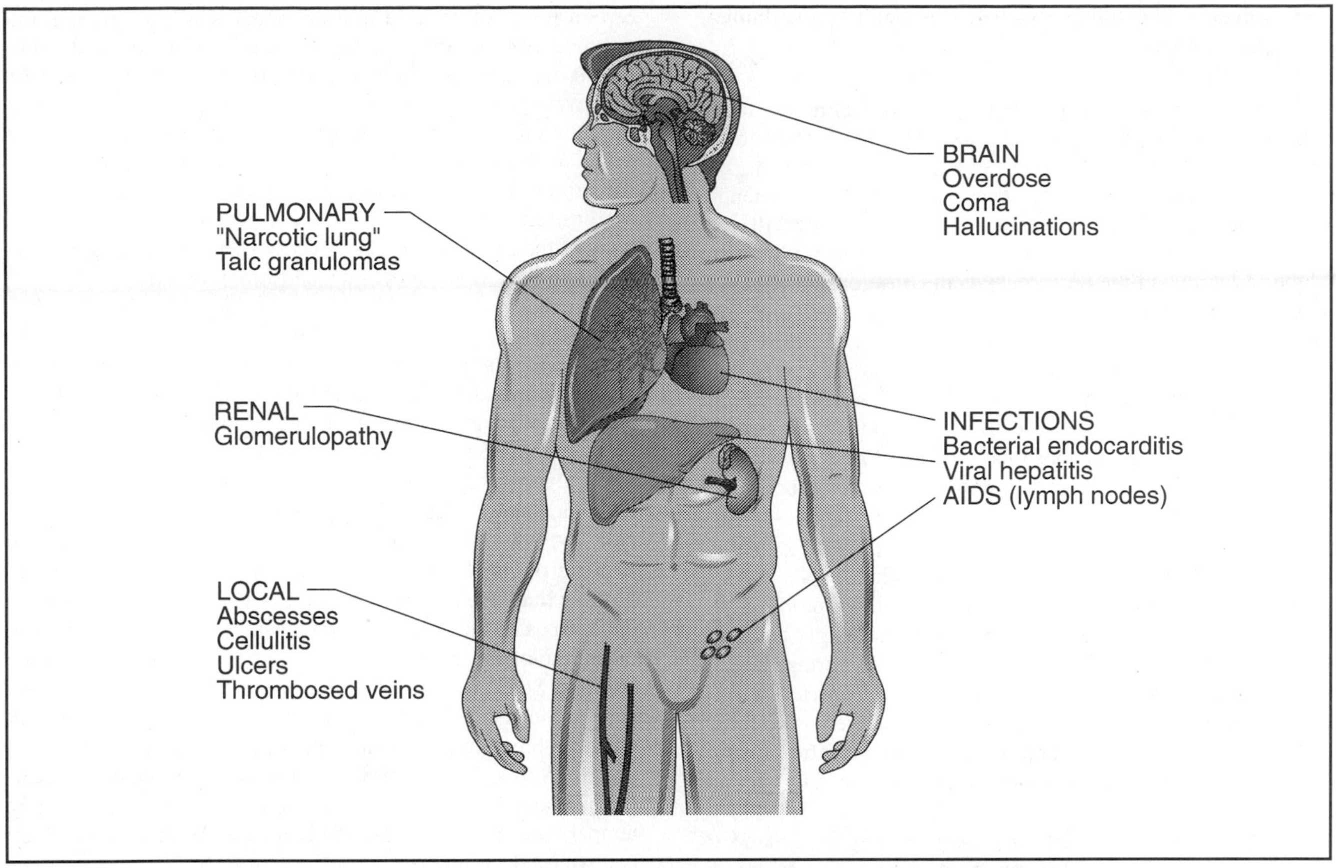

Substance abuse often causes a variety of medical abnormalities and conditions throughout the body, as shown in the illustration above. *(Illustration by Electronic Illustrators Group.)*

may need to be surgically removed. The accumulated liquid blood can be drained from holes drilled into the skull. The surgeon may need to open a section of skull to remove a large hematoma or to tie off a bleeding vein.

Corticosteroids and **diuretics** (water pills) can control brain swelling. After surgery, antiseizure drugs may help control or prevent seizures, which may start as long as two years after the head injury.

If treatment is provided soon enough, recovery is usually complete. Headache, **amnesia**, attention problems, anxiety, and giddiness may continue for some time after surgery. Most symptoms in adults usually disappear within six months, with further improvement over several years. Children tend to recover much faster.

SUBSTANCE ABUSE AND DEPENDENCE

Substance abuse involves the use of drugs, alcohol or other chemicals in a way that interferes with normal healthy functioning. Substance abuse cuts across all lines of race, culture, educational and socioeconomic status. Substance abuse is an enormous public health problem, with far-ranging effects. In addition to the health problems substance abuse can cuase, it is also considered to be an important factor in a wide variety of social problems, affecting rates of crime, domestic violence, **sexually transmitted diseases** (including HIV/**AIDS**), unemployment, homelessness, teen **pregnancy**, and failure in school. One study estimated that 20% of the total yearly cost of health care in the United States is spent on the effects of drug and alcohol abuse.

A wide range of substances can be abused. The most common classes include:

- Opioids (including such prescription pain killers as morphine and demerol, as well as illegal substances such as heroin)
- Benzodiazapines (including prescription drugs used for treating **anxiety**, such as Valium)
- Sedatives or ''downers'' (including prescription barbiturate drugs commonly referred to as tranquilizers)
- Stimulants or ''speed'' (including prescription amphetamine drugs used as weight loss drugs and in the treatment of attention deficit disorder)
- Cannabinoid drugs obtained from the hemp plant (including marijuana)
- Cocaine-based drugs
- Hallucinogenic or ''psychedelic'' drugs (including LSD, PCP or angel dust)

- Inhalants (including anesthetics as well as paint thinner, gas or glue)
- Alcohol

A number of important terms must be defined in order to have a complete discussion of substance abuse. Drug tolerance refers to a person's body becoming accustomed to the symptoms produced by a specific quantity of a substance. When a person first begins taking a substance, he/she will note various mental or physical reactions brought on by the drug (some of which are the very changes in consciousness that the individual is seeking through substance use). Over time, the same dosage of the substance will produce fewer of the desired feelings. In order to continue to feel the desired effect of the substance, progressively higher drug doses must be taken. Most substances of abuse tend to either slow or a speed up basic body functions such as breathing, heart rate, blood pressure. When a drug is stopped abruptly, the person's body will respond by over-reacting. Functions slowed by the abused substance will be suddenly speeded up, while previously stimulated functions will be suddenly slowed. This results in very unpleasant symptoms, known as withdrawal symptoms.

Scientists don't think there is just one single cause of substance abuse, although it does seem as if certain people have a genetic tendency to develop addictive behaviors. However, other social factors are most likely involved as well, including social problems and peer pressure. Other mental disorders can increase the chance that a person will become addicted.

The symptoms of substance abuse may be related to both its social effects and its physical effects. The social effects of substance abuse may include dropping out of school or losing a series of jobs, engaging in fighting and violence in relationships, and legal problems (ranging from driving under the influence to the commission of crimes designed to obtain the money needed to support an expensive drug habit).

Physical effects of substance abuse are related to the specific drug being abused:

- Opioid drug users may move slowly, lose weight, have mood swings, and have small pupils.
- Benzodiazapine and barbiturate users may appear sleepy and slowed, with slurred speech, small pupils, and occasional confusion.
- Amphetamine users may have excessively high energy, sleep problems, weight loss, rapid pulse, high blood pressure, occasional psychotic behavior and enlarged pupils.
- Marijuana users may be sluggish and slow to react, exhibiting mood swings and red eyes with dilated pupils.
- Cocaine users may have wide variations in their energy level, severe mood disturbances, and a constantly runny nose. ''Crack'' cocaine may cause aggressive or violent behavior.
- Hallucinogenic drug users may display bizarre behavior due to **hallucinations** and dilated pupils. LSD can cause flashbacks.

Other symptoms may depend on the type of substance being abused. For example, heroin, other opioid drugs, and certain forms of cocaine may be injected using a needle and a hypodermic syringe. A person abusing an injectable substance may have needle marks on arms or legs, with redness and swelling of the vein in which the substance was injected. Furthermore, poor judgment brought on by substance use can result in the injections being made under horrifyingly dirty conditions. These unsanitary conditions and the use of shared needles can cause infections of the injection sites, major infections of the heart, as well as infection with HIV, certain forms of hepatitis (a liver infection), and **tuberculosis**.

Cocaine is often taken as a powdery substance which is ''snorted'' through the nose. This can result in frequent nose bleeds, sores in the nose, and even an eating away of the nasal septum (the structure which separates the two nostrils). Other forms of cocaine include smokable or injectable forms of cocaine such as free base and crack cocaine.

Overdosing on a substance is a frequent complication of substance abuse. **Drug overdose** can be purposeful (with suicide as a goal), or due to carelessness, the unpredictable strength of substances purchased from street dealers, mixing of more than one type of substance or of a substance and alcohol, or as a result of the ever-increasing doses which a person must take of those substances to which he or she has become tolerant. Substance overdose can be a life-threatening emergency. Substances with depressive effects may dangerously slow the breathing and heart rate, drop the body temperature, and result in a general unresponsiveness. Stimulants may dangerously boost the heart rate and blood pressure, increase body temperature, and cause bizarre behavior. With cocaine, there is also a risk of **stroke**.

Still other symptoms may be caused by unknown substances mixed with street drugs in order to stretch a batch. A health care worker faced with a patient suffering extreme symptoms will have no idea what other substance that person may have unwittingly put into his or her body. Thorough drug screening can help with this problem.

The most difficult aspect of diagnosis involves overcoming the patient's refusal to acknowledge the problem. This may cause the person to completely deny the substance use or underestimate the degree of the problem and its effects.

One of the simplest and most commonly used screening tools used by doctors to diagnose substance abuse is called the CAGE questionnaire:

- Have you ever tried to Cut down on your substance use?
- Have you ever been Annoyed by people trying to talk to you about your substance use?
- Do you ever feel Guilty about your substance use?
- Do you ever need an Eye opener (use of the substance first thing in the morning) in order to start your day?

Other, longer lists of questions exist in order to try to determine the severity and effects of a person's substance abuse. A family history is another helpful tool in diagnosing substance abuse.

A physical exam may reveal signs of substance abuse in the form of needle marks, tracks, damage to the inside of the nostrils from snorting drugs, or unusually large or small pupils. Substance use also can be detected by examining the blood, urine, or hair in a laboratory. This drug testing is limited by sensitivity, specificity and the time elapsed since the person last used the drug.

Treatment has several goals, which include helping a person deal with the uncomfortable and possibly life-threatening symptoms associated with withdrawal from an addictive substance, helping a person deal with the social effects which substance abuse has had on his or her life, and efforts to prevent relapse. Individual or group psychotherapy is sometimes helpful.

Detoxification may take from several days to many weeks, and can either focus on ''cold turkey'' (complete and immediate ending of all substance use) or by slowly decreasing the dose which a person is taking to minimize the side effects of withdrawal. Some substances absolutely must be tapered, because ''cold turkey'' methods of detoxification are potentially deadly. Alternatively, a variety of medications may be used to combat the unpleasant and threatening physical symptoms of withdrawal. A substance (such as methadone in the case of heroine addiction) may be substituted for the original substance of abuse, with gradual tapering of this substituted drug. In practice, many patients may be maintained on methadone and lead a reasonably normal life style. Because of the rebound effects of wildly fluctuating blood pressure, body temperature, heart and breathing rates, as well as the potential for bizarre behavior and hallucinations, a person undergoing withdrawal must be carefully monitored.

Alternative treatments for substance abuse include treatments specifically designed to aid a person who is suffering from the effects of withdrawal and the toxicities of the abused substance, as well as treatments which are intended to decrease a person's **stress** level, thus hopefully decreasing the likelihood that he or she will relapse.

Treatments thought to improve a person's ability to stop substance use include **acupuncture** and hypnotherapy. Ridding the body of toxins is believed to be aided by **hydrotherapy** (bathing regularly in water containing baking soda, sea salt or Epsom salts). Herbs also may help, including milk thistle, burdock, and licorice. Anxiety brought on by substance withdrawal is thought to be lessened by using other herbs, which include valerian, vervain, skullcap and kava.

Other treatments aimed at reducing the stress during detox include **biofeedback**, **guided imagery**, and various meditations such as **yoga** and **tai chi**.

After a person has successfully withdrawn from substance use, the even more difficult task of recovery begins. Recovery refers to the life-long efforts of a person to avoid returning to substance use. The craving can be so strong, even years and years after initial withdrawal has been accomplished, that a previously addicted person is virtually forever in danger of slipping back into substance use. Triggers for such a relapse include any number of life stresses such as problems on the job or in the marriage, loss of a relationship, **death** of a loved one, financial stresses. While some people remain in counseling indefinitely, others find that various support groups or 12-Step Programs such as Narcotics Anonymous and Alcoholic Anonymous are the most helpful way of monitoring the recovery process and avoiding relapse.

Another important aspect of treatment is the involvement of close family members. Because substance abuse has severe effects on the functioning of the family, and because research shows that family members can accidentally develop behaviors which inadvertently serve to support a person's substance habit, most good treatment will involve all family members.

Prevention is best aimed at teenagers, who are at very high risk for substance experimentation. Data compiled in 1987 showed that 25% of high school seniors had used an illegal substance (other than marijuana) in the preceding year. Education regarding the risks and consequences of substance use, as well as teaching methods of resisting peer pressure, are both important components of a prevention program. Furthermore, it is important to identify children at higher risk for substance abuse including victims of physical or sexual abuse, children of parents who have a history of substance abuse, especially alcohol, and children with school failure and/or attention deficit disorder. These children will require a more intensive prevention program.

Sudden Cardiac Death

Sudden cardiac death (SCD) is an unexpected death due to heart problems which occurs within one hour from the start of any heart-related symptoms. SCD is sometimes called cardiac arrest.

When the heart suddenly stops beating effectively and breathing ends, a person is said to have experienced sudden cardiac death.

SCD is not the same as actual death, when the brain also dies. The important difference is that sudden cardiac death is potentially reversible, and if the heart can be started again, the brain won't die.

Sudden cardiac death is also not the same as a **heart attack**. A heart attack is caused by a block in an artery which feeds the heart, so the heart doesn't get enough oxygen. The part of the heart that has been starved of oxygen is damaged beyond repair, but the heart can still beat.

Sudden cardiac death usually happens when the lower chamber of the heart quivers instead of pumping in an organized rhythm (ventricular fibrillation). This disorganized type of heartbeat almost never returns to normal by itself, so the condition requires immediate intervention. An extremely rapid heartbeat (usually over 100 beats a minute) also can lead to sudden cardiac death. The risk for SCD is higher for anyone with heart disease.

When the heart stops beating effectively and the brain is being deprived of oxygenated blood, it's a medical emergency.

Sudden cardiac death is diagnosed when there is a sudden loss of consciousness, breathing stops, and there is no effective heartbeat.

When sudden cardiac death occurs, the first priority is to restore the flow of oxygen-rich blood to the brain. Next, normal heart rhythm must be restored. Forcing air into the mouth will get oxygen into the lungs, and compressing the chest will get some blood flowing to the lungs, brain, and coronary arteries. This process of forced breathing and chest compression is called **cardiopulmonary resuscitation (CPR)**. When trained help arrives, they will attempt to establish a normal heartbeat. To avoid brain death, CPR must begin within four to six minutes and advanced life support measures must begin within eight minutes. CPR requires no special medical skills and training is available nationwide.

Sudden cardiac death is reversible in most people if treatment is begun quickly. However, of the people who are resuscitated, 40% will have another SCD within two years if they don't get treatment for the underlying cause of the problem. Drugs and pacemakers may help.

Sudden Infant Death Syndrome

Sudden Infant Death Syndrome (SIDS) is defined as ''the sudden death of an infant under one year of age that remains unexplained after a thorough case investigation, including performance of a complete **autopsy**, examination of the death scene, and review of the clinical history.'' SIDS kills approximately 5,000-7,000 babies in the United States each year between the age of one week and one year, with the highest incidence from one to four months. SIDS strikes even healthy babies; more males than females; is more frequent in fall, winter, and early spring; and, while the rate is higher among African-American babies, it is no respecter of race, education, or socioeconomic factors. No one can predict which baby will die from SIDS and, while it is neither contagious nor hereditary, a baby whose sibling died from SIDS is at increased risk. **Death** is sudden and painless and occurs within seconds, usually during **sleep**.

SIDS, commonly called ''crib death'' or ''cot death,'' can be traced through history to at least Old Testament times yet today its cause remains a mystery. For decades, researchers looked for biological or physiological causes. Central **sleep apnea** (cessation of breathing during sleep), the focus of intense investigations over many years, has now been ruled out, as have suffocation, aspiration, and immunization. A turnaround developed in the late 1980s when studies determined that a baby placed on its stomach or side to sleep was at increased risk, probably because of rebreathing its own carbon dioxide resulting in asphyxiation. The U.S. Consumer Products Safety Commission estimates 30% of SIDS-related deaths may be due to unsafe sleeping environments or bedding, such as placing the baby on a soft mattress, waterbed, comforter, pillow, or in a crib with soft toys or bumpers. Babies of pregnant women who smoke, and young babies exposed to passive cigarette smoke, are at higher risk of SIDS. Babies kept too warm are also more susceptible.

Massive **public health** awareness campaigns in New Zealand, Australia, and Norway addressing the above risk factors, reduced the number of SIDS deaths by as much as 50%. Similar campaigns in the United States—particularly the ''Back to Sleep'' campaign which followed recommendations by the American Academy of Pediatrics that healthy babies be placed on their backs to sleep—saw a 20-30% decline from 1992 to 1994, and by 35% in 1996. In countries where the prone sleeping position has been reduced by as little as five to 10%, the SIDS death rate has declined by 70-80%. The higher incidence of SIDS among the African-American population may be because public awareness campaigns are not effectively reaching that population.

Several other theories encompass SIDS: In 1989, a British scientist implicated mould, flame retardants, and other fumes in cot mattresses—this controversial finding was ruled out in a *British Medical Journal* news release in May, 1998. Some experts believe infant-parent ''co-sleeping'' is beneficial in helping prevent SIDS—others say the opposite. While breast feeding increases a baby's natural immunity and provides psychological and physiological benefits to mother and baby, it has not been found to protect against SIDS. A paper published in the *British Medical Journal* in March, 1998 reported that two babies died of what was attributed to SIDS following a transcontinental flight—no scientific studies have been done to determine the safety of air travel for young infants. A case-control study reported that babies of pregnant women who drank more than four cups of coffee daily were more prone to SIDS—these results need to be confirmed by other studies.

Suicide

Suicide is the third leading cause of death among adolescents, occurring at a rate of 10.8 per 100,000 among 15-19 year olds in 1992. Suicide is much less common among 10-14 year olds, at 1.7 per 100,000, although the rate of suicide has increased dramatically since 1950 among all age groups. Suicide attempts are much more common, occurring in 2% of adolescent girls and 1% of adolescent boys per year. Significant suicidal ideation (with a plan to commit suicide or intent to die) is more common, occurring in 5-10% of children and adolescent youth.

The suicide completion rate is about four times higher in males than females, while the rate of attempt is two to three times higher in females than males. Completed suicide may be greater among males because of their tendency to utilize methods of more potential lethality. The rate of suicide also varies according to victims' race. Highest are Native Americans and whites. The suicide rate among African American males increased dramatically in the 1980s, and now approaches 80% of the white male suicide rate.

In the United States, the most common method for completed suicide is firearms, followed by hanging, carbon monoxide, and jumping. A gun in the house, particularly a loaded gun, appears to increase the risk for completed suicide, even in those youth without other obvious risk factors for suicide. Among suicide attempters, the two most common methods are overdose and wrist-cutting.

The most common precipitants for suicidal behavior among children and adolescents involve interpersonal conflict or loss, most frequently with parents or romantic attachment figures. Family discord, physical or sexual abuse, and an upcoming legal or disciplinary crisis are also commonly associated with completed and attempted suicide. Adolescents who complete suicide show relatively high suicidal intent (wish to die), although many are intoxicated at the time of death. The most serious suicide attempters leave suicide notes, show evidence of planning, and use an irreversible method. Most adolescent suicide attempts, though, are of relatively low intent and lethality, and only a minority actually want to die. Usually, suicide attempters want to escape psychological pain or unbearable circumstances, gain attention, influence others, or communicate strong feelings, such as anger or love.

The vast majority of both suicide attempters and completers have evidence of at least one major psychiatric disorder. These disorders are most often affective disorders, causing changes in moods or emotions. Major depressive disorder is the single biggest risk factor for attempted or completed suicide, with the risk heightened even further by comorbid anxiety, substance abuse, or **conduct disorder**. Bipolar affective disorder also conveys increased risk for completed and attempted suicide. There is an average of seven years between the onset of disorder and completed suicide in adolescence, so repeated suicide threats or attempts are common. Youths who attempt suicide feel hopeless, are impulsive, and have poor problem-solving and social skills. Children with other illnesses may also face an increased risk of suicidal behavior. For example, children with epilepsy have a higher suicide rate, which may be related to the side effects of the drug phenobarbital.

Family history and environment are also risk factors for suicide. The relatives of both suicide attempters and completers have high prevalences of affective disorder, substance abuse, assaultive behavior, suicide, and suicide attempts. The tendency for suicidal behavior appears to be passed on independently of the transmission of psychiatric disorders, and may be more closely related to the tendency for impulsive aggression. The family environments of suicide attempters and completers have been described as discordant, with greater exposure to family violence, including physical and **sexual abuse**. Both have also been exposed to suicidal behavior. Studies of friends and siblings of suicide victims show they tend not to imitate the act, suggesting that increased risk is related more to distant exposure. For example, media publicity about fictional or true suicides have been shown consistently to increase the risk for suicide and suicidal behavior.

Repeated suicide attempts are common, but rates vary. Follow-up studies ranging from one to 12 years found a reattempt rate among adolescents of between 6% and 15% per year, with the greatest risk within the first three months after the initial attempt. Factors associated with a higher reattempt rate included chronic and severe psychopathology (depression and substance abuse), hostility and **aggression**, noncompliance with treatment, poor level of social adaptation, family discord, abuse, or neglect, and parental psychopathology. The risk for completed suicide ranges from 0.7% per year among males and 0.1% per year among females seen in an emergency room for an overdose. Among psychiatric inpatients after a 10-15 year follow-up, the risks are higher, 10% for males and 2.9% for females.

Suicidal ideation, or thinking about suicide, is even more common than suicidal behavior. Suicidal ideation spans a continuum from non-specific thoughts, for example, ''life is not worth living,'' to specific ideation. Community surveys indicate that between 12 and 25% of primary and high school children have some form of suicidal ideation, whereas 5-10% have suicidal ideation with a plan or intent to make a suicide attempt. Not surprisingly, specific ideation is more closely associated with risk for attempted suicide, and frequently occurs with other risk factors.

Suicidal behavior is rare in prepubertal children, probably because of their relative inability to plan and execute a suicide attempt. Psychiatric risk factors, such as depression and substance abuse, become more frequent in adolescence, contributing to the increase in the frequency of suicidal behavior in older children. The emergence of conflicts with parents and with boy/girlfriends and legal or disciplinary problems are frequently associated with suicidal behavior. Some view the transition from primary to middle school as particularly stressful, especially for girls. Finally, parental monitoring and supervision decrease with increasing age, so that adolescents may be more likely to experience emotional difficulties without parents' knowledge.

The first step in the care of a suicidal patient is to determine the degree of suicidal risk and the appropriate level of care. It is critical to obtain a no-suicide contract with the patient and family, in which the patient promises to refrain from self-destructive behavior and to notify the professional or caregiver if he or she does feel suicidal again. Treatment of the suicidal youngster should proceed on four levels: (1) removal of firearms and dangerous medications from the home; (2) treatment of the underlying psychiatric disorders; (3) remediation of social and problem-solving skills; and (4) family education about psychiatric problems and suicidal risk.

See also Self-injury

SULFONAMIDES

Sulfonamides are medicines that prevent the growth of bacteria in the body. They are used to treat many kinds of infections caused by bacteria and certain other microorganisms. Doctors may prescribe these drugs to treat urinary tract infections, ear infections, frequent or long-lasting **bronchitis**, bacterial **meningitis**, certain eye infections, *Pneumocystis carinii* **pneumonia**, traveler's diarrhea, and a number of other kinds of infections. These drugs will *not* work for colds, flu, and other infections caused by viruses.

Sulfonamides (also called sulfa drugs) are available only by prescription in tablet and liquid forms. Some commonly-used sulfonamides are sulfisoxazole (Gantrisin) and the combination drug sulfamethoxazole and trimethoprim (Bactrim, Cotrim).

The recommended dosage depends on the type of sulfonamide, the strength of the medicine, and the medical problem for which it's being taken. Sulfonamides should always be taken exactly as directed and for the full course of medication to make sure the infection clears up completely.

Sulfonamides work best when they are at constant levels in the blood, so the medicine should be taken in evenly-spaced doses through the day and night. For best results, the medicine should be taken with a full glass of water. Drinking extra glasses of water throughout the day may help prevent side effects.

Although such side effects are rare, some people have had severe and life-threatening reactions to sulfonamides. These include sudden, severe liver damage, serious blood problems, breakdown of the outer layer of the skin, and a condition called Stevens-Johnson syndrome, in which people get blisters around the mouth, eyes, or anus. Call a doctor right away if any of these signs of a dangerous reaction occur:

- Skin rash or reddish or purplish spots on the skin
- Other skin problems, such as blistering or peeling
- **Fever**
- **Sore throat**
- **Cough**
- **Shortness of breath**
- Joint **pain**
- Pale skin
- Yellow skin or eyes

Because this medicine may cause **dizziness**, anyone who takes sulfonamides should not drive, use machines or do anything that might be dangerous until they have found out how the drugs affect them.

Sulfonamides may cause blood problems that can interfere with healing and lead to additional infections, so injuries should be avoided while taking this medicine. It's especially important not to damage the mouth when brushing or flossing the teeth or using a toothpick. Dental work should not be done until the blood is back to normal.

This medicine may increase sensitivity to sunlight. Since even brief exposure to sun can cause a severe **sunburn** or a rash, patients should avoid direct sunlight, especially between 10 a.m. and 3 p.m.; wear a hat and tightly woven clothing that covers the arms and legs; use a sunscreen with a skin protection factor (SPF) of at least 15; protect the lips with a sun block lipstick; and avoid tanning beds, tanning booths, or sunlamps.

Babies under 2 months should not be given sulfonamides unless their doctor has ordered the medicine. Older people may be especially sensitive to the effects of sulfonamides, increasing the chance of unwanted side effects, such as severe skin problems and blood problems. Patients who are taking water pills (diuretics) at the same time as sulfonamides may also be more likely to have these problems.

People with certain medical conditions or who are taking certain other medicines can have problems if they take sulfonamides:

Anyone who has had unusual reactions to sulfonamides, water pills (diuretics), diabetes medicines, or **glaucoma** medicine in the past should let his or her physician know before taking sulfonamides. The physician should also be told about any **allergies** to foods, dyes, preservatives, or other substances.

In studies of laboratory animals, some sulfonamides cause **birth defects**. The drugs' effects on unborn babies have not been studied, but pregnant women should not use this medicine near the time of labor and delivery because it may cause side effects in the baby. Women who are pregnant or who may become pregnant should check with their doctors about the safety of using sulfonamides during **pregnancy**.

Sulfonamides pass into breast milk and may cause liver problems, anemia, and other problems in nursing babies whose mothers take the medicine. Because of those problems, women should not breastfeed when they are taking this drug. Women who are breastfeeding and who need to take this medicine should check with their doctors to find out how long they need to stop breastfeeding.

Before using sulfonamides, people with any of these medical problems should make sure their physicians are aware of their conditions:

- Anemia or other blood problems
- Kidney disease
- Liver disease
- **Asthma** or severe allergies
- Alcohol abuse
- Poor nutrition
- Abnormal intestinal absorption
- **Porphyria** (a disorder of blood pigment)
- Folic acid deficiency
- Deficiency of the enzyme glucose-6-phosphate dehydrogenase (G6PD).

Taking sulfonamides with certain other drugs may affect the way the drugs work or may increase the chance of side effects. The most common side effects are mild **diarrhea**, **nausea**, vomiting, dizziness, **headache**, loss of appetite, and tiredness. These problems usually go away as the body adjusts to the drug and don't require medical treatment. More serious side effects aren't common, but any of the following should be reported to a doctor immediately:

- **Itching** or skin rash
- Reddish or purplish spots on the skin
- Other skin problems, such as redness, blistering, peeling
- Severe, watery or bloody diarrhea
- Muscle or joint aches
- Fever
- Sore throat
- Cough
- Shortness of breath
- Unusual tiredness or weakness
- Unusual bleeding or bruising
- Pale skin
- Yellow eyes or skin
- Swallowing problems.

Sulfonamides may interact with a large number of other medicines. When this happens, the effects of one or both of the drugs may change or the risk of side effects may be greater. Among the drugs that may interact with sulfonamides are:

- **Acetaminophen** (Tylenol)
- Medicine for overactive thyroid
- Male hormones (androgens)
- Female hormones (estrogens)
- Other medicines used to treat infections

- Birth control pills
- Medicines for diabetes such as glyburide (Micronase)
- Blood thinners such as warfarin (Coumadin)
- Disulfiram (Antabuse), used to treat alcohol abuse
- Amantadine (Symmetrel) used to treat flu and also **Parkinson's disease**
- Water pills (diuretics) such as hydrochlorothiazide (HCTZ, HydroDIURIL)
- The anticancer drug methotrexate (Rheumatrex)
- Antiseizure medicines such as valproic acid (Depakote, Depakene).

The list above does not include every drug that may interact with sulfonamides, so any patient taking this medicine should check with a doctor or pharmacist before combining sulfonamides with anything.

Sunburn

Sunburn is an inflammation of the skin caused by overexposure to the ultraviolet (UV) rays of the sun. There are two types of ultraviolet rays, UVA and UVB. UVA rays penetrate the skin more deeply than UVB rays, and can cause melanoma in susceptible people. UVB rays, on the other hand, cause sunburn and wrinkling.

Skin **cancer** from sun overexposure is a serious health problem in the United States, affecting almost a million Americans each year. One out of 87 will develop malignant melanoma, the most serious type of skin cancer, and 7,300 of them will die each year.

Fair-skinned people are most susceptible to sunburn, because their skin produces only small amounts of the protective pigment called melanin. People trying to get a tan too quickly in strong sunlight are also more vulnerable to sunburn.

Repeated sun overexposure and burning not only cause cancer; it also can prematurely age the skin, causing a yellow, wrinkled appearance.

The ultraviolet rays in sunlight destroy cells in the outer layer of the skin, damaging tiny blood vessels underneath. Once the skin is burned, blood vessels dilate and leak fluid. Skin cells stop making protein, and the cellular DNA is damaged by the ultraviolet rays; repeated DNA damage is what can lead to cancer. As the sun burns the skin, it triggers the body's immune defenses, which identify the burned skin as "foreign." At the same time, the sun transforms a substance on the skin so that it interferes with this immune response, protecting the skin from attack by the immune system. However, this also means that any malignant cells in the skin will be able to grow freely.

Once the skin is burned, it will turn red and blister. Several days later, the dead skin cells peel off.

Aspirin or anti-inflammatory drugs can ease the **pain**, swelling and inflammation of sunburn. Tender skin should be protected against the sun until it has healed. In addition, sunburned skin may feel better after applications of:

- Calamine lotion
- Sunburn cream or spray
- Cool tap water compress
- Colloidal oatmeal (Aveeno) baths
- Dusting powder to reduce chafing

People who are severely sunburned should see a doctor, who may prescribe corticosteroid cream to speed healing.

Over-the-counter preparations containing aloe are an effective treatment for sunburn, easing pain and inflammation while also relieving dryness of the skin. A variety of topical herbal remedies applied as lotions, poltices, or compresses may also help relieve the effects of sunburn. Calendula (*Calendula officinalis*) is one of the most often recommended herbal treatments to ease inflammation.

Moderately burned skin should heal within a week. However, while the skin will heal after a sunburn, the risk of skin cancer increases with each exposure and subsequent burns. Even one bad burn in childhood carries an increased risk of skin cancer.

Everyone over 6 months of age on should use a water-resistant sunscreen with a sun protective factor (SPF) of at least 15. To protect the skin, individuals should apply at least one ounce of sunscreen 30 minutes before going outside, reapplying every two hours (more often after swimming). Babies should be kept completely out of the sun for the first 6 months of life, because their skin is thinner than older children and thus more susceptible to sun damage. Moreover, sunscreens have not been approved for use on infants.

In addition, people should:

- Limit sun exposure to 15 minutes the first day, even if the weather is hazy, slowly increasing exposure daily.
- Reapply sunscreen every two hours (more often if sweating or swimming).
- Reapply waterproof sunscreen after swimming more than 80 minutes, after toweling off, or after perspiring heavily.
- Avoid the sun between 10 a.m. and 3 p.m.
- Use waterproof sunscreen on legs and feet, since the sun can burn even through water.
- Wear an opaque shirt in water, because reflected rays are intensified.

If using a sunscreen under SPF 15, simply applying more of the same SPF won't prolong allowed time in the sun. Instead, patients should use a higher SPF in order to lengthen exposure safely. A billed cap protects 70% of the face; a wide-brimmed hat is better. People at very high risk for skin cancer can wear clothing that blocks almost all UV rays, but most people can simply wear white cotton summer-weight clothing with a tight weave.

Sunscreens

Sunscreens are products applied to the skin to protect against the harmful effects of the sun's ultraviolet (UV) rays. While everyone needs a little sunshine (15 minutes a day helps the body make vitamin D), longer exposure may cause problems from wrinkles to **skin cancer**. Sunscreens help protect against the sun's damaging effects—but just how much protection they provide is a matter of debate.

The sun gives off two kinds of ultraviolet radiation—UV-A and UV-B. For many years, experts thought that only UV-B was harmful, but recent research suggests that UV-A may be just as dangerous, although its effects may take longer to show up. In particular, UV-A may have a role in causing a particularly deadly form of skin cancer called malignant melanoma, which has been on the rise in recent decades as tanning has become more popular. Over the same period, the thin layer of ozone that protects life on earth from the sun's ultraviolet (UV) radiation is being depleted. This allows more UV radiation to get through, adding to the risk of overexposure.

Most sunscreen products contain ingredients that provide adequate protection only against UV-B rays. Even those labeled as "broad spectrum" sunscreens may offer only partial protection against UV-A radiation. Those containing the ingredient avobenzone give the most protection against UV-A rays.

Some medical experts are concerned that sunscreens give people a false sense of security, allowing them to stay in the sun longer than they should. Although sunscreens protect the skin from burning, they may not protect against other kinds of damage. A number of studies suggest that people who use sunscreens may actually increase their risk of melanoma because they spend too much time in the sun. This does not mean that people should stop using sunscreens. It means that they should not rely on sunscreens alone for protection. According to the American Academy of Dermatology, sunscreens should be one part of sun protection, along with wide-brimmed hats and tightly-woven clothing that covers the arms and legs.

Many brands of sunscreens are available that contain a variety of active ingredients that work by absorbing, reflecting, or scattering some or all of the sun's rays. The U.S. Food and Drug Administration requires sunscreen products to carry a sun protection factor (SPF) rating on their labels. This number tells how well the sunscreen protects against burning. The higher the number, the longer a person can stay in the sun without burning. Sunscreen products are sold as lotions, creams, gels, oils, sprays, sticks, and lip balms, and can be bought without a physician's prescription.

Be sure to read the instructions that come with the sunscreen. Some need to be applied as long as one or two hours before sun exposure; others should be applied 30 minutes before exposure. It should be applied liberally to all exposed parts of the skin, including the hands, feet, nose, ears, neck, scalp (if the hair is thin or very short), and eyelids, but avoid the eyes. A lip balm containing sunscreen should be used to protect the lips. Sunscreen needs to be reapplied liberally every one or two hours, or more frequently when perspiring heavily. Sunscreen should also be reapplied after going in the water.

Sunscreen alone will not provide full protection from the sun. When possible, the body should be protected with a hat, long pants, long-sleeved shirt, and sunglasses. It's best to avoid the sun between 10 a.m. and 2 p.m. (11 a.m. to 3 p.m. Daylight Saving Time) when the sun's rays are strongest. The sun can damage the skin even on cloudy days, so sunscreen should be used every day. Be especially careful at high elevations or in areas with surfaces that reflect the sun's rays, such as sand, water, concrete, or snow.

Sunlamps, tanning beds, and tanning booths were once thought to be safer than the sun, because they give off primarily UV-A rays. In fact, UV-A rays cause serious skin damage and may increase the risk of melanoma, and health experts advise people not to use these tanning devices.

People with fair skin, blond, red or light brown hair, and light colored eyes are at greatest risk for developing skin cancer. Also at high risk are those with many large skin **moles**. These people should avoid exposure to the sun as much as possible. However, even dark skinned people may suffer skin damage from the sun and should be careful about exposure.

Sunscreens should not be used on children under 6 months because of the risk of side effects. Instead, children this young should be kept out of the sun. Children over 6 months should be protected with clothing and sunscreens of at least SPF 15, preferably lotions. Sunscreens containing alcohol should not be used on children because they may irritate the skin.

Older people who stay out of the sun and use sunscreens may not produce enough vitamin D in their bodies. They may need to increase the vitamin D in their **diets** by including foods such as fortified milk and salmon. A health care professional can help decide if this is necessary.

Anyone who has had unusual reactions to any sunscreen ingredients in the past should check with a physician or pharmacist before using a sunscreen. The doctor or pharmacist should also be told about any **allergies** to foods, dyes, preservatives, or other substances, especially the following:

- Artificial sweeteners
- Anesthetics such as benzocaine, procaine, or tetracaine
- Diabetes medicine taken by mouth
- Hair dyes
- Sulfa medicines
- Water pills
- Cinnamon flavoring

People with skin conditions or diseases should check with their doctors before using a sunscreen. This is especially true of people with conditions that get worse with exposure to light.

The most common side effects are drying or tightening of the skin. This problem doesn't need medical attention unless it doesn't improve. Other side effects are rare, but possible. If any of the following symptoms occur, check with a doctor as soon as possible:

- **Acne**
- Burning, **itching**, or stinging
- Redness or swelling
- Rash (with or without blisters) that oozes and crusts
- **Pain**
- Pus in hair follicles.

Anyone who uses a prescription or nonprescription drug that is applied to the skin should check with a doctor before using a sunscreen.

SUPPORT GROUPS

Support groups are groups of people who, often on a volunteer basis, help others in need of guidance, sympathy, and kindness. There are many different kinds of support groups such as **HIV** and **AIDS** support group, Alcoholics anonymous support group, different **cancer** support groups, Step-parents support group, New mom's support group, Twins support group and so on. The main purpose of these groups is to make moral support and information readily available to those individuals who need it, in order to live their lives to the fullest.

Many people with cancer, AIDS, and other life-threatening diseases face many challenges that may leave them feeling overwhelmed, afraid, and alone. Sometimes, it can be difficult to cope with these challenges or even to talk to supportive family and friends. Such people may find it therapeutic to meet with other people who have a problem similar to theirs and often this can be accomplished by joining a support group. Members of the support group may be able to help the person feel less alone and can improve their ability to deal with the uncertainties and challenges that life brings. However, support groups are not for everyone. Some people may actually find support groups stressful.

Most support groups are free. Some may collect voluntary donations, or charge modest membership dues to cover basic expenses. A useful support group, for example, a **breast cancer** support group, should include both newcomers and other patients who have survived the illness for long periods, in order to provide a balanced perspective for the group. The group should be stable and meet the needs of its members. There should be leaders who can empathize, gently draw out the shy members and distill the discussion into useful information.

Many organizations offer support groups for individuals with diseases such as cancer, AIDS, drugs and alcohol addictions etc. The doctor, nurse, or hospital social worker will have information about support groups such as their location, size, and type and how often they meet. In addition, many newspapers carry a special health supplement containing information about where to find support groups. Commercial on-line services have added a new dimension to the availability of support for people who need it. American Online, Prodigy, CompuServe all have bulletin boards where various groups regularly provide support and information to all of its members.

There are several kinds of support groups to meet individual needs. Support groups may be led by a professional such as a psychiatrist, psychologist, or social worker or by other patients. These groups may be for a particular disease, for teens or young adults, for family members, or for support that is more general. Support groups can vary in approach, size and how often they meet. It is important that individuals find an atmosphere that they are comfortable with and meets their individual needs.

SURGICAL INSTRUMENTS

The earliest surgical operations were probably circumcision (removal of the foreskin of the penis) and trepanation (making a hole in the skull, for release of pressure and/or spirits). Primitive surgical instruments consisted of flint or obsidian knives and saws. Stone Age skulls from around the world have been found with holes from trepanning. Primitive people used knives to remove fingers, and the ancient Mesopotamian cultures practiced surgery to some degree. Small copper Sumerian knives of about 3000 B.C. are believed to be surgical instruments. The Babylonian *Code of Hammurabi* of about 1700 B.C. mentions bronze lancets—sharp-pointed two-edged instruments used to make small incisions. The Code, however, provided harsh penalties for poor treatment outcomes, so surgery was practiced only sparingly. Likewise, ancient Chinese and Japanese cultures were opposed to cutting into the human body, so surgical instruments were used very little.

By contrast, the ancient Egyptians recorded surgical procedures as early as 2500 B.C. They fashioned sharper instruments with metal and copper, and designed special tools to remove the brain when preparing bodies for mummification. The ancient Hindus excelled at surgery. The great surgical textbook, ***Sushruta** Samhita*, probably dates back to the final centuries B.C. This work described 20 sharp and 101 blunt surgical instruments, including forceps, pincers, trocars (sharp-pointed instruments fitted with a small tube), and cauteries (irons to heat and sear tissue), mostly made of steel. The ancient Hindus used lancets for cataract surgery, scalpels to restore amputated noses via plastic surgery, and sharp knives to remove bladder stones. Ancient Peruvians performed trepanation and left behind various obsidian surgical instruments, including scalpels and chisels. The Greeks practiced surgery, mostly on external parts, using forceps, knives, and probes, among other instruments. Bronze Roman surgical instruments found at Pompeii include a scalpel with a steel blade, spring and scissor forceps, a sharp hook, and shears. **Celsus** in the first century A.D. described the use of ligatures to tie off blood vessels and reduce bleeding during operations. **Galen** (130-200) in the second century A.D. gave detailed instructions on the use of surgical instruments.

After ancient times, medical knowledge atrophied, and surgeons fell to a lowly status. In the absence of knowledge about **antiseptics**, surgery was highly risky, so only the simplest and most urgent operations, such as **amputation**s, were performed. A few physicians sought to spread knowledge of surgical procedures and published texts that illustrated surgical instruments. Among these were the Muslim Spaniard Albucasis (eleventh century—his favorite instrument was the cautery), the Germans Fabricius and Scultetus (1600s), and the Britons William Clowes (1591), Peter Lowe (1596), and John Woodall (1639). Most important was the Frenchman **Ambroise Paré** (1517-1590), the great surgeon of the Renaissance, who revived use of the ligature and invented many surgical procedures and instruments, among the latter being the ''crow's beak'' to hold blood vessels while tying them off. He also perfected an instrument for cataract removal.

The era of modern surgery began with the introduction of anesthesia and antiseptics/antisepsis in the mid-1800s. Louis Pasteur (1822-1895) suggested sterilizing surgical instruments in 1878, and the American doctor **William Halsted** (1852-1922) introduced sterile rubber gloves to surgery in the

1890s. The discovery of X-rays in 1895 gave surgeons an invaluable diagnostic tool. Refinements in surgery were made possible by the introduction of the operating microscope (microsurgery) in the mid-twentieth century and **laser surgery** in the 1970s. New uses for or processing of existing materials continually enhances surgical and diagnostic processes: glass in the form of optical fibre is used in the manufacture of the flexible endoscope, a thin tube with light source, camera, and tiny surgical tools that provides visual examination and allows non-invasive surgery through a natural body opening such as the throat or through a tiny incision; NiTi, bonded nickel and titanium, provides strong, biocompatible, and corrosive resistant metal for implantable devices such as the Mitek anchor used in orthopedic surgery; non-magnetic surgical tools utilizing titanium are durable and lightweight, and compatible with **magnetic resonance imaging**; and bendable handles on surgical instruments—which straighten with the heat of sterilization—allow precision in **open-heart surgery**.

Increasingly sophisticated technology makes ever-more-precise surgical tools possible, among them voice-activated operating microscopes and robotic surgical hands: NASA's Technology Commercialized Program unveiled a robotic "brain surgeon" in June 1997; their "Smart Probe," robotically guided through the brain, uses minute sensors to measure tissue density and blood flow and an endoscope to transmit real-time images and information to the surgeon via adaptable software that literally learns from experience. Also in 1997, the University of California at Berkeley developed a "millirobot" prototype—not yet used by a surgeon—which enters the body and differentiates between healthy and cancerous tissue. Looking much like a fountain pen, this little robot transmits data to the surgeon who directs the operation from a remote location using a television console and controls like joy sticks. Researchers predict that by the end of the first decade in the 2000s, surgeons miles away from an accident victim or battlefield casualty will be directing robotic surgery.

SUSHRUTA

The *Sushruta Samhita* is one of two early texts that form the cornerstone of the Indian medical tradition of Ayurveda (Ayurveda means science of life). The other treatise is called the *Charaka Samhita*. *Samhita* is Sanskrit for compendium, and Sushruta and Charaka are proper names. So the titles translate as "Sushruta's Compendium" and "Charaka's Compendium." Like the *Charaka Samhita*, the *Sushruta Samhita* made revisions and alterations to an earlier text on which it is based, in this case, the writings of Divodasa Dhanvantari, the author's teacher. The author, Sushruta, is identified as the son of the Vedic sage Visvamitra. The text is long, running over 1,700 pages in English translation. The exact date of its composition is unknown, but is generally thought to be around 100

Like the *Charaka Samhita*, the *Sushruta Samhita* refers to the eight branches of **Ayurvedic medicine**. *Sushruta* is organized similarly to *Charaka*, but in addition to emphasizing therapeutics, it also discusses **surgery**, which *Charaka* barely mentions. The text is divided into six sections and 184 chapters. In another major departure from *Charaka*, *Sushruta* describes the need for and way to conduct dissections on human cadavers to gain knowledge of anatomy. Students might practice on natural and artificial objects, for example, vegetables and leather bags full of water. Quartered sacrifical animals were used to study different kinds of anatomy.

Sushruta details about 650 drugs of animal, plant, and mineral origin. In addition, it describes more than 300 kinds of operations that call for 42 different surgical processes and 121 different types of instruments. Other chapters in *Sushruta* make clear the high value put on the well-being of children, and on that of expectant mothers. *Sushruta*'s coverage of toxicology (the study of poisons) is more extensive than that in *Charaka*, and goes into great detail regarding symptoms, first-aid measures, and long-term treatment, as well as classification of poisons and methods of poisoning.

In keeping with the Ayurvedic philosophy of preserving life and preventing the infirmity of old age, *Sushruta* extols the benefits of clean living, pure thinking, good habits and regular exercise, and special diets and drug preparations. A plant called soma that is described in the early texts but has never been clearly identified was recommended as a treatment for rejuvenating body and mind. *Sushruta* explains the need of all living creatures to sleep and to dream as a function of two principles of the mind that give glimpses of previous existences or warn of future ill health. When both principles are weakened, **coma** results.

Sushruta explains the origins of disease as imbalances of vital **humors** that occur either individually or in combination, and that originate from within the body or outside of it, or for no known reason. It discusses the use of surgical devices such as tourniquets and setting plasters, and surgical tools and procedures. Operations are described for amputations, hemorrhoids, **hernia** repair, **eye** surgery, and **Cesarean section**. An operation using skin flaps, for example, to repair a nose, was also described in *Sushruta*. The procedure was observed in India by a British surgeon in 1793 and published in London the following year, thus changing the course of plastic surgery in Europe.

Charaka restricts access to medical training to the three higher orders of society, but *Sushruta* also admits members of the lowest of the four classes. However, such persons would be excluded from special ceremonies accorded to students of more respectable parentage. *Sushruta* describes the day-to-day life of the physician in ancient India, who made the rounds of patients' residences and also maintained a consulting room in his own home, complete with a storeroom of drugs and equipment. Although doctors could command a good living, they might also treat learned brahmins — priests — and the poor for free. *Sushruta* describes the ideal qualities of a nurse, and suggests that doctors may have been required to have licenses.

The drugs described in *Sushruta* include 395 plant substances, 57 substances of animal origin, and 64 mineral substances, metals, and so on. Many of the complicated procedures for dissolving, macerating, extracting, and combusting a variety of solid, squashy, and liquid substances remain part of modern Ayurvedic pharmacological practice.

The conquest by Arabs of the Indian province of Sind (now a part of Pakistan) in the eighth century unleashed a scholarly exchange of scientific ideas. The *Sushruta samhita* was translated into Arabic and later into Persian. These translations, as well as those of *Charaka*, helped to spread the science of Ayurveda far beyond India.

See also Charaka; Pharmacy; Plastic, cosmetic, and reconstructive surgery

SUTHERLAND, EARL (1915-1974)

American biochemist

Earl Wilbur Sutherland, Jr., the fifth of six children in his family, was born on November 19, 1915, in Burlingame, Kansas. His father, Earl Wilbur Sutherland, a Wisconsin native, had attended Grinnell College for two years and farmed in New Mexico and Oklahoma before settling in Burlingame to run a dry-goods business, where Earl Wilbur, Jr., and his siblings worked. Sutherland's mother, Edith M. Hartshorn, came from Missouri. She had been educated at a "ladies college," and had received some nursing training. In 1933 Sutherland entered Washburn College in Topeka, Kansas. Supporting his studies by working as an orderly in a hospital, Sutherland graduated with a B.S. in 1937. Sutherland then entered Washington University Medical School in St. Louis, Missouri. There he enrolled in a pharmacology class taught by **Carl Ferdinand Cori**. Impressed by Sutherland's abilities, Cori offered him a job as a student assistant. This was Sutherland's first experience with research. The research on the sugar glucose that Sutherland undertook in Cori's laboratory started him on a line of inquiry that led to his later groundbreaking studies.

Sutherland received his M.D. in 1942, after which he worked for one year as an intern at Barnes Hospital while continuing to do research in Cori's laboratory. Sutherland was called into service during World War II as a battalion surgeon under General George S. Patton.

In 1945, Sutherland returned to Washington University in St. Louis where he decided to commit himself to a career in research. By 1953, Sutherland had advanced to the rank of associate professor at Washington University. During these years he came into contact with many leading figures in biochemistry, including **Arthur Kornberg**, **Edwin G. Krebs**, T. Z. Posternak, and others now recognized as among the founders of modern molecular biology. But Sutherland preferred, for the most part, to do his research independently. While at Washington University, Sutherland began a project to understand how an enzyme known as phosphorylase breaks down glycogen, a form of the sugar stored in the liver. He also studied the roles of the hormone adrenaline, also known as epinephrine, and glucagon, secreted by the pancreas, in stimulating the release of energy-producing glucose from glycogen.

Sutherland left Washington for Western Reserve (now Case Western) University in Cleveland in 1953. It was during the ten years he spent in Cleveland that Sutherland clarified an important mechanism by which hormones produce their effects. Scientists had previously thought that hormones acted on whole organs. Sutherland, however, showed that hormones stimulate individual cells in a process that takes place in two steps. First, a hormone attaches to specific receptors on the outside of the cell membrane. Sutherland called the hormone a "first messenger." The binding of the hormone to the membrane triggers release of a molecule known as cyclic AMP within the cell. Cyclic AMP then goes on to play many roles in the cell's metabolism, and Sutherland referred to the molecule as the "second messenger" in the mechanism of hormone action. In particular, Sutherland studied the effects of the hormone adrenaline, also called epinephrine, on liver cells. When adrenaline binds to liver cells, cyclic AMP is released and directs the conversion of sugar from a stored form into a form the cell can use.

Sutherland made two more important discoveries while at Western Reserve. He found that other hormones also spur the release of cyclic AMP when they bind to cells, in particular, the adrenocorticotropic hormone and the thyroid-stimulating hormone. This implied that cyclic AMP was a sort of universal intermediary in this process, and it explained why different hormones might induce similar effects. In addition, cyclic AMP was found to play an important role in the metabolism of one-celled organisms, such as the amoeba and the bacterium *Escherichia coli,* which do not have hormones. That cyclic AMP is found in both simple and complex organisms implies that it is a very basic and important biological molecule and that it arose early in evolution and has been conserved throughout millennia.

In 1963 Sutherland moved to Vanderbilt University in Nashville, Tennessee, where he was able to devote more of his time to research. At Vanderbilt, Sutherland continued his work on cyclic AMP. He and other researchers continued to discover physiological processes in different tissues and various animal species that are influenced by cyclic AMP, for example in brain cells and **cancer** cells. In the meantime, his pioneering studies had opened up a new field of research. By 1971, as many as two thousand scientists were studying cyclic AMP.

For most of his career Sutherland was well-known mainly to his scientific colleagues. In the early 1970s, however, a rush of awards gained him more widespread public recognition. Most notably, in 1971 he was awarded the Nobel Prize for "his long study of hormones, the chemical substances that regulate virtually every body function." In 1973 Sutherland moved to the University of Miami. Shortly thereafter, he suffered a massive esophageal hemorrhage, and he died on March 9, 1974, after surgery for internal bleeding, at the age of 58.

SUTURES, VASCULAR • See Carrel, Alexis

SWEATING

Sweating is the body's way of cooling itself and is a normal response to a hot environment or intense exercise. However, Hyperhidrosis (excessive sweating unrelated to these conditions)—as sweat retention syndrome—can be a problem for some people. Those with constantly moist hands may feel uncomfortable shaking hands or touching, while others with sweaty armpits and feet may have to contend with the unpleasant odor that results from the bacterial breakdown of sweat and cellular debris (bromhidrosis). People with hyperhidrosis often must change their clothes at least once a day, and their shoes can be ruined by the excess moisture. Hyperhidrosis may also contribute to such skin diseases as athlete's foot (tinea pedis) and contact dermatitis.

Sweat retention syndrome, or miliaria rubra, also known as prickly heat, is a common disorder of the sweat glands.

The skin contains two types of glands: one produces oil and the other produces sweat. Sweat glands are coil-shaped and extend deep into the skin. They are capable of plugging up at several different depths, producing four distinct skin **rashes**.

- Miliaria crystallina is the most superficial of the occlusions. At this level, only the thin upper layer of skin is effected. Little blisters of sweat that cannot escape to the surface form. A bad **sunburn** as it just starts to blister can look exactly like this.
- Deeper plugging causes miliaria rubra as the sweat seeps into the living layers of skin, where it irritates and itches.
- Miliaria pustulosais (a complication of miliaria rubra) when the sweat is infected with pyogenic bacteria and turns to pus.
- Deeper still is miliaria profunda. The skin is dry, and goose bumps may or may not appear.

There are two requirements for each of these phases of sweat retention: hot enough weather to induce sweating, and failure of the sweat to reach the surface.

Conditions or situations that can trigger hyperhidrosis are varied. They include stressful situations, eating spicy foods, consuming alcohol, the presence of underlying disorders (e.g. tuberculosis, malaria, lymphoma, and diabetes), menopause, hormonal imbalances, and the use of certain drugs. Physicians believe that hyperhidrosis can be linked to a breakdown in communication between the brain and the mechanisms that activate sweating. In addition, a genetic link may also exist: about 40% of people with the condition have a family history of it.

The best evidence to date suggests that bacteria form the plugs in the sweat glands. These bacteria are probably normal inhabitants of the skin, and why they suddenly interfere with sweat flow is still not known.

Infants are more likely to get miliaria rubra than adults. All the sweat retention rashes are also more likely to occur in hot, humid weather.

Besides **itching**, these conditions prevent sweat from cooling the body, which it is supposed to do by evaporating from the skin surface. Sweating is the most important cooling mechanism available in hot environments. If it does not work effectively, the body can rapidly become too hot, with severe and even lethal consequences. Before entering this phase of heat stroke, there will be a period of heat exhaustion symptoms—**dizziness**, thirst, weakness—when the body is still effectively maintaining its temperature. Then the temperature rises, often rapidly, to 104-5° F (40° C) and beyond. This is an emergency of the first order, necessitating immediate and rapid cooling. The best method is immersion in ice water.

The condition of excessive sweating is diagnosed by patient report and a **physical examination**.

The rash and dry skin in hot weather associated with sweat retention syndrome are sufficient usually to diagnose this condition.

Most over-the-counter antiperspirants are not strong enough to effectively prevent hyperhidrosis. To treat the disorder, doctors usually prescribe 20% aluminum chloride hexahydrate solution (Drysol), which the patient applies at night to the affected areas that are then wrapped in a plastic film until morning. Drysol works by blocking the sweat pores. Formaldehyde- and glutaraldehyde-based solutions can also be prescribed; however, formaldehyde may trigger an allergic reaction and glutaraldehyde can stain the skin (for this reason it is primarily applied to the soles). Anticolinergic drugs may also be used. In addition, an electrical device that emits low-voltage current can be held against the skin to reduce sweating. These treatments are usually conducted in a doctor's office on a daily basis for several weeks, followed by weekly visits. Dermatologists also recommend that patients wear clothing made of natural or absorbent fabrics, avoid high-buttoned collars, use talc or cornstarch, and keep underarms shaved.

The only permanent cure for hyperhidrosis of the palms is a surgical procedure. To treat severe excessive sweating, a surgeon can remove a portion of the nerve near the top of the spine that controls palm sweat. However, not very many neurosurgeons in the United States will perform the procedure. Alternatively, it is possible to remove the sweat gland-bearing skin of the armpits, but this is a major procedure that may require skin grafts.

The rash of sweat retention syndrome itself may be treated with topical anti-pruritics (itch relievers). Preparations containing aloe, menthol, camphor, eucalyptus oil, and similar ingredients are available commercially. Even more effective, particularly for widespread itching in hot weather, are cool baths with corn starch and/or oatmeal (about 0.5 lb [224 g] of each per bathtub-full).

Dermatologists can peel off the upper layers of skin using a special ultraviolet light. This will remove the plugs and restore sweating, but is not necessary in most cases.

Much more important, however, is to realize that the body cannot cool itself adequately without sweating. Careful monitoring for symptoms of heat disease is important. If they appear, some decrease in the ambient temperature must be achieved by moving to the shade, taking a cool bath or shower or turning up the air conditioner.

While hyperhidrosis cannot be cured without radical surgery, it can usually be controlled effectively.

The rash associated with sweat retention sayndrome disappears in a day with cooler temperatures, but the skin may not recover its ability to sweat for two weeks—the time needed to replace the top layers of skin with new growth from below.

Experimental application of topical **antiseptics** like hexachlorophene almost completely prevented these rashes.

Sydenham's Chorea

Also called St. Vitus' dance, Sydenham's chorea is a disorder of the central nervous system characterized by jerky, uncontrollable movements, either of the face or of the arms and legs. It occurs chiefly in children following an attack of **rheumatic fever** (an infectious disease caused by certain types of bacteria, usually beginning with a **strep throat** or **tonsillitis**).

Sydenham's chorea is rare in the United States today, although it is a common problem throughout the developing world.

Sydenham's chorea appears as uncontrollable twitching or jerking of any part of the body that gets worse if the patient tries to stop the movements, but disappears with sleep. The involuntary jerks are random, and voluntary movements are clumsy. Early signs of the problem include slurred speech and increasingly-poor handwriting.

Treatment includes bed rest and antibiotics; sedation may be needed if the involuntary movements are severe. Sydenham's chorea will go away as the patient recovers, and it doesn't usually require treatment, although it responds to mild sedatives. Typically, it lasts for several months before clearing up; there are no long-term problems associated with the condition.

It can be prevented only if rheumatic fever is prevented, by treating a bacterial infection with a full 10 days of **antibiotics** (penicillin or erythromycin).

Sydenham, Thomas (1624-1689)

English physician

Thomas Sydenham was born into a prominent family in Dorset, England. He received a bachelor of medicine degree from Magdalen Hall, Oxford in 1648, and a doctor of medicine degree from Cambridge in 1676. In 1655 he began practicing medicine in King Street, Westminster. Because he reintroduced into medicine the Hippocratic method of accurate bedside observation and the use of these observations in the classification and treatment of disease, he became known as the ''English **Hippocrates**.''

At the time of Sydenham's entry into medicine, the climate of his profession tended toward the theoretical. Many of his colleagues were *systematists* who believed that all physical phenomena could be explained by a single chemical cause. In contrast, Sydenham directed his attention toward his patients' particular symptoms. He saw a need to develop a general clinical description of individual diseases, and his eventual fame arose from the firsthand accounts he recorded at his patients' bedsides in pursuit of this goal.

An empiricist and a skeptic, he believed human understanding to be limited to experiencing and interpreting observable data. Applying his empiricism to the improvement of the

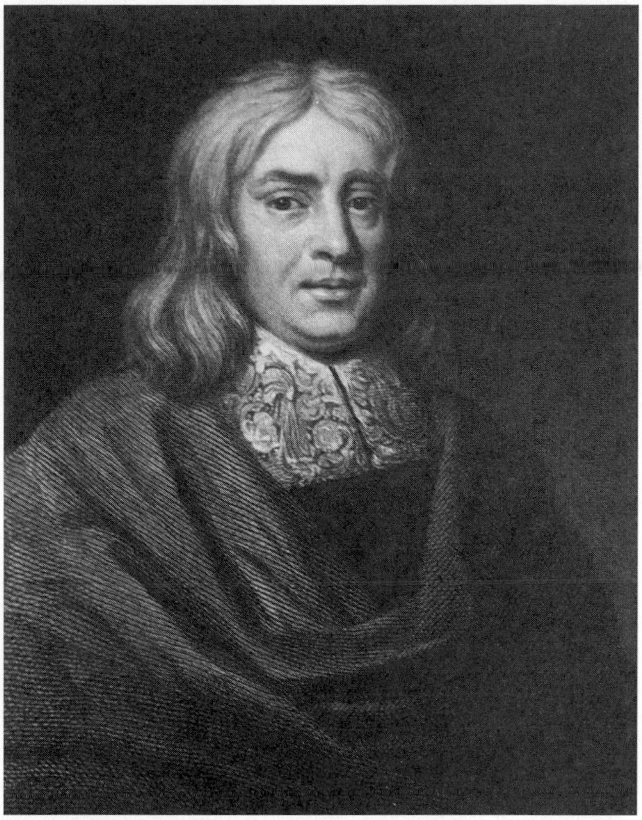

Thomas Sydenham

science of medicine, he made the results of his treatments the test of the truth in his observations of illness. Known also as an optimist for his understanding of nature as an orderly instrument of a benevolent God, he believed that nature cured patients; physicians were merely nature's assistants.

Sydenham's approach to the understanding of the natural world had much in common with that of his contemporary, philosopher John Locke (1632-1704). Locke assisted or collaborated with Sydenham on several medical texts. In his *Essay Concerning Human Understanding*, Locke placed Sydenham alongside Robert Boyle, Isaac Newton, and Christiaan Huygens, calling them ''master-builders'' in the new sciences.

Between the years of 1669 and 1674, Sydenham kept a notebook of clinical observations upon which he based his magnum opus: *Observationes medicae circa morborum acutorum historiam et curationem*, published in 1676. He was the first to describe Sydenham's chorea ('' St. Vitus' Dance''), but merely as an aside in a treatise on another subject. The first western physician to use quinine in the treatment of **malaria**, liquid opium (laudanum) in pain relief, and iron in the treatment of diseases of the blood, he is known also for the cooling regimen which revolutionized the treatment of **smallpox** and other fevers, and especially for the application of his medical principles in his treatise on gout, of which he eventually died in London, England.

Syphilis

Syphilis is a chronic, degenerative, **sexually transmitted disease**. Highly contagious— particularly during the early stages of its progression—syphilis can be cured in its primary and secondary stages with **penicillin** administered over a prolonged period, although treatment in the primary stage fails approximately two to 20% of the time. Left untreated, it continues, eventually causing serious damage to the nerves, brain, eyes, heart, and other organs. Although the incidence of syphilis has been reduced somewhat through education programs and medication, the incidence remains high and has risen dramatically in connection with the **AIDS** virus, making it a **public health** concern around the world.

Spread primarily by sexual contact, syphilis begins as a small, hard, painless sore, called a *primary* (or *Hunter's*) *chancre*, which disappears in one to five weeks after infection. Left untreated, the disease passes into the secondary stage, lodging in the lymph nodes. Within 6-12 weeks, discolored patches appear on the palms of the hands and soles of the feet; skin sores, mucous patches in the mouth, throat and cervix, and a body rash appear; along with patchy hair loss and flu-like symptoms. This second stage can last two to six weeks. Left untreated, syphilis goes into its latent stage, during which no symptoms are evident. One in every three people with latent syphilis develop third stage disease which becomes evident from 10-40 years after the primary stage, and can lead to paralysis and death. Pregnant women infected with the disease can transmit the infection to the unborn child, causing congenital syphilis. Approximately 40% of these babies die and most of those who live suffer serious abnormalities.

The earliest records of syphilis are those of Spanish physician, Rodrigo Ruiz de Isla, who wrote that he treated syphilis patients in Barcelona in 1493. He further claimed that the soldiers of explorer Christopher Columbus contracted the disease in the Caribbean and brought it back to Europe in 1492. However, others challenge this position. Some medical historians believe that syphilis has been present from ancient times but was often mislabeled or misdiagnosed.

Italian physician and writer, Girolamo Fracastoro, gave the disease its name in his poem ''Syphilis sive morbus Gallicus'' (Syphilis or the French Disease), published in 1530 during the height of a European epidemic. However, for centuries, the disease was called pox or the great pox. At that time, treatment was mercury, used in vapor baths, as an ointment, or taken orally. The mercury increased the flow of saliva and phlegm, supposedly to wash out the poisons, but it also caused discomfort such as loss of hair and teeth, abdominal pains, and mouth sores.

Through the centuries, a milder form of the disease evolved and often became confused with **gonorrhea**. In 1767, physician John Hunter infected himself with fluid from a patient who had gonorrhea to prove these were two different diseases. Unknown to Hunter, the patient also had syphilis. Hunter developed the sore indicative of syphilis that now bears his name. The distinction between the two diseases was made clear in 1879 when German bacteriologist, Albert Neisser, isolated the bacterium responsible for gonorrhea.

In 1903, Russian biologist **Elie Metchnikoff** and French scientist Pierre-Paul-Emile Roux demonstrated that syphilis could be transmitted to monkeys and then studied in the laboratory. They also showed that mercury ointment was an effective treatment in the early stages.

Two years later, German zoologist Fritz Schaudinn and his assistant Erich Hoffmann discovered the bacterium responsible for syphilis—the spiral-shaped spirochete called *Treponema pallidum*. The following year, German physician **August von Wassermann** (1866-1925) developed the first diagnostic test for syphilis based on new findings in immunology. The test involved checking for the syphilis antibody in a sample of blood. One drawback was that the test would take two days to complete.

In 1904, German research physician **Paul Ehrlich** began focusing on a safe, effective treatment for syphilis. Ehrlich had spent many years studying the effect of dyes on biological tissues and treatments for tropical diseases. His work in the emerging field of immunology earned him a Nobel Prize in 1908.

Ehrlich began working with the arsenic-based compound ''atoxyl'' as a possible treatment for syphilis. Japanese bacteriologist, Sahachiro Hata, came to study syphilis with Ehrlich. Hata tested hundreds of derivatives of atoxyl and finally found one that worked, number 606. Ehrlich called it ''Salvarsan.'' Following clinical trials, in 1911 Ehrlich and Hata announced the drug was an effective cure for syphilis. The drug attacked the disease germs but did not harm healthy **cells**; thus, Salvarsan ushered in the new field of **chemotherapy**. Ehrlich went on to develop two safer forms of the drug, including neosalvarsan in 1912 and sodium salvarsan in 1913.

Penicillin came into widespread use in treating bacterial diseases during World War II. It was first used against syphilis in 1943 by New York physician, John F. Mahoney, and it remains the treatment of choice today. Other **antibiotics** are also effective.

Meanwhile, Russian-American researcher Reuben Leon Kahn (1887-1979) developed a modified test for syphilis in 1923 which took only a few minutes to complete. Another test was developed by researchers **William A. Hinton** (1883-1959) and J. A. V. Davies. Today, syphilis is diagnosed either by signs and symptoms, microscopic examination of a lesion specimen, and fluorescent antibody blood tests. There is no inoculation against the disease.

Syringe

A pumplike device used for hypodermic or subcutaneous (beneath the skin) injections or to remove liquids by suction, the syringe consists of a tube—usually made of plastic—that is tapered at one end and has a plunger at the other that either creates suction when pulled back or forces out fluid when pushed forward. The syringe may be used for intravenous (going into the veins), intramuscular (into the muscle), or intradermal (between skin layers) injections to administer drugs or vaccines.

The conceptualization of the syringe is thought to have originated in fifteenth-century Italy, but it was not developed for practical use until several centuries later. In 1657, experiments were conducted on syringe-like devices by two Englishmen, Christopher Wren (1632-1723) and Robert Boyle. Dominique Anel, a surgeon to the seventeenth-century army of French King Louis XIV (1638-1715), is usually credited with the invention of the kind of syringe used today, which he devised to clean wounds with suction. The first true hypodermic syringe was created by Charles Pravaz, a French physician, in 1853; it was made entirely of silver and held one cubic centimeter of liquid. Around the same time, Scotsman Alexander Wood devised a subcutaneous injection method, allowing physicians to administer intravenous anesthesia for the first time. An Englishman named Fergusson used a syringe made partially of glass, thus allowing visual monitoring of injections. The all-glass syringe developed by a man named Luer in France in 1869 further reduced the risk of infection.

Today, increased public awareness about acquired immune deficiency syndrome (**AIDS**) and concern about halting the progress of the deadly human immunodeficiency virus (HIV) has led to the widespread use of disposable syringes, which are used only once and then discarded. In some cities, these syringes have been distributed free to users of illegal, injectable drugs, whose sharing of unsanitary needles containing traces of HIV-infected blood has made them among the most common victims of AIDS. Although many health practitioners and others believe this practice is in the public's best interest, it has met with resistance from those who feel it encourages, or at least communicates, tolerance of illegal drug use.

SYSTEMIC LUPUS ERYTHEMATOSUS

Systemic lupus erythematosus (also called lupus, or SLE) is a disease in which a person's **immune system** attacks and injures the body's own organs and tissues. Almost every system of the body can be affected by SLE.

The body's immune system is a network of cells and tissues responsible for fighting off invading foreign organisms such as bacteria, viruses, and fungi. Antibodies are special immune cells that recognize these foreign invaders, and begin a chain of events to destroy them. In an autoimmune disorder like SLE, a person's antibodies begin to recognize the body's own tissues as foreign, causing inflammation of the tissues. In SLE, some of the common antibodies that normally fight diseases are thought to be out of control, and begin to attack the cell's central structure that contains genetic material.

SLE can occur in both men and women of all ages, but 90% of patients are women and most are in their childbearing years. African Americans are more likely than Caucasians to develop SLE.

Occasionally, medications can cause a syndrome of symptoms very similar to SLE called drug-induced lupus. Medications that may cause this syndrome include hydralazine (used to treat high blood pressure) and procainamide (used for abnormal heartbeats). Drug-induced lupus almost always disappears after the patient stops taking the medications that caused it.

The cause of SLE is unknown, but it is likely there are many factors that influence its development. Because the vast majority of patients are women, scientists suspect the disease may be associated with female hormones. SLE also may have a genetic basis, although more than one gene is believed to be involved in the development of the disease. Because patients with the disease may suddenly get worse after exposure to a range of substances such as sunlight, alfalfa sprouts, and certain medications, researchers suspect that some environmental factors may also be at work.

The severity of a patient's condition changes over time. Patients may have periods with mild or no symptoms, followed by a sudden worsening as new organs become affected. Many SLE patients have **fevers**, fatigue, muscle **pain**, weakness, loss of appetite, and weight loss. The spleen and lymph nodes are often swollen and enlarged. The development of other symptoms in SLE varies, depending on the organs affected.

- Joints. About 90% of SLE patients have joint pain and problems such as arthritis.
- Skin. A number of skin **rashes** may occur, including a red butterfly-shaped rash that spreads across the nose and cheekbones or a coin-shaped rash of red, scaly bumps on the cheeks, nose, scalp, ears, chest, back, and the tops of the arms and legs. The roof of the mouth may develop sore, irritated ulcers. Hair loss is common. SLE patients tend to be very sensitive to the sun.
- Lungs. Inflammation of the lungs and tissues of the chest cavity causes a fluid build up in the lungs, with coughing and **shortness of breath**.
- Heart and circulatory system. The tissue surrounding the heart or the heart itself may become inflamed. These heart problems may result in abnormal beats (arrhythmias), problems in pumping the blood strongly enough or even sudden **death**. Blood clots often form in the blood vessels and may lead to complications.
- Nervous system. **Headaches**, seizures, personality changes, and confusion may occur.
- Kidneys. The kidneys may be damaged so that they can't filter the blood, which could lead to kidney failure.
- Gastrointestinal system. Patients may experience nausea, vomiting, **diarrhea**, and abdominal pain. The lining of the abdomen may become inflamed (peritonitis).
- Eyes. The eyes may become red, sore, and dry. Inflammation of the nerves responsible for eyesight may cause vision problems; inflammation of the blood vessels that serve the retina may lead to blindness.

Diagnosis of SLE is not easy, since there are no sure-fire tests for the condition. Many of the symptoms and test results of SLE patients are similar to those of patients with different diseases, including **rheumatoid arthritis**, **multiple sclerosis**, and various other nervous system and blood disorders.

Tests may check for a high level of certain antibodies or low numbers of red blood or white blood cells. Samples of tissue from affected skin and kidneys show characteristics of the disease.

The American Rheumatism Association developed a list of symptoms used to diagnose SLE. Research supports the idea that people who have at least four of the eleven criteria (not necessarily at the same time) are extremely likely to have SLE. The criteria are:

- Butterfly rash
- Discoid rash
- **Photosensitivity**
- Mouth ulcers
- Arthritis
- Inflammation of the lining of the lungs or the lining around the heart
- Kidney damage
- Seizures or psychosis
- Certain types of anemia and low counts of certain white blood cells
- Certain immune cells, anti-DNA antibodies, or a false-positive test for **syphilis**
- Antinuclear antibodies

Treatment depends on the organ systems affected by SLE and the severity of the disease. Some patients have a mild form of SLE which responds to **nonsteroidal anti-inflammatory drugs** like ibuprofen (Motrin, Advil) and **aspirin**. Severe skin rashes and joint problems may respond to a group of medications usually used to treat **malaria**. More severely ill patients with potentially life-threatening complications (including kidney disease, heart inflammation, or nervous system complications), need to be treated with stronger drugs such as steroids. Because steroids have serious side effects, they are reserved for more severe cases of SLE. Drugs that decrease the activity of the immune system also may be used for severely ill SLE patients.

Other treatments for SLE try to ease specific symptoms. Clotting disorders require blood thinners. Psychotic disorders require specific medications. Kidney failure may require either kidney dialysis (waste materials removed from the blood) or a kidney transplant.

A number of alternative treatments may help reduce the symptoms of SLE. These include **acupuncture** and **massage** for relieving the pain of sore joints and muscles. **Stress** management is important for people with SLE, including such techniques as **meditation**, hypnosis, and **yoga**. Dietary suggestions include reduced amounts of red meat and dairy products in order to decrease pain and inflammation. Food **allergies** are believed either to contribute to SLE or to occur as a result of the digestive problems. Wheat, dairy products, and soy are the major offenders. A diet rich in fish containing omega-3 fatty acids such as mackerel, sardines, and salmon may help. Because alfalfa sprouts have been associated with the onset of flares in SLE, they should be avoided.

Supplements may improve the health of SLE patients including **vitamins** B, C, and E, as well as selenium, zinc, magnesium, and a complete trace mineral supplement. Vitamin A is believed to help improve the coin-shaped skin rashes.

The prognosis for patients with SLE varies, depending on which organs are affected and how severe the inflammation is. Some patients have long periods of time with mild or no symptoms. Between 90% and 95% of patients are still living after 2 years and about 82-90% of patients are still living after 5 years. After 10 years, between 71% and 80% of patients are still alive; between 63% and 75% are still alive after 20 years.

The most likely causes of death during the first 10 years include infections and kidney failure. After that, the most likely cause of death involves the development of abnormal blood clots.

Because SLE frequently affects women of childbearing age, **pregnancy** is an important issue. About 30% of pregnant women with SLE will miscarry, and about 25% of all babies born to mothers with SLE are premature. While most babies born to mothers with SLE are normal, a rare condition called neonatal lupus causes a baby of an affected mother to develop a skin rash, liver or blood problems, and a serious heart condition.

There are no known ways to avoid getting SLE, but it's poissible to prevent the flareups by staying out of the sun, getting plenty of rest, eating a healthy diet, decreasing stress, and exercising regularly. It is important for a patient to try to identify the early signs of a flare-up (fever, increased fatigue, rash, headache) so that the person can try to prevent it from worsening.

SZENT-GYÖRGYI, ALBERT (1893-1986)

Hungarian-American biochemist

In 1893, Albert Szent-Györgyi was born in Budapest, Hungary, into a family of noted scientists. During World War I, he spent several years in the Austrian army but, although decorated for bravery, became increasingly convinced the war was a senseless one. Deliberately wounding himself, he returned to his studies and obtained his medical degree from the University of Budapest in 1917. A year later—in large part because the Austrian defeat left his family financially strained—Szent-Györgyi decided to seek further training in other countries. Restless and intellectually curious, he worked and studied in Berlin, Germany, the Netherlands and at the Mayo Clinic in the United States. Finally, in 1927, he obtained his Ph.D. at England's Cambridge University.

At Cambridge, Szent-Györgyi worked in **Frederick Gowland Hopkins**' laboratory and, for a time, concentrated on trying to determine the function of the body's adrenal gland. During that period, in an odd roundabout way, the restless scientist suddenly found himself taking up a new interest: fruits and vegetables. He had already noticed that when someone acquires Addison's disease, which causes the adrenal gland to wither, brownish spots typically appear on the patient's skin. These spots, he felt, were surprisingly similar to the brown spots that appear on plants damaged by oxidation. Intrigued, he asked himself: could oxidation affect the tissue of humans in the same way it affected that of plants?

To answer his own question, Szent-Györgyi first studied plants, like potatoes, that invariably turn brown when exposed to too much oxygen. Then he turned his attention to plants that did not turn brown in similar situations, suspecting that they might possess some kind of antioxidizing substance. Sure enough, Szent-Györgyi not only found such a substance in both oranges and cabbages, but he also found an identical substance in adrenal glands. Because the substance's molecule seemed to possess six carbon atoms, he named it hexuronic acid.

For several years, while working on other projects, Szent-Györgyi continued to investigate his newly discovered substance, (even sending a portion of it to his friend and fellow chemist Walter Norman Haworth (1883-1950), who was eventually to identify vitamin C's chemical structure). But not until 1931—when he had returned to Hungary and joined the faculty of the University of Szeged—could he devote his full attention to it. That year, working with a young American associate, S.L. Svirbely, he discovered that the substance had considerable antiscorbutic effect—it could, in other words, both prevent and counteract **scurvy**. For further research, though, he needed enormous amounts of the hexuronic acid, and he could no longer afford the sources he had been using. Almost in desperation, he turned to one of Hungary's best-known exports, the paprika, a fruit in the red pepper family. And to his intense relief, paprika proved to be an exceedingly rich source of the acid. With ample supplies at his disposal, Szent-Györgyi was able to prove that, as he had long suspected, hexuronic acid was really vitamin C. (He published his findings in 1932, just two weeks after an American team of researchers, headed by Charles G. King, made a similar announcement.) Szent-Györgyi and Haworth, decided to rename the acid, which from then on was called ascorbic acid.

For a few more years, Szent-Györgyi continued to study the activity of ascorbic acid in the body. His researches eventually led him to the isolation of a new catalyst that he called *cytoflave* and which was later identified as vitamin B2 or riboflavin. He also began an intense investigation into the oxygen uptake of minced muscle tissue, his work laying the foundation for the elucidation of the citric acid cycle by **Hans Krebs**.

For his various research projects, particularly those relating to vitamin C, Szent-Györgyi received the Nobel Prize in physiology or medicine in 1937. Later, the scientist switched his studies to the biochemical processes involved in muscle contractions. Active in the anti-Nazi underground during World War II, he was ordered killed by Adolf Hitler (1889-1945) himself, but was saved by friends who brought him to the Swedish Embassy (neutral territory in those days). He remained there until the danger passed. In 1947, he decided to immigrate to the United States and was immediately offered a position at the Marine Biological Laboratories at Woods Hole, Massachusetts.

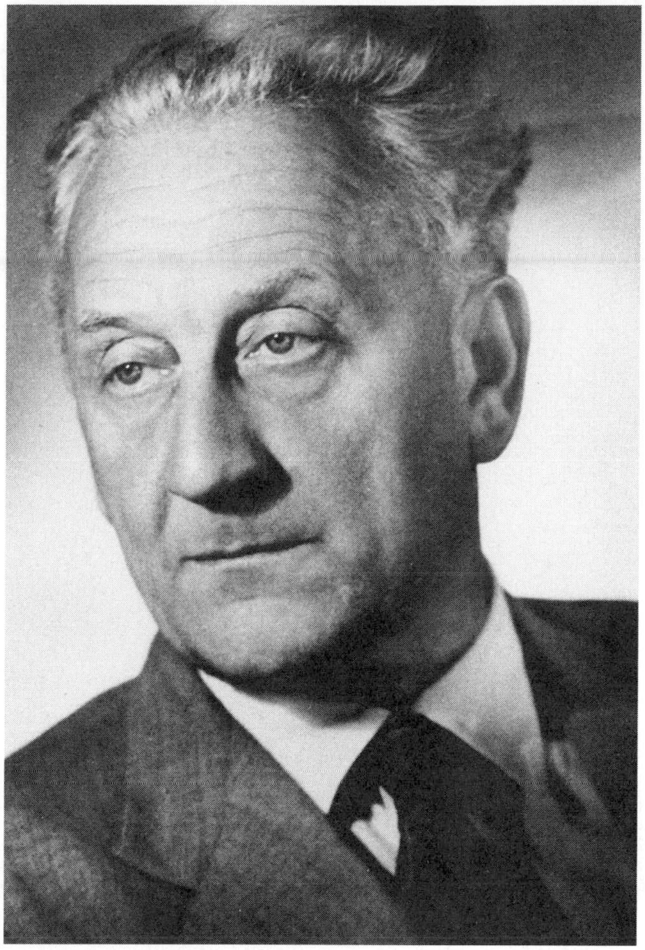

Albert Szent-Györgyi

T

TAI CHI

Tai chi is a Chinese **exercise** system which uses slow, smooth body movements to achieve a state of relaxation of both body and mind. It can help achieve a state of physical and mental relaxation while also strengthening the cardiovascular system.

As a very slow and gentle form of moving, tai chi has virtually no side effects. However, if a person has any doubts about joints, vertebrae, or heart, a doctor should be consulted.

Developed originally in China as a self-defense strategy, tai chi (the "supreme ultimate fist") is practiced in modern times primarily as a gentle exercise technique. Described as "**meditation** in motion," the tai chi practitioner performs a series of postures or bodily movements in a slow and graceful manner, with each movement flowing without pause to the next. According to Chinese legend, the technique was created by a Taoist monk who was inspired as he watched a crane and a snake do battle. Impressed by the snake's ability to subtly and swiftly avoid the bird's thrusts, he devised a series of self-defense techniques that don't involve force, but rather stresses evasion, causing the opponent's own momentum to work against him.

Tai chi is an ancient form of exercise that at one point had more than 100 separate movements or postures. Currently there are two popular versions of 18 and 37 movements respectively. In China, 10 million people practice some type of tai chi daily, making it one of the most popular forms of exercise in the world. In the United States, tai chi is learned in classes in which students (or "players," as they are called in China) wear loose, comfortable clothing and either go barefoot or wear only socks or soft shoes. In China, tai chi is almost always practiced outdoors at dawn, and ideally near trees. Unlike other martial arts, tai chi is not competitive. Classes usually begin with a few minutes of standing meditation to calm the mind and gather energy. Following warm-up exercises, students are taught the basics of a particular form or posture. Learning forms is not easy, and it takes some time to master what looks like a simple position. Properly-done postures are done in a relaxed way with the circular and rhythmic movements of one position flowing seamlessly into the next.

While strict attention to body position is critical, proper breathing is considered to be equally important. Just as movements are slow and continuous and without strain, breathing should be effortless yet deep. Finally, both mental and physical balance is considered essential to tai chi. The experienced practitioner of tai chi maintains perfect body balance throughout the exercise series. Altogether, the five essential qualities of tai chi are:

- Slowness (to develop awareness)
- Lightness (to make movements flow)
- Balance (to prevent body strain)
- Calmness (to maintain continuity)
- Clarity (to focus the mind)

Tai chi has both physical and mental benefits. If done regularly, it improves muscle tone, flexibility, balance, and coordination. Many older people find that it boosts their energy, stamina, and agility, sharpens their reflexes, and gives an overall sense of well-being. The calming and meditative aspects of tai chi allow many to experience its ability to relieve stress. Some claim tai chi to be a healing therapy, and it is often used to support other treatments for chronic conditions; arthritis and digestive disorders are just two examples. Like **yoga**, tai chi has several different styles to suit the individual. It can eventually be done daily by an individual, and ultimately becomes a very personal endeavor. Most Westerners find it best to practice tai chi in the same place and at the same time of day, and those who enjoy it most are those who are not seeking major, dramatic breakthroughs, but rather who can take pleasure in small gains that accumulate over a long period of time.

Tai chi is a safe exercise system for people of all ages and fitness levels. Done properly, without any over-stretching, tai chi should not leave a person feeling tired or sore. Besides its overall fitness benefits and **stress** reduction aspects, regular tai chi sessions are said to be especially helpful for seniors, as it lowers their blood pressure. The practice may help arthritis sufferers and patients recovering from an injury or heart problems. It also improves balance, and reduces the risk of falling, especially important for the elderly. Because of the low stress level of the exercises it is particularly attractive form of exercise to seniors.

Tapeworm diseases

Tapeworms are a group of parasitic worms that live in the intestinal tracts of some animals. Several different species of tapeworms can infect humans. Tapeworm disease or cestodiasis occurs most commonly after eating raw or undercooked meat or fish that contains the immature form of the tapeworm. Tapeworm infections pose a serious public health problem in many less developed countries due to poor sanitation conditions. The disease is most common where livestock, such as cattle and pigs, are raised in areas where human feces are not disposed of in a sanitary manner. Another common source of human tapeworms are certain species of freshwater fish. Tapeworm infections tend to occur more frequently in areas of the world where the people regularly eat raw or undercooked beef, pork, or fish. Persons of all ages and both sexes are susceptible to tapeworm infection, but children are generally not exposed until they are old enough to begin eating meat or fish.

In addition to the typical infection caused by eating undercooked meat or fish, people may also be directly infected by ingesting tapeworm eggs shed by the adult worm. This type of tapeworm infection can lead to a condition referred to as cysticercosis, where the larvae continue to develop within tissues other than the intestinal tract. One of the most serious forms of this disease occurs when the tapeworm larvae infect the central nervous system, a disease referred to as neurocysticercosis. In contrast to a typical tapeworm infection, which may not be associated with symptoms, neurocysticercosis is a serious condition that may cause seizures and is potentially life-threatening.

Identification of tapeworm segments or eggs in a stool sample is necessary for diagnosis of an adult tapeworm infection. In many cases, a tentative diagnosis may be made on the basis of a patient's description of short chains of tapeworm segments in their stool. Whenever possible, tapeworm segments should be carefully collected in water or salt solutions, using strict precautions to avoid contamination. Stool examination should be performed in a laboratory having experience in the diagnosis of intestinal parasites. It is recommended that at least three stool samples be collected on alternate days to increase the likelihood of being able to make an accurate diagnosis. **magnetic resonance imaging** (MRI) may be necessary to determine the exact location of the tapeworm larvae within the body.

Effective treatment of tapeworm infections involves administering compounds that are toxic to the adult worm. Many of the early treatments were also somewhat toxic to the patient, so treatment was often quite an ordeal. Newer medications are much more easily tolerated and are highly effective in eliminating the parasite from the body. It is recommended that follow-up stool samples be examined at one month and three months after treatment has been completed. Treatment can be considered successful if no eggs are present in several stool samples. It should be noted that the tapeworm medications do not kill the tapeworm eggs when they kill the adult worm, so the potential for infection with eggs still exists as the dead worm segments are passed. Proper personal hygiene in individuals receiving treatment will greatly reduce this potential.

The best way to prevent infection with tapeworms is to eliminate the exposure of livestock to the tapeworm eggs by properly disposing of human feces. The next best strategy is to thoroughly cook or freeze all meat and fish before it is eaten to prevent consumption of live tapeworm larvae in infected samples. Larval cysts in pork and beef are killed by moderate temperatures of 150°F (65°C) or if frozen for at least 12 hours. Proper cooking of freshwater fish could also eliminate the possibility of human infection with the fish tapeworm. Freezing fresh fish for 24 hours will also kill the larval form.

See also Diarrhea; Pernicious anemia

Taste

Taste is one of the five senses (the others being **smell**, **touch**, vision, and hearing) through which all animals interpret the world around them. Specifically, taste is the sense for determining the flavor of food and other substances. One of the two chemical senses (the other being smell), taste is stimulated through the contact of certain chemicals in substances with clusters of taste bud cells found primarily on the tongue. However, taste is a complex sensing mechanism that is also influenced by the smell and texture of substances. An individual's unique sense of taste is partially inherited, but factors such as culture and familiarity can help determine why one person's favorite food made be hot and spicy while another just can't get enough chocolate.

The primary organ for tasting is the mouth. Clusters of cells called taste buds (because under the microscope they look similar to plant buds) cover the tongue and are also found to a lesser extent on the cheek, throat, and the roof of the mouth. First discovered in the 19th century by German scientists Georg Meissner and Rudolf Wagner, taste buds lie on the elevated or ridged surface of the tongue (called the papillae) and have hairlike extensions (microvilli) to increase the receptor surface of the cells. For most foods and substances, saliva breaks down the chemical components that travel through the pores in the papillae to reach the taste buds, which specialize primarily in processing one of the four major taste groups: sweet, sour, salty, and bitter.

Taste occurs when specific proteins in the food bind to receptors on the taste buds. These receptors, in turn, send messages to the brain's cerebral cortex, which interprets the flavor. The actual chemical processes involved for each major taste group vary. For example, salty and sour flavors occur when saliva breaks down sodium or acids, respectively. The chemical constituents of foods that give bitter and sweet tastes, however, are much harder to specify because many chemical components are involved.

Although certain taste buds seemed to have an affinity for one of the four major flavors, continued research into this intricate biological process has revealed a complex neural and chemical network that precludes simple black and white explanations. For example, each taste bud actually has receptors for sweet, sour, salty, and bitter sensations, indicating that taste buds are sensitive to a complex flavor spectrum just like vision is sensitive to a broad color spectrum grouped into the four major colors of red, orange, yellow, and green. Particular proteins of taste are also under study, like gustducin, which may set off the plethora of chemical reactions that causes something to taste bitter.

Taste buds for all four taste groups can be found throughout the mouth, but specific kinds of buds are clustered together in certain areas. Think about licking an ice cream cone; taste buds for sweetness are grouped on the tip of our tongue. The buds for sour tastes are on the sides of the tongue and salty on the front. Bitter taste buds on the back of the tongue can make people gag, a natural defense mechanism to help prevent poisoning.

People constantly regenerate new taste buds every 3-10 days to replace the ones worn out by scalding soup, frozen yogurt, and the like. Unfortunately, as people grow older, their taste buds lose their fine tuning because they are replaced at a slower rate. As a result, middle-aged and older people require more of a substance to produce the same sensations of sweetness or spiciness, for example, than would be needed by a child eating the same food.

Scientists have also discovered that genetic makeup partially accounts for individual tasting abilities and preferences for specific foods. According to researchers at Yale University, some people are genetically programmed to have more taste buds and, as a result, taste more flavors in a particular food. (The number of taste buds varies in different animal species. For example, cows have 25,000 taste buds, rabbits 17,000, and adult people approximately 10,000.) In general, a person's ability to taste can lie anywhere in a spectrum from poor to exceptional, with the ability to sense tastes increasing in proportion to the number of taste buds present. The difference in the number of taste buds can be extreme. Researchers have found anywhere from 11 to 1,100 taste buds per square inch in various young people tested. They have also found that women tend to have more taste buds than men and, as a result, are often better tasters. How well people taste greatly affects what they like. Studies at Yale, for example, revealed that children with fewer taste buds who are classified as poor tasters liked cheese more often than exceptional tasters, who experienced a more bitter sensation, probably because of increased sensitivity to the combination of calcium and the milk protein casein found in cheese.

Despite the important role that taste buds play in recognizing flavors, they do not work alone in providing the experience of taste. For example, the amount of naturally occurring salt in saliva varies; the result being that those with less saliva can better taste the saltiness of certain foods than others, who may end up adding salt to get a similar flavor. The smell and texture of foods are also important contributing factors to how people perceive a food to taste and whether or not they like it. Food in the mouth produces an odor that reaches the nose through the nasopharynx (the opening that links the mouth and the nose). Since smell is much more sensitive to odors than taste is to flavors, people often first experience the flavor of a food by its odor. A cold or flu is probably the most common example of how important smell is to taste. People with congestion often experience a diminished ability to taste. The taste buds, however, are working fine; it's the lack of smell that hinders the brain's ability to process flavor. The texture and temperature of food also influences how it tastes. For example, many people would not think of drinking cold coffee, while others will not eat pears because of a dislike for the fruit's gritty texture.

The predilection for certain foods and tastes is not determined merely by biology. Culture and familiarity with foods greatly influence taste preferences. The Japanese have long considered raw fish, or sushi, to be a savory delicacy. But only a decade or so ago, few Americans would have enjoyed such a repast. But as the number of Japanese restaurants with sushi bars grew, so did American's familiarity with this delicacy and, as a result, their taste for it.

The inability to taste is so intricately linked with smell that it is often difficult to tell whether the problem lies in tasting or smelling. An estimated two to four million people in the United States suffer from some sort of taste or smell disorder. The inability to taste or smell not only robs an individual of certain sensory pleasures, it can also be dangerous. Without smell or taste, for example, people cannot determine whether food is spoiled, making them vulnerable to food poisoning. Also, some psychiatrists believe that the lack of taste and smell can have a profoundly negative affect on a person's quality of life, leading to depression or other psychological problems.

There are a variety of causes for taste and smell disorders, from a biological breakdown to the effects of environmental toxins. In addition to cold or flu, common physical ailments that can assault the sense of taste and smell include **allergies** and various viral or bacterial infections that produce swollen mucous membranes. Fortunately, most of these problems are temporary and treatable. However, neurological disorders due to brain injury or diseases like Parkinson's or Alzheimer's can cause more permanent damage to the intricate neural network that processes the sense of taste and smell. Some drugs can also cause these disorders by inhibiting certain enzymes, affecting the body's **metabolism**, and interfering with the neural network and receptors needed to taste and smell. Exposure to environmental toxins like lead, mercury, insecticides, and solvents can also wreak havoc on the ability to smell and taste by causing damage to taste buds and sensory cells in the nose or brain.

TATTOO

A tattoo is a permanent mark on the skin made by piercing the skin with needles and introducing pigment. Tattooing is considered generally safe when done by an experienced tattooist who sterilizes equipment and follows proper sanitary practices, and if appropriate care is taken during the healing process. However, getting a tattoo involves perforating the skin—one of the body's principal protections against disease. If not done safely, this can cause life-threatening infections. According to the U.S. **Centers for Disease Control**, human immunodeficiency virus (HIV), **hepatitis** B virus, and other blood-borne infections may be transmitted if blood-contaminated instruments are not properly sterilized or disinfected. The American Red Cross refuses donations of blood from anyone who has undergone tattooing during the previous year. There is also a risk of an allergic reaction to tattoo pigment. In some cases, large, thick scars (sarcoid-like granulomas) have formed at a tattoo site.

Tattooing has been practiced since ancient times. In 1992, a 4000-year-old body of a man with tattoos was found in a glacier in Austria. In ancient Egypt, a tattoo was considered a sign of nobility or fertility. In England and Europe, tattooing became popular among royal families in the late 1800s. The mother of Winston Churchill, Lady Randolph Churchill, had a tattoo of a snake on her wrist.

During most of the 20th century, tattoos had an unsavory reputation largely associated with motorcycle and street gangs, criminals, and military personnel. In the 1980s and 1990s, however, tattooing became more mainstream, with tattoos sported by musicians such as Cher and sports figures including Dennis Rodman.

Tattoos are applied using a small device that works like a sewing machine. A needle bar containing anywhere from one to 14 needles is moved across the skin. The needles penetrate the skin, injecting colored ink. This can produce **pain**, and a small amount of bleeding. You can expect the site to crust and peel during the first week.

Anyone considering a tattoo should visit a number of tattooists, observing the cleanliness of their establishments and asking about infection control. Reputable studios take pride in their sterilization practices and equipment. They should be happy to answer your questions. If a tattooist refuses to discuss safety issues, go somewhere else.

Questions to ask might include:

- Do you have an autoclave (a heat sterilization chamber regulated in the U.S. by the Food and Drug Administration)? This machine is a must.
- Do you require consent forms from customers? This should be filled out prior to tattooing.
- How often do you use needles? Needles should come in a sterile package, and should be used once, then disposed of in a leakproof, puncture-resistant biohazard container.
- Do you keep a record of the dyes used in each client's tattoo? This can be useful if the tattoo is removed at a later date.
- Do you wash hands and use latex gloves during the procedure? What do you do if you are interrupted, for example, to answer the phone or open a drawer? If telephones or other objects are touched, the gloves should be discarded and new ones used to complete the procedure.
- How often do you clean and disinfect the premises, including the bathroom?
- Do you serve clients who appear to be under the influence of alcohol or drugs?
- Do you tattoo minors? Many U.S. states prohibit this.
- What do you do with leftover ink? This should be discarded after each procedure. It should never be returned to the supply bottle.
- Are you a member of the Alliance of Professional Tattooists? This nonprofit group educates tattooists in infection control practices.

You should also check with city or county health officials to find out what local regulations apply to tattooing, and whether complaints have been made concerning the studio you are considering. Some states and municipal governments (for example, New York City) have outlawed tattooing.

Never tattoo yourself or allow it to be done by a friend or a 'scratcher' working out of a kitchen or van.

After receiving a tattoo, you must wait at least two weeks before swimming or exposing the site to direct sunlight. After that, sunscreen should be used to keep the pigments from fading. It is important to keep the site clean and moisturized to allow healing. After healing, you should put a bandage over the site if you visit a tanning salon.

It is important to remember that tattoos are intended to be permanent, and that removing them can be expensive and leave scars or permanent discoloration. methods to remove tattoos include:

- Surgical removal—in which the entire tattoo is cut away. The skin is then drawn together and stitched with sutures. This will leave a scar.
- Dermabrasion—sanding the skin with an abrasion device. This is likely to cause bleeding and scarring.
- Salabrasion—a centuries-old technique using a salt solution, followed by abrasion, often applied by a device such as that used in dermabrasion. This can leave a scar if the solution penetrates too deeply.
- Scarification—using an acid solution to remove the tattoo, leaving a scar in its place.
- Laser removal—a variety of lasers are available for this purpose. Often no anesthetic is needed, but the skin may scar, discolor, or thicken.

Besides being a fashion statement, tattooing can have more practical applications, such as covering hemangiomas (pink/red skin lesions also known as port wine stains), color changes in the lips after facial surgery, and masking the mottled-skin appearance of **vitiligo**. Tattooing can also be used to apply ''permanent'' eyeliner, although the iron oxide sometimes used for this purpose can cause injury if you later undergo **magnetic resonance imaging** (MRI).

TATUM, EDWARD LAWRIE (1909-1975)

American biochemist

Edward Lawrie Tatum's experiments with simple organisms demonstrated that cell processes can be studied as chemical reactions and that such reactions are governed by genes. With George Beadle, he offered conclusive proof in 1941 that each biochemical reaction in the cell is controlled via a catalyzing enzyme by a specific gene. The ''one gene-one enzyme'' theory changed the face of biology and gave it a new chemical expression. For the first time, the nature of life seemed within the grasp of science's quantitative methods. Tatum, collaborating with Joshua Lederberg, demonstrated in 1947 that bacteria reproduce sexually, thus introducing a new experimental organism into the study of molecular genetics. Spurred by Tatum's discoveries, other scientists worked to understand the precise chemical nature of the unit of heredity called the gene. This study culminated in 1953 with the description by James Watson and Francis Crick of the structure of DNA. Tatum's use of microorganisms and laboratory mutations for the study of biochemical genetics led directly to the biotechnology revolution of the 1980s. Tatum and Beadle shared the 1958 Nobel Prize in physiology or medicine with Joshua Lederberg for ushering in the new era of modern biology.

Tatum was born on December 14, 1909, in Boulder, Colorado, to Arthur Lawrie Tatum and Mabel Webb Tatum. He was the first of three children; a younger brother and sister would follow. Both of Edward's parents excelled academically. His father held two degrees, an M.D. and a Ph.D. in pharmacology. Edward's mother was one of the first women to graduate from the University of Colorado. Presumably an interest in science and medicine ran in the Tatum family: Edward would become a research scientist, his brother a physician, and his sister a nurse. As a boy, Edward played the French horn and trumpet; his interest in music lasted his whole life. He also enjoyed swimming and ice-skating.

In 1925, when Tatum was fifteen years old, his father accepted a position as a pharmacology professor at the University of Wisconsin. Tatum studied at the University of Chicago Experimental School and for two years at the University of Chicago before transferring and completing his undergraduate work at the University of Wisconsin. He almost became a geologist before deciding in his senior year to major in chemistry.

Tatum earned his A.B. degree in chemistry from the University of Wisconsin in 1931. In 1932 he earned his master's degree in microbiology. Two years later, in 1934, he received a Ph.D. in biochemistry for a dissertation on the cellular biochemistry and nutritional needs of a bacterium. Understanding the biochemistry of microorganisms such as bacteria, yeast, and molds would persist at the heart of Tatum's career.

After receiving his doctorate, Tatum remained at the University of Wisconsin for one year as a research assistant in biochemistry. He married the same year he completed his Ph.D. In Livingston, Wisconsin, Tatum wed June Alton, the daughter of a lumber dealer, on July 28, 1934. They eventually had two daughters, Margaret Carol and Barbara Ann.

From 1936 to 1937, Tatum studied bacteriological chemistry at the University of Utrecht in the Netherlands while on a General Education Board fellowship for postgraduate study. In Utrecht he worked in the laboratory of F. Kogl, who had identified the vitamin biotin. In Kogl's lab Tatum investigated the nutritional needs of bacteria and fungi. While Tatum was in Holland, he was contacted by geneticist George Beadle. Beadle, seven years older than Tatum, had done genetic studies with the fruit fly *Drosophila melanogaster* Drosophila melanogaster while in the laboratory of Thomas Hunt Morgan at the California Institute of Technology. Beadle, newly arrived at Stanford University, was now looking for a biochemist who could collaborate with him as he continued his work in genetics. He hoped to identify the enzymes responsible for the inherited eye pigments of *Drosophila*.

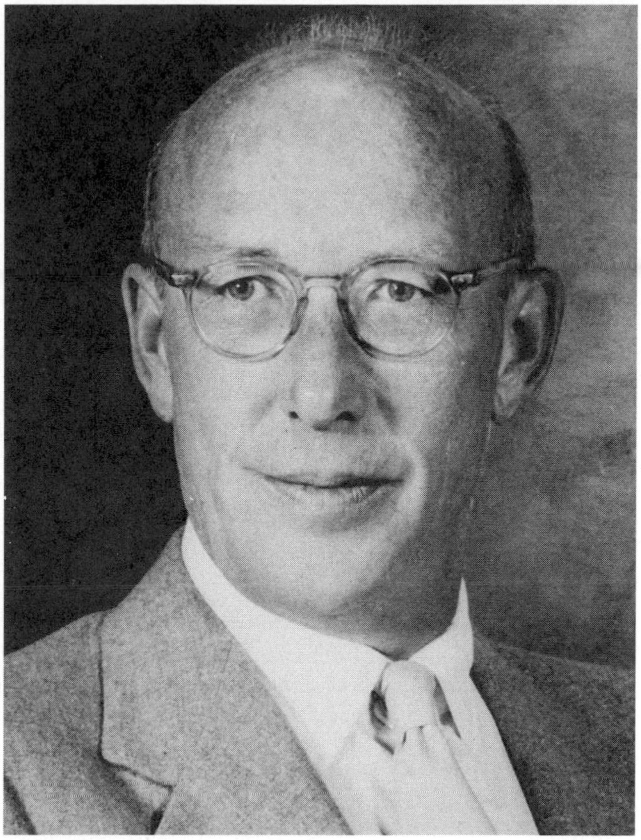

Edward Lawrie Tatum

Upon his return to the United States in the fall of 1937, Tatum was appointed a research associate at Stanford University in the department of biological sciences. There he embarked on the *Drosophila* project with Beadle for four years. The two men successfully determined that kynurenine was the enzyme responsible for the fly's eye color and that it was controlled by one of the eye-pigment genes. This and other observations led them to postulate several theories about the relationship between genes and biochemical reactions. Yet they realized that *Drosophila* was not an ideal experimental organism on which to continue their work.

Tatum and Beadle began searching for a suitable organism. After some discussion and a review of the literature, they settled on a pink mold that commonly grows on bread known as *neurospora crassa.* The advantages to working with *neurospora* were many: it reproduced very quickly, its nutritional needs and biochemical pathways were already well known, and it had the useful capability of being able to reproduce both sexually and asexually. This last characteristic made it possible to grow cultures that were genetically identical and also to grow cultures that were the result of a cross between two different parent strains. With neurospora, Tatum and Beadle were ready to demonstrate the effect of genes on cellular biochemistry.

The two scientists began their *neurospora* experiments in March 1941. At that time, scientists spoke of ''genes'' as the units of heredity without fully understanding what a gene might look like or how it might act. Although they realized that genes were located on the chromosomes, they didn't know what the chemical nature of such a substance might be. An understanding of DNA (deoxyribonucleic acid, the molecule of heredity) was still twelve years in the future. Nevertheless, geneticists in the 1940s had accepted Gregor Mendel's work with inheritance patterns in pea plants. Mendel's theory, rediscovered by three independent investigators in 1900, states that an inherited characteristic is determined by the combination of two hereditary units (genes), one each contributed by the parental cells. A dominant gene is expressed even when it is carried by only one of a pair of chromosomes, while a recessive gene must be carried by both chromosomes to be expressed. With *Drosophila*, Tatum and Beadle had taken genetic mutants—flies that inherited a variant form of eye color—and tried to work out the biochemical steps that led to the abnormal eye color. Their goal was to identify the variant enzyme, presumably governed by a single gene, that controlled the variant eye color. This proved technically very difficult, and as luck would have it, another lab announced the discovery of kynurenine's role before theirs did. With the neurospora experiments, they set out to prove their one gene-one enzyme theory another way.

The two investigators began with biochemical processes they understood well: the nutritional needs of *neurospora.* By exposing cultures of *neurospora* to X rays, they would cause genetic damage to some bread mold genes. If their theory was right, and genes did indeed control biochemical reactions, the genetically damaged strains of mold would show changes in their ability to produce nutrients. If supplied with some basic salts and sugars, normal *neurospora* can make all the amino acids and vitamins it needs to live except for one (biotin).

This is exactly what happened. In the course of their research, the men created, with X-ray bombardment, a number of mutated strains that each lacked the ability to produce a particular amino acid or vitamin. The first strain they identified, after 299 attempts to determine its mutation, lacked the ability to make vitamin B_6. By crossing this strain with a normal strain, the offspring inherited the defect as a recessive gene according to the inheritance patterns described by Mendel. This proved that the mutation was a genetic defect, capable of being passed to successive generations and causing the same nutritional mutation in those offspring. The X-ray bombardment had altered the gene governing the enzyme needed to promote the production of vitamin B_6.

This simple experiment heralded the dawn of a new age in biology, one in which molecular genetics would soon dominate. Nearly forty years later, on Tatum's death, Joshua Lederberg told the *New York Times* that this experiment ''gave impetus and morale'' to scientists who strived to understand how genes directed the processes of life. For the first time, biologists believed that it might be possible to understand and quantify the living cell's processes.

Tatum and Beadle were not the first, as it turned out, to postulate the one gene-one enzyme theory. By 1942 the work of English physician Archibald Garrod, long ignored, had been rediscovered. In his study of people suffering from a particular inherited enzyme deficiency, Garrod had noticed the disease seemed to be inherited as a Mendelian recessive. This suggested a link between one gene and one enzyme. Yet Tatum and Beadle were the first to offer extensive experimental evidence for the theory. Their use of laboratory methods, like X rays, to create genetic mutations also introduced a powerful tool for future experiments in biochemical genetics.

During World War II, the methods Tatum and Beadle had developed in their work with pink bread mold were used to produce large amounts of penicillin, another mold. Their basic research, unwittingly, thus had a very important practical effect as well. In 1944 Tatum served as a civilian staff member of the U.S. Office of Scientific Research and Development at Stanford. Industry, too, used the methods the men developed to measure vitamins and amino acids in foods and tissues.

In 1945, at the end of the war, Tatum accepted an appointment at Yale University as an associate professor of botany with the promise of establishing a program of biochemical microbiology within that department. Apparently the move was due to Stanford's lack of encouragement of Tatum, who failed to fit into the tidy category of biochemist or biologist or geneticist but instead mastered all three fields. In 1946 Tatum did indeed create a new program at Yale and became a professor of microbiology. In work begun at Stanford and continued at Yale, he demonstrated that the one gene-one enzyme theory applied to yeast and bacteria as well as molds.

In a second extremely fruitful collaboration, Tatum began working with Joshua Lederberg in March 1946. Lederberg, a Columbia University medical student fifteen years younger than Tatum, was at Yale during a break in the medical school curriculum. Tatum and Lederberg began studying the bacterium *Escherichia coli*. At that time, it was believed that *E. coli* reproduced asexually. The two scientists proved otherwise. When cultures of two different mutant bacteria were mixed, a third strain, one showing characteristics taken from each parent, resulted. This discovery of biparental inheritance in bacteria, which Tatum called genetic recombination, provided geneticists with a new experimental organism. Again, Tatum's methods had altered the practices of experimental biology. Lederberg never returned to medical school, earning instead a Ph.D. from Yale.

In 1948 Tatum returned to Stanford as professor of biology. A new administration at Stanford and its department of biology had invited him to return in a position suited to his expertise and ability. While in this second residence at Stanford, Tatum helped establish the department of biochemistry. In 1956 he became a professor of biochemistry and head of the department. Increasingly, Tatum's talents were devoted to promoting science at an administrative level. He was instrumental in relocating the Stanford Medical School from San Francisco to the university campus in Palo Alto. In that year Tatum also was divorced from his wife June. On December 16, 1956, he married Viola Kantor in New York City. Kantor was the daughter of a dentist in Brooklyn. Owing in part to these complications in his personal affairs, Tatum left the West Coast and took a position at the Rockefeller Institute for Medical Research (now Rockefeller University) in January 1957. There he continued to work through institutional channels to support young scientists, and served on various national committees. Unlike some other administrators, he emphasized nurturing individual investigators rather than specific kinds of projects. His own research continued in efforts to understand the genetics of neurospora and the nucleic acid metabolism of mammalian cells in culture.

In 1958, together with Beadle and Lederberg, Tatum received the Nobel Prize in physiology or medicine. The Nobel Committee awarded the prize to the three investigators for their work demonstrating that genes regulate the chemical processes of the cell. Tatum and Beadle shared one-half the prize and Lederberg received the other half for work done separately from Tatum. Lederberg later paid tribute to Tatum for his role in Lederberg's decision to study the effects of X-ray-induced mutation. In his Nobel lecture, Tatum predicted that "with real understanding of the roles of heredity and environment, together with the consequent improvement in man's physical capacities and greater freedom from physical disease, will come an improvement in his approach to, and understanding of, sociological and economic problems."

Tatum had a marked interest in social issues, including population control. In 1965 and 1966 Tatum organized other Nobel laureates in science to make public endorsements of family planning and birth control. These included statements to Pope Paul VI, whose encyclical against birth control for Catholics was issued at this time.

Tatum's second wife, Viola, died on April 21, 1974. Tatum married Elsie Bergland later in 1974 and she survived his death the following year, on November 5, 1975. Tatum died at his home on East Sixty-third Street in New York City after an extended illness. In a memoir written for the *Annual Review of Genetics,* Lederberg recalled that Tatum's last years were "marred by ill health, substantially self-inflicted by a notorious smoking habit." Lederberg noted, too, that Tatum's "mental outlook" was scarred by the painful death of his second wife.

In addition to the Nobel Prize, Tatum received the Remsen Award of the American Chemical Society in 1953 for his work in biparental inheritance and sexual reproduction in bacteria. In 1952 he was elected to the National Academy of Sciences. He was a founding member of the *Annual Review of Genetics* and joined the editorial board of *Science* in 1957. Tatum's collected papers occupy twenty-five feet of space in the Rockefeller University Archives and span the years from 1930 to 1975.

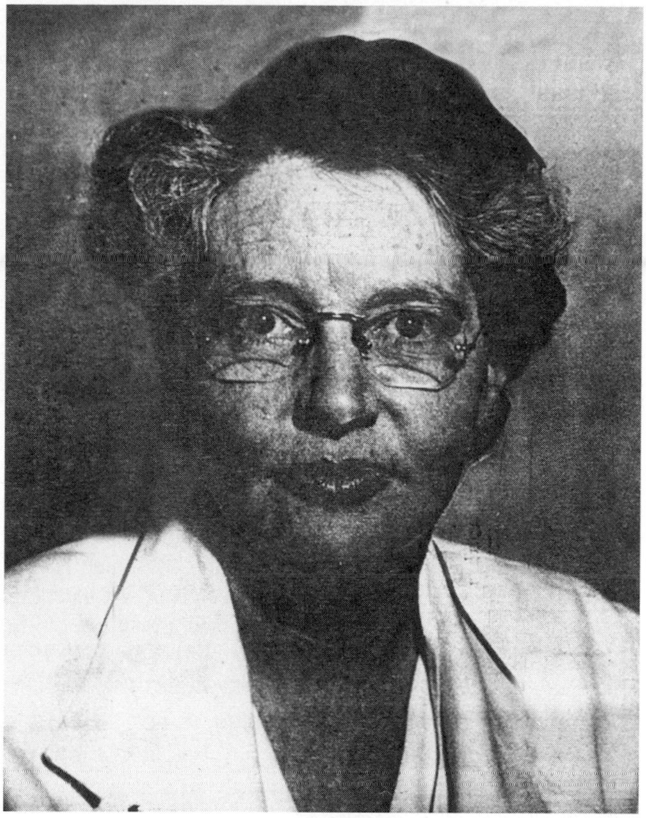

Helen Taussig

TAUSSIG, HELEN BROOKE (1898-1986)

American physician

Helen Taussig was the founder of pediatric cardiology and one of the first outstanding women in American medicine. Born in Cambridge, Massachusetts, to an academic family, Taussig's father was a Harvard economist and her mother one of the first students at Radcliffe College. Taussig also studied at Radcliffe, where she became a tennis champion, and then moved to the University of California at Berkeley to broaden her knowledge. After receiving her bachelor's degree in 1921, Taussig enrolled at Harvard Medical School—as a special student, because women were not admitted to the regular program then. She transferred to Boston University Medical School where she was directed toward specializing in the heart by Dr. Alexander Begg (1881-1940), who also encouraged her to complete her studies at Johns Hopkins Medical School in Baltimore, Maryland. After receiving her medical degree from Johns Hopkins in 1927, Taussig completed an internship in pediatrics and in 1930 became head of the Children's Heart Clinic of Johns Hopkins Hospital, a position she held until her retirement in 1963.

Taussig began to use fluoroscopy and X-rays to determine what caused "blue babies," infants born with insufficient oxygenation of their bloodstream. She developed a theory that the condition was caused by a nonfunctioning artery. When Alfred Blalock (1899-1964) became chief surgeon at Johns Hopkins, Taussig interested him in her theory, and together they developed what became known as the ''Blalock-Taussig Shunt,'' an operation that would save thousands of babies and initiated a major breakthrough in cardiac surgery that paved the way to **open-heart surgery**. Taussig continued to devote her career to pediatric heart disease, making important contributions in knowledge about acute **rheumatic fever** and congenital defects. Her two-volume *Congenital Malformations of the Heart*, published in 1947, became a standard in the field. In the early 1960's Taussig again saved untold thousands of children by going to Germany to investigate reported **birth defects** caused by the drug thalidomide. On her return, Taussig recommended to the **Food and Drug Administration** that the drug be banned in the United States.

In 1959, Taussig was made the first female full professor of the Johns Hopkins Medical School. She received the first Rivers Fellowship of the National Foundation-March of Dimes in 1963, a five-year cash award that allowed her to continue her research after her retirement. She continued patient follow-up studies and traveled widely, lecturing and teaching. In 1965 Taussig became the first woman president of the American Heart Association. At the time of her death in 1986 at the age of 87 in a car accident, Taussig was actively engaged in research on heart defects in birds.

Tay-Sachs disease

Tay-Sachs disease is an inherited **birth defect** which first becomes noticeable at about four to six months of age when an otherwise healthy baby gradually ceases to smile, crawl, turn over, or reach out, and ultimately becomes blind and paralyzed. **Death** occurs at about the age of five years. Tay-Sachs disease is among a number of genetic disorders that result from the body's inability to produce lipid-degrading enzymes. Lacking these enzymes, lipids accumulate in the cells, resulting in **kidney failure**, enlargement of the liver and spleen, **mental retardation**, blindness, skeletal deformities, and, eventually, the shut-down of the entire **nervous system**.

Tay-Sachs disease was the first of its type to be studied, and was first recognized by the British ophthalmologist, Warren Tay (1843-1927) in 1881. Tay noticed a cherry-red spot on the retina of a one-year-old child who exhibited many of the signs of the disorder. The child gradually deteriorated and died.

A similar report was published by Bernard Sachs (1858-1944), an American neurologist, who was the first person to describe the cellular changes that accompany the disease and to comment on its prevalence among Eastern European Jews. Today we know that Tay-Sachs disease is an autosomally recessive genetic disorder that occurs because of the body's failure to produce the enzyme (protein) *hexosaminidase A* (hex A). Approximately one in every 27 American Jews carries the Tay-Sachs gene. Also, non-Jewish descendants of French-Canadians from the East St. Lawrence River Valley in Quebec and Cajuns from Louisiana experience approximately 100 times the rate of the disorder than the general population. In this hereditary disorder, the carrier of the Tay-Sachs gene does not develop the illness, nor do their children who do, however, stand a 50 percent chance of inheriting the gene. When both parents carry the gene, each of their children has a one in four possibility of having the disease. Programs for DNA-based genetic testing were developed in the early 1980s, measurement of hex A enzyme in the blood will also identify a carrier, and prenatal testing called *amniocentesis* and *chronic villus sampling* (CVS) will diagnose Tay-Sachs before birth. There is no treatment to prevent the disease from progressing, nor is there a cure.

Carriers of Canavan disease, a similar yet less readily identifiable disease to Tay-Sachs, affects one in 37 Eastern European Jews. This disease can now also be identified through genetic testing. The defective gene can be passed from generation to generation before a baby is born with the disease. Therefore, even families with no known history of the disease can carry the gene.

Temin, Howard Martin (1934-)

American molecular biologist

Howard Temin proposed in the 1960s the provirus theory of how the ribonucleic acid (RNA) genes of retroviruses combine with the deoxyribonucleic acid (DNA) of host cells. As one of the first to discover the viral enzyme reverse transcriptase that copies the RNA, he largely proved that his theory was correct. For this discovery, he received part of the 1975 Nobel Prize in physiology or medicine.

Temin was born in Philadelphia, where his father was a lawyer and his mother was active in civic activities. He majored in biology at Swarthmore College, graduating in 1955. He began research on a tumor-producing virus called the Rous sarcoma virus while a graduate student at the California Institute of Technology, where he received his Ph.D. in 1959. While there he was a student of **Renato Dulbecco** (1914-), and also worked with **Max Delbrück** and Matthew Meselson, all of whom made major contributions to the understanding of cell mechanisms. Temin joined the faculty of the University of Wisconsin-Madison in 1960 and has spent his entire career there.

The ability of a virus to cause tumors was first described in 1911 by the American pathologist **Peyton Rous** (1879-1970), for whom the virus was later named. Further study had to await the genetic discoveries and techniques of the 1940s and 1950s. In 1960 Temin theorized that after being infected by the virus, the host cell made copies of the virus as well as itself. After other scientists showed in 1961 that the genetic material of the Rous virus was RNA, Temin also proposed that after the virus enters the cell it copies its RNA genes into DNA (the provirus). This DNA enters the cell's nucleus and becomes part of the cell's own DNA, where it directs production of the next generation of the virus and is inherited by future cell generations. In 1970, Temin and his co-worker, Satoshi Mizutani, showed that the Rous sarcoma virus contained an

RNA-copying enzyme (or polymerase) before it infected the cell. The enzyme, which directs DNA production from RNA, was later named reverse transcriptase.

In addition to his Nobel Prize, Temin received many other honors including the American Chemical Society Award in Enzyme Chemistry, the Gairdner International Award, and the Albert Lasker Award in Basic Medical Research. He was also a member of the American Academy of Arts and Sciences and the National Academy of Sciences.

Temporary Assistance for Needy Families

The federal government, through New Deal legislation in the 1930s, put in place a program that provided subsidies to state and local governments to provide economic support to the very poor. This program, colloquially referred to as **welfare**, was known until recently as the Aid to Families with Dependent Children (AFDC) program.

The AFDC, which actually dated to the 1910s and was implemented by most states, was originally intended to be a program to help widowed mothers and mothers whose husbands had left them. In its early years, the program was very small, and fairly successful. The AFDC program was replaced in 1996 by the TANF (Temporary Assistance to Needy Families) program, which is run by the states who must follow federal guidelines.

There are a number of restrictions on TANF benefits; for example, adults cannot receive TANF benefits for more than 5 years, and adults who receive TANF benefits must take jobs within 2 years. There is also a waiting period of 5 years before most new immigrants can receive TANF benefits.

In 1960, 3 million women and children were collecting AFDC benefits. That number doubled in five years and then doubled again by 1975. By 1995, 13.6 million women and children were receiving AFDC grants. In addition, the types of recipients had changed drastically. By 1991, widows, the group that AFDC was originally designed for, made up only 1.6% of all recipients. Mothers who were divorced, separated, or never married rose, however, from 37% of the rolls in 1950 to 85% in 1991.

The race and ethnicity of the recipients also changed. In 1939, more than 80% of recipients were white. By 1996, 60% of the recipients were women and children of color. In absolute numbers, however, there were slightly more whites on AFDC than blacks, and twice as many whites receiving public benefits than blacks.

There are a number of popular misconceptions about recipients of TANF grants. Although it is frequently assumed that more and more people are receiving welfare payments through TANF, the fact is that in 1993 5.5% of the total population received TANF supplements, but in 1997 only 3.9% of the total population did. Likewise, many Americans believe TANF grants are too generous; in fact, the average monthly TANF income for a household of three is $499, compared to a federal poverty level income of $1,043. Many people believe that most TANF parents are teenagers, but when one examines the ages of parents in TANF families, 6% are 19 years and under; 21% are between the ages of 20 and 24 years; 21% are between the ages of 25 and 29 years; 35% are between 30 and 39 years of age; and 17% are 40 years old and over.

In addition, many people fail to realize that TANF families tend to be small, with approximately 75% of the recipients having two or fewer children. TANF families are racially and ethnically diverse; about 37% are African American, 36% are White, and 20% are Hispanic. It is also not well known that most TANF mothers have prior work experience.

It is true, however, that most TANF mothers are single parents (only 13% are married with their husbands present); that recipients are more likely to remain on TANF rolls for long periods if they are single and have little formal education (nearly half of all TANF mothers have less than a high school education); and that many recipients find the absence of affordable, reliable **child care** an impediment to taking jobs.

See also Divorce; Welfare

Temporomandibular joint disorders

Temporomandibular joint disorder (TMJ) is the name given to a group of symptoms that cause **pain** in the head, face, and jaw. The symptoms include **headache**s, soreness in the chewing muscles, and clicking or stiffness of the joints. TMJ disorder, which is also sometimes called TMJ syndrome, results from pressure on the facial nerves due to muscle tension or abnormalities of the bones in the area of the hinge joint between the lower jaw and the temporal bone. This hinge joint is called the temporomandibular joint. There are two temporomandibular joints, one on each side of the skull just in front of the ear. The name of the joint comes from the two bones that make it up. The temporal bone is the name of the section of the skull bones where the jaw bone (the mandible) is connected. The temporomandibular joint also contains a piece of cartilage called a disc, which keeps the temporal bone and the jaw bone from rubbing against each other. The jaw pivots at the joint area in front of the ear. Anything that causes a change in shape or functioning of the temporomandibular joint will cause pain and other symptoms.

TMJ syndrome has several possible physical causes:

- Muscle tension. Muscle tightness in the temporomandibular joint usually results from overuse of muscles. This overuse in turn is often associated with psychological **stress**, and clenching or grinding of the teeth (**bruxism**).
- Injury. A direct blow to the jaw or the side of the head can result in bone fracture, soft tissue bruising, or a dislocation of the temporomandibular joint itself.
- Arthritis. Both **osteoarthritis** and **rheumatoid arthritis** can cause TMJ.
- Internal derangement. Internal derangement is a condition in which the cartilage disk lies in front of its proper position. In most cases of internal derangement, the disc

moves in and out of its correct location, making a clicking or popping noise as it moves. In a few cases, the disc is permanently out of position, and the patient's range of motion in the jaw is limited.

- Hypermobility. Hypermobility is a condition in which the ligaments that hold the jaw in place are too loose and the jaw tends to slip out of its socket.
- Birth abnormalities. These are the least frequent cause of TMJ but do occur in a minority of patients. In some cases, the top of the jawbone is too small; in others, the top of the jawbone outgrows the lower part.

TMJ disorders are most frequently diagnosed by dentists. The dentist can often diagnose TMJ based on **physical examination** of the patient's face and jaw. The examination might include pressing on (palpating) the jaw muscles for soreness or asking the patient to open and close the jaw in order to check for misalignment of the teeth in the upper and lower jaw. This condition is called **malocclusion**. The dentist might also gently move the patient's jaw in order to check for loose ligaments. If the dentist suspects that the patient has internal derangement of the disc, he or she can use a technique called arthrography to make the diagnosis. In an arthrogram, a special dye is injected into the joint, which is then x-rayed. Arthrography can be used to evaluate the movement of the jaw and the disc as well as size and shape, and to evaluate the effectiveness of treatment for TMJ.

In many cases, the cause of pain in the TMJ area is temporary and disappears without treatment. About 80% of patients with TMJ will improve in six months without medications or physical treatments. Patients with TMJ can be given **muscle relaxants** if their symptoms are related to muscle tension. Some patients may be given **aspirin** or nonsteriodal anti-inflammatory drugs (NSAIDs) for minor discomfort. If the TMJ is related to rheumatoid arthritis, it may be treated with **corticosteroids**, methotrexate (MTX, Rheumatrex) or gold sodium (Myochrysine).

Patients who have difficulty with bruxism are usually treated with splints. A plastic splint called a nightguard is given to the patient to place over the teeth before going to bed. Splints can also be used to treat some cases of internal derangement by holding the jaw forward and keeping the disc in place until the ligaments tighten. The splint is adjusted over a period of two to four months.

TMJ can also be treated with ultrasound, electromyographic **biofeedback**, stretching **exercises**, **stress management** techniques, or **massage**. Surgery is ordinarily used only to treat TMJ caused by birth deformities or certain forms of internal derangement caused by misshapen discs.

The prognosis for recovery from TMJ is excellent for almost all patients. Most patients do not need any form of long-term treatment. Surgical procedures to treat TMJ are quite successful. In the case of patients with TMJ caused by arthritis or infectious diseases, the progression of the arthritis or the success of eliminating infectious agents determines whether TMJ can be eliminated.

See also Bruxism; Malocclusion

Tendinitis

Tendinitis is the inflammation of a tendon, a tough rope-like tissue that connects muscle to bone, usually occuring in individuals in middle or old age as a result of overuse over a long period of time. Tendinitis does occur in younger patients as a result of acute overuse. Tendons that commonly become inflamed include those of the hand and of the upper arm that effect the shoulder. Achilles tendon, at the heel of the foot, and the tendon that runs across the top of the foot also may develop tendinitis.

Sudden stretching or repeated overuse causes injury to the connection between the tendon and its bone or muscle. The injury is largely mechanical, but when it appears, the body tries to heal it by initiating inflammation. Inflammation increases the blood supply, bringing nutrients to the damaged tissues along with immunogenic agents to combat infection. The result is swelling, tenderness, **pain**, heat, and redness if it is close to the skin.

Some tendon injuries are superficial and easy to identify. These include **tennis elbow** (extensor tendinitis) over the outside of the elbow, and Achilles' tendinitis just above the heel of the foot. There are several tendons in the shoulder that can be overused or stretched, and usually a shoulder will have more than one injury at a time. Tendonitis in the biceps may accompany a tear of the shoulder ligaments or an impingement of one bone or another. Careful pressure testing and movement of the parts is all that is necessary to identify the tendinitis.

Rest, ice, compression, and elevation (RICE) will treat the acute condition. The best way to apply ice is in a bag with water. The water applies the cold directly to the skin. Chemical ice packs can get too cold and cause frostbite. Compression using an elastic wrap minimizes swelling and bleeding in an acute sprain. Splinting may help rest the limb. Pain and anti-inflammatory medications (**aspirin**, naproxen, ibuprofen) will help. Sometimes the inflammation lingers and requires additional treatment. Injections of cortisone-like medicine often relieve chronic tendonitis, but should be reserved for resistant cases since cortisone can occasionally cause problems of its own. If tendinitis is persistent and unresponsive to nonsurgical treatment, a surgery to remove the afflicted portion of tendon can be performed. Surgery is also conducted to remove calcium buildup that comes with persistent tendinitis.

Increasing intake of antioxidant-rich foods and lowering intake of animal fats may help reduce the inflammation. **Acupuncture** has also been used to combat tendinitis. **Hydrotherapy**, such as a whirlpool bath, may also help relax the surrounding muscles. If given enough time, tendons will strengthen to meet the demands placed on them. They grow slowly because of their poor blood supply, so adequate time is required for good conditioning.

Tennis elbow

The classic tennis elbow is caused by repeated forceful contractions of wrist muscles located on the outer forearm. The stress created at a common muscle origin causes microscopic tears leading to inflammation of several structures of the elbow. These include muscles, tendons, bursa, periosteum, and epicondyle (bony projections on the outside and inside of the elbow, where muscles of the forearm attach to the bone of the upper arm). This overuse injury is common between ages 20-40.

People at risk for tennis elbow are those in occupations that require strenuous or repetitive forearm movement. Such jobs include mechanics or carpentry. Sport activities that require individuals to twist the hand, wrist, and forearm, such as tennis, throwing a ball, bowling, golfing, and skiing, can cause tennis elbow. Individuals in poor physical condition, who are exposed to repetitive wrist and forearm movements for long periods of time, may be prone to tennis elbow. This condition is also called epicondylitis, lateral epicondylitis, medial epicondylitis, or golfer's elbow, where **pain** is present at the inside epicondyle. If the condition becomes long-standing and chronic, a decrease in grip strength can develop.

Diagnosis of tennis elbow includes the individual observation and recall of symptoms, a thorough medical history, and physical examination by a physician. Diagnostic testing is usually not necessary unless there may be evidence of nerve involvement from underlying causes. X rays are usually always negative because the condition is primarily soft tissue in nature, in contrast to a bony disorder.

Heat or ice is helpful in relieving tennis elbow pain. Once acute symptoms have subsided, **heat treatments** are used to increase blood circulation and promote healing. The physician may recommend **physical therapy** to increase the thermal temperature of the tissues in order to address both pain and inflammation. Occasionally, a tennis elbow splint may be useful to help decrease stress on the elbow throughout daily activities. **Exercise**s become very important to improve flexibility to all forearm muscles, and will aid in decreasing muscle and tendon tightness that has been creating excessive pull at the common attachment of the epicondyle. The physician may also prescribe **nonsteroidal anti-inflammatory drugs** (NSAIDS) to reduce inflammation and pain. Injections of cortisone or anesthetics are often used if physical therapy is ineffective. Cortisone reduces inflammation, and anesthetics temporarily relieve pain. Physicians are cautious regarding excessive number of injections as this has recently been found to weaken the tendon's integrity. If conservative methods of treatment fail, surgical release of the tendon at the epicondyle may be a necessary form of treatment. However, surgical intervention is relatively rare.

Massage therapy has been found to be beneficial if symptoms are mild. Massage techniques are based primarily on increasing circulation to promote efficient reduction of inflammation. **acupuncture** and **acupressure** have been used as well. Contrast **hydrotherapy** (alternating hot and cold water or compresses, 3 minutes hot, 30 seconds cold, repeated 3 times, always ending with cold) applied to the elbow can help bring nutrient-rich blood to the joint and carry away waste products. Botanical medicine and **homeopathy** may also be effective therapies for tennis elbow. For example, cayenne (*Capsicum frutescens*) ointment or prickly ash (*Zanthoxylum americanum*) oil applied topically may help to increase blood flow to the affected area and speed healing.

Until symptoms of pain and inflammation subside, activities requiring repetitive wrist and forearm motion should be avoided. Once pain decreases to the point that return to activity can begin, the playing of sports, such as tennis, for long periods should not occur until excellent condition returns. Many times, choosing a different size or type of tennis racquet may help. Frequent rest periods are important despite what the wrist and forearm activity may be. Compliance to a stretching and strengthening program is very important in helping prevent recurring symptoms.

See also Tendonitis

Teratogen

Teratogens are substances that produce neurological and physical malformations in developing human fetuses. The word comes from the Greek *teras*, meaning "malformation" or "monstrosity." Certainly, ever since the first malformed baby was born, people have wondered what causes **birth defects**. Most early explanations referred to mystical forces: the influence of celestial bodies, divine intervention, even conception during the woman's menstrual period. The theory of maternal impression was widely accepted from the seventeenth to the early twentieth centuries. According to this concept, a specific, strong impression on the mother during **pregnancy** would produce a corresponding specific birth defect in her child; for instance, a mother who was startled by a hare might give birth to a child with a harelip.

During the nineteenth and early twentieth centuries, however, a number of researchers showed that exposure of animals (such as chickens and fish) to certain physical and chemical substances would produce birth defects in their offspring. While a few medical investigators conducted studies that showed similar effects in mammals, the scientific community as a whole embraced the concept that a woman's placenta acted as an impenetrable barrier preventing harmful substances from reaching the unborn child. This belief was shattered by the thalidomide tragedy.

Thalidomide, a synthetic developed by Chemie Grunenthal, was hailed as a "wonder drug" which enduced a sound sleep with no hangover effect the following morning and no fatal effects in overdose cases. Its use spread rapidly across Canada and Europe after its introduction in West Germany in 1958, and was considered so safe it was dispensed over the counter rather than by prescription. In 1959, twelve infants were born in West Germany with severe deformities—a very rare condition called phocomelia, in which the arms and legs developed into stubs resembling a seal's flippers. No link to thalidomide was considered, even after 83 more cases were reported in 1960. (Cases of such birth defects eventually climbed to 5,000 in Germany and 10,000 worldwide.)

In September 1960, the American drug firm William S. Merrell submitted to the **Food and Drug Administration** (FDA) an application to market thalidomide in the United States. The application, considered routine, was given to a new FDA employee, Dr. **Frances Kelsey** (1914-), who was expected to approve it within the usual sixty days. Kelsey, however, became concerned about some of the effects of thalidomide, repeatedly postponing approval while asking Merrell for further information. Meanwhile, cases of phocomelia continued to mount in Europe. Finally, in November 1961, a Hamburg pediatrician named Widukind Lenz, established that the mothers of many of the infants with severe birth defects at his clinic had taken thalidomide. The link was confirmed by Dr. William McBride in Australia and, by the end of November, thalidomide was withdrawn from the market. Early in 1962, Dr. **Helen Taussig** of Johns Hopkins University, traveled to Europe to investigate the phocomelia situation and, upon her return, she publicly warned American physicians about the dangers of thalidomide and urged the FDA to ban the drug. Media publicity galvanized public opinion, and a new, landmark law was passed in 1962 mandating much stricter procedures for testing and marketing all drugs. (Bendectin, an **antinausea drug** also marketed by Merrell, was voluntarily withdrawn by the firm from the market following several lawsuits claiming the drug caused birth defects, even though scientific evidence at the trials and subsequent laboratory tests could not confirm this.)

However, with dramatic proof of the potential effects of teratogens, investigations exploded and a wide variety of substances have now been shown to have the ability to produce birth defects. These include cocaine and crack cocaine—which cause severe problems including premature birth, low birth weight, physical defects, death at birth, and babies addicted at birth; alcohol—which can cause **Fetal Alcohol Syndrome**, **mental retardation**, and other defects; hormones (testosterone taken during pregnancy results in male genitalia on a female baby); doses of vitamin A above 8,000 IU per day and vitamin A derivatives such as isotretinoin and etretinate cause multiple congenital malformations; and many other substances including—but certainly not limited to—central **nervous system**-active drugs, **aspirin**, **caffeine**, **cigarette** and other types of smoke, food additives, pesticides, herbicides, toxins in the workplace, and viruses such as **rubella**. Virtually all drugs, including illegal, prescription, and over the counter drugs, have teratogenic possibilities. Researchers have found that damage depends upon the stage of pregnancy during which the fetus is exposed to the teratogen, duration of exposure, and the nature of the substance. For the first two weeks, the developing embryo is relatively impervious to teratogens; from then until the end of the second month, the rapidly developing organs and body parts are vulnerable to severe malformations from exposure to harmful substances; after that, teratogens can interfere with fetal growth, body function, and brain development.

In the early 1990s concerns were raised about the effect of teratogens on sperm. Studies have linked fathers' exposure to a number of substances—especially lead, pesticides, organic solvents, and heavy metal fumes—to birth defects in their offspring. Research continues in this area.

TESTICULAR CANCER

Testicular cancer is a cancerous growth occurring in the male gonads, or testes. The testes are located outside the body cavity, in the scrotum. Although testicular cancer is a rare type of cancer, it often grows very quickly. It is the most common type of cancer to occur in young males, with most cases occurring in men under the age of 30 years. Recent advances in treatment have made testicular cancer very manageable and curable. Testicular cancer is more prevalent in males whose testes have not descended into the scrotum.

Testicular cancer usually shows no early symptoms. It is suspected when a mass is felt in the testes, although a testicular mass does not necessarily mean cancer. It is important for men to perform periodic examinations of their testes in order to detect any mass at an early stage. In advanced cases, or metastatic testicular cancer, symptoms include lower back **pain** and discomfort, difficulty in urinating, a **cough**, and breathing difficulties. A feeling of heaviness in the testes is also common and there is sometimes pain.

No cause for testicular cancer has been identified. Exposure of the fetus to certain chemicals or an individual's exposure to environmental estrogens may cause changes in cells that could lead to testicular cancer. As of yet, however, there is no conclusive evidence to name a cause. Higher rates of testicular cancer occur in men with HIV infection, suggesting that the two may also be related. Studies examining the relationship of testicular trauma, such as may occur with bike riding, and the occurrence of testicular cancer found that trauma does not contribute to testicular cancer.

Once a mass is identified in the testes, the abdomen and other areas of the body are felt (palpated) to check for additional masses. A **computed tomography scan** (CT scan) of the abdomen and pelvis, as well as **chest x rays**, are performed to determine if the cancer has spread to other areas of the body. Sometimes the lymphatic vessels are also examined by x ray (lymphangiogram) and some blood tests that are also helpful. These tests will allow the oncologist to determine the type, extent, and severity of the cancer. Blood tests can also be used to monitor the progress of treatment and check for recurrences of testicular cancer. A tissue sample or **biopsy** will also be taken to confirm the diagnosis of cancer.

Treatment for testicular cancer depends upon the type and extent of the cancer. However, the first line of treatment is usually surgery to remove the mass. If the cancer has spread to other parts of the body, surgery is followed by **chemotherapy**. **Radiation therapy** may also be used to treat testicular cancer. **Alternative medicine** may be helpful to support the person undergoing conventional treatment for testicular cancer. Dietary modifications emphasizing whole foods and healthy fats, nutritional supplementation, **acupuncture**, Chinese and western botanical medicine, and **homeopathic medicine** can strengthen the person and assist with recovery from surgery, chemotherapy, or radiation.

The cure rate for testicular cancer that hasn't spread (non-metastatic) is 95%. This high cure rate for testicular cancer that is caught early makes self-examination extremely important. Patients cured of testicular cancer, however, need to be seen frequently because they are at a greater risk for developing additional cancers later in life.

Since the causes of testicular cancer are unknown, it is difficult to give specific measures to prevent it. One theory is that testicular cancer is related to exposure to environmental estrogens, such as insecticides and byproducts of the plastics industry. It is possible that avoidance of these products may decrease the risk of this type of cancer. Many types of cancers are associated with smoking. Stopping or cutting back on smoking decreases the risk of many cancers, and may also decrease the risk of testicular cancer. Other suspected causes for testicular cancer occur prenatally; one of these is smoking during **pregnancy**. Long term studies are underway to investigate this possibility.

TESTICULAR SELF-EXAMINATION

Testicular self-examination is one of the most important steps to take in detecting the early signs of **testicular cancer**. As the most common form of cancer in men ages 15-35, testicular cancer may be caught early through a monthly self-examination and an increased awareness of the symptoms of the disease. Testicular cancer, when detected in its early stages is highly curable.

The most effective time to perform a testicular self-examination is after a warm bath or shower when the scrotum is relaxed from the heat. Begin by standing in front of a mirror to look for any changes or swelling on the skin of the scrotum. Using both hands, examine each testicle by placing the index and middle fingers under the testicle with the thumbs placed on top. Gently roll the testicle between the thumbs and fingers. One testicle may appear slightly larger than the other. This is normal. At this point, locate the epididymis, which is the soft, tubelike structure behind the testicle responsible for collecting and distributing sperm. It is important to become familiar with the epididymis so as not to identify it as a suspicious lump. The spermatic cord branches up from the epididymis and can be checked for abnormalities by a gentle squeezing beginning above the right testicle, with the cord between the thumb and first two fingers of the right hand.

During each monthly self-examination, look for symptoms of testicular cancer, which include a small, painless lump in the testicle; a sensation of heaviness in the scrotum; a dull throb in the lower abdomen or groin; a distinct change in the way a testicle feels; or an abrupt collection of fluid in the scrotum. Typically appearing in the form of a small painless pea-size lump, cancerous lumps are usually found on the sides or front of the testicle.

If a suspicious lump or any other changes are found during a self-examination, it is important to see a doctor immediately. While the symptoms may not be cancerous, it is important to be examined to determine an early diagnosis of the disease and begin proper treatment if needed.

TESTICULAR TORSION

Testicular torsion is a disorder of the testicles caused by the twisting of the spermatic cord. In order to understand how this rare condition occurs, it is important to understand the structure of the testicles. Located just below the abdomen, the testicles are two, small oval organs that descend outside the body within a sac called the scrotum. Within the scrotum, the testicles are each suspended by a spermatic cord. If the cord becomes twisted, the blood supply is cut off to the testicle, resulting in the condition known as torsion. The testicles play a vital role for the human male body as the producer of sperm and the supplier of the male sex hormone testosterone.

While there is often no known cause for the torsion of the spermatic cord, the condition may occasionally be present at birth. Certain physical activity may also result in an injury or sudden, strong constriction of muscles attached to the testicle and spermatic cord that leads to torsion, which usually occurs in one testicle only. Additionally, it is the most common cause of scrotal or testicular pain in boys and nonsexually active adolescents.

As the most common cause of scrotal or testicular pain in boys and nonsexually active adolescents, testicular torsion is recognizable by sudden pain in one testicle; redness, tenderness, and swelling of the scrotum; nausea and vomiting; sweating; and if pain is severe, rapid heartbeat. While males of all ages are susceptible to torsion, it is most common in adolescents 12-20 years old. A manual examination, possibly along with an ultrasound, can confirm a diagnosis of torsion.

Upon noticing symptoms of testicular torsion or suspecting its presence, it is important to seek medical treatment immediately. While torsion may correct itself, surgery is usually needed to unravel the twisted spermatic cord and attach the affected testicle to the inside scrotal wall to prevent recurrence. If surgery is not used within three to four hours after symptoms begin, the testicle is usually injured beyond repair. To further reduce the occurrence of torsion, the unaffected testicle will usually be operated on as well. Complications of untreated testicular torsion include the death of testicular tissue due to an obstructed blood supply, resulting in the necessary removal of the affected testicle and spermatic cord. If the removal of one testicle is needed, the remaining healthy testicle will function normally, supplying enough testosterone for regular male maturation, sex life, and reproduction.

See also Adolescent health

TETANUS

Tetanus is a potentially fatal disease which causes severe contraction of the muscles. Historically called ''lockjaw,'' it usually begins with muscle spasms in the jaw making it difficult to open one's mouth, causes difficulty swallowing, and stiff and painful neck, shoulder, and back muscles which soon spreads to muscles of the abdomen, arms, and legs. (A baby born in unsanitary surroundings can develop neonatal tetanus.) If not treated, the disruption of muscular control may result in fatal interference with breathing. Tetanus is caused by the bacterium called *Clostridium tetani*, a microorganism which lives in soil, invades the body through breaks in the skin—especially deep puncture wounds—and produces a toxin called *tetanospasmin*. Although tetanus was widespread at the turn of the century, it can be prevented today through immunization.

Several important scientists made significant contributions to the control of tetanus. Arthur Nicolaier (1862-1942) discovered the tetanus bacterium in 1884. Three years later, while engaged in a study of disinfectants, German bacteriologist **Emil von Behring** noticed that the blood serum of tetanus-immune laboratory rats neutralized the **anthrax** bacteria. He set about isolating the substance that gave the rats resistance to the bacteria.

In the Berlin laboratory of scientist **Robert Koch**, Behring joined with Japanese bacteriologist **Shibasaburo Kitasato**, the first person to isolate the tetanus bacterium in pure culture in 1889. He later isolated and described the bacteria that cause **diphtheria**, anthrax, and **bubonic plague**. Behring and Kitasato discovered that the presence of tetanus and diphtheria toxins in blood cause the blood to produce *antitoxins* that neutralize the poisonous substances. When they injected small amounts of tetanus toxin into animals, the animals produced antitoxins, which gave them immunity from the disease. Furthermore, blood serum containing antitoxins extracted from these animals and injected into other animals gave the new animals immunity to tetanus, as well. They called this procedure "blood serum therapy."

Behring developed a way to produce antitoxin serum in guinea pigs, and later developed a toxin-antitoxin mixture which was an effective vaccine against tetanus. In 1893, French scientist, Pierre-Paul-Emile Roux (1853-1933), assistant to **Louis Pasteur** at the Pasteur Institute, developed improved procedures for using antitoxin serum to prevent as well as treat tetanus.

Today, the tetanus vaccine is included in the DPT vaccine, which also prevents diphtheria and pertussis (**whooping cough**). The DPT inoculation contains weak toxins that serve to stimulate the growth of antibodies to the diseases. It is given in three shots administered two months apart beginning about two months after birth. Booster shots are given at fifteen months, and four to six years. A tetanus booster is recommended every ten years, even for the elderly. If a person suffers a dangerous wound, an additional tetanus injection may be administered at that time.

TETRACYCLINES

Tetracyclines are medicines that kill certain infection-causing microorganisms. Tetracyclines are called broad-spectrum **antibiotics**, because they can be used to treat a wide variety of infections. Physicians may prescribe these drugs to treat eye infections, **pneumonia**, **gonorrhea**, Rocky Mountain spotted fever, **urinary tract infections**, and other infections caused by bacteria. The medicine is also used to treat **acne**. The tetracyclines will *not* work for colds, flu, and other infections caused by viruses.

Tetracyclines are available only with a physician's prescription. They are sold in capsule, tablet, liquid, and injectable forms. Some commonly used medicines in this group are tetracycline (Achromycin V, Sumycin) and doxycycline (Doryx, Vibramycin). The recommended dosage depends on the type of tetracycline, its strength, and the type and severity of infection for which it is being taken. Check with the physician who prescribed the drug or the pharmacist who filled the prescription for the correct dosage. To make sure the infection clears up completely, take the medicine for as long as it has been prescribed. Do not stop taking the drug just because symptoms begin to improve. Tetracycline works best when at a constant level in the blood. To help keep levels constant, take the medicine in doses spaced evenly through the day and night. Do not miss any doses.

This medicine works best when taken on an empty stomach, with a full glass of water. The water will help prevent irritation of the stomach and esophagus (the tube-like structure that runs from the throat to the stomach). If the medicine still causes stomach upset, it may be necessary to take it with food. However, tetracyclines should *never* be taken with milk or milk products, as these may prevent the medicine from working properly. Do not drink or eat milk or dairy products within 1-2 hours of taking tetracyclines (except doxycycline and minocycline). Do not take **antacids**, calcium supplements, salicylates such as Magan or Trilisate, magnesium-containing **laxatives**, or sodium bicarbonate (baking soda) within 1-2 hours of taking tetracyclines. Do not take any medicines that contain iron (including multivitamin and mineral supplements) within 2-3 hours of taking tetracyclines.

The most common side effects are stomach cramps or a burning sensation in the stomach, mild **diarrhea**, nausea, or vomiting. These problems usually go away as the body adjusts to the drug and do not require medical treatment. Less common side effects, such as sore mouth or tongue and **itching** of the rectal or genital areas also may occur and do not need medical attention unless they do not go away or they are bothersome. Some people feel dizzy when taking these drugs. The medicine may also cause blurred vision. Because of these possible effects, anyone who takes these drugs should not drive, use machines or do anything else that might be dangerous until they have found out how the drugs affect them.

This medicine may increase sensitivity to sunlight. Even brief exposure to sun can cause a severe **sunburn** or a rash. While being treated with this medicine, avoid being in direct sunlight, especially between 10 a.m. and 3 p.m.; wear a hat and tightly woven clothing that covers the arms and legs; use a sunscreen with a skin protection factor (SPF) of at least 15; protect the lips with a sun block lipstick; and do not use tanning beds, tanning booths, or sunlamps. The sensitivity to sunlight and sunlamps may continue for 2 weeks to several months after stopping the medicine, so continue to be careful about sun exposure.

Tetracyclines may permanently discolor the teeth of people who took the medicine in childhood. The drugs may also slow down the growth of children's bones. Do not give tetracyclines to infants or children under 8 years of age unless directed to do so by the child's physician. Pregnant women should not take tetracyclines during the last half of pregnancy. These drugs can prevent the baby's bones and teeth from developing properly and can cause the baby's adult teeth to be permanently discolored. The medicine can also cause liver problems in pregnant women. Women who are breastfeeding should not take tetracyclines. The drugs pass into breast milk and can affect the nursing baby's teeth and bones. They may also make the baby more sensitive to sunlight and may increase its risk of fungal infections. Birth control pills may not work properly when taken while tetracyclines are being taken. To prevent **pregnancy**, use additional methods of birth control while taking tetracyclines.

Taking outdated tetracyclines can cause serious side effects. Do not take this medicine if its color, appearance, or taste have changed or if the expiration date on its label has passed. Flush any such medicine down the toilet. If there is any question about whether the medicine is still good, check with a physician or pharmacist. Anyone who has had unusual reactions to tetracyclines in the past should let his or her physician know before taking the drugs again. Before using tetracyclines, people with diabetes, or diseases of the liver or kidneys should make sure their physicians are aware of their conditions.

See also Antibiotics

Tetralogy of Fallot

Tetralogy of Fallot is a common syndrome of congenital heart defects. This condition, present *in utero,* is caused by the narrowing of the pulmonary artery and a hole between the ventricles of the heart. When the baby is born and begins to breathe on its own, the baby turns cyanotic, or blue, due to the deoxygenated blood that bypasses the lungs as a result of this deformity.

Each defect acts in combination with the other to create a malfunction of the heart. The problem starts very early in the uterus with a narrowed pulmonary valve and a hole between the ventricles. This is not particularly a problem for a fetus because hardly any blood flows through the lungs until birth. It is only after birth that the defects pose a problem. The blood that is supposed to start flowing through the lungs cannot easily get there because of the narrowed valve, however the hole between the ventricles remains open. Because of the opening between ventricles, much of the blood that comes back to the heart needing oxygen is sent out without being properly oxygenated. In addition, the right heart has to pump at the same pressure as the left side. Several things follow. First, the baby turns blue (cyanotic) because of the deoxygenated blood that bypasses the lungs. Deoxygenated blood is darker and appears blue through the skin. Second, the right side of the heart (ventricle) hypertrophies (gets more muscular) from the extra **exercise** demanded of it. Next, the low oxygen causes the blood to get thicker and clot more easily. Clots in the veins can now pass through the hole in the heart and directly enter the aorta, where they can do much more damage than in the lungs—such as causing infarcts in the brain. In addition, these anomalies make the lining of the heart more susceptible to infection—**endocarditis**—which can damage valves and lead to blood poisoning (septicemia).

Tetralogy is a congenital defect with unknown causes. A complete evaluation of the circulation is required, including testing the blood for its oxygen content, ultrasound and x rays of the heart accompanied by a contrast agent to determine the amount of blood flowing in the wrong direction. A search for other **birth defects** is also necessary, because they tend to happen together.

Correction of the defects are done through surgery. Surgery must be carefully timed with attention to the progression of the disease process, the size of the infant, and the size of the various defects. There are temporary surgical procedures that can prolong the time before corrective surgery while the baby grows larger and stronger. During surgery, the pulmonary valve is widened, the ventricular septal defect is closed, and any interim fixes removed. Surgical correction has a high rate of success, returning the child to near normal health.

See also Birth defects

Thalassemia

Thalassemia is an inherited disorder that affects the production of hemoglobin and causes **anemia**. Hemoglobin is the substance in red blood cells that enables them to transport oxygen throughout the body. It is composed of a hem molecule and protein molecules called globins. Owing to an inherited genetic trait, lower-than-normal amounts of globins are manufactured in the bone marrow. If the trait is inherited from both parents, a globin may be entirely absent. Thalassemia causes varying degrees of anemia, which can range from insignificant to life threatening. The resulting anemia triggers a surge in red blood cell production, but the new cells are also defective. The bone marrow expands as it attempts to keep pace with the perceived need for new red blood cells, setting the stage for bone deformity and **pain**. **Jaundice**, indicated by yellowed skin, can result from high levels of bilirubin (the end product of hemoglobin degradation). The spleen can become abnormally large and effects on the immune system increase the vulnerability to infection. At the same time, a lot of energy is invested in red blood cell production, stunting development and growth.

Humans have the genes to construct six types of globins, but do not use all six at once. Different globins are produced depending on the stage of development: embryonic, fetal, or adult. There is a different gene for each type of globin, with the exception of alpha-globin, which has two genes. (Genes are inherited in pairs, one copy from each parent.) A gene mutation may lead to inadequate levels of the related globin, reduced hemoglobin formation, and anemia. Such mutations are the underlying cause of thalassemia. Thalassemia is classified according to the globin that is affected. The most common types of thalassemia are beta-thalassemia and alpha-thalassemia. Beta-thalassemia is caused by a mutation in the gene responsible for beta-globin. If a mutated beta-globin gene is inherited from both parents, the result is beta-thalassemia major, a severe, potentially life-threatening anemia. Beta-thalassemia major may also be referred to as Cooley's anemia or erythroblastic anemia. If only one mutated copy of the beta-globin gene is inherited, mild-to-nonexistent symptoms may appear; this condition is called beta-thalassemia minor. A person with one mutated copy of the beta-globin gene is referred to as a carrier of the beta-thalassemia trait.

The alpha-thalassemias are more complex because a person inherits two alpha-globin genes from each parent, yielding a total of two pairs of alpha-globin genes. Mutations in these genes can give rise to a range of symptoms. As long as adequate levels of alpha-globins are produced, the person—otherwise, called the carrier of the alpha-thalassemia trait—will have few, if any symptoms. In cases in which alpha-globin is severely reduced, or not produced at all, the consequences can be fatal during fetal development or shortly after birth.

People with Mediterranean (including North African), Middle Eastern, or southeast Asian ancestry are at higher risk of being carriers of or developing beta-thalassemia than are other populations. Alpha-thalassemia also is more likely to affect people of Mediterranean, African, Middle Eastern, and southeast Asian descent. In some areas, 1 in 150-200 children are born with thalassemia major. It has been estimated that 2 million people in America carry the thalassemia trait. When two carriers of the same type thalassemia produce a child, there is a 25% possibility that the child will inherit moderate or severe thalassemia.

Thalassemia may be diagnosed from the symptoms; however, with proper medical treatment, a diagnosis may be made before symptoms become life- or health-threatening. Basic information that is used in diagnosis includes race and ethnic background, family history, and age. Unexpectedly slow development, along with pallor, jaundice, enlarged spleen or liver, or deformed bones can be common signs of thalassemia.

Laboratory tests are used to confirm a diagnosis and determine the type of thalassemia. These tests can also be used to identify carriers. A **blood count** is done in which the numbers of red blood cells are calculated. The size of the blood cells and the ratio of mature to immature cells are also determined. A higher-than-normal presence of unusually small or immature red blood cells indicate a problem in red blood cell production. Further tests measure the amount of hemoglobin; a low concentration indicates anemia. Hemoglobin molecules can be separated based on the component globin molecules, which aids in diagnosing the type of thalassemia. This process is known as hemoglobin electrophoresis.

Thalassemia cannot be cured; therapy focuses on managing symptoms. Treatment is not necessary for individuals who are unaffected or only develop mild symptoms. The mainstays of thalassemia management are blood **transfusion**s and iron chelation therapy. Blood transfusions are typically given every 6-8 weeks, but may be more frequent in some cases. These transfusions have two purposes: to keep hemoglobin at or near normal levels and to prevent the bone marrow from producing ineffective red blood cells. Repeated transfusions carry the risk of iron loading, a condition in which the body accumulates too much iron. As the iron stores become too large, iron deposits form in the liver, heart, and endocrine glands. These iron deposits cause organ damage and, left unchecked, death. Iron chelation therapy begins between ages three to five with desferrioxamine. The desferrioxamine is administered under the skin of the abdomen or via an implanted venous (vein) port. Once the appropriate dose for an individual is determined, the drug must be administered on a daily or near-daily basis.

Thalassemia has been treated with **bone marrow transplantation**. However, bone marrow transplants are strictly limited by several factors, including the general health of the marrow recipient and whether a donor with compatible marrow can be found. Bone marrow transplants are risky—fatality rates range between 10-30%—and success cannot be guaranteed.

Once the genes that determine thalassemia are inherited, the disease cannot be prevented. Screening offers the opportunity of identifying thalassemia carriers. Carriers may decide to undergo **genetic testing and counseling** to assess potential risks to their children. Finally, prenatal testing, usually chorionic villus sampling or amniotic fluid testing, allows identification of thalassemia in unborn children.

See also Anemia

THEILER, MAX (1899-1972)

South African American virologist

Max Theiler (pronounced Tyler) was born on a farm near Pretoria, South Africa, on January 30, 1899. He enrolled in a two-year premedical program at the University of Cape Town in 1916. In 1919, soon after the conclusion of World War I, he sailed for England, where he pursued further medical training. Despite this rigorous training, Theiler never received the M.D. degree because the University of London refused to recognize his two years of training at the University of Cape Town.

Theiler was frustrated by the ineffectiveness of most medical procedures and the lack of cures for serious illnesses. After finishing his medical training in 1922, the 23-year-old Theiler obtained a position at Harvard Medical School. His early research focused on amoebic dysentery and rat-bite fever. From there, he developed an interest in the yellow-fever virus.

Yellow fever is a tropical viral disease that causes severe fever, slow pulse, bleeding in the stomach, jaundice, and the notorious symptom, black vomit. The disease is fatal in 10%—15% of cases, the cause of death being complete shutdown of the liver or kidneys. Most people recover completely, after a painful, extended illness, with complete immunity to reinfection. The first known outbreak of yellow fever devastated Mexico in 1648. The last major breakout in the continental U.S. claimed 435 lives in New Orleans in 1905. Despite the medical advances of the twentieth century, this tropical disease remains incurable.

By the 1920s, yellow-fever research shifted away from an all-out war on mosquitoes to attempts to find a vaccine to prevent the spread of the disease. Theiler's first big breakthrough was his discovery that mice could be used experimentally in place of the Rhesus monkey and that they had several practical research advantages. When yellow-fever virus was injected into their brains, the mice didn't develop human symptoms.

One unintended research discovery kept Theiler out of his lab and in bed for nearly a week. He accidentally contracted yellow fever from one of his mice, which caused a slight fever and weakness. Theiler was much luckier than some other yellow-fever researchers. Many had succumbed to the disease in the course of their investigations. However, this small bout of yellow fever simply gave Theiler an immunity to the disease. In effect, he was the first recipient of a yellow-fever vaccine.

In 1930, Theiler reported his findings on the effectiveness of using mice for yellow fever research in the respected journal *Science.* The initial response to his findings was overwhelmingly negative, even from his immediate supervisor. Undaunted, Theiler moved from Harvard University, where he was considered an upstart, to the Rockefeller Foundation in New York City. Eventually, yellow-fever researchers began to see the logic behind Theiler's use of the mouse and followed his lead. By passing the yellow-fever virus from mouse to mouse, he was able to shorten the incubation time and increase the virulence of the disease, which enabled research data to be generated more quickly and cheaply. He was now certain that an attenuated live vaccine, one weak enough to cause no harm yet strong enough to generate immunity, could be developed.

A colleague at the Rockefeller Foundation, Dr. Wilbur A. Sawyer, used Theiler's mouse strain, a combination of yellow fever virus and immune serum, to develop a human vaccine. Sawyer is often wrongly credited with inventing the first human yellow-fever vaccine. He simply transferred Theiler's work from the mouse to humans. Ten workers in the Rockefeller labs were inoculated with the mouse strain, with no apparent side effects. The mouse-virus strain was subsequently used by the French government to immunize French colonials in West Africa, a hot spot for yellow fever. This so-called ''scratch'' vaccine was a combination of infected mouse brain tissue and cowpox virus and could be quickly administered by scratching the vaccine into the skin. It was used throughout Africa for nearly 25 years and led to the near total eradication of yellow fever in the major African cities.

While he was somewhat pleased with the new vaccine, Theiler considered the mouse strain inappropriate for human use. In some cases, the vaccine led to encephalitis in a few recipients and caused less severe side effects, such as headache or nausea, in many others. Theiler believed that a ''killed'' vaccine, which used a dead virus, wouldn't produce an immune effect, so he and his colleagues set out to find a milder live strain. He began working with the Asibi yellow-fever strain, a form of the virus so powerful that it killed monkeys instantly when injected under the skin. The Asibi strain thrived in a number of media, including chicken embryos. Theiler kept this virus alive for years in tissue cultures, passing it from embryo to embryo, and only occasionally testing the potency of

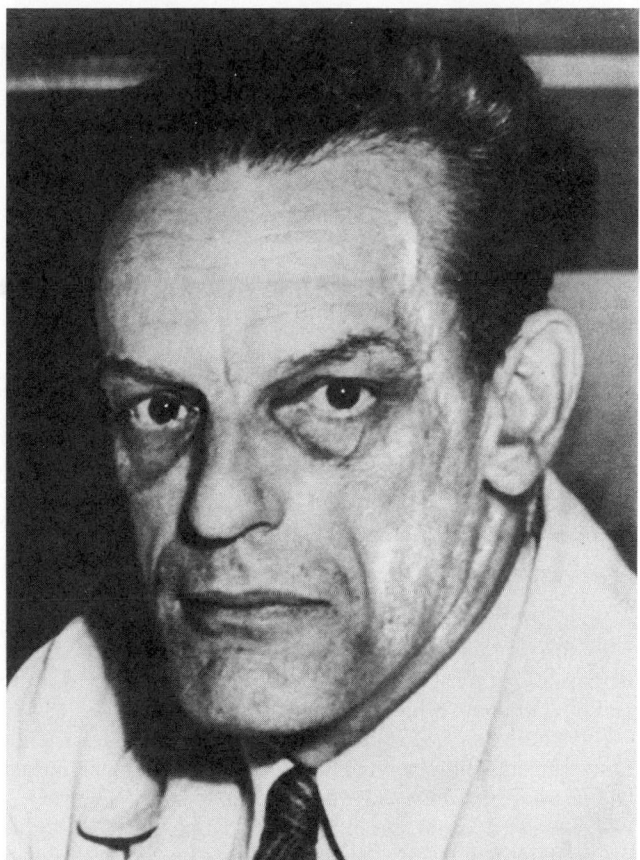

Max Theiler.

the virus in a living animal. He continued making subcultures of the virus until he reached strain number 176. Then, he tested the strain on two monkeys. Both animals survived and seemed to have acquired a sufficient immunity to yellow fever. In March 1937, after testing this new vaccine on himself and others, Theiler announced that he had developed a new, safer, attenuated vaccine, which he called 17D strain. This new strain was much easier to produce, cheaper, and caused very mild side effects.

From 1940 to 1947, with the financial assistance of the Rockefeller Foundation, more than 28 million 17D-strain vaccines were produced, at a cost of approximately two cents per unit, and given away to people in tropical countries and the U.S. The vaccine was so effective that the Rockefeller Foundation ended its yellow-fever program in 1949, safe in the knowledge that the disease had been effectively eradicated worldwide and that any subsequent outbreaks could be controlled with the new vaccine. Unfortunately, almost all yellow-fever research ended around this time and few people studied how to cure the disease. For people in tropical climates who live outside of the major urban centers, yellow fever is still a problem. A major outbreak in Ethiopia in 1960–62 caused 30,000 deaths. The World Health Organization still uses Theiler's 17D vaccine and is attempting to inoculate people in remote areas.

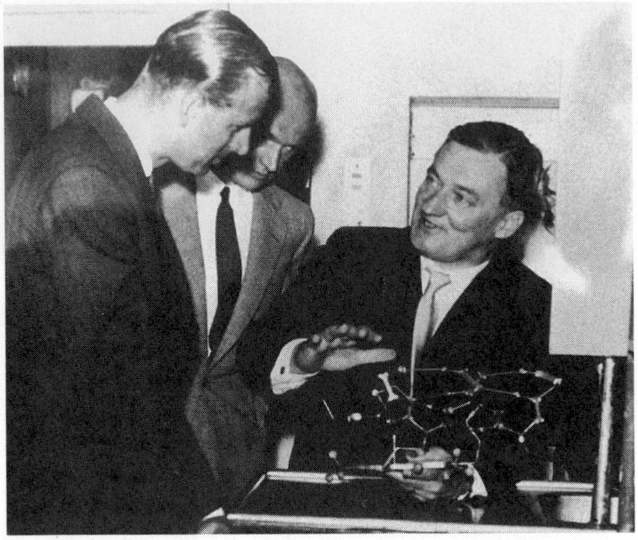

Axel Hugo Theorell

In 1951, Theiler received the Nobel Prize in medicine or physiology ''for his discoveries concerning yellow fever and how to combat it.''

After developing the yellow-fever vaccine, Theiler turned his attention to other viruses, including some unusual and rare diseases, such as Bwamba fever and Rift Valley fever. His other, less exotic research focused on polio and led to his discovery of a polio-like infection in mice known as encephalomyelitis or Theiler's disease. In 1964, he retired from the Rockefeller Foundation, having achieved the rank of associate director for medical and natural sciences and director of the Virus Laboratories. In that same year, he accepted a position as professor of epidemiology and microbiology at Yale University in New Haven, Connecticut. He retired from Yale in 1967. Theiler died on August 11, 1972, at the age of 73.

THEORELL, AXEL HUGO TEODOR (1903-1982)

Swedish biochemist

Axel Hugo Theorell was born in Linköping, Sweden, on July 6, 1903. He received his bachelor of medicine degree (1924) and his doctor of medicine (1930) from the Karolinska Institute in Stockholm. He also studied at the Pasteur Institute in Paris. When a crippling attack of **polio**myelitis made a career as a physician impractical, he decided instead to pursue research and teaching. His academic work while at Stockholm was an inquiry into the chemistry of plasma lipids (fatty acids) and their effect on red blood cells. A technique he developed at this time to separate the plasma proteins albumin and globulin was later to prove useful in his work on isolating enzymes (globular proteins) and coenzymes, which help to activate specific enzymes.

As professor of chemistry at Uppsala University from 1930–1936, Theorell expanded his research on plasma lipids to concentrate on myoglobin, a muscle protein whose oxygen-carrying capacities he compared to that of hemoglobin in the blood. By isolating (purifying) myoglobin, he was able to show its absorption and storage capacities, and to measure, using centrifugal force, its molecular weight. This determination of its physical properties showed that myoglobin was a separate protein from hemoglobin.

In 1933 Theorell received a grant from the Rockefeller Foundation that enabled him to further his study of enzymes with **Otto Warburg** at the Kaiser Wilhelm Institute (now the Max Planck Institute) in Berlin. Warburg had attempted without success to isolate the yellow enzyme. Using his own methods, Theorell accomplished the isolation. He further separated the yellow enzyme into two parts: the catalytic coenzyme and the pure protein apoenzyme. He also found that the main ingredient of the yellow enzyme is the plasma protein albumin. An important corollary to the research was Theorell's discovery of the chemical chain reaction necessary for cellular oxidation or respiration. These contributions brought a test-tube creation of life closer to reality, and advanced the study of the chemical differences between normal and cancerous cells.

Returning to Stockholm, Theorell became head of the biochemistry department at the Karolinska Institute, part of a Nobel Institute established for the purpose of providing Theorell with further research opportunities. Under his direction, the department acquired a reputation for excellence that attracted biochemists from all over the world. It was here that Theorell continued his research on cytochrome c, succeeding in his attempts to purify it by 1939. He furthered this study that same year in the United States with his colleague, Linus Pauling, who discovered the alpha spiral (protein molecules arranged in a twisted-atom chain).

After World War II, a collaboration with Britton Chance of the University of Pennsylvania elucidated steps in the oxidation (breakdown) of alcohol and gave the process a name—the Theorell-Chance mechanism. Theorell's study of the enzymes that catalyze the oxidation, alcohol dehydrogenases, provided a new method for determining the level of alcohol in the bloodstream—a technique that came to be used by Sweden and West Germany to test the sobriety of their citizens. From a different perspective, Theorell's alcohol enzyme research pinpointed several bacterial strains, knowledge of which was thought to be useful in the treatment of **tuberculosis**. Theorell was awarded the 1955 Nobel Prize in physiology or medicine for ''his discoveries concerning the nature and mode of action of oxidation enzymes.'' Theorell retired from the Nobel Institute in 1970. Afflicted with a stroke in 1974, his health deteriorated over the following years. He died on August 15, 1982, while vacationing on an island off the coast of Sweden.

THOMAS, E.DONNALL (1920-)

American physician

E. Donnall Thomas has pioneered techniques for transplanting bone marrow, an operation that has been utilized to treat patients with **cancers** of the blood, such as leukemia. For proving that such transplants could save the lives of dying patients, Thomas was awarded the Nobel Prize in physiology of medicine in 1990 (he shared the award with **Joseph E. Murray**).

E. Donnall Thomas was born on March 15, 1920, in the small town of Mart, Texas. After graduating from a high school class of approximately fifteen students, Thomas entered the University of Texas at Austin in 1937. He received a B.A. in 1941 and continued on for a master's degree, which was awarded in 1943.

After completing his master's degree, Thomas started medical school at the University of Texas Medical Branch in Galveston. After six months, however, he transferred to Harvard Medical School, where he received his M.D. in 1946. He became an intern and then a resident at Peter Bent Brigham Hospital in Boston and began to specialize in blood diseases. Thomas interrupted his formal medical training to serve as a physician in the United States Army (1948–1950). He then returned to the Boston area and did research on leukemia treatments for a year as a postdoctoral fellow at the Massachusetts Institute of Technology. In 1953 he worked as an instructor at Harvard Medical School.

Thomas moved to New York in 1955 to take the position of physician-in-chief at the Mary Imogene Bassett Hospital in Cooperstown. The next year he became, in addition, an associate clinical professor of medicine at the College of Physicians and Surgeons at Columbia University. During the next eight years Thomas had the opportunity to develop and research his ideas about bone marrow transplants, and he applied these concepts to treating cancers of the blood.

Leukemia is a type of cancer in which certain blood cells, known generally as white blood cells, are produced in abnormally large numbers by the bone marrow. In other kinds of cancer, the diseased cells pile up into a tumor, which can often be treated by simply cutting out the lump. Leukemic blood cells, however, circulate throughout the body, making them much more difficult to eliminate. Furthermore, the white blood cells that become abnormal in leukemia are an important part of the body's **immune system**. Even if they could be destroyed by a means such as radiation, without them the patient would be vulnerable to infections.

In the 1950s, researchers showed that inbred laboratory mice could be irradiated, thus destroying the production of white blood cells by their bone marrow, and then saved from infection by a transplant of bone marrow taken from healthy mice. Inspired by these experiments, Thomas began similar studies on dogs, but he faced two important obstacles. First, the recipient animal's immune system had to be prevented from attacking and destroying the transplanted bone marrow—such immune rejection has long been a problem for bone marrow as well as organ transplant surgery. And second, if the bone marrow transplant was successful and the donated marrow began to produce white blood cells, these cells were likely to attack the recipient's other tissues, perceiving them as foreign. Both of these problems had been avoided in the earlier studies with inbred mice because the mice were genetically identical, and hence, have identical immune systems. People are not so similar genetically, with the exception of identical twins. All attempts to graft bone marrow between a donor and recipient who were not identical twins failed. In 1956, Thomas performed the first bone marrow transplant to a leukemia patient from an identical twin. Although the patient's immune system did not reject the transplant, the cancer recurred.

Many researchers gave up working on organ transplants because the problems of immune rejection seemed insurmountable, but Thomas persisted. In 1963 he moved to Seattle to become a professor at the University of Washington Medical School. There he put together a team of expert researchers and began experimenting with new drugs that could suppress the recipient's immune system and thus prevent rejection of the new tissue. In the meantime, new methods were being developed by other researchers to identify people whose immune systems were similar, in order to match organ donors and recipients. The new methods of tissue typing were based on molecules known as histocompatibility antigens. Thomas's team performed the first bone marrow transplant to a leukemia patient from a matched donor in March 1969. During the 1970s they developed and perfected a comprehensive procedure for treating leukemia patients: first the patients receive radiation, both to kill cancer cells and to weaken the immune system so that it does not reject the transplant; then their bone marrow is replaced with marrow from a compatible donor. The patients also are given drugs that continue to suppress their immune systems. Many patients had been cured of leukemia using this technique by the late 1970s. Since then Thomas and his colleagues have improved their success rate from about 12–50%. In addition to leukemia and other cancers of the blood, bone marrow transplants are used to treat certain inherited blood disorders and to aid people whose bone marrow has been destroyed by accidental exposure to radiation.

It was in 1990 that Thomas was awarded the Nobel Prize in physiology or medicine in 1990, a commendation he shared with Joseph E. Murray, another American physician who has done important work in the area of transplants. The Nobel Prize came as a surprise. Thomas told reporters that the award is more often given to scientists who do basic research than to those that develop clinical treatments. As reported in *Time* magazine, both men were cited by the Nobel committee for discoveries ''crucial for those tens of thousands of severely ill patients who either can be cured or given a decent life when other treatment methods are without success.''

THREADWORM INFECTION

Threadworm infection is an intestinal disease, which occasionally spreads to the skin, caused by a type of parasitic roundworm (helminth). In untreated patients, the disease has a high rate of reinfection caused by worms already present in the body. This type of disease recurrence is called autoinfection. Because of autoinfection, threadworms can remain inside humans for as long as 45 years after the initial infestation.

Threadworm infection, which is also called strongyloidiasis, occurs in most countries of the world but is natural to (endemic in) tropical and subtropical climates. Strongyloidiasis is less common than other parasitic infections but may affect as much as 25% of the population in some developing countries. In the United States, threadworm infection is most likely to be found among immigrants; returning travelers or military personnel; people who live in parts of Appalachia and the southeastern states; and persons in homes for the retarded and similar institutions.

Human beings are universally susceptible to threadworm infection, although adults and older children are at greater risk of infection than younger children. The disease does not confer immunity. In addition to humans, threadworms can infect dogs, cats, horses, pigs, rats, and monkeys. The roundworm that lives in soil and can survive there for several generations. Mature threadworms may grow as long as 1-2 inches (2.5-5 cm). The larvae have two stages in their life cycle: a rod-shaped (rhabdoid) first stage, which is not infective; and a threadlike (filariform) stage, in which the larvae can penetrate intact human skin and internal tissues.

The infection is most commonly transmitted when a person comes into contact—usually by walking barefoot—with soil containing *S. stercoralis* larvae in their filariform stage. The threadlike larvae penetrate the skin, enter the lymphatic system, and are carried by the blood to the lungs. Once in the lungs, the larvae burst out of the capillaries into the patient's main respiratory system. They migrate upwards—usually without symptoms—to the patient's throat, where they are swallowed and carried down into the digestive tract. The filariform larvae settle in the small intestine. They mature into adults that deposit eggs that hatch—usually in the intestines—into noninfectious rhabdoid larvae. The rhabdoid larvae then migrate into the patient's large intestine and are excreted in the feces. The time from initial penetration of the skin to excretion is 17–28 days. The rhabdoid larvae metamorphose into the infective filariform stage in the soil.

Threadworms are unique among human parasites in having both free-living and parasitic forms. In the free-living life cycle, some rhabdoid larvae develop into adult worms that live in contaminated soil and produce eggs that hatch into new rhabdoid larvae. The adult worms may live as long as five years.

The signs and symptoms of threadworm infection vary according to the stage of the disease as the larvae migrate throughout the body. Patients who suffer from autoinfection may have chronic or intermittent symptoms for years after they are first infected. The filariform larvae usually enter the body through the skin of the feet. There may be swelling, **itching**, and **hives** at the point of entry that may be confused with insect bites. Patients with chronic threadworm infection may also develop an itchy rash on their buttocks, thighs, or abdomen.

Although some patients may notice only mild **diarrhea** and cramps, others may have **fever**, nausea, vomiting, general weakness, and blood or mucus in their stools. The **pain** may mimic a stomach ulcer. When the larvae migrate to the lungs and air passages, the patient may have symptoms ranging from a simple dry **cough** to fever, difficulty breathing, and coughing up blood or pus.

Hyperinfection syndrome is a potentially fatal set of complications resulting from the spread of filariform larvae to the lungs and other organ systems. It can include inflammation of the heart tissue, stomach **ulcers**, perforation of the intestines, blood poisoning, **meningitis**, **shock**, and eventual **death**. Hyperinfection syndrome is most likely to occur in patients with immune disorders or **malnutrition**, or in those taking anti-inflammatory or corticosteriod medications. It has been reported in only a few **AIDS** patients.

Threadworm autoinfection in humans follows two patterns. In internal autoinfection, some rhabdoid larvae in the lower bowel develop into filariform larvae that enter the bloodstream from the intestines and migrate to the lungs. In external autoinfection, the skin around the patient's anus is infected by larvae in the feces.

The doctor is likely to consider a diagnosis of threadworm infection when a patient has the symptoms described earlier and a history of travel or military service in areas where the disease is endemic. A definite diagnosis is made by finding rhabdoid or filariform larvae in the patient's body fluids. The larvae may be found in fresh stool specimens or in mucus coughed up when the infection has reached the lungs. Because the larvae cannot be detected in the stools of 25% of infected patients, the string test is often performed to confirm the diagnosis. In this test, the patient swallows a weighted string which is withdrawn after four hours. The digestive juices absorbed by the string are then examined for the presence of threadworm larvae.

Doctors can also use blood tests and diagnostic imaging to support the diagnosis. Between 85% and 95% of patients with threadworm infections will have a measurable level of antibodies in their blood, even though these antibodies do not prevent the disease from spreading. In addition, patients with severe infections often have unusually high levels of white cells in their blood. X rays of the intestines or the chest often help in locating specific areas of inflamed or ulcerated tissue.

Threadworm infections are treated with medications. The drugs most often given are ivermectin, thiabendazole (Mintezol), and albendazole. Ivermectin is generally preferred because it has fewer side effects than thiabendazole. These drugs, which are taken by mouth over a period of 2-7 days, work by preventing the development of eggs and new larvae. Patients with severe infections should be given protein replacement, blood **transfusion**s, and fluids to replace losses from nausea, vomiting, and diarrhea. Patients who are taking **corticosteroids** should be carefully evaluated if they have symptoms of threadworm infection, because these medications encourage the development of hyperinfection syndrome. The prognosis for complete recovery is good for most patients, except those with hyperinfection syndrome or severe protein loss.

There is no effective immunization against threadworm infection. Prevention of the disease requires careful attention to personal and institutional hygiene in endemic areas, including handwashing after defecating and before handling food. Other precautions include wearing shoes when visiting countries with high rates of threadworm infection, and monitoring close contacts of patients for signs of infection.

See also Diarrhea

Throat culture

A throat culture is a technique for identifying disease bacteria in material taken from the throat. Most throat cultures are done to rule out infections caused by beta-hemolytic streptococci, which cause **strep throat**. Hemolytic means that these streptococci destroy red blood cells. These organisms are Group A streptococci, specifically *Streptococcus pyogenes*. Since most **sore throats** are caused by viral infections rather than by *S. pyogenes*, a correct diagnosis is important to prevent unnecessary use of **antibiotics** and to begin treatment of strep infections as soon as possible. Group A **streptococcal infections** are potentially life-threatening, often involving other parts of the body in addition to the throat. Besides causing sore throat (pharyngitis), streptococci can also cause **scarlet fever**, **rheumatic fever**, kidney disease, or **abscesses** around the tonsils.

Throat cultures can also be used to identify other disease organisms that are present in the patient's throat; and to identify people who are carriers of the organisms that cause **meningitis** and **whooping cough**. Besides their use in diagnosis, throat cultures are sometimes used to test antibiotics for their effectiveness in treating different infections.

Throat cultures should be taken before the patient is given any antibiotic medications. In addition, the patient's immunization history should be checked to evaluate the possibility that diseases other than strep are causing the sore throat. The care provider should wash the hands carefully after taking the specimen to prevent the spread of any infectious organisms.

A throat culture test should be done on anyone who has symptoms of a strep throat. These symptoms include a sore throat that may be accompanied by a **fever**, body aches, and loss of appetite. Age is a consideration, in that strep throat is more common in children than in adults. The tonsils and the back of the throat often appear red, swollen, and streaked with pus. These symptoms usually appear 1-3 days after being exposed to group A strep. Because strep is highly contagious, family members and close contacts of patients diagnosed with strep throat should also have throat cultures performed if they show signs of the disease.

The specimen for throat culture is obtained by wiping the patient's throat with a cotton swab. The patient is asked to tilt the head back and open the mouth wide. With the tongue depressed and the patient saying "ah," the care provider wipes the back of the throat and the tonsils with a sterile swab. The swab is applied to any area that appears either very red or discharging pus. The swab is removed gently without touching the teeth, gums, or tongue. It is then placed in a sterile tube for immediate delivery to a laboratory. Obtaining the specimen takes less than 30 seconds. Laboratory results are usually available in two to three days. The swabbing procedure may cause gagging but is not **pain**ful. The doctor makes a note for the laboratory to indicate if any disease organisms other than strep are suspected, because some require special growth conditions in the laboratory. The patient does not need to avoid food or fluids before the test. Recent gargling or treatment with antibiotics, however, will affect the culture results. The laboratory should be notified if the patient has been recently taking antibiotic medications.

S. pyogenes is cultured on a growth medium called blood agar. Agar is a gel that is made from the cell walls of red algae. Blood agar is made from agar gel and sheep's blood. When the throat swab reaches the laboratory, it is wiped across a blood agar plate. The plate is allowed to incubate for 24-48 hours to allow the growth of bacteria. If the organism is a Group A hemolytic streptococcus, the area immediately around the bacterial colony will be cleared of red blood cells. Hemolytic streptococci dissolve (lyse) red blood cells, leaving a clear zone surrounding the colony.

So-called instant strep tests are now available to help diagnose strep throat. They can be used in the doctor's office and take about 10-30 minutes to perform. Instant tests detect an antigen associated with the streptococcus. If an instant throat test is negative, however, a standard throat culture can be performed to verify the results.

See also Sore throat; Strep throat

Thrombophlebitis

Thrombophlebitis is the inflammation of a vein with blood clot formation inside the vein at the site of inflammation. Thrombophlebitis is also known as phlebitis, phlebothrombosis, and venous thrombosis. If the inflammation component is minor, the disease is usually called venous or phlebothrombosis. Thrombophlebitis can occur in both deep veins and superficial veins, but most often occurs in the superficial veins of the legs. When thrombophlebitis occurs in a superficial vein, one that is near the surface of the skin and is visible to the eye, the disease is called superficial thrombophlebitis. Any form of injury to a blood vessel can result in thrombophlebitis. In the case of superficial thrombophlebitis, the blood clot usually attaches firmly to the wall of the affected blood vein. Since superficial blood veins do not have muscles that massage the veins, blood clots in superficial veins tend to remain where they form and seldom break loose.

When thrombophlebitis occurs in a deep vein, a vein that runs deep within muscle tissue, it is called deep venous thrombosis. Deep venous thrombosis presents the threat of producing blood clots that will break loose to form emboli. These can lodge in other tissues where they can block the blood supply, typically in the lungs. This results in tissue damage and can sometimes be serious or fatal, for example, **pulmonary embolism**.

The main symptoms are tenderness and **pain** in the area of the affected vein. Redness and/or swelling may also be seen. In the case of deep venous thrombosis, there is more swelling than is caused by superficial thrombophlebitis, and the patient may experience muscle stiffness in the affected area.

There are many causes of thrombophlebitis. The main causes can be grouped into three categories; injury to blood veins, increased blood clotting, and blood stasis. When blood veins are damaged, collagen in the blood vein wall is exposed. Platelets respond to collagen by initiating the clotting process. Damage to a vein can occur as a consequence of indwelling catheters, trauma, infection, or the injection of irritating substances. Increased tendency of the blood to clot can be caused by malignant tumors, genetic disorders, and **oral contraceptives**. Stasis, in which the blood clots due to decreased blood flow in an area, can happen following surgery, as a consequence of **varicose veins**, as a complication of postpartum states, and following prolonged bed rest. In the case of prolonged bed rest, blood clots form because of inactivity, which allows blood to move sluggishly and stagnate (collect) in blood veins. This can lead to blood clots. These clots (also called emboli) are sometimes released when the patient stands up and resumes activity. This can present a problem if the emboli lodge in vital organs. In the case of postpartum patients, a **fever** developing 4-10 days after delivery may indicate thrombophlebitis.

In superficial thrombophlebitis, the location of the clot can sometimes be seen by the unaided eye. Blood clots are hard and can usually be detected by a physician using palpation (massage). Deep venous thrombosis requires specialized diagnostic instruments to detect the blood clot. Among the instruments a physician may use are ultrasound and x ray, coupled with dye injection (venogram).

Superficial thrombophlebitis usually resolves without treatment. If treatment of superficial thrombophlebitis is given, it is usually limited to the application of heat or anti-inflammatory drugs, like **aspirin** or ibuprofen, which also help to relieve the pain. It can take from several days to several weeks for the clot to resolve and the symptoms to completely disappear. Rarely, **anticoagulant** drugs may be administered.

Deep venous thrombosis is a serious condition and is treated with anticoagulant drugs and by keeping the affected limb elevated. The primary objective in treating deep venous thrombosis is prevention of a pulmonary embolism. The patient usually is hospitalized during initial treatment. The prescribed anticoagulant drugs limits the ability of blood clots to grow and new clots to form. Sometimes, a drug that dissolves blood clots is administered. These drugs must be used with caution because as the clot dissolves, it may release from the site where it formed and becomes an embolus. Surgery may be used if the affected vein is likely to present a long term threat of producing blood clots that will release emboli.

Thrombocytopenia

Thrombocytopenia is an abnormal drop in the number of blood cells involved in forming blood clots. These cells are called platelets. The normal amount of platelets is usually between 150,000 and 450,000 cells per microliter of blood. A microliter is an amount equal to one one-millionth of a liter (a liter is almost equal to a quart). Platelet numbers are counted by having a blood sample collected and placing a measured amount of blood in a machine called a cell counter. When the platelet number drops below 150,000 cells per microliter of blood, this person is said to be thrombocytopenic.

Abnormal reductions in the number of platelets are caused when abnormalities occur in any of the following three processes: decreased platelet production by the bone marrow; increased trapping of platelets by the spleen; or a more rapid than normal destruction of platelets. Persons with this condition easily bruise and can have episodes of excess bleeding (a hemorrhage).

Platelets come from megakaryocytes, which are produced in the material located within the center cavity of the bones (bone marrow). When abnormalities develop in the marrow, the marrow cells can lose their ability to produce platelets in correct amounts. The result is a lower than normal level of platelets in the blood. Drugs used in **cancer chemotherapy** can cause the marrow to malfunction in this way, as can the presence of tumor cells in the marrow itself.

Normally, the spleen holds about one-third of the body's platelets as part of this organ's function to recycle aging or damaged red blood cells (the cells that carry oxygen in the blood). When liver disease or cancer of the spleen is present, the spleen can enlarge, resulting in a greater number of platelets staying in the organ. This condition results in abnormally low numbers of platelets in the blood.

Platelets can breakdown in unusually high amounts in persons with abnormalities in their blood vessel walls, with blood clots, or with man-made replacement heart valves. Devices placed inside blood vessels to keep them from closing (stents) due to weakened walls or fat build-up can also cause platelets to breakdown. In addition, infections and other changes in the immune system can speed up the removal of platelets from the circulation.

Thrombocytopenia is diagnosed by having a blood sample taken and counting the platelets present in the sample. However, accurately determining the medical reason for this conditions is complex. Once a low **platelet count** is verified, a careful evaluation of the function of the bone marrow and spleen are necessary. Improper functioning of either or both of these organs can cause thrombocytopenia. In addition, the causes for the abnormal spleen or marrow function must be investigated since different cancers, blood disorders, or liver disease can be the true cause for the drop in platelets found in the blood.

If low platelet counts are caused by an enlarged spleen, removal of the spleen can help raise the platelet level, since the spleen is no longer there to capture the platelets. However, proper treatment for what causes the enlarged spleen is necessary as well. Low platelet counts can indicate more serious conditions. If a dysfunctional immune system is found to be the cause for this condition, drugs like steroids or gamma globulin can be used to help maintain platelet levels in certain cases. If low platelet levels are due to an abnormally low level of platelet production, **transfusion**s of platelets can be given as well.

There is no known way to prevent thrombocytopenia.

See also Platelet count

Thrombocytosis

Thrombocytosis is a blood disorder, in which the body produces a surplus of platelets (thrombocytes). Platelets are blood cells that stick together, helping blood clot. The cause of essential thrombocytosis is unknown. Secondary thrombocytosis may have many causes, including acute hemorrhage, **anemia**, arthritis, **cancer**, and certain medications. Surgery, particularly removal of the spleen (splenectomy), may also be a causative factor.

Two of every three patients who have thrombocytosis do not have any symptoms of the disease at the time of diagnosis. Younger patients may remain symptom-free for years. Enlargement of the spleen is detected in 60% of patients with thrombocytosis. The liver may also be enlarged. As many as half of all patients experience bleeding from the skin, gums, or nose, and 20-50% have some blockage of veins or arteries.

Other symptoms of thrombocytosis include:

- Bloody stools
- Bruising
- **Dizziness**
- **Headache**
- Hemorrhage
- Prolonged bleeding after having surgery or after having a tooth pulled
- Redness or tingling of the hands and feet
- Weakness. In rare instances, the lymph nodes become enlarged.

The highest **platelet count**s usually produce the most severe symptoms. Younger patients (especially women) may not have symptoms, even though their platelet counts are very high. Complications of thrombocytosis include **stroke**, **heart attack**, and formation of blood clots in the arms and legs.

A doctor should be notified whenever bleeding is unexplained or prolonged or the patient develops:

- Chest or leg **pain**
- Confusion
- Numbness
- Weakness.

Any patient who has thrombocytosis should be encouraged not to smoke. In young people who have no symptoms, this condition can remain stable for many years. These patients should be monitored by a physician, but may not require treatment. Treatment for patients who do have symptoms focuses on controlling bleeding, preventing the formation of blood clots, and lowering platelet levels. Treatment for secondary thrombocytosis involves treating the condition or disease responsible for excess platelet production.

In 1997, the United States Food and Drug Administration (FDA) approved the use of anagrelide HCI (Agrylin) to reduce elevated platelet counts and decrease the risk of clot formation. Some patients have benefited from the use of hydroxyurea, an anti-cancer drug. Low doses of **aspirin** may prevent clotting, but can cause serious hemorrhages. If drug therapy does not bring platelet counts down to an acceptable level as rapidly as necessary, plateletpheresis may be performed. Usually combined with drug therapy and used primarily in medical emergencies, this procedure consists of:

- Withdrawing blood from the patient's body
- Removing platelets from the blood
- Returning the platelet-depleted blood to the patient.

Many patients with thrombocytosis remain free of complications for long periods. However, some patients may die as a result of blood clots or uncontrolled bleeding. There is no known way to prevent thrombocytosis.

See also Platelet count

Thyroid cancer

Thyroid cancer is a disease in which the thyroid cells become abnormal, grow uncontrollably, and form tumors. The thyroid is a butterfly-shaped gland, located at the base of the throat. It has two lobes, the left and the right. The thyroid gland makes hormones that regulate heart rate, blood pressure, body temperature, and **metabolism**. The hormones produced by the thyroid also affect the **nervous system**, muscles, and other organs, and play an important role in regulating childhood growth and development. The thyroid uses iodine, a mineral found in some foods, to make several of its hormones.

Thyroid cancers are grouped into four types, depending on how the cells look under the microscope. The four types are papillary, follicular, medullary, and anaplastic thyroid cancers. The cancers grow at different rates, so the aggressiveness of each **cancer** is different. Papillary and follicular cancer develops in the cells that produce **thyroid hormones** containing iodine. About 60-80% of all thyroid cancers are papillary cancers. Medullary cancers develop in the parafollicular cells (also known as the C cells) which produce the calcitonin hormone. These cancers have a tendency to spread to other parts of the body and hence are difficult to control. Anaplastic cancer is the fastest growing of all thyroid cancers and is usually fatal.

Exposure to radiation during childhood is a known risk factor for thyroid cancer. In areas of the world where people's **diets** are low in iodine, papillary and follicular cancers occur more frequently. In the United States, dietary iodine is plentiful because it is added to table salt and other foods.

The most frequent symptom of thyroid cancer is a lump or nodule that can be felt in the neck. The lymph nodes may be swollen and the voice may become hoarse because the tumor presses on the nerves leading to the voice box.

The doctor may use several tests to confirm a diagnosis of thyroid cancer. Blood tests, such as the thyroid stimulating hormone (TSH) test, may be ordered to check how well the patient's thyroid is functioning. An ultrasound scan, may be used to produce a picture of the thyroid. This test can determine whether the lumps found in the thyroid are fluid-filled cysts or solid malignant tumors.

A radioactive scan is used to identify abnormal areas in the thyroid. The patient is given a very small amount of radioactive iodine, which can either be taken by mouth or injected into the thyroid. Since the thyroid is the only gland in the body that absorbs iodine, the radioactive iodine accumulates there. A x-ray image can then be taken to identify areas in the thyroid that do not absorb iodine normally. These abnormal spots are called "cold spots" and further tests are performed to check whether the cold spots are benign or malignant tumors. The most accurate diagnostic tool for thyroid cancer is a biopsy. In this process, a sample of thyroid tissue is withdrawn and examined under a microscope.

Treatment for thyroid cancer depends on the type of cancer and its stage. Four types of treatment are used: surgical removal, **radiation therapy**, hormone therapy, and **chemotherapy**.

If the cancer has not spread to distant parts of the body, surgical removal is the usual treatment. The surgeon may remove the side or lobe of the thyroid where the cancer is found (lobectomy) or all of it (total thyroidectomy). Radiation therapy uses high-energy x rays to kill cancer cells and shrink tumors. Because the thyroid cells are the only cells of the body that take up iodine, the radioactive iodine collects in any thyroid tissue remaining in the body and kills the cancer cells. Chemotherapy is used if the cancer has spread to other parts of the body and surgery is not possible. This treatment is aimed at killing or slowing the growth of cancer cells throughout the body.

Hormone therapy uses hormones to stop the cancer cells from growing. When the thyroid gland is removed and levels of thyroid hormones fall, the pituitary gland starts producing a hormone called ''thyroid stimulating hormone'' (TSH). TSH stimulates the thyroid cells to grow. This stimulation would also induce growth of the cancerous thyroid cells. To prevent this, the natural hormones that are produced by the thyroid are taken in the form of pills. Thus, their levels remain normal and inhibit the pituitary from making TSH.

Like most cancers, cancer of the thyroid is best treated when it is found early. Patients who are treated for papillary, follicular cancer or medullary thyroid cancer have an excellent rate of survival. Eighty to 90% of patients will live for at least 10 years after surgery. The fourth type of thyroid cancer, anaplastic, is usually fatal. Only 3-17% of patients with this cancer survive for 5 years.

Because most people with thyroid cancer have no known risk factor, it is not possible to completely prevent this disease. The National Cancer Institute recommends that a doctor examine anyone who has received radiation to the head and neck during childhood at intervals of one or two years. The neck and the thyroid should be carefully examined for any lumps or enlargement of the nearby lymph nodes. Ultrasonography may be used for people at risk for thyroid cancer.

THYROID DISORDERS

Located in the front of the neck, the thyroid gland produces the hormones thyroxine (T_4) and triiodothyronine (T_3) that regulate the body's metabolic rate by helping to form protein ribonucleic acid (RNA) and increasing oxygen absorption in every cell. In turn, the production of these hormones are controlled by thyroid-stimulating hormone (TSH) that is produced by the pituitary gland. When production of the thyroid hormones increases despite the level of TSH being produced, hyperthyroidism occurs. The excessive amount of thyroid hormones in the blood increases the body's metabolism, creating both mental and physical symptoms.

Curiously, the thyroid gland is often enlarged whether it is making too much hormone, too little, or sometimes even when it is functioning normally. TSH increases the amount of thyroxin secreted by the thyroid and also causes the thyroid gland to grow.

- Hyperthyroid goiter—If the amount of stimulating hormone is excessive, the thyroid will both enlarge and secrete too much thyroxin. The result—hyperthyroidism with a goiter. Graves' disease is the most common form of this disorder.
- Euthyroid goiter—The thyroid is the only organ in the body to use iodine. If dietary iodine is slightly inadequate, too little thyroxin will be secreted, and the pituitary will sense the deficiency and produce more TSH. The thyroid gland will enlarge enough to make sufficient thyroxin.
- Hypothyroid goiter—If dietary iodine is severely reduced, even an enlarged gland will not be able to make enough thyroxin. The gland will keep growing under the influence of TSH, but it may never be able to make enough thyroxin.

The term hyperthyroidism covers any disease which results in overabundance of thyroid hormone. Other names for hyperthyroidism, or specific diseases within the category, include Graves' disease, diffuse toxic goiter, Basedow's disease, Parry's disease, and thyrotoxicosis. The disease is 10 times more common in women than in men, and the annual incidence of hyperthyroidism in the United States is about one per 1,000 women. Although it occurs at all ages, hyperthyroidism is most likely to occur after the age of 15. There is a form of hyperthyroidism called Neonatal Grave's disease, which occurs in infants born of mothers with Graves' disease. Occult hyperthyroidism may occur in patients over 65 and is characterized by a distinct lack of typical symptoms. Diffuse toxic goiter occurs in as many as 80% of patients with hyperthyroidism.

Hyperthyroidism is often associated with the body's production of autoantibodies in the blood which cause the thyroid to grow and secrete excess thyroid hormone. This condition, as well as other forms of hyperthyroidism, may be inherited. Regardless of the cause, hyperthyroidism produces the same symptoms, including weight loss with increased appetite, **shortness of breath** and fatigue, intolerance to heat, heart **palpitations**, increased frequency of bowel movements, weak muscles, **tremors**, **anxiety**, and difficulty sleeping. Women may also notice decreased menstrual flow and irregular menstrual cycles.

Patients with Graves' disease often have a goiter (visible enlargement of the thyroid gland), although as many as 10% do not. These patients may also have bulging eyes. Thyroid storm, a serious form of hyperthyroidism, may show up as sudden and acute symptoms, some of which mimic typical hyperthyroidism, as well as the addition of **fever**, substantial weakness, extreme restlessness, confusion, emotional swings or **psychosis**, and perhaps even **coma**.

Excess TSH (or similar hormones), cysts, and tumors will enlarge the thyroid gland. Of these, TSH enlarges the entire gland while cysts and tumors enlarge only a part of it.

The only symptom from a goiter is the large swelling just above the breast bone. Rarely, it may constrict the trachea (windpipe) or esophagus and cause difficulty breathing or swallowing. The rest of the symptoms come from thyroxin or the lack of it.

Physicians will look for physical signs and symptoms indicated by patient history. On inspection, the physician may note symptoms such as a goiter or eye bulging. Other symptoms or family history may be clues to a diagnosis of hyperthyroidism. An elevated body temperature (basal body temperature) above 98.6°F (37°C) may be an indication of a heightened metabolic rate (basal metabolic rate) and hyperthyroidism. A simple blood test can be performed to determine the amount of thyroid hormone in the patient's blood. The diagnosis is usually straightforward with this combination of clinical history, **physical examination**, and routine blood hormone tests. Radioimmunoassay, or a test to show concentrations of **thyroid hormones** with the use of a radioisotope mixed with fluid samples, helps confirm the diagnosis. A thyroid scan is a nuclear medicine procedure involving injection of a radioisotope dye which will tag the thyroid and help produce a clear image of inflammation or involvement of the entire thyroid. Other tests can determine thyroid function and thyroid-stimulating hormone levels. Ultrasonography, **computed tomography scans** (CT scan), and **magnetic resonance imaging** (MRI) may provide visual confirmation of a diagnosis or help to determine the extent of involvement.

The size, shape, and texture of the thyroid gland help the physician determine the cause of goiter. A battery of blood tests are required to verify the specific thyroid disease. Functional imaging studies using radioactive iodine determine how active the gland is and what it looks like.

Treatment will depend on the specific disease and individual circumstances such as age, severity of disease, and other conditions affecting a patient's health.

Antithyroid drugs are often administered to help the patient's body cease overproduction of thyroid hormones. This medication may work for young adults, pregnant women, and others. Women who are pregnant should be treated with the lowest dose required to maintain thyroid function in order to minimize the risk of hypothyroidism in the infant.

Radioactive iodine is often prescribed to damage cells that make thyroid hormone. The cells need iodine to make the hormone, so they will absorb any iodine found in the body. The patient may take an iodine capsule daily for several weeks, resulting in the eventual shrinkage of the thyroid in size, reduced hormone production and a return to normal blood levels. Some patients may receive a single larger oral dose of radioactive iodine to treat the disease more quickly. This should only be done for patients who are not of reproductive age or are not planning to have children, since a large amount can concentrate in the reproductive organs (gonads).

Some patients may undergo surgery to treat hyperthyroidism. Most commonly, patients treated with thyroidectomy, in the form of partial or total removal of the thyroid, suffer from large goiter and have suffered relapses, even after repeated attempts to address the disease through drug therapy. Some patients may be candidates for surgery because they were not good candidates for iodine therapy, or refused iodine administration. Patients receiving thyroidectomy or iodine therapy must be carefully monitored for years to watch for signs of hypothyroidism, or insufficient production of thyroid hormones, which can occur as a complication of thyroid production suppression.

Goiters of all types will regress with treatment of the underlying condition. Dietary iodine may be all that is needed. However, if an iodine deficient thyroid that has grown in size to accommodate its deficiency is suddenly supplied an adequate amount of iodine, it could suddenly make large amounts of thyroxin and cause a thyroid storm, the equivalent of racing your car motor at top speed.

Hyperthyroidism can be treated with medications, therapeutic doses of radioactive iodine, or surgical reduction. Surgery is much less common now than it used to be because of progress in drugs and radiotherapy.

Hyperthyroidism is generally treatable and carries a good prognosis. Most patients lead normal lives with proper treatment. Thyroid storm, however, can be life-threatening and can lead to heart, liver, or kidney failure.

Although goiters diminish in size, the thyroid may not return to normal. Sometimes thyroid function does not return after treatment, but thyroxin is easy to take as a pill.

There are no known prevention methods for hyperthyroidism, since its causes are either inherited or not completely understood. The best prevention tactic is knowledge of family history and close attention to symptoms and signs of the disease. Careful attention to prescribed therapy can prevent complications of the disease.

Euthyroid goiter and hypothyroid goiter are common around the world because many regions have inadequate dietary iodine, including some places in the United States. International relief groups are providing iodized salt to many of these populations. Because **mental retardation** is a common result of hypothyroidism in children, this is an extremely important project.

THYROID FUNCTION TESTS

Thyroid function tests are blood tests used to evaluate how effectively the thyroid gland is working. These tests include the thyroid-stimulating hormone test (TSH), the thyroxine test (T_4), the triiodothyronine test (T_3), the thyroxine-binding globulin test (TBG), the triiodothyronine resin uptake test (T_3RU), and the long-acting thyroid stimulator test (LATS).

Thyroid function tests are used to:

- Help diagnose an underactive thyroid (hypothyroidism) and an overactive thyroid (hyperthyroidism)
- Evaluate thyroid gland activity
- Monitor response to thyroid therapy.

Thyroid treatment must be stopped one month before blood is drawn for a thyroxine (T_4) test.Steroids, propranolol (Inderal), cholestryamine (Questran), and other medications that may influence thyroid activity are usually stopped before a triiodothyronine (T_3) test. Estrogens, anabolic steroids, phenytoin, and thyroid medications may be discontinued prior to a thyroxine-binding globulin (TBG) test. The laboratory analyzing the blood sample must be told if the patient cannot stop taking any of these medications. Some patients will be told to take these medications as usual so that the doctor can determine how they affect thyroxine-binding globulin. Patients are asked not to take estrogens, androgens, phenytoin (Dilantin), salicylates, and thyroid medications before having a triiodothyronine resin uptake (T_3RU) test. Prior to taking a long-acting thyroid stimulant (LATS) test, the patient will probably be told to stop taking all drugs that could affect test results.

Most doctors consider the sensitive thyroid-stimulating hormone (TSH) test to be the most accurate measure of thyroid activity. By measuring the level of TSH, doctors can determine even small problems in thyroid activity. Because this test is sensitive, abnormalities in thyroid function can be determined before a patient complains of symptoms.

TSH ''tells'' the thyroid gland to secrete the hormones thyroxine (T_4) and triiodothyronine (T_3). Before TSH tests were used, standard blood tests measured levels of T_4 and T_3 to determine if the thyroid gland was working properly. The triiodothyrine (T_3) test measures the amount of this hormone in the blood. T_3 is normally present in very small amounts, but has a significant impact on metabolism. It is the active component of thyroid hormone. The thyroxinc-binding globulin (TBG) test measures blood levels of this substance, which is manufactured in the liver. TBG binds to T_3 and T_4, prevents the kidneys from flushing the hormones from the blood, and releases them when and where they are needed to regulate body functions.

The triiodothyronine resin uptake (T_3RU) test measures blood T_4 levels. Laboratory analysis of this test takes several days, and it is used less often than tests whose results are available more quickly.

The long-acting thyroid stimulator (LATS) test shows whether blood contains long-acting thyroid stimulator. Not normally present in blood, LATS causes the thyroid to produce and secrete abnormally high amounts of hormones.

It takes only minutes for a nurse or medical technician to collect the blood needed for these blood tests. A needle is inserted into a vein, usually in the forearm, and a small amount of blood is collected and sent to a laboratory for testing. The patient will usually feel minor discomfort from the ''stick'' of the needle. Not all laboratories measure or record thyroid hormone levels the same way. Each laboratory will provide a range of values that are considered normal for each test.

See also Thyroid disorders

THYROID HORMONES

Thyroid hormones are artificially made hormones that make up for a lack of natural hormones produced by the thyroid gland. The thyroid gland, a butterfly-shaped structure in the lower part of the neck, normally produces a hormone called thyroxine. This hormone controls the rate of metabolism — all the physical and chemical processes that occur in cells to allow growth and maintain body functions. When the thyroid gland does not produce enough thyroxine, body processes slow down. People with underactive thyroid glands feel unusually tired and may gain weight, even though they eat less. They may also have trouble staying warm and may have other symptoms, such as dry skin, dry hair, and a puffy face. By making up for the lack of natural thyroxine and bringing the rate of metabolism back to normal, artificially made thyroid hormone improves these symptoms.

Thyroid hormones also may be used to treat goiter (enlarged thyroid gland) and certain types of **thyroid cancer**. Thyroid hormones, also called thyroid drugs, are available only with a physician's prescription. They are sold in tablet form. A commonly used thyroid hormone is levothyroxine (Synthroid, Levoxyl, Levothroid). For adults and teenagers, the usual starting dose of levothyroxine tablets is 0.0125 mg (12.5 micrograms) to 0.05 mg (50 micrograms) per day. The physician who prescribes the medicine may gradually increase the dose over time. For children, the dose depends on body weight and must be determined by a physician.

Taking thyroid hormones exactly as directed is very important. The physician who prescribes the medicine will figure out exactly how much of the medicine a patient needs. Taking too much or too little can make the thyroid gland overactive or underactive. This medicine should be taken at the same timc every day.

People who take thyroid hormones because their thyroid glands do not produce enough natural hormone may need to take the medicine for the rest of their lives. Seeing a physician regularly while taking this medicine is important. The physician will make sure that the medicine is working and that the dosage is correct.

Anyone who is taking thyroid hormones should be sure to tell the health care professional in charge before having any surgical or dental procedures or receiving emergency treatment. In patients with certain kinds of heart disease, this medicine may cause chest **pain**s and **shortness of breath** during **exercise**. People who have this problem should be careful not to exert themselves too much. This medicine is safe to take during **pregnancy**, but the dosage may need to be changed. Women who are pregnant should check with their physicians to make sure they are taking the proper dosage.

Anyone who has had unusual reactions to thyroid hormones in the past should let his or her physician know before taking the drugs again. The physician should also be told about any **allergies** to foods, dyes, preservatives, or other substances. Before using thyroid hormones, people with any of these medical problems should make sure their physicians are aware of their conditions:

- Heart disease
- High blood pressure
- Hardening of the arteries
- Diabetes
- History of overactive thyroid
- Underactive adrenal gland
- Underactive pituitary gland.

This medicine usually does not cause side effects if the dosage is right. Certain symptoms may be signs that the dose needs to be changed. Check with a physician if any of these symptoms occur:

- **Headache**
- **Fever**
- **Diarrhea**
- Vomiting
- Changes in appetite
- Weight loss
- Changes in menstrual period
- **Tremors** of the hands
- Leg cramps
- Increased sensitivity to heat
- Sweating
- Irritability
- Nervousness
- Sleep problems.

Other side effects are possible. Anyone who has unusual symptoms while taking thyroid hormones should get in touch with his or her physician.

Thyroid hormones may interact with other medicines. This may increase or decrease the effects of the thyroid medicine and may interfere with treatment. Anyone who takes thyroid hormones should not take any other prescription or nonprescription (over-the-counter) medicines without the approval of his or her physician. Among the drugs that may interact with thyroid hormones are:

- Medicine for colds, hay fever, and other allergies
- Medicine for **asthma** and other breathing problems
- Medicine for diabetes
- Blood thinners
- Amphetamines
- Diet pills (appetite suppressants)
- Cholesterol-lowering drugs such as cholestyramine (Questran) and colestipol (Colestid).

See also Thyroid function tests

TINBERGEN, NIKOLAAS (1907-1988)

Dutch English zoologist and ethologist

Nikolaas Tinbergen was born April 15, 1907, in The Hague, Netherlands. His older brother Jan studied physics but later turned to economics, winning the first Nobel Prize awarded in that subject in 1969. The Tinbergens lived near the seashore, where Tinbergen often went to collect shells, camp, and watch animals, many of which he would later formally research.

After high school, Tinbergen worked at the Vogelwarte Rossitten bird observatory and later began studying biology at the State University of Leiden, Netherlands. For his dissertation, Tinbergen studied bee-killer wasps and was able to experimentally demonstrate that the wasps use landmarks to orientate themselves. Tinbergen first established the traditional routes of the wasps near their burrows, then altered the landscape to see how the wasps' behavior would be affected. Tinbergen was awarded his Ph.D. in 1932.

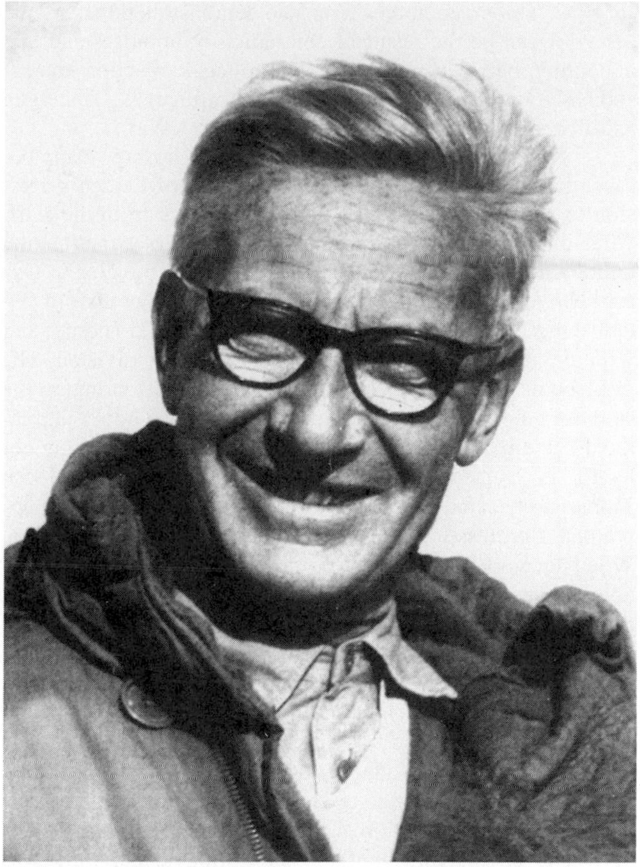

Nikolaas Tinbergen

Shortly after his 1932 wedding to Elisabeth Rutten, the Tinbergens embarked on an expedition to Greenland, where Tinbergen studied the role of evolution in the behavior of snow buntings, phalaropes, and Eskimo sled dogs. When he returned to the Netherlands in 1933, he became an instructor at the State University, where he organized an undergraduate course on animal behavior. Tinbergen's work had been recognized in the field of biology but it was not until after he met **Konrad Lorenz**—the acknowledged father of ethology—that his work began to form a directed body of research. Tinbergen took his family to Lorenz's home in Austria for a summer so the two men could work together. Although they published only one paper together, their collaboration lasted a number of years.

During 1936, Tinbergen and Lorenz began constructing a theoretical framework for the study of ethology, which was then a fledgling field. They hypothesized that instinct, as opposed to simply being a response to environmental factors, arises from an animal's impulses. This idea is expressed by the concept of a fixed-action pattern, a repeated, distinct set of movements or behaviors, which Tinbergen and Lorenz believed all animals have. A fixed-action pattern is triggered by something in the animal's environment. In some species of gull, for instance, hungry chicks will peck at a decoy with a red spot on its bill, a characteristic of the gull. Tinbergen showed that in some animals learned behavior is critical for survival. Tinbergen and Lorenz also demonstrated that animal behavior can be the result of contradictory impulses and that a conflict between drives may produce a reaction that is strangely unsuited to the stimuli. Unfortunately, Tinbergen and Lorenz's work was disrupted by World War II.

Tinbergen spent much of the war in a hostage camp because he had protested the State University of Leiden's decision to remove three Jewish faculty members from the staff. After the war ended, he became a professor of experimental biology at the University. In 1949, Tinbergen traveled to Oxford University in England to lecture. He stayed at Oxford, establishing the journal *Behavior* with W. H. Thorpe and working in the University's animal behavior division. His 1951 book *The Study of Instinct* is credited with bringing the study of ethology to many English readers. The book summarized some of the newest insights into the ways signaling behavior is created over the course of evolution. In 1955, Tinbergen became an English citizen, and in 1966 he was appointed a professor and fellow of Oxford's Wolfson College. When the work of Tinbergen, Lorenz, and von Frisch, who had demonstrated that honeybees communicate by dancing, received the Nobel Prize in 1973, it was the first time the Nobel Committee recognized work in sociobiology or ethology.

The ability of an organism to adapt to its environment is another element of Tinbergen's work. After he retired from Oxford in 1974, he and his wife attempted to explain autistic behavior in children to adaptability. The Tinbergens' assertion that autism may be caused by the behavior of a child's parents caused some consternation in the medical community. Tinbergen believed that much of the opposition to his work was caused by the unflattering view of human behavior it presented. Tinbergen died December 21, 1988, after suffering a stroke at his home in Oxford, England.

TINNITUS

Tinnitus affects as many as 40 million adults in the United States. Tinnitus is hearing ringing, buzzing, or other sounds, in one or both ears, or in the head, without external cause. It is defined as either objective or subjective. In objective tinnitus, the doctor can hear the sounds, as well as the patient. Objective tinnitus is typically caused by tumors, turbulent blood flow through malformed vessels, or by rhythmic muscular spasms. Most cases of tinnitus are subjective, which means that only the patient can hear the sounds.

Subjective tinnitus is frequently associated with **hearing loss**. About 90% of patients have sensorineural hearing loss; 5% suffer from conductive hearing loss; 5% have normal hearing. The causes of subjective tinnitus include:

- Impacted ear wax
- Ear infections
- Hardening of the structures of the inner ear
- Hearing loss related to age or excessive noise
- Ototoxic medications, including **aspirin**, quinine, some **diuretics**, heavy metals, alcohol, and certain **antibiotics**
- Meniere's syndrome
- Head trauma
- Systemic diseases, including **syphilis**, **hypertension**, hypothyroidism, or **anemia**.
- Tumors of the ear.

Diagnosis of tinnitus includes a **physical examination** of the patient's head and neck. The doctor will use an otoscope to examine the ears for wax, infection, or structural changes. He or she will also use a stethoscope to listen to the blood vessels in the neck. Additional tests may also utilized.

The Rinne and Weber tests are commonly used to evaluate the type and severity of hearing loss. In the Weber test, the doctor holds a tuning fork against the patient's forehead or front teeth. If the hearing loss is sensorineural, the sound radiates to the ear with better hearing; if the hearing loss is conductive, the sound will be louder in the damaged ear. In the Rinne test, the tuning fork is placed alternately on the mastoid bone (behind the ear) and in front of the ear. In conductive hearing loss, bone conduction (BC) is greater than air conduction (AC). In sensorineural hearing loss, AC is greater than BC.

Magnetic resonance **angiography** or venography (MRA and MRV) can be used to evaluate malformations of the blood vessels. **Computed tomography scans** (CT scans) or magnetic resonance imaging scans (MRIs) can be used to locate tumors or abnormalities of the brain stem.

The doctor may order a complete **blood count** (CBC) with specific antibody tests to rule out syphilis or immune system disorders.

Some cases of tinnitus can be treated by removal of the underlying cause. These include surgical treatment of impacted ear wax, tumors, head injuries, or malformed blood vessels; discontinuance of ototoxic medications; and antibiotic treatment of infections. Subjective tinnitus, especially that associated with age-related hearing loss, can be treated with **hearing aids**, noise generators or other masking devices, **biofeedback**, antidepressant medications, or lifestyle modifications (elimination of smoking, coffee, and aspirin).

A variety of alternative therapies may be helpful in the treatment of tinnitus. Dietary adjustments, including the elimination of coffee and other stimulants, may be useful, since stimulants can make tinnitus worse. In addition, reducing the amount of fat and cholesterol in the diet can help improve blood circulation to the ears. Nutritional supplementation with vitamin C, vitamin E, B **vitamins**, calcium, magnesium, potassium, and essential fatty acids is also recommended. Gingko (*Gingko biloba*) is often suggested, since it is believed to enhance circulation to the brain. **Acupuncture** treatments may help decrease the level of tinnitus sounds the patient hears, and constitutional homeopathic treatment may also be effective.

The prognosis depends on the cause of the tinnitus and the patient's emotional response. Most patients with subjective tinnitus do not find it seriously disturbing, but about 5% have strong negative feelings. These patients are frequently helped by instruction in relaxation techniques.

See also Hearing loss

TISSUE TYPING

Tissue typing is a group of procedures that determines the type of histocompatibility antigens on a person's cells or tissues. This procedure is typically used prior to transplantation of tissues or organs to ensure as close a match as possible between the donor and the recipient. If the histocompatibility antigens do not match well, there is a much greater chance that the recipient will reject the donated tissue.

Histocompatibility antigens are molecules on the surface of all cells in the body. The specific types of histocompatibility antigens present on a person's cells determine their identity and distinguish each person. They are a "fingerprint," as each person has a unique set of histocompatibility antigens. If the antigens on tissue or organs from a donor do not match that of the recipient, a rejection response can occur. The recipient's **immune system** will detect the difference between the two sets of antigen and start a rejection response to kill the donated tissue. Except in the case of identical twins, no two people are identical in terms of their histocompatibility antigen types. However, the closer two tissues come to matching, the more likely the recipient will accept the donated tissue or organ.

Human Lymphocyte Antigens (HLA) is the name given to the most commonly used histocompatibility antigens. The antigens can be grouped into two classes: class I antigens are found on almost all cells, and class II antigens are normally found only on B lymphocytes, macrophages, monocytes, dendritic cells, and endothelial cells.

Generally, typing is performed on blood cells because they are an easy sample to obtain. Blood is withdrawn from a vein in the forearm, and the cells are separated. There are a number of different techniques used to identify the antigens on the cells. Typically, specific antibodies react with the cells. Each antibody preparation is specific for one histocompatibility antigen. If the antigen is present, the antibody will bind to it. Laboratory instruments are used to detect antibody binding to the cells. Class II antigens are determined by the mixed lymphocyte reaction (MLR) or by a polymerase chain reaction (PCR). In the mixed lymphocyte reaction, lymphocyte replication occurs if there is a mismatch, and is detected by a specific assay. The PCR test is a DNA-based test that can detect the presence or absence of antigens by determining whether cells have the genes for the antigens.

One type of transplant does not require tissue typing. In the case of corneal transplants, tissue typing is not needed because cornea do not have their own blood supply. This greatly reduces the chance that immune cells will come in contact with the cornea and recognize it as foreign. For this reason, corneas can be transplanted from any person, and there is little chance of rejection.

See also Corneal transplantation

TONSILLECTOMY AND ADENOIDECTOMY

Tonsils may be removed (with or without the adenoids) when the child has obstruction of the upper airway, and/or **sleep apnea**. This is a condition in which the child snores loudly and stops breathing temporarily at intervals during sleep. Other indications include: inability to swallow properly because of enlarged tonsils; "hot potato" voice (breathy voice) and other speech abnormalities due to enlarged tonsils; recurrent or persistent **abscess**es or throat infections.

Doctors do not agree completely on the number of **sore throat**s that make a tonsillectomy necessary. Most would agree that four cases of **strep throat** in any one year; six or more episodes of **tonsillitis** in one year; or five or more episodes of tonsillitis per year for two years indicate that the tonsils should be removed.

Adenoids are removed (with or without the tonsils) when the child has any of the following conditions:

- Alteration of facial growth because of enlarged adenoids.
- Upper airway obstruction.
- Development of an irregular bite (dental **malocclusion**).
- Difficult speech or swallowing.

These surgeries are not performed as frequently today as they were in the past. One reason for a more conservative approach is that there is always some risk involved when a patient is put under general anesthesia. In some cases, a T & A may need to be modified or postponed:

- Children with cleft palates should not have the adenoids removed.
- Bleeding disorders. These must be brought under control before surgery.
- Acute tonsillitis. Surgery should be postponed—usually for three to four weeks—until the infection is gone.

Tonsillectomies are hospital procedures. In adults, they may be performed under local **anesthesia**. Children are usually placed under general anesthesia. The doctor depresses the tongue in order to see the throat and removes the tonsils with a scooplike instrument. The adenoids are usually removed through the nose.

After surgery, patients are turned on the side after the operation to prevent the possibility of blood being drawn into the lungs. The patient's vital signs are checked. After the patient is fully awake, he or she can drink water and other nonirritating liquids. Adult patients are usually warned to expect some bleeding after the operation and a very sore throat. **Antibiotics** are given to prevent infection. Medications to relieve **pain** may also be given. For at least the first 24 hours, the patient is fed soft or pureed foods and fluids. If the adenoids alone were removed, the patient may be allowed solid food the day after surgery.

Patients are usually sent home the next day, with instructions to call the doctor if there is bleeding, an earache, or a **fever** that lasts longer than three days. They are told to expect a white scab to form in the throat between five and 10 days after surgery.

About one in every fifteen thousand tonsillectomies ends in **death**, either from the anesthesia or from bleeding to death five to seven days after the operation. There is also a chance that children with previously normal speech will develop a nasal-sounding voice.

See also Sore throat; Strep throat; Tonsillitis

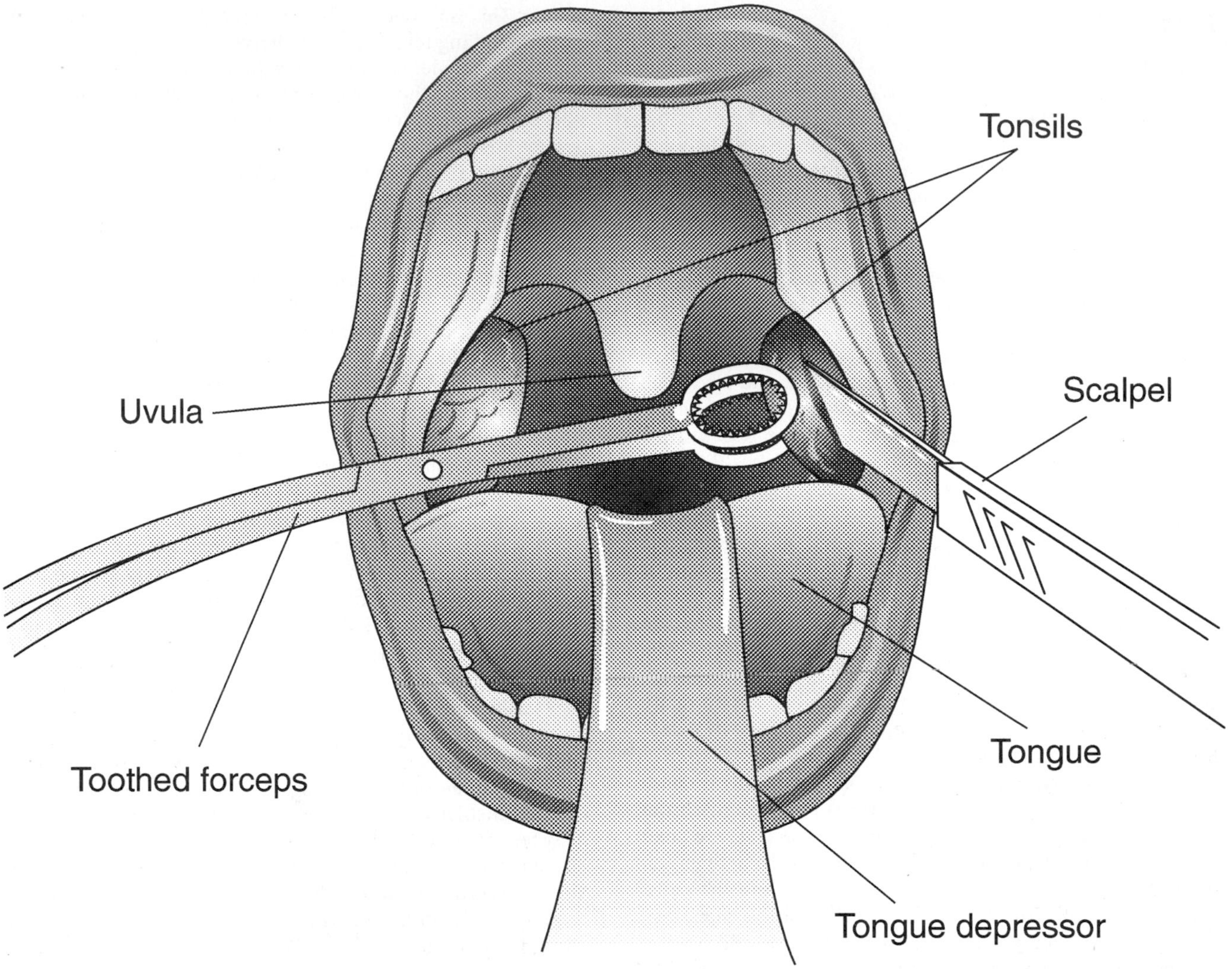

Tonsillectomy and adenoidectomy are surgical procedures performed to remove the tonsils or adenoids. Both operations are typically performed on children. The illustration above shows a tonsillectomy in progress. ***(Illustration by Electronic Illustrators Group.)***

TONSILLITIS

Tonsillitis is an infection and swelling of the tonsils, which are oval-shaped masses of lymph gland tissue located on both sides of the back of the throat. The tonsils normally help to prevent infections. They act like filters to trap bacteria and viruses entering the body through the mouth and sinuses. The tonsils also stimulate the immune system to produce antibodies to help fight off infections. Anyone of any age can have tonsillitis; however, it is most common in children between the ages of five and 10 years.

A mild or severe **sore throat** is one of the first symptoms of tonsillitis. Symptoms can also include **fever**, chills, tiredness, muscle aches, earache, **pain** or discomfort when swallowing, and swollen glands in the neck. Very young children may be fussy and stop eating. When a doctor or nurse looks into the mouth with a flashlight, the tonsils may appear swollen and red. Sometimes, the tonsils will have white or yellow spots or flecks or a thin coating. The doctor will also examine the eyes, ears, nose, and throat, looking at the tonsils for signs of swelling, redness, or a discharge. A careful examination of the throat is necessary to rule out **diphtheria** and other conditions that may cause a sore throat. Since most sore throats in children are caused by viruses rather than bacteria, the doctor may take a **throat culture** in order to test for the presence of streptococcal bacteria, verify the results, and wait for the laboratory report before prescribing **antibiotics**. A blood test may also be done to rule out a more serious infection or condition, and to check the white blood cell count to see if the body is responding to the infection. In some cases, the doctor may order blood tests for mononucleosis, since about a third of patients with mononucleosis develop **streptococcal infections** of the tonsils.

Treatment of tonsillitis also involves keeping the patient comfortable while the illness runs its course. This supportive care includes bed rest, drinking extra fluids, gargling with warm salt water, and taking pain relievers—usually

NSAIDs—to reduce fever. Frozen juice bars and cold fruit drinks can bring some temporary relief of sore throat pain; drinking warm tea or broth can be soothing. If the patient has several episodes of severe tonsillitis, the doctor may recommend a tonsillectomy, which is the surgical removal of the tonsils.

Strengthening the immune system is important whether tonsillitis is caused by bacteria or viruses. Naturopaths often recommend dietary supplements of vitamin C, bioflavonoids, and beta-carotenes—found naturally in fruits and vegetables—to ease inflammation and fight infection. A variety of herbal remedies also may be helpful in treating tonsillitis. As with any condition, the treatment and dosage should be appropriate for the particular symptoms and age of the patient.

Tonsillitis usually resolves within a few days with rest and supportive care. Treating the symptoms of sore throat and fever will make the patient more comfortable. If fever persists for more than 48 hours, however, or is higher than 102°F, the patient should be seen by a doctor. If antibiotics are prescribed to treat an infection, they should be taken as directed for the complete course of treatment, even if the patient starts to feel better in a few days. Prolonged symptoms may indicate that the patient has other upper respiratory infections, most commonly in the ears or sinuses. An **abscess** behind the tonsil (a peritonsillar abscess) may also occur. In rare cases, a persistent sore throat may point to more serious conditions, such as **rheumatic fever** or **pneumonia**.

The bacteria and viruses that cause tonsillitis are easily spread from person to person. It is not unusual for an entire family or several students in the same classroom to come down with similar symptoms, especially if *S. pyogenes* is the cause. The risk of transmission can be lowered by avoiding exposure to anyone who already has tonsillitis or a sore throat. Drinking glasses and eating utensils should not be shared and should be washed in hot, soapy water before reuse. Old toothbrushes should be replaced to prevent reinfection. People who are caring for someone with tonsillitis should wash their hands frequently, to prevent spreading the infection to others.

See also Sore throat; Strep throat

Toothache

A toothache is any **pain** or soreness within or around a tooth, indicating inflammation and possible infection. A toothache may feel like a sharp pain or a dull ache. The tooth may be sensitive to pressure, heat, cold, or sweets. In cases of severe pain, identifying the problem tooth is often difficult. Any patient with a toothache should see a dentist at once for diagnosis and treatment. Most toothaches get worse if not treated.

Toothaches may result from any of a number of causes:

- **Tooth decay** (dental caries)
- Inflammation of the tooth pulp (pulpitis)
- **Abscesses**
- Gum disease, including periodontitis
- Loose or broken filling
- Cracked or impacted tooth
- Exposed tooth root
- Food wedged between teeth or trapped below the gum line
- Tooth nerve irritated by clenching or grinding of teeth (**bruxism**)
- Pressure from congested sinuses
- Traumatic injury.

Diagnosis includes identifying the location of the toothache, as well as the cause. The dentist begins by asking the patient specific questions about the toothache, including the types of foods that make the pain worse, whether the tooth is sensitive to temperature or biting, and whether the pain is worse at night. The dentist then examines the patient's mouth for signs of swelling, redness, and obvious tooth damage. The presence of pus indicates an abscess or gum disease. The dentist may flush the sore area with warm water to dislodge any food particles and to test for sensitivity to heat. The dentist may then dry the area with gauze to determine sensitivity to touch and pressure. The dentist may probe tooth crevices and the edges of fillings with a sharp instrument, looking for areas of tooth decay. Finally, the dentist may take x rays, looking for evidence of decay between teeth, a cracked or impacted tooth, or a disorder of the underlying bone.

Toothaches should always be professionally treated by a dentist. Some methods of self-treatment, however, may help manage the pain until professional care is available:

- Rinsing with warm salt water
- Using dental floss to remove any food particles
- Taking **aspirin** or **acetaminophen** (Tylenol) to relieve pain. The drug should be swallowed—*never* placed directly on the aching tooth or gum.
- Applying a *cold* compress against the outside of the cheek. Do not use heat, because it will tend to spread infection.
- Using clove oil (*Syzygium aromaticum*) to numb the gums. The oil may be rubbed directly on the sore area or used to soak a small piece of cotton and applied to the sore tooth.

Treatment will depend on the underlying cause of the toothache. If the pain is due to tooth decay, the dentist will remove the decayed area and restore the tooth with a filling of silver amalgam or composite resin. Loose or broken fillings are removed, new decay cleaned out, and a new filling is placed. If the pulp of the tooth is damaged, root canal therapy is needed. The dentist or a specialist called an endodontist removes the decayed pulp, fills the space left behind with a soothing paste, and covers the tooth with a crown to protect and seal it. If the damage cannot be treated by these methods, or if the tooth is impacted, the tooth must be extracted.

Prompt dental treatment provides a positive outcome for toothache. In the absence of active infection, fillings, **root canal treatments**, or extractions may be performed with minimal discomfort to the patient. When a toothache is left untreated, a severe infection may develop and spread to the sinuses or jawbone, and eventually cause blood **poisoning**.

Maintaining proper **oral hygiene** is the key to preventing toothaches. The best way to prevent tooth decay is to brush at least twice a day, preferably after every meal and snack. Flossing once a day also helps prevent gum disease by removing food particles and bacteria at and below the gum line, as well as between teeth. People should visit their dentist at least every six months for oral examinations and professional cleaning.

See also Oral hygiene; Root canal treatment

Toothbrush and toothpaste

The earliest toothbrushes were simply small sticks mashed and frayed at one end to increase their cleaning surface. Ancient Roman patricians employed special slaves to clean their teeth, and toothbrushing formed part of some ancient religious rituals. The bristle brush was probably invented by the Chinese; it came to Europe during the seventeenth century and soon was widely used. French dentists, who were the most advanced in Europe at the time, advocated the use of toothbrushes in the seventeenth and early eighteenth centuries. In pre-Revolutionary America, dentists urged the use of bristle toothbrushes. Nylon has replaced natural bristles in modern brushes. Hard bristles, once recommended, are now thought to be too abrasive, and soft nylon bristles with rounded ends are preferred. Special brushes have also been designed to remove plaque and debris from relatively large spaces between teeth, or spaces between caps and bridges. Dr. Scott's Electric Toothbrush was marketed in 1880; its manufacturer claimed the brush was ''permanently charged with electro-magnetic current.'' The first real electric toothbrush was developed in Switzerland after World War II. This corded model was introduced to the United States market in 1960 by Squibb under the name Broxodent. General Electric followed in 1961 with its rechargeable cordless model. Although it seemed like an odd idea to many people, the electric toothbrush was an immediate success.

Like toothbrushes, compounds for cleaning teeth (and freshening breath) have been used since ancient times. Early Egyptian, Chinese, Greek, and Roman writings describe numerous mixtures for both pastes and powders. The more palatable ingredients included powdered fruit, burnt shells, talc, honey, ground shells, and dried flowers. The less appetizing ingredients included mice, the head of a hare, lizard livers, and urine. Powder and paste formulas continued to proliferate through the Middle Ages. Unfortunately, many of these recipes used agents that corroded or abraded the non-replaceable tooth enamel. Modern toothpastes began to appear in the 1800s. Peabody suggested adding soap to tooth cleaners in 1824, chalk was popularized by John Harris in the 1850s, and soon the well-known S. S. White Company introduced a paste in a collapsible tube. Dr. Washington W. Sheffield, a Connecticut dentist, put his popular Dr. Sheffield's Creme Dentifrice, in its collapsible tube, on the market in 1892. The toothpaste tube reigned supreme until 1984, when the pump dispenser—which originated in Europe—was introduced to the U.S. market. Fluoride was added to toothpaste in 1956 when Proctor & Gamble launched its Crest product. Home whitening solutions, which utilize hydrogen peroxide, are available to remove discoloring stains from tooth enamel. In 1996, the federal government approved the use of lasers for teeth whitening. This procedure uses laser energy to ''excite'' the hydrogen peroxide, causing it to expel free radical oxygen which ''attacks'' the organic composition of the stain. Still controversial because of its expense, and the lack of knowledge concerning long-term effect on tooth enamel, this procedure is fast and even has some success at lightening teeth discolored by antibiotic use during pregnancy.

See also Fluoride treatment

Tooth decay

Tooth decay, which is also called dental cavities or dental caries, is the destruction of the outer surface (enamel) of a tooth. Decay results from the action of bacteria that live in plaque, which is a sticky, whitish film formed by a protein in saliva (mucin) and sugary substances in the mouth. The plaque bacteria sticking to tooth enamel use the sugar and starch from food particles in the mouth to produce acid.

Tooth decay is a common health problem, second in prevalence only to the **common cold**. It has been estimated that 90% of people in the United States have at least one cavity and that 75% of people had their first cavity by the age of 5. Although anyone can have a problem with tooth decay, children and senior citizens are the two groups at highest risk. Other high-risk groups include people who eat a lot of starchy and sugary foods; people living in areas without a fluoridated water supply; and people who already have numerous dental restorations (fillings and crowns).

Baby bottle tooth decay is a dental problem that frequently develops in infants that are put to bed with a bottle containing a sweet liquid. Baby bottle tooth decay is also called nursing-bottle caries and bottle-mouth syndrome. Bottles containing liquids such as milk, formula, fruit juices, sweetened drink mixes, and sugar water continuously bathe an infant's mouth with sugar during naps or at night. The bacteria in the mouth use this sugar to produce acid that destroys the child's teeth. The upper front teeth are typically the ones most severely damaged; the lower front teeth receive some protection from the tongue. Pacifiers dipped in sugar, honey, corn syrup, or other sweetened liquid also contribute to bottle-mouth syndrome. The first signs of damage are chalky white spots or lines across the teeth. As decay progresses, the damage to the child's teeth becomes obvious.

Tooth decay requires the simultaneous presence of three factors: plaque bacteria, sugar, and a vulnerable tooth surface. Although several microorganisms found in the mouth can cause tooth decay, the primary disease agent appears to be *Streptococcus mutans*. The sugars used by the bacteria are simple sugars such as glucose, sucrose, and lactose. They are converted primarily into lactic acid. When this acid builds up on an unprotected tooth surface, it dissolves the **minerals** in the enamel, creating holes and weak spots (cavities). As the decay spreads inward into the middle layer (the dentin), the tooth becomes more sensitive to temperature and touch. When the

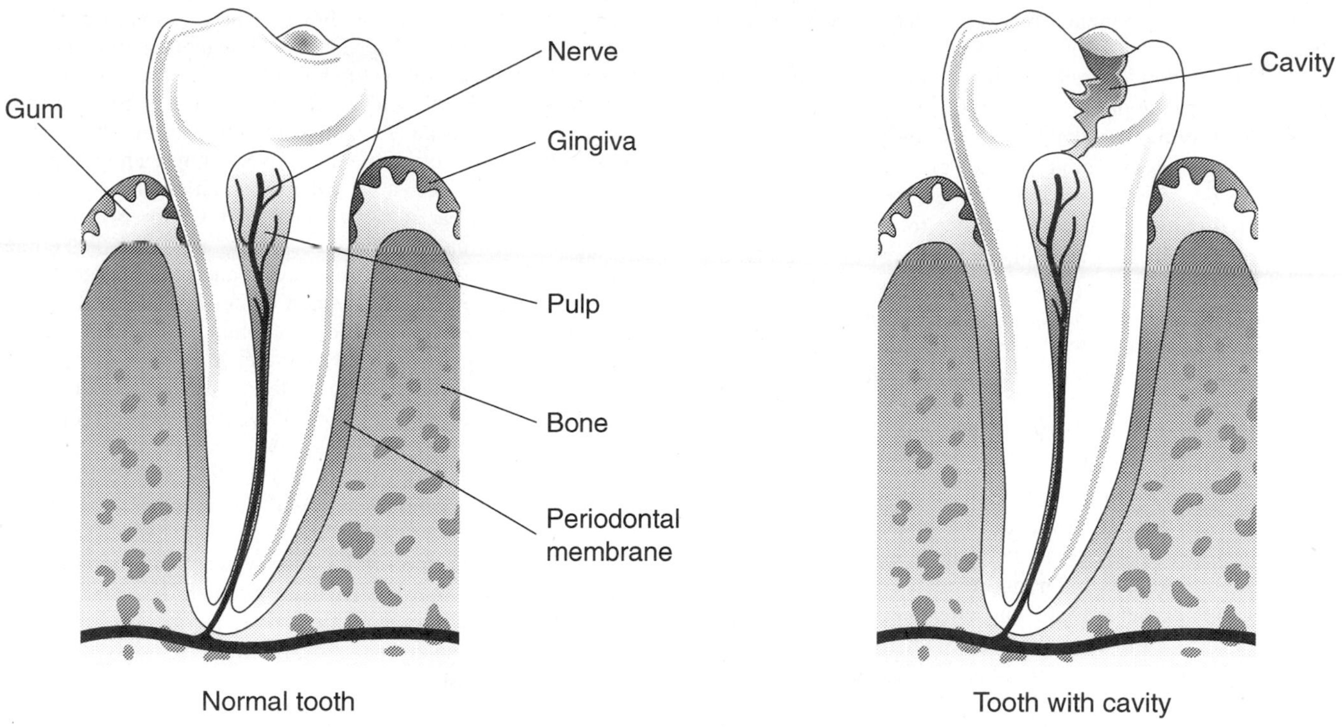

Tooth decay is the destruction of the outer surface, or enamel, of a tooth. It is caused by acid buildup from plaque bacteria, which dissolves the minerals in the enamel and creates cavities. ***(Illustration by Electronic Illustrators Group.)***

decay reaches the center of the tooth (the pulp), the resulting inflammation (pulpitis) produces a **toothache**.

Tooth decay develops at varying rates. It may be found during a routine six-month dental checkup before the patient is even aware of a problem. In other cases, the patient may experience common early symptoms, such as sensitivity to hot and cold liquids or localized discomfort after eating very sweet foods. The dentist or dental hygienist may suspect tooth decay if a dark spot or a pit is seen during a visual examination. Front teeth may be inspected for decay by shining a light from behind the tooth. This method is called transillumination. Areas of decay, especially between the teeth, will appear as noticeable shadows when teeth are transilluminated. X rays may be taken to confirm the presence and extent of the decay. The dentist then makes the final clinical diagnosis by probing the enamel with a sharp instrument.

Tooth decay in pits and fissures may be differentiated from dark shadows in the crevices of the chewing surfaces by a dye that selectively stains parts of the tooth that have lost mineral content. A dentist can also use this dye to tell whether all tooth decay has been removed from a cavity before placing a filling.

Damage caused by baby bottle tooth decay is often not diagnosed until the child has a severe problem, because parents seldom bring infants and toddlers in for dental check-ups. Dentists want to initially examine primary teeth between 12 and 24 months. Children still drinking from a bottle anytime after their first birthday are likely to have tooth decay.

To treat most cases of tooth decay in adults, the dentist removes all decayed tooth structure, shapes the sides of the cavity, and fills the cavity with an appropriate material, such as silver amalgam or composite resin. The filling is put in to restore and protect the tooth. If decay has attacked the pulp, the dentist or a specialist, called an endodontist, may perform **root canal treatment** and cover the tooth with a crown.

In cases of baby bottle tooth decay, the dentist must assess the extent of the damage before deciding on the treatment method. If the problem is caught early, the teeth involved can be treated with fluoride, followed by changes in the infant's feeding habits and better **oral hygiene**. Primary teeth with obvious decay in the enamel that has not yet progressed to the pulp need to be protected with stainless steel crowns. Fillings are not usually an option in small children because of the small size of their teeth and the concern of recurrent decay. When the decay has advanced to the pulp, pulling the tooth is often the treatment of choice. Unfortunately, loss of primary teeth at this age may hinder the young child's ability to eat and speak. It may also have bad effects on the alignment and spacing of the permanent teeth when they come in.

With timely diagnosis and treatment, the progression of tooth decay can be stopped without extended **pain**. If the pulp of the tooth is infected, the infection may be treated with **antibiotics** prior to root canal treatment or extraction. The longer decay goes untreated, however, the more destructive it becomes and the longer and more intensive the necessary treatment will be. In addition, a patient with two or more areas of tooth decay is at increased risk of developing additional cavities in the future. It is easier and less expensive to prevent tooth decay than to treat it. The four major prevention strategies include: proper oral hygiene; fluoride; sealants; and attention to diet.

The best way to prevent tooth decay is to brush the teeth at least twice a day, preferably after every meal and snack, and floss daily. Cavities develop most easily in spaces that are hard to clean. These areas include surface grooves, spaces between teeth, and the area below the gum line. Effective brushing cleans each outer tooth surface, inner tooth surface, and the horizontal chewing surfaces of the back teeth, as well as the tongue. Flossing once a day also helps prevent gum disease by removing food particles and plaque at and below the gum line, as well as between teeth. Patients should visit their dentist every six months for oral examination and professional cleaning.

Older adults who have lost teeth or had them removed still need to maintain a clean mouth. Bridges and dentures must be kept clean to prevent gum disease. Dentures should be relined and adjusted by a dentist whenever necessary to maintain proper fit. These adjustments help to keep the gums from becoming red, swollen, and tender.

Parents can easily prevent baby bottle tooth decay by not allowing a child to fall asleep with a bottle containing sweetened liquids. Bottles should be filled only with plain, unsweetened water. The child should be introduced to drinking from a cup around six months of age and weaned from bottles by twelve months. If an infant seems to need oral comfort between feedings, a pacifier specially designed for the mouth may be used. Pacifiers, however, should never be dipped in honey, corn syrup, or other sweet liquids. After the eruption of the first tooth, parents should begin routinely wiping the infant's teeth and gums with a moist piece of gauze or a soft cloth, especially right before bedtime. Parents may begin brushing a child's teeth with a small, soft toothbrush at about two years of age, when most of the primary teeth have come in. They should apply only a very small amount (the size of a pea) of toothpaste containing fluoride. Too much fluoride may cause spotting (fluorosis) of the tooth enamel. As the child grows, he or she will learn to handle the toothbrush, but parents should control the application of toothpaste and do the follow-up brushing until the child is about 7 years old.

Fluoride is a natural substance that slows the destruction of enamel and helps to repair minor tooth decay damage by remineralizing tooth structure. Toothpaste, mouthwash, fluoridated public drinking water, and vitamin supplements are all possible sources of fluoride. Children living in areas without fluoridated water should receive 0.5 mg/day of fluoride (0.25 mg/day if using a toothpaste containing fluoride) from three to five years of age, and 1 mg/day from 6-12 years.

While fluoride is important for protecting children's developing teeth, it is also of benefit to older adults with receding gums. It helps to protect their newly exposed tooth surfaces from decay. Older adults can be treated by a dentist with a fluoride solution that is painted onto selected portions of the teeth or poured into a fitted tray and held against all the teeth.

Because fluoride is most beneficial on the smooth surfaces of teeth, sealants were developed to protect the irregular surfaces of teeth. A sealant is a thin plastic coating that is painted over the grooves of chewing surfaces to prevent food and plaque from being trapped there. Sealant treatment is painless because no part of the tooth is removed, although the tooth surface is etched with acid so that the plastic will adhere to the rough surface. Sealants are usually clear or tooth-colored, making them less noticeable than silver fillings. They cost less than fillings and can last up to 10 years, although they should be checked for wear at every dental visit. Children should get sealants on their first permanent ''6-year'' molars, which come in between the ages of five and seven, and on the second permanent ''12-year'' molars, which come in between the ages of 11 and 14. Sealants should be applied to the teeth shortly after they erupt, before decay can set in. Although sealants have been used in the United States for about 25 years, one survey by the National Institute of Dental Research reported that fewer than 8% of American children have them.

The risk of tooth decay can be lowered by choosing foods wisely and eating less often. Foods high in sugar and starch, especially when eaten between meals, increase the risk of cavities. The bacteria in the mouth use sugar and starch to produce the acid that destroys the enamel. The damage increases with more frequent eating and longer periods of eating. For better dental health, people should eat a variety of foods, limit the number of snacks, avoid sticky and overly sweetened foods, and brush often after eating.

Drinking water is also beneficial for rinsing food particles from the mouth. Children can be taught to ''swish and swallow'' if they are unable to brush after lunch at school. Similarly, saliva stimulated during eating makes it more difficult for food and bacteria to stick to tooth surfaces. Saliva also appears to have a buffering effect on the acid produced by the plaque bacteria and to act as a remineralizing agent. Older patients should be made aware that some prescription medications may decrease salivary flow. Less saliva tends to increase the activity of plaque bacteria and encourage further tooth decay. Chewing sugarless gum increases salivation and thus helps to lower the risk of tooth decay.

See also Oral hygiene; Root canal treatment; Toothache

Tooth extraction

Tooth extraction is the removal of a tooth from its socket in the bone. Extraction is performed for positional, structural, or economic reasons. Teeth are often removed because they are impacted. Teeth become impacted when they are prevented from growing into their normal position in the mouth by gum tissue, bone, or other teeth. Impaction is a common reason for the extraction of wisdom teeth. Extraction is the only known method that will prevent further problems. Teeth may also be extracted to make more room in the mouth prior to straightening the remaining teeth (orthodontic treatment), or because they are so badly positioned that straightening is impossible. Extraction may be used to remove teeth that are so badly decayed or broken that they cannot be restored. In addition, patients sometimes choose extraction as a less expensive alternative to filling or placing a crown on a severely decayed tooth.

Tooth extraction can be performed with local **anesthesia** if the tooth is exposed and appears to be easily removable in one piece. An instrument called an elevator is used to loosen (luxate) the tooth, widen the space in the bone, and break the tiny elastic fibers that attach the tooth to the bone. Once the tooth is dislocated from the bone, it can be lifted and removed with forceps.

If the extraction is likely to be difficult, the dentist may refer the patient to an oral surgeon. Oral surgeons are specialists who are trained to give nitrous oxide, an intravenous sedative, or a general anesthetic to relieve **pain**. Extracting an impacted tooth or a tooth with curved roots typically requires cutting through gum tissue to expose the tooth. It may also require removing portions of bone to free the tooth. Some teeth must be cut and removed in sections. The extraction site may or may not require one or more stitches to close the cut (incision).

Before an extraction, the dentist will take the patient's medical history, noting **allergies** and prescription medications. A dental history is also taken, with particular attention to previous extractions and reactions to anesthetics. The dentist may then prescribe antibiotics or recommend stopping certain medications prior to the extraction. The tooth is x-rayed to determine its full shape and position, especially if it is impacted.

If the patient is going to have deep anesthesia, he or she should wear loose clothing with sleeves that are easily rolled up to allow for an intravenous line. The patient should not eat or drink anything for at least six hours before the procedure. Arrangements should be made for a friend or relative to drive the patient home after the surgery.

An important aspect of aftercare is encouraging a clot to form at the extraction site. The patient should put pressure on the area by biting gently on a roll or wad of gauze for several hours after surgery. Once the clot is formed, it should not be disturbed. The patient should not rinse, spit, drink with a straw, or smoke for at least 24 hours after the extraction and preferably longer. Vigorous **exercise** should not be done for the first three to five days.

For the first two days after the procedure, the patient should drink liquids without using a straw, and eat soft foods. Any chewing must be done on the side away from the extraction site. Hard or sticky foods should be avoided. The mouth may be gently cleaned with a toothbrush, but the extraction area should not be scrubbed. Wrapped ice packs can be applied to reduce facial swelling. Swelling is a normal part of the healing process. It is most noticeable in the first 48-72 hours. As the swelling subsides, the patient may experience muscle stiffness. Moist heat and gentle exercise will restore jaw movement. The dentist may prescribe medications to relieve the postoperative pain.

Potential complications of tooth extraction include postoperative infection, temporary numbness from nerve irritation, jaw fracture, and jaw joint pain. An additional complication is called dry socket. When a blood clot does not properly form in the empty tooth socket, the bone beneath the socket is painfully exposed to air and food, and the extraction site heals more slowly.

After an extraction, the wound usually closes in about two weeks. It takes three to six months for the bone and soft tissue to be restructured. Complications such as infection or dry socket may prolong the healing time.

See also Oral hygiene; Toothache; Tooth decay

Tooth replacements and restorations

A tooth restoration is any artificial substance or structure that replaces missing teeth or part of a tooth in order to protect the mouth's ability to eat, chew, and speak. Restorations include fillings, inlays, crowns, bridges, partial and complete dentures, and dental implants. Restorations have somewhat different purposes depending on their extensiveness. Fillings, inlays, and crowns are intended to repair damage to individual teeth. They replace tooth structure lost by decay or injury, protect the part of the tooth that remains, and restore the tooth's shape and function. Bridges, dentures, and implants are intended to protect the shape and function of the mouth as a whole.

Fillings are restorations that are done to repair damage caused by **tooth decay** (dental caries). To stop the decay process, the dentist removes the decayed portion of the tooth using a high-speed drill or an air abrasion system, shapes the cavity walls, and replaces the tooth structure with a filling of silver amalgam, composite resin, or gold. The filling is placed in the cavity as a liquid or soft solid. It sets within a few minutes and continues to harden over the next several hours. Silver amalgam is commonly used to fill cavities on the biting surfaces of the back teeth, because it is strong enough to withstand the tremendous pressures exerted by grinding and chewing. Composite resin is typically used to fill cavities in front teeth and any other teeth that are visible when the patient smiles, because its color can be matched to the tooth surface. Gold as a filling material is far less common, but is being increasingly used. Although it is more expensive and less easily applied, it does not trigger the sensitivity reactions that some patients have to silver amalgam.

An inlay resembles a filling in that it fills the space remaining after the decayed portion of a tooth has been removed. The difference is that an inlay is shaped outside the patient's mouth and then cemented into place. After the decay is removed and the cavity walls are shaped, the dentist makes a wax pattern of the space. A mold is cast from the wax pattern. An inlay, usually of gold, is made from this mold and sealed into the tooth with dental cement.

The crown of a tooth is the portion that is covered by enamel. A restorative crown replaces this outer part to protect the tooth. This protection becomes necessary when a tooth cracks or has its entire structure weakened by decay. As with a filling or inlay, the dentist first removes the decayed portion of the tooth. The tooth is then prepared for a crown. It may be tapered on the outside edges to a peg, reinforced with a cast metal core, or rebuilt with both a cast metal core and a post. A wax impression of the prepared tooth and the teeth next to it is made. The new crown is made to fit this mold. The crown may be made of gold or stainless steel alone, metal with a veneer of tooth-colored porcelain or resin, or of porcelain or resin alone. The finished crown is then placed over the prepared tooth, adjusted, and cemented into place.

Bridges are a type of restoration that is done when one or more permanent teeth are lost or pulled. Bridges are nonremovable appliances of one or more artificial teeth (pontics) anchored by crowns on the adjacent teeth (abutment teeth). The abutment teeth carry the pressure when the patient chews food.

A partial denture is similar to a bridge in that it fills a gap left by missing teeth with artificial teeth on a metal frame. A partial denture is removable, however. It attaches to a crown on the abutment tooth with a metal clasp or precision attachment. A partial denture is primarily used at the end of a row of natural teeth, where there is only one abutment tooth. The pressure exerted by chewing is shared by this abutment and the soft tissues of the gum ridge beneath the appliance.

Dental implants are a means of securing crowns, bridges, and dentures in the mouth. A hard plastic or metal fixture is implanted through the soft tissue into the bone. Over time, the bone grows around this fixture, firmly anchoring it. The exposed end of this fixture is covered with a crown and may serve as a stable abutment for a bridge or denture.

Complete dentures may be worn when all of the top or bottom teeth have been lost. A complete denture consists of artificial teeth mounted in a plastic base molded to fit the remaining oral anatomy. It may or may not be held in place with a denture adhesive. A partial or complete denture may take several weeks of getting used to. Inserting and removing the denture will take practice. Speaking clearly may be difficult at first—the patient may find it helpful to read out loud for practice. Eating may also feel awkward. The patient should begin by eating small pieces of soft foods. Very hard or sticky foods should be avoided. Patients with dentures must work on good **oral hygiene**. Specialty brushes and floss threaders may be used to remove plaque and food from around crowns and bridges. Dentures should be removed and brushed daily with a specially designed brush and a denture cleaner or other mild soap. The patient should see the dentist for an adjustment if there is any discomfort or irritation resulting from a restoration. Otherwise, the patient should see the dentist at least twice a year for an oral examination.

See also Oral hygiene; Tooth decay; Toothache

TORCH TEST

The TORCH test, which is sometimes called the TORCH panel, belongs to a category of blood tests called infectious-disease antibody titer tests. This type of blood test measures the presence of antibodies (protein molecules produced by the human immune system in response to a specific disease agent) and their level of concentration in the blood. The name of the test comes from the initial letters of the five disease categories. The TORCH test measures the levels of an infant's antibodies against five groups of chronic infections: **Toxoplasmosis**, Other infections, **Rubella**, Cytomegalovirus (CMV), and Herpes simplex virus (HSV). The ''other infections'' usually include **syphilis**, **hepatitis** B, coxsackie virus, Epstein-Barr virus, varicella-zoster virus, and human parvovirus.

Since the TORCH test is a screening or first-level test, the pediatrician may order tests of other body fluids or tissues to confirm the diagnosis of a specific infection. In the case of toxoplasmosis, rubella, and syphilis, cerebrospinal fluid may be obtained from the infant through a spinal tap in order to confirm the diagnosis. In the case of CMV, the diagnosis is confirmed by culturing the virus in a sample of the infant's urine. In HSV infections, tissue culture is the best method to confirm the diagnosis.

The five categories of organisms whose antibodies are measured by the TORCH test are grouped together because they can cause a cluster of symptomatic **birth defects** in newborns. This group of defects is sometimes called the TORCH syndrome. A newborn baby with these symptoms will be given a TORCH test to see if any of the five types of infection are involved. The symptoms of the TORCH syndrome include:

- Small size in proportion to length of the mother's **pregnancy** at time of delivery. Infants who are smaller than would be expected (below the 10th percentile) are referred to as small-for-gestational-age, or SGA.
- Enlarged liver and spleen
- Low level of platelets in the blood
- Skin rash. The type of skin rash associated with the TORCH syndrome is usually reddish-purple or brown and is caused by the leakage of blood from broken capillaries into the baby's skin.
- Involvement of the central nervous system. These defects can include **encephalitis**, calcium deposits in the brain tissue, and seizures.
- **Jaundice**. The yellowish discoloration of the skin and whites of the eyes due to liver disease.

In addition to these symptoms, each of the TORCH infections has its own characteristic symptom cluster in newborns:

The normal result would be normal levels of immunoglobulin M (IgM) antibody in the infant's blood. IgM is one of five types of protein molecules found in blood that function as antibodies. IgM is a specific class of antibodies that seeks out virus particles. In contrast to adults, IgM is the most common type of immunoglobulin in newborn children. It is, therefore, the most useful indicator of the presence of a TORCH infection. The general abnormal, or positive, finding would be high levels of IgM antibody. The test can be refined further for antibodies specific to given disease agents. The TORCH screen, however, can produce both false-positive and false-negative findings. Doctors can measure IgM levels in the infant's cerebrospinal fluid, as well as in the blood, if they want to confirm the TORCH results.

See also Rubella; Syphilus; Toxoplasmosis

TORTICOLLIS

Torticollis (cervical dystonia or spasmodic torticollis) is a type of movement disorder, in which the muscles controlling the neck cause sustained twisting or frequent jerking.

In torticollis, certain muscles controlling the neck undergo repetitive or sustained contraction, causing the neck to jerk or twist to the side. Cervical dystonia causes forward twisting, and is called antecollis. Backward twisting is known as retrocollis. The abnormal posture caused by torticollis is often debilitating, and is usually **pain**ful.

Torticollis most commonly begins between age 30-60, with females affected twice as often as males. According to the National Spasmodic Torticollis Association, torticollis affects 83,000 people in the United States. Dystonia tends to become more severe during the first months or years after onset, and may spread to other regions, especially the jaw, arm, or leg. Torticollis should not be confused with other causes of abnormal neck posture, such as orthopedic or congenital problems.

The nerve signals responsible for torticollis are thought to originate in the basal ganglia, a group of brain structures involved in movement control. The exact defect is unknown. Some cases of dystonia are due to the inheritance of a defective gene, whose function was unknown as of mid-1998. Other cases are correlated with neck or head trauma, such as from an automobile accident. Use of certain **antipsychotic drugs**, or neuroleptics, can induce dystonia.

There are three types of torticollis:

- Tonic, in which the abnormal posture is sustained
- Clonic, marked by jerky head movements.
- Mixed, a combination of tonic and clonic movements

Symptoms usually begin gradually, and may be intermittent at first, worsening in times of **stress**. Symptoms usually progress over two to five years, and then remain steady. Symptoms may be relieved somewhat when lying down. Many people with torticollis can temporarily correct their head position by sensory tricks, as touching the chin or cheek on the side opposite the turning. The reason for the effectiveness of this ''geste antagoniste,'' as it is called, is unknown.

Pain in the neck, back, or shoulder affects more than two-thirds of all people with torticollis. Pain may spread to the arm or hand.

Diagnosis of torticollis is aided by an electrical study (electromyography) that can detect overactive muscles. Imaging studies, including x rays, may be done to rule out other causes of abnormal posture. A detailed medical history is needed to determine possible causes, including trauma.

A variety of oral drugs are available to relax muscles, including baclofen. For a subgroup of patients, L-dopa provides effective relief. Denervation of the involved neck muscles may be performed with injection of alcohol or phenol on to the nerve.

Injection of botulinum toxin (BTX) is considered by many to be the treatment of choice. By preventing release of chemical messages from the nerve endings that stimulate the involved muscles, BTX partially paralyzes the muscles, therefore allowing more normal posture and range of motion. BTX treatment lasts several months, and may be repeated.

Physical therapy can help relieve secondary consequences of torticollis. Regular muscle stretching prevents contracture, or permanent muscle shortening. Pain and spasm may be temporarily lessened with application of heat or ice. Stress management techniques may help prevent worsening. An occupational therapist can suggest home or work modifications to reduce fatigue and improve function. Braces constructed to replace the patient's own sensory tricks may help reduce abnormal posture.

TOUCH

Touch is one of the five senses (the others being **smell**, **taste**, vision, and hearing) through which animals and people interpret the world around them. While the other senses are localized primarily in a single area (such as vision in the **eye**s or taste in the tongue), the sensation of touch (or contact with the outside world) can be experienced anywhere on the body, from the top of the head to the tip of the toe. Touch is based on nerve receptors in the skin that send electrical messages through the central nervous system to the cerebral cortex in the brain, which interprets these electrical codes. For the most part, the touch receptors specialize in experiencing either hot, cold, pain, or pressure. Arguably, touch is the most important of all the senses; without it animals would not be able to recognize pain (such as scalding water), which would greatly decrease their chances for survival. Research has also shown that touch has tremendous psychological ramifications in areas like **child development**, persuasion, healing, and reducing anxiety and tension.

Our sense of touch is based primarily in the outer layer of skin called the epidermis. Nerve endings that lie in or just below the epidermis cells respond to various outside stimuli, which are categorized into four basic stimuli: pressure, pain, hot, and cold. Animals experience one or a combination of these sensations through a complex neural network that sends electrical impulses through the spinal cord to the cerebral cortex in the brain. The cerebral cortex, in turn, contains brain cells (neurons) arranged in columns that specialize in interpreting specific types of stimuli on certain parts of the body.

The sensation of touch begins with various receptors in the skin. Although these receptors appear to specialize in reacting to certain sensations, there is some debate concerning this specificity because most touch stimuli are a combination of some or all of the four major categories.

Scientists have identified several types of touch receptors. Free nerve ending receptors, located throughout the body at the bases of hair, are associated primarily with light pressure (such as wind) and pain. Meissner corpuscles are nerve endings contained in tiny capsules and are found primarily in the fingertips and areas especially sensitive to touch (in the form of low-frequency vibrations), like the soles of the feet and the tongue. The Pacinian corpuscles look like the cross section of an onion and are found in deep tissues in the joints, the genitals, and the mammary glands. They are extremely sensitive to pressure and are also stimulated by rapid movement of the tissues and vibrating sensations. Ruffini endings, which are also located in the deeper layers of the skin, respond to continuous stimulation, like steady pressure or tension within the skin. Merkel disks are found near the base of the epidermis and respond to continuous stimulation or pressure. The skin also contains specific thermoreceptors for sensing hot and cold and nociceptors that identify high intensity stimulation in the form of pain.

Most, if not all of these receptors, are designed to adapt or become accustomed to the specific stimulation they interpret. In other words, the receptor does not continue to register a constant "feeling" with the same intensity as when it first begins and may even shut off the tactile experience. Imagine, for example, putting on a wool sweater over bare skin. The initial prickly sensation eventually abates, allowing the wearer to become accustomed to the feeling. Other examples include wearing jewelry such as rings, necklaces, and watches.

These receptors are also found in greater numbers on different parts of the body. For example, peoples' backs are the least sensitive to touch, while their lips, tongue, and fingertips are most sensitive to tactile activity. Most receptors for cold are found on the surface of the face while thermoreceptors for warmth usually lie deeper in the skin and are fewer in number. A light breeze on the arm or head is felt because there tend to be more sense receptors at the base of the hairs than anywhere else.

Touch has a tremendous impact on most animals' physical and psychological well being. Numerous studies of humans and other animals have shown that touch greatly influences how we develop physically and respond to the world mentally. For example, premature babies that receive regular massages will gain weight more rapidly and develop faster mentally than those who do not receive the same attention. When baby rats are separated from their mothers for only 45 minutes, they undergo physiological or biochemical changes, specifically a reduction in a growth hormone. Touching of premature babies can also stimulate growth hormones (such as the hormone needed to absorb food) that occur naturally in healthy babies.

A baby does not have to be premature or sickly to benefit from touch. Even healthy babies show benefits from touch in terms of emotional stability. Difficult children often have a history of abuse and neglect. The reason is that touch serves as a type of reassurance to infants that they are loved and safe, which translates into emotional well being. In general, babies who are held and touched more tend to develop better alertness and cognitive abilities over the long run.

Touch continues to have a great psychological impact throughout peoples' lives. Even adults who are hospitalized or sick at home seem to have less anxiety and tension headaches when they are regularly touched or caressed by caretakers or loved ones. Numerous studies have shown that touch also has a healing power. Researchers have found that touch reduces rapid heart beats and irregular heart beats (**arrhythmias**). Another study showed that baby rats who are touched often during infancy develop more receptors to control the production of biochemicals called glucocorticoids, which are known as stress chemicals because of their ability to cause muscle shrinkage, high blood pressure, elevated cholesterol, and more.

Touch's psychological impact goes beyond physical and mental health. Researchers have shown that touch is a powerful persuasive force. For example, studies have shown that touch can have a big impact in marketing and sales. Salespeople often use touch to establish a camaraderie and friendship that can result in better sales. In general, people are more likely to respond positively to a request if it is accompanied by a slight touch on the arm or hand. In a study of waiters and waitresses, for example, those that lightly touched a patron often received better tips.

Tourette syndrome

Tourette syndrome (TS) is an inherited disease of the nervous system, first described more than a century ago by the pioneering French neurologist, Dr. George Gilles de la Tourette. Before age 18, patients with TS develop *motor* tics, that is, repeated, jerky, stereotyped, purposeless muscle movements in almost any part of the body. *Vocal* tics occur in the form of loud grunting or "barking" noises or, in some cases, words or phrases. In most cases, the tics come and go, and they often are replaced by different types of sounds or movements, which may become more complex as the patient grows older.

TS is three times more common in men than in women. The motor tics, which usually occur in bouts several times a day, may make it very hard for the patient to perform simple acts like tying shoelaces, not to mention work-related tasks or driving. In addition, TS may be very detrimental socially. Some patients have an irresistible urge to curse or use offensive racial terms (a condition called coprolalia), though this is not under voluntary control. Other people may not wish to be with TS patients and, even if they are accepted, TS patients live in fear of shocking others and embarrassing themselves. In time, they may close themselves off from former friends and even relatives.

Research shows that, in TS, something is wrong with the way in which the brain produces or uses important substances called neurotransmitters, which control how signals are sent along the nerve cells. The neurotransmitters dopamine and serotonin have been implicated in TS; noradrenaline is thought to be the most important stimulant. Medications that mimic noradrenaline may cause tics in susceptible patients. Whatever the exact defect, it is handed down through the genes from parents to children. If one parent has TS, each child has a 50% chance of getting the abnormal gene. Seven of every ten girls who inherit the gene, and nearly all boys who inherit it, will develop symptoms of TS.

Patients with TS are more likely to have trouble controlling their impulses, to have **dyslexia** (or other learning problems), and to talk during sleep or wake frequently. Compulsive behavior, such as constantly washing the hands or repeatedly checking that a door is locked, is a common feature of TS, seen in 30-90% of all patients.

A number of examples will show why TS can be such a strange and dramatic disorder:

- Simple motor tics (blinking the eyes, pouting the lips, shaking or jerking the head, shrugging the shoulders, and grimacing or "making faces"). Rapid finger movements are common, as are snapping the jaws and clicking the teeth.

- Complex motor tics (jumping, touching part of the body or certain objects, smelling things over and over, stamping the feet, and twirling about). Some TS patients throw objects, others arrange things in a certain way. Biting, head-banging, writhing (snake-like) movements, rolling the eyes up or from side to side, and sticking out the tongue all may be seen. A child may write the same letter or word over and over, or may tear apart papers and books. Though they do not mean to, TS patients may make obscene gestures.
- Simple vocal tics (clearing the throat, **cough**ing, snorting, barking, grunting, yelping, clicking the tongue). They may repeat sounds such as "uh, uh," or "eee."
- Complex vocal tics and patterns. Older children with TS may repeat a phrase such as "Oh boy," "all right," or "what's that?" Or they may repeat everything they, or others, say a certain number of times. Some patients speak very rapidly or loudly, or in a strange tone or accent. Coprolalia (saying "dirty words" or phrases that are sexual or aggressive) is probably the best known feature of TS, but fewer than one-third of all patients actually do this.

Behavioral abnormalities that may be associated with TS include **attention-deficit/hyperactivity disorder** (ADHD) and disruptive behaviors, including **conduct disorder** and oppositional defiant disorder, with aggressive, destructive, antisocial, or negativistic behavior. Academic disorders, **learning disorders**, and sleep abnormalities (such as sleepwalking and nightmares) are also seen.

TS is diagnosed by observing the symptoms and asking whether relatives have had a similar condition. To qualify as TS, both motor and vocal tics should be present for at least a year and should begin before age 18 (or, some believe, age 21). There are no specific tests for TS. Often, the diagnosis is delayed because the patient is misunderstood not only at home and at school, but often in the doctor's office as well. It may take some time for the patient to trust the doctor enough not to suppress the strangest or most alarming tics. A test of the brain's electrical activity (**electroencephalograph** or EEG) is often abnormal, but not specific. Medication history is very important in making the diagnosis as well, because stimulant drugs may provoke tics or aggravate the symptoms of TS.

A majority of patients with TS do not need to take drugs, as their tics do not interfere much with their lives, and they develop normally. In serious cases, a drug used to treat severe mental illness, such as haloperidol (Haldol) or pimozide (Orap), is given, starting with a very low dose and increasing until the tics respond without side effects occurring. Researchers are developing new **antipsychotic drugs** that may be targeted to particular symptoms of TS.

TOXIC SHOCK SYNDROME

There are two types of Toxic Shock Syndrome: The first (TSS), identified in 1978, is caused by the bacteria *Staphylococcus aureus (staph)*. The second (STSS) and more recent discovery, is caused by a Group A *Streptococcus (strep)* bacteria. Although both are rare, both can be fatal. When either the staph or strep bacterium enter a wound, their growth causes a poison—or *toxin*, which enters the blood stream. Once this toxin enters the **nervous system**, it causes **headaches**, confusion, a drastic drop in blood pressure, and perhaps unconsciousness. Ultimately, the body goes into **shock**. Signs of shock include cold hands and feet; cool, moist skin; **shortness of breath**; rapid breathing; and **anxiety**. The toxin may also invade the heart or kidneys. Symptoms, which differ slightly between the two syndromes, begin suddenly and can be treated with **antibiotics**; shock may be treated with intravenous fluids, and medication to correct blood pressure.

TSS was identified in 1978 in relation to the use of tampons during **menstruation**, although anyone is susceptible to TSS if their **immune system** is unable to fight off staph invasion through an infected wound. The majority of women affected by tampon use are under the age of 30 and primarily between the ages of 15 and 19, 98% of cases occur in white women, and the death rate is about 6% of reported cases. This syndrome begins when the staph bacterium enter the system through the vagina—perhaps through a scratch from a tampon applicator. Highly absorbent tampons, particularly those containing rayon, appear to encourage the breeding of germs and thus increase the risk of TSS. Symptoms, which appear suddenly, may include a fever above 102 degrees Fahrenheit, a sunburn-like rash, peeling skin from the palms and soles, low blood pressure, vomiting or **diarrhea**, confusion or other mental changes, fatigue, thirst, and rapid breathing. Some women who have recovered from TSS have reported subsequent hair loss, loss of limbs, **paralysis**, and miscarriages; some people experience recurrence of the syndrome. Experts advise changing the tampon every four to six hours, alternating between sanitary napkins and tampons, ceasing the use of tampons in the presence of thrush, vaginal cuts or sores, or if vaginosis was present within the preceding year, avoiding tampons containing rayon, and paying particular attention to cleanliness. In the United States, TSS affects approximately 17 people in 100,000 and about 200 people per year.

STSS, a severe illness which proves fatal in more than 50% of cases, develops when the strep bacteria enters a cut, wound, surgical incision, or even **chickenpox** blisters. Seldom does strep throat cause STSS, however. Symptoms are similar to TSS, and the area surrounding the wound becomes red and swollen and sometimes necrotic (begins to die). STSS, classified as an "emerging" illness and related to the strain of strep called "**flesh-eating** bacteria," is reported in only one or two out of every 100,000 people in the U.S. As this infection is still not well understood, prevention advice focuses on thoroughly cleansing and covering the wound with a **bandage** as quickly as possible. Medical advice should be sought immediately the wound becomes red or swollen, or with the onset of **fever**.

See also Chickenpox

TOXOPLASMOSIS

Toxoplasmosis is an infectious disease caused by the one-celled protozoan parasite *Toxoplasma gondii.* Toxoplasmosis is caused by a one-celled protozoan parasite known as *Toxoplasm gondii.* Cats, the primary carriers of the organism, become infected by eating rodents and birds infected with the organism. Once ingested, the organism reproduces in the intestines of cats, producing millions of eggs, known as oocysts, which are excreted in cat feces daily for approximately two weeks. In the United States, it is estimated that approximately 30% of cats have been infected by *T. gondii.* Oocysts are not capable of producing infection until approximately 24 hours after being excreted, but they remain infective in water or moist soil for approximately one year. When cattle, sheep, or other livestock forage through areas with contaminated cat feces, these animals become carriers of the disease. Fruits and vegetables can also become contaminated when irrigated with untreated water that has been contaminated with cat feces. In humans and other animals, the organisms produce thick-walled, dormant structures, called cysts, in the muscle and other tissues of the body.

Most humans contract toxoplasmosis by eating cyst-contaminated raw or undercooked meat, vegetables, or milk products. Humans can also become infected when they come into contact with the *T. gondii* eggs while cleaning a cat's litterbox, gardening, or playing in a sandbox, for instance. Once infected, an individual is immune to reinfection. The incubation period or period between infection and the start of the disease ranges from several days to months.

Healthy individuals do not usually display symptoms. When symptoms do occur, they are usually mild, resembling **infectious mononucleosis**, and include the following:

- Enlarged lymph nodes
- Muscle **pain**s
- **Fever** that comes and goes
- General ill feeling.

While anyone can be infected by *T. gondii*, usually only those individuals with weakened immune systems (immunocompromised) develop severe symptoms of the disease. For them, toxoplasmosis can be debilitating, and fatal. Immunocompromised individuals at-risk include those with **AIDS**, **cancer**, or other chronic illnesses.

There is no person-to-person transmission, except from an infected mother to her child in the womb. Approximately six out of 1,000 women contract toxoplasmosis during **pregnancy**. Nearly half of these maternal infections are passed on to the fetus. Known as congenital toxoplasmosis, this form of the disease is acquired at birth by approximately 3,300 infants in the United States every year. The risk of fetal infection is estimated to be between one in 1,000 to one in 10,000. In children born with toxoplasmosis, symptoms may be severe and quickly fatal, or may not appear until several months, or even years, after birth.

The distinction is made between acquired toxoplasmosis, where an individual becomes infected, and neonatal congenital toxoplasmosis, where a fetus is born with the infection because the mother became infected during pregnancy. If a fetus becomes infected early in pregnancy, it can cause the fetus to spontaneously abort, and be stillborn. If full-term, the infant may die in infancy or suffer from central nervous system lesions. If the mother becomes infected in the last three months of pregnancy, however, the prognosis is good and the baby may not even display any symptoms.

In adults, if the infection continues for an extended period of time, chronic toxoplasmosis can cause an inflammation of the eyes, called retinochoroiditis, that can lead to blindness, severe yellowing of the skin and whites of the eyes (**jaundice**), easy bruising, and convulsions. Adults with weakened immune systems have a high risk of developing cerebral toxoplasmosis, including inflammation of the brain (**encephalitis**), one-sided weakness or numbness, mood and personality changes, vision disturbances, muscle spasms, and severe **headache**s. If untreated, cerebral toxoplasmosis can lead to **coma** and **death**. This form of encephalitis is the second most common AIDS-related nervous system infection that takes advantage of a person's weakened immune system (opportunistic infection).

A diagnosis of toxoplasmosis is made based on clinical signs and supporting laboratory results, including visualization of the protozoa in body tissue or **isolation** in animals and blood tests. Laboratory tests for toxoplasmosis are designed to detect increased amounts of a protein or antibody produced in response to infection with the toxoplasmosis organism. Antibody levels can be elevated for years, however, without active disease.

Most individuals who contract toxoplasmosis do not require treatment, because their immune systems are able to control the disease. Symptoms are not usually present. Mild symptoms may be relieved by taking over-the-counter medications, such as **acetaminophen** (Tylenol) and ibuprofen (Motrin, Advil). **Sore throat** lozenges and rest may also ease the symptoms. Although the treatment of women infected with toxoplasmosis during pregnancy is controversial, most physicians feel that treatment is justified. Transmission of toxoplasmosis from the mother to the fetus may be prevented if the mother takes the specific antibiotic therapy. AIDS patients who have not been infected may be given a drug called TMP/SMX (Bactrim or Septra) to prevent toxoplasmosis infection. To treat cases of toxoplasmosis in immunocompromised AIDS patients, antibiotic combinations may effectively treat the disease.

The prognosis is poor when congenital toxoplasmosis is acquired during the first three months of pregnancy. Afflicted children die in infancy or suffer damage to their central nervous systems that can result in physical and **mental retardation**. Infection later in pregnancy usually results in only mild symptoms, if any. The prognosis for acquired toxoplasmosis in adults with strong immune systems is excellent. The disease often disappears by itself after several weeks. However, the prognosis for immunodeficient patients is not as positive. These patients often relapse when treatment is stopped. The disease can be fatal to all immunocompromised patients, especially AIDS patients, and particularly if not treated. As a result, immunocompromised patients are typically placed on anti-toxoplasmosis drugs for the rest of their lives.

There are no drugs that can eliminate *T. gondii* cysts in animal or human tissues. Humans can reduce their risks of developing toxoplasmosis by practicing the following:

- Freezing (to 10.4°F/–12°C) and cooking foods to an internal temperature of 152°F/67°C will kill the cysts
- Practicing sanitary kitchen techniques, such as washing utensils and cutting boards that come into contact with raw meat
- Keeping pregnant women and children away from household cats and cat litter
- Disposing of cat feces daily, because the oocysts do not become infective until after 24 hours
- Helping cats to remain free of infection by feeding them dry, canned, or boiled food and by discouraging hunting and scavenging
- Washing hands after outdoor activities involving soil contact and wearing gloves when gardening.

Tracheotomy

A tracheotomy is a life-saving surgical procedure in which an opening is made in a patient's windpipe (trachea) and tube is inserted into the opening in the throat to allow breathing to continue in the event of airway obstruction. Once the emergency situation passes, the tube can be removed and the opening closed.

The first tracheotomy was performed in 1825 by French physician Pierre Bretonneau (1778-1862) on a four-year-old girl whose throat had become obstructed with the scar tissue that forms in the throats of diphtheria victims. Bretonneau had attempted two tracheotomies previously and failed, but his determination, skill, and dexterity finally paid off, saving the girl's life. Bretonneau, the son of a surgeon, became a physician at the hospital in Tours. Practicing medicine among the poor, he was the first to study such diseases as typhoid fever and diphtheria in detail and was the first to use the term ''diphtheria.'' Also a skilled craftsman, Bretonneau made hydraulic hammers, barometers, and thermometers.

Tracheotomies can be used for people who need long-term artificial airway support—such as poliomyelitis victims or people paralyzed from the neck down, people with respiratory infections, cancer, airway burns, upper airway obstruction, and even extreme cases of sleep apnea.

Traction

Traction is the use of a pulling force to treat muscle and skeleton disorders and is usually applied to the arms and legs, the neck, the backbone, or the pelvis. It is used to treat **fractures**, dislocations, and long-duration muscle spasms, and to prevent or correct deformities.

Traction serves several purposes:

- It aligns the ends of a fracture by pulling the limb into a straight position.
- It ends muscle spasm.
- It relieves **pain**.
- It takes the pressure off the bone ends by relaxing the muscle.

There are two main types of traction: skin traction and skeletal traction. Within these types, many specialized forms of traction have been developed to address problems in particular parts of the body. The application of traction is an exacting technique that requires training and experience, since incorrectly applied traction can cause harm. Positioning the extremity so that the angle of pull brings the ends of the fracture together is essential. Elaborate methods of weights, counterweights, and pulleys have been developed to provide the appropriate force, while keeping the bones aligned and preventing muscle spasm. The patient's age, weight, and medical condition are all taken into account when deciding on the type and degree of traction.

Skeletal traction is performed when more pulling force is needed than can be withstood by skin traction, or when the part of the body needing traction is positioned so that skin traction is impossible. Skeletal traction uses weights of 25-40 pounds. Skeletal traction requires the placement of tongs, pins, or screws into the bone so that the weight is applied directly to the bone. This is an invasive procedure that is done in an operating room under general, regional, or local anesthesia. Correct placement of the pins is essential to the success of the traction. The pin can be kept in place several months, and must be kept clean to prevent infection. Once the hardware is in place, pulleys and weights are attached to wires to provide the proper pull and alignment on the affected part. Specialized forms of skeletal traction include cervical traction used for fractures of the neck vertebrae, overhead arm traction used for certain types of upper arm fractures, and tibia pin traction used for some fractures of the femur, hip, or pelvis.

X rays are done prior to the application of both forms of traction, and may be repeated during treatment to assure that the affected parts are staying in alignment and healing properly. Aftercare for skin traction involves making sure the limb stays aligned, and caring for the skin so that it does not become sore and irritated. The patient should also be alert to any swelling or tingling in the limb that would suggest that the limb has been wrapped too tightly.

Aftercare for skeletal traction is more complex. The patient is likely to be immobile for an extended period. Deep breathing **exercise**s are taught so that respiratory function is maintained during this time of little activity. Patients are also encouraged to do range of motion exercises with the unaffected parts of the body. The patient is taught how to use a trapeze (an overhead support bar) to shift on and off a bedpan, since it is not possible to get up to use the toilet. In serious injuries, traction may be continued for several months until healing is complete.

The main risks associated with skin traction are that the traction will be applied incorrectly and cause harm, or that the skin will become irritated. There are more risks associated with skeletal traction. Bone inflammation may occur in response to the introduction of foreign material into the body. Infection can occur at the pin sites. If caught early, infection

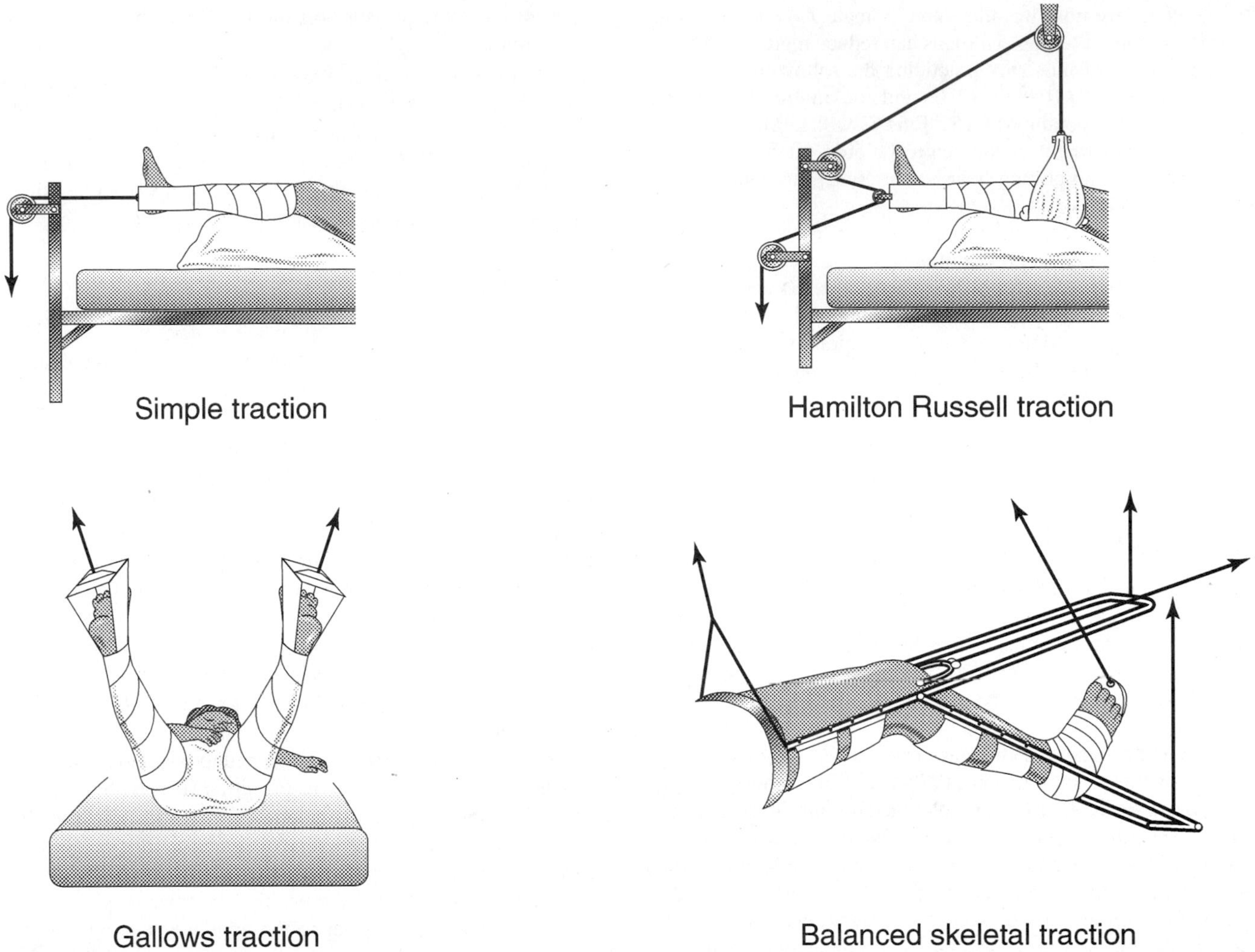

Traction refers to the usage of a pulling force and special devices, such as a cast or splint, to treat muscle and skeletal disorders. It is used to treat fractures, dislocations, and long-duration muscle spasms, and to prevent or correct deformities. The illustration above features several commonly used forms of traction. ***(Illustration by Electronic Illustrators Group.)***

can be treated with **antibiotics**, but if severe, it may require removal of the pin.

See also Fractures

TRANSFUSION

Transfusion is the process of transferring whole blood or blood components from one person (donor) to another (recipient), to restore lost blood, to improve clotting time, and to improve the ability of the blood to deliver oxygen to the body's tissues. Whole blood is used exactly as it was received from the donor. Blood components are parts of whole blood, such as red blood cells (RBCs), plasma, platelets, clotting factors, immunoglobulins, and white blood cells. Use of blood components is a more efficient way to use the blood supply, because blood that has been processed (fractionated) into components can be used to treat more than one person.

Whole blood is generally used when a person has lost a lot of blood by injury or surgical procedures and is given to help restore the blood volume, which is essential for maintaining blood pressure. Red blood cells are the blood component most frequently used for transfusion. As only cells in the body that transport oxygen, a transfusion of RBCs increases the amount of oxygen that can be carried to the tissues of the body. RBCs that have been separated from the liquid plasma (packed RBCs) are given to people who have anemia or who have lost a lot of blood. Platelets are another component frequently given by transfusion. Platelets are a key factor in blood clotting. The clear fluid that carries blood cells (plasma) also contains blood-clotting factors. The platelets and plasma clotting factors are extracted from donated blood and concentrated for use. These factors are used to treat people with clotting disorders, such as **hemophilia**.

For donors, the process of giving blood is very safe. Only sterile equipment is used and there is no chance of catching an infection from the equipment. There is a slight chance of infection at the puncture site if the skin is not properly washed before the collection needle is inserted. Some donors feel light-headed upon standing for the first time after donating. Occasionally, a donor will faint. Donors are advised to drink lots of liquids to replace the fluid lost with the donated blood. Strenuous **exercise** should be avoided for the rest of the day. Most patients have very slight symptoms or no symptoms at all after donating blood.

For recipients, a number of precautions must be taken. The blood given by transfusion must be matched with the recipient's blood type. Generally, patients are limited to receiving only blood of the exact same ABO and Rh type as their own. For example, a person with B+ blood can only receive blood or blood cells from another person with B+ blood. An exception is blood type O, called the universal donor, because people of all blood types can accept it. Incompatible blood types can cause a serious adverse reaction (transfusion reaction). Blood is introduced slowly by gravity flow directly into the veins (intravenous infusion) so that medical personnel can observe the patient for signs of adverse reactions. People who have received many transfusions can develop an immune response to some factors in foreign blood cells. Though many efforts are made to ensure a safe blood supply, infectious diseases can occasionally be transmitted through donated blood.

Each year in the United States, about 14,000,000 pints of blood are donated. Blood collection is strictly regulated by the Food and Drug Administration (FDA). The FDA has rules for the collection, processing, storage, and transportation of blood and blood products. In addition, the American Red Cross, the American Association of Blood Banks, and most states have specific rules for the collection and processing of blood. The main purpose of regulation is to ensure the quality of blood and to prevent the transmission of infectious diseases through donated blood. Before blood and blood products are used, they are extensively tested for infectious agents, such as hepatitis and **AIDS**.

Autologous transfusion is a procedure in which patients donate blood for their own use. Patients who are to undergo surgical procedures for which a blood transfusion might be required may elect to donate a store of blood for the purpose ahead of time. Directed donors are family or friends of the patient who needs a transfusion. Blood that is not used for the identified patient becomes part of the general blood supply.

TRAUMATIC AMPUTATIONS

Traumatic **amputation** is the accidental severing of some or all of a body part. A complete amputation totally detaches a limb or appendage from the rest of the body. In a partial amputation, some soft tissue remains attached to the site. Traumatic amputation most often affects limbs and appendages like the arms, ears, feet, fingers, hands, legs, and nose.

Trauma is the second leading cause of amputation in the United States. About 30,000 traumatic amputations occur in this country every year. Four of every five traumatic amputation victims are male, and most of them are between the ages of 15–30. Farm and factory workers have greater-than-average risks of suffering injuries that result in traumatic amputation. Automobile and motorcycle accidents and the use of lawnmowers, saws, and power tools are also common causes of traumatic amputation.

Blood loss may be massive or minimal, depending on the nature of the injury and the site of the amputation. Patients who lose little blood and have less severe injuries sometimes feel more **pain** than patients who bleed heavily and whose injuries are life-threatening.

When the patient and the amputated part(s) reach the hospital, an Emergency Department physician will assess the probability that the severed tissue can be successfully reattached. The Mangled Extremity Severity Score (MESS) assigns numerical values to such factors as body temperature, circulation, numbness, **paralysis**, tissue health, and the patient's age and general health. This is one of the diagnostic tools used to determine how successful reattachment surgery is apt to be. The total score is doubled if blood supply to the amputated part has been absent or diminished for more than six hours. A general, emergency, or orthopedic surgeon makes the final determination about whether surgery should be performed. The surgeon also considers the patient's wishes and lifestyle. Additional concerns are how and to what extent the amputation will affect the patient's quality of life and ability to perform everyday activities.

First aid or emergency care given immediately after the amputation has a critical impact on both the physicians' ability to salvage and reattach the severed part(s) and the patient's ability to regain feeling and function. Muscle tissue dies quickly, but a well-preserved part can be successfully reattached as much as 24 hours after the amputation occurs. Tissue that has not been preserved will not survive for more than six hours.

The most important steps to take when a traumatic amputation occurs are:

- Contact the nearest emergency services provider, clearly describe what has happened, and follow any instructions given.
- Make sure the victim can breathe; administer CPR if necessary.
- Control bleeding, using direct pressure but minimizing or avoiding contact with blood and other body fluids.
- Patients should not be moved if back, head, leg, or neck injuries are suspected or if motion causes pain. If none are found by the EMT, lie the victim flat, with the feet raised 12 inches above the surface.
- Cover the victim with a coat or blanket to prevent **shock**.

The injured site should be cleansed with a sterile solution and wrapped in a clean towel or other thick material that will protect the wound from further injury. Tissue that is still attached to the body should not be forced back into place. If it cannot be gently replaced, it should be held in its normal position and supported until additional care is available.

Saving the patient's life is always more important than recovering the amputated part(s). Transporting the patient to a hospital or emergency center should never be delayed until missing pieces are located. No amputated body part is too small to be salvaged. Debris or other contaminating material should be removed, but the tissue should not be allowed to get wet. An amputated body part should be wrapped in bandages, towels, or other clean, protective material and sealed in a plastic bag. Placing the sealed bag in a cooler or in a container that is inside a second container filled with cold water or ice will help prevent tissue deterioration.

Possible complications of traumatic amputation include:

- Excessive bleeding
- Infection
- Muscle shortening
- **Pulmonary embolism**.

About 80% of all amputees over the age of four experience tingling, **itching**, numbness, or pain in the place where the amputated part used to be. Phantom sensations may begin immediately after the amputation, or they may develop months or years later. They often occur after an injury to the site of the amputation.

These intermittent feelings may:

- Occur frequently or only once in a while
- Be mild or intense
- Last for a few minutes or several hours
- Help patients adjust more readily to an artificial limb (prosthesis).

The best way to prevent traumatic amputation is to observe common-sense precautions like using seat belts and obeying speed limits and other traffic regulations. It is important to take special precautions when using potentially dangerous equipment and make sure machinery is turned off and disconnected before attempting to service or repair it. Appropriate protective clothing should be worn at all times.

See also Amputation

TREMORS

Tremor is an unintentional (involuntary), rhythmical alternating movement that may affect the muscles of any part of the body. Tremor is caused by the rapid alternating contraction and relaxation of muscles and is a common symptom of diseases of the nervous system (neurologic disease). Occasional tremor is felt by almost everyone, usually as a result of fear or excitement. However, uncontrollable tremor or shaking is a common symptom of disorders that destroy nerve tissue such as **Parkinson's disease** or **multiple sclerosis**. Tremor may also occur after **stroke** or **head injury**. Other tremor appears without any underlying illness.

The cause of essential tremor not linked to any other problem, is not known, although it is an inherited problem in more than half of all cases. The genetic condition has an autosomal dominant inheritance pattern, which means that any children of an affected parent will have a 50% chance of developing the condition. Essential tremor most often appears when the hands are being used, whereas a person with Parkinson's disease will most often have a tremor while walking or while the hands are resting. People with essential tremor will usually have shaking head and hands, but the tremor may involve other parts of the body. The shaking often begins in the dominant hand and may spread to the other hand, interfering with eating and writing. Some people also develop a quavering voice. Essential tremor affects men and women equally. The shaking often appears at about age 45, although the disorder may actually begin in adolescence or early adulthood. Essential tremor that begins very late in life is sometimes called "senile tremor."

Several different classes of drugs can cause tremor as a side effect. These drugs include amphetamines, **antidepressant drugs**, **antipsychotic drugs**, **caffeine**, and lithium. Tremor also may be a sign of withdrawal from alcohol or street drugs.

Close attention to where and how the tremor appears can help provide a correct diagnosis of the cause of the shaking. The source of the tremor can be diagnosed when the underlying condition is found. Diagnostic techniques that make images of the brain, such as **computed tomography scan** (CT scan) or **magnetic resonance imaging** (MRI), may help form a diagnosis of multiple sclerosis or other tremor caused by disorders of the central nervous system. Blood tests can rule out metabolic causes such as thyroid disease. A family history can help determine whether the tremor is inherited.

Neither tremor nor most of its underlying causes can be cured. Most people with essential tremor respond to drug treatment, which may include propranolol, primidone, or a benzodiazepine. People with Parkinson's disease may respond to levodopa or other antiparkinson drugs.

Research has shown that about 70% of patients treated with botulinum toxin A (Botox) have some improvement in tremor of the head, hand, and voice. Botulinum is derived from the bacterium *Clostridium botulinum*. This bacterium causes **botulism**, a form of **food poisoning**. It is poisonous because it weakens muscles. A very weak solution of the toxin is used in cases of tremor and **paralysis** to force the muscles to relax. However, some patients experience unpleasant side effects with this drug and cannot tolerate effective doses. For other patients, the drug becomes less effective over time. About half of patients don't get relief of tremor from medications at all.

Tremor control therapy is a type of treatment using mild electrical pulses to stimulate the brain. These pulses block the brain signals that trigger tremor. Some patients experience complete relief with this technique, but for others it is of no benefit at all. About 5% of patients experience complications from the surgical procedure, including bleeding in the brain. The procedure causes some discomfort, because patients must be awake while the implant is placed. Batteries must be replaced by surgical procedure every three to five years.

A patient with extremely disabling tremor may find relief with a surgical technique called thalamotomy, in which the surgeon destroys part of the thalamus. However, the procedure is complicated by numbness, balance problems, or speech problems in a significant number of cases. Pallidotomy is another type of surgical procedure sometimes used to decrease tremors from Parkinson's disease. In this technique, the surgeon destroys part of a small structure within the brain called the globus pallidus internus. The globus is part of the basal ganglia, another part of the brain that helps control movement. This surgical technique also carries the risk of disabling permanent side effects.

See also Multiple sclerosis; Parkinson's disease

TRICHINOSIS

Trichinosis, a disease caused by the parasitic intestinal roundworm *Trichinella spiralis* (trichinae), is contracted by warm-blooded mammals through ingestion of raw or undercooked meat infected by trichinae. Pork and bear meat are primary sources of human infection; beaver, opossums, rats, walruses and whales can also carry the parasite. Infected animals remain asymptomatic; however, symptoms in humans—which can begin as soon as five or a late as 45 days after exposure—can range from asymptomatic to death. Symptoms include fluid retention in the upper eyelids, diarrhea, physical weakness, excessive thirst and sweating, chills, fever, muscle pain, anorexia, breathing difficulties, and perhaps even kidney and heart damage. Severity depends upon the number of parasites ingested. Although trichinosis is found in some grain-fed pigs, swine fed on garbage containing infected meat scraps is the primary source of human trichinosis. In 1954, a campaign to cook garbage before feeding it to swine was implemented in the United States. Inspection of meat in packing plants also helps prevent human infection.

Trichinosis was discovered in 1835 by James Paget, a 21-year-old, first-year medical student in London who, during an autopsy, noticed tiny specks in the muscle tissue of an Italian man. Under a microscope, they turned out to be tiny cysts housing worm larvae which were given their name by his professor. The first record of trichinae in meat for human consumption was in 1846 when Philadelphian physician, Joseph Leidy, noticed tiny specks in a slice of pork he was eating and recalled seeing similar specks in human muscle tissue just days earlier. Under the microscope, they were indeed trichinae. In the 1850s, German scientists Rudolf Leuckart and Rudolph Virchow found the parasite was transmitted animal-to-animal through ingestion of infected meat or feces. Not until 1860, however, was trichinosis found to cause severe illness and death in humans when German physician, Friedrich A. von Zenker, discovered the parasite during an autopsy of a young servant woman. Tracing her illness, he found she had tasted raw pork sausage before cooking it for Christmas dinner. Although her employers also became sick, the effect was less severe because cooking reduced the number of parasites. von Zenker sent samples of the girl's tissue to Leuckart and Virchow, who traced the complete life cycle of the parasites.

Trichinae larvae migrate to muscle tissue and form a housing, or cyst. The larvae in these cysts hatch into adult worms only after coming into contact with digestive juices in the stomach. The hatched larvae pass into the intestines, mate, and reproduce. One female adult worm can produce up to 1,500 larvae, which then penetrate the intestines, enter the blood stream, pass through the heart, and travel throughout the entire body. They invade the voluntary muscle tissue, feed for about three weeks, coil up tightly, develop their protective housing, and lie dormant—often for many years—until their host dies. If the host tissue is ingested by another animal or a human, contact with the digestive juices causes the larvae to hatch and the life cycle begins again. Although antiparasitic medications will kill adult worms and intestinal larvae, once larvae enter the muscle tissue, they are there for the life of the host and treatment can only relieve symptoms. Experimental studies of *Thiabendazole* in animals do show reduction in both muscle and intestinal infections, however, and the drug has been used in a few human cases. The only sure way to prevent infection is to cook meat—particularly pork—until the internal temperature is at least 171°F (76.4°C), or freeze it at -13 °F (-24.8°C) for 10 to 20 days.

TRICHOMONIASIS

Trichomoniasis refers to an infection of the genital and urinary tract caused by a protozoa (the smallest, single-celled members of the animal kingdom). *Trichomonas vaginalis*. This infection is passed almost 100% of the time through sexual contact and, occurs more often in individuals who have multiple sexual partners. The protozoan is passed to an individual by contact within the body fluids of an infected sexual partner. It often occurs simultaneously with other sexually transmitted diseases, especially **gonorrhea**.

In women, the symptoms of trichomoniasis include an unpleasant vaginal odor, and a heavy, frothy, yellow discharge from the vagina. The genital area (vulva) is often very itchy, and there is frequently **pain** with urination or with sexual intercourse. The labia (lips) of the vagina, the vagina itself, and the cervix (the narrowed, lowest segment of the uterus which extends into the upper part of the vagina) will be bright red and irritated.. A woman is most susceptible to infection just after having completed her menstrual period.

Men may carry the organism unknowingly, since infection in men may cause mild or no symptoms. Occasionally, a man will notice a small amount of yellowish discharge from his penis, usually first thing in the morning. There may be some mild discomfort while urinating.

Diagnosis is easily made by taking a sample of the discharge from the woman's vagina, or from the opening of the man's penis. The sample is put on a slide, and viewed under a microscope. The protozoa, which are able to move about, are easily viewed. Usual treatment is a single large dose of metronidazole or split doses over the course of a week. Sexual partners of an infected individual must all be treated, to prevent the infection being passed back and forth.

Cure of trichomoniasis may be difficult to achieve with alternative treatments. Some practitioners suggest eliminating sweets and carbohydrates from the diet and supplement with antioxidants, including **vitamins** A, C, and E, and zinc. Naturopaths may recommend treatment with two douches (a wash used inside the vagina), alternating one in the morning and one at bedtime. One douche contains the herbs calendula (*Calendula officinalis*), goldenseal (*Hydrastis canadensis*), and echinacea (*Echinacea* spp.); the other douche contains plain yogurt. The herbal douche helps to kill the protozoa, while the yogurt reestablishes healthy flora in the vagina. Acidifying the vagina by douching with boric acid or vinegar may also be useful.

Prognosis is excellent with appropriate treatment of the patient and all sexual partners. Without treatment, the infection can smolder on for a very long time, and can be passed to all sexual partners. All sexually transmitted diseases can be prevented by using adequate protection during sexual intercourse. Effective forms of protection include male and female **condoms**.

See also Gonorrhea; Sexually transmitted diseases

TRIGLYCERIDES TEST

Triglycerides test is a blood test to determine the amount of triglycerides, a form of fat, in the blood. The triglycerides test is one of the screening tests for excess lipids (fats) in the blood. It is usually part of an evaluation of risk factors for heart disease. High levels of triglycerides in the blood can mean that there is too much fat in the diet. Hypertriglyceridemia (high levels of triglycerides) is associated with coronary heart disease, especially since elevated triglycerides levels are often associated with unhealthy low levels of hyper-density lipoproteins (the ''good'' cholesterol), which are necessary for good health.

For triglycerides testing, blood is drawn from a vein in the arm. A vein at the inside of the elbow or on the back of the hand is usually selected. The area where the needle will be inserted is cleaned with antiseptic. A small needle is inserted through the skin and into the vein, allowing a small amount of blood to flow into a collection tube or syringe. Once the blood is collected, the needle is removed from the puncture site.

Before the blood test, the patient may be required to refrain from eating food for 8–12 hours. Patients should not drink alcohol for 24 hours before the test. Some drugs may affect the test and the patient may be asked to cease taking certain medications before the test. **Oral contraceptives**, estrogen, and cholestyramine (a drug used to treat high cholesterol) can increase triglyceride levels. Ascorbic acid (vitamin C), asparaginase (an enzyme), and various drugs used to treat high blood lipids, can decrease blood triglyceride levels. These substances should not be taken prior to this test.

After the blood sample has been taken and the needle withdrawn from the puncture site, a cotton ball or gauze pad may be placed over the site and direct pressure applied to reduce bleeding. A piece of surgical tape or gauze adhesive bandage strip may be secured over the site to prevent further bleeding.

The normal range of triglycerides in the blood depends on the age and gender of the patient. Women naturally have higher levels of triglycerides than men. **Pregnancy** can also increase triglyceride levels. As people age and gain weight, triglyceride levels generally increase. For adults, a normal level is considered to be less than 200 mg/dl (milligrams per deciliter). Levels from 200-400 mg/dL are considered borderline high. Triglyceride levels ranging from 400-1000 mg/dL are considered high and levels greater than 1000 mg/dL are considered very high. High levels of triglycerides may indicate liver disease (**cirrhosis**), an under-active thyroid problem, uncontrolled diabetes, an infection of the pancreas (**pancreatitis**), kidney disease, or a diet too low in protein and too high in carbohydrates.

Extremely low triglycerides levels (less than 10 mg/dL) can also indicate a problem. Low levels may indicate **malnutrition** (not enough nutrients in the diet), malabsorption (inadequate absorption of nutrients in the intestinal tract), a diet too low in fat, or an over-active thyroid problem.

TROPICAL MEDICINE

Tropical medicine has been notoriously difficult to define because so few illnesses are limited to the tropics, and so many are found there. Be that as it may, tropical medicine is concerned mainly with a number of parasitic and other infectious diseases that are responsible for major health problems in low-income tropical countries. For example, **malaria** causes one million deaths per year, mostly in children under five in Africa. In certain villages of Zaire and Angola, trypanosomiasis (**sleeping sickness**) affects 70-80% of inhabitants. **Leprosy** is synonymous with stigma, and new treatment regimens offer hope that it will soon be controlled. But it still afflicts between one and two million people in the world, mostly in Asia, Africa, and Latin America. Fifteen million poor people in 73 countries suffer from gross enlargement of the limbs, a symptom of chronic filarial disease.

Many of these so-called tropical diseases also existed in Europe and North America until relatively recently. In the Middle Ages leprosy was epidemic throughout Europe, and malaria was endemic in swampy regions in the United States and Europe into the 20th century. In the summer of 1793 an epidemic of **yellow fever** forced the United States government to relocate from Philadelphia to New York. Although other conditions, like epilepsy, can occur anywhere, in the tropics they are found at a higher rate as a result of parasitic infections. In addition, the changing epidemiology of diseases such as **polio**, now under control in temperate climates, emphasizes their importance in the tropics.

Tropical medicine as a discipline was established by colonial powers, mainly England, France, and the Netherlands, to protect their citizens in the colonies; it was essentially colonial medicine. Later, tropical medicine became concerned with the health of local populations in the tropics. This trend increased dramatically with the independence of the former colonies in the 1960s. Travel medicine, a branch of tropical medicine, continues the focus on the health of outsiders visiting the tropics. International health considers the broader questions that concern populations of the tropics, focusing on health and development, rather than the treatment of individual cases of particular diseases. Clinical tropical medicine is a subspecialty of infectious diseases dealing with selected parasitic and fewer bacterial (e.g., leprosy) and viral (e.g., yellow fever) pathogens. Outside tropical regions, clinical tropical medicine is mainly the concern of travel medicine and infectious disease specialists. Within the tropics, tropical medicine is for the most part indistinguishable from general medicine.

Research efforts in tropical medicine comprise both basic and applied research. Basic research concentrates on pathogens and vectors — that is, organisms that carry infectious agents from one host to another — in the disciplines of immunology, molecular biology, and other biological life sciences. Applied research aims to generate drugs, **vaccines**, and other approaches to treatment and prevention. Because of the respective level of investment required and anticipated returns, it is easier to find support for basic research than applied research for most tropical diseases. Whereas basic research yields important contributions to science, applied research requires major inputs that are less likely to earn financial rewards for investors from the impoverished affected populations.

Current priorities in tropical medicine and international health are focused on control or eradication (where possible) of tropical diseases with three basic approaches: (1) better treatments for clinical tropical medicine (e.g., drugs and surgery); (2) disease-specific **public health** interventions (e.g., vaccines, vector control, insected-impregnated bednets to kill the mosquitoes that carry malaria, and so on); and (3) general development efforts to reduce the burden of tropical diseases (e.g., **sanitation**, hygiene, and decreasing poverty). These last measures were most effective in eliminating tropical diseases from Europe and North America.

Although the role of ''tropical medicine'' as it is traditionally understood is presently the subject of a lively debate, an argument could be made for its viability on the following grounds: It continues to provide a focus on major diseases of low-income countries that would otherwise be neglected because applied research lacks commercial potential. Tropical diseases are closely linked to problems of international health and needs for general development. In the overall scope of the discipline, the initial focus on the health of outsiders is now less of a priority.

See also Epidemic and pandemic; Filariasis; Infection control; Preventive medicine

TUBAL LIGATION

Tubal ligation is a permanent voluntary form of birth control (**contraception**) in which a woman's Fallopian tubes are surgically cut or blocked off to prevent **pregnancy**. Tubal ligation is performed in women who definitely want to prevent future pregnancies. It is frequently chosen by women who do not want more children, but who are still sexually active and potentially fertile, and want to be free of the limitations of other types of birth control. Women who should not become pregnant for health concerns or other reasons may also choose this birth control method. Tubal ligation is one of the leading methods of contraception, having been chosen by over 10 million women in the United States— about 15% of women of reproductive age. The typical tubal ligation patient is over age 30, is married, and has had 2-3 children.

Tubal ligation should be postponed if the woman is unsure about her decision. While it is sometimes reversible, the procedure should be considered permanent and irreversible. Up to 10% of sterilized women regret having had the surgery, and about 1% seek treatment in attempts to restore fertility.

The Fallopian tubes, which are about 10 cm long and 0.5 cm in diameter, are found on the upper outer sides of the uterus, and open into the uterus through small channels. It is within the Fallopian tube that fertilization, the joining of the egg and the sperm, takes place. During tubal ligation, the tubes are cut or blocked in order to close off the sperm's access to the egg. Normally, tubal ligation takes about 20-30 minutes, and is performed under general **anesthesia**, spinal anesthesia, or local anesthesia with sedation. The surgery can be performed on either hospitalized patients within 24 hours after **childbirth** or on outpatients. The woman can usually leave the hospital the same day. Tubal ligation costs about $2,000 when performed by a private physician, but is less expensive when performed at a family planning clinic. Most insurance plans cover treatment costs.

Preparation for tubal ligation includes patient education and counseling. Before surgery, it is important that the woman understand the permanent nature of tubal ligation, and the risks of anesthesia and surgery. Her medical history is reviewed, and a **physical examination** and laboratory testing are performed. The patient is not allowed to eat or drink for several hours before surgery.

After surgery, the patient is monitored for several hours before she is allowed to go home. She is instructed on care of the surgical wound, and what signs to watch for, such as **fever**, nausea, vomiting, faintness, or **pain**. These signs could indicate that complications have occurred. While major complications are uncommon after tubal ligation, there are risks with any surgical procedure. Possible side effects include infection and bleeding. Rarely, **death** may occur as a complication of general anesthesia if a major blood vessel is cut. The death rate following tubal ligation is about 4 per 100,000 sterilizations.

After having her tubes ligated, a woman does not need to use any form of birth control to avoid pregnancy. Tubal ligation is almost 100% effective for the prevention of conception. The possibility for treatment failure is very low— fewer than 1 in 200 women (0.4%) will become pregnant during the first year after sterilization. Failure can happen if the cut ends of the tubes grow back together; if the tube was not completely cut or blocked off; if a plastic clip or rubber band is loose or comes off; or if the woman was already pregnant at the time of surgery.

See also Contraception

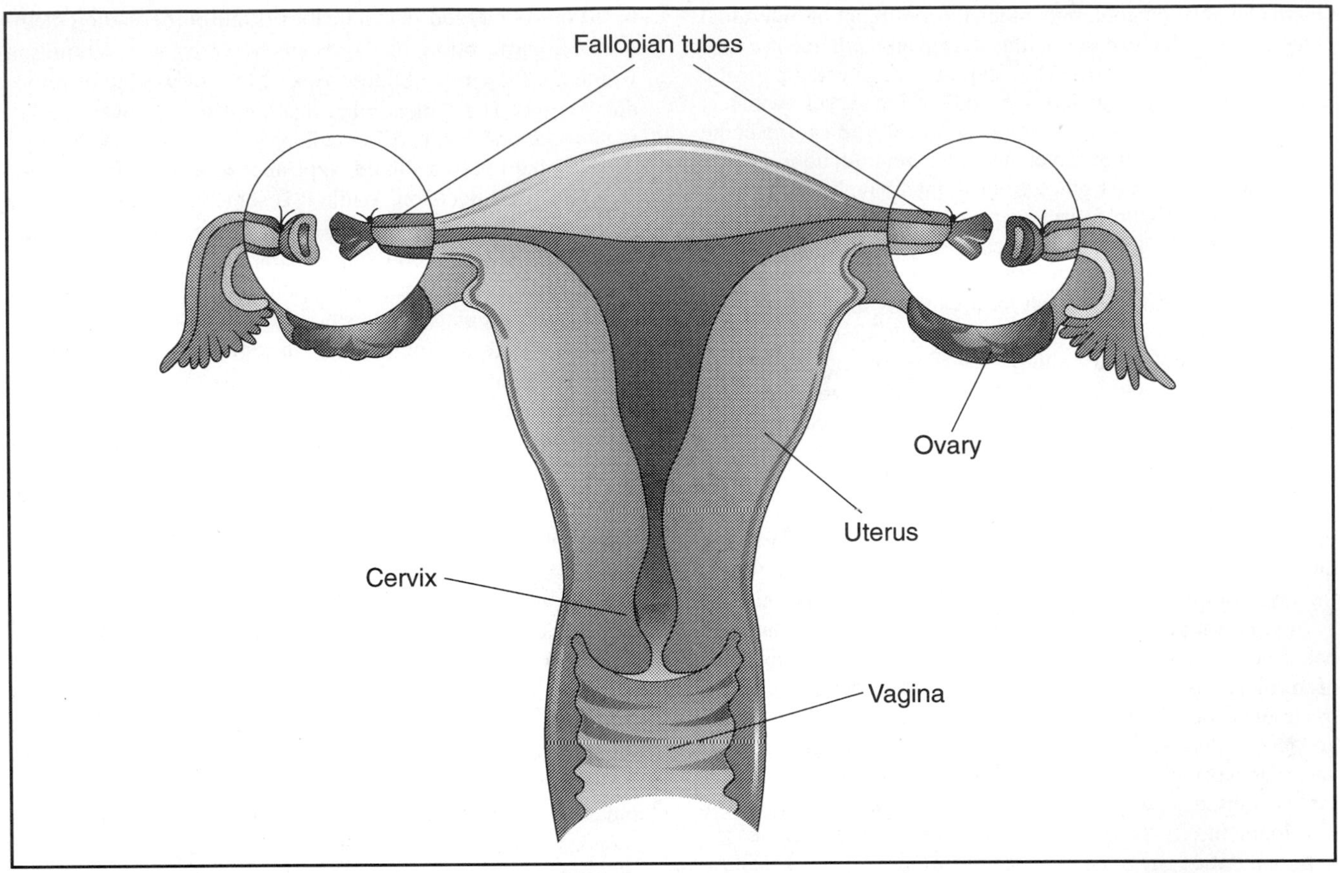

Tubal ligation is a permanent form of contraception in which a woman's Fallopian tubes are surgically cut, cauterized, tied, or blocked to prevent pregnancy. This procedure blocks the pathway sperm takes to fertilize an egg. ***(Illustration by Electronic Illustrators Group.)***

TUBE FEEDINGS

Nutrients, either a special liquid formula or pureed food, are delivered to a patient through a tube directly into the gastrointestinal tract, usually into the stomach or small intestine. Tube feeding provides nutrition to patients who are unable or unwilling to eat food. Conditions where tube feeding is considered include **protein-energy malnutrition**, liver or kidney failure, **coma**, or in patients who cannot chew or swallow (dysphagia) due to **stroke**, **brain tumor**, or **head injury**. Patients who are receiving radiation therapy or **chemotherapy** treatments for **cancer** may also be candidates for tube feedings.

A flexible, narrow tube is inserted into some portion of the digestive tract and liquid formulas or liquefied foods are placed into the tube to meet the patient's nutritional needs. The feeding may be pumped into the tube or allowed to drip into the tube continuously or at scheduled feeding times.

A feeding tube can be inserted by a surgical or nonsurgical procedure in several positions along the gastrointestinal tract. The tube may be inserted into the nose and passed down the throat and through the esophagus. A nasogastric tube is inserted through the nose with the end of the tube reaching into the stomach. A nasoduodenal or nasojejunal tube is inserted through the nose and ends in either the duodenum or jejunum, both of which are portions of the small intestine. This type of tube placement is usually used for short term feeding. Surgical placement of a feeding tube may be done if there will be a long term need for feeding that bypasses the upper digestive tract. An esophagostomy creates an opening in the esophagus, a gastrostomy creates an opening into the stomach, and a jejunostomy creates an opening into the jejunum. The feeding tube is then inserted through the surgically-created opening.

Tube feedings can be a mixture of regular foods which are blended with liquid to make a consistency which will pass through the tube. Nutritionally balanced liquid products are often more convenient to use and ensure a balance of proteins, fats, and carbohydrates along with **vitamins** and **minerals**. Specialized formulas are also available to meet almost any nutritional need. For example, patients with severe **burns**, protein-energy malnutrition, or slow wound healing may require formulas that are higher in protein. Patients with renal failure may require low protein formulas with lower concentrations of minerals and vitamins.

Patients with ostomy feeding tubes may have the tube positioned level with the surrounding skin. A cap or button can be placed over the opening so that it can be more comfortably concealed under clothing. The opening and surrounding tissue need to be cleaned and inspected regularly to prevent infec-

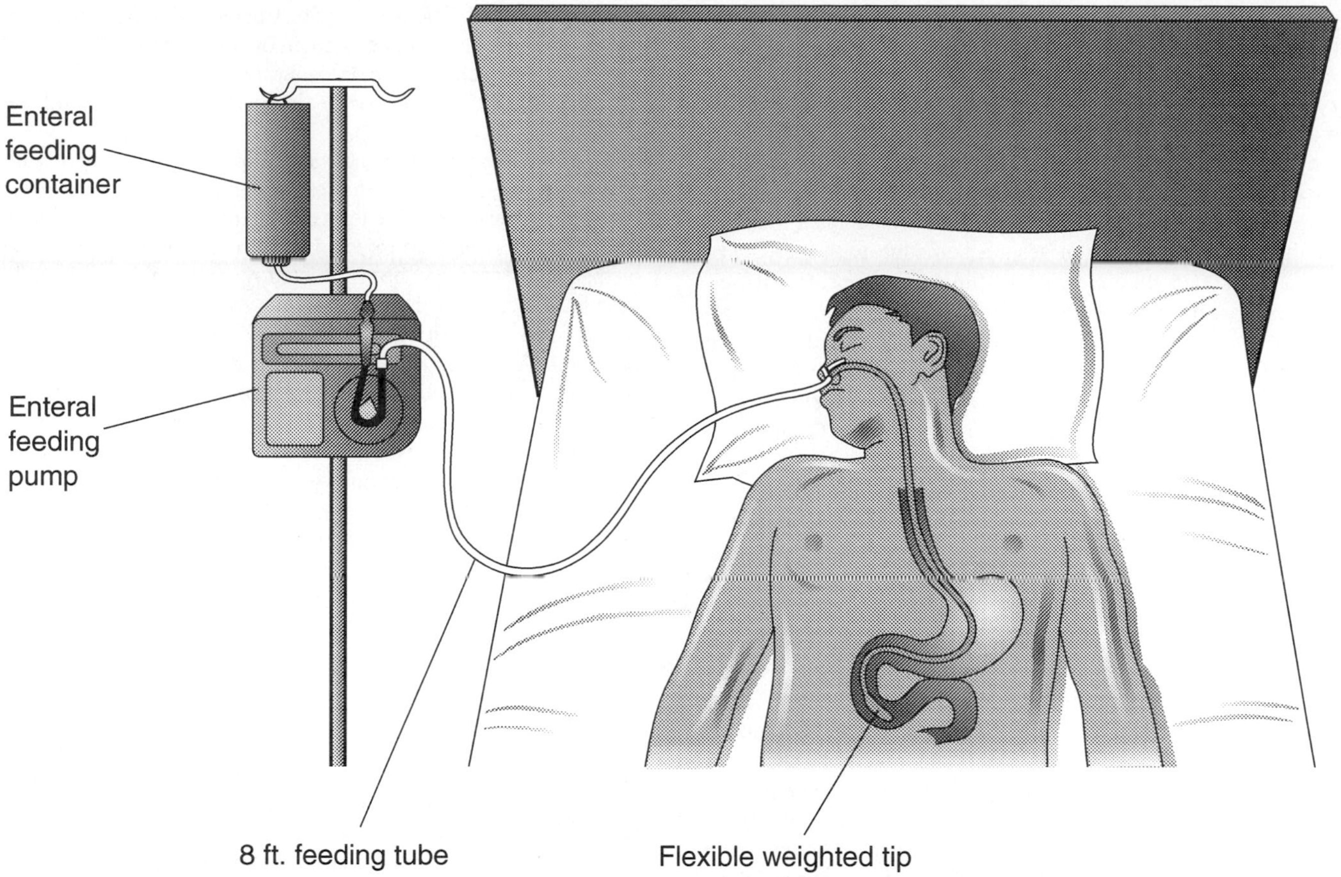

A feeding tube can be inserted by a surgical or nonsurgical procedure in several positions along the gastrointestinal tract to provide nutrition to patients who are unable or unwilling to eat food. The feeding may be pumped into the tube or allowed to drip into the tube continuously, or at scheduled feeding times. The illustration above features a nasojejunal tube which is inserted through the nose and ends in either the duodenum or jejunum. *(Illustration by Electronic Illustrators Group.)*

tion. For patients with a tube inserted through the nose, daily nasal hygiene is important and the mouth and lips should be kept moist. Good mouth care is necessary for any patient with a feeding tube.

Formula from the tube can back-up in the esophagus and be breathed into the trachea and lungs causing aspiration **pneumonia**. The placement of the tube should be checked frequently and the head of the bed elevated during and after feeding to prevent the solution from moving back up the digestive tract. Feeding tubes can also become clogged and need to be flushed regularly with water. If the feeding formula is too concentrated or given too fast, the patient may experience nausea, vomiting, cramping, and bloating. The feeding may need to be diluted with liquid or the rate at which it is given decreased. **Diarrhea** or **constipation** can occur if the feeding is not the right composition or does not provide enough liquid. The tube itself can irritate the nasal passage, esophagus, or surrounding tissues.

A patient may be able to transition back to a normal diet of solid foods after short term supplementation with formula through a feeding tube. In cases where long term nutritional therapy is required, all of the patient's nutritional needs will have to be provided by the formula. The balance of fluids, calories, proteins, fats, vitamins, and minerals may need to be adjusted periodically.

See also Malnutrition

Tuberculin skin test

Tuberculosis (TB) is an airborne infectious disease caused by the bacteria *Mycobacterium tuberculosis*. The two most common types of tests to screen for this disease are the Mantoux PPD tuberculin skin test, which is generally considered the most reliable, and the TB tine test. A diagnosis of tuberculosis is never made based on the results of a TB skin test, but requires further testing including a **sputum culture** and a **chest x ray**.

Because TB is spread through the air, especially in poorly ventilated areas, it is more commonly found among people living in crowded conditions, such as jails, nursing homes, and homeless shelters. Often, a TB skin test will be given as part of a **physical examination** when a person is hiring a new employee, particularly for those individuals seeking employment in the healthcare or food service professions.

People can be exposed to TB without showing any symptoms or necessarily developing the disease. Individuals with normally functioning immune systems generally prevent the spread of the bacteria by "walling off" or encysting the bacteria within the body. Anyone who has had close contact with someone who has active tuberculosis (such as a friend or family member); has been around someone with active TB; has a weakened immune system (immunocompromised), either from a chronic disease, such as HIV infection, or as a result of a tissue or organ transplant or other medical treatment designed to suppress the immune system; or displays symptoms of the disease should be tested. Symptoms include a persistent **cough**, **fever**, weight loss, night sweats, fatigue, and loss of appetite.

Although generally considered safe, it is important to inform the person conducting the test if you may be pregnant, have had a positive TB test in the past, or have had tuberculosis in the past. People who have had a positive TB test in the past will probably always have a positive test and should not be tested again. Also, anyone who is known to have active TB should not be tested because the local reaction to the test may be so severe that it requires surgical care.

TB skin tests are usually given at a clinic, hospital, or doctor's office. Sometimes the tests are given at schools or workplaces. Many cities provide free TB skin tests and follow-up care. The Mantoux PPD tuberculin skin test involves injecting a very small amount of a substance called PPD tuberculin just under the top layer of the skin (intracutaneously). Tuberculin is a mixture of antigens obtained from the culture of *M. tuberculosis*. Antigens are foreign particles or proteins that stimulate the immune system to produce antibodies. The test is usually given on the inside of the forearm about halfway between the wrist and the elbow, where a small bubble will form as the tuberculin is injected. The skin test takes just a minute to administer and feels more like a pinprick than a shot.

After 48-72 hours, the test site will be examined by a trained person for evidence of swelling. People who have been exposed to tuberculosis will develop an immune response, causing a slight redness or swelling at the injection site. Reactions may not peak until after 72 hours in elderly individuals or those who are being tested for the first time. If there is a lump or swelling, the health care provider will use a ruler to measure the size of the reaction.

The other method of TB skin test is called the multiple puncture test or tine test because the small test instrument has several small tines that lightly prick the skin. The small points of the instrument are either coated with dried tuberculin or are used to puncture through a film of liquid tuberculin. The test is read by measuring the size of the largest papule. Because it is not possible to precisely control the amount of tuberculin used in the tine test, a positive test should be verified using the Mantoux test. For this reason, the tine test is not as widely used as the Mantoux test and is considered to be less reliable.

After having a TB skin test, it is extremely important to make sure that the patient keeps the appointment to have the test reaction read. The patient is instructed to keep the test site clean, uncovered, and to not scratch or rub the area. Should severe swelling, **itching**, or **pain** occur, or if the patient has trouble breathing, the clinic or health care provider should be contacted immediately.

In people who have not been exposed to TB, there will be little or no swelling at the test site after 48-72 hours. This is a negative test. Negative tests can be interpreted to mean that the person has not been infected with the tuberculosis bacteria or that the person has been infected recently and not enough time has elapsed for the body to react to the skin test. Persons become sensitive between two and ten weeks after the initial infection. As a result, if the person has been in contact with someone with tuberculosis, the test should be repeated in three months. Also, because it may take longer than 72 hours for an elderly individual to develop a reaction, it may be useful to repeat the TB skin test after one week to adequately screen these individuals. Immunocompromised persons may be unable to react sufficiently to the Mantoux test, and either a chest x ray or sputum sample may be required.

TUBERCULOSIS

Tuberculosis (TB) is a potentially fatal contagious disease that can affect almost any part of the body but is mainly an infection of the lungs. It is caused by a bacterial microorganism, the tubercle bacillus or *Mycobacterium tuberculosis*. Although TB can be treated, cured, and can be prevented if persons at risk take certain drugs, scientists have never come close to wiping it out. Few diseases have caused so much distressing illness for centuries and claimed so many lives.

Tuberculosis was popularly known as consumption for a long time. In 1882, the microbiologist Robert Koch discovered the tubercle bacillus, at a time when one of every seven **death**s in Europe was caused by TB. Because **antibiotics** were unknown, the only means of controlling the spread of infection was to isolate patients in private sanitoriums or hospitals limited to patients with TB—a practice that continues to this day in many countries. When streptomycin, the first antibiotic effective against *M. tuberculosis*, was discovered in the early 1940s, the infection began to come under control. Although other more effective anti-tuberculosis drugs were developed in the following decades, the number of cases of TB in the United States began to rise again in the mid-1980s. This upsurge was in part again a result of overcrowding and unsanitary conditions in the poor areas of large cities, prisons, and homeless shelters. Infected visitors and immigrants to the United States also contributed to the resurgence of TB. An additional factor is the **AIDS** epidemic. AIDS patients are much more likely to develop tuberculosis because of their weakened immune systems.

Tuberculosis is more common in elderly persons. More than one-fourth of the nearly 23,000 cases of TB reported in the United States in 1995 developed in people above age 65. Many elderly patients developed the infection some years ago when the disease was more widespread. There are additional reasons for the vulnerability of older people: those living in nursing homes and similar facilities are in close contact with others who may be infected. The aging process itself may weaken the body's immune system, which is then less able to ward off the tubercle bacillus. Finally, bacteria that have lain dormant for some time in elderly persons may be reactivated and cause illness.

TB also is more common in blacks, who are more likely to live under conditions that promote infection. Alcoholics and intravenous drug abusers are also at increased risk of contracting tuberculosis. Until the economic and social factors that influence the spread of tubercular infection are remedied, there is no real possibility of completely eliminating the disease.

Tuberculosis spreads by droplet infection. This type of transmission means that when a TB patient exhales, **cough**s, or sneezes, tiny droplets of fluid containing tubercle bacilli are released into the air. This mist, or aerosol as it is often called, can be taken into the nasal passages and lungs of a susceptible person nearby. Unlike many other infections, TB is not passed on by contact with a patient's clothing, bed linens, or dishes and cooking utensils. The most important exception is **pregnancy**. The fetus of an infected mother may contract TB by inhaling or swallowing the bacilli in the amniotic fluid.

Once inhaled, tubercle bacilli may reach the small breathing sacs in the lungs (the alveoli), where they are taken up by cells called macrophages. The bacilli multiply within these cells and then spread through the lymph vessels to nearby lymph nodes. Sometimes the bacilli move through blood vessels to distant organs. At this point they may either remain alive but inactive (quiescent), or they may cause active disease. At least nine of ten patients who harbor *M. tuberculosis* do not develop symptoms or physical evidence of active disease, and their x-rays remain negative. They are not contagious; however, they do form a pool of infected patients who may get sick at a later date and then pass on TB to others.

Pulmonary tuberculosis is TB that affects the lungs. Its initial symptoms are easily confused with those of other diseases. An infected person may at first feel vaguely unwell or develop a cough blamed on smoking or a cold. A small amount of greenish or yellow sputum may be coughed up when the person gets up in the morning. In time, more sputum is produced that is streaked with blood. Persons with pulmonary TB do not run a high **fever**, but they often have a low-grade one. They may wake up in the night drenched with cold sweat when the fever breaks. The patient often loses interest in food and may lose weight. Chest **pain** is sometimes present. If the infection allows air to escape from the lungs into the chest cavity (**pneumothorax**) or if fluid collects in the pleural space (pleural effusion), the patient may have difficulty breathing. If a young adult develops a pleural effusion, the chance of tubercular infection being the cause is very high.

Although the lungs are the major site of damage caused by tuberculosis, many other organs and tissues in the body may be affected. The usual progression is for the disease to spread from the lungs to locations outside the lungs (extrapulmonary sites). In some cases, however, the first sign of disease appears outside the lungs. The many tissues or organs that tuberculosis may affect include the skin, bones, and joints; kidneys and female reproductive organs; abdominal cavity and intestines; and the meninges (tissues that cover the brain and the spinal cord). Miliary TB is a life-threatening condition that occurs when large numbers of tubercle bacilli spread throughout the body. Huge numbers of tiny tubercular lesions develop that cause marked weakness and weight loss, severe anemia, and gradual wasting of the body.

The diagnosis of TB is made on the basis of laboratory test results. Often, the first indication of TB is an abnormal chest x-ray or other test result rather than physical discomfort. On a chest x ray, evidence of the disease appears as numerous white, irregular areas against a dark background, or as enlarged lymph nodes. A PPD, the **tuberculin skin test** is always done to show whether the patient has been infected by the tubercle bacillus. To verify the test results, the physician obtains a sample of sputum or a tissue sample (biopsy) for culture.

The prognosis for recovery from TB is good for most patients, if the disease is diagnosed early and given prompt treatment with appropriate medications on a long-term regimen. Modern surgical methods have a good outcome in most cases in which they are needed. Miliary tuberculosis is still fatal in many cases but is rarely seen today in developed countries.

Vaccination is one major preventive measure against TB. A vaccine called BCG (Bacillus Calmette-Guérin, named after its French developers) is made from a weakened mycobacterium that infects cattle. Vaccination with BCG does not prevent infection by *M. tuberculosis* but it does strengthen the immune system of first-time TB patients. As a result, serious complications are less likely to develop.

See also Tuberculin skin test

TULAREMIA

Tularemia is an illness caused by a bacteria. It results in **fever**, rash, and greatly enlarged lymph nodes.

Tularemia infects a variety of wild animals, including rabbits, deer, squirrels, muskrat, and beaver. Humans can acquire the bacteria directly from contact with the blood or body fluids of these animals, from the bite of a tick or fly which has previously fed on the blood of an infected animal, or from contaminated food or water.

Tularemia occurs most often in the summer months. It is most likely to infect people who come into contact with infected animals, including hunters, furriers, butchers, laboratory workers, game wardens, and veterinarians. In the United States, the vast majority of cases of tularemia occur in the southeastern and Rocky Mountain states.

Five types of illness may occur, depending on where/how the bacteria enter the body:

- Ulceroglandular/Glandular tularemias comprise 75-85% of all cases. This type is contracted through the bite of an infected tick that has defecated bacteria-laden feces in the area of the bite wound. A tender red bump appears in the area of the original wound. Over a few weeks, the bump develops a punched-out center (ulcer). Nearby lymph nodes grow hugely swollen and very tender. The lymph nodes may drain a thick, pus-like material. Other symptoms include fever, chills, and weakness. In adults, the lymph nodes in the groin are most commonly affected; in children, the lymph nodes in the neck.

- Oculoglandular tularemia accounts for only about 1% of all cases of tularemia. It occurs when a person's contaminated hand rubs his or her eye. The lining of the eyelids and the surface of the white of the eye becomes red and severely **pain**ful, with multiple small yellow bumps and pitted sores (ulcers). Lymph nodes around the ears, under the jaw, or in the neck may swell and become painful.
- Oropharyngeal and Gastrointestinal tularemia occurs when contaminated meat is undercooked and then eaten, or when water from a contaminated source is drunk. Poor hygiene after skinning and cleaning an animal obtained through hunting can also lead to the bacteria entering through the mouth. Sores in the mouth and throat, as well as abdominal pain, nausea and vomiting, ulcers in the intestine, intestinal bleeding, and **diarrhea** may all occur.
- Pulmonary tularemia is rare, but it occurs when a person inhales a spray of infected fluid, or when the bacteria reach the lungs through the blood circulation. A severe **pneumonia** follows.
- Typhoidal tularemia is particularly hard to diagnose, because it occurs without the usual skin manifestations or swelling of lymph glands. Symptoms include continuously high fever, terrible **headache**, and confusion. The illness may result in a severely low blood pressure, with signs of poor blood flow to the major organs (**shock**).

To diagnose tularemia, samples are prepared from the **skin lesions** with special stains, to allow identification of the causative bacteria under the microscope. Other tests are available to demonstrate the presence of antibodies (special immune cells which the body produces in response to the presence of specific foreign invaders) which would be increasing over time in an infection with tularemia.

Streptomycin (given as a shot in a muscle) and gentamicin (given as either a shot in a muscle or through a needle in the vein) are both used to treat tularemia. Other types of **antibiotics** have been tested, but have often resulted in relatively high rates of relapse (20%).

With treatment, **death** rates from tularemia are under 1%. Without treatment, however, the death rate may reach 30%. The pneumonia and typhoidal types have the worst prognosis without treatment.

Prevention involves avoiding areas known to harbor ticks and flies, or the appropriate use of insect repellents. Hunters should wear gloves when skinning animals or preparing meat. Others (butchers, game wardens, veterinarians) who work with animals or carcasses should always wear gloves. A vaccine exists, but is usually only given to people at very high risk due to their profession or hobby (veterinarians, laboratory workers, butchers, hunters, game wardens).

TUMOR REMOVAL

Tumor removal is a surgical procedure to remove an abnormal growth.

A tumor can be either benign, like a wart, or malignant, in which case it is a **cancer**. Benign tumors are well circumscribed and are generally easy to remove completely. In contrast, cancers pose some of the most difficult problems in all of surgery.

Currently 40% of all cancers are treated with surgery alone. In 55%, surgery is combined with other treatments—usually radiation therapy or **chemotherapy**.

The doctor needs to decide if surgery should be done at all. Because cancers spread (metastasize) to normal tissues, sometimes at the other end of the body, the ability of surgery to cure must be addressed at the outset. As long as the cancer is localized, the initial presumption is that cure should be attempted by removing it as soon as possible.

Non-curative surgery may make other treatments more effective. ''Debulking'' a cancer—making it smaller—is thought to assist radiation and chemotherapy to get to the remaining pieces of the cancer and be more effective.

Another important function surgery performs in cancer treatment is accurately assessing the nature and extent of the cancer. Most cancers cannot be adequately identified without a piece being placed under a microscope. This piece is obtained by surgery. Surgery is also the only way to determine exactly how far the tumor has spread. There are a few standard methods of comparing one cancer to another for the purposes of comparing treatments and estimating outcomes. These methods are called ''staging.'' The most universal method is the TNM system.

- ''T'' stands for ''tumor'' and reflects the size of the tumor.
- ''N'' represents the spread of the cancer to lymph nodes, largely determined by those nodes removed at surgery that contain cancer cells. Since cancers spread mostly through the lymph system, this is a useful measure of their ability to disperse.
- ''M'' refers to the metastases, how far they are from the original cancer and how often they have multiplied.

Other methods of staging include Duke's method and similar systems, which add to the above criteria the degree of invasion of the cancer into the surrounding tissues.

Staging is particularly important with lymphomas such as **Hodgkin's disease**. These cancers may appear in many places in the lymphatic system. Because they are very radiosensitive, radiation treatment is often curative if all the cancer is irradiated. Therefore, it must all be located. Surgery is a common, usually essential, method of performing this staging. If the disease is too widespread, the staging procedure will dictate chemotherapy instead of radiation.

Curative cancer surgery demands special considerations. There is a danger of spreading or seeding the cancer during the process of removing it. Presuming the cancer cells can grow almost anywhere in the body they end up, the surgeon must not ''spill'' cells into the operating field or ''knock them loose'' into the blood stream. Special techniques called ''block resection'' and ''no touch'' are used. Block resection means taking the entire specimen out as a single piece. ''No touch'' means that only the normal tissue removed with specimen is handled; the cancer itself is never touched. This prevents ''squeezing'' cancer cells out into the circulation. Further, in this technique pains are taken to clamp off the blood supply first, preventing cells from leaving by that route later in the surgery.

To diagnose cancer, four types of biopsy techniques are used:

- Aspiration biopsy. A needle is inserted into the tumor and a sample is withdrawn.
- Needle biopsy. A special cutting needle is inserted into the core of the tumor and a core sample is cut out.
- Incisional biopsy. A portion of a large tumor is removed, usually before complete tumor removal.
- Excisional biopsy. A whole lesion is removed along with surrounding normal tissue.

Once surgical removal has been decided, an oncologic surgeon will remove the tumor whole, taking with it a large section of the surrounding normal tissue. The healthy tissue is removed to minimize the risk of possible seeding.

When surgical removal of a tumor is unacceptable as a sole treatment, a portion of the tumor is removed to ''debulk'' the mass. Debulking aids radiation and chemotherapy treatments.

Retesting and periodical examinations are necessary to ensure that a tumor has not reformed after total removal.

The possibility of mestastasis and seeding are risks that have to be considered in consultation with an oncologist.

TYPHOID FEVER

Typhoid fever is a life-threatening disease of the intestinal system caused by the typhoid bacillus, *Salmonella typhosa*, which lives only in humans who carry it in their bloodstream and intestinal tract. Typhoid fever is spread when the bacteria is ''shed'' by infected people who handle food or fluids without washing their hands, or when sewage carrying the bacteria contaminates water, milk, and other foods. Although relatively rare since the advent of vaccines and improvement of public sanitation (about 400 cases are reported annually in the United States, 70% of which are acquired through international travel), typhoid fever was once common and still arises in impoverished areas of the world where squalid conditions prevail and medical treatment is unavailable. Symptoms of the disease become evident within one to two weeks after infection and include sore throat, fever, headache, nausea, and loss of appetite, which are sometimes followed by the appearance of red spots on the chest and abdomen and, in severe cases, delirium and death. As the bacteria invade the intestines, they cause ulcerations and bleeding. This can lead to holes in the intestines and the bacteria can invade the bloodstream and sometimes spread to the bone marrow or spinal cord causing **meningitis**. The fever generally lasts three to four weeks and then subsides.

Treatment for typhoid includes cold sponge baths to lower the fever and plenty of liquids to avoid dehydration. **Antibiotics**, such as chloramphenicol, are also effective.

One of the first clinical descriptions of typhoid fever was made by English physician Thomas Willis (1621-1675). French physician Pierre-Fidèle Bretonneau (1778-1862) was the first to accurately describe the progression of the disease in 1819. He went on to detail a typhoid epidemic in France, and reported that the disease was transmitted by contact with other contaminated people. Bretonneau also distinguished between typhoid fever and a form of **typhus** that were often mistaken.

Almroth Edward Wright, an English physician, conducted research in blood coagulation and developed a vaccine against typhoid fever in 1889. The vaccine was effective when tested on soldiers during the Boer War. During World War I, British soldiers were the only ones vaccinated and their incidence of typhoid fever was greatly reduced. Wright went on to conduct important work in bacteriology and was knighted in 1906.

Scottish physician William Boog Leishman (1865-1926) is also credited with developing a vaccine against typhoid fever which was effectively used during the war. Much later, during the 1960s and 1970s, Margaret Pittman and others were involved with comparative studies of typhoid vaccines.

Researchers learned that the disease was spread through contaminated food and that, often, carriers of the disease showed no symptoms. Such was the case of Mary Mallon (1870?-1938), a cook who earned the nickname Typhoid Mary because she carried the bacillus for typhoid fever. Josephine Baker, a pioneer in public sanitation, succeeded in tracking down Mallon and from 1907 until 1910 the cook was hospitalized while experts attempted, unsuccessfully, to eradicate the bacillus. She was then released with the understanding that she would report for regular testing and also find a new profession. Mallon subsequently disappeared and, after a five-year hiatus, was once again apprehended and quarantined for the remainder of her life.

TYPHUS

Throughout history, battles and wars have been lost due to typhus epidemics that spread among soldiers fighting in unsanitary conditions. After World War I, 25 million people in the Soviet Union alone were infected with the disease. People forced to live in crowded, filthy, rodent-infested neighborhoods also suffered untimely deaths from the disease.

Howard Taylor Ricketts, an American pathologist born in Findlay, Ohio in 1871, is credited with discovering the genus Rickettsia, the cause of the disease, during his studies of Rocky Mountain spotted fever, which he noticed resembled typhus. In 1910, Ricketts traveled to Mexico City to study typhus, which he found was transmitted by a body louse. But his research had tragic results. Before he could return to the United States where he had accepted a position at the University of Pennsylvania, Ricketts died of typhus, the very disease he was studying.

At the same time, the curiosity of French physician Charles-Jean-Henri Nicolle's (1866-1936) was aroused by the contagious aspects of typhus, which he had witnessed while working at the Pasteur Institute in Tunis, Tunisia. Outside the hospital, the disease was caught on contact. Hospital admission employees also caught it, but once inside the hospital, the patient no longer seemed contagious.

He began to suspect body lice as the carriers when he realized the patients were stripped and scrubbed down when they entered the hospital. His work with animals proved his suspicions. Nicolle won the 1928 Nobel Prize in physiology or medicine for his work on typhus. Nicolle, the son of a Rouen physician, was born in 1866 and practiced medicine in Paris and Rouen until deafness began to interfere with his effectiveness in treating patients. In 1903, he moved to Tunis where he remained until his death in 1936.

Epidemic typhus is carried by lice. This disease, caused by *R. prowazekii*, was responsible for millions of deaths in eastern Europe and the Balkan countries after World War I and World War II. It devastated military troops during World War I, but during World War II, DDT was used to kill the lice carrying the disease. *R. prowazekii* also causes recrudescent epidemic typhus, a disease which is reactivated years after an initial bout of epidemic typhus.

After an incubation period of about one week, a person infected with typhus develops a headache, chills, prostration, and fever up to 104° F. Other symptoms include a rash, conjunctivitis (inflammation of the mucous membrane that lines the inner surface of the eyelids and covers the forepart of the eyeball), and a dry cough. In severe cases, there is renal failure and mental confusion. Death occurs in 10 to 50 percent of the cases, and the mortality rate increases if the victim is over 60 years old. However, under medical supervision, drug therapy can be very effective.

Murine endemic typhus is caused by *R. typhi*, a microorganism carried by a rat flea. It occurs worldwide and was once common in the southeastern United States. When the rat flea cannot find a natural host, it feeds on humans. During the feeding, it drops infected feces which, when rubbed into a break in the skin, give rise to the disease.

The incubation period of murine endemic typhus is one to two weeks. The infected person initially develops a headache, malaise, backache, and chills. Later, typhus causes shaking, chills, fever up to 103° F, severe headache, vomiting, and nausea. Eventually a rash appears in the armpits and inner surface of the upper arms and moves to the trunk, thighs and lower arms. After the rash disappears, a dry cough develops. Murine endemic typhus is fairly mild compared to other diseases caused by *rickettsia*. It can be treated with tetracyclines, but even untreated, death rarely results.

The typhus vaccine, developed by **Hans Zinsser** in 1932, is based on dead microorganisms which stimulate the body's **immune system** to produce antibodies to the antigens carried on the surfaces of the dead cells. The immune system also produces ''memory cells'' which remain in the body to trigger a rapid response in the event of reinfection. Since the vaccine uses dead organisms, the reaction is mild and there is no risk of the patient contracting the disease. Inoculation, **antibiotics** and control of rats and lice have combined to greatly reduce the incidence of typhus throughout the world.

U

ULCERS (DIGESTIVE)

In general, an ulcer is any eroded area of skin or a mucous membrane, marked by tissue disintegration. In common usage, however, ulcer is usually used to refer to disorders in the upper digestive tract. The terms ulcer, gastric ulcer, and peptic ulcer are often used loosely and interchangeably. Peptic ulcers can develop in the lower part of the esophagus, the stomach, the first part of the small intestine (the duodenum), and the second part of the small intestine (the jejunum).

It is estimated that 2% of the adult population in the United States has active peptic ulcers, and that about 10% will develop ulcers at some point in their lives. There are about 500,000 new cases of peptic ulcer in the United States every year, with as many as 4 million recurrences. The male/female ratio for ulcers of the digestive tract is 3:1.

The most common forms of peptic ulcer are duodenal and gastric. About 80% of all ulcers in the digestive tract are duodenal ulcers. This type of ulcer may strike people in any age group but is most common in males between the ages of 20 and 45. Gastric ulcers account for about 16% of peptic ulcers. They are most common in males between the ages of 55 and 70. The single most common cause of gastric ulcers is the use of **nonsteroidal anti-inflammatory drugs**, or NSAIDs. The widespread use of NSAIDs is thought to explain why the incidence of gastric ulcers in the United States is rising.

There are two major causes of peptic ulcers: *Helicobacter pylori*infection and certain types of medication.

Helicobacter pylori is a rod-shaped bacterium that lives in the mucous tissues that line the digestive tract. Infection with *H. pylori* is the most common cause of duodenal ulcers. About 95% of patients with duodenal ulcers are infected with *H. pylori*.

Nonsteroidal anti-inflammatory drugs, or NSAIDs, are painkillers that many people use for **headache**s, sore muscles, arthritis, menstrual cramps, and similar complaints. Many NSAIDs are available without prescriptions. Common NSAIDs include **aspirin**, ibuprofen (Advil, Motrin), flurbiprofen (Ansaid, Ocufen), ketoprofen (Orudis), and indomethacin (Indacin). Chronic NSAID users have 40 times the risk of developing a gastric ulcer as nonusers. Aspirin is most likely to cause ulcers.

Smoking increases a patient's chance of developing an ulcer, decreases the body's response to therapy, and increases the chances of dying from ulcer complications.

The symptoms of gastric ulcers include feelings of **indigestion** and heartburn, weight loss, and repeated episodes of gastrointestinal bleeding. Ulcer pain is often described as gnawing, dull, aching, or resembling hunger pangs. The patient may be nauseated and suffer loss of appetite.

The symptoms of duodenal ulcers include heartburn, stomach pain relieved by eating or **antacids**, weight gain, and a burning sensation at the back of the throat. The patient is most likely to feel discomfort two to four hours after meals, or after having citrus juice, coffee, or aspirin.

Not all digestive ulcers produce symptoms; as many as 20% of ulcer patients have so-called painless or silent ulcers. Silent ulcers occur most frequently in the elderly and in chronic NSAID users.

Between 10–20% of peptic ulcer patients develop complications at some time during the course of their illness. All of these are potentially serious conditions. Complications are not always preceded by diagnosis of or treatment for ulcers; as many as 60% of patients with complications have not had prior symptoms.

Bleeding is the most common complication of ulcers. It may result in anemia, vomiting blood, or the passage of bright red blood through the rectum. About half of all cases of bleeding from the upper digestive tract are caused by ulcers. The mortality rate from ulcer hemorrhage is 6–10%.

About 5% of ulcer patients develop perforations, which are holes in the duodenal or gastric wall through which the stomach contents can leak out into the abdominal cavity. The incidence of perforation is rising because of the increased use of NSAIDs, particularly among the elderly. The signs of an ulcer perforation are severe pain, **fever**, and tenderness when the doctor touches the abdomen. Most cases of perforation require emergency surgery. The mortality rate is about 5%.

The diagnosis of peptic ulcers is rarely made on the basis of a **physical examination** alone. The only significant finding may be mild soreness in the area over the stomach when the doctor presses it. The doctor is more likely to suspect an ulcer if the patient has one or more of the following risk factors:

- Male sex
- Age over 45
- Recent weight loss, bleeding, recurrent vomiting, **jaundice**, back pain, or anemia
- History of using aspirin or other NSAIDs
- History of heavy smoking
- Family history of ulcers or **stomach cancer**.

An endoscopy is considered the best procedure for diagnosing digestive ulcers and for taking samples of stomach tissue for biopsies. An endoscope is a slender tube-shaped instrument that allows the doctor to view the tissues lining the stomach and duodenum. Duodenal ulcers are rarely malignant.

Most doctors presently recommend treatment to eliminate *H. pylori* in order to prevent ulcer recurrences. Without such treatment, ulcers recur at the rate of 80% per year. The usual regimen used to eliminate the bacterium is a combination of tetracycline, bismuth subsalicylate (Pepto-Bismol), and metronidazole (Metizol).

The prognosis for recovery from ulcers is good for most patients. Very few ulcers fail to respond to the medications that are currently used to treat them.

Strategies for the prevention of ulcers or their recurrence include the following:

- Eradication of *H. pylori* in patients already diagnosed with ulcers
- Avoiding unnecessary use of aspirin and NSAIDs
- Giving up smoking
- Cutting down on alcohol, tea, coffee, and sodas containing **caffeine**.

ULTRASOUND TESTS

Ultrasound (or sonogram) technology allows doctors to ''see'' inside a patient without resorting to surgery. A transmitter sends high-frequency sound waves into the body, where they bounce off the different tissues and organs to produce a distinctive pattern of echoes. A receiver ''hears'' the returning echo pattern and forwards it to a special computer, which translates the data into an image on a television screen. Ultrasound is better than x rays at distinguishing subtle variations between soft, fluid-filled tissues, so it is particularly useful in providing diagnostic images of the abdomen, breast, eye, pelvis, scrotum, and thyroid. Unlike x rays, it does not damage tissues with ionizing radiation. Improvements in the technology, application, and interpretation of ultrasound continue. Its low cost, portability, versatility, safety, and speed have made it a popular medical imaging technique. Ultrasound remains faster and less expensive than **computed tomography scans** (CT), its primary rival.

Ultrasound technology can also be used for treatment purposes. The direct therapeutic value of ultrasonic waves lies in their mechanical nature. They are shock waves, just like audible sound, and vibrate the materials through which they pass. These vibrations are mild and virtually unnoticeable at the frequencies and intensities used for imaging. However, strongly focused, high-intensity, high-frequency ultrasound can also be used to destroy certain types of tumors, as well as gallstones. High-intensity ultrasound is useful for treating soft tissue injuries, such as strains, tears and associated scarring; the heating and agitation they cause are believed to promote rapid healing through increased circulation. Ultrasound is most frequently used therapeutically as a visual aid during surgical procedures—such as guiding needle placement to drain fluid from a cyst, or to extract tumor cells for analysis.

Ultrasound is valuable for finding the reason for abdominal pain, which can signal anything from organ malfunction or injury to malignant growths. In the case of abdominal trauma, such as after a car crash or a fall, ultrasound can pinpoint the location, cause, and severity of hemorrhaging or locate a foreign object, such as a bullet.

In breast ultrasound, the sound waves pass through the breast and bounce back or echo from various tissues to form a picture of the internal structures. Its most common application is to investigate a specific area of the breast where a problem is suspected. A palpable lump and/or an abnormality discovered on an x ray (mammogram) can be further evaluated by ultrasound. It is especially helpful in distinguishing between a fluid-filled cyst and a solid mass such as a tumor.

Breast ultrasound is often the first step taken to evaluate masses in women under 35 whose mammograms can be difficult to interpret because of their denser breast tissue. The lack of radiation used with ultrasound also makes it ideal for studying breast abnormalities in women who are pregnant, and it is effective in assessing breast implants for leakage or rupture. Breast inflammation, where pockets of infection or **abscess**es may form, can be diagnosed and monitored by ultrasound.

Ultrasound imaging equipment also allows eye specialists (ophthalmologists) to ''see'' the eye in great detail without the **pain** and risk of exploratory surgery or the limitations and uncertainty inherent in traditional visual examination. Ultrasound is used to detect and diagnose many eye diseases and injuries, to measure the eye prior to corrective surgery, and to treat problems. When presented with general symptoms, ultrasound can speed diagnosis if a serious condition is suspected. A special type of ultrasound, known as Doppler, can even perceive and measure circulation in the tiny blood vessels of the eye.

Ultrasound can reveal the exact type, extent, and location of damage in the eye, from deformations and ruptures to internal bleeding, and so can assist emergency care efforts. Ophthalmic ultrasound imaging is also used routinely to guide the precise placement of instruments during surgery, and can be used directly for the treatment of **glaucoma** and tumors of the eye.

Pelvic ultrasound is most commonly performed during **pregnancy**. Early in the pregnancy, it might be used to determine the size of the uterus or the fetus, to detect multiple or **ectopic pregnancy**, to confirm that the fetus is alive, or to confirm the due date. Toward the middle of the pregnancy, ultrasound can confirm fetal growth, reveal anatomical defects, and check the placenta. Toward the end of pregnancy, it can evaluate fetal size, position, and growth. Doctors may also use ultrasound to guide them during diagnostic procedures like amniocentesis and chorionic villus sampling. Both of these tests use long needles inserted through the mother's abdomen into the uterus or placenta to gather cells.

Scrotal ultrasound is an imaging technique used to diagnose suspected abnormalities of the scrotum. It is the primary imaging method used to evaluate disorders of the testicles and surrounding tissues, such as an absent or undescended testicle, an inflammation problem, a fluid collection, abnormal blood vessels, or a mass.

Thyroid ultrasound is an imaging technique used for diagnosing suspected thyroid disease, such as a goiter. The thyroid gland is an organ located in front of the neck that plays an important role in controlling the body's metabolism. Specialized thyroid ultrasounds, such as color Doppler flow studies, can add valuable information. By showing an image of the blood circulation in the gland, this study can assess some ambiguous masses in greater detail to further refine diagnosis.

Ultrasound studies may also be done periodically to assess the response of the thyroid gland to medical therapy. Patients who have received therapeutic radiation to the head or neck are also monitored at regular intervals using thyroid ultrasound, since they have a higher risk of **thyroid cancer** and other abnormalities.

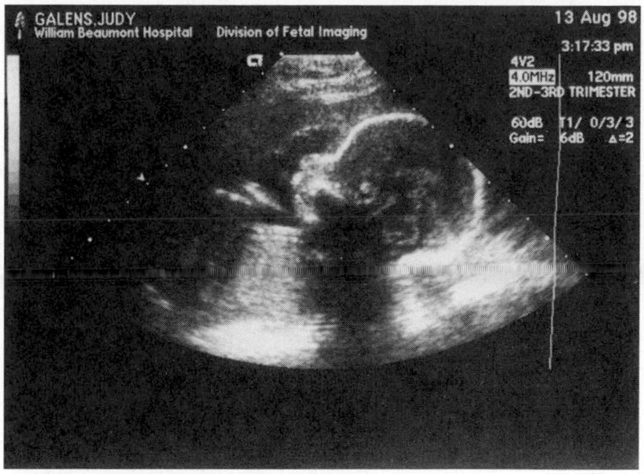

Ultrasound image of young Graham Galens Narins, in profile.

ULTRAVIOLET LIGHT TREATMENT

Ultraviolet light treatment uses a particular band of the nonvisible light spectrum to treat **psoriasis** and a variety of other skin diseases. It can be used alone or in combination with other medications applied directly to the skin or taken internally.

Ultraviolet (UV) light treatment is used primarily in cases of severe psoriasis that have not responded to other medications or in cases affecting large portions of the body. Patients will typically receive a series of 3–5 weekly treatments for a month or more to bring their psoriasis symptoms into check. They may also receive periodic maintenance treatments to prevent recurrence of their psoriasis. Other skin conditions treated with UV light treatments are **vitiligo**, a condition in which people lose pigmentation in large patches of their skin, and atopic dermatitis, an allergy-related skin condition that produces itchy, reddish, and scaly patches of skin.

Exposure to UV radiation is known to prematurely age the skin over time and increase the risk of skin **cancer**. These potential effects should be weighed against the potential benefits of the treatment. A history will be taken regarding sun exposure and burning, medications, such as **diuretics**, that may increase UV sensitivity exposure, and any history of skin cancers. Sometimes, UV light treatments are given in combination with photosensitizing agents, which maximize UV's effects on the skin. Patients who receive these agents, called psoralens, must take care to avoid exposure to sunlight, which also contains UV radiation. Exposure to UV radiation can also cause **cataracts** and other eye damage, so the patient's eyes must be adequately shielded during the treatments.

UV light treatment can employ one of two bands of the ultraviolet spectrum: ultraviolet A (UVA), and ultraviolet B (UVB). Patients receive full body treatments in special light boxes; smaller areas of the skin are sometimes treated with hand-held devices.

Psoriasis is the most common skin disease treated with UVB light treatment. Its mechanism of action remains unclear, but investigators speculate it may kill abnormal skin cells or alter immune system reactions in the skin. Most patients require 18–30 treatments before substantial improvement or complete clearing is seen. The intensity of the UV applied will vary depending on the patient's skin type. Fair-skinned patients will start with a relatively weaker dose; dark-skinned patients, a stronger dose.

The Goeckerman regimen, a treatment that combines UVB light with coal tar applied to the skin, is among the oldest and most frequently used treatments for patients with moderate to severe psoriasis. The coal tar is a photosensitizing agent, and, when it interacts with UVB, it appears to limit the abnormal turnover of skin cells characteristic of psoriasis.

Another kind of treatment involves psoralens, which are photosensitizing agents found in plants. They have been known since ancient Egypt but have only been available in a chemically synthesized form since the 1970s. Psoralens are taken systemically or can be applied directly to the skin. The psoralens allow a relatively lower dose of UVA to be used. When they are combined with exposure to UVA in PUVA, they are highly effective at clearing psoriasis.

Choosing the proper dose for PUVA is similar to the procedure followed with UVB. The physician can choose a dose based on the patient's skin type. Often, however, a small area of the patient's skin will be exposed to UVA after ingestion of psoralen. The dose of UVA that produces uniform redness 72 hours later becomes the starting dose for treatment.

Some patients experience nausea and **itching** after ingesting the psoralen compound. For these patients ''bath PUVA'' may be a good option.

No major preparation is required for UV light treatments. Areas of the skin that are especially sensitive to the effects of UV light, such as the groin, backside, or face, are shielded during the treatments. Areas not affected by psoriasis are also covered. Special goggles are worn to protect the eyes.

No major aftercare is required following UV light treatments. Patients, however, must take great care to limit or eliminate other exposures to UV radiation, such as from sunlight or tanning beds, because of the increased risk of premature aging of the skin and the development of skin cancers.

People who receive UV light treatments are at higher risk of premature aging of the skin, and of developing skin cancer. These risks should be balanced against the benefits of treatment.

Psoriasis will normally show significant improvement to complete healing with three to five UVB treatments a week for about four to five weeks. PUVA treatments may require a bit longer to take effect, but because the overall dosage of UV is lower, they are thought by some investigators to be a safer alternative to UVB treatments.

Modern light boxes carefully control the dosage of UV radiation and the exposure time. Overdose or overexposure is possible, however, and can lead to severe **burns**. It is important to choose a treatment provider who is experienced in the technique. It is also important to tell the physician about all medications being taken by the patient.

UNDESCENDED TESTES

Also known as cryptorchidism, undescended testes is a congenital condition characterized by testicles that do not extend to the scrotum.

In the fetus, the testes are in the abdomen. As development progresses, they migrate downward through the groin and into the scrotum. This event takes place late in fetal development, during the eighth month of gestation. Thirty percent of premature boys have testes that have not yet made the full descent. Only 3–4% of fullterm baby boys have undescended testes, and half of those complete the journey by the age of three months. Eighty percent of all undescended testes cases naturally correct themselves during the first year of life. Undescended testes that are not corrected can lead to sterility and an increased risk of **testicular cancer**.

The cause of undescended testes is presently unknown; however its symptoms are quite apparent. One or both of the testicles can be undescended, making the testicles appear missing or lopsided.

One form of diagnosis is the newborn examination, in which the doctor always checks for testes in the scrotum. If they are not found, a search will be conducted, but not necessarily right away. In most cases, the testes will drop into place later. If the testes are present at all, they can be anywhere within a couple inches of the appropriate spot. In 5% of cases, one testis is completely absent. In 10%, the condition occurs on both sides. Presence of undescended testes is indicated by measuring the amount of gonadotropin hormone in the blood.

Once doctors determined that the testes will not naturally descend, surgery becomes necessary. The procedure is called an orchiopexy and is relatively simple once the testes are located. The surgery is usually performed when the boy is between one to two years old.

Undescended testes must be treated to eliminate the increased risk of testicular cancer and the possibility of sterility. Undescended testes are twice as likely to develop **cancer**. Ten percent of all testicular cancers are in undescended testes.

URINALYSIS

Urinalysis is a diagnostic physical, chemical, and microscopic examination of a urine sample (specimen). Specimens can be obtained by normal emptying of the bladder (voiding) or by a hospital procedure called catheterization.

Urinalyses are performed for several reasons:

- General evaluation of health.
- Diagnosis of metabolic or systemic diseases that affect kidney function.
- Diagnosis of endocrine disorders. Twenty-four-hour urine studies are often ordered for these tests.
- Diagnosis of diseases or disorders of the kidneys or urinary tract.
- Monitoring of patients with diabetes.
- Testing for **pregnancy**.
- Screening for drug abuse.

Urinalysis should not be performed while a woman is menstruating or having a vaginal discharge. A woman who must have a urinalysis while she has a vaginal discharge or is having her period should insert a fresh tampon before beginning the test. She should also hold a piece of clean material over the entrance to her vagina to avoid contaminating the specimen.

Patients do not have to fast or change their food intake before a urine test. They should, however, avoid intense athletic training or heavy physical work before the test because it may result in small amounts of blood in the urine.

The following drugs can affect urinalysis results. The patient may be asked to stop taking them until after the test:

- Nitrofurantoin (Macrodantin, Furadantin). Nitrofurantoin is prescribed for infections of the urinary tract and other bacterial infections.
- Phenazopyridine (Pyridium). This medication is used to relieve burning and **pain** caused by urinary-tract infections.
- Rifampin (Rifadin). This medication is prescribed to treat **tuberculosis**, prevent the spread of **meningitis**, and treat other infections.

Bladder catheterization is sometimes used to collect urine samples from hospitalized patients. It should not, however, be used to collect specimens from males with acute inflammation of the prostate or from a patient of either sex with a fractured pelvis.

Collecting a urine sample from emptying the bladder takes about two or three minutes. The sample can be collected at home as well as in a doctor's office. Urine specimens are usually collected early in the morning before breakfast. Urine collected eight hours after eating and at least six hours after the most recent urination is more likely to indicate abnormalities. Some people may be asked to void into a clean container before getting out of bed in the morning.

The doctor or hospital will supply a sterile container for a specimen being collected for a colony count. A colony count is a test that detects bacteria in urine that has been cultured for 24–48 hours. It is used instead of a routine urinalysis when a patient's symptoms suggest a urinary tract infection. Nonsterile containers can be used for routine specimens that will not be tested immediately after being collected. An ordinary open-necked jar may be used after it and its lid have been soaked in very hot water for 15–20 minutes and then air-dried.

Urine specimens should not remain unrefrigerated for longer than two hours. A urine specimen that cannot be delivered to a laboratory within two hours should be stored in a refrigerator. The reason for this precaution is that urine samples undergo chemical changes at room temperature. Blood cells begin to dissolve and the urine loses its acidity.

A doctor, nurse, or laboratory technician will look at the specimen to see if the urine is red, cloudy, or looks unusual in any way. He or she will also note any unusual odor.

Urine samples are tested with a variety of different instruments and techniques. Some tests use dipsticks, which are thin strips of plastic that change color in the presence of specific substances. Dipsticks can be used to measure the acidity of the urine (its pH) or the presence of blood, protein, sugar, or substances produced during the breakdown of fatty acids (ketones). A urinometer is used to compare the density of the urine specimen with the density of plain water. This measurement is called specific gravity.

The urine specimen is also examined under a microscope to determine whether it contains blood cells, crystals, or small pieces of fibrous material (casts).

Most urine specimens from adults or older children are collected by the patient's voiding into a suitable container. Soaps and disinfectants may contaminate urine specimens and should not be used. The doctor or laboratory may supply a special antiseptic solution that won't irritate the skin. The method for collection varies somewhat according to age and sex.

Before collecting a urine sample, a woman or girl should use a clean cotton ball moistened with lukewarm water to cleanse the external genital area. Gently separating the folded skin (labia) on either side of her vagina, she should move the cotton ball from the front of the area to the back. After repeating this process several times, using a fresh piece of cotton each time, she should dry the area with a clean towel.

To prevent menstrual blood, vaginal discharge, or germs from the external genitalia from contaminating the specimen, a woman or girl should release some urine before she begins to collect her sample. A urine specimen obtained this way is called a midstream clean catch.

A man or boy should use a piece of clean cotton, moistened with antiseptic, to cleanse the head of his penis and the passage through which urine leaves his body (the urethral meatus). He should draw back his foreskin if he has not been circumcised. He should move the cotton in a circular motion away from the urinary opening, using a fresh piece of cotton each time. After repeating this process several times, he should use a fresh piece of cotton to remove the antiseptic. After the area has been thoroughly cleansed, he should begin urinating and collect a small sample in a container without interrupting the stream of urine.

A parent, nurse, or doctor should cleanse the child's genitals and as much of the surrounding area as will fit into the sterile urine-collection bag provided by the hospital. When the area has been thoroughly cleansed, the bag should be attached to the child's genital area and left in place until the child has urinated. It is important to remember not to touch the inside of the bag and to remove it as soon as a specimen has been obtained.

Bladder catheterization is a hospital procedure used to collect uncontaminated urine when the patient cannot void. A catheter is a thin flexible tube that the doctor inserts through the urethra into the bladder to allow urine to flow out. To minimize the risk of infecting the patient's bladder with bacteria, many doctors use a so-called Robinson catheter, which is a plain rubber or latex tube that is removed as soon as the specimen is collected.

Suprapubic bladder aspiration is a technique that is sometimes used to collect urine from infants younger than six months. The doctor withdraws urine from the bladder into a syringe through a needle inserted through the skin over the bladder. This technique is used only when the child cannot void because of an abnormal urethra or if he or she has a urinary tract infection that has not responded to treatment.

Normal urine is a clear straw-colored liquid. It has a slight odor. It contains some crystals, a small number of cells from the tissues that line the bladder, and transparent (hyaline) casts. Normal urine does *not* contain sugars, yeast cells, protein, ketones, bacteria, or parasitic organisms.

The time of day a urine sample is collected can make a difference in the appearance of the specimen. Some foods and medicines, including red beets, asparagus, and penicillin, can affect the color or smell of urine. Although most color variations are harmless, they sometimes indicate the presence of serious disease. A doctor, nurse, or laboratory technician should be notified if the urine is red or cloudy or looks unusual in any way.

Urine may be cloudy (turbid) because it contains red or white blood cells, bacteria, fat, mucus, digestive fluid (chyle), or pus from a bladder or kidney infection.

Foul-smelling urine is a common symptom of urinary-tract infection. A fruity odor is associated with **diabetes mellitus**, **starvation** and **dehydration**, or ketone formation. Other distinctive odors are present in the urine of patients with maple syrup urine disease or **phenylketonuria** (PKU).

URINARY ANTI-INFECTIVES

Urinary anti-infectives are medicines used to treat or prevent infections of the urinary tract—the passage through which urine flows from the kidneys out of the body.

Normally, no bacteria or other disease-causing organisms live in the bladder. Likewise, the urethra—the tube-like structure that carries urine from the bladder out of the body—usually has either no bacteria or not enough to cause problems. But the bladder, urethra, and other parts of the urinary tract may become infected when disease-causing organisms invade from other body regions or from outside the body. Urinary anti-infectives are used to treat such infections or to prevent them in people who get them often.

Commonly used urinary anti-infectives include methenamine (Urex, Hiprex, Mandelamine), nalidixic acid (NegGram) and nitrofurantoin (Macrobid, Furatoin, and other brands). These medicines are available only with a physician's prescription and come in capsule, tablet, granule, and liquid forms.

People with certain medical conditions must take precautions because they may have problems if they take methenamine, nalidixic acid, nitrofurantoin.

For example, people with severe liver disease who take methenamine may have worsened symptoms of their disease. And people who are dehydrated or who have severe kidney disease may be more likely to have side effects that affect the kidneys.

Some people feel drowsy, dizzy, or less alert than usual when using nalidixic acid. The medicine may also cause blurred vision or other vision changes. Because of these possible problems, anyone who takes nalidixic acid should not drive, operate machinery, or do anything else that might be dangerous until they have found out how the drugs affect them.

Nalidixic acid may increase sensitivity to sunlight. Even brief exposure to sun can cause a severe **sunburn** or a rash.

Women who are breastfeeding should check with their physicians before using nitrofurantoin. It passes into breast milk and could cause problems in nursing babies whose mothers take it. This is especially true of babies with glucose-6-phosphate dehydrogenase (G6PD) deficiency. The medicine also should not be given directly to babies up to 1 month of age.

Older people may be more likely to have side effects when taking nitrofurantoin, because they are more sensitive to the drug's effects.

There are some general precautions for all urinary anti-infectives. Symptoms should improve within a few days of starting to take a urinary anti-infective. If they do not, or if they become worse, check with a physician right away. Patients who need to take this medicine for long periods should see their physicians regularly, so that the physician can check their progress.

Anyone who has had unusual reactions to urinary anti-infectives in the past should let his or her physician know before taking the drugs again. The physician should also be told about any **allergies** to foods, dyes, preservatives, or other substances.

People who take urinary anti-infectives should be aware that side effects are possible. Anyone who has unusual symptoms while taking this type of medicine should get in touch with his or her physician.

All the drugs that may interact with a urinary anti-infective are not listed here. Be sure to check with a physician or pharmacist before combining a urinary anti-infective with any other prescription or nonprescription (over-the-counter) medicine.

URINARY CATHETERIZATION

Urinary catheterization is the insertion of a catheter into a patient's bladder. The catheter is used as a conduit to drain urine from the bladder into an attached bag or container.

Urinary catheterization is employed in hospital and nursing home settings to maintain urine output in patients who are undergoing surgery, or who are confined to the bed and physically unable to use a bedpan. Critically ill patients who require strict monitoring of urinary output are also frequently catheterized.

Intermittent insertion of a urinary catheter is a treatment option for patients with certain types of urinary **incontinence**. Patients who are unable to completely empty the bladder during urination (urinary retention), or patients who have a bladder obstruction, may also require intermittent urinary catheterization. Disabled individuals with neurological disorders that cause **paralysis** or a loss of sensation in the perineal area may also use regular intermittent catheter insertion to void their bladders.

Because urinary catheterization carries a risk of causing urinary tract infection (UTI), precautions should be used to keep the catheter clean and free of bacteria. Patients requiring intermittent catheterization should be well trained in the technique by a qualified health care professional.

Intermittent catheterization is performed a minimum of four times a day by the patient or a care giver. The genital area near the urethral opening is wiped with an antiseptic agent, such as iodine. A lubricant may be used to facilitate the entry of the catheter into the urethra, and a topical local anesthetic may be applied to numb the urethral opening during the procedure. One end of the catheter is placed in a container, and the other end is inserted into and guided up the urethra until urine flow begins. When urine flow stops, the catheter may be moved or rotated, or the patient may change positions to ensure that all urine has emptied from the bladder. The catheter is then withdrawn, cleaned, and sterilized for the next use. Recommended cleaning practices vary, from the use of soap and water to submersion in boiling water or a disinfectant solution. Some patients prefer to use a new catheter with each insertion.

Nonintermittent catheterization, which is initiated in a hospital or nursing home setting, uses the same basic technique for insertion of the urinary tract catheter. The catheter is inserted by a nurse or other health care professional, and remains in the patient until bladder function can be maintained independently. When the catheter is removed, patients will experience a pulling sensation and may feel some minor discomfort. If the catheter is required for an extended period of time, a long-term, indwelling catheter, such as a Foley catheter, is used. To prevent infection, it should be regularly exchanged for a new catheter every three to six weeks.

Use of indwelling catheters should be restricted to patients whose incontinence is caused by urinary tract obstruction that can not be treated, and for which alternative therapy is not feasible.

If a patient wishes to perform intermittent catheterization himself, training in the technique by a qualified health care professional is required. Basic instruction in the anatomy, antiseptic techniques, catheter insertion, and proper catheter care should be provided. Patients learning chronic intermittent urinary catheterization may also benefit from an ultrasound examination to verify that they are completely emptying their bladder during the procedure.

Patients using intermittent catheterization as a treatment for incontinence will experience a period of adjustment as they try to establish a catheterization schedule that is adequate for their normal level of fluid intake.

Antibiotics may be prescribed as a preventative measure in long-term urinary catheterization patients who are at risk for urinary tract infection.

A patient with an indwelling catheter must be reassessed periodically to determine whether alternative treatment may be more effective in treating the problem.

Trauma to the urethra and/or bladder may result from incorrect insertion of the catheter. Repeated irritation to the urethra during catheter insertion may cause scarring and/or stricture, or narrowing, of the urethra. The catheter may introduce bacteria into the urethra and bladder, resulting in urinary tract infection. UTI can cause **fever** and inflammation of the bladder and urethra. Patients who practice intermittent catheterization can reduce their risks for UTI by using antiseptic techniques for insertion and catheter care.

When used correctly, catheterization facilitates complete voiding of the bladder.

URINARY SYSTEM

The excretory system removes cellular wastes and helps maintain the salt-water balance in an organism. In providing these functions, excretion contributes to the body's homeostasis, the maintenance of constancy of the internal environment. When cells break down proteins, they produce nitrogenous wastes, such as urea. The excretory system serves to remove these nitrogenous waste products, as well as excess salts and water, from the body. When cells break down carbohydrates during cellular respiration, they produce water and carbon dioxide as a waste product. The **respiratory system** gets rid of carbon dioxide every time we exhale. The **digestive system** removes feces, the solid undigested wastes of digestion, by a process called elimination or defecation.

The main excretory system in humans is the urinary system. The skin also acts as an organ of excretion by removing water and small amounts of urea and salts (as sweat). The urinary system includes a pair of bean-shaped kidneys located in the back of the abdominal cavity. Each day, the kidneys filter about 162 quarts (180 liters) of blood, enough to fill a bathtub. They remove urea, toxins, medications, and excess ions and form urine. The kidneys also balance water and salts as well as acids and bases. At the same time, they return needed substances to the blood. Of the total liquid processed, about 1.3 quarts (1.5 liters) leaves the body as urine.

The size of an adult kidney is approximately 4 in (10 cm) long and 2 in (5 cm) wide. Urine leaves the kidneys in tubes at the hilus, a notch that occurs at the center of the concave edge. Blood vessels, lymph vessels, and nerves enter and leave the kidneys at the hilus. If we cut into a kidney, we see that the hilus leads into a space known as the renal sinus. We also observe two distinct kidney layers. There is the renal cortex, an outer reddish layer, and the renal medulla, a reddish brown layer. Within the kidneys, nephrons clear the blood of wastes, create urine, and deliver urine to a tube called a ureter, which carries the urine to the bladder. The urinary bladder is a hollow muscular structure that is collapsed when empty and pear-shaped and distended when full. The urinary bladder then empties urine into the urethra, a duct leading to outside the body. A sphincter muscle controls the flow of urine between the urinary bladder and the urethra.

Each kidney contains over one million nephrons, each of which consists of a tuft of capillaries surrounded by a capsule on top of a curving tube. The tuft of capillaries is called a glomerulus. Its capsule is cup-shaped and is known as Bowman's capsule. The glomerulus and Bowman's capsule form the top of a tube, the renal tubule. Blood vessels surround the renal tubule, and urine forms in it. The renal tubules of many nephrons join in collecting tubules, which in turn merge into larger tubes and empty their urine into the ureters in the renal sinus. The ureters exit the kidney at the hilus.

The job of clearing the blood of wastes in the nephrons occurs in three stages. They are filtration, reabsorption, and tubular secretion.

1. The first stage in clearing the blood is filtration, the passage of a liquid through a filter to remove impurities. Filtration occurs in the glomeruli. Blood pressure forces plasma, the liquid portion of the blood, through the capillary walls in the glomerulus. The plasma contains water, glucose, amino acids, and urea. Blood cells and proteins are too large to pass through the wall, so they stay in the blood. The fluid, now called filtrate, collects in the capsule and enters the renal tubule.

2. During reabsorption, needed substances in the filtrate travel back into the bloodstream. Reabsorption occurs in the renal tubules. There, glucose and other nutrients, water, and essential ions materials pass out of the renal tubules and enter the surrounding capillaries. Normally 100% of glucose is reabsorbed. (Glucose detected in the urine is a sign of diabetes mellitus, which is characterized by too much sugar in the blood due to a lack of insulin.) Reabsorption involves both diffusion and active transport, which uses energy in the form of ATP. The waste-containing fluid that remains after reabsorption is urine.

3. Tubular secretion is the passage of certain substances out of the capillaries directly into the renal tubules. Tubular se-

cretion is another way of getting waste materials into the urine. For example, drugs such as penicillin and phenobarbital are secreted into the renal tubules from the capillaries. Urea and uric acid that may have been reabsorbed are secreted. Excess potassium ions are also secreted into the urine. Tubular secretions also maintain the pH of the blood.

The volume of the urine varies according to need. Antidiuretic hormone (ADH), released by the posterior pituitary gland, controls the volume of urine. The amount of ADH in the bloodstream varies inversely with the volume of urine produced. If we perspire a lot or fail to drink enough water, special nerve cells in the hypothalamus, called osmoreceptors, detect the low water concentration in the blood. They then signal neurosecretory cells in the hypothalamus to produce ADH, which is transmitted to the posterior pituitary gland and released into the blood, where it travels to the renal tubules. With ADH present, the kidney tubules reabsorb more water from the urine and return it to the blood, and the volume of urine is reduced. If we take in too much water, on the other hand, the osmoreceptors detect the overhydration and inhibit the production of ADH. Reabsorption of water is reduced, and the volume of urine is increased. Alcohol inhibits ADH production and therefore increases the output of urine.

The liver also plays an important role in excretion. This organ removes the ammonia and converts it into the less toxic urea. The liver also chemically changes and filters out certain drugs such as penicillin and erythromycin. These substances are then picked up by the blood and transported to the kidneys, where they are put into the execretory system.

The urinary system must function properly to ensure good health. During a physical examination, the physician frequently performs a **urinalysis**. Urine testing can reveal diseases such as **diabetes mellitus**, **urinary tract infections**, **kidney stones**, and renal disease. Urography, taking X–rays of the urinary system, also helps diagnose urinary problems. In this procedure, an opaque dye is introduced into the urinary structures so that they show up in the X rays. **Ultrasound** scanning is another diagnostic tool. It uses high frequency sound waves to produce an image of the kidneys. Biopsies, samples of kidney tissue obtained in a hollow needle, are also useful in diagnosing kidney disease.

Disorders of the urinary tract include urinary tract infections (UTI). An example is cystitis, a disease in which bacteria infect the urinary bladder, causing inflammation. Most UTIs are treated with **antibiotics**. Sometimes kidney stones, solid salt crystals, form in the urinary tract. Kidney stones can obstruct the urinary passages and cause severe pain, and bleeding. If they do not pass out of the body naturally, the physician may use shock wave treatment. In this treatment, a shock wave focused on the stone from outside the body disintegrates it. Physicians also use surgery to remove kidney stones. Renal failure is a condition in which the kidneys lose the ability to function. Nitrogenous wastes build up in the blood, the pH drops, and urine production slows down. If left unchecked, this condition can result in death. In chronic renal failure, the urinary system declines, causing permanent loss of kidney function.

Hemodialysis and kidney transplant are two methods of helping chronic renal failure. In hemodialysis, an artificial kidney device cleans the blood of wastes and adjusts the composition of ions. During the procedure, blood is taken out of the radial artery in the patient's arm. It then passes through dialysis tubing, which is selectively permeable. The tubing is immersed in a solution. As the blood passes through the tubing, wastes pass out of the tubing and into the surrounding solution. The cleansed blood returns to the body. Kidney transplants also help chronic kidney failure. In this procedure, a surgeon replaces a diseased kidney with a closely matched donor kidney. Although about 23,000 people in the United States wait for donor kidneys each year, fewer than 8,000 receive kidney transplants. Current research aims to develop new drugs to help kidney failure better dialysis membranes for the artificial kidney.

URINARY TRACT INFECTIONS

Cystitis is defined as inflammation of the urinary bladder. Urethritis is an inflammation of the urethra, which is the passageway that connects the bladder with the exterior of the body. Sometimes cystitis and urethritis are referred to collectively as a lower urinary tract infection, or UTI. Infection of the upper urinary tract involves the spread of bacteria to the kidney and is called pyelonephritis.

The frequency of bladder infections in humans varies significantly according to age and sex. The male/female ratio of UTIs in children younger than 12 months is 4:1 because of the high rate of **birth defects** in the urinary tract of male infants. In adult life, the male/female ratio of UTIs is 1:50. After age 50, however, the incidence among males increases due to prostate disorders.

Cystitis is a common female problem. It is estimated that 50% of adult women experience at least one episode of dysuria (painful urination); half of these patients have a bacterial UTI. Between 2-5% of women's visits to primary care doctors are for UTI symptoms. About 90% of UTIs in women are uncomplicated but recurrent.

UTIs are uncommon in younger and middle-aged men, but may occur as complications of bacterial infections of the kidney or prostate gland.

In children, cystitis is often caused by congenital abnormalities (present at birth) of the urinary tract. Vesicoureteral reflux is a condition in which the child cannot completely empty the bladder. It allows urine to remain in or flow backward (reflux) into the partially empty bladder.

The causes of cystitis vary according to sex because of the differences in anatomical structure of the urinary tract.

Most bladder infections in women are so-called ascending infections, which means that they are caused by disease agents traveling upward through the urethra to the bladder. The relative shortness of the female urethra (1.2-2 inches in length) makes it easy for bacteria to gain entry to the bladder and multiply. The most common bacteria associated with UTIs in women include *Escherichia coli* (about 80% of cases), *Staphylococcus saprophyticus*, *Klebsiella*, *Enterobacter*, and *Proteus* species. Risk factors for UTIs in women include:

- Sexual intercourse. The risk of infection increases if the woman has multiple partners.

- Use of a diaphragm for **contraception**
- An abnormally short urethra
- Diabetes or chronic **dehydration**
- The absence of a specific enzyme (fucosyltransferase) in vaginal secretions. The lack of this enzyme makes it easier for the vagina to harbor bacteria that cause UTIs.
- Inadequate personal hygiene. Bacteria from fecal matter or vaginal discharges can enter the female urethra because its opening is very close to the vagina and anus.
- History of previous UTIs. About 80% of women with cystitis develop recurrences within two years.

The early symptoms of cystitis in women are dysuria, or pain on urination; urgency, or a sudden strong desire to urinate; and increased frequency of urination. About 50% of female patients experience **fever**, pain in the lower back or flanks, **nausea and vomiting**, or shaking chills. These symptoms indicate pyelonephritis, or spread of the infection to the upper urinary tract.

Most UTIs in adult males are complications of kidney or prostate infections. They are usually associated with a tumor or **kidney stones** that block the flow of urine and are often persistent infections caused by drug-resistant organisms. UTIs in men are most likely to be caused by *E. coli* or another gram-negative bacterium. *S. saprophyticus*, which is the second most common cause of UTIs in women, rarely causes infections in men. Risk factors for UTIs in men include:

- Lack of **circumcision**. The foreskin can harbor bacteria that cause UTIs.
- **Urinary catheterization**. The longer the period of catheterization, the higher the risk of UTIs.

The symptoms of cystitis and pyelonephritis in men are the same as in women.

Hemorrhagic cystitis, which is marked by large quantities of blood in the urine, is caused by an acute bacterial infection of the bladder. In some cases, hemorrhagic cystitis is a side effect of **radiation therapy** or treatment with cyclophosphamide. Hemorrhagic cystitis in children is associated with adenovirus type 11.

When cystitis is suspected, the doctor will first examine the patient's abdomen and lower back, to evaluate unusual enlargements of the kidneys or swelling of the bladder. In small children, the doctor will check for fever, abdominal masses, and a swollen bladder.

The next step in diagnosis is collection of a urine sample. The procedure differs somewhat for women and men. Laboratory testing of urine samples can now be performed with dipsticks that indicate immune system responses to infection, as well as with microscopic analysis of samples. Normal human urine is sterile. The presence of bacteria or pus in the urine usually indicates infection. The presence of hematuria, or blood in the urine, may indicate acute UTIs, kidney disease, kidney stones, inflammation of the prostate (in men), **endometriosis** (in women), or **cancer** of the urinary tract. In some cases, blood in the urine results from athletic training, particularly in runners.

Female patients require a pelvic examination as part of the procedure to obtain urine specimens. The patient lies on an obstetrical table with legs in the stirrups. The doctor first takes a vaginal culture smear. The patient is then asked to void while lying on the table. The first five to 10 ml are collected to test for urethral infection. A midstream urine sample of 200 ml is then collected to test for bladder infection.

In women, a vaginal bacterial count that is higher than those of the two urine samples indicates vaginitis. A high bacterial count in the first urine sample indicates urethritis. A count of more than 104 bacteria CFU/ml (colony forming units per milliliter) in the midstream sample indicates a bladder or kidney infection. A colony is a large number of microorganisms that grow from a single cell within a substance called a culture. Bacterial count can be given in CFU or colony forming units.

In male patients, the doctor will cleanse the opening to the urethra with an antiseptic before collecting the urine sample. The first 10 ml of specimen are collected separately. The patient then voids a midstream sample of 200 ml. Following the second sample, the doctor will massage the patient's prostate and collect several drops of prostatic fluid. The patient then voids a third urine specimen for prostatic culture.

A high bacterial count in the first urine specimen or the prostatic specimens indicates urethritis or prostate infections respectively. A bacterial count greater than 100,000 bacteria CFU/ml in the midstream sample suggests a bladder or kidney infection.

Women with recurrent UTIs can be given ultrasound tests of the kidneys and bladder together with a voiding cystourethrogram to test for structural abnormalities. (A cystourethrogram is an x-ray test in which an iodine dye is used to better view the urinary bladder and urethra.) Voiding cystourethrograms are also used to evaluate children with UTIs. In some cases, **computed tomography scans** (CT scans) can be used to evaluate patients for possible cancers in the urinary tract.

Uncomplicated cystitis is treated with **antibiotics**. These include penicillin, ampicillin, and amoxicillin; sulfisoxazole or sulfamethoxazole; trimethoprim; nitrofurantoin; **cephalosporins**; or fluoroquinolones. (Flouroquinolones are generally not used in children under 18 years of age.) Treatment for women is short-term; most patients respond within three days. Men do not respond as well to short-term treatment and require seven to 10 days of oral antibiotics for uncomplicated UTIs.

Patients of either sex may be given phenazopyridine or flavoxate to relieve painful urination.

Trimethoprim and nitrofurantoin are preferred for treating recurrent UTIs in women.

Over 50% of older men with UTIs also suffer from infection of the prostate gland. Some antibiotics, including amoxicillin and the cephalosporins, do not affect the prostate gland. Fluoroquinolone antibiotics or trimethoprim are the drugs of choice for these patients.

Patients with pyelonephritis can be treated with oral antibiotics or intramuscular doses of cephalosporins. Medications are given for 10-14 days, and sometimes longer. If the patient requires hospitalization because of high fever and dehydration caused by vomiting, antibiotics can be given intravenously.

A minority of women with complicated UTIs may require surgical treatment to prevent recurrent infections. Surgery is also used to treat reflux problems (movement of the urine backwards) or other structural abnormalities in children and anatomical abnormalities in adult males.

The prognosis for recovery from uncomplicated UTIs is excellent; however, complicated UTIs in males are difficult to treat because they often involve bacteria that are resistant to commonly used antibiotics.

Women with two or more UTIs within a six-month period are sometimes given prophylactic treatment, usually nitrofurantoin or trimethoprim for three to six months. In some cases the patient is advised to take an antibiotic tablet following sexual intercourse.

Other preventive measures for women include:

- Drinking large amounts of fluid
- Voiding frequently, particularly after intercourse
- Proper cleansing of the area around the urethra.

The primary preventive measure for males is prompt treatment of prostate infections. Chronic **prostatitis** may go unnoticed but can trigger recurrent UTIs. In addition, males who require temporary catheterization following surgery can be given antibiotics to lower the risk of UTIs.

U.S. Department of Health and Human Services

The U.S. Department of Health and Human Services (HHS) is the principal agency in this country devoted to protecting the health of Americans and to providing essential human services, especially for those who have difficulty helping themselves.

Milestones in the evolution of the U.S. Department of Health and Human Services date to the earliest years of this country's history. In 1798, the first Marine Hospital, a forerunner of today's **Public Health** Service, was established to care for seafarers. In 1862, President Abraham Lincoln established the Department of Agriculture, which became a forerunner to the **Food and Drug Administration**. In 1887, the federal government opened a small laboratory in New York for research on disease that eventually grew into the **National Institutes of Health**. In 1906, Congress passed the first Food and Drug Act, authorizing the government to monitor the purity of foods and the safety of medicines, now a responsibility of the Food and Drug Administration. In 1912, President Theodore Roosevelt urged the creation of a Children's Bureau to combat the exploitation of children. And in 1935, Congress passed the Social Security Act.

In 1999, the Department administered more than 300 programs that served the following areas: medical and social science research; infectious **disease prevention**; food and drug safety; **Medicare and Medicaid**; financial assistance for low-income families; child support enforcement; maternal and infant health; the Head Start program; **child abuse** and **domestic violence**; substance abuse treatment and prevention; services for older Americans; and health services for Native Americans.

Health and Human Services provides more grants each year than any other federal agency, providing some 60,000 grants annually. The Medicare program is the nation's largest health insurer, handling more than 900 million claims each year.

The Department of Health and Human Services works closely with state and local governments, and many HHS-funded services are administered at the local level by state or county agencies, or through private sector grants. In fiscal year 1999, the Health and Human Services budget stood at $387 billion, at which time there were 59,800 Health and Human Services employees.

Operating divisions of the Department of Health and Human Services include: the National Institutes of Health (supporting research projects nationwide in diseases like **cancer**, **Alzheimer's disease**, diabetes, arthritis, heart ailments, and **AIDS**); the Food and Drug Administration (overseeing the safety of foods and cosmetics, and the safety and efficacy of pharmaceuticals, biological products and medical devices); the **Centers for Disease Control** and Prevention (providing a system of health surveillance to monitor and prevent outbreak of diseases); the Agency for Toxic Substances and Disease Registry (preventing exposure to hazardous substances from waste sites); the Indian Health Service (handling Native American health services); the Health Resources and Services Administration (providing health resources for medically underserved populations); the Substance Abuse and Mental Health Services Administration (overseeing substance abuse prevention, addiction treatment, and mental health services); the Agency for Health Care Policy and Research (supporting research on health care systems, health care quality and cost issues, and effectiveness of medical treatments); the Health Care Financing Administration (administering the Medicare and Medicaid programs); the Administration for Children and Families (providing services and assistance to needy children and families); and the Administration on Aging (supporting a nationwide aging network and providing services so that the elderly can continue to live independently.

See also Aging; Independent living; Retirement

Uterine cancer

The endometrium is the tissue forming the inner lining of the uterus. Uterine cancer (also called endometrial **cancer**) develops when the cells of the endometrium become abnormal and grow uncontrollably. It is a common type of cancer among women and generally occurs in women who have gone through **menopause** and are 45 years old or older.

The uterus (also called the womb) is the hollow female organ that supports the development and nourishment of the unborn baby during **pregnancy**. It has a thick muscular wall and an inner lining called the endometrium. The endometrium is very sensitive to hormones and it changes daily during the woman's menstrual cycle. It is designed to provide an ideal environment for the fertilized egg to implant itself and begin to grow. If pregnancy does not occur, the endometrium is shed at the time of the menstrual period. The bleeding that occurs during a woman's period is the shedding of the endometrium along with the accompanying blood and tissue. More than 95% of uterine cancers arise in the endometrium.

Although the exact cause of endometrial cancer is unknown, there are several factors that increase a woman's risk of developing this particular cancer. Among them are age, obesity, and having diseases such as diabetes or hypertension. In addition, a woman who has irregular menstrual periods, or had their first period at a young age or are going through menopause at an advanced age have a slightly higher risk for developing endometrial cancer.

Endometrial cancers have a very good chance of being cured because there are symptoms that are evident very early on in the disease. The most common symptom of endometrial cancer is unusual bleeding or discharge. Especially in women who have gone through menopause, any vaginal bleeding should be brought to the attention of the doctor immediately. Any abnormal vaginal discharge should also be reported. **Pain** in the pelvic region and the presence of a lump (mass) are symptoms that occur late in the disease.

If the doctor suspects endometrial cancer, he/she will conduct a series of tests to confirm the diagnosis. The first step will involve taking a complete personal and family medical history. A **physical examination**, which will include a thorough pelvic examination, will also be done.

The doctor may order an endometrial **biopsy**. A small piece of endometrial tissue is removed and is sent to a laboratory for examination. If the biopsy tissue looks abnormal, but confirmation is needed, the doctor may perform another procedure known as dilatation and curettage (D & C).

The treatment and prognosis for cancer depends on the type and stage of the cancer The standard treatments available for endometrial cancer are surgery, **radiation therapy**, hormonal therapy, and **chemotherapy**.

Surgery is the best option when endometrial cancer is diagnosed at its very early stages. Radiation therapy uses high-energy radiation from x rays and gamma rays to kill the cancer cells. Side effects are common with radiation therapy. **Premature menopause** and some problems with urination may also occur. The decision to use radiation therapy depends on the stage of the disease. Chemotherapy uses **anticancer drugs** to kill the cancer cells. The drugs are given orally (by mouth) or intravenously. Generally, a combination of drugs is given since it is more effective than a single drug in treating cancer. Side effects with this treatment include stomach upset, vomiting, appetite loss, hair loss, mouth or vaginal sores, fatigue, menstrual cycle changes, and premature menopause. Chemotherapy is usually reserved for women with advanced (stage IV) or recurrent disease because this therapy is not as effective as surgery or radiation.

Hormonal therapy uses drugs like progesterone that will slow the growth of endometrial cells. These drugs are usually available as pills. This therapy is usually reserved for women with advanced or recurrent disease.

Since it is possible to detect endometrial cancer early, the chances of curing it are excellent. In fact, if the cancer is found in its very earliest stage, approximately 96% of patients survive five years or more.

In order to prevent endometrial cancer, women (especially postmenopausal women) should report any abnormal vaginal bleeding to the doctor. Early diagnosis is extremely important in this disease. Controlling **obesity**, blood pressure, and diabetes can help to reduce the risk of this disease. The use of birth control pills over a long period of time has been shown to reduce the risk of this cancer. There is some evidence that women on estrogen replacement therapy after menopause have a substantially reduced risk of endometrial cancer if progestins are taken along with estrogen. Doctors routinely prescribe estrogen and progesterone together unless there is a reason why a woman cannot take progesterone. Doctors should also pay very close attention to any abnormal vaginal bleeding in women after menopause.

UTERINE FIBROIDS

Uterine fibroids (also called leiomyomas or myomas) are benign growths of the muscle inside the uterus. They are not cancerous, nor are they related to cancer. Fibroids can cause a wide variety of symptoms, including heavy menstrual bleeding and pressure on the pelvis.

Uterine fibroids are extremely common. About 25% of women in their reproductive years have noticeable fibroids. There are probably many more women who have tiny fibroids that are undetected.

Fibroids develop between the ages of 30–50. They are never seen in women less than 20 years old. After **menopause**, if a woman does not take estrogen, fibroids shrink. It appears that African-American women are much more likely to develop uterine fibroids.

Fibroids are divided into different types, depending on the location. Submucous fibroids are found in the uterine cavity; intramural fibroids grow on the wall of the uterus; and subserous fibroids are located on the outside of the uterus. Many fibroids are so large that they fit into more than one category. The symptoms caused by fibroids are often related to their location.

No one knows exactly what causes fibroids. However, the growth of fibroids appears to depend on the hormone estrogen. Fibroids often grow larger when estrogen levels are high, as in **pregnancy**. Medications that lower the estrogen level can cause the fibroids to shrink.

The signs and symptoms of fibroids include:

- Heavy uterine bleeding. This is the most common symptom, occurring in 30% of women who have fibroids. The excess bleeding usually happens during the menstrual period. Flow may be heavier, and periods may last longer. Women who have submucous or intramural fibroids are most likely to have heavy uterine bleeding.
- Pelvic pressure and **pain**. Large fibroids that press on nearby structures such as the bladder and bowel can cause pressure and pain. Larger fibroids tend to cause worse symptoms.
- **Infertility**. This is a rare symptom of fibroids. It probably accounts for less than 3% of infertility cases. Fibroids

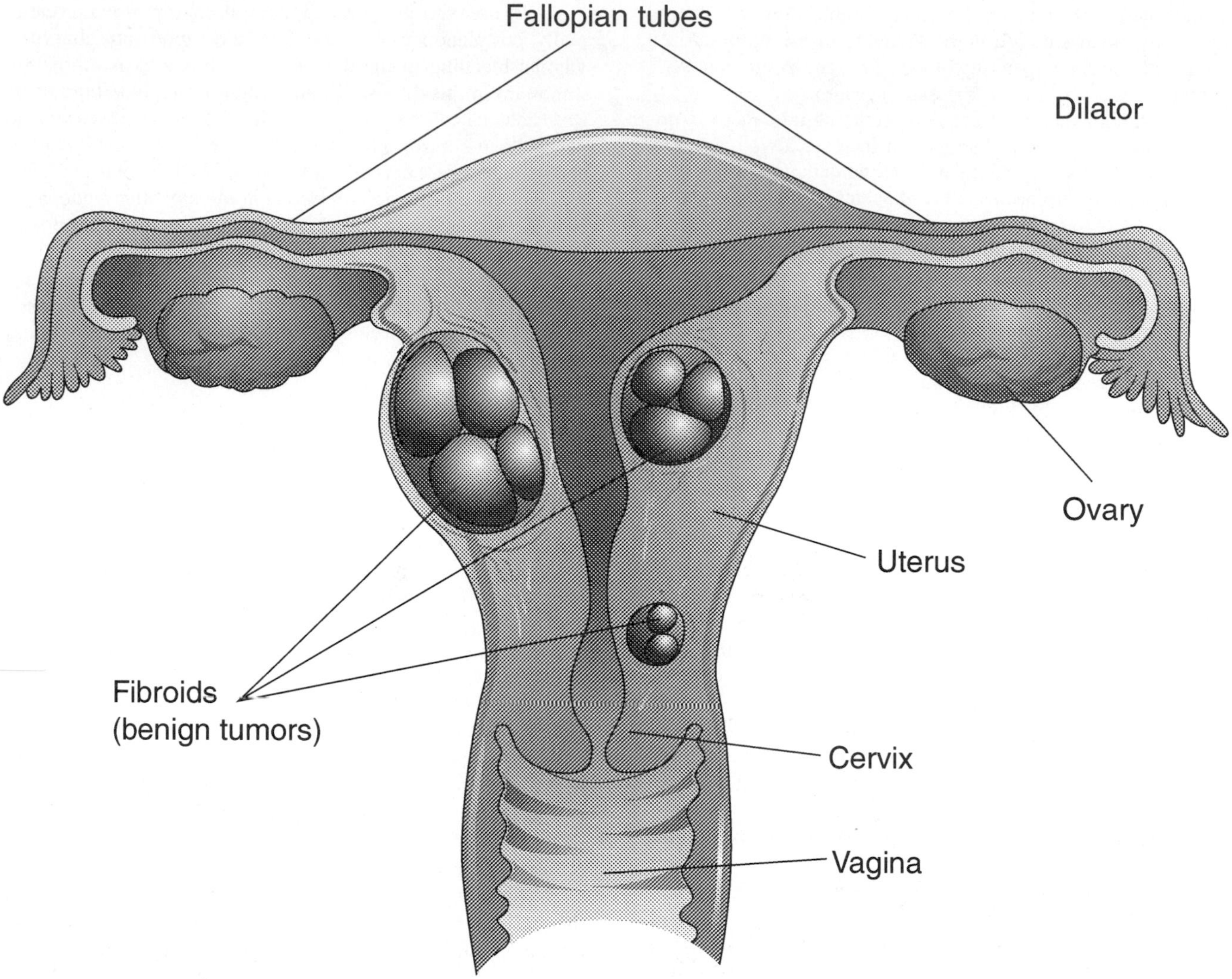

Common sites of uterine fibroids.

can cause infertility by compressing the uterine cavity. Submucous fibroids can fill the uterine cavity and interfere with implantation of the fertilized egg.

- Miscarriage. This is also an unusual symptom of fibroids, probably accounting for only a tiny fraction of the miscarriages that occur.
- Pregnancy complications. Fibroids can greatly increase in size during pregnancy, because of increased levels of estrogen. They can cause pain, and even lead to **premature labor**.

A health care provider can usually feel fibroids during a routine pelvic examination. Ultrasound can be used to confirm the diagnosis, but this is not necessary.

Not all fibroids cause symptoms. Even fibroids that do cause symptoms may not require treatment. In the majority of cases, the symptoms are inconvenient and unpleasant, but do not result in health problems.

Occasionally, fibroids lead to such heavy menstrual bleeding that the woman becomes severely anemic. In these cases, treatment of the fibroids may be necessary. Very large fibroids are much harder to treat. Therefore, many doctors recommend treatment for moderately-sized fibroids, in the hopes of preventing them from growing into large fibroids that cause worse symptoms.

The following are possible treatment plans:

- Observation. This is the most common plan. Most women already have symptoms at the time their fibroids are discovered, but feel that they can tolerate their symptoms. Therefore, no active treatment is given, but the woman and her physician stay alert for signs that the condition might be getting worse.
- **Hysterectomy**. This involves surgical removal of the uterus, and it is the only real cure for fibroids. In fact, 25% of hysterectomies are performed because of symptomatic fibroids. By the time a woman has a hysterecto-

my for fibroids, she has usually endured several years of worsening symptoms. That's because fibroids tend to grow over time. A gynecologist can remove a fibroid uterus during either an abdominal or a vaginal hysterectomy. The choice depends on the size of the fibroids and other factors such as previous births and previous surgeries.

- Myomectomy. In this surgical procedure only the fibroids are removed; the uterus is repaired and left in place. This is the surgical procedure many women choose if they are not finished with childbearing. At first glance, it seems that this treatment is a middle ground between observation and hysterectomy. However, myomectomy is actually a difficult surgical procedure, more difficult than a hysterectomy. Myomectomy often causes significant blood loss, and blood **transfusion**s may be required. In addition, some fibroids are so large, or buried so deeply within the wall of the uterus, that it is not possible to save the uterus, and a hysterectomy must be done, even though it was not planned. There are exceptions to this, however. Sometimes, fibroids grow on a stalk (pedunculated fibroids), and these are easy to remove.
- Medical treatment. Since fibroids are dependent on estrogen for their growth, medical treatments that lower estrogen levels can cause fibroids to shrink. A group of medications known as GnRH antagonists can dramatically lower estrogen levels. Women who take these medications for three to six months find that their fibroids shrink in size by 50% or more. They usually experience dramatic relief of their symptoms of heavy bleeding and pelvic pain.

Unfortunately, GnRH antagonists cause unpleasant side effects in over 90% of women. The therapy is usually used for only three months, and should not be used for more than six months because the risk of developing brittle bones (**osteoporosis**) begins to rise. Once the treatment is stopped, the fibroids begin to grow back to their original size. Within six months, most of the old symptoms return. Therefore, GnRH agonists cannot be used as long-term solution. At the moment, treatment with GnRH antagonists is used mainly in preparation for surgery (myomectomy or hysterectomy). Shrinking the size of the fibroids makes surgery much easier, and reducing the heavy bleeding allows a woman to build up her **blood count** before surgery.

Fibroids can cause problems during pregnancy because they often grow in size. Large fibroids can cause pain and lead to premature labor. Fibroids cannot be removed during pregnancy because of the risk of injury to the uterus and hemorrhage. GnRH antagonists cannot be used during pregnancy. Treatment is limited to pain medication and medication to prevent premature labor, if necessary.

Many women who have fibroids have no symptoms or have only minor symptoms of heavy menstrual bleeding or pelvic pressure. However, fibroids tend to grow over time, and gradually cause more symptoms. Many women ultimately decide to have some form of treatment. Currently, hysterectomy is the most popular form of treatment.

Uterine fibroids cannot be prevented.

V

VACCINATION

Vaccination is the use of vaccines to prevent specific diseases.

Many diseases that once caused widespread illness, disability, and death now can be prevented through the use of vaccines. Vaccines are medicines that contain weakened or dead bacteria or viruses. When a person takes a vaccine, his or her immune system responds by producing antibodies—substances that weaken or destroy disease-causing organisms. When the person is later exposed to live bacteria or viruses of the same kind that were in the vaccine, the antibodies prevent those organisms from making the person sick. In other words, the person becomes immune to the disease the organisms normally cause. The process of building up immunity by taking a vaccine is called immunization.

Vaccines are used in several ways. Some, such as the **rabies** vaccine, are given only when a person is likely to have been exposed to the virus that causes the disease—through a dog bite, for example. Others are given to travelers planning to visit countries where certain diseases are common. Vaccines such as the **influenza** vaccine, or ''flu shot,'' are given mainly to specific groups of people—older adults and others who are at high risk of developing influenza or its complications. Then, there are vaccines that are given to almost everyone, such as the one that prevents **diphtheria**.

Children routinely have a series of vaccinations that begins at birth. Given according to a specific schedule, these vaccinations protect against **hepatitis** B, diphtheria, **tetanus**, pertussis (**whooping cough**), **measles**, **mumps**, **rubella** (German measles), varicella (**chickenpox**), **polio**, and *Haemophilus influenzae* type b (Hib disease, a major cause of spinal **meningitis**). This series of vaccinations is recommended by the American Academy of Family Physicians, the American Academy of Pediatrics, and the Centers for Disease Control and Prevention and is required in all states before children can enter school.

In addition, vaccines are available for preventing **anthrax**, **cholera**, **hepatitis A**, Japanese encephalitis, meningococcal meningitis, **plague**, pneumococcal infection (meningitis, **pneumonia**), **tuberculosis**, **typhoid fever**, and **yellow fever**. Most vaccines are given as injections, but a few (such as the oral polio vaccine) are given by mouth.

Some vaccines are combined in one injection, such as the measles-mumps-rubella (MMR) or diphtheria-pertussis-tetanus (DPT) combinations.

Anyone planning a trip to another country should check to find out what vaccinations are needed. Some vaccinations must be given as much as 12 weeks before the trip, so getting this information early is important. Many major hospitals and medical centers have travel clinics that can provide this information. The Traveler's Health Section of the Centers for Disease Control and Prevention also has information on vaccination requirements.

Vaccines are not always effective, and there is no way to predict whether a vaccine will ''take'' in any particular person. To be most effective, vaccination programs depend on whole communities participating. The more people who are vaccinated, the lower everyone's risk of being exposed to a disease. Even people who do not develop immunity through vaccination are safer when their friends, neighbors, children, and coworkers are immunized.

Like most medical procedures, vaccination has risks as well as substantial benefits. Anyone who takes a vaccine should make sure that he or she is fully informed about both the benefits and the risks. Any questions or concerns should be discussed with a physician or other health care provider. The Centers for Disease Control and Prevention, located in Atlanta, Georgia, also is a good source of information.

Vaccines may cause problems for people with certain **allergies**. In general, anyone who has had an unusual reaction to a vaccine in the past should let his or her physician know before taking the same kind of vaccine again. The physician also should be told about any allergies to foods, medicines, preservatives, or other substances.

Anyone who takes a vaccine should let the physician know all other medicines he or she is taking and should ask

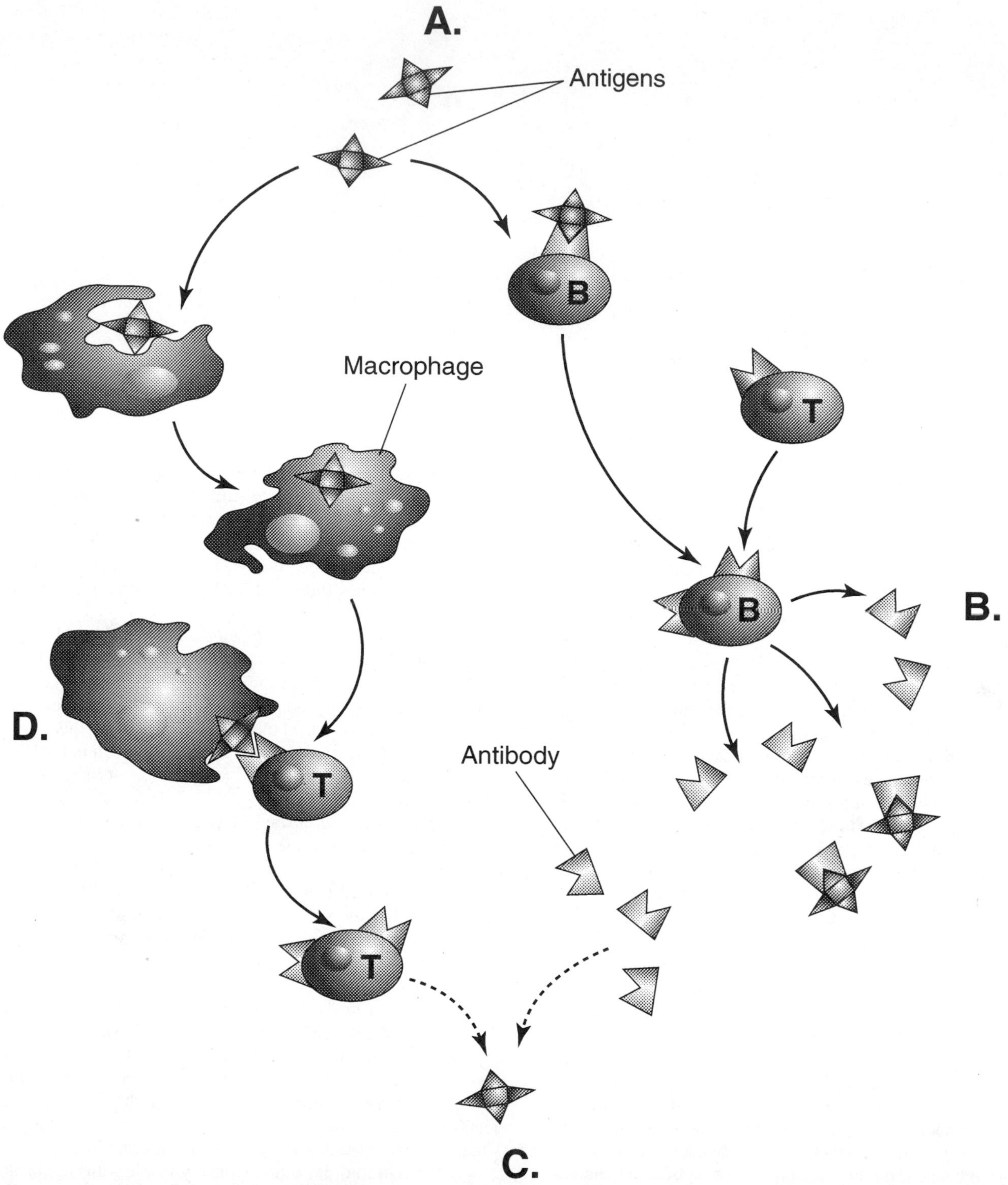

How vaccines work: A. Vaccines contain antigens (weakened or dead viruses, bacteria, and fungi that cause disease and infection). When introduced into the body, the antigens stimulate the immune system response by instructing B cells to produce antibodies, with assistance from T-cells. B. The antibodies are produced to fight the weakened or dead viruses in the vaccine. C. The antibodies "practice" on the weakened viruses, preparing the immune system to destroy real and stronger viruses in the future. D. When new antigens enter the body, white blood cells called macrophages engulf them, process the information contained in the antigens, and send it to the T-cells so that an immune system response can be mobilized. *(Illustration by Electronic Illustrators Group.)*

whether the possible interactions could interfere with the effects of the vaccine or the other medicines.

People with certain medical conditions should be cautious about taking vaccines. Influenza vaccine, for example, may reactivate **Guillain-Barré syndrome** (GBS) in people who have had it before. This vaccine also may worsen illnesses that involve the lungs, such as **bronchitis** or pneumonia. Vaccines that cause **fever** as a side effect may trigger seizures in people who have a history of seizures caused by fever.

Certain vaccines are not recommended for use during **pregnancy**, but some may be given to women at especially high risk of getting a specific disease such as polio. Vaccines also may be given to pregnant women to prevent medical problems in their babies. For example, vaccinating a pregnant woman with tetanus toxoid can prevent her baby from getting tetanus at birth. Women who are breastfeeding should check with their physicians before taking any vaccine.

Most side effects from vaccines are minor and easily treated. The most common are **pain**, redness, and swelling at the site of the injection. Anyone who has an unusual reaction after receiving a vaccine should get in touch with a physician right away.

Vane, John R. (1927-)

English pharmacologist

John Robert Vane was born March 29, 1927, in Tardebigge, Worcester. His parents' Christmas gift of a chemistry set sparked Vane's interest in science when he was twelve, and his home became the site of numerous experiments. However, upon entering the University of Birmingham in 1944, he found that the work given him was not as challenging as he anticipated. At the advice of a professor, he decided to go to Oxford University to study pharmacology after receiving his B.S. in chemistry from Birmingham in 1946. Vane became a fellow on Oxford's Therapeutic Research Council for the next two years. He obtained a B.S. in pharmacology from Oxford in 1949, and earned his doctorate in 1953. After leaving Oxford, Vane came to America to teach pharmacology at Yale University. He returned to England in 1955 as a senior lecturer in pharmacology at the Royal College of Surgeons, at its Institute of Basic Medical Sciences.

Vane became interested in prostaglandins in the late 1950s. Discovered in the 1930s, they were originally thought to be secreted by the prostate gland, which is how they got their name. Prostaglandins are natural compounds, developed from fatty acids, which control many bodily functions. Different prostaglandins regulate blood pressure and coagulation, allergic reactions to substances, the rate of **metabolism**, glandular secretions, and contractions in the uterus.

For many years after the discovery of prostaglandins, scientists were unaware of how they were produced and how they functioned. In the early 1960s Vane expanded upon the procedure known as biological assay (bioassay), by which the strength of a substance is measured by comparing its effects on an organism with those of a standard preparation. Vane developed the dynamic bioassay, which allows scientists to measure more than one substance in blood or body fluids. This method enabled Vane and his colleagues at the Royal College to prove that prostaglandins are produced by many tissues and organs in the body. Further research led the scientists to discover that, unlike hormones, certain prostaglandins are effective only in the areas where they were formed.

In 1966 Vane advanced to professor of experimental pharmacology at the Institute for Basic Medical Sciences and continued his studies. An experiment he conducted in 1969 resulted in the discovery of the methods by which aspirin alleviates pain and reduces inflammation. Using the lung tissue of guinea pigs, Vane found that aspirin inhibited the production of a certain prostaglandin that causes inflammation. He published the results in a June, 1971, issue of *Nature New Biology,* a science magazine.

In 1973 Vane resigned his post at the Institute to enter the business world as director of research and development at the Wellcome Foundation, a pharmaceutical company. Following up on research by the Swedish chemist Bengt Samuelsson (who found that a type of prostaglandin was responsible for allowing blood to clot), Vane discovered the existence of a prostaglandin with the opposite quality, which inhibits clot formation. With the assistance of the Upjohn Chemical Corporation, Vane isolated the secretion, which he named prostacyclin. This discovery proved to be of great assistance in dissolving clots blocking the blood supply in stroke and heart attack victims and is also useful for keeping blood from clotting during surgery. Scientists have discovered even more uses for prostaglandins, including the treatment of ulcers, alleviating pain from menstruation and gallstones, and stimulating contractions for childbirth.

Vane, along with Samuelsson and Swedish chemist Sune Bergström, was given the Albert Lasker Basic Medical Research Award in 1977 for his work on prostaglandins. Five years later, in 1982, the Nobel Committee gave the trio the Nobel Prize for medicine or physiology. After receiving the award, Vane predicted that future research on prostaglandins would create major breakthroughs in the areas of medicine. ''In the next 20 years we should see a substantial attack on the disease process,'' *Time* quoted him as saying. ''We will be able to find new drugs that have effects on cardiovascular disease, on asthma, on heart attack,'' and even health problems associated with old age, the magazine reported.

During the 1980s Vane embarked on a crusade for greater research on new drugs to fight both new diseases (such as acquired immunodeficiency syndrome, known as **AIDS**) and drug-resistant strains of old diseases, such as **malaria**. In articles for scientific and medical journals, he stressed the need for greater international cooperation in the search for a cure or vaccine for AIDS and advocated the creation of an Institute for Tropical Diseases to research new drugs to battle disease in the tropics.

Varicose veins

Varicose veins are dilated, tortuous, elongated superficial veins that are usually seen in the legs.

Varicose veins, also called varicosities, are seen most often in the legs, although they can be found in other parts of the body. Most often, they appear as lumpy, winding vessels just below the surface of the skin. There are three types of veins, superficial veins that are just beneath the surface of the skin, deep veins that are large blood vessels found deep inside muscles, and perforator veins that connect the superficial veins to the deep veins. The superficial veins are the blood vessels most often affected by varicose veins and are the veins seen by eye when the varicose condition has developed.

The inside wall of veins have valves that open and close in response to the blood flow. When the left ventricle of the heart pushes blood out into the aorta, it produces the high pressure pulse of the heartbeat and pushes blood throughout the body. Between heartbeats, there is a period of low blood pressure. During the low pressure period, blood in the veins is affected by gravity and wants to flow downward. The valves in the veins prevent this from happening. Varicose veins start when one or more valves fail to close. The blood pressure in that section of vein increases, causing additional valves to fail. This allows blood to pool and stretch the veins, further weakening the walls of the veins. The walls of the affected veins lose their elasticity in response to increased blood pressure. As the vessels weaken, more and more valves are unable to close properly. The veins become larger and wider over time and begin to appear as lumpy, winding chains underneath the skin. Varicose veins can develop in the deep veins also. Varicose veins in the superficial veins are called primary varicosities, while varicose veins in the deep veins are called secondary varicosities.

The predisposing causes of varicose veins are multiple, and lifestyle and hormonal factors play a role. Some families seem to have a higher incidence of varicose veins, indicating that there may be a genetic component to this disease. Varicose veins are progressive; as one section of the veins weakens, it causes increased pressure on adjacent sections of veins. These sections often develop varicosities. Varicose veins can appear following **pregnancy**, **thrombophlebitis**, congenital blood vessel weakness, or **obesity**, but is not limited to these conditions. **Edema** of the surrounding tissue, ankles, and calves, is not usually a complication of primary (superficial) varicose veins and, when seen, usually indicates that the deep veins may have varicosities or clots.

Varicose veins are a common problem; approximately 15% of the adult population in the United States have varicose veins. Women have a much higher incidence of this disease than men. The symptoms can include aching, **pain**, itchiness, or burning sensations, especially when standing. In some cases, with chronically bad veins, there may be a brownish discoloration of the skin or ulcers (open sores) near the ankles. A condition that is frequently associated with varicose veins is spider-burst veins. Spider-burst veins are very small veins that are enlarged. They may be caused by back-pressure from varicose veins, but can be caused by other factors. They are frequently associated with pregnancy and there may be hormonal factors associated with their development. They are primarily of cosmetic concern and do not present any medical concerns.

Varicose veins can usually be seen. In cases where varicose veins are suspected, but can not be seen, a physician may frequently detect them by palpation (pressing with the fingers). X rays or ultrasound tests can detect varicose veins in the deep and perforator veins and rule out blood clots in the deep veins.

There is no cure for varicose veins. Treatment falls into two classes; relief of symptoms and removal of the affected veins. Symptom relief includes such measures as wearing support stockings, which compress the veins and hold them in place. This keeps the veins from stretching and limits pain. Other measures are sitting down, using a footstool when sitting, avoiding standing for long periods of time, and raising the legs whenever possible. These measures work by reducing the blood pressure in leg veins. Prolonged standing allows the blood to collect under high pressure in the varicose veins. **Exercise** such as walking, biking, and swimming, is beneficial. When the legs are active, the leg muscles help pump the blood in the veins. This limits the amount of blood that collects in the varicose veins and reduces some of the symptoms. These measures reduce symptoms, but do not stop the disease.

Surgery is used to remove varicose veins from the body. It is recommended for varicose veins that are causing pain or are very unsightly, and when hemorrhaging or recurrent thrombosis appear. Surgery involves making an incision through the skin at both ends of the section of vein being removed. A flexible wire is inserted through one end and extended to the other. The wire is then withdrawn, pulling the vein out with it. This is called ''stripping'' and is the most common method to remove superficial varicose veins. As long as the deeper veins are still functioning properly, a person can live without some of the superficial veins. Because of this, stripped varicose veins are not replaced.

Injection therapy is an alternate therapy used to seal varicose veins. This prevents blood from entering the sealed sections of the vein. The veins remain in the body, but no longer carry blood. This procedure can be performed on an outpatient basis and does not require anesthesia. It is frequently used if people develop more varicose veins after surgery to remove the larger varicose veins and to seal spider-burst veins for people concerned about cosmetic appearance. Injection therapy is also called sclerotherapy. At one time, a method of injection therapy was used that did not have a good success rate. Veins did not seal properly and blood clots formed. Modern injection therapy is improved and has a much higher success rate.

Untreated varicose veins become increasingly large and more obvious with time. Surgical stripping of varicose veins is successful for most patients. Most do not develop new, large varicose veins following surgery. Surgery does not decrease a person's tendency to develop varicose veins. Varicose veins may develop in other locations after stripping.

VARMUS, HAROLD E. (1939-)

American microbiologist and virologist

Harold Eliot Varmus was born in Oceanside, New York, on December 18, 1939. He attended Amherst College, graduating with a B.A. degree in 1961 (twenty-three years later, Amherst would award him with an honorary doctorate). Varmus went on to perform graduate work at Harvard University, receiving an M.A. degree in 1962, then he studied medicine at Columbia University, receiving an M.D. in 1966.

Varmus practiced medicine as an intern and resident at the Presbyterian Hospital of New York City between 1966 and 1968. He then worked as a clinical associate at the National Institutes of Health in Bethesda, Maryland, from 1968 to 1970. Moving to California, Varmus served as a lecturer in the department of microbiology at the University of California in San Francisco, becoming an associate professor in 1974—the same year that he was named associate editor of *Cell and Virology*—then, in 1979, he was promoted to full professor of microbiology, biochemistry and biophysics. During the 1980s, Varmus began to accumulate a number of prestigious honors for his research, including the 1982 California Academic Scientist of the Year award and the 1983 Passano Foundation award; he was also the co-recipient of the Lasker Foundation award. In 1984, Varmus received both the Armand Hammer Cancer prize and the General Motors Alfred Sloan award, and the American Cancer Society made him an honorary professor of molecular virology. These honors were followed by the Shubitz Cancer prize and, in 1989, the Nobel Prize in physiology or medicine.

Varmus and J. Michael Bishop, his colleague from the University of California at San Francisco, were awarded the Nobel Prize in in honor of their 1976 discovery which showed that normal cells contain genes that can cause **cancer**. Varmus and Bishop, working with Dominique Stehelin and Peter Vogt, helped to prove the theory that cancer has a genetic component, demonstrating that oncogenes are actually normal genes that are altered in some way, perhaps due to carcinogen-induced mutations. Their research focused on Rous sarcoma, a virus which can produce tumors in chickens by attaching to a normal chicken gene as it duplicates within a cell. Since then, research has identified a number of additional ''proto-oncogenes'' which, when circumstances dictate, abandon their normal role of overseeing cell division and growth and turn potentially cancerous. Varmus's and Bishop's oncogene studies had a tremendous impact on the efforts to understand the genetic basis of cancer. The results of their work quickly found practical applications, especially in cancer diagnosis and prognosis.

Varmus was nominated by U.S. President Bill Clinton to the directorship of the National Institutes of Health and was confirmed in November 1993. The director of the NIH plays a vital part in setting the course for biomedical research in the United States. Varmus's nomination was strongly supported by biomedical scientists, but there was some opposition from **AIDS** activists. They—as well as others who were concerned with the health of women and members of minority groups—were concerned that Varmus would be more interested in basic biomedical research than in applied studies and feared that the medical research related to their specific concerns might be neglected. Varmus has argued that basic research in science, especially investigations of the fundamental properties of cells, genes, and tissues, could eventually lead to cures for many diseases, such as AIDS and cancer. As director, Varmus is also interested in revitalizing the intramural research program at NIH. He believes that science education in the United States needs to be improved and that students should be exposed to a science curriculum sooner, in smaller classes, by better-informed teachers.

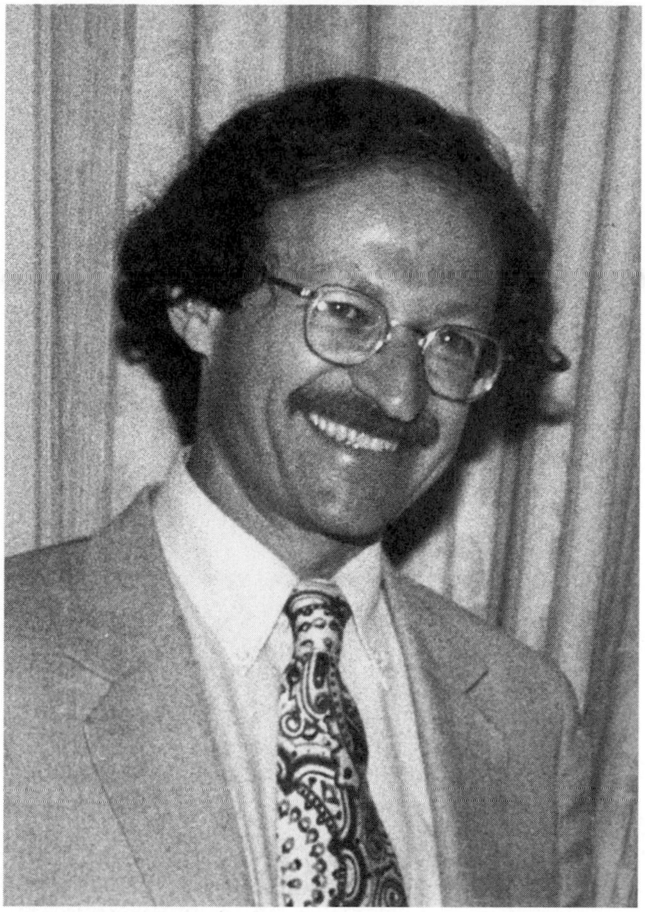

Harold Eliot Varmus

VASCULITIS

Vasculitis refers to a varied group of disorders which all share a common underlying problem of inflammation of a blood vessel or blood vessels. The inflammation may affect any size blood vessel, anywhere in the body. It may affect either arteries and/or veins. The inflammation may be focal, meaning that it affects a single location within a vessel; or it may be widespread, with areas of inflammation scattered throughout a particular organ or tissue, or even affecting more than one organ system in the body.

Inflammation is a process which occurs when the immune system of the body responds to either an injury or a foreign invader (virus, bacteria, or fungi). The immune system response involves sending a variety of cells and chemicals to the area in question. Inflammation causes blood vessels in the area to leak, causing swelling. The inflamed area becomes red, hot to the touch, and tender.

Antibodies are immune cells which recognize and bind to specific markers (called antigens) on other cells (including bacteria and viruses). These antibody-antigen complexes can then stimulate the immune system to send a variety of other cells and chemicals involved in inflammation to their specific location.

Some researchers believe that the damaging process of vasculitis is kicked off by such antibody-antigen complexes. These complexes are deposited along the walls of the blood vessels. The resulting inflow of immune cells and chemicals causes inflammation within the blood vessels.

The type of disease caused by vasculitis varies depending on a number of factors:

- The organ system or tissue in which the vasculitis occurs
- The specific type of inflammatory response provoked
- Whether the affected vessels are veins (which bring blood to the heart) or arteries (which carry blood and oxygen from the heart to the organs and tissues)
- The degree to which blood flow within the affected vessel is reduced.

Some types of vasculitis appear to be due to a type of allergic response to a specific substance (for example, a drug). Other types of vasculitis have no identifiable initiating event. Furthermore, researchers have not been able to consistently identify antibody-antigen complexes in all of the types of diseases caused by vasculitis. The types of antigens responsible for the initial immune response have often gone unidentified as well. Furthermore, not all people with such complexes deposited along the blood vessels go on to develop vasculitis. Some researchers believe that, in addition to the presence of immune complexes, an individual must have some other characteristics which make him or her susceptible to vasculitis. Many questions have yet to be answered to totally explain the development these diseases.

Symptoms of vasculitis depend on the severity of the inflammation and the organ system or systems affected. Some types of vasculitis are so mild that the only symptoms noted are small reddish-purple dots (called petechiae) on the skin due to tiny amounts of blood seeping out of leaky blood vessels. In more widespread types of vasculitis, the patient may have general symptoms of illness, including **fever**, achy muscles and joints, decreased appetite, weight loss, and loss of energy. The organ systems affected by vasculitis may include:

- The skin
- The joints
- The gastrointestinal system
- The heart
- The lungs
- The kidneys

Multiple types of disease are associated with vasculitis. Many autoimmune diseases have vasculitis as one of their complications. These include **systemic lupus erythematosus**, **rheumatoid arthritis**, **scleroderma**, and polymyositis. Other types of diseases which have vasculitis as their major manifestations include:

- Polyarteritis nodosa
- Kawasaki's disease
- Henoch-Schonlein purpura
- Serum sickness
- Temporal arteritis (also called giant cell arteritis)
- Takayasu's arteritis,
- Wegener's granulomatosis

Diagnosis of any type of vasculitis involves demonstrating the presence of a strong inflammatory process. Tests which reveal inflammation throughout the body include erythrocyte sedimentation rate, blood tests which may reveal anemia and increased white blood cells, and tests to demonstrate the presence of immune complexes and/or antibodies circulating in the blood. An x-ray procedure, called **angiography**, involves injecting dye into a major artery, and then taking x-ray pictures to examine the blood vessels, in order to demonstrate the presence of inflammation of the vessel walls. Tissue samples (biopsies) may be taken from affected organs to demonstrate inflammation.

Even though there are many different types of vasculitis, with many different symptoms based on the organ system affected, treatments are essentially the same. They all involve trying to decrease the activity of the immune system. Steroid medications (like prednisone) are usually the first types of drugs used. Steroids work by interfering with the chemicals involved in the inflammatory process. More potent drugs for severe cases of vasculitis have more serious side effects. These include drugs like cyclophosphamide. Cyclophosphamide works by actually killing cells of the patient's immune system.

The prognosis for vasculitis is quite variable. Some mild forms of vasculitis, such as those brought on by reactions to medications, may resolve totally on their own and not even require treatment. Temporal arteritis, serum sickness, Henoch-Schonlein purpura, and Kawasaki's disease usually have excellent prognoses, although when Kawasaki's affects the heart, there is a high **death** rate. Other types of vasculitis were always fatal, prior to the availability of prednisone and cyclophosphamide, and continue to have high rates of fatal complications. These include polyarteritis nodosa and Wegener's granulomatosis.

Because so little is known about what causes a particular individual to develop vasculitis, there are no known ways to prevent it.

Vasectomy

A vasectomy is a surgical procedure performed on males in which the vas deferens (tubes that carry sperm from the testicles to the seminal vesicles) are cut, tied, cauterized (burned or seared) or otherwise interrupted. The semen no longer contains sperm after the tubes are cut, so conception cannot occur. The testicles continue to produce sperm, but they die and are absorbed by the body.

The purpose of this operation is to provide reliable **contraception**. Research indicates that the level of effectiveness is 99.6%. Vasectomy is the most reliable method of contraception.

Vasectomies are often performed in the doctor's office using a local anesthesia. The patient's scrotum area will be shaved and cleaned with an antiseptic solution to reduce the chance of infection. A small incision is made into the scrotum (the sac containing the testicles that produce the sperm). Each of the vas deferens (one from each testicle) is tied in two places with nonabsorbable (permanent) sutures and the tube is severed between the ties. The ends may be cauterized (burned or seared) to decrease the chance that they will leak or grow back together.

Sterility does not occur immediately after the procedure is finished. Men must use other methods of contraception until two consecutive semen analyses confirm that there are no sperm present in the semen. This will take 4-6 weeks or 15-20 ejaculations to clear all of the sperm from the tubes.

''No scalpel'' vasectomies are gaining popularity. Instead of an incision, a small puncture is made into the scrotum. The vas deferens are cut and sealed in a manner similar to that described above. No stitches are necessary and the patient has less **pain**. Other advantages include less damage to the tissues, less bleeding, less risk of infection, and less discomfort after the procedure.

In some, cases vasectomies may be reversed. However, this procedure should be considered permanent as there is no guarantee of successful reversal.

No special physical preparation is required. The physician will first assess the patient's general health in order to identify any potential problems that could occur. The doctor will then explain possible risks and side effects. The patient is asked to sign a consent form which indicates that he understands the information he has received, and gives the doctor permission to perform the operation.

Following the surgery, ice packs are often applied to the scrotum to decrease pain and swelling. A dressing (or athletic supporter) which supports the scrotum can also reduce pain. Mild over-the-counter pain medication such as **aspirin** or **acetaminophen** (Tylenol) should be able to control any discomfort. Activities may be restricted for 1-2 days, and sexual intercourse for 3-4 days.

There are very few risks associated with vasectomy other than infection, bruising, epididymitis (inflammation of the tube that carries the sperm from the testicle to the penis), and sperm granulomas (collection of fluid that leaks from a poorly sealed or tied vas deferens). These are easily treated if they do occur. Patients do not experience difficulty achieving an erection, maintaining an erection, or ejaculating. There is no decrease in the production of the male hormone (testosterone), and sex drive and ability are not altered. Vasectomy is safer and less expensive than **tubal ligation** (sterilization of a female by cutting the fallopian tube to prevent conception).

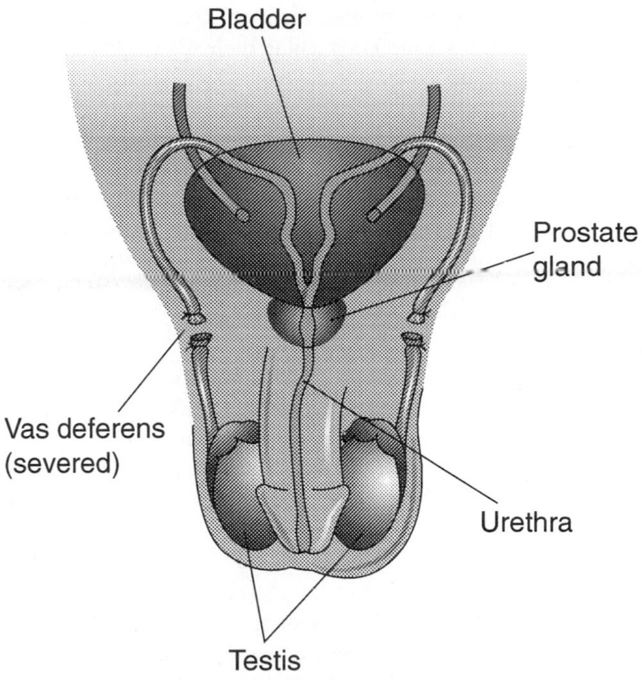

Vasectomy is a surgical procedure performed on males in which the vas deferens (tubes that conduct sperm from the testicles to the penis) are cut, tied, cauterized, or otherwise interrupted. Although the testicles still produce sperm, the sperm die and are absorbed by the body. Men who have had vasectomies may continue to ejaculate the same amount of semen as before the procedure. *(Illustration by Electronic Illustrators Group.)*

VASODILATORS

Vasodilators are medicines that act directly on muscles in blood vessel walls to make blood vessels widen (dilate).

Vasodilators are used to treat high blood pressure (**hypertension**). By widening the arteries, these drugs allow blood to flow through more easily, reducing blood pressure. Controlling high blood pressure is important because the condition puts a burden on the heart and the arteries, which can lead to permanent damage over time. If untreated, high blood pressure increases the risk of **heart attack**s, **heart failure**, **stroke**, or kidney failure. Vasodilators usually are prescribed with other types of blood pressure drugs and rarely are used alone.

Examples of vasodilators are hydralazine (Apresoline) and minoxidil (Loniten). The vasodilator hydralazine also may be used to control high blood pressure in pregnant women or to bring down extremely high blood pressure in emergency situations. In the forms used for treating high blood pressure (tablets or injections), these drugs are available only with a physician's prescription. A liquid form of minoxidil, used to promote hair growth in people with certain kinds of baldness and is applied directly to the scalp, is sold without a prescription.

Seeing a physician regularly while taking a vasodilator is important, especially during the first few months. The physician will check to make sure the medicine is working as it should and will watch for unwanted side effects. People who have high blood pressure often feel fine. But even when they feel well, patients should keep seeing their physicians and taking their medicine.

Vasodilators will not cure high blood pressure, but will help control the condition. To avoid the serious health problems that high blood pressure can cause, patients may have to take medicine for the rest of their lives. Furthermore, medicine alone may not be enough. People with high blood pressure may also need to avoid certain foods and keep their weight under control. The health care professional who is treating the condition can offer advice on what measures may be necessary.

Some people feel dizzy or have **headaches** while using this medicine. These problems are especially likely to occur in older people, who are more sensitive than younger people to the medicine's effects. Anyone who takes these drugs should not drive, use machines, or do anything else that might be dangerous until they know how the drugs affect them.

People who have certain medical conditions or who are taking certain other medicines may have problems if they take vasodilators. Before taking these drugs, be sure to let the physician know about any of these conditions:

Anyone who has had an unusual reaction to a vasodilator in the past should let his or her physician know before taking this type of drug again. The physician should also be told about any **allergies** to foods, dyes, preservatives, or other substances.

Several problems—from excess hair growth to blood abnormalities—have been reported in babies whose mothers take this vasodilators during **pregnancy**. In studies of laboratory animals, hydralazine causes **birth defects** in mice and rabbits, but not in rats. The effects of taking vasodilators during pregnancy have not been specifically studied in humans. Women who are pregnant or who may become pregnant should check with their physicians before using this medicine. Women who become pregnant while taking a vasodilator should tell their physicians right away.

Using a vasodilator to lower blood pressure may worsen the problems that result from heart disease, blood vessel disease, or a recent heart attack or stroke. This medicine may also make **angina** (chest **pain**) worse. And in people with pheochromocytoma (tumor of the adrenal medulla), vasodilators may make the tumor more active. Before using a vasodilator, people with any of these medical problems should make sure their physicians are aware of their conditions.

Anyone who has unusual symptoms while taking a vasodilator should get in touch with his or her physician.

Vasodilators may interact with other medicines. *Do not take any other medicine without the approval of the physician who prescribed the vasodilator.* In particular, avoid using over-the-counter medicines for appetite control, colds, cough, sinus problems, asthma, hay fever and other allergies, as these may increase blood pressure. At the other extreme, dangerously low blood pressure may result when drugs such as the blood pressure medicine guanethidine (Ismelin) or nitrates, used to treat chest pain, are combined with vasodilators.

VESALIUS, ANDREAS (1514-1564)

Flemish anatomist and physician

While still a young physician, Andreas Vesalius overturned the fourteen-centuries-old Galenic canon of medicine and founded modern scientific anatomy.

Born in Brussels in what is today Belgium to a family established in medicine for several generations, the young Andreas showed an early interest in anatomy. He attended the University of Louvain and then studied medicine at the University of Paris where he became skilled at dissection under teachers who were dedicated followers of **Galen**.

After a stint as a military surgeon, Vesalius enrolled at the University of Padua, Europe's preeminent medical school, receiving his doctor of medicine degree in 1537. Immediately assuming a post as lecturer in surgery and anatomy at Padua, Vesalius proved to be an innovative teacher. Contrary to prevailing practice, he performed dissections himself during the lectures and illustrated the lesson with large, detailed anatomical charts. The lectures were enormously popular and demand for the charts was so great that Vesalius had them printed as *Tabulae anatomicae sex* in 1538.

As Vesalius proceeded with his dissections, he increasingly noted obvious conflicts between what he saw in the human body and what Galen described. Galen's errors, Vesalius reasoned, arose because the ancient anatomist relied only on animal dissections, which often did not apply to human anatomy. Vesalius set down the principle that true, fundamental medical knowledge must come from human dissection, practiced by each individual physician.

To attract established physicians to the study of anatomy and promote the teaching of this new science, Vesalius devoted himself for five years to the production of his magnum opus, one of the most important books in medical history and the world's first textbook of anatomy: *De humani corporis fabrica*, published in 1543. Vesalius carefully supervised all aspects of the book's production. The *Fabrica* contained detailed anatomical descriptions of all parts of the human body, including directions for carrying out dissections; magnificent, meticulous illustrations, probably by students from Titian's studio; and a clear explanation of the objective, scientific method of conducting medical research.

Publication of the *Fabrica* rocked Galenism to its foundations. This shattering of the revered, supposedly infallible ideas of Galen provoked bitter controversy, which may have been why Vesalius abruptly quit anatomical research and became court physician to Emperor Charles V and, later, to Charles's son, Philip II of Spain. As in anatomy, Vesalius achieved renown as a medical practitioner. In 1564 he left Spain for a trip to the Holy Land, perhaps intending then to return to teaching at Padua. On the way back from Palestine, however, his ship was wrecked, and Vesalius died on the island of Zante at the age of fifty.

VIOLENCE AND VIOLENCE PREVENTION

Violence lies at the extreme of deviant behavior. The U.S. Bureau of Justice Statistics show that American teenagers experience the highest rates of violent crime, while blacks experience the highest rates of *serious* violent crime. The homicide rate is highest for teens and young adults. Victims of violent crimes have reported that juveniles age 12-17 committed about one-quarter of the serious violent crimes in 1997.

Domestic violence, primarily against women, occurs so often in the United States that the **American Medical Association** declared it to be **public health** hazard (1992). Women between the ages of 19 and 29 are particularly at risk. In 1994, violence against women was declared a federal crime. More women receive injuries at the hands of their intimate partners than from any other single cause. In New York City, it is the leading cause of death among women. Another way of looking at the problem is to note that, during the Vietnam War, there were 58,000 American soldiers killed in Southeast Asia; in the same period of time, 51,000 women were murdered by their domestic partners in America.

Child abuse and domestic violence frequently occur in the same family. Researchers estimate that 50-70% of men who assault their wives also abuse their children. Children are 1,500 times more likely to be abused in homes where domestic violence already occurs. Domestic violence may result in physical injury, psychological harm, or neglect of children. There is a documented relationship between family violence and juvenile delinquency. Abused children have a six times greater chance of committing suicide, 24% greater chance committing sexual assault crimes, and a 50% greater likelihood of abusing drugs and alcohol. Findings show, however, that children growing up in violent homes do not need to be physically abused to take on violent and delinquent behavior; it is simply enough to witness their mother's abuse. Studies have shown that adolescents who are exposed to high levels of violence in their neighborhoods are at increased risks of engaging in antisocial behavior and of suffering from anxiety, depression and psychosomatic illness. Disturbingly, a 1997 **Centers for Disease Control** and Prevention (CDC) study found that nationwide, 8.5% of all students carry a weapon to school, and 4% of all students missed one or more days of school in the month preceding the study because they felt unsafe at school or traveling to school.

While the overall mortality rate among U.S. children decreased 33.5% between 1979 and 1995, the number of homicides and suicides among American children have dramatically increased over the last two decades, according to a report issued in 1999 by the Public Health Policy Advisory Board. In 1995, the Commonwealth Fund Commission on **Women's Health** reported that an individual's response to an acute violent event is largely the same whether that person is experiencing trauma from war, incarceration in a concentration camp, or domestic assault. The commission noted that is not uncommon for the victim of a violent act to experience paralyzing terror, anxiety bordering on panic, loss of control, and sudden realizations of his/her own vulnerability, with reactions that can include nightmares, insomnia, poor concentration, amnesia, hypervigilance, and hypersensitivity to any association even remotely connected with violence, such as the slamming of a door.

A 1999 study sponsored by the Group for the Advancement of Psychiatry's Committee on Preventive Psychiatry proposed three preventive strategies focused on both communities and individuals to help reduce current levels of teen violence. The study concluded that prevention can take one of three forms: *universal* preventive measures aimed at the general population, for example, federal and state programs that enhance prenatal care, maternal/infant care and nutrition, and family management for preschool children and parents (this idea is based in part on an observed link of violence to poor **nutrition**); *selective* strategies focused on high-risk (usually urban) communities such as Head Start, gun-free zones around schools, job training programs aimed at high-risk youth, and midnight basketball leagues; and *indicated* programs consisting of efforts aimed at teens thought to be at especially high risk for violent behavior. In the case of indicated programs, the researchers cited the so-called *Boston miracle*, where a combination of well-funded efforts reduced the number of teens killed by guns to zero for a period of over 2 years. While some other researchers agree that more and better interventions are needed to mitigate the human suffering of perpetrators and victims alike, they fear the funding and political will for these efforts will be lacking in an era more concerned with punishment than prevention. At least one social observer has questioned whether attempts to end violence in America have any hope of succeeding as long as legislators continue to approve hundreds of millions of dollars in funds each year for weapons of mass destruction.

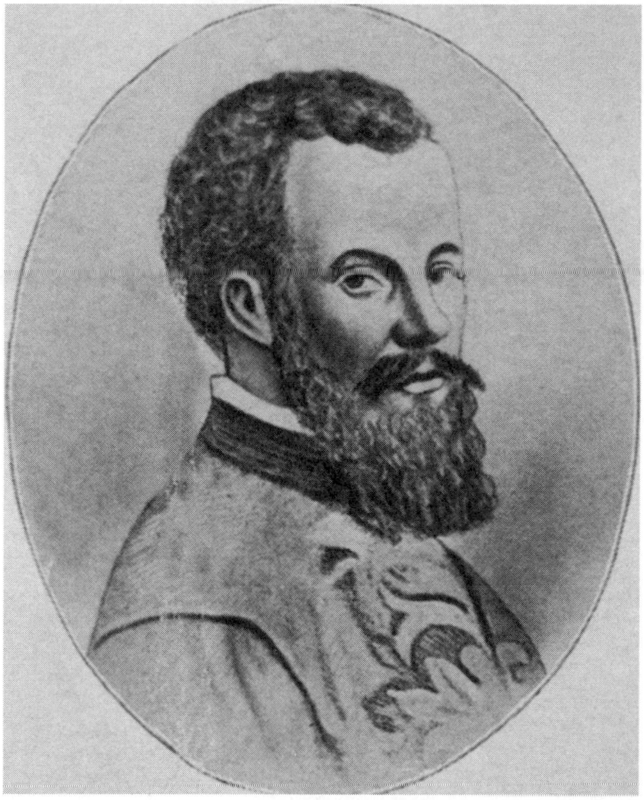

Andreas Vesalius

See also Mental illness

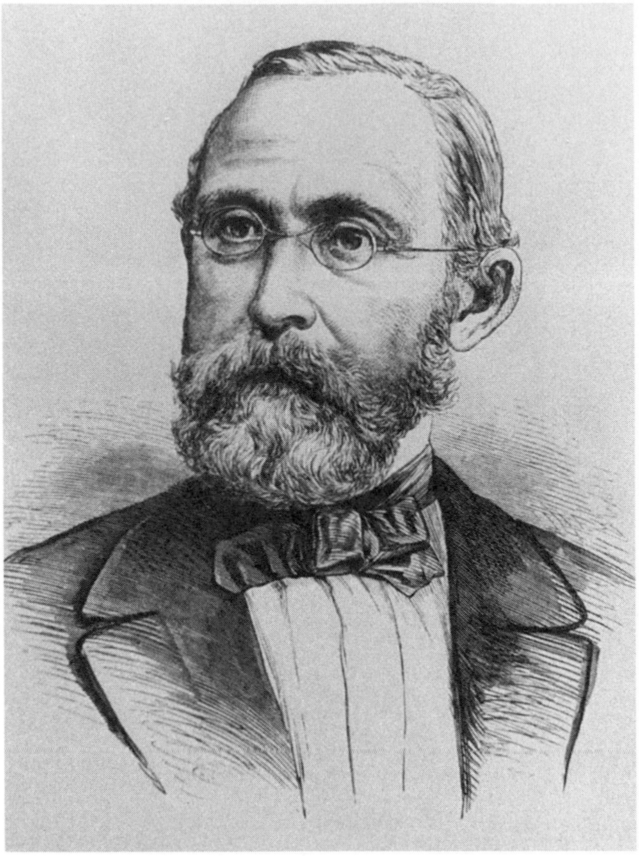

Rudolf Virchow

VIRCHOW, RUDOLF CARL (1821-1902)

German physician and anatomist

Rudolf Virchow, an only child, was born in a small rural town in Germany. His early interest in the natural sciences and broad humanistic training helped him get high marks throughout school. In 1839, his outstanding scholarly abilities earned him a military fellowship to study medicine at the Freidrich-Wilhelms Institut in Berlin, Germany. Virchow had the opportunity to study under Johannes Müller, gaining experience in experimental laboratory and diagnostic methods.

In 1843, he received his medical degree from the University of Berlin and went on to become company surgeon at the Charité Hospital in Berlin. In this post, he was one of the first to describe ''white blood'' (leukemia). As a young man, he became a powerful speaker for the new generation of German physicians. He viewed medical progress as coming from three main sources: clinical observations, including examination of the patient; animal experimentation to test methods and drugs; and pathological anatomy, especially at the microscopic level. He also insisted that life was the sum of physical and chemical actions and essentially the expression of cell activity. Although these views caused some older physicians to condemn Virchow, he received his medical license in 1846.

Two years later, Virchow was sent to Prussia to treat victims of a **typhus** epidemic. Seeing the desperate condition of the Polish minority, he recommended sweeping educational and economic reform and political freedom. From that point on, he was a firm believer that to do any good for sick people, one must treat the sick society. Acting on his convictions, Virchow fought in the uprisings of 1848 and became a member of the Berlin Democratic Congress. Unfortunately, his strong political and social conscience cost him his university post. Virchow finally left Berlin for the more liberal atmosphere of the University of Wurzburg. There he embarked on his highest level of scientific achievement—his development of cellular pathology.

In 1855, Virchow published his journal article on cellular pathology. ''*Omnis cellula e cellula*,'' he wrote, meaning all cells arise from cells. Essentially, his article generalized the concept of cell theory and modernized the entire medical field. The cell became the fundamental living unit in both healthy *and* diseased tissue. He used the microscope to bring the study of disease down to a more fundamental level; disease occurred because healthy living cells were altered or disturbed. However, he rejected the **germ theory** developed by **Louis Pasteur**, arguing instead that diseased tissue resulted from the breakdown of order within cells and not from the invasion of a foreign body. Scientists have since discovered that disease results from both circumstances.

VISION TRAINING

Vision training, also known as vision therapy or orthoptics, consists of a variety of programs to enhance visual performance. It includes treatments for focusing, binocularity, and eye movement problems. Vision training is generally provided by an optometrist (O.D.).

While visual acuity refers to how clearly each eye can see, vision training addresses how well the two eyes work together as a team. When looking at an object, the eyes must focus on the object (e.g., focusing for near or far objects). This involves the lens system of the eyes. The eyes must also work as a team and point at the same object so that the person does not see double. Aiming precisely at the same object will aid in depth perception (stereopsis) and seeing objects in three-dimensions (3D).

Although crossed eyes (**strabismus**) is an obvious condition, many defects in the coordination of eye movement are far less apparent. Even so, they can cause problems in reading, driving vehicles, and other complex tasks that require the integrated function of eyes and body. It is the goal of vision therapy to improve these subtle interactions using carefully devised **exercise**s and devices.

The discipline, called ''behavioral optometry,'' involves a careful evaluation of visual function, concentrating on complex skills such as rapid reading, distance perception, peripheral field awareness, accommodative facility, and the coordinated movement of each eye in relationship to the other. From that assessment the doctor goes on to design a course of exercises to correct the problems discovered. Like any other type of training, success requires practice and persistence until habits and reflexes can be retrained.

There are a number of different techniques and instruments used in vision therapy; the field is evolving rapidly in many directions. Some computerized exercises are being developed that promise better patient motivation. A device called the Dynavision apparatus, has produced positive results in retraining **stroke** victims to operate motor vehicles. And traditional forms of vision therapy have increased reading efficiency in an older age group (62 to 75 years).

Because the goal of vision training is to improve visual efficiency and visual processing, people having problems reading should consider a vision training evaluation. Children rubbing their eyes while reading, avoiding reading, or getting **headaches** while reading should be evaluated. Problems with sustaining focusing (accommodative insufficiency) or problems keeping words single (convergence or divergence problems) may be present. A full eye-health evaluation and vision training workup may reveal a problem. Vision training is also appropriate for people learning how to coordinate the eyes after surgery for strabismus. Vision training can also be used in lazy eye (**amblyopia**) and includes patching the eye and doing various exercises.

Dyslexia is a problem with following the flow of words when reading. Often the order of letters or words is reversed. It is a complex problem involving the way the brain processes the stream of information coming in from the eyes. While vision therapy is not a treatment for dyslexia or learning disabilities, there may be an underlying visual processing problem that may be present. Vision therapy can be part of a multidisciplinary approach to treating learning disabilities.

Sports vision deals with visual performance in sport-related activities. Protective eyewear is also a large consideration when participating in sports. Basketball, baseball, racquetball, and swimming (and other sports as well) can all cause injury to the eyes. Batting helmets with face shields, protective goggles with polycarbonate lenses, or something as simple as ultraviolet (UV) coatings on glasses to protect the eyes from the sun in outdoor sports such as golf can protect the eyes. Hitting a baseball or throwing a basketball into a hoop requires accurate fixation. Golfers need to see clearly and judge distance. Bifocals may need to be adjusted to allow for putting, driving, and reading the score card. While many of these issues (e.g., UV coatings) can be addressed at a regular eye exam, sports vision may be able to help with more specific, individual problems.

Behavioral optometry is a relatively new field of study. Results are mixed. Newer techniques, more refined evaluation methods, and newer pieces of apparatus are continuously being appraised. More study results are needed to define the scope and benefits of this discipline.

Vision therapy is individually tailored to the subject and the discovered problems. It can be a lengthy process with many variations that requires repetition until eye muscles, coordination, reflexes, habits, and the way the brain handles visual input are all retrained. Each program will be individualized. The patient should be aware of the time involved for treatment. Treatment can be from several weeks to several months depending upon the condition. Some insurance plans may cover vision training.

If vision therapy is recommended, the optometrist will discuss thoroughly what is expected and necessary for success. The patient must be prepared to perform some eye exercises at home.

Even after the treatment is successful, it may be necessary to continue the exercises to maintain the benefits. It may be necessary to repeat treatment in the future.

No risk is involved. The treatment is safe.

A carefully and individually tailored program of vision therapy should result in a gradual improvement in whatever complex visual function is being addressed. This progress ought to be measurable by using the same tests that were used to diagnose it. If the patient had symptoms, such as headaches or double vision while reading, they should be alleviated.

Because the treatment is safe, the only abnormal result is failure. At the start of treatment, the optometrist should provide a reasonable estimate of what improvement to expect and how long it will take. Should this prove incorrect, either the treatment needs to be modified or the problem deemed untreatable by that method.

VISUAL IMPAIRMENT AND BLINDNESS

Total blindness is the inability to tell light from dark, or the total inability to see. Visual impairment or low vision is a severe reduction in vision that can't be corrected with standard glasses or contact lenses and reduces a person's ability to function at certain or all tasks. Legal blindness (which is actually a severe visual impairment) refers to a best-corrected central vision of 20/200 or worse in the better eye or a visual acuity of better than 20/200 but with a visual field no greater than 20° (e.g., side vision that is so reduced that it appears as if the person is looking through a tunnel).

Vision is normally measured using a Snellen chart. A Snellen chart has letters of different sizes that are read, one eye at a time, from a distance of 20 ft. People with normal vision are able to read the 20 ft line at 20 ft—20/20 vision—or the 40 ft line at 40 ft, the 100 ft line at 100 ft, and so forth. If at 20 ft the smallest readable letter is larger, vision is designated as the distance from the chart over the size of the smallest letter that can be read.

Eye care professionals measure vision in many ways. Clarity (sharpness) of vision indicates how well a person's central visual status is. The diopter is the unit of measure for refractive errors such as nearsightedness, farsightedness, and **astigmatism** and indicates the strength of corrective lenses needed. People do not just see straight ahead; the entire area of vision is called the visual field. Some people have good vision (e.g., see clearly) but have areas of reduced or no vision (blind spots) in parts of their visual field. Others have good vision in the center but poor vision around the edges (peripheral visual field). People with very poor vision may be able only to count fingers at a given distance from their eyes. This distance becomes the measure of their ability to see.

The World Health Organization (WHO) defines impaired vision in five categories:

- Low vision 1 is a best corrected visual acuity of 20/70.
- Low vision 2 starts at 20/200.
- Blindness 3 is below 20/400.
- Blindness 4 is worse than 5/300
- Blindness 5 is no light perception at all
- A visual field between 5° and 10° (compared with a normal visual field of about 120°) goes into category 3; less than 5° into category 4, even if the tiny spot of central vision is perfect.

Color blindness is the reduced ability to perceive certain colors, usually red and green. It is a hereditary defect and affects very few tasks. Contrast sensitivity describes the ability to distinguish one object from another. A person with reduced contrast sensitivity may have problems seeing things in the fog because of the decrease in contrast between the object and the fog.

According to the WHO there are over forty million people worldwide whose vision is category 3 or worse, 80% of whom live in developing countries. Half of the blind population in the United States is over 65 years of age.

The leading causes of blindness include:

- **Macular degeneration**
- **Glaucoma**
- **Cataracts**
- Diabetes mellitus.

Other possible causes include infections, injury, or nutrition.

Most infectious eye diseases have been eliminated in the industrialized nations by sanitation, medication, and public health measures. Viral infections are the main exception to this statement. Some infections that may lead to visual impairment include:

- Herpes simplex **keratitis.**
- Trachoma.
- **Leprosy** (Hansen's disease).
- River blindness.

Exposure of a pregnant woman to certain diseases (e.g., **rubella** or **toxoplasmosis**) can cause congenital eye problems. Injuries to the eyes can result in blindness. Very little blindness is due to disease in the brain or the optic nerves. **Multiple sclerosis** and similar nervous system diseases, **brain tumor**s, diseases of the eye sockets, and head injuries are rare causes of blindness.

Vitamin A deficiency is a widespread cause of corneal degeneration in children in developing nations. As many as five million children develop xerophthalmia from this deficiency each year. Five percent end up blind.

A low vision exam is slightly different from a general exam. While a case history, visual status, and eye health evaluation are common to both exams, some things do differ. Eye charts other than a Snellen eye chart will be used. Testing distance will vary. A trial frame worn by the patient is usually used instead of the instrument containing the lenses the patient sits behind (phoropter). Because the low vision exam is slightly more goal oriented than a general exam, for example, what specifically is the patient having trouble with (reading, seeing street signs, etc.), different optical and nonoptical aids will generally be tried. Eye health is the last thing to be checked so that the lights necessary to examine the eyes won't interfere with the rest of the testing.

There are many options for patients with visual impairment. There are optical and nonoptical aids. Optical aids include:

- Telescopes
- Hand magnifiers
- Stand magnifiers
- Prisms
- Closed circuit television (CCTV)

Nonoptical aids can include large print books and magazines, check-writing guides, large print dials on the telephone, and more.

For those who are blind, there are enormous resources available to improve the quality of life. For the legally blind, financial assistance for help may be possible. Braille and audio books are increasingly available. Guide dogs provide well-trained eyes and independence. Orientation and mobility training is available. There are special schools for blind children and access to disability support through Social Security and private institutions.

The prognosis generally relates to the severity of the impairment and the ability of the aids to correct it. A good low vision exam is important to be aware of the latest low vision aids.

VITAMIN A DEFICIENCY

Vitamin A deficiency exists when the chronic failure to eat sufficient amounts of vitamin A or beta-carotene results in levels of blood-serum vitamin A that are below a defined range. Beta-carotene is a form of pre-vitamin A, which is readily converted to vitamin A in the body. Night blindness is the first symptom of vitamin A deficiency. Prolonged and severe vitamin A deficiency can produce total and irreversible blindness.

Vitamin A (called retinol in mammals) is a fat-soluble vitamin. The recommended dietary allowance (RDA) for vitamin A is 1.0 mg/day for the adult man and 0.8 mg/day for the adult woman. Since beta-carotene is converted to vitamin A in the body, the body's requirement for vitamin A can be supplied entirely by beta-carotene. Six mg of beta-carotene are considered to be the equivalent of 1 mg of vitamin A. The best sources of vitamin A are eggs, milk, butter, liver, and fish, such as herring, sardines, and tuna. Beef is a poor source of vitamin A. Plants do not contain vitamin A, but they do contain beta-carotene and other carotenoids. The best sources of beta-carotene are dark-green, orange, and yellow vegetables; spinach, carrots, oranges, and sweet potatoes are excellent examples. Cereals are poor sources of beta-carotene.

Vitamin A is used for two functions in the body. Used in the eye, it is a component of the eye's light-sensitive parts, containing rods and cones, that allow for night-vision or for seeing in dim-light circumstances. Vitamin A (retinol) occurs in the rods. Another form of Vitamin A, retinoic acid, is used in the body for regulating the development of various tissues, such as the cells of the skin, and the lining of the lungs and intestines. Vitamin A is important during embryological development, since, without vitamin A, the fertilized egg cannot develop into a fetus.

Vitamin A deficiency occurs with the chronic consumption of diets that are deficient in both vitamin A and beta-carotene. When vitamin A deficiency exists in the developed world, it tends to happen in alcoholics or in people with diseases that affect the intestine's ability to absorb fat. Examples of such diseases are **celiac disease** (chronic nutritional disorder), **cystic fibrosis**, and cholestasis (bile-flow failure or interference). Vitamin A deficiency occurred in infants during the early 1900s in Denmark. The deficiency resulted when milk fat was made into butter for export, leaving the by-product (skimmed milk) for infant feeding. Vitamin A deficiency has taken place in infants in impoverished populations in India, where the only foods fed to the infants were low in beta-carotene. Vitamin A deficiency is also common in areas like Southeast Asia, where polished rice, which lacks the vitamin, is a major part of the diet.

The earliest symptom of vitamin A deficiency is night blindness. Prolonged deficiency results in drying of the conjunctiva (the mucous membrane that lines the inner surface of the eyelids and extends over the forepart of the eyeball). With continued vitamin A deficiency, the drying extends to the cornea (xerophthalamia). The cornea eventually shrivels up and becomes ulcerated (keratinomalacia). Superficial, foamy gray triangular spots may appear in the white of the eye (Bitot's spots). Finally, inflammation and infection occur in the interior of the eye, resulting in total and irreversible blindness.

Vitamin A status is measured by tests for retinol. Blood-serum retinol concentrations of 30-60 mg/dl are considered in the normal range. Levels that fall below this range indicate vitamin A deficiency. Night blindness is measured by a technique called electroretinography. Xerophthalamia, keratinomalacia, and Bitot's spots are diagnosed visually by trained medical personnel.

Vitamin A deficiency can be prevented or treated by taking vitamin supplements or by getting injections of the vitamin. The specific doses given are oral retinyl palmitate (110 mg), retinyl acetate (66 mg), or injected retinyl palmitate (55 mg) administered on each of two successive days, and once a few weeks later if symptoms are not relieved.

The prognosis for correcting night blindness is excellent. Xerophthalamia can be corrected with vitamin A therapy. Ulcerations, tissue death, and total blindness, caused by severe vitamin A deficiency, cannot be treated with vitamin A.

Vitamin A deficiency can be prevented by including foods rich in vitamin A or beta-carotene as a regular component of the diet; liver, meat, eggs, milk, and dairy products are examples. Foods rich in beta-carotene include red peppers, carrots, pumpkins, as well as those just mentioned. Margarine is rich in beta-carotene, because this chemical is used as a coloring agent in margarine production. In Africa, Indonesia, and the Philippines, vitamin A deficiency is prevented by public health programs that supply children with injections of the vitamin.

VITAMIN B_6 DEFICIENCY

Vitamin B_6 is used by the body as a catalyst in reactions that involve amino acids. Vitamin B_6 deficiency is rare, since most foods eaten contain the vitamin.

Vitamin B_6 is a water-soluble vitamin. The recommended dietary allowance (RDA) for vitamin B_6 is 2.0 mg/day for the adult man and 1.6 mg/day for the adult woman. Vitamin B_6 in the diet generally occurs as a form called pyridoxal phosphate. In this form, it cannot be absorbed by the body. During the process of digestion, the phosphate group is removed, and pyridoxal is produced. However, the body readily absorbs pyridoxal, and converts it back to the active form of the vitamin (pyridoxal phosphate).

Poultry, fish, liver, and eggs are good sources of vitamin B_6, comprising about 3-4 mg vitamin/kg food; meat and milk contain lesser amounts of the vitamin. The vitamin also occurs, at about half this level, in a variety of plant foods, including beans, broccoli, cabbage, and peas. Vitamin B_6 tends to be destroyed with prolonged cooking, with storage, or with exposure to light.

As mentioned, vitamin B_6 takes various forms. One of these forms, called pyridoxine, is relatively stable. For this reason, pyridoxine is the form of vitamin B_6 that is used in vitamin supplements, or when foods are fortified. Apples and other fruits are poor sources of the vitamin, containing only 0.2-0.6 mg vitamin/kg food.

Vitamin B_6, used mainly in the body for the processing of amino acids, performs this task along with certain enzymes. The enzyme that participates in this type of complex is aminotransferase. Several types of aminotransferase exist. With vitamin B_6 deficiency, while aminotransferase continues to occur in the various organs of the body, there is an abnormally low level of the active vitamin B_6/aminotransferase complex present. Thus, this vitamin deficiency results in the impairment of a variety of activities in the body. With supplement correction of the vitamin B_6 deficiency, the aminotransferase then readily forms the active complex, and normal metabolism is restored.

Vitamin B_6 converts certain amino acids (glutamic acid, aspartic acid, glycine) to energy. This allows the body to process all dietary protein, even when the dietary protein is in excess of the body's needs. Vitamin B_6 also allows the body to synthesize certain amino acids. For example, if the diet is deficient or low in certain amino acids, such as glycine or serine, vitamin B_6 enables the body to make them from sugar. Vitamin B_6 is used also for the synthesis of certain hormones, such as adrenaline.

Vitamin B_6 deficiency occurs rarely. When it does, it is usually associated with poor absorption of nutrients in the gastrointestinal tract (as in alcoholism, or with chronic **diarrhea**), the taking of certain drugs (as isoniazid, hydrolazine, penicillamine) that inactivate the vitamin, with genetic disorders that inhibit metabolism of the vitamin, or in cases of **starvation**.

The symptoms of vitamin B_6 deficiency in adults are only vaguely defined. These include nervousness, irritability, **insomnia**, muscle weakness, and difficulty in walking. Vitamin B_6 deficiency may produce fissures and cracking at the corners of the mouth. The deficiency occurred in infants fed early versions of commercial canned infant formula, when the vitamin had been inadvertently omitted from the formula. This error resulted in infants failing to grow, in irritability, and in seizures.

Vitamin B_6 status is measured by the transaminase stimulation test. This test requires extraction of red blood cells, and placement of the cells in two test tubes. Special chemicals (reagents) are added to both test tubes to allow for measurement of aminotransferase. This enzyme requires pyridoxal phosphate. A known quantity of pure pyridoxal phosphate is added to one of the test tubes. The activity level of the enzyme is measured, and compared, in both test tubes. If the added pyridoxal phosphate did not stimulate activity, the patient is considered not to be deficient in vitamin B_6. Neither is the patient considered deficient if only slight stimulation occurred. But if a stimulation of four-fold or more occurred, a vitamin B_6 deficiency is present.

Vitamin B_6 deficiency can be prevented or treated with consumption of the recommended dietary allowance, as supplied by food or by vitamin supplements.

The prognosis for correcting vitamin B_6 deficiency is excellent.

Vitamin B_6 deficiency is not a major concern for most people. The deficiency can be prevented with consumption of a mixed diet that includes poultry, fish, eggs, meat, vegetables, and grains.

VITAMIN D DEFICIENCY

Vitamin D deficiency exists when the concentration of 25-hydroxy-vitamin D (25-OH-D) in the blood serum occurs at 12 ng/ml (nanograms/milliliter), or less. The normal concentration of 25-hydroxy-vitamin D in the blood serum is 25-50 ng/ml. When vitamin D deficiency continues for many months in growing children, the disease commonly referred to as rickets will occur. A prolonged deficiency of the vitamin in adults results in osteomalacia. Both diseases involve defects in bones.

Vitamin D is a fat-soluble vitamin, meaning it is able to be dissolved in fat. While some vitamin D is supplied by the diet, most of it is made in the body. To make vitamin D, cholesterol, a sterol that is widely distributed in animal tissues and occurs in the yolk of eggs, as well as in various oils and fats, is necessary. Once cholesterol is available in the body, a slight alteration in the cholesterol molecule occurs, with one change taking place in the skin. This alteration requires the energy of sunlight (or ultraviolet light). Vitamin D deficiency, as well as rickets and osteomalacia, tends to occur in persons who do not get enough sunlight and who fail to eat foods that are rich in vitamin D.

Once consumed, or made in the body, vitamin D is further altered to produce a hormone called 1,25-dihydroxy-vitamin D (1,25-diOH-D). The conversion of vitamin D to 1,25-diOH-D does not occur in the skin, but in the liver and kidney. First, vitamin D is converted to 25-OH-D in the liver; it then enters the bloodstream, where it is taken-up by the kidneys. At this point, it is converted to 1,25-diOH-D. Therefore, the manufacture of 1,25-diOH-D requires the participation of various organs of the body—the liver, kidney, and skin.

The purpose of 1,25-diOH-D in the body is to keep the concentration of calcium at a constant level in the bloodstream. The maintenance of calcium at a constant level is absolutely required for human life to exist, since dissolved calcium is required for nerves and muscles to work. One of the ways in which 1,25-diOH-D accomplishes this mission is by stimulating the absorption of dietary calcium by the intestines.

The sequence of events that can lead to vitamin D deficiency, then to bone disease, is as follows: a lack of vitamin D in the body creates an inability to manufacture 1,25-diOH-D, which results in decreased absorption of dietary calcium and increased loss of calcium in the feces. When this happens, the bones are affected. Vitamin D deficiency results in a lack of bone mineralization (calcification) in growing persons, or in an increased demineralization (decalcification) of bone in adults.

Vitamin D deficiency can be caused by conditions that result in little exposure to sunlight. These conditions include: living in northern countries; having dark skin; being elderly or an infant, and having little chance to go outside; and covering one's face and body, such as for religious reasons. Many Arab women cover the entire body with black cloth, and wear a veil and black gloves when they go outside. These women may acquire vitamin D deficiency, even though they live in a sunny climate.

Most foods contain little or no vitamin D. As a result, sunshine is often a deciding factor in whether vitamin D deficiency occurs. Although fortified milk and fortified infant formula contain high levels of vitamin D, human breast milk is rather low in the vitamin. The term fortified means that **vitamins** are added to the food by the manufacturer.

No harm is likely to result from vitamin D deficiency that occurs for only a few days a year. If the deficiency occurs for a period of many months or years, however, rickets or osteomalacia may develop. The symptoms of rickets include bowed legs and bowed arms. The bowed appearance is due to the softening of bones, and their bending if the bones are weight-bearing. Bone growth occurs through the creation of new cartilage, a soft substance at the ends of bones. When the mineral calcium phosphate is deposited onto the cartilage, a hard structure is created. In vitamin D deficiency, though, calcium is not available to create hardened bone, and the result is soft bone. Other symptoms of rickets include particular bony bumps on the ribs called rachitic rosary (beadlike prominences at the junction of the ribs with their cartilages) and knock-knees. Seizures may also occasionally occur in a child with rickets, because of reduced levels of dissolved calcium in the bloodstream.

Although osteomalacia is rare in the United States, symptoms of this disease include reduced bone strength, an increase in bone **fractures**, and sometimes bone **pain**, muscle weakness, and a waddling walk.

Rickets and osteomalacia are almost always treated with oral supplements of vitamin D, with the recommendation to acquire daily exposure to direct sunlight. An alternative to sunlight is the use of an ultraviolet (UV) lamp. When using UV lamps, the eyes must be covered to protect them against damage. Many types of sunglasses allow UV light to pass through, so only those that are opaque to UV light should be used. Attempts to acquire sunlight through glass windows fail to help the body make vitamin D. This is because UV light does not pass through window glass.

The prognoses for correcting vitamin D deficiency, rickets, and osteomalacia are excellent. Vitamin D treatment results in the return of bone mineralization to a normal rate, the correction of low plasma calcium levels, the prevention of seizures, and a recovery from bone pain. On the other hand, deformities such as bowed legs and the rachitic rosary persist throughout adult life.

Food fortification has almost completely eliminated rickets in the United States. Vitamin D deficiency can be prevented by acquiring the RDA through drinking fortified milk and eating fortified cereals. For those who cannot drink milk, supplements of pills might be considered. In some older people, a 400 IU supplement may not be enough to result in the normal absorption of calcium; therefore, daily doses of 10,000 IU per day may be needed. For infants who are fed only breast milk (and rarely exposed to sunshine), a daily supplement of 200-300 IU is recommended.

Vitamin E deficiency

Vitamin E deficiency is a very rare problem that results in damage to nerves. When vitamin E deficiency does occur, it strikes people with diseases that prevent the absorption of dietary fats and fat-soluble nutrients. Since vitamin E is a fat-soluble vitamin, it has some of the properties of fat.

The recommended dietary allowance (RDA) for vitamin E is 10 mg/day for the adult man, 8 mg/day for the adult woman, and 3 mg/day for the infant. Vitamin E occurs in foods in a variety of related forms. The most potent and useful form of vitamin E is called alpha-tocopherol. The best sources of vitamin E are vegetable oils, such as corn oil, soy oil, and peanut oil. Animal fats, such as butter and lard, contain lower levels of the vitamin. Corn oil contains about 16 mg of alpha-tocopherol per 100 g oil. Wheat-germ oil contains 120 mg alpha-tocopherol per 100 g oil. Fish, eggs, and beef contain relatively low levels of the vitamin, with about 1 mg per 100 g food.

Vitamin E seems to have only one function in the body: the prevention of the natural and continual process of deterioration of all body tissues. This deterioration is provoked by a number of causes; one of these is toxic oxygen. During the body's metabolism of atmospheric oxygen, toxic oxygen is produced continuously in the body by the formation of by-products. These toxic by-products include hydrogen peroxide, superoxide, and hypochlorite.

Hypochlorite is a natural product, produced by cells of the immune system. It is also the active component of bleach. Once formed, toxic oxygen can damage various parts of the body, such as the membranes which form the boundaries of every cell. Vitamin E serves the body in protecting membranes from toxic oxygen damage. In contrast, vitamin C serves to protect the aqueous, or watery, regions of the cell from toxic oxygen damage. The membranes that are most sensitive to toxic oxygen damage are the membranes of nerves; therefore, the main symptom of vitamin E deficiency is damage to the nervous system.

As mentioned, when vitamin E deficiency occurs, it strikes people with diseases that prevent the absorption of dietary fats and fat-soluble nutrients. These diseases include **cystic fibrosis**, cholestasis (bile-flow obstruction). Bile salts, produced in the liver, are required for the absorption of fats. Cholestasis causes a decrease in the formation of bile salts and the consequent failure of the body to absorb dietary fats. For this reason, this disease may result in vitamin E deficiency. Premature infants may be at risk for vitamin E deficiency because they may be born with low tissue levels of the vitamin, and because they have a poorly developed capacity for absorbing dietary fats. Infants suffering from fat-malabsorption diseases can develop symptoms of vitamin E deficiency by age two. In adults, the onset of a fat-malabsorption disease can provoke vitamin E deficiency after a longer period, as an example, ten years.

Vitamin E deficiency in humans results in ataxia (poor muscle coordination with shaky movements), decreased sensation to vibration, lack of reflexes, and **paralysis** of eye muscles. One particularly severe symptom of vitamin E deficiency is the inability to walk.

Vitamin E status is measured by assessment of the content of alpha-tocopherol in the blood plasma, using a method called high-pressure liquid chromatography. Blood plasma levels of alpha-tocopherol that are 5.0 mg/l, or above, indicate normal vitamin E status; levels below 5.0 mg/l indicate vitamin E deficiency.

Vitamin E deficiency that occurs with cholestatic liver disease, or other **malabsorption syndromes**, can be treated with weekly injections of 100 mg alpha-tocopherol that may continue for six months. Vitamin E deficiency in premature infants may require treatment for only a few weeks.

The prognosis for correcting the neurological symptoms of vitamin E deficiency is fair to excellent.

The prevention of vitamin E deficiency should not be a concern for most people, since the vitamin is found in a wide variety of foods. Attention has been given to the theory that vitamin E serves to protect against **cancer** and **atherosclerosis**. The evidence that normal levels of vitamin E protect against atherosclerosis is fairly convincing. However, there is little or no proof that vitamin E intake, above and beyond the recommended daily allowance (RDA), can prevent cancer or atherosclerosis.

Vitamin K deficiency

Vitamin K deficiency exists when chronic failure to eat sufficient amounts of vitamin K results in a tendency for spontaneous bleeding or in prolonged and excessive bleeding with trauma or injury. Vitamin K deficiency occurs also in newborn infants, as well as in people treated with certain **antibiotics**. The protein in the body most affected by vitamin K deficiency is a blood-clotting protein called prothrombin.

Vitamin K is a fat-soluble vitamin. The recommended dietary allowance (RDA) for vitamin K is 80 mg/day for the adult man, 65 mg/day for the adult woman, and 5 mg/day for the newborn infant. The vitamin K present in plant foods is called phylloquinone; while the form of the vitamin present in animal foods is called menaquinone. Both of these **vitamins** are absorbed from the diet and converted to an active form called dihydrovitamin K.

Spinach, lettuce, broccoli, brussels sprouts, and cabbage are good sources of vitamin K, containing about 8 mg vitamin K/kg food. Cow milk is also a good source of the vitamin.

A portion of the body's vitamin K is supplied by bacteria living in the intestine rather than by dietary sources.

Vitamin K plays an important role in blood clotting. Without the vitamin, even a small cut would cause continuous bleeding in the body, and **death**. Blood clotting is a process that begins automatically when any injury produces a tear in a blood vessel. The process of blood clotting involves a collection of molecules, which circulate continuously through the bloodstream. When an injury occurs, these molecules rapidly assemble and form the blood clot. The clotting factors are proteins, and include proteins called Factor II, Factor VII, Factor IX, and Factor X. Factor II is also called prothrombin. These proteins require vitamin K for their synthesis in the body. The blood-clotting process also requires a dozen other proteins that do not need vitamin K for their synthesis.

Newborns are especially prone to vitamin K deficiency. A nursing-mother's milk is low in the vitamin; breast milk can supply only about 20% of the infant's requirement. Infants are born with low levels of vitamin K in their body; they do not have any vitamin K-producing bacteria in their intestines. Their digestive tracts are sterile. As a result, a form of vitamin K deficiency, called hemorrhagic disease of the newborn, may develop. This disease involves spontaneous bleeding beneath the skin or elsewhere in the infant's body, and occurs in about 1% of all infants. In rare cases, it causes death due to spontaneous bleeding in the brain.

Vitamin K deficiency in adults is rare. When it occurs, it is found in people with diseases that prevent the absorption of fat. These diseases include **cystic fibrosis**, **celiac disease**, and cholestasis. Vitamin K deficiency can exist in adults treated with antibiotics that kill the bacteria that normally live in the digestive tract. As mentioned, the intestine-bacteria supply part of our daily requirement of vitamin K. Vitamin K deficiency can result in bleeding gums, and in skin that is easily bruised.

Vitamin K status is measured by the prothrombin time test. The normal prothrombin time is about 13 seconds. With vitamin K deficiency, the prothrombin time can be several minutes. The test involves taking a sample of blood, placing it in a machine called a fibrometer, and measuring the time it takes for blood-clot formation. Blood-clotting problems can also be caused by a rare genetic disease called **hemophilia**. Hemophilia is not related to vitamin K deficiency. Once vitamin K deficiency is suspected, further tests must be used to distinguish it from possible hemophilia. Where a bleeding disorder can be corrected by vitamin K treatment, the diagnosis of vitamin K deficiency is proven to be correct.

Vitamin K deficiency in newborn infants is treated and prevented with a single injection of phylloquinone (5 mg). Adults with vitamin K deficiency are treated with daily oral doses of 10 mg phylloquinone for one week.

The prognosis for correcting vitamin K deficiency, and associated blood-clotting problems, is excellent.

Aside from newborns and young infants, vitamin K deficiency is not a concern for the general population. Vitamin K deficiency can be prevented by assuring that the diet contains foods such as spinach, cabbage, brussels sprouts, and eggs. Soybean oil, canola oil, and olive oil are good sources of the vitamin, while corn oil and peanut oil are very poor sources.

Vitamin toxicity

Vitamin toxicity is a condition in which a person develops symptoms as side effects from taking massive doses of **vitamins**. Vitamins vary in the amounts that are required to cause toxicity and in the specific symptoms that result. Vitamin toxicity, which is also called hypervitaminosis or vitamin **poisoning**, is becoming more common in developed countries because of the popularity of vitamin supplements. Many people treat themselves for minor illnesses with large doses (megadoses) of vitamins.

Vitamins are organic molecules in food that are needed in small amounts for growth, reproduction, and the maintenance of good health. Some vitamins can be dissolved in oil or melted fat. These fat-soluble vitamins include vitamin D, vitamin E, vitamin A (retinol), and vitamin K. Other vitamins can be dissolved in water. These water-soluble vitamins include folate (folic acid), vitamin B_{12}, biotin, vitamin B_6, niacin, thiamin, riboflavin, pantothenic acid, and vitamin C (ascorbic acid). Taking too much of any vitamin can produce a toxic effect. Vitamin A and vitamin D are the most likely to produce hypervitaminosis in large doses, while riboflavin, pantothenic acid, biotin, and vitamin C appear to be the least likely to cause problems.

Vitamin supplements are used for the treatment of various diseases or for reducing the risk of certain diseases. For example, moderate supplements of folic acid appear to reduce the risk for certain **birth defects** (neural tube defects), and possibly reduce the risk of **cancer**. Therapy for diseases brings with it the risk for irreversible vitamin toxicity only in the case of vitamin D.

With the exception of folic acid supplements, the practice of taking vitamin supplements by healthy individuals has little or no relation to good health. Most adults in the United States can obtain enough vitamins by eating a well-balanced diet. It has, however, become increasingly common for people to take vitamins at levels far greater than the RDA. These high levels are sometimes called vitamin megadoses. Megadoses are harmless for most vitamins. But in the cases of a few of the vitamins— specifically vitamin D, vitamin A, and vitamin B_6— megadoses can be harmful or fatal. Some experts think that megadoses of vitamin C may protect people from cancer. On the other hand, other researchers have gathered indirect evidence that vitamin C megadoses may cause cancer.

Vitamin D and vitamin A are the most toxic of the fat-soluble vitamins. The symptoms of vitamin D toxicity are nausea, vomiting, **pain** in the joints, and loss of appetite. Toxic doses of vitamin D taken over a prolonged period of time result in irreversible deposits of calcium crystals in the soft tissues of the body that may damage the heart, lungs, and kidneys.

Vitamin A toxicity can occur with long-term consumption of 20 mg of retinol or more per day. The symptoms of vitamin A overdosing include accumulation of water in the brain (**hydrocephalus**), vomiting, tiredness, constipation, bone pain, and severe **headaches**.

Megadoses of vitamin E may produce headaches, tiredness, double vision, and diarrhea in humans. Studies with animals fed large doses of vitamin E have revealed that this vitamin may interfere with the absorption of other fat-soluble vitamins.

Prolonged consumption of megadoses of vitamin K (menadione) results in anemia, which is a reduced level of red blood cells in the bloodstream. When large doses of menadione are given to infants, they result in the deposit of pigments in the brain, nerve damage, the destruction of red blood cells (hemolysis), and **death**.

Folate occurs in various forms in food. There are over a dozen related forms of folate. The folate in oral vitamin supplements occurs in only one form, however— folic acid. Large doses of folic acid (20 grams/day) can result in eventual kidney damage.

Vitamin B_{12} is important in the treatment of pernicious anemia. Pernicious anemia is more common among middle-aged and older adults; it is usually detected in patients between the ages of 40 and 80. Although vitamin B_{12} toxicity is not an issue for patients being treated for pernicious anemia, treatment of these patients with folic acid may cause problems. Specifically, pernicious anemia is often first detected because the patient feels weak or tired. If the anemia is not treated, the patient may suffer irreversible nerve damage. The problem with folic acid supplements is that the folic acid treatment prevents the anemia from developing, but allows the eventual nerve damage to occur.

Vitamin B_6 is clearly toxic at doses about 1000 times the RDA. When the patient stops taking high doses of this vitamin, recovery begins after two months. Complete recovery may take two to three years.

Large doses of vitamin C are considered to be toxic in persons with a family history of or tendency to form **kidney stones** or gallbladder stones.

Niacin comes in two forms, nicotinic acid and nicotinamide. Either form can satisfy the adult requirement for this vitamin. Nicotinic acid, however, is toxic at levels of 100 times the RDA. It can cause flushing of the skin, nausea, diarrhea, and liver damage.

In all cases, treatment of vitamin toxicity requires discontinuing vitamin supplements. Vitamin D toxicity needs additional action to reduce the calcium levels in the bloodstream because it can cause abnormally high levels of plasma calcium (hypercalcemia). Severe hypercalcemia is a medical emergency and may be treated by infusing a solution of 0.9% sodium chloride into the patient's bloodstream. The infusion consists of two to three liters of salt water given over a period of one to two days.

The prognosis for reversing vitamin toxicity is excellent for most patients. Side effects usually go away as soon as overdoses are stopped. The exceptions are severe vitamin D toxicity, severe vitamin A toxicity, and severe vitamin B_6 toxicity. Too much vitamin D leads to deposits of calcium salts in the soft tissue of the body, which cannot be reversed. Birth defects due to vitamin A toxicity cannot be reversed. Damage to the nervous system caused by megadoses of vitamin B_6 can be reversed, but complete reversal may require a recovery period of over a year.

VITAMINS

Vitamins are organic components in food that are needed in very small amounts for growth and for maintaining good health. The vitamins include vitamin D, vitamin E, vitamin A, and vitamin K, or the fat-soluble vitamins, and folate (folic acid), vitamin B_{12}, biotin, vitamin B_6, niacin, thiamin, riboflavin, pantothenic acid, and vitamin C (ascorbic acid), or the water-soluble vitamins. Vitamins are required in the diet in only tiny amounts, in contrast to the energy components of the diet. The energy components of the diet are sugars, starches, fats, and oils, and these occur in relatively large amounts in the diet.

Most of the vitamins are closely associated with a corresponding vitamin deficiency disease. **Vitamin D deficiency** causes rickets, a disease of the bones. **Vitamin E deficiency** occurs only very rarely, and causes nerve damage. **Vitamin A deficiency** is common throughout the poorer parts of the world, and causes night blindness. Severe vitamin A deficiency can result in xerophthalamia, a disease which, if left untreated, results in total blindness. **Vitamin K deficiency** results in spontaneous bleeding. Mild or moderate folate deficiency is common throughout the world, and can result from the failure to eat green, leafy vegetables or fruits and fruit juices. Folate deficiency causes megaloblastic anemia, which is characterized by the presence of large abnormal cells called megaloblasts in the circulating blood. The symptoms of megaloblastic anemia are tiredness and weakness. Vitamin B_{12} deficiency occurs with the failure to consume meat, milk or other dairy products. Vitamin B_{12} deficiency causes megaloblastic anemia and, if severe enough, can result in irreversible nerve damage. Niacin deficiency results in **pellagra**. Pellagra involves skin **rashes** and scabs, **diarrhea**, and mental depression. Thiamin deficiency results in beriberi, a disease resulting in atrophy, weakness of the legs, nerve damage, and **heart failure**. Vitamin C deficiency results in **scurvy**, a disease that involves bleeding. Specific diseases uniquely associated with deficiencies in vitamin B_6, riboflavin, or pantothenic acid have not been found in the humans, though persons who have been starving, or consuming poor diets for several months, might be expected to be deficient in most of the nutrients, including vitamin B_6, riboflavin, and pantothenic acid.

Some of the vitamins serve only one function in the body, while other vitamins serve a variety of unrelated functions. Hence, some vitamin deficiencies tend to result in one type of defect, while other deficiencies result in a variety of problems.

People are treated with vitamins for three reasons. The primary reason is to relieve a vitamin deficiency, when one has been detected. Chemical tests suitable for the detection of all vitamin deficiencies are available. The diagnosis of vitamin deficiency is often aided by visual tests, such as the examination of blood cells with a microscope, the x ray examination of bones, or a visual examination of the eyes or skin.

A second reason for vitamin treatment is to prevent the development of an expected deficiency. Here, vitamins are administered even with no test for possible deficiency. One example is vitamin K treatment of newborn infants to prevent bleeding.

A third reason for vitamin treatment is to reduce the risk for diseases that may occur even when vitamin deficiency cannot be detected by chemical tests. One example is folate deficiency. The risk for cardiovascular disease can be slightly reduced for a large fraction of the population by folic acid supplements. And the risk for certain **birth defects** can be sharply reduced in certain women by folic acid supplements.

Vitamin treatment is important during specific diseases where the body's normal processing of a vitamin is impaired. In these cases, high doses of the needed vitamin can force the body to process or utilize it in the normal manner. One example is **pernicious anemia**, a disease that tends to occur in middle age or old age, and impairs the absorption of vitamin B_{12}. Surveys have revealed that about 0.1% of the general population, and 2-3% of the elderly, may have the disease. If left untreated, pernicous anemia leads to nervous system damage. The disease can easily be treated with large oral daily doses of vitamin B_{12} (hydroxocobalamin) or with monthly injections of the vitamin.

Vitamin supplements are widely available as over-the-counter products. But whether they work to prevent or curtail certain illnesses, particularly in people with a balanced diet, is a matter of debate and ongoing research. For example, vitamin C is not proven to prevent the **common cold**. Yet, millions of people take it for that reason. Ask a physician or pharmacist for more information on the appropriate use of multivitamin supplements.

Vitamin A and vitamin D can be toxic in high doses. Side effects range from dizziness to kidney failure. Ask a physician or pharmacist about the correct use of a multivitamin supplement that contains these vitamins.

Vitamin treatment is usually done in three ways: by replacing a poor diet with one that supplies the recommended dietary allowance, by consuming oral supplements, or by injections. Injections are useful for persons with diseases that prevent absorption of fat-soluble vitamins. Oral vitamin supplements are especially useful for persons who otherwise cannot or will not consume food that is a good vitamin source, such as meat, milk or other dairy products. For example, a vegetarian who will not consume meat may be encouraged to consume oral supplements of vitamin B_{12}.

Treatment of genetic diseases which impair the absorption or utilization of specific vitamins may require megadoses of the vitamin throughout one's lifetime. Megadose means a level of about 10-1000 times greater than the RDA. Pernicious anemia, homocystinuria, and biotinidase deficiency are three examples of genetic diseases which are treated with megadoses of vitamins.

Few risks are associated with vitamin treatment. Any possible risks depend on the vitamin and the reason why it was prescribed. Ask a physician or pharmacist about how and when to take vitamin supplements, particularly those that have not been prescribed by a physician.

VITILIGO

Vitiligo is a condition in which a loss of cells that give color to the skin (melanocytes) results in smooth, white patches in the midst of normally pigmented skin.

Vitiligo is a common, often inherited disorder characterized by areas of well-defined, milky white skin. People with vitiligo may have eye abnormalities and also have a higher incidence of thyroid disease, **diabetes mellitus**, and **pernicious anemia**. Vitiligo affects about 1-2% of the world's population. It is more easily observed in sun-exposed areas of the body and in darker skin types, but it affects any area of the body and all races. Vitiligo seems to affect men and women equally, although women more frequently seek treatment for the disorder.

Vitiligo may appear as one or two well-defined white patches or it may appear over large portions of the body. Typical sites for generalized vitiligo are areas surrounding body openings, bony areas, fingers, and toes. It can begin at any age but about 50% of the time it starts before the age of 20.

Vitiligo is a disorder with complex causes. People with vitiligo seem to inherit a genetic predisposition for the disorder, and the appearance of disorder can be brought on by a variety of precipitating causes. Many people report that their vitiligo first appeared following a traumatic or stressful event, such as an accident, job loss, **death** of a family member, severe **sunburn**, or serious illness. There are at least three theories about the underlying mechanism of vitiligo. One theory says nerve endings in the skin release a chemical that is toxic to the melanocytes. A second theory states that the melanocytes simply self-destruct. The third explanation is that vitiligo is a type of autoimmune disease in which the immune system targets the body's own cells and tissues.

The primary symptom of vitiligo is the loss of skin color. Hair growing from the affected skin areas also lacks color. In addition, people with vitiligo may have pigment abnormalities of the retina or iris of the eyes. A minority of patients also may have inflammation of the retina or iris, but vision is not usually impaired.

The diagnosis of vitiligo is usually made by observation. Progressive, white areas found at typical sites point to a diagnosis of vitiligo. If the diagnosis is not certain, the doctor will test for other conditions which can mimic vitiligo, such as chemical leukoderma or **systemic lupus erythematosus**. If the tests rule out other conditions, vitiligo is confirmed.

Vitiligo cannot be cured, but it can be managed. Cosmetics can be used to improve the appearance of the white areas not covered by clothing. **Sunscreens** prevent burning of the affected areas and also prevent the normal skin around the patches from becoming darker. Skin creams and oral medications are available for severe cases, but they have side effects that may make them undesirable. Autologous transplantation of skin is an option for those who are severely affected. Bleaching or depigmentation of the normal skin is another option.

In addition to treating the skin, attention should be paid to the psychological well-being of the individual. Extreme cases of vitiligo can be unattractive and may affect a person's outlook and social interactions.

The condition is usually gradually progressive. Sometimes the patches grow rapidly over a short period, and then the condition remains stable for many years.

No measures are currently known to prevent vitiligo.

Vivisection

Vivisection is the dissection of living animals for scientific research and is sometimes more broadly used to describe all types of animal research. The dissection of living animals to learn more about how the body functions dates back to ancient times. **Galen** (ca 130-ca 200 A.D.) conducted numerous animal experiments (principally using the Barbary ape) to investigate animal physiology. For example, he would cut nerves to determine which nerves were associated with paralysis in different parts of the body. In the seventeenth century, **William Harvey** (1578-1657) conducted famous animal experiments that demonstrated how the blood circulates through the body. Despite the many advances made in medicine through vivisection, many people oppose animal experimentation. As a result, an ethical debate over animal experimentation has been ongoing for more than 200 years.

As the science of medicine grew so did the use of vivisection. In the mid-nineteenth century, **Louis Pasteur** (1822-1895) isolated the microbe that causes anthrax and then developed a vaccine against the deadly disease through his studies on rabbits and guinea pigs. Following in the footsteps of Pasteur, many other scientists began experimenting with animals to develop vaccines and antibiotics. This vein of research continues today in the study of diseases such as AIDS, malaria, and other infectious diseases. Vivisection has also been of vital importance in many other areas, including advances in open-heart surgery, treatments for kidney failure, and the development of drugs and transplantation. Keen insights and life-saving advances in medicine gained through vivisection have propelled animal experimentation to the forefront of modern scientific research.

In addition to medical experiments, vivisection has been used in other types of research, such as testing cosmetics and household cleaning products. Many of these experiments focus on a substance's toxicity, such as how it may irritate the eyes. However, growing sentiments against this type of "non-necessary" research has led most industries to abandon animal testing. But medical vivisection remains a hotly debated issue. On the one hand, proponents say that helping cure diseases justify vivisection. However, animal rights' activists (or anti-vivisectionists) do not believe animals should be harmed to help humans. Many also question the validity of scientific results based on animal experimentation, pointing out that animals' bodies and physiology often differ greatly from human beings. They add that alternatives can and should be developed for vivisection. These alternatives include more test-tube (in vitro), clinical, and epidemiological studies and greater use of mod odern medical technology such as magnetic resonance imaging (MRI) scans, which provide detailed images of the body and its inner workings.

In 1966, the United States passed the Animal Welfare Act, which sets standards for housing, handling, feeding, and transportation of experimental animals. However, the act places no restrictions on the types of experiments that can be performed.

Vivisection remains a prominent component of medical research today. Researchers and others point to past advances in medicine made through the use of vivisection and say that many more disease that cause wide-spread suffering among humans may be cured through animal research. For example, recent animal research has indicated that nerve regeneration is possible, which could lead to treatments and cures for spinal cord injuries that cause paralysis.

The English writer Samuel Johnson (1709-1784) reflected the anti-vivisectionist's belief succinctly in 1758 when he wrote: "And if the knowledge of physiology has been somewhat increased, he surely buys knowledge dear...at the expense of his humanity." The pro-vivisectionists counter that many future advances in healing diseases and healing the body can not be achieved without animal experimentation. The ethical debate over vivisection is unlikely to abate in near the future.

See also Galen; William Harvey; Louis Pasteur

Volkmann, Richard von (1830-1889)

German surgeon

Von Volkmann pioneered antiseptic procedures and was especially known for his advances in **orthopedic surgery**.

Von Volkmann was born in Leipzig, Germany and attended medical schools in Giessen, Halle, and Berlin. Starting in 1867, he worked as a professor of surgery at the University of Halle, also directing its medical clinic.

Near the beginning of his illustrious medical career, von Volkmann and a partner discovered a method for operating effectively on joints and the extremities. From 1865 to 1872, he contributed sections to the *Pitha-Billroth Handbook of Surgery*, while from 1870 to 1889 he served as editor of *The Collection of Clinical Lectures*. Von Volkmann also wrote *Contributions on Surgery* in 1873. An avid writer of nonclinical prose as well, the surgeon (using the pen name Richard Leander) enjoyed crafting fairy tales and poems that were sometimes accompanied by his artist son's professional illustrations.

Unlike many of his colleagues, Von Volkmann firmly believed in the benefits of maintaining a sterile environment during surgery and other clinical procedures when infection was possible. His status as a surgeon encouraged the acceptance of antiseptic practices. In 1878 Von Volkmann became the first surgeon to excise a cancerous rectum, while several years earlier, he discovered that long exposure to tar and paraffin can precipitate **skin cancer**. In 1881, he provided the first clinical description of a contraction of the fingers, now known as Volkmann's contracture, caused by pressure or injury. The surgeon died in Jena, Germany, in 1889.

von Helmholtz, Hermann • See Helmholtz, Hermann von

Vulvar cancer

Vulvar cancer refers to an abnormal, cancerous growth in the external female genitalia.

Vulvar cancer is a rare disease that occurs mainly in elderly women. The vulva refers to the external female genitalia, which includes the labia (Latin for lips), the opening of the vagina, the clitoris, and the space between the vagina and anus (perineum). Vulvar cancer can affect any part of the female genitalia, but usually affects the labia. There are two pairs of labia. The labia meet to protect the openings of the vagina and urethra (the tube that connects to the bladder). The outer, most prominent folds of skin are called labia majora, and the smaller, inner skin folds are called labia minora.

Most vulvar cancers are squamous cell carcinomas. Squamous cells are the main cell type of the skin. Squamous cell carcinoma often begins at the edges of the labia majora or labia minora or the area around the vagina. This type of cancer is usually slow growing and may begin with a precancerous condition referred to as vulvar intraepithelial neoplasia (VIN), or dysplasia. This means that precancerous cells are present in the surface layer of skin.

Other, less common, types of vulvar cancer are melanoma, basal cell carcinoma, adenocarcinomas, Paget's disease of the vulva, and tumors of the connective tissue under the skin. Melanoma, a cancer that develops from the cells that produce the pigment that determines the skin's color, can occur anywhere on the skin, including the vulva. It is the second most common type of vulvar cancer, and accounts for about 4% of cases. Basal cell carcinoma, which is the most common type of cancer that occurs on parts of the skin exposed to the sun, very rarely occurs on the vulva. Adenocarcinomas develop from glands, including the glands at the opening of the vagina that produce a mucus-like lubricating fluid.

Vulvar cancer is most common in women over 50 years of age. Additional risk factors for vulvar cancer include having multiple sexual partners, **cervical cancer**, and the presence of chronic vaginal and vulvar inflammations. This type of cancer is often associated with **sexually transmitted diseases**.

Cancer is caused when the normal mechanisms that control cell growth become disturbed, causing the cells to continually grow without stopping. This is usually the result of damage to the DNA in the cell. Studies have indicated several risk factors for vulvar cancer that include:

- Infection with human papillomavirus (HPV). This virus is a sexually transmitted disease that can cause **genital warts**.
- Cigarette smoking. Smoking in combination with HPV was found to be a particularly strong risk factor for vulvar cancer.
- Infection with human **immunodeficiency** virus (HIV). This virus, associated with **AIDS**, decreases the body's immune ability, leaving it vulnerable to a variety of diseases, including vulvar cancer.
- Herpes virus. This sexually transmitted virus (HSV2) is also associated with increased risk for vulvar cancer.
- Chronic vulvar inflammation. Long term irritation and inflammation of the vulva and vagina, which may be caused by poor hygiene, can increase the risk of vulvar cancer.
- Vulvar intraepithelial neoplasia (VIN). This abnormal growth of the surface cells of the vulva can sometimes progress to cancer.

If squamous cell vulvar cancer is present, it may appear as a raised red, pink, or white nodule. It is often accompanied by **itching**, **pain**, bleeding, vaginal discharge, and painful urination. Malignant melanoma of the vulva usually appears as a pigmented, ulcerated growth. Other types of vulvar cancer may appear as a distinct mass of tissue, sore and scaly areas, or cauliflower-like growths that look like **warts**. Any abnormalities should be reported to a gynecologist for examination.

A gynecological examination will be used to observe the suspected area. During this examination, the physician may use a special magnifying instrument called a colposcope to see the area better. Additionally, the area may be treated with a dilute vinegar solution, which causes some abnormal areas to turn white, making them easier to see. During this examination, if any area is suspected of being abnormal, a tissue sample (biopsy) will be taken. The diagnosis of cancer depends on a microscopic analysis of this tissue by a pathologist.

The diagnosis for vulvar cancer will determine how advanced the cancer is and how much it has spread. This is determined by the size of the tumor and how deep it has invaded the surrounding tissue and organs, such as the lymph nodes. It will also be determined if the cancer has metastasized, which means it has spread to other organs. This part of the diagnosis will be described by rating the cancer as stage I, II, III, or IV; with I being the least severe and IV being the most severe.

Tests used to determine the stage include x ray and computed tomography scan (CT scan).

Treatment for vulvar cancer will depend on its stage and the patient's general state of health. The primary treatment for vulvar cancer is surgery to remove the affected vulvar area and possibly the associated lymph nodes. The surgery may be done by laser, to burn off a minimal amount of tissue, or scalpel, to remove more of the tissue. The choice will depend on the severity of the cancer. If a large area of the vulva is removed, it is called a vulvectomy. A vulvectomy may require skin grafts from other areas of the body to cover the wound. Surgery may also be followed by **chemotherapy** and **radiation therapy** to kill additional cancer cells. All three of these procedures have risks associated with them, which should be discussed with the care giver.

Survival depends strongly on how advanced the disease is, meaning what stage it is in. If diagnosed and treated early, the 5-year survival rate is 91%, it drops to only 15% in the advanced stage (stage IV).

The risk of cancer of the vulva can be decreased by reducing the risk factors for the cancer, most of which involve lifestyle factors. Specifically, to reduce the risk of vulvar cancer, women should not smoke and should refrain from engaging in risky sexual behavior. Good hygiene of the genital area to prevent infection and inflammation may also reduce the risk of vulvar cancer.

Regular gynecological examinations are necessary to detect precancerous conditions that can be treated before the cancer becomes invasive. Since some vulvar cancer is a type of skin cancer, the American Cancer Society also recommends self-examination of the vulva using a mirror. If **moles** are present in the genital area, use the ABCD rule:

- Asymmetry. A cancerous mole may have two halves of unequal size.
- Border irregularity. A cancerous mole may have ragged or notched edges.
- Color. A cancerous mole may have variations in color.
- Diameter. A cancerous mole may have a diameter wider than 6 millimeters (1/4 inch).

VULVOVAGINITIS

Inflammation of the vagina and vulva are most often caused by a bacterial, fungal, or parasitic infection.

Vulvovaginitis, vulvitis, and vaginitis are general terms that refer to the inflammation of the vagina and/or vulva (the external genital organs of a woman).These conditions can be caused by bacterial, fungal, or parasitic infections. Also, vulvovaginitis can be caused by low estrogen levels (called ''atrophic vaginitis'') or any type of allergic or irritation response from things such as spermicidal products, **condom**s, soaps, and bubble bath.

In general, vulvovaginitis causes vaginal discharge, irritation, and **itching**. One of the most common reasons why women visit their doctor is because there has been a change in vaginal discharge. It is completely normal for a woman to have a vaginal discharge, the amount and consistency of which varies during the course of the menstrual cycle. Each of the three most common types of vulvovaginitis will be described separately.

Bacterial vaginosis is the most common cause of vaginitis during the childbearing years. Forty percent to 50% of vaginitis cases are caused by bacterial vaginosis. The occurrence of bacterial vaginosis is difficult to determine but studies have proposed that 10% to 41% of women have had it at least once. The occurrence of bacterial vaginosis in the United States is highest among African-American women and women who have had multiple sexual partners and lowest among Asian women and women with no history of sexual contact with men. Bacterial vaginosis is not considered a sexually transmitted disease although it can be acquired by sexual intercourse.

Bacterial vaginosis is not caused by a particular organism but is a change in the balance of normal vaginal bacteria. Ninety percent of the bacteria found in a healthy vagina belong to the *Lactobacillus* family. For unknown reasons, there is a shift in the bacterial population that results in overgrowth of other bacteria. Patients suffering from bacterial vaginosis have very high numbers of bacteria such as *Gardnerella vaginalis*, *Mycoplasmahominis*, *Bacteroides* species, and *Mobiluncus* species. These bacteria can be found at numbers 100 to 1000 times greater than found in the healthy vagina. In contrast, *Lactobacillus* bacteria are in very low numbers or completely absent from the vagina of women with bacterial vaginosis.

Candida vulvovaginitis also has been called ''vulvovaginal **candidiasis**,'' ''candidal vaginitis,'' ''monilial infection,'' or ''vaginal yeast infection.'' Twenty to 25% of the vaginitis cases are candida vulvovaginitis. It has been estimated that about 75% of all women get a vaginal yeast infection at least once. In 80-90% of the cases, candida vulvovaginitis is caused by an overgrowth of the yeast *Candida albicans*. The remaining cases are caused by other species of *Candida*. It is not known what causes the yeast overgrowth. However, **antibiotics** can inadvertently kill normal bacteria in the vagina and cause an overgrowth of *Candida*. Candida vulvovaginitis is not considered a sexually transmitted disease because *Candida* species are commonly found in the healthy vagina. It is a rare disease in girls before **puberty** and in celibate women. Vaginal yeast infections tend to occur more frequently in women who are pregnant, diabetic and not controlling their disease, taking birth control pills, or taking antibiotics. Some women have four or more attacks per year which is called ''recurrent vaginal candidiasis.''

Trichomoniasis, which is sometimes called ''trich,'' accounts for 15-20% of the cases of vaginitis. It is estimated that two million to three million American women get trichomoniasis each year. Unlike the previous two causes of vulvovaginitis, trichomoniasis is a sexually transmitted disease. This means that the disease is passed from person-to-person only by sexual contact. Trichomoniasis occurs in both men and women and is caused by an infection with the single-celled parasite *Trichomonas vaginalis*. Infection with *Trichomonas vaginalis* is frequently associated with other sexually transmitted diseases and assists the spread of the **AIDS** virus.

Vulvovaginitis is most often caused by a bacterial, fungal, or parasitic infection as described above. Other microorganisms may cause vulvovaginitis, or it may be caused by allergic reaction, irritation, injury, low estrogen levels, and certain diseases. Risk factors for bacterial vaginosis include using an intrauterine device (**IUD**), being of a non-white race, prior **pregnancy**, first sexual activity at an early age, having multiple sexual partners, and having a history of **sexually transmitted diseases**. Persons at an increased risk for candida vulvovaginitis include those who have had previous candida infections, frequent sexual intercourse, use birth control pills, have AIDS, are pregnant, are taking antibiotics or **corticosteroids**, are diabetic, use douches, use perfumed feminine hygiene sprays, wear tight clothing, or use vaginal sponges or an IUD.

The typical symptoms of vulvovaginitis are: vaginal discharge, itching, and irritation. Some women may have few or no symptoms, while others may have pronounced symptoms. The main symptom of bacterial vaginosis is a fishy-smelling, thin, milky-white or gray vaginal discharge but itching and burning may also be present. The fishy smell is stronger after sexual intercourse. The symptoms of candida vulvovaginitis are itching, soreness, **pain**ful sexual intercourse, and a thick, curdy, white (like cottage cheese) vaginal discharge. Trichomoniasis symptoms are: painful urination, painful sexual intercourse, and a yellow-green to gray, foul smelling, sometimes frothy, vaginal discharge.

To diagnose vulvovaginitis, the doctor will examine the vagina (using a speculum to keep the vagina open) and take a sample of the vaginal discharge for tests and microscopic analysis. Diagnosis may be difficult because there are many different causes of vulvovaginitis.

There are four signs that indicate that a woman has bacterial vaginosis. These signs (called ''Amsel's criteria'') are: a thin, milky white discharge that clings to the walls of the vagina, presence of a fishy odor, a vaginal pH of greater than 4.5, and the presence of ''clue cells'' in the vagina. Clue cells are vaginal cells that are covered with small bacteria. A diagnosis of candida vulvovaginitis is made after finding a normal vaginal pH (4 to 4.5) and the presence of many yeast cells in the sample of vaginal discharge or growth of yeast on laboratory media. A trichomoniasis diagnosis is made when the parasites are found in the vaginal discharge either by microscopic examination or in laboratory cultures.

Both bacterial vaginosis and trichomoniasis must be treated with prescription medication. Candida vulvovaginitis may be treated with either prescription or over-the-counter medicines (not recommended in the absence of a confirmed diagnosis).

Vulvovaginitis is a disease with minor symptoms and most women respond well to medications. It is believed that certain vaginal infections, if left untreated, can lead to more serious conditions such as **pelvic inflammatory disease**, endometritis, postsurgical infections, and spread of the AIDS virus.

W

Wagner-Jauregg, Julius (1857-1940)

Austrian physician

Wagner-Jauregg was born Julius Wagner on March 7, 1857, in the village of Wels, Austria. He was the oldest son of Ludovika Ranzoni and Adolf Johann Wagner, a government official. The family name became ''Wagner von Jauregg'' when Adolf Johann was raised to the nobility, but following the collapse of the Austro-Hungarian empire in 1918, the ''von'' was dropped.

While attending medical school at the University of Vienna, Wagner-Jauregg received thorough training in experimental biology and met the father of psychoanalysis, Sigmund Freud, who was studying at the Institute of General and Experimental Pathology. Despite Wagner-Jauregg's lack of interest in psychoanalysis, the two remained lifelong friends. In 1880 Wagner-Jauregg was awarded a medical degree for his thesis on the heart under conditions of acceleration.

Originally, Wagner-Jauregg hoped to practice general medicine, but when Vienna's two teaching hospitals turned him down, he reluctantly accepted a position as an assistant in the university's psychiatric clinic. Although he had little training in mental illness, he quickly became a qualified instructor in psychiatry and neurology. Wagner-Jauregg was a clinician, skilled in detailed observation and careful case analysis. Using the latest techniques of animal experimentation, he spent his life working to advance the biological understanding of mental illness. His first research entailed the investigation of how certain chemicals stimulate breathing after strangulation.

In 1889 Wagner-Jauregg was appointed professor of psychiatry at the University of Graz and for the next four years studied the effect of the thyroid gland on behavior. An ardent vivisectionist, he discovered that when the thyroid was removed from a cat, the animal's behavior became convulsive and violent. Cretinism in humans, Wagner-Jauregg put forth in an early paper, was due to a malfunction of the thyroid. During his years in Graz, he travelled frequently in central and southeastern Austria studying peasants with goiter and found that small amounts of **iodine** reduced their hugely swollen necks. He urged the sale of iodized salt in alpine regions, a measure the Austrian government undertook belatedly in 1923.

In 1893 Wagner-Jauregg was made a full professor at the University of Vienna and appointed director of the Hospital for Nervous and Mental Diseases and the State Mental Asylum. As a member of the Austrian Board of Health, he helped draft important legislation protecting the rights of the mentally ill and regulating the certification of the insane. At his urging, psychiatry became a compulsory subject in the undergraduate curriculum.

While still only a medical assistant, Wagner-Jauregg had studied the beneficial effect of high fever on psychotic patients. For a monograph that he published in 1888, he surveyed instances where epidemics of typhoid, malaria, **small pox**, and **scarlet fever** had swept through mental asylums. In 30 cases reaching back to antiquity, he described how bouts of high fever had brought dramatic relief in cases of melancholy, mania, and paresis. At the end of his monograph, Wagner-Jauregg suggested that malaria might be used experimentally to induce a ''fever cure'' in psychotic patients, although at the time he lacked the authority to undertake so radical a treatment.

The monograph received little notice when it was published. In it, Wagner-Jauregg had formulated two bold hypotheses: first, that some psychoses were organic in nature, and second, that one disease might be employed to eradicate another disease. In Graz, he had produced fever with injections of tuberculin, a protein used to treat **tuberculosis**, until it was learned that tuberculin was unsafe. In Vienna, he injected paralytic patents with typhus vaccine and staphylococci but was disappointed by the results. Most of the cures proved to be temporary, and patients soon relapsed.

It was not until World War I that conditions were ripe for a radical trial. By then a series of important discoveries had confirmed the link between paresis and syphilis. In 1905 re-

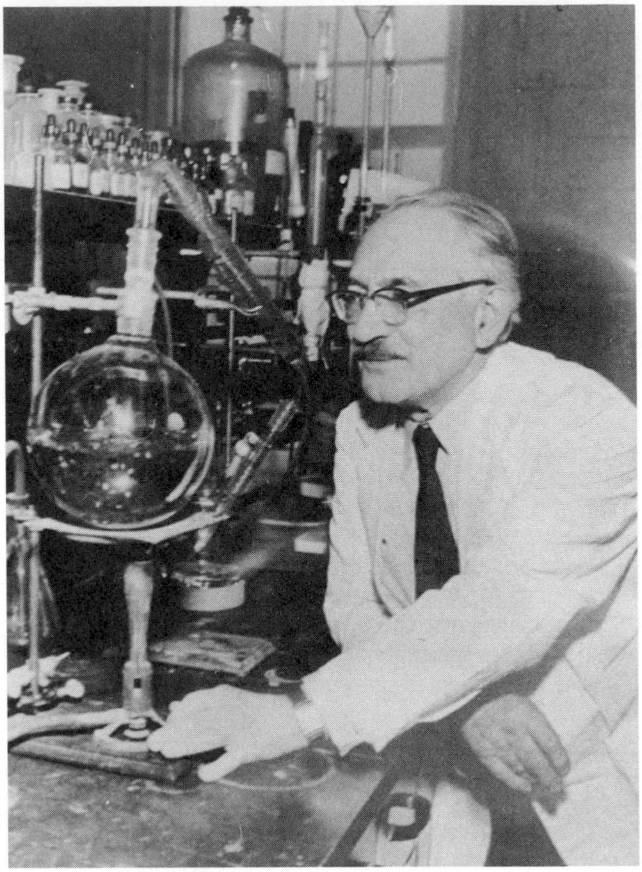

Selman Abraham Waksman

searchers had identified the syphilis bacillus, *Spirochaete pallida.* A year later, the Wasserman test for syphilis revealed that paresis was a progressive disease of the brain caused by untreated syphilis. In Wagner-Jauregg's time, paresis accounted for 15% of the patients confined to mental hospitals. The disease was thought to be incurable and invariably ended in insanity, paralysis, and death within three to four years.

In the final years of World War I, Wagner-Jauregg was treating victims of shell shock when he encountered a soldier suffering from malaria. On June 14, 1917, Wagner-Jauregg used blood drawn from the malarial soldier to infect nine patients suffering from paresis. Quinine, the medicine used to treat malaria, was withheld until each patient had endured seven to eleven attacks of fever. The results were astonishing. Six patients experienced a dramatic remission of symptoms, and three were able to return to normal life. In 1919 Wagner-Jauregg began full-scale clinical trials.

At first, Wagner-Jauregg's reports were greeted with considerable skepticism by the medical community. Some physicians considered it unethical to deliberately induce a disease as serious as malaria. Others feared the outbreak of malaria epidemics in major metropolitan centers. But trials elsewhere produced similar results. Employing only a mild strain of malaria easily cured by quinine, mortality remained low while complete recovery was experienced by thirty to forty percent of all patients. Patients who had only recently contracted syphilis could be cured completely when the ''malaria cure'' was used in conjunction with injections of Salvarsan and Neosalvarsan, two drugs used to treat early syphilis. In 1927 Wagner-Jauregg became the first psychiatrist to be awarded the Nobel Prize in physiology or medicine.

Safer methods of inducing fever were tried—preparations of colloidal sulfur, hot-water baths, and ''fever cabinets''—but none had the high rates of success typical of malaria. Until the discovery of penicillin during World War II, malaria remained the preferred treatment for advanced syphilis. Medical opinion differed on just how the fever cure worked since it seemed unlikely that the fever killed all of the spirochete bacteria, which cause syphilis. Instead, it was believed that the stress produced by the malaria attack in some way strengthened the body's defenses against the syphilitic infection. Stress treatments such as electroshock continue to play a role in the treatment of psychiatric disorders.

In 1928, one year after receiving the Nobel Prize, Wagner-Jauregg retired at the age of seventy-one. He died on September 27, 1940, in Vienna at age eighty-four, shortly before the discovery of penicillin made his fever cure obsolete.

WAKSMAN, SELMAN ABRAHAM (1888-1973)

American microbiologist

Waksman focused his research on the study of agents that kill microorganisms. He coined the term ''**antibiotic**'' and discovered streptomycin, which was the first effective treatment for **tuberculosis**.

Born in Priluki, Russia, Waksman emigrated to the United States after graduating from high school. He earned his graduate degree at Rutgers University and continued his studies at University of California, returning to Rutgers as a member of the faculty. Waksman specialized in the study of soil-living microorganisms. One of his students, René Jules Dubos (1901-1981), noticed that a number of antibacterial substances could be found in soil. One of these substances, gramicidin, was found to be active against **pneumonia**, but it was too toxic to use in humans. Dubos's work inspired Waksman to turn to the search for such antibacterial substances.

In the following decades, he found and tested dozens of antibiotics. One of them, actinomycin A, was more powerful than **penicillin**, but also highly toxic. Waksman had been culturing a mold of the genus *Streptomyces* in his laboratory for years and in 1943, he isolated a chemical from it which destroyed *gram-negative* bacteria, a type of bacteria even the newly discovered penicillin could not kill.

Streptomycin, as he called the chemical, was being tested on humans by 1945. The tests were successful in treating bacterial **meningitis** and in destroying the tubercle bacillus—the cause of tuberculosis and the most difficult to treat of all infectious diseases. The initial tests of streptomycin were so promising that within three years, the drug was being mass-produced for extensive clinical trials directed at various forms of tuberculosis. Once again, the drug worked wonders. By 1950, streptomycin had been proven effective against seventy microorganisms that did not respond to penicillin and was one of the most important drugs available to physicians in the battle against bacterial infections. Further research on microorganisms in soil led to the discovery of yet another group of powerful antibiotics, the tetracyclines. Waksman was awarded the 1952 Nobel Prize in medicine and physiology for his work.

WALD, GEORGE (1906-1997)

American biochemist

A born and bred New Yorker, George Wald graduated from New York University in 1927 and received his Ph.D. five years later from Columbia University. For the next two years, Wald studied in Europe, working with two of the continent's most eminent chemists, Berlin's **Otto Warburg** and, in Zurich, Switzerland, Paul Karrer (1889-1971), a pioneer in vitamin A research. He then returned to the United States and, in 1934, joined the faculty of Harvard University, where he remained for the rest of his career.

From the start, Wald was primarily interested in the photochemistry of vision. In 1933, he had already discovered that vitamin A was a vital ingredient in the eye's retina, specifically in the pigments contained in the retina's rods and cones. The rods—the tiny rod-shaped cells that allow the eye to see in dim light—contained a pigment called rhodopsin. What exactly was the relationship between rhodopsin and the vitamin A it contained? Wald wasn't certain but during his first quarter century at Harvard, he and his co-workers, in particular, Paul K. Brown (1919-), did their best to find out.

The group's first task was to break down rhodopsin—until then, generally considered one large, lumpy, and exceedingly complicated molecule—into its component parts. Rhodopsin, Wald soon demonstrated, was in reality composed of two substances: a colorless protein, opsin, and a yellow *carotenoid*, retinal (or *retinene*) that was actually the aldehyde form of vitamin A. Rhodopsin's role in the visual cycle was a crucial one. When stimulated by light rays, Wald discovered, the rhodopsin molecule promptly splits into its two component parts and the retinal fraction is transformed back into vitamin A by an enzyme. In the dark, the process is reversed: vitamin A becomes retinal, the components come back together and once again form rhodopsin. Most important of all: the various biochemical changes trigger an electrical activity that excites both the retina's nerves and the optic nerve resulting in vision.

In the course of working out this complex scenario, Wald answered the question that had long puzzled scientists: why is night blindness an early sign of vitamin A deficiency? Because, Wald explained, as the light-dark changes take place, some retinal is invariably lost and more must be formed from the body's supply of vitamin A. If, over time, this supply becomes exhausted, no more retinal can be made, the rods no longer function normally—and the eye no longer sees in dim light. In the 1950s and 1960s, Wald and his Harvard associates went on to identify the pigments in the retina's cones—all also

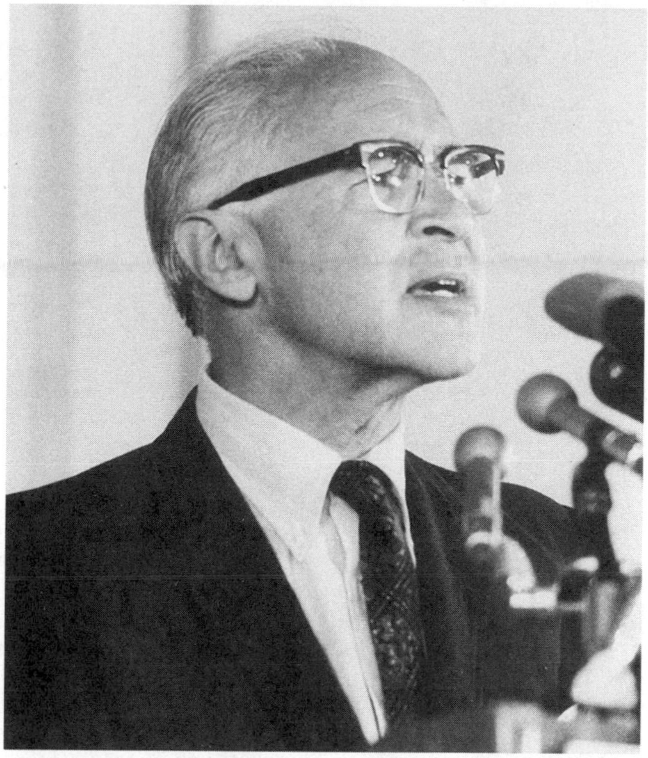

George Wald

related to vitamin A—that detect red, yellow-green and blue light and showed how the absence of one of these pigments can result in **color blindness**. For these and his earlier discoveries, Wald shared the Nobel Prize in physiology and medicine in 1967.

WALD, LILLIAN (1867-1940)

American nurse and social worker

Lillian Wald was born on March 10, 1867 in Cincinnati, Ohio; she died on September 1, 1940 in Westport, Connecticut. She was the daughter of Max D. Wald, a merchant, and Minnie Wald; she never married. Wald is remembered for her dedication to the cause of public health, and for establishing important social reforms to accommodate the needs of the turn-of-the-century immigrant population in New York City. During her career, Wald was a public health nurse, settlement leader, and social reformer. In 1891, she graduated from New York Hospital for nurses, and in 1893 from Women's Medical College (N.Y.). In 1892, she worked as a nurse at the New York Juvenile Asylum.

Wald's achievements were considerable; she founded public health **nursing** in the United States. With Mary Brewster, she opened the Henry Street Settlement on Manhattan's Lower east Side, providing visiting nurse service and settlement services to the poor residents of that community; she also inspired the organization of similar services elsewhere. From

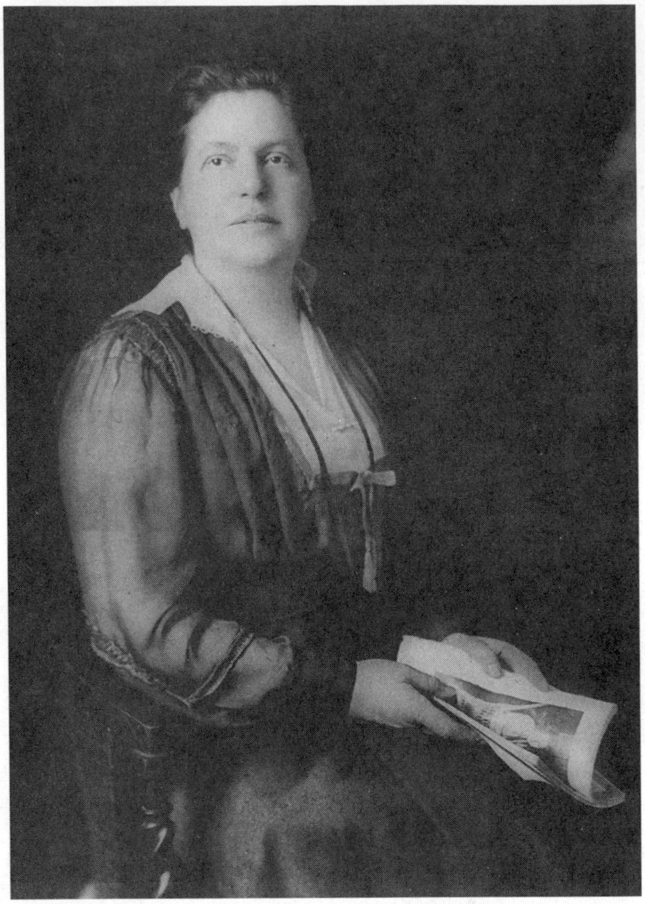

Lillian Wald

1893 to 1933, she was the co-founder and head of the Settlement, which under Wald's directorship acquired worldwide attention and respect. (It is particularly noteworthy that this neighborhood center provided opportunities for recreation and artistic expression, as well as medical services.) With Lina Rogers, she began the first public school nursing service in the world (New York City, 1902). She persuaded life insurance companies, starting with the Metropolitan Life Insurance Company in 1909, to organize nursing programs for their policyholders. Wald was also a pioneer in the field of child welfare, introducing the idea that it is the responsibility of the community to see that children are provided for. Toward this end, she conceived the idea of a United States Children's Bureau, which was later established at her urging (1912). She originated the plan for the American Red Cross' town and country nursing program. Wald was instrumental in the founding of the National Organization for Public Health Nursing, and served as that organization's first president in 1912. Wald wrote two autobiographical works, *The House on Henry Street* (1915), and *Windows on Henry Street* (1934).

WARBURG, OTTO HEINRICH (1883-1970)

German biochemist

Otto Warburg, an outstanding biochemist, was born in Freiburg, Germany. His Jewish father was a physics professor from an old family of bankers, philanthropists, scholars, and businessmen. The family of his Christian mother was filled with public officials, lawyers, and soldiers. When Warburg was twelve, the family moved to Berlin; Germany's leading scientists, musicians, and artists were frequent visitors to their home. Warburg studied chemistry under Emil Fischer at the University of Berlin, earning his Ph.D. in 1906, and then received a medical degree from the University of Heidelberg in 1911.

In 1913 Warburg became head of his own laboratory at the Kaiser Wilhelm (later Max Planck) Institute for Biology in Berlin. Here he devoted himself entirely to research topics of his own choosing. A tireless and innovative experimenter, Warburg made a number of important biochemical discoveries during his long career at the Institute; the Dictionary of Scientific Biography lists an extraordinary fifty-nine ''major discoveries and fields of interest'' for this man.

Warburg left the Institute during World War I to serve as a cavalry officer on the Russian front, where he was wounded. In 1918, he resumed his work in Berlin at the urging of Albert Einstein. During World War II, Warburg was allowed to remain at the Institute in spite of being part Jewish, probably because of his important research on **cancer**, a disease that Hitler greatly feared. Remaining remarkably fit, Warburg was an avid horseback rider until he broke his leg at age 85. He died two years later in Berlin.

Warburg's three major fields of interest during his more than fifty years of laboratory research were intracellular respiration, photosynthesis, and cancer. Studying respiration in the early 1920s, he devised a way to use thin slices of living tissue to test **oxygen** consumption and invented a manometer to measure this oxygen uptake. He discovered the respiratory enzyme iron oxygenase and identified its active group (iron); this work earned Warburg the 1931 Nobel Prize for Physiology or Medicine.

Warburg went on to further enzyme and coenzyme study, isolating a number of enzymes important in respiration and **metabolism**, clarifying the functioning of vitamins and developing important spectrophotometric techniques for metabolic research. Working on photosynthesis, Warburg showed that it could occur with almost perfect thermodynamic efficiency. He discovered the electron carrier ferredoxin in green plants, and how light energy is converted to chemical energy during photosynthesis.

Warburg also spent many years researching cancer. During his studies of respiration, he discovered that cancerous cells extract energy by metabolizing glucose rather than by absorbing molecular oxygen from the blood. In Warburg's opinion, it was this faulty respiration that caused cells to become cancerous. Because certain substances can inhibit oxygen uptake in cells, Warburg advocated eating untreated foods grown without pesticides or artificial fertilizers. To prevent and treat cancer, Warburg recommended a diet of **iron** and B vitamins that are rich sources of active respiratory enzymes. Warburg was considered for the 1926 Nobel Prize for his findings on tumor metabolism.

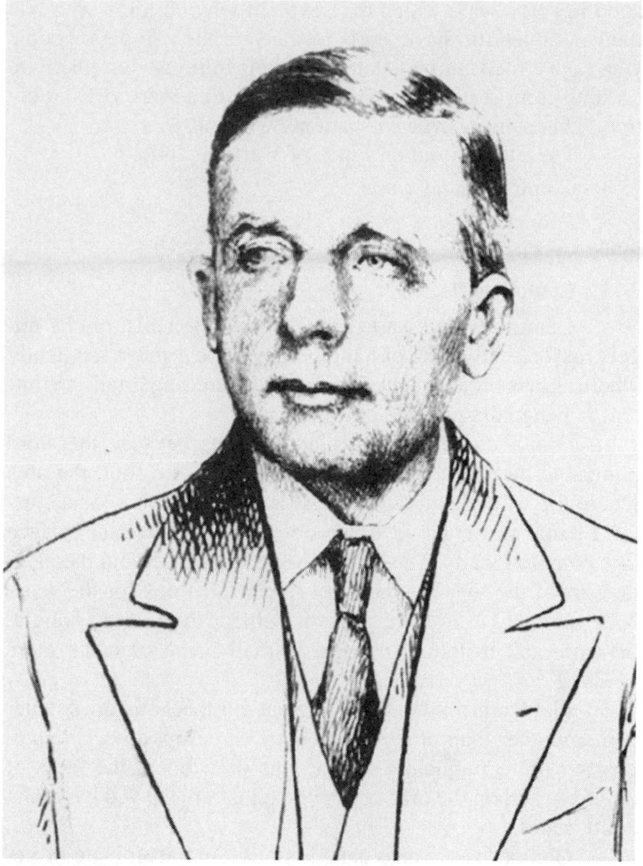

Otto Heinrich Warburg

Warren, John (1753-1815)

American surgeon

John Warren was born on July 27, 1753 in Roxbury, Massachusetts, and died on April 4, 1815 in Boston. He was the son of Joseph Warren, a prosperous farmer, and Mary Warren. In 1777, he married Abigail Collins, with whom he had 17 children. He is remembered as a physician, anatomist, surgeon, and medical educator. Warren graduated with an A.B. degree in 1771 from Harvard College. He subsequently studied medicine with his brother Joseph, a Revolutionary War hero, and in 1786 received an honorary M.D. degree from Harvard University. From 1774 to 1775, he had a brief and not entirely successful medical practice at Salem, Massachusetts. From 1775 to 1777, he served as hospital surgeon during the siege of Boston and the New York-New Jersey campaign. From 1777 to 1782, he was in charge of the Continental Army hospital in Boston. Between 1780 and 1782, he delivered three series of anatomical lectures, the last two sponsored by the Boston Medical Society. From 1783 to 1815, he was a member of the (original) faculty of Harvard Medical School, where he became the first Hersey Professor of Anatomy and Surgery. From 1804 to 1815, he served as seventh president of the Massachusetts Medical Society. He was active in community affairs, serving as grand master of the Massachusetts Lodge of Free and Accepted Masons. He was a founder and president of the Massachusetts Humane Society; a founder of the Anthology Club; a trustee and manager of the Massachusetts Charitable Society; a trustee of the Massachusetts Agricultural Society; a member of the editorial board of *Boston Magazine*; and a fellow of the American Academy of Arts and Sciences. Although gifted as an anatomist, surgeon, and teacher, John Warren is also remembered as being ambitious to the point of harshness and self-righteous to the point of disagreeability.

Warren was the single most important person in the early institutionalization of Boston medicine. He gave public lectures on anatomy toward the end of the Revolution. As a surgeon, Warren successfully amputated at the shoulder joint (1781), performed an abdominal resection (1785); and excised the parotid gland (1804). Upon his death in 1815, John Warren was succeeded as Harvard's Professor of Surgery by his son, John Collins Warren, who would later become the first American to operate under ether anesthesia. Warren's writings include *A View of the Mercurial Practice in Febrile Diseases* (1813).

See also Military medicine

Warts

Warts are small, benign growths caused by a viral infection of the skin or mucous membrane. The virus infects the surface layer. The viruses that cause warts are members of the human papilloma virus (HPV) family. Warts are not **cancer**ous but some strains of HPV, usually not associated with warts, have been linked with cancer formation. Warts are contagious from person to person and from one area of the body to another on the same person.

Particularly common among children, young adults, and women, warts are a problem for 7-10% of the population. There are close to 60 types of HPV that cause warts, each preferring a specific skin location. For instance, some types of HPV cause warts to grow on the skin, others cause them to grow inside the mouth, while still others cause them to grow on the genital and rectal areas. However, most can be active anywhere on the body. The virus enters through the skin and produces new warts after an incubation period of one to eight months. Warts are usually skin-colored and feel rough to the touch, but they also can be dark, flat, and smooth.

Warts are passed from person to person, directly and indirectly. Some people are continually susceptible to warts, while others are more resistant to HPV and seldom get them. The virus takes hold more readily when the skin has been damaged in some way, which may explain why children who bite their nails tend to have warts located on their fingers. People who take a medication to suppress their immune system or are on long-term steroid use are also prone to a wart virus infection. This same is true for patients with **AIDS**.

The more common types of warts include:

- Common hand warts
- Foot warts
- Flat warts
- **Genital warts.**

Common hand warts grow around the nails, on the fingers, and on the backs of hands. They appear more frequently where skin is broken, such as in areas where fingernails are bitten or hangnails picked.

Foot warts are called plantar warts because the word plantar is the medical term for the sole of the foot, the area where the wart usually appears as a single lesion or as a cluster. Plantar warts, however, do not stick up above the surface like common warts. The ball of the foot, the heel and the plantar part of the toes are the most likely locations for the warts because the skin in those areas is subject to the most weight, pressure and irritation, making a small break or crack more likely.

Flat warts tend to grow in great numbers and are smaller and smoother than other warts. They can erupt anywhere, appearing more frequently on the legs of women, the faces of children, and on the areas of the face that are shaved by young adult males.

Genital warts, also called condyloma acuminata or venereal warts, are one of the most common causes of sexually transmitted disease (STD) in this country. According to the *Journal of the American Medical Association's* STD Information Center, they are contracted by sexual contact with an infected person who carries HPV and are more contagious than other warts. It is estimated that two-thirds of the people who have sexual contact with a partner with genital warts will develop the disease within three months of contact. As a result, about one million new cases of genital warts are diagnosed in the United States each year.

Genital warts tend to be small flat bumps or they may be thin and tall. They are usually soft and not scaly like other warts. In women, genital warts appear on the genitalia, within the vagina, on the cervix, and around the anus or within the rectum. In men, genital warts usually appear on the tip of the penis but may also be found on the scrotum or around the anus. Genital warts can also develop in the mouth of a person who has had oral sexual contact with an infected person. Patients who notice warts in their genital area should see a doctor. The doctor may be able to diagnose the warts with a simple examination. If the warts are small, the doctor may put a vinegar-like liquid on the skin, which makes the warts turn white and easier to see, and then use a magnifying glass to look for them.

Many of the nonprescription wart remedies available at drug stores will remove simple warts from hands and fingers. These medications may be lotions, ointments, or plasters and work by chemically removing the skin that was affected by the wart virus. The chemicals are strong, however, and should be used with care since they can remove healthy as well as infected skin. These solutions should be avoided by diabetics and those with cardiovascular or other circulatory disorders whose skin may be insensitive and not appreciate irritation.

Physicians should be consulted if there are no signs of progress after a month of self treatment. Doctors have many ways of removing warts, including using stronger topically applied chemicals than those available in drugstores. A second method of removal is freezing or cryosurgery on the wart using liquid nitrogen. **Cryotherapy** is relatively inexpensive, does not require anesthesia, and usually does not result in scarring.

Genital warts are the most difficult to treat. They can be removed, but the viral infection itself cannot be cured. Often, because the warts are so small, more than one treatment may be needed. The virus continues to live in the deeper skin, which is why warts often return after they have been removed. Strong chemicals may be applied as well as surgical excision with or without electrocautery.

Wassermann, August von (1866-1925)

German bacteriologist

August von Wassermann discovered a blood serum test that enabled doctors to find out if a patient had syphilis, a potentially lethal disease which, in some patients, has a very long latency period during which no symptoms are detectable.

Wassermann was born in Bamberg, Germany, on February 21, 1866, to Dora (Bauer) and Angelo Wassermann, a banker. He received his secondary education in Bamberg and studied medicine at several German and Austrian universities. Wassermann married Alice von Taussig in 1895. They had two sons. He received his M.D. degree in 1888 at the University of Strasbourg. In 1890, Wassermann began work at the Institute for Infectious Diseases in Berlin, which was directed by **Robert Koch**.

Although Wassermann did important work on tetanus, cholera, diphtheria, and tuberculosis, he is best known for his discovery of a blood serum test (now called the Wassermann test) that enabled doctors to find out if a patient was infected by syphilis. The bacterium that causes syphilis, *Treponema pallidum*, can lay dormant in a person's body for many years, even a lifetime, without ever manifesting overt symptoms. Syphilis can be spread by sexual intercourse or from a pregnant mother to her fetus. Therefore, people who are infected with the bacterium need to be identified, so they can be treated and do not spread the disease unintentionally.

In 1906, Wassermann and Albert Neisser developed a syphilis test for the blood serum of patients. Serum is the pale yellow fluid that is one of the constituents of blood. People with syphilis produce an antibody, which is a molecule in the blood serum produced by the body's immune system to attack the syphilis bacterium. When a patient's blood serum with the syphilis antibody is introduced into a mixture of beef heart extract, animal blood serum, and washed red blood cells, the patient's antibody combines with parts of the mixture to create visible clumps of cells, which demonstrate the presence of the antibody and thus the presence of the syphilis bacterium. Wassermann's test helped doctors detect syphilis in babies and adults in order to treat the disease more effectively at an earlier stage in its development. The test is a very useful, inexpensive screening procedure. However, if positive, it must be confirmed with a more specific blood test

From 1903 to 1909, in collaboration with Wilhelm Kolle, Wassermann wrote the six-volume *Handbuch der pathogenen Mikroorganismen*, a book about disease-producing microorganisms. Wassermann was named the director of the department of experimental therapy at the Kaiser-Wilhelm Institute in Berlin in 1913. In 1924, he was diagnosed with kidney disease, and he died in Berlin on March 16, 1925. He continued to direct the department of experimental therapy up until his death.

See also Robert Koch

Waterhouse, Benjamin (1754-1846)

American physician

Benjamin Waterhouse was born March 4, 1754 in Newport, Rhode Island; he died on October 2, 1846 in Boston. He was the son of Timothy Waterhouse, a maker of chairs who is said to have been a judge of the Court of Common Pleas and on the Governor's Council, and Hannah Waterhouse. In 1788 he married Elizabeth Oliver, with whom he had six children; in 1819 he married Louisa Lee, with no children resulting from the second marriage. He attended the academy founded by Bishop Berkeley. Between 1775 and 1178, he studied medicine with Dr. John Halliburton and judge Robert Lightfoot in Newport. In 1780, he studied medicine and science at Edinburgh for nine months and in London with his relative John Fothergill. In 1780, he obtained the M.D. degree in Leyden, where he spent another year studying history and the law of nations. In 1786, he received an honorary M.D. degree from Harvard University. He began practicing medicine in Newport in 1782, and was elected to the Board of Fellows, College of Rhode Island (Brown). From 1783 to 1812, he was a member of the original faculty of Harvard Medical School. He was the first Hersey Professor of the Theory and Practice of Physic. (He was later forced to resign because of incompatibility with the rest of the medical faculty, and also because of his role in trying to establish a new medical society that probably would have to led to the founding of another medical school.) From 1807 to 1809, he served as chief physician of the U.S. Marine Hospital in Charlestown, Massachusetts. (Although he was instrumental in introducing substantial improvements there, he was dismissed amidst charges of petty graft.) From 1813 to 1820, he served first as a hospital surgeon and later as medical superintendent of all military posts in New England. During the 1820s, Waterhouse strongly supported Samuel Thomson and his medical system. His later life was largely devoted to literary pursuits.

Supported by President Thomas Jefferson, Benjamin Waterhouse was instrumental in introducing Edward Jenner's method of cowpox **vaccination** in the United States (1799 to 1802), during which time he attempted to maintain a monopoly over the cowpox vaccine (partly for selfish reasons and partly to keep the vaccine out of the hands of incompetent or fraudulent hands). In July, 1800 Waterhouse made the first vaccinations in the United States on his four children. He induced the Boston Board of Health to sponsor a controlled experiment in which 19 vaccinated and 2 unvaccinated boys were exposed to smallpox under the same conditions; the result was that the vaccinated individuals demonstrated immunity and the unvaccinated persons succumbed to the disease. Waterhouse was more interested in science than medicine, and lectured on natural history (biology and minerology), first at Rhode Isalnd College (1786 to 1787) and later at Harvard (1788 to 1806). Waterhouse's lectures were the first to systematically treat these subjects at Harvard. Waterhouse was a strong moralist, and published (on November 20, 1804) a warning against the increased use of alcohol and tobacco. Essentially a displaced philosopher, Waterhouse constantly stirred up trouble wherever he went, but is nevertheless considered to have done much more good than harm in the course of his life.

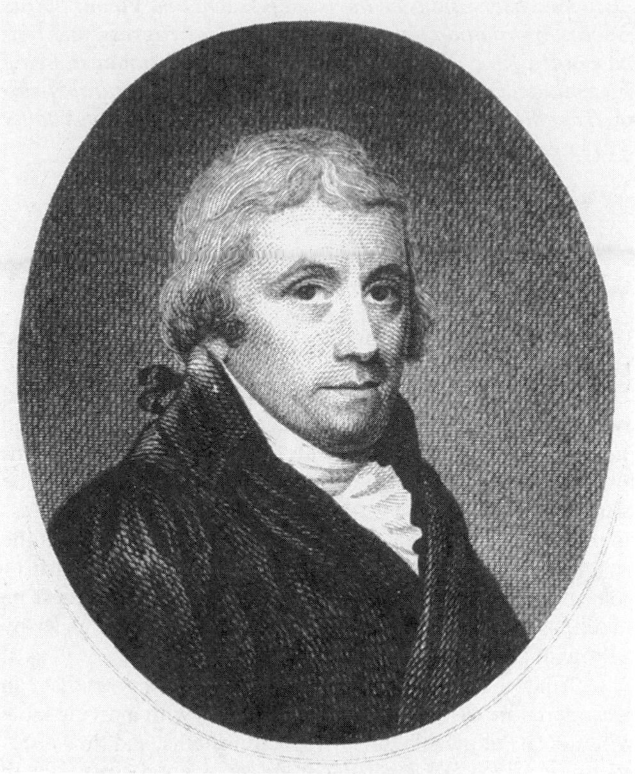

Benjamin Waterhouse.

Among his writings are *A Synopsis of a Course on the Theory and Practice of Medicine. In Four Parts* (1786); *The Rise, Progress, and Present State of Medicine* (1792); *A Prospect of Exterminating the Small Pox, Part I* (1880), *Part II* (1802); *Cautions to Young Persons Concerning Health...Showing the Evil Tendency of the Use of Tobac-*

co...with Observations on the Use of Ardent and Vinous Spirits (1805); *Information Respecting the Origin, Progress, and Efficacy of the Kine Pock Inoculation* (1810); *The Botanist, Being the Botanical Part of a Course of Lectures on Natural History...Together with a Discourse on the Principles of Vitality* (1811).

See also Military medicine; Cigarette smoking

WATER SAFETY

There are several important rules that apply to all water sports. The sportsman/woman should have the right equipment and the right instruction; engage in the sport with a buddy; and avoid the use of alcohol or medication that may cause impaired judgment. Nonswimmers account for two thirds of all drowning victims annually; swimming is an important life skill to be learned from an early age. Children should never swim unsupervised. If a swimmer gets into trouble, efforts to reach the victim should be made by extending an oar, tree branch or pole. If the victim cannot be reached, qualified help must be called, as even a competent swimmer can be pulled under by a drowning person.

Underwater diving or skin diving is not a sport that can be undertaken casually. Planning carefully with a diving table will indicate allowable times at specific depths, and time needed to resurface. Divers should utilize a good timer, depth gauge, and fly a diving flag and/or use a surface marker buoy. Caution must be taken to equalize pressure on the eardrums as the diver goes down, to prevent eardrum rupture at about 30 feet. Diving should be avoided with colds or flu, that may prevent clearing of the Eustachian tubes. ''The bends,'' or **decompression sickness**, the fundamental mechanism of which is a too-rapid reduction in pressure, such as might occur from too rapid an ascent from deep-sea diving. The result is that the increased nitrogen in the blood, and especially in lipid stores, that has occurred under the influence of the increased pressure, effervesces into the various tissues, producing gas emboli in the bones, joints, central nervous system, and blood, frequently with fatal consequences. Slow decompression permits the dissolved nitrogen to diffuse gradually into the blood and be eliminated by the lungs.

Surfing is a physically demanding sport, that requires the participant to be a competent swimmer in good physical condition. Care must be taken in handling the board out of the water, to avoid injury to bystanders. The board should be carried under the arm with the fin turned inward. Before taking a wave, the surfer should stay clear of swimmers and other surfers; the first surfer on a wave has the right of way.

Safety in water-skiing depends as much on those in the skiboat as on the skier. Two people in the boat allows one to concentrate on navigation, while the other translates the skier¤s hand signals. Both skiers and boaters should be competent swimmers, and wear a lifejacket and clothing to suit the weather conditions. Water skiing should be enjoyed in daylight hours only, and never in unfamiliar or shallow water.

Boaters should be competent swimmers and wear a personnel flotation device (PFD). All motorized boats must carry a fire extinquisher and, and every member of the crew must know how to operate the equipment. Before boating, a responsible person should be informed of destination and expected return time. The use of Personal Watercraft (PWC) has increased significantly over recent years, and so, unfortunately has the number of PWC-related accidents reported to the U. S. Coast Guard. More than 26 states have adapted PWC laws, as developed by the National Association of State Boating Law Administrators. These laws address minimum operator age to 16 years, require all operators and passengers to wear life jackets, and prohibit nighttime and reckless operation. Additional laws are being developed to address specific issues of unsafe operating patterns, including jumping wakes closely behind large vessels. Several states are requiring completion of a boater education course before use of a PWC. Continued vigilance and attention to the general rules of water safety can help assure enjoyable experiences in water sports.

WATKINS, JR., LEVI (1945-)

African American cardiac surgeon

Levi Watkins, Jr., the first black graduate of Vanderbilt University School of Medicine, has conducted research on congestive heart failure and also performed the first implantation of the automatic defibrillator in February 1980 at Johns Hopkins Hospital in Baltimore. The Automatic Implantation Defibrillator (AID) is designed to restore the heart's normal rhythm during an attack of ventricular fibrillation or arrhythmia, an irregularity of the heartbeat caused by coronary scar tissue or hardening of the coronary artery. When arrhythmia occurs, the heart is unable to pump blood and, unless corrected by devices such as the AID, the sufferer can die.

Watkins was born on June 13, 1945, in Parsons, Kansas, to Levi Watkins, Sr., an educator who became the president of Alabama State University, and Lillian Bernice Varnado. He graduated from Tennessee State University with honors in 1966. Watkins received his medical degree from the Vanderbilt University School of Medicine in Nashville in 1970 and completed his residency at the Johns Hopkins University Hospital, where he was the first black chief resident of cardiac surgery.

After his residency, Watkins was appointed assistant professor and then professor of surgery at Johns Hopkins. Watkins also spent two years conducting research at Harvard Medical School's Department of Physiology, investigating the relationship between congestive heart failure and the renin angiotensin system. Within the renin angiotensin system, a kidney enzyme is associated with the production of a hormone that causes dilation of blood vessels and contraction of muscles. Watkins's research led to the use of angiotensin blockers to treat congestive heart failure.

In 1982, discussing the ground-breaking AID device in *Ebony,* Watkins observed that ''Now we can give patients the ultimate protection from this sudden death.'' At that time, it was estimated that 500,000 people died from arrhythmia annually, making the disorder one of the leading causes of death in the United States. Invented by Michel Mirowski, the director of the coronary care unit at Sinai Hospital in Baltimore, the AID is a small, battery-operated generator that is implanted in the patient's abdomen. One electrode leading from the AID is inserted into the right chamber of the heart; a second electrode is affixed to the tip of the heart. When the AID senses an abnormal heart rhythm, it administers mild shocks to restore the normal rhythm. The success of the device means a positive prognosis for patients who do not respond to medication for the disorder (about twenty-five percent). Watkins's initial AID surgical procedure was soon followed by dozens of successful implantations, and representatives of medical centers throughout the country applied to be trained for the procedure.

In addition to his work with cardiac arrhythmia at Johns Hopkins, Watkins has been a pioneer in the application of lasers to heart surgery, and has directed research on heart disease, particularly as it affects minorities, through Maryland's Minority Health Commission and Panel for Coronary Artery Bypass Surgery. An aggressive recruiter of black students for Johns Hopkins Medical School, he was appointed in 1979 to the university's admissions committee. In 1983, Watkins joined the national board of the Robert Wood Johnson Minority Faculty Development Program. His other professional affiliations include the American Board of Surgery and the American Board of Thoracic Surgery.

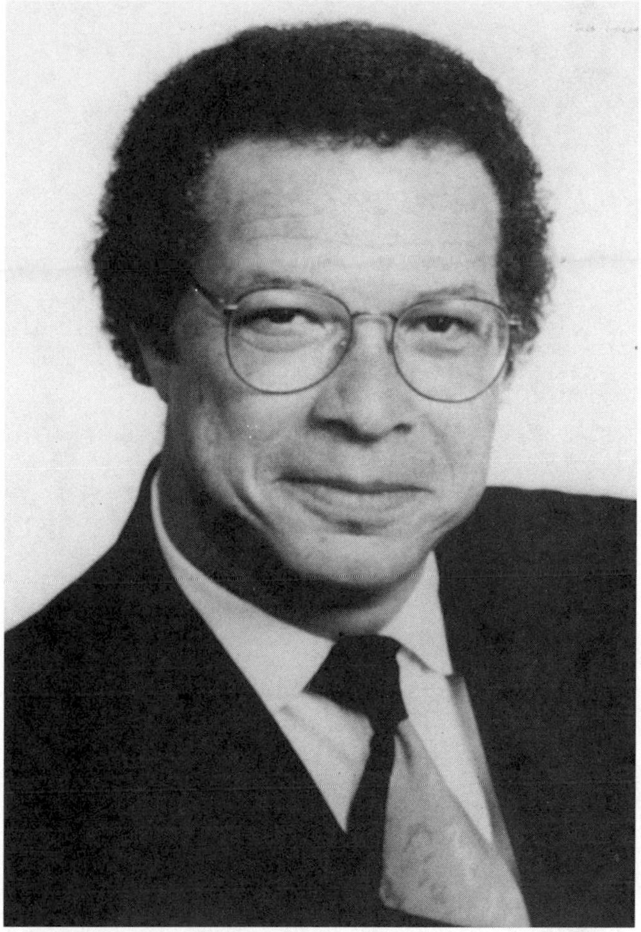
Levi Watkins, Jr.

WATSON, JOHN BROADUS (1878-1958)
American psychologist

Watson was an important leader of the behaviorist school of psychology who laid out its basic principles, publicized it, and influenced many people to enter the field of psychology.

Watson was born on January 9, 1878, in Greenville, South Carolina. His mother, Emma Kesiah Watson, was a devout Christian, and his father, Pickens Butler Watson, abused alcohol and abandoned his family when Watson was 12. In high school, Watson was an indifferent student, and he was arrested twice. He received his Master's degree from Furman College in 1900 and his Ph.D. from the University of Chicago in 1903 when he was 25. A year later he married Mary Amelia Ickes, one of his students. They had two children, Mary and John. Because Watson was a womanizer, this consequently ruined the marriage.

After he graduated from the University of Chicago, Watson stayed on to teach and to study the behavior of rats. In 1908, he moved to the Johns Hopkins University in Baltimore, where he soon became department chair when the man who hired him was caught in a bordello during a police raid. At Johns Hopkins, Watson set up a laboratory to run psychological experiments, and he continued his studies of animal behavior. He also began to study the behavior of small children.

In 1913, Watson published a famous article, "Psychology as a Behaviorist Views It," in *Psychological Review*. His article distinguished behaviorism from other schools of psychology and codified its main beliefs. Behaviorists studied observable animal and human behaviors, not states of consciousness which were difficult to verify. Behaviorists were objective, instead of relying on subjective descriptions of an individual's mental states. Behaviorists also tried to predict and control animal and human behaviors. Watson's article was a described as lucid and eloquent manifesto for behaviorism. In 1914, he published a major work, *Behavior: An Introduction to Comparative Psychology*. He became president of the American Psychological Association in 1915.

With a student collaborator, Rosalie Rayner, Watson conducted one of his best-known experiments on Albert B., an eleven-month-old child. Watson and Rayner conditioned the child to fear rats and other furry animals. They placed a white rat by Albert B., and when he reached for it, they scared him with a loud noise. They repeated this sequence of actions several times, which conditioned Albert to cry every time he saw the rat. Albert also began to associate the scary noise with any furry thing, including dogs, rabbits, fur coats, and cotton balls. Based on this experiment and others like it, Watson claimed in 1924 that he could take a child at random and, by controlling the environment, he could condition the child to grow up to be a doctor, artist, or thief. Later in his life, Watson would be less optimistic about the powers of behaviorism.

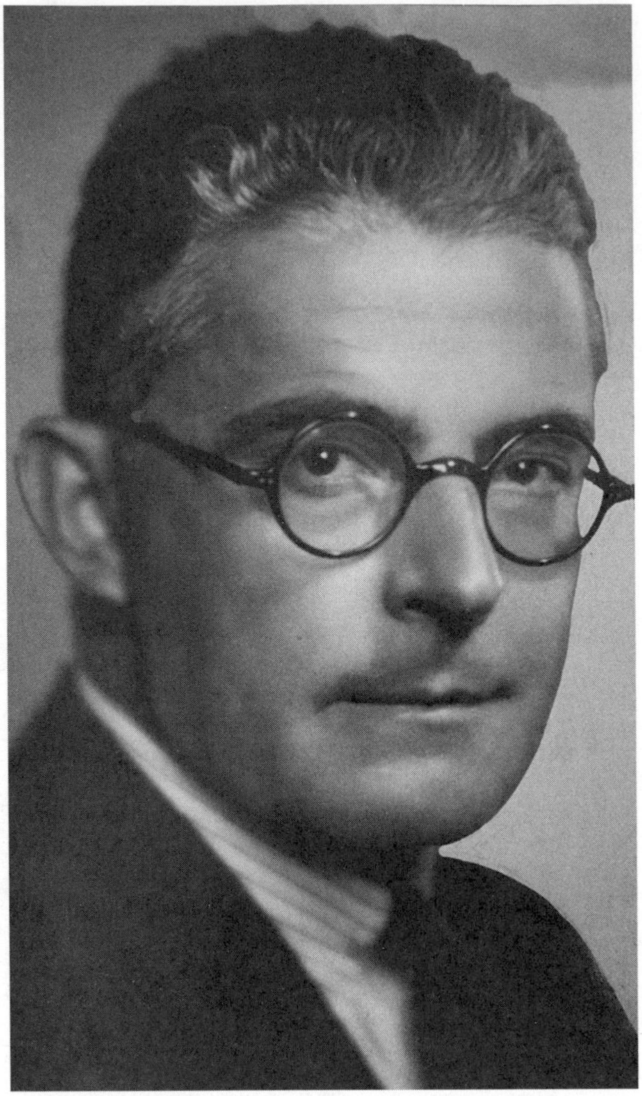

John Broadus Watson

Watson's womanizing caught up with him in 1920. His wife, Mary, found a love letter from Rosalie Rayner in one of his pockets, and she later obtained a number of his love letters to Rayner. Mary had suffered Watson's love affairs before, so she confronted her husband, telling him to stop seeing Rayner. Watson refused. Mary filed for divorce with irrefutable evidence of his philandering. In the resulting scandal, Watson had to resign his position at Johns Hopkins, an action that left him bitter.

Watson landed on his feet, however. He moved to New York City, became a vice president in the J. Walter Thompson advertising agency, and made a huge salary that enabled him to live on a country estate. He also married Rosalie Rayner, and they had two sons, William and James. He continued to publish, and in 1925 he published a popular book, *Behaviorism*, and in 1928, he published *Psychological Care of Infant and Child.*

In 1935, Rosalie died at the age of 35. One of his sons said that Watson never recovered from her death. In that same year, he left J. Walter Thompson for another company, where he worked until he retired in 1946. In 1957, Watson received the gold medal from the American Psychological Association for his contributions to psychology. He died in New York City on September 25, 1958, at the age of 80.

WATSON, JAMES DEWEY (1928-)

American biologist

James Watson is undoubtedly one of the most famous scientists of the twentieth century. He is recognized as co-discoverer of the structure of *deoxyribonucleic acid* (DNA) and was co-recipient of the 1962 Nobel Prize in physiology and medicine for his work in genetics. He has authored several books in recent years, including a light-hearted and informal account of his research appropriately titled *The Double Helix.* This successful book created celebrity status for Dr. Watson among the general public and added to his popularity in the scientific community. James Watson is still actively participating in several projects at an age when most other people are considering retirement.

Watson was born on April 6, 1928, in Chicago, Illinois. He was an extremely intelligent child who used his photographic memory to his advantage. By age 10, he was a regular contestant on a popular radio show called "The Quiz Kids." He studied zoology at the University of Chicago when he was only 15 years old. By age 19, he was conducting postgraduate research on viruses at the University of Indiana. It was here that he earned his Ph.D. degree in 1950. He continued his virus work in Denmark for a short period of time before several scientists convinced him to concentrate on genetics and molecular biology. This new direction lead him to Cavendish Laboratory at Cambridge University in 1951. It was here that he first met **Francis Crick**.

A friendship soon developed between Watson and Crick. It didn't take long before Watson's enthusiastic approach to genetic research persuaded Crick to assist him in developing a DNA model. During this time, DNA research was not a high priority for most scientists. Furthermore, Watson and Crick entered the race to find the structure of DNA rather late. Linus Pauling had already announced that he believed DNA was a single-stranded molecule and **Maurice Hugh Frederick Wilkins** had already completed several years of work in this area. Some fellow scientists thought that Watson lacked the mathematical and genetic background necessary to take on such a demanding project. With the odds stacked against them, Watson and Crick proceeded to develop their own unique hypothesis. They believed the DNA structure was actually made of two parallel strands. They obtained structural working models and attempted to fit the pieces together using proven chemical laws and prior studies. Many times, the model, which resembled a large tinker-toy ladder, fell apart or simply did not fit previously established evidence. Their tedious task was somewhat like trying to put together a model airplane with only a small portion of the instruction sheet and no picture of how the assembled plane should look.

Finally, two major clues fell into place. Watson and Crick knew that the amounts of the base pairs (adenine, thymine, cytosine, and guanine), which connect the two strands of the DNA molecule, were nearly equivalent. Crystallographic evidence supplied by Maurice Wilkins and **Rosalind Elsie Franklin** also suggested that the sugar-phosphate component was on the outside of the model. Watson saw that the shape of the structure formed by the bonding of adenine to thymine was identical to that of the cytosine and guanine pair. These base pairs fit neatly into the overall twisted ladder, or double helix, form without any distortion. It also meant that each side of the ladder was complementary to the other. This explained how DNA could be precisely copied and synthesized each time a cell divides.

The completed model consisted of a double backbone of sugar and phosphate molecules arranged in repeating units. Between these, like rungs in a ladder, were the flat pairs of bases. In 1953, when Watson was only 25 years old, he and Crick announced their discovery. Almost 10 years later, after numerous tests confirmed their results, they shared the Nobel Prize with Maurice Wilkins. Today we know that DNA is the molecule that contains the essential set of directions that each cell needs to perform vital life functions. The details of the DNA molecule are so precise that differences in the microstructure could mean the difference between a man and a mouse, or between life and death.

After such an important discovery at such a young age, Watson could have chosen to take a long vacation. In reality, much has happened in his life since then. Watson has published numerous papers, written several genetics textbooks, and taught at the California Institute of Technology and Harvard University. Today, Watson is director of the prestigious Cold Spring Harbor Laboratory in New York. This institution is involved in genetic and **cancer** research. From 1988-1992, he also was director of the National Center for Human Genome Research, where he helped lead the Human Genome Project. The goal of this endeavour is to eventually identify all of the 50,000 to 100,000 human genes. Watson believes that this will make it easier to screen DNA and identify individuals who are at risk of developing a variety of genetically caused diseases. Someday people with defective genes may be helped by some form of gene therapy.

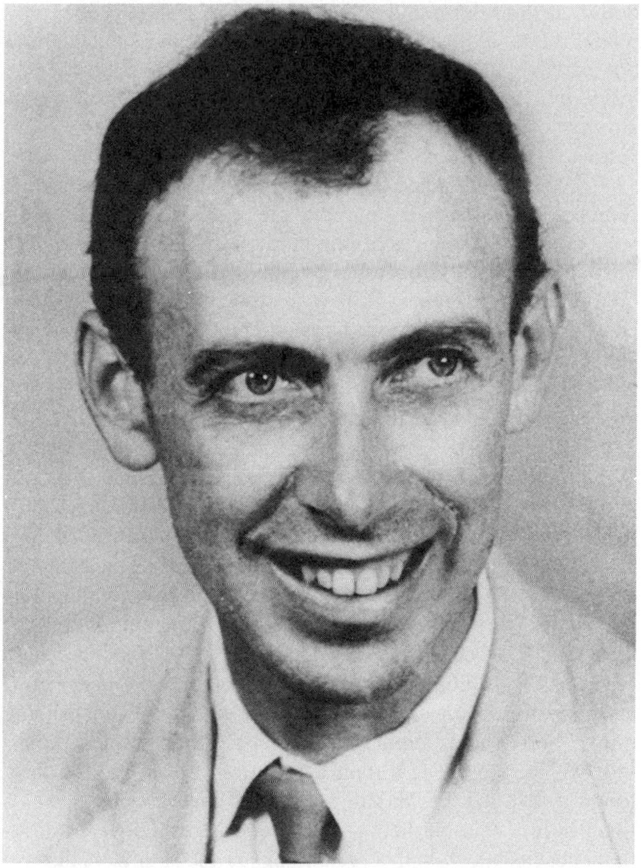

James Dewey Watson

WEBER, ERNST HEINRICH (1795-1878)

German anatomist and physiologist

Ernst Heinrich Weber made important discoveries about the sense of touch and invented the idea of the just-noticeable difference between two similar physical stimuli. He founded psychophysics, the branch of psychology that studies the relations between physical stimuli and mental states.

Weber, the third of 13 children, was born June 24, 1795, in Wittenburg, Germany. His father was Michael Weber, a professor of theology. Weber learned Latin in secondary school, and began to study medicine in 1811 at the University of Wittenberg. He received his doctor of medicine degree in 1815, specializing in comparative anatomy. Weber became a lecturer at the University of Leipzig in 1817 and was promoted to professor of anatomy the following year. He remained at the University of Leipzig until his retirement.

Weber made his name studying touch, pain, sight, hearing, taste, and smell. He was one of the first psychologists to experiment. He did not just sit at a desk and speculate about human mental states and perceptions. Instead, he tested human subjects to discover how they actually reacted to physical stimuli, publishing the results of many of his experiments about touch in *De Tactu* in 1834.

Weber developed the concept of the just-noticeable difference. He had his subjects lift one weight and then another to see if they could detect a difference between the two. If the differences were small, the subjects could not tell the two weights apart. If the differences were large, the subjects noticed them. Weber then searched for the smallest perceivable difference between a standard weight and a different weight. He discovered that the just-noticeable difference was best described as a ratio. For lifting weights, the ratio was one to 40. That is, for any standard unit of 40, subjects would notice a difference if one more unit were added to the weight. This ratio applied if Weber used 20, 40, or 80 ounces. If Weber only added half a unit, subjects would not notice the difference. The one-to-40 ratio applied when subjects lifted a weight using both their muscles and their sense of touch. When Weber only rested the weights on a subject's skin, and the subject could not use his muscles to sense the weight, then the ratio became lower, one to 30. The difference in perception meant that sensitivity to change was sharper if a person used two or more senses.

Weber conducted experiments about just-noticeable differences in vision, pain, auditory pitch, smell, and taste. Subjects noticed differences of one-sixtieth in light intensity, one-thirtieth in pain differences, one-tenth in pitch perception, one-quarter in smell, and one-third in taste. The ratios in all of these senses did not hold up at extremes. Thus, if a weight was too small, a subject would not recognize the difference. At the other extreme, if another candle were added to a well-lit room, the subject would not recognize its difference either.

Weber also tested to see if subjects would recognize when they were being touched by one or two points of an object. Weber would close the legs of a drafting compass until their points were almost together, and then touch them to a blindfolded subject's back or cheek. If the legs of the compass were close together, then the subject would perceive them as one touch. Weber then pulled the legs of the compass further apart and touched them again to the subject's back or cheek, to see at what point the subject would notice two touches rather than one. Using this method, Weber discovered that the human body had different sensitivities to touch. Subjects could tell two touches in less than a twentieth of an inch on their tongues, two touches in half an inch on their cheeks, and two touches in 2 = in on their backs. Weber's results were important decades later when nerve endings in the skin were discovered. Fingertips, which have many nerve endings, make very subtle distinctions, but the human back, which has far fewer nerve endings, makes coarser distinctions.

Weber retired from his university professorship in 1871, and he died in Leipzig, Germany, on January 26, 1878.

WELFARE

More than 35 million Americans have incomes that fall below the poverty line, and more than one in five American children are poor. In 1994, nearly half of all poor children under the age of six lived in families with incomes falling below half of the poverty line. That figure doubled over the 20 years preceding 1994. The number of people who work full time and are still poor has risen sharply as well. In 1975, 6% of young children who lived in families with one full-time worker were poor. By 1994, that figure had gone up to 15%. Despite these trends, there has been a decline in recent years in the number of recipients needing welfare assistance. In January 1993, for example, 5.5% of the total population was on welfare, but in January 1997, only 3.9% of the total population was receiving welfare payments.

Contrary to popular opinion, welfare payments are not overly generous: a U.S. Department of Labor report published in 1998 showed that the average monthly income for a household of three on welfare was $499, compared with the federal poverty level of $1,043.

The roots of modern American compassion for the poor can be traced back to colonial times when it was not uncommon for one family to care for another, and to the establishment of local poorhouses. The role of government in the public sector dates back to the founding of public schools in the nineteenth century, and has included the expansion of Civil War pensions, programs to aid mothers, and the creation of social security. The federal government, through New Deal legislation in the 1930s, put in place a program that provided subsidies to state and local governments to provide economic support to the very poor. This program, colloquially referred to as welfare, was known until recently as the Aid to Dependent Families (AFDC) program.

The AFDC, which actually dated to the 1910s, was originally intended to be a program to help widowed mothers and mothers whose husbands had left them. In its early years, the program was very small, however fairly successful. The AFDC program was replaced in 1996 by the TANF (Temporary Assistance to Needy Families) program, which is run by the states, following federal guidelines. The various welfare programs that were put into place by the federal government in the 1930s never entirely eliminated the role that the private sector played in helping the poor. There are still many examples of partnerships between government sectors and private charities like the Salvation Army or the Catholic Charities, or other various religious groups.

Critics of public welfare programs have long claimed that welfare is degrading to the recipient, discourages work, discourages family formation, and encourages family disintegration. Although it is true that most welfare mothers are single parents, recent government statistics show that over one-third of welfare families stay on welfare for one year or less. This is not to say that there are not binds for many welfare recipients; for example, if they stay home and apply for welfare, they can get a Medicaid card that allows them to take their children to the doctor, but if they are working long hours at minimum wage, their employer will probably not provide them with health insurance.

Over the past 30 years, there have been changes in family structures, and in what the economy has been doing for unskilled workers. At the time that the New Deal legislators designed the welfare system, it was felt that mothers should be encouraged to stay home, because what they did at home constituted work. Current thinking is that mothers need to be in the workforce. In addition, the racial composition of the people being helped has changed. Originally the majority of welfare recipients were white, now less than 36% are. Controversies about welfare tend to have more to do with major social changes and not simply the amount spent on welfare programs. These social changes have almost overwhelmed a welfare program that was based on different premises when it was started.

WELL-BABY EXAMINATION

Well-baby examinations are held regularly during the first two years of a baby's life. They allow the pediatrician to monitor and advise on the baby's growth and development. The American Academy of Pediatrics (AAP) recommends the newborn infant see a doctor for a check-up at birth, one, two, four, six, nine, 12, 15, 18, and 24 months, and annually thereafter. Most pediatricians follow this schedule, or some variation of it, in prescribing a check-up regimen for their patients. The features of a well-baby examination or ''check-up'' include: Taking a history. During this stage, the **physician** or an assistant will ask the parents a number of questions. Topics include developmental milestones, interactions with peers and adults, sleeping patterns, and eating habits. Typical questions include, ''Are there any changes or concerns that have come up since the last visit?''; ''How is the child functioning in child-care?''; ''How is the relationship with peers?'' The pediatrician (or an assistant) will observe the parents and the infant for signs of distress or difficulties with adjustment. In addition, they will be alert for any signs of **child abuse**. Performing a physical examination. At every visit, the child will be examined by the physician, usually conducted while the child is undressed to his or her diaper or underwear. Parents should discuss this aspect of the routine with the older infant and toddler prior to the visit, so that he or she is prepared to remove his or her clothes. The child will be measured, weighed, and have temperature and blood pressure recorded. Infants will have head circumference measured as well. The pediatrician will also check the eyes, ears, mouth, and throat; heart and lung rates; abdomen for unusual masses or enlargements; genitalia for anything unusual; arm and leg movement; and reflexes. Answering parents' questions. The pediatrician may solicit questions by asking the parent if they have any concerns. Some parents bring written questions so that they will not forget to ask something they want more information about. Explaining expected developmental pattern to parents. The pediatrician can help parents understand their child's next stage of development by explaining what stages are coming next, and by forewarning parents of difficulties that typically arise. The pediatrician also discusses behavior, nutrition, and safety issues, recommending childproofing strategies and emphasizing car seat use, for example. Administering developmental and medical tests and immunizations. Many pediatricians order various tests, such as **urinalysis**, tuberculin test, and blood tests during the first two years. The AAP recommends cholesterol screening of children over age two whose parents have a history of cardiovascular disease before age 55, or have blood cholesterol levels above 240mg/dl. Because there are a number of controversial factors influencing the value of cholesterol screening, as of the late 1990s the AAP did not recommend universal cholesterol screening.

See also Child care

WELLER, THOMAS (1915-)

American virologist

Thomas Huckle Weller was born on June 15, 1915, in Ann Arbor, Michigan, where his father was chairman of the pathology department at the University of Michigan Medical School.

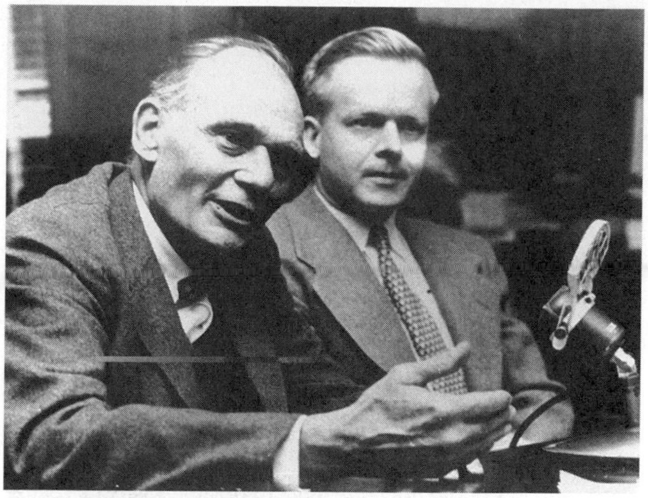

Thomas Weller

Weller showed an interest in biology from an early age. He attended the University of Michigan for his bachelor's and master's degrees, then entered Harvard Medical School in 1936, where he studied parasitology. Weller did research under **John Enders**, who was then studying methods of growing animal cells outside the body.

While in medical school, Weller began working on tissue-culture techniques and also took up an interest in viruses that cause infectious diseases. After medical school, he began work at Children's Hospital in Boston, but this was soon interrupted by service in the Army Medical Corps during World War II. Because he was stationed in Puerto Rico, Weller worked on tropical diseases, such as one caused by the tropical liver parasite Schistosoma. After returning to Children's Hospital, he began perfecting ways of keeping cells alive by changing the medium instead of transferring the cells. He used this method to study the **mumps** virus, then began working on the varicella virus, which causes chickenpox.

Along with Enders and another colleague, Frederick C. Robbins (his roommate in medical school), Weller worked with the poliomyelitis virus, developing a technique that allowed them to grow a virus in culture for many generations. This method made it easier to eventually culture a variant, an attenuated virus that could multiply without being dangerous—the kind of virus that is ideal for a vaccine. Although Weller did not work on a **polio** vaccine (later developed by **Jonas Salk** and **Albert Sabin**), this lab technique enabled others to do so, earning Weller, Enders, and Robbins the 1954 Nobel Prize for physiology or medicine.

Weller began studying the virus that causes chickenpox and showed that it is the same virus that causes the skin disease known as **shingles** (herpes zoster). He also isolated cytomegalovirus, and in 1962, he isolated the virus that causes **rubella** (German measles).

Weller left Children's Hospital in 1954 and spent his subsequent years as chairman of Harvard's Department of Tropical Public Health. He married Kathleen Fahey in 1945; they have two sons and two daughters.

Wells, Horace • See Nitrous oxide

Wheezing

Wheezing is a high-pitched whistling sound associated with labored breathing.

Wheezing occurs when a child or adult tries to breathe deeply through air passages that are narrowed or filled with mucus as a result of:

- Allergy
- Infection
- Illness
- Irritation.

Wheezing is most common when exhaling. It is sometimes accompanied by a mild sensation of tightness in the chest. Anxiety about not being able to breathe easily can cause muscle tension that makes matters worse.

Wheezing is the symptom most associated with **asthma**. It can be caused by:

- Exposure to allergens (food, pollen, and other substances, that cause a person to have an allergic reaction)
- Fumes
- Ice-cold drinks, or very cold air
- Medication
- Strenuous **exercise**
- Weather changes.
- **Foreign objects** trapped in the airway
- **Cystic fibrosis**, and other genetic disorders
- Respiratory illnesses like **pneumonia**, **bronchitis**, congestive **heart failure**, and emphysema.

To make a diagnosis, a family physician, allergist, or pulmonary specialist takes a medical history that includes questions about **allergies**, or unexplained symptoms that may be the result of allergic reactions. If the pattern of the patient's symptoms suggests the presence of allergy, skin and blood tests are performed to identify the precise nature of the problem.

A pulmonary function test may be ordered to measure the amount of air moving through the patient's breathing passages. X rays are sometimes indicated for patients whose wheezing seems to be caused by chronic bronchitis or emphysema.

Mild wheezing may be relieved by drinking plenty of juice, water, weak tea, and broth. Ice-cold drinks should be avoided.

A vaporizer can help clear air passages. A steam tent, created by lowering the face toward a sink filled with hot water, placing a towel over the head and sink, and inhaling the steam, can do likewise.

Bronchodilators (medications that help widen narrowed airways) may be prescribed for patients whose wheezing is the result of asthma.

Antibiotics are generally used to cure acute bronchitis and other respiratory infections. **Expectorants** (cough-producing medications) or bronchodilators are prescribed to remove excess mucus from the breathing passages.

If wheezing is caused by an allergic reaction, **antihistamines** will probably be prescribed to neutralize body chemicals that react to the allergen.

Breathing problems can be life-threatening. Immediate medical attention is required whenever an individual:

- Turns blue or gray and stops breathing
- Becomes extremely short of breath, and is unable to speak
- Coughs up bubbly-pink or white phlegm
- Seems to be suffocating
- Develops a **fever** of 101°F (38.3°C) or higher
- Wheezes most of the time, and coughs up gray or greenish phlegm.

Certain **yoga** positions (Bridge, Cobra, Pigeon, and Sphinx) may relieve wheezing by improving breathing control and reducing stress. Patients whose wheezing is related to asthma, chronic bronchitis, emphysema, or a severe allergic reaction may benefit from these techniques, but must continue to have their condition monitored by a conventional physician.

Mild wheezing caused by infection or acute illness usually disappears when the underlying cause is eliminated.

Some doctors believe that childhood respiratory infections may activate parts of the immune system that prevent asthma from developing.

Stopping smoking can eliminate wheezing. So can reducing or preventing exposure to other substances that cause the problem.

Whiplash

Whiplash is a sudden, moderate-to-severe strain affecting the bones, discs, muscles, nerves, or tendons of the neck.

The neck is composed of seven small bones. Known as the cervical spine, these bones:

- Support the head
- Help maintain an unobstructed enclosure for the spinal cord
- Influence the shape and structure of the spine
- Affect posture and balance.

About 1,000,000 whiplash injuries occur in the United States every year. Most are the result of motor vehicle accidents or collisions involving contact sports. When unexpected force jerks the head back, and then forward, the bones of the neck snap out of position and irritated nerves can interfere with flow of blood and transmission of nerve impulses. Pinched nerves can damage or destroy the function of body parts whose actions they govern.

Osteoarthritis of the spine increases the risk of whiplash injury. So do poor driving habits, driving in bad weather, or driving when tired, tense, or under the influence of alcohol or other drugs.

Tension shortens and tightens muscles. Fatigue relaxes them. Either condition increases the likelihood that whiplash will occur and the probability that the injury will be severe.

Sometimes symptoms of whiplash appear right away. Sometimes they do not develop until hours, days, or weeks after the injury occurs. Symptoms of whiplash include:

- **Pain** or stiffness in the neck, jaw, shoulders, or arms
- **Dizziness**
- Headache
- Loss of feeling in an arm or hand
- **Nausea and vomiting**.

Depression and vision problems are rare symptoms of this condition.

Whiplash is difficult to diagnose because x rays and other imaging studies do not always reveal changes in bone structure. Organs affected by nerve damage or reduced blood supply may generate symptoms not clearly related to whiplash.

Diagnosis is based on observation of the patient's symptoms, medical history, **physical examination**, and neurological studies to determine whether the spine has been injured.

Medication, physical therapy, and supportive measures are used to treat whiplash. Chiropractors gently realign the spine to relax pinched nerves or improve blood flow. A patient whose symptoms are severe may wear a soft, padded collar (Thomas collar or cervical collar) until the pain diminishes.

When pressure on the root of the nerve causes loss of strength or sensation in a hand or arm, a cervical **traction** apparatus may be recommended.

Inflammation and cramping can be alleviated by wrapping ice or an ice pack in a thin towel and applying it to the injured area for 10-20 minutes every hour. After the first 24 hours, painful muscle spasms can be prevented by alternating cold packs with **heat treatments**. Letting a warm shower run on the neck and shoulders for 10-20 minutes twice a day is recommended. Between showers, warm towels or a heat lamp should be used to warm and soothe the neck for 10-15 minutes several times a day.

Improving posture is important, and gentle **massage** can be beneficial. Sleeping without a pillow promotes healing, and a cervical collar or small rolled towel pinned under the chin can provide support and prevent muscle fatigue.

Alcohol should be avoided. A chiropractor, primary care physician, or orthopedic specialist should be notified whenever a painful neck injury occurs. Another situation requiring attention is if the face or arm weakens or becomes painful or numb following a neck injury.

With treatment, whiplash can usually be cured in one week to three months after injury occurs. If nerve roots are damaged, numbness and weakness may last until recovery is complete.

Chiropractors can recommend diet and **exercise** techniques to reduce stress and tension. Careful, defensive driving, wearing seatbelts, and using padded automobile headrests can lessen the likelihood of whiplash.

WHIPPLE, GEORGE HOYT (1878-1976)

American pathologist

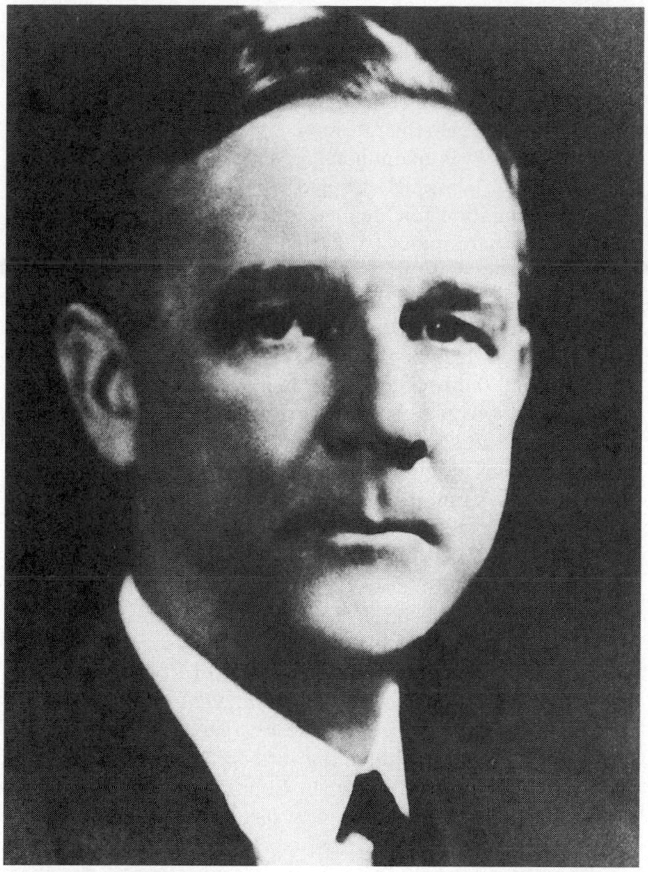

George Hoyt Whipple

George Whipple was born on August 28, 1878, in Ashland, New Hampshire, the son of Frances Anna Hoyt Whipple and Ashley Cooper Whipple, a general practitioner. At the age of fourteen Whipple entered Phillips Academy in Andover, Massachusetts, and enrolled at Yale College (now Yale University) as a premedical student four years later. After graduating with high standing in 1900, Whipple spent a year teaching and coaching at Holbrook Military Academy in New York to earn money for medical studies, and in 1901 he entered Johns Hopkins University's School of Medicine.

When Whipple received his M.D. in 1905, he joined the Johns Hopkins staff as an assistant in pathology, working under the renowned pathologist William Henry Welch. It was as a 29-year-old assistant performing an autopsy on a missionary doctor that Whipple made his first notable medical contribution: he described a rare condition in the intestinal tissues, which has since come to be called Whipple's disease. A year spent at a hospital in the Panama Canal Zone led to further notable advances in **malaria** and **tuberculosis** research.

When he returned to Johns Hopkins in 1908, Whipple turned his attention to studies in liver damage and the way in which liver cells repair themselves. Studies with dogs led Whipple to realize the importance of bile, a substance manufactured in the liver by the breakdown of hemoglobin, a complex pigment in red corpuscles. Beginning his assistant professorship at Johns Hopkins in 1911, Whipple came to focus on the interrelationship of bile, hemoglobin, and the liver. In 1913, along with a talented medical student, Charles W. Hooper, Whipple was able to show that bile pigments could be produced outside of the liver, solely from the breakdown of hemoglobin in the **blood**. Using this experiment as a starting point, Whipple set a new course for his studies. Since bile pigments are formed from hemoglobin, Whipple reasoned that he should tackle the question of hemoglobin itself, beginning with how it is manufactured. It was a fateful decision.

In 1914, Whipple accepted a position as director of the Hooper Foundation for Medical Research at the University of California in San Francisco. In that same year he also married his long-time sweetheart, Katharine Ball Waring, and the couple moved to California. His assistant, Hooper, also came with him to California and together with a new assistant, Frieda Robscheit-Robbins, they began experiments which would lead to a major breakthrough. By systematically bleeding laboratory dogs, Whipple and his team were able to induce a controlled anemic condition. They then tested various foods and their effects upon hemoglobin regeneration, finding that a diet of liver produced a pronounced increase in hemoglobin regeneration. While such short term effects were encouraging, they were still far from conclusive.

In 1920 Whipple was named dean of the University of California Medical School. However, he remained in California for just a year after before accepting a similar position at a new medical complex at the University of Rochester in New York. In his new position, Whipple directed the building and staffing of the University of Rochester School of Medicine and Dentistry, all the while directing further hemoglobin research. In 1925, Whipple and Robscheit-Robbins were able to prove conclusively that a liver diet was successful in counteracting its effects by increasing the production of hemoglobin, and his results were published. With Whipple's cooperation, the pharmaceutical firm of Eli Lilly began producing a commercially available liver extract within a year. Whipple refused to patent his findings, anddirected all royalties from the sales of the extract to fund additional research. Whipple's experiments paved the way for further studies by two Boston researches, **George Richards Minot** and William P. Murphy, who used liver therapy to successfully treat **pernicious anemia** in 1926.

In 1934, Whipple, along with Minot and Murphy, was awarded the Nobel Prize for Physiology or Medicine for their separate work in liver therapy. After receiving the prize, Whipple continued his hemoglobin experiments, turning now to the study of iron in the body and utilizing the new technology of radioisotope elements to follow the distribution of iron in the body. He also made important contributions to the study of an anemic disorder peculiar to people of Mediterranean extraction, a disorder for which Whipple suggested the name *thalassemia.*

Whipple never forgot his students, and took real pleasure in teaching. When in later years he was offered the position of Director of the Rockefeller Institute, he politely but adamantly declined, preferring his classes and his research. Whipple finally relinquished his chair as dean in 1953 at the age of 75, but remained on the faculty of the University of Rochester, teaching pathology until 1955. In 1963 he established a medical and dental library for the university valued at $750,000.

Whipple's life was long and productive. He was an active outdoorsman well into his ninth decade. With his wife Katharine, he had two children: a son, Hoyt, who followed in the Whipple tradition of medicine, and a daughter, Barbara. He died in Rochester on February 1, 1976, in the hospital he had helped to build.

Whooping cough

Whooping cough, also known as pertussis, is a highly contagious disease which causes classic spasms (paroxysms) of uncontrollable coughing, followed by a sharp, high-pitched intake of air which creates the characteristic ''whoop'' of the disease's name.

Whooping cough is caused by a bacteria called *Bordatella pertussis. B. pertussis* causes its most severe symptoms by attaching itself to those cells in the respiratory tract which have cilia. Cilia are small, hair-like projections that beat continuously, and serve to constantly sweep the respiratory tract clean of such debris as mucus, bacteria, viruses, and dead cells. When *B. pertussis* interferes with this normal, janitorial function, mucus and cellular debris accumulate and cause constant irritation to the respiratory tract, triggering coughing and increasing further mucus production.

Whooping cough is a disease which exists throughout the world. While people of any age can contract whooping cough, children under the age of two are at the highest risk for both the disease and for serious complications and **death**. Apparently, exposure to *B. pertussis* bacteria earlier in life gives a person some immunity against infection with it later on. Subsequent infections resemble the **common cold**.

Whooping cough has four somewhat overlapping stages: incubation, catarrhal stage, paroxysmal stage, and convalescent stage.

An individual usually acquires *B. pertussis* by inhaling droplets infected with the bacteria coughed into the air by someone already suffering with the infection. Incubation is the symptomless period of 7-14 days after breathing in the *B. pertussis* bacteria, and during which the bacteria multiply and penetrate the lining tissues of the entire respiratory tract.

The catarrhal stage is often mistaken for an exceedingly heavy cold. The patient has teary eyes, sneezing, fatigue, poor appetite, and an extremely runny nose (rhinorrhea). This stage lasts about 10-14 days.

The paroxysmal stage, lasting two to four weeks, begins with the development of the characteristic whooping cough. Spasms of uncontrollable coughing, the ''whooping'' sound of the sharp inspiration of air, and vomiting are all hallmarks of this stage. The whoop is believed to occur due to inflammation and mucous which narrow the breathing tubes, causing the patient to struggle to get air into his/her lungs; the effort results in intense exhaustion. The paroxysms (spasms) can be induced by overactivity, feeding, crying, or even overhearing someone else cough.

The mucus which is produced during the paroxysmal stage is thicker and more difficult to clear than the more watery mucus of the catarrhal stage, and the patient becomes increasingly exhausted attempting to clear the respiratory tract through coughing. Severely ill children may have great difficult maintaining the normal level of oxygen in their systems, and may appear somewhat blue after a paroxysm of coughing, due to the low oxygen content of their blood. Such children may also suffer from swelling and degeneration of the brain (encephalopathy), which is believed to be caused both by lack of oxygen to the brain during paroxysms, and also by bleeding into the brain caused by increased pressure during coughing. Seizures may result from decreased oxygen to the brain. Some children have such greatly increased abdominal pressure during coughing that **hernia**s result (hernias are the abnormal protrusion of a loop of intestine through a weak area of muscle). Another complicating factor during this phase is the development of **pneumonia** from infection with another bacterial agent; the bacteria takes hold due to the patient's already-weakened condition.

If the patient survives the paroxysmal stage, recovery occurs gradually during the convalescent stage, usually taking about three to four weeks. However, spasms of coughing may continue to occur over a period of months, especially when a patient contracts a cold, or other respiratory infection.

Diagnosis based just on the patient's symptoms is not particularly accurate, as the catarrhal stage may appear to be a heavy cold, a case of the flu, or a simple **bronchitis**. Other viruses and **tuberculosis** infections can cause symptoms similar to those found during the paroxysmal stage. The presence of a pertussis-like cough along with an increase of certain specific white blood cells (lymphocytes) is suggestive of pertussis (whooping cough). However, cough can occur from other pertussis-like viruses. The most accurate method of diagnosis is to culture (grow on a laboratory plate) the organisms obtained from swabbing mucus out of the nasopharynx (the breathing tube continuous with the nose). *B. pertussis* can then be identified by examining the culture under a microscope.

Treatment with the antibiotic erythromycin is helpful only at very early stages of whooping cough, during incubation and early in the catarrhal stage. After the cilia and the cells bearing those cilia, are damaged, the process cannot be reversed. Such a patient will experience the full progression of whooping cough symptoms; symptoms will only improve when the old, damaged lining cells of the respiratory tract are replaced over time with new, healthy, cilia-bearing cells. However, treatment with erythromycin is still recommended, to decrease the likelihood of *B. pertussis* spreading. In fact, all members of the household where a patient with whooping cough lives should be treated with erythromycin to prevent the spread of *B. pertussis* throughout the community. The only other treatment is supportive, and involves careful monitoring of fluids to prevent **dehydration**, rest in a quiet, dark room to decrease paroxysms, and suctioning of mucus.

Just under one percent of all cases of whooping cough cause death. Children who die of whooping cough usually have one or more of the following three conditions present:

- Severe pneumonia, perhaps with accompanying encephalopathy
- Extreme weight loss, weakness, and metabolic abnormalities due to persistent vomiting during paroxysms of coughing
- Other pre-existing conditions, so that the patient is already in a relatively weak, vulnerable state (such conditions may include low birth weight babies, poor nutrition, infection with the **measles** virus, presence of other respiratory or gastrointestinal infections or diseases).

The mainstay of prevention lies in programs similar to the mass immunization program in the United States which begins immunization inoculations when infants are two months old. The pertussis vaccine, most often given as one immunization together with **diphtheria** and **tetanus**, has greatly reduced the incidence of whooping cough.

Wiener, Alexander (1907-1976)

American physician and immunohematologist

Alexander Wiener was a physician who, along with fellow scientist Karl Landsteiner, discovered the Rh factor in blood. He also discovered a number of other antigens (substances in the blood that cause the development of antibodies). The Rh factor is an antigen named after the rhesus monkey, the animal in which it was first discovered. Blood that contains the factor is called Rh-positive, whereas blood that lacks it is labeled Rh-negative. The discovery of the Rh factor led to an understanding of adverse reactions to blood transfusions that occurred inexplicably in some patients even though compatibility of blood type (A, B, AB, and O) in donor and recipient had been observed. The discovery of the Rh factor also brought about an understanding of the possible adverse reactions when an Rh-negative mother carried an Rh-positive fetus. Wiener developed a life-saving method of replacing the damaged blood of new-born infants who had erythroblastosis fetalis, the infant blood disease that sometimes results from Rh incompatibility. He was also instrumental in getting the results of his research applied to legal issues such as disputed paternity, and to cases involving crimes such as homicide and assault. Author or co-author of more than five hundred scientific articles, he also wrote several books, including what for years was the standard textbook on the subject, *Blood Groups and Transfusion.* His many awards include the Lasker Award of the American Public Health Association, which he received in 1946, and the Passano Foundation Award, received in 1951.

Alexander Solomon Wiener was born March 16, 1907, in Brooklyn, New York, the son of George Wiener, an attorney who had emigrated from Russia in 1903, and Mollie (Zuckerman) Wiener. He attended Brooklyn public schools, graduating from Brooklyn Boys' High School at the age of 15. He was awarded scholarships to attend Cornell University, where he was elected to Phi Beta Kappa in his senior year. Both in high school and in college he pursued an interest in mathematics. In high school he took courses in analytic geometry and calculus and was a member of the mathematics team and president of the mathematics club. He continued his study of mathematics at Cornell University, and contributed mathematical problems to the *American Mathematical Monthly.* He majored in biology, however, receiving his A.B. in 1926. He then entered the Long Island College of Medicine (now the SUNY College of Medicine) and was awarded an M.D. in 1930.

While he was in medical school, Wiener began his first research on blood groups at the Jewish Hospital of Brooklyn, where he would also intern from 1930 to 1932 and with which he would be affiliated for his entire professional career. From 1933 to 1935 he served as the head of the Division of Genetics and Biometrics, from 1932 to 1952 as head of the blood transfusion division, and thereafter as attending immunohematologist. From 1949 he was also affiliated with Adelphi Hospital, including three years (1949–1952) as the head of the blood transfusion division. In addition, he began a private medical practice in 1932, but three years later he founded Wiener Laboratories, where he limited his practice to clinical pathology and blood grouping. In 1938 he joined the faculty of the Department of Forensic Medicine of New York University School of Medicine, moving up the academic ranks to professor by 1968. In 1938 he also began his long-time association with the Office of the Chief Medical Examiner of New York City. He married Gertrude Rodman in 1932. They had two daughters, Jane Helen and Barbara Rae. Wiener died of leukemia in New York on November 6, 1976.

The background to the discovery of the Rh factor lay in earlier discoveries concerning the nature of blood. In 1901 Karl Landsteiner had distinguished four main human blood groups: A, B, AB, and O. These classifications refer to antigens (substances that produce antibodies) on the surface of the red blood cells. Blood type A contains the A antigen, B contains the B antigen, AB contains both, and O contains neither. However, in the 1920s other blood factors or antigens were discovered—M, N, and P.

In the 1930s Wiener began collaborating with Landsteiner, who was affiliated with the Rockefeller Institute for Medical Research in New York. In 1937 Landsteiner and Wiener were studying the M factor in apes and monkeys, focussing on its action as an agglutinogen (its ability to clump red blood cells together). They showed that different anti-M sera (blood sera samples with antibodies opposing the M antigen) produced differing reactions, and concluded that there were at least five distinct M blood factors. This led to further experimentation in which they tested the sera of rabbits immunized with rhesus monkey blood cells. The antibodies produced by rabbit blood in response to rhesus monkey antigens led them to believe that unknown blood factors might be discovered in human blood by the same method. They began experiments using human blood and the anti-sera from rhesus blood, and thereby discovered a new antigen that they called the Rh factor. The importance of this discovery in transfusions was recognized in 1939 when it was understood that although the first transfusion of Rh-positive blood into an Rh-negative person may be harmless, the sensitization that resulted meant that a second transfusion could cause a dangerous hemolytic reaction involving the damage or destruction of red blood cells.

Wiener then studied the sera from Rh negative patients who had hemolytic transfusion reactions, and the sera from Rh-negative mothers of erythroblastotic babies. These babies have Rh positive blood, some of which enters the mother's blood, usually shortly before or during birth. The mother's blood forms an antibody to the Rh factor and crosses back to the fetal blood supply. The result is the damage or destruction of the fetal red blood cells containing the Rh antigen. He discovered that the expected Rh antibodies often could not be found. He hypothesized that there must be two different forms of Rh antibodies, one that caused the agglutination of cells (which he called bivalent antibodies), the other capable of coating the red blood cells without clumping them (which he called univalent or blocking antibodies). In 1944 and 1945 he developed tests for both types of antibodies.

Wiener noted the fallacy of assuming a one-to-one correspondence between antigens and antibodies. One antigen could produce multiple blood specificities. He soon discovered additional Rh factors that were related to the original one. In the human Rh system (now known as the Rh-Hr system), Wiener and others established as many as 25 different blood factors that form the basis of a large number of blood types.

Wiener's research had many practical implications. It led to an understanding of erythroblastosis fetalis, for which Wiener himself devised (1944–1946) a treatment by means of a complete exchange transfusion replacing the damaged Rh-positive blood of the infant with Rh-negative blood. This treatment led to a significant decline in the rate of infant mortality. Knowledge of Rh factors also made blood transfusions far safer. Other implications of Wiener's research derived from the fact that all blood factors are inherited in predictable fashion, and that they combine in a highly specific way in individuals, allowing a sophisticated method of "fingerprinting." Blood factor analysis became important in legal matters (such as establishing paternity), as well as criminal matters, such as the use of blood for identification in homicide and assault. It also facilitated advances in physical anthropology—different groups of people have different proportions of various blood factors, so that tribal movements can sometimes be traced by analysis of blood factor percentages in populations.

Wiener's research had significant legal implications. He was a member of the American Medical Association legal committee that sponsored blood test laws in all states, and he was the co-author of its 1935 report. He was instrumental in the passage of the New York State law allowing blood tests in disputed paternity cases. He and his father, attorney George Wiener, assisted in drafting a number of laws concerning blood testing that became part of the New York State domestic relations, civil, and criminal codes.

Wiener liked playing the piano, going to the movies, and playing cards. He also enjoyed tennis and gulf. In addition, he continued his life-long interest in mathematics and physics by avidly reading in these areas. A member of many professional organizations, he was also an honorary member of the Mystery Writers of America.

WIESCHAUS, ERIC F. (1947-)

American biologist

Wieschaus was born in South Bend, Indiana, in 1947 but grew up in Alabama. He received his bachelor's degree in biology from the University of Notre Dame in 1969 and his doctorate from Yale in 1974. His doctoral dissertation involved using genetic methods to label the progeny (offspring) of single cells in fly embryos. He showed that even at the earliest cellular stages, cells were already determined to form specific regions of the body called segments.

Wieschaus began his Nobel-winning work in the latter part of the 1970s. The Alabama native spent three years with **Christiane Nüsslein-Volhard** in the European Molecular Biology Lab at the University of Heidelberg, Germany, tackling the question of why individual cells in a fertilized egg develop into various specific tissues. They elected to study *Drosophila*, or fruit flies, because of their extremely fast embryonic development. New generations of fruit flies can be bred in a week. In addition, fruit flies have only one set of genes controlling development compared to the four sets humans possess. This means that testing each fruit fly gene individually takes one-fourth the time it would involve to test human genes.

To begin their experiment, Nüsslein-Volhard and Wieschaus damaged male fruit fly deoxyribonucleic acid (DNA) by applying ultraviolet light to the genes or by feeding the flies sugar water laced with chemicals. Then the team ''knocked out'' one gene from the fly, breeding generations of fruit flies without that particular piece of code. In this way, Nüsslein-Volhard and Wieschaus were able to isolate all the genes crucial to the early stages of embryonic development. When the flies were bred, the females produced dead embryos. These lifeless embryos resulted from only 150 different mutations of the 40,000 mutations applied. These 150 genes proved to be essential to the proper development of the fly embryo because, when damaged, the genes caused extraordinary deformities that killed the embryo. By viewing the fly embryos with a two-person microscope, Wieschaus and Nüsslein-Volhard were able to simultaneously view and classify a large quantity of malformations caused by gene mutations. Next, they identified 15 different genes, that, when mutated, eliminate specific body segments in the fly embryos. Wieschaus also established that systematic categorizing of genes that control the various stages of development could be accomplished.

Their first research results reported that the number of genes controlling early development was not only limited, but could also be classified into specific functional groups. They also identified genes that cause severe congenital defects in flies. After additional experimentation, the principles involved with the fruit fly genes were found to apply to higher animals and humans. This led to the realization that many similar genes control human development, and this finding could have a tremendous impact on the medical world. The applications of their research extend to in vitro fertilization, identifying congenital **birth defects**, and increased knowledge of substances that can endanger early stages of **pregnancy**.

It wasn't until 1995, however, that he won the Nobel Prize in Physiology or Medicine, along with Edward B. Lewis and Christaine Nüsslein-Volhard, for his work on identifying key genes that make a fertilized fruit fly egg develop into a segmented embryo. His research could help improve knowledge of how genes control embryonic development in higher organisms, including identifying genes that cause human birth defects.

WIESEL, TORSTEN (1924-)

Swedish American neurophysiologist

Torsten Nils Wiesel was born on June 3, 1924, in Uppsala, Sweden, the son of Anna-Lisa Bentzer Wiesel and Fritz S. Wiesel, the chief psychiatrist at the Beckomberga Mental Hospital in Stockholm. Wiesel entered medical school at the Karolinska Institute in Stockholm in 1941 and studied neurophysiology and psychiatry. In 1954, he received his medical degree, becoming an instructor at the institute as well as an assistant in the Department of Child Psychiatry at Karolinska Hospital. Wiesel then came to the United States in 1955 to do postdoctoral work at the Wilmer Institute of Johns Hopkins School of Medicine.

At Johns Hopkins, Wiesel worked under Stephen Kuffler, whose exhaustive work had proved that the vision of mammals is distinctly different from that of non-mammals. Wiesel became interested in the idea that the critical level of visual perception must take place in the brain of mammals. In 1958, Wiesel set off with **David Hubel** on the research that would result in a new theory of visual perception.

Wiesel and Hubel studied the striate or visual cortex which is located at the back of the brain. They discovered which cells in the cortex responded to which pattern or level of light. They also conducted experiments to map the striate cortex by injecting the eyes of experimental animals with radioactively labeled amino acid. These amino acids would be taken up by the cell bodies of the retina and transported to cells in the visual cortex. In some cases, the visual cortexes were dissected in order to see, by the use of autoradiographs or X-ray like photos, where the labeled amino acids actually ended up. Such experiments, begun in 1959, used both cats and macaque monkeys. That same year Kuffler was appointed a professor at the Harvard University Medical School, and Wiesel and Hubel joined him there. Wiesel was appointed assistant professor of physiology, and became a full professor in 1964.

The Wiesel-Hubel team soon began publishing the results of their experimental method, and it was clear that they had uncovered new complexities to the visual process. Within the visual cortex itself, Wiesel and Hubel made two important discoveries. First they showed that there is a hierarchy of types of cells in the cortex, ranking from simple to complex to hypercomplex, depending on the information each is able to process. They termed the process of putting the millions of building blocks of visual information back together into a picture ''convergence.'' Their second major discovery was a further organization of the cortical cells into roughly vertical divisions of two types: orientation columns and ocular dominance columns. Within these columns are simple, complex, and hypercomplex cells working toward a progressive convergence of visualization. Until the time of Wiesel's and Hubel's work, it was assumed that all cells of the cerebral cortex were more or less uniform. Wiesel and Hubel showed that the visual cortex is constituted of a cell pattern, which appears to be designed specifically for vision. As a result of their discovery, current theory now posits that the rest of the cerebral cortex may follow this form-follows-function rule.

Wiesel and Hubel researched another experimental model in which they used kittens to study the effect of various visual impairments on development. They discovered that if one eye were deprived of certain or all visual stimuli at three to five weeks of age, the central functioning of that eye would always be suppressed from cortical processing. Kittens, and by extension mammals in general, though born with a complete visual cortex, must still "learn" to see. Even if an early impairment is later corrected, the repaired eye will still remain functionally impaired as far as the visual cortex is concerned. The realization that there is a critical stage for visual development revolutionized the field of pediatric ophthalmology, calling for the earliest possible intervention in cases of strabismus, or crossed eyes, and congenital cataracts.

By 1973 Wiesel succeeded Kuffler as chair of the Department of Neurobiology at Harvard, and was named the Robert Winthrop Professor of Neurobiology in 1974. In 1981, Wiesel and Hubel were awarded the Nobel Prize for Physiology or Medicine, sharing it with Sperry from Caltech. The Karolinska Institute in Stockholm, which administers the prize and where Wiesel began his professional career, praised Hubel and Wiesel for their discoveries concerning information processing in the visual system. Wiesel and Hubel continued their close working relationship until Wiesel left Harvard in 1984 to head the neurobiology lab at Rockefeller University where he continued his researches on vision. In 1992 he was named president of Rockefeller University.

Weisel's first marriage, to Teiri Stenhammer, ended in divorce after 14 years in 1970. Wiesel was married again in 1973, to Grace Yee. The couple had one child, Sara Elisabet. His second marriage also ended in divorce in 1981. Wiesel became a naturalized U.S. citizen in 1990.

WILKINS, MAURICE HUGH FREDERICK (1916-)

British biophysicist

Maurice Wilkins was born on December 15, 1916, at Pongaroa, New Zealand. At the age of six, he was brought to England. His career began as a nuclear physicist. Wilkins earned a Ph.D. from the University of Birmingham in 1940. During World War II, he applied his background toward the development of the atomic bomb. After the war ended, Wilkins was troubled by the application of the atomic bomb and focused on solving biological problems with physical methods. He initially studied *deoxyribonucleic acid*(DNA) because it was a relatively large molecule that could be easily isolated for use in a wide variety of studies.

In the 1940s, scientists had yet to realize the importance of DNA as a carrier molecule of life's genetic code. One day, Wilkins noticed that, when a gel preparation of DNA was touched with a glass stirring rod and observed under the microscope, a thin fiber of DNA was drawn out. This chance observation implied that the molecules of the DNA were arranged in some regular fashion. Wilkins and one of his colleagues, **Rosalind Elsie Franklin**, developed X-ray diffraction photographs of DNA. They did this by studying how light patterns bend or diffract when crystalline materials are exposed to X-rays. From the photos, Wilkins was able to determine the distance across the double helix and the length of one turn of this helix.

Wilkins proceeded to demonstrate that the structure was not merely an artifact resulting in the isolation of DNA from the cell. X-ray diffraction photographs of complete biological systems closely resembled those taken from isolated DNA. This proved that DNA had the same organization both before and after isolation. These small bits of evidence, when combined with chemical data, confirmed that DNA was shaped like a twisted ladder, or double helix. Franklin and Wilkins also showed that the phosphate groups of the DNA were located on the outside of the molecule. Wilkins later showed the X-ray diffraction photos to **James Dewey Watson**, who was working with **Francis Crick** to develop a complete model of the DNA structure at Cambridge University. Watson was excited about the photos, because they confirmed his and Crick's proposed DNA structure. Watson and Crick incorporated the work of Wilkins, Franklin, and other scientists to ultimately build a series of accurate models. They eventually used all the known features of DNA to produce a model that gave the same diffraction pattern that Wilkens founded.

After these findings were published in 1953, Wilkins continued to develop his X-ray diffraction patterns to demonstrate the unique character of Watson and Crick's model. He also applied X-ray techniques to help determine the structure of *ribonucleic acid* (RNA). In 1962, Wilkins was awarded the Nobel Prize in physiology and medicine along with James Watson and Francis Crick. Wilkins's work was used as a guide to develop the DNA structure and later helped to prove that the structure proposed by Watson and Crick was correct.

WILLIAMS, ANNA WESSELS (1863-1954)

American bacteriologist and public health pioneer

During a long professional career doing research at the New York City Department of Health Laboratory, Anna Williams pioneered laboratory techniques for the diagnosis of many diseases. Dr. Williams also wrote and lectured about her findings in an era when women in science were few and very rarely recognized for their contributions.

Anna Wessels Williams was born in 1863 in Hackensack, New Jersey and graduated from the Women's Medical College in New York City in 1891. She studied in Europe for a time, during which she visited **Robert Koch**, the discoverer of **tuberculosis** bacteria. When she returned to New York she began work for the Department of Health, where her first research assignment was in the diagnosis and treatment of **diphtheria**, a bacterial disease that was on the rise during the mid-1890s. Dr. Williams successfully isolated one strain of diphtheria bacteria, *Corynebacterium diphtheriae*, although her work went uncredited at the time. The strain became known as "Park 8," named after the director of the laboratory, Dr. W. H. Park, who was on vacation at the time of the discovery. During this period also, Williams worked with Dr. Alexander Lambert to develop a standardized test for **typhoid fever**.

In 1896 Dr. Williams briefly visited Paris where she learned valuable laboratory techniques for the diagnosis of rabies. Several years later, while examining microscope slides of smears taken from the brains of rabid animals, Dr. Williams discovered unusual "bodies" that appeared in all the cells. These characteristic features were named Negri bodies for an Italian scientist working at the same time in a laboratory in Italy. The two bacteriologists, Williams and Negri, communicated their findings, and Williams pioneered a technique that led to a faster diagnosis of rabies based on the appearance of the stained slides.

In 1904 New York City was experiencing an epidemic of **pneumonia**. In response, Williams and Park examined specimens from hundreds of pneumonia patients and observed that *pneumococcus bacteria* were present. Their findings occurred several years before discovery of the bacteria by Oswald T. Avery and others, who are usually credited with the diagnosis of the disease. Williams was also involved in tests for typhoid fever and helped to give laboratory confirmation of the diagnosis of "Typhoid Mary," a carrier of the disease who was subsequently apprehended and confined.

Williams worked closely with another pioneer in public health, Josephine Baker, who headed the Department of Children's Hygiene where great efforts were made to report and eradicate the children's diseases that often ran rampant in the city's slums. It was thought that *trachoma*, a chronic eye disease that can lead to a reduction in vision, was affecting thousands of New York City children. However, in her study from 1912 to 1913, Dr. Williams concluded that most cases had been misdiagnosed and that the children were suffering from the more common infection, conjunctivitis.

During the **polio** outbreak of 1916, Williams began research on that disease. 1918, however, marked the beginning of the "flu years" and much of her research time was devoted to finding the cause of **influenza**. In only two months of 1918 there were close to 11,000 reported deaths caused by influenza and almost 10,000 from pneumonia. Williams and others at their New York City laboratory set to work on the variety of bacterial agents that could cause flu. But their work was inconclusive and Williams made reference in her report of the difficulties in trying to look for a possible viral cause. Identification of viruses, which indeed cause the flu, remained elusive during this period of research.

In the 1920s, Williams did extensive studies on **scarlet fever**. The Dick test, which had just recently been developed by George and Gladys Dick, had been used to test thousands of school children for the disease. Williams surveyed hundreds of scarlet fever cases that had been positively diagnosed for the antitoxin that had been used.

In the 1930s Williams published a compilation of her work on bacterial diseases entitled *Streptococci in Relation to Man in Health and Disease*. She received honors for her pioneering work as a woman of science, but spoke of the difficulty and bias women faced in a field dominated by men. She retired in 1934 and was 91 when she died.

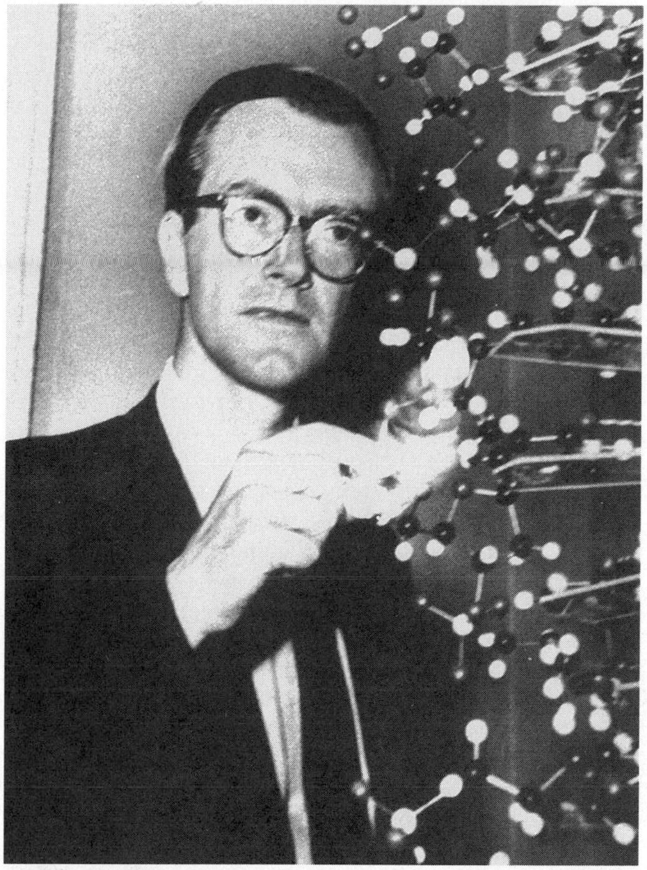

Maurice Hugh Frederick Wilkins

WILLIAMS, DANIEL HALE (1858-1931)

American physician

Daniel Williams, a meticulous, knowledgeable surgeon and founder of the first interracial hospital in the United States, advanced further in medicine than any other African-American doctor of his time. Among his many achievements, Williams is credited with having performed the first emergency **open-heart surgery**.

Williams was born the fifth of seven children of Daniel and Sarah Ann Price Williams on January 18, 1858 in Hollidaysburg, Pennsylvania. At the age of eleven, he was left an orphan after his father, a prosperous barber, died of tuberculosis and his mother deserted him. First apprenticed to a cobbler, he rebelled against repetitive, menial labor and moved to Edgerton, Wisconsin, to live with his sister Sally. He boarded with a foster family and found work as a barber and guitarist in a string band so that he could attend Haire's Classical Academy in Janesville, from which he graduated in 1877.

Following the example of his older brother, he studied law for a time. After a year, intrigued by the work of the town doctor, he requested a position as doctor's assistant. To increase his knowledge of medicine, he read journals and texts. After two years apprenticeship, working as a laborer on a lake steamer, and borrowing money from friends and family to pay his tuition, he completed a medical degree from Chicago Medical College in 1883. Because African-American doctors were denied privileges at white hospitals, he worked as a surgeon at the South Side Dispensary in a ghetto area until 1892.

Under primitive conditions—either in his office or in the patient's hom—Williams performed necessary surgery without an anesthesiologist or X-rays, either in his office or in the patient's home. To improve surgical standards and his patients' chances for survival, he founded Provident Hospital, a twelve-bed facility which accepted patients of all races, augmenting his meager funds by organizing donations of linen, beds, cleaning supplies, and kitchenware. Fundraisers, including abolitionist Frederick Douglass, provided the money for medical instruments and drugs.

Williams took a personal interest in his community hospital by working lengthy stints and ended his day by disinfecting floors and instruments. He evolved high standards for employees, including his nurse's training program, which accepted only qualified applicants. By maintaining strict standards and because of his skills as a surgeon, he achieved a better mortality ratio than other hospitals. Because of his reputation, patients from surrounding states requested his services.

In 1893, under the supervision of six associates, Williams saved a stockyard laborer suffering from a knife wound to the pericardium by administering only local anesthesia, cleansing with a saline solution, and performing open-chest surgery, a dramatic departure from standard protocol. The success of the procedure rated headlines in the *Chicago Daily Inter-Ocean*, although many people doubted that a African-American doctor could evolve such an innovation.

From this major breakthrough came offers of positions at other institutions. He chose to serve as chief surgeon of Washington's Freedmen's Hospital, revamping its surgical program with the same antiseptic controls and nurse's training he had instituted at Provident. To modernize Freemen's further, he staffed the hospital with qualified specialists and created departments for each specialty. So successful were his innovations that he held training sessions at Howard University.

After a shift in the political climate reduced Williams's effectiveness, he opted to return to Chicago. Having married teacher Alice Johnson Williams, he settled in as staff associate of Mercy and St. Luke's hospitals, taking time to serve as the first African-American member of the Illinois board of health in 1889 and again in 1891 and as surgeon for the City Railway Company, a rare opportunity for a African-American man. He also helped organize the National Medical Association for Black Doctors and taught at Meharry Medical College and Howard University.

Williams received an LL.D. degree from Wilberforce University in 1908 and was named a fellow of the American College of Surgeons and a member of the Chicago Surgical Society. Always interested in the training of African-American medical professionals, he immersed himself in the work of the NAACP as well as in the creation of schools that gave African-Americans an opportunity to develop medical skills. He retired from medicine in 1920. After his wife's death, he attended a few private patients, gardened and swam in his spare time. Already a victim of diabetes, he suffered a paralyzing stroke in 1925 and died at his summer home in Idlewild, Michigan, on August 4, 1931.

Wilms' tumor

Wilms' tumor is a cancerous tumor of the kidney that usually occurs in young children.

When an unborn baby is developing, the kidneys are formed from primitive cells. Over time, these primitive cells become more specialized. The cells mature and organize into the normal kidney structures. Sometimes, clumps of these cells remain in their original, primitive form. If these cells begin to multiply after birth, they may ultimately form a large mass of abnormal cells. This is known as a Wilms' tumor.

Wilms' tumor is a type of malignant tumor. This means that it is made up of cells that are significantly immature and abnormal. These cells are also capable of invading nearby structures within the kidney and traveling out of the kidney into other structures. Malignant cells can even travel through the body to invade other organ systems, most commonly the lungs and brain. These features of Wilms' tumor make it a type of cancer that, without treatment, would eventually cause **death**. However, advances in medicine during the last 20 years have made Wilms' tumor a very treatable form of cancer.

Wilms' tumor occurs almost exclusively in young children. The average patient is about three years old. Females are only slightly more likely than males to develop Wilms' tumors. Wilms' tumors are found more commonly in patients with other types of **birth defects**. These defects include:

- Absence of the colored part (the iris) of the eye (aniridia)
- Enlargement of one arm, one leg, or half of the face (hemihypertrophy)
- Certain birth defects of the urinary system or genitals
- Certain genetic syndromes (WAGR syndrome, Denys-Drash syndrome, and Beckwith-Wiedemann syndrome).

The cause of Wilms' tumor is not totally understood. Because 15% of all patients with this type of tumor have other genetic defects, it seems clear that at least some cases of Wilms' tumor may be due to a genetic defect. It appears that the tendency to develop a Wilms' tumor can run in families. In fact, about 1-2% of all children with a Wilms' tumor have family members who have also had a Wilms' tumor.

Some patients with Wilms' tumor experience abdominal **pain**, nausea, vomiting, high blood pressure, or blood in the urine. However, the parents of many children with this type of tumor are the first to notice a firm, rounded mass in their child's abdomen. This discovery is often made while bathing or dressing the child, and frequently occurs before any other symptoms appear. Rarely, a Wilms' tumor is diagnosed after there has been bleeding into the tumor, resulting in sudden swelling of the abdomen and a low red blood cell count (anemia).

Initial diagnosis of Wilms' tumor is made by looking at the tumor using various imaging techniques. Ultrasound and

computed tomography scans (CT scans) are helpful in diagnosing Wilms' tumor. Intravenous pyelography, where a dye injected into a vein helps show the structures of the kidney, can also be used in diagnosing this type of tumor. Final diagnosis, however, depends on obtaining a tissue sample from the mass (biopsy), and examining it under a microscope in order to verify that it has the characteristics of a Wilms' tumor. This biopsy is usually done during surgery to remove or decrease the size of the tumor. Other studies (**chest x rays**, CT scan of the lungs, bone marrow biopsy) may also be done in order to see if the tumor has spread to other locations.

Treatment for Wilms' tumor almost always begins with surgery to remove or decrease the size of the kidney tumor. Except in patients who have tumors in both kidneys, this surgery usually will require complete removal of the affected kidney. During surgery, the surrounding lymph nodes, the area around the kidneys, and the entire abdomen will also be examined. Additional biopsies of these areas may be done to see if the cancer has spread. The next steps of treatment depend on whether/where the cancer has spread. Samples of the tumor are also examined under a microscope to determine particular characteristics of the cells making up the tumor.

Information about the tumor cell type and the spread of the tumor is used to decide the best kind of treatment for a particular patient. Treatment is usually a combination of surgery, medications used to kill cancer cells (**chemotherapy**), and x rays or other high energy rays used to kill cancer cells (**radiation therapy**).

The prognosis for patients with Wilms' tumor is quite good, compared to the prognosis for most types of cancer. The patients who have the best prognosis are usually those who have a small-sized tumor, a "favorable" cell type, are young (especially under two years old), and have an early stage of cancer that has not spread. The average two-year survival rate for children with Wilms' tumor is 92%.

There are no known ways to prevent a Wilms' tumor, although it is important that children with birth defects associated with Wilms' tumor be carefully monitored.

Witchcraft and medicine

The origins of medicine are closely linked to the supernatural. The primitive view of medicine had more to do with magic than with what is considered medicine today. Witchcraft, or the practice of magic, could be used to inflict illness or to take it away. **Hippocrates** and later physicians tried to separate medicine from magical thinking, but the two remained connected until at least the 17th century. Until this time, physicians themselves might be just as likely to explain illness as due to supernatural influences as the common man. Their use of astrology is a case in point. In some cultures, the link between magic and medicine persists to today, and people throughout the world use divination, astrology, and other practices to diagnose and treat illness.

The practice of witchcraft is tied to the supposed ability of the witch to manipulate nature to his or her own ends. Those ends might be good or evil. Alongside the belief in magical causes and cures of disease existed a more practical side of the so-called witchcraft. Healers both in the past and present use traditional medicines which often include effective herbal and other remedies. The rituals that accompany the remedies can be supportive by providing emotional and psychological comfort to an ill person and those around him.

The modern perception that witches are associated with evil began in Europe during the medieval period (13th century). Most of the so-called witches were likely well-meaning healers such as midwives. Such people were said to practice white magic. However, there were others who used, or at least had the reputation for using, magic with bad intentions. These people were accused of practicing black magic. Although most so-called witches were harmless, their knowledge and activities drew on the primitive, pagan roots of medicine. Church authorities were suspicious. Authorities believed that witches manipulated natural events with the aid of demons. Soon, they virtually ceased to distinguish between black magic and white magic, and witch hunts claimed the lives of tens of thousands of people over the following centuries.

Witches today mostly fall into two classes: those in native cultures and people who practice a neopagan religion called Wicca. Wicca centers on a reverence for nature and the desire to harm no one; it is far removed from the medieval concept of witchcraft. The medieval concept persists to some extent through modern satanism, or the worship of evil, but it is uncommon.

See also Midwifery

Withering, William (1741-1799)

English physician

William Withering was born at Wellington, Shropshire, England on March 17, 1741; he died in Birmingham, England on October 6, 1799. Withering was the son of an **apothecary** at Wellington. He is considered to have been one of the most capable clinicians of his time. He also acquired considerable distinction as a botanist, which earned him the sobriquet "the flower of physicians." He is particularly memorable for his pioneering work in the use of digitalis. After graduating form Edinburgh Medical School in 1766, he served as physician at Stafford Infirmary from 1776 to 1775. On the death of William Small (1734 to 1775), one of the founders of the Lunar Society of Birmingham, Erasmus Darwin invited Withering to take over Small's medical practice in Birmingham. (Withering also became a member of the Lunar society, and several of its members became his patients.) Withering went on to establish a successful practice, and became physician to the General Hospital in Birmingham. In the last ten years of his life, Withering suffered a great deal from pulmonary disease. To combat his ill health, he lived in thermostatically controlled rooms, a way of life that inspired the pun "the flower of Physic is Withering."

Withering's career was marked by exceptional versatility. He described the scarlatina and scarlatina sore throat epidemics of 1771 and 1778, and in 1793 recommended a remarkably modern treatment for phthisis. His *Botanical Arrangement of all the Vegetables* (1776) is considered a masterpiece; it remained a standard work for over a century. Other endeavors embraced the fields of minerology (the mineral witherite, or barium carbonate, is named after him), climatology, chemistry (he opposed the phlogiston theory), and music (he played the flute and harpsichord); he also was a breeder of cattle and dogs. In 1776, Withering learned from an elderly woman of Shropshire that foxglove is effective in treating dropsy. In Withering's time, dropsy was considered to be a primary disease, and as he did not know the distinction between cardiac and renal dropsy, he soon began experimenting with its use in heart diseases. Although he was disappointed to find that cerebral dropsy (hydrocephalus) and ovarian (cystic) dropsy did not yield to the drug, he began recommending foxglove wherever he could. By 1783, foxglove was included in the Edinburgh Pharmacopoeia. Withering's views on foxglove were supported by Cullen, but disputed by Lettsom. In 1785, he published his *Account of the Foxglove*, in which he described the proper use of digitalis in scientifically controlled dosage for the treatment of dropsy; in it he also hinted at its possible use in heart disease, for which it is still widely prescribed. Withering also included a protest in his book against certain abuses of digitalis that were then beginning to arise. He became a Fellow of the Royal Society in 1785, and contributed five papers to that Society's *Philosophical Transactions* (three of these are concerned with minerology). When he died, Withering was buried in the old church at Edgbaston; the monument over his grave is adorned with foxglove.

WOMEN'S HEALTH

The field of women's health is concerned with health issues and aging changes relating to postpubescent females. During adolescence (ages 12-20), a young woman's health begins to involve menstrual cycles and body changes, as well as new **nutrition**al needs, susceptibility to diseases, and other concerns. The onset of adolescence may carry with it an emotional impact to health that could give rise to **eating disorders**, unprotected sex, and substance abuse. It is not uncommon for some young women to experience a drop in self-esteem due to **peer pressure**s and the biological changes they are experiencing.

In addition to the four teenage health epidemics, which are **AIDS**, drug addiction, early pregnancy, and violence, problems confronting a young woman include the abuse of tobacco, alcohol, and illicit drugs; overexposure to the sun; the establishment of poor nutritional habits; and eating disorders.

During the adulthood years (ages 20-45), a woman must integrate the roles of woman, worker, wife, and mother. Health issues now tend to reflect career and marital decisions, as well as the special health needs associated with **pregnancy** and childbirth. The multiple roles that a woman must assume leave her particularly susceptible to chronic fatigue syndrome and depression. This is also the time when women are most susceptible to immune system disorders such as lupus and **rheumatoid arthritis**. They also may be at risk for **diabetes** and other chronic conditions due to persistent lack of **exercise** and poor diet. Finally, a woman may fall victim to **domestic violence** at this time of her life. Additional health concerns for adult women include weight gain, breast cancer, **ovarian cancer**, and **skin cancer**. Unlike men, who experience no sudden cessation in testicular function, women experience an abrupt decline in estrogen levels with a concomitant change in their physical and mental health at the time when their menses stop (**menopause**). At menopause, a woman must contend with associated changes in her cardiovascular system, bones, and central nervous system, as well as with the emotional trauma associated with the menopause. In anticipating menopause, a woman may experience a sense of urgency in making life decisions, such as bearing a child or making **retirement** plans. She may also have to make decisions about undergoing **hormone replacement therapy** to treat menopausal symptoms, and about managing risks associated with estrogen deficiency such as heart disease and **osteoporosis**. Besides heart disease, diabetes, colon cancer, skin cancer, and **cataracts** and **glaucoma**, women between the ages of 45 and 65 must also be concerned with their susceptibility to breast cancer and ovarian cancer.

In the postmenopausal phase of life (ages 65 and up), a woman's health largely depends on freedom from conditions that can largely be controlled through continued good nutrition and exercise, which include heart disease, osteoporosis, and cancer. Because women statistically outlive men, many postmenopausal women experience bereavement due to the loss of their spouses. Many women become burdened by the accumulation of chronic ailments at this time, which may make them dependent upon more than one medical specialist. Ailments that postmenopausal woman frequently experience include **osteoarthritis**, loss of hearing orvision; accidental falls; **influenza** and **pneumonia**; gastrointestinal ailments; inability to adapt to heat and cold; incontinence; and thyroid problems.

See also Adolescent health; Adolescent pregnancy; Puberty; Reproductive system; Sexually transmitted diseases

WONG-STAAL, FLOSSIE (1947-)

Chinese-American Virologist

Wong is considered one of the world's top experts in viruses and a codiscoverer of the human immunodeficiency virus (HIV) that causes **AIDS**, but her interest in science did not come naturally.

Born as Yee Ching Wong in communist mainland China, she fled with her family in 1952 to Hong Kong, where she entered an all-girls Catholic school. When students there achieved good grades, they were steered into scientific studies. The young Wong had excellent marks, but initially had no plans of becoming a scientist. Against her expectations, she gradually fell in love with science. Another significant result of attending the private school was the changing of her name. The school encouraged Wong to adopt an English name. Her father, who did not speak English, chose the name Flossie from newspaper accounts of Typhoon Flossie, which had struck Hong Kong the previous week. For many years, the name was an embarrassment to her.

Even though none of Wong's female relatives had ever gone to college or university (all were housewives), her family enthusiastically supported her education and in 1965 she went to the United States to study at the University of California at Los Angeles. In 1968, Wong graduated magna cum laude with a B.A. in bacteriology, also obtaining a doctorate in molecular biology in 1972.

During postgraduate work at the university's San Diego campus in 1971–72, Wong married and added Staal to her name. The marriage eventually ended in divorce.

In 1973, Wong-Staal moved to Bethesda, Maryland, where she worked at the National Cancer Institute (NCI) with AIDS pioneer Robert Gallo, studying retroviruses—the mysterious family of viruses to which HIV belongs. Searching for a cause for the newly discovered AIDS epidemic, Gallo, Wong-Staal and other NCI colleagues identified HIV in 1983, simultaneously with a French researcher. In 1985, Wong-Stall was responsible for the first cloning of HIV. Her efforts also led to the first genetic mapping of the virus, allowing eventual development of tests that screen patients and donated blood for HIV.

In 1990, the Institute for Scientific Information declared Wong-Staal as the top woman scientist of the previous decade, and the fourth-ranked scientist under the age of 45.

That same year, Wong-Staal returned to the University of California at San Diego to continue her AIDS research. Four years later, the university created a new Center for AIDS Research, headed by Wong-Staal. There, she has worked to find both vaccines against HIV and a cure for AIDS, using the new technology of **gene therapy**.

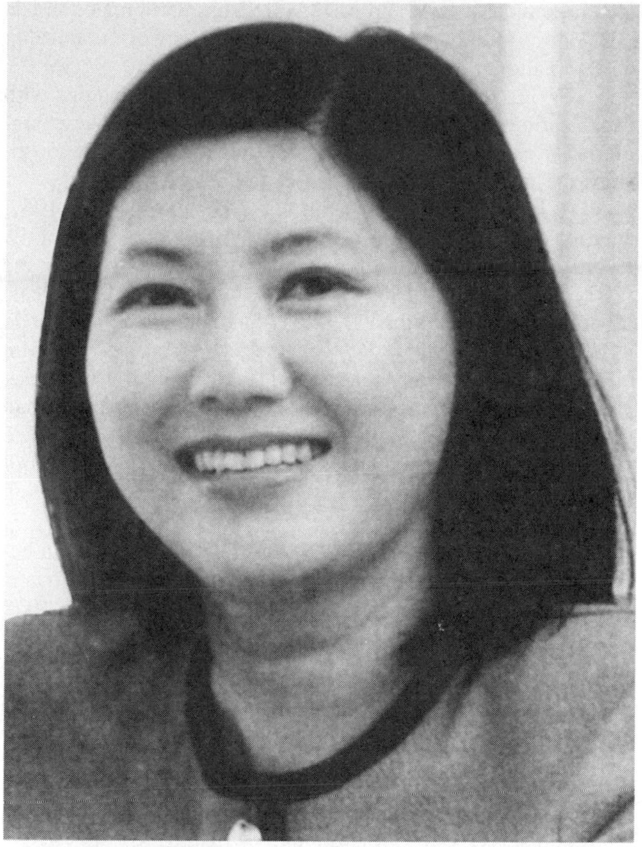
Flossie Wong-Staal

World Health Organization

A specialized agency of the United Nations, the World Health Organization (WHO) was founded on April 7, 1948. WHO is chartered to promote technical cooperation for health among nations, to carry out programs to control and eradicate disease, and to improve the quality of human life.

In 1973, the governing World Health Assembly decided that WHO should collaborate with, rather than assist, its member states in developing practical guidelines for national health care systems. As of 1999, WHO had 191 member states.

All countries that are members of the United Nations are eligible to become members of WHO. The World Health Assembly, which meets in May of each year in Geneva, determines the policies of WHO, elects the Director-General, and reviews and approves WHO's budget.

Attempts at international collaboration in the field of **public health** date back to the mid-19th century. In 1851, the First International Sanitary Conference was held in Paris with the goal of producing an international sanitary convention; unfortunately, it failed. In 1892, however, the International Sanitary Convention was adopted, but it addressed only **cholera**. The year 1902 saw the establishment of the International Sanitary Bureau, which now serves as the World Health Organization's regional office for the Americas. In 1907, the Office International d'Hygeine Publique (OIHP) was established in Paris. The League of Nations, established in 1919, set up a Health Organization to work with OIHP. The International Sanitary Convention was revised in 1926 to include provisions against **typhus** and **smallpox**. The last International Sanitary Convention was held in Paris in 1938. In 1945, the United Nations Conference on International Organization in San Francisco unanimously approved a proposal by Brazil and China to establish a new, autonomous, internal health organization, which would become the World Health Organization in 1948.

The four functions of WHO are to provide worldwide guidance in the field of health; to set global health standards; to cooperate with governments in strengthening health programs; and to develop and transfer health technology, information, and standards. WHO defines health as "a state of complete physical, mental, and social well-being and not merely the absence of disease."

WHO works closely with other organizations within the United Nations (UN). WHO has teamed up with UNICEF to promote **breast-feeding**. Together with UNICEF, UNESCO, the World Bank, and several other UN departments, WHO has participated in a program coordinating the global effort to control the spread of HIV and **AIDS**. WHO has participated in UN efforts to promote chemical safety, and it has work to develop an international food standards program.

WHO also maintains close working relationships with organizations not affiliated with the United Nations. An example is its collaboration with Rotary International to work toward the worldwide eradication of **polio**.

WHO has achieved a number of successes. In 1967, smallpox was endemic in 31 countries. Largely because of the efforts of WHO, this disease has not appeared anywhere in the world since October 1977. It has been estimated that at least 20 million people would have died of smallpox since 1977 had it not been eradicated. One of the first scourges to claim WHO's attention was the crippling and disfiguring disease, **yaws**. With the support of WHO, 46 million yaws patients had been treated in 49 countries. WHO has sought to eradicate river blindness (onchocerciasis), a parasitic disease of the tropics, by spraying the breeding sites of the disease-carrying blackflies.

WHO has set as a top priority the eradication of infectious diseases, and it counts among its achievements the lowering of child mortality from 134 per 1000 live births in 1970 to about 80 in 1995. Other accomplishments include providing health care services, reducing mortality and increasing life expectancy, delivering essential drugs, introducing environmental **sanitation** measures, and providing guidelines for healthier cities.

Specific targets for the year 2000 include the eradication of dracunculiasis, poliomyelitis, **leprosy**, neonatal **tetanus**, Chagas disease, and iodine deficiency disorders.

Wounds

A wound occurs when the integrity of any tissue is compromised (e.g. skin breaks, muscle tears, burns, or bone fractures). A wound may be caused by an act, such as a gunshot, fall, or surgical procedure; by an infectious disease; or by an underlying condition.

Types and causes of wounds are wide ranging, and health care professionals have several different ways of classifying them. They may be chronic, such as the skin ulcers caused by diabetes mellitus, or acute, such as a gunshot wound or animal bite. Wounds may also be referred to as open, in which the skin has been compromised and underlying tissues are exposed, or closed, in which the skin has not been compromised, but trauma to underlying structures has occurred (e.g. a bruised rib or cerebral contusion). Emergency personnel and first-aid workers generally place acute wounds in one of eight categories:

- Abrasions. Also called scrapes, they occur when the skin is rubbed away by friction against another rough surface (e.g. rope burns and skinned knees).
- Avulsions. Occur when an entire structure or part of it is forcibly pulled away, such as the loss of a permanent tooth or an ear lobe. Explosions, gunshots, and animal bites may cause avulsions.
- Contusions. Also called bruises, these are the result of a forceful trauma that injures an internal structure without breaking the skin. Blows to the chest, abdomen, or head with a blunt instrument (e.g. a football or a fist) can cause contusions.
- Crush wounds. Occur when a heavy object falls onto a person, splitting the skin and shattering or tearing underlying structures.
- Cuts. Slicing wounds made with a sharp instrument, leaving even edges. They may be as minimal as a paper cut or as significant as a surgical incision.
- Lacerations. Also called tears, these are separating wounds that produce ragged edges. They are produced by a tremendous force against the body, either from an internal source as in **childbirth**, or from an external source like a punch.
- Missile wounds. Also called velocity wounds, they are caused by an object entering the body at a high speed, typically a bullet.
- Punctures. Deep, narrow wounds produced by sharp objects such as nails, knives, and broken glass.

Acute wounds have a wide range of causes. Often, they are the unintentional results of motor vehicle accidents, falls, mishandling of sharp objects, or sports-related injury. Wounds may also be an intentional result of violence involving assault with weapons, including fists, knives, or guns.

The general symptoms of a wound are localized **pain** and bleeding.

Treatment of wounds involves stopping any bleeding, then cleaning and dressing the wound to prevent infection. Additional medical attention may be required if the effects of the wound have compromised the body's ability to function effectively.

Most bleeding may be stopped by direct pressure. Direct pressure is applied by placing a clean cloth or dressing over the wound and pressing the palm of the hand over the entire area. This limits local bleeding without disrupting a significant portion of the circulation. The cloth absorbs blood and allows clot formation; the clot should not be disturbed, so if blood soaks through the cloth, another cloth should be placed directly on top rather than replacing the original cloth.

If the wound is on an arm or leg that does not appear to have a broken bone, the wound should be elevated to a height above the person's heart while direct pressure is applied. Elevating the wound allows gravity to slow down the flow of blood to that area.

Once the bleeding has been stopped, cleaning and dressing the wound is important for preventing infection. Although the flowing blood flushes debris from the wound, running water should also be used to rinse away dirt. Embedded particles such as wood slivers and glass splinters, if not too deep, may be removed with a needle or pair of tweezers that has been sterilized in rubbing alcohol or in the heat of a flame. Once the wound has been cleared of foreign material and washed, it should be gently blotted dry, with care not to disturb the blood clot. An antibiotic ointment may be applied. The wound should then be covered with a clean dressing and bandaged to hold the dressing in place.

Additional medical attention is necessary in several instances. Wounds which penetrate the muscle beneath the skin should be cleaned and treated by a doctor. Such a wound may require stitches to keep it closed during healing. Some deep wounds which do not extend to the underlying muscle may only require butterfly bandages to keep them closed during healing. Wounds to the face and neck, even small ones, should always be examined and treated by a doctor to preserve sensory function and minimize scarring. Deep wounds to the hands and wrists should be examined for nerve and tendon damage. Puncture wounds may require a **tetanus** shot to prevent serious infection. Animal bites should always be examined and the possibility of **rabies** infection determined.

Wounds which develop signs of infection should also be brought to a doctor's attention. Signs of infection are swelling, redness, tenderness, throbbing pain, localized warmth, **fever**, swollen lymph glands, the presence of pus either in the wound or draining from it, and red streaks spreading away from the wound.

With even as little as one quart of blood lost, a person may lose consciousness and go into traumatic **shock**. Because this is life-threatening, emergency medical assistance should be called immediately. If the person stops breathing, artificial respiration (also called mouth-to-mouth resuscitation or rescue breathing) should be administered. In the absence of a pulse, **cardiopulmonary resuscitation (CPR)** must be performed. Once the person is breathing unassisted, the bleeding may be attended to.

Without the complication of infection, most wounds heal well with time. Depending on the depth and size of the wound, it may or may not leave a visible scar.

Wright, Louis Tompkins (1891-1952)

American physician

A brilliant medical doctor and specialist in fractures and head injuries, Louis Wright made strides in multiple directions in the field of medicine. His greatest accomplishments include his perfection of an intradermal **smallpox vaccination**, the use of Aureomycin for *lymphogranuloma venereum* (a viral venereal disease), the treatment of humans with antibiotic chlortetracycline, the invention of a brace to cushion head and neck injuries, a blade plate for the treatment of knee fractures, and drug therapy for **cancer**. The son of Dr. Ceah Ketcham and Lulu Tompkins Wright, he was born in LaGrange, Georgia, on July 23, 1891. His father died in 1895, leaving the family penniless. To support her children, Wright's mother worked as a dormitory matron.

Influenced by his stepfather, Dr. William Fletcher Penn, Wright decided to study medicine. He earned a B.A. from Clark University in Atlanta in 1911 and graduated valedictorian of his class. While studying for his M.D. from Harvard University, he worked as a field hand to earn his tuition. A staunch civil rights advocate, he interrupted class attendance to picket showings of D. W. Griffith's movie *The Birth of a Nation* and challenged and eventually defeated a rule denying African American medical students access to white patients.

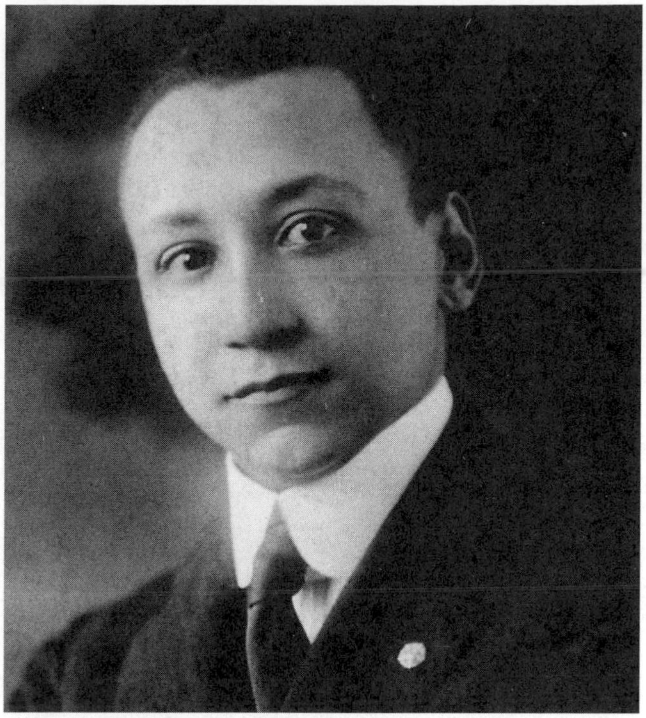

Louis Tompkins Wright

Although Wright graduated cum laude and fourth in his class, he was denied a place at any Boston hospital. After interning at Freedmen's Hospital and distinguishing himself with a research article concerning application of the Schick test to African Americans, he was licensed in three states and practiced in Atlanta before joining the U. S. Medical Corps in 1917. It was during his wartime service that he perfected the intradermal injection of smallpox vaccine to lessen side effects. Stationed in France, he became the youngest surgeon to superintend a hospital.

Shortly after marrying Corinne Cooke, Wright set up a surgical practice in New York City in 1919. The next year he joined the staff of Harlem Hospital, where he advanced from the lowest level to surgical director and began an open-door policy toward people of color. Among his other associations were surgeon for the New York police, president of Crisis Publishing Company, board member of the New York department of hospitals, and lieutenant colonel in the Medical Corps Reserves. He also served as a director of the NAACP and vigorously opposed the establishment of separate veterans' hospitals for African Americans.

In 1948, with grants from the Damon Runyon Fund and the Cancer Institute, Wright changed directions and inaugurated research on chemotherapy for cancer patients by starting the Harlem Hospital Cancer Research Foundation. His fifteen articles on the effects of teropterin, triethylene melamine, hormones, and **folic acid** on tumors detailed breakthroughs in cancer treatment. His daughter, Dr. Jane Wright Jones, joined his staff and continued his work after his death.

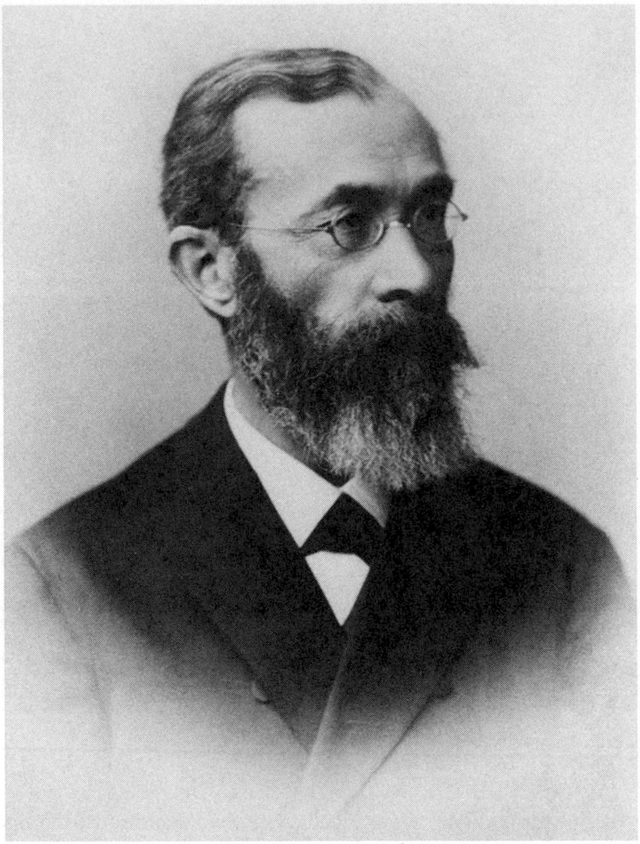

Wilhelm Wundt

Wright's awards include a purple heart for his service in World War I, the NAACP's Springarn Medal, and honors from the American College of Surgeons. He published eighty-nine articles, mainly concerning his experiments with Aureomycin and Terramycin, and with accident injuries. He also contributed a chapter to Scudder's *Treatment of Fractures*. Wright suffered a heart attack and died on October 8, 1952.

WUNDT, WILHELM (1832-1920)

German physiologist and psychologist

Wilhelm Wundt is famous for founding experimental psychology, establishing the first experimental psychology laboratory, and training several generations of important American and European psychologists.

Wundt was born on August 16, 1832, in Neckarau, Germany. He was the youngest of four children born to a Lutheran minister and his wife. As a child, Wundt was very lonely, and spent much of his time as a companion to a retarded boy. Wundt was an indifferent student who daydreamed a lot and earned poor grades. One school he attended suggested that he drop out and become a mailman. He ultimately graduated from high school, but with a poor record. He went to medical school at the University of Tübingen for a year but did not do well. After his father died, Wundt finally realized that he had to change his ways or he would not finish medical school. In an amazing turnaround, he enrolled at the medical school at Heidelberg, studied hard, received his M.D., and in 1855 received the highest scores in the state medical examinations.

After graduation, Wundt studied at the University of Berlin, and then, in 1857, he became a lecturer in physiology at the University of Heidelberg. A year later, Hermann Helmholtz, the famous physiologist and physicist, came to Heidelberg, and Wundt worked as his lab assistant. From 1858 to 1862, Wundt published his theories of sense perception, the *Beiträge zur Theorie der Sinneswahrnehmung*. Beginning in 1862, Wundt taught the first course in history about scientific psychology.

Wundt's ideas are difficult to summarize because he was involved in so many areas, because he changed his views about many subjects in his 68 years of writing, and because his writing has no single, common theme. He was interested in introspection, but he scorned the kind of introspection that involved vague, subjective thinking about thinking. Instead, Wundt focused some of his research on reaction times, the time it takes between the first impression of a stimulus on a subject's senses and the subject's perceptions based on the stimulus. Wundt was also a great systematizer, creating a set of categories into which he could place his ideas about attention, stimuli, feelings, volition, impulses, memory, judgment, causality, and creativity.

In 1871, Helmholtz stepped down as head of the physiology department at Heidelburg. He continued to write, and in 1873-1874 he published a ground-breaking two-volume book on the principles of physiological psychology, *Grundzüge der physiologischen Psychologie*. This book roughly outlined Wundt's system of psychology. In 1875, Wundt became a professor at the University of Leipzig where, in 1879, he established the first laboratory devoted to experimental psychology.

Wundt remained at Leipzig until his retirement. He worked in his laboratory, published many books, and taught hundreds of students from Europe and the United States. By the end of his career, he had directed almost 200 doctoral dissertations. He was a fine lecturer, and people from around the world came to Leipzig to study under him. Many of the most famous psychologists of the early twentieth century were his students.

Although Wundt had many distinctions, he was felt to have many faults. He was very narrow-minded and dictatorial. He told his doctoral students what they were to write on for their dissertations, and he was strongly opposed to child psychology, animal experimentation, and any practical applications of psychology. Wundt could be very scornful to psychologists who did not do things his way, and he often rejected new ideas that became very important in the history of psychology. By the end of his career, he had made his fair share of enemies, even though his psychological laboratory had many imitators and his books and lectures were much admired.

Wundt retired in 1917, but continued writing until shortly before his death in Grossbothen, Germany, on August 31,

1920. By the time he died, this daydreamer who had been told to drop out of school and become a mailman had published 53,735 pages of scholarly research.

X

X-RAY MACHINE

The very first x-ray device was discovered accidentally by the German scientist **Wilhelm Röntgen** (1845-1923) in 1895. He found that a cathode-ray tube emitted certain invisible rays that could penetrate paper and wood and, the first person in the world to see through human flesh, even saw a perfectly clear outline of the bones in his own hand. Röntgen studied these new rays—which he called x rays—for several weeks before publishing his findings in December of 1895. For his great discovery, he was given the honorary title of Doctor of Medicine and awarded the 1901 Nobel Prize for physics. Adamant his discovery was free for the benefit of humankind, Röntgen refused to patent it.

X rays are waves of *electromagnetic energy* which behave in much the same way as light rays, but at wavelengths approximately 1000 times shorter than the wavelength of light. X rays can pass uninterrupted through low-density substances such as tissue, whereas higher-density targets reflect or absorb the x rays because there is less space between the atoms for the short waves to pass through. Thus, an x-ray image shows dark areas where the rays traveled completely through the target (such as with flesh) and light areas where the rays were blocked by dense material (such as bone). Following the discovery of x rays in 1895, this scientific wonder was seized upon by sideshow entertainers who allowed patrons to view their own skeletons and gave them pictures of their own bony hands wearing silhouetted jewelry.

The most important application of the x ray, however, was in medicine, an importance recognized almost immediately after Röntgen's findings were published. Within weeks of its first demonstration, an x-ray machine was used in America to diagnose bone fractures. Thomas Alva Edison invented an x-ray fluoroscope in 1896, which was used by American physiologist Walter Cannon (1871-1945) to observe the movement of barium sulfate through the digestive system of animals and, eventually, humans. In 1913 the first x-ray tube designed specifically for medical purposes was developed by American chemist William Coolidge. X rays have since become the most reliable method for internal diagnosis.

At the same time, a new science was being founded on the principles introduced by German physicist Max von Laue (1879-1960), who theorized that crystals could be to x rays what diffraction gratings were to visible light. He conducted experiments in which the interference pattern of x rays passing through a crystal were examined; these patterns revealed a great deal about the internal structure of the crystal. William Henry Bragg and his son William Lawrence Bragg took this field even farther, developing a system of mathematics that could be used to interpret the interference patterns. This method, known as x-ray crystallography, allowed scientists to study the structures of crystals with unsurpassed precision and is an important tool for scientists, particularly those striving to synthesize chemicals. By analyzing the information within a crystal's interference pattern, enough can be learned about that substance to create it artificially in a laboratory, and in large quantities. This technique was used to isolate the molecular structures of penicillin, insulin, and DNA.

Modern medical x-ray machines are grouped into two categories: ''hard'' or ''soft'' x rays. Soft x rays, which operate at a relatively low frequency, are used to image bones and internal organs and, unless repeated excessively, cause little tissue damage. Hard x rays, very high frequencies designed to destroy molecules within specific cells thus destroying tissue, are used in radiotherapy, particularly in the treatment of cancer. The high voltage necessary to generate hard x rays is usually produced using cyclotrons or synchrotrons (variations of particle accelerators, or atom smashers).

In 1996, *Amorphous silicon x-ray detectors* were introduced which produce real-time, high resolution images by converting x-rays into light, the light into electrical signals which are interpreted by a computer, which produces digital data displayed as digital images, which can be enlarged to target a specific area. Images are filmless and instantly available, formatted for electronic storage and/or transmission. First applied to **mammography**, this technology reduces radiation, cost of film and storage, and can be used in industrial applications. Also in 1996, researchers at NASA's Marshall Space Flight Center developed the *high resolution* or *high brilliance* x ray which generates beams 100 times more intense than conventional x rays. These beams can be controlled and focused by reflecting them through tens of thousands of tiny curved capillaries, much as light is directed through fiberoptics. NASA is using this instrument to define the atomic structure of proteins for use as blueprints in designing drugs. It may also initiate smaller, less expensive, and safer x-ray sources.

A familiar use for x rays is the security scanner for examining baggage at airports, while a new application for the Advanced Photon Source (APS)—the worlds largest x-ray device valued at $800 million—is in archaeology. The University of Chicago plans to utilize the machine—designed to provide biologists, chemists, physicists, and materials scientists with information into molecular structures—to analyze ancient tools. Not only harmless to these ancient artifacts, it is 10,000,000 times more accurate than other methods of determining chemical content. Meanwhile, the timber industry hopes to save millions of dollars with new technology known as the *Glass Log Technique* developed at Monash University in Australia. This x-ray tube produces cross-section images of logs and, combined with **computerized tomography**, constructs three-dimensional images of the wood inside log, revealing its quality without having to saw the log open.

X-RAY STUDIES

X-ray crystallography is a process by which the extremely fine atomic structure of many crystals can be examined and recorded. It was first developed not as a research tool but as a means of determining the nature of x rays themselves.

X rays were discovered—quite accidentally—in 1895 by Wilhelm Röntgen (1845-1923). Although his intensive research revealed much about the properties of these new rays, such as their ability to penetrate certain substances, Röntgen could not ascertain whether x rays consisted of particles or longitudinal waves. This question puzzled scientists until 1912, when German physicist Max von Laue (1879-1960) directed an x-ray beam through a crystal. As the x ray struck the lattice-like pattern of atoms within the crystal, an interference (or diffraction) pattern was formed—an effect that could only occur if x rays were waves, like light.

Laue's experiment proved to his fellow scientists the longitudinal nature of x rays. However, it was an Australian professor, William Henry Bragg, and his son William Lawrence Bragg who realized the significance of Laue's discovery. They surmised that the structure of the crystal on a molecular level could be deduced from a study of the interference pattern. In order to prove their theory they also designed an x-ray spectrometer to measure the specific wavelengths of x rays, and devised a mathematical system for analyzing the information. In 1915 the father-son team shared the Nobel Prize for Physics for the establishment of a new scientific method, x-ray crystallography.

In crystallography, x rays are used to probe the structure of a variety of crystals. The pattern of diffracted x rays is analogous to an atomic ''shadow''—by examining where the x rays are blocked by the crystal's atoms, scientists can define the structure of those atoms. This was first seen by the Braggs, who found that crystals consist not of molecules, but rather of groups of layered ions; for example, a sodium chloride crystal is formed from sodium ions and chlorine ions. X-ray crystallography quickly became an important tool for validating many of Danish physicist Niels Bohr's (1885-1962) theories of atomic structure.

Perhaps the most important application of x-ray crystallography is its use in synthesizing substances, particularly in medicine. Many of the medicinal chemicals that have been discovered by scientists are very difficult to produce naturally in large amounts. In this case, it becomes necessary to create the chemicals in the laboratory through synthesis. However, before a chemist can synthesize a substance, a very specific map of its atomic structure must be obtained, a map that can only be drawn by using x-ray crystallography. Few scientists have been more successful at this than the British chemist Dorothy Hodgkin (1910-). During World War II, Hodgkin and her colleagues determined the structure of penicillin, whose synthesis was necessary to supply army hospitals. Since then, Hodgkin's team has worked on the crystallographic cartography of vitamin B_{12} (prescribed to prevent pernicious anemia) and insulin (used in the treatment of diabetes). Other researchers have used x-ray technologies to record the structures of proteins, hemoglobin, and the now-familiar double-helix of DNA (deoxyribonucleic acid).

The development of x-ray crystallography also created the science of mineralogy. Once they were able to examine in detail the inner structure of many minerals, mineralogists were able to define the major mineral groups. The understanding that stems from crystallography has also allowed scientists to construct the man-made minerals used in industry.

Y

YALOW, ROSALYN S. (1921-)

American biophysicist

Rosalyn S. Yalow is the co-developer of **radioimmunoassay** (RIA), an extremely sensitive isotopic method of measuring hormones and other substances in blood. Her work earned her part of the 1977 Nobel prize in physiology or medicine.

Rosalyn Sussman was born in New York, New York where her father owned a small paper and twine business. Neither of her parents had attended high school, but they encouraged her studies. Interested in mathematics from childhood, she graduated from Hunter College in 1941, the first woman to receive a degree in their recently established physics department, and was the only woman in her entering class of 400 at the University of Illinois College of Engineering, earning her Ph.D. in nuclear physics there in 1945. There, also, she met her future husband, fellow physics student Aaron Yalow.

In 1947, Yalow established the radioisotope laboratory at the Bronx (New York) Veterans Administration Hospital, where she spent her entire career. Until 1950, she also taught physics full-time at Hunter College. That year, Solomon A. Berson, a resident in internal medicine at the hospital, became interested in her work. They worked together for twenty-two years, until his untimely death in 1972 (making him ineligible to share the Nobel prize). Their first research was using isotopes to study blood volume and diagnose thyroid diseases by measuring iodine metabolism. Yalow and Berson then adapted the same method to hormones, including insulin, which was widely available. By 1959 they had perfected their method, which they called *radioimmunoassay* (RIA), so that it was sensitive enough to detect one thousand billionths of a gram of material per milliliter of blood. In the process, they discovered that hormones bind with antibodies and also that, contrary to the prevailing theory, Type II (adult onset) diabetes is caused by the body's inefficient use of insulin, not by failure to produce the hormone.

RIA rapidly became a standard laboratory technique. Medical uses include diagnosis of cancer and measurement of blood levels of hormones, **vitamins**, and other substances. It is also used in forensic work, for example, to determine narcotics and poison levels in blood.

Besides being a pioneer in her own field, Yalow is a strong supporter of women in science. Among her honors is the 1976 Albert Lasker Basic Medical Research Award, of which she was the first woman recipient.

YAWS

Yaws is a chronic illness that first affects the skin, and later the bones.

Yaws tends to strike children, particularly between the ages of two and five. It is common in areas where poverty and overcrowding interfere with good hygiene. It is most prevalent in rural areas throughout Africa, Southeast Asia, and in locations bordering the equator in the Americas.

Yaws is caused by a spiral-shaped bacterium (spirochete) called *Treponema pertenue*. This bacterium belongs to the same family as the bacterium that causes **syphilis**.

Yaws is passed among people by direct skin contact. The bacterium requires a scratch or insect bite to actually settle in and cause infection. An injury on the leg is the most common part of the body through which the bacteria enter. Young children, who are constantly bumping themselves in play, who wear little clothing, who do not wash their hands often, and who frequently put their hands in their mouths, are particularly susceptible to yaws.

The first symptom of this disease occurs three to four weeks after bacterial infection. The area where the bacteria originally entered the skin becomes a noticeable bump (papule). The papule grows larger and develops a punched-out center (ulcer), covered with a yellow crust. Adjacent lymph nodes may become swollen and tender. The first papule may take as long as six months to heal. Secondary soft, gummy growths then appear on the face, arms and legs, and buttocks. These

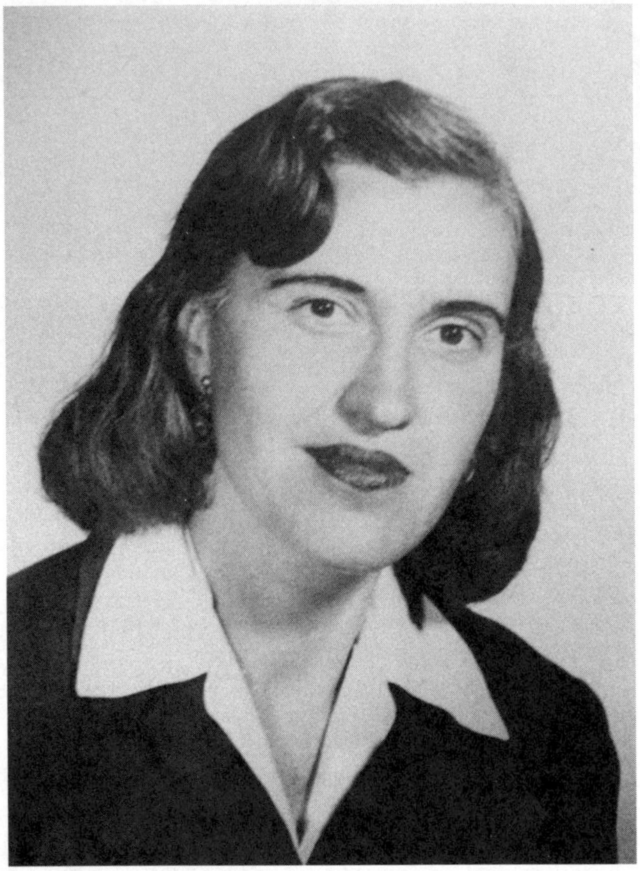

Rosalyn S. Yalow

soft, tumor-like masses may also grow on the soles of the feet, causing the patient to walk in an odd and characteristic fashion on the sides of his or her feet (nicknamed "crab yaws"). More destructive tumors may then disrupt the bones of the face, the jaw, and the lower leg. Ulcers around the nose and on the face may be very mutilating.

Samples taken from the first papules may be examined using a technique called dark-field microscopy. This often allows the spirochetes to be identified. They may also be identified in fluid withdrawn from swollen lymph nodes. Various tests can also be run on blood samples to determine if an individual is producing antibodies (special immune cells) in response to the presence of these spirochetes.

A single penicillin injection in a muscle is sufficient to completely end the disease.

Without treatment, yaws is a terribly disfiguring chronic illness. With appropriate treatment, progression of the disease can be completely halted.

The World Health Organization (WHO) has been working to totally eradicate yaws, just as **smallpox** was successfully eradicated. This has not occurred, however. WHO continues to work to identify and respond to outbreaks quickly, in an effort to at least slow the spread of yaws.

YELLOW FEVER

Yellow fever is a severe infectious disease, caused by a virus called a "flavivirus." This flavivirus has caused outbreaks of epidemic proportions throughout Africa and tropical America. The first written evidence of such an epidemic occurred in the Yucatan in 1648. Since that time, much has been learned about the interesting transmission patterns of this devastating illness.

In order to understand how yellow fever is passed, several terms need to be defined. The word "host" refers to an animal that can be infected with a particular disease. The term "vector" refers to an organism which can carry a particular disease-causing agent (such as a virus or bacteria) without actually developing the disease. The vector can then pass the virus or bacteria on to a new host.

Many of the common illnesses in the United States (including the **common cold**, many viral causes of **diarrhea**, and **influenza** or "flu") are spread via direct passage of the causative virus between human beings. Yellow fever, however, cannot be passed directly from one infected human being to another. Instead, the virus responsible for yellow fever requires an intermediate vector, a mosquito, which carries the virus from one host to another.

The hosts of yellow fever include both humans and monkeys. The cycle of yellow fever transmission occurs as follows: an infected monkey is bitten by a tree-hole breeding mosquito. This mosquito acquires the virus, and can pass the virus on to any number of other monkeys that it may bite. When a human is bitten by such a mosquito, the human may acquire the virus. In the case of South American yellow fever, the infected human may return to the city, where an urban mosquito (*Aedes aegypti*) serves as a viral vector, spreading the infection rapidly by biting humans.

Once a mosquito has passed the yellow fever virus to a human, the chance of disease developing is about 5-20%. Infection may be fought off by the host's immune system, or may be so mild that it is never identified.

In human hosts who develop the disease yellow fever, there are five distinct stages through which the infection evolves. These have been termed the periods of incubation, invasion, remission, intoxication, and convalescence.

Yellow fever's incubation period (the amount of time between the introduction of the virus into the host and the development of symptoms) is three to six days. During this time, there are generally no symptoms identifiable to the host.

The period of invasion lasts two to five days, and begins with an abrupt onset of symptoms, including **fever** and chills, intense headache and lower backache, muscle aches, nausea, and extreme exhaustion. The patient's tongue shows a characteristic white, furry coating in the center, surrounded by a swollen, reddened margin. While most other infections that cause a high fever also cause an increased heart rate, yellow fever results in an unusual finding, called Faget's sign. This is the simultaneous occurrence of a high fever with a slowed heart rate. Throughout the period of invasion, there are still live viruses circulating in the patient's blood stream. Therefore, a mosquito can bite the ill patient, acquire the virus, and continue passing it on to others.

The next phase is called the period of remission. The fever falls, and symptoms decrease in severity for several hours to several days. In some patients, this signals the end of the disease; in other patients, this proves only to be the calm before the storm.

The period of intoxication represents the most severe and potentially fatal phase of the illness. During this time, lasting three to nine days, a type of degeneration of the internal organs (specifically the kidneys, liver, and heart) occurs. This fatty degeneration results in what is considered the classic triad of yellow fever symptoms: **jaundice**, black vomit, and the dumping of protein into the urine. Jaundice causes the whites of the patient's eyes and the patient's skin to take on a distinctive yellow color. This is due to liver damage, and the accumulation of a substance called bilirubin, which is normally processed by a healthy liver. The liver damage also results in a tendency toward bleeding; the patient's vomit appears black due to the presence of blood. Protein, which is normally kept out of the urine by healthy, intact kidneys, appears in the urine due to disruption of the kidney's healthy functioning.

Patients who survive the period of intoxication enter into a relatively short period of convalescence. They recover with no long term effects related to the yellow fever infection. Further, infection with the yellow fever virus results in lifelong immunity against repeated infection with the virus.

Diagnosis of yellow fever depends on the examination of blood by various techniques in order to demonstrate either yellow fever viral antigens (the part of the virus that stimulates the patient's immune system to respond) or specific antibodies (specific cells produced by the patient's immune system which are directed against the yellow fever virus). The diagnosis can be strongly suspected when Faget's sign is present. When the classic triad of symptoms is noted yellow fever is strongly suspected.

There are no current anti-viral treatments available to combat the yellow fever virus. The only treatment of yellow fever involves attempts to relieve its symptoms. Fevers and **pain** should be relieved with **acetaminophen**, not **aspirin** or ibuprofen, both of which could increase the already-present risk of bleeding. **Dehydration** (due to fluid loss both from fever and bleeding) needs to be carefully avoided. This can be accomplished by increasing fluids. The risk of bleeding into the stomach can be decreased through the administration of **antacids** and other medications. Hemorrhage may require blood **transfusion**s. Kidney failure may require dialysis (a process that allows the work of the kidneys in clearing the blood of potentially toxic substances to be taken over by a machine, outside of the body).

Five to ten percent of all diagnosed cases of yellow fever are fatal. Jaundice occurring during a yellow fever infection is an extremely grave predictor. Twenty to fifty percent of these patients die of the infection. **Death** may occur due to massive bleeding (hemorrhage), often following a lapse into a **coma**tose state.

A very safe, very effective yellow fever vaccine exists. About 95% of vaccine recipients acquire long-term immunity to the yellow fever virus. Careful measures to decrease mosquito populations in both urban areas and jungle areas in which humans are working, along with programs to vaccinate all people living in such areas, are necessary to avoid massive yellow fever outbreaks.

YOGA

Yoga is a system that benefits the body, mind, and spirit by teaching self-control through a series of **exercises**, as well as through breathing, relaxation, and **meditation** techniques.

The goal of yoga is to help the practitioner attain his or her complete physical, emotional, mental, and spiritual potential. Yoga also attempts to restore the whole person to balance and to improve and maintain good health.

Yoga is an ancient practice that has undergone a major revival in the late 20th century, especially in the West. The recovery of seals from the Indus Valley that date to around 2000 BC, showing people in recognizable yoga positions, suggests that yoga was practiced at least that early; however, some scholars believe yoga was practiced as early as 4000 BC. Yoga did not gain much attention in the United States until the 1893 World's Fair in Chicago when the charismatic Swami Vivekananda gave a much-publicized talk at the World Parliament of Religions. Interest in yoga has increased steadily since the 1960s; by the 1990s, some aspect of yoga could be found as part of nearly all exercise and fitness regimens.

The word "yoga" derives from the Sanskrit language and means "union" or "yoke." Altogether, there are six major yogic paths or schools: these are Hatha yoga, Raja yoga, Karma yoga, Bhakti yoga, Jnana yoga, and Tantra yoga. Despite the different focus of each, all paths emphasize proper breathing techniques and meditation, and all are grounded in the belief that internal balance of mind and body is essential to good health.

The most popular form of yoga in the West in Hatha yoga, which uses a series of physical exercises, called asanas, to help the student achieve emotional and physical balance. The asanas were originally developed to help the early yogis maintain long periods of sitting meditation. And because the respiratory system links the body and the mind, breathing exercises are an essential part of doing the asanas.

Reasons for the renewed interest in yoga in the West include the following:

- Yoga is an inner-directed regimen that does not emphasize performance or competition.
- Whereas many exercise programs are based on the concept of "no pain, no gain," in yoga, pain is taken as a message to stop and try a different position.
- Yoga teaches relaxation and alertness at the same time.
- Yoga teaches concentration.

Many persons with physical, mental or emotional problems have found yoga beneficial. In 1996, the American Yoga Association identified fifteen separate conditions that that the asanas had been observed to help. They are as follows:

- **Addiction**, by flushing out toxins and stimulating the brain's pleasure-giving chemicals.
- Anxiety, by reducing the severity of panic attacks.

- Arthritis, by reducing stiffness and pain and maintaining joint mobility.
- Asthma and breathing disorders, by strengthening respiratory muscles and capacity.
- Back and neck problems, by healing, preventing injury, and improving flexibility.
- **Chronic fatigue syndrome**, by restoring energy to the body.
- Depression, by counteracting feelings of lethargy and poor self-esteem.
- Diabetes, by complementing needed lifestyle changes and improving circulation.
- **Headaches**, by relieving tension and migraine headaches by relaxation and stress-management techniques.
- Heart disease, by improving the circulatory system by stretching muscles, nerves, and blood vessels.
- **Infertility**, by improving the health of the reproductive system by relaxation.
- **Insomnia**, by improving sleep by bringing balance to life.
- **Pain management**, by reducing pain and serving as a distraction from it.
- **Premenstrual syndrome** and **menopause**, by reducing the discomfort of hormonal changes and toning the glandular system.
- Weight management, by toning muscles and improving concentration, willpower, and self-esteem.

Yoga should be considered as complementary to, rather than as a substitution for, medical treatment. Although most yoga exercise is safe for nearly everyone, certain positions should not be done by individuals with special physical problems. Those with health or fitness concerns should consult a qualified health practitioner before taking up the practice of yoga.

Z

ZINKERNAGEL, ROLF M. (1944-)

Swiss immunologist and virologist

Rolf M. Zinkernagel was born on January 6, 1944, in Basel, Switzerland. In 1962, he attended the University of Basel, deciding to study medicine rather than chemistry—his other great interest—because the former profession offered the possibility of clinical or private practice as well as research. He passed his final boards in 1968 and in 1970, the university accepted his M.D. dissertation.

In 1969, Zinkernagel's work in the surgery department of a hospital in Basel failed to spark his interest. He began looking around for other possible career paths. From 1970 to 1973 he worked as a postdoctoral fellow at the University of Lausanne, Switzerland, in a laboratory studying the process by which the **immune system** kills virus-infected cells. Zinkernagel's project, trying to monitor the destruction of bacterial cells preloaded with radioactive chromium-51, was frustrating because the method never worked properly on the bacteria—but it gave him experience with a number of experimental techniques that were to prove crucial for his Nobel-winning research.

In 1972, Robert Blanden of the John Curtin School of Medical Research, Canberra, Australia, came to the Swiss university to teach a **World Health Organization** course on immunology. Intrigued by the course and encouraged by senior researchers at Lausanne, Zinkernagel applied for a fellowship with Blanden at the Curtin school. Thanks to a two-year Swiss Foundation for Biomedical Fellowships grant, Zinkernagel and his young family moved to Australia in 1973. While at the Curtin school, Zinkernagel earned a Ph.D. in immunology, finishing his dissertation in 1975.

A fortuitous accident led Zinkernagel to team up with another young postdoctoral fellow at the Curtin school, **Peter Doherty**. While the Blanden laboratory was cramped for space, Doherty had room in his assigned lab. Thanks in part to their shared love of operatic music—and Zinkernagel's penchant for singing it aloud while working—Zinkernagel began to work with Doherty on how white blood cells called killer T cells identify virus-infected host cells to attack. ''He was tolerable, but loud,'' according to Doherty.

At the time, immunologists were very interested in a group of genes collectively called the major histocompatibility complex, or MHC. These genes, clustered together in the DNA sequence, encode a series of proteins called the MHC antigens, which determine whether a transplanted organ will be accepted or rejected by a recipient. If the MHC genes of the donor and the recipient match, the organ survives; if they do not, the organ is attacked by the recipient's immune system and dies.

A number of researchers had guessed that the rejection of MHC-mismatched organs was essentially the same process as the killing of virus-infected cells by killer T cells. Zinkernagel and Doherty demonstrated that this was true, and that the MHC antigens were necessary for killer T cells to tell friend from foe. But when they investigated further, they found something very unexpected; most immunologists had expected that when virus-infected cells and killer cells were poorly MHC matched, the immune cells' killing response would be strongest, much as in badly matched transplants. But the opposite was true. In order to get proper T-cell killing of the virus-infected cells, Zinkernagel and Doherty discovered, the cells' MHC regions had to match.

The two had discovered that T cells—indeed, the immune response in general—can only recognize viral proteins when they are displayed in the context of properly matched MHC antigens. The immune system, which had evolved to recognize ''self'' from ''other'' did not react most strongly to ''other,'' but to a third state, ''altered self.'' This discovery finally put transplant rejection into biological context. The body does not purposely reject mismatched organs because they are different, it rejects them because it mistakenly identifies the mismatched MHC antigens as ''self'' antigens that have been altered by interaction with viral proteins. The finding also opened the way to better methods for heading off transplant rejection, for creating vaccines, and for further unraveling the workings of immunity as well as understanding vulnerability to certain infections and autoimmune disease, where the body mistakenly attacks its own tissues.

Zinkernagel's and Doherty's work together took place in a fairly short amount of time between 1973 and 1974. By 1976, both were moving on, with Zinkernagel going to the Scripps Clinic Research Institute in La Jolla, California, as an associate—a rank roughly equal to an assistant professor at a university. There he studied whether or not the thymus gland—long known to play a role in the "maturation" of infection-fighting white blood cells—used MHC antigens to select which white blood cells would mature and which would die before being released to the bloodstream. The work once again proved seminal, providing the first evidence that the thymus only allows killer cells that react against slightly altered self MHC antigens to survive. This helped explain how and why killer T cells recognize altered-self antigens most strongly. The thymus prevents autoimmune disease by killing off killer cells that would otherwise attack healthy tissues and prevents a too-weak immune response by destroying those that would fail to attack any but the most profoundly changed self antigens.

Zinkernagel became a member—the equivalent of a full professor—at Scripps in 1979. But later that year he returned to Switzerland to take an associate professorship at the University of Zurich, followed by a full professorship in 1988. During that period, his work with Doherty began to receive growing international recognition, with an Ehrlich Prize in Germany in 1983 and a Gairdner Foundation International Award in Canada in 1986. In 1992 Zinkernagel was named head of the Institute of Experimental Immunology in Zurich and also received the Christoforo Colombo Award in Italy, to be followed by an Albert Lasker Medical Research Award—often a prelude to a Nobel—in 1995.

In 1996, Zinkernagel joined the ranks of the Nobel laureates because of his relatively early work with Doherty defining the system by which the immune system identifies friend and foe. His work since then has built upon this discovery, revealing how the thymus gland selects only white blood cells that react properly to virus-infected cells and investigating the complex interplay by which viruses and their hosts co-evolve.

ZINSSER, HANS (1878-1940)

American bacteriologist and immunologist

Hans Zinsser was the youngest son of a German immigrant who owned a chemical products company in New York, New York. After a privileged childhood including private schooling, study abroad, and European travel, Zinsser attended Columbia College where his poetic imagination flourished along with his scientific curiosity. When it came time for him to decide on a profession, he chose science and earned an M.D. and M.A. from the College of Physicians and Surgeons of Columbia University in 1903. He became a professor of bacteriology and immunology at Stanford University in 1911, moved to Columbia in 1913, and then to Harvard Medical School in 1923.

Zinsser's interest in the epidemiology of infectious diseases led him to join the American Red Cross Sanitary Commission on its mission to Serbia in 1915 where a **typhus** epidemic had broken out. His investigations of typhus also took him to the Soviet Union in 1923, Mexico in 1931, and China in 1938, studying a group of organisms called Rickettsia—the cause of typhus—which are carried by a louse or a rat flea and transmitted to humans by a bite from the parasites. The diseases spread rapidly in areas of poor sanitation and overcrowding. If left untreated, typhus (from a Greek word meaning cloudy or misty, referring to the altered mental state the disease causes) can result in death in 9-18 days. Zinsser wrote about his research in a lively yet scientifically accurate book which he referred to as a "biography of the life history of typhus." The book, *Rats, Lice and History*, was published in 1935 and dedicated to Charles Nicolle (1866-1936), the French bacteriologist who won the 1928 Nobel Prize in physiology or medicine for his work on the transmission by body lice of typhus fever from rats to humans. Zinsser's research on typhus proved that there actually are three types of this disease caused by two distinct agents—one carried by lice and the other by rodents. After studying cases in New York and Boston, Massachusetts, Zinsser noted that sporadic typhus, or Brill's disease (named after Dr. Nathan Brill [1860-1925] of New York City who found the disease among immigrants in New York and first described it in 1898), seemed to occur primarily in immigrants from the Soviet Union, and that cases of this disease were mild. Therefore, he hypothesized that these cases were recrudescent or reactivated typhus contracted abroad rather than new infections. The causative organism was found to be *R. prowazekii*, the same louse-borne organism that causes the more severe epidemic typhus. Endemic, or murine (rodent-associated) typhus, caused by *R. typhi*, (formerly known as *R. mooseri* and named for Hermann Mooser) is transmitted by the rat flea. Symptoms are milder than those of epidemic typhus.

In the search for an immunization against typhus, Zinsser and M. Ruiz Castañeda in 1932 discovered antibodies in the blood serum of typhus patients. The scientists knew they needed large quantities of microorganisms to produce a vaccine, so they infected chick embryo yolk sac tissue with *Rickettsia.* This tissue was used to inoculate normal chick tissue which was then grown on the surface of agar in flasks. Zinsser's work led to new tissue culture methods still used today as standard laboratory procedures. The typhus vaccine developed by Zinsser and his coworkers contains dead *Rickettsia* which carry markers called antigens. These antigens spark an **immune system** reaction whether they are alive, weakened, or dead. When detected by the human immune system, a response is triggered that sends macrophages and B cells to destroy the antigens. The B cells also produce memory cells which initiate offensive attacks if the antigens are rediscovered in the blood during a future infection. Since the vaccine contains weakened or dead organisms, the person experiences a mild reaction, but does not develop typhus.

In addition to his groundbreaking work on Rickettsial diseases, Zinsser also made important contributions to the knowledge of the nature of antigen-antibody reactions, the causes of **rheumatic fever** and the measurement of virus size. Zinsser's autobiography, *As I Remember Him*, was published in 1940. He died in New York City that same year.

Sources Consulted

Acheson, E.D. "Edwin Chadwick and the W orld We Live In." *The Lancet* 336 (December 15, 1993): 1482-85.

Ackernecht, Erwin H. *A Short History of Medicine.* New York: Ronald Press, Inc., 1968.

American Academy of Orthopaedic Surgeons. *Athletic Training and Sports Medicine.* 2nd ed. Rosemont, IL: American Academy of Orthopaedic Surgeons, 1991.

American Medical Association. "Nathan Smith Davis, MD: 1817-1904." May 1, 1999 <http://www.ama-assn.org/about/1847_99.htm#davis>.

American Men & Women of Science 1998-99: A Biographical Directory of Today's Leaders in Physical, Biological, and Related Sciences. 20th Ed. 8 Vols. New York: R. R. Bowker, 1998.

Asimov, Isaac. *Asimov's Biographical Dictionary of Science and Technology.* Garden City, NY: Doubleday & Company, Inc. 1982.

Associated Press. "Study: McGwire's Supplement Does Nothing for Strength, May Cause Harm" (June 2, 1999). July 7, 1999 <http://www.intelihealth.com/IH/ihtIH?t=333&st=333&r=EMIHC000&c=227767>.

Astrand, Per-Olof. "Introduction—Man as an Athlete." In *Oxford Textbook of Sports Medicine.* 2nd ed. New York: Oxford University Press, 1998.

Baker, Robert. "Resistance to Medical Ethics Reform in the Nineteenth Century." The Centre for Bioethics Virtual Library. July 26, 1999 <http://www.med.upenn.edu/bioethic/library/papers/baker/Resistance.html>.

——, Arthur Caplan, Linda Emanuel, and Stephan R. Latham. "Crisis, Ethics, and the American Medical Association." *Journal of the American Medical Association* (July 9, 1997). July 27, 1999 <http://www.ama-assn.org/sci-pubs/journals/archive/jama/vol_278/no_2/ed71005.htm>.

Bean, William B. "William Osler: The Egerton Yorrick Davis Alias," in *Humanism in Medicine.* Springfield: Charles C. Thomas, 1973.

Bendiner, Elmer, and Jessica Bendiner. *Biographical Dictionary of Medicine.* New York: Facts on File, 1990.

Benedictine Monks of St. Augustine's Abbey, Ramsgate. *The Book of Saints.* 6th ed. London: A & C Black, 1989.

"Biography of Dr. David Satcher." Office of the U. S. Surgeon General. 1999 <http://www.surgeongeneral.gov/osg/sgbio.htm>.

Brazelton, T. Berry, M.D. *Touchpoints: The Essential Reference.* New York: Addison-Wesley Publishing Company, 1992.

Bryan, Charles S. *Osler: Inspirations from a Great Physician.* New York: Oxford University Press, 1997.

Bynum, W. F. and Roy Porter. *Companion Encyclopedia of the History of Medicine.* Vol. 2. New York: Routledge, 1993.

Campbell, G. A. "A Brief History of Inflammation." VMED 5264—General Pathology. May 9, 1999 <http://aeb.cvm.okstate.edu/vmed5264/Reference/inflamm2.htm>.

Canning, Claire D., and Siegfried M. Pueschel. "Developmental Expectations: An Overview." In *A Parent's Guide to Down Syndrome: Toward a Brighter Future,* edited by Sigfried M. Pueschel. Paul H. Brookes, 1990. Reprint, "Motor Development and Self-Help Skills Milestones." Riverbend Down Syndrome Parent Support Group (November 24, 1998). July 17, 1999 <http://www.altonweb.com/cs/downsyndrome/motormi.html>.

Caplan, Arthur. "Organ Procurement and Transplantation: Ethical and Practical Issues," vol. 2, no. 5 (September 1995). July 24, 1999 <http://www.upenn.edu/ldi/issuebrief2_5.html>.

Carr, Ian. "The Lesion." May 9, 1999 <http://www.umanitoba.ca/faculties/medicine/units/history/lesion/lesion11.html>.

The Catholic Encyclopedia. Electronic version, New Advent, Inc., 1997 <http://www.knight.org/advent/cathen/>.

Centers for Disease Control and Prevention National Center for Infectious Diseases. "Helicobacter Pylori." DBMD Disease Listing (September 1997). June 8, 1999 <http://www.cdc.gov/ncidod/dbmd/md.htm>.

——. "Helicobacter Pylori Infections." DBMD Disease Listing (January 1998). June 8, 1999 <http://www.cdc.gov/ncidod/dbmd/diseaseinfo/hpylori_t.htm>.

Centers for Disease Control and Prevention Division of Bacterial and Mycotic Diseases. "Helicobacter Pylori Infections: Frequently Asked Questions." DBMD Disease Listing (April 1999). June 8, 1999 <http://www.cdc.gov.ncidod/dbmd/diseaseinfo/hpylori_g.htm>.

Centers for Disease Control and Prevention. National Center for HIV, STD, and TB Prevention. "Can I Get HIV from Getting a Tattoo or through Body Piercing?" (November 1998). July 14, 1999 <http://www.cdc.gov/nchstp/hiv_aids/pubs/faq/faq27.htm>.

Clendening, Logan. *The Source Book of Medical History.* New York: Paul B. Hoeber, Inc., 1942.

Colliers Encyclopedia [CD-ROM], s.v. "child development," "health screening."

Concise Dictionary of Scientific Biography, s.v. "Bowman, William"; "Bretonneau, Pierre Fidele"; "Celsus, Aulus Cornelius."

Conomy, John P. "Dr. George Sumner Huntington and the Disease Bearing His Name." Huntington's Disease Society of America, Northeast Ohio Chapter Home Page. July 13, 1999 <http://www.lkwdpl.org/hdsa/conomy.htm>.

Current Biography Yearbook, 1997. New York: H. W. Wilson, 1997.

Daintith, John, Sarah Mitchell, Elizabeth Tootill, and Derek Gjertsen (editors). *Biographical Encyclopedia of Scientists.* 2nd ed. Vol. I. Bristol and Philadelphia: Institute of Physics Publishing, 1994.

de la Garza, Amanda, *American Science Leaders* [CD-ROM]. Goleta, CA: ABC-Clio, 1998.

Debus, Allen G. (editor). *World Who's Who in Science.* Chicago, IL: Marquis Who's Who, 1968.

Delaney, John J. *Dictionary of Saints.* New York: Doubleday, 1980.

Dobson, Jessie, and R. Milnes Walker. *Barbers and Barber-Surgeons of London.* Oxford: Blackwell Scientific Publications, 1979.

Doby, T. *Discoverers of Blood Circulation.* New York: Abelard-Shuman, 1963.

"Dr. James Parkinson (1755-1828)." July 13, 1999 <http://www.uic.edu/depts/mcne/founders/page0071.html>.

The Electronic Nobel Museum. The Nobel Foundation. "John Carew Eccles" (August 11, 1998). June 9, 1999 <http://www.nobel.se/laureates/medicine-1963-1-bio.html>.

——. The Nobel Foundation. "Press Release: The 1998 Nobel Prize in Physiology or Medicine" (October 12, 1998). July 14, 1999 <http://nobel.sdsc.edu/laureates/medicine-1998-press.html>.

Encyclopedia Britannica Online <http://members.eb.com/>.

Encyclopedia.com <http://www.encyclopedia.com>.

Faiver, Christopher. *The Counselor Intern's Handbook.* New York: Brooks/Cole Publishing, 1994.

"Fitness and Sports Medicine Zone: Sports Medicine Timeline." *InteliHealth—Home to Johns Hopkins Health Information: The History of Sports Medicine* (December 6, 1998). May 20, 1999 <http://www.intelihealth.com/IH/ihtIH?t=8902&c=203646&p=~br,IHW|~st,7165|~r,WSIHW000|~b,*|&d=dmtContent>.

"Flossie Wong-Staal." *Notable Asian Americans.* Gale Research, 1995. Reproduced in *Biography Resource Center.* Farmington Hills, MI: The Gale Group. August 1999. <http://www.galenet.com/servlet/BioRC>.

Freyenberger, Barbara. "Tattooing and Body Piercing: Decision Making for Teens." Iowa Health Book: Dermatology (November 1998). July 14, 1999 <http://www.vh.org/Patients/IHB/Derm/Tattoo/>.

General Assembly of South Carolina. *House Bill 3662: A Concurrent Resolution* (1998). July 14, 1999 <http://www.leginfo.state.sc.us/sessions/113/text/1133662t.html>.

Georgia Civil Justice Foundation. "Quick Facts on Medical Malpractice." July 21, 1999 <http://www.civiljustice.org/medical.htm>.

German, William McKee. *Doctors Anonymous: The Story of Laboratory Medicine.* New York: Duell, Sloan and Pearce. 1941.

Gillispie, Charles Coulston (editor). *Dictionary of Scientific Biography.* NY: Charles Scribner's Sons, 1970.

Goldman, Erik L. "AAD Takes Stand Against Body Piercing." Skin and Alergy News (January 1999). July 14, 1999 <http://patient.medscape.com/IMNG/SkinAllergyNews/1999/v.30.n01/san3001.09.01.html>.

Gordon, Richard. *Great Medical Disasters* New York: Stein and Day, 1983.

——. *An Alarming History of Famous and Difficult Patients.* New York: St. Martin's Press, 1997.

Granit, Ragnar. "Nobel Prize in Physiology or Medicine 1963: Presentation Speech by Professor R. Granit, member of the Nobel Committee for Physiology or Medicine of the Royal Caroline Institute" (1963). June 9, 1999. <http://www.nobel.se/laureates/medicine-1963-press.html>.

Haas, L. F. "Pieter Camper (1721-89)." *Journal of Neurology, Neurosurgery, and Psychiatry* 69 (1993): 844.

Hales, Dianne, and Robert E. Hales. *Caring for the Mind: The Comprehensive Guide to Mental Health.* New York: Bantam Books, 1995.

Hamlin, Christopher. "Edwin Chadwick and the Engineers, 1842-1854," *Technology and Culture* 33 (October 1992): 680-709.

Harney, David M. "Selecting Medical Malpractice Defendants." Lecttric Law Library (1993). July 21, 1999 <http://www.lectlaw.com/files/med33.htm>.

Hershenson, David B. *Community Counseling: Contemporary Theory and Practice.* Philadelphia: Allyn & Bacon, 1996.

Hussey-Gardner, Brenda. "Motor Development." *Parenting to Make a Difference* (September 1997). July 19, 1999 <http://www.parentingme.com/motordev.htm>.

Ingram, D. G. W., and C. N. L. Brooke. "History of the College: John Caius—Our Second Founder" (April 1995). April 29, 1999 <http://www.cai.cam.ac.uk/caius/history/#Caius>.

Ivory, Phil. "The Legacy of Guillaume Duchenne." *Quest,* vol. 5, no. 5 (October 1998). July 13, 1999 <http://www.mdausa.org/publications/Quest/q55duchenne.html>.

Jerome, Saint. "Letter LXXVII to Oceanus." Christian Classics Ethereal Library (August 14, 1996). <http://ccel.wheaton.edu/fathers/NPNF2-06/letters/letter77.htm>.

Karolinska Institute. "Press Release October 12, 1998: The Nobel Assembly at the Karolinska Institute has today decided to award the 1998 Nobel Prize in Physiology or Medicine jointly to Robert F Furchgott, Louis J Ignarro, and Ferid Murad for their discoveries concerning 'nitric oxide as a signalling molecule in the cardiovascular system.'" July 14, 1999 <http://www.nobel.se/announcement-98/medicine98.html>

Kirsch, J.P. "St. Fabiola." *The Catholic Encylcopedia.* NY: The Encyclopedia Press, 1913. Electronic version, New Advent, Inc., 1997. June 9, 1999 <http://www.csn.net/advent/cathen/05743a.htm>.

Knight, James A. "The Relevance of Osler for Today's Humanity-Oriented Medical Student." In *Humanism in Medicine.* Springfield: Charles C. Thomas, 1973.

Koenig, Harold G. *Is Religion Good for Your Health?* New York: Haworth Press, 1997.

Kraut, Alan M. *Silent Travelers: Germs, Genes, and the "Immigrant Menace."* New York: BasicBooks, 1994.

Kunz, Jeffrey R. M., M.D., and Asher J. Finkel, M.D. *The American Medical Association Family Medical Guide.* New York: Random House, 1997.

Larkin, Marilyn. "Tattoos and Permanent Makeup." U.S. Food and Drug Administration (October 1993). July 14, 1999 <http://www.vm.cfsan.fda.gov/~dms/cos-204.html>.

Lasker Foundation Living Library. "Award Citation: Robert Furchgott" (1998). July 14, 1999 <http://www.laskerfoundation.org/library/furchgott/citation1.html>.

——. "Award Citation: Ferid Murad" (1998). July 14, 1999 <http://www.laskerfoundation.org/library/murad/citation1.html>.

Leache, Penelope. *Your Baby & Child: From Birth to Age Five.* New York: Alfred A. Knopf, 1988.

Lindahl, Sten. "Presentation Speech—1998 Nobel Prize in Medicine." The Electronic Nobel Museum. The Nobel Foundation (December 14, 1998). July 14, 1999 <http://www.nobel.se/festivities/98/speeches/medicine-presentation.html>.

Link, Eugene Perry. *The Social Ideas of American Physicians (1776-1976).* Selinsgrove: Susquehanna University Press, 1992.

Lukas, Susan. *Where to Start and What to Ask.* New York: W. W. Norton & Co., 1993.

Lyons, Albert S., and R. Joseph Petrucelli. *Medicine: An Illustrated History.* New York: Harry N. Abrams, Inc., 1978.

Magill, Frank N. (editor). *The Great Scientists.* Danbury: Grolier Educational Corp., 1989.

Malloch, Archibald. Introduction to *A Boke or Counseill against the Disease called the SWEATE,* by John Caius. 1552. Reprint, New York: Scholars' Facsimiles & Reprints, 1937.

Malone, Patrick S., Torsten B. Neilands, and Robert L. Helmreich. "Conformity Behavior Shows a Curvilinear Effect of Cognitive Load" (1995). June 8, 1999 <http://uts.cc.utexas.edu/~neilands/psych/research/conformity>.

Marcus, Rachel. "Just Say NO." *Challenge* (spring 1997). July 14, 1999 <http://www.research.ucla.edu/chal/25.htm>.

Maulitz, Russell C. "The Pathological Tradition." *Companion Encyclopedia of the History of Medicine,* edited by W. F. Bynum and Roy Porter. New York: Routledge, 1993.

Mayo Clinic Health Oasis. "Body Piercing: It's More Than Skin Deep" (March 24, 1997). July 14, 1999 <http://www.mayohealth.org/mayo/9703/htm/pierce.htm>.

——. "You Get Under My Skin" (May 29, 1996). July 14, 1999 <http://www.mayohealth.org/mayo/9605/htm/tattoos.htm>.

Mazur, James E. *Learning and Behavior.* 4th ed. Upper Saddle River, NJ: Prentice Hall, 1998.

McFarland, Edward G. "Sports Enhancers: The Good, the Questionable, and the Dangerous." *InteliHealth* (July 15, 1998). May 20, 1999 <http://www.intelihealth.com/IH/ihtIH?d=dmtContent&c=191998&p=~br,IHW|~st,408|~r,WSIHW000|~b,*|>.

McGee, Glenn. "Ethical Issues in Genetics in the Next 100 Years." The Center for Bioethics Virtual Library. July 26, 1999 <http://www.med.upenn.edu/bioethics/library/papers/glenn/100years.html>.

McIntyre, Neil. "Osler and Medical Education." In *Oslerian Anniversary: Incorporating the Fitzpatrick Lecture for 1975.* London: The Osler Club of London, 1976.

McMinn, R. M. H., and R. T. Hutchings. *The Color Atlas of Human Anatomy.* 2nd ed. Chicago: Year Book Medical Publishers, 1988.

"Medical Malpractice." Court TV Legal Cafe (1997). July 21, 1999 <http://www.courttv.com/legalcafe/health/misdiag/misdiag_background.html>.

Meldrum, Marcia. "Sir John Carew Eccles." In *Nobel Laureates in Medicine or Physiology: A Biographical Dictionary,* edited by Daniel M. Fox, Marcia Meldrum, and Ira Rezak. NY: Garland Publishing, 1990.

Miller, Benjamin Frank, and Claire Brackman Keane. *Miller-Keane Encyclopedia & Dictionary of Medicine, Nursing & Allied Health.* 6th ed. Philadelphia: Saunders, 1997.

Mitka, Mike. "1998 Nobel Prize Winners Are Announced: Three Discoverers of Nitric Oxide Activity." *The Journal of the American Medical Association* (November 18, 1998). July 14, 1999 <http://www.ama-assn.org/sci-pubs/journals/archive/jama/vol_280/no_19/jmn80155.htm>.

Moeller, Dade W. *Environmental Health.* Cambridge, MA: Harvard University Press, 1992.

National Institute of Environmental Health Sciences. "Environmental Health Questions and Answers: Tattoo" (April 1999). July 14, 1999 <http://www.niehs.nih.gov/external/faq/tatoo.htm>.

National Institutes of Health Office of Alternative Medicine. "Fields of Practice: Mind/Body Control, Prayer and Mental Healing." *InteliHealth* (June 17, 1998). June 8, 1999 <http://www.intelihealth.com/IH/ihtIH?t=8513&c=190009&p=~br,IHC|~st,9273|~r,EMIHC000|~b,*|&d=dmtContent>.

National Museum of Health and Medicine. 1999 <http://natmedmuse.afip.org/home.html>

The National Organ and Tissue Donation Initiative. "Frequently Asked Questions." July 24, 1999 <http://www.organdonor.gov/faq.html>.

Newman, C. E. "Osler as a Physician." *Oslerian Anniversary: Incorporating the Fitzpatrick Lecture for 1975.* London: The Osler Club of London, 1976.

Nottridge, Rhoda. *Care for Your Body.* New York: Crestwood House, 1993.

Nuttall, Paul. "Infant Development." National Network for Child Care (July 1995). July 19, 1999 <http://www.nncc.org/Child.Dev/infant.dev.html>.

Oriel, J. D. "Eminent Venereologists 5: Carl Credé." *Genitourinary Medicine* 67 (1991): 67-69.

Parry, Melanie (editor). *Chambers Biographical Dictionary.* 6th ed. New York: Larousse Kingfisher Chambers, 1997.

Penfield, Wilder. "Osler's Voice." *Humanism in Medicine.* Springfield, IL: Charles C. Thomas, 1973.

Porter, Dorothy. "Public Health." In *Companion Encyclopedia of the History of Medicine,* edited by W. F. Bynum and Roy Porter. London: Routledge, 1993.

Porter, Roy. "Religion and Medicine." In *Companion Encyclopedia of the History of Medicine,* edited by W. F. Bynum and Roy Porter. Vol. 2. New York: Routledge. 1993.

—— (editor). *The Cambridge Illustrated History of Medicine.* New York: Cambridge University Press, 1996.

——. *The Greatest Benefit to Mankind.* New York: Norton, 1997.

Renstrom, Per A. F. H. "An Introduction to Chronic Overuse Injuries." In *Oxford Textbook of Sports Medicine,* 2nd ed., edited by Mark Harries, et al. New York: Oxford University Press, 1998.

Robak, Warren. "UCLA Pharmacologist Wins Nobel Prize in Medicine for Work on Nitric Oxide as an Important Signaling Chemical" (October 12, 1998). July 14, 1999 <http://www.uclanews.ucla.edu/docs/wr457.html>.

Robb-Smith, A. H. T. "Osler's Sense of Humour." In *Oslerian Anniversary: Incorporating the Fitzpatrick Lecture for 1975.* London: The Osler Club of London, 1976.

The Royal College of Surgeons of England. "History of the Royal College of Surgeons of England" (June 18, 1999). May 17, 1999 <http://www.rcseng.ac.uk/public/collmed/history.htm>.

Rubsamen, David S. "Medical Malpractice Case of the Month: An 'Epidemic' of Medical Malpractice?: A Commentary on the Harvard Medical Practice Study" (October 1998). July 21, 1999 <http://www.hookman.com/mp9810.htm>.

Sarafino, Edward P. *Health Psychology: Biopsychosocial Interactions.* 2nd. ed. Toronto: John Wiley & Sons, 1994.

Savage-Smith, Emile. "Europe and Islam." In *Western Medicine: An Illustrated History,* edited by Irvine Louden. New York: Oxford University Press, 1997.

The School of Medicine of the University of California, San Diego. "UCSD School of Medicine Catalog—Faculty

Profiles: Dr. Flossie Wong-Staal" (March 1999). July 14, 1999 <http://cybermed.ucsd.edu/Catalog/Profiles/wong.html>.

Stanish, William D. "Introduction—Acute Sports Injuries." In *Oxford Textbook of Sports Medicine,* 2nd ed., edited by Mark Harries, et al. New York: Oxford University Press, 1998.

Sussman, Carole. "Flossie Wong-Staal, Ph.D." Center for AIDS Research (November 1998). July 14, 1999 <http://hsrd.ucsd.edu/CFAR/FWS_Homepage/FWS.HTML>.

Talbott, John H. *A Biographical History of Medicine: Excerpts and Essays on the Men and Their Work.* New York: Grune & Stratton, 1970.

Taylor, Robert B. (editor). *Family Medicine: Principals and Practice.* 5th ed. New York: Springer, 1997.

Ten Doesschate, G. Introduction to *Optical Dissertation on Vision,* by Pieter Camper. 1746. Reprint, Nieuwkoop: B. De Graaf, 1962.

The University of Texas Houston Health Sciences Center. "Biosketch: 1998 Nobel Prize in Physiology or Medicine Winner, Dr. Ferid Murad" (October 1998). <http://www.uth.tmc.edu/uth_orgs/pub_affairs/news/releases/bio.html>.

———. "New Department Chairman Named to National Academy of Sciences" (May 1997). July 14, 1999 <http://www.uth.tmc.edu/uth_orgs/pub_affairs/news/releases/murad.html>.

———. "Quotes from Ferid 'Fred' Murad, M.D., Ph.D., Co-winner of the Nobel Prize in Physiology or Medicine, October 12, 1998" (May 7, 1999). July 14, 1999 <http://www.uth.tmc.edu/uth_orgs/pub_affairs/news/releases/quotes.html>.

Thomas, Clayton L. (editor). *Taber's Cyclopedic Medical Dictionary.* 17th ed. Philadelphia: F. A. Davis Company, 1993.

Thomas, Joseph. *Lippincott's Pronouncing Biographic Dictionary.* Philadelphia: J. B. Lippincott Company, 1930.

ThriveOnline: Your Health Resource. <http://www.thriveonline.com>.

Trotter, Robert T. II, Anne M. Bowen, and James M. Potter, Jr. "Network Models for HIV Outreach and Prevention Programs for Drug Users." In *Social Networks, Drug Abuse, and HIV Transmission,* edited by Richard H. Needle, et al. Rockville MD: National Institute on Drug Abuse, 1995.

United Network for Organ Sharing. "UNOS Critical Data: Milestones" (1999). July 24, 1999 <http://www.unos.org/Newsroom/critdata_milestones.htm>.

——. "UNOS Critical Data: Waiting List Snapshots" (1999). July 24, 1999 <http://www.unos.org/Newsroom/critdata_wait.htm>.

——. "UNOS—Number One Issue: The Critical Organ Shortage" (1999). July 24, 1999 <http://www.unos.org./About/NumOne_main.htm>.

——. "Top 10 Myths about Donation" (1999). July 24, 1999 <http://www.unos.org/Newsroom/myth_main.htm>.

Walsh, James J. "Mateo Realdo Colombo." *The Catholic Encyclopedia.* 1913. Electronic version, New Advent, Inc., 1998. April 29, 1999 <http://www.csn.net/advent/cathen/04125a.htm>.

Westfall, Richard S. "Colombo, Realdo." The Galileo Project (October 3, 1997). April 29, 1999 <http://es.rice.edu/ES/humsoc/Galileo/Catalog/FilesBAK1/colombo.html>.

Williams, Trevor I. (editor). *A Biographical Dictionary of Scientists.* 3rd ed. New York: Halsted Press, John Wiley & Sons, 1982.

World Health Organization. "Fact Sheet N149: Typhoid Fever" (March 1997). April 28, 1999 <http://www.who.int/inf-fs/en/fact149.html>.

Zero to Three: National Center for Infants, Toddlers, and Families. "Birth to 8 Months: Young Infants" (July 7, 1999). July 19, 1999 <http://www.zerotothree.org/birth_18.html>.

——. "8 to 18 Months: Explorers" (July 7, 1999). July 19, 1999 <http://www.zerotothree.org/8_18months.html>.

——. "18 Months to 3 Years: Toddlers and Two-Year-Olds" (July 7, 1999). July 19, 1999 <http://www.zerotothree.org/18_3years.html>.

Historical Chronology

c. 5000 B.C.
Earliest evidence found for the practice of trepanation (trephining), an operation whereby an opening is made in the skull without damage to the brain. Comparative anthropological evidence indicates that trepanation may have been used for both medical and magical purposes (exorcism), as there was no clear dividing line between medicine and magic.

c. 2700 B.C.
Emperor Shen-Nung, the second of China's three legendary rulers, establishes a variety of medical practices. According to tradition, he is the inventor of acupuncture.

c. 2600 B.C.
Emperor Huang-ti, the third of China's legendary monarchs, rules. According to tradition, he is the author *Neiching* ("Book of Medicine"), a standard Chinese text on internal diseases.

c. 2500 B.C.
Surgical operations are depicted on the tomb of the Pharaohs at Saqquarah (part of the ancient city of Memphis, southwest of Cairo).

c. 1800 B.C.
Medical practice in the Babylonian Empire is governed by the Code of Hammurabi.

c. 1550 B.C.
The Ebers papyrus (named for its discoverer, German archaeologist Georg Ebers), a written compendium of about 700 magical remedies and descriptions of folk medicine, is written in Egypt.

c. 1500 Vedic medicine in India first begins.

c. 1000 Hindu physicians exhibit broad clinical knowledge of tuberculosis. In India, the Laws of Manu view it as an unclean, incurable disease, and an impediment to marriage.

c. 700 B.C.
Athara-Veda, the famous Indian medical text, is written.

522 B.C. Democedes, Greek physician, founds a medical school at Athens.

c. 500 B.C.
Brahmanic medicine first begins in India.

430 B.C. Earliest recorded plague in Europe is an epidemic that breaks out in Athens, Greece.

c. 400 B.C.
Hippocrates (460-370 B.C.). Greek physician, provides the first detailed description of tuberculosis (called *phthusis*). He is considered the "father of medicine" and the first to treat medicine as a science.

c. 350 B.C.
Praxagoras, Greek physician, first distinguishes between veins and arteries, recognizing that these are two different kinds of vessels.

c. 350 B.C.
Aristotle (384-322 B.C.), Greek philosopher, is one of the first embryologists and is considered the founder of comparative anatomy.

c. 300 B.C.
Herophilus, Greek anatomist, establishes himself as the first careful anatomist and the first to perform dissections in public.

c. 250 B.C.
Erasistratus (c.304-c.250), Greek physician, describes the brain as being divided into a larger cerebrum and a smaller cerebellum part and discov-

ers the sinuses of the dura mater. He also first notes cirrhosis of the liver.

206 B.C. Chinese medicine is consolidated at the beginning of the Han dynasty.

c. 200 B.C. Chinese physicians base their healing methods on a number of fundamental Chinese medico-philosophical principles, including the duality of yin and yang, and qi, or life-energy

c. 160 B.C. First record is made of a woman practicing medicine in China.

91 B.C. Greek scientific medicine takes hold in Rome when the physician Asclepiades (c.130-40 B.C.) of Bythinia settles in the West. Bythinia is an important geographic connection between East and West and so is Asclepiades.

c. 1 B.C./1 A.D. Ancient Chinese medical practices described in the *Yellow Emperor's Inner Canon of Medicine*, composed in the form of a dialogue between Huang-ti and his prime minister.

30 Aulus Cornelius Celsus, Roman encyclopedist, writes his influential book *De re medicina* (*On Medicine*). This work contains good descriptions of many conditions and operations, and is probably drawn from the collections of writings of the school of Hippocrates. Rediscovered in the fifteenth century, it becomes highly influential.

c. 75 Dioscorides, Greek physician, writes the first systematic pharmacopoeia. His *De materia medica* in five volumes provides accurate botanical and pharmacological information. Preserved by the Arabs, translated into Latin, and printed in 1478, it becomes a standard botanical reference.

c. 100 Rufus of Ephesus, active during Trajan's (98-117) reign, first describes the hyaloid membrane of the crystalline lens of the eye.

c. 100 Soranus of Ephesus, Greek physician, writes *Gynaecology*, a treatise on midwifery and women's diseases. His work contains rational precepts concerning infant hygiene.

c. 120 Aretaeus of Cappadocia (c.81-138), Greek physician, describes epilepsy, tuberculosis, tetanus, diphtheria, and diabetes.

169 Claudius Galenus (129.-c.199), also known as Galen, Greek physician, becomes imperial physician, first serving Commodus, the son of Roman Emperor Marcus Aurelius (121-180). He founds experimental physiology and writes many medical texts that become authoritative for many centuries. He is regarded as one of the earliest physicians to understand the diagnostic value of the pulse.

176 Stabiae, a popular health resort for tuberculosis patients is established near Naples, Italy. It is believed that fumes from the nearby Mt. Vesuvius are beneficial for lung ulcers.

c. 280 The twelve-volume *Mei Ching* ("Book of the Pulse") is compiled in China

c. 300 Sts. Cosmas and Damian, two Syrian brother physicians, are martyred during Roman Emperor Diocletian's (245-313) final effort to suppress Christianity in the Roman Empire. They are revered as the protectors of Christian physicians.

313 Roman Emperor Constantine (274-337) issues an edict (Edict of Milan) recognizing Christianity as a legal religion.

c. 370 Basil of Caesarea (330-379) founds and organizes a large hospital at Caesarea (in Palestine).

c. 375 Oribasius (325-403), Byzantine physician and pupil of Zeno, first describes the membrana tympani of the ear and the salivary glands.

c. 400 St. Fabiola, a Christian noblewoman, founds the first nosocomium, or hospital, in the West. After establishing the first hospital in Rome, she founds a hospice for pilgrims in Porto, Italy.

c. 500 Chinese Taoist philosopher Tao Hung-ching (451-526) compiles a fundamental text of materia medica that is the basis of Chinese pharmacology for centuries.

c. 525 Aetius of Amida, physician to Byzantine Emperor Justinian I (ruled 527-565), is the first to ascribe medicinal powers to magnets.

540 First documented outbreak of bubonic plague,

c. 600 A medical school flourishes in Jandishapur, Persia, bringing together Greek, Persian, Indian, and Syrian influences.

644 Rotharus, king of Lombardy, issues an edict ordering the segregation of lepers.

c. 650 Paul of Aegina (625-690), Byzantine physician, is the first to practice obstetrics as a specialty. His seven-volume *Epitome* collects the writings of ancient authors.

c. 700 St. Benedictus Crispus, archbishop of Milan from 681 to 730, writes his *Commentarium medicinale*, an elementary practical manual in verse.

758 First hospital in Japan is founded.

785 Theophilos of Eddessa dies. Astrologer to al-Mahdi, the third Abbasid caliph, he translates Galen's writings into Syriac.

c. 825 Mesue the Elder (d. 857), also known as Ibn-Massawaih, writes a treatise entitled *Disorder of the Eye*. Ophthalmology flourishes in Islamic medicine.

c. 830 In the Byzantine Empire, Leo the Iatrophysycist, also known as Leo of Theassalonica, compiles a medical encyclopedia which contains a large section on surgery.

c. 849 Walahrfid Strabo writes his *Hortulus* ("Little Garden"), which describes a number of plants and their therapeutic properties.

c. 850 Ali Rabban al-Tabari writes *Firdaws al-hikma* ("The Paradise of Wisdom"), which provides Islamic medicine with its basic principles.

c. 850 Islamic philosopher al-Kindi writes his *De medicinarum compositarum gradibus* ("On the Dosages of Mixed Medicines"), which attempts to base dosages of medicines on mathematical measurements.

c. 850 Christian physician Sabur ibn-Sahl of Jandishapur compiles a twenty-two volume work on antidotes, a work which will dominate Islamic medicine for four centuries.

c. 875 Bertharius, the abbot of Monte Casino from 857 to 884, writes two treatises, *De innumeris remediorum utilitatibus* ("On the Uses of Many Remedies") and *De innumeris morbis* ("On Many Diseases"), describing the practices of medicine in monasteries.

896 Rhazes (c.865-c.930), as he is known in the West, namely Abu-Bakr Muhammad ibn Zakariyya al-Razi, Persian physician and alchemist, distinguishes between the specific characteristics of smallpox and measles. He is also regarded as the first to classify all substances into animal, vegetable, and mineral entities.

c. 900 First medical books written in Old English appear. *Lacnunga* and the *Leech* (Healer's) *Book of Bald* also include sections on botany.

918 Caliph al-Muqtadir founds a hospital in Baghdad and chooses Rhazes (c.865-c.930), Persian physician and alchemist, as its director.

c. 955 Jewish "Prince of Medicine," called Isaac Judaeus (Isaac the Jew) in the West, and whom the Islamic world knows as Ishaq ibbn Sulaiman al-Isra'ili, dies. Born c. 880, he writes classic works on fever and uroscopy, as well as a *Guide of the Physicians.*

c. 975 Abu Mansur al-Muwaffaq writes his *Liber fundamentorum pharamacologiae* ("Foundations of Pharmacology"), which gathers and classifies almost 600 cures.

c. 1000 The greatest Islamic surgeon Abu'l-Qasim Khalaf ibn Abbas (936-1013), whom the West knows as Albucasis, writes his famous *Al-Tasrif li-man 'ajaza al-ta'lif* ("The Recourse of Him Who Cannot Compose a Medical Work of His Own"), a compendium of medicine, including a valuable section on surgery.

c. 1010 The School of Salerno flourishes in Italy. Begun around the start the of the ninth century, it reaches its pinnacle, preserving its fame until the end of the fourteenth century. This medical school in southern Italy grants the first medical diplomas and attracts students from Europe, Asia, and northern Africa,

1021 "Dancing Mania," or St. Vitus's Dance, breaks out in Europe. Named after the chapel of St. Vitus, who, according to tradition, healed the disease, this is a convulsive, neurological condition, also called chorea, and is usually associated with rheumatic fever.

1037 The great Persian physician and philosopher Avicenna (b. 980) dies. Known in the West as Avicenna, Abi Ali al-Husayn ibn 'Abdallah ibn Sinna is known for his *Kitab al-Qanun* ("Canon"), a comprehensive, encyclopedic synthesis of the principal medical tradition. Avicenna's work becomes one of the accepted authorities for European physicians for several centuries.

1137 St. Bartholomew's Hospital is founded in London.

1140 Roger II of Sicily introduces a compulsory examination for medical doctors and grants the School of Salerno official status and his protection.

c. 1140 Bologna, Italy, starts developing as a major European medical center. In the next century, the Italian physician Taddeo Alderotti (c.1223-1295) opens a school of medicine there.

c. 1150 Ibn Zuhr, known in the West as Avenzoar (c.1090-1162), Arabian physician, flourishes in Andalusia and emphasizes the value of experience over tradition.

c. 1150 Hildegard of Bingen (1099-1179), the abbess of Rupertsberg, mystic, scientist, and musician, writes her *Liber simplicis medicinae* ("Book of Simple Medicine"), which describes the healing power of plants, minerals, and animals.

1169 Averroës, as he is known in the West, or, in the Islamic world, Abu-l-Walid Muhammad ibn Ahnad Ibn Rushd, the great Arabian philosopher and scientist primarily known for his commentaries on Aristotle, completes his *al-Kulliyat* ("The Book of

General Principles"), an influential survey of the entire field of medicine.

c. 1180 Rabbi Moshe ben Maimun (1135-1204), known in the West as Moses Maimonides, writes his *Regimen of Health*, in which the eminent Jewish philosopher, known among Arabs as Abu 'Imran ibn 'Ubdaidalla Musa ibn Maimun, offers practical advice to people with health problems.

1181 Medical school at Montpellier, France, is founded.

1224 Frederick II (1194-1250), Holy Roman Emperor, king of Sicily, and grandson of Roger II of Sicily, issues laws regulating the study of medicine. His requirement of proper examinations elevates the status of physicians. He also founds the University of Messina.

1240 Frederick II founds the University of Naples.

1241 Frederick II issues a law allowing the dissection of cadavers. The law also regulates surgery and pharmacy.

c. 1270 Syrian physician 'Ala' al-Din ibn al-Nafis correctly describes pulmonary circulation in his *Sharh Tashrih al-Qanun*, a commentary on Avicenna's anatomy.

c. 1285 Invention of spectacles (eyeglasses) is attributed to Salvino degli Armati (d. 1317). A rival claim is also made for the monk, Alessandro della Spina, around 1305. Although neither claim can be proven absolutely, there is little doubt that spectacles were invented in Venice, a city renowned for its master glass makers.

1296 Lanfranc of Milan (c.1250-1306), Italian surgeon active in Paris, is the first to describe a cerebral concussion. Also called Lanfranchi or Lanfranco, he is the first to differentiate between hypertrophy and cancer of the breast. His *Chirurgia magna* introduces into France the operating techniques of the Italian schools.

1319 First criminal prosecution for body-snatching is conducted.

1316 Italian anatomist, Mondino de Luzzi (c.1270-c.1326) publishes his first book devoted entirely to anatomy. His book remains authoritative until Andreas Vesalius publishes his anatomy text in 1543.

1333 Botanical garden is established in Venice for the cultivation of medicinal herbs.

1345 First apothecary shop opens in London.

1348 Europe is ravaged by the plague. Some physicians, namely the prominent French surgeon Guy de Chauliac (c.1300-1368), oppose the prevailing supernatural and superstitious interpretations of the disease, arguing for effective prevention. Between the fall of 1347, when the plague came to Europe, and 1350, when the epidemic had largely run its course, about one in three Europeans died of this disease.

1374 As the plague spreads, the Republic of Ragusa (now Dubrovnik, Croatia) imposes a thirty-day period of isolation on people coming from plague-stricken areas. The isolation period is eventually extended to forty days: *quarantenaria*, which is the origin of the modern term "quarantine."

1450 Nicholas Krebs of Cues (1401-1464), known as Nicholas Cusanus, German prelate, theologian, mathematician, and philosopher, suggests that the pulse and respiration be timed with a water-clock and that a patient's blood and urine be weighed.

1473 First printing of Avicenna's *Canon*, which becomes one of the most famous texts in the history of medicine.

1483 Giovanni Arcolani (d. 1484), Italian surgeon, publishes his book, *Practica*, in which he is the first to recommend the filling of teeth with gold.

1490 First Latin edition of Galen's works is published. His anatomical writings will dominate the field of medicine until Vesalius.

1500 First recorded successful Cesarean section operation is performed. Jacob Nufer, who is employed to neuter animals, performs this emergency surgical procedure on his wife, who lives to bear more children.

1500 Leonardo da Vinci (1452-1519), Italian artist and scientist, begins his serious anatomical investigations, which he continues until his death. He studies the structure of muscles and bones by dissecting cadavers. Unpublished until modern times, his findings are unknown to his contemporaries.

1507 Antonio Benivieni (c.1440-1502), Italian physician, founds pathological anatomy with his *De abditis nonullis ac mirandis morborum et sanationum causis* ("On the Causes of Some Internal and Remarkable Diseases and Recoveries"), published posthumously. In this work, he explains for the first time how dissection of cadavers can facilitate the study of internal disease and also help determine the cause of death.

1508 Guaiac wood is brought to Europe from America. Also called *lignum vitae* (wood of life), the tree has a resin, obtained by distilling its wood, that is used to treat respiratory disorders.

1513 Eucharius Rösslin publishes his *Der Swangern Frauen under Hebammen Rosengarten* ("Garden of Roses for Pregnant Women and Midwives"), which is the earliest manual for midwives.

1514 Giovanni da Vigo (1460-1525), Italian physician and surgeon to Pope Julius II, published his *Practica copiosa in arte chirurgica* ("Practice of the Art of Surgery, Fully Explained"). In his work, he endorses the excruciating practice of using hot oil and cautery on gunshot wounds.

1518 College of Physicians is established in London.

1519 Thomas Linacre's English translation of Galen's *Methodus medendi* ("Method of Healing") is published.

1521 Giacomo Berengario da Carpi (c.1460-1530), Italian surgeon, publishes his *Commentaria*, which includes the first published anatomical drawings made from nature. Berengario da Carpi completes a detailed study of the brain and is the first to discuss the action of cardiac valves. A reformer of anatomy, he is regarded as a precursor of Vesalius.

1524 First hospital in the New World is built by the Spanish conqueror Hernando Cortez (1485-1547) in Mexico.

1527 Paracelsus (1493-1541), Swiss physician and alchemist, publicly burns the writings of Galen at Basel. He rejects traditional, academic medicine as irrational, and founds iatrochemistry, or medical chemistry, declaring that the human body is somehow connected to the laws of chemistry.

1530 Girolamo Fracastoro (1478-1553), Italian physician and humanist, writes his poem called *Syphilis sive morbus gallicus* ("Syphilis or the French Disease"), which gives the definitive name to the sexually-transmitted disease that is spreading throughout Europe.

1535 Mariano Santo di Barletta (1490-1550), Italian physician, gives the first account of a median lithotomy, in which a surgeon makes an incision into the urinary bladder to remove a kidney stone.

1536 Paracelsus, Swiss physician and alchemist, publishes his great surgical treatise *Chirurgia magna*. He stresses the importance of using minerals to treat diseases, thus effectively founding chemotherapy.

1536 Ambroise Paré (1510-1590), surgeon to Henri II of France (1519-1559), performs the first exarticulation of the elbow joint. He is also the first to popularize the use of a truss for a hernia.

1543 Andreas Vesalius (1514-1564), Flemish anatomist, publishes his epoch-making *De humani corporis fabrica*, the first accurate book on human anatomy. Its illustrations are of the highest level of realism as well as artistic achievement, and the result is a masterpiece that is both a triumph of Renaissance printing and one of the greatest medical works ever written.

1545 Ambroise Paré, French surgeon, publishes his *Method of Treating Wounds*. He emphasizes cleanliness and the use of soothing ointments when treating gunshot wounds.

1546 Girolamo Fracastoro, Italian physician and humanist, writes his *De contagione et contagiosis morbis* ("On Contagion and Contagious Diseases"), which contains new ideas on the transmission of contagious diseases. This work marks the beginning of the scientific study of contagion.

1546 Giovanni Ingrassia discovers the tube between the throat and the middle ear. The discovery was later attributed to Bartolommeo Eustachio, also known as Eustachius.

1551 Gabriele Fallopia (1523-1563), also known as Fallopio, or Fallopius, succeeds Vesalius to the chair of anatomy at Padua. He describes the inner ear and the tubes that lead the human ovum from the ovary to the uterus (now called Fallopian tubes).

1553 Michael Servetus (1516-1559), Spanish physician and theologian, rediscovers pulmonary (or lesser) circulation.

1558 Matteo Realdo Colombo (1516-1559), Italian anatomist, is the first to use living animals in laboratory experiments (especially to study the function of the heart and lungs). He is also the first to describe the mediastinum (the mass of tissue and organs separating the two lungs).

1559 Matteo Realdo Colombo, Italian anatomist, publishes his *De re anatomica* ("On Anatomy") in Venice. Strongly influenced by Vesalius, this work contains Colombo's discovery of the pulmonary (lesser) circulation of the blood.

1562 Bartolomeo Eustachio (1520-1574), Italian anatomist, is appointed professor of medicine in the Collegio della Sapienza in Rome. He discovers the narrow canal connecting the ear and the throat, which becomes known as the Eustachian tube.

1563 Bartolommeo Eustachio, Italian anatomist, publishes his *Libellus de dentibus* ("Book on Teeth"), in which it is stated for the first time that the second teeth have their own dental sac, and do not originate, as Vesalius believed, from the roots of the milk teeth.

1563 Garcia da Orta (c.1500-c.1568), Portuguese botanist, compiles the first good compendium on the materia medica of East Indians, as well as the first European manual on tropical medicine.

1564 Ambroise Paré (1510-1590), The French surgeon best known for his improvements in battlefield surgery, publishes his *Dix livres de la chirurgie* ("Ten Books of Surgery"), in which he discusses some of his important surgical innovations, including the tying-off of blood vessels during amputations. He becomes known as the father of modern surgery.

1566 Guillaume Rondelet (1507-1566), French naturalist and physician, builds the first anatomy amphitheater in Rome. This facility allows the observing students to surround the instructor.

1575 Juan Huarte de San Juan (c.1530-1592), Spanish physician, publishes his *Examen de Ingenios para las Ciencias* ("The Scientific Study of the Mind"), which is considered the first modern attempt at systematically studying the functions of the brainand establishing a link between psychology and physiology.

1584 Sir Walter Raleigh (1554-1618), English explorer and writer, brings curare from Guiana. Obtained from a plant, this drug is a skeletal-muscle relaxant that can cause paralysis.

1586 Marcello Donati (c.1538-1602) of Italy gives the first description of a gastric ulcer.

1595 Andreas Libavius (1560-1616), German alchemist, publishes his *Alchymia* in Frankfurt, Germany. Many scholars regard it as the first chemical textbook. Libavius believes there is an important link between medicine and chemistry.

1597 Gasparo Tagliacozzi (1545-1599), Italian surgeon, performs rhinoplasty (plastic surgery of the nose) a procedure known to the ancient Hindus. Tagliacozzi's work is based on solid anatomical knowledge.

c. 1600 Invention of the first obstetrical forceps, credited to a member of the Chamberlen family. Designed for difficult deliveries this instrument is known to have been suggested by the Frenchman Pierre Franco in 1561, and it is believed that William Chamberlen (c.1540-1596) took the secret of its design with him when he fled to England from France in 1576. Both of his sons were named Peter, and one of them is often credited with the invention. The family kept the design of the forceps a closely guarded secret for more than a century.

1603 Hieronymus Fabricius ab Aquapendente (1537-1619), an Italian physician also known as Girolamo Fabrici, discovers the one-way valve in veins, but fails to realize its significance.

1604 Johann Kepler (1571-1630), German astronomer, publishes his book *Ad Vitellionem, paralipomena.* He describes for the first time how the retina is essential to sight. He also details the part the lens plays in refraction and establishes that myopia is caused by the convergence of luminous rays before they reach the retina. In a later work (*Dioptrica*, 1637), he compares the eye to a camera obscura.

1609 Louise Bourgeois (1563-1636), French midwife, publishes her book on obstetrics and gynecology. She attended the French aristocracy and delivered the future king, Louis XIII, whom she reportedly saved from asphyxia.

1619 Christoph Scheiner (1575-1650), German astronomer, publishes his *Oculus* ("The Eye"), in which he gives an experimental demonstration of the role of the retna, describes the eye's adjustment reflexes, and correctly explaines the function of the crystalline lens.

1621 Johannes Baptista van Helmont (1577-1635), Flemish physician and alchemist, writes his *Ortus medicinae* ("The Garden of Medicine"), in which he discusses the anatomical changes that occur in disease. Van Helmont is regarded as the founder of modern pathology.

1624 Adriaan van den Spigelius (1578-1625), Dutch anatomist, publishes the first account of malaria.

1628 William Harvey (1578-1657), English physician, publishes his *Exercitatio de motu cordis et sanguinis in animalibus* ("An Anatomical Essay Concerning the Movement of the Heart and the Blood in Animals"), in which he announces his discovery of the circulation of the blood. His arguments are based on his brilliant, clearly described experiments. It becomes a classic of science.

1628 First definite description of blood transfusion is published by Giovanni Colle (1558-1630), Italian physician, in his *Methodus facile procurandi tuta et nova medicamenta* ("A Method of Safely Administering New Medications").

1632 Marco Aurelio Severino (1580-1656), Italian surgeon, also known as Severinus, publishes his *De recondita abscessum natura* ("On Hidden Abscesses"), which is regarded as the first modern manual of surgical pathology.

1633 Stephen Bradwell publishes his *Help in Suddain Accidents*, which is the first book on first aid.

1637 René Descartes (1594-1650), French philosopher and mathematician, publishes his *Discours de la méthode.* This landmark work applies a mechanistic view to science and medicine, establishing a world view which dominates the life sciences for some time.

1640 Juan del Vigo introduces cinchona into Spain. Native to the Andes, the bark of this tree is processed to obtain quinine, used in treatment of malaria.

1642 Johan Georg Wirsung (1600-1643), German anatomist, discovers the pancreatic duct while performing a dissection in Padua.

1642 The first Western account of beriberi, a disease caused by a deficiency of vitamin B_1, is made in *De medicina Indorum* ("On Medicine in the Indies") written by the Dutch physician, J. Brontius.

1648 Jean Pecquet (1622-1674), French physician, discovers the thoracic duct and the receptaculum chyli while dissecting a dog. He announces this in his book *Experimenta nova anatomica* ("New Anatomical Research").

1648 Willem Piso (1611-1678), Dutch physician and botanist, also called Le Pois, points out the effectiveness of ipecac against dysentery in his book *De medicina brasielieni* ("On Brazilian Medicine"). He is among the first to become acquainted with tropical diseases, distinguishing between yaws and syphilis.

1648 Giovanni Alfonso Borelli (1608-1679), Italian mathematician and physiologist, publishes his *Delle cagioni delle febri maligni nella Sicilia negi anni 1647 e 1648* ("On the Causes of the Malignant Fevers in Sicily in the Years 1647 and 1648"), which contains the first full description of the iatromechanical system. Borelli explains every aspect of the body using mechanics.

1653 Olof Rudbeck (1630-1702), Swedish naturalist, discovers lymphatic vessels in a dog.

1654 Francis Glisson (1597-1677), English anatomist and physiologist, keeps excellent clinical records and is able to give an accurate description of rickets. He also breaks new ground with his study of the liver.

1656 Guerner Rolfinck (1599-1673), German physician and chemist, demonstrates that a cataract is a clouding of the lens.

1658 Johann Jakob Wepfer (1620-1695), Swiss physician, shows that stroke is caused by cerebral hemorrhage (bleeding in the brain).

1660 Using a microscope, Marcello Malpighi (1628-1699), Italian physician, discovers tiny vessels connecting the arteries and veins of the circulatory system. He calls these tiny vessels capillaries.

1662 Lorenzo Bellini (1643-1704), Italian anatomist, publishes his *Exercitatio anatomica de structura et usu renum* ("Study of the Structure and Functions of the Kidney") at age nineteen, and discovers the tubules, or excretory ducts, of the kidneys.

1664 Jan Swammerdam (1637-1680), Dutch naturalist and microscopist, discovers the valves of the lymphatics.

1664 Thomas Willis (1621-1675), English physician, writes his *Cerebri anatome* ("Anatomy of the Brain"), which gives a complete account of the nervous system. He also first describes the spinal accessory nerve. His influential book is illustrated by the famous English architect and scientist, Christopher Wren (1632-1723).

1665 Robert Hooke (1635-1703), English physicist, publishes his landmark book on microscopy called *Micrographia.* Containing some of the most beautiful drawings of microscopic observations ever made. his book leads to many discoveries in related fields.

1665 Bubonic plague in London kills 75,000 people.

1665 Marcello Malpighi (1628-1694), Italian physician, describes the brain's white matter in his *De cerebro* ("On the Brain").

1666 Jean-Baptiste Denis (1643-1704), physician to French King Louis XIV (1638-1715), first transfuses blood from an animal (lamb) to a human subject. The patient temporarily improves but then dies.

1666 Marcello Malpighi, Italian physician, provides the first description of red blood corpuscles in his *De polypo cordis* ("On the Polyps of the Heart").

1667 Walter Needham (c.1631-c.1691), French physician, publishes his important work on obstetrics. In his *Traité des maladies des femmes grosses* he is the first to refer to tubal pregnancy and to correct the ancient view that the pelvic bones separate during labor.

1668 First successful intravenous injection on a human is made by the German physician, Johann Daniel Major (1634-1693). At about the same time, another German medical doctor, Johann Sigmund Elsholtz (1623-1688), also performs a successful injection.

1669 Richard Lower (1631-1691), English physician, shows that blood takes up air in the lungs. He concludes correctly that the dark venous blood changes to bright red when it absorbs some of the air passing through the lungs.

1672 Thomas Willis, English physician, describes creeping paralysis and dementia praecox.

1673 Antoni Leeuwenhoek (1632-1723), Dutch biologist and microscopist, contacts the Royal Society of London, and they begin publishing, in the form of letters, the important discoveries he makes using his simple but powerful microscope. He makes microscopic observations of the blood and gives a precise description of red corpuscles.

1674 French physician Morel de Villiers invents the tourniquet for stopping major hemorrhages.

1680 *De motu animalium* ("On Animal Motion") by Giovanni Alfonso Borelli (1608-1679), Italian mathematician and physician, is published posthumously. He considers the body a machine whose structure and functions are entirely reducible to mechanical laws and describes the muscles and bones of the human body as a system of levers.

1683 Thomas Sydenham (1624-1684), English physician, publishes his masterful treatise on gout. He greatly influences the practice of internal medicine with his revival of the Hippocratic methods of observation and experimentation.

1684 Raymond Vieussens (1641-1715), French physician and anatomist, publishes his *Neurographia universalis*, which contains the first description of the brain's "centrum ovale" (the central white matter of the cerebellum)and sheds light on the structure of the nervous system.

1688 Johan Hofer (1669-1752) coins the word "nostalgia" to describe the somatic ailment provoked by homesickness.

1690 John Locke (1623-1704), English philosopher and physician, publishes his *Essay Concerning Humane Understanding*, which includes his empirical philosophy of medicine.

1697 Antonio Pacchioni (1665-1726), Italian anatomist, discovers the brain's dura mater, the tough outer membrane covering the brain and spinal cord.

1700 Bernardo Ramazzini (1633-1714), Italian physician, publishes the first systematic treatment of occupational illnesses. His book, *De morbis artificum* ("Diseases of Artisans"), opens a new field of modern medicine—trade diseases and industrial hygiene.

1700 Giorgio Baglivi (1668-1706), Italian anatomist, publishes his *De fibra motrice* ("On Motor Fibers"), which is based on microscopic observations. He is the first to distinguish between smooth and striated muscles.

1704 Antonio Maria Valsalva (1666-1723), Italian anatomist, introduces the terms "external," "middle," and "internal" to describe the anatomy of the ear in his *De aure humana tractatus* ("A Treatise on the Human Ear").

1708 Hermann Boerhaave (1668-1738), Dutch physician, publishes his *Institutiones medicae* ("The Institutes of Medicine"). Arguably the most eminent physician in Europe since Galen, he is known as the "Dutch Hippocrates." This textbook on physiology goes through a huge number of editions and is translated into many languages.

1723 The first modern English hospital medical school, Guy's Hospital, is founded in London by the philanthropist bookseller, Thomas Guy (1664-1724).

1732 Philadelphia Hospital is founded.

1735 Gaspar Casal (1679-1759), Spanish physician, gives the earliest description of pellagra, caused by a deficiency of niacin in the diet.

1736 Claudius Amyand (c.1680-1740), English surgeon, performs the first successful appendectomy.

1741 Emanuel Swedenborg (1688-1772), Swedish scientist, philosopher, and theologian, publishes his *Oeconomia regni animalis*. This work, which was ignored by his contemporaries, includes Swedenborg's remarkably advanced studies of the brain.

1749 Jean-Baptiste Sénag (1693-1770), French physician, begins the study of cardiology as an independent discipline within the field of medical pathology with his study titled *Traité de la structure du coeur* ("Treatise on the Structure of the Heart").

1752 René-Antoine Ferchault de Réaumur (1683-1757), French physicist and physiologist, studies the physiology of digestion and obtains digestive juice.

1753 James Lind (1716-1794), Scottish physician, first publishes his *Treatise of the Scurvy.* This vitamin-deficiency disease, which killed more sailors on long voyages than did battle with the enemy, was finally eliminated in the British Navy some years after the publication of Lind's book. Because the Navy gave their crews lime juice, British sailors were nicknamed "Limeys."

1757 Alexander Monro (1697-1767), English physician, distinguishes between the lymphatic and the circulatory systems.

1759 Kaspar Friedrich Wolff (1734-1794), German physiologist, launches modern embryology with his *Theoria generationis* ("Theory of Generation").

1761 Leopold Edler von Auenbrugger (1722-1809), Austrian physician, first describes his percussion method, which becomes a major contribution to the diagnosis and prognosis of diseases of the chest. Ever since, physicians use this thumping-on-the-chest method to diagnose the condition of a patient's chest.

1761 Giovanni Battista Morgagni (1682-1771), Italian anatomist, publishes his great *De sedibus et causis morborum* ("On the Sites and Causes of Disease"), which founds pathological anatomy. Based on 640 dissections that Morgagni had performed, this books establishes pathology as a genuine branch of modern medicine.

1764 Antoine Louis (1723-1792), French surgeon, introduces digital compression for hemorrhage,

1768 William Heberden (1710-1801), English physician, first introduces the term "angina pectoris" to describe the painful heart condition caused by an oxygen deficiency.

1768 Tuberculosis and meningitis in children are described in a posthumously published book by Robert Whytt (1714-1766), Scottish physician.

1770 William Hunter (1718-1783), English anatomist, founds a school of anatomy in London. It is here that the best British anatomist and surgeons of the period, including his brother John, are trained.

1770 First medical degree in the American colonies is conferred by King's College.

1771 John Hunter (1728-1793), English surgeon, founds scientific dentistry with his treatise *The Natural History of the Human Teeth.*

1773 Medical Society of London is founded.

1773 Human Society is founded in England. Its goals include providing first aid to survivors of suicide attempts, as well as general medical advice to the general population.

1773 First insane asylum in the American colonies is founded in Williamsburg, Virginia.

1776 William Cumberland Cruikshank (1752-1840), Scottish surgeon and chemist, discovers that severed nerves can grow back together.

1777 American general George Washington (1732-1799) orders the inoculation of the Continental Army to prevent smallpox.

1783 Harvard Medical School is established.

1784 Domenico Cotugno (1736-1822), Italian physician, discovers cerebrospinal fluid.

1785 William Withering (1741-1799), English physician, uses digitalis as a cure for dropsy (abnormal increase of fluid).

1785 John Hunter, English surgeon, discovers collateral circulation and introduces ligation in the artery for the treatment of aneurysm. Hunter is a founder of experimental and surgical pathology, as well as a pioneer in experimental morphology.

1786 Samuel Hahnemann (1755-1833), founder of modern homeopathic medicine, publishes his *Über die Arsenikvergiftung: ihre Hilfe und gerichtliche Ausmittelung* ("On Poisoning by Arsenic: Its Treatment and Forensic Detection"), in which he discusses the toxic effects of drugs.

1793 Thomas Young (1773-1829), English physician, describes the mechanism of accommodation in the eye, namely, the eye's automatic adjustment to objects viewed from different distances. He says that this is accomplished by the curvature of the lens.

1793 Philippe Pinel (1745-1826), French physician, is put in charge of an insane asylum where he begins the first systematic studies of the conditions of the inmates. Pinel believed that insanity was a disease of the mind and that those suffering from it deserved humane treatment.

1794 John Dalton (1766-1844), English chemist, first describes color-blindness. Dalton himself is colorblind.

1796 English physician Edward Jenner (1749-1823) successfully carries out the first vaccination against smallpox. He inoculates a boy, James Phipps, with cowpox to protect him from the more serious disease smallpox.

1797 William Hyde Wollaston (1766-1828), English physician and chemist, discovers uric acid in gouty joints.

1798 Thomas Malthus (1766-1828), English clergyman and economist, publishes his influential *Essay on Population*, in which he projects a number of imminent catastrophes resulting from overpopulation.

1799 Tuberculosis reaches its pinnacle as a cause of death in Europe. According to estimations, it cause 1 out of 3.8 deaths.

1799 Marie-François-Xavier Bichat (1771-1802), publishes his *Traité des membranes* ("Treatise on Membranes"), effectively founding the field of histology

1800 Bartolomeo Ruspini of Italy invents the first dental mirror.

1800 Humphry Davy (1778-1829), English chemist, discovers the anesthetic effect of nitrous oxide, or laughing gas. It becomes the first chemical anesthetic.

1801 Thomas Young (1773-1829), English physician, is the first to describe astigmatism.

1802 Marie-François-Xavier Bichat, French physician, and his colleague Friedrich Burdach (1776-1847), are the first to use the term "biology" to describe the science of the general properties of living beings.

1805 Friedrich Wilhelm Adam Sertürner (1783-1841), German chemist, first isloates morphine, the active principle of opium. In doing so, he lays the groundwork for alkaloid chemistry.

1806 Gaspard Vieusseux (1746-1814) of Switzerland describes cerebrospinal meningitis.

1807 Jean-Nicolas Corvisart (1755-1821), French physician, publishes what eventually becomes an important treatise on the lesions of the heart and large vessels.

1809 Ephraim McDowell (1771-1830), American surgeon, performs the first ovariotomy (to remove an ovarian cyst) on a 47-year-old woman. The operation is successful, and she lives to be 78. His success refutes the notion that it is impossible to cut into the abdomen without causing death, thus paving the way for abdominal surgery.

1810 Samuel Hahnemann (1755-1843), German physician, publishes his *Organon der rationellen Heilkunde* ("Handbook of Rational Healing"), which offers the first systematic exposition of the homeopathic method of healing.

1811 Charles Bell (1774-1843), Scottish surgeon, publishes his findings on the motor and sensory nerves. Now called "Bell's Law," they state that the anterior spinal roots of the brain are for motor responses, whereas the posterior roots are for sensory responses.

1812 Benjamin Rush (1745-1813), American physician, publishes his *Medical Inquiries and Observations upon the Diseases of the Mind*, which is the first American treatise on psychiatry.

1817 James Parkinson (1755-1824), English physician, publishes his *Essay on the Shaking Palsy*, the first description of the condition that comes to be known as Parkinson's disease.

1818 The heart beat is perceived in the fetus.

1818 Valentine Mott (1785-1865), American surgeon, is first to ligate the innominate artery. This huge artery in the chest provides blood to the right arm, as well as to the right side of the head and neck. In order to prevent bleeding to death during surgery, this area needs to be tied off.

1819 René-Théophile-Hyacinthe Laënnec (1781-1826), French physician, invents the stethoscope and develops diagnosis by auscultation. Although initially resisted by the medical community, Laënnec's invention eventually revolutionizes diagnostic medicine.

1820 Pierre-Joseph Pelletier (1788-1842) and Joseph-Bienaimé Caventou (1795-1877), both of France, first isolate quinine, the active principle of cinchona bark used to treat malaria.

1825 American surgeon William Beaumont (1785-1853) begins his studies of human digestion. In 1822, Beaumont treats a young French Canadian named Alexis St. Martin for a gun shot wound in the abdomen. The wound heals leaving a permanent opening (fistula) into St. Martin's stomach. This allows Beaumont to actually see a working human stomach and he carries out more than 200 experiments with St. Martin to study digestion. As a result of these experiments, Beaumont concludes that the stomach acts on food chemically.

1826 Johannes Peter Müller (1802-1858), German physiologist, discovers that sensory nerves can interpret impulses in only one manner. For example, the optic nerve registers a flash of light however it is stimulated (by light or otherwise).

1827 Richard Bright (1789-1858), English physician, publishes his *Reports of Medical Cases*, which contains the first complete description of a kidney disease called nephritis. He also describes a chronic kidney disorder that becomes known as Bright's disease.

1831 Justus von Liebig (1803-1873), German chemist, Eugène Soubeiran (1793-1858), French pharmacologist, and Samuel Guthrie (1782-1848), American chemist, independently discover the anesthetic chloroform.

1832 British Medical Association is founded.

1833 Philipp Lorenz Geiger (1785-1836), German pharmaceutist, and his colleague, Hesse, first isolate atropine from belladonna.

1836 Theodore Schwann (1810-1882), German physiologist, discovers the fermentive property of the stomach enzyme pepsin.

1838 Isaac Ray (1807-1881), American physician, writes the first book on the medical jurisprudence of insanity. In this work, he describes a form of insanity that he says impairs the moral sense, rendering a person less responsible for his action. It becomes known as Ray's mania.

1838 Jean-Etienne-Dominique Esquirol (1772-1840), French physician, publishes his seminal *Des maladies mentales* ("Mental Maladies").

1839 Caspar Wistar Pennock (1799-1867) of the U.S. invents the first flexible-tube stethoscope. This replaces the awkward wooden tube invented by Laënnec.

1840 William Bowman (1816-1892), English anatomist, publishes his classic paper "On the Minute Structure and Movement of Voluntary Muscle." This eventually becomes the definitive study of muscle histology.

1841 Friedrich Gustav Jacob Henle (1809-1885), German pathologist and anatomist, publishes his *Allgemeine Anatomie* ("General Anatomy"), regarded as the first systematic textbook of anatomy.

1842 William Bowman (1816-1892), English anatomist, first demonstrates that urine is the product of superfiltration by the Malpighian bodies of the kidney's cortex.

1842 First successful use of ether as an anesthetic during a tooth extraction is conducted by American dentist, Elijah Pope, under the direction of William E. Clarke, a medical student.

1842 Crawford Williamson Long (1815-1878), American physician, successfully and painlessly removes a small tumor from a friend's neck, using ether as an anesthetic. Long waits until 1849 to publicize this procedure.

1842 Oliver Wendell Holmes (1809-1894), American author and physician, discovers that puerperal (childbed) fever is contagious.

1843 Gabriel Andral (1797-1876), French physician, is the first to urge that blood be examined in cases of disease.

1844 Horace Wells (1815-1848), American dentist, is the first to use nitrous oxide as an anesthetic in dentistry.

1844 Antoine-Jérôme Ballard (1802-1876), French chemist, discovers amyl nitrate. This drug will be used in the treatment of angina pectoris.

1846 Claude Bernard (1813-1878), French physiologist, discovers the digestive function of the pancreas.

1846 James Marion Sims (1813-1883), American surgeon, invents the vaginal speculum. Sims uses his new tool, which resembles a bent spoon, to correct a displaced uterus of a woman who had fallen from a horse. It soon becomes indispensable for other gynecological procedures.

1846 Oliver Wendell Holmes, American author and physician, first suggests the use of the terms "anaesthesia" and "anaesthetic" in a letter to William Thomas Green Morton (1819-1868), American dentist. Morton used ether as an anesthetic on a patient during a tooth extraction in September 1846.

1847 John Collins Warren (1778-1856), American surgeon, introduces ether as an anesthetic for general surgery. It soon becomes an essential part of surgery worldwide.

1847 James Young Simpson (1811-1870), Scottish obstetrician, introduces the use of chloroform anesthesia during labor and delivery. However, the use of anesthesia during childbirth does not gain wide acceptance until it is administered to Queen Victoria during the birth of Prince Leopold in 1853.

1847 Ignaz Philipp Semmelweis (1818-1865), Hungarian physician, observes correctly that puerperal (childbed) fever is directly related to doctors' uncleanliness. He begins a campaign to convince physicians to practice basic antiseptic measures, such as hand washing, but he is ridiculed and largely ignored by his colleagues.

1847 Claude Bernard, French physiologist, finds that chemicals are generated in the body, and goes on to promote the idea of "internal environment."

1847 American Medical Association is founded.

1848 Guillaume-Benjamin-Amand Duchenne (1806-1875), French physician and pioneer in physiology, makes use of electrodiagnosis and electrotherapy.

1848 First medical school solely for women, The Women's Medical College of Pennsylvania, is founded. It is incorporated in 1850 as the Female Medical College of Pennsylvania.

1849 John Snow (1813-1858), English physician, first states the theory that cholera is a water-borne disease, and that it is usually contracted by drinking contaminated water.

1849 First woman to receive a medical degree in the U.S. is Elizabeth Blackwell (1821-1910).

1849 Thomas Addison (1793-1860), English physician, describes pernicious anemia and is the first to give an accurate description of the hormone deficiency disease that results from the deterioration of the adrenal cortex. It comes to be known as Addison's disease.

1850 Rudolf Albert von Kölliker (1814-1905), Swiss anatomist and physiologist, publishes his *Mikroskopische Anatome* ("Microscopical Anatomy"). With its emphasis on cell structure, this work sets the stage for the emergence of cytology.

1850 Guillaume-Benjamin-Amand Duchenne, French physician and neurologist, gives the first description of the progressive muscular atropht called ataxia.

1851 Hermann von Helmholtz (1821-1894), German physiologist and physicist, perfects the first ophthalmoscope. This new instrument enables the physician to see into the eye, making ophthalmology an exact science.

1852 Mount Sinai Hospital, the first Jewish hospital in the U.S., is founded in New York City.

1852 George P. Cammann, American physician, develops the modern (two-ear) stethoscope.

1852 Magnus Huss (1807-1890) of Sweden coins the term "alcoholism" to define addiction to alcohol as a disease.

1853 Charles-Gabriel Pravaz (1791-1853), French physician, first publishes his description of a hypodermic syringe.

1854 Florence Nightingale, English nurse, takes charge of a barracks hospital when the Crimean War breaks out. Her compassion and common-sense approach to nursing set new standards and greatly advance nursing as a profession.

1854 Jules Baillarger (1810-1890), French physician, describes manic depression or bipolar disorder, which he defines as *folie à double forme* ("insanity with two manifestations").

1855 Albrecht von Graefe (1828-1870), German surgeon, first introduces the operation of iridectomy in the treatment of iritis, iridochoroiditis, and glaucoma. Regarded as the creator of modern eye surgery, he trains some of the greatest ophthalmologists of the nineteenth century.

1855 Manuel Garcia, a singing coach working in Paris, invents the laryngoscope.

1856 Hermann von Helmholtz (1821-1894), German physiologist and physicist, publishes the first part of his *Handbuch der Physiologischen Optik* ("Handbook of Physiological Optics"). In this work he unites morphology, physics, and physiology into a single conceptual synthesis.

1857 Bacteriology is founded with the publication of French chemist Louis Pasteur's (1822-1895) observations on lactic fermentation.

1858 Guillaume Benjamin Amand Duchenne (1806-1875), French physician and neurologist, gives the classic description of tabes dorsalis, a form of muscular dystrophy named after him.

1858 Henry Gray (1827-1862), English anatomist, publishes *Gray's Anatomy, Descriptive and Applied.*

1859 Hermann Brehmer (1826-1889), German physician, establishes the first successful sanatorium for tuberculosis at Gorbersdorf in Silesia, Germany. The therapies used include exercise, fresh air, hydrotherapy, and rest.

1859-60 Albert Niemann (1806-1877) of Germany prepares cocaine by isolating the active principle of *Erythroxylon coca*, a plant known to ancient cultures. Until its addictive properties are recognized, cocaine is used by physicians as a pain reliever and stimulant.

1860 Jakob von Heine (1800-1879), German orthopedist, first describes "infantile spinal paralysis," which becomes known as poliomyelitis.

1861 E. B. Wolcott (1804-1880), American surgeon, performs the first recorded surgical removal of the kidney (nephrectomy).

1862 Jules Péan (1830-1898), French surgeon, first devises the hemostatic forceps. This pincer-shaped instrument enables surgeons to stop hemorrhages by temporarily closing off an artery.

1862 Jean-Marie Charcot (1825-1893), French neurologist, starts teaching at the Salpêtrière Hospital. The greatest neurologist of his time, Charcot influences many disciples including Sigmund Freud.

1863 Albert von Bezold (1836-1868), German physiologist, discovers the accelerator nerve fibers of the heart, and shows that they originate in the spinal cord.

1863 Adolf von Baeyer (1836-1884), German chemist, discovers barbituric acid, the parent compound of a family of chemicals called barbiturates.

1864 Jean-Henri Dunant, Swiss humanitarian, founds the Red Cross.

1865 Joseph Lister (1827-1912), English surgeon, uses carbolic acid spray on a compound fracture to prevent infection, thus laying the groundwork for antiseptic surgery.

1865 Gregor Johann Mendel (1822-1884), Austrian botanist and monk, publishes the first of a series of papers in which he carefully documents his discovery of the laws of heredity. Mendel's work is ignored for more than thirty years, but he is now recognized as the founder of genetics.

1867 John S. Bobbs (1809-1870), American surgeon, performs the first cholecystomy—the surgical removal of stones from the gallbladder by an incision in the abdomen.

1868 Carl August Wunderlich (1815-1877), German physician, publishes his major work on the relation of fever to disease. He is the first to recognize that fever is not itself a disease but a symptom, and his writing forms the basis of modern clinical thermometry.

1868 Thomas Moreno y Maiz, French pharmacologist, suggests that cocaine be used as an anesthetic.

1868 Jean-Antoine Villemin (1827-1892), French physician, first demonstrates that tuberculosis does not occur spontaneously, but is an infection caused by a transmitted agent.

1869 Friedrich von Esmarch (1823-1908), German physician, first introduces the first-aid bandage, a package for use on the battlefield to control hemorrhage.

1869 Johann Friedrich Mieschner (1844-1895), Swiss biochemist, discovers a universal cell substance that is later named "nucleic acid."

1870 Christian Albert Theodor Billroth (1829-1894), Austrian surgeon, conducts the first complete removal of the larynx on a human patient. He is also considered the founder of modern abdominal surgery.

1871 Carl Friedrich Otto Westphal (1833-1890), German neurologist, first describes and introduces the term "agoraphobia" as the morbid fear of open spaces. He also introduces the term "paranoia."

1873 Gerhard Henrik Armauer Hansen (1841-1912), Norwegian physician, discovers the specific bacteria that causes leprosy.

1874 DDT is synthesized.

1875 William Pepper (1843-1898), American physician, first describes the abnormal changes in the bone marrow that occur in pernicious anemia.

1876 Adolf Wilhelm Hermann Kolbe (1818-1884), German chemist, accomplishes one of the earliest syntheses of an organic compound from inorganic substances. His work on the electrolysis of the salts of fatty acids enables him to first isolate salicylic acid, which becomes a building block of aspirin.

1877 Patrick Manson (1844-1922), Scottish physician, identifies filaria—a kind of parasitic worm—as the cause of the tropical disease elephantiasis. He later shows it is transmitted by a mosquito, and discovers that an insect can be host to a developing parasite that causes a human disease.

1877 Louis Pasteur (1822-1895), French chemist, first distinguishes between aerobic and anaerobic bacteria.

1878 Robert Koch (1843-1910), German bacteriologist, first publishes his landmark findings on the causes of traumatic infectious disease. On the basis of his findings, Koch establishes his rules for properly identifying the causative agent of a disease. Koch states that the microorganism must be located in a diseased animal, and that after it is cultured, or grown, it must be capable of causing disease in a healthy animal. Finally, the newly infected animal must yield the same bacteria as those found in the original animal. Koch goes on to isolate the specific bacteria that causes a number of diseases, the most famous being tuberculosis.

1878 Louis Pasteur, French chemist, defends the germ theory of disease before the French Academy of Medicine. He maintains that specific organisms cause specific diseases and that once these organisms are known, ways to prevent or cure a disease could be developed.

1879 Albert Ludwig Sigesmund Neisser (1855-1916), German dermatologist, discovers Gonococcus, the pus-producing bacterium that causes gonorrhea.

1880 Louis Pasteur, French chemist, first isolates and describes Streptococcus and Staphylococcus (both in puerperal septicemia).

1880 Karl Joseph Eberth (1835-1926), German pathologist, first isolates the typhoid bacillus.

1880 Carl Weigert (1845-1904) offers a classic description of a heart attack.

1880 Robert Lawson Tait (1845-1899) performs the first appendectomy in England.

1880 Charles-Louis-Alphonse Laveran (1845-1922), French physician and parasitologist, discovers the parasite that causes malaria fever.

1881 Clara Barton (1821-1912) organizes the American Red Cross in Washington, D.C.

1881 Anton Wolfler (1850-1817) of Bohemia first introduces gastroenterostomy (a surgical linking between the stomach and the bowel), a procedure usually necessitated by cancer.

1882 Robert Koch, German bacteriologist, announces his discovery of the tuberculosis bacillus, proving the existence of a pathogen.

1882 Ilya Ilich Mechnikov (1845-1916), Russian-French bacteriologist, begins research that results in his discovery of phagocytosis. He demonstrates that white corpuscles in animal blood flock to the site of any infection and are able to ingest the invading bacteria. He calls them "phagocytes," from the Greek meaning "devouring cells."

1882 Carlo Forlanini (1847-1918), Italian physician, first introduces the use of artificial pneumothorax (collapsing the lung) as a means of treating pulmonary tuberculosis.

1882 Edwin Klebs (1843-1913), German pathologist, discovers the diphtheria bacillus.

1883 Giulio Bizzozero (1846-1901), Italian pathologist, demonstrates that platelets are a constant element of blood.

1884 Arthur Nicolaier (1862-1942), German physician and bacteriologist, discovers the tetanus bacillus.

1884 Etienne-Stéphane Tarnier (1828-1897), French obstetrician, invents an incubator for the care of prematurely born infants,

1884 Robert Koch (1843-1910), German bacteriologist, discovers the cholera bacillus.

1884 Carl Koller (1857-1944), Bohemian-American opthamologist, first uses cocaine as a local anesthetic during eye surgery.

1885 Louis Pasteur (1822-1895), French chemist, first uses a successful vaccine for rabies to treat Joseph Meister, a boy badly mauled by a rabid dog.

1886 Ernst von Bergmann (1836-1907), German surgeon, first introduces steam sterilization for surgery and establishes the modern standardized aseptic ritual.

1886 Franz von Soxhlet first suggests that milk given to infants be sterilized.

1886 Richard von Krafft-Ebing (1840-1902), German neurologist, publishes his landmark case history study of sexual abnormalities, *Psychopathia sexualis.*

1886 Reginald Heber Fitz (1843-1913), American surgeon, first describes the pathology and clinical features of appendicitis. He details how a physician can diagnose the condition and prescribes when an operation is required. It is Fitz who names the disease.

1887 Oskar Medin (1847-1927), Swedish pediatrician, is the first to recognize the epidemic nature of poliomyelitis.

1887 Anton Weichselbaum (1845-1920), Austrian pathologist, first demonstrates that meningococcus in the spinal fluid is the cause of the epidemic cerebrospinal meningitis.

1887 Augustus Desiré Waller (1865-1922), French physiologist, first records the electrical activity of the human heart and lays the foundation for electrocardiography.

1889 Hans Buchner (1850-1902), German bacteriologist, first establishes the bactericidal effect of blood serum.

1889 The Johns Hopkins Hospital in Baltimore, Maryland, first opens.

1890 Emil Adolf von Behring (1854-1917), German bacteriologist, discovers antitoxins. He is able to produces an immunity against tetanus in an animal by injecting it with graded doses of serum from an animal suffering from tetanus. He uses his discovery of antitoxins to develop an antitoxin for diphtheria, a disease that was usually lethal in children.

1890 William Stewart Halsted (1852-1922), American surgeon, first introduces the use of sterile rubber gloves in the operating room.

1891 First child is treated with diphtheria antitoxin.

1891 Paul Ehrlich (1864-1915), German bacteriologist, discovers that methyl blue dye immobilizes the malaria bacterium and begins searching for other, more potent, microbial dyes.

1891 Paul Eugen Bleiler (1857-1939), Swiss psychiatrist, publishes his *Die Gruppe der Schizophrenien* ("The Schizopohrenia Group"), in which he reorganizes the varius syndromes known as dementia praecox, or early dementia, and designates the new disease "schizophrenia."

1892 Dmitrie Iosifovich (1864-1920), Russian botanist, demonstrates the existence of viruses for the first time.

1893 Sigmund Freud (1856-1939), Austrian neurologist and psychiatrist, describes paralysis caused by purely mental factors.

1894 First major epidemic of poliomyelitis in the U.S. breaks out.

1894 Shibasaburo Kitasato (1856-1931), Japanese bacteriologist, and Alexandre Emile John Yersin (1863-1943), Swiss bacteriologist, independently discover the plague bacillus.

1895 Richard Friedrich Johann Pfeiffer (1858-1945), German physician and bacteriologist, introduces bacteriolysis, or the concept of antibodies, when he discovers that the abdominal fluids of immunized guinea pigs dissolve cholera bacilli that had been introduced into the abdomen.

1895 Wilhelm Konrad Röntgen (1845-1923), German physicist, discovers x rays in his laboratory. One of the earliest applications of x rays is in medical diagnosis and therapy.

1895 Heinrich Irenaeus Quincke (1842-1922), German physician, conducts the first spinal tap or lumbar puncture to study cerebrospinal fluid and for diagnosis and treatment.

1896 Max von Gruber (1835-1927), German bacteriologist, and Herbert Edward Durham (1866-1945), English bacteriologist, discover agglutination. This phenomenon of blood clumping together occurs when the antibodies it contains react to an introduced agent, such as a bacterium.

1896 Joseph-François-Félix Babinski (1857-1932), French physician, discovers the large toe reflex that comes to bear his name. The lack of this involuntary backward-bending of the big toe after the sole of the foot has been stimulated indicates a neurological disorder.

1896 Christiann Eijkmann (1858-1930), Dutch physician, first produces a deficiency disease experimentally (beriberi in birds). This becomes an important step toward the discovery of vitamins.

1896 Hermann Strauss, German physician, first uses x rays to investigates a patient's gastrointestinal tract.

1896 Ludwig Rehn (1849-1930), German surgeon, is credited with being the first to suture a heart wound successfully.

1896 Scipione Reva-Rocci (1863-1903) of Italy invents the mercury sphygonomanometer, the precursor of the modern blood-pressure instrument.

1897 Kiyoshi Shiga (1870-1957), Japanese bacteriologist, discovers the dysentery bacillus.

1897 First whole-body xray of a living person taken in a single exposure is made by William James Morton (1845-1920), American neurologist.

1897 Ronald Ross (1857-1932), English physician, discovers the malaria parasite in the Anopheles mosquito. He is awarded the Nobel Prize for Physiology or Medicine for his work on malaria in 1902.

1898 Emil Herman Fischer (1852-1919), German chemist, isolates the purine nucleus of uric compounds and elucidates their structure. This turns out to be highly significant, for purines are an important part of a group of substances called nucleic acids.

1899 Aspirin is marketed by the German pharmaceutical firm Bayer.

1899 First documented cure of cancer by x-ray treatment is the accomplishment of Tage Anton Ultimus Sjögren (1859-1939), Swedish surgeon. The patient's squamous carcinoma of the cheek is cured following x-ray treatment and minor surgery.

1900 Ernest Wertheim (1864-1920), German surgeon, performs a radical hysterectomy for the cancer of the cervix.

1900 Karl Landsteiner (1868-1943), Austrian-American physician, discovers the different types of human blood. He finds there are different blood groups (A, B, AB, and O), which differ in the capacity of their serum to clump together. With the ability to blood-type both patient and donor, blood transfusions become safe.

1901 Emil Adolf von Behring (1854-1917), German bacteriologist, is the first recipient of the Nobel Prize for Physiology or Medicine. He is honored for his work on serum therapy, particularly its application against diphtheria.

1901 Walter Reed (1851-1932), American military surgeon, proves that yellow fever is transmitted by a mosquito.

1902 Harvey Cushing (1869-1939), American surgeon, performs the first nerve suture.

1903 Svante August Arrhenius (1859-1927), Swedish chemist, first uses the term "immunochemistry."

1903 Willem Einthoven (1860-1927) invents the electrocardiograph.

1904 First radical operation for prostate cancer is performed by Hugh Hampton Young (1870-1945), American urologist.

1904 Paul Ehrilch (1854-1915), German bacteriologist, discovers a microbial dye called trypan red that helps destroy the trypanosomes which cause diseases such as sleeping sickness.

1904 Ivan Petrovich Pavlov (1849-1936), Russian physiologist, is awarded the Nobel Prize for Physiology or Medicine for establishing the connections between the nervous system and digestion.

1905 Alfred Einhorn, German chemist, discovers procaine (Novocaine), which becomes a widely-used local anesthetic.

1905 Jules-Jean-Baptiste-Vincent Bordet (1870-1961), Belgian bacteriologist, and his his colleague, Octave Gengou (1875-1957), discover the bacillus of whooping cough. Bordet later discovers a method of immunization against this dreaded childhood disease,

1905 John Winter of England resuscitates a heart by injecting epinephrine.

1905 Robert Koch (1843-1910), German bacteriologist, receives the Nobel Prize for Physiology or Medicine for his work on tuberculosis. He is one of the founders of bacteriology.

1905 Fritz Richard Schaudinn (1871-1906), German zoologist, discovers *Spirocheta pallida* (later renamed *Treponema pallidum*), the parasite which causes syphilis.

1906 August von Wasserman (1866-1925), German bacteriologist, first develops a diagnostic blood test for syphilis.

1906 Frederick Gowland Hopkins (1861-1947), English biochemist, first argues that certain "accessory" factors in food are necessary to sustain life. This theory of trace substances becomes the starting of point of further work on vitamin requirements, which leads to the discovery of what come to be called vitamins.

1906 Howard Taylor Ricketts (1871-1910), American pathologist, proves that a wood tick transmits Rocky Mountain spotted fever. He locates the microorganism that causes the disease and finds it has both bacteria- and virus-like qualities. It eventually is called rickettsia.

1907 Clemens Peter Pirquet von Cesenatico (1874-1929), Austrian physician, first introduces the skin reaction tet for the diagnosis of tubercolosis.

1907 Clemens Peter Pirquet von Cesenatico, Austrian physician, and Bela Schick (1877-1967), Hungarian pediatrician, introduces the notion and term "allergy."

1908 Bela Schick, Hungarian pediatrician, devises the first skin test to determine a patient's susceptibility to diphtheria.

1908 G. Ghedini, Italian physician, introduces the biopsy of bone marrow as a clinical procedure.

1908 Reuben Ottenberg, American physician, reports the first transfusion in which blood tests for compatibility are done.

1909 Charles-Jules-Henri Nicolle (1866-1936), French bacteriologist, proves that typhus fever is transmitted by the body louse.

1910 Francis Peyton Rous (1879-1970), American pathologist, experiments with transmitting sarcomas in hens and discovers the first cancer-inducing virus.

1910 Paul Ehrlich (1854-1915), German bacteriologist, and Sahachiro Hata (1872-1938), Japanese bacteriologist, announce their discovery of an effective treatment for syphilis. Ehrlich names the new drug "Salvarsan." This discovery marks the beginning of modern chemotherapy.

1910 Albrecht Kossel (1853-1927), German biochemist, is awarded the Nobel Prize for Physiology or Medicine for his outstanding discoveries concerning the chemistry of the cell and the cell nucleus.

1910 James Bryan Herrick (1861-1954), American physician, first describes sickle-cell anemia, a disease caused by a blood cell anomaly. Thsi type of anemia occurs mostly in people of African descent.

1910 Charles-Jules-Henri Nicolle, French bacteriologist, discovers the viral origin of influenza.

1911 Hideyo Noguchi (1876-1928), Japanese bacteriologist, first introduces the skin test for syphilis.

1911 R. A. Lambert and F. M. Hanes perform the first successful in vitro cultivation of tumor cells. This technique proves very useful for the advancement of cancer researche

1912 Elmer Verner McCollum (1879-1967) and Marguerite Davis (1887-1967), both American chemists, discover vitamin A in butter and egg yolk. This fat-soluble vitamin is necessary for normal bone development and the health of certain tissues, especially the retina of the eye.

1912 Friedrich A. Paneth (1887-1958), German-British chemist, and Georg von Hevesy (1885-1966), Hungarian chemist, first use radioactive indicators experimentally in living bodies.

1912 James Bryan Herrick, American physician, first describes a myocardial infarction, commonly known as a heart attack.

1912 Alexis Carrel (1873-1944), French-American surgeon, succeeds in producing the first true cell culture chick embryo fibroblasts). Since he is able to keep the tissue alive, his research enables scientists to monitor cell development.

1912 Researchers discover that phenobarbital is effective against epileptic seizures.

1913 Johannes Andreas Grib Fibiger (1876-1928), Danish pathologist, produces the first nonviral tumor in a laboratory experiment with on rats. This shows that cancers can be caused by purely chemical agents.

1914 Henry Hallett Dale (1875-1968), English biologist, first isolates acetylcholine—a substance that will prove crucial to the discovery of the chemical transmission of nerve impulse.

1914 Louis Anatole La Garde (1849-1920), American surgeon, publishes *Gunshot Injuries*, a work which becomes a classic source. He demonstrates that bullet wounds are not sterile, and that, contrary to prevalent views, microorganisms survive the bullet's heat and enter the wound.

1916 Jay McLean (1890-1957), American physiologist, first isolated the anticoagulant heparin.

1918 An influenza pandemic breaks out. The incredibly high mortality rates are attributed to the rapidity with which the disease develops into pneumonia and other secondary complications. The estimated worldwide toll is 25 million.

1918 First blood and serum banks are established in Europe during World War I.

1919 Mercurochrome is first introduced by Hugh Hampton Young (1870-1945), American urologist, and is used an an antiseptic and germicide.

1919 Francis Gilman Blake (1887-1952), and James Dowling Trask (1890-1942), American physicians, first demonstrate that measles is caused by a virus.

1921 Jules Gonin (1870-1035), Swiss ophthalmologist, performs an operation for retinal detachment.

1922 Insulin is administered for the first time to a patient with diabetes mellitus. This becomes possible after the Canadian physiologists Frederick Grant Banting (1891-1941) and Charles Best (1899-1978) develop a method of extracting insulin from the pancreas in 1921.

1922 Fernando E. Rodriguez, working at the U.S. Army Dental School, demonstrates the cycle of tooth decay, laying the foundation for modern preventive dentistry.

1923 Carlos Williamson describes the rejection phenomenon.

1923 Georg von Hevesy (1885-1966), Hungarian chemist, first uses radioactive tracers to follow the path of a substance in an organism.

1923 Ernest Henry Starling (1866-1927), English physiologist, publishes *Wisdom of the Body* in which he emphasizes the importance of the endocrine system in regulating the homeostasis of an organism.

1924 Albert-Léon Calmette (1863-1933), French bacteriologist, develops an antituberculosis vaccine using attenuated live bacilli.

1924 Willem Einthoven (1860-1927), Dutch physiologist, is awarded the Nobel Prize for Physiology or Medicine for his discovery of the mechanism of the electrocardiogram.

1924 George Frederick Dick (1881-1967) and Gladys R. H. Dick (1881-1963), American physicians, discover that hemolytic streptococcus causes scarlet fever. They also develop a skin test to determine susceptibility to this disease.

1925 Florence Rena Sabin (1871-1953), American anatomist and biologist, becomes the first woman member of the National Academy of Sciences.

1926 George Richards Minot (1885-1950) and William Parry Murphy (1892-1987), both American physicians, first introduce their raw liver diet in the treatment of perniceous anemia. Their treatment was suggested by earlier research conducted by American pathologist George Hoyt Whipple (1875-1976). While studying the effects of various foods on anemic dogs, Whipple discovered that liver was the best stimulator of hemoglobin production.

1926 Peter Muhlens (1874-1943) of Germany, and colleagues, introduce the first synthetic anti-malarial drug, Plasmoquin.

1926 Barend C. P. Jansen and Willem F. Donath, Dutch biochemists, first isolate thiamine (vitamin B_1).

1926 Joseph Goldberger (1874-1929), American pathologist, and colleagues, discover that pellagra is caused by a diet totally deficient in niacin, one of the B-complex vitamins.

1926 Johannes Andreas Grib Fibiger (1867-1928), Danish bacteriologist, is awarded the Nobel Prize for Physiology or Medicine for his discovery of the Spiropter carcinoma. He is the first scientist to induce cancer in laboratory animals.

1926 Otto Heinrich Warburg (1883-1970), German biochemist, is the first to determine that cancer cells derive energy from lactic acid fermentation, and can therefore be damaged by radiation.

1928 Alexander Fleming (1881-1955), Scottish bacteriologist, discovers penicillin, the first antibiotic.

1928 George Nicholas Papanicolaou (1883-1962), Greek-American physician, invents the Pap test, a painless and simple smear procedure for the early detection of cervical and uterine cancer.

1928 Albert Szent-Györyi (1893-1986), Hungarian-American biochemist, first isolates and describes ascorbic acid, which he later shows to be identical with vitamin C.

1928 Charles-Jules-Henri Nicolle (1866-1936), French physician, is awarded the Nobel Prize for Physiology or Medicine for proving that typhus is transmitted to humans by the louse.

1929 Philip Drinker (1893-1977), American industrial hygienist, invents the iron lung. This machine performs the function of the muscles that control breathing allowing people who are unable to breathe to be kept alive. This device saves the lives of polio patients where breathing muscles are paralyzed.

1929 Werner Forssmann (1904-1979), German surgeon, invents the first practical system for heart catheterization. By inserting a tube containing radio-opaque dye into the heart, physicians are able to improve accuracy of heart diagnosis without surgery.

1929 Karl Lohmann discovers adenosine triphosphate, the molecule that acts as an energy converter in all living things.

c. 1930 The technique of using a needle to obtain samples of amniotic fluid (in which a fetus floats) from a mother's womb is developed.

1931 Kenneth Merrill Lynch, American pathologist, reports what is believed to be the first fatal cases of asbestosis in the United States.

1932 Charles Scott Sherrington (1857-1952), English neurologist, and Edgar Douglas Adrian (1889-1977), English physiologist, are awarded the Nobel Prize for Physiology or Medicine for their discoveries regarding the functions of neurons.

1932 Gerhard Domagk (1895-1964), German bacteriologist, discovers the antibacterial effects of Prontosil, the first of the suffronamede drugs.

1932 Hans Adolf Krebs (1900-1981), German-British biochemist, first describes and names the citric acid cycle (Krebs cycle). This chemical sequence explains the metabolic pathways that carbohydrates, fats, and even proteins follow. The cycle also plays a fundamental role in virtually all cell metabolism.

1933 First blood bank in the United States is founded by American bacteriologist Earl W. Flosdorff (1904-1958) and American microbiologist Stuart Mudd.

1933 Christopher Howard Andrewes (1896-1988), English pathologist, Wilson Smith (1897-1965), English bacteriologist, and Patrick Playfair Laidlaw (1881-1940), English physician, demonstrate the viral nature of the human influenza agent by transmitting it to a ferret and then transferring it onto a suitable culture medium.

1934 L. D. Felton discovers the phenomenon of immunization paralysis caused by excessive antigens. Later called immunization tolerance, it will become a central problem in organ transplants.

1935 António Caetano de Abreu Freire Egas Moniz (1874-1955), Portuguese surgeon, performs the first lobotomy. This operation, which severs the nerve fibers connecting the patient's thalamus with the prefrontal lobes of the brain, opens the field of psychosurgery. Used as a last resort, it is later replaced by drug therapy.

1935 John Heysham Gibbon, Jr. (1903-1973), American surgeon, demonstrates for the first tme that life can be maintained by an external pump acting as an artificial heart. He accomplishes this during surgery on a dog.

1936 Tadeusz Reichstein (1897-1996), Polish-Swiss chemist, first isolates cortisone. This organic compound, present in small amounts in the human body, is found to have anti-inflammatory properties.

1936 Frank Macfarlane Burnet (1899-1065), Australian immunologist, isolates the first mutant bacteriophage—a bacteriolytic virus. This discovery is important for the development of genetic theory.

1937 Daniel Bovet (1907-1992), Swiss-French-Italian pharmacologist, discovers amphetaimes—compounds that neutralize certain symptoms of allegric reactions. Later, he synthesizes curare and develops a method to use it during surgery as a muscle relaxer.

1937 Lung cancer in cigarette smokers is first described by American surgeons Alton Ochsner (1896-1981) and Michael Ellis DeBakey (1908-), who suggest that smoking causes cancer.

1937 Max Theiler (1899-1972), South African-American microbiologist, develops a safe, effective vaccine against yellow fever.

1938 Howard W. F. Florey (1898-1968), Austrian-English biochemist and Ernst Boris Chain (1906-1979), German-English biochemist, first isolate and purify penicillin. making it potentially available for general use.

1938 Albert Hoffman of Switzerland first synthesizes lysergic acid diethylamide, known as LSD-25. A mind-altering chemical, it eventually becomes a trendy (and illegal) drug in the 1960s and 1970s.

1938 Ugo Cerletti (1877-1963), Italian physician, starts treating severely depressed patients with electric shocks (ECT).

1939 Paul H. Müller (1899-1965), Swiss chemist, discovers the insect-repelling properties of DDT (dichlorodiphenyltrichloroethane), which was first synthesized in 1873. Extremely effective for agricultural purposes and in controlling typhus epidemics, it is eventually identified as a powerful environmental pollutant and banned by many countries.

1940 Karl Landsteiner (1868-1943), Austrian-American physician, and Alexander S. Wiener, American immunohematologist, discover the Rhesus factor in blood, shedding light on erythroblastosis fetalis, a disease of newborns.

1940 Selman Abraham Waksman (1888-1973), Russian American microbiologist, discovers streptomycia, the first antibiotic effective against tuberculosis. Streptomycia, derived from a fungus is found to be active against the 70 different bacteria that did not respond to penicillin.

1941 Norman M. Gregg (1892-1966) of Australia discovers that rubella during pregnancy can cause congenital abnormalities.

1941 Penicillin is first used to treat pneumonia.

1942 C. Auerbach in England discovers yperite, the first known chemical mutagen. The identification of this and of other substances that can cause structural changes in genes offers science a new tool for investigating the structure of genes via induced mutations.

1943 Carl Ferdinand Cori (1896-1984) and Gerty Theresa Radnitz Cori (1896-1957), Czech-American biochemists, first achieve the test-tube synthesis of glycogen. They later (1947) win a Nobel Prize for Medicine or Physiology for determining the role sugar plays in the metabolism of animals.

1943 Penicillin is first used on a large scale by the U.S. Army in the North African campaigns. Data obtained from these studies show that early expectations for the drug are realistic, and the groundwork is laid for the massive use of penicillin in civilian medicine after the war.

1943 DDT is given its first major test by the U.S. Army in Naples, Italy, where it stops a typhus epidemic by killing the typhus-carrying lice.

1944 First successful operation to remedy the "blue baby" syndrome is conducted by the American surgeon Alfred Blalock (1899-1964). He uses a technique based on the research by the American pediatric cardiologist Helen Brooke Taussig (1898-1986).

1945 First kidney dialysis machine is invented by Willem J. Kolff (1911-). His system keeps patients with kidney failure alive by filtering out urea from their blood.

1945 Guy Henry Faget (1892-1947), American physician, first introduces promin, a drug which proves effective against leprosy.

1945 Alexander Fleming (1881-1955), Scottish bacteriologist, Ernst Boris Chain (1906-1979), German-English biochemist, and Howard Walter Florey (1898-1968), Austrian-English pathologist, are awarded the Nobel Prize for Physiology or Medicine for the discovery of penicillin and its curative effect in various infective diseases.

1946 Edward Mills Purcell (1912-1995), American physicist, and Felix Bloch (1905-1983), Swiss American physicist, independently develop nuclear magnetic resonance, a technique that has a wide range of applications including studying the interior of living things noninvasively.

1947 Theodore E. Woodward, American physician, reports the first specific cure of typhoid fever with chloraphenicol one of the earliest antibiotics, during a trip to Malaya.

1948 Seymour Morgan Farber (1912-1995), American physician, uses the first antimetabolite (a substance that disrupts the metabolism of cancer cells) in cancer chemotherapy. He uses methotrexate (aminopterin) to treat leukemia.

1948 Philip Showalter Hench (1896-1965), American physician, uses cortisone to successfully treat rheumatoid arthritis.

1948 Alfred Charles Kinsey (1894-1956), American zoologist and student of sexual behavior, publishes *Sexual Behavior in the Human Male*. This landmark study of sexuality is followed by his 1953 book, *Sexual Behavior in the Human Female.*

1949 Walter Rudolf Hess (1881-1973), Swiss physiologist, is awarded the Nobel Prize for Physiology or Medicine for his discovery of the functional organization of the interbrain as a coordinator of the activities of the internal organs.

1949 First use of lithium as a drug for manic depression.

1950 John H. Gibbon, Jr. (1903-1973), American surgeon, creates the heart-lung machine.

1951 First kidney transplant operation attempted in the U.S.

1951 First successful oral contraceptive introduced. Gregory Pincus (1903-1967), American biologist discovers a synthetic hormone that renders a woman infertile. It is soon marketed in pill form. The "pill" enables people to think of sexual intercourse as an act that is not by definition connected to pregnancy.

1951 Scientists discover that fluoride can prevent tooth decay.

1951 Joseph E. Smadel, Kenneth Goodner, Fred R. McCrumb, Jr., and Theodore E. Woodward, American physicians, are the first to demonstrate that broad spectrum antibiotics can cure septicemmic and pneumonic types of human plague.

1952 Paul M. Zoll (1911-1999), American physician, introduces the first practical cardiac pacemaker.

1952 Paul M. Zoll, American physician, first develops the technique of external stimulation by electric shock in cases of cardiac arrest.

1952 J. Delay of France discovers the antipsychotic action of Largactyl (chloropromazine). This breakthrough is later followed by further progress in psychotherapeutic drug research.

1952 Douglas Bevis, English physician, publishes an article describing his use of amniocentesis in Rh-factor cases. This process uses a needle to obtain samples of amniotic fluid from a mothers womb. This is the first use of amniocentesis for a fetal diagnosis.

1952 First mechanical heart pump is used successfully on a human being undergoing heart surgery. Designed by the American surgeon Forest D. Dodrill (1902-1997), with help from General Motors engineers, the portable electric pump performs the heart's function while surgery is performed.

1952 Charles Hufnagel (1916-1989), American surgeon, of the U.S. inserts the first artificial heart valve.

1952 Robert Wallace Wilkins (1906-), American physician, studies the drug reserpine, and finds it has a sedative effect without causing drowsiness.

Reserpine and other drugs of this type become known as tranquilizers.

1953 Michael Ellis DeBakey, (1908-) American surgeon, performs the first successful carotid endarterectomy (the removal of plaque build-up from within the lining of an artery).

1953 First successful open-heart operation supported by a heart-lung machine is conducted the American surgeon John Heysham Gibbon, Jr. (1903-1973).

1954 Jonas Edward Salk (1914-1995), American virologist, produces the first safe and effective vaccine that prevents paralytic polio.

1954 Joseph Edward Murray, American surgeon, conducts the first successful organ transplant as he transfers a kidney from one twin to another.

1954 First measles vaccine is developed by John Franklin Enders (1897-1985), American micrologist, and Thomas Pebbles, American pediatrician. Although an immunization program using this vaccine is started, a truly successful and practical vaccine is not achieved until 1963.

1955 Chlorpromazin, also called Thorazine, is first used to treat psychiatric disorders, primarily schizophrenia.

1956 Joe-Hin Tjio, Indonesian-American biologist, and Johann Albert Levan, Swiss cytologist, show that the human species does not have 48 chromosomes, as believed, but rather 46.

1956 Niels Kai Jerne (1911-1994), Danish physician, proposes the clonal selection theory of antibody selection to explain how white blood cells are able to produce a large range antibodies.

1957 Alick Isaacs (1921-1967), Scottish virologist, demonstrates that antibodies act only against bacteria. This means that antibodies are not one of the bodies natural forms of defense against viruses. This knowledge leads, also in 1957, to the discovery of interferon by Isaacs and his colleague Jean Lindenmann of Switzerland. They find that the generation of a small amount of protein is the body's first line of defense against a virus and describe this protein as an "interfering protein" or interferon.

1958 Ultrasound first used in obstetrics to examine an unborn fetus.

1958 The human chemical called dopamine is identified as a neurotransmitter.

1958 Denis Burkitt, Irish physician, publishes his first account of what becomes known as "Burkitt's lymphoma," a cancer of the lymphatic system.

1958 George Wells Beadle (1903-1989), American geneticist, and Edward Lawrie Tatum (1909-1975), American biochemist, are awarded the Nobel Prize for Physiology or Medicine for their discovery that genes act by regulating definite chemical events. Joshua Lederberg (1925-), American geneticist, is also awarded the Nobel Prize for Physiology or Medicine for his discoveries concerning genetic recombination and the organization of genetic material of bacteria.

1959 Severo Ochoa (1905-1993), Spanish-American biochemist, and Arthur Kornberg (1918-), American biochemist, are awarded the Nobel Prize for Physiology or Medicine for their discovery of the mechanisms in the biological synthesis of RNA and DNA.

1959 Albert Bruce Sabin (1906-1993), Polish American virologist, announces successful results from testing live attenuated polio vaccine. His vaccine eventually is preferred over the Salk (killed) vaccine, since it can be administered orally and offers protection with a single dose.

1960 Frank Macfarlane Burnet (1899-1985), Australian immunologist, and Peter Brian Medawar (1915-1987), English biologist, are awarded the Nobel Prize in Physiology or Medicine for the discovery of acquired immunological tolerance.

1962 Francis Compton Crick (1916-), English biochemist, James Dewey Watson (1928-), American biochemist, and Maurice Hugh Frederick Wilkins (1916-), New Zealand-English physicist, are awarded the Nobel Prize for Physiology or Medicine for their discoveries concerning the molecular structure of nucleic acids and their significance for information transfer in living matter.

1963 Thomas E. Starzl (1926-), American surgeon, performs the first human liver transplant. The recipient survives for 23 days.

1963 James Hardy, American surgeon, performs the first lung transplant.

1963 Valium, the world's most widely used tranquilizer, is first developed.

1964 U.S. National Library of Medicine introduces a computer-based system for the analysis and retrieval of medical literature (MEDLARS).

1964 Rh-negative mothers who are injected with Rh antibodies deliver babies unaffected by Rh incompatibility.

1966 Michael Ellis DeBakey, American surgeon, designs an artificial left ventricle, which he implants in a patient's heart.

1967 Mammography, a form of x-ray procedure for the detection of breast cancer, is introduced as a widely used diagnostic tool.

1967 First successful human hear transplant is performed by the South African surgeon Christiaan Neethling Barnard (1922-). The recipient, Louis Washkansky, lives for 18 days.

1967 René Favolaro (1923-), Argentinian American surgeon, performs the first coronary bypass operation using a vein.

1968 Carlo Valenti, American physician, determines whether a fetus is affected by Down's syndrome, a genetic disorder, by analyzing cells taken from the mother's amniotic fluid.

1968 Ion Gresser, American virologist, and Kari Cantell, Finnish virologist, develop a way of producing interferon in useful amounts from human blood cells.

1968 Har Gobind Khorana (1922-), Indian American chemist, and Marshall Warren Nirenberg (1927-), American biochemist, are awarded the Nobel Prize for Physiology or Medicine for their interpretation of the genetic code and its function in protein synthesis.

1969 Allan MacLeod Cormack (1924-1998), South African-born American physicist, constructs the first computerized axial tomography (CAT) scanner. His initial model uses a thin beam of x rays aimed at a section of the body but repeated from many different angles. However, he lacks a system to process the large amount of data produced.

1969 Max Delbrück (1906-1981), German-American microbiologist, Alfred Day Hershey (1908-1997), American microbiologist, and Salvador Edward Luria (1912-1991), Italian-American microbiologist, are awarded the Nobel Prize for Physiology or Medicine for their discoveries concerning the replication mechanism and genetic structure of viruses.

1969 First artificial heart is implanted in a human being. Denton A. Cooley (1920-), American surgeon, implants a mechanical heart made of silicon. This temporary device keeps a patient alive for 65 hours until a human heart is implanted to replace it. The patient dies 38 hours after the second operation as a result of kidney failure.

1970 Patrick Steptoe (1913-1988) and Robert G. Edwards, both English physicians, accomplish in-vitro fertilization in humans.

1970 The first cardiac pacemaker is implanted in a patient's chest.

1971 First computerized axial tomography (CAT) machine is installed in England. It incorporates the new design by Godfrey Newbold Hounsfield (1919-), English electrical engineer, who uses computers to collate the x-ray data and create a tomographic image that offers a detailed, sharp map of a particular cross-section of the body.

1972 Robert C. Gallo (1937-), American cell biologist, and his colleagues indentify interleukin 2, which is a factor that stimulates growth in human T-cells.

1972 John Charnley (1911-1982), English orthopedic surgeon, designs the first satisfactory artificial hip.

1974 The Heimlich maneuver, developed by Henry J. Heimlich (1920-), American surgeon, is introduced as first aid for choking.

1975 David Baltimore (1938-), American biochemist, Renato Dulbecco (1914-), Italian American virologist, and Howard Martin Temin (1934-1994), American oncologist, are awarded the Nobel Prize for Physiology or Medicine for their discoveries concerning the interaction between viruses and the genetic material of the cell.

1976 Jean-François Borel, a microbiologist at the Swiss pharmaceutical firm Sandoz, publishes the structures and properties of a new immunosuppressant called cyclosporin.

1976 Roger Guillemin (1924-), French-born American physiologist, discovers a new class of hormonal substances endorphins that are produced in the central nervous system. Endorphins have the natural ability to relieve pain.

1977 Earliest known AIDS patients in the United States are two homosexual men in New York who are diagnosed with Kaposi's sarcoma.

1977 Andreas R. Grüntzig (1939-1985), Swiss physician, develops a method of unclogging diseased coronary arteries called angioplasty.

1978 First test-tube baby, Louise Brown, is born in England on July 25. This is the birth of the first human being conceived outside the human body. Implanted in the mother's uterus by English physicians Patrick Steptoe and Robert G. Edwards, the fertilized egg developed normally.

1978 Smallpox is eliminated worldwide.

1978 David Botstein, Ronald W. Davis, and Mark H. Skolnick announce the potential for using DNA sequencing to develop markers for certain genetic diseases.

1980 The lithotripter, a device that pulverizes kidney stones with sound waves (without any surgery), is invented in Germany by researchers at Dornier Medical Systems

.1980 Charles Weissman of Switzerland produces the first genetically engineered human interferon, making large-scale production possible.

1981 AIDS (Acquired Immune Deficiency Syndrome) is officially recognized by the U.S. Centers for Disease Control, and the first clinical description of this disease is made. It is soon recognized that AIDS is an infectious disease caused by a virus that spreads virtually exclusively by blood and other body fluids.

1982 First brain tissue transplants are used for Parkinson's disease. The therapy is unsuccessful.

1982 First product of genetic engineering is approved by the U.S. Food and Drug Administration. Eli Lilly & Company is permitted to market human insulin (Humulin) produced by bacteria.

1982 Oncogenes, or cancer-causing genes, are discovered.

1982 First Jarvik 7 artificial heart is implanted by William DeVries, American surgeon. The patient, Barney Clark, lives for 112 days.

1983 Researchers discover a gene marker for Duchenne muscular dystrophy.

1983 Nancy Wexler (1945-), American neuropsychologist, and James Gusella (1952-) discover a marker for Huntington's chorea, a rare and fatal hereditary disease that results in degeneration of brain tissue.

1983 Researchers discover that a bacterium causes ulcers of the stomach and small intestine. This leads to a major reevaluation of such factors as stress and diet in the treatment of ulcers.

1984 First successful gene therapy is accomplished in a mammal. A normal gene is successfully introduced to compensate for a defective one.

1984 First baby is born from a frozen embryo.

1984 William H. Clewall, American surgeon, performs the first successful surgery on a fetus in the uterus.

1985 Surgically implantable defibrillator is approved by the U.S. Food and Drug Administration. This regulatory device is used to maintain a correct heartbeat.

1985 Gene marker for cystic fibrosis is found on chromosome 7.

1985 Lasers are used for the first time to unblock clogged arteries.

1986 First genetically engineered vaccine approved for human use is the hepatitis B vaccine.

1986 AIDS virus is isolated. Called the Human Immune Deficiency Virus, it is part of a group of viruses known as retroviruses. No cure or vaccine is yet available.

1987 Ignacio Navarro Madrazo implants cells from the adrenal gland and alleviates Parkinson's disease.

1987 Defective genes are linked to colon cancer.

1987 Artificial chromosomes are produced.

1987 Michael Zasloff announces the discovery the discovery of new antibiotics from the skin of the African clawed frog. He names them magainins.

1988 First patent is issued for a "transgenic non-human mammal"—a genetically alterted mouse that is predisposed to cancer.

1988 National Institutes of Health approves the injection of genetically-altered cells into humans.

1989 John Michael Bishop (1936-) and Harold Elliot Varmus (1939-), American virologists, are awarded the Nobel Prize for Physiology or Medicine for their discovery of the cellular origin of retroviral oncogenes.

1990 Human Genome Project begins in the U.S. with the selection of six participating institutions. The project's goal is to map the entire human genetic code.

1990 First patient to receive gene therapy is a four-year-old girl suffering from ADA deficiency (a genetic disorder that makes the immune system unable to fight infection). She receives a series of intravenous infusions of here own immune cells that have been "gene-corrected" by the introduction of normal genes encoding functional human ADA.

1991 U.S. National Institutes of Health begins a new type of cancer gene therapy using genes from a natural tumor-fighting substance in cells called TNF (tumor necrosis factor).

1991 Research in the U.S. produces evidence that drug treatment with GM-1 ganglioside helps patients suffering from spinal cord injury.

1991 The safety of silicon breast implants continues to be questioned, with problems such as silicon leakage, allergic reactions, and interference with detection of breast cancer occurring in as much as 30 percent of the 2,000,000 women in the U.S. who received implants.

1992 An astonishing resurgence of pulmonary tuberculosis occurs in large urban areas in the U.S. and Europe.

1992 The era of animal-to-human transplants begins with the transplantation of a baboon's liver into a man whose liver had been almost destroyed by hepatitis B. The patient dies 70 days after the surgery of a hemorrhage caused by an infection.

1992 Researchers at Harvard Medical School investigate 15 male schizophrenics using MRI (magnetic resonance imaging) and find that compared to 15 normal control subjects, the patients had significant reduction (13-19%) in the volume of gray matter in three specific regions of the left temporal lobe of the brain.

1992 James Dewey Watson (1928-), American biochemist, leader of the Human Genome Project, resigns. Many believe that his resignation is due to disagreements about gene patenting.

1993 Researchers in France announce they have constructed the first rough map of all the human chromosomes.

1993 American Heart Association confirms that taking aspirin can prevent some cardiovascular problems and treat others.

1993 Teams of researchers in the U.S. and Europe discover the gene for Huntington's chorea on chromosome 4.

1994 Researchers identify the gene responsible for certain breast cancers. Twenty-two coding defects where found in the gene, which was named BRCA1.

1994 Raul Andino and colleagues at the University of California, San Francisco, detect an immune response in animals injected with a polio vaccine with added HIV-1 proteins.

1995 Australian researchers learn that a weakened form of the HIV virus does not cause AIDS. According to Nicholas J. Deacon of the National Center for HIV Research, such mutated viruses may provide the basis for a vaccine.

1996 Richard M. Meyers and Len A. Pennacchio of Stanford University, and Finnish scientists discover the gene responsible for epilepsy.

1996 Maxine Papadakis of the Department of Veterans Affairs Medical Center in San Francisco and colleagues find that GFH (growth hormone factor) does not reverse the aging process.

1996 Scientists identify the hepatitis G virus.

1996 Researchers at the National Cancer Institute claim that beta carotene provides no protection against cancer and heart disease.

1997 Researchers discover that abnormal accumulation of proteins in the cell's nucleus may be responsible for a variety of brain disorders, including Huntington's disease.

1997 Surgical repositioning of the retina, radiation to stop blood flow, and the introduction of photochemical dyes to attack new blood vessels are among the new procedures used to treat macular degeneration, a scarring of the retina caused by blood vessel growth in the eye.

1997 Researchers find that antibodies can transport radioactive atoms to cancerous cells. This procedure destroys the cancerous cells, but only minimally damages healthy tissue.

1998 Scientists find that cancer vaccines including cells from a patient's own body provide a boost to the patient's immune system.

1998 Researchers at the Fulda Medical Center in Germany demonstrate that FGF (fibroblast growth factor), a human protein, enables the heart to create new blood vessels, providing relief for patients with blocked coronary arteries.

1998 Researchers find that T-20, an experimental drug, protects immune cells from HIV.

1998 Carl G. Hellerquist of Vanderbilt University and his research group find that CM101, a bacterial toxin suggested as a cancer drug, heals spinal cord injuries in mice.

1998 Scientists develop a vaccine that protects guinea pigs from the Ebola virus.

1998 Studies indicate that both chemotherapy and radiation therapy are needed for the treatment of cervical cancer.

1999 Physicians inject laboratory-grown neurons into a patient's brain in an effort to reverse stroke-induced brain damage.

1999 U.S. Army and American Red Cross researchers develop a bandage that uses a natural clotting factor to prevent massive bleeding.

1999 The Institute of Medicine, a federal advisory panel, declares marijuana has a number of significant medicinal properties.

1999 Salvatore V. Pizzo, American physician, announces that malignant tumors would be unable to grow without ATP (adenosine triphosphate), a nucleotide that acts as a conduit for chemical energy in cells. A fundamental element of the life process, ATP also provides energy to malignant cells.

1999 Researchers announce that a study of World War II veterans indicates that late-onset (after age 50) Parkinson's disease does not have a genetic cause.

1999 Beatrice H. Hahn of the University of Alabama at Birmingham announces that genetic studies confirm the roots of the AIDS virus (HIV) can be traced to viruses affecting chimpanzees living in west-central Africa.

General Index

A

B

D

E

G

H

I

J

K

L

M

N

O

P

Q

R

S

U

V

W

X

Y

Z